Brief Contents

Review Extracts

Nursing students face the challenge of becoming familiar with the language used in A&P. Most of the students that enter the nursing program here lack a strong scientific background. Therefore, it is important to utilize textbooks that have key features such as glossaries and definitions to allow them to become familiar with the language as they are working through the text. I really like the way this book is divided with the *Language of Science* and the *Language of Medicine*.

We encourage students to use online resources accompanying core texts to supplement their revision material. Most of the programs utilize MCQs as all or part of the assessment. Students are encouraged to use self-test sections of online resources and textbooks to test their understanding and knowledge as part of the review process. This also is advantageous in their preparation for their exams. Students always want more MCQ practice. Having a resource such as this would provide this practice and allow appropriate and timely feedback.

Senior Lecturer in Physiology, University of Manchester

In terms of learning challenges, the greatest one that our students face is the volume of work they need to understand in a short space of time. We are therefore reliant on students completing a significant amount of self-study to meet learning outcomes. Students frequently state that they are unsure as to how much depth they need when it comes to physiology knowledge, so it is refreshing to see a text that provides detail and context, with case examples and chapter summaries. The online self-assessment quizzes would help students to gauge their knowledge level.

The accompanying *Brief Atlas and Quick Guide* is an excellent adjunct to the main text. The final section in this text is exceptionally useful as an introduction but also a revision guide to the *Language of Science and Medicine*. In the early part of the course, students often state that they are confused by terminology and feel they are learning a new language. Although being immersed in this language seems to bring them up to speed quickly, a tangible guide would facilitate this learning.

The online resources that accompany the main text offer many varied resources and activities to supplement learning. The self-assessment quizzes are helpful and quick to complete, being multiple choice in nature. Using these alongside the questions and chapter summaries in the main text would offer students good opportunities to consolidate their understanding.

We have started to introduce more opportunities for blended learning within our programme to encourage students to engage online as well as appreciate the tangible resources and learning opportunities of face-to-face learning. I think having textbooks and associated resources that encourage students to participate in simple activities to consolidate their learning would be a great help to us when attempting to further continue with blended learning environments. With numbers of healthcare students expected to increase over the next few years in the UK higher education sector, I feel that there will be a continued push to move learning and teaching away from the lecture theatre and towards the blended learning market. Developing concrete resources that can be used alongside healthcare programmes will be essential.

Physiotherapy Lecturer, Cardiff University

I think this book is at a good level; it has plenty of detail, but the language isn't too complicated. The writing style is easy to understand.

I really liked the animations. I'm a visual learner and I felt they really helped deepen my understanding. I also really enjoyed the online post-test questions because it was good to be able to check my understanding and look for gaps in my knowledge. The approach is also very similar to my multiple-choice exam and would be a great revision tool.

I love the accompanying human body atlas. I really enjoy having anatomical photos to look at and would have even bought the atlas as a stand-alone.

3rd Year Student Nurse, University of Dundee

In relation to A&P, I find that I'm a visual learner and pictures help me to understand processes. The structure of the Patton & Thibodeau book is very clear. The book is also at the appropriate level of understanding and is very visually appealing, with pictures to help add context.

The online material will be of great use for me to test my knowledge around different structures and functions of the body. An online approach to the different topics makes learning anatomy and physiology more exciting!

3rd Year Student Nurse, University of Dundee

I find this book to be very informative and at a level that I can understand. I felt that the information was consistent throughout and that I was able to learn a lot from it.

All of the online content that I have been provided with through the various EVOLVE resources has been very relevant and helpful. I really like the activities, as these always help to prepare me before I begin revision. The quiz is also very useful, as this is the way that my assessment is set out at university. Furthermore, the quick review was a really pleasant surprise, as this is such a great way of learning information quickly and testing how much I know. From this I am able to recap what I need to know as well as feeling content with my knowledge. The videos are also really useful because it's good to reinforce knowledge in different ways.

The post-test questions are the exact same layout as the one that my university uses. This means that I can sit in the comfort of my halls and practice the conditions of the test months before it takes place. I am also guaranteed that the content that I am answering questions on will be relevant to my anatomy and physiology exam. Also, as there are only 15 questions, this makes for a quick summary of what I have revised while helping me to see where I could improve. By continually participating in these tests, I can see if I have improved over time.

What a brilliant price for this book! When I first received this package, I instantly thought that it was worth around £100 or so as it's packed with so many amazing elements. Not only the content, but the images make it look so expensive and professional. I also love the atlas. The high-quality photographs really help to cement knowledge, as I know what the relevant organs look like depending on what ward I am working on as a nursing student. Moreover, EVOLVE is really helpful 'on the go' in case I want to quickly review information. All of this for such a great price? That's so worth it and I wouldn't hesitate to recommend this book at all!

1st Year Student Nurse, Keele University

ANATOMY & PHYSIOLOGY

ANATOMY & PHYSIOLOGY

Adapted International Edition

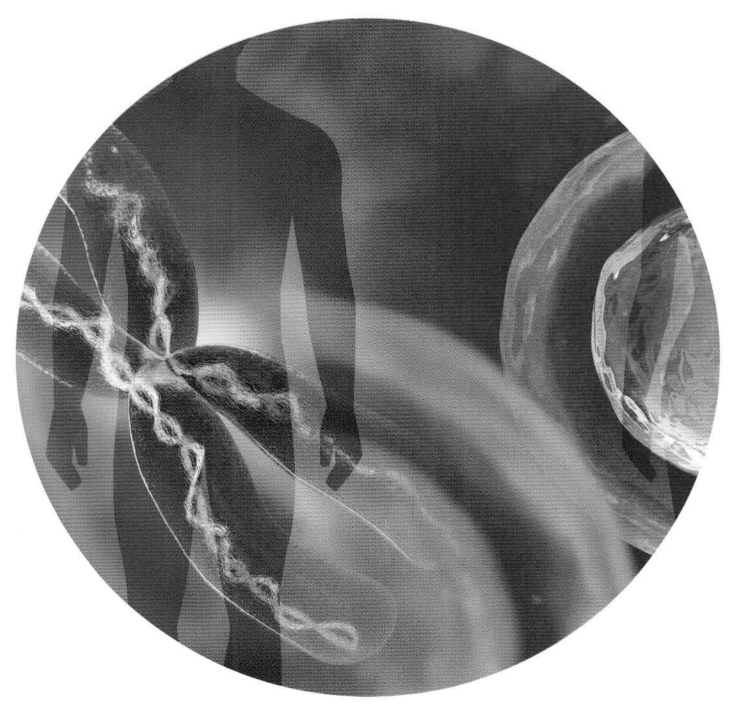

KEVIN T. PATTON PhD
Professor of Anatomy & Physiology Instruction
New York Chiropractic College
Seneca Falls, New York

Professor Emeritus of Life Sciences
St. Charles Community College
Cottleville, Missouri

Assistant Professor Emeritus of Physiology
Course Director Emeritus in Human Physiology
St. Louis University Medical School
St. Louis, Missouri, USA

GARY A. THIBODEAU PhD
Chancellor Emeritus
Professor Emeritus of Biology
University of Wisconsin—River Falls
River Falls, Wisconsin, USA

Adapted by
ANDREW HUTTON BSc MSc
Lecturer in Life Science
Edinburgh, UK

ELSEVIER

ELSEVIER

Anatomy & Physiology by Patton and Thibodeau

Ninth edition © 2016 by Mosby, an imprint of Elsevier Inc.
Eighth edition © 2013 by Mosby, an imprint of Elsevier Inc.
Seventh edition © 2010 by Mosby, an imprint of Elsevier Inc.
First published in 1987 © Mosby, an imprint of Elsevier Inc.
ISBN: 978-0323298834

This adaptation of Anatomy & Physiology by Kevin Patton and Gary Thibodeau was undertaken by Elsevier Ltd and is published by arrangement with Elsevier Inc.

Anatomy & Physiology, Adapted International Edition

ISBN: 978-0-7020-7860-6
Part ISBN: 978-0-7020-7601-5 (not available for individual sale)

Printed in China
Last digit is the print number: 9 8 7 6 5 4 3 2 1

Senior Content Strategist: Alison Taylor
Senior Content Development Specialist: Helen Leng
Project Manager: Julie Taylor
Design: Brian Salisbury

About the Authors

Kevin Patton has taught anatomy and physiology (A&P) to high school, community college, and university students from various backgrounds for more than 3 decades. Kevin found that the work that led him to a PhD in vertebrate anatomy and physiology instilled in him an appreciation for the "Big Picture" of human structure and function. This experience has helped him produce a text that will be easier to understand for all students. He has earned several citations for teaching A&P, including the Missouri Governor's Award for Excellence in Teaching. "One thing I've learned," says Kevin, "is that most of us learn scientific concepts more easily when we can see what's going on." His talent for using imagery to teach is evident throughout this edition, with its extensive array of visual resources. Kevin's interest in promoting excellence in teaching anatomy and physiology has led him to take an active role in the Human Anatomy and Physiology Society (HAPS), where he is a President Emeritus, was the founding director of the HAPS Institute, and was awarded the HAPS President's Medal for outstanding contributions in promoting the mission of excellence in A&P teaching and learning. Kevin also teaches graduate courses to prospective and current A&P professors and produces online resources for A&P students and teachers, including *theAPstudent.org* and *theAPprofessor.org*. His blog *PattonAP.org* provides insights and teaching notes for faculty using this textbook.

To my family and friends, who never let me forget the joys of discovery, adventure, and good humor.

To the many teachers who taught me more by who they were than by what they said.

To my students who help me keep the thrill of learning fresh and exciting.

Kevin T. Patton

Gary Thibodeau has been teaching anatomy and physiology (A&P) for more than 3 decades. Since 1975, *Anatomy & Physiology* has been a logical extension of his interest and commitment to education. Gary's teaching style encourages active interaction with students, and he uses a wide variety of teaching methodologies—a style that has been incorporated into every aspect of this edition. He is considered a pioneer in the introduction of collaborative learning strategies to the teaching of A&P. Conferral of Emeritus status in the University of Wisconsin System has provided him with additional time to interact with students and teachers across the country and around the world. His focus continues to be successful student-centered learning—leveraged by text, Web-based, and ancillary teaching materials. Over the years, his success as a teacher has resulted in numerous awards from both students and professional colleagues. Gary is active in numerous professional organizations, including the Human Anatomy and Physiology Society (HAPS), the American Association for the Advancement of Science, and the American Association of Clinical Anatomists. His biography is included in numerous publications, including *Who's Who in America, Who's Who in American Education, Outstanding Educators in America, American Men and Women of Science*, and *Who's Who in Medicine and Healthcare*. While earning master's degrees in both zoology and pharmacology, as well as a PhD in physiology, Gary says that he became "fascinated by the connectedness of the life sciences." That fascination has led to this edition's unifying themes that focus on how each concept fits into the "Big Picture" of the human body.

To my parents, M.A. Thibodeau and Florence Thibodeau, who had a deep respect for education at all levels and who truly believed that you never give up being a student.

To my wife, Emogene, an ever-generous and uncommonly discerning critic, for her love, support, and encouragement over the years.

To my children, Douglas and Beth, for making it all worthwhile.

To my grandchildren, Allan Gary Foster and Johanna Lorraine Foster, for proving to me that you really can learn something new every day.

Gary A. Thibodeau

About the Adapter

Andrew R. Hutton, BSc MSc

After graduating from the University of Hull in 1968 Andrew worked in the pharmaceutical industry for *The Wellcome Foundation* contributing to the introduction of chemotherapeutic agents into the National Health Service. He then decided to change career and trained to lecture in further education. In the UK Andrew taught anatomy and physiology to sixth-formers in international schools and technical colleges. On moving to the Middle East he lectured and tutored medical students, nurses and allied health students in scientific English in the Faculty of Medicine at Kuwait University. Most recently he taught anatomy and physiology, biochemistry and medical terminology to nurses entering Napier University in the Scottish higher education system.

During his teaching career, which lasted over three decades, Andrew motivated students to understand the principles of science rather than the rote learning of facts. He encouraged students to become independent thinkers through relevant practical hands-on activities, thought provoking questions and problem solving.

Retired from full-time teaching, he now devotes time to the development of interactive medical terminology courses, dictionaries and A&P animations via websites and mobile applications.

He is the author of *An Introduction to Medical Terminology for Health Care*, now in its 5th edition, and *Pocket Medical Terminology* both published by Elsevier. His current interests include the history of biology and medicine, and he is an active member of the Royal Scottish Society of Arts (RSSA).

Adapted International Edition Contributors

Professor Donald R.J. Singer, BMedBiol, MD, FRCP, FBPhS

President, Fellowship of Postgraduate Medicine

Professor Donald Singer was awarded Bachelor of Medical Biology and Bachelor of Medicine and Surgery degrees from the University of Aberdeen in 1975 and 1978 respectively, followed by the MD degree in 1995. He served as senior lecturer/consultant and then reader at St George's Hospital Medical School from 1996–2003, having previously trained at the Aberdeen Teaching Hospitals, Hammersmith Hospital, the Royal Postgraduate Medical School, and the Charing Cross and Westminster Medical School. While at St George's, he held honorary research posts at the Harefield Heart Science Centre, a research facility of the National Heart and Lung Institute, a division of the Faculty of Medicine of Imperial College. He was appointed professor of clinical pharmacology and therapeutics at the graduate medical school of the University of Warwick in 2003. In 2007, Professor Singer was elected president of the Fellowship of Postgraduate Medicine. In 2014, he was on the Faculty of Yale University School of Medicine.

Dr Daniel J. Matusiak, BS, MA, EdD

Life Science Instructor, St Dominic High School, O'Fallon, Missouri; Adjunct Professor, St Charles Community College, Cottleville, Missouri

Daniel J. Matusiak, EdD is currently a life science teacher at St. Dominic High School in O'Fallon, Missouri. In addition to teaching in the St. Louis Archdiocese, he spent twenty-six years as an adjunct professor at St. Charles Community College located in Cottleville, Missouri, outside the St. Louis, Missouri metropolitan area.

Over the past forty-five years, Dan has taught anatomy and physiology, human biology, and general biology. Since 2001, Dan has worked as an ancillary and contributing author for many titles including Kevin Patton's titles: *Anatomy and Physiology*, *Structure and Function of the Human Body*, and *The Human Body in Health and Disease*. Most of this work was in developing online resources. In 2010, Dan developed the first edition of *Anatomy and Physiology Review Cards*, published by Elsevier/Mosby and now in its third edition.

Adapted International Edition Reviewers

John Clarke, BEd, MEd
Lecturer in Nursing
Robert Gordon University
Aberdeen
UK

Thomas H. Gillingwater, BSc (Hons), MBA, PhD, FAS, FRSB
Professor of Anatomy
College of Medicine & Veterinary Medicine
University of Edinburgh
UK

Jill Morgan, MSc, MCSP, FHEA
Lecturer (Physiotherapy)
School of Healthcare Sciences
College of Biomedical and Life Sciences
Cardiff University
UK

Elizabeth Sheader, BSc (Hons), PhD, PGCE, SFHEA
Senior Lecturer (Physiology)
Faculty of Biology, Medicine and Health
University of Manchester
UK

Rhys Thatcher, BSc (Hons), MSc, SFHEA, FBASES
Reader in Exercise Physiology
Institute of Biological Environmental and Rural Sciences
Aberystwyth University
UK

US Edition Reviewers

The Department of Physiology and The Department of Anatomy & Structural Biology
Otago School of Medical Sciences University of Otago
Dunedin, New Zealand

Mohammed Abbas
Wayne County Community College

Laura Anderson
Elk County Catholic High School

Bert Atsma
Union County College

John Bagdade
Northwestern University

Mary K. Beals
Southern University and A&M College

Rachel Venn Beecham
Mississippi Valley State University

Brenda Blackwelder
Central Piedmont Community College

Richard Blonna
William Paterson College

Claude Bouchei
INSERM

Charles T. Brown
Barton County Community College

Laurence Campbell
Florida Southern College

Patricia W. Campbell
Carolinas College of Health Sciences

Geralyn M. Caplan
Owensboro Community and Technical College

Roger Carroll
University of Tennessee School of Medicine

Melvin Chambliss
Alfred State College
SUNY College of Technology

Pattie Clark
Abraham Baldwin College

Richard Cohen
Union County College

Barbara A. Coles
Wake Technical Community College

Harry W. Colvin, Jr.
University of California–Davis

Teresa Cowan
Baker College of Auburn Hills

Dorwin Coy
University of North Florida

Douglas M. Dearden
General College of University of Minnesota

Cheryl Donlon
Northeast Iowa Community College

J. Paul Ellis
St. Louis Community College

Frank G. Emanuele
Mercyhurst University

Cammie Emory
Bossier Parish Community College

Julie Fiez
Washington University School of Medicine

Beth A. Forshee
Lake Erie College of Osteopathic Medicine

Laura Frost
Florida Gulf Coast University

Debbie Gantz
Mississippi Delta Community College

Christy Gee
South College–Asheville

Becky Gesler
Spalding University

Norman Goldstein
California State University–Hayward

Zully Villanueva Gonzalez
Dona Ana Branch Community College

John Goudie
Kalamazoo Area Mathematics & Science Center

Charles J. Grossman
Xavier University

Monica L. Hall-Woods
St. Charles Community College

Rebecca Halyard
Clayton State College

Ann T. Harmer
Orange Coast College

Linden C. Haynes
Hinds Community College

Lois Jane Heller
University of Minnesota School of Medicine

Lee E. Henderson
Prairie View A&M University

Angela R. Hess
Bloomsburg University

Paula Holloway
Ohio University

Julie Hotz-Siville
Mt. San Jacinto College

Gayle Dranch Insler
Adelphi University

Patrick Jackson
Canadian Memorial Chiropractic College

Carolyn Jaslow
Rhodes College

Gloria El Kammash
Wake Technical Community College

Murray Kaplan
Iowa State University

Kathy Kath
Henry Ford Hospital School of Radiologic Technology

Brian H. Kipp
Grand Valley State University

Johanna Krontiris-Litowitz
Youngstown State University

William Langley
Butler County Community College

Michael Levitzky
Louisiana State University School of Medicine

Clifton Lewis
Wayne County Community College

Jerri Lindsey
Tarrant County Junior College

Eddie Lunsford
Southwestern Community College

Bruce Luon
University of Texas Medical Branch

Melanie S. MacNeil
Brock University

Susan Marshall
St. Louis University School of Medicine

Gary Massaglia
Elk County Christian High School

Bruce S. McEwan
The Rockefeller University

Jeff Mellenthin
The Methodist Debakey Heart Center

Lanette Meyer
Regis University/Denver Children's Hospital

Donald Misumi
Los Angeles Trade–Technical Center

Susan Moore
New Hampshire Community Technical College

Rose Morgan
Minot State University

Jeremiah Morrissey
Washington University School of Medicine

Greg Mullen
South Louisiana Community College/ National EMS Academy

Robert Earl Olsen
Briar Cliff College

Susan M. Caley Opsal
Illinois Valley Community College

Juanelle Pearson
Spalding University

Nicole Pinaire
St. Charles Community College

Wanda Ragland
Macomb Community College

Saeed Rahmanian
Roane State Community College

Robert S. Rawding
Gannon University

Carolyn Jean Rivard
Fanshawe College of Applied Arts and Technology

Mary F. Ruh
St. Louis University School of Medicine

Jenny Sarver
Sarver Chiropractic

Henry M. Seidel
The Johns Hopkins University School of Medicine

Gerry Silverstein
University of Vermont–Burlington

Charles Singhas
East Carolina University

Marci Slusser
Reading Area Community College

Paul Keith Small
Eureka College

William G. Sproat, Jr.
Walters State Community College

Snez Stolic
Griffith University

Aleta Sullivan
Pearl River Community College

Kathleen Tatum
Iowa State University

Reid Tatum
St. Martin's Episcopal School

Kent R. Thomas
Wichita State University

Todd Thuma
Macon College

Stuart Tsubota
St. Louis University

Judith B. Van Liew
State University of New York College at Buffalo

Karin VanMeter
Iowa State University/Des Moines Area Community College

Gordon Wardlaw
Ohio State University

Amy L. Way
Lock Haven University of Pennsylvania

Anthony J. Weinhaus
University of Minnesota

Cheryl Wiley
Andrews University

Clarence C. Wolfe
Northern Virginia Community College

Preface

This textbook relates the story of the human body's structure and function. More than simply a collection of facts, it is both a teaching tool and a learning tool. It was written to help students unify information, stimulate critical thinking, and acquire a taste for knowledge about the wonders of the human body. The story related in this textbook will help students avoid becoming lost in a maze of facts while navigating a complex learning environment. It will encourage them to explore, to question, and to look for relationships, not only between related facts in a single discipline, but also between fields of academic inquiry and personal experience.

This edition of the text has been extensively revised to better tell the story of the human body. Because pictures are important in telling our story, we have significantly upgraded our art program. Many of the longer chapters were split into smaller chapters to improve comprehension and better organize study. We also improved our execution of a page design and layout that maximizes learning effectiveness. As with each new edition, we added carefully selected new information on both anatomy and physiology to provide an accurate and up-to-date presentation. We have retained the basic philosophy of personal and interactive teaching that characterized previous editions. Essential, accurate, and current information continues to be presented in a comfortable storytelling style. Emphasis is placed on concepts rather than descriptions, and the "connectedness" of human structure and function is repeatedly reinforced by unifying themes.

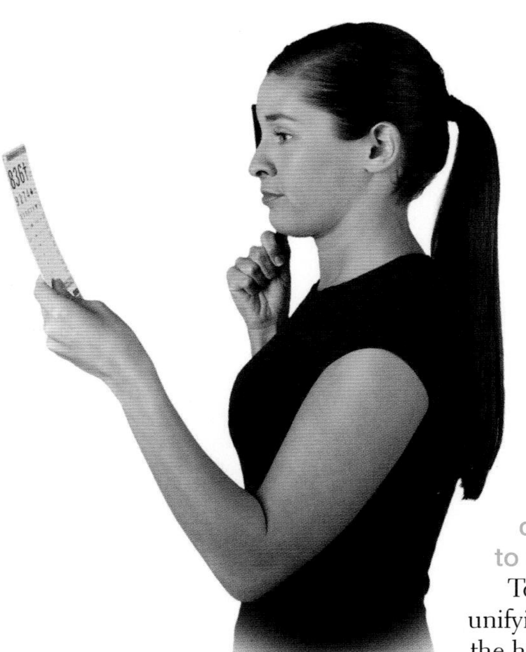

UNIFYING THEMES

Anatomy and physiology encompasses a body of knowledge that is large and complex. Students are faced with the need to know and understand a multitude of individual structures and functions that constitute a bewildering array of seemingly disjointed information. Ultimately, the student of anatomy and physiology must be able to "pull together" this information to view the body as a whole—to see the "Big Picture." If a textbook is to be successful as a teaching tool in such a complex learning environment, it must help unify information, stimulate critical thinking, and motivate students to master a new vocabulary.

To accomplish this synthesis of information, unifying themes are required to tell the story of the human body effectively. In addition, a mechanism to position and implement these themes must be an integral part of each chapter. Unit 1 begins with "Seeing the Big Picture," an overview that encourages students to place individual structures or functions into an integrated framework. Then, a special "The Big Picture" section wraps up the story of each chapter so that its significance in the overall function of the body can easily be seen. *Anatomy & Physiology* is dominated by two major unifying themes: (1) the complementarity of normal structure and function and (2) homeostasis. The student is shown, as our story unfolds, how organized anatomical structures of a particular size, shape, form, or placement serve unique and specialized functions. The integrating principle of homeostasis is used to show how the "normal" interaction of structure and function is achieved and maintained by counterbalancing forces within the body. Repeated emphasis of these principles encourages students to integrate otherwise isolated factual information into a cohesive and understandable whole. "The Big Picture" summarizes the larger interaction between structures and functions of the different body systems. As a result, the story of anatomy and physiology emerges as a living and dynamic topic of personal interest and importance to students.

AIMS OF THE REVISION

As in past editions, our revision efforts focused on identifying the need for new or revised information and for additional visual presentations that clarify important, yet sometimes difficult, content areas.

In this edition, we have included information on new concepts in many areas of anatomy and physiology. For example, new data on the role of the human microbiome and updates in terminology have been included. Most of these changes are subtle adjustments to our current understanding of human science. However, the accumulation of all of these subtle changes makes this edition the most up-to-date textbook available.

We have also added information on calculating mean arterial pressure, the role of autonomic receptors in pharmacology, the nature of head trauma, assessing acid-base balance using arterial blood gases, and other clinically relevant topics. This material, scattered throughout the book, better prepares students for their clinical courses.

One of the most apparent changes that you will notice in this edition is a continuation of the reorganization of chapters begun in the previous edition. A hallmark of our textbook has been its effective "chunking" of material into manageable bite-size pieces. These changes reflect our continuing commitment to that approach. Most noticeable is the splitting of eleven of the longest chapters into smaller, more compact narratives that students can read easily in one sitting. This reorganization offers an opportunity to provide more clarity and emphasis to topics such as *homeostasis,* which is now covered in its own chapter (Chapter 2). Likewise, *nerve signalling* (Chapter 19), *ventilation* (Chapter 36), *gas exchange and transport* (Chapter 37), and other topics benefit by being the focus of their own easily digestable chapters.

As we chunked the chapters, we also carefully clarified and added subheadings to improve the telling of our story. Besides providing graphic scaffolding to help students construct a clear understanding of concepts as the story unfolds, these subheadings also help students find relevant material as they later "raid" their textbook for specific help in clarifying difficult concepts—or concepts they missed or forgot after their first reading.

Another aim of this revision has been the expansion of our use of online ***Connect It!*** articles. More than two dozen new articles have been added in this edition, some of them expanded versions of boxed sidebars that previously appeared in the textbook proper. Besides providing interesting asides that help spark interest in a topic and motivate deeper learning, these articles provide an opportunity to integrate diverse topics scattered throughout the book. For example, the new article *The Human Microbiome* is called out in many different chapters, helping readers see the numerous connections that characterize human structure and function. Such "integrative" use of the articles has been expanded and improved in this edition.

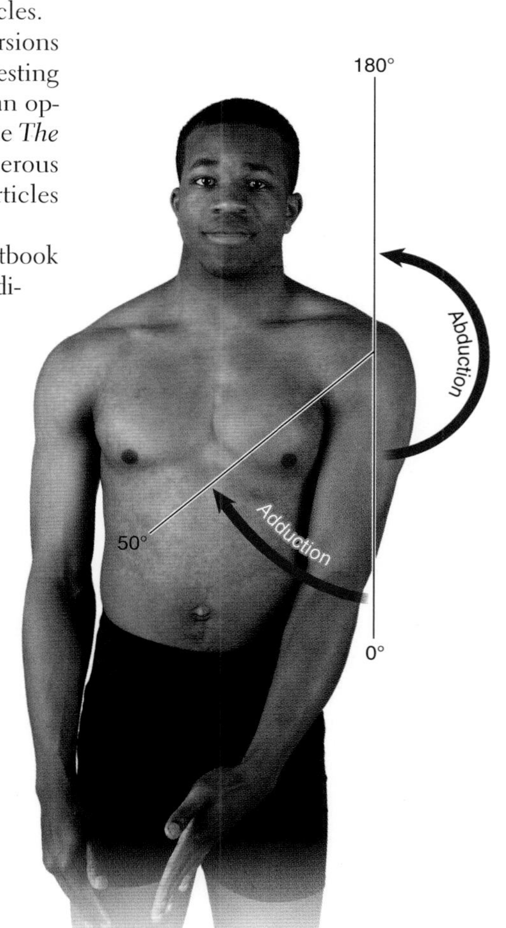

Previous editions have featured what is now our signature page design that makes the textbook easier to use by putting the illustrations, graphs, and tables closer to the related text. In this edition, we have worked hard to make the page layout even more effective for telling our story. Our extensive set of summary tables helps students visually organize important concepts and complements the improved design to provide a multisensory learning tool. We have improved the art program by adopting a new style for graphs, which not only clarify concepts but also provide the practice in graph interpretation needed for professional courses in health careers. Many photographs featuring live anatomical models were replaced with a coordinated set of new photographs (some of which appear on this page). Several new illustrations maintain the use of a consistent Colour Key (pp. xxxii-xxxiii) for certain cell parts, tissue types, and biomolecules to help make learning easier for beginning students.

In this edition, we continue our effort to make this text accessible to students whose first language is not English. After consulting with ESL specialists and ESL learners, we have continued to enhance our word lists and improve our readability to make the concepts of human structure and function more understandable for all students.

As teachers of anatomy and physiology, we know that to be effective a text must be clear and readable, and it must challenge and excite the student. This text remains one that students will read—one designed to help the teacher teach and the student learn. To accomplish this end, we facilitated the comprehension of difficult material for students with thorough, consistent, and nonintimidating explanations that are free of unnecessary terminology and extraneous information. This easy access to complex ideas remains the single most striking hallmark of our textbook.

ILLUSTRATIONS AND DESIGN

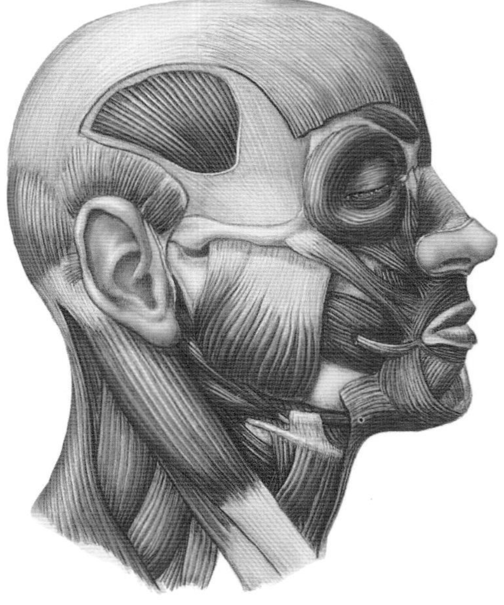

A major strength of this text has always been the exceptional quality, accuracy, and beauty of the illustration program. It is the original "visual" anatomy and physiology textbook. We have worked very closely with scientific illustrators to provide attractive and colourful images that clearly and accurately portray the major concepts of anatomy and physiology.

The truest test of any illustration is how effectively it can complement and strengthen the written information in the text and how successfully it can be used by the student as a learning tool. Each illustration is explicitly referred to in the text in bold type and is designed to support the text discussion. Careful attention has been paid to placement and sizing of the illustrations to maximize usefulness and clarity. Each figure and all labels are relevant to—and consistent with—the text discussion. Each illustration has a boldface title for easy identification. Most illustrations also include a concise explanation that guides the student through the image as a complement to the nearby text narrative.

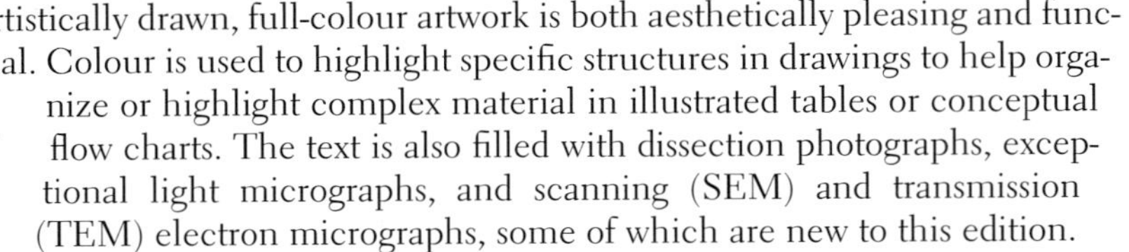

The artistically drawn, full-colour artwork is both aesthetically pleasing and functional. Colour is used to highlight specific structures in drawings to help organize or highlight complex material in illustrated tables or conceptual flow charts. The text is also filled with dissection photographs, exceptional light micrographs, and scanning (SEM) and transmission (TEM) electron micrographs, some of which are new to this edition.
In addition, examples of medical imagery, including CT scans, PET scans, MRIs, and x-ray photographs, are used throughout the text to show structural detail, explain medical procedures, and enhance the understanding of differences that distinguish pathological conditions from normal structure and function. All illustrations used in the text are an integral part of the learning process and should be carefully studied by the student.

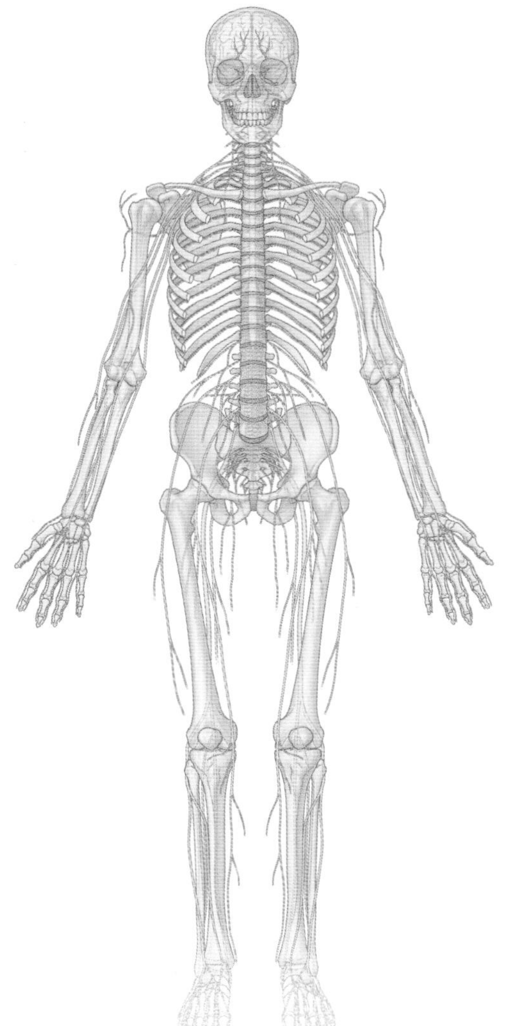

LEARNING AIDS

Anatomy & Physiology is a student-oriented text. Written in a readable style that tells a coherent story, the text is designed with many different pedagogical aids to motivate and maintain interest. The special features and learning aids listed below are intended to facilitate learning and retention of information in the most effective and efficient manner.

No textbook can replace the direction and stimulation provided by an enthusiastic teacher to a curious and involved student. However, a full complement of innovative pedagogical aids that are carefully planned and implemented can contribute a great deal to the success of a text as a learning tool. An excellent textbook can and should be enjoyable to read and should be helpful to both student and teacher. We hope you agree that the learning aids in *Anatomy & Physiology* meet the high expectations we have set.

Unit Introductions

Each of the six major units of the text begins with a brief overview statement. The general content of the unit is discussed, and the chapters and their topics are listed. Before beginning the study of material in a new unit, students are encouraged to scan the introduction and each of the chapter outlines in the unit to understand the relationship and "connectedness" of the material to be studied. Each unit has a colour-coded tab at the outside edge of every page to help you quickly find the information you need.

Chapter Learning Aids

Study Hints *give specific suggestions for using many of the learning aids found in each chapter.* Because many readers have never learned the special skills needed to make effective use of pedagogical resources found in science textbooks, helpful tips are embedded within each Chapter Outline, Language of Science & Medicine list, Case Study, Chapter Summary, Review Questions set, and Critical Thinking section. Answers for the Quick Check and Case Study questions are available for students on the Evolve website (*evolve.elsevier.com/Patton/AP/international/*), and answers for these plus the Review and Critical Thinking Exercises are available for instructors in the TEACH Instructor's Resource.

Hint

Chapter Outline *summarizes the contents of a chapter at a glance.* An overview outline introduces each chapter and enables the student to preview the content and direction of the chapter at the major concept level before beginning a detailed reading. Page references enable students to quickly locate topics in the chapter.

Language of Science *introduces you to new scientific terms in the chapter.* A comprehensive list of new terms is presented at the beginning of the chapter. Each term in the list has an easy-to-use pronunciation guide to help the learner easily "own" the word by being able to say it. Literal translations of each term's word parts are included to help students learn how to deduce the meaning of new terms on their own. The listed terms are defined in the text body, where they appear in boldface type, and are also in the Glossary at the back of the book. The boldface type feature enables students to scan the text for new words before beginning their first detailed reading of the material, so they may read without having to disrupt the flow to grapple with new words or phrases. The Language of Science word list includes terms related to the essential anatomy and physiology presented in the chapter. Another word list near the end of the chapter, a feature described on the next page as the Language of Medicine, is an inventory of all the new clinical terms introduced in the chapter.

Colour-coded illustrations *help beginning students appreciate the "Big Picture" of human structure and function.* A special feature of the illustrations in this text is the careful and consistent use of colour to identify important structures and substances that recur throughout the book. Consistent use of a colour key helps beginning students appreciate the "Big Picture" of human structure and function each time they see a familiar structure in a new illustration. For an explanation of the colour scheme, see the Colour Key on pp. xxxii-xxxiii.

Anatomical compass rosettes *help students learn the orientation of anatomical structures.* Where appropriate, small orientation diagrams and directional anatomical compass rosettes are included as part of an illustration to help students locate a structure with reference to the body as a whole or orient a small structure in a larger view.

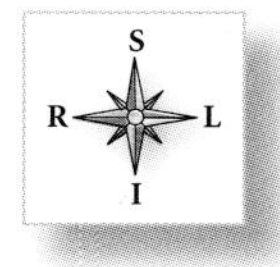

Quick Check questions *test your knowledge of material you've just read.* Short objective-type questions are located immediately following major topic discussions throughout the body of the text. These questions cover important information presented in the preceding section. Students unable to answer the questions should reread that section before proceeding. This feature therefore enhances reading comprehension. Quick Check items are numbered by chapter, and a numerical listing of their answers can be found on the Evolve website (*evolve.elsevier.com/Patton/AP/international/*).

Quick CHECK

1. List the major subdivisions of the human nervous system.
2. What two organs make up the central nervous system?
3. Contrast the somatic nervous system with the autonomic nervous system.

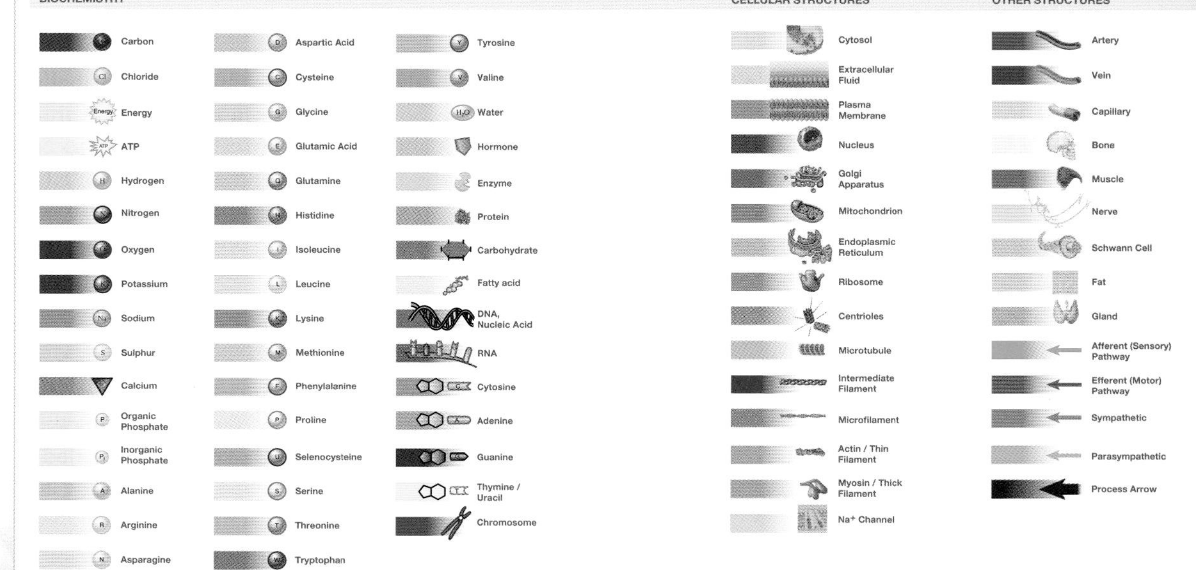

Connect It! features *call the reader's attention to online articles that illustrate, clarify, and apply concepts encountered in the text.* Embedded within the text narrative, these boxes connect you with interesting, brief online articles that stimulate thinking, satisfy your curiosity, and help you apply important concepts. **Connect It!** articles also help you understand connections among structures and functions throughout the body, integrating concepts into a "Big Picture" of human function. They are often illustrated with micrographs, medical images, and medical illustrations.

CONNECT IT! 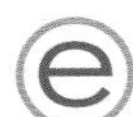

Tiny, barrel-shaped organelles called *vaults* may also assist with transport of molecules to and from the nucleus. To learn more about these little transport shuttles, check out ***Vaults*** online at ***Connect It!.***

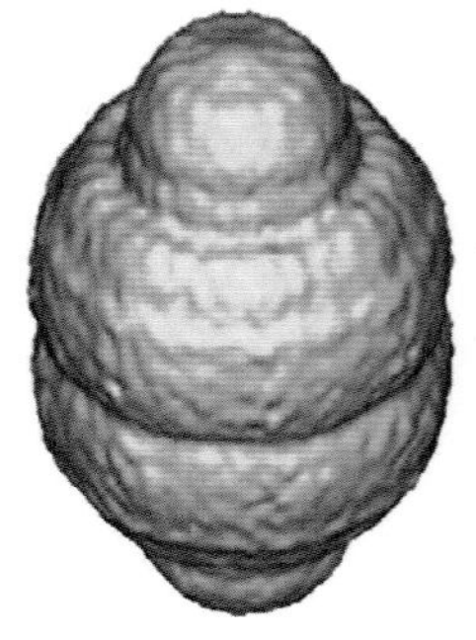

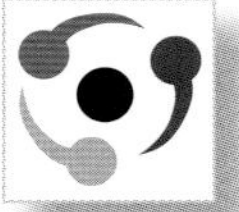

Cycle of Life *describes major changes that occur over a person's lifetime.* In many body systems, changes in structure and function are frequently related to a person's age or state of development. In appropriate chapters of the text, these changes are highlighted in this special section.

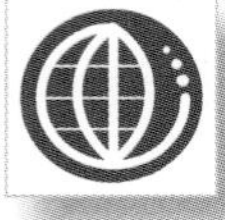

The Big Picture *explains the interactions of the system discussed in a particular chapter with the body as a whole.* This helps students relate information about body structures or functions that are discussed in the chapter to the body as a whole. The Big Picture feature helps you improve critical thinking by focusing on how structures and functions relate to one another on a bodywide basis.

Mechanisms of Disease *helps you understand the basic principles of human structure and function by showing what happens when things go wrong.* Examples of pathology, or disease, are included in many chapters of the book to stimulate student interest and to help students understand that the disease process is a disruption in homeostasis, a breakdown of normal integration of form and function. The intent of the Mechanisms of Disease section is to reinforce the normal structures and mechanisms of the body while highlighting the general causes of disorders for a particular body system. These sections are heavily illustrated with diagrams and medical photographs that bring pathology concepts to life.

LANGUAGE OF SCIENCE

isotonic contraction
(eye-soh-TON-ik kon-TRAK-shun)
[*iso-* **equal,** *ton-* **stretch or tension,** *-ic* **relating to,** *con-* **together,** *-tract-* **drag or draw,** *-tion* **process**]

lactate (LAK-tayt)
[*lact-* **milk,** *-ate* **salt of an acid**]

M line
[*M mittel* **middle**]

motor endplate
[*mot-* **move,** *-or* **agent**]

UNIT 2

Language of Medicine *introduces you to new clinical terms in the chapter.* A brief list of clinical terms is presented near the end of each chapter. As in the Language of Science list at the beginning of the chapter, each term has a phonetic pronunciation guide and translations of word parts. The listed terms are defined in the text body, where they appear in boldface type.

Case Study *challenges you with "real-life" clinical or other practical situations so you can creatively apply what you have learned.* Case studies precede the chapter summaries. The case study consists of a description of a real-life situation and a series of questions that require the student to use critical thinking skills to determine the answers.

Chapter Summary *outlines essential information in a way that helps you organize your study.* Detailed end-of-chapter summaries provide excellent guides for students as they review the text materials before examinations. Many students also find the summaries to be useful as a chapter preview in conjunction with the chapter outline.

Audio Chapter Summaries *allow you to listen and learn wherever you may be.* These summaries are available in MP3 format for download at the Evolve website (*evolve.elsevier.com/Patton/AP/international/*).

Review Questions *help you determine whether you have mastered the important concepts of each chapter.* Review questions at the end of each chapter give students practice in using a narrative format to discuss the concepts presented in the chapter.

Critical Thinking Questions *actively engage and challenge you to evaluate and synthesize the chapter content.* Critical thinking questions require students to use their higher level reasoning skills and demonstrate their understanding of, not just their repetition of, complex concepts.

Boxed Sidebars

As always, we made every effort to update factual information and incorporate the most current anatomy and physiology research findings in this edition. Although there continues to be an incredible explosion of knowledge in the life sciences, not all new information is appropriate for inclusion in a fundamental-level textbook. Therefore we were selective in choosing new clinical, pathological, or special-interest material to include in this edition. This text remains focused on normal anatomy and physiology. The addition of new boxed content is intended to stimulate student interest and provide examples that reinforce the immediate personal relevance of anatomy and physiology as important disciplines for study.

General Interest Boxes *provide an expanded explanation of specific chapter content.* Many chapters contain boxed essays, occasionally clinical in nature, that expand on or relate to material covered in the text. Examples of subjects include the Brainbow visualization of neural networks and the enteric nervous system.

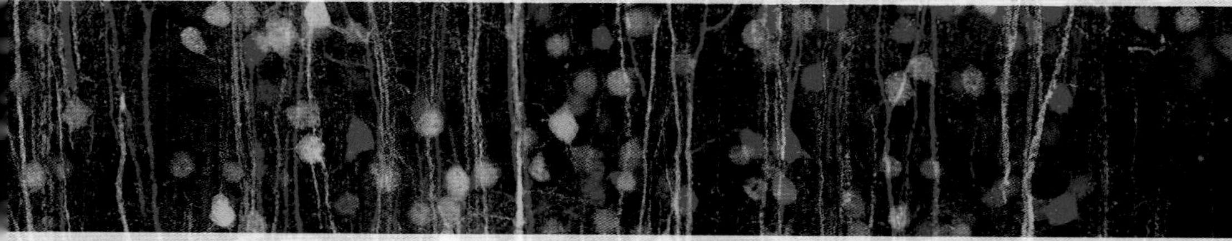

Health Matters *presents current information on diseases, disorders, clinical applications, and other health issues related to normal structure and function.* In some instances, examples of structural anomalies or pathophysiology are presented. Information of this type is often useful in helping students understand the mechanisms involved in maintaining the "normal" interaction of structure and function.

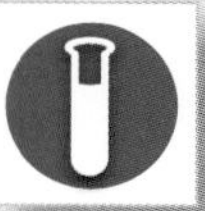

Diagnostic Study *keeps you abreast of developments in diagnosing diseases and disorders.* These boxes deal with specific diagnostic tests used in clinical medicine or research. Lumbar puncture, angiography, and antenatal diagnosis and treatment are examples.

FYI *gives you more in-depth information on interesting topics mentioned in the text.* Topics of current interest, such as new advances in anatomy and physiology research, are covered in these "for your information" boxes.

Sports and Fitness *highlights sports-related topics.* Exercise physiology, sports injury, and physical education applications are highlighted in these boxes.

Glossary

A comprehensive glossary of terms is located at the end of the text. An expanded list of accurate, concise definitions and phonetic pronunciation guides is provided, along with word parts and their literal translations.

Learning Supplements for Students

Brief Atlas and Quick Guide

This comprehensive supplement is packaged with every new copy of this edition of *Anatomy & Physiology*. One section features a full-colour ***Brief Atlas of Human Anatomy*** containing cadaver dissections, osteology, organ casts, histology specimens, and surface anatomy photographs. This helpful supplement serves as a handy reference for students as they study the human body in class and in the laboratory—and even later on in clinical and career contexts. Also included is the ***Quick Guide to the Language of Science & Medicine***, which provides the foundation for learning the terminology of A&P. This quick guide features basic principles of terminology and lists of common roots, prefixes, suffixes, acronyms, Roman numerals, and the Greek alphabet.

Clear View of the Human Body

This edition again features a student favorite—a full-colour, semitransparent model of the body called the ***Clear View of the Human Body.*** Found after the end of Chapter 13, this feature permits the virtual dissection of male and female human bodies along several different planes of the body. Developed by Kevin Patton and Paul Krieger, this tool helps learners assimilate their knowledge of the complex structure of the human body. It also provides a unique learning resource that helps students visualize human anatomy in the manner of today's clinical body imaging technology.

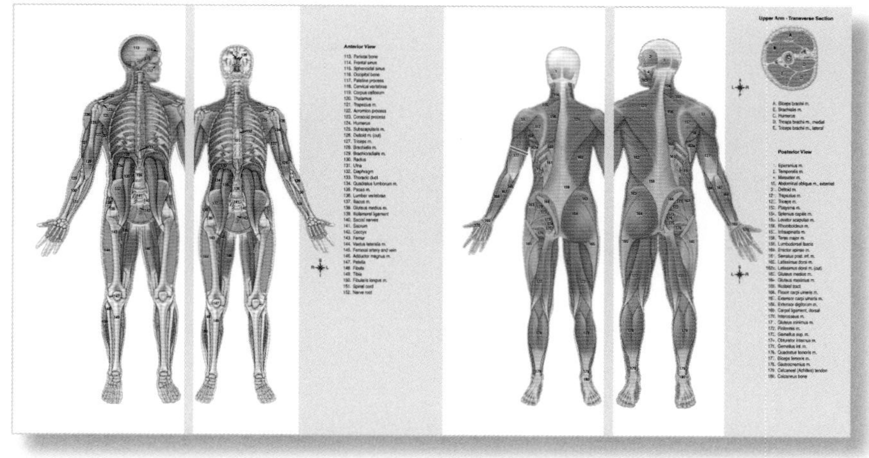

evolve

EVOLVE.ELSEVIER.COM/PATTON/AP/INTERNATIONAL/

This edition of *Anatomy & Physiology* is supported by an expanded multimedia Evolve website, featuring:

- Audio Summaries for each chapter available for streaming or download in convenient MP3 form.
- Answers to all of the Quick Check and Case Study questions found in the textbook.
- Quick access to all Connect It! articles cited in the textbook.
- The Body Spectrum Electronic Anatomy Colouring Book, which offers dozens of anatomy illustrations that can be coloured online or printed out and coloured by hand.

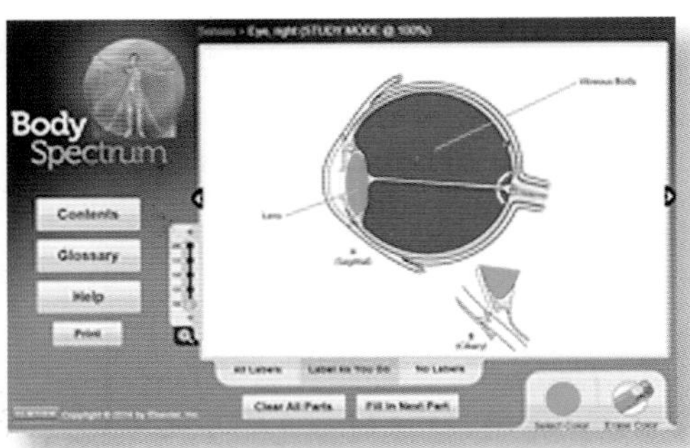

- More than 500 Student Post-Test questions that allow you to get instant feedback on what you've learned in each chapter.
- State-of-the-art 3-D animations, which show and describe physiological processes by body system.
- WebLinks to provide students with access to hundreds of important sites simply by clicking on a subject in the book's table of contents.

You can visit the Evolve site by pointing your browser to *evolve.elsevier.com/Patton/AP/international/*.

Lecturer Information

This well-established and highly successful publication—which is the original 'visual' A&P textbook—is hallmarked by its clarity of approach. Given the volume of information now available at even the introductory level of the study of A&P, emphasis is placed on *concepts* rather than descriptions, which enables students to acquire a firm understanding of the working of the human body without being overwhelmed by vast amounts of detailed information.

Furthermore, given the challenge for many readers who are new to the language of science and medicine, the content has been prepared in conjunction with ESL specialists and learners to ensure that it is as direct and unambiguous as possible. This simplicity of approach makes the book ideal for students who may be new to the life sciences, and/or those for whom English may not be their first language.

Of all the A&P titles available for undergraduate students of this type, *Patton and Thibodeau's Anatomy & Physiology* is designed to be the easiest to assimilate in other ways, and continual improvement in approach and design has given rise to what is arguably the most robust 'pedagogic scaffold' in any A&P textbook to date. Precise details of this development, and other characteristics of the book, are given by the editors within the preface.

For this new *Adapted International Edition*, the publishers have taken the 9th edition of *Anatomy & Physiology* and supplemented it with relevant changes from the 10th edition. This approach was taken for reasons of the publication cycle, but we are confident that this volume will perfectly meet the needs of undergraduate students outside of the USA and Canada wherever they reside.

Anatomy & Physiology is also supported by the popular EVOLVE website. For lecturers who are unfamiliar with this resource, this unique offering provides a range of learning and teaching materials for both students and faculty, a feature that has found wide appeal in many countries. If you are unfamiliar with EVOLVE, we feel confident that you will find the additional content to be of value to your activities and those of your students, particularly in the context of self-directed learning and the blended learning environment.

The EVOLVE resource contains a series of PowerPoint presentations, which have been prepared to accompany each chapter within the book. There are two types of presentation: the first provides 'lecture outlines' to guide the instructor on the key points of the subject area as he/she presents to a student group. The second type complements the first and is designed for use, if desired, with audience response systems such as i-Clicker, thereby allowing the lecturer to quickly assess how well the group is understanding the topic area and where areas of additional explanation may be required. Of course, both sets of PowerPoint files may be freely edited to meet the needs of local teaching and assessment requirements.

We are also pleased to offer a test bank that contains over 7000 multiple choice, true/false, short answer, and challenge questions designed for use with software such as ExamView, a facility that allows you to create, administer and manage questions for formative and summative assessment. When you register as an instructor on EVOLVE, you will automatically receive access to the ExamView software or, alternatively, the content can be used with quizzing engines found with standard learning management systems such as Moodle and Blackboard.

EVOLVE also comes with *TEACH* lesson plans, one for each chapter, which are designed to help instructors make best use of their time by providing pre-prepared topic objectives, teaching 'focal points,' and even suggested assignments. Each lesson plan also includes a selection of formative assessment Q&As, *Instructor Preparation* for the classroom, a 50-minute PowerPoint lecture (with recommended 'talking points'), and suggestions for classroom activities (with approximate timings).

Kevin Patton also offers his personal 'teaching tips' to help colleagues optimise their teaching sessions and avoid some of the pitfalls that newcomers can readily encounter. Examples include the use of 'CATS,' or classroom assessment techniques, such as the 'one-minute essay' at the end of the lecture in which students outline the most important thing they have learned in the session, or the 'muddiest point,' in which the students leave an index card with the lecturer at the end of the lecture identifying the topic they found the most difficult. Tips are also given on helping students take notes effectively and the use of 'double' quizzing, a means of motivating students to focus on what they need to know and of identifying those who are struggling with the course.

As with many Elsevier textbooks, an EVOLVE lecturer resource image bank is also provided. The online art comes with and without labels, or even 'leader lines,' for lecturers who require plain images, and can be downloaded as JPG files or within PowerPoint for ease of use.

Finally, the online student resource facility gives access to a broad selection of animations that you may also find helpful in your teaching programme. Topics covered range from principles of basic science, such as molecule formation, to anatomical features and physiological processes, the latter of which cover a broad range of subjects ranging from renal filtration through metabolic acidosis and bone formation and growth.

We hope you will appreciate this extensive range of online resources. To access this material please register as an instructor by logging on to evolve.elsevier.com/Patton/AP/international/. Although the material is easy to use, if at any point you need technical support it can be provided via the following URL https://service.elsevier.com/app/overview/evolve/ or by calling 001-800-401-9962.

Acknowledgements

Over the years, many people have contributed to the development and success of *Anatomy & Physiology*. We extend our thanks and deep appreciation to all of the students and classroom instructors who have provided us with helpful suggestions. We also thank the many contributors and reviewers who have, over the last several editions, provided us with extraordinary insights and useful features that we have added to our textbook.

Paul Krieger helped us design the *Clear View of the Human Body*, for which we are grateful. Thanks to Betsy Brantley, who contributed many of the case studies found in this edition.

A special thanks goes to Dan Matusiak, who has contributed in many ways to the last few editions.

Also, a very special thanks to Dr. Joanne Wagner, PT, PhD, Richard Hawkins of MMS Medical, and Jeff Wilsman of Southampton Medical for help securing medical supplies for our photo shoot, and to the crew and staff at Meoli Digital for a great shoot!

To those at Elsevier who put their best efforts into producing this edition, we are indebted. We are also grateful to our friends at Graphic World, who helped us improve and execute our integrated design, layout, and art program.

Kevin T. Patton
Gary A. Thibodeau

Contents

Colour Key

BIOCHEMISTRY

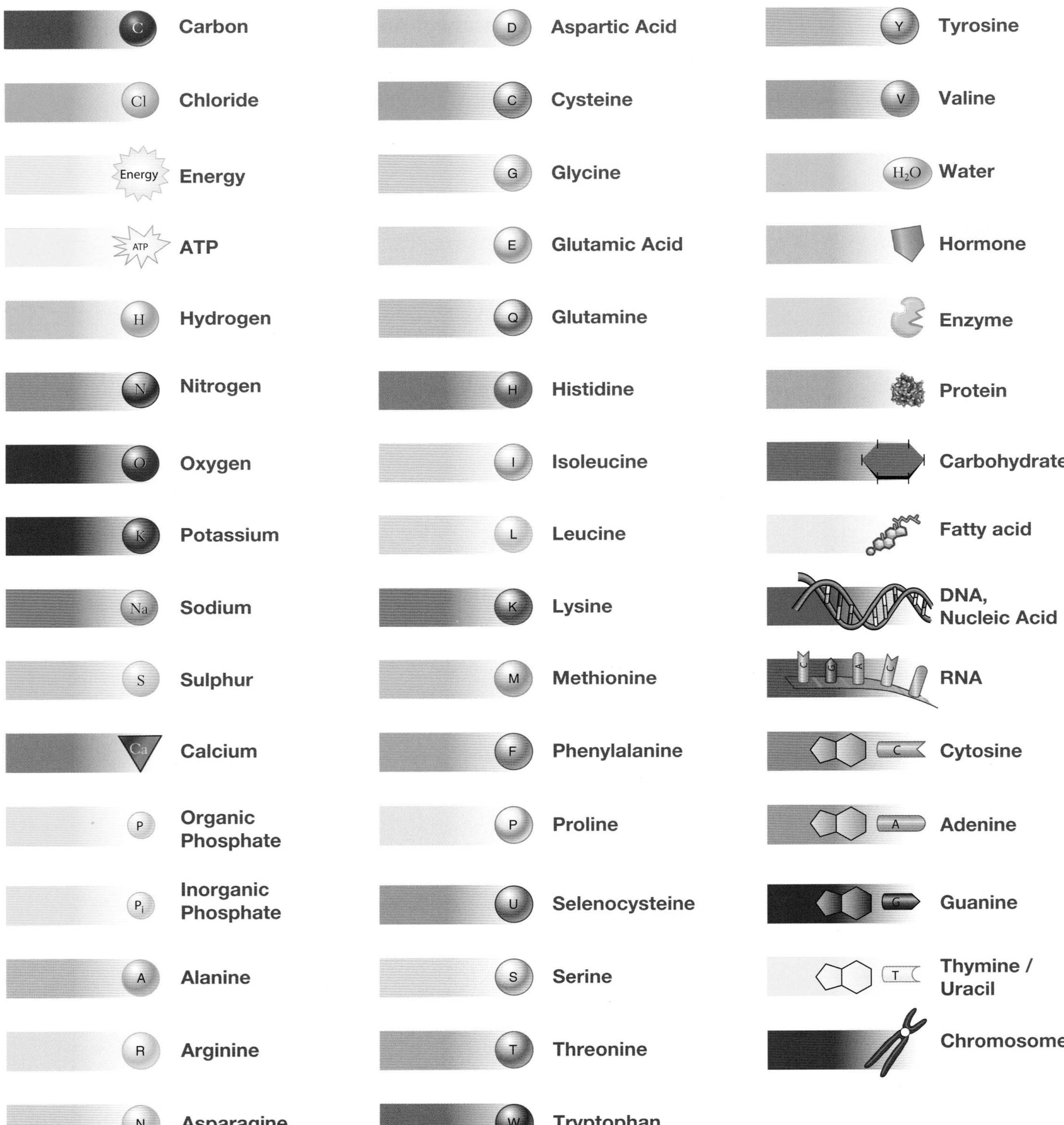

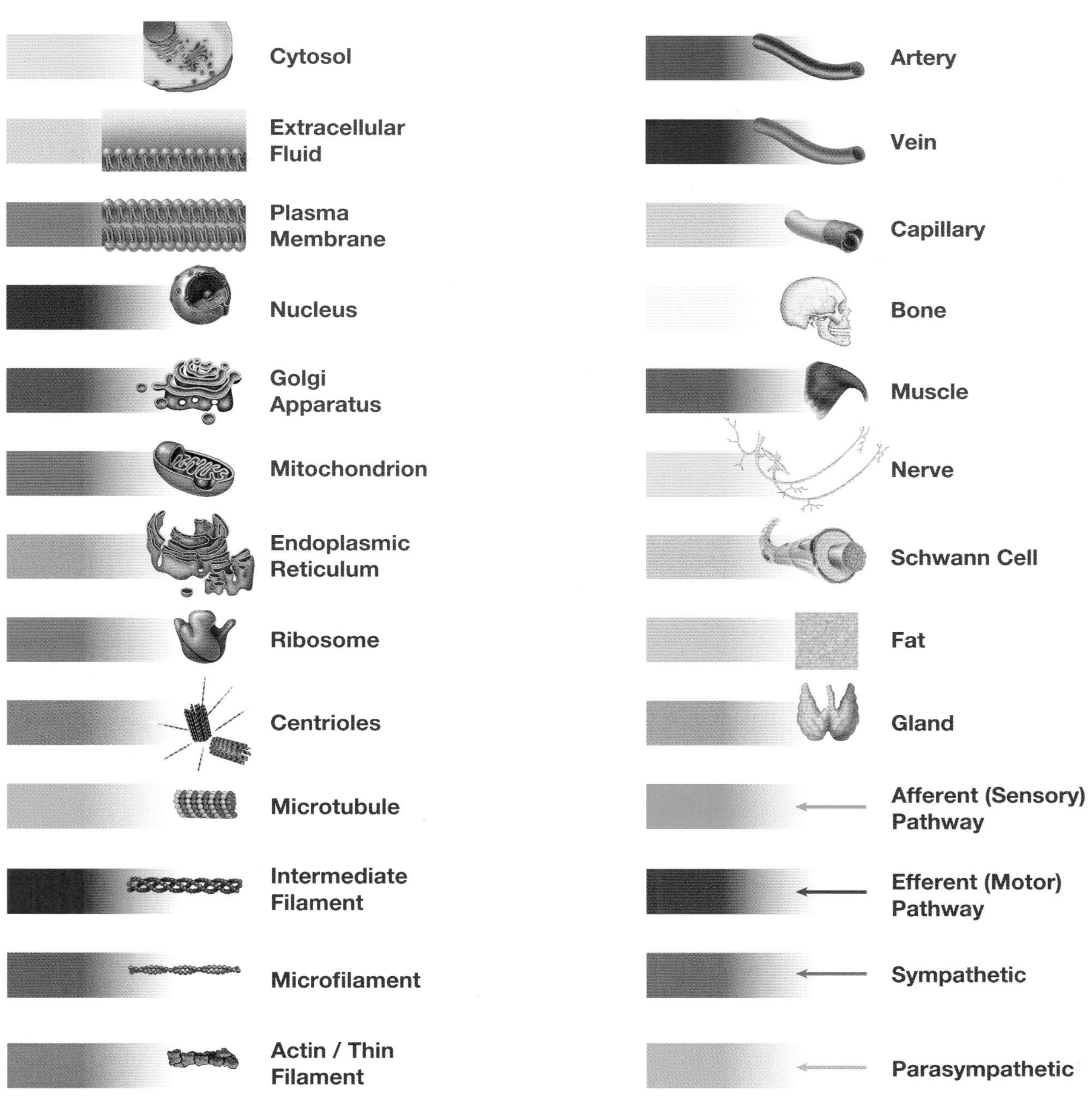
CELLULAR STRUCTURES
Cytosol
Extracellular Fluid
Plasma Membrane
Nucleus
Golgi Apparatus
Mitochondrion
Endoplasmic Reticulum
Ribosome
Centrioles
Microtubule
Intermediate Filament
Microfilament
Actin / Thin Filament
Myosin / Thick Filament
Na+ Channel
OTHER STRUCTURES
Artery
Vein
Capillary
Bone
Muscle
Nerve
Schwann Cell
Fat
Gland
Afferent (Sensory) Pathway
Efferent (Motor) Pathway
Sympathetic
Parasympathetic
Process Arrow

Illustration and Photograph Credits

COVER AND FRONT MATTER

Shutterstock.com

UNIT 1

Seeing the Big Picture box: Copyright Kevin Patton, Lion Den Inc, Weldon Spring, MO.

Chapter 1

1-2: De Humani Corporis Fabrica (On the Structure of the Human Body), in 1543. **1-3, 1-8, 1-9:** Courtesy Barbara Cousins. **1-10:** Redrawn from Muscolino JE: *Know the body: muscle, bone, and palpation essentials*, St. Louis, 2012, Mosby. **1-11, A:** Courtesy Vidic B, Suarez RF: *Photographic atlas of the human body*, St. Louis, 1984, Mosby. **1-11, B:** Suarez RF: *Photographic atlas of the human body*, St. Louis, 1984, Mosby. **Connect It! box:** From Goldman L, Ausiello D: *Cecil textbook of medicine*, ed 22, Philadelphia, 2004, Saunders.

Chapter 2

2-6: Data from Schwartz WJ: A clinician's primer on the circadian clock: its localization, function, and resetting. *Adv Intern Med*, 38:81-106, 1993. In (redrawn from) Koeppen B, Stanton B: *Berne & Levy physiology*, ed 6, Mosby, 2010. **2-8, 2-9, B:** From Patton KT, Thibodeau G: *Human body in health & disease*, ed 6, St. Louis, 2014, Mosby. **2-9, A:** From Donne DG, Viles JH, Groth D, Melhorn I: Structure of the recombinant full-length hamster prion protein PRp (29-231): the N terminus is highly flexible, *Proc Natl Acad Sci USA*, 94:13452-13457, 1997. Copyright National Academy of Sciences, USA.

Chapter 3

3-1: From Patton KT, Thibodeau G: *Human body in health & disease*, ed 6, St. Louis, 2014, Mosby. **3-4:** From Sugimoto Y, Pou P, Abe M et al: Chemical identification of individual surface atoms by atomic force microscopy, *Nature*, 466:64-67, 2007. **3-8, C:** Michael Godomski/Tom Stack & Associates. **Case Study box:** From Potter P, Perry A: *Basic nursing: essentials for practice*, ed 6, St. Louis, 2006, Mosby.

Chapter 4

4-13: From Patton KT, Thibodeau GA: *Mosby's handbook of anatomy & physiology*, ed 2, St. Louis, 2014, Elsevier. **4-14:** From Patton K, Thibodeau G, Douglas M: *Essentials of anatomy and physiology*, Mosby, 2012. **4-15, Box 4-4 (photo):** From National Institute of General Medical Sciences, *The structures of life*, July 2007, retrieved November 2008 from http://www.nigms.nih.gov/news/science_ed/structlife/. **Box 4-2 (photo):** Copyright Kevin Patton, Lion Den Inc, Weldon Spring, MO.

Chapter 5

5-1, B: Courtesy A. Arlan Hinchee. **5-2, 5-9, 5-10, 5-13, 5-15 (electron micrographs), 5-17:** From Pollard T, Earnshaw W: *Cell biology*, revised reprint, international edition, ed 1, Philadelphia, 2004, Saunders. **5-7, B, 5-12, B, 5-18, B:** Courtesy Charles Flickinger, University of Virginia. **5-11, B:** Courtesy Brenda Russell. **5-14:** From Patton KT, Thibodeau GA: *Mosby's handbook of anatomy & physiology*, ed 2, St. Louis, 2014, Elsevier. **5-15 (fluorescence light micrographs [right panel]), 5-15, A:** Courtesy I. Herman, Tufts University. **5-15, B:** Courtesy E. Smith and E. Fuchs, University of Chicago. **5-15, C:** Courtesy G. Borisy, University of Wisconsin, Madison. **5-16, B:** With permission of Dr. Conly Rieder, Wadsworth Center, Albany, NY. **5-18, A:** Susumu Ito. **Table 5-4 (figures):** From Patton KT, Thibodeau GA: *Mosby's handbook of anatomy & physiology*, ed 2, St. Louis, 2014, Elsevier. **Connect It! box (figure):** From Kong LB et al: Structure of the vault, a ubiquitous cellular component, *Structure*, 7:371-379, 1999.

Chapter 6

6-9: Adapted from McCance K, Huether S: *Pathophysiology*, ed 4, St. Louis, 2002, Mosby. **6-11 (electron micrographs):** Courtesy M.M. Perry and A.B. Gilbert, Edinburgh Research Centre. **Box 6-1, B:** From Goldman L, Ausiello D: *Cecil textbook of medicine*, ed 22, Philadelphia, 2004, Saunders.

Chapter 7

7-1 (photo): Cold Spring Harbor Laboratory. **7-4:** Adapted from Pollard T, Earnshaw W: *Cell biology*, revised reprint, international edition, ed 1, Philadelphia, 2004, Saunders. **7-10, A-F:** Dennis Strete. **7-12:** Wikimedia Commons.

Chapter 8

8-1: From Patton KT, Thibodeau GA: *Mosby's handbook of anatomy & physiology*, ed 2, St. Louis, 2014, Elsevier. **8-4 (bottom image):** Modified from Pollard TD, Earnshaw W: *Cell biology*, ed 2, Philadelphia, 2007, W.B. Saunders Company. **8-5:** From Gartner LP, Hiatt JL: *Color textbook of histology*, ed 3, Philadelphia, 2007, Saunders. **8-7:** From Callen J, Greer K, Hood A et al: *Color atlas of dermatology*, Philadelphia, 1993, Saunders. **8-10, A, B:** From Samuelson DA: *Textbook of veterinary histology*, W.B. Saunders Company, 2007. **8-10, C:** Will Murray (Willscrit), http://wilmurraymedia.com. **8-12:** Reprinted with permission from Gregor Reid, PhD, Lawson Health

Research Institute. **8-13:** From Gartner L, Hiatt J: *Color textbook of histology*, ed 3, Philadelphia, 2007, Saunders.

Chapter 9

9-2, 9-4, 9-6, 9-7, 9-8, 9-9, 9-14, 9-16, 9-17, 9-18, 9-23, 9-25, 9-26, 9-27, 9-29, 9-30, 9-31, 9-32, 9-33: Dennis Strete. **9-3 (drawing):** Barbara Cousins. **9-3 (electron micrograph), 9-10, 9-15, B:** From Erlandsen SL, Magney J: *Color atlas of histology*, St. Louis, 1992, Mosby. **9-5:** Ed Reschke **9-20, 9-28:** From Gartner L, Hiatt J: *Color textbook of histology*, ed 3, Philadelphia, 2007, Saunders. **9-21, 9-24:** From Kerr J: *Atlas of functional histology*, London, 1999, Mosby. **9-22:** Courtesy Gary Thibodeau. **Box 9-1:** From Zitelli B, Davis H: *Atlas of pediatric physical diagnosis*, ed 3, Philadelphia, 1997, Mosby.

UNIT 2

Chapter 10

10-1 (photo): Ed Reschke. **10-1 (drawing), 10-6, 10-29:** Barbara Cousins. **10-3:** Copyright Kevin Patton, Lion Den Inc, Weldon Spring, MO. **10-10:** From Rouzaud F, Kadekaro A, Abdel-Malek Za, Hearing VJ: MC1R and the response of melanocytes to ultraviolet radiation, *Mutat Res*, 571:136, 2005. **10-11:** From Regezi J, Sciubba JJ, Jordan RCK: *Oral pathology: clinical pathologic correlations*, ed 5, St. Louis, 2008, Saunders. **10-12:** From Epstein O, Perkin GD, Cookson J, de Bono D: *Clinical examination*, ed 3, St. Louis, 2003, Mosby. **10-13 (gradient):** From McCance K, Huether S: *Pathophysiology*, ed 5, St. Louis, 2005, Mosby. **10-17, C:** Copyright © by David Scharf, 1986, 1993. **10-18:** Copyright Kevin Patton, Lion Den Inc, Weldon Spring, MO. **10-20:** Courtesy Christine Olekyk. **10-21, 10-24, 10-25:** From Habif TP: *Clinical dermatology*, ed 4, St. Louis, Mosby, 2004. **10-22:** From Habif TP: *Clinical dermatology*, ed 2, St. Louis, 1990, Mosby. **10-26:** From Potter P, Perry A: *Basic nursing: essentials for practice*, ed 5, St. Louis, 2003, Mosby. **10-27:** From James WD, Berger TG, Elston DM: *Andrew's diseases of the skin: clinical dermatology*, ed 10, London, 2000, Saunders. **10-28, A:** From Goldman L, Ausiello D: *Cecil textbook of medicine*, ed 23, Philadelphia, 2003, Saunders. **10-28, B:** From Noble J: *Textbook of primary care medicine*, ed 3, Philadelphia, 2001, Mosby. **10-28, C:** From Townsend C, Beauchamp RD, Evers BM, Mattox K: *Sabiston textbook of surgery*, ed 18, Philadelphia, 2008, Saunders. **10-28, D:** From Rakel R: *Textbook of family medicine*, ed 7, Philadelphia, 2007, Saunders. **Box 10-1:** Courtesy James A. Ischen, MD, Baylor College of Medicine. **Box 10-4:** From Emond R: *Color atlas of infectious diseases*, ed 4, Philadelphia, 2003, Mosby. **Box 10-5 (figure):** Courtesy Photo Researchers, Inc. http://images.sciencesource.com/search/SB1498. **Box 10-7 (figure):** From Callen JP et al: *Color atlas of dermatology*, ed 2, Philadelphia, 2000, Saunders. **Case Study (figure):** Copyright Kevin Patton, Lion Den Inc.

Chapter 11

11-3, B: From White T: *Human osteology*, ed 2, Philadelphia, 2000, Academic Press. **11-4, B:** From Moses K, Nava P, Banks J, Petersen D: *Moses atlas of clinical gross anatomy*, Philadelphia, 2005, Mosby. **11-6, B, 11-24, A, B:** Dennis Strete. **11-8, 11-16:** From Williams P: *Gray's anatomy*, ed 38, Philadelphia, 1996, Churchill Livingstone. **11-9, A:** From Muscolino J: *Kinesiology*, St. Louis, 2006, Mosby. **11-9, B:** From Erlandsen SL, Magney J: *Color atlas of histology*, St. Louis, 1992, Mosby. **11-10:** Wikimedia Common. **11-13:** From Patton K, Thibodeau G, Doublas M: *Essentials of anatomy and physiology*, St. Louis, 2012, Mosby. **11-14:** From Pollard TD, Earnshaw W: *Cell biology*, ed 2, Philadelphia, 2007, Saunders. **11-17:** From Zitelli B, Davis H: *Atlas of pediatric physical diagnosis*, ed 4, Philadelphia, Mosby, 2002. **11-18:** Ed Reschke. **11-20:** From Booher JM, Thibodeau Ga: *Athletic injury assessment*, St. Louis, 1985, Mosby. **11-24, 11-25:** From Kumar V, Abbas A, Fausto N: *Robbins and Cotran pathologic basis of disease*, ed 7, Philadelphia, 2005, Saunders.

Chapter 12

12-2 (photo), 12-3 (photo), 12-4 (photo), 12-5 (photo), Courtesy Vidic B, Suarez FR: *Photographic atlas of the human body*, St. Louis, 1984, Mosby. **12-6 (photo), 12-11, 12-16, 12-13 (inset):** From Williams P: *Gray's anatomy*, ed 38, Philadelphia, Churchill Livingstone, 1996. **12-14, A-H:** From Gosling J, Harris P, Whitmore I, Willan P: *Human anatomy*, ed 4, Philadelphia, 2002, Mosby. **12-17:** Courtesy Dr. N. Blevins, New England Medical Center, Boston.

Chapter 13

13-2, D, 13-3, C, 13-4, C, 13-5, 13-6, 13-7, 13-8, D, E, 13-9, B (photos): Courtesy Vidic B, Suarez FR: *Photographic atlas of the human body*, St. Louis, 1984, Mosby. **13-7, 13-11, B, D:** From Abrahams P, Marks S, Hutchings R: *McMinn's color atlas of human anatomy*, ed 5, Philadelphia, 2003, Mosby. **13-10 (drawings):** From Yvonne Wylie Walston. **13-10 (photo inset):** From Seidel HM, Ball JW, Dains JE, Benedict GW: *Mosby's guide to physical examination*, ed 5, St. Louis, 2003, Mosby. **Case Study box:** From Browner B, Jupiter J, Trafton P: *Skeletal trauma: basic science, management, and reconstruction*, ed 3, Philadelphia, 2003, Saunders.

Chapter 14

14-3, B, 14-6, 14-7, A, B, 14-8, 14-11: From Gosling J, Harris P, Whitmore I, Willan PI: *Human anatomy*, ed 4, Philadelphia, 2002, Mosby. **14-5, B, D, 14-7, C, 14-9, B, D, 14-10, B, D:** Courtesy Vidic B, Suarez FR: *Photographic atlas of the human body*, St. Louis, 1984, Mosby. **14-26:** From Seidel HM, Ball JW, Dains JE, Benedict GW: *Mosby's guide to physical examination*, ed 5, St. Louis, 2003, Mosby. **14-27:** From Swartz MH: *Textbook of physical diagnosis*, ed 4, Philadelphia, 2002, Saunders. **14-28:** Courtesy Lanny L. Johnson, MD, East Lansing, MI. **Box 14-1 (photo):** From Cummings N, Stanley-Green S, Higgs P: *Perspectives in athletic training*, St. Louis, 2009, Mosby. **Box 14-3:** From Canale ST: *Campbell's operative orthopaedics*, ed 9, St Louis, 1998, Mosby. **Case Study box:** From Goldman L, Ausiello D: *Cecil textbook of medicine*, ed 23, Philadelphia, 2007, Saunders.

Chapter 15

15-4: Adapted from Muscolino J: *Kinesiology*, St. Louis, 2006, Mosby. **15-14:** From Gosling J, Harris P, Whitmore I, Willan P: *Human anatomy*, ed 4, Philadelphia, 2002, Mosby. **Box 15-1 (photo):** From Harkreader H: *Fundamentals of nursing: caring and clinical judgment*, ed 3, St. Louis, 2007, Saunders.

Chapter 16

Box 16-1: Shutterstock.com

Chapter 17

17-4, A: Courtesy Dr. J.H. Venable, Department of Anatomy, Colorado State University, Fort Collins, CO. **17-4, B,** Courtesy Dr. H.E. Huxley. **17-6:** From Leeson CR, Leeson T, Paparo A: *Text/atlas of histology*, St. Louis, 1988, Saunders. **17-7, A:** Courtesy of Don Fawcett, Harvard Medical School, Boston, Massachusetts. In Pollard TD: Earnshaw W: *Cell biology*, ed 2, St. Louis, 2007, Saunders. **17-10, 17-11, 17-15:** From Lodish H: *Molecular cell biology*, ed 4, New York, 2000, WH Freeman. **17-12, B:** Courtesy H.E. Huxley, Brandeis University, Waltham, Ma. **17-18, B:** Courtesy Dr. Paul C. Letourneau, Department of Anatomy, Medical School, University of Minnesota, MN. **17-22:** Adapted from Pollard T, Earnshaw W: *Cell biology*, ed 2, Philadelphia, 2008, Saunders. **17-30 (photos):** Courtesy Dr. Frederic S. Fay, Department of Physiology, University of Massachusetts, Worschester, Ma. **17-32 (photo):** Courtesy Kellie White. **Box 17-6, A:** From Kumar V, Abbas A, Fausto N: *Robbins and Cotran pathologic basis of disease*, ed 7, Philadelphia, 2005, Saunders. **Box 17-7 (photo):** From Fritz S: *Mosby's fundamentals of therapeutic massage*, ed 5, St. Louis, 2013, Mosby.

UNIT 3

Chapter 18

18-1: From Patton KT, Thibodeau G: *Human body in health & disease*, ed 6, St. Louis, 2014, Mosby. 18-13: Redrawn from FitzGerald MJT, Gruener G, Mtui E: *Clinical neuroanatomy and neuroscience*, ed 6, Edinburgh, Saunders, 2011. **18-14:** From Feldman M, Friedman L, Brandt L: *Sleisenger & Fordtran's gastrointestinal and liver disease*, ed 8, Philadelphia, 2006, Saunders. **Box 18-1, A:** Courtesy Marie Simar Couldwell, MD, and Maiken Nedergaard.

Chapter 19

Box 19-1 (photo): From Christensen GJ: *A consumer's guide to dentistry*, ed 2, St. Louis, 2002, Mosby. **Box 19-2:** Copyright Kevin Patton, Lion Den Inc., Weldon Spring, MO. **Box 19-3 (photo):** Courtesy Tamily Weissman and Jean Livet.

Chapter 20

20-2, B, 20-10, C, Box 20-3: From Abrahams P, Marks S, Hutchings R: *McMinn's color atlas of human anatomy*, ed 5, Philadelphia, 2003, Mosby. **20-5, C:** Redrawn from FitzGerald MJT, Gruener G, Mtui E: *Clinical neuroanatomy and neuroscience*, ed 6, Saunders, 2011. **20-7 (photo):** From Gosling J, Harris P, Whitmore I, Willan P: *Human anatomy*, ed 4, Philadelphia, 2002. **20-9, B:** Courtesy Vidic B, Suarez FR: *Photographic atlas of the human body*, St. Louis, 1984, Mosby. **20-16, C:** From Gigandet X, Hagmann P, Kurant M, et al: Estimating the confidence level of white matter connections obtained with MRI tractography, *PLoS ONE*, 3(12):e4006, 2008. **20-25:** Courtesy Walter Schreider, University of Pennsylvania. **20-26:** Courtesy D.N. Markand. **Box 20-1 (photos):** From Forbes CD, Jackson WD: *Color atlas and text of clinical medicine*, ed 3, London, 2003, Mosby. **Box 20-6 (photo):** From Chipps EM, Clanin NJ, Campbell VG: *Neurologic disorders*, St. Louis, 1992, Mosby-Year Book, Inc. **Table 20-3:** Redrawn from FitzGerald MJT, Gruener G, Mtui E: *Clinical neuroanatomy and neuroscience*, ed 6, Saunders, 2011.

Chapter 21

21-1: From Drake RL et al: *Gray's atlas of anatomy*, Philadelphia, 2008, Churchill Livingstone/Elsevier. **Box 21-3 (photo):** From Habif TP: *Clinical dermatology*, ed 2, St. Louis, 1990, Mosby. **Box 21-4:** From Perkin GD: *Mosby's color atlas and text of neurology*, London, 1998, Times Mirror International Publishers. **Box 21-5:** From Beare P, Myers J: *Adult health nursing*, ed 3, St. Louis, 1998, Mosby.

Chapter 22

Case Study box (photo): Courtesy Flickr, Photo Sharing.

Chapter 23

23-1: Adapted from Guyton A, Hall J: *Textbook of medical physiology*, ed 11, Philadelphia, 2006, Saunders. **23-3, A:** From Seidel HM, Ball JW, Dains JE, Benedict GW: *Mosby's guide to physical examination*, ed 6, St. Louis, 2006, Mosby. **23-3, B:** From Swartz MH: *Textbook of physical diagnosis*, ed 4, Philadelphia, 2002, Saunders. **23-4:** Adapted from Boron W, Boulpaep E: *Medical physiology*, updated version, ed 1, Philadelphia, 2005, Saunders.

Chapter 24

24-3, D: Omikron/Photo Researchers. **24-8, B:** Adapted from Guyton A, Hall J: *Textbook of medical physiology*, ed 11, Philadelphia, 2006, Saunders. **24-11:** Copyright Kevin Patton, Lion Den Inc, Weldon Spring, MO. **24-13:** From Newell FW: *Ophthalmology: principles and concepts*, ed 7, St. Louis, 1992, Mosby. **24-18, C:** Courtesy Dr. Scott Mittman, Johns Hopkins Hospital, Baltimore, MD. **24-23:** From Seidel HM, Ball JW, Dains JE, Benedict GW: *Mosby's guide to physical examination*, ed 3, St. Louis, 2003, Mosby. **24-25:** Adapted from Boron W, Boulpaep E: *Medical physiology*, updated version, ed 1, Philadelphia, 2005, Saunders. **24-27:** From Bingham BJG, Hawke M, Kwok P: *Atlas of clinical otolaryngology*, St. Louis, 1992, Mosby–Year Book. **24-29, 24-30, A:** From Swartz MH: *Textbook of physical diagnosis*, ed 4, Philadelphia, 2002, Saunders. **Box 24-3 (figure):** From *Ishihara's tests for colour deficiency*, Tokyo, Japan, 1973, Kanehara Trading Co, Copyright Isshinkai Foundation.

Chapter 25

25-13: Adapted from Hinson J, Raven P: *The endocrine system*, Edinburgh, 2007, Churchill Livingstone.

Chapter 26

26-2: From Erlandsen SL, Magney J: *Color atlas of histology*, St. Louis, 1992, Mosby. **26-7:** Adapted from Boron W, Boulpaep E: *Medical physiology*, updated version, ed 1, Philadelphia, 2005, Saunders. **26-9, B:** From Jacob S: *Atlas of human anatomy*, Edinburgh, 2002, Churchill Livingstone. **26-12, B:** From Abrahams P, Marks S, Hutchings R: *McMinn's color atlas of human anatomy*, ed 3, Philadelphia, 2003, Mosby. **26-13:** Dennis Strete. **26-15:** From Gosling J, Harris P, Whitmore I, Willan P: *Human anatomy*, ed 4, Philadelphia, 2002, Mosby. **26-17:** From Kierszenbaum A: *Histology and cell biology*, Philadelphia, 2002, Mosby. **Box 26-4, A:** From Swartz MH: *Textbook of physical diagnosis*, ed 4, Philadelphia, 2002, Saunders. **Box 26-4, B:** From Goldman L, Schafer AI: *Goldman's Cecil medicine*, ed 24, Vol. 2, Philadelphia, 2012, Saunders. **Box 26-6 (figures):** Courtesy Gower Medical Publishers. **Box 26-1 (photo A):** Courtesy

Robert F. Gagel, MD and Ian McCutcheon, MD, University of Texas MD Anderson Cancer Center, Houston. In Black JM, Hawks JH: *Medical-surgical nursing: clinical management for positive outcomes,* ed 8, St. Louis, 2009, Saunders. **Box 26-1 (photo B):** From Forbes CD, Jackson WF: *Color atlas and text of clinical medicine,* ed 3, 2003, Mosby, Elsevier Science Ltd.

UNIT 4

Chapter 27

27-3, D: From Zakus SM: *Clinical procedures for medical assistants,* ed 3, St. Louis, 1995, Mosby. **27-4:** From Shiland BJ: *Mastering healthcare terminology,* ed 3, St. Louis, 2010, Mosby. **27-5:** Patton KT, Thibodeau G: *Human body in health & disease,* ed 6, St. Louis, 2014, Mosby. **27-8 (inset):** From Carr J, Rodak B: *Clinical hematology atlas,* St. Louis, 1999, Elsevier. **27-11 (inset):** From Belcher AE: *Blood disorders,* St. Louis 1993, Mosby. **27-13, 27-14, 27-15, 27-16, 27-17:** Dennis Strete. **27-18:** From Turgeon M: *Linne & Ringsud's clinical laboratory science,* ed 5, St. Louis, 2007, Mosby. **27-19:** From Carr JH, Rodak BF: *Clinical hematology atlas,* ed 2, St. Louis, 2004, Elsevier. **27-20, B:** Copyright Dennis Kunkel Microscopy Inc. **27-23:** From Cotran R, Kumar V, Collins T: *Robbins pathologic basis of disease,* ed 6, Philadelphia, Saunders, 1999. **27-24, 27-25:** From Kumar V, Abbas A, Fausto N: *Robbins and Cotran pathologic basis of disease,* ed 7, Philadelphia, 2005, Saunders. **Table 27-2:** Adapted from Pagana KD, Pagana TJ: *Mosby's manual of diagnostic and laboratory tests,* ed 5, St. Louis, 2013, Mosby. **Case Study box:** From Stevens ML: *Fundamentals of clinical hematology,* Philadelphia, 1997, Saunders.

Chapter 28

28-1: Courtesy Patricia Kane, Indiana University Medical School. **28-9 (drawing):** From Wilson SF, Giddens JF: *Health assessment for nursing practice,* ed 2, St. Louis, 2001, Mosby. **28-9 (inset):** From Seidel HM, Ball JW, Dains JE, Benedict GW: *Mosby's guide to physical examination,* ed 6, St. Louis, 2006, Mosby. **28-17:** From Noble A, Johnson R, Thomas A, Bass P: *The cardiovascular system,* Edinburgh, 2005, Churchill Livingstone. **28-20:** From Kumar V, Abbas A, Fausto N: *Robbins and Cotran pathologic basis of disease,* ed 7, Philadelphia, 2005, Saunders. **28-24:** Courtesy Guzzetta and Dossey, 1984. **28-25:** From Aehlert B: *ACLS quick review study cards,* ed 2, St. Louis, 2004, Mosby. **28-26:** From Cotran R, Kumar V, Collins T: *Robbins pathologic basis of disease,* ed 6, Philadelphia, 1999, Saunders. **Box 28-1:** From Goldman L, Ausiello D: *Cecil textbook of medicine,* ed 23, Philadelphia, 2008, Saunders. **Case Study box:** From Hicks GH: *Cardiopulmonary anatomy and physiology,* Philadelphia, 2000, Saunders.

Chapter 29

29-5: Adapted from McCance K, Huether S: *Pathophysiology,* ed 5, St. Louis, 2006, Mosby. **29-9, C, 29-11, A, C, 29-13, B, C:** From Abrahams P, Marks S, Hutchings R: *McMinn's color atlas of human anatomy,* ed 5, Philadelphia, 2003, Mosby. **29-26 (photo):** From Swartz MH: *Textbook of physical diagnosis,* ed 4, Philadelphia, 2002, Saunders. **29-29:** From Cotran R, Kumar V, Collins T: *Robbins pathologic basis of disease,* ed 6, Philadelphia, 1999, Saunders. **Box 29-1:** Courtesy Simon C, Janner M: *Color atlas of pediatric diseases with differential diagnosis,* ed 2, Hamilton, Ontario, 1990, BC Decker. **Case Study box:** Courtesy Dr. Daniel Simon and Mr. Paul Zambino

Chapter 30

30-1: From Harvey W: *The anatomical exercises,* London, 1995, Dover Publishing. **30-6:** From Rhoades R, Pflanzer R: *Human physiology,* ed 3, Philadelphia, 1995, Perennial. **30-9:** Adapted from Guyton A, Hall J: *Textbook of medical physiology,* ed 11, Philadelphia, 2006, Saunders. **30-11, 30-19, B:** Adapted from Boron W, Boulpaep E: *Medical physiology,* updated version, ed 1, Philadelphia, 2005, Saunders. **30-25:** Adapted from Canobbio MM: *Cardiovascular disorders,* St. Louis, 1990, Mosby. **30-28:** Adapted from the Guidelines of the European Society of Hypertension and of the European Society of Cardiology.

Chapter 31

31-6: Courtesy Ballinger P, Frank E: *Merrill's atlas of radiographic positions and radiologic procedures,* vol 1, ed 10, St. Louis, 2003, Mosby. **31-7:** Adapted from McCance K, Huether S: *Pathophysiology,* ed 4, St. Louis, 2002, Mosby. **31-8:** Adapted from Boron W, Boulpaep E: *Medical physiology,* updated version, ed 1, Philadelphia, 2005, Saunders. **31-9, A:** Adapted from Mathers L, Chase R, Dolph J, Glasgow E: *CLASS clinical anatomy principles,* Philadelphia, 1996, Mosby. **31-9, B:** From Nielsen M: *Human anatomy lab manual and workbook,* ed 4, Dubuque, IA, 2002, Kendall/Hunt Publishing Company. **31-10, B, 31-18, B:** Dennis Strete. **31-15:** From National Institute of Allergy and Infectious Diseases, National Institutes of Health, Bethesda, MD. **31-16, 31-25:** From Seidel HM, Ball JW, Dains JE, Benedict GW: *Mosby's guide to physical examination,* ed 6, St. Louis, 2006, Mosby. **31-17, B:** Courtesy Dr. Edward L. Applebaum, Head, Department of Otolaryngology, University of Illinois Medical Center, Chicago, IL. **31-19:** Adapted from Rhoades R, Pflanzer R: *Human physiology,* ed 3, Philadelphia, 1995, Perennial. **31-20:** Courtesy Vidic B, Suarez FR: *Photographic atlas of the human body,* St. Louis, 1984, Mosby. **31-22:** Courtesy Walter Tunnesen, MD, The American Board of Pediatrics, Chapel Hill, NC. **31-23:** From Goldstein B, editor: *Practical dermatology,* ed 2, St. Louis, 1997, Mosby. **31-24:** From Stone DR, Gorbach SL: *Atlas of infectious diseases,* Philadelphia, 2000, Saunders. **Case Study box:** From Cohen J, Powderly WG: *Infectious diseases,* ed 2, St. Louis, 2004, Mosby.

Chapter 32

32-1, 32-8, Box 32-1, B: From Abbas A, Lichtman A: *Cellular and molecular immunology,* ed 5, Philadelphia, 2003, Saunders. **32-4:** From Roitt IM, Brostoff, Male DK: *Immunology,* ed 3, St. Louis, 1993, Mosby. **32-6:** Adapted from McCance K, Huether, S: *Pathophysiology,* ed 5, St. Louis, 2006, Mosby. **32-10:** From McCance K, Huether S: *Pathophysiology: the biologic basis for disease in adults and children,* ed 7, Mosby, 2014. **Box 32-1, A:** From Copstead-Kirkhorn L, Banasik J: *Pathophysiology,* ed 2, St. Louis, 1999, Saunders.

Chapter 33

33-1: Copyright Dennis Kunkel Microscopy Inc. **33-3, 33-4, 33-5, 33-9, 33-14, 33-15, 33-16, 33-17, 33-18, 33-20, Box 32-1, B, Box 33-6:** From Abbas A, Lichtman A: *Cellular and molecular immunology,* ed 5, Philadelphia, 2003, Saunders. **33-13, 33-21:** From Copstead-Kirkhorn L, Banasik J: *Pathophysiology,* ed 2, St. Louis, 1999, Saunders. **Box 33-3:** From Stinchcombe JC, Griffiths GM: The role of the secretory immunological synapse in killing by CD8+

CTL, *Semin Immunol,* 15(6):301-305, 2003. **Box 33-5:** Adapted from McCance K, Huether S: *Pathophysiology,* ed 4, St. Louis, 2002, Elsevier. **Case Study box:** From Mason DJ, Leavitt J, Chaffee M: *Policy and politics in nursing and health care,* ed 5, St. Louis, 2007, Saunders.

Chapter 34

34-1, A: Julie Dermansky/Science Source. **34-1, B:** Ria Novosti/Science Source. **34-1, C:** Mauro Fermariello/Science Source. **34-1, D:** Global Warming Art. **34-8:** Copyright Kevin Patton, Lion Den Inc, Weldon Spring, MO (courtesy National Tiger Sanctuary).

UNIT 5

Chapter 35

35-4: From Stevens A, Lowe J: *Human histology,* ed 3, Philadelphia, 2005, Mosby. **35-8, B:** Custom Medical Stock Photo Inc. **35-9:** Adapted from Thompson JM, Wilson SF: *Health assessment for nursing practice,* St. Louis, 1996, Mosby. **35-13, B:** From Erlandsen SL, Magney J: *Color atlas of histology,* St. Louis, 1992, Mosby. **35-12:** From Hutchings RT, McMinn RM: *McMinn's color atlas of human anatomy,* ed 2, Chicago, 1988, Year Book Medical Publishers. **35-14:** From Epstein O, Perkin GD, Cookson J, de Bono D: *Clinical examination,* ed 3, Philadelphia, 2003, Mosby. **35-16:** Courtesy Vidic B, Suarez RF: *Photographic atlas of the human body,* St. Louis, 1984, Mosby. **35-19:** From Zitelli B, Davis H: *Atlas of pediatric physical diagnosis,* ed 4, Philadelphia, 2002, Mosby. **35-20, 35-21:** From Kumar V, Abbas A, Fausto N: *Robbins and Cotran pathologic basis of disease,* ed 7, Philadelphia, 2005, Saunders.

Chapter 36

36-6: From Drake R, Vogl AW, Mitchell A: *Gray's anatomy for students,* Philadelphia, 2005, Churchill Livingstone. **36-9, A, 36-16:** Adapted from Boron W, Boulpaep E: *Medical physiology,* updated version, ed 1, Philadelphia, 2005, Saunders. **39-9, B:** Antonia Reeve/Science Source. **36-12, Box 36-2:** Adapted from Davies A, Moores C: *The respiratory system,* Edinburgh, 2004, Churchill Livingstone. **36-14:** Patton KT, Thibodeau G: *Human body in health & disease,* ed 6, St. Louis, 2014, Mosby. **Box 36-6:** Copyright Kevin Patton, Lion Den Inc, Weldon Spring, MO. **Box 36-7:** Adapted from Guyton A, Hall J: *Textbook of medical physiology,* ed 11, Philadelphia, 2006, Saunders.

Chapter 37

37-4, 37-13: Adapted from Boron W, Boulpaep E: *Medical physiology,* updated version, ed 1, Philadelphia, 2005, Saunders. **37-5:** From Rhoades R, Pflanzer R: *Human physiology,* ed 3, Philadelphia, 1995, Perennial. **37-6:** From Patton KT, Thibodeau G: *Human body in health & disease,* 6th edition, Mosby, 2014.

Chapter 38

38-4, B: Copyright Kevin Patton, Lion Den Inc, Weldon Spring, MO. **38-5:** Dennis Strete. **38-6, B:** From Zitelli B, Davis H: *Atlas of pediatric physical diagnosis,* ed 3, Philadelphia, 1997, Mosby. **38-10 (inset):** From Weir J, Abrahams P: *Imaging atlas of the human anatomy,* ed 2, Philadelphia, 1997, Mosby. **38-12, B:** From Stevens A, Lowe J: *Human histology,* ed 3, Philadelphia, Mosby, 2005. **38-16:** From Emond R, Welsby P, Rowland H: Colour atlas of infectious diseases, ed 4, Edinburgh, 2003, Mosby. **38-18, A:** Wilson SF, Giddens JF: *Health assessment for nursing practice,* ed 2, St. Louis, 2001, Mosby. **38-18, B:** From Greig JD, Garden OJ: *Color atlas of surgical diagnosis,* London, 1996, Times Mirror International Publishers. **38-19, D:** Courtesy Kevin Patton, Weldon Spring, MO. **38-21, B, 38-22, Box 38-2:** From Daffner DH: *Clinical radiology: the essentials,* ed 3, Baltimore, 1992, Lippincott, Williams & Wilkins.

Chapter 39

39-2, B: From Abrahams P, Marks S, Hutchings R: *McMinn's color atlas of human anatomy,* ed 5, Philadelphia, 2003, Saunders. **39-4, B:** From Erlandsen SL, Magney J: *Color atlas of histology,* St. Louis, 1992, Mosby. **39-5:** SPL/Photo Researchers. **39-10, A:** Courtesy Baylor Regional Transplant Institute, Baylor University Medical Center, Dallas, TX. **39-14:** Courtesy Thompson JM, Wilson SF: *Health assessment for nursing practice,* St. Louis, 1996, Mosby. **39-20:** From Cotran R, Kumar V, Collins T: *Robbins pathologic basis of disease,* ed 6, Philadelphia, 1999, Saunders. 39-17: From Doughty DB, Jackson D: *Gastrointestinal disorders,* St. Louis, 1993, Mosby.

Chapter 40

40-4, Box 40-1: Adapted from Boron W, Boulpaep E: *Medical physiology,* updated version, ed 1, Philadelphia, 2005, Saunders. **40-19, B:** Courtesy Dr. Andrew Evan, Indiana University. **Box 40-2, B:** Adapted from Smith M, Morton D: *The digestive system,* Edinburgh, 2001, Churchill Livingstone. **Box 40-4, B, C:** From Stevens A, Lowe J: *Human histology,* ed 3, Philadelphia, 2005, Mosby.

Chapter 41

41-1: © Public Health England in association with the Welsh Government, Food Standards Scotland and the Food Standards Agency in Northern Ireland. © Crown copyright 2016. **41-13, B:** Courtesy Brenda Russell, PhD, University of Illinois at Chicago. **41-17, B:** Adapted from Carroll R: *Elsevier's integrated physiology,* Philadelphia, 2007, Mosby. **41-19:** Adapted from *Report of the Expert Panel for Population Strategies for Blood Cholesterol Reduction,* Bethesda, MD, November 1990, The National Cholesterol Education Program, National Heart Lung and Blood Institute, Public Health Service, US Department of Health and Human Services, NIH Publication No. 90-3046. **41-24, 41-25, 41-28, 41-31, Box 41-9, B:** Adapted from Mahan LK, Escott-Stump S: *Krause's food, nutrition and diet therapy,* ed 11, St. Louis, 2004, Saunders. **41-30:** Adapted from Guyton A, Hall J: Textbook of medical physiology, ed 11, Philadelphia, 2006, Saunders. **41-32:** From Zitelli B, Davis H: *Atlas of pediatric physical diagnosis,* ed 3, Philadelphia, 1997, Mosby. **Box 41-2:** Courtesy Bevelander G, Ramalay J: *Essentials of histology,* ed 8, St. Louis, 1979, Mosby.

Chapter 42

42-1, A: Barbara Cousins. **42-1, B, 42-2, B:** From Abrahams P, Marks S, Hutchings R: *McMinn's color atlas of human anatomy,* ed 5, Philadelphia, 2003, Mosby. **42-2, A, 42-10:** Adapted from Brundage DJ: *Renal disorders,* Mosby's clinical nursing series, St. Louis, 1992, Mosby. **42-3, B:** From Weir J, Abrahams P: *Imaging atlas of the human anatomy,* ed 2, Philadelphia, 1997, Mosby. **42-6:** From

Heylings D, Spence R, Kelly B: *Integrated anatomy*, Edinburgh, 2007, Churchill Livingstone. **42-7, 42-11, 42-16:** From Stevens A, Lowe J: *Human histology*, ed 3, Philadelphia, 2005, Mosby. **42-8:** From Gosling J, Harris P, Whitmore I, Willan P: *Human anatomy*, ed 4, Philadelphia, 2002, Mosby. **42-9:** Adapted from Guyton A, Hall J: *Textbook of medical physiology*, ed 11, Philadelphia, 2006, Saunders. **42-14, 42-15, B:** From Boron W, Boulpaep E: *Medical physiology*, updated version, ed 1, Philadelphia, 2005, Saunders. **42-29:** From Kumar V, Abbas A, Fausto N: *Robbins and Cotran pathologic basis of disease*, ed 7, Philadelphia, 2005, Saunders. **Table 42-2:** From Bonewit-West K: *Clinical procedures for medical assistants*, ed 8, St. Louis, Saunders, 2011.

Chapter 43

43-7: Copyright Kevin Patton, Lion Den Inc, Weldon Spring, MO. **43-18:** Adapted from Mahan LK, Escott-Stump S: *Krause's food, nutrition and diet therapy*, ed 12, St. Louis, 2007, Saunders. **43-11:** From Bloom A, Ireland J: *Color atlas of diabetes*, ed 2, St. Louis, 1992, Mosby.

Chapter 44

Box 44-1: Courtesy Kevin Patton, Lion Den Inc, Weldon Spring, MO.

UNIT 6

Chapter 45

45-3, A, 45-8, E: Lennart Nilsson. **45-4, 45-8, F:** From Stevens A, Lowe J: *Human histology*, ed 3, Philadelphia, 2005, Mosby. **45-5:** Courtesy Dr. Mark Ludvigson, US Army Medical Corps, St Paul, MN. **45-9, 45-10, 45-13:** From Erlandsen SL, Magney J: *Color atlas of histology*, St. Louis, 1992, Mosby. **45-11:** Barbara Cousins. **45-12:** From Abrahams P, Marks S, Hutchings R: *McMinn's color atlas of human anatomy*, ed 5, Philadelphia, 2003, Mosby. **45-14, B:** Courtesy Vidic B, Suarez RF: *Photographic atlas of the human body*, St. Louis, 1984, Mosby. **45-15:** Adapted from Guyton A, Hall J: *Textbook of medical physiology*, ed 11, Philadelphia, 2006, Saunders. **45-16:** Adapted from Boron W, Boulpaep E: *Medical physiology*, updated version, ed 1, Philadelphia, 2005, Saunders. **45-17, Box 45-1:** From Seidel HM, Ball JW, Dains JE, Benedict GW: *Mosby's guide to physical examination*, ed 6, St. Louis, 2006, Mosby.

Chapter 46

46-1, B: From Moses K, Nava P, Banks J, Petersen D: *Moses atlas of clinical gross anatomy*, Philadelphia, 2005, Mosby. **46-3, B, 46-6, 46-7:** From Gosling J, Harris P, Whitmore I, Willan P: *Human anatomy*, ed 4, Philadelphia, 2002, Mosby. **46-5C:** From Familiari G, et al: Ultrastructural dynamics of human reproduction, from ovulation to fertlization and early embryo development, *Int Rev Cytol*, 249:53-141, 2006. **46-10:** From Stevens A, Lowe J: *Human histology*, ed 3, Philadelphia, Mosby, 2005. **46-11:** From McKee GT: *Cytopathology*, London, 1997, Mosby-Wolfe. **46-12:** Courtesy Dr. Richard Blandau, Department of Biological Structure, University of Washington School of Medicine, Seattle, WA, from his film *Ovulation and egg transport in mammals*, 1973. **46-18:** Adapted from Boron W, Boulpaep E: *Medical physiology*, updated version, ed 1, Philadelphia, 2005, Saunders. **46-21, 46-23:** From Mettler F: *Essentials of radiology*, ed 2, Philadelphia, 2005, Saunders. **46-22, A:** From Abrahams P, Marks S, Hutchings R: *McMinn's color atlas of human anatomy*, ed 5, Philadelphia, 2003, Saunders. **46-22, B:** From Symonds EM, MacPherson MB: *Color atlas of obstetrics and gynecology*, London, 1994, Mosby Wolfe. **46-24:** From Kumar V, Abbas A, Fausto N: *Robbins and Cotran pathologic basis of disease*, ed 7, Philadelphia, 2005, Saunders. **46-25, B, C,** From Cotran R, Kumar V, Collins T: *Robbins pathologic basis of disease*, ed 6, Philadelphia, 1999, Saunders. **Box 46-6 (photo):** Ferri FF: *Ferri's color atlas and text of clinical medicine*, 2009, Saunders/Elsevier. **Box 46-7:** Michael Donne, Science Photo Library, Science Source.

Chapter 47

47-5 (photo), 47-13: Lennart Nilsson. **47-7:** Courtesy Lucinda L. Veeck, Jones Institute for Reproductive Medicine, Norfolk, Va. **47-11, B:** From Cotran R, Kumar V, Collins T: *Robbins pathologic basis of disease*, ed 6, Philadelphia, 1999, Saunders. **47-12, B:** Adapted from Hinson J, Raven P: *The endocrine system*, Edinburgh, 2007, Churchill Livingstone. **47-14:** From Moore KL, Persand TV: *The developing human*, ed 6, Philadelphia, 1998, Saunders. **46-17, 46-18, 47-25:** Adapted from Boron W, Boulpaep E: *Medical physiology*, updated version, ed 1, Philadelphia, 2005, Saunders. **47-23:** Courtesy Ron Edwards, Chesterfield, MO. **47-24:** Copyright Kevin Patton, Lion Den Inc, Weldon Spring, MO. **47-26:** Adapted from Mahan LK, Escott-Stump S: *Krause's food, nutrition and diet therapy*, ed 12, St. Louis, 2007, Saunders. **47-27:** Adapted from McCance K, Huether S: *Pathophysiology*, ed 5, St. Louis, 2005, Mosby. **47-29, B:** Adapted from Ignatavicius D, Bayne MV: *Medical-surgical nursing: a nursing process approach*, Philadelphia, 1991, Saunders. **47-30:** From Andersen JL, Schjerling P, Saltin B: Muscle, genes, and athletic performance, *Sci Am*, 283(3):49-55, 2000. **47-31:** From Goldman L, Ausiello D, *Cecil textbook of medicine*, ed 23, Philadelphia, 2003, Saunders. **47-32:** Data from YouGov and the Office for National Statistics, UK. **Table 47-1:** Data published by the Office for National Statistics, UK. **Box 47-2, B:** Courtesy Kevin Patton, Lion Den Inc, Weldon Spring, MO. **Box 47-3 (photo):** Courtesy of the Progeria Research Foundation. Peabody, Massachusetts, http://www.progeriaresearch.org. **Case Study box:** From Hagen-Ansert SL: *Textbook of diagnostic ultrasonography*, vol 2, ed 6, St. Louis, 2007, Mosby.

Chapter 48

48-1: Adapted from Boron W, Boulpaep E: *Medical physiology*, updated version, ed 1, Philadelphia, 2005, Saunders. **48-5:** From Jorde L, Carey J, Bamshad M: *Medical genetics*, ed 3, Philadelphia, 2004, Saunders. **48-10:** From McCance K, Huether S: *Pathophysiology*, ed 4, St. Louis, 2002, Mosby. **48-13, B:** From Kumar V, Abbas A, Fausto N: *Robbins and Cotran pathologic basis of disease*, ed 7, Philadelphia, 2005, Saunders. **48-14, A:** Courtesy Lois McGavran, Denver Children's Hospital. **48-14, B:** From Zitelli: *Atlas of pediatric physical diagnosis*, ed 6, St. Louis, 2012, Mosby. **48-15, 48-16, B, 48-17, B:** Courtesy Nancy S. Wexler, PhD, Columbia University.

UNIT 1

The Body as a Whole

The nine chapters in Unit 1 "set the stage" for the study of human anatomy and physiology. They provide the unifying information required to understand the "connectedness" of human structure and function. They will help you understand how organized anatomical structures of a particular size, shape, form, or placement serve important functions. The illustration that opens this unit shows the body not as a jumble of isolated parts but as an integrated whole.

In Chapter 1, the concept of levels of organization in the body is presented. Chapter 2 introduces the unifying theme of homeostasis to explain how the interaction of structure and function is achieved and maintained by dynamic counterbalancing forces within the body. The material presented in Chapters 3 and 4—Chemical Basis of Life and Biomolecules—provides an understanding of the basic chemical interactions that influence the control, integration, and regulation of these counterbalancing forces in every organ system of the body.

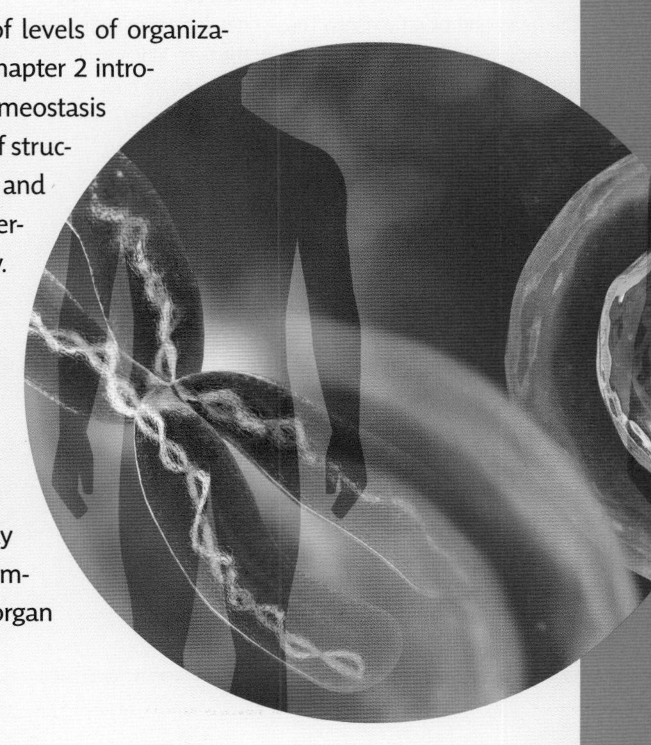

Unit 1 concludes with information that builds on the organizational and biochemical information presented in the first four chapters. The structure and function of cells presented in Chapters 5, 6, and 7 explain why physiologists often state that "all body functions are cellular functions". Grouping similar cells into functioning tissues is accomplished in Chapters 8 and 9. Subsequent chapters of the text focus on the remaining organ systems of the body. •

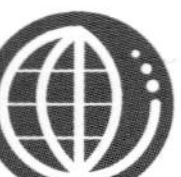

the big picture | Seeing the BIG picture

Before reading this introduction, you probably spent a few minutes flipping through this book. Naturally, you are curious about your course in human anatomy and physiology, and you want to see what lies ahead. It is more than that. You are curious about the human body—about yourself, really. We all have that desire to learn more about how our bodies are put together and how all the parts work. Unlike many other people, though, you now have the opportunity to gain an understanding of the underlying scientific principles of human structure and function.

To truly understand the nature of the human body requires an ability to appreciate "the parts" and "the whole" at the same time. As you flipped through this book for the first time, you probably looked at many different body parts. Some were microscopic—such as muscle cells—and some were very large—such as arms and legs. In looking at these parts, however, you gained very little insight about how they worked together to allow you to sit here, alive and breathing, and read and comprehend these words.

Think about it for a moment. What does it take to be able to read these words and understand them? You might begin by thinking about the eye. How do all of its many intricate parts work together to form an image? The eye is not the only organ you are using right now. What about the bones, joints, and muscles you are using to hold the book, to turn the pages, and to move your eyes as they scan this paragraph? Let's not forget the nervous system. The brain, spinal cord, and nerves are receiving information from the eyes, evaluating it, and using it to coordinate the muscle movements. The squiggles we call letters are being interpreted near the top of the brain to form complex ideas. In short, you are *thinking* about what you are reading.

But that does not cover everything. How are you getting the energy to operate your eyes, muscles, brain, and nerves? Energetic chemical reactions inside each cell of these organs require oxygen and nutrients captured by the lungs and digestive tract and delivered by the heart and blood vessels. These chemical reactions produce wastes that are handled by the liver, kidneys, and other organs. All of these functions must be coordinated, a feat accomplished by regulation of body organs by hormones, nerves, and other mechanisms.

Learning to name the various body parts, to describe their detailed structure, and to explain the mechanisms that produce their functions is an essential step that leads to the goal of understanding the human body. To actually reach that goal, however, you must be able to draw together isolated facts and concepts. In other words, understanding the nature of individual body parts becomes more meaningful when you understand how the parts work together in a living, whole person.

Many textbooks are written like reference books—dictionaries, for example. They provide detailed descriptions of the structure and function of individual body parts, often in logical groupings, while rarely stopping to step back and look at the whole person. In this book, however, we have incorporated the "whole body" aspect into the discussion of every major topic. In chapter and unit introductions, in appropriate paragraphs within each section, and in specific sections near the end of each chapter, we have stepped back from the topic at hand and refocused attention to the broader view.

We are confident that the "whole body" approach will help you put each new fact or concept you learn into its proper place within a larger framework of understanding. You may also better appreciate why it is important to learn some detailed facts that may at first seem to have no practical value to you. When you have finished learning the many details covered in this course, however, you will have also gained a more complete understanding of the essential nature of the human body.

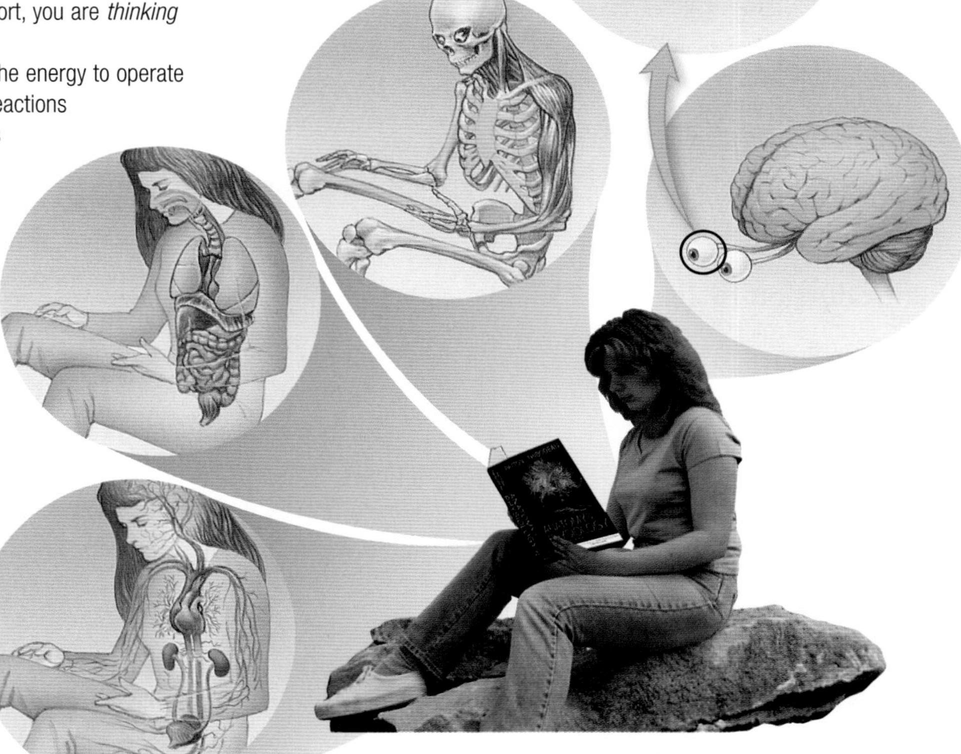

1 Organization of the Body

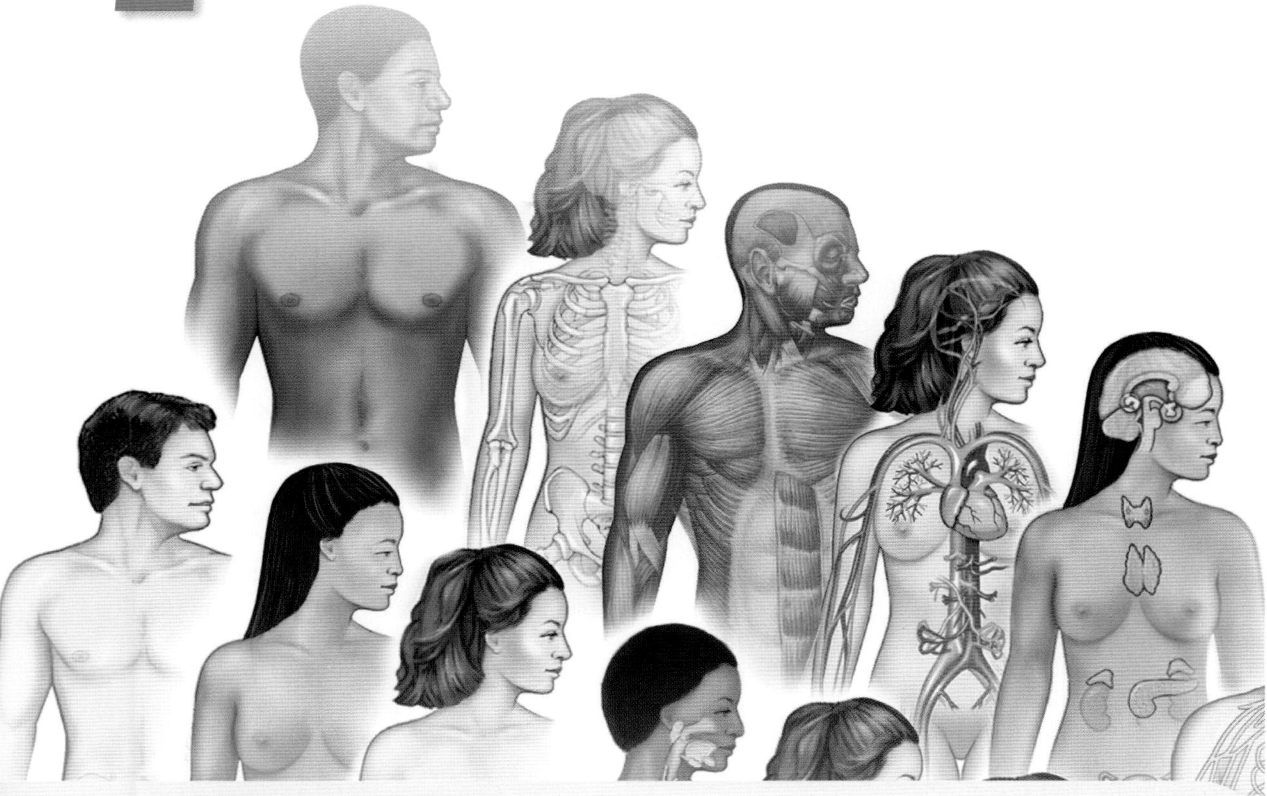

CHAPTER OUTLINE

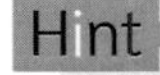
Hint ▸ *Scan this outline before you begin to read the chapter, as a preview of how the concepts are organized.*

LANGUAGE OF SCIENCE

Hint ▸ *Use this list to aid your pronunciation of unfamiliar words.*

abdominopelvic cavity (ab-DOM-i-no-PEL-vik KAV-i-tee) [*abdomin-* **belly,** *-pelv-* **basin,** *cav-* **hollow,** *-ity* **state**]

anatomical position (an-ah-TOM-i-kal po-ZISH-un) [*ana-* **apart,** *-tom-* **cut,** *-ical-* **relating to,** *posit-* **place,** *-tion* **state**]

anatomy (ah-NAT-o-mee) [*ana-* **apart,** *-tom-* **cut,** *-y* **action**]

anterior (an-TEER-ee-or) [*ante-* **front,** *-er-* **more,** *-or* **quality**]

apical (AY-pik-al) [*apic-* **tip,** *-al* **relating to**]

autopoiesis (aw-toe-poy-EE-sis) [*auto-* **self,** *-poiesis* **making**]

basal (BAY-sal) [*bas-* **base,** *-al* **relating to**]

bilateral symmetry (bye-LAT-er-al SIM-e-tree) [*bi-* **two,** *-later-* **side,** *-al* **relating to,** *sym-* **together,** *-metr-* **measure,** *-ry* **condition of**]

body plane (BOD-ee playn)

cadaver (kah-DAV-er) [*cadaver* **dead body**]

cell (sell) [*cell* **storeroom**]

cell theory (sell THEE-o-ree) [*cell* **storeroom,** *theor-* **look at,** *-y* **act of**]

central (SEN-tral) [*centr-* **centre,** *-al* **relating to**]

contralateral (kon-trah-LAT-er-al) [*contra-* **against**, *-later-* **side**, *-al* **relating to**]

coronal plane (ko-RO-nal plane) [*corona-* **crown,** *-al* **relating to,** *plan-* **flat surface**]

cortical (KOR-tik-al) [*cortic-* **cortex (bark),** *-al* **relating to**]

cross-section (kraws SEK-shun) [*cross-* **across**, *sect-* **cut**, *-tion* **process**]

distal (DIS-tal) [*dist-* **distance,** *-al* **relating to**]

dorsal cavities (DOR-sal KAV-i-teez) [*dors-* **back,** *-al* **relating to,** *cav-* **hollow,** *-ity* **state**]

eponym (EP-o-nim) [*epo-* **above,** *-nym* **name**]

continued on p. 18

You have just begun the study of one of nature's most wondrous structures—the human body. **Anatomy** and **physiology** are branches of biology that are concerned with the form and functions of the body. Anatomy is the study of body structure, whereas physiology deals with body function. As you learn about the complex interdependence of structure and function in the human body, you become, in a very real sense, the subject of your own study.

Regardless of your field of study or your future career goals, acquiring and using information about your body structure and functions will enable you to live a more knowledgeable, involved, and healthy life in this science-conscious age. Your study of anatomy and physiology provides a unique and fascinating understanding of self, and this knowledge allows for more active and informed participation in your own personal health care decisions. If you are pursuing a health-, science-, or athletic-related career, your study of anatomy and physiology takes on added significance. It provides the necessary concepts you will need to understand your professional courses and succeed in clinical experiences.

SCIENCE AND SOCIETY

Before we get to the details, we should emphasize that everything you will read in this book is in the context of a broad field of inquiry called *science*. Science is a style of inquiry that attempts to understand nature in a rational, logical manner. Using detailed observations and vigorous tests, or *experiments*, scientists winnow out each element of an idea or **hypothesis** until a reasonable conclusion about its validity can be made. Rigorous experiments that eliminate any influences or biases not being directly tested are called *controlled experiments*. If the results of observations and experiments are repeatable, they may verify a hypothesis and eventually lead to enough confidence in the concept to call it a *theory*. Theories in which scientists have an unusually high level of confidence are sometimes called *laws*. Experiments may disprove a hypothesis, a result that often leads to the formation of new hypotheses to be tested.

Figure 1-1 summarizes some of the basic concepts of how new scientific principles are developed. As you can see, science is a dynamic process of getting closer and closer to the truth about nature, including the nature of the human body. Science is definitely not a set of unchanging facts as many people in our culture often assume.

We should also take this opportunity to point out the social and cultural context of the science presented in this book. Scientists drive the process of science, but our culture drives the kinds of questions we ask about nature and how we attempt to answer them. For example, cutting apart human *cadavers* (dead bodies) for the purpose of studying them has not always been an acceptable activity in all cultures. Today the debate faced by our culture concerns the acceptability of using live animals in scientific experiments. Because our culture does not condone most experiments involving living humans, we have until now often conducted testing on animals that are similar to humans. In fact, most of the theories presented in this book are based on animal experimentation, but cultural influences now are pulling scientists in other experimental directions they otherwise may not have taken.

Similarly, science affects culture. Recent advances in understanding human genes and technological advances in our ability to use so-called *stem cells* and other tissues from human embryos, human cadavers, and living donors to treat devastating diseases have sparked new debates concerning how our culture defines what it means to be a human being.

As you study the concepts presented in this book, keep in mind that they are not set in stone. Science is a rapidly changing set of ideas and processes that not only is influenced by our cultural biases but also affects our cultural awareness of who we are.

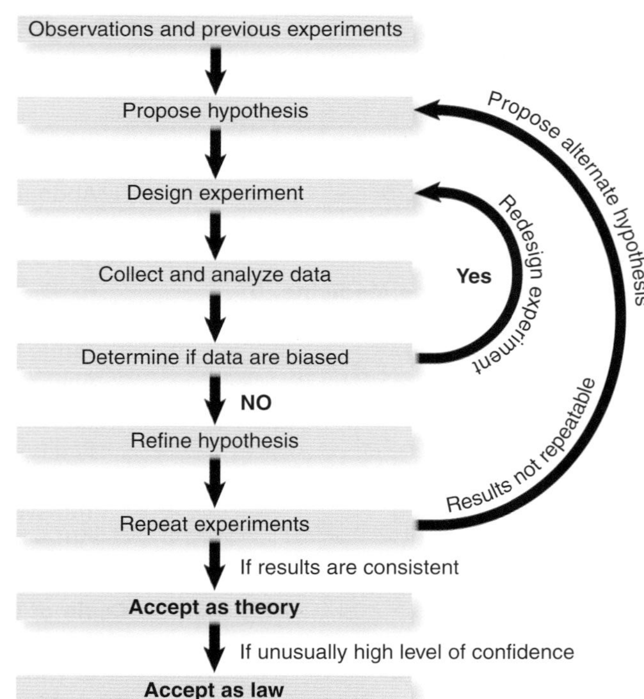

FIGURE 1-1 The scientific method. This flowchart summarizes the classic ideal of how new principles of science are developed. Initial observations or results from other experiments may lead to the formation of a new hypothesis. As more testing is performed to eliminate outside influences or biases and ensure consistent results, scientists begin to have more confidence in the principle and call it a *theory* or *law*.

CONNECT IT! 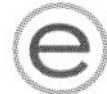

For a quick peek at the major scientific breakthroughs that have changed our lives—and serve as the core concepts of this book—check out ***The Nobel Legacy*** online at ***Connect It!***

ANATOMY AND PHYSIOLOGY

ANATOMY

Anatomy is often defined as study of the structure of an organism and the relationships of its parts. The word *anatomy* is derived from Greek word parts that mean "to cut apart". Students of anatomy still learn about the structure of the human body by literally cutting it apart. This process, called *dissection*, remains a principal technique used to isolate and study the structural components or parts of the human body.

Biology is defined as the scientific study of life. Both anatomy and physiology are subdivisions of this very broad area of inquiry. Each of these subdivisions can be further divided into smaller areas of study. For example, the term **gross anatomy** is used to describe the study of body parts visible to the naked eye. Before invention of the microscope, anatomists had to study human structure relying only on the eye during dissection. These early anatomists could make only a gross, or whole, examination, as you can see in **Figure 1-2**. With the use of modern microscopes, many anatomists now specialize in **microscopic anatomy**, including the study of cells, called *cytology* (sye-TOL-o-jee), and tissues, called *histology* (hiss-TOL-o-jee).

Other branches of anatomy include the study of human growth and development (*developmental anatomy*) and the study of diseased body structures (*pathological anatomy*). In the chapters that follow, you will study the body by systems—a process called *systemic anatomy.* Systems are groups of organs that have a common function, such as the bones in the skeletal system and the muscles in the muscular system.

PHYSIOLOGY

Physiology is the science that deals with the functions of the living organism and its parts. The term is a combination of two Greek words (*physis*, "nature," and *logos*, "words or study"). Simply stated, it is the study of physiology that helps us understand how the body works. Physiologists attempt to discover and understand the intricate control systems that permit the body to operate and survive in changing and often hostile environments.

As a scientific discipline, physiology can be subdivided according to (1) the type of organism involved, such as human physiology or plant physiology; (2) the organizational level studied, such as molecular or cellular physiology; or (3) a specific or *systemic* function being studied, such as neurophysiology, respiratory physiology, or cardiovascular physiology.

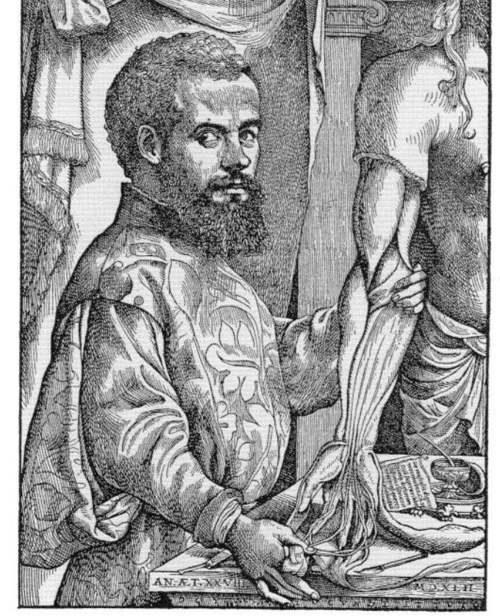

FIGURE 1-2 Gross anatomy. This famous woodcut of a gross dissection appeared in the world's first modern anatomy textbook, *De Humani Corporis Fabrica (On the Structure of the Human Body),* in 1543. This woodcut features the book's author, Andreas Vesalius, who is considered to be the founder of modern anatomy. The body being dissected is called a *cadaver.*

In the chapters that follow, both anatomy and physiology are studied by dividing the human body into specific organ systems. This unit begins with an overview of the body as a whole. In subsequent chapters the body is dissected and studied, both structurally (anatomy) and functionally (physiology), into "levels of organization" so that its component parts can be more easily understood and then "fit together" into a living and integrated whole. It is knowledge of anatomy and physiology that allows us to understand how nerve impulses travel from one part of the body to another; how muscles contract; how light energy can be transformed into visual images; how we breathe, digest food, reproduce, excrete wastes, and sense changes in our environment; and even how we think and reason.

Quick CHECK

1. Describe how science develops new principles.
2. Define *anatomy* and *physiology.*
3. List the three ways in which physiology can be subdivided as a scientific discipline.
4. What name is used to describe the study of the body that focuses on groups of organs that have a common function?

LANGUAGE OF SCIENCE AND MEDICINE

You may have noticed by now that many scientific terms, such as anatomy and physiology, are made up of non-English word parts. Many such terms make up the core of the language used to communicate ideas in science and medicine. Learning in science thus begins with learning a new vocabulary, just as when you learn a new language to help you understand and communicate in a region of the world other than the one you call home.

To help you learn the vocabulary of anatomy and physiology, we have provided several helpful tools for you. Within each chapter, lists of new terms titled *Language of Science* and *Language of Medicine* give you each new key (boldface) term that you will be learning in that chapter. Each term in the list has a pronunciation guide and an explanation (or meaning) of each of the word parts that make up the term.

We have also included a separate compact reference called QUICK GUIDE TO THE LANGUAGE OF SCIENCE AND MEDICINE with this textbook. Take a moment now to locate it. After you have finished reading this chapter, quickly review the tips for learning scientific language. Then keep it nearby so that you will have a handy list of commonly used word parts at your fingertips.

You will see that most scientific terms are made up of word parts from Latin or Greek. Most Western scientists first began corresponding with one another in these languages, because they were commonly the first written languages learned by educated people. Other languages such as German, French, and Japanese are also sources of some scientific word parts.

As with any language, scientific language changes constantly. This is useful because we often need to fine-tune our terminology to reflect changes in our understanding of science and to accommodate new discoveries. But it also sometimes leads to confusion. In an attempt to clear up some of the confusion, the International Federation of Associations of Anatomists (IFAA) formed a worldwide committee to publish a list of "universal" or standard anatomical terminology. The list for *gross anatomy*, the structure we can see without magnification, was published in 1998 as *Terminologia Anatomica (TA)*. In 2008 the *Terminologia Histologica (TH)* was published for *microscopic anatomy*—the study of body structure requiring significant magnification for the purpose of visualization.

Although there remain some alternate (and newer) terms used in anatomy, the lists are useful standard references. The lists show each term in Latin and English (based on the Latin form), along with a reference number. In this textbook we use the English terms from the published lists as our standard reference, but we do occasionally refer to the pure Latin form or an alternate term when appropriate for beginning students.

TABLE 1-1 Characteristics of Human Life

CHARACTERISTIC	DESCRIPTION
Responsiveness	Ability of an organism to sense, monitor, and respond to changes in both its external and internal environments
Conductivity	Capacity of living cells to transmit a wave of electrical disturbance from one point to another within the body
Growth	Organized increase in the size and number of cells and therefore an increase in size of the individual or a particular organ or part
Respiration	Exchange of respiratory gases (oxygen and carbon dioxide) between an organism and its environment
Digestion	Process by which complex food products are broken down into simpler substances that can be absorbed and used by individual body cells
Absorption	Movement of molecules, such as respiratory gases or digested nutrients, through a membrane and into the body fluids for transport to cells for use
Secretion	Production and release of important substances, such as digestive juices and hormones, for diverse body functions
Excretion	Removal of waste products from the body
Circulation	Movement of body fluids containing many substances from one body area to another in a continuous, circular route through hollow vessels
Reproduction	Formation of new individual offspring

One of the basic principles of the standardized terminology is the avoidance of **eponyms**, or terms that are based on a person's name. Instead, a more descriptive Latin-based term is always preferred. Thus the term *eustachian tube* (tube connected to the middle ear, named after the famed Italian anatomist Eustachius) is now replaced with the more descriptive *auditory tube*. Likewise, the *islets of Langerhans* (in the pancreas) are now simply *pancreatic islets*. In the rare cases where eponyms do appear in a standard list, we now avoid the possessive form. Thus *Bowman's capsule* (in kidney tissue) is now either *glomerular capsule* or *Bowman capsule*.

There are no such standard lists of physiological terms. However, many principles used in anatomical terminology are used in physiology. For example, most terms have an English spelling but are based on Latin or Greek word parts. And, as in anatomy, eponyms are less favoured than descriptive terms.

A Quick Guide to the Language of Science and Medicine accompanies this book. It offers a handy summary of the basic principles of using your new "A&P language". The quick guide also lists common roots, prefixes, and suffixes—along with acronyms, abbreviations, Greek letters, Roman numerals, and much more.

This may all seem like a lot more than you want to know right now. However, if you focus on learning the new words as you begin each new topic, as though you are in a foreign land and need to pick up a few phrases to get by, you will find your study of anatomy and physiology easy and enjoyable.

CHARACTERISTICS OF LIFE

Anatomy and physiology are important disciplines in biology—the study of life. But what is life? What is the quality that distinguishes a vital and functional being from a dead body? We know that a living organism is endowed with certain characteristics not associated with inorganic matter. However, it is sometimes hard to find a single criterion to define life.

One could say that living organisms are self-organizing or self-maintaining and nonliving structures are not. This concept is called **autopoiesis**, which literally means "self making". Another idea, called the *cell theory*, states that any independent structure made up of one or more microscopic units called *cells* is a living organism.

Instead of trying to find a single difference that separates living and nonliving things, scientists sometimes define life by listing what are often called *characteristics of life*. Lists of characteristics of life may differ from one physiologist to the next, depending on the type of organism being studied and the way in which life functions are grouped and defined. Attributes that characterize life in bacteria, plants, or animals may vary. Characteristics of life that are considered most important in humans are described in **Table 1-1**.

Each characteristic of life is related to the sum total of all the physical and chemical reactions occurring in the body. The term **metabolism** is used to describe these various processes. They include the steps involved in the breakdown of nutrient materials to produce energy and the transformation of one material into another. For example, if we eat and absorb more sugar than needed for the body's immediate energy requirements, it is converted into an alternate form, such as fat, that can be stored in the body. Metabolic reactions are also required for making complex compounds out of simpler ones, as in tissue growth, wound repair, or manufacture of body secretions.

Each characteristic of life—its functional manifestation in the body, its integration with other body functions and structures, and its mechanism of control—is the subject of study in subsequent chapters of the text.

Quick CHECK

5. What is an *eponym*?
6. What single criterion might be used to define life?
7. Define the term *metabolism* as it applies to the characteristics of life.

LEVELS OF ORGANIZATION

Before you begin the study of the structure and function of the human body and its many parts, it is important to think about how the parts are organized and how they might logically fit together and function effectively. The differing levels of organization that influence body structure and function are illustrated in **Figure 1-3**.

CHEMICAL LEVEL—BASIS FOR LIFE

Note that organization of the body begins at the chemical level (see **Figure 1-3**). There are more than 100 different chemical building blocks of nature called *atoms*—tiny spheres of matter so small they are invisible. Every material thing in our universe, including the human body, is composed of atoms.

Combinations of atoms form larger chemical groupings, called *molecules*. Molecules, in turn, often combine with other atoms and molecules to form larger and more complex chemicals, called *macromolecules*.

The unique and complex relationships that exist between atoms, molecules, and macromolecules in living material form a gel-like material made of fluids, particles, and membranes called *cytoplasm*—the essential material of human life. Unless proper relationships among chemical elements are maintained, death results. Maintaining the type of chemical organization in cytoplasm required for life requires the expenditure of energy. In Chapters 3 and 4 important information related to the chemistry of life is discussed in more detail.

ORGANELLE LEVEL

Chemical structures may be organized within larger units called *cells* to form various structures called **organelles,** the next level of organization (see **Figure 1-3**). An organelle may be defined as a structure made of molecules organized in such a way that it can perform a specific function. Organelles are the "tiny organs" that allow each cell to live. Organelles cannot survive outside the cell, but without organelles the cell itself could not survive either.

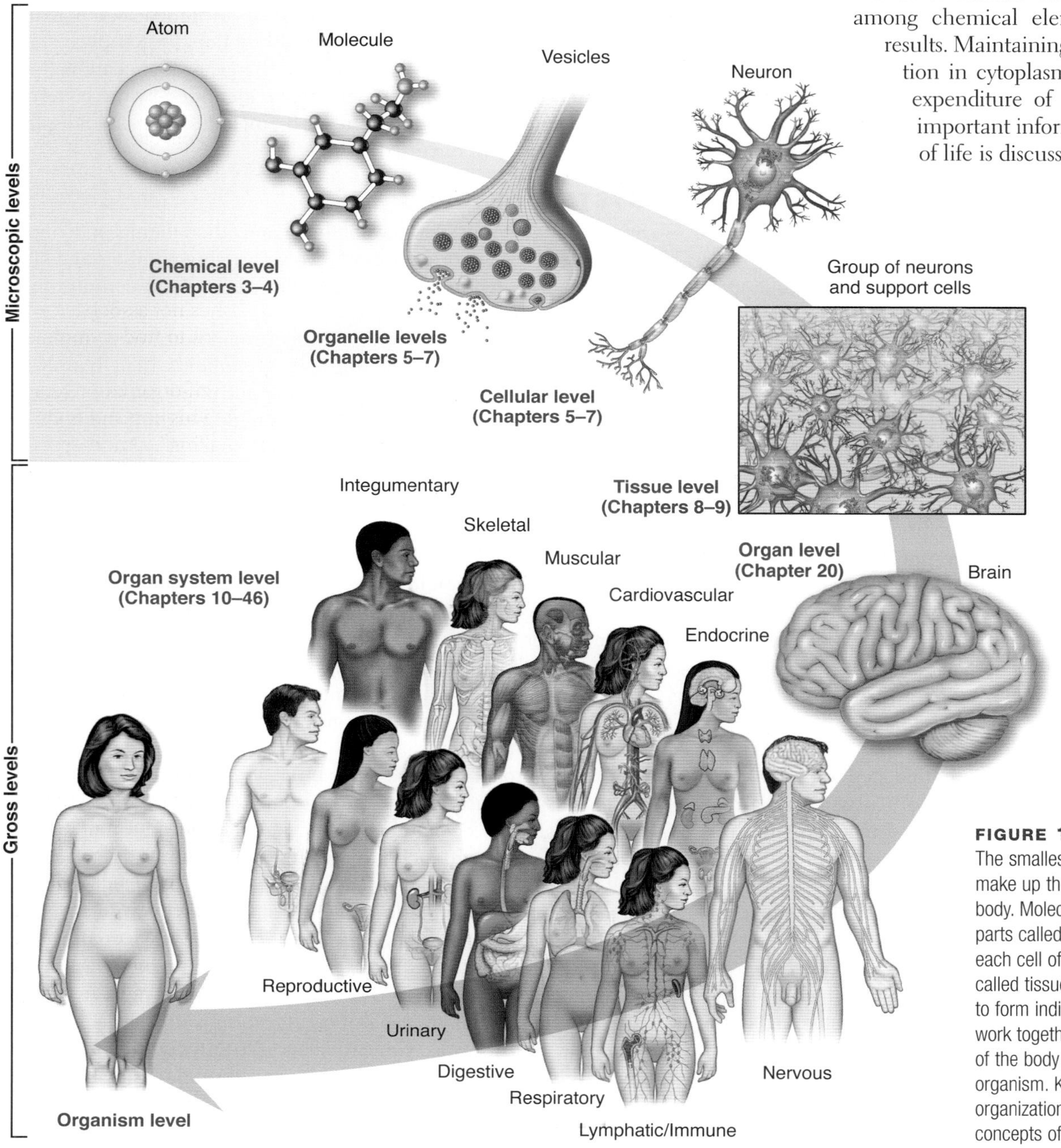

FIGURE 1-3 Levels of organization. The smallest parts of the body are the atoms that make up the chemicals, or molecules, of the body. Molecules, in turn, make up microscopic parts called organelles that fit together to form each cell of the body. Groups of similar cells are called tissues, which combine with other tissues to form individual organs. Groups of organs that work together are called systems. All the systems of the body together make up an individual organism. Knowledge of the different levels of organization will help you understand the basic concepts of human anatomy and physiology.

Dozens of different kinds of organelles have been identified. A few examples:

- *Mitochondria* (my-toe-KON-dree-ah)—the "powerhouses" of cells that provide energy needed by the cell to carry on day-to-day functioning, growth, and repair
- *Golgi* (GOL-jee) *apparatus*—set of sacs that provides a "packaging" service to the cell by storing material for future internal use or for export from the cell
- *Endoplasmic reticulum (ER)*—network of channels within the cell that act as "highways" for the movement of chemicals and as sites for chemical processing

Chapter 5 contains a more complete discussion of important organelles and their functions.

Cellular Level

The characteristics of life ultimately result from a hierarchy of structure and function that begins with the organization of atoms, molecules, and macromolecules. Further organization that results in organelles is the next step. However, in the view of the anatomist, the most important function of the chemical and organelle levels of organization is that of furnishing the basic building blocks required for the next higher level of body structure—*the cellular level.*

Cells are the smallest and most numerous structural units that possess and exhibit the basic characteristics of living matter. How many cells are there in the body? One estimate places the number of cells in a 70-kg adult human body at 3.72×10^{13} or 37 trillion!

Each cell is surrounded by a membrane and is characterized by a single nucleus surrounded by cytoplasm that includes the numerous organelles required for the normal processes of living.

Although all cells have certain features in common, they specialize or *differentiate* to perform unique functions. Fat cells, for example, are structurally modified to permit the storage of fats, whereas other cells, such as cardiac muscle cells, are able to contract with great force (see **Figure 1-3**). Muscle, bone, nerve, and blood cells are other examples of structurally and functionally unique cells.

Tissue Level

The next higher level of organization beyond the cell is the *tissue level* (see **Figure 1-3**). Tissues represent another step in the progressive organization of living matter. By definition, a **tissue** is a group of a great many similar cells that all developed together from the same part of the embryo and all perform a certain function. Tissue cells are surrounded by varying amounts and kinds of nonliving, intercellular substances, or the *matrix*. Tissues are the "fabric" of the body.

There are four major or principal tissue types: *epithelial, connective, muscle,* and *nervous.* Considering the complex nature of the human body, this is a surprisingly short list of major tissues. Each of the four major tissues, however, can be subdivided into several distinct subtypes. Together the body tissues are able to meet all the structural and functional needs of the body.

The tissue used as an example in **Figure 1-3** is nervous tissue. Note how the cells are branching and interconnected. The details of tissue structure and function are covered in Chapters 8 and 9.

Organ Level

Organ units are more complex than tissues. An **organ** is defined as a structure made up of several different kinds of tissues arranged so that, together, they can perform a special function.

If tissues are the "fabric" of the body, an organ is like an item of clothing with a specific function made up of different fabrics. The heart is an example of the *organ level:* muscle and connective tissues give it shape and pump blood; epithelial tissues line the cavities, or chambers; and nervous tissues permit control of the pumping contractions of the heart.

Tissues seldom exist in isolation. Instead, joined together, they form organs that represent discrete, but functionally complex, operational units. Each organ has a unique shape, size, appearance, and placement in the body, and each can be identified by the pattern of tissues that form it. The lungs, heart, brain, kidneys, liver, and spleen are all examples of organs.

System Level

Systems are the most complex of the organizational units of the body. The **system** level of organization involves varying numbers and kinds of organs arranged so that, together, they can perform complex functions for the body.

Eleven major systems compose the human body: integumentary, skeletal, muscular, nervous, endocrine, cardiovascular, lymphatic/immune, respiratory, digestive, urinary, and reproductive. Systems that work together to accomplish the general needs of the body are summarized in **Table 1-2**.

Take a few minutes to read through **Table 1-2**. The left column points out that several different systems often work together to accomplish some overall goal. For example, the first three systems listed (integumentary, skeletal, muscular) make up the framework of the body and therefore provide support and movement. Note also that this table corresponds to the organization of this book. Once we get to the system level of organization, we will study each system one by one, chapter by chapter. To help you navigate through the book, we have organized the chapters into units of several systems each—units that group the systems by common or overlapping functions.

You are probably aware that some systems can be grouped together or split apart. We use those groupings that are most useful to us. For example, because both the skeletal and muscular systems work together to produce athletic movements, an athletic trainer may study them together as the *musculoskeletal system.* A physiotherapist may also include concepts of nervous control of movement and study the *neuromusculoskeletal system.* On the other hand, a neurologist may find it useful to keep in mind a distinction between the sensory nervous system and the motor nervous system. In any case, the idea of levels of organization is universal, and once you know how it works, you can adapt it to suit your own changing needs. The plan of dividing the body into 11 major systems is widely used among biologists, so we will use it as the basis of our study too.

CONNECT IT!

The many important roles of the *microbial systems* of the body, or human **microbiome,** have come to the forefront of human biology. The complex interactions of microorganisms (such as bacteria) in our body with one another, and with our own cells, tissues, and organs, have proven to be critical to maintaining normal structure and function of the body. Learn more in ***The Human Microbiome*** at ***Connect It!***

Organism Level

The living human **organism** is certainly more than the sum of its parts. It is a marvellously coordinated team of interactive structures that is able to survive and flourish in an often hostile environment. Not only can the human body reproduce itself (and its genetic information) and maintain ongoing repair and replacement of worn or damaged parts, it can also maintain—in a constant and predictable way—an incredible number of variables required for a human to lead a healthy, productive life.

We are able to maintain a "normal" body temperature and fluid balance in widely varying environmental extremes. We maintain constant blood levels of many important chemicals and nutrients. We experience effective protection against disease, elimination of waste products, and coordinated movement. We correctly and quickly interpret sound, visual images, and other external stimuli with great regularity. These are a few examples of how the different levels of organization in the human organism permit expression of the characteristics associated with life.

As you study the structure and function of the human body, it is too easy to think of each part or function in isolation from the body as a whole. Always remember that you are ultimately dealing with information related to the entire human organism—not information limited to an understanding of the structure and function of a single organelle, cell, tissue, organ, or organ system. Do not limit your learning to the memorization of facts. Instead, connect and integrate factual information so that your understanding of human structure and function is related not to a part of the body but to the body as a whole.

Quick CHECK

8. List the seven levels of organization.
9. Identify three organelles.
10. List the four major tissue types.
11. List the 11 major organ systems.

ANATOMICAL POSITION

Discussions about the body, how it moves, its posture, or the relationship of one area to another, assume that the body as a whole is in a specific position called the **anatomical position.** In this reference position the body is in an erect, or standing, posture with the arms at the sides and palms turned forward (**Figure 1-4**). The head and feet are also pointing forward. The anatomical position is a reference position that gives meaning to the directional terms used to describe the body parts and regions.

Bilateral symmetry is one of the most obvious of the external organizational features in humans. The person shown in **Figure 1-4** is divided by a line into bilaterally symmetrical sides. To say that humans are bilaterally symmetrical simply means that the right and left sides of the body are mirror images of each other and only one plane can divide the body into left and right halves. One of the most important features of bilateral symmetry is balanced proportions. There is a remarkable correspondence in size and shape when comparing similar anatomical parts or external areas on opposite sides of the body. Take a moment to look at the bilateral external symmetry of the body in Figures 1-1 and 1-2 in the Brief Atlas of the Human Body.

TABLE 1-2 Body Systems (with Unit and Chapter References)

FUNCTIONAL CATEGORY	SYSTEM	PRINCIPAL ORGANS	PRIMARY FUNCTIONS
Support and movement (Unit Two)	Integumentary (Chapter 10)	Skin	Protection, temperature regulation, sensation
	Skeletal (Chapters 11–14)	Bones, ligaments	Support, protection, movement, mineral and fat storage, blood production
	Muscular (Chapters 15–17)	Skeletal muscles, tendons	Movement, posture, heat production
Communication, control, and integration (Unit Three)	Nervous (Chapters 18–24)	Brain, spinal cord, nerves, sensory organs	Control, regulation, and coordination of other systems, sensation, memory
	Endocrine (Chapters 25–26)	Pituitary gland, adrenals, pancreas, thyroid, parathyroids, and other glands	Control and regulation of other systems
Transportation and defence (Unit Four)	Cardiovascular (Chapters 27–30)	Heart, arteries, veins, capillaries	Exchange and transport of materials
	Lymphatic immune (Chapters 31–34)	Lymph nodes, lymphatic vessels, spleen, thymus, tonsils	Immunity, fluid balance
Respiration, nutrition, and excretion (Unit Five)	Respiratory (Chapters 35–37)	Lungs, bronchial tree, trachea, larynx, nasal cavity	Gas exchange, acid–base balance
	Digestive (Chapters 38–41)	Stomach, small and large intestines, oesophagus, liver, mouth, pancreas	Breakdown and absorption of nutrients, elimination of waste
	Urinary (Chapters 42–44)	Kidneys, ureters, bladder, urethra	Excretion of waste, fluid and electrolyte balance, acid–base balance
Reproduction and development (Unit Six)	Reproductive (Chapters 45–48)	*Male:* Testes, vas deferens, prostate, seminal vesicles, penis	Reproduction, continuity of genetic information, nurturing of offspring
		Female: Ovaries, fallopian tubes, uterus, vagina, breasts	

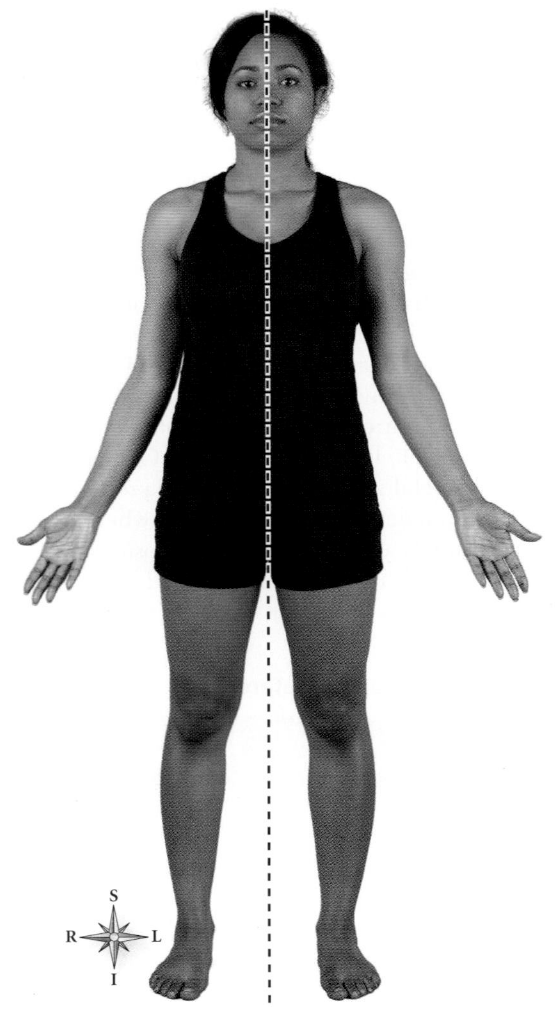

FIGURE 1-4 Anatomical position and bilateral symmetry. In the anatomical position, the body is in an erect, or standing, posture with the arms at the sides and palms forward. The head and feet are also pointing forward. The *dotted line* shows the axis of the body's bilateral symmetry. As a result of this organizational feature, the right and left sides of the body are mirror images of each other.

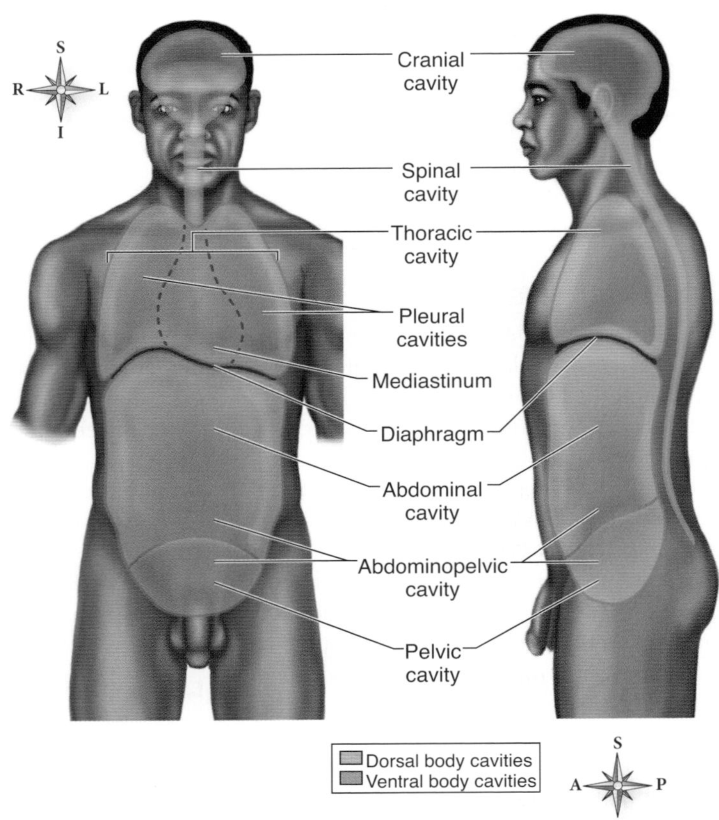

FIGURE 1-5 Major body cavities. The dorsal body cavities are in the dorsal (back) part of the body and include a cranial cavity above and a spinal cavity below. The ventral body cavities are on the ventral (front) side of the trunk and include the thoracic cavity above the diaphragm and the abdominopelvic cavity below the diaphragm. The thoracic cavity is subdivided into the mediastinum in the centre and pleural cavities to the sides. The abdominopelvic cavity is subdivided into the abdominal cavity above the pelvis and the pelvic cavity within the pelvis.

The terms *ipsilateral* and *contralateral* are often used to identify the placement of one body part with respect to another on the same or opposite side of the body. **Ipsilateral** simply means "same side", and **contralateral** means "opposite side". These terms may be used in describing injury to an extremity, for example. If the right knee were injured and swollen, one could say that "the right knee is enlarged compared with the *contralateral knee*".

Supine and *prone* are terms used to describe the position of the body when it is not in the anatomical position. In the supine position the body is lying face upward, and in the prone prosition the body is lying face downward.

BODY CAVITIES

The body contains many hollows or *cavities* that each house compact arrangements of internal organs. The location and outlines of major body cavities are illustrated in **Figure 1-5**.

VENTRAL CAVITIES

During early development, a huge internal body cavity subdivides into two major **ventral cavities**—the thoracic cavity (chest cavity) and the abdominopelvic cavity. The **thoracic cavity** has a mid-portion called the **mediastinum**, which contains the heart and other structures surrounded by fibrous tissue. On the left and right sides of the mediastinum are spaces called **pleural cavities** in which the lungs reside.

The mediastinum houses the heart, the trachea, right and left bronchi, the oesophagus, the thymus, various blood vessels (e.g., thoracic aorta, superior vena cava), the thoracic duct and other lymphatic vessels, various lymph nodes, and nerves (such as the phrenic and vagus nerves).

The heart is surrounded by a fibrous sac lined with a thin, slippery membrane that doubles back on itself to form a lubricating, fluid-filled pocket around the heart. **Figure 1-6** demonstrates how this structure resembles a water-filled balloon with a fist thrust into it. Like the fist surrounded by a double wall of balloon, the heart is surrounded by a double-walled pericardial membrane filled with a small amount of watery pericardial fluid.

This structural pattern, seen commonly within body cavities, will be revisited often throughout your study of human anatomy. Often,

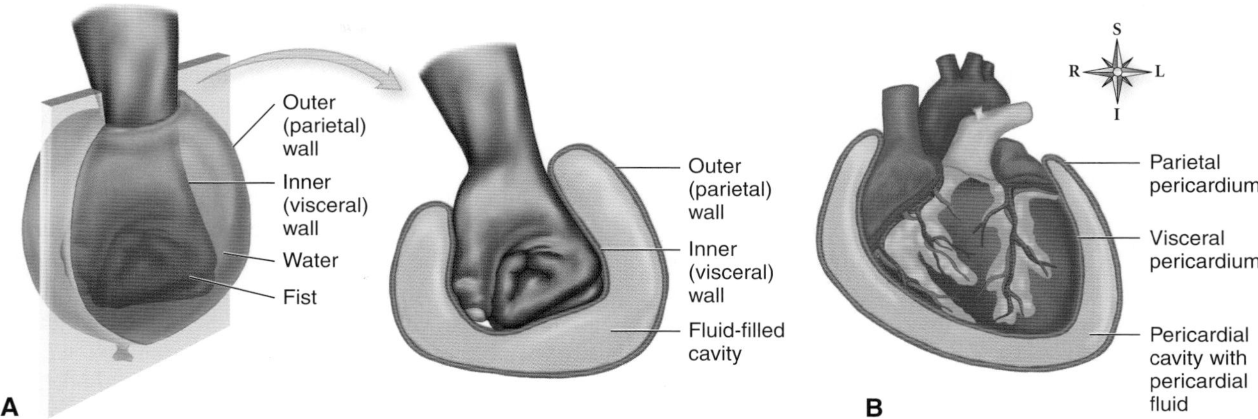

FIGURE 1-6 Membranes that line cavities. A, The analogy of a fist thrust into a water-filled balloon demonstrates how a membrane can form a double-walled structure made up of an outer parietal layer and an inner visceral layer separated by a thin pocket of fluid. **B,** The heart is surrounded by a thin, fluid-producing pericardial membrane that likewise forms a parietal and visceral layer, creating a flattened pericardial cavity filled with pericardial fluid.

one layer of the membrane called the **parietal** layer lines the cavity and doubles back on itself to form a **visceral** layer covering the organs. The "space" of the cavity is thus reduced to the flattened pocket of fluid between the parietal and visceral layers.

This pattern also occurs in each pleural cavity, where a *parietal pleura* hugs the inside of the thoracic wall and doubles back to cover the lung—thus forming a *visceral pleura*. The term ***pleural cavity*** can refer to the entire space to the side of the mediastinum or to just the potential space left surrounding the lung between the parietal and visceral pleura. Peek ahead to **Figure 8-8** on p. 145 to see the double-layer structure of the pleurae.

The **abdominopelvic cavity** has an upper portion, the *abdominal cavity*, and a lower portion, the *pelvic cavity*. The abdominal cavity contains the liver, gallbladder, stomach, pancreas, intestines, spleen, kidneys, and ureters. The bladder, certain reproductive organs (uterus, uterine tubes, and ovaries in females; prostate gland, seminal vesicles, and part of the vas deferens in males), and part of the large intestine (namely, the sigmoid colon and rectum) lie in the pelvic cavity (**Table 1-3**).

The membrane lining the inside of the abdominal cavity is called the *parietal peritoneum*. The membrane that covers the organs within the abdominal cavity is called the *visceral peritoneum*. If you skip ahead to **Figure 1-11**, you will see that there is a space or opening between the two membranes in the abdomen. This is called the *peritoneal cavity*. Body membranes are discussed in greater detail in Chapter 8.

Dorsal Cavities

The **dorsal cavities** form along the dorsum or back of the body early in development as bones grow around the tube that eventually forms our central nervous system. The dorsal cavities include the *cranial cavity* and *spinal cavity*.

The cranial cavity is the space within the skull that houses the brain. The spinal cavity, the location of the spinal cord, lies within the hollow spinal canal formed by a stacked column of doughnut-like vertebrae (see **Figure 1-5**).

TABLE 1-3 Organs in Ventral Body Cavities

AREAS	ORGANS
Thoracic Cavity	
Right pleural cavity	Right lung
Mediastinum	Heart Trachea Right and left bronchi Oesophagus Thymus gland Aortic arch and thoracic aorta Venae cavae Various lymph nodes and nerves Thoracic duct
Left pleural cavity	Left lung
Abdominopelvic Cavity	
Abdominal cavity	Liver Gallbladder Stomach Pancreas Intestines Spleen Kidneys Ureters
Pelvic cavity	Urinary bladder Female reproductive organs Uterus Uterine tubes Ovaries Male reproductive organs Prostate gland Seminal vesicles Part of vas deferens Part of large intestine, namely, sigmoid colon and rectum

Other Cavities

In anatomy, the term *cavity* can also refer to any hollow within the body or its organs. We will eventually explore smaller cavities within the eyeball, heart, long bones, skull, and other parts of the body.

BODY REGIONS

Identification of an object begins with overall recognition of its structure and form. Initially, it is in this way that the human form can be distinguished from other creatures or objects. Recognition occurs as soon as you can identify the overall shape and basic outline. For more specific identification to occur, details of size, shape, and appearance of individual body areas must be described. Individuals differ in overall appearance because specific body areas, such as the face or torso, have unique identifying characteristics. Detailed descriptions of the human form require that specific regions be identified and appropriate terms be used to describe them (**Figure 1-7** and **Table 1-4**).

The body as a whole can be subdivided into two major portions or components: *axial* and *appendicular*. The axial portion of the body consists of the head, neck, and torso, or trunk. The appendicular portion of the body consists of the upper and lower extremities and their connections to the axial portion.

Each major area is subdivided as shown in **Figure 1-7**. Note, for example, that the trunk is composed of the thoracic, abdominal, and pelvic areas. The *upper extremity*, or upper limb, is divided into shoulder, arm, forearm, wrist, and hand components. The *lower extremity*, or lower limb, is divided into hip, thigh, leg, ankle, and foot.

Although most terms used to describe gross body regions are familiar, misuse is common. The term *leg* is a good example. To an anatomist, *leg* refers to the area of the lower extremity between the knee and ankle, not to the entire lower limb. Also, some terms can have more

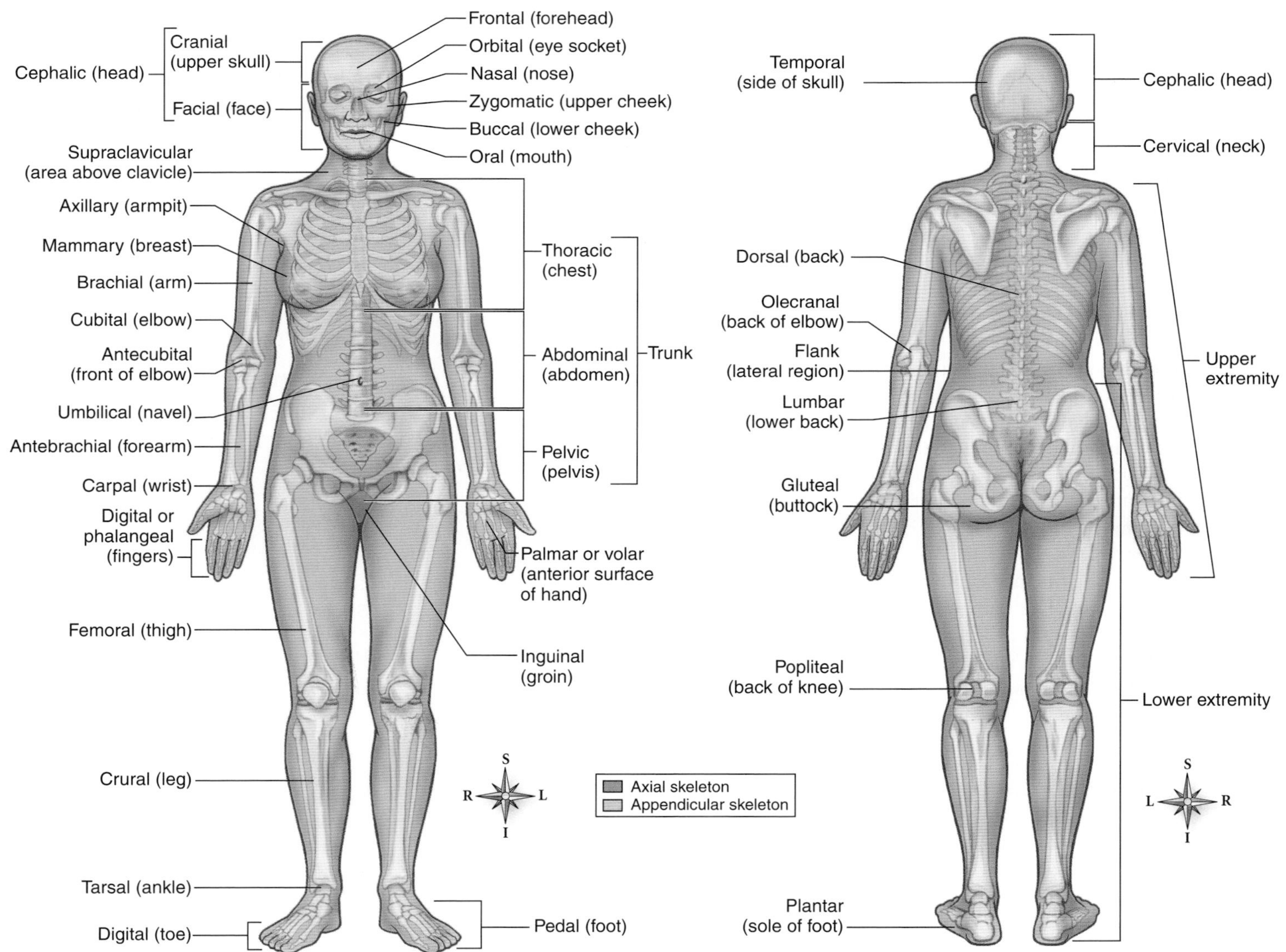

FIGURE 1-7 Specific body regions. Note that the body as a whole can be subdivided into two major portions: axial (along the middle, or *axis,* of the body) and appendicular (the arms and legs, or *appendages*). Names of specific body regions follow the Latin form, with the English equivalent in parentheses.

TABLE 1-4 Latin-Based Descriptive Terms for Body Regions*

BODY REGION	AREA OR EXAMPLE	BODY REGION	AREA OR EXAMPLE
Abdominal (ab-DOM-in-al)	Anterior torso below diaphragm	**Mammary** (MAM-er-ee)	Breast
Acromial (ah-KRO-mee-al)	Shoulder	**Manual** (MAN-yoo-al)	Hand
Antebrachial (an-tee-BRAY-kee-al)	Forearm	**Mental** (MEN-tal)	Chin
Antecubital (an-tee-KYOO-bi-tal)	Depressed area just in front of elbow (cubital fossa)	**Nasal** (NAY-zal)	Nose
Axillary (AK-si-lair-ee)	Armpit (axilla)	**Navel** (NAY-vel)	Area around navel, or umbilicus
Brachial (BRAY-kee-al)	Arm	**Occipital** (ok-SIP-i-tal)	Back of lower part of skull
Buccal (BUK-al)	Cheek (inside)	**Olecranal** (o-LECK-ra-nal)	Back of elbow
Calcaneal (cal-CANE-ee-al)	Heel of foot	**Oral** (OR-al)	Mouth
Carpal (KAR-pal)	Wrist	**Orbital** or **ophthalmic** (OR-bi-tal *or* op-THAL-mik)	Eyes
Cephalic (se-FAL-ik)	Head	**Otic** (O-tik)	Ear
Cervical (SER-vi-kal)	Neck	**Palmar** (PAHL-mar)	Palm of hand
Coxal (KOK-sal)	Hip	**Patellar** (pa-TELL-ar)	Front of knee
Cranial (KRAY-nee-al)	Skull	**Pedal** (PEED-al)	Foot
Crural (KROO-ral)	Leg	**Pelvic** (PEL-vik)	Lower portion of torso
Cubital (KYOO-bi-tal)	Elbow	**Perineal** (pair-i-NEE-al)	Area (perineum) between anus and genitals
Cutaneous (kyoo-TANE-ee-us)	Skin (or body surface)	**Plantar** (PLAN-tar)	Sole of foot
Digital (DIJ-i-tal)	Fingers or toes	**Pollex** (POL-lex)	Thumb
Dorsal (DOR-sal)	Back or top	**Popliteal** (pop-li-TEE-al)	Area behind knee
Facial (FAY-shal)	Face	**Pubic** (PYOO-bik)	Pubis
Femoral (FEM-or-al)	Thigh	**Supraclavicular** (soo-pra-cla-VIK-yoo-lar)	Area above clavicle
Frontal (FRON-tal)	Forehead	**Sural** (SUR-al)	Calf
Gluteal (GLOO-tee-al)	Buttock	**Tarsal** (TAR-sal)	Ankle
Hallux (HAL-luks)	Great toe	**Temporal** (TEM-por-al)	Side of head
Inguinal (ING-gwi-nal)	Groin	**Thoracic** (tho-RAS-ik)	Chest
Lumbar (LUM-bar)	Lower part of back between ribs and pelvis	**Zygomatic** (zye-go-MAT-ik)	Cheek (outside)

*The left column lists English adjectives based on Latin terms that describe the body parts listed in English in the right column.

than one meaning. For example, *cubital* can refer to the elbow or to the forearm. Likewise, *crural* can refer to just the leg, or to just the thigh, or to the thigh and leg together. When you encounter such terms, it is best to determine which meaning is being used. In this book we consistently employ the commonly used meanings listed in **Table 1-4**.

Abdominopelvic Regions

For convenience in locating abdominopelvic organs, anatomists divide the abdominopelvic cavity like a tic-tac-toe grid into nine imaginary regions. The following is a list of the nine regions (**Figure 1-8**) identified from right to left and from top to bottom:

Upper Region

1. Right hypochondriac region
2. Epigastric region
3. Left hypochondriac region

Middle Region

4. Right lumbar (flank) region
5. Umbilical region
6. Left lumbar (flank) region

Lower Region

7. Right iliac (inguinal) region
8. Hypogastric (pubic) region
9. Left iliac (inguinal) region

The most superficial organs located in each of the nine abdominopelvic regions are shown in **Figure 1-8** (p. 14) and Figure 1-18 of the Brief Atlas of the Human Body.

The term *hypochondriac* means "under cartilage", and it refers to the rib cartilage. In the right hypochondriac region, the right lobe of the liver and the gallbladder are visible. Viewed superficially, only a portion of the stomach and a small portion of the large intestine are visible in the left hypochondriac region.

Epigastric literally means "upon (over) the stomach". In the epigastric region, parts of the right and left lobes of the liver and a large portion of the stomach can be seen.

Note that the right lumbar region includes parts of the large and small intestines (see **Figure 1-8**). The superficial organs seen in the umbilical region include a portion of the transverse colon and loops of the small intestine. Additional loops of the small intestine and a part of the colon can be seen in the left lumbar region.

The term *iliac* refers to the hip region, it contains the ileum which is the lowest part of the small intestine. The right iliac region contains the caecum and parts of the small intestine. The left iliac region shows portions of the colon and the small intestine.

Hypogastric means "below the stomach". Only loops of the small intestine, the urinary bladder, and the appendix are seen in the hypogastric region.

Abdominopelvic Quadrants

Physicians and other health professionals often use a simpler method and divide the abdomen into four quadrants to describe the site of abdominopelvic pain or locate some type of internal pathologic condition such as a tumour or abscess. One horizontal line and one vertical line passing through the umbilicus (navel) divide the abdomen into *right upper quadrant (RUQ)* and *left upper quadrant (LUQ)* and *right lower quadrant (RLQ)* and *left lower quadrant (LLQ)*.

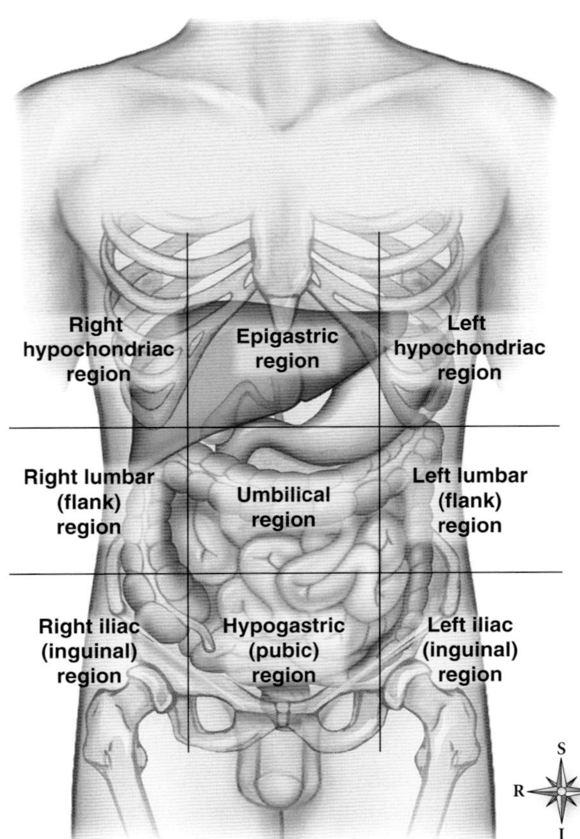

FIGURE 1-8 Nine regions of the abdominopelvic cavity. Only the most superficial structures of the internal organs are shown here.

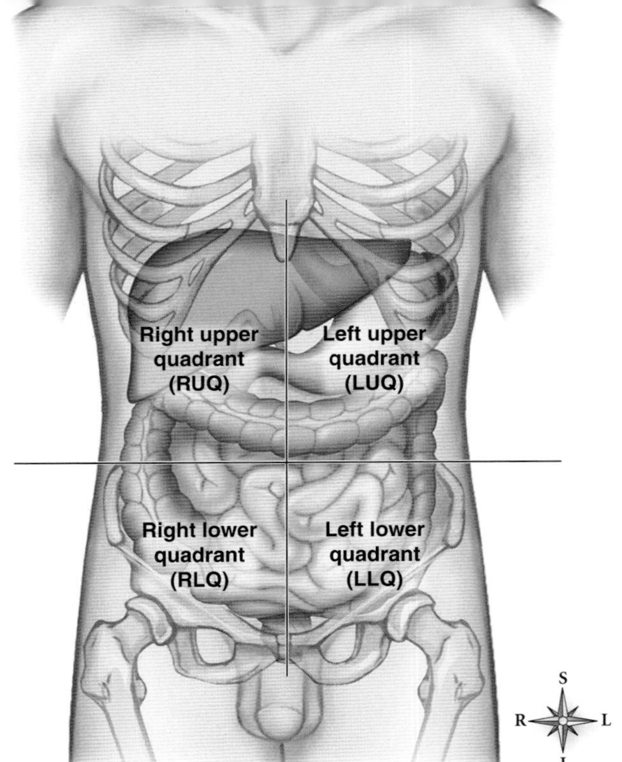

FIGURE 1-9 Division of the abdomen into four quadrants. The diagram shows the relationship of internal organs to the four abdominopelvic quadrants.

Figure 1-9 (at right) and Figure 1-17 of the Brief Atlas of the Human Body show the four abdominal quadrants.

Quick CHECK

12. Define the term *anatomical position* and explain its importance.
13. Name the two major subdivisions of the body as a whole.
14. Identify the two major body cavities and the subdivisions of each.
15. List the nine abdominopelvic regions and four abdominopelvic quadrants.

TERMS USED IN DESCRIBING BODY STRUCTURE

Directional Terms

To minimize confusion when discussing the relationship between body areas or the location of a particular anatomical structure, specific terms must be used. When the body is in the anatomical position, the following directional terms can be used to describe the location of one body part with respect to another (**Figure 1-10**).

Superior and Inferior

Superior means "toward the head", and **inferior** means "toward the feet". *Superior* also means "upper" or "above", and *inferior* means "lower" or "below". For example, the lungs are located superior to the diaphragm, whereas the stomach is located inferior to it.

Anterior and Posterior

Anterior means "front" or "in front of"; **posterior** means "back" or "in back of". In humans—who walk in an upright position—*ventral* (toward the belly) can be used in place of anterior, and *dorsal* (toward the back) can be used for posterior. For example, the nose is on the anterior surface of the body, and the shoulder blades are on its posterior surface.

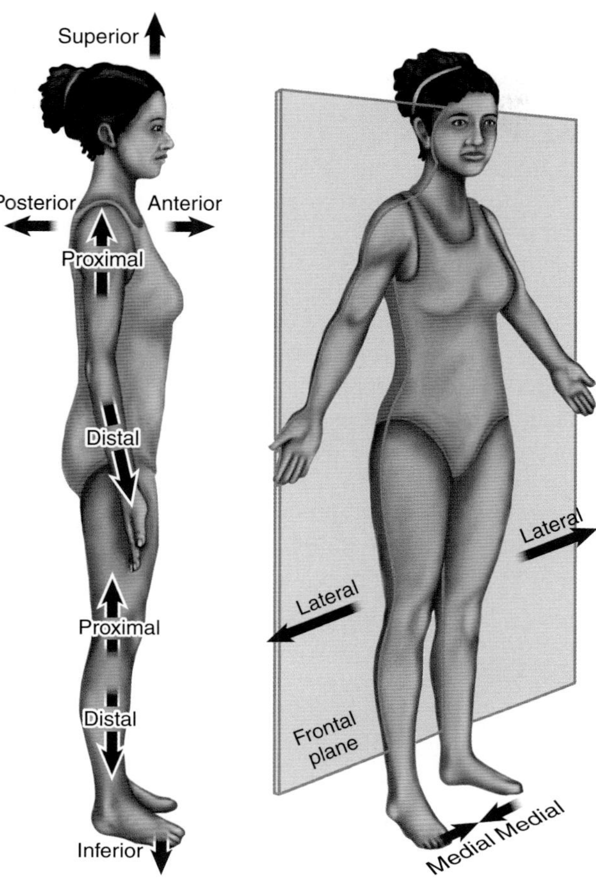

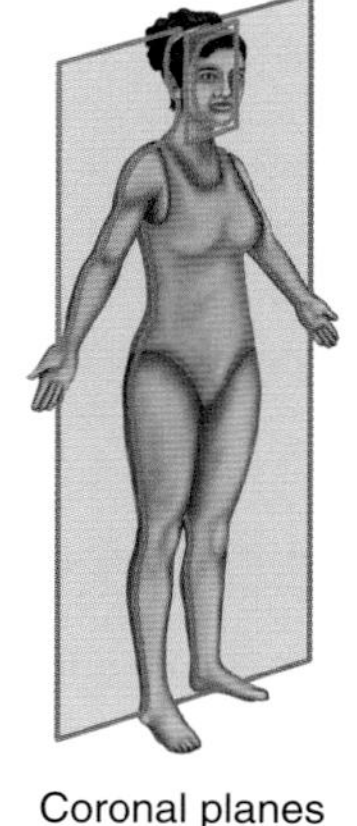

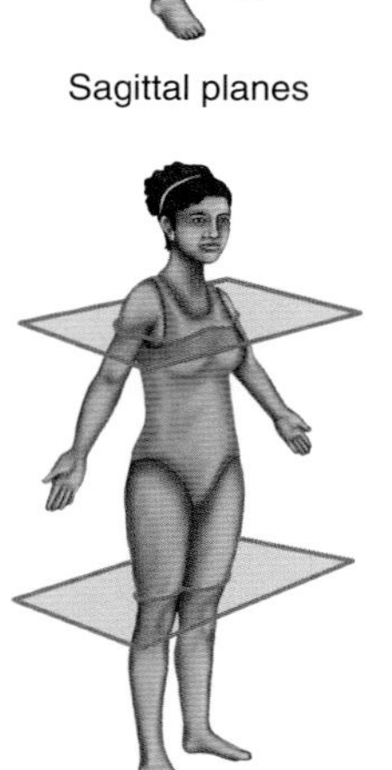
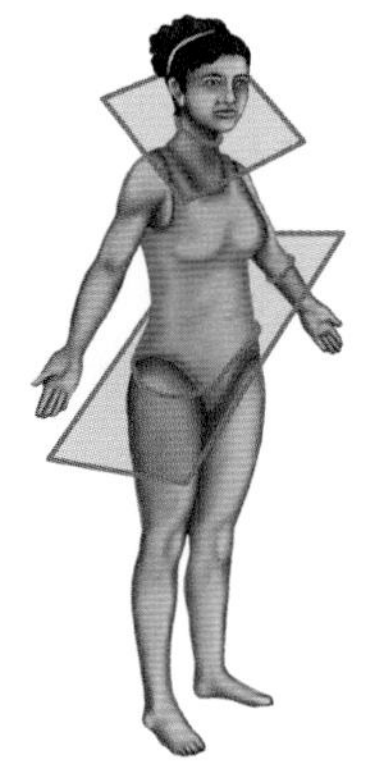

FIGURE 1-10 Directions and planes of the body.

Medial and Lateral

Medial means "toward the midline of the body"; **lateral** means "toward the side of the body, or away from its midline". For example, the great toe is at the medial side of the foot, and the little toe is at its lateral side. The heart lies medial to the lungs, and the lungs lie lateral to the heart.

Proximal and Distal

Proximal means "toward or nearest the trunk of the body, or nearest the point of origin of one of its parts"; **distal** means "away from or furthest from the trunk or the point of origin of a body part". For example, the elbow lies at the proximal end of the forearm, whereas the hand lies at its distal end.

Superficial and Deep

Superficial means "nearer the surface"; **deep** means "further away from the body surface". For example, the skin of the arm is superficial to the muscles below it, and the bone of the upper part of the arm is deep to the muscles that surround and cover it. Refer often to the table of anatomical directions on the inside front cover. It is intended to serve as a useful and ready reference for review.

Terms Related to Organs

When discussing anatomical relationships among organs in a system or region, or anatomical relationships within an organ, additional terms are often useful.

Lumen

Many organs of the body are hollow, such as the stomach, small intestine, airways of the lungs, blood vessels, urinary organs, and so on. The hollow area of any of these organs is called the **lumen.** The term *luminal* means "of or near the lumen". For example, blockage of the respiratory airway may be called a *luminal obstruction.*

Central and Peripheral

Central is plain English and means "near the centre". **Peripheral** means "around the boundary". For example, the central nervous system includes the brain and spinal cord, which are near the centre of the body. The peripheral nervous system, on the other hand, includes the nerves of the muscles, skin, and other organs that are nearer the periphery, or outer boundaries, of the body.

Medullary and Cortical

Medullary refers to an inner region or core of an organ. **Cortical** refers to an outer region or layer of an organ. For example, the inner region of the kidney is the *medulla,* and any structures there are described as medullary. Similarly, the term *cortical* describes structures found in the outer layer of kidney tissue (the *cortex* of the kidney).

Basal and Apical

Some organs, such as the heart and each lung, are somewhat cone-shaped. Thus we borrow terms that describe the point or *apex* of a cone and the flat part or *base* of a cone. **Basal** refers to the base or widest part of an organ. **Apical** refers to the narrow tip of an organ. For example, in the heart the term *apical* refers to the "point" of the heart that rests on the diaphragm. *Basal* and *apical* may also refer to individual cells: the apical surface faces the lumen of a hollow organ, and the basal surface of the cell faces away from the lumen. Many of the more common directional terms that you will use in this course are listed in a handy table inside the front cover of the book.

Anatomical Compass Rosette

To make the reading of anatomical figures a little easier, an *anatomical compass rosette* is used throughout this book. On many figures, you will notice a small compass rosette similar to those on geographical maps. Rather than being labelled N, S, E, and W, the anatomical compass rosette is labelled with abbreviated anatomical directions:

A = Anterior	**P** (opposite A) = Posterior
D = Distal	**P** (opposite D) = Proximal
I = Inferior	**S** = Superior
L (opposite M) = Lateral	**M** = Medial
L (opposite R) = Left	**R** = Right

The anatomical compass rosette sometimes instead uses terms such as *basal* and *apical* if that makes the illustration clearer. For your convenience, the anatomical compass rosette and its possible directions, a helpful diagram of the planes and directions of the body, and a summary table are found on the inside back cover of this book. Refer to it frequently until you are familiar enough with anatomy to do without it.

BODY PLANES AND SECTIONS

The transparent glasslike plates in **Figure 1-10** that divide the body into parts represent different *planes* of the body. In geometry, a plane is an imagined flat surface or plate with no thickness. In anatomy, we often section (cut) the body or an organ along such an imagined flat surface—a **body plane.** The resulting cut is called a **section** of the body or organ. An infinite number of sections can be made along an infinite number of planes, and each section made is named after the particular plane along which it occurs.

There are three major body planes that lie at right angles to one another. They are called the *sagittal*, *coronal*, and *transverse* planes.

Sagittal Planes

Any lengthwise plane running from front to back and top to bottom, dividing the body or any of its parts into right and left sides, is called a **sagittal plane.** A flat cut made along a sagittal plane is called a *sagittal section*.

If a sagittal section is made in the exact midline of the body, resulting in equal and symmetrical right and left halves, the section is called a *median sagittal section* or *midsagittal section* (see **Figure 1-10**).

Coronal Planes

Any lengthwise plane running from side to side and top to bottom, dividing the body or any of its parts into anterior and posterior portions, is called a **coronal plane.** A coronal plane may also be called a *frontal plane*. A cut made along a coronal plane is called a *coronal section* or a *frontal section*.

Transverse Planes

Any crosswise plane that divides the body or any of its parts into upper and lower parts is called a **transverse plane.** A transverse plane is sometimes called a *horizontal plane.* A cut along any transverse plane of the body or an organ may be called a *transverse section* or *horizontal section*.

Figure 1-11 shows the organs of the abdominal cavity as they would appear in the transverse plane or "cut" through the abdomen represented in **Figure 1-10**. In addition to the actual photograph, a simplified line diagram helps in identifying the primary organs. Note that organs near the bottom of the photo or line drawing are in a posterior position. The cut vertebra of the spine, for example, can be identified in its position behind, or posterior, to the stomach. The kidneys are located on either side of the vertebra—they are *lateral* and the vertebra is *medial.*

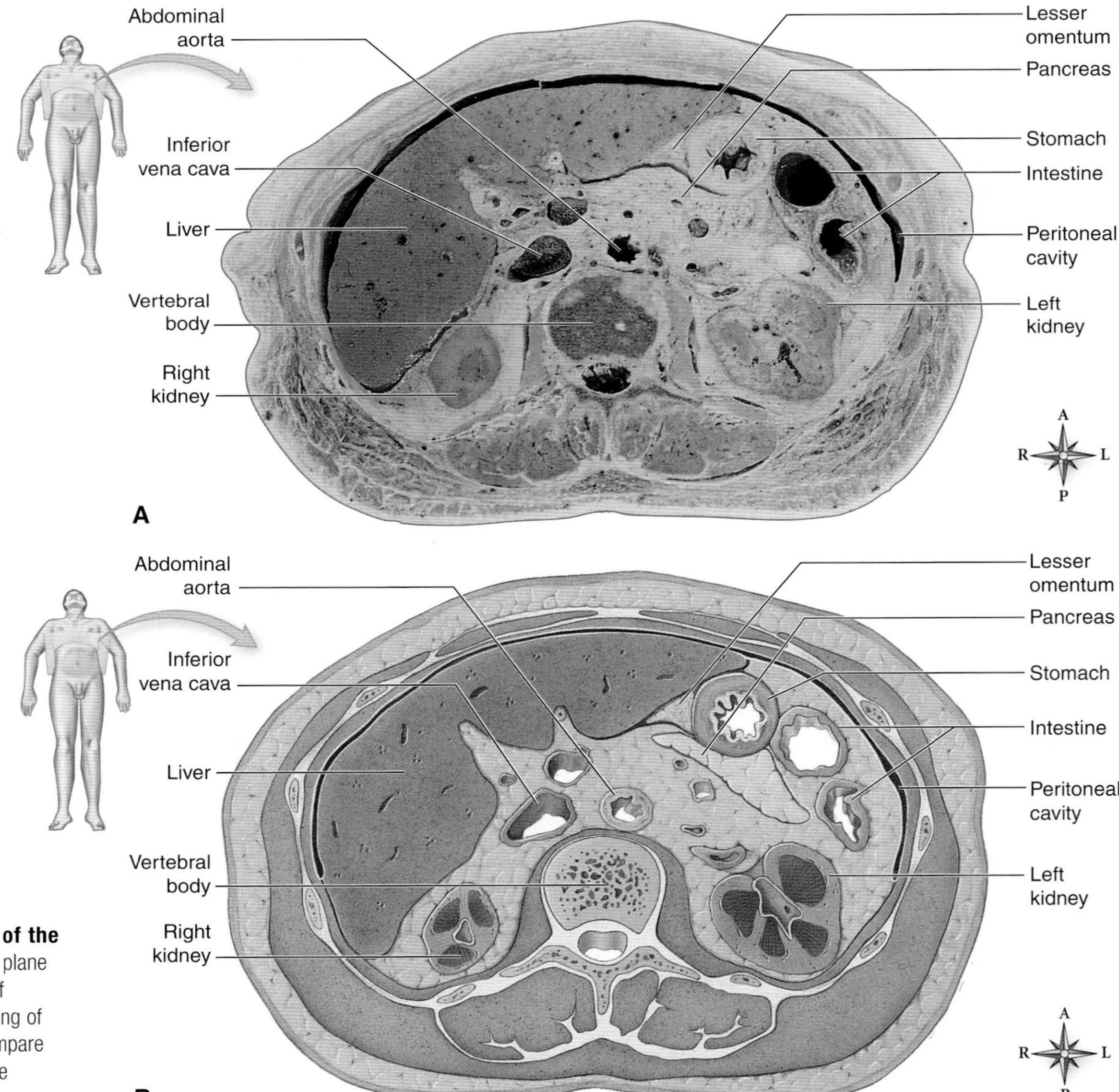

FIGURE 1-11 Transverse section of the abdomen. A, A transverse, or horizontal, plane through the abdomen shows the position of various organs within the cavity. **B,** A drawing of the photograph helps clarify the photo. Compare these views, both seen from below, with the medical image shown in the box on p. 17.

Note also in **Figure 1-11** that the transverse sections are viewed *from below*. This may be at odds with your natural tendency to think of viewing sections from above, so it is important to remember that it is common in anatomical and medical images to show transverse sections from below.

Other Planes and Sections

In anatomy, it is common to use additional terms to help clarify the plane of cutting. For example, a cut along a plane parallel with the short axis of an organ is called a **cross-section.** A cross-section of the whole body would be a transverse section. A cut along the long axis of an organ is called a **longitudinal section.** If you cut off the tip of the finger, you have made a cross-section. If instead you have split a finger down the middle, from the fingertip to the hand, you have made a longitudinal section.

Sometimes it is helpful to make a cut along a plane that is not at right angles to the planes we have already mentioned. Such diagonal cuts are called **oblique sections.**

Quick CHECK

16. Define and contrast each term in these pairs: superior/inferior, anterior/posterior, medial/lateral, dorsal/ventral.
17. How is anatomical left different from your left?
18. Explain how an anatomical compass rosette is used in anatomical illustrations.
19. List and define the three major planes that are used to divide the body into parts.

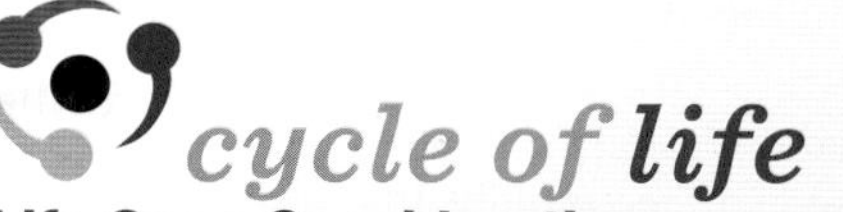

Life Span Considerations An important generalization about body structure is that every organ, regardless of location or function, undergoes change over the years. In general, the body performs its functions least well at both ends of life—in infancy and in old age. Organs develop and grow during the years before maturity, and body functions gradually become more and more efficient and effective. In a healthy young adult all body systems are mature and fully operational.

After maturity, effective repair and replacement of the body's structural components often decrease. The term **atrophy** is used to describe the wasting effects of advancing age. Atrophy can result from disuse, as we slow down in our advanced years, or from the processes of ageing itself that reduce our ability to repair or replace worn tissue.

The changes in functions that occur during the early years are called *developmental processes.* Those that occur during the late years are called *ageing processes.* The study of ageing processes and other changes that occur in our lives as we get older is called *gerontology.* Many specific age changes are noted in the chapters that follow. •

INTERACTION OF STRUCTURE AND FUNCTION

One of the most unifying and important concepts of the study of anatomy and physiology is the principle of *complementarity of structure and function.* In the chapters that follow, you will note again and again that anatomical structures are adapted to perform specific functions. Each structure has a particular size, shape, form, or placement in the body that makes it especially efficient at performing a unique and important activity.

The relationships between the levels of structural organization will take on added meaning as you study the various organ systems in the chapters that follow. For example, as you study the respiratory system in Chapter 36, you will learn about a special chemical substance secreted by cells in the lungs that helps to keep tiny air sacs in these organs from collapsing during respiration. Hereditary material called DNA (a macromolecule) "directs" the differentiation of specialized cells in the lungs during development so that they can

CONNECT IT!

Why bother to learn about planes and sections of the body? In the short term, you'll need to understand how to interpret the many illustrations like **Figure 1-11** in this book—or the series of photographs in Part 4 of the Brief Atlas of the Human Body. In the long term, you will use the concept of planes and sections in clinical settings—as in medical imaging.

Cadavers (preserved human bodies used for scientific study) can be cut into sagittal, frontal, or transverse sections for easy viewing of internal structures, but living bodies, of course, cannot. This fact has been troublesome for medical professionals who must determine whether internal organs are injured or diseased. In some cases the only sure way to detect a lesion or variation from normal is extensive exploratory surgery. Fortunately, advances in medical imaging allow physicians to visualize internal structures of the body without risking the trauma or other complications associated with extensive surgery. This figure shows a CT (computed tomography) scan similar to the perspective of **Figure 1-11**. CT scanning and some of the other widely used techniques are illustrated and described in ***Medical Imaging of the Body*** online at ***Connect It!***

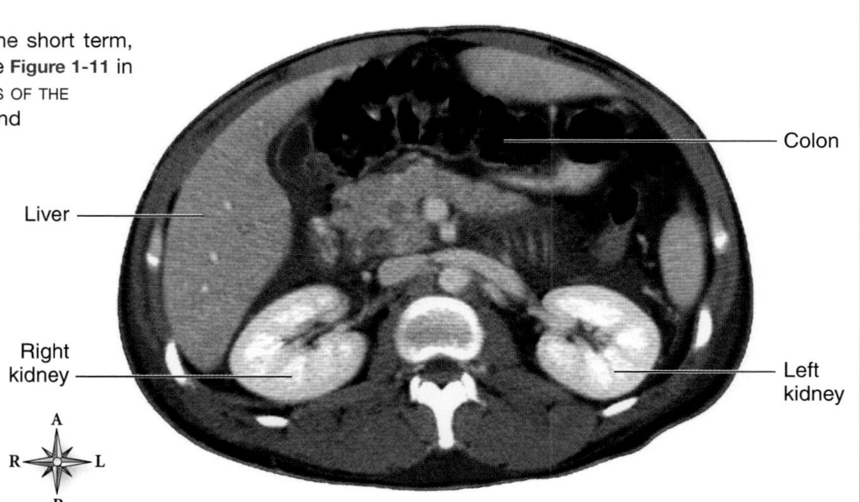

effectively contribute to respiratory function. As a result of DNA activity, special chemicals are produced, cells are modified, and tissues appear that are uniquely suited to this organ system. The cilia (organelles), which cover the exposed surface of cells that form the tissues lining the respiratory passageways, help detect, trap, and eliminate inhaled contaminants such as dust. The structures of the respiratory tubes and lungs assist in efficient and rapid movement of air and also make possible the exchange of critical respiratory gases such as oxygen and carbon dioxide between the air in the lungs and the blood. Working together as the respiratory system, specialized chemicals, organelles, cells, tissues, and organs supply every cell of the human body with necessary oxygen and constantly remove carbon dioxide.

Structure determines function, and function influences the actual anatomy of an organism over time. Structure and function are thus complementary—they are like two sides of a coin. Understanding this fact helps students better understand the mechanisms of disease and the structural abnormalities often associated with pathology. Current research in the study of human biology is now focused in large part on integration, interaction, development, modification, and control of functioning body structures.

By applying the principle of complementarity of structure and function as you study the structural and functional levels of the body's organization in each organ system, you will be able to integrate otherwise isolated factual information into a cohesive and understandable whole. A memorized set of individual and isolated facts is soon forgotten—the parts of an anatomical structure that can be related to its function are not.

CONNECT IT! 

One example of the relationship among body structure, function, and disease relates to how a person's body shape or **somatotype** can be an indicator of either wellness or risk of disease. To see **ectomorph**, **mesomorph**, and **endomorph** somatotypes and learn how they may correlate with health, check out ***Body Types and Disease*** at ***Connect It!***

Quick CHECK

20. Define what is meant by "complementarity of structure and function".
21. Give an example of how the chemical macromolecule DNA can have an influence on body structure.

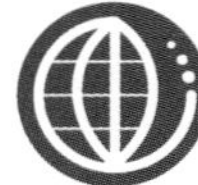

the big picture | Organization of the Body

Ultimately, your success in the study of anatomy and physiology, your ability to see the "big picture", will require understanding, synthesis, and integration of structural information and functional concepts. After you have completed your study of the individual organ systems of the body presented in the chapters that follow, you must be able to reassemble the parts and view the body in a holistic, integrated way.

The body is truly more than the sum of the parts, and understanding the connectedness of human structure and function is the real challenge—and the greatest reward—in the study of anatomy and physiology. Your ability to integrate otherwise isolated factual information about bones, muscles, nerves, and blood vessels, for example, will allow you to view anatomical components of the body and their functions in a more cohesive and understandable way. This chapter introduces the principle of homeostasis as the glue that integrates and explains how the normal interaction of structure and function is achieved and maintained and how a breakdown of this integration results in disease. Furthermore, it provides the basis for understanding and integrating the body of knowledge, both factual and conceptual, that anatomy and physiology encompass.

Mastery of any academic discipline or achieving success in any health care–related work environment requires the ability to communicate effectively. The ability to understand and appropriately use the vocabulary of anatomy and physiology allows you to accurately describe the body itself, the orientation of the body in its surrounding environment, and the relationships that exist between its component parts in both health and disease. This chapter provides you with information necessary to be successful in seeing "the big picture" as you master the details of each organ system, which, although presented separately in subsequent chapters of the text, are in reality part of a marvellously integrated whole. •

LANGUAGE OF SCIENCE *(continued from p. 3)*

gross anatomy (grohs ah-NAT-o-mee)
[*gross* **large**, *ana-* **apart**, *-tom-* **cut**, *-y* **action**]

hypothesis (hye-POTH-eh-sis)
[*hypo-* **under or below**, *-thesis* **placing or proposition**]; *pl.*, **hypotheses** (hye-POTH-eh-seez)

inferior (in-FEER-ee-or)
[*infer-* **lower**, *-or* **quality**]

ipsilateral (ip-si-LAT-er-al)
[*ipsi-* **same**, *-later* **side**, *-al* **relating to**]

lateral (LAT-er-al)
[*later-* **side**, *-al* **relating to**]

longitudinal section (lon-ji-TYOO-dih-nal SEK-shun)
[*longitud-* **length**, *-al* **relating to**, *sect-* **cut**, *-tion* **process**]

lumen (LOO-men)
[*lumen* **light**]; *pl.*, **lumina**

medial (MEE-dee-al)
[*media-* **middle**, *-al* **relating to**]

mediastinum (MEE-dee-as-TYE-num)
[*mediastin-* **midway**, *-um* **thing**]

medullary (meh-DUL-ar-ee)
[*medula-* **marrow or pith (middle)**, *-ary* **relating to**]

metabolism (me-TAB-o-liz-im)
[*meta-* **over**, *-bol-* **throw**, *-ism* **action**]

microbiome (my-kroh-BYE-ohm)
[*micro-* **small**, *-bio-* **life**, *-ome* **entire collection**]

microscopic anatomy (my-kroh-SKOP-ik ah-NAT-o-mee)
[*micro-* **small**, *-scop-* **see**, *-ic* **relating to**, *ana-* **apart**, *-tom-* **cut**, *-y* **action**]

oblique section (o-BLEEK SEK-shun)
[*obliq-* **slanted**, *sect-* **cut**, *-tion* **process**]

organ (OR-gan)
[*organ* **instrument**]

organelle (or-gah-NELL)
[*organ-* **tool or instrument,** *-elle* **small**]

organism (OR-gah-niz-im)
[*organ-* **instrument,** *-ism* **condition**]

parietal (pah-RYE-i-tal)
[*parie-* **wall,** *-al* **relating to**]

peripheral (pe-RIF-er-al)
[*peri-* **around,** *-phera-* **boundary,** *-al* **relating to**]

physiology (fiz-ee-OL-o-jee)
[*physio-* **nature (function),** *-o-* **combining form,** *-log-* **words (study of),** *-y* **activity**]

posterior (pos-TEER-ee-or)
[*poster-* **behind,** *-or* **quality**]

proximal (PROK-si-mal)
[*proxima-* **near,** *-al* **relating to**]

sagittal plane (SAJ-i-tal plane)
[sagitta- **arrow,** *-al* **relating to,** *plan-* **flat surface**]

section (SEK-shun)
[*sect-* **cut,** *-tion* **process**]

superficial (soo-per-FISH-al)
[*super-* **over or above,** *-fici-* **face,** *-al* **relating to**]

superior (soo-PEER-ee-or)
[*super-* **over or above,** *-or* **quality**]

system (SIS-tem)
[*system* **organized whole**]

thoracic cavity (thoh-RASS-ik)
[*thorac-* **chest (thorax),** *-ic* **relating to**]

tissue (TISH-yoo)
[*tissue* **fabric**]

transverse plane (TRANZ-vers plane)
[*trans-* **across or through,** *-vers* **turn,** *plan-* **flat surface**]

ventral cavities (VEN-tral KAV-ih-teez)
[*ventr-* **belly,** *-al* **relating to,** *cav-* **hollow,** *-ity* **state**]

viscera, visceral (VISS-er-ah) (VISS-er-al)
[*visc-* **internal organ,** *-al* **relating to**; *sing.,* **viscus**]

LANGUAGE OF MEDICINE

atrophy (AT-ro-fee)
[*a-* **without,** *-troph* **nourishment,** *-y* **state**]

ectomorph (EK-toh-morf)
[*ecto-* **outside,** *-morph* **form**]

endomorph (EN-doh-morf)
[*endo-* **within,** *-morph* **shape**]

mesomorph (MEZ-oh-morf)
[*meso-* **middle,** *-morph* **form**]

somatotype (so-MAT-o-type)
[*soma-* **body,** *-type* **kind**]

case study

Laura is about to complete her final year at the local sixth-form college and is considering applying for a degree course in adult nursing. Her career advisor has arranged for her to shadow a nurse for a day at the local hospital in the Accident and Emergency department to see what the job involves.

For the first hour the nurse was busy with administration, signing in patients, and taking their blood pressure, weight, and temperature—not the exciting job Laura had envisaged. Then an ambulance arrived, and Laura heard the paramedics report to the nurse, "Stab wound to the right upper quadrant, cuts to the brachial region, and a large contusion on his right, lower extremity proximal to the knee."

Laura was unsure what had happened to the patient. Now try to interpret what the paramedic said to the nurse.

1. Where was the patient stabbed?
   a. In his thoracic cavity
   b. In his abdominopelvic cavity
   c. In his pericardial cavity
   d. In his pleural cavity
2. What organ is most likely to have been damaged by the knife attack?
   a. His heart
   b. His lungs
   c. His liver
   d. His spleen
3. Where is the contusion (bruise) on the patient's body?
   a. Near his right groin
   b. Just above his right ankle
   c. His lower right thigh
   d. Behind his right knee
4. Where is the patient's brachial region?
   a. His armpit
   b. His lower leg
   c. His cheek
   d. His upper arm

Hint To solve a case study, you may have to refer to the glossary or index, other chapters in this textbook, **Connect It!,** and other resources.

CHAPTER SUMMARY

To download an MP3 version of the chapter summary for use with your mobile device, access the ***Audio Chapter Summaries*** *online at evolve.elsevier.com.*

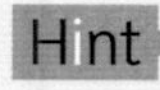

Scan this summary after reading the chapter to help you reinforce the key concepts. Later, use the summary as a quick review before your class or before a test.

Science and Society

A. Science involves logical inquiry based on experimentation (**Figure 1-1**)
   1. Hypothesis—idea or principle to be tested in experiments
   2. Experiment—series of tests of a hypothesis; a controlled experiment eliminates biases or outside influences

3. Theory—a hypothesis that has been supported by experiments and thus shown to have a high degree of confidence
4. Law—a theory that has an unusually high level of confidence

B. The process of science is active and changing as new experiments add new knowledge
C. Science is affected by culture and culture is affected by society

Anatomy and Physiology

A. Anatomy and physiology are branches of biology concerned with the form and functions of the body
B. Anatomy—science of the structure of an organism and the relationship of its parts
   1. Gross anatomy—study of the body and its parts relying only on the naked eye as a tool for observation (**Figure 1-2**)
   2. Microscopic anatomy—study of body parts with a microscope
      a. Cytology—study of cells
      b. Histology—study of tissues
   3. Developmental anatomy—study of human growth and development
   4. Pathological anatomy—study of diseased body structures
   5. Systemic anatomy—study of the body by systems
C. Physiology—science of the functions of organisms; subdivisions named according to:
   1. Organism involved—human or plant physiology
   2. Organizational level—molecular or cellular physiology
   3. Systemic function—respiratory physiology, neurophysiology, or cardiovascular physiology

Language of Science and Medicine

A. Scientific terms are often based on Latin or Greek word parts
B. Terminology tools are provided in the BRIEF ATLAS OF THE HUMAN BODY packaged with this book
C. *Terminologia Anatomica (TA)* and *Terminologia Histologica (TH)*
   1. Official lists of anatomical terms (*TA*, gross anatomy; *TH*, microscopic anatomy)
   2. Terms listed in Latin, English, and by number
   3. Avoids use of eponyms (terms based on a person's name)
D. Physiology terms do not have an official list but follow the same principles as *TA* and *TH*

Characteristics of Life

A. A single criterion may be adequate to describe life, for example:
   1. Autopoiesis—living organisms are self-organized and self-maintaining
   2. Cell theory—if it is made of one or more cells, it is alive
B. Characteristics of life considered most important in humans are summarized in **Table 1-1**
C. Metabolism—sum total of all physical and chemical reactions occurring in the living body

Levels of Organization (Figure 1-3)

A. Chemical level—basis for life
   1. Organization of chemical structures separates living material from nonliving material
   2. Organization of atoms, molecules, and macromolecules results in living matter—a gel called *cytoplasm*
B. Organelle level
   1. Chemical structures organized to form organelles that perform individual functions
   2. It is the functions of the organelles that allow the cell to live
   3. Dozens of organelles have been identified, including:
      a. Mitochondria
      b. Golgi apparatus
      c. Endoplasmic reticulum
C. Cellular level
   1. Cells—smallest and most numerous units that possess and exhibit characteristics of life
   2. Each cell has a nucleus surrounded by cytoplasm within a limiting membrane
   3. Cells differentiate to perform unique functions
D. Tissue level
   1. Tissue—an organization of similar cells specialized to perform a certain function
   2. Tissue cells are surrounded by nonliving matrix
   3. Four major tissue types
      a. Epithelial tissue
      b. Connective tissue
      c. Muscle tissue
      d. Nervous tissue
E. Organ level
   1. Organ—organization of several different kinds of tissues to perform a special function
   2. Organs represent discrete and functionally complex operational units
   3. Each organ has a unique size, shape, appearance, and placement in the body
F. System level
   1. Systems—most complex organizational units of the body
   2. System level involves varying numbers and kinds of organs arranged to perform complex functions (**Table 1-2**):
      a. Support and movement
      b. Communication, control, and integration
      c. Transportation and defence
      d. Respiration, nutrition, and excretion
      e. Reproduction and development
   3. Microbiome—set of interacting communities of bacteria and other microorganisms that inhabit the human body; microbial systems influence normal body functions
G. Organism level
   1. The living human organism is greater than the sum of its parts
   2. All of the components interact to allow the human to survive and flourish

Anatomical Position (Figure 1-4)

A. Primary anatomical reference position
   1. Body erect with arms at sides and palms forward
   2. Head and feet pointing forward
B. *Bilateral symmetry*—a term meaning that right and left sides of the body are mirror images
   1. Bilateral symmetry confers balanced proportions
   2. Remarkable correspondence of size and shape between body parts on opposite sides of the body

3. Ipsilateral structures are on the same side of the body in anatomical position
4. Contralateral structures are on opposite sides of the body in anatomical position

C. Other major body positions
1. Supine—body lying face upward
2. Prone—body lying face downward

Body Cavities (Figure 1-5; Table 1-3)

A. Ventral cavities
1. Thoracic cavity
   a. Mediastinum contains the heart and surrounding structures
   b. Right and left pleural cavities contain lungs
2. Abdominopelvic cavity
   a. Abdominal cavity
   b. Pelvic cavity
3. Ventral cavities are lined with slippery double-layered membranes (Figure 1-6)
   a. Parietal layer—covers inside wall of cavity
   b. Visceral layer—covers internal organ(s)
   c. *Cavity* can refer either to the potential space between these two layers or to the entire space in which the organs reside

B. Dorsal cavities
1. Cranial cavity
2. Spinal cavity

C. Other cavities are hollows found in many organs throughout the body

Body Regions (Figure 1-7; Table 1-4)

A. Axial subdivision
1. Head
2. Neck
3. Torso, or trunk, and its subdivisions

B. Appendicular subdivision
1. Upper extremity and subdivisions
2. Lower extremity and subdivisions

C. Abdominopelvic regions (Figure 1-8)
1. Upper
   a. Right hypochondriac region
   b. Epigastric region
   c. Left hypochondriac region
2. Middle
   a. Right lumbar region
   b. Umbilical region
   c. Left lumbar region
3. Lower
   a. Right iliac (inguinal) region
   b. Hypogastric region
   c. Left iliac (inguinal) region

D. Abdominopelvic quadrants (Figure 1-9)
1. Right upper quadrant
2. Left upper quadrant
3. Right lower quadrant
4. Left lower quadrant

Terms Used In Describing Body Structure

A. Directional terms (Figure 1-10)
1. Superior and inferior
2. Anterior (ventral) and posterior (dorsal)
3. Medial and lateral
4. Proximal and distal
5. Superficial and deep

B. Terms related to organs
1. Lumen (luminal)
2. Central and peripheral
3. Medullary (medulla) and cortical (cortex)
4. Apical (apex) and basal (base)

C. Anatomical compass rosette—a compass rosette that signifies anatomical directions rather than geographic directions, as on a map

D. A list of directional terms and a guide to using the anatomical compass rosette are found inside the back cover of the book

Body Planes and Sections (Figures 1-10 and 1-11)

A. Planes are lines of orientation along which cuts or sections can be made to divide the body, or a body part, into smaller pieces

B. There are three major body planes, which lie at right angles to each other:
1. Sagittal plane runs front to back so that sections through this plane divide the body (or body part) into right and left sides
   a. If section divides the body (or part) into symmetrical right and left halves, the plane is called *midsagittal* or *median sagittal*
2. Frontal (coronal) plane runs lengthwise (side to side) and divides the body (or part) into anterior and posterior portions
3. Transverse (horizontal) plane is a "crosswise" plane and divides the body (or part) into upper and lower parts

C. Other planes and sections
1. Cross-section runs along a plane parallel with the short axis of an organ
2. Longitudinal section follows a plane parallel with the long axis of an organ
3. Oblique sections run along diagonal (slanted) planes

Interaction of Structure and Function

A. Complementarity of structure and function is an important and unifying concept in the study of anatomy and physiology

B. Anatomical structures are adapted to perform specific functions because of their unique size, shape, form, or body location

C. Understanding the interaction of structure and function assists in the integration of otherwise isolated factual information

Cycle of Life: Life Span Considerations

A. Structure and function of body undergo changes over the early years (developmental processes) and late years (ageing processes)

B. Infancy and old age are periods when the body functions least well

C. Young adulthood is period of greatest homeostatic efficiency

D. *Atrophy*—term to describe the wasting effects of advancing age

REVIEW QUESTIONS

Hint

Write out the answers to these questions after reading the chapter and reviewing the Chapter Summary. Note—writing out your answers will consolidate learning and provide a valuable resource of information.

1. Define the terms *anatomy* and *physiology*.
2. List and briefly describe the levels of organization that relate the structure of an organism to its function. Give examples characteristic of each level.
3. Give examples of each system level of organization in the body and briefly discuss the function of each.
4. What is meant by the term *anatomical position*? How do the specific anatomical terms of position or direction relate to this body orientation?
5. What is bilateral symmetry? What terms are used to identify placement of one body part with respect to another on the same or opposite sides of the body?
6. What does the term *somatotype* mean? Name the three major somatotypes and briefly describe the general characteristics of each. (Hint: Review ***Body Types and Disease*** online at ***Connect It!***)
7. Define briefly each of the following terms: *anterior, distal, sagittal plane, medial, dorsal, coronal plane, organ, parietal peritoneum, superior, tissue.*
8. Locate the mediastinum.
9. Discuss in general terms the principle of complementarity of structure and function.

CRITICAL THINKING QUESTIONS

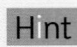

After finishing the Review Questions, write out the answers to these more in-depth questions to help you apply your new knowledge. Go back to sections of the chapter that relate to concepts that you find difficult.

1. Each characteristic of life is related to body metabolism. Explain how digestion, circulation, and growth are metabolically related.
2. What diseases may result in a patient with an endomorph somatotype and a waist-to-hip ratio of 1:2? (Hint: Review ***Body Types and Disease*** online at ***Connect It!***)
3. An x-ray technician has been asked to take radiographs of the entire large intestine (colon), including the appendix. Which of the nine abdominopelvic regions must be included in the radiograph?
4. Body cavities can be subdivided into smaller and smaller sections. Identify, from largest to smallest, the cavities in which the urinary bladder can be placed.

2 Homeostasis

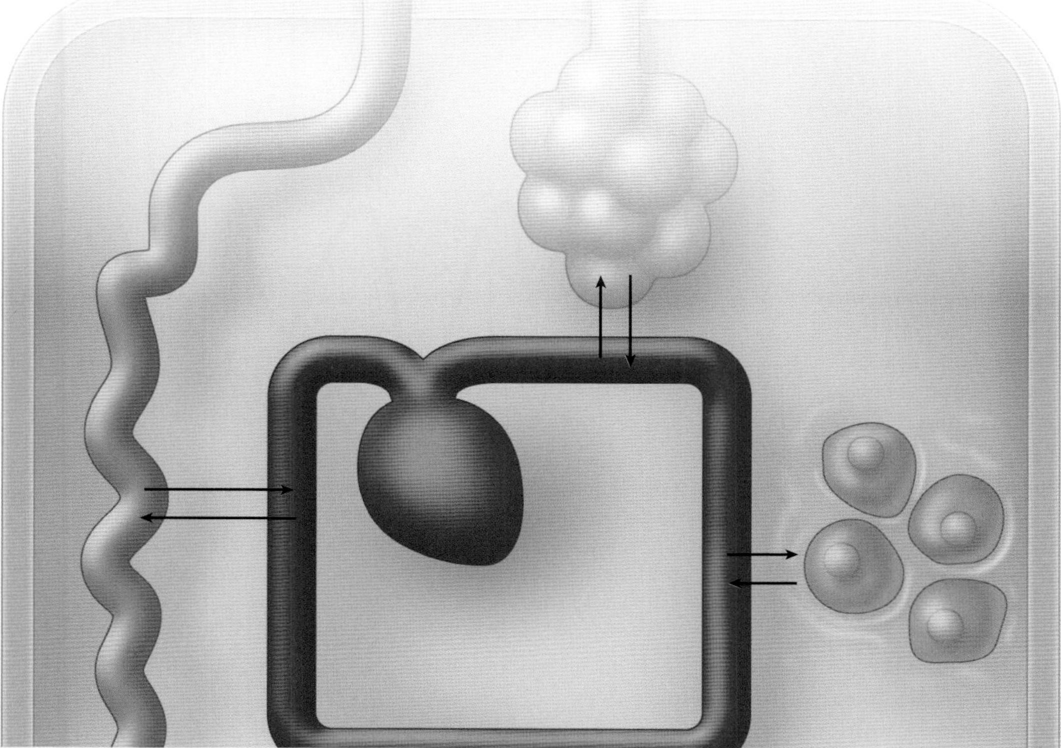

CHAPTER OUTLINE

Hint Scan this outline before you begin to read the chapter, as a preview of how the concepts are organized.

A central principle of human function is that we maintain relatively constant conditions inside our body. Unless our body is able to maintain about the same temperature, pressure, oxygen level, acidity, moisture, and so on, all the time, our cells cannot function properly. We will get sick and we will die unless proper conditions are restored. Any of the functions of the organs and systems of the body we will study throughout the rest of this book are all explained by their impact on maintaining relatively constant conditions inside our body. This concept of internal stability is called homeostasis and is the focus of this chapter. After studying this chapter, you will have a basic understanding of homeostatic balance and how it is maintained in the body. Your

LANGUAGE OF SCIENCE

Hint Use this list to aid your pronunciation of unfamiliar words.

afferent (AF-fer-ent)
[*a[d]-* **toward,** *-fer-* **carry,** *-ent* **relating to**]

circadian (sir-KAY-dee-en)
[*circa-* **around,** *-di-* **day,** *-an* **relating to**]

effector (ef-FEK-tor)
[*effect-* **accomplish,** *-or* **agent**]

efferent (EF-fer-ent)
[*e-* **away,** *-fer-* **carry,** *-ent* **relating to**]

extrinsic control
(eks-TRIN-sik kon-TROL)
[*extr-* **outside or beyond,** *-insic* **beside**]

feedback control loop
(FEED-bak kon-TROL loop)

homeostasis (ho-mee-o-STAY-sis)
[*homeo-* **same or equal,** *-stasis* **standing still**]

hypothalamus
(hye-poh-THAL-ah-muss)
[*hypo-* **under or below,** *-thalamus* **inner chamber**] *pl.,* **hypothalami**

integrator (IN-te-gray-ter)
[*integr-* **whole,** *-at(e)-* **process,** *-or* **agent**]

internal environment
(in-TERN-al en-VIR-ro[n]-ment)
[*intern-* **inside,** *-al* **relating to,** *environ-* **surround,** *-ment* **condition**]

intracellular control
(in-tra-SELL-yoo-lar kon-TROL)
[*intra-* **inside or within,** *-cell* **storeroom**]

intrinsic control
(in-TRIN-sik kon-TROL)
[*intr-* **inside or within,** *-insic* **beside**]

negative feedback
(NEG-ah-tiv FEED-bak)
[*negat-* **deny,** *-ive* **relating to**]

oxytocin (OT) (ock-see-TOH-sin)
[*oxy-* **sharp (oxygen),** *-toc-* **birth,** *-in* **substance**]

pathology (pah-THOL-o-jee)
[*patho-* **disease,** *-o-* **combining form,** *-log-* **words (study of),** *-y* **activity**]

positive feedback
(POZ-ih-tiv FEED-bak)
[*posit-* **put or place,** *-ive* **relating to**]

continued on p. 34

understanding will deepen as you move forward in your studies, as you encounter example after example of body functions maintaining constantly high oxygen levels, normal fluid pressure, low waste levels, high nutrient levels, and so on. You will also encounter examples of disorders that occur when organs fail and our body cannot maintain normal internal conditions.

HOMEOSTASIS

THE INTERNAL ENVIRONMENT

More than a century ago a great French physiologist, Claude Bernard (1813–1878), made a remarkable observation. He noted that body cells survived in a healthy condition only when the temperature, pressure, and chemical composition of their fluid environment remained relatively constant. He called the environment of cells the **internal environment**, or *milieu intérieur.* Bernard realized that although many elements of the external environment in which we live are in a constant state of change, important elements of the internal environment, such as body temperature, remain remarkably stable. For example, Bernard's neighbour, who travels from his Paris home heated with a fireplace to the snowy slopes of the Alps in January, is exposed to dramatic changes in air temperature within a few hours.

Fortunately, in a healthy individual, body temperature will remain at or very near normal regardless of temperature changes that may occur in the external environment. Just as the external environment surrounding the body as a whole is subject to change, so too is the fluid environment surrounding each body cell. The remarkable fluid that bathes each cell contains literally dozens of different substances. Good health, indeed life itself, depends on the correct and constant amount of each substance in the blood and other body fluids. The precise and constant chemical composition of the internal environment must be maintained within very narrow limits ("normal ranges"), or sickness and death will result.

RELATIVE STABILITY

In 1932 a famous American physiologist, Walter B. Cannon, suggested the name **homeostasis** for the relatively constant states maintained by the body. Homeostasis is a key word in modern physiology. It comes from two Greek words (*homoios,* "the same", and *stasis,* "standing"). "Standing or staying the same", then, is the literal meaning of homeostasis. In his classic publication titled *The Wisdom of the Body,* Cannon advanced one of the most unifying and important themes of physiology. He suggested that every regulatory mechanism of the body exists to maintain homeostasis, or constancy, of the body's internal fluid environment.

However, as Cannon emphasized, homeostasis does not mean something set and immobile that stays exactly the same all the time. In his words, homeostasis "means a condition that may vary, but which is relatively constant". It is the maintenance of relatively constant internal conditions despite changes in either the internal or the external environment that characterizes homeostasis. For example, even if external temperatures vary, homeostasis of body temperature means that it remains relatively constant at about 37°C, although it may vary slightly above or below that point and still be "normal". The fasting concentration of blood glucose, an important nutrient, can also vary somewhat and still remain within normal limits (**Figure 2-1**).

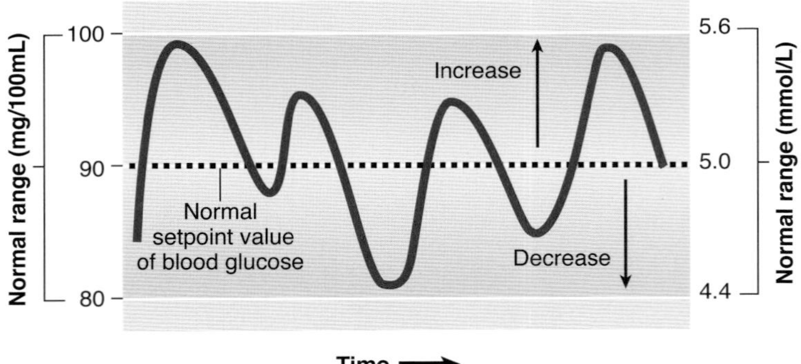

FIGURE 2-1 Homeostasis of blood glucose. The range over which a given value, such as the blood glucose concentration, is maintained is accomplished through homeostasis. Note that the concentration of glucose fluctuates above and below a normal setpoint value 5 mmol/L (90 mg/100 mL) within a normal setpoint range 4.4 to 5.6 mmol/L (80 to 100 mg/100 mL).

SET POINT

This normal reading or range of normal is called the **set point** or **setpoint range.** A value between 4.4 and 5.6 mmol of glucose per litre of blood, depending on dietary intake and timing of meals, is typical. Although levels of the important gases oxygen and carbon dioxide also vary with the respiratory rate, these substances, like body temperature and blood glucose levels, must be maintained within very narrow limits.

CONNECT IT!

What are the normal setpoint values for the concentration of clinically important substances found in the body? Check out ***Clinical and Laboratory Values*** online at ***Connect It!***

Specific regulatory mechanisms are responsible for adjusting body systems to maintain homeostasis. This ability of the body to "self-regulate", or "return to normal" to maintain homeostasis, is a critically important concept in modern physiology and also serves as a basis for understanding mechanisms of disease. Each cell of the body, each tissue, and each organ system plays an important role in homeostasis. Each of the diverse regulatory systems described in subsequent chapters of the text is explained as a function of homeostasis. You will learn how specific regulatory activities such as temperature control or carbon dioxide elimination are accomplished. In addition, an understanding of the relationship of homeostasis to healthy survival helps explain why such mechanisms are necessary.

Models of Homeostasis

Take a moment to study **Figure 2-2**. This diagram is a classic way of envisioning the idea of the body as a "bag of fluid". The fluid inside the bag is our internal environment, and it is this fluid that must be kept at a relatively constant temperature, glucose level, and so on, if the cells that make up the body are to survive. It is like a big, walking fishbowl, and our cells are the fish. All the little tubes and gizmos you see in **Figure 2-2** are the systems that keep the "water in the fishbowl"—your internal fluid environment—stable. For example, the tube representing the digestive tract is a way for food in the external environment to be absorbed into the internal environment. So, just as you feed your goldfish every day, keeping the nutrient level in the fishbowl relatively constant over the years, your digestive tract keeps your body's nutrient levels relatively constant over the years.

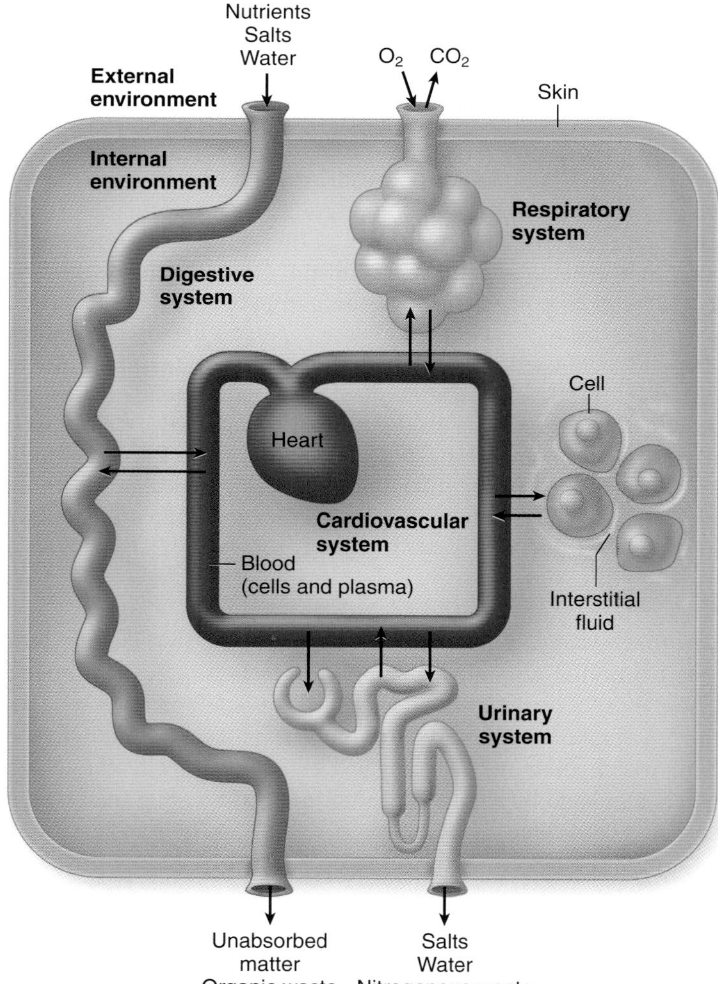

FIGURE 2-2 Diagram of the body's internal environment. The human body is like a bag of fluid separated from the external environment. Tubes, such as the digestive tract and respiratory tract, bring the external environment to deeper parts of the bag where substances may be absorbed into the internal fluid environment or excreted into the external environment. All the "accessories" somehow help maintain a constant environment inside the bag that allows the cells that live there to survive.

TABLE 2-1 Homeostatic Functions of Body Systems

SYSTEM	SUMMARY OF FUNCTION
Integumentary	Separates internal environment from external environment, providing stability of internal fluid volume
Skeletal	Supports and protects internal environment, allowing movement; stores minerals that can be moved into and out of internal fluid
Muscular	Powers and directs movements; provides heat
Nervous	Regulates homeostatic mechanisms, sensing changes, integrating information, sending signals to effectors
Endocrine	Homeostatic regulation by secreting signalling hormones that travel through internal environment to effector cells
Cardiovascular	Maintains internal constancy by transporting nutrients, water, oxygen, hormones, wastes, and other materials and heat within the internal environment
Lymphatic	Maintains constant fluid pressure by draining excess fluid from tissues, cleaning it, and recycling it to bloodstream
Immune	Defends internal environment against harmful agents
Respiratory	Maintains stable O_2 and CO_2 levels in body by exchanging these gases between external and internal environments; provides vocal communication with others for protection, hunting, etc.
Digestive	Maintains relatively constant nutrient level in body by digesting food and absorbing nutrients into internal environment
Urinary	Maintains constantly low level of waste and regulates pH of internal environment; helps maintain constancy of internal water volume and balance of ions and other substances
Reproductive	Passes genetic code containing information for forming a body and maintaining homeostasis to offspring

O_2, oxygen; *CO_2*, carbon dioxide; *pH*, acidity.

All the other "accessories" in **Figure 2-2** are like the accessories you may use in your fishbowl. The urinary system is like a filter that keeps waste levels constantly low. The respiratory system is like an aquarium's air pump and gets oxygen deep into the body to keep oxygen levels high for your cells. Throughout the book, we will regularly refer back to this diagram and the idea it represents—because this idea is the foundation for understanding all of physiology. If you know that everything functions to keep your "fishbowl" of a body relatively constant so that your "fish", or cells, will stay alive, you can understand the basic function of every organ of every system! **Table 2-1** lists the homeostatic functions of each of the major body systems.

There are many different ways to visualize the concept of homeostasis and processes involved in maintaining homeostatic balance. For example, homeostatic balance is often compared to a circus acrobat maintaining balance on a high wire—the so-called *Wallenda model* of homeostasis. It is also common to compare the body's homeostatic mechanisms to a home heating system controlled by a thermostat. Keep in mind that each of these models or representations emphasizes only one or two aspects of the overall concept and does not impart a complete understanding of homeostasis. Such deep understanding will come only with continued study of the many models and many examples you will encounter in this chapter and throughout the book.

Quick CHECK

1. Describe what is meant by "the body's internal environment".
2. Define the term *homeostasis.*
3. Summarize the concept of a *set point.*
4. Describe how a bag of fluid or a fishbowl can be a model for a stable human body.

HOMEOSTATIC CONTROL MECHANISMS

FEEDBACK LOOPS

Maintaining homeostasis means that the cells of the body are in an environment that meets their needs and permits them to function normally in changing external conditions. Processes for maintaining or restoring homeostasis are known as *homeostatic control mechanisms.* They involve virtually all of the body's organs and systems. If circumstances occur that require changes or more active regulation in some aspect of the internal environment, the body must have appropriate control mechanisms available that respond to these changing needs and then restore and maintain a healthy internal environment. For example, exercise increases the need for oxygen and results in accumulation of the waste product carbon dioxide. By increasing our breathing rate above its average of about 17 breaths per minute, we can maintain an adequate blood oxygen level and also increase the elimination of carbon dioxide. When exercise stops, the need for an increased respiratory rate no longer exists and the frequency of breathing returns to normal.

To accomplish this self-regulation, a highly complex and integrated communication control system or network is required. This type of network is called a **feedback control loop.** Different networks in the body control such diverse functions as blood carbon dioxide levels, temperature, heart rate, sleep cycles, and thirst. Regulatory networks usually make use of feedback control loops. Information, or feedback, may be transmitted in these control loops by nervous impulses or by specific chemical messengers called *hormones,* which are secreted into the blood. Regardless of the body function being regulated or the mechanism of information transfer (nerve impulse or hormone secretion), these feedback control loops have the same basic components and work in the same way.

BASIC COMPONENTS OF CONTROL SYSTEMS

There is a minimum of four basic components in every feedback control loop:

1. Sensor mechanism
2. Integrator or control centre
3. Effector mechanism
4. Feedback

The terms *afferent* and *efferent* are important directional terms commonly used in physiology. In this case, they are used to describe movement of a signal from a sensor mechanism to a particular integrating or control centre and, in turn, movement of a signal from that centre to some type of effector mechanism. **Afferent** means that a signal is travelling toward a particular centre or point of reference, and **efferent** means that the signal is moving away from a centre or other point of reference. These terms are of particular importance in the study of the nervous and endocrine systems in Unit 3.

Sensor

The process of regulation and the concept of return to normal require that the body be able to "sense" or identify the variable being controlled. A physiological **variable** is any state or condition in the body that can change or vary. Sensory nerve cells or hormone-producing (endocrine) glands frequently act as homeostatic sensors. To function in this way, a **sensor** must be able to identify the characteristic or condition being controlled. It must also be able to respond to any changes that may occur from the normal setpoint range. If deviations from the normal setpoint range occur, the sensor generates an afferent signal (nerve impulse or hormone) to transmit that information to the second component of the feedback loop—the integrator.

Integrator

The **integrator** is often called the *integration centre* or *control centre* of the feedback loop. Often a discrete area of the brain, the integrator receives input from a homeostatic sensor. That information is analyzed and integrated with input from other sensors. Thus the actual value of a variable is compared with the setpoint value of the variable. Depending on the result of this comparison, an efferent signal may travel from the centre to some type of effector mechanism, where a specific action is initiated, if necessary, to maintain homeostasis. First, the level or magnitude of the variable being measured by the sensor is compared with the normal setpoint level that must be maintained for homeostasis. If significant deviation from that predetermined level exists, the integration or control centre sends its own signal to the third component of the control loop—the effector mechanism.

Effector

Effectors are organs, such as muscles or glands, that directly influence controlled physiological variables. For example, it is effector action that increases or decreases variables such as body temperature, heart rate, blood pressure, or blood sugar concentration to keep them within their normal range. The activity of effectors is ultimately regulated by feedback of information regarding their own effects on a controlled variable.

Feedback

Many physiologists use the example of an electric heater controlled by a thermostat to explain how feedback control systems work. This analogy is a good one because it parallels the homeostatic mechanism used to control body temperature. In this example, changes in room temperature (the controlled variable) are detected by a thermometer (sensor) attached to the thermostat (integrator) (**Figure 2-3**, A). The thermostat contains a switch that controls the electric heater (effector). When cold weather causes a decrease in room temperature, the change is detected by the thermometer and relayed to the thermostat. The thermostat compares the actual room temperature with the setpoint temperature. After the integrator determines that the actual

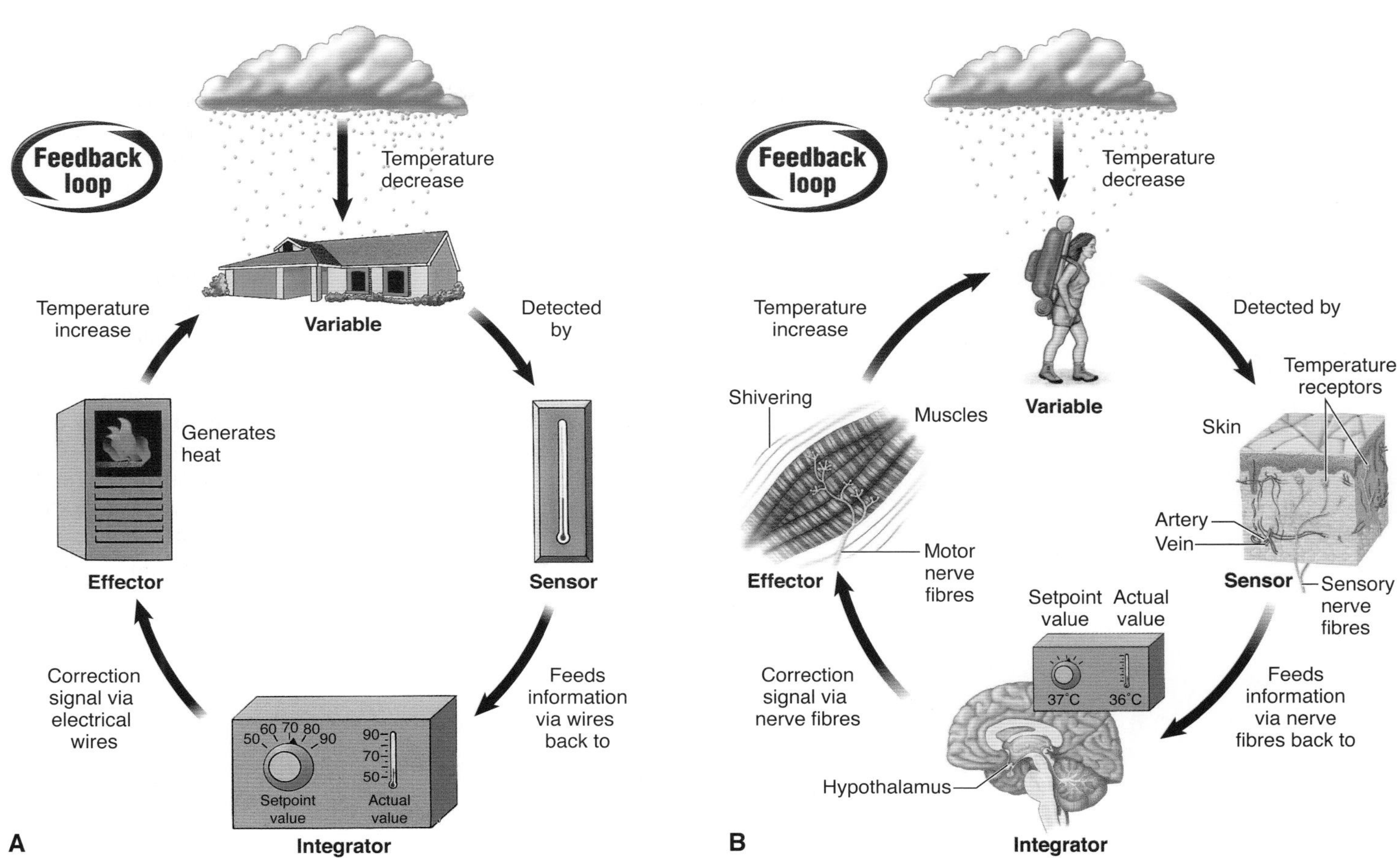

FIGURE 2-3 Basic components of homeostatic control mechanisms. A, Heat regulation by a heater controlled by a thermostat. **B,** Homeostasis of body temperature. Note that in both examples **A** and **B,** a stimulus (drop in temperature) activates a sensor mechanism (thermostat or body temperature receptor) that sends input to an integrating, or control, centre (on–off switch or hypothalamus), which then sends input to an effector mechanism (heater or contracting muscle). The resulting heat that is produced maintains the temperature in a "normal range". Feedback of effector activity to the sensor mechanism completes the control loop. Both are examples of negative feedback loops.

temperature is too low, it sends a "correction" signal by switching on the heater. The heater produces heat and thus increases room temperature back toward normal. As the room temperature increases above normal, feedback information from the thermometer causes the thermostat to switch off the heater. Thus by intermittently switching the heater off and on, a relatively constant room temperature can be maintained.

Body temperature can be regulated in much the same way as room temperature is regulated by the heating system just described (**Figure 2-3**, *B*). Here, sensory receptors in the skin and other tissues act as sensors by monitoring body temperature. When cold weather causes the body temperature to decrease, feedback information is relayed through the nerves to the "thermostat" in a part of the brain called the **hypothalamus.** An integrator in the hypothalamus compares the actual body temperature with the "built-in" setpoint body temperature and subsequently sends a nerve signal to effectors.

In this example, the skeletal muscles act as effectors by shivering and thus producing heat. Shivering increases body temperature back to normal, at which point it stops as a result of feedback information that causes the hypothalamus to shut off its stimulation of the skeletal muscles. More specifics of body temperature control are discussed in Chapter 10.

The impact of effector activity on sensors may be positive or negative. Therefore, homeostatic control mechanisms are categorized as negative or positive feedback systems. By far the most important and numerous of the homeostatic control mechanisms are negative feedback systems.

Negative Feedback in Control Systems

The example of temperature regulation by action of a thermostatically regulated heater is a classic example of **negative feedback.** Negative feedback control systems are inhibitory. They oppose or "negate" a change (such as a drop in temperature) by creating a response (production of heat) that is opposite in direction to the initial disturbance (fall in temperature below a normal set point).

All negative feedback mechanisms in the body respond in this way regardless of the variable being controlled. They produce an action that is opposite to the change that activated the system, as discussed in **Box 2-1**. It is important to emphasize that negative feedback control systems *stabilize* physiological variables. They keep variables from straying too far outside their normal ranges. Negative feedback systems are responsible for maintaining a constant internal environment.

Sometimes such feedback loops are described in terms of *stimulus* and *response*. A **stimulus** is a change in a variable that elicits a

BOX 2-1 *sports and fitness* | **Negative Feedback During Exercise**

In our first example of a negative feedback loop, we saw that when body temperature decreases below the setpoint value, the response is to shiver and produce heat—thus returning the body temperature back to the set point (**Figure 2-3**, *B*). Another example occurs when body temperature increases above the set point—as may happen when exercising. The hypothalamus receives feedback from temperature sensors and responds to the high body temperature by triggering the activity of sweat glands (the effectors). As sweat evaporates from the skin, it carries heat away from the body and thus reduces the body's temperature back toward the set point. Peek ahead to **Figure 10-16** on p. 194 to see an illustration of this example.

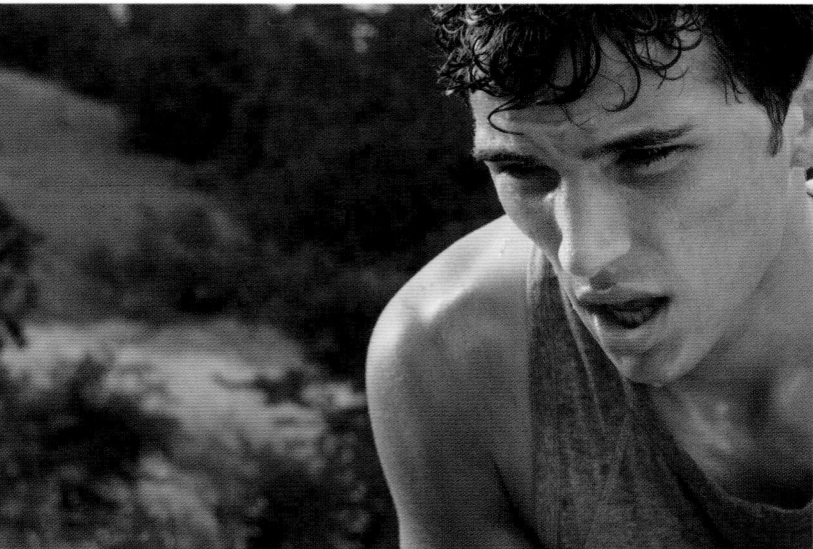

Yet another example of negative feedback that occurs during exercise helps maintain relatively stable oxygen and carbon dioxide levels in the blood. As our muscles work, they remove a large amount of oxygen from the blood, thus lowering the blood oxygen level below its set point. At the same time, blood carbon dioxide levels climb dramatically above its set point. Chemical sensors in blood vessels send feedback to the brainstem through sensory nerves. Integrators in the brain respond by increasing the rate and depth of breathing, which increases the rate of adding oxygen to and removing carbon dioxide from the bloodstream. All of which brings the "blood gases" back toward their set points—and brings the body back toward its normal conditions.

Many other negative feedback mechanisms operate during exercise to maintain normal acid levels in the blood, maintain normal water content in body tissues, and more. •

reaction in a feedback loop. The **response** is the reaction—the operation of the effector in a feedback loop.

Quick CHECK

1. List the basic components of every feedback control system.
2. Describe how a thermostat-controlled heating system is a feedback loop.
3. What makes a negative feedback loop negative?

Positive Feedback in Control Systems

Positive feedback is also possible in control systems. However, because positive feedback does not operate to help the body maintain a stable, or homeostatic, condition, it is often harmful, even disastrous, to survival. Positive feedback control systems are stimulatory. Instead of opposing a change in the internal environment and causing a return to normal, positive feedback tends to amplify or reinforce the change that is occurring.

In the example of the electric heater controlled by a thermostat, a positive feedback loop continues to increase the temperature. It does so by stimulating the electric heater to produce more and more heat. Each increase in heat production is followed by a positive stimulation to increase the temperature even more. Typically, such responses result in instability and disrupt homeostasis because the variable in question continues to deviate further and further away from its normal range.

Only a few examples of positive feedback operate in the body in normal conditions. In each case, positive feedback accelerates the process in question. The feedback causes an ever increasing rate of events to occur until something stops the process. In other words, positive feedback loops tend to amplify or accelerate a change—in contrast to negative feedback loops, which reverse a change. Strictly speaking, positive feedback is not homeostatic because it does not promote constancy of the internal environment. However, in some cases it can quickly amplify a process in a way that ultimately restores stability and protects the body from harm.

Although positive feedback is not the usual type of feedback in the body, it is no less important. Events that lead to a simple sneeze, the birth of a baby, an immune response to an infection, or the formation of a blood clot are all examples of helpful positive feedback.

One of the mechanisms that operates during delivery of a newborn illustrates that positive feedback can be helpful to survival. As delivery begins, the fetus is pushed from the *womb*, or *uterus*, into the birth canal, or *vagina*. Stretch receptors in the wall of the reproductive tract detect the increased stretch caused by the head pushing outward (**Figure 2-4**). Information regarding increased stretch is fed back to the brain, which triggers the pituitary gland to secrete a hormone called **oxytocin (OT)**.

Oxytocin travels through the bloodstream to the uterus, where it stimulates stronger contractions. Stronger contractions push the fetus further along the birth canal, thereby increasing stretch and stimulating the release of more oxytocin. Uterine contractions quickly get stronger and stronger until the baby is pushed out of the body and the positive feedback loop is broken. OT can also be injected therapeutically by a physician to stimulate labour contractions.

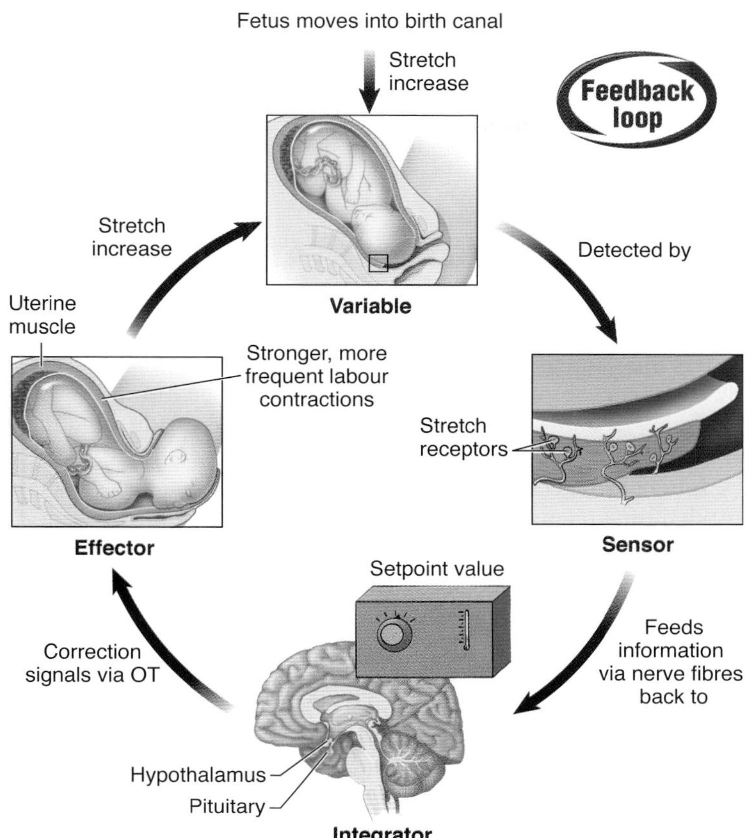

FIGURE 2-4 Positive feedback loop. An example of positive feedback occurs during labour when stretch of the uterus and birth canal beyond the set point is detected and triggers the release of oxytocin (OT). OT stimulates stronger and more frequent uterine muscle contractions, pushing the baby forward and thus stretching the tract even further beyond setpoint range. That triggers the release of more OT and thus even stronger and more frequent contractions. Labour contractions get stronger and more frequent until finally the baby is delivered, relieving stretch of the reproductive tract and thus breaking the positive feedback loop.

The positive-feedback amplification of labour contractions speeds up the delivery of a newborn and thus lowers the risk of hazardous complications for both the mother and child.

Another example of positive feedback occurs when a blood vessel is damaged and platelets stick together to form a plug to slow the loss of blood. As platelets stick, they release chemicals that attract more platelets to the injury and trigger them to stick—until eventually a clot is formed. In this case, the positive feedback allows a blood clot to form very rapidly and thus minimize blood loss from the damaged vessel.

Changing the Set Point

Like the set point on an electric heater's thermostat, the physiological set points in your body can be changed. Your body's setpoint temperature is a good example. First, not everyone's set point, or "normal", body temperature is the same. **Figure 2-5** shows the difference in body temperatures observed in a group of healthy students. You can see that temperatures varied widely. This explains why some people are comfortable at a temperature that is too cold for others around them—their temperature set point must be naturally lower.

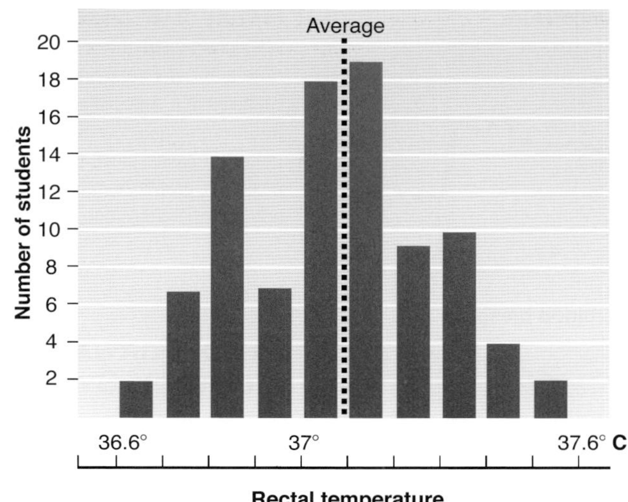

FIGURE 2-5 Range of normal body temperatures. In a well-controlled experiment, a group of healthy students show a wide range of normal rectal temperatures. The average (mean) temperature of this group is 37.1°C.

However, your set point can also change in varying circumstances. For example, we know a man who once turned up the thermostat in his house to get the temperature warm enough to get some unwelcome visitors to leave. Likewise, during a bacterial infection, your immune system sends chemicals to signal the brain's hypothalamus to "turn up the setpoint temperature". Your body shivers, and you may ask for a blanket as your body tries to reach this new higher set point. You now have a fever. The bacteria that have invaded your body did so because they liked the temperature of your body. When you are experiencing a fever, your body becomes uncomfortably warm for the bacteria, and they slow down their reproductive rate, which slows the infection. At the same time, the warmer temperature helps improve the immune system's function as it deals with the bacteria. After the infection is over, the hypothalamus returns to its usual set point. You may sweat to lower the temperature back down to the lower "normal" set point and your fever goes away.

The body naturally changes some set points to different values at different times of the day. **Figure 2-6** shows some examples of variables that normally exhibit a daily rhythm of highs and lows. Daily cycles are called **circadian** rhythms or cycles. Depending on the time of day or night, the body's internal clock mechanisms can raise or lower some of the set points for physiological variables in the body such as hormone concentration in the blood plasma, body temperature, and blood pressure. Note in **Figure 2-6**, A, that a person's body temperature usually drops at night. For this reason, many of us feel comfortable with a lower room temperature at night—perhaps even programming our home's thermostat to lower its setpoint temperature at night.

CONNECT IT!

For a brief summary of an important mechanism of timekeeping in the body, review ***The Timekeeping Hormone*** online at ***Connect It!***

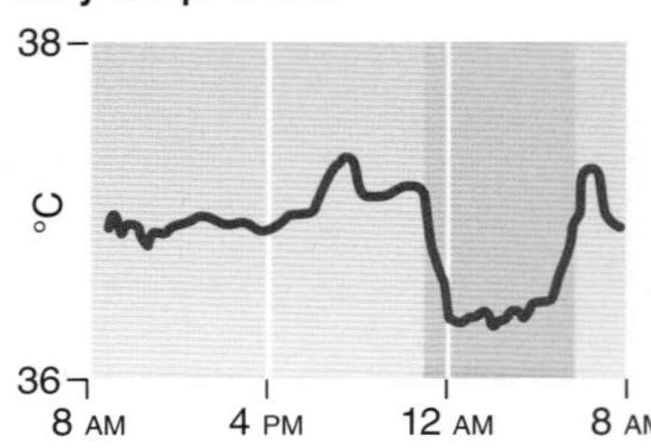

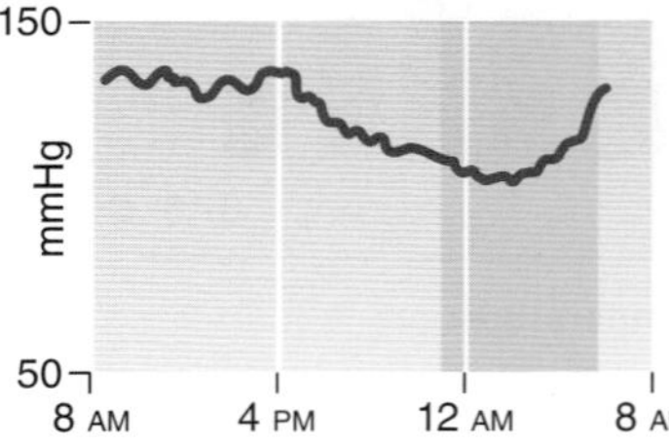

Plasma GH
10
ng/mL
0
8 AM
4 PM
12 AM
8 AM

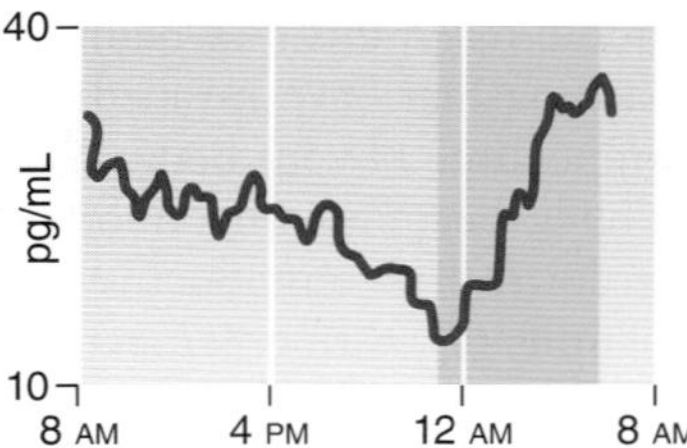

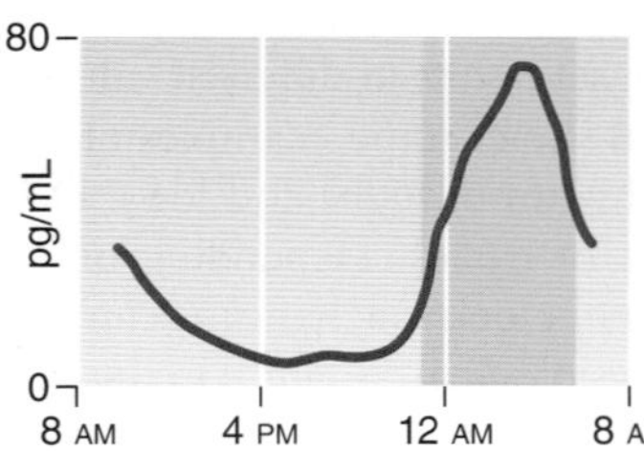

FIGURE 2-6 Circadian cycles. The body's internal clock mechanisms raise and lower set points for some variables in a daily high-low rhythm, as these examples show. Shaded areas represent typical sleep times. (*Systolic*, peak; *GH*, growth hormone; *ACTH*, adrenocorticotropic hormone.)

Feed-Forward in Control Systems

As you study the complexity of control systems throughout the body, you will no doubt run into cases of **feed-forward** in control systems. Feed-forward is the concept that information may flow ahead to another process to trigger a change in anticipation of an event that will follow.

For example, when you eat a meal, the stomach stretches and this triggers stretch sensors in the stomach wall. As you would expect, the stretch sensors trigger a feedback response that causes the release of digestive juices and contraction of stomach muscles. This is normal negative feedback because secretion and muscle activity eventually get rid of the food and bring the stretch of the stomach back down to normal. It will continue as long as there is food to stretch the stomach. At the same time, the stretch stimulus is triggering the small intestine and related organs to increase secretion there as well—*before* the food has arrived. In other words, information from one feedback loop (in the stomach) has leaped ahead to the next logical feedback loop (in the intestines) to get the second loop ready ahead of time.

Another example of feed-forward control occurs when you see or smell food and your salivary glands respond by secreting saliva and your stomach starts to contract rhythmically as it secretes its own juices in anticipation of food being eaten.

Feed-forward causes a feedback loop to anticipate a stimulus before it actually happens.

LEVELS OF HOMEOSTATIC CONTROL

One of the first principles that will occur to you as you study human physiology is that the functions of cells, tissues, organs, and systems are integrated into a coordinated whole. This is accomplished by many different feedback loops and feed-forward systems operating at many different levels of organization within the body (**Figure 2-7**).

Intracellular control mechanisms operate at the cell level. These mechanisms regulate functions within the cell, often by means of genes and enzymes. The role of genes and enzymes is discussed further in Chapters 6 and 7.

Intrinsic control mechanisms operate at the tissue and organ levels. Sometimes also called local control or *autoregulation*, intrinsic mechanisms often make use of chemical signals. For example, prostaglandins are molecules sent as signals to other nearby cells. Intrinsic regulation may also be "built into" the tissue or organ. For instance, when cardiac muscle in the heart is stretched, the muscle automatically contracts with more force. Prostaglandins are discussed further in Chapters 4 and 25. Many other examples of intrinsic control are discussed throughout the book.

Extrinsic control means "outside" control and operates at the system and organism levels. Extrinsic control usually involves nervous and endocrine (hormonal) regulation. It is called "extrinsic" control because the nerve signals and hormones originate outside the controlled organ. Nervous regulation is introduced in more detail in Chapters 18 through 23, and endocrine regulation is introduced in Chapter 25.

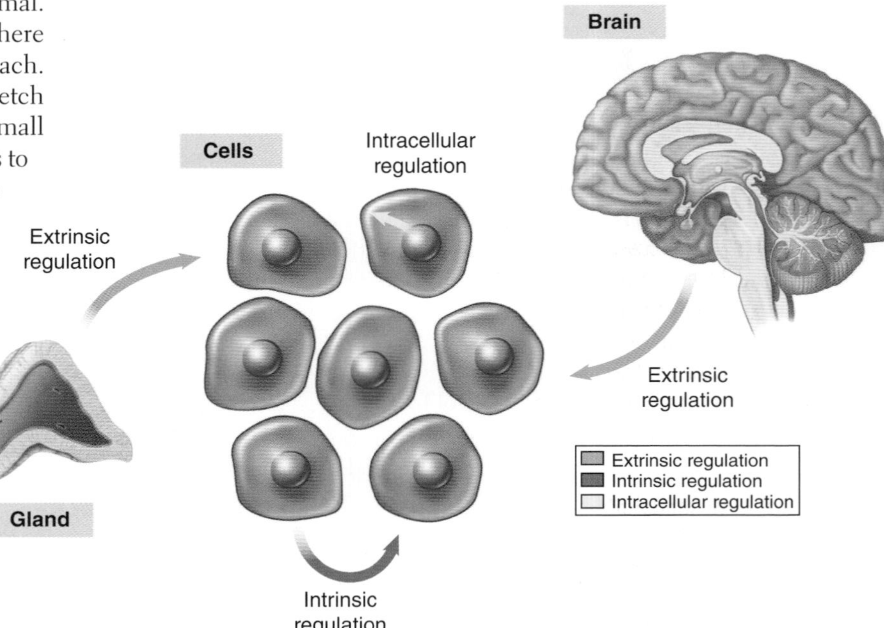

FIGURE 2-7 Levels of control. The many complex processes of the body are coordinated at multiple levels: intracellular (within cells), intrinsic (within tissues and organs), and extrinsic (organ to organ).

SUMMARY OF HOMEOSTASIS

In summary, homeostasis is the relative constancy of the body's fluid internal environment. It is regulated by a complex network of mechanisms that includes feedback loops. When the body is healthy, internal conditions fluctuate but usually stay within a set point or "normal" range. Most homeostatic mechanisms operate on the negative feedback principle. They are activated, or turned on, by changes in the environment that surround every body cell. Negative feedback systems are inhibitory. They reverse the change that initially activated the homeostatic mechanism. By reversing the initial change, a homeostatic mechanism tends to maintain or restore internal constancy.

Occasionally, a positive (stimulatory) feedback mechanism helps promote survival. Such positive or stimulatory feedback systems may be required to bring specific body functions to swift completion.

The set point of some variables can be set to a higher or lower value, allowing the variable to be held at different setpoint ranges in different circumstances. For example, body temperature is maintained at a higher set point during some infections. There is also a daily lowering of the body temperature set point during nightly sleep.

Feed-forward occurs when sensory information "jumps ahead" to a feedback loop to get it started before the stimulus actually changes the controlled physiological variable. This happens when we salivate in anticipation of eating food.

Homeostatic control systems can operate at any (or all) of several different levels: within the cell, from cell to cell within a tissue, and throughout the body. This layering of regulation allows for precise coordination of functions within organs as well as in the whole body.

Quick CHECK

1. How does a *positive* feedback loop differ from a *negative* feedback loop?
2. In what circumstances could the set point for a variable change normally?
3. Define *circadian rhythm.*
4. Describe an example of *feed-forward* in a physiological control system.
5. Contrast intracellular, intrinsic, and extrinsic levels of control.

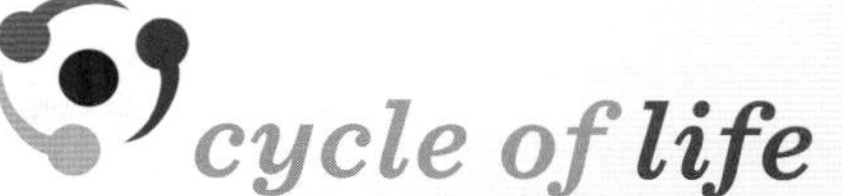

cycle of life

Life Span Considerations During infancy and early childhood, some homeostatic mechanisms—such as maintaining stable glucose concentrations in the blood plasma—may not be as efficient as they are in adulthood. Therefore, babies and young children may have more difficulty maintaining normal blood glucose levels when fasting. Homeostatic mechanisms may also lose some of their efficiency and precision in regulating some physiological variables in advanced old age. Some of this loss of homeostatic efficiency associated with ageing results from the decreasing ability of ageing effectors to function well because of degeneration of organs. •

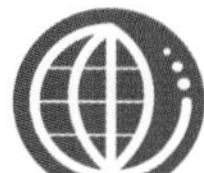

the big picture | Homeostasis

The relative constancy of the body's internal fluid environment is regulated by many complex mechanisms. Nearly every function of the human body—the function of every system, organ, tissue, and cell—can be understood more clearly as part of a process of maintaining such constancy. Thus this chapter has laid out a central idea of physiology that will guide us through the remaining chapters of the book. Principles of homeostasis will explain for us the workings of the heart, the brain, the lungs, the kidneys, the gut, and more. Nearly everything we will study from now on in physiology will simply be more examples of homeostatic function. •

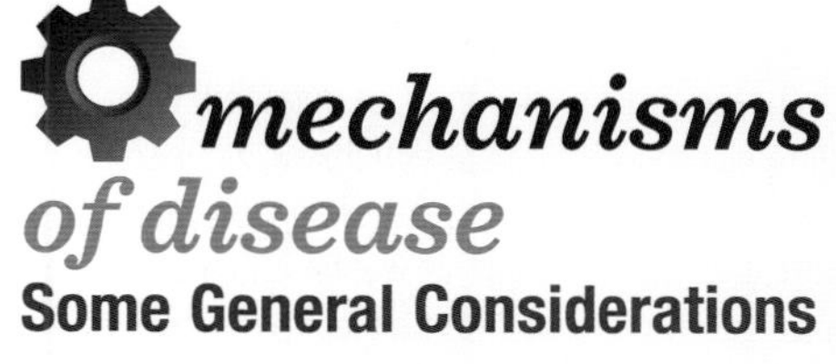

mechanisms of disease

Some General Considerations A clearer understanding of the normal function of the body often comes from our study of disease (**Box 2-2**). **Pathophysiology** is the organized study of the underlying physiological processes associated with disease. Pathophysiologists attempt to understand the mechanisms of a disease and its course of development, or *pathogenesis.* Near the end of each chapter of this book we briefly describe some important disease mechanisms that illustrate the breakdown of normal functions described in that chapter.

Many diseases are best understood as disturbances to homeostasis, the relative constancy of the body's internal environment (**Figure 2-8**). If homeostasis is

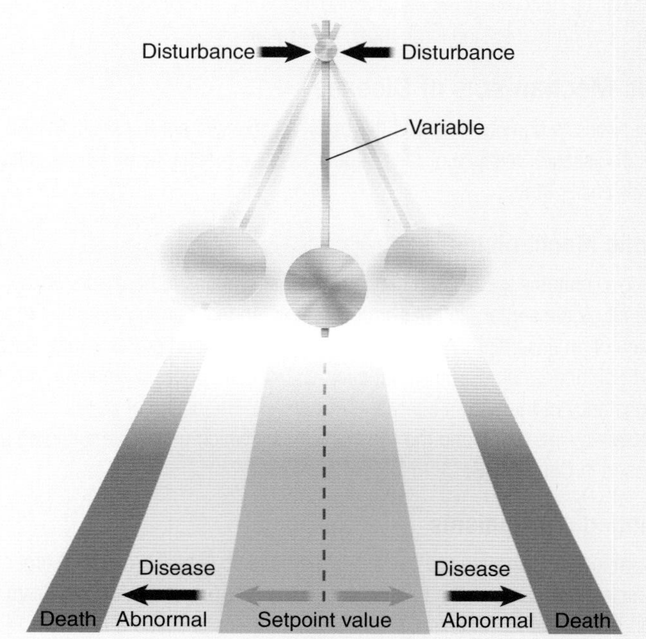

FIGURE 2-8 Model of homeostatic balance and disease. Movement of the variable in question, away from the setpoint value, is depicted as normal fluctuations. Sometimes a physiological disturbance pushes the body beyond its capacity to maintain homeostasis and into the abnormal range for a given physiological parameter—resulting in disease. Disturbances in the extreme may result in death.

H

BOX 2-2 *health matters* | **Disease Terminology**

Everyone is interested in **pathology**—the study of disease. Researchers want to know the scientific basis of abnormal conditions. Health practitioners want to know how to prevent and treat various diseases. Every one of us, when we suffer from the inevitable head cold or something more serious, want to know what is going on and how best to deal with it. Pathology has its own terminology, as in any specialized field. Just as with other scientific terms, most disease-related terms are derived from Latin and Greek word parts. For example, *patho-* comes from the Greek word for disease (*pathos*) and is used in many terms, including *pathology* itself.

Disease conditions are usually *diagnosed* or identified by **signs** and **symptoms.** Signs are objective abnormalities that can be seen or measured by someone other than the patient, whereas symptoms are the subjective abnormalities that are felt only by the patient. Although *sign* and *symptom* are distinct terms, we often use them interchangeably. A **syndrome** is a collection of different signs and symptoms that occur together. When signs and symptoms appear suddenly, persist for a short time, and then disappear, we say that the disease is **acute.** On the other hand, diseases that develop slowly and last for a long time (perhaps for life) are labelled **chronic** diseases. The term *subacute* refers to diseases with characteristics somewhere between acute and chronic.

The study of all the factors involved in causing a disease is its **aetiology.** The aetiology of a skin infection often involves a cut or abrasion and subsequent invasion and growth of a bacterial colony. Diseases with undetermined causes are said to be **idiopathic. Communicable** diseases are those that can be transmitted from one person to another.

The term *aetiology* refers to the theory of a disease's cause, but the actual pattern of a disease's development is called its **pathogenesis.** The common cold, for example, begins with a *latent,* or "hidden", stage during which the cold virus establishes itself in the patient. No signs of the cold are yet evident. In infectious diseases, the latent stage is also called **incubation.** The cold may then manifest itself as a mild nasal drip and trigger a few sneezes. It subsequently progresses to its full fury and continues for a few days. After the cold infection has run its course, a period of *convalescence,* or recovery, occurs. During this stage, body functions return to normal. Some chronic diseases, such as cancer, exhibit a temporary reversal that seems to be a recovery. Such reversal of a chronic disease is called a **remission.** If a remission is permanent, we say that the person is "cured".

Epidemiology is the study of the occurrence, distribution, and transmission of diseases in human populations. A disease that is native to a local region is called an **endemic** disease. If the disease spreads to many individuals in a relatively short time, the situation is called an **epidemic. Pandemics** are epidemics that affect large geographic regions, perhaps spreading worldwide. Because of the speed and availability of modern air travel, pandemics are more common than they once were. Almost every flu season we see a new strain of influenza virus quickly spreading from continent to continent.

Names of specific diseases are often descriptive, such as *rheumatoid arthritis* (meaning "autoimmune inflammation of joints"). Some disease names are eponyms, with a person's name incorporated into the term, as in *Parkinson disease (PD).* For linguistic simplicity and technical advantages, the nonpossessive form of eponyms is used in this textbook. For example, Down Syndrome is used in preference to Down's Syndrome. Note also that some disease names are abbreviated with an acronym such as *DMD* (for *Duchenne muscular dystrophy*). •

disturbed, various negative feedback mechanisms usually return the body to normal. When a disturbance goes beyond the normal fluctuation of everyday life, we can say that a disease condition exists. In acute conditions the body recovers its homeostatic balance quickly. In chronic diseases a normal state of balance may never be restored. If the disturbance keeps the body's internal environment too far from normal for too long, death may result.

Basic Mechanisms of Disease

Disturbances to homeostasis and the body's responses are the basic mechanisms of disease. Because of their variety, disease mechanisms can be categorized for easier study.

Genetic Mechanisms

Altered, or mutated, genes can cause abnormal proteins to be made. These abnormal proteins often do not perform their intended function, resulting in the absence of an essential function. On the other hand, such proteins may instead perform an abnormal, disruptive function. Either case poses a potential threat to the constancy of the body's internal environment. The action of genes is first discussed in Chapter 7, and the mechanisms by which genes are inherited are discussed in Chapter 48.

Pathogenic Organisms

Many important disorders are caused by pathogenic (disease-causing) organisms or particles that damage the body in some way (**Figure 2-9**). Any organism that lives in or on another organism to obtain its nutrients is called a *parasite.* The presence of microscopic or larger parasites may interfere with normal body functions of the host and cause disease. Besides parasites, there are organisms that poison or otherwise damage the human body to cause disease. Some of the major pathogenic organisms and particles include the following:

Prions (proteinaceous infectious particles) are proteins that may cause misfolding of protein molecules, thus converting normal proteins of the cell into different proteins. The altered form of the protein may then be inherited. For example, they can alter some brain-cell proteins into abnormal tangles, thereby causing loss of nervous system function. Prion protein (also called *PrP*) molecules are a newly discovered type of pathogen, and not much is known about how the prion works to cause such diseases as bovine spongiform encephalopathy (BSE; "mad cow disease") or variant Creutzfeldt–Jakob disease (vCJD). However, not all prions cause disease. Some are now known to be involved in memory formation and the normal maintenance of the insulating sheath around many nerve fibres.

Viruses are intracellular parasites that consist of a DNA or RNA core surrounded by a protein coat and, sometimes, a lipoprotein envelope. They are particles that invade human cells and cause them to produce viral components. Sometimes, the term *virion* is used to designate the complete virus particle as it exists outside the host cell.

Bacteria are tiny, primitive cells that lack nuclei. They cause infection by parasitizing tissues or otherwise disrupting normal function.

Fungi are simple organisms similar to plants but lack the chlorophyll pigments that allow plants to make their own food. Because they cannot make their own food, fungi must parasitize other tissues, including those of the human body.

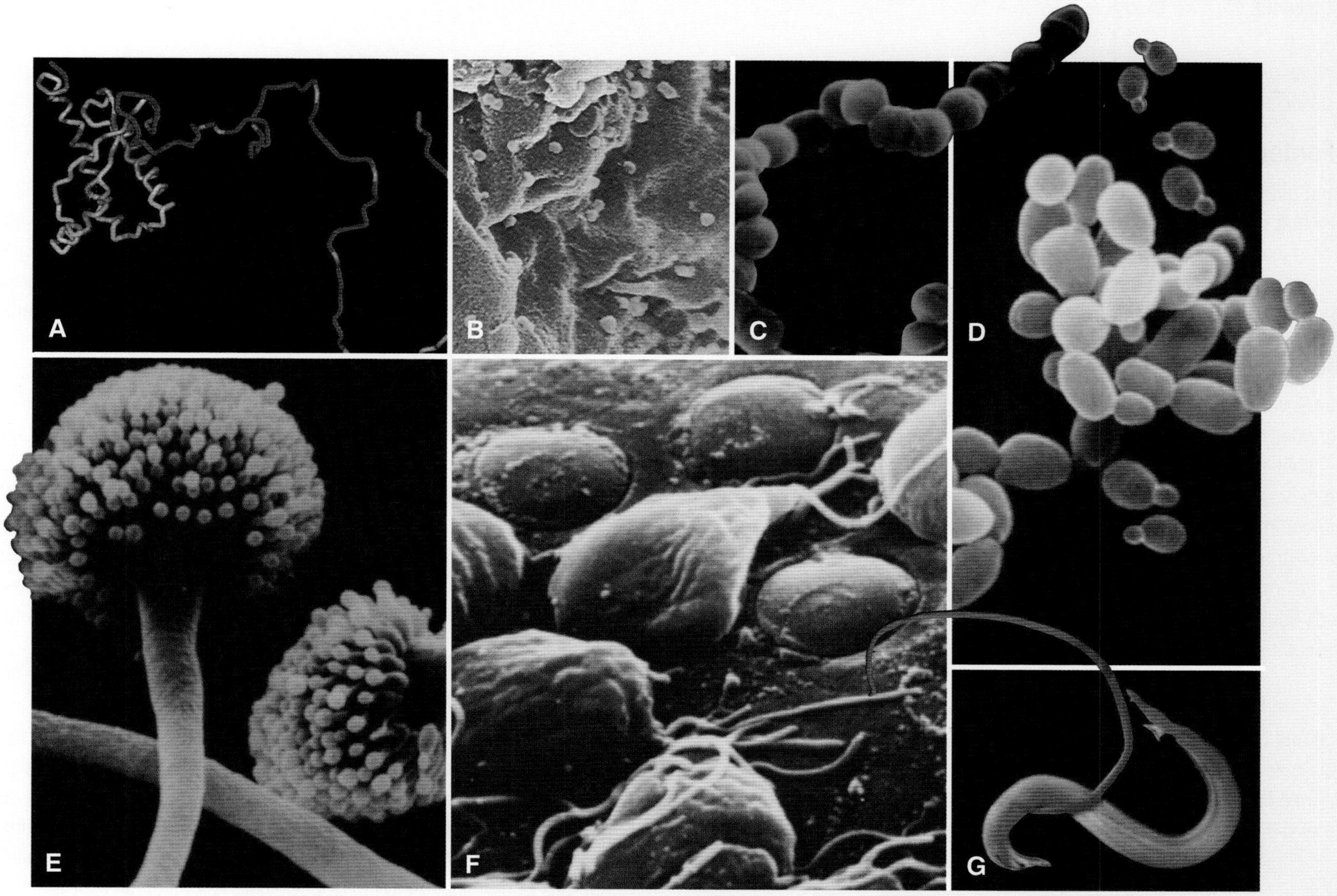

FIGURE 2-9 Pathogenic organisms. A, Prion (cause of variant Creutzfeldt–Jakob disease). **B,** Viruses (the human immunodeficiency virus [HIV], which causes AIDS). **C,** Bacteria (*Streptococcus* bacteria, which cause strep throat and other infections). **D,** Fungi (yeast cells that commonly infect the urinary and reproductive tracts). **E,** Fungi (the mould that causes aspergillosis). **F,** Protozoans (the flagellated cells that sometimes cause traveller's diarrhoea). **G,** Pathogenic animals (the parasitic worms that cause schistosomiasis).

Protozoa are protists, one-celled organisms larger than bacteria whose DNA is organized into a nucleus. Many types of protozoa parasitize human tissues.

Pathogenic animals are large, multicellular organisms such as insects and worms. Such animals can parasitize human tissues, bite or sting, or otherwise disrupt normal body function.

CONNECT IT! 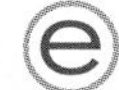

Although we usually first think of disease when we think of bacteria or fungi, our bodies normally team with complex communities of microbes. This human microbiome normally helps us fend off disease and maintain wellness. It is often an imbalance in, or invasion of, our microbiome that allows pathogens to cause disease. Review this concept in ***The Human Microbiome*** at ***Connect It!***

Examples of infections or other conditions caused by pathogenic organisms are given in many chapters throughout this book.

Tumours and Cancer

Abnormal tissue growths, or neoplasms, can cause various physiological disturbances, as described in Chapter 8.

Physical and Chemical Agents

Agents such as toxic or destructive chemicals, extreme heat or cold, mechanical injury, and radiation can each affect the normal homeostasis of the body. Examples of healing of tissues damaged by physical agents are discussed in Chapters 8, 10, and a few other chapters.

Malnutrition

Insufficient or imbalanced intake of nutrients causes various diseases; these are outlined in Chapters 40 and 41.

Autoimmunity

Some diseases result from the immune system attacking one's own body (*autoimmunity*) or from other mistakes or overreactions of the immune response. Autoimmunity, literally "self-immunity", is discussed in Chapters 32 and 33 along with other disturbances of the immune system.

Inflammation

The body often responds to disturbances with an *inflammatory response*. The inflammatory response, which is described in Chapters 8, 9, and 32, is a normal mechanism that usually speeds recovery from an infection or injury. However, when the inflammatory response occurs at inappropriate times or is abnormally prolonged or severe, normal tissues may become damaged. Thus some disease symptoms are caused by the inflammatory response.

Degeneration

By means of many still unknown processes, tissues sometimes break apart or *degenerate.* Although a normal consequence of ageing, degeneration of one or more tissues resulting from disease can occur at any time. The degeneration of tissues associated with ageing is discussed in nearly every chapter of this book.

Risk Factors

Other than direct causes or disease mechanisms, certain predisposing conditions may exist that make a disease more likely to develop. Usually called *risk factors,* they often do not actually cause a disease but just put one "at risk" for it. Risk factors can combine and increase a person's chance for contracting a specific disease even more. Some of the major types of risk factors are as follows.

Genetic Factors

There are several types of genetic risk factors. Sometimes an inherited trait puts one at greater than normal risk for development of a specific disease. For example, light-skinned people are more at risk for certain forms of skin cancer than are dark-skinned people. This occurs because light-skinned people have less pigment in their skin to protect them from cancer-causing ultraviolet radiation (see Chapter 10). Membership in a certain ethnic group, or *gene pool,* involves the "risk" of inheriting a disease-causing gene that is common in that gene pool. For example, certain Africans and their descendants are at greater than average risk of inheriting *sickle cell anaemia*—a serious blood disorder.

Age

Biological and behavioural variations during different phases of the human life cycle put us at greater risk for certain diseases at certain times in our life. For example, middle ear infections are more common in infants than in adults because of the difference in ear structure at different ages.

Lifestyle

The way we live and work can put us at risk for some diseases. People whose work or personal activity puts them in direct sunlight for long periods have a greater chance for development of skin cancer because this puts them in more frequent contact with ultraviolet radiation from the sun. Tobacco use increases the risk of cancer, respiratory disease, and other ailments. A high-fat, low-fibre diet may increase the risk for certain types of cancer.

Stress

Physical, psychological, or emotional stress can put one at risk for problems such as chronic high blood pressure (hypertension), peptic ulcers, and headaches. Conditions caused by psychological factors are sometimes called *psychogenic* (mind-caused) disorders. Chapter 34 discusses the concept of stress and its effect on health.

Environmental Factors

Although environmental factors such as climate and pollution can actually cause injury or disease, some environmental situations simply put us at greater risk for getting certain diseases. For example, because some parasites survive only in tropical environments, we are not at risk of being infected with them if we live in a temperate climate.

Microorganisms

Different types of pathological organisms, such as viruses and bacteria, are now suspected of being "infectious cofactors" in the development of certain noninfectious diseases that in the past were not considered to result directly from their presence in the body. For example, we now have very strong evidence to link infections caused by hepatitis B virus with liver cancer and human papillomavirus with cervical cancer. We also know that the bacterium *Helicobacter pylori,* which causes ulcers, is in some way also a factor in the development of certain types of stomach cancer.

Preexisting Conditions

A preexisting condition can adversely affect our capacity to defend ourselves against an entirely different condition or disease. Thus the *primary* (preexisting) condition can put a person at risk for development of a *secondary* condition. For example, in individuals with AIDS the primary condition is characterized by a suppressed immune system. As a result, secondary or "opportunistic" infections such as pneumonia often develop. Obesity is a risk factor for many conditions, including heart disease, diabetes, stroke, some forms of cancer, and high blood pressure.

CONNECT IT! 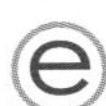

World events have shown us that the intentional transmission of disease can be used as a weapon of terror. For example, the bacterial infection anthrax usually infects grazing animals, such as sheep, but has been used as a weapon against people. For more, check out ***Disease as a Weapon*** online at ***Connect It!***

LANGUAGE OF SCIENCE *(continued from p. 23)*

response (ree-SPONS)
[respons- **reply**]

sensor (SEN-ser)
[*sens-* **feel,** *-or* **agent**]

stimulus (STIM-yoo-lus)
[*stimulus* **incitement**]

variable (VAIR-ee-ah-bil)
[*vari-* **change,** *-able* **capable**]

LANGUAGE OF MEDICINE

acute (ah-KYOOT)
[*acute* **sharp**]

aetiology (e-tee-OL-o-jee)
[*aetio-* **cause,** *-o-* **combining form,** *-log-* **words (study of),** *-y* **activity**]

bacterium (bak-TEE-ree-um)
[*bacterium* **small staff**]; *pl.,* **bacteria**

chronic (KRON-ik)
[*chron-* **time,** *-ic* **relating to**]

communicable (kom-MYOO-ni-kah-bil)
[*communic-* **common,** *-able* **capacity for**]

endemic (en-DEM-ik)
[*en-* **in,** *-dem-* **people,** *-ic* **relating to**]

epidemic (ep-i-DEM-ik)
[*epi-* **upon,** *-dem-* **people,** *-ic* **relating to**]

epidemiology (EP-i-dee-mee-OL-o-jee)
[*epi-* **upon,** *-dem-* **people,** *-o-* **combining form,** *-log-* **words (study of),** *-y* **activity**]

fungus (FUNG-us)
[*fungus* **mushroom**]; *pl.,* **fungi** (FUNG-eye)

idiopathic (id-ee-o-PATH-ik)
[*idio-* **peculiar,** *-path-* **disease,** *-ic* **relating to**]

incubation (in-kyoo-BAY-shun)
[*in-* **in or on,** *-cuba-* **lie,** *-tion* **condition of**]

pandemic (pan-DEM-ik)
[*pan-* **all,** *-dem-* **people,** *-ic* **relating to**]

pathogenesis (path-o-JEN-e-sis)
[*patho-* **disease,** *-gen-* **produce,** *-esis* **process**]

pathogenic animal (path-o-JEN-ik)
[*patho-* **disease,** *-gen-* **produce,** *-ic* **condition of**]

pathophysiology (path-o-fiz-ee-OL-o-jee)
[*patho-* **disease,** *-physio-* **nature (function),** *-o-* **combining form,** *-log-* **words (study of),** *-y* **activity**]

prion (PREE-on)
[**condensed from proteinaceous infectious particle**]

protozoan (pro-toe-ZO-an)
[*proto-* **first,** *-zoan* **animal**]; *pl.,* **protozoa**

remission (ree-MISH-un)
[*re-* **back or again,** *-miss-* **to send,** *-sion* **condition of**]

sign (syn)
[*sign* **mark**]

symptom (SIMP-tum)
[*sym-* **together,** *-tom* **fall**]

syndrome (SIN-drome)
[*syn-* **together,** *-drome* **running or (race)course**]

virus (VYE-rus)
[*virus* **poison**]

case study

Caroline is an accomplished track and field athlete. Today she is participating in the 1500-metre run. As she prepares for her race, Caroline is calm and relaxed. Her heart rate is 65 beats per minute and her breathing rate is 12 breaths per minute. Just before the race, Caroline drinks a substantial amount of water, stretches, and completes several warm-up exercises.

From the start of the race and through its duration, Caroline's body incurs changes that upset her homeostatic balance. These physiological demands require her body to respond in order to successfully complete this physical challenge.

1. Before the race, Caroline's body begins to respond to the challenge of the 1500-metre run. Which of these homeostatic mechanisms are set in place before she even begins to run?
   a. Breathing rate and heart rate decrease to offset the initial expenditure of energy.
   b. Breathing rate and heart rate increase as a result of epinephrine preparing her body for the competition.
   c. Sweat glands are inhibited to reduce water loss.
   d. Any water taken in is transported to skeletal muscles.
2. During the race, what physiological changes occur in her body that upset her homeostatic balance?
   a. Skeletal muscle demands deplete energy (adenosine triphosphate, or ATP) reserves.
   b. Increased muscle contraction increases core body temperature.
   c. Profuse sweating results in water loss.
   d. All of these are physiological changes that upset homeostatic balance.
3. As Caroline competes in the 1500-metre run, osmoreceptors in her hypothalamus detect a fall in the amount of water in her blood. This results in the secretion of antidiuretic hormone (ADH) from the posterior pituitary gland in the brain. ADH stimulates the kidney collecting ducts to reabsorb more water into the blood so less water passes into her urine. After the race, she replenishes her water by drinking, ADH secretion decreases and the amount of water in the blood returns to the normal level. This is an example of what type of feedback mechanism?
   a. Positive feedback
   b. Negative feedback
   c. Physiological feedback
   d. Feed-forward control system

Hint To solve a case study, you may have to refer to the glossary or index, other chapters in this textbook, **Connect It!,** and other resources.

CHAPTER SUMMARY

To download an MP3 version of the chapter summary for use with your mobile device, access the ***Audio Chapter Summaries*** *online at evolve.elsevier.com.*

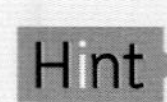

Scan this summary after reading the chapter to help you reinforce the key concepts. Later, use the summary as a quick review before your class or before a test.

Homeostasis

A. Term *homeostasis* coined by American physiologist Walter B. Cannon
B. *Homeostasis* is used to describe the relatively constant states maintained by the body—internal environment around body cells remains constant
C. Body adjusts important variables from a normal set point in an acceptable or normal range; fluctuation with limits is normal
D. Examples of homeostasis
   1. Temperature regulation
   2. Regulation of blood carbon dioxide level
   3. Regulation of blood glucose level (**Figure 2-1**)
E. Natural variability of body function to maintain relative constancy is normal, but abnormal variability may be a sign of disease.
F. Models of homeostasis
   1. The body can be envisioned as a bag of fluid (**Figure 2-2**)
   2. In the *fishbowl model* of homeostasis, the body is the bowl of fluid that must be kept constant, the cells of the body are like fish, and the organ systems are like the accessories used to maintain stability

3. In the *Wallenda model* of homeostasis, the body is compared to a circus highwire walker
4. In the *heating system model*, the body is like a home with a thermostat acting as a control centre to regulate the electric heater and keep the interior constantly warm
5. Each different model of homeostasis emphasizes different aspects of the overall concept

Homeostatic Control Mechanisms

A. Feedback loops
   1. Communication networks for maintaining or restoring homeostasis by self-regulation through feedback
   2. Afferent communication goes toward a control centre or other point of reference
   3. Efferent communication goes away from a control centre or other point of reference
B. Basic components of control mechanisms (**Figure 2-3**)
   1. Sensor mechanism—specific sensors detect and react to any changes from normal in a physiological variable
   2. Integrating, or control, centre—information is analyzed and integrated, and then if needed, a specific action is initiated
   3. Effector mechanism—effectors directly influence controlled physiological variables
   4. Feedback—process of information about a variable constantly flowing back from the sensor to the integrator
C. Negative feedback in control systems
   1. Are inhibitory; they negate changes in a variable
      a. Stabilize physiological variables
      b. Produce an action that is opposite to the change that activated the system
   2. Are responsible for maintaining homeostasis
   3. Are much more common than positive feedback in control systems
   4. Can be described in terms of stimulus and response
   5. Examples—shivering in response to a drop in body temperature, sweating in response to elevated body temperature
D. Positive feedback in control systems (**Figure 2-4**)
   1. Are stimulatory
      a. Amplify or reinforce the change that is occurring
      b. Tend to produce destabilizing effects and disrupt homeostasis
   2. Can sometimes bring specific body functions to swift completion. Examples include:
      a. Increased labour contractions in response to stretching of the birth canal
      b. Blood clotting
E. Changing the set point
   1. Like the set point on an electric heater's thermostat, physiological set points can change
   2. Not all individuals have the same set points, so "normal" is really a range of different values among humans (**Figure 2-5**)
   3. Fever is an example of the body changing a set point temporarily to fight infection
   4. There are circadian (daily) patterns of changes in set points; e.g., nightly increase in blood melatonin levels (**Figure 2-6**)
F. Feed-forward in control systems occurs when information flows ahead to another process or feedback loop to trigger a change in anticipation of an event that will follow

Levels of Control (Figure 2-7)

A. Intracellular control
   1. Regulation within cells
   2. Genes or enzymes can regulate cell processes
B. Intrinsic control (autoregulation)
   1. Regulation within tissues or organs
   2. May involve chemical signals (e.g., prostaglandins)
   3. May involve other "built-in" mechanisms
C. Extrinsic control
   1. Regulation from organ to organ
   2. May involve nerve signals
   3. May involve endocrine signals (hormones)

Summary of Homeostasis

A. Homeostatic mechanisms generally operate on the negative feedback principle
B. Occasionally, positive (stimulatory) feedback mechanisms promote homeostasis by bringing specific body functions to swift completion
C. Set points exhibit ranges that can change with changing circumstances
D. Feed-forward occurs when we react to disturbances in variables before they actually occur
E. Homeostatic control occurs at different levels: within the cell, from cell to cell within a tissue, and throughout the body

Cycle of Life: Life Span Considerations

A. Structure and function of body undergo changes over the early years (developmental processes) and late years (ageing processes)
B. Infancy and old age are periods when the body functions least well
C. Young adulthood is period of greatest homeostatic efficiency
D. *Atrophy*—term to describe the wasting effects of advancing age

REVIEW QUESTIONS

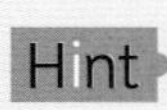

Write out the answers to these questions after reading the chapter and reviewing the Chapter Summary. Note—writing out your answers will consolidate learning and provide a valuable resource of information.

1. What does the term *homeostasis* mean? Illustrate some generalizations about body function using homeostatic mechanisms as examples.
2. Contrast *homeostatic control mechanisms* and *feedback control loops*.
3. Name the four basic components of a control loop.
4. What is the difference between a negative feedback loop and a positive feedback loop?
5. Describe what happens in the body to counteract a drop in body temperature in terms of *stimulus* and *response*.
6. Identify three examples of negative feedback control in the body.

7. Identify two examples of normal positive feedback control in the body.
8. Define the term *circadian rhythm*. Describe how circadian rhythm operates in a typical day for you.
9. Describe what *feed-forward* is in a control system.
10. Classify the three levels of homeostatic control in the body.
11. Categorize health and disease in terms of homeostasis.
12. List the major types of risk factors that may increase a person's chance of developing a specific disease.
13. Define *pathogen* and give examples of six types of pathogens.

CRITICAL THINKING QUESTIONS

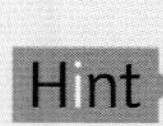

After finishing the Review Questions, write out the answers to these more in-depth questions to help you apply your new knowledge. Go back to sections of the chapter that relate to concepts that you find difficult.

1. Use the *fishbowl model* of homeostasis to describe how the kidneys help maintain homeostasis.
2. When driving in traffic, it is important to stay in your own lane. If you see that you are drifting out of your lane, your brain tells your arms and hands to move in such a way that you get back in your lane. Identify the three components of a control loop in this example. Classify this as a positive or negative feedback loop.
3. As your blood glucose drops below the setpoint value, what strategies might the body employ to raise the glucose concentration back toward the set point?
4. When muscle cells become starved for oxygen, they will send a chemical signal to nearby blood vessels to dilate (expand) and thereby increase blood flow. Is this an example of negative feedback or positive feedback? Is this an example of intracellular, intrinsic, or extrinsic control? Explain your answer.
5. Why are expectant mothers comforted by knowing that childbirth is a positive feedback control mechanism?
6. You are charged with explaining homeostasis to a group of sixth-formers. Develop an analogy of tightrope walking as an example of homeostasis. Concentrate on the movement and balance of the walker's body.

3 Chemical Basis of Life

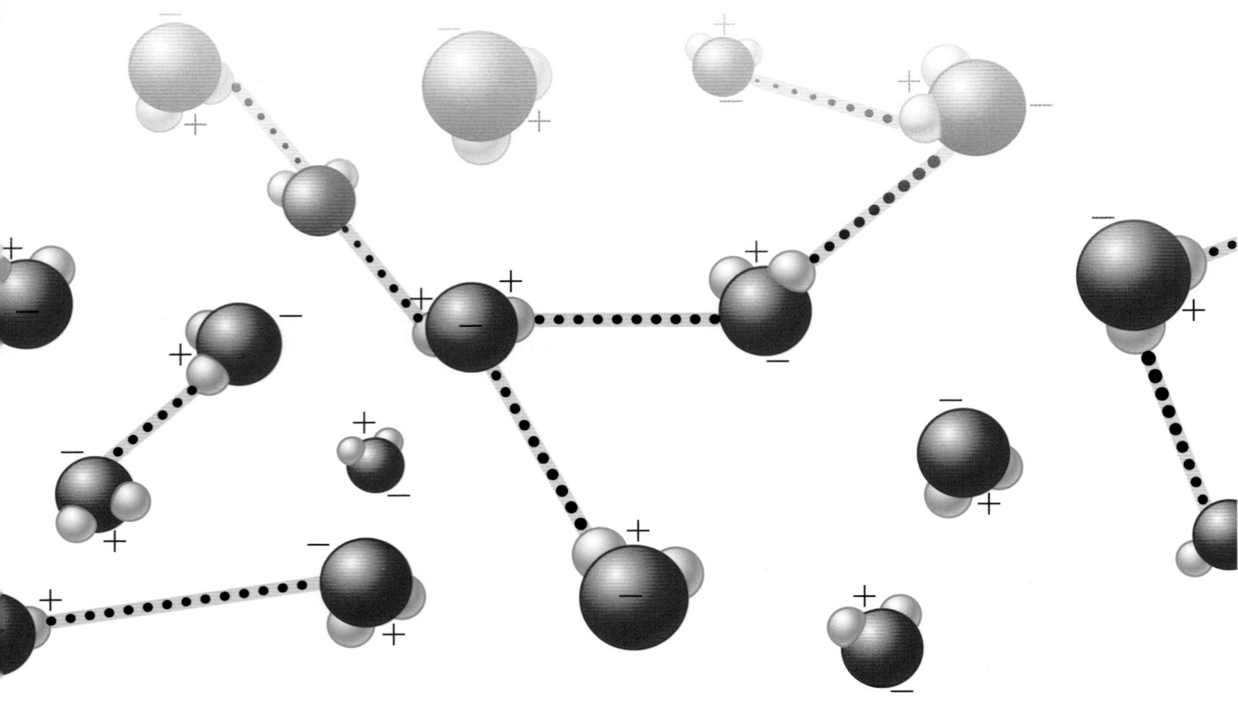

CHAPTER OUTLINE

Hint ▸ *Scan this outline before you begin to read the chapter, as a preview of how the concepts are organized.*

LANGUAGE OF SCIENCE

Hint ▸ *Use this list to aid your pronunciation of unfamiliar words.*

acid (ASS-id)
[*acid* **sour**]

adenosine triphosphate (ATP) (ah-DEN-o-seen try-FOS-fate)
[blend of *adenine* and *ribose; tri-* **three,** *-phosph-* **phosphorus,** *-ate* **oxygen**]

anabolism (ah-NAB-ol-iz-im)
[*anabol-* **build up,** *-ism* **action**]

atom (AT-om)
[*atom* **indivisible**]

base (BAYS)
[*bas* **base**]

biomolecule (bye-oh-MOL-eh-kyool)
[*bio-* **life,** *-molec-* **mass,** *-ule* **small**]

buffer (BUFF-er)
[*buffe-* **cushion,** *-er* **actor**]

catabolism (kah-TAB-ol-iz-im)
[*catabol-* **throw down,** *-ism* **action**]

compound (KOM-pownd)
[*compoun-* **put together**]

covalent bond (ko-VAYL-ent bond)
[*co-* **with,** *-valen-* **power,** *bond* **band**]

decomposition reaction (dee-kom-poh-SIH-shun ree-AK-shun)
[*de-* **opposite of,** *-compo-* **to assemble,** *-tion* **process,** *re-* **again,** *-action* **action**]

dehydration synthesis (dee-hye-DRAY-shun SIN-the-sis
[*de-* **from,** *-hydr-* **water,** *-ation* **process,** *synthesis* **putting together**]

electrolyte (eh-LEK-troh-lyte)
[*electro-* **electricity,** *-lyt-* **loosening**]

element (eh-leh-ment)
[*element* **first principle**]

energy level
[*en-* **in,** *-erg-* **work,** *-y* **state**]

exchange reaction
[*ex-* **from,** *-change* **to change,** *re-* **again,** *-action* **action**]

hydrolysis (hye-DROL-i-sis)
[*hydro-* **water,** *-lysis* **loosening**]

ion (EYE-on)
[*ion* **to go**]

ionic bond
[*ion* **to go,** *bond* **band**]

isotope (EYE-so-tohp)
[*iso-* **equal,** *-tope* **place**]

metabolism (meh-TAB-ol-iz-im)
[*meta-* **over,** *-bol-* **throw,** *-ism* **action**]

continued on p. 51

Anatomy and physiology are subdivisions of biology—the study of life. To best understand the characteristics of life, what living matter is, how it is organized, and what it can do, we must appreciate and understand certain basic principles of chemistry that apply to the life process.

Life itself depends on proper levels and proportions of chemical substances in the cytoplasm of cells. The various structural levels of organization described in Chapter 1 are ultimately based on the existence and interrelationships of atoms and molecules. Chemistry, like biology, is a very broad scientific discipline. It deals with the structure, arrangement, and composition of substances and the reactions they undergo. Just as biology may be subdivided into many subdisciplines or branches, such as anatomy and physiology, chemistry may also be divided into focused areas. Biochemistry is the field of chemistry that deals with living organisms and life processes. It deals directly with the chemical composition of living matter and the processes that underlie life activities such as growth, muscle contraction, and transmission of nervous impulses.

This chapter provides a foundation in the basic principles of chemistry we will need to understand the concepts revealed in later chapters. The next chapter is a survey of several important classes of large biomolecules that will also be important in our later studies. •

UNITS OF MATTER

Elements and Compounds

Chemists use the term *matter* to describe in a general sense all of the materials or substances around us. Anything that has mass and occupies space is matter.

Substances are either **elements** or **compounds.** An element is said to be "pure" in the sense that it cannot be broken down or decomposed into two or more different substances. Carbon and oxygen are good examples of elements. In most living material, elements do not exist alone in their pure state. Instead, two or more elements are joined to form chemical combinations called *compounds.* Compounds can be broken down or decomposed into the elements that are contained within them. Water is a compound (H_2O). It can be broken down into atoms of hydrogen and atoms of oxygen in a 2 : 1 ratio.

Other examples of elements include phosphorus, copper, and nitrogen (**Figure 3-1**). For convenience in writing chemical formulas

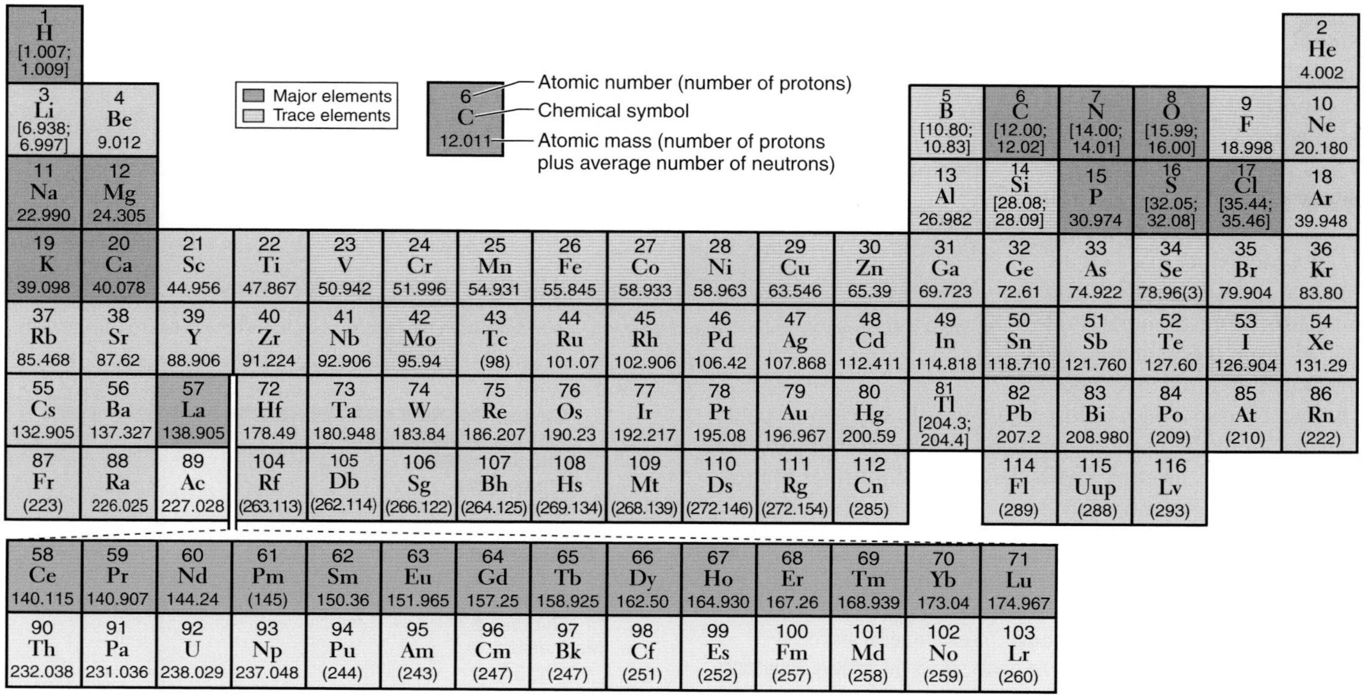

Major elements / Trace elements

6 — Atomic number (number of protons); C — Chemical symbol; 12.011 — Atomic mass (number of protons plus average number of neutrons)

1	2	3	4	5	6	7	8	9	10	11	12	13	14	15	16	17	18
1 H [1.007; 1.009]																	2 He 4.002
3 Li [6.938; 6.997]	4 Be 9.012											5 B [10.80; 10.83]	6 C [12.00; 12.02]	7 N [14.00; 14.01]	8 O [15.99; 16.00]	9 F 18.998	10 Ne 20.180
11 Na 22.990	12 Mg 24.305											13 Al 26.982	14 Si [28.08; 28.09]	15 P 30.974	16 S [32.05; 32.08]	17 Cl [35.44; 35.46]	18 Ar 39.948
19 K 39.098	20 Ca 40.078	21 Sc 44.956	22 Ti 47.867	23 V 50.942	24 Cr 51.996	25 Mn 54.931	26 Fe 55.845	27 Co 58.933	28 Ni 58.963	29 Cu 63.546	30 Zn 65.39	31 Ga 69.723	32 Ge 72.61	33 As 74.922	34 Se 78.96(3)	35 Br 79.904	36 Kr 83.80
37 Rb 85.468	38 Sr 87.62	39 Y 88.906	40 Zr 91.224	41 Nb 92.906	42 Mo 95.94	43 Tc (98)	44 Ru 101.07	45 Rh 102.906	46 Pd 106.42	47 Ag 107.868	48 Cd 112.411	49 In 114.818	50 Sn 118.710	51 Sb 121.760	52 Te 127.60	53 I 126.904	54 Xe 131.29
55 Cs 132.905	56 Ba 137.327	57 La 138.905	72 Hf 178.49	73 Ta 180.948	74 W 183.84	75 Re 186.207	76 Os 190.23	77 Ir 192.217	78 Pt 195.08	79 Au 196.967	80 Hg 200.59	81 Tl [204.3; 204.4]	82 Pb 207.2	83 Bi 208.980	84 Po (209)	85 At (210)	86 Rn (222)
87 Fr (223)	88 Ra 226.025	89 Ac 227.028	104 Rf (263.113)	105 Db (262.114)	106 Sg (266.122)	107 Bh (264.125)	108 Hs (269.134)	109 Mt (268.139)	110 Ds (272.146)	111 Rg (272.154)	112 Cn (285)		114 Fl (289)	115 Uup (288)	116 Lv (293)		

58 Ce 140.115	59 Pr 140.907	60 Nd 144.24	61 Pm (145)	62 Sm 150.36	63 Eu 151.965	64 Gd 157.25	65 Tb 158.925	66 Dy 162.50	67 Ho 164.930	68 Er 167.26	69 Tm 168.939	70 Yb 173.04	71 Lu 174.967
90 Th 232.038	91 Pa 231.036	92 U 238.029	93 Np 237.048	94 Pu (244)	95 Am (243)	96 Cm (247)	97 Bk (247)	98 Cf (251)	99 Es (252)	100 Fm (257)	101 Md (258)	102 No (259)	103 Lr (260)

FIGURE 3-1 Periodic table of elements. The major elements found in the body are highlighted in pink. The trace elements, found in very tiny quantities in the body, are highlighted in orange. (Atomic mass numbers in brackets show the natural range of isotopes; those in parentheses are uncertain or theoretical.)

and in other types of notation, chemists assign a symbol to each element, usually the first letter or two of the English or Latin name of the element: P, phosphorus; Cu, copper (Latin *cuprum*); N, nitrogen (see **Figure 3-1**). Note in **Table 3-1** that 26 elements are listed as being present in the human body. Although all are important, 11 are called *major elements.* Four of these major elements—carbon, oxygen, hydrogen, and nitrogen—make up about 96% of the material in the human body (**Figure 3-2**). The 15 remaining elements are present in amounts that are less than 0.1% of body weight and are called *trace elements.* The unique "aliveness" of a living organism does not depend on a single element or mixture of elements but on the complexity, organization, and interrelationships of all elements required for life.

TABLE 3-1 Elements in the Human Body

ELEMENT	SYMBOL	HUMAN BODY WEIGHT (%)	IMPORTANCE OR FUNCTION
Major Elements			
Oxygen	O	65.0	Necessary for cellular respiration; component of water
Carbon	C	18.5	Backbone of organic molecules
Hydrogen	H	9.5	Component of water and most organic molecules; necessary for energy transfer and respiration
Nitrogen	N	3.3	Component of all proteins and nucleic acids
Calcium	Ca	1.5	Component of bones and teeth; triggers muscle contraction
Phosphorus	P	1.0	Principal component in the backbone of nucleic acids; important in energy transfer
Potassium	K	0.4	Principal positive ion within cells; important in nerve function
Sulphur	S	0.3	Component of many energy-transferring enzymes
Sodium	Na	0.2	Important positive ion surrounding cells
Chlorine	Cl	0.2	Important negative ion surrounding cells
Magnesium	Mg	0.1	Component of many energy-transferring enzymes
Trace Elements			
Silicone*	Si	<0.1	Uncertain
Aluminium*	Al	<0.1	Uncertain
Iron	Fe	<0.1	Critical component of haemoglobin in the blood
Manganese	Mn	<0.1	Component of many energy-transferring enzymes
Fluorine	F	<0.1	Hardens crystals that form teeth and bones
Vanadium*	V	<0.1	Uncertain
Chromium	Cr	<0.1	Alters insulin (hormone) effects that regulate carbohydrate lipid and protein metabolism
Copper	Cu	<0.1	Key component of many enzymes
Boron	B	<0.1	May strengthen cell membranes; plays a role in brain and bone development
Cobalt	Co	<0.1	Component of vitamin B_{12}
Zinc	Zn	<0.1	Key component of some enzymes
Selenium	Se	<0.1	Component of an antioxidant enzyme
Molybdenum	Mo	<0.1	Key component of some enzymes
Tin	Sn	<0.1	Uncertain
Iodine	I	<0.1	Component of thyroid hormone

**Ultratrace* elements (occur in extraordinarily low concentrations in the human body but still have biological functions).

ATOMS

The most important of all chemical theories was advanced in 1805 by the English chemist John Dalton. He proposed the concept that matter is composed of **atoms** (from the Greek *atomos,* "indivisible"). His idea was revolutionary and yet simple—that all matter, regardless of the form it may assume (liquid, gas, or solid), is composed of units he called *atoms.*

Dalton conceived of atoms as solid, indivisible particles, and for about 100 years this was believed to be true. We now know that atoms are divisible into even smaller or *subatomic* particles, some of which exist in a "cloud" surrounding a dense central core called a *nucleus.* More than 100 million atoms of even very dense and heavy substances, if lined up, would measure barely 25 mm and would consist mostly of empty space! Our knowledge about the number and nature of subatomic particles and the central nucleus around which they move continues to grow as a result of ongoing research.

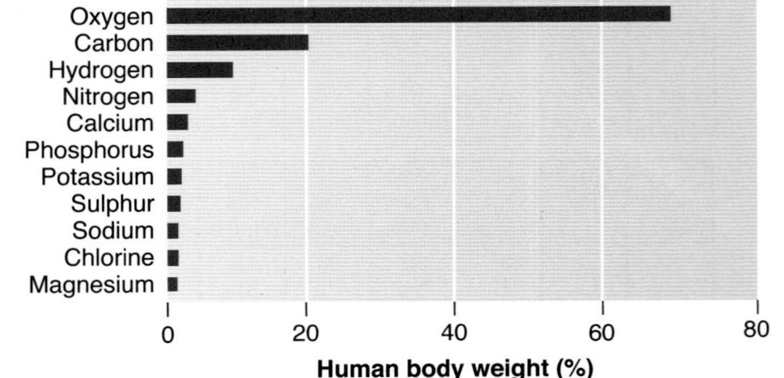

FIGURE 3-2 Major elements of the body. These elements are found in great quantity in the body (see **Figure 3-1**). The graph shows the relative abundance of each in the body. Notice that oxygen (O), carbon (C), hydrogen (H), and nitrogen (N) predominate.

Quick CHECK

1. What is biochemistry?
2. What is the difference between an element and a compound?
3. What elements make up 96% of the material in the human body?

ATOMIC STRUCTURE

Cloud Model

Atoms contain several different kinds of smaller or subatomic particles that are found in either a central nucleus or its surrounding "electron cloud" or "field". **Figure 3-3**, A, shows an atomic model of carbon illustrating the most important types of subatomic particles:

- Protons (p^+)
- Neutrons (n^0)
- Electrons (e^-)

Note that the carbon atom in **Figure 3-3** has a central corelike *nucleus*. It is located deep inside the atom and is made up of six positively charged *protons* (p^+) and six uncharged *neutrons* (n^0). Note also that the nucleus is surrounded by a cloud or field of six negatively charged *electrons* (e^-). Because protons are positively charged and neutrons are neutral, the nucleus of an atom bears a positive electrical charge equal to the number of protons that are present in it.

Electrons move around the atom's nucleus in what can be represented as an electron cloud or field (**Figure 3-3**, *B*). The number of negatively charged electrons moving around an atom's nucleus equals the number of positively charged protons in the nucleus. The opposite charges therefore cancel or neutralize each other, which means atoms are electrically neutral particles.

The so-called electron clouds are really just areas where the electrons are most likely to be found moving about rapidly. However, they can sometimes be visualized with a special form of microscope, as you can see in **Figure 3-4**.

Atomic Number and Mass Number

Elements differ in their chemical and physical properties because of differences in the number of protons in their atomic nuclei. The number of protons in an atom's nucleus, called its *atomic number*, is therefore critically important—it identifies the kind of element it is.

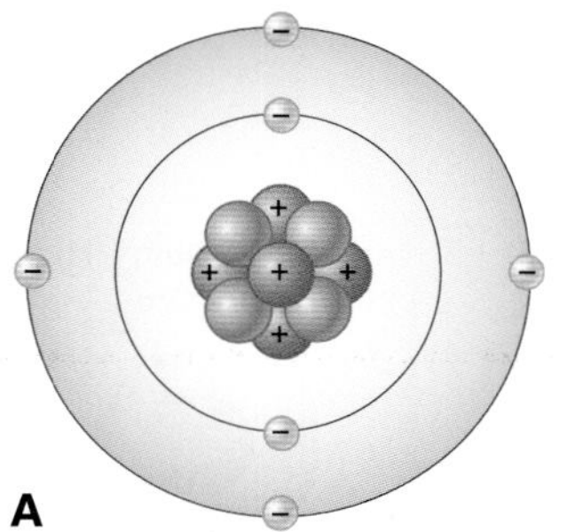

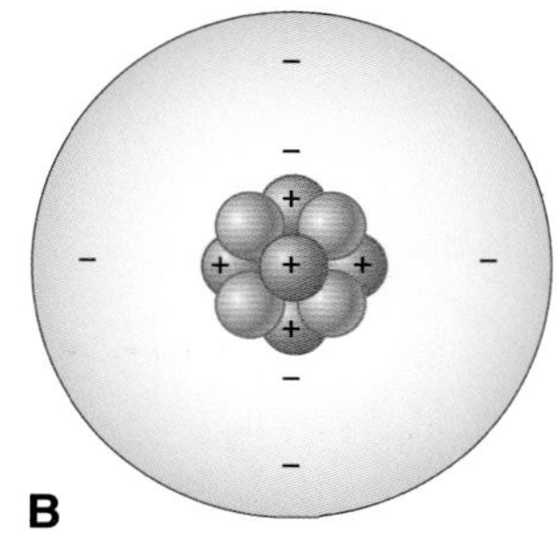

FIGURE 3-3 Models of the atom. The nucleus—protons (+) and neutrons—is at the core. Electrons inhabit outer regions called electron *shells* or energy levels **(A)** or probability distributions called electron clouds **(B)**. This drawing depicts a carbon atom. All carbon atoms (and *only* carbon atoms) have six protons. (Not all of the protons in the nucleus are visible in this illustration.)

FIGURE 3-4 Atoms. The cloudlike structures seen here were recorded using an atomic force microscope (AFM) and represent the outer surfaces of individual atoms along the flat surface of a crystal. Different colours are added to represent different kinds of atoms.

Look again at the elements important in living organisms listed in **Table 3-1**. Each element is identified by its symbol and atomic number. Hydrogen, for example, has an atomic number of 1; this means that all hydrogen atoms—and *only* hydrogen atoms—have one proton in their nucleus. All carbon atoms—and *only* carbon atoms—contain six protons and have an atomic number of 6. All oxygen atoms, and only oxygen atoms, have eight protons and an atomic number of 8. In short, each element is identified by its own unique number of protons, that is, by its own unique atomic number. If two atoms contain a different number of protons, they are different elements.

There are 92 elements that occur naturally on earth. Because each element is characterized by the number of protons in its atoms (atomic number), there are atoms that contain from 1 to 92 protons. Additional elements have been discovered as a result of sophisticated research in the area of particle physics.

The term *mass number* refers to the mass of a single atom. The mass number is sometimes called the *atomic mass*. It equals the number of protons plus the number of neutrons in the atom's nucleus. The weight of electrons is, for practical purposes, negligible. Because protons and neutrons weigh almost exactly the same, the equation for determining mass number is as follows:

$$\text{Mass number} = (p^+ + n^0)$$

The largest naturally occurring atom is uranium. It has a mass number of 238, with a nucleus containing 92 protons and 146 neutrons. In contrast, hydrogen, which has only one proton and no neutrons in its nucleus, has a mass number of 1.

Energy Levels

The total number of electrons in an atom equals the number of protons in its nucleus (see **Figure 3-3**). These electrons are known to exist in regions surrounding the atom's nucleus.

No single model of the atom sufficiently explains all we know about atomic structure. However, two simple models of atoms may be useful here to begin our discussion.

The cloud model suggests that any one electron cannot be exactly located at a specific point at any particular time. This concept is called a *probability distribution* and refers to the probability of finding an electron at any specific location outside the nucleus. Earlier models based on the work of a Danish physicist, Niels Bohr, who won the 1922 Nobel Prize in Physics for his groundbreaking contributions, suggested that electrons move in regular patterns around the nucleus much like the planets in our solar system move around the sun. A simplified version of the Bohr model of the atom (see

Figure 3-3, A) is perhaps most useful in visualizing the structure of atoms as they enter into chemical reactions.

In the Bohr model, the electrons are shown in shells or concentric circles. The different shells show the relative distances of the electrons from the nucleus. The electrons surrounding the atom's nucleus are seen in this model as existing in simple rings or shells. Each ring represents a different **energy level,** and each can hold only a certain maximum number of electrons (**Figure 3-5**). The number and arrangement of electrons orbiting in an atom's energy levels are important because they determine whether the atom is chemically reactive.

In chemical reactions between atoms, it is the electrons in the outermost energy level that participate in the formation of chemical bonds. In each energy level, electrons tend to group in pairs. As a rule, an atom can be listed as chemically stable and unable to react with another atom if its outermost energy level has four pairs of electrons, or a total of eight. Such an atom is said to have a stable electron configuration. The pairing of electrons is important. If the outer energy level contains single, unpaired electrons, the atom will be chemically reactive. Atoms with fewer than eight electrons in the outer energy level will attempt to lose, gain, or share electrons with other atoms to achieve stability. This tendency is called the **octet rule.**

Consider an atom of oxygen, which has a total of six electrons in its outer energy level. As you can see in **Figure 3-6**, it has two unpaired electrons so it is two electrons short of satisfying the octet rule. Oxygen is likely to enter into chemical reactions to gain or share electrons with other atoms. By doing so, the oxygen atom will fill in its outer energy level and thus satisfy the octet rule.

The octet rule holds true except for atoms that are limited to a single energy level that is filled by a maximum of two electrons. For example, hydrogen has but one electron in its single energy level. It therefore has an incomplete energy level with an unpaired electron. The result is a highly reactive tendency of hydrogen to enter into many chemical reactions. Helium, however, has two electrons in its single energy level. Because this is the maximum number for this energy level, no chemical activity is possible, and no naturally occurring compound containing helium exists. Helium is an *inert*, or stable, element.

The atoms shown in **Figure 3-6** illustrate several of the most important facts related to energy levels. Note that even in the hydrogen atom with its very basic structure, positive and negative charges balance. Hydrogen, carbon, and oxygen will react chemically because they do not satisfy the octet rule.

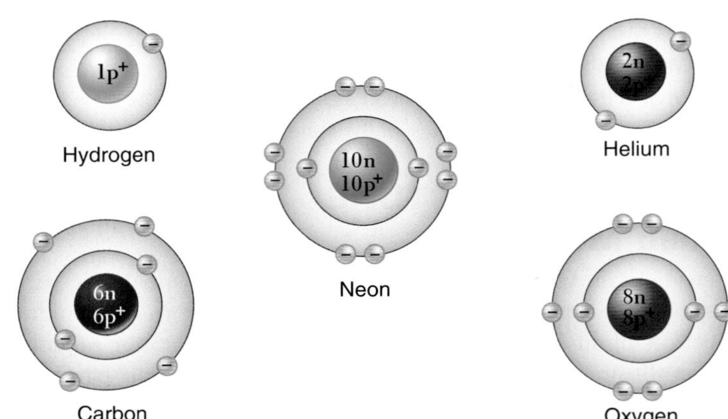

FIGURE 3-6 Energy levels (shells) of five common elements. All atoms are balanced with respect to positive and negative charges as in these examples of five common elements. In atoms with a single energy level, two electrons are required for stability. Hydrogen with its single electron is reactive, whereas helium with its full energy level is not. In atoms with more than one energy level, eight electrons in the outermost energy level are required for stability. Neon is stable because its outer energy level has eight electrons. Oxygen and carbon, with six and four electrons, respectively, in their outer energy levels, are chemically reactive.

ISOTOPES

All atoms of the same element contain the same number of protons but do not necessarily contain the same number of neutrons. **Isotopes** of an element contain the same number of protons but different numbers of neutrons.

Isotopes have the same basic chemical properties as any other atom of the same element, and they also have the same atomic number. However, because they have a different number of neutrons, they differ in mass number. Usually a hydrogen atom has only one proton and no neutrons (atomic number, 1; mass number, 1). **Figure 3-7** illustrates this most common type of hydrogen and two of its isotopes. Note that the isotope of hydrogen called *deuterium* (^2H) has one proton and one neutron (mass number, 2). *Tritium* (^3H) is the isotope of hydrogen that has one proton and two neutrons (mass number, 3).

The term *atomic weight* refers to the average mass number for a particular element based on the typical proportion of different

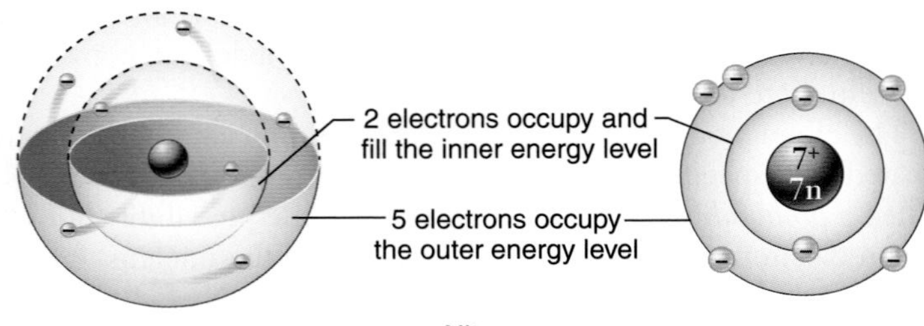

FIGURE 3-5 Energy levels (electron shells) surrounding the nucleus of an atom. Each concentric shell represents a different electron energy level surrounding the nucleus of an atom.

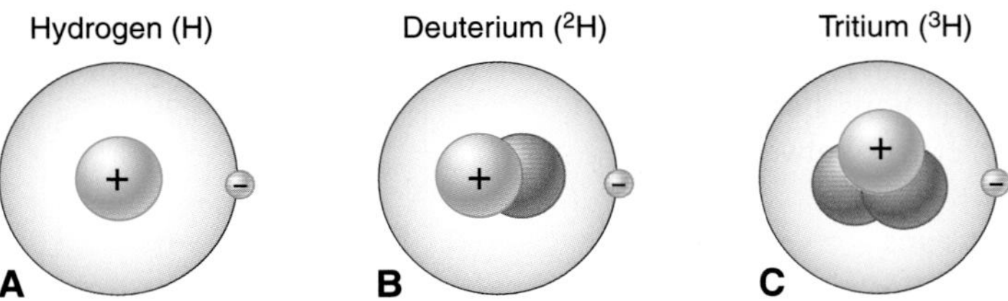

FIGURE 3-7 Structure of hydrogen and two of its isotopes. A, The most common form of hydrogen. **B,** An isotope of hydrogen called *deuterium* (^2H). **C,** The hydrogen isotope *tritium* (^3H). Note that isotopes of an element differ only in the number of its neutrons.

isotopes found in nature. Atomic weights are shown in the periodic table of elements illustrated in **Figure 3-1**, below each chemical symbol. Note that the atomic weights for some elements, such as hydrogen and carbon, are listed as ranges instead of averages. For elements with isotope proportions that vary widely in nature, chemists find ranges more useful than averages.

The atomic nuclei of more than 99% of all carbon atoms in nature have six protons and six neutrons (atomic number, 6; mass number, 12). An important isotope of carbon has seven neutrons instead of six and is called *carbon-13* (^{13}C). Carbon-13 makes up about 1% of the world's carbon atoms. The presence of carbon-13 in human tissues is useful in molecular studies of metabolic processes in the body. Another important carbon isotope has eight neutrons instead of six; it is called *carbon-14* (^{14}C). Carbon-14 is an example of a special type of isotope that is unstable and undergoes nuclear breakdown—it is designated as a *radioactive isotope*, or **radioisotope.** During breakdown, radioactive isotopes emit nuclear particles and radiation—a process called *decay*.

CONNECT IT! 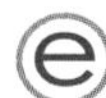

Radioactivity is the emission of radiation from an atom's nucleus. Alpha particles, beta particles, and gamma rays are the three kinds of radiation.

Alpha particles are relatively heavy particles consisting of two protons plus two neutrons. They shoot out of a radioactive atom's nucleus at a reported speed of 30,000 kilometres per second. *Beta particles* are electrons formed in a radioactive atom's nucleus by one of its neutrons breaking down into a proton and an electron. The proton remains behind in the nucleus, and the electron is ejected from it as a beta particle. Beta particles, because they are electrons, are much smaller than alpha particles, which consist of two protons and two neutrons. In addition, beta particles travel at a much greater speed than alpha particles do. *Gamma rays* are electromagnetic radiation, a form of light energy.

Radioactivity differs from chemical activity because it can change the number of protons in an atom, thus changing the atom from one element to another!

Check out ***Radioactivity*** online at ***Connect It!*** to find out how radioactivity affects the human body.

Quick **CHECK**

4. List and define the three most important types of subatomic particles.
5. How are the atomic number and atomic weight of an atom defined?
6. What is an energy level?
7. Explain what is meant by the *octet rule.*
8. What is an isotope?

ATTRACTIONS BETWEEN ATOMS

CHEMICAL BONDS

Interactions between two or more atoms occur largely as a result of activity between electrons in their outermost energy level. The result, called a *chemical reaction*, most often involves unpaired electrons.

Ultimately, in atoms with fewer or more than eight electrons in the outer energy level, reactions will occur that result in the loss, gain, or sharing of one atom's unpaired electrons with those of another atom to satisfy the octet rule for both atoms. The result of such reactions between atoms is the formation of larger chemical structures such as *crystals* and **molecules.** For example, two atoms of oxygen can combine with one carbon atom to form molecular carbon dioxide, or CO_2. If atoms of more than one element combine, the result, as defined earlier, is a compound. In other words, oxygen exists as a molecule (O_2) and is an element. Water exists as a molecule (H_2O) and is a compound. Reactions that hold atoms together do so by the formation of *chemical bonds.* There are two types of chemical bonds that unite atoms into larger structures: ionic (or electrovalent) bonds and covalent bonds.

Ionic Bonds

A chemical bond formed by the transfer of electrons from one atom to another is called an *ionic*, or *electrovalent, bond.* Such a bond occurs as a result of the attraction between atoms that have become electrically charged by the loss or gain of electrons. When dissolved in water (**Figure 3-8**), such atoms separate into **ions.** It is important to remember that ions can be positively or negatively charged and that ions with opposite charges are attracted to each other.

Note in **Figure 3-8**, A, that in the outer energy level of the sodium atom there is a single unpaired electron. If this electron were "lost", the outer ring would be stable because it would have a full outer octet (four pairs of electrons). The loss of the electron would result in the formation of a sodium ion (Na^+) with a positive charge. This is because there is now one more proton (+) than electron (–).

The chlorine atom, in contrast, has one unpaired electron plus three paired electrons, or a total of seven electrons, in its outer energy level. By the addition of another electron, chlorine would satisfy the octet rule—its outer energy level would have a full complement of four paired electrons. The addition of another electron would result in the formation of a negatively charged chloride ion (Cl^-).

Sodium transfers or donates its one unpaired electron to chlorine and becomes a positively charged sodium ion (Na^+). Chlorine accepts the electron from sodium and pairs it with its one unpaired electron, thereby filling its outer energy level with the maximum of four electron pairs and becoming a negatively charged chloride ion (Cl^-). The positively charged sodium ion (Na^+) is attracted to the negatively charged chloride ion (Cl^-), and the formation of NaCl crystals, ordinary table salt, results. This process illustrates ionic or electrovalent bonding.

The electron transfer changed the two atoms of the elements sodium and chlorine into ions. An **ionic bond** is simply the strong electrostatic force that binds the positively and negatively charged ions together in a crystal.

Covalent Bonds

Just as atoms can be held together in crystals by ionic bonds formed when atoms gain or lose electrons, atoms can also be bonded together into molecules by *sharing* electrons. A chemical bond formed by the sharing of one or more pairs of electrons between the outer energy levels of two atoms is called a **covalent bond.** This type of chemical bonding is of great significance in physiology.

The major elements of the body (carbon, oxygen, hydrogen, and nitrogen) almost always share electrons to form covalent bonds. For example, if two atoms of hydrogen are bound together by the sharing of one electron pair, a *single* covalent bond is said to exist, and a molecule of hydrogen gas results (**Figure 3-9**, A). Covalent bonds

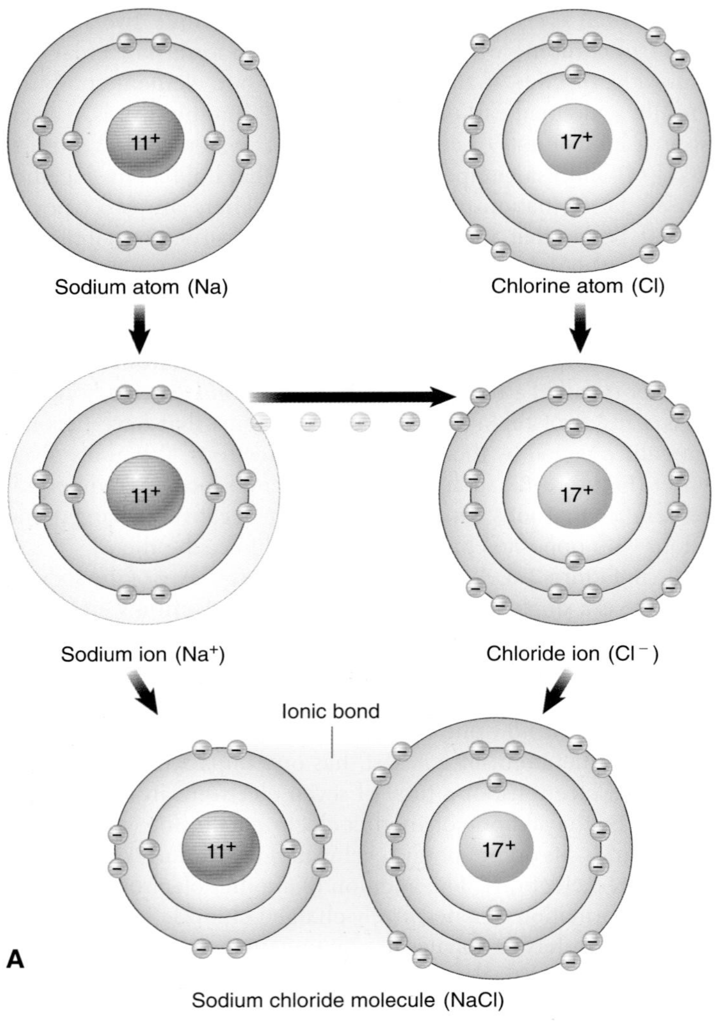

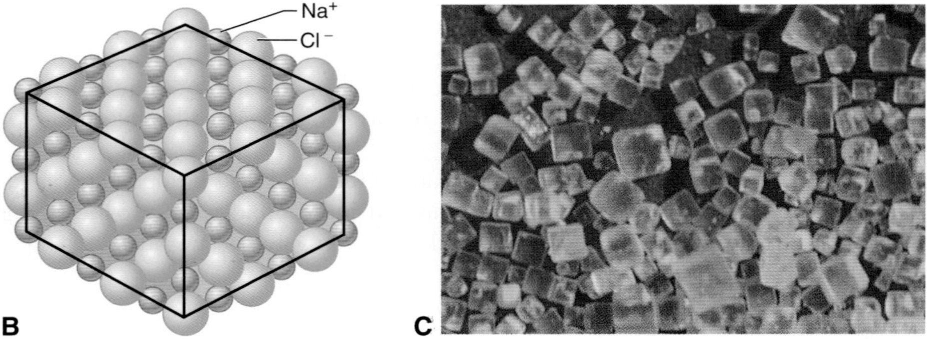

FIGURE 3-8 Example of an ionic bond. **A,** Energy-level models show the steps involved in forming an ionic bond between atoms of sodium and chlorine within the internal fluid environment of the body (water). Sodium "donates" an electron to chlorine, thereby forming a positive sodium ion and a negative chloride ion. The electrical attraction between the now oppositely charged ions forms an ionic bond. **B,** The space-filling model shows a crystal of sodium chloride (table salt) in the typical cube-shaped formation. **C,** Photomicrograph showing cubic crystals of sodium chloride after the removal of water.

that bind atoms together by sharing *two* pairs of electrons are called *double bonds* (**Figure 3-9**, *B*). The example shown illustrates two atoms of oxygen, each sharing two electrons with a carbon atom to acquire a complete outer energy level of eight electrons and thus satisfy the octet rule. A molecule of carbon dioxide results.

An often-asked question is which type of bond is stronger: ionic or covalent? The answer is not simple. Factors such as how many nearby bonds exist, the spatial arrangement of atoms, and amount of electrical attraction between atoms, all play a role in determining the amount of energy needed to break a particular bond. In the fluid internal environment of the human body, however, we often generalize that ionic bonds—which often dissociate readily in water—are weaker than covalent bonds.

ATTRACTIONS BETWEEN MOLECULES

Hydrogen Bonds

In addition to ionic and covalent bonds, another type of attractive force, called a *hydrogen bond*, can exist between biologically important molecules. Hydrogen bonds are much weaker forces than ionic or covalent bonds because they require less energy to break. Although an individual hydrogen bond is weak, large numbers of these bonds can collectively exert a strong attractive force. Instead of forming as a result of transfer or sharing of electrons between atoms, hydrogen bonds result from unequal charge distribution on a molecule. Such molecules are said to be **polar.**

Water is a good example of a polar molecule. Note in **Figure 3-10** that although an atom of water is electrically neutral (the number of negative charges equals the number of positive charges), it has a partial positive charge (the hydrogen side) and a partial negative charge (the oxygen side). That is, the water molecule has a positive pole and a negative pole. The partial charges result from the electrons having a higher probability of being found nearer the highly positive oxygen nucleus than either hydrogen nucleus. That is, the electrons are not shared equally within the molecule. Thus water is said to be "polar" because it has regions with different partial charges. Hydrogen bonds serve to weakly attach the partially negative (oxygen) side of one water molecule to the partially positive (hydrogen) side of an adjacent water molecule.

Figure 3-11 illustrates hydrogen bonding between water molecules. Depending on how many of these hydrogen bonds are intact at one instant, the water may be either liquid (few bonds) or solid (many bonds). If the water molecules are too far apart to form any hydrogen bonds, then the water is a gas, such as steam.

Hydrogen bonds form only between H atoms that are covalently bonded to an oxygen, nitrogen, or fluorine atom. In water molecules H is bonded to O, thus producing the polarity that permits the formation of hydrogen bonds between water molecules.

The ability of water molecules to form hydrogen bonds between molecules accounts for many of the unique properties of water that make it an ideal medium for the chemistry of life. Hydrogen bonds are also important in maintaining the three-dimensional structure of proteins and nucleic acids, also described later in the chapter. In contrast to water, many lipids such as oils and fats are **nonpolar.** Nonpolar molecules have electrons that are shared equally among atoms and therefore have no **polarity**—that is, no difference in charge among regions of the molecule. Thus, when water and oil

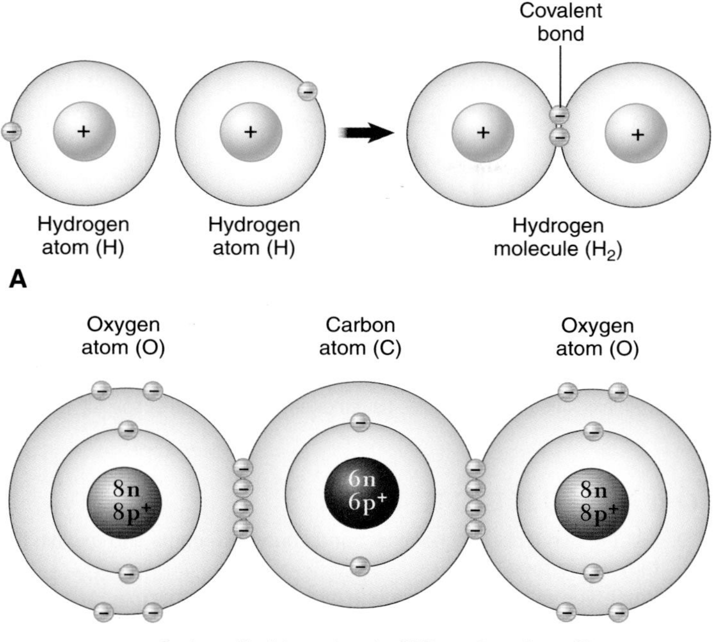

FIGURE 3-9 Types of covalent bonds. A, A single covalent bond formed by the sharing of one electron pair between two atoms of hydrogen results in a molecule of hydrogen gas. **B,** A double covalent bond (double bond) forms by the sharing of two pairs of electrons between two atoms. In this case, two double bonds form—one between carbon and each of the two oxygen atoms forming a molecule of carbon dioxide.

come together they do not form bonds with each other. Even when mixed, oil and water eventually separate because polar water molecules are attracted to one another and move together to form H bonds—leaving the unbound nonpolar oil molecules behind in a separate pool.

Other Weak Attractions

Other weak attractions sometimes attract molecules to each other, even if only temporarily. Shifts in the locations of electrons within each molecule result in fleeting changes in the partial electrical charge of some regions of the molecule. This change in electrical charge may result in attraction to oppositely charged regions of another molecule. In the scope of our course, however, we will not concern ourselves with the different varieties of weak attractions or how they are produced. It is important to know only that they exist and sometimes play an underlying role in holding the material of the body together.

CHEMICAL REACTIONS

Chemical reactions involve interactions between atoms and molecules, which in turn involve the formation or breaking of chemical bonds. Three basic types of chemical reactions that you will learn to recognize as you study physiology are the following:

1. Synthesis reactions
2. Decomposition reactions
3. Exchange reactions

To the chemist, reactions can be symbolized by variations on a simple formula. In *synthesis reactions,* two or more substances called *reactants* combine to form a different, more complex substance called a *product.* **Synthesis** literally means "putting together". The process can be summarized by the following formula:

$$\underset{\text{(Reactants)}}{A + B} \xrightarrow{\text{Energy}} \underset{\text{(Product)}}{AB}$$

Synthesis reactions result in the formation of new bonds, and energy is required for the reaction to occur and the new product to form. Many such reactions occur in the body. Every cell, for example,

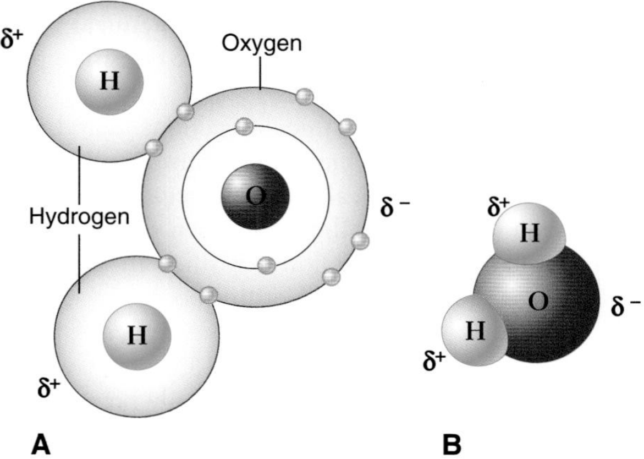

FIGURE 3-10 Water—example of a polar molecule. The polar nature of water is represented in an energy-level model **(A)** and a space-filling model **(B)**. The two hydrogen atoms are nearer one end of the molecule and give that end a partial positive charge (δ+). The "oxygen end" of the molecule attracts the electrons more strongly and thus has a partial negative charge (δ–). Notice that a lowercase Greek letter delta (δ) represents a partial charge.

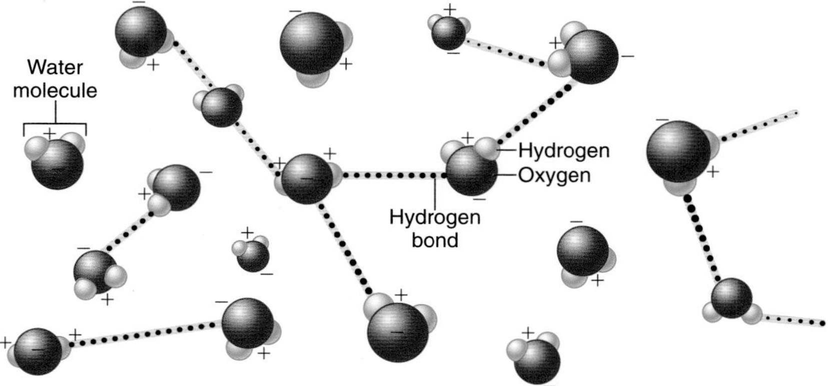

FIGURE 3-11 Hydrogen bonds between water molecules. Hydrogen bonds serve to weakly attach the negative (oxygen) side of one water molecule to the positive (hydrogen) side of a nearby water molecule. This diagram depicts a few bonded molecules, as one would expect in liquid water. Ice would instead have more hydrogen bonds; steam would have no such bonds.

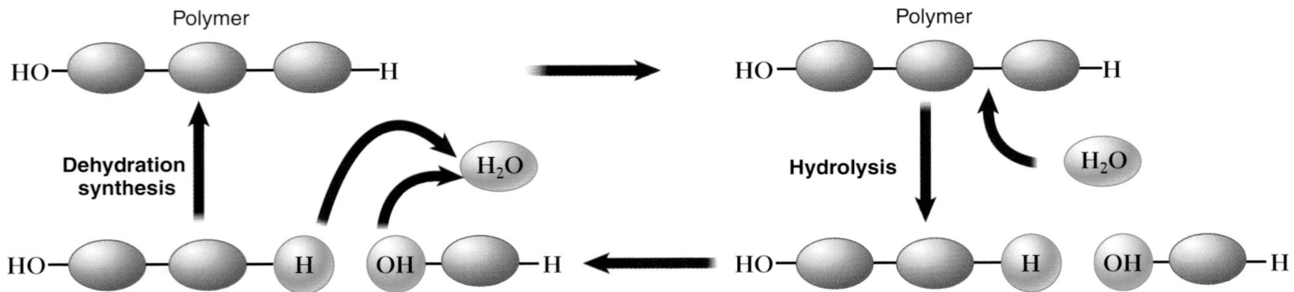

FIGURE 3-12 Metabolic reactions. Hydrolysis (right) is a catabolic reaction that adds water to break down large molecules into smaller molecules, or subunits. Dehydration synthesis (left) is an anabolic reaction that operates in the reverse fashion: small molecules are assembled into large molecules by removing water. Note that specific examples of dehydration synthesis are shown in **Figures 4-6** and **4-13**.

combines amino acid molecules as reactants to form complex protein compounds as products. The ability of the body to synthesize new tissue in wound repair is a good example of this type of reaction.

Decomposition reactions result in the breakdown of a complex substance into two or more simpler substances. In this type of reaction, chemical bonds are broken and energy is released. Energy can be released in the form of heat, or it can be captured for storage and future use. Decomposition reactions can be summarized by the following formula:

$$AB \longrightarrow A + B + Energy$$

Decomposition reactions occur when a complex nutrient is broken down in a cell to release energy for other cellular functions. The products of such a reaction are ultimately waste products. Decomposition and synthesis are opposites. Synthesis builds up; decomposition breaks down. Synthesis forms chemical bonds; decomposition breaks chemical bonds. Decomposition and synthesis reactions are often coupled with one another in such a way that the energy released by a decomposition reaction can be used to drive a synthesis reaction.

The nature of **exchange reactions** permits two different reactants to exchange components and, as a result, form two new products. An exchange reaction is often symbolized by the following formula:

$$AB + CD \longrightarrow AD + CB$$

Exchange reactions break down, or decompose, two compounds and, in exchange, synthesize two new compounds. Certain exchange reactions take place in the blood. One example is the reaction between lactic acid and sodium bicarbonate. The decomposition of both substances is exchanged for the synthesis of sodium lactate and carbonic acid. These changes can be seen more easily in the following equation:

$$H \cdot Lactate + NaHCO_3 \rightarrow Na \cdot Lactate + H \cdot HCO_3$$

The formula *H · Lactate* represents lactic acid; $NaHCO_3$ is the formula for sodium bicarbonate; *Na · Lactate* represents sodium lactate; and $H \cdot HCO_3$ represents carbonic acid.

Reversible reactions, as the name suggests, proceed in both directions. A great many synthesis, decomposition, or exchange reactions are reversible, and a number of them are cited in later chapters of this book. An arrow pointing in both directions is used to denote a reversible reaction:

$$A + B \rightleftharpoons AB$$

Quick CHECK

9. List the two types of chemical bonds between atoms and explain how they are formed.
10. What type of bonds attracts one molecule to another?
11. Diagram the three basic types of chemical reactions.

METABOLISM

Body Chemistry

The term **metabolism** is used to describe all the chemical reactions that occur in body cells. Informally, metabolism may be called *body chemistry*.

The important topics of nutrition and metabolism are discussed fully in Chapter 41. Nutrition and metabolism are described together because the total of all the chemical reactions or metabolic activity occurring in cells is associated with the use the body makes of foods after they have been digested, absorbed, and circulated to cells. The terms catabolism and anabolism are used to describe the two major types of metabolic activity.

Catabolism describes chemical reactions that break down larger food molecules into smaller chemical units and, in so doing, often *release energy*. The release of energy is related to the disruption of chemical bonds. This breakdown of bonds in the chemical compounds contained in the foods and beverages that we consume provides the energy to power all of our activities.

Anabolism involves the many chemical reactions that build larger and more complex chemical molecules from smaller subunits (**Figure 3-12**). Anabolic chemical reactions *require energy*—energy most often made available by the breakdown of **adenosine triphosphate (ATP).** ATP will be explored further in the next chapter—and will appear in most chapters of this book.

Catabolism

Catabolism consists of chemical reactions that not only break down relatively complex compounds into simpler ones but also release energy from them. This breakdown process represents a type of chemical reaction called **hydrolysis** (see **Figure 3-12**). As a result of hydrolysis occurring during catabolism, a water molecule is added to break a larger compound into smaller subunits. For example, hydrolysis of a fat molecule breaks it down into its subunits—glycerol and fatty acid molecules; a disaccharide such as sucrose breaks down into its monosaccharide subunits—glucose and fructose; and the subunits of protein hydrolysis are amino acids.

Ultimately, catabolic reactions will further degrade these building blocks of food compounds—glycerol, fatty acids, monosaccharides, and amino acids—into the end products carbon dioxide, water, and other waste products. During this process, energy is released. Some of the energy released by catabolism is heat energy, the heat that keeps our bodies warm. However, more than half the energy released is immediately recaptured and transferred to a molecule called *ATP*, which transfers the energy to cell components that need it to do work. ATP is discussed in more detail later in the next chapter.

ANABOLISM

Anabolism is the term used to describe chemical reactions that join simple molecules together to form more complex biomolecules—notably, carbohydrates, lipids, proteins, and nucleic acids. Literally thousands of anabolic reactions take place continually in the body. The type of chemical reaction responsible for this joining together of smaller units to form larger molecules is called *condensation* or **dehydration synthesis** (see **Figure 3-12**). It is a key reaction during anabolism. As a result of dehydration synthesis, water is removed as smaller subunits are fused together.

Anabolism requires energy, which is transferred from ATP molecules. Anabolic reactions use energy to join monosaccharide units to form larger carbohydrates, fuse amino acids into peptide chains, and form fat molecules from glycerol and fatty acid subunits.

Quick CHECK

12. What does the term *metabolism* mean?
13. What is the difference between *anabolism* and *catabolism*?
14. What is the role of *ATP* in the body?

ORGANIC AND INORGANIC COMPOUNDS

In living organisms, there are two kinds of compounds: *organic* and *inorganic*. Organic compounds are generally defined as compounds composed of molecules that contain carbon–carbon (C—C) covalent bonds or carbon–hydrogen (C—H) covalent bonds—or both kinds of bonds. Few inorganic compounds have carbon atoms in them, and none have C—C or C—H bonds. Organic molecules are generally larger and more complex than inorganic molecules. Large organic molecules important in living organisms are often called **biomolecules.**

The human body has inorganic and organic compounds because both are equally important to the chemistry of life. This chapter focuses mainly on inorganic chemistry. The next chapter focuses on organic chemistry.

INORGANIC MOLECULES

IMPORTANCE OF WATER

Although water is an inorganic compound, it has been called the "cradle of life" because all living organisms require water to survive. Each body cell is bathed in fluid, and it is only in this precisely regulated and homeostatically controlled environment that cells can function. In addition to water surrounding the cell, the basic substance of each cell, cytoplasm, is itself largely water. Water is certainly the body's most abundant and important compound. Fifty percent or more of a normal adult's body weight is water, which serves a host of vital functions. Because of water's pervasive importance in all living organisms, an understanding of the basics of water chemistry is important. In a very real sense, water chemistry forms the basis for the chemistry of life.

Properties of Water

The chemist views water as a simple and stable compound. It has an atomic structure that results from the combination of two covalent bonds between a single oxygen atom and two hydrogen atoms.

Recall that water molecules are polar molecules and interact with one another because they have a partial positive charge at one end and a partial negative charge at their other end. Take a moment to go back and review **Figure 3-10**. This simple chemical property, called *polarity*, allows water to act as a very effective *solvent* into which solutes can dissolve. Proper functioning of a cell requires the presence of many chemical substances. Many of these compounds are quite large and must be broken into smaller and more reactive particles (ions) for reactions to occur. Because of its polar nature, water tends to dissociate ionic compounds in solution and surround any molecule that has an electrical charge (**Figure 3-13**). The 'coat' of water that thus forms around charged solutes is often called a hydration shell. The fact that so many substances dissolve in water is of utmost importance in the life process.

The critical role that water plays as a solvent permits the *transportation* of many essential materials within the body. By dissolving nutrient molecules in blood, for instance, water enables these materials to enter and leave the blood capillaries in the digestive organs and eventually enter cells in every area of the body. In turn, waste products are transported from where they are produced to excretory organs for elimination from the body.

Another important function of water stems from the fact that water both absorbs and gives up heat slowly. These properties of

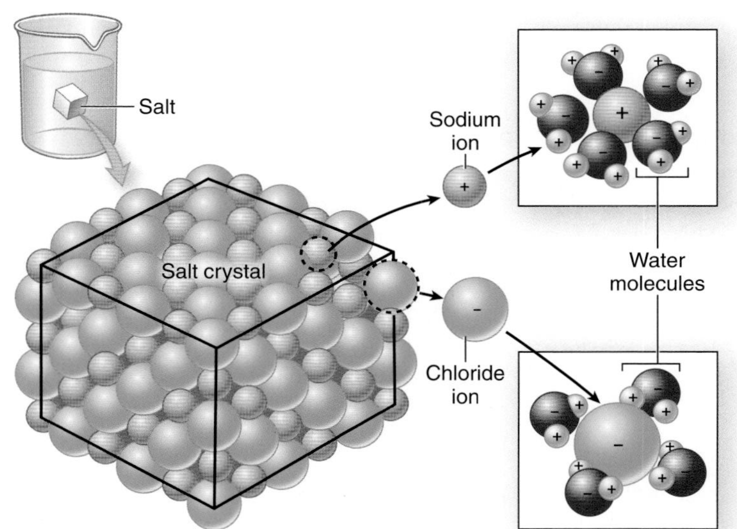

FIGURE 3-13 Water as a solvent. The polar nature of water *(red and blue)* favours ionization of substances in solution. Sodium (Na^+) ions *(pink)* and chloride (Cl^-) ions *(green)* dissociate in the solution.

water enable it to maintain a relatively constant temperature. This allows the body, which has a large water content, to resist sudden changes in temperature. Chemists describe this property by saying that water has a high *specific heat;* that is, water can lose and gain large amounts of heat with little change in temperature. As a result, excess body heat produced by the contraction of muscles during exercise, for example, can be transported by blood to the body surface and dissipated into the environment with little actual change in core temperature.

Chemists and biologists recognize water's high *heat of vaporization* as another important physical quality. This characteristic requires the absorption of significant amounts of heat to change water from a liquid to a gas. The energy is required to break the many hydrogen bonds that hold adjacent water molecules together in the liquid state. Thus the body can dissipate excess heat and maintain a normal temperature by evaporation of water (sweat) from the skin surface whenever excess heat is being produced.

Understanding and appreciating the importance of water in the life process are critical. Water does more than act as a solvent, produce ionization, and facilitate chemical reactions. It has essential chemical roles of its own in addition to the many important physical qualities it brings to body function (**Table 3-2**). It plays a key role in such processes as cell permeability, active transport of materials, secretion, and membrane potential, to name a few.

Oxygen and Carbon Dioxide

Oxygen (O_2) and carbon dioxide (CO_2) are important inorganic substances that are closely related to cellular respiration.

Molecular oxygen in the body is present as two oxygen atoms joined by a double covalent bond. Oxygen is required to complete the decomposition reactions required for the release of energy from nutrients burned by the cell.

Carbon dioxide is considered one of a group of very simple carbon-containing inorganic compounds. It is an important exception to the "rule of thumb" that inorganic substances do not contain carbon. Like oxygen, carbon dioxide is involved in cellular respiration. It is produced as a waste product during the breakdown of complex nutrients and also serves an important role in maintaining the appropriate acid–base balance in the body.

TABLE 3-2 Properties of Water

PROPERTY	DESCRIPTION	EXAMPLE OF BENEFIT TO THE BODY
Strong polarity	Polar water molecules attract other polar compounds, which causes them to dissociate	Many kinds of molecules can dissolve in cells, thereby permitting a variety of chemical reactions and allowing many substances to be transported
High specific heat	Hydrogen bonds absorb heat when they break and release heat when they form, thereby minimizing temperature changes	Body temperature stays relatively constant; body chemistry facilitated
High heat of vaporization	Many hydrogen bonds must be broken for water to evaporate	Evaporation of water in perspiration cools the body
Cohesion	Hydrogen bonds hold molecules of water together	Water works as lubricant or cushion to protect against damage from friction or trauma

Electrolytes

Other inorganic substances include acids, bases, and salts. These substances belong to a large group of compounds called **electrolytes.** Electrolytes are substances that break up, or *dissociate,* in solution to form charged particles, or ions. Sometimes the ions themselves are also called electrolytes. Ions with a positive charge are called *cations,* and those with a negative charge are called *anions.* **Figure 3-13** shows the way in which water molecules work to dissociate a common electrolyte, sodium chloride (NaCl), into Na^+ cations and Cl^- anions.

Acids and Bases

Acids and bases are common and very important chemical substances in the body. Early chemists categorized acids and bases by such characteristics as taste or the ability to change the colour of certain dyes. Acids, for example, taste sour and bases taste bitter. The dye litmus will turn blue in the presence of a base and red when exposed to an acid. These and other observations illustrate a fundamental point, namely, that acids and bases are chemical opposites. Although acids and bases dissociate in solution, both release different types of ions. The unique chemical properties of acids and bases when they are in solution are perhaps the best way to differentiate them.

Acids

By definition, an **acid** is any substance that will release a hydrogen ion (H^+) when in solution. A hydrogen ion is simply a bare proton—the nucleus of a hydrogen atom. Therefore, acids are often called *proton donors.* It is the concentration of hydrogen ions that accounts for the chemical properties of acids. The level of "acidity" of a solution depends on the number of hydrogen ions a particular acid will release.

One particular point should be understood about water. Water molecules dissociate continually in a reversible reaction to form hydrogen ions (H^+) and hydroxide ions (OH^-):

$$H_2O \rightleftharpoons H^+ + OH^-$$

Recall from our discussion of ionic bonds (p. 43) that having a single unpaired electron in the outer energy level makes an atom unstable and that losing that electron results in a more stable structure. This is precisely the reason dissociation of water occurs. In pure water, the balance between these two ions is equal. However, when an acid such as hydrochloric acid (HCl) dissociates into H^+ and Cl^-, it shifts the H^+/OH^- balance in favour of excess H^+ ions, thus increasing the level of acidity. The more hydrogen ions (H^+) produced, the stronger the acid.

A *strong acid* is an acid that completely, or almost completely, dissociates to form H^+ ions. A *weak acid,* on the other hand, dissociates very little and therefore produces few excess H^+ ions in solution. There are many important acids in the body, and they perform many functions. Hydrochloric acid, for example, is the acid produced in the stomach to aid the digestive process.

Bases

Bases, or *alkaline* compounds, are electrolytes that, when dissociated in solution, shift the H^+/OH^- balance in favour of OH^-. This can be accomplished by increasing the number of hydroxide ions (OH^-) in solution or decreasing the number of H^+ ions present. The fact that bases will combine with or accept H^+ ions (protons) is the reason the term *proton acceptor* is used to describe these substances. The dissociation of a common base, sodium hydroxide, yields the cation Na^+ and the OH^- anion.

Like acids, bases are classified as strong or weak, depending on how readily and completely they dissociate into ions. Important bases in the body, such as the bicarbonate ion (HCO_3^-), play critical roles in the transportation of respiratory gases, in maintaining normal pH balance, and in the elimination of waste products from the body.

The pH scale

The term **pH** is literally an abbreviation for a phrase meaning "the power of hydrogen" and is used to mean the relative H^+ ion concentration of a solution. As you can see at the left side of **Figure 3-14**, the pH value is the negative of the base-10 logarithm of the H^+ ion concentration. The pH indicates the degree of *acidity* or *alkalinity* of a solution. As the concentration of H^+ ions increases, the pH goes down and the solution becomes more acidic; a decrease in H^+ ion concentration makes the solution more alkaline and the pH goes up:

- A pH of 7 indicates neutrality (equal amounts of H^+ and OH^-)
- A pH of less than 7 indicates acidity (more H^+ than OH^-)
- A pH greater than 7 indicates alkalinity (more OH^- than H^+)

The overall pH range is often expressed numerically on a logarithmic scale of 1 to 14. Keep in mind that a change of 1 pH unit on this

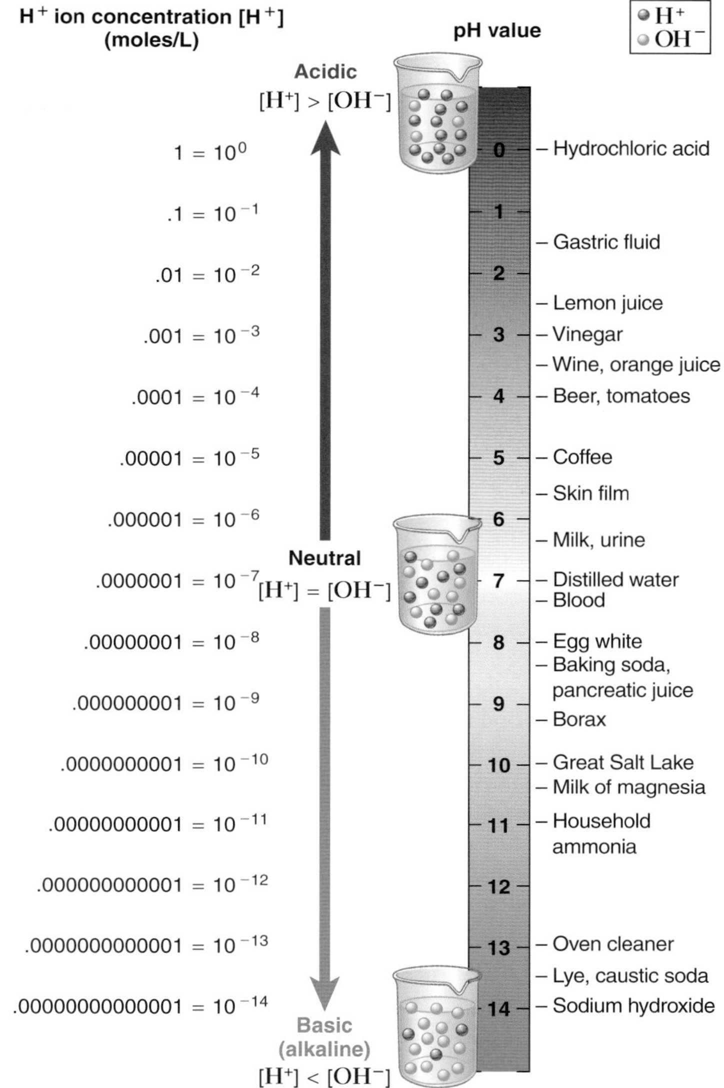

FIGURE 3-14 The pH scale. Note that as the concentration of H^+ increases, the solution becomes increasingly acidic and the pH value decreases. As the H^+ concentration decreases, the pH value increases, and the solution becomes more and more basic, or alkaline. (The scale on the left side of the diagram shows the actual concentrations of H^+ in moles per litre, or molar concentration, as an ordinary number and expressed as an exponent [logarithm] of 10. You can see that the pH scale is simply the negative of the exponent of 10.)

BOX 3-1 *fyi* | The pH Unit

A pH value of 7, for example, means that a solution with that measurement contains 10^{-7} grams of hydrogen ions per litre. Translating this logarithm into a number, a pH of 7 means that such a solution contains 0.0000001 (i.e., 1/10,000,000) gram of hydrogen ions per litre. A solution with a measurement of pH 6 contains 0.000001 (1/1,000,000) gram of hydrogen ions per litre, and one of pH 8 contains 0.00000001 (1/100,000,000) gram of hydrogen ions per litre. Note that a solution with pH 7 contains *10 times* as many hydrogen ions as a solution with pH 8 and that pH decreases as the hydrogen ion concentration increases.

The photo shows a test strip being used to verify placement of a patient's feeding tube by measuring the pH of gastric juice (in the cup) removed through the feeding tube by a syringe. A reading of pH 1 to pH 4 shows that the tube is likely to still be in the stomach, rather than further along in the intestines—where the pH would be closer to neutral. Gastric juice with a pH of 1 has an H^+ concentration that is a *million times* the H^+ concentration of a neutral solution! •

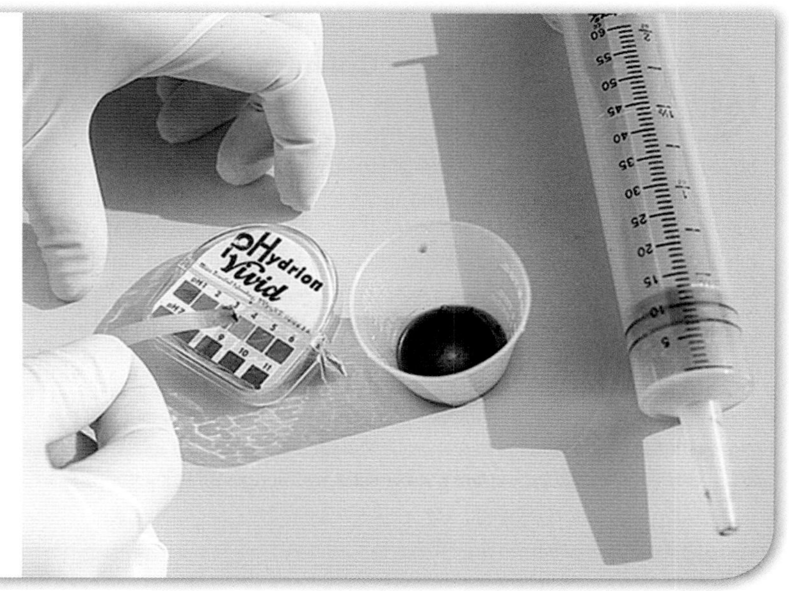

type of scale represents a 10-fold difference in actual concentration of H^+ ions (**Box 3-1**).

Buffers

The normal pH range of blood and other body fluids is extremely narrow. For example, venous blood (pH 7.36) is only slightly more acidic than arterial blood (pH 7.41). The difference results primarily from carbon dioxide entering venous blood as a waste product of cellular metabolism. Carbon dioxide is carried as carbonic acid (H_2CO_3) and therefore lowers the pH of venous blood. More than 30 *litres* of carbonic acid is transported in venous blood each day and eliminated as carbon dioxide by the lungs, and yet 1 litre of venous blood contains only about 1/100,000,000 gram more H^+ ions than 1 litre of arterial blood does!

The incredible constancy of the pH homeostatic mechanism relies partly on the presence of substances, called **buffers,** that minimize changes in the concentrations of H^+ and OH^- ions in our body fluids. Buffers are said to act as a "reservoir" for H^+ ions. They donate, or remove, H^+ ions to or from a solution if that becomes necessary to maintain a constant pH. Examples of important buffer systems and specifics of buffer action are discussed in Chapter 44.

Salts

A salt is any compound that results from the chemical interaction of an acid and a base. Salts, like acids and bases, are electrolyte compounds and dissociate in solution to form positively and negatively charged ions. Ions exist in solution. If the water is removed, the ions will crystallize and form salt. When mixed and allowed to react, the positive ion (cation) of a base and the negative ion (anion) of an acid will join to form a salt and additional water in the manner of a typical exchange reaction. The reaction between an acid and a base to form a salt and water is called a *neutralization reaction:*

$$\begin{array}{ccccccc} AB & + & CD & \longrightarrow & CB & + & AD \\ HCl & + & NaOH & \longrightarrow & NaCl & + & H_2O \\ \text{Acid} & & \text{Base} & & \text{Salt} & & \text{Water} \end{array}$$

TABLE 3-3 Inorganic Salts Important in Body Functions

SALT	FORMULA	IONS
Sodium chloride	$NaCl$	$Na^+ + Cl^-$
Calcium chloride	$CaCl_2$	$Ca^{++} + 2Cl^-$
Magnesium chloride	$MgCl_2$	$Mg^{++} + 2Cl^-$
Sodium bicarbonate	$NaHCO_3$	$Na^+ + HCO_3$
Potassium chloride	KCl	$K^+ + Cl^-$
Sodium sulphate	Na_2SO_4	$2Na^+ + SO_4^=$
Calcium carbonate	$CaCO_3$	$Ca^{++} + CO_3^=$
Calcium phosphate	$Ca_3(PO_4)_2$	$3Ca^{++} + 2PO_4^{\equiv}$

Note that the sodium and the chloride join to form the salt, whereas the hydroxide ion "accepts" or combines with a hydrogen ion to form water.

The sources of many of the major and trace mineral elements listed in **Table 3-1** are inorganic salts, which are common in many body fluids and certain tissues such as bone. These elements often exert their full physiological effects only when present as charged atoms or ions in solution.

The proper amount and concentration of such mineral ions as potassium (K^+), calcium (Ca^{++}), and sodium (Na^+) are required for proper functioning of nerves and for contraction of muscle tissue. See Chapter 43 for specific homeostatic control mechanisms that regulate electrolyte balance in blood and other body fluids. **Table 3-3** lists several inorganic salts that, on dissociation in body fluids, contribute important ions required for numerous body functions.

Quick CHECK

15. Discuss the properties of water that make it so important in living organisms.
16. What is an electrolyte?
17. How do acids and bases react with each other when in solution?
18. What is pH?

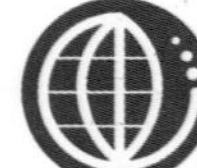

the big picture | Chemical Basis of Life

The importance of the concept of organization at all levels of body structure and function was introduced in Chapters 1 and 2 and will be reinforced as you study the individual organ systems of the body in subsequent chapters of the text. Understanding the information in this chapter is a critical first step in connecting the chemistry of life with a real understanding of how the body functions and the relationships that exist between differing functions and body structures.

How the basic chemical building blocks of the body are organized and how they relate to one another are key determinants in understanding normal structure and function, as well as understanding pathological anatomy and disease.

Consider the following questions. Each one relates to the study of one or more organ systems covered in subsequent chapters. Your ability to answer these and many other questions correctly will require knowledge of basic chemistry.

- How do common antacids work?
- How do proton-pump inhibitors work?
- Is an electrolyte-rich sports drink better than plain water in replacing fluids lost during prolonged, vigorous exercise?
- How does a change in Ca^{++} concentration in the blood affect heart function?
- Why do electrons have a critical role in providing energy for muscle contraction?
- Why does breathing oxygen at the end of a marathon run help an athlete recover more quickly?
- What roles do ions play in triggering muscle contractions and producing nerve impulses?

These are the types of real-world, end-of-chapter questions that you will encounter throughout the text that require the application of basic chemistry.

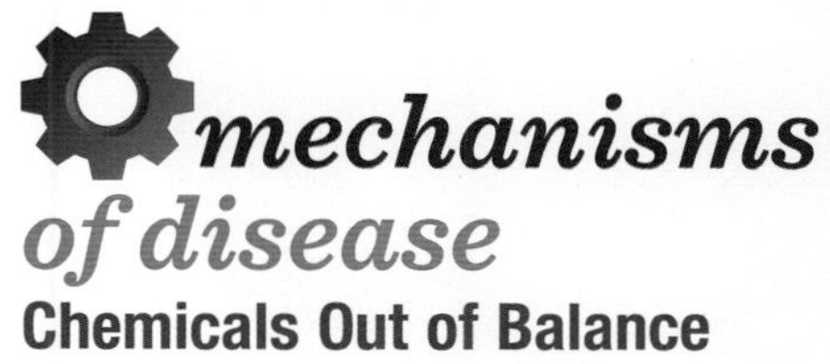

mechanisms of disease

Chemicals Out of Balance

As we have learned in this chapter, all the various classes of chemicals in the body each have their particular functions in maintaining the life of the body. If the balances among various groups of chemicals fluctuate too far from their setpoint values, the homeostatic balance of the body is threatened.

Let's examine just one common example of such an imbalance. The carbon dioxide (CO_2) concentration in the blood will climb too high, a condition called **hypercapnia,** when the respiratory system fails to remove it from the blood at the normal rate. Thus we have a CO_2 imbalance. This will have several effects. For one, the high CO_2 levels will inhibit cell metabolism and thus reduce the normal activity of the body. For another, because CO_2 tends to form an acid, the pH of the body's internal environment will drop to below the setpoint level—a condition called **acidosis.** Acidosis, in turn, may disrupt the shapes of proteins throughout the body and thus interfere with the normal structure and function of the body. Unless CO_2 balance is restored quickly, a person will die.

Various elements of the scenario we just described are touched on later in appropriate places in the book. However, this is just one of many examples of chemical imbalances that can serve as a mechanism of disease. Nutrient imbalances, ion imbalances, and so on, can all be life-threatening.

CONNECT IT! 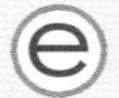

Review ***Radioactivity*** online at ***Connect It!*** for more on radiation and its adverse effect on health.

Some chemicals called **toxins** that enter the body can cause damage to our own molecules. Toxins, or poisons, cause their damage by destroying our molecules, combining with our molecules to render them useless, or otherwise disrupting the normal chemical balance and chemical activity of our bodies. For example, *carbon monoxide (CO)* is a gas that binds to haemoglobin in our blood so tightly that the haemoglobin can no longer carry the oxygen needed for life. Mercury (Hg), a toxic metal that was once commonly used in industry and health care, can enter cells and bind to sulphur-containing molecules in the organelles. Mercury can thus damage cell functions throughout the body.

Most diseases are ultimately chemical disorders—missing or malfunctioning molecules. Watch for these chemical problems as we explore mechanisms of disease in later chapters.

LANGUAGE OF SCIENCE *(continued from p. 38)*

molecule (MOL-eh-kyool)
[*mole-* **mass,** *-cule* **small**]

nonpolar (non-PO-lar)
[*non-* **not,** *-pol-* **pole,** *-ar* **relating to**]

octet rule (ok-TET rool)
[*octet* **group of eight**]

pH (pee AYCH)
[abbreviation for *potenz* **power,** *hydrogen* **hydrogen**]

polar (PO-lar)
[*pol-* **pole,** *-ar* **relating to**]

polarity (poh-LAIR-ih-tee)
[*pol-* **pole,** *-ar-* **relating to,** *-ity* **state**]

radioactivity (ray-dee-o-ak-TIV-it-ee)
[*radio* **send out rays**]

radioisotope (ray-dee-oh-EYE-so-tohp)
[*radio-* **send out rays,** *-iso-* **equal,** *-tope* **place**]

reversible reaction (ree-VER-si-bul ree-AK-shun)
[*re-* **again,** *-vers-* **turn,** *-ible* **able to,** *re-* **again,** *-action* **action**]

synthesis (SIN-the-sis)
[*synthes-* **put together,** *-is* **process**]

LANGUAGE OF MEDICINE

acidosis (ass-i-DOE-sis)
[*acid-* **sour,** *-osis* **condition**]

hypercapnia (hye-per-KAP-nee-ah)
[*hyper-* **above,** *-capn-* **vapour (CO_2),** *-ia* **condition**]

toxin (TOK-sin)
[*tox-* **poison,** *-in* **substance**]

case study

This year, during her college's spring break, Kylie is visiting France for the first time. On the first night of her vacation, she and her friends go out to dinner. Feeling rather adventurous, Kylie eats raw oysters as an appetizer. Unfortunately, the oysters contain a high concentration of pathogenic bacteria, and 24 hours later, Kylie is experiencing the "adventure" of food poisoning. Among her symptoms are nausea, vomiting, abdominal pain and diarrhoea.

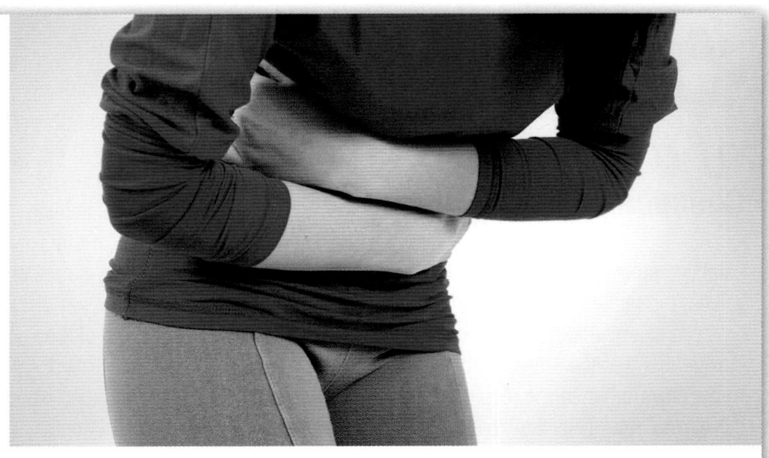

1. Select an answer that best fits the missing words. With continued vomiting, Kylie keeps losing ________ from her stomach, that could make her entire body too ________.
   a. acid; acidic
   b. base; basic
   c. acid; basic
   d. base; acidic
2. When we talk about measuring the pH of a substance, we are measuring the concentration of what ions in that substance?
   a. Oxygen ions
   b. Carbon ions
   c. Phosphate ions
   d. Hydrogen ions

   Finally after 48 hours, Kylie is able to keep clear liquids down.
3. Why should she not drink just plain water?
   a. Water cannot replenish the electrolytes she has lost.
   b. Flavoured liquids will more effectively stimulate her appetite.
   c. Water can irritate the stomach lining.
   d. Plain water is just fine; it will quickly replace her body's lost fluid.

   When Kylie feels well enough to try eating something, her first food items should provide energy but be easy to digest.
4. Which organic molecule best fits that description—high energy, easily digested?
   a. Protein
   b. Carbohydrates
   c. Triglycerides
   d. Nucleic acids

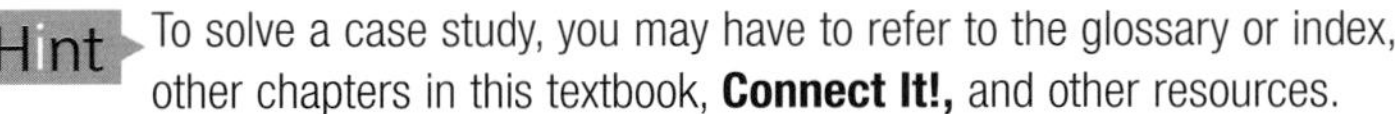
Hint To solve a case study, you may have to refer to the glossary or index, other chapters in this textbook, **Connect It!,** and other resources.

CHAPTER SUMMARY

To download an MP3 version of the chapter summary for use with your mobile device, access the ***Audio Chapter Summaries*** *online at evolve.elsevier.com.*

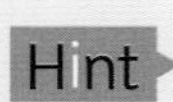
Hint *Scan this summary after reading the chapter to help you reinforce the key concepts. Later, use the summary as a quick review before your class or before a test.*

Units of Matter

A. Elements and compounds (**Figure 3-1**)
   1. Matter—anything that has mass and occupies space
   2. Element—simple form of matter, a substance that cannot be broken down into two or more different substances
      a. There are 26 elements in the human body
      b. There are 11 *major elements*, 4 of which (carbon, oxygen, hydrogen, and nitrogen) make up 96% of the human body (**Figure 3-2**)
      c. There are 15 *trace elements* that make up less than 2% of body weight
   3. Compound—atoms of two or more elements joined to form chemical combinations

B. Atoms (**Figure 3-3**)
   1. The concept of an atom was proposed by the English chemist John Dalton

Atomic Structure

A. Cloud model—nucleus surrrounded by electron cloud

B. Atoms contain several different kinds of subatomic particles; the most important are:
   1. Protons (p^+)—positively charged subatomic particles found in the nucleus
   2. Neutrons (n^0)—neutral subatomic particles found in the nucleus
   3. Electrons (e^-)—negatively charged subatomic particles found in the electron cloud (**Figure 3-4**)

C. Atomic number and mass number
   1. Atomic number (**Table 3-1**)
      a. Number of protons in an atom's nucleus
      b. Critically important; atomic number identifies the kind of element
   2. Mass number
      a. Mass of a single atom
      b. Equal to the number of protons plus the number of neutrons in the nucleus ($p^+ + n^0$)

D. Energy levels (**Figures 3-5** and **3-6**)
   1. Total number of electrons in an atom equals the number of protons in the nucleus (in a stable atom)
   2. Electrons form a "cloud" around the nucleus

3. *Bohr model*—a model resembling planets revolving around the sun; useful in visualizing the structure of atoms
   a. Exhibits electrons in concentric circles showing relative distances of the electrons from the nucleus
   b. Each ring or shell represents a specific energy level and can hold only a certain number of electrons
   c. Number and arrangement of electrons determine whether an atom is chemically stable
   d. An atom with eight, or four pairs, of electrons in the outermost energy level is chemically stable
   e. An atom without a full outermost energy level is chemically reactive
4. *Octet rule*—atoms with fewer or more than eight electrons in the outer energy level will attempt to lose, gain, or share electrons with other atoms to achieve stability

D. Isotopes (**Figure 3-7**)
1. Isotopes of an element contain the same number of protons but different numbers of neutrons
2. Isotopes have the same atomic number and therefore the same basic chemical properties as any other atom of the same element, but they have a different mass number
3. Atomic weight—the average mass number of isotopes typically found among atoms in nature
4. Radioactive isotope (radioisotope)—an unstable isotope that undergoes nuclear breakdown and emits nuclear particles and radiation

Attractions Between Atoms

A. Chemical reaction—interaction between two or more atoms that occurs as a result of activity between electrons in their outermost energy levels
B. Molecule—two or more atoms covalently joined together
C. Compound—consists of groupings of atoms of two or more elements
D. Chemical bonds—two types unite atoms into groupings such as crystals and molecules
1. Ionic, or electrovalent, bond (**Figure 3-8**)—formed by transfer of electrons; strong electrostatic force that binds positively and negatively charged ions together
2. Covalent bond (**Figure 3-9**)—formed by sharing of electron pairs between atoms

Attractions Between Molecules

A. Hydrogen bonds
1. Form when electrons are unequally shared
   a. Example: water molecule
   b. Polar molecules have regions with partial electrical charges resulting from unequal sharing of electrons among atoms (i.e., they exhibit polarity)
2. Areas of different partial charges on nearby molecules attract one another and form hydrogen bonds
3. Occur between a hydrogen bonded to an O, N, or F, and another hydrogen bonded to an O, N, or F
4. Polar water will not remain mixed with nonpolar lipids (oils and fats) because water groups together by H bonding, thus leaving the unbound lipid molecules behind in a separate group

B. Other weak attractions—molecules are attracted to each other through differences in electrical charge

Chemical Reactions

A. Involve the formation or breaking of chemical bonds
B. Three basic types of chemical reactions are involved in physiology:
1. Synthesis reaction—combining of two or more substances to form a more complex substance; formation of new chemical bonds: $A + B \rightarrow AB$
2. Decomposition reaction—breaking down of a substance into two or more simpler substances; breaking of chemical bonds: $AB \rightarrow A + B$
3. Exchange reaction—decomposition of two substances and, in exchange, synthesis of two new compounds from them: $AB + CD \rightarrow AD + CB$
4. Reversible reactions—occur in both directions

Metabolism

A. Metabolism—all of the chemical reactions that occur in body cells; informally called *body chemistry* (**Figure 3-12**)
B. Catabolism
1. Chemical reactions that break down complex compounds into simpler ones and release energy; hydrolysis is a common catabolic reaction
2. Ultimately, the end products of catabolism are carbon dioxide, water, and other waste products
3. Some of the energy released is transferred to ATP, which is then used to do cellular work

C. Anabolism
1. Chemical reactions that join simple molecules together to form more complex molecules
2. Chemical reaction responsible for anabolism is dehydration synthesis (condensation)

Organic and Inorganic Compounds

A. Inorganic compounds—few have carbon atoms and none have C—C or C—H bonds
B. Organic compounds—have at least one carbon atom and at least one C—C or C—H bond in each molecule; will be explored further in next chapter

Inorganic Molecules

A. Water
1. Most abundant and important compound in the body
2. Properties of water (**Table 3-2**)
   a. Polarity—allows water to act as an effective solvent in the body; ionizes substances in solution (**Figure 3-10**)
   b. Solvent allows transportation of essential materials throughout the body (**Figure 3-13**)
   c. High specific heat—water can lose and gain large amounts of heat with little change in its own temperature; enables the body to maintain a relatively constant temperature
   d. High heat of vaporization—water requires the absorption of significant amounts of heat to change it from a liquid to a gas; allows the body to dissipate excess heat

B. Oxygen and carbon dioxide—closely related to cellular respiration
   1. Oxygen—required to complete decomposition reactions necessary for the release of energy in the body
   2. Carbon dioxide—produced as a waste product and also helps maintain the appropriate acid–base balance in the body

C. Electrolytes
   1. Large group of inorganic compounds that includes acids, bases, and salts
   2. Substances that dissociate in solution to form ions (the resulting ions are also sometimes called *electrolytes*)
   3. Positively charged ions are cations; negatively charged ions are anions
   4. Acids and bases—common and important chemical substances that are chemical opposites
      a. Acids
         (1) Any substance that releases a hydrogen ion (H^+) when in solution—*proton donor*
         (2) Level of *acidity* depends on the number of hydrogen ions a particular acid will release
      b. Bases
         (1) Electrolytes that dissociate to yield hydroxide ions (OH^-) or other electrolytes that combine with hydrogen ions (H^+)
         (2) Described as *proton acceptors*
      c. pH scale—assigns a value to measures of acidity and alkalinity (**Figure 3-14**)
         (1) pH indicates the degree of acidity or alkalinity of a solution
         (2) pH of 7 indicates neutrality (equal amounts of H^+ and OH^-); a pH less than 7 indicates acidity; a pH higher than 7 indicates alkalinity
   5. Buffers
      a. Maintain the constancy of pH
      b. Minimize changes in the concentrations of H^+ and OH^- ions
      c. Act as a *reservoir* for hydrogen ions
   6. Salts (**Table 3-3**)
      a. Compounds that result from chemical interaction of an acid and a base
      b. Reaction between an acid and a base to form a salt and water is called a *neutralization reaction*

REVIEW QUESTIONS

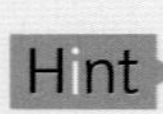

Write out the answers to these questions after reading the chapter and reviewing the Chapter Summary. Note—writing out your answers will consolidate learning and provide a valuable resource of information.

1. Define the following terms: element, compound, atom, molecule.
2. Compare early nineteenth century and present-day concepts of atomic structure.
3. Create a table identifying the three kinds of subatomic particles. Include name, charge, and location of each particle.
4. Are atoms electrically charged particles? Give the reason for your answer.
5. What four elements make up approximately 96% of the body's weight? List them in order of decreasing occurrence.
6. How does the atomic number of an element differ from the atomic mass of the element?
7. Explain the general rule by which an atom can be listed as chemically stable and unable to react with another atom.
8. Define and give an example of an isotope.
9. Explain what the term radioactivity means.
10. How does an atom's radioactivity differ from its chemical activity?
11. Define these terms: alpha particles, beta particles, and gamma rays.
12. Explain how radioactive atoms become transformed into atoms of a different element.
13. Explain what the term chemical reaction means.
14. Identify and differentiate between the three basic types of chemical reactions.
15. Define the term inorganic.
16. Explain why water is said to be polar. List four functions of water that are crucial to survival.
17. What are electrolytes? How are they formed?
18. Define cation, anion and ion. Give an example of each.
19. Define the terms acid, base, salt, and buffer.
20. What does the pH of a solution measure? Relate your answer to the concentration of hydrogen ions and hydroxide ions.
21. What is catabolism? What function does it serve?
22. Distinguish between catabolism, anabolism, and metabolism.

CRITICAL THINKING QUESTIONS

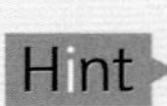

After finishing the Review Questions, write out the answers to these more in-depth questions to help you apply your new knowledge. Go back to sections of the chapter that relate to concepts that you find difficult.

1. Identify the specific areas of chemistry that would be of interest to a biochemist.
2. In modern airships, the gas of choice used to inflate them is helium rather than hydrogen. Hydrogen would be lighter, but helium is safer. Compare and contrast the atomic structure of hydrogen and helium. What characteristics of the atomic structure of helium make it so much less reactive than hydrogen? Speculate what could happen to an airship filled with hydrogen.
3. Contrast single covalent bonds, double covalent bonds, and ionic bonds.
4. If an adult has a body weight of 77 kg, how much of that weight consists of water?

4 Biomolecules

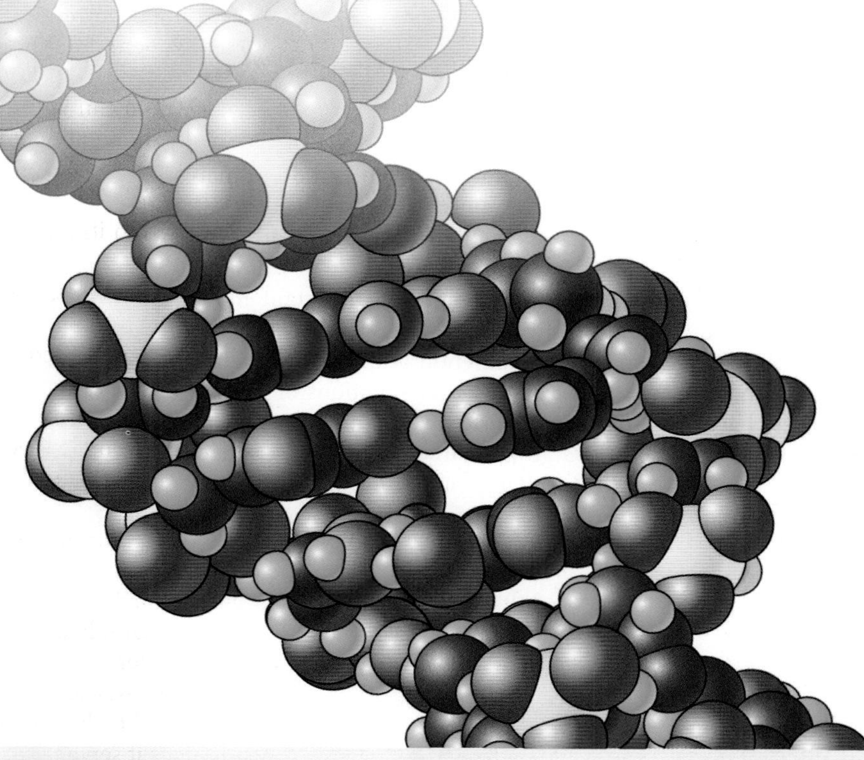

CHAPTER OUTLINE

Hint *Scan this outline before you begin to read the chapter, as a preview of how the concepts are organized.*

In the previous chapter, we explored the basic units of matter—atoms and molecules—and how they interact with one another. In this chapter, we continue that story with a survey of some of the larger biomolecules—molecules made in the body. You are already familiar with most of these substances: carbohydrates, lipids, and proteins, for example. Here we will learn more about the chemical nature of these classes of molecules, as well as examples of various types of each commonly encountered in the human body.

LANGUAGE OF SCIENCE

Hint *Use this list to aid your pronunciation of unfamiliar words.*

adenosine triphosphate (ATP) (ah-DEN-o-seen try-FOS-fate)
[blend of *adenine* and *ribose, tri-* **three,** *-phosph-* **phosphorus,** *-ate* **oxygen**]

amino acid (ah-MEE-no ASS-id)
[*amino* **NH_2,** *acid* **sour**]

carbohydrate (kar-bo-HYE-drate)
[*carbo-* **carbon,** *-hydr-* **hydrogen,** *-ate* **oxygen**]

cholesterol (koh-LESS-ter-ol)
[*chole-* **bile,** *-stero-* **solid,** *-ol* **alcohol**]

denature (de-NAYT-shur)
[*de-* **remove,** *-nature* **nature**]

disaccharide (dye-SAK-ah-ride)
[*di-* **two,** *-sacchar-* **sugar,** *-ide* **chemical**]

enzyme (EN-zime)
[*en-* **in,** *-zyme* **ferment**]

fatty acid (FAT-tee AS-id)
[*fat-* **fat,** *-ty* **state,** *acid* **sour**]

free radical (RAD-i-kal)
[*radic-* **root,** -al **relating to**]

functional group (FUNK-shun-al groop)
[*function-* **perform,** *-al* **relating to**]

functional protein (FUNK-shun-al PRO-teen)
[*function-* **perform,** *-al* **relating to,** *prote-* **primary,** *-in* **substance**]

glucose (GLOO-kohs)
[*gluco-* **sweet,** *-ose* **carbohydrate (sugar)**]

glycerol (GLIS-er-ol)
[*glyce-* **sweet,** *-ol* **alcohol**]

glycogen (GLYE-koh-jen)
[*glyco-* **sweet,** *-gen* **produce**]

high-energy bond
[*en-* **in,** *-erg* **work,** *-y* **state,** *bond* **band**]

hydrophilic (hye-dro-FIL-ik)
[*hydro-* **water,** *-phil-* **love,** *-ic* **relating to**]

hydrophobic (hye-droh-FOH-bik)
[*hydro-* **water,** *-phob-* **fear,** *-ic* **relating to**]

lipid (LIP-id)
[*lipi-* **fat,** *-id* **form**]

macromolecule (mak-roh-MOL-eh-kyool)
[*macro-* **large,** *-molec-* **mass,** *-ule* **small**]

continued on p. 71

This survey will serve as a foundation for later explorations in which we will learn how genetic information is stored and retrieved, how cells, tissues, and organs are constructed, how our body stores and retrieves energy, how regulatory signals are sent, how nutrients are obtained and used by the body—and much more. In fact, every remaining chapter of this book will include the activity of some of these large biomolecules.

ORGANIC MOLECULES

The term *organic* is used to describe the enormous number of compounds that contain carbon—specifically C—C or C—H bonds.

Recall that carbon atoms have only four electrons in their outer energy level (see **Figure 3-3**, A); four electrons are required to satisfy the octet rule. As a result, each carbon atom can join with up to four other atoms to form literally thousands of molecules of varying size and shape. Although some organic molecules are small and have only one or two subunits, the large **macromolecules** often have many subunits attached to one another or to other chemical compounds (**Figure 4-1**).

In the human body, the following four major groups of organic substances are very important:

1. Carbohydrates
2. Lipids
3. Proteins
4. Nucleic acids and related molecules

Although most of these large organic molecules are synthesized in the cells of our body, many of the subunits come from the food we eat. In later chapters, we will see how the digestive system breaks large molecules into their component subunits, then absorbs them into the bloodstream to make them available for cells to rebuild into human biomolecules.

Figure 4-1 shows examples of the four major organic substances represented by three-dimensional models. Many macromolecules are composed of basic building blocks, such as glucose or amino acids, that are joined in chains of varying length by covalent bonds.

The term **functional groups** is often used to describe certain arrangements of atoms attached to the carbon core of many organic molecules. Functional groups—also called *radicals*—often go into and out of combination with large organic molecules. Organic radicals are often designated simply as *R*. A **free radical** is a functional group that is temporarily unattached and is highly reactive because of unpaired electrons. Because it is ready to form a covalent bond, it will combine with another molecule within a small fraction of a second after it is free. Different radicals or functional groups confer unique chemical properties. Our later discussions will occasionally involve some of these functional groups. Take a moment now to preview the examples shown in **Figure 4-2**.

CARBOHYDRATES

All **carbohydrate** compounds contain the elements carbon, hydrogen, and oxygen—usually in the ratio of 1 to 2 to 1. The carbon atoms link to one another in chains or rings. Carbohydrates include the substances commonly called *sugars* and *starches.*

Carbohydrates provide the primary source of chemical energy needed by every body cell. In addition, carbohydrates serve a structural role as components of such critically important molecules as RNA and DNA, which are involved in cell reproduction and protein synthesis. These and other functions of carbohydrates are listed in **Table 4-1**.

As a group, carbohydrates are divided into three types or classes that are characterized by the length of their carbon chains. The three types are named as follows:

1. Monosaccharides (simple sugars)
2. Disaccharides (double sugars)
3. Polysaccharides (complex sugars)

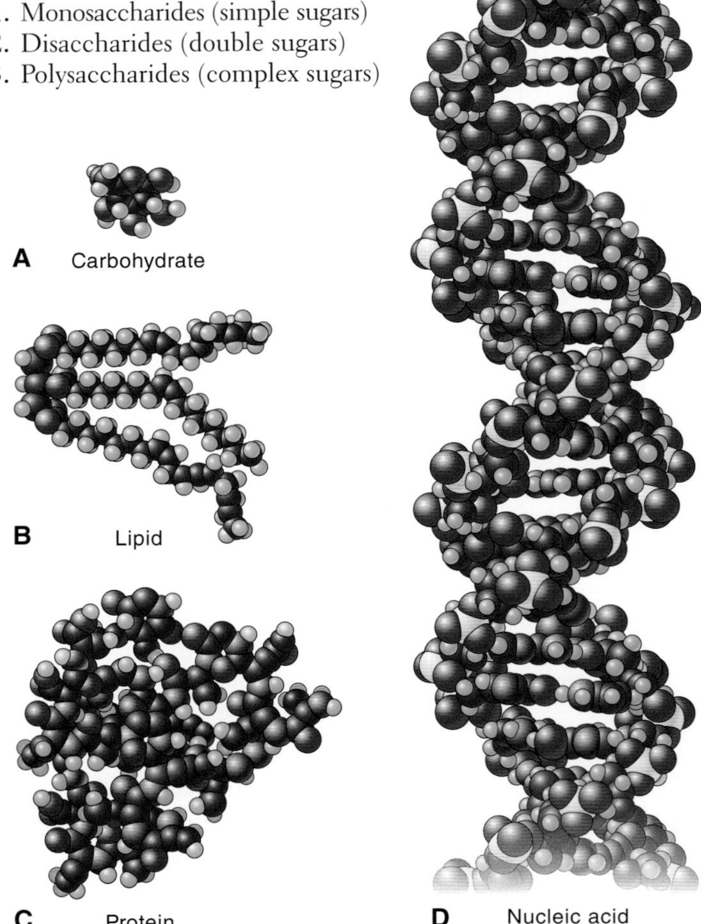

FIGURE 4-1 Important organic molecules. Molecular models showing examples of the four major groups of organic substances: **A,** carbohydrate; **B,** lipid; **C,** protein; **D,** nucleic acid.

Functional Group	Structural Formula	Models
Hydroxyl	–OH	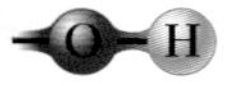
Carbonyl	–C– ‖ O	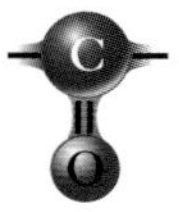
Carboxyl	O // –C \\ OH	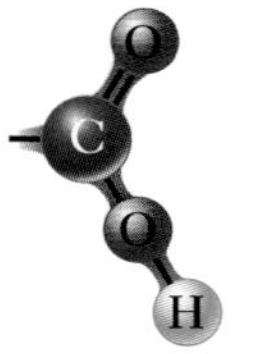
Methyl	H | –C–H | H	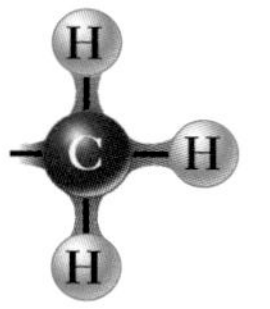
Amino	H / –N \\ H	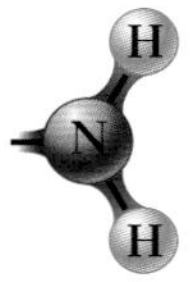
Sulphhydryl	–SH	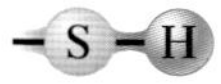
Phosphate	OH | –O–P–OH ‖ O	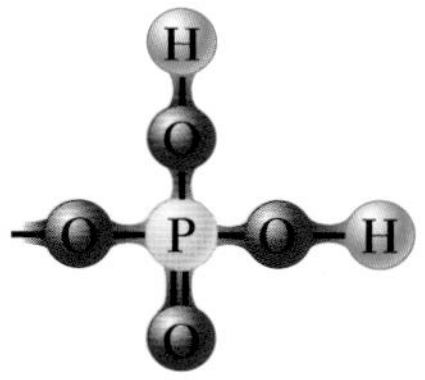
Acetyl	O H ‖ | –C–C–H | H	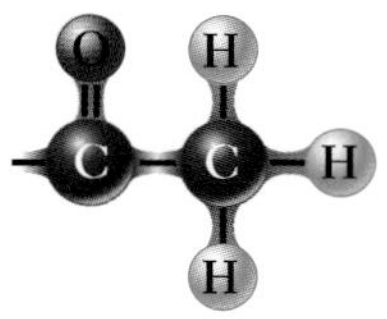

FIGURE 4-2 The principal functional chemical groups. Each functional group or *radical (R)* confers specific chemical properties on the molecules that possess them.

MONOSACCHARIDES

Monosaccharides, or simple sugars, are relatively small carbohydrates. The most important simple sugar is **glucose**. It is a six-carbon sugar with the formula $C_6H_{12}O_6$. The chemical formula indicates that each molecule of glucose contains 6 atoms of carbon, 12 atoms of hydrogen, and 6 atoms of oxygen. Because it has six carbon atoms, it is called a *hexose* (*hexa*, "six"). Glucose is present in the dry state as a *straight chain* but curls into a *cyclic* compound (ring) when dissolved in water. In **Figure 4-3** the straight chain and cyclic arrangements are shown with a three-dimensional model of the molecule. However, it is important to remember that all forms of glucose represented in models or illustrations are the same molecule.

In addition to glucose, other important hexoses, or six-carbon simple sugars, include fructose and galactose. Not all monosaccharides, however, are hexoses. Some are *pentoses* (from *penta*, five), so named because they contain five carbon atoms. *Ribose* and *deoxyribose* are pentose monosaccharides of great importance in the body—they are covered further when we study nucleic acids later in this chapter. Like all monosaccharides, ribose and deoxyribose are simple sugars—but strange sugars in that they are not sweet.

TABLE 4-1 Major Functions of Human Carbohydrate Compounds

FUNCTION	EXAMPLE
Energy	Simple sugars provide the main source of energy for cells; complex carbohydrates may provide temporary energy storage
Molecular structure	Ribose and deoxyribose sugars serve as components of RNA and DNA subunits
Cell membrane components	Sugars on cell membranes may act as signals or identification tags, as in immune system identification of cell types
Extracellular matrix	Carbohydrates make up important functional materials within the substance found between cells of some tissues
Dietary fibre	Carbohydrates that make up plant fibres promote digestive health

DISACCHARIDES AND POLYSACCHARIDES

Substances classified as **disaccharides** (double sugars) or **polysaccharides** (complex sugars) are carbohydrates composed of two or more simple sugars that are bonded together through a dehydration synthesis reaction that involves the removal of water. *Sucrose* (table sugar), *maltose*, and *lactose* are all disaccharides. Each consists of two monosaccharides linked together.

Figure 4-4 shows the formation of sucrose from glucose and fructose. Note that a hydrogen atom from the glucose molecule combines with a hydroxyl group (OH) from the fructose molecule to form water, with an oxygen atom left to bind the two subunits together. Lactose is likewise synthesized from glucose and galactose. Two glucose molecules join to form maltose.

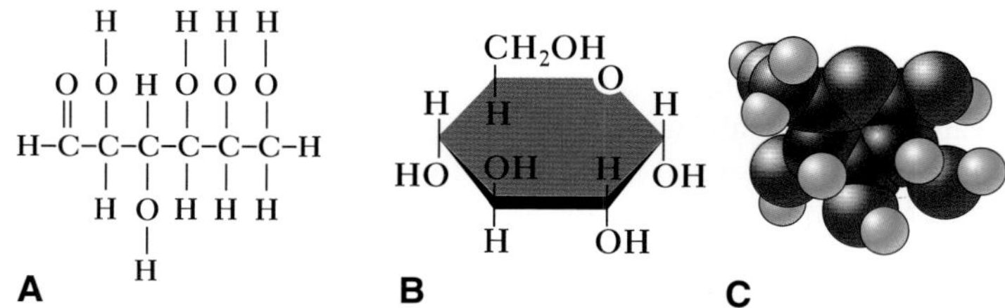

FIGURE 4-3 Structure of glucose. A, Straight chain, or linear model, of glucose. **B,** Ring model representing glucose in solution. **C,** Three-dimensional, or space-filling, model of glucose.

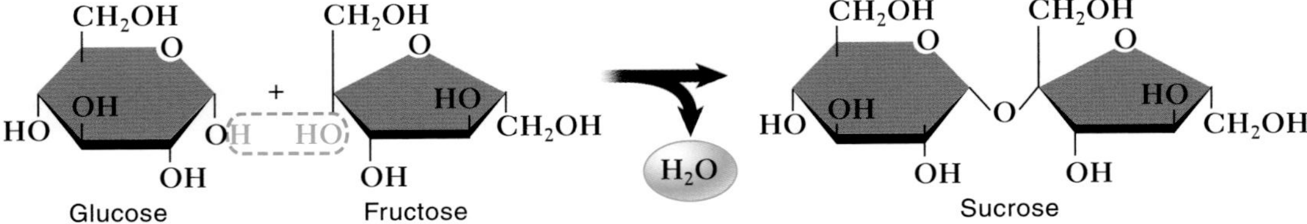

FIGURE 4-4 Formation of sucrose. Glucose and fructose are joined in a synthesis reaction that involves the removal of water.

Polysaccharides consist of many monosaccharides chemically joined to form straight or branched chains. Once again, water is removed as the many monosaccharide subunits are joined. Any large molecule made up of many identical small molecules is called a *polymer.* Polysaccharides are polymers of monosaccharides. **Glycogen,** a polymer of glucose, is sometimes referred to as *animal starch.* It is the main polysaccharide in the body and has an estimated molecular weight of several million—truly a macromolecule.

Quick CHECK

1. List the four major groups of organic substances.
2. Identify the most important monosaccharide, or simple sugar.
3. Identify a carbohydrate polymer and explain how it is formed.

CONNECT IT! 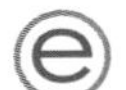

Detecting sugars in our food may be critical for our survival. Review ***Sensing Food*** online at ***Connect It!*** to find out more about how this is part of the ongoing chemical analysis of every bite we take.

LIPIDS

Lipids, according to one definition, are water-insoluble organic biomolecules. Lipids ordinarily do not dissolve in water because lipid molecules are generally **nonpolar.** Because electrons are shared equally within a molecule, there are no partially charged regions and thus lipids do not cling to the partially charged areas of the polar water molecules. Although insoluble in water, most lipids, many with an oil-like consistency and greasy feel, dissolve readily in some organic solvents such as ether, alcohol, or benzene.

Like the carbohydrates, lipids are composed largely of carbon, hydrogen, and oxygen. However, the proportion of oxygen in lipids is much lower than that in carbohydrates. Many lipids also contain other elements such as nitrogen and phosphorus. As a group, lipids include a large assortment of compounds that have been classified in several ways. Classification of lipids includes triglycerides or fats, phospholipids, steroids, and prostaglandins (PGs).

Lipids are critically important biological compounds and have several major roles in the body (**Table 4-2**). Many are used for energy purposes, whereas others serve a structural role and function as integral parts of cell membranes. Other important lipid compounds serve as vitamins or protect vital organs by serving as "fat pads", or shock absorbers, in certain body areas. One type of lipid material actually serves as "insulator material" around nerves, thus serving to prevent "short circuits" and speed nervous impulse transmissions.

TABLE 4-2 Major Functions of Human Lipid Compounds

FUNCTION	EXAMPLE
Energy	Lipids can be stored and broken down later for energy; they yield more energy per unit of weight than carbohydrates or proteins do
Structure	Phospholipids and cholesterol are required components of cell membranes
Vitamins	Lipid-soluble vitamins: vitamin A forms retinal (necessary for night vision); vitamin D increases calcium uptake; vitamin E promotes wound healing; and vitamin K is required for the synthesis of blood-clotting proteins
Protection	Fatty tissue surrounds and protects organs
Insulation	Fatty tissue under the skin minimizes heat loss; lipid tissue (containing myelin) covers nerve cells and electrically insulates them
Regulation	Steroid hormones regulate many physiological processes; for example, oestrogen and testosterone are responsible for many of the differences between females and males; prostaglandins help regulate inflammation and tissue repair; some phospholipids regulate cell functions

TRIGLYCERIDES OR FATS

Triglycerides (triacylglycerols), or fats, are the most abundant lipids, and they function as the body's most concentrated source of energy. Two types of building blocks are needed to synthesize or build a fat molecule: **glycerol** and **fatty acids.** Each glycerol unit is joined to three fatty acids, and the glycerol building block is the same in each fat molecule. Therefore, it is the specific type of fatty acid molecule or component that identifies and determines the chemical nature of any fat.

Types of Fatty Acids

Fatty acids vary in the length of their carbon chains (number of carbon atoms) and in the number of hydrogen atoms that are attached to, or "saturate", the available bonds around each carbon in the chain. Naturally occurring fatty acids have an even number of carbons, usually numbering between 12 and 18. **Figure 4-5** shows a structural formula and three-dimensional model for a saturated (palmitic) and unsaturated (linolenic) fatty acid.

By definition, a *saturated fatty acid* is one in which all available bonds of its hydrocarbon chain are filled—that is, saturated—with hydrogen atoms. The chain contains no double bonds (**Figure 4-5**, *A*). In contrast, an *unsaturated fatty acid* has one or more double bonds in its hydrocarbon chain because not all the chain's carbon atoms are saturated with hydrogen atoms. Looking at **Figure 4-5**, *B*, you can easily see that some of the hydrogens are missing from the carbon backbone of the unsaturated fatty acid.

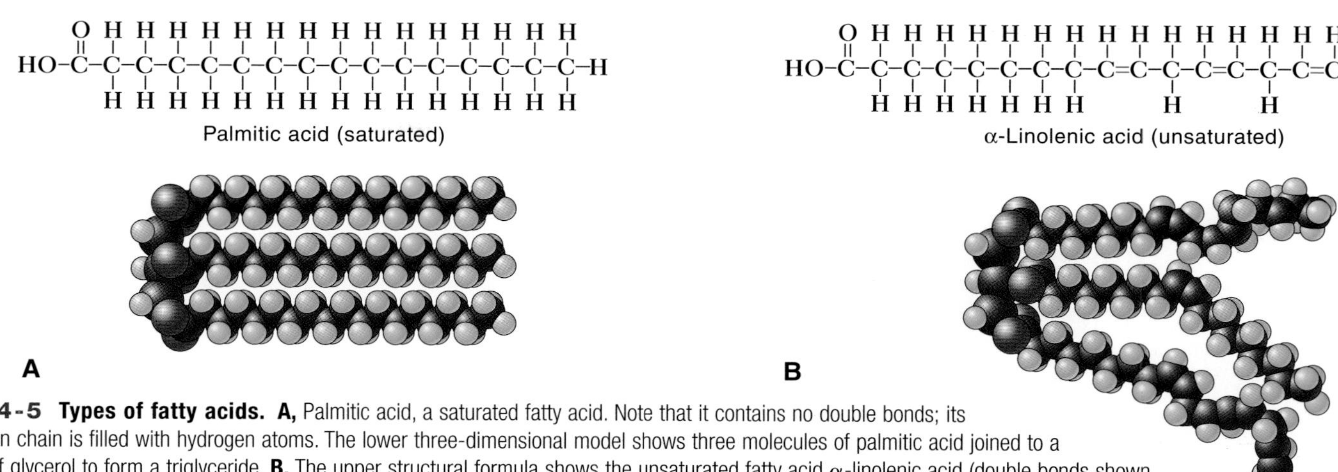

FIGURE 4-5 Types of fatty acids. A, Palmitic acid, a saturated fatty acid. Note that it contains no double bonds; its hydrocarbon chain is filled with hydrogen atoms. The lower three-dimensional model shows three molecules of palmitic acid joined to a molecule of glycerol to form a triglyceride. **B,** The upper structural formula shows the unsaturated fatty acid α-linolenic acid (double bonds shown in *red*). The lower three-dimensional model shows triglyceride exhibiting "kinks" caused by the presence of double bonds in the component fatty acids.

Monounsaturated fatty acids have only one double carbon bond in their chain and *polyunsaturated* fatty acids have more than one double bond.

The degree of saturation is the most important factor in determining the physical and chemical properties of fatty acids. For example, animal fats such as tallow and lard are solids at room temperature, whereas vegetable oils are typically liquids. The difference lies in the extent of unsaturation—animal fats are mostly saturated, whereas most vegetable oils are not. Note in **Figure 4-5**, *B*, that the presence of double bonds in a fatty acid molecule will cause the chain to kink or bend.

Fats become more oily and liquid as the number of unsaturated double bonds increases. The kinks and bends in the unsaturated molecules keep them from fitting closely together. In contrast, the lack of kinks in saturated fatty acids allows the molecules to fit tightly together to form a solid mass at higher temperatures.

Formation of Triglycerides

Figure 4-6 shows the formation of a triglyceride. Its name, *glycerol tricaproate*, suggests that it contains three molecules of the six-carbon fatty acid *caproic acid* attached to a glycerol molecule. Note that the three caproic acid building blocks attach by their carboxyl groups (COOH) to the three hydroxyl groups (OH) of the glycerol molecule to form the triglyceride and three molecules of water. The process is one you are now familiar with—it is a dehydration synthesis reaction. Keep in mind that although some fats, such as glycerol tricaproate, contain three molecules of the same fatty acid, others may have two or three different fatty acids attached to glycerol. Caproic acid is considered to be a *short-chain* fatty acid; some triglycerides contain fatty acids with a carbon backbone several times longer, thus forming *long-chain* fatty acids.

Phospholipids

Phospholipids are lipid compounds similar to triglycerides. They are modified, however, in that one of the three fatty acids attached to glycerol in a triglyceride is replaced in a phospholipid by another type of chemical structure containing phosphorus and nitrogen. The structural formula of a phospholipid is shown in **Figure 4-7**. Observe that the phospholipid molecule contains glycerol. Joined to the glycerol at one end of the molecule are two fatty acids. Attached to glycerol but extending in the opposite direction is the phosphate group, which is attached to a nitrogen-containing compound.

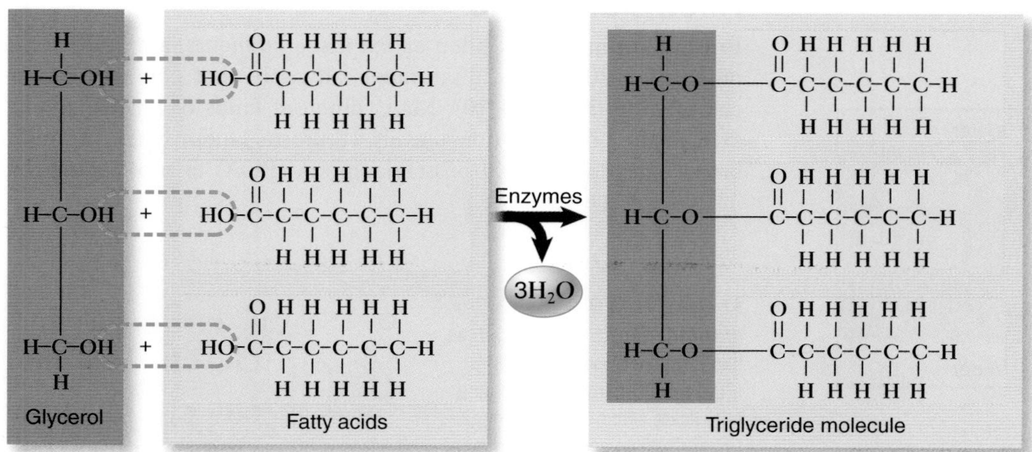

FIGURE 4-6 Formation of triglyceride. Glycerol tricaproate is a composite molecule made up of three molecules of caproic acid (a six-carbon fatty acid) coupled in a dehydration synthesis reaction to a single glycerol backbone. In addition to the triglyceride, this process results in the formation of three molecules of water.

The head, or end of the molecule containing the phosphorus group, in a phospholipid molecule is polar and is therefore water soluble. The term **hydrophilic,** meaning "water loving", also applies to the phospholipid head. The end formed by the two fatty acids is nonpolar and is therefore lipid soluble or **hydrophobic** ("water fearing"). This unique property means that phospholipid molecules can bridge, or join, two different chemical environments—a water environment on one side and a lipid environment on the other. Thus in water they often form bilayers (double layers) with the fatty tails facing toward one another and the heads forming sheets that face the water on

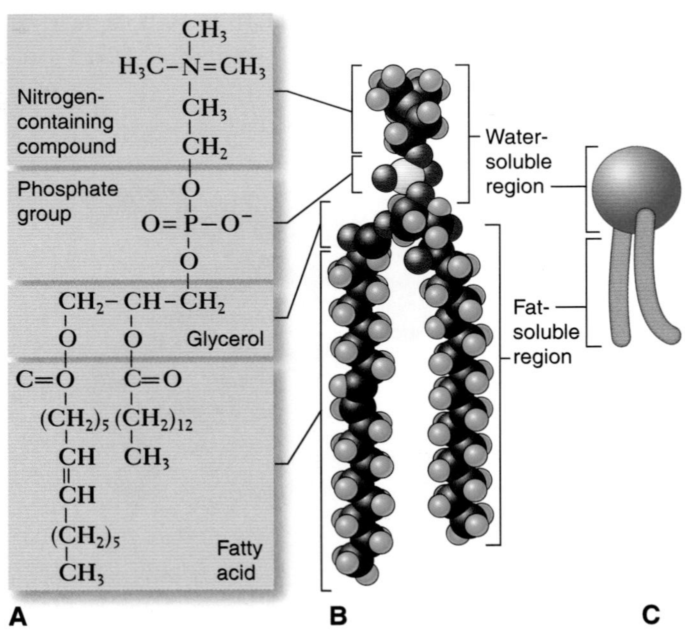

FIGURE 4-7 Phospholipid molecule. A, Chemical formula of a phospholipid molecule. **B,** Molecular model showing water- and lipid-soluble regions. **C,** Cartoon often used to represent the double-tailed phospholipid molecule.

either side of the bilayer (**Figure 4-8**). For this reason, phospholipids are a primary component of cell membranes (which are bilayers); they are discussed further in Chapter 5.

A small number of phospholipids in each cell of the body play a completely different role: they are regulatory molecules. Called *phosphoinositides (PIs)*, these phospholipids have a huge impact on the complex functions of the cell. Malfunctions of PIs are sometimes involved in causing cancer, obesity, infections, and other diseases.

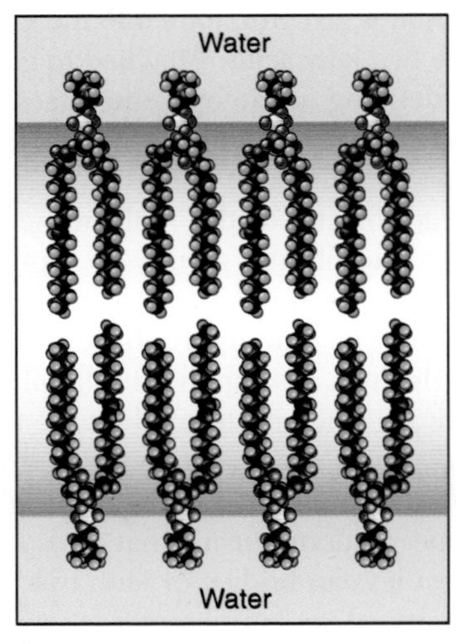

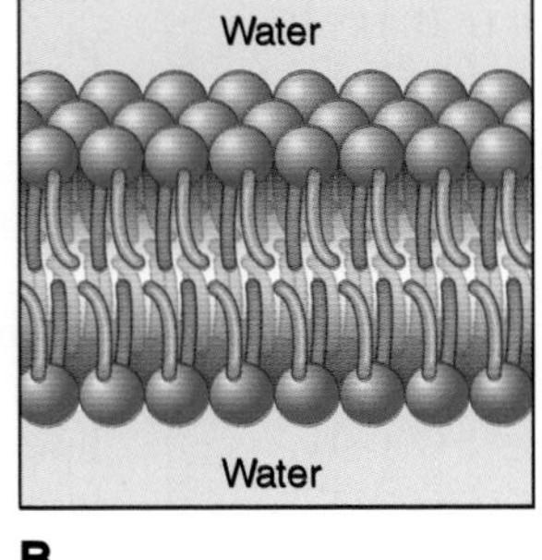

FIGURE 4-8 Phospholipid bilayer. A, Orientation of phospholipid molecules when surrounded by water and forming a bilayer. **B,** Cartoon commonly used to depict a phospholipid bilayer.

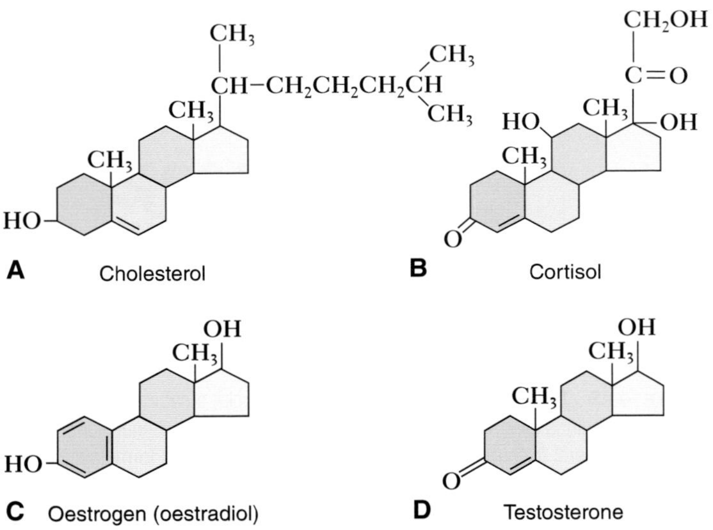

A Cholesterol

B Cortisol

C Oestrogen (oestradiol)

D Testosterone

FIGURE 4-9 Steroid compounds. The steroid nucleus—highlighted in *yellow*—found in cholesterol **(A)** forms the basis for many other important compounds such as cortisol **(B)**, oestradiol (an oestrogen) **(C)**, and testosterone **(D)**.

Steroids

Steroids are a large and important class of lipids whose molecules have as their main feature the *steroid nucleus* (**Figure 4-9**). The steroid nucleus is composed of four attached rings that are structurally similar but may have widely diverse functions related to the differing functional groups that are attached to them.

Steroids, some of which are called *sterols*, are widely distributed in the body and are involved in many important structural and functional roles. **Cholesterol** is a steroid found in the plasma membrane surrounding every body cell (see Chapter 5 and **Box 4-1**). Its presence helps stabilize this important cellular structure and is required for many reactions that cells must perform to survive. In addition, the body slightly modifies cholesterol molecules to form such important hormones as cortisone, oestrogen, and testosterone. It is also used to make the bile salts needed for digestion. The steroid nucleus is also a part of the active hormone form of vitamin D called *calcitriol*.

Prostaglandins

Prostaglandins (PGs), often called *tissue hormones*, are lipids composed of a 20-carbon unsaturated fatty acid that contains a five-carbon ring (**Figure 4-10**). Many different kinds of prostaglandins exist in the body. We now classify 16 prostaglandin types into nine broad categories, called prostaglandin A (PGA) to prostaglandin I

FIGURE 4-10 Prostaglandin. Prostaglandins such as this example of prostaglandin E (PGE) are 20-carbon unsaturated fatty acids with a 5-carbon ring. Prostaglandins act as local regulators in the body.

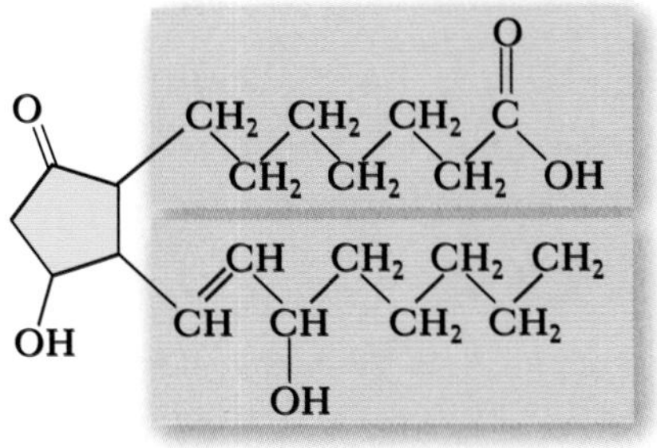

BOX 4-1 *health matters* | **Blood Lipoproteins**

A lipid such as cholesterol can travel in the blood only after it has attached to a protein molecule—forming a lipoprotein. Some of these molecules are called *high-density lipoproteins (HDLs)* because they have a higher proportion of dense protein than low-density cholesterol. Another type of molecule contains less protein than cholesterol, so it is called *low-density lipoprotein* (LDL). The composite nature of a lipoprotein molecule is shown in the figure.

The cholesterol in LDLs is often called "bad" cholesterol because high blood levels of LDL are associated with *atherosclerosis,* a life-threatening blockage of arteries. LDLs carry cholesterol to cells, including the cells that line blood vessels. HDLs, on the other hand, carry so-called "good" cholesterol *away from cells* and toward the liver for elimination from the body. A low proportion of LDL in the blood is associated with a low risk for atherosclerosis. •

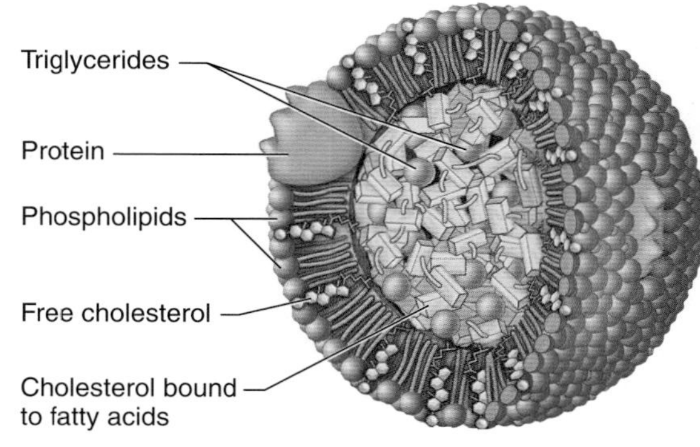

(PGI). Each major grouping of prostaglandins can be further subdivided according to chemical structure and function.

Prostaglandins were first associated with prostate tissue and were named accordingly. Subsequent discoveries, however, have shown that these biologically powerful chemical substances are produced by cell membranes located in almost every body tissue. They are formed and then released from cell membranes in response to a particular stimulus. Once released, they have a very local effect and are then inactivated.

The effects of prostaglandins in the body are many and varied. They play a crucial role in regulating the effects of several hormones, influence blood pressure and the secretion of digestive juices, enhance the body's immune system and inflammatory response (**Box 4-2**), and have an important role in blood clotting and respiration, to name a few. The use of prostaglandins and prostaglandin inhibitors as drugs is an exciting and rapidly growing area in clinical medicine.

We discuss the regulatory roles of prostaglandins and related compounds in Chapter 25, as we explore the hormonal regulation of body function.

Quick **CHECK**

4. What are the building blocks of a triglyceride, or fat?
5. What is a phospholipid, and why is it an important type of molecule?
6. Identify the important steroid that stabilizes cellular structure.

PROTEINS

All **proteins** have four elements: carbon, oxygen, hydrogen, and nitrogen. Many proteins also contain small amounts of sulphur, iron, magnesium, zinc, and other trace metals. Some also contain phosphorus. Proteins (from word parts meaning "first-rank substance") are the most abundant of the organic compounds in the body. As their name implies, their functions are of first-rank importance. Protein molecules are among the giant macromolecules, along with many of the polysaccharides and nucleic acids.

The many roles played by proteins in the body can be divided into two broad categories: *structural* and *functional.* Structural proteins form the structure of the cells, tissues, and organs of the body. Various unique shapes and compositions such as flexible strands, elastic strands, and waterproof layers allow structural proteins to form the

BOX 4-2 *fyi* | **Aspirin and Prostaglandins**

In the presence of an appropriate stimulus such as irritation or injury, fatty acids required for prostaglandin synthesis are released by cell membranes. If a specific type of enzyme, *cyclooxygenase (COX),* is present to interact with these fatty acids, prostaglandins will be synthesized and released from the cell membrane into the surrounding tissue fluid.

Prostaglandins sometimes serve as inflammatory agents. They cause local dilation of blood vessels with resulting heat (fever), swelling, redness, and pain. Aspirin (acetylsalicylic acid [ASA]) is a *COX inhibitor* and thus works to relieve these symptoms by blocking the activity of the COX-1 and COX-2 enzymes. If these enzymes cannot function properly, prostaglandin synthesis will be inhibited and symptoms will be relieved.

Prostaglandins sometimes serve to regulate blood clotting. Again, aspirin can inhibit prostaglandin synthesis and play a therapeutic role in preventing abnormal blood clots or reducing abnormal clots that have already begun forming. For this reason, some people at risk for a heart attack triggered by abnormal blood clots are advised to take daily low-dose aspirin to reduce the formation of abnormal clots. If a heart attack has already begun, full-dose aspirin taken immediately may stop the clotting and thus increase a person's chances of surviving the episode by about 25%.

The functions of prostaglandins and the actions of other COX enzyme inhibitors are discussed further in Chapter 25. •

Aspirin. Acetylsalicylic acid (aspirin) is a commonly used cyclooxygenase (COX) inhibitor that reduces prostaglandin effects in the body such as inflammation, fever, and blood clotting.

FIGURE 4-11 Basic structural formula for an amino acid. Note relationship of the functional or radical group (R), amino group, and carboxyl group to the alpha carbon. The amino group (NH_2) is depicted in the figure as H_2N to show that the *nitrogen* atom of the group bonds to the alpha carbon.

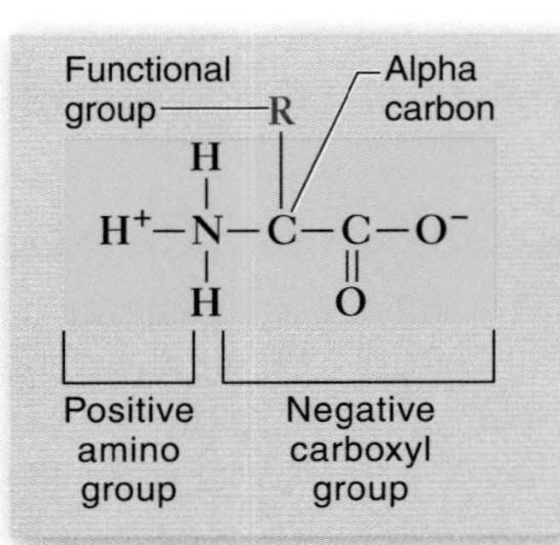

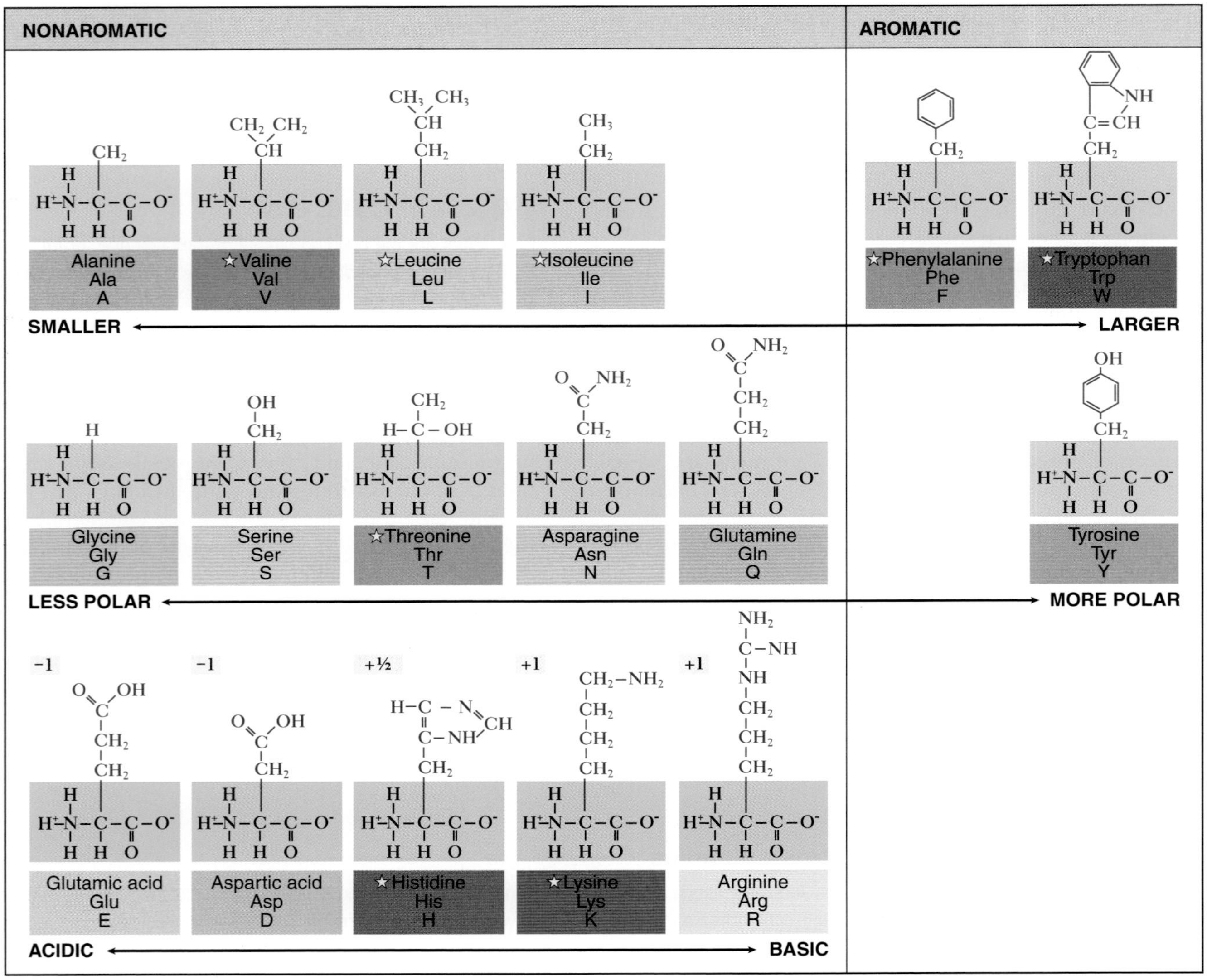

	NONAROMATIC					AROMATIC	
NONPOLAR	Alanine Ala A	☆Valine Val V	☆Leucine Leu L	☆Isoleucine Ile I		☆Phenylalanine Phe F	☆Tryptophan Trp W
	SMALLER ←						→ LARGER
POLAR UNCHARGED	Glycine Gly G	Serine Ser S	☆Threonine Thr T	Asparagine Asn N	Glutamine Gln Q		Tyrosine Tyr Y
	LESS POLAR ←						→ MORE POLAR
IONIZABLE	-1 Glutamic acid Glu E	-1 Aspartic acid Asp D	+½ ☆Histidine His H	+1 ☆Lysine Lys K	+1 Arginine Arg R		
	ACIDIC ←				→ BASIC		

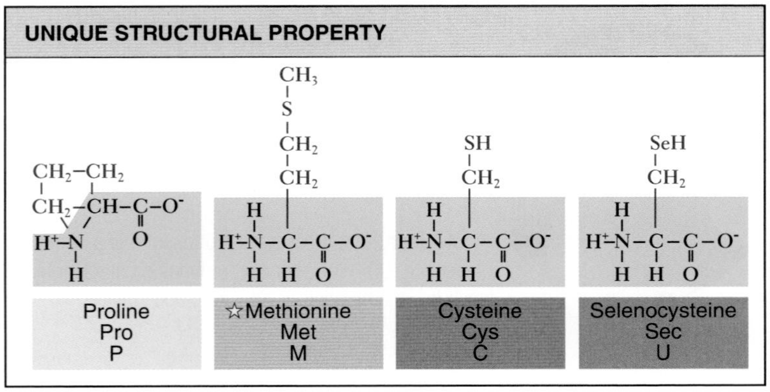

UNIQUE STRUCTURAL PROPERTY			
Proline Pro P	☆Methionine Met M	Cysteine Cys C	Selenocysteine Sec U

FIGURE 4-12 The standard amino acids of the human body. The full name for each is given, followed by the three-letter abbreviation and the one-letter symbol. The structural formulas show that each amino acid has the same chemical backbone *(green highlight)* but differs from the others in the functional group or radical (R) that it possesses *(red)*. Essential amino acids are indicated by a star preceding the name. Notice the great variety of sizes among the amino acids, the different polarities or charges, the different levels of acidity, and the other differing chemical characteristics. Like different kinds of blocks in a set of toy blocks, this makes it possible to build different proteins with a wide variety of chemical characteristics and functions. (Additional types of amino acids may be added to proteins after their initial structure is formed.)

many different building blocks of the body. Functional proteins are chemists. The unique shape of each functional protein allows it to fit with certain other chemicals and cause some change in the molecules. For example, **enzymes** are functional proteins that bring molecules together or split them apart in chemical reactions. Protein hormones such as insulin trigger chemical changes in cells to produce the hormone's effects.

It is the *shape* or conformation of a protein that determines how it performs. The main principle in understanding how proteins work is that form and function go hand in hand—the right shape for the right job.

Compared with water with a total mass number of 18, giant protein molecules may have a total mass number of several million! However, all protein molecules, regardless of size, have a similar basic structure. They are chainlike polymers composed of multiple subunits, or building blocks, linked end to end. The building blocks of all proteins are called *amino acids.*

Amino Acids

The elements that make up a protein molecule are bonded together to form chemical units called **amino acids.** Proteins are composed of 21 naturally occurring amino acids, and nearly all of the 21 amino acids are usually present in every protein. Of these 21, 8 are known as *essential amino acids.* They cannot be produced by the body and must be included in the adult diet. The 13 remaining *nonessential amino acids* can be produced from other amino acids or from simple organic molecules readily available to the body cells.

CONNECT IT!

Some scientists state that there are 20 amino acids making up proteins, and others 21 or 22. Why is this? Find out in ***Amazing Amino Acids*** online at ***Connect It!***

The basic structural formula for an amino acid is shown in **Figure 4-11**. As you can see, it consists of a *carbon atom* (called the *alpha* carbon) to which are bonded a positive *amino group* (NH_3^+), a negative *carboxyl group* (COO^-), a *hydrogen atom,* and a *functional group* or *radical (R).* It is this functional group that constitutes the unique, identifying part of an amino acid.

The 21 amino acids that make up most human proteins are shown in **Figure 4-12**. You can see that each individual amino acid has its own chemical nature because of its unique functional group. Some are more acidic, some more basic. Some tend to ionize and thus have an electric charge. Others have regions of different partial charges and are therefore polar. On the other hand, some amino acids tend to be nonpolar. Some are large and some are small. Individual amino acids are often compared with the letters of the alphabet. Just as combinations of individual letters form word combinations, different amino acids form protein chains. Think of amino acids as the alphabet of proteins.

The ability of amino acids to "link up" in all possible combinations allows the body to build or synthesize an almost infinite variety of different protein "words" or chains that may contain a dozen, several hundred, or even thousands of amino acids. Each of these chains can have different regions with different chemical characteristics.

Amino acids often become joined by peptide bonds. A **peptide bond** is one that binds the carboxyl group of one amino acid to the amino group of another amino acid. O from the negative carboxyl group of one amino acid and two H atoms from the positive amino group of another amino acid split off to form water plus a new compound called a *peptide.* A peptide made up of only two amino acids linked by a peptide bond is a *dipeptide.* A *tripeptide* consists of three amino acids linked by two bonds. The linkage of four amino acids by these peptide bonds is shown in **Figure 4-13**, A. A long sequence or chain of amino acids—usually 100 or more—linked by peptide

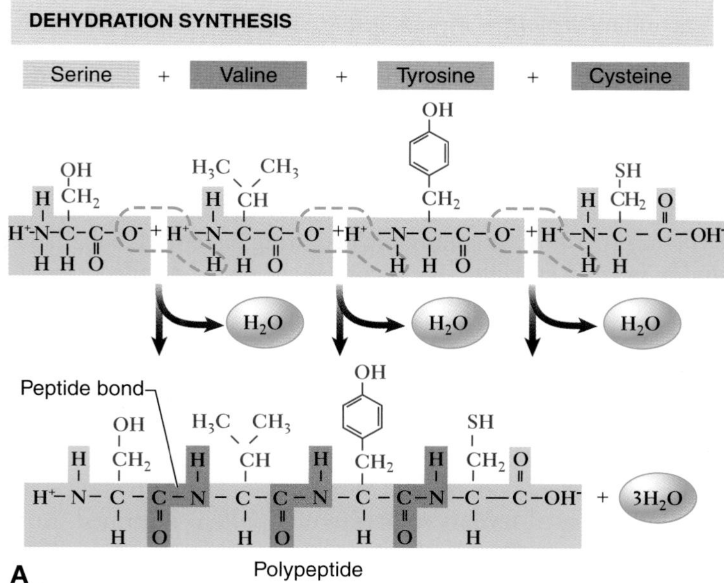

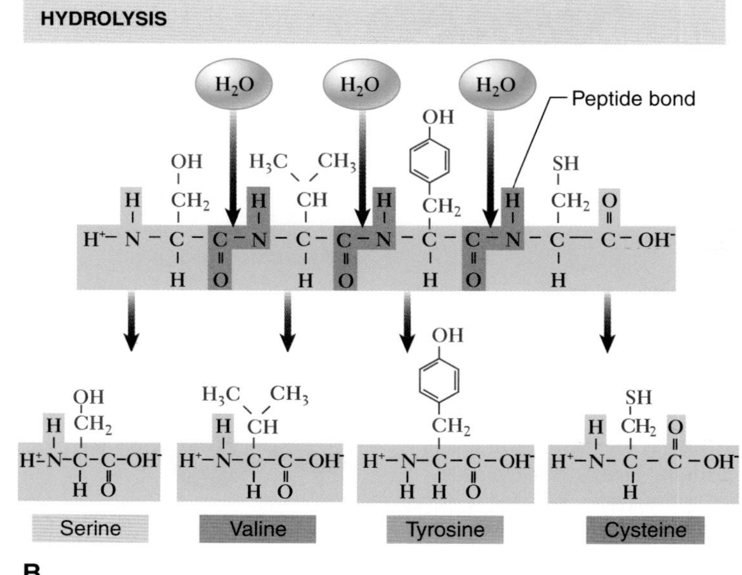

FIGURE 4-13 Formation (dehydration synthesis) and decomposition (hydrolysis) of a polypeptide. A, Linkage of four amino acids by three peptide bonds resulting in the dehydration synthesis of a polypeptide chain and three molecules of water. **B,** Decomposition (hydrolysis) reaction resulting from the addition of three molecules of water. Peptide bonds are broken and individual amino acids are released.

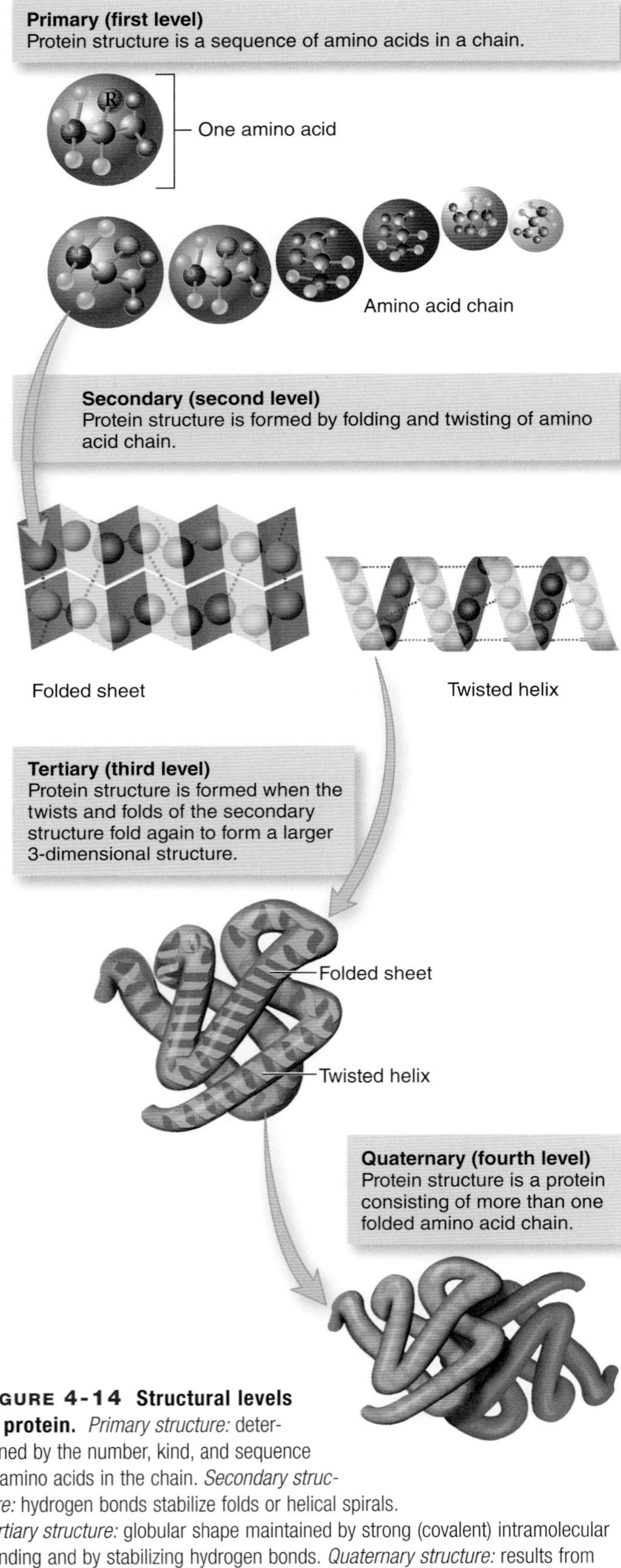
Primary (first level)
Protein structure is a sequence of amino acids in a chain.
One amino acid
Amino acid chain
Secondary (second level)
Protein structure is formed by folding and twisting of amino acid chain.
Folded sheet
Twisted helix
Tertiary (third level)
Protein structure is formed when the twists and folds of the secondary structure fold again to form a larger 3-dimensional structure.
Folded sheet
Twisted helix
Quaternary (fourth level)
Protein structure is a protein consisting of more than one folded amino acid chain.

FIGURE 4-14 Structural levels of protein. *Primary structure:* determined by the number, kind, and sequence of amino acids in the chain. *Secondary structure:* hydrogen bonds stabilize folds or helical spirals. *Tertiary structure:* globular shape maintained by strong (covalent) intramolecular bonding and by stabilizing hydrogen bonds. *Quaternary structure:* results from bonding between more than one polypeptide unit.

bonds constitutes a *polypeptide*. When the length of the polymer chain exceeds about 100 amino acids, the molecule is called a *protein* rather than a polypeptide.

Do you see a similarity between the formation of a polysaccharide, such as glycogen, from simple sugar "building blocks" and the formation of a polypeptide from amino acid building blocks? In both processes, many subunits are joined together, resulting in the loss of water molecules. Thus both are examples of the *condensation* or *dehydration synthesis* reactions that are very common in living organisms. A decomposition reaction called *hydrolysis* requires the addition of a water molecule to break a bond. During hydrolysis of a peptide chain, the peptide linkages between adjacent amino acids in the sequence are broken by the addition of water, and individual amino acids are released (**Figure 4-13**, *B*).

Levels of Protein Structure

Biochemists often describe four levels of increasing complexity in protein organization:

1. Primary (first level)
2. Secondary (second level)
3. Tertiary (third level)
4. Quaternary (fourth level)

These four levels of protein structure are illustrated in **Figure 4-14**.

Primary Protein Structure

The **primary structure** of a protein refers simply to the number, kind, and sequence of amino acids that make up the polypeptide chain. The hormone of the human parathyroid gland, parathyroid hormone (PTH), is a protein that retains its primary structure—it is a noodle-like molecule consisting of only one polypeptide chain of 84 amino acids.

Secondary Protein Structure

Most polypeptides do not exist as a straight chain. Instead, they show a **secondary structure** in which the chains are coiled or bent into pleated sheets. The most common type of coil takes a clockwise direction and is called an alpha helix. In this type of secondary structure, the coils of the protein chain resemble a spiral staircase, with the coils stabilized by hydrogen bonds between successive turns of the spiral. Pleated beta sheets are likewise stabilized by hydrogen bonds. This stabilizing function of hydrogen bonding in protein structure is critical. A commonly occurring pattern of alpha helices and/or beta sheets within the secondary structure is called a *motif*. A motif often imparts a specific function to each protein in which it appears.

Tertiary Protein Structure

Just as a primary structure polypeptide chain can pleat or bend into a helical secondary structure, so too can a secondary structure protein chain undergo other contortions and be further twisted so that a globular-shaped **tertiary structure** of a protein is formed. In this structure, the polypeptide chain is so twisted that its coils touch one another in many places, and "spot welds", or interlocking connections, occur. Some of these linkages may be strong covalent bonds between amino acid units that exist in the same chain (**Box 4-3**).

BOX 4-3 *fyi* | Disulphide Linkages

Hair contains a threadlike fibrous protein called *keratin* that is rich in the sulphur-containing amino acid cysteine. The protein chains in keratin are linked in numerous places by S—S bonds that form between cysteines within each hair shaft. These bonds are called *disulphide linkages.*

The object of a "permanent wave" is to change the arrangement of these bonds by breaking the naturally occurring disulphide linkages and then causing them to reform in another pattern. Strong chemicals are applied to the hair that break the existing or "natural" disulphide linkages. The hair is then curled on some type of roller and then another chemical is applied that causes the disulphide bridges to become reestablished in the new or reoriented configuration. •

Disulphide linkage. The yellow highlighted area shows a disulphide linkage in a folded protein. Other forces maintaining the folded protein structure are also shown.

Most of the linkages are ionic bonds. Hydrogen bonds and other weak attractions also help stabilize the twisted and convoluted loops of the structure. A tertiary structure may include several complicated "knots" called *domains*. Each specific type of domain has specific functions that contribute to the overall function of a protein.

The red muscle protein myoglobin, which is discussed in Chapter 17, is an example of a protein with a tertiary structure.

Quaternary Protein Structure

A **quaternary structure** protein is one that contains clusters of more than one polypeptide chain, all linked together into one giant molecule. Antibody molecules that protect us from disease (see Chapter 33) and haemoglobin molecules in red blood cells (see Chapter 27) are examples.

A group of proteins called *chaperones*, which are present in every body cell, acts to direct the steps required for many proteins to fold into the twisted and convoluted shape required for them to function properly (**Box 4-4**). Some of these chaperone proteins are called *chaperonins*. Inappropriate folding of some proteins is known to be associated with certain diseases.

The critically important chemical reactions that permit chaperonins to organize proteins into the different organizational levels required for a particular function can occur only within a very narrow pH range. Maintaining acid–base balance and normal pH in body cells and fluids is discussed in depth in Chapter 44.

Importance of Protein Shape

Properly folded protein molecules are highly organized in their structure and show a very definite relationship between their shape and their function. The final, functioning shape for a protein is often called its *native state*. The native states of the strong **structural proteins** found in tendons and ligaments are fibrous, or threadlike, insoluble, and very stable (**Figure 4-15**). In contrast, **functional proteins** such as enzymes, certain protein hormones, antibodies, albumin, and haemoglobin have native states that are globular (ball shaped), often soluble, and have chemically reactive regions. **Table 4-3** summarizes some of the important roles played by proteins.

Simply stated, proteins perform their roles by having the right shape for their job—whatever that job is. Given the nearly infinite variety of different amino acid sequences and the complexity of how proteins are folded, you can see that the body can make just about any tool or building block it needs for a variety of jobs. Consider also that if one of the body's proteins loses its shape, or **denatures**, it will lose its function (**Figure 4-16**). Factors that can cause a protein to denature include changes in temperature, changes in pH, radiation,

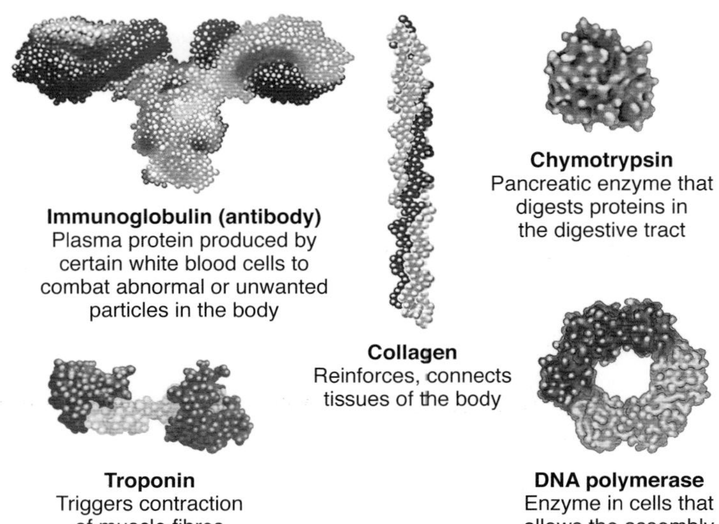
Immunoglobulin (antibody)
Plasma protein produced by certain white blood cells to combat abnormal or unwanted particles in the body
Chymotrypsin
Pancreatic enzyme that digests proteins in the digestive tract
Collagen
Reinforces, connects tissues of the body
Troponin
Triggers contraction of muscle fibres
DNA polymerase
Enzyme in cells that allows the assembly of DNA strands

FIGURE 4-15 Variety of protein shapes. These images of folded protein structures provide examples of the wide variety of shapes that proteins have in the human body.

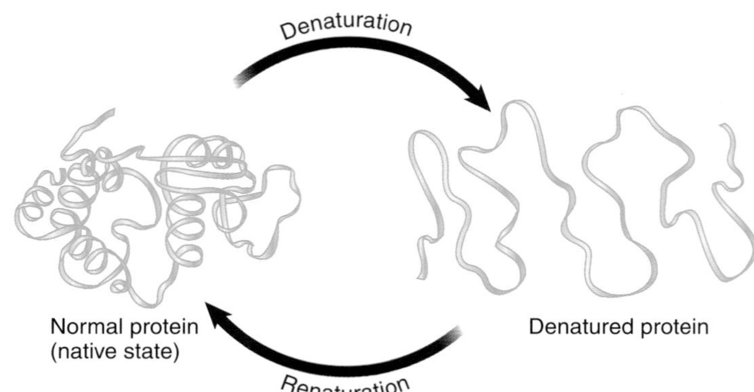

FIGURE 4-16 Denatured protein. When a protein loses its normal folded organization and thus loses its functional shape, it is called a *denatured protein.* Denatured proteins are not able to function normally. However, if the protein shape is restored, the *renatured protein* may resume its normal function.

and the presence of certain hazardous chemicals. Depending on the circumstances, restoring the proper chemical environment of a protein may allow it to *renature* to its native state and begin functioning normally once again.

One last thing to remember about protein shape is that it is often dynamic—that is, proteins often move as they perform their functions. Besides the occasional bend or twist, many proteins have moving parts that resemble hinges, spinning rotors, and grabbing pinchers that permit proteins to move in interesting and useful ways—as you shall see in later chapters.

CONNECT IT!

If a protein is built incorrectly or it denatures, its shape is abnormal and the whole body may be in peril. For an example of a genetic disorder caused by such abnormal proteins, check out ***Phenylketonuria (PKU)*** online at ***Connect It!***

BOX 4-4 *fyi* Visualizing Proteins

Only a few decades ago, the usual way for a biochemist to demonstrate the three-dimensional structure of a protein molecule was by building wooden ball-and-stick models. These models were less than ideal because they took a long time to build, often fell apart, and were not easy to handle. Now there are many sophisticated, but easy-to-use, computer programs that can "build" protein molecules on the monitor screen. These *virtual protein molecules* can be rotated and viewed from nearly any angle. They can also be changed when trying to design a new protein molecule for therapeutic or other purposes. Here, three common types of protein models are shown. The *ribbon model* shows the areas where alpha helices and folded sheets form within the molecule. The *space-filling model* shows each atom as a "cloud" filling up the space occupied by that atom. The *surface-rendering model* shows the three-dimensional boundaries of the whole protein molecule and often colour-coding for charged regions on the surface of the protein. •

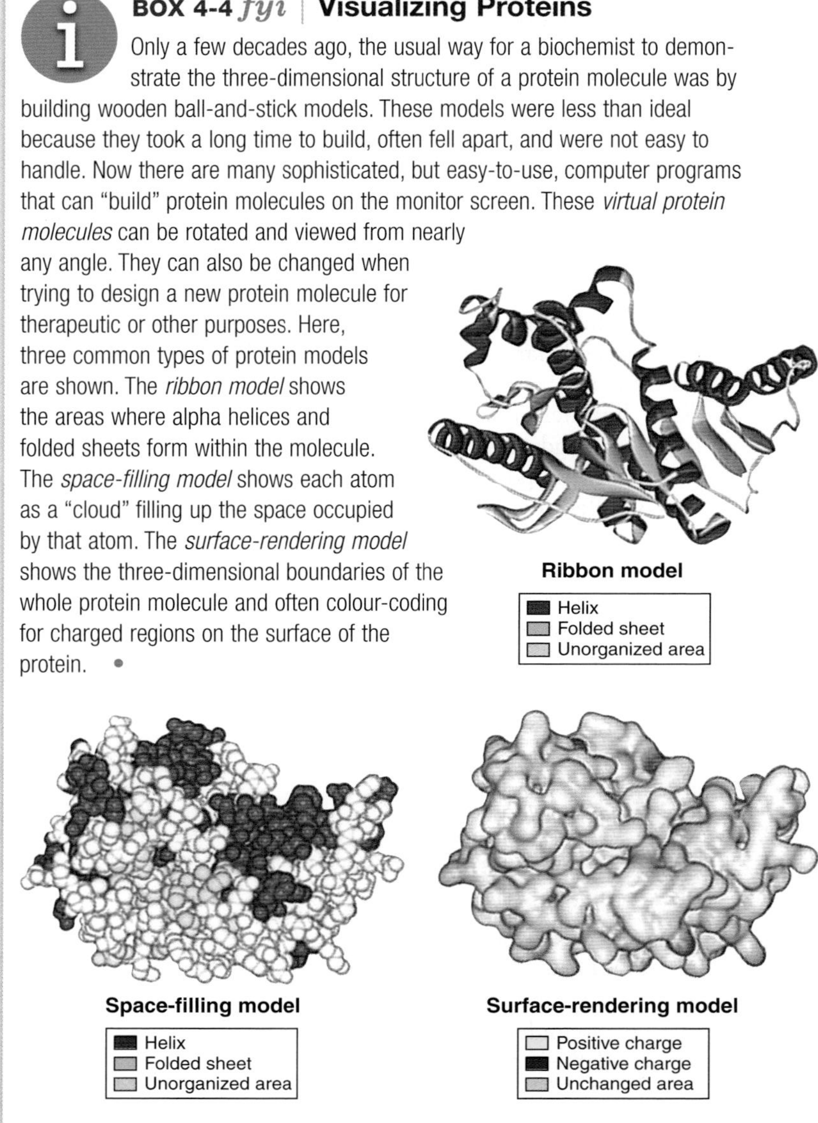

TABLE 4-3 Major Functions of Human Protein Compounds

FUNCTION	EXAMPLE
Provide structure	Structural proteins include keratin of skin, hair, and nails; parts of cell membranes; tendons
Catalyze chemical reactions	Lactase (enzyme in intestinal digestive juice) catalyzes chemical reaction that changes lactose to glucose and galactose
Transport substances in blood	Proteins classified as albumins combine with fatty acids to transport them in the form of lipoproteins
Communicate information to cells	Insulin, a protein hormone, serves as a chemical messenger from islet cells of the pancreas to cells all over the body
Act as receptors	Binding sites of certain proteins on surfaces of cell membranes serve as receptors for insulin and various other hormones
Defend body against many harmful agents	Proteins called *antibodies* or *immunoglobulins* combine with various harmful agents to render those agents harmless
Provide energy	Proteins can be metabolized for energy

Quick CHECK

7. What element is present in all proteins but not in carbohydrates?
8. Identify the building blocks of proteins and explain what common chemical features they all share.
9. Explain the four levels of protein structure.

NUCLEIC ACIDS AND RELATED MOLECULES

DNA AND RNA

Survival of humans as a species—and survival of every other species—depends largely on two kinds of **nucleic acid** molecules. Almost everyone has heard or seen their abbreviated names, DNA and RNA, but their full names are much less familiar. They are deoxyribonucleic and ribonucleic acids (i.e., DNA and RNA). Nucleic acid molecules are polymers of thousands and thousands of smaller molecules called **nucleotides**—deoxyribonucleotides in DNA molecules and ribonucleotides in RNA molecules.

A *deoxyribonucleotide* consists of the pentose sugar named *deoxyribose,* a nitrogenous base (either adenine, cytosine, guanine, or thymine), and a phosphate group (**Figure 4-17**). *Ribonucleotides* are similar but contain the sugar ribose instead of deoxyribose and the nitrogenous base uracil instead of thymine (**Table 4-4**).

Two of the bases in a deoxyribonucleotide, specifically adenine and guanine, are called *purine bases* because they derive from *purine.* Purines have a double ring structure. Cytosine and thymine derive from *pyrimidine,* so they are known as *pyrimidine bases.* Pyrimidines have a single ring structure. The pyrimidine base uracil replaces thymine in RNA. More about the differences between DNA and RNA is discussed in Chapter 7.

DNA molecules, the largest molecules in the body, are very large polymers composed of many nucleotides. The nucleotides are joined together, saccharide group to phosphate group, by dehydration synthesis (condensation) to form a long sugar-phosphate backbone. Two of these long polynucleotide chains compose a single DNA molecule. The chains coil around each other to form a double helix. A helix is a spiral shape similar to the shape of a wire in a spring. **Figure 4-17** is a diagram of the double-helix DNA.

Each helical chain in a DNA molecule has its phosphate-sugar backbone toward the outside and its bases pointing inward toward the bases of the other chain. More than that, each base in one chain is joined to a base in the other chain by means of either two or three hydrogen bonds to form what is known as a *base pair.* The two polynucleotide chains of a DNA molecule are thus held together by hydrogen bonds between the two members of each base pair (see **Figure 4-17**).

TABLE 4-4 Comparison of DNA and RNA Structure

	DNA	RNA
Polynucleotide strands	Double; very long	Single or double; short
Sugar	Deoxyribose	Ribose
Base pairing	Adenine–thymine (A–T)	Adenine–uracil (A–U)
	Guanine–cytosine (G–C)	Guanine–cytosine (G–C)

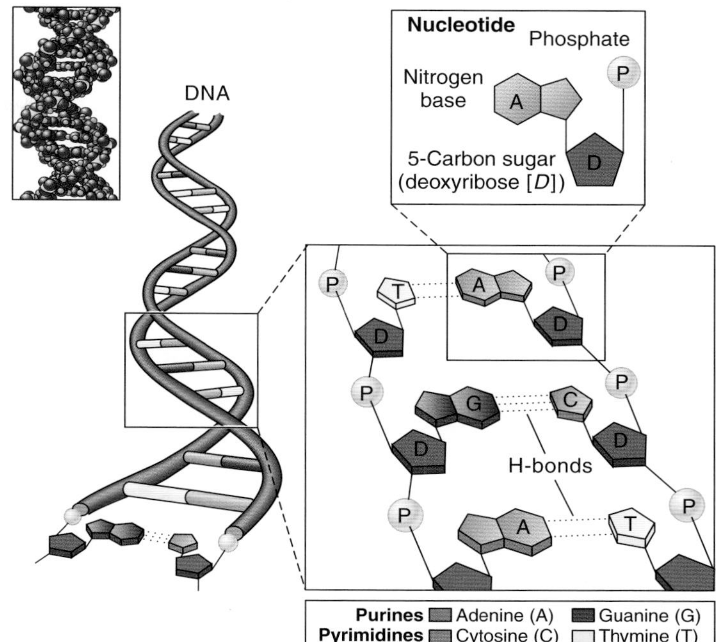

FIGURE 4-17 The DNA molecule. Representation of the DNA double helix showing the general structure of a nucleotide and the two kinds of *base pairs:* adenine (A) *(blue)* with thymine (T) *(yellow)* and guanine (G) *(purple)* with cytosine (C) *(red).* Note that the G–C base pair has three hydrogen bonds and an A–T base pair has two. Hydrogen bonds are extremely important in maintaining the structure of this molecule.

One important principle to remember is that only two kinds of base pairs are present in DNA. What are they? Symbols used to represent them are A::::T and G::::C. Although a DNA molecule contains only these two kinds of base pairs, it contains millions of them—more than 100 million pairs estimated in one human DNA molecule! Two other impressive facts are that the millions of base pairs occur in the same sequence in all the millions of DNA molecules in one individual's body but in a slightly different sequence in the DNA of all other individuals. In short, the base pair sequence in DNA is unique to each individual. This fact has momentous significance because DNA functions as the molecule of heredity. It has a weighty responsibility: that of passing the traits of one generation to the next. DNA accomplishes this feat by acting as an "information molecule" that stores the master code of all the recipes (the *genes*) needed to make the various RNA and protein molecules of the body.

The details of how the information is stored and retrieved by the cells is introduced in Chapter 7, and then Chapter 48 features even more discussion of the processes of heredity.

Most types of RNA molecules consist of a single strand, but the strand often folds on itself to form a compact folded structure. Each RNA strand is a sequence of ribonucleotides that is essentially copied from a portion of a DNA molecule. Thus RNA molecules act as "temporary copies" of the master code of hereditary information in the DNA molecules. These RNA "copies" are involved in the process of protein synthesis.

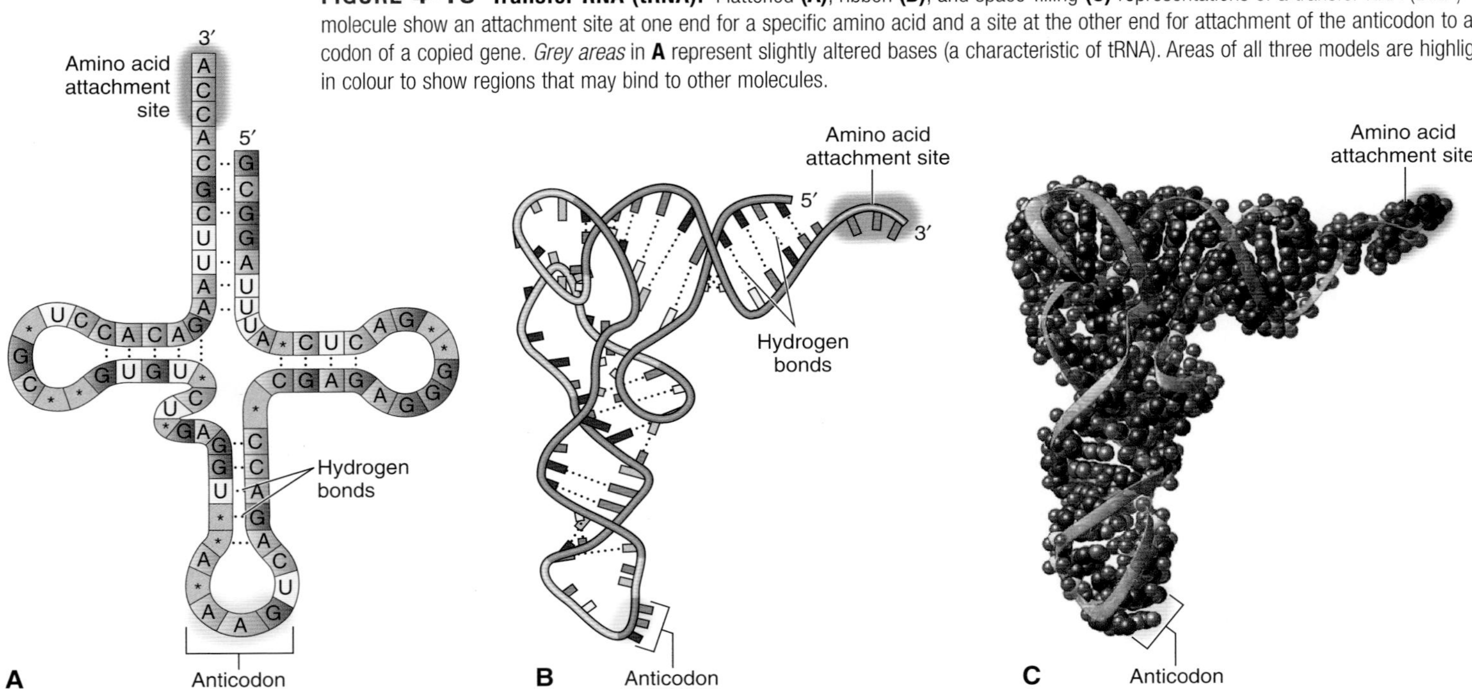

FIGURE 4-18 Transfer RNA (tRNA). Flattened **(A)**, ribbon **(B)**, and space-filling **(C)** representations of a transfer RNA (tRNA) molecule show an attachment site at one end for a specific amino acid and a site at the other end for attachment of the anticodon to a codon of a copied gene. *Grey areas* in **A** represent slightly altered bases (a characteristic of tRNA). Areas of all three models are highlighted in colour to show regions that may bind to other molecules.

Figure 4-18 shows a type of RNA called *transfer RNA (tRNA)*. tRNA is used by the cell to "grab" a specific amino acid and place it in the correct sequence when building a primary protein strand. The correct location in the sequence is guaranteed by matching tRNA's three-base *anticodon* to the complementary *codon* copied from a gene (a "protein recipe" in the genetic code). Chapter 7 outlines the process by which all of this takes place in the cell.

Instead of acting as "information molecules", some RNA molecules regulate cell function. For example, a type of RNA enzyme sometimes called a *ribozyme* is involved in editing the code of RNA strands by removing sections of the code and joining the remaining pieces. A recently discovered type of *double-strand RNA (dsRNA)* is now known to regulate cell function by silencing gene expression in a process called *RNA interference (RNAi)*. These processes are discussed further in Chapter 7.

Thus we can say that RNA can act as either an "information molecule" or as a regulatory molecule that helps cells properly use encoded information.

Nucleotides and Related Molecules

Besides joining together to form nucleic acids, nucleotides and related molecules also play other important roles in the body.

Adenosine triphosphate (ATP) is a very important molecule composed of an adenine and ribose sugar (a combination called *adenosine*) to which are attached a string of three phosphate groups (**Figure 4-19**, A). Thus ATP is really an adenine ribonucleotide with two "extra" phosphate groups attached. The "squiggle" lines indicate covalent bonds that link the phosphate groups. These bonds are called **high-energy bonds** because when they are broken during catabolic chemical reactions, the energy released is used to form

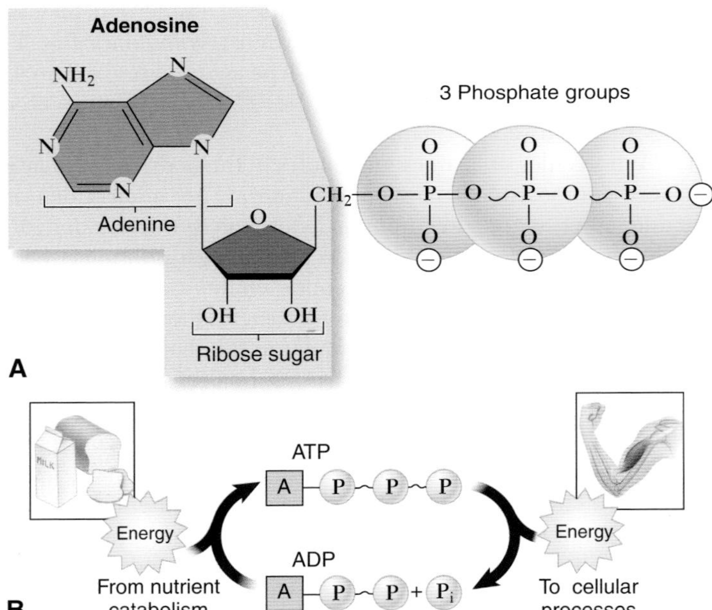

FIGURE 4-19 Adenosine triphosphate (ATP). A, Structure of ATP. A single adenosine group *(A)* has three attached phosphate groups *(P)*. High-energy bonds between the phosphate groups can release chemical energy to do cellular work. **B,** General scheme of the ATP energy cycle. ATP stores energy in its last high-energy phosphate bond. When that bond is later broken, energy is transferred as important intermediate compounds are formed. The adenosine diphosphate (ADP) and phosphate groups that result can be resynthesized into ATP, thereby capturing additional energy from nutrient catabolism. Note that energy is transferred from nutrient catabolism to ADP, thus converting it to ATP, and energy is transferred *from* ATP to provide the energy required for anabolic reactions or cellular processes as it reverts back to ADP.

new compounds. The energy carried by ATP can thus be used in doing the body's work—the work of muscle contraction and movement, of active transport, and of biosynthesis (**Figure 4-19**, *B*).

Because ATP is the form of energy that cells generally use, it is an especially important organic molecule. ATP is a molecule that can pick up energy and give it to another chemical process; therefore, it is often called the *energy currency* of cells. A set of enzyme reactions releases the energy that is stored in ATP by splitting it into *adenosine diphosphate (ADP)* and an inorganic phosphate group. It is also possible to split ADP into *adenosine monophosphate (AMP)* and phosphate, with the release of energy. In this case the bond between the second and third phosphate groups is broken.

In prolonged or intense exercise, when ATP is in short supply, muscles turn to *creatine phosphate (CP)* for extra energy. Creatine phosphate is another high-energy molecule made up of an amino acid derivative and a phosphate connected with a high-energy bond. When CP releases its phosphate group, the energy can be used to add a phosphate to ADP, thus "recharging" ATP. In extreme cases, a cell may use ADP for energy by breaking another phosphate bond.

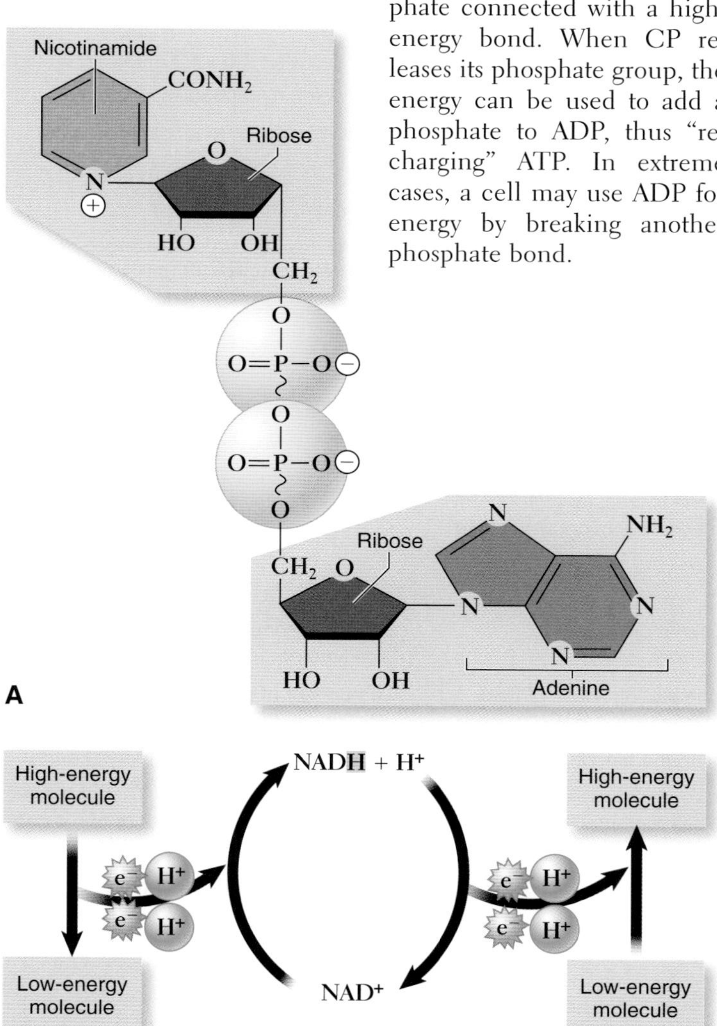

FIGURE 4-20 Nicotinic adenine dinucleotide (NAD^+). NAD^+ is made up of two different ribonucleotides **(A)** and acts as a coenzyme to pick up high-energy particles released from the catabolism of food molecules and shuttle them to another chemical pathway where the energy can be transferred to another molecule **(B)**.

Chapters 6 and 41 discuss in detail the metabolic pathways that are involved in ATP synthesis and breakdown. A cell at rest has a relatively high ATP concentration, whereas an active cell has less ATP but is constantly rebuilding its stores. An exhausted cell has a high ADP concentration and very low levels of ATP. It must resynthesize needed ATP to sustain its activity over time. Fortunately, cells at rest can recycle ADP and ATP and then reverse the cycle, thus reusing small amounts of ATP on a continuing basis. Exercise physiologists estimate that the body can use up to 0.5 kilograms of ATP per minute during very strenuous physical activity. If reuse were impossible, we would require about 40 kilograms of ATP per day to remain active.

Other energy-transferring nucleotides such as nicotinamide adenine dinucleotide (NAD^+) and flavin adenine dinucleotide (FAD) are also used by cells to transfer energy among molecules (**Figure 4-20**, *A*). NAD^+ and FAD act as coenzymes to shuttle energy-carrying particles (electrons) from one metabolic pathway to another during the many complicated steps of transferring energy from food molecules to ATP (**Figure 4-20**, *B*). The entire process of energy transfer, including the role of NAD^+ and FAD, is discussed in detail in Chapter 41.

Nucleotides are also sometimes used as a signal inside the cell. ATP is used throughout the body as a signal between cells. ATP can also break down to a one-phosphate molecule called *cAMP (cyclic adenosine monophosphate)* that is used as an intracellular signal within cells. This role of cAMP is outlined in Chapters 19 and 25.

COMBINED FORMS

You have already noticed that large molecules can be joined together to form even larger molecules. Sometimes, only a small addition or alteration is made. For example, in the case of ATP, two extra phosphate groups are added to an adenine-containing RNA nucleotide. This gives the nucleotide a completely different function. Instead of becoming involved in storing or transmitting genetic information, the ATP molecule transfers energy from one chemical pathway to another. We will learn much more about ATP later. The point now is that macromolecules can be joined to other molecules to make them even larger and to change their functions.

Table 4-5 lists some of the combined or altered macromolecules you will encounter in your study. Note also the many different important functions performed by these molecules. The names of the combined molecules usually tell you what is in them. *Lipoproteins* contain lipid and protein groups combined into a single molecule. *Glycoproteins* contain carbohydrate (*glyco*, "sweet") and protein. Often, the base word (*protein* in this case) indicates which component is dominant. The prefix represents the component found in a lesser amount. Thus glycoproteins have more protein than they do carbohydrate.

Table 4-5 also reviews examples of all the various types of important biomolecules we have discussed in this chapter. It shows the type of subunit present, gives a typical function, and lists one or more examples of each. Bookmarking this table for future reference will help you as you encounter these substances in the remaining chapters of this book.

TABLE 4-5 Examples of Important Biomolecules

MACROMOLECULE	SUBUNIT	FUNCTION	EXAMPLE
Carbohydrates			
Glucose	Simple sugar (hexose: $C_6H_{12}O_6$)	Stores energy	Blood glucose
Ribose	Simple sugar (pentose: $C_5H_{10}O_5$)	Plays role in expression of hereditary information	Component of RNA
Deoxyribose	Simple sugar (pentose: $C_5H_{10}O_4$)	Plays role in storage and transmission of hereditary information	Component of DNA
Glycogen	Glucose	Stores energy	Liver glycogen
Lipids			
Triglycerides	Glycerol + 3 fatty acids	Store energy	Body fat
Phospholipids	Glycerol + phosphate + 2 fatty acids	Make up cell membranes	Plasma membrane of cell
Steroids	Steroid nucleus (4-carbon ring)	Make up cell membranes Hormone synthesis	Cholesterol, various steroid hormones Oestrogen
Prostaglandins	20-carbon unsaturated fatty acid containing 5-carbon ring	Regulate hormone action; enhance immune system; affect inflammatory response	Prostaglandin E, prostaglandin A
Proteins			
Functional proteins	Amino acids	Regulate chemical reactions	Haemoglobin, antibodies, enzymes
Structural proteins	Amino acids	Component of body support tissues	Muscle filaments, tendons, ligaments
Nucleic Acids			
DNA	Nucleotides (sugar, phosphate, base)	Encodes hereditary information	Chromatin, chromosomes
RNA	Nucleotides (sugar, phosphate, base)	Helps decode hereditary information; acts as "RNA enzyme"; silencing of gene expression	Transfer RNA (tRNA), messenger RNA (mRNA), double-strand RNA (dsRNA)
Nucleotides and Related Molecules			
Adenosine triphosphate (ATP)	Phosphorylated nucleotide (adenine + ribose + 3 phosphates)	Transfers energy from fuel molecules to working molecules	ATP present in every cell of the body
Creatine phosphate (CP)	Amino acid derivative + phosphate	Transfers energy from fuel to ATP	CP present in muscle fibre as "backup" to ATP
Nicotinic adenine dinucleotide (NAD^+)	Combination of two ribonucleotides	Acts as coenzyme to transfer high-energy particles from one chemical process to another	NAD^+ present in every cell of the body
Combined or Altered Forms			
Glycoproteins	Large proteins with small carbohydrate groups attached	Similar to functional proteins	Some hormones, antibodies, enzymes, cell membrane components
Proteoglycans	Large polysaccharides with small polypeptide chains attached	Lubrication; increase thickness of fluid	Component of mucous fluid and many tissue fluids in the body
Lipoproteins	Protein complex containing lipid groups	Transport lipids in the blood	LDLs (low-density lipoproteins); HDLs (high-density lipoproteins)
Glycolipids	Lipid molecule with attached carbohydrate group	Component of cell membranes	Component of membranes of nerve cells
Ribonucleoprotein	Combination of RNA nucleotide and protein	Enzyme-like actions such as splicing mRNA	Small nuclear ribonucleoproteins (snRNPs or "snurps") that make up the spliceosome structure in a cell

Quick CHECK

10. Name two important nucleic acids.
11. What is a nucleotide?
12. What is meant by the term *base pair?*
13. What are some roles of nucleotides in the body?

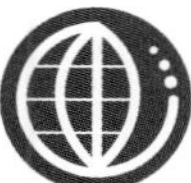

the big picture | Biomolecules

How the basic chemical building blocks of the body are organized and how they relate to one another were outlined in the previous chapter. In this chapter, we applied those principles in our survey of the large biomolecules that play central roles in subsequent chapters.

As we continue our exploration of human structure and function, our knowledge of the key biomolecules will help us answer these questions:

- Why are dieticians concerned with saturated and unsaturated fatty acids?
- How do we digest our food?
- What role do protein molecules play in muscle contraction?
- Should athletes be concerned about their intake of amino acids?
- Why must individuals with diabetes restrict their intake of sugars and other sweets?
- Why do some people inherit a particular disease and others do not?
- What food substances produce the most energy?
- Why do steroid hormones work differently than nonsteroid hormones?

These are the types of real-world, end-of-chapter questions that you will encounter throughout the text that require basic knowledge of biomolecules. Refer often to the information in this chapter as you formulate your answers. Think of chemistry as an important part of the Big Picture in your study of anatomy and physiology.

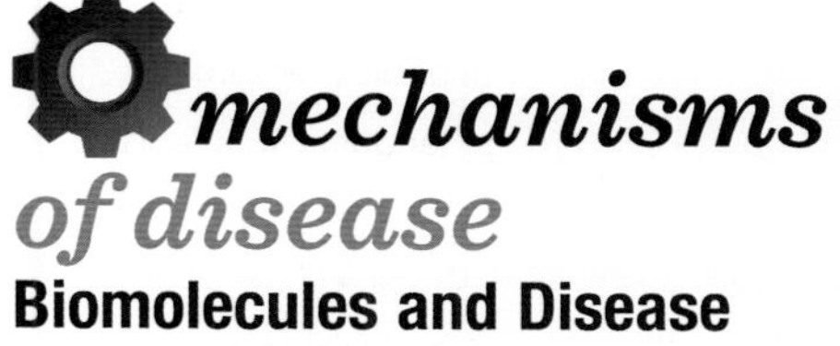

mechanisms of disease

Biomolecules and Disease

Abnormalities and deficiencies of biomolecules are the core of many diseases. Many of these disorders are better discussed in the context of later chapters, where we will be better informed about the functions of the tissues, organs and systems involved. For now, we will briefly survey some basic mechanisms to set the stage for more in-depth discussions in later chapters.

Disorders Involving Carbohydrates

One of the most important and widespread chronic diseases of our time is **diabetes mellitus (DM)**, a disorder of carbohydrate use in the body. In DM, the body cannot always use glucose efficiently for energy because cells fail to sufficiently transport glucose from the blood to be used inside the cells. Various aspects of DM's mechanisms will be explored in later chapters.

Disorders Involving Lipids

Among leading causes of death are heart disease and stroke, both often linked with abnormally high blood concentrations of cholesterol (**hypercholesterolaemia**) and triglycerides (**hypertriglyceridaemia**). Both these conditions are forms of **hyperlipidaemia**—abnormally high lipid concentration in the blood. **Box 4-1** begins the discussion of these mechanisms that will continue in later chapters.

Disorders Involving Proteins

As we discussed earlier in this chapter, misfolding of proteins can cause many diseases. Protein folding—and what happens when it goes awry—is a relatively new and very active area of biomedical research. Other mistakes in protein structure, such as the absence or substitution of amino acids in the primary structure of a protein, can also cause severe disease**. Phenylketonuria (PKU)** is one of these disorders that appeared earlier in this chapter. We will see more examples in later chapters.

Disorders Involving Nucleic Acids

Most of us are aware that mistakes in our genetic code can lead to disease—often called genetic disorders. Many examples of such disorders appear in many later chapters, culminating in a detailed exploration of genetic disorders in Chapter 48.

LANGUAGE OF SCIENCE *(continued from p. 55)*

monosaccharide (mon-oh-SAK-ah-ride)
[*mono-* **one,** *-sacchar-* **sugar,** *-ide* **chemical**]

nonpolar (non-PO-lar)
[*non-* **not,** *-pol-* **pole,** *-ar* **relating to**]

nucleic acid (nyoo-KLAY-ik ASS-id)
[*nucle-* nut **kernel,** *-ic* **relating to,** *acid* **sour**]

nucleotide (NYOO-klee-oh-tide)
[*nucleo-* **nut or kernel,** *-ide* **chemical**]

peptide bond (PEP-tyde bond)
[*pept-* **digest,** *-ide* **chemical**]

phospholipid (fos-fo-LIP-id)
[*phospho-* **phosphorus,** *-lip-* **fat,** *-id* **form**]

polysaccharide (pahl-ee-SAK-ah-ride)
[*poly-* **many,** *-sacchar-* **sugar,** *-ide* **chemical**]

primary protein structure (PRY-mair-ee PRO-teen STRUK-cher)
[*prim-* **first,** *-ary* **relating to,** *prote-* **primary,** *-in* **substance,** *structur-* **arrangement**]

prostaglandin (PG) (pross-tah-GLAN-din)
[*pro-* **before,** *-sta-* **stand,** *-gland-* **acorn,** *-in* **substance**]

protein (PRO-teen)
[*prote-* **primary,** *-in* **substance**]

secondary protein structure (SEK-on-dayr-ee PRO-teen STRUK-cher)
[*second-* **second,** *-ary* **relating to,** *prote-* **primary,** *-in* **substance,** *structur-* **arrangement**]

steroid (STAYR-oid)
[*ster-* **sterol,** *-oid* **like**]

structural protein (STRUK-cher-al PRO-teen)
[*structur-* **arrangement,** *-al* **relating to,** *prote-* **primary,** *-in* **substance**]

tertiary protein structure (TER-shee-air-ee PRO-teen STRUK-cher)
[*tert-* **third,** *-ary* **relating to,** *prote-* **primary,** *-in* **substance,** *structur-* **arrangement**]

triglyceride (try-GLISS-er-yde)
[*tri-* **three,** *glycer-* **sweet (glycerine),** *-ide* **chemical**]

LANGUAGE OF MEDICINE

diabetes mellitus (DM) (dye-ah-BEE-teez mell-EYE-tus)
[*diabetes* **pass-through or siphon,** *mellitus* **honey-sweet**]

hypercholesterolaemia (hye-per-koh-les-ter-ohl-EE-mee-ah)
[*hyper-* **excessive,** *-chole-* **bile,** *-stero-* **solid,** *-ol-* **alcohol,** *-(h)aem-* **blood,** *-ia* **condition**]

hyperlipidaemia (hye-per-lip-id-EE-mee-ah)
[*hyper-* **excessive,** *-lipi-* **fat,** *-id-* **form,** *-aem-* **blood,** *-ia* **condition**]

hypertriglyceridaemia (hye-per-try-gliss-er-yde-EE-mee-ah)
[*hyper-* **excessive,** *-tri-* **three,** *glycer-* **sweet (glycerine),** *-id-* **chemical,** *-aem-* **blood,** *-ia* **condition**]

phenylketonuria (PKU) (fen-il-kee-toh-NOO-ree-ah)
[*phen-* **shining (phenol),** *-yl-* **chemical,** *-keton-* **acetone,** *-ur-* **urine,** *-ia* **condition**]

case study

As a 22–year old man, Danny knew he was slightly overweight and not in the physical condition he was in 4 years ago when he played football at school. His new job required a physical examination complete with blood tests. The results of his blood tests indicated that Danny's total cholesterol value was 5.8 mmol/L. His good cholesterol (HDL) was low 1.0 mmol/L, and his bad cholesterol (LDL) was high 3.5 mmol/L.

Danny's doctor recommended he should reduce his dietary fat intake and increase his physical activity by beginning an exercise programme. The doctor stated that it was important to lower his total cholesterol value below 5 mmol/L, raise his good cholesterol (HDL) level and reduce his bad cholesterol (LDL) level.

1. What is the significance of a high total cholesterol value?
   a. High blood concentrations of cholesterol in the body are toxic
   b. Total cholesterol levels that exceed 5 mmol/L can denature proteins
   c. High blood concentrations of cholesterol are associated with a high risk of atherosclerosis
   d. Total cholesterol levels that exceed 5 mmol/L can alter the structure of the plasma membrane
2. Why are high-density lipoproteins (HDLs) considered "good cholesterol"?
   a. HDLs carry cholesterol to cells, including cells that line blood vessels
   b. HDLs have fewer proteins than low-density (LDLs)
   c. HDLs have more cholesterol than protein
   d. HDLs carry cholesterol away from cells and toward the liver for elimination from the body
3. Because Danny needs to reduce his intake of food that is high in cholesterol, which of the following would you recommend as part of his diet?
   a. Food of plant origin
   b. Liver
   c. Egg yolks
   d. Any food of animal origin

Hint To solve a case study, you may have to refer to the glossary or index, other chapters in this textbook, **Connect It!,** and other resources.

CHAPTER SUMMARY

To download an MP3 version of the chapter summary for use with your mobile device, access the ***Audio Chapter Summaries*** *online at evolve.elsevier.com.*

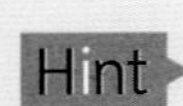

Scan this summary after reading the chapter to help you reinforce the key concepts. Later, use the summary as a quick review before your class or before a test.

Organic Molecules

A. Organic molecules
   1. Molecules that contain C—C or C—H bonds (**Figure 4-1**; **Table 4-5**)
   2. Often have functional groups (radicals [R]) attached to the carbon-containing core of the molecule (**Figure 4-2**)
      a. Free radical—temporarily unattached, highly reactive, chemical group
      b. Functional groups confer unique chemical properties to the molecules on which they are attached

Carbohydrates

A. Carbohydrates—organic compounds containing carbon, hydrogen, and oxygen (usual ratio 1:2:1); commonly called *sugars* and *starches* (**Table 4-1**)
  1. Monosaccharides—simple sugars with short carbon chains; those with six carbons are hexoses (e.g., glucose), whereas those with five are pentoses (e.g., ribose, deoxyribose) (**Figure 4-3**)
  2. Disaccharides and polysaccharides—two (di-) or more (poly-) simple sugars that are bonded together through a dehydration synthesis (condensation) reaction (**Figure 4-4**)

Lipids (Table 4-2)

A. Water-insoluble organic molecules that are critically important biological compounds
B. Major roles:
  1. Energy source
  2. Structural role
  3. Integral parts of cell membranes
C. Triglycerides or fats (**Figures 4-5** and **4-6**)
  1. Most abundant lipids and most concentrated source of energy
  2. Building blocks of triglycerides are glycerol (the same for each fat molecule) and fatty acids (different for each fat, determining its chemical nature)
    a. Types of fatty acids—saturated fatty acid (all available bonds are filled) and unsaturated fatty acid (has one or more double bonds)
      (1) Monounsaturated—only one double bond
      (2) Polyunsaturated—more than one double bond
    b. Triglycerides are formed by dehydration synthesis (condensation)
D. Phospholipids (**Figure 4-7**)
  1. Lipid compounds similar to triglycerides
  2. One end of the phospholipid is water-soluble (hydrophilic); the other end is lipid soluble (hydrophobic)
  3. Phospholipids can join two different chemical environments
  4. Phospholipids may form double layers called *bilayers* that make up cell membranes (**Figure 4-8**)
  5. Phosphoinositides (PIs) are regulatory molecules
E. Steroids (**Figure 4-9**)
  1. Main component is steroid nucleus
  2. Involved in many structural and functional roles
F. Prostaglandins (**Figure 4-10**)
  1. Commonly called *tissue hormones*; produced by cell membranes throughout the body
  2. Effects are many and varied; however, they are released in response to a specific stimulus and are then inactivated

Proteins (Table 4-3)

A. Most abundant organic compounds
B. Chainlike polymers of amino acids held together by peptide bonds to form a polypeptide
C. Amino acids—building blocks of proteins (**Figures 4-11 to 4-13**)
  1. Essential amino acids—eight amino acids that cannot be produced by the adult human body
  2. Nonessential amino acids—13 amino acids that can be produced from molecules available in the adult human body
  3. Amino acids consist of a carbon atom, an amino group, a carboxyl group, a hydrogen atom, and a functional group or radical (R)
D. Levels of protein structure (**Figure 4-14**)
  1. Protein molecules are highly organized and show a definite relationship between structure and function
  2. Four levels of protein organization
    a. Primary structure—refers to the number, kind, and sequence of amino acids that make up the polypeptide chain held together by peptide bonds
    b. Secondary structure—polypeptide is coiled or bent into helices (spirals) and pleated sheets stabilized by hydrogen bonds; may include recurring patterns of helices and/or sheets called motifs
    c. Tertiary structure—a secondary structure can be further twisted and converted to a complex globular shape
      (1) The helices and pleated sheets touch in many places and are "welded" by covalent disulphide bonds, hydrogen bonds, and other attractive forces
      (2) May include regions called domains that act as functional units
    d. Quaternary structure—highest level of organization occurring when protein contains more than one polypeptide chain
E. Importance of protein shape—shape of protein molecules determines their function (**Figure 4-15**)
  1. Final functional shape of the protein molecule is called its *native state*
  2. Structural proteins form the structures of the body
  3. Functional proteins cause chemical changes in the molecules
  4. Denatured proteins have lost their shape and therefore their function (**Figure 4-16**)
  5. Proteins can be denatured by changes in pH, temperature, radiation, and other chemicals
  6. If the chemical environment is restored, proteins may be renatured and function normally
  7. Proteins often have parts that move to perform their functions

Nucleic Acids and Related Molecules

A. DNA (deoxyribonucleic acid)
  1. Composed of deoxyribonucleotides—that is, structural units composed of the pentose sugar (deoxyribose), phosphate group, and nitrogenous base (cytosine, thymine, guanine, or adenine)
  2. DNA molecule consists of two long chains of deoxyribonucleotides coiled into a double-helix shape (**Figure 4-17**)
  3. Alternating deoxyribose and phosphate units form the backbone of the chains
  4. Base pairs hold the two chains of DNA molecule together by hydrogen bonding
    a. Adenine binds to thymine (two hydrogen bonds)
    b. Cytosine binds to guanine (three hydrogen bonds)

5. Specific sequence of more than 100 million base pairs constitutes one human DNA molecule; all DNA molecules in one individual are identical and different from those of all other individuals
6. DNA functions as the molecule of heredity

B. RNA (ribonucleic acid) (**Figure 4-18**, **Table 4-4**)
1. Composed of the pentose sugar (ribose), phosphate group, and a nitrogenous base
2. Nitrogenous bases for RNA are adenine, uracil, guanine, or cytosine (uracil replaces thymine)
3. Some RNA molecules are temporary copies of segments (genes) of the DNA code and are involved in synthesizing proteins
4. Some RNA molecules are regulatory and act as enzymes (ribozymes) or silence gene expression (RNA interference)

C. Nucleotides
1. Nucleotides have other important roles in the body
2. ATP (**Figure 4-19**)
   a. Composition
      (1) Adenosine
         (a) Ribose—a pentose sugar
         (b) Adenine—a nitrogen-containing molecule
      (2) Three phosphate subunits
         (a) High-energy bonds present between phosphate groups
         (b) Cleavage of high-energy bonds releases energy during catabolic reactions
   b. Energy stored in ATP is used to do the body's work
   c. ATP often called the *energy currency* of cells
   d. ATP splits into adenosine diphosphate (ADP) and an inorganic phosphate group by special enzymes
   e. If ATP is depleted during prolonged exercise, creatine phosphate (CP) or ADP can be used for energy
3. NAD^+ and FAD (**Figure 4-20**)
   a. Used as coenzymes to transfer energy from one chemical pathway to another
4. cAMP (cyclic AMP)
   a. Made from ATP by removing two phosphate groups to form a monophosphate
   b. Used as an intracellular signal

Combined Forms

A. Large molecules can be joined together to form even larger molecules

B. Give the molecules a completely different function

C. Names of combined molecules tell you what is in them
1. Base word tells which component is dominant
2. Prefix is the component found in a lesser amount

D. Examples
1. Adenosine triphosphate (ATP)—two extra phosphate groups to a nucleotide
2. Lipoproteins—lipid and protein groups combined into a single molecule
3. Glycoproteins—carbohydrate (*glyco*, "sweet") and protein
4. Examples of combined forms and their functions in the body listed in **Table 4-5**

REVIEW QUESTIONS

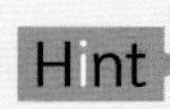

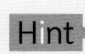

Write out the answers to these questions after reading the chapter and reviewing the Chapter Summary. Note—writing out your answers will consolidate learning and provide a valuable resource of information.

1. What are the structural units, or building blocks of proteins, carbohydrates, triglycerides and DNA?
2. Explain what a protein molecule's binding site is. What function does it serve in enzymes?
3. Describe some of the functions proteins perform.
4. Create a table that compares carbohydrates, proteins, lipids and nucleic acids. Use these benchmarks: (a) solubility in water; (b) contains nitrogen; (c) contains carbon; (d) an energy source; (e) subunits; (f) major types.
5. What groups make up a nucleotide? How many nucleotide bases are found in DNA and RNA?
6. What pentose sugar is present in a deoxyribonucleotide?
7. Describe the size, shape, and chemical structure of the DNA molecule.
8. What base is thymine always paired with in the DNA molecule? What other two bases are always paired?
9. You meet someone who has never heard of DNA. Explain its function and relevance to our society.

CRITICAL THINKING QUESTIONS

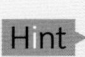

After finishing the Review Questions, write out the answers to these more in-depth questions to help you apply your new knowledge. Go back to sections of the chapter that relate to concepts that you find difficult.

1. Amylase is an enzyme present in saliva that begins the breakdown of starch. As with all enzymes, amylase is specific to this particular chemical reaction. Explain how a change in the shape of this protein might affect this reaction.
2. Amino acids are the building blocks of proteins. Less than a dozen amino acids make up most of our proteins. Explain how so few amino acids are responsible for the billions of proteins that are used by the body.
3. How does ATP supply the cells with the energy they need to work? Outline the general scheme of the ATP energy cycle.
4. One can say that all of the DNA in the animal kingdom is the same. Bears, dogs, dinosaurs and fruit flies have essentially the same DNA that we have. Explain how the genetic uniqueness of a species arises.

5 Cell Structure

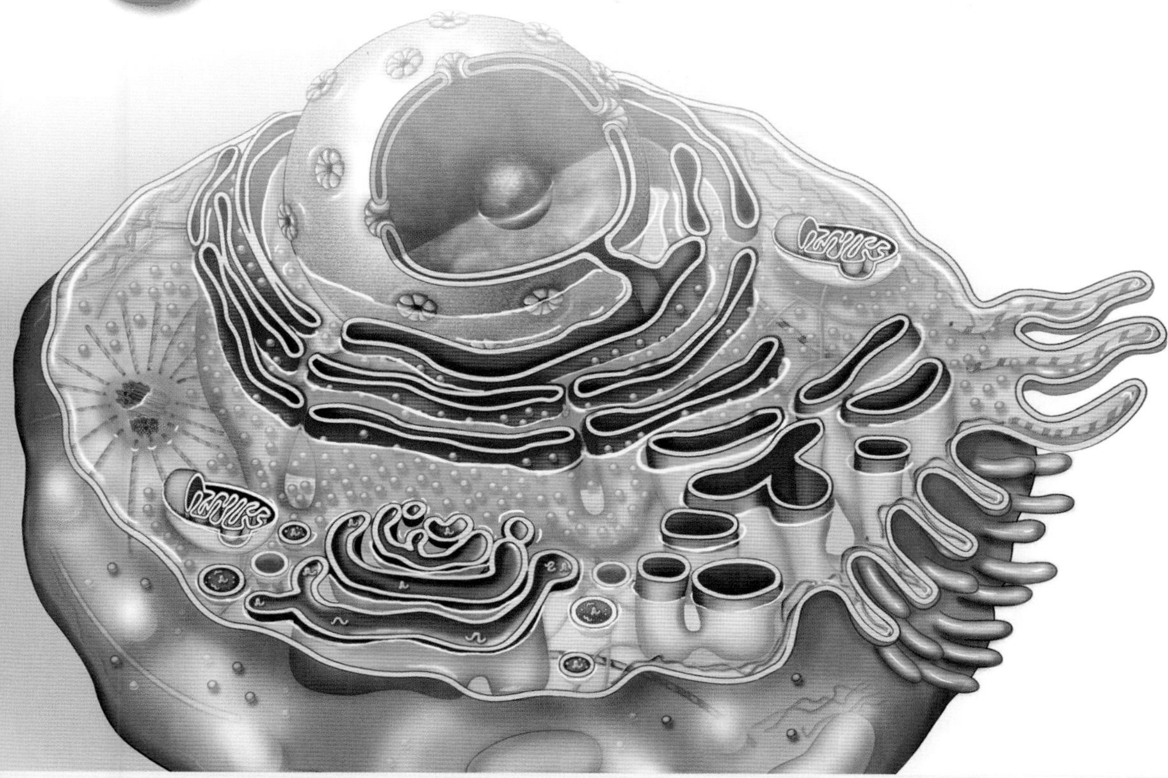

CHAPTER OUTLINE

Hint Scan this outline before you begin to read the chapter, as a preview of how the concepts are organized.

In the 1830s, two German scientists, Matthias Schleiden (SHLY-den) and Theodor Schwann, advanced one of the most important and unifying concepts in biology—the cell theory. It states simply that the cell is the fundamental organizational unit of life. Although earlier scientists had seen cells, Schleiden and Schwann were the first to suggest that all living things are composed of cells. Some 37 trillion of them make up the human body. Actually, the study of cells has captivated

LANGUAGE OF SCIENCE

Hint Use this list to aid your pronunciation of unfamiliar words.

aster (AS-ter)
[*aster,* **star**]

centriole (SEN-tree-ohl)
[*centr-* **centre,** *-ole* **small**]

centrosome (SEN-troh-sohm)
[*centr-* **centre,** *-som-* **body**]

chromatin (KROH-mah-tin)
[*chrom-* **colour,** *-in* **substance**]

chromosome (KROH-meh-sohm)
[*chrom-* **colour,** *-som-* **body**]

chromosome territory (CT)
(KROH-meh-sohm TAIR-it-or-ee)
[*chrom-* **colour,** *-som-* **body,** *terri-* **land,** *-ory* **place**]

cilium (SIL-ee-um)
[*cili-* **eyelid,** *-um* **thing (eyelash)**]
pl., cilia

composite cell (KOM-pah-zit sell)
[*composite* **to assemble,** *cell* **storeroom**]

crista
[*crista* **crest or fold**] *pl.,* cristae

cytoplasm (SYE-toh-plaz-em)
[*cyto-* **cell,** *-plasm* **substance**]

cytoskeleton (sye-toh-SKEL-e-ton)
[*cyto-* **cell,** *-skeleto-* **dried body**]

desmosome (DES-mo-sohm)
[*desmos-* **band,** *-som-* **body**]

endoplasmic reticulum (ER)
(en-doh-PLAZ-mik reh-TIK-yoo-lum)
[*endo-* **inward or within,** *-plasm-* **substance,** *-ic* **relating to,** *ret-* **net,** *-ic-* **relating to,** *-ul-* **little,** *-um* **thing**] *pl.,* endoplasmic reticula

flagellum (flah-JEL-um)
[*flagellum* **whip**] *pl.,* flagella

fluid mosaic model
(FLOO-id mo-ZAY-ik MOD-el)

gap junction (gap JUNK-shen)

Golgi apparatus
(GOL-jee ap-ah-RA-tus)
[*Camillo Golgi* **Italian histologist**]

hydrophilic (hye-dro-FIL-ik)
[*hydro-* **water,** *-phil-* **love,** *-ic* **relating to**]

hydrophobic (hye-droh-FOH-bik)
[*hydro-* **water,** *-phob-* **fear,** *-ic* **relating to**]

continued on p. 94

the interest of countless scientists for more than 300 years. However, these small structures have not yet yielded all their secrets, not even to the probing tools of present-day researchers.

To introduce you to the world of cells, three brief chapters summarize the essential concepts of cell structure and function. This chapter begins the discussion by describing the functional anatomy of common cell structures. The term *functional anatomy* refers to the study of structures as they relate to function. Chapter 6, Cell Function, continues the discussion by outlining in more detail some important and representative cellular processes. Chapter 7 goes on to discuss the growth and reproduction of cells. •

CONNECT IT! 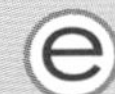

What *are* the probing tools available to today's cell scientists? Mostly, they are the tools used in various forms of **microscopy.** Check out ***Tools of Microscopic Anatomy*** online at ***Connect It!*** to see explanations and examples of *light microscopy (LM), scanning* and *transmission electron microscopy (SEM and TEM),* and *atomic force microscopy (AFM)* that are used throughout this book.

FUNCTIONAL ANATOMY OF CELLS

The principle of complementarity of structure and function was introduced in Chapter 1 and is evident in the relationships that exist between cell size, shape, and function. Almost all human cells are microscopic in size (**Table 5-1**). Their diameters range from 7.5 micrometres (μm) (for example, red blood cells) to about 150 μm (for example, female sex cell or ovum). The full stop at the end of this sentence measures about 100 μm—roughly 13 times as large as our smallest cells and two thirds the size of the human ovum. Like other anatomical structures, cells exhibit a particular size or form because they perform a certain activity. A nerve cell, for example, may have threadlike extensions over a metre in length! Such a cell is ideally suited to transmit nervous impulses from one area of the body to another. Muscle cells are adapted to contract—that is, to shorten or lengthen with pulling strength. Other types of cells may serve protective or secretory functions (**Table 5-2**).

CONNECT IT! 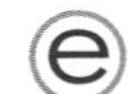

Are you a little confused by the metric size units used in science? Check out ***Metric Measurements and Their Equivalents*** online at ***Connect It!***

TABLE 5-1 Units of Size

UNIT	SYMBOL	EQUAL TO	USED TO MEASURE
Centimetre	cm	1/100 metre	Objects visible to the eye
Millimetre	mm	1/1,000 metre (1/10 cm)	Very large cells; groups of cells
Micrometre (micron)	μm	1/1,000,000 metre (1/1000 mm)	Most cells; large organelles
Nanometre	nm	1/1,000,000,000 metre (1/1,000 μm)	Small organelles; large biomolecules

The Typical Cell

Despite their distinctive anatomical characteristics and specialized functions, the cells of your body have many similarities. There is no cell that truly represents or contains all the various components found in the many types of human body cells. As a result, students

TABLE 5-2 Example of Cell Types

TYPE	STRUCTURAL FEATURES	FUNCTIONS
Nerve cells	Surface that is sensitive to stimuli Long extensions	Detect changes in internal or external environment Transmit nerve impulses from one part of the body to another
Muscle cells	Elongated, threadlike Contain tiny fibres that slide together forcefully	Contract (shorten) to allow movement of body parts
Red blood cells	Contain haemoglobin, a red pigment that attracts, then releases, oxygen	Transport oxygen in the bloodstream (from lungs to other parts of the body)
Gland cells	Contain sacs that release a secretion to the outside of the cell	Release substances such as hormones, enzymes, mucus, and sweat
Immune cells	Some have outer membranes able to engulf other cells Some have systems that manufacture antibodies Some are able to destroy other cells	Recognize and destroy "nonself" cells such as cancer cells and invading bacteria

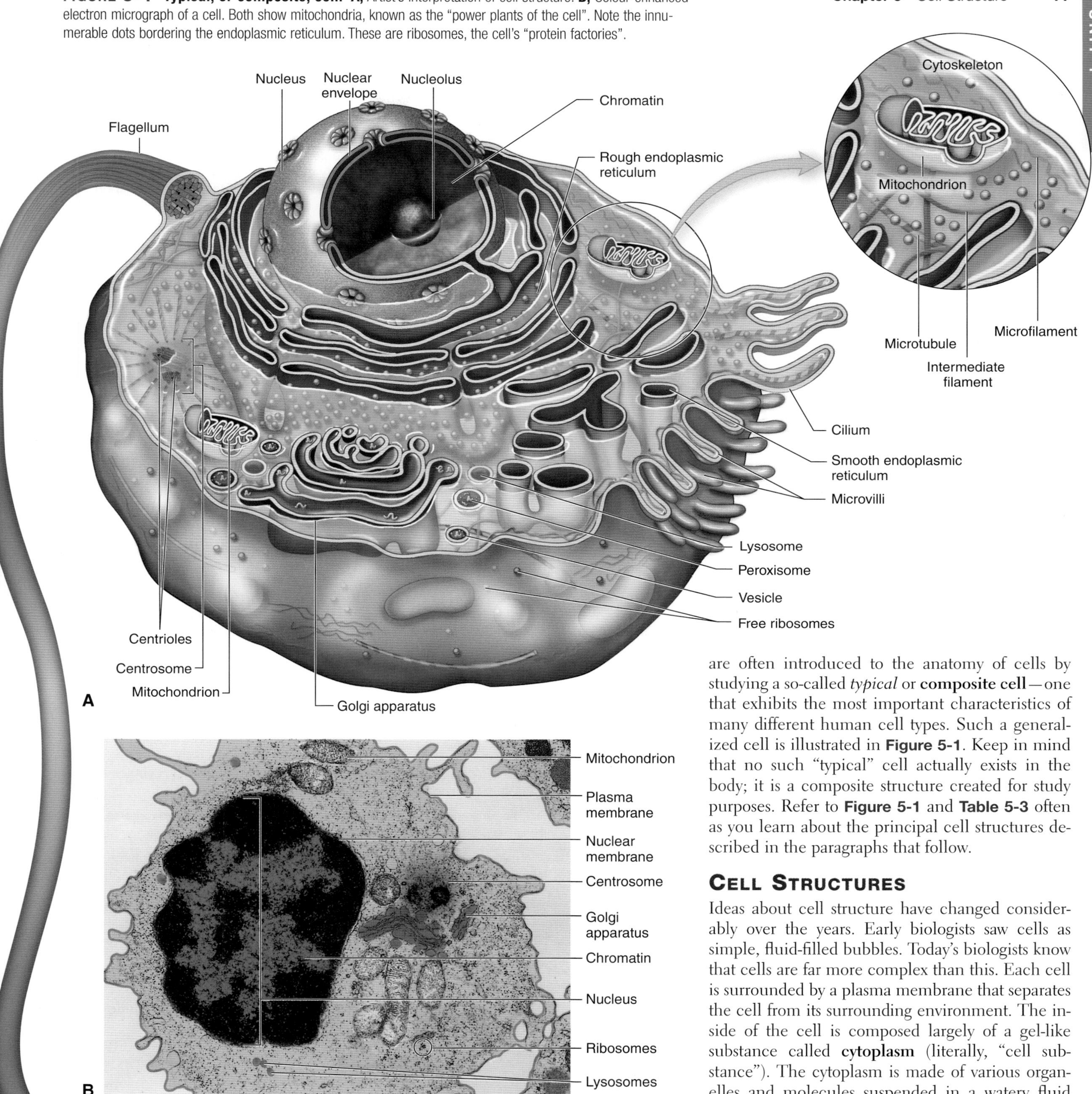

FIGURE 5-1 Typical, or composite, cell. A, Artist's interpretation of cell structure. **B,** Colour-enhanced electron micrograph of a cell. Both show mitochondria, known as the "power plants of the cell". Note the innumerable dots bordering the endoplasmic reticulum. These are ribosomes, the cell's "protein factories".

are often introduced to the anatomy of cells by studying a so-called *typical* or **composite cell**—one that exhibits the most important characteristics of many different human cell types. Such a generalized cell is illustrated in **Figure 5-1**. Keep in mind that no such "typical" cell actually exists in the body; it is a composite structure created for study purposes. Refer to **Figure 5-1** and **Table 5-3** often as you learn about the principal cell structures described in the paragraphs that follow.

Cell Structures

Ideas about cell structure have changed considerably over the years. Early biologists saw cells as simple, fluid-filled bubbles. Today's biologists know that cells are far more complex than this. Each cell is surrounded by a plasma membrane that separates the cell from its surrounding environment. The inside of the cell is composed largely of a gel-like substance called **cytoplasm** (literally, "cell substance"). The cytoplasm is made of various organelles and molecules suspended in a watery fluid

TABLE 5-3 Some Major Cell Structures and Their Functions

CELL STRUCTURE	DESCRIPTION	FUNCTIONS
Membranous		
Plasma membrane	Phospholipid bilayer reinforced with cholesterol and embedded with proteins and other organic molecules	Serves as the boundary of the cell, maintains its integrity; protein molecules embedded in plasma membrane perform various functions; for example, they serve as markers that identify cells of each individual, as receptor molecules for certain hormones and other molecules, and as transport mechanisms
Endoplasmic reticulum (ER)	Network of canals and sacs extending from the nuclear envelope; may have ribosomes attached	Ribosomes attached to rough ER synthesize polypeptides that enter rough ER for folding and finishing, then move on to smooth ER; ER synthesizes IMPs and membrane lipids incorporated in cell membranes, steroid hormones, detoxification enzymes, glycogen-regulating enzymes, and carbohydrates used to form glycoproteins—also removes and stores Ca^{++} from the cell's interior
Golgi apparatus	Stack of flattened sacs (cisternae) surrounded by vesicles	Synthesizes carbohydrate, combines it with protein, and packages the product as globules of glycoprotein
Vesicles	Tiny membranous bags	Temporarily contain molecules for transport or later use
Lysosomes	Tiny membranous bags containing enzymes	Digestive enzymes break down defective cell parts (autophagy) and ingested particles; a cell's "digestive system"; some lysosomes are involved in membrane repair or secretion
Peroxisomes	Tiny membranous bags containing enzymes	Enzymes detoxify harmful substances in the cell
Mitochondria	Tiny membranous capsule surrounding an inner, highly folded membrane embedded with enzymes; has small, ringlike chromosome (DNA)	Catabolism; adenosine triphosphate (ATP) synthesis; a cell's "power plants"
Nucleus	A usually central, spherical double-membrane container of chromatin (DNA); has large pores	Houses the genetic code, which in turn dictates protein synthesis, thereby playing an essential role in other cell activities, namely, cell transport, metabolism, and growth
Nonmembranous		
Ribosomes	Small particles assembled from two tiny subunits of rRNA and protein	Site of protein synthesis; a cell's "protein factories"
Proteasomes	Hollow protein cylinders with embedded enzymes	Destroys misfolded or otherwise abnormal proteins manufactured by the cell; a "quality control" mechanism for protein synthesis
Cytoskeleton	Network of interconnecting flexible filaments, stiff tubules, and molecular motors within the cell	Supporting framework of the cell and its organelles; functions in cell movement (using molecular motors); forms cell extensions (microvilli, cilia, flagella)
Centrosome	Region of cytoskeleton that includes two cylindrical groupings of microtubules called centrioles	Acts as the microtubule-organizing centre (MTOC) of the cell; centrioles assist in forming and organizing microtubules
Microvilli	Short, fingerlike extensions of plasma membrane; supported internally by microfilaments	Tiny, fingerlike extensions that increase a cell's absorptive surface area
Cilia and flagella	Moderate (cilia) to long (flagella) hairlike extensions of plasma membrane; supported internally by cylindrical formation of microtubules, sometimes with attached molecular motors	Cilia move substances over the cell surface or detect changes outside the cell; flagella propel sperm cells
Nucleolus	Dense area of chromatin and related molecules within nucleus	Site of formation of ribosome subunits

called *cytosol*, or sometimes *intracellular fluid*. As **Figure 5-2** shows, the cytoplasm is crowded with large and small molecules—and various organelles. This dense crowding of molecules and organelles actually helps improve the efficiency of chemical reactions in the cell.

The nucleus, which is not usually considered to be part of the cytoplasm, is generally at the centre of the cell. Each different cell part is structurally suited to perform a specific function within the cell—much as each of your organs is suited to a specific function within your body. In short, the main cell structures are (1) the plasma membrane; (2) cytoplasm, including the organelles; and (3) the nucleus (see **Figure 5-1**).

Quick CHECK

1. What important concept in biology was proposed by Schleiden and Schwann?
2. Give an example of how cell structure relates to its function.
3. List the three main structural components of a typical cell.

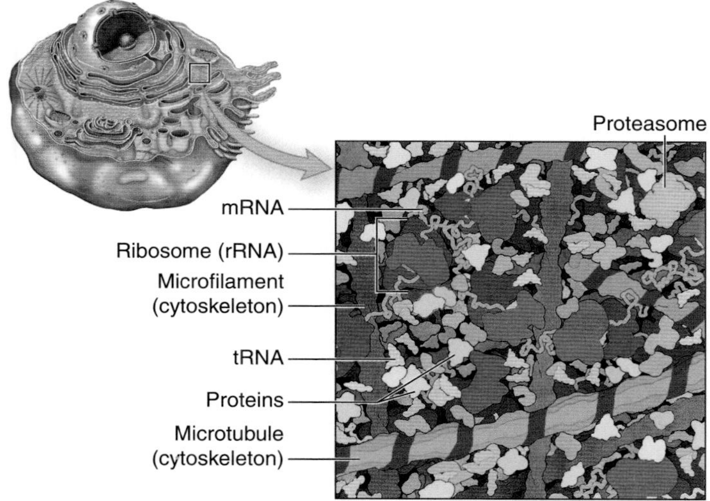

FIGURE 5-2 Cytoplasm. This drawing shows that the cytoplasm is made up of a dense arrangement of fibres, protein molecules, organelles, and other structures, suspended in the liquid cytosol. Such crowding helps molecules interact with one another and thus improves the efficiency of cellular metabolism.

CELL MEMBRANES

Figure 5-1 shows that a typical cell contains a variety of membranes. The outer boundary of the cell, or **plasma membrane,** is just one of these membranes. Each cell also has various *membranous organelles.* Membranous organelles are sacs and canals made of the same type of membrane material as the plasma membrane. This membrane material is a very thin sheet—averaging only about 7.5 nm thick—made of lipid, protein, and other molecules (see **Table 5-1**).

MEMBRANE STRUCTURE

Figure 5-3 shows a simplified view of the evolving model of cell membrane structure. This concept of cell membranes is called the **fluid mosaic model.** Like the tiles in an art mosaic, the different molecules that make up a cell membrane are arranged in a sheet. Unlike art mosaics, however, this mosaic of molecules is fluid; that is, the molecules are able to slowly float around the membrane like icebergs in the ocean. The fluid mosaic model shows us that the molecules of a cell membrane are bound tightly enough to form a

FIGURE 5-3 Plasma membrane. The plasma membrane is made of a bilayer of phospholipid molecules arranged with their nonpolar "tails" pointing toward each other. Cholesterol molecules help stabilize the flexible bilayer structure to prevent breakage. Protein molecules (integral membrane proteins or IMPs) and protein-hybrid molecules may be found on the outer or inner surface of the bilayer—or extending all the way through the membrane.

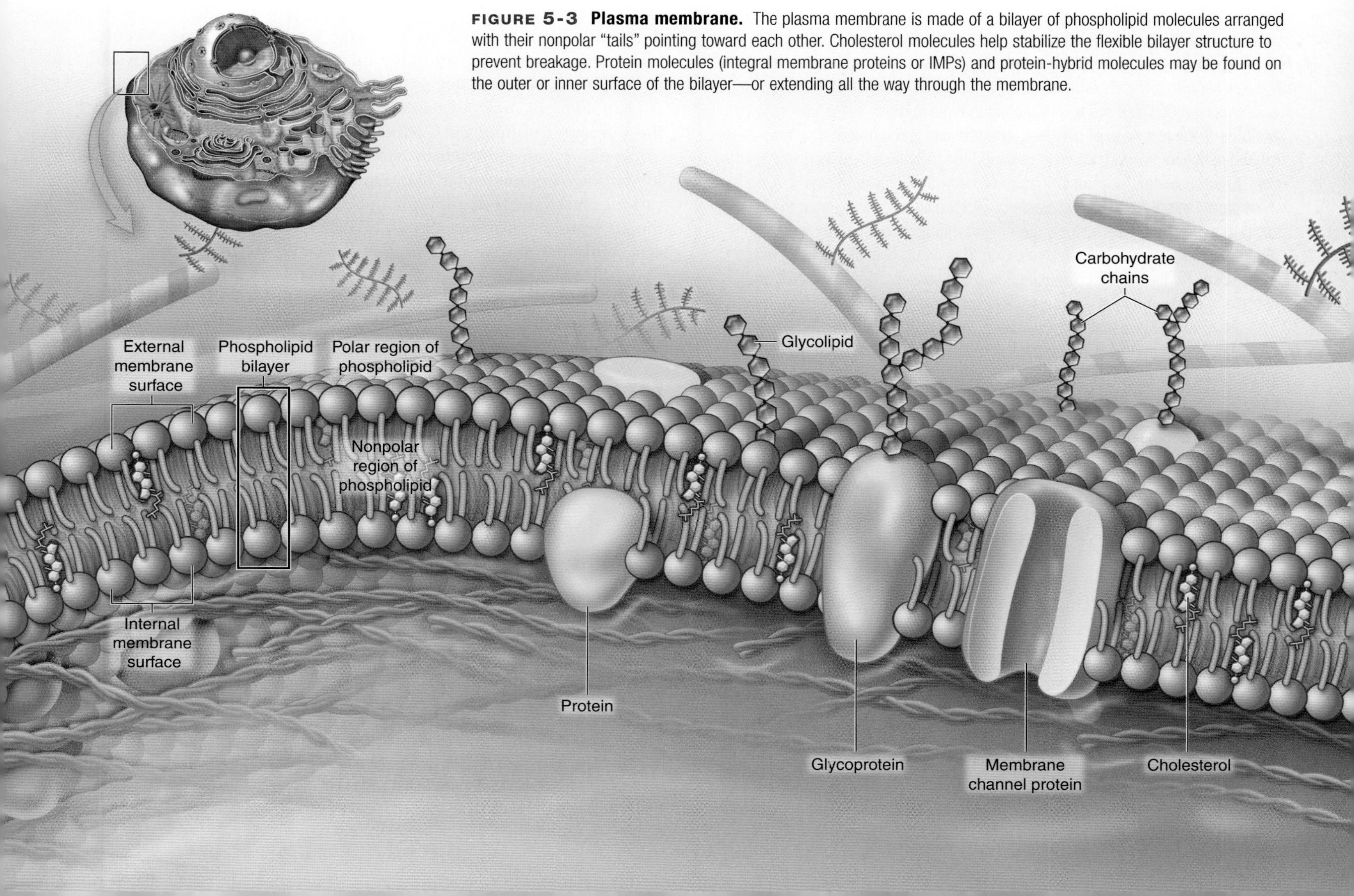

continuous sheet but loosely enough that the molecules can slip past one another.

What are the forces that hold a cell membrane together? The short answer to that question is chemical attractions. The primary structure of a cell membrane is a double layer of phospholipid molecules. Recall from Chapter 4 that phospholipid molecules have "heads" that are water soluble and double "tails" that are lipid soluble (see **Figure 4-7** on p. 60). Because their heads are **hydrophilic** ("water loving") and their tails are **hydrophobic** ("water fearing"), phospholipid molecules naturally arrange themselves into double layers, or *bilayers,* in water. This allows all the hydrophilic heads to face toward water and all the hydrophobic tails to face away from water (see **Figure 4-8** on p. 60).

Because the internal environment of the body is simply a water-based solution, phospholipid bilayers appear wherever phospholipid molecules are scattered among the water molecules. Cholesterol is a steroid lipid that mixes with phospholipid molecules to form a blend of lipids that stays just fluid enough to function properly at body temperature. Without cholesterol, cell membranes would break far too easily.

Each human cell manufactures various kinds of phospholipid and cholesterol molecules, which then arrange in a bilayer to form a natural "fencing" material of varying thickness that can be used throughout the cell. This "fence" allows many lipid-soluble molecules to pass through easily—just like a picket fence allows air and water to pass through easily. However, because most of the phospholipid bilayer is hydrophobic, cell membranes do not allow water or water-soluble molecules to pass through easily. This characteristic of cell membranes is ideal because most of the substances in the internal environment are water soluble. What good is a membrane boundary if it allows just about everything to pass through it?

Just as there are different fencing materials for different kinds of fences, cells can make any of a variety of different phospholipids for different areas of a cell membrane. For example, some areas of a membrane are stiff and less fluid; others are somewhat flimsy. Many cell membranes are packed more densely with proteins than seen in **Figure 5-3**; other membranes have less protein.

Some membrane lipids combine with carbohydrates to form glycolipids, and some unite with protein to form lipoproteins easily. Recall from Chapter 4 that proteins are made up of many amino acids, some of which are polar, some nonpolar (see **Figure 4-12**, p. 62). By having different kinds of amino acids in specific locations, protein molecules may become anchored within the bilayer of phospholipid heads and tails or attached to one side or the other of the membrane.

The different molecular interactions within the membrane allow the formation of lipid **rafts,** which are stiff groupings of membrane molecules (often very rich in cholesterol) that travel together like a log raft on the surface of a lake (**Figure 5-4**). Rafts help organize the various components of a membrane. Rafts play an important role in the pinching of a parent cell into two daughter cells during cell division. Rafts may also sometimes allow the cell to form depressions that pouch inward and then pinch off as a means of carrying substances into the cell (**Box 5-1**). Human immunodeficiency virus (HIV), for example, enters cells by first connecting to a raft protein in the plasma membrane and then subsequently being pulled into the cell.

BOX 5-1 *caveolae*

The list of organelles inside human cells that have been identified with new techniques of cell imaging (see ***Tools of Microscopic Anatomy*** online at ***Connect It!***) and biochemical analysis has continued to grow. Among the more recently discovered organelles are the "little caves", or *caveolae* (*singular,* caveola). Caveolae are tiny indentations of the plasma membrane that indeed resemble tiny caves (see the figure). Caveolae appear to form from rafts of lipid and protein molecules in the plasma membrane that pinch in and move inside the cell. Caveolae can capture extracellular material and shuttle it inside the cell or even all the way across the cell (see the figure). Although there is much yet to understand about the many functions of caveolae, one possible problem that they may cause has already been outlined. Some caveolae in the cells that line blood vessels may have CD36 cholesterol receptors that attract low-density lipoproteins (LDLs, which carry the so-called *bad cholesterol*). As the figure shows, once the LDLs attach to the receptor, the caveola closes and migrates to the other side of the cell. There, the LDL molecules are released to build up behind the lining of the blood vessel. As the LDLs accumulate, the blood vessel channel narrows and obstructs the flow of blood—a major cause of stroke and heart disease.

Researchers believe that other diseases, such as certain forms of diabetes, cancer, and muscular dystrophy, may also result from inappropriate actions taken by caveolae. •

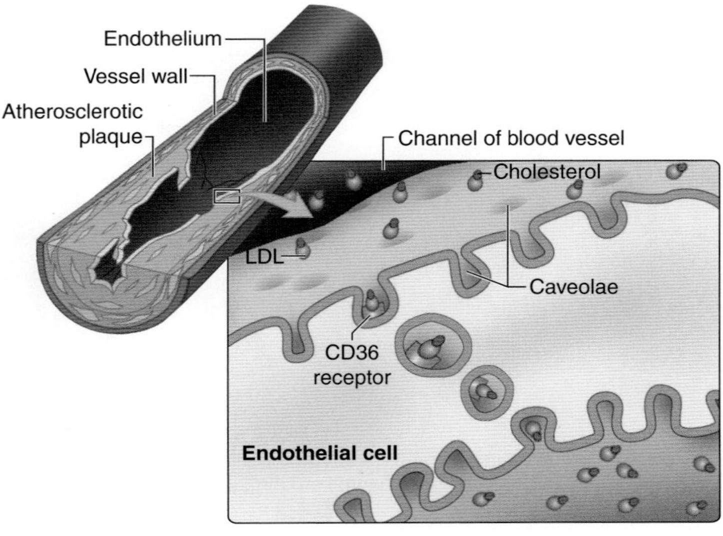

MEMBRANE FUNCTION

Embedded within the phospholipid bilayer are a variety of **integral membrane proteins (IMPs).** As their name implies, they are

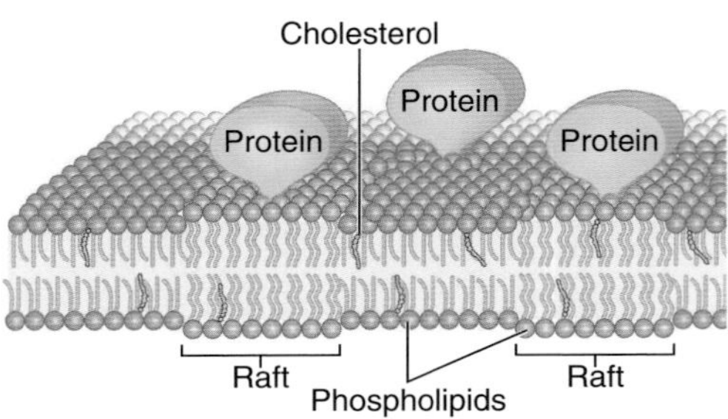

FIGURE 5-4 Rafts. The raft phospholipids have a richer supply of cholesterol than surrounding regions do and, along with attached integral membrane proteins, form rather rigid floating platforms in the surface of the membrane. Rafts help organize functions at the surfaces of cells and organelles.

integrated into the structure of the membrane itself. Proteins that have some functional regions or *domains* that are hydrophilic and other domains that are hydrophobic can be integrated into a phospholipid bilayer and remain stable. IMPs have many different structural forms that allow them to serve various functions (see **Table 5-3**).

Transport

A cell can control what moves through any section of membrane by means of IMPs that act as transporters (see **Figure 5-3**). Many of these transporters have domains forming openings that, like gates in a fence, allow water-soluble molecules to pass through the membrane. Specific kinds of transporters allow only certain kinds of molecules to pass through—and the cell can determine whether these "gates" are open or closed at any particular time. We consider this function of integral membrane proteins again in Chapter 6 when we study transport mechanisms in the cell.

Identification

Some IMPs have carbohydrates attached to their outer surface—forming *glycoprotein* molecules—that act as identification markers. Such markers, which are recognized by other molecules, act as signs on a fence that identify the enclosed area. Cells and molecules of the immune system can thus distinguish between normal "self" cells and abnormal or "nonself" cells. Not only does this mechanism allow us to attack cancer or bacterial cells, it also prevents us from receiving blood donations from people who don't have cell markers similar to our own. Some membrane proteins are enzymes that catalyze cellular reactions. Some IMPs bind to other IMPs to form connections between cells or bind to support filaments within the cell to anchor them.

Signalling

Other IMPs are **receptors** that can react to the presence of hormones or other regulatory chemicals and thereby trigger metabolic changes in the cell. The process by which cells translate the signal received by a membrane receptor into a specific chemical change in the cell is called **signal transduction.** The word *transduction* means "carry across", as a message being carried across a membrane.

Recent discoveries continue to show the vital importance of signal transduction in the normal function of cells and therefore the whole body. Being one of the most active areas of biomedical research, the study of signal transduction has provided many answers to the causes of diseases, which in turn has led to effective treatments and cures. As you continue your study of human structure and function, try to find instances of signal transduction in cells that provide a vital link in important processes throughout the body. By doing so, you will better understand the "big picture" of human structure and function.

Connection

Some IMPs connect the cell membrane to another membrane, as when two cells join together to form a larger mass of tissue. Other IMPs connect a membrane to the framework of fibres inside the cell or to the mass of fibres and other molecules that make up the extracellular matrix (ECM).

Table 5-4 summarizes the functional anatomy of cell membranes.

TABLE 5-4 Functional Anatomy of Cell Membranes

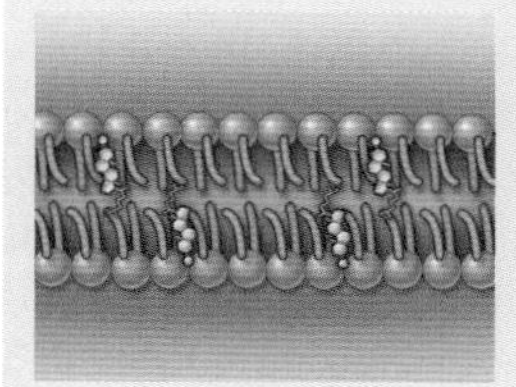	**Structure:** Sheet (bilayer) of phospholipids stabilized by cholesterol **Function:** Maintains boundary (integrity) of a cell or membranous organelle
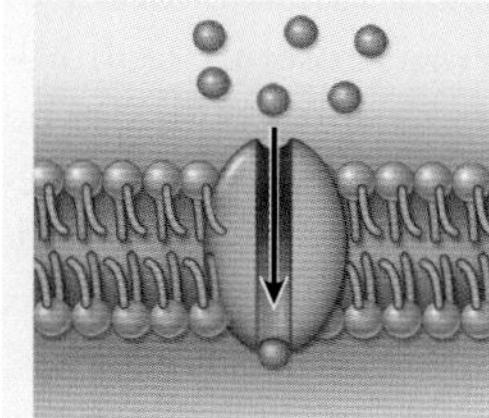	**Structure:** Integral membrane proteins that act as channels or carriers of molecules **Function:** Controlled transport of water-soluble molecules from one compartment to another
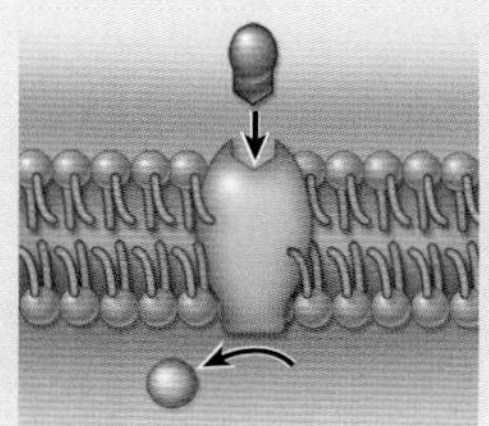	**Structure:** Receptor molecules that trigger metabolic changes in membrane (or on other side of membrane) **Function:** Sensitivity to hormones and other regulatory chemicals; involved in signal transduction
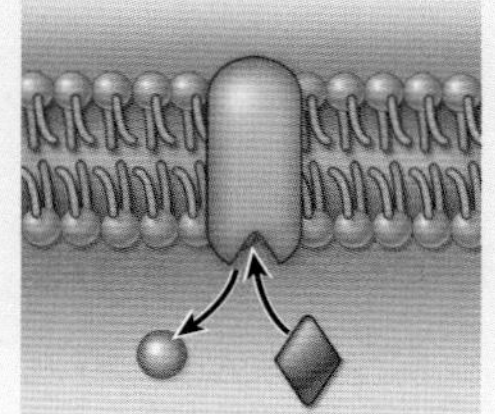	**Structure:** Enzyme molecules that catalyze specific chemical reactions **Function:** Regulation of metabolic reactions
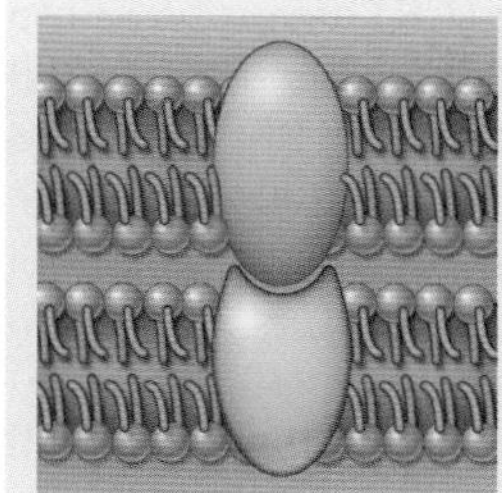	**Structure:** Integral membrane proteins that bind to molecules outside the cell **Function:** Form connections between one cell and another
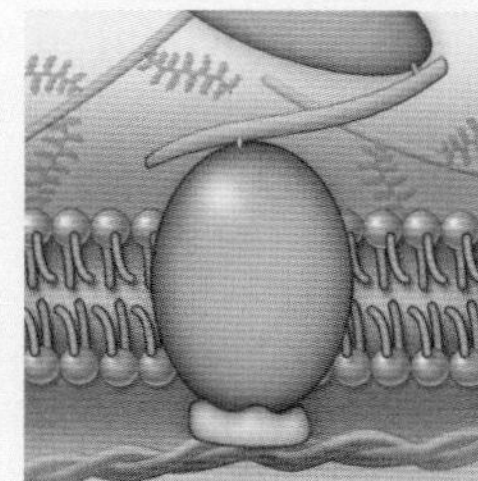	**Structure:** Integral membrane proteins that bind to support structures **Function:** Support and maintain the shape of a cell or membranous organelle; participate in cell movement; bind to fibres of the extracellular matrix (ECM)
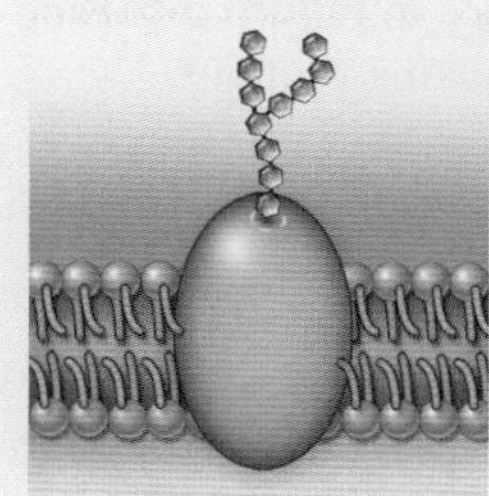	**Structure:** Glycoproteins or proteins in the membrane that act as markers **Function:** Recognition of cells or organelles

CYTOPLASM AND ORGANELLES

Cytoplasm is the gel-like internal substance of cells that contains many tiny suspended structures. Early cell scientists believed cytoplasm to be a rather uniform fluid filling the space between the plasma membrane and the nucleus. We now know that the cytoplasm of each cell is actually a watery solution called *cytosol* plus hundreds or even thousands of "little organs", or **organelles,** that thicken the cytoplasm and result in its gel-like consistency. **Table 5-3** lists some of the major types of organelles that we will encounter in this book. Until relatively recently, when newer microscope technology became available, many of these organelles simply could not be seen. Those that could be seen were simply called *inclusions* because their roles as integral parts of the cell were not yet recognized. Undoubtedly, some of the cellular structures we now call inclusions will eventually be recognized as organelles and given specific names.

Many types of organelles have been identified in various cells of the body. To make it easier to study them, they have been classified into two major groups: *membranous organelles* and *nonmembranous organelles.* Membranous organelles are those that are described as sacs or canals made of cell membrane. Nonmembranous organelles are not made of membrane; they are made of microscopic filaments or other particles. As you read through the following sections, be sure to note whether the organelle being discussed is membranous or nonmembranous (see **Table 5-3**). Then try to identify these organelles in Figure 5-1 of the BRIEF ATLAS OF THE HUMAN BODY.

ENDOPLASMIC RETICULUM (ER)

Endoplasm is the cytoplasm located toward the centre of a cell. *Reticulum* means small network. Therefore, the name **endoplasmic reticulum (ER)** means literally a small network located deep inside the cytoplasm. When first seen, it appeared to be just that. Later on, however, more highly magnified views under the electron microscope showed the ER to be distributed throughout the cytoplasm (see **Figure 5-1**). ER consists of membranous-walled canals and flat, curving sacs that are arranged in parallel sheets. Like many other organelles, the ER is in constant motion within the cell, often contacting other organelles in the cell to form temporary "partnerships".

The endoplasmic reticulum can serve a variety of functions in a cell. A common way of describing ER identifies two main types of ER: rough ER (RER) and smooth ER (SER).

Rough ER (RER)

Rough ER is made up of broad, flattened sacs that extend outward from the boundary of the nucleus. RER sacs are dotted with innumerable small granules called *ribosomes.* The granules give rough ER the "rough" appearance of sandpaper, as you can see in **Figure 5-5**. Ribosomes are themselves distinct organelles for making proteins.

As new polypeptide strands are released from the ribosomes that "dock" at the RER surface, they enter the lumen (cavity) of the RER network. Once inside, the polypeptide strands fold with the help of chaperone molecules. The folded proteins sometimes unite with other proteins to form larger molecules.

Many of the proteins formed in the RER facilitate the production of phospholipids. These phospholipids immediately join the bilayer that forms the RER's membrane boundary—thus "making more membrane".

The proteins made in the RER move through the lumen of the ER network, or become embedded in the cell membrane (phospholipid bilayer) that forms the wall of each sac. Many of these molecules eventually move toward the Golgi apparatus, where they are processed further, and some of them eventually leave the cell.

Smooth ER (SER)

No ribosomes border the membranous wall of the smooth ER—hence its smooth appearance and its name. The SER part of the network is usually more tubular in structure than the flattened sacs of the RER, as you can see in **Figure 5-5**.

Although the smooth ER does not receive new polypeptides from ribosomes, it continues the chemical processing started in the RER. The SER thus contains enzymes and other molecules processed in both the RER and SER. Some of the enzymes alter polypeptides already present and some synthesize other molecules such as lipids and carbohydrates. Included among

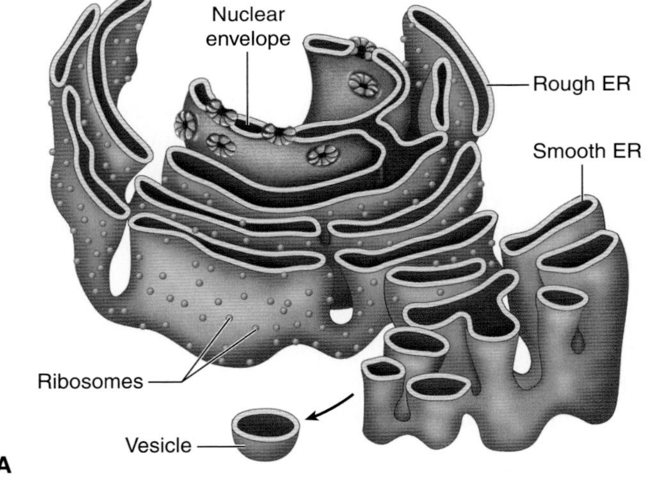

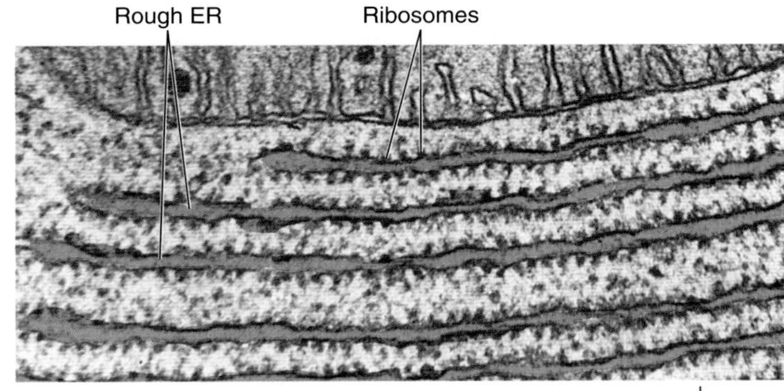

FIGURE 5-5 Endoplasmic reticulum (ER). In both the drawing **(A)** and the transmission electron micrograph **(B)**, the rough ER (RER) is distinguished by the presence of tiny ribosomes dotting the boundary of flattened membrane sacs. The smooth ER (SER) is more tubular in structure and lacks ribosomes on its surface. Note also that the ER is continuous with the outer membrane of the nuclear envelope.

these are the steroid hormones and some of the carbohydrates used to form glycoproteins.

Some SER enzymes help cells destroy toxins, such as drugs. Other SER enzymes help regulate the breakdown of glycogen into glucose when the cells need energy.

Although started in the RER, most of the phospholipids and cholesterol that form cell membranes are synthesized in the SER. As these membrane lipids are made, they simply become part of the smooth ER's wall. Integral membrane proteins—such as transporters and receptors—synthesized in the ER are also added to the membrane. Bits of the ER break off from time to time and travel to other membranous organelles—even to the plasma membrane—and become part of the membrane of those organelles. The smooth ER, then, is the organelle that makes membrane for use throughout the cell.

Smooth ER also transports calcium ions (Ca^{++}) from the cytosol into the sacs of the ER, thus helping maintain a low concentration of Ca^{++} in a cell's interior. Knowing that Ca^{++} is moved into the ER and stored there is a fact that will prove useful in helping you understand the information in later chapters.

Ribosomes

Every cell contains thousands of **ribosomes.** Many of them are attached to the rough endoplasmic reticulum, and many of them lie free, scattered throughout the cytoplasm. Find them in both locations in **Figure 5-1**. Because ribosomes are too small to be seen with a light microscope, no one knew they existed until the electron microscope revealed them in 1955. We now know that each ribosome is a nonmembranous structure made of two tiny, interlocking pieces. One piece is a *large subunit* and the other a *small subunit* (**Figure 5-6**).

Each subunit of the ribosome is composed of ribonucleic acid (RNA) bonded to protein. Ribosomal RNA is often abbreviated as rRNA. Other types of ribonucleic acid in the cell include messenger RNA (mRNA) and transfer RNA (tRNA), among others. **Figure 5-6** shows a threadlike mRNA molecule moving through a ribosome, providing the "recipe" for a polypeptide strand. You can also see a tiny tRNA particle inside the cavity between the ribosomal subunits. tRNA's job is to bring (i.e., transfer) an amino acid to the correct location in the mRNA recipe sequence. The major types of RNA and their roles in the cell are discussed in more detail in Chapter 7.

The function of ribosomes is protein synthesis. Ribosomes are the molecular machines that translate the genetic code to make proteins, or to use a popular term, they are the cell's "protein factories". They make both its structural and its functional proteins (enzymes).

A ribosome is a temporary structure. The two ribosomal subunits link together only when there is an mRNA present and ready to direct the formation of a new polypeptide strand. When the polypeptide is finished, the subunits fall away from each other. The subunits may be used again in another round of protein synthesis.

Working ribosomes usually function in groups called *polyribosomes* or *polysomes*. Polyribosomes form when more than one ribosome begins translating the same long, threadlike mRNA molecule. Under the electron microscope, polyribosomes look like short strings of beads.

In Chapter 7, after you have learned a little more about cell structures, you will be ready to look at the details of how ribosomes carry out protein synthesis.

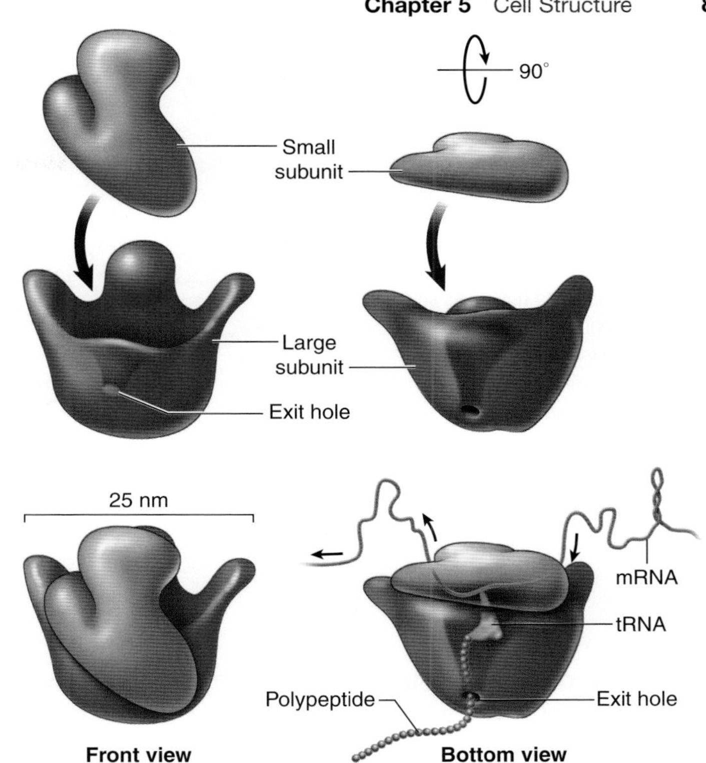

FIGURE 5-6 Ribosome. A ribosome is composed of a small subunit and a large subunit, shown here from two different perspectives. After the small subunit attaches to a messenger RNA (mRNA) strand containing the genetic "recipe" for a polypeptide strand, the subunits come together to form a complete ribosome. Transfer RNA (tRNA) brings amino acids into the cavity between subunits, where they are assembled into a strand according to the mRNA code. As the polypeptide strand elongates, it moves out through a tunnel and a tiny exit hole in the large subunit.

Golgi Apparatus

The **Golgi apparatus** is a membranous organelle consisting of separate tiny sacs, or *cisternae*, stacked on one another and located near the nucleus (**Figure 5-7**; see also **Figure 5-1**). Sometimes also called the *Golgi complex,* it was first noticed in the nineteenth century by the Italian biologist Camillo Golgi. Like the endoplasmic reticulum, the Golgi apparatus processes molecules within its membranes. The Golgi apparatus seems to be part of the same system that prepares protein molecules for export from the cell.

The role of the Golgi apparatus in processing and packaging protein molecules for export from the cell is summarized in **Figure 5-8**. First, proteins synthesized by ribosomes and transported to the end of an endoplasmic reticulum canal are packaged into tiny membrane bubbles, or **vesicles,** that break away from the endoplasmic reticulum.

The vesicles then move to the Golgi apparatus and fuse with the first cisterna. Protein molecules thus released into the cisterna are then chemically altered by enzymes present there. For example, the enzymes may attach carbohydrate molecules synthesized in the Golgi apparatus to form glycoproteins.

The processed and sorted molecules are then "pinched off" in another vesicle. Each such *Golgi vesicle* moves to the next cisterna for further processing. The proteins and glycoproteins eventually end up in the outermost cisterna, from which vesicles pinch off and move to another part of the cell. Often, the final destination is the plasma membrane.

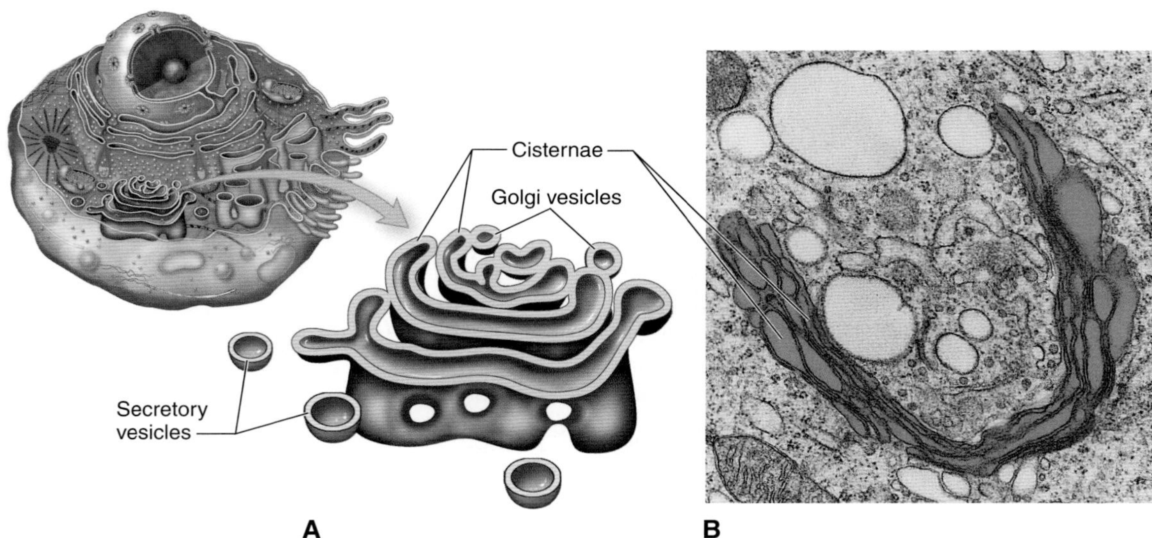

FIGURE 5-7 Golgi apparatus. **A,** Sketch of the structure of the Golgi apparatus showing a stack of flattened sacs, or *cisternae,* and numerous small membranous bubbles, or *secretory vesicles.* **B,** Transmission electron micrograph (TEM) showing the Golgi apparatus highlighted with colour.

FIGURE 5-8 The cell's protein export system. The Golgi apparatus processes and packages protein molecules delivered from the endoplasmic reticulum by small vesicles. After entering the first cisterna of the Golgi apparatus, a protein molecule undergoes a series of chemical modifications, is sent (by means of a vesicle) to the next cisterna for further modification, and so on, until it is ready to exit the last cisterna. When it is ready to exit, a molecule is packaged in a membranous secretory vesicle that migrates to the surface of the cell and "pops open" to release its contents into the space outside the cell. The vesicle membrane, including any integral membrane proteins, then becomes part of the plasma membrane. Some vesicles remain inside the cell for some time and serve as storage vessels for the substance to be secreted.

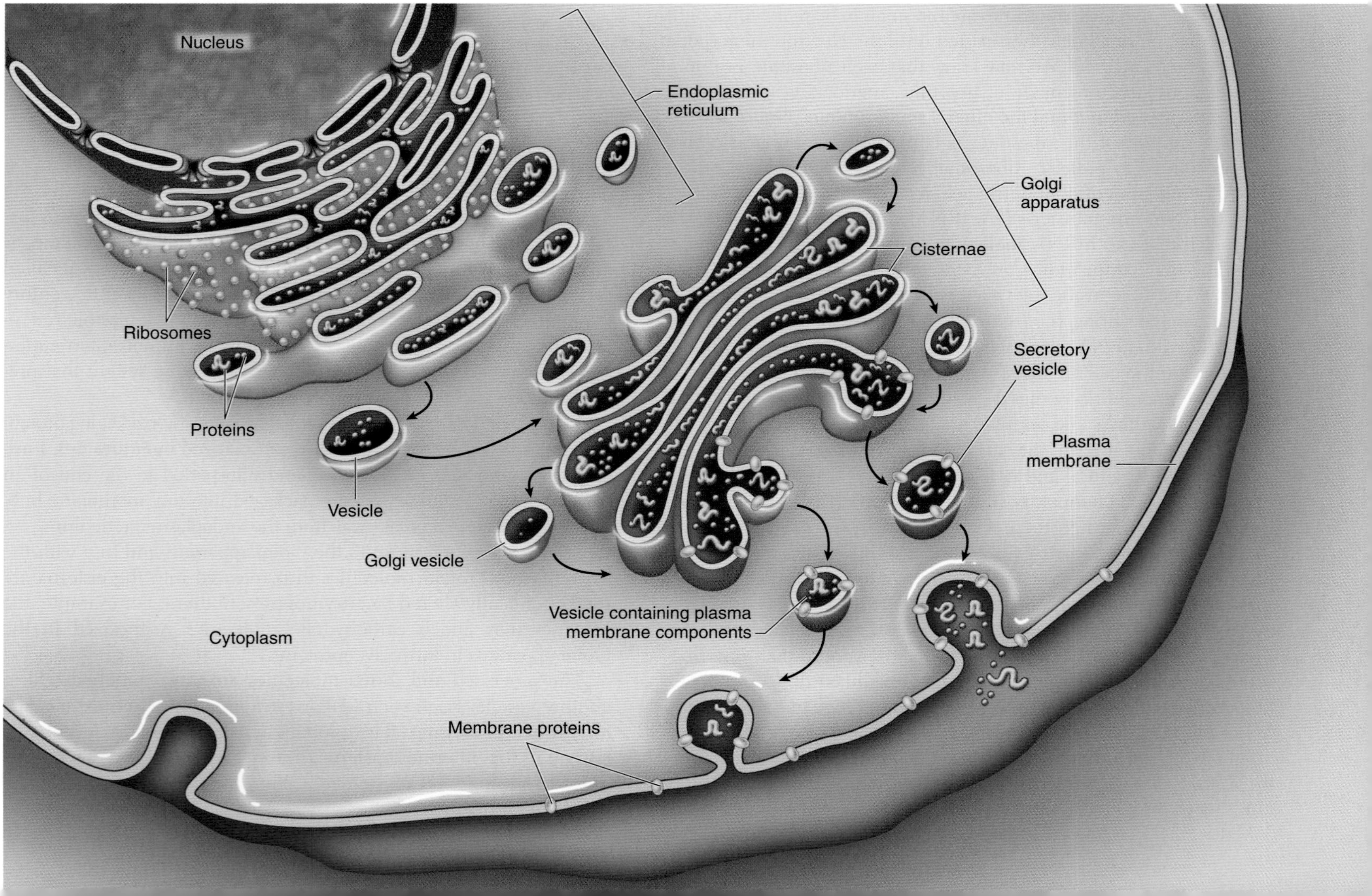

At the plasma membrane, the vesicles release their contents outside the cell in a process called *secretion*. Other protein and glycoprotein molecules may instead be incorporated into the membrane of a Golgi vesicle. This means that these molecules eventually become part of the plasma membrane, as seen in **Figure 5-8** and **Table 5-2**.

CONNECT IT!

Scientists are using their knowledge of the Golgi apparatus to mimic the cell's chemical-making functions in order to manufacture therapeutic treatments more efficiently. Check out ***Biomimicry*** online at ***Connect It!***

Lysosomes

Like the endoplasmic reticulum and Golgi apparatus, **lysosomes** have membranous walls—indeed, they are vesicles that have pinched off from the Golgi apparatus. The size and shape of lysosomes change with the stage of their activity. In their earliest, inactive stage, they look like mere granules. Later, as they become active, they take on the appearance of small vesicles or sacs (see **Figure 5-1**). The interior of the lysosome contains various kinds of enzymes capable of breaking down all the protein components of cells.

Lysosomal enzymes have several important functions in cells. Chiefly, they help the cell break down proteins and cytoplasm that are not needed to get them out of the way. This process of "self eating" is called autophagy. The amino acids and other products resulting from the breakdown process can be reused by the cell. In the process illustrated in **Figure 5-9**, defective or unneeded organelles can be thus recycled. Integral membrane proteins from the plasma membrane that pinch off inside the cell can be recycled in the same manner. Likewise, cells may engulf bacteria or other extracellular particles and destroy them with lysosomal enzymes. Thus lysosomes deserve their nicknames of "digestive bags" and because of their involvement in breakdown of old, worn out cells, "suicide bags". Scientists are also discovering the roles of some lysosomes in repairing plasma membranes and releasing important substances from the cell.

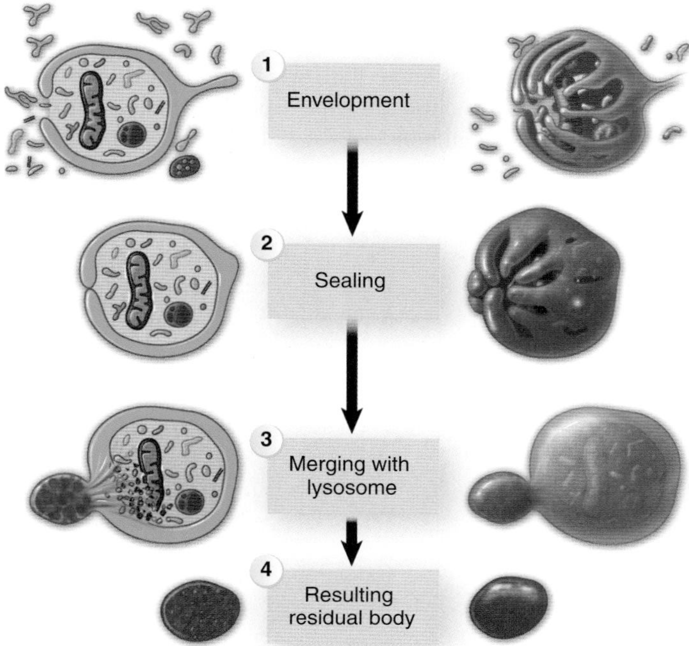

FIGURE 5-9 Lysosome. The process of destroying old cell parts (autophagy) follows these steps: (1) Membrane from the endoplasmic reticulum (ER) or Golgi apparatus encircles the material to be destroyed. (2) A membrane capsule completely traps the material. (3) A lysosome fuses with the membrane capsule, and digestive enzymes from the lysosome enter the capsule and destroy the contents. (4) Undigested material remains in a compact *residual body.*

Proteasomes

The **proteasome** is another protein-destroying organelle in the cell. As **Figure 5-10** shows, the proteasome is a hollow, cylindrical "drum" made up of protein subunits. Found throughout the cytoplasm, the proteasome is responsible for breaking down abnormal and misfolded proteins released from the ER, as well as destroying normal regulatory proteins in the cytoplasm that are no longer needed. But unlike the lysosome, which destroys large groups of protein molecules all at once, the proteasome destroys protein molecules one at a time.

Before a protein enters the hollow interior of the proteasome, it must be tagged with a chain of very small proteins called *ubiquitins.* The ubiquitin chain then enters the proteasome and subsequently "pulls" the rest of the protein in after it. As it passes through the cap of the proteasome, the protein is unfolded. Then active sites inside the central chamber break apart the peptide bonds. The resulting short peptide chains, 4 to 25 amino acids long, exit through the other end of the proteasome. The short peptides are easily broken down into their component amino acids for recycling by the cell.

Proper functioning of proteasomes is important in prevention of abnormal cell function and possibly severe disease. For example, in *Parkinson disease (PD)* the proteasome system fails, and consequently, the still intact improperly folded proteins kill nerve cells in the brain that are needed to regulate muscle tension.

Peroxisomes

The **peroxisome** is another type of vesicle containing enzymes that is present in the cytoplasm of some cells. These organelles, which pinch off from the SER, detoxify harmful substances that may enter

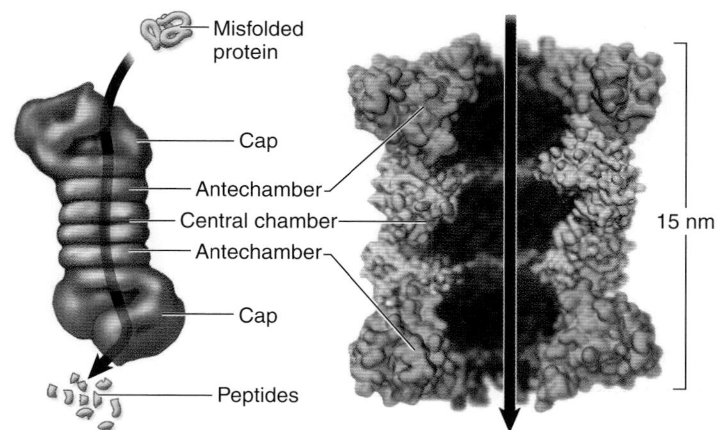

FIGURE 5-10 Proteasome. Made up of protein subunits, the proteasome is a hollow cylinder with regulatory end caps. Following the path shown by *arrows,* a ubiquitin-tagged protein molecule unfolds as it enters the cap and is then broken down into small peptide chains (4 to 25 amino acids), which leave through the other end of the proteasome. The peptides are subsequently broken down into amino acids, which are recycled by the cell. The proteasome is a little over half the size of a ribosome.

cells. They are often seen in kidney and liver cells and serve important detoxification functions in the body. Peroxisomes contain the enzymes *peroxidase* and *catalase,* which are important in detoxification reactions involving hydrogen peroxide (H_2O_2). Hydrogen peroxide is the chemical that gives this organelle its name.

MITOCHONDRIA

Find the cell's little "power plants" called **mitochondria** shown in **Figure 5-1** and **Figure 5-11**. Magnified thousands of times, as they are there, they look like small, partitioned sausages—if you can imagine sausages only 1.5 μm (1500 nm) long and half as wide. Yet, like all organelles, even as tiny as they are, mitochondria have a highly organized molecular structure.

Their membranous walls consist of not one but two delicate membranes. They form a sac within a sac. The inner membrane is contorted into folds called **cristae.** The large number and size of these folds gives the inner membrane a comparatively huge surface area for such a small organelle.

Embedded in the inner membrane are enzymes that are essential for assembling a chemical vital for life: *adenosine triphosphate (ATP).* ATP was first introduced in Chapter 4 as the molecule that transfers energy from food to cellular processes. It is the job of each mitochondrion to extract energy from food molecules and use it to build ATP molecules. Then the ATP molecules leave the mitochondrion and break apart to release the energy in a variety of specific chemical reactions throughout the cell. Thus each mitochondrion acts as a tiny "power plant" that converts energy from a stored form to a more directly usable form (temporarily stored in ATP). Chapters 6 and 41 present more detailed information about this vital process that provides usable energy for the cell.

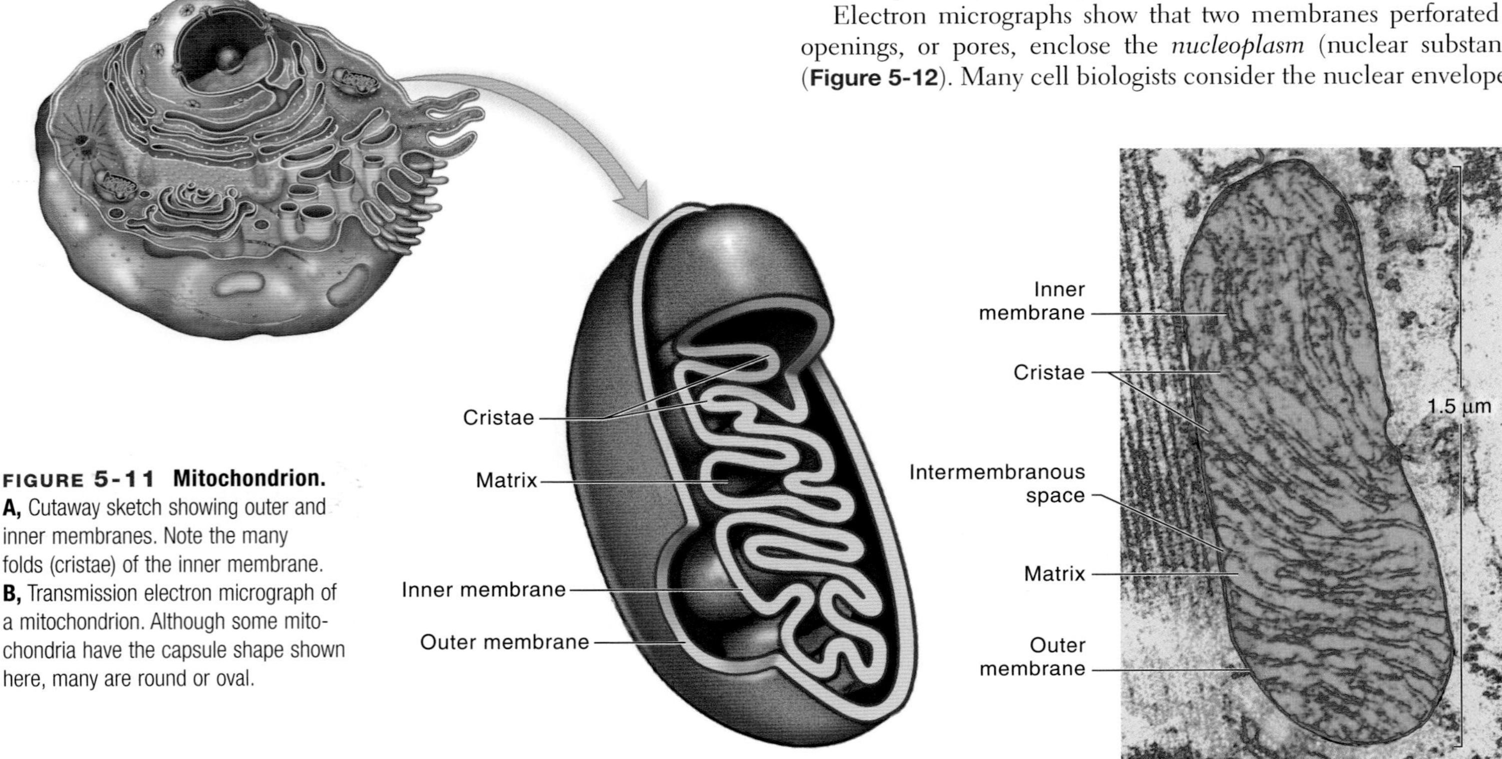

FIGURE 5-11 Mitochondrion. **A,** Cutaway sketch showing outer and inner membranes. Note the many folds (cristae) of the inner membrane. **B,** Transmission electron micrograph of a mitochondrion. Although some mitochondria have the capsule shape shown here, many are round or oval.

Both the inner and outer membranes of the mitochondrion have essentially the same molecular structure as the cell's plasma membrane. All evidence gathered so far indicates that the functional proteins in the membranes of the cristae are arranged precisely in the order of their functioning. This is another example, but surely an impressive one, of the principle stressed in Chapter 1—self-organization is a foundation stone and a vital characteristic of life.

The fact that mitochondria generate most of the power for cellular work suggests that the number of mitochondria in a cell might be directly related to its amount of activity. This principle does seem to hold true. In general, the more work a cell does, the more mitochondria its cytoplasm contains. Liver cells, for example, do more work and have more mitochondria than sperm cells do. A single liver cell contains 1000 or more mitochondria, whereas only about 25 mitochondria are present in a single sperm cell. The mitochondria in some cells multiply when energy consumption increases. For example, frequent aerobic exercise can increase the number of mitochondria inside skeletal muscle cells.

Each mitochondrion has its own DNA molecule, a very surprising discovery indeed! This enables each mitochondrion to make some of its own enzymes. Having its own DNA also enables each mitochondrion to divide and produce genetically identical daughter mitochondria. Scientists believe that mitochondria are bacteria that have become part of our cells—a concept that has several useful applications discussed more thoroughly in Chapter 48.

NUCLEUS

The **nucleus,** one of the largest cell structures (see **Figure 5-1**), usually occupies the central portion of the cell. The shape of the nucleus and the number of nuclei present in a cell vary. One spherical nucleus per cell, however, is common.

Electron micrographs show that two membranes perforated by openings, or pores, enclose the *nucleoplasm* (nuclear substance) (**Figure 5-12**). Many cell biologists consider the nuclear envelope to

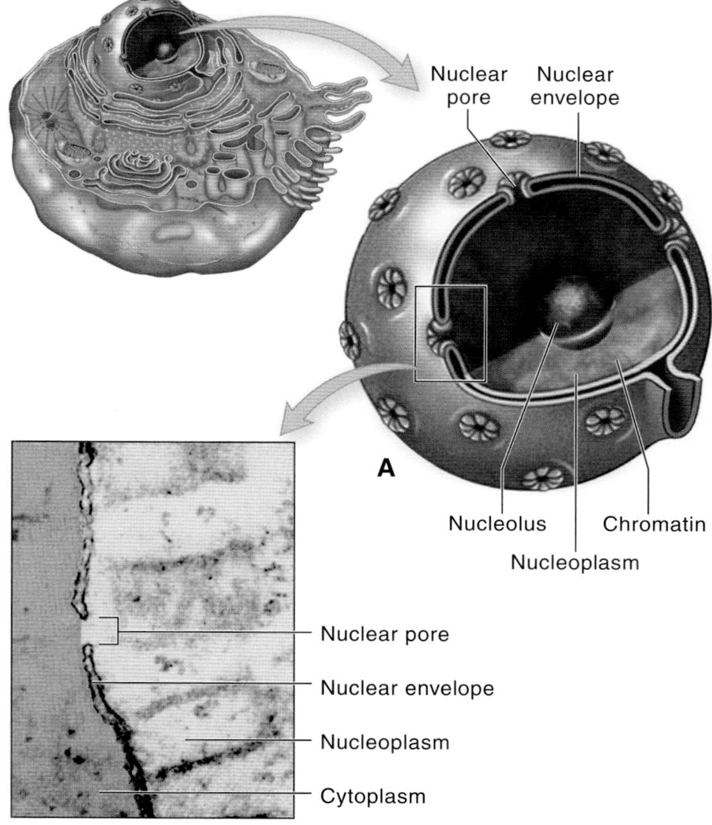

FIGURE 5-12 Nucleus. A, An artist's rendering of the nucleus cut to see the interior. Note the cut-off connection to the ER. **B,** Electron micrograph showing that the nuclear envelope is composed of two separate membranes and is perforated by large openings, or nuclear pores.

be part of the ER because, as you can see in **Figure 5-5**, it is continuous with the innermost portion of the ER. *Nuclear pores* are intricate structures often called *nuclear pore complexes (NPCs)* (**Figure 5-13**). Nuclear pore complexes act as gatekeepers and transport mechanisms that selectively permit molecules and other structures to enter or leave the nucleus.

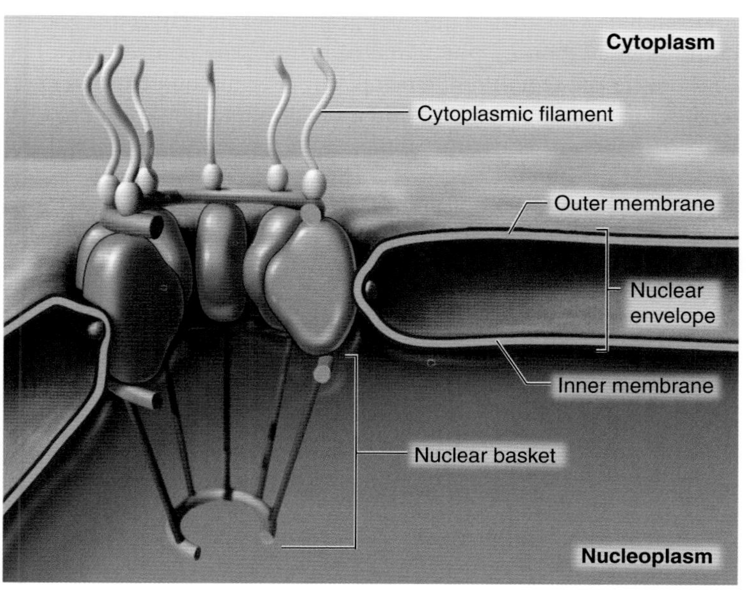

FIGURE 5-13 Nuclear pore complex (NPC). The elaborate structure of the nuclear pore complex hints at its many roles in regulating the movement of small particles between the inside and outside of the nucleus.

CONNECT IT! 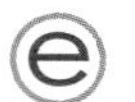

Tiny, barrel-shaped organelles called *vaults* may also assist with transport of molecules to and from the nucleus. To learn more about these little transport shuttles, check out ***Vaults*** online at ***Connect It!***

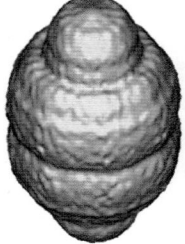

The two nuclear membranes, together called the nuclear envelope, have essentially the same type of structure as other cell membranes. The membranous walls of the endoplasmic reticulum extend outward from the membranes of the nuclear envelope.

Probably the most important fact to remember about the nucleus is that it contains DNA molecules, the well-known heredity molecules often referred to in news stories. In nondividing cells, the DNA molecules appear as tiny bunches of tangled threads sprinkled with granules. This material is named **chromatin.** Chromatin is from the Greek *chroma*, "colour", so named because it readily takes the colour of stains. These chromatin tufts are not randomly spread throughout the nucleus. They continually move like dancers into various positions within the nucleus as the DNA performs its functions.

When the process of cell division begins, DNA molecules become more tightly coiled. They become so compact that they look like short, rodlike structures and are then called **chromosomes.** All normal human cells (except mature sex cells) contain 46 chromosomes, and each chromosome consists of one DNA molecule plus some protein molecules.

The functions of the nucleus are primarily functions of DNA molecules. In brief, DNA molecules contain the master code for making all the RNA plus the many enzymes and other proteins of a cell. Therefore, DNA molecules ultimately dictate both the structure and the function of cells. Chapter 7 briefly discusses how a cell transcribes and translates the master code to synthesize specific proteins. DNA molecules are inherited, so DNA plays a pivotal role in the process of heredity—a concept we explore further in Chapter 48.

CONNECT IT! 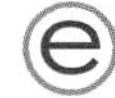

In nondividing cells, chromosomes are found in the form of chromatin strands that occupy specific **chromosome territories (CTs)** within the nucleus. See an example of a CT map in ***Chromosome Territories*** online at ***Connect It!***

The most prominent structure visible in the nucleus is a small nonmembranous body that stains densely when studied in the laboratory setting and is called the **nucleolus** (see **Figure 5-12**, A). Like chromosomes, it consists chiefly of a nucleic acid, but the nucleic acid is not DNA. It is RNA, or ribonucleic acid (see pp. 67–68).

The nucleolus functions to synthesize ribosomal RNA (rRNA) and combine it with protein to form the subunits that will later combine to form ribosomes, the protein factories of cells (see **Figure 5-6**). You might guess, therefore, and correctly so, that the more protein a cell makes, the larger its nucleolus appears. Cells of the pancreas, to cite just one example, make large amounts of protein and have large nucleoli.

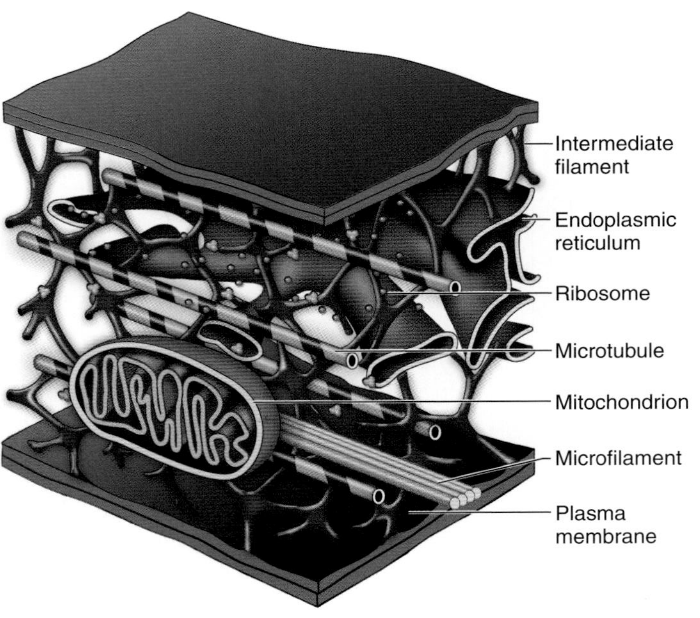

FIGURE 5-14 The cytoskeleton. Artist's interpretation of the cell's internal framework. Notice that the "free" ribosomes and other organelles are not really *freely* floating in the cell.

Quick **CHECK**

4. List at least three functions of the plasma membrane.
5. Define the term *organelle.*
6. Identify three organelles by name and give one function of each.
7. Distinguish between membranous and nonmembranous organelles.

CYTOSKELETON

As its name implies, the **cytoskeleton** is the cell's internal supporting framework. Like the bony skeleton of the body, the cytoskeleton is made up of rather rigid, rodlike pieces that not only provide support but also allow movement. Like the body's musculoskeletal framework, the cytoskeleton has musclelike groups of fibres and other mechanisms that move the cell, or parts of the cell, with great strength and mobility. In this section, we take a look at the basic characteristics of the cell's internal skeleton, as well as several organelles that are associated with it.

Cell Fibres

No one knew much about *cell fibres* until the development of two new research methods: one with fluorescent molecules and the other with stereomicroscopy—that is, three-dimensional pictures of whole, unsliced cells made with high-voltage electron microscopes. Using these techniques, investigators discovered intricate arrangements of fibres of varying widths. The smallest fibres seen have a width of about 3 to 6 nm! Of particular interest is their arrangement. They form a three-dimensional, chaotic lattice, a kind of scaffolding in the cell. These fibres appear to support parts of the cell formerly thought to float free in the cytoplasm—the endoplasmic reticulum, mitochondria, and "free" ribosomes (**Figure 5-14**; see also **Figures 5-1** and **5-2**). Cytoskeletal fibres may even "fence in" regions of the plasma membrane to prevent free-floating movement of embedded proteins.

The smallest cell fibres are called **microfilaments.** Microfilaments often serve as part of our "cellular muscles". They are made of thin, twisted strands of protein molecules (**Figure 5-15**, *A*). In some microfilaments, the proteins can be pulled by little "motors" and slide past one another to cause shortening of the cell. The most obvious example of such shortening occurs in muscle cells, where many bundles of microfilaments are pulled together to shorten the cells with great force.

Cell fibres called **intermediate filaments** are twisted protein strands that are slightly thicker than microfilaments (**Figure 5-15**, *B*). Their twisted structure allows them to stretch without breaking. Intermediate filaments are thought to form much of the supporting framework in many types of cells. They act as the tendons and ligaments of the cell, holding the cell together as it is pushed and pulled. For example, the protective cells in the outer layer of skin are filled with a dense arrangement of tough intermediate filaments.

The thickest of the cell fibres are tiny, hollow tubes called **microtubules.** As **Figure 5-15**, *C*, shows, microtubules are made of protein subunits arranged in a spiral fashion. Microtubules are sometimes called the "engines" of the cell because they often move things around in the cell—or even cause movement of the entire cell. For example, both the movement of vesicles within the cell and the movement of chromosomes during cell division are thought to be accomplished by microtubules.

Just as the body's musculoskeletal system helps us sense our body's position and environmental impacts, the cell's cytoskeleton can detect changes in the cell's position and impacts that affect the cell.

In addition to the "bones" and "muscles" that make up the cytoskeleton, there are many types of functional proteins that allow the various parts to interact with one another. For example, receptor molecules help parts link to one another and may even permit signals to be sent between parts. Molecular motors, described later, move parts. Other functional proteins such as enzymes keep everything running smoothly too.

Centrosome

An example of an area of the cytoskeleton that is very active and requires coordination by functional proteins is the **centrosome.** The centrosome is a region of the cytoplasm near the nucleus that coordinates the building and breaking apart of microtubules in the cell. For this reason, this nonmembranous structure is often called the *microtubule-organizing centre (MTOC).*

Look for the tiny yellow-green centrosome in **Figure 5-15**, *C* (right panel). You can see, radiating out from the centrosome in this micrograph, the green-stained microtubules organized around it.

The boundaries of the centrosome are rather indistinct because it lacks a membranous wall. However, the general location of the centrosome is easy to find because of a pair of cylindrical structures called **centrioles.**

Under the light microscope, centrioles appear as two dots located near the nucleus. The electron microscope, however, reveals them to be not mere dots but tiny cylinders (**Figure 5-16**). The walls of the cylinders consist of nine bundles of microtubules, with three tubules

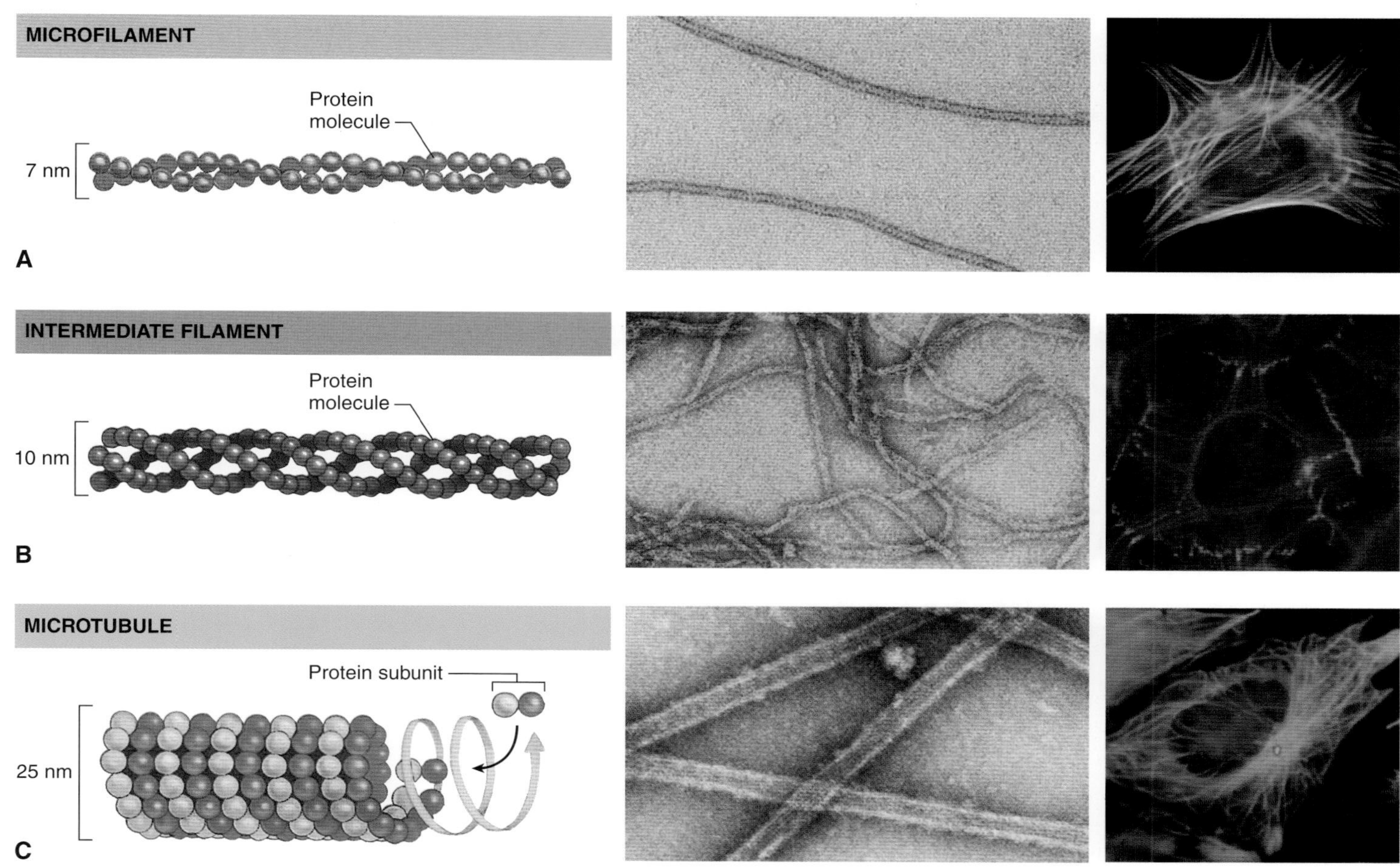

FIGURE 5-15 Cell fibres. The left panel of each part is a sketch, the middle panel is a transmission electron micrograph (TEM), and the right panel is a light micrograph using fluorescent stains to highlight specific molecules within each cell. **A,** *Microfilaments* are thin, twisted strands of protein molecules. **B,** *Intermediate filaments* are thicker, twisted protein strands. **C,** *Microtubules* are hollow fibres that consist of a spiral arrangement of protein subunits. Note the bright yellow-green microtubule-organizing centre (centrosome) near the large purple nucleus in the bottom right panel.

in each bundle. A curious fact about these two tubular-walled cylinders is that they are tethered by tiny fibres and sit at right angles to each other. This special arrangement occurs when the centrioles separate in preparation for cell division (see **Table 7-5** on p. 129). Before separating, a daughter centriole is formed perpendicular to each member of the original pair (both become "mother" centrioles) so that a complete pair may be distributed to each new cell.

A cloudlike mass of material surrounding the centrioles is called the *pericentriolar material (PCM)*. The PCM is active in starting the growth of new microtubules. The distal and subdistal appendages on the mother centriole that you can see in **Figure 5-16**, A, are anchor points for microtubules.

The microtubule organizing function of the centrosome plays an important role during cell division, when a special "spindle" of microtubules is constructed for the purpose of pulling chromosomes apart and toward each daughter cell. As this spindle forms, the centrosome is anchored by an **aster,** which is a formation of microtubules radiating outward from the centrioles.

In addition to their involvement in forming the spindle that appears during cell division and other key components of the cytoskeleton, the centrosome is involved in the formation of microtubular cell extensions (discussed in Cell Extensions on p. 90).

Molecular Motors

Have you wondered as you've read along how all the little vesicles, organelles, and molecules always seem to be able to move on their own power to where they need to go in a cell? Vesicles don't have feet! So how do they move from place to place in an organized way? The answer is surprising: cellular movement *does* rely on "foot" power! The cell's internal "feet" are actually little protein structures called **molecular motors.** As you can see in **Figure 5-17**, these little motors are like tiny feet that pull huge loads along the microtubules and microfilaments of the cytoskeleton. The loads may be vesicles or other small organelles, fibres, or large molecules. The tiny *motor proteins* transport organelles along a microtubule or fibre as if they were railway carriages being pulled along a track. This system provides rapid, orderly movement of structures and materials around the cell. It also allows the cell's framework to move with force, extending and contracting to create movements of the cell. In fact, muscles in your body are able to contract with force because of the action of

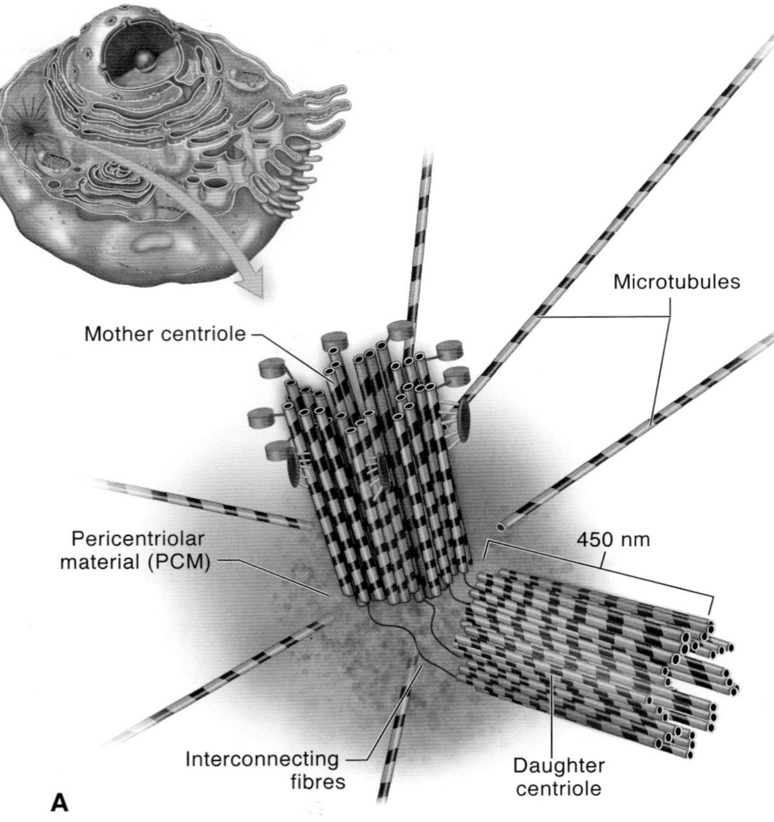

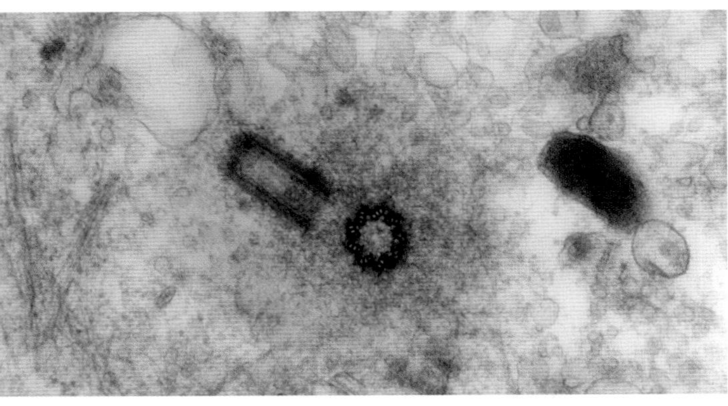

FIGURE 5-16 Centrosome. Sketch **(A)** and transmission electron micrograph (TEM) **(B)** showing the structure of the centrosome, which acts as a microtubule-organizing centre for the cell's cytoskeleton.

many myosin molecules (see **Figure 5-17**) pulling together overlapping rows of microfilaments within each muscle cell, as mentioned earlier.

The cell attaches motor molecules to the ends of cisternae in the Golgi apparatus and pulls these sacs outward into their characteristic flattened shape. This action eventually pulls vesicles off the Golgi cisternae.

FIGURE 5-17 Motor proteins. Molecular motors include the proteins myosin, kinesin, and dynein. They move along a track—microtubules or microfilaments—and pull larger structures such as vesicles, fibres, or particles. Such movement can be used for intracellular transport or movement of the cell's entire framework.

Other types of molecular motors can be used to generate power by converting mechanical energy to chemical energy, like the motor of a hybrid automobile—an example that we explore in Chapter 41.

Cell Extensions

In some cells the cytoskeleton forms projections that extend the plasma membrane outward to form tiny, fingerlike processes. These processes, *microvilli*, *cilia*, and *flagella*, are present only in certain types of cells—depending, of course, on a cell's particular functions.

Microvilli

Microvilli are found in epithelial cells that line the intestines and other areas where absorption is important (**Figure 5-18**, A). Like tiny fingers crowded against each other, microvilli cover part of the surface of a cell (see **Figure 5-1**). A single microvillus measures about 0.5 μm long and only 0.1 μm or less across. Inside each microvillus are microfilament bundles that provide both structural support and the ability to move. Because one cell has hundreds of these projections, the surface area of the cell is increased manyfold—a structural feature that enables the cell to perform its function of absorption at a faster rate.

Cilia

Cilia and flagella are cell processes that have cylinders made of microtubules at their core. Each cylinder is composed of nine double microtubules arranged around two single microtubules in the centre—a slightly different

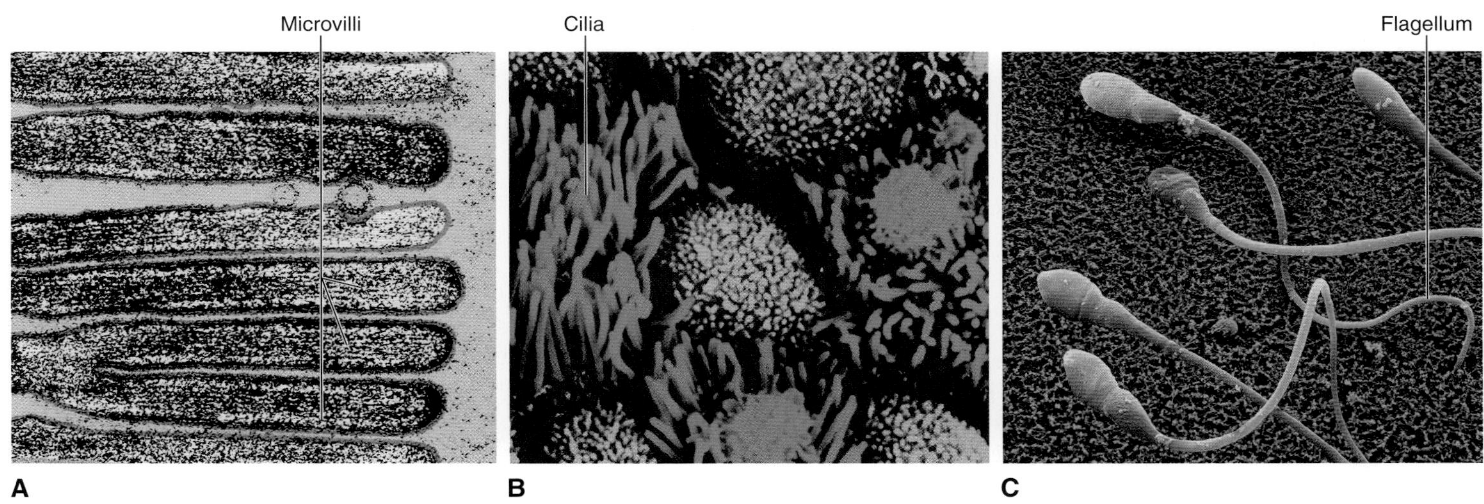

FIGURE 5-18 Cell processes. A, *Microvilli* are numerous, fingerlike projections that increase the surface area of absorptive cells. This electron micrograph shows a longitudinal section of microvilli from a cell lining the small intestine. Note the bundles of microfilaments that support the microvilli. **B,** *Cilia* are numerous, fine processes that transport fluid across the surface of the cell. This electron micrograph shows cilia (long projections) and microvilli (small bumps) on cells lining the lung airways. **C,** In humans, *flagella* are single, elongated processes on sperm cells that enable these cells to "swim".

arrangement than in centrioles. With the addition of molecular motors, this particular arrangement is suited to movement. Dynein, a type of motor protein (see **Figure 5-17**), moves the microtubule pairs so they slip back and forth past one another to produce a "wiggling" movement.

Among human cells, what distinguishes cilia from flagella are their size, number, and pattern of movement. Human cilia are shorter and more numerous than flagella (**Figure 5-18**, *B*). Under low magnification, cilia look like tiny hairs. The cilia often move in a rhythmic, coordinated way to push substances such as mucus along the cell surface, as explained in **Figure 5-19**. In the lining of the respiratory tract, the movement of cilia keeps contaminated mucus on cell surfaces moving toward the throat, where it can be swallowed. In the lining of the female reproductive tract, cilia keep the ovum moving toward the uterus. Cilia also have a sensory function, detecting changes in the mucus being moved.

Except for blood cells, most cell types have a single *primary cilium*. The primary cilium lacks the centre pair of microtubules and certain motor molecules, such as dynein (see **Figure 5-17**). Therefore, the primary cilium cannot move like other types of cilia. However, they have other important functions. For example, primary cilia often act as sensory organelles that permit sensations such as vision, hearing, balance, and so on, as you will learn in Chapter 24. In the kidney, primary cilia monitor urine flow and, if damaged, can cause kidney failure. Primary cilia also play a critical role in centriole replication and regulation of cell reproduction (see Chapter 7).

Flagella

Flagella are single, long structures in the only type of human cell that has this feature: the human sperm cell (see **Figure 5-18**, *C*). A sperm cell's flagellum moves like the tail of an eel (as you can see in **Figure 5-19**) to allow the cell to "swim" toward the female sex cell (ovum).

Each year brings with it the discovery of new types of cytoskeletal components. As we tease out their functions, we find that the cytoskeleton is an amazingly rich network that is literally the

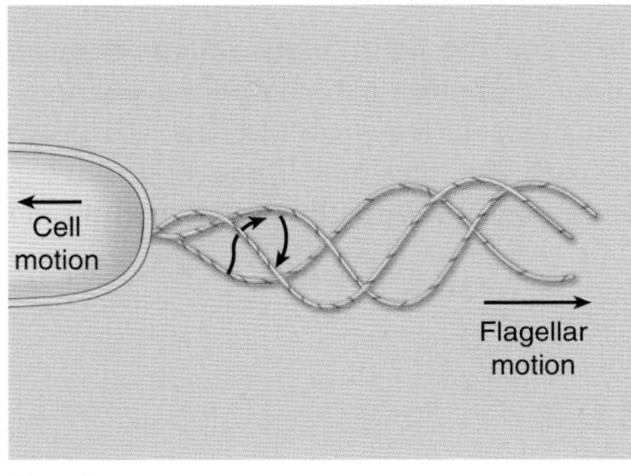

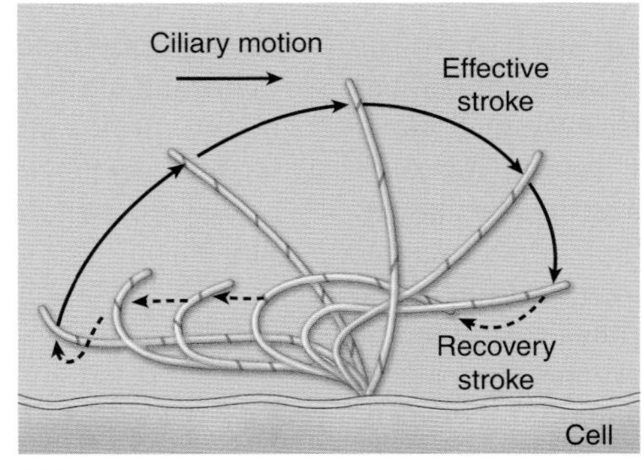

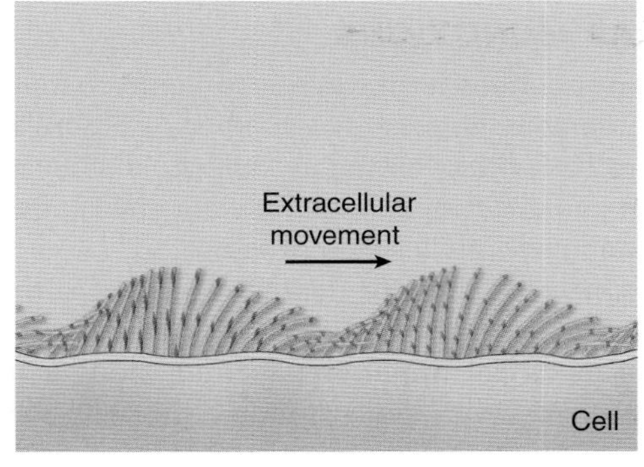

FIGURE 5-19 Movement patterns. A flagellum *(left)* produces wavelike movements, which propels a sperm cell forward—like the tail of an eel. In humans, cilia (*middle* and *right*) found in groups on stationary cells beat in a coordinated oarlike pattern to push fluid and particles in the extracellular fluid along the outer cell surface.

"bones and muscles" of the cell. It provides a variety of many different types of cell movement, both internal and external, depending on the cell and the circumstances. It provides many different kinds of structural support for the cell and its parts—and even becomes involved in connections with other cells. Most amazing of all, the cytoskeleton has the ability to organize itself by means of a complex set of signals and reactions so that it can quickly respond to the needs of the cell.

CELL CONNECTIONS

The tissues and organs of the body must be held together, so they must, of course, be connected in some way. Many cells attach directly to the extracellular material, or *matrix*, that surrounds them. A group of integral membrane proteins called *integrins* helps hold cells in their place in a tissue. Some integrin molecules span the plasma membrane and often connect the fibres of the cytoskeleton inside the cell to the extracellular fibres of the matrix, thereby anchoring the cell in place. In this manner, also, some cells are held to one another indirectly by fibrous nets that surround groups of cells. Certain muscle cells are held together this way.

Cells may form direct connections with each other. Integrins are sometimes involved in direct cell connections, but other connecting proteins, such as *selectins*, *cadherins*, and *immunoglobulins*, help form most cell-to-cell connections. Not only do such connections hold the cells together, they sometimes also allow direct communication between the cells. The major types of direct cell connections are summarized in **Figure 5-20**.

DESMOSOMES

Desmosomes sometimes have the appearance of small "spot welds" that hold adjacent cells together. Adjacent skin cells are held together this way. Note in **Figure 5-20** that fibres on the outer surface of each *spot desmosome* interlock with each other. This arrangement resembles Velcro, which holds things together tightly when tiny plastic hooks become interlocked with fabric loops. Note also that the desmosomes are anchored internally by intermediate filaments of the cytoskeleton.

Some cells have a beltlike version of the desmosome structure that completely encircles the cell. This form may be called a *belt desmosome* to distinguish it from a spot desmosome. The belt desmosome is sometimes also called an *adhesive belt* or *zona adherens*.

GAP JUNCTIONS

Gap junctions form when membrane channels of adjacent plasma membranes connect to each other. As **Figure 5-20** shows, such junctions have the following two effects: (1) they form gaps or "tunnels" that join the cytoplasm of two cells, and (2) they fuse the two plasma membranes into a single structure.

One advantage of this arrangement is that certain molecules can pass directly from one cell to another. Another advantage is that electrical impulses travelling along a membrane can travel over many cell membranes in a row without stopping in between separate membranes because they have "run out of membrane". Heart muscle cells are joined by gap junctions so that a single impulse can travel to, and thus stimulate, many cells at the same time.

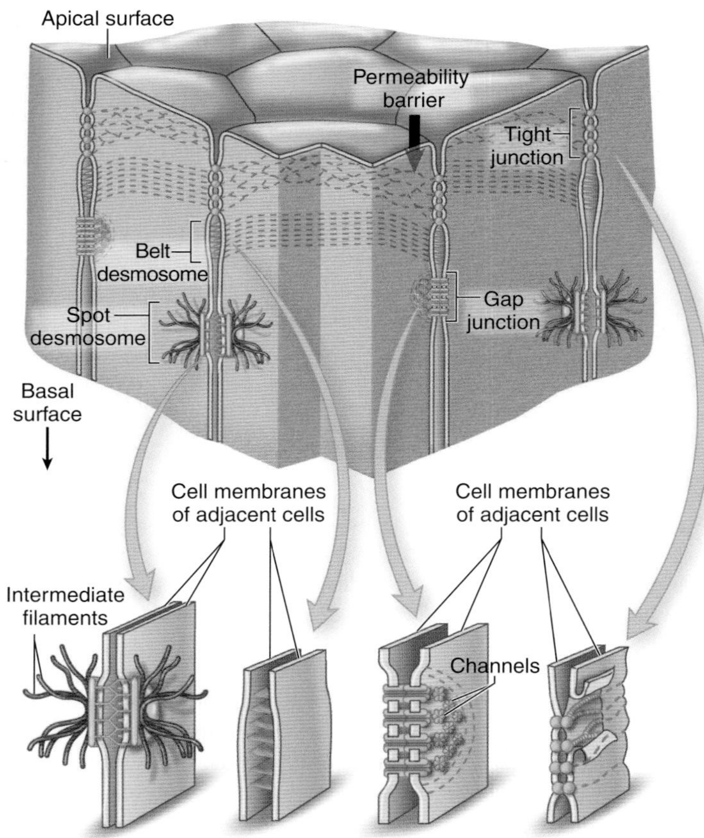

FIGURE 5-20 Cell connections. Spot and belt desmosomes, gap junction, and tight junction.

TIGHT JUNCTIONS

Tight junctions occur in cells that are joined near their apical surfaces by "collars" of tightly fused membrane. As you can see in **Figure 5-20**, rows of integral membrane proteins that extend all the way around a cell fuse with similar integral membrane proteins in neighbouring cells. An entire sheet of cells can be bound together the way soft drink cans are held in a six-pack by plastic collars—only more tightly. When tight junctions hold a sheet of cells together, molecules cannot easily *permeate*, or spread through, the cracks between the cells. Tight junctions occur in the lining of the intestines and other parts of the body, where it is important to control what gets past a sheet of cells. The only way for a molecule to get past the intestinal lining is through controlled channel, or carrier, molecules in the plasma membranes of the cells.

Quick **CHECK**

8. Describe the three types of fibres in the cytoskeleton.
9. What is the function of the centrosome?
10. Name each of the three typical types of cell junctions and describe them.

the big picture | Cell Anatomy and the Whole Body

Probably one of the most difficult things to do when first exploring the microscopic world of the cell is to appreciate the structural significance a single cell has to the whole body. Where are these unseen cells? How does each relate to this big thing I call my body?

One useful way to approach the structural role of cells in the whole body is to think of a large, complicated building. For example, the building in which you take your anatomy and physiology course is made up of thousands, perhaps hundreds of thousands, of structural subunits. Bricks, blocks, metal or wood studs, boards, and so on are individual structures within the building that all have specific parts, or organelles, that somehow contribute to overall function. A brick often has sides of certain dimensions that allow it to fit easily with other bricks or with other building materials. Three or four surfaces are usually textured in an aesthetically pleasing manner, and holes in two of the brick surfaces lighten the weight of the brick, allow other materials such as wires or reinforcing rods to pass through, and permit mortar to form a stronger joint with the brick. The material from which each brick is made has been formulated with certain ratios of sand, clay, pigments, or other materials. Each structural feature of each brick has a functional role to play. Likewise, each brick and other structural subunits of the building have an important role to play in supporting the building and making it a pleasing, functional place to study.

Like the structural features of a brick, each organelle of each cell has a functional role to play within the cell. In fact, you can often guess a cell's function by the proportion and variety of different organelles it has. Each cell, like each brick in a building, has a role to play in providing its tiny portion of the overall support and function of the whole body. Where are these cells? In the same place you would find bricks and other structural subunits in a building—everywhere! Like bricks and mortar, everything in your body is made of cells and the extracellular material surrounding them. How do cells relate to the whole body? Like bricks that are held together to form a building, cells form the body.

Just as a brick building is made of many different materials, the human body includes many structural subunits, each with its own structural features or organelles that contribute to the function of the cell—and therefore to the whole body.

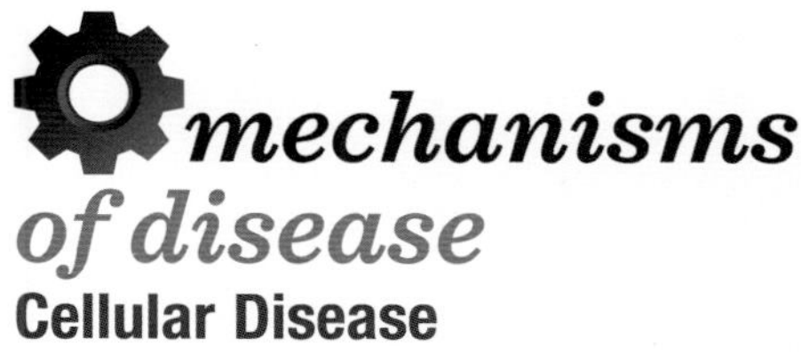

mechanisms of disease

Cellular Disease

The more that we learn about the mechanisms of disease, the more apparent it becomes that most diseases known to medicine involve abnormalities of cells. Even a few abnormal cells can so disrupt the internal environment of the body that a person's health can be in immediate danger. The following paragraphs list several important categories of disease that are caused by cell abnormalities. Specific diseases belonging to these categories are discussed further in later chapters. The sampler here and in the next couple of chapters about cell function will start you off with a basic understanding of cellular mechanisms of disease.

Disorders Involving Cell Membranes

Disorders involving cell membrane receptors are being actively investigated by biologists. One such particularly common disorder is a form of **diabetes mellitus (DM)** called *type 2 diabetes.* This condition is often produced by a cellular response to obesity that triggers a reduction in the number of functioning membrane receptors for the hormone *insulin.* Cells throughout the body thus become less sensitive to insulin, the hormone that allows glucose molecules to enter the plasma membrane. Without sufficient stimulation by insulin, the cells literally starve for energy-rich glucose, even though it is available outside the cell.

Duchenne muscular dystrophy (DMD), a severe inherited condition, results from "leaky" membranes in muscle cells. *Dystrophin,* a protein that normally helps connect a muscle cell's cytoskeleton to the plasma membrane and to the surrounding extracellular matrix, is missing (**Figure 5-21**). Muscle contractions pull at the weakened connections to the plasma membrane and rip holes that allow calcium ions (Ca^{++}) to enter the cell. This flood of Ca^{++} triggers chemical reactions that destroy the muscle, causing life-threatening paralysis.

Disorders Involving Organelles

Any abnormality of any of the organelles is likely to produce disease. Knowing the functions of the organelles helps health professionals understand the nature and symptoms of these disorders.

Failure of mitochondria reduces the cell's ability to produce enough energy for normal function. Mitochondrial abnormalities resulting from chemical damage are known to be a factor in many significant degenerative diseases, such as **Parkinson disease (PD).** PD affects the areas of the brain that control muscles, progressively making effective movement more difficult. Mitochondrial dysfunction is also thought to be involved in the normal degeneration associated with ageing.

Some degenerative diseases may also involve the breakdown of the microtubules of the cytoskeleton, which often happens in PD.

Failure of the protein-making system of the ribosomes, ER, and Golgi apparatus can produce many types of diseases that are caused by the absence of one or more proteins critical for body function. Failure of the quality control system provided by proteasomes has been implicated in the buildup of abnormal proteins that form the plaques that characterize **Alzheimer disease (AD)** and other degenerative disorders.

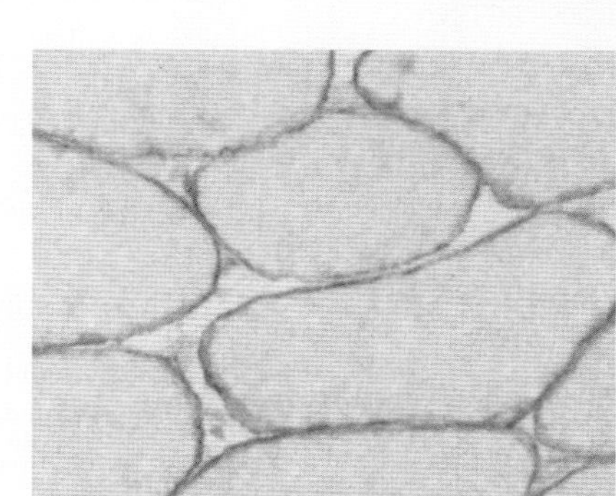

FIGURE 5-21 Dystrophin. This cross-section of muscle fibres has been stained for the presence of dystrophin (seen along each cell's plasma membrane). In Duchenne muscular dystrophy (DMD), this protein would be completely absent, thus causing damage to the membranes of muscle fibres that results in destruction of muscle tissue.

LANGUAGE OF SCIENCE (continued from p. 75)

integral membrane protein (IMP) (IN-te-grel MEM-brayn PROH-teen) [*integr-* **whole,** *-al* **relating to,** *membran-* **thin skin,** *prote-* **primary,** *-in* **substance**]

intermediate filament (in-ter-MEE-dee-it FIL-ah-ment) [*inter-* **between,** *-mediate* **divide,** *fila-* **threadlike,** *–ment* **process**]

lysosome (LYE-so-sohm) [*lyso-* **loosen,** *-som-* **body**]

microfilament (my-kroh-FIL-ah-ment) [*micro* **small,** *-fila-* **threadlike,** *-ment* **thing**]

microscopy (my-KROS-kah-pee) [*micro-* **small,** *-scop-* **see,** *-y* **activity**]

microtubule (my-kroh-TYOOB-yool) [*micro-* **small,** *-tubule* **little tube**]

microvillus (my-kroh-VIL-us) [*micro-* **small,** *-villus* **shaggy hair**] *pl.,* microvilli

mitochondrion (my-toh-KON-dree-on) [*mito-* **thread,** *-chondrion-* **granule**] *pl.,* mitochondria

molecular motor (mo-LEK-yoo-lar MO-ter) [*mole-* **mass,** *-cul-* **small,** *-ar* **relating to,** *mot-* **move,** *-or* **agent**]

nucleolus (nyoo-klee-OH-lus) [*nucleo-* **nucleus (kernel),** *-olus* **little**] *pl.,* nucleoli

nucleus (NYOO-klee-us) [*nucleus* **kernel**] *pl.,* nuclei

organelle (org-an-EL) [*organ-* **tool or organ,** *-elle* **small**]

peroxisome (pe-ROKS-ih-sohm) [*peroxi-* **hydrogen peroxide,** *-soma* **body**]

plasma membrane (PLAZ-mah MEM-brayne) [*plasma* **substance,** *membran-* **thin skin**]

proteasome (PROH-tee-ah-sohm) [*protea-* **protein,** *-som-* **body**]

receptor (ree-SEP-tor) [*recept-* **receive,** *-or* **agent**]

ribosome (RYE-boh-sohm) [*ribo-* **ribose or RNA,** *-som-* **body**]

signal transduction (SIG-nal tranz-DUK-shen) [*trans-* **across,** *-duc-* **transfer,** *-tion* **process**]

tight junction (tite JUNK-shen)

vesicle (VES-i-kul) [*vesic-* **blister,** *-cle* **little**]

LANGUAGE OF MEDICINE

Alzheimer disease (AD) (AHLZ-hye-mer) [*Alois Alzheimer* **German neurologist**]

diabetes mellitus (DM) (dye-ah-BEE-teez mell-EYE-tus) [*diabetes* **pass-through or siphon;** *mellitus* **honey-sweet**]

Duchenne muscular dystrophy (DMD) (doo-SHEN MUSS-kyoo-lar DISS-troh-fee) [*Duchenne* Guillaume B.A. Duchenne de Boulogne; **French neurologist;** *muscul-* **little mouse (muscle),** *-ar* **relating to;** *dys-* **bad,** *-troph-* **nourishment,** *-y* **state**]

Parkinson disease (PD) (PAR-kin-son) [*James Parkinson* **English physician**]

case study

Tom, a trainee laboratory technician, decided to specialize in electron microscopy. He spent the first two weeks of his training learning how to fix, stain and section a range of tissues for use in the transmission electron microscope (TEM). Once his first preparation was ready, the senior research technician scanned the image and assessed the results with Tom. The senior technician explained that the processing of cells for examination in the vacuum created by the TEM damages the structure of delicate plasma membranes. Tom would not be able to see the pores and structures that allow hydrophilic molecules into the cell, but he could expect to see many organelles in great detail.

1. Which membrane structures that transport hydrophilic molecules had been damaged in the processing of Tom's cells?
   a. Phospholipids
   b. Glycolipids
   c. Transmembrane cholesterols
   d. Channel proteins
2. Tom then moved the specimen and could immediately see a network of membranes that appeared to form channels with small dark particles attached to their outer surface. In some areas, the channels appeared smooth with no dark particles. What was Tom observing?
   a. The Golgi apparatus
   b. Endoplasmic reticulum
   c. A mitochondrion
   d. Microtubules
3. What were the dark particles observed by Tom?
   a. Lysosomes
   b. Peroxisomes
   c. Ribosomes
   d. Mitochondria
4. After looking at many specimens, Tom noticed fibrous structures within some cells, and they were different sizes. The larger fibres sometimes appeared in bundles, and the senior technician told him they form part of the cell's cytoskeleton.
   What were the large fibrous structures observed by Tom?
   a. Microtubules
   b. Microfilaments
   c. Microvilli
   d. Intermediate filaments

Hint To solve a case study, you may have to refer to the glossary or index, other chapters in this textbook, **Connect It!,** and other resources.

CHAPTER SUMMARY

To download an MP3 version of the chapter summary for use with your mobile device, access the **Audio Chapter Summaries** *online at evolve.elsevier.com.*

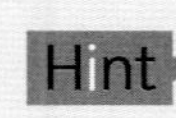

Scan this summary after reading the chapter to help you reinforce the key concepts. Later, use the summary as a quick review before your class or before a test.

Functional Anatomy of Cells

A. The typical cell (**Figure 5-1**)
   1. Also called composite cell
   2. Vary in size; all are microscopic (**Table 5-1**)
   3. Vary in structure and function (**Table 5-2**)

B. Cell structures
   1. Plasma membrane—separates the cell from its surrounding environment
   2. Cytoplasm—thick gel-like substance inside the cell composed of numerous organelles suspended in watery cytosol; each type of organelle is suited to perform particular functions (**Figure 5-2**)
   3. Nucleus—large membranous structure near the centre of the cell

Cell Membranes

A. Each cell contains a variety of membranes
   1. Plasma membrane (**Figure 5-3**)—outer boundary of cell
   2. Membranous organelles—sacs and canals made of the same material as the plasma membrane

B. Fluid mosaic model—theory explaining how cell membranes are constructed
   1. Molecules of the cell membrane are arranged in a sheet
   2. The mosaic of molecules is fluid; that is, the molecules are able to float around slowly
   3. This model illustrates that the molecules of the cell membrane form a continuous sheet
   4. Chemical attractions are the forces that hold membranes together

C. Phospholipid bilayer
   1. Primary structure of a cell membrane is a double layer of phospholipid molecules
      a. Heads are hydrophilic (“water loving”)
      b. Tails are hydrophobic (“water fearing”)
      c. They arrange themselves in bilayers in water
   2. Cholesterol molecules are scattered among the phospholipids to allow the membrane to function properly at body temperature
   3. Most of the bilayer is hydrophobic; therefore water or water-soluble molecules do not pass through easily
   4. Rafts—groupings of membrane molecules that float as a unit in the membrane (**Figure 5-4**); rafts may pinch inward to bring material into the cell or organelle

D. Integral membrane proteins (IMPs) (**Table 5-4**)
   1. A cell controls what moves through the membrane by means of IMPs embedded in the phospholipid bilayer
   2. Some IMPs have carbohydrates attached to them and as a result form glycoproteins that act as identification markers
   3. Some IMPs are receptors that react to specific chemicals, sometimes permitting a process called *signal transduction*
   4. Some IMPs connect the cell membrane to another membrane to form a larger mass of tissue

Cytoplasm and Organelles

A. Cytoplasm—gel-like internal substance of cells that includes many organelles suspended in watery intracellular fluid called *cytosol*

B. Two major groups of organelles (**Table 5-3**)
   1. Membranous organelles are sacs or canals made of cell membranes
   2. Nonmembranous organelles are made of microscopic filaments or other nonmembranous materials

C. Endoplasmic reticulum (ER) (**Figure 5-5**)
   1. Made of membranous-walled canals and flat, curving sacs arranged in parallel rows throughout the cytoplasm; extend from the plasma membrane to the nucleus
   2. Proteins move through the canals
   3. Two types of endoplasmic reticulum
      a. Rough endoplasmic reticulum (RER)
         (1) Ribosomes dot the outer surface of the membranous walls
         (2) Ribosomes synthesize proteins, which fold within the RER and move toward the Golgi apparatus, then eventually leave the cell
         (3) Functions in protein synthesis, membrane synthesis, and intracellular transportation
      b. Smooth endoplasmic reticulum (SER)
         (1) No ribosomes border the membranous wall
         (2) Functions more varied than for the rough endoplasmic reticulum
            (a) Makes enzymes that detoxify the cell
            (b) Makes enzymes that regulate conversion of glycogen to glucose (for energy)
            (c) Synthesizes certain lipids and carbohydrates and creates membranes for use throughout the cell
            (d) Removes and stores Ca^{++} from the cell’s interior

D. Ribosomes (**Figure 5-6**)
   1. Many are attached to the rough endoplasmic reticulum and many lie free, scattered throughout the cytoplasm
   2. Each ribosome is a nonmembranous structure made of two pieces, a large subunit and a small subunit; each subunit is composed of rRNA and protein
   3. Ribosomes in the endoplasmic reticulum make proteins for “export” or to be embedded in the plasma membrane; free ribosomes make proteins for the cell’s domestic use

E. Golgi apparatus
   1. Membranous organelle consisting of cisternae stacked on one another and located near the nucleus (**Figure 5-7**)
   2. Processes protein molecules from the endoplasmic reticulum (**Figure 5-8**)
   3. Processed proteins leave the final cisterna in a vesicle; contents may then be secreted outside the cell

F. Lysosomes (**Figure 5-9**)
   1. Made of microscopic membranous sacs that have “pinched inward” from the plasma membrane and become filled with digestive enzymes from the ER and Golgi apparatus

2. The cell's own digestive system; enzymes in lysosomes digest the protein structures of unneeded or defective cell parts (autophagy), including integral membrane proteins, and particles that have become trapped in the cell; some lysosomes help repair cell membranes and release important substances from the cell

G. Proteasomes (**Figure 5-10**)
  1. Hollow, protein cylinders found throughout the cytoplasm
  2. Break down abnormal/misfolded proteins and normal proteins no longer needed by the cell (and which may cause disease)
  3. Break down protein molecules one at a time by tagging each one with a chain of ubiquitin molecules, unfolding it as it enters the proteasome, and then breaking apart peptide bonds

H. Peroxisomes
  1. Small membranous sacs containing enzymes that detoxify harmful substances that enter the cells
  2. Often seen in kidney and liver cells

I. Mitochondria (**Figure 5-11**)
  1. Made up of microscopic sacs; wall composed of inner and outer membranes separated by fluid; thousands of particles make up enzyme molecules attached to both membranes
  2. The "power plants" of cells; mitochondrial enzymes catalyze series of oxidation reactions that provide nearly most of a cell's energy supply
  3. Each mitochondrion has a DNA molecule, which allows it to produce its own enzymes and replicate copies of itself

Nucleus

A. Definition—spherical body in centre of cell; enclosed by an envelope with many pores

B. Structure (**Figure 5-12**)
  1. Consists of a nuclear envelope (composed of two membranes, each with essentially the same molecular structure as the plasma membrane) surrounding nucleoplasm
     a. Can be considered part of the ER
     b. Nuclear envelope has holes called *nuclear pores*
     c. Nuclear pore complexes (NPCs) are elaborate gateways into and out of the nucleus (**Figure 5-13**)
  2. Contains DNA (heredity molecules), which appear as:
     a. Chromatin threads or granules in nondividing cells
     b. Chromosomes in early stages of cell division

C. Functions of the nucleus are functions of DNA molecules; DNA determines both the structure and function of cells and heredity

Cytoskeleton

A. The cell's internal supporting framework (**Figure 5-14**)
  1. Made up of tiny, flexible fibres and rigid, rodlike pieces
  2. Provides support for cell shape
  3. Can move the cell or its parts
  4. Detects changes inside and outside the cell

B. Cell fibres
  1. Intricately arranged fibres of varying length that form a three-dimensional, irregularly shaped lattice
  2. Fibres appear to support the endoplasmic reticulum, mitochondria, and "free" ribosomes
  3. Microfilaments (**Figure 5-15**)—smallest cell fibres
     a. Serve as "cellular muscles"
     b. Made of thin, twisted strands of protein molecules that lie parallel to the long axis of the cell
     c. Can slide past each other and cause shortening of the cell
  4. Intermediate filaments—twisted protein strands slightly thicker than microfilaments; form much of the supporting framework in many types of cells
  5. Microtubules—tiny, hollow tubes that are the thickest of the cell fibres
     a. Made of protein subunits arranged in a spiral fashion
     b. Their function is to move things around inside the cell

C. Centrosome (**Figure 5-16**)
  1. An area of the cytoplasm near the nucleus that coordinates the building and breaking apart of microtubules in the cell
  2. Nonmembranous structure also called the *microtubule organizing centre (MTOC)*
  3. Plays an important role during cell division
  4. The general location of the centrosome is identified by the centrioles

D. Molecular motors
  1. Motor proteins (**Figure 5-17**) include dynein, myosin, and kinesin
  2. Molecular motors can pull larger structures along microtubules and microfilaments as if along a track, providing intracellular transport and movements of the entire cell

E. Cell extensions
  1. Cytoskeleton forms projections that extend the plasma membrane outward to form tiny, fingerlike processes
  2. There are three types of these processes; each has specific functions (**Figure 5-18**)
     a. Microvilli—found in epithelial cells that line the intestines and other areas where absorption is important; they help increase the surface area manyfold
     b. Cilia and flagella—cell processes that have cylinders made of microtubules and molecular motors at their core (**Figure 5-19**)
        (1) Cilia are shorter and more numerous than flagella; some cilia found in groups have coordinated oarlike movements that brush material past the cell's surface; all cilia have sensory functions
        (2) Flagella are found only on human sperm cells; flagella move with a tail-like movement that propels the sperm cell forward

Cell Connections

A. Cells are held together by fibrous nets that surround groups of cells (e.g., muscle cells), or cells have direct connections to each other

B. Three types of direct cell connections (**Figure 5-20**)
  1. Desmosome
     a. Fibres on the outer surface of each desmosome interlock with each other; anchored internally by intermediate filaments of the cytoskeleton

b. Spot desmosomes are like "spot welds" at various points connecting adjacent membranes
c. Belt desmosomes encircle the entire cell; also called *adhesive belt* or *zona adherens*

2. Gap junctions—membrane channels of adjacent plasma membranes that adhere to each other—have two effects:
   a. Form gaps or "tunnels" that join the cytoplasm of two cells
   b. Fuse two plasma membranes into a single structure
3. Tight junctions
   a. Occur in cells that are joined by "collars" of tightly fused material
   b. Molecules cannot permeate the cracks of tight junctions
   c. Occur in the lining of the intestines and other parts of the body where it is important to control what gets through a sheet of cells

REVIEW QUESTIONS

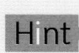

Write out the answers to these questions after reading the chapter and reviewing the Chapter Summary. Note—writing out your answers will consolidate learning and provide a valuable resource of information.

1. What is the range in human cell diameters?
2. List the three main cell structures.
3. Describe the molecular structure of the plasma membrane. What is the width of the plasma membrane?
4. Summarize the communication function of the plasma membrane, its transportation function, and its identification function.
5. Prepare a table classifying the following cellular structures/organelles: endoplasmic reticulum, ribosomes, Golgi apparatus, mitochondria, lysosomes, proteasomes, peroxisomes, cytoskeleton, cell fibres, centrosome, centrioles and cell extensions. Include the following columns: organelle name, function and structure. Include a column indicating whether the structure is membranous or nonmembranous.
6. Describe the three types of intercellular junctions. What are the special functional advantages of each?
7. Outline the functions of the nucleus and the nucleoli. What are the unique features of the nuclear envelope?
8. Name three kinds of micrography used in this book to illustrate cell structures. What perspective does each give that the other two do not? (See ***Connect It!***, p. 76.)

CRITICAL THINKING QUESTIONS

After finishing the Review Questions, write out the answers to these more in-depth questions to help you apply your new knowledge. Go back to sections of the chapter that relate to concepts that you find difficult.

1. Using the complementarity principle that cell structure is related to its function, discuss how the shapes of the nerve cell and muscle cell are specific to their respective functions.
2. What is the relationship among ribosomes, endoplasmic reticulum, Golgi apparatus, and plasma membrane? How do they work together as a system?
3. Develop a descriptive nickname for the following organelles: rough endoplasmic reticulum, smooth endoplasmic reticulum, ribosomes, Golgi apparatus, lysosomes, nucleus, nucleolus, vesicles and cytoskeleton. The nickname should summarize the primary function. Several are listed throughout the chapter. For example: the mitochondrion is regarded as the powerhouse; the nucleus is the control centre. Try to create names other than those listed.

6 Cell Function

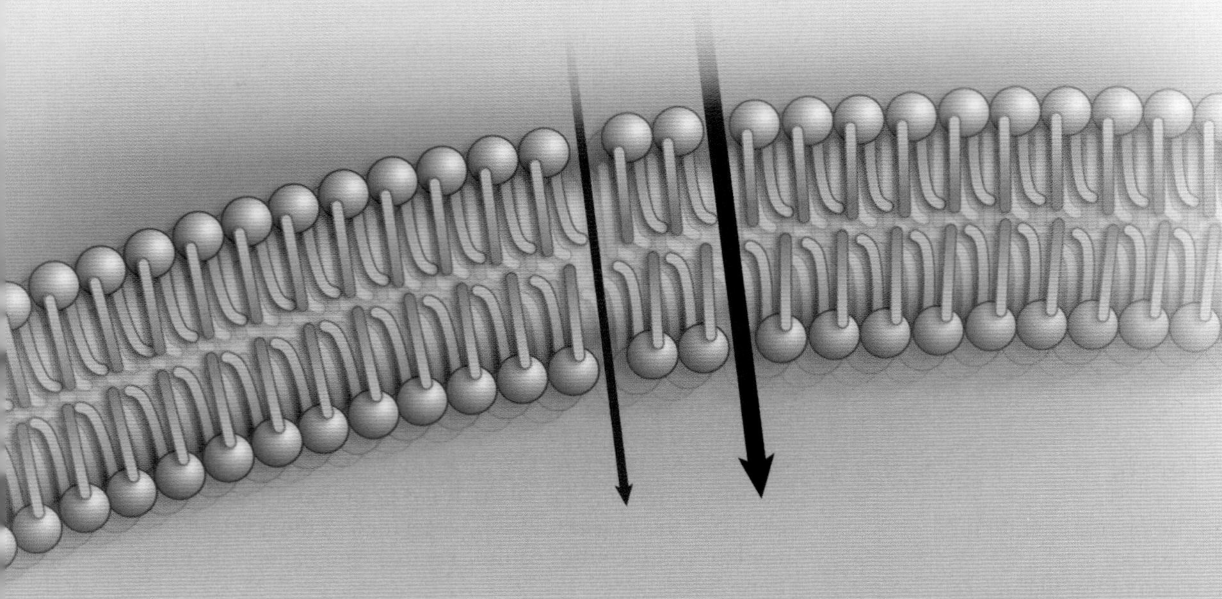

CHAPTER OUTLINE

Hint ▸ *Scan this outline before you begin to read the chapter, as a preview of how the concepts are organized.*

The cell is the basic functional unit of the body, so it is no wonder that a good understanding of human physiology begins with an overview of cell function. In Chapter 5, you were introduced to the basic structures of the cell. That discussion also included an introduction to some of the important functions of the cell. In this chapter, we take that a step further.

We begin with a brief study of cell membrane transport—a concept that is the foundation for understanding the function of muscles, nerves, glands, hormones, and most other concepts of human physiology. Then, an overview of cell metabolism will set the stage for understanding the "body chemistry" of the whole human organism. That will lead us into Chapter 7, where we explore concepts of cell growth and reproduction.

LANGUAGE OF SCIENCE

Hint ▸ *Use this list to aid your pronunciation of unfamiliar words.*

actual osmotic pressure (actual os-MOT-ik PRESH-ur) [*osmo-* **impulse,** *-ic* **relating to**]

aerobic (air-OH-bik) [*aer-* **air,** *-bi-* **life,** *-ic* **relating to**]

allosteric effector (al-o-STEER-ik ee-FECKT-or) [*allo-* **another,** *-ster-* **solid,** *-ic* **relating to;** *effect* **accomplish**]

anabolism (ah-NAB-oh-liz-im) [*anabol-* **build up,** *-ism* **condition**]

anaerobic (an-air-OH-bik) [*an-* **without,** *-aer-* **air,** *-bi-* **life,** *-ic* **relating to**]

catabolism (kah-TAB-oh-liz-im) [*cata-* **against,** *-bol-* **to throw,** *-ism* **condition**]

catalyst (KAT-ah-list) [*cata-* **lower,** *-lys-* **loosen,** *-st* **actor**]

cellular respiration (SELL-yoo-lar res-pih-RAY-shun) [*cell* **storeroom,** *-ular* **relating to;** *respire-* **breathe,** *-ation* **process**]

citric acid cycle (SIT-rik ASS-id SYE-kul) [*citr-* **lemony,** *-ic* **relating to;** *acid* **sour,** *cycle* **circle**]

coenzyme (koh-EN-zyme) [*co-* **together,** *-en-* **in,** *-zyme* **ferment**]

concentration gradient (kon-sen-TRAY-shun GRAY-dee-ent) [*con-* **together,** *-centr-* **centre,** *-ation* **process;** *gradi-* **step,** *-ent* **state**]

cotransport (koh-TRANZ-port) [*co-* **together,** *-trans-* **across,** *-port* **carry**]

countertransport [*counter-* **against,** *-trans-* **across,** *-port* **carry**]

dialysis (dye-AL-i-sis) [*dia-* **apart,** *-lysis* **loosening**]

diffusion (dih-FYOO-shun) [*diffus-* **spread out,** *-sion* **process**]

electron transport system (ETS) (eh-LEK-tron TRANZ-port SIS-tem) [*electro-* **electricity,** *-on* **subatomic particle;** *trans-* **across,** *-port* **carry**]

continued on p. 116

MOVEMENT OF SUBSTANCES THROUGH CELL MEMBRANES

If a cell is to survive, it must be able to move substances to where they are needed. We already know one way that cells move organelles within the cytoplasm: pushing or pulling performed by the cytoskeleton. A cell must also be able to move various ions and molecules in and out through the plasma membrane, as well as from one membranous compartment to another within the cell. In this first part of the chapter, we explore some of the basic mechanisms a cell uses to move substances across its membranes.

Before beginning a discussion of individual processes, we must realize that membrane transport processes can be labelled as *passive* or *active*. Passive processes do not require any energy expenditure or "activity" of the cell membrane—the particles move by using energy that they already have. Active processes, on the other hand, do require the expenditure of metabolic energy by the cell. In active processes the transported particles are actively "carried" across the membrane. Keep this distinction in mind as we explore the basic mechanisms of cell membrane transport.

Passive Transport Processes

Diffusion

Often, molecules simply spread or diffuse through the membranes. The term **diffusion** refers to a natural phenomenon caused by the tendency of small particles to spread out evenly within any given space. All molecules in a solution bounce around in short, chaotic paths. As they collide with one another, they tend to spread out, or diffuse. Think of the example of a lump of sugar dissolving in water (**Figure 6-1**). Right after the lump is placed in the water, the sugar molecules are very close to one another—the sugar concentration in the lump is very high. As the sugar dissolves, the molecules begin colliding with one another and thus push each other away. Given enough time, the sugar eventually diffuses evenly throughout the water.

Note that during diffusion, molecules move from an area of higher concentration to an area of lower concentration. Another way of stating this principle is to say that diffusion occurs down a **concentration gradient.** A concentration gradient is simply a measurable difference in concentration from one area to another.

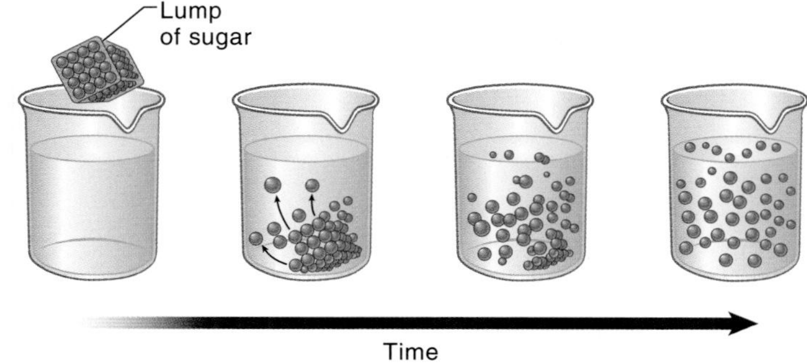

FIGURE 6-1 Diffusion. The molecules of a lump of sugar are very densely packed when they enter the water. As sugar molecules collide frequently in the area of higher concentration, they gradually spread away from each other—toward the area of lower concentration. Eventually, the sugar molecules become evenly distributed.

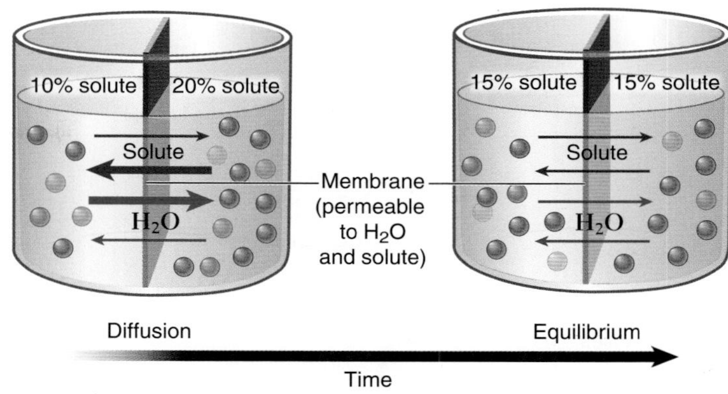

FIGURE 6-2 Diffusion through a membrane. Note that the membrane allows solute (a dissolved particle) and water to pass and that it separates a 10% solution from a 20% solution. The container on the left shows the two solutions separated by the membrane at the start of diffusion. The container on the right shows the result of diffusion after time.

Because molecules spread from the area of *higher* concentration to the area of *lower* concentration, they spread down the concentration gradient. The greater the difference in concentration from one area to another (that is, the larger or steeper the gradient), the greater is the movement of molecules.

Perhaps the best way to learn the principle of diffusion across a membrane is to look at the example illustrated in **Figure 6-2**. Here we have different mixtures of a *solute* (dissolved substance) in water. Suppose a 10% solute mixture is separated from a 20% solution by an artificial membrane. Suppose further that the membrane has pores in it that allow solute and solvent molecules to pass through. Solute particles and water molecules darting about the solution collide with each other and with the membrane. Some inevitably hit the membrane pores from the 20% solute side, and some hit the membrane pores from the 10% side. Just as inevitably, some pass through the pores in both directions. For a while, more solute particles enter the pores from the 20% side simply because they are more numerous there than on the 10% side. More of these particles, therefore, move through the membrane from the 20% solute solution into the 10% solute solution than diffuse through it in the opposite direction. In other words, the overall direction of diffusion is from the side where the concentration is higher (20%) to the side where the concentration is lower (10%).

During the time that diffusion of solute particles is taking place, diffusion of water molecules is also going on. Remember, the direction of diffusion of any substance is always down that substance's concentration gradient. Water molecules are more concentrated on the 10% solute solution side because the solution is more dilute—or watery—on that side. Thus water molecules move from the 10% solute solution side to the 20% solute solution side. As **Figure 6-2** shows, diffusion of both kinds of molecules eventually produces a dynamic form of equilibrium in which both solutions have equal concentrations. We say that *equilibration* has occurred.

Dynamic equilibrium is not a static state with no movement of molecules across the membrane. Instead, it is a balanced state in which the number of molecules of a substance bouncing to one side of the membrane exactly equals the number of molecules of that substance that are bouncing to the other side. Once equilibration has occurred, overall diffusion may have stopped, but balanced diffusion of small numbers of molecules may continue.

Simple Diffusion

Now that we know that concentration gradients drive diffusion, we can explore how the molecules actually find a way through a cell membrane (**Table 6-1**). Sometimes molecules diffuse directly through the bilayer of phospholipid molecules that forms most of a cell membrane. As discussed in Chapter 5, lipid-soluble molecules can pass through easily. As **Figure 6-3** shows, small hydrophobic molecules such as oxygen (O_2) and carbon dioxide (CO_2) can diffuse directly through the phospholipid bilayer. Small, uncharged particles such as water (H_2O) and urea can diffuse only slightly. Such molecules simply dissolve in the phospholipid fluid, diffuse through this fluid, and then move into the water solution on the other side of the membrane. When molecules pass directly through the phospholipid membrane, the process is called **simple diffusion.**

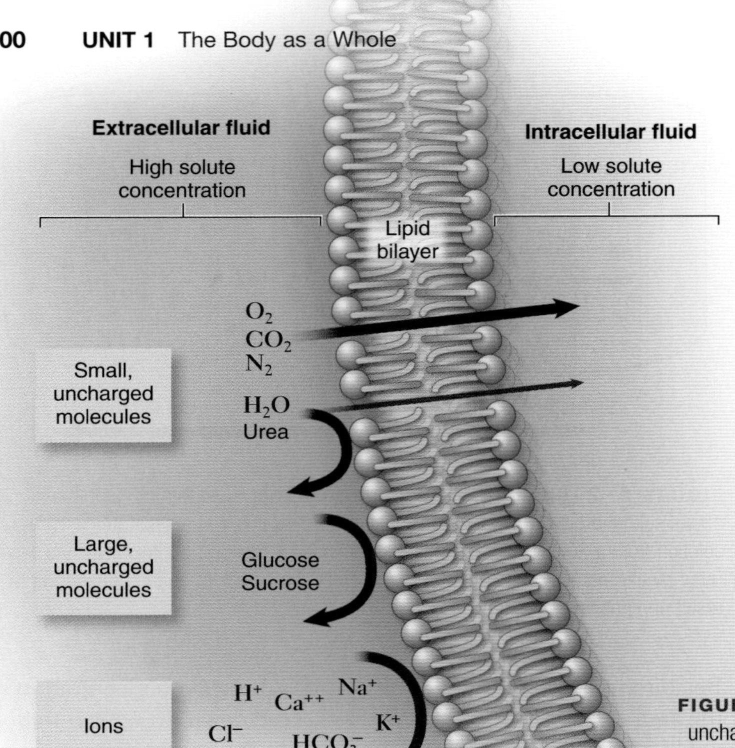

FIGURE 6-3 Simple diffusion through a phospholipid bilayer. Some small, uncharged molecules can easily pass through the phospholipid membrane, but water and urea (a waste product of protein catabolism) rarely get through the membrane. Larger uncharged molecules and ions (charged molecules) may not pass through the phospholipid membrane at all.

TABLE 6-1 Passive Transport Processes

PROCESS		DESCRIPTION	EXAMPLES
Simple diffusion		Movement of particles through the phospholipid bilayer or through channels from an area of high concentration to an area of low concentration—that is, down the concentration gradient	Movement of carbon dioxide out of all cells
Osmosis		Passive transport of water through a selectively permeable membrane in the presence of at least one impermeant solute	Osmosis of water molecules into and out of cells to correct imbalances in water concentration
Channel-mediated passive transport (facilitated diffusion)		Diffusion of particles through a membrane by means of channel structures in the membrane (particles move down their concentration gradient)	Diffusion of sodium ions into nerve cells during a nerve impulse
Carrier-mediated passive transport (facilitated diffusion)		Diffusion of particles through a membrane by means of carrier structures in the membrane (particles move down their concentration gradient)	Diffusion of glucose molecules into most cells

When molecules are allowed to cross a membrane, they are said to *permeate* the membrane. Thus a membrane is *permeable* to a molecule only if it can pass through that membrane. We say that a molecule is *permeant* if it is able to diffuse across a membrane, and it is *impermeant* if it is unable to diffuse across the membrane.

Box 6-1 shows how the process of diffusion can be harnessed to "clean up" the blood after a person's kidneys fail.

Osmosis

A special case of "diffusion" is called **osmosis.** Osmosis is the movement of water through a selectively permeable membrane. Often, water is able to move across a living membrane that does not allow movement of one or more other substances. Thus water is permeant and therefore can equilibrate its concentration on both sides of the membrane, but the impermeant solutes cannot. Technically, osmosis is a bit different than true diffusion—but we will use the classic diffusion model for osmosis here to provide a simple and clear introduction to osmosis.

How can water move through cell membranes? If you look at **Figure 6-3**, you see that water barely passes through phospholipid membranes! In 1988 Peter Agre solved this mystery by proving the existence of small water channels in cell membranes called *aquaporins* (meaning "water pores"). It is the presence of aquaporins that makes membranes permeable to water. We will see how such channels allow other substances to move easily across membranes later. For now, let us focus on osmosis—a very important type of passive transport in the body.

BOX 6-1 *dialysis*

In certain circumstances, a type of diffusion called **dialysis** may occur. Dialysis is a form of diffusion in which the selectively permeable nature of a membrane causes the separation of smaller solute particles from larger solute particles. *Solutes* are the particles dissolved in a *solvent* such as water. Together, the solutes and solvents form a mixture called a *solution.*

Part *A* of the figure illustrates the principle of dialysis. A bag made of dialysis membrane—material with microscopic pores—is filled with a solution containing glucose, water, and albumin (protein) molecules and immersed in a container of pure water. Both water and glucose molecules are small enough to pass through the pores in the dialysis membrane. Albumin molecules, like all protein molecules, are very large and do not pass through the membrane's pores. Because of differences in concentration, glucose molecules diffuse out of the bag as small water molecules diffuse into the bag. Despite a concentration gradient, the albumin molecules do not diffuse out of the bag. Why not? Because they simply will not fit through the tiny pores in the membrane. After some time has passed, the large solutes are still trapped within the bag, but most of the smaller solutes are outside of it.

The principle of dialysis can be used in medicine to treat patients with kidney failure. In **haemodialysis** (part *B* of the figure), blood pumped from a patient is exposed to a dialysis membrane that separates the blood from a clean, osmotically balanced dialysis fluid. Small solutes such as urea and various ions can diffuse through the membrane to reach an equilibrium, thus removing them from the blood. The larger plasma proteins (including albumin) and blood cells remain in the blood, which is returned to the patient's body. In haemodialysis, the process of dialysis is used to "clean up" the patient's blood because the kidneys have failed to perform this task. •

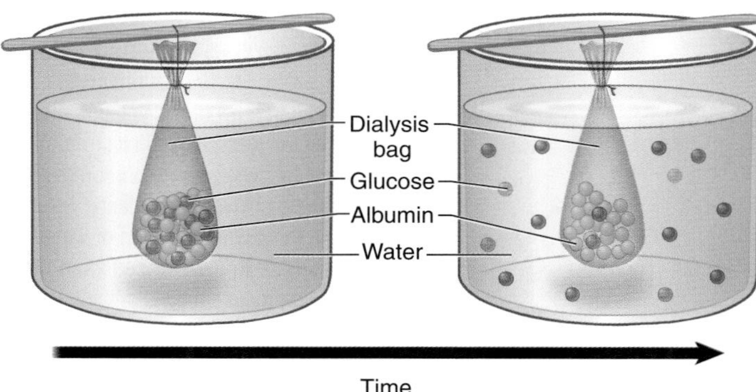

Dialysis. A, A dialysis bag containing glucose, water, and albumin (protein) molecules is suspended in pure water. Over time, the smaller solute molecules (glucose) diffuse out of the bag. The larger solute molecules (albumin) remain trapped in the bag because the bag is impermeable to them. Thus dialysis is diffusion that results in separation of small and large solute particles.

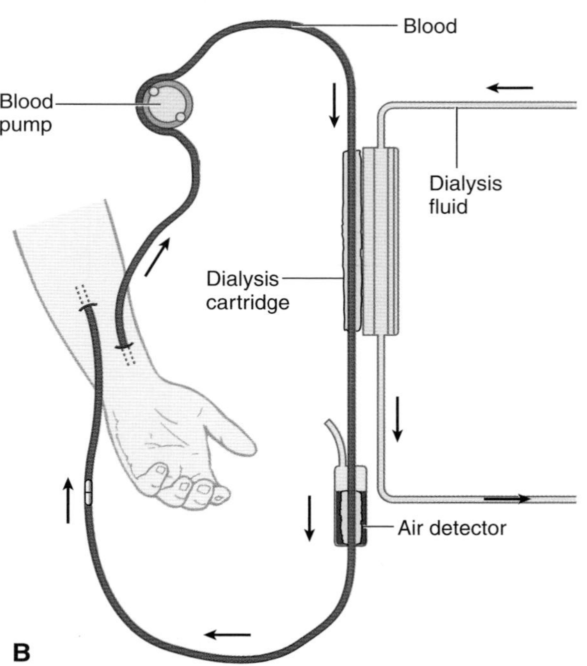

Haemodialysis. B, In haemodialysis, the patient's blood is pumped through a dialysis cartridge, which has a semipermeable membrane that separates the blood from the clean dialysis fluid. As dialysis occurs, some of the urea and other small solutes in the blood diffuse into the dialysis fluid, whereas the larger solutes (plasma proteins) and blood cells remain in the blood.

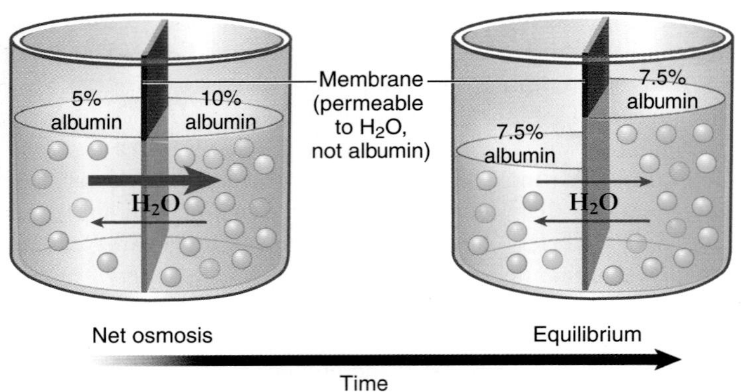

FIGURE 6-4 Osmosis. Osmosis is the passive movement of water through a selectively permeable membrane. The membrane shown in this diagram is permeable to water but not to albumin. Because there are relatively more water molecules in 5% albumin than 10% albumin, more water molecules osmose from the more dilute into the more concentrated solution (as indicated by the larger arrow in the left diagram) than osmose in the opposite direction. The overall direction of osmosis, in other words, is toward the more concentrated solution. Net osmosis produces the following changes in these solutions: (1) their concentrations equilibrate, (2) the volume and pressure of the originally more concentrated solution increase, and (3) the volume and pressure of the other solution decrease proportionately.

First, let us look at an example of osmosis. Imagine that you have a 10% albumin solution separated by a membrane from a 5% albumin solution (**Figure 6-4**). Assume that the membrane has water pores and is freely permeable to water but impermeable to albumin. The water molecules move or *osmose* through the membrane from the area of high water concentration to the area of low water concentration. That is, the water moves from the more dilute 5% albumin solution to the less dilute 10% albumin solution. Although equilibrium is eventually reached, the albumin does not diffuse across the membrane. Only the water moves. Because of this osmosis, one solution loses volume and the other solution gains volume (see **Figure 6-4**).

Unlike the open container pictured in **Figure 6-4**, cells are closed containers. They are enclosed by their plasma membranes. Actually, most of the body is composed of closed compartments such as cells, blood vessels, tubes, and bladders. In closed compartments, such as a toy water balloon, changes in volume also mean changes in pressure. Adding volume to a cell by osmosis increases its pressure, just as adding volume to a water balloon increases its pressure. Water pressure that develops in a solution as a result of osmosis into that solution is called **osmotic pressure.** Taking this principle a step further, we can state that osmotic pressure develops in the solution that originally has the higher concentration of impermeant solute. It is this pressure that ultimately drives osmosis—and what makes it a bit different from ordinary diffusion.

Potential osmotic pressure is the maximum osmotic pressure that *could develop* in a solution when it is separated from pure water by a selectively permeable membrane. **Actual osmotic pressure,** on the other hand, is pressure that *already has developed* in a solution by means of osmosis. Actual osmotic pressure is easy to measure because it is already there.

Because potential osmotic pressure is a *prediction* of what the actual osmotic pressure would be, it cannot be measured directly. What determines a solution's potential osmotic pressure? The answer, simply put, is the concentration of particles of impermeant solutes dissolved in the solution. Thus one can predict the direction of osmosis and the amount of pressure it will produce by knowing the concentrations of impermeant solutes in two solutions.

The concept of osmosis and osmotic pressure has very important practical consequences in human physiology and medicine. Homeostasis of volume and pressure is necessary to maintain the healthy functioning of human cells. The volume and pressure of body cells tend to remain fairly constant because intracellular fluid (fluid inside the cell) is maintained at about the same potential osmotic pressure as extracellular fluid (fluid outside the cell).

A fluid that has the same potential osmotic pressure as a cell is said to be **isotonic** to the cell (**Figure 6-5**, *B*). Isotonic comes from the word parts *iso-*, meaning "same", and *-tonic*, referring to "pressure". The isotonic solution and cytosol have the same potential osmotic pressure because they have the same concentration of impermeant solutes.

A human cell placed in a concentrated solution of impermeant solutes will shrivel up. Look at the example of a red blood cell in **Figure 6-5**, *C*. The pictured cell is in a solution with a higher concentration of impermeant solutes than that found in the cell and, therefore, has a higher potential osmotic pressure. The extracellular solution is said to be **hypertonic** (higher pressure) to the intracellular solution (cytosol). Cells placed in solutions that are hypertonic to intracellular fluid always shrivel.

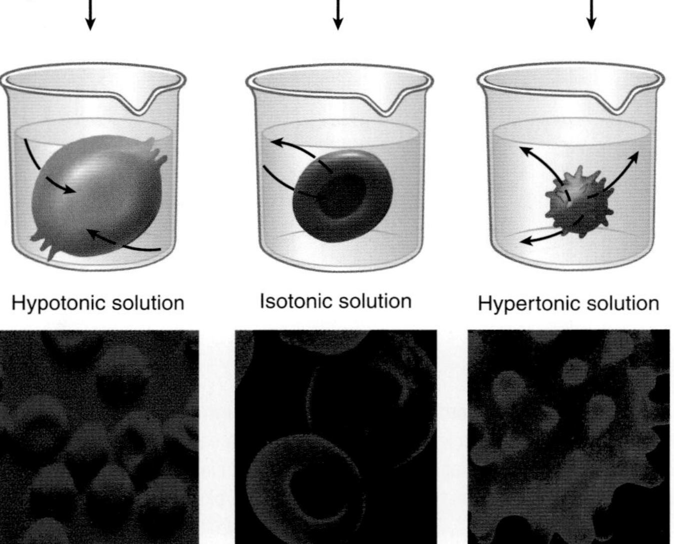

FIGURE 6-5 Effects of osmosis on cells. A, Normal red blood cells placed in a hypotonic solution may swell (as the scanning electron micrograph shows) or even burst (as the drawing shows). This change results from the inward diffusion of water (osmosis). **B,** Cells placed in an isotonic solution maintain constant volume and pressure because the potential osmotic pressure of the intracellular fluid matches that of the extracellular fluid. **C,** Cells placed in a solution that is hypertonic lose volume and pressure as water osmoses out of the cell into the hypertonic solution. The "spikes" seen in the scanning electron micrograph are rigid microtubules of the cytoskeleton. These supports become visible as the cell "deflates", giving them a bumpy or *crenated* appearance.

If cells shrivel too much, they may become permanently damaged—or even die. Obviously, this fact is medically important. Large amounts of solutes cannot be introduced into the body without considering the effect they will have on the concentration of impermeant solutes in the extracellular fluid. If a treatment or procedure causes extracellular fluid to become hypertonic to the cells of the body, serious damage may occur.

If a human cell is placed in a very dilute solution, such as pure water, the cell may swell. If it expands enough, the cell may burst, or *lyse*. Look at the example of a red blood cell in **Figure 6-5**, A. This cell is placed in a solution that is **hypotonic** (lower pressure) to the intracellular fluid. Hypotonic solutions tend to lose pressure because they have a lower concentration of impermeant solutes, and thus a higher water concentration, than the opposite solution. Water always osmoses from the hypotonic solution to the cytosol.

In summary, we can state that osmosis is the movement of water across a membrane that limits the movement of at least some of the solute molecules.

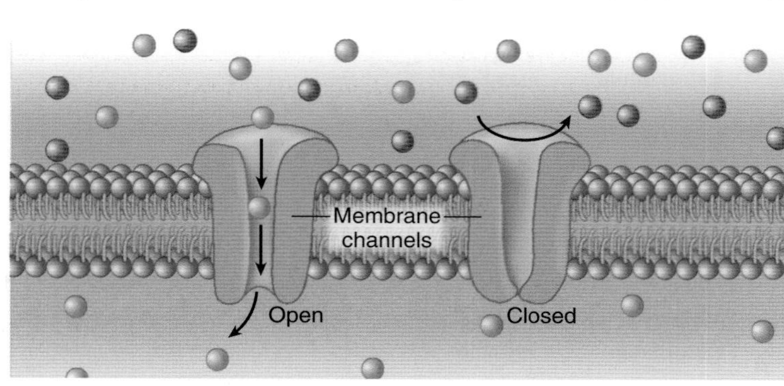

FIGURE 6-6 Membrane channels. Gated channel proteins form tunnels through which only specific molecules may pass—as long as the "gates" are open. Ions or molecules that do not have a specific shape and charge are never permitted to pass through the channel. Notice that the transported ions or molecules move from an area of high concentration to an area of low concentration. The cell membrane is said to be permeable to the type of molecule in question. Filtration, another type of passive transport process, is discussed in **Box 6-2** on p. 104.

CONNECT IT! 

Do you want to know how to calculate the osmotic pressure of any solution? Check out ***Osmotic Pressure of a Solution*** online at ***Connect It!***

Facilitated Diffusion

For a long time, biologists thought that simple diffusion was the only way that molecules could diffuse through a cell membrane. They found that water-soluble ions such as sodium ions (Na^+) and small water soluble molecules such as glucose could not pass through an artificial phospholipid bilayer easily (see **Figure 6-3**). However, they also found that these water-soluble molecules could pass through living cell membranes quickly. Even water molecules, which pass through the thin phospholipid membrane only rarely, diffuse very rapidly through most living cell membranes. It was not until the presence of various transport proteins, such as membrane channels and membrane carriers, was discovered that we understood how these ions and molecules crosss cell membranes. These membrane transporters enable a kind of mediated passive transport that is often called **facilitated diffusion** because the diffusion is facilitated or helped by the transporters.

Channel-Mediated Passive Transport

As you already know, cell membranes possess protein "tunnels", better known as *membrane channels* (see **Table 5-4**, p. 81, and **Figure 6-6**). Membrane channels are pores through which water molecules, specific ions, or other small, water-soluble molecules can pass. For example, sodium ions (Na^+) pass only through *sodium channels* and chloride ions (Cl^-) pass only through *chloride channels*. Recall that water moves through aquaporins, which are water-specific channels, during osmosis. Aquaporin channels may also be called aquapores. Membrane channels can exhibit such *specificity* because their molecular structure prevents molecules of the wrong shape and the wrong pattern of charges to pass through the channel. Thus living membranes can be permeable to some molecules but not to others, depending on the type of channels present.

As **Figure 6-6** shows, the permeability of a membrane can also be affected by the opening and closing of membrane channels. Because channels can open or close, they are sometimes called *gated channels*. The active or "open" state can be almost immediately changed to the "closed" state, or changed from closed to open, by various triggering mechanisms. Some gated channels are triggered by electrical changes (voltage), others by light, and still others by mechanical or chemical stimuli. We will look at these various types of triggering mechanisms in later chapters. Open-gated channels may in certain conditions become inactive, stopping the flow of molecules and becoming insensitive to trigger stimuli, before actually closing and resuming sensitivity to stimuli.

Because a living cell membrane can limit the diffusion of some molecules by opening or closing channels in different situations, we say the membrane is *selectively permeable*. Membrane channel structure often permits diffusion in only one direction. So the cell can also determine whether to allow certain molecules to pass in either direction (depending on the concentration gradient, of course) or in only one direction (when the concentration gradient permits).

Aquaporins are among the more recently discovered types of membrane channels. As their name suggests, these channels permit water molecules to diffuse through a cell membrane much more rapidly than by simple diffusion. Aquaporins are thought to be responsible for the very rapid changes in blood cell volume during osmosis illustrated in **Figure 6-5**.

Because ions move down their concentration gradients as they pass through channels, this type of facilitated diffusion is passive and thus called *channel-mediated passive transport*.

Carrier-Mediated Passive Transport

Molecules may move down their concentration gradient by passing through a different type of membrane transporter called a *membrane carrier*. Thus the carrier may facilitate diffusion in a process called *carrier-mediated passive transport*.

As **Figure 6-7** shows, the carrier structure attracts a solute to a binding site, changes its shape, and then releases the solute to the other side of the membrane. This mechanism differs from channel-mediated transport, which does not involve binding the solute molecule and changing shape to release the bound solute. Carrier reactions are reversible and may thus transport molecules in either direction, depending on the concentration gradient.

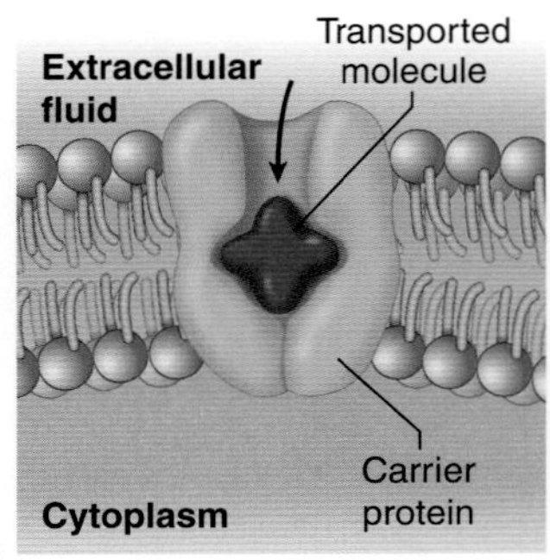

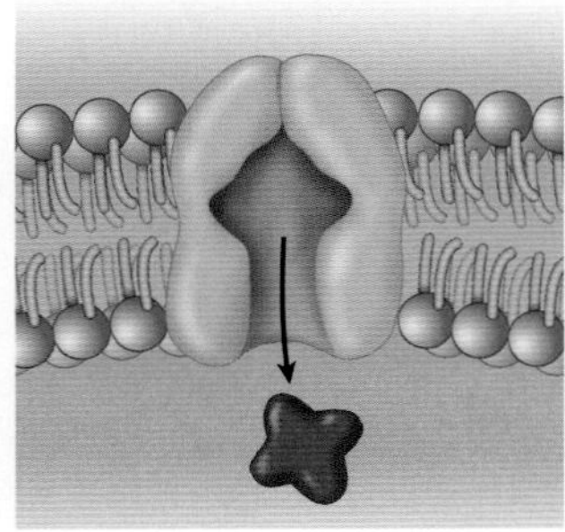

FIGURE 6-7 Membrane carrier. In carrier-mediated transport, a membrane-bound carrier protein attracts a solute molecule to a binding site **(A)** and changes shape in a manner that allows the solute to move to the other side of the membrane **(B)**. Passive carriers may transport molecules in either direction, depending on the concentration gradient.

As in channel-mediated and simple diffusion, carrier-mediated diffusion also transports substances down a concentration gradient (that is, from high to low concentration). An example is the adenosine diphosphate–adenosine triphosphate (ADP-ATP) carrier found in the membranes of the mitochondrion. This carrier moves ADP into the mitochondrion because the ADP concentration inside is kept low by constant conversion to ATP. Because ATP is thus kept constantly high inside the mitochondrion, ATP passes down its concentration gradient through the ADP-ATP carrier to the outside, where ATP is continually dropping (through use by cell processes).

Role of Passive Transfer Processes

Diffusion of any type is a passive process. In other words, the energy for transport through a membrane does not come from the membrane but from the energy of collision already possessed by the moving molecule. The only requirement of the cell is that it be permeable to the type of molecule in question. Because substances are moved down their concentration gradients, such passive transport tends to maintain an equilibrium of these substances.

We have explored many varieties of diffusion across a membrane, summarized in **Table 6-1**. Simple diffusion occurs when molecules dissolve directly through the phospholipid bilayer. Facilitated diffusion requires transport proteins in the membrane. The transporters could be channels, such as the water channels needed for osmosis or the ion channels needed to move sodium or potassium ions. The transporters could instead be carriers, such as those needed to move ADP and ATP into and out of the mitochondrion. Filtration, yet another type of passive transport process, is discussed in **Box 6-2**.

All of these passive transport mechanisms are needed to move critical substances into or out of cells and organelles to maintain an equilibrium. Considering the importance of homeostatic balance, you can see that passive transport is critical to human function. As you will discover in the last part of the chapter, many diseases and even death can result from malfunctions of these passive transport processes.

ACTIVE TRANSPORT PROCESSES

All the membrane transport processes that we have seen so far are passive processes. The force of movement comes from the concentration gradient—that is, from a physical force of nature. The driving force for active transport processes, on the other hand, comes from the cell itself. Energy of metabolism must be used by cells to force particles across a membrane that otherwise would not move across.

Transport by Pumps

Membrane transporters called *membrane pumps* carry out a transport process in which cellular energy is used to move molecules

BOX 6-2 *filtration*

Another important passive process for transport in the body is **filtration.** This form of transport involves the passing of water and permeable solutes through a membrane by the force of hydrostatic pressure. *Hydrostatic pressure* is the force, or weight, of a fluid pushing against a surface.

Filtration is movement of molecules through a membrane from an area of high hydrostatic pressure to an area of low hydrostatic pressure—that is, down a hydrostatic pressure gradient. Filtration most often transports substances through a sheet of cells. The force of pressure pushes the molecules through or between the cells that form the sheet. Because the filtration membrane does not allow larger particles through, filtration results in the separation of large and small particles, as you can see in the figure. This is similar to dialysis (see **Box 6-1**, p. 101), except that dialysis is driven by a *concentration gradient.* Filtration is instead driven by a *hydrostatic pressure gradient.*

A simple model of filtration is found in many drip-type coffee makers. Ground coffee is placed in a porous paper filter cup in an upper container and boiling water is added. Gravity pulls downward on the mixture in the upper container, generating hydrostatic pressure against the bottom of the filter. The pores in the paper filter are large enough to let water molecules and other small particles pass through to a coffee pot below the filter. Most of the coffee grounds are too large to pass through the filter. The coffee in the pot below is called the *filtrate.*

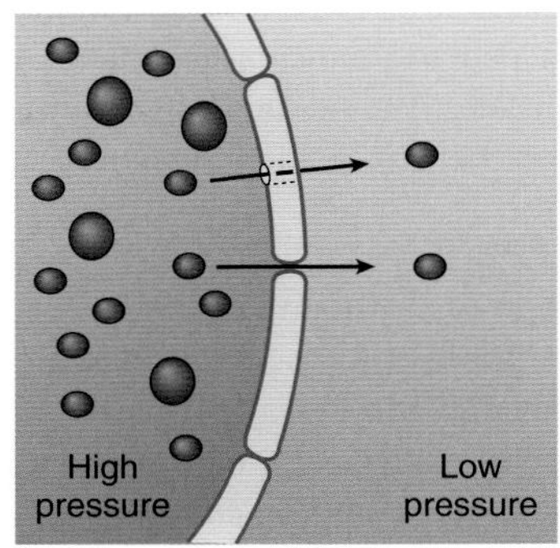

Filtration. Particles small enough to fit through the pores in the filtration membrane move from the area of high hydrostatic pressure to the area of low hydrostatic pressure. This results in separation of small particles from larger particles.

How and where does filtration occur in the body? Most often, it occurs in tiny blood vessels called *capillaries,* which are found throughout the body. Hydrostatic pressure of the blood (blood pressure) generated by heart contractions, gravity, and other forces pushes water and small solutes out of the capillaries and into the interstitial spaces of a tissue. Blood cells and large blood proteins are too large to fit through pores in the capillary wall; therefore, they cannot be filtered out of the blood. Capillary filtration allows the blood vessels to supply tissues with water and other essential substances quickly and easily without losing its cells and blood proteins. Capillary filtration is also the first step used by the kidney to form urine. •

BOX 6-3 *transport of different solutes*

In looking at different types of carriers and pumps in the body, we see that some transport only one type of molecule at a time. This type of transporter is often called a *uniporter.* For example, the GLUT uniporters in many cells passively move glucose from blood plasma into cells. *GLUT* is an acronym for *GLU*cose *T*ransporter. **Figure 6-8** shows uniport of two Ca^{++} ions by a calcium pump.

Symporters instead move two or more types of molecule in the same direction through a membrane. For example, the SGLT1 symporter in the digestive tract transports sodium ions and glucose together into absorptive cells. *SGLT1* is the acronym for *S*odium–*GL*ucose *T*ransporter *1.* Symport can also be called **cotransport.**

Antiporters, on the other hand, are transporters that move two different types of molecules in opposite directions at the same time. For example, *Band 3* antiporters in red blood cells passively exchange bicarbonate ions (HCO_3^-) for chloride ions (Cl^-) in opposite directions at the same time. Na-K ATPase (sodium–potassium pump) actively antiports sodium ions and potassium ions in all cells of the body. Antiport can also be called **countertransport.**

Sometimes, active transport of one type of solute creates a concentration gradient that drives the passive transport of another solute. For example, in part B of the figure the active transport of sodium ions creates a concentration gradient that drives the cotransport of glucose along with sodium by a symport mechanism. In this case, the movement of sodium is an example of *primary active transport.* The movement of glucose, which depends on the sodium concentration gradient created by primary active transport, is an example of *secondary active transport.* This particular example of secondary active transport is often referred to as *sodium cotransport of glucose.* •

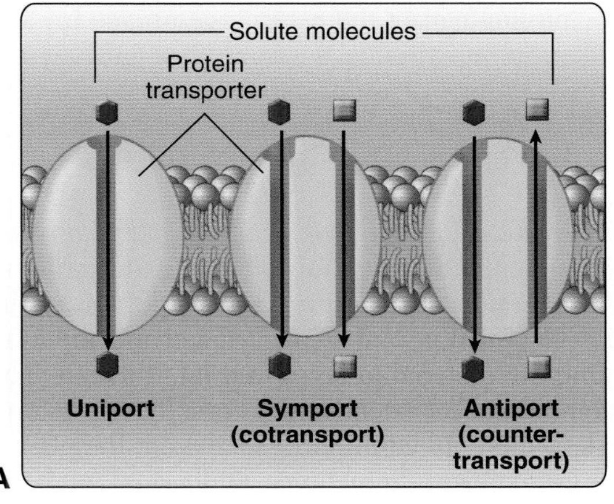

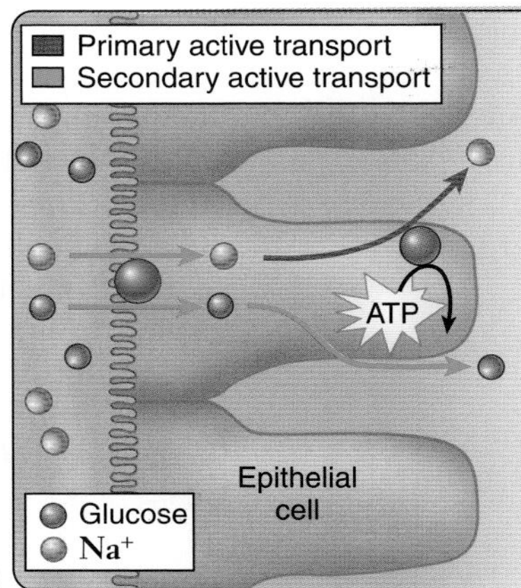

A, Direction of transport. Movement of one solute (uniport), movement of two or more solute types in the same direction (symport or cotransport), and movement of two or more solute types in opposite directions (antiport or countertransport). **B,** Primary and secondary active transport. In this example, primary active transport of sodium by a sodium pump creates a concentration gradient that drives the passive cotransport of glucose along with sodium. Because it depends on the sodium gradient, sodium cotransport of glucose is an example of secondary active transport. *ATP,* Adenosine triphosphate.

"uphill" through a cell membrane. By "uphill", we mean that the substance moves from an area of low concentration to an area of higher concentration. An actively transported substance moves *against* its concentration gradient. This is exactly the opposite of diffusion, in which a substance is transported *down* its concentration gradient—or "downhill". It is important to remember that molecules will not travel uphill on their own, any more than a ball will roll uphill by itself. Molecules will travel uphill only when they are forced by pump mechanisms powered by cellular energy. Moving solutes in different directions is discussed in **Box 6-3**.

Active pumping is an extremely important process. It allows cells to move certain ions or other water-soluble particles to specific areas. For example, active *calcium pumps* in the membranes of muscle cells allow the cell to force nearly all the intracellular calcium ions (Ca^{++}) into special compartments—or out of the cell entirely (**Figure 6-8**). This is important because a muscle cell cannot operate

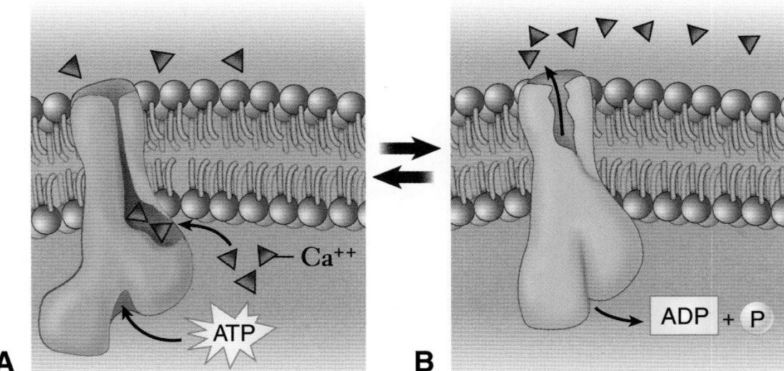

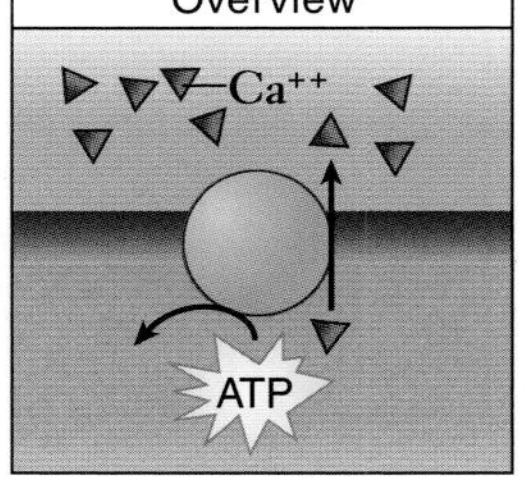

FIGURE 6-8 Calcium pump. A, Two calcium ions (Ca^{++}) enter the pump, and then adenosine triphosphate (ATP) associates with the activating centre of the pump. **B,** As the energy released from ATP (forming adenosine diphosphate [ADP] + phosphate [P]) changes the shape of the pump, the Ca^{++} ions are released on the opposite side of the membrane. The small inset shows a simplified view of a calcium pump's action.

properly unless the intracellular Ca^{++} concentration is kept low during rest. Other cells use active transport pumps for similar purposes—that is, to create a concentration gradient of a particular solute.

One type of active transport pump, the *sodium–potassium pump*, operates in the plasma membrane of all human cells (**Figure 6-9**). It is essential for healthy cell survival. As its name suggests, the sodium–potassium pump actively transports sodium ions (Na^+) and potassium ions (K^+)—but in opposite directions. It transports sodium ions *out* of cells and potassium ions *into* cells. By so doing, the sodium–potassium pump maintains a lower sodium concentration in intracellular fluid than in the surrounding extracellular fluid. At the same time, this pump maintains a higher potassium concentration in the intracellular fluid than in the surrounding extracellular fluid. Both ions bind to the same membrane transporter, a molecule known as *sodium–potassium adenosine triphosphatase (Na-K ATPase)*. **Figure 6-9** shows that three Na^+ ions bind to sodium-binding sites on the pump's inner face. At the same time, an energy-containing ATP molecule produced by the cell's mitochondria binds to the pump. The ATP breaks apart, and its stored energy is transferred to the pump. The pump then changes shape, releases the three Na^+ ions to the outside of the cell, and attracts two K^+ ions to its potassium-binding sites. The pump then returns to its original shape and releases the two K^+ ions and the remnant of the ATP molecule to the inside of the cell.

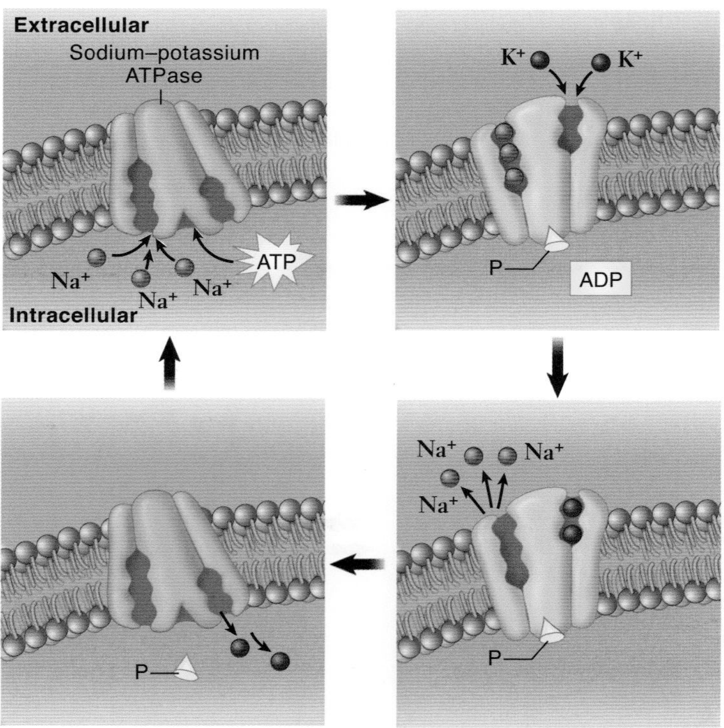

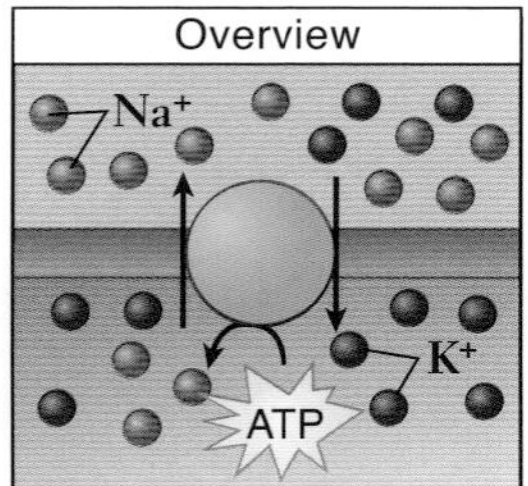

FIGURE 6-9 Sodium–potassium pump. Three sodium ions (Na^+) bind to sodium binding sites on the pump's inner face. At the same time, an energy-containing ATP molecule produced by the cell's mitochondria binds to the pump. The ATP breaks apart, and its stored energy is transferred to the pump. The pump then changes shape, releases the three Na^+ ions to the outside of the cell, and attracts two potassium ions (K^+) to its potassium binding sites. The pump then returns to its original shape, and the two K^+ ions and the remnant of the ATP molecule are released to the inside of the cell. The pump is now ready for another pumping cycle. *ATPase,* Adenosine triphosphatase. The small inset is a simplified view of Na-K pump activity. *ATP,* Adenosine triphosphate.

Transport by Vesicles

Like active transport pumps, mechanisms that carry large groups of molecules into or out of the cell by means of vesicles require the expenditure of metabolic energy by the cell. Such bulk transport mechanisms differ from pump mechanisms in that they allow substances to enter or leave the interior of a cell without actually moving through its plasma membrane (**Figure 6-10**).

Endocytosis

In **endocytosis** the plasma membrane "traps" some extracellular material and brings it into the cell. The basic mechanism of endocytosis is summarized in **Figure 6-10**. In endocytosis, the cytoskeleton does all the work by pulling part of the plasma membrane inward, thereby forming a depression, while at the same time pushing the membrane at the edges to form a sort of trap for extracellular material. When the extended edges of membrane fuse, a vesicle is formed. The cytoskeleton then pulls the vesicle containing extracellular material inward.

In a type of endocytosis called *receptor-mediated endocytosis*, receptors in the plasma membrane first bind to specific molecules in the extracellular fluid (**Figure 6-11**). This causes a portion of the plasma membrane to be pulled inward by the cytoskeleton and form a small pocket around the material to be moved into the cell. The edges of the membranous pocket extend and eventually fuse to form a vesicle. The vesicle is then pulled inward—away from the plasma membrane—by the cytoskeleton. Sometimes, endocytosis picks up various molecules and other particles along with receptor-bound molecules.

There are two basic forms of endocytosis: *phagocytosis* and *pinocytosis*. In **phagocytosis,** microorganisms or other large particles are engulfed by the plasma membrane and enter the cell in vesicles that have pinched off from the membrane. Once inside, they fuse with the membranous walls of lysosomes. Enzymes from the lysosomes then digest the particles into their component molecules. The products of digestion may subsequently diffuse through the membranous wall of the vesicle into the cytoplasm. The term *phagocytosis* means "condition of the cell eating" (from the word parts *phago-*, meaning "eat", *-cyto-*, meaning "cell", and *-osis*, meaning "condition").

Pinocytosis, or "condition of the cell drinking", is a similar process in which fluid and the substances dissolved in it enter a cell. Besides providing a way for a cell to bring fluids and solutes into the

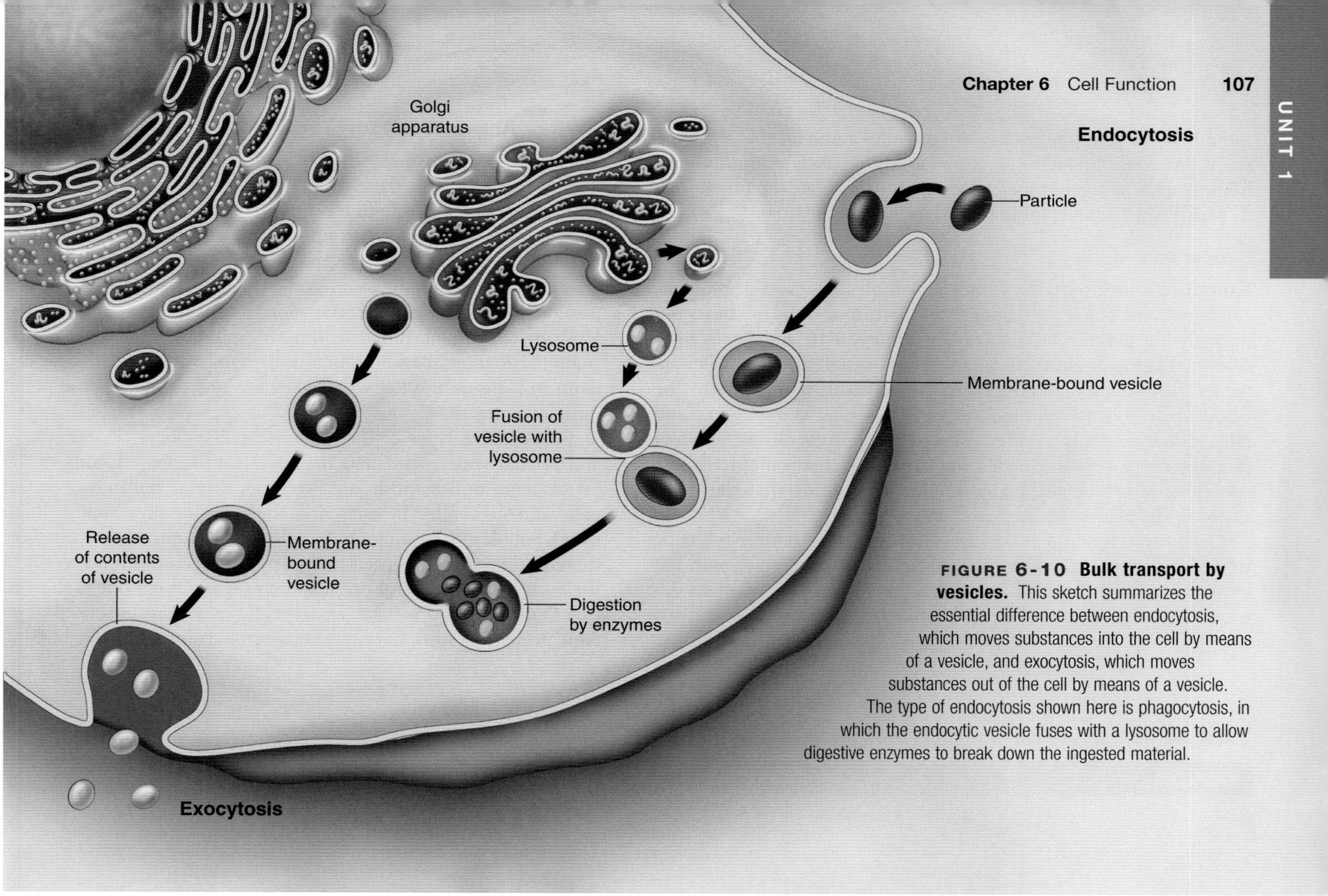

Endocytosis

Particle

Golgi apparatus

Lysosome

Membrane-bound vesicle

Fusion of vesicle with lysosome

Release of contents of vesicle

Membrane-bound vesicle

Digestion by enzymes

Exocytosis

FIGURE 6-10 Bulk transport by vesicles. This sketch summarizes the essential difference between endocytosis, which moves substances into the cell by means of a vesicle, and exocytosis, which moves substances out of the cell by means of a vesicle. The type of endocytosis shown here is phagocytosis, in which the endocytic vesicle fuses with a lysosome to allow digestive enzymes to break down the ingested material.

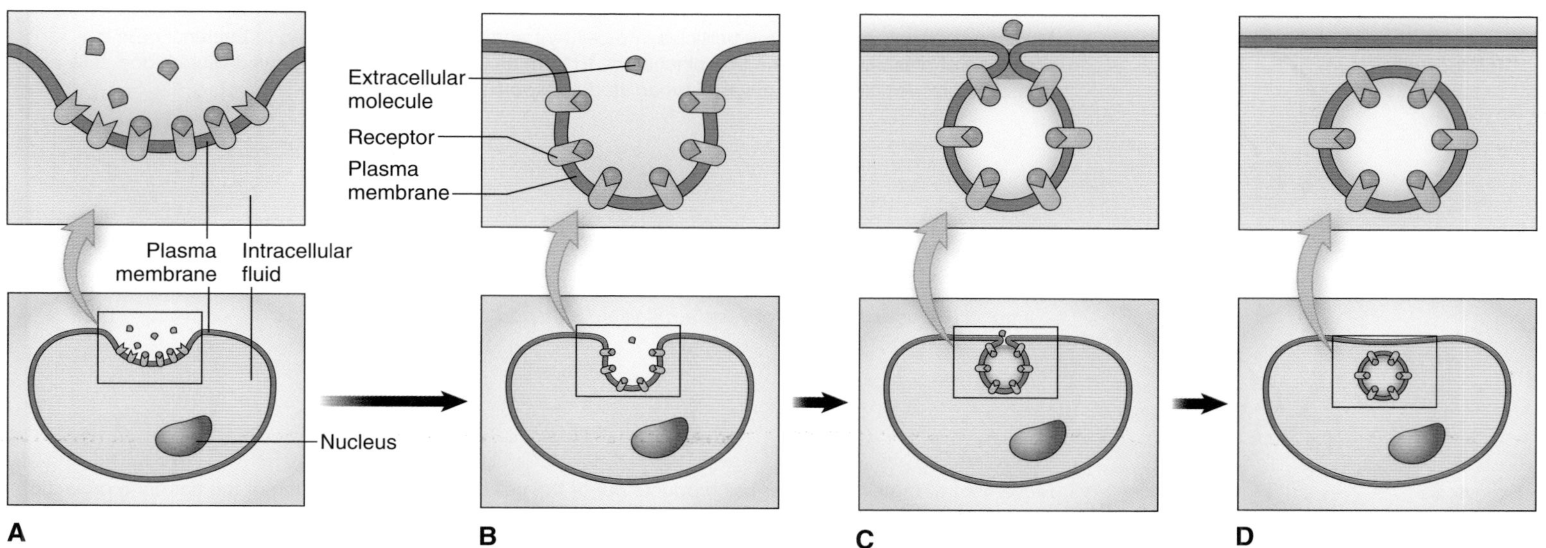

FIGURE 6-11 Receptor-mediated endocytosis. A, Membrane receptors bind to specific molecules in the extracellular fluid. **B,** A portion of the plasma membrane is pulled inward by the cytoskeleton and forms a small pocket around the material to be moved into the cell. **C,** The edges of the pocket eventually fuse and form a vesicle. **D,** The vesicle is then pulled inward—away from the plasma membrane—by the cytoskeleton. In this example, only the receptor-bound molecules enter the cell. In some cases, some free molecules or even entire cells may also be trapped within the vesicle and transported inward.

interior of the cell, pinocytosis also provides a way for the cell to remove material, including membrane receptors and transporters, from the plasma membrane. A cell can thus regulate the function of its plasma membrane (**Table 6-2**).

Exocytosis

Exocytosis is the process by which large molecules, notably proteins, can leave the cell even though they are too large to move out through the plasma membrane (see **Figure 6-10** and **Table 6-2**). After first being enclosed in membranous vesicles by the Golgi apparatus, the vesicles are pulled out to the plasma membrane by the cytoskeleton. The vesicles then fuse with the plasma membrane and release their contents outside the cell. Some gland cells secrete their products by exocytosis. Besides providing a mechanism of transport, exocytosis also provides a way for new membrane material to be added to the plasma membrane.

Cells may also "pinch off" an entire vesicle—thereby releasing substances contained within an extracellular vesicle or *exosome*. For example, cells in the skin manufacture pigments that are then distributed to other nearby cells in exosomes. Sometimes cells' waste is removed by exosomes.

Role of Active Transport Processes

Active transport processes include any mechanism that moves substances across a membrane using cellular energy—thus giving the membrane an active role in transport.

Major mechanisms of active transport in the body are ion pumps, which move ions against their concentration gradients and thus create a concentration of these ions on one side or the other. A cell can use ion pumps to keep a certain ion at an unusually high or low level, or concentrate them within an organelle. For example, the smooth ER (endoplasmic reticulum) membrane concentrates calcium ions inside the ER where they are stored for later use (as in muscle contraction).

Other active types of transport include endocytosis, exocytosis, and related vesicle-mediated processes within cells. Efforts of the cytoskeleton pull or push large volumes of material into or out of cells and organelles by wrapping them in (or unwrapping them from) bubbles of membrane (vesicles). In Chapter 5, we saw how these processes can be used to transport molecules from the ER to the Golgi apparatus, and eventually to secrete them out of the cell (see **Figure 5-8**). As you can imagine, this mechanism is used to secrete everything from hormones to neurotransmitters in the body.

TABLE 6-2 Active Transport Processes

PROCESS		DESCRIPTION	EXAMPLES
Pumping	ATP	Movement of solute particles from an area of low concentration to an area of high concentration (up the concentration gradient) by means of an energy-consuming pump structure in the membrane	In muscle cells, pumping of nearly all calcium ions to special compartments—or out of the cell
Phagocytosis (endocytosis)		Movement of cells or other large particles into cell by trapping it in a section of plasma membrane that pinches off to form an intracellular vesicle; a type of *vesicle-mediated transport*	Trapping of bacterial cells by phagocytic white blood cells
Pinocytosis (endocytosis)		Movement of fluid and dissolved molecules into a cell by trapping them in a section of plasma membrane that pinches off to form an intracellular vesicle; a type of *vesicle-mediated transport*	Trapping of large protein molecules by some body cells
Exocytosis		Movement of proteins or other cell products out of the cell by fusing a secretory vesicle with the plasma membrane; a type of *vesicle-mediated transport*	Secretion of the hormone prolactin by pituitary cells

Quick **CHECK**

1. Name as many passive processes that transport substances across a cell membrane as you can. How are they alike? How are they different?
2. What causes osmotic pressure to develop in a cell?
3. Describe three different active processes that transport substances across a cell membrane. What distinguishes them from passive processes?

CELL METABOLISM

METABOLISM

Chapter 3 (pp. 46–47) introduced the concept of **metabolism:** the chemical reactions that occur in the body. *Cell metabolism,* then, refers to the chemical reactions of the cell. This section of Chapter 6 picks up the important theme of human body chemistry and applies it to cell physiology. Later chapters also continue to bring up this theme because after all, body chemistry is the basis for all human functions.

Cell metabolism involves many different kinds of chemical reactions that often occur in a sequence of reactions called a **metabolic pathway.** A metabolic pathway can be described as being *catabolic* if its net effect is to break large molecules down into smaller ones. Recall that **catabolism** is the kind of metabolism that breaks down molecules, usually nutrient molecules, and thereby releases energy from the broken molecules. On the other hand, some metabolic pathways build larger molecules from smaller ones and are thus called *anabolic pathways.* Recall that **anabolism** is the kind of metabolism that builds large, complex molecules from smaller ones. Anabolic pathways usually require a net input of energy, whereas catabolic pathways usually produce a net output of energy.

ROLE OF ENZYMES

Enzymes, which are classified as *functional proteins,* were introduced on p. 63 in Chapter 4. We are now ready for a more comprehensive introduction to enzymes.

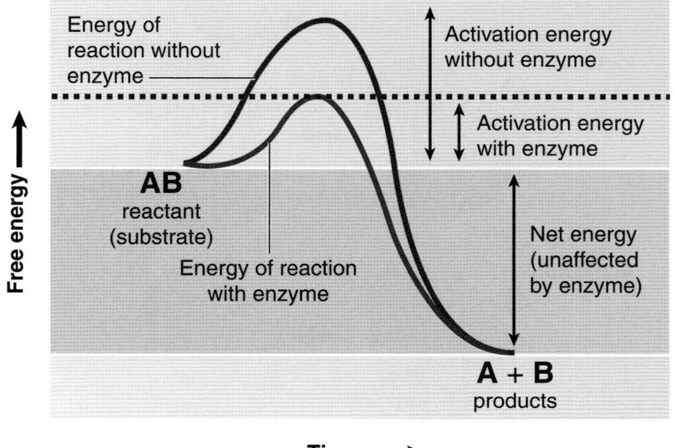

FIGURE 6-12 Enzymes as catalysts. A catalyst is a chemical that reduces the activation energy of a reaction—the energy needed to get a reaction started. Enzymes thus allow reactions to occur at the low level of free energy available at normal human body temperatures.

The series of chemical reactions that make up a metabolic pathway in a cell do not usually just happen on their own. At normal body temperatures, the *activation energy* needed to start a chemical reaction is too great for many molecules to react by themselves. What is needed to make essential chemical reactions happen is a **catalyst**—a chemical that reduces the amount of activation energy needed to start a chemical reaction (**Figure 6-12**). Catalysts participate in chemical reactions but are not themselves changed by the reaction. This is the role of enzymes in the cell—to act as chemical catalysts that allow metabolic reactions to occur. So important are they that life has been defined as the "orderly functioning of hundreds of enzymes" by one scientist.

Chemical Structure of Enzymes

Enzymes are proteins and have the chemical properties of proteins. Enzymes are usually tertiary or quaternary proteins of complex shape. Often, their molecules contain a nonprotein part called a *cofactor.* Inorganic ions or vitamins may make up part of a cofactor. If the cofactor is an organic nonprotein molecule, it is called a **coenzyme.**

A very important structural attribute of enzymes is the **active site.** The active site is the portion of the enzyme molecule that chemically "fits" the substrate molecule or molecules. Recall that a *substrate* is the molecule acted on by an enzyme molecule.

Since the enzyme acts on a substrate because the shape and electrochemical attractions of the active site complement some portion of the substrate or substrates, biochemists often use a modern variation of the **lock-and-key model** to describe the action of enzymes. As **Figure 6-13** shows, the active site of an enzyme chemically fits a portion of the substrate just as a key fits into a lock. Like a key in a lock, the enzyme can bind substrates together ("locking" them together) or can unbind components of a substrate ("unlocking" them). And, as with a key, some movement of the enzyme shape is often required to "open the lock" or alter the substrate. As shown in **Figure 6-13**, such dynamic movements are critical to proper enzyme function.

Classification and Naming of Enzymes

Two systems used for naming enzymes are as follows: the suffix *-ase* is used with the root name of the substance whose chemical reaction is catalyzed (the substrate chemical, that is) or with the word that describes the kind of chemical reaction catalyzed. Thus, according to the first method, sucrase is an enzyme that catalyzes a chemical reaction in which sucrose takes part. According to the second method, sucrase might also be called a *hydrolase* because it catalyzes the hydrolysis of sucrose. Enzymes investigated before these methods of nomenclature were adopted are still called by older names, such as *pepsin* and *trypsin.*

Classified according to the kind of chemical reactions catalyzed, enzymes fall into several groups:

Oxidation-reduction enzymes. These are known as oxidases, hydrogenases, and dehydrogenases. Energy release for muscular contraction and all physiological work depends on these enzymes.

Hydrolyzing enzymes, or hydrolases. Digestive enzymes belong to this group. The hydrolyzing enzymes are named after the substrate acted on, for example, lipase, sucrase, and maltase.

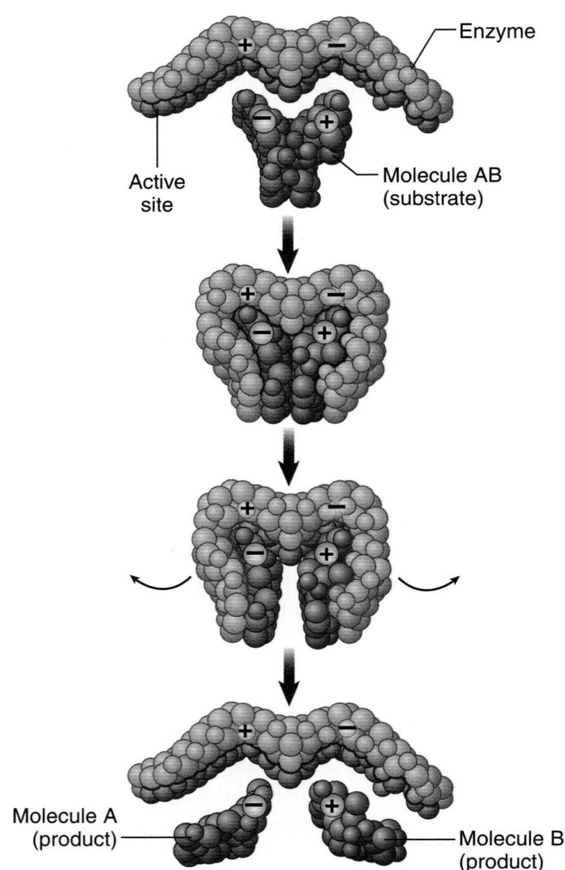

FIGURE 6-13 Model of enzyme action. Enzymes are functional proteins whose molecular shape allows them to catalyze chemical reactions. Substrate molecule AB is acted on by a digestive enzyme to yield simpler molecules A and B as products of the reaction. Notice how the active site of the enzyme chemically fits the substrate—the *lock-and-key* model of biochemical interaction. Notice also how the enzyme molecule bends its shape in performing its function, which is a *dynamic* variation of the classic lock-and-key model.

Phosphorylating enzymes. These add or remove phosphate groups and are known as phosphorylases or phosphatases.
Enzymes that add or remove carbon dioxide. These are known as carboxylases or decarboxylases.
Enzymes that rearrange atoms within a molecule. These are known as mutases or isomerases.
Hydrases. These add water to a molecule without splitting it, as do hydrolases.

Enzymes are also classified as intracellular or extracellular, depending on whether they act within cells or outside them in the surrounding medium. Most enzymes act intracellularly in the body; an important exception is the digestive enzymes. All digestive enzymes are classified as hydrolases because they catalyze the hydrolysis of food molecules.

General Function of Enzymes

In general, enzymes regulate cell functions by regulating metabolic pathways (**Figure 6-14**). As stated earlier, each reaction of a metabolic pathway requires one or more types of enzymes to permit that reaction to occur. An entire metabolic pathway can be turned on or off by the activation or inactivation of any one of the enzymes that catalyze reactions in that particular pathway. A few general principles of enzyme function will help you understand their role in regulating cell metabolism more clearly.

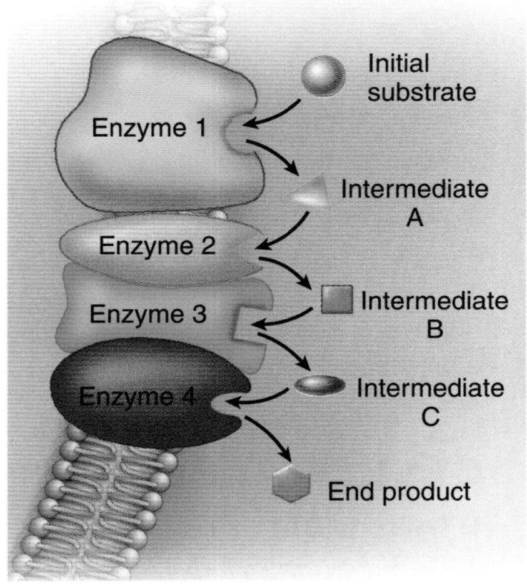

FIGURE 6-14 Enzyme regulation of a metabolic pathway. In a metabolic pathway, the product of one enzyme-regulated reaction becomes the substrate for the next reaction. Thus a whole series of enzymes is required to keep the pathway functioning. Notice that these enzymes are embedded in a cell membrane whereas other types of enzymes are mobile in the cytosol or extracellular in location.

Most enzymes are *specific in their action;* that is, they act only on a specific substrate. This is attributed to their "key-in-a-lock" kind of action, the configuration of the enzyme molecule fitting the configuration of some part of the substrate molecule (see **Figure 6-13**). This also means that every reaction that occurs in a metabolic pathway requires one or more specific enzymes—or else the reaction will not occur and the entire pathway will be disrupted.

Various physical and chemical agents activate or inhibit enzyme action by changing the shape of enzyme molecules. A molecule or other agent that alters enzyme function by changing its shape is

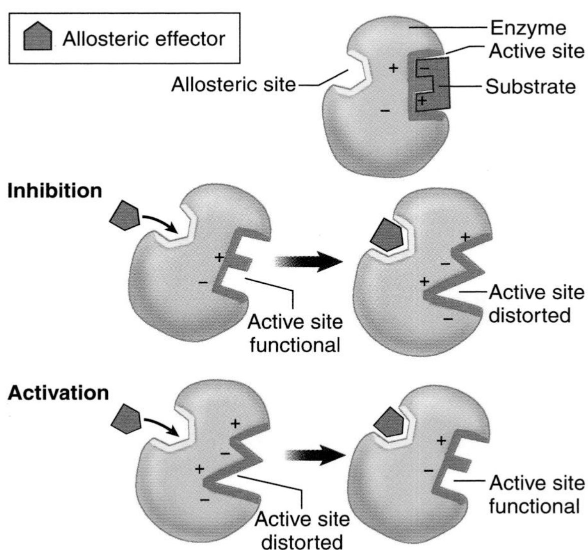

FIGURE 6-15 Allosteric effect. The allosteric effect occurs when some agent, in this case an allosteric effector molecule, binds to the enzyme at an allosteric site and thereby changes the shape of the enzyme's active site. Such an allosteric effect may inhibit enzyme action (by distorting the active site) or activate the enzyme (by giving the active site its functional shape).

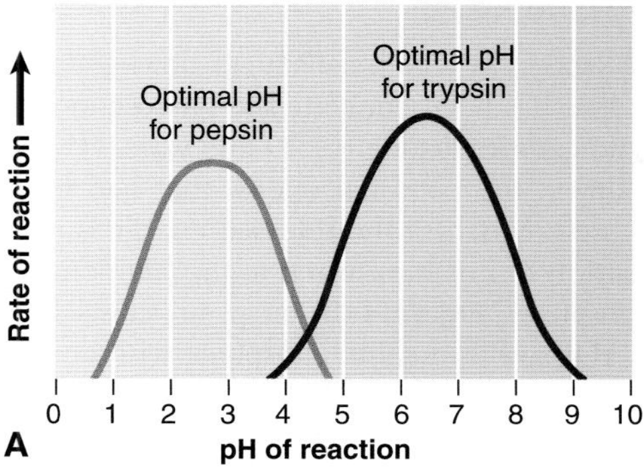

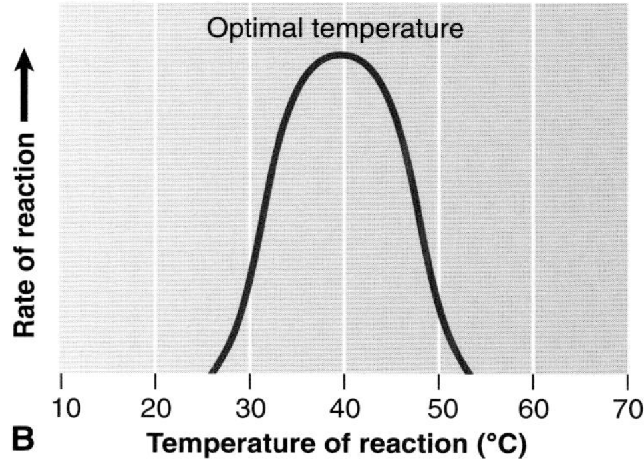

FIGURE 6-16 Effects of pH and temperature on enzyme function. The rate of reactions catalyzed can be affected by the allosteric effects of the chemical or physical properties of the surrounding medium. **A,** Enzymes catalyze chemical reactions with greatest efficiency within a narrow range of pH. For example, pepsin (a protein-digesting enzyme in gastric juice) operates within a low pH range, whereas trypsin (a protein-digesting enzyme in pancreatic juice) operates within a higher pH range. **B,** Most enzymes in the human body work best within a narrow range of temperatures near 40°C.

called an **allosteric effector.** An *effector* is an agent that accomplishes something, and *allosteric* literally means "relating to a change in three-dimensional shape". Thus an allosteric effector is simply an agent that changes the shape of a molecule. Remember the principle you learned about the shape of proteins in Chapter 4: When the shape changes, so does the function. This certainly applies to enzymes.

Some allosteric effectors are molecules that attach to an *allosteric site* on the enzyme molecule and thereby change the shape of the active site on a different part of the enzyme. As **Figure 6-15** shows, allosteric effectors of this type may inhibit or activate enzymes by altering the shape of the active site.

Other types of allosteric effectors include certain antibiotic drugs, changes in pH, or changes in temperature. The allosteric effect of pH is produced by the fact that changes in the concentration of hydrogen ions (H^+) influence the chemical attractions that hold molecules—including enzymes—in their complex, multidimensional shapes. Temperature has a similar allosteric, or shape-changing, effect on enzymes. As **Figure 6-16** shows, changing the pH or temperature alters the shape of the active sites of enzyme molecules enough to affect their function. Cofactors, when they are added to or removed from an enzyme molecule, also have an allosteric effect.

Feedback loop

In the process known as **end-product inhibition**, a chemical product at the end of a metabolic pathway binds to the allosteric site of one or more enzymes along the pathway that produced it and thereby inhibits the synthesis of more product (**Figure 6-17**). This is a type of automatic negative feedback mechanism in the cell that prevents the accumulation of an extreme amount of a metabolic product.

Most enzymes catalyze a chemical reaction in both directions, the direction and rate of the reaction being governed by the law of mass action. An accumulation of a product slows the reaction and tends to reverse it.

Enzymes are continually being destroyed and therefore have to be continually synthesized, even though they are not used up in the reactions they catalyze.

Many enzymes are synthesized as inactive **proenzymes.** Substances that convert proenzymes to active enzymes are often called **kinases.** Kinases usually do their job of activating enzymes by means of an allosteric effect (see **Figure 6-15**). For example, enterokinase changes inactive trypsinogen into active trypsin by changing the shape of the molecule. Within cells, a type of kinase called simply *kinase* A has been shown to activate enzymes that regulate certain pathways after a hormonal signal is received by the cell.

Quick CHECK

4. Describe the structure of an enzyme. How does its structure determine its function?
5. What is an allosteric effector? Give examples.

CATABOLISM

There are many catabolic pathways that operate inside human cells. Perhaps the most important for a basic understanding of cell catabolism is the pathway known as **cellular respiration.** This section briefly outlines the basic concepts of the cellular respiratory pathway. Details of this pathway are further outlined in Chapter 41.

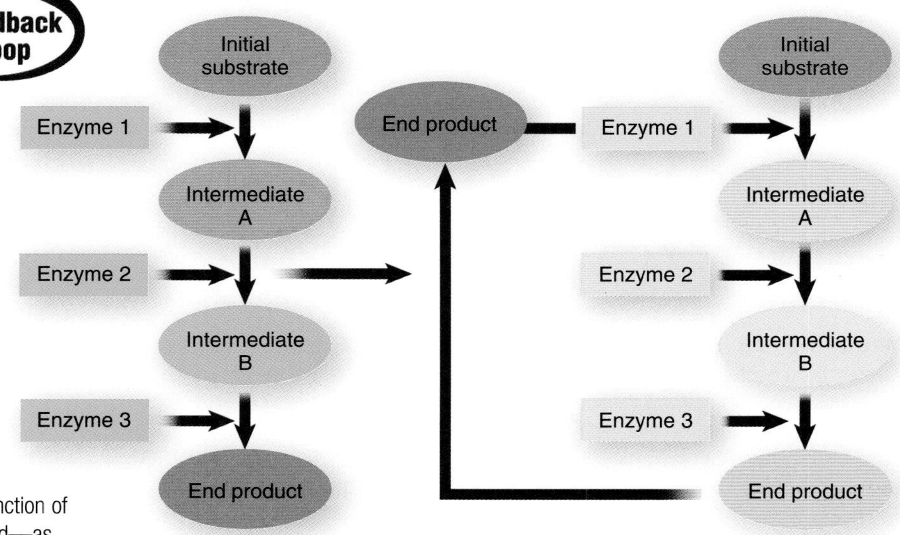

FIGURE 6-17 Feedback inhibition of enzymes. Formation of an excessive amount of end product can be inhibited by a negative feedback mechanism. In this example, the end product itself inhibits the function of an enzyme needed early in the pathway. Thus the entire pathway is inhibited—as long as there is an excess of the end product.

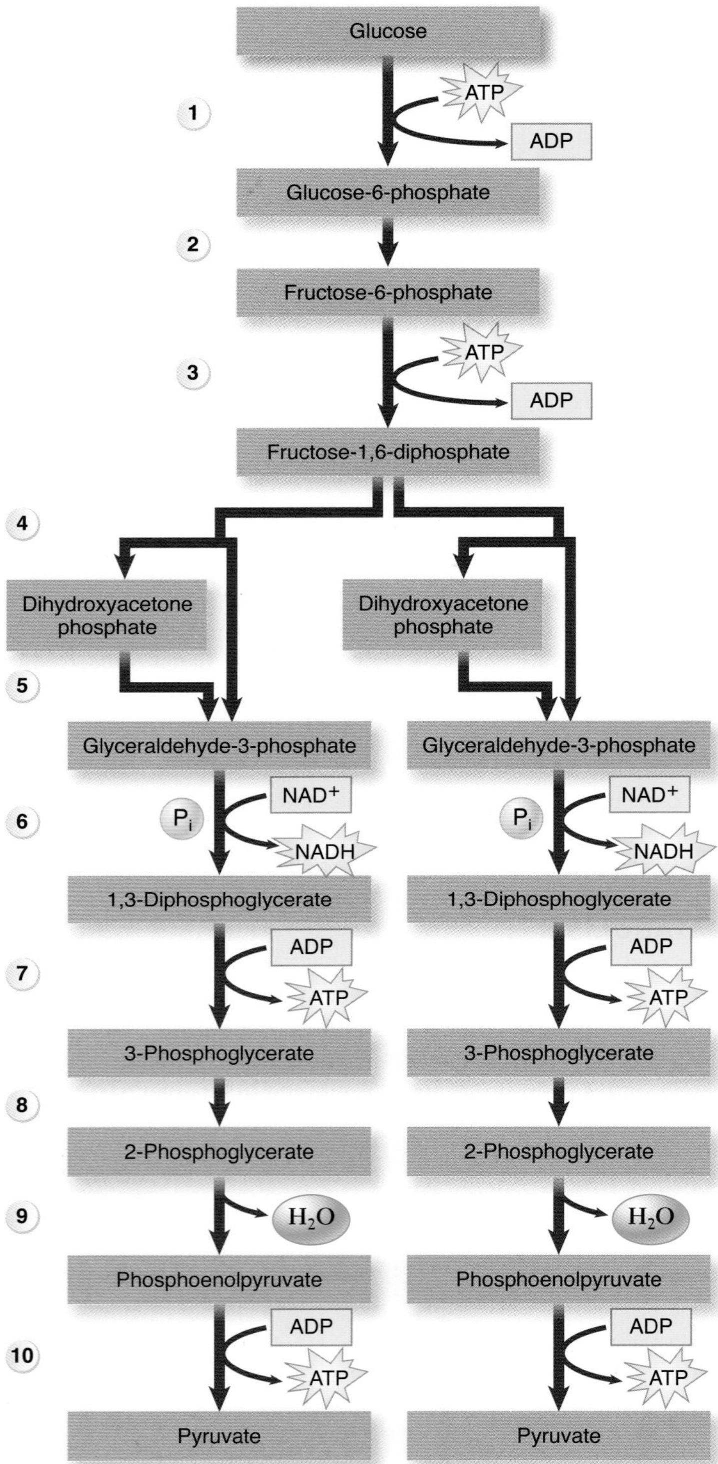

FIGURE 6-18 Glycolysis. This diagram of the reactions involved in glycolysis represents a classic example of a catabolic pathway. Note that each of the ten chemical reactions in this pathway cannot proceed until the previous step has occurred. Recall from our discussion that each step also requires the presence of one or more specific enzymes. *ADP,* Adenosine diphosphate; *ATP,* adenosine triphosphate; *NAD*$^+$ and *NADH,* forms of nicotinamide adenine dinucleotide; *P*$_i$, inorganic phosphate.

Overview of Cellular Respiration

Cellular respiration is the process by which cells break down glucose ($C_6H_{12}O_6$), or a nutrient that has been converted to glucose or one of its simpler products, into carbon dioxide (CO_2) and water (H_2O). As the molecule breaks down, the potential energy that had been stored in its bonds is released. Much of the released energy is converted into heat, but a portion of it is transferred to the high-energy bonds of adenosine triphosphate. **Figure 4-19** on p. 68 shows how ATP is synthesized from ADP and inorganic phosphate with energy obtained from cellular respiration.

Three smaller pathways are chemically linked together to form the larger catabolic pathway known as *cellular respiration*:

1. Glycolysis
2. Citric acid cycle
3. Electron transport system

The paragraphs that follow briefly introduce these three basic processes.

Glycolysis

Glycolysis is a catabolic pathway that begins with glucose, which contains six carbon atoms per molecule, and ends with pyruvate, which contains only three carbon atoms per molecule. As **Figure 6-18** shows, each glucose molecule that enters this pathway is eventually broken in half. In fact, the name *glycolysis* literally means "breaking glucose".

Glycolysis occurs in the cytosol of cells, outside any particular organelle. The cytosol, then, must contain all the enzymes necessary to catalyze each of the reactions that make up the glycolysis pathway. Because the reactions of glycolysis require no oxygen, glycolysis is said to be **anaerobic.** This type of pathway is classified as fermentation.

Glycolysis releases a small portion of the potential energy stored in the glucose molecule. Some of this energy is transferred to ATP, a molecule that can then transfer the energy to any of a large number of energy-consuming reactions in the cell. Some of the energy is transferred to another energy transfer molecule, a form of nicotinamide adenine dinucleotide (NADH). NADH may eventually transfer its energy to ATP in the electron transport system, a later step of cellular respiration that is discussed shortly.

Once pyruvate is formed by glycolysis, there is a fork in the metabolic pathway. That is, the molecule could enter one of two pathways linked to glycolysis (see **Figure 6-18**). If oxygen is available, the pyruvate molecule will follow the *aerobic pathway* and enter the citric acid cycle. This type of respiration is called **aerobic** respiration because oxygen (O_2) is required for this sequence of reactions to occur. If oxygen is unavailable for a particular pyruvate molecule to enter the aerobic pathway, it will continue along an anaerobic pathway to form a molecule called *lactate.* Lactate is later converted back to pyruvate or glucose in an energy- and oxygen-requiring pathway.

When the anaerobic pathway is followed, a small amount of the total energy stored in glucose is made available to the cell. However, if enough oxygen is not available to maintain a setpoint level of ATP by means of the aerobic pathway, the anaerobic pathway can help maintain adequate ATP levels for cellular functions to continue. Because oxygen is later used to process the lactate formed by anaerobic processes, biochemists say that an *oxygen debt* has been incurred.

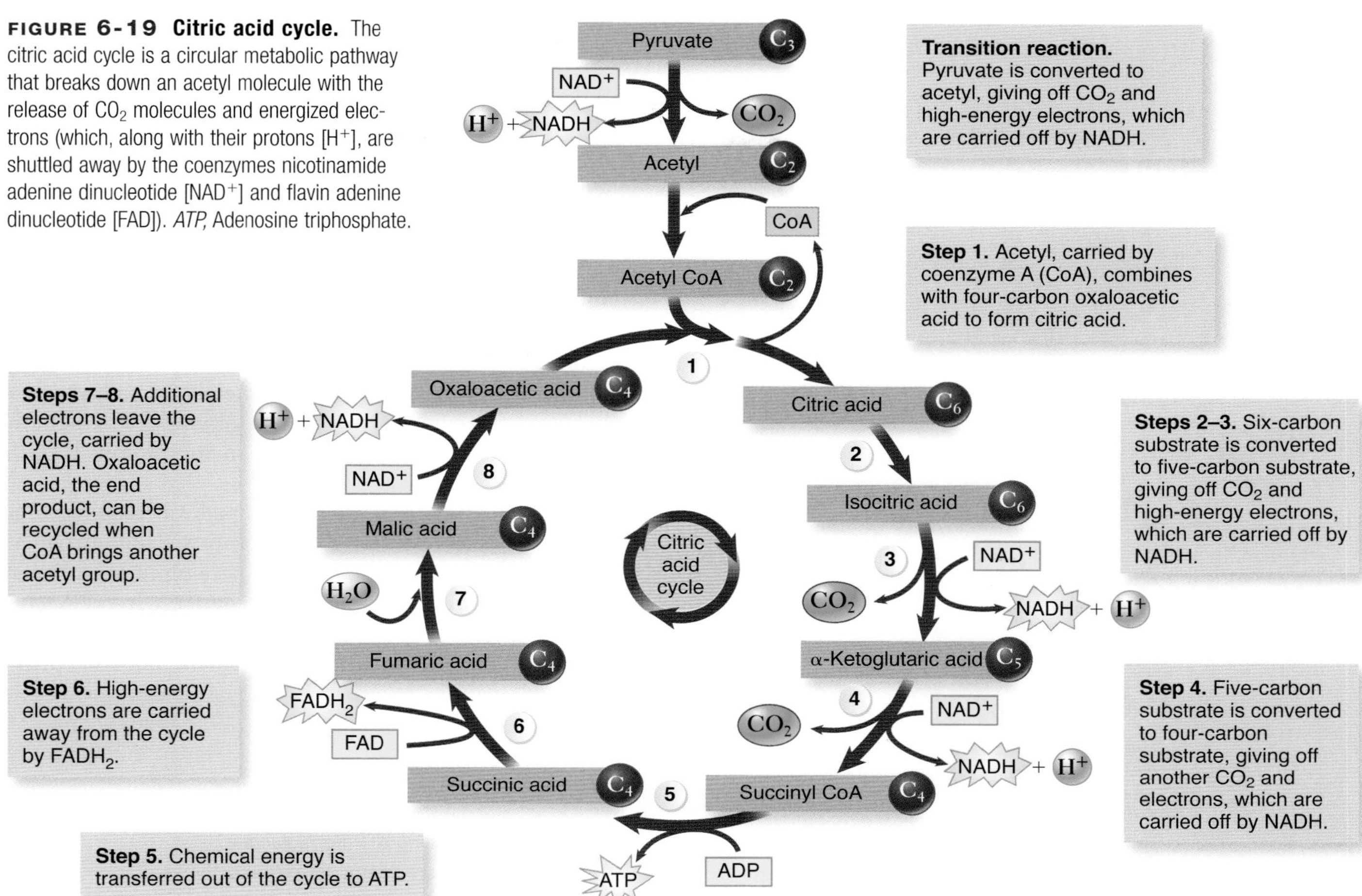

FIGURE 6-19 Citric acid cycle. The citric acid cycle is a circular metabolic pathway that breaks down an acetyl molecule with the release of CO_2 molecules and energized electrons (which, along with their protons [H^+], are shuttled away by the coenzymes nicotinamide adenine dinucleotide [NAD^+] and flavin adenine dinucleotide [FAD]). *ATP,* Adenosine triphosphate.

The additional oxygen that is taken in to process the extra lactate is now referred to as excess post-exercise oxygen consumption (EPOC) rather than oxygen debt. Much of the lactate diffuses out of the cell that formed it and is later processed in liver cells, which are adapted to perform this function efficiently.

Citric Acid Cycle

If oxygen is available, the pyruvate molecules formed by glycolysis are prepared to enter the next major phase of aerobic cellular respiration—the **citric acid cycle.** This cyclic (repeating) sequence of reactions is still sometimes called the *Krebs cycle* after Sir Hans Krebs, who discovered this pathway in the first part of the twentieth century. **Figure 6-19** shows that pyruvate is converted to acetyl that combines with coenzyme A (CoA) before it moves into the citric acid cycle. During this transition into the citric acid cycle, the molecule loses one of its carbons, along with some oxygen, producing waste carbon dioxide (CO_2). This cycle also produces some available energy that is transferred to NADH and then to the electron transport system, as explained later.

The citric acid cycle, like glycolysis, is a sequence of many chemical reactions (see **Figure 6-19**). As in glycolysis, each reaction of the citric acid cycle requires one or more specific enzymes. These enzymes are located in the inner chamber of the mitochondrion, so that is the cell location in which the citric acid cycle occurs.

In the citric acid cycle, the two-carbon acetyl group that breaks away from its escort, CoA, is further broken down to yield its stored energy. A small amount of this energy is transferred directly to ATP molecules, but most of the available energy is transferred in the form of energized electrons (e^-) and their accompanying protons (H^+) to the coenzyme NAD^+ or flavin adenine dinucleotide (FAD). NAD^+ then becomes NADH and FAD becomes the reduced form of FAD ($FADH_2$). More information on how these coenzymes pick up energy released from a metabolic pathway is found in Chapter 41 on p. 932. The energized electrons (along with their protons) then move into the next phase of cellular respiration—the electron transport system.

Electron Transport System

As **Figure 6-20** shows, NADH (and $FADH_2$) transfer the energized electrons to a set of special molecules embedded in the cristae of the inner mitochondrial membrane. These special electron-accepting molecules make up the **electron transport system (ETS).** As energized electrons leap from one of these molecules to the next, their energy is used to pump their accompanying protons (H^+) from the inner chamber of the mitochondrion to the outer chamber. As the protons build up in the outer chamber, a concentration gradient of protons develops. Protons then begin passive movement through the

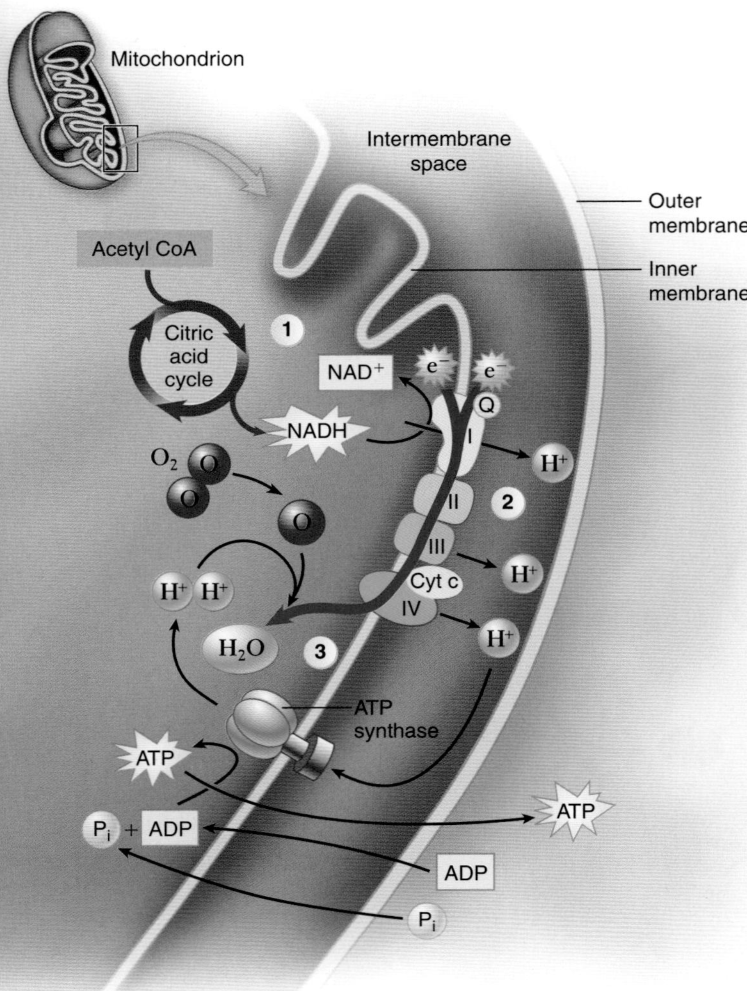

FIGURE 6-20 Electron transport system (ETS). 1, Pairs of high-energy electrons (e^-) and their protons (H^+) are shuttled from the citric acid cycle by coenzymes NAD and FAD to protein complexes (I, II, III, IV) embedded in the inner membrane of the mitochondrion. **2,** As the electrons are transported from molecule to molecule (*red path*), their energy is used to pump the protons (H^+) to the intermembrane space. **3,** As the proton gradient increases, passive movement of protons back across the membrane (through the ATP synthase carrier) provides the energy needed to "recharge" ADP and P to form ATP. Notice that oxygen (from O_2) is required as the final acceptor of the electrons and protons transported through the system, thus forming H_2O as a byproduct. *ADP,* Adenosine diphosphate; *ATP,* adenosine triphosphate; *FAD,* flavin adenine dinucleotide; *NAD,* nicotinamide adenine dinucleotide.

inner mitochondrial membrane into the inner chamber by way of "reverse pump" carriers (*ATP synthase*). These ATP synthase carriers convert the energy of passive proton flow into chemical energy, which is transferred to ATP molecules. In short, the energy transferred from the citric acid cycle is used to put protons behind a sort of dam, and then the energy of protons flowing back through "energy generators" from behind the dam is transferred to ATP. In most cells, aerobic respiration transfers enough energy from each glucose molecule to form 36 ATP molecules—2 directly from glycolysis and 34 from the rest of the pathway.

The low-energy electrons that come away from the electron transport system are accepted by oxygen molecules. This is why oxygen molecules are required for this metabolic pathway—to act as final electron acceptors. Once they combine with oxygen, the electrons are reunited with their accompanying protons (H^+) to form water (H_2O).

In summary, the aerobic respiratory pathway requires an input of glucose and oxygen and, by the action of specific enzymes, coenzymes, and other molecules, produces an output of carbon dioxide, water, and the real biochemical prize—energy in ATP. The major steps in cellular respiration are summarized in **Figure 6-21**. For an expanded discussion of cellular respiration, refer to Chapter 41, pp. 933–944.

Quick CHECK

6. What are the three catabolic pathways that together make up the process of generating ATP from glucose?
7. Which extracts more energy for cell use, the aerobic or anaerobic pathway?
8. To what molecule must energy be transferred before it can be used by most cell processes?
9. Briefly outline each of the major steps of cellular respiration.

ANABOLISM

Many anabolic or "building" pathways occur in human cells. Perhaps the most important for the beginning student to understand is the process of protein synthesis. Why is protein synthesis considered the central anabolic process of the cell? How is protein synthesis accomplished? These questions are answered as the story of cell function continues in the next chapter.

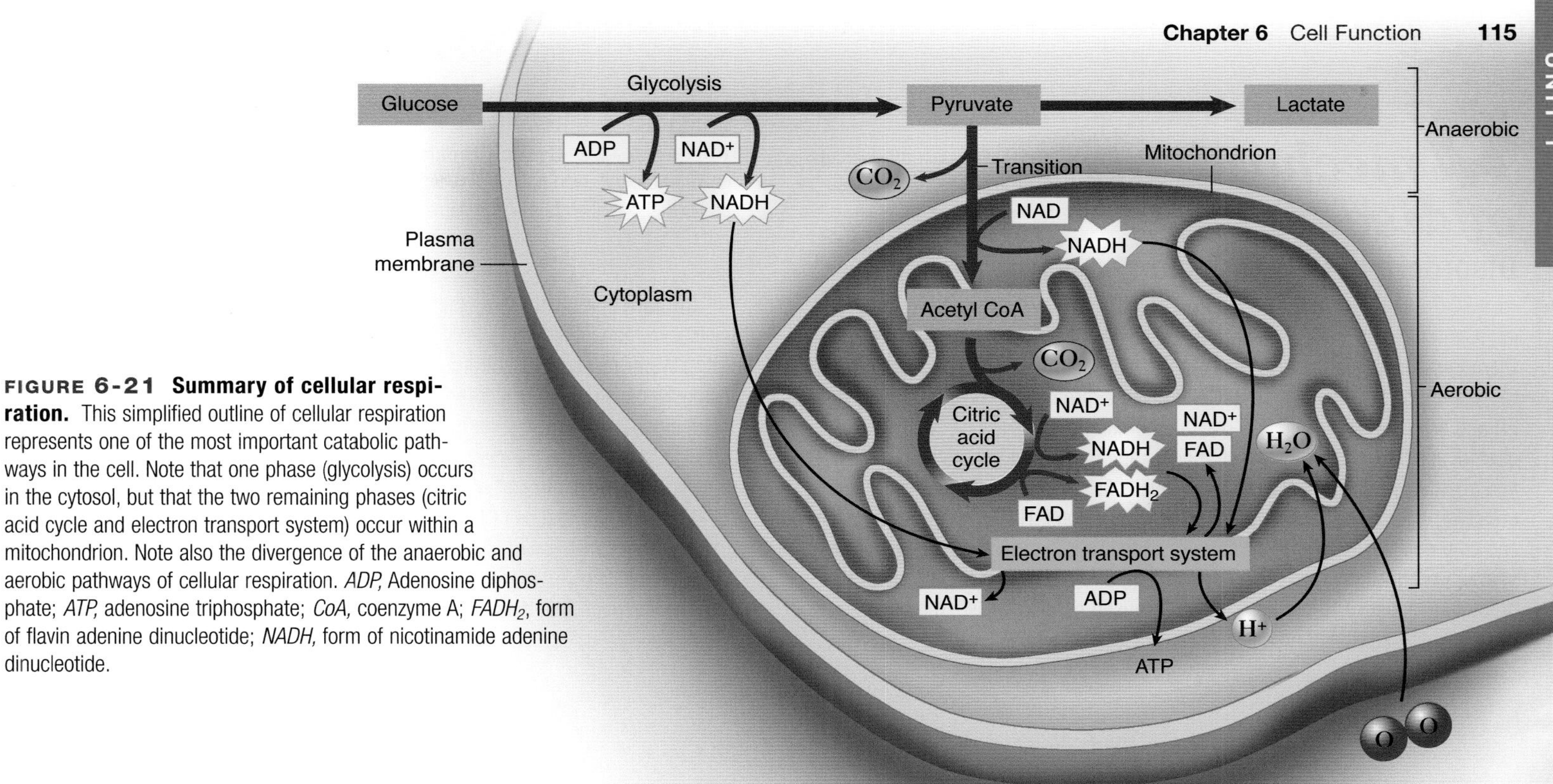

FIGURE 6-21 Summary of cellular respiration. This simplified outline of cellular respiration represents one of the most important catabolic pathways in the cell. Note that one phase (glycolysis) occurs in the cytosol, but that the two remaining phases (citric acid cycle and electron transport system) occur within a mitochondrion. Note also the divergence of the anaerobic and aerobic pathways of cellular respiration. *ADP,* Adenosine diphosphate; *ATP,* adenosine triphosphate; *CoA,* coenzyme A; *$FADH_2$,* form of flavin adenine dinucleotide; *NADH,* form of nicotinamide adenine dinucleotide.

the big picture | Cell Physiology and the Whole Body

When exploring the microscopic world of cells, it is easy to get caught up in the intricate mechanisms that operate in each specific organelle. Once you feel comfortable with these mechanisms, try to put them together into a bigger picture of cell function. For example, most of the processes that we explored in this chapter are going on at about the same time within each and every cell of your body. Each cell is transcribing genes and synthesizing polypeptides, which are then dumped into the ER and transported to the Golgi apparatus for processing and packaging before being sent off to become a lysosome or being secreted by exocytosis. At the same time, energy for this and other cell work is being transferred from nutrient molecules to ATP molecules, which act as energy storage batteries for the cell. The cytoskeleton and the cell membrane are transporting materials into, out of, and around the cytoplasm. Studying cell structure and function is like looking at the score of a symphony for the first time. All the individual parts look unrelated and somewhat confusing, but with a little effort you can combine them to form a coherent whole. The "symphony" of normal cell function results from a coordinated combination of many processes dictated by the cell's "musical score"—the genetic code.

However, there is a larger symphony playing out in the body. There are trillions of cells all performing together in concert to produce normal human function. How do cells grow and reproduce to form a whole, healthy body? Chapter 7 picks up our story to answer that question.

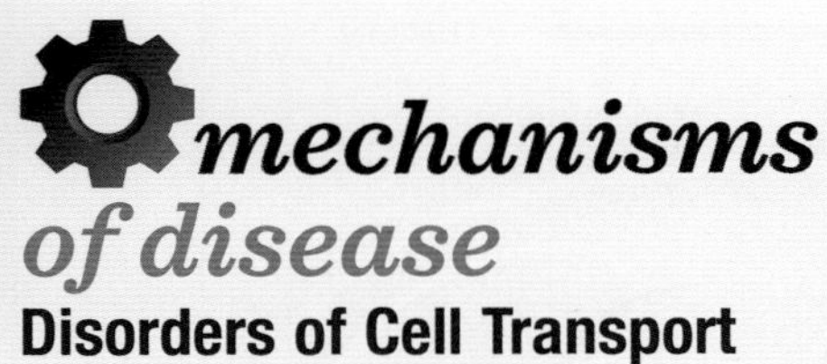

mechanisms of disease

Disorders of Cell Transport

Several very severe diseases result from damage to cell transport mechanisms. **Cystic fibrosis (CF),** for example, is an inherited condition in which chloride ion (Cl^-) channels in the plasma membrane called *CTFRs (cystic fibrosis transmembrane conductance regulators)* are defective. In the most common form of CF, this happens when abnormal CTFR channel proteins become misfolded in the ER and are thus not sent to the plasma membrane. Because Cl^- transport is altered, secretions such as sweat, mucus, and pancreatic juice are very salty—and often very thick. Abnormally thick mucus in the lungs impairs normal breathing and often leads to recurring lung infections. Thick pancreatic secretions can plug ducts that carry important enzymes to the digestive tract. **Figure 6-22** shows a child with CF next to a healthy child of the same age. Because of the breathing, digestive, and other problems caused by the disease, the affected child has not developed normally.

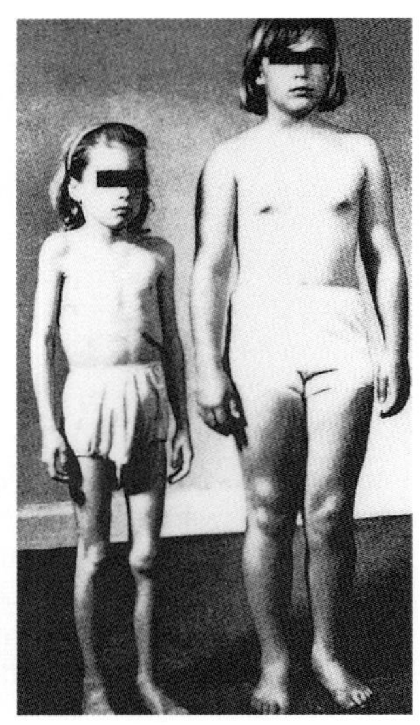

FIGURE 6-22 Cystic fibrosis (CF). The child on the left, who has CF, has failed to develop as normally as the child of the same age on the right.

Cholera is a bacterial infection that causes cells lining the intestines to leak chloride ions (Cl^-). Water follows Cl^- out of the cells by osmosis, causing severe diarrhoea and the resulting loss of water by the body. Death can occur in a few hours if treatment is not received. Interestingly, carriers of the defective CTFR gene that produces CF are resistant to cholera infections. Having defective Cl^- transport mechanisms apparently protects a person from an infection that disrupts normal Cl^- transport. This is one of many examples where so-called disease genes have turned out to have beneficial effects.

LANGUAGE OF SCIENCE *(continued from p. 98)*

endocytosis (en-doh-sye-TOH-sis)
[*endo-* **inward or within,** *-cyto-* **cell,** *-osis* **condition**]

end-product inhibition
(end-PROD-ukt in-hib-ISH-un)

enzyme (EN-zyme)
[*en-* **in,** *-zyme* **ferment**]

exocytosis (eks-o-sye-TOH-sis)
[*exo-* **outside or outward,** *-cyto* **cell,** *-osis* **condition**]

facilitated diffusion
(fah-SIL-i-tay-ted di-FYOO-zhun)
[*facili-* **easy,** *-ate* **act of,** *diffuse-* **spread out,** *-sion* **process**]

filtration (fil-TRAY-shun)
[*filtr-* **strain,** *-ation* **process**]

hypertonic (hye-per-TON-ik)
[*hyper-* **excessive,** *-ton-* **tension,** *-ic* **relating to**]

hypotonic (hye-poh-TON-ik)
[*hypo-* **under or below,** *-ton-* **tension,** *-ic* **relating to**]

isotonic (eye-soh-TON-ik)
[*iso-* **equal,** *-ton-* **tension,** *-ic* **relating to**]

kinase (KYE-nayz)
[*kin-* **motion,** *-ase* **enzyme**]

lock-and-key model
(lok and kee MOD-el)

metabolic pathway
(met-ah-BOL-ik PATH-way)
[*meta-* **over,** *-bol-* **throw,** *-ic* **relating to**]

metabolism (meh-TAB-oh-liz-im)
[*meta-* **over,** *-bol-* **throw,** *-ism* **action**]

osmosis (os-MO-sis)
[*osmos-* **push,** *-osis* **condition**]

osmotic pressure
(os-MOT-ik PRESH-ur)
[*osmo-* **push,** *-ic* **relating to**]

phagocytosis (fag-oh-sye-TOH-sis)
[*phago-* **eat,** *-cyto-* **cell,** *-osis* **condition**]

pinocytosis (pin-oh-sye-TOE-sis)
[*pino-* **drink,** *-cyto-* **cell,** *-osis* **condition**]

potential osmotic pressure
(po-TEN-shal os-MOT-ik PRESH-ur)
[*potent-* **power,** *-ial* **relating to,** *osmo-* **push,** *-ic* **relating to**]

proenzyme (pro-EN-zime)
[*pro-* **first,** *-en-* **in,** *-zyme* **ferment**]

simple diffusion
(simple di-FYOO-zhun)
[*diffus-* **spread out,** *-sion* **process**]

LANGUAGE OF MEDICINE

cholera (KOL-er-ah)
[*chole-* **bile,** *-a* **state**]

cystic fibrosis (CF)
(SIS-tik fye-BRO-sis)
[*cyst-* **sac,** *-ic* **relating to;** *fibr-* **thread or fibre,** *-osis* **condition**]

haemodialysis (he-mo-dye-AL-i-sis)
[*haemo-* **relating to blood,** *-dia-* **apart,** *-lysis* **loosening**]

case study

Toby, a student on a radiotherapy degree course, was very late for his work experience day and had to pedal his bike as fast as he could to make up time. The increased rate of respiration in Toby's muscle cells released more carbon dioxide into his bloodstream. After a few minutes the pH of his blood began to fall. Negative feedback mechanisms then operated to increase his breathing rate to vent off the extra carbon dioxide and maintain homeostasis.

1. The movement of carbon dioxide through Toby's muscle cell membranes into the blood capillaries is an example of:
   a. Active transport by vesicles in the membranes
   b. Facilitated diffusion
   c. Simple diffusion
   d. Active transport by membrane 'pumps'

Toby had been asked by his supervisor to investigate the uptake of iodine by the thyroid gland for a tutorial. He was surprised to learn that the concentration of iodide inside the follicular cells of the thyroid gland is 20–50 times that of the blood plasma. This is brought about by the sodium–iodide symporter, a type of membrane protein that moves iodide and sodium ions against their concentration gradient.

2. The movement of iodide ion into the thyroid follicle cells is an example of:
   a. Active transport by vesicles
   b. Facilitated diffusion
   c. Simple diffusion
   d. Active transport by membrane "pumps"

It was a hot day, and after his tutorial Toby cycled home. He has missed his lunch and afternoon breaks because he had to catch up with his work; he felt he could drink at least a litre of water.

3. If Toby did drink a large volume of water in a short time, what would happen to the tonicity of his blood?
   a. His blood would become hypertonic
   b. His blood would become hypotonic
   c. His blood would become isotonic
   d. The water would have no effect on his blood

Hint To solve a case study, you may have to refer to the glossary or index, other chapters in this textbook, **Connect It!,** and other resources.

CHAPTER SUMMARY

To download an MP3 version of the chapter summary for use with your mobile device, access the ***Audio Chapter Summaries*** *online at evolve.elsevier.com.*

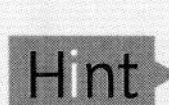

Scan this summary after reading the chapter to help you reinforce the key concepts. Later, use the summary as a quick review before your class or before a test.

Movement of Substances through Cell Membranes

A. Passive transport processes—do not require any energy expenditure of the cell membrane (**Table 6-1**)
  1. Diffusion—a passive process (**Figure 6-1**)
     a. Molecules spread through the membranes
     b. Molecules move from an area of high concentration to an area of low concentration, down a concentration gradient (**Figure 6-2**)
     c. As molecules diffuse, a state of equilibrium will occur
  2. Simple diffusion (**Figure 6-3**)
     a. Molecules cross through the phospholipid bilayer
     b. Solutes permeate the membrane; therefore we call the membrane permeable
  3. Osmosis (**Figure 6-4**)
     a. Movement or "diffusion" of water through a selectively permeable membrane; movement of at least some of the solute particles (the impermeant solutes) is limited
     b. Water pressure that develops as a result of osmosis is called *osmotic pressure*
     c. Potential osmotic pressure is the maximum pressure that could develop in a solution when it is separated from pure water by a selectively permeable membrane; knowledge of potential osmotic pressure allows prediction of the direction of osmosis and the resulting change in pressure
        (1) Isotonic—describes a fluid having the same potential osmotic pressure as cytosol (**Figure 6-5**)
        (2) Hypertonic—"higher pressure"; cells placed in solutions that are hypertonic always shrivel as water flows out of them; this has great medical importance: if medical treatment causes the extracellular fluid to become hypertonic, serious damage may occur
        (3) Hypotonic—"lower pressure"; cells placed in a hypotonic solution may swell as water flows into them; water always osmoses from the hypotonic solution into the cytosol
     d. Osmosis results in gain of volume on one side of the membrane and loss of volume on the other side of the membrane
  4. Facilitated diffusion (mediated passive transport)
     a. A special kind of diffusion in which movement of molecules is made more efficient by the action of transporters embedded in a cell membrane
     b. Transports substances down a concentration gradient
     c. Energy required comes from the collision energy of the solute

d. Channel-mediated passive transport (**Figure 6-6**)
   (1) Channels are specific—allow only one type of solute to pass through
   (2) Gated channels may be open or closed (or inactive)—may be triggered by any of a variety of stimuli
   (3) Channels allow membranes to be selectively permeable
   (4) Aquaporins are water channels that permit rapid osmosis
e. Carrier-mediated passive transport (**Figure 6-7**)
   (1) Carriers attract and bind to the solute, change shape, and release the solute out the other side of the carrier
   (2) Carriers are usually reversible, depending on the direction of the concentration gradient

5. Role of passive transport processes
   a. Move substances down their concentration gradient, thus maintaining equilibrium—and homeostatic balance
   b. Types of passive transport—simple and facilitated diffusion (channels and carriers); osmosis is a special example of channel-mediated passive transport of water

B. Active transport processes—require the expenditure of metabolic energy by the cell (**Table 6-2**)
   1. Transport by pumps
      a. Pumps are membrane transporters that move a substance against their concentration gradient—opposite of diffusion
      b. Examples: calcium pumps (**Figure 6-8**) and sodium-potassium pumps (**Figure 6-9**)
   2. Transport by vesicles—allow substances to enter or leave the interior of a cell without actually moving through its plasma membrane
      a. Endocytosis—the plasma membrane "traps" some extracellular material and brings it into the cell in a vesicle
         (1) Two basic types of endocytosis (**Figure 6-10**)
            (a) Phagocytosis—"condition of cell eating"; large particles are engulfed by the plasma membrane and enter the cell in vesicles; the vesicles fuse with lysosomes, which digest the particles
            (b) Pinocytosis—"condition of cell drinking"; fluid and the substances dissolved in it enter the cell
         (2) Receptor-mediated endocytosis—membrane receptor molecules recognize substances to be brought into the cell (**Figure 6-11**)
      b. Exocytosis
         (1) Process by which large molecules, notably proteins, can leave the cell even though they are too large to move out through the plasma membrane
         (2) Large molecules are enclosed in membranous vesicles and then pulled to the plasma membrane by the cytoskeleton, where the contents are released
         (3) Exocytosis also provides a way for new material to be added to the plasma membrane
         (4) Exosome—extracellular vesicle that may pinch off a cell during exocytosis
   3. Role of active transport processes
      a. Active transport requires energy use by the membrane
      b. Pumps—concentrate substances on one side of membrane, as when storing an ion inside an organelle
      c. Vesicle-mediated (endocytosis, exocytosis)—move large volumes of substances at once, as in secretion of hormones and neurotransmitters

Cell Metabolism

A. Metabolism is the set of chemical reactions in a cell
   1. Catabolism—breaks large molecules into smaller ones; usually releases energy
   2. Anabolism—builds large molecules from smaller ones; usually consumes energy

B. Role of enzymes
   1. Enzymes are chemical catalysts that reduce the activation energy needed for a reaction (**Figure 6-12**)
   2. Enzymes regulate cell metabolism
   3. Chemical structure of enzymes
      a. Proteins of a complex shape
      b. The active site is where the enzyme molecule fits the substrate molecule—a type of lock-and-key model (**Figure 6-13**)
   4. Classification and naming of enzymes
      a. Enzymes usually have an *-ase* ending, with the first part of the word signifying the substrate or the type of reaction catalyzed
      b. Oxidation-reduction enzymes—known as oxidases, hydrogenases, and dehydrogenases; energy release depends on these enzymes
      c. Hydrolyzing enzymes—hydrolases; digestive enzymes belong to this group
      d. Phosphorylating enzymes—phosphorylases or phosphatases; add or remove phosphate groups
      e. Enzymes that add or remove carbon dioxide—carboxylases or decarboxylases
      f. Enzymes that rearrange atoms within a molecule—mutases or isomerases
      g. Hydrases add water to a molecule without splitting it
   5. General functions of enzymes
      a. Enzymes regulate cell functions by regulating metabolic pathways (**Figure 6-14**)
      b. Enzymes are specific in their actions
      c. Various chemical and physical agents known as allosteric effectors affect enzyme action by changing the shape of the enzyme molecule; examples of allosteric effectors include (**Figure 6-15**):
         (1) Temperature (**Figure 6-16**, *B*)
         (2) Hydrogen ion (H^+) concentration (pH) (**Figure 6-16**, *A*)
         (3) Cofactors
         (4) End products of certain metabolic pathways (**Figure 6-17**)
      d. Most enzymes catalyze a chemical reaction in both directions

   e. Enzymes are continually being destroyed and continually being replaced
   f. Many enzymes are first synthesized as inactive proenzymes

C. Catabolism
   1. Cellular respiration, the pathway by which glucose is broken down to yield its stored energy, is an important example of cell catabolism; cellular respiration has three pathways that are chemically linked (**Figure 6-21**)
      a. Glycolysis (**Figure 6-18**)
      b. Citric acid cycle (**Figure 6-19**)
      c. Electron transport system (ETS) (**Figure 6-20**)
   2. Glycolysis (**Figure 6-18**)
      a. Pathway in which glucose is broken apart into two pyruvate molecules to yield a small amount of energy (which is transferred to ATP and NADH)
      b. Includes many chemical steps (reactions that follow one another), each regulated by specific enzymes
      c. Is anaerobic (requires no oxygen)
      d. Occurs within cytosol (outside the mitochondria)
      e. Enzymes may convert some of the pyruvate into lactate, which pools until it can be converted back to pyruvate and used in the aerobic pathway to generate ATP
   3. Citric acid cycle (Krebs cycle) (**Figure 6-19**)
      a. Pyruvate (from glycolysis) is converted into acetyl, which is picked up by CoA and enters the citric acid cycle after losing CO_2 and transferring some energy to NADH, ATP amd $FADH_2$
      b. Citric acid cycle is a repeating (cyclic) sequence of reactions that occur inside the inner chamber of a mitochondrion; acetyl splits from CoA and is broken down to yield waste CO_2 and energy (in the form of energized electrons), which is transferred to ATP, NADH, and $FADH_2$
   4. Electron transport system (ETS) (**Figure 6-20**)
      a. Energized electrons are carried by NADH and $FADH_2$ from glycolysis and the citric acid cycle to electron acceptors embedded in the cristae of the mitochondrion
      b. As electrons are shuttled along a chain of electron-accepting molecules in the cristae, their energy is used to pump accompanying protons (H^+) into the space between mitochondrial membranes
      c. Protons flow back into the inner chamber through pump molecules in the cristae, and their energy of movement is transferred to ATP
      d. Low-energy electrons coming off the ETS bind to oxygen and rejoin their protons to form water (H_2O)

D. Anabolism
   1. Protein synthesis is a central anabolic pathway in cells, to be covered in more detail in Chapter 7

The Big Picture: Cell Physiology and the Whole Body

A. Most cell processes are occurring at the same time in all of the cells throughout the body
B. Functions of individual cells are understood in the context of the trillions of cells of the body, to be explored further in Chapter 7

REVIEW QUESTIONS

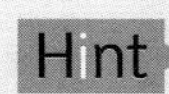

Write out the answers to these questions after reading the chapter and reviewing the Chapter Summary. Note—writing out your answers will consolidate learning and provide a valuable resource of information.

1. Define the terms diffusion, dialysis, facilitated diffusion, osmosis, and filtration.
2. Explain how a concentration gradient relates to the process of diffusion.
3. Describe and give an example of a membrane channel.
4. Construct a table comparing the terms hypotonic, isotonic and hypertonic. In the columns, define the terms and draw an illustration of how water moves into and out of a red blood cell in each solution.
5. State the principle that describes what conditions in a solution must exist for osmotic pressure to develop.
6. State the principle about the direction of active transport.
7. Name and describe the active transport pump that operates in the plasma membrane of all human cells.
8. Explain the processes of endocytosis and exocytosis. Define pinocytosis and phagocytosis.
9. Describe the classification of enzymes.
10. Discuss three general principles of enzyme function.
11. What is metabolism? catabolism? anabolism?
12. Describe briefly each of the three pathways that make up the process of cellular respiration.

CRITICAL THINKING QUESTIONS

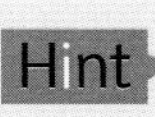

After finishing the Review Questions, write out the answers to these more in-depth questions to help you apply your new knowledge. Go back to sections of the chapter that relate to concepts that you find difficult.

1. The process of dialysis and the process of a white blood cell trapping bacteria by phagocytosis are both transport processes. Compare and contrast these processes and identify them as active or passive.
2. Which type of osmotic pressure can be more easily measured? Explain your answer.
3. Intravenous solutions can be isotonic to blood cells. Therefore, it is very important to know whether sugar, a nonelectrolyte, or salt (NaCl), an electrolyte, is being given in the solution so that the proper amount can be added. What would result if the tonicity of the solution is not isotonic to the blood cells?
4. White blood cells engulf bacteria and solutions that contain dissolved proteins. How would you summarize the processes that allow them to ingest both solids and liquids?
5. Explain how the shape of an enzyme determines its function. What would result if an allosteric effector changed the shape of the enzyme?
6. Compare and contrast aerobic and anaerobic pathways.
7. Why is the mitochondrion such an important organelle for survival of the cell? Explain why some cells, such as skeletal muscle cells, have more mitochondria than others do.

7 Cell Growth and Development

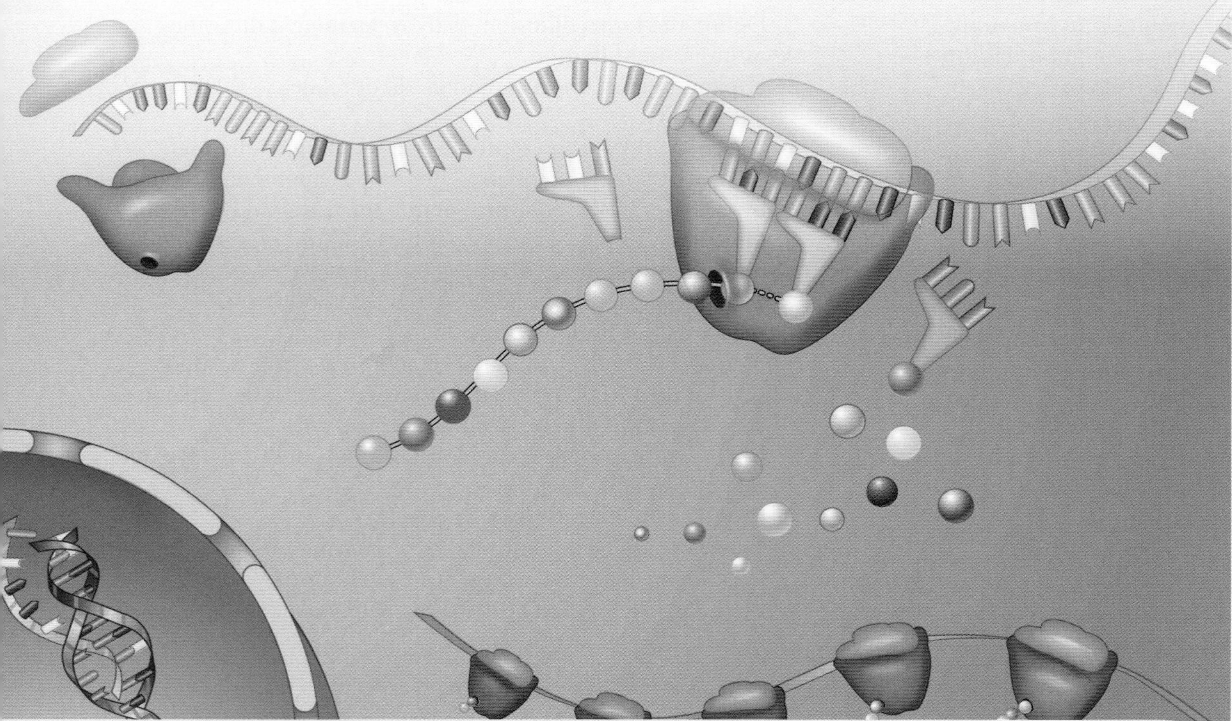

CHAPTER OUTLINE

Hint ▶ *Scan this outline before you begin to read the chapter, as a preview of how the concepts are organized.*

Cell growth and reproduction are the most fundamental of all living functions. These two processes together constitute the cell life cycle. On these processes depend the continued survival of all organisms already living and the creation of all new organisms. Cell growth depends on using genetic information in DNA to make the structural and functional proteins needed for cell survival. Cell reproduction ensures that the genetic information is passed from one generation of cells to the next and from one generation of organisms to the next. Mistakes in these processes can cause lethal genetic disorders, cancer, and other conditions. Advances in our ability to manipulate the genetic code, and thus cell growth and reproduction, now present us with ethical implications more far-reaching than those accompanying the birth of the atomic age. All this makes the cell life cycle a worthy and fascinating topic of study.

LANGUAGE OF SCIENCE

Hint ▶ *Use this list to aid your pronunciation of unfamiliar words.*

anaphase (AN-ah-fayz)
[*ana-* **apart,** *-phase* **stage**]

apoptosis
(app-o-TOH-sis or app-op-TOH-sis)
[*apo-* **away,** *-pto-* **fall,** *-osis* **condition or process**]

complementary pairing
(kom-pleh-MEN-tah-ree PAIR-ing)
[*comple-* **complete,** *-ment-* **process,** *-ary* **relating to**]

cyclin (SYE-klin)
[*cycl-* **circle,** *-in* **substance**]

cyclin-dependent kinase (CDK)
(SYE-klin dee-PEND-ent KI-nays)
[*cycl-* **circle,** *-in* **substance;** *de-* **from,** *-pend-* **hang,** *-ent* **relating to;** *kin-* **motion,** *-ase* **enzyme**]

cytokinesis (sye-toe-kin-EE-sis)
[*cyto-* **cell,** *-kinesis* **movement**]

deoxyribonucleic acid (DNA)
(dee-OK-see-rye-boh-nyoo-KLAY-ik ASS-id)
[*de-* **removed,** *-oxy-* **sharp (oxygen),** *-ribo-* **ribose,** *-nucle-* **nucleus (kernel),** *-ic* **relating to;** *acid* **sour**]

differentiate (dif-er-EN-shee-ayt)
[*different-* **difference,** *-iate* **act of**]

diploid (DIP-loid)
[*diplo-* **double,** *-oid* **form**]

exon (EKS-on)
[*exo-* **outside,** *-on* **unit**]

gamete (GAM-eet)
[*gamet* **sexual union**]

haploid (HAP-loid)
[*haplo-* **single,** *-oid* **form**]

interphase (IN-ter-fayz)
[*inter-* **between,** *-phase* **stage**]

intron (IN-tron)
[*intra-* **within,** *-on* **unit**]

meiosis (my-OH-sis)
[*meiosis* **becoming smaller**]

metaphase (MET-ah-fayz)
[*meta-* **change or middle,** *-phase* **stage**]

mitosis (my-TOH-sis)
[*mitos-* **thread,** *-osis* **condition**]

obligatory base pairing
(o-BLIG-ah-tor-ee base PAIR-ing)

polyribosome (POL-ee-RYE-bo-sohm)
[*poly-* **many,** *-som-* **body**]

continued on p. 133

PROTEIN SYNTHESIS

As stated in the previous chapter, the most important anabolic pathway for the student beginning the study of anatomy and physiology to understand is the process of protein synthesis. Protein synthesis is important for several reasons. First of all, protein synthesis is required for cell growth and maintenance. Protein synthesis begins with reading of the genetic "master code" in the cell's DNA. The genetic code dictates the structure of each protein produced during the growth process of each cell. A basic understanding of how the genetic code is used by the cell is essential for understanding modern concepts of human biology, including the study of disease processes.

Protein synthesis is also an important process because it influences all cell structures and functions. Proteins synthesized by the cell either are structural elements themselves or are enzymes or other functional proteins that direct the synthesis of other structural and functional molecules such as carbohydrates, lipids, and nucleic acids. In short, protein synthesis is the central building process for cell growth and maintenance.

Deoxyribonucleic Acid (DNA)

In 1953, American scientist James Watson, and three British scientists, Francis Crick, Maurice Wilkins, and Rosalind Franklin, won the race to solve the puzzle of DNA's molecular structure (**Figure 7-1**). Nine years later, Watson, Crick, and Wilkins received the Nobel Prize for their brilliant and significant work—hailed as the greatest biological discovery of our time. (Franklin died before the Nobel Prize was awarded.)

Since the original discovery of DNA's structure, we have seen a new branch of biology called *molecular genetics* emerge from our rapidly growing knowledge of DNA and how it works. Indeed, we have seen a revolution in human biology as we witness the continuing application of molecular genetics transform every single aspect of anatomy, physiology, and medicine. We begin our outline of protein synthesis with a discussion of DNA because it truly is, as Watson called it, "the most golden of all molecules".

The **deoxyribonucleic acid (DNA)** molecule is a giant among molecules. Its size and the complexity of its shape exceed those of most molecules. The importance of its function—in a word, information—surpasses that of any other molecule in the world. To visualize the shape of the DNA molecule, picture an extremely long, narrow ladder made of a pliable material (see **Figure 7-1**). Now imagine it twisting around and around on its axis and taking on the shape of a steep spiral staircase millions of turns long. This is the shape of the DNA molecule—a double spiral or *double helix*.

The DNA molecule is a *polymer*, which means that it is a large molecule made up of many smaller molecules joined together in sequence. DNA is a polymer of millions of pairs of nucleotides. A nucleotide is a compound formed by combining phosphoric acid with a sugar and a nitrogenous base. The DNA molecule has four different kinds of nucleotides. Each consists of a phosphate group that attaches to the sugar deoxyribose, which attaches to one of four bases. Nucleotides differ, therefore, in their nitrogenous base component—containing either adenine or guanine (purine bases) or cytosine or thymine (pyrimidine bases). (Deoxyribose is a sugar that is not sweet and one whose molecules contain only five carbon atoms.) Note what the name *deoxyribonucleic acid* tells you—that this compound contains deoxyribose, that it occurs in the nucleus, and that it is an acid.

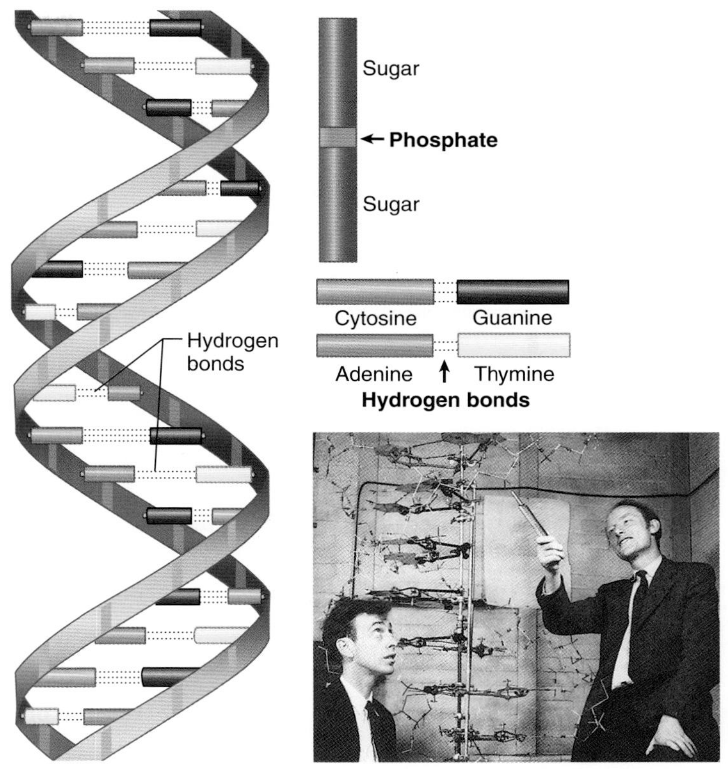

FIGURE 7-1 Watson–Crick model of the DNA molecule. The DNA structure illustrated here is based on that published by James Watson (photograph, *left*) and Francis Crick (photograph, *right*) in 1953. Note that each side of the DNA molecule consists of alternating sugar and phosphate groups. Each sugar group is united to the sugar group opposite it by a pair of nitrogenous bases (adenine–thymine or cytosine–guanine). The sequence of these pairs constitutes a genetic code that determines the structure and function of a cell.

Figure 7-1 reveals additional and highly significant facts about DNA's molecular structure. First, observe which compounds form the sides of the DNA spiral staircase—a long line of phosphate and deoxyribose units joined alternately one after the other. Look next at the stair steps. Note two facts about them: two bases join (loosely bound by hydrogen bonds) to form each step, and only two combinations of bases occur. The same two bases invariably pair off with each other in a DNA molecule. Adenine always goes with thymine (or vice versa, thymine with adenine), and guanine always goes with cytosine (or vice versa). This aspect of DNA molecular structure is called **obligatory base pairing.** Pay particular attention to this base pairing, for it is the key to understanding how a DNA molecule is able to duplicate itself. DNA duplication, or *replication* as it is usually called, is one of the most important of all biological phenomena because it is an essential and crucial part of the mechanism of genetics.

Another aspect of DNA's molecular structure that has great functional importance is the sequence of its base pairs. Although the kinds of base pairs possible in all DNA molecules are the same, the *sequence* of these base pairs is not the same in all DNA molecules. For instance, the sequence of the base pairs composing the seventh, eighth, and ninth steps of one DNA molecule might be cytosine–guanine, adenine–thymine, and thymine–adenine. Such a sequence

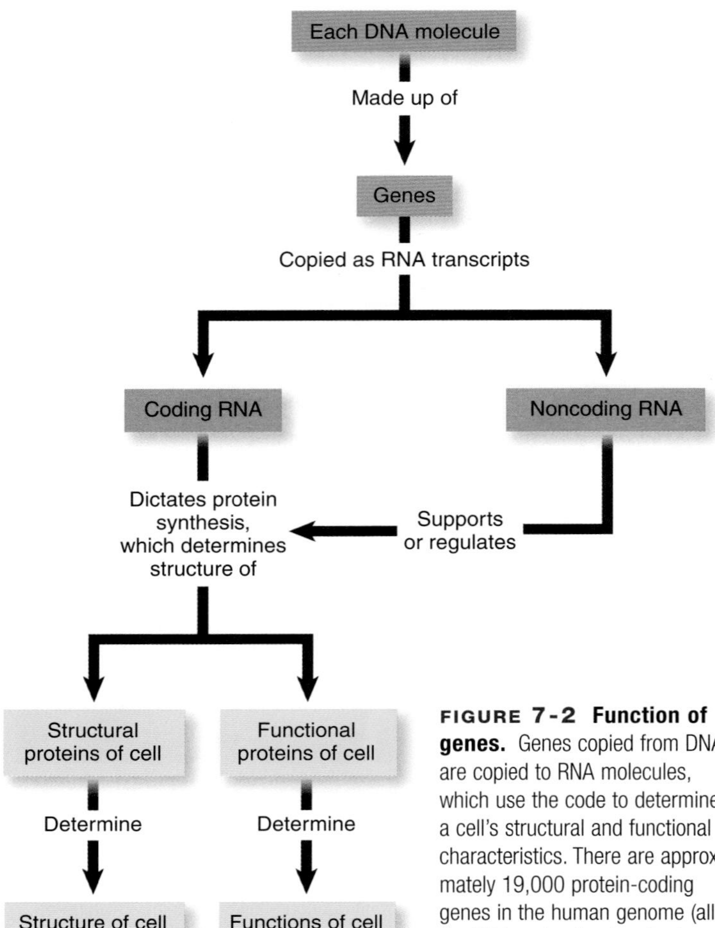

FIGURE 7-2 Function of genes. Genes copied from DNA are copied to RNA molecules, which use the code to determine a cell's structural and functional characteristics. There are approximately 19,000 protein-coding genes in the human genome (all the DNA molecules together).

of three bases forms a code word or "triplet" called a *codon*. In another DNA molecule the coding sequence of the base pairs making up these same steps might be entirely different, perhaps thymine–adenine, guanine–cytosine, and cytosine–guanine. Perhaps these seem to be minor details, but nothing could be further from the truth, because it is the sequence of the base pairs in the nucleotides that make up the DNA molecules that identifies each gene. Therefore, it is the sequence of base pairs that determines all hereditary traits.

A human *gene* is a segment of a DNA molecule. One gene consists of a chain of up to several thousand pairs of nucleotides joined one after the other in a precise sequence. Each gene in DNA is a code. As **Figure 7-2** shows, a gene is the code for building a short strand of RNA (ribonucleic acid).

Ribonucleic Acid (RNA)

To make a protein, the gene code in DNA is first copied to a messenger ribonucleic acid (mRNA) molecule, or transcript. Each mRNA transcript of a gene may then be translated by the cell and used to build one polypeptide chain. Because it is a copy of a gene's code, we call mRNA *coding RNA*. A few RNA transcripts are instead used to support or regulate polypeptide production. We call such RNA molecules *noncoding RNAs*. Examples of noncoding RNAs are rRNA (ribosomal RNA) and tRNA (transfer RNA). **Table 7-1** summarizes the major types of RNA.

One or more polypeptides made using RNA are used by the cell to make up each of a cell's structural proteins and the many functional proteins that regulate cellular processes. Therefore, as **Figure 7-2** shows, the 19,000 or so protein-coding genes that make up a cell's genome (DNA set) determine the cell's structure and its functions.

Transcription

Protein synthesis begins when a single strand of RNA (ribonucleic acid) forms along a segment of one strand of a DNA molecule. **Figure 7-3** summarizes how this process happens. Recall from Chapter 4 that RNA differs from DNA in certain respects (see **Table 4-4**, p. 67). Its molecules are smaller than those of DNA, and RNA contains ribose instead of deoxyribose. In addition, one of the four bases in RNA is uracil instead of thymine. As a strand of RNA is forming along a strand of DNA, uracil attaches to adenine, and guanine attaches to cytosine. The process is known as **complementary pairing.** Thus a single-strand molecule of messenger RNA (mRNA) is formed.

TABLE 7-1 Major Types of RNA

ACRONYM	NAME	DESCRIPTION	ROLE IN CELL FUNCTION
RNA Involved in Protein Synthesis			
mRNA	Messenger RNA	Single, unfolded strand of nucleotides	Serves as working copy of one protein-coding gene
rRNA	Ribosomal RNA	Single, folded strand of nucleotides	Component of the ribosome (along with proteins); attaches to mRNA and participates in translation
tRNA	Transfer RNA	Single, folded strand of nucleotides; has an anticodon at one end and an amino acid–binding site at the other end	Carries a specific amino acid to a specific codon of mRNA at the ribosome during translation
snRNP	Small nuclear ribonucleo-protein	Single, folded strand of RNA (combined with polypeptide chains)	Component of the spliceosome (see **Box 7-1**); attaches to an mRNA transcript to facilitate editing (removal of introns; splicing of exons) into the final version of mRNA
RNA Involved in Gene Silencing			
dsRNA	Double-strand RNA	Double strand of nucleotides (may be up to several hundred nucleotides long)	Involved in RNA interference; *see* siRNA, which is a type of dsRNA
siRNA	Short interfering RNA	Short segment of double-strand RNA (only 20–25 nucleotides long)	Forms part of the RNA-induced silencing complex (RISC) during RNA interference

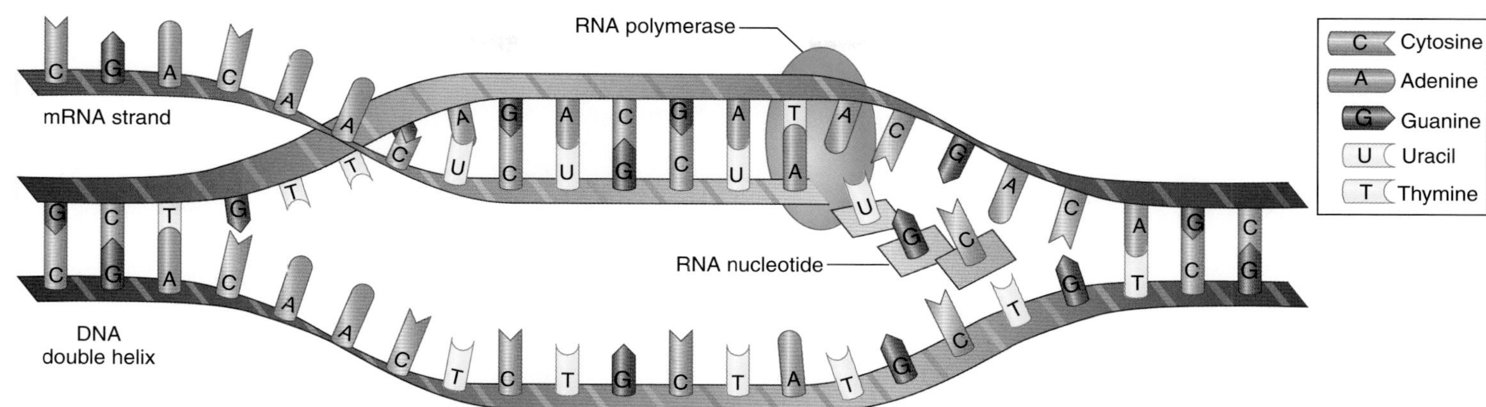

FIGURE 7-3 Transcription of messenger RNA (mRNA). A DNA molecule "unzips" in the region of the gene to be transcribed. RNA nucleotides already present in the nucleus temporarily attach themselves to exposed DNA bases along one strand of the unzipped DNA molecule according to the principle of complementary pairing. As the RNA nucleotides attach to the exposed DNA, they bind to each other and form a chainlike RNA strand called a *messenger RNA (mRNA)* molecule. Note that the new mRNA strand is an exact copy of the base sequence on the opposite side of the DNA molecule. As in all metabolic processes, the formation of mRNA is controlled by an enzyme—in this case, the enzyme is called *RNA polymerase.*

The name "messenger RNA" describes its function. As soon as it is formed, it separates from the DNA strand, is edited, moves out of the nucleus, and carries a "message" to a ribosome in the cell's cytoplasm to direct the synthesis of a specific polypeptide. Synthesis of any RNA molecule is often called **transcription** because it actually copies or "transcribes" a portion of the DNA code—just like you "transcribe" your class notes when you make a copy of them.

Other forms of RNA, such as transfer RNA (tRNA) and ribosomal RNA (rRNA) are constructed by mechanisms similar to mRNA transcription.

Editing the Transcript

After the preliminary version of the mRNA molecule is formed, its message is "edited" into a final version before it reaches a ribosome (**Figure 7-4**). Just as you may edit your class notes by rearranging them for clarity after you transcribe them, the editing process allows the cell to arrange the code so that it will work in making a specific, needed polypeptide.

To begin editing, a modified guanine (G) nucleotide caps one end of the mRNA strand. At about the same time, a string of 50 to 200 adenine (A) nucleotides attaches to the opposite end of the mRNA strand. This string of A nucleotides is sometimes called the *poly A tail.* The cap and poly A tail both assist in the next step of mRNA editing. The cap and poly A tail also eventually help transport the mRNA strand out of the nucleus and assist in starting and stopping the translation process described in the next section.

Some segments of the RNA transcript represent noncoding parts of DNA called **introns.** These intron segments are removed by a complicated process involving small nuclear structures called *spliceosomes* (**Box 7-1**). This leaves behind segments that are copies of the DNA's **exons.** Many of these exons encode the functional domains within protein molecules. Only these exon copies will be used in the final recipe for the protein. All the RNA segments representing exons are then *spliced* (joined) together by enzymes to form the final edited form of mRNA. It is this edited version of RNA that leaves the nucleus and participates in the next step of protein synthesis.

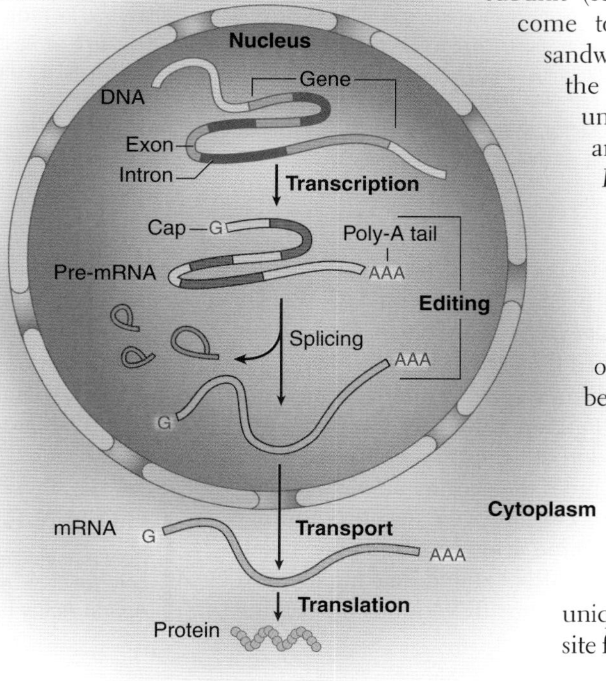

FIGURE 7-4 Editing of an mRNA transcript. After the preliminary mRNA strand is transcribed from a gene in DNA, it is capped with a modified G nucleotide at one end. At the same time, a poly A string is attached at the other end. The intron sections of the transcript are then removed and the remaining exons joined, or spliced, together to form the final version of mRNA. The edited mRNA transcript then moves out of the nucleus to participate in translation (see **Figure 7-3**).

Translation

In the cytoplasm, the edited mRNA molecule attracts first a small ribosome subunit and then a large subunit (see **Figure 5-6**). As the subunits come together, they form an "mRNA sandwich" with the mRNA molecule in the middle. Recall that the two subunits of the now-complete ribosome are composed largely of *ribosomal RNA* (rRNA). The cell is now ready to interpret or "translate" the genetic code and form a specific sequence of amino acids in a process called **translation.**

In translation, yet another type of RNA—*transfer RNA* (tRNA)—becomes involved in protein synthesis (**Figure 7-5**). As the name implies, tRNA molecules carry or "transfer" amino acids to the ribosome for placement in the prescribed sequence. This function is determined by a unique molecular structure: a binding site for a specific amino acid at one end

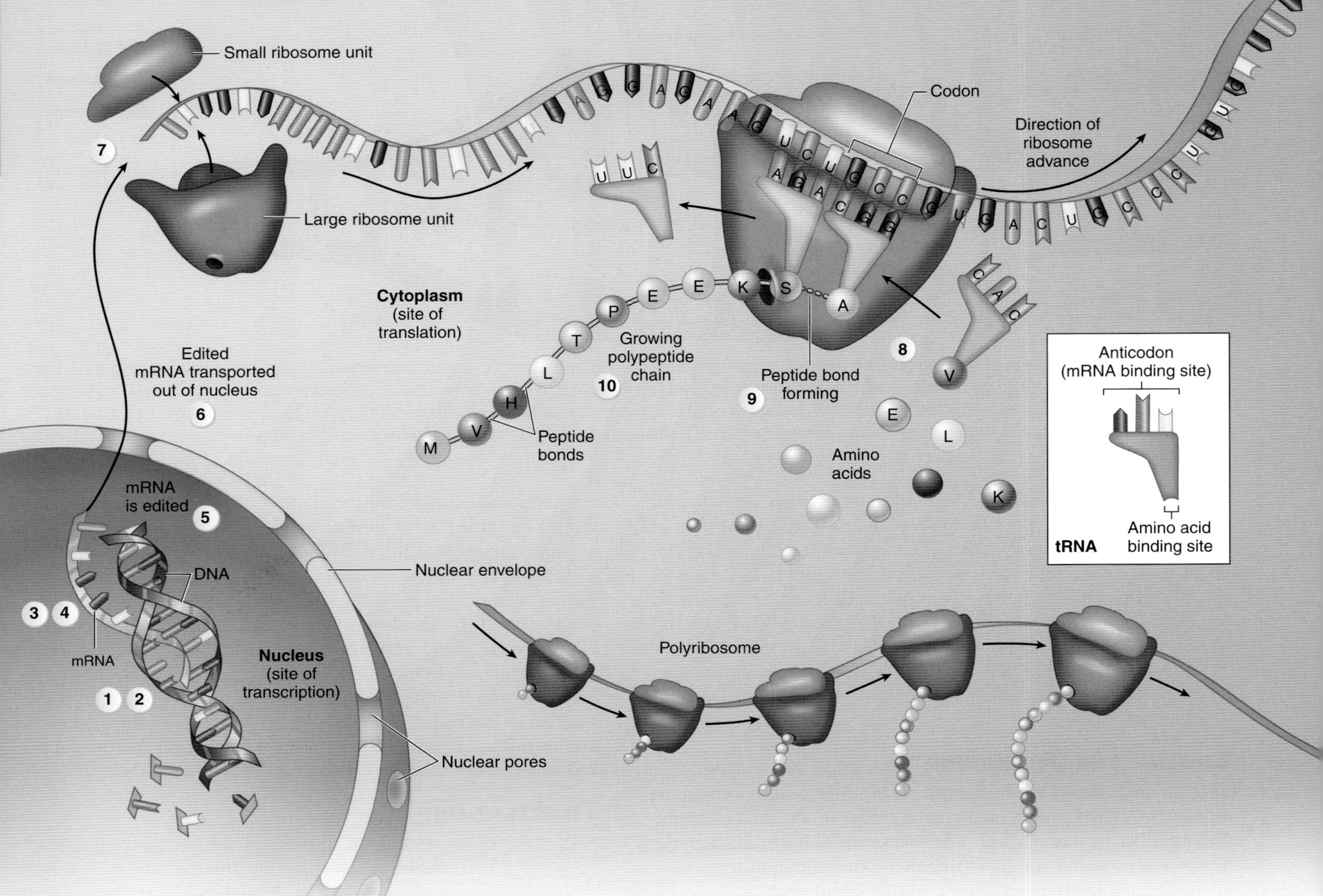

FIGURE 7-5 Protein synthesis. Each of the numbered steps in the figure is further summarized in **Table 7-2**. Protein synthesis begins with transcription, a process in which an mRNA molecule forms along one gene sequence of a DNA molecule within the cell's nucleus *(1–3)*. As it is formed, the mRNA molecule separates from the DNA molecule *(4)*, is edited *(5)*, and leaves the nucleus through the large nuclear pores *(6)*. Outside the nucleus, ribosome subunits attach to the beginning of the mRNA molecule and begin the process of translation *(7)*. In translation, transfer RNA (tRNA) molecules bring specific amino acids—encoded by each mRNA codon—into place at the ribosome site *(8)*. As the amino acids are brought into the proper sequence, they are joined together by peptide bonds *(9)* to form long strands called polypeptides *(10)*. Several polypeptide chains may be needed to make a complete protein molecule. Amino acids are identified by colour codes and abbreviations (see **Figure 4-12** on p. 62). See **Table 7-2** for further clarification of protein synthesis.

and a binding site for a specific mRNA codon (base triplet) at the other end (see **Figure 4-18** on p. 68). Because tRNA's binding site for mRNA contains the three bases that exactly complement one mRNA codon, this binding site is often called the *anticodon.*

After picking up its amino acid from a pool of different types of amino acids floating free in the cytoplasm, a tRNA molecule moves to the ribosome. There, its anticodon attaches to a complementary mRNA codon—the codon that signifies the specific amino acid carried by that tRNA molecule (**Figure 7-6**). After the next tRNA brings its amino acid into place, the two amino acids form a peptide bond. The ribosome then moves down the mRNA strand, making the next mRNA codon available for a complementary tRNA molecule bearing the appropriate amino acid. More tRNA molecules, one after the other in rapid sequence, bring more amino acids to the ribosome and fit them into their proper position in the growing chain of amino acids. As **Figure 7-5** shows, the ribosome is all the while moving down the mRNA strand—until it reaches the end, where the ribosome subunits fall away.

CONNECT IT!

How many different amino acids can be used to make proteins? Is this the only function of amino acids in the human body? Find out in ***Amazing Amino Acids*** online at ***Connect It!***

BOX 7-1 *spliceosome*

The noncoding *intron* segments of the mRNA initially transcribed from a DNA gene are removed by a complicated process involving small structures called **spliceosomes.** Found inside the nucleus, spliceosomes are about the size of a ribosome. Spliceosomes are made up of subunits consisting of *small nuclear ribonucleoproteins* (*snRNPs,* pronounced "snurps").

During mRNA editing, a snRNP subunit will attach at the beginning of an intron and another snRNP will attach at a spot in the intron called the "branch point". Eventually, several different subunits will all assemble on the intron in this manner to form a complete spliceosome. As the figure shows, the assembled spliceosome then breaks the strand as it bends the intron into a loop called a *lariat.* The intron lariat breaks completely away from the strand, and the spliceosome splices the ends of the remaining coding *exon* segments together. Only the spliced exons remain in the final, edited version of mRNA, which is later translated into the polypeptide encoded by the gene.

The intron may later break down into individual nucleotides, which are then recycled by the cell and used again for transcription. The intron may instead be processed to form a noncoding RNA strand with regulatory functions (see ***The RNA Revolution*** at ***Connect It!***). After splicing is accomplished, the snRNP subunits of the spliceosome are free to reassemble on another intron and repeat the process. •

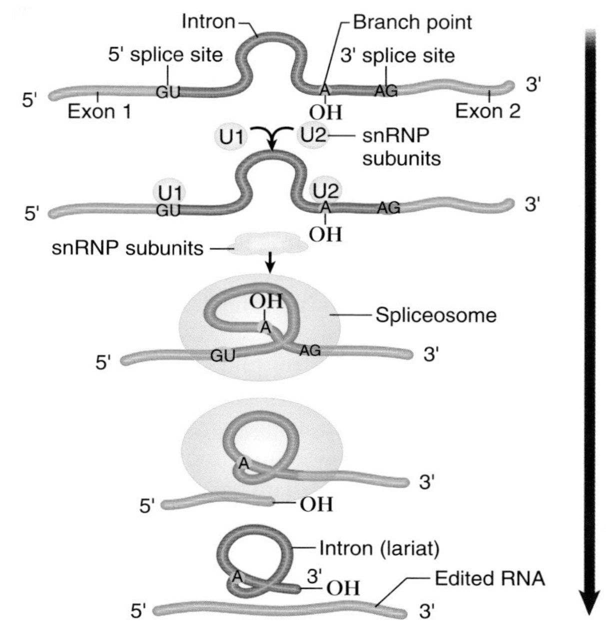

Editing of mRNA by the spliceosome. A simplified view of the complex splicing process.

Each of the tools needed for translation—mRNA, tRNA, and ribosome subunits—can be reused again and again to form copies of the same polypeptide. As a matter of fact, one ribosome can follow another along the same mRNA strand, each making its own polypeptide. Cell biologists often observe a whole train of ribosomes positioned along a single mRNA strand, each making an identical copy of the encoded polypeptide. Such a **polyribosome** is pictured in **Figure 7-5**.

CONNECT IT!

Translation can be inhibited or prevented by a process called **RNA interference (RNAi).** The illustrated article ***The RNA Revolution***—available online at ***Connect It!***—details the concept of *gene silencing* by interfering with the process of translating the genes. RNAi can be used by cells to protect against virus infections.

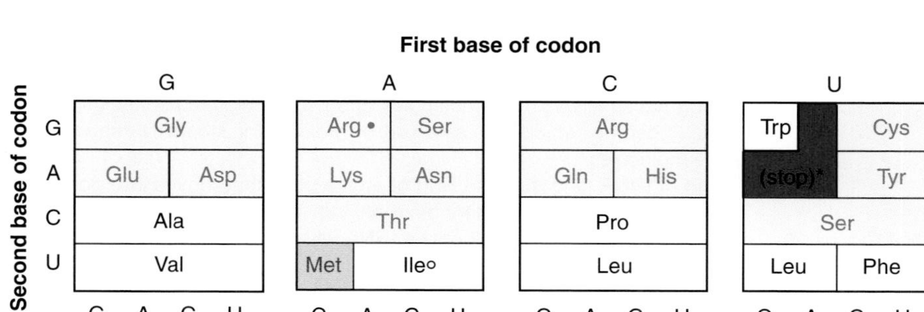

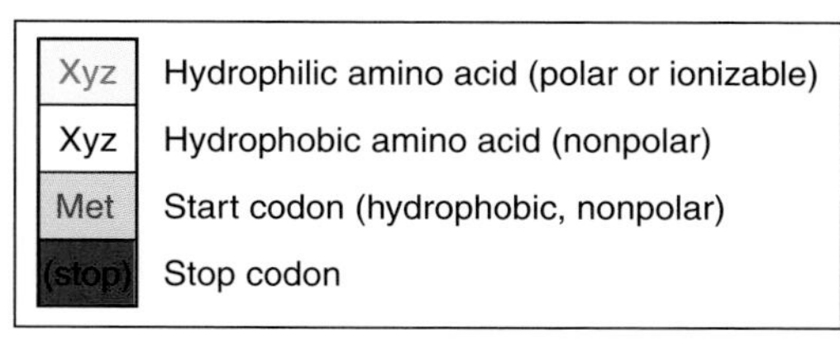

FIGURE 7-6 The genetic code. The first graphic "phrasebook" or "decoder" of the genetic language of the cell was developed in 1966 to summarize the amino acids encoded by various codons (three-base sequences of nucleotides) in RNA. To read this more recent decoder adapted for human biology, start with any codon (for example, CGA). Find the first base along the top of the decoder to find the correct box to use (C is the third box). The second base is found in each row of that box, labelled on the left (G is the first row). Then use the third base to find the correct column, labelled at the bottom of each box (A is the second column, showing that arginine [Arg] is the amino acid encoded by CGA; the bluish colour tells us that arginine is a hydrophilic amino acid). •AGG, AGA act as stop codons in mitochondria. ○AUA codes for methionine (Met) in mitochondria. *UGA, a stop codon, instead encodes selenocysteine (Sec) in the cytoplasm when a certain pattern appears in the surrounding codons; in mitochondria UGA instead encodes tryptophan.

Post-Translation Processing

As specific polypeptides are formed, chaperone proteins and other enzymes in the endoplasmic reticulum (ER), Golgi apparatus, or cytosol assist them in folding and linking to form secondary, tertiary, and perhaps quaternary protein molecules (see **Figure 5-8**). In some polypeptides, enzymes remove or insert additional amino acids or other chemical groups. Enzymes may also catalyze the formation of hybrid molecules such as lipoproteins or glycoproteins.

If any of the proteins formed during this process fail to fold or are misfolded, they will not function properly. Chaperone molecules may be able to refold them into the proper shape. But if not, then the cell risks serious problems. Recall from Chapter 5 that proteasomes break down unfolded and misfolded proteins, allowing the cell to recycle the amino acids and "start over again" (see **Figure 5-10**, p. 85). If this "quality control" program fails to take care of all the defective proteins, they may clump together and form dense masses called *plaques* that could damage or kill the cell. Several degenerative diseases such as Alzheimer disease (AD) and Parkinson disease (PD) involve such a mechanism.

Protein anabolism is one of the major kinds of cellular work. One human cell is estimated to synthesize thousands of different enzymes! In addition to this staggering workload, the cell produces many different protein compounds that help form its own structures, and many cells also synthesize special functional proteins for use in other parts of the body. Liver cells are an example; they synthesize proteins such as prothrombin, fibrinogen, albumin, and globulin for blood plasma.

The complete set of proteins synthesized by a cell is called the **proteome** of the cell. The human proteome is the complete set of proteins synthesized by all the cells of the human body. The human proteome is much larger than the human genome (entire set of genes). How can that be, if genes are codes for the polypeptides that make up proteins? It is because each polypeptide may be used in a variety of different combinations with other polypeptides, enabling the production of a huge variety of different proteins.

For your convenience, **Table 7-2** gives a detailed, step-by-step outline of this important process of protein synthesis.

TABLE 7-2 Summary of Protein Synthesis

STEP	LOCATION IN THE CELL	DESCRIPTION
Transcription		
1	Nucleus	One region, or gene, of a DNA molecule "unzips" to expose its bases
2	Nucleus	According to the principles of complementary base pairing, RNA nucleotides already present in the nucleoplasm temporarily attach themselves to the exposed bases along one side of the DNA molecule
3	Nucleus	As RNA nucleotides align themselves along the DNA strand, they bind to each other and thus form a chainlike strand called *messenger RNA* (mRNA); this binding of RNA nucleotides is controlled by the enzyme RNA polymerase
Preparation of mRNA		
4	Nucleus	As the preliminary mRNA strand is formed, it peels away from the DNA strand This mRNA strand is a copy, or *transcript,* of a gene
5	Nucleus	The spliceosome edits the mRNA molecule by removing noncoding portions of the strand (introns) and splicing the remaining pieces (exons)
6	Nuclear pores	The edited mRNA strand is transported out of the nucleus through pores in the nuclear envelope
Translation		
7	Cytoplasm	Two subunits sandwich the end of the mRNA molecule to form a ribosome
8	Cytoplasm	Specific transfer RNA (tRNA) molecules bring specific amino acids into place at the ribosome, which acts as a sort of "holder" for the mRNA strand and tRNA molecules The kind of tRNA (and thus the kind of amino acid) that moves into position is determined by complementary base pairing: each mRNA codon exposed at the ribosome site will permit only a tRNA with a complementary *anticodon* to attach
9	Cytoplasm	As each amino acid is brought into place at the ribosome, an enzyme in the ribosome binds it to the amino acid that arrived just before it The chemical bonds formed, called *peptide bonds,* link the amino acids together to form a long chain called a *polypeptide*
10	Cytoplasm	As the ribosome moves along the mRNA strand, more and more amino acids are added to the growing polypeptide chain in the sequence dictated by the mRNA codons (each codon represents a specific amino acid to be placed in the polypeptide chain) When the ribosome reaches the end of the mRNA molecule, it drops off the end and separates into large and small subunits again; often, enzymes later link two or more polypeptides together to form a whole protein molecule

Quick CHECK

1. How does DNA act as a "master molecule" of a cell?
2. Where in the cell does transcription occur? Editing (splicing)? Translation?
3. What determines the primary sequence in which amino acids are assembled to form a specific polypeptide?

Cell Growth

As stated earlier, one of the two major phases of the cell life cycle is the growth phase (**Figure 7-7** and **Table 7-3**). It is during this phase that a newly formed cell produces new molecules, from which it constructs the additional cell membrane, cell fibres, and other structures necessary for growth. And as just stated, all the structural proteins, plus the enzymes needed to make lipids, carbohydrates, and other substances, are made by the cell with information contained in the genes of DNA molecules. First, we will review a simplified account of how these proteins are made and how additional organelles are produced. Later, we explore how the cell replicates its DNA molecules in anticipation of reproduction.

Production of Cytoplasm

As a cell grows, it must produce additional cytoplasm and the plasma membrane necessary to contain it. One mechanism by which additional cytoplasm is produced is protein synthesis. Recall from the

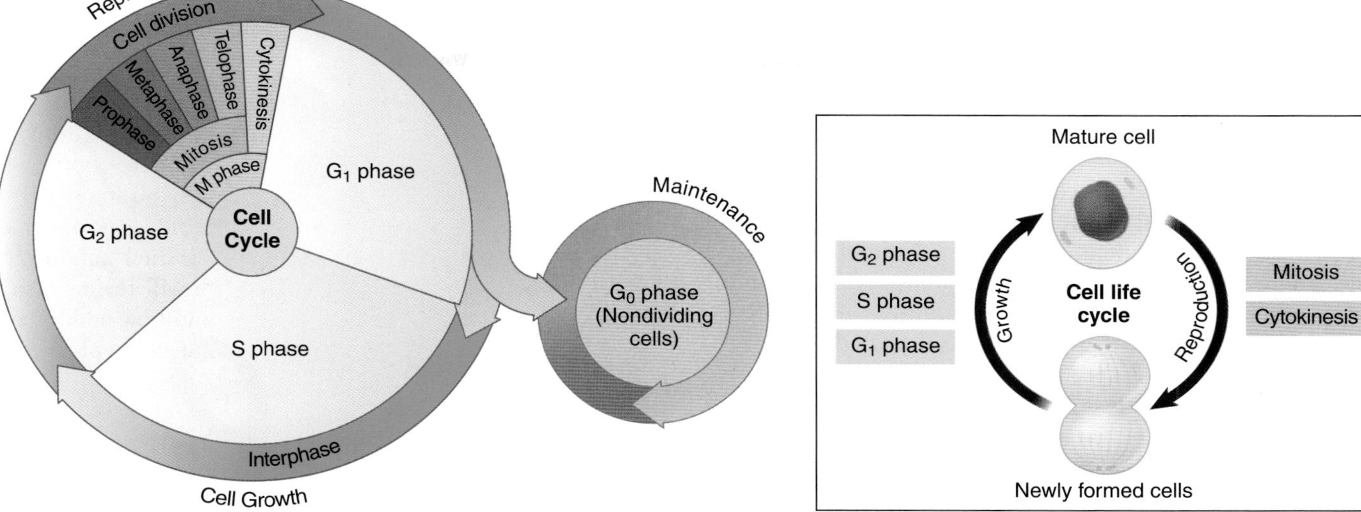

FIGURE 7-7 Life cycle of the cell. The processes of growth and reproduction of successive generations of cells exhibit a cyclic pattern. Newly formed cells grow to maturity by synthesizing new molecules and organelles (*G_1* and *G_2 phases*), including the replication of an extra set of DNA molecules (*S phase*) in anticipation of reproduction. Mature cells reproduce (*M phase*) by first distributing the two identical sets of DNA (produced during the S phase) in the orderly process of mitosis, then by splitting the plasma membrane, cytoplasm, and organelles of the parent cell into two distinct daughter cells (cytokinesis). Daughter cells that do not go on to reproduce are in a maintenance phase (*G_0*).

previous section that protein synthesis is an anabolic process, which means that small molecules are joined together to form large molecules. Amino acids are strung together in a specific sequence to form polypeptide chains. Two or more folded polypeptide chains may then be linked to form larger, more complex protein molecules. In the previous paragraphs, we briefly described how the cell "copies" information from genes and interprets it to form specific polypeptides. Refer again to **Table 7-2** to review the process of protein synthesis.

Production of additional proteins means not only that more structural proteins are available to contribute to growth of the cytoplasm but also that more enzymes are available to catalyze the production of other organic compounds. Enzymes produced by protein synthesis are used to make additional carbohydrates, lipids, and nucleic acids—as well as more protein molecules.

Products of cell anabolism during the growth phase of the cell life cycle may be used in the production of additional organelles and plasma membrane. This is a good opportunity to go back to Chapter 5 and review the process by which the cell membrane—and thus membranous organelles and plasma membrane—is made by the ER and Golgi apparatus.

TABLE 7-3 Summary of the Cell Life Cycle

PHASE OF CELL LIFE CYCLE	DESCRIPTION
Cell Growth	***Interphase***
Protein synthesis	Proteins are manufactured according to the cell's genetic code; functional proteins, the enzymes, direct the synthesis of other molecules in the cells and thus the production of more and larger organelles and plasma membrane; sometimes called the *first growth phase* or *G_1 phase* of interphase
DNA replication	Nucleotides, influenced by newly synthesized enzymes, arrange themselves along the open sides of an "unzippered" DNA molecule, thereby creating two identical daughter DNA molecules; produces two identical sets of the cell's genetic code, which enables the cell to later split into two different cells, each with its own complete set of DNA; sometimes called the *(DNA) synthesis* stage or *S phase* of interphase
Protein synthesis	After DNA is replicated, the cell continues to grow by means of protein synthesis and the resulting synthesis of other molecules and various organelles; this *second growth phase* is also called the *G_2 phase*
Cell Reproduction	***M Phase***
Mitosis or meiosis	The parent cell's replicated set of DNA is divided into two sets and separated by an orderly process into distinct cell nuclei; mitosis is subdivided into at least four phases: *prophase, metaphase, anaphase,* and *telophase*
Cytokinesis	The plasma membrane of the parent cell "pinches in" and eventually separates the cytoplasm and two daughter nuclei into two genetically identical daughter cells

Most of the membranous organelles and plasma membrane increase in size or number (or both) by the membrane-producing processes referred to in Chapter 5. One notable exception is the mitochondrion. Each mitochondrion is capable of replicating itself in a process similar to that used by some one-celled organisms such as bacteria. Mitochondria often replicate themselves during the cell growth phase so that their total number is very large by the time the cell is ready to reproduce. Nonmembranous organelles grow by anabolic processes associated with the centrosome, or microtubule-organizing centre, and other cell components, such as ribosomes, that manufacture elements of the cytoskeleton.

DNA Replication

As a cell becomes larger, mechanisms that are just now beginning to be understood trigger the synthesis of a complete copy of the nucleus's set of DNA molecules. Replication of the entire set of DNA molecules, or genome, prepares the cell for reproduction, when one set will go to one daughter cell and the other set to the other daughter cell. The mechanics of DNA replication resemble those of RNA synthesis—as we shall see.

In the first step of DNA replication, the tightly coiled DNA molecules uncoil except for small segments. (Because these remaining tight little coils are denser than the thin, elongated sections, they absorb more stain and appear as chromatin granules under the microscope. The thin, uncoiled sections, in contrast, are invisible because they absorb so little stain.) As the DNA molecule uncoils, its two strands come apart. Then, along each of the two separated strands of nucleotides, a complementary strand forms. Intracellular fluid contains many DNA nucleotides. By the mechanism of obligatory base pairing and with the work of specific enzymes, nucleotides become attached at their correct places along each DNA strand (**Figure 7-8**). This means that new thymine—that is, from the intracellular fluid—attaches to the "old" adenine in the original DNA strand. Conversely, new adenine attaches to old thymine. Also, new guanine joins old cytosine, and new cytosine joins old guanine.

Note in **Figure 7-8** that the DNA nucleotides are added in different directions in each of the two strands of the mother DNA molecule. This results in the end of one mother strand not being copied. The loss of useful code is prevented by the presence of **telomeres** (literally, "end roots"), which are strands of "extra" nucleotides that can be lost without affecting the coding part of the chromosome. As telomeres shorten, they eventually disappear unless rebuilt by the enzyme *telomerase*. Telomerase contains a bit of RNA that provides the code for rebuilding the telomere sequence.

By the end of this part of the growth phase, each of the two DNA strands of the original DNA molecule has a complete new complementary strand attached to it. Each half of the DNA molecule, or strand, in other words, has duplicated itself to create a whole new DNA molecule. Thus two new chromosomes now replace each original chromosome. However, at this stage (before cell reproduction has actually begun), each daughter chromosome is called a *chromatid* instead of a chromosome. The two chromatids formed from each original chromosome contain duplicate copies of DNA and, therefore, the same genes as the chromosome from which they were formed. Chromatids are present as attached pairs. Their point of attachment is called the *centromere*. **Table 7-4** gives a detailed, step-by-step account of the process of DNA replication.

Because DNA replication is really the synthesis of new DNA, this part of a cell's growth phase is sometimes called the *synthesis phase* or, simply, the *S phase*. The portions of the growth phase before and after the S phase are simply called the *first growth* (G_1) *phase* and the *second growth* (G_2) *phase*. The first and second growth phases are characterized by a great deal of cytoplasm growth caused by a general increase in the anabolism of protein and other substances, as well as the production of new organelles and plasma membrane. The growth phases are also called *gap phases* because they represent a gap between major reproductive events.

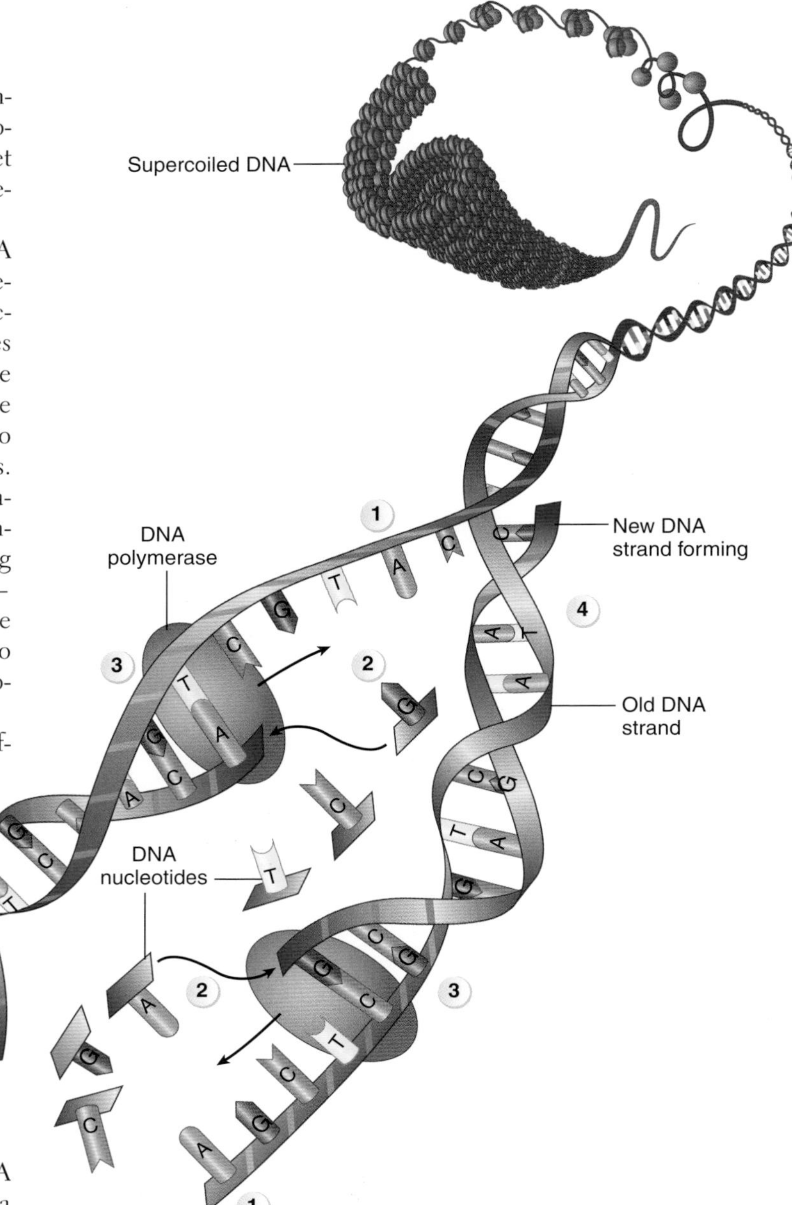

FIGURE 7-8 DNA replication When a DNA molecule makes a copy of itself, it "unzips" to expose its nucleotide bases. Through the mechanism of obligatory base pairing, coordinated by the enzyme DNA polymerase, new DNA nucleotides bind to the exposed bases (in an opposite direction on each strand). This forms a new "other half" to each half of the original molecule. After all the bases have new nucleotides bound to them, two identical DNA molecules will be ready for distribution to the two daughter cells. Numbers refer to steps described in **Table 7-4**.

CELL REPRODUCTION

Now that we have briefly looked at the growth phase, it is time to turn to the other major phase of the cell life cycle: cell reproduction (sometimes called the *M phase*). Simply put, cells reproduce by splitting themselves into two separate cells. One *parent cell* thus becomes two smaller *daughter cells*.

Splitting of the plasma membrane and cytoplasm into two is called **cytokinesis** (meaning "cell movement"). This name is apt because the cell's cytoskeleton moves the plasma membrane and

TABLE 7-4 Summary of DNA Replication*

STEP	DESCRIPTION
1	DNA molecules uncoil and "unzip" to expose their bases
2	Nucleotides already present in the intracellular fluid of the nucleus attach to the exposed bases according to the principle of obligatory base pairing
3	As nucleotides attach to complementary bases along each DNA strand, the enzyme *DNA polymerase* causes them to bind to each other
4	As new nucleotides fill in the spaces left open on each DNA strand, two identical *daughter molecules* are formed; as the parent DNA molecule completely unzips, the two daughter molecules coil to become distinct, but genetically identical, DNA double helices called *chromatids*

*These steps are illustrated in **Figure 7-8**.

internal structures in a way that pinches it in half, thereby forming two equivalent daughter cells.

Of course, each daughter cell must possess all the resources necessary for survival if the cycle of life is to remain unbroken. That means that besides sufficient cytoplasm, including mitochondria and other organelles, each cell must also have a complete set of genetic information (DNA) needed to run a cell properly. This aspect of cell reproduction or *cell division* is accomplished by a process called **mitosis.** During mitosis, the cell organizes replicated DNA into two identical sets and then distributes one complete set to each daughter cell.

MITOSIS

Mitosis, the process of organizing and distributing nuclear DNA during cell division, is a continuous process (**Table 7-5**) consisting of four distinct phases:

1. Prophase
2. Metaphase
3. Anaphase
4. Telophase

When the cell is not experiencing mitosis—during the growth phase between cell divisions—it is said to be in **interphase** (meaning "between phase"). A cell is not actively reproducing during interphase, but it is actively *preparing for* reproduction. Not just the DNA molecules replicate; the centrosomes replicate as well. The centriole pairs in the parent centrosome split, and each single centriole produces a daughter centriole to produce a new pair of centrioles surrounded by a starlike formation of microtubules called an *aster* radiating outward. Go back to p. 90 and look at **Figure 5-16** to review the details of centrosome structure. Additional cytoplasm, membrane, and other cell structures are likewise being constructed in anticipation of cell division.

Prophase

The cell enters **prophase** when it begins to divide, usually before cytokinesis, or "pinching in half," becomes apparent. During prophase, which literally means "before phase", the nuclear envelope falls apart as the paired chromatids coil up to form dense, compact *chromosomes* (**Figure 7-9**). By the end of prophase, each chromosome consists of a pair of short, thick bodies joined together at a

TABLE 7-5 The Major Events of Mitosis

PROPHASE	METAPHASE	ANAPHASE	TELOPHASE
1. Chromosomes shorten and thicken (from coiling of the DNA molecules that compose them); each chromosome consists of two chromatids attached at the centromere	1. Chromosomes align across the equator of the spindle fibre at its centromere	1. Each centromere splits, thereby detaching two chromatids that compose each chromosome from each other, elongating in the process (DNA molecules start uncoiling)	1. Changes occurring during telophase essentially reverse those taking place during prophase; new chromosomes start elongating (DNA molecules start uncoiling)
2. Centrosomes move to opposite poles of the cell; spindle fibres appear and begin to orient between opposing poles		2. Sister chromatids (now called *chromosomes*) move to opposite poles; there are now twice as many chromosomes as there were before mitosis started	2. A nuclear envelope forms again to enclose each new set of chromosomes
3. Nucleoli and the nuclear membrane disappear			3. Spindle fibres disappear

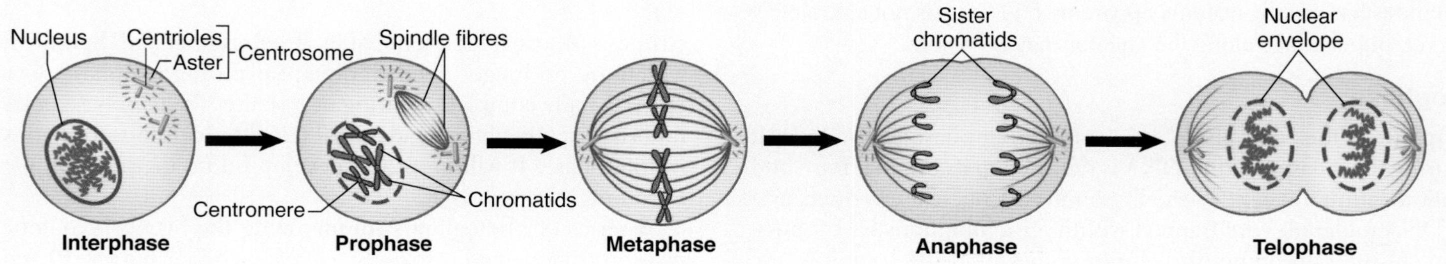

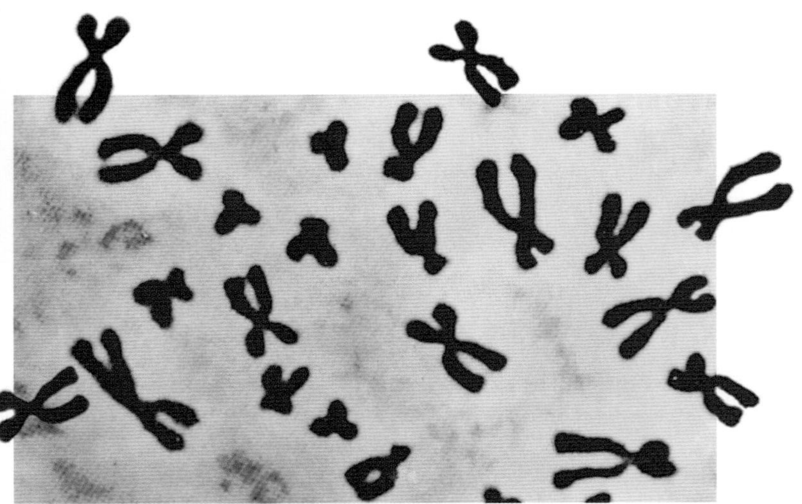

FIGURE 7-9 Chromosomes. Light micrograph showing chromosomes of a normal human cell before cell division is complete (metaphase). Additional detailed views of chromosome structure are found in Chapter 48.

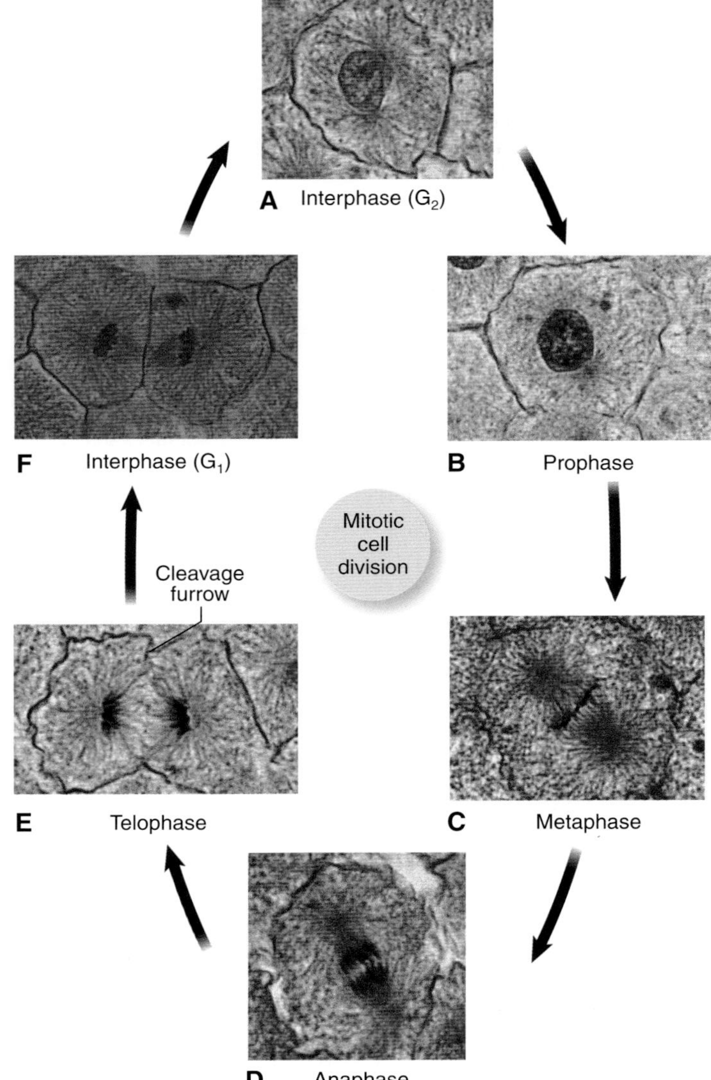

FIGURE 7-10 Mitotic cell division. Series of photomicrographs showing animal cells undergoing a cycle of mitotic cell division. **A,** Interphase—division begins at the end of interphase (G_2), after the cell has already replicated the DNA in its nucleus and increased its cytoplasm sufficiently for division. **B,** Prophase—chromosomes form from the nuclear chromatin material as the nuclear envelope disappears. **C,** Metaphase—chromosomes line up along the cell's equatorial plate, with spindle fibres distinctly visible on either side. **D,** Anaphase—spindle fibres pull each of the two chromatids (now called chromosomes) toward opposite poles of the cell. **E,** Telophase—chromosomes are now at opposite poles, nuclear envelopes begin forming around each group, and the cleavage furrow of cytokinesis becomes apparent. **F,** Interphase—after mitosis and cytokinesis are complete, the two daughter cells begin the first growth (G_1) of interphase. When they are ready, each daughter cell may continue the life cycle by undergoing mitotic division.

centromere. At the same time that chromosomes are forming, the replicated centrosomes move away from each other and toward opposite ends, or "poles", of the parent cell. As the centrosomes move apart, a parallel arrangement of microtubules, or *spindle fibres*, is constructed between them. Aster fibres radiating from each centrosome anchor the spindle at each pole of the cell.

Metaphase

The term **metaphase** literally means "position-changing phase" or "in-the-middle phase". This name is appropriate because during this phase the chromosomes, no longer trapped within a nucleus, are moved by the cytoskeleton into an orderly pattern. The chromosomes are aligned along a plane at the "equator" of the cell about midway between the centriole pairs at opposite poles of the cell (the *equatorial plate*). One chromatid of each chromosome faces one pole of the cell, and its identical sister chromatid faces the opposite pole. Each chromatid then attaches to a spindle fibre.

Anaphase

Anaphase, or the "apart phase", begins as soon as all the chromosomes have aligned along the cell's equator. During this phase of mitosis, the centromere of each chromosome splits to form two chromosomes, each consisting of a single DNA molecule. Each chromosome is pulled toward the nearest pole (i.e., toward the nearest centrosome) by a spindle fibre. The effect of this movement is that one set of DNA molecules reaches one end of the cell and another set reaches the other end of the cell—forming two separate but identical pools of genetic information. By the time a dividing cell has reached anaphase, cytokinesis has usually become apparent. The cell has not completely split yet, but cleavage along the equator may be visible.

Telophase

Telophase is the "end phase", or "completion phase", of mitosis. It is during this phase that the DNA is returned to its original form and location within the cell. The cell rebuilds the nuclear envelope, and the DNA molecules are trapped within a membranous basket once again. At the same time, the chromosomes elongate back into the chromatin form. Recall that DNA cannot participate in protein synthesis unless at least some of its length is uncoiled. Spindle fibres, which are no longer needed, disappear during telophase. Cytokinesis is usually completed during or just after the telophase portion of mitosis. Each genetically identical daughter cell thus formed is now in interphase. It will grow and develop into a mature cell, perhaps becoming a parent itself.

A series of photographs summarizing the events of mitotic cell division (mitosis and cytokinesis) are shown in **Figure 7-10** and Figure 5-2 of the Brief Atlas of the Human Body.

CONNECT IT! 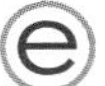

See an image of how chromosomes unwind during telophase to form specific areas of chromatin called *chromosome territories* in ***Chromosome Territories*** online at ***Connect It!***

MEIOSIS

Meiosis is the type of cell division that occurs only in primitive sex cells during the process of becoming mature sex cells. As a result of meiosis, the primitive sex cells (*spermatogonia* in the male and *oogonia* in the female) become mature sex cells called **gametes.** Male gametes are named *spermatozoa* but usually are called *sperm.* Female gametes are named *ova* (singular, *ovum*). In humans, all somatic cells contain 46 chromosomes. This total of 46 chromosomes per cell is known as the **diploid** number of chromosomes. *Diploid* comes from the Greek *diploos,* meaning "two" or "pair". In somatic cells the 46 chromosomes are present in 22 homologous pairs—the remaining 2 being the sex chromosomes XY (male) or XX (female). During meiosis, or *reduction division,* the diploid chromosome number (46) of the primitive spermatogonium or oogonium is reduced to the **haploid** number of 23 found in mature sex cells, or gametes. **Figure 7-11** shows that meiotic division occurs in two steps: *meiosis I,* during which the number of chromosomes is halved but the chromatid pairs remain together, and *meiosis II,* during which the chromatids finally split apart.

The end result of fertilization is the fusion of two gametes, each containing the haploid number (23) of chromosomes. Fertilization results in formation of a zygote, which is a diploid cell having 46 chromosomes, 23 chromosomes being contributed by each parent. The zygote is the first cell of the human offspring. It will then undergo mitotic division to form 2 cells, then 4, and so on until 37 trillion cells are eventually formed.

During development, the new daughter cells will specialize, or **differentiate,** to become specific cell types, which in turn will form specific organs. In mature tissues, some cells may opt out of the cycle and remain in a growth and maintenance phase called the G_0 *phase.* We will have a little more to say about the development and maintenance of different tissue types in Chapters 8 and 9. More detailed information about meiosis and the formation of sex cells, fertilization, and development is explored in Chapters 45 through 48.

REGULATING THE CELL LIFE CYCLE

Table 7-3 summarizes the main phases of the cell life cycle, including the growth and reproductive phases. You may wonder what mechanisms control when and how a cell moves from one stage to another in its cycle of growth and reproduction. Experiments in the late twentieth century revealed the activity of regulatory proteins known as **cyclins** and **cyclin-dependent kinases (CDKs)** and the genes that produce them. The number of CDK enzyme molecules stays about the same throughout the cell's life cycle, but the number of cyclin molecules varies widely. A variety of factors cause cyclin levels to increase over time, until the numbers are sufficient to trigger the CDK enzymes to get to work to drive the cell cycle forward.

Cells also regulate the cell life cycle through *tumour suppressor genes,* such as the *p53* gene, that trigger inhibition of the cell cycle. This allows cell division to slow or stop when cells become crowded, for example. In many cancers, the *p53* gene is abnormal and therefore allows cells to continue to grow beyond their normal boundaries (**Box 7-2**).

Diploid parent cell
(46 chromosomes)
Mitosis
Primary sex cells
(DNA replicated
before division)
Meiosis I
Secondary sex cells
(DNA not replicated
before division)
Meiosis II
Haploid gametes
(23 chromosomes)

FIGURE 7-11 Meiosis. Meiotic cell division takes place in two steps: meiosis I and meiosis II. Meiosis I is called *reduction division* because the number of chromosomes is reduced by half (from the diploid number to the haploid number). A more detailed diagram of meiosis is presented in **Figure 47-1** on p. 1092.

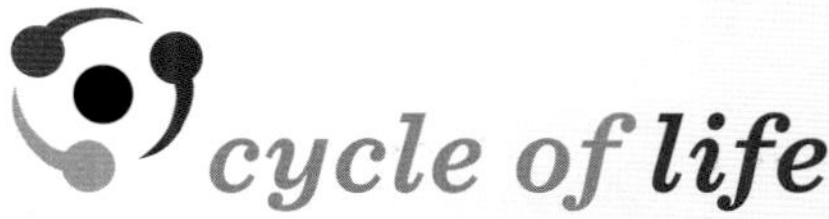

cycle of life

Cells Different types of cells have highly variable life cycles. The active life span of a single cell may vary from a few minutes to years, depending on its function and level of activity. Some cells may remain dormant or inactive for years. Then, when they are "activated" by some biological need and become functional, their life span may be shortened dramatically.

One example involves cells in the immune system that are programmed to produce antibodies against a specific disease. Other examples include the female sex cells, or ova, which are present from birth. They mature throughout the reproductive life span of the individual so that each month at least one cell will become fully developed and provide an opportunity for fertilization to occur.

Structure follows function at every level of organization in the body. Often, function decreases with advancing age, and resulting changes occur in cell numbers and their ability to function effectively. As a result, we lose functional capacity in every body organ system. Our muscles may atrophy, the skin will lose its elasticity, and our respiratory, cardiovascular, and skeletal systems will become affected because of cellular changes that accompany ageing. •

BOX 7-2 *changes in cell growth, reproduction, and survival*

Cells have the ability to adapt to changing conditions. Cells may alter their size, reproductive rate, or other characteristics to adapt to changes in the internal environment. Such adaptations usually allow cells to work more efficiently. However, sometimes cells alter their characteristics abnormally—thereby decreasing their efficiency and threatening the health of the body. Common types of changes in cell growth and reproduction are summarized here.

Cells may respond to changes in function, hormone signals, or the availability of nutrients by increasing or decreasing in size. The term **hypertrophy** refers to an increase in cell size, and the term **atrophy** refers to a decrease in cell size.

Either type of adaptive change can occur easily in muscle tissue. When a person continually uses muscle cells to pull against heavy resistance, as in weight training, for example, the cells respond by increasing in size. Body builders thus increase the size of their muscles by hypertrophy—increasing the size of muscle cells. Atrophy often occurs in underused muscle cells. For example, when a broken arm is immobilized in a cast for a long period, muscles that move the arm often atrophy. Because the muscles are temporarily out of use, muscle cells decrease in size. Atrophy may also occur in tissues whose nutrient or oxygen supply is diminished.

Sometimes cells respond to changes in the internal environment by increasing their rate of reproduction—a process called **hyperplasia**. The ending *-plasia* comes from a Greek word that means "formation"—referring to the formation of new cells. Because *hyper-* means "excessive", *hyperplasia* means excessive cell reproduction. Like hypertrophy, hyperplasia causes an increase in the size of a tissue or organ. However, hyperplasia is an increase in the *number of cells* rather than an increase in the size of each cell. A common example of hyperplasia occurs in the milk-producing glands of the female breast during pregnancy. In response to hormone signals, the glandular cells reproduce rapidly to prepare the breast for milk production and nursing.

If the body loses its ability to control mitosis normally, abnormal hyperplasia may occur. Sometimes, this results from a failure to properly regulate the rate of the cell cycle. For example, abnormalities of *tumour suppressor* mechanisms governed by the *p53* gene can permit cell division beyond normal limits. The new mass of cells thus formed is a tumour, or **neoplasm.** Neoplasms may be relatively harmless growths called **benign** tumours. If tumour cells can break away and travel through the blood or lymphatic vessels to other parts of the body, the neoplasm is a **malignant tumour,** or cancer. Cells in malignant neoplasms often exhibit a characteristic called **anaplasia.** Anaplasia is a condition in which cells fail to *differentiate* into a specialized cell type. **Dysplasia** is an abnormal change in shape, size, or organization of cells in a tissue and is often associated with neoplasms.

Part *A* of the figure summarizes a few of the changes that can occur in cell growth and reproduction.

Cells also die sometimes. In **necrosis,** cells die because of an injury or pathological condition, often causing nearby cells to die and triggering an immune response called *inflammation,* which removes the debris if possible.

Nonpathological cell death, often called **apoptosis,** occurs frequently in the cells of your body. Apoptosis is a type of programmed cell death in which organized biochemical steps within the cell lead to fragmentation of the cell and removal of the pieces by phagocytic cells. Apoptosis occurs when cells are no longer needed or when they have certain malfunctions that could lead to cancer or some other potential problem. Apoptosis is the normal process by which our tissues and other groups of cells remodel themselves throughout the life span. Although apoptosis is a normal cell function, it can be abnormally triggered in some conditions. •

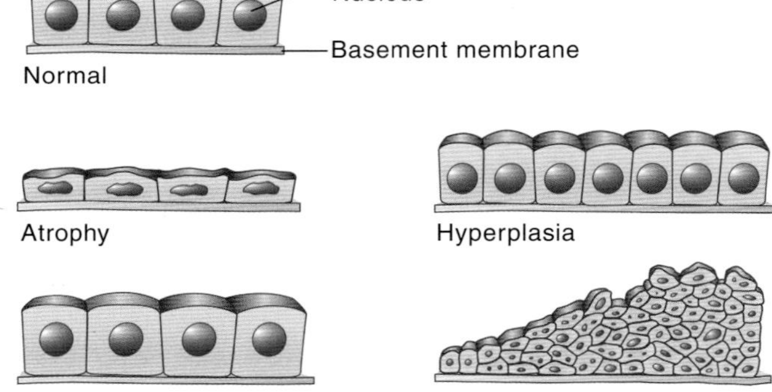

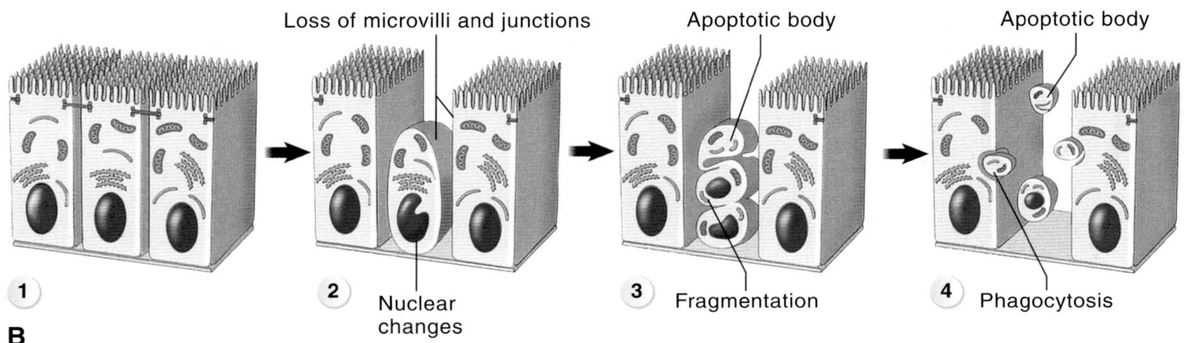

A, Alterations in cell growth and reproduction. **B,** Apoptosis. *1,* Early in apoptosis, the cell begins making the enzymes needed to break down the cell, but no structural changes yet occur. *2,* As apoptosis proceeds, surface features such as microvilli and cell junctions are lost, and nuclear DNA condenses and is broken into fragments. *3,* The cell then rapidly splits into apoptotic bodies. Note that the nucleus has also fragmented. *4,* Apoptotic bodies may then be digested by adjacent cells, by extracellular enzymes, or (not shown) by nearby phagocytic cells.

Scientists often compare the CDK molecules with an engine that drives the cell forward through the phases of its life cycle. Cyclins act like a gear box that "shifts" the CDK into "drive" and thus moves the cell into the reproductive phase of the cycle. Suppressor mechanisms such as those regulated by the *p53* gene act as "brakes" that slow or stop cell division at appropriate times.

The molecular mechanisms that interact to regulate the cell life cycle are complex and not yet completely understood. Discoveries about how these molecules and their genes work continue to help us better understand the mechanisms of cancer and other cellular disorders.

Quick CHECK

4. What are the two major phases of the cell life cycle? During which of these phases does mitosis occur?
5. How does the cytoplasm of a cell grow?
6. What is the difference between mitotic cell division and meiotic cell division?

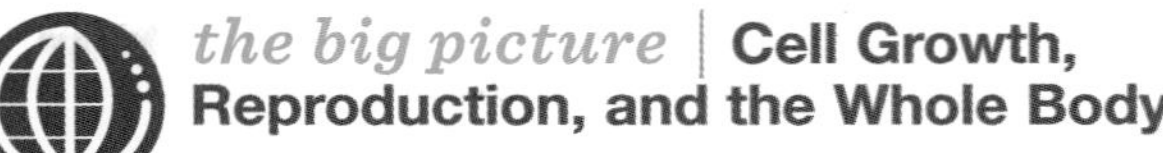

the big picture | Cell Growth, Reproduction, and the Whole Body

In previous chapters, we considered the cell as a whole living unit in which many dynamic processes keep an individual cell alive and functioning. Let's take another step back from our mental image of a cell. Picture a huge "society" of trillions of cells—the human body. We now understand more fully how we develop from a single cell to that huge society of cells. We have seen that the growth of cytoplasm, the accurate replication of the genetic code, and cell division are all necessary to the growth and maintenance of the entire human body.

Looking back on the last few chapters, we can now better appreciate that each cell contributes to the survival of its society (the body)—and itself—by specializing in functions that help maintain the relative constancy of the internal environment. When we think of that relative constancy, homeostasis, we should appreciate that it is all accomplished by the action of many individual cells. How are individual cells grouped together? How do they function as groups to promote homeostasis? These questions are answered, at least in part, in Chapters 8 and 9.

mechanisms of disease
Cell Growth and Reproduction Disorders

Disorders Involving DNA and Protein Synthesis

Genetic disorders are pathological conditions caused by mistakes, or **mutations,** in a cell's genetic code. Abnormal genes cause the production of abnormal enzymes or other proteins. Abnormal proteins, in turn, cause abnormalities in cellular function—producing a specific disease. Many diseases are known to be caused by this mechanism, including some diseases such as infections or cancer that also involve other pathological mechanisms. Another example is **sickle cell anaemia,** a blood disease caused by the production of abnormal haemoglobin (the protein in red blood cells that carries oxygen). Mistakes in enzyme production can cause a whole group of metabolic disorders called **inborn errors of metabolism.**

Disorders Involving Cell Reproduction

As mentioned earlier in this chapter (see p. 131), abnormalities in mitotic division can cause tumours to arise. **Cancers** are tumours that tend to spread, often disrupting vital functions and eventually killing those with the disease. Even noncancerous tumours can cause significant health impairment—or death—depending on their size and location.

Infections

Bacteria and viruses can infect cells and thus damage them in ways that produce disease. Bacteria, tiny one-celled organisms, may parasitize cells directly and thus destroy them by stealing the cells' proteins and other substances needed for cell survival. The bacteria may produce toxins that damage cells or interrupt cell functions. These toxins may also elicit violent reactions of the immune system. Viruses are microscopic particles that contain DNA or RNA. Viruses cause disease by taking over the genetic apparatus of a cell to force a cell to produce viral DNA or RNA and synthesize viral proteins. Thus viral infections use the cell's resources to produce viral products—or even new viruses. If enough cells are damaged during a bacterial or viral infection to disrupt vital functions, death may result (**Figure 7-12**).

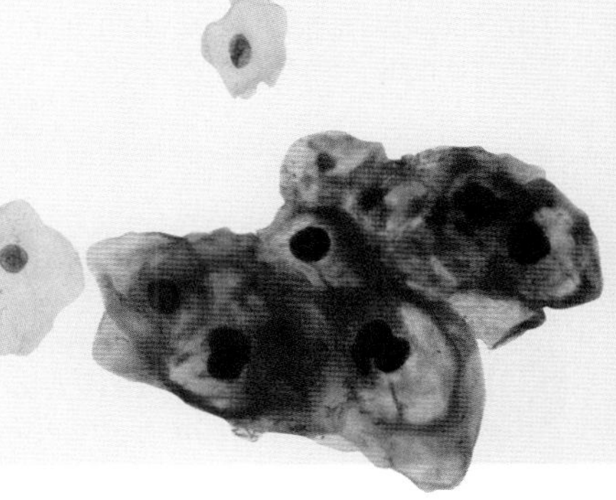

FIGURE 7-12 Viral infection. The pink cells have been infected by human papillomavirus (HPV) and show abnormal structure that is quite different than normal cells (blue).

LANGUAGE OF SCIENCE *(continued from p. 120)*

prophase (PRO-fayz)
[*pro-* **first,** *-phase* **stage**]

proteome (PRO-tee-ome)
[*prote-* **protein,** *-ome* **body (whole set)**]

RNA interference (RNAi)

spliceosome (SPLISE-oh-sohm)
[*splice-* **cut rope and join remaining ends,** *-som-* **body**]

telomere (TEL-oh-meer)
[*telo-* **end,** *-mer-* **root**]

telophase (TEL-oh-fayz)
[*telo-* **end,** *-phase* **stage**]

transcription (tran-SKRIP-shun)
[*trans-* **across,** *-script-* **write,** *-tion* **process**]

translation (tranz-LAY-shun)
[*translat-* **bring across,** *-tion* **process**]

LANGUAGE OF MEDICINE

anaplasia (an-ah-PLAY-zha)
[*ana-* **without,** *-plas(m)-* **substance or form,** *-ia* **condition**]

atrophy (AT-ro-fee)
[*a-* **without,** *-trophy* **nourishment,** *-y* **state**]

benign (be-NYNE)
[*benign* **kind**]

dysplasia (diss-PLAY-zha)
[*dys-* **disordered,** *-plas(m)-* **substance or form,** *-ia* **condition**]

hyperplasia (hye-per-PLAY-zha)
[*hyper-* **excessive,** *-plas(m)-* **substance or form,** *-ia* **condition**]

hypertrophy (hye-PER-tro-fee)
[*hyper-* **excessive,** *-troph-* **nourishment,** *-y* **state**]

malignant tumour
(mah-LIG-nant TYOO-mer)
[*malign* **bad,** *-ant* **state;** *tumour* **swelling**]

mutation (myoo-TAY-shun)
[*mutat-* **change,** *-tion* **state**]

necrosis (ne-KROH-sis)
[*necro-* **death,** *-osis* **condition**]

neoplasm (NEE-o-plazm)
[*neo-* **new,** *-plasm* **tissue or substance**]

sickle cell anaemia
(SIK-ul sell ah-NEE-mee-ah)
[*sickle* **crescent;** *cell* **storeroom;** *an-* **without,** *-aem-* **blood,** *-ia* **condition**]

case study

Catherine had been experiencing abdominal pain. She was referred by her GP to a consultant in gynaecological oncology. Following physical examination and an ultrasound scan, the consultant informed Catherine that she had a mass on her left ovary. After further tests, she was advised that her left ovary be surgically removed. Catherine was visibly upset, but the consultant assured her it was more likely to be a benign neoplasm and would not be as serious as she imagined.

1. Catherine's consultant explained that she had a neoplasm. What is a neoplasm?
   a. A neoplasm is a tumour that could be relatively harmless (benign)
   b. A neoplasm is a tumour that could be harmful (malignant)
   c. A neoplasm is composed of cells that increase in size, and therefore it is relatively harmless
   d. A neoplasm is an abnormal change in the shape of cells, and thus it is relatively harmless

2. The surgeon who removed the neoplasm noticed that some of the ovarian cells had undergone apoptosis. What is apoptosis?
   a. Apoptosis is when cells die as a result of an injury or pathological condition
   b. Apoptosis is normal cell death, and it occurs frequently in the cells of the body
   c. Apoptosis is an increase in the size of cells and may not have a pathological origin
   d. Apoptosis is an increase in the mass of cells, which is often a benign tumour

3. Had Catherine's surgeon found ovarian cells that exhibited a characteristic called anaplasia, he would treat her condition as a cancer. What is anaplasia?
   a. Anaplasia is a type of programmed cell death in which the cells have mutated and metastasized
   b. Anaplasia is a term that describes cells increasing their rate of reproduction and thus metastasizing throughout the body
   c. Anaplasia is a condition in which cells fail to differentiate into specialized cells, and this condition is often a characteristic of malignant neoplasms
   d. *Anaplasia* is a term that describes cells that decrease in size and thus fail to carry out normal functions

Hint To solve a case study, you may have to refer to the glossary or index, other chapters in this textbook, **Connect It!**, or other resources.

CHAPTER SUMMARY

To download an MP3 version of the chapter summary for use with your mobile device, access the **Audio Chapter Summaries** *online at evolve.elsevier.com.*

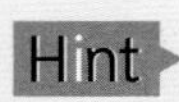

Scan this summary after reading the chapter to help you reinforce the key concepts. Later, use the summary as a review before your class or before a test.

Growth and Reproduction of Cells

A. Cell growth and reproduction of cells are the most fundamental of all living functions and together constitute the cell life cycle
   1. Cell growth—depends on using genetic information in DNA to make the structural and functional proteins needed for cell survival
   2. Cell reproduction—ensures that genetic information is passed from one generation to the next

Protein Synthesis

A. Protein synthesis is a central anabolic pathway in cells (**Table 7-2**)
B. Deoxyribonucleic acid (DNA)
   1. A double-helix polymer (composed of nucleotides) that functions to transfer information, encoded in genes, to direct the synthesis of proteins (**Figure 7-1**)
   2. Gene—a segment of a DNA molecule that consists of up to several thousand pairs of nucleotides and contains the code for synthesizing one RNA molecule, which then may be translated into one polypeptide (**Figure 7-2**)

C. Ribonucleic acid (RNA) (**Table 7-1**)
   1. Coding RNA—mRNA, which is a transcript of a code for one polypeptide
   2. Noncoding RNA—rRNA and tRNA, which are each copies of a DNA gene but regulate processes rather than code for a polypeptide
D. Transcription—mRNA forms along a segment of one strand of DNA (**Figure 7-3**); tRNA and rRNA are formed by a similar mechanism
E. Editing the transcript (**Figure 7-4**)
   1. Noncoding introns are removed and the remaining exons are spliced together to form the final, edited version of the mRNA copy of the DNA segment
   2. Spliceosomes are ribosome-sized structures in the nucleus that splice mRNA transcripts (**Box 7-1**)
F. Translation (**Figure 7-5**)
   1. After leaving the nucleus and being edited, mRNA associates with a ribosome in the cytoplasm
   2. tRNA molecules bring specific amino acids to the mRNA at the ribosome; the type of amino acid is determined by the fit of a specific tRNA's anticodon with mRNA's codon (**Figure 7-6**)
   3. As amino acids are brought into place, peptide bonds join them—eventually producing an entire polypeptide chain
   4. Translation of genes can be inhibited by RNA interference (RNAi), which protects the cell against viral infection
G. Post-translation processing
   1. Chaperone molecules and other enzymes in the cytosol, ER, and Golgi apparatus help fold polypeptides
   2. Polypeptides may combine into larger protein molecules or hybrid molecules
   3. Proteome
      a. All the proteins synthesized by a cell make up the cell's proteome
      b. All the proteins synthesized in the whole body is called the *human proteome*

Cell Growth

A. Newly formed cells produce a variety of molecules and other structures necessary for growth by using the information contained in the genes of DNA molecules; this stage is known as *interphase* (**Figure 7-7**)
B. Production of cytoplasm
   1. More cell material is made, a largely anabolic process
   2. Growth and/or replication of organelles and plasma membrane
   3. Replication of centrosomes and DNA in anticipation of cell division
C. DNA replication (**Table 7-4**)
   1. Replication of the genome prepares the cell for reproduction; the mechanics are similar to RNA synthesis
   2. DNA base pairing (**Figure 7-8**)
      a. The DNA strand uncoils and the strands come apart
      b. Along each separate strand, a complementary strand forms
         (1) Because the strands are rebuilt in opposite directions, one strand is not completely rebuilt
         (2) Telomeres are noncoding, protective segments of DNA at the ends of a chromosome; they are used up during DNA replication to prevent loss of needed DNA code; telomeres can be rebuilt by the enzyme telomerase
      c. The two new strands are called *chromatids* instead of chromosomes
      d. Chromatids are attached pairs; the point of attachment is called the centromere
D. The growth phase of the cell life cycle can be subdivided into the first growth phase (G_1), the [DNA] synthesis phase (S), and the second growth phase (G_2)

Cell Reproduction

A. Cells reproduce by splitting themselves into two smaller daughter cells (**Table 7-5**)
B. Mitotic cell division—the process of organizing and distributing nuclear DNA during cell division has four distinct phases (**Figure 7-10**)
   1. Prophase—"before phase"
      a. After the cell has prepared for reproduction during interphase, the nuclear envelope falls apart as the chromatids coil up to form chromosomes that are joined at the centromere (**Figure 7-9**)
      b. As chromosomes form, centrosomes (centrioles/aster) move away from each other toward the poles of the parent cell and spindle fibres are constructed between them
   2. Metaphase—"position-changing phase" or "in-the-middle phase"
      a. Chromosomes align along a middle "equatorial" plane, with one chromatid of each chromosome facing its respective pole
      b. Each chromatid attaches to a spindle fibre
   3. Anaphase—"apart phase"
      a. The centromere of each chromosome splits to form two chromosomes, each consisting of a single DNA molecule
      b. Each chromosome is pulled toward the nearest pole to form two separate, but identical, pools of genetic information
   4. Telophase—"end phase"
      a. DNA returns to its original form and location within the cell
      b. After completion of telophase, each daughter cell begins interphase to develop into a mature cell
C. Meiosis (**Figure 7-11**; see also **Figure 47-1**)

Regulating the Cell Life Cycle

A. Cyclin-dependent kinases (CDKs) are activating enzymes that drive the cell through the phases of its life cycle
B. Cyclins are regulatory proteins that control the CDKs and "shift" them to start the next phase

Cycle of Life: Cells

A. Different types of cells have different life cycles
B. Advancing age creates changes in cell numbers and in their ability to function effectively
   1. Examples of decreased functional ability include muscle atrophy, loss of elasticity of the skin, and changes in the cardiovascular, respiratory, and skeletal systems

The Big Picture: Cell Physiology and the Whole Body

A. Most cell processes are occurring at the same time in all of the cells throughout the body
B. The processes of normal cell function result from the coordination dictated by the genetic code

REVIEW QUESTIONS

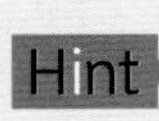

Write out the answers to these questions after reading the chapter and reviewing the Chapter Summary. Note—writing out your answers will consolidate learning and provide a valuable resource of information.

1. Describe the size and shape of a DNA molecule.
2. Where is most of a cell's DNA located? Is DNA located in any other organelle? If so, where?
3. Briefly outline the steps of protein synthesis.
4. As a cell grows, how is additional cell material added?
5. What are the steps involved in DNA replication and when does it occur?
6. Define *mitosis*.
7. Briefly describe the four distinct phases of mitosis.
8. Define *meiosis* and discuss its four distinct stages. What is the significance of meiosis? Why is it limited to sex cells?
9. When does the reduction of chromosomes from the diploid to the haploid number take place?
10. Give examples of normal and abnormal hyperplasia.

CRITICAL THINKING QUESTIONS

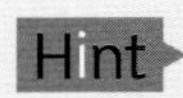

After finishing the Review Questions, write out the answers to these more in-depth questions to help you apply your new knowledge. Go back to sections of the chapter that relate to concepts that you find difficult.

1. Certain antibiotics can damage ribosomes in normal human body cells. People taking these antibiotics need to be carefully monitored. Summarize the result of fewer ribosomes on the process of transcription and translation.
2. DNA is often called the "blueprint of life". However, DNA is composed of only four nitrogen bases as part of its nucleotide structure. Explain how these four nitrogen bases can influence the genetic makeup of an individual. Hypothesize how these same bases also comprise the DNA of the entire living world.
3. Watson called DNA "the most golden of all molecules" primarily because of its role in protein synthesis. How would you describe the importance of the process of protein synthesis in the functioning of a cell?
4. A cast is commonly used to immobilize a broken bone. When the cast is removed, the muscles on that limb are usually smaller and weaker than the muscles on the other limb. How would you explain the difference between the two limbs?
5. Compare and contrast hypertrophy and hyperplasia.
6. The nucleus has been called the "brain" or the "control centre" of the cell. By applying what you have learned, describe how the nucleus can control growth, development, and day-to-day functions of a cell.

8 Introduction to Tissues

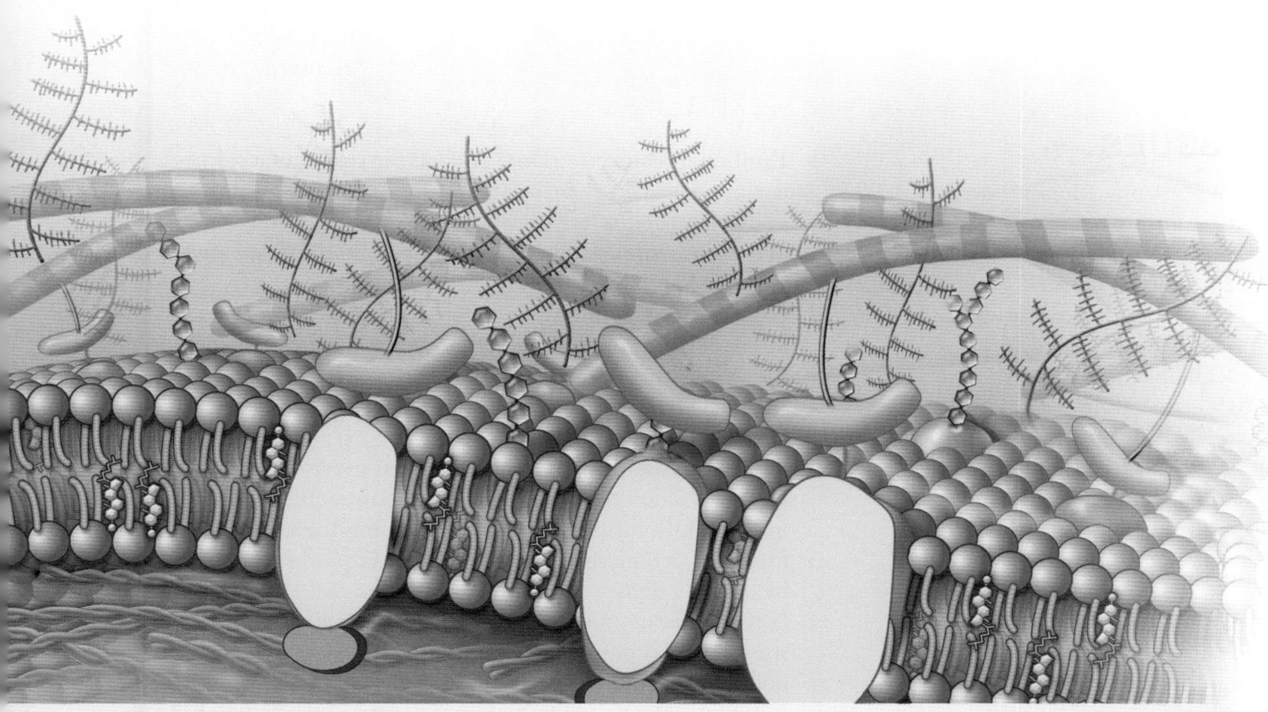

CHAPTER OUTLINE

Hint Scan this outline before you begin to read the chapter, as a preview of how the concepts are organized.

LANGUAGE OF SCIENCE

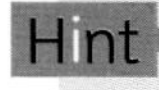 *Use this list to aid your pronunciation of unfamiliar words.*

basement membrane (BM)
[*base-* **base,** *-ment* **thing,** *membran-* **thin skin**]

collagen (KOL-ah-jen)
[*colla-* **glue,** *-gen* **produce**]

connective tissue
(kon-NEK-tiv TISH-yoo)
[*con-* **together,** *-nect-* **bind,** *-ive* **relating to,** *tissu-* **fabric**]

cutaneous membrane
(kyoo-TAYN-ee-us)
[*cut-* **skin,** *-aneous* **relating to,** *membran-* **thin skin**]

ectoderm (EK-toh-derm)
[*ecto-* **outside,** *-derm* **skin**]

elastin (e-LAS-tin)
[*elast-* **drive or propel,** *-in* **substance**]

endoderm (EN-doh-derm)
[*endo-* **inward or within,** *-derm* **skin**]

epithelial membrane
(ep-i-THEE-lee-al)
[*epi-* **on or upon,** *-theli-* **nipple,** *-al* **relating to,** *membran-* **thin skin**]

epithelial tissue (ep-i-THEE-lee-al)
[*epi-* **on or upon,** *-theli-* **nipple,** *-al* **relating to,** *tissu-* **fabric**]

extracellular matrix (ECM)
(eks-trah-SEL-yoo-lar MAY-triks)
[*extra-* **beyond,** *-cell-* **storeroom,** *-ular* **relating to,** *matrix* **womb**]
pl., matrices

goblet cell (GOB-let sel)
[*gobl-* **bowl,** *-et* **small,** *cell* **storeroom**]

histogenesis (his-toh-JEN-eh-sis)
[*histo-* **tissue,** *gen-* **produce,** *-esis* **process**]

histology (his-TOL-oh-jee)
[*histo-* **tissue,** *-o-* **combining form,** *-log-* **words (study of),** *-y* **activity**]

interstitial fluid (IF) (in-ter-STISH-al)
[*inter-* **between,** *-stit-* **stand,** *-al* **relating to**]

matrix (MAY-triks)
[*matrix* **womb**] *pl.,* matrices

membrane
[*membran-* **thin skin**]

mesoderm (MEZ-oh-derm)
[*meso-* **middle,** *-derm* **skin**]

mucus (MYOO-kus)
[*mucus* **slime**]

continued on p. 151

A tissue is a group of similar cells that perform a common function. Tissues can be thought of as the fabric of the body, which is "sewn together" to form the organs of the body and to hold all the organs together as a whole. In fact, the term tissue literally means "fabric".

To understand the fabric of the body, we begin in this chapter with an overview of the general organization and development of tissues. In Chapter 9, we then outline the chief characteristics of the various tissue types that you will encounter later in your study of human anatomy and physiology. •

INTRODUCTION TO TISSUES

Each tissue specializes in performing at least one unique function that helps maintain homeostasis, ensuring the survival of the whole body. Cells in one tissue may form a thin sheet only one cell deep, whereas the cells of another tissue may form huge masses containing millions of cells. Regardless of the size, shape, or arrangement of cells in a tissue, they all are surrounded by or embedded in a complex extracellular material that often is called simply **matrix.**

The four major types of human tissue that were introduced in Chapter 1 are described in more detail in this and the following chapter. An understanding of the major tissue types will help you understand the next higher levels of organization in the body—organs and organ systems. Eventually, your knowledge of **histology** (the biology of tissues) will give you a better appreciation for the nature of the whole body.

PRINCIPAL TYPES OF TISSUE

Although a number of subtypes are present in the body, all tissues can be classified by their structure and function into four principal types:

1. **Epithelial tissue** covers and protects the body surface, lines body cavities, specializes in moving substances into and out of the body or particular organs (secretion, excretion, and absorption), and forms many glands. The cells in epithelial tissue are usually very close together, with very little extracellular matrix (ECM).
2. **Connective tissue** functions to support the body and its parts, connect and hold them together, transport substances through the body, and protect it from foreign invaders. The cells in connective tissue are often relatively far apart and separated by large quantities of matrix.
3. **Muscle tissue** produces movement; it moves the body and its parts. Muscle cells are adapted for contractility and produce movement by shortening or lengthening the contractile units found in cytoplasm. Muscle tissue also produces most of the heat of the body.
4. **Nervous tissue** may be the most complex tissue in the body. It specializes in communication among the various parts of the body and in integration of their activities. This tissue's major function is the generation of complex messages that coordinate the body functions.

BOX 8-1 *sports and fitness*

Tissues and Fitness

Achieving and maintaining ideal body weight is a health-conscious goal. However, a better indicator of health and fitness is **body composition.** Exercise physiologists assess body composition to identify the percentage of the body made of lean tissue and the percentage made of fat. Body fat percentage is often determined by using calipers to measure the thickness of skin folds at certain locations on the body (see figures). The thickness measurements, which reflect the volume of adipose tissue under the skin, are then used to estimate the percentage of fat in the entire body. A much more accurate method is to weigh a subject totally immersed in a tank of water. Fat has very low density and therefore increases the buoyancy of the body. When in water, a person's measured weight is relatively low if the body fat percentage is high and the measured weight is high if the body fat percentage is low.

A person with low body weight may still have a high ratio of fat to muscle, an unhealthy condition. In this case the individual is "underweight" but "overfat". In other words, fitness depends more on the percentage and ratio of specific tissue types than on the overall amount of tissue present. Therefore, one goal of a good fitness program is a desirable body fat percentage. For men, the ideal is 15% to 18%, and for women, the ideal is 20% to 22%.

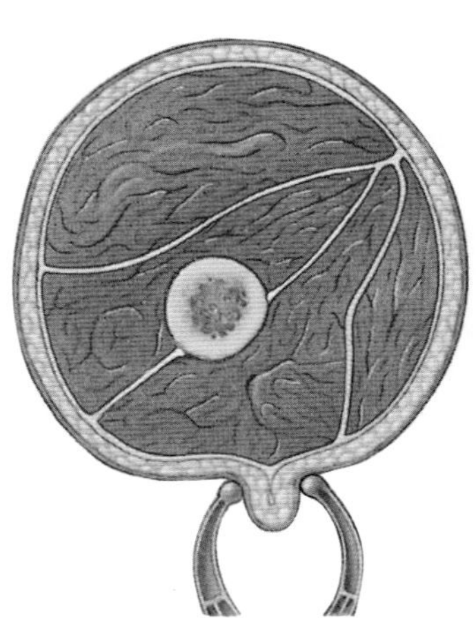

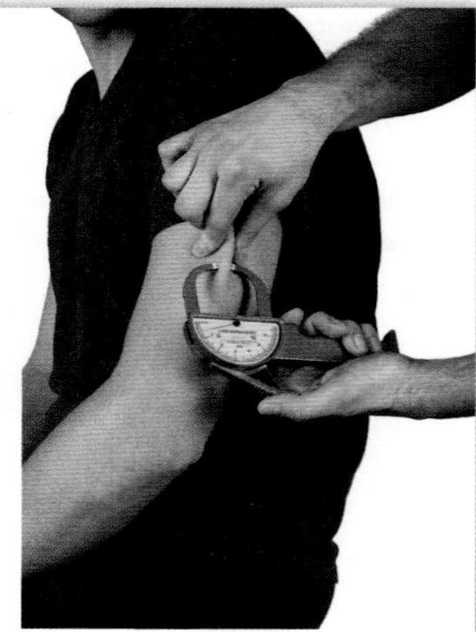

Because fat contains stored energy (measured in calories or kilojoules), a low fat percentage means a low energy reserve. High body fat percentages are associated with several life-threatening conditions, including cardiovascular disease. A balanced diet and an exercise program ensure that the ratio of fat to muscle tissue stays at a level appropriate for maintaining homeostasis. •

TABLE 8-1 Major Tissues of the Body

TISSUE TYPE	STRUCTURE	FUNCTION	EXAMPLES IN THE BODY
	Epithelial tissue		
	One or more layers of densely arranged cells with very little extracellular matrix May form either sheets or glands	Covers and protects the body surface Lines body cavities Transport of substances (absorption, secretion, excretion) Glandular activity	Outer layer of skin Lining of the respiratory, digestive, urinary, reproductive tracts Glands of the body
	Connective tissue		
	Sparsely arranged cells surrounded by a large proportion of extracellular matrix often containing structural fibres (and sometimes mineral crystals)	Supports body structures Transports substances throughout the body	Bones Joint cartilage Tendons and ligaments Blood Fat
	Muscle tissue		
	Long fibrelike cells, sometimes branched, capable of pulling loads; extracellular fibres sometimes hold muscle fibre together	Produces body movements Produces movements of organs such as the stomach, heart Produces heat	Heart muscle Muscles of the head/neck, arms, legs, trunk Muscles in the walls of hollow organs such as the stomach, intestines
	Nervous tissue		
	Mixture of many cell types, including several types of neurons (conducting cells) and neuroglia (support cells)	Communication between body parts Integration and regulation of body functions	Tissue of brain and spinal cord Nerves of the body Sensory organs of the body

The major tissue types are also summarized in **Table 8-1**.

Box 8-1 shows how the ratio of different tissues in body—and their distribution—are related to overall wellness and fitness.

Development of Tissues

The four major tissues of the body appear early in the embryonic period of development. Within the first 2 weeks after conception, cells of the offspring move and regroup in an orderly way into three **primary germ layers** called **endoderm, mesoderm,** and **ectoderm** (**Figure 8-1**). During this process the cells in each germ layer become increasingly more differentiated to form specific tissues—a set of processes that are together called **histogenesis** (**Box 8-2**). Remodelling themselves by a combination of new growth, differentiation, and apoptosis, these early layers eventually give rise to the various organs of the body. Embryonic development is discussed more thoroughly in Chapter 47.

EXTRACELLULAR MATRIX

Fluid Environment of the Body

Recall from Chapter 2 that a central principle of human physiology is homeostasis—the relative constancy of the internal fluid environment. This fluid environment fills the spaces between the cells of the body. Tissues differ in the amount and kind of fluid material between the cells—the **extracellular matrix (ECM).**

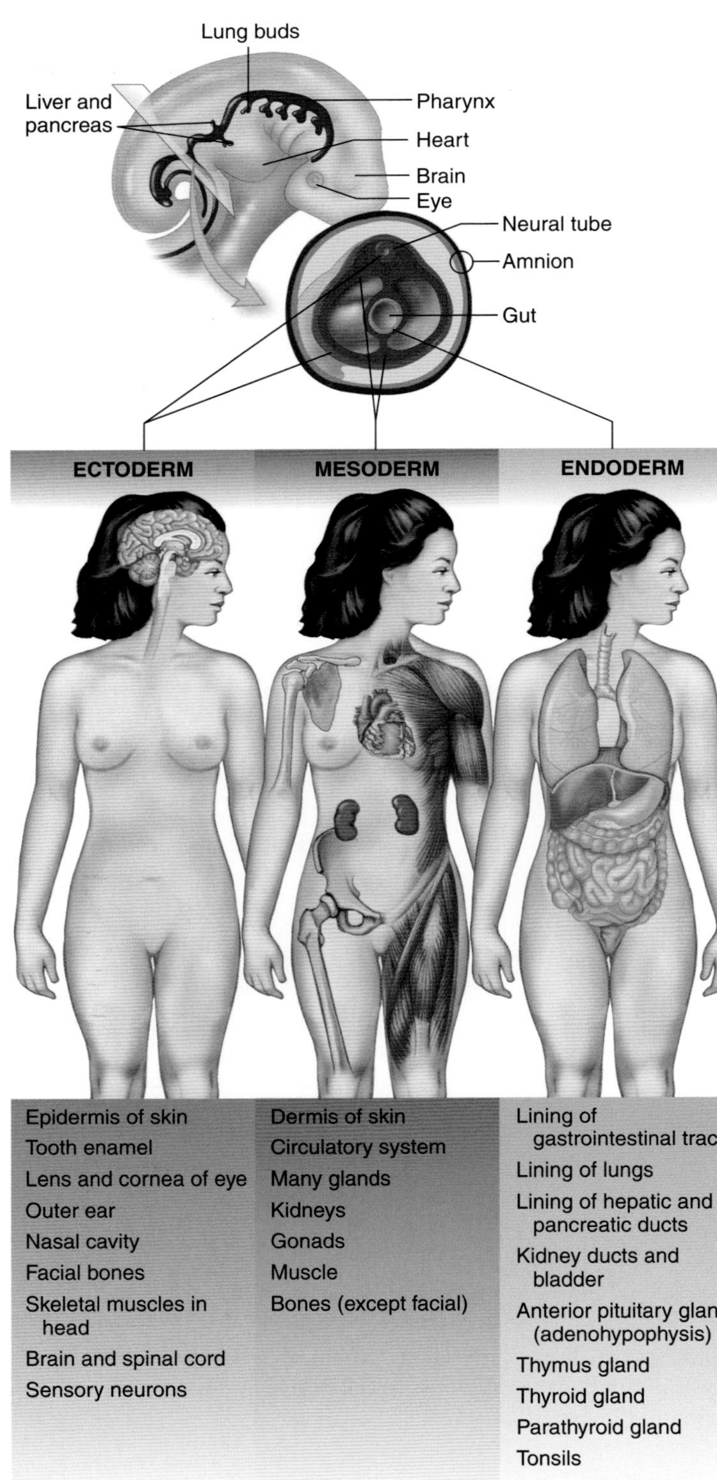

FIGURE 8-1 Primary germ layers. The primary germ layers that form during embryonic development eventually give rise to specific tissues by way of processes collectively called *histogenesis.*

BOX 8-2 *stem cells*

During embryonic development, new kinds of cells can be formed from a special kind of undifferentiated cell called a **stem cell.**

Embryonic stem cells have the potential to reproduce many different kinds of daughter cells, including more stem cells—thus populating the body with all the different cells and tissues needed for body function. Sometimes controversial research is now under way to learn the secrets of embryonic stem cells and develop therapies in which embryonic stem cells might be used to repair or replace damaged tissue in adults.

Adult stem cells are undifferentiated cells found scattered within a differentiated, mature tissue. Many different tissues contain adult stem cells—we may soon find that all adult tissues have some stem cells. Adult stem cells can usually produce any of the specialized cell types within their particular tissue. However, recent research shows that some adult stem cells can be coaxed into producing a variety of different types of cells. For example, blood cell–producing stem cells from bone marrow have been used to help repair damaged muscle tissue in laboratory animals. Already, therapies for treating degenerative diseases of muscles, the heart, and the brain—and even baldness—are being proposed by medical scientists. •

The ECM is not "just" water, or even water with a few solutes. It is more accurate to think of the ECM as a gel that in many tissues is a bit like jelly. Jelly is mostly water but has a network of microscopic, interlocking fibres that thicken it. In addition to water, the ECM of tissues also has a variety of different proteins and **proteoglycans** that give it a range of different consistencies, depending on the specific tissue. **Figure 8-2** and **Table 8-2** hint at the complex nature of the ECM.

The particular makeup of the extracellular matrix in bone and cartilage, for example, results in a solid or very firm gel that contributes to the strength and resiliency of the body. The ECM of blood tissue—the blood *plasma*—is mostly water and solutes and therefore flows easily. However, the blood *can* form interlocking fibres under specific circumstances, as it does during blood clotting, to form a more solid substance (a clot).

Some tissues have very little ECM. Other tissues are almost entirely extracellular matrix—with only a few cells present. Some types of ECM contain large numbers of structural protein fibres that make them flexible or elastic, some contain many mineral crystals that make them rigid, and others are very fluid.

Components of the Extracellular Matrix

Proteins in the extracellular matrix include various types of structural protein fibres such as *collagen* and *elastin,* both of which are discussed frequently throughout this book. Most tissues also include complex arrangements of protein–carbohydrate hybrid molecules such as *glycoproteins* and *proteoglycans.* In some tissues, such as bone, there may also be calcium-containing mineral crystals that make the ECM rigid.

Collagen

Collagenous fibres are made of the protein **collagen** and often occur in twisted bundles—an arrangement that provides great tensile

FIGURE 8-2 Extracellular matrix (ECM). A, The extracellular matrix is made up of water, proteins/glycoproteins, and proteoglycans that often form large bundles or complexes that bind together and to the cells of the tissue. Although the makeup of ECM varies from tissue to tissue, it usually includes some connections to integrins in the plasma membranes, thereby allowing for structural integrity, as well as communication and coordination within the tissue. **B,** A detailed view of a proteoglycan complex shows many proteoglycans, each with a protein backbone and attached carbohydrate subunits—all held together by a polysaccharide chain. **C,** Detailed view of a collagen bundle showing the individual collagen fibres within it.

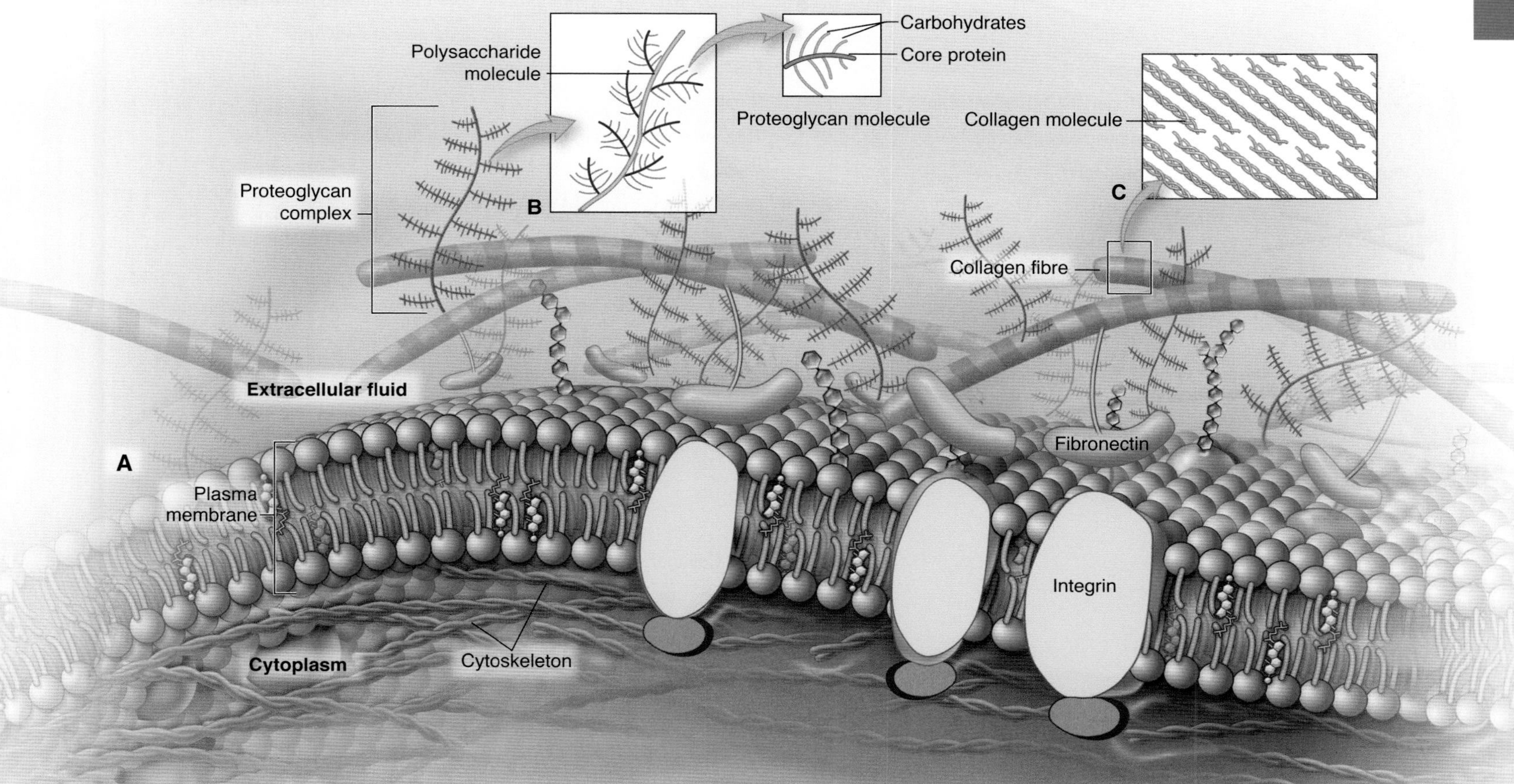

strength (**Figure 8-3**). Because collagenous fibres look white in living tissue, they are sometimes called *white fibres.* However, they often appear pink in stained microscopic specimens.

Of all the hundreds of different protein compounds in the body, collagen is the most abundant. Biologists estimate that it constitutes somewhat more than one fourth of all the protein in the body. And interestingly, one of the most basic factors in the ageing process, according to some researchers, is the change in the molecular structure of collagen that occurs gradually with the passage of years. In its hydrated form, collagen is also known as *gelatin.* Perhaps you have eaten some flavoured gelatin made from animal collagen.

Reticular fibres, in contrast to collagenous fibres, occur in three-dimensional networks and, although delicate, support small structures such as capillaries, nerve fibres, and lymphoid structures such as lymph nodes and tonsils. Reticular fibres are made of a special type of collagen called *reticulin* or *collagen III.*

Epithelial cells secrete another special type of collagen called *collagen IV.* Thin, kinked collagen IV fibres form a two-dimensional network that serves as the base layer—or *basal lamina*—under a sheet of epithelial cells. **Figure 8-4** shows how the collagen IV forms a flat framework within the basal lamina. Reticulin-producing cells in the connective tissue below the basal lamina produce a thin *fibroreticular lamina* of reticular tissue. The union of basal and fibroreticular laminae together forms the **basement membrane (BM)**—a thin, gluelike connection between a sheet of epithelial cells and the underlying fibrous connective tissue.

Besides forming a connecting layer between tissues, the loose networks of fibres within the basement membrane also serve as filters or screens to regulate movement of particles by size. This ability is important in controlling which particles can move across the walls of blood capillaries, air sacs of the lungs, and filtering tubules of the kidneys.

Elastin

Elastic fibres are made of a protein called **elastin,** which returns to its original length after being stretched (**Figure 8-5**). Elastin is a rubbery substance that is held in a fibrous shape by long, thin microfilaments—as you can see in **Figure 8-5**, *B.* Elastic fibres are found in "stretchy" tissues, such as the cartilage of the external ear and the walls of arteries. Because elastin fibres look yellowish in living tissue, they are sometimes called *yellow fibres.*

TABLE 8-2 **Components of the Extracellular Matrix (ECM)***

COMPONENT	EXAMPLE	DESCRIPTION
Water		Water molecules along with a small number of ions (mostly Na^+ and Cl^-)
Proteins	Collagen	Strong, flexible structural protein fibre that forms ropelike bundles
	Collagen IV	Thin, kinked fibres that form two-dimensional networks
	Elastin	Flexible, elastic structural protein fibre
	Nidogen (NID-1 or entactin)	Small protein
	Reticulin (collagen III)	Thin structural protein that forms three-dimensional networks
Glycoproteins	Fibronectin	Rodlike glycoprotein
	Laminin	Glycoproteins arranged as a three-pronged fork or cross
Proteoglycans	Chondroitin sulphate	Protein backbone with attached chains of various polysaccharides
	Heparan sulphate	
Polysaccharides	Hyaluronic acid (hyaluronate)	Long chain of saccharide subunits; form backbone for proteoglycan attachment

BM, Basement membrane.

*Not all components are present in all ECM; examples of only some of the many major ECM components are provided.

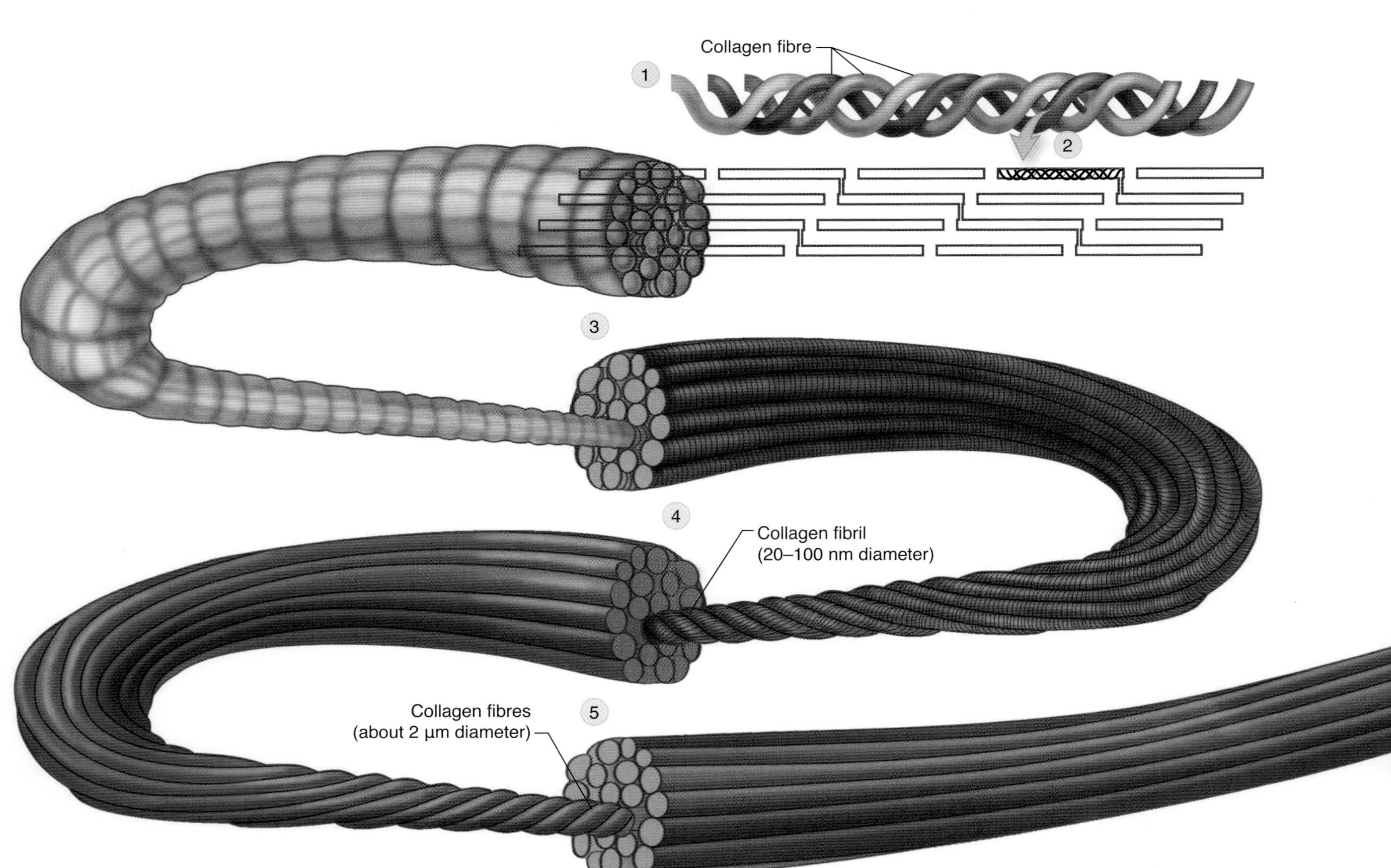

FUNCTION	EXAMPLE OF LOCATION
Solvent for dissolved ECM components; provides fluidity of ECM	All tissues of the body
Provides flexible strength to tissues	Tendons, ligaments, bones, cartilage, many tissues
Provides a thin, flat framework connected to nearby cells	In basal lamina (of BM) beneath epithelial tissues
Allows flexibility and elastic recoil of tissues	Skin, cartilage of ear, walls of arteries
Forms links to strengthen and communicate within networks of fibres	In basal lamina (of BM) beneath epithelial tissues
Forms supportive networks within or around small structures	Capillaries, nerves, lymphoid structures
Binds ECM to cells; communicates with cells through integrins	Many tissues of the body; for example, connective tissues
Binds ECM components together and to cells; communicates with cells through integrins	In basal lamina (of BM) beneath epithelial tissues
Shock absorber	Cartilage, bone, heart valves
Regulates various tissue functions (e.g., blood vessel formation, blood clotting)	In basal lamina (of BM) beneath epithelial tissues
Thickens fluid; lubricates; supports proteoglycan molecules	Loose fibrous connective tissue, joint fluids

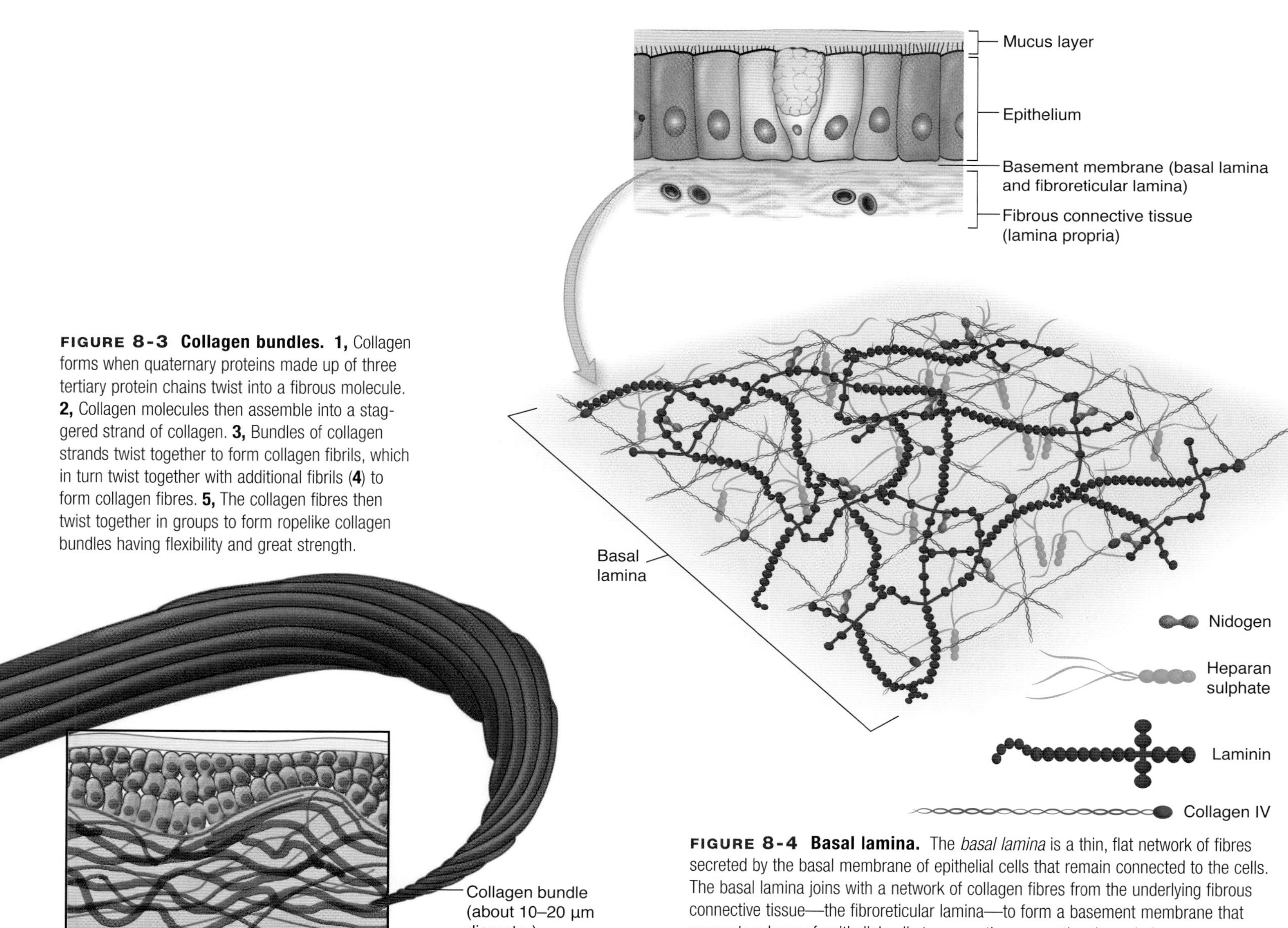

FIGURE 8-3 Collagen bundles. 1, Collagen forms when quaternary proteins made up of three tertiary protein chains twist into a fibrous molecule. **2,** Collagen molecules then assemble into a staggered strand of collagen. **3,** Bundles of collagen strands twist together to form collagen fibrils, which in turn twist together with additional fibrils (**4**) to form collagen fibres. **5,** The collagen fibres then twist together in groups to form ropelike collagen bundles having flexibility and great strength.

FIGURE 8-4 Basal lamina. The *basal lamina* is a thin, flat network of fibres secreted by the basal membrane of epithelial cells that remain connected to the cells. The basal lamina joins with a network of collagen fibres from the underlying fibrous connective tissue—the fibroreticular lamina—to form a basement membrane that connects a layer of epithelial cells to supportive connective tissue below.

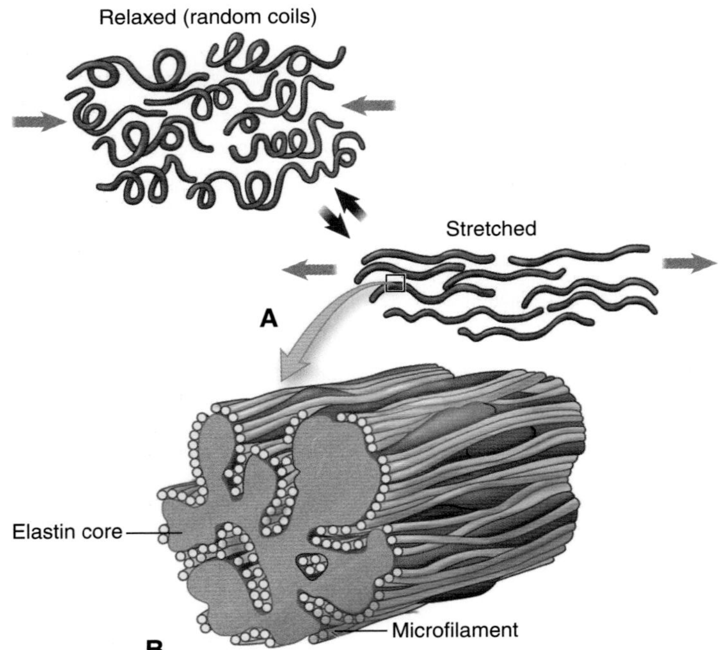

FIGURE 8-5 Elastin fibres. A, Elastin fibres form random coils within the extracellular matrix (ECM) that may easily be stretched. When released, the elastin fibres will recoil to a relaxed formation. **B,** Each elastin fibre is made of stretchy, formless elastin that is held in a fibrous shape by an arrangement of microfibrils.

Glycoproteins and Proteoglycans

The ECM also contains many glycoproteins, which are mainly protein molecules with attached carbohydrate subunits. For example, fibronectin and laminin in the basal lamina under epithelial cells help connect collagen and proteoglycans to cells by attaching to integrin protein molecules embedded in the plasma membrane of cells and connected internally to the cytoskeleton (see **Figures 8-2** and **8-4**). This arrangement thus unites the cells and their surroundings into a strong, integral structure. It also provides a communication mechanism between the ECM and the cell that allows coordination of cell and tissue development, as well as guidance of cell movement and shape changes.

Proteoglycans are hybrid molecules made up mostly of carbohydrates attached to a protein backbone, as you can see in **Figure 8-2**, *B*. Many of the sugars attached to the protein backbone of a proteoglycan molecule are *N-acetylglucosamine (NAG)*. Examples of proteoglycans are *chondroitin sulphate* and *heparan sulphate* (see **Table 8-2**).

Considering the makeup of ECM, it's no wonder that many dietary supplements that claim to improve the health of bones and joints include calcium, glucosamine, and/or chondroitin sulphate—all are important components of the ECM of cartilage and bone tissues.

Holding Tissues Together

In some tissues, it is the ECM that holds the tissue in a single mass. For example, in skeletal muscles, it is mostly a network of structural protein fibres in the ECM that holds skeletal muscle tissue together. In such cases, components of the ECM bind to the integrins in the outer membranes of the cells, and the integrins bind to components of the internal cytoskeleton.

In other tissues, it is primarily the intercellular junctions, such as the *desmosomes* and *tight junctions* described in a previous chapter (see Chapter 5, p. 92), that hold groups of cells together to form tissues found in sheets or other continuous masses of cells. The tissue that forms the outer layer of skin is held together this way. In some tissues, the ECM does not bind to tissue cells. For example, the fluid nature of the blood's matrix (plasma) does not hold blood tissue in a solid mass at all.

Quick **CHECK**

1. Name the four basic tissue types and give the major function of each.
2. What is a primary germ layer?
3. What is the ECM? What is it made of?
4. How do elastic fibres differ from collagenous fibres?

TISSUE REPAIR

When damaged by mechanical or other injuries, tissues have varying capacity to repair themselves. Damaged tissue regenerates or is replaced by tissue we know as scars. Tissues usually repair themselves by allowing phagocytic cells to remove dead or injured cells and then filling in the gaps that are left. This growth of functional new tissue is called **regeneration.**

Epithelial and connective tissues have the greatest capacity to regenerate (**Figure 8-6**). When a break in an epithelial membrane occurs, as in a cut, cells quickly divide to form daughter cells that fill the wound. In connective tissues, cells that form collagen fibres become active after an injury and fill in a gap with an unusually dense mass of fibrous connective tissue. If this dense mass of fibrous tissue is small, it may be replaced by normal tissue later. If the mass is deep

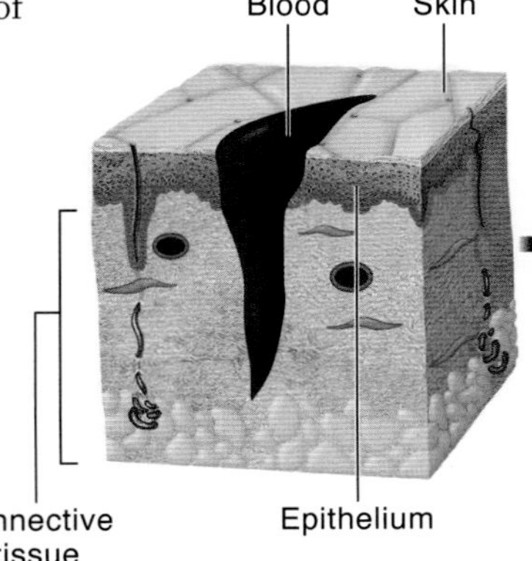

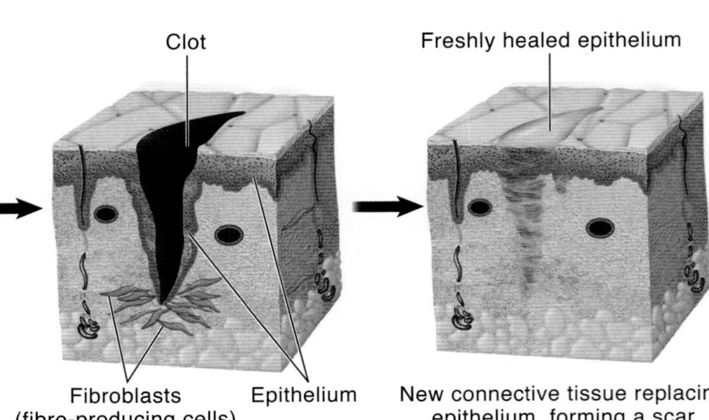

FIGURE 8-6 Healing of a minor wound. When a minor injury damages a layer of epithelium and the underlying connective tissue (as in a minor skin cut), the epithelial tissue and the connective tissue can self-repair.

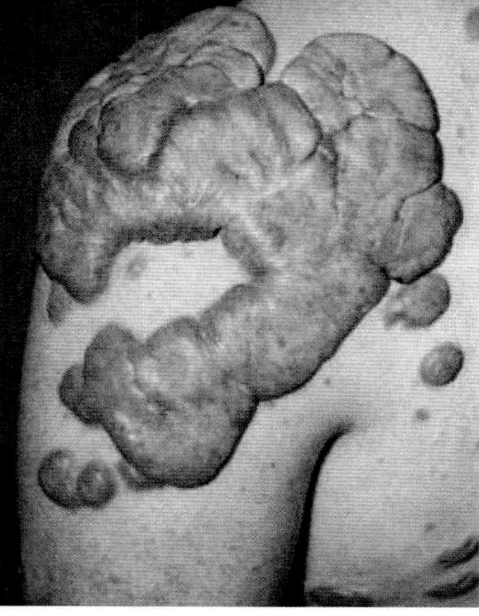

FIGURE 8-7 Keloid. Keloids are thick scars that form in the lower layer of the skin in predisposed individuals.

or large or if cell damage was extensive, it may remain as a dense fibrous mass, called a **scar.** An atypical and unusually thick scar that may develop in the lower layer of the skin, such as that shown in **Figure 8-7**, is called a **keloid.**

Muscle tissue, on the other hand, has a limited capacity to regenerate and thus heal itself. Scientists are just now learning about the abilities of muscle fibres to be replaced in adults. Damaged muscle is sometimes replaced with fibrous connective tissue instead of muscle tissue. When this happens, the organ involved loses some or all of its ability to function.

CONNECT IT!

Crushing injuries of skeletal muscle can release massive amounts of intracellular substances into the blood stream that can have life-threatening consequences, as in the condition rhabdomyolysis. Learn more in the article ***Rhabdomyolysis*** online at ***Connect It!***

Like muscle tissue, nerve tissue also has a limited capacity to regenerate. Neurons can sometimes regenerate, but very slowly and only if certain neuroglia are present to "pave the way". In the normal adult brain and spinal cord, a few new neurons are regularly produced in certain regions. However, adult brain neurons do not often grow back when injured. Thus serious brain and spinal cord injuries often result in at least some permanent damage. Fortunately, research on *nerve growth factors* produced by neuroglia offers the promise of treating brain damage. Research on adult stem cells present in both muscle and nerve tissue also holds hope for such therapies.

CONNECT IT!

One of the natural processes that reacts to injuries and helps promote healing is **inflammation**. We will explore this process in more detail when we discuss immunity. For now, you may want to check out ***Inflammation*** online at ***Connect It!***

BODY MEMBRANES

The term **membrane** refers to a thin, sheetlike structure that may have many important functions in the body. Membranes cover and protect the body surface, line body cavities, and cover the inner surfaces of hollow organs such as the digestive, reproductive, and respiratory passageways. Some membranes anchor organs to each other or to bones, and others cover the internal organs. In certain areas of the body, membranes secrete lubricating fluids that reduce friction during organ movements such as beating of the heart or lung expansion and contraction. Membrane lubricants also decrease friction between bones and joints. Two major categories, or types, of body membranes exist (**Figure 8-8**):

1. **Epithelial membranes,** composed of epithelial tissue glued by a basement membrane to an underlying layer of supportive connective tissue
2. **Connective tissue membranes,** composed exclusively of various types of connective tissue; no epithelial cells are present in this type of membrane

EPITHELIAL MEMBRANES

There are three types of epithelial tissue membranes in the body: (1) cutaneous membrane, (2) serous membranes, and (3) mucous membranes (**Figure 8-9**).

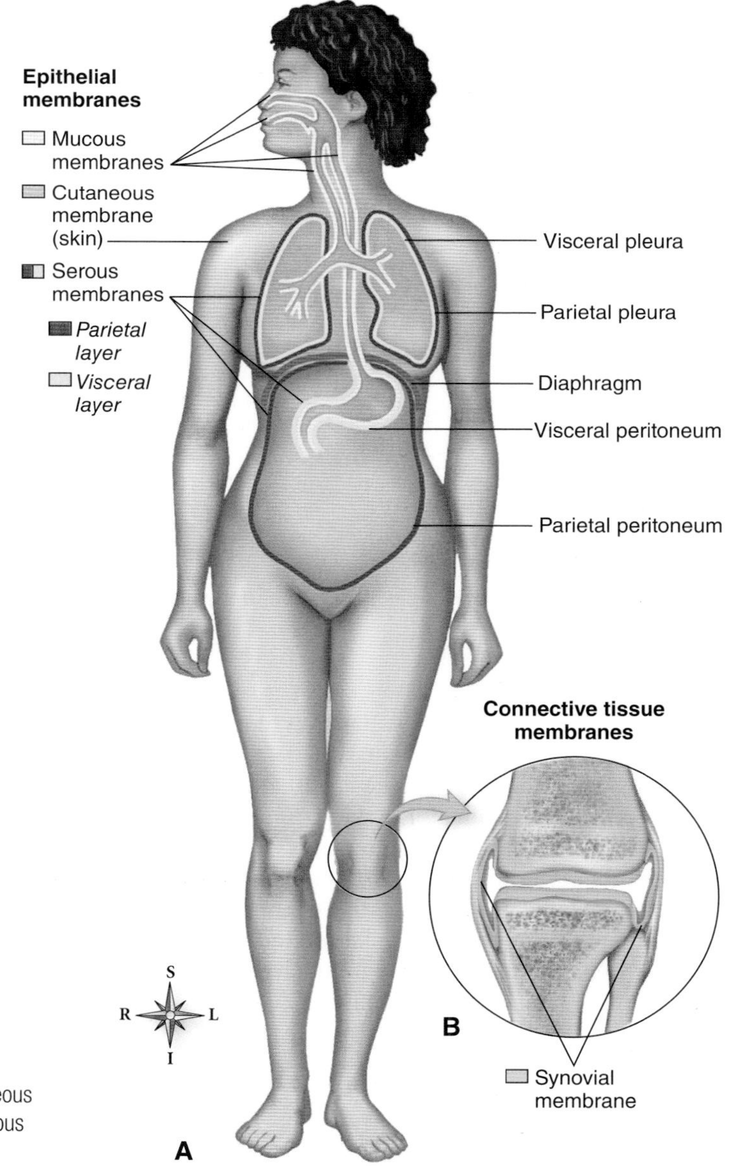

FIGURE 8-8 Types of body membranes. A, Epithelial membranes, including cutaneous membrane (skin), serous membranes (parietal and visceral pleura and peritoneum), and mucous membranes. **B,** Connective tissue membranes, including synovial membranes.

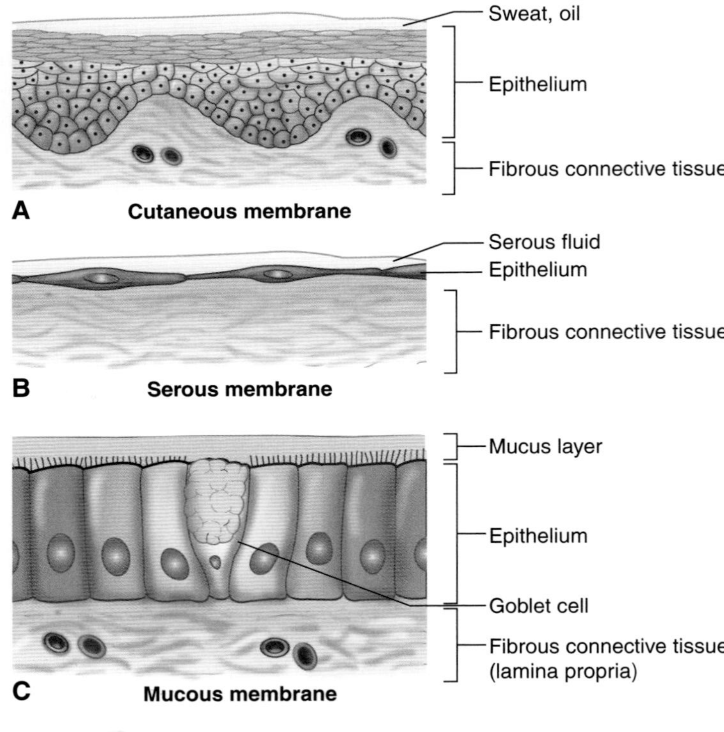

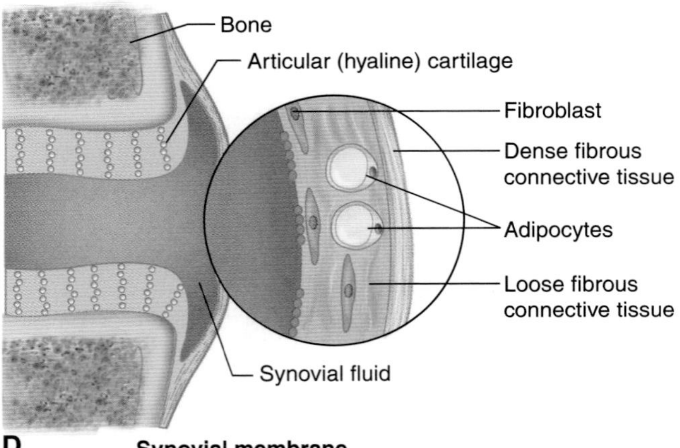

FIGURE 8-9 Microscopic structure of body membranes.

Cutaneous Membrane

The **cutaneous membrane** covers body surfaces that are exposed to the external environment. The cutaneous membrane, or **skin**, is the primary organ of the integumentary system. It is one of the most important and certainly one of the largest and most visible organs of the body. In most individuals the skin composes approximately 16% of body weight. It fulfils the requirements necessary for an epithelial tissue membrane in that it has a superficial layer of epithelial cells and an underlying layer of supportive connective tissue. It also contains many sweat and oil glands that produce a *surface film* over the skin. The structure of the skin is uniquely suited to its many functions. The skin is discussed in depth in Chapter 10.

Serous Membranes

Serous membrane lines cavities that are not open to the external environment and covers many of the organs inside these cavities. Serous membranes are sometimes called by their Latin name, *serosa.*

Like all epithelial membranes, a serous membrane is composed of two distinct layers of tissue. One of the layers, the epithelial sheet, is a thin layer of simple squamous epithelium. The other layer, the connective tissue layer, forms a very thin sheet that holds and supports the epithelial cells.

Serous membranes secrete a thin, watery fluid that lubricates organs as they rub against one another and against the walls of cavities.

The serous membrane that lines body cavities and covers the surfaces of organs in these cavities is in reality a single, continuous sheet covering two different surfaces. As first described in Chapter 1, the *parietal membrane* is the portion that lines the wall of the cavity like wallpaper and the *visceral membrane* covers the surface of the viscera (organs within the cavity). Go back to **Figure 1-6** on p. 11 to see how this double-layer structure resembles the wall of a water-filled balloon after a fist is thrust into it.

Two important serous membranes are shown in **Figure 8-8**: the *pleura,* which surrounds a lung and lines the thoracic cavity, and the *peritoneum,* which covers the abdominal viscera and lines the abdominal cavity. Another example is the *pericardium,* which surrounds the heart (**Box 8-3**).

Mucous Membranes

Mucous membranes are epithelial membranes that line body surfaces opening directly to the exterior. Mucous membranes are sometimes called by their Latin name, *mucosa.* Examples of mucous membranes include those lining the respiratory, digestive, urinary, and reproductive tracts. The epithelial component of the mucous membrane varies, depending on its location and function, an application of the principle of structure fits function. In the oesophagus, for example, a tough, abrasion-resistant stratified squamous epithelium is found. A thin layer of simple columnar epithelium covers the walls of the lower segments of the digestive tract. The fibrous connective tissue underlying the epithelium in mucous membranes is called the lamina propria.

Mucous membranes get their name from the fact that they produce a film of **mucus** that coats and protects the underlying cells. In addition to protection, mucus also serves other purposes. For example, mucus acts as a lubricant for food as it moves along the digestive tract. In the respiratory tract, it serves as a sticky trap for contaminants.

Mucus is a watery secretion that contains a mixture of *mucins,* which are a group of about two dozen different proteoglycans.

H

BOX 8-3 *health matters*

Inflammation of Serous Membranes

Pleurisy (also called *pleuritis*) is a very painful pathological condition characterized by inflammation of the serous membranes (pleurae) that line the chest cavity and cover the lungs. Pain is caused by irritation and friction as the lungs rub against the walls of the chest cavity. In severe cases the inflamed surfaces of the pleura fuse, and permanent damage may develop. The term **peritonitis** is used to describe inflammation of the serous membranes in the abdominal cavity. Peritonitis is sometimes a serious complication of an infected appendix. Inflammation of the serous membranes (serous pericardia) that surround the heart is a condition called **pericarditis**. See ***Inflammation*** online at ***Connect It!*** for more about the inflammatory response. •

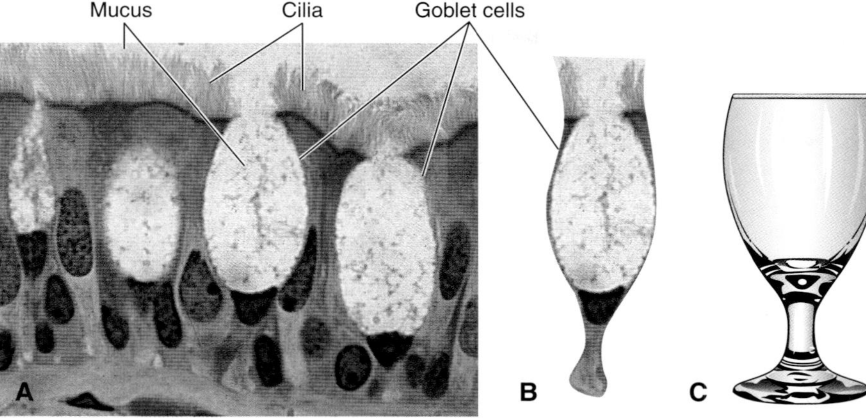

FIGURE 8-10 Goblet cells. Mucus-producing goblet cells (**A**) can be identified by the large vesicles of mucus ready for release into the extracellular matrix. An isolated goblet cell in the process of secreting mucus (**B**) is shown next to a water goblet (**C**), which it resembles.

Different mucins are found in different locations in the body. Some mucins are attached directly to the plasma membranes of the epithelial cells to form a protective coat. Other mucins are released by **goblet cells** and form a protective, sometimes lubricating blanket of gel (**Figure 8-10**). Thus mucous membranes have two layers of protective coating. A detailed diagram of the structure of a goblet cell is shown in Figure 5-6 in the Brief Atlas of the Human Body.

Some mucous membranes are populated with epithelial cells covered with a dense coat of motile cilia. Recall from Chapter 5 (**Figure 5-19** on p. 91) that these cilia can move as a coordinated team. **Figure 8-11** shows how such teams of cilia can propel a blanket of mucus in a particular direction along the surface of the mucous membrane. This mechanism can move contaminated mucus out of the airways and can help move ova (eggs) along the tubes of the female reproductive tract.

The mucous membrane is clinically important because it is the place where our body will most likely interact with microorganisms from the external environment. In fact, a very active area of research is attempting to understand the microbial colonization of mucous membranes in the digestive tract, respiratory tract, urinary tract, and reproductive tract (**Figure 8-12**). As researchers learn more about how mucus defends our internal environment from attack, the better able they will be to develop new strategies to avoid life-threatening infections. Chapter 33 discusses the role of mucous membranes in immunity.

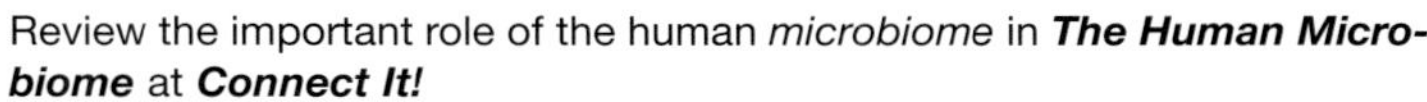

CONNECT IT!

Review the important role of the human *microbiome* in ***The Human Microbiome*** at ***Connect It!***

Connective Tissue Membranes

Unlike cutaneous, serous, and mucous membranes, connective tissue membranes do not contain epithelial components. The **synovial membranes** lining the spaces between bones and joints that move are classified as connective tissue membranes. These membranes are smooth and slick and secrete a thick and colourless lubricating fluid called **synovial fluid.** The membrane itself, with its specialized fluid,

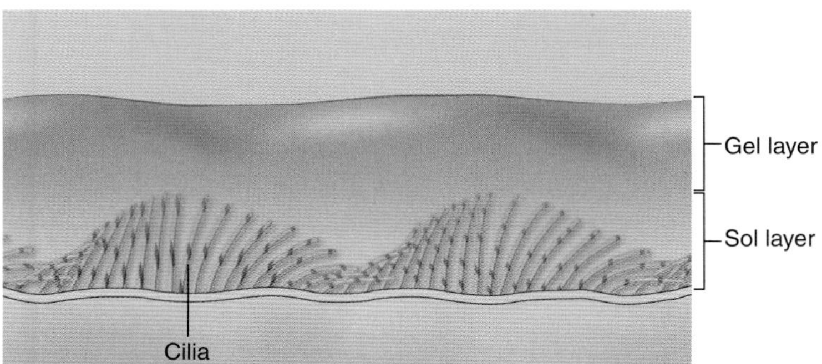

FIGURE 8-11 Movement of mucus. Mucus secreted by goblet cells (see **Figure 8-10**) forms a continuous blanket with an inner watery region (*sol layer*) and an outer dense layer (*gel layer*) that is moved along by the action of motile cilia. Coordinated movement of cilia, powered by molecular motors in epithelial cells, pushes the mucus blanket along with any particles that become embedded in the gel layer.

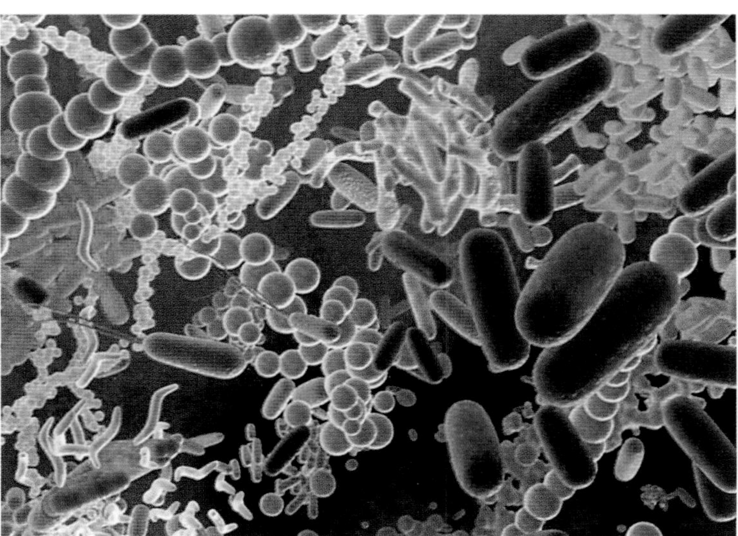

FIGURE 8-12 Colonization of mucous membranes by microbes. This colourized scanning electron micrograph shows many different types of bacteria that colonize the mucous membranes of the digestive tract and urinary tract within a short time after birth (*yellow,* bifidobacteria; *red,* coliform bacteria; *purple,* lactobacilli; *light blue,* streptococci; *green,* other coccal bacteria).

TABLE 8-3 Membranes of the Body

TYPE	SUPERFICIAL LAYER	DEEP LAYER	LOCATION	FLUID SECRETION	FUNCTION
Epithelial					
Cutaneous (skin)	Keratinized stratified squamous epithelium (epidermis)	Dense irregular fibrous connective tissue (dermis)	Directly exposed to external environment	Sweat; sebum (skin oil)	Protection, sensation, thermoregulation
Serous	Simple squamous epithelium	Fibrous connective tissue	Lines body cavities that are not open to the external environment	Serous fluid	Lubrication
Mucous	Various types of epithelium	Fibrous connective tissue (lamina propria)	Lines tracts that open to the external environment	Mucus	Protection, lubrication
Connective					
Synovial	Dense fibrous connective tissue	Loose fibrous connective tissue	Lines joint cavities (in movable joints)	Synovial fluid	Helps hold joint together, lubricates, cushions

BOX 8-4 *imagining cross-sections*

When you look at photomicrographs of membranes or other structures that are tubelike, saclike, or folded into complex shapes, it is sometimes hard to imagine what you are really looking at.

As diagram *A* shows, when you cut a tube on a cross-section, the slice looks like a ring (if cut at a right angle) or oval (if cut at an oblique, or slanted, angle). Diagram *A* also shows that if the tube is bent where the cut is made, it can also look like an oval on your slide. Diagram *B* shows what happens when you have many tubes next to one another—your slice has many round or oval rings (depending on the angle of the cut).

Diagram *C* shows what can happen when a membrane such as the intestinal lining is folded into complex shapes. The slice may look like a sort of zigzag line of cells, or if it is at a high magnification, it may just look like a series of parallel rows.

Imagining such cross-sections will help you in the remaining chapters as you look at diagrams and micrographs of various membranes of the body in cross-section. •

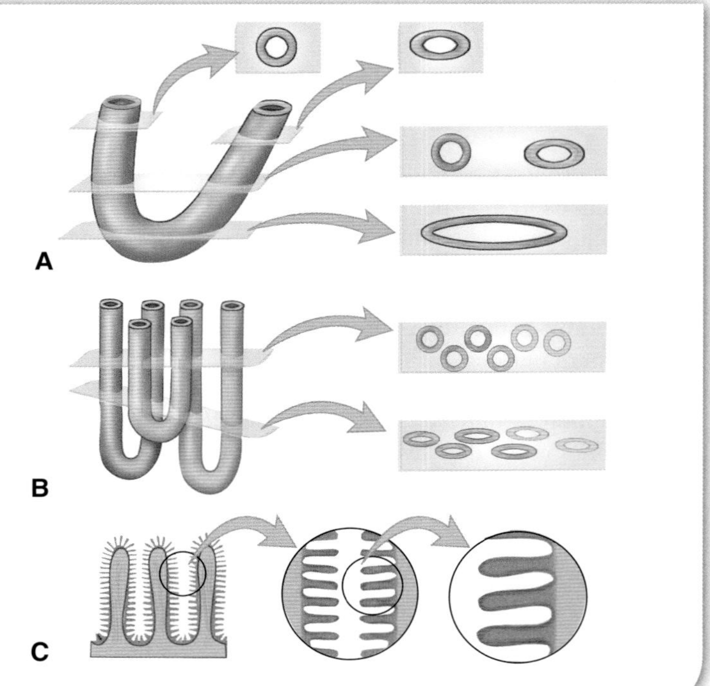

helps reduce friction between the opposing surfaces of bones in movable joints. Synovial membranes also line the small, cushionlike sacs called *bursae* found between some moving body parts.

Table 8-3 summarizes the main characteristics of the four major types of membranes in the body. **Box 8-4** shows how to imagine how membranes found in folds or tubes look in microscopic cross-sections—a useful skill as you survey specific tissue types in the next chapter.

Quick CHECK

5. Which two of the four major tissue types have the greatest capacity to regenerate after an injury?
6. Why does damaged muscle often lose some or all of its ability to function?
7. Name the four principal types of body membranes. Which are epithelial membranes?
8. Define *mucus* and describe its function in the body.

the big picture | Tissues, Membranes, and the Whole Body

Tissues and body membranes are sometimes called "the fabric of the body". Like the pieces of fabric in a garment, tissues and body membranes are portions of a larger integrated structure. Just as each type of fabric in a complex garment has a different functional role determined by its structural characteristics, so does each type of tissue within the body. One of the ultimate functional goals of most tissues and membranes is maintenance of relative constancy in the body: homeostasis.

How do the major tissue types help maintain homeostasis? Epithelial tissues promote constancy of the body's internal environment in several ways. They form membranes that contain and protect the internal fluid environment, they absorb nutrients and other substances needed to maintain an optimum concentration in the body, and they secrete various products that regulate body functions involved in homeostasis. Connective tissues hold organs and systems together to form a whole, connected body. They also form structures that support the body and permit movement, such as the components of the skeleton.

Some connective tissues, such as blood, transport nutrients, wastes, and other substances within the internal environment. Some blood cells help protect the internal environment by participating in the body's immune system. Muscle tissues work in conjunction with connective tissues (for example, bones and tendons) to permit movement (a function needed to avoid injury); to communicate; and to find food, shelter, and other requirements. Nervous tissue works with glandular epithelial tissue to regulate various body functions in a way that maintains homeostatic balance.

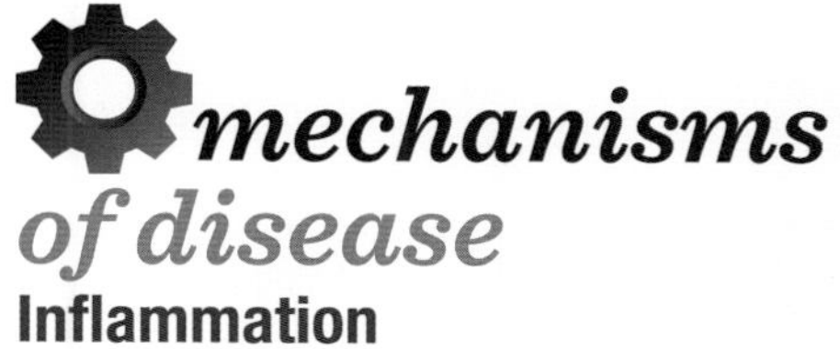

Inflammation

Inflammation—also called the inflammatory response—is a set of reactions to tissue injury. We discuss it in more detail in ***Inflammation*** online at **Connect It!** As a brief introduction, we list the four main signs of inflammation and how each represents an adaptive response of the body to promote healing.

- Redness—produced by increased blood flow to the injury site, which dilutes the injuring agent and delivers needed immune cells
- Heat—produced by the increased blood flow, it may inhibit the reproduction of some harmful microbes
- Swelling—produced by increased permeability of blood vessels, causing shift of fluid into ECM that helps dilute the injuring agent and permits immune cells and chemical agents to move freely
- Pain—often caused by the increased pressure in tissues from swelling, pain alerts the body to the injury so the tissue will be immobilized during healing and possibly treated medically

Tumours and Cancer

The concept of tumours and cancer was introduced in Chapter 2, then expanded in **Box 7-2** on p. 132. Because tumours are tissue abnormalities, we resume our discussion here. Keep in mind that these and other tissue abnormalities continue to be important in later chapters as well.

Neoplasms

The term **neoplasm** literally means "new matter" and refers to any abnormal growth of cells: another name for a neoplasm is **tumour.** Neoplasms can be distinct lumps of abnormal cells or, in blood tissue, can be diffuse. Neoplasms are often classified as **benign** or **malignant.** Benign tumours are called that because they do not spread to other tissues and they usually grow very slowly. Their cells are often well differentiated, unlike the undifferentiated cells typical of malignant tumours. Cells in a benign tumour tend to stay together, and they are often surrounded by a capsule of dense tissue. Benign tumours are not usually life-threatening but can be if they disrupt the normal function of a vital organ. Malignant tumours, or **cancers,** on the other hand, are not encapsulated and tend to spread to other regions of the body. For example, cells from malignant breast tumours usually form new (secondary) tumours in bone, brain, and lung tissues. The cells migrate by way of lymphatic or blood vessels. This manner of spreading is called **metastasis.**

Metastasis can occur long before a tumour becomes detectable during cancer screening, which explains why cancer screening is only one of many tools for preventing death from cancer.

Cells that do not **metastasize** can spread another way: they grow rapidly and extend the tumour into nearby tissues (**Figure 8-13**). Malignant tumours may replace part of a vital organ with abnormal, undifferentiated tissue—a life-threatening situation.

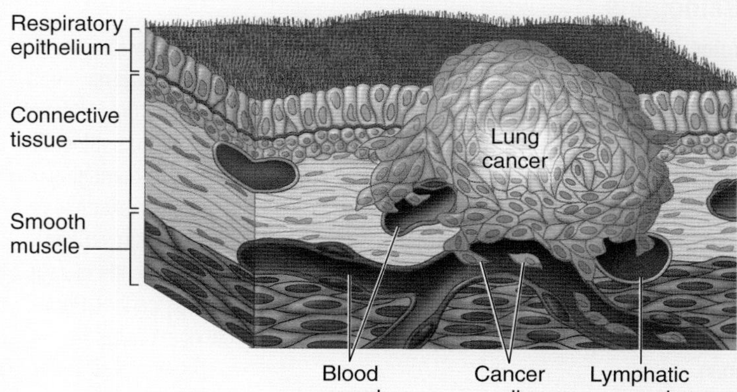

FIGURE 8-13 Cancer. This abnormal mass of proliferating cells in the lining of lung airways is a malignant tumour—lung cancer. Note how some cancer cells are leaving the tumour and entering the blood and lymph vessels.

Neoplasms are classified further into subgroups, depending on the tissue in which they originate. Both benign and malignant tumours can be divided into three types: epithelial tumours, connective tissue tumours, and miscellaneous tumours. Benign tumour types that arise from epithelial tissues include *papilloma* (a fingerlike projection), *adenoma* (glandular tumour), and *naevus* (small, pigmented skin tumours). Benign tumour types that arise from connective tissues include *lipoma* (adipose tumour), *osteoma* (bone tumour), and *chondroma* (cartilage tumour). Malignant tumours that arise from epithelial tissues are generally called **carcinomas.** Examples include *melanoma* (cancer of skin pigment cells) and *adenocarcinoma* (glandular cancer).

Malignant tumours that arise from connective tissues are generally called **sarcomas.** Examples include *lymphoma* (lymphatic cancer), *osteosarcoma* (bone cancer), and *fibrosarcoma* (cancer of fibrous connective tissue). Miscellaneous tumours are those that do not fit any of the previous categories. For example, an *adenofibroma* is a benign neoplasm formed by epithelial and connective tissues. Another example is *neuroblastoma,* a malignant tumour that arises from nerve tissue.

The aetiologies (origins) of various forms of cancer puzzle medical science no less today than a hundred years ago. We do know that cancer involves uncontrolled cell division: **hyperplasia** (too many cells) and/or **anaplasia** (abnormal, undifferentiated cells). Thus the mechanism of all cancers is a mistake or problem in cell division. What we are uncertain of is the cause of the abnormal cell division. Currently, several factors are known to play a role.

Genetic Factors

Many forms of cancer are known to be inherited directly, perhaps involving abnormal "cancer genes" called **oncogenes.** Another type of gene, called a **tumour suppressor gene,** may fail to operate and thus allow cancer to develop. As we learned in Chapter 7, such regulator genes limit the cell life cycle so that tissues do not become overcrowded. Exactly how these genes work is still being investigated. For example, the regulator gene called *p53* springs into action at the first sign of cancer and initiates a chain reaction that stops or slows the cell life cycle and may even cause the cell's death—before it can develop into full-blown cancer.

Presumably, many cancers involve a genetic predisposition (risk factor) coupled with other cancer-causing mechanisms. Cancers with known genetic risk factors include basal cell carcinoma (a type of skin cancer), breast cancer, and neuroblastoma (a cancer of nerve tissue).

Carcinogens

Carcinogens (cancer makers) are agents that affect genetic activity in some way and cause abnormal cell reproduction. Some carcinogens are **mutagens** (mutation makers) that cause changes or mutations in a cell's DNA structure. Although many industrial products are known to be carcinogens, various natural mineral, vegetable, and animal materials are also carcinogenic. Exposure to damaging types of radiation or other physical injuries can be carcinogenic. For example, sunburns or chronic exposure to sunlight can cause skin cancer. Even viruses have been known to cause cancer, perhaps by altering the genetic code of cells during an infection or by damaging the body's ability to suppress cancer. Papilloma (wart) viruses have been blamed for many cases of cervical cancer in women.

Age

Certain cancers are found primarily in young people (e.g., leukaemia) and others primarily in older adults (e.g., colon cancer). The age factor may result from changes in the genetic activity of cells over time or from the accumulated effects of cell damage.

Metabolic Factors

People with metabolic disorders such as *diabetes mellitus* and *obesity* are often at a greater risk of developing cancer. Such disruptions of normal body chemistry could cause signals to tissues that promote mistakes in cell reproduction that lead to cancer.

CONNECT IT! 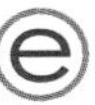

A person's body shape or *somatotype* can be an indicator of cancer risk. To learn more about this, check out ***Body Types and Disease*** at ***Connect It!***

Detection and Treatment of Cancer

Signs of cancer are those one would expect of a malignant neoplasm: the appearance of abnormal, rapidly growing tissue. Cancer specialists, or *oncologists,* have stressed that early detection of cancer is important because it is in the early stages of development of primary tumours that many cancers are most treatable. Some methods used to detect the presence of cancer include the following:

Self-examination for the early signs of cancer previously described is one method for detection of cancer. For example, women are encouraged to perform a monthly breast self-examination. Likewise, men are encouraged to perform a monthly testicular self-examination. If an abnormality is found, it can be further investigated with one of the following described methods.

Medical imaging techniques that visualize deep tissues for medical study are often used to detect cancers. Radiography (x-ray photography) often is used to detect the presence of tumours. *Mammography,* x-ray photography of a breast, is considered an important detection tool for this type of cancer. *Computed tomography (CT)* (x-ray scanning), *magnetic resonance imaging (MRI)* (electromagnetic scanning), and *ultrasonography* (ultrasound scanning) produce cross-sectional images of body regions suspected of having tumours.

CONNECT IT! 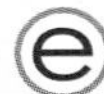

Check out ***Medical Imaging of the Body*** online at ***Connect It!*** to see diagrams of medical imaging technology and examples of the images produced by them.

Blood tests to determine the concentration of ions, enzymes, or other blood components are useful in detecting cancer when the results show abnormalities associated with particular forms of cancer. Cancer cells may also produce or trigger the production of substances often referred to as *tumour markers.* For example, tests for a number of cancer markers are now being used in conjunction with other diagnostic tests.

Biopsy is the removal and examination of living tissue. Microscopic examination of tumour tissue removed surgically or through a needle sometimes reveals whether it is malignant or benign.

The information gained from these techniques can be used to *stage* and *grade* malignant tumours. Staging involves classifying a tumour based on its size and the extent of its spread. Grading is an assessment of what the tumour is likely to do based on the degree of abnormality of the cells—a useful basis for making a prognosis (statement of probable outcome).

Without treatment, cancer usually results in death. The progress of a particular type of cancer depends on the type of cancer and its location. Many cancer patients develop *cachexia,* a syndrome involving loss of appetite, weight loss, and general weakness. Various anatomical or functional abnormalities may arise as a result of damage to particular organs. The ultimate causes of death in cancer patients include secondary infection by pathogenic microorganisms, organ failure, haemorrhage (blood loss), and in some cases, undetermined factors.

Of course, once cancer has been identified, every effort is made to treat it and thus prevent or delay its progress. Surgical removal of cancerous tumours is sometimes performed, but the probability that malignant cells have been left behind must be addressed. **Chemotherapy,** or "chemical therapy" with *cytotoxic* (cell-killing) compounds or antineoplastic drugs, can be used after surgery to destroy any remaining malignant cells. **Radiation therapy,** also called *radiotherapy,* involves the use of destructive x-ray or gamma radiation alone or with chemotherapy to destroy any remaining cancer cells. **Laser therapy,** in which an intense beam of light destroys a tumour, is also sometimes coupled with chemotherapy or radiation therapy.

CONNECT IT! 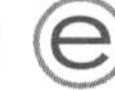

Immunotherapy is a cancer treatment that bolsters the body's own defences against cancer cells or introduces cancer antibodies into the body. Because viruses cause some types of cancer, oncologists hope that vaccines against certain forms of cancer will greatly reduce cancer risk. Learn more about this topic at ***Immunotherapy*** online at ***Connect It!***

Perhaps the most promising research area in the battle against cancer is *molecular oncology.* This rapidly growing medical specialty attempts to use advances in molecular biology and genetics to develop so-called *rational drugs* that, unlike conventional chemotherapy agents, target only those specific molecules, enzymes, receptors, or other features unique to cancer cells or tumour growth. Ideally, such treatments would affect only the cancer and spare normal cells and body functions, thus increasing efficiency and reducing side effects. Three of the most promising new classes of "rational" drugs used to treat various types of cancer include the following:

Monoclonal antibodies, for example, trastuzumab for breast cancer and cetuximab for colorectal cancer

Antiangiogenesis (anti–blood vessel formation) *agents,* for example, vascular endothelial growth factor (VEGF) for various solid tumours

Tyrosine kinase inhibitors (enzyme inhibitors), for example, imatinib for chronic myeloid leukaemia

Some oncologists believe that future advances in rational drug design could mean for cancer what antibiotics meant for infectious diseases.

LANGUAGE OF SCIENCE *(continued from p. 137)*

mucous membrane (MYOO-kus)
[*muc-* **slime,** *-ous* **characterized by;** *membran-* **thin skin**]

muscle tissue (MUSS-el TISH-yoo)
[*mus-* **mouse,** *-cle* **small;** *tissu-* **fabric**]

nervous tissue (NERV-us TISH-yoo)
[*nervous* **relating to nerves;** *tissu-* **fabric**]

proteoglycan (PRO-tee-oh-GLYE-kan)
[*proteo-* **protein,** *-glycan* **polysaccharide** (from *-glyc-* **sweet**)]

serous membrane (SEE-rus)
[*sero-* **watery body fluid,** *-ous* **characterized by;** *membran-* **thin skin**]

synovial fluid (si-NO-vee-all)
[*syn-* **together,** *-ovi-* **egg (white),** *-al* **relating to;** *fluid* **flow**]

synovial membrane (si-NO-vee-all)
[*syn-* **together,** *-ovi-* **egg (white),** *-al* **relating to;** *membran-* **thin skin**]

LANGUAGE OF MEDICINE

anaplasia (an-ah-PLAY-zee-ah)
[*ana-* **without,** *-plas(m)-* **substance or form,** *-ia* **condition**]

benign (bee-NYNE)
[benign **kind**]

biopsy (BYE-op-see)
[*bio-* **life,** *-ops-* **view,** *-y* **act of**]

carcinogen (kar-SIN-oh-jen)
[*carcino-* **cancer,** *-gen* **produce**]

carcinoma (kar-si-NO-mah)
[*carcin-* **cancer,** *-oma* **tumour**]

chemotherapy (kee-moh-THAYR-ah-pee)
[*chemo-* **chemical,** *-therapy* **treatment**]

hyperplasia (hye-per-PLAY-zee-ah)
[*hyper-* **excessive,** *-plas(m)-* **substance or form,** *-ia* **condition**]

immunotherapy (im-yoo-no-THAYR-ah-pee)
[*immuno-* **free,** *-therapy* **treatment**]

keloid (KEE-loyd)
[*kel-* **claw,** *-oid* **like**]

laser therapy (LAY-zer THAYR-ah-pee)
[*laser* **shortened "light amplification by stimulated emission of radiation"**]

malignant (mah-LIG-nant)
[*malign* **bad**]

metastasis (meh-TAS-tah-sis)
[*meta-* **change,** *-stasis* **standing**]

metastasize (meh-TAS-tah-size)
[*meta-* **change,** *-stas-* **standing,** *-ize* **make**]

mutagen (MYOO-tah-jen)
[*muta-* **change,** *-gen* **produce**]

neoplasm (NEE-oh-plaz-em)
[*neo-* **new,** *-plasm* **formation**]

oncogene (ON-koh-jeen)
[*onco-* **tumour,** *-gen-* **produce**]

pericarditis (pair-ih-kar-DYE-tis)
[*peri-* **around,** *-cardi-* **heart,** *-itis* **inflammation**]

peritonitis (pair-i-toh-NYE-tis)
[*peri-* **around,** *-ton-* **to stretch,** *-itis* **inflammation**]

pleurisy (PLOOR-i-see)
[*pleur-* **side of body,** *-isy* **condition**]

radiation therapy (ray-dee-AY-shun THAYR-ah-pee)
[*radiat-* **to emit rays,** *-tion* **process;** *therapy* **treatment**]

regeneration (ree-jen-er-AY-shun)
[*re-* **again,** *generat-* **produce,** *-tion* **process**]

rhabdomyolysis (RAB-doh-mye-OL-ih-sis)
[*rhabdo-* **rod,** *-myo-* **muscle,** *-lysis* **loosening**]

sarcoma (sar-KOH-mah)
[*sarco-* **flesh,** *-oma* **tumour**]

tumour (TYOO-mer)
[*tumour* **swelling**]

tumour suppressor gene (TYOO-mer soo-PRESS-or jeen)
[*tumour* **swelling;** *suppress-* **press down,** *-or* **agent;** *gen-* **produce** or **generate**]

case study

Nathan had been mountain biking for about 2 hours, winding his way up and down the familiar trails with a devil-may-care attitude. Pedalling at a breakneck speed, he swerved around a fallen branch as he headed down the last steep incline, and suddenly he lost control and went flying off his bike. After rolling over a couple of times, he stopped hard, jamming his foot against a boulder. His friends helped him limp the rest of the way down the hill and back to their car; then they drove him to Accident and Emergency at the local hospital.

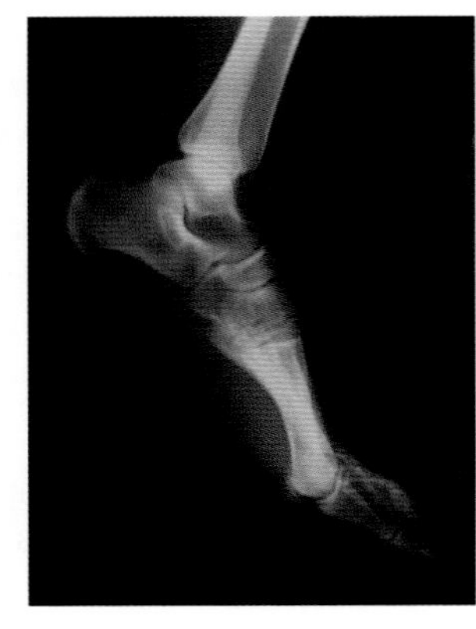

The specialty registrar ordered an x-ray film of Nathan's leg and foot to confirm no break in the bones. She came back soon with the results and told Nathan that there was no break, just "soft tissue damage" (i.e., a sprained ankle). By "soft tissue", she meant the tendons and ligaments (connective tissues) that hold all the bones of the foot and ankle together.

1. Nathan was fortunate that his tissue damage was limited to epithelial and connective tissue. Had he incurred damage to muscle or nerve tissue, how would that have affected his recovery?
   a. Haemorrhaging would be reduced thereby aiding recovery
   b. Keloids would develop if there were muscle and nerve damage
   c. Muscle and nerve tissue have limited regenerative capabilities, thus causing permanent damage
   d. No rehabilitation would be required as nerve and muscle tissue heals rapidly

In addition to spraining his ankle, Nathan cut his arm in the fall. He had a deep gash that required five stitches to close.

2. What type of membrane did the stitches go through?
   a. Cutaneous
   b. Serous
   c. Mucous
   d. Epidermal
3. In the membrane through which the stitches passed, which layer connects the epithelial layer to the connective tissue layer?
   a. Membrane glue
   b. Basement membrane
   c. Intercellular membrane
   d. Epithelial-connective lamina
4. The specialty registrar informed Nathan that because of his medical history and depth of the gash, he may develop a keloid rather than a normal scar. How does a keloid differ from a normal scar?
   a. A keloid is an inflamed region around an existing fibrous mass (scar)
   b. Keloids result from minor scratches on the skin's surface, whereas a scar is the result of damage to the lower layer of the skin
   c. A scar typically forms a limited, slightly raised area at the wound site, whereas a keloid is an unusually thick scar that may expand well beyond the original injury site
   d. Keloids are mucous excretions that develop from normal scars

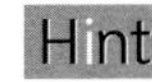
To solve a case study, you may have to refer to the glossary or index, other chapters in this textbook, ***Connect It!,*** and other resources.

CHAPTER SUMMARY

To download an MP3 version of the chapter summary for use with your mobile device, access the ***Audio Chapter Summaries*** *online at evolve.elsevier.com.*

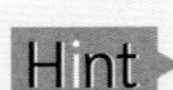

Scan this summary after reading the chapter to help you reinforce the key concepts. Later, use the summary as a quick review before your class or before a test.

Introduction to Tissues

A. Tissue—group of similar cells that perform a common function
B. Matrix—nonliving intercellular material
C. Principal types of tissue (**Table 8-1**)
   1. Epithelial tissue
   2. Connective tissue
   3. Muscle tissue
   4. Nervous tissue
D. Embryonic development of tissues (**Figure 8-1**)
   1. Primary germ layers
      a. Endoderm
      b. Mesoderm
      c. Ectoderm
   2. Histogenesis—the process of the primary germ layers differentiating into different kinds of tissue

Extracellular Matrix (ECM)

A. Fluid environment of the body—complex, nonliving material between cells in a tissue (**Figure 8-2**)
   1. Some tissues have a large amount of ECM; other tissues have hardly any ECM
   2. Different kinds of components give ECM in different tissues a variety of characteristics
B. Components of the ECM (**Table 8-2**)
   1. Water
   2. Proteins and proteoglycans
      a. Collagen
         (1) Collagenous fibres—twisted ropes of collagen that form strong, flexible bundles (**Figure 8-3**)
         (2) Reticular fibres—thin reticulin (collagen III) fibres form a delicate 3D network to support structures
         (3) Basal lamina—collagen IV forms a flat, screenlike framework that links to the base of epithelial cells and to the fibroreticular fibres (collagen) in the underlying connective tissue to form a gluelike basement membrane

b. Elastin—stretchy elastic fibres made of elastin that impart the ability to recoil (**Figure 8-5**)
c. Glycoproteins and proteoglycans
(1) Glycoproteins are proteins with a few carbohydrate attachments
(2) Fibronectin and laminin help connect the ECM components to cells by binding with integrins in plasma membranes
(3) Glycoprotein attachments also allow local communication within a tissue
(4) Proteoglycans are hybrid molecules that are mostly carbohydrates attached to a protein backbone
(5) Examples of proteoglycans: chondroitin sulphate, heparan sulphate, and hyaluronate
(6) Different proteoglycans give different characteristics to ECM, such as thickness and shock absorption (**Table 8-2**)

C. Holding tissues together
1. ECM helps bind tissues together structurally
a. ECM components bind to each other and to integrins in plasma membranes of cells
b. In some tissues, it is primarily intercellular junctions that hold cells together
2. ECM element provides local communication among ECM components and various cells—through connection via integrins in plasma membranes

Tissue Repair

A. Tissues have a varying capacity to repair themselves; damaged tissue regenerates or is replaced by scar tissue
B. Regeneration—growth of new tissue (**Figure 8-6**)
C. Scar—dense, fibrous mass; unusually thick scar is a keloid (**Figure 8-7**)
D. Epithelial and connective tissues have the greatest ability to regenerate
E. Muscle and nervous tissues have limited capacity to regenerate

Body Membranes

A. Thin tissue layers that cover surfaces, line cavities, and divide spaces or organs (**Figure 8-8**, **Table 8-3**)
B. Epithelial membranes are most common type (**Figure 8-9**)
1. Cutaneous membrane (skin)
a. Primary organ of integumentary system
b. One of the most important organs
c. Comprises approximately 16% of body weight
2. Serous membrane (serosa)
a. Parietal membranes—line closed body cavities
b. Visceral membranes—cover visceral organs
c. Pleura—surrounds a lung and lines the thoracic cavity
d. Peritoneum—covers the abdominal viscera and lines the abdominal cavity
3. Mucous membrane (mucosa)
a. Lines and protects organs that open to the exterior of the body
b. Found lining ducts and passageways of the respiratory, digestive, and other tracts
c. Lamina propria—fibrous connective tissue underlying mucous epithelium
d. Mucus
(1) Made up mostly of water and mucins—proteoglycans that form a double-layer protection against environmental microbes (**Figure 8-12**)
(2) Produced by goblet cells (**Figure 8-10**)
(3) Propelled by motile cilia (**Figure 8-11**)

C. Connective tissue membranes
1. Do not contain epithelial components
2. Synovial membranes—line the spaces between bone in joints
3. Have smooth and slick membranes that secrete synovial fluid
4. Help reduce friction between opposing surfaces in a movable joint
5. Synovial membranes also line bursae

The Big Picture: Tissues, Membranes, and the Whole Body

A. Tissues and membranes maintain homeostasis
1. Epithelial tissues
a. Form membranes that contain and protect the internal fluid environment
b. Absorb nutrients
c. Secrete products that regulate functions involved in homeostasis
2. Connective tissues
a. Hold organs and systems together
b. Form structures that support the body and permit movement
3. Muscle tissues
a. Work with connective tissues to permit movement
4. Nervous tissues
a. Work with glandular epithelial tissue to regulate body function

REVIEW QUESTIONS

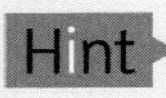

Write out the answers to these questions after reading the chapter and reviewing the Chapter Summary. Note—writing out your answers will consolidate learning and provide a valuable resource of information.

1. Define the term *tissue* and identify the four principal tissue types.
2. What is the function of the primary germ layers? Name them.
3. Describe the regenerative capacity of muscle and nerve tissues.
4. Name the two major categories or types of body membranes. Give examples of each.
5. What is a neoplasm?
6. Compare epithelial to connective tissue. Use these criteria: cell spacing, blood supply, presence of matrix, ability to regenerate.

CRITICAL THINKING QUESTIONS

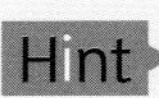

After finishing the Review Questions, write out the answers to these more in-depth questions to help you apply your new knowledge. Go back to sections of the chapter that relate to concepts that you find difficult.

1. A baby was born with congenital problems in the skeletal and muscular system. From what primary germ layers do these systems arise? What is the earliest possible developmental stage during which a problem could have affected just one primary germ layer?
2. Many athletes work to reduce their body fat to the lowest possible percentage. What would happen if too little body fat were present?
3. Develop a flowchart or other diagram to describe the process by which tissues respond to injury.
4. If a small but deep cut involving skin and muscle occurs, predict which tissue will probably heal first and which will heal more completely. Explain your answer.
5. When a joint swells, sometimes it is necessary to remove a thick colourless liquid from the joint. What is it, where did it come from, and what is its normal function?
6. The zygote ultimately gives rise to all cells in your body, including the highly specialized cells of your nervous system. Decribe this transition, discussing the steps and processes that lead to these specialized cells.

9 Tissue Types

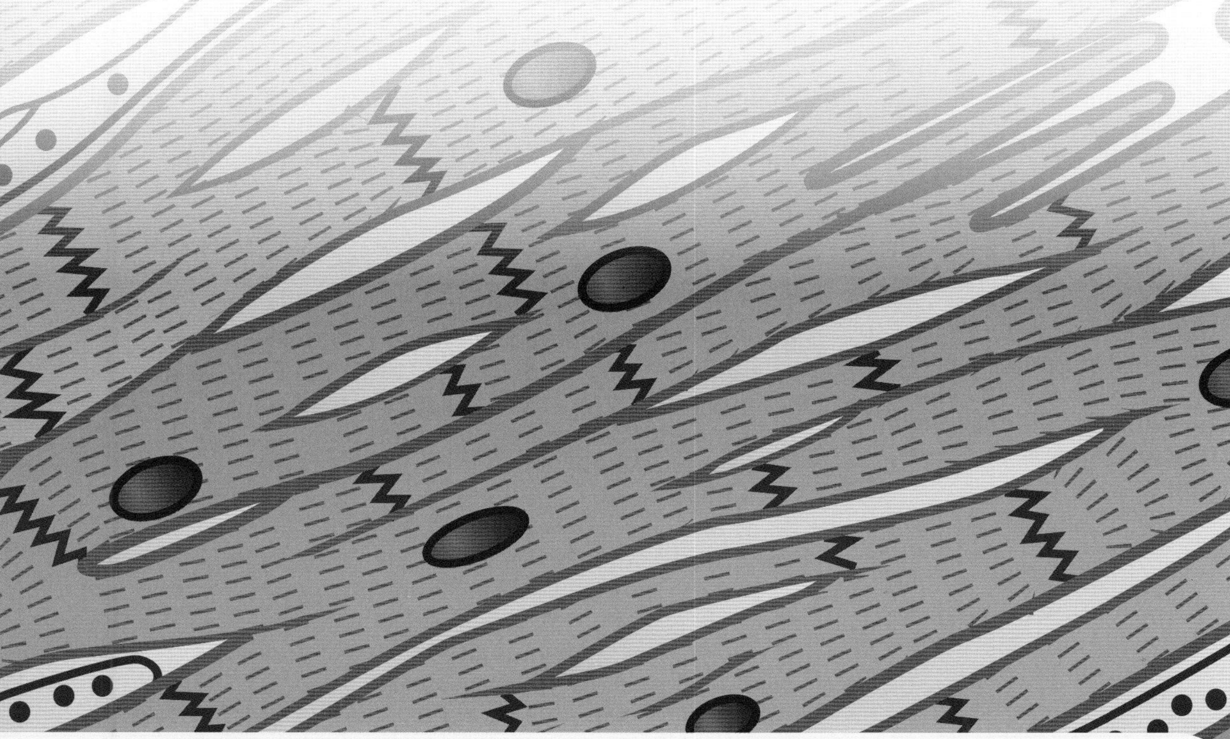

CHAPTER OUTLINE

Hint ▸ *Scan this outline before you begin to read the chapter, as a preview of how the concepts are organized.*

In the previous chapter, you learned that tissues can be thought of as the fabric of the body, which is "sewn together" to form the organs of the body and to hold all the organs together as a whole. Now that you understand the role of tissues in the body and general characteristics of the four main tissue types, you are ready to survey the specific subtypes that you will encounter later in your study of human anatomy and physiology. Learning the essential characteristics of these human tissue types now will make it far easier to understand concepts that you will explore in later chapters.

CONNECT IT! 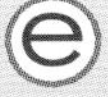

This brief survey of histology involves many images made with microscopes of various types. Refer to ***Tools of Microscopic Anatomy*** online at ***Connect It!*** for an overview of the types of microscopy used in this chapter.

LANGUAGE OF SCIENCE

Hint ▸ *Use this list to aid your pronunciation of unfamiliar words.*

absorption (ab-SORP-shun)
[*ab-* **from,** *-sorp-* **suck,** *-tion* **process**]

adipocyte (AD-i-poh-syte)
[*adipo-* **fat,** *-cyte* **cell**]

adipose tissue (AD-i-pohs)
[*adipo-* **fat,** *-ose* **full of,** *tissu-* **fabric**]

alveolar (al-VEE-oh-lar)
[*alveo-* **hollow,** *-ola-* **little,** *-ar* **relating to**]

areolar (ah-REE-oh-lar)
[*are-* **open space,** *-ola-* **little,** *-ar* **relating to**]

avascular (ah-VAS-kyoo-lar)
[*a-* **without,** *-vas-* **vessel,** *-ula-* **little,** *-ar* **relating to**]

axon (AK-son)
[*axon* **axle**]

canaliculus (kan-ah-LIK-yoo-lus)
[*canal-* **channel,** *-iculi* **little**]
pl., canaliculi

cancellous bone tissue (KAN-seh-lus)
[*cancel-* **lattice,** *-ous* **characterized by,** *tissu-* **fabric**]

cardiac muscle tissue (KAR-dee-ak)
[*cardia-* **heart,** *-ac* **relating to,** *mus-* **mouse,** *-cle* **small,** *tissu-* **fabric**]

chondrocyte (KON-droh-syte)
[*chondro-* **cartilage,** *-cyte* **cell**]

cilium (SIL-ee-um)
[*cili-* **eyelid,** *-um* **thing (eyelash)**]
pl., cilia

collagenous dense fibrous tissue (koh-LAJ-eh-nus dense FYE-brus TISH-yoo)
[*colla-* **glue,** *-gen* **produce,** *dense* **thick,** *fibr-* **thread or fibre,** *-ous* **relating to,** *tissu-* **fabric**]

columnar (koh-LUM-nar)
[*column-* **column,** *-ar* **relating to**]

compact bone tissue (kom-PAKT)
[*compact* **to put together,** *tissu-* **fabric**]

compound
[*compound* **put together**]

connective tissue (koh-NEK-tiv TISH-yoo)
[*con-* **together,** *-nect-* **bind,** *-ive* **relating to,** *tissu-* **fabric**]

cuboidal (KYOO-boyd-al)
[*cub-* **cube,** *-oid* **like,** *-al* **relating to**]

dendrite (DEN-dryte)
[*dendr-* **tree,** *-ite* **part (branch) of**]

continued on p. 173

EPITHELIAL TISSUE

Types and Locations of Epithelial Tissue

Epithelial tissue, or **epithelium,** often is subdivided into two types: (1) **membranous** (covering or lining) epithelium and (2) **glandular** epithelium. Membranous epithelium covers the body and some of its parts and lines the serous cavities (pleural, pericardial, and peritoneal), the blood and lymphatic vessels, and the respiratory, digestive, and genitourinary tracts. Membranous epithelium is often called *surface epithelium*. Glandular epithelium is grouped in solid cords or hollow follicles and tubes that form the secretory units of endocrine and exocrine glands.

Functions of Epithelial Tissue

Epithelial tissues have a widespread distribution throughout the body and serve several important functions:

Protection. Generalized protection is the most important function of membranous epithelium. It is the relatively tough and impermeable epithelial covering of the skin that protects the body from mechanical and chemical injury and also from invading bacteria and other disease-causing microorganisms.

Sensory functions. Epithelial structures adapted for sensory functions are found in the skin, nose, eye, and ear.

Secretion. Glandular epithelium is adapted for secretory activity. Secretory products include hormones, mucus, digestive juices, and sweat.

Absorption. The lining epithelium of the gut and respiratory tract allows for the absorption of nutrients from the gut and the exchange of respiratory gases between air in the lungs and the blood.

Excretion. The unique epithelial lining of kidney tubules makes the excretion and concentration of excretory products in the urine possible.

Generalizations About Epithelial Tissue

Most epithelial tissues are characterized by extremely limited amounts of intercellular, or matrix, material. This explains their characteristic appearance, when viewed under a light microscope, of a continuous sheet of cells packed tightly together. With the electron microscope, however, narrow spaces—about 20 nm wide—can be seen around the cells. These spaces, like other intercellular spaces, contain **interstitial fluid (IF).**

Epithelial tissues generally renew themselves throughout life. The presence of stem cells in most epithelial tissues allows epithelium to continuously produce new cells of various types.

Sheets of epithelial cells make up the surface layer of skin and mucous and serous membranes. Epithelial cells exhibit a characteristic called **polarity,** meaning that they have two opposite faces. The *basal* pole faces underlying connective tissue and the *apical* pole at the free surface of the sheet faces outward. The basal poles of epithelial cells adhere to an underlying layer of connective tissue by means of an adhesive, permeable layer of extracellular matrix (ECM) called the *basement membrane (BM)* (see **Figure 8-4** on p. 143).

Epithelial tissues contain no blood vessels. As a result, epithelium is said to be **avascular** (*a,* "without"; *vascular,* "vessels"). Hence oxygen and nutrients must diffuse from capillaries in the underlying connective tissue through the permeable basement membrane to reach living epithelial cells.

At intervals between adjacent epithelial cells, their plasma membranes are modified to hold the cells together. These complex intercellular structures, such as **desmosomes** and **tight junctions,** are described in Chapter 5.

Epithelial cells can reproduce themselves. They frequently go through the process of cell division. Because epithelial cells in many locations undergo considerable wear and tear, this fact has practical importance. It means, for example, that new cells can replace old or destroyed epithelial cells in the skin or in the lining of the gut or respiratory tract.

Classification of Epithelial Tissue

Membranous Epithelium

Classification Based on Cell Shape

The shape of membranous epithelial cells may be used for classification purposes. Four cell shapes, called **squamous, cuboidal, columnar,** and **pseudostratified columnar,** are used in this classification scheme (**Figure 9-1**).

Squamous (Latin, "scaly") cells are flat and platelike. Cuboidal cells, as the name implies, are cube-shaped and have more cytoplasm than the scalelike squamous cells do. Columnar epithelial cells have more height than width and thus appear narrow and cylindrical.

Pseudostratified columnar epithelium has only one layer of oddly shaped columnar cells. Although each cell touches the basement membrane, the tops of some pseudostratified cells do not fully extend to the surface of the membrane. Also, some nuclei are near the "top" of the cell and some near the "bottom" of the cell—rather than all nuclei being near the bottom. The result is a false *(pseudo)* appearance of layering, or stratification, when only a single layer of cells is present.

Classification Based on Layers of Cells

In most cases the location and function of membranous epithelium determine whether its cells will be stacked and layered or arranged

TABLE 9-1 Classification Scheme for Membranous Epithelial Tissues

SHAPE OF CELLS*	TISSUE TYPE
One Layer	
Squamous	Simple squamous
Cuboidal	Simple cuboidal
Columnar	Simple columnar
Pseudostratified columnar	Pseudostratified columnar
Several Layers	
Squamous	Stratified squamous
Cuboidal	Stratified cuboidal
Columnar	Stratified columnar
(Varies)	Transitional

*In the top layer (if more than one layer is present in the tissue).

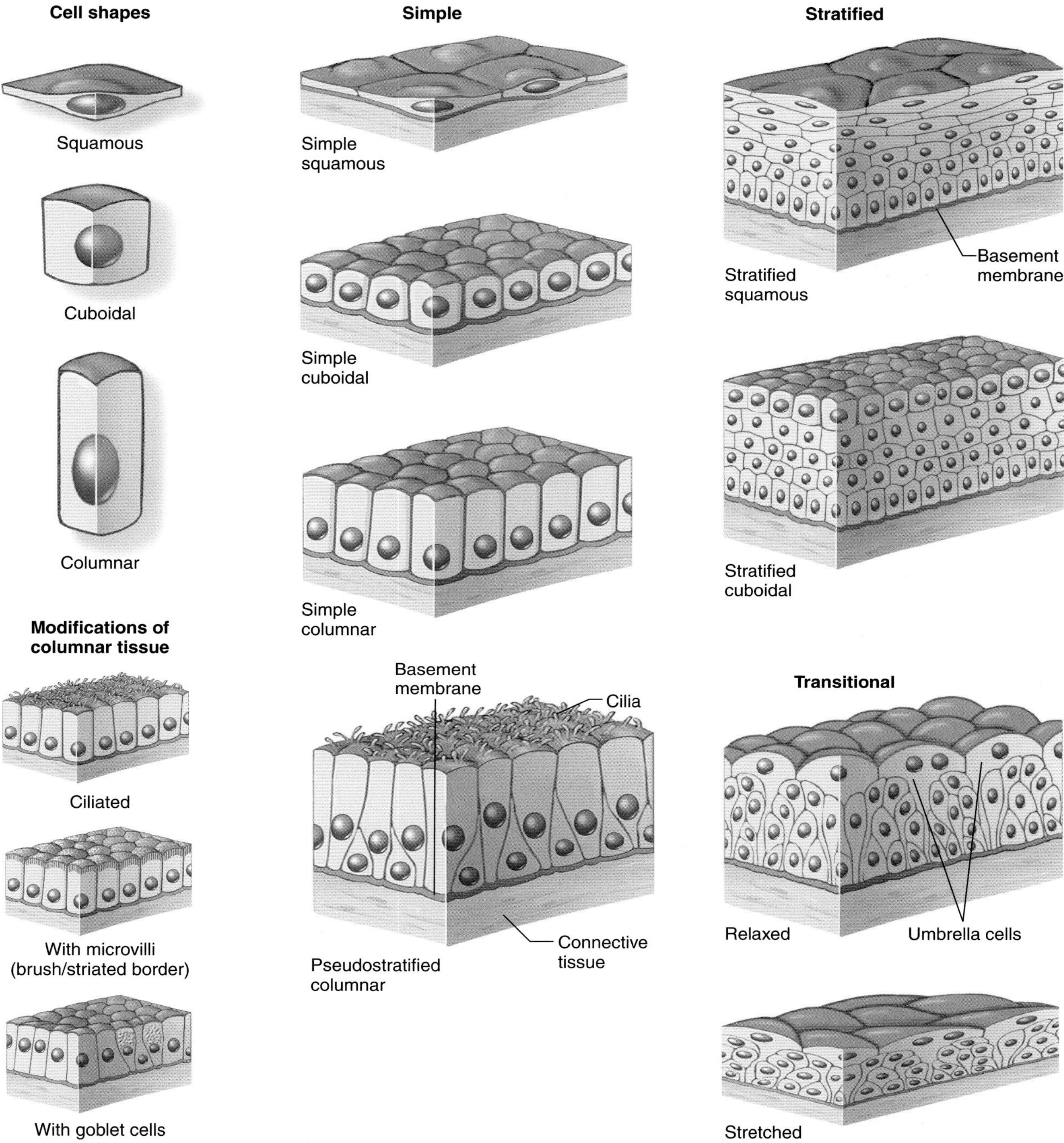

FIGURE 9-1 Classification of epithelial tissues. The tissues are classified according to the shape and arrangement of cells. The colour scheme of these drawings is based on a common staining technique used by histologists called *haematoxylin and eosin (H&E)* staining. H&E staining usually renders the cytoplasm pink and the chromatin inside the nucleus a purplish colour. The cellular membranes, including the plasma membrane and nuclear envelope, do not usually pick up any stain and thus may be transparent. (See **Box 8-4** for information on cross-sections of membranous tissues.)

in a sheet one cell layer thick. An arrangement of epithelial cells in a single layer is called **simple epithelium.** If epithelial cells are layered one on another, the tissue is called **stratified epithelium. Transitional epithelium** (described later) is a unique arrangement of differing cell shapes in a stratified, or layered, epithelial sheet.

If membranous or covering epithelium is classified by the shape and layering of its cells, the specific types listed in **Table 9-1** are possible. Note that stratified tissue types are named for the shape of cells in their top layer only. Each type is described in the paragraphs that follow, and selected examples are illustrated in **Figures 9-2** to **9-9**. Additional examples can be found in Part 5 of the Brief Atlas of the Human Body.

Simple Epithelium. **Simple squamous epithelium** consists of only one layer of flat, scalelike cells (**Figure 9-2**). Consequently, substances can readily diffuse or filter through this type of tissue. The

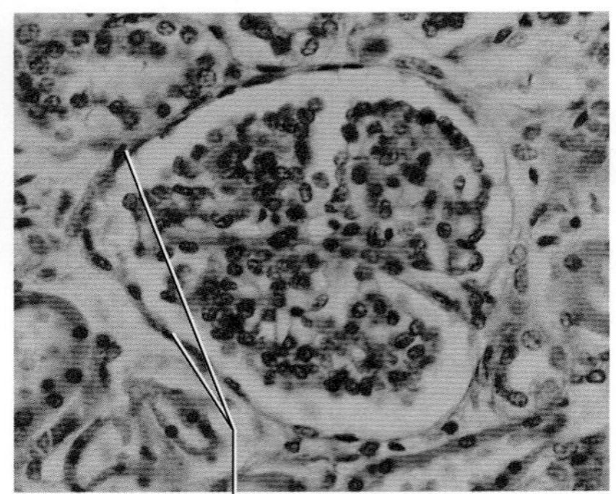

FIGURE 9-2 Simple squamous epithelium. Photomicrograph of the Bowman (glomerular) capsule of the kidney showing thin simple squamous epithelium. Note how the haematoxylin and eosin (H&E) staining (see **Figure 9-1**) renders the cytoplasm of each cell pink and each nucleus a purplish colour. The outlines of cellular membranes are transparent in the photomicrograph.

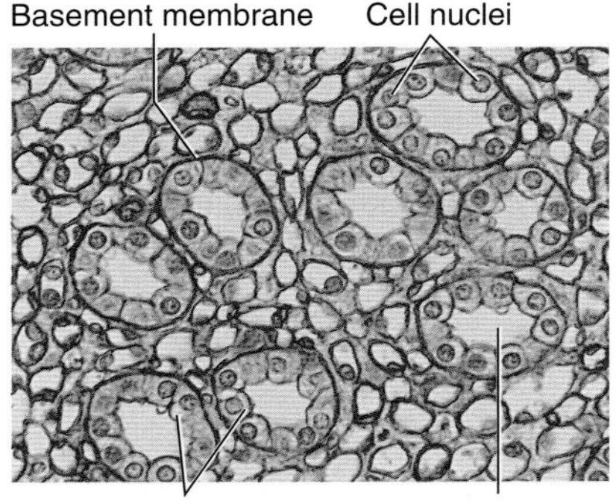

FIGURE 9-4 Simple cuboidal epithelium. Photomicrograph of kidney tubules showing the single layer of cuboidal cells touching a basement membrane. Note the cuboidal cells that enclose the tubule opening (lumen).

microscopic air sacs (alveoli) of the lungs, for example, are composed of this kind of tissue, as are the linings of blood and lymphatic vessels and the surfaces of the pleura, pericardium, and peritoneum (**Figure 9-3**). (Blood and lymphatic vessel linings are called **endothelium,** and the surfaces of the pleura, pericardium, and peritoneum are called **mesothelium.** Some histologists classify these linings as connective tissue because of their embryological origin.)

Simple cuboidal epithelium is composed of one layer of cuboidal cells resting on a basement membrane (**Figure 9-4**). This type of epithelium is seen in many types of glands and their ducts. It is also found in the ducts and tubules of other organs, such as the kidney.

Simple columnar epithelium composes the surface of the mucous membrane that lines the stomach, intestine, uterus, uterine tubes, and parts of the respiratory tract (**Figure 9-5**). It consists of a single layer of cells, many of which have a modified structure. Three common modifications are goblet cells, cilia, and microvilli (see **Figure 9-1**).

Goblet cells have large, secretory vesicles that give them the appearance of a goblet. Compare the goblet cells labelled in **Figure 9-5** with those in **Figure 8-10** and in Figures 5-6, 5-7, and 5-8 in the Brief Atlas of the Human Body. The vesicles contain **mucus,** which goblet cells produce in great quantity and secrete onto the surface of the epithelial membrane. Mucus is a solution of water, electrolytes, and proteoglycans that can have many different functions, such as lubrication and protection.

Recall from Chapter 5 that **cilia** are microscopic cell extensions, each supported internally by a cylindrical arrangement of microtubules. Cilia are sensory organs of a cell that detect changes, such as the presence of certain chemicals, outside the cell. The microtubule system inside the cilia can also produce movement by the action of molecular motors.

In the intestine, for example, the plasma membranes of many columnar cells extend out in hundreds and hundreds of microscopic fingerlike projections called **microvilli.** Microvilli are much shorter and much more numerous than cilia. By greatly increasing the surface area of the intestinal mucosa, microvilli make it especially well suited for absorbing nutrients and fluids from the intestine.

Pseudostratified columnar epithelium is found lining the air passages of the respiratory system and certain segments of the male reproductive system, such as the urethra (**Figure 9-6**). Although appearing to be stratified, only a single layer of irregularly shaped columnar cells touches the basement membrane. The cells are of differing heights, and many are not tall enough to reach the upper surface of the epithelial sheet. This fact, coupled with placement of cell nuclei at odd and irregular levels in the cells, gives a false (pseudo) impression of stratification. Mucus-secreting goblet cells are numerous, and cilia are present.

In the respiratory system, the cilia of simple columnar and pseudostratified epithelium lining air passages detect the presence of contaminants in a thin layer of tacky mucus. In response, the cilia

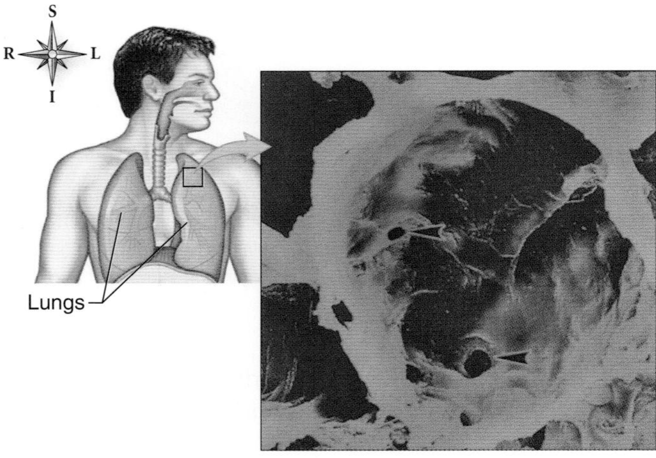

FIGURE 9-3 Simple squamous lining of the lung. The tiny air sacs of the lung, which are called *alveoli,* are lined with a thin layer of simple squamous epithelium. This thin epithelium, shown clearly in the scanning electron micrograph in the inset, allows for easy diffusion of oxygen and carbon dioxide across the walls of the alveoli. *Arrowheads* indicate pores that allow air to pass from one alveolus to another.

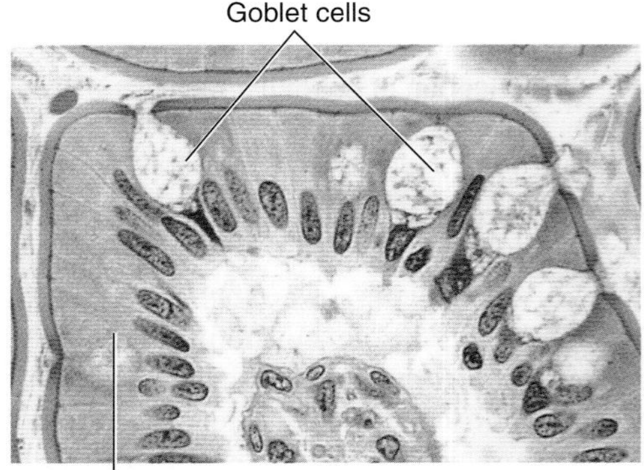

FIGURE 9-5 Simple columnar epithelium. Photomicrograph of simple columnar epithelium. Note the goblet, or mucus-producing, cells present.

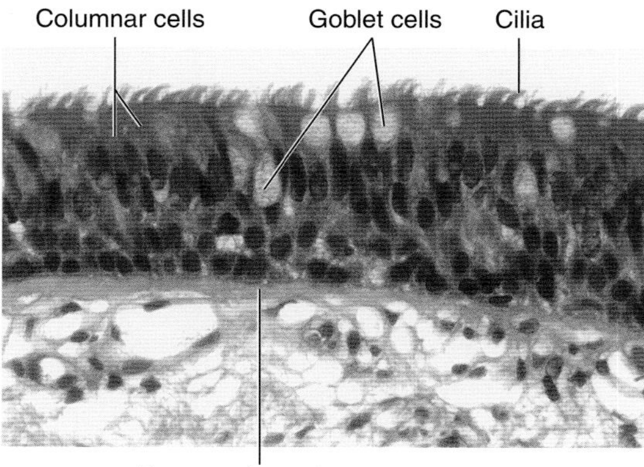

FIGURE 9-6 Pseudostratified columnar epithelium. This photomicrograph from the respiratory system shows that each irregularly shaped columnar cell touches the underlying basement membrane. Placement of cell nuclei at irregular levels in the cells gives a false (pseudo) impression of stratification. This tissue is ciliated—note the "fuzz" along the outer edge of the cells.

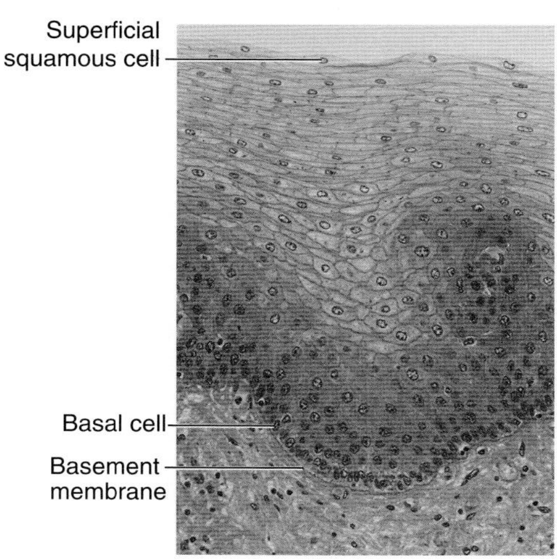

FIGURE 9-8 Nonkeratinized stratified squamous epithelium. Photomicrograph of the lining of the oesophagus. Each cell in the layer is flattened near the surface and attached to the sheet. No flaking of dead cells from the surface occurs. All cells have nuclei. Compare with **Figure 9-7**.

move together in the same direction over the free surface of the epithelium—pushing the mucus film. As a result, dust particles and other contaminants in the inspired air trapped by the mucus are moved toward the mouth and away from the delicate lung tissues.

Stratified Epithelium. **Stratified squamous epithelium** is characterized by multiple layers of cells with typically flattened squamous cells at the free, or outer, surface of the epithelial sheet (**Figure 9-7**).

In *keratinized* stratified squamous epithelium, the presence of tough keratin fibres in the squamous cells contributes to the protective qualities of skin covering the body surface. Details of the histology of this type of epithelium are presented in Chapter 10.

Nonkeratinized stratified squamous epithelium is found lining the vagina, mouth, and oesophagus (**Figure 9-8**). Its free surface is moist, and the outer epithelial cells, unlike those found in the skin, do not contain keratin. This type of epithelium serves a protective function.

Stratified cuboidal epithelium also serves a protective function. Typically, two or more rows of low cuboidal cells are arranged randomly over a basement membrane. Stratified cuboidal epithelium can be located in the sweat gland ducts, in the pharynx, and over parts of the epiglottis.

Stratified columnar epithelium has multiple layers of columnar cells, with only the most superficial cells being obviously columnar in appearance. It is a protective type of epithelium found in only a few places in the human body. It is located in segments of the male urethra and in the mucous layer near the anus.

Transitional epithelium is a stratified tissue typically found in body areas that are subjected to stress and tension changes, such as the wall of the urinary bladder (**Figure 9-9**). Because it lines part of the urinary tract, it is also called *urothelium*.

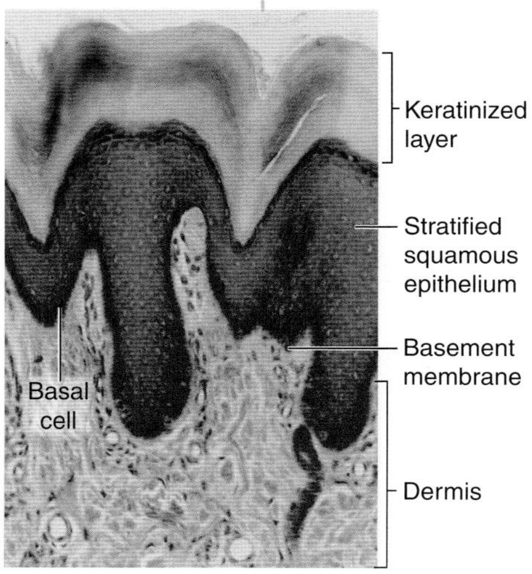

FIGURE 9-7 Keratinized stratified squamous epithelium. Photomicrograph of the thick skin showing cells becoming progressively flattened and scalelike as they approach the surface and are lost. The outer surface (keratinized layer) of this epithelial sheet contains many flattened cells that have lost their nuclei.

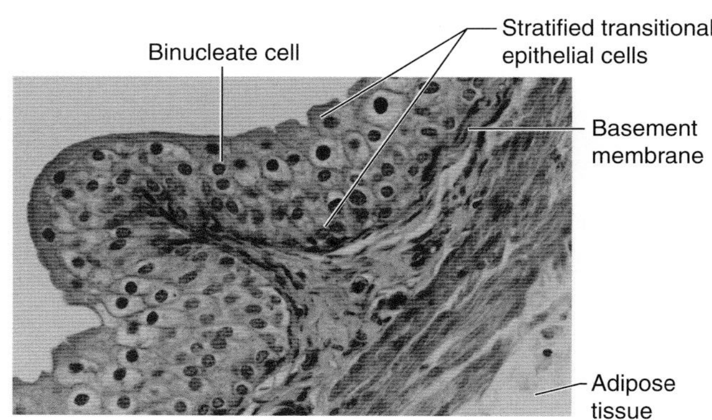

FIGURE 9-9 Transitional epithelium. Photomicrograph from the urethra showing that its cell shape is variable from cuboidal to squamous. Several layers of cells are present. Intermediate and surface cells do not touch the basement membrane.

TABLE 9-2 Epithelial Tissues

TISSUE	LOCATION	FUNCTION
Membranous		
Simple squamous	Alveoli of lungs	Absorption by diffusion of respiratory gases between alveolar air and blood
	Lining of blood and lymphatic vessels (called endothelium; classified as connective tissue by some histologists)	Absorption by diffusion, filtration, and osmosis
	Surface layer of the pleura, pericardium, and peritoneum (called *mesothelium*; classified as connective tissue by some histologists)	Absorption by diffusion and osmosis; also, secretion
Stratified squamous (Nonkeratinized; Keratinized)	*Nonkeratinized:* Surface of the mucous membrane lining the mouth, oesophagus, and vagina	Protection
	Keratinized: Surface of the skin (epidermis)	Protection
Transitional (Relaxed; Stretched)	Surface of the mucous membrane lining the urinary bladder and ureters	Permits stretching Protection
Simple columnar (Without surface specialization; With microvilli (brush/striated border); Ciliated; With goblet cells)	Surface layer of the mucous lining of the stomach, intestines, and part of the respiratory tract	Protection Secretion Absorption Moving of mucus (by ciliated columnar epithelium)
Pseudostratified columnar	Surface of the mucous membrane lining the trachea, large bronchi, nasal mucosa, and parts of the male reproductive tract (epididymis and vas deferens); lines the large ducts of some glands (e.g., parotid)	Protection
Simple cuboidal	Ducts and tubules of many organs, including the exocrine glands and kidneys	Secretion Absorption
Stratified cuboidal/columnar	Ducts of the sweat glands and mammary glands; lining of the pharynx; covering some of the epiglottis; lining portions of the male urethra	Protection
Glandular		
	Glands	Secretion

In many instances, 10 or more layers of cuboidal cells of varying shapes are present in the absence of stretching or tension. Cells in the apical (surface) layer are often called *umbrella cells* because of their wide, curving apical surface. Umbrella cells may have more than one nucleus. As tension increases, the epithelial sheet is expanded, the number of observable cell layers decreases, and cell shape changes from roughly cuboidal to squamous in appearance. Note in **Figure 9-1** how the umbrella cells flatten out when stretched. This ability of transitional epithelium to stretch protects the bladder wall and other distensible structures that it lines from tearing when stretched with great force.

The major types of epithelium are summarized in **Table 9-2**.

Glandular Epithelium

Epithelium of the glandular type is adapted for secretory activity. Regardless of the secretory product produced, glandular activity depends on complex and highly regulated cellular activities requiring the expenditure of stored energy.

Unlike the single or layered cells of membranous epithelium typically found in protective coverings or linings, glandular epithelial cells may function singly as **unicellular glands,** or they may function in clusters, solid cords, or hollow follicles as **multicellular glands.** Glandular secretions may be discharged into ducts, into the lumen of hollow visceral structures, onto the body surface, or directly into the blood.

All **glands** in the body can be classified as either exocrine or endocrine glands. **Exocrine glands,** by definition, discharge their secretion products into ducts. The salivary glands are typical exocrine glands. The secretion product (saliva) is produced in the gland and then discharged into a duct that transports it to the mouth. **Endocrine glands** are often called *ductless glands* because they discharge their secretion products (hormones) directly into blood or interstitial fluid. The pituitary, thyroid, and adrenal glands are typical endocrine glands.

Structural Classification of Exocrine Glands

Multicellular exocrine glands are most often classified by structure, with the shape of their ducts and the complexity (branching) of their duct systems used as distinguishing characteristics. Shapes include **tubular** and **alveolar** (saclike). Simple exocrine glands have only one duct leading to the surface, and **compound** exocrine glands have two or more ducts. **Table 9-3** describes some of the major structural types of exocrine glands. **Figure 9-10** shows examples of exocrine glands in the lining of the stomach.

Functional Classification of Exocrine Glands

In addition to structural differences, exocrine glands also differ in the method by which they discharge their secretion products from the cell. Using these functional criteria, three types of exocrine glands may be identified (**Figure 9-11**):

1. Apocrine
2. Holocrine
3. Merocrine

Apocrine glands collect their secretory products near the apical face of the cell and then release them into a duct by pinching

TABLE 9-3 Structural Classification of Multicellular Exocrine Glands

SHAPE*	COMPLEXITY†	TYPE	EXAMPLE
Tubular (single, straight) (Duct; Secretory cells)	Simple	Simple tubular	Intestinal glands
Tubular (coiled)	Simple	Simple coiled tubular	Sweat glands
Tubular (multiple)	Simple	Simple branched tubular	Gastric (stomach) glands
Alveolar (single)	Simple	Simple alveolar	Sebaceous (skin oil) glands
Alveolar (multiple)	Simple	Simple branched alveolar	Sebaceous glands
Tubular (multiple)	Compound	Compound tubular	Mammary glands
Alveolar (multiple)	Compound	Compound alveolar	Mammary glands
Some tubular; some alveolar	Compound	Compound tubulo-alveolar	Salivary glands

*Shape of the distal secreting units of the gland.

†Number of ducts reaching the surface.

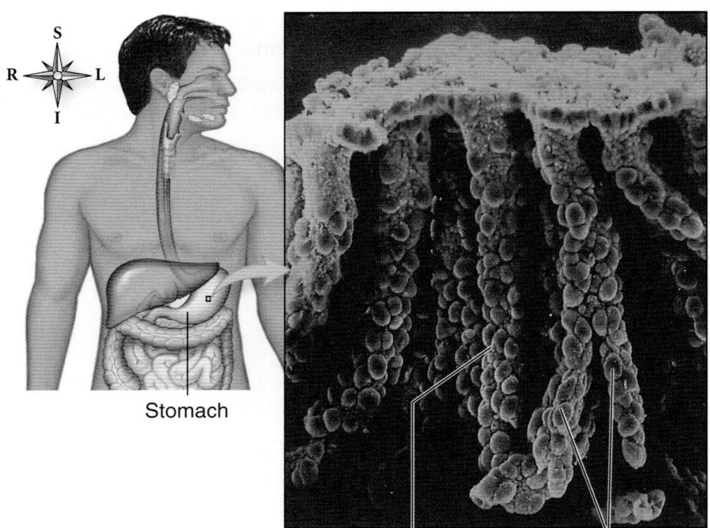

FIGURE 9-10 Exocrine glands in the stomach. The inset shows a scanning electron micrograph of exocrine glands, called gastric glands, in the lining of the stomach. These glands produce gastric juice—a mixture of water, mucus, enzymes, acid, and other substances.

a vesicle off the distended end. This process results in some loss of cytoplasm and damage to the cell. Recovery and repair of cells are rapid, however, and continued secretion occurs. The milk-producing mammary glands are examples of apocrine-type glands, as are some sweat glands.

Holocrine glands—such as the sebaceous glands that produce oil to lubricate the skin—collect their secretory product inside the cell and then rupture completely to release it. These cells literally self-destruct to complete their function.

Merocrine glands discharge their secretion product directly through the cell or plasma membrane. This discharge process is completed without injury to the plasma membrane and without loss of cytoplasm. Only the secretion product passes from the glandular cell into the duct. Most secretory cells are of this type. The salivary glands are examples of merocrine-type exocrine glands.

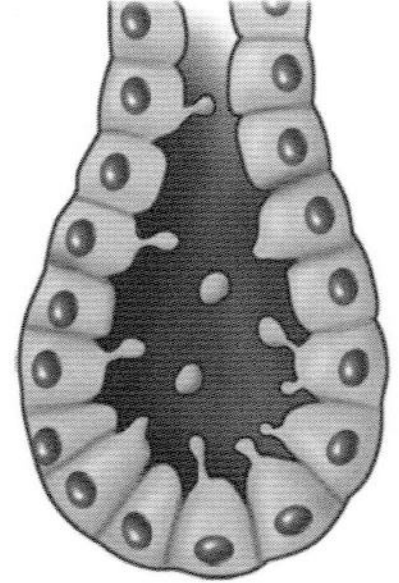

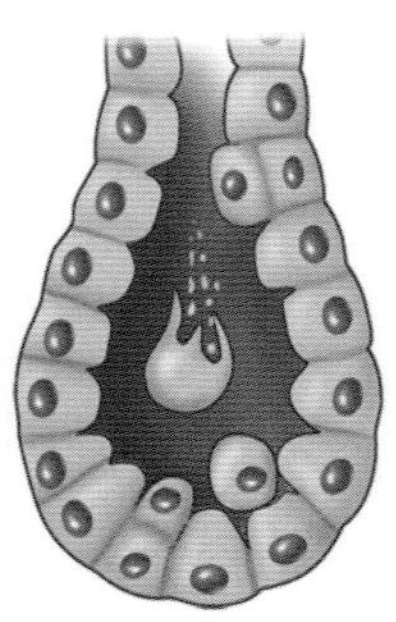

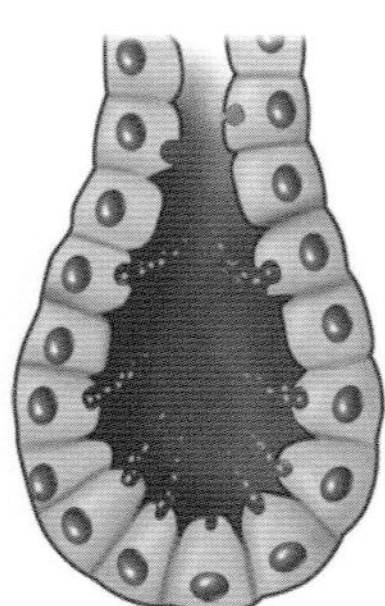

FIGURE 9-11 Three types of exocrine glands. Exocrine glands may be classified by the method of secretion.

Quick CHECK

1. List at least three functions of epithelial tissue.
2. What are the three basic shapes of epithelial cells?
3. Distinguish between a simple epithelial tissue and a stratified epithelial tissue.
4. How do exocrine glands secrete their products?

CONNECTIVE TISSUE

Connective tissue is one of the most widespread and diverse tissues in the body and is found in or around nearly every organ of the body. Connective tissue arises during embryonic development from stem cell tissue called *mesenchyme,* most of which originates in the mesoderm (primary germ layer). Connective tissue exists in more varied forms than the other three basic tissues do. Among the types that we will discuss are delicate tissue paper webs, tough resilient cords, rubbery elastic sheets, rigid bones, and a fluid (blood).

Functions of Connective Tissue

Connective tissue connects, supports, transports, and defends. It connects tissues to each other, for example. It also connects muscles to muscles, muscles to bones, and bones to bones. It forms a supporting framework for the body as a whole and for its organs individually. One kind of connective tissue—blood—transports a large array of substances between parts of the body. And finally, several kinds of connective tissue cells even defend us against microorganisms and other invaders.

Characteristics of Connective Tissue

Connective tissue consists predominantly of extracellular matrix (ECM). Embedded in the matrix are relatively few cells. The ECM of connective tissues is made up of varying numbers and kinds of fibres, fluid, and perhaps other material sometimes called *ground substance.* The qualities of the ECM's fibres and other components largely determine the structural characteristics of each type of connective tissue. The matrix of blood, for example, is a fluid (plasma). It contains numerous blood cells but no fibres, except when it coagulates. Some connective tissues have the consistency of a soft gel, some are firm but flexible, some hard and rigid, some tough, others delicate—and in each case it is their matrix and extracellular fibres that make them so.

A connective tissue's extracellular matrix contains one or more of the following kinds of fibres: collagenous (or white), reticular, or elastic (or yellow). Fibroblasts and some other cells produce these protein fibres. Collagenous fibres are tough and strong (see **Figure 8-3** on p. 143), reticular fibres are delicate, and elastic fibres are extensible and elastic (see **Figure 8-5** on p. 144).

In addition to protein fibres, the matrix of connective tissues contains a number of *proteoglycans* made up of polysaccharide chains often containing *glucosamine* and bound to a protein core (see **Figure 8-2**). These chemicals make the matrix fluid thick enough to be a barrier to bacteria and other microbes. They also form a transparent lubricant and help hold the tissue together. Among the more notable of these compounds are *hyaluronic acid* and *chondroitin sulphate.*

Classification of Connective Tissue

Connective tissues have been classified by histologists in several different ways. Usually they are placed in different categories or types according to the structural characteristics of the intercellular material. The classification scheme we have adopted here is widely used and includes most of the major types:

1. Fibrous (connective tissue proper)
   a. Loose fibrous (areolar)
   b. Adipose
   c. Reticular
   d. Dense
      (1) Irregular
      (2) Regular
         (a) Collagenous
         (b) Elastic
2. Bone
   a. Compact
   b. Cancellous (spongy)
3. Cartilage
   a. Hyaline
   b. Fibrocartilage
   c. Elastic
4. Blood

Fibrous tissues, also called *connective tissue proper,* such as loose fibrous connective, adipose, reticular, and dense fibrous tissues have many fibres in the ECM as their predominant feature. The type and arrangement of extracellular fibres are what distinguish members of the group from one another. Bone is considered a separate category of connective tissue because it has fibres and a hard mineralized ECM. Cartilage is yet another category because besides fibres, it has a type of ECM that traps water to form a firm gel. Blood, the last category listed, is characterized by the lack of fibres in its matrix.

These major types of connective tissues are described further in the following pages and in **Table 9-4**. Illustrations of many of these connective tissue types can be found adjacent to their descriptions and in Part 5 of the Brief Atlas of the Human Body.

Fibrous Connective Tissue

Loose Fibrous Connective Tissue (Areolar)

Loose fibrous connective tissue, shown in **Figure 9-12**, is sometimes called *areolar tissue.* It is loose because it is stretchable and ordinary because it is one of the most widely distributed of all tissues. *Areolar* was the early name for the loose fibrous connective tissue that connects many adjacent structures of the body. It acts like a glue spread between them—but an elastic glue that permits movement. The word **areolar** means "like a small space" and refers to the bubbles that appear as areolar tissue is pulled apart during dissection.

The matrix of loose fibrous connective tissue is a soft, thick gel mainly because it contains hyaluronic acid (see **Table 8-2** on p. 142). An enzyme, hyaluronidase, can change the matrix from its thick gel state to a watery consistency. Physicians have made use of this knowledge for many years. They often inject a commercial preparation of hyaluronidase with drugs or fluids. By decreasing the viscosity (thickness) of intercellular material, the enzyme hastens diffusion and absorption of the injected material and lessens tissue tension and pain. Some bacteria, notably *pneumococci* and *streptococci,* spread through connective tissues by secreting hyaluronidase.

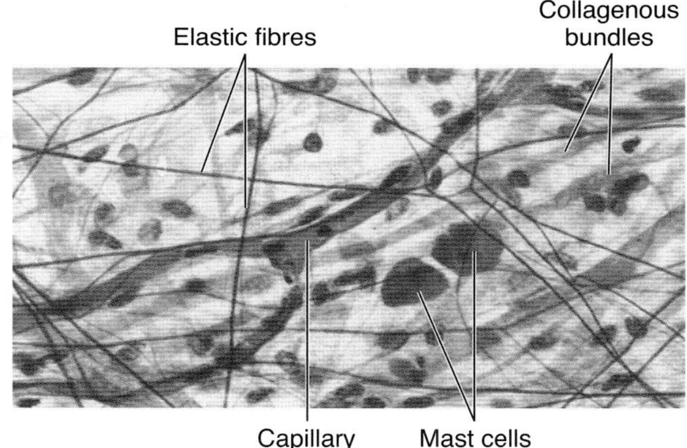

FIGURE 9-12 Loose fibrous (areolar) connective tissue. Note how the haematoxylin and eosin (H&E) staining (see **Figure 9-1**) renders the bundles of collagen fibres a pinkish colour and the elastin fibres and cell nuclei a darker, purplish colour. Compare the loose arrangement of fibres here with fibres in **Figures 9-17**, **9-18**, and **9-20**.

The matrix of loose fibrous connective tissue contains numerous fibres and cells, typically many interwoven collagenous and elastic fibres and about a half dozen kinds of cells (**Figure 9-13**). **Fibroblasts** are usually present in the greatest numbers in loose fibrous connective tissue, and **macrophages** are second. Fibroblasts synthesize the gel-like ground substance and the fibres present in it. Macrophages carry

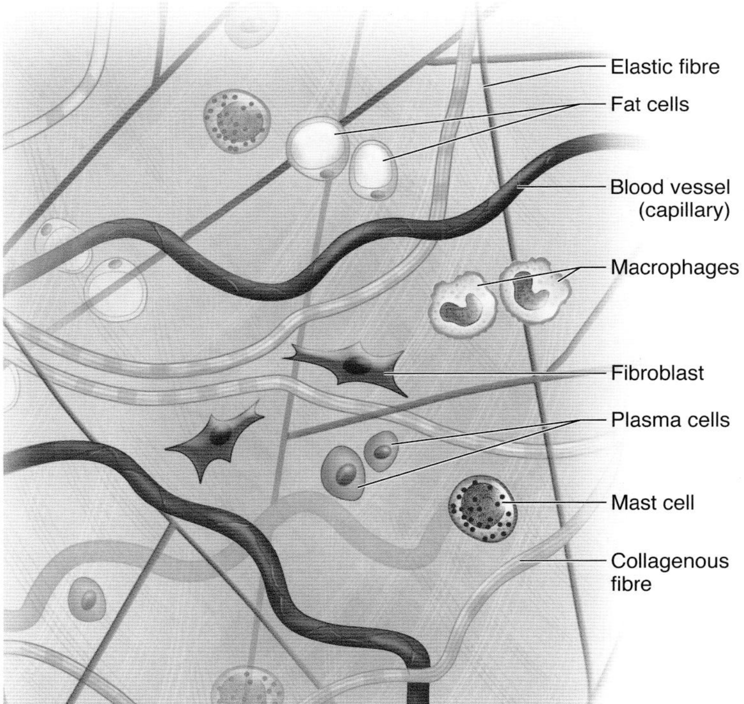

FIGURE 9-13 Diagram of loose fibrous (areolar) connective tissue. This artist's sketch illustrates the fact that loose fibrous connective tissue includes a number of different extracellular matrix (ECM) components such as collagenous fibres and elastic fibres, as well as a variety of different cell types.

TABLE 9-4 Connective Tissues

TISSUE	LOCATION	FUNCTION
Fibrous		
Loose fibrous (areolar) 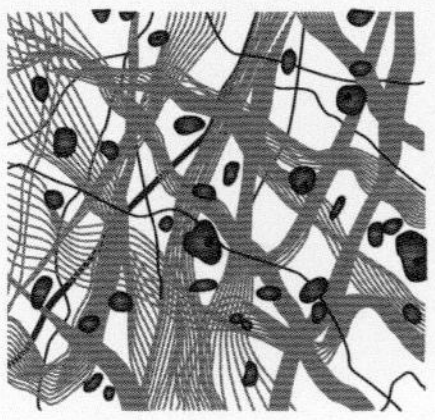	Between other tissues and organs Superficial fascia	Connection
Adipose (fat) 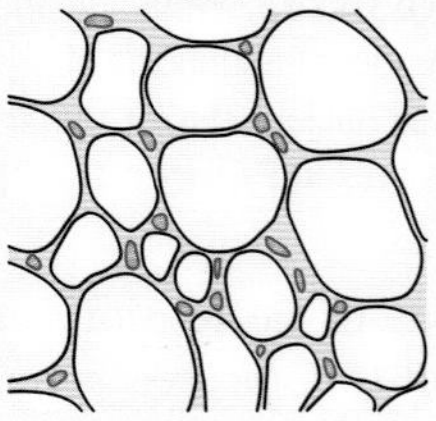	Under skin Padding at various points	Protection Insulation Support Energy reserves Heat production Regulation of other tissues
Reticular 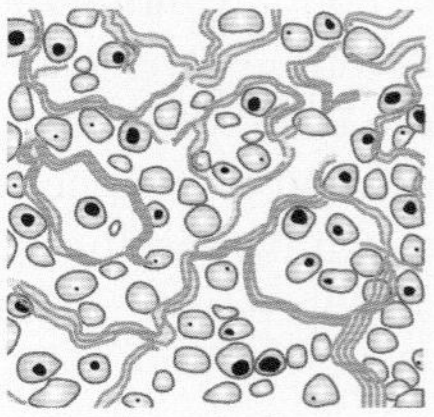	Inner framework of spleen, lymph nodes, bone marrow	Support Filtration Blood production Immunity
Dense Fibrous		
Irregular 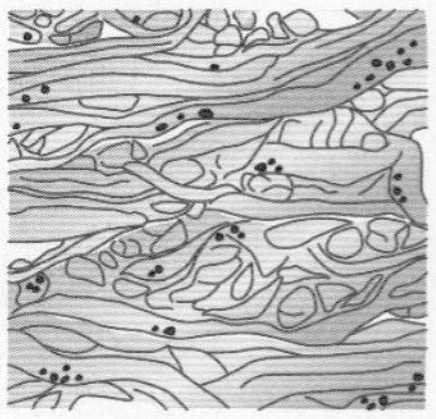	Deep fascia Dermis Scars Capsule of kidney, spleen, lymph nodes, etc.	Connection Support
Regular collagenous 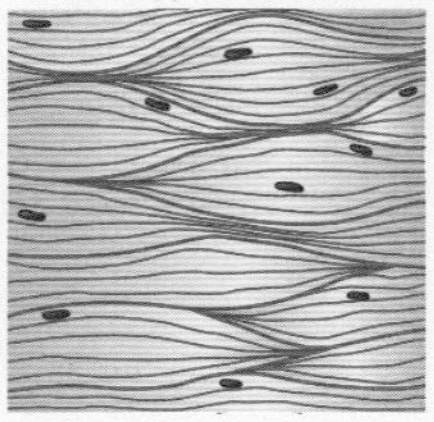	Tendons Ligaments Aponeuroses	Flexible but strong connection
Elastic 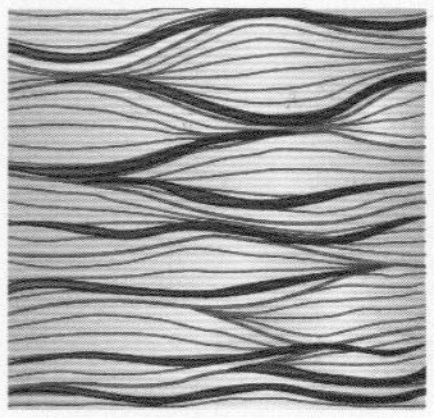	Walls of some arteries	Flexible, elastic support
Bone		
Compact bone 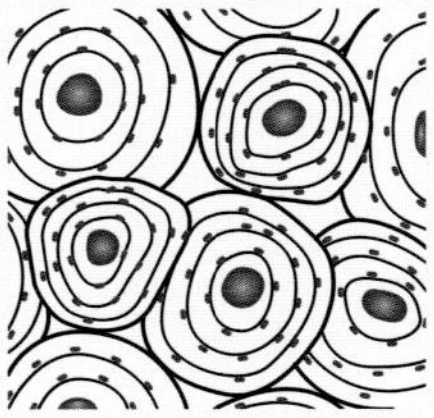	Skeleton (outer shell of bones)	Support Protection Calcium reservoir
Cancellous (spongy) bone 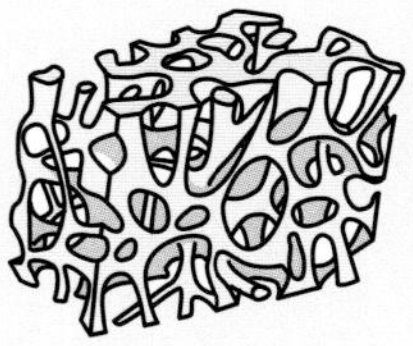	Skeleton (inside bones)	Support Provides framework for blood production
Cartilage		
Hyaline 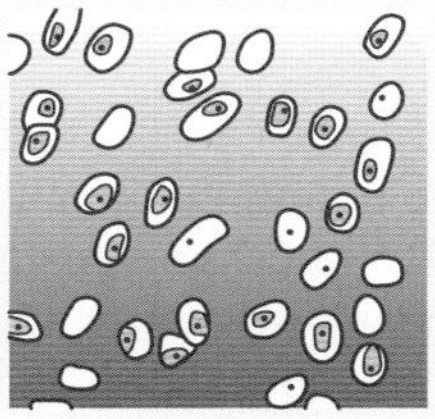	Part of nasal septum Covering articular surfaces of bones Larynx Rings in trachea and bronchi	Firm but flexible support; connection between structures
Fibrocartilage 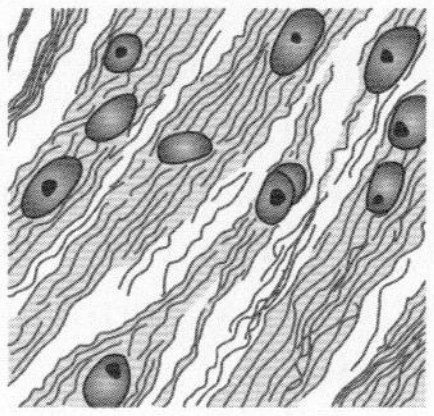	Discs between vertebrae Pubic symphysis	
Elastic 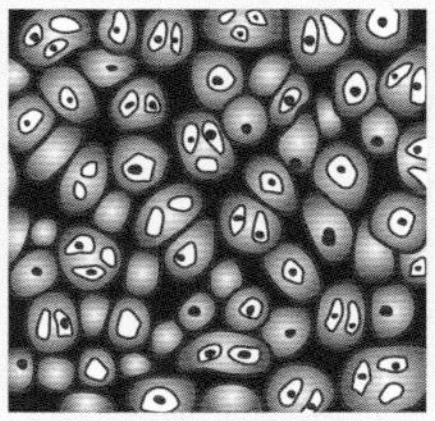	External ear Eustachian or auditory tube	
Blood		
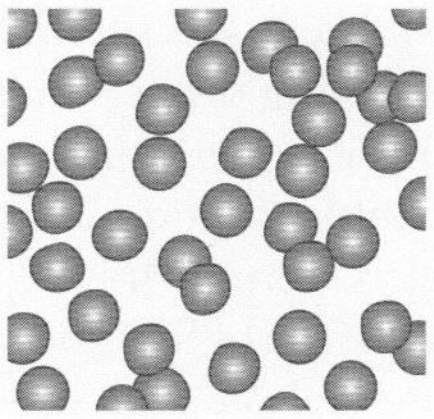	In the blood vessels	Transportation Protection

BOX 9-1 *health matters* | **Hay Fever and Asthma**

Mast cells in loose fibrous connective tissues are often involved in *allergic,* or *hypersensitivity,* reactions in local tissues. This is a type of inflammation (see ***Connect It!: Inflammation*** online) in response to *allergens,* which are substances that trigger such allergic responses. For example, the inflammation that you experience after a bee sting or when your skin is exposed to poison ivy are both examples of allergic or hypersensitivity reactions. Such reactions are triggered when mast cells encounter an allergen and release any of a group of chemical mediators.

For example, in hay fever (allergies to grasses and other plants), mast cells release the chemical **histamine.** Histamine increases the permeability of blood vessels in the nasal membranes, which in turn causes swelling in the lining of the nose. This gives us a "stuffy" feeling because the swelling makes it difficult to breathe easily. Histamine can also cause itchiness of the nose and eyes (see figure). The stuffiness and itchy eyes of hay fever can be relieved by antihistamines such as loratidine and fexofenadine, which block histamine's action.

On the other hand, a different mast cell product is responsible for the breathing difficulties in an asthma attack. In asthma, chemicals called *leukotrienes* trigger muscles in the walls of the respiratory tract to contract—thereby constricting the airways. Thus, leukotriene-blocking drugs such as montelukast and zileuton are used as third line agents when first line (inhaled beta 2 agonists) and second line (inhaled corticosteroids) are insufficient.

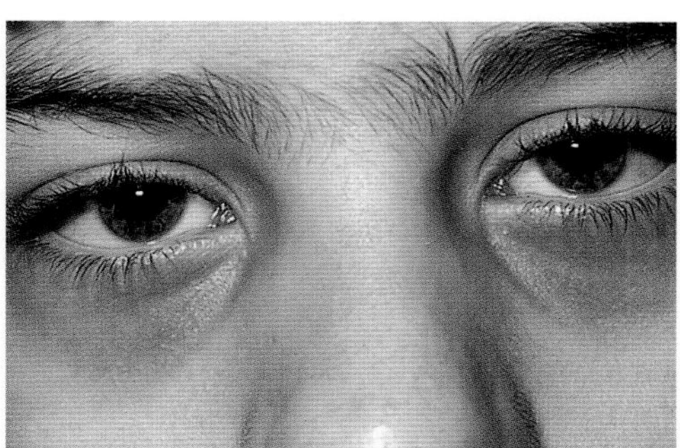

Allergic eyes. Some allergies cause itchiness and watering of the eyes, which may trigger frequent rubbing of the eyes, which produces these reddened features.

on *phagocytosis*, hence their name, which means "large eater". Phagocytosis is part of the body's vital collection of defence mechanisms.

Mast cells, also found in loose fibrous connective tissue, are capable of releasing a variety of molecules such as *histamine*, *heparin sulphate*, *leukotrienes*, and *prostaglandins*. These chemical mediators are released in response to exposure to substances from outside the body and produce a type of inflammation response (**Box 9-1**).

Other kinds of cells found in loose fibrous connective tissue are various forms of white blood cells (leucocytes) and some fat cells.

Adipose Tissue

Adipose tissue differs from loose fibrous connective tissue mainly in that it contains predominantly fat cells, also called **adipocytes,** and many fewer fibroblasts, macrophages, and mast cells (**Figure 9-14**). Each adipocyte typically has one large vesicle filled with stored triglycerides. This fat vesicle is so large that it pushes the cytoplasm of the cell outward against the plasma membrane as it stores more and more fat. This fat vesicle expands the entire cell to a huge size.

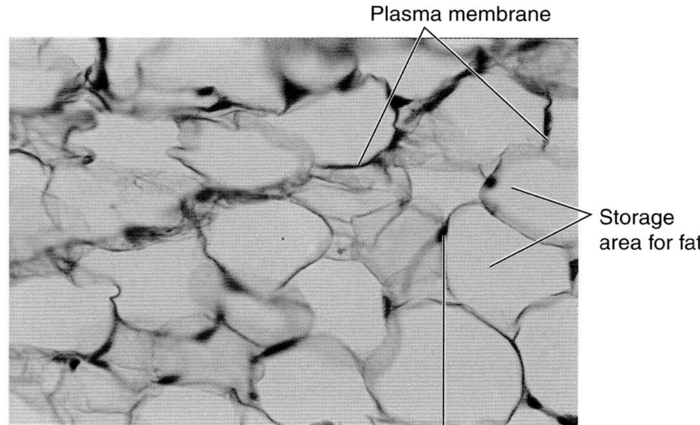

FIGURE 9-14 Adipose tissue. Note the large storage spaces for fat inside the adipose tissue cells in white fat.

The hormone *leptin* is released from adipocytes as they expand, signalling the brain and other tissues regarding how much fat is stored and ready to use for energy. The role of leptin is described further in Chapters 26 and 41.

The predominant form of adipose tissue is *white fat,* which serves mainly as an energy-storage depot for the body. White fat also acts as an insulating material to conserve body heat. Another role of white fat is to provide supporting, protective pads around the kidneys and various other structures. Because it is less dense than water, white fat increases buoyancy of the body when floating or swimming in water.

Brown fat is a far less abundant form of adipose tissue. The small polygon-shaped adipocytes in brown fat are able to use fat stored in many small vesicles to generate heat with their numerous mitochondria. This function is vital to the survival of newborns, who do not have enough muscle to generate enough heat by shivering. In adults, this fat-burning function may help regulate overall fat content of the body.

Beige fat is a region of white fat in which some of the adipocytes have "browned" or converted to the brown fat form. Near white fat adipocytes can detect changes in body temperature and signal the brown fat adipocytes to generate heat—thus supplementing the nervous system's feedback loop that helps maintain normal body temperature.

Figure 9-15 shows the location of the main fat storage areas in adults and how fat distribution varies between males and females. **Box 8-1** on p. 138 discusses body composition.

Reticular Tissue

A three-dimensional web—that is, a reticular network—identifies **reticular tissue** (**Figure 9-16**). The word *reticular* means "like a net". Slender, branching reticulin fibres with reticular cells overlying them compose the reticular meshwork. Branches of the cytoplasm of reticular cells follow the branching reticular fibres.

Reticular tissue forms the framework of the spleen, lymph nodes, and bone marrow. It is often called *marrow tissue* or *lymphoid tissue* in these locations. Reticular tissue functions as part of the body's

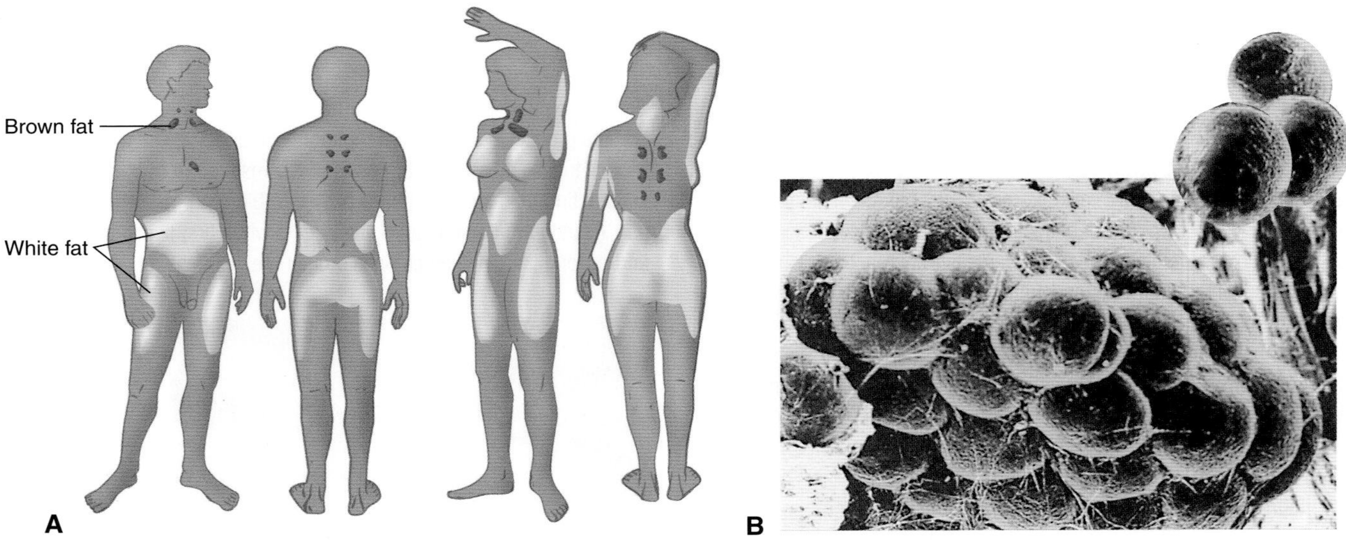

FIGURE 9-15 Fat distribution. A, The different distribution of fat in adult male and female bodies. **B,** Electron micrograph of a cluster of adipose cells in white fat held together by a network of fine reticular fibres (×150).

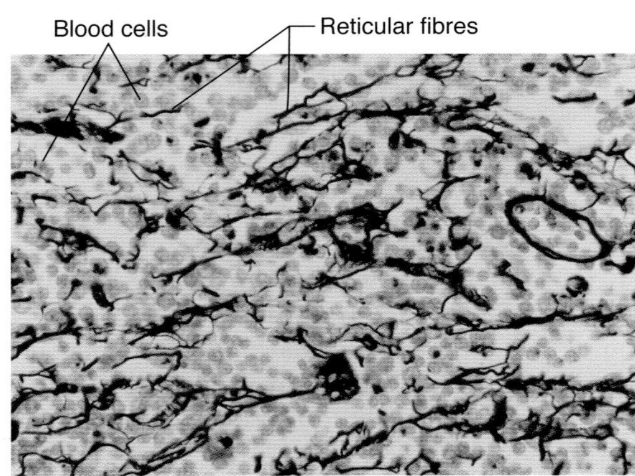

FIGURE 9-16 Reticular connective tissue. The supporting framework of reticular fibres are stained black in this section of lymph node.

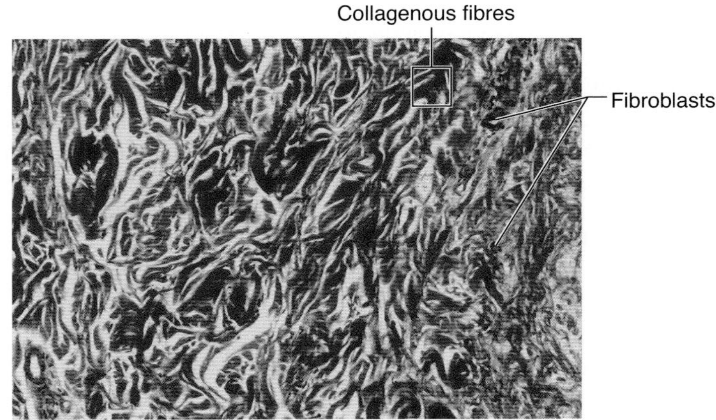

FIGURE 9-17 Dense irregular fibrous connective tissue. Section of skin (dermis) showing arrangements of collagenous fibres (pink) and purple-staining fibroblast cell nuclei.

complex mechanisms for producing blood cells and for defending itself against microorganisms and injurious substances. The reticular meshwork filters injurious substances out of the blood and lymph. Various types of reticular cells then phagocytose (engulf and destroy) the trapped substances. Another function of some reticular cells is to make reticular fibres.

Dense Fibrous Tissue

Dense fibrous tissue consists mainly of fibres packed densely in the matrix. It contains relatively few fibroblast cells. Some dense fibrous tissues are designated as *regular* and others are designated as *irregular*, depending on the arrangement of fibres.

Dense Irregular Fibrous Tissue

In dense irregular fibrous tissues, the bundles of collagenous fibres intertwine in irregular, swirling arrangements (**Figure 9-17**). This irregular pattern forms a thick mat of strong connective tissue that can withstand stresses applied from any direction. Dense irregular fibrous tissue forms the strong inner skin layer called the *dermis*. It also forms the outer capsule of such organs as the kidney and the spleen, as well as much of the fascia that surrounds muscles (**Box 9-2**).

Dense Regular Fibrous Tissue

In dense regular fibrous tissues, the bundles of fibres are arranged in regular, parallel rows. One form of dense regular fibrous tissue is predominantly bundles of collagenous fibres and may be called **collagenous dense regular fibrous tissue** (**Figure 9-18**). This type of fibrous tissue is flexible but possesses great tensile strength when pulled from either or both ends. These characteristics are desirable in structures that anchor muscle to bone, such as tendons (**Figure 9-19**). Ligaments (which connect bone to bone) instead have a predominance of elastic fibres. Hence ligaments exhibit some degree of elasticity.

Another form of dense (regular) fibrous tissue contains mostly elastic fibres and may be called **elastic dense regular fibrous tissue.**

BOX 9-2 *fascia*

The term **fascia** is a general name for the fibrous connective tissue masses that can be seen by the unaided eye in many locations throughout the body. The word *fascia* is Latin for "band". This literal translation is helpful because it summarizes the general structure and function of fascia: fibrous tissue that binds together the structures of the body.

Fascia is always some form of fibrous connective tissue and almost always features many collagenous fibres that are interwoven in an irregular arrangement. In some areas of the body, for example under the skin, fascia is mostly adipose tissue. In other areas, such as around some of the muscles, it is dense, irregular fibrous tissue. Often some of the fibres of fascia extend into the tissue of nearby organs, thus strongly binding to them.

For convenience, anatomists often distinguish between *superficial fascia,* which is just under the skin, and *deep fascia,* which extends well into the body and surrounds muscles, blood vessels, and other organs (see the figure). •

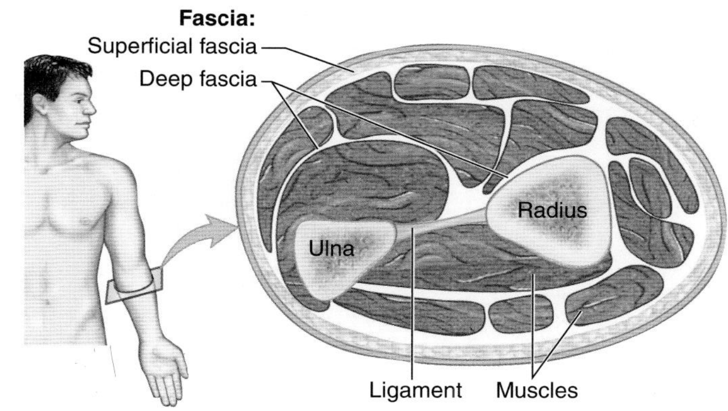

Fascia. Horizontal section of the forearm showing the superficial fascia under the skin and deep fascia below that, extending to surround the individual muscles.

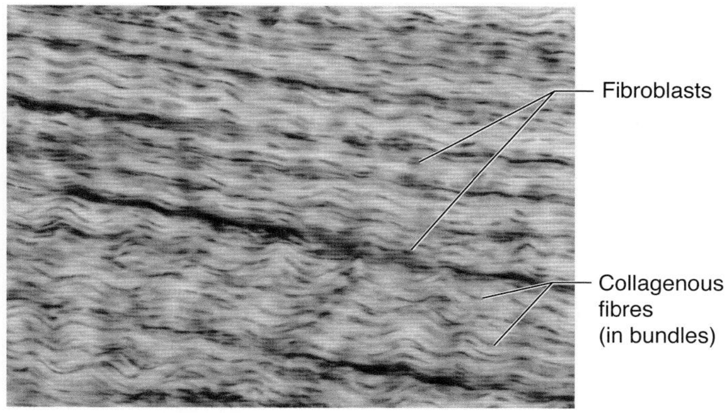

FIGURE 9-18 Collagenous dense regular fibrous connective tissue. Photomicrograph of tissue in a tendon. Note the multiple (regular) bundles of collagenous fibres arranged in parallel rows.

As you can see in **Figure 9-20**, elastic fibres in this type of tissue are in a parallel arrangement. In the walls of arteries, this arrangement permits the walls to be pushed out by blood pressure without breaking and then recoil to a smaller diameter when the blood pressure decreases.

Bone Tissue

Bone, or *osseous tissue,* is a rather unique form of very hard connective tissue. The mature cells of bone, **osteocytes,** are embedded in a unique matrix material containing both collagen fibres and mineral salt crystals. The inorganic mineral crystals make up about 66% of the total extracellular matrix. These mineral crystals are responsible for the hardness of bone.

Bones are the organs of the skeletal system. They provide support and protection for the body and serve as points of attachment for muscles. In addition, the calcified matrix of bones serves as a mineral reservoir for the body. A lattice made of bone also serves as the support for **red bone marrow,** which produces new blood cells.

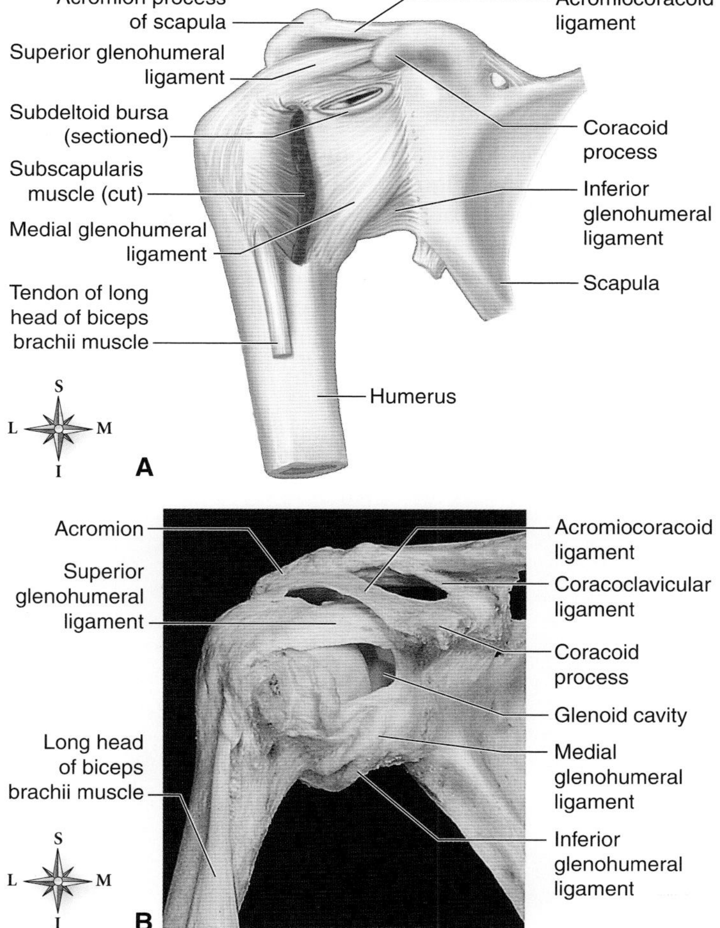

FIGURE 9-19 Tendons and ligaments. A, Tendons and ligaments of the shoulder are examples of dense fibrous connective tissue. **B,** Photo of cadaver dissection. Note the many strong connections needed to keep this important joint functioning properly.

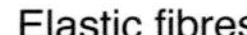

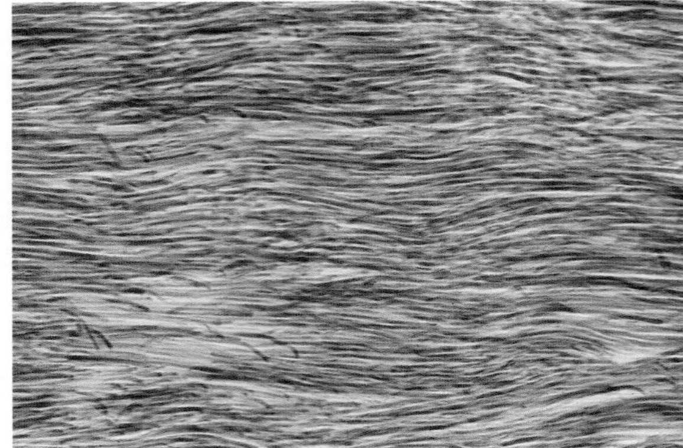

FIGURE 9-20 Elastic dense regular fibrous connective tissue. Note the roughly parallel arrangement of short, darkly stained elastic fibres.

Certain bones called **membrane bones** (e.g., flat bones of the skull) are formed within membranous tissue, whereas others (e.g., long bones such as the humerus) are formed indirectly through replacement of cartilage in a process called **endochondral ossification** (**Figure 9-21**). The details of bone formation are presented in Chapter 11.

Compact Bone Tissue

The type of bone tissue that forms the hard shell of a bone is called **compact bone tissue** (**Figure 9-22**). The basic organizational or structural unit of compact bone is the microscopic **osteon,** or *haversian system* (**Figure 9-23**). Osteocytes, or bone cells, are located in small spaces, or **lacunae,** which are arranged in concentric layers of bone matrix called **lamellae.** Small canals called **canaliculi** connect each lacuna and osteocyte with nutrient blood vessels found in the central, or haversian, canal.

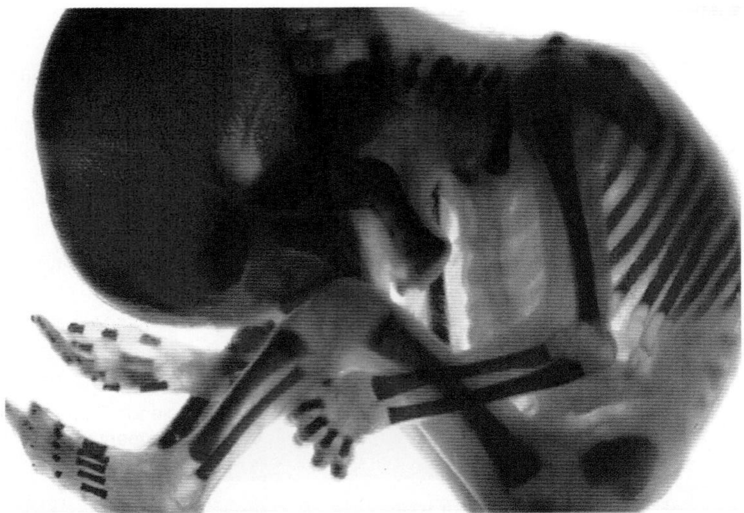

FIGURE 9-21 Ossification of the skeleton. The darkly stained areas of mineralization seen in this 14-week-old fetus show how the cartilage and membrane skeleton is beginning to develop into bone.

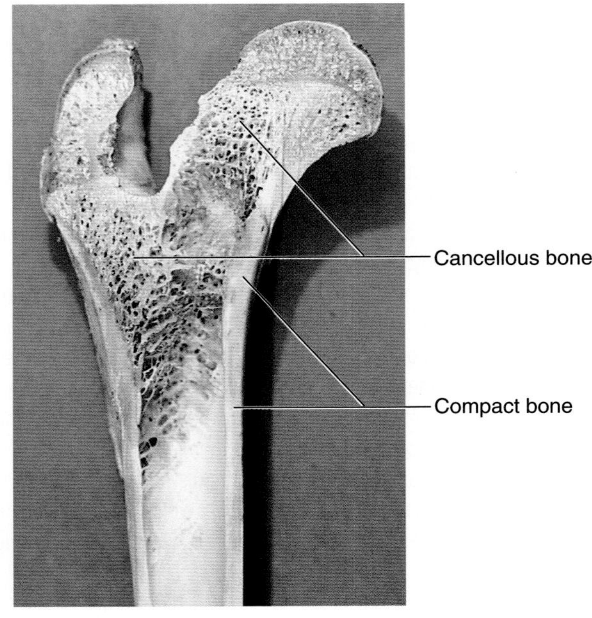

FIGURE 9-22 Types of bone tissue. Compact bone is found forming most of the hard shell of a bone. Cancellous (spongy) bone forms a network of hard beams of bone tissue inside many bones.

Mature osteocytes are actually trapped in hard bone matrix. At one time they were active, bone-forming cells called **osteoblasts.** However, as they surround themselves with bone, they become trapped and cease making new bone matrix. Another type of bone cell, the **osteoclast,** or bone-destroying cell, may dissolve the bone away from the mature osteocyte and release it to again become an active osteoblast. Mature bone can thus grow and be reshaped by the simultaneous activity of osteoclasts breaking down and removing existing bone tissue as osteoblasts lay down new bone.

Cancellous (Spongy) Bone Tissue

Inside many bones is a lattice of thin beams of **cancellous bone tissue** (**Figure 9-24**). These thin beams, or **trabeculae,** form a framework that supports a softer tissue—*red bone marrow.* Red bone marrow is also called *myeloid tissue* (the term *myeloid* literally means "of

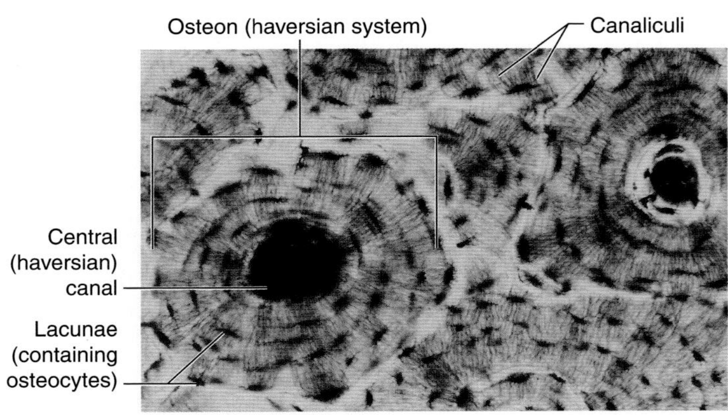

FIGURE 9-23 Compact bone tissue. Photomicrograph of ground compact bone. Many wheel-like structural units of bone, known as *osteons* or *haversian systems,* are apparent in this section.

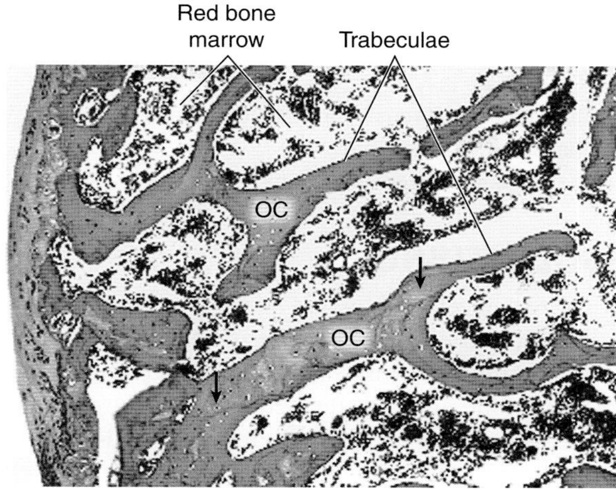

FIGURE 9-24 Cancellous bone tissue. Photomicrograph of cancellous (spongy or trabecular) bone. The pink-stained mineralized bone tissue forms a lattice of irregular beams, or trabeculae, that support the softer reticular tissue of the bone marrow. The darkly stained nuclei of osteocytes (OC) are visible, as well as the dark boundaries *(arrows)* of mineralized bone layers or lamellae.

marrow"). Myeloid tissue is a type of reticular tissue that contains the stem cells responsible for producing the various types of blood cells. It also contains fat-storing *adipocytes.*

The lattice of trabeculae also gives internal support to the bone, much as the crisscrossing pattern of the roof trusses of a building help support the weight of a roof. Because cancellous bone looks somewhat like a sponge at first glance, it is sometimes called *spongy bone tissue.* This type of bone is also called *trabecular bone* because of its many trabeculae.

CONNECT IT! 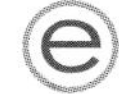

For a closer look at myeloid tissue and its location in the human skeleton, check out the illustrations in ***Sites of Haematopoiesis*** online at ***Connect It!***

Cartilage Tissue

Cartilage differs from other connective tissues in that only one cell type, the **chondrocyte,** is present. Chondrocytes produce the fibres and the tough, rubbery ground substance of cartilage. Chondrocytes, like bone cells, are found in small openings called *lacunae.* Cartilage is avascular (lacking blood vessels), so nutrients must reach the cells by diffusion. Movement is through the matrix from blood vessels located in a connective tissue membrane called the **perichondrium,** which surrounds the cartilage mass. Injuries to cartilage heal slowly, if at all, because of this inefficient method of nutrient delivery.

Hyaline Cartilage Tissue

Hyaline cartilage takes its name from the Greek word *hyalos* or "glass". The name is appropriate because the low amount of collagen in the matrix gives hyaline cartilage a shiny and translucent appearance. This is the most prevalent type of cartilage and is found in the support rings of the respiratory tubes and covering the ends of bones that articulate at joints (**Figure 9-25**).

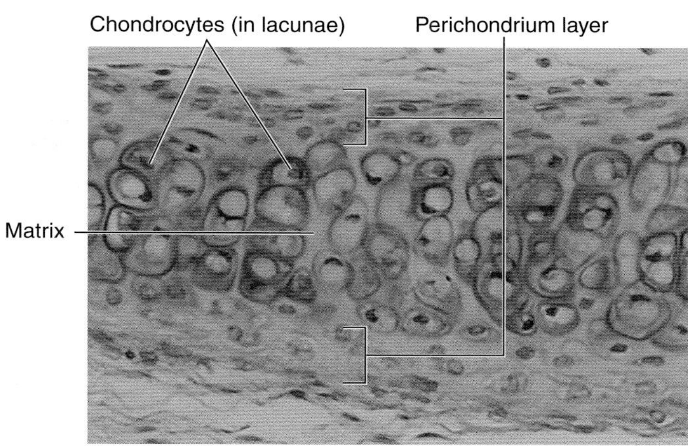

FIGURE 9-25 Hyaline cartilage. Photomicrograph of the trachea. Note the many spaces, or lacunae, in the gel-like matrix.

Fibrocartilage Tissue

Fibrocartilage is the strongest and most durable type of cartilage (**Figure 9-26**). The matrix is rigid and filled with a dense packing of strong white collagen fibres. Fibrocartilage discs serve as shock absorbers between adjacent vertebrae (intervertebral discs) and in the knee joint. Damage to the fibrocartilage pads or joint menisci (curved pads) in the knee occurs commonly as a result of sports-related injuries.

Elastic Cartilage Tissue

Elastic cartilage contains few collagen fibres but large numbers of very fine elastic fibres that give the matrix material a high degree of flexibility (**Figure 9-27**). This type of cartilage is found in the external ear and in the voice box, or larynx.

Blood Tissue

Blood is perhaps the most unusual connective tissue because it exists in a liquid state and contains neither ground substance nor fibres (**Figure 9-28**).

Whole blood is often divided into a matrix, or *liquid fraction,* called **plasma** and **formed elements,** or blood cells. Blood cells may

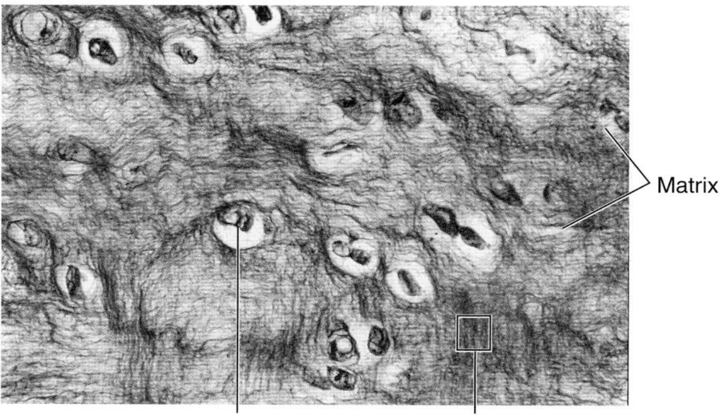

FIGURE 9-26 Fibrocartilage. Photomicrograph of the pubic symphysis joint. The strong, dense fibres that fill the matrix convey shock-absorbing qualities.

be divided into three classes: red blood cells, or **erythrocytes;** white blood cells, or **leucocytes;** and **thrombocytes,** or platelets. The liquid fraction makes up about 55% of whole blood, and the formed elements comprise about 45%.

Blood performs many body transport functions, including movement of respiratory gases (oxygen and carbon dioxide), nutrients, and waste products. In addition, blood plays a critical role in maintaining a constant body temperature and regulating the pH of body fluids. White blood cells function in destroying harmful microorganisms.

Circulating blood tissue is formed in the *red marrow* of bones and in other tissues by a process of differentiation called *haematopoiesis.* This blood-forming tissue is sometimes given the status of a separate connective tissue type: **haematopoietic tissue.**

Blood and its formation are described in detail in Chapter 27.

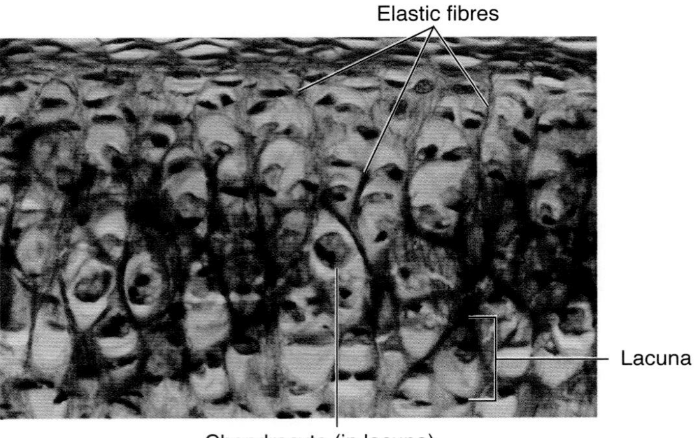

FIGURE 9-27 Elastic cartilage. Photomicrograph of the epiglottis (lid) of the voice box (larynx). Note the cartilage cells in the lacunae surrounded by matrix and dark-staining elastic fibres.

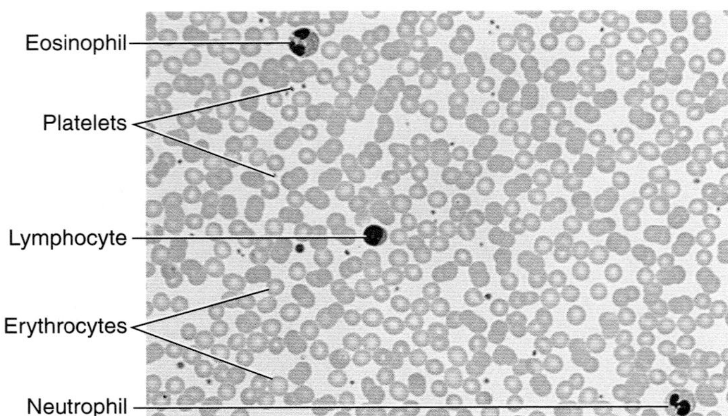

FIGURE 9-28 Blood. Photomicrograph of a human blood smear (×270) showing three white blood cells, or leucocytes, surrounded by numerous smaller red blood cells and platelets.

Quick CHECK

5. Name three kinds of fibres that may be present in a connective tissue ECM. Of what are they made?
6. Name four types of fibrous connective tissue and briefly describe each.
7. What makes bone tissue hard?
8. What is unique about the matrix of blood tissue?

MUSCLE TISSUE

Three types of **muscle tissue** are present in the body—skeletal muscle, smooth muscle, and cardiac muscle (**Table 9-5**). Their names suggest their locations. **Skeletal muscle tissue** (**Figure 9-29**) makes up most of the muscles attached to bones; these are the organs that we think of as our muscles. **Smooth muscle tissue,** also sometimes called *visceral muscle tissue* (**Figure 9-30**), is found in the walls of the viscera (hollow internal organs, e.g., the stomach, intestines, and blood vessels; **Figure 9-31**). **Cardiac muscle tissue** makes up the wall of the heart (**Figure 9-32**).

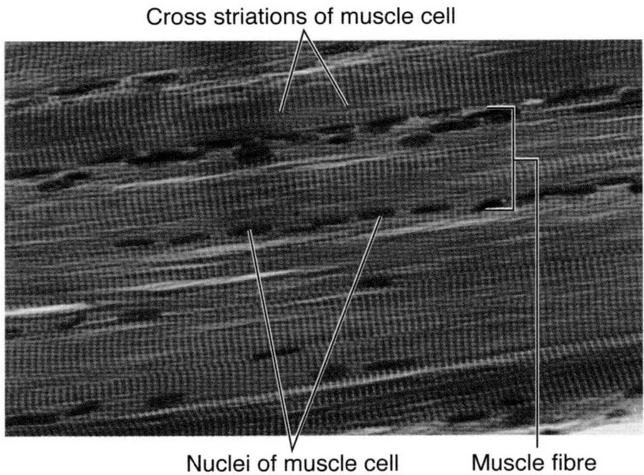

FIGURE 9-29 Skeletal muscle. Note the striations of the muscle cell fibres in longitudinal section.

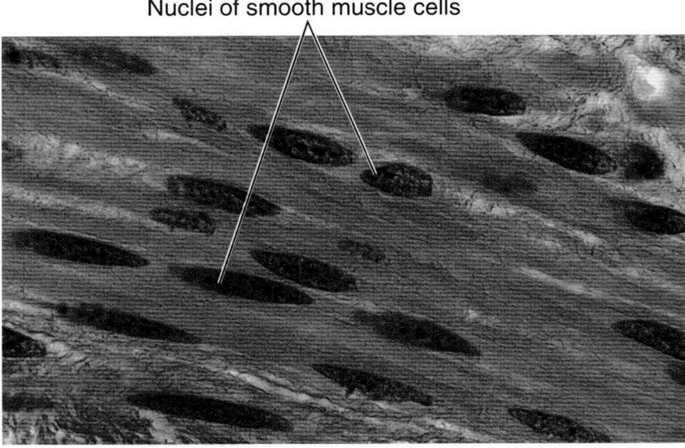

FIGURE 9-30 Smooth muscle. Photomicrograph, longitudinal section. Note the central placement of nuclei in the spindle-shaped smooth muscle fibres.

Another name for skeletal muscle is *striated voluntary* muscle. The term *striated* refers to cross striations (stripes) visible on microscopic slides of the tissue. The term *voluntary* indicates that voluntary or willed control of skeletal muscle contractions is possible. Another name for smooth muscle is *nonstriated involuntary*. Smooth muscle has no cross striations and cannot ordinarily be controlled by the will. Another name for cardiac muscle is *striated involuntary* muscle. Like skeletal muscle, cardiac muscle has cross striations, and like smooth muscle, its contractions cannot ordinarily be controlled by will.

Look now at **Figure 9-29** and observe the following structural characteristics of skeletal muscle cells: many cross striations, many nuclei per cell, and long, narrow, threadlike shape of the cells. Skeletal muscle cells may have a length of more than 3.75 cm, but they have diameters of only 10 to 100 μm. Because this gives them a threadlike appearance, muscle cells are often called *muscle fibres*. Chapter 17 gives more detailed information about the structure of skeletal muscle tissue.

Smooth muscle cells are also long, narrow fibres, but not nearly as long as striated fibres. One can see the full length of a smooth muscle fibre in a microscopic field, but only a small part of a striated fibre. According to one estimate, the longest smooth muscle fibres measure about 500 μm and the longest striated fibres about 40,000 μm.

TABLE 9-5 Muscle and Nervous Tissues

TISSUE	LOCATION	FUNCTION
Muscle		
Skeletal (striated voluntary)	Muscles that attach to bones	Movement of bones Heat production
	Extrinsic eyeball muscles	Eye movements
	Upper third of the oesophagus	First part of swallowing
Smooth (nonstriated, involuntary, or visceral)	In the walls of tubular viscera of the digestive, respiratory, and genitourinary tracts	Movement of substances along the respective tracts
	In the walls of blood vessels and large lymphatic vessels	Change diameter of blood vessels, thereby aiding in regulation of blood pressure
	In the ducts of glands	Movement of substances along ducts
	Intrinsic eye muscles (iris and ciliary body)	Change diameter of pupils and shape of the lens
	Arrector muscles of hairs	Erection of hairs (gooseflesh)
Cardiac (striated involuntary)	Wall of the heart	Contraction of the heart
Nervous		
	Brain Spinal cord Nerves	Excitability Conduction

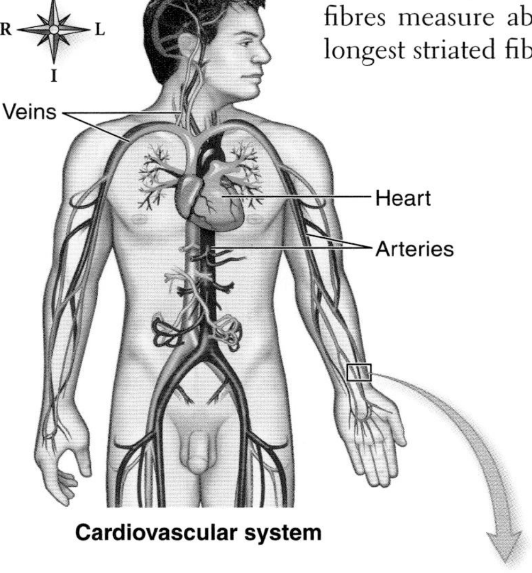

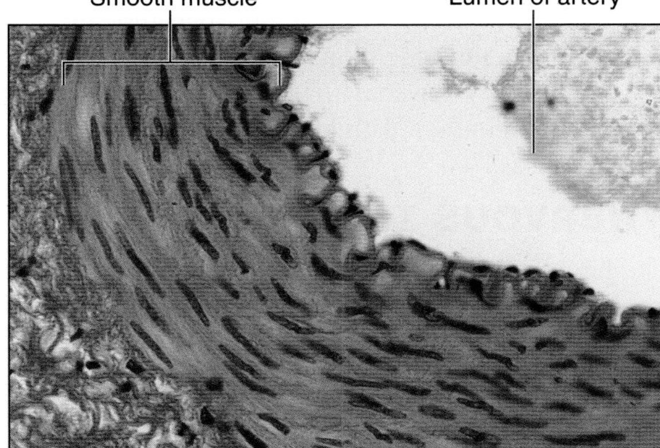

FIGURE 9-31 Location of smooth muscle. Smooth muscle is found in the walls of most internal hollow organs such as the stomach, intestines, and blood vessels. For example, the cross-section of an artery shown in the inset reveals that the arterial wall has a thick layer of smooth muscle, which contracts or relaxes to control the diameter of the artery—thus controlling the flow of blood through this vessel.

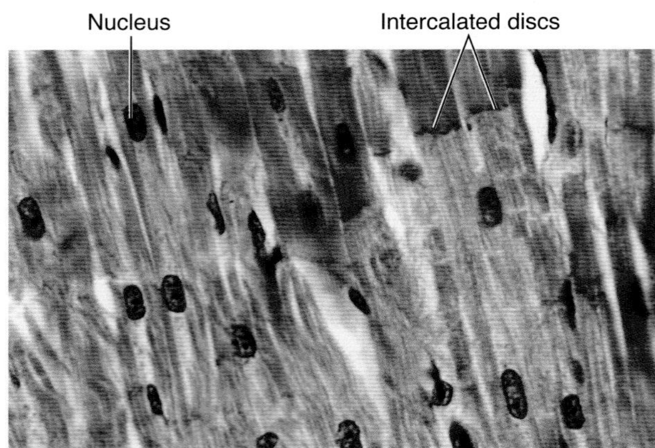

FIGURE 9-32 Cardiac muscle. The dark bands, called *intercalated discs,* which are characteristic of cardiac muscle, are easily identified in this tissue section.

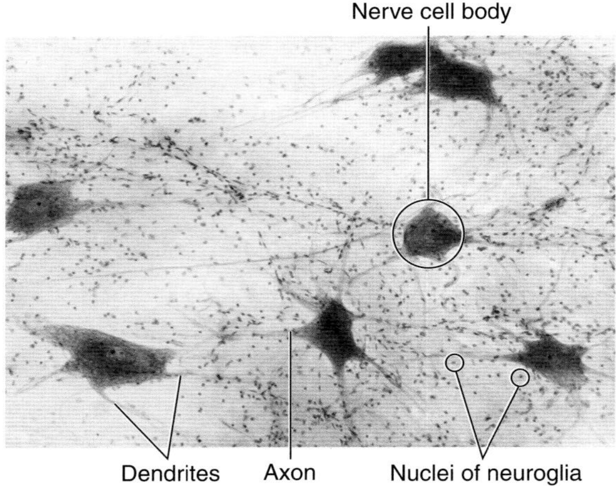

FIGURE 9-33 Nervous tissue. Photomicrograph showing multipolar neurons surrounded by smaller neuroglia in a smear of spinal cord tissue. All the large neurons in this photomicrograph show characteristic soma, or cell bodies, and multiple cell processes.

As **Figure 9-30** shows, smooth muscle fibres have only one nucleus per fibre and are nonstriated or smooth in appearance. Smooth muscle fibres are shaped like a spindle—that is, they are cylinders that taper at both ends.

Under the light microscope, cardiac muscle fibres (see **Figure 9-32**) have cross striations and unique dark bands (intercalated discs) that join together the untapered ends of fibres. The electron microscope, however, reveals that the intercalated discs are actually places where the plasma membranes of two cardiac fibres abut end-to-end. They also seem to be incomplete cells that branch into each other to form a big continuous mass of cytoplasm. Cardiac fibres branch in and out, but a complete plasma membrane encloses each cardiac fibre—around its end (at intercalated discs) and its sides. Because gap junctions are included among the connections at each intercalated disc, however, tiny "tunnels" functionally connect the cytoplasm of all the cardiac fibres into a network called a *syncytium* that acts as a coordinated unit.

Additional illustrations of the three major muscle tissue types can be found in Part 5 of the Brief Atlas of the Human Body.

Muscle cells are the movement specialists of the body. Because their cytoskeletons include bundles of microfilaments capable of movement, they have a higher degree of contractility (ability to shorten and lengthen with force) than cells of any other tissue.

NERVOUS TISSUE

The basic function of the nervous system is to rapidly regulate, and thereby integrate, the activities of the different parts of the body. Functionally, rapid communication is possible because **nervous tissue** has much more developed excitability and conductivity characteristics than any other type of tissue does.

The organs of the nervous system are the brain, the spinal cord, and the nerves. Actual nerve tissue is ectodermal in origin and consists of two basic kinds of cells. The "nerve cells", or **neurons,** are the conducting units of the nervous system. Numerous surrounding cells called **neuroglia** connect, support, and regulate the function of the neurons. For examples, see **Table 9-5**, **Figure 9-33**, and Part 5 of the Brief Atlas of the Human Body.

All neurons are characterized by a cell body called the **soma** and, generally, at least two processes: one **axon,** which transmits nerve impulses away from the cell body, and one or more **dendrites,** which carry nerve signals toward the axon. Most neurons are located within the organs of the central nervous system—the brain and spinal cord.

There are many types of neuroglia, all with different structures and functions. For example, *astrocytes* help regulate neuron function, including protection from harmful toxins. *Microglia* help destroy pathogens and damaged tissue cells in the brain. *Schwann cells* and *oligodendrocytes* electrically insulate axons to increase their speed of conduction. In addition to physically supporting neurons, neuroglia are known to have important coordinating roles in the nervous system—a concept that we explore further in Chapter 18.

The anatomy and physiology of the nervous system are presented in Chapters 18 through 24.

Quick CHECK

9. Name the two types of involuntary muscle. Where is each found in the body?
10. What are the two principal types of cell in nervous tissue? What is the function of each?

the big picture | Tissue Types and the Whole Body

Now that you have a basic knowledge of the various types of body "fabric"—the various specialized human tissues—you are ready to study the structure and function of specific organs and systems. As you take this next step in your studies, pay close attention to the tissue types that make up each organ. Think about the unique structure and function of each tissue type. If you do, you will find it easier to understand the characteristics of a particular organ, and you will also improve your understanding of the integrated nature of the whole body.

LANGUAGE OF SCIENCE *(continued from p. 155)*

dense fibrous tissue (dense FYE-brus TISH-yoo)
[*dense* **thick,** *fibr-* **thread or fibre,** *-ous* **relating to,** *connect-* **bind,** *-ive* **relating to,** *tissu-* **fabric**]

desmosome (DES-moh-sohm)
[*desmo-* **band,** *-som-* **body**]

elastic cartilage (eh-LAS-tik KAR-ti-lij)
[*elast-* **drive or propel,** *-ic* **relating to,** *cartilag* **cartilage**]

elastic dense fibrous tissue (eh-LAS-tik dense FYE-brus TISH-yoo)
[*elast-* **drive or propel,** *-ic* **relating to,** *dense* **thick,** *fibr-* **fibre,** *tissu-* **fabric**]

endochondral ossification (en-doh-KON-dral os-i-fi-KAY-shun)
[*endo-* **inward or within,** *-chondr-* **cartilage,** *-al* **relating to,** *oss-* **bone,** *-fic-* **make,** *-ation* **process**]

endocrine gland (EN-doh-krin)
[*endo-* **inward or within,** *-crin-* **secrete,** *gland* **acorn**]

endothelium (en-doh-THEE-lee-um)
[*endo-* **inward or within,** *-theli-* **nipple,** *-um* **thing**] *pl.,* endothelia

epithelium (ep-i-THEE-lee-um)
[*epi-* **on or upon,** *theli-* **nipple,** *-um* **thing**] *pl.,* epithelia

erythrocyte (eh-RITH-roh-syte)
[*erythro-* **red,** *-cyte* **cell**]

excretion (eks-KREE-shun)
[*excret-* **to separate,** *-tion* **process**]

exocrine gland (EK-soh-krin)
[*exo-* **outside or outward,** *-crin* **secrete,** *gland* **acorn**]

fascia (FASH-ee-ah)
[*fascia* **band**]

fibroblast (FYE-broh-blast)
[*fibr-* **thread or fibre,** *-blast* **bud**]

fibrocartilage (fye-broh-KAR-ti-lij)
[*fibr-* **thread or fibre,** *-cartilage* **cartilage**]

formed element (formd EL-eh-ment)
[*element* **first principle**]

gland
[*gland* **acorn**]

glandular (GLAN-dyoo-lar)
[*gland-* **acorn (gland),** *-ula-* **little,** *-ar* **relating to**]

goblet cell (GOB-let sel)
[*gobl-* **bowl,** *-et* **small,** *cell* **storeroom**]

haematopoietic tissue (hee-mah-toh-poy-ET-ik)
[*haemato-* **blood,** *-poie-* **to make,** *-ic* **relating to,** *tissu-* **fabric**]

histamine (HIS-tah-meen)
[*hist-* **tissue,** *-amine* **ammonia compound**]

hyaline cartilage (HYE-ah-lin KAR-ti-lij)
[*hyaline* **of glass,** *cartilag* **cartilage**]

interstitial fluid (IF) (in-ter-STISH-al)
[*inter-* **between,** *-stit-* **stand,** *-al* **relating to**]

lacuna (lah-KOO-nay)
[*lacuna* **pit**] *pl,.* lacunae

lamella (lah-MEL-ah)
[*lam-* **plate,** *-ella* **little**] *pl.,* lamellae

leucocyte (LOO-koh-syte)
[leuco- **white,** -cyte **cell**]

loose fibrous connective tissue (LOOS FYE-brus kon-NEK-tiv TISH-yoo)
[*fibr-* **thread or fibre,** *-ous* **relating to,** *con-* **together,** *-nect-* **bind,** *-ive* **relating to,** *tissu-* **fabric**]

macrophage (MAK-roh-fayj)
[*macro-* **large,** *-phag-* **eat**]

mast cell
[*mast* **fattening,** *cell* **storeroom**]

membrane bone
[*membran-* **thin skin**]

membranous (MEM-brah-nus)
[*membran-* **thin skin,** *-ous* **characterized by**]

mesothelium (mez-oh-THEE-lee-um)
[*meso-* **middle or median,** *-theli-* **nipple,** *-um* **thing**] *pl.,* mesothelia

microvillus (my-kroh-VIL-us)
[*micro-* **small,** *-villus* **shaggy hair**] *pl.,* microvilli

muscle tissue (MUSS-el TISH-yoo)
[*mus-* **mouse,** *-cle* **small,** *tissu-* **fabric**]

mucus (MYOO-kus)
[*mucus* **slime**]

multicellular gland
[*multi-* **many,** *-cell-* **storeroom,** *-ular* **relating to,** *gland* **acorn**]

neuroglia (nyoo-ROG-lee-ah)
[*neuro-* **nerve,** *-glia* **glue**] *sing.,* neuroglial cell

neuron (NYOO-ron)
[*neuron* **string** or **nerve**]

osteoblast (OS-tee-oh-blast)
[*osteo-* **bone,** *-blast* **bud**]

osteoclast (OS-tee-oh-klast)
[*osteo-* **bone,** *-clast* **break**]

osteocyte (OS-tee-oh-syte)
[*osteo-* **bone,** *-cyte* **cell**]

osteon (OS-tee-on)
[*osteo-* **bone,** *-on* **unit**]

perichondrium (pair-i-KON-dree-um)
[*peri-* **around,** *-chondr-* **cartilage,** *-um* **thing**] *pl.,* perichondria

plasma (PLAZ-mah)
[*plasma* **substance**]

polarity (poh-LAIR-ih-tee)
[*pol-* **pole,** *-ar-* **relating to,** *-ity* **state**]

pseudostratified columnar epithelium (SOOD-oh-STRAT-i-fyed koh-LUM-nar ep-i-THEE-lee-um)
[*pseudo-* **false,** *-strati-* **layer,** *-fied* **made,** *column-* **column,** *-ar* **characterized by**] *pl.,* epithelia

red marrow (MAIR-oh)
[*marrow* **pith (middle)**]

reticular tissue (reh-TIK-yoo-lar)
[*ret-* **net,** *-ic-* **relating to,** *-ul-* **little,** *-ar* **characterized by,** *tissu-* **fabric**]

secretion (se-KREE-shun)
[*secret-* **separate,** *-tion* **process**]

simple epithelium (ep-i-THEE-lee-um)
[*simple* **not mixed,** *epi-* **on,** *-theli-* **nipple,** *-um* **thing**] *pl.,* epithelia

skeletal muscle tissue (SKEL-eh-tal)
[*skeleto-* **dried body,** *-al* **relating to,** *mus-* **mouse,** *-cle* **small,** *tissu-* **fabric**]

smooth muscle tissue
[*mus-* **mouse,** *-cle* **small,** *tissu-* **fabric**]

soma (soh-mah)
[*soma* **body**]

squamous (SKWAY-muss)
[*squam-* **scale,** *-ous* **characterized by**]

stratified epithelium (STRAT-i-fyde ep-i-THEE-lee-um)
[*strati-* **layer,** *-fied* **made,** *epi-* **on,** *-theli-* **nipple,** *-um* **thing**] *pl.,* epithelia

thrombocyte (THROM-boh-syte)
[*thrombo-* **clot,** *-cyte* **cell**]

tight junction (tyte JUNK-shun)

trabecula (trah-BEK-yoo-la)
[*trab-* **beam,** *-ula* **little**] *pl.,* trabeculae

transitional epithelium (tran-ZISH-en-al ep-i-THEE-lee-um)
[*trans-* **across,** *-tion* **process,** *epi-* **on,** *-theli-* **nipple,** *-um* **thing**] *pl.,* epithelia

tubular (TYOOB-yoo-lar)
[*tub-* **tube,** *-ul-* **little,** *-ar* **relating to**]

unicellular gland (yoon-ih-SEL-yoo-lar)
[*uni-* **one,** *-cell-* **storeroom,** *-ular* **relating to,** *gland* **acorn**]

case study

Mark is a forensic pathologist working in a university laboratory that provides an independent pathology service to the local police force. As he specializes in histopathology, Mark was consulted about four tissue samples recovered from a crime scene. He was asked to analyze the samples and identify the organs from which they came.

1. Sample 1 had cells with large vesicles. Each vesicle within the cells of this tissue was so large that it pushed the cytoplasm of the cell outward towards the plasma membrane. Mark identified this tissue as:
   a. Epithelial tissue
   b. Skeletal muscle
   c. Adipose tissue
   d. Reticular tissue
2. Sample 2 was a dense, fibrous tissue that contained bundles of collagenous fibres arranged in regular, parallel rows. Which structure contains a large amount of this type of tissue?
   a. The urinary bladder
   b. A tendon
   c. The bladder
   d. The stomach
3. Sample 3 was a calcified tissue that contained thin structures that formed a crisscross pattern. It looked somewhat like a sponge with spaces filled with red marrow. Mark quickly identified this tissue as:
   a. Cancellous bone
   b. Compact bone
   c. Cartilage
   d. Loose fibrous connective tissue
4. The final sample contained chondrocytes within small openings called lacunae. Mark knew immediately that this was cartilage. However, the challenge was to identify the specific type. This tissue contained a small amount of collagen in the matrix and appeared shiny and translucent. Identify the type of cartilage and the region of the body where it is found.
   a. Hyaline cartilage from the external ear
   b. Hyaline cartilage found at the ends of bones in a synovial joint
   c. Fibrocartilage found in intervertebral discs
   d. Elastic cartilage found in the larynx

Hint To solve a case study, you may have to refer to the glossary or index, other chapters in this textbook, **Connect It!,** and other resources.

CHAPTER SUMMARY

*To download an MP3 version of the chapter summary for use with your mobile device, access the **Audio Chapter Summaries** online at evolve.elsevier.com.*

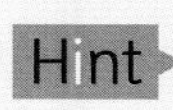

Scan this summary after reading the chapter to help you reinforce the key concepts. Later, use the summary as a quick review before your class or before a test.

Epithelial Tissue

A. Types and locations
  1. Epithelium is divided into two types:
     a. Membranous (covering or lining) epithelium
     b. Glandular epithelium
  2. Locations
     a. Membranous (surface) epithelium—covers the body and some of its parts; lines the serous cavities, blood and lymphatic vessels, and respiratory, digestive, and genitourinary tracts
     b. Glandular epithelium—secretory units of endocrine and exocrine glands

B. Functions
  1. Protection
  2. Sensory functions
  3. Secretion
  4. Absorption
  5. Excretion

C. Generalizations about epithelial tissue
  1. Limited amount of matrix material
  2. Membranous type attached to a basement membrane; cells have apical–basal polarity
  3. Avascular
  4. Cells are in close proximity, with many desmosomes and tight junctions
  5. Capable of reproduction

D. Classification of epithelial tissue
  1. Membranous (covering or lining) epithelium (**Table 9-1**)
     a. Classification based on cell shape (**Figure 9-1**)
        (1) Squamous
        (2) Cuboidal
        (3) Columnar
        (4) Pseudostratified columnar
     b. Classifications based on layers of cells (**Table 9-2**)
        (1) Simple epithelium
           (a) Simple squamous epithelium (**Figures 9-2** and **9-3**)
              (i) One-cell layer of flat cells
              (ii) Permeable to many substances
              (iii) Examples: endothelium—lines blood vessels; mesothelium—pleura
           (b) Simple cuboidal epithelium (**Figure 9-4**)
              (i) One-cell layer of cuboidal cells
              (ii) Found in many glands and ducts
           (c) Simple columnar epithelium (**Figure 9-5**)
              (i) Single layer of tall, column-shaped cells
              (ii) Cells often modified for certain functions such as goblet cells (secretion), cilia (sensation and movement), microvilli (absorption)
              (iii) Often lines hollow visceral structures
           (d) Pseudostratified columnar epithelium (**Figure 9-6**)
              (i) Columnar cells of differing heights
              (ii) All cells rest on basement membrane but may not reach the free surface above
              (iii) Cell nuclei at odd and irregular levels
              (iv) Line the air passages and segments of male reproductive system
              (v) Motile cilia and mucus are important modifications
        (2) Stratified epithelium
           (a) Keratinized stratified squamous epithelium
              (i) Multiple layers of flat, squamous cells (**Figure 9-7**)
              (ii) Cells filled with keratin
              (iii) Covering outer skin on body surface
           (b) Nonkeratinized stratified squamous epithelium (**Figure 9-8**)
              (i) Lines the vagina, mouth, and oesophagus
              (ii) Free surface is moist
              (iii) Primary function is protection
           (c) Stratified cuboidal epithelium
              (i) Two or more rows of cells are typical
              (ii) Basement membrane is indistinct
              (iii) Located in sweat gland ducts and pharynx
           (d) Stratified columnar epithelium
              (i) Multiple layers of columnar cells
              (ii) Only most superficial cells are typical in shape
              (iii) Rare
              (iv) Located in segments of male urethra and near anus
           (e) Transitional epithelium (**Figure 9-9**)
              (i) Located in lining of hollow viscera subjected to stress (e.g., urinary bladder)
              (ii) Stratified—often 10 or more layers thick
              (iii) Protects organ walls from tearing
  2. Glandular epithelium
     a. Specialized for secretory activity
     b. Exocrine glands—discharge secretions into ducts
     c. Endocrine glands—“ductless” glands; discharge secretions directly into blood or interstitial fluid
     d. Structural classification of exocrine glands (**Figure 9-10**; **Table 9-3**)
        (1) Multicellular exocrine glands are classified by the shape of their ducts and the complexity of their duct system
        (2) Shapes include tubular and alveolar

(3) Simple exocrine glands—only one duct leads to the surface
(4) Compound exocrine glands—have two or more ducts
e. Functional classification of exocrine glands (**Figure 9-11**)
(1) Apocrine glands
(a) Secretory products collect near apex of cell and are secreted by pinching off the distended end
(b) Secretion process results in some damage to cell's plasma membrane and some loss of cytoplasm
(c) Mammary glands and some sweat glands are good examples of this secretory type
(2) Holocrine glands
(a) Secretion products, when released, cause rupture and death of the cell
(b) Sebaceous glands are holocrine
(3) Merocrine glands
(a) Secrete directly through cell membrane
(b) Secretion proceeds with no damage to plasma membrane and no loss of cytoplasm
(c) Most numerous gland type

Connective Tissue

A. Functions, characteristics, and types
1. General function—connects, supports, transports, and protects
2. General structure
a. Extracellular matrix (ECM) predominates in most connective tissues and determines their physical characteristics
b. ECM consists of fluid, gel, or solid matrix, with or without extracellular fibres (collagenous, reticular, and elastic) and proteoglycans or other compounds that thicken and hold together the tissue (**Figure 9-12**)
3. Four main types (**Table 9-4**)
a. Fibrous (connective tissue proper)
(1) Loose fibrous (areolar)
(2) Adipose
(3) Reticular
(4) Dense
(a) Irregular
(b) Regular (collagenous and elastic)
b. Bone
(1) Compact bone
(2) Cancellous bone
c. Cartilage
(1) Hyaline
(2) Fibrocartilage
(3) Elastic
d. Blood
B. Fibrous connective tissue
1. Loose fibrous (areolar) connective tissue (**Figure 9-12**)
a. One of the most widely distributed of all tissues
b. Intercellular substance is prominent and consists of collagenous and elastic fibres loosely interwoven and embedded in soft viscous ground substance
c. Several kinds of cells present, notably, fibroblasts and macrophages, also mast cells, plasma cells, fat cells, and some white blood cells (**Figure 9-13**)
d. Function—stretchy, flexible connection
2. Adipose tissue (**Figures 9-14** and **9-15**)
a. Similar to loose fibrous connective tissue but contains mainly fat cells
b. Functions
(1) Acts as food (energy) reserve, support, protection, insulation (white fat), and heat generation (brown fat)
(2) White fat in which some cells have "browned" is called beige fat; white adipocytes can detect body temperature changes and signal brown adipocytes to generate heat
(3) Produces the hormone leptin, which signals the brain how much fat is stored
3. Reticular tissue (**Figure 9-16**)
a. Forms framework of spleen, lymph nodes, and bone marrow
b. Consists of network of branching reticular fibres with reticular cells overlying them
c. Functions—defence against microorganisms and other injurious substances; reticular meshwork filters out injurious particles and reticular cells phagocytose them
4. Dense fibrous tissue
a. Matrix consists mainly of fibres packed densely and relatively few fibroblast cells
(1) Irregular—fibres intertwine irregularly to form a thick mat (**Figure 9-17**)
(2) Regular—bundles of fibres are arranged in regular parallel rows
(a) Collagenous—mostly collagenous fibres in ECM (**Figures 9-18** and **9-19**)
(b) Elastic—mostly elastic fibres in ECM (**Figure 9-20**)
b. Locations—composes structures that need great tensile strength, such as tendons and ligaments; also dermis and the outer capsule of the kidney and spleen
c. Function—furnishes flexible connections that are strong or stretchy
C. Bone tissue
1. Uniquely hard and strong connective tissue type
a. Cells—osteocytes—embedded in a calcified matrix
b. Inorganic component of matrix accounts for 66% of total bone tissue
2. Functions
a. Support
b. Protection
c. Point of attachment for muscles
d. Reservoir for minerals
e. Supports blood-forming tissue
3. Compact bone (**Figures 9-22** and **9-23**)
a. Osteon (haversian system)
(1) Structural unity of bone
(2) Spaces for osteocytes called *lacunae*

(3) Matrix present in concentric rings called *lamellae*
(4) Canaliculi are canals that join lacunae with the central haversian canal

b. Cell types
(1) Osteocyte—mature, inactive bone cell
(2) Osteoblast—active bone-forming cell
(3) Osteoclast—bone-destroying cell

c. Formation (ossification) (**Figure 9-21**)
(1) In membranes—e.g., flat bones of skull
(2) From cartilage (endochondral)—e.g., long bones, such as the humerus

4. Cancellous bone (**Figures 9-22** and **9-24**)
a. Trabeculae—thin beams of bone
b. Supports red bone marrow
(1) Myeloid tissue—a type of reticular tissue
(2) Produces blood cells
c. Called spongy bone because of its spongelike appearance

D. Cartilage
1. Chondrocyte is the only cell type present
2. Lacunae house cells as in bone
3. Avascular—therefore nutrition of cells depends on diffusion of nutrients through matrix
4. Heals slowly after injury because of slow nutrient transfer to cells
5. Perichondrium is membrane that surrounds cartilage
6. Types
a. Hyaline (**Figure 9-25**)
(1) Appearance is shiny and translucent
(2) Most prevalent type of cartilage
(3) Located on ends of articulating bones
b. Fibrocartilage (**Figure 9-26**)
(1) Strongest and most durable type of cartilage
(2) Matrix is semirigid and filled with strong white fibres
(3) Found in intervertebral discs and pubic symphysis
(4) Serves as shock-absorbing material between bones at the knee (menisci)
c. Elastic (**Figure 9-27**)
(1) Contains many fine elastic fibres
(2) Provides strength and flexibility
(3) Located in external ear and larynx

E. Blood
1. A liquid tissue (**Figure 9-28**)
2. Contains neither ground substance nor fibres
3. Composition of whole blood
a. Liquid fraction (plasma) is the matrix—55% of total blood volume
b. Formed elements contribute 45% of total blood volume
(1) Red blood cells, erythrocytes
(2) White blood cells, leucocytes
(3) Platelets, thrombocytes
4. Functions
a. Transportation
b. Regulation of body temperature
c. Regulation of body pH
d. White blood cells destroy bacteria
5. Circulating blood tissue is formed in the red bone marrow by a process called *haematopoiesis*; the blood-forming tissue is sometimes called *haematopoietic tissue*

Muscle Tissue

A. Types (**Table 9-5**)
1. Skeletal, or striated voluntary (**Figure 9-29**)
2. Smooth, or nonstriated involuntary, or visceral (**Figures 9-30** and **9-31**)
3. Cardiac, or striated involuntary (**Figure 9-32**)

B. Microscopic characteristics
1. Skeletal muscle—threadlike cells with many cross striations and many nuclei per cell
2. Smooth muscle—elongated narrow cells, no cross striations, one nucleus per cell
3. Cardiac muscle—branching cells with intercalated discs (formed by end-to-end connection of plasma membranes of adjacent cells)

Nervous Tissue

A. Functions—rapid regulation and integration of body activities

B. Special characteristics
1. Excitability
2. Conductivity

C. Organs
1. Brain
2. Spinal cord
3. Nerves

D. Cell types (**Table 9-5**)
1. Neuron—conducting unit of system (**Figure 9-33**)
a. Cell body, or soma
b. Processes
(1) Axon (single process)—transmits nerve impulse away from the cell body
(2) Dendrite (one or more)—transmits nerve impulse toward the cell body and axon
2. Neuroglia—special connecting, supporting, coordinating cells that surround neurons

The Big Picture: Tissue Types and the Whole Body

A. Specific tissue types determine the structure and function of organs and systems

REVIEW QUESTIONS

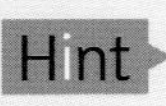

Write out the answers to these questions after reading the chapter and reviewing the Chapter Summary. Note—writing out your answers will consolidate learning and provide a valuable resource of information.

1. What are the five most important functions of epithelial tissue?
2. Which of the following best describes the number of blood vessels in epithelial tissue: none, very few, very numerous? Considering their blood supply, how do epithelial cells generally acquire important nutrients and exchange gases?
3. Explain how the shape of epithelial cells is used for classification purposes. Identify the four types of epithelium described in this classification process.
4. Classify epithelium according to the layers of cells present.
5. List the types of simple and stratified epithelium and give examples of each. Recalling the principle of complementarity of structure and function, how is the structure of a simple squamous epithelium well suited for its function?
6. What is glandular epithelium? Give examples.
7. Discuss the structural classification of exocrine glands. Give examples of each type.
8. Describe loose fibrous connective tissue.
9. How do the types of dense fibrous connective tissue differ from one another?
10. Discuss and compare the microscopic anatomy of bone and cartilage tissue. Include in the discussion a description of the matrix of each. How does the matrix of bone tissue support its function? How does the matrix of cartilage support its function?
11. Construct a table comparing the structure of the three major types of cartilage. Include in columns: location of specific cartilage, composition of the matrix, concentration of chondrocytes, strength of tissue. Cite a minimum of two locations for each.
12. List the components of whole blood and discuss the basic function of each fraction or cell type.
13. List the three major types of muscle tissue. Indicate if each type can initiate or conduct an electrical impulse.
14. Identify the two basic types of cells in nervous tissue. Of the two types of cells, which one is most abundant?
15. Based on basic tissue type, which of the following terms should not be grouped with the others?
    a. muscle
    b. ligament
    c. cartilage
    d. blood

CRITICAL THINKING QUESTIONS

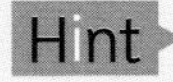

After finishing the Review Questions, write out the answers to these more in-depth questions to help you apply your new knowledge. Go back to sections of the chapter that relate to concepts that you find difficult.

1. Summarize the structural characteristics of epithelial tissues that enable them to perform their specific functions.
2. Does the production of saliva, milk, or oil cause the most damage to the cell that produces it? Explain.
3. Describe the role of fibres in the classification of connective tissue. What examples can you find of these various types?
4. Based on your knowledge of tissues, explain how sufficient dietary intake of calcium could ensure the normal development of bone.
5. Defend this statement: Bone tissue is a dynamic tissue, constantly being remodelled.
6. If a tendon is badly damaged, it may need to be replaced surgically. Based on what you know about the structural and functional differences, explain why a tendon rather than a ligament must replace it.
7. A tissue viewed under the microscope displays cells in little holes, densely packed fibres, and no blood vessels. This describes which connective tissue—dense regular connective tissue, hyaline cartilage, fibrocartilage or adipose tissue?

UNIT 2

Support and Movement

The eight chapters in Unit 2 describe the outer covering of the body, as well as the bones, muscles, and articulations, or joints, of the body. The skin is selected in Chapter 10 as the first organ system to be studied. Chapter 11, Skeletal Tissues, provides information on the types of skeletal tissues and how they are formed, grown, and repaired if injured and how they function. Skeletal tissues protect and support body structures and function as storage sites for important mineral elements vital to many body functions. Blood cell formation also occurs within the red marrow of bones.

The organs of the skeletal system, bones, are organized into major subdivisions and described in Chapters 12 and 13. Movement between bones occurs at joints, or articulations, which are classified in Chapter 14 according to both structure and potential for movement.

Anatomy of the major muscle groups, organized by location in the body, is surveyed in Chapters 15 and 16. Discussion of muscle groups in Chapters 15 and 16 focuses on how muscles function, how they attach to bones, how they are named, and how they are integrated functionally with other body organ systems. Then the basic concepts of muscle physiology are discussed in Chapter 17. The microscopic and molecular structure of muscle cells and tissues is related to function, as is the gross structure of individual muscles.

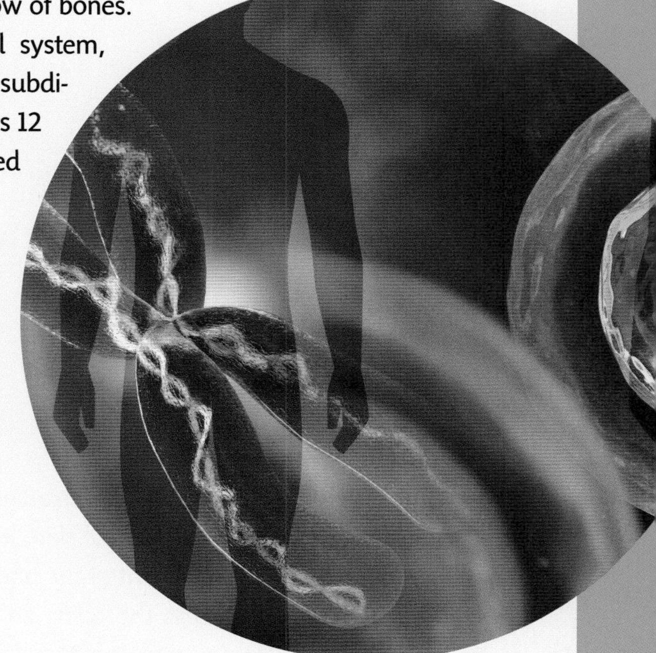

10 Skin

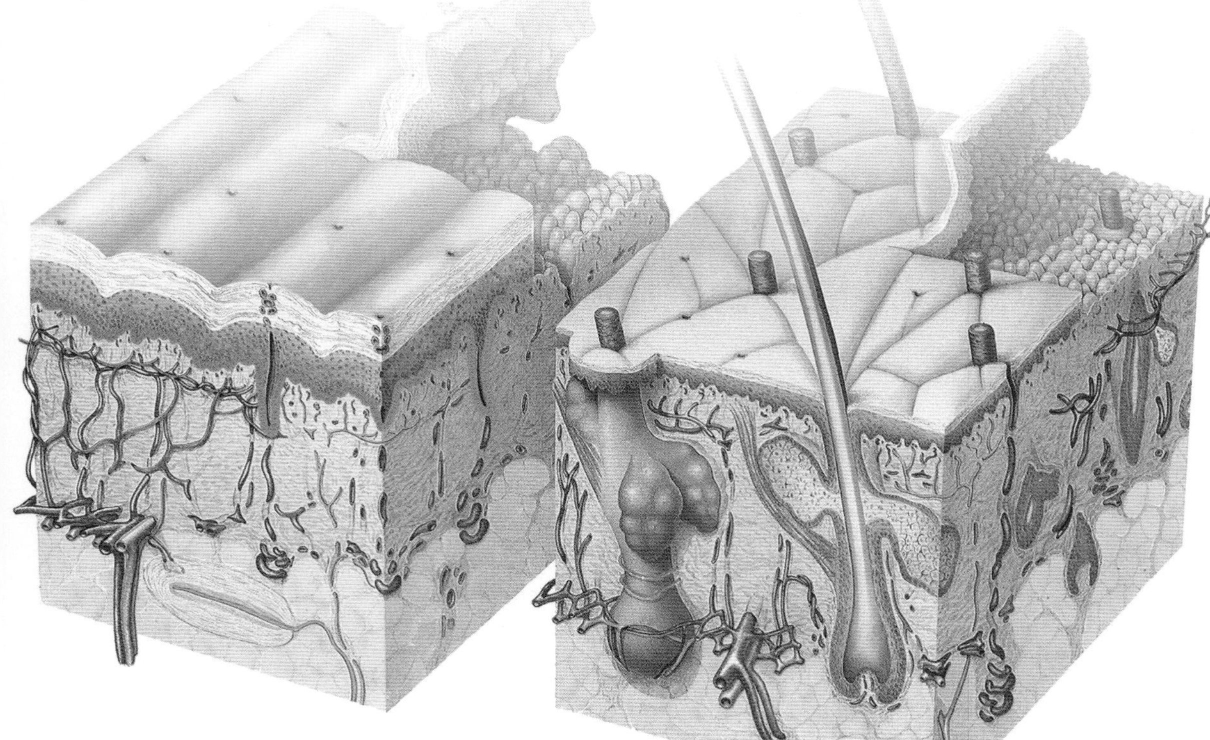

CHAPTER OUTLINE

Hint: *Scan this outline before you begin to read the chapter, as a preview of how the concepts are organized.*

Vital, diverse, complex, extensive—these adjectives describe the body's largest, thinnest, and one of its most important organs, the skin. It forms a self-repairing and protective boundary between the internal environment of the body and an often hostile external world.

The skin's surface is as large as the body, an area in average-sized adults of roughly 1.6 to 1.9 m^2. Its thickness varies from slightly less than 0.05 cm to slightly more than 0.5 cm.

As you know, the body is characterized by a "nested", or hierarchical, type of organization. Complexity progresses from cells to tissues and then to organs and organ systems. This chapter

LANGUAGE OF SCIENCE

Hint: *Use this list to aid your pronunciation of unfamiliar words.*

albinism (AL-bi-niz-em)
[*alba-* **white,** *-ism* **condition**]

apocrine sweat gland (AP-oh-krin)
[*apo-* **from,** *-crin-* **secrete,** *gland* **acorn**]

arrector pili muscle
(ah-REK-tor PYE-lye)
[*arrector* **raiser,** *pili* **of hair,** *mus-* **mouse,** *-cle* **small**]

callus (KAL-us)
[*callus* **hard skin**]

cerumen (seh-ROO-men)
[*cer(a)-* **wax**, *-men* **formed of**]

ceruminous gland (seh-ROO-mi-nus)
[*cer(a)-* **wax**, *-min-* **formed of,** *-ous* **relating to,** *gland* **acorn**]

cleavage line (KLEE-vij)

cortex (KOHR-teks)
[*cortex* **bark**] *pl.*, cortices

cutaneous membrane
(kyoo-TAYN-ee-us)
[*cutis* **skin,** *-ous* **made of**]

cuticle (KYOO-ti-kul)
[*cut-* **skin,** *-icle* **little**]

dendritic cell (DC) (den-DRIH-tik)
[*dendr-* **tree,** *-it-* **part (branch) of,** *-ic* **relating to,** *cell* **storeroom**]

dermal papilla (DER-mal pah-PIL-ah)
[*derma-* **skin,** *-al* **relating to,** *papilla* **nipple**] *pl.*, papillae

dermis (DER-mis)
[*dermis* **skin**]

dermoepidermal junction (DEJ)
(DER-mo-EP-i-der-mal JUNK-shun)
[*derm-* **skin,** *epi-* **on or upon**]

desquamation (des-kwah-MAY-shun)
[*de-* **to remove,** *-squama-* **scale,** *-tion* **process**]

eccrine sweat gland (EK-rin)
[*ec-* **out,** *-crin-* **secrete,** *gland* **acorn**]

eleidin (eh-LEE-din or eh-LEE-ih-din)
[*elei-* **olive tree,** *-in* **substance**]

epidermis (ep-i-DER-mis)
[*epi-* **on or upon,** *-dermis* **skin**]

eumelanin (yoo-MEL-ah-nin)
[*eu-* **true,** *-melan-* **black,** *-in* **substance**]

friction ridge (friK-SHUN ridj)

germinal matrix
(JER-mi-nal MAY-triks)
[*germ* **sprout,** *-al* **relating to,** *matrix* **womb**] *pl.*, matrices

continued on p. 203

discusses the skin and its appendages—hair, nails, and skin glands—as an organ system. Ideally, by studying the skin and its appendages before you proceed to the more complex organ systems in the chapters that follow, you will improve your understanding of how structure is related to function. **Integument** is another name for the skin and the connective tissue just beneath it. **Integumentary system** is a term used when considering the integument as an organ system consisting of the skin, hair, nails, and exocrine glands.

STRUCTURE OF THE SKIN

The skin is a thin, relatively flat organ classified as a membrane—the **cutaneous membrane.** As **Figure 10-1** shows, two primary layers comprise the skin:

1. Epidermis—the superficial, thinner layer
2. Dermis—the deep, thicker layer

The epidermis is an epithelial layer derived from the ectodermal germ layer of the embryo. By the seventeenth week of gestation, the epidermis of the developing fetus has all the essential characteristics of the adult. The deeper dermis is derived from the mesoderm.

CONNECT IT! 

To briefly review the primary germ layers, check out ***Embryonic Development of Tissues*** online at ***Connect It!***

The **dermis** is a relatively dense and vascular connective tissue layer that may average more than 4 mm in thickness in some body areas. The area where the cells of the epidermis meet the connective tissue cells of the dermis is called the **dermoepidermal junction (DEJ)** (**Figure 10-2**). Beneath the dermis lies a soft **hypodermis** rich in fat and loose fibrous connective tissue. The hypodermis is not considered to be part of the skin proper but is still considered to be part of the integumentary system.

THIN AND THICK SKIN

Most of the body surface is covered by skin that is classified as *thin skin*. The hairless skin covering the palms of the hands (and fingertips), soles of the feet, and other body areas subject to friction is classified as *thick skin*. These terms refer only to the epidermal layer and not to overall or total skin thickness, which includes the epidermis and dermis. Total skin thickness varies from 0.5 mm in areas such as the eyelids to more than 5 mm over the back, with most of the difference accounted for by variation in depth of the dermis.

In thick skin, each of the five strata, or layers, of the epidermis described below are present, and each stratum is generally several cell layers thick. The outermost stratum—the stratum corneum—is especially noticeable in thick skin and is generally composed of many cell layers. Hair is not found in thick skin.

In thick skin, the underlying dermal papillae are raised in curving parallel *epidermal ridges*—or **friction ridges**—to form fingerprints or footprints that are visible on the overlying epidermis. As their name implies, friction ridges increase friction—similar to the function of the ridges of tyre treads. These ridges help us pick up and manipulate small objects with the hands and provide slip resistance to the soles of the feet. The epidermal ridges also act as sensory aids that amplify vibrations as we lightly swipe across a textured surface. When thick skin soaks in water, it often wrinkles significantly—a response regulated by nerves that may enhance our ability to grip surfaces. The surface of thick skin is shown in **Figure 10-3**, *A*. Several micrographs of thick skin are found in Part 5 of the BRIEF ATLAS OF THE HUMAN BODY.

In thin skin, the number of cell layers in each epidermal stratum is less than in thick skin, and one or more strata may be absent entirely. Raised parallel ridges are not present in the dermis of thin skin (**Figure 10-3**, *B*). Instead, the dermal papillae project upward individually and therefore no "fingerprints" are formed on the more superficial epidermis above.

EPIDERMIS

Cell Types

The epidermis is composed of several types of epithelial cells (**Figure 10-4**).

Keratinocytes eventually become filled with a tough, fibrous protein called **keratin.** These cells, arranged in distinct strata, or layers,

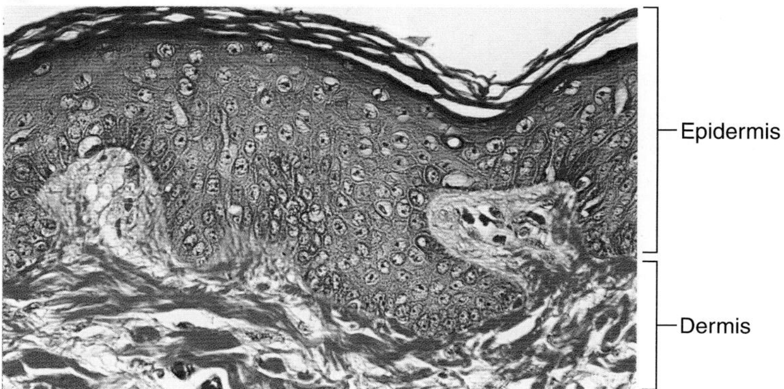

FIGURE 10-1 Photomicrograph of the skin. The staining of this cross-section of skin clearly shows the red superficial epidermis and the bluish dermis below it. This photograph has been cropped; the dermis is actually quite thick in comparison to the epidermis.

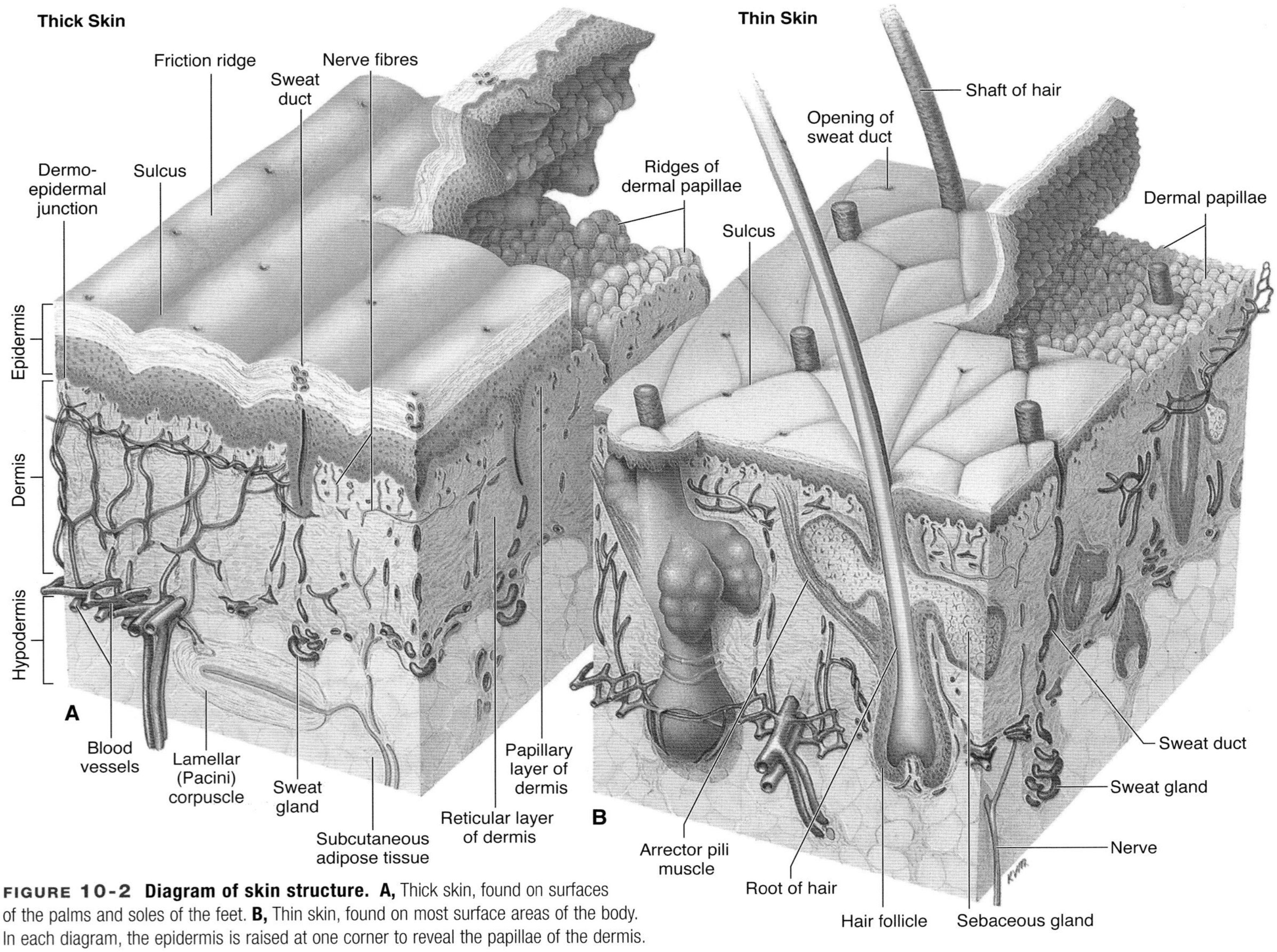

FIGURE 10-2 Diagram of skin structure. A, Thick skin, found on surfaces of the palms and soles of the feet. **B,** Thin skin, found on most surface areas of the body. In each diagram, the epidermis is raised at one corner to reveal the papillae of the dermis.

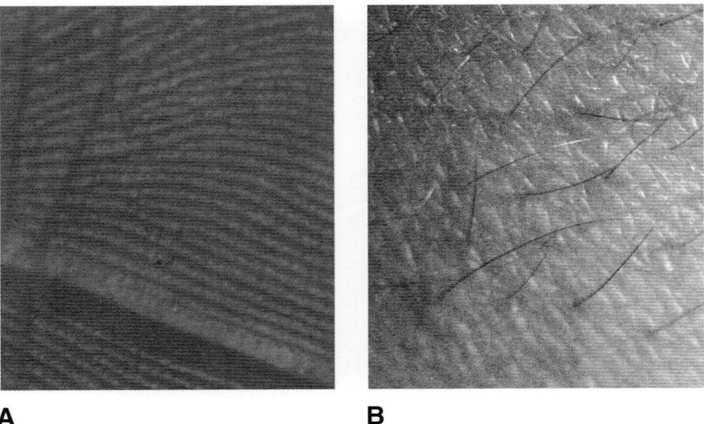

FIGURE 10-3 Thick and thin skin. A, The surface of thick skin is hairless and features regular, deep sulci and friction ridges, which form the "prints" of the palmar and plantar surfaces of the hands and feet. **B,** The surface of thin skin features irregular sulci (grooves) and hairs.

are by far the most important cells in the epidermis. They make up more than 90% of the epidermal cells and form the principal structural element of the outer skin. After they are dead and fully keratinized, the flattened keratinocytes are sometimes called *corneocytes*.

Melanocytes contribute coloured pigments to the skin and serve to decrease the amount of ultraviolet (UV) light that can penetrate into the deeper layers of the skin. Although they often make up more than 5% of the epidermal cells, melanocytes may also be completely absent from the skin in certain nonlethal conditions (**Box 10-1**).

Epidermal **dendritic cells (DCs)** of the skin, also called *Langerhans cells*, are branched cells that play a role in immunity. As a type of *antigen-presenting cell (APC)*, each dendritic cell finds markers (antigens) on bacteria and other invaders and presents them to other immune system cells for recognition and destruction—an important defensive function. These cells originate in the bone marrow but migrate to the deep cell layers of the epidermis early in life. Dendritic cells and other APCs are discussed further in Chapters 32 and 33.

Tactile epithelial cells, also called *Merkel cells*, are located in the deepest layer of the epidermis. As **Figure 10-4** shows, they

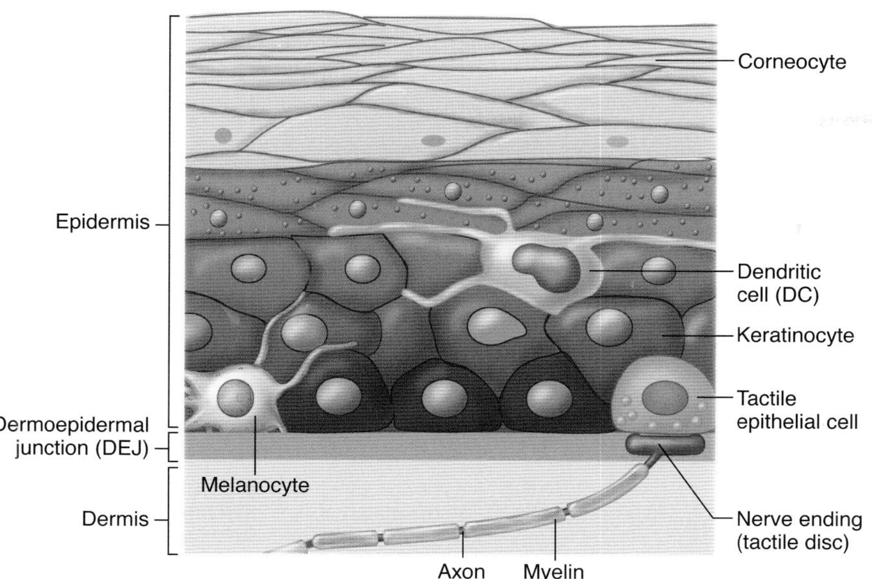

FIGURE 10-4 Epidermal cell types. Keratinocytes, most of the cells seen here, begin their life in the deepest layer of the epidermis and are pushed upward as more keratinocytes are formed. Melanocytes produce pigments. Epidermal dendritic cells *(DCs)* have a function in immunity. Tactile epithelial cells (Merkel cells) attach to sensory nerve endings to form "light touch" receptors.

BOX 10-1 *health matters*

Vitiligo

An acquired condition called **vitiligo** results in loss of pigment in certain areas of the skin. The patches of depigmented white skin that characterize this condition contain melanocytes, but for unknown reasons they no longer produce pigment.

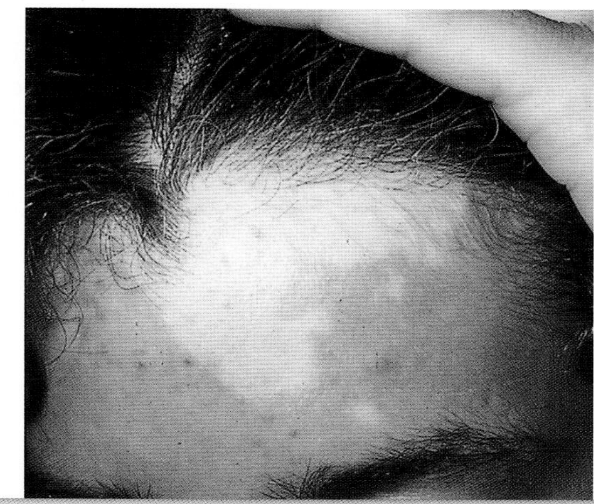

UNIT 2

connect to sensory nerve endings to form structures that serve as light touch receptors.

Cell Layers

The cells of the epidermis are found in up to five distinct layers, or **strata.** Each stratum (meaning "layer") is named for its structural or functional characteristics. The strata of the epidermis are listed here in order from deepest to most superficial.

1. **Stratum basale** (base layer). The stratum basale is a single layer of columnar cells. Only the cells in this deepest stratum of the epithelium undergo mitosis. As a result of this regenerative activity, cells transfer or migrate outward from the basal layer through the other layers until they are shed from the skin surface. The term *stratum germinativum* (growth layer) is often used to designate stratum basale (or sometimes, stratum basale and stratum spinosum together).
2. **Stratum spinosum** (spiny layer). The stratum spinosum layer of the epidermis is formed from 8 to 10 layers of irregularly shaped cells with very prominent intercellular bridges, or desmosomes. When viewed under a microscope, the desmosomes appear to pull points of the plasma membranes of adjoining cells toward one another. This gives cells of this layer a spiny or prickly appearance. Cells in this epidermal layer are rich in ribonucleic acid (RNA) and are therefore well equipped to initiate the protein synthesis required for the production of keratin.
3. **Stratum granulosum** (granular layer). The process of surface keratin formation begins in the stratum granulosum of the epidermis. Cells are arranged in a sheet two to four layers deep and are filled with intensely staining granules called **keratohyalin,** which are required for surface keratin formation. At this stage, the keratinocytes also form small bodies of *glycophospholipids* (part sugar, part phospholipid) built up in multiple layers. Stratum granulosum cells are packed very tightly together, each taking on a complex, many-sided shape. All those many surfaces against one another allow formation of numerous tight junctions. The tight packing and the tight junctions together help give the epidermis its leak-proof qualities by acting as a barrier to water and solutes. This structure also allows cells to migrate up and out of the layer without breaking the continuity of the leak barrier. Even though there is some important biochemical activity at this stage, cells in the stratum granulosum have started to degenerate. As a result, high levels of lysosomal enzymes are present in the cytoplasm, and the nuclei are in the process of breaking down. In thin skin, not many cells at this stage are present, so this layer of the epidermis may not be visible.
4. **Stratum lucidum** (clear layer). The keratinocytes in the stratum lucidum are very flat, closely packed, and clear. Typically, nuclei are absent and the cell outlines are now indistinct. These dying cells are filled with a substance called **eleidin,** which will eventually be transformed to keratin. This layer is absent in thin skin but is apparent in sections of thick skin from the soles of the feet and the palms of the hands.
5. **Stratum corneum** (horny layer). The stratum corneum is the most superficial layer of the epidermis. It is composed of very thin squamous (flat) cells, which at the skin surface are dead and continually being shed and replaced. Much of the cytoplasm in these cells has been replaced by a dense network of keratin fibres. The glycophospholipids from the multilayer bodies cement the keratin fibres into a strong, waterproof barrier. The desmosomes that hold adjacent keratinocytes together strengthen this layer even more and permit it to withstand considerable wear and tear. The process by which cells in this layer are formed from cells in deeper layers of the epidermis and then filled with keratin and moved to the surface is called **keratinization.**

The stratum corneum is sometimes called the outer *barrier area* of the skin because it functions as a barrier to water loss and to many incoming environmental threats ranging from microorganisms and harmful chemicals to physical trauma. Once this barrier layer is damaged, the effectiveness of the skin as a protective covering is greatly reduced, and many contaminants can easily pass through the lower layers of the cellular epidermis. If the glycophospholipid barrier is washed away by prolonged soaking in water (especially if the water contains lipid-dissolving detergents), the keratin may absorb water and make the skin appear a bit puffy and wrinkled—most easily seen in thick skin because of its high water content. Nerve regulation often adds a wrinkling effect in fingers and toes that helps us keep a grip on objects or on the ground when they are wet. Certain diseases of the skin cause the stratum corneum layer of the epidermis to thicken far beyond normal limits—a condition called **hyperkeratosis.** The result is a thick, dry, scaly skin that is inelastic and subject to painful fissures.

Table 10-1 clearly shows each of these layers of the epidermis.

Epidermal Growth and Repair

The most important function of the integument—protection—largely depends on the special structural features of the epidermis and its ability to create and repair itself after injury or disease.

Turnover time and *regeneration* time are terms used to describe the period required for a population of cells to mature and

TABLE 10-1 Structure of the Skin

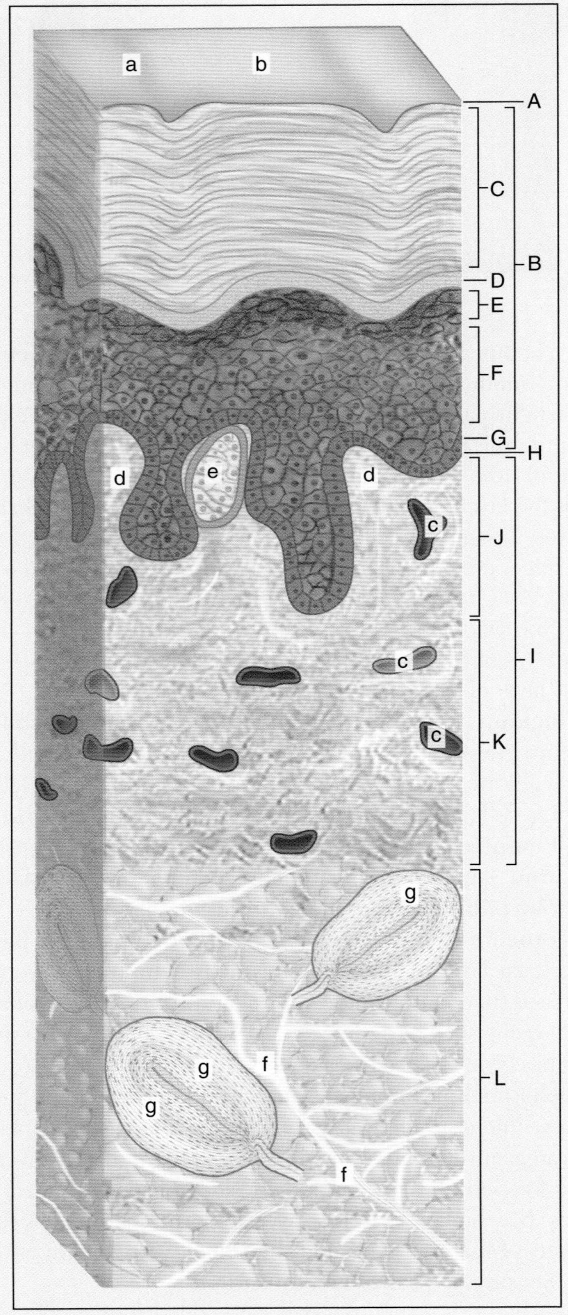

	STRUCTURE	DESCRIPTION
A	Surface film	Thin film coating the skin; made up of a mixture of sweat, sebum, desquamated cells and fragments, various chemicals, microorganisms; protects the skin
B	**Epidermis**	Superficial primary layer of the skin; made up entirely of keratinized stratified squamous epithelium; derived from the ectoderm; also includes hairs, sweat glands, sebaceous glands
C	Stratum corneum (horny layer)	Several layers of flakelike dead cells (or *corneocytes*) mostly made up of dense networks of *keratin* fibres cemented by *glycophospholipids* and forming a tough, waterproof barrier; the keratinized layer **a,** sulcus (groove) **b,** friction ridge
D	Stratum lucidum (clear layer)	A few layers of squamous cells filled with *eleidin*—a keratin precursor that gives this layer a translucent quality (not visible in thin skin)
E	Stratum granulosum (granular layer)	2–5 layers of dying, somewhat flattened cells filled with darkly staining keratohyalin granules and multilayered bodies of glycophospholipids; nuclei disappear in this layer
F	Stratum spinosum (spiny layer)	8–10 layers of cells pulled by desmosomes into a spiny appearance
G	Stratum basale (base layer)	Single layer of mostly columnar cells capable of mitotic cell division; it is from this layer that all cells of superficial layers are derived; includes keratinocytes and some melanocytes
H	Dermoepidermal junction (DEJ)	The basement membrane, a unique and complex arrangement of adhesive components that glue the epidermis and dermis together
I	Dermis	Deep primary layer of the skin; made up of fibrous tissue; also includes some blood and lymphatic vessels **(c),** muscles, and nerves; derived from mesoderm
J	Papillary layer	Loose fibrous tissue with collagenous and elastic fibres; forms nipplelike bumps (papillae, **d**); includes tactile corpuscles (touch receptors, **e**) and other sensory receptors
K	Reticular layer	Tough network (reticulum) of collagenous dense irregular fibrous tissue (with some elastic fibres); forms most of the dermis
L	Hypodermis (subcutaneous layer; superficial fascia)	Loose fibrous (areolar) connective tissue and adipose tissue; under the skin (not part of the skin); includes fibrous bands or *skin ligaments* **(f)** that connect the skin strongly to underlying structures; includes lamellar corpuscles (pressure receptors, **g**) and other sensory receptors

reproduce. Obviously, as the surface cells of the stratum corneum are lost, replacement of keratinocytes by mitotic activity must occur. New cells must be formed at the same rate that old keratinized cells flake off from the stratum corneum to maintain a constant thickness of the epidermis. Cells push upward from the stratum basale into each successive layer, die, become keratinized, and eventually desquamate (fall away), as did their predecessors. This fact illustrates a physiological principle: While life continues, the body's work is never done. Even at rest it is producing millions upon millions of new cells to replace old ones.

A cell-signalling protein called *epidermal growth factor (EGF)* plays a role in regulating the regeneration and repair of the epidermis, as its name suggests. Discovery of EGF has led to its use as a therapy to stimulate skin repairs in diabetic and pressure ulcers and other conditions. EGF requires the hormone *insulin-like growth factor 1 (IGF-1)* to have its full effect in stimulating skin growth and repair. *Growth hormone (GH)* also has a growth-promoting effect on epidermal cells. The cooperative actions of hormones are explored further in Chapters 25 and 26.

Research suggests that the regeneration time required for completion of mitosis, differentiation, and movement of new keratinocytes from the stratum basale to the surface of the epidermis is about 35 days. The process can be accelerated by abrasion of the skin surface, which tends to peel off a few of the cell layers of the stratum corneum. The result is an intense stimulation of mitotic activity in the stratum basale and a shortened turnover period. If abrasion continues over a prolonged period, the increase in mitotic activity and shortened turnover time will result in an abnormally thick stratum corneum and the development of **calluses** at the point of friction or irritation. Although callus formation is a normal and protective response of the skin to friction, several skin diseases are also characterized by abnormally high mitotic activity in the epidermis. In such conditions, the thickness of the corneum is dramatically increased. As a result, scales accumulate and skin lesions often develop.

Normally, about 10% to 12% of all cells in the stratum basale enter mitosis each day. Cells migrating to the surface proceed upward in vertical columns from discrete groups of 8 to 10 of these basal cells undergoing mitosis. Each group of active basal cells, together with its vertical columns of migrating keratinocytes, is called an *epidermal proliferating unit*, or EPU. Keratinization proceeds as the cells migrate toward the stratum corneum. As mitosis continues and new basal cells enter the column and migrate upward, fully keratinized "dead" cells are sloughed off at the skin surface. Numerous skin diseases are characterized by an abnormally high rate of keratinization.

Quick CHECK

1. Identify the two main or primary layers of skin. What tissue type dominates each layer?
2. The terms *thin* and *thick* skin refer to which primary layer of skin? How do thin and thick skin differ?
3. Identify the two main cell types found in the epidermis.
4. List the five layers, or strata, of the epidermis.

DERMOEPIDERMAL JUNCTION

Electron microscopy and histochemical studies have demonstrated the existence of a rather unique area between the epidermis and dermis called the *dermoepidermal junction (DEJ)*.

The DEJ is a unique kind of basement membrane (BM) that includes special fibrous elements and a unique polysaccharide gel that strongly cement the superficial epidermis to the dermis below. The junction "glues" the two layers together and provides mechanical support for the epidermis, which is attached to its upper surface. **Box 10-2** shows what happens when this "skin glue" fails.

In addition, the DEJ serves as a partial barrier to the passage of some cells and large molecules. Certain dyes, for example, if injected into the dermis cannot passively diffuse upward into the

BOX 10-2 *health matters* | Blisters

Blisters (see figures) may result from injury to cells in the epidermis or from separation of the dermoepidermal junction (DEJ). For example, repeated rubbing of the skin against the inside of a shoe or when gripping a tool can pull cells off the DEJ and create a space that fills with interstitial fluid. Regardless of cause, blisters represent a basic reaction of skin to injury. Any irritant that damages the physical or chemical bonds that hold adjacent skin cells or layers together, such as poison ivy, initiates blister formation.

The cell-to-cell junctions (desmosomes) that hold adjacent cells in the epidermis together are essential for integrity of the skin. If these intercellular bridges, sometimes described as "spot welds" between adjacent cells, are weakened or destroyed, the skin literally falls apart and away from the body. Damage to the DEJ produces similar results.

Blister formation follows burns, friction injuries, exposure to primary irritants, or accumulation of toxic breakdown products after cell injury or death in the layers of the skin. Typically, chemical agents that break disulphide linkages or hydrogen bonds cause blisters. Because both types of these chemical bonds are the functional connecting links in intercellular bridges (or desmosomes), their involvement in blister formation serves as a good example of the relationship between structure and function at the chemical level of organization.

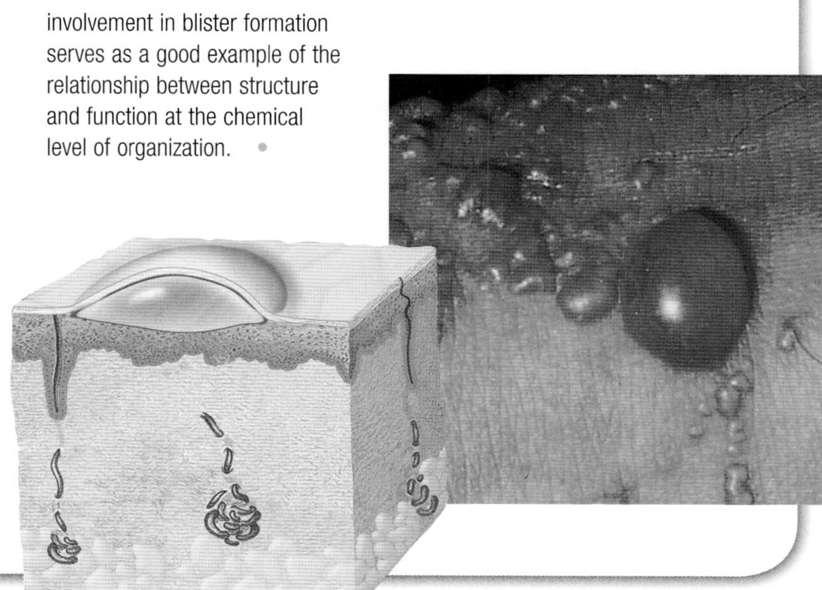

epidermis unless the junctional barrier is damaged by heat, enzymes, or other chemicals that change its permeability characteristics. Although the junction is remarkably effective in preventing separation of the two skin layers, even when they are subjected to relatively high shear force, this barrier is thought to have only a limited role in preventing passage of harmful chemicals or disease-causing organisms through the skin from the external environment. Any widespread detachment of a large area of epidermis from the dermis is an extremely serious condition that may result in overwhelming infection and death.

DERMIS

The dermis, or corium, is sometimes called the "true skin". It is composed of two layers—a thin *papillary layer* and a thicker *reticular layer*. The dermis is much thicker than the epidermis and may exceed 4 mm on the soles and palms. It is thinnest on the eyelids and penis, where it seldom exceeds 0.5 mm. As a rule of thumb, the dermis on the ventral surface of the body and over the appendages is generally thinner than on the dorsal surface. The mechanical strength of the skin is in the dermis. In addition to serving a protective function against mechanical injury and compression, this layer of the skin provides a reservoir storage area for water and important electrolytes. A widespread network of nerves and nerve endings in the dermis called *somatic sensory receptors* also processes sensory information such as pain, pressure, touch, and temperature. Sensory receptors found in skin are discussed in detail in Chapter 23. At various levels of the dermis extend a variety of muscle fibres, hair follicles, sweat and sebaceous glands, and many lymphatic and blood vessels. It is the rich vascular supply of the dermis that plays a critical role in regulation of body temperature—a function described later in the chapter.

Papillary Layer

Note in **Figure 10-2** that the thin superficial layer of the dermis forms bumps, called **dermal papillae,** that project into the epidermis. *Papilla* (plural, *papillae*) is the Latin word for "nipple" and is used often in anatomy to name any small, nipplelike bump. The **papillary** layer takes its name from the papillae on its surface. Between the sculptured surface of the papillary layer and the stratum basale lies the important dermoepidermal junction.

The papillary layer and its papillae are composed essentially of loose fibrous connective tissue elements and a fine network of thin collagenous and elastic fibres. The thin epidermal layer of the skin conforms tightly to the ridges of dermal papillae. As a result, the epidermis also has characteristic ridges on its surface. Epidermal ridges are especially well defined on the tips of the fingers and toes. In each of us they form a unique pattern—an anatomical fact made famous by the art of fingerprinting. Dermal ridges perform a function that is very important to human survival; they allow us to grip surfaces well enough to walk upright on slippery surfaces and to grasp and use tools. For that reason, they are usually called *friction ridges*.

Reticular Layer

The thick **reticular** layer of the dermis consists of a much more dense *reticulum*, or network of fibres, than is seen in the papillary layer above it. It is this dense layer of tough and interlacing white collagenous fibres that, when commercially processed from animal skin, results in leather. Although most of the fibres in this layer are of the collagenous type, which gives toughness to the skin, elastic fibres are also present. These fibres make the skin stretchable and elastic (able to rebound).

The dermis serves as a point of attachment for numerous skeletal (voluntary) and smooth (involuntary) muscle fibres. Several skeletal muscles are attached to the skin of the face and scalp. These muscles permit a variety of facial expressions and are also responsible for voluntary movement of the scalp. The distribution of smooth muscle fibres in the dermis is much more extensive than the skeletal variety. Each hair follicle has a small bundle of involuntary muscles attached to it. These are the **arrector pili muscles.** Contraction of these muscles makes the hair "stand on end"—as in extreme fright, for example, or from cold. As the hair is pulled into an upright position, shown in **Figure 10-5**, it raises the skin around it into what we commonly call "goose bumps". In the dermis of the skin of the scrotum and in the pigmented skin called the *areolae* surrounding the nipples, smooth muscle cells form a loose network. Contraction of these smooth muscle cells wrinkles the skin and causes elevation of the testes or erection of the nipples.

Millions of somatic sensory receptors are located in the dermis of all skin areas (**Figure 10-6**; see also **Figure 10-2**). They permit the skin to serve as a sense organ transmitting sensations of pain, pressure, touch, and temperature to the brain.

Hair follicles and various skin glands, made up of epithelial tissues that extend from the surface of the epidermis, have most of their structures within the reticular layer of the dermis.

Dermal Growth and Repair

Unlike the epidermis, the dermis does not continually shed and regenerate. It does maintain itself, but rapid regeneration of connective tissue in the dermis occurs only during unusual circumstances, as in the healing of wounds (see **Figure 8-6**, p. 144). In the healing of a wound such as a surgical incision, fibroblasts in the dermis quickly reproduce and begin forming an unusually dense mass of new connective tissue fibres. If this dense mass is not replaced by normal tissue, it remains as a *scar*.

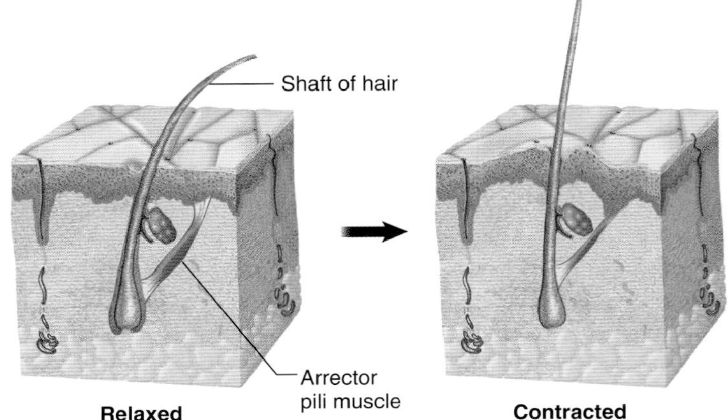

FIGURE 10-5 Arrector pili muscle. When the arrector pili muscle contracts, it pulls the follicle and hair into a more perpendicular position, thus "fluffing up" the hair. Note how a "goose bump" is raised around the hair shaft.

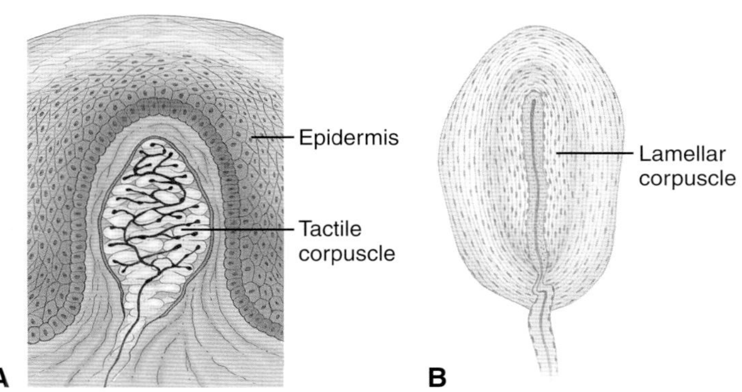

FIGURE 10-6 Skin receptors. Receptors are sensitive nerve endings that make it possible for the skin to act as a sense organ. **A,** This *tactile (Meissner) corpuscle* is capable of detecting deep touch (deep pressure). **B,** Another skin receptor is the *lamellar corpuscle,* also called a *Pacini corpuscle,* which also detects sensations of deep pressure.

The dense bundles of white collagenous fibres that characterize the reticular layer of the dermis tend to orient themselves in patterns that differ in appearance from one body area to another. The result is formation of patterns called **cleavage lines** (**Figure 10-7**). If surgical incisions are made parallel to the cleavage lines, or *Langer lines,* the resulting wound will have less tendency to gape open and will tend to heal with a thin and less noticeable scar.

If the elastic fibres in the dermis are stretched too much—for example, by a rapid increase in the size of the abdomen during pregnancy or as a result of great obesity—these fibres will weaken and tear. The initial result is the formation of pinkish or slightly bluish depressed furrows with jagged edges. These tiny linear markings *(stretch marks)* are really tiny tears. When they heal and lose their colour, the *striae* (Latin, "furrows") that remain appear as glistening silver-white scar lines.

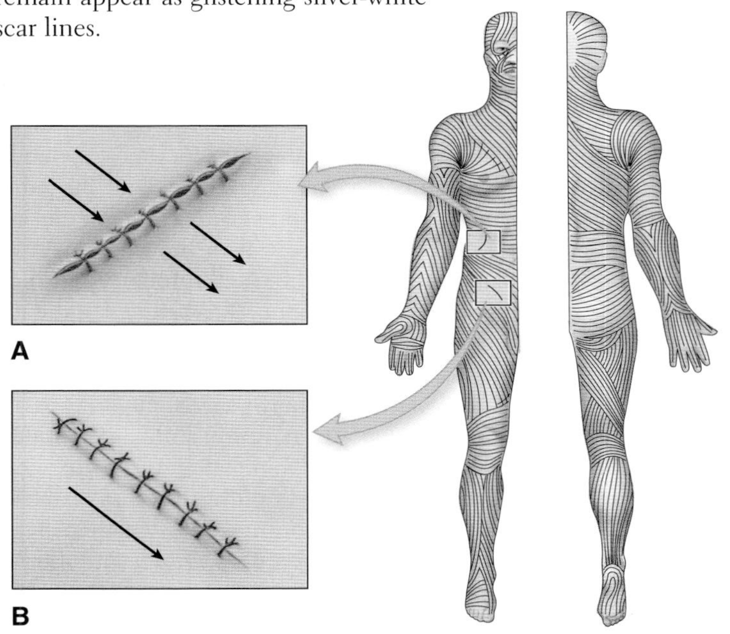

FIGURE 10-7 Cleavage lines. A, If an incision "cuts across" cleavage lines (Langer lines), stress tends to pull the cut edges apart and may retard healing. **B,** Surgical incisions parallel to cleavage lines are subjected to less stress and tend to heal more rapidly.

HYPODERMIS

The hypodermis is sometimes called the **subcutaneous layer,** or **superficial fascia** (see **Box 9-2**, p. 167). It is not considered to be part of the skin proper, but it is still included in part of the integument. This layer lies deep to the dermis and thus forms a connection between the skin and the underlying structures of the body. Thus the hypodermis is often discussed along with the skin because of the close structural and functional association of these two superficial body structures. **Box 10-3** discusses one reason why it is important to know about the location and structure of the hypodermis.

The hypodermis is mostly loose fibrous and adipose tissue, along with nerves, blood vessels, and lymphatic vessels.

The fat content of the hypodermis varies with the state of nutrition and in obese individuals may exceed 10 cm in thickness in certain areas. The density and arrangement of fat cells and collagen fibres in this area determine the relative mobility of the skin. Bands of fibres called *skin ligaments* running through the hypodermis help hold the skin to underlying structures such as deep fascia and muscles (**Table 10-1**, *f*). When skin is removed from an animal by blunt dissection, separation occurs in the "cleavage plane" that exists between the superficial fascia and the underlying structures.

Some scientists hypothesize that acupuncture needles "grab and twist" fibres in the hypodermis as they are rotated, which pulls on the local network of interconnected fibres and cells. This is thought to trigger cell-to-cell signals that can produce pain-relieving or other therapeutic effects.

The relationship between the skin and hypodermis can be seen in many of the cross-sections of the body shown in Part 4 of the BRIEF ATLAS OF THE HUMAN BODY.

UNIT 2

BOX 10-3 *health matters* Subcutaneous and Intradermal Injections

Although the hypodermis, or subcutaneous layer, is not part of the skin itself, it carries the major blood vessels and nerves to the skin above. The rich blood supply and loose spongy texture of this area make it an ideal site for the rapid and relatively pain-free absorption of injected material. Liquid medicines, such as insulin, and pelleted implant materials are often administered by *subcutaneous (SQ) injection* with a *hypodermic needle* into this spongy and porous layer beneath the skin. *Intradermal (ID) injections,* on the other hand, place the medication in the skin proper. ID injections, which are ideal for some vaccines, are hard to administer with a typical needle because it is so easy to punch through to the hypodermis. Therefore, this type of injection is sometimes given with special needle-free injectors.

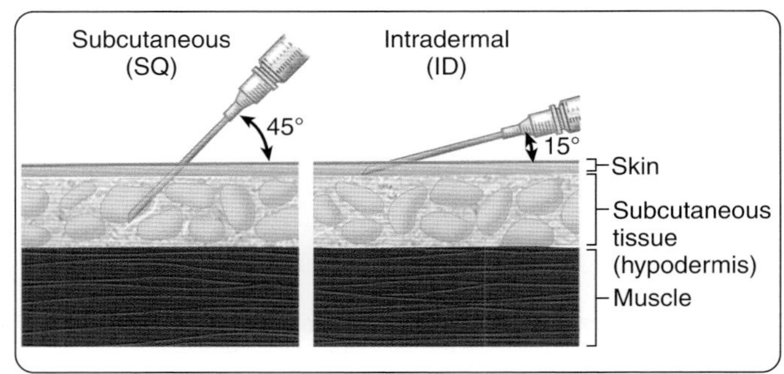

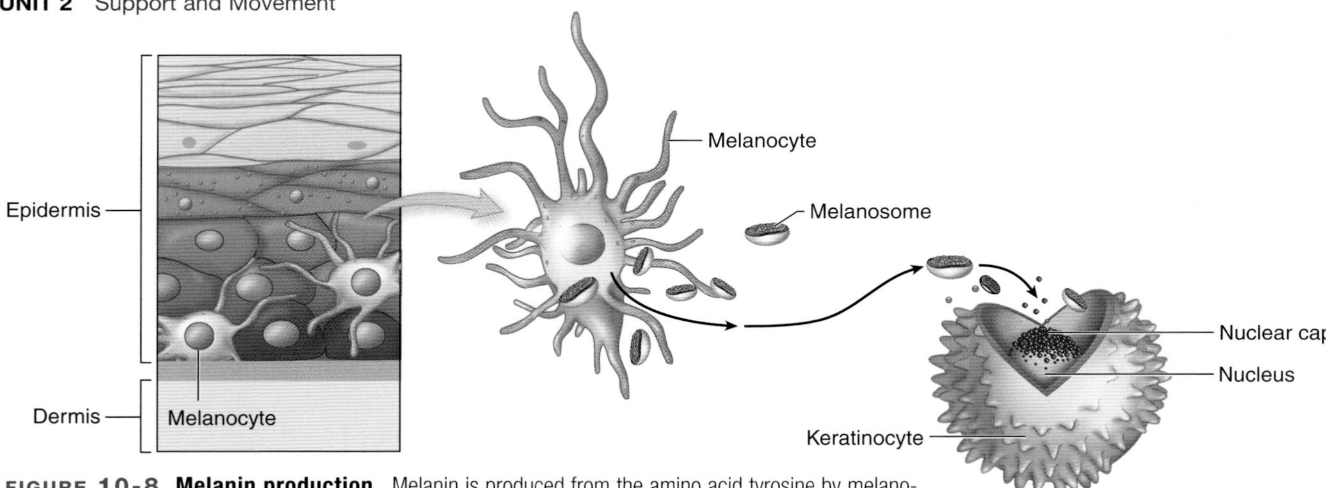

FIGURE 10-8 Melanin production. Melanin is produced from the amino acid tyrosine by melanocytes in the stratum basale. Melanocytes have long projections that reach between the keratinocytes and release packets of pigment called *melanosomes.* By endocytosis, the melanosomes are brought into the keratinocytes, where they are arranged as a cap over the nucleus—protecting it from UV radiation from above.

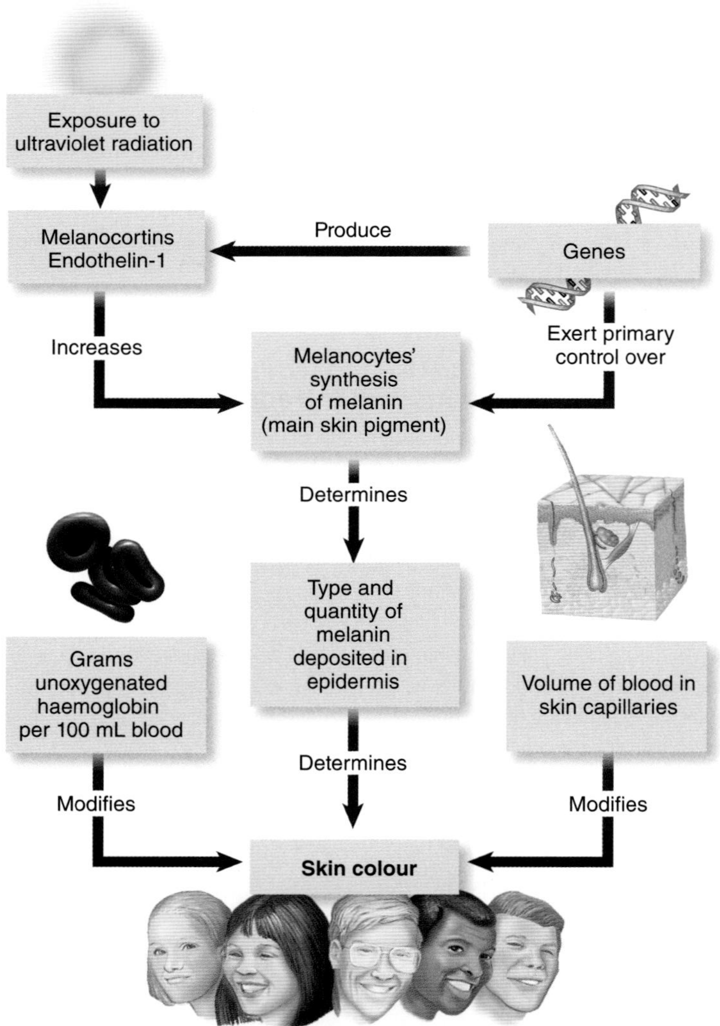

FIGURE 10-9 How genes affect skin colour. Genes determine an individual's basic skin colour by controlling the amount and type of melanin synthesized and deposited in the epidermis. However, as the diagram shows, other factors may modify the basic skin colour.

Quick **CHECK**

5. What is the name of the gluelike layer separating the dermis from the epidermis?
6. Which layer of the dermis forms the bumps that produce ridges on the palms and soles?
7. Which layer is vascular: the epidermis or dermis?
8. What is the main function of the hypodermis?

SKIN COLOUR

MELANIN

Human skin ranges widely in colour. The main determinant of skin colour is the quantity and type of **melanin** deposited in the cells of the epidermis by melanocytes. The number of pigment-producing melanocytes scattered throughout the stratum basale of the epidermis in most body areas is about the same in all humans. It is the amount and type of melanin pigment actually produced by these cells that account for the majority of skin colour variations among families.

Two groups of melanin are made by the melanocytes of the body. One group of these pigments is called **eumelanin** and the other group is called **pheomelanin.** The word *eumelanin* literally means "true black substance" because it is very dark brown, sometimes nearly black. *Pheomelanin* means "dusky black substance"—which hints at its lighter reddish or orange colour. Dark-skinned and dark-haired people produce large quantities of eumelanin. On the other hand, people with very light skin with red-orange freckles and red hair produce pheomelanin—and little if any eumelanin—in the skin.

Of all body cells, only melanocytes have the ability to routinely convert the amino acid *tyrosine* into melanin pigments. The pigment granules are produced and then released in tiny exosomes (extracellular vesicles) called **melanosomes.** The melanins are then transferred to surrounding keratinocytes, where they form a sort of light-absorbing protective cap over the nucleus (**Figure 10-8**). The pigment-producing process is regulated in the cell by the enzyme *tyrosinase*. But this conversion process depends on several metabolic factors that can alter the rate of conversion (**Figure 10-9**).

Heredity is a major factor in melanin production. Geneticists tell us that several genes exert primary control over the amount of melanin formed by melanocytes. These genes may affect any part of the chemical pathway that produces the two types of melanin. For example, if the enzyme tyrosinase is absent from birth because of a genetic mutation, the melanocytes cannot form melanin and a condition called **albinism** results. Albino individuals have a characteristic absence of pigment in their hair, skin, and eyes. Thus heredity determines how dark or light one's skin colour will be (see Chapter 48).

Other factors can influence the expression of the genes for melanin production. Sunlight is an obvious example. Prolonged exposure to the ultraviolet (UV) radiation in sunlight causes melanocytes to increase melanin production and darken skin colour (**Figure 10-10**). Note in **Figure 10-8** that the melanosomes form a cap over the top of the nucleus in each keratinocyte. The melanin in this nuclear cap absorbs UV radiation before it can reach the DNA inside the nucleus, where it can cause severe damage that can lead to skin cancer and other problems. Unless the cells are protected by melanin, UV radiation can also break down other important molecules, such as the vitamin *folic acid* (B_9). Eumelanin absorbs more UV radiation than pheomelanin does—which explains why very dark-skinned individuals have less risk of developing skin cancer than very light-skinned, reddish-freckled individuals do.

Research shows that dark skin pigmentation also facilitates apoptosis (programmed cell death) of any cells that do sustain damage to their DNA structure. Removal of DNA-damaged cells prevents them from becoming cancerous.

Melanin production is stimulated when *melanocortin* receptors are triggered at the surface of a melanocyte. Melanocortins are a family of hormones produced from a single gene that codes for a large polypeptide that breaks into distinct hormones. One product of the gene is adrenocorticotropic hormone (ACTH), some of which breaks down further to form *alpha melanocyte-stimulating hormone* (*α-MSH*). Although tiny amounts of melanocortins are released by the anterior pituitary gland, they can also be made by keratinocytes in response to UV radiation—thus triggering nearby melanocytes to produce more melanin. Other local regulatory proteins, such as *endothelin-1 (ET-1)*, act with melanocortins to produce this "tanning" effect. Some people with light skin, red hair, and freckles inherit

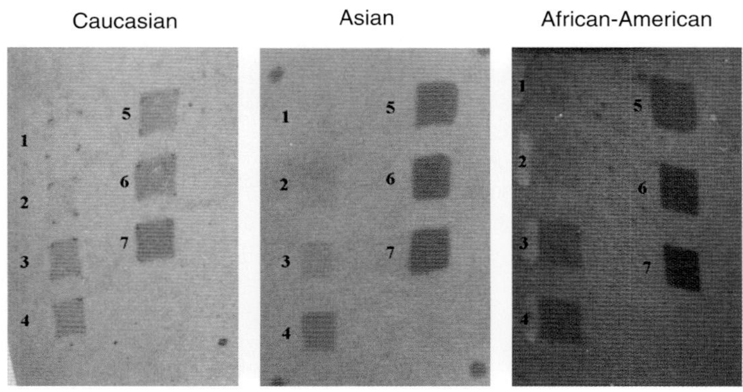

FIGURE 10-10 Tanning effects in skin. Photos showing skin effects of ultraviolet (UV) radiation on day 8 after exposure to increasing doses (1 through 7) in three skin types. Note that the Caucasian skin involves more redness (from burning) than the darker skin types, which become even darker in response to higher doses of UV radiation.

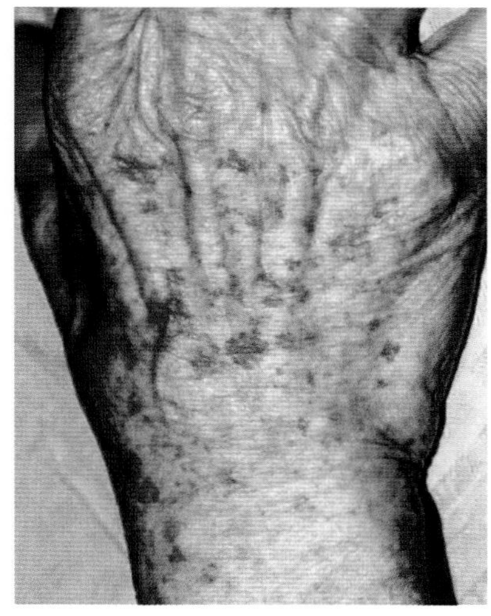

FIGURE 10-11 Age spots. Hyperpigmentations from the cumulative effects of ultraviolet (UV) exposure over the years can produce a dark type of "age spots" that are also called "liver spots". Note the skin also wrinkles with age.

malfunctioning melanocyte receptors or melanocortin genes and thus fail to produce melanin in response to UV exposure.

Increasing age may also influence melanocyte activity. In many individuals, apoptosis of melanocyte stem cells in hair follicles produces the greying of the hair often associated with age. Cumulative exposure to UV radiation over the years can also trigger excess production of melanin. This may result in a collection of dark "age spots" on the skin (**Figure 10-11**).

OTHER PIGMENTS

In addition to melanin, other pigments such as the yellow pigment beta-carotene (β-carotene) found in many vegetables and roots (for example, carrots) also contribute to skin colour. Because β-carotenes can be converted by the body into vitamin A—a critically important nutrient for skin growth—they are stored in skin tissue. Extremely high consumption of carrot juice or sweet potatoes, in infants especially, may cause an orange or yellow colouration of the skin. Yellowish discolouration can also be caused by jaundice (**Box 10-4**) or can be seen after a bruise begins to heal (see **Figure 10-13**).

As epidermal cells age and stop undergoing mitosis, they often accumulate a brown-yellow pigment called *lipofuscin*. Aged skin often shows a mottling of brown-yellow age spots as a result.

An individual's basic skin colour can also change temporarily when the volume of blood flowing through skin capillaries increases or decreases. The reason is that blood contains the reddish pigment haemoglobin (Hb) that carries oxygen or carbon dioxide. If blood vessels in the skin dilate, as they do during blushing, the skin appears to be redder than usual because of additional haemoglobin flowing through the dermis. If skin blood vessels constrict, on the other hand, skin blood volume decreases, and the skin may turn paler (less red) than usual.

In general, the sparser the pigments in the epidermis, the more transparent the skin and therefore the more vivid the change in skin colour with a change in skin blood volume. Conversely, the richer the pigmentation, the more opaque the skin and therefore the less the change in skin colour with a change in skin blood volume.

In some abnormal conditions, skin colour changes because of an excess amount of haemoglobin that is low in oxygen and high in carbon dioxide. If skin contains relatively little melanin, it will appear bluish—that is, *cyanotic*—when its blood has a high proportion of unoxygenated haemoglobin. The blue colouration results from the fact that haemoglobin changes from a bright red to a deep maroon when it loses oxygen and gains carbon dioxide. Light reflecting from the dark red haemoglobin and diffused by fibres in the

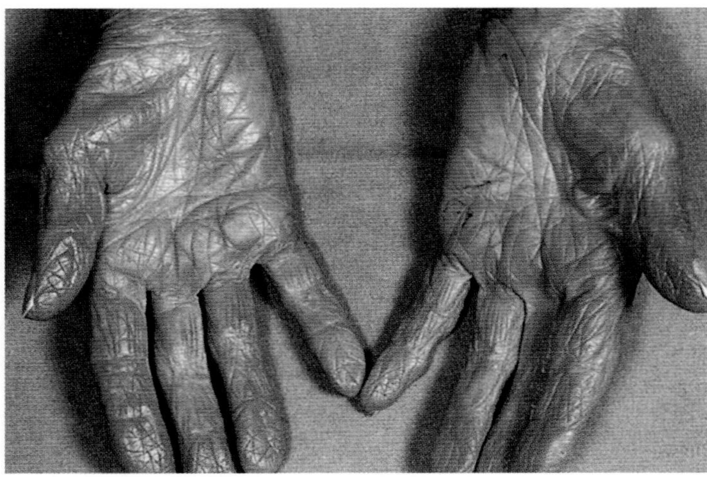

FIGURE 10-12 Cyanosis. The blue discolouration of the fingers of this light-skinned individual is caused by the diffusion of light reflected off dark, unoxygenated haemoglobin in the blood vessels of the skin. The fingertips have an especially high volume of blood and thus look bluer than other regions of the skin.

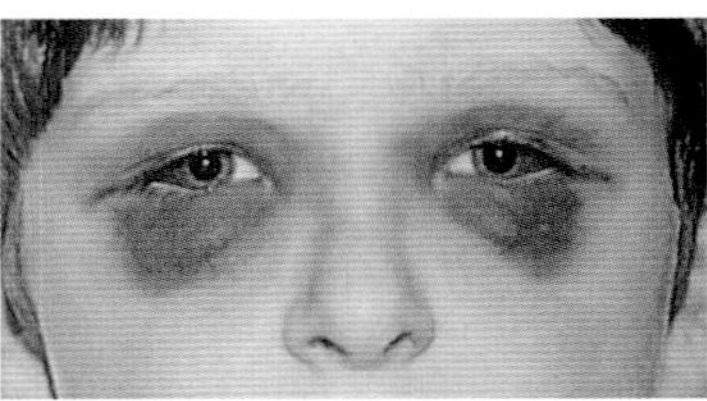

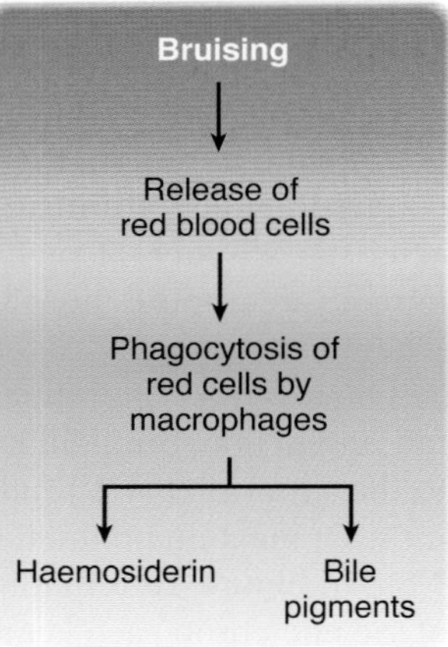

FIGURE 10-13 Colour changes in a bruise. In this light-skinned individual, different colours appear in the bruised area of the skin as haemoglobin becomes unoxygenated and turns bluish (see **Figure 10-12**) and perhaps even black as the blood clots. As macrophages consume the haemoglobin, it is broken down into brownish, greenish, and yellowish pigments—sometimes producing a rainbow of skin colours.

skin may appear blue—as you can see in **Figure 10-12**. In general, the darker the skin pigmentation, the greater the amount of unoxygenated haemoglobin that must be present before **cyanosis** ("condition of blueness") becomes visible.

Bruising can cause a variety of different skin colours to appear in light-skinned individuals, as you can see in **Figure 10-13**. When damage to blood vessels in the skin permits the release of red blood cells, their reddish colour begins to darken and produce the bluish colours described previously when haemoglobin loses oxygen and gains carbon dioxide. As the blood clots, it may begin to appear darker blue or even black. Macrophages remove the haemoglobin and break it down into iron-containing *haemosiderin* (a brownish pigment) and several iron-free *bile pigments* that are greenish and yellowish.

Pigments from cosmetics or from tattoos can also change the colouring of the skin. Most cosmetics simply add layers of pigment on top of the skin. Some temporary tattoos also add layers of pigment on top of the skin. Henna tattoos stain epidermal cells, which are later shed—making their brown colour temporary. Permanent tattoos are made by using a needle to insert pigments into the dermis of the skin. Because these pigments eventually diffuse to deeper layers of the dermis, such a tattoo may fade or become less distinct after several decades. Some permanent tattoos are made by cutting the skin and rubbing in pigments, producing coloured scar tissue.

FUNCTIONS OF THE SKIN

Skin functions are crucial to maintenance of homeostasis and thus to survival itself. They are diverse and include such different processes as protection, sensation, growth, synthesis of important chemicals and hormones (such as vitamin D), excretion, temperature regulation, and immunity. Because of its structural flexibility, the skin permits body growth and movement to occur without injury. We also know that certain substances can be absorbed through the skin, including the lipid-soluble vitamins (A, D, E, and K), oestrogens and

BOX 10-4 *health matters* | Jaundice

Yellowish discolouration of the skin and other tissues, such as the "white" or sclera of the eye, can be caused by bile pigments. Bile pigments are a natural breakdown product when old red blood cells are destroyed. Ordinarily, bile pigments are excreted from the liver into the digestive tract, where they become part of the faeces and are eliminated by the body. However, in some cases the liver is unable to remove bile from the blood efficiently—thus allowing the bile to stain the tissues of the body. An example of a condition that can cause **jaundice** is a liver infection, as illustrated in the photograph.

Jaundice also often occurs just after birth. In about half of all full-term newborns, jaundice occurs when old red blood cells containing an immature fetal form of haemoglobin are rapidly replaced with red blood cells containing the mature form of haemoglobin. Often, a baby's liver is simply too immature to handle the removal of such a large amount of bile pigment all at once. This form of jaundice is temporary and usually disappears without treatment. UV light breaks down bile pigments in the skin and can help speed recovery in infants with moderate to severe cases of jaundice.

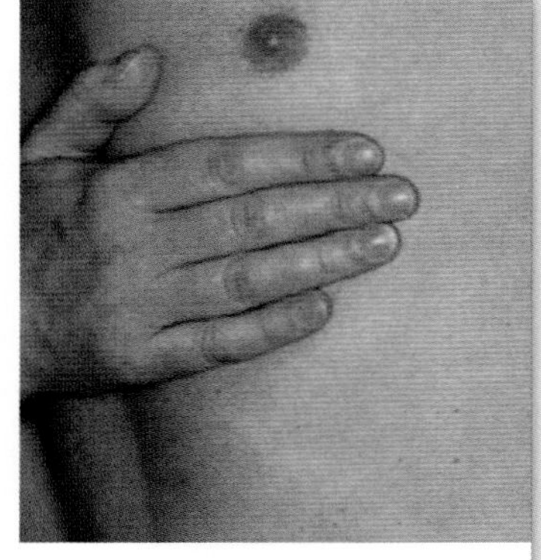

Jaundice. Yellowish discolouration of the skin and other tissues by bile pigments was, in the case seen here, caused by a liver infection. The yellow tinge of the skin can be best seen by comparing the patient's skin colour with that of the physician's hand.

TABLE 10-2 Functions of the Skin

FUNCTION	EXAMPLE	MECHANISM
Protection	Against microorganisms	Surface film/mechanical barrier
	Against dehydration	Keratin
	Against ultraviolet radiation	Melanins
	Against mechanical trauma	Tissue strength
Sensation	Pain Heat and cold Pressure Touch	Somatic sensory receptors
Permits movement and growth without injury	Body growth and change in body contours during movement	Elastic and recoil properties of skin and subcutaneous tissue
Endocrine	Vitamin D production	Activation of precursor compound in skin cells by ultraviolet light
Excretion	Water Urea Ammonia Uric acid	Regulation of sweat volume and content
Immunity	Destruction of microorganisms and interaction with immune system cells (helper T cells)	Phagocytic cells and epidermal dendritic cells
Temperature regulation	Heat loss or retention	Regulation of blood flow to the skin and evaporation of sweat

other sex hormones, corticoid hormones, and certain drugs such as nicotine and nitroglycerin.

The skin also produces melanin—the pigment that serves as an extremely effective screen to potentially harmful ultraviolet light—and keratin—one of nature's most flexible yet enduring protective proteins. Refer to **Table 10-2** as you read about the seven functions of the skin described in the paragraphs that follow.

PROTECTION

The keratinized stratified squamous epithelial cells that cover the epidermis make the skin a formidable barrier. It protects underlying tissues against invasion by hordes of microorganisms, bars entry of most harmful chemicals, and minimizes mechanical injury to underlying structures that might otherwise be harmed by even the relatively minor types of trauma experienced on a regular basis.

In addition to protection from microbiological entry, chemical hazards, and mechanical trauma, the skin also protects us from dehydration caused by loss of internal body fluids and from unwanted entry of fluids from the external environment. The ability of the pigment melanin to protect us from the harmful effects of overexposure to ultraviolet light is yet another protective function of the skin.

Surface Film

The ability of the skin to act as a protective barrier against an array of potentially damaging assaults from the environment begins with the proper functioning of a thin film of emulsified material spread over its surface. The **surface film** is produced by the mixing of residue and secretions from sweat and sebaceous glands with epithelial cells constantly being cast off from the epidermis. The shedding of epithelial elements from the skin surface is called **desquamation.** A variety of microbial cells are another important part of the mixture (**Box 10-5**).

Functions of surface film include the following:

- Antibacterial and antifungal activity
- Lubrication
- Hydration of the skin surface
- Buffering of caustic irritants
- Blockade of many toxic agents

The chemical composition of surface film includes (1) amino acids, sterols, and complex phospholipids from the breakdown of sloughed epithelial cells; (2) fatty acids, triglycerides, and waxes from sebum; (3) water, ammonia, lactate, urea, and uric acid from sweat;

UNIT 2

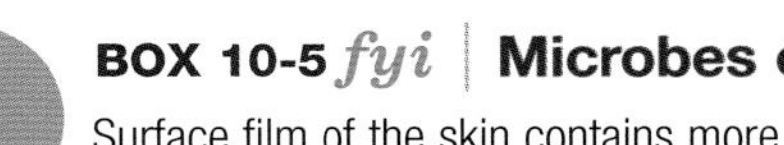

BOX 10-5 *fyi* **Microbes of the Skin**

Surface film of the skin contains more than just the mixed secretions of various glands and the sloughed-off keratinized cells of stratum corneum. It is teaming with a variety of microbes—microscopic organisms such as bacteria and fungi (see **Figure 8-12** on p. 147). They range in size from tiny virus particles that are much smaller than a cell to multicellular animals such as the "face" mite shown in the figure. This mite lives harmlessly in hair follicles—mostly on the face. There are up to ten times as many tiny organisms on your body's skin and mucous membranes as there are human cells in your body! These microbes act as a set of interactive ecosystems—a **microbiome.**

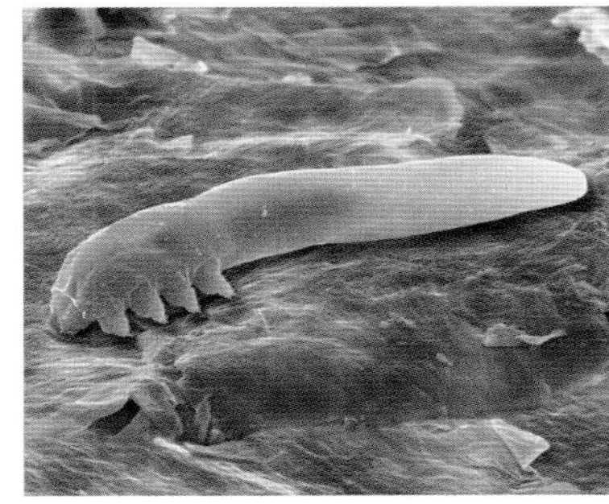

There are always some pathogenic bacteria and yeasts in the body's microbiome, but when you are healthy they are kept in check by an overwhelming majority of nonpathogenic microorganisms. If the healthy ecological balance is upset, however, the pathogens can take over in local areas and cause disease. Sometimes, even microorganisms that normally do no harm can get out of control and cause disease.

Scientists have been mapping out the widely varied microbial communities that inhabit different locations of our skin in hopes of preventing or curing skin disorders. They have already discovered that the microbiome of each person has unique characteristics. We may soon be able to identify individuals by their microbiome as easily as we do by using fingerprints!

CONNECT IT! 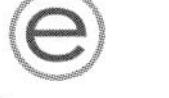

Review the concept of microbiomes and see a map showing the diversity of different bacterial communities on the human skin in ***The Human Microbiome*** at ***Connect It!***

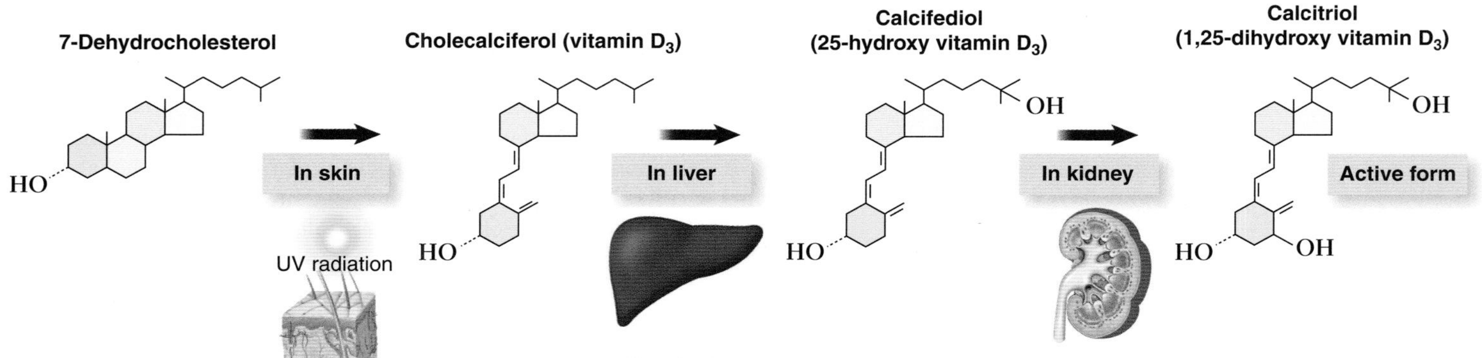

FIGURE 10-14 Vitamin D production. The essential first step in producing the active form of vitamin D in the body occurs in the presence of ultraviolet (UV) light in the skin.

and (4) antimicrobial agents that help regulate the skin's microbiome and prevent or reduce infections. The specific chemical composition of surface film is variable, and samples taken from skin covering one body area often have a different "mix" of chemical components than film covering skin in another area does. This difference helps explain the unique and localized distribution patterns of certain skin diseases and also explains why the skin covering a particular area of the body is sometimes more susceptible to attack by certain bacteria or fungi.

Sensation

The widespread placement of the millions of different somatic sensory receptors found in the skin enables it to function as a sophisticated sense organ covering the entire body surface (see **Figures 10-1** and **10-3**). Skin receptors serve as antennas that detect stimuli, which eventually produce the general, or somatic, senses, including pressure, touch, temperature, pain, and vibration. When these receptors are activated by their respective stimuli, they make it possible for the body to respond to changes occurring in both the external and internal environments. A full discussion of the anatomy and physiology of the somatic sense receptors is provided in Chapter 23.

Flexibility

Contraction of our muscles produces the purposeful movement that serves as one of the most easily observed "Characteristics of Life" discussed in Chapter 1. For movement of the body to occur without injury, the skin must be supple and elastic. It grows as we grow and exhibits stretch and recoil characteristics that permit changes in body contours to occur without tearing or laceration.

Excretion

By regulating the volume and chemical content of sweat, the body, through a function of the skin, can influence both its total fluid volume and the amounts of certain waste products, such as uric acid, ammonia, and urea that are excreted. In most circumstances the skin plays only a minor role in the overall excretion of body wastes. However, it can become a more important function in certain disease states or pathological conditions.

Hormone (Vitamin D) Production

The first step in the production of vitamin D in the body occurs when the skin is exposed to ultraviolet light. When this occurs, molecules of a chemical called *7-dehydrocholesterol*, which is normally found in skin cells, are converted into a precursor substance called *cholecalciferol* (**Figure 10-14**). This chemical is then transported in the blood to the liver and kidneys where it is converted into an active form of vitamin D—a compound that influences several important chemical reactions in the body. In this respect, vitamin D fulfils the requirements required for a substance to be classified as a *hormone*. In general, any chemical substance produced in one body area and then transported in the blood to another location where it has its effect is called a *hormone*. Hormones are critically important regulators of homeostasis and are discussed in detail in Chapters 25 and 26.

Melanin in the skin must be dark enough to protect the skin from damage from UV radiation, destruction of folic acid, and other adverse health effects. However, if there is too much melanin, the body cannot synthesize enough vitamin D for normal function. In such a case, vitamin D from outside the body is necessary to compensate for the failure of skin to make enough vitamin D. Research shows that various human populations often have just enough melanin to protect them from harm by the UV radiation levels in their native region—and not so much that it prevents vitamin D production.

Immunity

Important defensive cells that attach to and destroy pathogenic microorganisms are found in the skin and play an important role in immunity. In addition, epidermal dendritic cells function with helper T cells to trigger helpful immune reactions in certain diseases.

Homeostasis of Body Temperature

Despite sizable variations in environmental temperature, humans maintain a remarkably constant core body temperature. The functioning of the skin in homeostasis of body temperature is critical to survival and is examined in some detail.

In most people, body temperature moves up and down very little in the course of a day. It hovers close to a set point of about 37°C, perhaps increasing to 37.6°C by late afternoon and decreasing to around 36.2°C by early morning. This homeostasis of body temperature is of the utmost importance. Why? Because healthy survival depends on biochemical reactions taking place at certain rates—and these rates depend on normal enzyme functioning, which depends on body temperature staying within the narrow range of normal.

To maintain an even temperature, the body must balance the amount of heat it produces with the amount it loses. This means that if extra heat is produced in the body, this same amount of heat must be lost from it. Obviously, if this does not occur, if increased heat loss does not closely follow increased heat production, body temperature climbs steadily upward. If body temperature increases above normal for any reason, the skin plays a critical role in heat loss by the physical phenomena of evaporation, radiation, conduction, and convection.

Heat Production

Heat is produced by one means—metabolism of foods. Because the muscles, brown fat and glands (especially the liver) are the most active tissues, they carry on more metabolism and therefore produce more heat than any of the other tissues. The chief determinant of how much heat the body produces is the amount of muscular work it does. During exercise and shivering, for example, metabolism and heat production increase greatly. But during sleep, when very little muscular work is being done, metabolism and heat production decrease. The skin does produce a small amount of heat in the brown fat of the hypodermis, especially in newborns, but the skin's major role is retaining and dissipating heat to maintain homeostasis of body temperature.

Heat Loss

As already stated, one mechanism the body uses to maintain relative constancy of internal temperature is to regulate the amount of heat loss. Some 80% or more of this transfer of heat occurs through the skin; the remainder takes place in mucous membranes. As **Figure 10-15** shows, heat loss can be regulated by altering the flow of blood in the skin. If heat must be conserved to maintain a constant body temperature, dermal blood vessels constrict (vasoconstriction) to keep most of the warm blood circulating deeper in the body. If heat loss must be increased to maintain a constant temperature, dermal blood vessels widen (vasodilation) to increase the skin's supply of warm blood from deeper tissues. Heat transferred from the warm blood to the epidermis can then be lost to the external environment through the physical processes of evaporation, radiation, conduction, and convection.

Evaporation

Heat energy must be expended to evaporate any fluid. Evaporation of water constitutes one method by which heat is lost from the body, especially from the skin. Evaporation is especially important in high environmental temperatures, when it is the only method by which heat can be lost from the skin. A humid atmosphere necessarily retards evaporation and therefore lessens the cooling effect derived from it—the explanation for the fact that the same degree of temperature seems hotter in humid climates than in dry ones. At moderate temperatures, evaporation accounts for about half as much heat loss as radiation does.

Radiation

Radiation is the transfer of heat from the surface of one object to that of another without actual contact between the two. Heat radiates from the body surface to nearby objects that are cooler than the skin and radiates to the skin from those that are warmer than the skin. This is the principle of heating and cooling systems. In cool environmental temperatures, radiation accounts for a greater percentage of heat loss from the skin than conduction and evaporation combined do. In hot environments, no heat is lost by radiation but may be gained by radiation from warmer surfaces to the skin.

Conduction

Conduction means the transfer of heat to any substance actually in contact with the body—to clothing or jewelry, for example, or even to cold foods or liquids ingested. This process accounts for a relatively small amount of heat loss.

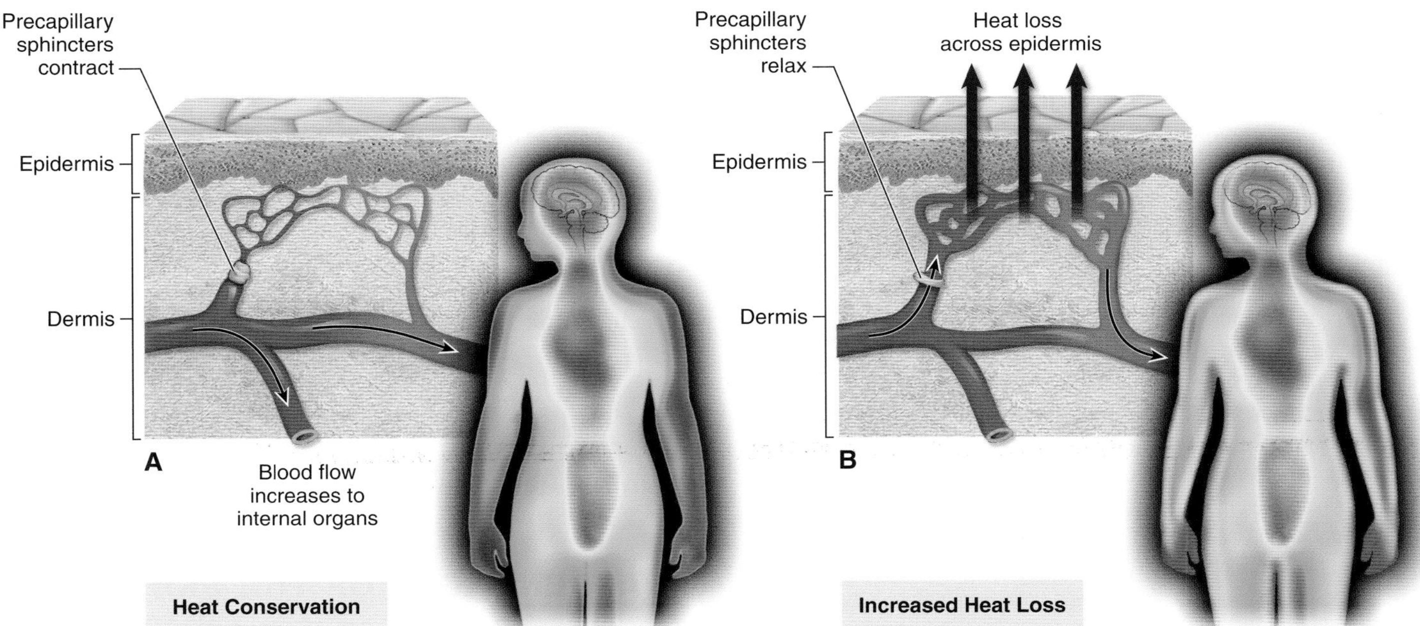

FIGURE 10-15 The skin as a thermoregulatory organ. When homeostasis requires that the body conserve heat, blood flow in the warm organs of the body's core increases. **A,** When heat must be lost to maintain stability of the internal environment, flow of warm blood to the skin increases. **B,** Heat can be lost from the blood and skin by means of radiation, conduction, convection, and evaporation. The head, hands, and feet are major areas of heat loss.

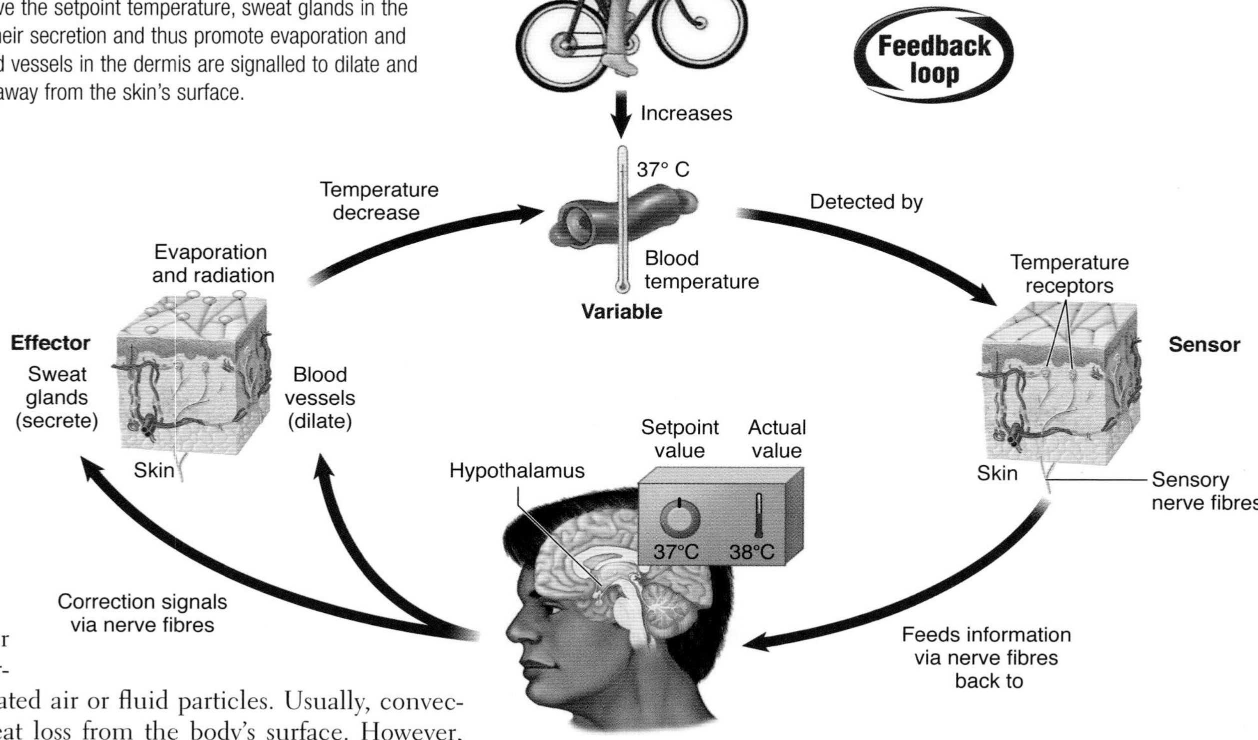

FIGURE 10-16 Role of skin in homeostasis of body temperature. Body temperature is continually monitored by nerve receptors in the skin and other parts of the body. These receptors feed information back to the hypothalamus of the brain, which compares the actual temperature with the setpoint temperature and then sends out an appropriate correction signal to effectors. If actual body temperature is above the setpoint temperature, sweat glands in the skin are signalled to increase their secretion and thus promote evaporation and cooling. At the same time, blood vessels in the dermis are signalled to dilate and thus promote radiation of heat away from the skin's surface.

Convection

Convection is the transfer of heat away from a surface by movement of heated air or fluid particles. Usually, convection causes very little heat loss from the body's surface. However, under certain conditions, it can account for considerable heat loss, as you know if you have ever stepped from your shower into even slightly moving air from an open window.

Homeostatic Regulation of Heat Loss

The operation of the skin's blood vessels and sweat glands must be coordinated carefully and must take into account moment-by-moment fluctuations in body temperature. Like most homeostatic mechanisms, heat loss by the skin is controlled by a negative feedback loop (**Figure 10-16**). Temperature receptors in a part of the brain, called the *hypothalamus*, detect changes in the body's internal temperature. If some disturbance, such as exercise, increases body temperature above the setpoint value of 37°C, the hypothalamus acts as an integrator and sends a nervous signal to the sweat glands and blood vessels of the skin. The sweat glands and blood vessels (the effectors) respond to the signal by acting in ways that promote heat loss. Sweat glands increase their output of sweat (increasing heat loss by evaporation), and blood vessels increase their diameter (increasing heat loss by radiation and other means). This process continues until the homeostatic set point for normal body temperature is reached (**Box 10-6**).

BOX 10-6 *sports and fitness*
Exercise and the Skin

Excess heat produced by the skeletal muscles during exercise increases the core body temperature far beyond the normal range. Because blood in vessels near the skin's surface dissipates heat well, the body's control centres adjust blood flow so that more warm blood from the body's core is sent to the skin for cooling. During exercise, blood flow in the skin can be so high that the skin takes on a redder colouration.

To help dissipate even more heat, sweat production increases to as high as 3 L per hour during exercise. Although each sweat gland produces very little of this total, more than 3 million individual sweat glands are found throughout the skin. Sweat evaporation is essential to keeping body temperature in balance, but excessive sweating can lead to a dangerous loss of fluid. Because the usual intake of fluids may not replace the water lost through sweating, it is important to increase fluid consumption during and after any type of exercise to avoid *dehydration*. •

Quick **CHECK**

9. What is the one means of heat production in the body? In what type of organs does most heat production occur?
10. Name three of the four physical processes by which heat is lost from the body.

APPENDAGES OF THE SKIN

Appendages of the skin consist of *hair*, *nails*, and *skin glands*. In addition to illustrations of these appendages here, see also the micrographs of hair and skin glands in Part 5 of the BRIEF ATLAS OF THE HUMAN BODY.

HAIR

We have about 5 million hairs on the skin of our body. About 150,000 hairs are on our heads, with the rest scattered all over the skin. Only a few areas of the skin are hairless—notably the palms of the hands and the soles of the feet. Hair is also absent from the lips, nipples, and some areas of the genitals.

Development of Hair

Many months before birth, tiny tubular pockets called **hair follicles** begin to develop in most parts of the skin. By about the sixth month of pregnancy the developing fetus is all but covered by an extremely fine and soft hair coat, called **lanugo.** Most of the lanugo hair is lost before birth. Soon after birth, any lanugo hair that remains is lost and then replaced by **vellus** hair, which is stronger, fine, and usually less pigmented (see **Figure 10-3**, *B*).

The replacement hair growth after birth first appears on the scalp, eyelids, and eyebrows, and the coarse pubic and axillary hair that develops at puberty is called **terminal hair.** In the adult male, terminal hair replaces 80% to 90% of the vellus hair on the chest and extremities and also makes up the beard. In the female, far less vellus hair is replaced with the coarser terminal variety except in the pubic and axillary areas.

Hair growth begins at the base of the follicle (**Figure 10-17**). The follicle wall consists of two primary layers: (1) an outer dermal root sheath and (2) an epithelial root sheath, which is subdivided into external and internal layers (**Figure 10-17**, *B*). At the bottom of the follicle is a cap-shaped cluster of cells known as the **germinal matrix.** Protruding into the germinal matrix is a small mound of the dermis, called the **hair papilla,** which is an important structure because it contains the blood capillaries that nourish the germinal matrix (see **Figure 10-17**). Cells of the germinal matrix are responsible for forming hairs. They undergo repeated mitosis, push upward in the follicle, and become keratinized to form a hair. As long as cells of the germinal matrix remain alive, hair regenerates even though it is cut, plucked, or otherwise removed.

Part of the hair, namely, the root, lies hidden in the follicle. The visible part of a hair is called the **shaft.** The inner core of a hair is known as the **medulla,** the more superficial portion around it is called the **cortex,** and the covering layer is called the *cuticle.* If hair is plucked from the follicle, the internal epithelial root sheath will be torn free as well and appears as a whitish layer adherent to the hair cuticle. Layers of keratinized cells make up the cortex.

Besides being a structure to grow and support hair, the hair follicle wall also serves as a primary location of adult stem cells for various types of skin cells such as melanocytes and keratinocytes.

Appearance of Hair

Deposited in the cells of the hair are varying amounts of melanins, the pigments responsible for hair colour. Although reflections of light can affect hair colour somewhat, it is largely the amount, type, and distribution of melanin that determine the colour of hair. Varying amounts of eumelanins in the cortex and/or medulla can produce

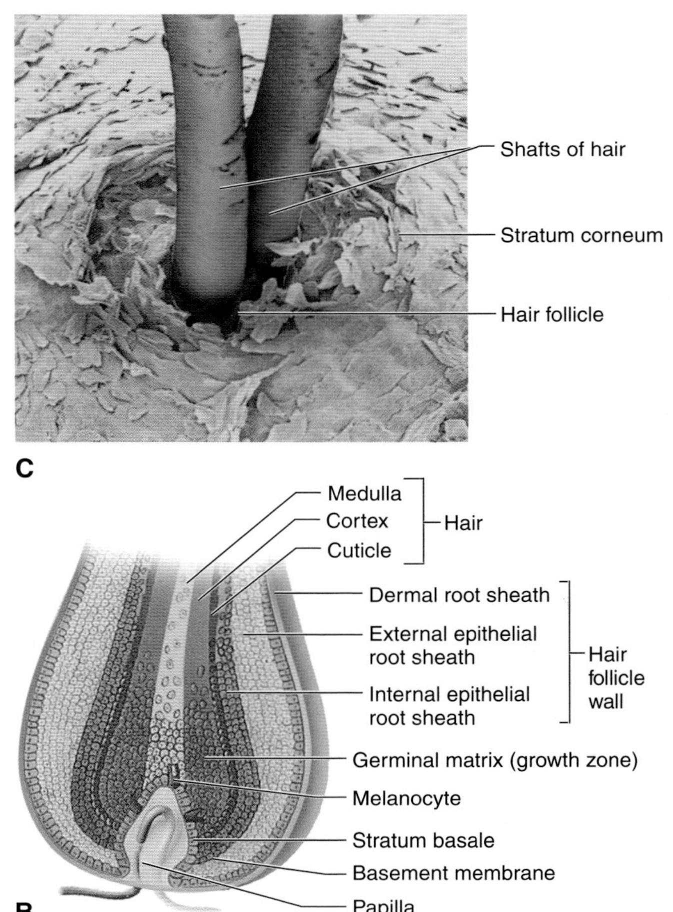

FIGURE 10-17 Hair follicle. A, Relationship of a hair follicle and related structures to the epidermal and dermal layers of the skin. **B,** Enlargement of a hair follicle wall and hair bulb. **C,** Scanning electron micrograph showing shafts of hair extending from their follicles.

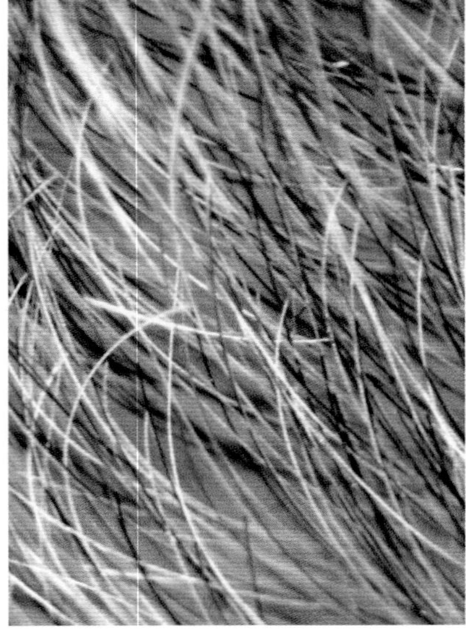

FIGURE 10-18 Grey hair. Grey hair results from a scattered arrangement of both white (pigmentless) hairs and darker (pigmented) hairs.

many shades of blonde and brunette hair. Pheomelanins give hair a reddish tint. Advancing age often produces an increasing smattering of white hairs—the proverbial "crown of glory". White hairs have no pigments at all but appear white because of the diffusion of light through the translucent hair shaft. White hair results from the accumulation of oxygen *free radicals*—highly reactive forms of oxygen that increase as we age. The free radicals damage stem cells in the hair follicle. We fail to maintain the production of new melanocytes and thus lose the ability to produce pigment in the hair. Grey hair, seen in **Figure 10-18**, is usually a "salt-and-pepper" mixed arrangement of white and dark hairs. Besides adding colour, melanin also imparts strength to the hair shaft.

Whether hair is straight or wavy depends mainly on the shape of the shaft. Straight hair has a round, cylindrical shaft. Wavy hair, in contrast, has a flat shaft that is not as strong. As a result, it is more easily broken or damaged than is straight hair. Two or more small **sebaceous glands** secrete **sebum**, an oily substance, into each hair follicle (see **Figure 10-17**). The sebaceous gland secretions lubricate and condition the hair and surrounding skin to keep it from becoming dry, brittle, and easily damaged. Lipid-containing hair and skin conditioners can add to this damage-reducing effect.

Hair alternates between periods of growth and rest. On average, hair on the head grows a little less than 12 mm per month, or about 13 cm a year. Body hair grows more slowly. Head hairs reportedly live between 2 and 6 years, then die and are shed. Normally, however, new hairs replace those lost. But baldness, also called *alopecia*, can develop.

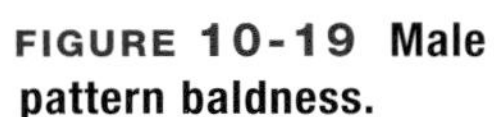

FIGURE 10-19 Male pattern baldness.

A common type of baldness occurs only when two requirements are met: genes for baldness must be inherited and the male sex hormones (*androgens*) must be present. When the right combination of these causative factors exists, *androgenic alopecia* or **male pattern baldness** (**Figure 10-19**) inevitably results. An available treatment that may slow or stop the development of male pattern baldness is the drug minoxidil. Unfortunately, the treatment is expensive, must be continued for life if new hair growth is to be retained, and does not always produce as dramatic an effect as hoped.

Contrary to what many people believe, hair growth is not stimulated by frequent cutting or shaving. In addition, stories about hair or beard growth continuing after death are also false. What may appear to be continuing beard growth after death is in reality only a more visible beard in a skin surface dehydrated by environmental conditions or the embalming process.

NAILS

Heavily keratinized epidermal cells compose fingernails and toenails. The visible part of each nail is called the **nail body.** The rest of the nail, namely, the **root,** lies in a flat sinus hidden by a fold of skin bordered by the **cuticle** (**Figure 10-20**).

Under the nail lies a layer of epithelium called the **nail bed**. The nail bed nearest the root has a crescent-shaped white area known as the *lunule* or **lunula,** or "little moon", that is often visible under the proximal end of the nail body.

Because it contains abundant blood vessels, the nail bed normally appears pink through the translucent part of the nail bodies. Clinically, this is useful to know. Cyanosis (blueness) often appears under the nails first (see **Figure 10-12**), and thus nail beds are often monitored closely during surgery or other procedures in which oxygenation of the blood may suddenly drop. Sometimes, lightly pigmented streaks appear in the nail beds of dark-skinned individuals (**Figure 10-21**).

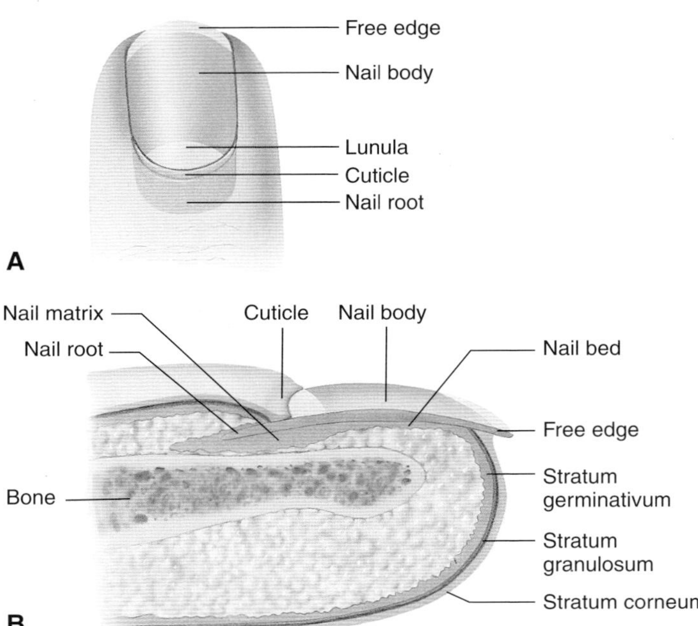

FIGURE 10-20 Structure of nails. A, Fingernail viewed from above. **B,** Sagittal section of a fingernail and associated structures.

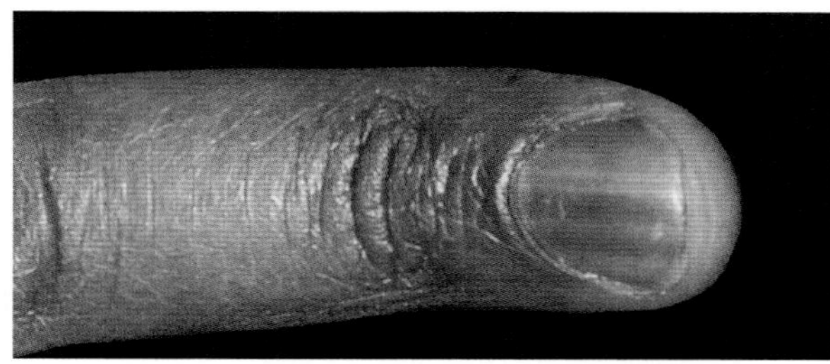

FIGURE 10-21 Pigmented nails. In light-skinned individuals, the nail bed is usually free of pigmentation. In very dark-skinned individuals, yellowish or brown pigmented bands (seen in the photograph) are common.

Nails grow by mitosis of cells in the stratum basale beneath the lunula and root. On average, nails grow about 0.5 mm a week. Fingernails, however, as you may have noticed, grow faster than toenails, and both grow faster in the summer than in the winter. Even minor trauma to long fingernails can sometimes result in loosening of the nail from the nail bed with a resulting separation that starts at the distal or free edge of the affected nail (**Figure 10-22**). The condition, called **onycholysis,** is common.

Bruising under a nail can cause discolouration as the bruise forms, then heals. Fungal infections can also cause discolouration of nails, often turning them yellow or even black. Fungal infections also often weaken the nail structure, causing a nail to flake, split, or break more easily.

Artificial nails made of plastic can be used to help repair broken nails or simply to enhance the nails' appearance. However, health care workers are discouraged from using artificial nails because they tend to transmit bacterial infection more easily. In surgical patients, artificial nails obscure signs of cyanosis, which is a helpful clinical sign of oxygen deficiency.

Quick CHECK

11. Identify the pigment that determines hair colour.
12. List seven functions of the skin.
13. How does surface film contribute to the protective function of the skin?
14. List the appendages of the skin.

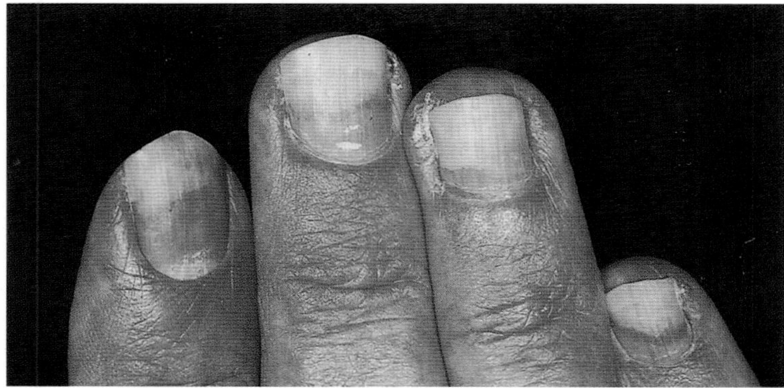

FIGURE 10-22 Onycholysis. In the photo, note that separation of the nails from the nail bed begins at the free edge. Minor trauma to long fingernails is the most common cause.

SKIN GLANDS

The skin glands include three kinds of microscopic exocrine glands: sweat, sebaceous, and ceruminous (**Figure 10-23**).

Sweat Glands

Sweat or **sudoriferous glands** are the most numerous of the skin glands. They can be classified into two groups—*eccrine* and *apocrine*—based on the type of secretion, location, and nervous system connections.

Eccrine sweat glands are by far the most numerous, important, and widespread sweat glands in the body. They are small, with a secretory portion less than 0.4 mm in diameter, and are distributed over the total body surface with the exception of the lips, ear canal, glans penis, and nail beds. Eccrine sweat glands are a simple, coiled, tubular type of gland.

Eccrine sweat glands function throughout life to produce a transparent watery liquid (*perspiration*, or *sweat*) rich in salts, ammonia, uric acid, urea, and other wastes. In addition to elimination of waste, sweat plays a critical role in helping the body maintain a constant core temperature.

Histologists estimate that a single square centimetre of skin on the palms of the hands contains about 500 sweat glands. Eccrine sweat glands are also numerous on the soles of the feet, forehead, and upper part of the torso. With a good magnifying glass you can locate the openings of these sweat gland ducts on the skin ridges of the palms and on the skin of the palmar surfaces of the fingers. Although the ducts of eccrine glands travel through both the dermis and epidermis to open on the skin surface, the actual secretory portion is located in the subcutaneous tissue.

Apocrine sweat glands are located deep in the subcutaneous layer of the skin in the armpit (axilla), the areola of the breast, and the pigmented skin areas around the anus. They are much larger than eccrine glands and often have secretory units that reach 5 mm or more in diameter. They are connected to hair follicles and are classified as simple, branched tubular glands.

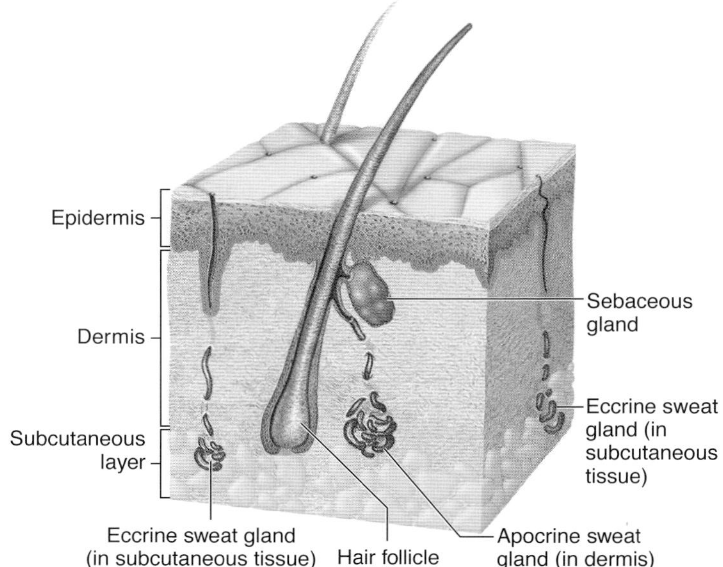

FIGURE 10-23 Skin glands. Several types of exocrine glands occur in the skin.

UNIT 2

Apocrine glands enlarge and begin to function at puberty; they produce a more viscous and coloured secretion than eccrine glands do. In the female, apocrine gland secretions show cyclic changes linked to the menstrual cycle. The odour often associated with apocrine gland secretion is not caused by the secretion itself. Instead, it is caused by decomposition of the secretion by skin bacteria.

CONNECT IT! 

Apocrine sweat contains a class of molecules called **pheromones,** which are signalling molecules detected by other individuals. They may be used as a territorial marker, but in humans they seem to serve mainly as social or sexual signals. Want to know more about these "sex molecules"? Check out ***Pheromones and the Vomeronasal Organ*** online at ***Connect It!***

cycle of life

Skin Everyone is aware of the dramatic changes in skin that each person experiences from birth through the mature years. Infants and young children have relatively smooth and unwrinkled skin characterized by the elasticity and flexibility associated with extreme youth. Because the skin tissues are in an active phase of new growth, healing of skin injuries is often rapid and efficient. Young children have fewer sweat glands than adults do, so their bodies rely more on increased blood flow to maintain normal body temperature. This explains why preschoolers often become "red-faced" while playing outdoors on a warm day.

As adulthood begins, at puberty, hormones stimulate the development and activation of sebaceous glands and sweat glands. After the sebaceous glands become active, especially during the initial years, they often overproduce sebum and thus give the skin an unusually oily appearance. Sebaceous ducts may become clogged or infected and form acne pimples or other blemishes on the skin (**Box 10-7**). Activation of apocrine sweat glands during puberty causes increased sweat production—an ability needed to maintain an adult body properly—and also the possibility of increased "body odour." Body odour is caused by wastes produced by bacteria that feed on the organic compounds found in apocrine sweat and on the surface of the skin.

As one continues past early adulthood, the sebaceous and sweat glands become less active. Although this can provide a welcome relief to those with acne or other problems associated with overactivity of these glands, it can affect normal function of the body. For example, the reduction of sebum production can cause the skin and hair to become less resilient and therefore more likely to wrinkle or crack. Wrinkling can also be caused by an overall degeneration in the skin's ability to maintain itself as efficiently as it did during the early years of life (**Figure 10-24**).

Loss of function in sweat glands as adulthood advances adversely affects the body's ability to cool itself during exercise or when the external temperature is high. Thus elderly individuals are more likely to develop severe problems during hot weather than are young adults.

Figure 10-11 shows the hyperpigmented "age spots" seen in the elderly after years of sun exposure. •

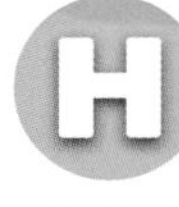

BOX 10-7 *health matters* | **Acne**

Common *acne,* or *acne vulgaris,* occurs most often in the adolescent years as a result of overactive secretion by the sebaceous glands, with blockage and inflammation of their ducts.

The rate of sebum secretion increases more than fivefold between 10 and 19 years of age. As a result, sebaceous gland ducts may become plugged with sloughed skin cells and sebum contaminated with bacteria. The inflamed plug is called a *comedo* and is the most characteristic sign of acne. Pus-filled *pimples* or *pustules* result from secondary infections within or beneath the epidermis, often in a hair follicle or sweat pore. •

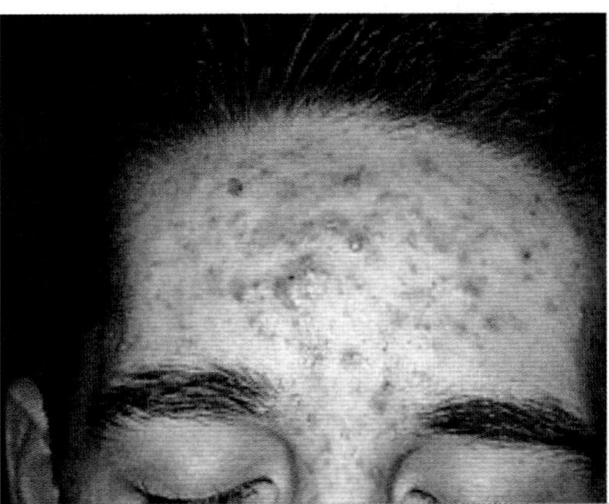

Sebaceous Glands

Sebaceous glands secrete oil for the hair and skin. Wherever hairs grow from the skin, there are sebaceous glands, at least two for each hair. The oil, or **sebum**, keeps the hair supple and the skin soft and pliant. It is nature's own protective skin cream that prevents excessive water loss from the epidermis. Because sebum is rich in chemicals that have an antifungal effect, such as triglycerides, waxes, fatty acids, and cholesterol, it also contributes to reducing fungal activity on the skin surface. This property of sebum increases the effectiveness of the skin's surface film and helps protect the skin from numerous types of fungal infections.

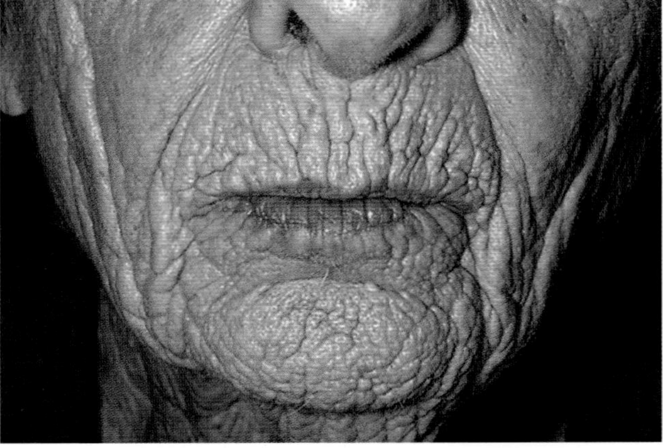

FIGURE 10-24 Aged skin. In late adulthood, wrinkles in the skin often develop—especially in areas of frequent movement such as on the hands, around the mouth, and around the eyelids.

Sebaceous glands are simple branched glands of varying size that are found in the dermis, except in the skin of the palms and soles. Although almost always associated with hair follicles, some sebaceous glands do open directly onto the skin surface in such areas as the glans penis, lips, and eyelids. Sebum secretion increases during adolescence because it is stimulated by increased blood levels of sex hormones. Often sebum accumulates in and enlarges some of the ducts of the sebaceous glands, thereby forming white pimples. With oxidation, this accumulated sebum darkens and forms a **blackhead.**

Ceruminous Glands

Ceruminous glands are a special variety or modification of apocrine sweat glands. Histologically, they appear as simple coiled tubular glands with excretory ducts that open onto the free surface of the skin in the external ear canal or with sebaceous glands into the necks of hair follicles in this area. The mixed secretions of sebaceous and ceruminous glands form a brown waxy substance called **cerumen.** Although it serves a useful purpose in protecting the skin of the ear canal from dehydration, excess cerumen can harden and cause blockage in the ear, resulting in loss of hearing.

Quick **CHECK**

15. What are the two types of sweat glands? How do they differ?
16. List two functions of sebum.
17. What substances make up the skin's surface film?

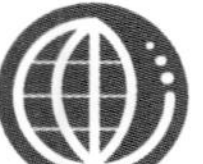

the big picture | **Skin and the Whole Body**

The skin is one of the major components of the body's structural framework. It is continuous with the connective tissues that hold the body together, including the fascia, bones, tendons, and ligaments. The integumentary, skeletal, and muscular systems work together to protect and support the whole body.

As stated several times in this chapter, the skin is a barrier that separates the internal environment from the external environment. Put another way, the skin *defines* the internal environment of the body. The barrier formed by the skin is a formidable one indeed; the skin possesses numerous mechanisms for protecting internal structures from the sometimes harsh external environment. Without these protective mechanisms, the internal environment could not maintain a relative constancy that is independent of the external environment.

First, the dermis and epidermis work together to form a tough, waterproof envelope that protects us from drying out and from the dangers of chemical or microbial contamination. The sebaceous secretions of the skin, along with other components of the skin's surface film, enhance the skin's ability to protect the internal environment. Protection against mechanical injuries is provided by hair, calluses, and the layers of the skin itself. Pigmentation in the skin and our ability to regulate its concentration protect us from the harmful effects of solar radiation.

Although its primary functions are support and protection, the skin has other important roles in maintaining homeostasis. For example, the skin is also an important agent in the regulation of body temperature—it serves as a sort of "radiator" that can be activated or deactivated as needed. It helps maintain a constant level of calcium in the body by producing vitamin D, which is necessary for normal absorption of calcium in the digestive tract. Ridges on the palms and fingers allow us to make and use tools for getting food, building shelters, and conducting other survival tasks. The skin's flexibility and elasticity permit the free movement required to perform such tasks. Sensory nerve receptors in the dermis allow the skin to be a "window on the world". Information about the external environment is relayed from skin receptors to nervous control (integration) centres, where it is used to coordinate the function of other organs.

As you continue your study of the various organ systems of the body, keep in mind that none of them could operate properly without the structural and functional assistance of the integumentary system.

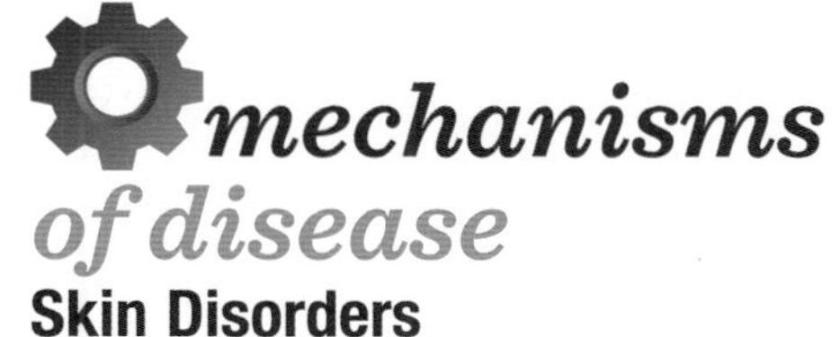

Skin Disorders

Any disorder of the skin can be called a **dermatosis,** which means "skin condition". Many dermatoses involve inflammation of the skin, or **dermatitis.** Various disorders involving the skin have already been discussed in this chapter. A few more representative disorders are described here.

Skin Infections

The skin is the first line of defence against microorganisms that might invade the body's internal environment. It is no wonder that the skin is a common site of infection. In adults, the antimicrobial characteristics of sebum in the skin's surface film often inhibit skin infections. In children, the lack of sebum in surface film makes the skin less resistant to infection.

Many different viruses, bacteria, and fungi cause skin conditions. Here are a few examples of skin infections caused by different types of pathogenic (disease-causing) organisms:

1. **Impetigo.** This highly contagious bacterial condition results from *Staphylococcus* or *Streptococcus* infection and occurs most often in young children. Impetigo starts as a reddish discolouration, or *erythema,* but soon develops into vesicles (blisters) and yellowish crusts. Occasionally the infection becomes systemic (bodywide) and thus is life-threatening.
2. **Tinea.** Tinea is the general name for many different *mycoses* (fungal infections) of the skin. Ringworm, jock itch, and athlete's foot are all classified as tinea. Signs of tinea include erythema, scaling, and crusting. Occasionally, fissures, or cracks, in the epidermis develop at creases in the epidermis. **Figure 10-25** shows a case of ringworm, a tinea infection that typically forms a round rash that heals in the centre to form a ring. Antifungal agents usually stop the acute infection but are unable to completely destroy the

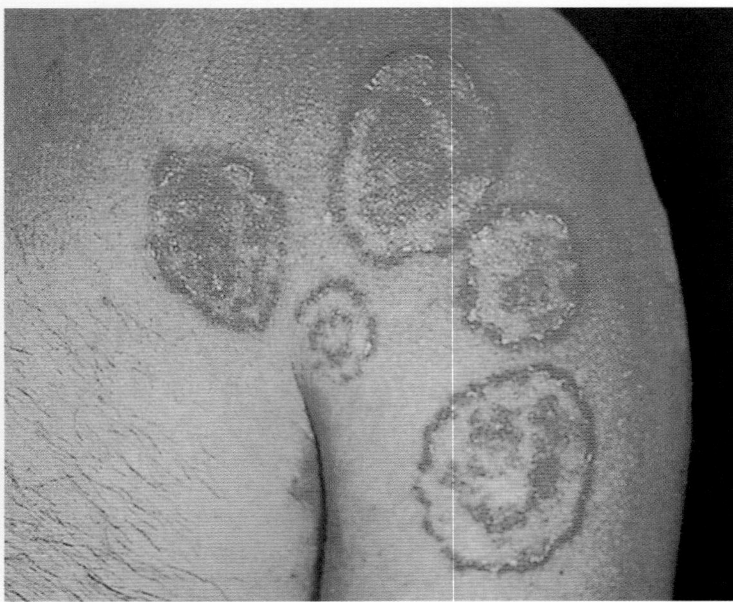

FIGURE 10-25 Tinea infection (ringworm). Note that the lesions heal in the centre, with inflamed rings left on the skin's surface.

fungus. Recurrence of tinea can be avoided by keeping the skin dry because fungi require a moist environment to grow.

3. **Warts.** Caused by papillomaviruses, warts are nipple-like neoplasms of the skin. Although they are usually benign, some warts transform to become malignant. Transmission of warts generally occurs through direct contact with warts on the skin of an infected person. Warts can be removed by freezing, drying, laser therapy, or the application of chemicals.
4. **Boils.** Also called *furuncles,* boils are local *Staphylococcus* infections of hair follicles characterized by large, inflamed, pus-filled lesions. A group of untreated boils may fuse into even larger lesions called *carbuncles.*

Vascular and Inflammatory Skin Disorders

Everyone who might ever be called on to provide care to a bedridden or otherwise immobilized individual should be aware of the causes and nature of pressure sores, or **decubitus ulcers** (**Figure 10-26**). *Decubitus* means "lying down", a name that hints at a common cause of pressure sores: lying in one position for long periods. Also called *bedsores,* these lesions appear after blood flow to a local area of skin slows because of pressure on skin covering bony prominences such as the ankles. Ulcers form and infections develop as lack of blood flow causes tissue damage. Frequent changes in body position and soft support cushions help prevent decubitus ulcers.

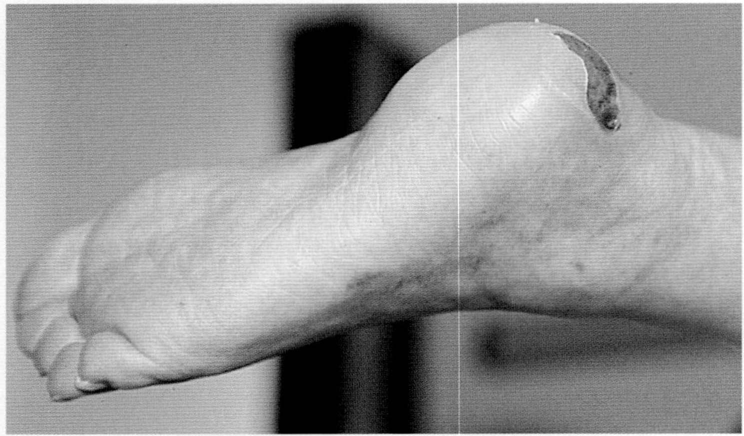

FIGURE 10-26 Decubitus ulcer. The skin forms craterlike lesions when the blood supply is diminished and skin tissue cannot be maintained in the area of reduced blood flow.

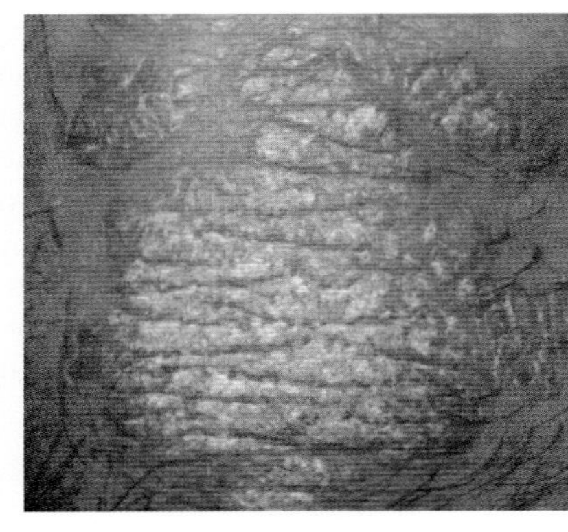

FIGURE 10-27 Psoriasis. Inflammation and scaling are characteristic of this skin disorder.

A common type of skin disorder that involves blood vessels is **urticaria,** or *hives.* This condition is characterized by raised red lesions, called *wheals,* caused by leakage of fluid from the skin's blood vessels. Urticaria is often associated with severe itching. Hypersensitivity or allergic reactions, physical irritants, and systemic diseases are common causes.

Scleroderma is an autoimmune disease that affects the blood vessels and connective tissues of the skin. The name *scleroderma* comes from the word parts *sclera-,* which means "hard", and *derma,* which means "skin". Hard skin is a good description of the lesions characteristic of scleroderma. Scleroderma begins as a mild inflammation that later develops into a patch of yellowish, hardened skin. Scleroderma most commonly remains a mild, localized condition. Very rarely, localized scleroderma progresses to a systemic form that affects large areas of the skin and other organs. Persons with advanced systemic scleroderma seem to be wearing a mask because skin hardening prevents them from moving their mouths freely. Both forms of scleroderma occur more commonly in women than in men.

Psoriasis is a chronic inflammatory disorder of the skin thought to have a genetic basis. This common skin problem is characterized by cutaneous inflammation accompanied by silver-coloured, scaly lesions that develop from an excessive rate of epithelial cell growth (**Figure 10-27**).

Eczema is the most common inflammatory disorder of the skin. This condition is characterized by inflammation often accompanied by papules (bumps), vesicles (blisters), and crusts. Eczema is not a distinct disease but rather a sign or symptom of an underlying condition. For example, an allergic reaction called *contact dermatitis* can progress to become eczematous. Poison ivy is a form of contact dermatitis—occurring on *contact* with chemicals produced by the poison ivy plant.

Skin Cancer

Each year in the United Kingdom more than 140,000 new cases of skin cancer are diagnosed. These *neoplasms,* or abnormal growths, result from cell changes in the epidermis and are among the most common forms of cancer in humans.

Two forms of the disease, called **basal cell carcinoma** and **squamous cell carcinoma,** account for more than 90% of all reported cases of skin cancer (**Figure 10-28**, *A* and *B*). Both types are very responsive to treatment and seldom *metastasize,* or spread to other body areas. However, if left untreated, these cancers can cause significant damage to adjacent tissues that results in disfigurement and loss of function.

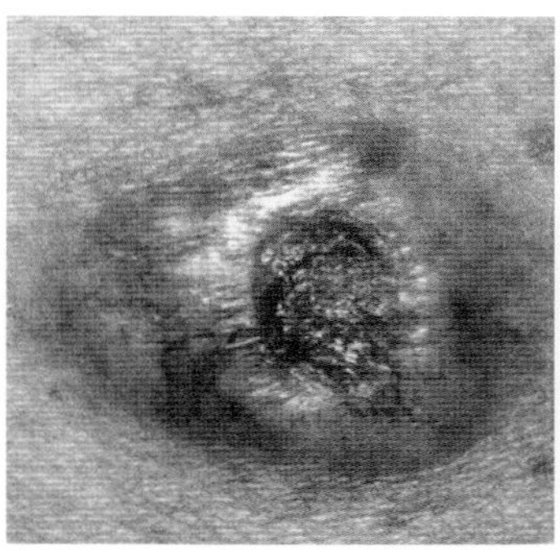

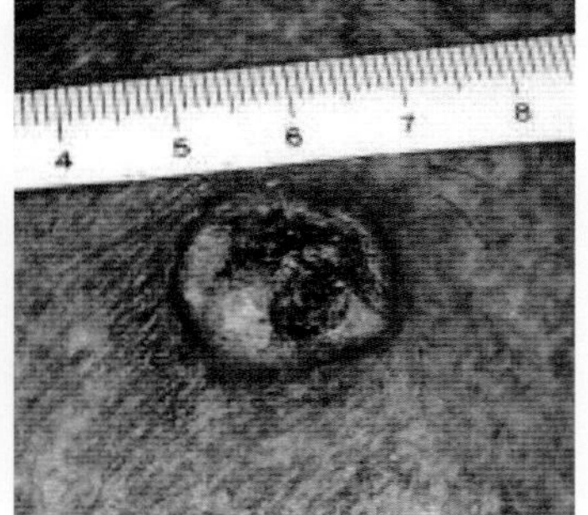

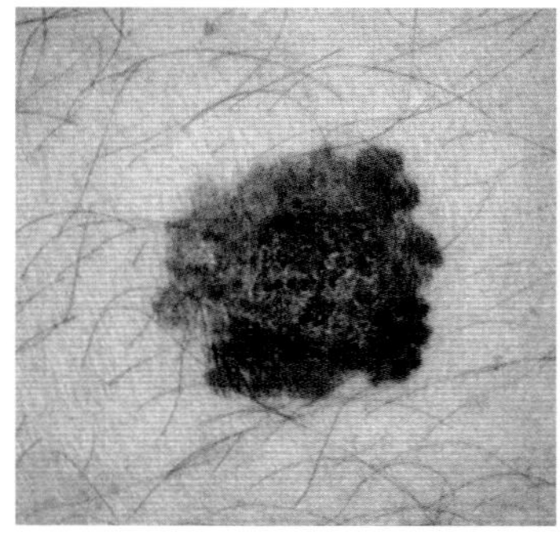

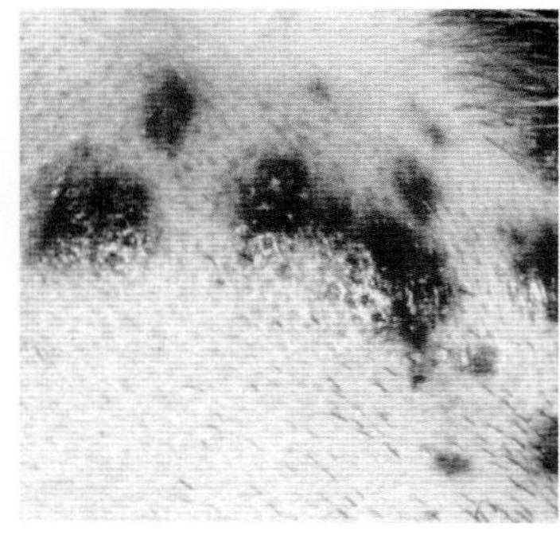

FIGURE 10-28 Skin cancers.

A third type of skin cancer called **malignant melanoma** has a tendency to spread to other body areas and is a much more serious form of the disease than either the basal cell or squamous cell varieties (**Figure 10-28**, *C*). About 15,000 new cases of malignant melanoma are reported each year in the UK, and of that number more than 2500 people die of the disease.

Kaposi sarcoma (KS) appears in immune deficiencies such as AIDS. It produces purple papules on the skin (**Figure 10-28**, *D*) and quickly spreads to the lymph nodes and internal organs.

CONNECT IT! 

How can you tell the difference between a normal mole and skin cancer? Find out at ***Skin Cancer*** online at ***Connect It!***

Abnormal Body Temperature

Maintenance of body temperature within a narrow range is necessary for normal functioning of the body. **Figure 10-29** shows that straying too far out of the normal range of body temperatures can have very serious physiological consequences. A few important conditions related to body temperature follow.

1. **Fever,** or a *febrile* state, is an unusually high body temperature associated with a systemic inflammatory response. In the case of infections, chemicals called **pyrogens** (literally "fire makers") cause the thermostatic control centres of the hypothalamus to produce a fever. Because the body's "thermostat" is reset to a higher setting, a person feels a need to warm up to this new temperature and often experiences "chills" as the febrile state begins. The high body temperature associated with infectious fever is thought to enhance the body's immune responses to eliminate the pathogen. Strategies aimed at reducing the temperature of a febrile person are normally counteracted by the body's heat-generating mechanisms and have the effect of further weakening the infected person. In ordinary circumstances, it is best to let the fever "break" on its own after the pathogen is destroyed.
2. **Malignant hyperthermia (MH),** an inherited condition, is characterized by abnormally increased body temperature (hyperthermia) and muscle rigidity when exposed to certain anaesthetics or muscle relaxants (suxamethonium, for example). The drug *dantrolene,* which inhibits heat-producing muscle contractions, has been used to prevent or relieve the effects of this condition.
3. **Heat exhaustion** occurs when the body loses a large amount of fluid from heat loss mechanisms. This usually happens when environmental temperatures are high. Although normal body temperature is maintained, the loss of water and electrolytes can cause weakness, dizziness, nausea, and possibly loss of consciousness. Heat exhaustion may also be accompanied by skeletal muscle cramps often called *heat cramps.* Heat exhaustion is treated with rest (in a cool environment) accompanied by fluid replacement.
4. **Heat stroke,** or *sunstroke,* is a severe, sometimes fatal condition resulting from the inability of the body to maintain normal temperature in an extremely warm environment. Such thermoregulatory failure may result from factors such as old age, disease, drugs that impair thermoregulation, or simply overwhelming

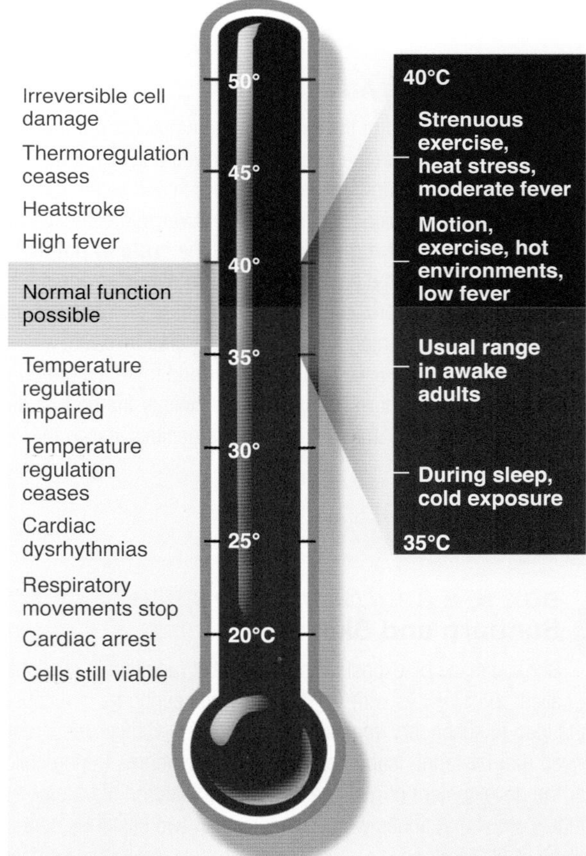

FIGURE 10-29 Body temperature. This diagram, modelled after a thermometer, shows some physiological consequences of abnormal body temperature. The inset shows a range of body temperatures at which normal function is possible. Ideally, body temperature should be near 37°C, but the body can operate normally within the range shown if conditions are not ideal.

elevated environmental temperatures. Heat stroke is characterized by body temperatures of 41°C or higher, tachycardia (rapid heart rate), headache, and hot, dry skin. Confusion, convulsions, or loss of consciousness may occur. Unless the body is cooled and body fluids are replaced immediately, death may result.

5. **Hypothermia** is the inability to maintain normal body temperature in extremely cold environments. Hypothermia is characterized by body temperatures lower than 35°C, shallow and slow respirations, and a faint, slow pulse. Hypothermia is usually treated by slowly warming the affected person's body.
6. **Frostbite** is local damage to tissues caused by extremely low temperatures. Damage to tissues results from the formation of ice crystals accompanied by a reduction in local blood flow. **Necrosis** (tissue death) and even **gangrene** (decay of dead tissue) can result from frostbite.

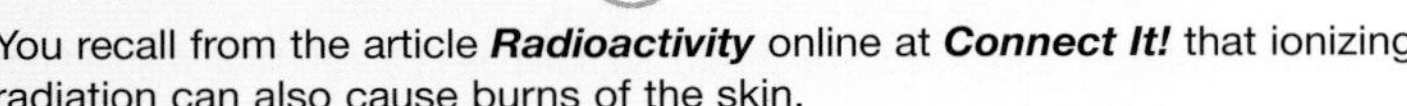

CONNECT IT!

You recall from the article ***Radioactivity*** online at ***Connect It!*** that ionizing radiation can also cause burns of the skin.

Burns

Typically we think of a burn as a thermal injury or lesion caused by contact of the skin with some hot object or fire. In addition, overexposure to ultraviolet light (sunburn) (**Box 10-8**) or contact with an electric current or corrosive chemicals causes injury or death to skin cells. The injuries that result can all be classified as *burns.*

Estimating Body Surface Area

When burns involve large areas of the skin, treatment and the prognosis for recovery depend in large part on the total area involved and the severity of the burn. The severity of a burn is determined by the depth and extent (percentage of body surface burned) of the lesion. There are several ways to estimate the extent of body surface area burned. One method is called the **"rule of palms"** and is based on the assumption that the palm size of a burn patient is about 1% of the total body surface area. Therefore, estimating the number of "palms" that are burned approximates the percentage of body surface area involved.

The "**rule of nines**" (**Figure 10-30**) is another and more accurate method of determining the extent of a burn injury. In this technique the body is divided into 11 areas of 9% each, with the area around the genitals, called the *perineum,* representing the additional 1% of body surface area. As **Figure 10-30** shows, 9% of the skin covers the head and each upper extremity, including the front and back surfaces. Twice as much, or 18%, of the total skin area covers the front and back of the trunk and each lower extremity, including the front and back surfaces. The rule of nines works well with adults but does not reflect the differences in body surface area in small children. Special tables called *Lund–Browder charts,* which take the large surface area of certain body areas (such as the head) in a growing child into account, are used by physicians to estimate burn percentages in children.

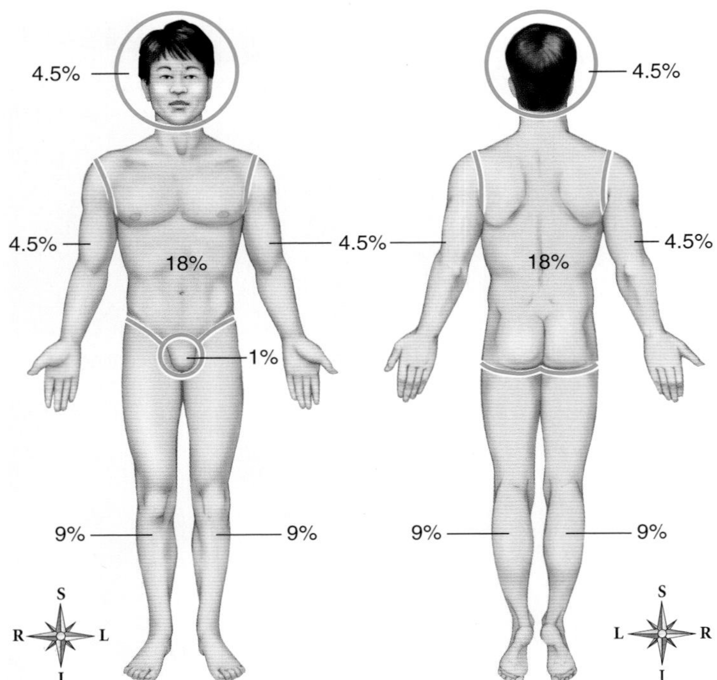

FIGURE 10-30 "Rule of nines". The "rule of nines" is one method used to estimate amount of skin surface burned in an adult.

Besides estimating the proportion of the body affected by a burn, the depth of the injury is also determined.

A **superficial epidermal** burn involves the epidermis but not the dermis as in typical sunburn. The burn causes minor discomfort and some reddening of the skin. Although the surface layers of the skin may peel in 1 or 2 days, no blistering occurs and the actual tissue destruction is minimal.

Partial thickness, superficial dermal burns involve the epidermis and part of the papillary layer of the dermis. The skin is pink and painful with blistering.

Partial thickness, deep dermal burns involve the epidermis and entire papillary dermis down to the reticular dermis. There may be damage to sweat glands, hair follicles and sebaceous glands. The skin appears dry or moist, blotchy and cherry-red. The burn may be painful or painless, with or without blisters.

Full thickness burns involve the entire thickness of the skin and possibly subcutaneous tissue. The skin is dry and white, brown or black in colour with no blisters and is usually painless. The skin in the burned area is described as waxy or leathery and has no healing capacity; the patient always needs to be referred to surgery.

Full thickness+ burns indicate the entire skin and underlying structures such as muscle and bone are involved.

Knowledge of burn depth and the percentage of the body affected helps to determine treatment, healing time and the potential for complications such as infection and scarring. (See **Figure 10-31**).

BOX 10-8 *health matters*
Sunburn and Skin

Burns caused by exposure to harmful UV radiation in sunlight are commonly called *sunburns.* As with any burn, serious sunburns can cause tissue damage and lead to secondary infections and fluid loss. Cancer researchers have theorized that blistering (superficial epidermal) sunburns during childhood may trigger the development of malignant melanoma later in life. Some epidemiological studies show that adults who had more than two blistering sunburns before the age of 20 years have a greater risk for melanoma than someone who experienced no such burns. If this theory is true, it could explain the dramatic increase in skin cancer rates in the UK in recent decades. Those who grew up as sunbathing and "suntans" became popular in the 1950s through the 1980s are now, as adults, exhibiting melanoma at a much higher rate than in previous generations.

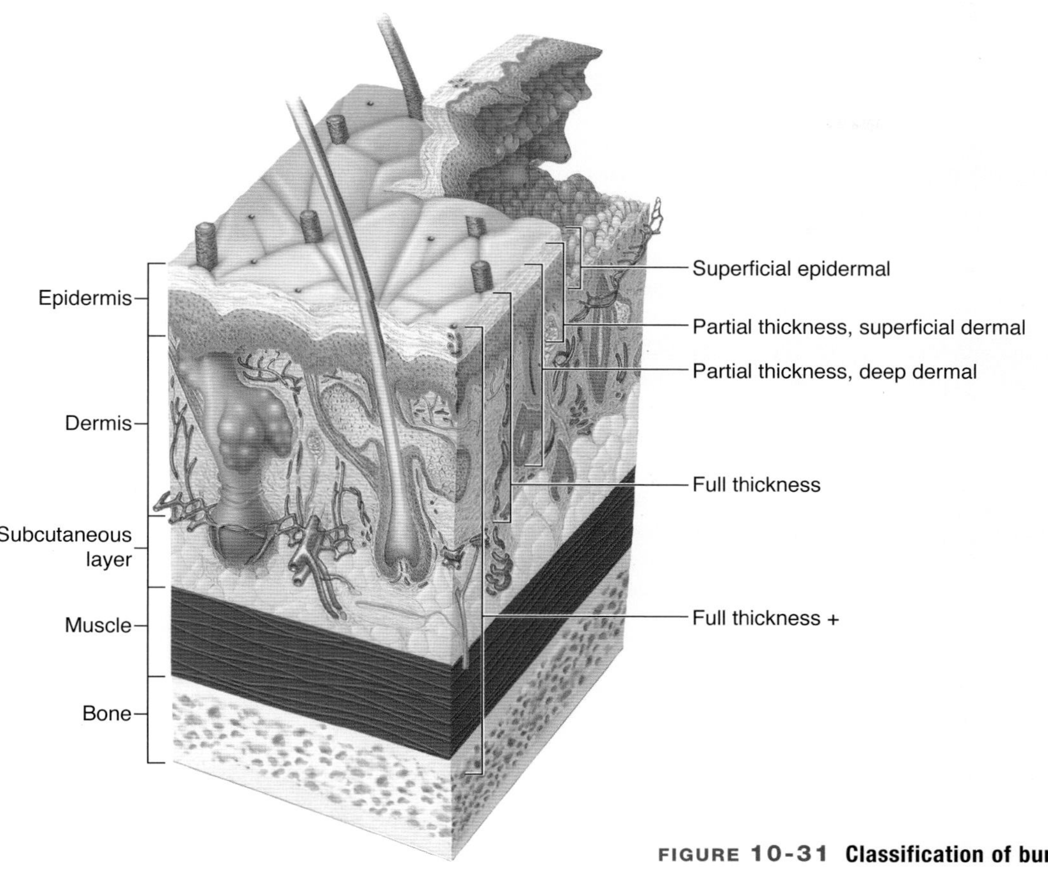

FIGURE 10-31 **Classification of burns.**

LANGUAGE OF SCIENCE *(continued from p. 180)*

hair follicle (FOHL-i-kul)
[*foll-* **bag,** *-icle* **little**]

hair papilla (pah-PIL-ah)
[*papilla* **nipple**] *pl.,* papillae

hyperkeratosis (hye-per-ker-ah-TOH-sis)
[*hyper-* **excessive,** *-kera-* **horn,** *-osis* **condition**]

hypodermis (hye-poh-DER-mis)
[*hypo-* **under or below,** *-dermis* **skin**]

integument (in-TEG-yoo-ment)
[*integument* **covering**]

integumentary system (in-teg-yoo-MEN-tar-ee)
[*integument* **covering,** *-ary* **relating to**]

keratin (KER-ah-tin)
[*kera-* **horn,** *-in* **substance**]

keratinization (ker-ah-tin-i-ZAY-shun)
[*kera* **horn,** *-in-* **substance,** *-iz-* **to cause,** *-ation* **process**]

keratinocyte (keh-RAT-i-no-syte)
[*kera-* **horn,** *-in-* **substance,** *-cyte* **cell**]

keratohyalin (ker-ah-toh-HYE-ah-lin)
[*kera-* **horn,** *-hyal-* **glass,** *-in* **substance**]

lanugo (lah-NOO-go)
[*lanugo* **down**]

lunula (LOO-nyoo-lah)
[*luna-* **moon,** *-ula* **small**]

medulla (meh-DUL-ah)
[*medulla* **marrow or pith (middle)**]
pl. medullae or medullas

melanin (MEL-ah-nin)
[*melan-* **black,** *-in* **substance**]

melanocyte (MEL-ah-no-syte)
[*melan-* **black,** *-cyte* **cell**]

melanosome (MEL-ah-no-sohm)
[*melan-* **black,** *-som-* **body**]

microbiome (my-kroh-BYE-ohm)
[*micro-* **small,** *-bio-* **life,** *-ome* **entire collection**]

papillary (PAP-i-lair-ee)
[*papilla-* **nipple,** *-ary* **relating to**]

pheomelanin (fee-oh-MEL-ah-nin)
[*pheo-* **dusky,** *-melan-* **black,** *-in* **substance**]

pheromone (fair-o-mohn)
[*pher-* **carry,** *-mone* **hormone (excite)**]

reticular (reh-TIK-yoo-lar)
[*ret-* **net,** *-ic-* **relating to,** *-ul-* **little,** *-ar* **relating to**]

sebaceous gland (seh-BAY-shus)
[*seb-* **tallow (hard animal fat),** *-ous* **relating to,** *gland* **acorn**]

sebum (SEE-bum)
[*sebum* **tallow (hard animal fat)**]

stratum (STRAH-tum)
[*stratum* **layer**] *pl.,* strata

stratum basale (STRAH-tum bay-SAH-lee)
[*stratum* **layer,** *bas-* **base,** *-ale* **relating to**] *pl.,* strata

stratum corneum (STRAH-tum KOR-nee-um)
[*stratum* **layer,** *corneum* **horn**] *pl.,* strata

stratum granulosum (STRAH-tum gran-yoo-LOH-sum)
[*stratum* **layer,** *gran-* **grain,** *-ul-* **little,** *-osum* **thing**] *pl.,* strata

stratum lucidum (STRAH-tum LOO-see-dum)
[*stratum* **layer,** *lucid-* **clear,** *-um* **thing**]
pl., strata

stratum spinosum (STRAH-tum spi-NO-sum)
[*stratum* **layer,** *spino-* **spine,** *-um* **thing**]
pl., strata

subcutaneous layer (sub-kyoo-TAY-nee-us)
[*sub-* **beneath,** *-cut-* **skin,** *-ous* **relating to**]

sudoriferous gland (soo-doh-RIF-er-us)
[*sudo-* **sweat,** *-fer-* **bear or carry,** *-ous* **relating to,** *gland* **acorn**]

superficial fascia (soo-per-FISH-all FAH-shah)
[*super-* **over or above,** *-fici-* **face,** *-al* **relating to,** *fascia* **band**]

vellus (VEL-us)
[*vellus* **wool**]

LANGUAGE OF MEDICINE

basal cell carcinoma
(BAY-sal cell kar-si-NOH-mah)
[*bas-* **base,** *-al* **relating to,** *cell* **storeroom,** *carcin-* **cancer,** *-oma* **tumour**]

cyanosis (sye-ah-NO-sis)
[*cyan-* **blue,** *-osis* **condition**]

decubitus ulcer
(deh-KYOO-bi-tus UL-ser)
[*decubitus* **lying-down position,** *ulcer* **sore**]

dermatitis (der-mah-TYE-tis)
[*derma-* **skin,** *-itis* **inflammation**]

dermatosis (der-mah-TOH-sis)
[*derma-* **skin,** *-osis* **condition**]

eczema (EK-zeh-mah)
[*ec-* **out,** *-zema* **boiling**]

hypothermia (hye-poh-THER-mee-ah)
[*hypo-* **under or below,** *-therm-* **heat,** *-ia* **abnormal condition**]

impetigo (im-peh-TYE-go)
[*impetigo* **an attack**]

jaundice (JAWN-dis)
[*jaun-* **yellow,** *-ice* **state**]

Kaposi sarcoma (KS)
(KAH-poh-see sar-KOH-mah)
[**Moritz K. Kaposi, Hungarian dermatologist,** *sarco-* **flesh,** *-oma* **tumour**]

malignant hyperthermia (MH)
(mah-LIG-nant hye-per-THERM-ee-ah)
[*malign-* **bad,** *-ant* **state,** *hyper-* **excessive,** *-therm-* **heat,** *-ia* **abnormal condition**]

malignant melanoma
(mah-LIG-nant mel-ah-NO-mah)
[*malign-* **bad,** *-ant* **state,** *melan-* **black,** *-oma* **tumour**]

necrosis (neh-KROH-sis)
[*necro-* **death,** *-osis* **condition**]

onycholysis (on-ik-oh-LYE-sis)
[*onycho-* **nail,** *-lysis* **loosen**]

psoriasis (so-RYE-ah-sis)
[*psor-* **itching,** *-iasis* **condition**]

pyrogen (PYE-roh-jen)
[*pyro-* **heat,** *-gen* **produce**]

scleroderma (skleer-oh-DER-mah)
[*sclero-* **hard,** *-derma* **skin**]

squamous cell carcinoma
(SKWAY-muss sell kar-si-NO-mah)
[*squam-* **scale,** *-ous* **characterized by,** *cell* **storeroom,** *carcin-* **cancer,** *-oma* **tumour**]

tinea (TIN-ee-ah)
[*tinea* **worm**]

urticaria (er-ti-KAIR-ee-ah)
[*urtica-* **nettle,** *-ia* **abnormal condition**]

vitiligo (vit-i-LYE-go)
[*vitiligo* **blemish**]

case study

One afternoon, James (12 years old) was playing in his tree house. While running his fingers along the railing, he suddenly yelled, snatching his hand back off the rail. When he looked down, he saw a small sliver of wood sticking out of his middle finger. The splinter hurt, but his finger wasn't bleeding.

1. What primary layer or layers of the cutaneous membrane had the splinter gone through? (Hint: There was no bleeding.)
   a. Epidermis only
   b. Dermis only
   c. Both epidermis and dermis
   d. Stratum basale only

2. If the splinter had gone into James's arm instead of his finger, which of these layers would the splinter NOT have pierced?
   a. Stratum corneum
   b. Stratum granulosum
   c. Stratum spinosum
   d. Stratum lucidum

The puncture had broken James's intact skin barrier allowing bacteria and other pathogens to enter.

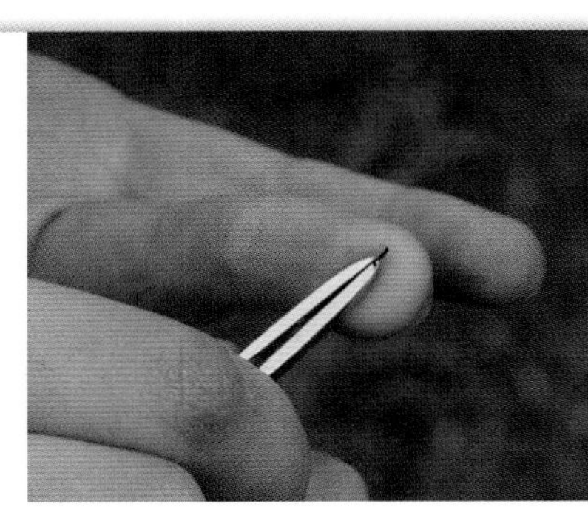

3. What cells in the skin help identify pathogens and mark them for destruction?
   a. Keratinocytes
   b. Melanocytes
   c. Dendritic cells (Langerhans cells)
   d. Lamellar (Pacini) corpuscles

Hint To solve a case study, you may have to refer to the glossary or index, other chapters in this textbook, ***Connect It!,*** and other resources.

CHAPTER SUMMARY

To download an MP3 version of the chapter summary for use with your mobile device, access the ***Audio Chapter Summaries*** *online at evolve.elsevier.com.*

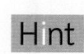

Scan this summary after reading the chapter to help you reinforce the key concepts. Later, use the summary as a quick review before your class or before a test.

Introduction

A. Skin (integument) is body's largest organ
B. Skin measures approximately 1.6 to 1.9 m^2 in average-sized adult
C. Integumentary system describes the skin and its appendages—the hair, nails, and skin glands

Structure of the Skin

A. Skin classified as a cutaneous membrane
B. Two primary layers—epidermis and dermis; joined by dermoepidermal junction (**Figures 10-1** and **10-2**)
C. Hypodermis lies beneath dermis
D. Thin and thick skin (**Figure 10-3**)
  1. "Thin skin"—covers most of body surface (1 to 3 mm thick); has hair and smooth surface
  2. "Thick skin"—soles and palms (4 to 5 mm thick); ridged surface with no hair
E. Epidermis
  1. Cell types (**Figure 10-4**)
    a. Keratinocytes—constitute over 90% of cells present; principal structural element of the outer skin; sometimes called *corneocytes* after they are fully keratinized
    b. Melanocytes—pigment-producing cells (5% of the total); contribute to skin colour; filter ultraviolet light
    c. Epidermal dendritic cells—branched antigen-presenting cells (APCs); they play a role in immune response; also called *Langerhans cells*
    d. Tactile epithelial cells (Merkel cells)—attach to sensory nerve endings to form "light touch" receptors
  2. Cell layers
    a. Stratum basale (base layer)—single layer of columnar cells; only these cells undergo mitosis and then migrate through the other layers until they are shed; *stratum germinativum* (growth layer) is another name for stratum basale (or stratum spinosum and stratum basale together)
    b. Stratum spinosum (spiny layer)—cells arranged in 8 to 10 layers with desmosomes that pull cells into spiny shapes; cells rich in RNA
    c. Stratum granulosum (granular layer)—cells arranged in two to four layers and filled with keratohyalin granules; contain high levels of lysosomal enzymes; helps form a leak-proof barrier
    d. Stratum lucidum (clear layer)—cells filled with keratin precursor called *eleidin;* absent in thin skin
    e. Stratum corneum (horny layer)—most superficial layer; dead cells filled with keratin (barrier area)
  3. Epidermal growth and repair
    a. Turnover or regeneration time refers to time required for epidermal cells to form in the stratum basale and migrate to the skin surface—about 35 days
    b. Several hormones support normal growth and repair of the epidermis: epidermal growth factor (EGF), insulin-like growth factor 1 (IGF-1), and growth hormone (GH)
    c. Shortened turnover time will increase the thickness of the stratum corneum and result in callus formation
    d. Normally 10% to 12% of all cells in stratum basale enter mitosis daily
    e. Each group of 8 to 10 basal cells in mitosis with their vertical columns of migrating keratinocytes is called an *epidermal proliferating unit,* or *EPU*
F. Dermoepidermal junction (DEJ)
  1. A basement membrane, with unique fibrous elements, and a polysaccharide gel serve to "glue" the epidermis to the dermis below
  2. The junction serves as a partial barrier to the passage of some cells and large molecules
G. Dermis
  1. Sometimes called "true skin"—much thicker than the epidermis and lies beneath it
  2. Gives strength to the skin
  3. Serves as a reservoir storage area for water and electrolytes
  4. Contains various structures
    a. Arrector pili muscles and hair follicles (**Figure 10-5**)
    b. Sensory receptors (**Figure 10-6**)
    c. Sweat and sebaceous glands
    d. Blood vessels
  5. Rich vascular supply plays a critical role in temperature regulation
  6. Layers of dermis
    a. Papillary layer—composed of dermal papillae that project into the epidermis; contains fine collagenous and elastic fibres; contains the dermoepidermal junction; forms a unique pattern that gives individual fingerprints
    b. Reticular layer—contains dense, interlacing white collagenous fibres and elastic fibres to make the skin tough yet stretchable; when processed from animal skin, produces leather
  7. Dermal growth and repair
    a. The dermis does not continually shed and regenerate itself as does the epidermis
    b. During wound healing, fibroblasts begin forming an unusually dense mass of new connective fibres; if not replaced by normal tissue, this mass remains a scar
    c. Cleavage lines (**Figure 10-7**)—patterns formed by the collagenous fibres of the reticular layer of the dermis; also called *Langer lines*
    d. Dermal adipocytes—active in scarring, ageing and fighting infection

H. Hypodermis
1. Also called the subcutaneous layer or superficial fascia
2. Located deep to the dermis; forms connection between skin proper and other structures
3. Usually included in the integument but not the skin proper
4. Mostly loose fibrous and adipose tissue along with nerves, blood vessels and lymphatic vessels

Skin Colour

A. Melanin
1. Basic determinant is quantity, type, distribution of melanin
2. Types of melanin
   a. Eumelanin—group of dark brown (almost black) melanins
   b. Pheomelanin—group of reddish and orange melanins
3. Melanin formed from tyrosine by melanocytes (**Figure 10-8**)
   a. Melanocytes release melanin in packets called *melanosomes*
   b. Melanosomes are ingested by surrounding keratinocytes and form a cap over the nucleus
4. Albinism—congenital absence of melanin
5. Process regulated by tyrosinase, exposure to sunlight (UV radiation), and certain hormones, including melanocortins (ACTH, α-MSH) and ET-1 (**Figures 10-9** and **10-10**)
6. Cumulative effects of UV exposure may produce age spots (**Figure 10-11**)

B. Other pigments
1. Beta-carotene (group of yellowish pigments from food) can also contribute to skin colour
2. Lipofuscin—accumulates in cells that have ceased mitosis in ageing skin, producing brown-yellow age spots
3. Haemoglobin—colour changes also occur as a result of changes in blood flow
   a. Redder skin colour when blood flow to skin increases
   b. Cyanosis—bluish colour caused by darkening of haemoglobin when it loses oxygen and gains carbon dioxide (**Figure 10-12**)
   c. Bruising can cause a rainbow of different colours to appear in the skin (**Figure 10-13**)
4. Other pigments—from cosmetics, tattoos, bile pigments in jaundice (**Box 10-4**)

Functions of the Skin (Table 10-2)

A. Protection
1. Physical barrier and immune barrier to microorganisms
2. Barrier to chemical hazards
3. Reduces potential for mechanical trauma
4. Prevents dehydration
5. Protects against excess UV exposure (melanin function)
6. Surface film
   a. Emulsified protective barrier formed by mixing of residue and secretions of sweat and sebaceous glands with sloughed epithelial cells from skin surface; shedding of epithelial elements is called *desquamation*
   b. Functions
      (1) Antibacterial, antifungal activity
      (2) Lubrication
      (3) Hydration of skin surface
      (4) Buffer of caustic irritants
      (5) Blockade of toxic agents
   c. Chemical composition
      (1) From epithelial elements—amino acids, sterols, and complex phospholipids
      (2) From sebum—fatty acids, triglycerides, and waxes
      (3) From sweat—water, ammonia, urea, and lactic and uric acids

C. Sensation
1. Skin acts as a sophisticated sense organ
2. Somatic sensory receptors detect stimuli that permit us to detect pressure, touch, temperature, pain, and other general senses

D. Flexibility
1. Skin is supple and elastic, thus permitting change in body contours without injury

E. Excretion
1. Water
2. Urea/ammonia/uric acid

F. Hormone (vitamin D) production (**Figure 10-14**)
1. Exposure of skin to UV light converts 7-dehydrocholesterol to cholecalciferol—a precursor to vitamin D
2. Blood transports precursor to liver and kidneys where vitamin D is produced

G. Immunity
1. Phagocytic cells destroy bacteria
2. Epidermal dendritic cells trigger helpful immune reaction working with “helper T cells”

H. Homeostasis of body temperature
1. To maintain homeostasis of body temperature, heat production must equal heat loss; skin plays a critical role in this process
2. Heat production
   a. By metabolism of foods in skeletal muscles, brown fat and liver
   b. Chief determinant of heat production is the amount of muscular work being performed
3. Heat loss—approximately 80% of heat loss occurs through the skin; remaining 20% occurs through the mucosa of the respiratory, digestive, and urinary tracts (**Figure 10-15**)
   a. Evaporation—to evaporate any fluid, heat energy must be expended; this method of heat loss is especially important at high environmental temperatures when it is the only method by which heat can be lost from the skin
   b. Radiation—transfer of heat from one object to another without actual contact; important method of heat loss in cool environmental temperatures
   c. Conduction—transfer of heat to any substance actually in contact with the body; accounts for relatively small amounts of heat loss
   d. Convection—transfer of heat away from a surface by movement of air; usually accounts for a small amount of heat loss

4. Homeostatic regulation of heat loss (**Figure 10-16**)
   a. Heat loss by the skin is controlled by a negative feedback loop
   b. Receptors in the hypothalamus monitor the body's internal temperature
   c. If body temperature is increased, the hypothalamus sends a nervous signal to the sweat glands and blood vessels of the skin
   d. The hypothalamus continues to act until the body's temperature returns to normal

Appendages of the Skin

A. Hair (**Figure 10-17**)
   1. Development of hair
      a. Distribution—over entire body except palms of hands and soles of feet and a few other small areas
      b. Fine and soft hair coat existing before birth called *lanugo*
      c. Coarse pubic and axillary hair that develops at puberty called *terminal hair*
      d. Hair follicles and hair develop from epidermis; mitosis of cells of germinal matrix forms hairs
      e. Papilla—cluster of capillaries under germinal matrix
      f. Root—part of hair embedded in follicle in dermis
      g. Shaft—visible part of hair
      h. Medulla—inner core of hair; cortex—outer portion
   2. Appearance of hair
      a. Colour—result of different amounts, distribution, types of melanin in cortex of hair (**Figure 10-18**)
      b. Growth—hair growth and rest periods alternate; hair on head averages 13 cm of growth per year
      c. Sebaceous glands—attach to and secrete sebum (skin oil) into follicle
      d. Male pattern baldness (androgenic alopecia) results from combination of genetic tendency and male sex hormones (**Figure 10-19**)

B. Nails (**Figure 10-20**)
   1. Consist of epidermal cells converted to hard keratin
   2. Nail body—visible part of each nail
   3. Root—part of nail in groove hidden by fold of skin, the cuticle
   4. Lunula—moon-shaped white area nearest root
   5. Nail bed—layer of epithelium under nail body; contains abundant blood vessels
      a. Appears pink under translucent nails
      b. Nails may have pigmented streaks (**Figure 10-21**)
      c. Separation of a nail from the nail bed is called *onycholysis* (**Figure 10-22**)
   6. Growth—nails grow by mitosis of cells in stratum basale beneath the lunula; average growth about 0.5 mm per week, or slightly over 2.5 cm per year

C. Skin glands (**Figure 10-23**)
   1. Two types of sweat glands
      a. Eccrine glands
         (1) Most numerous sweat glands; quite small
         (2) Distributed over total body surface with exception of a few small areas
         (3) Simple, coiled, tubular glands
         (4) Function throughout life
         (5) Secrete perspiration or sweat; eliminate wastes and help maintain a constant core temperature
      b. Apocrine glands
         (1) Located deep in subcutaneous layer
         (2) Limited distribution—axilla, areola of breast, and around anus
         (3) Large (often more than 5 mm in diameter)
         (4) Simple, branched, tubular glands
         (5) Begin to function at puberty
         (6) Secretion shows cyclic changes in female with menstrual cycle
   2. Sebaceous glands
      a. Secrete sebum—oily substance that keeps hair and skin soft and pliant; prevents excessive water loss from skin
      b. Lipid components have antifungal activity
      c. Simple, branched glands
      d. Found in dermis except in palms and soles
      e. Secretion increases in adolescence; may lead to formation of pimples and blackheads
   3. Ceruminous glands
      a. Modified apocrine sweat glands
      b. Simple, coiled, tubular glands
      c. Empty contents into external ear canal alone or with sebaceous glands
      d. Mixed secretions of sebaceous and ceruminous glands called *cerumen* (wax)
      e. Function of cerumen to protect area from dehydration; excess secretion can cause blockage of ear canal and loss of hearing

Cycle of Life: Skin

A. Children
   1. Skin is smooth, unwrinkled, and characterized by elasticity and flexibility
   2. Few sweat glands
   3. Rapid healing

B. Adults
   1. Development and activation of sebaceous and sweat glands
   2. Increased sweat production; can result in body odour
   3. Increased sebum production; can result in acne

C. Old age
   1. Decreased sebaceous and sweat gland activity
      a. Wrinkling (**Figure 10-24**)
      b. Decrease in body's ability to cool itself

The Big Picture: Skin and the Whole Body

A. Skin is a major component of the body's structural framework
B. Skin defines the internal environment of the body
C. Primary functions are support and protection

REVIEW QUESTIONS

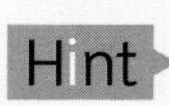

Write out the answers to these questions after reading the chapter and reviewing the Chapter Summary. Note—writing out your answers will consolidate learning and provide a valuable resource of information.

1. List and briefly discuss several of the different functions of the skin.
2. List three cell types found in the epidermis.
3. List and describe the cell layers of the epidermis from superficial to deep.
4. What layer of the epidermis is sometimes called the *barrier area*?
5. Discuss the process of epidermal growth and repair.
6. What is keratin? Where is it found and how is it formed?
7. What part of the skin contains blood vessels? Why do paper cuts rarely bleed?
8. Why is the process of blister formation a good example of the relationship between the skin's structure and function?
9. Describe the two layers of the dermis. Which layer helps make the skin stretchable and able to rebound?
10. What are arrector pili muscles? Speculate on the role they play in maintaining body temperature.
11. List the appendages of the skin.
12. Identify each of the following: hair papilla, germinal matrix, hair root, hair shaft, follicle.
13. List the three primary types of skin glands.
14. What is the difference between eccrine and apocrine sweat glands?
15. Discuss the importance of the surface film of the skin.
16. How is the "rule of nines" used in determining the extent of a burn injury?
17. What are the differences between a superficial epidermal burn, partial thickness superficial dermal burn and a full thickness burn? Why do some victims of severe life-threatening burns show no signs of experiencing intense pain?

CRITICAL THINKING QUESTIONS

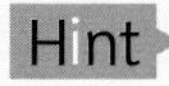

After finishing the Review Questions, write out the answers to these more in-depth questions to help you apply your new knowledge. Go back to sections of the chapter that relate to concepts that you find difficult.

1. The stratum corneum, hair follicle, nails, sweat glands, oil glands, and stratum basale are all discussed in this chapter. Make a distinction regarding whether these structures are part of the integumentary system only or both the integumentary system and the integument?
2. Identify what affects the thickness of the skin (dermis and epidermis). What is the relationship between what affects the thickness of the skin and the thickness of the hypodermis?
3. What is the dermoepidermal junction (DEJ)? By analyzing its anatomical components, what inference can you make regarding how it functions?
4. In terms of leaving a less noticeable scar, why should an incision on the front of the thigh be made at a different angle than an incision on the back of the thigh?
5. Concern about skin cancer is causing people to reduce the amount of time they spend in the sun. If this caution is carried to the extreme, explain how it would impact skin function.
6. Explain why a light-skinned individual would be more susceptible to malignant melanoma.
7. An individual running a marathon expends a great deal of energy. Much of this energy generates heat, which increases core body temperature. What is the role of sweat glands in balancing body temperature during this strenuous exercise? With inevitable loss of fluid during exercise what suggestions do you have for avoiding dehydration?

11 Skeletal Tissues

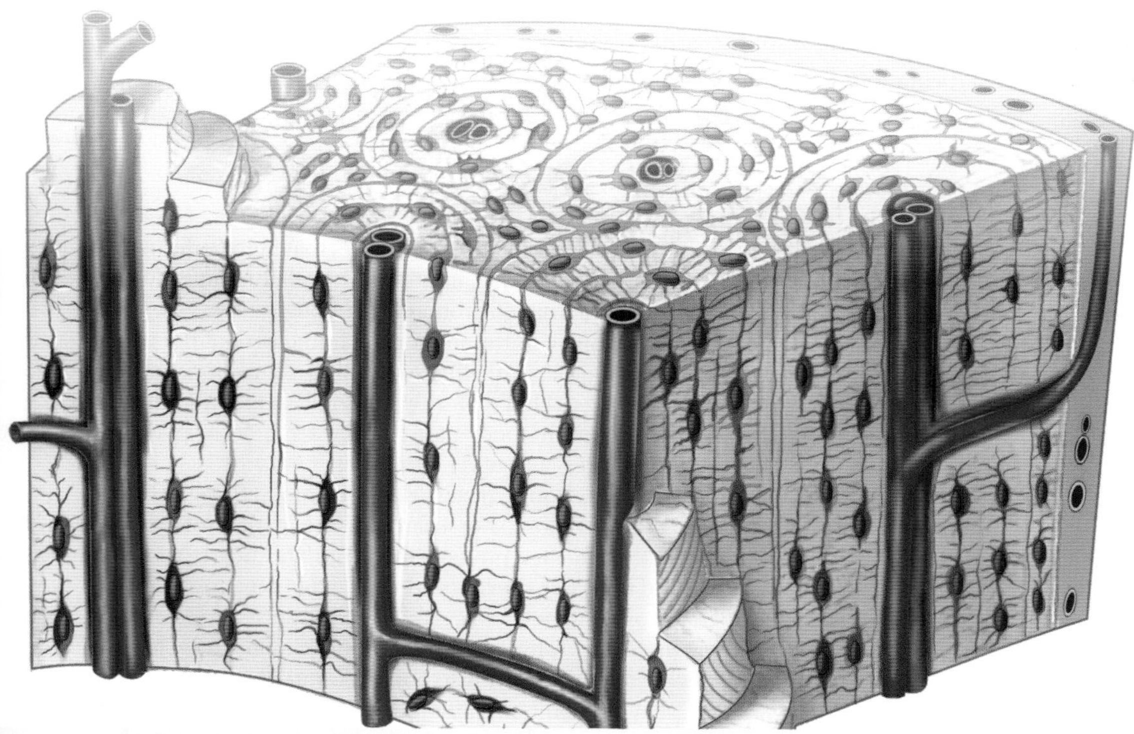

CHAPTER OUTLINE

Hint ▸ *Scan this outline before you begin to read the chapter, as a preview of how the concepts are organized.*

LANGUAGE OF SCIENCE

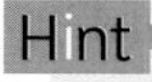 *Use this list to aid your pronunciation of unfamiliar words.*

appositional growth (ap-oh-ZISH-un-al) [*ap-* **toward,** *-posit-* **put or place,** *-ion* **process,** *-al* **relating to**]

articular cartilage (ar-TIK-yoo-lar KAR-ti-lij) [*artic-* **joint,** *-ul-* **little,** *-ar* **relating to,** *cartilag-* **cartilage**]

bone matrix (MAY-triks) [*matrix* **womb**] *pl.,* matrices

cancellous bone (KAN-seh-lus) [*cancel-* **lattice,** *-ous* **characterized by**]

cartilage (KAR-ti-lij)

central canal (SEN-tral kah-NAL)

chondrification centre (kon-dri-fi-KAY-shun) [*chondr-* **cartilage,** *-fic-* **make,** *-ation* **process**]

chondrocyte (KON-droh-syte) [*chondro-* **cartilage,** *-cyte* **cell**]

compact bone (KOM-pakt bohn)

diaphysis (dye-AF-i-sis) [*dia-* **through or apart,** *-physis* **growth**] *pl.,* diaphyses

diploe (DIP-lo-EE) [*diploe* **folded over (doubled)**]

elastic cartilage (eh-LAS-tik KAR-ti-lij) [*elast-* **to drive or propel,** *-ic* **relating to,** *cartilag-* **cartilage**]

endochondral ossification (en-doh-KON-dral os-i-fi-KAY-shun) [*endo-* **within,** *-chondr-* **cartilage,** *-al* **relating to,** *os-* **bone,** *-fic-* **make,** *-ation* **process**]

endosteum (en-DOS-tee-um) [*end-* **within,** *-osteum* **bone**]

epiphyseal plate (ep-i-FEEZ-ee-al) [*epi-* **on,** *-phys-* **growth,** *-al* **relating to,** *plate* **flat**]

epiphysis (eh-PIF-i-sis) [*epi-* **on,** *-physis* **growth**] *pl.,* epiphyses

fibrocartilage (fye-broh-KAR-ti-lij) [*fibr-* **thread or fibre,** *-cartilag-* **cartilage**]

hyaline cartilage (HYE-ah-lin KAR-ti-lij) [*hyaline* **glass,** *cartilag-* **cartilage**]

continued on p. 228

This is the first of four chapters on the skeletal system, or more simply, the skeleton (**Figure 11-1**). This chapter focuses mainly on two highly adapted types of connective tissues that make up the skeleton—bone and cartilage. We also briefly discuss the fibrous connective, blood, nervous, epithelial, lymphatic, marrow, and fatty tissues found in the skeleton.

Chapters 12 and 13 then go on to discuss the overall organization of the skeleton. Individual bones, which are considered separate, discrete organs, are also discussed in these chapters. Then Chapter 14 outlines the articulations, or joints. Articulations are the points of contact between bones that either stabilize the parts of the skeleton or make movement possible.

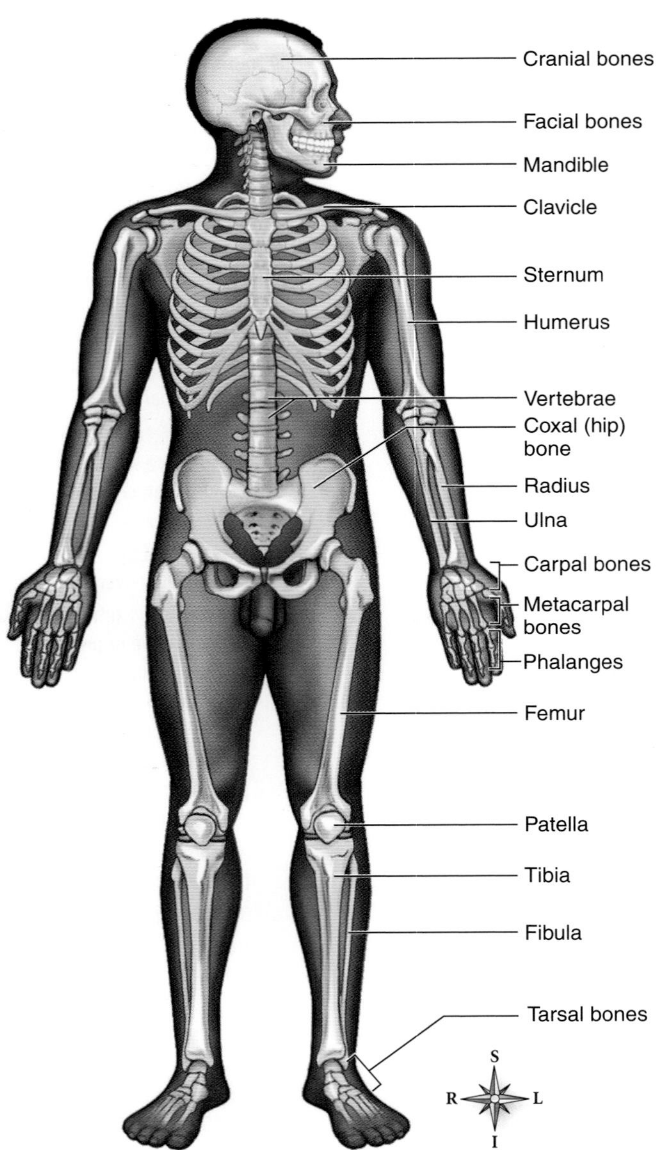

FIGURE 11-1 The skeleton.

FUNCTIONS OF BONE

A good place to begin a study of the skeletal system is with the overall functions of its organs, the bones and ligaments. **Ligaments** are fibrous bands that help hold the various bones together into an organized skeleton. **Bones** are rigid, mineralized structures that help perform five major roles in the body. Each is important for maintaining overall stability of the body's internal environment, or homeostasis.

1. *Support.* Bones serve as the supporting framework of the body, much as steel girders are the supporting framework of our modern buildings. They contribute to the shape, alignment, and positioning of the body parts. Bones are held in place by ligaments, muscles, and other structures.
2. *Protection.* Hard, bony "boxes" serve to protect the delicate structures they enclose. For example, the skull protects the brain, and the rib cage protects the lungs and heart. You can also use the bones of your arm to help defend against injuries to the face or abdomen.
3. *Movement.* Bones along with their joints constitute levers. Muscles are anchored firmly to bones. As muscles contract and shorten, they pull on bones, thereby producing movement at a joint. This process is discussed further in Chapter 14.
4. *Mineral storage.* Bones serve as the major reservoir for calcium, phosphorus, and certain other minerals. Homeostasis of the blood calcium concentration—essential for healthy survival—depends largely on changes in the rate of calcium movement between blood and bones. If, for example, the blood calcium concentration increases above normal, calcium moves more rapidly out of blood into bones and more slowly in the opposite direction. The result? Blood calcium concentration decreases—usually to its homeostatic level. Hormonal control of blood calcium is discussed further in Chapter 26.
5. *Haematopoiesis. Haematopoiesis*, or blood cell formation, is a vital process carried on by red bone marrow, or *myeloid tissue.* Myeloid tissue, in the adult, is located primarily in the ends, or epiphyses, of certain long bones, in the flat bones of the skull, in the pelvis, and in the sternum and ribs. The process of haematopoiesis is discussed further in Chapter 27.

TYPES OF BONES

Structurally, a simple way to categorize the 206 or more bones of the skeleton is by shape. Usually they are divided into five categories: long bones, short bones, flat bones, irregular bones, and sesamoid bones. **Figure 11-2** shows an example of each type. The size, shape, and appearance of bones vary according to the role of each bone in the skeleton. Some bones must bear great weight; others serve a protective function or serve as delicate support structures, such as for the fingers and toes.

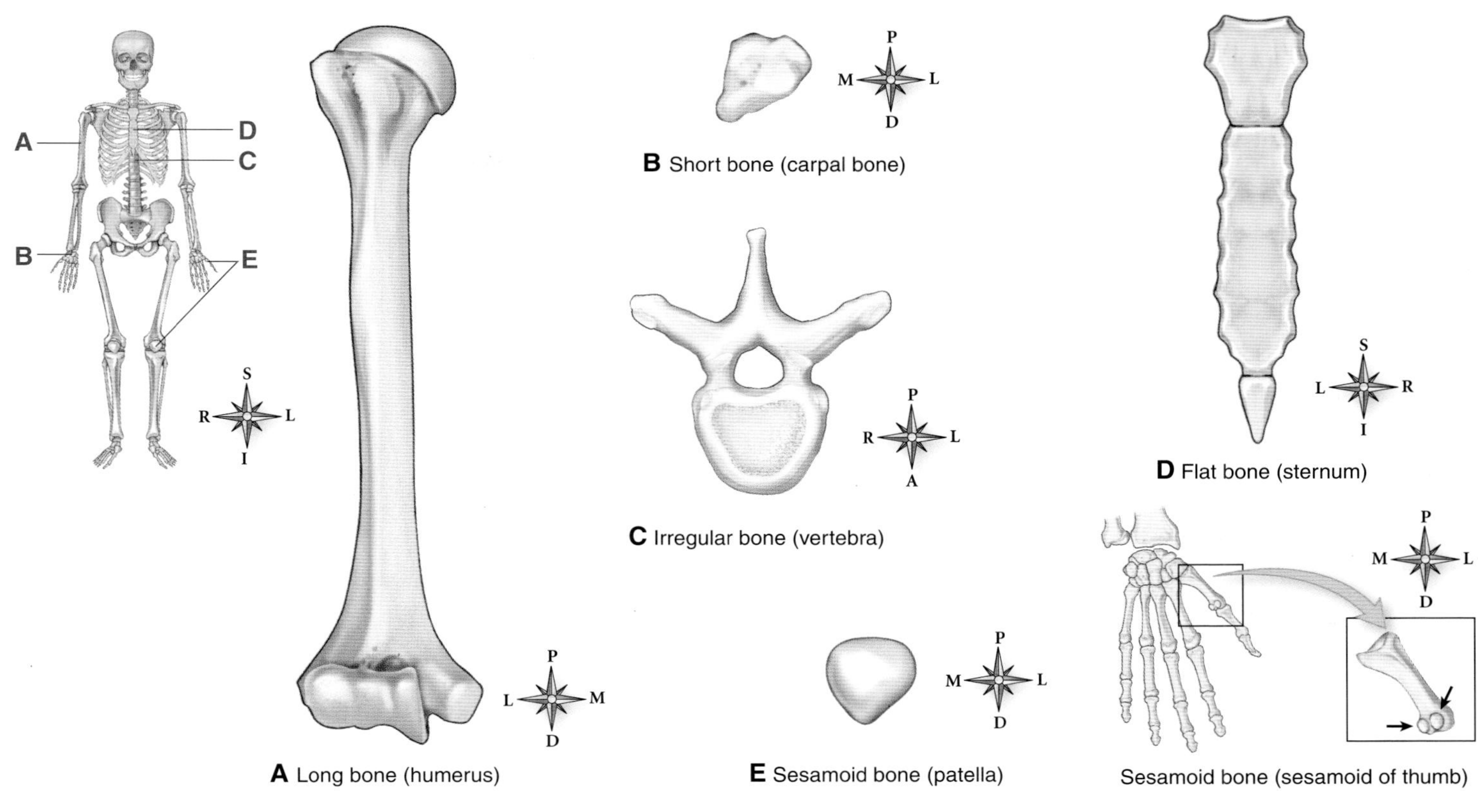

FIGURE 11-2 Types of bones. Examples of bone types include the following: **A,** long bones (humerus); **B,** short bones (carpal bone); **C,** irregular bones (vertebra); **D,** flat bones (sternum); and **E,** sesamoid bones (patella and sesamoid of thumb).

Bones differ in size and shape and also in the amount and proportion of the two different types of bone tissue that compose them. **Compact bone** is dense and "solid" in appearance. **Cancellous bone,** on the other hand, is characterized by open space with a network of thin, branched crossbeams. Recall from Chapter 9 that cancellous bone is also called *spongy bone* or *trabecular bone.* Both compact and cancellous bone types are discussed when the microscopic structure of bone is described later in the chapter, and micrographs of these tissues appear in Part 5 of the BRIEF ATLAS OF THE HUMAN BODY.

All five shape categories of bone discussed here have varying amounts of cancellous and compact bone in their structure.

Long bones are easily identified by their roughly cylindrical shape that is longer than it is wide. They also have enlarged and often uniquely shaped ends that articulate with other bones. The femur of the thigh and humerus of the arm are examples. Other examples include the radius, ulna, tibia, fibula, metacarpal bones, metatarsal bones, and phalanges.

Short bones are often described as cube- or box-shaped structures that are about as broad as they are long. Examples include each of the wrist (carpal) and ankle (tarsal) bones.

Flat bones are generally broad and thin with a flattened and often curved surface. Certain bones of the skull, the shoulder blades (scapulae), ribs, and breastbone (sternum) are typical flat bones.

Irregular bones are often clustered in groups and come in various sizes and shapes. The vertebral bones that form the spine and the facial bones of the skull are good examples.

Sesamoid bones, which are sometimes grouped with the irregular bones, often appear singly rather than in groups. The name comes from "sesame seed" because these bones often resemble sesame seeds in size and shape. The number of sesamoid bones in the body can be many or only a few—the number and size vary from one person to the next. Sesamoid bones usually develop in the tendons close to the joints. The patella (kneecap) is the largest sesamoid bone—one of the few that consistently appear in the human skeleton.

Quick CHECK

1. Name the two major types of connective tissue found in the skeletal system.
2. Name the two different types of bone tissue.

PARTS OF A LONG BONE

A long bone consists of the following structures visible to the naked eye: diaphysis, epiphyses, articular cartilage, periosteum, medullary (marrow) cavity, and endosteum. Identify each of these structures in the tibia shown in **Figure 11-3**, A. The tibia is the longer, stronger, and more medially located of the two leg bones.

1. **Diaphysis**—main shaftlike portion. Its hollow, cylindrical shape and the thick compact bone that composes it adapt the diaphysis well to its function of providing strong support without adding cumbersome weight.
2. **Epiphyses**—the proximal and distal ends of a long bone. Epiphyses have a bulbous shape that provides generous space near

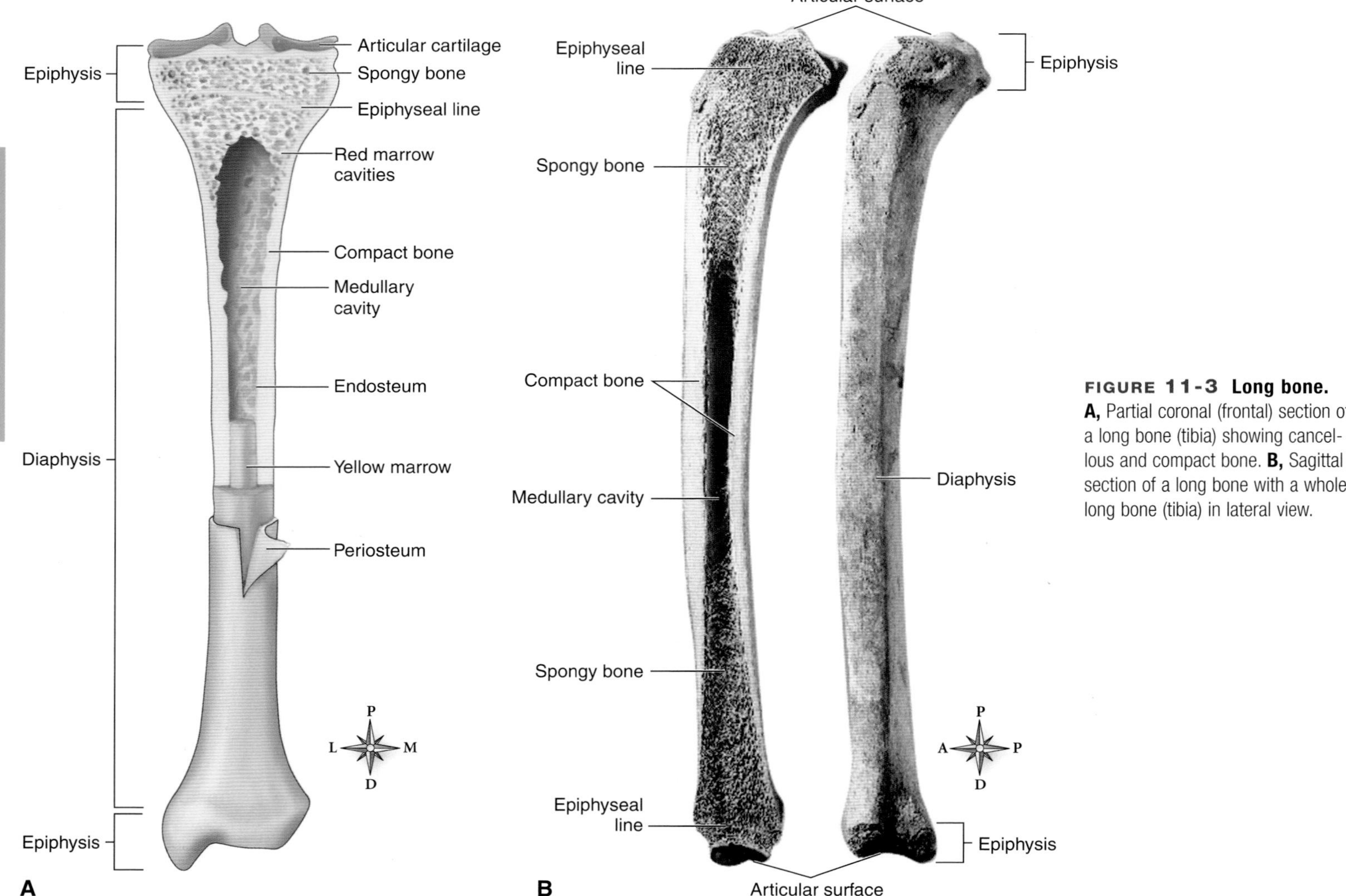

FIGURE 11-3 Long bone. **A,** Partial coronal (frontal) section of a long bone (tibia) showing cancellous and compact bone. **B,** Sagittal section of a long bone with a whole long bone (tibia) in lateral view.

joints for muscle attachments and also gives stability to joints. Look at **Figure 11-3** to note the innumerable small spaces in the bone of the epiphysis. They make this kind of bone look a little like a sponge—hence its name, spongy, or cancellous, bone. A soft connective tissue called *red marrow* fills the spaces within this spongy bone. Early in development, epiphyses are separated from the diaphysis by a layer of cartilage, the *epiphyseal plate.* The cartilage layer is eventually replaced by bone, forming an *epiphyseal line.* The region between the epiphyses and diaphysis (in a mature bone) or the epiphyseal plate region (in a growing bone) is called the **metaphysis.**

3. **Articular cartilage**—thin layer of hyaline cartilage that covers the articular or joint surfaces of epiphyses. The resiliency of this material cushions jolts and blows.
4. **Periosteum**—dense, white fibrous membrane that covers bone except at joint surfaces, where articular cartilage forms the covering. Many of the periosteum fibres penetrate the underlying bone and weld these two structures to each other. In addition, muscle tendon fibres interlace with periosteal fibres, thereby anchoring muscles firmly to bone. The periosteum is a critically important membrane that, depending on its location, also contains bone-forming and bone-destroying cells and blood vessels that become incorporated into bones during their initial growth or subsequent remodelling and repair. This important membrane is essential for bone cell survival and for bone formation, a process that continues throughout life.
5. **Medullary cavity**—a tubelike hollow space in the diaphysis of a long bone, also called a *marrow cavity.* In the adult the medullary cavity is filled with connective tissue rich in fat—a substance called **yellow marrow.**
6. **Endosteum**—a thin, fibrous membrane that lines the medullary cavity of long bones. The endosteum lines the spaces of spongy bone as well. Like the periosteum, the endosteum has various types of bone cells and the stem cells that produce them.

Parts of Flat Bones and Other Bones

The structure of the flat bone is very similar to that of a long bone but simpler. As you can see in **Figure 11-4**, a flat bone of the cranium has outer and inner walls made of compact bone. These hard

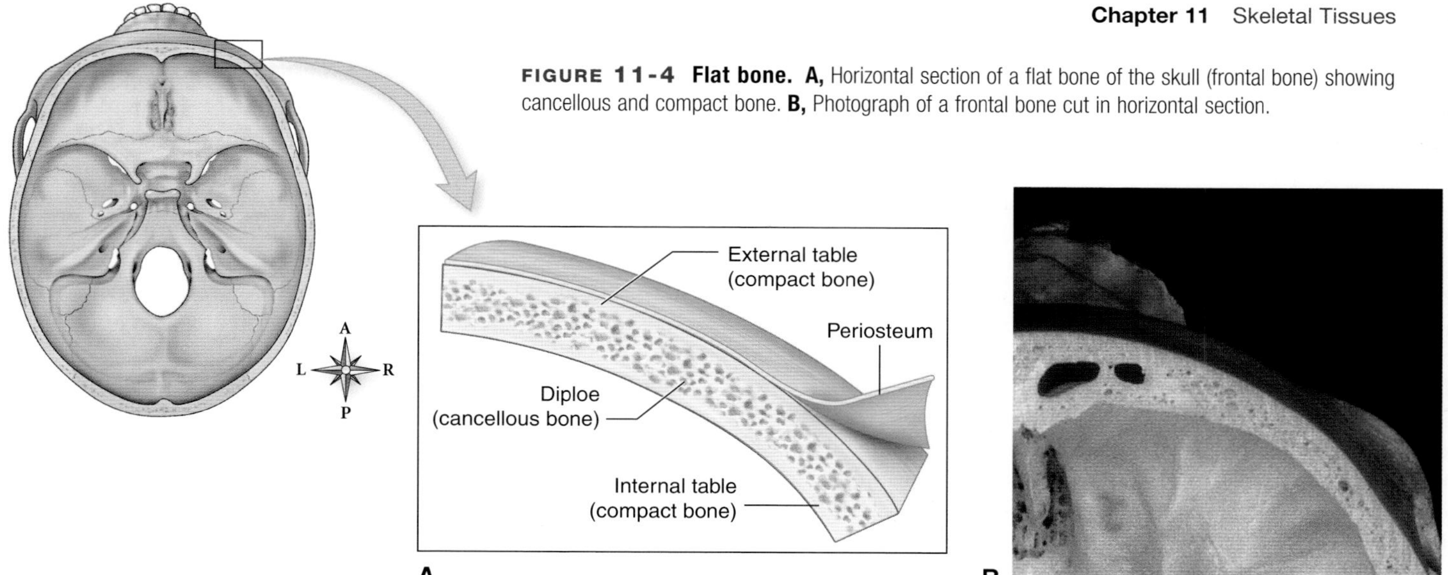

FIGURE 11-4 Flat bone. A, Horizontal section of a flat bone of the skull (frontal bone) showing cancellous and compact bone. **B,** Photograph of a frontal bone cut in horizontal section.

walls are called the **internal table** and **external table.** Between is a region called the **diploe,** which is made up of cancellous bone. Other flat bones, such as the ribs and sternum, have a similar overall structure. Like long bones, flat bones are covered in a periosteum and the inner spaces are lined with endosteum.

Red marrow fills the spaces of the cancellous bone inside many flat bones. The sternum, which contains red marrow even in adulthood, is one example. To help in the diagnosis of leukaemia and certain other diseases, a physician may decide to perform a needle puncture of one of these bones. In this type of diagnostic procedure, a needle is inserted through the skin and compact bone into the red marrow, and a small amount of the marrow is then aspirated and examined under the microscope for evidence of normal or abnormal blood cells. The procedure, called *aspiration biopsy cytology (ABC)*, is discussed on p. 629.

Short bones, irregular bones, and sesamoid bones all have features similar to those of flat bones.

BONE TISSUE

Bone tissue, sometimes called osseous tissue, is perhaps the most distinctive form of connective tissue in the body. It is typical of other connective tissues in that it consists of cells, fibres, and extracellular material, or matrix. However, its extracellular components are hard and calcified. In bone the extracellular material, or matrix, predominates. It is much more abundant than the bone cells, and it contains many fibres of collagen (the body's most abundant protein). The rigidity of bone enables it to serve supportive and protective functions.

As a tissue, bone is ideally suited to its functions. You can easily see the concept that structure and function are interrelated in bone tissue! It has a tensile strength nearly equal to that of cast iron but at less than one third the weight. Bone is organized so that its great strength and minimal weight result from the interrelationships of its structural components. The relationship of structure to function is seen all the way through the chemical, cellular, tissue, and organ levels of organization.

Composition of Bone Matrix

The extracellular matrix (ECM) of bone, or **bone matrix,** can be subdivided into two principal chemical components: *inorganic salts* and *organic matrix*. About two thirds of the matrix by dry weight analysis consists of inorganic salts and one third, organic material. You may find it helpful to review the section describing the unique characteristics of ECM in Chapter 8 on p. 141 and illustrated in **Figure 8-2** on the same page.

Inorganic Salts

The calcified nature and thus the hardness of bone result from the deposition of rocklike crystals of calcium and phosphate. Chemists call them *hydroxyapatite* crystals. The process of forming these crystals within a softer tissue is called *calcification*. The tiny, needlelike hydroxyapatite crystals make up about 85% of the total inorganic matrix and are found oriented in the microscopic spaces between collagen fibres so that they can most effectively resist stress and mechanical deformation.

In addition to hydroxyapatite and about 10% calcium carbonate, other mineral constituents such as magnesium, sodium, sulphate, and fluoride are also found in bone. Unfortunately, harmful elements can become incorporated into bone matrix as well and result in loss of normal function or active disease. For example, radioactive elements such as radium, strontium-90, uranium, or plutonium can become concentrated in bone and continue to emit radiation, which can lead to various types of cancer and other serious disease.

CONNECT IT!

To learn more about the effects of radiation in the body and how it can be used in imaging bones, check out the articles ***Radioactivity*** and ***Bone Scans*** online at ***Connect It!***

Organic Matrix

The organic matrix of bone and other connective tissues is a composite of collagenous fibres and a mixture of protein and polysaccharides called *ground substance*. Connective tissue cells secrete the gel-like ground substance. The ground substance of bone provides support and adhesion between cellular and fibrous elements and also serves an active role in many cellular metabolic functions necessary for growth, repair, and remodelling.

Chondroitin sulphate and **glucosamine** are the names of chemical substances that many people recognize as components of over-the-counter dietary supplements. Taken alone or together they are widely thought to facilitate healing and reduce the "wear and tear" pain of osteoarthritis. However, research has yet to fully support that claim. Chondroitin sulphate and glucosamine are found naturally in the body and are important constituents of the ground substance in both bone and cartilage. Chemically, chondroitin sulphate is a large protein molecule that helps cartilage remain compressible and elastic and may slow its destruction. Glucosamine is an amino sugar important in cartilage formation, maintenance, and repair. Go back to **Figure 8-2** (p. 141) to see how such molecules are incorporated into the ECM of a tissue.

Components of the organic matrix help cartilage maintain a smooth surface and springy consistency. They add to overall strength and also give bone some degree of plasticlike resilience so that applied stress—within reasonable limits—does not result in frequent crush or fracture injuries.

Quick **CHECK**

3. List the six structural components of a typical long bone that are visible to the naked eye.
4. Identify the two principal chemical components of bone matrix.
5. Why is it important that cartilage in the skeleton have some "give" or spring to it?

MICROSCOPIC STRUCTURE OF BONE

The basic structural components and cell types of bone were described briefly in Chapter 9. In the paragraphs that follow, additional information about bone structure and cell types will serve as a basis for learning the functional characteristics of this important tissue. Understanding how a bone forms and grows, how it repairs itself after injury, and how it interacts with other tissues and organs in maintaining various important homeostatic mechanisms is based on a knowledge of its basic structure—a structure as unique as its chemical composition.

Compact Bone

Compact bone constitutes about 80% of the total bone mass in the adult human body. It contains many cylinder-shaped structural units called **osteons,** or *haversian systems.* Note in **Figure 11-5** that each osteon surrounds a **central canal** that runs lengthwise through the bone. Living bone cells in these units are literally cemented together to constitute the structural framework of compact bone. The unique structure of the osteon permits delivery of nutrients and removal of waste products from metabolically active, but imprisoned, bone cells.

Several simple structures make up each osteon: lamellae, lacunae, canaliculi, and a central canal. As you read the following descriptions, identify each structure in **Figure 11-5**.

Lamellae. *Concentric lamellae* are cylinder-shaped layers of calcified matrix in the osteon. Lamellae (layers) of hard bone matrix are also present outside the osteon. *Interstitial lamellae* are layers of calcified matrix between osteons. They are the remnants of older osteons that have been altered by bone growth or remodelling. A few layers of bone matrix also run around the outer boundary of compact bone, encircling all the osteons. These layers that run along the inner circumference (along the endosteum) and outer circumference (along the periosteum) of a bone are called *circumferential lamellae.*

Lacunae. These are small spaces in bone matrix that contain tissue fluid and in which bone cells lie imprisoned between the hard layers of the lamellae.

Canaliculi. These ultra-small canals radiate in all directions from the lacunae and connect them to one another and to a larger canal, the central canal.

Central canal. Also called an *osteonal canal* or *haversian canal,* the central canal extends lengthwise through the centre of each osteon. The central canal is lined with endosteum and contains blood vessels, lymphatic vessels, and nerves. Nutrients and oxygen move from the central canal through canaliculi to the lacunae and their bone cells—a short distance of about 0.1 mm or less.

Parallel central canals are connected to each other by **transverse canals** (*Volkmann canals*). These communicating canals contain nerves and vessels that carry blood and lymph from the exterior surface of the bone to the osteons.

Cancellous Bone

Cancellous, or spongy, bone constitutes about 20% of the total bone mass and differs in microscopic structure from compact bone. As you recall, the structural unit of compact bone is the highly organized osteon. There are no osteons in cancellous bone. Instead, it consists of crisscrossing bony branches called **trabeculae.** Bone cells are found within the trabeculae. Nutrients are delivered to the cells and waste products are removed by diffusion through tiny canaliculi that extend to the surface of the very thin bony branches. Cancellous bone is often called **trabecular bone.**

Note that the cancellous bone shown in **Figure 11-6** lies between two layers of compact bone, much like the filling in a sandwich. Recall that the middle layer of spongy bone is called the *diploe.* This layered organization is typical of flat bones such as those found in the skull. Cancellous bone is also found inside short and irregular bones, as well as inside the epiphyses (see **Figure 11-3**) and lining the medullary cavities of long bones (see **Figure 11-5**, A).

The placement of trabeculae in spongy bone is not as random and unorganized as it might first appear. They are *fractal* in nature, meaning that they appear random, but there is really an underlying, complex organization to them. The bony branches are actually arranged along lines of stress, and their size and orientation will therefore differ among individual bones according to the nature and magnitude of the applied load (**Figure 11-7**). This feature greatly enhances a bone's strength and is yet another example of how structure fits function in the human body.

Locked within a seemingly lifeless calcified matrix, bone cells are active metabolically. They must, like all living cells, continually

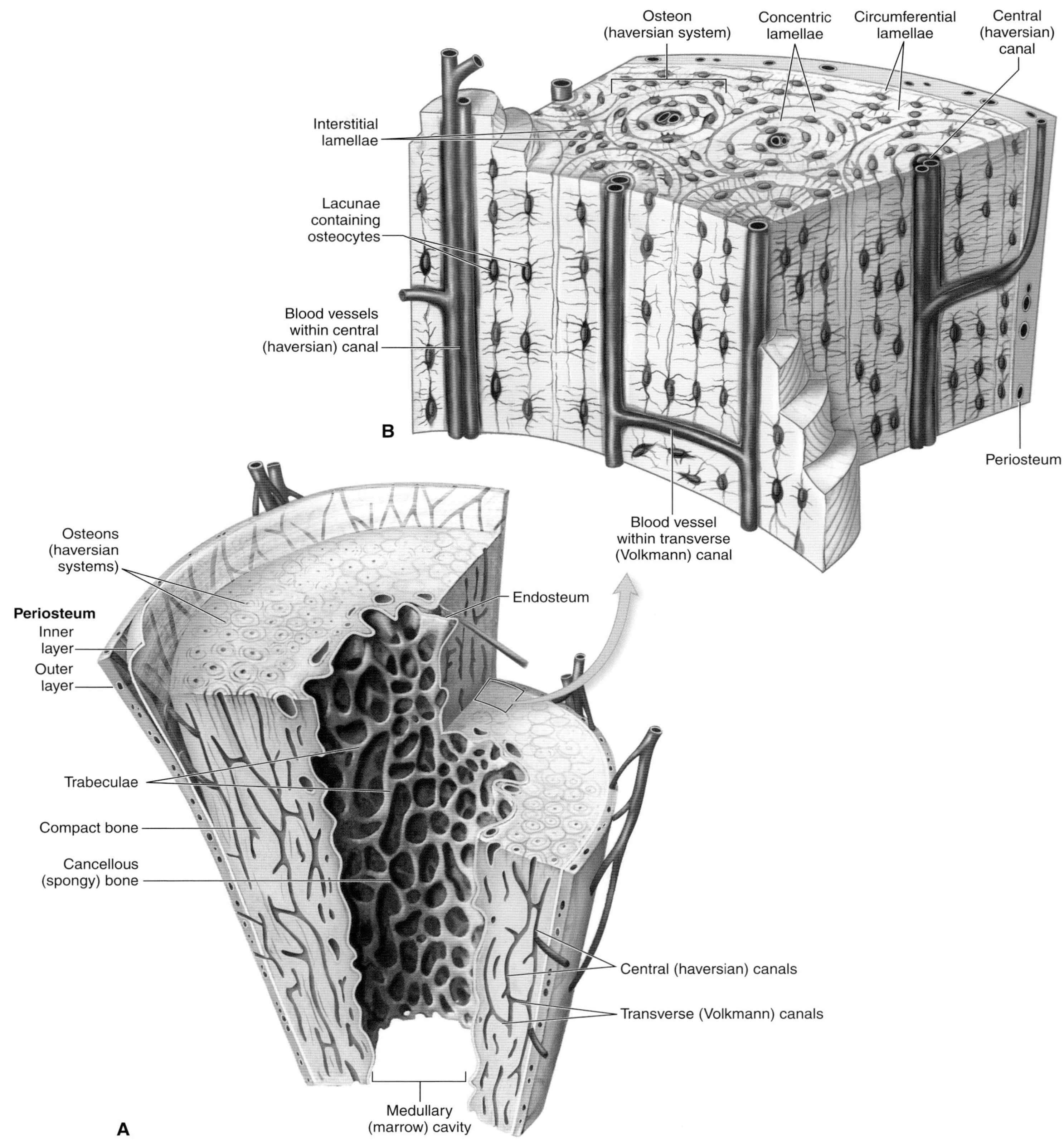

FIGURE 11-5 Compact and cancellous bone in a long bone. A, Longitudinal section of a long bone showing both cancellous and compact bone. **B,** Magnified view of compact bone.

receive food and oxygen and excrete their wastes, so blood supply to bone is both important and abundant.

One or more arteries supply the bone marrow in the internal medullary cavity and provide nutrients to areas of cancellous bone. In addition, blood vessels from the periosteum, when they eventually become covered by new bone in the development process, become incorporated into the bone itself and then, by way of the transverse canals and by connections with other vessels in adjacent osteons, ultimately serve the nutrient needs of cells that, because of their own secretions, have become surrounded by calcified matrix in compact bone. The mechanism by which periosteal blood vessels become "imprisoned" by the deposition of new bone during growth and remodelling is described later in this chapter.

Quick CHECK

6. Identify the main structures that form the osteon.
7. Name the canals that connect blood vessels between adjacent, parallel osteons.
8. Name the tiny branches of hard bone present in cancellous bone.

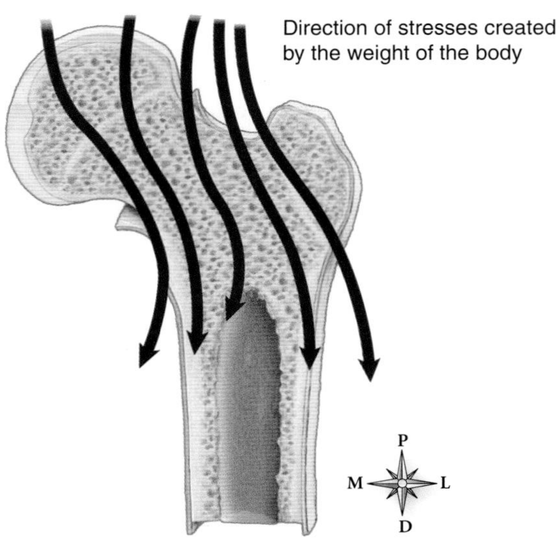

FIGURE 11-7 Orientation of trabeculae. Longitudinal section of a long bone showing trabeculae oriented along lines of stress.

Types of Bone Cells

Three major types of cells are found in bone: *osteoblasts* (bone-forming cells), *osteoclasts* (bone-reabsorbing cells), and *osteocytes* (mature bone cells). All bone surfaces are covered with a continuous layer of cells that is critical to the survival of bone. This layer is composed of relatively large numbers of osteoblasts interspersed with a much smaller population of osteoclasts.

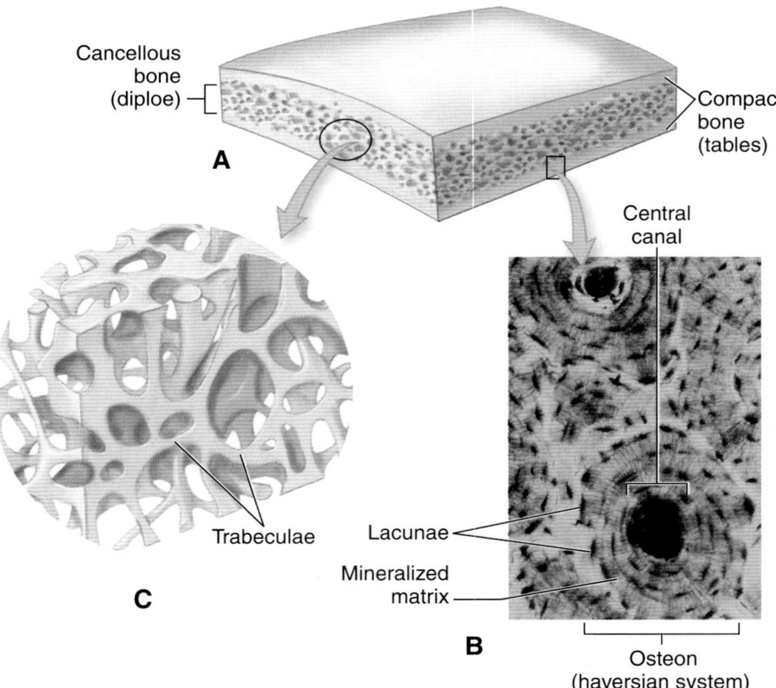

FIGURE 11-6 Compact and cancellous bone in a flat bone. A, Section of a flat bone. (See also **Figure 11-4**.) Outer layers of compact bone surround cancellous bone. Note the fine structure of compact **(B)** and cancellous **(C)** bone.

Osteoblasts are small cells that synthesize and secrete an organic matrix called *osteoid.* Collagen strands in the osteoid serve as a framework for the formation of hydroxyapatite crystals, which mineralizes the bone tissue. *Osteogenic stem cells,* found in the endosteum and lining the central canals, undergo cell division to form osteoblasts.

Osteoclasts are giant multinucleate cells (**Figure 11-8**) that are responsible for the active erosion of bone minerals. They are formed by the fusion of several precursor cells and contain large numbers of mitochondria and lysosomes. Osteoclasts erode bone by releasing *hydrochloric acid (HCl)* that dissolves the hard mineral crystals and *collagenase*, which is an enzyme that breaks the peptide bonds in collagen proteins. The dissolved mineral ions and amino acids that result from bone erosion are reabsorbed by the bloodstream and recycled for use by fibroblasts, osteoblasts, or other cells of the body.

Each 24-hour period sees an alternation of primarily osteoblast, then osteoclast activity. Note in **Figure 11-8** how a branchlike piece of bone is being "sculpted" by an osteoclast eroding existing bone

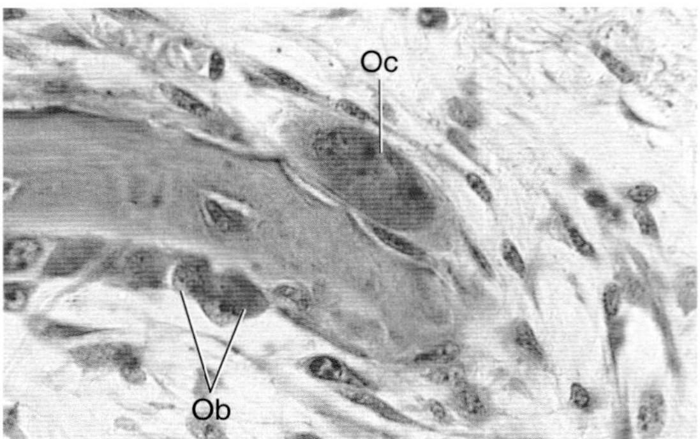

FIGURE 11-8 Bone-forming and bone-eroding cells. Note the large multinucleate osteoclast cell *(Oc)* dissolving bone on the upper surface of a developing branch of bone while smaller osteoblast cells *(Ob)* on the undersurface of the bone are secreting new osteoid.

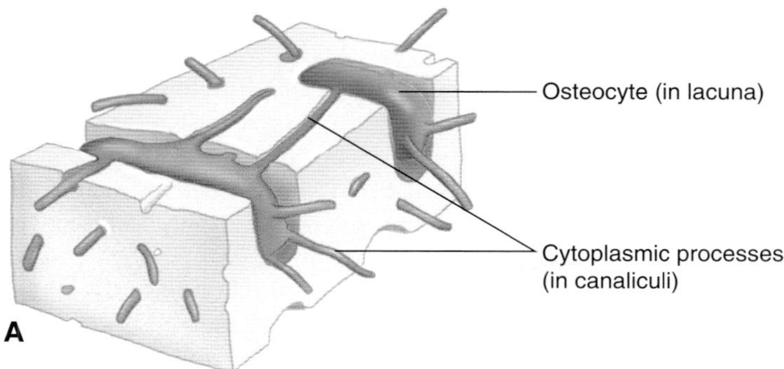

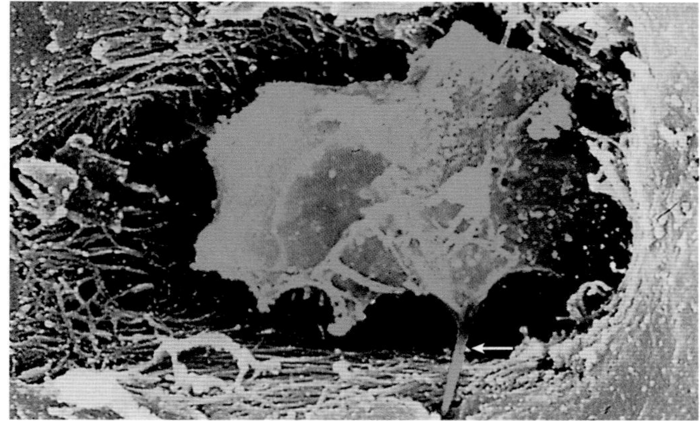

FIGURE 11-9 Osteocyte. A, Sketch showing osteocytes trapped inside hollow lacunae within hard bone matrix. **B,** Scanning electron micrograph showing an osteocyte within a lacuna. Note the cytoplasmic process *(arrow)* extending into a canaliculus below. The cell is surrounded by collagen fibres and mineralized bone.

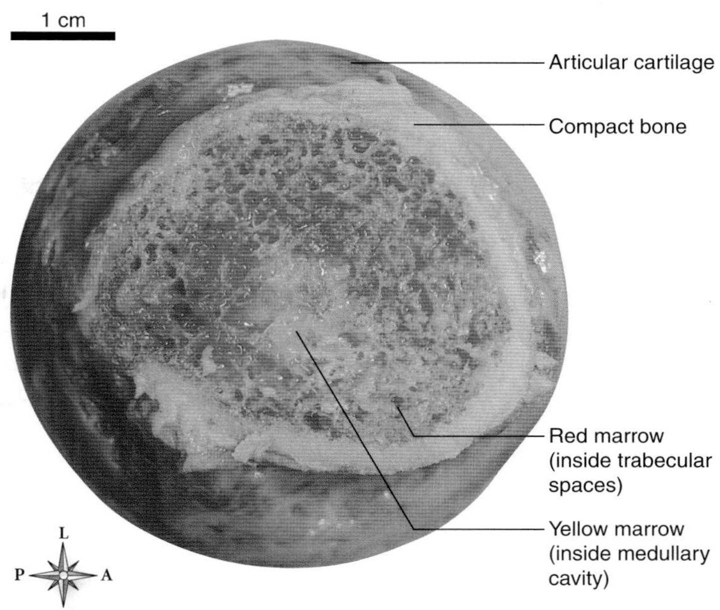

FIGURE 11-10 Bone marrow. Photograph of the head of the femur removed during a hip replacement surgery. A wedge has been removed from the bone to show the marrow spaces inside. Compare with **Figure 11-3**.

mineral from its upper surface while osteoblasts are simultaneously depositing new osteoid on its under surface. As minerals are dissolved during bone erosion, they are reabsorbed back into the blood, their original source.

The process of bone formation and reabsorption characterizes bone as a dynamic tissue that undergoes continuous change and remodelling.

Osteocytes are mature, nondividing osteoblasts that have become surrounded by matrix and now lie within lacunae. **Figure 11-9** includes an illustration and a scanning electron micrograph showing a mature osteocyte within a lacuna. Note that a cytoplasmic process from the cell is extending into a canaliculus below. Cytoplasmic processes from neighbouring cells are connected by gap junctions, which allow the cells to share water and nutrients. Numerous collagen fibres are seen in the ground substance and mineralized bone surrounding the osteocyte.

The way in which these cell types work together to produce bone is described in detail when the development of bone is discussed later in this chapter.

BONE MARROW

Bone marrow is a type of soft, diffuse connective tissue called **myeloid tissue.** It serves as the site for production of blood cells and is found in the medullary cavities of certain long bones and in the spaces of spongy bone in some areas (**Figure 11-10**).

During the lifetime of an individual, two types of marrow exist. In an infant's or child's body, virtually all the bones contain *red marrow.* This is named for its function in the production of red blood cells. As an individual ages, the red marrow is gradually replaced by *yellow marrow.* In yellow marrow, the increasing population of *adipocytes* (fat cells) begins to replace haematopoietic stem cells. The adipocytes also signal the remaining stem cells to reduce blood cell production. With advancing age, yellow marrow becomes almost rust-coloured, less fatty, and more gelatinous in consistency.

The main bones in an adult that still contain red marrow include the ribs, bodies of the vertebrae, and ends of the humerus in the upper part of the arm, the pelvis, and the femur, or thigh bone. During times of decreased blood supply, yellow marrow in an adult can alter to become red marrow. Such a transition may occur during periods of prolonged anaemia caused by chronic blood loss, exposure to radiation or toxic chemicals, and certain diseases.

If the bone marrow is severely diseased or damaged, a **bone marrow transplant** can be a lifesaving treatment. In this procedure, red marrow from a compatible donor is introduced into the recipient intravenously. If the recipient's immune system does not reject the new tissue, which is always a danger in tissue transplants, the donor cells may establish a colony of new, healthy tissue in the bone marrow.

CONNECT IT! 

Where in the body are the sources of new blood cells? The illustrations in ***Sites of Haematopoiesis*** online at ***Connect It!*** will help you visualize the many locations of blood cell production.

REGULATION OF BLOOD CALCIUM LEVELS

The bones of the skeletal system serve as a storehouse for about 98% of the body's calcium reserves. As the major reservoir for this physiologically important body mineral, bones play a key role in maintaining the constancy of blood calcium levels.

To maintain homeostasis of blood calcium levels within a very narrow range, calcium is mobilized and moves into and out of blood during the continuous remodelling of bone. It is the balance between deposition of bone by osteoblasts and breakdown and reabsorption of bone matrix by osteoclasts that helps regulate blood calcium levels. During bone formation, osteoblasts serve to remove calcium from blood, thus lowering its circulating levels. However, when osteoclasts are active and breakdown of bone predominates, calcium is released into blood and circulating levels will increase.

Homeostasis of the calcium ion concentration is essential not only for bone formation, which is described later, but also for normal blood clotting, transmission of nerve impulses, and maintenance of skeletal and cardiac muscle contraction. The primary homeostatic mechanisms involved in the regulation of blood calcium levels involve the secretion of two hormones: (1) *parathyroid hormone (PTH)* by the parathyroid glands and (2) *calcitonin (CT)* by the thyroid gland.

Mechanisms of Calcium Homeostasis

Parathyroid Hormone

The actions of parathyroid hormone (PTH) are fully discussed in Chapter 26. However, the importance of this hormone as the primary regulator of calcium homeostasis and its effect on bone remodelling call for a brief description here.

Feedback loop

When the level of calcium in blood passing through the parathyroid glands decreases below its normal homeostatic setpoint level, osteoclasts are stimulated to initiate increased breakdown of bone matrix, which results in the release of calcium into blood and the return of calcium levels to normal (**Figure 11-11**). In addition, parathyroid hormone also increases renal absorption of calcium from urine, thus reducing its loss from the body.

Another effect of parathyroid hormone is to stimulate vitamin D synthesis, which increases the efficiency of absorption of calcium from the intestine. If blood passing through the parathyroid glands has an elevated calcium level, osteoclast activity will be suppressed, thus reducing the breakdown of bone matrix and the level of calcium circulating in blood. The multiple effects of this type of hormonal control permit the body to precisely regulate a number of homeostatic mechanisms that have an effect both directly and indirectly on the blood levels of this important mineral.

Parathyroid hormone is the most critical factor in homeostasis of blood calcium levels. As a result of its actions and the ability of the body to regulate its formation and release, bones remain strong and calcium levels are maintained within normal limits during both bone formation and bone reabsorption.

Calcitonin

Calcitonin, also discussed in Chapter 26, is a protein hormone produced by endocrine cells in the thyroid gland. It is produced in response to high blood calcium levels and functions to stimulate bone deposition by osteoblasts and inhibit osteoclast activity. As a result, calcium will move into the bones from the blood and circulating levels will decrease. Bisphosphonate (BP) drugs treat postmenopausal osteoporosis by similarly inhibiting osteoclast activity. Alternatively, nasal spray containing calcitonin is available.

Although calcitonin does play a role in the homeostasis of blood calcium levels, it is far less important than parathyroid hormone.

Other Mechanisms

Additional regulatory mechanisms also play a role in calcium homeostasis by affecting mineral storage in the bone. For example, *growth hormone (GH)* secreted from the anterior pituitary gland stimulates the development of new bone and can thus reduce calcium in the blood. On the other hand, the neurotransmitter *serotonin*, produced in the nerves of the gut, may act as a hormone to inhibit osteoblast activity and thus raise blood calcium level.

Research also shows that osteoblasts themselves are able to monitor extracellular calcium levels and react to changes.

DEVELOPMENT OF BONE

When the skeleton begins to form before birth, it consists not of bones but of cartilage and fibrous structures shaped like bones. Gradually, these cartilage "models" become transformed into real bones when the cartilage is replaced with calcified bone matrix (see **Figure 9-21** on p. 168). This process of constantly "remodelling" a growing bone as it changes from a small cartilage model to the characteristic shape and proportion of the adult bone requires continuous activity by the bone-forming osteoblasts and bone-resorbing osteoclasts.

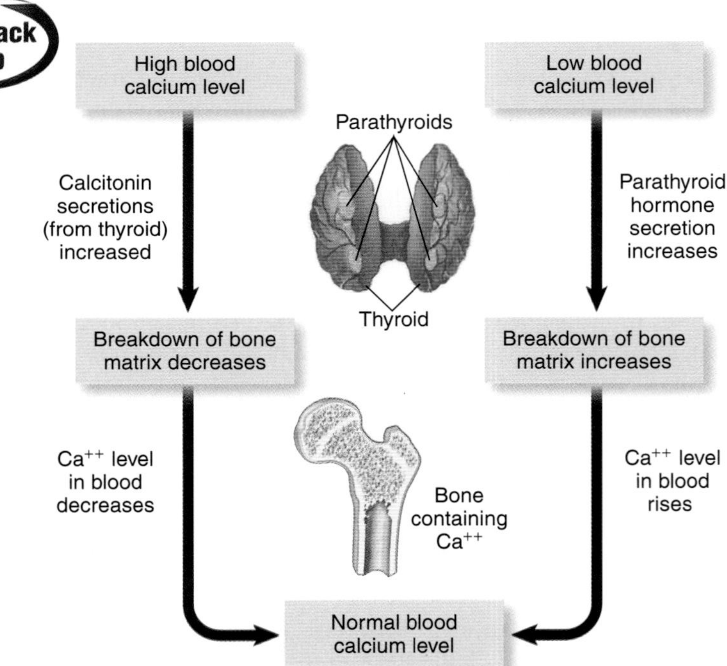

FIGURE 11-11 Calcium homeostasis. Calcitonin and parathyroid hormones have antagonistic (opposing) effects that help to maintain a homeostatic balance of calcium in the blood.

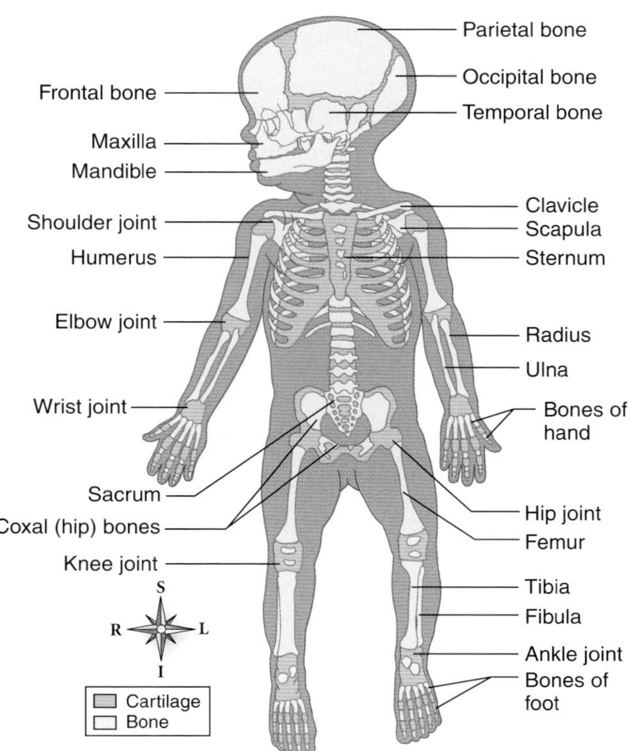

FIGURE 11-12 Bone development. Diagram showing osseous development at birth.

The laying down of calcium salts in the gel-like matrix of the forming bones is an ongoing process. This calcification process is what makes bones as "hard as bone". The combined action of osteoblasts and osteoclasts sculpts bones into their adult shape. The term **osteogenesis** is used to describe this process.

"Sculpting" by the bone-forming and bone-resorbing cells allows bones to respond to stress or injury by changing size, shape, and density. The stress placed on certain bones during exercise increases the rate of bone deposition. For this reason, athletes or dancers may have denser, stronger bones than less active people.

Most bones of the body are formed from cartilage models in a process called **endochondral ossification,** meaning "bone formation in cartilage". A few flat bones are formed within fibrous membrane, rather than cartilage, in the process of **intramembranous ossification.**

Figure 11-12 illustrates osseous development of an infant at birth.

CONNECT IT!

Patterns of bone-forming activity in the skeleton often can be visualized with a *bone scan.* To see a bone scan image and learn how it is produced, check out ***Bone Scans*** online at ***Connect It!***

Intramembranous Ossification

Intramembranous ossification takes place, as its name implies, within a connective tissue membrane. The flat bones of the skull, for example, begin to take shape when groups of osteogenic stem cells within the membrane differentiate into osteoblasts.

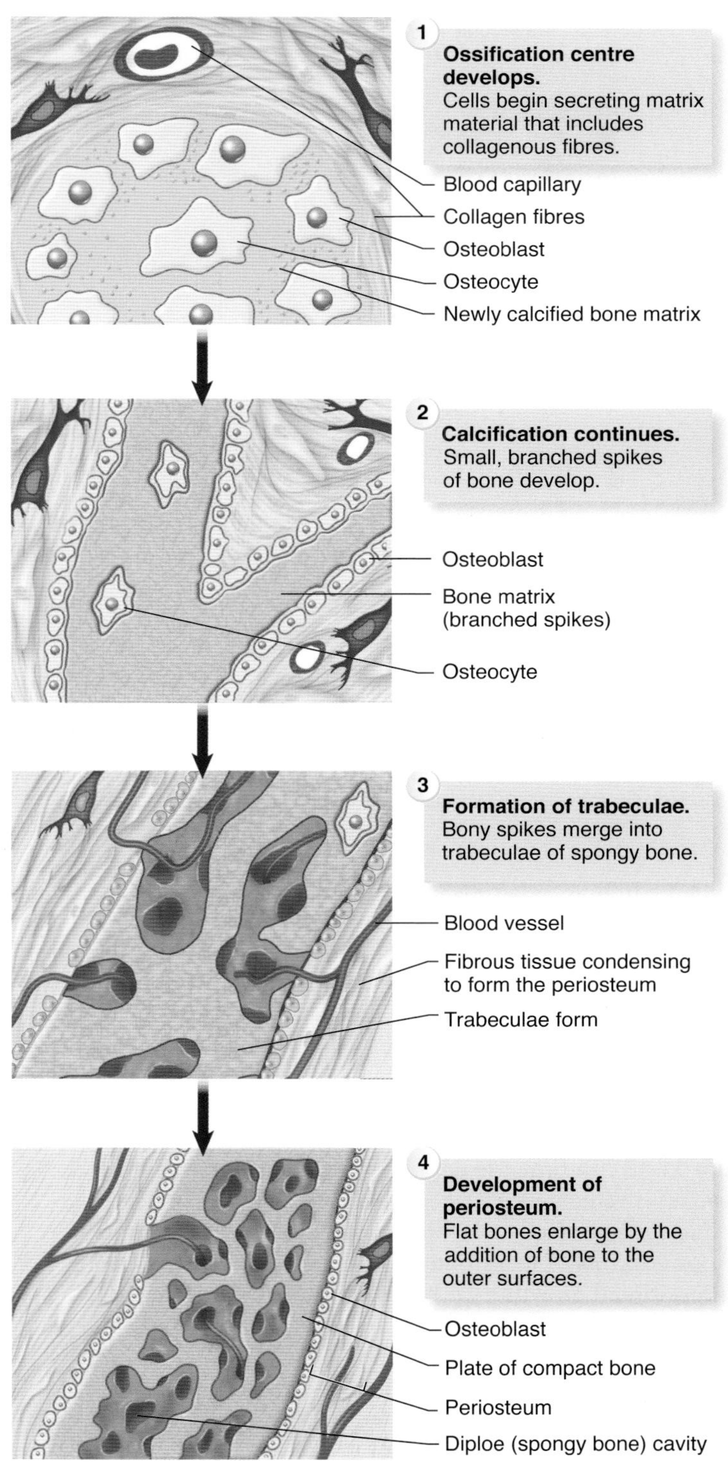

FIGURE 11-13 Intramembranous bone formation. A simplified overview of the steps in forming flat bones. Note that in each succeeding step, the view "zooms out" to a lower magnification. Compare with **Figure 11-6**.

These clusters of osteoblasts are called **ossification centres.** They secrete matrix material and collagenous fibres (**Figure 11-13**). The Golgi apparatus in an osteoblast specializes in synthesizing and secreting carbohydrate compounds of the type called *mucopolysaccharides,* and its endoplasmic reticulum makes and secretes collagen, a

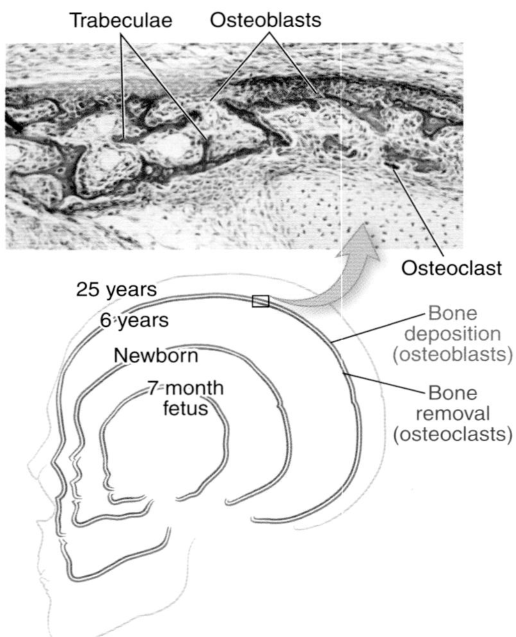

FIGURE 11-14 Flat bone growth in the skull. The micrograph inset shows appositional growth during intramembranous formation of skull bones. Note that *osteoblasts* near the superficial surface of the bone add more bone trabeculae while *osteoclasts* near the deep surface remove bony trabeculae—allowing the skull to increase in size in a way that leaves space for the developing brain.

protein. In time, relatively large amounts of the mucopolysaccharide substance, or *ground substance*, accumulate around each osteoblast. Numerous bundles of collagenous fibres then become embedded in the ground substance. Together, the ground substance and collagenous fibres constitute the organic bone matrix. Calcification of the organic bone matrix occurs when complex calcium salts are deposited in it.

As calcification of bone matrix continues, the trabeculae appear and join in a network to form spongy bone (see **Figure 11-13**). In time the core layer of spongy bone (diploe) will be covered on each side by plates of compact, or dense, bone. Once formed, a flat bone grows in size by the addition of osseous tissue to its outer surface. The process is called **appositional growth.** Flat bones cannot grow by interior expansion as is the case with endochondral bone growth described in the following section.

Figure 11-14 shows appositional growth in the flat bones of the skull during development.

Endochondral Ossification

Most bones of the body are formed from cartilage models, with bone formation spreading essentially from the centre to the ends. The steps of endochondral ossification are illustrated in **Figure 11-15**.

The cartilage model of a typical long bone, such as the tibia, can be identified early in embryonic life (**Figure 11-15**, *A*). The cartilage model then develops a periosteum (**Figure 11-15**, *B*) that soon enlarges and produces a ring, or collar, of bone. Bone is deposited by osteoblasts, which differentiate from cells on the inner surface of the covering periosteum. Soon after appearance of the ring of bone, the cartilage begins to calcify (**Figure 11-15**, *C*), and a **primary ossification centre** forms when a blood vessel enters the rapidly changing cartilage model at the midpoint of the diaphysis.

Endochondral ossification progresses from the diaphysis toward each epiphysis (**Figure 11-15**, *D*), and the bone grows in length. The process is called *interstitial growth*. Eventually, **secondary ossification centres** appear in the epiphyses (**Figure 11-15**, *E*), and bone growth proceeds toward the diaphysis from each end (**Figure 11-15**, *F*).

Until bone growth in length is complete, a layer of the cartilage, known as the **epiphyseal plate,** remains between each epiphysis and the diaphysis. During periods of growth, proliferation of epiphyseal cartilage cells brings about a thickening of this layer. Ossification of the additional cartilage nearest the diaphysis follows—that is, osteoblasts synthesize organic bone matrix, and the matrix undergoes calcification (**Figure 11-16**). As a result, the bone becomes longer (**Figure 11-17**). It is the epiphyseal plate that allows the diaphysis of a long bone to increase in length.

The epiphyseal plate shown in **Figure 11-18** is composed of many layers of cells. Several layers of cells closest to the epiphysis (not visible in the micrograph) are "resting" cartilage cells. These cells are

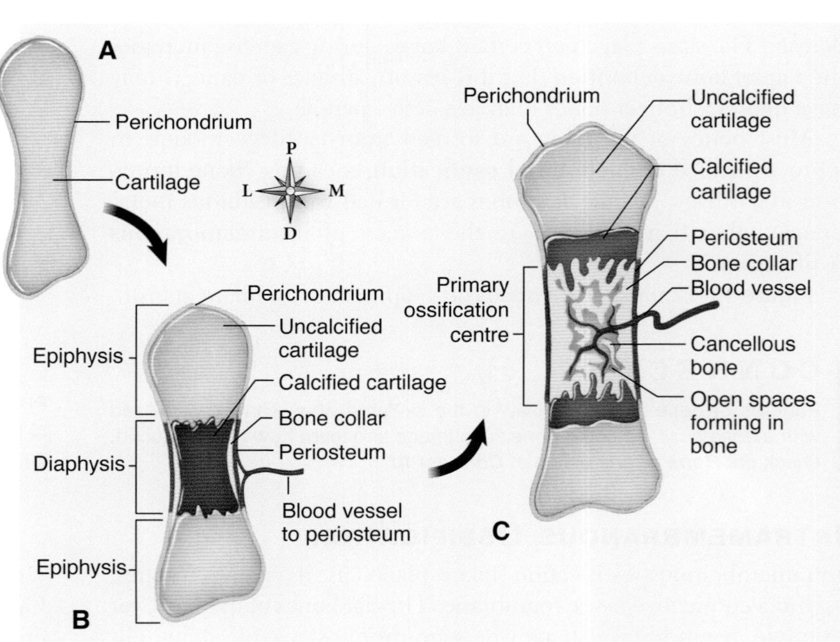

FIGURE 11-15 Endochondral bone formation. A, Cartilage model. **B,** Bone collar formation under the periosteum. **C,** Development of the primary ossification centre and entrance of a blood vessel. **D,** Prominent medullary cavity with thickening and lengthening of the collar. **E,** Development of secondary ossification centres in epiphyseal cartilage. **F,** Enlargement of secondary ossification centres, with bone growth proceeding toward the diaphysis from each end. **G,** With cessation of bone growth, the lower, then upper, epiphyseal plates disappear (only the epiphyseal lines remain).

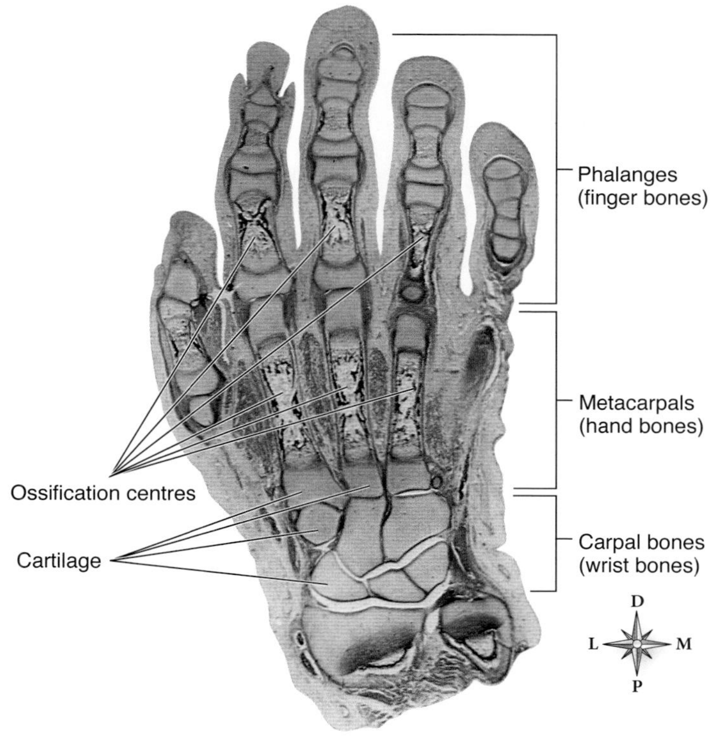

FIGURE 11-16 Fetal ossification centres. Photograph of a specially prepared fetal hand specimen showing primary ossification centres in the bones of the hand (metacarpal bones) and fingers (phalanges). Note that none of the wrist (carpal) bones show any evidence of ossification.

not proliferating or undergoing change. This *resting zone* serves as a point of attachment firmly joining the outer end, or epiphysis, of a bone to the shaft.

The topmost layers of cells shown in **Figure 11-18** make up the *proliferating zone.* The proliferating zone is composed of cartilage cells that are undergoing active mitosis. As a result of mitotic division and increased cellular activity, the layer thickens and the plate as a whole increases in length (**Figure 11-19**).

The next set of cell layers, called the *zone of hypertrophy,* is composed of older, enlarged cells that are undergoing degenerative changes associated with calcium deposition.

The layer closest to the diaphysis is a thin *ossification zone* composed of dead or dying cartilage cells undergoing rapid calcification. As the process of calcification progresses, this layer becomes fragile and disintegrates. The resulting space is soon filled with new bone tissue, and the bone as a whole grows in length.

When epiphyseal cartilage cells stop multiplying and the cartilage has become completely ossified, bone growth ends. Radiographs can reveal any epiphyseal cartilage still present. When bones have grown their full length, the epiphyseal cartilage disappears—bone has replaced it and is then continuous between epiphysis and diaphysis.

The point of articulation between the epiphysis and diaphysis of a growing long bone, however, is susceptible to injury if overstressed—especially in a young child or preadolescent athlete. In these individuals the epiphyseal plate can be separated from the diaphysis or epiphysis, resulting in **epiphyseal fracture** (**Figure 11-20**).

The relationship between interstitial growth (growth in length) and appositional growth (growth in diameter) during endochondral ossification of a long bone is shown in **Figure 11-21**.

Quick CHECK

9. Name the three major types of bone cells.
10. Name the two types of bone marrow.
11. What are the five functions of bone?
12. Identify the two types of bone formation.

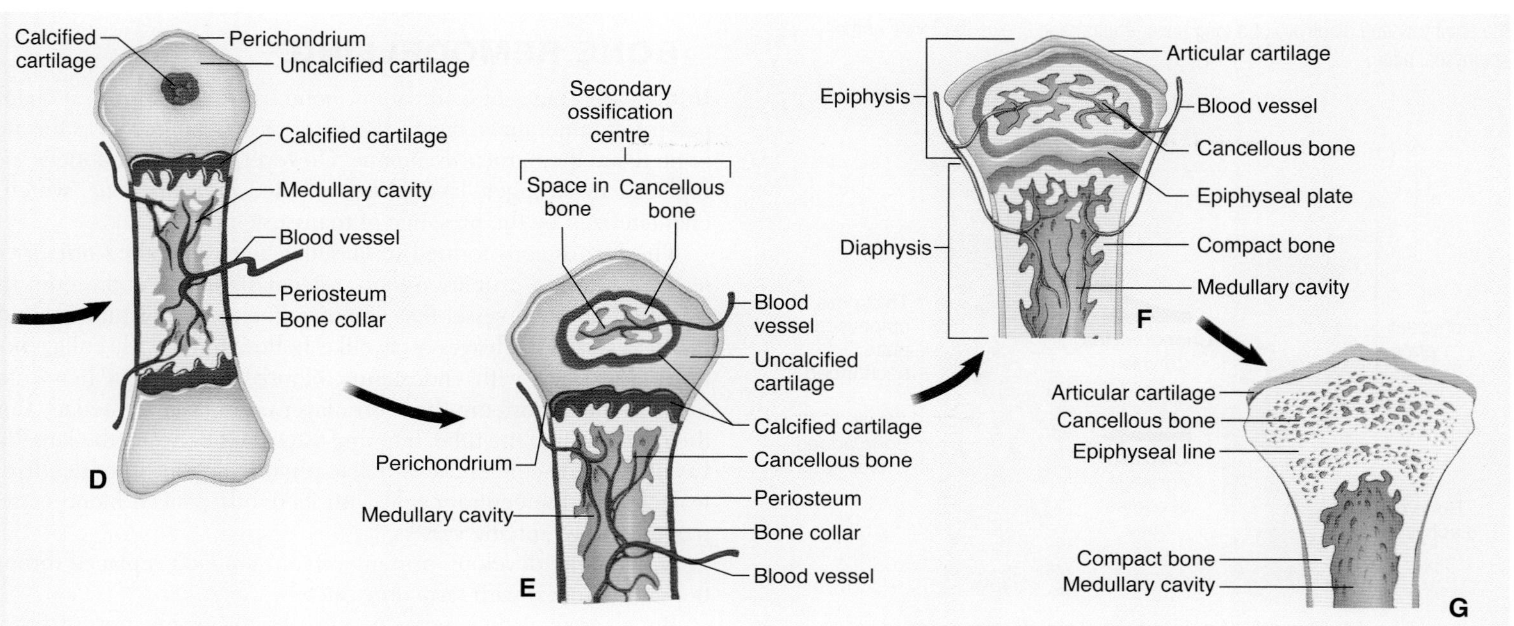

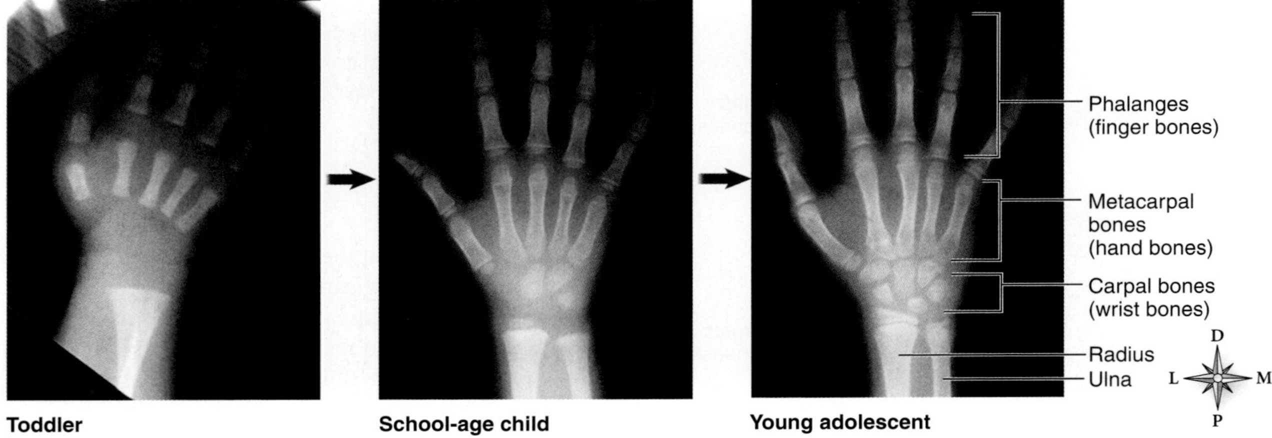

FIGURE 11-17 Endochondral ossification of the hand and wrist. Radiographs showing increasing numbers of ossification centres becoming visible as bright white areas in the wrist with increasing age.

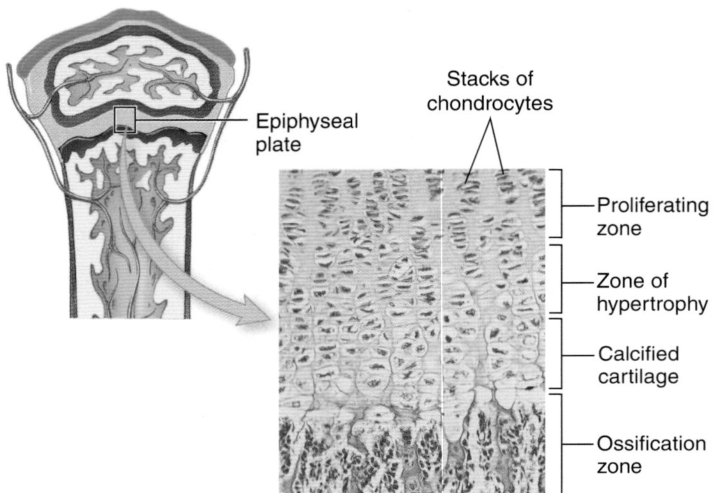

FIGURE 11-18 Epiphyseal plate structure. An epiphyseal plate between the epiphysis and diaphysis of a long bone. Photograph shows the zones of the epiphyseal plate.

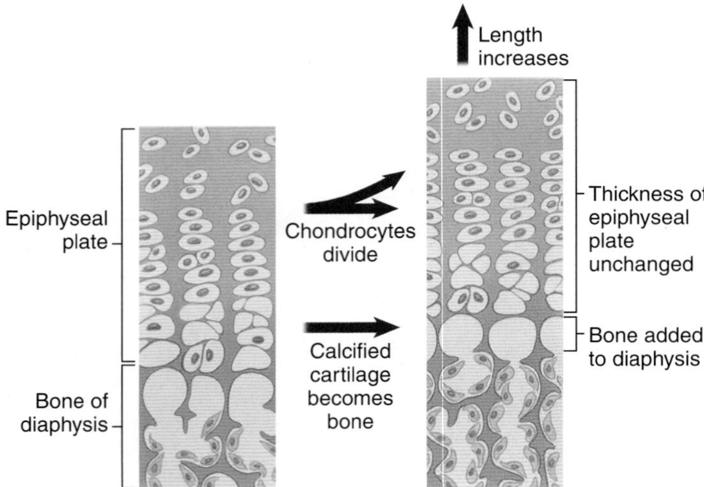

FIGURE 11-19 Growth of epiphyseal plate. Diagrams showing steps in ossification on either side of the epiphyseal plate.

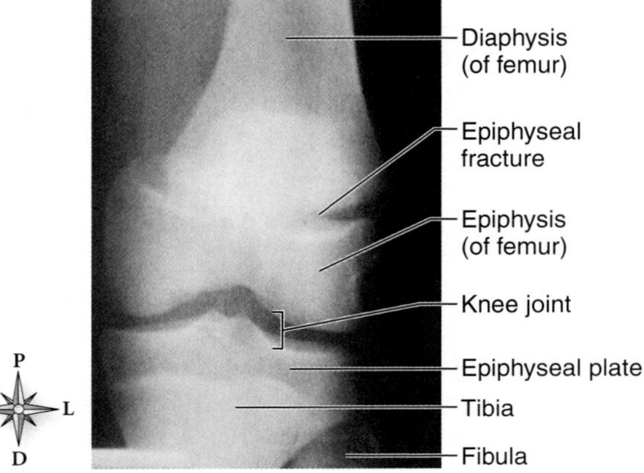

FIGURE 11-20 Epiphyseal fracture. Radiograph showing an epiphyseal fracture of the distal end of the femur in a young athlete. Note the separation of the diaphysis and epiphysis at the level of the growth plate.

BONE REMODELLING

In the early stages of ossification, bone tissue develops in a chaotic pattern of mineralized layers. Its crisscross appearance gives this new bone tissue the name *woven bone*. However, the woven bone is soon replaced by stronger, layered bone called *lamellar bone*, which is characterized by the presence of many osteons.

The first osteons formed in lamellar bone are called *primary osteons*. To form a primary osteon, osteoclasts in the endosteum that surrounds a blood vessel first demineralize a cone or tube around a blood vessel. This leaves a cavelike hollow filled with collagenous fibres and lined with endosteum. **Figure 11-22** shows how osteoblasts in the endosteum then form layer upon layer (lamellae) along the inside wall of the tube, trapping osteocytes between the lamellae. Eventually, the concentric lamellae run out of space to mineralize—leaving only the central canal with its tightly packed blood vessels, nerves, and lymphatic vessels.

As the bone develops, primary osteons are later replaced through the same process with *secondary osteons*.

Bones grow at their outer margins by the ossification of fibrous tissue by osteoblasts. Long bones grow in diameter by the combined

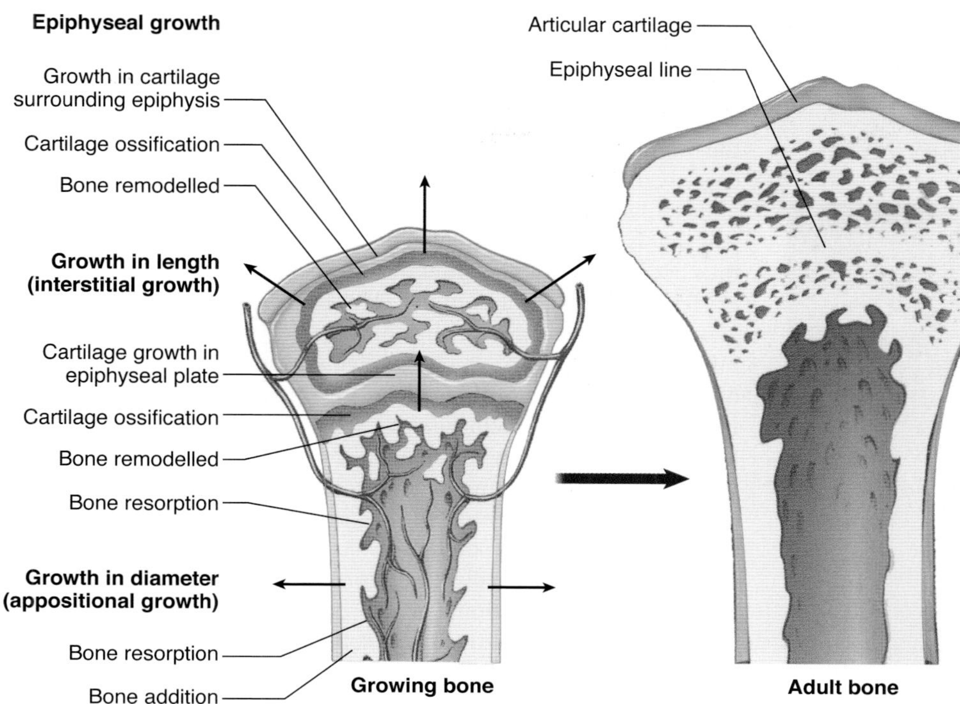

FIGURE 11-21 Bone remodelling. Bone formation on the outside of the shaft coupled with bone reabsorption on the inside increases the bone's diameter. Endochondral growth during bone remodelling increases the length of the diaphysis and causes the epiphysis to enlarge. Intramembranous ossification under the periosteum of the diaphysis increases the diameter of a long bone's shaft.

action of osteoblasts and osteoclasts. Osteoclasts enlarge the diameter of the medullary cavity by eating away the bone of its walls. At the same time, osteoblasts from the periosteum build new bone around the outside of the bone. By this dual process, a bone with a larger diameter and larger medullary cavity is produced from a smaller bone with a smaller medullary cavity.

The remodelling activity of osteoclasts (removal of old bone) and osteoblasts (deposition of new bone) is important in homeostasis of blood calcium levels. It also permits bones to grow in length and diameter and to change their overall shape and the size of the marrow cavity (see **Figure 11-21**).

The formation of bone tissue continues long after bones have stopped growing. Throughout life, bone formation (ossification) and bone destruction (reabsorption) proceed concurrently. These opposing processes balance each other during the early to middle years of adulthood. The rate of bone formation equals the rate of bone destruction. Bones, therefore, neither grow nor shrink. They stay constant in size.

Not so in the earlier years. During childhood and adolescence, ossification occurs at a faster rate than bone reabsorption does. Bone gain outstrips bone loss, and bones grow larger. But between the ages of 35 and 40 years, the process reverses, and from that time on, bone loss exceeds bone gain. Bone gain occurs slowly at the outer, or periosteal, surfaces of bones. Bone loss, on the other hand, occurs at the inner, or endosteal, surfaces and takes place at a somewhat faster pace. More bone is lost on the inside than gained on the outside, and inevitably bones become remodelled as the years go by.

Recall that under mechanical stress cancellous bone remodels its trabeculae in different directions and thicker diameters to better withstand the stress (see **Figure 11-7**). Remodelling in compact bone involves the formation of new (secondary) osteons when bones are stressed. The higher the mechanical load on a bone, the narrower the tube hollowed out by osteoclasts as they prepare for the new osteon. Thus bones that bear the greatest weight have the narrowest osteons. These narrower osteons also have denser mineralization. The dense mineralization along with more numerous, narrower osteons give the bone great strength to resist

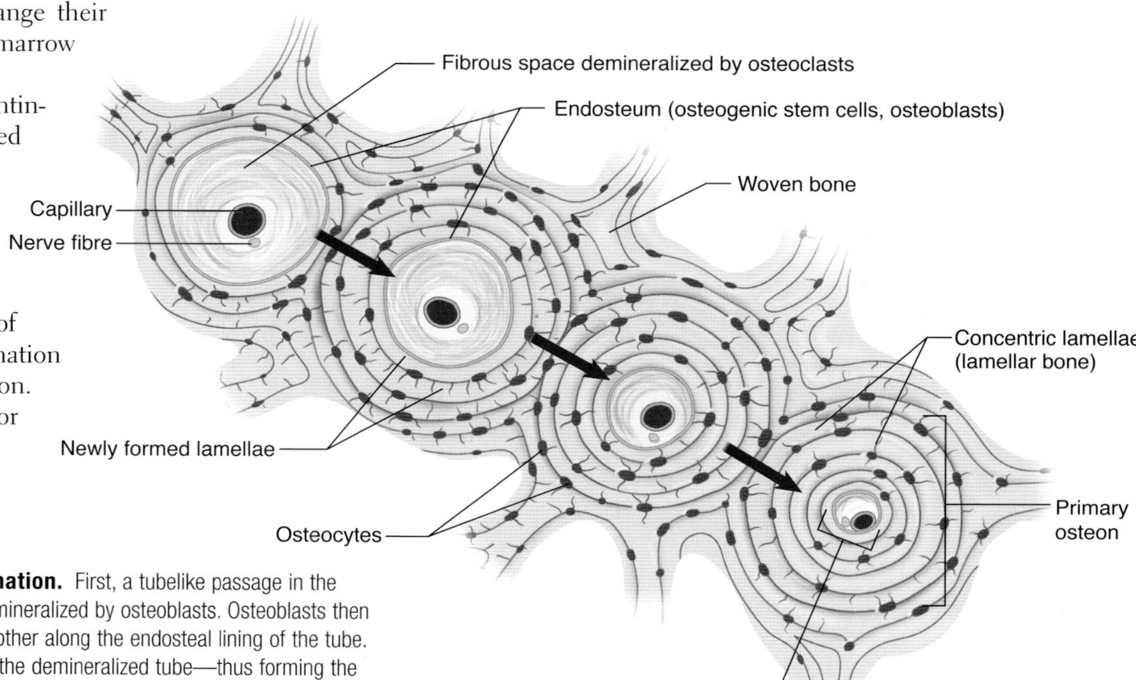

FIGURE 11-22 Primary osteon formation. First, a tubelike passage in the woven bone surrounding a blood vessel is demineralized by osteoblasts. Osteoblasts then begin laying down one layer (lamella) after another along the endosteal lining of the tube. As layers build up, they eventually fill most of the demineralized tube—thus forming the concentric lamellae around a central canal that characterize an osteon.

UNIT 2

BOX 11-1 *sports and fitness*

Exercise and Bone Density

Walking, jogging, and other forms of exercise subject bones to stress. They respond by laying down more collagen fibres and mineral salts in the bone matrix. This, in turn, makes bones stronger. But inactivity and lack of exercise tend to weaken bones because of decreased collagen formation and excessive calcium withdrawal. To prevent these changes, as well as many others, astronauts regularly perform special exercises in space because of the lack of gravity. Regular weight-bearing exercise is also an important part of the prevention and treatment of osteoporosis. •

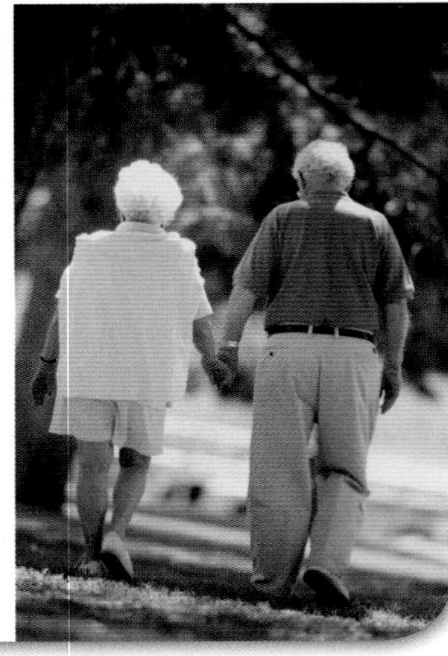

Physical activity increases bone density.

the stress. It is clear then why physical activity, which increases the various loads on bones throughout the body, tends to increase the density and strength of the skeleton (**Box 11-1**).

REPAIR OF BONE FRACTURES

The term *fracture* is defined as a break in the continuity of a bone. *Fracture healing* is the process that results in bone repair. The complex bone tissue repair process that follows a fracture is apparently initiated by bone death or by damage to periosteal and osteon blood vessels.

A bone fracture invariably tears and destroys blood vessels that carry nutrients to osteocytes. It is this vascular damage that initiates the highly regulated and generally very successful repair process described later. When uncomplicated fractures occur in healthy children and young adults, the healing process often results in a repair that is all but impossible to detect 6 months after injury. Healing thus becomes a simple matter of adjusting normal bone remodelling processes to repair the injury. However, especially in older age groups, fracture repair may be complicated by underlying disease or other health problems, such as osteoporosis, diabetes, infection, or diminished blood supply to the injured area. In these cases, delayed healing, instability, deformity, or even nonunion of the fractured bone can result in very serious medical complications.

The process of fracture healing is shown in **Figure 11-23**, *A* to *E*. Vascular damage occurring immediately after a fracture results in haemorrhage and the pooling of blood at the point of injury. The resulting blood clot is called a *fracture haematoma* (see **Figure 11-23**, *B*). The fracture haematoma quickly becomes "organized", develops a fibrin mesh, and transforms into a soft mass of *granulation tissue* containing inflammatory cells, fibroblasts, bone- and cartilage-forming cells, and new capillaries. Soon, islands of cartilaginous tissue called *procallus* form, and although they offer no structural rigidity for weight bearing, they help anchor the ends of the fractured bone more firmly (see **Figure 11-23**, *C*).

Growing numbers of osteoblasts continue the healing process with the formation of bony *callus* tissue. It serves to bind the broken ends of the fracture on both the outside surface and along the marrow cavity internally. The rapidly growing callus tissue effectively "collars" or "splints" the broken ends and stabilizes the fracture so that healing can proceed (see **Figure 11-23**, *D*). If the fracture is properly aligned and immobilized and if complications do not develop, callus tissue will be actively "modelled" and eventually

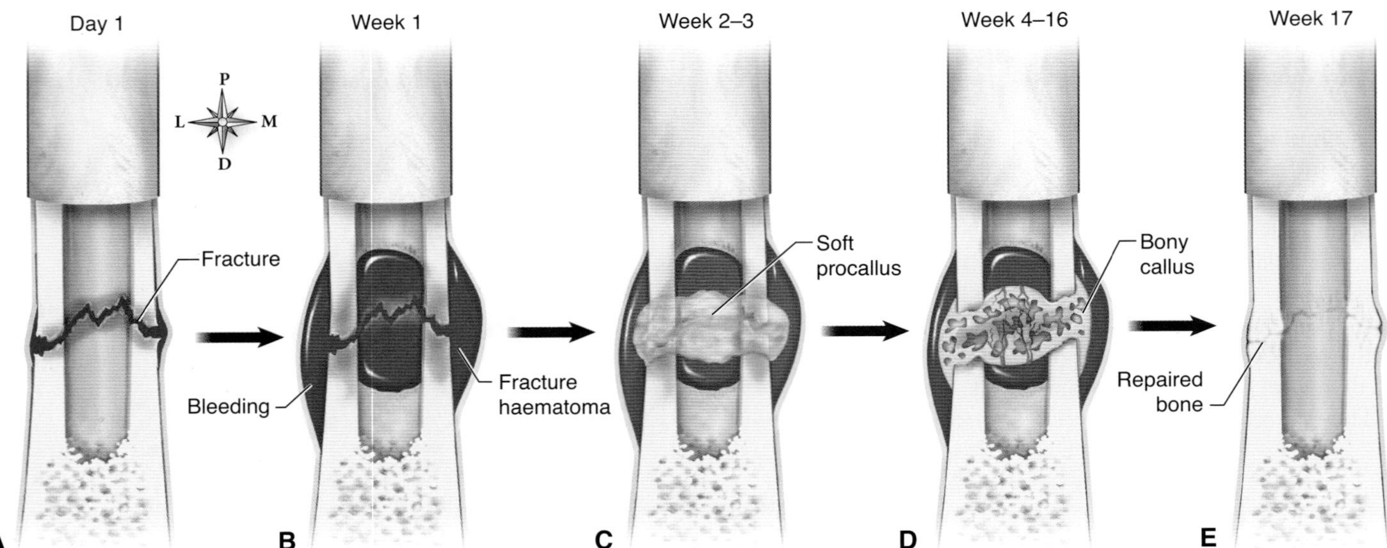

FIGURE 11-23 Bone fracture healing. A, Fracture of the femur. **B,** Formation of a fracture haematoma. **C,** Formation of a soft, cartilaginous procallus. **D,** Formation of internal and external bony callus. **E,** Bone remodelling complete. Time frames are approximate and can vary with age, health, nutrition, and so on. This process can be supplemented with external splints, casts and/or surgical use of supportive pins, plates or other devices.

replaced with normal bone as the injury heals completely (see **Figure 11-23**, *E*).

CONNECT IT!

What are the types of bone fractures? How are they treated? Learn more about bone fractures in Chapter 13, p. 279, and in ***Bone Fractures*** online at ***Connect It!***

CARTILAGE

TYPES OF CARTILAGE

Cartilage is classified as connective tissue and is classified into three types called **hyaline cartilage, elastic cartilage,** and **fibrocartilage.** As a tissue, cartilage resembles bone in some ways but differs from bone in other ways. Innumerable collagenous fibres reinforce the matrix of both tissues, and as with bone, cartilage consists more of extracellular substance than cells. However, in cartilage the fibres are embedded in a firm gel instead of a calcified cement substance. Hence cartilage has the flexibility of a firm plastic material, whereas bone has the rigidity of cast iron.

Another difference is that no canal system and no blood vessels penetrate the cartilage matrix. Cartilage is avascular and bone is abundantly vascular. Nevertheless, cartilage cells, as with bone cells, lie in lacunae. However, because no canals and blood vessels interlace cartilage matrix, nutrients and oxygen can reach the scattered, isolated **chondrocytes** (cartilage cells) only by diffusion. They diffuse through the matrix gel from capillaries in the fibrous covering of the cartilage—the **perichondrium**—or from synovial fluid in the case of articular cartilage.

The three cartilage types differ from one another largely by the relative amounts of elastic and collagenous fibres that are embedded in the matrix material. *Hyaline* is the most abundant type, and both elastic cartilage and fibrocartilage are considered modifications of the hyaline type. Collagenous fibres are present in all three types but are most numerous in *fibrocartilage.* Hence it has the greatest tensile strength. *Elastic cartilage* matrix contains elastic fibres in addition to collagenous fibres and thus has elasticity as well as firmness.

Cartilage is an excellent skeletal support tissue in the developing embryo. It forms rapidly and yet retains a significant degree of rigidity, or stiffness. A majority of the bones that eventually form the axial and the appendicular skeleton described in Chapters 12 and 13 first appear as cartilage models. Skeletal maturation involves replacement of the cartilage models with bone.

After birth there is a decrease in the total amount of cartilage tissue present in the body. However, it continues to play an important role in the growth of long bones until skeletal maturity and is found throughout life as the material that covers the articular surfaces of bones in joints. The three types of cartilage also serve other important functions throughout the body.

Hyaline Cartilage

Hyaline, in addition to being the most common type of cartilage, serves many functions. It resembles milk glass in appearance (**Figure 11-24**, *A*). In fact, its name is derived from the Greek word meaning "glassy". Sometimes called *gristle*, it is semitransparent and often has a bluish, opalescent cast.

In the embryo, hyaline cartilage forms from differentiation of mesenchymal cells that become crowded together in so-called **chondrification centres.** As the cells enlarge, they secrete matrix material that surrounds the delicate collagen fibrils. Eventually, the continued production of matrix separates and isolates the cells, or chondrocytes, into compartments, which, as in bone, are called *lacunae.* Like bone, the organic matrix of hyaline cartilage is a mixture of ground substance and collagenous fibres. The ground substance is rich in both chondroitin sulphate and a unique gel-like polysaccharide. Both substances are secreted from chondrocytes in much the same way protein and carbohydrates are secreted from glandular cells.

In addition to covering the articular surfaces of bones, hyaline cartilage forms the costal cartilages that connect the anterior ends of the ribs with the sternum, or breastbone. It also forms the cartilage rings in the trachea, bronchi of the lungs, and tip of the nose.

Elastic Cartilage

Elastic cartilage gives form to the external ear, the epiglottis that covers the opening of the respiratory tract when swallowing, and the

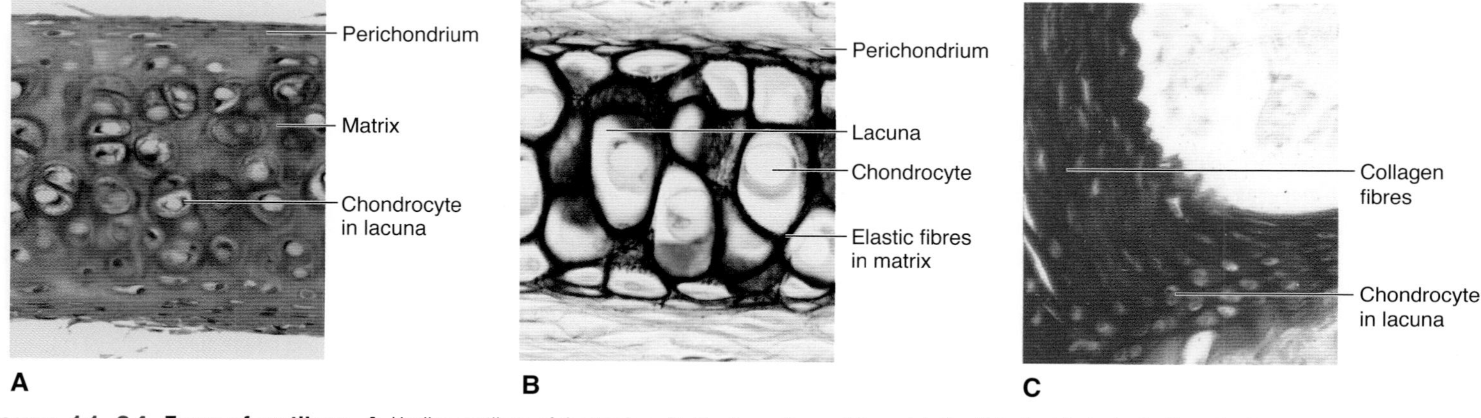

FIGURE 11-24 Types of cartilage. A, Hyaline cartilage of the trachea. **B,** Elastic cartilage of the epiglottis. Note the black elastic fibres in the cartilage matrix and the perichondrium layers on both surfaces. **C,** Fibrocartilage of an intervertebral disc.

eustachian, or auditory, tubes that connect the middle ear and nasal cavity. The collagenous fibres of hyaline cartilage are also present—but in fewer numbers—in elastic cartilage. Large numbers of darkly stained elastic fibres confer the elasticity and resiliency typical of this form of cartilage (**Figure 11-24**, *B*).

Fibrocartilage

Fibrocartilage—or *fibrous cartilage*—is characterized by abundant fibrous elements within the matrix (**Figure 11-24**, *C*). It is strong, rigid, and most often associated with regions of dense connective tissue in the body. It occurs in the pubic symphysis, in intervertebral discs, and near the points of attachment of some large tendons to bones.

Function of Cartilage

The tough, rubberlike nature of cartilage permits it to sustain great weight when covering the articulating surfaces of bones. It also may serve as a shock-absorbing pad between articulating bones in the spine. In other areas, such as the external ear, nose, or respiratory passages, cartilage provides a strong, yet pliable support structure that resists deformation or collapse of tubular passageways. Cartilage permits growth in the length of long bones and is largely responsible for their adult shape and size.

Growth of Cartilage

Growth of cartilage occurs in two ways:

1. Interstitial growth
2. Appositional growth

During interstitial growth, cartilage cells within the substance of the tissue mass divide and begin to secrete additional matrix (see **Figure 11-19** on p. 222). Internal division of chondrocytes is possible because of the soft, pliable nature of cartilage tissue. This form of growth is most often seen during childhood and early adolescence, when a majority of cartilage is still soft and capable of expansion from within. Interstitial growth may be referred to as *endogenous growth* because it occurs *within* the cartilage tissue.

Appositional growth occurs when chondrocytes in the deep layer of the perichondrium begin to divide and secrete additional matrix. The new matrix is then deposited on the surface of the cartilage, which causes it to increase in size. Appositional growth is unusual in early childhood but, once initiated, continues beyond adolescence and throughout an individual's life. Appositional growth may be referred to as *exogenous growth* because it occurs on the *outer* surfaces of cartilage tissue.

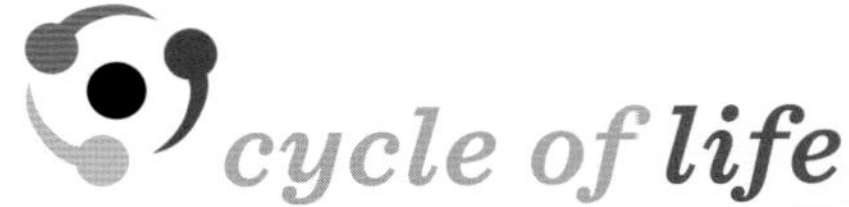

Skeletal Tissues This chapter focused on the changes that occur in bone and cartilage tissue from the time before birth to advanced old age. For instance, we have outlined in some detail the process by which the soft cartilage and membranous skeleton become ossified over a period of years. By the time a person is a young adult in their mid-20s, the skeleton has become fully ossified. A few areas of soft tissue—the cartilaginous areas of the nose and ears, for example—may continue to grow and ossify very slowly throughout adulthood so that by advanced old age, some structural changes are apparent.

Changes in skeletal tissue that occur during adulthood usually result from specific conditions. For example, the mechanical stress of weight-bearing exercise can trigger dramatic increases in the density and strength of bone tissue. Pregnancy, nutritional deficiencies, and illness can all cause loss of bone density accompanied by loss of structural strength.

In advanced adulthood, degeneration of bone and cartilage tissue becomes apparent. Replacement of hard bone matrix by softer connective tissue results in a loss of strength that increases susceptibility to injury. This is especially true in older women who suffer from osteoporosis. Fortunately, even very light exercise by elderly individuals can counteract some of the skeletal tissue degeneration associated with old age.

Quick CHECK

13. Name three major types of cartilage.
14. Identify the primary type of cartilage cell.
15. List the two mechanisms of cartilage growth.

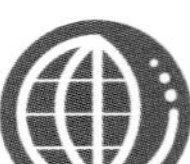

the big picture | Skeletal Tissues

Skeletal tissues influence many important body functions that are crucial to the "big picture" of overall health and survival of the individual. The pervasive importance of the protective and support functions of skeletal tissues is immediately apparent. Bone and cartilage tissues are organized and grouped to protect the body and its internal organs from injury.

In addition to providing a supporting and protective framework, these tissues also contribute to the shape, alignment, and positioning of the body and its myriad parts. Also, because of the organization of skeletal tissues into bones and the articulation of these bones in joints, we are able to engage in purposeful and coordinated movement. Bone remodelling permits ongoing change to occur in both structure and related functions throughout the cycle of life.

The homeostatic function of skeletal tissues is beautifully illustrated by the role they play in mineral storage and release. For example, regulation of blood calcium levels is important in such diverse areas as nerve transmission, muscle contraction, and normal clotting of blood. Because they contain red marrow, the bones also serve in the important role of haematopoiesis, or blood cell formation. This function ties skeletal tissues to such diverse homeostatic functions as regulation of body pH and the transport of respiratory gases and vital nutrients. By viewing skeletal tissues in such a broad and interrelated functional context, you can more readily sense the "connectedness" that unites these otherwise seemingly isolated body structures to the "big picture" of overall health and survival.

mechanisms of disease

Diseases of Skeletal Tissues: Malignant Tumours of Bone and Cartilage

Osteosarcoma (osteogenic sarcoma) is the most common primary malignant tumour of skeletal tissue and is often the most fatal. It appears more commonly in males, with a peak age of incidence between 10 and 25 years. Common sites of involvement are the tibia, femur, and humerus. Roughly 10% of patients experience metastases to the lungs, and if left untreated, the course can involve widespread metastases and death within 1 year. Therapy commonly involves surgery followed by chemotherapy.

Chondrosarcoma is a malignant tumour of hyaline cartilage that arises from chondroblasts. It is a large, bulky, slow-growing tumour occurring most often in middle-aged persons. Common sites of involvement include the humerus, femur, spine, pelvis, ribs, and scapula. Large excisions or amputation of the affected extremity can improve survival rates. Chemotherapy has not been proven to be effective.

Metabolic Bone Diseases

Metabolic bone diseases are disorders of bone remodelling.

As a serious and very common bone disease, especially in older age groups, **osteoporosis** has been the subject of intense scientific research and widespread public interest and concern. Characterized by increased bone porosity and reduced mineral density and mass, osteoporotic bones fracture easily. Some bones, such as the vertebral bodies in the spinal column, are particularly susceptible to damage. These bones have a large percentage of cancellous bone with trabeculae that become less numerous and weak in osteoporosis. The result is extensive and progressive microfracture of many of the remaining trabeculae and eventual vertebral collapse (**Figure 11-25**). Over time, increasing numbers of vertebral compression fractures result in a shortened stature and cause an abnormal backward curvature of the spine called "dowager's hump". The condition is, unfortunately, a common sign of long-standing osteoporosis in many untreated older women. Although osteoporosis can occur in both men and women, one of every two women who survive 40 years after menopause will suffer an osteoporosis-related fracture, in contrast to one in 40 men of similar age.

In most women, a majority of the bone loss characteristic of osteoporosis occurs during the decade after menopause and beyond. However, significant loss can occur much earlier—even during adolescence. Therefore, health care providers are suggesting earlier screening for the disease and lifestyle changes that include weight-bearing exercise and a diet adequate in calcium and vitamin D.

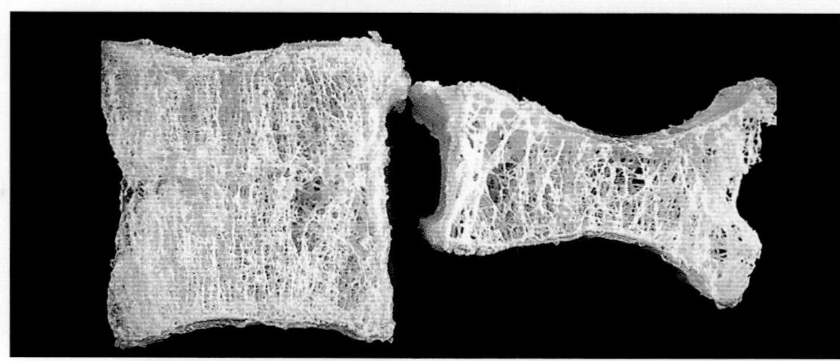

A

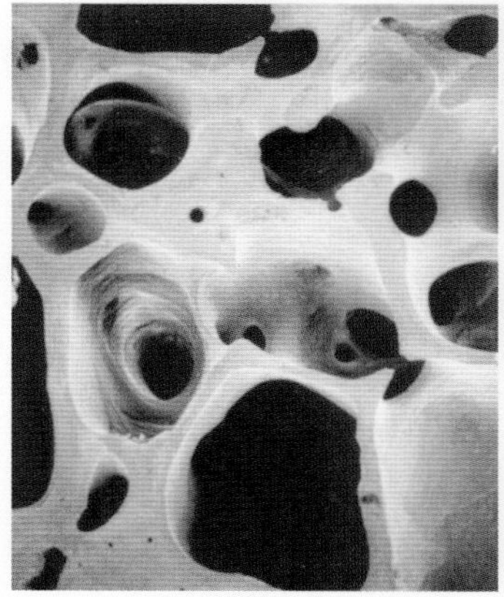

B

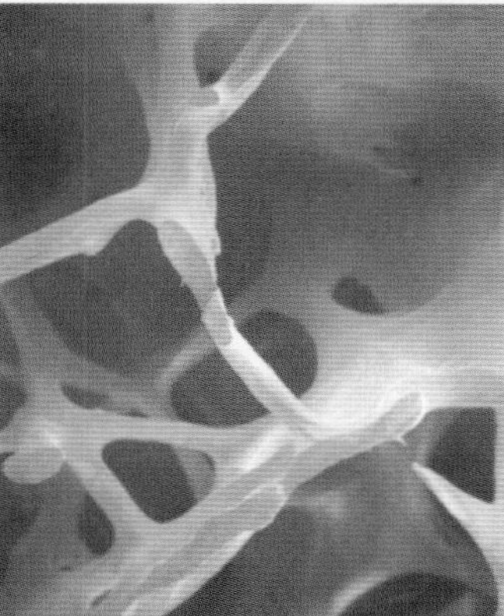

C

FIGURE 11-25 Osteoporosis. A, Compare the normal vertebral body (*left*) with the osteoporotic specimen (*right*). Note that the osteoporotic vertebral body has been shortened by compression fractures. **B,** Scanning electron micrograph (SEM) of normal bone. **C,** SEM of osteoporotic bone. Note the loss of trabeculae and appearance of enlarged pores caused by osteoporosis.

CONNECT IT!

How can you tell if you have osteoporosis? View ***Measuring Bone Mineral Density*** at ***Connect It!*** to learn how bone density is measured.

Rickets and Osteomalacia

Rickets in young children and **osteomalacia** in adults are metabolic skeletal diseases that affect significant numbers of individuals worldwide. Both diseases are characterized by demineralization or loss of minerals from bone related to vitamin D deficiency. The loss of minerals is coupled with increased production of unmineralized matrix. Rickets involves demineralization of developing bones in infants and young children before skeletal maturity. In osteomalacia, mineral content is lost from bones that have already matured. In rickets, the lack of rigidity caused by the demineralization of developing bones results in gross skeletal changes, including the classic "bowing of the legs" symptom (**Figure 11-26**). The demineralization of bones in osteomalacia does not generally affect overall skeletal contours but does result in increased susceptibility to fractures, especially in the vertebral bodies and femoral necks. **Box 11-2** discusses how nutritional deficiencies affect cartilage as well as bone tissue.

BOX 11-2 *health matters*

Cartilage and Nutritional Deficiencies

Certain nutritional deficiencies and other metabolic disturbances have an immediate and very visible effect on cartilage. It is for this reason that changes in cartilage often serve as indicators of inadequate vitamin, mineral, or protein intake. Vitamin A and protein deficiency, for example, will decrease the thickness of epiphyseal plates in the growing long bones of young children—an effect immediately apparent on x-ray examination. The opposite effect occurs in vitamin D deficiencies. As the epiphyseal cartilage increases in thickness but fails to calcify, the growing bones become deformed and bend under weight bearing. The bent long bones are a sign of rickets (see **Figure 11-26**).

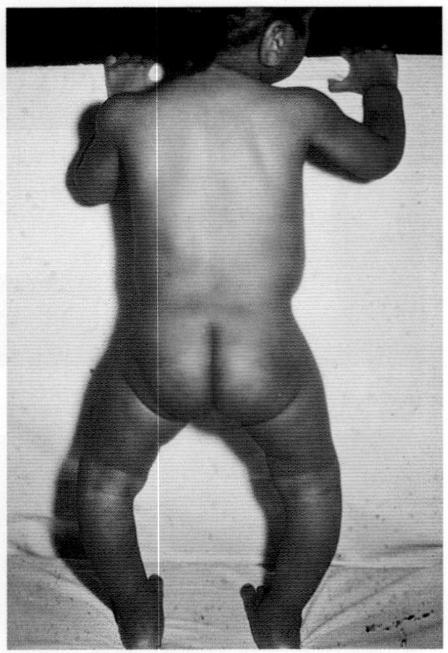

FIGURE 11-26 Rickets. Bowing of legs in this toddler is due to poorly mineralized bones from rickets.

Osteitis deformans, also known as *Paget disease,* is a disorder affecting older adults. It is characterized by proliferation of osteoclasts and compensatory increased osteoblastic activity. The result is rapid and disorganized bone remodelling. The bones formed are poorly constructed and weakened. It commonly affects the skull, humerus, femur, vertebra, and pelvic bones. Clinical manifestations may include bone pain, tenderness, and fractures. However, the majority of patients experience minimal changes and never know they have the disease. No treatment is recommended in an asymptomatic patient.

Osteomyelitis is a bacterial infection of the bone and marrow tissue. Infections of bone are often more difficult to treat than soft tissue infections because of the decreased blood supply and density of the bone. Bacteria, viruses, fungi, and other pathogens may cause osteomyelitis. *Staphylococcus* bacteria are the most common pathogens. Osteomyelitis is associated with extension of another infection (e.g., bacteraemia, urinary tract infection, vascular ulcer) or direct bone contamination (e.g., gunshot wound, open fracture). Patients who are elderly, poorly nourished, or diabetic are also at risk. Thrombosis of blood vessels in osteomyelitis often results in ischaemia and bone necrosis. As a result, infection can extend under the periosteum and spread to adjacent soft tissues and joints. Signs and symptoms may include an area that is swollen, warm, tender to touch, and painful. Early recognition of infection and aggressive antimicrobial management are required. Sometimes patients may require many weeks of antibiotic therapy.

LANGUAGE OF SCIENCE *(continued from p. 209)*

intramembranous ossification (in-trah-MEM-brah-nus os-i-fi-KAY-shun)
[*intra-* **within,** *-membran-* **thin skin,** *-ous* **characterized by,** *os-* **bone,** *-fication* **to make**]

ligament (LIG-ah-ment)
[*liga-* **bind,** *-ment* **result of action**]

medullary cavity (meh-DULL-air-ee)
[*medulla-* **marrow or pith (middle),** *-ary* **relating to,** *cav-* **hollow,** *-ity* **state**]

metaphysis (meh-TAF-i-sis)
[*meta-* **middle,** *-physis* **growth**]

myeloid tissue (MY-eh-loyd)
[*myel-* **marrow,** *-oid* **of or like,** *tissu-* **fabric**]

ossification centre (os-i- fi-KAY-shun SEN-ter)
[*os-* **bone,** *-fic-* **make,** *-ation* **process**]

osteoblast (OS-tee-oh-blast)
[*osteo-* **bone,** *-blast* **bud**]

osteoclast (OS-tee-oh-klast)
[*osteo-* **bone,** *-clast* **break**]

osteocyte (OS-tee-oh-syte)
[*osteo-* **bone,** *-cyte* **cell**]

osteogenic stem cell (os-tee-oh-JEN-ik stem sel)
[*osteo-* **bone,** *-gen-* **produce,** *-ic* **relating to**]

osteon (OS-tee-on)
[*osteo-* **bone,** *-on* **unit**]

perichondrium (pair-i-KON-dree-um)
[*peri-* **around,** *-chondr-* **cartilage,** *-um* **thing**] *pl.,* perichondria

periosteum (pair-ee-OS-tee-um)
[*peri-* **around,** *-osteum* **bone**]

primary ossification centre (os-i-fi-KAY-shun)
[*primary* **first order,** *os-* **bone,** *-fic-* **make,** *-ation* **process**]

secondary ossification centre (SEK-on-dair-ee os-i-fih-KAY-shun)
[*secondary* **second order,** *os-* **bone,** *-fic-* **make,** *-ation* **process**]

sesamoid bone (SES-ah-moyd)
[*sesam-* **sesame seed,** *-oid* **like**]

trabecula (trah-BEK-yoo-la)
[*trab-* **beam,** *-ula* **little**] *pl.,* trabeculae

trabecular bone (trah-BEK-yoo-lar)
[*trab-* **beam,** *-ula-* **little,** *-ar* **relating to**]

transverse canal (tranz-vers kah-NAL)
[*trans-* **across,** *-vers-* **turn**]

yellow marrow (YEL-oh MAIR-oh)

LANGUAGE OF MEDICINE

bone marrow transplant (MAIR-oh TRANZ-plant)

chondroitin sulphate (kon-DROY-tin SUHL-fayt)
[*chondr-* **cartilage,** *-oid* **of or like,** *-in* **substance,** *sulph-* **sulphur,** *-ate* **oxygen**]

epiphyseal fracture (ep-i-FEEZ-ee-al)
[*epi-* **on,** *-phys-* **growth,** *-al* **relating to,** *fracture* **to break**]

glucosamine (gloo-KOHS-ah-meen)
[*glucos-* **sweetness or glucose,** *-amine* **ammonia compound**]

osteogenesis (os-tee-oh-JEN-eh-sis)
[*osteo-* **bone,** *-gen-* **produce,** *-esis* **process**]

osteomalacia (os-tee-oh-mah-LAY-shah)
[*osteo-* **bone,** *-malacia* **softening**]

osteoporosis (os-tee-oh-poh-ROH-sis)
[*osteo-* **bone,** *-poro-* **pore,** *-osis* **condition**]

rickets (RIK-ets)
[**unknown origin**]

case study

Eleanor stepped off the curb to cross the road, just as she had done thousands of times before. But this time, her hip gave way, and she suddenly found herself on the ground, unable to get back up. An x-ray film at the hospital showed a fracture in the neck of her femur. Eleanor wondered how she could have broken a bone by simply stepping off a curb. The doctor was talking about surgery and a 6-month recovery time. She would definitely have to reschedule the cruise she had booked to celebrate retirement.

1. Which of the following conditions likely caused Eleanor's broken hip?
   a. Osteosarcoma
   b. Rickets
   c. Osteoporosis
   d. Osteomyelitis
2. What type of bone did Eleanor fracture?
   a. Long bone
   b. Short bone
   c. Flat bone
   d. Irregular bone
3. What type of cartilage would you find covering the ends of that bone?
   a. Elastic cartilage
   b. White fibrous cartilage
   c. Fibrocartilage
   d. Hyaline cartilage

After her surgery, Eleanor received a prescription from her doctor for a bisphosphonate (BP) drug.

4. What is the primary effect of a bisphosphonate drug?
   a. Inhibits osteoclasts
   b. Stimulates osteoblasts
   c. Stimulates osteocytes
   d. All of the above

Hint To solve a case study, you may have to refer to the glossary or index, other chapters in this textbook, ***Connect It!,*** and other resources.

UNIT 2

CHAPTER SUMMARY

To download an MP3 version of the chapter summary for use with your mobile device, access the ***Audio Chapter Summaries*** *online at evolve.elsevier.com.*

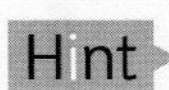

Scan this summary after reading the chapter to help you reinforce the key concepts. Later, use the summary as a quick review before your class or before a test.

Functions of Bone

A. Support—bones form the framework of the body and contribute to the shape, alignment, and positioning of body parts; ligaments help hold bones together (**Figure 11-1**)
B. Protection—bony "boxes" protect the delicate structures they enclose
C. Movement—bones with their joints constitute levers that move as muscles contract
D. Mineral storage—bones are the major reservoir for calcium, phosphorus, and other minerals
E. Haematopoiesis—blood cell formation is carried out by myeloid tissue

Types of Bones

A. Structurally, there are five major types of bones (**Figure 11-2**)
   1. Long bones—cylindrical
   2. Short bones—boxlike
   3. Flat bones—broad, sheetlike
   4. Irregular bones—various shapes
   5. Sesamoid bones—seedlike
B. Size, shape, and appearance of bones vary to meet the various needs served
C. Bones vary in the proportion of compact and cancellous (spongy) bone
   1. Compact bone—dense and solid in appearance
   2. Cancellous bone—characterized by open space partially filled with a lattice of thin branched structures supporting soft tissue
D. Parts of a long bone (**Figure 11-3**)
   1. Diaphysis
      a. Main shaft of a long bone
      b. Hollow, cylindrical shape and thick compact bone
      c. Function—to provide strong support without cumbersome weight
   2. Epiphyses
      a. Both ends of a long bone; made of cancellous bone filled with marrow
      b. Bulbous shape
      c. Function—to provide attachments for muscles and give stability to joints
   3. Articular cartilage
      a. Layer of hyaline cartilage that covers the articular surface of epiphyses
      b. Function—to cushion jolts and blows
   4. Periosteum
      a. Dense, white fibrous membrane that covers bone
      b. Attaches tendons firmly to bones
      c. Contains cells that form and destroy bone
      d. Contains blood vessels important in growth and repair
      e. Contains blood vessels that send branches into bone
      f. Essential for bone cell survival and bone formation
   5. Medullary (or marrow) cavity
      a. Tubelike, hollow space in the diaphysis
      b. Filled with yellow marrow in adults
   6. Endosteum—thin fibrous membrane that lines the medullary cavity

E. Parts of a flat bone and other bones
   1. Inner portion is cancellous bone covered on the outside with compact bone
      a. Cranial flat bones have an internal and external table of compact bone and an inner cancellous region called the *diploe* (**Figure 11-4**)
      b. Bones are covered with periosteum and lined with endosteum, as in a long bone
      c. Other flat bones, short bones, and irregular bones have features similar to the cranial bones
   2. Spaces inside the cancellous bone of short, flat, irregular, and sesamoid bones are filled with red marrow

Bone Tissue

A. Most distinctive form of connective tissue
B. Extracellular components are hard and calcified
C. Rigidity of bone allows it to serve its supportive and protective functions
D. Tensile strength nearly equal to that of cast iron at less than one third the weight
E. Composition of bone matrix
   1. Inorganic salts
      a. Hydroxyapatite—crystals of calcium and phosphate contribute to bone hardness
      b. Slender needlelike crystals are oriented to most effectively resist stress and mechanical deformation
      c. Magnesium, sodium, sulphate, and fluoride are also found in bone
   2. Organic matrix
      a. Composite of collagenous fibres and an amorphous mixture of protein and polysaccharides called *ground substance*
      b. Ground substance—secreted by connective tissue cells
      c. Adds to overall strength of bone and gives some degree of resilience to bone

Microscopic Structure of Bone

A. Compact bone (**Figure 11-5**)
   1. Contains many cylinder-shaped structural units called *osteons*, or *haversian systems* (**Figure 11-6**)
   2. Osteons surround central (osteonal or haversian) canals that run lengthwise through bone and are connected by transverse (Volkmann) canals
      a. Living bone cells located in these units
      b. Constitute the structural framework of compact bone
   3. Osteons permit delivery of nutrients and removal of waste products
   4. Structure of osteon
      a. Lamellae
         (1) Concentric—cylinder-shaped layers of calcified matrix around the central canal
         (2) Interstitial—layers of bone matrix *between* the osteons; left over from previous osteons or woven bone
         (3) Circumferential—few layers of bone matrix that surround all the osteons; run along the outer circumference of a bone and inner circumference (boundary of medullary cavity) of a bone
      b. Lacunae—small spaces containing tissue fluid in which bone cells are located between hard layers of the lamella
      c. Canaliculi—ultra-small canals radiating in all directions from the lacunae and connecting them to each other and to the central canal
      d. Central canal (osteonal or haversian canal)—extends lengthwise through the centre of each osteon and contains blood vessels and lymphatic vessels

B. Cancellous bone—also called *spongy bone* or *trabecular bone* (**Figure 11-6**)
   1. No osteons in cancellous bone; instead, it has trabeculae
   2. Nutrients are delivered and waste products removed by diffusion through tiny canaliculi
   3. Lattice of bony branches (trabeculae) are arranged along lines of stress to enhance the bone's strength (**Figure 11-7**)
   4. Blood supply
      a. Bone cells receive blood supply from the bone marrow in the internal medullary cavity of cancellous bone
      b. Blood vessels from the periosteum become incorporated into the bone and serve nutrient needs of cells by way of transverse (Volkmann) canals, connected with vessels in the central canals of osteons

C. Types of bone cells
   1. Osteoblasts (**Figure 11-8**)
      a. Bone-forming cells found in all bone surfaces
      b. Small cells synthesize and secrete osteoid, an important part of the ground substance
      c. Collagen fibrils line up in osteoid and serve as a framework for the deposition of calcium and phosphate
   2. Osteoclasts (**Figure 11-8**)
      a. Giant multinucleated cells containing many mitochondria and lysosomes
      b. Responsible for the active erosion of bone minerals
         (1) Hydrochloric acid (HCl) dissolves hard bone minerals, releasing ions
         (2) Collagenase is an enzyme that breaks collagen proteins into amino acids
         (3) Ions and amino acids are reabsorbed by blood and recycled
   3. Osteocytes—mature, nondividing osteoblasts surrounded by matrix and lying within lacunae (**Figure 11-9**)

Bone Marrow

A. Type of soft, diffuse connective tissue; called *myeloid tissue*
B. Site for the production of blood cells
C. Found in the medullary cavities of long bones and in the spaces of spongy bone
D. Two types of marrow occur during a person's lifetime (**Figure 11-10**)
   1. Red marrow
      a. Found in virtually all bones in an infant's or child's body
      b. Functions to produce red blood cells
   2. Yellow marrow
      a. As an individual ages, red marrow is replaced by yellow marrow
      b. Marrow cells become saturated with fat and are no longer active in blood cell production

E. Main bones in an adult that still contain red marrow include the ribs, bodies of the vertebrae, humerus, pelvis, and femur
F. Yellow marrow can change to red marrow during times of decreased blood supply, such as anaemia, exposure to radiation, and certain diseases

Regulation of Blood Calcium Levels

A. Bone is a calcium depot and serves as a storehouse for about 98% of body calcium reserves
   1. Helps maintain constancy of blood calcium levels
      a. Calcium is mobilized and moves into and out of blood during bone remodelling
      b. During bone formation, osteoblasts remove calcium from blood and lower circulating levels
      c. During breakdown of bone, osteoclasts release calcium into blood and increase circulating levels
   2. Homeostasis of calcium ion concentration essential for the following:
      a. Bone formation, remodelling, and repair
      b. Blood clotting
      c. Transmission of nerve impulses
      d. Maintenance of skeletal and cardiac muscle contraction
B. Mechanisms of calcium homeostasis (**Figure 11-11**)
   1. Parathyroid hormone (PTH)
      a. Primary regulator of calcium homeostasis
      b. Stimulates osteoclasts to initiate breakdown of bone matrix and increase blood calcium levels
      c. Increases renal absorption of calcium from urine
      d. Stimulates vitamin D synthesis
   2. Calcitonin (CT)
      a. Protein hormone produced in the thyroid gland
      b. Produced in response to high blood calcium levels
      c. Stimulates bone deposition by osteoblasts
      d. Inhibits osteoclast activity
      e. Far less important in homeostasis of blood calcium levels than is parathyroid hormone
   3. Other mechanisms
      a. Growth hormone (GH)—increases bone growth, thus reducing blood calcium
      b. Serotonin—inhibits osteoblast activity, thus increases blood calcium

Development of Bone

A. Osteogenesis—development of bone from small cartilage or membrane model to adult bone (**Figure 11-12**)
B. Intramembranous ossification (**Figure 11-13**)
   1. Occurs within a connective tissue membrane
   2. Flat bones begin when groups of cells differentiate into osteoblasts
   3. Osteoblasts are clustered together in ossification centres
   4. Osteoblasts secrete matrix material and collagenous fibrils
   5. Large amounts of ground substance accumulate around each osteoblast
   6. Collagenous fibres become embedded in the ground substance and constitute the bone matrix
   7. Bone matrix calcifies when calcium salts are deposited
   8. Trabeculae appear and join in a network to form spongy bone
   9. Appositional growth occurs by adding osseous tissue (**Figure 11-14**)
C. Endochondral ossification (**Figure 11-15**)
   1. Most bones begin as a cartilage model with bone formation spreading essentially from the centre to the ends
   2. Periosteum develops and enlarges to produce a collar of bone
   3. Primary ossification centre forms (**Figure 11-16**)
   4. Blood vessel enters the cartilage model at the midpoint of the diaphysis
   5. Bone grows in length as endochondral ossification progresses from the diaphysis toward each epiphysis (**Figure 11-17**)
   6. Secondary ossification centres appear in the epiphysis, and bone growth proceeds toward the diaphysis
   7. Epiphyseal plate remains between the diaphysis and each epiphysis until bone growth in length is complete
   8. Epiphyseal plate is composed of four layers (**Figures 11-18** and **11-19**)
      a. "Resting" cartilage cells—point of attachment joining the epiphysis to the shaft
      b. Zone of proliferation—cartilage cells undergoing active mitosis, which causes the layer to thicken and the plate to increase in length
      c. Zone of hypertrophy—older, enlarged cells undergoing degenerative changes associated with calcium deposition
      d. Zone of calcification—dead or dying cartilage cells undergoing rapid calcification
   9. Epiphyseal plate can be a site for bone fractures in young people (**Figure 11-20**)
   10. Long bones grow in both length and diameter (**Figure 11-21**)

Bone Remodelling

A. Primary osteons develop within early woven bone (**Figure 11-22**)
   1. Conelike or tubelike space is hollowed out by osteoclasts
   2. Osteoblasts in the endosteum that lines the tube begin forming layers (lamellae) that trap osteocytes between layers.
   3. A central canal is left for the blood and lymphatic vessels and nerves
   4. Primary osteons can be replaced later by secondary osteons in a similar manner
B. Bones grow in length and diameter by the combined action of osteoclasts and osteoblasts
   1. Osteoclasts enlarge the diameter of the medullary cavity
   2. Osteoblasts from the periosteum build new bone around the outside of the bone
C. Mechanical stress, as from physical activity, strengthens bone

Repair of Bone Fractures

A. Fracture—break in the continuity of a bone
B. Fracture healing (**Figure 11-23**)
   1. Fracture tears and destroys blood vessels that carry nutrients to osteocytes

2. Vascular damage initiates repair sequence
3. Callus—special repair tissue that binds the broken ends of the fracture together
4. Fracture haematoma—blood clot occurring immediately after the fracture, which is then resorbed and replaced by callus

Cartilage

A. Characteristics
  1. Avascular connective tissue
  2. Fibres of cartilage are embedded in a firm gel
  3. Has the flexibility of firm plastic
  4. No canal system or blood vessels
  5. Chondrocytes receive oxygen and nutrients by diffusion
  6. Perichondrium—fibrous covering of the cartilage
  7. Cartilage types differ because of the amount of matrix present and the amounts of elastic and collagenous fibres

B. Types of cartilage (**Figure 11-24**)
  1. Hyaline cartilage
    a. Most common type
    b. Covers the articular surfaces of bones
    c. Forms the costal cartilages, cartilage rings in the trachea, bronchi of the lungs, and the tip of the nose
    d. Forms from special cells in chondrification centres, which secrete matrix material
    e. Chondrocytes are isolated into lacunae
  2. Elastic cartilage
    a. Forms external ear, epiglottis, and eustachian tubes
    b. Large number of elastic fibres confers elasticity and resiliency
  3. Fibrocartilage (fibrous cartilage)
    a. Occurs in pubic symphysis and intervertebral discs
    b. Small quantities of matrix and abundant fibrous elements
    c. Strong and rigid

C. Function of cartilage
  1. Tough, rubberlike nature permits cartilage to sustain great weight or serve as a shock absorber
  2. Strong yet pliable support structure
  3. Permits growth in length of long bones

D. Growth of cartilage
  1. Interstitial or endogenous growth
    a. Cartilage cells divide and secrete additional matrix
    b. Seen during childhood and early adolescence while cartilage is still soft and capable of expansion from within
  2. Appositional or exogenous growth
    a. Chondrocytes in the deep layer of the perichondrium divide and secrete matrix
    b. New matrix is deposited on the surface, thereby increasing its size
    c. Unusual in early childhood, but once initiated, continues throughout life

Cycle of Life: Skeletal Tissues

A. Skeleton fully ossified by mid-20s
  1. Soft tissue may continue to grow—ossifies more slowly

B. Adults—changes occur from specific conditions
  1. Increased density and strength from exercise
  2. Decreased density and strength from pregnancy, nutritional deficiencies, and illness

C. Advanced adulthood—apparent degeneration
  1. Hard bone matrix replaced by softer connective tissue
  2. Exercise can counteract degeneration

REVIEW QUESTIONS

Write out the answers to these questions after reading the chapter and reviewing the Chapter Summary. Note—writing out your answers will consolidate learning and provide a valuable resource of information.

1. Describe the microscopic structure of bone and cartilage. What similarities do they possess?
2. Describe the structure of a long bone.
3. Explain the functions of the periosteum.
4. Describe the two principal chemical components of extracellular bone.
5. List and discuss each of the major anatomical components that together constitute an osteon.
6. Compare and contrast the three major types of cells found in bone.
7. Discuss and discriminate between the sequence of steps characteristic of fracture healing.
8. Compare and contrast the basic structural elements of bone and cartilage.
9. Compare the structure and function of the three types of cartilage.
10. What type of bone growth is responsible for an increase in the diameter of bones?

CRITICAL THINKING QUESTIONS

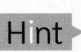

After finishing the Review Questions, write out the answers to these more in-depth questions to help you apply your new knowledge. Go back to sections of the chapter that relate to concepts that you find difficult.

1. Cancer treatment may precipitate the need for a bone marrow transplant. Osteoporosis is a condition characterized by an excessive loss of calcium in bone. These two conditions are disruptions or failures of two bone functions. Identify these two functions and explain what their normal functioning should be.
2. Compare and contrast bone formation in intramembranous and endochondral ossification.
3. Make a distinction between the growth processes of cartilage and bone? Explain.
4. Explain why a bone fracture along the epiphyseal plate may have serious implications in children and young adults.
5. During the ageing process, adults face the issue of a changing skeletal framework. Describe these changes and explain how these skeletal framework changes affect the health of older adults.

12 Axial Skeleton

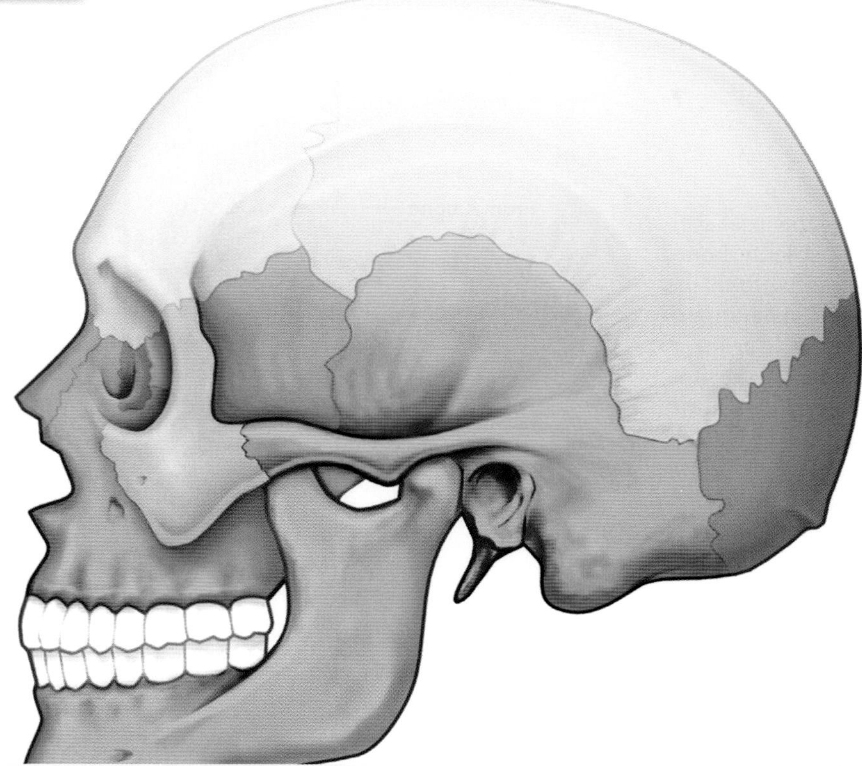

CHAPTER OUTLINE

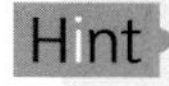 *Scan this outline before you begin to read the chapter, as a preview of how the concepts are organized.*

Just as skeletal tissues are organized to form bones, the bones are organized or grouped to form the skeletal system. The rigid bones lie buried within soft tissues, providing support and shape to the body. Understanding the relationship of bones to one another and to other body structures provides a basis for understanding the function of many other organ systems. Coordinated movement, for example, is possible only because of the way bones are joined in joints and the way muscles are attached to those bones.

The adult skeleton is composed of 206 named bones. Variations in the total number of bones in the body occur as a result of certain anomalies, such as extra ribs, or from failure of certain small bones to fuse in the course of development.

LANGUAGE OF SCIENCE

Hint *Use this list to aid your pronunciation of unfamiliar words.*

appendicular skeleton
(ah-pen-DIK-yoo-lar SKEL-eh-ton)
[*append-* **hang upon,** *-ic-* **relating to,** *-ul-* **little,** *-ar* **relating to**]

axial skeleton
(AK-see-all SKEL-eh-ton)
[*axi-* **axis,** *-al* **relating to**]

cervical vertebra
(SER-vi-kal VER-teh-bra)
[*cervi-* **neck,** *-al* **relating to,** *vertebra* **that which turns**] *pl.,* vertebrae

cranium (KRAY-nee-um)
[*cranium* **skull**]

cribriform plate (KRIB-ri-form)
[*cribri-* **sieve,** *-form* **shape**]

ethmoid (ETH-moyd)
[*ethmo-* **sieve,** *-oid* **like**]

fontanelle (FON-tah-nel)
[*fontan-* **fountain,** *-elle* **little**]

frontal bone (FRON-tal)
[*front-* **forehead,** *-al* **relating to**]

inferior nasal concha
(in-FEER-ee-or NAY-zal KONG-kah)
[*infer-* **lower,** *-or* **quality,** *nas-* **nose,** *-al* **relating to,** *concha* **sea shell**]
pl., conchae

lacrimal bone (LAK-ri-mal)
[*lacrima-* **tear,** *-al* **relating to**]

lumbar vertebra
(LUM-bar VER-teh-bra)
[*lumb-* **loin,** *-ar* **relating to,** *vertebra* **that which turns**] *pl.,* vertebrae

mandible (MAN-di-bal)
[*mandi-* **chew,** *-ble* **capable**]

maxilla (mak-SIH-lah)
[*maxilla* **upper jaw**] *pl.,* maxillae

nasal bone (NAY-zal)
[*nas-* **nose,** *-al* **relating to**]

occipital bone (awk-SIP-it-al)
[*occipit-* **back of head,** *-al* **relating to**]

palatine bone (PAL-ah-tyne)
[*palat-* **palate (roof of mouth),** *-ine* **relating to**]

parietal bone (pah-RYE-i-tal)
[*parie-* **wall,** *-al* **relating to**]

sinus (SYE-nus)
[*sinus* **hollow**]

sphenoid bone (SFEE-noyd)
[*spheno-* **wedge,** *-oid* **like**]

continued on p. 261

In Chapter 11 the basic types of skeletal tissue, including bone and cartilage, provide the background for study in this chapter of individual bones and their interrelationships in the skeleton. We begin here with a survey of the bones of the central or axial skeleton, then continue in Chapter 13 with a survey of the bones of the peripheral or appendicular skeleton. Chapter 14 then explores articulations—that is, how the bones form joints.

UNIT 2

DIVISIONS OF THE SKELETON

The human skeleton consists of two main divisions—the axial skeleton and the appendicular skeleton (**Figure 12-1**). Eighty bones make up the **axial skeleton.** This includes 74 bones that form the upright axis of the body and 6 tiny middle ear bones. The **appendicular skeleton** consists of 126 bones—more than half again as many as in the axial skeleton. Bones of the appendicular skeleton form the appendages to the axial skeleton: the shoulder girdles, arms, forearms, wrists, and hands and the hip girdles, thighs, legs, ankles, and feet.

One of the first things you should do in studying the skeleton is to familiarize yourself with the names of the individual bones listed in **Table 12-1**. Next, look at **Table 12-2**, which lists some terms often used to name or describe bone markings—specific features on an individual bone. After this preparation, begin a step-by-step exploration of the skeletal system by studying the illustrations, text, and tables that constitute the rest of this chapter. To help you learn to distinguish between the names of bones and the names of their markings, the bone names are highlighted in a boldface font and the markings are shown in a normal font in illustrations and tables throughout this chapter.

Many of the names of bones and markings follow Latin rules of pluralization, not the usual English rules. For example, the plural form of *vertebra* is *vertebrae*—not *vertebras*, as it would be in ordinary English. Review examples of Latin pluralization in the QUICK GUIDE TO THE LANGUAGE OF SCIENCE AND MEDICINE.

A picture is worth a thousand words. The illustrations and tables contained in this chapter were carefully selected and compiled to assist you in visualizing and organizing the material discussed. Part 2 of the BRIEF ATLAS OF THE HUMAN BODY has a large collection of labelled photographs of the bones and markings of the skeleton. If in addition to your textbook and brief atlas, you have access to individual bones or an articulated skeleton in a laboratory setting, frequent reference to these illustrations and tabular material will prove immensely helpful in your study efforts.

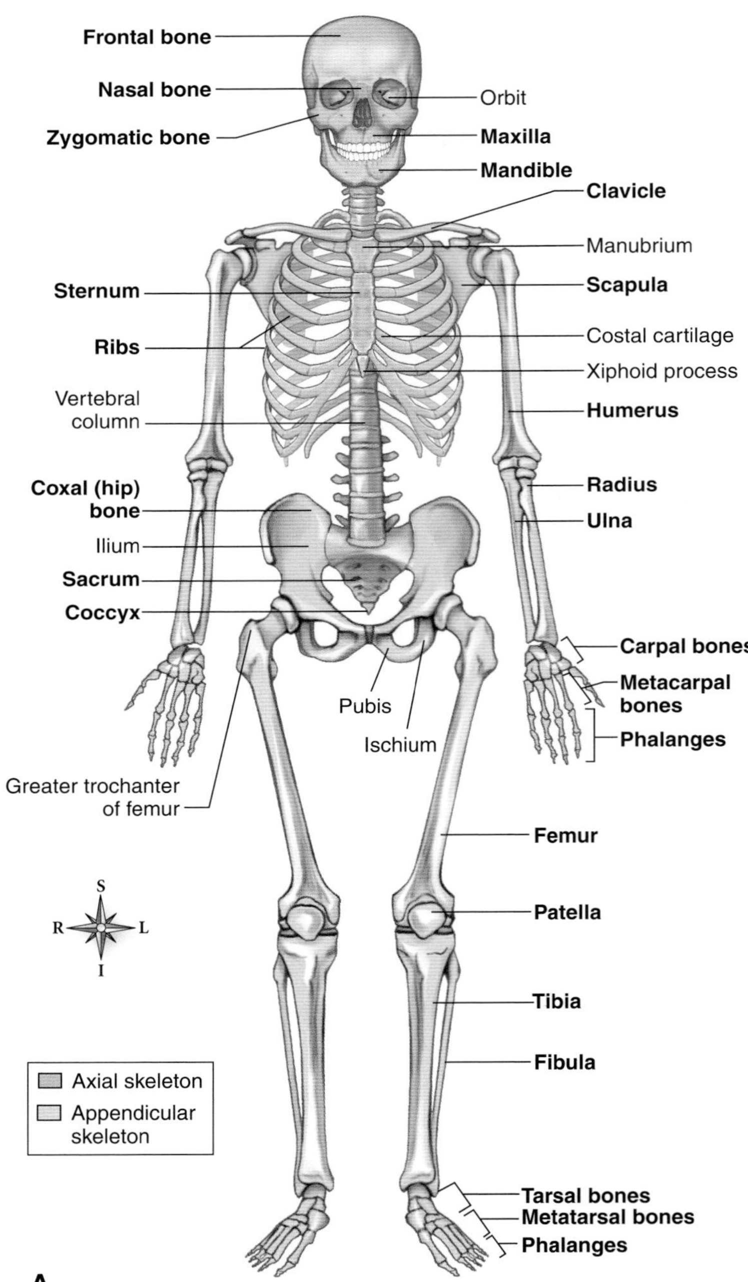

FIGURE 12-1 Skeleton. A, Anterior view. **B,** Posterior view. **C,** Lateral view.

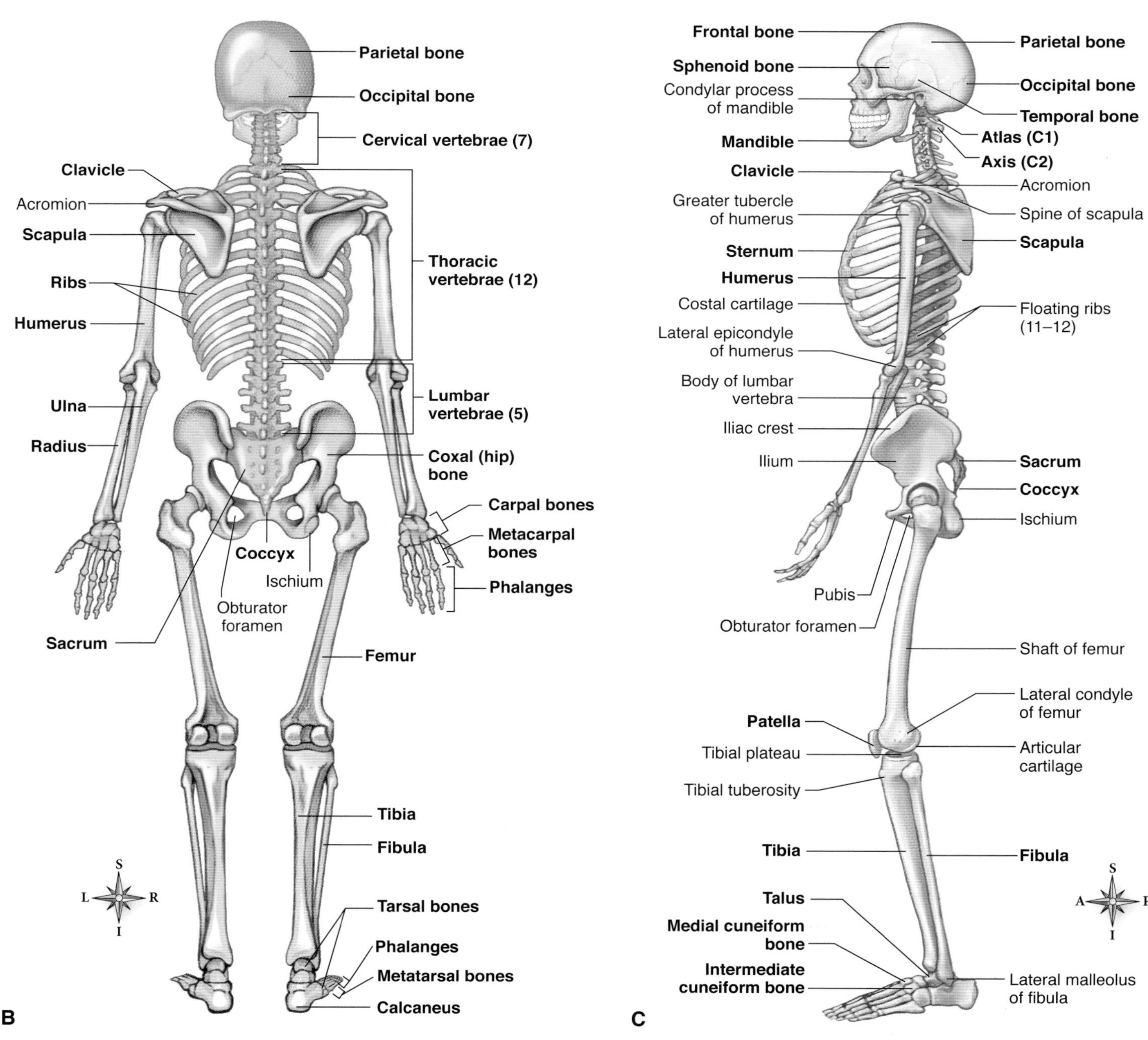
Parietal bone
Occipital bone
Cervical vertebrae (7)
Clavicle
Acromion
Scapula
Ribs
Humerus
Thoracic vertebrae (12)
Ulna
Radius
Lumbar vertebrae (5)
Coxal (hip) bone
Carpal bones
Metacarpal bones
Phalanges
Coccyx
Ischium
Obturator foramen
Sacrum
Femur
Tibia
Fibula
Tarsal bones
Phalanges
Metatarsal bones
Calcaneus
S
L
R
I
B
Frontal bone
Sphenoid bone
Condylar process of mandible
Mandible
Clavicle
Greater tubercle of humerus
Sternum
Humerus
Costal cartilage
Lateral epicondyle of humerus
Body of lumbar vertebra
Iliac crest
Ilium
Pubis
Obturator foramen
Patella
Tibial plateau
Tibial tuberosity
Tibia
Talus
Medial cuneiform bone
Intermediate cuneiform bone
Parietal bone
Occipital bone
Temporal bone
Atlas (C1)
Axis (C2)
Acromion
Spine of scapula
Scapula
Floating ribs (11–12)
Sacrum
Coccyx
Ischium
Shaft of femur
Lateral condyle of femur
Articular cartilage
Fibula
S
A
P
I
Lateral malleolus of fibula
C

TABLE 12-1 Bones of the Skeleton (206 Total)*

PART OF BODY	NAME OF BONE
Axial Skeleton (80 Bones Total)	
Skull (28 bones total)	
Cranium (8 bones)	Frontal (1) Parietal (2) Temporal (2) Occipital (1) Sphenoid (1) Ethmoid (1)
Face (14 bones)	Nasal (2) Maxillary (2) Zygomatic (malar) (2) Mandible (1) Lacrimal (2) Palatine (2) Inferior nasal conchae (turbinates) (2) Vomer (1)
Ear bones (6 bones)	Malleus (hammer) (2) Incus (anvil) (2) Stapes (stirrup) (2)
Hyoid bone (1)	
Vertebral column (26 bones)	Cervical vertebrae (7) Thoracic vertebrae (12) Lumbar vertebrae (5) Sacrum (1) Coccyx (1)
Sternum and ribs (25 bones)	Sternum (1) True ribs (14) False ribs (10)
Appendicular Skeleton (126 Bones Total)	
Upper extremities (including shoulder girdle) (64 bones)	Clavicle (2) Scapula (2) Humerus (2) Radius (2) Ulna (2) Carpal bones (16) Metacarpal bones (10) Phalanges (28)
Lower extremities (including hip girdle) (62 bones)	Innominate (2) Fibula (2) Femur (2) Patella (2) Tibia (2) Tarsal bones (14) Metatarsal bones (10) Phalanges (28)

*An inconstant number of small, flat, round bones known as *sesamoid bones* (because of their resemblance to sesame seeds) are found in various tendons in which considerable pressure develops. Because the number of these bones varies greatly between individuals, only two of them, the patellae, have been counted among the 206 bones of the body. Generally, two of them can be found in each thumb (in the flexor tendon near the metacarpophalangeal and interphalangeal joints) and great toe, plus several others in the upper and lower extremities. *Sutural bones (wormian bones),* the small islets of bone commonly found in some of the cranial sutures, have not been counted in this list of 206 bones because of their variable occurrence. The numeral after each bone name is the typical number of bones found in the adult skeleton.

TABLE 12-2 Terms Used to Describe Bone Markings

TERM	MEANING
Angle	A corner
Body	The main portion of a bone
Border	Edge of a bone
Condyle	Rounded bump; usually fits into a fossa on another bone to form a joint
Crest	Moderately raised ridge; generally a site for muscle attachment
Epicondyle	Bump near a condyle; often gives the appearance of a "bump on a bump"; for muscle attachment
Facet	Flat surface that forms a joint with another facet or flat bone
Fissure	Long, cracklike hole for blood vessels and nerves
Foramen	Round hole for vessels and nerves (*pl.,* foramina)
Fossa	Depression; often receives an articulating bone (*pl.,* fossae)
Head	Distinct epiphysis on a long bone, separated from the shaft by a narrowed portion (or neck)
Line	Similar to a crest but not raised as much (is often rather faint)
Margin	Edge of a flat bone or flat portion of the edge of a flat area
Meatus	Tubelike opening or channel (*pl.,* meatus or meatuses)
Neck	A narrowed portion, usually at the base of a head
Notch	A V-like depression in the margin or edge of a flat area
Process	A raised area or projection
Ramus	Curved portion of a bone, like a ram's horn (*pl.,* rami)
Sinus	Cavity within a bone
Spine	Similar to a crest but raised more; a sharp, pointed process; for muscle attachment
Sulcus	Groove or elongated depression (*pl.,* sulci)
Trochanter	Large bump for muscle attachment (larger than a tubercle or tuberosity)
Tuberosity	Oblong, raised bump, usually for muscle attachment; also called a *tuber*; a small tuberosity is called a *tubercle*

SKULL

Twenty-eight irregularly shaped bones form the skull (**Figure 12-2** to **Figure 12-8**). **Figures 12-2** through **12-7** show the articulated bones of the skull in full or sectioned views.

Figure 12-8 is a multipart series highlighting the individual bones and shows their relationship to the skull as a whole. As you study the skull, refer often to the illustrations and the descriptive information contained in **Table 12-3** to **Table 12-5**.

The skull consists of two major divisions: the **cranium,** or brain case, and the **face.** The cranium is formed by eight bones, namely, the frontal, two parietal, two temporal, the occipital, the sphenoid,

(continued on page 242)

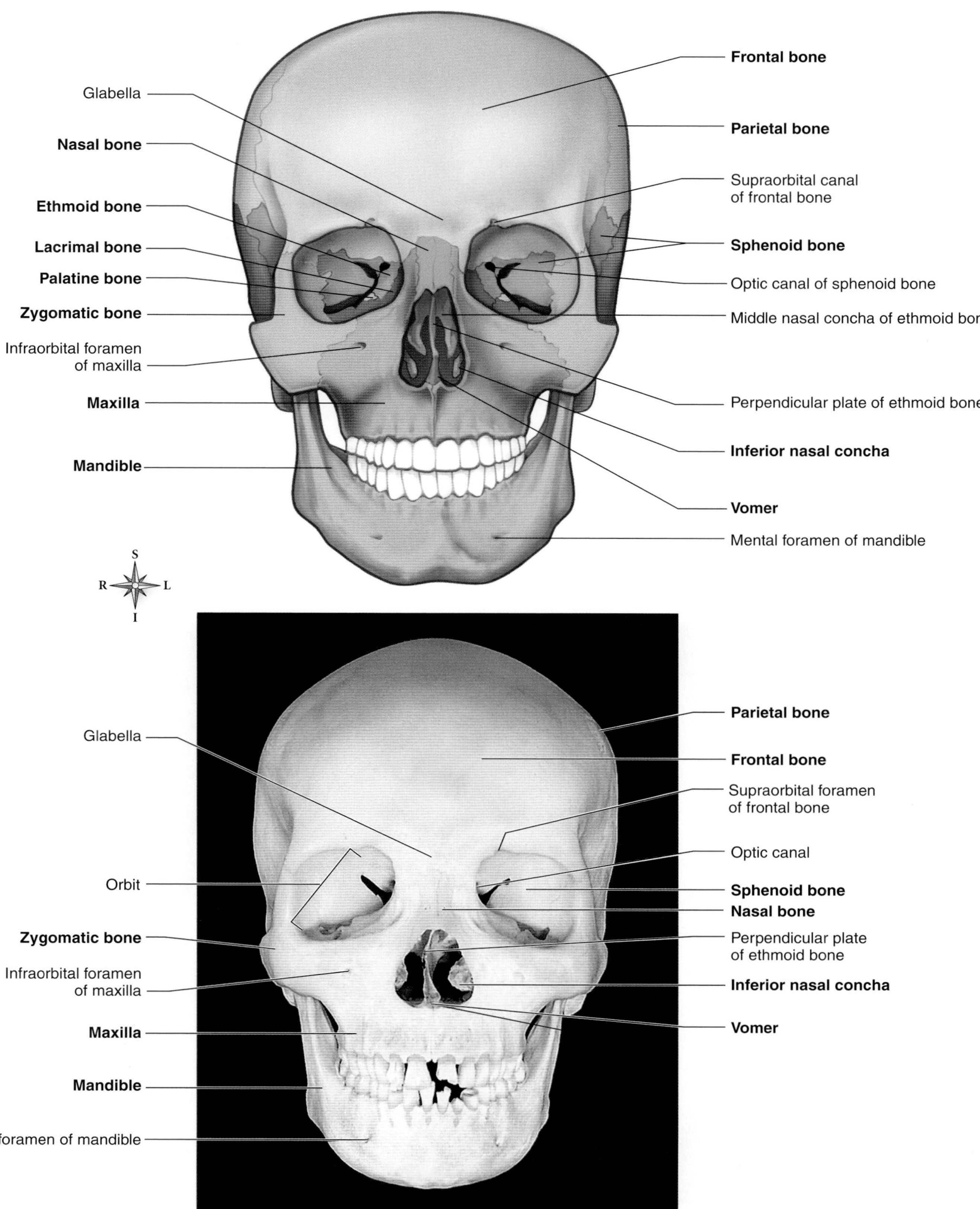

FIGURE 12-2 **Anterior view of the skull.**

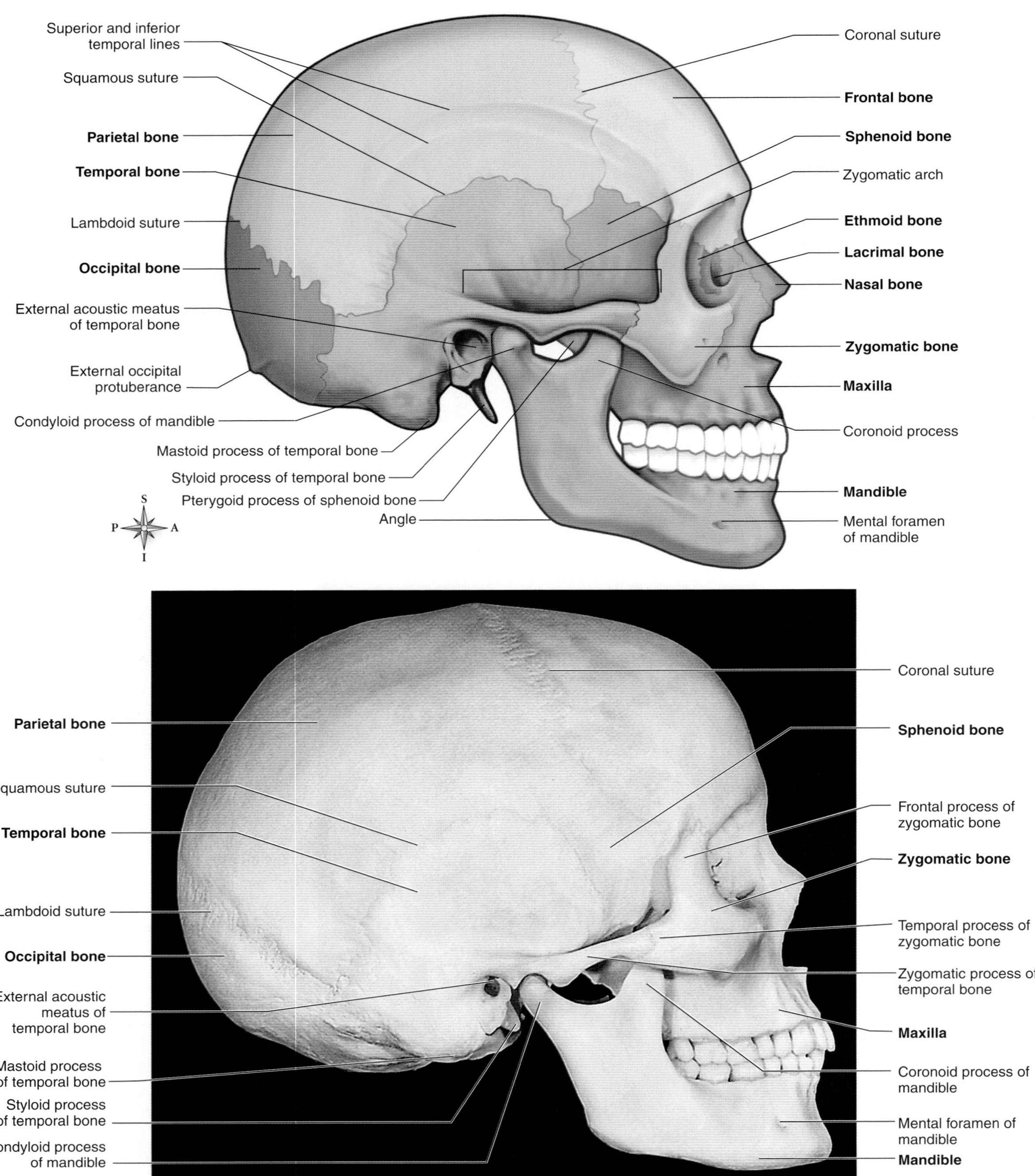

FIGURE 12-3 **Skull viewed from the right side.**

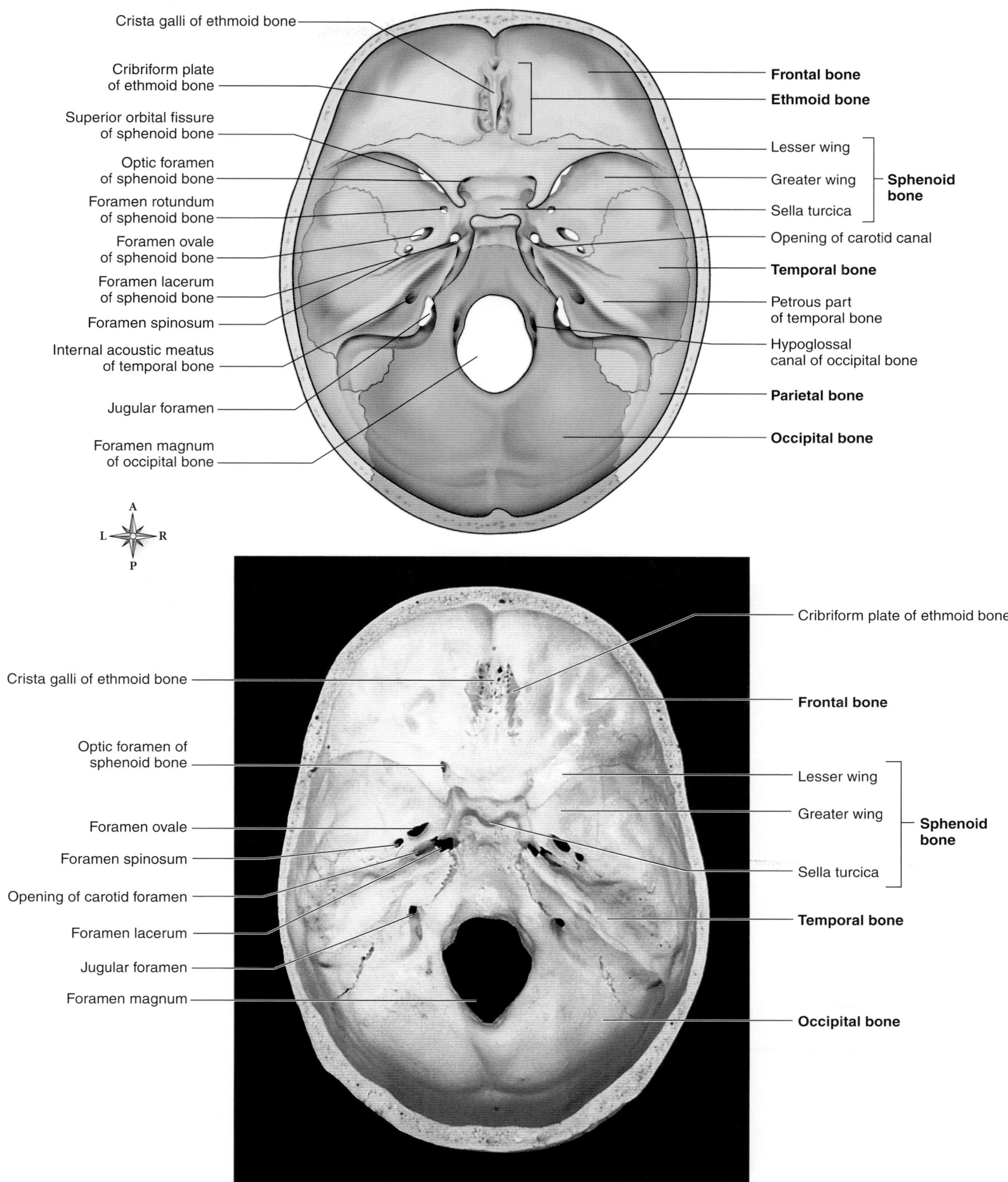
Crista galli of ethmoid bone
Cribriform plate of ethmoid bone
Superior orbital fissure of sphenoid bone
Optic foramen of sphenoid bone
Foramen rotundum of sphenoid bone
Foramen ovale of sphenoid bone
Foramen lacerum of sphenoid bone
Foramen spinosum
Internal acoustic meatus of temporal bone
Jugular foramen
Foramen magnum of occipital bone
Frontal bone
Ethmoid bone
Lesser wing
Greater wing
Sella turcica
Sphenoid bone
Opening of carotid canal
Temporal bone
Petrous part of temporal bone
Hypoglossal canal of occipital bone
Parietal bone
Occipital bone
A
L
R
P
Cribriform plate of ethmoid bone
Crista galli of ethmoid bone
Frontal bone
Optic foramen of sphenoid bone
Lesser wing
Greater wing
Sphenoid bone
Foramen ovale
Foramen spinosum
Sella turcica
Opening of carotid foramen
Foramen lacerum
Temporal bone
Jugular foramen
Foramen magnum
Occipital bone

FIGURE 12-4 Floor of the cranial cavity viewed from above.

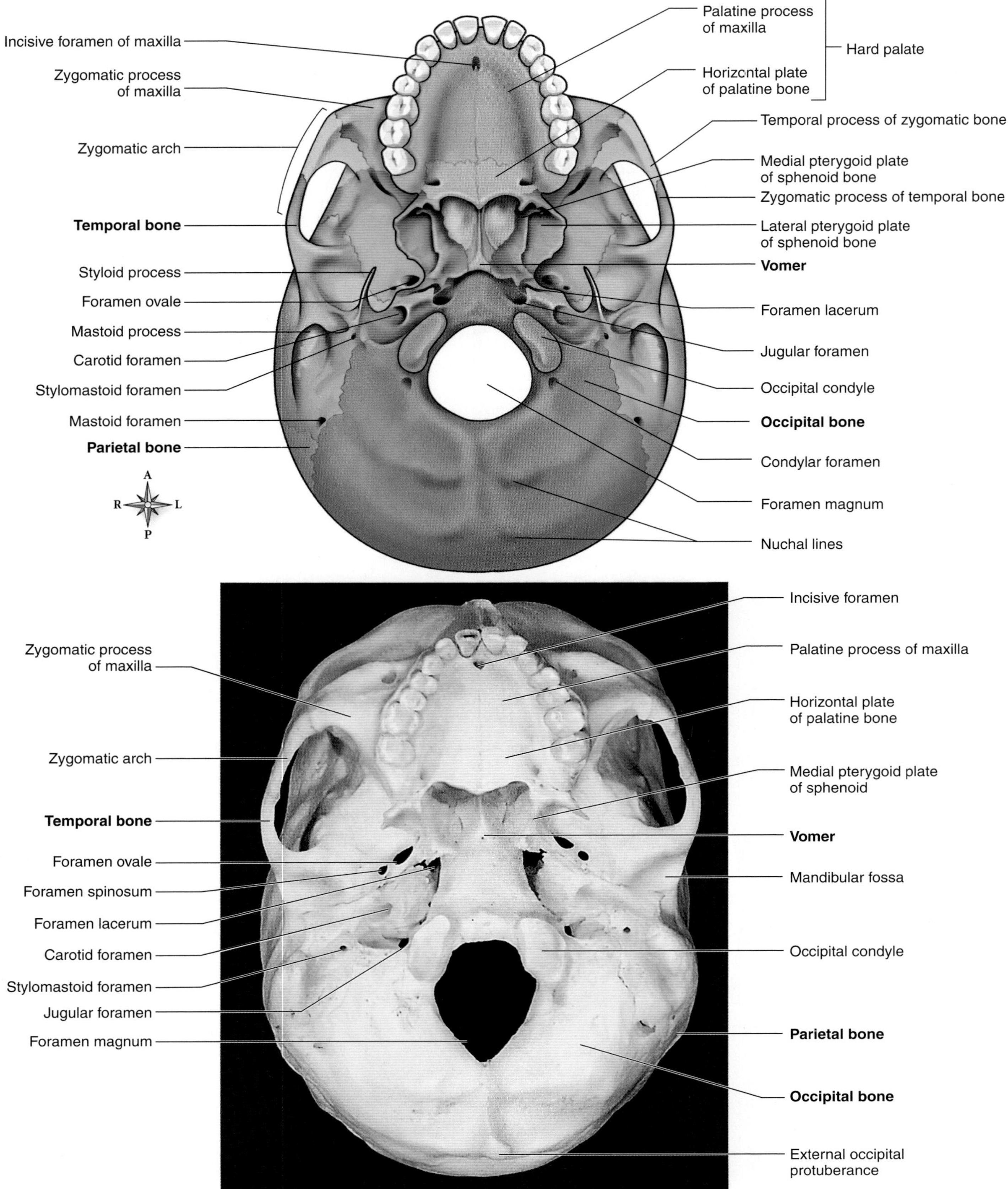
Incisive foramen of maxilla
Zygomatic process of maxilla
Zygomatic arch
Temporal bone
Styloid process
Foramen ovale
Mastoid process
Carotid foramen
Stylomastoid foramen
Mastoid foramen
Parietal bone
A
R
L
P
Palatine process of maxilla
Horizontal plate of palatine bone
Hard palate
Temporal process of zygomatic bone
Medial pterygoid plate of sphenoid bone
Zygomatic process of temporal bone
Lateral pterygoid plate of sphenoid bone
Vomer
Foramen lacerum
Jugular foramen
Occipital condyle
Occipital bone
Condylar foramen
Foramen magnum
Nuchal lines
Zygomatic process of maxilla
Zygomatic arch
Temporal bone
Foramen ovale
Foramen spinosum
Foramen lacerum
Carotid foramen
Stylomastoid foramen
Jugular foramen
Foramen magnum
Incisive foramen
Palatine process of maxilla
Horizontal plate of palatine bone
Medial pterygoid plate of sphenoid
Vomer
Mandibular fossa
Occipital condyle
Parietal bone
Occipital bone
External occipital protuberance

FIGURE 12-5 **Skull viewed from below.**

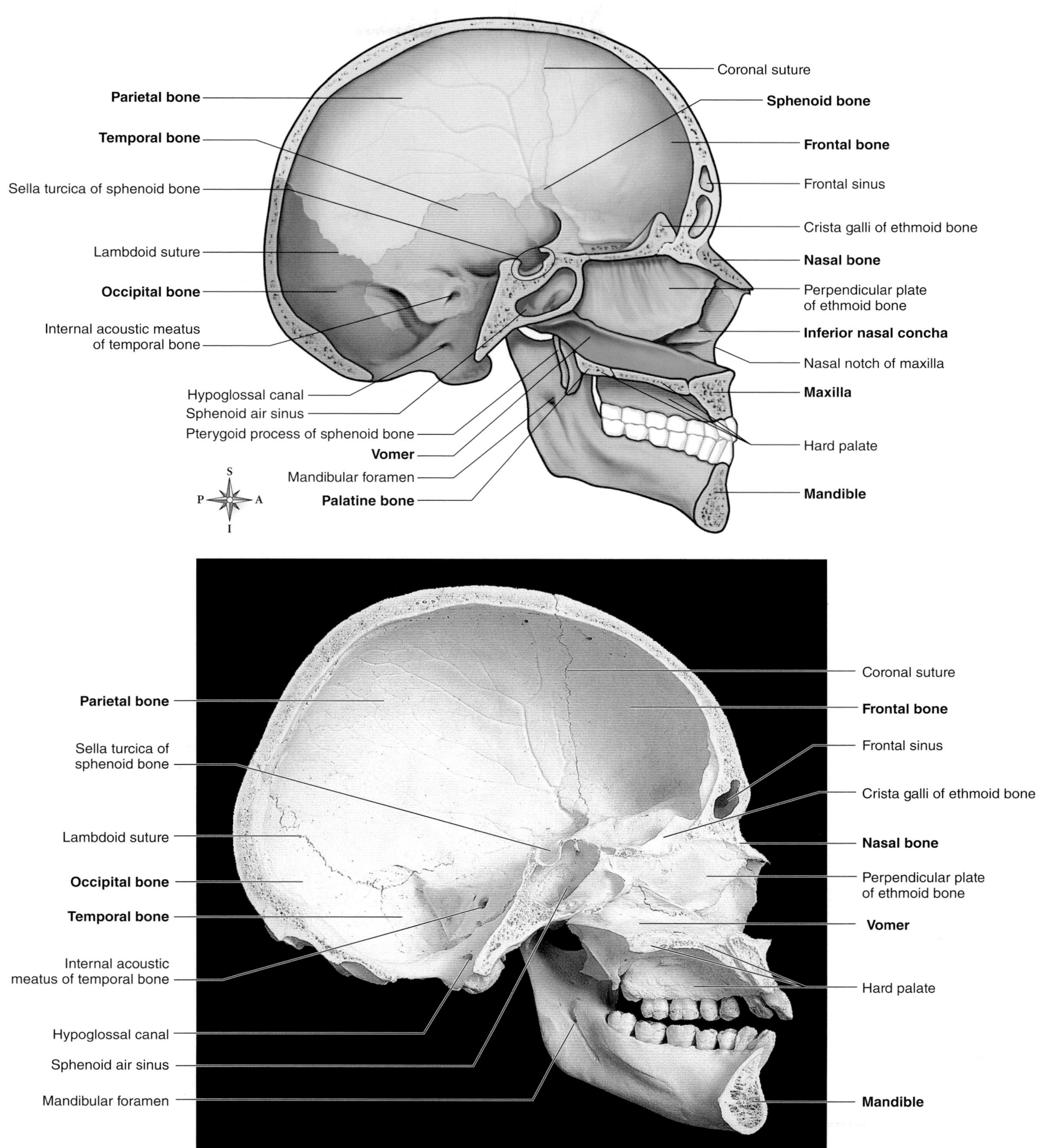

FIGURE 12-6 **Left half of the skull viewed from within.**

and the ethmoid (see **Table 12-3**). The 14 bones that form the face are the two maxillae, two zygomatic (malar), two nasal, the mandible, two lacrimal, two palatine, two inferior nasal conchae (turbinates), and the vomer (see **Table 12-4**). Note that all the facial bones are paired except for the mandible and vomer. All the cranial bones, on the other hand, are single (unpaired) except for the parietal and temporal bones, which are paired. The frontal and ethmoid bones of the skull help shape the face but are not numbered among the facial bones.

(continued on page 248)

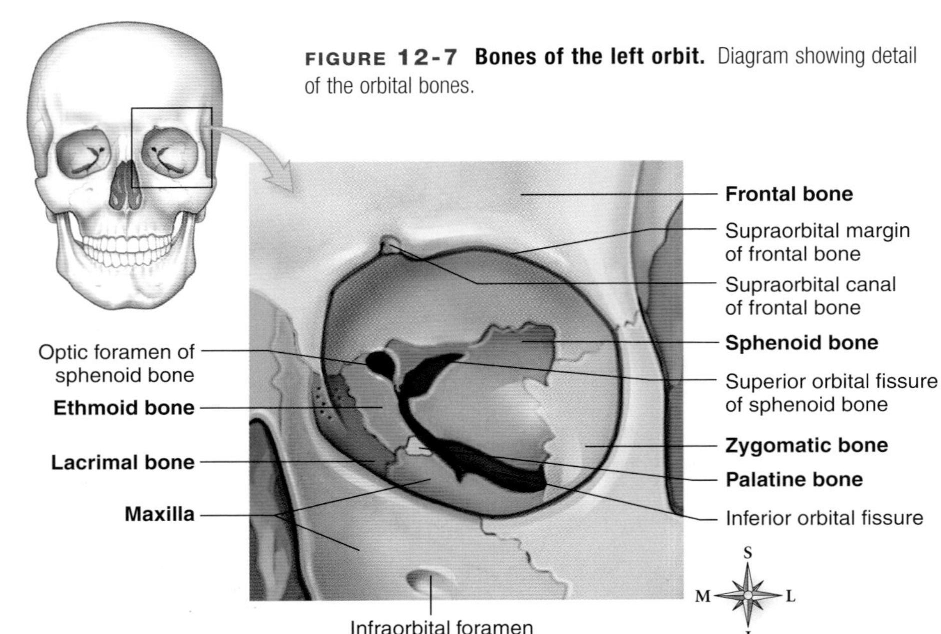

FIGURE 12-7 Bones of the left orbit. Diagram showing detail of the orbital bones.

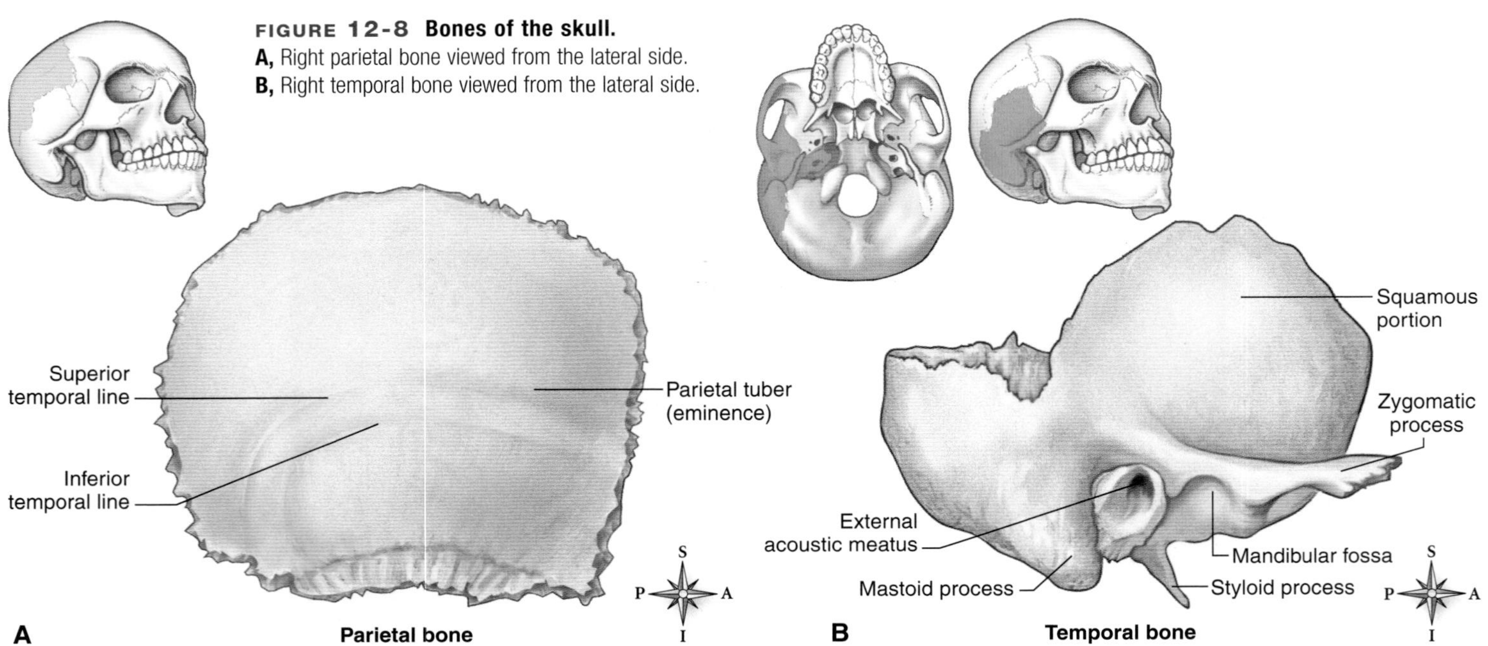

FIGURE 12-8 Bones of the skull. **A,** Right parietal bone viewed from the lateral side. **B,** Right temporal bone viewed from the lateral side.

TABLE 12-3 Cranial Bones and Their Markings

BONES AND MARKINGS	DESCRIPTION
Parietal	Prominent, bulging bones behind the frontal bone; form the top sides of the cranial cavity
Superior temporal line	Superior of two very faint curving lines across parietal and frontal bones
Inferior temporal line	Inferior of two very faint curving lines across parietal and frontal bones; sometimes more pronounced than superior line
Temporal	Form the lower sides of the cranium and part of the cranial floor; contain the middle and inner ear structures
Squamous portion	Thin, flaring upper part of the bone
Mastoid portion	Rough-surfaced lower part of the bone posterior to the external acoustic meatus
Petrous portion	Wedge-shaped process that forms part of the centre section of the cranial floor between the sphenoid and occipital bones; name derived from the Greek word for stone because of the extreme hardness of this process; houses the middle and inner ear structures
Mastoid process	Protuberance just behind the ear
Mastoid air cells	Mucosa-lined, air-filled spaces within the mastoid process
External acoustic meatus (or canal)	Tube extending into the temporal bone from the external ear opening to the tympanic membrane

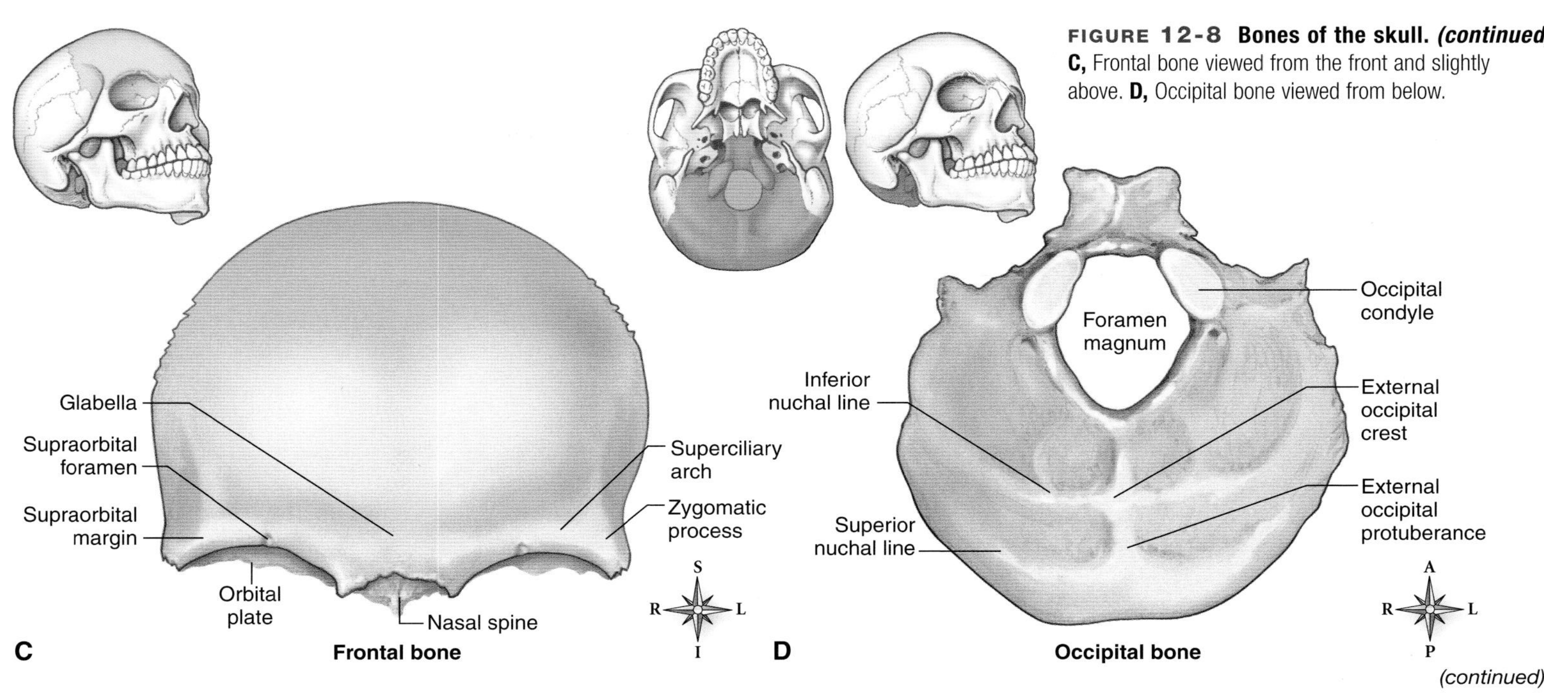

FIGURE 12-8 Bones of the skull. *(continued)* **C,** Frontal bone viewed from the front and slightly above. **D,** Occipital bone viewed from below.

(continued)

TABLE 12-3 Cranial Bones and Their Markings—cont'd

BONES AND MARKINGS	DESCRIPTION
Zygomatic process	Projection that articulates with the zygomatic (or malar) bone
Internal acoustic meatus	Fairly large opening on the posterior surface of the petrous part of the bone; transmits the eighth cranial nerve to the inner ear and the seventh cranial nerve on its way to the facial structures
Mandibular fossa	Oval-shaped depression anterior to the external acoustic meatus; forms the socket for the condyle of the mandible
Styloid process	Slender spike of bone extending downward and forward from the undersurface of the bone anterior to the mastoid process; often broken off in a dry skull; several neck muscles and ligaments attach to the styloid process
Stylomastoid foramen	Opening between the styloid and mastoid processes where the facial nerve emerges from the cranial cavity
Jugular fossa	Depression on the undersurface of the petrous part; dilated beginning of the internal jugular vein lodged here
Jugular foramen	Opening in the suture between the petrous part and occipital bone; transmits the lateral sinus and ninth, tenth, and eleventh cranial nerves
Carotid foramen (or canal)	Channel in the petrous part; best seen from the undersurface of the skull; transmits the internal carotid artery
Frontal	Forehead bone; also forms most of the roof of the orbits (eye sockets) and the anterior part of the cranial floor
Supraorbital margin	Arched ridge just below eyebrow; forms the upper edge of the orbit
Frontal sinuses	Cavities inside the bone just above supraorbital margin; lined with mucosa; contain air
Frontal tuberosities (tubers or eminences)	Bulge above each orbit; most prominent part of forehead
Superciliary arches (ridges)	Curved ridges caused by projection of the frontal sinuses; eyebrows lie superficial to these ridges
Supraorbital foramen (sometimes notch)	Foramen or notch in the supraorbital margin slightly medial to its midpoint; transmits supraorbital nerve and blood vessels
Glabella	Smooth area between the superciliary ridges and above the nose
Occipital	Forms the posterior part of the cranial floor and walls
Foramen magnum	Hole through which the spinal cord enters the cranial cavity
Occipital condyles	Convex, oval processes on either side of the foramen magnum; articulate with depressions on the first cervical vertebra
External occipital protuberance	Prominent projection on the posterior surface in the midline a short distance above the foramen magnum; can be felt as a definite bump
Superior nuchal line	Curved ridge extending laterally from the external occipital protuberance
Inferior nuchal line	Less well defined ridge paralleling the superior nuchal line a short distance below it
Internal occipital protuberance	Projection in the midline on the inner surface of the bone; grooves for the lateral sinuses extend laterally from this process and one for sagittal sinus extends upward from it

(continued)

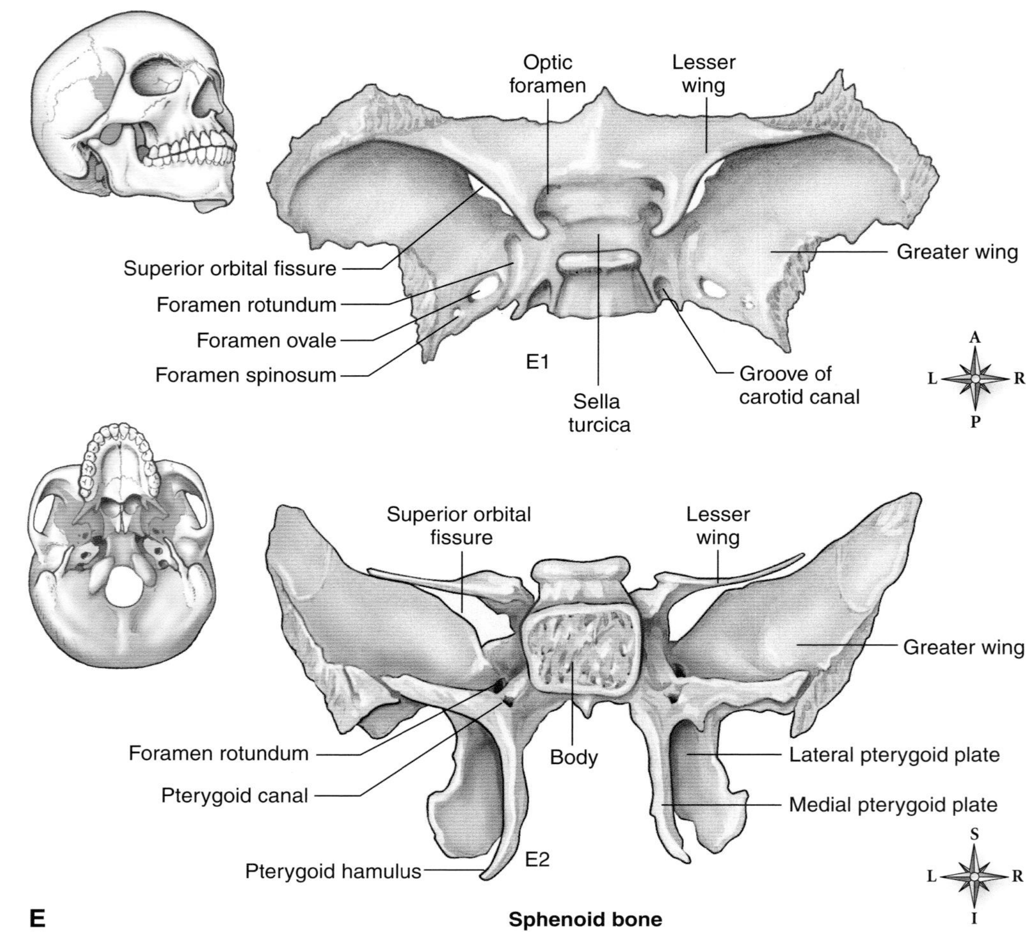

FIGURE 12-8 Bones of the skull. *(continued)* **E,** Sphenoid bone. **E1,** Superior view; **E2,** posterior view.

TABLE 12-3 Cranial Bones and Their Markings—cont'd

BONES AND MARKINGS	DESCRIPTION
Sphenoid	Keystone of the cranial floor; forms its midportion; resembles a bat with wings outstretched and legs extended downward posteriorly; lies behind and slightly above the nose and throat; forms part of the floor and sidewalls of the orbit
Body	Hollow, cubelike central portion
Greater wings	Lateral projections from the body; form part of the outer wall of the orbit
Lesser wings	Thin, triangular projections from the upper part of the sphenoid body; form the posterior part of the roof of the orbit
Sella turcica	Saddle-shaped depression on the upper surface of the sphenoid body; contains the pituitary gland; literally "Turkish chair"
Sphenoid sinuses	Irregular mucosa-lined, air-filled spaces within the central part of the sphenoid
Pterygoid processes	Downward projections on either side where the body and greater wing unite; comparable to the extended legs of a bat if the entire bone is likened to this animal; form part of the lateral nasal wall
Optic foramen	Passage that transmits the optic nerve into the orbit (at the base of the lesser wing); also called *optic canal*
Superior orbital fissure	Slitlike opening into the orbit; lateral to the optic foramen; transmits the third, fourth, and part of the fifth cranial nerves
Inferior orbital fissure	Slitlike opening between the sphenoid and maxilla into the orbit; transmits infraorbital and zygomatic nerves
Foramen rotundum	Opening in the greater wing that transmits the maxillary division of the fifth cranial nerve
Foramen ovale	Opening in the greater wing that transmits the mandibular division of the fifth cranial nerve
Foramen lacerum	Opening at the junction of the sphenoid, temporal, and occipital bones; transmits a branch of the ascending pharyngeal artery
Foramen spinosum	Opening in the greater wing that transmits the middle meningeal artery to supply the meninges

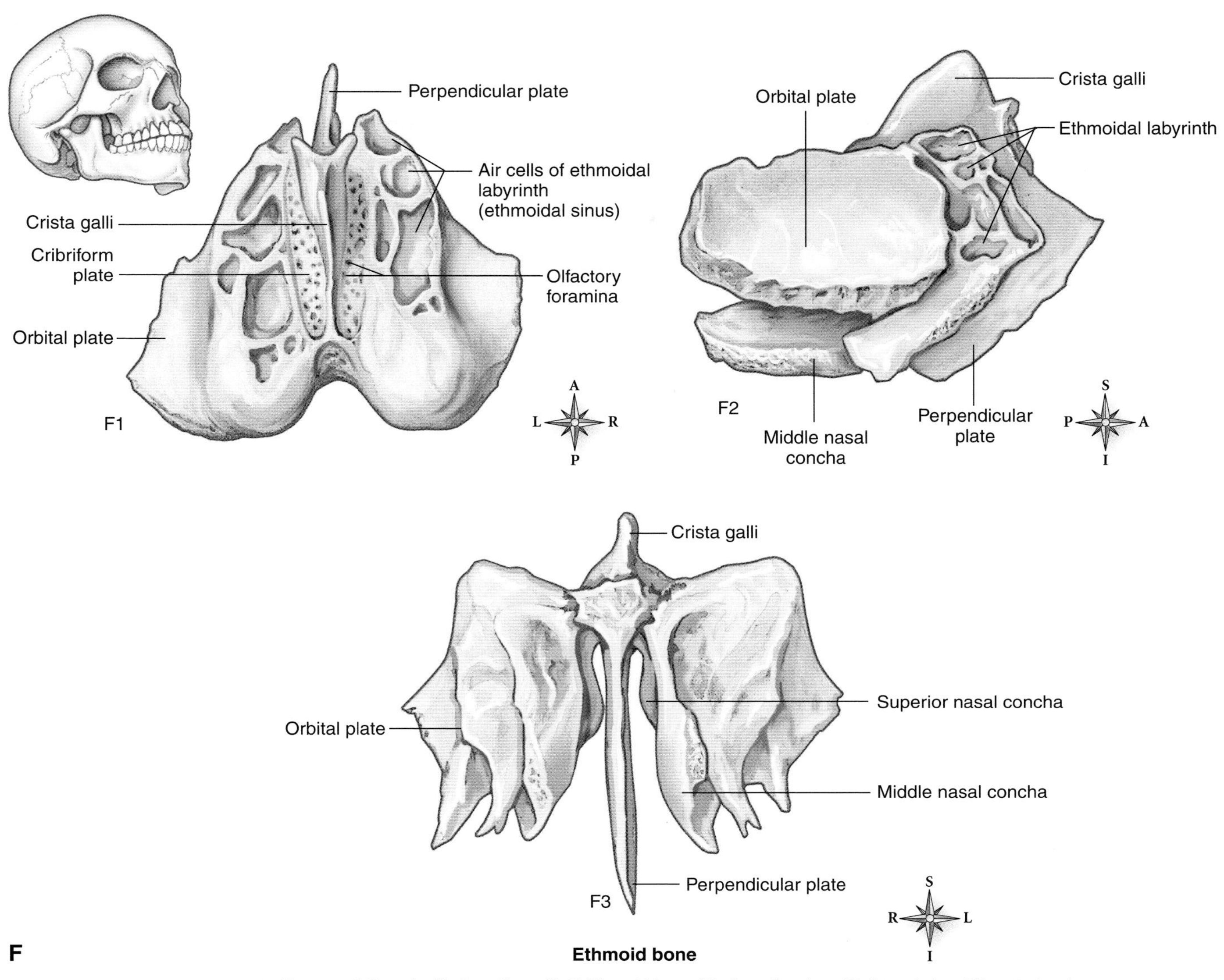

FIGURE 12-8 Bones of the skull. *(continued)* **F,** Ethmoid bone. **F1,** Superior view; **F2,** lateral view; **F3,** anterior view.

(continued)

TABLE 12-3 Cranial Bones and Their Markings—cont'd

BONES AND MARKINGS	DESCRIPTION
Ethmoid	Complex irregular bone that helps make up the anterior portion of the cranial floor, medial wall of the orbits, upper parts of the nasal septum, and sidewalls and part of the nasal roof; lies anterior to the sphenoid and posterior to the nasal bones
Cribriform plate	Olfactory nerves pass through numerous holes in this horizontal plate
Crista galli	Meninges (membranes around the brain) attach to this process
Perpendicular plate	Forms the upper part of the nasal septum
Ethmoid sinuses	Honeycombed, mucosa-lined air spaces within the lateral masses of the bone
Superior and middle nasal conchae (turbinates)	Help form the lateral walls of the nose
Ethmoidal labyrinth	Hollow lateral masses of the ethmoid; contain many air spaces (ethmoid cells or sinuses); the inner surface forms the superior and middle conchae

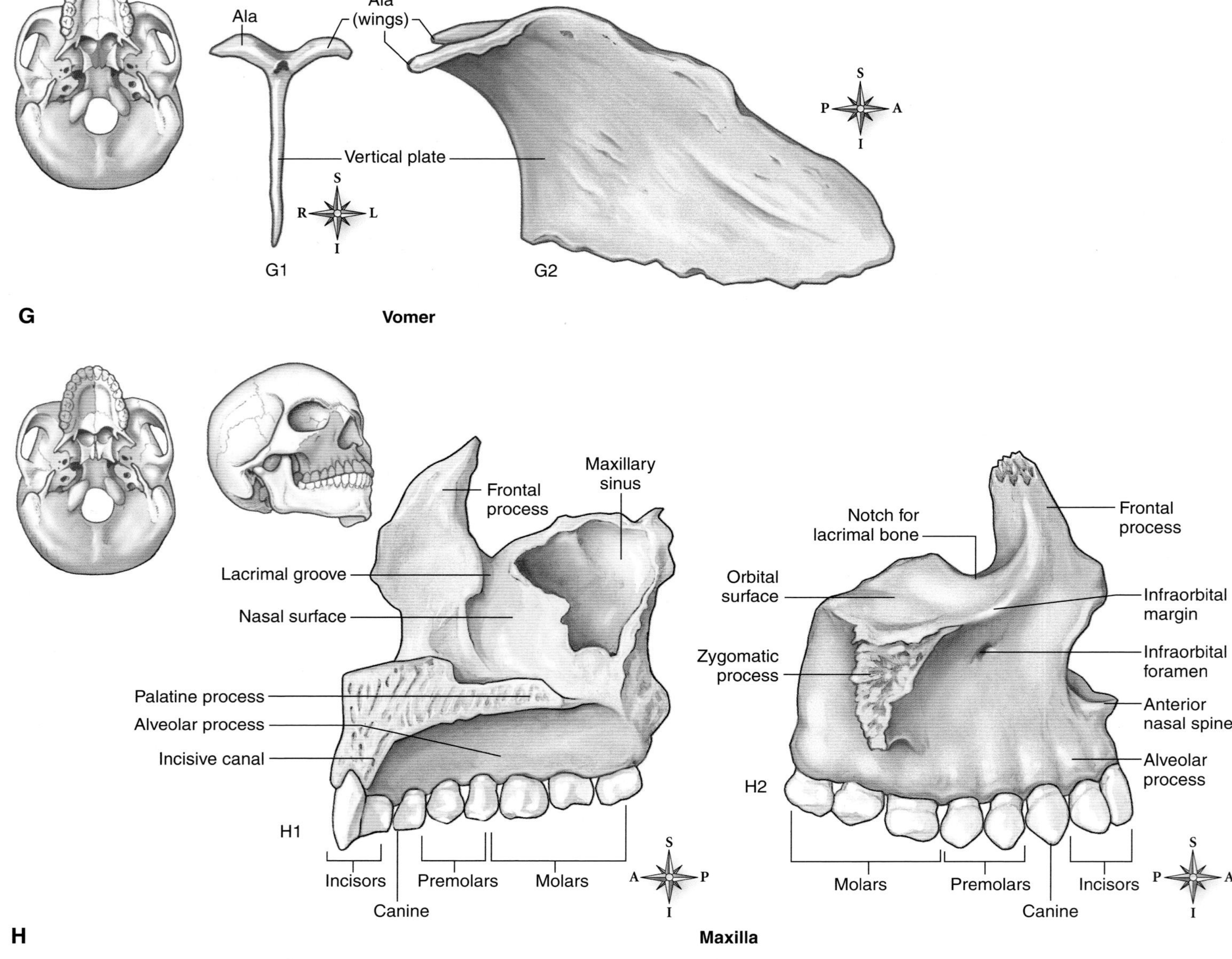

FIGURE 12-8 Bones of the skull. *(continued)* **G,** Vomer. **G1,** Anterior view; **G2,** lateral view. **H,** Right maxilla. **H1,** Medial view; **H2,** lateral view.

TABLE 12-4 Facial Bones and Their Markings

BONES AND MARKINGS	DESCRIPTION
Vomer	Forms inferior and posterior part of nasal septum; shaped like the blade of a plough
Ala	Flared (winglike) process; articulates with sphenoid and palatine bones
Maxilla	Upper jaw bones; form part of the floor of the orbit, anterior part of the roof of the mouth, and floor of the nose and part of the sidewalls of the nasal cavity
Alveolar process	Archlike process that holds the tooth sockets
Maxillary sinus	Large, air-filled cavity within body of maxilla; lined with mucous membrane; largest of paranasal sinuses
Zygomatic process	Extension (corner) that articulates with zygomatic bone
Palatine process	Horizontal plate that projects inward from the alveolar process; forms anterior and larger part of hard palate
Infraorbital margin	Curved ridgelike margin forming the lower edge of the orbit
Infraorbital foramen	Hole on external surface of lower edge of orbit; transmits vessels and nerves: also called *infraorbital canal*
Lacrimal groove	Groove on inner surface; joined by similar groove on lacrimal bone to form bony space for the nasolacrimal duct

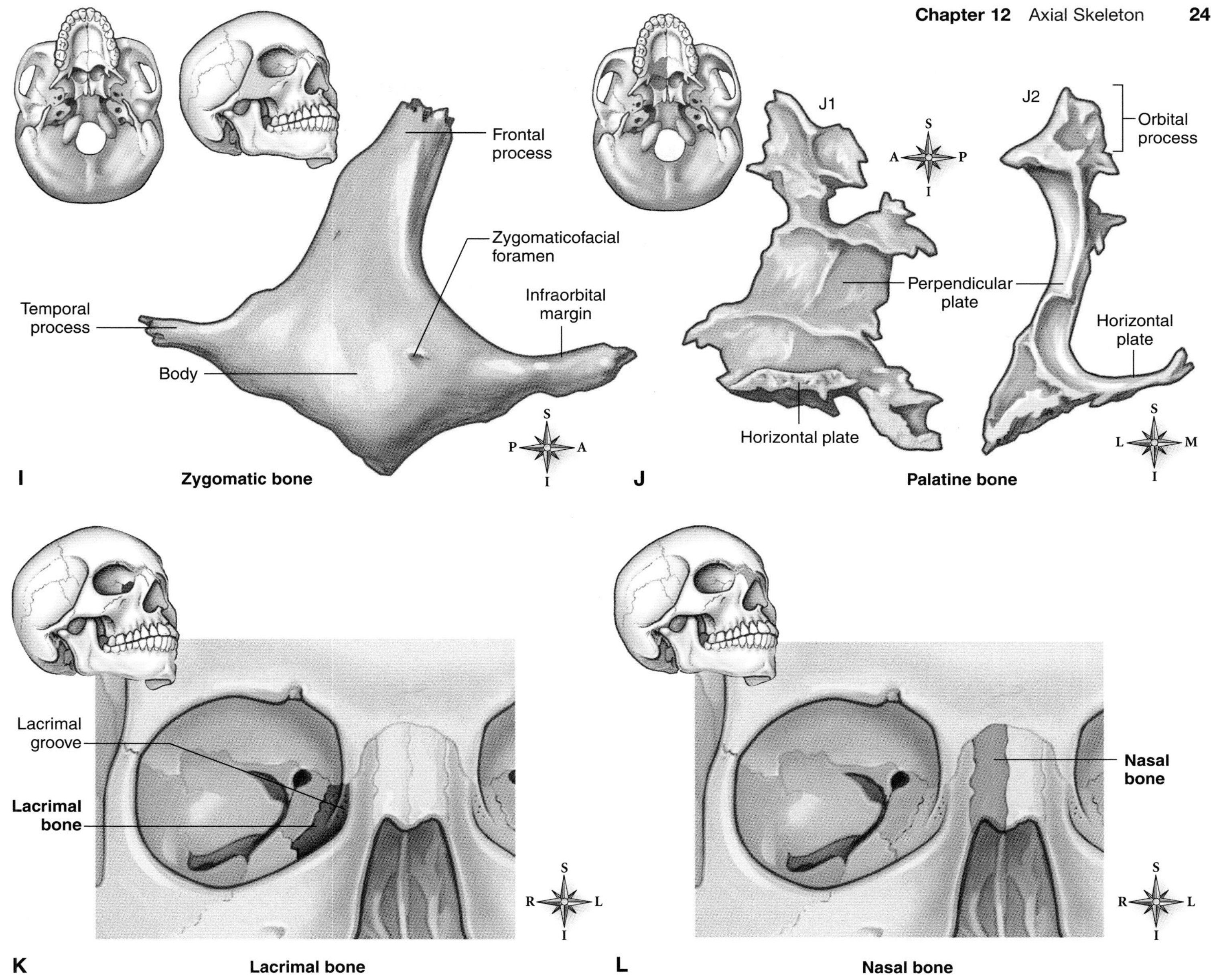

UNIT 2

FIGURE 12-8 Bones of the skull. ***(continued)*** **I,** Right zygomatic bone viewed from the lateral side. **J,** Right palatine bone. **J1,** Medial view; **J2,** anterior view. **K,** Right lacrimal bone viewed from the lateral side. **L,** Right nasal bone viewed from the lateral side. *(continued)*

TABLE 12-4 Facial Bones and Their Markings—cont'd

BONES AND MARKINGS	DESCRIPTION
Zygomatic	Cheekbones; form part of floor and sidewall of eye orbit; also called *malar bone*
Infraorbital margin	Curved, ridgelike margin forming the lower edge of the orbit
Temporal process	Projection that articulates with the temporal bone
Zygomatic arch	Curve formed by union of temporal process (of zygomatic bone) and zygomatic process (of temporal bone)
Palatine	Form the posterior part of the hard palate, floor, and part of the sidewalls of the nasal cavity and floor of orbit
Horizontal plate	Joined to the palatine processes of the maxillae to complete part of the hard palate
Lacrimal	Thin, platelike bones; posterior and lateral to nasal bones in medial wall of eye orbit; help form sidewall of nasal cavity (often missing in dry skull specimen)
Lacrimal groove	Depression for nasolacrimal (tear) duct; has widened, inferior *lacrimal fossa*
Nasal	Pair of small bones that form the upper part of bridge of nose
Inferior nasal conchae (turbinates)	Thin scroll of bone forming shelf along inner surface of sidewall of nasal cavity; lies above roof of mouth

(continued)

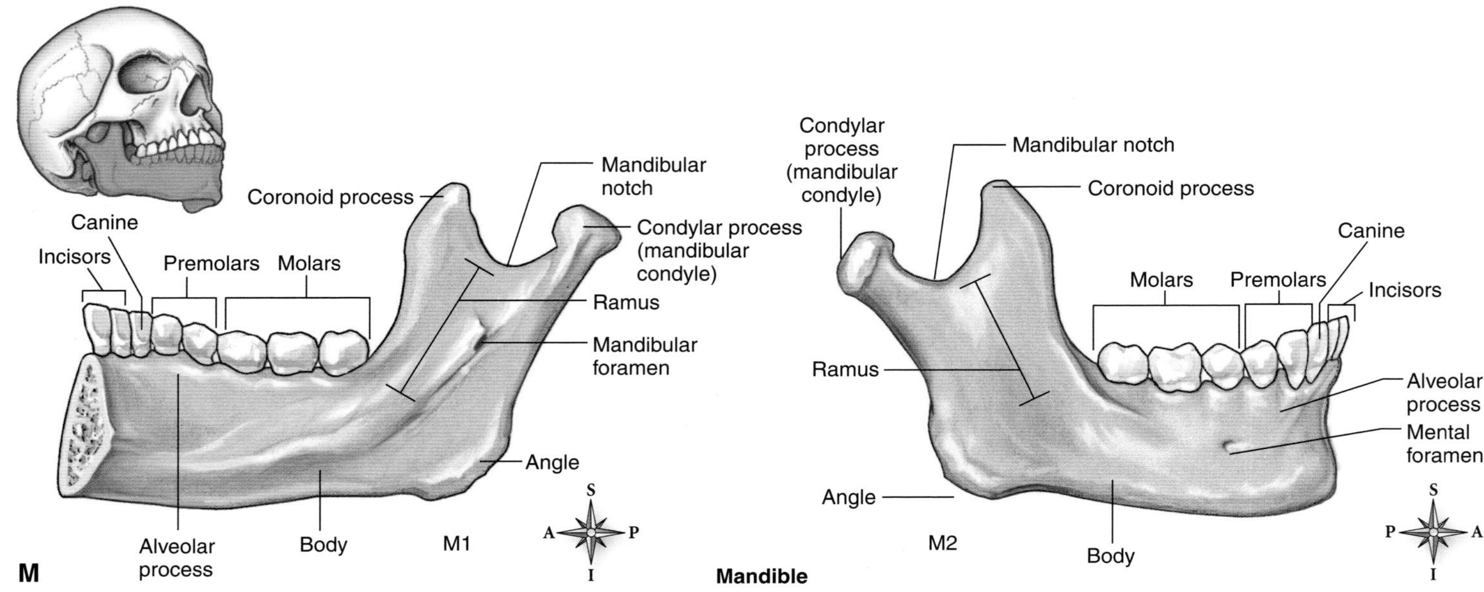

FIGURE 12-8 **Bones of the skull.** ***(continued)*** **M,** Right half of the mandible. **M1,** Medial view; **M2,** lateral view.

TABLE 12-4 Facial Bones and Their Markings—cont'd

BONES AND MARKINGS	DESCRIPTION
Mandible	Lower jawbone; largest, strongest bone of the face
Body	Main part of the bone; forms the chin
Ramus	Process, one on either side, that projects upward from the posterior part of the body
Condylar process	Part of each ramus that articulates with the mandibular fossa of the temporal bone
Neck	Constricted part just below the condyles
Alveolar process	Teeth set into this arch
Mandibular foramen	Opening on the inner surface of the ramus; transmits nerves and vessels to the lower teeth
Mental foramen	Opening on the outer surface below the space between the two bicuspids; transmits the terminal branches of the nerves and vessels that enter the bone through the mandibular foramen; dentists inject anaesthetics through these foramina
Coronoid process	Projection upward from the anterior part of each ramus; the temporal muscle inserts here
Angle	Juncture of posterior and inferior margins of ramus

Cranial Bones

The **frontal bone** forms the forehead and the anterior part of the calvaria or top of the cranium (see **Figure 12-8**, *C*). It contains mucosa-lined, air-filled spaces, or **sinuses**—the frontal sinuses. The frontal sinuses, with similar sinuses in the sphenoid, ethmoid, and maxillae, are often called paranasal sinuses because they have narrow channels that open into the nasal cavity (**Figure 12-9**). The paranasal sinuses are also discussed in Chapter 35, p. 804. A portion of the frontal bone forms the upper part of the orbits. It unites with the two parietal bones posteriorly in an immovable joint, or **suture**—the *coronal suture*. Several of the more prominent frontal bone markings are described in **Table 12-3**.

The two **parietal bones** give shape to the bulging topside of the cranium (see **Figure 12-8**, *A*). They form immovable joints with several bones: the *lambdoid suture* with the occipital bone, the *squamous suture* with the temporal bone and part of the sphenoid, and the *coronal suture* with the frontal bone.

The lower sides of the cranium and part of its floor are fashioned from two **temporal bones** (see **Figure 12-8**, *B*). They house the middle and inner ear structures and contain the *mastoid sinuses*, notable because of the occurrence of **mastoiditis,** an inflammation of the mucous lining of these spaces (see Mechanisms of Disease, pp. 260–261). For a description of several other temporal bone markings, see **Table 12-3**.

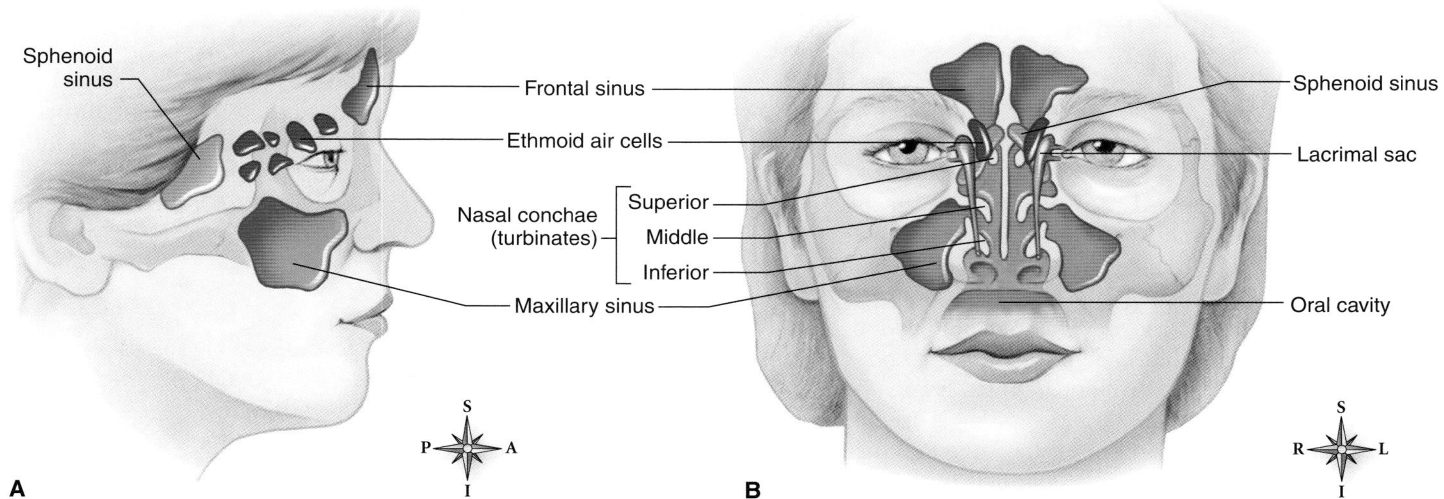

FIGURE 12-9 The paranasal sinuses. A, Lateral view. **B,** Frontal view.

The **occipital bone** creates the framework of the lower, posterior part of the skull (see **Figure 12-8**, *D*). It forms immovable joints with three other cranial bones—the parietal, temporal, and sphenoid—and a movable joint with the first cervical vertebra. **Table 12-3** lists a description of some of its markings.

The shape of the **sphenoid bone** resembles a bat with its wings outstretched and legs extended down and back. Note in **Figure 12-4** and **Figure 12-8**, *E*, the location of the sphenoid bone in the central portion of the cranial floor. Here it serves as the keystone in the architecture of the cranium and anchors the frontal, parietal, occipital, and ethmoid bones. The sphenoid bone also forms part of the lateral wall of the cranium and part of the floor of each orbit (see **Figure 12-2** and **Figure 12-3**). The sphenoid bone contains fairly large mucosa-lined, air-filled spaces—the sphenoid sinuses (see **Figure 12-6**). Several prominent sphenoid markings are described in **Table 12-3**.

The **ethmoid,** a complex, irregular bone, lies anterior to the sphenoid but posterior to the nasal bones. It helps fashion the anterior part of the cranial floor (see **Figures 12-4** and **12-8**, *F*), the medial walls of the orbits (see **Figure 12-2** and **Figure 12-7**), the upper parts of the nasal septum (see **Figure 12-2**) and the sidewalls of the nasal cavity (**Figure 12-10**), and the part of the nasal roof (the **cribriform plate**) perforated by small foramina through which olfactory nerve

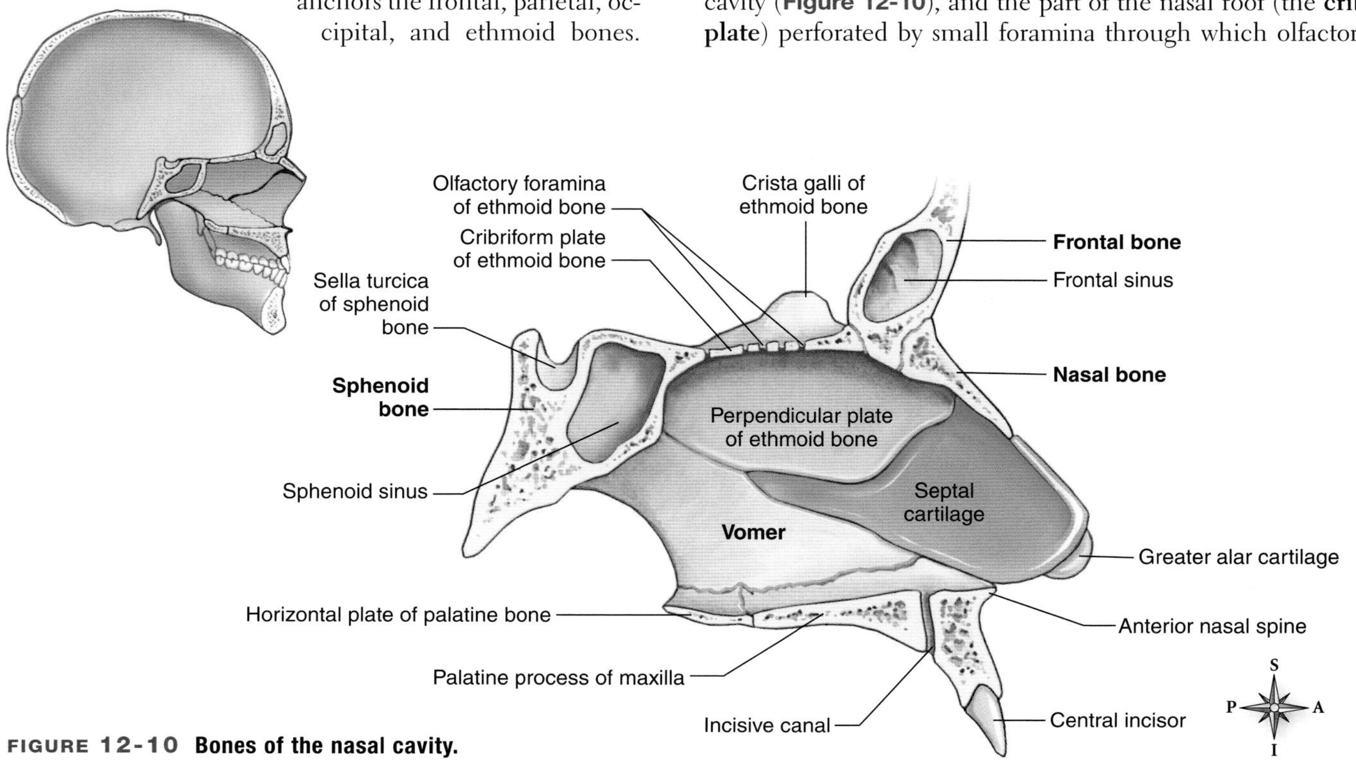

FIGURE 12-10 Bones of the nasal cavity.

branches reach the brain (**Box 12-1**). The lateral masses of the ethmoid bone are honeycombed with sinus spaces called *ethmoid air cells* (see **Figure 12-9**). For more ethmoid bone markings, see **Table 12-3**.

Facial Bones

The two **maxillae** serve as the keystone in the architecture of the face, just as the sphenoid bone acts as the keystone of the cranium. Each maxilla articulates with the other maxilla and also with a nasal, a zygomatic, an inferior concha, and a palatine bone (see **Figure 12-8**, *H*). Of all the facial bones, only the mandible does not articulate with the maxillae. The maxillae form part of the floor of the orbits, part of the roof of the mouth, and part of the floor and sidewalls of the nose. Each maxilla contains a mucosa-lined space, the *maxillary sinus* (see **Figure 12-9**). This sinus is the largest of the paranasal sinuses—that is, sinuses connected by channels to the nasal cavity. For other markings of the maxillae, see **Table 12-4**.

Unlike the upper jaw, which is formed by the articulation of the two maxillae, the lower jaw, because of fusion of its halves during infancy, consists of a single bone, the **mandible** (see **Figure 12-8**, *M*). It is the largest, strongest bone of the face. It articulates with the temporal bone in the only movable joint of the skull. Its major markings are identified in **Table 12-4**.

The cheek is shaped by the underlying **zygomatic bone** or *malar bone* (see **Figure 12-8**, *I*). This bone also forms the outer margin of the orbit and, with the zygomatic process of the temporal bone, makes the zygomatic arch. It articulates with four other facial bones: the maxillary, temporal, frontal, and sphenoid bones.

Shape is given to the nose by the two **nasal bones**, which form the upper part of the bridge of the nose (see **Figure 12-8**, *L*), and by the *septal cartilage*, which forms the lower part (see **Figure 12-10**). Although small, the nasal bones enter into several articulations: with the perpendicular plate of the ethmoid bone, the cartilaginous part of the nasal septum, the frontal bone, the maxillae, and each other.

An almost paper-thin bone, shaped and sized about like a fingernail, lies just posterior and lateral to each nasal bone. It helps form the sidewall of the nasal cavity and the medial wall of the orbit. Because it contains a groove for the nasolacrimal (tear) duct, this bone is called the **lacrimal bone** (see **Figure 12-8**, *K*). It joins the maxilla, frontal bone, and ethmoid bone.

CONNECT IT! 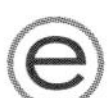

The sinuses of the skull are often visible in x-ray images and other radiographs, as you can see in ***Skeletal Radiography*** online at ***Connect It!***

The two **palatine bones** join to each other in the midline like two Ls facing each other. Their united horizontal portions form the posterior part of the hard palate (see **Figure 12-8**, *J*). The vertical portion of each palatine bone forms the lateral wall of the posterior part of each nasal cavity. The tip of the vertical portion is the *orbital process*, which forms part of the eye orbit (see **Figure 12-7**). The palatine bones articulate with the maxillae and the sphenoid bone.

There are two **inferior nasal conchae** (*turbinates*). Each concha is scroll-shaped and forms a kind of ledge projecting into the nasal cavity from its lateral wall. Each nasal cavity has three such ledges. The superior and middle conchae (which are projections of the ethmoid bone) form the upper and middle ledges. The inferior concha (which is a separate bone) forms the lower ledge. They are covered by mucosa and divide each nasal cavity into three narrow, irregular channels, the nasal meatus. The inferior nasal conchae form immovable joints with the ethmoid, lacrimal, maxilla, and palatine bones.

Two structures that are involved in the formation of the nasal septum have already been mentioned—the perpendicular plate of the ethmoid bone and the septal cartilage. One other structure, the **vomer bone**, completes the septum posteriorly (see **Figures 12-8**, *G*, and **12-10** and **Table 12-5**). It forms immovable joints with four bones: the sphenoid, ethmoid, palatine, and maxillae.

Eye Orbits

The right and left orbital cavities of the skull contain not only the eyes and associated muscles but also the lacrimal apparatus and important blood vessels and nerves. These structures are separated from the cranial cavity, nose, paranasal sinuses, and mouth by the often very thin and fragile orbital walls (see **Figures 12-2** and **12-7**).

CONNECT IT! 

The fragile bones of the eye orbit can fracture easily, causing a dramatic condition called ***panda eyes.*** See for yourself in ***Bone Fractures*** online at ***Connect It!***

BOX 12-1 *health matters* | The Cribriform Plate

Separation of the nasal and cranial cavities by the cribriform plate of the ethmoid bone has great clinical significance. The cribriform plate is perforated by many small openings that permit branches of the olfactory nerve responsible for the special sense of smell to enter the cranial cavity and reach the brain. Separation of these two cavities by a thin, perforated plate of bone presents real hazards. If the cribriform plate is damaged as a result of trauma to the nose, it is possible for potentially infectious material to pass directly from the nasal cavity into the cranial fossa. If fragments of a fractured nasal bone are pushed through the cribriform plate, they may tear the coverings of the brain or enter the substance of the brain itself.

TABLE 12-5 Special Features of the Skull

FEATURE	DESCRIPTION
Sutures	Immovable joints between skull bones
Squamous	Line of articulation along the top curved edge of the temporal bone
Coronal	Joint between the parietal bones and frontal bone
Lambdoid	Joint between the parietal bones and occipital bone
Sagittal	Joint between the right and left parietal bones
Fontanelles	"Soft spots" where ossification is incomplete at birth; allow some compression of the skull during birth; also important in determining the position of the head before delivery; six such areas located at angles of the parietal bones
Anterior (or frontal)	At the intersection of the sagittal and coronal sutures (juncture of the parietal bones and frontal bone); diamond shaped; largest of the fontanelles; usually closed by 11.2 years of age
Posterior (or occipital)	At the intersection of the sagittal and lambdoid sutures (juncture of the parietal bones and occipital bone); triangular; usually closed by the second month
Sphenoid (or anterolateral)	At the juncture of the frontal, parietal, temporal, and sphenoid bones
Mastoid (or posterolateral)	At the juncture of the parietal, occipital, and temporal bones; usually closed by the second year
Air sinuses	Spaces, or cavities, within bones; those that communicate with the nose are called *paranasal sinuses* (frontal, sphenoidal, ethmoidal, and maxillary); mastoid cells communicate with the middle ear rather than the nose, so are not included among the paranasal sinuses
Orbits formed by	
Frontal bone	Roof of the orbit
Ethmoid bone	Medial wall
Lacrimal bone	Medial wall
Sphenoid bone	Lateral wall
Zygomatic bone	Lateral wall
Maxilla	Floor
Palatine bone	Floor
Nasal septum formed by	Partition in the midline of the nasal cavity; separates the cavity into right and left halves
Perpendicular plate of the ethmoid bone	Forms the upper part of the septum
Vomer	Forms the lower, posterior part of the septum
Cartilage	Forms the anterior part of the septum
Sutural (wormian) bones	Small islets of bone in sutures; vary greatly from person to person
Malleus, incus, stapes	Tiny bones, referred to as *auditory ossicles,* in the middle ear cavity in the temporal bones; resemble, respectively, a miniature hammer, anvil, and stirrup

Fetal Skull

The skulls of both a fetus and a newborn infant have unique anatomical features not seen in an adult. For example, placement of the cranial bones in the fetal skull allows it to change shape during the birth process. During infancy and childhood, differential growth and development of certain areas of the skull produce changing proportions of the cranium and face. As you will learn in Chapter 47, the face at birth forms a relatively smaller proportion of the cranium (about one eighth) than in the adult (about one half). Also, whereas an infant's head is approximately one fourth the total height of the body, an adult's head is only about one eighth the total height (see **Figure 47-22** on p. 1111).

The **fontanelles,** visible in **Figure 12-11** and described in **Table 12-5**, are perhaps the best known of the unique features in the infant

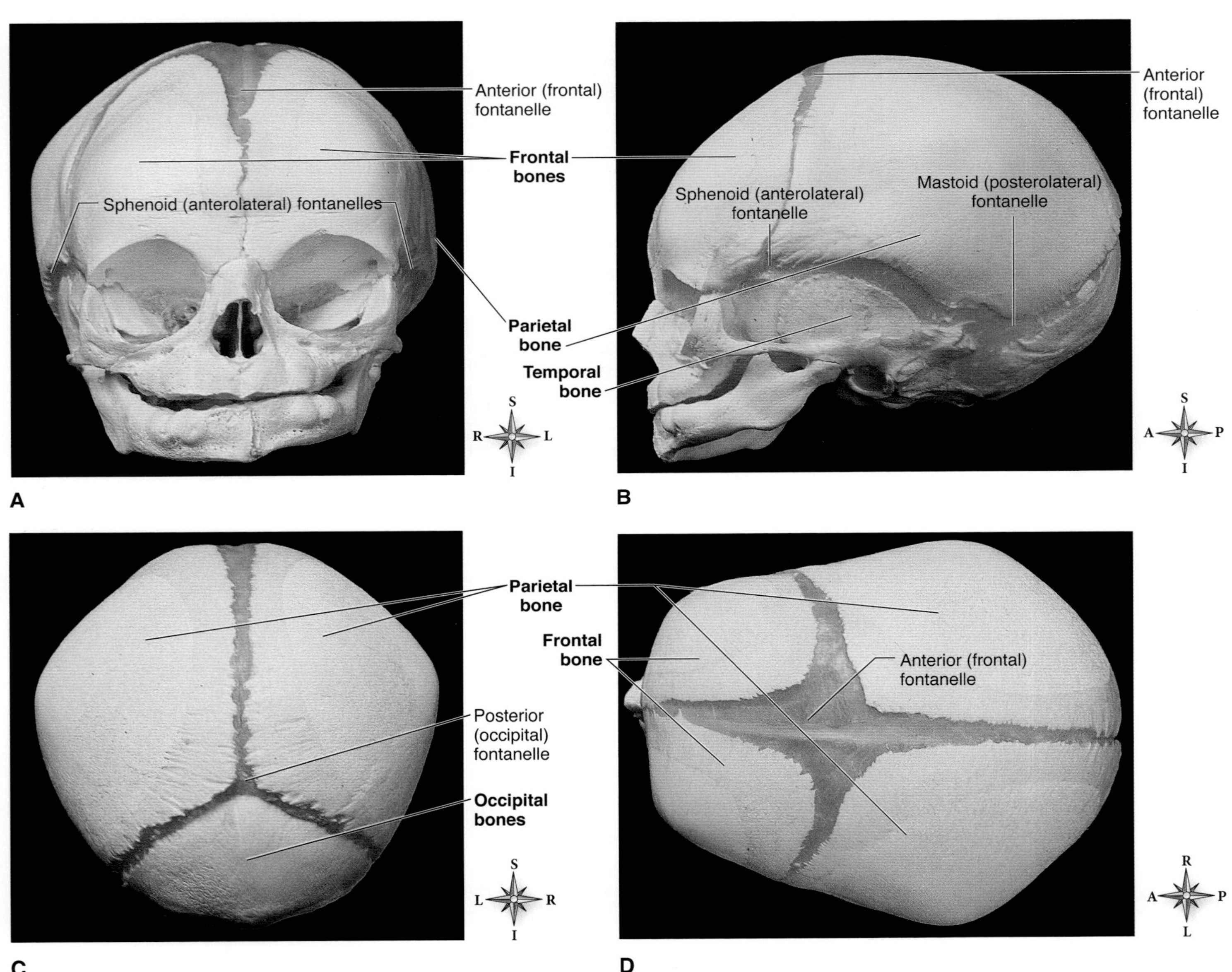

FIGURE 12-11 Skull at birth. A, Viewed from the front. **B,** Viewed from the left and slightly below. **C,** Viewed from behind. **D,** Viewed from above.

skull. Without the additional space between skull bones provided by the fontanelles, moulding of head shape as the baby passes through the birth canal could result in fracture of one or more cranial bones. Fontanelles also allow rapid brain growth to occur in infancy without causing damaging increases in intracranial pressure. When the fontanelles close and the cranial bones grow together as they reach adult size and shape, they fuse together and form the adult suture lines that remain visible throughout life (see **Table 12-5**).

Numerous other changes occur as the skull of the newborn undergoes skeletal ageing processes that prepare it for adult functions. For example, the paranasal sinuses, shown in **Figure 12-6** and described in detail in Chapter 35, undergo dramatic changes in size and placement during the time between birth and skeletal maturity. They are listed as special features of the skull in **Table 12-5**. In **Figure 12-11**, elevations that cover the developing deciduous, or baby, teeth can be seen in the body of the mandible. Over time these teeth will erupt and eventually be replaced by the adult dentition. These and other anatomical changes in the skull are possible because of the orderly sequence of ageing processes that occur between fetal life and skeletal maturity.

Special features of the skull, including the eye orbits, nasal septum, sutures, fontanelles, sutural (wormian) bones, and the auditory ossicles, are briefly described in **Table 12-5**.

CONNECT IT!

The skull changes quite a bit over the life span, a fact that helps anthropologists and forensic scientists determine the age of a person simply by examining the skeleton or skeletal remains. You can see examples of these changes in ***Skeletal Variations*** online at ***Connect It!***

HYOID BONE

The hyoid bone is a single bone in the neck—a part of the axial skeleton (**Table 12-6**). Its U shape may be felt just above the larynx (voice box) and below the mandible, where it is suspended from the styloid processes of the temporal bones (**Figure 12-12**). Several muscles attach to the hyoid bone. Among them are an extrinsic tongue muscle and certain muscles of the floor of the mouth. The hyoid claims the distinction of being the only bone in the body that articulates with no other bones.

Quick CHECK

1. Name the eight bones of the cranium and describe how they fit together.
2. Name the 14 bones of the face and describe how they fit together.
3. Which bone is the only bone that normally does not form a joint with any other bone of the skeleton?

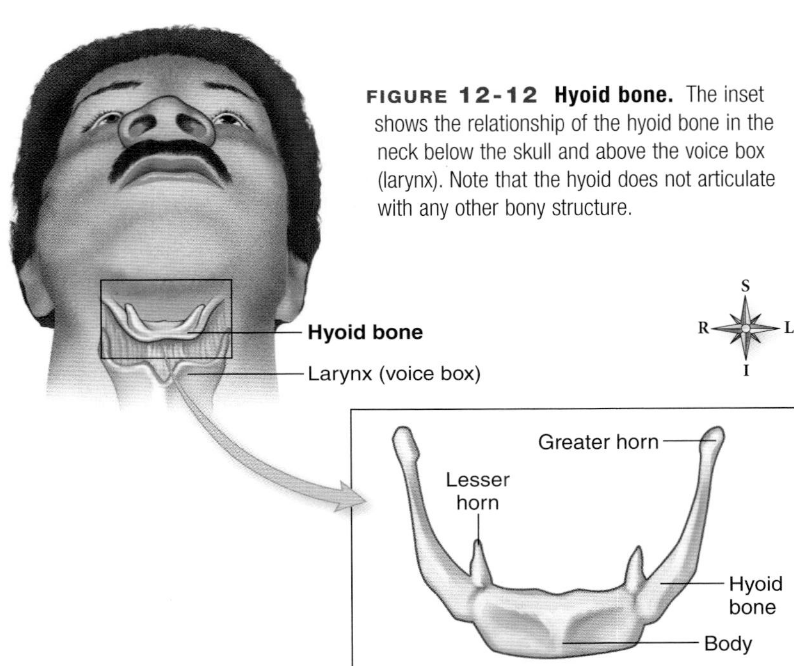

FIGURE 12-12 Hyoid bone. The inset shows the relationship of the hyoid bone in the neck below the skull and above the voice box (larynx). Note that the hyoid does not articulate with any other bony structure.

TABLE 12-6 Hyoid, Vertebrae, and Thoracic Bones and Their Markings

BONES AND MARKINGS	DESCRIPTION
Hyoid	U-shaped bone in the neck between the mandible and upper part of the larynx; distinctive as the only bone in the body not forming a joint with any other bone; suspended by ligaments from the styloid processes of the temporal bones
Body	Central part (apex of U)
Lesser horn	Tiny, anterior horn on each lateral end of body
Greater horn	Posterior horns (arms of U)

(continued)

UNIT 2

TABLE 12-6 **Hyoid, Vertebrae, and Thoracic Bones and Their Markings—cont'd**

BONES AND MARKINGS	DESCRIPTION
Vertebral column	Not actually a column, but a flexible, segmented curved rod; forms the axis of the body; head balanced above, ribs and viscera suspended in front, and lower extremities attached below; encloses the spinal cord *General features:* Anterior part of each vertebra (except the first two cervical) consists of the body; posterior part of the vertebrae consists of the neural arch, which in turn consists of two pedicles, two laminae, and seven processes projecting from the laminae
Body	Main part; flat, round mass located anteriorly; supporting or weight-bearing part of the vertebra
Pedicles	Short projections extending posteriorly from the body
Lamina	Posterior part of the vertebra to which pedicles join and from which processes project
Neural arch	Formed by the pedicles and laminae; protects the spinal cord posteriorly; congenital absence of one or more neural arches is known as *spina bifida* (the cord may protrude right through the skin)
Spinous process (spine)	Sharp process projecting inferiorly from laminae in the midline
Transverse processes	Right and left lateral projections from laminae
Superior articulating processes	Project upward from laminae; have smooth *superior articular facets*
Inferior articulating processes	Project downward from laminae; articulate with the superior articulating processes of vertebrae below; have smooth *inferior articular facets*
Spinal foramen	Hole in the centre of the vertebra formed by union of the body, pedicles, and laminae; spinal foramina, when vertebrae are superimposed on one another, form the spinal cavity that houses the spinal cord
Intervertebral foramina	Openings between the vertebrae through which the spinal nerves emerge
Cervical vertebrae	First or upper seven vertebrae; the foramen in each transverse process for transmission of the vertebral artery, vein, and plexus of nerves; short bifurcated spinous processes except on the seventh vertebra, where it is extra long and may be felt as a protrusion when head is bent forward; the bodies of these vertebrae are small, whereas spinal foramina are large and triangular
Atlas	First cervical vertebra; lacks a body and spinous process; superior articulating processes are concave ovals that act as rockerlike cradles for the condyles of the occipital bone; named *atlas* because it supports the head as Atlas supports the world in Greek mythology
Axis (epistropheus)	Second cervical vertebra, so named because the atlas rotates about this bone in rotating movements of the head; the *dens,* or odontoid process, is a peglike projection extending upward from the body of the axis that forms a pivot for rotation of the atlas
Thoracic vertebrae	Next 12 vertebrae; 12 pairs of ribs attached to these vertebrae; stronger, with more massive bodies than the cervical vertebrae; no transverse foramina; two sets of facets for articulations with the corresponding rib: one on the body, the second on the transverse process; the upper thoracic vertebrae have elongated spinous processes
Lumbar vertebrae	Next five vertebrae; strong, massive; superior articulating processes directed medially instead of upward; inferior articulating processes, laterally instead of downward; short, blunt spinous processes
Sacrum	Five separate vertebrae until about 25 years of age; then fused to form one wedge-shaped bone
Sacral promontory	Protuberance from the anterior, upper border of the sacrum into the pelvis; of obstetrical importance because its size limits the anteroposterior diameter of the pelvic inlet
Sacral canal	Inferior part of the vertebral (spinal) canal
Anterior (sacral) foramina	Pairs of holes along anterior (pelvic) surface of sacrum for passage of spinal nerves; sometimes called *pelvic foramina*
Posterior (sacral) foramina	Pairs of holes along posterior (dorsal) surface of sacrum for passage of spinal nerves; sometimes called *dorsal foramina*
Sacral hiatus	Gap in posterior wall of sacral canal in the bottom segment(s) of sacrum
Superior articular facet	Flat joint surface on each side of superior entrance to sacral canal
Medial sacral crest	Bumpy ridge along middle of posterior surface, similar to spinous processes of vertebrae
Intermediate sacral crest	Bumpy ridge just medial to the posterior foramina
Lateral sacral crest	Bumpy ridge just lateral to the posterior foramina
Apex	Inferior tip of sacrum
Auricular surface	Ear-shaped surface that articulates with ilium of pelvic bone
Coccyx	Three to five separate vertebrae in a child but fused into one in an adult

(continued on page 258)

VERTEBRAL COLUMN

The vertebral column is also called the *spinal column* or more simply the spine. It forms the longitudinal axis of the skeleton. It is a flexible rather than a rigid column because it is segmented. As **Figure 12-13** shows, the vertebral column consists of 24 **vertebrae** plus the sacrum and coccyx. Joints between the vertebrae permit forward, backward, and sideways movement of the column.

Consider too these additional facts about the vertebral column. The head is balanced on top, the ribs are suspended in front, the lower extremities are attached below, and the spinal cord is enclosed within. It is indeed the structural "backbone" of the body.

The seven **cervical vertebrae** constitute the skeletal framework of the neck (see **Figure 12-13**). The next 12 vertebrae are called **thoracic vertebrae** because of their location in the posterior part of the chest, or the thoracic region. The next five, the **lumbar vertebrae,** support the small of the back. Below the lumbar vertebrae lie the sacrum and coccyx. In an adult the sacrum is a single bone that has formed from the fusion of five separate vertebrae, and the coccyx is a single bone that has formed from the fusion of three to five vertebrae.

All the vertebrae resemble one another in certain features and differ in others. For example, all except the first cervical vertebra have a flat, rounded body placed anteriorly and centrally, plus a sharp or blunt *spinous process* projecting inferiorly in the posterior midline and two transverse processes projecting laterally (**Figure 12-14**). All but the sacrum and coccyx have a central opening, the *vertebral foramen*. An upward projection (the *dens*) from the body of the second cervical vertebra furnishes an axis for rotating the head. A long, blunt spinous process, which can be felt at the back of the base of the neck, characterizes the seventh cervical vertebra. Each thoracic vertebra has articular facets for the ribs. More detailed descriptions of the individual vertebrae, sacrum and coccyx are given in **Table 12-6**. The vertebral column, as a whole, articulates with the head, ribs, and iliac bones. Individual vertebrae articulate with each other in joints between their bodies and between their articular processes.

SPINAL CURVATURES

Have you ever noticed the four curves in your spine? To increase the carrying strength of the vertebral column and to make balance possible in the upright position, the vertebral column is curved.

When you look at the spine from the rear, you will see the thoracic (kyphotic) curvature and sacral (lordotic) curvature (see **Figure 12-13**, A). These are called convex curvatures because they round outward. The inward-curving curvatures of the spine are called concave curvatures. They are the cervical curvature and lumbar curvature.

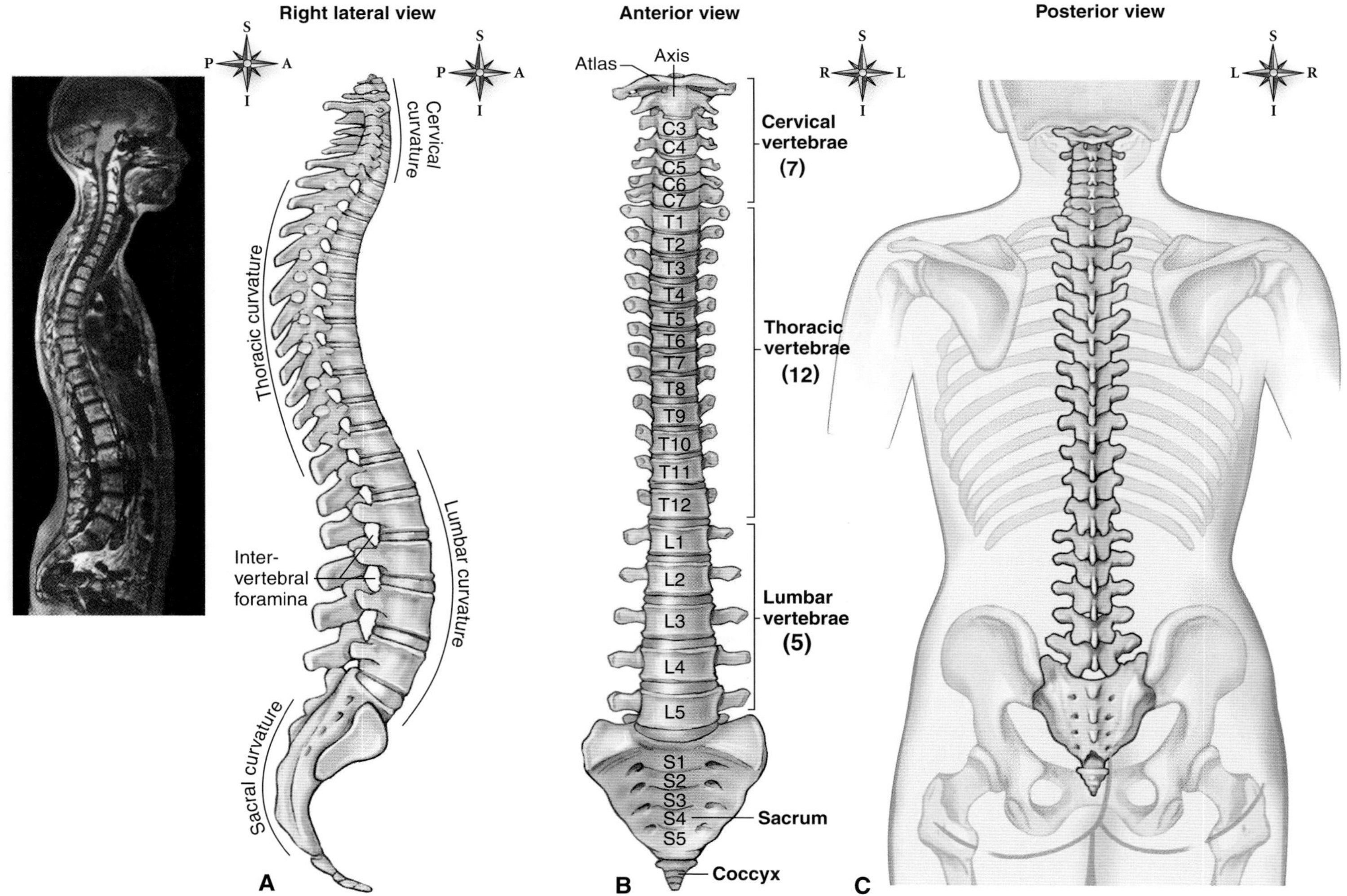

FIGURE 12-13 The vertebral column. A, Right lateral view. **B,** Anterior view. **C,** Posterior view. The photo inset shows a midline sagittal magnetic resonance image (MRI) of the vertebral column.

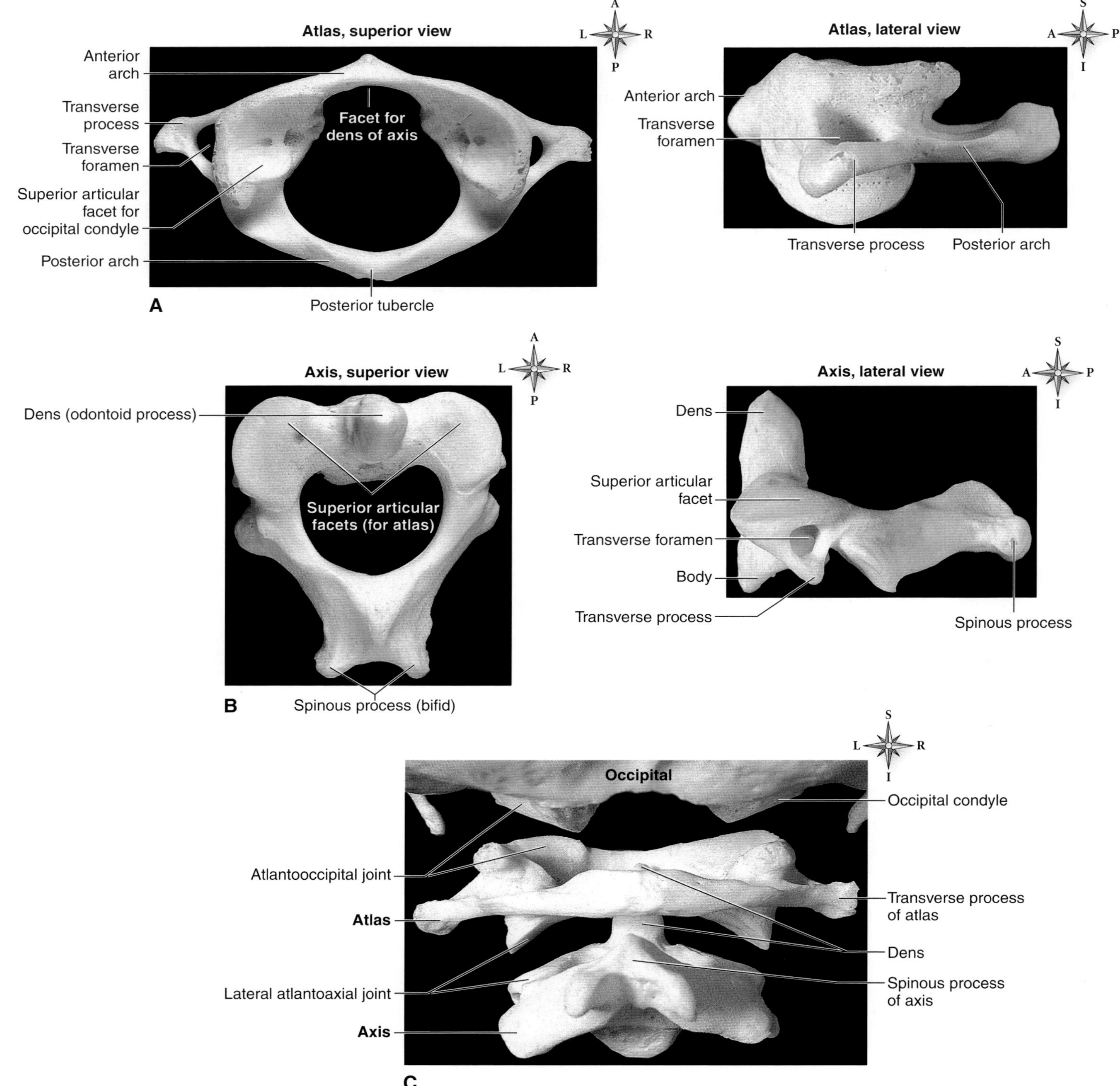

FIGURE 12-14 Vertebrae. A, Superior and lateral views of C1, the *atlas.* **B,** Superior and lateral views of C2, the axis. **C,** Base of the skull showing C1 (atlas) and C2 (axis) in posterior view. **D,** Lateral and superior views of a cervical vertebra, C7 (note the prominent spinous process). **E,** Superior and lateral views of a thoracic vertebra, T10. **F,** Superior and lateral views of a lumbar vertebra, L3. **G,** Lumbar vertebra L5 and the upper portion of the sacrum in an expanded anterior view. **H,** Oblique view of the sacrum and coccyx, showing the right coxal (hip) bone for reference.

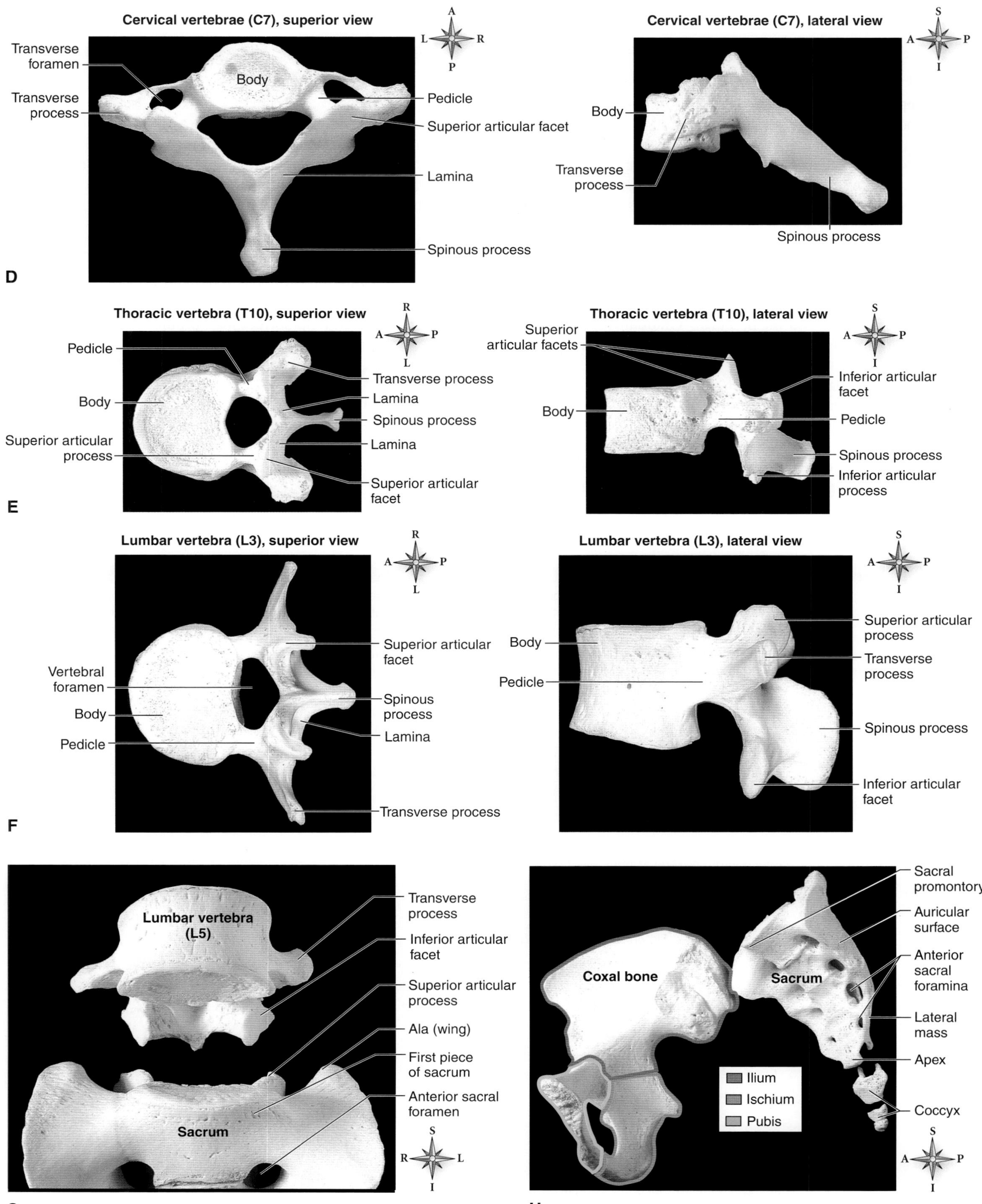
Cervical vertebrae (C7), superior view
Transverse foramen
Transverse process
Body
Pedicle
Superior articular facet
Lamina
Spinous process
D
Cervical vertebrae (C7), lateral view
Body
Transverse process
Spinous process
Thoracic vertebra (T10), superior view
Pedicle
Body
Superior articular process
Transverse process
Lamina
Spinous process
Lamina
Superior articular facet
E
Thoracic vertebra (T10), lateral view
Superior articular facets
Body
Inferior articular facet
Pedicle
Spinous process
Inferior articular process
Lumbar vertebra (L3), superior view
Vertebral foramen
Body
Pedicle
Superior articular facet
Spinous process
Lamina
Transverse process
F
Lumbar vertebra (L3), lateral view
Body
Pedicle
Superior articular process
Transverse process
Spinous process
Inferior articular facet
Lumbar vertebra (L5)
Sacrum
Transverse process
Inferior articular facet
Superior articular process
Ala (wing)
First piece of sacrum
Anterior sacral foramen
G
Coxal bone
Sacrum
Sacral promontory
Auricular surface
Anterior sacral foramina
Lateral mass
Apex
Coccyx
Ilium
Ischium
Pubis
H

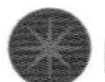

BOX 12-2 *balloon kyphoplasty*

Balloon kyphoplasty is an orthopaedic procedure used to treat the vertebral compression fractures that occur in osteoporosis, as a result of certain tumours, or after prolonged use of steroid drugs. Fractured (collapsed) vertebrae (see **Figure 11-23** on p. 224) result in shortened height and spinal deformity and may be the cause of chronic pain. The balloon kyphoplasty procedure involves the insertion of an inflatable balloonlike device called a **bone tamp** through a small incision in the skin and then through a channel drilled into the body of the fractured vertebra. Expansion of the balloon restores the vertebra to a normal height. The balloon is then deflated and removed, and the surgeon uses the needle to fill the cavity with a type of "super glue" bone cement that quickly hardens and thus stabilizes and seals the fracture. Another procedure, called **vertebroplasty,** also involves injecting bone cement, but without using a balloon. •

This is not true, however, of a newborn baby's spine. It forms a continuous convex curve—called the primary curvature—from top to bottom (see **Figure 47-23** on p. 1112). Gradually, as the baby learns to hold up his or her head, a reverse or concave curve develops in the neck (cervical region).

Later, as the baby learns to stand, the lumbar region of his or her spine also becomes concave (see **Figure 47-24** on p. 1112). The concave cervical and lumber curvatures are sometimes called secondary curvatures because they appear later in development than the primary (convex) curvatures. If individual vertebrae cannot bear the weight put on them, compression fractures may occur. Such fractures may cause the vertebrae to partially collapse and thus affect spinal curvature and overall stature. **Box 12-2** describes medical procedures that can help correct such problems.

THORAX

Twelve pairs of ribs, together with the vertebral column and sternum, form most of the bony cage known as the *thoracic cage* or, simply, the **thorax.** The posterior part of the thorax also includes the thoracic vertebrae.

TABLE 12-6 Hyoid, Vertebrae, and Thoracic Bones and Their Markings—cont'd

BONES AND MARKINGS	DESCRIPTION
Curvatures	Curvatures have great structural importance because they increase the carrying strength of the vertebral column, make balance possible in an upright position (if the column was straight, the weight of the viscera would pull the body forward), absorb jolts from walking (a straight column would transmit jolts straight to the head), and protect the column from fracture
Primary curvatures Thoracic curvature Sacral curvature	Column curves at birth from the head to the sacrum with the convexity posteriorly; after the child stands, the convexity persists only in the *thoracic* and *sacral* regions, which are therefore called *primary curvatures*
Secondary curvatures Cervical curvature Lumbar curvature	Concavities in the *cervical* and *lumbar* regions; the cervical concavity results from the infant's attempts to hold the head erect (2 to 4 months); the lumbar concavity, from balancing efforts in learning to walk (10 to 18 months)
Sternum	Breastbone; flat dagger-shaped bone; the sternum, ribs, and thoracic vertebrae together form a bony cage known as the *thorax*
Body	Main central part of the bone
Manubrium	Flaring, upper part
Xiphoid process	Projection of cartilage at the lower border of the bone
Ribs	
Types	
True ribs	Upper seven pairs; fasten to the sternum by costal cartilages
False ribs	False ribs do not attach to the sternum directly; the upper three pairs of false ribs attach by means of the costal cartilage of the seventh ribs
Floating ribs	The last two pairs of false ribs do not attach to the sternum at all and are therefore called "floating" ribs
Parts	
Head	Projection at the posterior end of a rib; articulates with the corresponding thoracic vertebra and one above, except the last three pairs, which join the corresponding vertebrae only
Neck	Constricted portion just below the head
Tubercle	Small knob just below the neck; articulates with the transverse process of the corresponding thoracic vertebra; missing in the lowest three ribs
Body or shaft	Main part of a rib
Costal cartilage	Cartilage at the sternal end of true ribs; attaches ribs (except floating ribs) to the sternum

Sternum

The medial part of the anterior chest wall is supported by the **sternum,** a somewhat dagger-shaped bone consisting of three parts: the upper handle part, the *manubrium*; the middle blade part, the *body*; and a blunt cartilaginous lower tip, the *xiphoid process*. The last ossifies during adult life. The manubrium articulates with the clavicle and first rib, whereas the next nine ribs join the body of the sternum, either directly or indirectly, by means of the *costal cartilages* (**Figure 12-15**).

Ribs

Ribs are elongated flat bones that form parallel curves resembling bars of a cage. Each rib articulates with both the body and the transverse process of its corresponding thoracic vertebra. The head of each rib articulates with the body of the corresponding thoracic vertebra, and the tubercle of each rib articulates with the vertebra's transverse process (**Figure 12-16**). In addition, the second through ninth ribs articulate with the body of the vertebra above. From its vertebral attachment, each rib curves outward, then forward and

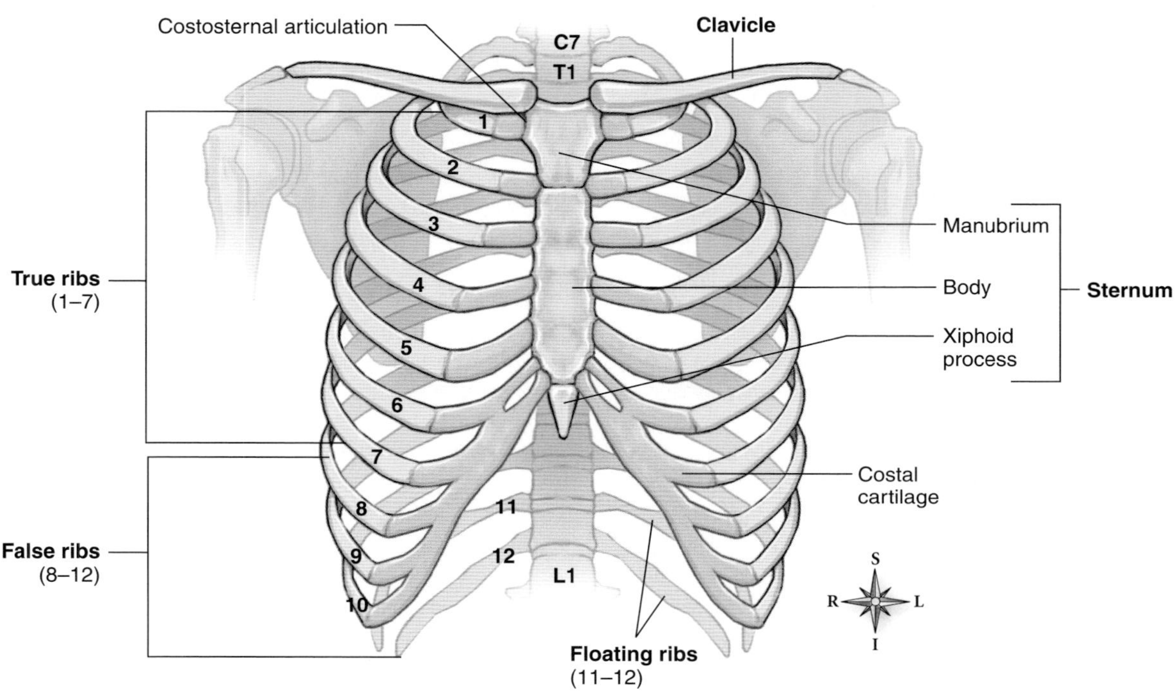

FIGURE 12-15 Thoracic cage. Note the costal cartilages and their articulations with the body of the sternum.

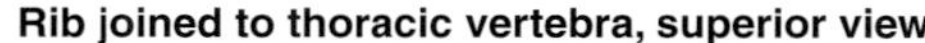

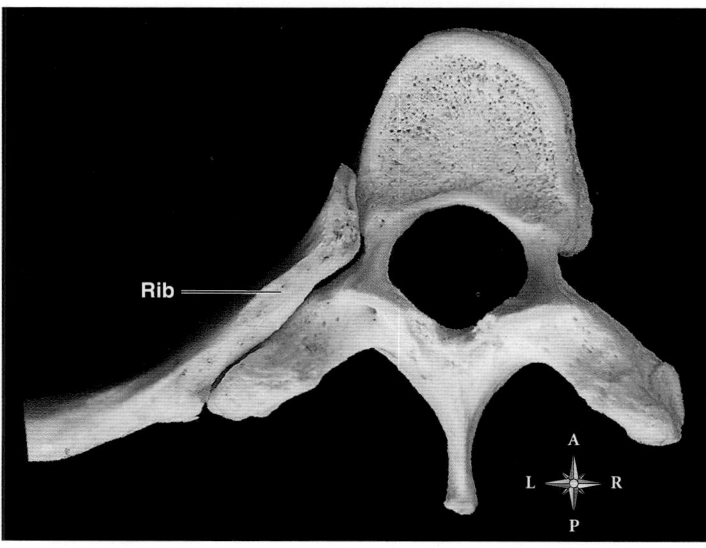

A

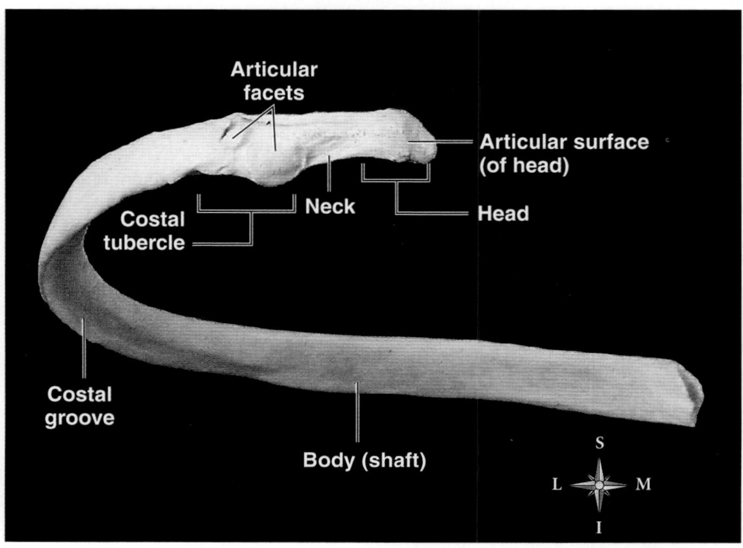

B

FIGURE 12-16 Articulation of a rib and vertebra. A, Note the head of the rib articulating with the vertebral body and the tubercle of the rib articulating with the transverse process of the vertebra. **B,** Anatomical components of a typical rib (fifth rib) viewed from behind.

downward (see **Figures 12-1** and **12-16**), a mechanical fact important for breathing.

Anteriorly, each rib of the first seven pairs joins a costal cartilage that attaches to the sternum. For this reason, these ribs are often called the *true ribs*. Ribs of the remaining five pairs, the *false ribs*, do not attach directly to the sternum. Instead, each costal cartilage of pairs 8, 9, and 10 attaches to the costal cartilage of the rib above it—indirectly attaching it to the sternum. Ribs of the last two pairs of false ribs are designated *floating ribs* because they do not attach even indirectly to the sternum (see **Figure 12-15**).

Quick CHECK

4. Name the three types of vertebrae and how many of each type are found in the vertebral column.
5. What bones make up the bony cage known as the thorax? How do these bones fit together to form this structure?
6. What is a floating rib?

mechanisms of disease

Disorders of the Axial Skeleton

Mastoiditis

Mastoiditis is inflammation of the air spaces within the mastoid portion of the temporal bone. Infectious material may find its way into the mastoid air cells from middle ear infections and, unless treated promptly and successfully, can produce very serious medical problems. The mastoid air cells do not drain into the nose, as do the paranasal sinuses. As a result, infectious material that accumulates may erode the bony partition that separates the air cells from the cranial cavity. If such erosion develops, the inflammation may spread to the brain or its covering membranes. Infection and an accumulation of pus (abscess) may then develop in or on the surface of the brain. Should this occur, a localized infection within the middle ear and mastoid air cells in the substance of the temporal bone escalates into a life-threatening medical emergency involving the central nervous system. Externally, clinical signs of mastoiditis include redness and swelling of the external ear and the skin overlying the mastoid process. The area is very painful when touched. In severe cases, the external ear may be pushed forward and downward by the underlying swelling (**Figure 12-17**).

Prompt treatment of middle ear infection, or **otitis media,** with antibiotics has made life-threatening cases of mastoiditis rare. Exceptions occur in instances of antibiotic resistance or in cases of inadequate or untreated chronic middle ear infections. If intensive antibiotic therapy fails and the subsequent accumulation of infectious material that fills the middle ear and mastoid air cells threatens extension into the cranial cavity, surgical intervention may be required. A surgical incision of the eardrum is often performed to reduce pressure and release pus from the middle ear. Although rarely performed today, surgical removal of part of the diseased mastoid portion of the temporal bone, a procedure called **mastoidectomy,** may also be necessary to drain trapped infectious material from the air cells. Fortunately, modern antibiotics and prompt medical treatment have dramatically reduced the need for this procedure with its attendant scarring and hearing loss.

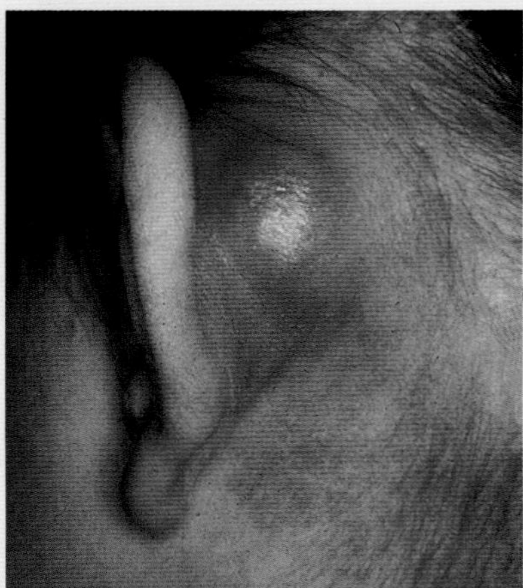

FIGURE 12-17 **Mastoiditis.** Note redness and swelling over the mastoid process of the temporal bone and extending up to the temporal region behind ear.

Abnormal Spinal Curvatures

The normal curvature of the spine is convex through the thoracic region and concave through the cervical and lumbar regions (see **Figure 12-13**). This gives the spine strength to support the weight of the rest of the body and makes it possible to also balance the weight of the body, which is necessary to stand and walk. A curved structure has more strength than does a straight one of the same size and material. Poor posture or disease may cause the lumbar curve to be abnormally accentuated—a condition known as "swayback", or **lordosis** (**Figure 12-18**, *A*). This condition is often seen during pregnancy as the woman adjusts to changes in her centre of gravity. It may also be secondary to traumatic injury or a degenerative process of the vertebral bodies.

Kyphosis, or "hunchback", is an abnormally increased roundness in the thoracic curvature (**Figure 12-18**, *B*). It is often seen in elderly people with osteoporosis or chronic arthritis, those with neuromuscular diseases, or individuals with compression fractures of the thoracic vertebrae. In a condition called **Scheuermann disease,** kyphosis can develop in children at puberty.

Abnormal side-to-side curvature is called **scoliosis** (**Figure 12-18**, *C*). This too may be idiopathic or a result of damage to the supporting muscles along the spine. It is a relatively common condition that appears before adolescence.

All three abnormal curvatures can interfere with normal breathing, posture, and other vital functions. The degree of abnormal curvature and resulting deformity of the vertebral column determine the various treatments instituted. The traditional treatment of scoliosis is the use of a supportive brace, called the

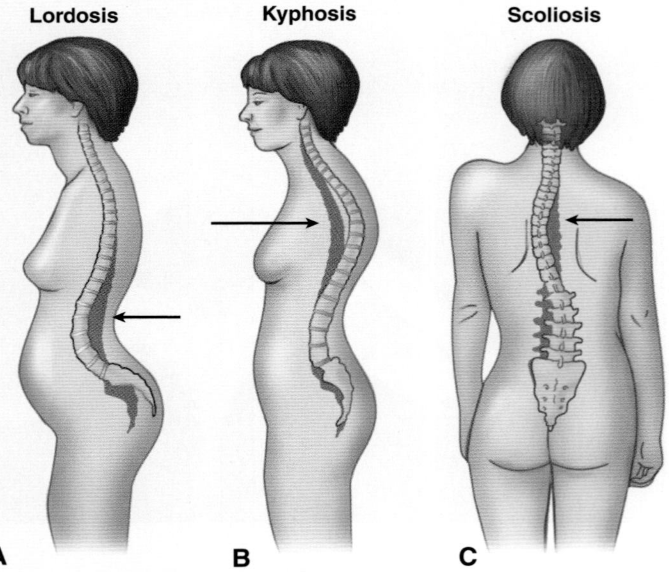

FIGURE 12-18 **Abnormal spine curvatures. A,** Lordosis. **B,** Kyphosis. **C,** Scoliosis. *Black arrows* highlight areas of abnormal curvature. Grey shadows show normal curvatures.

Milwaukee brace, that is worn on the upper part of the body 23 hours per day for up to several years. A newer approach to straightening abnormal curvature is **transcutaneous stimulation.** In this method, muscles on one side of the vertebral column are electrically stimulated to contract and pull the vertebrae into a more normal position. If these methods fail, correction may be achieved by surgical intervention in which pieces of bone from elsewhere in the skeleton, synthetic or natural materials, or metal rods, are grafted to (or inserted into) the deformed vertebrae to hold them in proper alignment. If treated early enough, kyphosis resulting from poor posture can be corrected with special exercises and instructions for appropriate posture. Kyphosis resulting from pathological causes may also require special braces or surgical intervention.

LANGUAGE OF SCIENCE *(continued from p. 233)*

sternum (STER-num)
[*sternum* **breastbone**] *pl.,* sterna or sternums

suture (SOO-chur)
[*sutur-* **seam**]

temporal bone (TEM-poh-ral)
[*tempora-* **temple (of head),** *-al* **relating to**]

thoracic vertebra (thoh-RASS-ik VER-teh-bra)
[*thorac-* **chest,** *-ic* **relating to,** *vertebra* **that which turns**] *pl.,* vertebrae

thorax (THOH-raks)
[*thorax* **chest**] *pl.,* thoraces

vertebra (VER-teh-bra)
[*vertebra* **that which turns**] *pl.,* vertebrae

vomer bone (VOH-mer)
[*vomer* **plowshare**]

zygomatic bone (zye-goh-MAT-ik)
[*zygo-* **union or yoke,** *-ic* **relating to**]

LANGUAGE OF MEDICINE

balloon kyphoplasty (KYE-foh-plas-tee)
[*kypho-* **hump,** *-plasty* **surgical repair**]

bone tamp (bohn tamp)

kyphosis (kye-FOH-sis)
[*kypho-* **hump,** *-osis* **condition**]

lordosis (lor-DOH-sis)
[*lordos-* **bent backward,** *-osis* **condition**]

mastoidectomy (mass-toyd-EK-toh-mee)
[*mast-* **breast,** *-oid-* **like,** *-ec-* **out,** *-tom-* **cut,** *-y* **action**]

mastoiditis (mass-toyd-EYE-tis)
[*mast-* **breast,** *-oid-* **like,** *-itis* **inflammation**]

Milwaukee brace (mil-WAWK-ee)
[*Milwaukee* **after the city in Wisconsin, U.S.A.**]

otitis media (o-TYE-tis MEE-dee-ah)
[*oti-* **ear,** *-itis* **inflammation**]

Scheuermann disease (SHOY-er-man)
[*Holger W. Scheuermann,* **Danish surgeon**]

scoliosis (skoh-lee-OH-sis)
[*scolio-* **twisted or crooked,** *-osis* **condition**]

transcutaneous stimulation (tranz-kyoo-TAYNE-ee-us)
[*trans-* **across,** *-cut-* **skin,** *-ous* **made of**]

vertebroplasty (ver-tee-broh-PLAS-tee)
[*vertebra* **that which turns,** *-plasty* **surgical repair**]

case study

While working an archaeological dig, Jennifer unearthed several bones that appeared to be the remains of a human skull. The skull was disarticulated. She carefully removed and cleaned each bone. Her task was to identify the bones and determine if the bones were those of an adult skull or an infant skull.

1. Among the bones she found was an irregularly shaped bone that resembled a bat. What is the name of this bone?
   a. Ethmoid
   b. Occipital
   c. Lacrimal
   d. Sphenoid
2. Jennifer could not reconstruct the entire cranium. She found only one frontal bone, two parietal bones, two temporal bones, one sphenoid bone, and one ethmoid bone. Which cranial bone was missing?
   a. Lacrimal
   b. Zygomatic
   c. Occipital
   d. Mandible
3. After reconstructing the skull, Jennifer noticed that the face formed about 1/8 of the entire skull. She also noticed that there were significant gaps between the cranial bones and concluded it belonged to:
   a. An adult
   b. A newborn infant
   c. A male
   d. A female

Hint To solve a case study, you may have to refer to the glossary or index, other chapters in this textbook, ***Connect It!,*** and other resources.

CHAPTER SUMMARY

To download an MP3 version of the chapter summary for use with your mobile device, access the ***Audio Chapter Summaries*** *online at evolve.elsevier.com.*

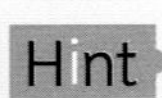

Scan this summary after reading the chapter to help you reinforce the key concepts. Later, use the summary as a quick review before your class or before a test.

Introduction

A. Skeletal tissues form bones—the organs of the skeletal system
B. The relationship of bones to one another and to other body structures provides a basis for understanding the function of other organ systems
C. The adult skeleton is composed of 206 separate bones

Divisions of the Skeleton (Figure 12-1; Table 12-1)

A. Axial skeleton—the 80 bones of the head, neck, and torso; composed of 74 bones that form the upright axis of the body and six tiny middle ear bones
B. Appendicular skeleton—the 126 bones that form the appendages to the axial skeleton; the upper and lower extremities

Axial Skeleton

A. Skull—made up of 28 bones in two major divisions: cranial bones and facial bones (**Figures 12-2** to **12-7**; **Table 12-3**)
  1. Cranial bones
    a. Frontal bone (**Figure 12-8**, *C*)
      (1) Forms the forehead and anterior part of the top of the cranium
      (2) Contains the frontal sinuses
      (3) Forms the upper portion of the orbits
      (4) Forms the coronal suture with the two parietal bones
    b. Parietal bones (**Figure 12-8**, *A*)
      (1) Form the bulging top of the cranium
      (2) Form several sutures: lambdoid suture with the occipital bone; squamous suture with the temporal bone and part of the sphenoid; and coronal suture with the frontal bone
    c. Temporal bones (**Figure 12-8**, *B*)
      (1) Form the lower sides of the cranium and part of the cranial floor
      (2) Contain the inner and middle ears
    d. Occipital bone (**Figure 12-8**, *D*)
      (1) Forms the lower, posterior part of the skull
      (2) Forms immovable joints with three other cranial bones and a movable joint with the first cervical vertebra
    e. Sphenoid bone (**Figure 12-8**, *E*)
      (1) A bat-shaped bone located in the central portion of the cranial floor
      (2) Anchors the frontal, parietal, occipital, and ethmoid bones and forms part of the lateral wall of the cranium and part of the floor of each orbit (**Figure 12-7**)
      (3) Contains the sphenoid sinuses
    f. Ethmoid bone (**Figure 12-8**, *F*)
      (1) A complex, irregular bone that lies anterior to the sphenoid and posterior to the nasal bones
      (2) Forms the anterior cranial floor, medial orbit walls, upper parts of the nasal septum, and sidewalls of the nasal cavity
      (3) The cribriform plate is located in the ethmoid
  2. Facial bones (**Table 12-4**)
    a. Maxilla (upper jaw) (**Figure 12-8**, *H*)
      (1) Two maxillae form the keystone of the face
      (2) Maxillae articulate with each other and with the nasal, zygomatic, inferior concha, and palatine bones
      (3) Forms parts of the orbital floors, roof of the mouth, and floor and sidewalls of the nose
      (4) Contains maxillary sinuses
    b. Mandible (lower jaw) (**Figure 12-8**, *M*)
      (1) Largest, strongest bone of the face
      (2) Forms the only movable joint of the skull with the temporal bone
    c. Zygomatic bone (**Figure 12-8**, *I*)
      (1) Shapes the cheek and forms the outer margin of the orbit
      (2) Forms the zygomatic arch with the zygomatic process of the temporal bones
    d. Nasal bone (**Figures 12-8**, *L* and **12-10**)
      (1) Both nasal bones form the upper part of the bridge of the nose, whereas cartilage forms the lower part
      (2) Articulates with the ethmoid, nasal septum, frontal bone, maxillae, and the other nasal bone
    e. Lacrimal bone (**Figure 12-8**, *K*)
      (1) Paper-thin bone that lies just posterior and lateral to each nasal bone
      (2) Forms the nasal cavity and medial wall of the orbit
      (3) Contains a groove for the nasolacrimal (tear) duct
      (4) Articulates with the maxilla, frontal, and ethmoid bones
    f. Palatine bone (**Figure 12-8**, *J*)
      (1) Two bones form the posterior part of the hard palate
      (2) Vertical portion forms the lateral wall of the posterior part of each nasal cavity
      (3) Articulates with the maxillae and the sphenoid bone
    g. Inferior nasal conchae (turbinates)
      (1) Form the lower edge projecting into the nasal cavity and form the nasal meatus
      (2) Articulate with ethmoid, lacrimal, maxillary, and palatine bones
    h. Vomer bone (**Figure 12-8**, *G*)
      (1) Forms the posterior portion of the nasal septum
      (2) Articulates with the sphenoid, ethmoid, palatine, and maxillae

B. Eye orbits (**Figure 12-7**)
  1. Right and left eye orbits
    a. Contain eyes, associated eye muscles, lacrimal apparatus, blood vessels, and nerves
    b. Thin and fragile orbital walls separate orbital structures from the cranial and nasal cavities and paranasal sinuses

C. Fetal skull (**Figure 12-11**)
   1. Characterized by unique anatomical features not seen in adult skull
   2. Fontanelles or "soft spots" (4) allow the skull to "mould" during the birth process and also allow for rapid growth of the brain (**Table 12-5**)
   3. Permits differential growth or appearance of skull components over time
      a. Face—smaller proportion of total cranium at birth (⅛) than in adult (½)
      b. Head at birth is ¼ the total height; at maturity about ⅛ body height
      c. Sutures appear with skeletal maturity (**Table 12-5**)
      d. Paranasal sinuses—change in size and placement with skeletal maturity (**Figure 12-9**)
      e. Appearance of deciduous and, later, permanent teeth

D. Hyoid bone (**Figure 12-12**)
   1. U-shaped bone located just above the larynx and below the mandible
   2. Suspended from the styloid processes of the temporal bone
   3. Only bone in the body that articulates with no other bones

E. Vertebral column (**Figure 12-13**)
   1. Forms the flexible longitudinal axis of the skeleton
   2. Consists of 24 vertebrae plus the sacrum and coccyx
   3. Segments of the vertebral column:
      a. Cervical vertebrae, 7
      b. Thoracic vertebrae, 12
      c. Lumbar vertebrae, 5
      d. Sacrum—in adults, results from the fusion of five separate vertebrae
      e. Coccyx—in adults, results from the fusion of three to five separate vertebrae
   4. Characteristics of the vertebrae (**Figure 12-14**; **Table 12-6**)
      a. All vertebrae, except the first, have a flat, rounded body anteriorly and centrally, a spinous process posteriorly, and two transverse processes laterally
      b. All but the sacrum and coccyx have a vertebral foramen
      c. Second cervical vertebra has an upward projection, the dens, to allow rotation of the head
      d. Seventh cervical vertebra has a long, blunt spinous process
      e. Each thoracic vertebra has articular facets for the ribs
   5. Vertebral column as a whole articulated with the head, ribs, and iliac bones
   6. Individual vertebrae articulate with one another in joints between their bodies and between their articular processes

F. Sternum (**Figure 12-15**)
   1. Dagger-shaped bone in the middle of the anterior chest wall made up of three parts:
      a. Manubrium—the upper handle part
      b. Body—middle blade part
      c. Xiphoid process—blunt cartilaginous lower tip, which ossifies during adult life
   2. Manubrium articulates with the clavicle and first rib
   3. Next nine ribs join the body of the sternum, either directly or indirectly, by means of the costal cartilages

G. Ribs (**Figures 12-15** and **12-16**)
   1. Twelve pairs of ribs, with the vertebral column and sternum, form the thorax
   2. Each rib articulates with the body and transverse process of its corresponding thoracic vertebra
   3. Ribs 2 through 9 articulate with the body of the vertebra above
   4. From its vertebral attachment, each rib curves outward, then forward and downward
   5. Rib attachment to the sternum:
      a. True ribs—pairs 1 through 7 join a costal cartilage that attaches it to the sternum
      b. False ribs—pairs 8 through 12
         (i) Pairs 8, 9 and 10 have costal cartilage that joins the cartilage of the rib above to be indirectly attached to the sternum
         (ii) Floating ribs—11 and 12 do not attach (even indirectly) to the sternum

REVIEW QUESTIONS

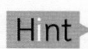

Write out the answers to these questions after reading the chapter and reviewing the Chapter Summary. Note—writing out your answers will consolidate learning and provide a valuable resource of information.

1. Describe the skeleton as a whole and identify its two major subdivisions.
2. Identify and differentiate between the bones in the cranium and face. List the bones of each.
3. Name and locate the fontanelles and sutures of the skull.
4. Name the five pairs of bony sinuses in the skull.
5. Discuss the clinical (medical) importance of the cribriform plate of the ethmoid bone and the mastoid air cells in the temporal bone.
6. Identify and discuss the normal primary and secondary curves of the spine. When in a child's life do the cervical and lumbar curves develop?
7. Identify the bony components of the thorax.
8. Describe vertebroplasty.
9. What are some of the functions of foramina in the skeleton?

CRITICAL THINKING QUESTIONS

After finishing the Review Questions, write out the answers to these more in-depth questions to help you apply your new knowledge. Go back to sections of the chapter that relate to concepts that you find difficult.

1. What are some functional advantages of the fontanelles of a baby's skull during the birth process?
2. Which part of the cranium is likely to be the thinnest? Give a reason for your answer.
3. What is the functional advantage of having air spaces in skull bones? What is a disadvantage to having these spaces lined with mucous membrane?

13 Appendicular Skeleton

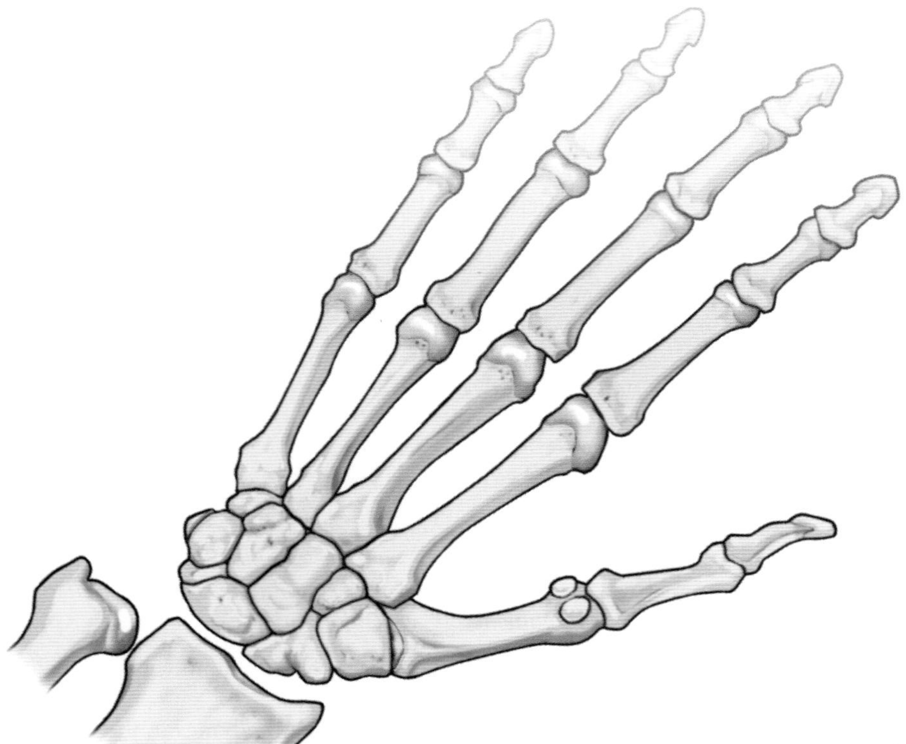

CHAPTER OUTLINE

Hint Scan this outline before you begin to read the chapter, as a preview of how the concepts are organized.

In the previous chapter we began our survey of the central or axial skeleton. This chapter continues the survey of bones of the human skeleton by exploring the peripheral or appendicular skeleton. The term *appendicular* literally means "relating to appendages", which are the upper extremity and the lower extremity. The upper extremity includes the bones of the shoulder girdle, arm, forearm, wrist, and hand (including fingers). The lower extremity includes the bones of the pelvic (hip) girdle, thigh, leg, ankle, and foot (including toes). The extremities or appendages involve many of the movable joints of the body—a topic that will be explored next, in Chapter 14.

LANGUAGE OF SCIENCE

Hint *Use this list to aid your pronunciation of unfamiliar words.*

carpal bone (KAR-pul bohn)
[*carp-* **wrist,** *-al* **relating to**]

chronological age (kroh-nah-LODJ-i-kul ayj)
[*chrono-*, **time,** *-log-* **words (study of),** *-ical* **relating to**]

clavicle (KLAV-i-kul)
[*clavi-* **key,** *-cle* **little**]

coxal bone (KOK-sal bohn)
[*coxa-* **hip,** *-al* **relating to**]

false pelvis (fals PEL-vis)
[*pelvis* **basin**]

femur (FEE-mur)
[*femur* **thigh**]

fibula (FIB-yoo-lah)
[*fibula* **clasp**] *pl.*, fibulae or fibulas

humerus (HYOO-mer-us)
[*humerus* **arm**] *pl.*, humeri

ilium (IL-ee-um)
[*ilium* **flank**] *pl.*, ilia

ischium (IS-kee-um)
[*ischium* **hip joint**] *pl.*, ischia

lateral longitudinal arch (LAT-er-al lon-jih-TYOO-di-nal)
[*later-* **side,** *-al* **relating to,** *longitud-* **length,** *-al* **relating to**]

longitudinal arch (lon-ji-TYOO-di-nal)
[*longitud-* **length,** *-al* **relating to**]

medial longitudinal arch (MEE-dee-al lon-ji-TYOO-dih-nal)
[*medi-* **middle,** *-al* **relating to,** *longitud-* **length,** *-al* **relating to**]

metacarpal bone (met-ah-KAR-pal)
[*meta-* **beyond,** *-carp-* **wrist,** *-al* **relating to**]

palpable (PAL-pah-bul)
[*palp-* **touch gently,** *-able* **capable**]

patella (pah-TEL-ah)
[*pat-* **dish,** *-ella* **small**] *pl.*, patellae

pelvic girdle (PEL-vic GER-dul)
[*pelvi-* **basin,** *-ic* **relating to,** *girdle* **belt**]

pubis (PYOO-biss)
[*pubis* **groin**] *pl.*, pubes

radius (RAY-dee-us)
[*radius* **ray**] *pl.*, radii

scapula (SKAP-yoo-lah)
[*scapula* **shoulder blade**] *pl.*, scapulae

continued on p. 280

UPPER EXTREMITY

The upper extremity—also called the *upper limb*—consists of the bones of the shoulder girdle, upper part of the arm, forearm, wrist, and hand (**Figure 13-1**).

Shoulder Girdle

Two bones, the **clavicle** and **scapula,** compose the **shoulder girdle** or *pectoral girdle.* Contrary to appearances, this belt or girdle of bone forms only one bony joint with the trunk: the sternoclavicular joint between the manubrium of the sternum and the clavicle. At its outer end, the clavicle articulates with the scapula, which attaches to the ribs by muscles and tendons, not by a true joint. All shoulder movements therefore involve the sternoclavicular joint. Various markings of the scapula are described in **Table 13-1** (see also **Figure 13-2**).

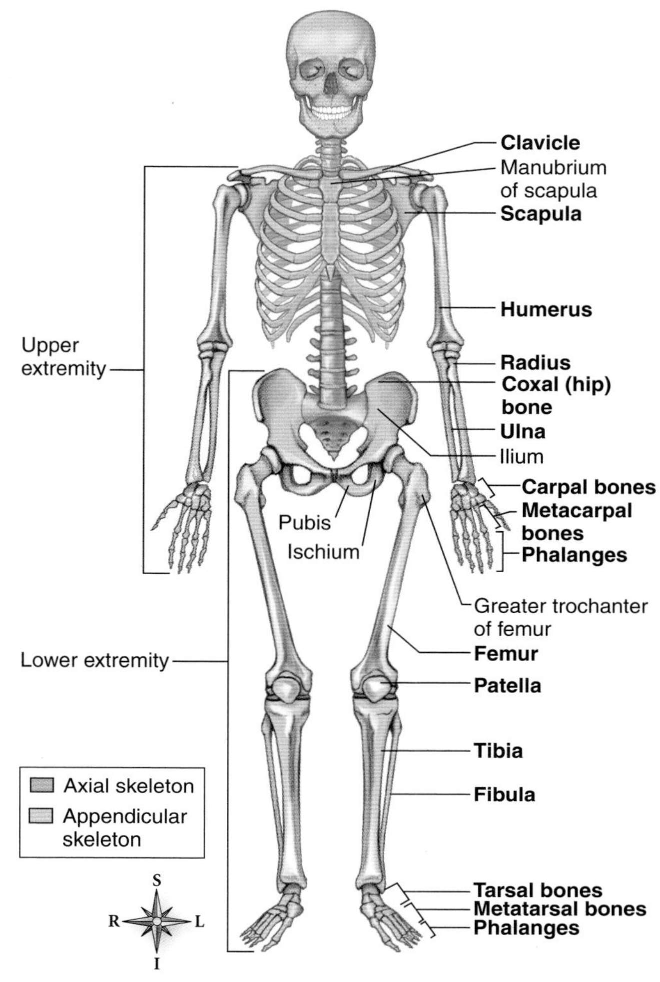

FIGURE 13-1 Appendicular skeleton. Overview of the upper extremity and lower extremity.

TABLE 13-1 Upper Extremity Bones and Their Markings

BONES AND MARKINGS	DESCRIPTION
Clavicle	Collar bones; the shoulder girdle is joined to the axial skeleton by articulation of the clavicles with the sternum (the scapula does not form a joint with the axial skeleton)
Scapula	Shoulder blades; the scapulae and clavicles together make up the shoulder girdle
Borders	Outer edges or margins of the scapula
Superior	Upper margin
Medial (vertebral)	Margin toward the vertebral column
Lateral (axillary)	Lateral margin, toward axilla
Angles	Corners of scapula where the borders meet
Inferior angle	Corner where lateral and medial border meet at bottom of scapula
Lateral angle	Corner where lateral and superior border meet at glenoid cavity
Superior (medial) angle	Corner where medial and superior border meet at top of scapula
Spine	Sharp ridge running diagonally across the posterior surface of the shoulder blade
Acromion	Slightly flaring projection at the lateral end of the scapular spine; may be felt at the tip of the shoulder; articulates with the clavicle
Coracoid process	Projection on the anterior surface from the upper border of the bone; may be felt in the groove between the deltoid and pectoralis major muscles, about 25 mm below the clavicle
Glenoid cavity	Arm socket

(continued on page 267)

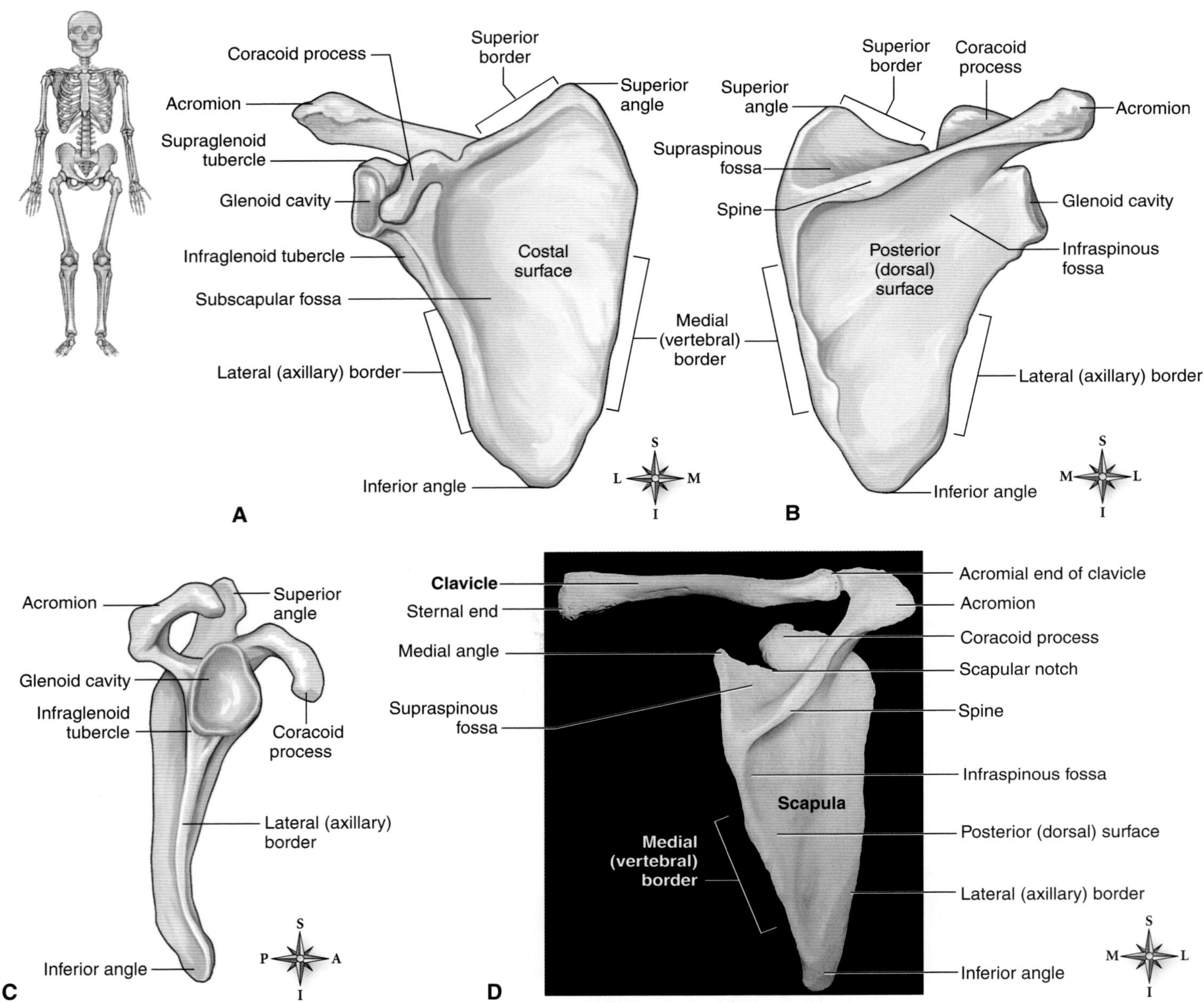

FIGURE 13-2 Right scapula. **A,** Anterior view. **B,** Posterior view. **C,** Lateral view. **D,** Posterior view showing articulation of the right scapula with the clavicle. (The skeleton inset shows the relative position of the right scapula within the entire skeleton.)

Arm

The **humerus,** or arm bone, like other long bones, consists of a shaft, or diaphysis, and two ends, or epiphyses (**Figure 13-3** and **Figure 13-4**).

The upper epiphysis bears several identifying structures: the head, anatomical neck, greater and lesser tubercles, intertubercular groove, and surgical neck. On the diaphysis are found the deltoid tuberosity and the radial groove. The distal epiphysis has four projections—the medial and lateral epicondyles, the capitulum, and the trochlea—and two depressions—the olecranon and coronoid fossae. For descriptions of all of these markings, see **Table 13-1**.

The humerus articulates proximally with the scapula and distally with the radius and the ulna.

Forearm

Two bones form the framework for the forearm: the **radius** on the thumb side and the **ulna** on the little finger side.

At the proximal end of the ulna, the olecranon projects posteriorly and the coronoid process projects anteriorly. There are also two depressions: the semilunar notch on the anterior surface and the radial notch on the lateral surface. The distal end has two projections: a rounded head and a sharper styloid process. For more detailed identification of these markings, see **Table 13-1**. The ulna articulates proximally with the humerus and radius and distally with a fibrocartilaginous disc, but not with any of the carpal bones.

The radius has three projections: two at its proximal end, the head and radial tuberosity, and one at its distal end, the styloid process (see

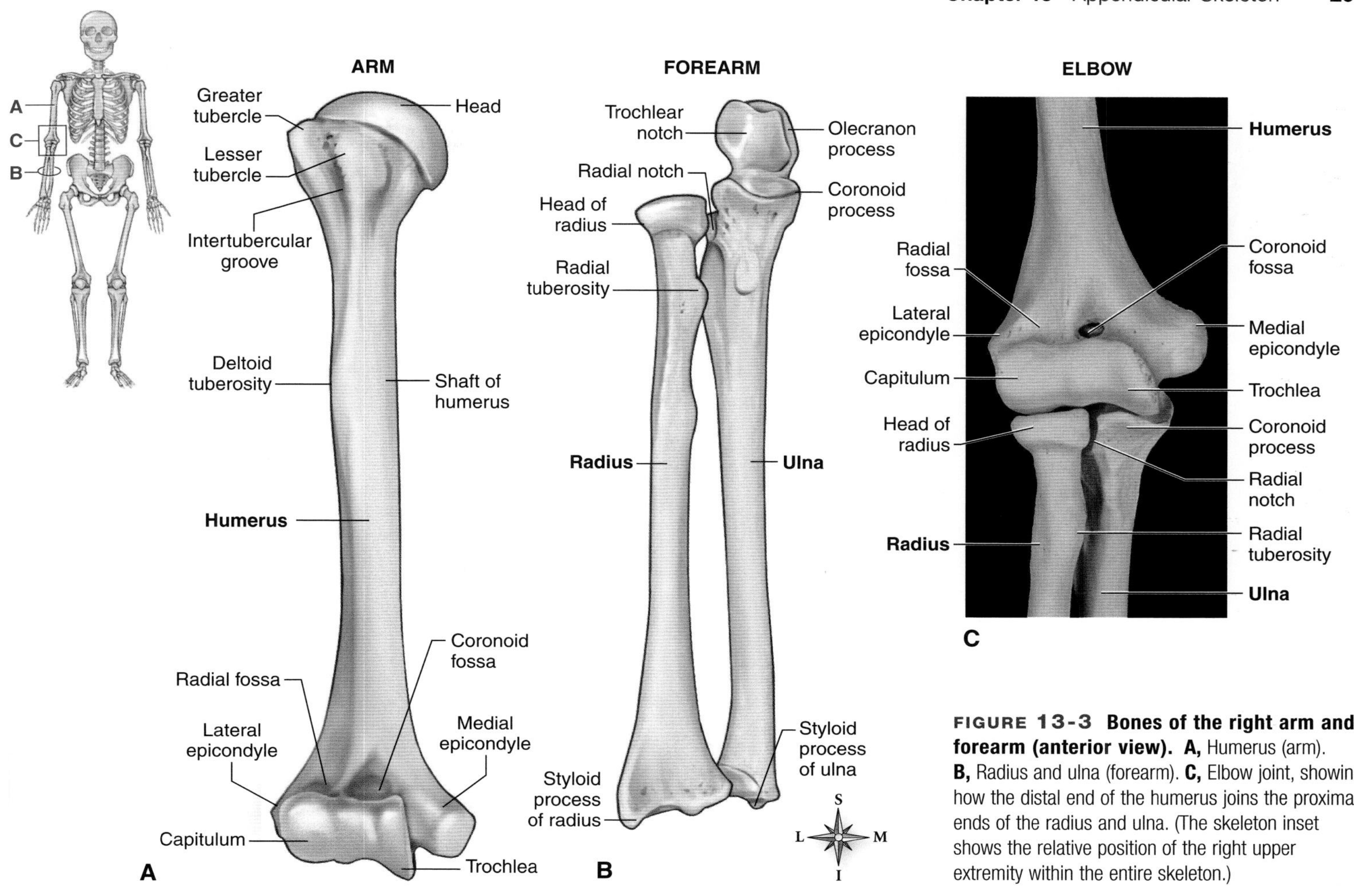

FIGURE 13-3 Bones of the right arm and forearm (anterior view). A, Humerus (arm). **B,** Radius and ulna (forearm). **C,** Elbow joint, showing how the distal end of the humerus joins the proximal ends of the radius and ulna. (The skeleton inset shows the relative position of the right upper extremity within the entire skeleton.)

TABLE 13-1 Upper Extremity Bones and Their Markings—cont'd

BONES AND MARKINGS	DESCRIPTION
Humerus	Long bone of the arm
Head	Smooth, hemispherical enlargement at the proximal end of the humerus
Anatomical neck	Oblique groove just below the head
Greater tubercle	Rounded projection lateral to the head on the anterior surface
Lesser tubercle	Prominent projection on the anterior surface just below the anatomical neck
Intertubercular groove	Deep groove between the greater and lesser tubercles; the long tendon of the biceps muscle lodges here
Surgical neck	Region just below the tubercles; so named because of its liability to fracture
Deltoid tuberosity	V-shaped, rough area about midway down the shaft where the deltoid muscle inserts
Radial groove	Groove running obliquely downward from the deltoid tuberosity; lodges the radial nerve
Epicondyles (medial and lateral)	Rough projections at both sides of the distal end
Capitulum	Rounded knob below the lateral epicondyle; articulates with the radius; sometimes called the *radial* head of the humerus
Trochlea	Projection with a deep depression through the centre similar to the shape of a pulley; articulates with the ulna
Olecranon fossa	Depression on the posterior surface just above the trochlea; receives the olecranon of the ulna when the forearm extends
Coronoid fossa	Depression on the anterior surface above the trochlea; receives the coronoid process of the ulna in flexion of the forearm

(continued)

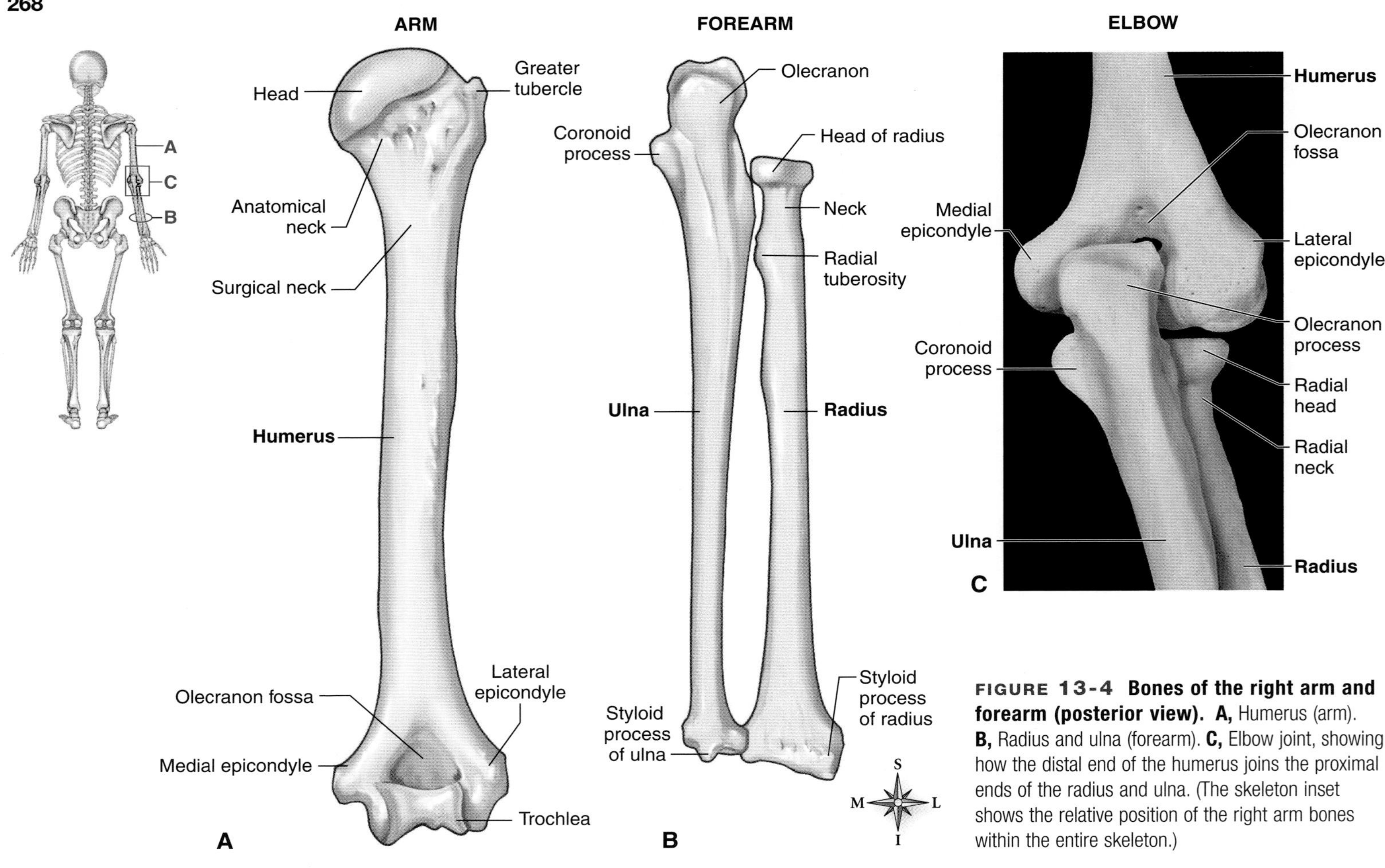

FIGURE 13-4 Bones of the right arm and forearm (posterior view). A, Humerus (arm). **B,** Radius and ulna (forearm). **C,** Elbow joint, showing how the distal end of the humerus joins the proximal ends of the radius and ulna. (The skeleton inset shows the relative position of the right arm bones within the entire skeleton.)

TABLE 13-1 Upper Extremity Bones and Their Markings—cont'd

BONES AND MARKINGS	DESCRIPTION
Radius	Bone of the thumb side of the forearm
Head	Disc-shaped process forming the proximal end of the radius; articulates with the capitulum of the humerus and with the radial notch of the ulna
Radial tuberosity	Roughened projection on the ulnar side, a short distance below the head; the biceps muscle inserts here
Styloid process	Protuberance at the distal end on the lateral surface (with the forearm in the anatomical position)
Ulna	Bone of the little finger side of the forearm; longer than the radius
Olecranon	Scooplike process that joins the trochlea of the humerus at the elbow
Coronoid process	Projection on the anterior surface of the proximal end of the ulna; the trochlea of the humerus fits snugly between the olecranon and coronoid processes
Trochlear notch	Curved notch between the olecranon and coronoid processes into which the trochlea fits; also called *semilunar notch*
Radial notch	Curved notch lateral and inferior to the trochlear notch; the head of the radius fits into this concavity
Head	Rounded process at the distal end; does not articulate with the wrist bones but with the fibrocartilaginous disc
Styloid process	Sharp protuberance at the distal end; can be seen from outside on the posterior surface
Carpal bones	Wrist bones; arranged in two rows at the proximal end of the hand; proximal row (from the little finger toward the thumb)—**pisiform, triquetrum, lunate**, and **scaphoid**; distal row—**hamate, capitate, trapezoid**, and **trapezium**
Metacarpal bones	Long bones forming the framework of the palm of the hand; numbered (from lateral side) **I, II, III, IV, V**
Phalanges	Miniature long bones of the fingers, three in each finger, two in each thumb; numbered (from medial/thumb side), each with a *base*, *shaft*, and *head,* lined up like a military parade formation (phalanx)
Proximal (I, II, III, IV, V)	
Middle (II, III, IV, V)	
Distal (I, II, III, IV, V)	

Figures 13-3 and **13-4**). There are two proximal articulations: one with the capitulum of the humerus and the other with the radial notch of the ulna. The three distal articulations are with the scaphoid and lunate carpal bones and with the head of the ulna.

Hand

The eight **carpal bones** (**Figure 13-5**) form what most people think of as the wrist but what, anatomically speaking, is the upper part of the hand. Only one of the carpal bones is evident from the outside, the pisiform bone, which projects posteriorly on the little finger side as a small rounded elevation. The pisiform bone is an example of a sesamoid bone.

Ligaments bind the carpal bones closely and firmly together in two rows of four each: proximal row (from the little finger toward the thumb)—pisiform, triquetrum, lunate, and scaphoid bones; distal row—hamate, capitate, trapezoid, and trapezium bones. The joints between the carpal bones and radius permit wrist and hand movements.

Of the five **metacarpal bones** that form the framework of the hand, the thumb metacarpal forms the most freely movable joint with the carpal bones. This fact has great significance. Because of the wide range of movement possible between the thumb metacarpal and the trapezium, particularly the ability to oppose the thumb to the fingers, the human hand has much greater dexterity than the

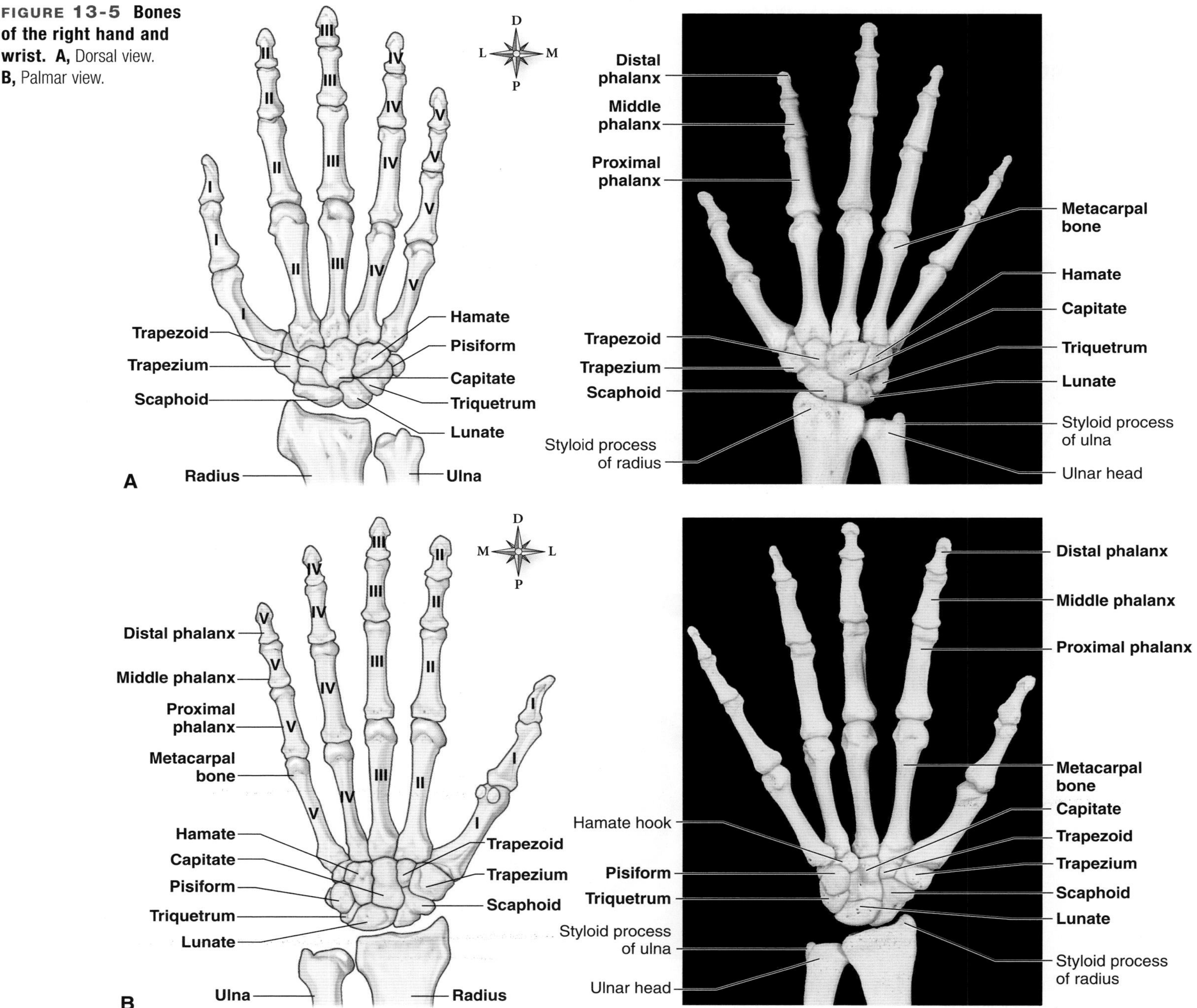

FIGURE 13-5 Bones of the right hand and wrist. A, Dorsal view. **B,** Palmar view.

forepaw of any animal, which has enabled humans to manipulate even small objects in their environment effectively.

The heads of the metacarpal bones, prominent as the proximal knuckles of the hand, articulate with the phalanges.

Quick CHECK

1. What bones make up the shoulder girdle? Where does the shoulder girdle form a joint with the axial skeleton?
2. What are the two bones of the forearm? In the anatomical position, which one is lateral?
3. Name the bones of the hand and wrist.

LOWER EXTREMITY

Bones of the hip, thigh, leg, ankle, and foot constitute the lower extremity or *lower limb* (**Table 13-2**).

Pelvic Girdle

Strong ligaments bind each **coxal bone** (*pelvic* or *hip bone*) to the sacrum posteriorly and to each other anteriorly to form the **pelvic girdle** (see **Figure 13-6** and **Figure 13-11**). The pelvic girdle serves as a stable, circular base that supports the trunk and attaches the lower extremities to it. (The coxal bone was formerly called the os coxae or innominate bone.)

In early life, each coxal bone is made up of three separate bones. Later, they fuse into a single, massive irregular bone that is broader than any other bone in the body. The largest and uppermost of the three bones is the **ilium,** the strongest and lowermost is the **ischium,** and the most anteriorly placed is the **pubis.** Numerous markings are present on the three bones (see **Table 13-2** and **Figure 13-6** and **Figure 13-7**).

The pelvis can be divided into two parts by an imaginary plane called the *pelvic inlet.* The edge of this plane, outlined in **Figure 13-6**, is called the *pelvic brim,* or *brim of the true pelvis.* The structure above the pelvic inlet, termed the **false pelvis,** is bordered by muscle in the front and by bone along the sides and back. The structure below the pelvic inlet, the so-called *true pelvis,* creates the boundary of another imaginary plane called the *pelvic outlet.* It is through the pelvic outlet that the digestive tract empties. The female reproductive tract also passes through the pelvic outlet; this is a fact of great importance in childbirth. The pelvic outlet is often just large enough for the passage of a baby during delivery; however, careful

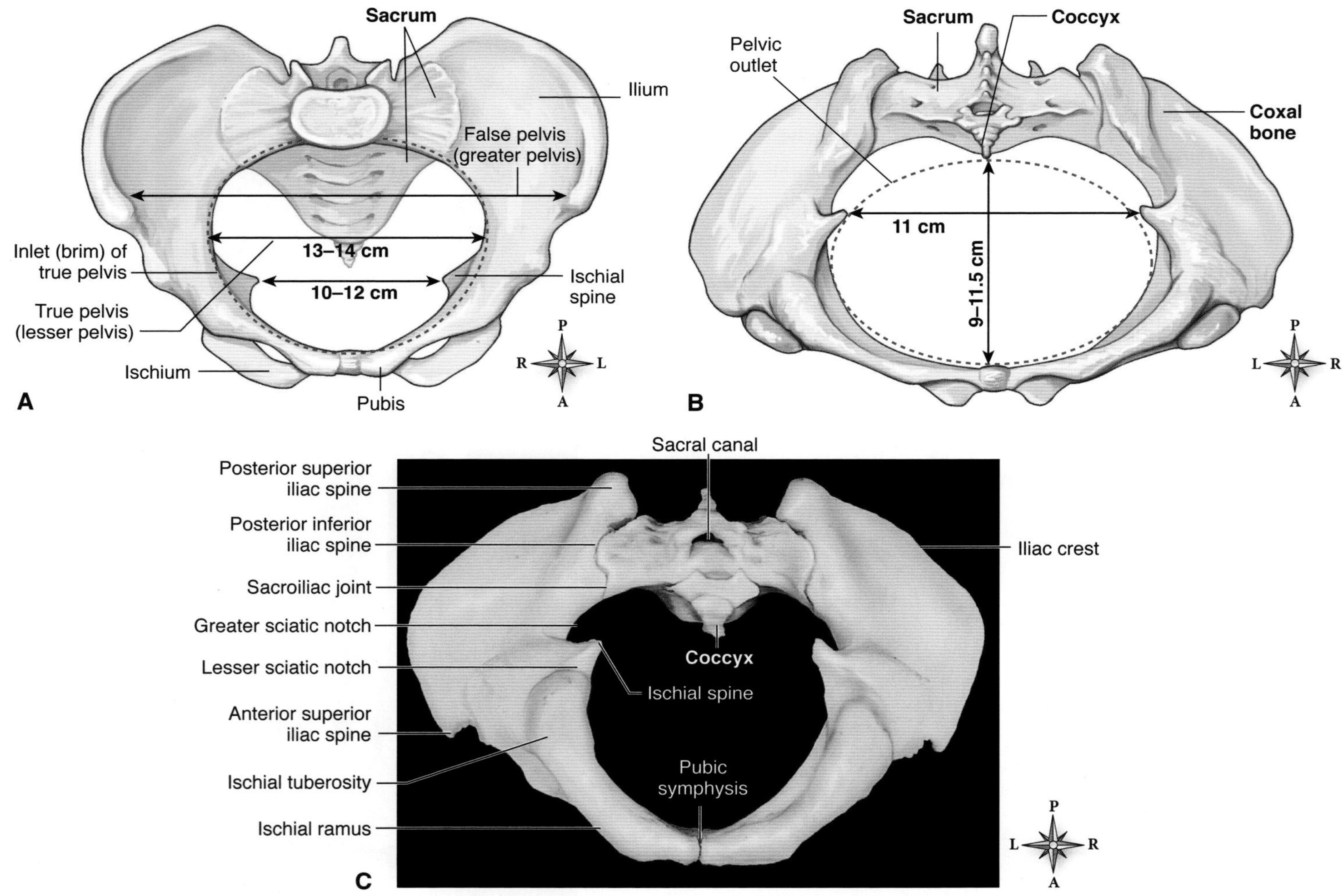

FIGURE 13-6 The female pelvis. A, Pelvis viewed from above. Note that the brim of the true pelvis (*dotted line*) marks the boundary between the superior false pelvis (*pelvis major*) and the inferior true pelvis (*pelvis minor*). **B** and **C,** Pelvis viewed from below. A comparison of the male pelvis and female pelvis is shown in **Figure 13-11**.

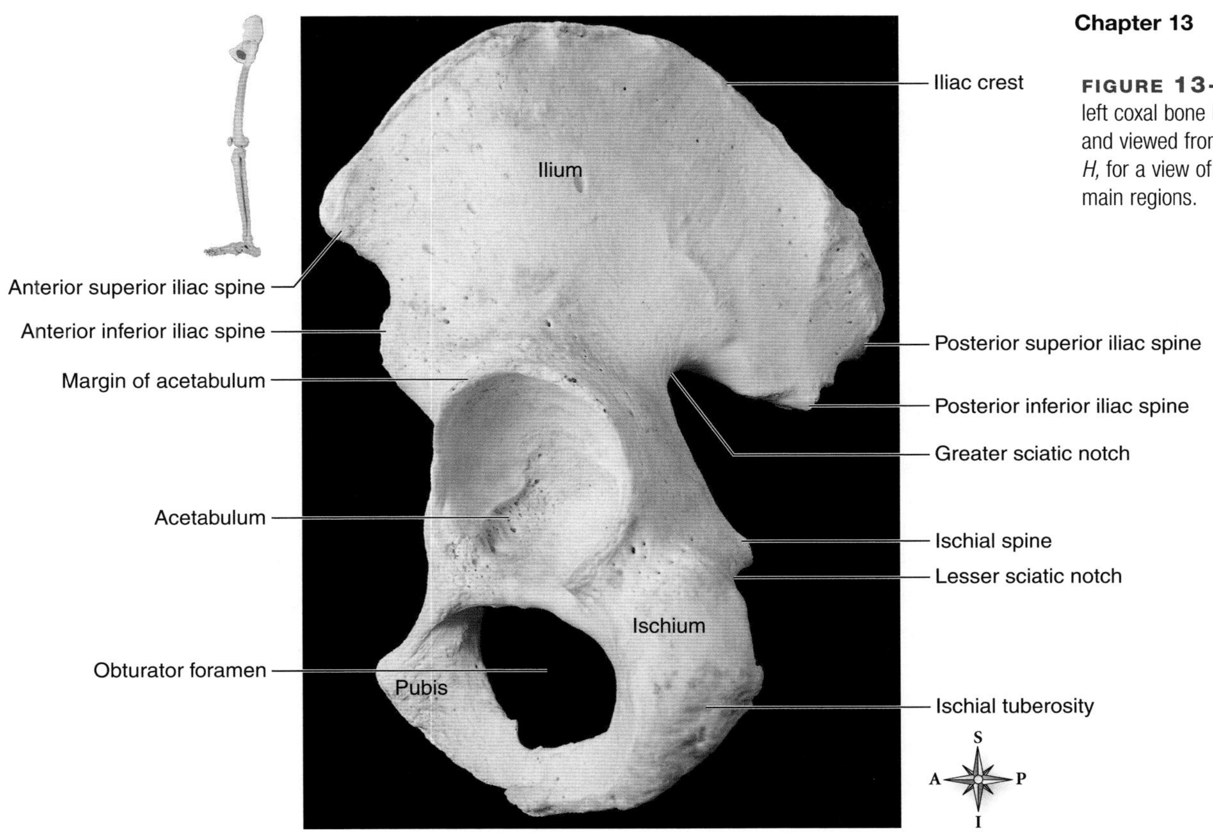

FIGURE 13-7 Left coxal (hip) bone. The left coxal bone is disarticulated from the bony pelvis and viewed from the side. Also see **Figure 12-14**, *H,* for a view of the right coxal bone outlining its three main regions.

UNIT 2

TABLE 13-2 Lower Extremity Bones and Their Markings

BONES AND MARKINGS	DESCRIPTION
Coxal	Large hip bone (pelvic bone); with the sacrum and coccyx, forms the basinlike pelvic cavity; lower extremities attached to the axial skeleton by the coxal bones
Ilium	Upper, flaring portion
Ischium	Lower, posterior portion
Pubis	Medial, anterior portion
Acetabulum	Hip socket; formed by union of the ilium, ischium, and pubis
Iliac crests	Upper, curving boundary of the ilium
Iliac spines	
Anterior superior	Prominent projection at the anterior end of the iliac crest; can be felt externally as the "point" of the hip
Anterior inferior	Less prominent projection short distance below anterior superior spine
Posterior superior	At the posterior end of the iliac crest
Posterior inferior	Just below the posterior superior spine
Greater sciatic notch	Large notch on the posterior surface of the ilium just below the posterior inferior spine
Ischial tuberosity	Large, rough, quadrilateral process forming the inferior part of the ischium; in an erect sitting position the body rests on these tuberosities
Ischial spine	Pointed projection just above the tuberosity
Pubic symphysis	Cartilaginous, amphiarthrotic joint between the pubic bones
Superior pubic ramus	Part of the pubis lying between the symphysis and acetabulum; forms the upper part of the obturator foramen
Inferior pubic ramus	Part extending down from the symphysis; unites with the ischium
Pubic arch	Curve formed by the two inferior rami
Subpubic angle	Angle formed under the inferior pubic rami; generally larger in women than in men
Pubic crest	Upper margin of the superior ramus
Pubic tubercle	Rounded process at the end of the crest

(continued)

TABLE 13-2 Lower Extremity Bones and Their Markings—cont'd

BONES AND MARKINGS	DESCRIPTION
Coxal—cont'd	
Obturator foramen	Large hole in the anterior surface of the coxal bone; formed by the pubis and ischium; largest foramen in the body
Pelvic inlet (or brim)	Boundary of the aperture leading into the true pelvis; formed by the pubic crests, iliopectineal lines, and sacral promontory; the size and shape of this inlet have obstetrical importance because if any of its diameters are too small, the infant's skull cannot enter the true pelvis for natural birth (or lesser pelvis)
True pelvis (or greater pelvis)	Space below the pelvic brim; true "basin" with bone and muscle walls and a muscle floor; pelvic organs located in this space
False pelvis (or lesser pelvis)	Broad, shallow space above the pelvic brim, or the pelvic inlet; name "false pelvis" is misleading because this space is actually part of the abdominal cavity, not the pelvic cavity
Pelvic outlet	Irregular circumference marking the lower limits of the true pelvis; bounded by the tip of the coccyx and two ischial tuberosities
Pelvic girdle (or bony pelvis)	Complete bony ring; composed of two hip bones (ossa coxae), the sacrum, and the coccyx; forms a firm base by which the trunk rests on the thighs and for attachment of the lower extremities to the axial skeleton
Femur	Thigh bone; largest, strongest bone of the body
Head	Rounded upper end of the bone; fits into the acetabulum
Neck	Constricted portion just below the head
Greater trochanter	Protuberance located inferiorly and laterally to the head
Lesser trochanter	Small protuberance located inferiorly and medially to the greater trochanter
Intertrochanteric line	Line extending between the greater and lesser trochanter
Linea aspera	Prominent ridge extending lengthwise along the concave posterior surface
Supracondylar ridges	Two ridges formed by division of the linea aspera at its lower end; the medial supracondylar ridge extends inward to the inner condyle, the lateral ridge to the outer condyle
Condyles	Large, rounded bulges at the distal end of the femur; one medial and one lateral
Epicondyles	Blunt projections from the sides of the condyles; one on the medial aspect and one on the lateral aspect
Adductor tubercle	Small projection just above the medial condyle; marks the termination of the medial supracondylar ridge
Trochlea	Smooth depression between the condyles on the anterior surface; articulates with the patella
Intercondylar fossa (notch)	Deep depression between the condyles on the posterior surface; the cruciate ligaments, which help bind the femur to the tibia, lodge in this notch
Patella	Kneecap; largest sesamoid bone of the body; embedded in the tendon of the quadriceps femoris muscle
Tibia	Shin bone
Condyles	Bulging prominences at the proximal end of the tibia; upper surfaces concave for articulation with the femur
Intercondylar eminence	Upward projection on the articular surface between the condyles
Crest	Sharp ridge on the anterior surface
Tibial tuberosity	Projection in the midline on the anterior surface
Medial malleolus	Rounded downward projection at the distal end of the tibia; forms the prominence on the medial surface of the ankle
Fibula	Long, slender bone of the lateral side of the leg
Lateral malleolus	Rounded prominence at the distal end of the fibula; forms the prominence on the lateral surface of the ankle

(continued on page 276)

positioning of the baby's head is required. Measurements such as those shown in **Figure 13-6** are routinely made via medical imaging by obstetricians to ensure successful delivery.

Despite its apparent rigidity, the joint between the pubic portions of each coxal bone, the *pubic symphysis*, softens before delivery. This softening allows the pelvic outlet to expand to accommodate the newborn's head as it passes out of the birth canal. The tiny coccyx bone, which protrudes into the pelvic outlet, sometimes breaks when the force of labour contractions pushes the newborn's head against it.

Thigh

The two thigh bones, or **femurs,** have the distinction of being the longest and heaviest bones in the body. Several prominent markings characterize them. For example, three projections are conspicuous at each epiphysis: the head and greater and lesser trochanters proximally and the medial and lateral condyles and adductor tubercle distally (**Figure 13-8**). Both condyles and the greater trochanter may be felt externally.

For a description of the various femur markings, see **Table 13-2**.

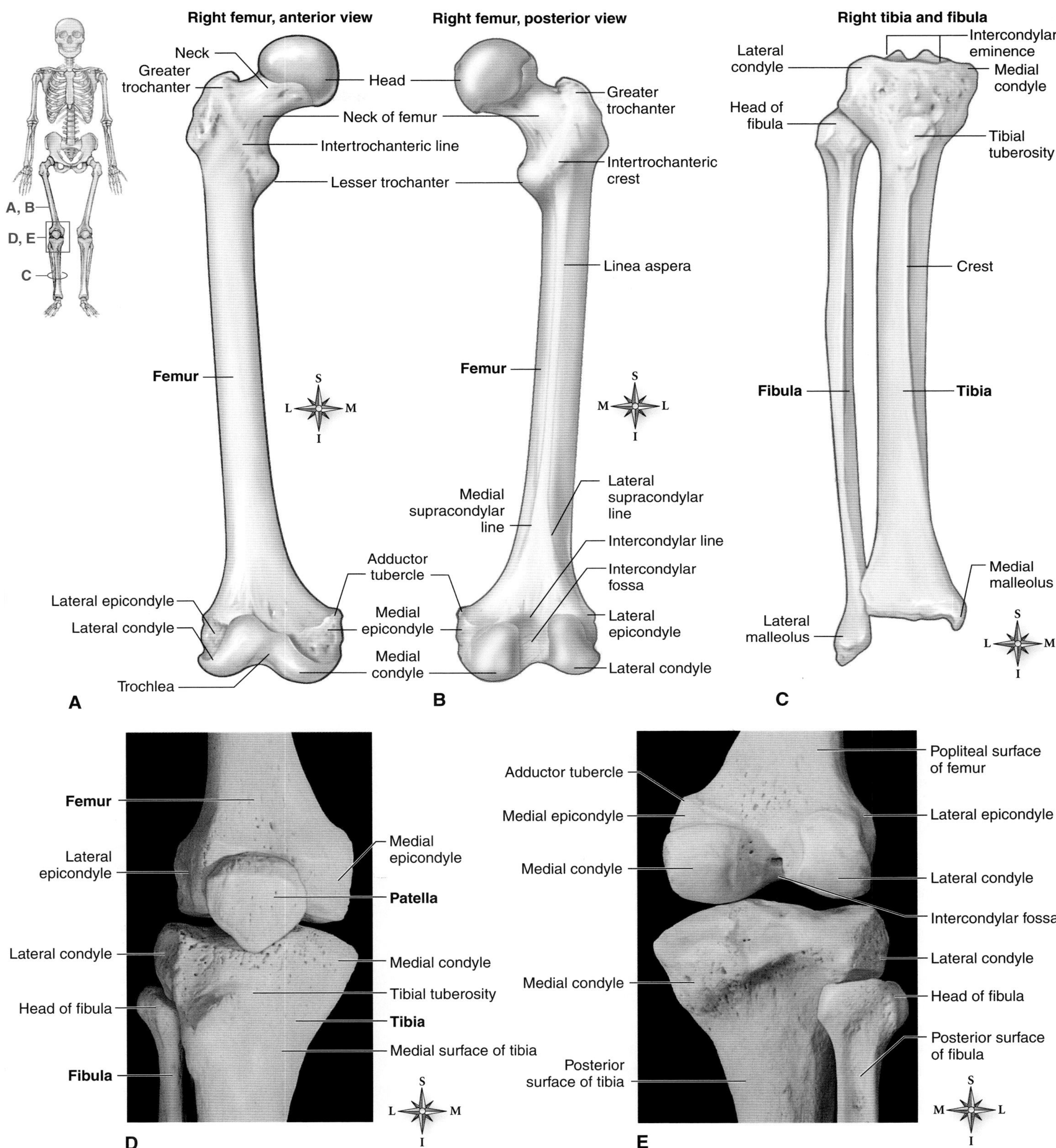

FIGURE 13-8 Bones of the thigh and leg. **A,** Right femur, anterior surface. **B,** Right femur, posterior view. **C,** Right tibia and fibula, anterior surface. **D,** Anterior aspect of the right knee skeleton. **E,** Right tibia and fibula, posterior aspect. (The skeleton inset shows the relative position of the bones of the thigh and leg within the entire skeleton.)

BOX 13-1 *sports and fitness* | **Chondromalacia Patellae**

Chondromalacia patellae is a degenerative process that results in softening (degeneration) of the articular surface of the patella. The symptoms associated with chondromalacia of the patella are a common cause of knee pain in many individuals—especially young athletes. The condition is usually caused by irritation of the patellar groove, with subsequent changes in the cartilage on the underside of the patella. The most common complaint is of pain arising from behind or beneath the kneecap, especially during activities that require flexion of the knee, such as climbing stairs, kneeling, jumping, or running. •

The largest sesamoid bone in the body, and one of the few that is almost universally present, is the **patella,** or kneecap, located in the tendon of the quadriceps femoris muscle as a projection to the underlying knee joint. Although some individuals have sesamoid bones in the tendons of other muscles, lists of bone names do not usually include them because they are not always present, are not found in any particular tendons, and are less important. (See the footnote in **Table 12-1** on p. 236.)

When the knee joint is extended, the patellar outline may be distinguished through the skin, but as the knee flexes, it sinks into the intercondylar notch of the femur and can no longer be easily distinguished.

Box 13-1 describes a condition that may cause patellar pain in young athletes.

Leg

The **tibia** is the larger and stronger and more medially and superficially located of the two leg bones. The **fibula** is smaller and more laterally and deeply placed.

At its proximal end, the fibula articulates with the lateral condyle of the tibia. The proximal end of the tibia, in turn, articulates with the femur to form the knee joint, the largest and one of the most complex and frequently injured joints of the body.

Distally, the tibia articulates with the fibula and also with the talus. The latter fits into a boxlike socket (ankle joint) formed by the medial and lateral malleoli, projections of the tibia and fibula, respectively. For other tibial markings, see **Table 13-2** and **Figure 13-8**. **Box 13-2** explains how the malleoli and other bony prominences can be palpated through the skin.

BOX 13-2 *fyi* | **Palpable Bony Landmarks**

Health professionals often identify externally palpable bony landmarks when dealing with the sick and injured. **Palpable** bony landmarks are bones that can be touched and identified through the skin. They serve as reference points in identifying other body structures.

Externally palpable bony landmarks are present throughout the body. Many skull bones, such as the zygomatic bone, can be palpated. The medial and lateral epicondyles of the humerus, the olecranon of the ulna, and the styloid process of the ulna and the radius at the wrist can be palpated on the upper extremity. The highest corner of the shoulder is the acromion process of the scapula.

When you put your hands on your hips, you can feel the superior edge of the ilium, called the iliac crest. The anterior end of the crest, called the anterior superior iliac spine, is a prominent landmark often used as a clinical reference. The sacral promontory is a prominent anteriorly projecting ridge or border on the superior aspect of the sacrum. Commonly, it serves as a palpable reference point when measuring the pelvis during obstetrical examinations.

The medial malleolus of the tibia and the lateral malleolus of the fibula are prominent at the ankle. The calcaneus, or heel bone, is easily palpated on the posterior aspect of the foot. On the anterior aspect of the lower extremity, examples of palpable bony landmarks include the patella, or kneecap; the anterior border of the tibia, or shin bone; and the metatarsal bones and phalanges of the toes.

Try to identify as many of the externally palpable bones of the skeleton as possible on your own body. Using these as points of reference will make it easier for you to visualize the placement of other bones that cannot be touched or palpated through the skin. •

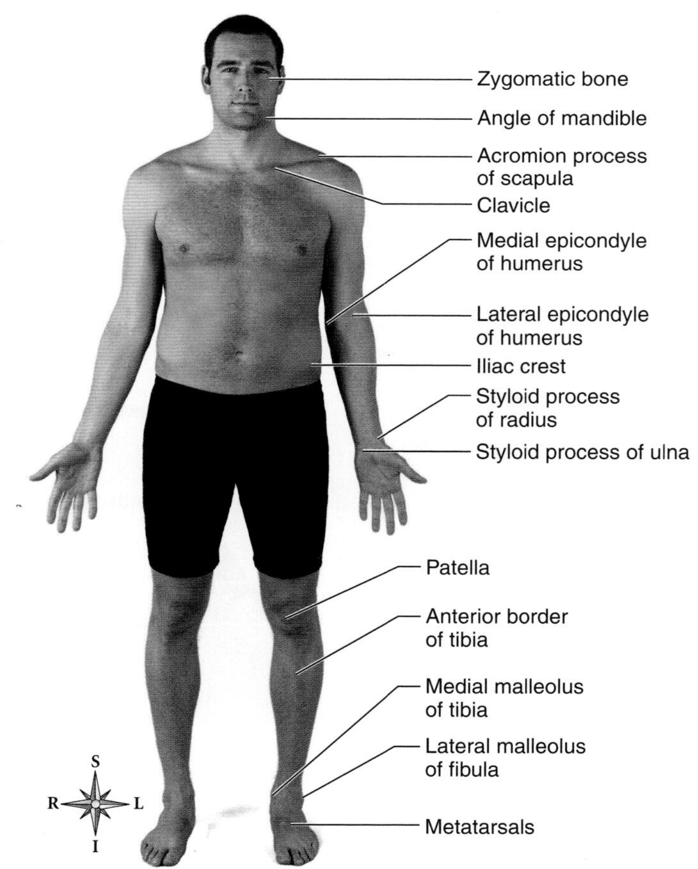

Foot

The structure of the **foot** is similar to that of the hand, with certain differences that adapt it for supporting weight (**Figure 13-9**). One example is the much greater solidity and the more limited mobility of the great toe compared with the thumb. Then, too, the foot bones are held together in such a way that they form springy lengthwise and crosswise arches (**Figure 13-10**). This arrangement is architecturally sound because arches furnish more supporting strength per given amount of structural material than does any other type of construction. Hence the two-way arch construction makes a highly stable base.

The **longitudinal arch** of the foot has an inner, or medial, portion and an outer, or lateral, portion. Both are formed by the placement of the tarsal and metatarsal bones. Specifically, some of the tarsal bones (calcaneus, talus, navicular, and cuneiforms) and the first three metatarsal bones (starting with the great toe) form the **medial longitudinal arch.** The calcaneus and cuboid tarsal bones plus the fourth and fifth metatarsal bones shape the **lateral longitudinal**

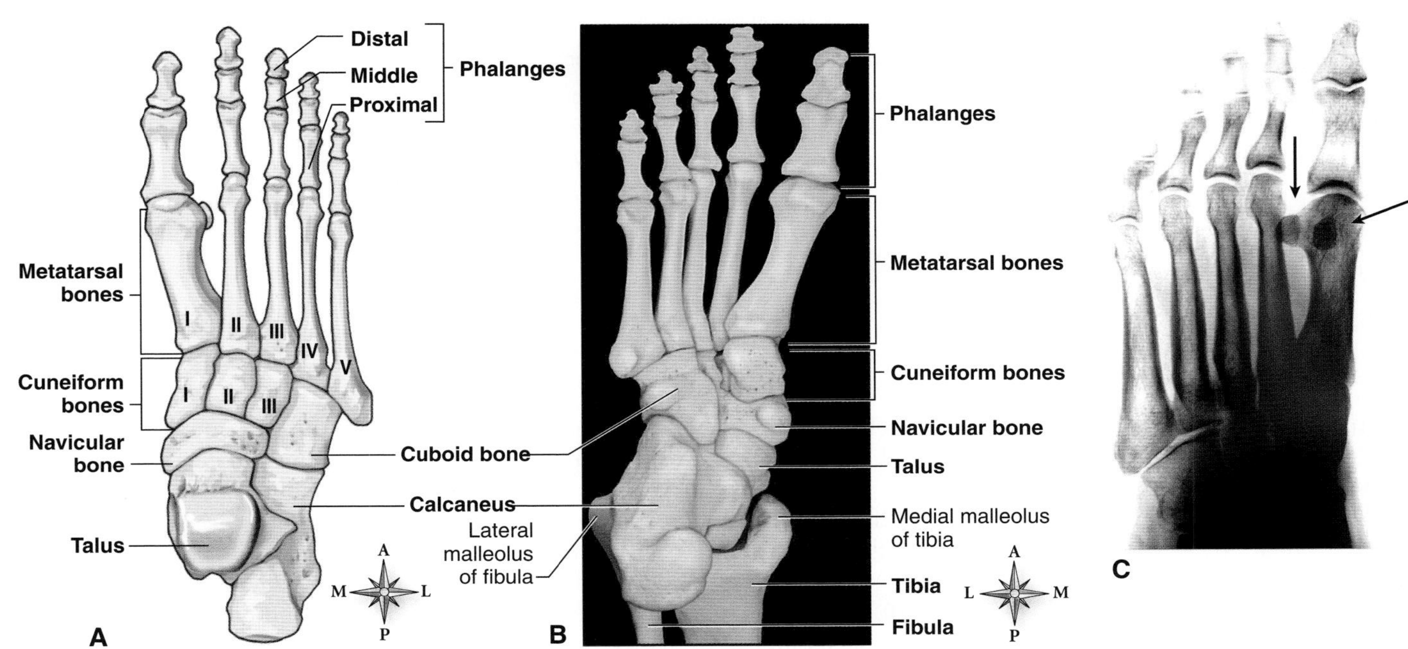

FIGURE 13-9 The foot. A, Bones of the right foot viewed from above. The tarsal bones consist of the cuneiforms, navicular, talus, cuboid, and calcaneus. **B,** Posterior aspect of the right ankle skeleton and inferior aspect of the right foot skeleton. **C,** X-ray film of the left foot showing prominent sesamoid bones (*arrows*) near the distal end (head) of the first metatarsal bone of the great toe.

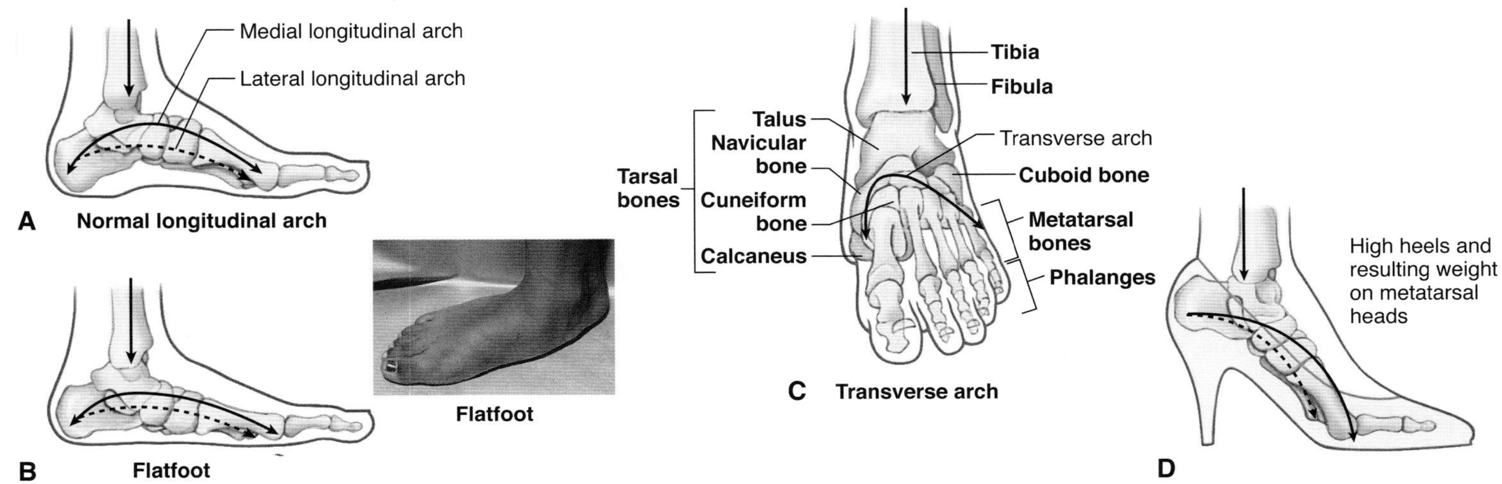

FIGURE 13-10 Arches of the foot. A, Longitudinal arch. The medial portion is formed by the calcaneus, talus, navicular, cuneiforms, and three metatarsal bones; the lateral portion is formed by the calcaneus, cuboid, and two lateral metatarsal bones. **B,** "Flatfoot" results when the tendons and ligaments attached to the tarsal bones are weakened. Downward pressure by the weight of the body gradually flattens out the normal arch of the bones. The photo shows the clinical appearance of a flatfoot. **C,** Transverse arch in the metatarsal region of the left foot. **D,** High heels throw the weight forward and cause the heads of the metatarsal bones to bear most of the body's weight. (*Arrows* show direction of force.)

TABLE 13-2 **Lower Extremity Bones and Their Markings—cont'd**

BONES AND MARKINGS	DESCRIPTION
Tarsal bones	Bones that form the heel and proximal or posterior half of the foot; include **calcaneus, talus, navicular, cuboid, medial cuneiform (I), intermediate cuneiform (II),** and **lateral cuneiform (III)**
Calcaneus	Heel bone
Talus	Uppermost of the tarsal bones; articulates with the tibia and fibula; boxed in the medial and lateral malleoli
Arches of foot	Curves of the bones of the foot and ankle that, along with muscles and other soft tissues, efficiently support the mass of the skeleton
Longitudinal arches	Tarsal and metatarsal bones so arranged as to form an arch from the front to the back of the foot
Medial	Formed by the calcaneus, talus, navicular, cuneiforms, and three medial metatarsal bones
Lateral	Formed by the calcaneus, cuboid, and two lateral metatarsal bones
Transverse (or metatarsal) arch	Metatarsal and distal row of tarsal bones (cuneiforms and cuboid) articulated so as to form an arch across the foot; bones kept in two arched positions by means of powerful ligaments in the sole of the foot and by muscles and tendons
Metatarsal bones	Long bones of the feet; numbered (from medial side) **I, II, III, IV, V**
Phalanges	Miniature long bones of the toes; two in each great toe; three in the other toes; numbered (from medial/thumb side), each with a *base*, *shaft*, and *head*
Proximal (I, II, III, IV, V)	
Middle (II, III, IV, V)	
Distal (I, II, III, IV, V)	

arch. The **transverse arch** of the foot results from the relative placement of the distal row of tarsals and the five metatarsal bones. (See **Table 13-2** for specific bones of different arches.)

Strong ligaments and leg muscle tendons normally hold the foot bones firmly in their arched positions. Not infrequently, however, these structures weaken and cause the arches to flatten—a condition aptly called **fallen arches,** or **flatfoot** (see **Figure 13-10**, *B*). Look at **Figure 13-10**, *D*, to see what shoes with high heels do to the position of the foot. They give a forward thrust to the body, which forces an undue amount of weight on the heads of the metatarsal bones. The resulting shift from the normal weight-bearing position of the feet may cause injury and chronic pain.

Normally, the tarsal and metatarsal bones have the major role in functioning of the foot as a supporting structure, with the phalanges being relatively unimportant. The reverse is true for the hand. Here, manipulation is the main function rather than support. Consequently, the phalanges of the fingers are all important, and the carpal and metacarpal bones are subsidiary.

In Chapter 11 the sesamoid bones were described as small rounded bones generally found embedded in the substance of tendons close to joints. The kneecap, or patella, is the largest of the sesamoid bones, as described previously. Other much smaller sesamoid bones are often found in tendons near the distal end (head) of the first metatarsal bone of the big toe (see **Figure 13-9**, *C*).

SKELETAL DIFFERENCES BETWEEN MEN AND WOMEN

General and specific differences exist between male and female skeletons. The general difference is one of size and weight, the male skeleton being larger and heavier. The specific differences most obviously concern the shape of the pelvic bones and cavity.

Whereas the male pelvis is deep and funnel shaped with a narrow subpubic angle (usually less than 90 degrees), the female pelvis, as **Figure 13-11** shows, is shallow, broad, and flaring, with a wider subpubic angle (usually greater than 90 degrees). The childbearing function obviously explains the necessity for these and certain other modifications of the female pelvis. These and other differences between the skeletons of the male and female are summarized in **Table 13-3**. More subtle specific differences between male and female skeletal structure are visible in the axial skeleton, particularly in the skull. Males tend to have larger skulls with more pronounced features such as the mastoid process, temporal lines, and superciliary arches. Female skulls tend to have rounder mandibles and eye orbits.

It is important to realize that averages are one thing, but individual variations are another. Genetic, environmental, and developmental factors also play a role in determining skeletal structure. Although any individual skeleton of either sex is likely to have a mix of typically "male" and "female" characteristics, most exhibit a clear tendency toward one or the other end of the male–female spectrum.

CONNECT IT! 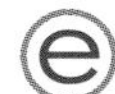

Check out the pictures of other specific skeletal differences between men and women in ***Skeletal Variations*** online at **Connect It!**

Quick **CHECK**

4. Which three bones fuse during skeletal development to form the coxal (hip) bone?
5. List the bones of the lower extremity and indicate their positions in the skeleton.
6. What is the functional advantage of foot arches?
7. Name two differences between typical male and female skeletons.

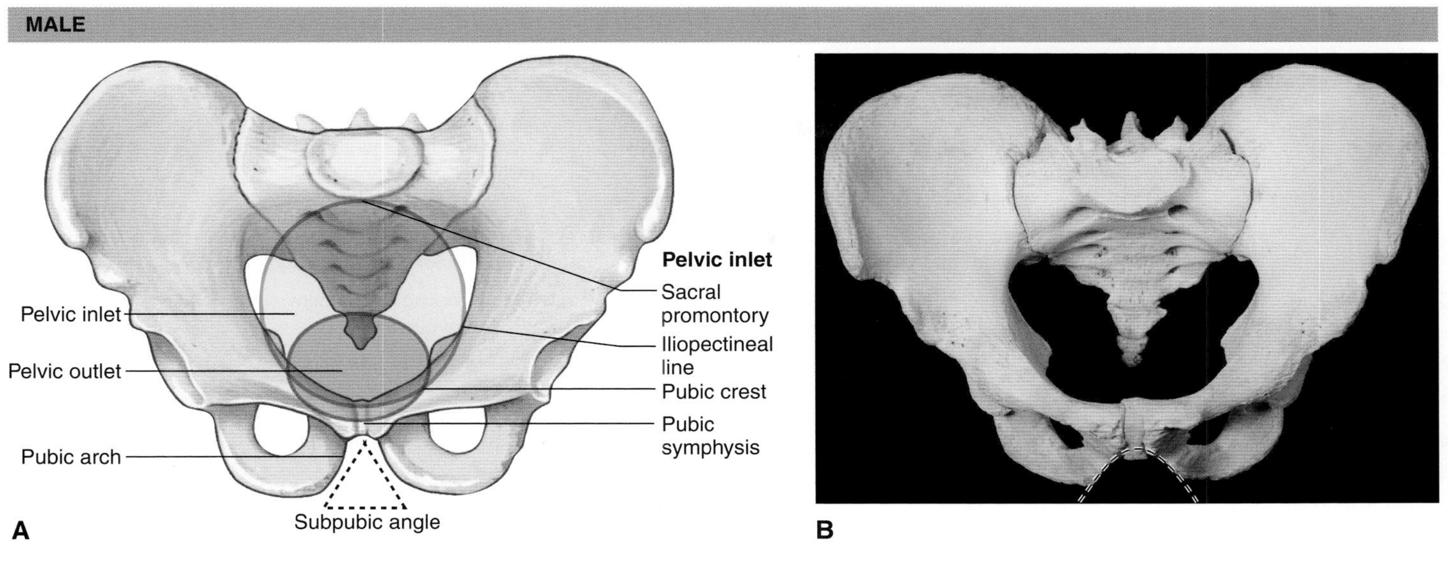

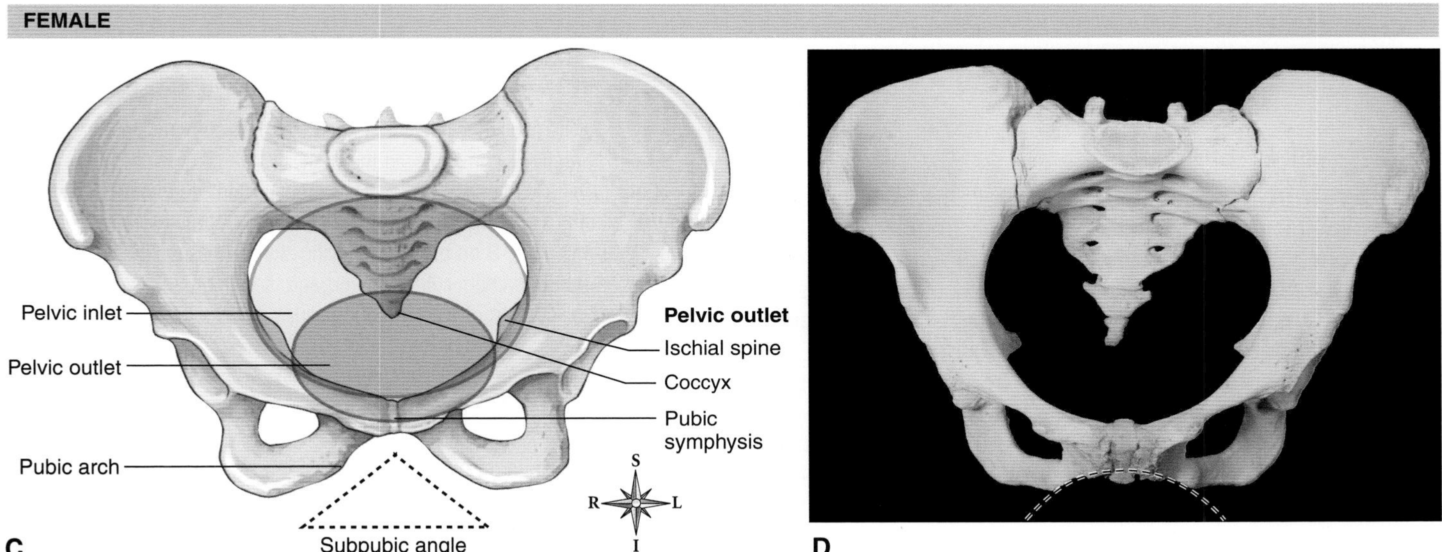

FIGURE 13-11 Comparison of the bony pelvis of the male and female skeletons. **A** and **C,** Diagrams showing components of the bony pelvis of the male and female. **B** and **D,** Photographs showing the bony pelvis of the male and female from in front and above. A dashed line in each image traces the subpubic angle.

TABLE 13-3 Comparison of Male and Female Skeletons

PORTION OF SKELETON	MALE	FEMALE
General form	Bones heavier and thicker	Bones lighter and thinner
	Muscle attachment sites more massive	Muscle attachment sites less distinct
	Joint surfaces relatively large	Joint surfaces relatively small
Skull	Forehead shorter vertically, with more prominent superciliary arches	Forehead more elongated vertically, with less prominent superciliary arches
	Mandible and maxillae relatively larger	Mandible and maxillae relatively smaller
	Facial area more pronounced	Facial area rounder, with less pronounced features
	Processes more pronounced	Processes less prominent

(continued)

TABLE 13-3 **Comparison of Male and Female Skeletons—cont'd**

PORTION OF SKELETON	MALE	FEMALE
Pelvis		
Pelvic cavity	Narrower in all dimensions Deeper Pelvic outlet relatively small	Wider in all dimensions Shorter and roomier Pelvic outlet relatively large
Sacrum	Long, narrow, with a smooth concavity (sacral curvature); sacral promontory more pronounced	Short, wide, flat concavity more pronounced in a posterior direction; sacral promontory less pronounced
Coccyx	Less movable	More movable and follows the posterior direction of the sacral curvature
Pubic arch	60- to 90-degree angle	90- to 120-degree angle
Pubic symphysis	Relatively deep	Relatively shallow
Ischial spine, ischial tuberosity, and anterior superior iliac spine	Turned more inward	Turned more outward and further apart
Greater sciatic notch	Narrow	Wide

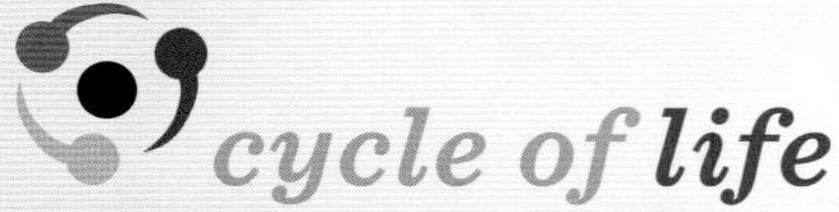

Skeletal System The changes that occur in the body's skeletal framework over the course of life result primarily from structural changes in bone, cartilage, and muscle tissues. For example, the resilience of incompletely ossified bone in young children allows their bones to withstand the mechanical stresses of childbirth and learning to walk with relatively little risk of fracturing.

Physicians often compare an individual's **bone age,** which is determined by the number of ossification centres visible on a radiograph, with **chronological age.** This type of information can prove useful in the diagnosis or treatment of many genetic, metabolic, or inflammatory skeletal diseases characterized by abnormally rapid or delayed skeletal maturity.

The density of bone and cartilage in a young to middle-aged adult permits the carrying of great loads. Loss of bone density in later adulthood can make a person so prone to fractures that simply walking or lifting with moderate force can cause bones to crack or break. Loss of skeletal tissue density may result in a compression of weight-bearing bones that causes a loss of height and perhaps an inability to maintain a standard posture. Degeneration of skeletal muscle tissue in late adulthood may also contribute to postural changes and loss of height. •

CONNECT IT! ⓔ

Check out ***Skeletal Variations*** online at ***Connect It!*** for graphic representations of changes in the skeleton throughout the life span.

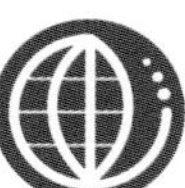

the big picture | **Skeletal System**

The skeletal system is a good example of increasing structural hierarchy or complexity in the body.

Recall from Chapter 1 that "levels of organization" characterize body structure so that all of our anatomical components logically fit together and function effectively (see **Figure 1-3** on p. 7). In studying skeletal tissues in Chapter 11, we proceeded from the chemical level of organization (inorganic salts and organic matrix) to a discussion of the cells and tissues of bone and cartilage.

In these two chapters on the skeleton, we have grouped skeletal tissues into discrete organs (bones) and then joined groups of individual bones together with varying numbers and kinds of other structures, such as blood vessels and nerves, to form a complex operational unit—the skeletal system. The "big picture" becomes more apparent when we integrate the skeletal system with other organ systems, which ultimately allows us to respond in a positive way to disruptions in homeostasis. The skeletal system, for example, plays a key role in purposeful movement, which in turn allows us to move away from potentially harmful stimuli. This organ system is much more than a collection of individual bones—it is a complex and interdependent functional unit essential for life. •

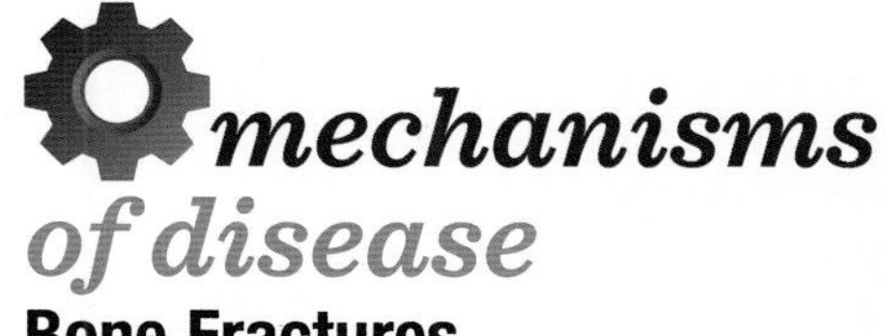

Bone Fractures

A *bone fracture* is defined as a partial or complete break in the continuity of a bone that most often occurs under mechanical stress. The most common cause of a fracture is traumatic injury. However, bone cancer, cysts, or metabolic bone disorders such as osteoporosis can also cause what are described as **pathological** or **spontaneous fractures.** In these types of fractures, the bone is so weak that it fractures under very little stress and in the absence of any significant trauma.

Most fractures can be identified visually during physical examination or on a standard radiograph. One exception is the so-called **stress fracture,** which often occurs in the absence of any clinically visible damage to bone or surrounding tissue. In addition, most x-ray images appear normal with this type of fracture. The microscopic bone damage typical of a stress fracture often appears in one or more bones of the leg or foot after repetitive trauma. Long-distance (marathon) runners and ballet dancers are notoriously "at risk". Often called hidden or occult fractures because they often remain unseen on regular radiographs, they are clearly visible on bone scans.

CONNECT IT! 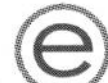

Check out ***Bone Scans*** online at ***Connect It!***

A **displaced fracture** or **open fracture,** also known as a *compound fracture* (**Figure 13-12**, *A*), is one in which broken bone projects through surrounding tissue and skin, thereby inviting the possibility of osteomyelitis (see p. 228) or other types of infection. A **nondisplaced fracture** or **closed fracture,** also known as a simple fracture (**Figure 13-12**, *B*) does not produce a break in the skin and therefore does not pose an immediate danger of bone infection. A closed fracture that results in one end of the broken bone being driven into the marrow cavity or diaphysis of the other bone segment is called an **impacted fracture.** As **Figure 13-12**, *C*, shows, fractures also are classified as "complete" or "incomplete". A **complete fracture** involves a break across the entire section of bone, whereas an **incomplete fracture** involves only a partial break, with the bone fragments still being partially joined. One type of incomplete fracture common in children is the **greenstick fracture,** in which a bone bends and breaks only along one side.

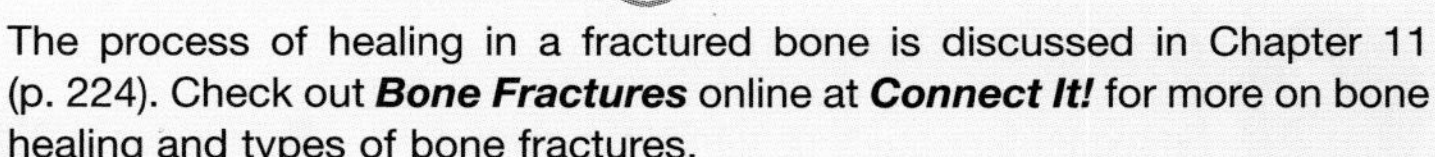

The process of healing in a fractured bone is discussed in Chapter 11 (p. 224). Check out ***Bone Fractures*** online at ***Connect It!*** for more on bone healing and types of bone fractures.

UNIT 2

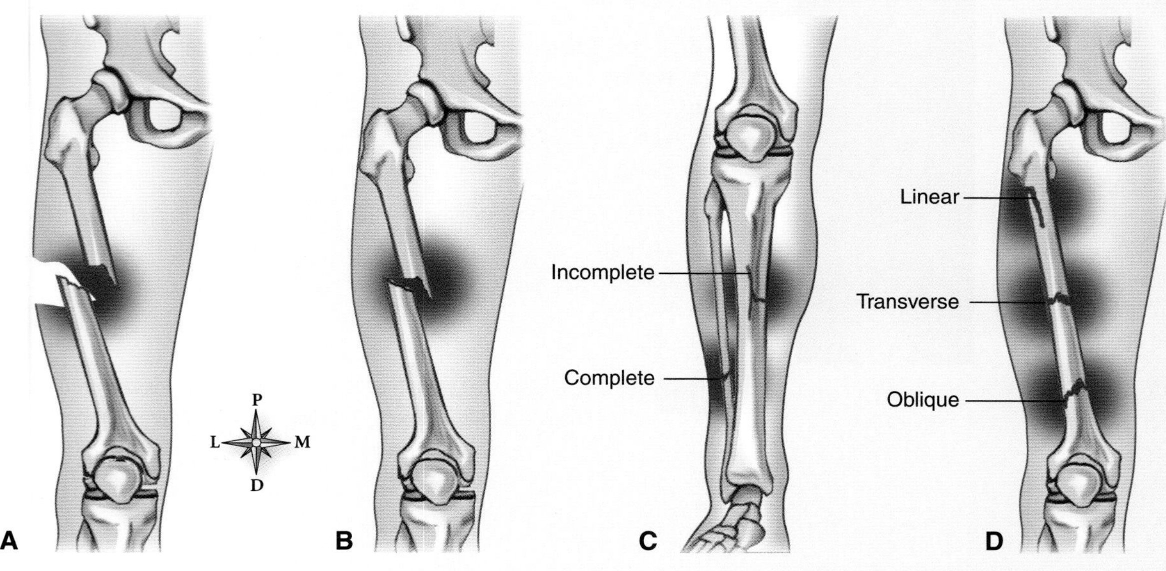

FIGURE 13-12 Bone fractures. A, Open. **B,** Closed. **C,** Incomplete and complete. **D,** Linear, transverse, and oblique.

LANGUAGE OF SCIENCE (continued from p. 264)

shoulder girdle (SHOHL-der GER-dul)
[*girdle* **belt**]

tibia (TIB-ee-ah)
[*tibia* **shin bone**] *pl.,* tibiae or tibias

transverse arch (tranz-VERS)

ulna (UL-nah)
[*ulna* **elbow**] *pl.,* ulnae or ulnas

LANGUAGE OF MEDICINE

chondromalacia patellae
(kon-droh-mah-LAY-shee-ah pah-TEL-ah)
[*chondro-* **cartilage,** *-malacia* **softening,** *pat-* **dish,** *-ella* **small**]

complete fracture
(kom-PLEET FRAK-chur)

displaced (open) fracture
(dis-PLAYSD [OH-pen] FRAK-chur)

fallen arches (flatfoot)
(FAHL-en ARCH-ez [flat-FOOT])

greenstick fracture
(GREEN-stik FRAK-chur)

impacted fracture
(im-PAK-ted FRAK-chur)

incomplete fracture
(in-kom-PLEET FRAK-chur)

nondisplaced (closed) fracture
(non-dis-PLAYSD [klohzd] FRAK-chur)

pathological (spontaneous) fracture
(path-o-LOJ-ik-al [spon-TAY-nee-us] FRAK-chur)

stress fracture (stres FRAK-chur)

case study

No matter how much he turned the steering wheel, Robert's car just kept veering directly toward the guardrail as it slid across the black ice. The impact from the car slamming against an immovable object was horrendous. Even though he was wearing his seat belt, Robert was thrown violently forward and sideways as the car and railing collided. After the car came to a jolting stop, Robert's first thought was to unbuckle his seat belt so he could get out of the car, but a severe pain in his chest kept him from moving. Thankfully, the paramedics were on the scene in a matter of minutes. They gently moved Robert from his car to a backboard and strapped his head in place.

In the Accident and Emergency department, a nurse gave Robert the news: his spine was fractured at "T6"; his fourth and fifth ribs were cracked; and he had a broken mandible and a shattered tibia and fibula.

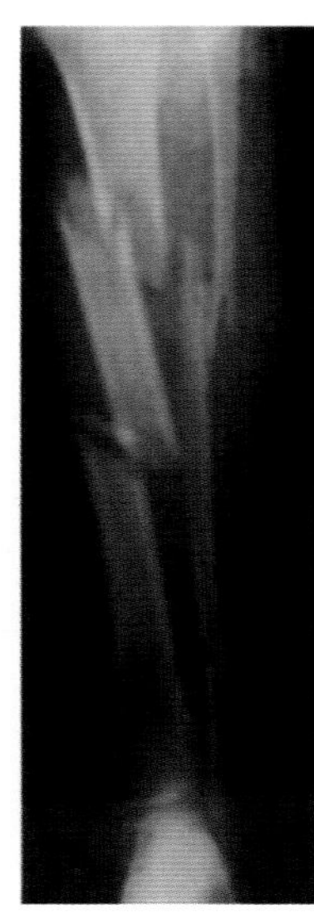

1. Which bone in the spine was fractured?
   a. Thyroid vertebra
   b. Tibia
   c. Tarsal
   d. Thoracic vertebra

2. What is another name for the fourth and fifth ribs that were cracked in the accident?
   a. Floating ribs
   b. False ribs
   c. True ribs
   d. Costal ribs

3. What daily activity will be affected most by his broken mandible?
   a. Walking
   b. Eating
   c. Writing
   d. Sitting

4. What daily activity will be affected most by his shattered tibia and fibula?
   a. Walking
   b. Eating
   c. Writing
   d. Sitting

Hint To solve a case study, you may have to refer to the glossary or index, other chapters in this textbook, ***Connect It!,*** and other resources.

CHAPTER SUMMARY

To download an MP3 version of the chapter summary for use with your mobile device, access the ***Audio Chapter Summaries*** *online at evolve.elsevier.com.*

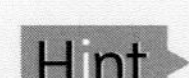

Scan this summary after reading the chapter to help you reinforce the key concepts. Later, use the summary as a quick review before your class or before a test.

Upper Extremity

A. Consists of the bones of the shoulder girdle, upper and lower parts of the arm, wrist, and hand (**Table 13-1**)
B. Shoulder girdle (**Figure 13-2**)
   1. Made up of the scapula and clavicle
   2. Clavicle forms the only bony joint with the trunk, the sternoclavicular joint
   3. At its distal end, the clavicle articulates with the acromion process of the scapula

C. Humerus (**Figures 13-3** and **13-4**)
   1. The long bone of the upper part of the arm
   2. Articulates proximally with the glenoid fossa of the scapula and distally with the radius and ulna
D. Ulna
   1. The long bone found on the little finger side of the forearm
   2. Articulates proximally with the humerus and radius and distally with a fibrocartilaginous disc
E. Radius
   1. The long bone found on the thumb side of the forearm
   2. Articulates proximally with the capitulum of the humerus and the radial notch of the ulna; articulates distally with the scaphoid and lunate carpal bones and with the head of the ulna
F. Carpal bones (**Figure 13-5**)
   1. Eight small bones that form the wrist
   2. Carpal bones are bound closely and firmly by ligaments and form two rows of four carpals each
      a. Proximal row is made up of the pisiform, triquetrum, lunate, and scaphoid
      b. Distal row is made up of the hamate, capitate, trapezoid, and trapezium
   3. The joints between the radius and carpal bones allow wrist and hand movements
G. Metacarpal bones
   1. Form the framework of the hand
   2. The thumb metacarpal forms the most freely movable joint with the carpal bones
   3. Heads of the metacarpal bones (the knuckles) articulate with the phalanges

Lower Extremity

A. Consists of the bones of the hip, thigh, leg, ankle, and foot (**Table 13-2**)
B. Pelvic girdle is made up of the sacrum and the two coxal bones bound tightly by strong ligaments (**Figure 13-6**)
   1. A stable circular base that supports the trunk and attaches the lower extremities to it
   2. Each coxal bone is made up of three bones that fuse together (**Figure 13-7**):
      a. Ilium—largest and uppermost
      b. Ischium—strongest and lowermost
      c. Pubis—most anterior
C. Femur—longest and heaviest bone in the body (**Figure 13-8**)
D. Patella—largest sesamoid bone in the body
E. Tibia
   1. The larger, stronger, and more medially and superficially located of the two leg bones
   2. Articulates proximally with the femur to form the knee joint
   3. Articulates distally with the fibula and talus
F. Fibula
   1. The smaller, more laterally and deeply placed of the two leg bones
   2. Articulates with the tibia
G. Foot (**Figures 13-9** and **13-10**)
   1. Structure is similar to that of the hand with adaptations for supporting weight
   2. Foot bones are held together to form spring arches
      a. Medial longitudinal arch is made up of the calcaneus, talus, navicular, cuneiforms, and medial three metatarsal bones
      b. Lateral longitudinal arch is made up of the calcaneus, cuboid, and fourth and fifth metatarsal bones

Skeletal Differences Between Men and Women

A. Male skeleton is larger and heavier than female skeleton
B. Pelvic differences (**Figure 13-11**; **Table 13-3**)
   1. Male pelvis—deep and funnel shaped, with a narrow pubic arch
   2. Female pelvis—shallow, broad, and flaring, with a wider pubic arch
C. Skull differences (**Table 13-3**)
   1. Male skull—larger with more prominent processes
   2. Female skull—rounded features
D. Individuals have a mix of male and female skeletal characteristics, but most commonly show an overall tendency to one or the other type

Cycle of Life: Skeletal System

A. Changes in the skeleton begin at fertilization and continue over a lifetime; changes can be positive or negative
B. Incompletely ossified skeleton in children provides the resiliency needed to withstand stress without breaking easily
C. Dense bone structure in young and middle adulthood permits bearing heavy loads
D. In later adulthood, reduced bone density makes fractures more likely and causes changes in posture and overall height
E. Details of ageing effects are found in Mechanisms of Disease section

The Big Picture: Skeletal System

A. Skeletal system is a good example of increasing structural hierarchy in the body
   1. Skeletal tissues grouped into discrete organs—bones
   2. Skeletal system consists of bones, blood vessels, nerves, and other tissues grouped to form a complex operational unit
   3. Integration of skeletal system with other body organ systems permits homeostasis to occur
   4. Skeletal system more than a collection of individual bones—it represents a complex and interdependent functional unit of the body

REVIEW QUESTIONS

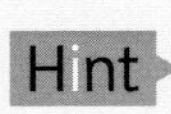

Write out the answers to these questions after reading the chapter and reviewing the Chapter Summary. Note—writing out your answers will consolidate learning and provide a valuable resource of information.

1. Describe and distinguish between the different kinds of bone fractures and discuss symptoms and treatments of broken bones.
2. Identify the bones of the shoulder and pelvic girdles.
3. Describe the difference between the *false* pelvis and *true* pelvis.
4. Identify, compare, and organize the bones of the arm, forearm, wrist, and hand with those of the thigh, leg, ankle, and foot.
5. Name the largest sesamoid bone in the body and give its function.
6. Discuss the arches of the foot and point out the functional importance of each.
7. Describe the role of the pubic symphysis during childbirth.
8. Identify features of the appendicular skeleton by applying the use of anatomical directions.
   a. Name the hook-like bony structure of the scapula that projects anteriorly.
   b. Name the bony landmark located on the lateral side of the humerus.
   c. Name the region of the humerus that articulates with the radius as part of the elbow joint.
   d. Which is the most lateral carpal bone of the proximal row?
   e. Name the region of the pelvis that supports the body's weight when sitting.

CRITICAL THINKING QUESTIONS

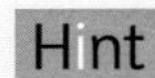

After finishing the Review Questions, write out the answers to these more in-depth questions to help you apply your new knowledge. Go back to sections of the chapter that relate to concepts that you find difficult.

1. Of the five metacarpal bones that form the framework of the hand, the thumb metacarpal forms the most freely movable joint with the carpals. Explain the significance of this anatomical structure.
2. Interpret the advantage of an additional bone in the carpal region over the tarsal region.
3. Compare and contrast the differences between the skeletal structure of males and females. What are the physiological reasons for these differences?
4. Explain how the shoulder and pelvic girdles stabilize the appendages.
5. Why do many bones of the skeleton have prominent bumps? What is their purpose?

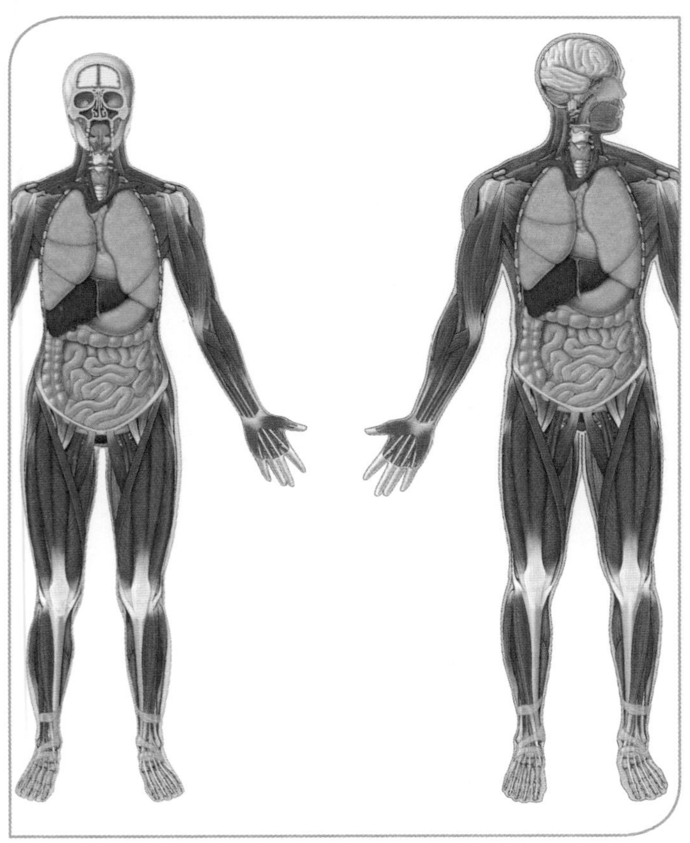

Clear View of the Human Body

Developed by
KEVIN PATTON and PAUL KRIEGER
Illustrated by
Dragonfly Media Group

INTRODUCTION

A complete understanding of human anatomy and physiology requires an appreciation for how structures within the body relate to one another. Such appreciation for anatomical structure has become especially important in the twenty-first century with the explosion in the use of diverse methods of medical imaging that rely on the ability to interpret sectional views of the human body.

The best way to develop your understanding of overall anatomical structure is to carefully dissect a large number of male and female human cadavers—then have those dissected specimens handy while reading and learning about each system of the body. Obviously, such multiple dissections and constant access to specimens are impractical for nearly everyone. However, the experience of a simple dissection can be approximated by layering several partially transparent, two-dimensional anatomical diagrams in a way that allows a student to "virtually" dissect the human body simply by paging through the layers.

This **Clear View of the Human Body** provides a handy tool for dissecting simulated male and female bodies. It also provides views of several different parts of the human body in a variety of cross-sections. The many different anterior and posterior views also give you a perspective on body structure that is not available with ordinary anatomical diagrams. This Clear View is an always-available tool to help you learn the three-dimensional structure of the body in a way that allows you to see how they relate to each other in a complete body. It will always be right here in your textbook, so place a bookmark here and refer to the Clear View frequently as you study each of the systems of the human body.

HINTS FOR USING THE CLEAR VIEW OF THE BODY

1. Starting at the first page of the Clear View, slowly lift the page as you look at the anterior view of the male and female bodies. You will see deeper structures appear, as if you had dissected the body. As you lift each successive layer of images, you will be looking at deeper and deeper body structures. A key to the labels is found in the grey sidebar.
2. Starting with the second section of the Clear View, notice that you are looking at the posterior aspect of the male and female body. Lift each layer from the edge to reveal body structures in successive layers from the back to the front. This very unique view will help you understand structural relationships even better.
3. On each page of the Clear View, look at the transverse section represented in the sidebar. The section you are looking at on any one page is from the location shown in the larger diagram as a red line. In other words, if you cut the body at the red line and tilted the upper part of the body toward you, you would see what is shown in the section diagram. Notice that each section has its own labelling system that is separate from the labels used in the larger images.

KEY

1. Epicranius m.
2. Temporalis m.
3. Orbicularis oculi m.
4. Masseter m.
5. Orbicularis oris m.
6. Pectoralis major m.
7. Serratus anterior m.
8. Basilic vein
9. Brachial fascia
10. Cephalic vein
11. Rectus sheath
12. Linea alba
13. Rectus abdominis m.
14. Umbilicus
15. Abdominal oblique m., external
16. Abdominal oblique m., internal
17. Transverse abdominis m.
18. Inguinal ring, external
19. Fossa ovalis
20. Fascia of the thigh
21. Great saphenous vein
22. Parietal bone
23. Frontal bone
24. Temporal bone
25. Zygomatic bone
26. Maxilla
27. Mandible
28. Sternocleidomastoid m.
29. Sternohyoid muscle
30. Omohyoid muscle
31. Deltoid m.
32. Pectoralis minor m.
33. Sternum
34. Rib (costal) cartilage
35. Rib
36. Greater omentum
37. Frontal lobe
38. Parietal lobe
39. Temporal lobe
40. Cerebellum
41. Nasal septum
42. Brachiocephalic vein
43. Superior vena cava
44. Thymus gland
45. Right lung
46. Left lung
47. Pericardium
48. Liver
49. Gallbladder
50. Stomach
51. Transverse colon
52. Small intestines
53. Biceps brachii m.
54. Brachioradialis m.
55. Adductor longus m.
56. Sartorius m.
57. Quadriceps femoris m.
58. Patellar ligament
59. Tibialis anterior m.
60. Sup. extensor retinaculum
61. Inf. extensor retinaculum
62. Cerebrum of brain
63. Cerebellum
64. Brainstem
65. Maxillary sinus
66. Nasal cavity
67. Tongue
68. Thyroid gland
69. Heart
70. Hepatic veins
71. Oesophagus
72. Spleen
73. Coeliac artery
74. Portal vein
75. Duodenum
76. Pancreas
77. Mesenteric artery
78. Ascending colon
79. Transverse colon
80. Descending colon
81. Sigmoid colon
82. Mesentery
83. Appendix
84. Inguinal ligament
85. Pubic symphysis
86. Extensor carpi radialis m.
87. Pronator teres m.
88. Flexor carpi radialis m.
89. Flexor digitorum profundus m.
90. Quadriceps femoris m.
91. Extensor digitorum longus m.
92. Thyroid cartilage
93. Trachea
94. Aortic arch
95. Right lung
96. Left lung
97. Pulmonary artery
98. Right atrium
99. Right ventricle
100. Left atrium
101. Left ventricle
102. Coracobrachialis m.
103. Inferior vena cava
104. Descending aorta
105. Right kidney
106. Left kidney
107. Right ureter
108. Rectum
109. Urinary bladder
110. Prostate gland
111. Iliac artery and vein
112. Uterus
113. Parietal bone
114. Frontal sinus
115. Sphenoidal sinus
116. Occipital bone
117. Palatine process
118. Cervical vertebrae
119. Corpus callosum
120. Thalamus
121. Trapezius m.
122. Acromion process
123. Coracoid process
124. Humerus
125. Subscapularis m.
126. Deltoid m. (cut)
127. Triceps m.
128. Brachialis m.
129. Brachioradialis m.
130. Radius
131. Ulna
132. Diaphragm
133. Thoracic duct
134. Quadratus lumborum m.
135. Psoas m.
136. Lumbar vertebrae
137. Iliacus m.
138. Gluteus medius m.
139. Iliofemoral ligament
140. Sacral nerves
141. Sacrum
142. Coccyx
143. Femur
144. Vastus lateralis m.
145. Femoral artery and vein
146. Adductor magnus m.
147. Patella
148. Fibula
149. Tibia
150. Fibularis longus m.
151. Spinal cord
152. Nerve root
153. Platysma m.
154. Splenius capitis m.
155. Levator scapulae m.
156. Rhomboideus m.
157. Infraspinatus m.
158. Teres major m.
159. Lumbodorsal fascia
160. Erector spinae m.
161. Serratus post. inf. m.
162. Latissimus dorsi m.
163. Gluteus medius m.
164. Gluteus maximus m.
165. Iliotibial tract
166. Flexor carpi ulnaris m.
167. Extensor carpi ulnaris m.
168. Extensor digitorum m.
169. Carpal ligament, dorsal
170. Interosseous m.
171. Gluteus minimus m.
172. Piriformis m.
173. Gemellus sup. m.
174. Obturator internus m.
175. Gemellus inf. m.
176. Quadratus femoris m.
177. Biceps femoris m.
178. Gastrocnemius m.
179. Calcaneal (Achilles) tendon
180. Calcaneus bone
181. Subcutaneous fat
182. Corpus spongiosum
183. Corpora cavernosa
184. Umbilical ligaments
185. Epigastric artery and vein
186. Right testis
187. Transverse thoracic m.
188. Parietal pleura
189. Common bile duct
190. Lesser omentum
191. Flexor digitorum profundus
192. Epiglottis

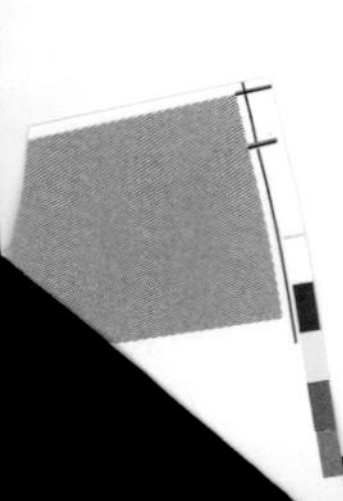

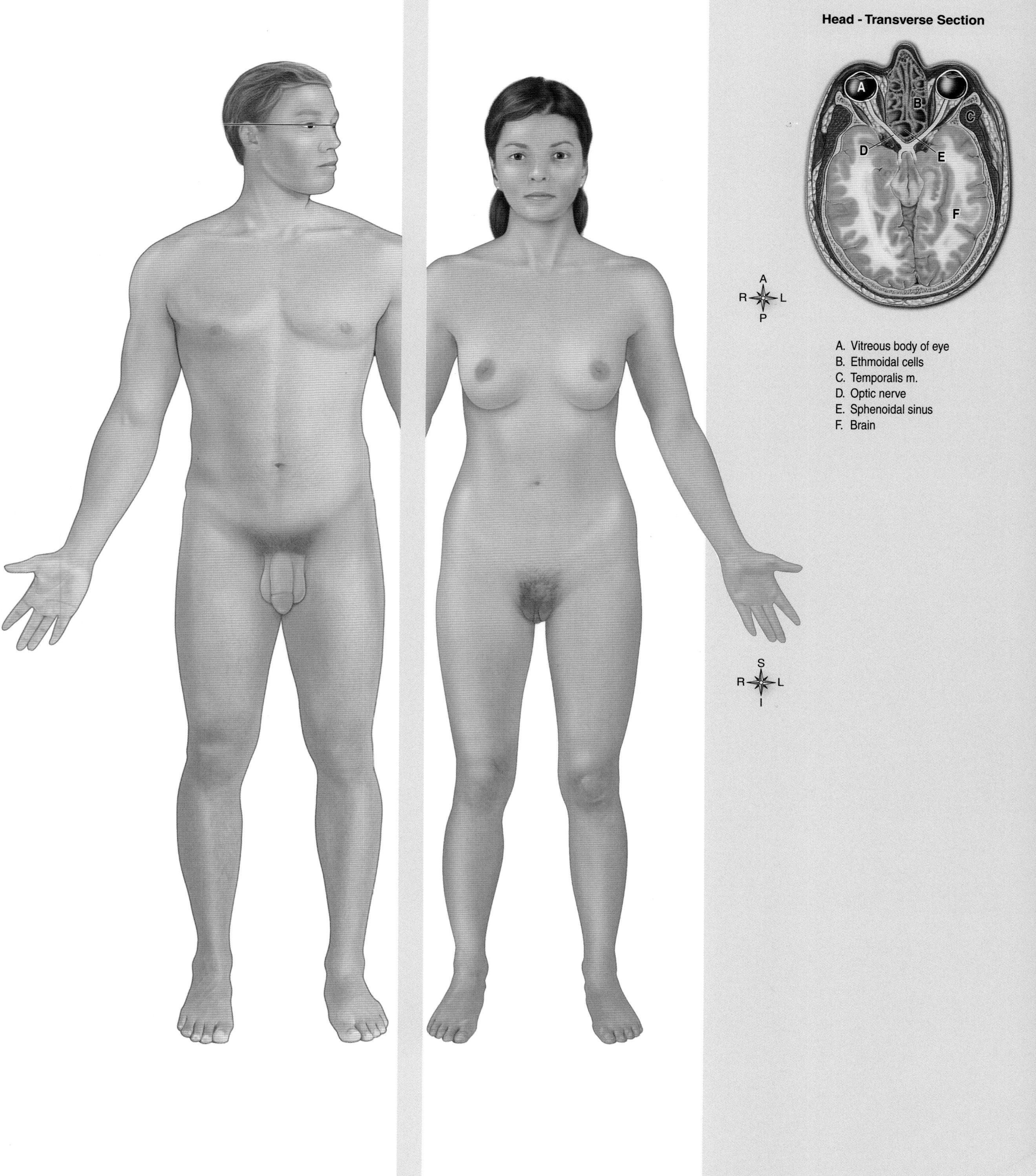
Head - Transverse Section
A
B
C
D
E
F
A
R
L
P
A. Vitreous body of eye
B. Ethmoidal cells
C. Temporalis m.
D. Optic nerve
E. Sphenoidal sinus
F. Brain
S
R
L
I

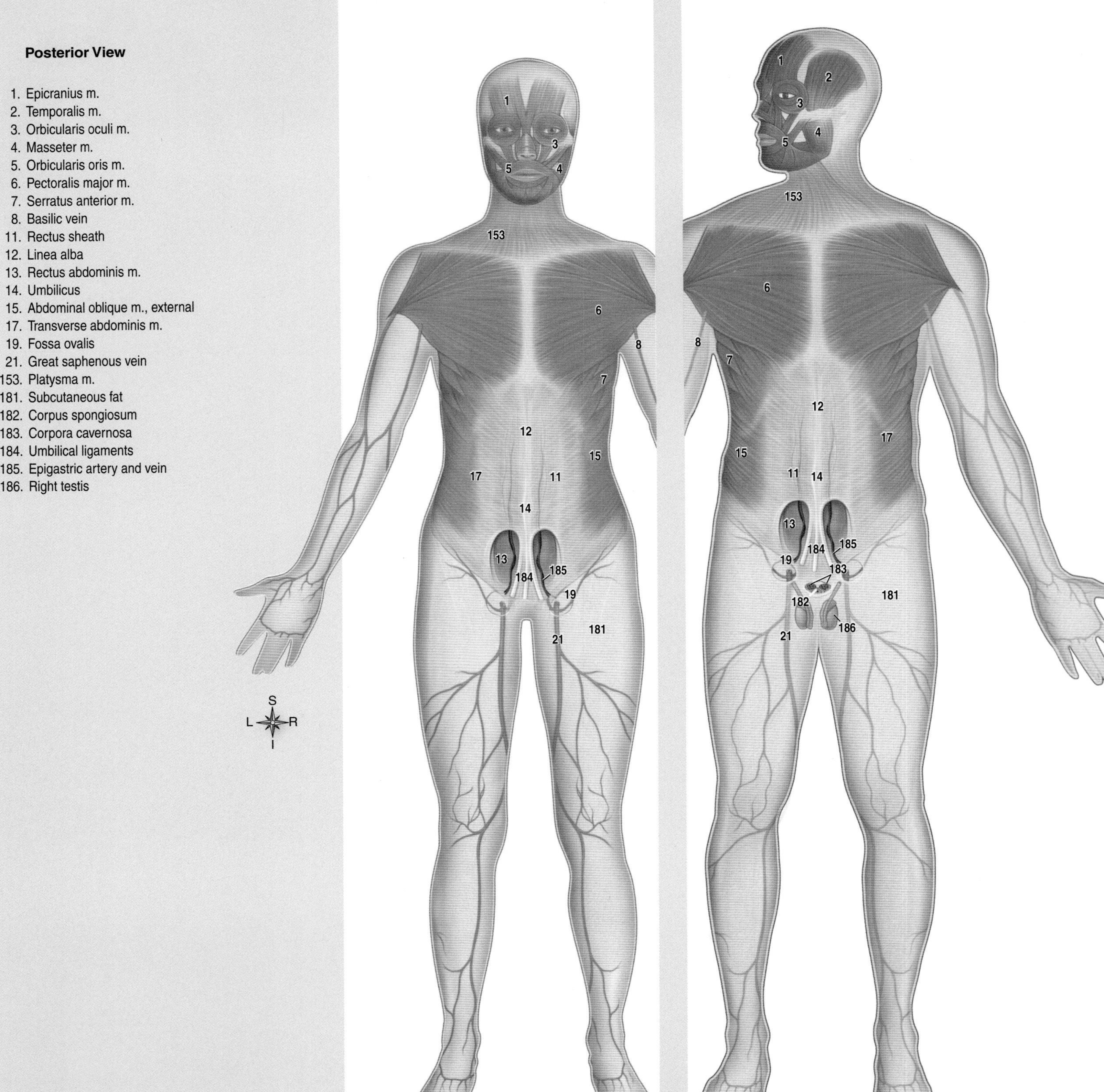
Posterior View
1. Epicranius m.
2. Temporalis m.
3. Orbicularis oculi m.
4. Masseter m.
5. Orbicularis oris m.
6. Pectoralis major m.
7. Serratus anterior m.
8. Basilic vein
11. Rectus sheath
12. Linea alba
13. Rectus abdominis m.
14. Umbilicus
15. Abdominal oblique m., external
17. Transverse abdominis m.
19. Fossa ovalis
21. Great saphenous vein
153. Platysma m.
181. Subcutaneous fat
182. Corpus spongiosum
183. Corpora cavernosa
184. Umbilical ligaments
185. Epigastric artery and vein
186. Right testis
S
L
R
I

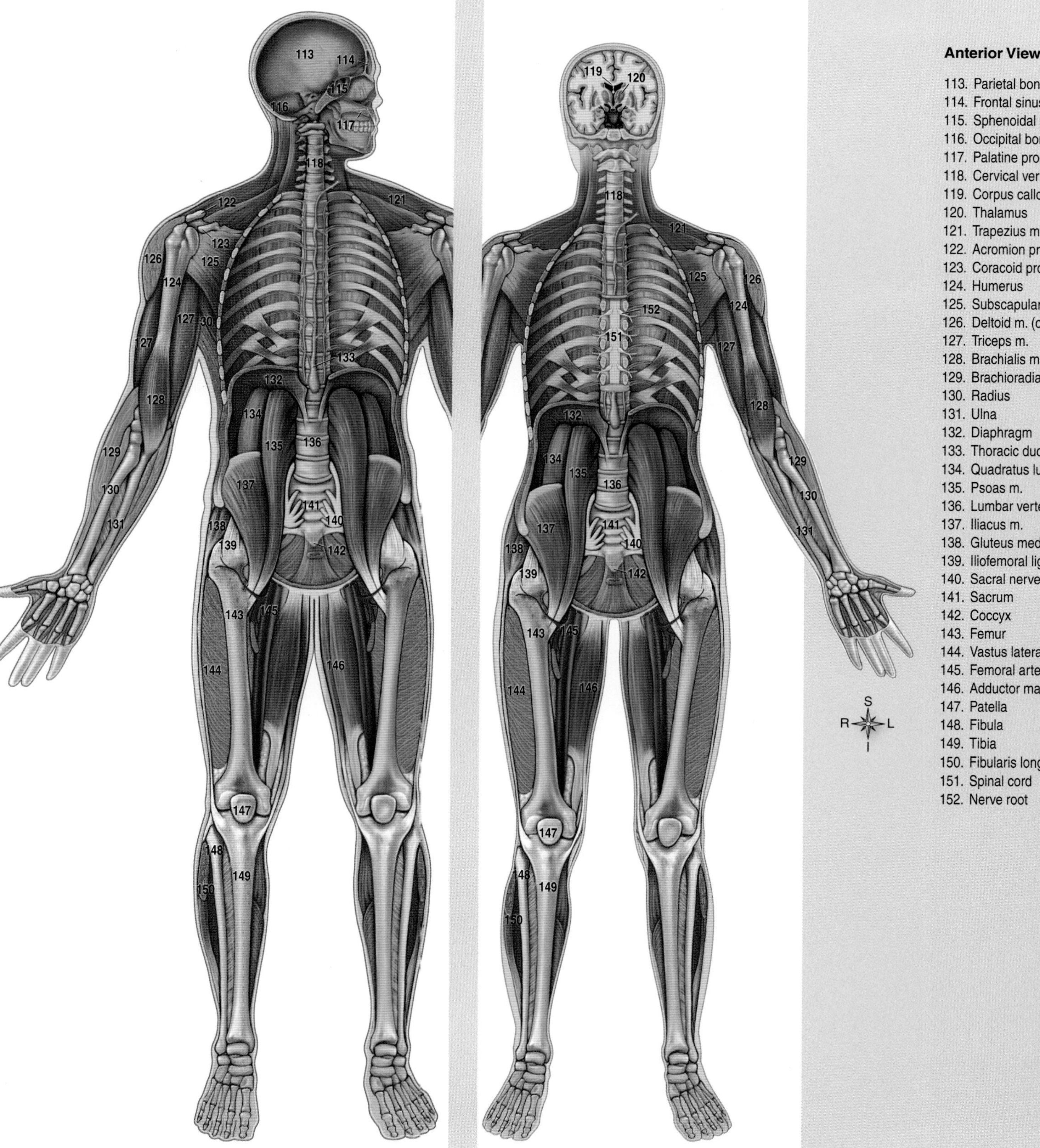

Anterior View

113. Parietal bone
114. Frontal sinus
115. Sphenoidal sinus
116. Occipital bone
117. Palatine process
118. Cervical vertebrae
119. Corpus callosum
120. Thalamus
121. Trapezius m.
122. Acromion process
123. Coracoid process
124. Humerus
125. Subscapularis m.
126. Deltoid m. (cut)
127. Triceps m.
128. Brachialis m.
129. Brachioradialis m.
130. Radius
131. Ulna
132. Diaphragm
133. Thoracic duct
134. Quadratus lumborum m.
135. Psoas m.
136. Lumbar vertebrae
137. Iliacus m.
138. Gluteus medius m.
139. Iliofemoral ligament
140. Sacral nerves
141. Sacrum
142. Coccyx
143. Femur
144. Vastus lateralis m.
145. Femoral artery and vein
146. Adductor magnus m.
147. Patella
148. Fibula
149. Tibia
150. Fibularis longus m.
151. Spinal cord
152. Nerve root

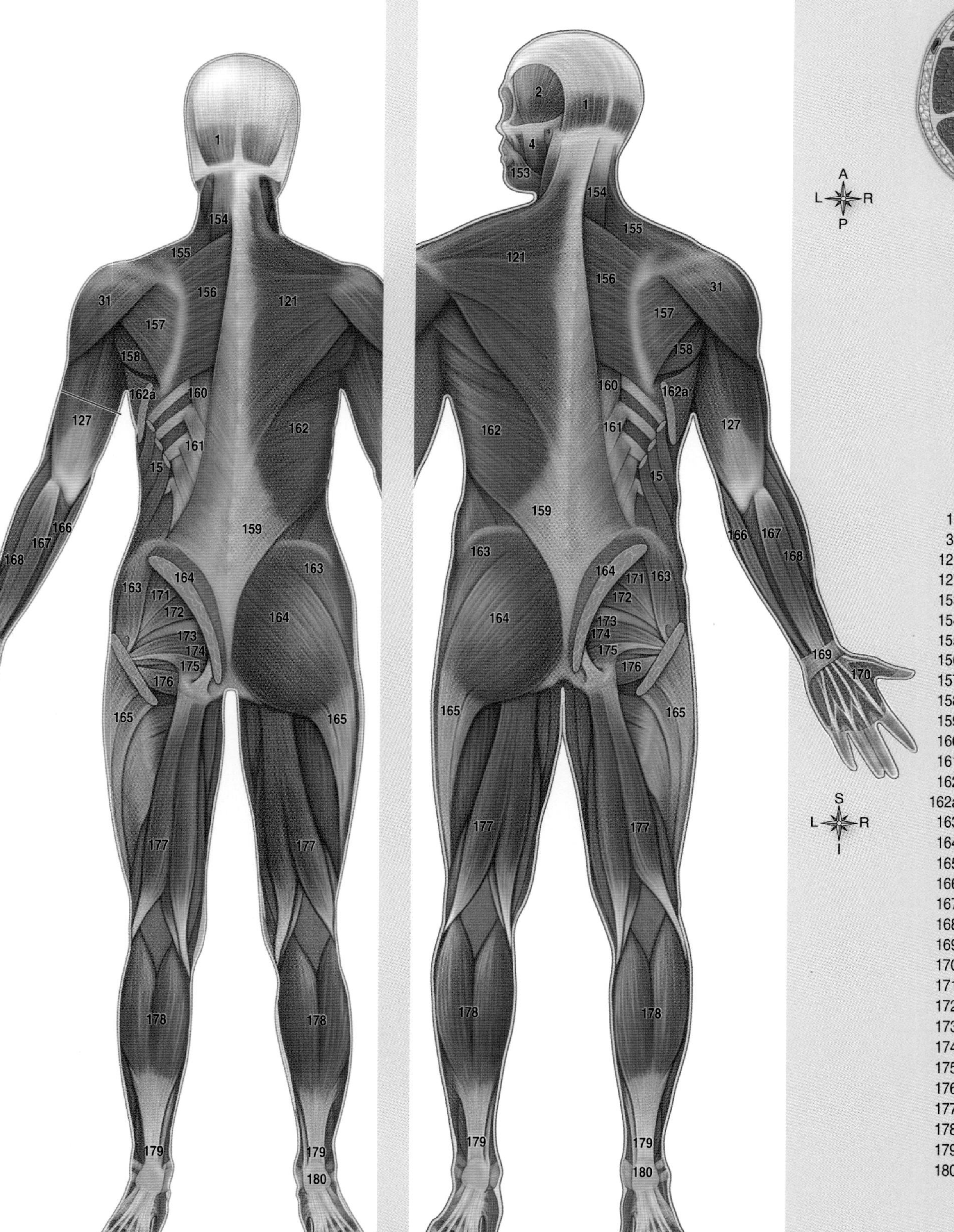

Upper Arm - Transverse Section

A. Biceps brachii m.
B. Brachialis m.
C. Humerus
D. Triceps brachii m., medial
E. Triceps brachii m., lateral

Posterior View

1. Epicranius m.
2. Temporalis m.
4. Masseter m.
15. Abdominal oblique m., external
31. Deltoid m.
121. Trapezius m.
127. Triceps m.
153. Platysma m.
154. Splenius capitis m.
155. Levator scapulae m.
156. Rhomboideus m.
157. Infraspinatis m.
158. Teres major m.
159. Lumbodorsal fascia
160. Erector spinae m.
161. Serratus post. inf. m.
162. Latissimus dorsi m.
162a. Latissimus dorsi m. (cut)
163. Gluteus medius m.
164. Gluteus maximus m.
165. Iliotibial tract
166. Flexor carpi ulnaris m.
167. Extensor carpi ulnaris m.
168. Extensor digitorum m.
169. Carpal ligament, dorsal
170. Interosseus m.
171. Gluteus minimus m.
172. Piriformis m.
173. Gemellus sup. m.
174. Obturator internus m.
175. Gemellus inf. m.
176. Quadratus femoris m.
177. Biceps femoris m.
178. Gastrocnemius m.
179. Calcaneal (Achilles) tendon
180. Calcaneus bone

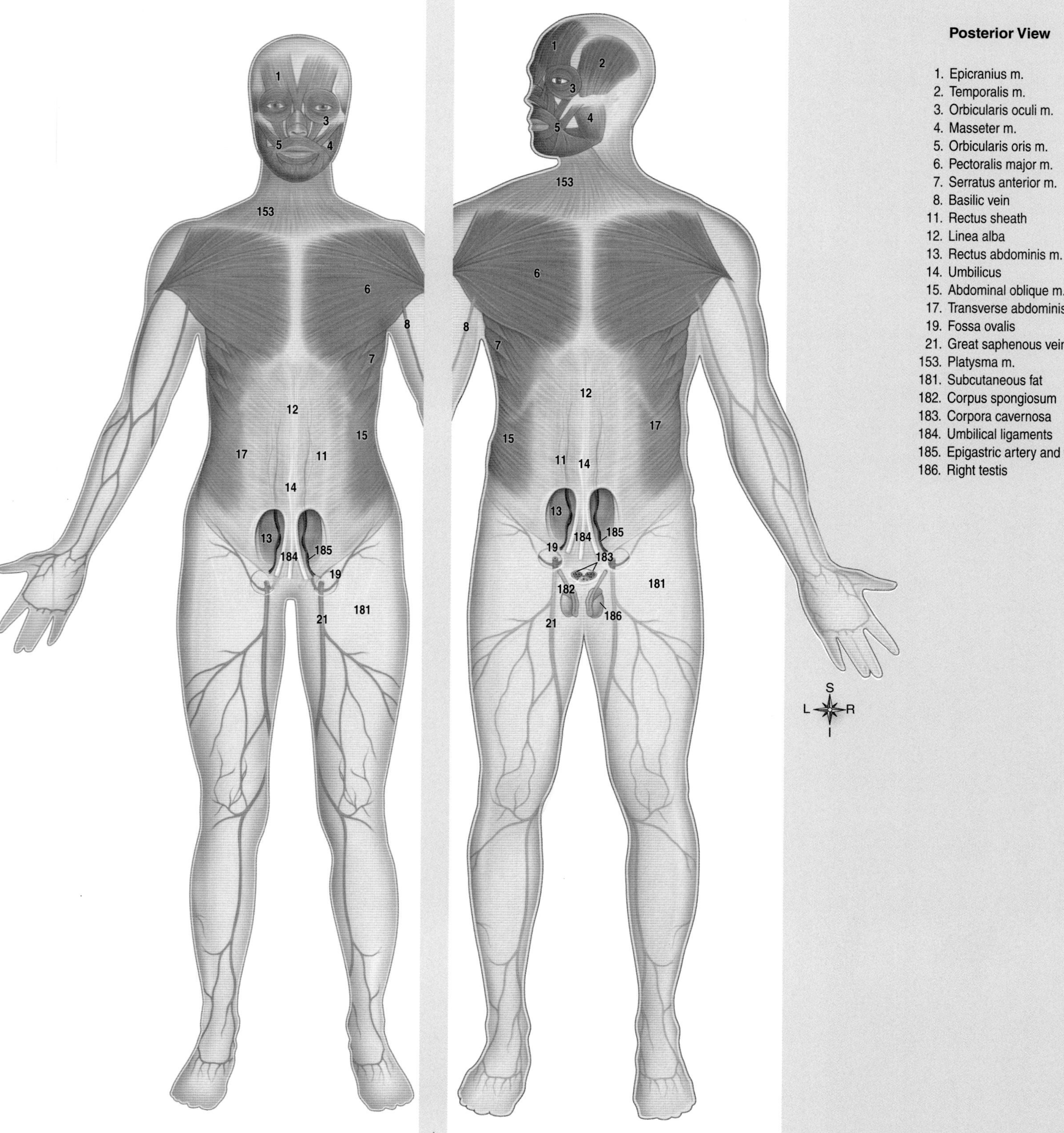
Posterior View
1. Epicranius m.
2. Temporalis m.
3. Orbicularis oculi m.
4. Masseter m.
5. Orbicularis oris m.
6. Pectoralis major m.
7. Serratus anterior m.
8. Basilic vein
11. Rectus sheath
12. Linea alba
13. Rectus abdominis m.
14. Umbilicus
15. Abdominal oblique m., external
17. Transverse abdominis m.
19. Fossa ovalis
21. Great saphenous vein
153. Platysma m.
181. Subcutaneous fat
182. Corpus spongiosum
183. Corpora cavernosa
184. Umbilical ligaments
185. Epigastric artery and vein
186. Right testis
S
L
R
I

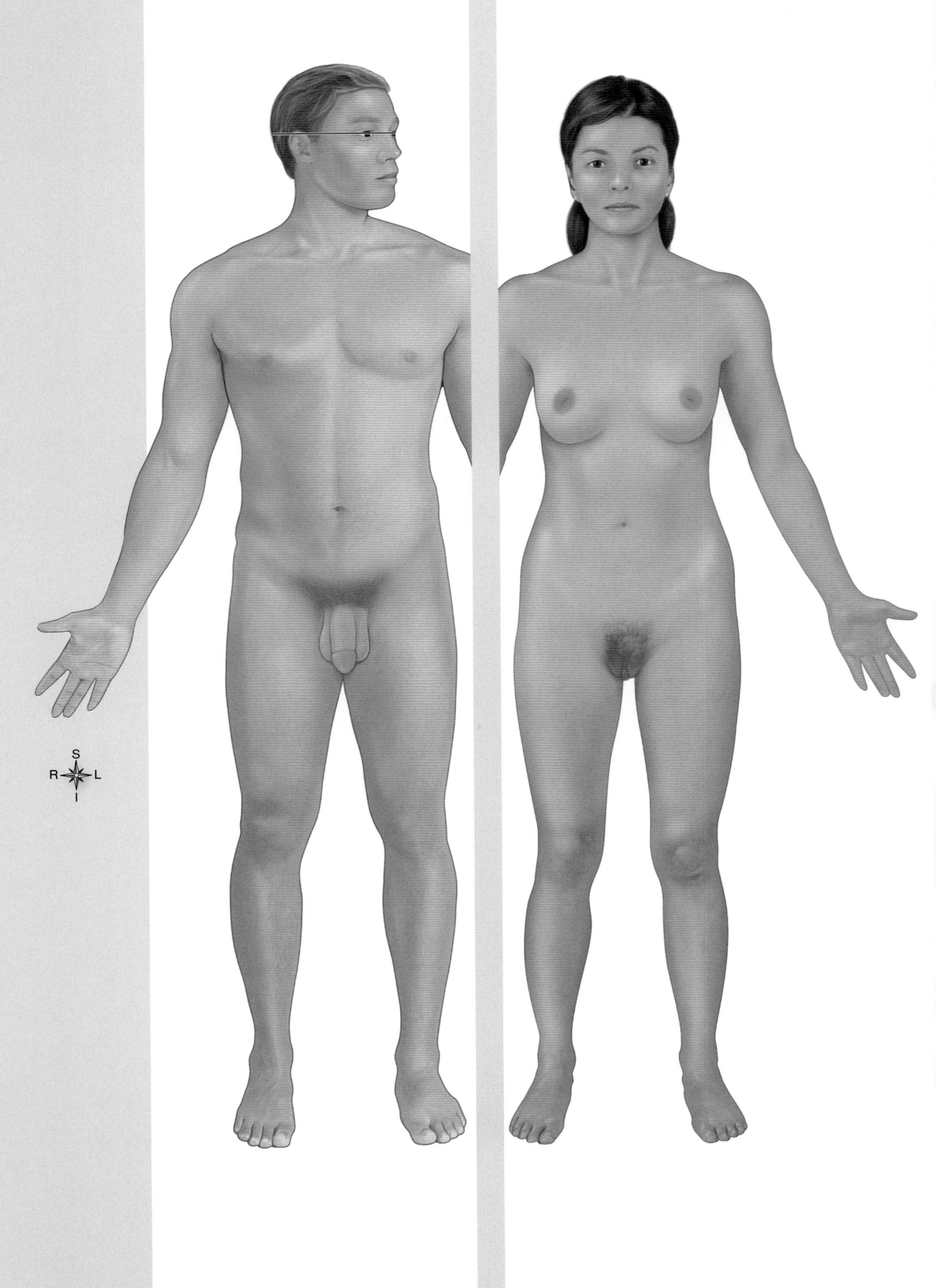
S
R
L
I

14 Articulations

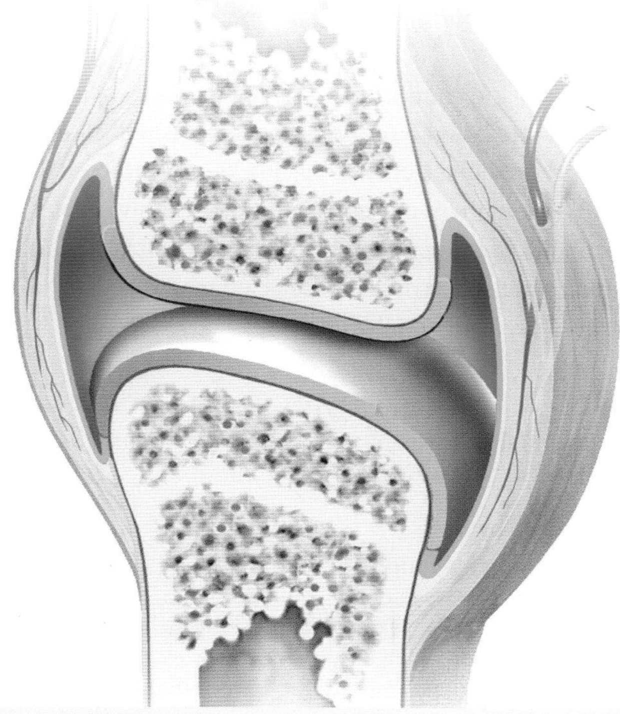

CHAPTER OUTLINE

Hint ▸ *Scan this outline before you begin to read the chapter, as a preview of how the concepts are organized.*

LANGUAGE OF SCIENCE

Hint ▸ *Use this list to aid your pronunciation of unfamiliar words.*

abduction (ab-DUK-shun)
[*ab-* **away,** *-duct-* **lead,** *-tion* **process**]

adduction (ad-DUK-shun)
[*ad-* **toward,** *-duct-* **lead,** *-tion* **process**]

amphiarthrosis
(am-fee-ar-THROH-sis)
[*amphi-* **both sides,** *-arthr-* **joint,** *-osis* **condition**] *pl.,* amphiarthroses

angular movement
(ANG-gyoo-lar MOOV-ment)

articular cartilage
(ar-TIK-yoo-lar KAR-ti-lij)
[*artic-* **joint,** *-ul-* **little,** *-ar* **relating to,** *cartilag-* **cartilage**]

articulation (ar-tik-yoo-LAY-shun)
[*artic-* **joint,** *-ul-* **little,** *-ation* **state**]

biaxial joint (bye-AK-see-al joynt)
[*bi-* **two,** *-axi-* **axle,** *-al* **relating to**]

bursa (BER-sah)
[*bursa* **purse**] *pl.,* bursae

carpometacarpal joint
(kar-po-met-ah-KAR-pal joynt)
[*carpo-* **wrist,** *-meta-* **beyond,** *-carp-* **wrist,** *-al* **relating to**]

circumduction (sir-kum-DUK-shun)
[*circum-* **around,** *-duct-* **lead,** *-tion* **process**]

depression
[*de-* **down,** *-press-* **press,** *-sion* **process**]

diarthrosis (dye-ar-THROH-sis)
[*dia-* **between,** *-arthr-* **joint,** *-osis* **condition**] *pl.,* diarthroses

distal interphalangeal (DIP)
(DIS-tal inter-fah-LAN-gee-al)
[*dist-* **distance,** *-al* **relating to,** *inter-* **between,** *-phalang-* **finger bones (ref. from rows of soldiers),** *-al* **relating to**]

dorsiflexion (dor-si-FLEK-shun)
[*dorsi-* **back,** *-flex-* **bend,** *-ion* **process**]

elevation
[*e(x)-* **up,** *-lev-* **raise,** *-at-* **perform,** *-tion* **process**]

eversion (ee-VER-shun)
[*e(x)-* **outward,** *-ver-* **turn,** *-sion* **process**]

continued on p. 308

An **articulation,** or joint, is a point of contact between bones. Although most joints in the body allow considerable movement, some are completely immovable or permit only limited motion or motion in only one plane or direction. In the case of immovable joints, such as the sutures of the skull, adjacent bones are bound together into a strong and rigid protective plate. In other joints, movement is possible but highly restricted. For example, joints between the bodies of the spinal vertebrae perform two seemingly contradictory functions. They help firmly bind the components of the spine to one another and yet permit normal but restricted movement to occur. Most joints in the body allow considerable movement to occur as a result of skeletal muscle contractions. It is the existence of such joints that permits us to execute complex, highly coordinated, and purposeful movements. Functional articulations between bones in the extremities, such as the shoulder, elbow, hip, and knee, contribute to controlled and graceful movement and provide a large measure of our enjoyment of life. This chapter begins by classifying joints and describing their identifying features. Coverage of joint classification and structure is followed by a discussion of body movements and a description of selected major joints. The chapter concludes by describing life cycle changes and some common joint diseases.

CLASSIFICATION OF JOINTS

Joints may be classified into three major categories by using a structural or a functional scheme.

If a *structural classification* is used, joints are named according to the type of connective tissue that joins the bones together (fibrous or cartilaginous joints) or by the presence of a fluid-filled joint capsule (synovial joints).

If a *functional classification* scheme is used, joints are divided into three classes according to the degree of movement they permit: **synarthroses** (immovable), **amphiarthroses** (slightly movable), and **diarthroses** (freely movable).

Table 14-1 classifies joints according to structure, function, and range of movement. Refer often to this table and to the illustrations that follow as you read about each of the major joint types in this chapter.

Fibrous Joints (Synarthroses)

The articulating surfaces of bones that form fibrous joints fit closely together. The different types and amount of connective tissue joining bones in this group may permit very limited movement in some fibrous joints, but most are fixed. There are three subtypes of fibrous joints: *syndesmoses*, *sutures*, and *gomphoses*.

Syndesmoses

Syndesmoses are joints in which fibrous bands (ligaments) connect two bones. The joint between the distal ends of the radius and ulna is joined by the *radioulnar interosseous ligament* (**Figure 14-1**). Although this joint is classified as a fibrous joint, some movement is possible because of ligament flexibility.

Sutures

Sutures are found only in the skull. In most sutures, teethlike projections jut out from adjacent bones and interlock with each other with only a thin layer of fibrous tissue between them. Sutures become ossified in older adults and form extremely strong lines of fusion between opposing skull bones (see **Figure 14-1**).

Gomphoses

Gomphoses are unique joints that occur between the root of a tooth and the alveolar process of the mandible or maxilla (see **Figure 14-1**). The fibrous tissue between the tooth's root and the alveolar process is a sheet made up of tiny ligaments and called the *periodontal membrane.*

Cartilaginous Joints (Amphiarthroses)

The bones that articulate to form cartilaginous joints are joined together by either hyaline cartilage or fibrocartilage. Joints characterized by the presence of hyaline cartilage between articulating bones are called *synchondroses,* and those joined by fibrocartilage are called *symphyses.* Cartilaginous joints permit only very limited movement between articulating bones in certain circumstances. During childbirth, for example, slight movement at the pubic symphysis facilitates the baby's passage through the pelvis.

TABLE 14-1 Primary Joint Classifications

FUNCTIONAL NAME	STRUCTURAL NAME	DEGREE OF MOVEMENT PERMITTED	EXAMPLE
Synarthroses	Fibrous	Immovable	Sutures of the skull
	Cartilaginous	Immovable	Synchondrosis between rib and sternum
Amphiarthroses	Fibrous	Slightly movable	Syndesmoses between radius and ulna
	Cartilaginous	Slightly movable	Pubic symphysis
Diarthroses	Synovial	Freely movable	Shoulder joint

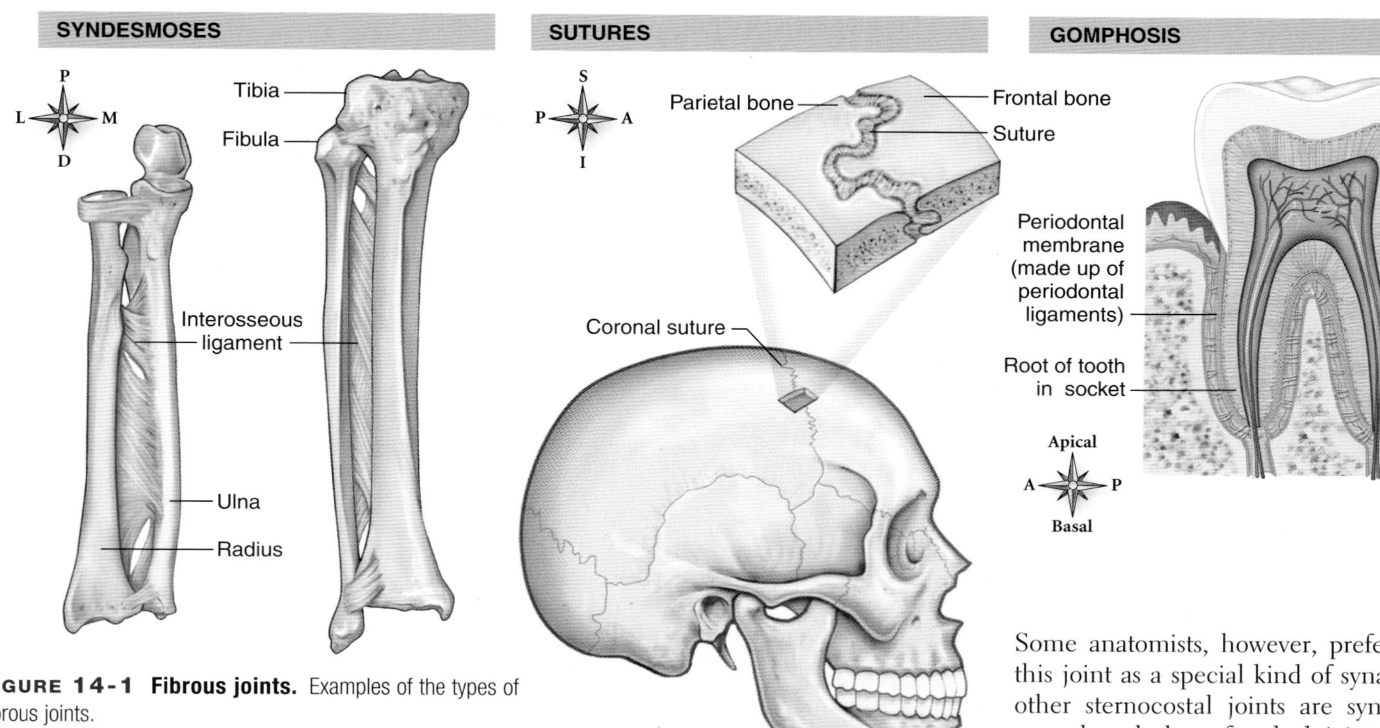

FIGURE 14-1 Fibrous joints. Examples of the types of fibrous joints.

Synchondroses

Note that joints identified as **synchondroses** have hyaline cartilage between articulating bones. One example of a synchondrosis is the joint between the sphenoid bone and the occipital bone (see **Figure 12-4** on p. 239).

Another commonly cited example is the articulation between the first rib and sternum (a *costosternal synchondrosis*; **Figure 14-2**). Some anatomists, however, prefer to classify this joint as a special kind of synarthrosis. All other sternocostal joints are synovial joints, even though they often lack joint capsules.

The best example of a synchondrosis is the joint present during the growth years between the epiphyses of a long bone and its diaphysis (see **Figure 14-2**). The epiphyseal plate between the epiphysis and diaphyses of a long bone is a temporary synchondrosis that normally does not move. The plate of hyaline cartilage is totally replaced by bone at skeletal maturity. Most synchondroses are present only in the immature skeleton as epiphyseal plates—they eventually disappear as the bones fuse together.

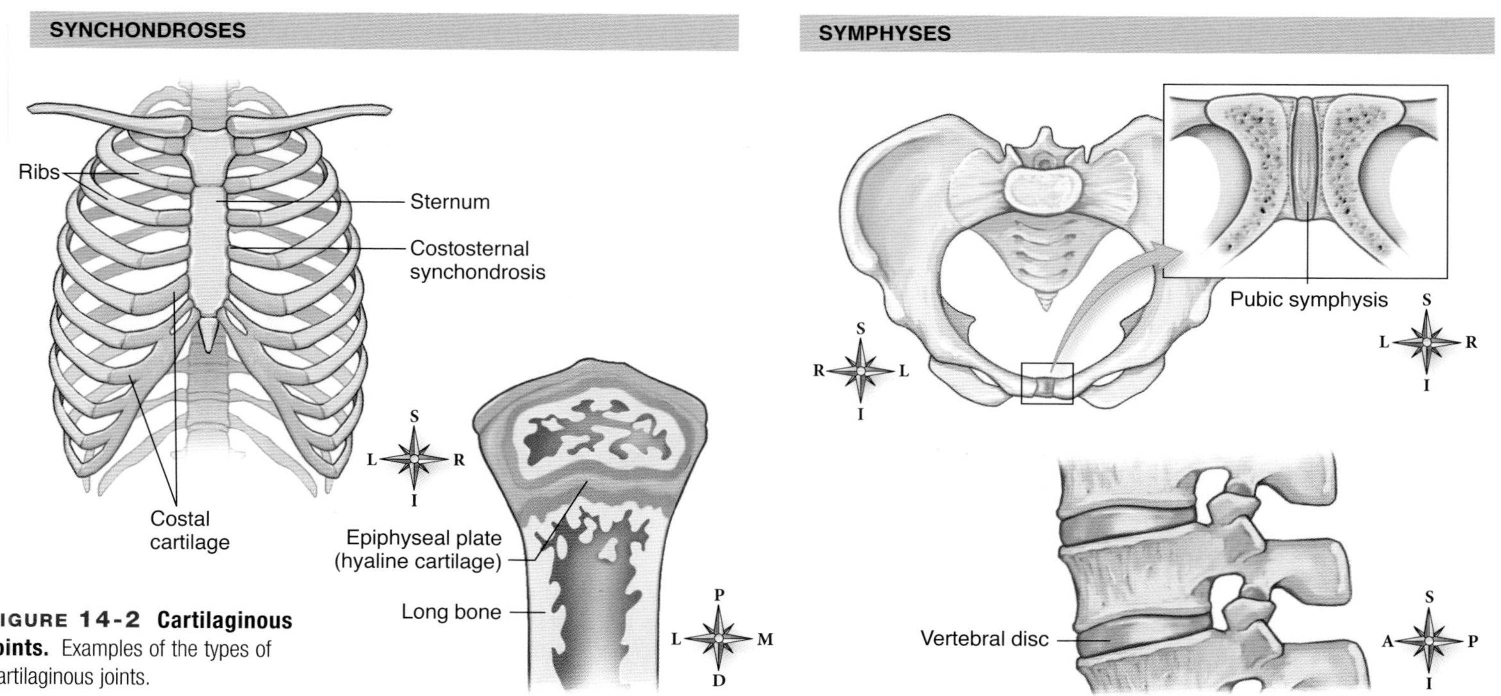

FIGURE 14-2 Cartilaginous joints. Examples of the types of cartilaginous joints.

TABLE 14-2 Classification of Fibrous and Cartilaginous Joints

TYPES	EXAMPLES	STRUCTURAL FEATURES	MOVEMENT
Fibrous Joints			
Syndesmoses	Joints between the distal ends of the radius and ulna	Fibrous bands (ligaments) connect articulating bones	Slight
Sutures	Joints between the skull bones	Teethlike projections of articulating bones interlock with a thin layer of fibrous tissue connecting them	None
Gomphoses	Joints between the roots of the teeth and the jawbones	Fibrous tissue connects the roots of the teeth to the alveolar processes	None
Cartilaginous Joints			
Synchondroses	Costal cartilage attachments of the first rib to the sternum; epiphyseal plate between the diaphysis and epiphysis of a growing long bone	Hyaline cartilage connects articulating bones	Slight
Symphyses	Pubic symphysis; joints between *bodies* of vertebrae	Fibrocartilage between articulating bones	Slight

Symphyses

A **symphysis** is a joint in which a pad or disc of fibrocartilage connects two bones. The tough fibrocartilage discs in these joints may permit slight movement when pressure is applied between the bones.

Most symphyses are located in the midline of the body. Examples of symphyses include the pubic symphysis and the articulation between the *bodies* of adjacent vertebrae (see **Figure 14-2**). The intervertebral disc in these joints is composed of tough and resilient fibrocartilage that absorbs shock and permits limited movement. The bones of the vertebral column have numerous points of articulation between them. Collectively, these joints permit limited motion of the spine in a very restricted range. The articulation between the *bodies* of adjacent vertebrae is classified as a cartilaginous joint. The points of contact between the *articular facets* of adjacent vertebrae are, however, considered synovial joints and are described later in the chapter.

Table 14-2 summarizes the different kinds of fibrous and cartilaginous joints.

Quick CHECK

1. Define the term *joint,* or *articulation.*
2. List the three major classes of joints according to both a structural and a functional scheme.
3. Name the three types of fibrous joints and give one example of each.
4. Identify the two types of cartilaginous joints and give one example of each.

SYNOVIAL JOINTS (DIARTHROSES)

Synovial joints are freely movable joints. They are not only the body's most mobile but also its most numerous and anatomically most complex joints. A majority of the joints between bones in the appendicular skeleton are synovial joints.

Structure of Synovial Joints

The following seven structures characterize synovial, or freely movable, joints (**Figure 14-3**):

1. **Joint capsule.** Sleevelike extension of the periosteum of each of the articulating bones. The capsule forms a complete cas-

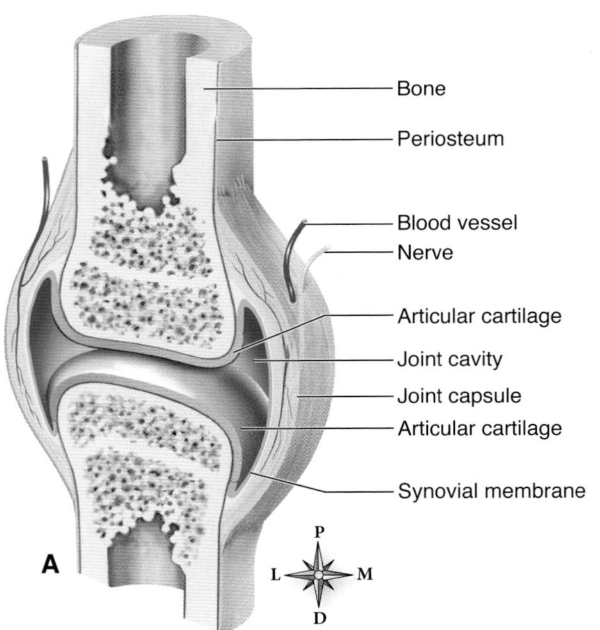

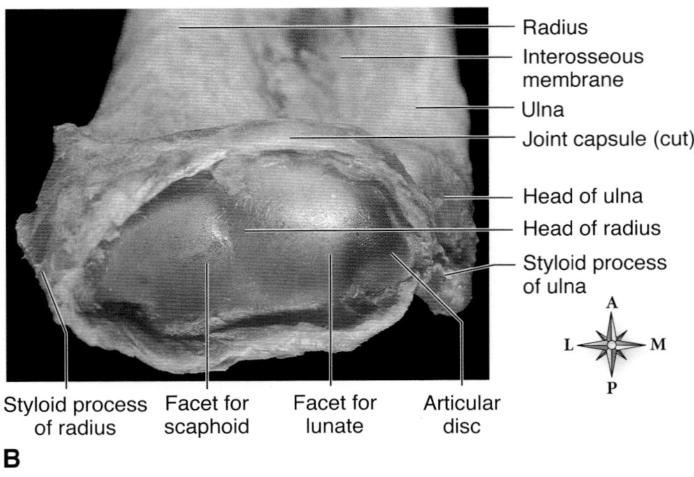

FIGURE 14-3 Structure of synovial joints. A, Artist's interpretation (composite drawing) of a typical synovial joint. **B,** Dissection photo showing the articular surface of a typical synovial joint—the distal radiocarpal joint (the joint capsule has been cut). See pp. 291–292 for a description of this joint.

ing around the ends of the bones, thereby binding them to each other.

2. **Synovial membrane.** Moist, slippery membrane that lines the inner surface of the joint capsule. It attaches to the margins of the articular cartilage. It also secretes synovial fluid, which lubricates and nourishes the inner joint surfaces.
3. **Articular cartilage.** Thin layer of hyaline cartilage covering and cushioning the articular surfaces of bones.
4. **Joint cavity.** Small space between the articulating surfaces of the two bones of the joint. Absence of tissue between articulating bone surfaces permits extensive movement. Synovial joints are therefore diarthroses, or freely movable joints.
5. **Menisci (articular discs).** Pads of fibrocartilage located between the articulating ends of bones in some diarthroses. Usually these pads divide the joint cavity into two separate cavities. The knee joint contains two menisci (see **Figure 14-10**).
6. **Ligaments.** Strong cords of dense, white fibrous tissue at most synovial joints. They grow between the bones, and lash them even more firmly together than is possible with the joint capsule alone.
7. **Bursae.** Some synovial joints contain a closed pillowlike structure called a **bursa,** which consists of a synovial membrane filled with synovial fluid. Bursae tend to be associated with bony prominences (such as in the knee or the elbow), where they function to cushion the joint and facilitate movement of tendons.

Types of Synovial Joints

Synovial joints are divided into three main groups: uniaxial, biaxial, and multiaxial. Each is subdivided further into two subtypes as follows:

1. **Uniaxial joints.** Synovial joints that permit movement around only one axis and in only one plane. Hinge and pivot joints are types of uniaxial joints (**Figure 14-4**, *A* and *B*).
   a. *Hinge joints.* Those in which the articulating ends of the bones form a hinge-shaped unit. Like a common door hinge, hinge joints permit only back-and-forth movements, namely, flexion and extension. If you have access to an articulated skeleton, examine the articulating end of the humerus (the trochlea) and the ulna (the semilunar notch). Observe their interaction as you flex and extend the forearm. Do you see why you can flex and extend your forearm but cannot move it in any other way at this joint? The shapes of the trochlea and the semilunar notch (see **Figure 13-3**, p. 267, and **Figure 13-4**, p. 268) permit only the uniaxial, horizontal-plane movements of flexion and extension at the elbow. Other hinge joints include the knee and interphalangeal joints.
   b. *Pivot joints.* Those in which a projection of one bone articulates with a ring or notch of another bone. Examples include a projection (dens) of the second cervical vertebra articulating with a ring-shaped portion of the first cervical vertebra and the head of the radius articulating with the radial notch of the ulna.

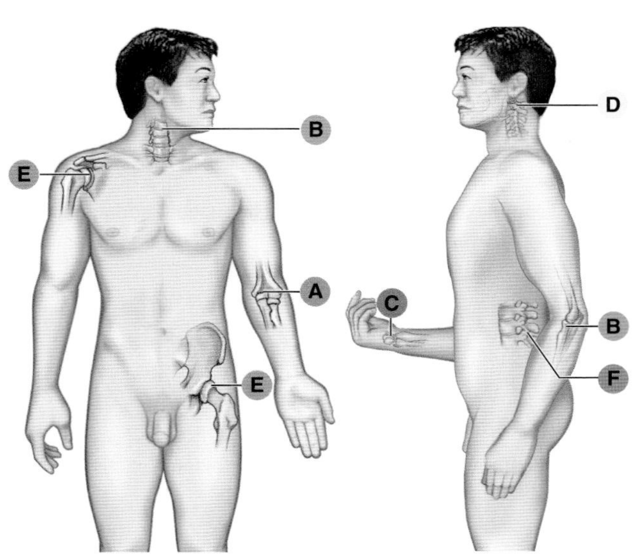

UNIAXIAL JOINTS

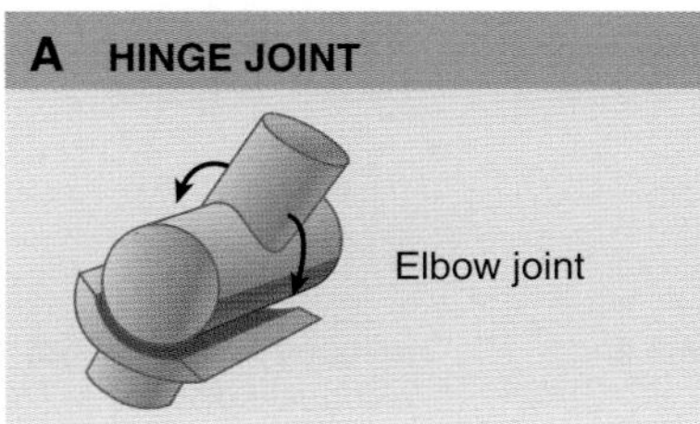

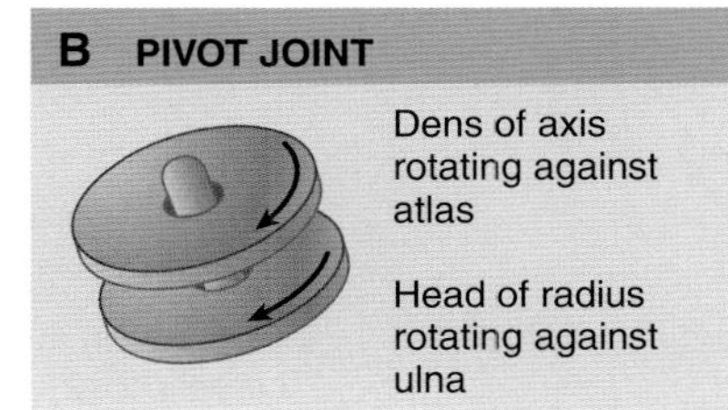

BIAXIAL JOINTS

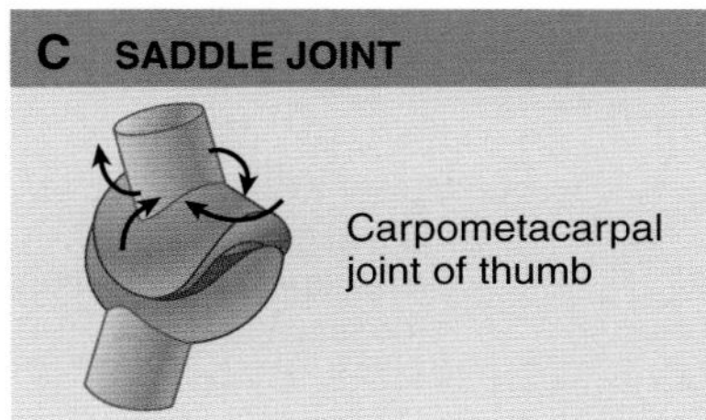

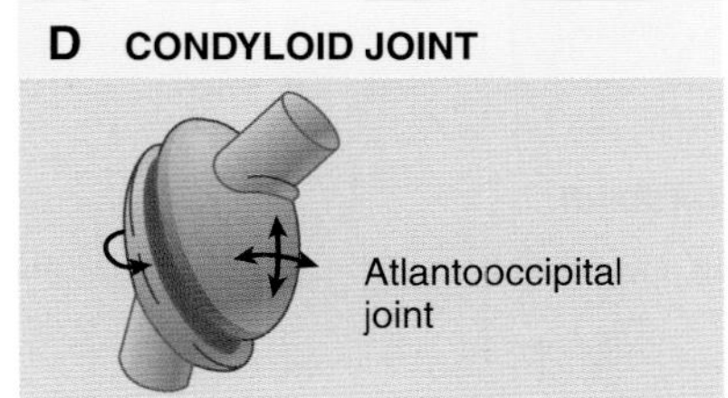

MULTIAXIAL JOINTS

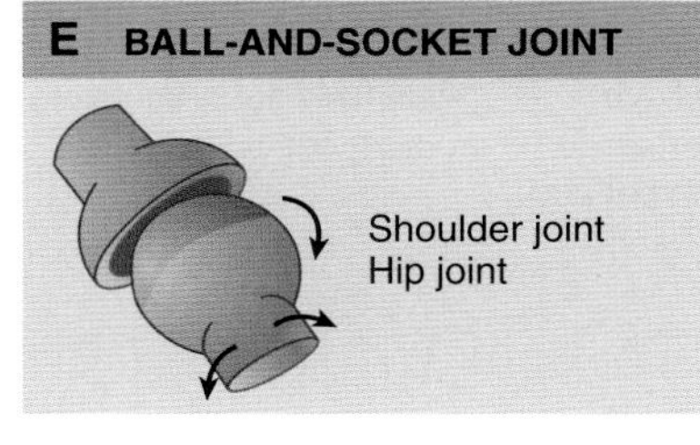

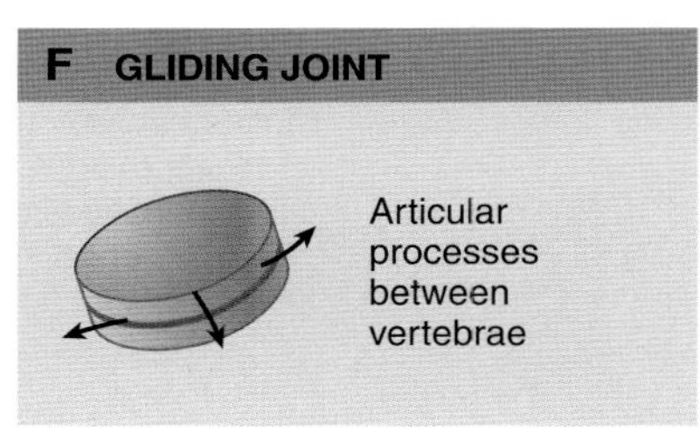

FIGURE 14-4 Types of synovial joints. Uniaxial: **A,** hinge, and **B,** pivot. Biaxial: **C,** saddle, and **D,** condyloid. Multiaxial: **E,** ball and socket, and **F,** gliding.

2. **Biaxial joints.** Diarthroses that permit movement around two perpendicular axes in two perpendicular planes. Saddle and condyloid joints are types of biaxial joints (**Figure 14-4**, *C* and *D*).
   a. *Saddle joints.* Those in which the articulating ends of the bones resemble reciprocally shaped miniature saddles. Only two saddle joints—one in each thumb—are present in the body. The thumb's metacarpal bone articulates in the wrist with a carpal bone (trapezium). The saddle-shaped articulating surfaces of these bones make it possible for the thumb to swing in an arc to touch the tips of the fingers—that is, to oppose the fingers. How important is this? To answer this for yourself, consider the following. Opposing the thumb to the fingers enables us to grip small objects. Were it not for this movement, we would have much less manual dexterity. A surgeon could not grasp a scalpel or suture needle effectively, and none of us could easily hold a pen or pencil for writing.
   b. *Condyloid (ellipsoidal) joints.* Those in which a condyle fits into an elliptical socket. Examples include condyles of the occipital bone fitting into elliptical depressions of the atlas and the distal end of the radius fitting into depressions of the carpal bones (scaphoid, lunate, and triquetrum).
3. **Multiaxial joints.** Joints that permit movement around three or more axes and in three or more planes (**Figure 14-4**, *E* and *F*).

TABLE 14-3 Classification of Synovial Joints

TYPES	EXAMPLES	STRUCTURE	MOVEMENT
Uniaxial			*Around one axis; in one place*
Hinge	Elbow joint	Spool-shaped process fits into a concave socket	Flexion and extension only
Pivot	Joint between the first and second cervical vertebrae	Arch-shaped process fits around a peglike process	Rotation
Biaxial			*Around two axes, perpendicular to each other; in two planes*
Saddle	Thumb joint between the first metacarpal and carpal bone	Saddle-shaped bone fits into a socket that is concave–convex–concave	Flexion, extension in one plane; abduction, adduction in the other plane; opposing the thumb to the fingers
Condyloid (ellipsoidal)	Joint between the radius and carpal bones	Oval condyle fits into an elliptical socket	Flexion, extension in one plane; abduction, adduction in the other plane
Multiaxial			*Around many axes*
Ball and socket	Shoulder joint and hip	Ball-shaped process fits into a concave socket	Widest range of movement: flexion, extension, abduction, adduction, rotation, circumduction
Gliding	Joints between the articular facets of adjacent vertebrae; joints between the carpal and tarsal bones	Relatively flat articulating surfaces	Gliding movements without any angular or circular movements

a. *Ball-and-socket joints (spheroid joints).* Our most movable joints. A ball-shaped head of one bone fits into a concave depression on another, thereby allowing the first bone to move in many directions. Examples include the shoulder and hip joints.
b. *Gliding joints.* Characterized by relatively flat articulating surfaces that allow limited gliding movements along various axes. Examples include the joints between the articular surfaces of successive vertebrae. (Articulations between the bodies of successive vertebrae are symphysis-type cartilaginous joints.) As a group, gliding joints are the least movable of the synovial joints.

Table 14-3 summarizes the classes of synovial joints.

Quick CHECK

5. List the seven structures that characterize synovial joints.
6. Name the three main categories of synovial joints grouped according to axial movement and list the two subtypes of joints found in each category.
7. Name one specific joint as an example of each of the six types of synovial joints.

UNIT 2

REPRESENTATIVE SYNOVIAL JOINTS

HUMEROSCAPULAR JOINT

The joint between the head of the humerus and the glenoid cavity of the scapula is the one we usually refer to as the shoulder joint (**Figure 14-5**). It is our most mobile joint. One anatomical detail, the

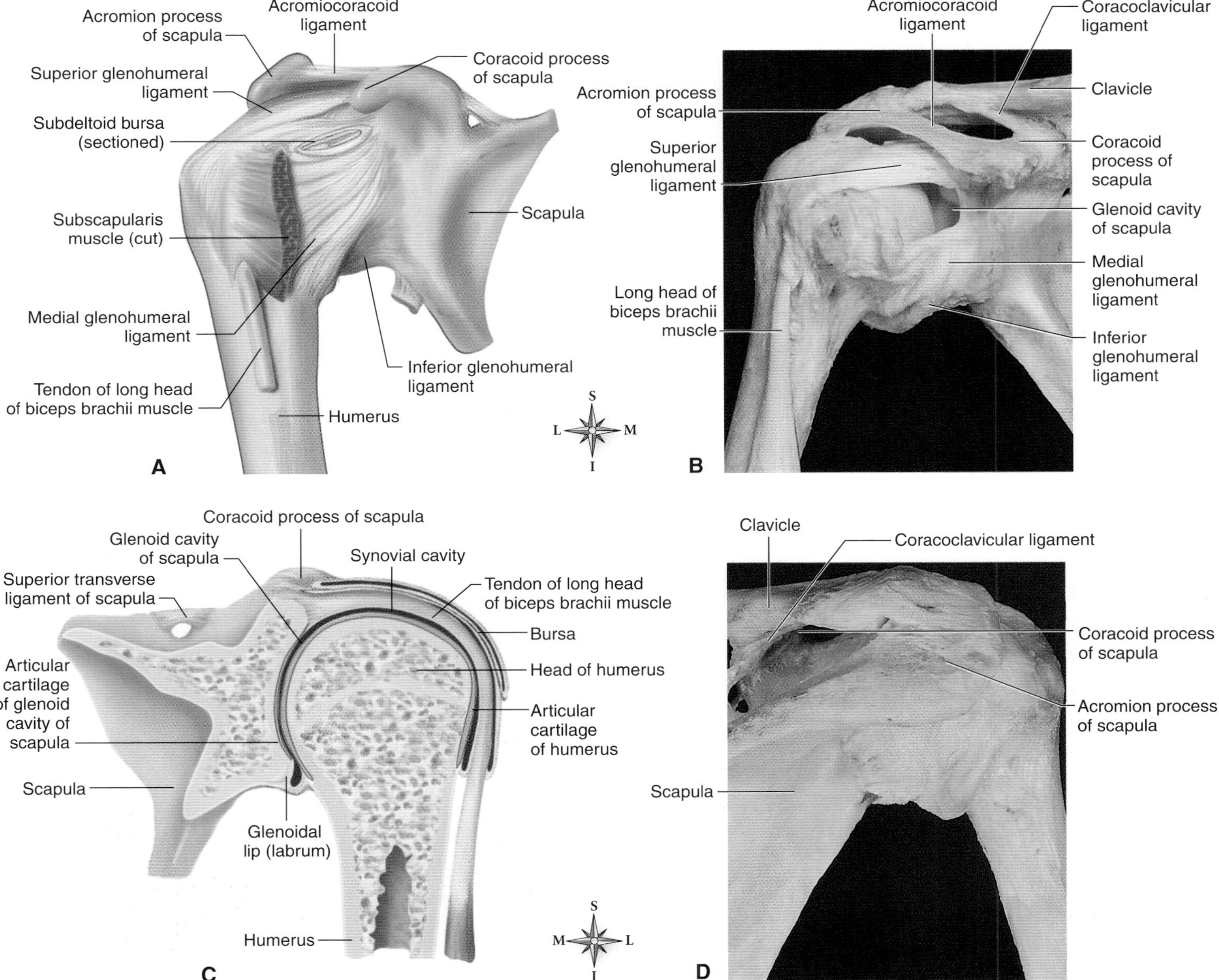

FIGURE 14-5 The shoulder joint. A, Artist's diagram, and **B,** dissection photo (anterior views). **C,** Artist's diagram, and **D,** dissection photo (viewed from behind through shoulder joint).

shallowness of the glenoid cavity, largely accounts for this mobility. The shallowness offers little interference to movement of the head of the humerus. Were it not for the glenoidal lip (see **Figure 14-5**, *C*), a narrow rim of fibrocartilage around the glenoid cavity, it would have scarcely any depth at all.

Some structures strengthen the shoulder joint and give it a degree of stability, notably several ligaments, muscles, tendons, and bursae. Note in **Figure 14-5**, *A*, for example, the superior, medial, and inferior glenohumeral ligaments. Each of these ligaments is a thickened portion of the joint capsule. Also in this figure, identify the subscapularis muscle, the tendon of the long head of the biceps brachii muscle, and a bursa.

Shoulder muscles and tendons form a cufflike arrangement around the joint. It is called the *rotator cuff.* Injuries to the rotator cuff are common in people participating in throwing and racket sports. The main bursa of the shoulder joint is the *subdeltoid bursa.* It lies wedged between the inferior surface of the deltoid muscle and the superior surface of the joint capsule. Other bursae of the shoulder joint are the subscapular, subacromial, and subcoracoid bursae. All in all, the shoulder joint is more mobile than stable. Dislocations of the head of the humerus from the glenoid cavity occur commonly.

CONNECT IT! 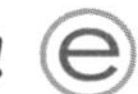

An x-ray photograph of the shoulder joint seen in ***Skeletal Radiography*** online at ***Connect It!*** clearly shows the bony structures and their anatomical relationships in a living body. Other joints of the body are also illustrated there.

Elbow Joint

The elbow joint (**Figure 14-6**) is a classic hinge joint formed by two articulations occurring between the distal end of the humerus and the proximal ends of the radius and ulna. Laterally it is the capitulum of the humerus that articulates with the head of the radius in the *humeroradial joint.* Medially, the trochlea of the humerus articulates with the trochlear notch of the ulna in the *humeroulnar joint.* Both of these joint components are surrounded by a single joint capsule and by ligaments on either side, called *collateral ligaments*, that fuse with the capsule to stabilize the joint and help prevent disarticulation.

The articulation between the proximal ends of the radius and ulna just below the joint capsule is called the *proximal radioulnar joint.* The point of articulation is between the head of the radius and the radial notch of the ulna and is stabilized by the *annular ligament.* Although it is not a part of the elbow joint involved in hinge movements, it does permit rotation of the forearm as the radial head moves on the ulna.

Dislocation of the radial head, called a "pulled elbow", is seen more often in young children than adults. The reason? The disc-shaped head of the radius does not attain its conical shape until late in childhood and therefore slips more easily from under the annular ligament. **Figure 14-6**, *B*, shows the annular ligament attached to the proximal end of the ulna in an adult. It firmly holds the head of the radius against the articular surface of the radial notch on the ulna, thus allowing the radius to rotate freely.

A number of other anatomical or clinical "points of interest" are associated with the elbow joint. The medial and lateral epicondyles are palpable bony landmarks (see **Box 13-2** on p. 274) on either side of the joint, and the **olecranon bursa,** which helps cushion the joint, is found just under the skin on its posterior surface overlying the olecranon of the ulna. **Olecranon bursitis** is inflammation of the bursa associated with prolonged pressure.

One of the most common sites for *venipuncture* (piercing a vein) to obtain blood is the median cubital vein located in the fossa just anterior to the joint.

Perhaps one of the most important structures near the joint is the ulnar nerve. It courses along the groove, sometimes called the "funny bone", between the olecranon and the medial epicondyle. Blows to this area produce unpleasant sensations in the hand and fingers supplied by the nerve. More severe injuries may result in

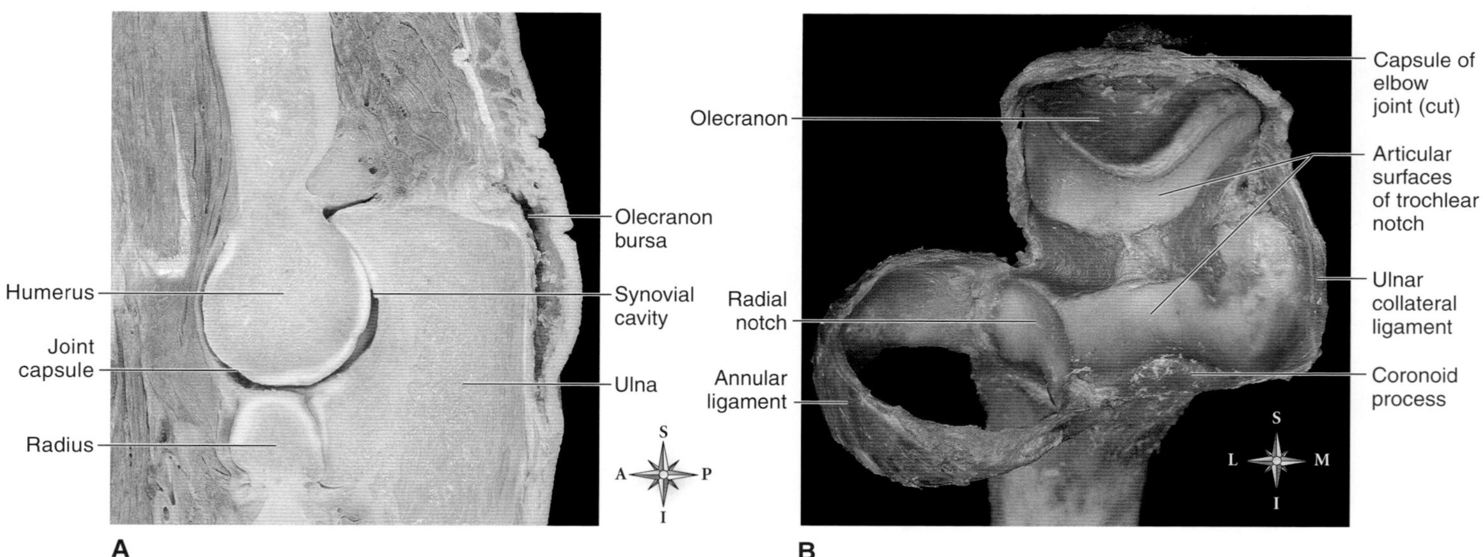

FIGURE 14-6 The elbow joint. A, Sagittal section through the elbow joint. **B,** Dissection photo showing the anterior view of the proximal end of the ulna with attached annular ligament.

paralysis of hand muscles and produce "clawhand" or a reduction in wrist movements.

Forearm, Wrist, Hand, and Finger Joints

Proper function of the forearm, wrist, hand, and fingers, as well as the joints that permit movement in these areas, is often said to be the functional "reason" for the upper extremity. Our ability to grasp and manipulate small objects, to properly focus the movement and strength of our upper extremities, and to perform the many movements required to coordinate or restore balance and equilibrium are only a few examples of activities that require normal functioning of our forearms, wrists, hands, and fingers.

In clinical medicine, treatment or repair of injuries to these important functional areas constitutes a highly specialized area of surgical practice. In addition to bones and joints, the relatively small area of the wrist and hand, especially, is packed with many other anatomical structures, such as muscles, ligaments, blood vessels, and nerves. Hand surgery, like many other forms of specialized surgery, requires both a mastery of complex techniques and an in-depth understanding of the anatomy involved.

There are seven categories of synovial joints between the bones of the forearm, wrist, hand, and fingers. They are named after the bones that touch or articulate with one another in the joints involved. Some of the movements produced are slight and subtle, whereas others are more apparent. All are important functionally and are illustrated later in the chapter.

Radioulnar Joints

The head of the radius and the radial notch of the ulna articulate just below the elbow joint to form the *proximal radioulnar joint* described earlier. Together with the *distal radioulnar joint,* which is the point of articulation between the ulnar notch of the radius and head of the ulna just above the wrist, the two **radioulnar joints** permit pronation and supination of the forearm.

Radiocarpal (Wrist) Joints

As the name in the heading implies, only the radius articulates directly with the wrist or carpal bones distally. The point of articulation between the head of the radius and the scaphoid and lunate carpal bones forms a typical synovial joint—in this case, a **radiocarpal joint**—and is shown in **Figure 14-7**. A full range of motions occurs at the joint and is illustrated later in the chapter.

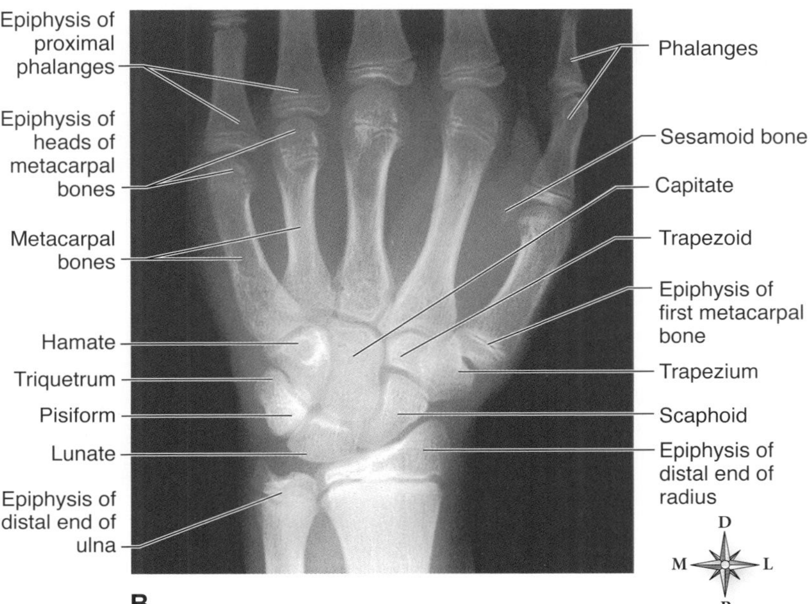

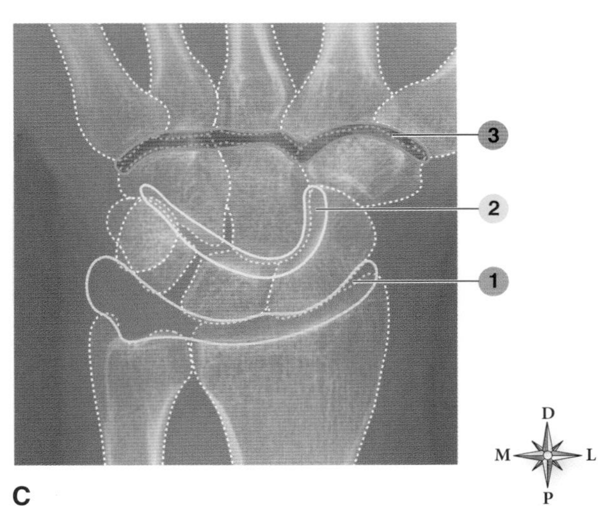

FIGURE 14-7 Joints of the wrist. A, Coronal section of the hand showing the joints of the wrist. Note that the thumb and little finger are not in the plane of section. **B,** Radiograph of an adolescent hand and wrist. Note that the epiphyseal plates are present. **C,** Major synovial spaces of the wrist: *1,* proximal; *2,* intermediate; *3,* distal.

Falls on an outstretched hand often result in fractures of the scaphoid bone. It is the scaphoid that transmits a majority of the applied force to the radial head. Unfortunately, loss of blood supply to a portion of the fractured scaphoid may result in necrosis of the broken fragment, which requires surgical removal or other specialized treatment. Note that a disc separates the distal part of the ulna from direct contact with the carpal bones.

Intercarpal Joints

The **intercarpal joints** occur at points of articulation between the eight carpal bones. Arranged in two rows (proximal and distal) of four bones each, the carpal bones and the joints between them are supported and stabilized by numerous ligaments. They are also stabilized by forearm muscle tendons acting on the wrist and digits that wrap around the wrist to form a sort of cuff.

The joint spaces usually communicate with each other, forming large joint spaces. You can see the three largest of these joint spaces in **Figure 14-7**, *C*. The relationships between the intercarpal joints are illustrated in **Figure 14-7**. Functionally, movements at the intercarpal joints are generally gliding with some abduction and flexion.

Carpometacarpal Joints

There are a total of three **carpometacarpal joints,** one for the thumb and two for the fingers. The thumb carpometacarpal joint is unique in having both a loose-fitting joint capsule and a saddle-shaped articular surface between the first metacarpal bone and the trapezium. Movements possible at this joint include flexion, extension, adduction, abduction, and circumduction. In addition, because of the special anatomical features of this joint, a combination movement called *opposition* of the thumb (see p. 303) is possible. Opposition allows us to touch the tips of any of the fingers with the tip of the thumb. It is this unique movement that permits us to grasp and manipulate small objects—a functional movement of immense practical significance.

The remaining two carpometacarpal joints are much less mobile than the saddle-shaped one for the thumb and are limited to essentially gliding-type movements.

Metacarpophalangeal Joints

In **metacarpophalangeal joints** the rounded heads of the metacarpal bones and the concave bases of the proximal phalanges articulate with each other (**Figure 14-8**). The capsule surrounding each joint is strengthened by collateral ligaments on both sides. The shape of the articular surfaces in these joints permits only limited adduction and abduction—and only when the fingers are extended. Much more extensive flexion and extension movements are possible.

Interphalangeal Joints

Interphalangeal joints are typical hinge-type synovial joints capable of flexion and extension. They exist between the heads of the phalanges and the bases of the more distal phalanges. In the fingers, two types of interphalangeal joints can be identified. The joints between the proximal and middle phalanges are called **proximal interphalangeal (PIP) joints,** whereas those between the middle and distal phalanges are called the **distal interphalangeal (DIP) joints.**

Understanding the relationship of articulations between the phalanges will help in understanding the various finger movements discussed later in the chapter (see **Figure 14-22**).

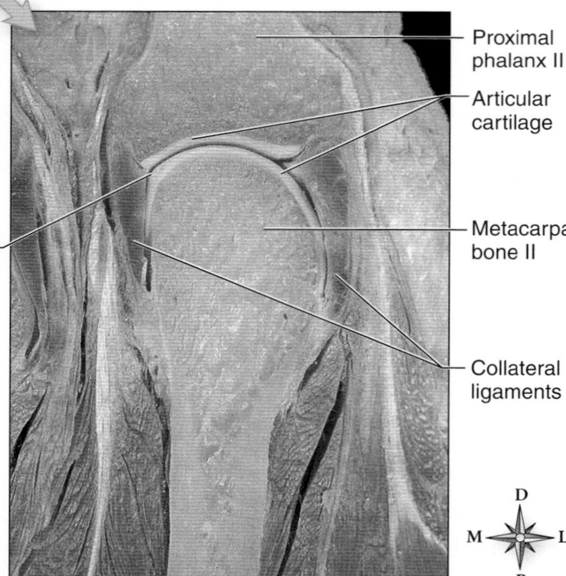

FIGURE 14-8 Joints of the hand and fingers. Radiograph of an adult hand shows the absence of epiphyseal plates. All the phalanges and metacarpal bones are easily seen. The inset shows a dissected specimen in a coronal section through the second metacarpophalangeal joint. The collateral ligaments are simply thickenings of the walls of the joint capsule.

Hip Joint

The first characteristic to remember about the hip joint is stability; the second is mobility (**Figure 14-9**). The stability of the hip joint derives largely from the shapes of the head of the femur and the acetabulum, the socket of the hip bone into which the femur head fits.

Turn to **Figure 13-7** and note the deep, cuplike shape of the acetabulum, and then observe the ball-like head of the femur in **Figure 13-8**, *A*. Compare these with the shallow, almost saucer-shaped glenoid cavity (see **Figure 13-2**, *C*) and the head of the humerus (see **Figure 13-3**). From these observations, note why the hip joint necessarily has a somewhat more limited range of movement than does the shoulder joint? Both joints, however, allow multiaxial movements. Both permit flexion, extension, abduction, adduction, rotation, and circumduction.

A joint capsule and several ligaments hold the femur and hip bones together and contribute to the hip joint's stability. The iliofemoral ligament connects the ilium with the femur, and the ischiofemoral and pubofemoral ligaments join the ischium and pubic bone to the femur. The iliofemoral ligament is one of the strongest ligaments in the body.

Knee Joint

The knee, or *tibiofemoral joint*, is the largest and one of the most complex and most commonly injured joints in the body

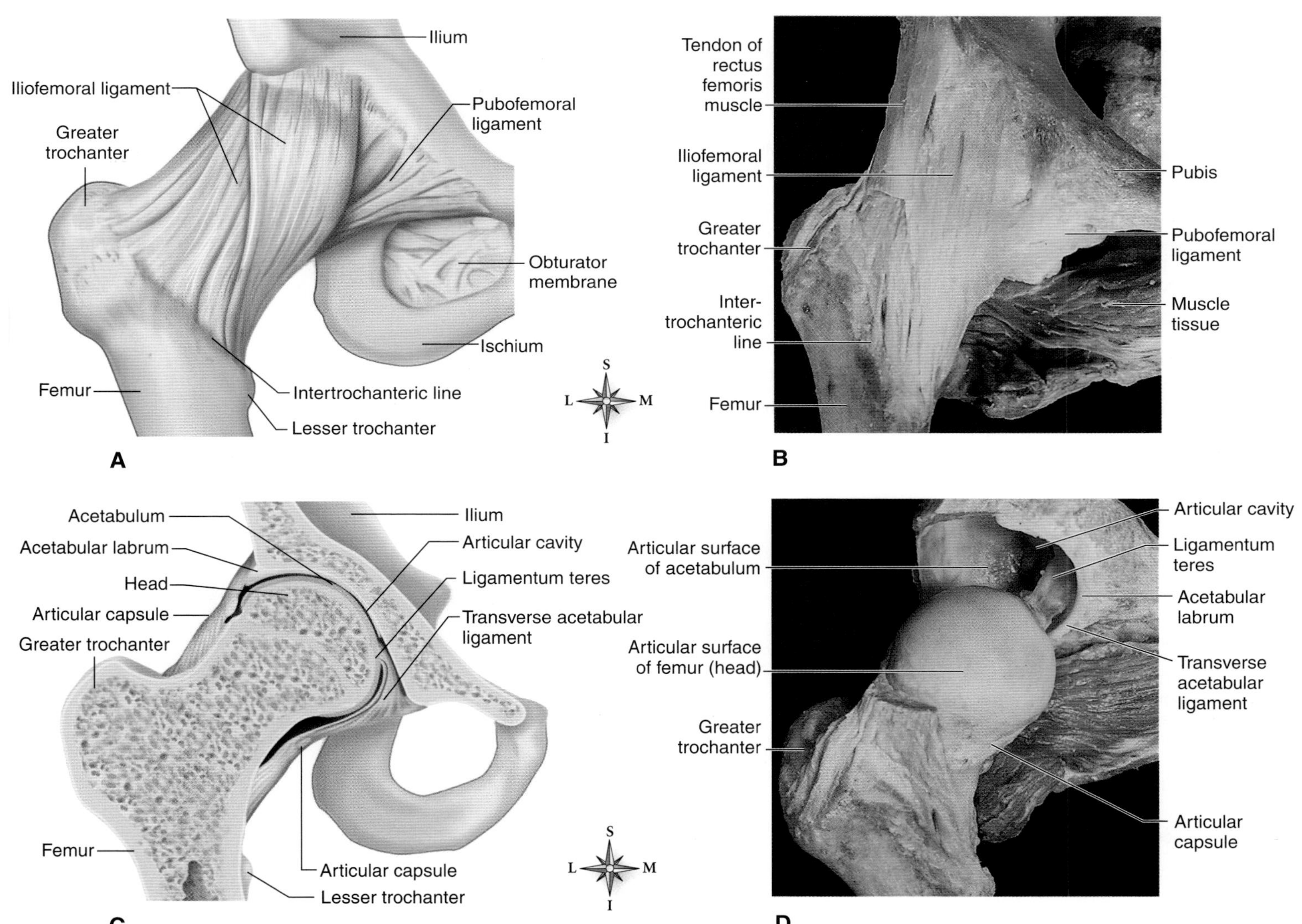

FIGURE 14-9 The hip joint. A, Artist's diagram, and **B,** dissection photo (anterior views). **C,** Artist's diagram, and **D,** dissection photo (coronal [frontal] section).

(**Figure 14-10** and **Figure 14-11**; **Box 14-1**). The condyles of the femur articulate with the flat upper surface of the tibia. Although this arrangement is precariously unstable, counteracting forces are supplied by a joint capsule, cartilages, and numerous ligaments and muscle tendons. Note, for example, in **Figure 14-10** the shape of the two cartilages labelled *medial meniscus* and *lateral meniscus*. They attach to the flat top of the tibia and, because of their concavity, form a kind of shallow socket for the condyles of the femur.

Of the many ligaments that hold the femur bound to the tibia, five can be seen in **Figure 14-10**. The *anterior cruciate ligament (ACL)* attaches to the anterior part of the tibia between its condyles, then crosses over and backward and attaches to the posterior part of the lateral condyle of the femur. The *posterior cruciate ligament (PCL)* attaches posteriorly to the tibia and lateral meniscus, then crosses over and attaches to the front part of the femur's medial condyle.

The *posterior meniscofemoral ligament* (Wrisberg ligament) attaches posteriorly to the lateral meniscus and extends up and over to attach to the medial condyle of the femur behind the attachment of the posterior cruciate ligament (**Figure 14-10**, *C*). The *transverse ligament* connects the anterior margins of the two menisci. Strong ligaments, the *fibular* and *tibial collateral ligaments*, located at the sides of the knee joint can be seen in **Figure 14-10**, *C*.

An *anterolateral ligament (ALL)*, connecting the lateral femoral epicondyle to the anterolateral part of the tibia at the lateral meniscus, has been proposed. Some consider the ALL to be part of the joint capsule rather than a distinct ligament.

Thirteen bursae serve as pads around the knee joint: four in front, four located laterally, and five medially. Of these, the largest is the *prepatellar bursa* (see **Figure 14-11**) inserted in front of the patellar ligament, between it and the skin. The painful ailment prepatellar

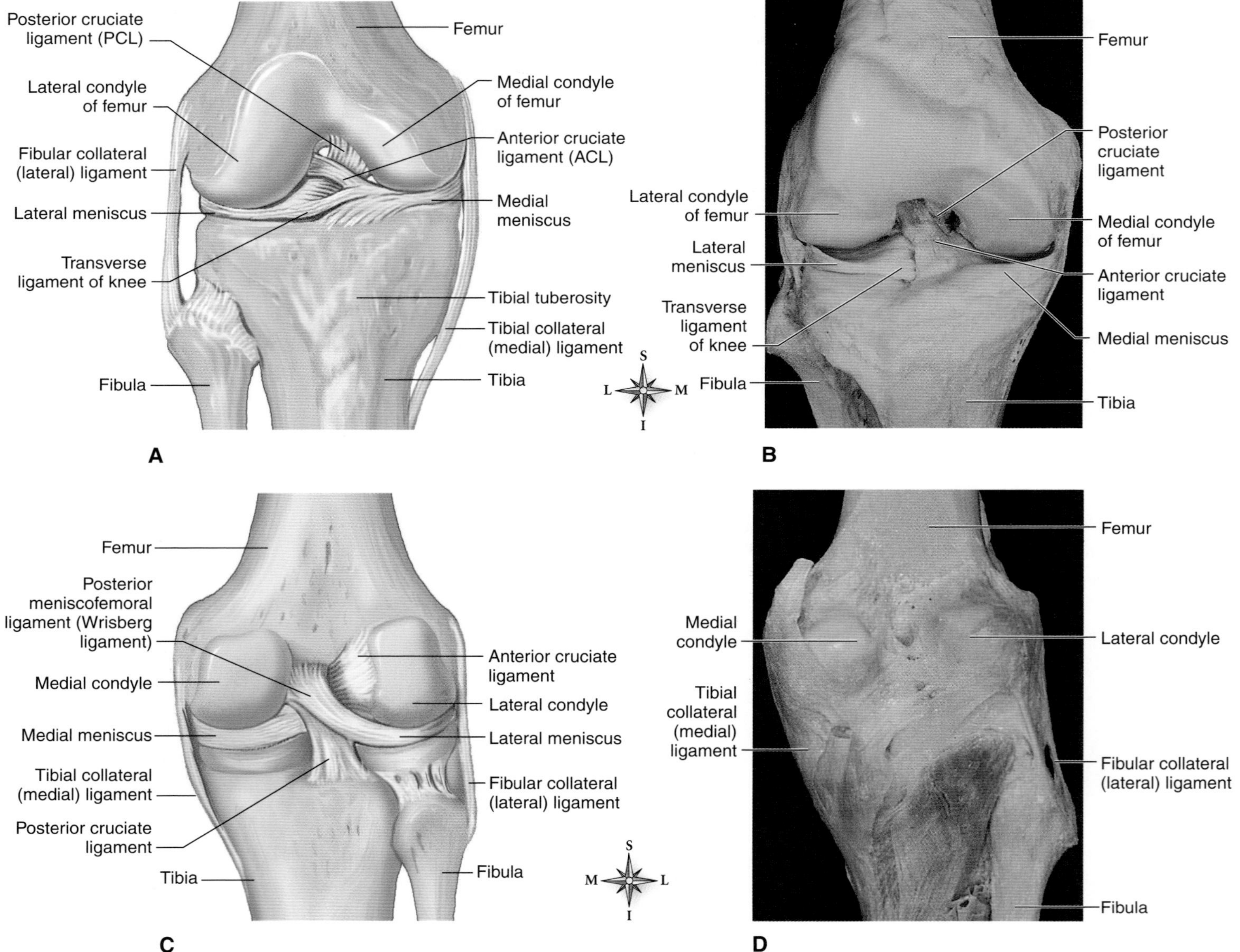

FIGURE 14-10 The right knee joint. A and **B,** Labelled dissection of the right knee viewed from in front. **C** and **D,** Viewed from behind.

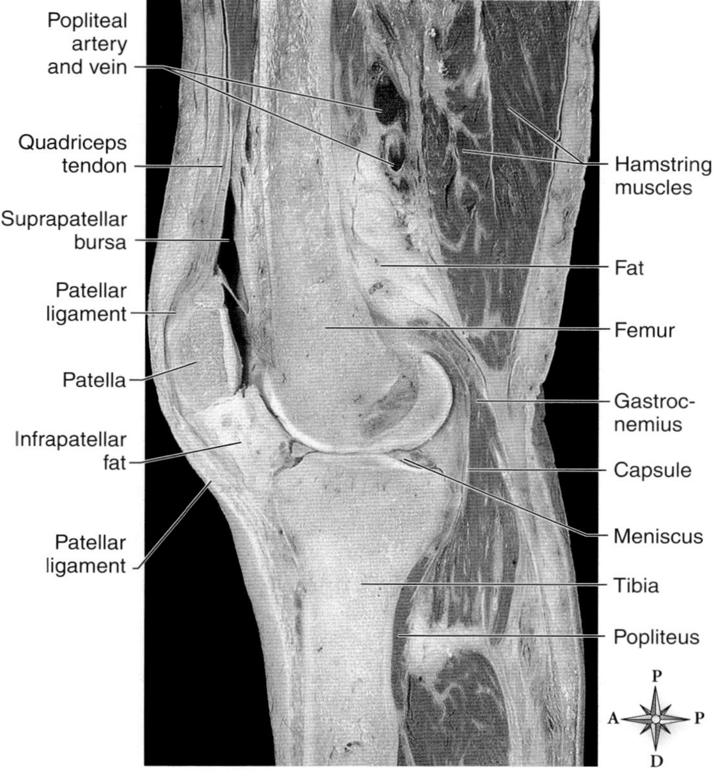

FIGURE 14-11 Knee joint (sagittal section). Cadaver dissection showing the articular surfaces and related structures.

bursitis, commonly called "housemaid's knee", is prevalent in people who spend long periods of time kneeling.

When compared with the hip joint, the knee joint is relatively unprotected by surrounding muscles. Consequently, the knee, more often than the hip, is injured by blows or sudden stops and turns. Athletes, for example, are prone to tearing a knee cartilage, specifically, one of the menisci (see **Figure 14-11**).

The structure of the knee joint permits the hingelike movements of flexion and extension. Also, with the knee flexed, some internal and external rotation can occur. In most of our day-to-day activities—even such ordinary ones as walking, going up and down stairs, and getting into and out of chairs—our knees bear the brunt of the load; they are the main weight-bearers. Knee injury or disease can therefore be crippling.

Ankle Joint

Anatomical comparisons of the wrist, hand, and fingers are often made with the ankle, foot, and toes. Although many anatomical similarities do exist, functional differences abound. Hand anatomy is a marvel of functional construction that permits flexibility and, especially with the presence of a saddle joint between the first metacarpal bone and the trapezium, discrete and precisely controlled movement. The bony structure of the ankle and foot, as well as the joints that exist between them, enhance stability and weight bearing rather than flexibility and a wide range of different movements.

Compare the articulating bones, joint types, and movements in each area listed in **Table 14-4**. Note in **Figure 14-12**, *B*, that the lateral malleolus of the ankle joint is lower than the medial and contributes to a wedge or so-called *mortise-shaped* articulation with the talus below. The combination of a uniquely shaped articular surface and strong supporting ligaments results in an excellent platform for weight bearing during standing and walking. However, so-called rotational ankle injuries do occur—especially in certain types of dance or during athletic activity.

The most common type of **sprained ankle** is caused by an internal rotation injury to the anterior talofibular ligament, seen in **Figure 14-12**. Symptoms include pain and swelling over the lateral

UNIT 2

BOX 14-1 *sports and fitness* | Knee Joint Injuries

The knee is the largest movable joint in the body and also one of the most vulnerable to injury. Because the knee is often subjected to sudden, strong forces during athletic activity, knee injuries are among the most common type of athletic injury. Sometimes the concave discs of articular cartilage on the tibia, called menisci, become torn when the knee twists while bearing weight. The ligaments holding the tibia and femur together and the medial and lateral menisci also can be injured in this way. Knee injuries also may occur when a weight-bearing knee collides with another person, especially from the side, as sometimes happens in sporting events. •

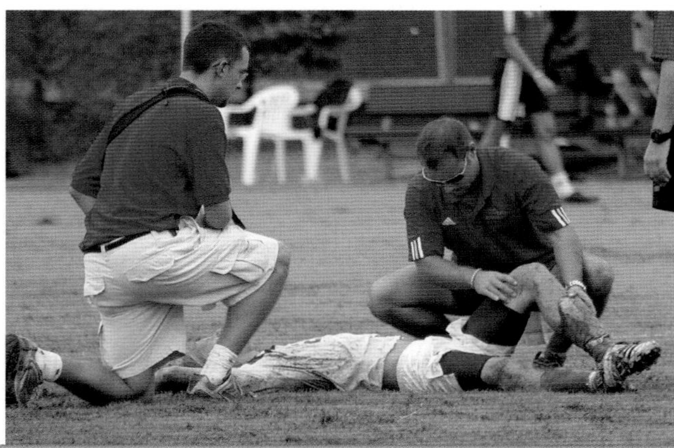

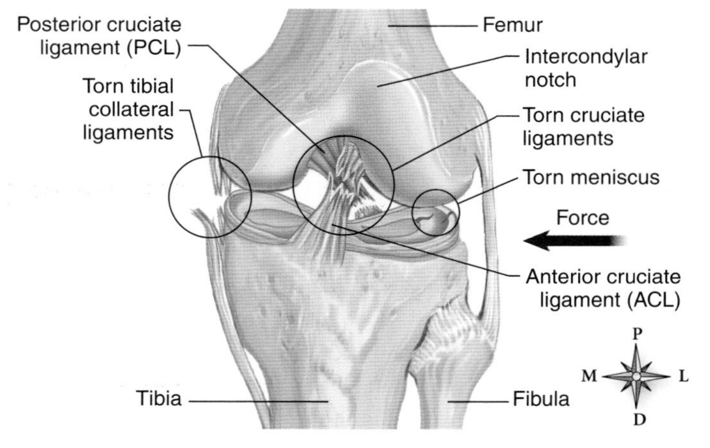

TABLE 14-4 Major Synovial and Cartilaginous Joints

NAME	ARTICULATING BONES	TYPE	MOVEMENTS
Atlantoepistropheal	Anterior arch of the atlas rotates about the dens of the axis (epistropheus)	Synovial (pivot)	Pivoting or partial rotation of the head
Vertebral	Between bodies of vertebrae	Cartilaginous (symphyses)	Slight movement between any two vertebrae but considerable motility for the column as a whole
	Between articular processes	Synovial (gliding)	Gliding
Sternoclavicular	Medial end of the clavicle with the manubrium of the sternum	Synovial (gliding)	Gliding
Acromioclavicular	Distal end of the clavicle with the acromion of the scapula	Synovial (gliding)	Gliding; elevation, depression, protraction, and retraction
Thoracic	Heads of ribs with bodies of vertebrae	Synovial (gliding)	Gliding
	Tubercles of ribs with transverse processes of vertebrae	Synovial (gliding)	Gliding
Costosternal	First rib with sternum	Cartilaginous (synchondrosis); sometimes classified as a special fibrous (synarthrosis)	Slight movement allows some expansion of thorax
Sternocostal	Ribs 2–14 with sternum	Synovial (gliding); lacks joint capsule	Slight movement allows some expansion of thorax
Shoulder	Head of the humerus in the glenoid cavity of the scapula	Synovial (ball and socket)	Flexion, extension, abduction, adduction, rotation, and circumduction of the upper part of the arm
Elbow	Trochlea of the humerus with the semilunar notch of the ulna; head of the radius with the capitulum of the humerus	Synovial (hinge)	Flexion and extension
	Head of the radius in the radial notch of the ulna	Synovial (pivot)	Supination and pronation of the forearm and hand; rotation of the forearm on the upper extremity
Wrist	Scaphoid, lunate, and triquetral bones articulate with the radius and articular disc	Synovial (condyloid)	Flexion, extension, abduction, and adduction of the hand
Carpal	Between various carpal bones	Synovial (gliding)	Gliding
Hand	Proximal end of the first metacarpal bone with the trapezium	Synovial (saddle)	Flexion, extension, abduction, adduction, and circumduction of the thumb and opposition to the fingers
	Distal end of the metacarpal bones with the proximal end of the phalanges	Synovial (hinge)	Flexion, extension, limited abduction, and adduction of the fingers
	Between phalanges	Synovial (hinge)	Flexion and extension of finger sections
Sacroiliac	Between the sacrum and two ilia	Synovial (gliding)	None or slight
Pubic symphysis	Between two pubic bones	Cartilaginous (symphysis)	Slight, particularly during pregnancy and delivery
Hip	Head of the femur in the acetabulum of the coxal bone	Synovial (ball and socket)	Flexion, extension, abduction, adduction, rotation, and circumduction
Knee	Between the distal end of the femur and proximal end of the tibia	Synovial (hinge)	Flexion and extension; slight rotation of the tibia
Tibiofibular (proximal)	Head of the fibula with the lateral condyle of the tibia	Synovial (gliding)	Gliding
Ankle	Distal end of the tibia and fibula with the talus	Synovial (hinge)	Flexion (dorsiflexion) and extension (plantar flexion)
Foot	Between tarsal bones	Synovial (gliding)	Gliding; inversion and eversion
	Between metatarsal bones and phalanges	Synovial (hinge)	Flexion, extension, slight abduction, and adduction
	Between phalanges	Synovial (hinge)	Flexion and extension

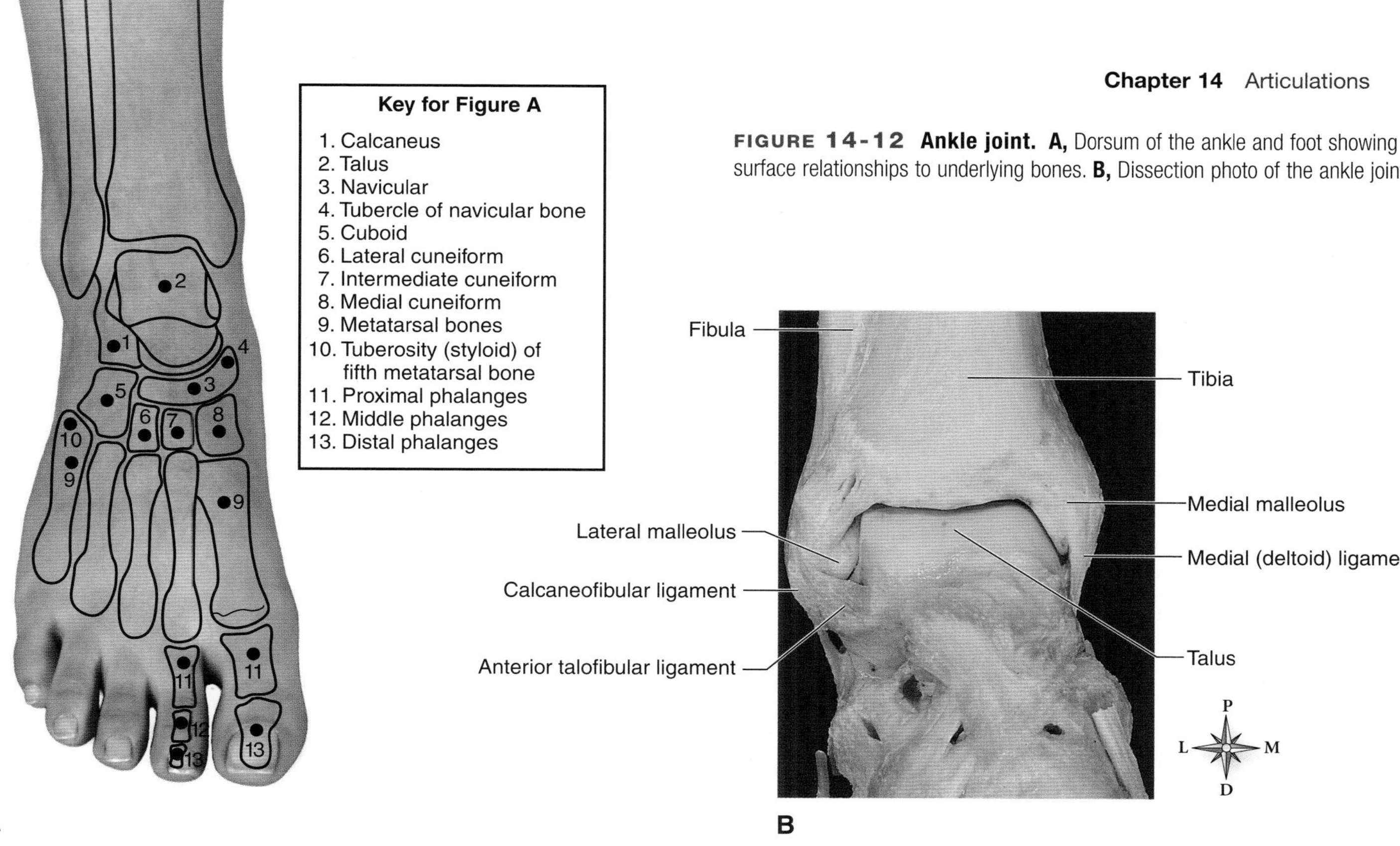

FIGURE 14-12 Ankle joint. A, Dorsum of the ankle and foot showing surface relationships to underlying bones. **B,** Dissection photo of the ankle joint.

side of the ankle with severe "point tenderness" just anterior to the lateral malleolus. External ankle rotation injuries generally result in fractures rather than ligament tears. In monomalleolar ankle injuries the lateral malleolus is broken. Bimalleolar injuries result in fracture of both malleoli, and in trimalleolar injuries both malleoli and the articular surface of the tibia are fractured. (OUCH!) The strong deltoid ligament, which helps maintain the medial longitudinal arch of the foot (see **Figure 13-10** on p. 275), is also commonly injured in severe twisting injuries affecting the ankle.

Vertebral Joints

One vertebra connects to another by several joints—between their *bodies*, as well as between their articular, transverse, and spinous *processes.* Recall that the cartilaginous (amphiarthrotic) joints between the *bodies* of adjacent vertebrae permit only very slight movement and are classified as symphyses. However, the synovial (diarthrotic) joints between the articulating surfaces of the vertebral *processes* are more movable and are classified as **gliding joints.** These joints hold the vertebrae firmly together so that they are not easily dislocated, but these joints also form a flexible column. Consider how many ways you can move the trunk of your body. You can flex it forward or laterally, you can extend it, and you can circumduct or rotate it (see **Figure 14-18**).

The bodies of adjacent vertebrae are connected by intervertebral discs and strong ligaments. Fibrous tissue and fibrocartilage form a disc's outer rim (called the *annulus fibrosus*). Its central core (the *nucleus pulposus*), in contrast, consists of a pulpy, elastic substance (**Figure 14-13**, A). With age, the nucleus loses some of its resiliency.

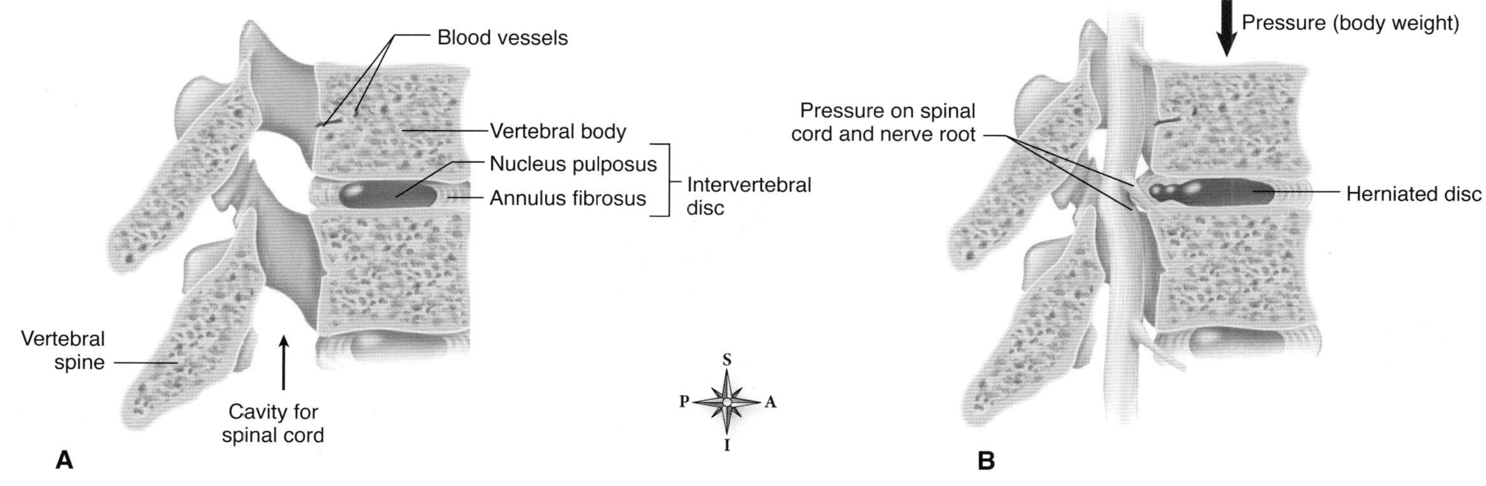

FIGURE 14-13 Vertebrae. Sagittal section of vertebrae showing normal **(A)** and herniated **(B)** discs.

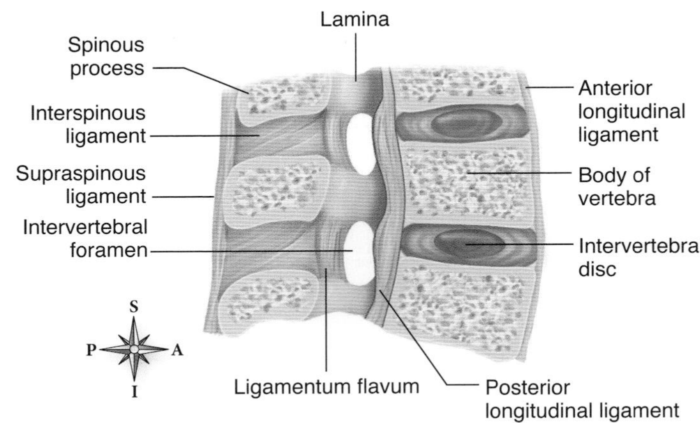

FIGURE 14-14 Vertebrae and their ligaments. Sagittal section of two lumbar vertebrae and their ligaments.

It may then be suddenly compressed by exertion or trauma and pushed through the annulus, with the herniating part protruding into the spinal canal and pressing on spinal nerves or the spinal cord itself. Severe pain results. In medical terminology, this is called a **herniated disc** or *herniated nucleus pulposus (HNP)*; in popular language, it is called a "slipped disc" (**Figure 14-13**, *B*).

In **Figure 14-14** the following ligaments that bind the vertebrae together can be identified: The *anterior longitudinal ligament*, a strong band of fibrous tissue, connects the anterior surfaces of the vertebral bodies from the atlas down to the sacrum. Connecting the posterior surfaces of the bodies is the *posterior longitudinal ligament*. The *ligamenta flava* bind the laminae of adjacent vertebrae firmly together. Spinous processes are connected by *interspinous ligaments*. In addition, the tips of the spinous processes of the cervical vertebrae are connected by the *ligamentum nuchae*; its extension, the *supraspinous ligament*, connects the tips of the rest of the vertebrae down to the sacrum. And finally, *intertransverse ligaments* connect the transverse processes of adjacent vertebrae.

Table 14-4 summarizes the entire chapter with descriptions of most of the individual joints of the body.

Quick CHECK

8. Which joint is the largest, most complex, and most commonly injured in the body?
9. List the two anatomical components of an intervertebral disc.

MOVEMENT AT SYNOVIAL JOINTS

The types of movement possible at synovial joints depend on the shapes of the articulating surfaces of the bones and on the positions of the joints' ligaments and nearby muscles and tendons (see **Figure 14-4**). All synovial joints, however, permit one or more of the following types of movements:

1. Angular
2. Circular
3. Gliding
4. Special

As you look at various examples of these types of movement, keep in mind that in the human body, more than one joint is involved with many movements of the body. We can *focus* on one joint as we observe normal movements, but more than one joint may actually be moving.

RANGE OF MOTION

Measuring **range of motion (ROM)** is often one of the first assessment techniques used by a health care provider to determine the degree of damage in an injured joint. In the absence of disease or injury, major synovial joints should function within a normal ROM.

Joint ROM can be measured actively or passively. In active movements the individual moves the joint or body part through its ROM, and in passive movements the physician or other health care provider moves the part with the patient's muscles in a relaxed state. Normally, both active and passive ROM should be about equal.

If a joint has an obvious increase or limitation in its range of motion, an instrument called a **goniometer** is used to measure the angle (**Figure 14-15**). A goniometer consists of two rigid shafts that intersect at a hinge joint. A protractor is fixed to one shaft so that motion can be read directly from the scale in degrees. The starting position is defined as the point at which the movable segment is at 0 degrees (usually the anatomical position). Measuring joint ROM provides a physician, nurse, athletic trainer, or therapist with information required to assess normal joint function, accurately measure dysfunction, or gauge treatment and rehabilitative progress after injury or disease.

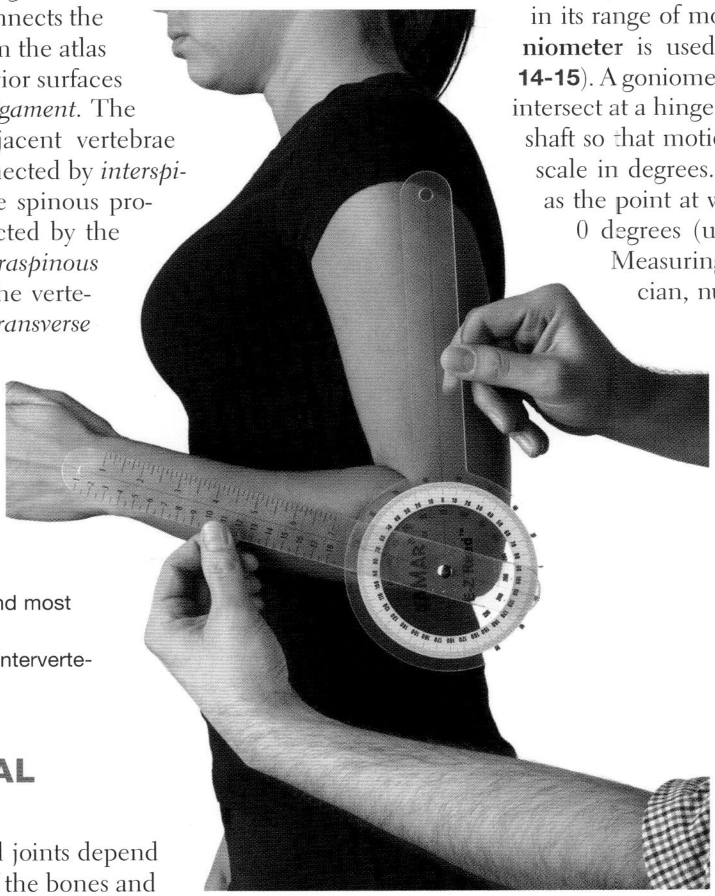

FIGURE 14-15 Use of a goniometer. Using a goniometer to measure range of motion (ROM) at the elbow.

Angular Movements

Angular movements change the size of the angle between articulating bones. Flexion, extension, abduction, and adduction are some of the different types of angular movements.

Flexion

Flexion decreases the angle between bones. It bends or folds one part on another. For example, if you bend your head forward on your chest, you are flexing it. If you bend your arm at the elbow, you are flexing the forearm (see **Figure 14-20**, *A*). Flexion, in short, is bending, folding, or withdrawing a part. Flexion can also occur when an extended structure is returned to the anatomical position.

Extension and Hyperextension

Extension increases the angle between bones. It returns a part from its flexed position to its anatomical position. Extensions are straightening or stretching movements. Extending a part beyond its anatomical position is sometimes called **hyperextension.** Hyperextension of the shoulder is illustrated in **Figure 14-19**, *A*, and of the knee in **Figure 14-24**. Clinically, *hyperextension* often refers to abnormal extension beyond a part's normal range of motion.

Plantar Flexion and Dorsiflexion

Plantar flexion occurs when the foot is stretched down and back (see **Figure 14-25**, *A*). This movement increases the angle between the top of the foot and the front of the leg. Recall that the definition of *extension* refers to an increase in the angle between articulating bones. Therefore, plantar flexion of the foot can also be described as extension. Look again at **Figure 14-25**, *A*, and note how the angle between the leg and the foot increases during plantar flexion.

Dorsiflexion occurs when the foot is tilted upward, thus decreasing the angle between the top of the foot and the front of the leg (see **Figure 14-25**, *A*).

Abduction and Adduction

Abduction moves a part away from the median plane of the body, as in moving the leg straight out to the side or fingers away from the midline of the hand. **Adduction** moves a part toward the median plane. Examples include bringing the arm back to the side or moving fingers toward the midline of the hand. Opposing movements in the shoulder can be seen in **Figure 14-19**, *B*.

Circular Movements

Circular movements result in the arclike rotation of a structure around an axis. The primary circular movements are rotation, circumduction, supination, and pronation.

Rotation and Circumduction

Rotation consists of pivoting a bone on its own axis. An example is moving the head from side to side as in indicating "no" (see **Figure 14-16**, *D*). **Circumduction** moves a part so that its distal end moves in a circle (**Figure 14-19**, *C*).

Supination and Pronation

Supination and **pronation** of the hand are shown in **Figure 14-20**, *B*. Pronation twists the forearm, moving the palm so that the thumbs point medially. Supination twists the forearm in the opposite rotation, moving the palm so that the thumbs point laterally.

Gliding Movements

Gliding movements are the simplest of all movements. The articular surface of one bone moves over the articular surface of another without any angular or circular movement. Gliding movements occur between the carpal and tarsal bones and between the articular facets of adjoining spinal vertebrae.

UNIT 2

Special Movements

Special movements are often unique or unusual movements that occur only in a very limited number of joints. These movements do not fit well into other movement categories and are generally described separately. Special movements include inversion, eversion, protraction, retraction, elevation, and depression.

Inversion and Eversion

Inversion turns the sole of the foot inward, whereas **eversion** turns it outward (see **Figure 14-25**, *B*).

Protraction and Retraction

Protraction moves a part forward, whereas **retraction** moves it back. For instance, if you stick out your jaw, you protract it, and if you pull it back, you retract it (see **Figure 14-17**, *A*).

Elevation and Depression

Elevation moves a part up, as in closing the mouth (see **Figure 14-17**, *B*). **Depression** lowers a part, moving it in the opposite direction from elevation.

Examples of Joint Movements

Illustrations in **Figures 14-16** through **14-25** provide examples of types of movement at selected synovial joints. Refer to these illustrations frequently as you read about the various types of movement possible at synovial joints.

You will notice that the movements can often be classified as opposites: flexion is the opposite of extension, protraction is the opposite of retraction, and so on. Remembering this concept will be useful to you in the next chapters when learning how opposing actions of different muscles both provide normal movements and help stabilize the body.

Quick CHECK

10. Name one example of each of the following types of movement at a synovial joint: angular, circular, gliding, and special.
11. Describe the difference between flexion and extension.
12. List the types of movement that are classified as *special movements*.

(continued on page 305)

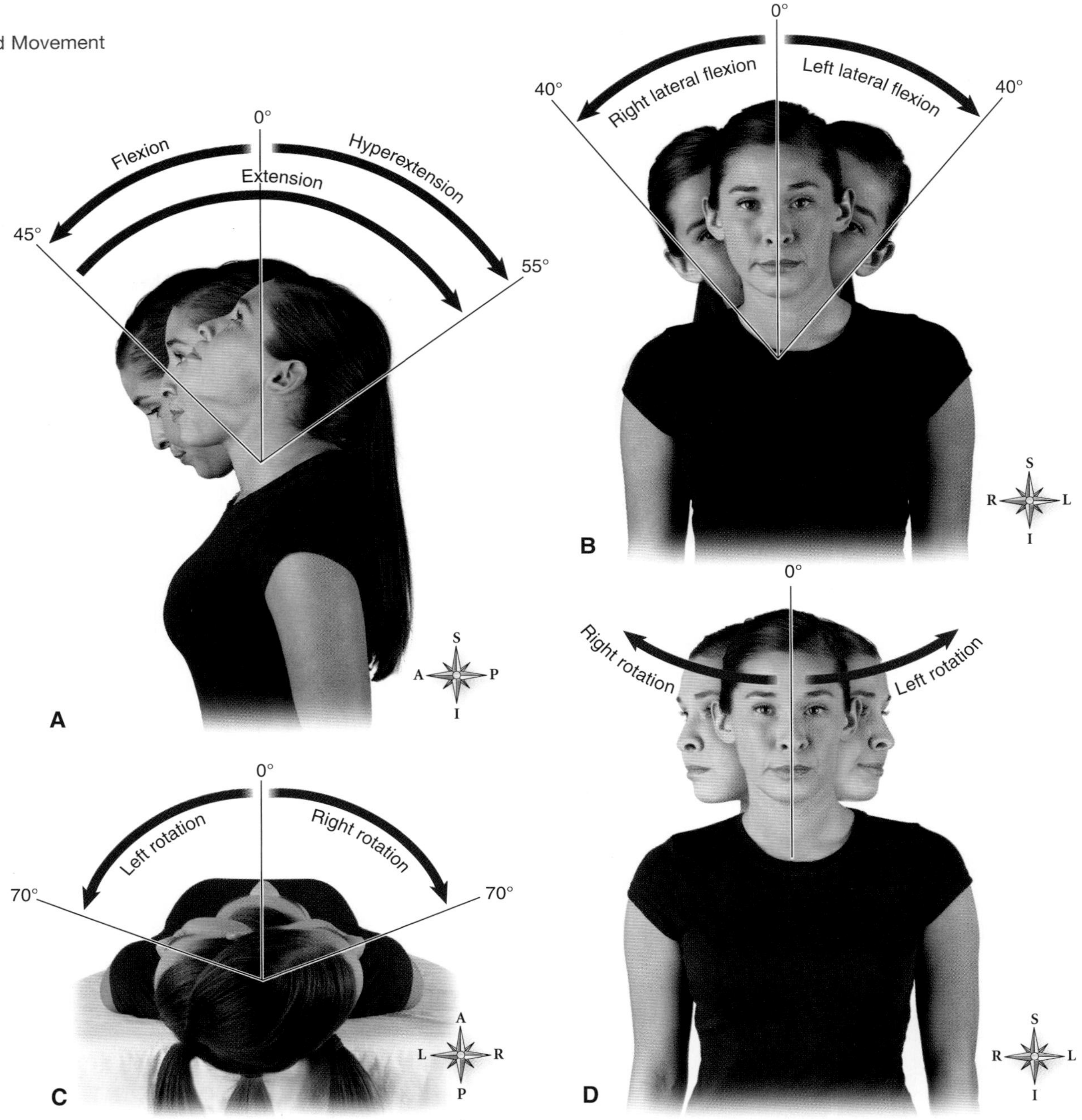

FIGURE 14-16 Movements and range of motion (ROM) of neck. A, Flexion and extension. Extension beyond the anatomical position is sometimes called *hyperextension.* **B,** Lateral bending. **C,** Rotation (supine position). **D,** Rotation (standing position).

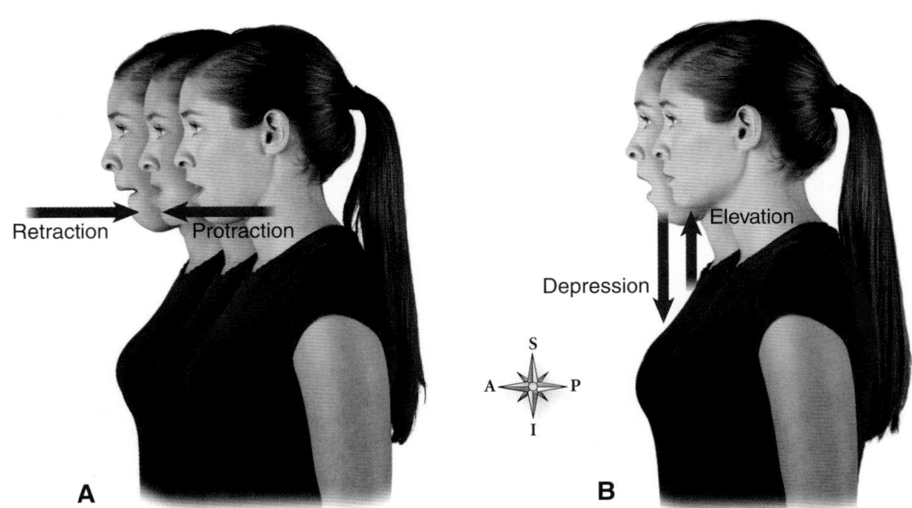

FIGURE 14-17 Movements of the jaw. A, Retraction and protraction. **B,** Elevation and depression.

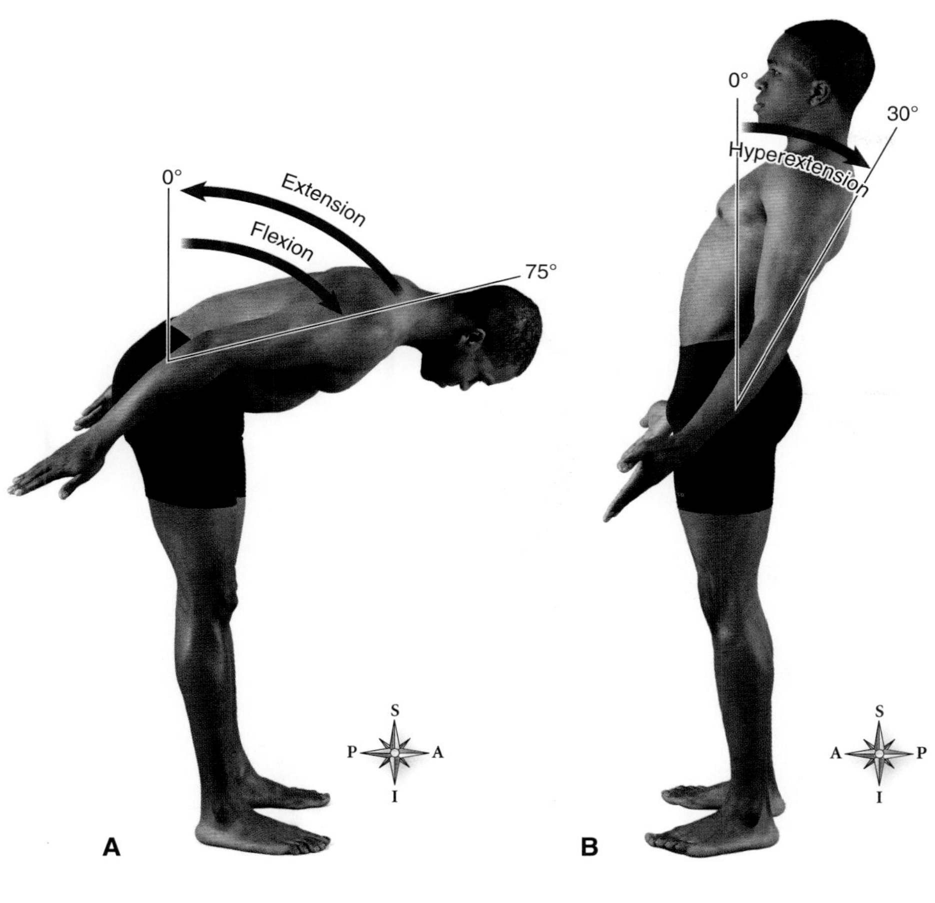

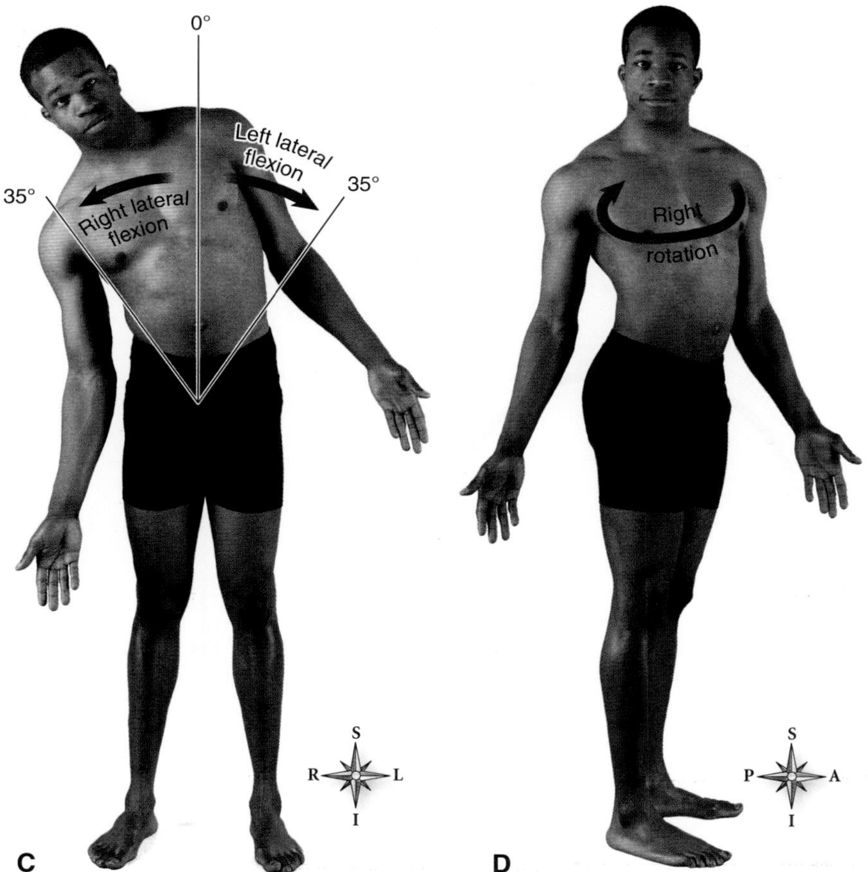

FIGURE 14-18 Movements and range of motion (ROM) of the thoracic and lumbar spine. A, Flexion and extension. **B,** Hyperextension. **C,** Lateral flexion (bending). **D,** Rotation of the upper part of the trunk.

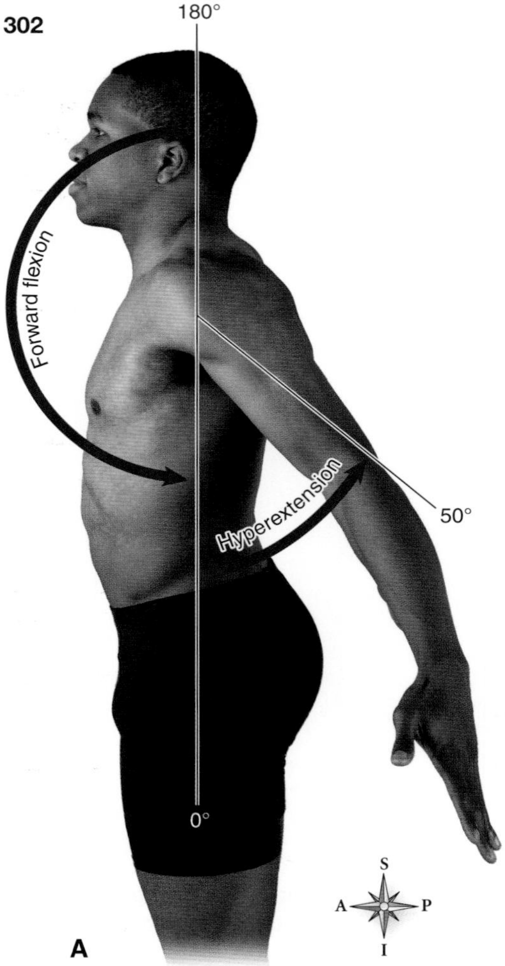

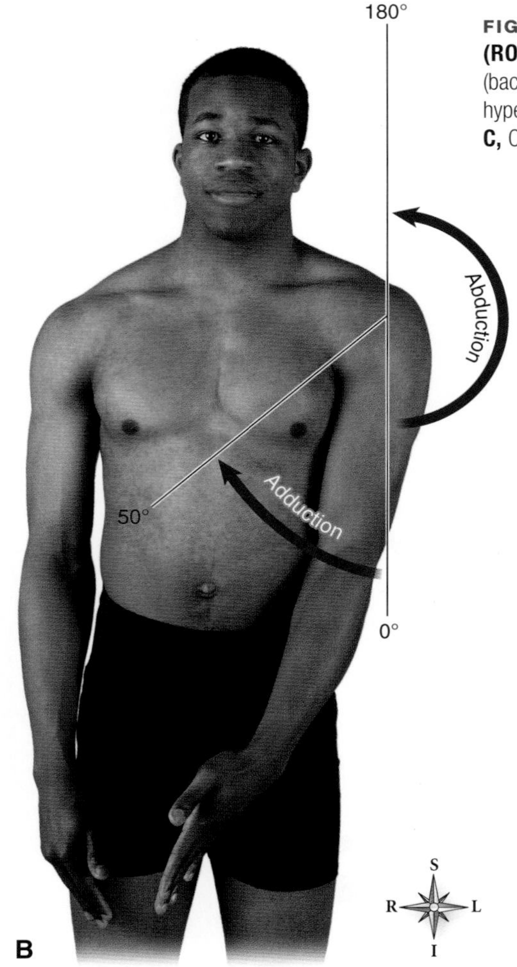

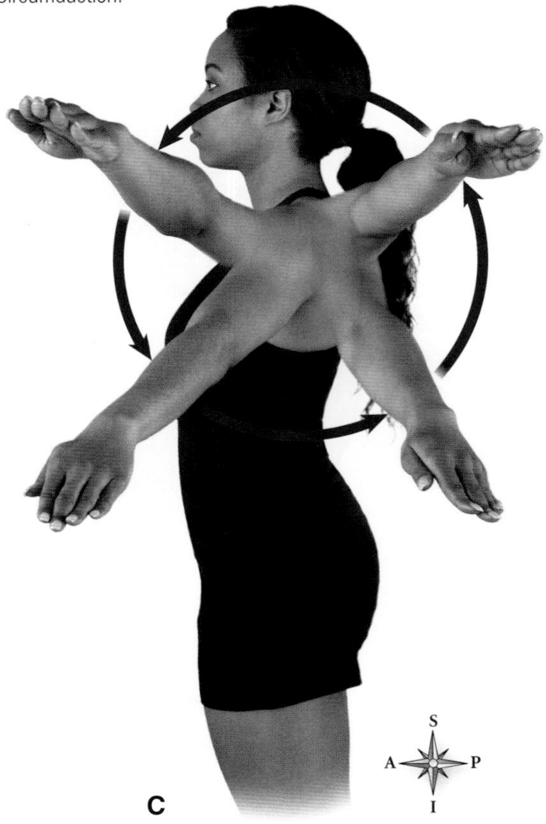

FIGURE 14-19 Movements and range of motion (ROM) of the shoulder. A, Forward flexion, extension (back to the anatomical position of 0 degrees), and backward hyperextension up to 50 degrees. **B,** Abduction and adduction. **C,** Circumduction.

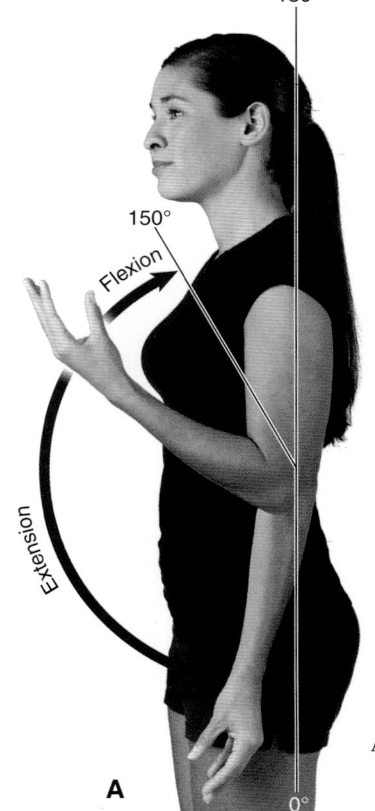

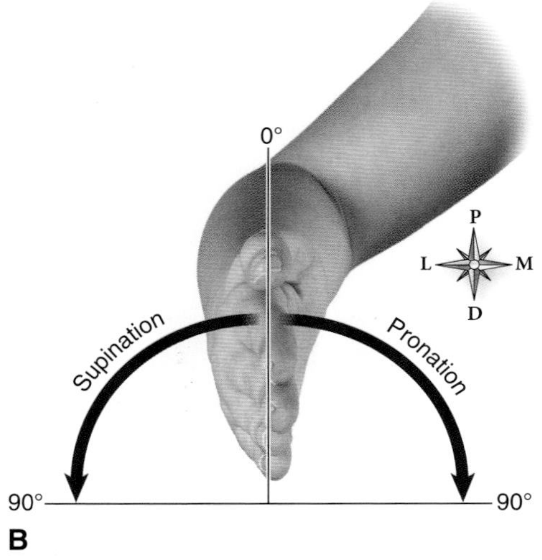

FIGURE 14-20 Movements and range of motion (ROM) of the elbow. A, Flexion and extension of the elbow. **B,** Supination and pronation of forearm.

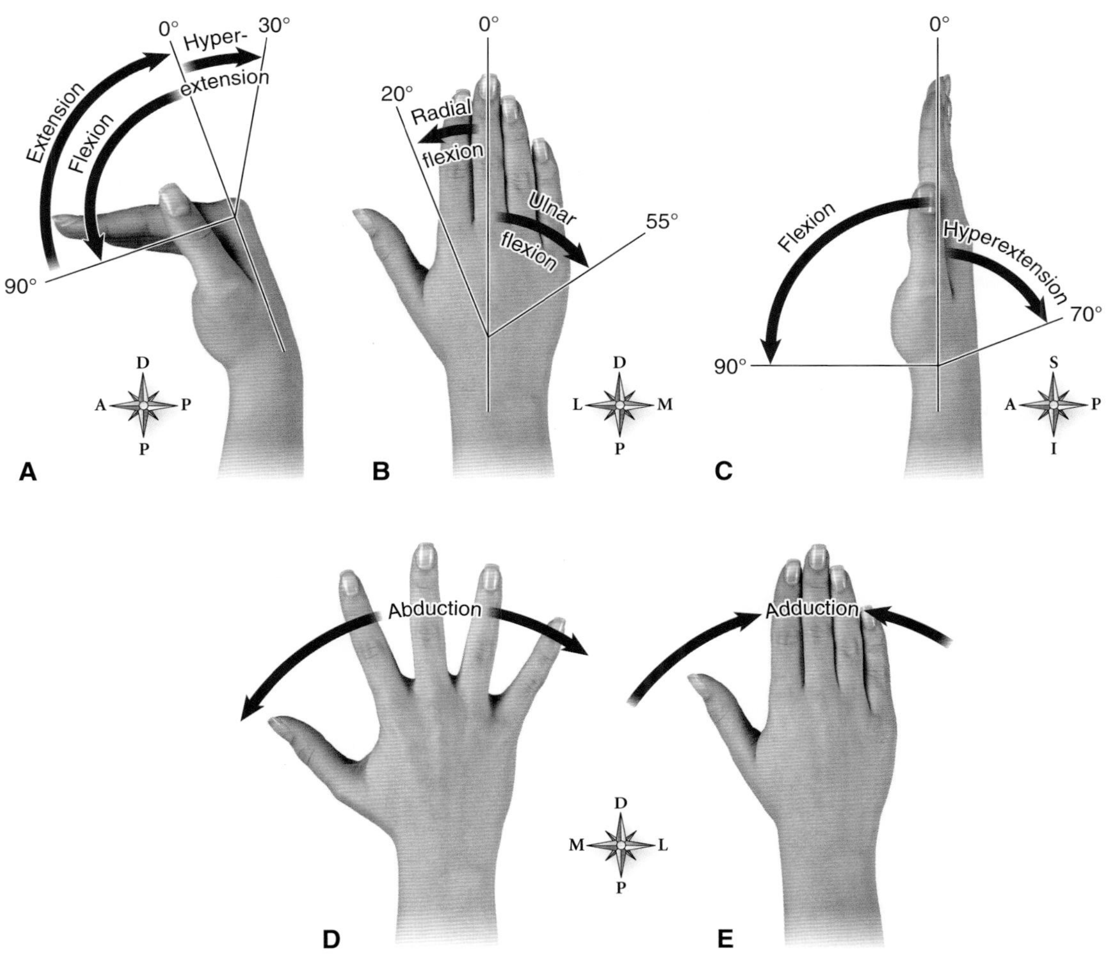

FIGURE 14-21 Movements and range of motion (ROM) of hand and wrist. A, Metacarpophalangeal flexion and hyperextension. **B,** Wrist radial and ulnar movement. **C,** Wrist flexion and hyperextension. **D,** Finger abduction. **E,** Finger adduction.

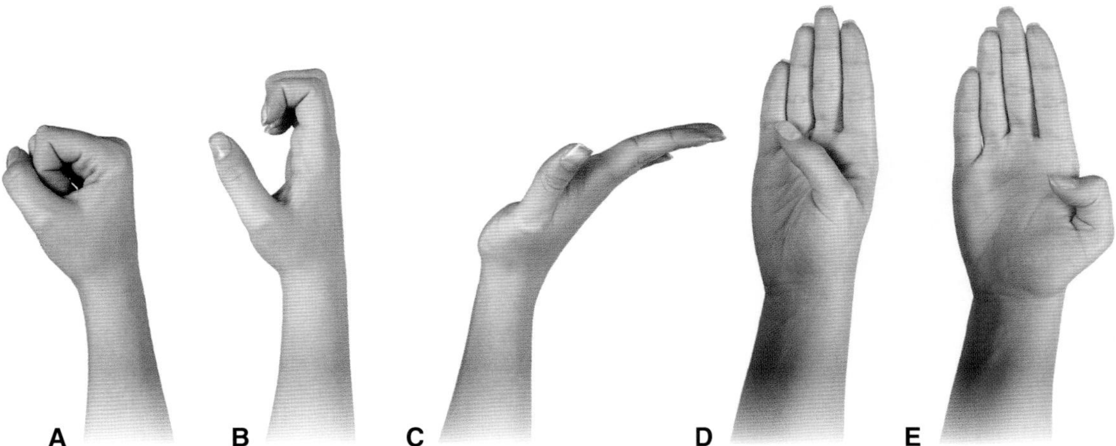

FIGURE 14-22 Movements of the fingers and thumb. A, Flexion of the metacarpophalangeal (MCP) joints and flexion of the interphalangeal (IP) joints. **B,** Extension of the metacarpophalangeal joints and flexion of the interphalangeal joints. **C,** Extension of the metacarpophalangeal and interphalangeal joints. **D,** Opposition of the thumb. **E,** Flexion of the thumb.

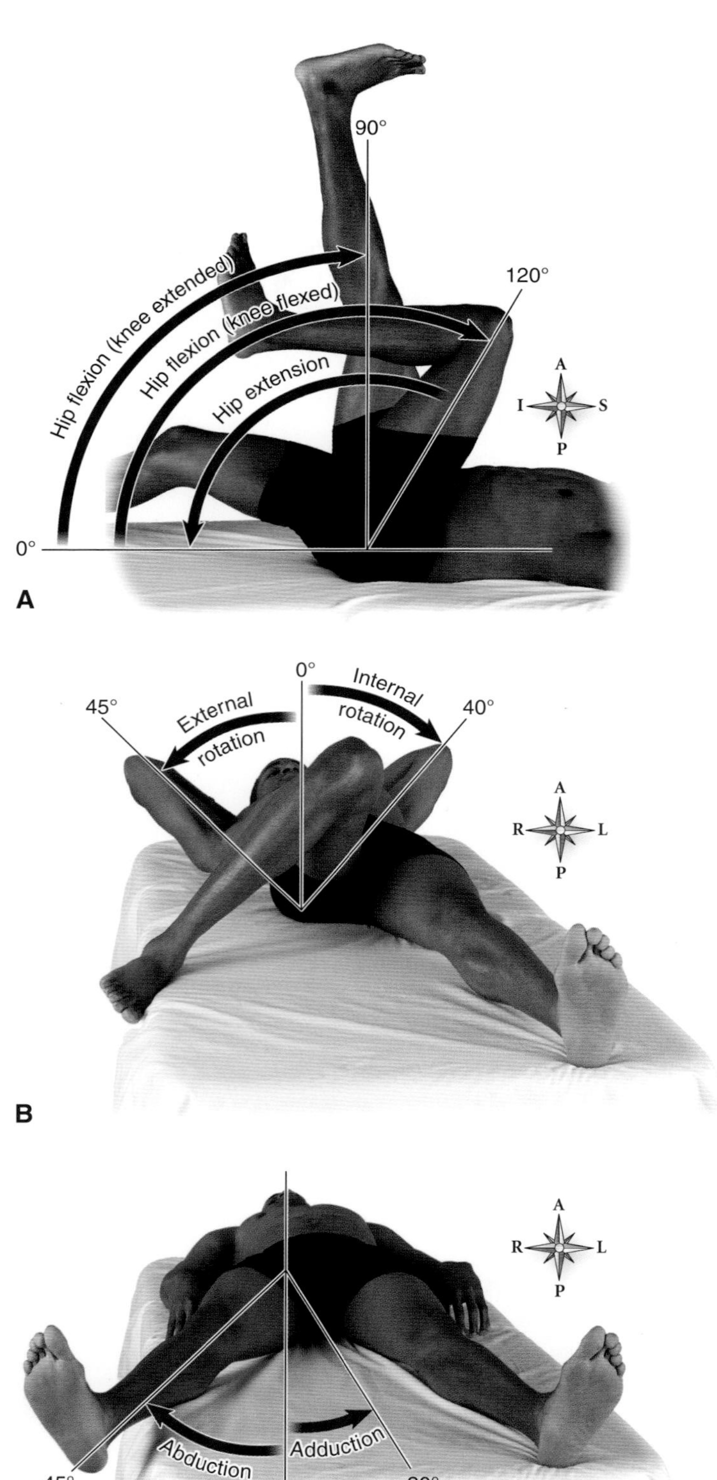

FIGURE 14-23 Movements and range of motion (ROM) of the hip. **A,** Hip flexion (knee extended 90 degrees; knee flexed 120 degrees) and hip extension. **B,** Internal rotation. **C,** Abduction and adduction.

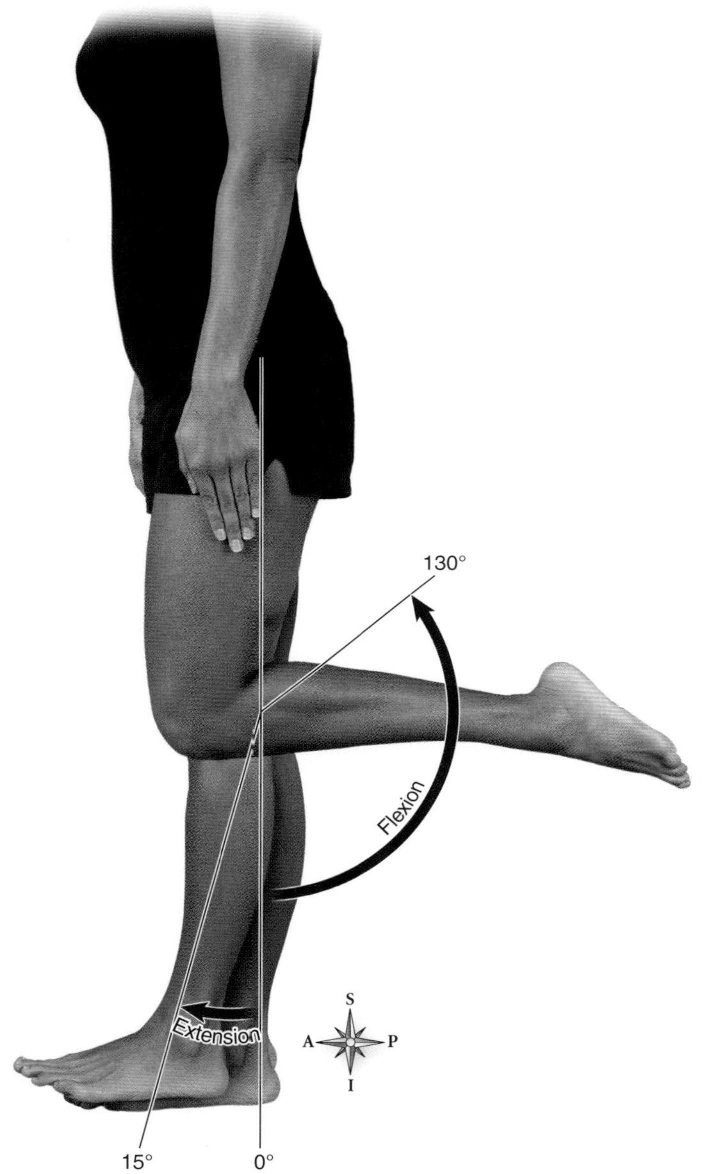

FIGURE 14-24 Movements and range of motion (ROM) of the knee. Flexion may reach 130 degrees. Extension occurs with movement from a 130-degree flexed position back to the 0-degree position. Hyperextension of 0 degrees to 15 degrees is possible in many individuals.

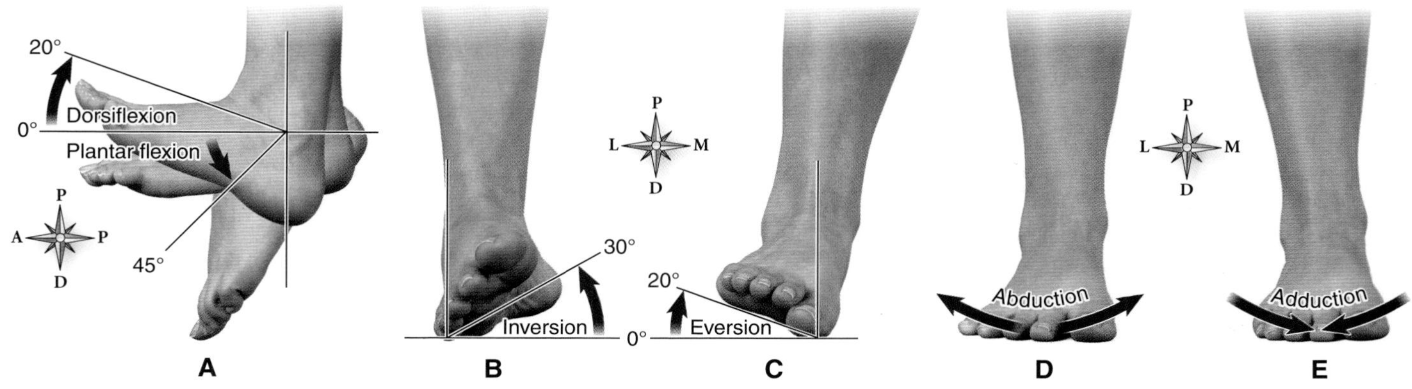

FIGURE 14-25 Movements and range of motion (ROM) of the foot and ankle. **A,** Dorsiflexion and plantar flexion. **B,** Inversion. **C,** Eversion. **D,** Abduction. **E,** Adduction.

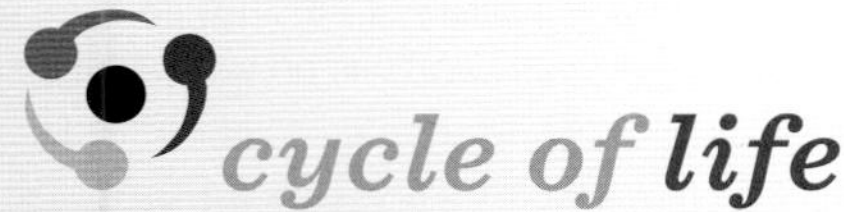

Articulations This chapter discusses the types of articulations that occur between bones and presents information on the common types of diseases that affect joints during the life cycle.

Changes in the way bones develop and in the sequence of ossification that occurs between birth and skeletal maturity also affect our joints. Fontanelles, which exist between bones of the cranium, disappear with increasing age, and the epiphyseal plates, which serve as points of articulation between the epiphyses and diaphyses of growing long bones, ossify at skeletal maturity.

Range of motion at synovial joints is typically greater early in life. With advancing age, joints are often described as being "stiff", range of motion decreases, and changes in gait are common. The difficulty with locomotion that affects many elderly individuals may result from disease conditions that involve the functional unit comprising muscles, bones, and joints.

Some skeletal diseases have profound effects that manifest as joint problems. Abnormal bone growth, or "lipping", which results in bone spurs, or sharp projections, on the articular surfaces of bones, dramatically influences joint function. Many of these disease conditions are associated with specific developmental periods, including early childhood, adolescence, and adulthood. •

the big picture | Articulations

Anatomists sometimes refer to the hand as "the reason for the upper extremity" and the thumb as "the reason for the hand". Statements such as these, when they are used in a functional context, underscore the relationship that exists between structure and function. Furthermore, they serve as examples of how "big picture" thinking is helpful in examining the interaction between body structures and the rationale for how and why they function as they do. Proper functioning of the joints is crucial for meaningful, controlled, and purposeful movement to occur—movement that permits human beings to respond to and control their environment in ways that other animals are not capable of doing. The joints of the upper extremity are good examples.

The great mobility of the upper extremity is possible because of the following: (1) the arrangement of the bones in the shoulder girdle, arm, forearm, wrist, and hand; (2) the location and method of attachment of muscles to these bones; and (3) proper functioning of the joints involved. We give up a great deal of stability in the upper extremity (especially the shoulder joint) to achieve mobility. We need that mobility and extensive range of motion to position the entire upper extremity, and especially the hand, in ways that permit us to interact with objects in our physical environment effectively. It is the proper functioning of the thumb that allows us to grasp and manipulate objects with great dexterity and control. Although loss of mobility in the upper extremity as a whole presents a significant functional problem, loss of thumb function can present equally serious and disabling problems by dramatically decreasing the overall ability to manipulate and grasp objects. By enabling us to effectively interact with our external environment, the joints of the upper extremity contribute in a significant way to maintenance of homeostasis. It is in the "big picture" context that the hand and thumb are truly functional "reasons" for the upper extremity and the hand, respectively. •

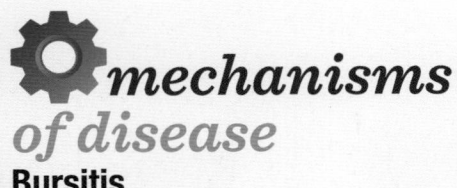

mechanisms of disease

Bursitis

Bursitis, or inflammation of a bursa, is a relatively common disorder. It is most often caused by prolonged pressure, excessive or repetitive exercise, or sudden trauma that involves one of these fluid-filled sacs. Although bursae are often associated with joints, where they may serve to cushion the joint or facilitate the movement of tendons over bony prominences, such as the olecranon of the elbow joint, the bursa itself is often completely separate from the joint space. Look again at Figure 14-6, *A.* It clearly shows the placement of the olecranon bursa just below the skin and independent of the joint space of the elbow. Therefore, inflammation of the olecranon bursa (Figure 14-26) may occur in the absence of any elbow joint inflammation or pathology. Bursitis near the knee joint is also common, especially in carpet layers, roofers, and others who work on their knees.

Joint Disorders

Joint disorders may be classified as **noninflammatory joint disease** or **inflammatory joint disease.** Serving as fulcrums, the joints permit smooth and precise movement to occur when a muscle contracts and pulls on bones. Because joints, bones, and muscles act together as a functional unit, joint disorders, regardless of type or classification, have profound effects on body mobility.

Noninflammatory Joint Disease

Noninflammatory types of joint disease can be distinguished from inflammatory joint conditions because they do not involve inflammation of the synovial membrane. Furthermore, noninflammatory joint diseases do not produce systemic signs or symptoms, such as fever, or damage other body organs such as the heart and lungs.

Osteoarthritis, known also as *degenerative joint disease (DJD),* is the most common noninflammatory disorder of movable joints. It is characterized by "wear and tear" degeneration and fracturing of articular cartilage (Box 14-2) and by abnormal formation of new bone ("bone spurs") at joint surfaces. In DJD the articular cartilage no longer acts as a "shock absorber", the joint space narrows, the synovial membrane thickens, and the ligaments calcify.

Large weight-bearing joints, such as the hips and knees, are often involved first, followed by involvement of joints in the fingers. Swelling deformities of the *distal* interphalangeal joints called **Heberden nodes** and of the *proximal* interphalangeal joints called **Bouchard nodes** are common. Figure 14-27, *A,* shows the hands of a woman with osteoarthritis. The cause of osteoarthritis is unknown, but obesity, ageing, and the "wear and tear" of mechanical stresses on joints over time are known to play a major role.

Unfortunately, no treatment is available to stop the degenerative joint disease process completely.

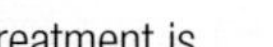

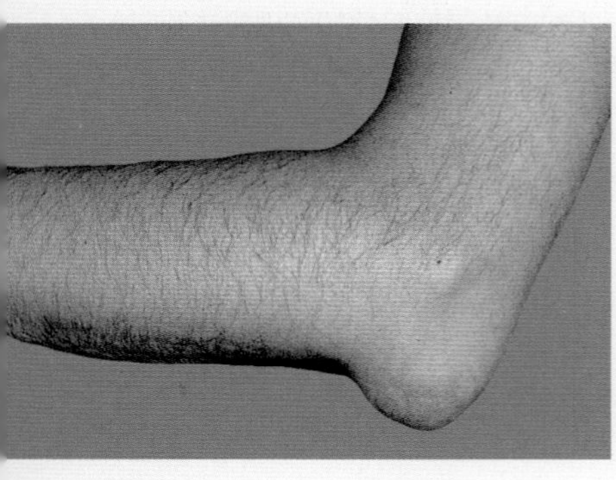

FIGURE 14-26 Olecranon bursitis. Pain, inflammation, and swelling of the bursa may limit motion, although the elbow joint itself may not be affected.

BOX 14-2 *health matters* | **Joint Mice**

The thin layer of cartilage that covers the articulating surfaces of bones in synovial joints may become cracked as a result of traumatic injury—especially to the knee. Such injuries are called **chondral fractures.** They result in fissuring of the articular cartilage, which can be likened to the cracking of an egg shell. If such an injury occurs, small fragments may become detached from the damaged layer of cartilage and enter the joint cavity. These fragments are called "loose bodies" or *joint mice* because they often cause clicking sounds or catching and locking sensations during joint movement. Symptoms often vary over time as cartilage fragments move about the joint cavity in the synovial fluid. Pain and loss of motion will occur if the fragments become lodged between opposing bone surfaces.

Symptoms, which appear in many people in their 50s and 60s, include morning stiffness, deep "achy" pain on movement that worsens with use, and limited joint motion. In many cases, symptoms can be treated effectively with standard **nonsteroidal antiinflammatory drugs (NSAIDs),** such as aspirin or ibuprofen, or by nutritional supplements such as glucosamine or chondroitin sulphate (see Chapter 11, p. 214). Injection into the joint space, especially of the knee, of a gelatinous type of lubricating fluid containing *hyaluronic acid* has proved useful in some cases. If the disease is more advanced, various types of prescription medications or partial or total joint replacements may be necessary (Box 14-3). Although the severity of symptoms may plateau or stabilize for varying periods, the disease is generally progressive once established and will continue over a lifetime. Osteoarthritis is the leading cause of long-term disability in ageing, but otherwise healthy, individuals.

Traumatic injury is often the cause of non-inflammatory joint problems. Dislocation occurs when the articular surfaces of bones forming the joint are no longer in proper contact with each other. A subluxation is a partial or minor dislocation in which bones are slightly misaligned. This displacement of bone alters the normal contour

A

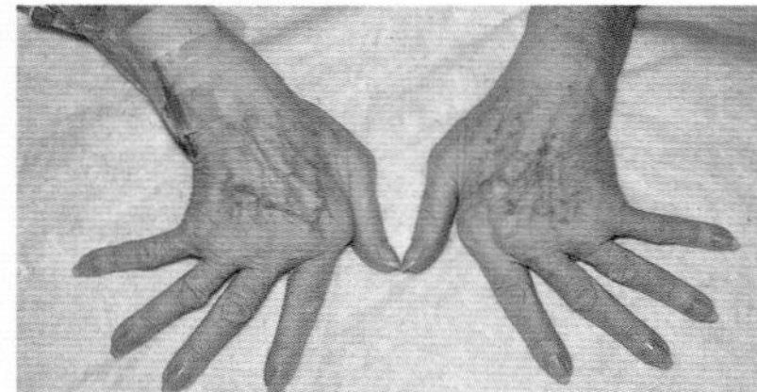

B

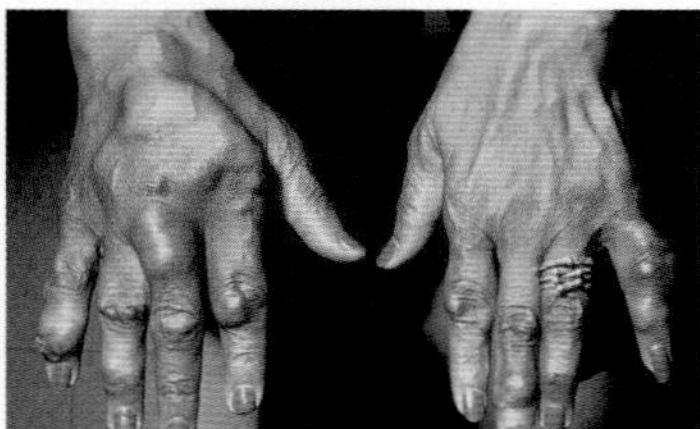

C

FIGURE 14-27 Types of arthritis. A, Osteoarthritis. Note Heberden nodes (*H*) on the distal interphalangeal joints and Bouchard nodes (*B*) on the proximal interphalangeal joints. **B,** Rheumatoid arthritis. Note the marked ulnar deviation of the fingers. **C,** Gouty arthritis. Note the tophi filled with sodium urate crystals.

BOX 14-3 *sports and fitness* | Joint Replacement

Arthroplasty is the total or partial replacement of a diseased joint with an artificial device called a **prosthesis.** Prosthetic joints or joint components must allow for considerable mobility and be durable, strong, and compatible with surrounding tissues. Development of new prosthetic materials and surgical techniques to replace diseased joints gained momentum with the first successful total hip replacement (THR) procedure. It was performed by noted English orthopaedic surgeon Sir John Charnley in 1963. Currently, hip and knee replacements are performed in nearly equal numbers and are the most common orthopaedic operations performed on older persons, performed more than 160,000 times each year in the UK. In addition, large numbers of elbow, shoulder, finger, and other joint replacement procedures are performed annually. Osteoarthritis and other types of degenerative bone disease often destroy or severely damage joints and cause unremitting pain. Total joint replacement is often the only effective treatment option available.

The THR procedure involves replacement of the femoral head by a metallic alloy prosthesis and the acetabular socket with a high-density polyethylene cup. In the past, both pieces were generally cemented into place with methyl methacrylate adhesive. Many of the newer prostheses, however, are "porous coated" to permit natural ingrowth of bone for stability and retention. The advantage of bone ingrowth is prevention of loosening that occurs if the cement bond weakens. With advanced surgical techniques and newer metal prostheses fabricated from alloys of titanium, cobalt/chrome, and surgical steel, 15–20 year THR and total knee replacement success rates have risen to approximately 90% in older patients. However, even more durable metal and plastic components are necessary to extend the life span of most hip and knee prostheses currently in use. At the present time, younger patients who stress artificial joints more than older adults are encouraged to delay replacement and rely instead on evolving therapies, which are intended to heal or regenerate diseased joint tissues. The x-ray illustration shows placement of a noncemented, porous-coated femoral prosthesis made of titanium alloy and a cemented acetabular socket made of high-density plastic. •

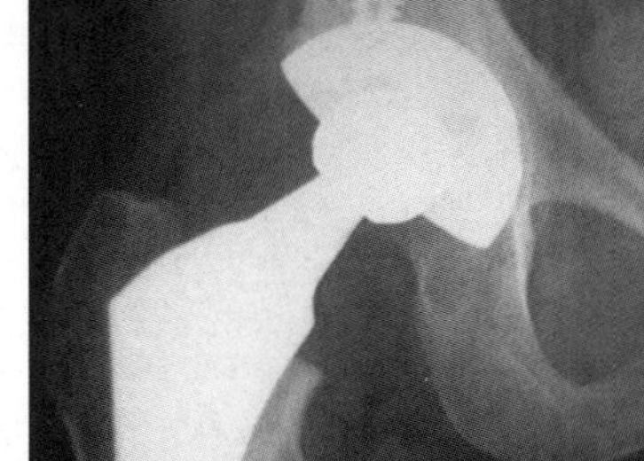

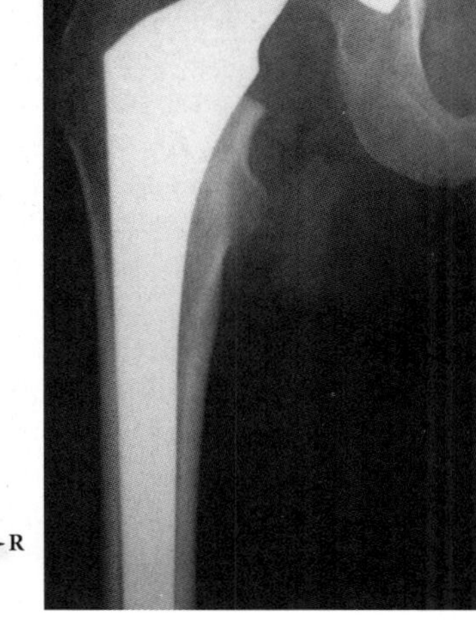

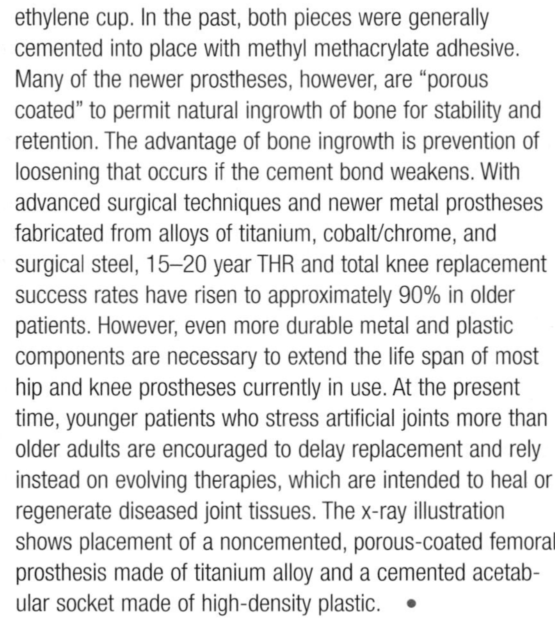

of the joint and can pull on or even tear surrounding ligaments. Refer once again to **Figure 14-6**, *B.* Recall that the annular ligament is intended to hold the head of the radius firmly against the radial notch of the ulna at the proximal radioulnar joint. Functionally, it is this anatomic relationship that allows the radius to rotate freely without dislocation during pronation and supination of the forearm. In children younger than 5 years especially, dislocation of the radial head, called a "pulled elbow", is a common traumatic joint injury. Pain and soft tissue swelling are associated with dislocation injuries. Effective treatment involves early reduction or realignment.

One of the most common traumatic joint injuries associated with athletic activity involves damage to the cartilaginous menisci of the knee. Because the menisci act as shock absorbers and stabilize the knee, severe tears may produce oedema, pain, instability, and limited motion. Arthroscopic surgical procedures are often used in both the diagnosis and treatment of this type of knee injury (**Figure 14-28**).

Arthroscopy is an imaging technique that allows a physician to examine the internal structure of a joint without the use of extensive surgery (see **Figure 14-28**, *A*). A narrow tube with lenses and a fibre-optic light source is inserted into the joint space through a small puncture. Isotonic saline (salt) solution is injected through a needle to expand the volume of the synovial space. This spreads the joint structures and makes viewing easier (see **Figure 14-28**, *B*).

Although arthroscopy is often used as a diagnostic procedure, it also can be used to perform joint surgery. While the surgeon views the internal structure of the joint through the arthroscope or on an attached video monitor, instruments can be inserted through puncture holes and used to repair or remove damaged tissue. Arthroscopic surgery is much less traumatic than previous methods in which the joint cavity was completely opened.

A **sprain** is an acute musculoskeletal injury to the ligamentous structures surrounding a joint that disrupts the continuity of the synovial membrane. A common cause is a twisting or wrenching movement often associated with "whiplash"-type injuries. Blood vessels may be ruptured, and bruising and swelling may occur. Limitation of joint motion is common in all sprain injuries. Ankle rotation sprain injuries are discussed on pp. 295–297.

A

Posterior cruciate ligament

Femur

Tibia

B

FIGURE 14-28 Arthroscopy. A, Fibre-optic light source inserted into a joint. **B,** Internal view of the joint.

Inflammatory Joint Disease

Arthritis is a general name for many different inflammatory joint diseases. Arthritis can be caused by a variety of factors, including infection, injury, genetic factors, and autoimmunity. Following is a brief list of the major types of arthritis.

Rheumatoid arthritis (RA) is a form of systemic autoimmune disease that involves chronic inflammation of many different tissues and organs of the body. Although organs such as the heart, lungs, skin, and muscles may become involved, the disease generally attacks joints first—and affects them most severely. A wide range of pathological joint changes are associated with RA. Initially, the synovial membrane becomes inflamed, thickened, and oedematous. Soon, the diseased synovial membrane produces an aggregation of inflammatory cells, granulation tissue, and fibroblasts called **pannus** that adhere to the articular cartilage. It is the continued growth and spreading of pannus tissue that destroys articular cartilage and bridges the opposing bones.

Eventually, the bones fuse together, movement ceases, and permanent crippling occurs. Small joints in the hands and feet are generally affected first. As the disease progresses, the wrists, ankles, elbows, knees, and cervical spine may also be involved. Because the disease is systemic, most patients experience symptoms such as anaemia, weight loss, fever, fatigue, and generalized muscle pain, as well as symptoms associated with specific types of joint pathology.

A characteristic deformity of the hands in RA is **ulnar deviation** of the fingers (**Figure 14-27**, *B*). A number of other common signs and symptoms are related to inflammation and loss of articular surface. They include reduction in joint mobility, pain, nodular swelling, and generalized aching and stiffness.

In the past, treatment for many patients was often limited to NSAIDs and other pain or antiinflammatory-type medication, corticosteroids, and so-called disease-modifying antirheumatic drugs such as methotrexate. Newer drugs influencing the altered immune system response in RA, called **TNF blockers,** are showing promise in many individuals with this disease. *Tumour necrosis factor (TNF)* is a substance made in excess by the body's immune system in RA. It is involved in pannus formation, destruction of articular cartilage, and pain and swelling of joints. By blocking the effects of this substance, people with moderate RA often experience significant relief from symptoms and from continued damage to bone and joints.

Juvenile rheumatoid arthritis (JRA) is often more severe than the adult form but involves similar deterioration and deformity of joints. Onset is generally systemic and associated with rash, high fever, and swelling of the liver and spleen. Targeted joints, which include the wrists, elbows, knees, and ankles, are generally warm and swollen. The joint inflammatory process often destroys the growth of epiphyseal cartilage, and the growth of long bones is arrested. This form begins during childhood and is more common in girls. In addition to articular damage, JRA also affects the heart, lungs, muscles, and kidneys in many young patients.

Gouty arthritis is another type of inflammatory arthritis. It is a metabolic disorder in which excess blood levels of uric acid, a nitrogenous waste, are deposited as sodium urate crystals within the synovial fluid of joints and in other tissues. These deposits, called **tophi,** are often obvious in the soft tissues of patients with gouty arthritis (see **Figure 14-27**, *C*). They trigger the chronic inflammation and tissue damage seen with the disease. Swelling, tenderness, or pain typically appears in the fingers, wrists, elbows, ankles, and knees. Non-steroidal anti-inflammatory drugs (NSAIDs) are used as first line treatment for an acute attack of gouty arthritis. Colchicine, a secondary metabolite originally extracted from plants, is also used, but only if NSAIDs are ineffective or not well tolerated.

Allopurinol and febuxostat are xanthine oxidase inhibitors commonly used for prophylaxis of chronic gout. They act to prevent the formation of uric acid.

Psoriatic arthritis is an inflammatory type of arthritis of varying severity that can progress from skin psoriasis.

LANGUAGE OF SCIENCE *(continued from p. 283)*

extension
[*ex-* **outward**, *-tens-* **stretch,** *-sion* **process**]

flexion (FLEK-shun)
[*flex-* **bend,** *-ion* **process**]

gliding joint (GLYDE-ing joynt)

gliding movement
(GLYDE-ing MOOV-ment)

gomphosis (gom-FOH-sis)
[*gomphos-* **bolt,** *-osis* **condition**]
pl., gomphoses

goniometer (gon-ee-OM-eh-ter)
[*gonio-* **angle,** *-meter* **measure**]

hyperextension
(hye-per-ek-STEN-shun)
[*hyper-* **excessive,** *-ex-* **out,** *-ten-* **stretch,** *-sion* **process**]

intercarpal joint (in-ter-KAR-pal joynt)
[*inter-* **between,** *-carp-* **wrist,** *-al* **relating to**]

interphalangeal joint
(in-ter-fah-LAN-jee-al joynt)
[*inter-* **between,** *-phalang-* **finger bones (ref. from rows of soldiers),** *-al* **relating to**]

inversion (in-VER-zhun)
[*in-* **inward,** *-ver-* **turn,** *-sion* **process**]

joint capsule (joynt KAP-sool)
[*joint* **a joining,** *caps-* **box,** *-ule* **little**]

joint cavity (joynt KAV-i-tee)
[*joint* **a joining,** *cav-* **hollow,** *-ity* **state**]

ligament (LIG-ah-ment)
[*liga-* **bind,** *-ment* **result of action**]

meniscus (meh-NIS-kus)
[*meniscus* **crescent**] *pl.*, menisci

metacarpophalangeal joint
(met-ah-KAR-poh-fah-LAN-jee-al joynt)
[*meta-* **beyond,** *-carpo-* **wrist,** *-phalang-* **finger bones (ref. from rows of soldiers),** *-al* **relating to**]

multiaxial joint (mul-tee-AK-see-al joynt)
[*multi-* **many,** *-axon* **axle**]

nonsteroidal antiinflammatory drug (NSAID) (non-STAYR-oyd-al an-ti-in-FLAM-ah-toh-ree drug [EN-SAYD or EN-SED])
[*non-* **not,** *-stero-* **solid,** *-oid* **like,** *-al* **relating to,** *anti-* **against,** *-inflam-* **set afire,** *-ory* **relating to**]

olecranon bursa
(o-LEK-rah-non BER-sah)
[*olecranon* **elbow,** *bursa* **purse**]
pl., bursae

plantar flexion (PLAN-tar FLEK-shun)
[*planta-* **sole,** *-ar* **relating to,** *flex-* **bend,** *-ion* **process**]

pronation (proh-NAY-shun)
[*pronat-* **bend forward,** *-tion* **process**]

protraction (proh-TRAK-shun)
[*pro-* **forward**, *-tract-* **drag,** *-tion* **process**]

proximal interphalangeal (PIP)
(PROK-si-mal in-ter-fah-LAN-gee-al)
[*proxima-* **near,** *-al* **relating to,** *inter-* **between,** *-phalang-* **finger bones (ref. from rows of soldiers),** *-al* **relating to**]

radiocarpal joint
(RAY-dee-oh-KAR-pal joynt)
[*radi-* **ray,** *-carp-* **wrist,** *-al* **relating to**]

radioulnar joint
(RAY-dee-oh-UL-nur joynt)
[*radi-* **ray,** *-ulna-* **elbow or arm,** *-ar* **relating to**]

retraction (re-TRAK-shun)
[*re-* **back,** *-tract-* **drag,** *-tion* **process**]

rotation (roh-TAY-shun)
[*rot-* **turn,** *-ation* **process**]

special movement (SPESH-ul MOOV-ment)
[*speci-* **form or kind,** *-al* **relating to**]

supination (soo-pi-NAY-shun)
[*supin-* **lying on the back,** *-ation* **process**]

suture (SOO-chur)
[*suture* **seam**]

symphysis (SIM-fi-sis)
[*sym-* **together,** *-physis* **growth**]
pl., symphyses

synarthrosis (sin-ar-THROH-sis)
[*syn-* **together,** *-arthr-* **joint,** *-osis* **condition**] *pl.*, synarthroses

synchondrosis (SIN-kon-DROH-sis)
[*syn-* **together,** *-chondr-* **cartilage,** *-osis* **condition**] *pl.*, synchondroses

syndesmosis (SIN-dez-MO-sis)
[*syn-* **together,** *-desmo-* **bond,** *-osis* **condition**] *pl.*, syndesmoses

synovial membrane (si-NO-vee-al)
[*syn-* **together,** *-ovi-* **egg (white),** *-al* **relating to,** *membran-* **thin skin**]

uniaxial joint (yoo-nee-AK-see-al joynt)
[*uni-* **one,** *-axi-* **axle,** *-al* **relating to**]

LANGUAGE OF MEDICINE

arthritis (ar-THRY-tis)
[*arthr-* **joint,** *-itis* **inflammation**]

Bouchard node (boo-SHAR nohd)
[*Charles J. Bouchard* **French physician,** *nod-* **knot**]

bursitis (ber-SYE-tis)
[*bursa-* **purse,** *-itis* **inflammation**]

chondral fracture (KON-dral FRAK-shur)
[*condr-* **cartilage,** *-al* **relating to,** *fracture* **a breaking**]

dislocation (dis-low-KAY-shun)
[*dis-* **apart,** *-locat-* **to place,** *-tion* **process**]

gouty arthritis (gow-tee ar-THRY-tis)
[*gout-* **drop,** *-y* **of or like,** *arthr-* **joint,** *-itis* **inflammation**]

Heberden node (HEB-er-den nohd)
[*William Heberden* **English physician,** *nod-* **knot**]

herniated disc (HER-nee-ayt-ed)
[*hernia-* **rupture,** *-ate* **act of**]

inflammatory joint disease (in-FLAM-ah-toh-ree joynt DIS-eez)
[*inflam-* **set afire,** *-ory* **relating to,** *joint* **a joining,** *dis-* **opposite of,** *-ease* **comfort**]

juvenile rheumatoid arthritis (JRA) (JOO-veh-neyel ROO-mah-toyd ar-THRY-tis)
[*juven-* **youth,** *-ile* **of or like,** *rheuma-* **flow,** *-oid* **like,** *arthr-* **joint,** *-itis* **inflammation**]

noninflammatory joint disease (non-in-FLAM-ah-toh-ree joynt DIS-eez)
[*non-* **not,** *-inflam-* **set afire,** *-ory* **relating to,** *joint* **a joining,** *dis-* **opposite of,** *-ease* **comfort**]

olecranon bursitis (o-LEK-rah-nohn ber-SYE-tis)
[*olecranon* **elbow,** *burs-* **purse,** *-itis* **inflammation**]

osteoarthritis (os-tee-oh-ar-THRY-tis)
[*osteo-* **bone,** *-arthr-* **joint,** *-itis* **inflammation**]

pannus (PAN-us)
[*pannus* **tattered cloth**]

prepatellar bursitis (pree-pah-TEL-er ber-SYE-tis)
[*pre-* **in front of,** *-pat-* **dish,** *-ella* **small,** *-ar* **relating to,** *bursa-* **purse,** *-itis* **inflammation**]

prosthesis (pros-THEE-sis)
[*prosthesis* **addition**] *pl.*, prostheses

rheumatoid arthritis (RA) (ROO-mah-toyd ar-THRY-tis)
[*rheuma-* **flow,** *-oid* **like,** *arthr-* **joint,** *-itis* **inflammation**]

sprain (sprayn)

sprained ankle (spraynd ANG-kul)

TNF (tumour necrosis factor) blocker (TEE-EN-EF [TYOO-mer ne-KRO-sis FAK-tor] BLOK-er)

tophus (TOH-fus)
[*tophus* **porous rock**] *pl.*, tophi

ulnar deviation (UL-nur dee-vee-AY-shun)
[*ulna-* **elbow,** *-ar* **relating to,** *de-* **out of,** *-via-* **road or path,** *-ation* **process**]

case study

While sprinting after the football, Julia was so intensely concentrating on scoring a goal that she didn't see the opposing team player coming at her from the side. The two players collided, and Julia felt a "pop" in her right knee followed by intense pain. In the Accident and Emergency department of the local hospital the specialty registrar informed her that she had torn her ACL.

1. What knee structure is referred to as the "ACL"?
   a. Anterior cruciate ligament
   b. Anatomical connecting ligament
   c. Anterior collateral ligament
   d. Arthroscopic collateral ligament

2. Which articulating bones form the knee joint?
   a. Femur and fibula
   b. Humerus and ulna
   c. Tibia and femur
   d. Fibula and tibia

Julia's immediate concern was whether she would be able to play football again. Unfortunately further tests verified that Julia had also damaged the medial meniscus in her right knee.

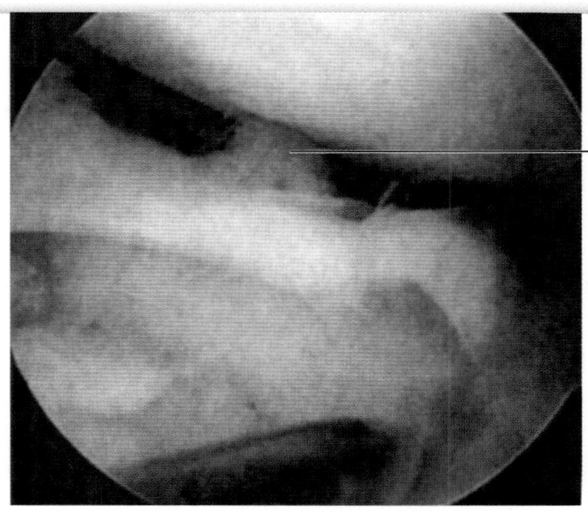

3. Which choice best describes a meniscus?
   a. A ligament
   b. A piece of cartilage
   c. A portion of bone
   d. A tendon

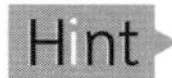
Hint: To solve a case study, you may have to refer to the glossary or index, other chapters in this textbook, ***Connect It!,*** and other resources.

CHAPTER SUMMARY

*To download an MP3 version of the chapter summary for use with your mobile device, access the **Audio Chapter Summaries** online at evolve.elsevier.com.*

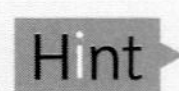

Scan this summary after reading the chapter to help you reinforce the key concepts. Later, use the summary as a quick review before your class or before a test.

Introduction

A. Articulation—point of contact between bones
B. Joints are mostly very movable, but some are immovable or allow only limited motion
C. Movable joints allow complex, highly coordinated, and purposeful movements to be executed

Classification of Joints

A. Joints may be classified by using a structural or functional scheme (**Table 14-1**)
   1. Structural classification—joints are named according to:
      a. Type of connective tissue that joins bones together (fibrous or cartilaginous joints)
      b. Presence of a fluid-filled joint capsule (synovial joint)
   2. Functional classification—joints are named according to the degree of movement allowed
      a. Synarthroses—immovable joints
      b. Amphiarthroses—slightly movable
      c. Diarthroses—freely movable
B. Fibrous joints (synarthroses)—bones of joints fit together closely, thereby allowing little or no movement (**Figure 14-1**)
   1. Syndesmoses—joints in which ligaments connect two bones
   2. Sutures—found only in the skull; teethlike projections from adjacent bones interlock with each other
   3. Gomphoses—between the root of a tooth and the alveolar process of the mandible or maxilla
C. Cartilaginous joints (amphiarthroses)—bones of joints are joined together by hyaline cartilage or fibrocartilage; allow very little motion (**Figure 14-2**)
   1. Synchondroses—hyaline cartilage present between articulating bones
   2. Symphyses—joints in which a pad or disc of fibrocartilage connects two bones
D. Synovial joints (diarthroses)—freely movable joints (**Figure 14-3**)
   1. Structures of synovial joints
      a. Joint capsule—sleevelike casing around the ends of the bones that binds them together
      b. Synovial membrane—membrane that lines the joint capsule and also secretes synovial fluid
      c. Articular cartilage—hyaline cartilage covering the articular surfaces of bones
      d. Joint cavity—small space between the articulating surfaces of the two bones of the joint
      e. Menisci (articular discs)—pads of fibrocartilage located between articulating bones
      f. Ligaments—strong cords of dense white fibrous tissue that hold the bones of a synovial joint more firmly together
      g. Bursae—synovial membranes filled with synovial fluid; cushion joints and facilitate movement of tendons
   2. Types of synovial joints (**Figure 14-4**)
      a. Uniaxial joints—synovial joints that permit movement around only one axis and in only one plane
         (1) Hinge joints—articulating ends of bones form a hinge-shaped unity that allows only flexion and extension
         (2) Pivot joints—a projection of one bone articulates with a ring or notch of another bone
      b. Biaxial joints—synovial joints that permit movements around two perpendicular axes in two perpendicular planes
         (1) Saddle joints—synovial joints in which the articulating ends of the bones resemble reciprocally shaped miniature saddles; only example in the body is in the thumbs
         (2) Condyloid (ellipsoidal) joints—synovial joints in which a condyle fits into an elliptical socket
      c. Multiaxial joints—synovial joints that permit movements around three or more axes in three or more planes
         (1) Ball-and-socket (spheroid) joints—most movable joints; the ball-shaped head of one bone fits into a concave depression
         (2) Gliding joints—relatively flat articulating surfaces that allow limited gliding movements along various axes

Representative Synovial Joints

A. Humeroscapular joint (**Figure 14-5**)
   1. Shoulder joint
   2. Most mobile joint because of the shallowness of the glenoid cavity
   3. Glenoid labrum—narrow rim of fibrocartilage around the glenoid cavity that lends depth to the glenoid cavity
   4. Structures that strengthen the shoulder joint are ligaments, muscles, tendons, and bursae
B. Elbow joint (**Figure 14-6**)
   1. Humeroradial joint—lateral articulation of the capitulum of the humerus with the head of the radius
   2. Humeroulnar joint—medial articulation of the trochlea of the humerus with the trochlear notch of the ulna
   3. Both components of the elbow joint are surrounded by a single joint capsule and stabilized by collateral ligaments
   4. Classic hinge joint
   5. Medial and lateral epicondyles are externally palpable bony landmarks
   6. Olecranon bursa independent of elbow joint space
      a. Inflammation called *olecranon bursitis*
      b. Trauma to nerve results in unpleasant sensations in the fingers and part of the hand supplied by the nerve
      c. Severe injury may cause paralysis of hand muscles or reduction in wrist movements

C. Proximal radioulnar joint—between the head of the radius and the medial notch of the ulna
   1. Stabilized by the annular ligament
   2. Permits rotation of the forearm
   3. Dislocation of the radial head called a "pulled elbow"
D. Distal radioulnar joint—point of articulation between the ulnar notch of the radius and the head of the ulna
   1. Acts with the proximal radioulnar joint
   2. Permits pronation and supination of the forearm
E. Radiocarpal (wrist) joints (**Figure 14-7**)
   1. Only the radius articulates directly with the carpal bones distally (scaphoid and lunate)
   2. Joints are synovial
   3. Scaphoid bone is fractured frequently
   4. Portion of the fractured scaphoid may become avascular
F. Intercarpal joints (**Figure 14-7**)
   1. Present between eight carpal bones
   2. Stabilized by numerous ligaments
   3. Joint spaces usually communicate
   4. Movements generally gliding with some abduction and flexion
G. Carpometacarpal joints—total of three joints
   1. One joint for the thumb—wide range of movements
   2. Two joints for the fingers—movements largely gliding type
   3. Thumb carpometacarpal joint is unique and important functionally
      a. Loose-fitting joint capsule
      b. Saddle-shaped articular surface
      c. Movements—extension, adduction, abduction, circumduction, and opposition
      d. Opposition—ability to touch the tip of the thumb to the tip of other fingers—movement of great functional significance
H. Metacarpophalangeal joints (**Figure 14-8**)
   1. Rounded heads of metacarpal bones articulate with concave bases of the proximal phalanges
   2. Capsule surrounding joints strengthened by collateral ligaments
   3. Primary movements are flexion and extension
I. Interphalangeal joints
   1. Typical diarthrotic, hinge-type, synovial joints
   2. Exist between heads of phalanges and bases of more distal phalanges
   3. Two categories:
      a. PIP joints—proximal interphalangeal joints (between proximal and middle phalanges)
      b. DIP joints—distal interphalangeal joints (between middle and distal phalanges)
J. Hip joint (**Figure 14-9**)
   1. Stable joint because of the shape of the head of the femur and the acetabulum
   2. A joint capsule and ligaments contribute to the joint's stability
K. Knee joint (**Figures 14-10** and **14-11**)
   1. Largest and one of the most complex and most frequently injured joints
   2. Tibiofemoral joint is supported by a joint capsule, cartilage, and numerous ligaments and muscle tendons
   3. Permits flexion, extension, and, with the knee flexed, some internal and external rotation
L. Ankle joint (**Figure 14-12**)
   1. Synovial-type hinge joint
   2. Articulation between the lower ends of the tibia and fibula and the upper part of the talus
   3. Joint is "mortise" or wedge-shaped
      a. Lateral malleolus lower than medial malleolus
   4. Internal rotation injury results in common "sprained ankle"
      a. Involves anterior talofibular ligament
   5. Other ankle ligaments also may be involved in sprain injuries—example is deltoid ligament
   6. External ankle rotation injuries generally involve bone fractures rather than ligament tears
      a. Monomalleolar ankle injury—lateral malleolus fractured
      b. Bimalleolar ankle injury—both malleoli fractured
      c. Trimalleolar ankle injury—fracture of both malleoli and articular surface of tibia
M. Vertebral joints (**Figures 14-13** and **14-14**)
   1. Vertebrae are connected to one another by several joints to form a strong flexible column
   2. Bodies of adjacent vertebrae are connected by intervertebral discs and ligaments
   3. Intervertebral discs are made up of two parts
      a. Annulus fibrosus—disc's outer rim, made of fibrous tissue and fibrocartilage
      b. Nucleus pulposus—disc's central core, made of a pulpy, elastic substance

Movement at Synovial Joints

A. Measuring range of motion (**Figure 14-15**)
   1. Range of motion (ROM) assessment used to determine extent of joint injury
   2. ROM can be measured actively or passively; both are generally about equal
   3. ROM measured by instrument called a *goniometer*
B. Angular movements—change the size of the angle between articulating bones
   1. Flexion—decreases the angle between bones; bends or folds one part on another (**Figures 14-16**, A; **14-18**; and **14-19**)
   2. Extension and hyperextension (**Figure 14-18**)
      a. Extension—increases the angle between bones, returns a part from its flexed position to its anatomical position
      b. Hyperextension—stretching or extending part beyond its anatomical position (**Figures 14-19**, **14-21**, and **14-23**)
   3. Plantar flexion and dorsiflexion (**Figure 14-25**)
      a. Plantar flexion—increases the angle between the top of the foot and the front of the leg
      b. Dorsiflexion—decreases the angle between the top of the foot and the front of the leg
   4. Abduction and adduction (**Figures 14-19** and **14-23**)
      a. Abduction—moves a part away from the median plane of the body
      b. Adduction—moves a part toward the median plane of the body

C. Circular movements
   1. Rotation and circumduction
      a. Rotation—pivoting a bone on its own axis (**Figure 14-16**, *D*)
      b. Circumduction—moves a part so that its distal end moves in a circle (**Figure 14-19**, *C*)
   2. Supination and pronation (**Figure 14-20**, *B*)
      a. Supination—turns the hand palm side up
      b. Pronation—turns the hand palm side down
D. Gliding movements—simplest of all movements; articular surface of one bone moves over the articular surface of another without any angular or circular movement
E. Special movements
   1. Inversion and eversion (**Figure 14-25**, *B* and *C*)
      a. Inversion—turning the sole of the foot inward
      b. Eversion—turning the sole of the foot outward
   2. Protraction and retraction (**Figure 14-17**, *A*)
      a. Protraction—moves a part forward
      b. Retraction—moves a part backward
   3. Elevation and depression (**Figure 14-17**, *B*)
      a. Elevation—moves a part up
      b. Depression—lowers a part

Cycle of Life: Articulations

A. Bone development and the sequence of ossification between birth and skeletal maturity affect joints
   1. Fontanelles between cranial bones disappear
   2. Epiphysial plates ossify at maturity
B. Older adults
   1. ROM decreases
   2. Changes in gait
C. Skeletal diseases manifesting as joint problems
   1. Abnormal bone growth (lipping)—influences joint motion
   2. Disease conditions can be associated with specific developmental periods

The Big Picture: Articulations

A. Hand—"reason for the upper extremity"; thumb—"reason for the hand"
   1. Examples of "big picture" type of thinking when used in functional context
B. Mobility of the upper extremity is extensive because of the following:
   1. Arrangement of bones in the shoulder girdle, arms, forearm, wrist, and hand
   2. Location and method of attachment of muscles to bones
   3. Proper functioning of joints
C. Mobility and extensive ROM needed to position upper extremity and hand to permit grasping and manipulation of objects, thus enabling effective interaction with objects in the external environment

REVIEW QUESTIONS

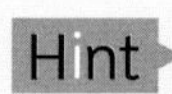

Write out the answers to these questions after reading the chapter and reviewing the Chapter Summary. Note—writing out your answers will consolidate learning and provide a valuable resource of information.

1. Classify joints and specify each group according to function and structure.
2. Define the terms *fibrous joints, cartilaginous joints*, and *synovial joints*.
3. Describe three types of fibrous joints. Give an example of each.
4. Name and define two types of cartilaginous joints. Give an example of each.
5. List and describe the different types of synovial joints. Give an example of each.
6. Name and define four kinds of angular movements permitted by some synovial joints.
7. Define and give an example of the following: rotation, circumduction, pronation, supination.
8. Describe the function of a goniometer. Name the medical professionals who may use this instrument.
9. What joint makes possible much of the dexterity of the human hand? Describe it and the movements it permits.
10. Describe vertebral joints.
11. Describe and differentiate between the following joints: humeroscapular, hip, knee.
12. How do loose bodies, or cartilaginous "joint mice", differ from menisci?
13. Outline the surgical procedure of total hip replacement (THR).
14. Name the two classifications of joint disorders and give examples of each.
15. Compare the range of movement at different joints.

CRITICAL THINKING QUESTIONS

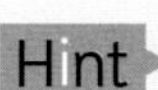

After finishing the Review Questions, write out the answers to these more in-depth questions to help you apply your new knowledge. Go back to sections of the chapter that relate to concepts that you find difficult.

1. The elbow, the joint between the bodies of vertebrae, and the root of a tooth in the jaw are all joints given different functional names. What are these names and what characteristic distinguishes them from one another?
2. A synovial joint is the most freely moving type of joint in the body, but joints require stability and protection also. Evaluate the seven structural characteristics of a synovial joint as primarily necessary for stability, movement, and protection.
3. Football players often sustain lateral blows to their extended knees, causing medial separation. Which of their ligaments is most likely to be damaged as a result of this type of injury?
4. Describe the anatomical structure of the knee and explain why the knee joint is the most commonly injured joint in the body.
5. Name an inflammatory autoimmune disorder that attacks articulations, and report on its symptoms.
6. What classification of synovial joints allows multiaxial movement?

15 Axial Muscles

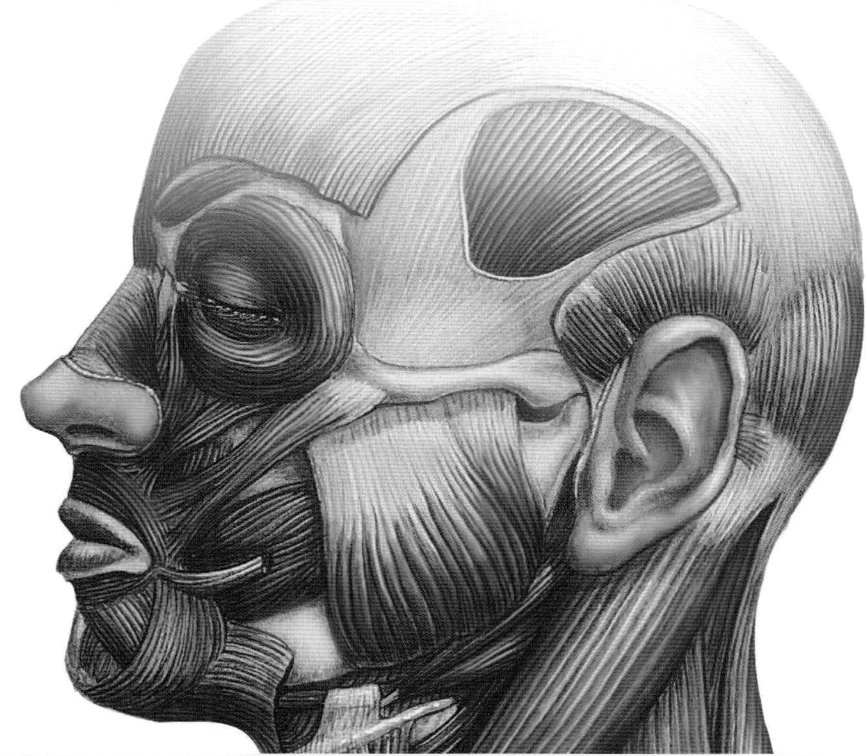

CHAPTER OUTLINE

Hint *Scan this outline before you begin to read the chapter, as a preview of how the concepts are organized.*

LANGUAGE OF SCIENCE

Hint *Use this list to aid your pronunciation of unfamiliar words.*

agonist (AG-ah-nist)
[*agon-* **struggle,** *-ist* **agent**]

anal triangle
[*an-* **ring (anus),** *-al* **relating to**]

antagonist (an-TAG-oh-nist)
[*ant-* **against,** *-agon-* **struggle,** *-ist* **agent**]

aponeurosis (ap-oh-nyoo-ROH-sis)
[*apo-* **from,** *-neur-* **sinew,** *-osis* **condition**] *pl.,* aponeuroses

buccinator muscle (BUK-si-NAY-tor)
[*buccinator* **trumpeter,** *mus-* **mouse,** *-cle* **little**]

bulbospongiosus muscle (bul-boh-spun-jee-OH-ses)
[*bulbo-* **bulb,** *-spongiosus* **spongy,** *mus-* **mouse,** *-cle* **little**]

coccygeus muscle (kohk-SIJ-ee-us)
[*coccygeus* **coccyx,** *mus-* **mouse,** *-cle* **little**]

convergent muscle (kon-VER-jent)
[*con-* **together,** *-verg-* **incline,** *-ent* **state,** *mus-* **mouse,** *-cle* **little**]

corrugator supercilii muscle (KOR-uh-gay-tor soo-per-SIL-ee-eye)
[*corrugator* **wrinkler,** *super-* **above,** *-cilli-* **eyelash,** *mus-* **mouse,** *-cle* **little**]

diaphragm (DYE-ah-fram)
[*dia-* **across,** *-phrag-* **enclose,** *-(u)m* **thing**]

endomysium (en-doh-MEE-see-um)
[*endo-* **within,** *-mys-* **muscle,** *-um* **thing**]

epimysium (ep-i-MIS-ee-um)
[*epi-* **upon,** *-mys-* **muscle,** *-um* **thing**]

erector spinae muscle (eh-REK-tor SPYNE-ee)
[*erect-* **upright,** *-or* **agent,** *spinae* **of the spine,** *mus-* **mouse,** *-cle* **little**]

external anal sphincter muscle (eks-TER-nal AY-nal SFINGK-ter)
[*extern-* **outside,** *-al* **relating to,** *an-* **ring (anus),** *-al* **relating to,** *sphinc-* **bind tight,** *-er* **agent,** *mus-* **mouse,** *-cle* **little**]

continued on p. 333

UNIT 2

Survival depends on the ability to maintain a relatively constant internal environment. Such stability often requires movement of the body. Although many different systems of the body have some role in accomplishing movement, it is the skeletal and muscular systems acting together that actually produce most body movements. We have investigated the architectural plan of the skeleton and have seen how its firm supports and joint structures make movement possible. However, bones and joints cannot move themselves. They must be moved by something. Our subject for now, then, is the large mass of skeletal muscle that moves the framework of the body: the **muscular system.**

Movement is one of the most distinctive and easily observed "characteristics of life". When we walk, talk, run, breathe, or engage in a multitude of other physical activities that are under the "willed" control of the individual, we do so by contraction of skeletal muscle.

There are more than 600 skeletal muscles in the body. Collectively, they constitute 40% to 50% of our body weight. And, together with the scaffolding provided by the skeleton, muscles also determine the form and contours of our body.

Contraction of individual muscle cells is ultimately responsible for purposeful movement. In Chapter 17 the physiology of muscular contraction is discussed. In this preliminary chapter, however, we will learn how contractile units are grouped into unique functioning organs—or muscles.

The manner in which muscles are grouped, the relationship of muscles to joints, and how muscles attach to the skeleton determine purposeful body movement. A discussion of muscle shape and how muscles attach to and move bones is followed by information on specific muscles and muscle groups. This chapter surveys major muscles of the *axial* region of the body, and the next chapter continues with a survey of major *appendicular* muscles.

SKELETAL MUSCLE STRUCTURE

Connective Tissue Components

The skeletal muscle cells, or *muscle fibres*, are covered by a delicate connective tissue membrane called the **endomysium** (**Figure 15-1**). Groups of skeletal muscle fibres, called *fascicles*, are then bound together into bundles by a tougher connective tissue envelope called the **perimysium.** The muscle as a whole is covered by a coarse sheath called the **epimysium.**

Because all three of these fibrous membranes are continuous with the fibrous structures that attach muscles to bones or other structures, muscles are firmly harnessed to the structures they pull on during contraction. The epimysium, perimysium, and endomysium of a muscle, for example, may be continuous with fibrous tissue that extends from the muscle as a **tendon,** a strong tough cord continuous at its other end with the fibrous periosteum covering a bone. Alternatively, the fibrous wrapping of a muscle may extend as a broad, flat sheet of connective tissue called an **aponeurosis,** which usually merges with the fibrous wrappings of another muscle. So tough and strong are tendons and aponeuroses that they are not often torn, even by injuries forceful enough to break bones or tear muscles. They are, however, occasionally pulled away from bones.

Fibrous connective tissue surrounding the muscle organ and located outside the epimysium and tendon is called **fascia.** *Fascia* is a general term for the fibrous connective tissue found under the skin and surrounding many deeper organs, including skeletal muscles and bones. Fascia just under the skin (the hypodermis) is sometimes called *superficial fascia,* and the fascia around muscles and bones is sometimes called *deep fascia.*

Sheets of fibrous connective tissue form double-walled tubes called **tendon sheaths** that enclose certain tendons, notably those of the wrist and ankle (**Figure 15-2**). Like bursae, the walls of tendon sheaths have a lining of synovial membrane. The moist, smooth surfaces that face each other within the double wall of a tendon sheath enable the tendon to move easily, almost without friction. Tendon sheaths that surround tendons of the fingers and wrists can be seen in cross section in Figures 4-11 and 4-12 of the Brief Atlas of the Human Body.

Table 15-1 clarifies the arrangement of the fibrous coverings of a muscle organ.

TABLE 15-1 Fibrous Coverings of Muscle Organs

FIBROUS STRUCTURE*	PART COVERED
Fascia	External to muscles, bones, other organs
Superficial fascia	Under the skin
Deep fascia	Surrounds deeper organs, including epimysium of muscle
Tendon sheath	Tubelike tunnel around tendon of muscle; lined with synovial membrane
Epimysium†	Surrounds entire muscle organ
Perimysium†	Surrounds a fascicle (bundle) of muscle fibres
Endomysium†	Surrounds an individual muscle fibre

*Listed here from superficial to deep; all of these fibrous structures are continuous with one another (that is, their fibres blend together).

†Continue and fuse together to form a tendon or aponeurosis.

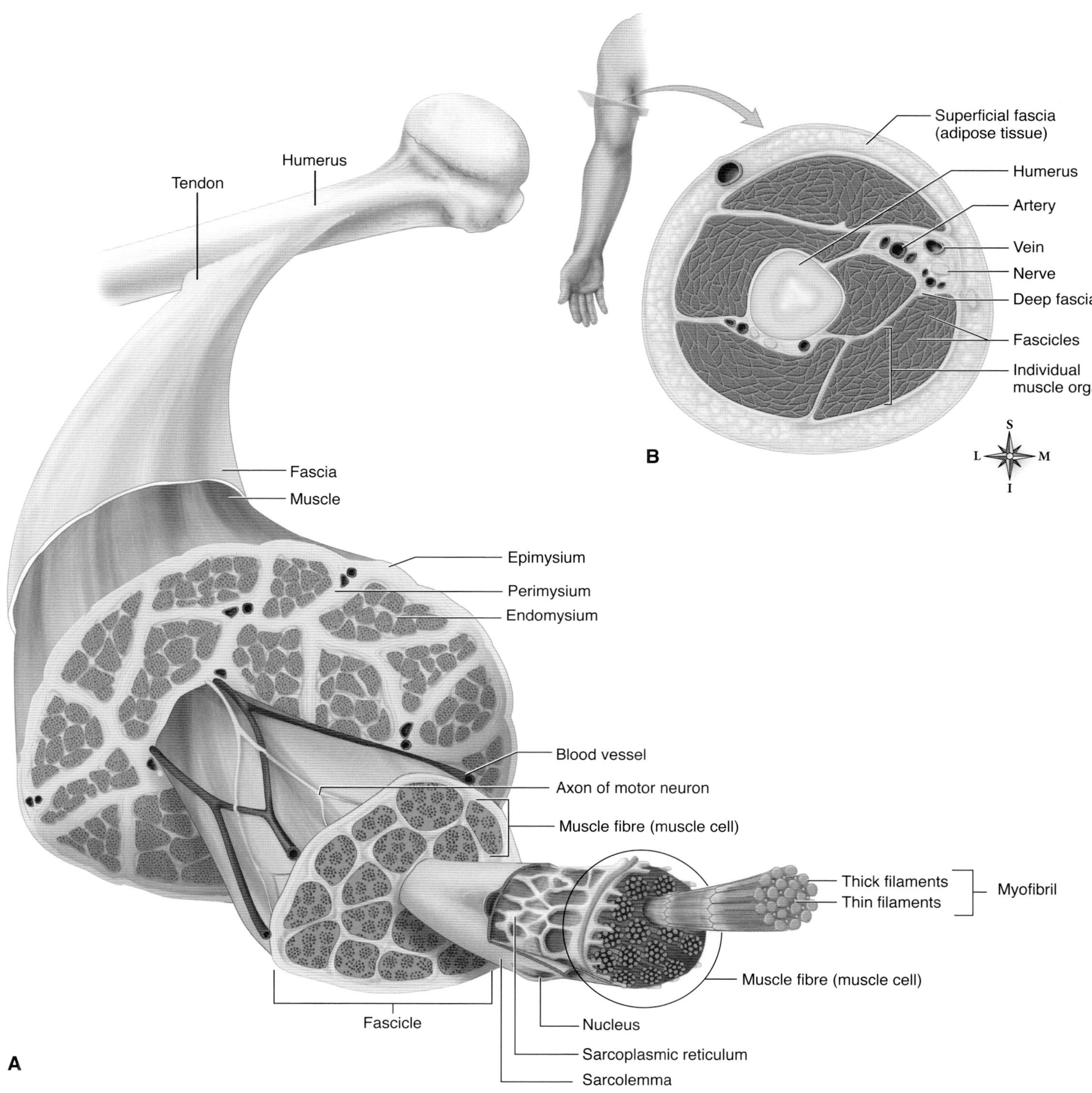

FIGURE 15-1 Structure of a muscle organ. A, Note that the connective tissue coverings (*epimysium, perimysium,* and *endomysium*) are continuous with one another and with the tendon. Note also that muscle fibres are held together by the perimysium in groups called *fascicles.* **B,** Diagram showing the arm in cross-section. Note the relationships of superficial and deep fascia to individual muscles and other structures in the plane of section.

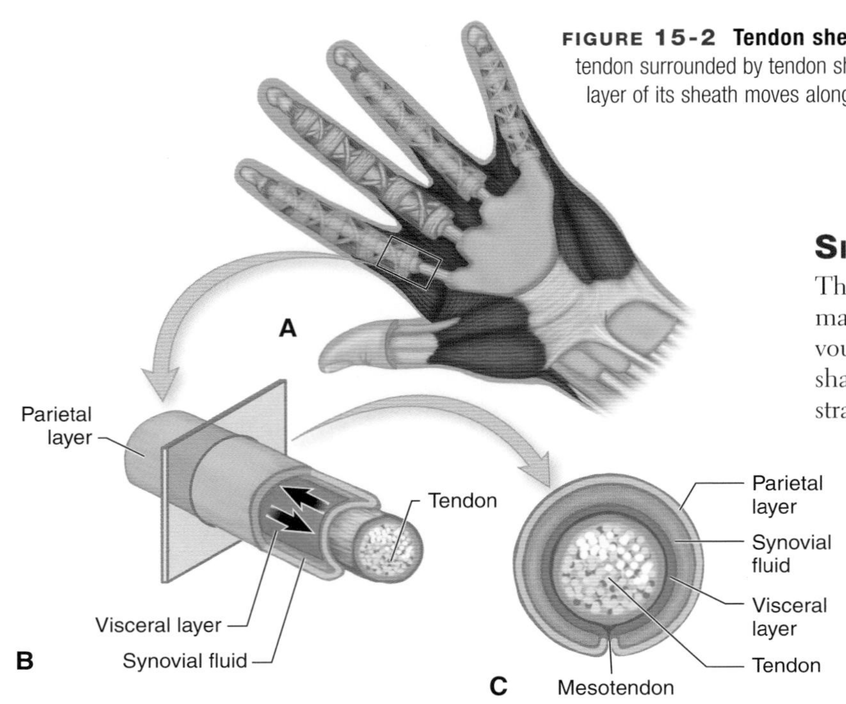

FIGURE 15-2 Tendon sheath. A, Many tendon sheaths are visible in this dissected hand. **B,** Segment of tendon surrounded by tendon sheath. **C,** Cross-section of tendon and its sheath. As a tendon moves, the visceral layer of its sheath moves along with it, sliding past the parietal layer and lubricated by synovial fluid.

Size, Shape, and Fibre Arrangement

The structures called *skeletal muscles* are organs. They consist mainly of skeletal muscle tissue plus important connective and nervous tissue components. Skeletal muscles vary considerably in size, shape, and arrangement of fibres. They range from extremely small strands, such as the stapedius muscle of the middle ear, to large masses, such as the muscles of the thigh. Some skeletal muscles are broad in shape and some are narrow. Some are long and tapering and some are short and blunt. Some are triangular, some quadrilateral, and some irregular. Some form flat sheets and others form bulky masses.

The strength and type of movement produced by the shortening of a muscle are related to the orientation of its fibres and overall shape, as well as its attachments to bone and involvement in joints. This is yet another example of the relationship

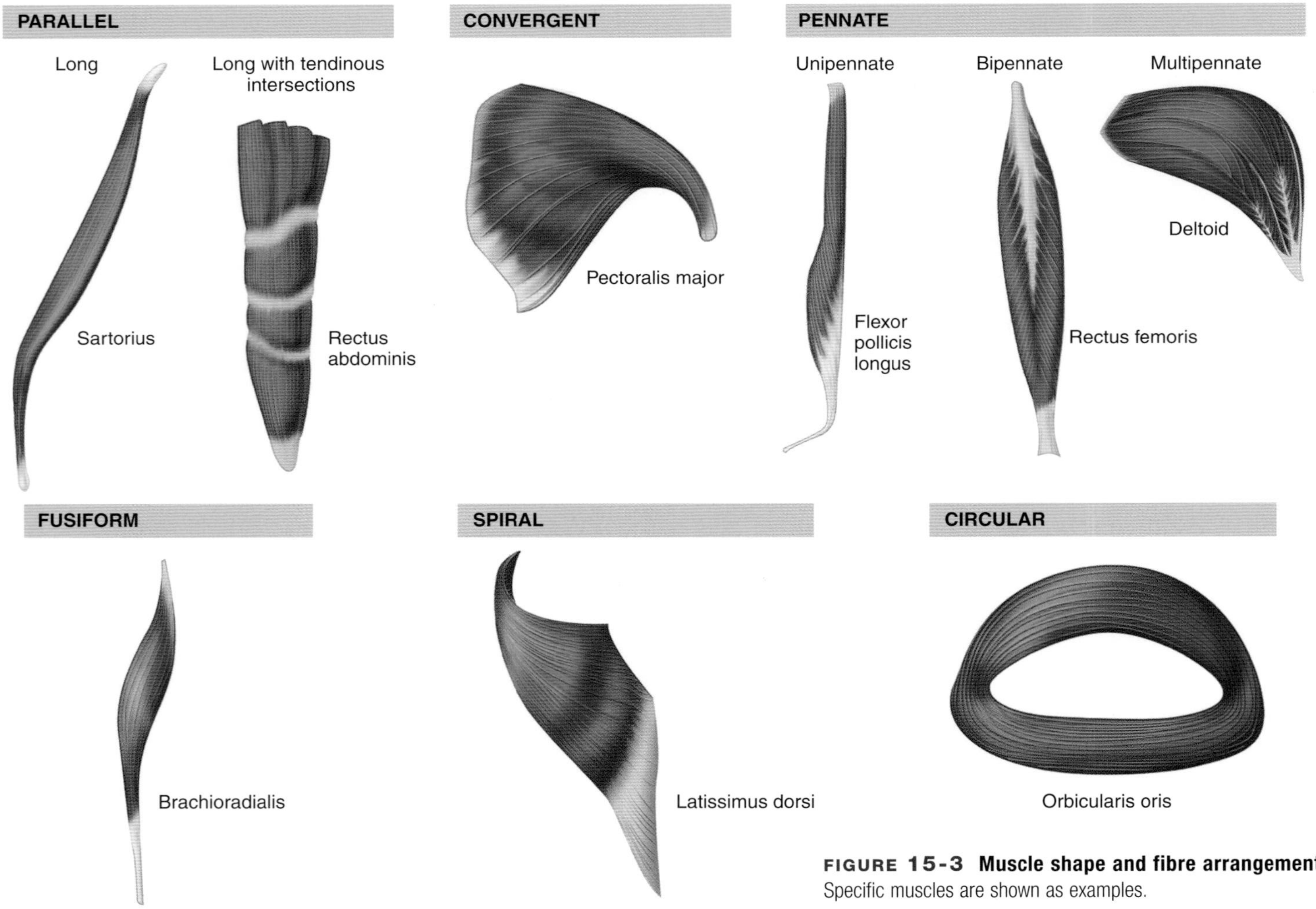

FIGURE 15-3 Muscle shape and fibre arrangement. Specific muscles are shown as examples.

between structure and function. Six muscle shapes are often used to describe and categorize skeletal muscles (**Figure 15-3**).

1. **Parallel muscles** can vary in length, but long straplike muscles with parallel fascicles are perhaps most typical. The sartorius muscle of the leg is a good example. The rectus abdominis muscles, which run the length of the anterior abdominal wall, have parallel muscle fascicles that are "interrupted" by transverse intersections.
2. **Convergent muscles** have fascicles that radiate out from a small to a wider point of attachment, much like the blades in a fan. The pectoralis major muscle is a good example.
3. **Pennate muscles** are said to be "featherlike" in appearance. Three categories of these muscles have uniquely different types of fascicle attachments that in some ways resemble the feathers in an old-fashioned plume pen. *Unipennate muscles*, such as the soleus, have fascicles that anchor to only one side of the connective tissue shaft. *Bipennate muscles*, such as the rectus femoris in the thigh, have a type of double-feathered attachment of fascicles. In *multipennate muscles*, such as the deltoid, the numerous interconnecting quill-like fascicles converge on a common point of attachment.
4. **Fusiform muscles** have fascicles that may be close to parallel in the centre, or "belly", of the muscle but converge to a tendon at one or both ends. The brachioradialis is a good example.
5. **Spiral muscles,** such as the latissimus dorsi, have fibres that twist between their points of attachment.
6. **Circular muscles,** sometimes called *orbicular muscles* and *sphincters*, often circle body tubes or openings. The orbicularis oris around the mouth is an example. The external anal sphincter around the anus is another example.

Quick CHECK

1. Identify (a) the connective tissue membrane that covers individual muscle fibres, (b) the membrane that surrounds groups of skeletal muscle fibres (fascicles), and (c) the membrane that covers the muscle as a whole.
2. Name the tough connective tissue cord that serves to attach a muscle to a bone.
3. Name three types of fibre arrangements seen in skeletal muscle.

ATTACHMENT OF MUSCLES

Most of our muscles span at least one joint and attach to both articulating bones. When contraction occurs, one bone usually remains fixed and the other moves. The points of attachment are called the *origin* and *insertion*.

The **origin** is the point of attachment that does not move when the muscle contracts. Therefore, the origin bone is the more stationary of the two bones at a joint when contraction occurs. The **insertion** is the point of attachment that moves when the muscle contracts (**Figure 15-4**). The insertion bone therefore moves along a "line of force" toward the origin bone when the muscle shortens. In case you are wondering why both bones do not move because both are pulled on by the contracting muscle, the answer is that one of them is normally stabilized by isometric contractions of other muscles or by certain features of its own that make it less mobile.

The terms *origin* and *insertion* provide us with useful points of reference. Many muscles have multiple points of origin or insertion. Understanding the functional relationship of these attachment points during muscle contraction helps in deducing muscle actions. The attachment points of the brachialis muscle of the arm shown in **Figure 15-4** help provide functional information. Distal insertion on the ulna in the forearm causes flexion to occur at the elbow when contraction occurs.

It should be realized, however, that origin and insertion are points that may change in certain circumstances. For example, not only can you grasp an object above your head and pull it down, but you can also pull yourself up to the object. Although

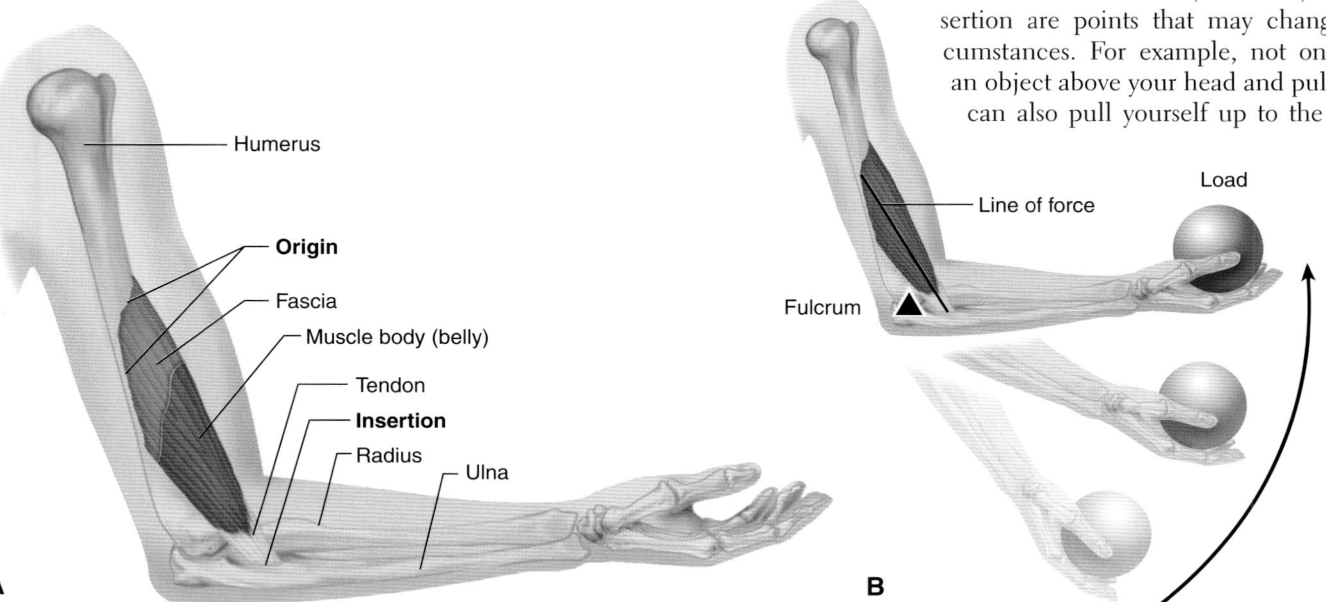

FIGURE 15-4 Attachments of a skeletal muscle. A, Origin and insertion of a skeletal muscle. A muscle originates at a relatively stable part of the skeleton (origin) and inserts at the skeletal part that is moved when the muscle contracts (insertion). **B,** Movement of the forearm during weightlifting. Muscle contraction moves bones, which serve as levers, and by acting on joints, which serve as fulcrums for those levers. See the text for discussion and review **Figure 15-6**, which illustrates types of levers.

UNIT 2

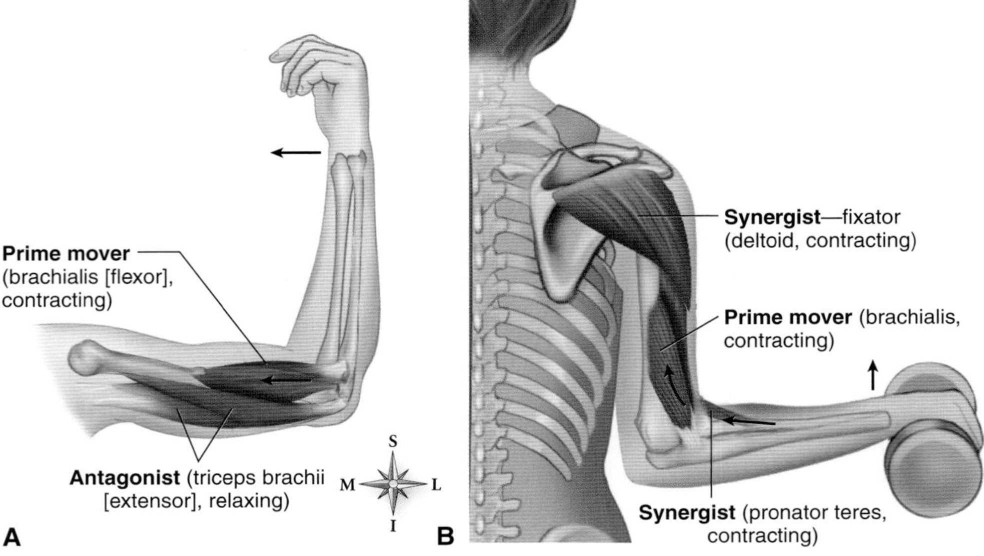

FIGURE 15-5 Muscle actions. A, The flexor muscle (brachialis) is the prime mover in flexing the elbow. The extensor muscle (triceps brachii) is the antagonist, which in this case must relax to permit easy flexion of the elbow. The pronator teres muscle acts as a synergist by also flexing the elbow. **B,** Here the brachialis is again the prime mover of flexion of the elbow. The pronator teres muscle acts as a synergist by also flexing the elbow. To prevent the biceps from also moving the shoulder while straining against a heavy weight, the posterior portion of the deltoid muscle tenses to stabilize the shoulder joint—thus acting as a fixator muscle in this action.

origin and insertion are convenient terms, they do not always provide the necessary information needed to understand the full functional potential of muscle action.

Muscle Actions

Skeletal muscles almost always act in groups rather than singly. As a result, most movements are produced by the coordinated action of several muscles. Some of the muscles in the group contract while others relax. The result is a movement pattern that allows for the functional classification of muscles or muscle groups. Several terms are used to describe muscle action during any particular movement pattern. The terms *prime mover (agonist)*, *antagonist*, *synergist*, and *fixator* are especially important and are discussed in the following paragraphs. Each term suggests an important concept that is essential to understanding such functional muscle patterns as flexion, extension, abduction, adduction, and other movements discussed in Chapter 14.

Any muscle that performs an action is a "mover". The term **prime mover** is used to describe a muscle that directly performs a specific movement. The movement produced by a muscle acting as a prime mover is described as the "action" or "function" of that muscle. For example, the brachialis shown in **Figure 15-4** and **Figure 15-5** is acting as a prime mover during flexion of the forearm. The term **agonist** can be applied to the prime mover, or any other "mover" muscle that directly contributes to the same action as the prime mover.

Antagonists are muscles that, when contracting, directly oppose prime movers (or agonists). They are relaxed while the prime mover is contracting to produce movement (see **Figure 15-5**). Simultaneous contraction of a prime mover and its antagonist muscle results in rigidity and lack of motion. The term *antagonist* is perhaps unfortunate because muscles cooperate, rather than oppose, in normal movement patterns. Antagonists are important in providing precision and control during contraction of prime movers.

Synergists are muscles that contract at the same time as the prime mover. They facilitate or complement prime mover actions so that the prime mover produces a more effective movement.

Fixator muscles generally function as joint stabilizers (see **Figure 15-5**, *B*). They frequently serve to maintain posture or balance during contraction of prime movers acting on joints in the arms and legs. Because fixator muscles assist the prime mover in performing an action, they are a type of synergist.

Movement patterns are complex, and most muscles function not only as prime movers but also at times as antagonists, synergists, or fixators. A prime mover in a particular movement pattern, such as flexion, may be an antagonist during extension or a synergist or fixator in other types of movement.

Quick CHECK

4. Identify the point of attachment of a muscle to a bone that (a) does not move when the muscle contracts and (b) one that does move when the muscle contracts.
5. What name is used to describe a muscle that directly performs a specific movement?
6. What muscle type helps maintain overall body posture when prime movers produce motion in the extremities?
7. Name the type of muscles that generally function as joint stabilizers.

Lever Systems

When a muscle shortens, the central body portion, called the **belly,** contracts. The type and extent of movement are determined by the load or resistance that is moved, the attachment of the tendinous extremities of the muscle to bone (origin and insertion), and the particular type of joint involved. In almost every instance, muscles that move a part do not lie over that part. Instead, the muscle belly lies proximal to the part moved. Thus muscles that move the forearm lie proximal to it—that is, in the upper part of the arm.

Knowledge of lever systems is important in understanding muscle action. By definition, a **lever** is any rigid bar free to turn about a fixed point called its *fulcrum.* Bones serve as levers, and joints serve as fulcrums of these levers. A contracting muscle applies a pulling force on a bone lever at the point of the muscle's attachment to the bone (**Box 15-1**). This force causes the insertion bone to move about its joint fulcrum.

A **lever system** is a simple mechanical device that makes the work of moving a weight or other load easier in some way. Lever systems are composed of four component parts:

1. A rigid rod or bar (bone) called a *lever*
2. A fixed pivot, or fulcrum (F), around which the lever moves (joint)
3. A load (L), or resistance, that is moved
4. A force, or pull (P), which produces movement (muscle contraction). The pull or force is also called the effort.

BOX 15-1 *sports and fitness*
Assessing Muscle Strength

Physiotherapists, certified athletic trainers, and other health care providers are often required to assess muscle strength. A basic principle of muscle action in a lever system is called the *optimum angle of pull.* An understanding of this principle is required for correct assessment of muscle strength.

In general, the optimum angle of pull for any muscle is a right angle to the long axis of the bone to which it is attached. When the angle of pull departs from a right angle and becomes more parallel to the long axis, the strength of contraction decreases dramatically. Contraction of the brachialis muscle demonstrates this principle very well. The brachialis crosses the elbow from the humerus to the ulna. In the anatomical position the elbow is extended and the angle of pull of the brachialis is parallel to the long axis of the ulna (see **Figures 15-4** and **15-5**). Contraction of the brachialis at this angle is very inefficient. As the elbow is flexed and the angle of pull approaches a right angle, the contraction strength of the muscle is greatly increased. Therefore, to test brachialis muscle strength correctly, the forearm should be flexed at the elbow (see figure).

Understanding the optimum angle of pull for any given muscle makes possible a rational approach to correct assessment of functional strength in that muscle. •

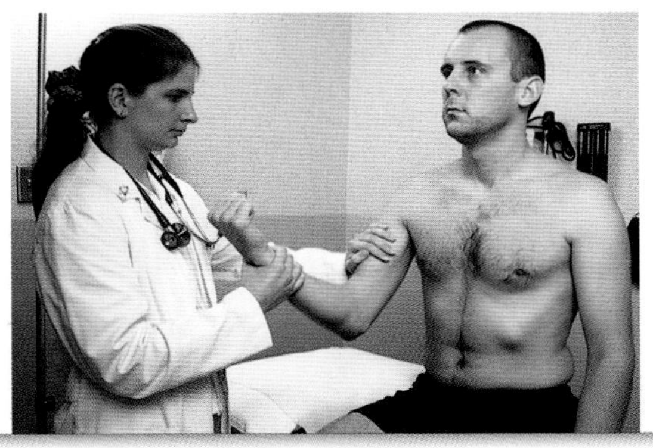

Figure 15-6 shows the three different types of lever arrangements. All three types are found in the human body.

First-Class Levers

As you can see in **Figure 15-6**, *A*, the fulcrum in a first-class lever lies between the effort, or pull (P), and the resistance, or load (W), as in a set of scales, a pair of scissors, or a child's seesaw. In the body the head being raised or tipped backward on the atlas is an example of a first-class lever in action. The facial portion of the skull is the load, the joint between the skull and atlas is the fulcrum, and the muscles of the back produce the pull. In the human body first-class levers are not abundant. They generally serve as levers of stability.

Second-Class Levers

In second-class levers the load lies between the fulcrum and the joint at which the pull is exerted. The wheelbarrow is often used as an example. The presence of second-class levers in the human body is a controversial issue. Some authorities interpret the raising of the body on the toes as an example of this type of lever (see **Figure 15-6**, *B*). In this example the point of contact between the toes and the ground is the fulcrum, the load is located at the ankle, and pull is

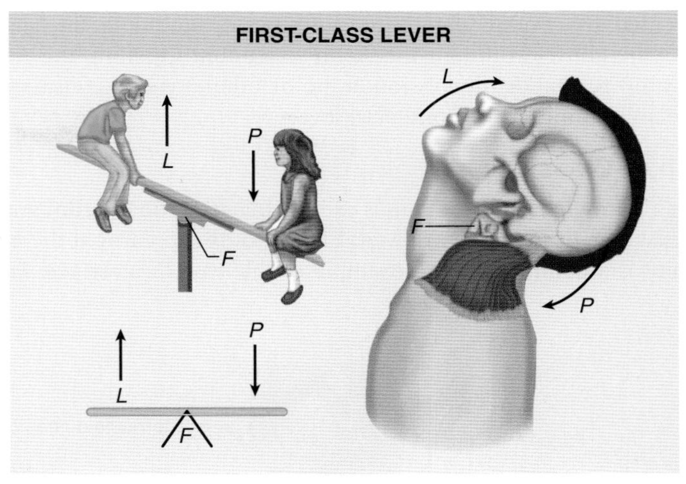

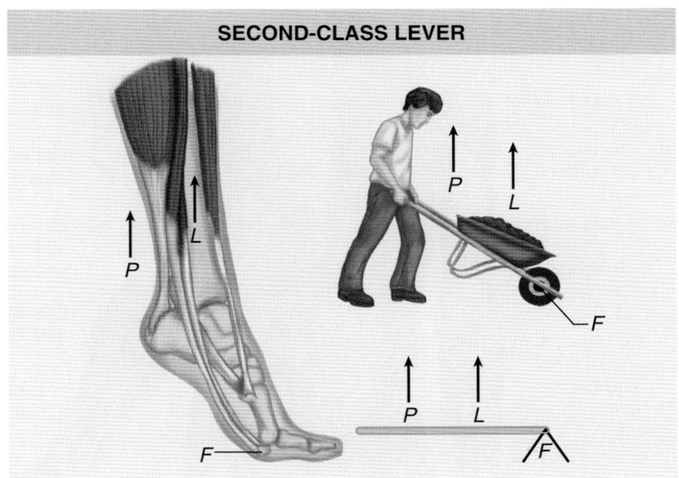

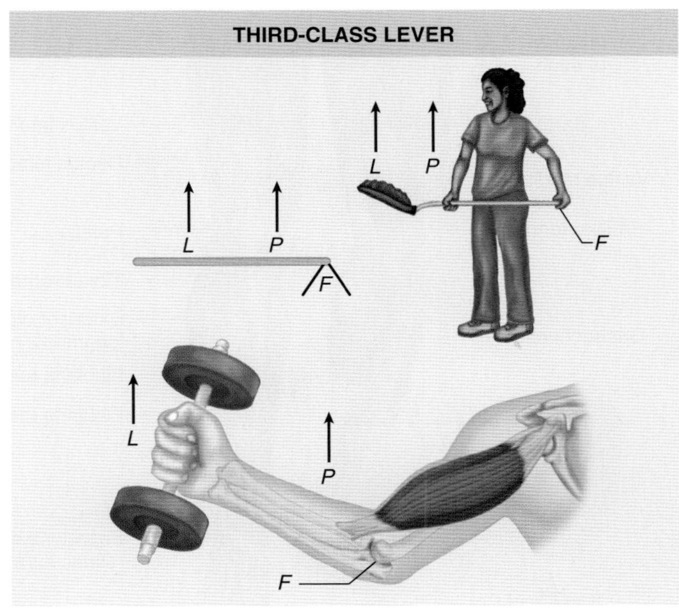

FIGURE 15-6 Lever classes. A, First class: fulcrum (F) between the load (L) and force or pull (P). **B,** Second class: load (L) between the fulcrum (F) and force or pull (P). **C,** Third class: force or pull (P) between the fulcrum (F) and the load (L). The lever rod is *yellow* in each drawing. Note the pull (P) is also called the effort.

exerted by several plantar flexor muscles, including the gastrocnemius muscle through the Achilles tendon. Opening the mouth against resistance (depression of the mandible) is also considered to be an example of a second-class lever.

Third-Class Levers

In a third-class lever the pull is exerted between the fulcrum and the resistance or load to be moved. Flexing of the forearm at the elbow joint is a commonly used example of this type of lever (see **Figure 15-6**, *C*). Third-class levers permit rapid and extensive movement and are the most common type found in the body. They allow insertion of a muscle very close to the joint that it moves.

CONNECT IT! 

Leverage is the change in effort needed when using a lever to do work. Want to know more about how muscles power the levers of the body? Check it out in ***Leverage*** online at ***Connect It!***

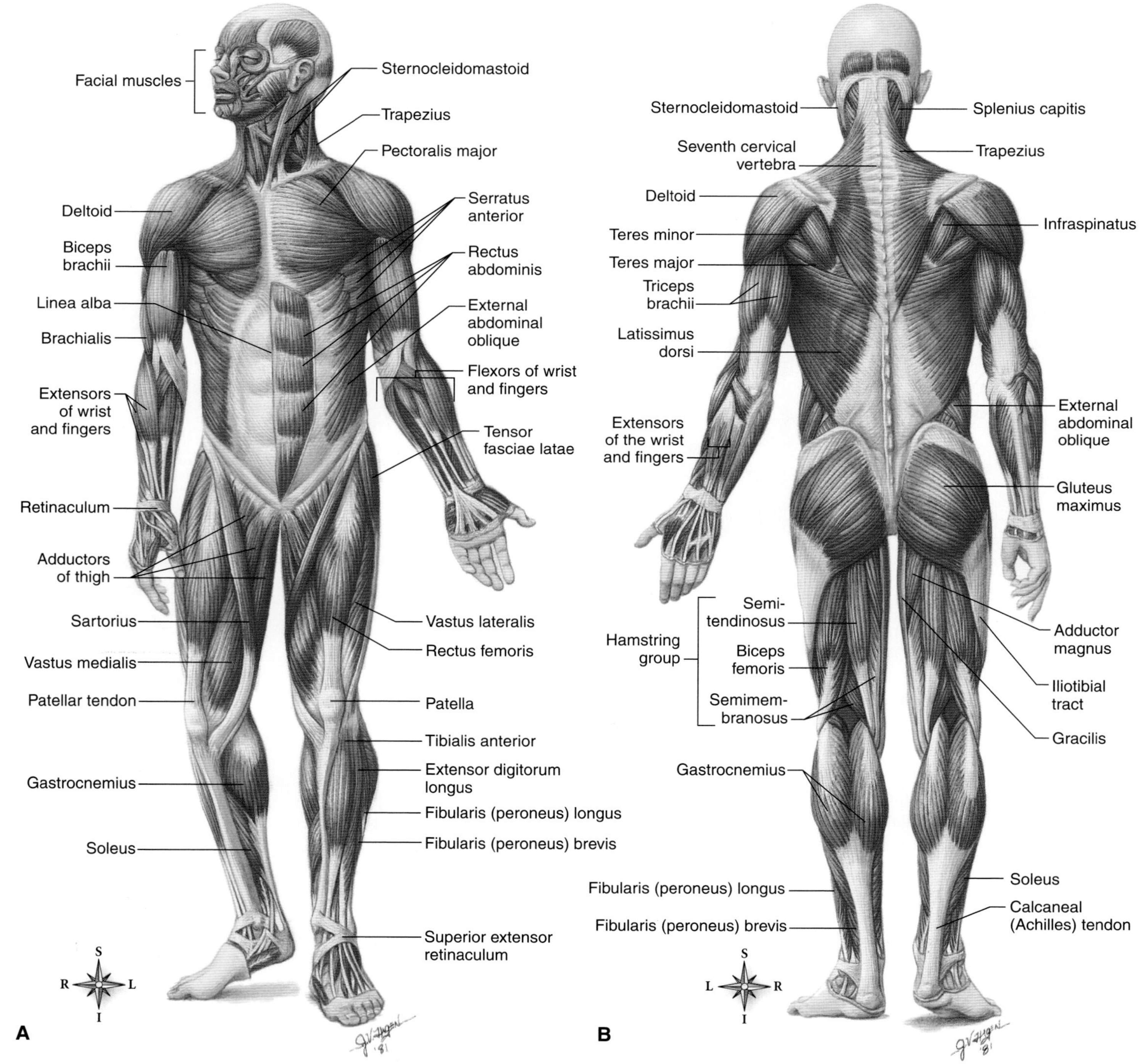

FIGURE 15-7 **General overview of the body's musculature. A,** Anterior view. **B,** Posterior view. **C,** Lateral view.

HOW MUSCLES ARE NAMED

The first thing you may notice as you start studying the muscles of the body is that many of the names seem difficult and foreign. The terms are less difficult if you keep in mind that most anatomical terms come from Latin.

Although we have strived to use only English names in this edition, some Latin terms still remain in common usage—especially in anatomy. This is certainly true in the health-related disciplines. For example, in some texts the deltoid muscle is called the *deltoideus* (Latin) and in others the *deltoid* (English). To minimize confusion, the terms used here will be the English versions from the *Terminologia Anatomica* (see Chapter 1). Even so, you will soon discover that the English versions are often the same or similar to the Latin versions!

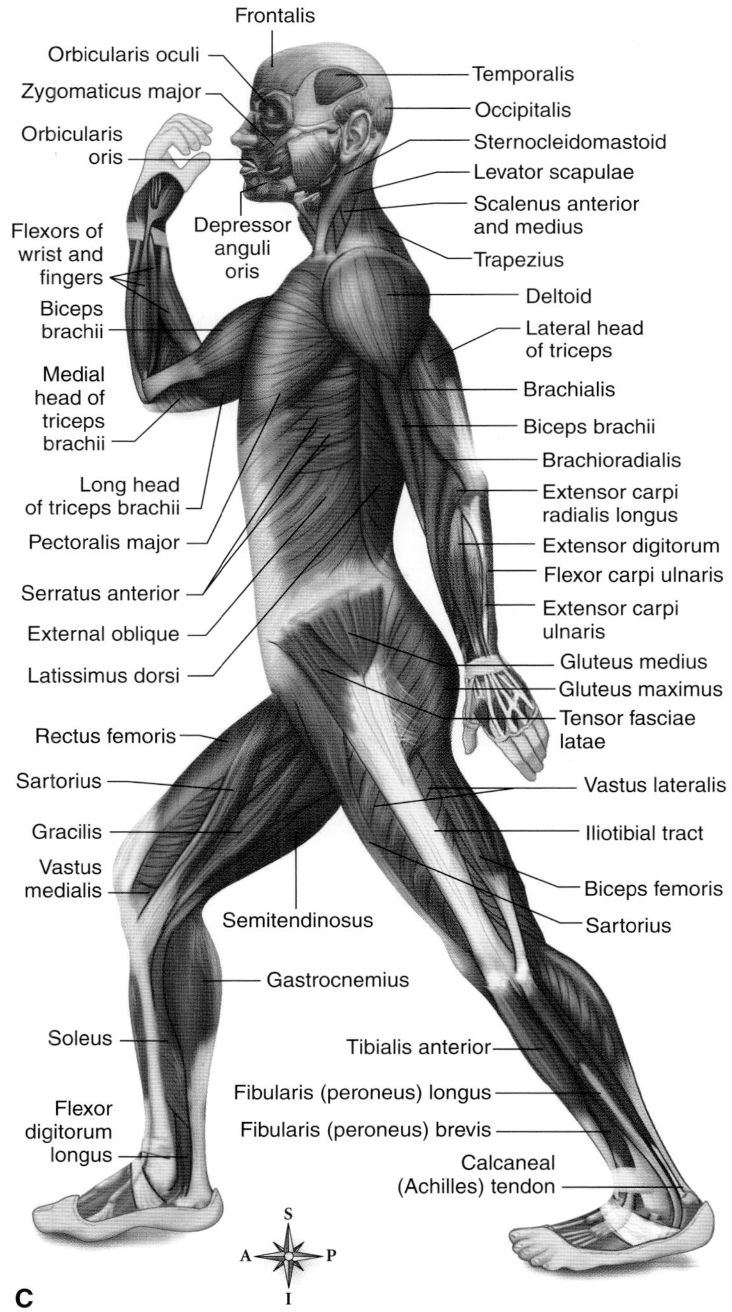

Regardless of the muscle name used, when one understands the reasons for the term used, it will seem more logical and be easier to learn and understand. Many of the muscles of the body shown in **Figure 15-7** or listed in **Tables 15-2** through **15-6** are named according to one or more of the following features:

Location. Many muscles are named as a result of location. The *brachialis* (arm) muscle and *gluteus* (buttock) muscles are examples. **Table 15-2** gives a listing of some major muscles grouped by location.

Function. The function of a muscle often is a part of its name. The *adductor* muscles of the thigh adduct, or move, the leg toward the midline of the body. **Table 15-3** lists selected muscles grouped according to function.

TABLE 15-2 Selected Muscles Grouped by Location

LOCATION	MUSCLES
Axial Muscles	
Neck	Sternocleidomastoid
Back	Trapezius Latissimus dorsi
Chest	Pectoralis major Serratus anterior
Abdominal wall	External oblique
Pelvic floor	Levator ani Coccygeus
Appendicular Muscles	
Shoulder	Deltoid
Arm	Biceps brachii Triceps brachii Brachialis
Forearm	Brachioradialis Pronator teres
Buttocks	Gluteus maximus Gluteus minimus Gluteus medius Tensor fasciae latae
Thigh	
Anterior thigh	Quadriceps femoris group Rectus femoris Vastus lateralis Vastus medialis Vastus intermedius
Medial thigh	Gracilis Adductor group (brevis, longus, magnus)
Posterior thigh	Hamstring group Biceps femoris Semitendinosus Semimembranosus
Leg	
Anterior leg	Tibialis anterior
Posterior leg	Gastrocnemius Soleus

Shape. Shape is a descriptive feature used for naming many muscles. The *deltoid* (triangular) muscle covering the shoulder is deltoid, or triangular, in shape (**Table 15-4**).

Direction of fibres. Muscles may be named according to the orientation of their fibres. The term *rectus* means straight. The fibres of the *rectus abdominis* muscle run straight up and down and are parallel to each other (**Table 15-5**).

Number of heads or divisions. The number of divisions or heads (points of origin) may be used to name a muscle. The word part *-cep-* means "head". *Biceps* (two), *triceps* (three), and *quadriceps* (four) refer to multiple heads, or points of origin. The *biceps brachii* is a muscle having two heads located in the arm (see **Table 15-5**).

Points of attachment. Origin and insertion points may be used to name a muscle. For example, the *sternocleidomastoid* has its origin on the sternum and clavicle and inserts on the mastoid process of the temporal bone.

Size of muscle. The relative size of a muscle can be used to name a muscle, especially if it is compared with the size of nearby muscles (**Table 15-6**). For example, the *gluteus maximus* is the largest

TABLE 15-3 Selected Muscles Grouped by Function

PART MOVED	EXAMPLE OF FLEXOR	EXAMPLE OF EXTENSOR	EXAMPLE OF ABDUCTOR	EXAMPLE OF ADDUCTOR
Head	Sternocleidomastoid	Semispinalis capitis	—	—
Arm	Pectoralis major	Trapezius Latissimus dorsi	Deltoid	Pectoralis major with latissimus dorsi
Forearm	With forearm supinated: biceps brachii With forearm pronated: brachialis With semisupination or semipronation: brachioradialis	Triceps brachii	—	—
Hand	Flexor carpi radialis and ulnaris Palmaris longus	Extensor carpi radialis, longus, and brevis Extensor carpi ulnaris	Flexor carpi radialis	Flexor carpi ulnaris
Thigh	Iliopsoas Rectus femoris (of quadriceps femoris group)	Gluteus maximus	Gluteus medius and minimus	Adductor group
Leg	Hamstrings	Quadriceps femoris group	—	—
Foot	Tibialis anterior	Gastrocnemius Soleus	*Evertors* Fibularis longus Fibularis brevis	*Invertor* Tibialis anterior
Trunk	Iliopsoas Rectus abdominis	Erector spinae	—	—

TABLE 15-4 Selected Muscles Grouped by Shape

NAME	MEANING	EXAMPLE
Deltoid	Triangular	Deltoid
Gracilis	Slender	Gracilis
Trapezius	Trapezoid	Trapezius
Serratus	Notched	Serratus anterior
Teres	Round	Pronator teres
Rhomboid	Rhomboidal	Rhomboid major
Orbicularis	Round or circular	Orbicularis oris
Pectinate	Comblike	Pectineus
Piriformis	Wedge-shaped	Piriformis
Platys	Flat	Platysma
Quadratus	Square	Quadratus femoris
Lumbrical	Wormlike	Lumbricals

TABLE 15-5 Selected Muscles Grouped by Heads and Fibre Direction

NAME	MEANING	EXAMPLE
Number of Heads		
Biceps	Two heads	Biceps brachii
Triceps	Three heads	Triceps brachii
Quadriceps	Four heads	Quadriceps
Digastric	Two bellies	Digastric
Direction of Fibres		
Oblique	Diagonal	External oblique rectus
Rectus	Straight	Rectus abdominis
Transverse	Transverse	Transversus abdominis
Circular	Around	Orbicularis oris
Spiral	Oblique	Supinator

TABLE 15-6 **Selected Muscles Grouped by Size**

NAME	MEANING	EXAMPLE
Major	Large	Pectoralis major
Maximus	Largest	Gluteus maximus
Minor	Small	Pectoralis minor
Minimus	Smallest	Gluteus minimus
Longus	Long	Adductor longus
Brevis	Short	Extensor pollicis brevis
Latissimus	Very wide	Latissimus dorsi
Longissimus	Very long	Longissimus
Magnus	Very large	Adductor magnus
Vastus	Vast or huge	Vastus medialis

muscle of the gluteal (from Greek *glautos*, meaning "buttock") region. Nearby, there is a small gluteal muscle, the *gluteus minimus*, and a midsize gluteal muscle, the *gluteus medius*.

Quick CHECK

8. Name the four major components of any lever system.
9. Identify the three types of lever systems found in the human body and give one example of each.
10. What type of lever system permits rapid and extensive movement and is the most common type found in the body?
11. List six criteria that may determine a muscle's name, and give an example of a specific muscle named according to each criterion.

Hints on How to Deduce Muscle Actions

To understand muscle actions, you first need to know certain anatomical facts, such as which bones muscles attach to and which joints they pull across. Then, if you relate these structural features to functional principles, you may find your study of muscles more interesting and less difficult than you may anticipate. Some specific suggestions for deducing muscle actions follow:

1. Start by making yourself familiar with the names, shapes, and general locations of the larger muscles by using **Table 15-2** as a guide.
2. Try to deduce which bones the two ends of a muscle attach to from your knowledge of the shape and general location of the muscle. For example, look carefully at the deltoid muscle as illustrated in **Figures 15-7** and **15-3**. To which bones does it seem to attach? Check your answer with **Table 16-2**, p. 340.
3. Next, determine which bone moves when the muscle shortens. (The bone moved by a muscle's contraction is its insertion bone; the bone that remains relatively stationary is its origin bone.) In many cases you can tell which is the insertion bone by trying to move one bone and then another. In some cases either bone may function as the insertion bone. Although not all muscle attachments can be deduced as readily as those of the deltoid, they can all be learned more easily by using this deduction method than by relying on rote memory alone.
4. Deduce a muscle's actions by applying the principle that its insertion moves toward its origin. Check your conclusions with the text. Here, as in steps 2 and 3, the method of deduction is intended merely as a guide and is not adequate by itself for determining muscle actions.
5. To deduce which muscle produces a given action (instead of which action a given muscle produces, as in step 4), start by inferring the insertion bone (the bone that moves during the action). The body and origin of the muscle will lie on one or more of the bones toward which the insertion moves—often a bone, or bones, proximal to the insertion bone. Couple these conclusions about origin and insertion with your knowledge of muscle names and locations to deduce the muscle that produces the action.

For example, if you wish to determine the prime mover for the action of raising the upper parts of the arms straight out to the sides, you infer that the muscle inserts on the humerus because this is the bone that moves. It moves toward the shoulder—that is, the clavicle and scapula—so the muscle probably has its origin on these bones. Because you know that the deltoid muscle fulfils these conditions, you conclude, and rightly so, that it is the muscle that raises the upper parts of the arms sideways.

AXIAL MUSCLES

Recall from Chapter 1, **Figure 1-7** (p. 12), that the body can be organized into a central or axial region and a peripheral or *appendicular* region. This concept was reinforced in Chapters 12 and 13 in the axial-appendicular organization of the human skeleton. Because skeletal muscles are attached to the skeleton, this organizational approach is useful here as well. For now, the focus is on the axial muscles. Chapter 16 surveys the major appendicular muscles.

The major axial muscles are listed, grouped, and illustrated in the tables and figures that follow. Begin your study with an overview of important superficial muscles, shown in **Figure 15-7**. The remaining figures in this chapter illustrate individual axial muscles or important muscle groups. Refer also to Part 1 of the Brief Atlas of the Human Body, where you will find a series of illustrations showing the position of major muscles relative to the surface of the body. Part 4 of the Brief Atlas shows many of the major muscles in cross-sectional views of the body.

Basic information about many muscles is given in **Tables 15-7** to **15-12** and in the tables of Chapter 16. Each table has a description of a group of muscles that move one part of the body. The actions listed for each muscle are those for which it is a prime mover. Remember, however, that a single muscle acting alone rarely accomplishes a given action. Instead, muscles act in groups as prime movers, synergists, antagonists, and fixators to bring about movements.

TABLE 15-7 Muscles of Facial Expression and Mastication

MUSCLE	ORIGIN	INSERTION	FUNCTION	NERVE SUPPLY
Muscles of Facial Expression				
Occipitofrontalis (part of epicranius)				
Frontal belly	Epicranial aponeurosis	Tissues of eyebrows and bridge of nose	Raises eyebrows, wrinkles forehead horizontally	CN VII
Occipital belly	Occipital bone (highest nuchal line)	Epicranial aponeurosis	Draws scalp backward	CN VII
Corrugator supercilii	Frontal bone (superciliary ridge)	Skin of eyebrow	Wrinkles forehead vertically	CN VII
Orbicularis oculi	Encircles eyelid		Closes eye	CN VII
Zygomaticus major	Zygomatic bone	Angle of mouth	Laughing (elevates angle of mouth)	CN VII
Orbicularis oris	Encircles mouth		Draws lips together	CN VII
Buccinator	Maxillae	Skin of sides of mouth	Facilitates smiling; blowing, as in playing trumpet	CN VII
Depressor anguli oris	Mandible	Angle of mouth	Draws ends of mouth downward, as when frowning	CN IV
Muscles of Mastication				
Masseter	Zygomatic arch	Mandible (external surface)	Elevates mandible, closing jaw	CN V
Temporalis	Temporal bone	Mandible	Elevates mandible; closing jaw	CN V
Pterygoids (lateral and medial)	Undersurface of skull	Mandible (medial surface)	Grates teeth	CN V

CN, Cranial nerve.

MUSCLES OF THE HEAD AND NECK

Muscles of Facial Expression

The muscles of facial expression (**Table 15-7** and **Figures 15-8** and **15-9**) are unique in that at least one of their points of attachment is to the deep layers of the skin over the face or neck. Contraction of these muscles produces a variety of facial expressions.

The **occipitofrontalis** is in reality two muscles. One portion lies over the forehead (frontal bone); the other covers the occipital bone in back of the head. The two muscular parts, or bellies, are joined by a connective tissue aponeurosis (the *epicranial aponeurosis*) that covers the top of the skull. The two occipitofrontalis bellies, along with the epicranial aponeurosis, are together called the *epicranius muscle.*

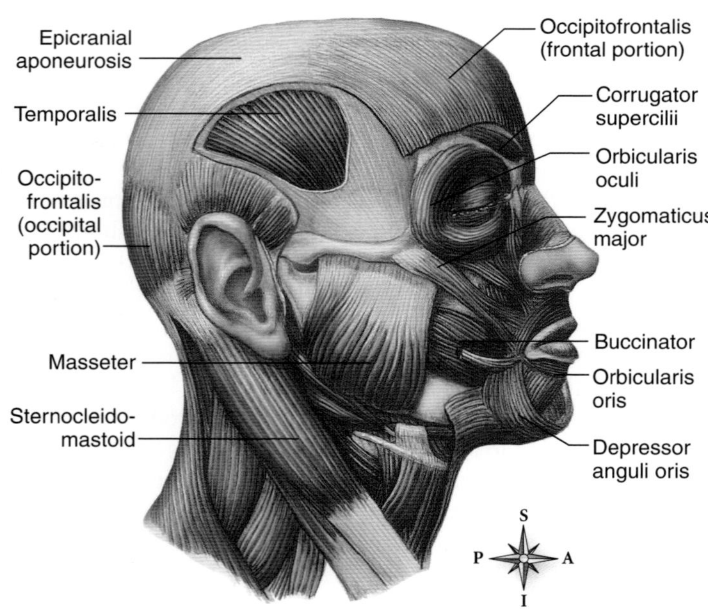

FIGURE 15-8 Muscles of facial expression and mastication. Lateral view.

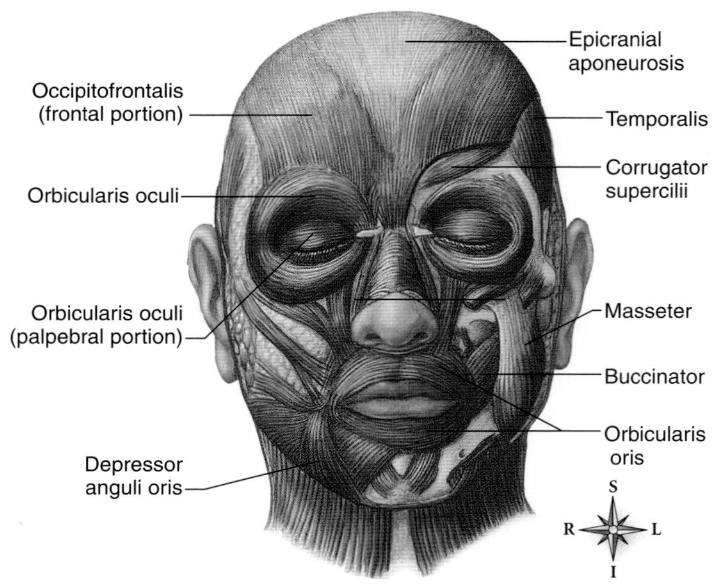

FIGURE 15-9 Muscles of facial expression and mastication. Anterior view.

The frontal belly of the occipitofrontalis raises the eyebrows (surprise) and wrinkles the skin of the forehead horizontally. The posterior belly draws the scalp back toward the posterior neck.

The **corrugator supercilii** draws the eyebrows together and produces vertical wrinkles above the nose (frowning). The **orbicularis oculi** encircles and closes the eye (blinking), whereas the **orbicularis oris** and **buccinator** pucker the mouth (kissing) and press the lips and cheeks against the teeth. The **zygomaticus major** draws the corner of the mouth upward (laughing).

Muscles of Mastication

The muscles of **mastication** shown in **Figure 15-10** are responsible for chewing movements. These powerful muscles (see **Table 15-7**) either elevate and retract the mandible (**masseter** and **temporalis**) or open and protrude it while causing sideways movement (**pterygoids**). The pull of gravity helps open the mandible during mastication, and the buccinator muscles play an important function by holding food between the teeth as the mandible moves up and down and from side to side.

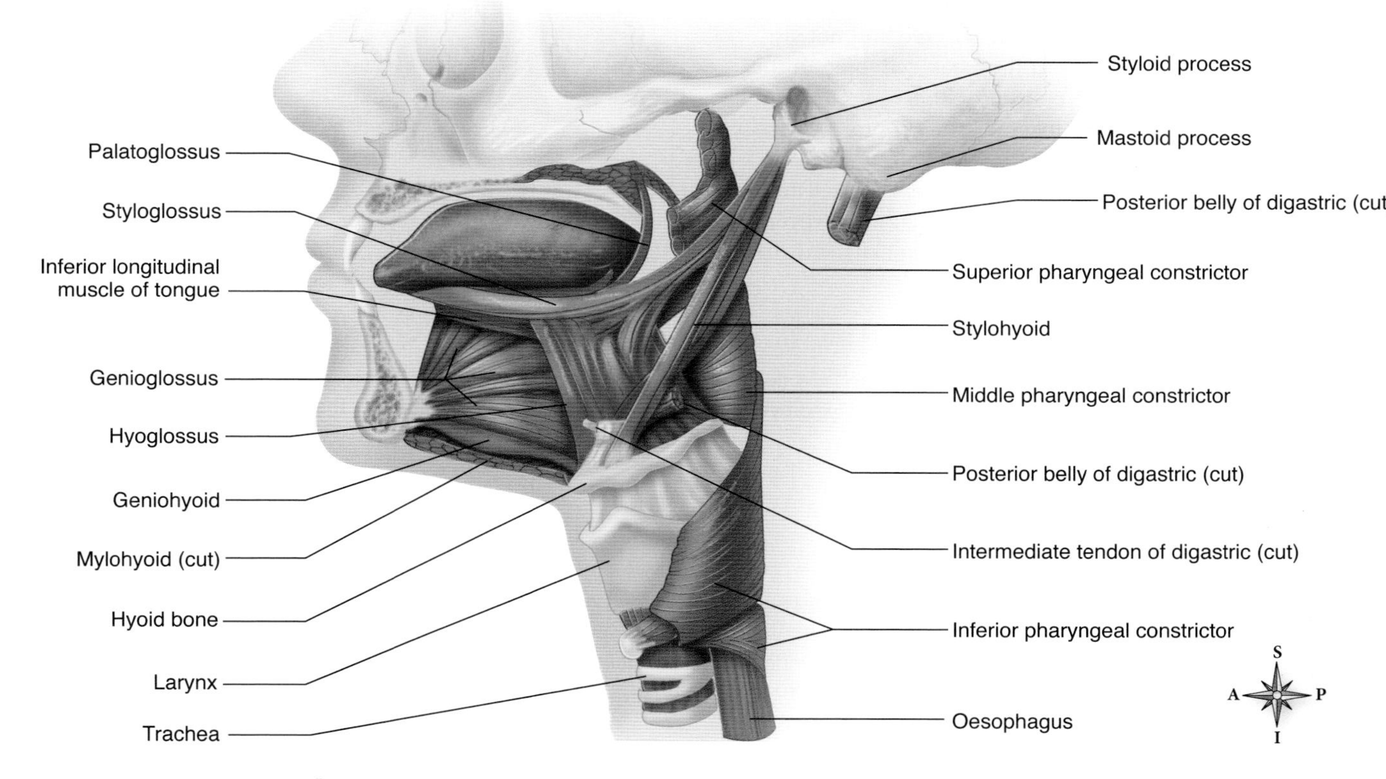

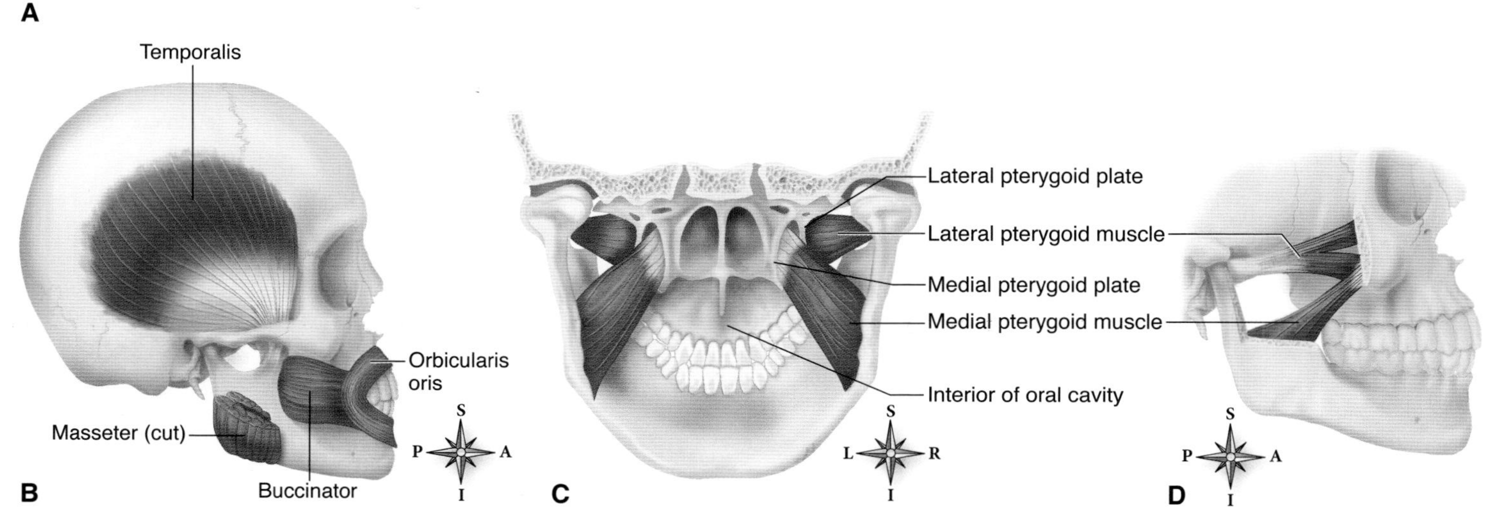

FIGURE 15-10 Muscles of mastication. **A,** Muscles of the tongue and pharynx. **B,** Right lateral dissection view showing the insertion of the temporalis muscle on the mandible—the masseter muscle is cut and part of the zygomatic arch has been removed. **C,** View of the pterygoids in a posterior dissection view. **D,** Lateral and medial pterygoid muscles viewed from the right side after removal of the zygomatic arch.

MUSCLES THAT MOVE THE HEAD

Paired muscles on either side of the neck are responsible for head movements (**Figure 15-11**). Note the points of attachment and functions of important muscles in this group listed in **Table 15-8**. When both **sternocleidomastoid** muscles (see **Figure 15-7**) contract at the same time, the head is flexed on the thorax—hence the name "prayer muscle". If only one muscle contracts, the head and face are turned to the opposite side.

The broad **semispinalis capitis** is an extensor of the head and helps flex it laterally. Acting together, the **splenius capitis** muscles serve as strong extensors that return the head to the upright position after flexion. When either muscle acts alone, contraction results in rotation and tilting toward that side. The bandlike **longissimus capitis** muscles are covered and not visible in **Figure 15-11**. They run from the neck vertebrae to the mastoid process of the temporal bone on either side and cause extension of the head when acting together. One contracting muscle will bend and rotate the head toward the contracting side.

The main function of the trapezius muscle in the neck and across the shoulders is to move the shoulders (scapulae). However, when the occipital bone acts as the insertion, the trapezius can help extend the neck.

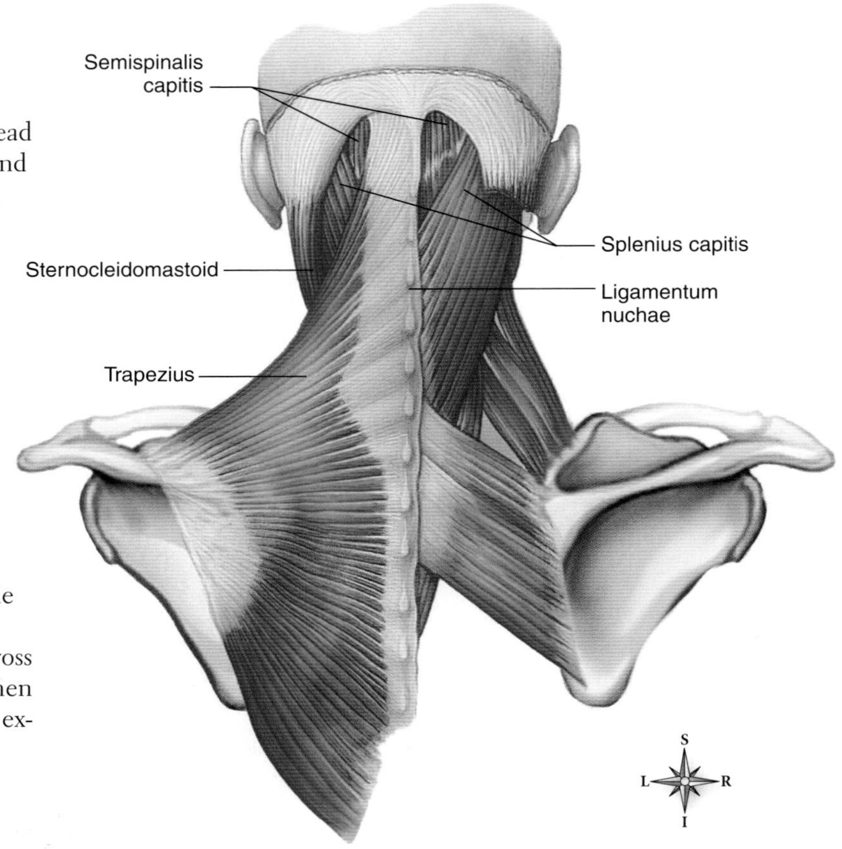

FIGURE 15-11 Muscles that move the head. Posterior view of muscles of the neck and the back.

Quick CHECK

12. List the steps you would take when deducing a muscle's action.
13. Which muscle of facial expression has two parts, one lying over the forehead and the other covering the back of the skull?
14. What group of muscles facilitates chewing movements?
15. What is the action of the sternocleidomastoid muscle?

TABLE 15-8 Muscles That Move the Head

MUSCLE	ORIGIN	INSERTION	FUNCTION	NERVE SUPPLY
Sternocleidomastoid	Sternum	Temporal bone (mastoid process)	Flexes head and neck (prayer muscle)	Accessory nerve
	Clavicle	—	One muscle alone, rotates head toward opposite side; spasm of this muscle alone or associated with trapezius called *torticollis,* or wryneck	—
Trapezius	Occipital bone (protruberance)	Clavicle	Raises or lowers the shoulders and shrugs them	Spinal accessory, second, third and fourth cervical nerves
	Vertebrae (cervical and thoracic)	Scapula (spine and acromion)	Extends the head and neck when the occiput acts as the insertion	
Semispinalis capitis	Vertebrae (transverse processes of upper six thoracic, articular processes of lower four cervical)	Occipital bone (between superior and inferior nuchal lines)	Extends head and neck; bends it laterally	First five cervical nerves
Splenius capitis	Ligamentum nuchae	Temporal bone (mastoid process)	Extends head and neck	Second, third, and fourth cervical nerves
	Vertebrae (spinous processes of upper three or four thoracic)	Occipital bone	Bends and rotates head toward same side as contracting muscle	
Longissimus capitis	Vertebrae (transverse processes of upper six thoracic, articular processes of lower four cervical)	Temporal bone (mastoid process)	Extends head and neck Bends and rotates head toward contracting side	Multiple innervation

TRUNK MUSCLES

Muscles of the Thorax

The muscles of the thorax are of critical importance in respiration (discussed in Chapter 36). Note in **Figure 15-12** and **Table 15-9** that the **internal** and **external intercostal muscles** attach to the ribs at different places and their fibres are oriented in different directions. As a result, contraction of the external intercostals elevates and contraction of the internal intercostals depresses the ribs—important in the breathing process. During inspiration the dome-shaped **diaphragm** flattens, thus increasing the size and volume of the thoracic cavity. As a result, air enters the lungs. Other muscles, such as the sternocleidomastoid muscles, serratus anterior muscles, and pectoralis major muscles can also assist in expanding the volume of the thorax during deep breathing—as may occur during moderate to heavy exercise (see **Figure 36-6** on p. 830).

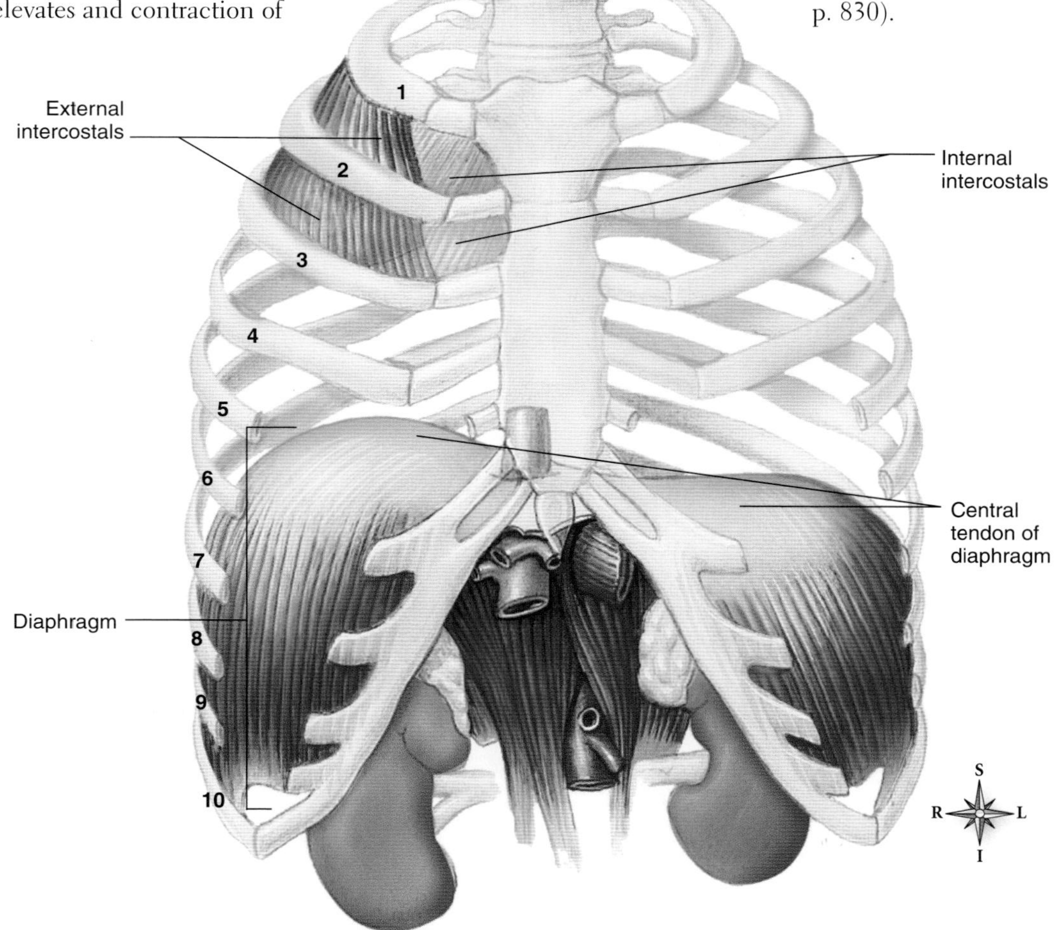

FIGURE 15-12 Muscles of the thorax. Anterior view. Note the relationship of the internal and external intercostal muscles and placement of the diaphragm.

TABLE 15-9 Muscles of the Thorax

MUSCLE	ORIGIN	INSERTION	FUNCTION	NERVE SUPPLY
External intercostals	Rib (lower border; forward fibres)	Rib (upper border of rib below origin)	Elevate and spread ribs	Intercostal nerves
Internal intercostals	Rib (inner surface, lower border; backward fibres)	Rib (upper border of rib below origin)	Depress ribs, pulling them together	Intercostal nerves
Diaphragm	Lower circumference of thorax (of ribcage)	Central tendon of diaphragm	Enlarges thorax, thereby causing inspiration	Phrenic nerves

Muscles of the Abdominal Wall

The muscles of the anterior and lateral abdominal wall (**Figure 15-13** and **Figure 15-14**; **Table 15-10**) are arranged in three layers, with the fibres in each layer running in different directions much like the layers of wood in a sheet of plywood. The result is a very strong "girdle" of muscle that covers and supports the abdominal cavity and its internal organs.

The fibres in the three layers of muscle in the anterolateral wall are arranged to provide maximum strength. In the **external oblique** the muscle fascicles or fibres extend inferiorly and medially, whereas the fibres of the middle muscle layer, the **internal oblique,** run almost at right angles to those of the external oblique above it. The fibres of the **transversus abdominis,** the innermost muscle layer, are, as the name implies, directed transversely.

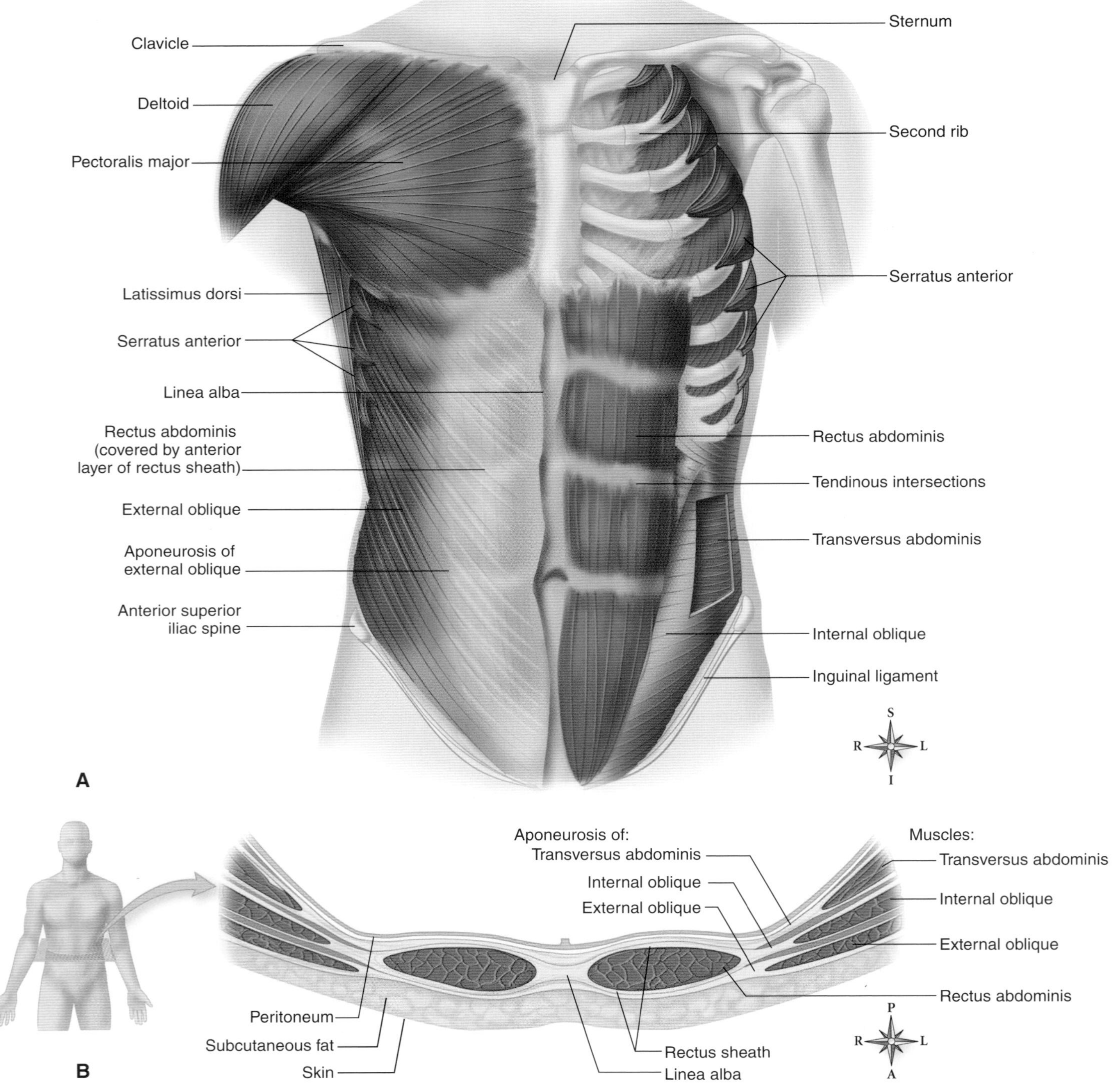

FIGURE 15-13 Muscles of the trunk and abdominal wall. A, Superficial muscles are visible on the right side of the body and deeper muscles on the left side of the body. **B,** Transverse section of the anterior wall above the umbilicus (see inset for location).

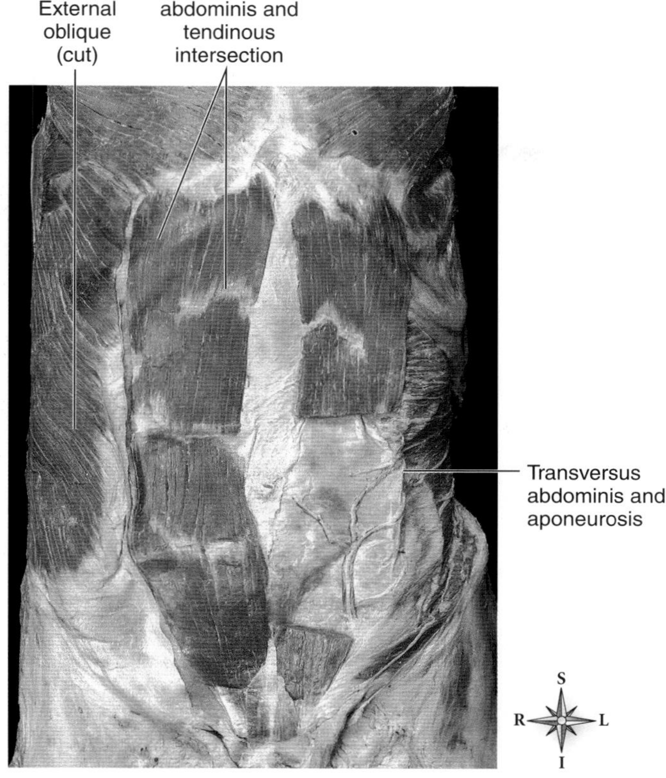

FIGURE 15-14 Dissection photo of the abdominal wall. The covering rectus sheaths, the left oblique muscles, and part of the left rectus have been removed.

In addition to these sheetlike muscles, the band- or strap-shaped rectus abdominis muscle runs down the midline of the abdomen from the thorax to the pubis. Note in **Figure 15-13** that its parallel running fibres are "interrupted" by three tendinous intersections.

When a surgeon "opens" or "closes" an incision through the anterolateral wall, attempts are made to maintain the inherent strength of the wall after surgery by sparing important nerves and blood vessels and by using suturing techniques during closure that will restore the direction of fibres in the cut layers of muscle.

In **Figure 15-14**, a number of superficial structures have been cut or partially removed. For example, part of the internal oblique has been removed to expose the underlying transversus abdominis, and the anterior (superficial) layer of the **rectus sheath** has been removed to better visualize the **rectus abdominis muscle** and its tendinous intersections.

Note also in **Figure 15-13**, *B*, that the aponeuroses of the external oblique, internal oblique, and transversus abdominis muscles form the rectus sheaths that cover the rectus abdominis muscles and then fuse in the midline to form a tough band of connective tissue called the **linea alba** ("white line"), which extends from the xiphoid process to the pubis. Occasionally, a surgical procedure will permit an incision through the linea alba rather than through abdominal musculature. Because the linea alba is essentially avascular in some areas, blood loss in such procedures is generally less than what may occur in other approaches.

Working as a group, the abdominal muscles not only protect and hold the abdominal viscera in place, but are responsible for a number of vertebral column movements, including flexion, lateral

TABLE 15-10 Muscles of the Abdominal Wall

MUSCLE	ORIGIN	INSERTION	FUNCTION	NERVE SUPPLY
External oblique	Ribs (lower eight)	Pelvis (iliac crest and pubis by way of the inguinal ligament)	Compresses abdomen	Lower seven intercostal nerves and iliohypogastric nerves
		Linea alba by way of an aponeurosis	Rotates trunk laterally	
Internal oblique	Pelvis (iliac crest and iliopsoas fascia)	Ribs (lower three)	Important postural function of all abdominal muscles is to pull the front of the pelvis upward, thereby flattening the lumbar curve of the spine; when these muscles lose their tone, common figure faults of protruding abdomen and lordosis develop	Last three intercostal nerves; iliohypogastric and ilioinguinal nerves
	Lumbodorsal fascia	Linea alba		
Transversus abdominis	Ribs (lower six)	Pubic bone	Same as external oblique	Last three intercostal nerves; iliohypogastric and ilioinguinal nerves
	Pelvis (iliac crest, iliopsoas fascia)	Linea alba		
	Lumbodorsal fascia	Ribs (costal cartilage of fifth, sixth, and seventh ribs)	Same as external oblique	Last five intercostal nerves; iliohypogastric and ilioinguinal nerves
Rectus abdominis	Pelvis (pubic bone and pubic symphysis)	Sternum (xiphoid process)	Same as external oblique; because abdominal muscles compress the abdominal cavity, they aid in straining, defaecation, forced expiration, childbirth; abdominal muscles are antagonists of the diaphragm, relaxing as it contracts and vice versa Flexes trunk	Last six intercostal nerves
Quadratus lumborum	Iliolumbar ligament; iliac crest	Last rib; transverse process of vertebrae (L1–L4)	Flexes vertebral column laterally; depresses last rib	Lumbar

bending, and some rotation. These important muscles are also involved in respiration and in helping "push" a baby through the birth canal during delivery. They also play a role in assisting in urination, defaecation, and vomiting.

Muscles of the Back

Considering the large number of us who experience back pain, strain, and injury either occasionally or chronically, you can imagine the importance of the back muscles to health and fitness. Statistics show that 80% of the population in most areas of the world experience backache at some time in their lives. Although symptoms may vary from mild to disabling, "back problems" continue to plague large numbers of individuals and pose significant financial, social, and health care problems.

The superficial back muscles play a major role in moving the head and limbs and are illustrated in **Figure 15-15**, A. The deep

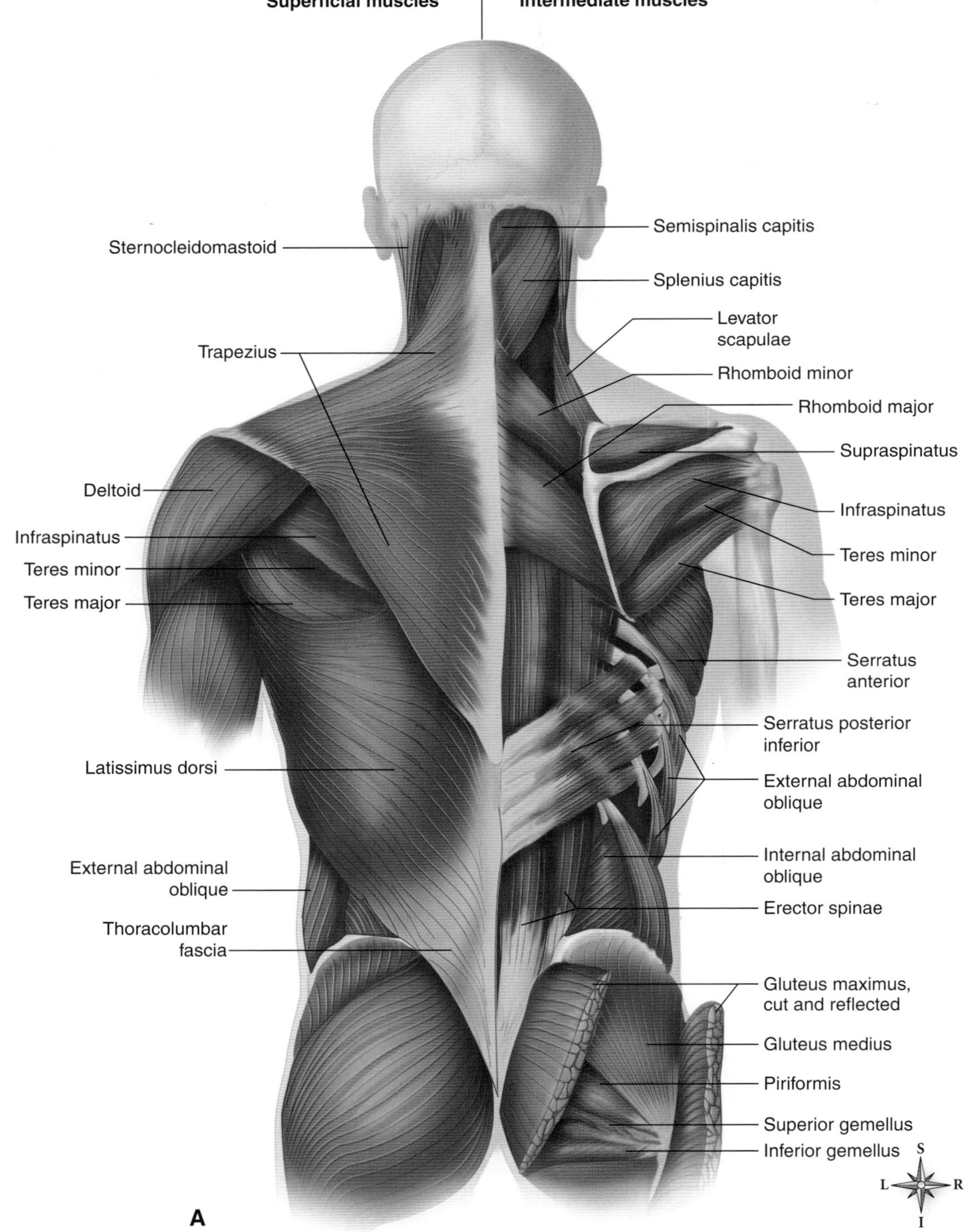

FIGURE 15-15 Muscles of the back. A, Superficial *(left)* and intermediate *(right)* muscle dissection of the back—posterior view. **B,** Deep muscle dissection of the back—posterior view. The superficial and intermediate muscles have been removed. The muscles in the gluteal region have been removed to expose the pelvic insertion of the multifidus.

back muscles (**Figure 15-15**, *B*) not only allow us to move our vertebral column, thus helping us bend this way and that, but also stabilize our trunk so that we can maintain a stable posture. These muscles really get a workout when we lift something heavy because they have to hold the body straight while the load is trying to bend the back.

The **erector spinae muscle** group consists of a number of long, thin muscles that travel all the way down our backs (see **Figure 15-15**). These muscles extend (straighten or pull back) the vertebral column and also flex the back laterally and rotate it a little. Even deeper than the erector spinae muscles are several additional back muscles. The **interspinales** and **multifidus groups,** for example, each connect one vertebra to the next; they also help extend the back and neck or flex them to the side. **Table 15-11** and **Figure 15-15**, *B*, summarize some of the important deep back muscles.

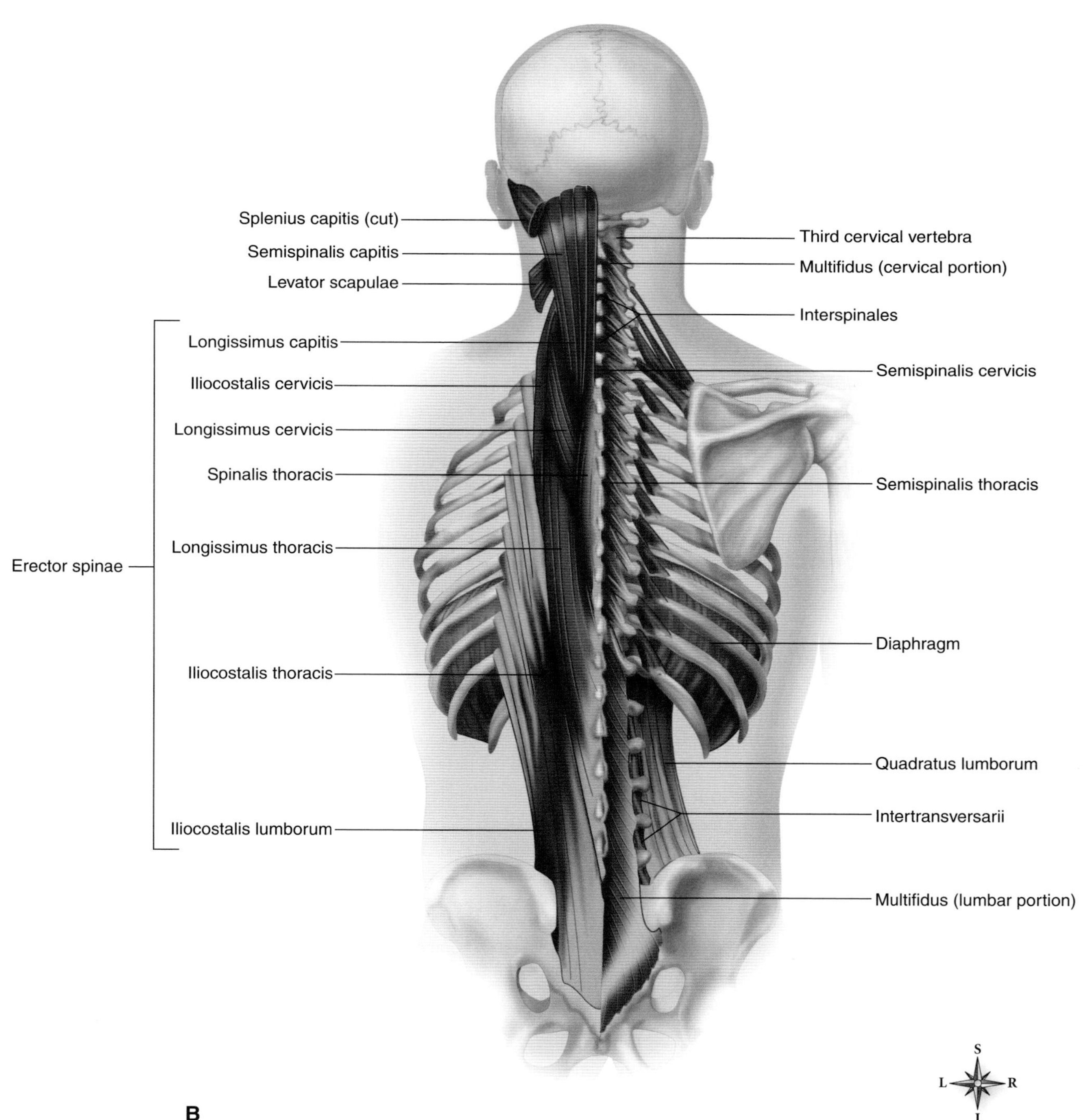

TABLE 15-11 Muscles of the Back

MUSCLE	ORIGIN	INSERTION	FUNCTION	NERVE SUPPLY
Erector spinae group				
Iliocostalis group	Various regions of the pelvis and ribs	Ribs and vertebra (superior to the origin)	Extends, laterally flexes the vertebral column	Spinal, thoracic, or lumbar nerves
Longissimus group	Cervical and thoracic vertebrae, ribs	Mastoid process, upper cervical vertebrae, or upper lumbar vertebrae	Extends head, neck, or vertebral column	Cervical or thoracic and lumbar nerves
Spinalis group	Lower cervical or lower thoracic/ upper lumbar vertebrae	Upper cervical or middle/upper thoracic vertebrae (superior to the origin)	Extends the neck or vertebral column	Cervical or thoracic nerves
Transversospinalis group				
Semispinalis group	Transverse processes of vertebrae (T2–T11)	Spinous processes of vertebrae (C2–T4)	Extends neck or vertebral column	Cervical or thoracic nerves
Multifidus group	Transverse processes of vertebrae; sacrum and ilium	Spinous processes (of next superior vertebra)	Extends, rotates vertebral column	Spinal nerves
Rotatores group	Transverse processes of vertebrae	Spinous processes (of next superior vertebra)	Extends, rotates vertebral column	Spinal nerves
Splenius	Spinous processes of vertebrae (C7–T1 or T3–T6)	Lateral occipital/mastoid or transverse processes of vertebrae (C1–C4)	Rotates, extends neck and flexes neck laterally	Cervical nerves
Interspinales group	Spinous processes of vertebrae	Spinous processes (of next superior vertebra)	Extends back and neck	Spinal nerves

Muscles of the Pelvic Floor

Structures in the pelvic cavity are supported by a reinforced muscular floor that guards the outlet below. The muscular pelvic floor filling the diamond-shaped outlet is called the **perineum.** Passing through the floor are the anal canal and urethra in both sexes and the vagina in the female.

The two **levator ani** and **coccygeus muscles** form most of the pelvic floor. They stretch across the pelvic cavity like a hammock. This diamond-shaped outlet can be divided into two triangles by a line drawn from side to side between the ischial tuberosities. The **urogenital triangle** is anterior to this line (above) and extends to the pubic symphysis, and the **anal triangle** is posterior (behind it) and ends at the coccyx.

Note in **Figure 15-16** that structures in the urogenital triangle include the **ischiocavernosus** and **bulbospongiosus muscles** associated with the penis in the male and the vagina in the female. Constriction of muscles called the **urethral sphincter,** which encircle the urethra in both sexes, helps control urine flow.

The anal triangle allows passage of the anal canal. The terminal portion of the canal is surrounded by the **external anal sphincter,** which regulates defaecation.

The origin, insertion, function, and innervation of important muscles of the pelvic floor are listed in **Table 15-12**. The coccygeus muscles lie behind the levator ani and are not visible in **Figure 15-16**.

Quick CHECK

16. Name the skeletal muscles that produce respiratory movements.
17. Name two functions of the rectus abdominis muscle.
18. What is the perineum?

TABLE 15-12 Muscles of the Pelvic Floor

MUSCLE	ORIGIN	INSERTION	FUNCTION	NERVE SUPPLY
Levator ani	Pubis and spine of the ischium	Coccyx	Together with the coccygeus muscles form the floor of the pelvic cavity and support the pelvic organs	Pudendal nerve
Ischiocavernosus	Ischium	Penis or clitoris	Compress the base of the penis or clitoris	Perineal nerve
Bulbospongiosus				
Male	Bulb of the penis	Perineum and bulb of the penis	Constricts the urethra and erects the penis	Pudendal nerve
Female	Perineum	Base of the clitoris	Erects the clitoris	Pudendal nerve
Deep transverse perineal	Ischium	Central tendon (median raphe)	Supports the pelvic floor	Pudendal nerve
Urethral sphincter	Pubic ramus	Central tendon (median raphe)	Constricts the urethra	Pudendal nerve
External anal sphincter	Coccyx	Central tendon (median raphe)	Closes the anal canal	Pudendal and S4

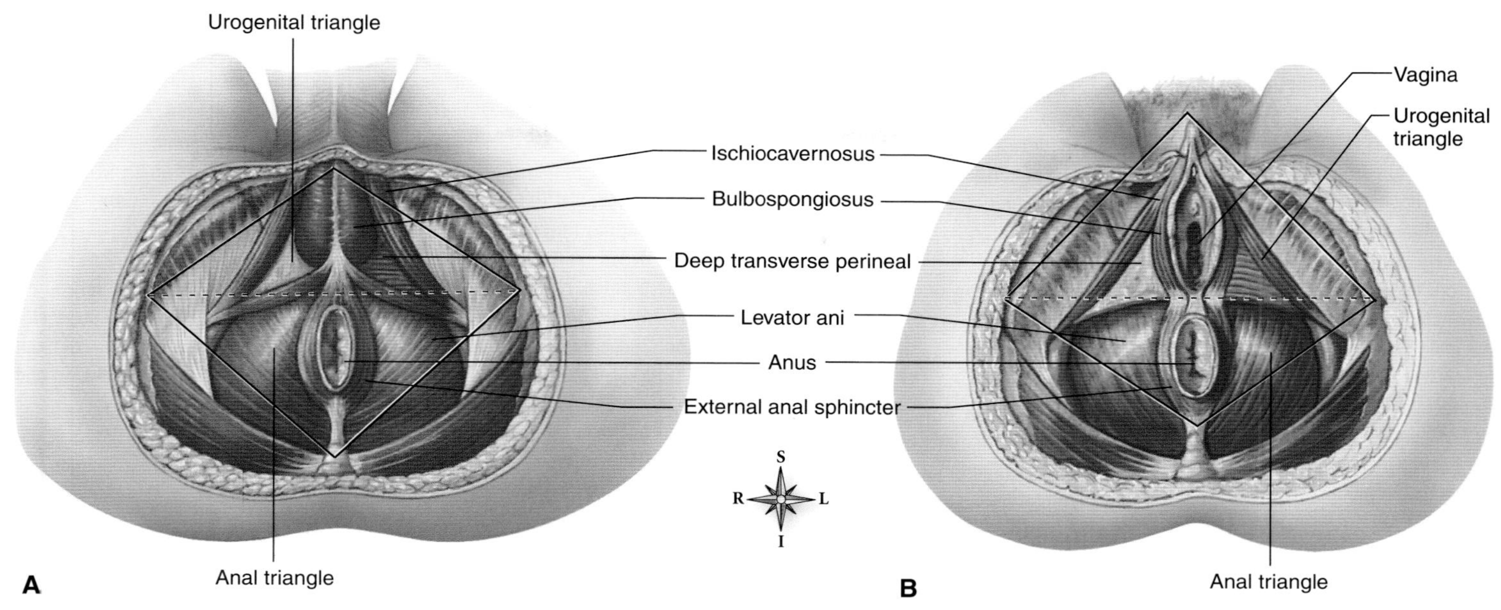

FIGURE 15-16 Muscles of the pelvic floor. A, Male, inferior view. **B,** Female, inferior view. Note the diamond-shaped outline of the perineum formed by the urogenital and anal triangles.

UNIT 2

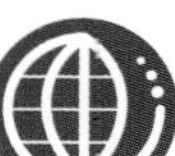

the big picture | Axial Muscles and the Whole Body

As you read through this chapter, what struck you most was probably the large number of individual muscles and their many actions. Although learning the names, locations, origins, insertions, and other details of the major muscles is a worthwhile endeavor, such an activity can cause you to lose sight of the "big picture". Step back from the details a moment to appreciate that the muscles work as coordinated teams of biological engines that move the various components of the flexible skeleton.

As a matter of fact, in this chapter you learned that the fibrous wrappings of each muscle are continuous with its tendons, which in turn are continuous with the fibrous structure of the bone to which they are attached. Thus we can see that the muscular and skeletal systems are in essence a single structure. This fact is very important in seeing a "big picture" comprising many individual muscles and bones. The entire skeletomuscular system, as it is often called, is actually a single, continuous structure that provides a coordinated, dynamic framework for the body.

Our "big picture" of the muscles of the body will become more complete as we move through the next chapter, which explores the appendicular muscles and the concept of posture.

LANGUAGE OF SCIENCE *(continued from p. 313)*

external intercostal muscle (eks-TER-nal in-ter-KOS-tal) [*extern-* **outside,** *-al* **relating to,** *inter-* **between,** *-costa-* **rib,** *-al* **relating to,** *mus-* **mouse,** *-cle* **little**]

external oblique muscle (eks-TER-nal oh-BLEEK) [*extern-* **outside,** *-al* **relating to,** *obliq-* **slanted,** *mus-* **mouse,** *-cle* **little**]

fascia (FASH-ee-ah) [*fascia* **band or bundle**]

fixator muscle (fik-SAY-tor) [*fixator* **fastener,** *mus-* **mouse,** *-cle* **little**]

fusiform muscle (FYOO-si-form) [*fusi-* **spindle,** *-form* **shape,** *mus-* **mouse,** *-cle* **little**]

insertion [*in-* **in,** *-ser-* **join,** *-tion* **process**]

internal intercostal muscle (in-TER-nal in-ter-KOS-tal) [*intern-* **inside,** *-al* **relating to,** *inter-* **between,** *-cost-* **rib,** *-al* **relating to,** *mus-* **mouse,** *-cle* **little**]

internal oblique muscle (in-TER-nal oh-BLEEK) [*intern-* **inside,** *-al* **relating to,** *obliq-* **slanted,** *mus-* **mouse,** *-cle* **little**]

interspinales group (in-ter-spy-NAH-leez) [*inter-* **between,** *-spina-* **spine,** *-al* **relating to**]

ischiocavernosus muscle (iss-kee-oh-KAV-er-no-sus) [*ischio-* **hip joint,** *-cavern-* **hollow space,** *-osus* **relating to,** *mus-* **mouse,** *-cle* **little**]

levator ani muscle (leh-VAY-tor AY-nye) [*levator* **lifter,** *ani* **of the anus,** *mus-* **mouse,** *-cle* **little**]

lever [*lev-* **lift,** *-er* **agent**]

lever system [*lev-* **lift,** *-er* **agent**]

linea alba (LIN-ee-ah AL-bah) [*linea* **line,** *alba* **white**]

longissimus capitis muscle (lon-JIS-i-mus KAP-i-tis) [*longissimus* **longest or very long,** *capit-* **head,** *mus-* **mouse,** *-cle* **little**]

masseter (mah-SEE-ter) [*masseter* **chewer**]

mastication (mass-ti-KAY-shun) [*mastica-* **chew,** *-ation* **process**]

multifidus muscle group (mul-TIF-i-dus) [*multi-* **many,** *-fidus* **split (into pieces),** *mus-* **mouse,** *-cle* **little**]

occipitofrontalis (ok-sip-i-toh-fron-TAL-is) [*occipit-* **back of head,** *front-* **forehead,** *-al* **relating to,** *-is* **thing**]

orbicularis oculi muscle (or-bik-yoo-LAIR-is OK-yoo-lye) [*orbi-* **circle,** *-cul-* **little,** *-ar* **relating to,** *-is* **thing,** *ocul-* **eye,** *mus-* **mouse,** *-cle* **little**]

orbicularis oris muscle (or-bik-yoo-LAIR-is OR-iss) [*orbi-* **circle,** *-cul-* **little,** *-ar* **relating to,** *-is* **thing,** *oris* **mouth,** *mus-* **mouse,** *-cle* **little**]

origin (OR-i-jin)

parallel muscle [*para-* **beside,** *-llel* **one another,** *mus-* **mouse,** *-cle* **little**]

pennate muscle (PEN-ayt) [*penn-* **feather,** *-ate* **of or like,** *mus-* **mouse,** *-cle* **little**]

perimysium (pair-i-MEE-see-um) [*peri-* **around,** *-mys-* **muscle,** *-um* **thing**]

perineum (pair-i-NEE-um) [*peri-* **around,** *-ine-* **excrete,** *-um* **thing**] *pl.,* perinea

prime mover [*prime* **first order**]

pterygoid muscle (TER-i-goid) [*ptery-* **wing,** *-oid* **like,** *mus-* **mouse,** *-cle* **little**]

rectus abdominis muscle (REK-tus ab-DOM-i-nus) [*rectus* **straight or upright,** *abdominis* **abdomen,** *mus-* **mouse,** *-cle* **little**]

rectus sheath (REK-tus sheeth) [*rectus* **straight or upright**]

semispinalis capitis muscle (sem-ee-spi-NAL-is KAP-i-tis) [*semi-* **half,** *spin-* **thorn (spine),** *-al-* **relating to,** *-is* **thing,** *capit-* **head,** *-is* **thing,** *mus-* **mouse,** *-cle* **little**]

spiral muscle [*mus-* **mouse,** *-cle* **little**]

splenius capitis muscle (SPLEH-nee-us KAP-i-tis) [*splenius* **patch,** *capit-* **head,** *-is* **thing,** *mus-* **mouse,** *-cle* **little**]

sternocleidomastoid muscle (STERN-oh-KLYE-doh-MAS-toyd) [*sterno-* **breastbone (sternum),** *-cleid-* **key (clavicle),** *-masto-* **breast (mastoid process),** *-oid* **like,** *mus-* **mouse,** *-cle* **little**]

synergist (SIN-er-jist) [*syn-* **together,** *-erg-* **to work,** *-ist* **agent**]

temporalis muscle (tem-poh-RAL-is) [*tempo-* **temple of head,** *-al* **relating to,** *-is* **thing,** *mus-* **mouse,** *-cle* **little**]

tendon [*tend-* **pulled tight,** *-on* **unit**]

tendon sheath (sheeth) [*tend-* **pulled tight,** *-on* **unit**]

transversus abdominis muscle (tranz-VERS-us ab-DOM-in-us) [*trans-* **across,** *-vers-* **turn,** *abdomin-* **belly**]

urethral sphincter (yoo-REE-thral SFINGK-ter) [*ure-* **urine,** *-thr-* **agent or channel (urethra),** *-al* **relating to,** *mus-* **mouse,** *-cle* **little,** *sphinc-* **bind tight,** *-er* **agent**]

urogenital triangle (YOO-roh-JEN-ih-tal) [*uro-* **urine,** *-genit-* **reproduction,** *-al* **relating to,** *tri-* **three,** *-angle* **corner**]

zygomaticus major muscle (zye-goh-MAT-ik-us) [*-zygo-* **union or yoke,** *-ic* **relating to,** *major* **greater,** *mus-* **mouse,** *-cle* **little**]

case study

At the sound of the starting pistol, Jeremy burst forward out of the blocks, sprinting down the track. About 20 metres into the race, he suddenly felt a sharp pain along the side of his abdomen. Wincing, he slowed down and hobbled to a stop.

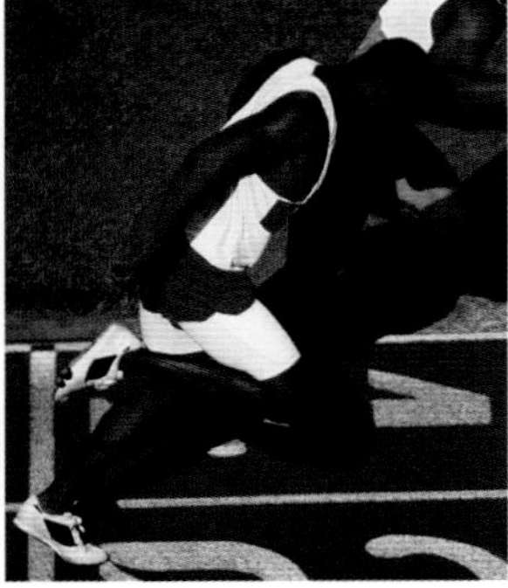

1. What muscle or muscle group had Jeremy likely injured?
   a. Pectoralis
   b. External intercostals
   c. External oblique
   d. Rectus abdominis

2. What muscle did Jeremy use when he closed his eyes in pain?
   a. Orbicularis oris
   b. Masseter
   c. Buccinator
   d. Orbicularis oculi

Jeremy made his way over to the grassy area beside the track and collapsed onto his side. In an effort to control the pain, he concentrated on taking deep, slow breaths in and out.

3. Which of the following muscles did Jeremy NOT use in breathing?
   a. Diaphragm
   b. External intercostals
   c. Sternocleidomastoid
   d. Internal intercostals

After several minutes, Jeremy rolled onto his back and tried to sit up.

4. Which of the following muscles would contract to pull him to a sitting position?
   a. Rectus abdominis
   b. Masseter
   c. Splenius capitis
   d. Temporalis

Hint To solve a case study, you may have to refer to the glossary or index, other chapters in this textbook, ***Connect It!,*** and other resources.

CHAPTER SUMMARY

To download an MP3 version of the chapter summary for use with your mobile device, access the ***Audio Chapter Summaries*** *online at evolve.elsevier.com.*

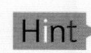

Scan this summary after reading the chapter to help you reinforce the key concepts. Later, use the summary as a quick review before your class or before a test.

Introduction

A. There are more than 600 skeletal muscles in the body (**Figure 15-7**)
B. From 40% to 50% of our body weight is skeletal muscle
C. Muscles fill in the form and contour of the body

Skeletal Muscle Structure (Figure 15-1)

A. Connective tissue components (**Table 15-1**)
 1. Endomysium—delicate connective tissue membrane that covers skeletal muscle fibres
 2. Perimysium—tough connective tissue binding together fascicles
 3. Epimysium—coarse sheath covering the muscle as a whole
 4. These three fibrous components continue and fuse to become a tendon or aponeurosis; a tendon sheath (lined with synovial membrane) covers some longer tendons (**Figure 15-2**)
B. Size, shape, and fibre arrangement (**Figure 15-3**)
 1. Vary considerably in size, shape, and fibre arrangement
 2. Size—range from extremely small to large masses
 3. Shape—variety of shapes, such as broad, narrow, long, tapering, short, blunt, triangular, quadrilateral, irregular, flat sheets, or bulky masses
 4. Arrangement—variety of arrangements, such as parallel to a long axis, converging to a narrow attachment, oblique, pennate, bipennate, or curved; the direction of fibres is significant because of its relationship to function
C. Attachment of muscles (**Figure 15-4**)
 1. Origin—point of attachment that does not move when the muscle contracts
 2. Insertion—point of attachment that moves when the muscle contracts
D. Muscle actions (**Figure 15-5**)
 1. Most movements are produced by the coordinated action of several muscles; some muscles in the group contract while others relax
  a. Prime mover—a muscle that directly performs a specific movement
  b. Agonist—any "mover" muscle that directly performs a movement, including the prime mover
  c. Antagonist—muscles that, when contracting, directly oppose prime movers; relax while the prime mover (agonist) is contracting to produce movement; provide precision and control during contraction of prime movers
  d. Synergists—muscles that contract at the same time as the prime movers; they facilitate prime mover actions to produce a more efficient movement
  e. Fixator muscles—joint stabilizers (type of synergist)
E. Lever systems
 1. In the human body, bones serve as levers and joints serve as fulcrums; contracting muscle applies a pulling force on a bone lever at the point of the muscle's attachment to the bone, which causes the insertion bone to move about its joint fulcrum
 2. Lever system—composed of four component parts (**Figure 15-6**)
  a. Rigid bar (bone)
  b. Fulcrum (F) around which the rod moves (joint)
  c. Load (L) that is moved
  d. Pull (P) that produces movement (muscle contraction), also called the effort
 3. First-class levers
  a. Fulcrum lies between the pull and the load
  b. Not abundant in the human body; serve as levers of stability
 4. Second-class levers
  a. Load lies between the fulcrum and the joint at which the pull is exerted
  b. Presence of these levers in the human body is a controversial issue
 5. Third-class levers
  a. Pull is exerted between the fulcrum and load
  b. Permit rapid and extensive movement
  c. Most common type of lever found in the body

How Muscles Are Named

A. Muscle names can be in Latin or English (this book uses English)
B. Muscles are named according to one or more of the following features:
 1. Location, function, shape (**Tables 15-2**, **15-3**, and **15-4**)
 2. Direction of fibres—named according to fibre orientation (**Table 15-5**)
 3. Number of heads or divisions (**Table 15-5**)
 4. Points of attachment—origin and insertion points
 5. Relative size—small, medium, or large (**Table 15-6**)

Axial Muscles

A. Muscles can be grouped according to axial (central) and appendicular (peripheral)
B. This chapter focuses on axial muscles; the following chapter focuses on appendicular muscles

Muscles of the Head and Neck

A. Muscles of facial expression—unique in that at least one point of attachment is to the deep layers of the skin over the face or neck (**Figures 15-8** and **15-9**; **Table 15-7**)
B. Muscles of mastication—responsible for chewing movements (**Figure 15-10**)
C. Muscles that move the head—paired muscles on either side of the neck are responsible for head movements (**Figure 15-11**; **Table 15-8**)

Trunk Muscles

A. Muscles of the thorax—of critical importance in respiration (**Figure 15-12**; **Table 15-9**)
B. Muscles of the abdominal wall—arranged in three layers, with fibres in each layer running in different directions to increase strength (**Figure 15-13**; **Table 15-10**)
C. Muscles of the back—bend or stabilize the back (**Figure 15-15**; **Table 15-11**)
D. Muscles of the pelvic floor—support the structures in the pelvic cavity (**Figure 15-16**; **Table 15-12**)

REVIEW QUESTIONS

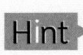

Write out the answers to these questions after reading the chapter and reviewing the Chapter Summary. Note—writing out your answers will consolidate learning and provide a valuable resource of information.

1. Define the terms *endomysium*, *perimysium*, and *epimysium*.
2. Identify/describe the most common type of lever in the body.
3. Give an example of a muscle named by location, function, shape, fibre direction, number of heads, and points of attachment.
4. Name the main muscles of the back, chest, abdomen, neck, and pelvic floor.
5. Name the main muscles that flex, extend, abduct, and adduct the head.
6. Name the main muscles that move the abdominal wall; that move the chest wall.
7. Identify the muscles of facial expression. What muscles facilitate smiling and frowning?

CRITICAL THINKING QUESTIONS

After finishing the Review Questions, write out the answers to these more in-depth questions to help you apply your new knowledge. Go back to sections of the chapter that relate to concepts that you find difficult.

1. Identify a muscle where the insertion is superior to the origin. Describe the appearance of a person upon contraction of the muscle with this arrangement.
2. How do the origin and insertion of a muscle relate to each other in regard to actual movement?
3. When the biceps brachii contracts, the elbow flexes. When the triceps brachii contracts, the elbow extends. Explain the role of both muscles in terms of agonist and antagonist in both of these movements.

16 Appendicular Muscles

CHAPTER OUTLINE

Hint Scan this outline before you begin to read the chapter, as a preview of how the concepts are organized.

This chapter continues the survey of major skeletal muscles that started in the previous chapter. Now that we have explored the basic structure of muscle organs and have surveyed major muscles of the axial region of the body, we are ready to explore the appendicular muscles. These muscles allow us to walk, run, climb, and swim; to make and use tools; to build shelter and build fires; and to defend ourselves against harm. Without such muscular abilities, we could not maintain the relative constancy of our internal environment—homeostasis—and therefore could not survive. Think of how you use each of the muscles surveyed in your day-to-day living.

LANGUAGE OF SCIENCE

Hint *Use this list to aid your pronunciation of unfamiliar words.*

calcaneal tendon (kal-KAY-nee-al)
[*calcane-* **heel,** *-al* **relating to,** *tend-* **pulled tight,** *-on* **unit**]

deltoid (DEL-toyd)
[*delta-* **triangle or (Δ) fourth letter of Greek alphabet,** *-oid* **like**]

extensor digitorum longus muscle (ek-STEN-ser dij-i-TOH-rum LONG-gus)
[*extensor* **stretcher,** *digit-* **finger or toe,** *-orum* **relating to,** *longus* **long,** *mus-* **mouse,** *-cle* **little**]

extrinsic foot muscle (eks-TRIN-sik)
[*extrins-* **outside,** *-ic* **relating to,** *mus-* **mouse,** *-cle* **little**]

extrinsic muscle (eks-TRIN-sik)
[*extrins-* **outside,** *-ic* **relating to,** *mus-* **mouse,** *-cle* **little**]

fibularis tertius muscle (fib-yoo-LAR-is TER-shee-us)
[*fibula-* **clasp (fibula),** *-ar-* **relating to,** *-is* **thing,** *tertius* **third,** *mus-* **mouse,** *-cle* **little**]

gastrocnemius muscle (GAS-trok-NEE-mee-us)
[*gastro-* **belly,** *-cnemius* **leg,** *mus-* **mouse,** *-cle* **little**]

gluteal muscle (GLOO-tee-al)
[*glut-* **buttocks,** *-al* **relating to,** *mus-* **mouse,** *-cle* **little**]

infraspinatus muscle (IN-frah-spy-nah-tus)
[*infra-* **below,** *-spina-* **spine,** *mus-* **mouse,** *-cle* **little**]

interosseous muscle (in-ter-OSS-ee-us)
[*inter-* **between,** *-os-* **bone,** *-ous* **relating to,** *mus-* **mouse,** *-cle* **little**]

intrinsic foot muscle (in-TRIN-sik)
[*intrins-* **inward,** *-ic* **relating to,** *mus-* **mouse,** *-cle* **little**]

intrinsic muscle (in-TRIN-sik)
[*intrins-* **inward,** *-ic* **relating to,** *mus-* **mouse,** *-cle* **little**]

levator scapulae (leh-VAY-tor SCAP-yoo-lee)
[*levator* **lifter,** *scapulae* **of the shoulder blade**]

lumbrical muscle (LUM-bri-kal)
[*lumbric-* **earthworm,** *-al* **relating to,** *mus-* **mouse,** *-cle* **little**]

continued on p. 359

APPENDICULAR MUSCLES

This chapter continues our survey of the major muscles of the body by focusing on the appendicular muscles. These are the muscles of the *appendages* or the extremities—the *upper extremity* (upper limb) and *lower extremity* (lower limb).

The major appendicular muscles are listed, grouped, and illustrated in the tables and figures that follow. Begin your study with an overview of important superficial muscles, shown in **Figure 16-1** and **Figure 15-7** (p. 320). Many of the figures in this chapter illustrate individual appendicular muscles or important muscle groups. Refer also to Part 1 of the Brief Atlas of the Human Body, where you will find a series of illustrations showing the position of major muscles relative to the surface of the body. Part 4 of the Brief Atlas shows many of the major muscles in cross-sectional views of the body.

Basic information about many appendicular muscles is given in **Tables 16-1** to **16-7**. Each table has a description of a group of muscles that move one part of the body. The actions listed for each muscle are those for which it is a prime mover. Remember, however, that a single muscle acting alone rarely accomplishes a given action. Instead, muscles act in groups as prime movers, synergists, antagonists, and fixators to bring about movements.

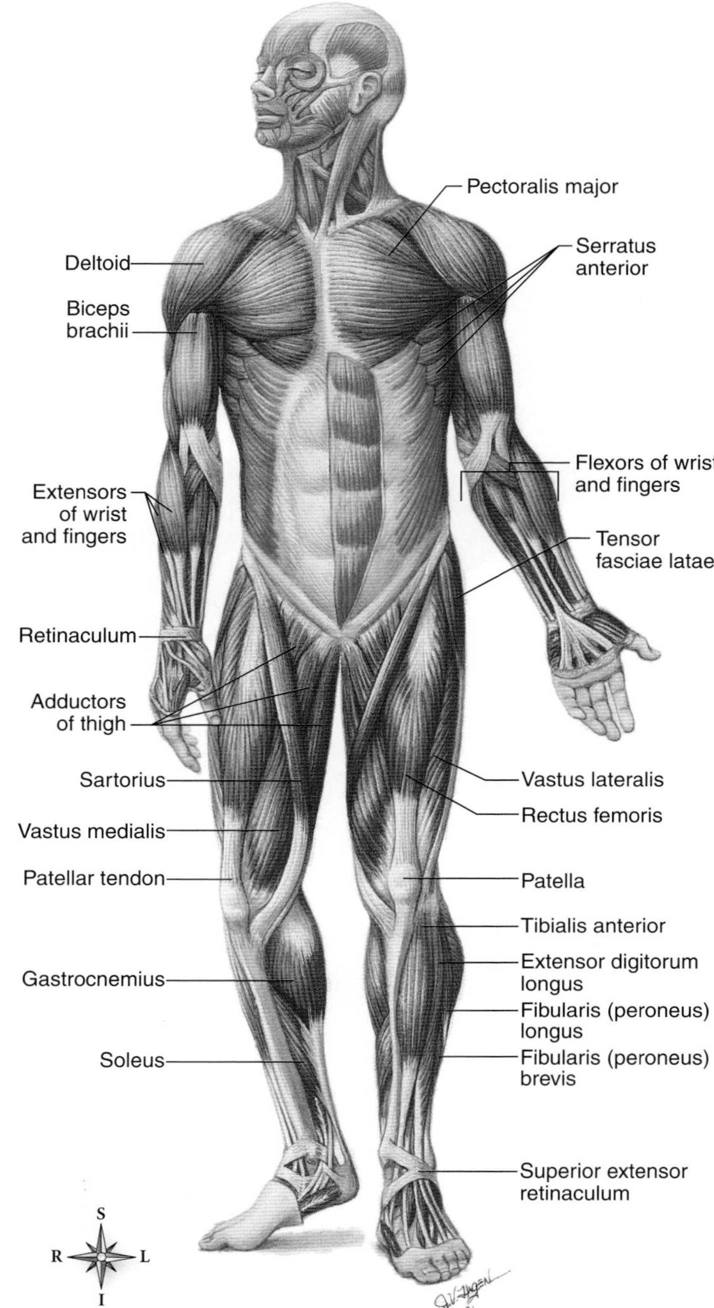

FIGURE 16-1 Appendicular muscles. Anterior view. Appendicular muscles are shown in red; axial muscles are shown in grey.

UPPER EXTREMITY MUSCLES

The muscles of the upper extremity include those acting on the shoulder or pectoral girdle and muscles located in the arm, forearm, and hand.

Muscles Acting on the Shoulder Girdle

Attachment of the upper extremity to the torso is by muscles that have an anterior location (chest) or posterior placement (back and neck). Six muscles (**Table 16-1**; **Figure 16-2**) that pass from the axial skeleton to the shoulder or pectoral girdle (scapula and clavicle) serve not only to "attach" the upper extremity to the body but also to do so in such a way that extensive movement is possible. The clavicle can be elevated and depressed and moved forward and back. The scapula is capable of an even greater variety of movements.

The **pectoralis minor** lies under the larger pectoralis major muscle on the anterior chest wall. It helps "fix" or stabilize the scapula against the thorax and also raises the ribs during forced inspiration. Another anterior chest wall muscle—the **serratus anterior**—helps hold the scapula against the thorax to prevent "winging" and is a strong abductor that is useful in pushing or punching movements.

The posterior muscles acting on the shoulder girdle include the **levator scapulae**, which elevates the scapula; the **trapezius**, which is used to "shrug" the shoulders; and the **rhomboid major** and **minor muscles,** which serve to adduct and elevate the scapula.

TABLE 16-1 Muscles Acting on the Shoulder Girdle

MUSCLE	ORIGIN	INSERTION	FUNCTION	NERVE SUPPLY
Trapezius	Occipital bone (protuberance)	Clavicle	Raises or lowers the shoulders and shrugs them	Spinal accessory; second, third, and fourth cervical nerves
	Vertebrae (cervical and thoracic)	Scapula (spine and acromion)	Extends the head and neck when the occiput acts as the insertion	
Pectoralis minor	Ribs (second to fifth)	Scapula (coracoid)	Pulls the shoulder girdle down and forward; can also pull ribs upward	Medial and lateral anterior thoracic nerve
Serratus anterior	Ribs (upper eight or nine)	Scapula (anterior surface, vertebral border)	Pulls the shoulder down and forward; abducts and rotates it upward	Long thoracic nerve
Levator scapulae	C1–C4 (transverse processes)	Scapula (superior angle)	Elevates and retracts the scapula and abducts the neck	Dorsal scapular nerve
Rhomboid				
Major	T1–T4	Scapula (medial border)	Retracts, rotates, and fixes the scapula	Dorsal scapular nerve
Minor	C6–C7	Scapula (medial border)	Retracts, rotates, elevates, and fixes the scapula	Dorsal scapular nerve

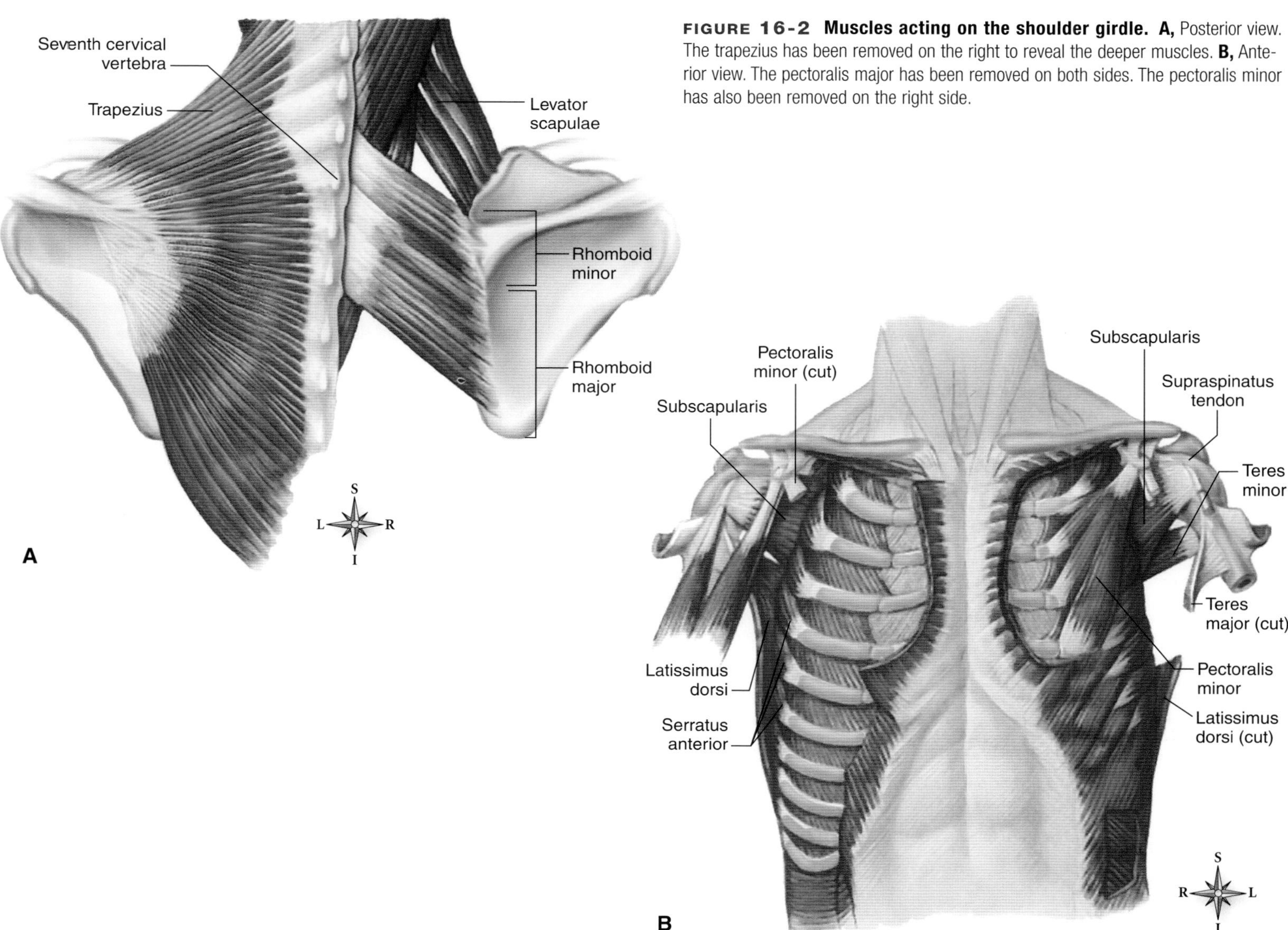

FIGURE 16-2 Muscles acting on the shoulder girdle. A, Posterior view. The trapezius has been removed on the right to reveal the deeper muscles. **B,** Anterior view. The pectoralis major has been removed on both sides. The pectoralis minor has also been removed on the right side.

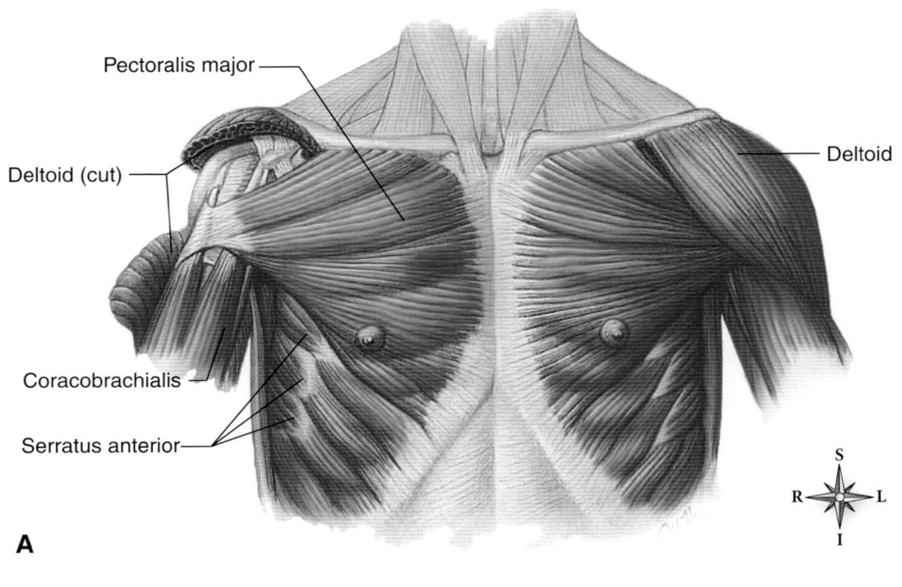

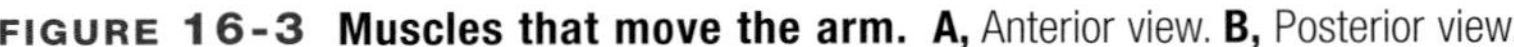

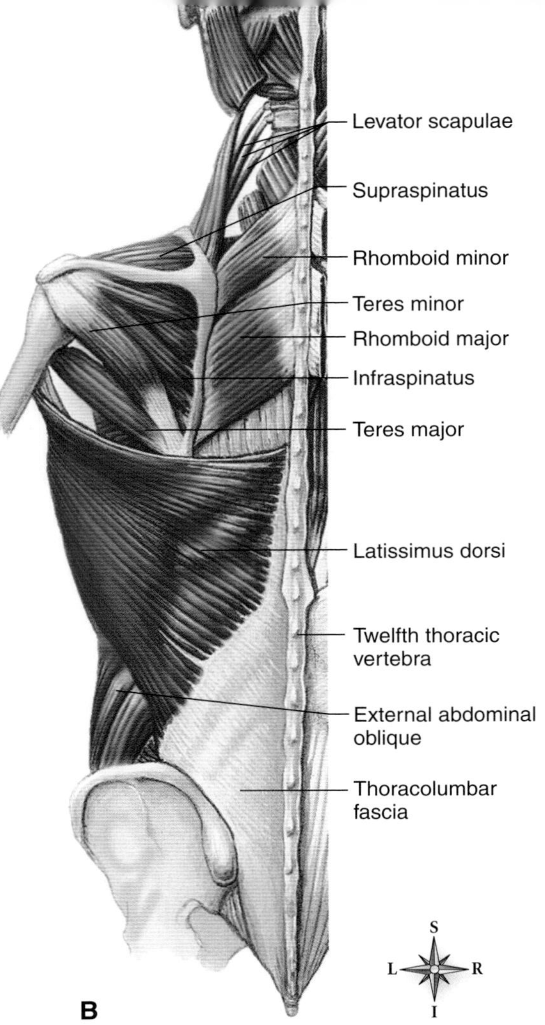

FIGURE 16-3 Muscles that move the arm. **A,** Anterior view. **B,** Posterior view.

TABLE 16-2 Muscles That Move the Arm

MUSCLE	ORIGIN	INSERTION	FUNCTION	NERVE SUPPLY
Axial*				
Pectoralis major	Clavicle (medial half) Sternum Costal cartilages of the true ribs	Humerus (greater tubercle)	Flexes the arm Adducts the arm anteriorly; draws it across the chest	Medial and lateral anterior thoracic nerves
Latissimus dorsi	Vertebrae (spines of the lower thoracic, lumbar, and sacral) Ilium (crest) Lumbodorsal fascia	Humerus (intertubercular groove)	Extends the arm Adducts the arm posteriorly	Thoracodorsal nerve
Scapular*				
Deltoid	Clavicle Scapula (spine and acromion)	Humerus (lateral side about halfway down—deltoid tubercle)	Abducts the arm Assists in flexion and extension of the arm	Axillary nerve
Coracobrachialis	Scapula (coracoid process)	Humerus (middle third, medial surface)	Adduction; assists in flexion and medial rotation of the arm	Musculocutaneous nerve
Supraspinatus†	Scapula (supraspinous fossa)	Humerus (greater tubercle)	Assists in abducting the arm	Suprascapular nerve
Teres minor†	Scapula (axillary border)	Humerus (greater tubercle)	Rotates the arm outward	Axillary nerve
Teres major	Scapula (lower part, axillary border)	Humerus (upper part, anterior surface)	Assists in extension, adduction, and medial rotation of the arm	Lower subscapular nerve
Infraspinatus†	Scapula (infraspinatus border)	Humerus (greater tubercle)	Rotates the arm outward	Suprascapular nerve
Subscapularis†	Scapula (subscapular fossa)	Humerus (lesser tubercle)	Medial rotation	Suprascapular nerve

**Axial* muscles originate on the axial skeleton. *Scapular* muscles originate on the scapula.

†Muscles of the rotator cuff (SITS muscles).

Muscles That Move the Arm

The shoulder is a synovial joint of the ball-and-socket type. As a result, extensive movement is possible in every plane of motion (**Box 16-1**). Muscles that move the upper part of the arm can be grouped by function as flexors, extensors, abductors, adductors, and medial and lateral rotators (**Table 16-2**; **Figure 16-3**). The actions listed in **Table 16-2** include primary actions and important secondary functions.

The **deltoid** is a good example of a multifunction muscle. It has three groups of fibres and may act as three separate muscles. Contraction of the anterior fibres will flex the arm, whereas the lateral fibres abduct and the posterior fibres serve as extensors. Four other muscles serve as both a structural and functional cuff around the shoulder joint and are referred to as the **rotator cuff muscles** (**Figure 16-4**). They include the **supraspinatus, infraspinatus, teres minor,** and **subscapularis**—the so-called *SITS muscles*.

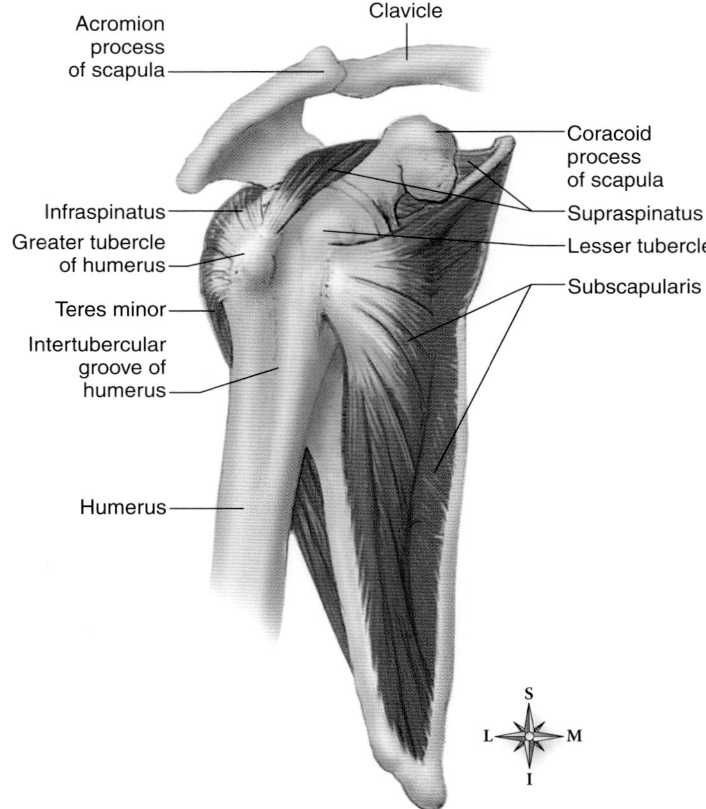

FIGURE 16-4 Rotator cuff muscles. Anterior view of the right shoulder showing the tendons of the teres minor, infraspinatus, supraspinatus, and subscapularis muscles surrounding the head of the humerus.

BOX 16-1 *sports and fitness* | Shoulder Joint Stability

The disparity in size between the large and nearly hemispheric head of the humerus and the much smaller and shallow glenoid cavity of the scapula is of great clinical significance. Because the head of the humerus is more than two times larger than the shallow glenoid concavity that receives it, only about a quarter of the articular surface of the humeral head is in contact with the fossa in any given position of the joint. This anatomical fact helps explain the inherent instability of the shoulder—our most mobile joint. The soft tissues surrounding the shoulder, such as the joint capsule, ligaments, and adjacent muscles, provide the primary restraint against excessive motion and potential dislocation.

Unfortunately, only a thin articular capsule surrounds the shoulder joint. It is extremely loose and does not function to keep the articulating bones of the joint in contact. This fact is obviously correlated with both the great range of motion (ROM) possible at this articulation and its tendency to dislocate as a result of athletic injury or other trauma. The tendons of the supraspinatus, infraspinatus, teres minor, and subscapularis muscles (called the *SITS muscles*) all blend with and strengthen the articular capsule. The musculotendinous cuff resulting from this fusion is called the **rotator cuff** (see **Figure 16-4**). The rotator cuff provides the necessary strength to help prevent anterior, superior, and posterior displacement of the humeral head during most types of activity. •

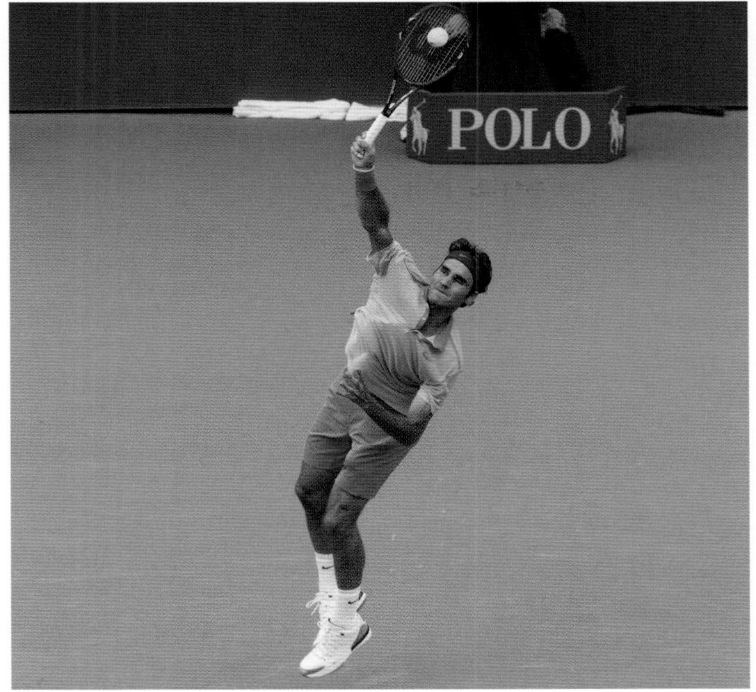

The rotator cuff stabilizes the shoulder during athletic activities.

Muscles That Move the Forearm

Selected superficial and deep muscles of the upper extremity are shown in **Figure 16-5** and **Figure 16-6**. Recall that most muscles acting on a joint lie proximal to that joint. Muscles acting directly on the forearm, therefore, are found proximal to the elbow and attach the bones of the forearm (ulna and radius) to the humerus or scapula above.

Table 16-3 lists the muscles acting on the forearm and gives the origin, insertion, function, and innervation of each. **Figure 16-7** shows the detail of attachment of several important muscles in this group.

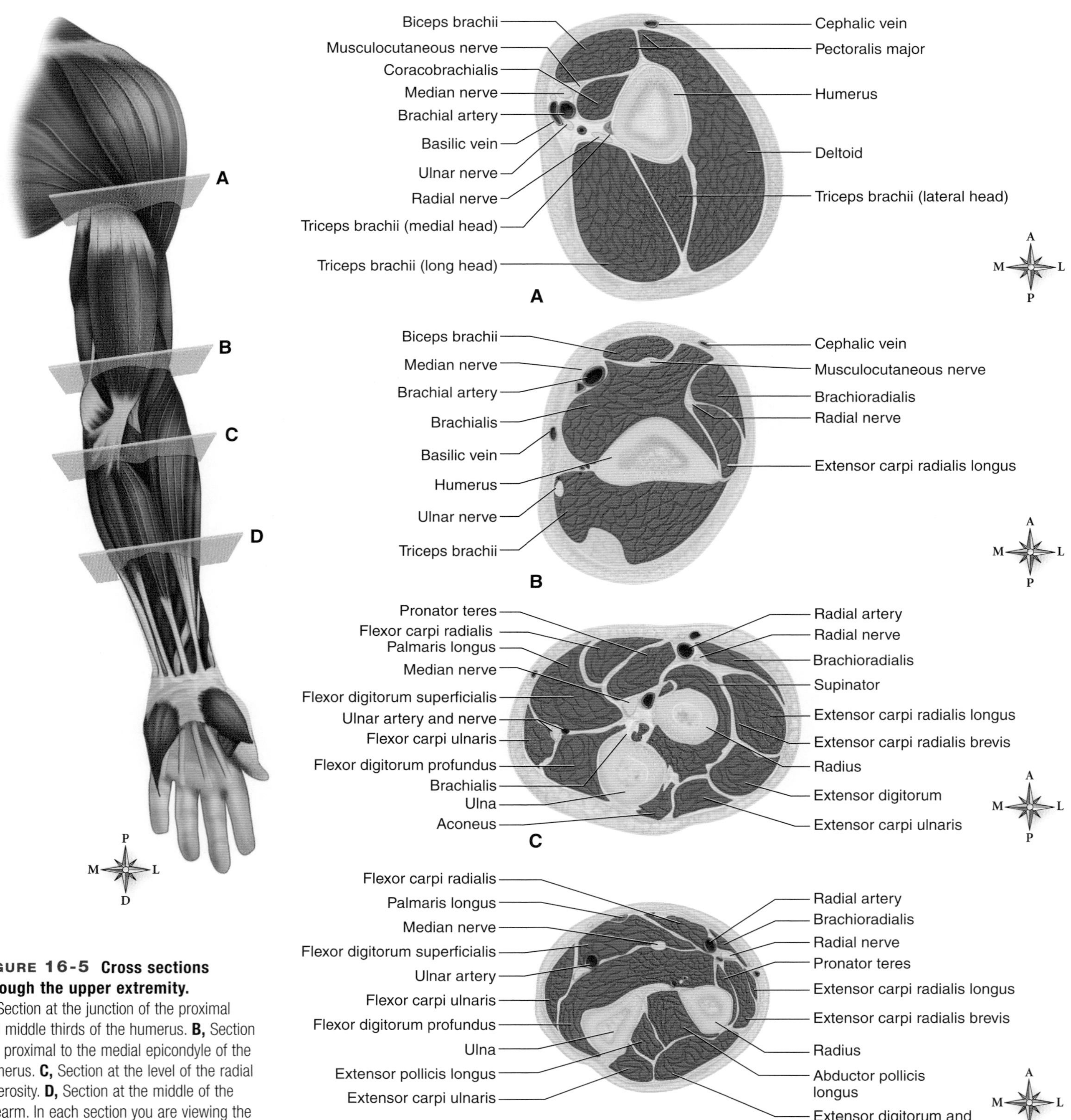

FIGURE 16-5 Cross sections through the upper extremity.
A, Section at the junction of the proximal and middle thirds of the humerus. **B,** Section just proximal to the medial epicondyle of the humerus. **C,** Section at the level of the radial tuberosity. **D,** Section at the middle of the forearm. In each section you are viewing the superior (proximal) aspect of the specimen.

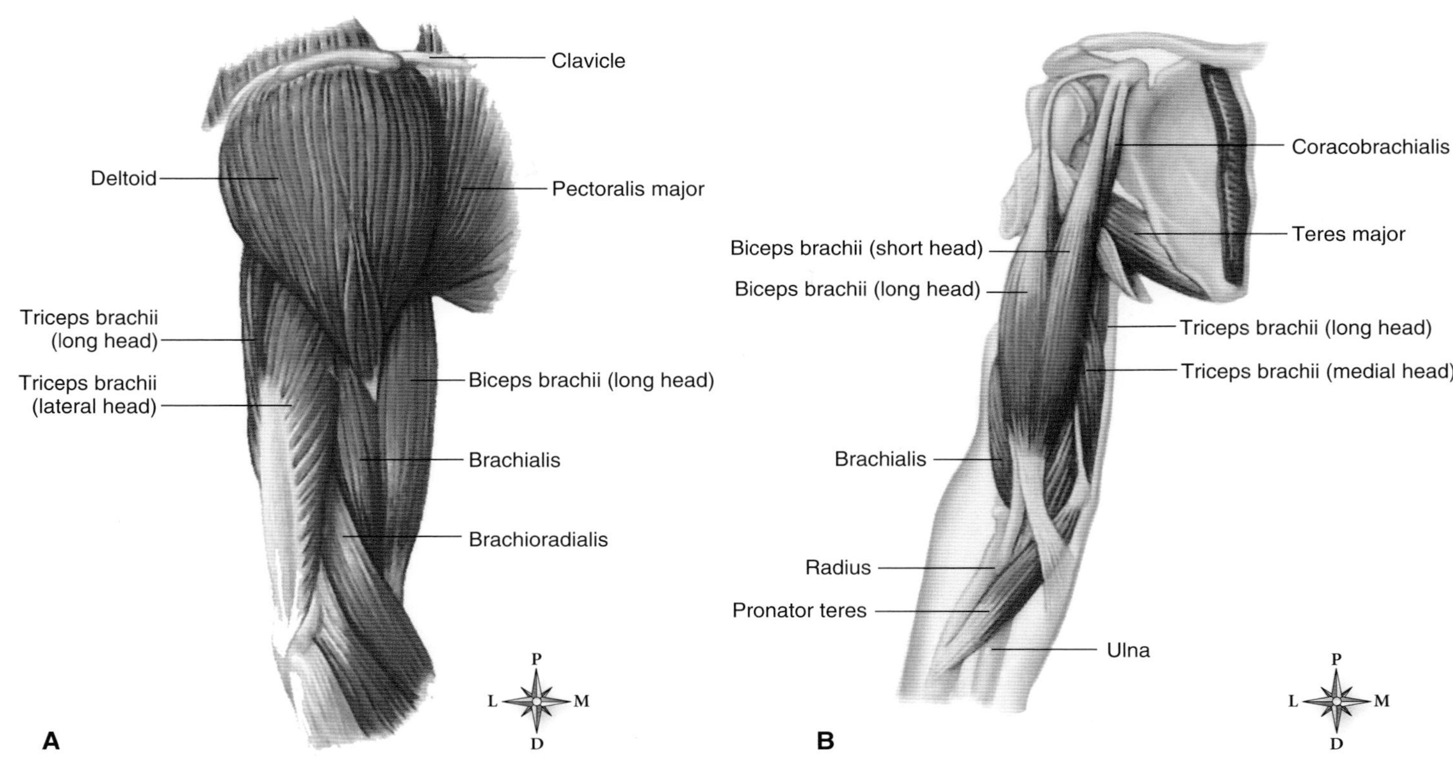

FIGURE 16-6 Muscles acting on the forearm. A, Lateral view of the right shoulder and arm. **B,** Anterior view of the right shoulder and arm (deep). The deltoid and pectoralis major muscles have been removed to reveal deeper structures.

TABLE 16-3 Muscles That Move the Forearm

MUSCLE	ORIGIN	INSERTION	FUNCTION	NERVE SUPPLY
Flexors				
Biceps brachii	Scapula (supraglenoid tuberosity) Scapula (coracoid)	Radius (tuberosity at the proximal end)	Flexes the supinated forearm Supinates the forearm and hand	Musculocutaneous nerve
Brachialis	Humerus (distal half, anterior surface)	Ulna (front of the coronoid process)	Flexes the forearm	Musculocutaneous nerve
Brachioradialis	Humerus (above the lateral epicondyle)	Radius (styloid process)	Flexes the semipronated or semisupinated forearm	Radial nerve
Extensor				
Triceps brachii	Scapula (infraglenoid tuberosity) Humerus (posterior surface—lateral head above the radial groove; medial head, below)	Ulna (olecranon)	Extends the lower arm	Radial nerve
Pronators				
Pronator teres	Humerus (medial epicondyle) Ulna (coronoid process)	Radius (middle third of the lateral surface)	Pronates and flexes the forearm	Median nerve
Pronator quadratus	Ulna (distal fourth, anterior surface)	Radius (distal fourth, anterior surface)	Pronates the forearm	Median nerve
Supinator				
Supinator	Humerus (lateral epicondyle) Ulna (proximal fifth)	Radius (proximal third)	Supinates the forearm	Radial nerve

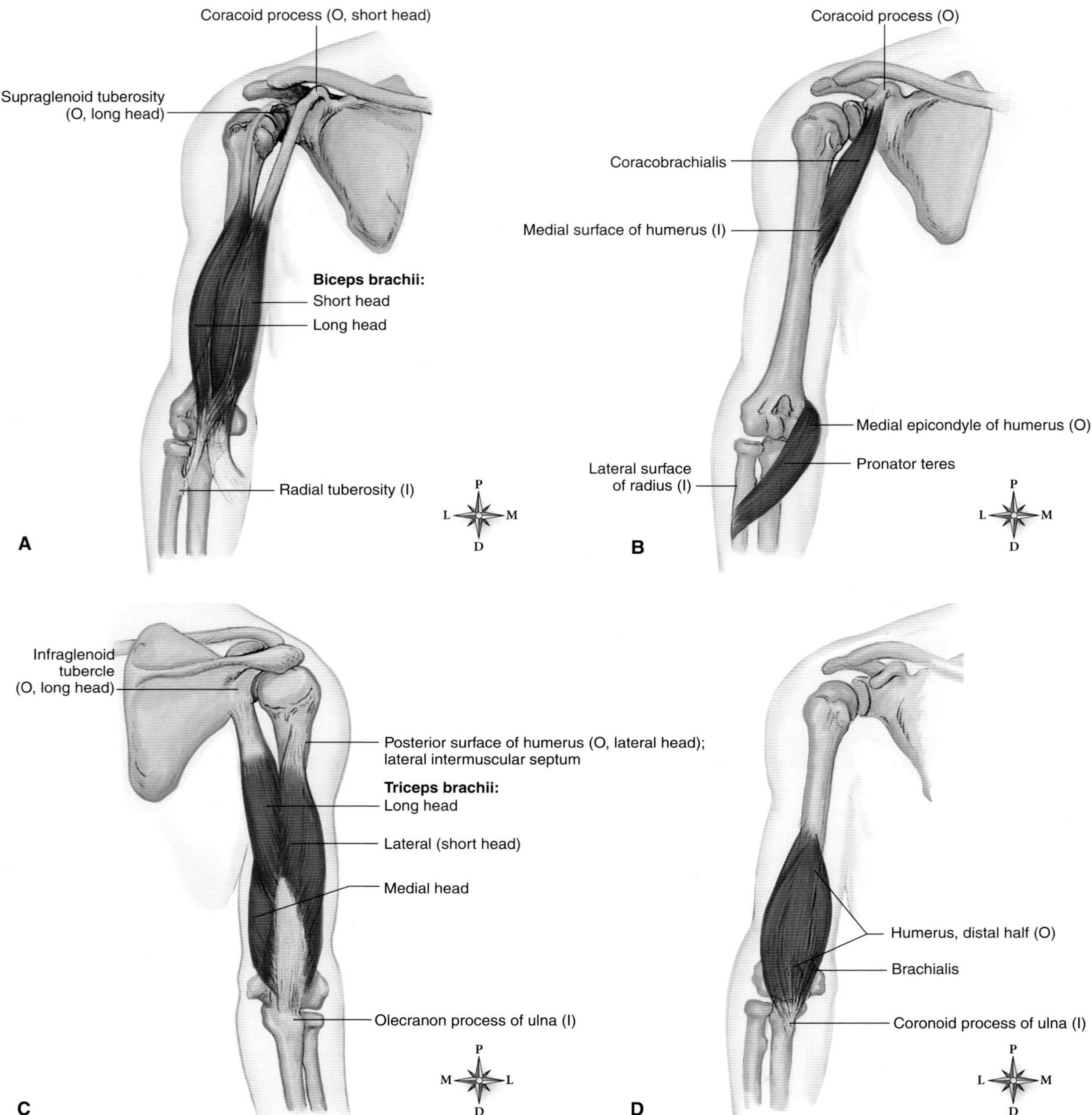

FIGURE 16-7 Muscles acting on the forearm. **A,** Biceps brachii. **B,** Coracobrachialis and pronator teres. **C,** Triceps brachii. **D,** Brachialis. *O,* Origin; *I,* insertion.

Muscles That Move the Wrist, Hand, and Fingers

Muscles that move the wrist, hand, and fingers can be **extrinsic muscles** or **intrinsic muscles.** The term *extrinsic* means "from the outside" and refers to muscles originating outside the part of the skeleton moved. Extrinsic muscles originating in the forearm can pull on their insertions in the wrist, hand, and fingers to move them. The term *intrinsic,* meaning "from within", refers to muscles that are actually within the part moved. Muscles that begin and end at different points within the hand can produce fine finger movements, for example.

Extrinsic muscles acting on the wrist, hand, and fingers are located on the anterior or the posterior surfaces of the forearm (**Figure 16-8**). In most instances, the muscles located on the anterior surface of the forearm are flexors and those on the posterior surface are extensors of the wrist, hand, and fingers (**Table 16-4**).

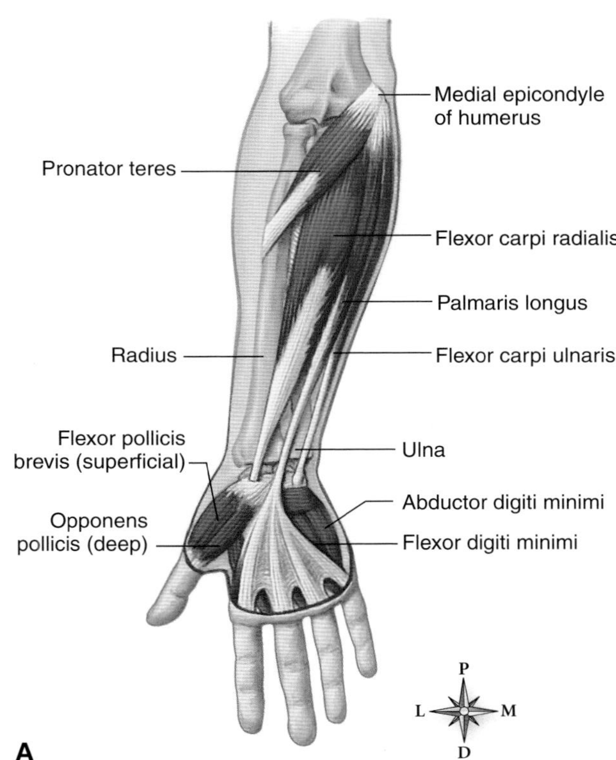

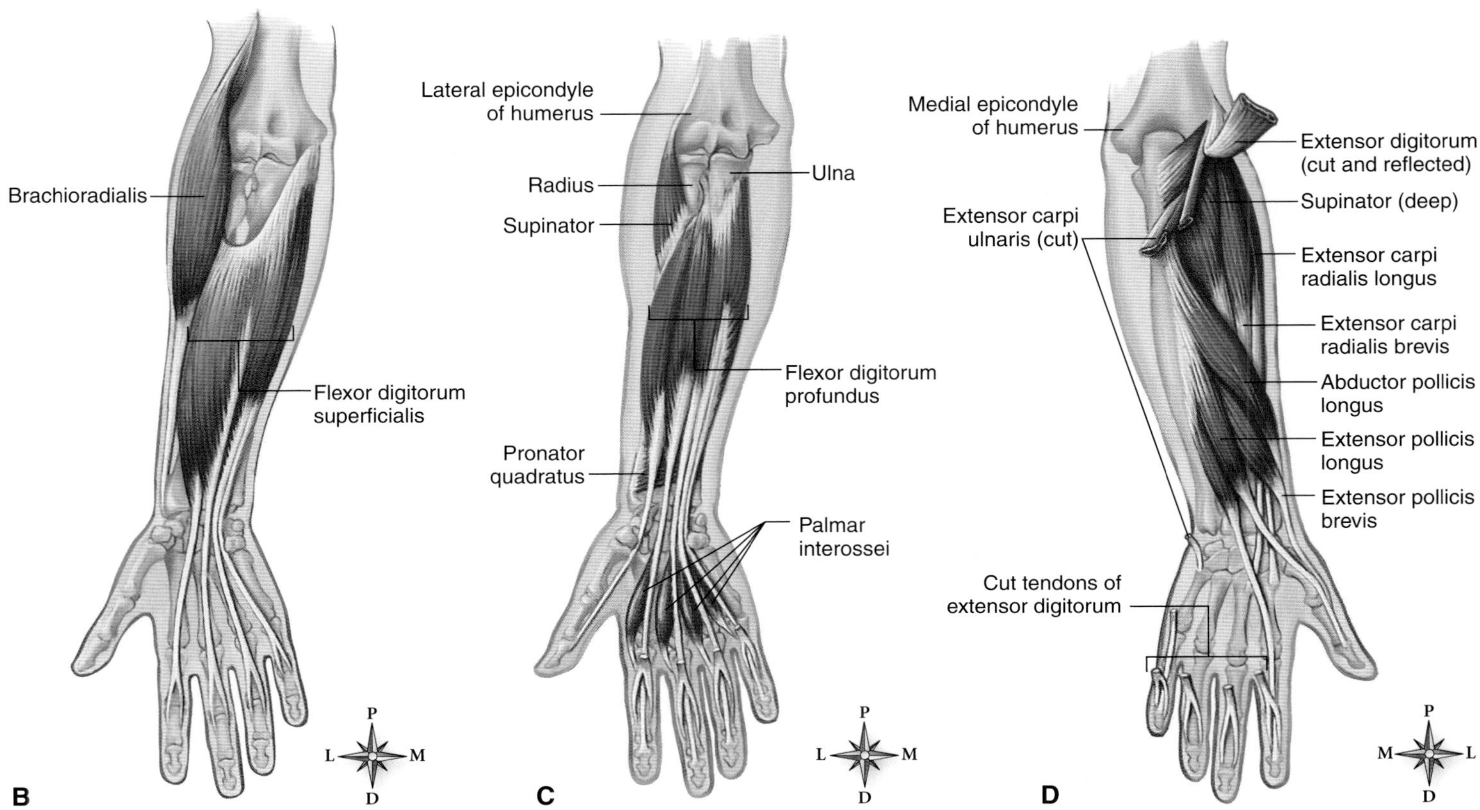

FIGURE 16-8 Muscles of the forearm. A, Anterior view showing the right forearm (superficial). The brachioradialis muscle has been removed. **B,** Anterior view showing the right forearm (deeper than **A**). The pronator teres, flexor carpi radialis and ulnaris, and palmaris longus muscles have been removed. **C,** Anterior view showing the right forearm (deeper than **A** or **B**). The brachioradialis, pronator teres, flexor carpi radialis and ulnaris, palmaris longus, and flexor digitorum superficialis muscles have been removed. **D,** Posterior view showing the deep muscles of the right forearm. The extensor digitorum, extensor digiti minimi, and extensor carpi ulnaris muscles have been cut to reveal deeper muscles.

TABLE 16-4 Muscles That Move the Wrist, Hand, and Fingers

MUSCLE	ORIGIN	INSERTION	FUNCTION	NERVE SUPPLY
Extrinsic				
Flexor carpi radialis	Humerus (medial epicondyle)	Second metacarpal (base of)	Flexes the hand Flexes the forearm	Median nerve
Palmaris longus	Humerus (medial epicondyle)	Fascia of the palm	Flexes the hand	Median nerve
Flexor carpi ulnaris	Humerus (medial epicondyle)	Pisiform bone	Flexes the hand	Ulnar nerve
	Ulna (proximal two thirds)	Third, fourth, and fifth metacarpals	Adducts the hand	
Extensor carpi radialis longus	Humerus (ridge above the lateral epicondyle)	Second metacarpal (base of)	Extends the hand Abducts the hand (moves toward the thumb side when the hand is supinated)	Radial nerve
Extensor carpi radialis brevis	Humerus (lateral epicondyle)	Second, third metacarpals (bases of)	Extends the hand	Radial nerve
Extensor carpi ulnaris	Humerus (lateral epicondyle) Ulna (proximal three fourths)	Fifth metacarpal (base of)	Extends the hand Adducts the hand (moves toward the little finger side when the hand is supinated)	Radial nerve
Flexor digitorum profundus	Ulna (anterior surface)	Distal phalanges (fingers 2 to 5)	Flexes the distal interphalangeal joints	Median and ulnar nerves
Flexor digitorum superficialis	Humerus (medial epicondyle) Radius Ulna (coronoid process)	Tendons of the fingers	Flexes the fingers	Median nerve
Extensor digitorum	Humerus (lateral epicondyle)	Phalanges (fingers 2 to 5)	Extends the fingers	Radial nerve
Intrinsic				
Opponens pollicis	Trapezium	Thumb metacarpal	Opposes the thumb to the fingers	Median nerve
Abductor pollicis brevis	Trapezium	Proximal phalanx of the thumb	Abducts the thumb	Median nerve
Adductor pollicis	Second and third metacarpals Trapezoid Capitate	Proximal phalanx of the thumb	Adducts the thumb	Ulnar nerve
Flexor pollicis brevis	Flexor retinaculum	Proximal phalanx of the thumb	Flexes the thumb	Median and ulnar nerves
Abductor digiti minimi	Pisiform	Proximal phalanx of the fifth finger (base of)	Abducts the fifth finger Flexes the fifth finger	Ulnar nerve
Flexor digiti minimi brevis	Hamate	Proximal and middle phalanx of the fifth finger	Flexes the fifth finger	Ulnar nerve
Opponens digiti minimi	Hamate Flexor retinaculum	Fifth metacarpal	Opposes the fifth finger slightly	Ulnar nerve
Interosseous				
Palmar interossei	Metacarpals	Proximal phalanges	Adducts the second, fourth, and fifth fingers	Ulnar nerve
Dorsal interossei	Metacarpals	Proximal phalanges	Abducts the second, third, and fourth fingers	Ulnar nerve
Lumbricals	Tendons of the flexor digitorum profundus	Phalanges (2 to 5)	Flexes the proximal phalanges (2 to 5) Extends the middle and distal phalanges (2 to 5)	Median nerve (phalanges 2 and 3) Ulnar nerve (phalanges 4 and 5)

BOX 16-2 *health matters* | Carpal Tunnel Syndrome

Some epidemiologists specialize in the field of occupational health, the study of health matters related to work or the workplace. Many problems seen by occupational health experts are caused by repetitive motions of the wrists or other joints. Meat cutters and workers who use word processors, for example, are at risk for conditions caused by repetitive motion injuries.

One common problem often caused by such repetitive motion is **tenosynovitis**—inflammation of a tendon sheath. Tenosynovitis can be painful, and the swelling characteristic of this condition can limit movement in affected parts of the body. For example, swelling of the tendon sheath around tendons in an area of the wrist known as the *carpal tunnel* can limit movement of the wrist, hand, and fingers.

The figure shows the relative positions of the tendon sheath and median nerve within the carpal tunnel. The carpal tunnel is formed as a fibrous band called the *flexor retinaculum* wraps over the tendons of the flexor muscles that lie within an arch formed by the carpal bones. If swelling, or any other lesion within the carpal tunnel, presses on the *median nerve,* a condition called **carpal tunnel syndrome** may result. Because the median nerve connects to the palm and radial side (thumb side) of the hand, carpal tunnel syndrome is characterized by weakness, pain, and tingling in this part of the hand. The pain and tingling may also radiate to the forearm and shoulder. Prolonged or severe cases of carpal tunnel syndrome may be relieved by injection of antiinflammatory agents. A permanent cure is sometimes accomplished by surgically cutting the flexor retinaculum to relieve the pressure on the median nerve.

The procedure called *carpal tunnel release* is one of the most common hand operations in the UK. Such operations are performed more than 52,000 times every year. When the procedure was first introduced in 1933, it was performed as an "open" procedure. A less invasive endoscopic approach was introduced in 1989; that and many other innovative surgical techniques and advances are now being used.

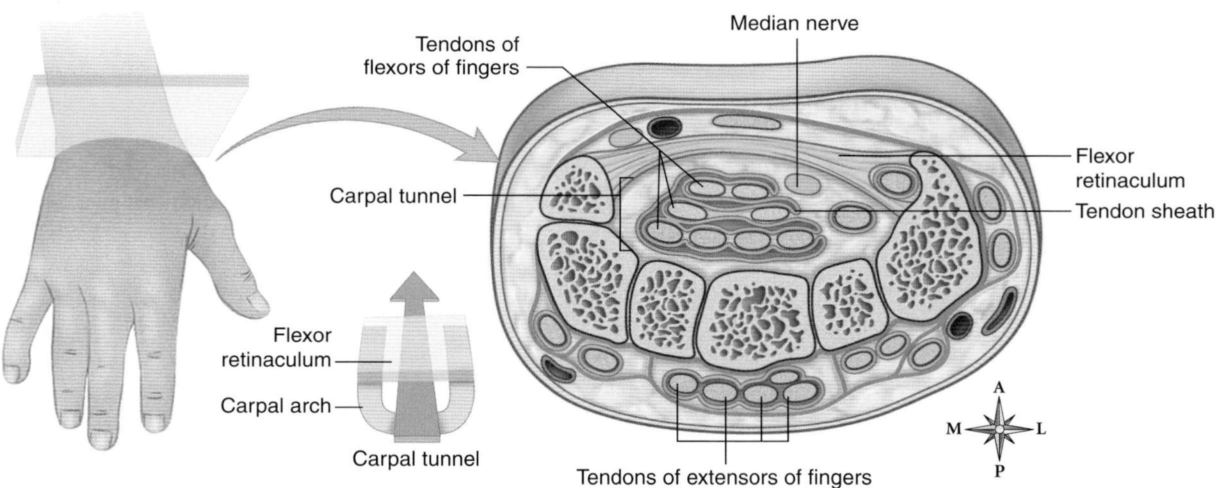

The carpal tunnel. The median nerve and muscles that flex the fingers pass through a concavity in the wrist called the *carpal tunnel.* Figure 4-12 in the Brief Atlas of the Human Body shows a detailed photograph of the carpal tunnel and surrounding structures.

Many of the flexors of the wrist and hand pass through a curve formed by the carpal bones called the *carpal tunnel.* The long tendons of these muscles slide through the carpal tunnel more easily because tendon sheaths lined with synovial membrane are present. **Box 16-2** discusses the importance of the carpal tunnel in occupational health.

A number of intrinsic muscles are responsible for precise movements of the hand and fingers. Examples include the **lumbrical** and **interosseous muscles,** which originate from and fill the spaces between the metacarpal bones and then insert on the phalanges of the fingers. As a group, the intrinsic muscles abduct and adduct the fingers and aid in flexing them.

Eight additional muscles serve the thumb and enable it to be placed in opposition to the fingers in tasks requiring grasping and manipulation. The **opponens pollicis** is a particularly important thumb muscle. It allows the thumb to be drawn across the palm to

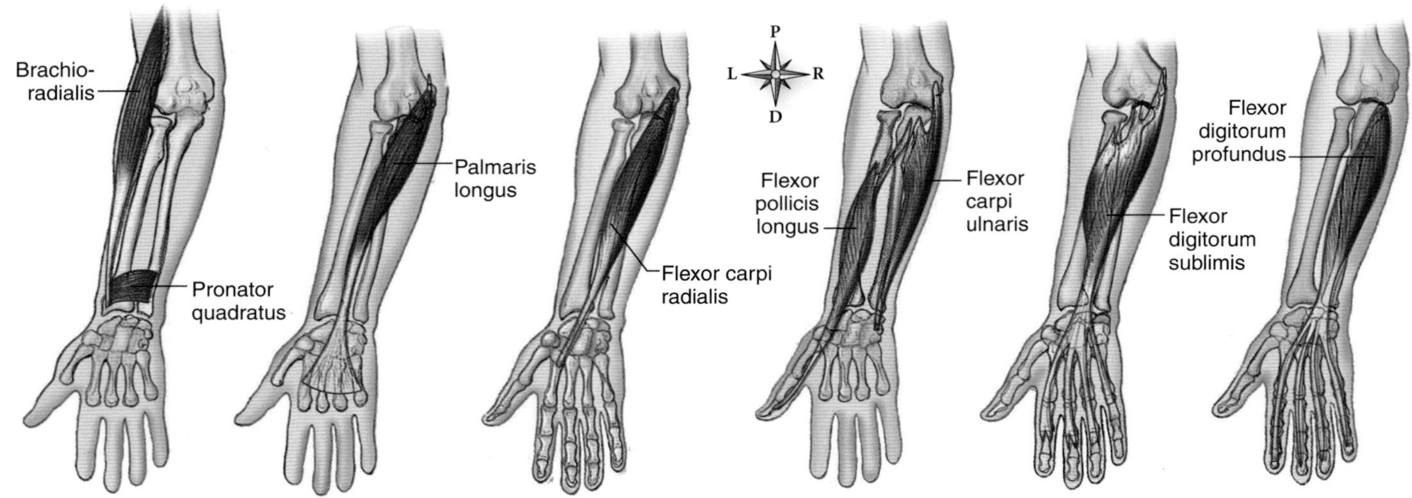

FIGURE 16-9 Selected forearm muscles. Right arm, anterior view.

touch the tip of any finger (opposition)—a critical movement for many manipulative-type activities (see **Figure 14-22** on p. 303).

Figure 16-8 and **Figure 16-9** show the placement and points of attachment for various individual extrinsic muscles acting on the wrist, hand, and fingers. **Figure 16-10** provides a detailed illustration of many of the intrinsic muscles of the hand.

Quick CHECK

1. What are the functions of the deltoid muscle?
2. What is the function of the biceps brachii muscle?
3. Distinguish the extrinsic from the intrinsic muscles of the hand and wrist.

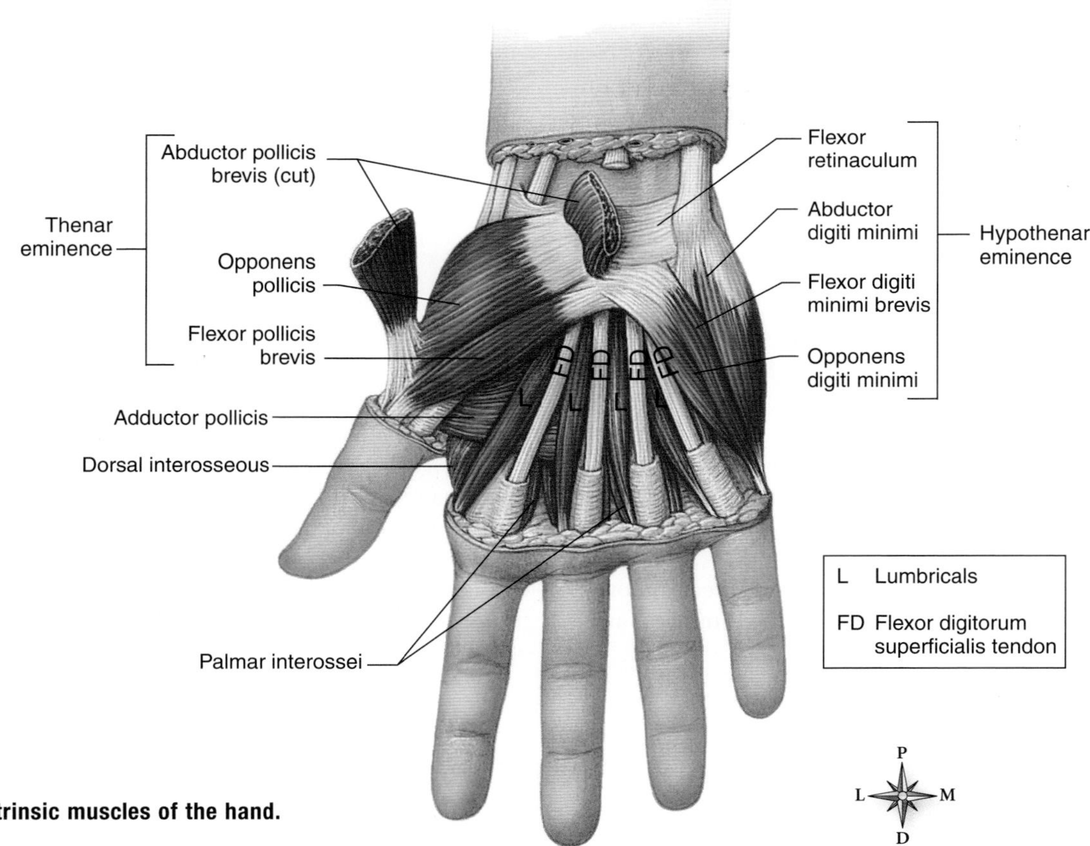

FIGURE 16-10 Intrinsic muscles of the hand. Anterior (palmar) view.

TABLE 16-5 Muscles That Move the Thigh

MUSCLE	ORIGIN	INSERTION	FUNCTION	NERVE SUPPLY
Iliopsoas (iliacus, psoas major, and psoas minor)	Ilium (iliac fossa)	Femur (lesser trochanter)	Flexes the thigh	Femoral and second to fourth lumbar nerves
	Vertebrae (bodies of twelfth thoracic to fifth lumbar)		Flexes the trunk (when the femur acts as the origin)	
Rectus femoris	Ilium (anterior, inferior spine)	Tibia (by way of the patellar tendon)	Flexes the thigh Extends the leg	Femoral nerve
Gluteal group				
Maximus	Ilium (crest and posterior surface) Sacrum and coccyx (posterior surface) Sacrotuberous ligament	Femur (gluteal tuberosity) Iliotibial tract	Extends the thigh—rotates outward	Inferior gluteal nerve
Medius	Ilium (lateral surface)	Femur (greater trochanter)	Abducts the thigh—rotates outward; stabilizes the pelvis on the femur	Superior gluteal nerve
Minimus	Ilium (lateral surface)	Femur (greater trochanter)	Abducts the thigh; stabilizes the pelvis on the femur Rotates the thigh medially	Superior gluteal nerve
Tensor fasciae latae	Ilium (anterior part of the crest)	Tibia (by way of the iliotibial tract)	Abducts the thigh Tightens the iliotibial tract	Superior gluteal nerve
Adductor group				
Brevis	Pubic bone	Femur (linea aspera)	Adducts the thigh	Obturator nerve
Longus	Pubic bone	Femur (linea aspera)	Adducts the thigh	Obturator nerve
Magnus	Pubic bone	Femur (linea aspera)	Adducts the thigh	Obturator nerve
Gracilis	Pubic bone (just below the symphysis)	Tibia (medial surface behind the sartorius)	Adducts the thigh and flexes and adducts the leg	Obturator nerve

LOWER EXTREMITY MUSCLES

The musculature, bony structure, and joints of the pelvic girdle and lower extremity function in locomotion and maintenance of stability. Powerful muscles at the back of the hip, at the front of the thigh, and at the back of the leg also serve to raise the full body weight from a sitting to a standing position. The muscles of the lower extremity include those acting on the hip or pelvic girdle, as well as muscles located in the thigh, leg, and foot.

Unlike the highly mobile shoulder girdle, the pelvic girdle is essentially fixed. Therefore, our study of muscles in the lower extremity begins with those arising from the pelvic girdle and passing to the femur; they produce their effects at the hip joint by moving the thigh.

Muscles That Move the Thigh and Leg

Table 16-5 identifies muscles that move the thigh and lists the origin, insertion, function, and nerve supply of each (**Figure 16-11**). Refer to **Figure 16-1** and **Figure 16-10** through **Figure 16-15**, which show individual muscles, as you study the information provided in the table.

Muscles acting on the thigh can be divided into three groups: (1) muscles crossing the front of the hip, (2) the three **gluteal muscles** and the **tensor fasciae latae**, and (3) the thigh adductors. One of the gluteal muscles, the gluteus medius muscle, is often the site of intramuscular injections (**Box 16-3**).

Table 16-6 identifies muscles that move the leg. Note that the quadriceps femoris group is made up of four large muscles that flex the thigh and extend the leg. The hamstring group, innervated by branches of the sciatic nerve, is made up of three muscles that extend the thigh and flex the leg. Again, see **Figure 16-1** and refer to **Figure 16-16** and **Figure 16-17** as you study the table.

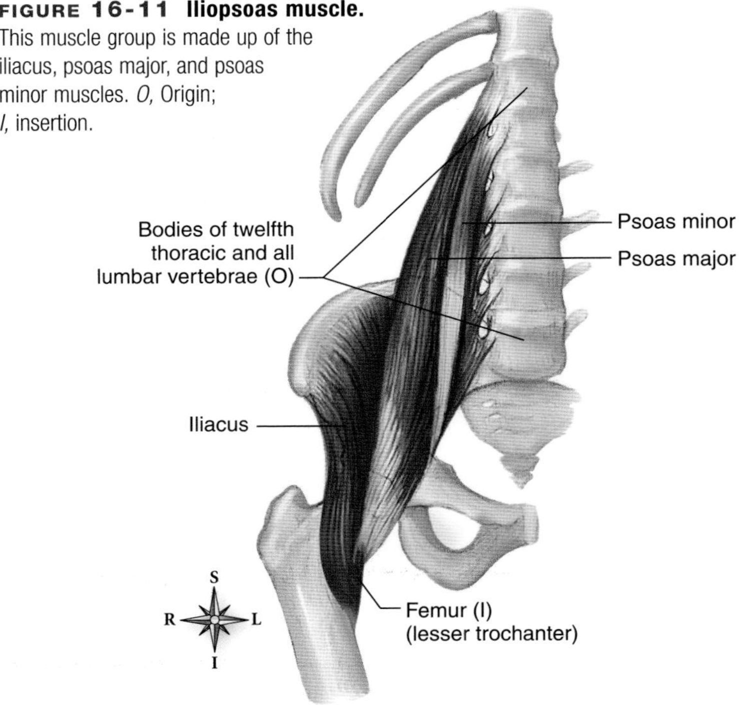

FIGURE 16-11 Iliopsoas muscle. This muscle group is made up of the iliacus, psoas major, and psoas minor muscles. *O,* Origin; *I,* insertion.

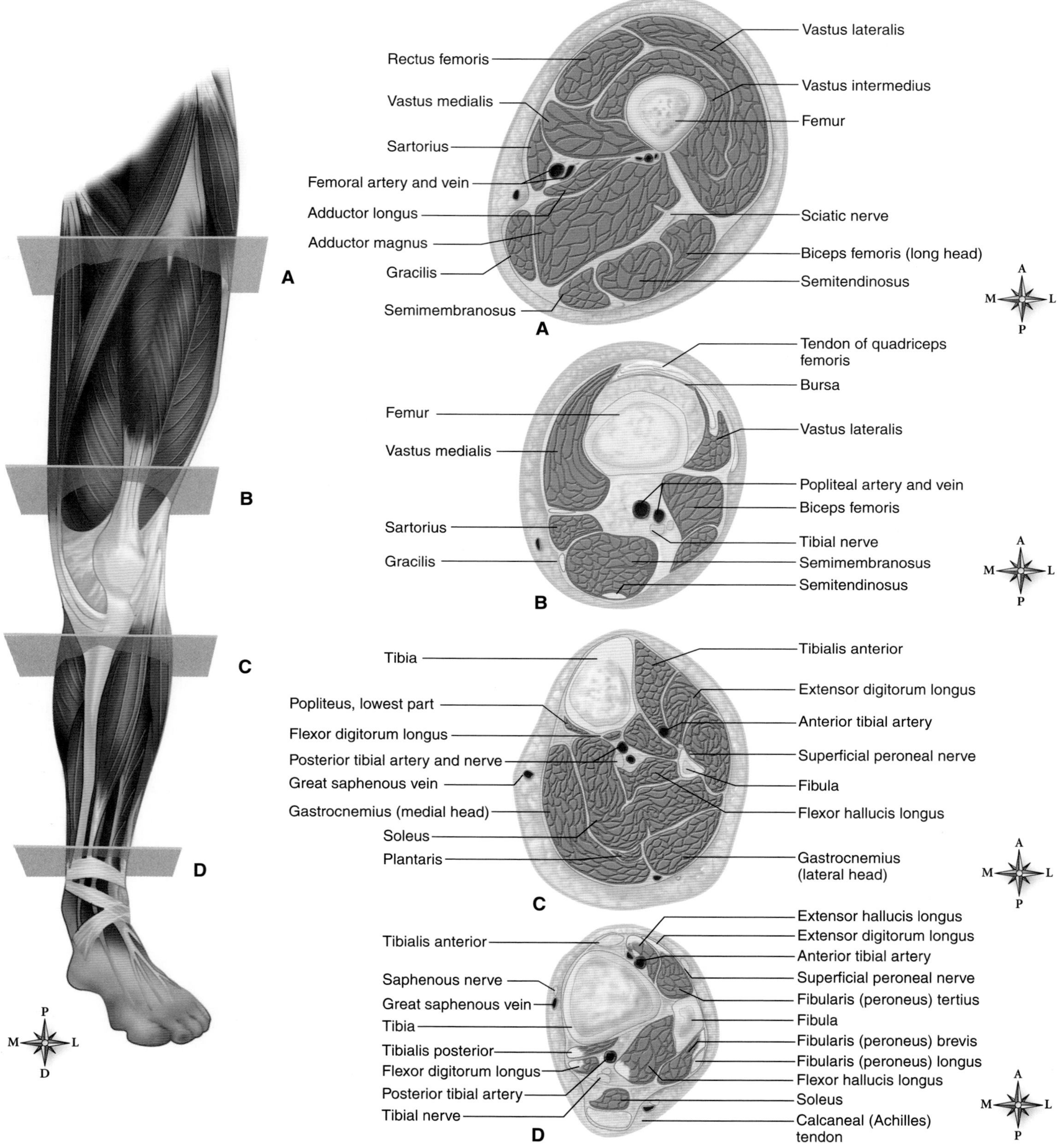

FIGURE 16-12 Cross-sections through the lower extremity. A, Section through the middle of the femur. **B,** Section about 4 cm above the adductor tubercle of the femur. **C,** Section about 10 cm distal to the knee joint. **D,** Section about 6 cm above the medial malleolus. In each section you are viewing the superior (proximal) aspect of the specimen.

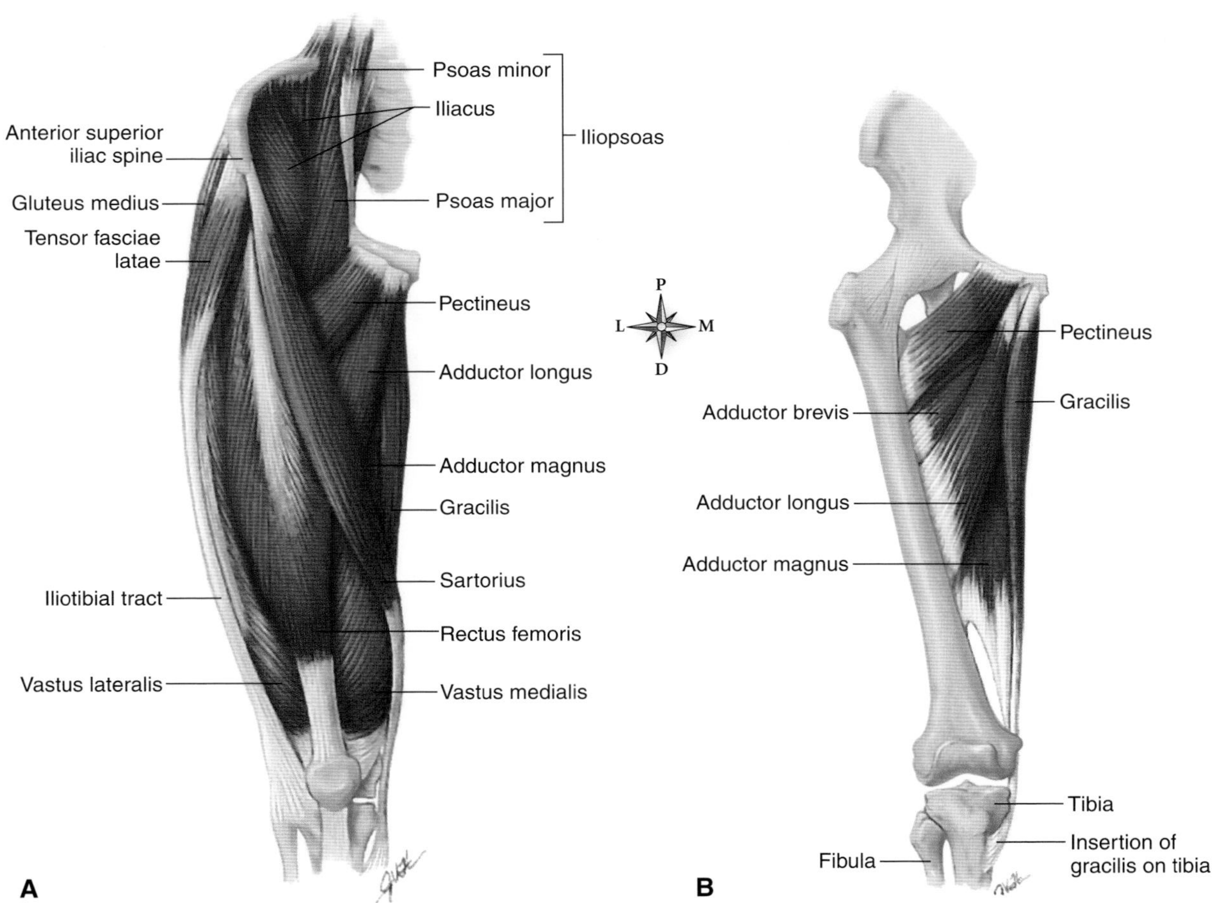

FIGURE 16-13 Muscles of the anterior aspect of the thigh. A, Anterior view of the right thigh. **B,** Adductor region of the right thigh. The tensor fasciae latae, sartorius, and quadriceps muscles have been removed.

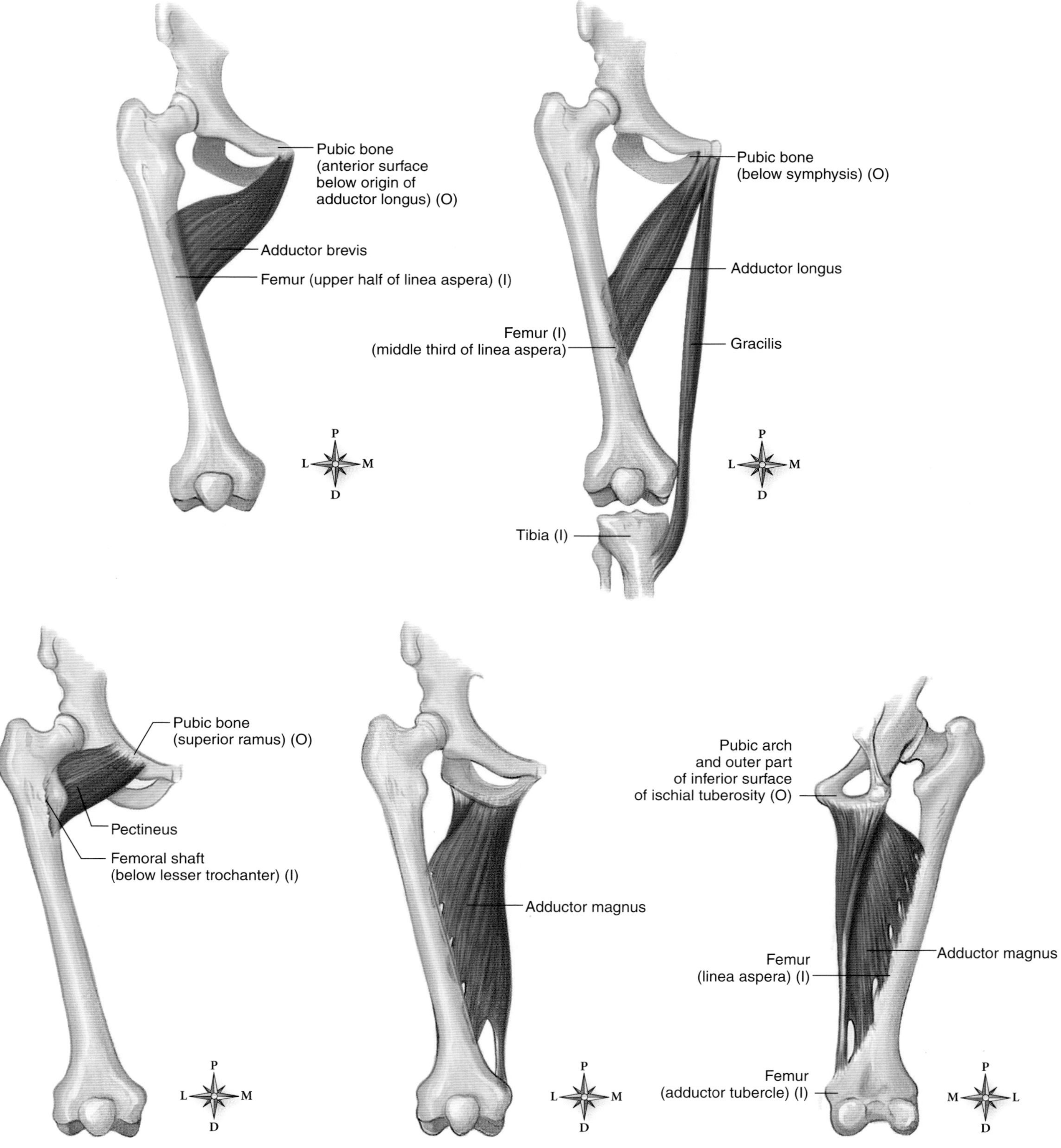

FIGURE 16-14 Muscles that adduct the thigh. *O,* Origin; *I,* insertion.

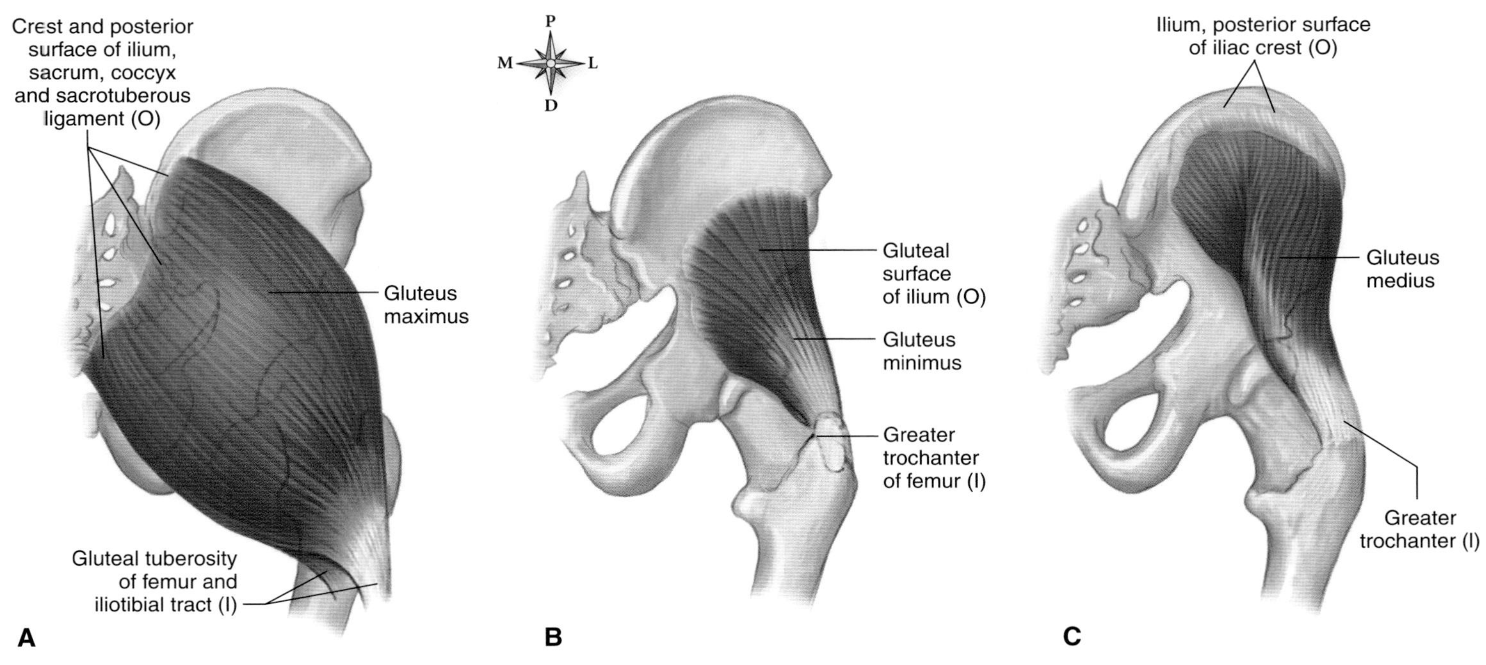

FIGURE 16-15 Gluteal muscles. A, Gluteus maximus. **B,** Gluteus minimus. **C,** Gluteus medius. *O,* Origin; *I,* insertion.

UNIT 2

BOX 16-3 *health matters* | Intramuscular Injections

Many drugs are administered by **intramuscular injection.** If the amount to be injected is 2 mL or less, the deltoid muscle is often selected as the site of injection. Note that in Figure A, the needle is inserted into the muscle about two fingerbreadths below the acromion process of the scapula and lateral to the tip of the acromion.

If the amount of medication to be injected is 2 to 3 mL, the gluteal area shown in Figure B is often used. Injections are made into the gluteus medius muscle near the centre of the upper outer quadrant.

Another technique of locating the proper injection site is to draw an imaginary diagonal line from a point of reference on the back of the bony pelvis (posterior superior iliac spine) to the greater trochanter of the femur. The injection is given about three fingers' breadth above and one third of the way down the line. It is important to avoid the sciatic nerve and the superior gluteal blood vessels during administration of the injection. Proper technique requires knowledge of the underlying anatomy.

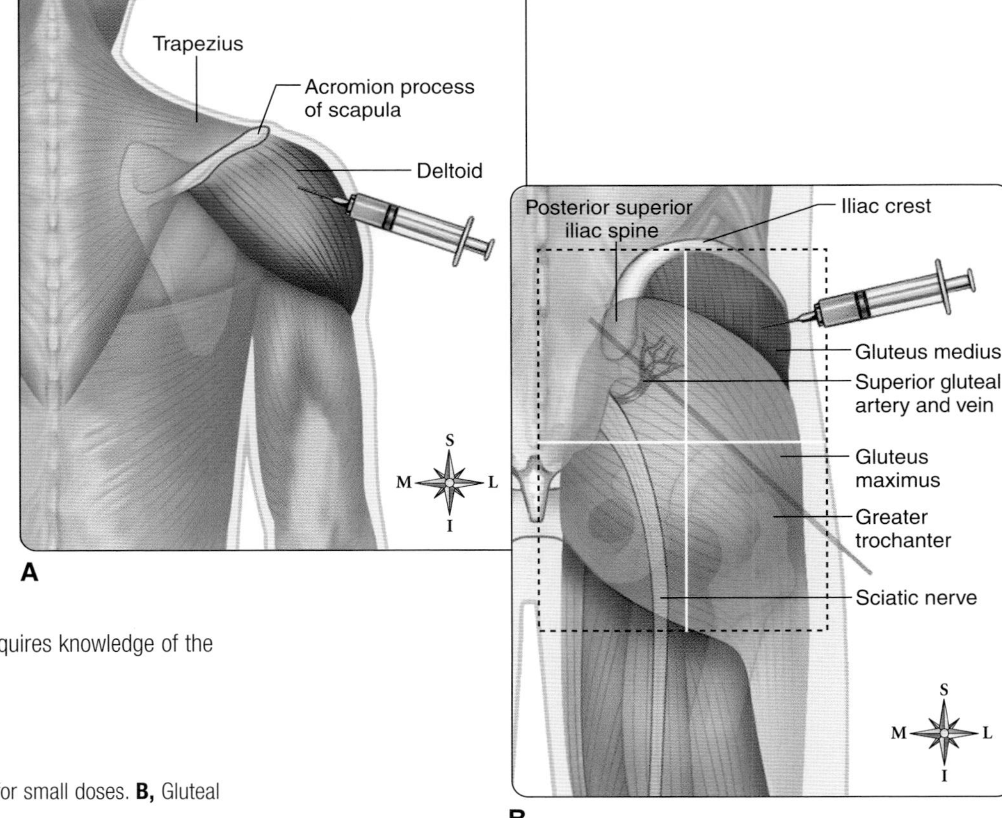

Intramuscular injection sites. A, Deltoid injection site for small doses. **B,** Gluteal injection site for larger doses.

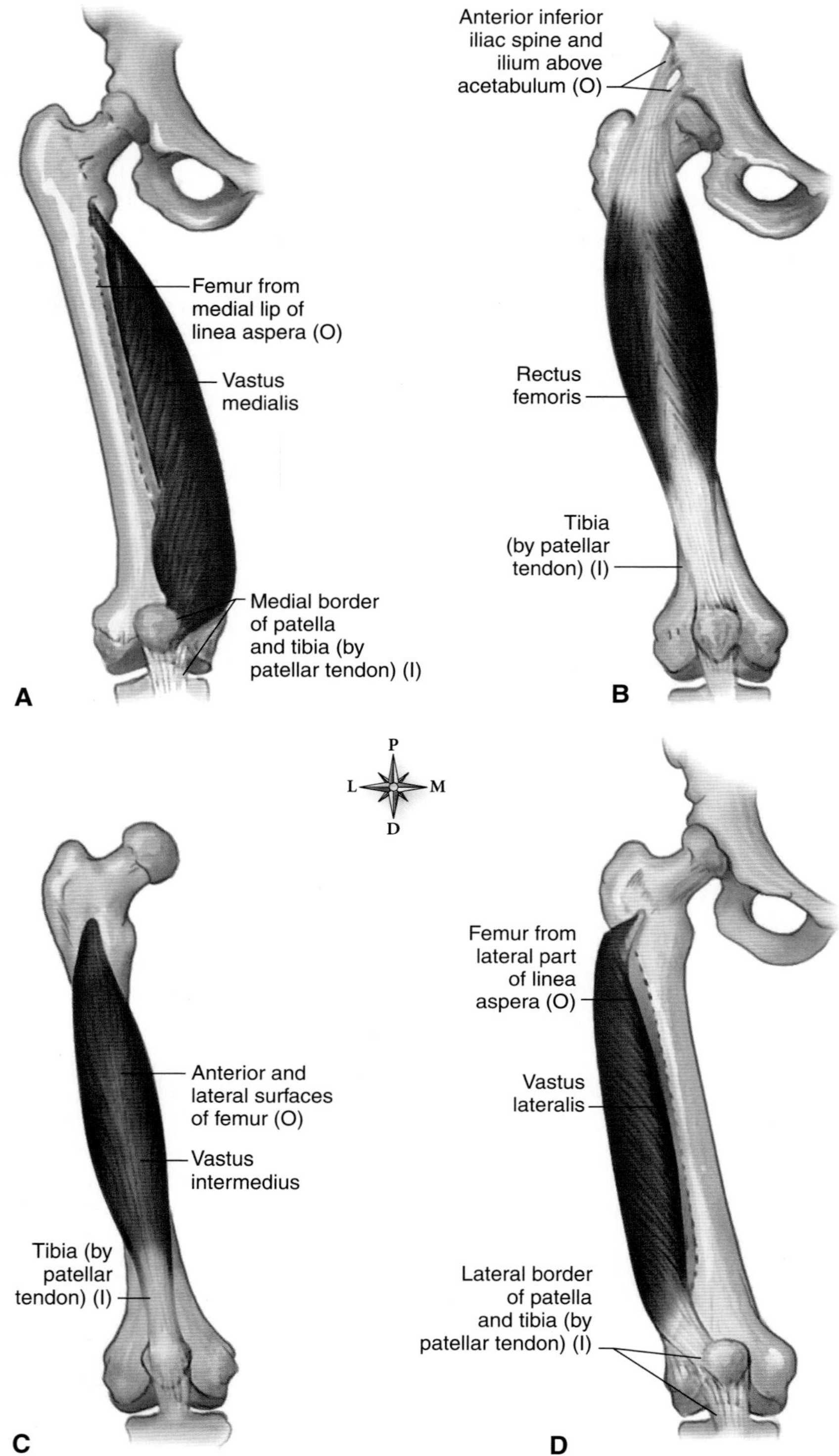

FIGURE 16-16 Quadriceps femoris group of thigh muscles. A, Vastus medialis. **B,** Rectus femoris. **C,** Vastus intermedius. **D,** Vastus lateralis. *O,* Origin; *I,* insertion.

TABLE 16-6 Muscles That Move the Leg

MUSCLE	ORIGIN	INSERTION	FUNCTION	NERVE SUPPLY
Quadriceps femoris group				
Rectus femoris	Ilium (anterior inferior spine)	Tibia (by way of patellar tendon)	Flexes the thigh Extends the leg	Femoral nerve
Vastus lateralis	Femur (linea aspera)	Tibia (by way of the patellar tendon)	Extends the leg	Femoral nerve
Vastus medialis	Femur	Tibia (by way of the patellar tendon)	Extends the leg	Femoral nerve
Vastus intermedius	Femur (anterior surface)	Tibia (by way of the patellar tendon)	Extends the leg	Femoral nerve
Sartorius	Coxal (anterior superior iliac spines)	Tibia (medial surface of the upper end of the shaft)	Adducts and flexes the leg Permits crossing of the legs tailor fashion	Femoral nerve
Hamstring group				
Biceps femoris	Ischium (tuberosity)	Fibula (head of)	Extends the thigh; flexes the leg	Common fibular nerve
	Femur (linea aspera)	Tibia (lateral condyle)	Flexes the leg	Tibial nerve
Semitendinosus	Ischium (tuberosity)	Tibia (proximal end, medial surface)	Extends the thigh; flexes the leg	Tibial nerve
Semimembranosus	Ischium (tuberosity)	Tibia (medial condyle)	Extends the thigh; flexes the leg	Tibial nerve

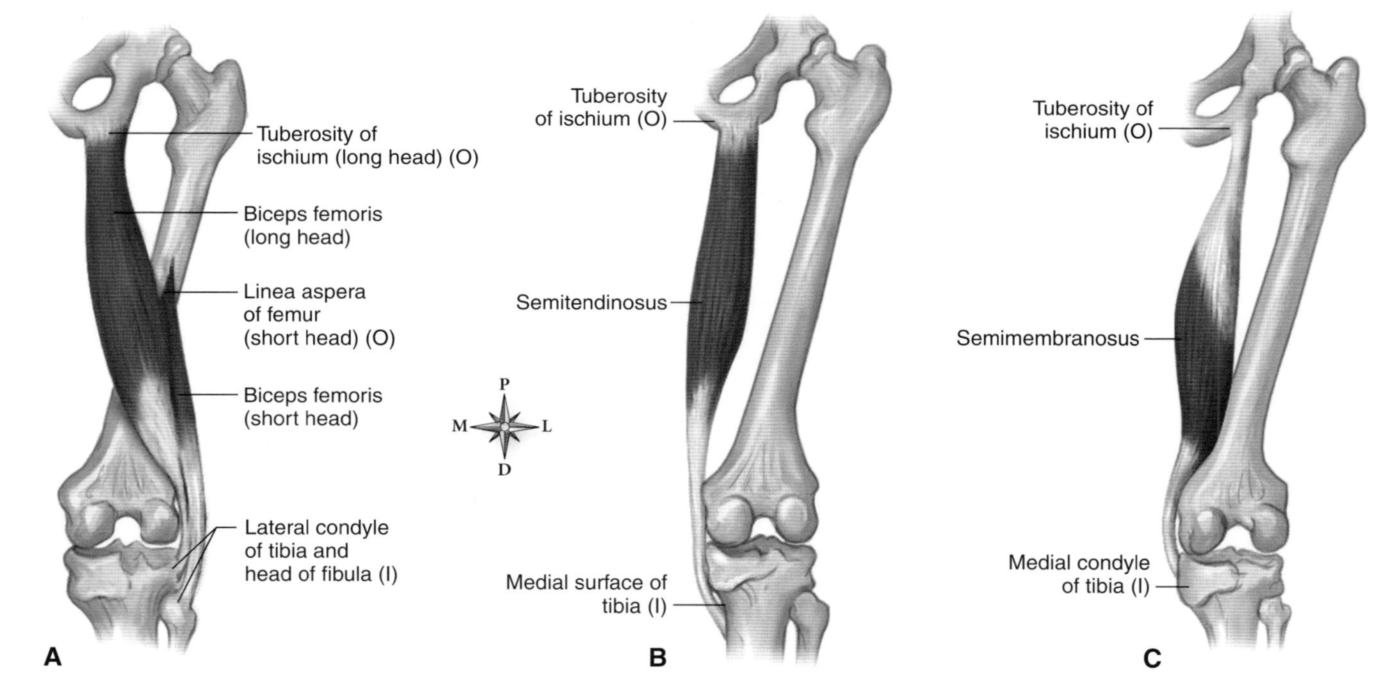

FIGURE 16-17 Hamstring group of thigh muscles. A, Biceps femoris. **B,** Semitendinosus. **C,** Semimembranosus. *O,* Origin; *I,* insertion.

Muscles That Move the Ankle and Foot

The muscles listed in **Table 16-7** and shown in **Figure 16-18** are responsible for movements of the ankle and foot. These muscles, called **extrinsic foot muscles,** are located in the leg but exert their actions by pulling on tendons that insert on bones in the ankle and foot. Extrinsic foot muscles are responsible for such movements as dorsiflexion, plantar flexion, inversion, and eversion of the foot. Muscles located within the foot itself are called **intrinsic foot muscles** (**Figure 16-19**). They are responsible for flexion, extension, abduction, and adduction of the toes.

The extrinsic muscles listed in **Table 16-7** may be divided into four functional groups: (1) dorsal flexors, (2) plantar flexors, (3) invertors, and (4) evertors of the foot.

The superficial muscles located on the posterior surface of the leg form the bulging "calf". The common tendon of the **gastrocnemius** and **soleus** is called the **calcaneal,** or *Achilles,* **tendon.** It inserts into the calcaneus, or heel bone. By acting together, these muscles serve as powerful flexors (plantar flexion) of the foot.

Dorsal flexors of the foot, located on the anterior surface of the leg, include the **tibialis anterior, fibularis tertius**, and **extensor digitorum longus.** In addition to functioning as a dorsiflexor of the foot, the extensor digitorum longus also everts the foot and extends the toes. Note in **Table 16-7** that the fibularis muscles are also called **peroneus muscles.**

Quick CHECK

4. Name the three gluteal muscles.
5. What is the function of the gastrocnemius muscle?

TABLE 16-7 Muscles That Move the Foot

MUSCLE	ORIGIN	INSERTION	FUNCTION	NERVE SUPPLY
Extrinsic				
Tibialis anterior	Tibia (lateral condyle of the upper body)	Tarsal (first cuneiform) Metatarsal (base of first)	Flexes the foot Inverts the foot	Common and deep peroneal nerves
Gastrocnemius	Femur (condyles)	Tarsal (calcaneus by way of the Achilles tendon)	Extends the foot Flexes leg	Tibial nerve (branch of the sciatic nerve)
Soleus	Tibia (underneath the gastrocnemius) Fibula	Tarsal (calcaneus by way of the Achilles tendon)	Extends the foot (plantar flexion)	Tibial nerve
Fibularis longus (peroneus longus)	Tibia (lateral condyle)	First cuneiform	Extends the foot (plantar flexion)	Common peroneal nerve
	Fibula (head and shaft)	Base of the first metatarsal	Everts the foot	
Fibularis brevis (peroneus brevis)	Fibula (lower two thirds of the lateral surface of the shaft)	Fifth metatarsal (tubercle, dorsal surface)	Everts the foot Flexes the foot	Superficial peroneal nerve
Fibularis tertius (peroneus tertius)	Fibula (distal third)	Fourth and fifth metatarsals (bases of)	Flexes the foot Everts the foot	Deep peroneal nerve
Extensor digitorum longus	Tibia (lateral condyle) Fibula (anterior surface)	Second and third phalanges (four lateral toes)	Dorsiflexion of the foot; extension of the toes	Deep peroneal nerve
Intrinsic				
Lumbricals	Tendons of the flexor digitorum longus	Phalanges (2 to 5)	Flex the proximal phalanges Extend the middle and distal phalanges	Lateral and medial plantar nerve
Flexor digiti minimi brevis	Fifth metatarsal	Proximal phalanx of the fifth toe	Flexes the fifth (small) toe	Lateral plantar nerve
Flexor hallucis brevis	Cuboid Medial and lateral cuneiform	Proximal phalanx of the first (great) toe	Flexes the first (great) toe	Medial and lateral plantar nerve
Flexor digitorum brevis	Calcaneus Plantar fascia	Middle phalanges of the toes (2 to 5)	Flexes toes 2 through 5	Medial plantar nerve
Abductor digiti minimi	Calcaneus	Proximal phalanx of the fifth (small) toe	Abducts the fifth (small) toe Flexes the fifth toe	Lateral plantar nerve
Abductor hallucis	Calcaneus	First (great) toe	Abducts the first (great) toe	Medial plantar nerve

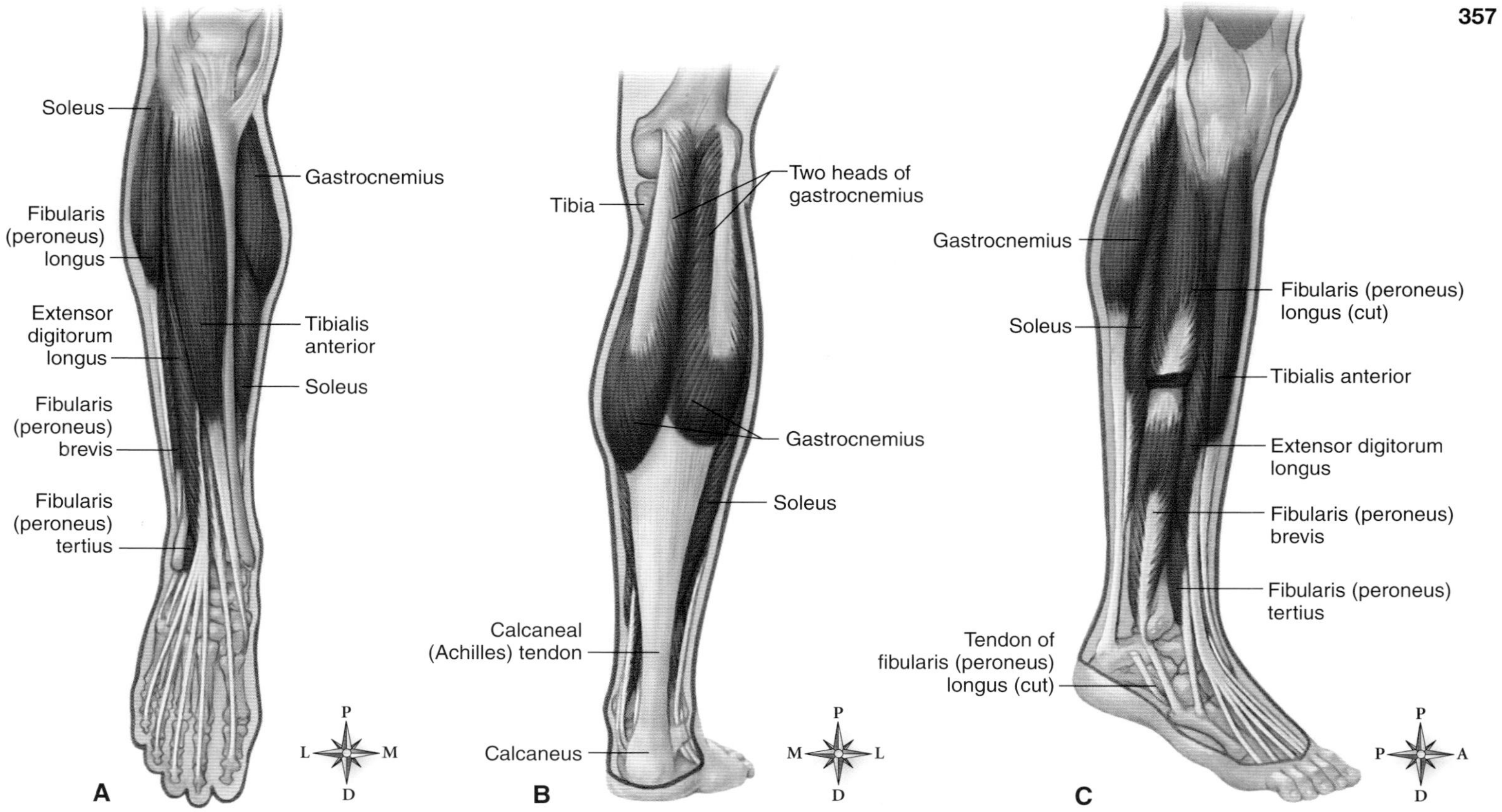

Soleus
Gastrocnemius
Fibularis (peroneus) longus
Extensor digitorum longus
Tibialis anterior
Soleus
Fibularis (peroneus) brevis
Fibularis (peroneus) tertius
A
Tibia
Two heads of gastrocnemius
Gastrocnemius
Soleus
Calcaneal (Achilles) tendon
Calcaneus
B
Gastrocnemius
Soleus
Fibularis (peroneus) longus (cut)
Tibialis anterior
Extensor digitorum longus
Fibularis (peroneus) brevis
Fibularis (peroneus) tertius
Tendon of fibularis (peroneus) longus (cut)
C

FIGURE 16-18 Superficial muscles of the leg. **A,** Anterior view. **B,** Posterior view. **C,** Lateral view.

Lumbricals
Flexor digiti minimi brevis
Abductor digiti minimi
Flexor hallucis brevis
Flexor digitorum brevis
Abductor hallucis
Plantar fascia (cut)

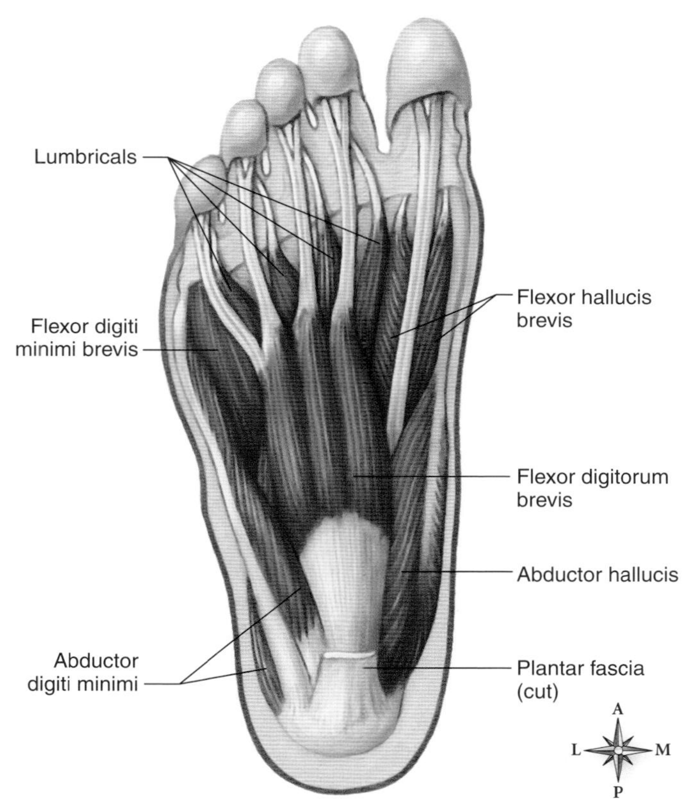

FIGURE 16-19 Intrinsic muscles of the foot. Inferior (plantar) view.

POSTURE

We have already discussed the major role of muscles in movement and heat production. We now turn our attention to a third way in which muscles serve the body as a whole—that of maintaining the posture of the body. Let us consider a few aspects of this important function.

The term **posture** means simply maintaining optimal body position.

"Good posture" means many things. It means body alignment that most favours function; it means the position that requires the least muscular work to maintain, specifically, the position that places the least strain on muscles, ligaments, and bones; and often it means keeping the body's centre of gravity over its base.

Good posture in the standing position, for example, means the head and chest held high; the chin, abdomen, and buttocks pulled in; the knees bent slightly; and the feet placed firmly on the ground about 15 cm apart. Good posture in a sitting position varies with the position that one is trying to maintain. Good posture during exercise, such as riding a horse or dribbling a basketball, means moving or tensing different parts of the body frequently to avoid falling.

How Posture Is Maintained

Gravity pulls on the various parts of the body at all times. Because bones are too irregularly shaped to balance themselves on each other, the only way the body can be held in any particular position is for muscles to exert a continual pull on bones. The muscles must pull in the opposite direction from gravity or other forces that pull on body parts.

When the body is in a standing position, gravity tends to pull the head and trunk forward and downward. Extensor muscles must therefore pull backward and upward on the head and trunk. Likewise, as gravity pulls the lower jaw downward; muscles must pull upward on it—to keep the mouth closed.

Muscles exert their pull against gravity by virtue of a property called **tonicity.** Tonicity, or **muscle tone,** literally means *tension* and refers to the continuous, low level of sustained contraction maintained by all skeletal muscles. Because tonicity is absent during deep sleep, muscle pull does not then counteract the pull of gravity. Hence, we cannot sleep standing up. Interestingly, astronauts in the low-gravity conditions of space station missions *can* sleep in a standing position, as long as they are secured inside special sleeping bags on the wall of the space station.

Many structures other than muscles and bones play a part in the maintenance of posture. The nervous system triggers skeletal muscle contractions and is thus responsible for the existence of muscle tone. The nervous system regulates and coordinates the amount of pull exerted by the individual muscles. Breathing in the respiratory system, abdominal activity by the digestive system, and other systemic activities all can affect posture. This is one of many examples of the important principle that body functions are interdependent.

The importance of posture can perhaps be best evaluated by considering some of the effects of poor posture. Poor posture throws more work on muscles to counteract the pull of gravity and therefore leads to fatigue more quickly than does good posture. Poor posture puts more strain on ligaments. It puts abnormal strain on bones and may eventually produce deformities. It also interferes with various functions such as respiration, heart action, and digestion.

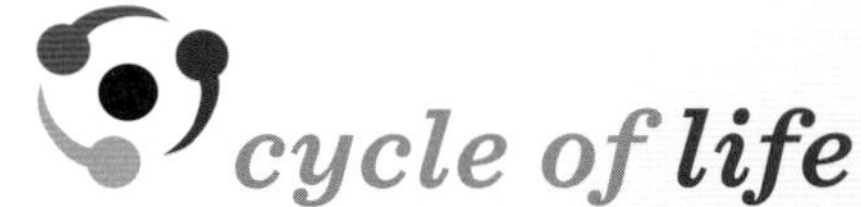

Muscular System Acting together, the muscular, skeletal, and nervous systems make it possible for us to move in a coordinated and controlled way. However, it is the contraction, or shortening, of muscles that ultimately provides the actual movement necessary for physical activity. Dramatic changes occur in the muscular system throughout the cycle of life. Muscle cells may increase or decrease in size and in their ability to shorten most effectively at different periods in life. In addition to age-related changes, many pathological conditions occurring at different ages may also affect the muscular system.

Because of the functional interdependence of the musculoskeletal and nervous systems, life cycle changes affecting the muscles often manifest in other components of the functional unit. During infancy and childhood, the ability to coordinate and control the strength of muscle contraction permits a sequential series of developmental steps to occur. A developing youngster learns to hold the head up, roll over, sit up, stand alone, and then walk and run as developmental changes permit better control and coordination of muscular contraction.

Degenerative changes associated with advancing age often result in replacement of muscle cell volume with nonfunctional connective tissue. As a result, the strength of muscular contraction diminishes. Recent findings show that much, if not all, of this age-related decrease in muscle strength actually results from disuse atrophy (see **Box 17-6** in Chapter 17) and may thus be avoidable. Pathological conditions associated with specific age ranges can also affect one or more components of the functional unit that permits us to move smoothly and effortlessly. •

CONNECT IT! ⓔ

As we discussed several times in the last two chapters, it is important to remember that muscles, tendons, and fascia work in teams to maintain posture and produce movement. Explore one of the ways that they work together in ***Whole-Body Muscle Mechanics*** online at ***Connect It!***

Quick CHECK

6. Define the term posture.
7. How does muscle tone relate to posture?
8. What effect might bad posture have on the body?

the big picture | Appendicular Muscles and the Whole Body

In the last two chapters, we saw how groups of muscles act as teams to move the skeleton in ways that allow normal function of the body. In this chapter, we explored the appendicular muscles that allow us to move our body around, to make things, and to use things. Getting food, water, shelter, and warmth require the actions of our arms and legs. Defending ourselves from predators or other dangers also requires the use of our extremity muscles. We also learned about the role of skeletal muscles in helping us maintain safe, stable positions as we live our daily lives.

Taking another step back, an even bigger picture comes into focus. Other systems of the body must play a role in the actions of the skeletomuscular system. For example, the nervous system senses changes in body position and degrees of movement—thereby permitting integration of feedback loops that ultimately regulate the muscular contractions that maintain posture and produce movements. The cardiovascular system maintains blood flow in the muscles, and the urinary and respiratory systems rid the body of wastes produced in the muscles. The respiratory and digestive systems bring in the oxygen and nutrients necessary for muscle function.

The picture is still not complete, however. We will see even more when Chapter 17 continues the story of muscle function by delving into the details of how each muscle works as an engine to drive the movement of the body. •

LANGUAGE OF SCIENCE *(continued from p. 337)*

muscle tone
[*mus-* **mouse,** *-cle* **little,** *ton-* **tension**]

opponens pollicis muscle
(o-POH-nenz POL-ih-sis)
[*opponens* **opposing,** *pollicis* **pole,** *mus-* **mouse,** *-cle* **little**]

pectoralis minor (pek-toh-RAL-is)
[*pector-* **breast,** *-al* **relating to,** *minor* **lesser**]

peroneus muscle (per-oh-NEE-us)
[*peroneus* **pin (of brooch or buckle)**]

posture (POS-chur)
[*postur-* **position**]

rhomboid major/minor muscles
(ROM-boyd)
[*rhombo-* **flatfish or equilateral parallelogram (rhombus),** *-oid* **like,** *major* **greater,** *minor* **lesser,** *mus-* **mouse,** *-cle* **little**]

rotator cuff muscle (roh-TAY-tor)
[*rot-* **turn,** *-ator* **agent,** *mus-* **mouse,** *-cle* **little**]

serratus anterior muscle
(ser-RAY-tus an-TEER-ee-or)
[*serra-* **saw teeth,** *-us* **thing,** *ante-* **front,** *-er-* **more,** *-or* **quality,** *mus-* **mouse,** *-cle* **little**]

soleus muscle (SOH-lee-us)
[*soleus* **sole of foot,** *mus-* **mouse,** *-cle* **little**]

subscapularis muscle
(sub-skap-yoo-LAR-is)
[*sub-* **beneath,** *-scapula-* **shoulder blades,** *-ar* **relating to,** *mus-* **mouse,** *-cle* **little**]

supraspinatus muscle
(SOO-prah-spy-nah-tus)
[*supra-* **above,** *-spina-* **spine,** *mus-* **mouse,** *-cle* **little**]

tensor fasciae latae muscle
(TEN-sor FASH-ee LAT-tee)
[*tensor* **stretcher,** *fascia* **band or bundle,** *lat-* **side,** *mus-* **mouse,** *-cle* **little**]

teres minor (TER-eez)
[*teres* **rounded,** *minor* **lesser**]

tibialis anterior muscle (tib-ee-AL-is)
[*tibia* **shinbone,** *-al* **relating to,** *ante-* **front,** *-er-* **more,** *-or* **quality,** *mus-* **mouse,** *-cle* **little**]

tonicity (toh-NIS-i-tee)
[*ton-* **stretch or tension,** *-ic* **relating to,** *-ty* **state**]

trapezius muscle (trah-PEE-zee-us)
[*trapezi-* **small table,** *mus-* **mouse,** *-cle* **little**]

LANGUAGE OF MEDICINE

carpal tunnel syndrome
(KAR-pul TUN-el SIN-drohm)
[*carp-* **wrist,** *-al* **relating to,** *syn-* **together,** *-drome* **running or (race) course**]

intramuscular injection
(in-trah-MUSS-kyoo-lar in-JEK-shun)
[*intra-* **within,** *mus-* **mouse,** *-cle* **little,** *-ar* **relating to,** *in-* **in,** *-ject-* **throw,** *-tion* **process**]

tenosynovitis (ten-oh-sin-oh-VYE-tis)
[*teno-* **pulled tight (tendon),** *-syn-* **together,** *-ovi-* **egg white (joint fluid),** *-itis* **inflammation**]

case study

Jack is a 15-year-old boy who enjoys playing football. He has been playing for almost 8 years, and until now he had not been hampered by any serious injuries. During his last game he collided with another player and incurred a severe injury to his posterior lower leg. Immediately after the collision, Jack's father took him to Accident and Emergency at the local hospital. X-ray examination ruled out any broken bones and the specialty registrar prescribed rest and physiotherapy for the injured muscles.

1. Which of these muscles did Jack likely injure?
   a. Biceps femoris
   b. Tibialis anterior
   c. Gastrocnemius
   d. Vastus medialis
2. Jack complained that although his lower leg hurt, he was also having difficulty moving his foot. Why would an injury to the lower leg affect the movement of his foot?
   a. The extrinsic muscles located in the lower leg exert their actions by pulling on tendons that insert on bones in the ankle and foot.
   b. The intrinsic muscles located in the lower leg exert their actions by pulling on tendons that insert on bones in the ankle and foot.
   c. The antagonistic muscles in the lower leg control the movement of the foot by contracting the intrinsic muscles of the ankle and foot.
   d. The prime mover of the ankle and the foot is located in the lower leg.
3. Fortunately, Jack had not damaged his calcaneal (Achilles) tendon. This is a common tendon to which muscles?
   a. Tibialis anterior and fibularis tertius
   b. Tibialis anterior and extensor digitorum longus
   c. Gastrocnemius and peroneus tertius
   d. Gastrocnemius and soleus
4. Had Jack injured his calcaneal tendon, how would this have affected his movement?
   a. He would not have been able to extend his foot.
   b. Dorsiflexion of the foot would have been limited.
   c. He would have had difficulty flexing the knee.
   d. Plantar flexion of the foot would have been limited.

Hint To solve a case study, you may have to refer to the glossary or index, other chapters in this textbook, ***Connect It!,*** and other resources.

CHAPTER SUMMARY

To download an MP3 version of the chapter summary for use with your mobile device, access the ***Audio Chapter Summaries*** *online at evolve.elsevier.com.*

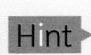

Scan this summary after reading the chapter to help you reinforce the key concepts. Later, use the summary as a quick review before your class or before a test.

Appendicular Muscles

A. Muscles can be grouped according to axial (central) and appendicular (peripheral) location in the body
B. This chapter focuses on appendicular muscles; the previous chapter focused on axial muscles

Upper Extremity Muscles

A. Muscles acting on the shoulder girdle—muscles that attach the upper extremity to the torso are located anteriorly (chest) or posteriorly (back and neck); these muscles also allow extensive movement (**Figure 16-2**; **Table 16-1**)
B. Muscles that move the arm—the shoulder is a synovial joint allowing extensive movement in every plane of motion (**Figure 16-3**; **Table 16-2**)
C. Muscles that move the forearm—found proximal to the elbow and attach to the ulna and radius (**Figures 16-5**, **16-6**, and **16-7**; **Table 16-3**)
D. Muscles that move the wrist, hand, and fingers—these muscles are located on the anterior or posterior surfaces of the forearm (**Figures 16-8** through **16-10**; **Table 16-4**)

Lower Extremity Muscles

A. The pelvic girdle and lower extremity function in locomotion and maintenance of stability
B. Muscles that move the thigh and leg (**Figures 16-1** and **16-11** through **16-17**; **Tables 16-5** and **16-6**)
C. Muscles that move the ankle and foot (**Figures 16-18** and **16-19**; **Table 16-7**)
   1. Extrinsic foot muscles in the leg pull on tendons that insert on bones in the ankle and foot; responsible for dorsiflexion, plantar flexion, inversion, and eversion
   2. Intrinsic foot muscles are located within the foot; responsible for flexion, extension, abduction, and adduction of the toes

Posture

A. Maintaining body posture is a major role of muscles
B. "Good posture"—body alignment that most favours function; achieved by keeping the body's centre of gravity over its base and requires the least muscular work to maintain
C. How posture is maintained
   1. Muscles exert a continual pull on bones in the opposite direction from gravity
   2. Structures other than muscle and bones have a role in maintaining posture
      a. Nervous system—responsible for the existence of muscle tone and also for regulation and coordination of the amount of pull exerted by individual muscles
      b. Respiratory, digestive, excretory, and endocrine systems all contribute to maintain posture

Cycle of Life: Muscular System

A. Muscle cells—increase or decrease in number, size, and ability to shorten at different periods
B. Pathological conditions at different periods of the life cycle may affect the muscular system
C. Life cycle changes—manifest in other components of the functional unit
   1. Infancy and childhood—coordination and control of muscle contraction permit sequential development steps
D. Degenerative changes of advancing age result in replacement of muscle cells with nonfunctional connective tissue

REVIEW QUESTIONS

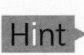

Write out the answers to these questions after reading the chapter and reviewing the Chapter Summary. Note—writing out your answers will consolidate learning and provide a valuable resource of information.

1. Name the main muscles of the shoulder, the arm, forearm, thigh, and leg.
2. Name the main muscles that flex, extend, abduct, and adduct the arm; that raise and lower the shoulder.
3. Name the main muscles that flex and extend the forearm; that flex and extend the wrist and hand.
4. Which muscle allows the thumb to be drawn across the palm to touch the tip of any finger?
5. Name the main muscles that flex, extend, abduct, and adduct the thigh; that flex and extend the leg and thigh; that flex and extend the foot.
6. Of the gluteal muscles, which one is often the site of intramuscular injections?
7. Identify a pair of muscles that are both synergist and antagonist with regard to the arm. Suggest which attachment allows them to be connected in this way.

CRITICAL THINKING QUESTIONS

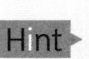

After finishing the Review Questions, write out the answers to these more in-depth questions to help you apply your new knowledge. Go back to sections of the chapter that relate to concepts that you find difficult.

1. Describe how the body maintains posture.
2. Describe the clinical significance of the difference in size between the large head of the humerus and the small and shallow glenoid cavity of the scapula.
3. If a person working as a word processor complained of weakness, pain, and tingling in the palm and thumb side of the hand, what type of problem might that person be experiencing? Explain specifically what would be happening to cause this discomfort.
4. Tennis players and cricket bowlers often incur rotator cuff injuries. List the muscles that make up the rotator cuff and explain the importance of these muscles and their role in joint stability.
5. Many drugs are administered by intramuscular injection. If the amount to be injected is 2 to 3 mL, which area is used?
6. Which muscle is used to "shrug" the shoulders? Identify another action of the muscle you have named. Speculate what key factor must change for this action to occur.

17 Muscle Contraction

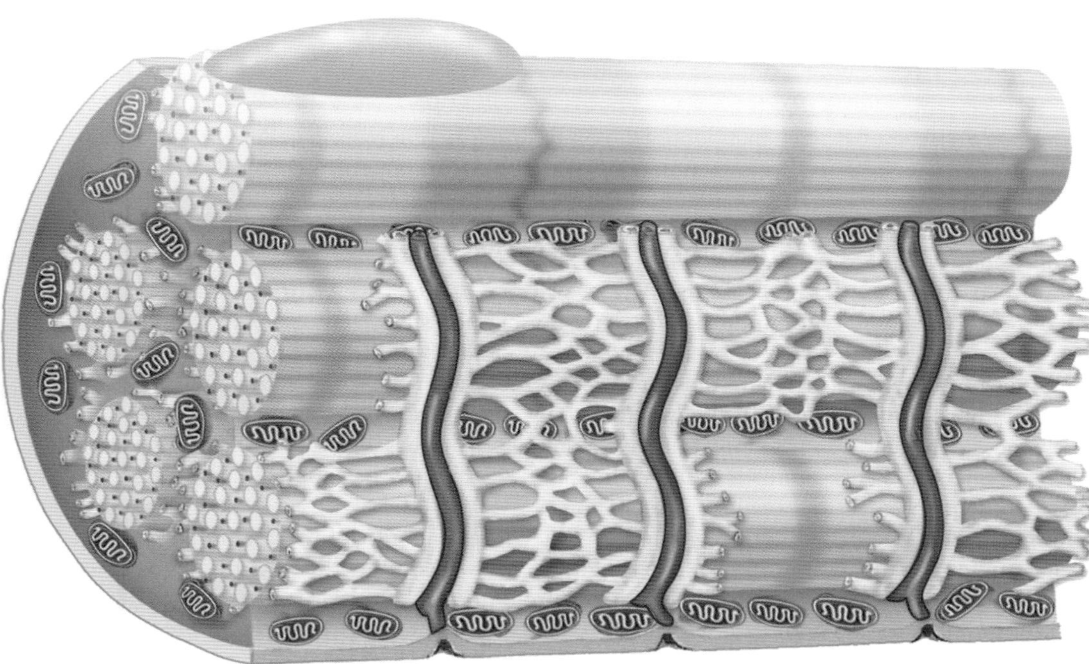

CHAPTER OUTLINE

Hint *Scan this outline before you begin to read the chapter, as a preview of how the concepts are organized.*

LANGUAGE OF SCIENCE

Hint *Use this list to aid your pronunciation of unfamiliar words.*

A band
[*A* **anisotropic**]

acetylcholine (ACh)
(ass-ee-til-KOH-leen)
[*acetyl-* **vinegar,** *-chol-* **bile,** *-ine* **made of**]

actin (AK-tin)
[*act-* **act or do,** *-in* **substance**]

concentric contraction
(kon-SEN-trik kon-TRAK-shun)
[*con-* **together,** *-centr-* **centre,** *-ic* **relating to,** *con-* **together,** *-tract-* **drag or draw,** *-tion* **process**]

contractility (kon-trak-TIL-i-tee)
[*con-* **together,** *-tract-* **drag or draw,** *-il-* **of or like,** *-ity* **quality of**]

creatine phosphate (CP)
(KREE-ah-tin FOS-fayt)
[*creat-* **flesh,** *-ine* **relating to,** *phosph-* **phosphorus,** *-ate* **oxygen**]

eccentric contraction
(ek-SENT-rik kon-TRAK-shun)
[*ec-* **out of,** *-centr-* **centre,** *-ic* **relating to,** *con-* **together,** *-tract-* **drag or draw,** *-tion* **process**]

elastic filament
(eh-LAS-tik FIL-ah-ment)
[*elas-* **drive or propel,** *-ic* **relating to,** *fila-* **thread,** *-ment* **thing**]

excitability (ek-syte-eh-BIL-i-tee)
[*excit-* **arouse,** *-abil-* **capable,** *-ity* **state**]

extensibility (ek-STEN-si-BIL-i-tee)
[*ex-* **outward,** *-tens-* **stretch,** *-abil-* **capable,** *-ity* **state**]

H band
[*H heller* **bright**]

hypertrophy (hye-PER-troh-fee)
[*hyper-* **excessive,** *-troph-* **nourishment,** *-y* **state**]

I band
[*I* **isotropic**]

intermediate fibre (in-ter-MEE-dee-it)
[*inter-* **between,** *-medi-* **middle,** *-ate* **of or like**]

isometric contraction
(eye-soh-MET-rik kon-TRAK-shun)
[*iso-* **equal,** *-metr-* **measure,** *-ic* **relating to,** *con-* **together,** *-tract-* **drag or draw,** *-tion* **process**]

continued on p. 386

In Chapters 15 and 16, we explored the anatomy of skeletal muscle organs and how they work together to accomplish specific body movements. In this chapter, we continue our study of the muscular system by examining the basic characteristics of skeletal muscle tissue. We uncover the mechanisms of contraction that permit skeletal muscle tissue to move the body's framework, as well as perform other functions vital to maintaining a constant internal environment. We also briefly examine smooth and cardiac muscle tissues and contrast them with skeletal muscle tissue.

GENERAL FUNCTIONS

If you have any doubts about the importance of muscle function to normal life, think about what it would be like without it. It is hard to imagine what life would be like if this matchless power were lost. However, as cardinal as it is, movement is not the only contribution muscles make to healthy survival. They also perform two other essential functions: production of a large proportion of body heat and maintenance of posture.

1. **Movement.** Skeletal muscle contractions produce movement of the body as a whole (locomotion) or movement of its parts.
2. **Heat production.** Muscle cells, like all cells, produce heat by the process known as catabolism (discussed in Chapters 6 and 41). The heat produced by just one cell is inconsequential, but because skeletal muscle cells are both highly active and numerous, together they produce a major share of total body heat. Skeletal muscle contractions therefore constitute one of the most important parts of the mechanism for maintaining homeostasis of temperature.
3. **Posture.** The continued partial contraction of many skeletal muscles makes possible standing, sitting, and maintaining a relatively stable position of the body while walking, running, or performing other movements.

FUNCTION OF SKELETAL MUSCLE TISSUE

FUNCTIONAL CHARACTERISTICS OF MUSCLE

Skeletal muscle cells have several characteristics that permit them to function as they do. One such characteristic is the ability to be stimulated, often called **excitability** or *irritability*. Because skeletal muscle cells are excitable, they can respond to regulatory mechanisms such as nerve signals.

Contractility of muscle cells, the ability to contract or shorten, allows muscle tissue to pull on bones and thus produce body movement. Sometimes muscle fibres do work by steadily resisting a load without actually becoming shorter. In such a case, the muscle cell is still said to be contracting. The term *contraction*, when applied to muscles, is meant in a broad sense of pulling the ends together—regardless of whether the cell actually gets shorter.

Extensibility, the ability to extend or stretch, allows muscles to return to their resting length after having contracted. Muscles may also extend while still exerting force, as when lowering a heavy object in your hand.

All of these characteristics of muscle cells are related to the microscopic structure of skeletal muscle cells. In the following passages, we first discuss the basic structure of a muscle cell. We then explain how a muscle cell's structural components allow it to perform its unique functions.

OVERVIEW OF THE MUSCLE CELL

Look at **Figure 17-1**. As you can see, a skeletal muscle is composed of bundles of skeletal muscle fibres that generally extend the entire length of the muscle. Muscle cells or *myocytes* are most frequently called "muscle fibres". One reason they are often called *fibres* instead of *cells* is their long, thin, threadlike shape. They are 1 to 40 mm long but have a diameter of only 10 to 100 μm. The gastrocnemius muscle of the calf, for example, has approximately a million threadlike muscle fibres.

During muscle tissue development, individual precursor cells fuse together to form a new, combined structure with many nuclei—the mature muscle fibre. That is why muscle fibres do not follow the general rule of one nucleus per cell: each fibre is made up of several cells that are combined into one. Some adult muscle fibres have one of these tiny precursor cells hugging their outer boundary. These *satellite cells* are stem cells that fuse with myocytes during strength training to make bigger muscle fibres. The satellite cells can also become active after a muscle injury to produce more muscle fibres. Scientists are now trying to understand this mechanism better in the hope of developing new therapies for replacing lost muscle tissues.

Skeletal muscle fibres have many of the same structural parts as other cells. Several of these parts, however, are referred to by different names with regard to muscle fibres. For example, **sarcolemma** is a name often used for the plasma membrane of a muscle fibre. **Sarcoplasm** is its cytoplasm.

Muscle fibres contain many more mitochondria than usually found in other types of cells (**Figure 17-2**), and as we have already learned, each fibre has several nuclei. Muscle cells contain networks of tubules and sacs known as the **sarcoplasmic reticulum (SR)**—the muscle fibre's version of smooth endoplasmic reticulum. The function of the SR is to temporarily store calcium ions (Ca^{++}). The membrane of the SR continually pumps Ca^{++} from the sarcoplasm and stores the ions within its sacs.

A structure unique to muscle cells is a system of transverse tubules, or **T tubules.** This name derives from the fact that these tubules extend transversely across the sarcoplasm, at a right angle to the long axis of the cell. As **Figures 17-1**, *B*, and **17-2** show, T tubules are formed by inward extensions of the sarcolemma. The chief function of T tubules is to allow electrical signals, or *impulses*, travelling along the sarcolemma to move deeper into the cell.

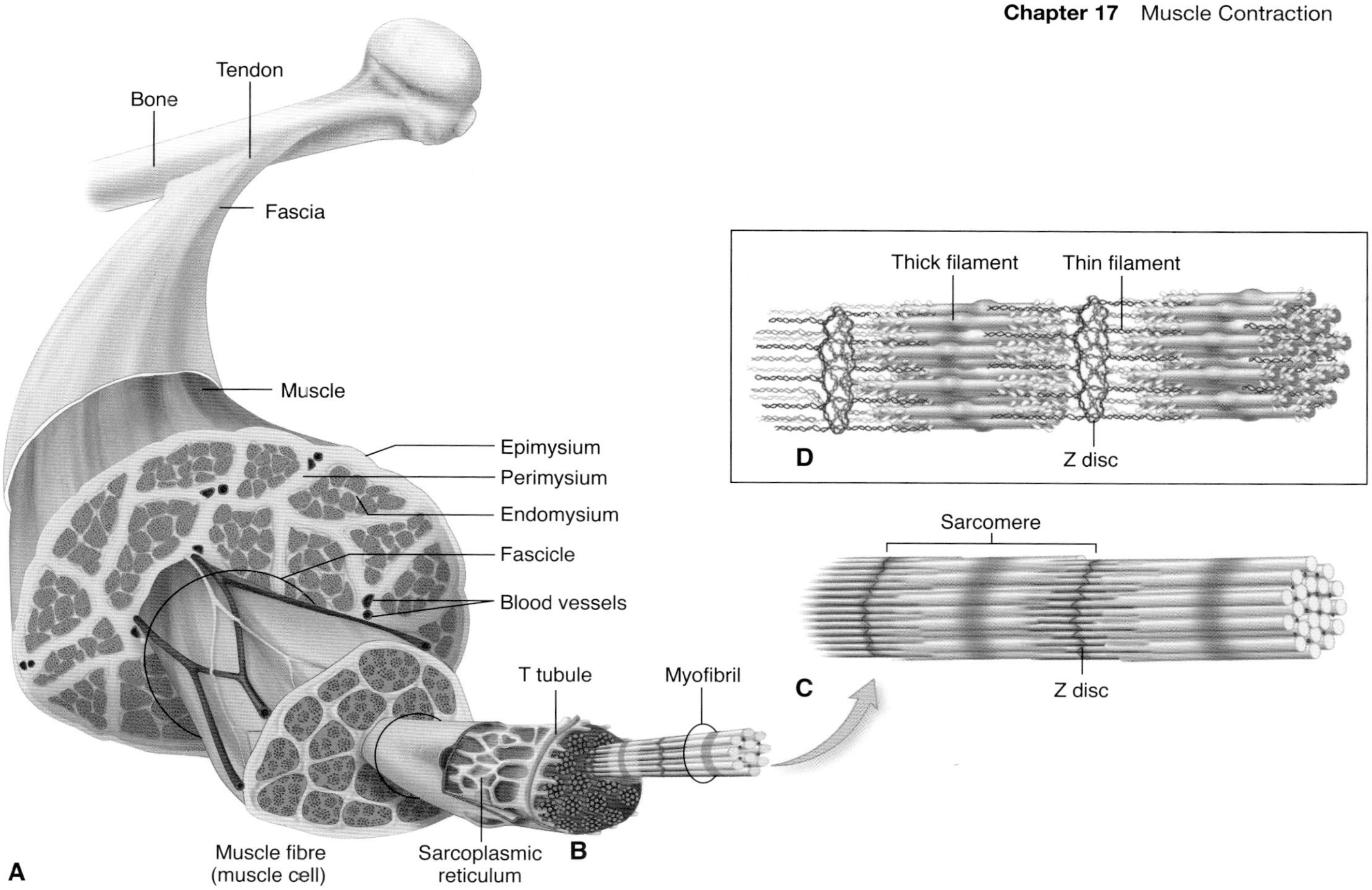

Tendon
Bone
Fascia
Muscle
Epimysium
Perimysium
Endomysium
Fascicle
Blood vessels
T tubule
Myofibril
Muscle fibre (muscle cell)
Sarcoplasmic reticulum
A
B
Thick filament
Thin filament
Z disc
D
Sarcomere
Z disc
C

FIGURE 17-1 Structure of skeletal muscle. A, Skeletal muscle organ composed of bundles of contractile muscle fibres held together by connective tissue. **B,** Greater magnification of a single fibre showing smaller fibres—myofibrils—in the sarcoplasm. Note the sarcoplasmic reticulum and T tubules forming a three-part structure called a *triad.* **C,** Myofibril magnified further to show a sarcomere between successive Z discs (Z lines). Cross striae are visible. **D,** Molecular structure of a myofibril showing thick myofilaments and thin myofilaments.

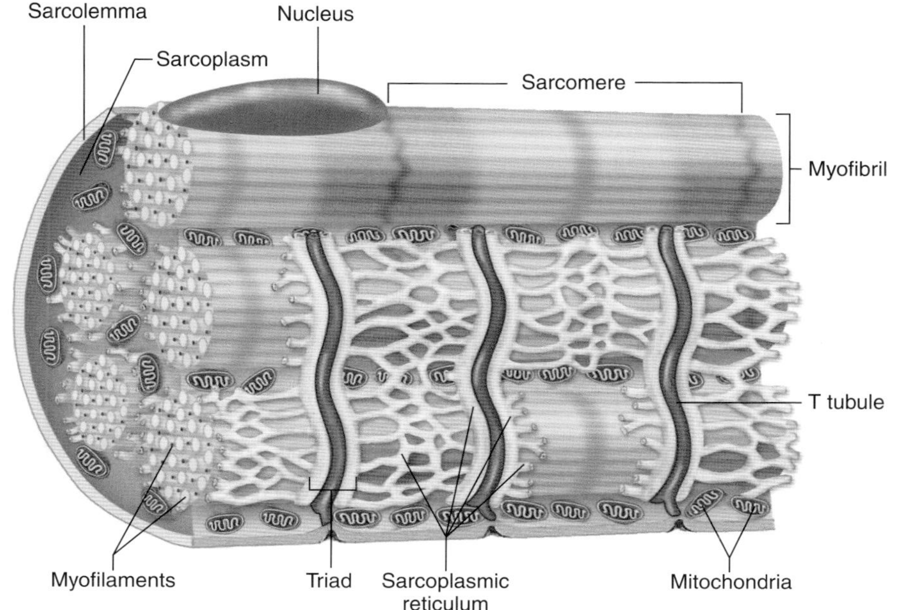

FIGURE 17-2 Unique features of the skeletal muscle cell. Note especially the T tubules, which are extensions of the plasma membrane, or sarcolemma, and the sarcoplasmic reticulum (SR), a type of smooth endoplasmic reticulum that forms networks of tubular canals and sacs containing stored calcium ions. A triad is a triplet of adjacent tubules: a terminal (end) sac of the SR, a T tubule, and another terminal sac of the SR.

Note in **Figures 17-1**, *B*, and **17-2** that a tubular sac of the SR butts up against each side of every T tubule in a muscle fibre. This triplet of tubules (a T tubule sandwiched between sacs of the SR) is called a **triad.** The triad is an important feature of the muscle cell because it allows an electrical impulse travelling along a T tubule to stimulate the membranes of adjacent sacs of the SR. **Figure 17-3** shows how this works. At rest, calcium ion pumps in the SR membrane pump Ca^{++} into the terminal sacs of the SR. However, when an electrical impulse travels along the sarcolemma and down the T tubule, gated Ca^{++} channels in the SR open in response to the voltage fluctuation. This floods the sarcoplasm with calcium ions—an important step in initiating muscle contraction, as we shall see.

Additional structures not found in other cells are present in skeletal muscle fibres. For instance, the cytoskeleton of the muscle fibre is quite unique. **Myofibrils** are bundles of very fine cytoskeletal filaments that extend lengthwise along skeletal muscle fibre and almost fill the sarcoplasm. A typical muscle fibre may have as many as a thousand or more myofibrils tightly packed inside it.

Myofibrils, in turn, are made up of still finer fibres called **myofilaments.** Note in **Figure 17-1**, *D*, that there are two types of myofilaments in the myofibril: *thick filaments* and *thin filaments.* You can see at a glance that some of the filaments are much thicker than others. Although they appear in contrasting colours in the diagram, they are actually colourless.

A **sarcomere** is a segment of the myofibril between two successive **Z discs** (Z lines) (**Box 17-1**). Find the label *sarcomere* in **Figure 17-1**, C. You will note that each myofibril consists of a lineup of many sarcomeres. Each sarcomere functions as a contractile unit. The A bands of sarcomeres appear as relatively wide, dark stripes (cross striae) under the microscope, and they alternate with narrower, lighter-coloured stripes formed by the I bands (see the figure in **Box 17-1**). Because of its cross striations (or *striae*), skeletal muscle is sometimes called *striated muscle.* Electron microscopy of skeletal muscle (**Figure 17-4**) reveals details that help us understand concepts of its structure and function.

Quick CHECK

1. What are the three major functions of the skeletal muscles?
2. Name some features of the muscle cell that are not found in other types of cells.
3. What causes the striations observed in skeletal muscle fibres?
4. Why is the triad relationship between T tubules and the SR important?

MYOFILAMENTS

Each muscle fibre contains a thousand or more parallel myofibrils that are only about 1 μm thick. Lying side by side in each myofibril are approximately 15,000 sarcomeres, each made up of hundreds of thick and thin filaments. The molecular structure of these

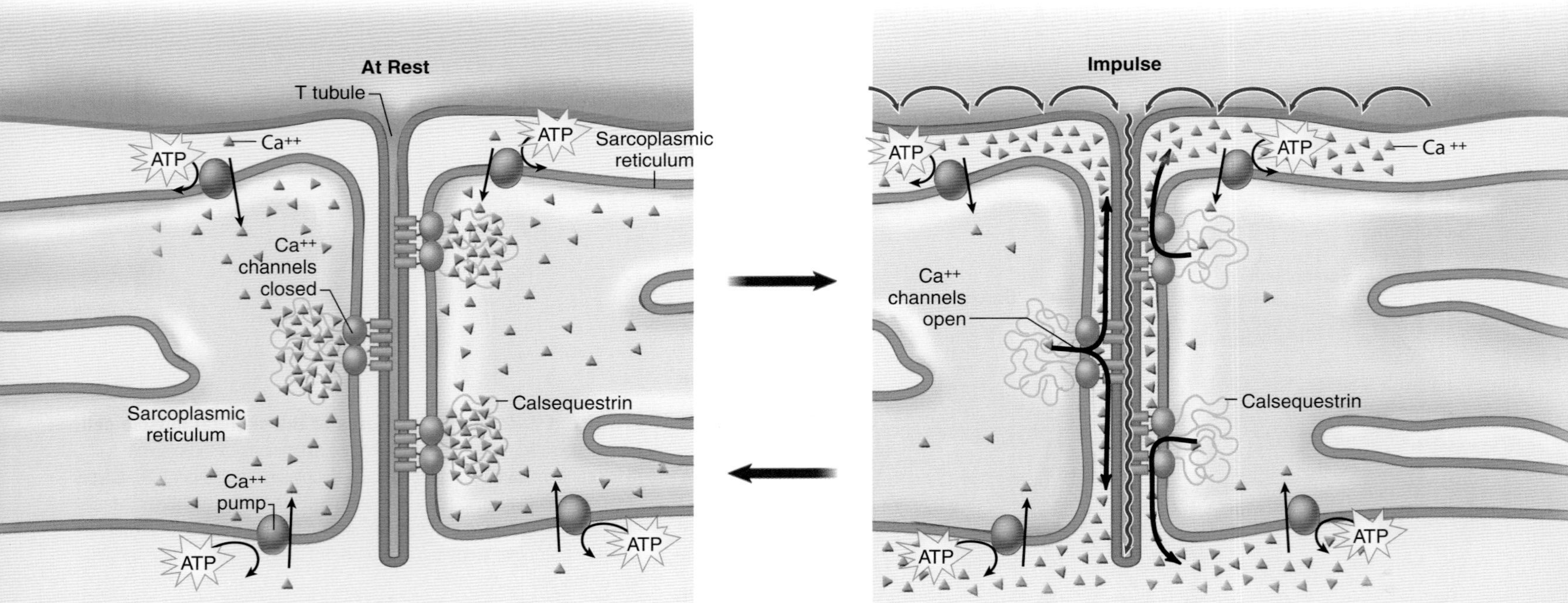

FIGURE 17-3 Storage and release of calcium ions at the triad. At rest *(left),* calcium ion pumps in the sarcoplasmic reticulum (SR) membrane actively pull Ca^{++} into the SR—thus creating a concentration gradient with very little Ca^{++} left in the sarcoplasm. Note that the Ca^{++} is sequestered by protein filaments *(calsequestrin)* in "bunches" just inside the closed Ca^{++} channels. When the fibre is stimulated *(right),* an electrical impulse travels from the sarcolemma and down the T tubule, where the voltage fluctuation triggers the opening of voltage-gated calcium channels. This allows passive diffusion of the Ca^{++} inside the SR out to the sarcoplasm, where it will trigger the contraction process. Almost immediately after stimulation releases Ca^{++}, the calcium channels close and the Ca^{++} is once again pumped into the sacs of the SR *(left). ATP,* Adenosine triphosphate.

BOX 17-1 *a more detailed look at the sarcomere*

The sarcomere is the basic contractile unit of the muscle cell. As you read the explanation of the sarcomere's structure and function, you might wonder what the Z disc, M line, and other components really are—and what they do for the muscle cell.

First of all, it is important that you appreciate the three-dimensional nature of the sarcomere. You can then realize that the Z disc (Z line), which often looks like a zigzag line in a flat diagram, is really a dense plate or disc to which the thin (actin) filaments directly anchor. Besides being an anchor for myofibrils, the Z disc is useful as a landmark separating one sarcomere from the next. The name Z disc comes from the German word *zwischen,* meaning "between".

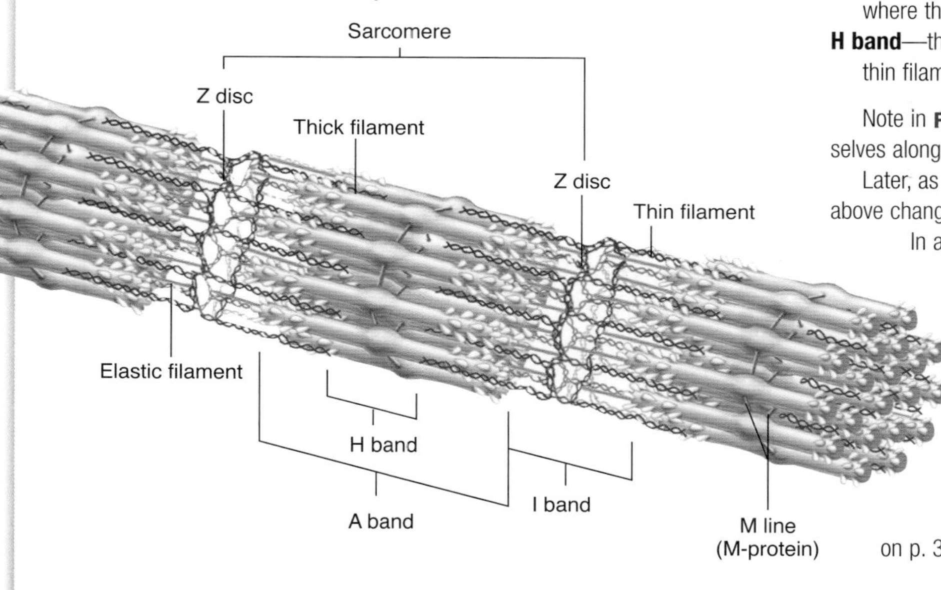

Detailed analysis of the sarcomere also shows that the thick (myosin) filaments are held together and stabilized by *M-protein* molecules that form a middle line called the **M line.** Note that the regions of the sarcomere are identified by specific zones or bands:

A band—the segment that runs the entire length of the thick filaments (also called *anisotropic band*)

I band—the segment that includes the Z disc and the ends of the thin filaments where they do not overlap the thick filaments (also called *isotropic band*)

H band—the middle region of the thick filaments where they do not overlap the thin filaments (H is from the German word *heller* "bright")

Note in **Figure 17-2** that the T tubules in human muscle fibres align themselves along the borders between the A band and I band.

Later, as you review the process of contraction, note how the regions listed above change during each step of the process.

In addition to thin and thick filaments, each sarcomere has numerous **elastic filaments.** Elastic filaments, composed of a protein called *titin (connectin),* anchor the thick filaments to the Z disc, as the figure shows. The elastic filaments are believed to give myofibrils, and thus muscle fibres, their characteristic elasticity. *Dystrophin,* not shown here, is a protein that holds the actin filaments to the sarcolemma. Dystrophin and a complex of connected molecules anchor the muscle fibre to surrounding matrix so that the muscle does not break during a contraction. Dystrophin and its role in muscular dystrophy are discussed further on p. 385. •

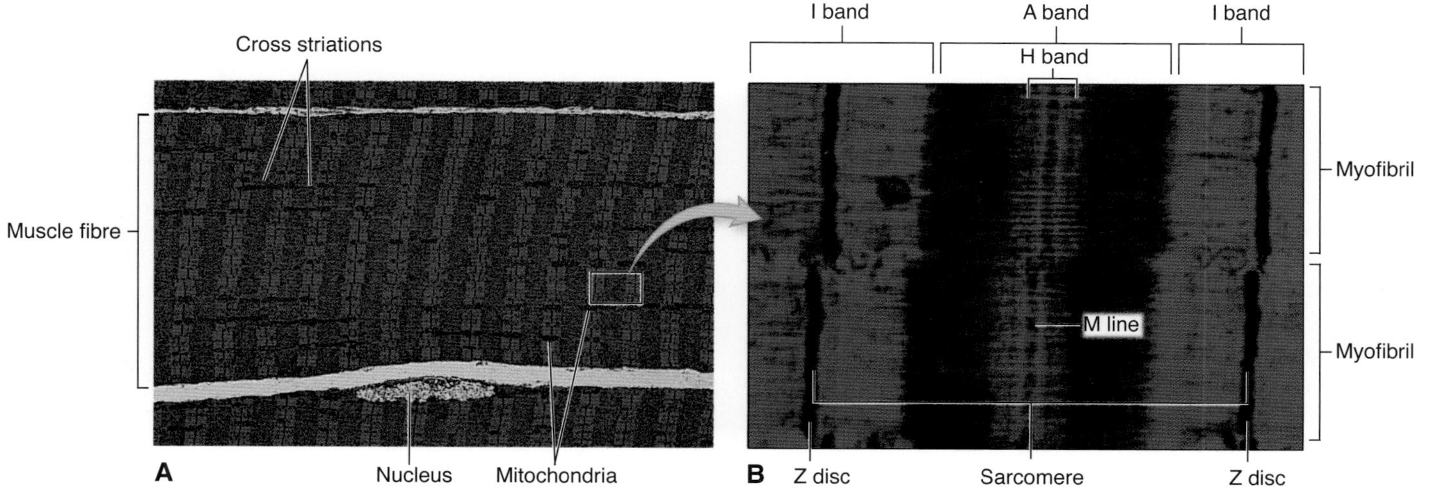

FIGURE 17-4 Skeletal muscle striations. Colour-enhanced scanning electron micrographs (SEMs) showing longitudinal views of skeletal muscle fibres. **B** shows detail of **A** at greater magnification. Note that the myofilaments of each myofibril form a pattern that, when viewed together, produces the striated (striped) pattern typical of skeletal muscle.

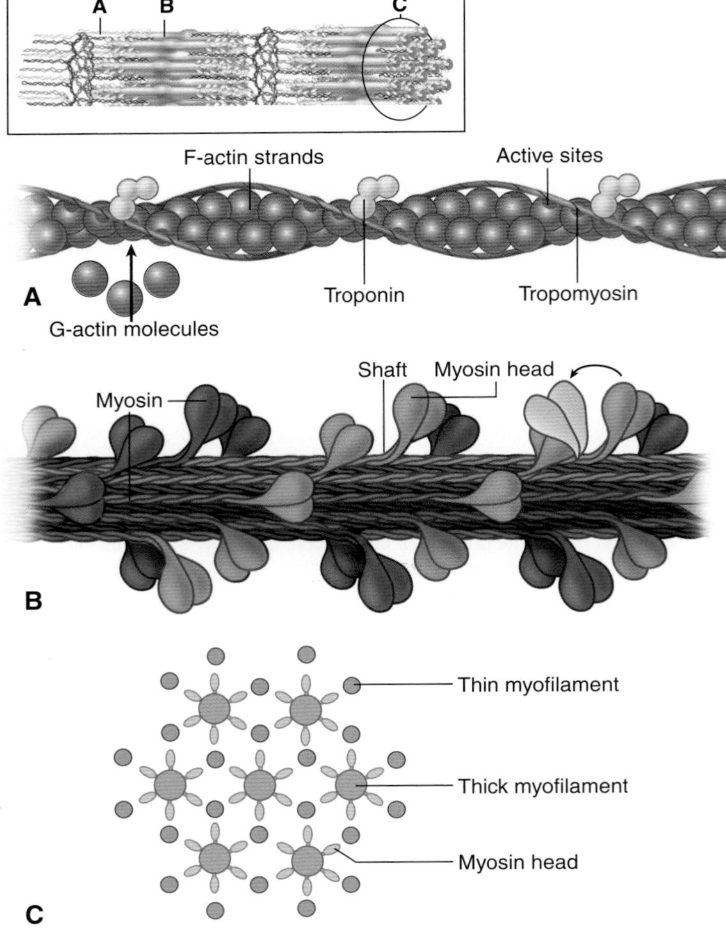

FIGURE 17-5 Structure of myofilaments. A, Thin myofilament. **B,** Thick myofilament. **C,** Cross-section of several thick and thin myofilaments showing the relative positions of myofilaments and the myosin heads that will form cross bridges between them.

myofilaments reveals the mechanism of how muscle fibres contract and do so powerfully. It is wise, therefore, to take a moment to first study the structure of myofilaments before discussing the detailed mechanism of muscle contraction.

First of all, four different kinds of protein molecules make up myofilaments: **myosin, actin, tropomyosin,** and **troponin.** The thin filaments are made of a combination of three proteins: actin, tropomyosin, and troponin. **Figure 17-5**, *A*, shows that globular actin molecules (*G-actin*) are strung together like beads to form two fibrous strands (*F-actin*) that twist around each other to form the bulk of each thin filament. Actin and myosin molecules have a chemical attraction for one another, but at rest, the active sites on the actin molecules are covered by long tropomyosin molecules. The tropomyosin molecules seem to be held in this blocking position by troponin molecules spaced at intervals along the thin filament (see **Figure 17-5**, *A*).

As **Figure 17-5**, *B*, shows, the thick filaments are made almost entirely of myosin molecules. Note that the myosin molecules are shaped like two golf clubs twisted together. Their long shafts bundle together to form a thick filament and their doubled "heads" stick out from the bundle. The myosin heads are chemically attracted to the actin molecules of the nearby thin filaments, so they angle toward the thin filaments. When they bridge the gap between adjacent myofilaments, the myosin heads are usually called **cross bridges.**

Recall from **Figure 5-17** (p. 90) that myosin acts as a molecular motor. The myosin in thick filaments can actively pull on actin when adenosine triphosphate (ATP) is available.

Within a myofibril, the thick and thin filaments alternate, as shown in **Figure 17-1**, *D*. They are also very close to one another, as you can see in the cross-section in **Figure 17-5**, *C*, and **Figure 17-6**. This arrangement is crucial for contraction. Another fact important for contraction is that the thin filaments attach to both Z discs (Z lines) of a sarcomere and that they extend in from the Z discs partway toward the centre of the sarcomere. When the muscle fibre is relaxed, the thin filaments terminate at the outer edges of the H bands. In contrast, the thick myosin filaments do not attach directly to the Z discs, and they extend only to the length of the A bands of the sarcomeres.

Mechanism of Contraction

To accomplish the powerful shortening, or contraction, of a muscle fibre, several processes must be coordinated in a stepwise fashion. These steps are summarized in the following sections and in **Box 17-2**.

Excitation of the Sarcolemma

In normal circumstances, a skeletal muscle fibre remains "at rest" until it is stimulated by a signal from a special type of nerve cell called a **motor neuron.** As **Figure 17-7** shows, motor neurons connect to the sarcolemma of a muscle fibre at a folded **motor endplate** to form a junction called a *neuromuscular junction.*

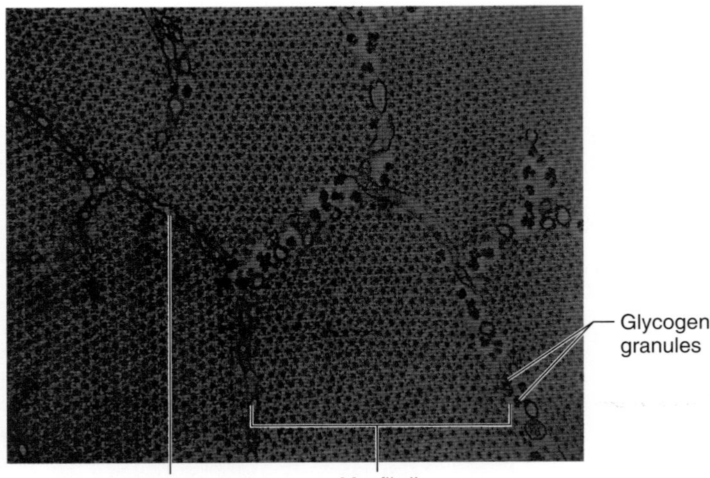

FIGURE 17-6 Cross-section of myofibrils. Colour-enhanced scanning electron micrographs (SEMs) showing a cross-section from a skeletal muscle fibre. Note the dense arrangement of thick and thin filaments, seen here in cross-section as mere dots. Note also the dark glycogen granules and sarcoplasmic reticulum tubules sandwiched between the myofibrils.

BOX 17-2 *major events of muscle contraction and relaxation*

Excitation and Contraction

1. A nerve impulse reaches the end of a motor neuron and triggers release of the neurotransmitter acetylcholine (ACh).
2. ACh diffuses rapidly across the gap of the neuromuscular junction and binds to ACh receptors on the motor endplate of the muscle fibre.
3. Stimulation of ACh receptors initiates an impulse that travels along the sarcolemma, through the T tubules, to the sacs of the sarcoplasmic reticulum (SR).
4. Ca^{++} is released from the SR into the sarcoplasm, where it binds to troponin molecules in the thin myofilaments.
5. Tropomyosin molecules in the thin myofilaments shift and thereby expose actin's active sites.
6. Energized myosin cross bridges of the thick myofilaments bind to actin and use their energy to pull the thin myofilaments toward the centre of each sarcomere. This cycle repeats itself many times per second, as long as adenosine triphosphate is available.
7. As the filaments slide past the thick myofilaments, the entire muscle fibre shortens.

Relaxation

1. After the impulse is over, the SR begins actively pumping Ca^{++} back into its sacs.
2. As Ca^{++} is stripped from troponin molecules in the thin myofilaments, tropomyosin returns to its position and blocks actin's active sites.
3. Myosin cross bridges are prevented from binding to actin and thus can no longer sustain the contraction.
4. Because the thick and thin myofilaments are no longer connected, the muscle fibre may return to its longer, resting length.

FIGURE 17-7 Neuromuscular junction (NMJ). A, Scanning electron micrograph showing several neuromuscular junctions (NMJs). *N,* Nerve fibres; *M,* Muscle fibres. **B,** This sketch shows a cutaway side view of the NMJ. Note how the distal end of a motor neuron fibre forms a synapse, or "chemical junction", with an adjacent muscle fibre. Neurotransmitter molecules (specifically, acetylcholine, or ACh) are released from the neuron's synaptic vesicles and diffuse across the synaptic cleft. There they stimulate receptors in the motor endplate region of the sarcolemma.

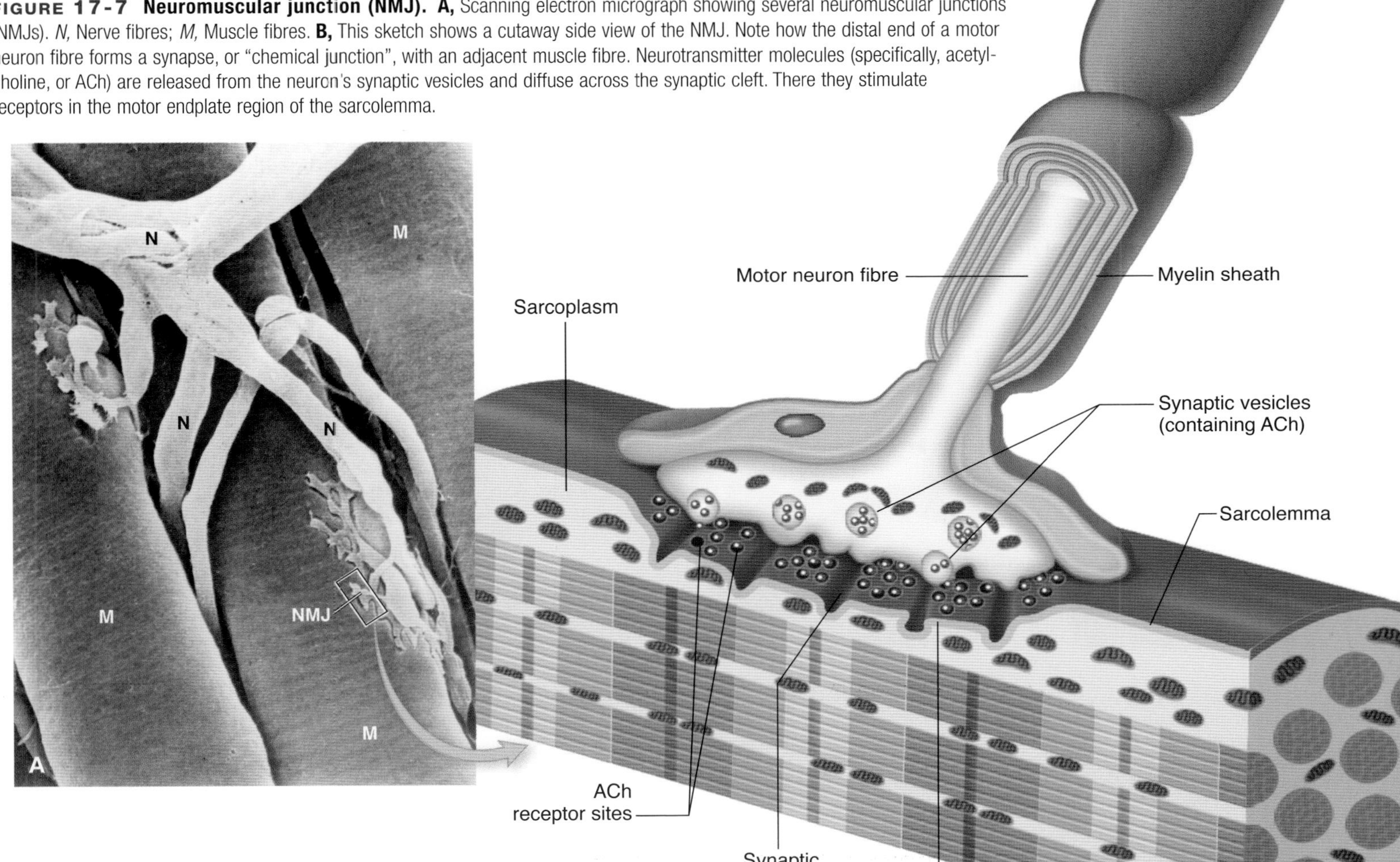

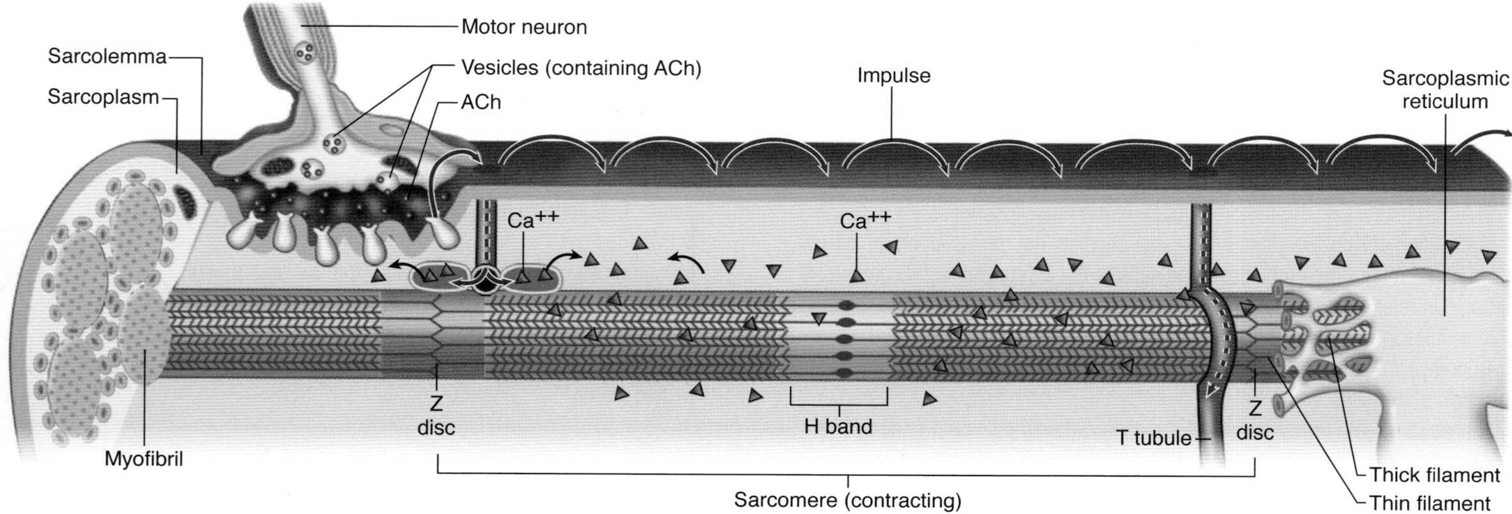

FIGURE 17-8 Effects of excitation on a muscle fibre. Excitation of the sarcolemma by a nerve impulse initiates an impulse in the sarcolemma. The impulse travels across the sarcolemma and through the T tubules, where it triggers adjacent sacs of the sarcoplasmic reticulum to release a flood of calcium ions (Ca^{++}) into the sarcoplasm. Ca^{++} is then free to bind to troponin molecules in the thin filaments. This binding, in turn, initiates the chemical reactions that produce a contraction.

A **neuromuscular junction (NMJ)** is a type of connection called a *synapse* and is characterized by a narrow gap, or synaptic cleft, across which *neurotransmitter* molecules transmit signals. When nerve impulses reach the end of a motor neuron fibre, small vesicles release a neurotransmitter, **acetylcholine (ACh),** into the synaptic cleft. Diffusing swiftly across this microscopic gap, acetylcholine molecules contact the sarcolemma of the adjacent muscle fibre. There they stimulate acetylcholine receptors and thereby initiate an electrical impulse in the sarcolemma. The process of synaptic transmission and induction of an impulse—a process often called *excitation*—is discussed in detail in Chapter 19.

Contraction

The impulse, a temporary electrical voltage imbalance, is conducted over the muscle fibre's sarcolemma and inward along the T tubules (**Figure 17-8**). The impulse in the T tubules triggers the release of a flood of calcium ions from the adjacent sacs of the SR (see **Figures 17-3** and **17-8**).

In the sarcoplasm, the calcium ions combine with troponin molecules in the thin filaments of the myofibrils (**Figure 17-9**). Recall that troponin normally holds tropomyosin strands in a position that blocks the chemically active sites of actin. When calcium binds to troponin, however, the tropomyosin shifts to expose active binding sites on the actin molecules (**Figure 17-10**).

Once the active sites are exposed, energized myosin heads of the thick filaments bind to actin molecules in the nearby thin filaments. The myosin head temporarily forms a *cross bridge* between the thick and thin filaments (**Figure 17-11**). After forming cross bridges, the myosin heads bend with great force, literally pulling the thin filaments past them. This is often called the "power stroke" of myosin.

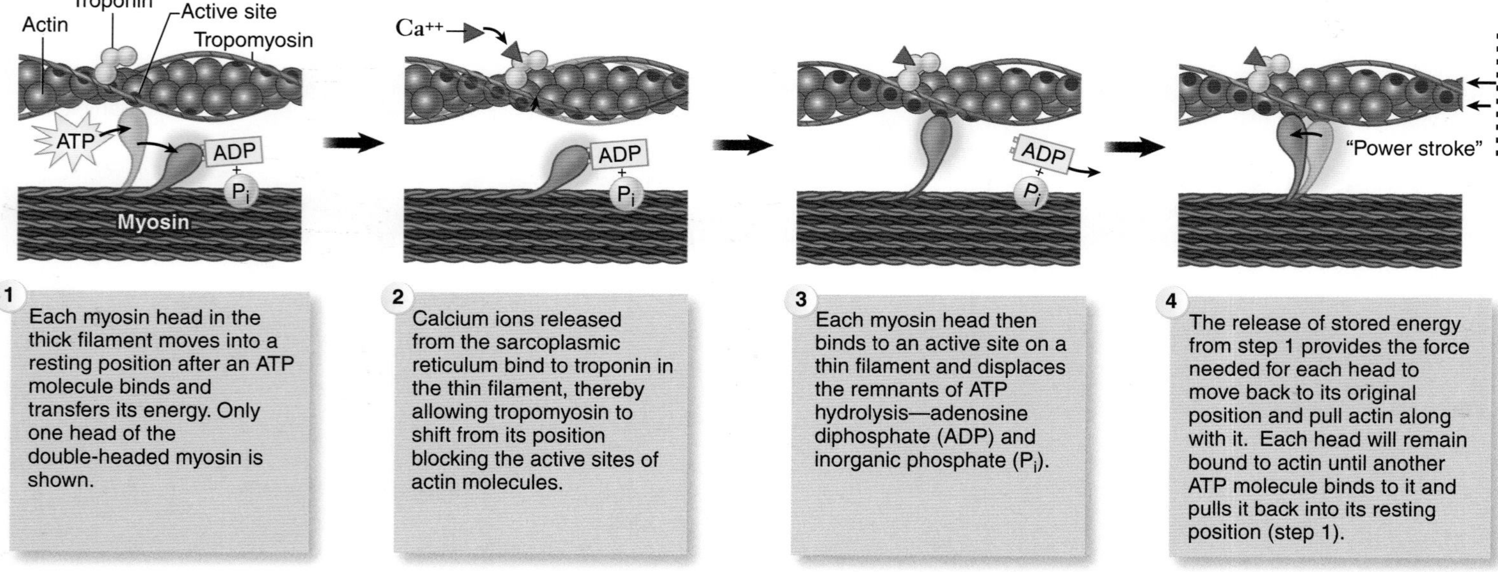

Troponin
Actin
Active site
Tropomyosin
ATP
ADP
+
P_i
Myosin
Ca^{++}
ADP
+
P_i
ADP
+
P_i
"Power stroke"
1
Each myosin head in the thick filament moves into a resting position after an ATP molecule binds and transfers its energy. Only one head of the double-headed myosin is shown.
2
Calcium ions released from the sarcoplasmic reticulum bind to troponin in the thin filament, thereby allowing tropomyosin to shift from its position blocking the active sites of actin molecules.
3
Each myosin head then binds to an active site on a thin filament and displaces the remnants of ATP hydrolysis—adenosine diphosphate (ADP) and inorganic phosphate (P_i).
4
The release of stored energy from step 1 provides the force needed for each head to move back to its original position and pull actin along with it. Each head will remain bound to actin until another ATP molecule binds to it and pulls it back into its resting position (step 1).

FIGURE 17-9 The molecular basis of muscle contraction.

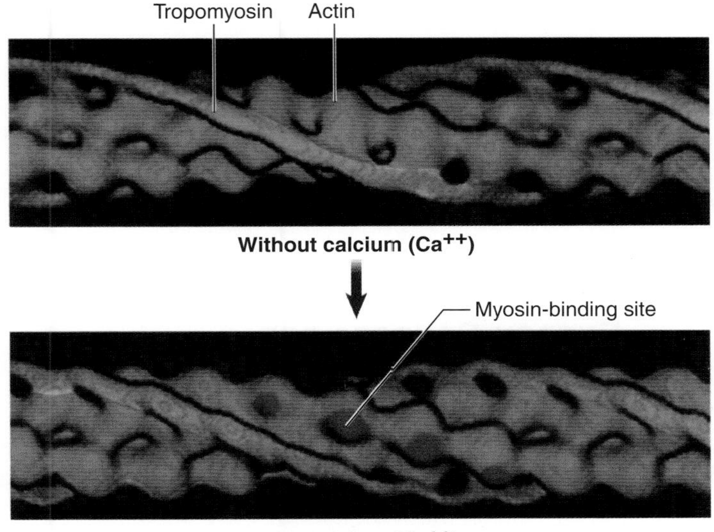

FIGURE 17-10 Role of calcium in muscle contraction. Colour-enhanced scanning electron micrograph (SEM) of a thin filament. When calcium is absent, the active myosin binding sites on actin are covered by tropomyosin. However, after calcium becomes available and binds to troponin, the tropomyosin is pulled out of its blocking position and reveals the active binding sites on actin.

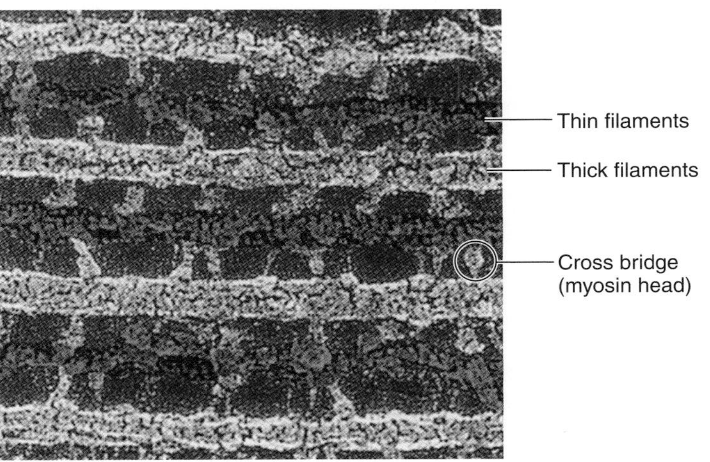

FIGURE 17-11 Cross bridges. Colour-enhanced scanning electron micrograph (SEM) showing the myosin heads functioning as cross bridges that connect the thick filaments to the thin filaments, pulling on the thin filaments and causing them to slide.

Each head then releases itself, binds to the next active site, and pulls again. **Figure 17-12** shows how sliding of the thin filaments toward the centre of each sarcomere quickly shortens the entire myofibril—and thus the entire muscle fibre. This model of muscle contraction has been called the **sliding-filament model.** Perhaps a better name might be *ratcheting-filament model* because the myosin heads actively ratchet the thin filaments toward the centre of the sarcomere with great force.

Muscle fibres usually contract to about 80% of their starting length—rarely to 60% or 70%. Some muscle fibres contract hardly at all because they are pulling on an unmoving load. Even so, such muscle fibres are still said to be "contracting" in a broad sense. Their sarcomeres are still working hard to pull the ends toward one another, as though they are at a steady "draw" in a game of tug-of-war

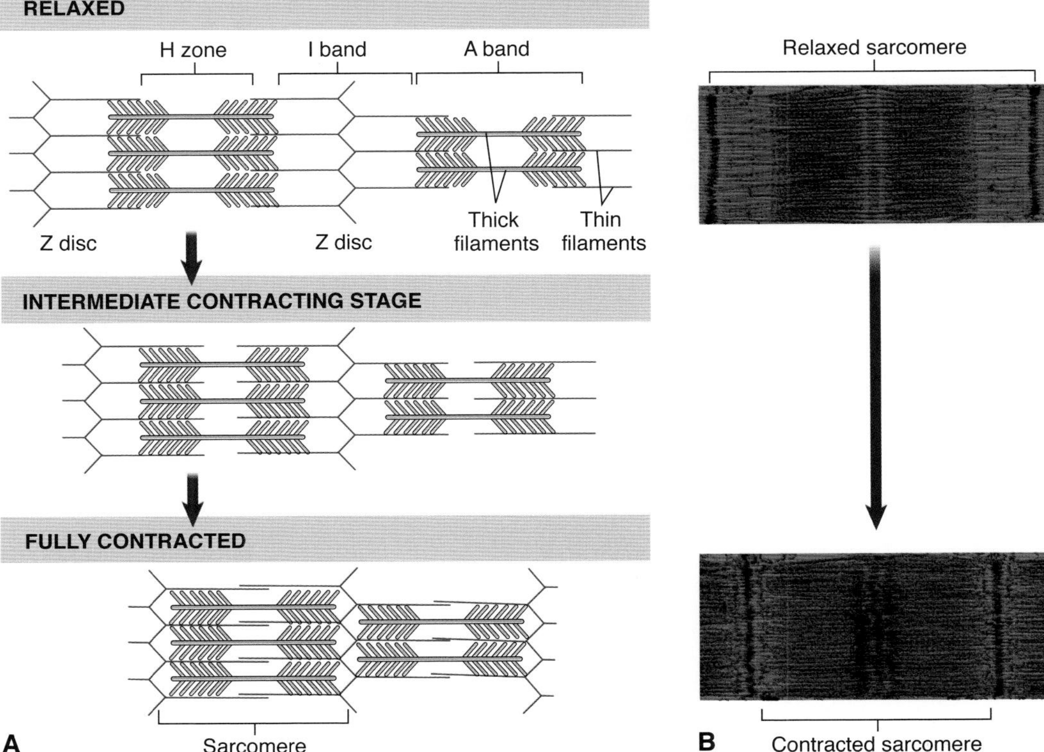

FIGURE 17-12 Sliding-filament model. **A,** During contraction, myosin cross bridges pull the thin filaments toward the centre of each of two sarcomeres, thus shortening the myofibril and the entire muscle fibre. **B,** Colour-enhanced transmission electron micrographs (TEMs) showing the shortening of a single sarcomere caused by the sliding of filaments during muscle contraction.

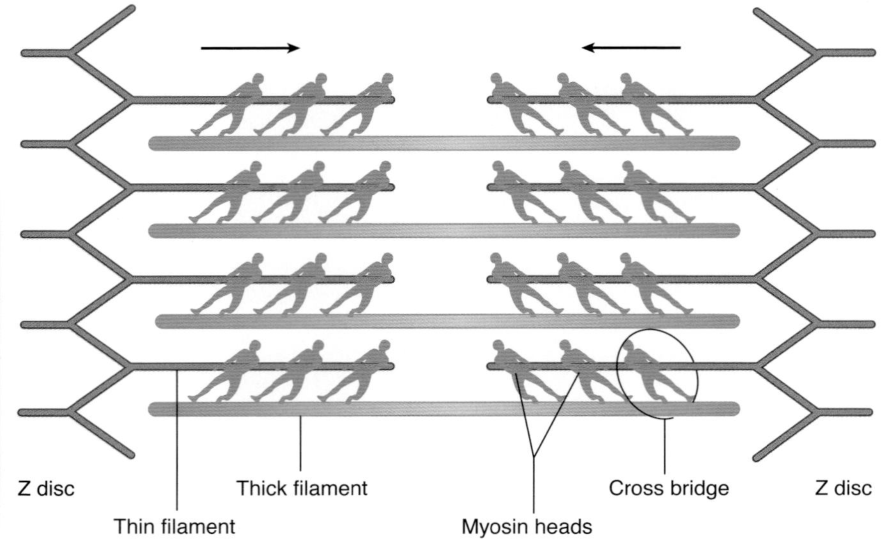

FIGURE 17-13 Simplified contracting sarcomere. This diagram illustrates the concept of muscle contraction as a sort of tug-of-war game in which the myosin heads (shown here as little people) hold onto thin filament "ropes"—thus forming cross bridges. As the myosin heads pull on the thin filaments, the Z discs (Z lines) get closer together—thus shortening the sarcomere. Likewise, the short length of a sarcomere may be held in position by the continued effort of the myosin heads.

(**Figure 17-13**). Because the actin–myosin bond is not permanent, the sarcomere cannot "lock up" once it has shortened to hold its position passively. Thus it takes energy to actively maintain a shortened position—by continually repeating the actin–myosin reaction as long as necessary.

Relaxation

Almost immediately after the SR releases its flood of calcium ions into the sarcoplasm, it begins actively pumping them back into its sacs once again. Within a few milliseconds, much of the calcium is recovered. Because the active transport carriers of the SR have greater affinity for calcium than the troponin molecules do, the calcium ions are stripped off the troponin molecules and returned to the sacs of the SR. As you might suspect, the removal of calcium ions from the thin filaments shuts down the entire process of contraction. Troponin without its bound calcium allows the tropomyosin to once again block actin's active sites. Myosin heads reaching for the next active site on actin are blocked, and thus the thin filaments are no longer being held—or pulled—by the thick filaments.

If no new nerve impulse immediately follows, the muscle fibre relaxes. The relaxed muscle fibre may remain at its contracted length, but forces outside the muscle fibre are likely to pull it back to its longer resting length.

As we have seen, the contraction process in a skeletal muscle fibre automatically shuts itself off within a small fraction of a second after the initial stimulation. However, a muscle fibre may sustain a contraction for some time if there are many stimuli in rapid succession. Rapidly occurring stimuli permit calcium ions to remain available in the sarcoplasm for a longer period, thereby sustaining the actin–myosin reaction.

> ***Quick* CHECK**
>
> 5. Describe the structure of thin and thick myofilaments, and name the kinds of proteins that compose them.
> 6. What is a neuromuscular junction (NMJ)? How does it work?
> 7. What is the role of calcium ions (Ca^{++}) in muscle contraction?

ENERGY SOURCES FOR MUSCLE CONTRACTION

ATP

The energy required for muscular contraction, or any other kind of work by the cell, is obtained by hydrolysis of a nucleotide called *adenosine triphosphate*, or *ATP*. Recall from Chapter 4 (**Figure 4-19**, p. 68) that this molecule has an adenine and ribose group (together called *adenosine*) attached to three phosphate groups. Two of the three phosphate groups in ATP are attached to the molecule by *high-energy bonds*. Breaking one of these high-energy bonds provides the energy necessary to pull the thin myofilaments during muscle contraction.

As **Figure 17-9**, *Step 1*, shows, before contraction occurs, each myosin cross-bridge head moves into a resting position when an ATP molecule binds to it. The ATP molecule breaks its outermost high-energy bond, thereby releasing inorganic phosphate (P_i) and transferring the energy to the myosin head. In a way, this is like pulling back the elastic band of a slingshot—the apparatus is "at rest" but ready to spring. When myosin binds to actin, the stored energy is released, and the myosin head does indeed spring back to its original position. Thus the energy transferred from ATP is used to do the work of pulling the thin filaments during contraction.

Another ATP molecule then binds to the myosin head, which then releases actin and moves into its resting position again—all set for the next "pull". This cycle repeats as long as ATP is available and actin's active sites are unblocked.

Muscle fibres must continually resynthesize ATP because they can keep only small amounts of it. There is only enough ATP in a muscle fibre for about 2 to 4 seconds of maximum contraction. However, energy for the resynthesis of ATP can be quickly supplied by the breakdown of another high-energy compound, **creatine phosphate (CP)**, as you can see in **Figure 17-14**. CP is a sort of backup energy molecule that provides enough energy for about 20 additional seconds of maximal contraction. Both ATP and CP are continually resynthesized—or "recharged"—by cellular respiration. Ultimately, energy for both ATP and CP synthesis comes from the catabolism of nutrients from food.

If a cell runs out of ATP completely and cannot resynthesize more, contraction stops—possibly resulting in stiffness caused by the inability of myosin heads to disengage from actin (see **Figure 17-9**). When this happens after death, it is called *rigor mortis* (**Box 17-3**).

Glucose and Oxygen

Continued, efficient nutrient catabolism by muscle fibres requires two essential ingredients: glucose and oxygen.

Glucose is a nutrient molecule that contains many chemical bonds. The potential energy stored in these chemical bonds is released during catabolic reactions in the sarcoplasm and mitochondria and

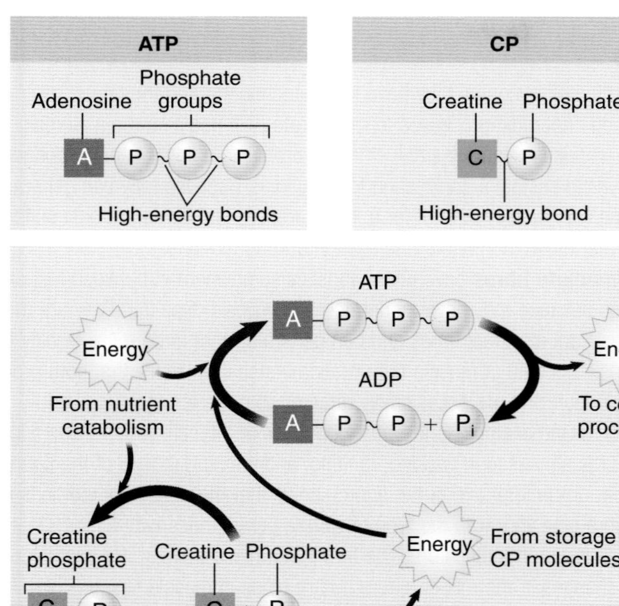

FIGURE 17-14 Energy sources for muscle contraction. A, A basic model of two high-energy molecules in the sarcoplasm: adenosine triphosphate (ATP) and creatine phosphate (CP). **B,** This diagram shows how energy released during the catabolism of nutrients can be transferred to the high-energy bonds of ATP directly or, instead, stored temporarily in the high-energy bond of CP. During contraction, ATP is hydrolyzed and the energy of the broken bond is transferred to a myosin head.

transferred to ATP or CP molecules. Ultimately, all the glucose needed by muscle fibres comes from the blood. Skeletal muscle fibres are surrounded by a network of blood capillaries, the tiny "exchange" vessels that allow molecules to enter or leave the blood (**Figure 17-15**). Some muscle fibres ensure an uninterrupted supply of glucose by storing it in the form of *glycogen*. Recall from Chapter 4 that glycogen is a polysaccharide made up of thousands of glucose subunits.

BOX 17-3 *fyi* | Rigor Mortis

The term **rigor mortis** is a Latin phrase that means "stiffness of death". In a medical context the term *rigor mortis* refers to the stiffness of skeletal muscles sometimes observed shortly after death. What causes rigor mortis? At the time of death, stimulation of muscle cells ceases. However, the muscle fibres of postural muscles may have been in midcontraction at the time of death—when the myosin–actin cross bridges are still intact. In addition, the sarcoplasmic reticulum (SR) releases much of the Ca^{++} it had been storing, thereby causing even more cross bridges to form. Adenosine triphosphate (ATP) is required to release the cross bridges and "energize" the myosin heads for their next attachment. Because the last of a cell's ATP supply is used up at the time it dies, many cross bridges may be left "stuck" in the contracted position. Thus muscles in a dead body may be stiff because individual muscle fibres ran out of the ATP required to "turn off" a muscle contraction. •

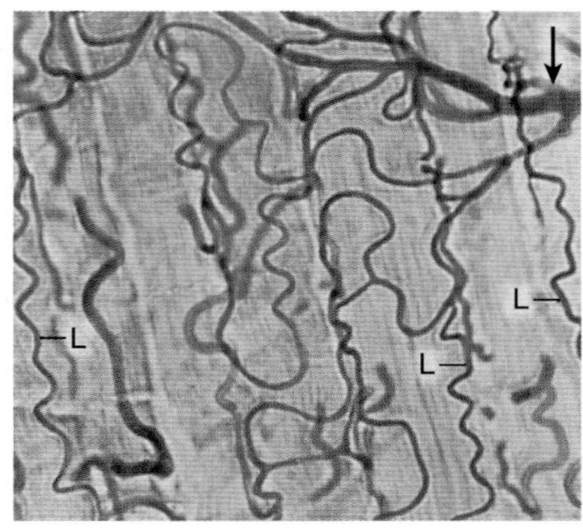

FIGURE 17-15 Blood supply of muscle fibres. Tiny "exchange" vessels called *capillaries* branch out longitudinally *(L)* from small arteries *(arrow)* to form a network that supplies muscle fibres with glucose and oxygen and removes carbon dioxide and lactate. In this micrograph, the muscle fibres appear translucent and the blood vessels appear reddish.

Oxygen, which is needed for a catabolic process known as the aerobic pathway, also ultimately comes from the blood. Most of the oxygen carried in the blood is temporarily bound to *haemoglobin* molecules—a reddish pigment inside red blood cells.

Oxygen can also be stored by cells to ensure an uninterrupted supply. During rest, excess oxygen molecules in the sarcoplasm are attracted to a large protein molecule called **myoglobin.** Like haemoglobin, myoglobin is a reddish pigment with iron (Fe) groups that attract oxygen molecules and hold them temporarily. When the oxygen concentration inside a muscle fibre decreases rapidly—as it does during exercise—it can be quickly resupplied from myoglobin. Muscle fibres that contain large amounts of myoglobin take on a deep red appearance and are often called *red fibres.* Muscle fibres with little myoglobin in them are light pink and are often called *white fibres.* Most muscle tissues contain a mixture of red and white fibres (**Box 17-4**).

Catabolic Pathways

The *aerobic* (oxygen-requiring) *pathway* is a catabolic process that produces the maximum amount of energy available from each glucose molecule. However, because the aerobic pathway is rather slow, muscle fibres can shift toward increased use of another catabolic process: the *anaerobic pathway.* As its name implies, the anaerobic pathway does not require the immediate use of oxygen. Besides its ability to produce ATP without oxygen, the anaerobic pathway has the added advantage of being very rapid. Muscle fibres that generate a great deal of force very quickly may rely heavily on the anaerobic pathway to resynthesize their ATP molecules. Anaerobic processes may allow the body to generate rapid bursts of energy in the short term, but it is aerobic respiration that usually dominates long-term energy production (**Figure 17-16**).

The anaerobic process, also called *fermentation,* results in the formation of an incompletely catabolized molecule called *lactate* because oxygen cannot be supplied quickly enough for pyruvate to be utilized through the Krebs cycle (review Chapter 6, page 113). When aerobic conditions return (following cessation of exercise), lactate may be converted back to glucose and thus "start again" in the catabolic pathway that begins with glycolysis. Or it may be converted back only so far as pyruvate and immediately enter the aerobic pathway.

Any lactate not converted in the muscle fibre may eventually diffuse into the blood and be delivered to the kidney and liver, where an oxygen-consuming process later converts it back into glucose.

BOX 17-4 *sports and fitness* | Types of Muscle Fibres

Skeletal muscle fibres can be classified into three types by their structural and functional characteristics: (1) *slow* (red) *fibres,* (2) *fast* (white) *fibres,* and (3) *intermediate fibres.* Each type is best suited to a particular type or style of muscular contraction—a fact that is useful in considering how different muscles are used during different athletic activities. Although each muscle organ contains a mix of all three fibre types (part *A* of the figure), different organs have these fibres in different proportions, depending on the types of contraction that they most often perform (part *B* of the figure).

Slow fibres are also called *red fibres* because they contain a high concentration of myoglobin, the reddish pigment used by muscle cells to store oxygen. They are called *slow fibres* because their thick myofilaments are made of a type of myosin (type I) that reacts at a slow rate. Because they contract so slowly, slow fibres are usually able to produce ATP quickly enough to keep pace with the energy needs of the myosin and thus avoid fatigue. This effect is enhanced by the larger number of mitochondria, more than found in other fibre types, and the rich oxygen store provided by the myoglobin. The slow, nonfatiguing characteristics of slow fibres make them especially well suited to the sustained contractions exhibited by postural muscles. Postural muscles containing a high proportion of slow fibres can hold the skeleton upright for long periods without fatigue.

Fast fibres are also called *white fibres* because they contain very little myoglobin. Fast fibres can contract much more rapidly than slow fibres because they have a faster type of myosin (type IIx) and because their system of T tubules and sarcoplasmic reticulum (SR) is more efficient at quickly delivering Ca^{++} to the sarcoplasm. The price of a rapid contraction mechanism is rapid depletion of ATP. Despite the fact that fast fibres typically contain a high concentration of glycogen, they have few mitochondria and thus must rely primarily on anaerobic processes to regenerate ATP. Because the anaerobic pathway produces relatively small amounts of ATP, fast fibres cannot produce enough ATP to sustain a contraction for very long. Because they can generate great force very quickly but not for a long duration, fast fibres are best suited for muscles that move the fingers and eyes in darting motions.

Intermediate fibres have characteristics somewhere in between fast and slow fibres because they have moderately fast myosin (type IIa). They are more fatigue resistant than fast fibres and can generate more force more quickly than slow fibres. This type of muscle fibre predominates in muscles that both provide postural support and are occasionally required to generate rapid, powerful contractions. One example is the *gastrocnemius* of the calf, which helps support the leg but is also used in walking, running, and jumping (part *B* of the figure).

The bar graph in part *C* of the figure shows that the relative proportions of muscle fibre type vary with the type of work a person does with his or her muscles. This graph underscores the fact that athletic training, for example, can produce changes in the mix of different fibre types in muscle tissue. •

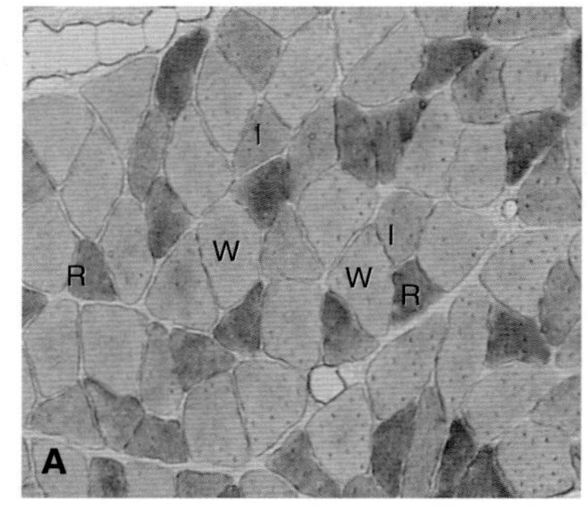

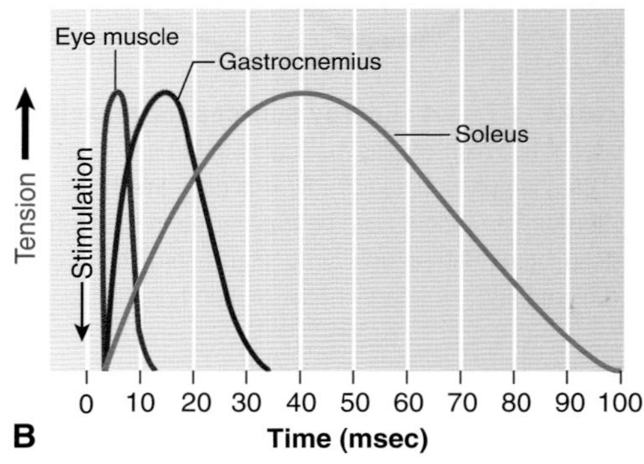

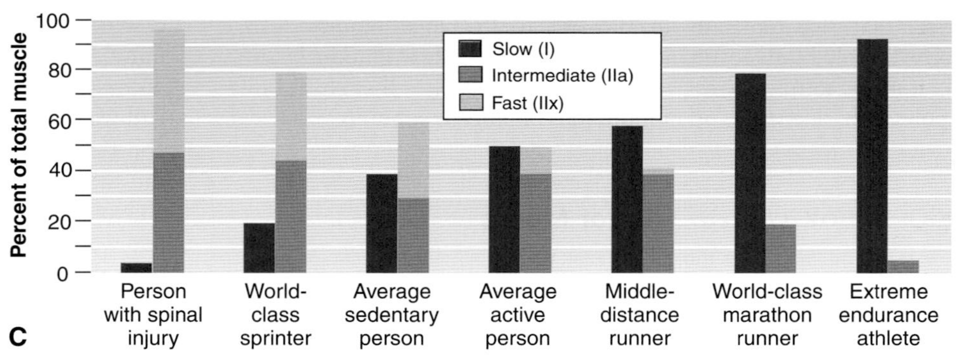

A, Types of muscle fibres. Using a special staining technique, this micrograph of a cross-section of skeletal muscle tissue shows a mix of fibre types: *R,* red (slow) fibres; *W,* white (fast) fibres; and *I,* intermediate fibres. **B,** Three styles of twitch contraction. Different muscle organs have different proportions of slow, fast, and intermediate fibres and thus produce different styles of twitch contractions in a myogram. **C,** Proportions of fibre types in muscle tissue. A person with a spinal cord injury eventually loses nearly all of the postural slow fibres while retaining mostly intermediate and fast fibres. In an extreme endurance athlete, on the other hand, the slow fibres develop so much that they greatly dominate the faster fibre types.

The accumulation of lactate in muscle fibres and blood was proposed as one of the reasons why, after vigorous exercise, a person may continue to breathe rapidly and deeply. The lactate was believed to be stimulating the respiratory control centres in the brain to increase the rate of breathing and thereby take in more oxygen. The body was said to repay the so-called *oxygen debt* by using the extra oxygen gained to process the lactate that was produced during exercise. However, we now know that lactate production is not the cause of deep, rapid breathing after exercise. Instead, it is due to a combination of many physiological factors that collectively cause excess post-exercise oxygen consumption (EPOC).

CONNECT IT! 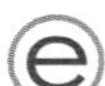

What are the factors that trigger rapid, deep breathing after exercise? Check out the brief illustrated article ***Deep Breathing After Exercise*** online at ***Connect It!***

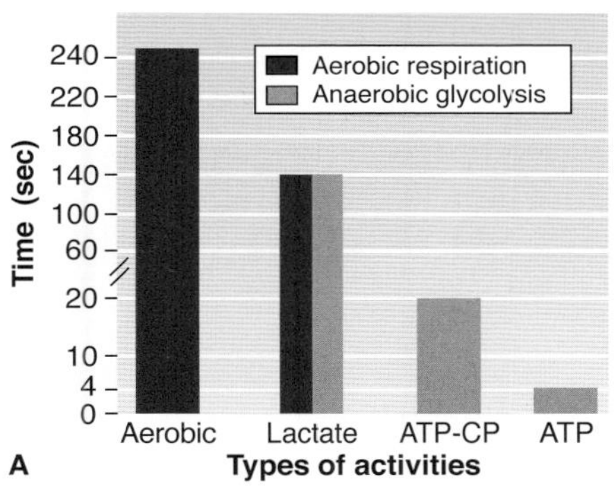

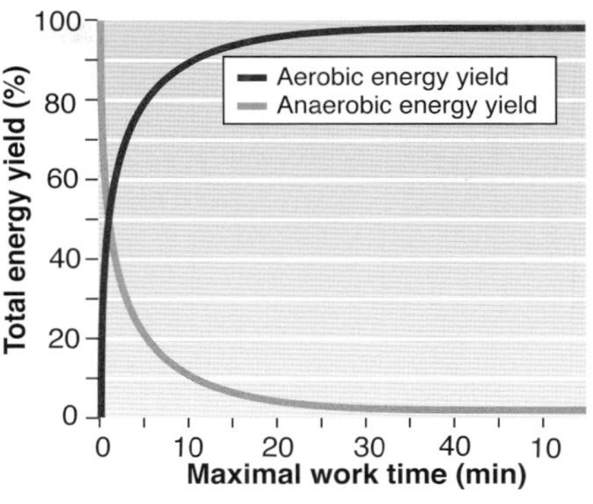

Duration of maximal exercise

	Seconds			Minutes					
	10	30	60	2	4	10	30	60	120
Anaerobic (%)	90	80	70	50	35	15	5	2	1
Aerobic (%)	10	20	30	50	65	85	95	98	99

B

FIGURE 17-16 Aerobic and anaerobic pathways during muscular activity. A, The aerobic pathway *(dark bars)* can supply energy for muscle contraction for a longer time than can the anaerobic pathway *(light bars).* **B,** The lines show that 100% of the energy used at the beginning of maximal exercise comes from anaerobic processes. However, the muscles soon switch to aerobic sources of energy so after 1 hour of maximal exercise, nearly 100% of the energy comes from aerobic respiration in the muscle fibres. More information on aerobic and anaerobic energy metabolism is found in Chapter 41.

Heat Production

Because the catabolic processes of cells are never 100% efficient, some of the energy released is lost as heat. Because skeletal muscle tissues produce such a massive amount of heat—even when they are doing hardly any work—they have a great effect on body temperature. Heat production or **thermogenesis** is an important function of skeletal muscles, especially in adults.

Recall from Chapter 10 that various heat loss mechanisms of the skin can be used to cool the body when it becomes overheated (see **Figure 10-15**, p. 193). Skeletal muscle tissues can likewise be used when the body's temperature falls below the setpoint value determined by the "thermostat" in the hypothalamus of the brain. As **Figure 17-17** shows, a low external temperature can reduce body temperature below the set point. Temperature sensors in the skin and other parts of the body feed this information back to the hypothalamus, which compares the actual value with the setpoint value (usually about 37°C). The hypothalamus responds to a decrease in body temperature by signaling skeletal muscles to contract. The shivering contractions that result produce enough waste heat to warm the body back to the setpoint temperature—and homeostatic balance is maintained. This strategy of using muscles to provide heat is sometimes called *shivering thermogenesis*.

Recall from Chapter 9 that brown fat is also capable of thermogenesis by "burning fuel" through catabolism—or *nonshivering thermogenesis*. Nonshivering thermogenesis in brown fat is especially important in newborns, who have not yet developed precision of the feedback loop that regulates shivering of muscles.

The subject of energy metabolism is discussed more thoroughly in Chapter 41.

Quick CHECK

8. Where does the energy stored in ATP come from?
9. Contrast the aerobic pathway and anaerobic pathway in muscle fibres.
10. What is the role of myoglobin in muscle fibres?

FIGURE 17-17 The role of skeletal muscle tissues in maintaining a constant body temperature. This diagram shows that a drop in body temperature caused by cold weather can be corrected by a negative feedback mechanism that triggers shivering (muscle contraction), which in turn produces enough heat to warm the body.

FUNCTION OF SKELETAL MUSCLE ORGANS

Although each skeletal muscle fibre is distinct from all other fibres, it operates as part of the large group of fibres that form a skeletal muscle organ. Skeletal muscle organs, often simply called *muscles*,

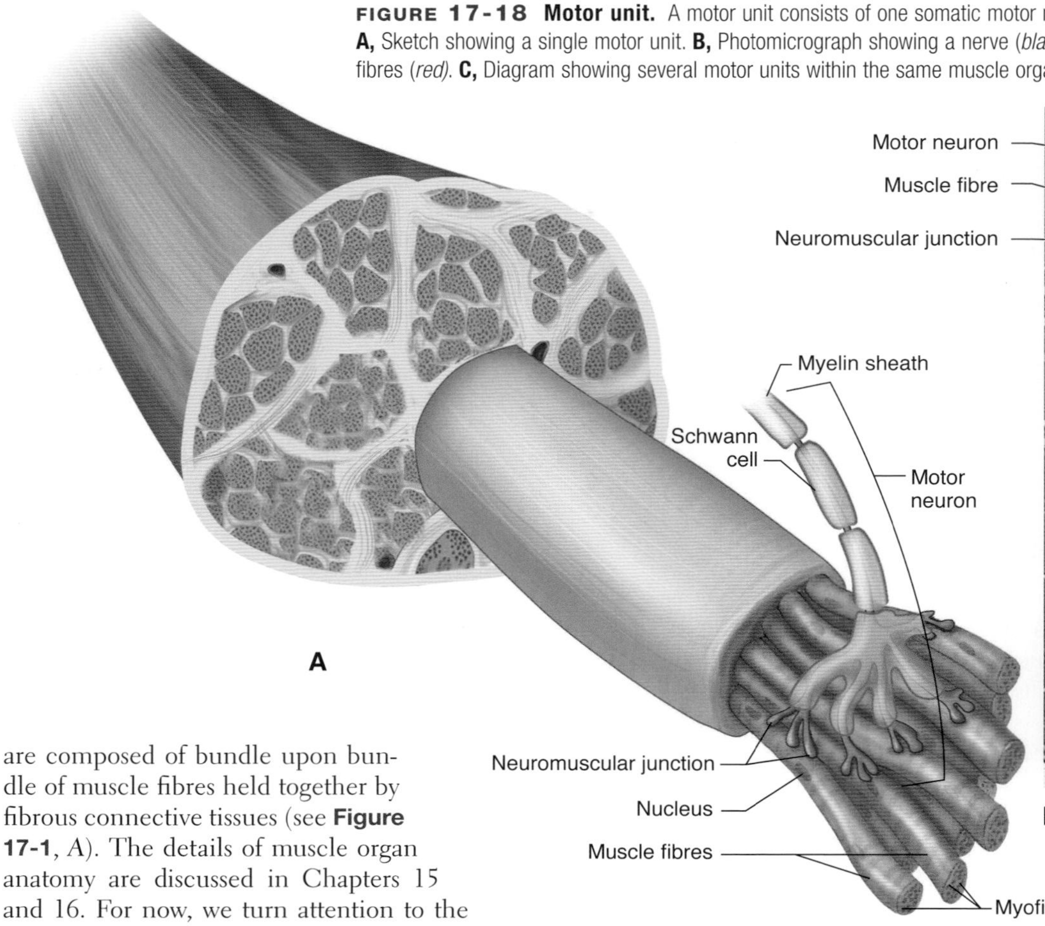

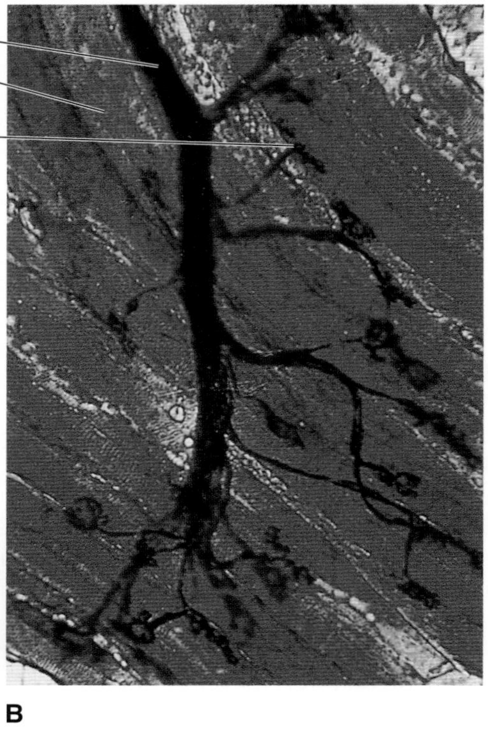

FIGURE 17-18 Motor unit. A motor unit consists of one somatic motor neuron and the muscle fibres supplied by its branches. **A,** Sketch showing a single motor unit. **B,** Photomicrograph showing a nerve (*black*) branching to supply several dozen individual muscle fibres (*red*). **C,** Diagram showing several motor units within the same muscle organ.

are composed of bundle upon bundle of muscle fibres held together by fibrous connective tissues (see **Figure 17-1**, A). The details of muscle organ anatomy are discussed in Chapters 15 and 16. For now, we turn attention to the matter of how skeletal muscle organs function as a single unit.

Motor Unit

Recall that each muscle fibre receives its stimulus from a motor neuron. This neuron, often called a *somatic motor neuron,* is one of several nerve cells that enter a muscle organ together in a bundle called a *motor nerve.* One of these motor neurons, plus the muscle fibres to which it attaches, constitutes a functional unit called a **motor unit** (**Figure 17-18**).

The single fibre of a somatic motor neuron divides into a variable number of branches on entering the skeletal muscle. The neuron branches of some motor units terminate in only a few dozen muscle fibres, whereas others terminate in a few thousand fibres. Consequently, impulse conduction by one motor unit may stimulate only a small part of a muscle organ, whereas conduction by another motor unit may activate a much larger portion of a muscle organ. This variability in the numbers of fibres supplied by a motor unit relates to the function of the muscle as a whole. As a rule, the fewer the number of fibres supplied by a skeletal muscle's individual motor units, the more precise the movements that muscle can produce. For example, in certain small muscles of the hand, each motor unit includes only a few muscle fibres, and these muscles produce precise finger movements. In contrast, motor units in large abdominal muscles that do not produce precise movements may have thousands of muscle fibres.

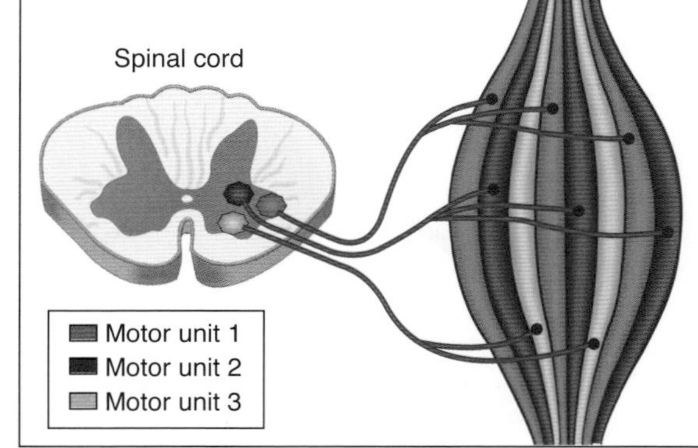

Myography

Many experimental methods have been used to study the contractions of skeletal muscle organs. They vary from relatively simple procedures, such as observing or palpating muscles in action, to the more complicated method of *electromyography* (recording electrical impulses from muscles as they contract). One method of studying muscle contraction that is particularly useful for the purposes of our discussion is called simply *myography,* a term that means "muscle graphing". This is a procedure in which the force or tension from the contraction of an isolated muscle is recorded as a line that rises

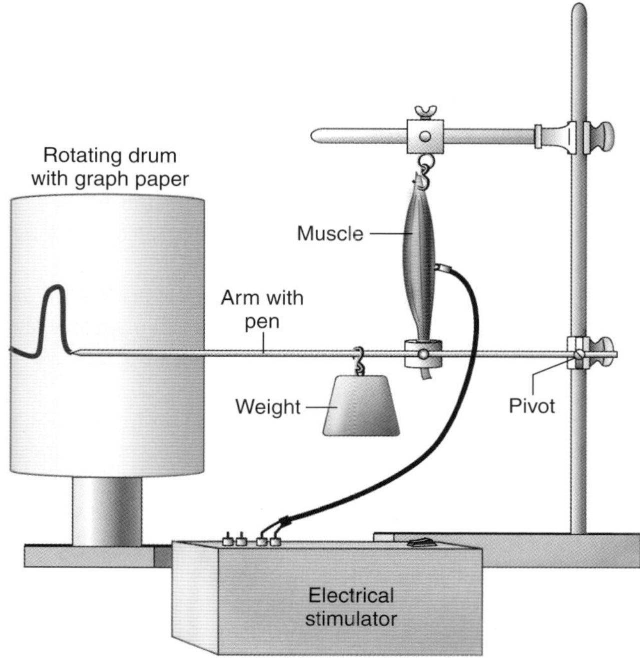

FIGURE 17-19 Myography. This classic type of myograph, called a *kymograph,* records muscle contractions as graphs showing changes in length. An isolated muscle moves the pen upward during contraction, and the weight pulls the muscle and pen downward as the muscle relaxes. A change in tension produces this change in length. Electrical voltage simulates a nerve impulse to stimulate the fibres in the muscle. Modern myography often uses computer-based systems that record similar muscle tension graphs.

and falls as the muscle contracts and relaxes (**Figure 17-19**). To get the muscle to contract, an electrical stimulus of sufficient intensity (the **threshold stimulus**) is applied to the muscle. A single, brief threshold stimulus produces a quick jerk of the muscle, called a **twitch contraction.**

The Twitch Contraction

The quick, jerky twitch contraction seen in a myogram serves as the fundamental model for how muscles operate. The myogram of a twitch contraction shown in **Figure 17-20** shows that the muscle does not begin to contract at the instant of stimulation but rather a fraction of a second later. The muscle then increases its tension (or shortens) until a peak is reached, after which it gradually returns to its resting state. These three phases of the twitch contraction are called, respectively, the *latent period,* the *contraction phase,* and the *relaxation phase.* The entire twitch usually lasts less than one tenth of a second.

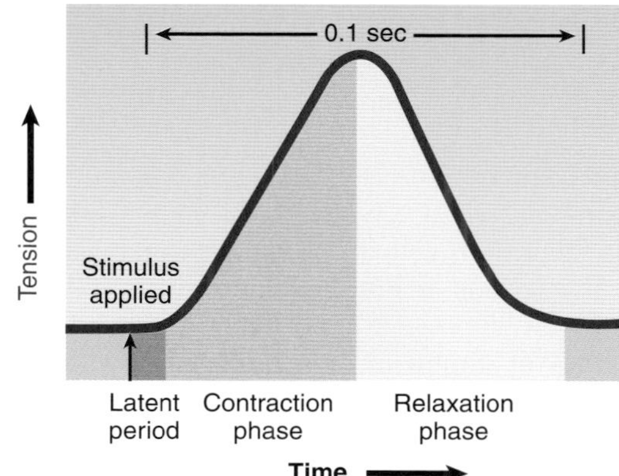

FIGURE 17-20 The twitch contraction. Three distinct phases are apparent: **(1)** the latent period, **(2)** the contraction phase, and **(3)** the relaxation phase.

During the latent period, the impulse initiated by the stimulation travels through the sarcolemma and T tubules to the SR, where it triggers the release of calcium ions into the sarcoplasm. It is not until the calcium binds to troponin and sliding of the myofilaments begins that contraction is observed. After a few milliseconds, the forceful sliding of the myofilaments ceases and relaxation begins. By the end of the relaxation phase, all of the myosin–actin reactions in all the fibres have ceased.

Twitch contractions of muscle organs rarely happen in the body. Even if we try to make our muscles twitch voluntarily, they won't. Instead, our nervous system subconsciously "smoothes out" the movements by briefly sustaining them. This process prevents injury and makes our movements more useful. Sustaining a smooth contraction is something that we will discuss a little later. But, to begin our discussion, a look at the twitch contraction gives us important insight about the mechanisms of more typical types of muscle organ contractions.

Treppe: The Staircase Phenomenon

One interesting effect that can be seen in myographic studies of the twitch contraction is called **treppe,** or the *staircase phenomenon.* Treppe is a gradual, steplike increase in the strength of contraction that can be observed in a series of twitch contractions that occur about 1 second apart (**Figure 17-21**, *B*).

In other words, a muscle contracts more forcefully after it has contracted a few times than when it first contracts—a principle used by athletes when they warm up. Several factors contribute to this phenomenon. For example, in warm muscle fibres, calcium ions diffuse through the sarcoplasm more efficiently and more actin–myosin reactions occur. In addition, calcium ions accumulate in the sarcoplasm of muscles that have not had time to relax and pump much of the calcium back into their SR. Thus, up to a point, a warm fibre contracts more strongly than does a cool fibre. After the first few stimuli, muscle responds to successive stimuli with maximal contractions. Eventually, though, it will respond with less and less strong contractions. The relaxation phase becomes shorter and finally disappears entirely. In other words, the muscle stays partially contracted—an abnormal state of prolonged contraction called *contracture.*

Repeated stimulation of muscle in time lessens its excitability and contractility and may result in **muscle fatigue,** a condition in which the muscle does not respond to the strongest stimuli. Complete muscle fatigue can be readily induced in an isolated muscle in a laboratory but very seldom occurs in the body (**Box 17-5**).

Tetanus

The concept of the simple twitch can help us understand the smooth, sustained types of contraction that are commonly observed in the body. Such smooth, sustained contractions are called *tetanic contractions* or, simply, **tetanus.**

Figure 17-21, *C*, shows that if a series of stimuli come in a rapid enough succession,

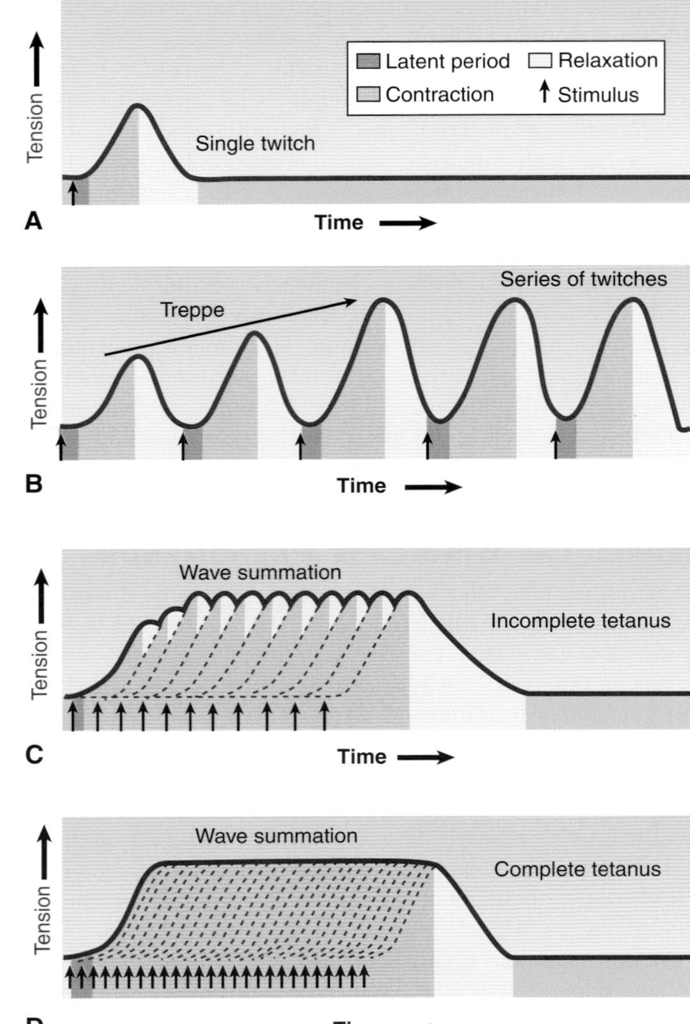

FIGURE 17-21 Myograms of various types of muscle contractions. **A,** A single twitch contraction. **B,** The treppe phenomenon, or "staircase effect", is a steplike increase in the force of contraction over the first few in a series of twitches. **C,** Incomplete tetanus occurs when a rapid succession of stimuli produces "twitches" that seem to add together (wave summation) to produce a rather sustained contraction. **D,** Complete tetanus is a smoother sustained contraction produced by the summation of "twitches" that occur so close together that the muscle cannot relax at all.

the muscle does not have time to relax completely before the next contraction phase begins. Muscle physiologists describe this effect as *multiple wave summation*—so named because it seems as though multiple twitch waves have been added together to sustain muscle tension for a longer time. The type of tetanus produced when very short periods of relaxation occur between peaks of tension is called *incomplete tetanus.* It is "incomplete" because the tension is not sustained at a completely constant level.

Figure 17-21, *D*, shows that when the frequency of stimuli increases, the distance between peaks of tension decreases to a point at which they seem to fuse into a single, sustained peak. This produces a very smooth type of tetanic contraction called *complete tetanus.*

Figure 17-22 shows the role of calcium in maintaining tetanus. Recall that it is a surge in intracellular calcium (from the SR) that triggers contraction (see **Box 17-2**, p. 367). When there is a single stimulus, there is a single surge in intracellular calcium and thus a single, rapid contraction. When there is a series of stimuli, close together in time, the intracellular calcium surges overlap and maintain a high level of calcium availability for a longer time. The force of contraction can be maintained as long as the calcium remains at a high enough level in the muscle fibres.

In a normal body, sustained muscle contraction results from two factors working at the same time. One factor is the rapid-fire stimulation of nerve fibres that permits wave summation to occur in each fibre. Another factor is the coordinated contractions of different motor units within the muscle organ. These motor units fire in an asynchronous, overlapping time sequence to produce a "relay team" effect that results in a relatively sustained contraction.

This brief description of twitch, treppe, and tetanus in myographic studies of isolated muscles gives us a model for understanding the basic principles of muscle action in ordinary life.

BOX 17-5 *sports and fitness*
Muscle Fatigue

Broadly defined, *muscle fatigue* is simply a state of exhaustion (a loss of strength or endurance) produced by strenuous muscular activity.

Physiological muscle fatigue is caused by any combination of local failure in the steps of muscle contraction (see **Box 17-2** on p. 367).

For example, failure of the sodium–potassium pumps to maintain the ion concentration gradients needed to produce action potentials may cause fatigue. Individual muscle fibres become less contractile until the proper Na^+ and K^+ gradients can be restored.

Depending on the muscle fibre type and the kind of activity, the cause may be a relative lack of adenosine triphosphate (ATP), which renders the myosin heads incapable of producing the force required for further muscle contractions. The low levels of ATP that produce fatigue may result from depletion of oxygen or glucose in muscle fibres or from an inability to regenerate ATP quickly enough. Thus depletion of glycogen in the muscle often produces fatigue.

Accumulation of phosphate molecules (from the breakdown of ATP) may further interfere with contraction by binding to calcium ions that would otherwise be participating in the contraction process.

Buildup of lactate in muscle tissue during exercise has been blamed for fatigue and the burning sensation sometimes associated with it, but this role of lactate has been disproven by recent experimental evidence.

Muscle tissue can limit physiological fatigue by increasing blood flow, thus bringing in additional oxygen and glucose—and taking away more CO_2. Muscle tissue also produces hormones that trigger the release of more glucose and other nutrients into the bloodstream. But eventually a muscle may not be able to sustain its work.

In ordinary circumstances, however, complete physiological fatigue rarely occurs. It is usually *psychological fatigue* that produces the exhausted feeling that stops us from continuing a muscular activity. Such fatigue is regulated by feedback loops that increase our feelings of fatigue as muscles work hard and thus protect the muscles from reaching a point where they could become seriously impaired.

In physiological muscle fatigue we *cannot* contract our muscles, but in psychological muscle fatigue we simply *will not* contract our muscles because we feel tired. •

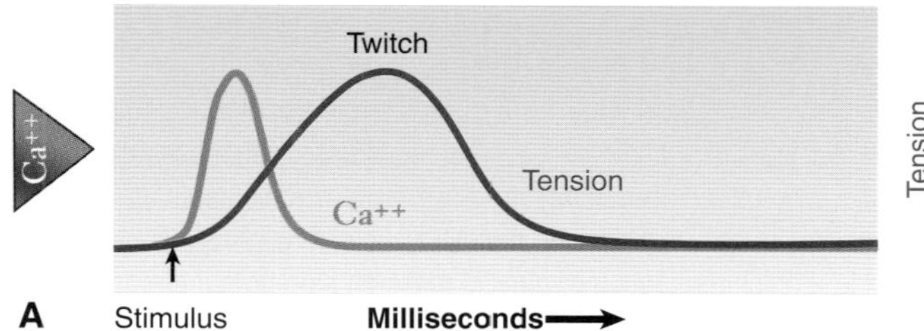

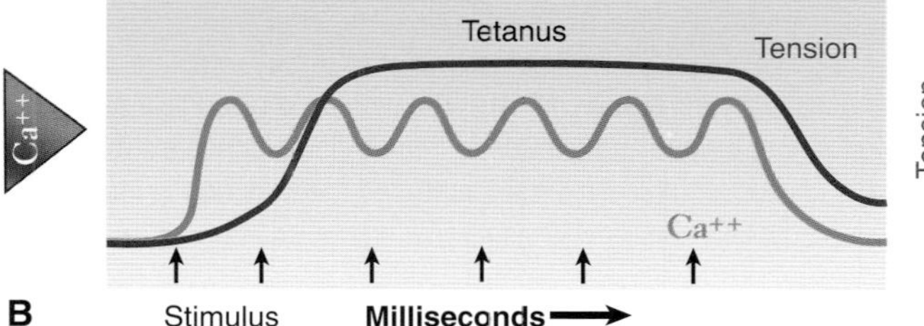

FIGURE 17-22 Role of calcium in twitch and tetanus. A, A single, sudden increase in calcium (Ca^{++}) availability triggers the twitch contraction. **B,** Repeated stimuli maintain a high level of calcium, permitting sustained (tetanic) contraction.

Quick **CHECK**

11. What are the three phases of a twitch contraction? What molecular events occur during each of these phases?
12. What is the difference between a twitch contraction and a tetanic contraction?
13. How does the treppe effect relate to the warm-up exercises of athletes?
14. What is tetanus? Is it normal?

Muscle Tone

A **tonic contraction** is a continual, partial contraction in a muscle organ. At any one moment a small number of the total fibres in a muscle contract and produce tautness of the muscle rather than a recognizable contraction and movement. Different groups of fibres scattered throughout the muscle contract in relays. Tonic contraction, or **muscle tone**, is the low level of continuous contraction characteristic of the muscles of normal individuals when they are awake.

Muscle tone is particularly important for maintaining posture. A striking illustration of this fact is the following: when a person loses consciousness, muscles lose their tone, and the person collapses in a heap, unable to maintain a sitting or standing posture. Muscles with less tone than normal are described as *flaccid*, and those with more than normal tone are called *spastic*.

Muscle tone is maintained by negative feedback mechanisms centred in the nervous system, specifically in the spinal cord. Stretch sensors in the muscles and tendons detect the degree of stretch in a muscle organ and feed this information back to an integrator mechanism in the spinal cord. When the actual stretch (detected by the stretch receptors) deviates from the setpoint stretch, signals sent via the somatic motor neurons adjust the strength of tonic contraction. This type of subconscious mechanism is often called a *spinal reflex* (discussed further in Chapters 19 to 21).

GRADED STRENGTH PRINCIPLE

Grades of Muscle Strength

Skeletal muscles contract with varying degrees of strength at different times—a fact called the **graded strength principle.** Because muscle organs can generate different grades of strength, we can match the force of a movement to the demands of a specific task (**Box 17-6**).

Metabolic Condition

Various factors contribute to the phenomenon of graded strength. We have already discussed some of these factors. For example, we stated that the metabolic condition of individual fibres influences their capacity to generate force. Thus, if many fibres of a muscle organ are unable to maintain a high level of ATP and become fatigued, the entire muscle organ suffers some loss in its ability to generate maximum force of contraction. On the other hand, the improved metabolic conditions that produce the treppe effect allow a muscle organ to increase its contraction strength.

Recruitment of Motor Units

Another factor that influences the grade of strength exhibited by a muscle organ is the number of fibres contracting simultaneously. Obviously, the more muscle fibres contracting at the same time, the stronger the contraction of the entire muscle organ. How large this number is depends on how many motor units are activated or **recruited.**

Recruitment of motor units, in turn, depends on the intensity and frequency of stimulation. In general, the more intense and the more frequent a stimulus, the more motor units that are recruited and the stronger the contraction. **Figure 17-23** shows that increasing the strength of the stimulus beyond the threshold level of the most sensitive motor units causes an increase in the strength of contraction. As the threshold level of each additional motor unit is reached, the strength of contraction increases. This process continues as the strength of stimulation increases until the maximal level

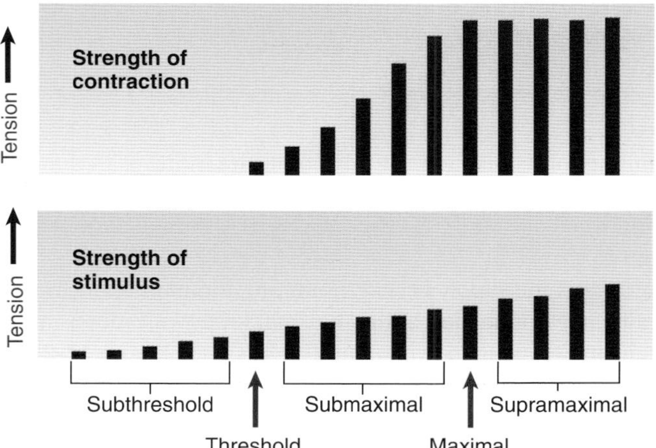

FIGURE 17-23 The strength of muscle contraction compared with the strength of the stimulus. After the threshold stimulus is reached, a continued increase in stimulus strength produces a proportional increase in muscle strength until the maximal level of contraction strength is reached.

BOX 17-6 *effects of exercise on skeletal muscles*

Most of us believe that exercise is good for us, even if we have no idea what or how many specific benefits can come from it. Some of the good consequences of regular, properly practised exercise are greatly improved muscle tone, better posture, more efficient heart and lung function, less fatigue, longer life, and a sense of looking and feeling better.

Skeletal muscles undergo changes that correspond to the amount of work that they normally do. During prolonged inactivity, muscles usually shrink in mass, a condition called **disuse atrophy** (part *A* of the figure). Disuse atrophy may result from general lack of use, but it is most often seen when a body part is immobilized by a cast or when the motor nerves are damaged. Exercise, on the other hand, may cause an increase in muscle size called **hypertrophy.**

Muscle hypertrophy can be enhanced by **strength training,** which involves contracting muscles against heavy resistance. Isometric exercises and weight-lifting are common strength-training activities. This type of training results in increased numbers of satellite cells merging with muscle fibres to form additional myofilaments in each muscle fibre. Although the number of muscle fibres stays the same, the increased number of myofilaments greatly increases the mass of the muscle. When strength training stops, the extra myofilaments are dismantled and the muscle atrophies. However, the extra nuclei may remain for years and thus enable a quick restoration of muscle mass and strength if strength training resumes.

Endurance training, often called **aerobic training** (part *B* of the figure), does not usually result in as much muscle hypertrophy as strength training does. Instead, this type of exercise program increases a muscle's ability to sustain moderate exercise over a long period. Aerobic activities such as running, bicycling, or other primarily isotonic movements increase the number of blood vessels in a muscle (see **Figure 17-15**). The increased blood flow allows more efficient delivery of oxygen and glucose to muscle fibres during exercise. Aerobic training also causes an increase in the number of mitochondria in muscle fibres. This allows production of more ATP as a rapid energy source. •

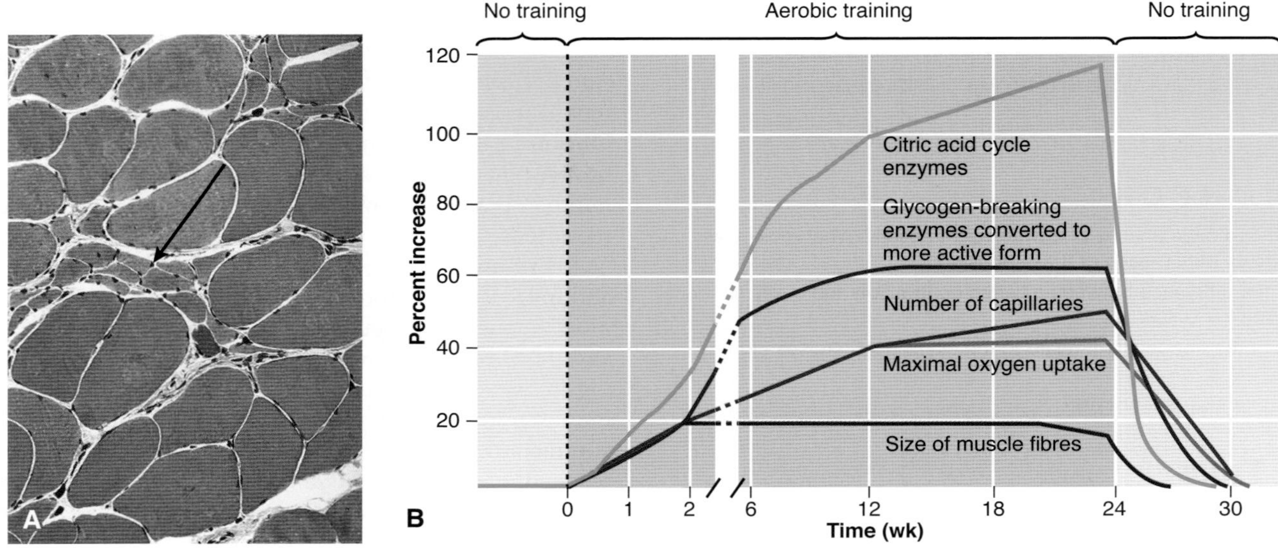

A, Disuse atrophy. The *arrow* points to a group of muscle fibres that have atrophied from disuse (in this case from nerve damage). Note how much smaller they are than the surrounding, normal fibres. **B, Effects of aerobic training.** The graph shows that aerobic training increases the metabolic condition of muscles mainly by increasing levels of enzymes and the availability of oxygen. Only moderate increases in muscle fibre size occur.

of contraction is reached. At this point, the limits of the muscle organ to recruit new motor units have been reached. Even if stimulation increases above the maximal level, the muscle cannot contract any more strongly.

As long as the supply of ATP holds out, the muscle organ can sustain a tetanic contraction at the maximal level, with motor units contracting and relaxing in overlapping "relays" (see **Figure 17-21**, *D*).

Effect of Muscle Length on Strength

The maximal strength that a muscle can develop is directly related to the initial length of its fibres—this is the *length–tension relationship* (**Figure 17-24**).

A muscle that begins a contraction from a short initial length cannot develop much tension because its sarcomeres are already compressed. Conversely, a muscle that begins a contraction from an overstretched initial length cannot develop much tension because the thick myofilaments are too far away from the thin myofilaments to effectively pull them and thus compress the sarcomeres. The strongest maximal contraction is possible only when the muscle organ has been stretched to an optimal initial length.

To illustrate this point, extend your elbow fully and try to contract the *brachialis* and *biceps brachii* muscles on the ventral side of the upper part of your arm. Now flex the elbow just a little and contract the brachialis and biceps again. Try it a third time with the elbow completely flexed. The greatest tension—seen as the largest "bulge" of the brachialis and biceps—occurs when the elbow is partly flexed and the flexor muscles only moderately stretched.

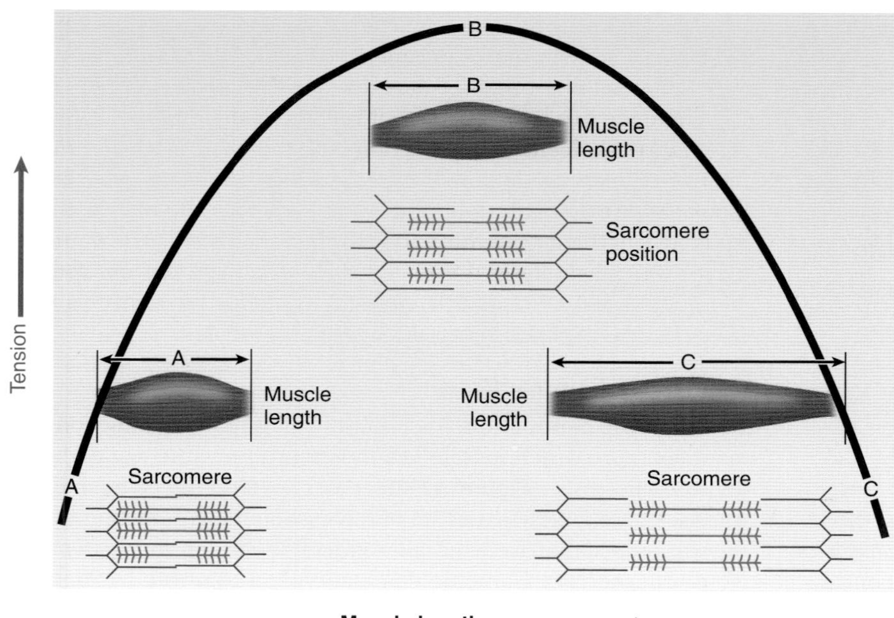

FIGURE 17-24 The length–tension relationship. As this graph of muscle tension shows, the maximum strength that a muscle can develop is directly related to the initial length of its fibres. At a short initial length, the sarcomeres are already compressed, and thus the muscle cannot develop much tension (position *A*). Conversely, the thick and thin myofilaments are too far apart in an overstretched muscle to generate much tension (position *C*). Maximum tension can be generated only when the muscle has been stretched to a moderate, optimal length (position *B*).

Effect of Load on Strength

Another factor that influences the strength of a skeletal muscle contraction is the amount of load imposed on the muscle. Within certain limits, the heavier the load, the stronger the contraction.

Lift your hand with palm up in front of you and then put this book in your palm. You can feel your arm muscles contract more strongly as the book is placed in your hand. This occurs because of a *stretch reflex*, a response in which the body tries to maintain constancy of muscle length (**Figure 17-25**).

An increased load threatens to stretch the muscle beyond the setpoint length that you are trying to maintain. Your body exhibits a negative feedback response when it detects the increased stretch caused by an increased load, feeds the information back to an integrator in the nervous system, and increases its stimulation of the muscle to counteract the stretch. This reflex maintains a relatively constant muscle length as load is increased up to a maximum sustainable level. When the load becomes too heavy and thus threatens to cause injury to the muscle or skeleton, the body abandons this reflex and forces you to relax and drop the load.

The major factors involved in the graded strength principle are summarized in **Figure 17-26**.

Mobilizing and Stabilizing Contractions

Isotonic Contractions

The term *isotonic* literally means "same tension" (*iso-*, "equal", *-tonic*, "relating to tension"). An **isotonic contraction** is a contraction in which the tone or tension within a muscle remains the same

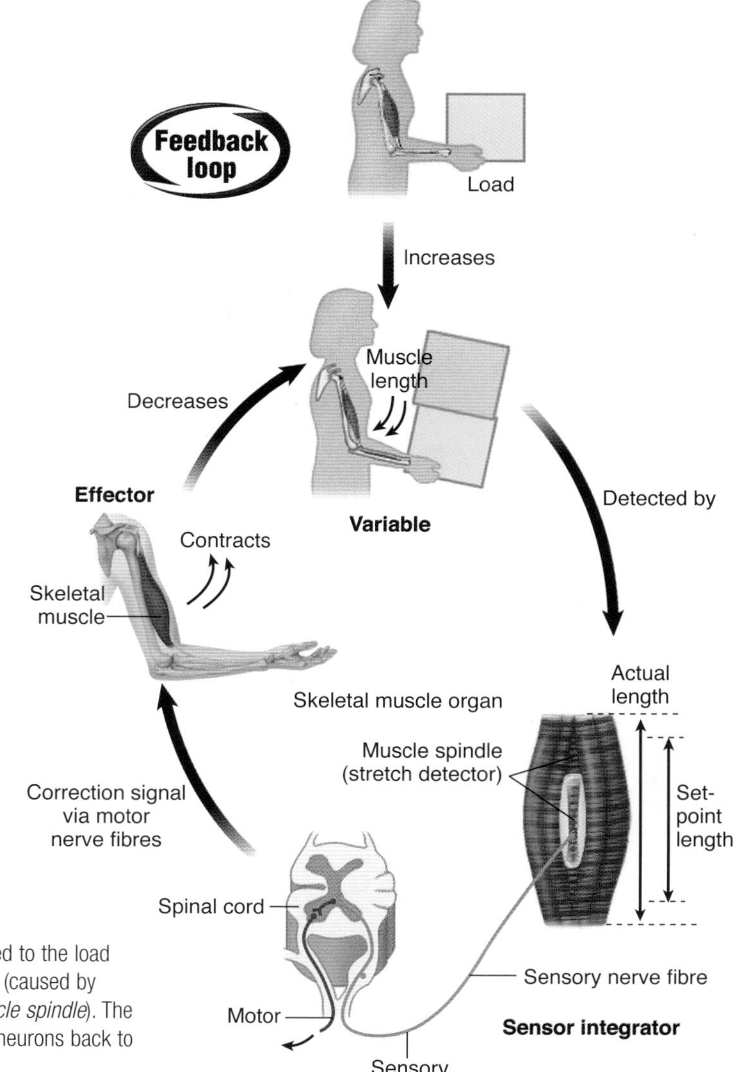

FIGURE 17-25 The stretch reflex. The strength of a muscle organ can be matched to the load imposed on it by a negative feedback response centred in the spinal cord. Increased stretch (caused by increased load) is detected by a sensory nerve fibre attached to a muscle cell (called a *muscle spindle*). The information is integrated in the spinal cord and a correction signal is relayed through motor neurons back to the same muscle, which increases tension to return to the setpoint muscle length.

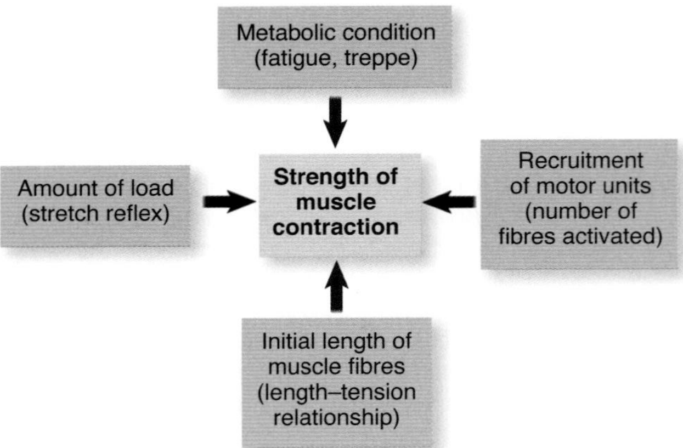

FIGURE 17-26 Factors that influence the strength of muscle contraction.

as the length of the muscle changes (**Figure 17-27**, *A*). Because the muscle is moving against its resistance (load) in an isotonic contraction, the energy of contraction is used to pull on the thin myofilaments and thus change the length of a fibre's sarcomeres. Put another way, in isotonic contractions the myosin cross bridges "win" the tug-of-war against a light load and are thus able to pull the thin myofilaments.

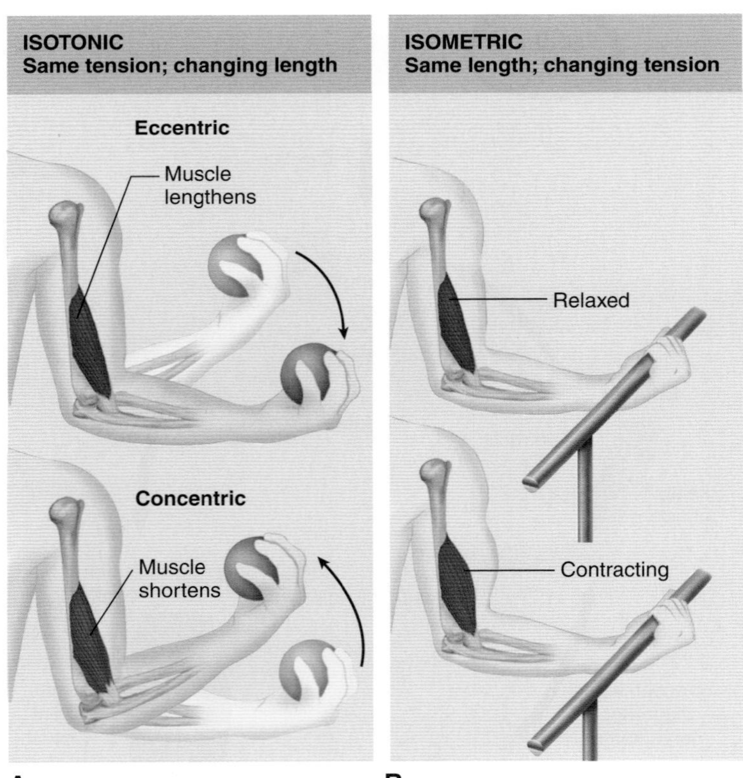

FIGURE 17-27 Isotonic and isometric contraction. A, In isotonic contraction the muscle shortens and produces movement. Concentric contractions occur when the muscle shortens during the movement. Eccentric contractions occur when the contracting muscle lengthens. **B,** In isometric contraction the muscle pulls forcefully against a load but does not shorten because it cannot overcome the resistance.

An isotonic contraction is a *mobilizing contraction* because it causes the body to move. Because the muscle is moving in an isotonic contraction, it is also called *dynamic tension*.

There are two basic varieties of isotonic contractions (see **Figure 17-27**, *A*). **Concentric contractions** are those in which the movement results in shortening of the muscle, as when you pick up this book. **Eccentric contractions** are those in which the movement results in lengthening of the muscle being contracted. For example, when you slowly lower the book you have just picked up, you are contracting the same muscle you just used to lift it—but this time you are lengthening the muscle, not shortening it.

Isometric Contractions

An **isometric contraction,** in contrast to an isotonic contraction, is a contraction in which muscle length remains the same while muscle tension increases (**Figure 17-27**, *B*). The term *isometric* literally means "same length". You can observe isometric contraction by lifting up on a stationary handrail and feeling the tension increase in your arm muscles. Isometric contractions can do work by "tightening" to resist a force, but they do not produce movements.

In isometric contractions, the tension produced by the power stroke of the myosin cross bridges cannot overcome the load placed on the muscle. Using the tug-of-war analogy, we can say that in isometric contractions the myosin cross bridges reach a "draw"—they hold their own against the load placed on the muscle but do not make any progress in sliding the thin myofilaments.

In contrast to an isotonic contraction, which mobilizes the body, an isometric contraction is a *stabilizing contraction* because it holds the body in a stable position. Because muscles remain stable during isometric contraction, it is also called *static tension*.

Box 17-7 explains the benefits of massaging muscles after vigorous isotonic or isometric exercise.

BOX 17-7 *sports and fitness*

Muscle Massage

Research shows that massaging muscles after exercise reduces the inflammation that can cause soreness after a workout or athletic competition. Massaging muscles for just 10 minutes immediately after exercise can decrease the chemicals that trigger the pain and swelling that sometimes follow vigorous use of skeletal muscles. Massaging muscles also increases the number of mitochondria in each muscle fibre—resulting in more energy being available for future contractions. •

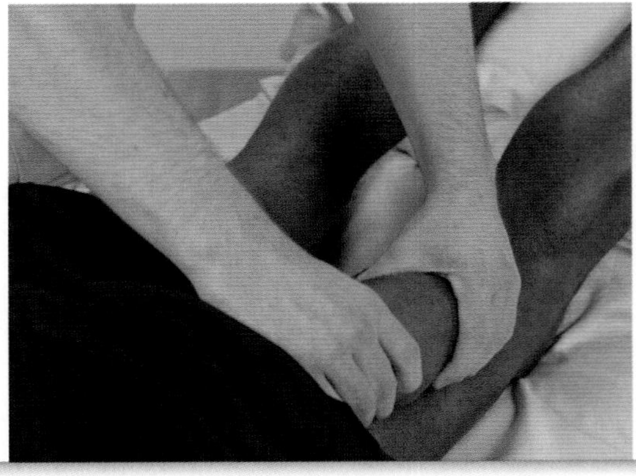

Quick CHECK

15. What is meant by the term *muscle tone?*
16. Name four factors that influence the strength of a skeletal muscle contraction.
17. What is meant by the phrase "recruitment of motor units"?
18. What is the difference between isotonic and isometric contractions? Concentric and eccentric?

FUNCTION OF CARDIAC AND SMOOTH MUSCLE TISSUE

Cardiac and smooth muscle tissues operate by mechanisms similar to those in skeletal muscle tissues. Detailed study of cardiac and smooth muscle function will be set aside until we discuss specific smooth and cardiac muscle organs in later chapters. However, it may be helpful to preview some of the basic principles of cardiac and smooth muscle physiology so that we can compare them with those that operate in skeletal muscle tissue. **Table 17-1** summarizes the characteristics of the three major types of muscle.

CARDIAC MUSCLE

Cardiac muscle, also known as *striated involuntary muscle*, is found in only one organ of the body: the heart. Forming the bulk of the wall of each heart chamber, cardiac muscle contracts rhythmically and continuously to provide the pumping action necessary to maintain a relative constancy of blood flow through the internal environment. As you shall see, its physiological mechanisms are well adapted to this function.

The functional anatomy of cardiac muscle tissue resembles that of skeletal muscle to a degree, but it exhibits certain unique features related to its role of continuously pumping blood. As **Figure 17-28** shows, each cardiac muscle fibre contains parallel myofibrils. Each myofibril includes sarcomeres that give the whole fibre a striated appearance.

Cardiac muscle fibre does not taper like skeletal muscle fibre but instead forms strong, electrically coupled junctions (intercalated discs) with other fibres. Besides having desmosomes joining the abutting ends of cardiac fibres, intercalated discs also feature gap junctions. Recall from **Figure 5-20** (p. 92) that gap junctions form little tunnels that functionally couple the membranes and cytoplasm of adjacent cells. This arrangement allows electrical impulses to flow directly from one cardiac fibre to the next.

The presence of intercalated discs, along with the branching exhibited by individual cells, allows cardiac fibres to form a continuous, electrically coupled mass called a **syncytium** (meaning "unit of combined cells"). Cardiac muscles thus form a continuous, contractile band around the heart chambers that conducts a single impulse across a virtually continuous sarcolemma—features necessary for an efficient, coordinated pumping action. The cardiac syncytium is yet another example of the principle that structure fits function.

Unlike skeletal muscle, in which a nervous impulse excites the sarcolemma to produce its own impulse, cardiac muscle is self-exciting. Cardiac muscle cells thus exhibit a continuing rhythm of excitation and contraction on their own, although the rate of self-induced impulses can be altered by nervous or hormonal input.

Figure 17-29 shows that impulses triggering cardiac muscle contractions are much more prolonged than those triggering skeletal muscle contractions. Because the sarcolemma of cardiac muscle sustains each impulse longer than in skeletal muscle, Ca^{++} remains in the sarcoplasm longer. This means that even though many adjacent cardiac muscle cells contract simultaneously, they exhibit a

TABLE 17-1 Characteristics of Muscle Tissues

	SKELETAL	CARDIAC	SMOOTH
Principal location	Skeletal muscle organs	Wall of heart	Walls of many hollow organs
Principal functions	Movement of bones, heat production, posture	Pumping of blood	Movement in walls of hollow organs (peristalsis, mixing of fluids)
Type of control	Voluntary	Involuntary	Involuntary
Structural features			
Striations	Present	Present	Absent
Nucleus	Many near the sarcolemma	Single (sometimes double); near the centre of the cell	Single; near the centre of the cell
T tubules	Narrow; form triads with the SR	Large diameter; form diads with the SR, regulate Ca^{++} entry into the sarcoplasm	Absent
Sarcoplasmic reticulum	Extensive; stores and releases Ca^{++}	Less extensive than in skeletal muscle	Very poorly developed
Cell junctions	No gap junctions	Intercalated discs (gap junctions and desmosomes)	*Single-unit*:* many gap junctions *Multiunit:* few gap junctions
Contraction style	Rapid twitch contractions of motor units usually summate to produce sustained tetanic contractions; must be stimulated by a neuron	Syncytium of fibres compress the heart chambers in slow, separate contractions (does not exhibit tetanus or fatigue); exhibits autorhythmicity	*Single-unit:* electrically coupled sheets of fibres contract autorhythmically and produce peristalsis or mixing movements *Multiunit:* individual fibres contract when stimulated by a neuron

SR, Sarcoplasmic reticulum.

*Also referred to as *visceral smooth muscle tissue*.

UNIT 2

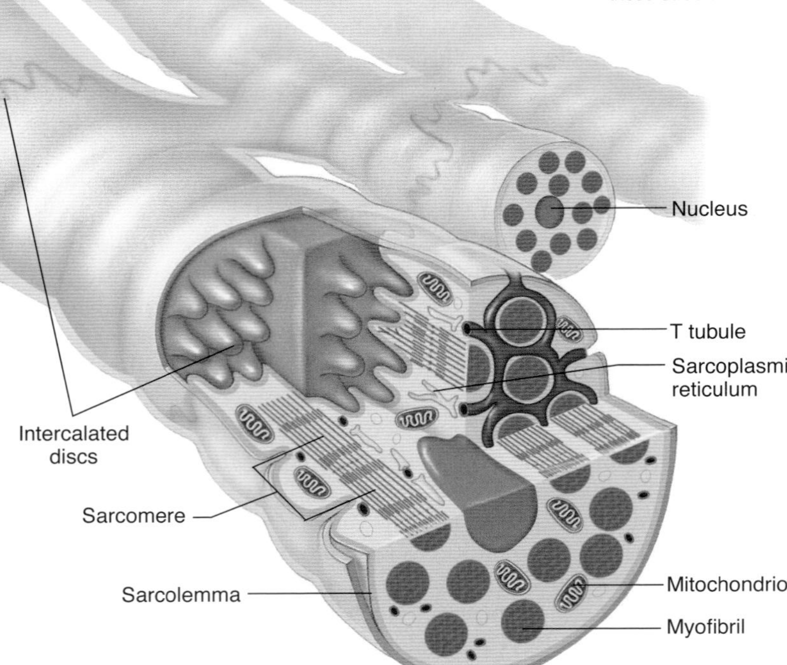

FIGURE 17-28 Cardiac muscle fibre. Unlike other types of muscle fibres, cardiac muscle fibre is typically branched and forms junctions, called *intercalated discs,* with adjacent cardiac muscle fibres. Like skeletal muscle fibres, cardiac muscle fibres contain sarcoplasmic reticula and T tubules—although these structures are not as highly organized as in skeletal muscle fibres.

prolonged contraction rather than a rapid twitch. It also means that impulses cannot come rapidly enough to produce tetanus. Because it cannot sustain long tetanic contractions, cardiac muscle does not normally run low on ATP and thus does not experience fatigue. Obviously, this characteristic of cardiac muscle is vital to keeping the heart continuously pumping.

Although cardiac muscle fibre has T tubules and SR, they are arranged a little differently than in skeletal muscle fibres. The T tubules are larger, and they form diads (double structures) rather than triads (triple structures), with a rather sparse SR. Much of the calcium that enters the sarcoplasm during contraction enters from outside the cells through the T tubules rather than from storage in the SR.

The structure and function of the heart are discussed further in Chapter 28.

Smooth Muscle

As we mentioned in Chapter 9, smooth muscle is composed of small, tapered cells with single nuclei. Smooth muscle cells do not have T tubules and have only loosely organized sarcoplasmic reticula. The calcium required for contraction comes from outside the cell and binds to a protein called *calmodulin,* rather than to troponin, to trigger a contraction event.

The lack of striations in smooth muscle fibres results from the fact that the thick and thin myofilaments are arranged quite differently than in skeletal or cardiac muscle fibres. As **Figure 17-30** shows, thin arrangements of myofilaments crisscross the cell and attach at their ends to the cell's plasma membrane. When cross bridges pull the thin filaments together, the muscle "balls up" and thus contracts the cell. Because the myofilaments are not organized into sarcomeres, they have more freedom of movement and as a result can contract a smooth muscle fibre to shorter lengths than in skeletal and cardiac muscle.

There are two types of smooth muscle tissue: *single-unit* and *multiunit* (**Figure 17-31**) smooth muscle.

In *visceral,* or **single-unit, smooth muscle,** gap junctions join individual smooth muscle fibres into large, continuous sheets—much like the syncytium of fibres observed in cardiac muscle. This type of smooth muscle is the most common, and it forms a muscular layer in the walls of many hollow structures such as the digestive, urinary, and reproductive tracts. Like cardiac muscle, single-unit smooth muscle commonly exhibits a rhythmic self-excitation, or *autorhythmicity* (meaning "self-rhythm"), that spreads across the entire tissue. When these rhythmic, spreading waves of contraction become strong enough, they can push the contents of a hollow organ progressively along its lumen. This phenomenon, called

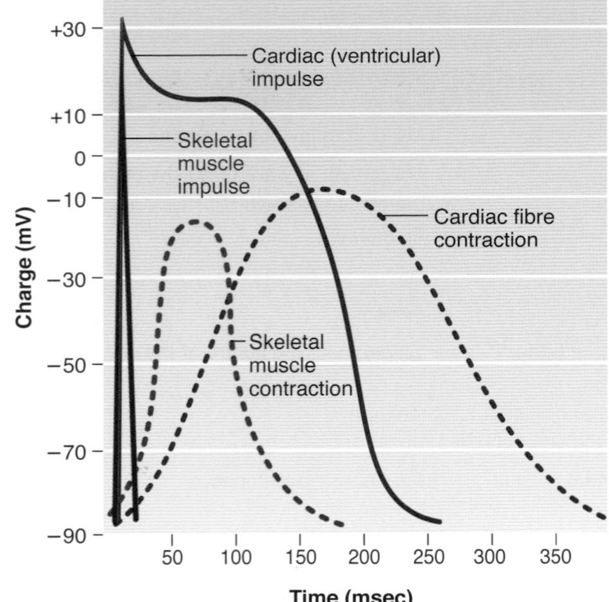

FIGURE 17-29 Cardiac and skeletal muscle contractions compared. A brief nerve impulse triggers a brief twitch contraction in skeletal muscle *(blue),* but a prolonged impulse in the heart tissue produces a rather slow, drawn-out contraction in cardiac muscle *(red).*

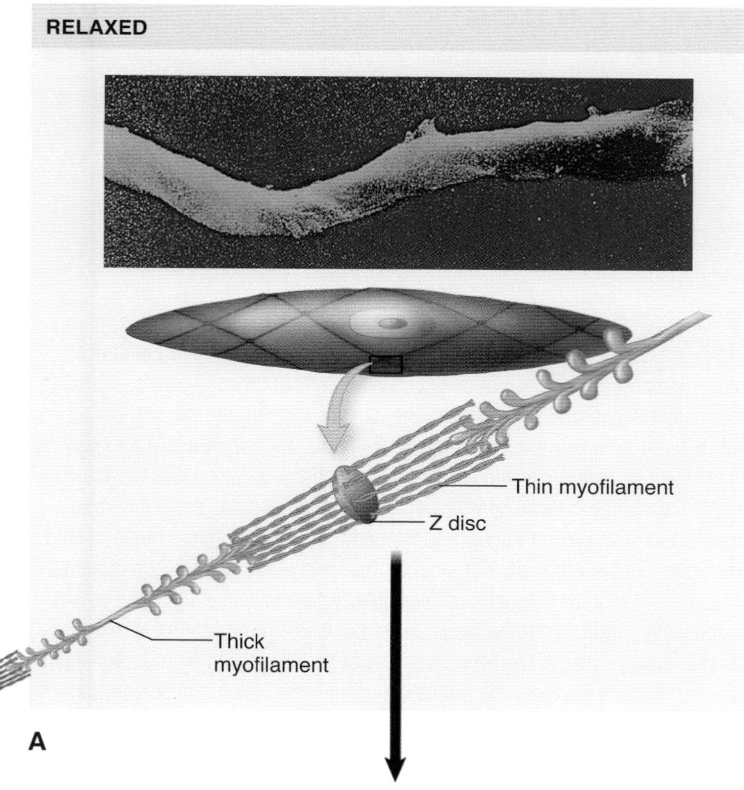

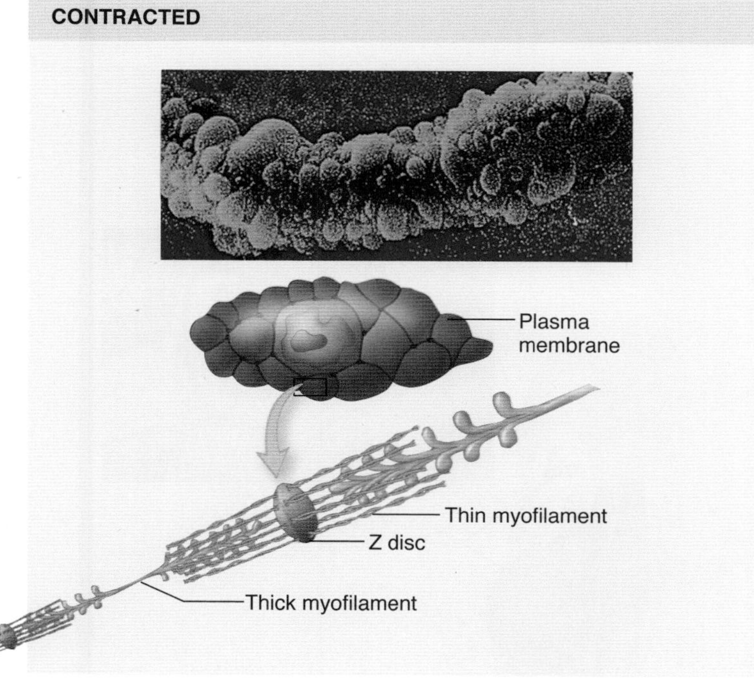

FIGURE 17-30 Smooth muscle fibre. A, Thin bundles of myofilaments span the diameter of a relaxed fibre. The scanning electron micrograph *(above)* shows that the surface of the cell is rather flat when the fibre is relaxed. **B,** During contraction, sliding of the myofilaments causes the fibre to shorten by "balling up". The SEM shows that the fibre becomes shorter and thicker and exhibits "dimples" where the myofilament bundles are pulling on the plasma membrane.

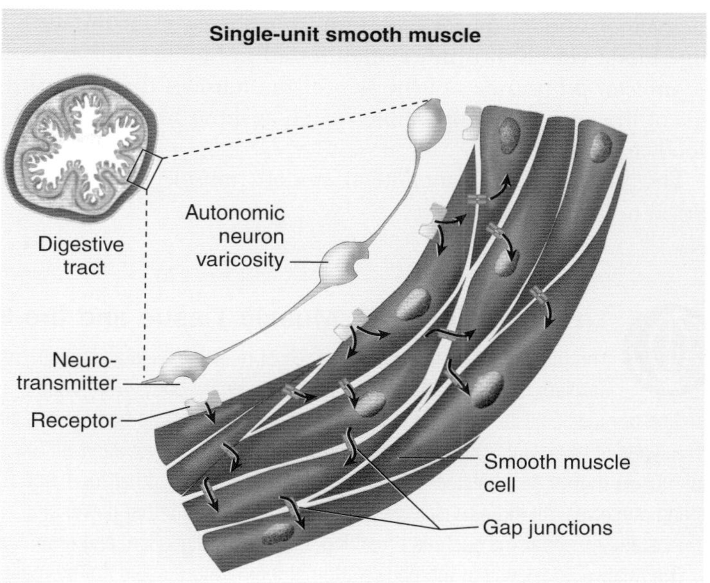

Multiunit smooth muscle

Eye

Varicosity

Neuron

B

FIGURE 17-31 Types of smooth muscle. A, Single-unit (visceral) smooth muscle. Neurotransmitters released from varicosities (bulges) in the nerve fibre trigger impulses in the smooth muscle membranes—an event that is transmitted to adjacent muscle fibres through gap junctions. Thus a large mass of muscle fibres acts as a single unit. **B,** Multiunit smooth muscle. Each muscle fibre is triggered independently by nerve stimulation.

peristalsis, moves food along the digestive tract, assists the flow of urine to the bladder, and pushes a baby out of the womb during labour. Such contractions can also be coordinated to produce mixing movements in the stomach and other organs.

Multiunit smooth muscle tissue does not act as a single unit (as in visceral muscle) but instead is composed of many independent single-cell units. Each independent fibre does not usually generate its own impulse but rather responds only to nervous input. Although this type of smooth muscle can form thin sheets, as in the walls of large blood vessels, it is more often found in bundles (for example, the *arrector pili* muscles of the skin or the muscles that control the lens of the eye) or as single fibres (such as those surrounding small blood vessels).

The structure and function of smooth muscle organs are discussed in later chapters.

Quick CHECK

19. How do slow, separate, autorhythmic contractions of cardiac muscle make it well suited to its role in pumping blood?
20. What produces the striations in cardiac muscle?
21. How are myofilaments arranged in a smooth muscle fibre?
22. What is the difference between single-unit and multiunit smooth muscle?

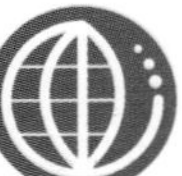

the big picture | Muscle Tissue and the Whole Body

The function of all three major types of muscle (skeletal, smooth, and cardiac) is integral to the function of the entire body. What does the function of muscle tissue contribute to homeostasis of the whole body? First, all three types of muscle tissue provide the movement necessary for survival. Skeletal muscle moves the skeleton so that we can seek shelter, gather food, and defend ourselves. All three muscle types produce movements that power vital homeostatic mechanisms such as breathing, blood flow, digestion, and urine flow.

The relative constancy of the body's internal temperature could not be maintained in a cool external environment if not for the "waste" heat generated by muscle tissue—especially the large mass of skeletal muscle found throughout the body. Maintenance of a relatively stable body position—posture—is also a primary function of the muscular system. Posture, specific body movements, and other contributions of the skeletal muscular system to homeostasis of the whole body were discussed in Chapters 15 and 16. The homeostatic roles of smooth muscle organs and the cardiac muscle organ (the heart) are examined in later chapters.

Like all tissues of the body, muscle tissue gives and takes. A number of systems support the function of muscle tissues. Without these systems, muscle would cease to operate. For example, the nervous system directly controls the contraction of skeletal muscle and multiunit smooth muscle. It also influences the rate of rhythmic contractions in cardiac muscle and visceral smooth muscle. The endocrine system produces hormones that assist the nervous system in regulation of muscle contraction throughout the body. The blood delivers nutrients and carries away waste products. Nutrients for the muscle are ultimately procured by the respiratory system (oxygen) and digestive system (glucose and other foods). The respiratory system also helps get rid of the waste of muscle metabolism, as does the urinary system. The liver processes lactate produced by muscles and converts it back to glucose. The immune system helps defend muscle tissue against infection and cancer—as it does for all body tissues. The fibres that make up muscle tissues, then, are truly members of the large, interactive "society of cells" that forms the human body.

mechanisms of disease Major Muscular Disorders

As you might expect, muscle disorders, or **myopathies,** generally disrupt the normal movement of the body. In mild cases, these disorders vary from inconvenient to slightly troublesome. Severe muscle disorders, however, can impair the muscles used in breathing—a life-threatening situation.

Muscle Injury

Injuries to skeletal muscles caused by overexertion or trauma usually result in a muscle **strain. Figure 17-32** shows an unusually severe muscle strain that resulted in a massive tear in the entire muscle organ. Muscle strains are characterized by muscle pain, or **myalgia,** and involve overstretching or tearing of muscle fibres. If an injury occurs in the area of a joint and a ligament is damaged, the injury may be called a **sprain.** Any muscle inflammation, including that caused by a muscle strain, is termed **myositis.** If tendon inflammation occurs with myositis, the condition is termed **fibromyositis.** A common injury of this type is *plantar fasciitis*, which occurs when the flat ligaments on the bottom of the foot—the plantar fascia—develop numerous small tears when the longitudinal arch of the foot is stressed (**Figure 13-10** on p. 275).

Although inflammation associated with such injuries may subside in a few hours or days, it usually takes weeks for damaged muscle fibres to repair. Some damaged muscle cells may be replaced by fibrous tissue, thereby forming scars. Occasionally, hard calcium is deposited in the scar tissue.

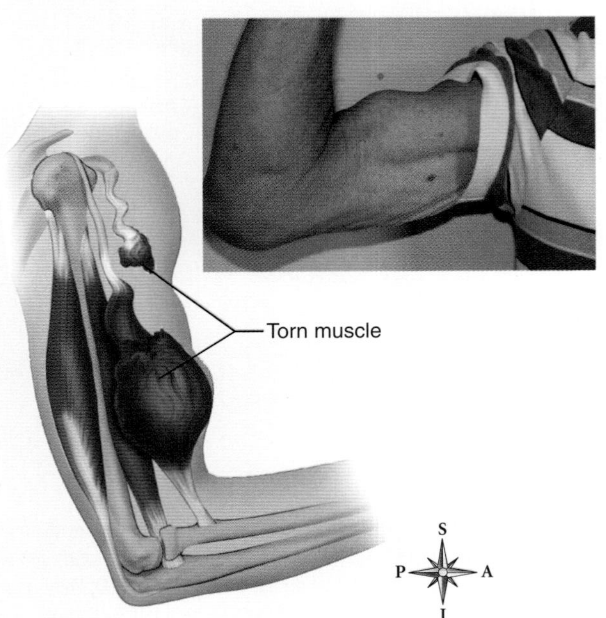

FIGURE 17-32 Muscle strain. Severe strain of the biceps brachii muscle. In a severe muscle strain, a muscle may break in two pieces, which results in a visible gap in muscle tissue under the skin. Note how the broken ends of the muscle reflexively contract (spasm) to form a knot of tissue.

Cramps often result from mild myositis or fibromyositis, but they can be a symptom of any irritation or an ion and water imbalance. **Box 17-8** outlines a few types of abnormal muscle contractions.

Minor trauma to the body, especially a limb, may cause a muscle bruise, or **contusion.** Muscle contusions involve local internal bleeding and inflammation. Severe trauma to a skeletal muscle may cause a *crush injury.* Crush injuries greatly damage the affected muscle tissue, and the release of muscle fibre contents into the bloodstream can be life-threatening. For example, the reddish muscle pigment myoglobin can accumulate in the blood and cause kidney failure.

Stress-induced muscle tension can result in myalgia and stiffness in the neck and back and is thought to be one cause of "stress headaches". Headache and back pain clinics use various strategies to treat stress-induced muscle tension. These treatments include massage, biofeedback, and relaxation training.

CONNECT IT! 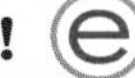

Review the article ***Rhabdomyolysis*** online at ***Connect It!***

Muscle Infections

Several bacteria, viruses, and parasites may infect muscle tissue—often producing local or widespread myositis. For example, in trichinosis, widespread myositis is common. The muscle pain plus stiffness that sometimes accompanies influenza is another example.

One bacterial infection you have probably heard of is called *tetanus*—a confusing name because that word also refers to normal, sustained muscle contractions (see **Figure 17-21**). However, tetanus *the infection* is an abnormal condition caused by infection of the central nervous system with the bacterium *Clostridium tetani.* This bacterium releases a toxin called *tetanospasmin* that triggers overactivity of the nervous system, often involving painful spasms of the muscles throughout the body. Because the spasms frequently begin in the head and cause the jaw muscles to tense involuntarily, the infection is often called "lockjaw".

Once a tragically common disease, **poliomyelitis** is a viral infection of the nerves that control skeletal muscle movement. Although the disease can be asymptomatic, it often causes paralysis that may progress to death. Poliomyelitis has been eliminated from the UK as a result of a comprehensive vaccination programme. There remains a very small risk it could be brought back into the UK, as it is still present in some parts of the world.

BOX 17-8 *health matters* | Abnormal Muscle Contractions

Cramps are painful muscle spasms (involuntary twitches). Cramps often occur when a muscle organ is fatigued or mildly inflamed, but they can be a symptom of any irritation or ion and water imbalance.

Convulsions are abnormal, uncoordinated tetanic contractions of varying groups of muscles. Convulsions may result from a disturbance in the brain, or seizure, in which the output along motor nerves increases and becomes disorganized.

Fibrillation is an abnormal type of contraction in which individual fibres contract asynchronously rather than at the same time. This produces a flutter of the muscle but no effective movement. Fibrillation can also occur in cardiac muscle, where it reduces the heart's ability to pump blood. •

Muscular Dystrophy

Muscular dystrophy is not a single disorder but a group of genetic diseases characterized by atrophy (wasting) of skeletal muscle tissues. Some, but not all, forms of muscular dystrophy can be fatal.

The common form of muscular dystrophy is **Duchenne muscular dystrophy (DMD).** This form of the disease is also called *pseudohypertrophy* (meaning "false muscle growth") because the atrophy of muscle is masked by excessive replacement of muscle by fat and fibrous tissue. DMD is characterized by mild leg muscle weakness that progresses rapidly to include the shoulder muscles. The first signs of DMD are apparent at about 3 years of age, and the stricken child is usually severely affected within 5 to 10 years. Death from respiratory or cardiac muscle weakness may occur by the time the individual is 21 years old.

DMD is caused by a mutation in the X chromosome, although other factors may be involved. DMD occurs primarily in boys. Because girls have two X chromosomes and boys only one, genetic diseases involving X chromosome abnormalities are more likely to occur in boys. This is true because girls with one damaged X chromosome may not exhibit an "X-linked" disease if their other X chromosome is normal (see Chapter 48).

The X-chromosome gene involved in DMD normally codes for the protein **dystrophin,** which forms strands in each skeletal muscle fibre and helps hold the cytoskeleton to the sarcolemma (see **Figure 5-21** on p. 93). Dystrophin thus helps keep the muscle fibre from breaking during contractions. Normal dystrophin is missing in those with DMD because a deletion or mutation of part of the dystrophin gene causes the resulting protein to be nonfunctional (it has the wrong shape to do the job). Therefore, in DMD muscle fibres break apart more easily—causing the symptoms of progressive muscle weakness.

Myasthenia Gravis

Myasthenia gravis is a chronic disease characterized by muscle weakness, especially in the face and throat. Most forms of this disease begin with mild weakness and chronic muscle fatigue in the face, then progress to wider muscle involvement. An acute episode of widespread and severe muscle weakness is called a *myasthenic crisis.* A person in myasthenic crisis is in danger of dying of respiratory failure because of weakness in the respiratory muscles.

Myasthenia gravis is an autoimmune disease in which the immune system attacks the acetylcholine receptors in the sarcolemma of muscle cells and results in a defect in the conduction of nerve impulses at the neuromuscular junction. Nerve impulses from motor neurons are then unable to fully stimulate the affected muscle (see **Figures 17-7** and **17-8**).

Hernias

Weakness of abdominal muscles can lead to a *hernia,* or protrusion, of an abdominal organ (commonly the small intestine or stomach) through an opening in the abdominal wall. There are several types of hernias.

CONNECT IT! 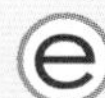

If you have not experienced a hernia before now, there is a good chance that one day you may. Hernias are quite common. See some examples of the common hernia types in ***Hernias*** online at ***Connect It!***

LANGUAGE OF SCIENCE (continued from p. 361)

isotonic contraction
(eye-soh-TON-ik kon-TRAK-shun)
[*iso-* **equal,** *ton-* **stretch or tension,** *-ic* **relating to,** *con-* **together,** *-tract-* **drag or draw,** *-tion* **process**]

lactate (LAK-tayt)
[*lact-* **milk,** *-ate* **salt of an acid**]

M line
[*M mittel* **middle**]

motor endplate
[*mot-* **move,** *-or* **agent**]

motor neuron (NYOO-ron)
[*mot-* **move,** *-or* **agent,** *neuron* **string or nerve**]

motor unit
[*mot-* **move,** *-or* **agent**]

multiunit smooth muscle
[*multi-* **many,** *mus-* **mouse,** *-cle* **little**]

muscle fatigue (fah-TEEG)
[*mus-* **mouse,** *-cle* **little**, *fatig-* **tire**]

muscle tone
[*mus-* **mouse,** *-cle* **little,** *ton-* **stretch or tension**]

myofibril (my-oh-FYE-bril)
[*myo-* **muscle,** *-fibr-* **thread or fibre,** *-il* **little**]

myofilament (my-oh-FIL-ah-ment)
[*myo-* **muscle,** *-fila-* **thread,** *-ment* **thing**]

myoglobin (my-oh-GLOH-bin)
[*myo-* **muscle,** *-glob-* **ball,** *-in* **substance**]

myosin (MY-oh-sin)
[*myos-* **muscle,** *-in* **substance**]

neuromuscular junction (NMJ)
(nyoo-roh-MUSS-kyoo-lar JUNK-shun)
[*neuro-* **nerve,** *-mus-* **mouse,** *-cul-* **little,** *-ar* **relating to**]

posture (POS-chur)
[*pos(i)t-* **place or put,** *-ure* **state**]

recruit
[*re-* **again,** *-cruit* **grow**]

sarcolemma (sar-koh-LEM-ah)
[*sarco-* **flesh,** *-lemma* **sheath**]
pl., sarcolemmae

sarcomere (SAR-koh-meer)
[*sarco-* **flesh,** *-mere* **part**]

sarcoplasm (SAR-koh-plaz-em)
[*sarco-* **flesh,** *-plasm* **substance**]

sarcoplasmic reticulum (SR)
(sar-koh-PLAZ-mik reh-TIK-yoo-lum)
[*sarco-* **flesh,** *-plasm-* **substance,** *-ic* **relating to,** *ret-* **net,** *-ic-* **relating to,** *-ul-* **little,** *-um* **thing**] *pl.*, reticula

single-unit smooth muscle
[*mus-* **mouse,** *-cle* **little**]

sliding-filament model
(SLY-ding FILL-ah-ment MOD-uhl)

slow fibre
[*fibr-* **thread or fibre**]

syncytium (sin-SISH-ee-em)
[*syn-* **together,** *-cyt-* **cell,** *-um* **a thing**]
pl., syncytia

T tubule (TEE TYOOB-yool)
[*T* **transverse,** *tub-* **tube,** *-ul-* **little**]

tetanus (TET-ah-nus)
[*tetanus* **tension**]

thermogenesis (ther-moh-JEN-eh-sis)
[*thermo-* **heat,** *-gen-* **produce,** *-esis* **process**]

threshold stimulus
(THRESH-hold STIM-yoo-lus)
[*stimul-* **excite,** *-us* **thing**] *pl.*, stimuli

tonic contraction (TON-ik)
[*ton-* **stretch,** *-ic* **relating to,** *con-* **together,** *-tract-* **drag or draw,** *-tion* **process**]

treppe (TREP-ee)
[*treppe* **staircase**]

triad (TRY-ad)
[*triad* **group of three**]

tropomyosin (troh-poh-MY-oh-sin)
[*tropo-* **turn,** *-myo-* **muscle,** *-in* **substance**]

troponin (troh-POH-nin)
[*tropo-* **turn,** *-in* **substance**]

twitch contraction
[*con-* **together,** *-tract-* **drag or draw,** *-tion* **process**]

Z disc (also called Z line) (ZED disc)
[*Z zwischen* **between**]

LANGUAGE OF MEDICINE

aerobic training (air-OH-bik)
[*aero-* **air,** *-ic* **relating to**]

contusion (kon-TOO-zhun)
[*contus-* **bruise,** *-sion* **result**]

convulsion (kon-VUL-shun)
[*convuls-* **pull violently,** *-sion* **result**]

cramp (kramp)
[*cramp* **bent**]

disuse atrophy (DIS-yoos AT-roh-fee)
[*dis-* **absence of,** *a-* **without,** *-troph* **nourishment**]

Duchenne muscular dystrophy (DMD)
(doo-SHEN MUSS-kyoo-lar DISS-troh-fee)
[*Guillaume B.A. Duchenne de Boulogne* **French neurologist,** *mus-* **mouse,** *-cul-* **little,** *-ar* **relating to,** *dys-* **bad,** *-troph-* **nourishment,** *-y* **state**]

dystrophin (DIS-trof-in)
[*dys-* **bad,** *-troph-* **nourishment,** *-in* **substance**]

fibrillation (fi-bri-LAY-shun)
[*fibr-* **thread or fibre,** *-illa-* **little,** *-ation* **process**]

fibromyositis (fye-broh-my-oh-SYE-tis)
[*fibr-* **thread or fibre,** *-myos-* **muscle,** *-itis* **inflammation**]

muscular dystrophy
(MUSS-kyoo-lar DISS-troh-fee)
[*mus-* **mouse,** *-cul-* **little,** *-ar* **relating to,** *dys-* **bad,** *-troph-* **nourishment,** *-y* **state**]

myalgia (my-AL-jee-ah)
[*my-* **muscle,** *-algia* **pain**]

myasthenia gravis
(my-es-THEE-nee-ah GRAH-vis)
[*my-* **muscle,** *-asthenia* **weakness,** *gravis* **severe**]

myopathy (my-OP-ah-thee)
[*myo-* **muscle,** *-path-* **disease,** *-y* **state**]

myositis (my-oh-SYE-tis)
[*myos-* **muscle,** *-itis* **inflammation**]

poliomyelitis (pol-ee-oh-my-eh-LYE-tis)
[*polio-* **grey,** *-mye-* **marrow,** *-itis* **inflammation**]

rigor mortis (RIG-or MOR-tis)
[*rigor* **stiffness,** *mortis* **of death**]

case study

It was snowing heavily again. Isabel was tired of shovelling snow from the entrance to her house, and it was only the beginning of December with several more weeks of winter to go. As she pushed the snow shovel across the driveway and tossed the snow onto an ever-growing mountain, she felt her muscles begin to ache.

1. By what process would Isabel's muscles first get their energy for contraction?
   a. Anaerobic pathway
   b. Aerobic pathway
   c. Recruitment
   d. Breakdown of creatine phosphate

2. The oxygen concentration inside Isabel's muscle fibres decreased rapidly as she shovelled snow. What molecule within her muscles quickly resupplied the oxygen?
   a. Haemoglobin
   b. Myoglobin
   c. Lactate
   d. Glycogen
3. Which protein molecules interact to allow Isabel's muscles to contract?
   a. Myosin and troponin
   b. Actin and myosin
   c. Actin and tropomyosin
   d. Troponin and tropomyosin

After several minutes of shovelling, Isabel stopped and took off her coat. She was surprised to find she was sweating even though the temperature was below freezing.

4. What caused Isabel's increased body temperature?
   a. Contraction of cardiac muscle cells
   b. Her increased respirations
   c. Contraction of skeletal muscle cells
   d. Conversion of ATP to glucose
5. To pick up a heavier shovelful of snow, Isabel would have to recruit more ______.
   a. Motor units
   b. Myoglobin
   c. Individual muscle fibres
   d. Myosin

Hint ▶ To solve a case study, you may have to refer to the glossary or index, other chapters in this textbook, ***Connect It!,*** and other resources.

UNIT 2

CHAPTER SUMMARY

To download an MP3 version of the chapter summary for use with your mobile device, access the **Audio Chapter Summaries** *online at evolve.elsevier.com.*

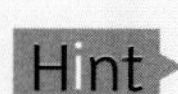

Scan this summary after reading the chapter to help you reinforce the key concepts. Later, use the summary as a quick review before your class or before a test.

Introduction

A. Muscular system is responsible for moving the framework of the body
B. In addition to movement, muscle tissue performs various other functions

General Functions

A. Movement of the body as a whole or movement of its parts
B. Heat production
C. Posture

Function of Skeletal Muscle Tissue

A. Characteristics of skeletal muscle cells
   1. Excitability (irritability)—ability to be stimulated
   2. Contractility—ability to contract, or shorten, and produce body movement
   3. Extensibility—ability to extend, or stretch, thereby allowing muscles to return to their resting length
B. Overview of the muscle cell (**Figures 17-1** and **17-2**)
   1. Muscle cells are called *fibres* because of their threadlike shape
   2. Sarcolemma—plasma membrane of muscle fibres
   3. Muscle fibres contain many mitochondria and several nuclei
   4. Sarcoplasmic reticulum (SR)
      a. Network of tubules and sacs found within muscle fibres
      b. Membrane of the SR continually pumps calcium ions from the sarcoplasm and stores the ions within its sacs for later release (**Figure 17-3**)
   5. T tubules
      a. Transverse tubules extend across the sarcoplasm at right angles to the long axis of the muscle fibre
      b. Formed by inward extensions of the sarcolemma
      c. Membrane has ion pumps that continually transport Ca^{++} ions inward from the sarcoplasm
      d. Allow electrical impulses travelling along the sarcolemma to move deeper into the cell
   6. Triad
      a. Triplet of tubules; a T tubule sandwiched between two sacs of sarcoplasmic reticulum
      b. Allows an electrical impulse travelling along a T tubule to stimulate the membranes of adjacent sacs of the sarcoplasmic reticulum
   7. Myofibrils—numerous fine fibres packed close together in sarcoplasm
   8. Sarcomere
      a. Segment of myofibril between two successive Z discs
      b. Each myofibril consists of many sarcomeres
      c. Contractile unit of muscle fibres
   9. Striated muscle (**Figure 17-4**)
      a. Dark stripes called A *bands;* light H band runs across the midsection of each dark A band
      b. Light stripes called *I bands;* dark Z disc extends across the centre of each light I band
C. Myofilaments (**Figures 17-5** and **17-6**)
   1. Each myofibril contains thousands of thick and thin myofilaments

2. Four different kinds of protein molecules make up myofilaments
   a. Myosin
      (1) Makes up almost all the thick filament
      (2) Myosin "heads" are chemically attracted to actin molecules
      (3) Myosin "heads" are known as *cross bridges* when attached to actin
   b. Actin—globular protein that forms two fibrous strands twisted around each other to form the bulk of the thin filament
   c. Tropomyosin—protein that blocks the active sites on actin molecules
   d. Troponin—protein that holds tropomyosin molecules in place
3. Thin filaments attach to both Z discs (Z lines) of a sarcomere and extend part way toward the centre
4. Thick myosin filaments do not attach to the Z discs

D. Mechanism of contraction
1. Excitation and contraction (**Figures 17-7** through **17-13**; **Table 17-1**)
   a. A skeletal muscle fibre remains at rest until stimulated by a motor neuron
   b. Neuromuscular junction—motor neurons connect to the sarcolemma at the motor endplate (**Figure 17-7**)
   c. Neuromuscular junction is a synapse where neurotransmitter molecules transmit signals
   d. Acetylcholine—the neurotransmitter released into the synaptic cleft that diffuses across the gap, stimulates the receptors, and initiates an impulse in the sarcolemma
   e. Nerve impulse travels over the sarcolemma and inward along the T tubules, which triggers the release of calcium ions
   f. Calcium binds to troponin, which causes tropomyosin to shift and expose active sites on actin
   g. Sliding filament model (**Figures 17-12** and **17-13**)
      (1) When active sites on actin are exposed, myosin heads bind to them
      (2) Myosin heads bend and pull the thin filaments past them
      (3) Each head releases, binds to the next active site, and pulls again
      (4) The entire myofibril shortens
2. Relaxation
   a. Immediately after the Ca^{++} ions are released, the sarcoplasmic reticulum begins actively pumping them back into the sacs (**Figure 17-3**)
   b. Ca^{++} ions are removed from the troponin molecules, thereby shutting down the contraction
3. Energy sources for muscle contraction (**Figure 17-14**)
   a. Hydrolysis of ATP yields the energy required for muscular contraction
   b. ATP binds to the myosin head and then transfers its energy to the myosin head to perform the work of pulling the thin filament during contraction
   c. Muscle fibres continually resynthesize ATP from the breakdown of creatine phosphate (CP)
   d. Catabolism by muscle fibres requires glucose and oxygen
   e. Glucose and oxygen supplied to muscle fibres by blood capillaries (**Figure 17-15**)
   f. At rest, excess O_2 in the sarcoplasm is bound to myoglobin (**Box 17-4**)
      (1) Red fibres—muscle fibres with high levels of myoglobin
      (2) White fibres—muscle fibres with little myoglobin
   g. Catabolic pathways
      (1) Aerobic pathway
         (a) Occurs when adequate O_2 is available from blood (**Figure 17-15**)
         (b) Slower than anaerobic pathway, thus supplies energy for the long term rather than the short term
      (2) Anaerobic pathway (**Figure 17-16**)
         (a) Very rapid, providing energy during first minutes of maximal exercise (**Figure 17-16**)
         (b) May occur when low levels of O_2 are available
         (c) Results in the formation of lactate, which requires energy and oxygen to convert back to glucose
         (d) Outdated term "oxygen debt" replaced by excess post-exercise oxygen consumption (EPOC), which results from a combination of factors (not lactate production)
   h. Heat production
   i. Skeletal muscle contraction produces waste heat that can be used to help maintain the setpoint body temperature, as in shivering thermogenesis (**Figure 17-17**)

Function of Skeletal Muscle Organs

A. Muscles are composed of bundles of muscle fibres held together by fibrous connective tissue
B. Motor unit (**Figure 17-18**)
1. Motor unit—motor neuron plus all muscle fibres to which it attaches
2. Some motor units consist of only a few muscle fibres, whereas others consist of numerous fibres
3. In general, the smaller the number of fibres in a motor unit, the more precise the movements available; the larger the number of fibres in a motor unit, the more powerful the contraction available

C. Myography—method of graphing the changing tension of a muscle as it contracts (**Figure 17-19**)
D. Twitch contraction (**Figure 17-20**)
1. A quick jerk of a muscle that is produced as a result of a single, brief threshold stimulus (generally occurs only in experimental situations)
2. The twitch contraction has three phases
   a. Latent phase—nerve impulse travels to the sarcoplasmic reticulum to trigger release of Ca^{++}
   b. Contraction phase—Ca^{++} binds to troponin and sliding of filaments occurs
   c. Relaxation phase—sliding of filaments ceases

E. Treppe—the staircase phenomenon (**Figure 17-21**, *B*)
 1. Gradual, steplike increase in the strength of contraction that is seen in a series of twitch contractions that occur 1 second apart
 2. Eventually, the muscle responds with less forceful contractions, and the relaxation phase becomes shorter
 3. If the relaxation phase disappears completely, a contracture occurs

F. Tetanus—smooth, sustained contractions
 1. Multiple wave summation—multiple twitch waves are added together to sustain muscle tension for a longer time
 2. Incomplete tetanus—very short periods of relaxation occur between peaks of tension (**Figure 17-21**, *C*)
 3. Complete tetanus—the stimulation is such that twitch waves fuse into a single, sustained peak (**Figure 17-21**, *D*)
 4. The availability of calcium determines whether a muscle will contract; if the calcium is continuously available, then contraction will be sustained (**Figure 17-22**)

G. Muscle tone
 1. Tonic contraction—continual, partial contraction of a muscle
 2. At any one time, a small number of muscle fibres within a muscle contract and produce a tightness or muscle tone
 3. Muscles with less tone than normal are flaccid
 4. Muscles with more tone than normal are spastic
 5. Muscle tone is maintained by negative feedback mechanisms

Graded Strength Principle

A. Graded strength principle—skeletal muscles contract with varying degrees of strength at different times

B. Factors that contribute to the phenomenon of graded strength (**Figure 17-26**)
 1. Metabolic condition of individual fibres
 2. Number of muscle fibres contracting simultaneously; the greater the number of fibres contracting, the stronger the contraction
 3. Number of motor units recruited
 4. Intensity and frequency of stimulation (**Figure 17-23**)
 5. Length–tension relationship (**Figure 17-24**)
  a. Maximal strength that a muscle can develop bears a direct relationship to the initial length of its fibres
  b. A shortened muscle's sarcomeres are compressed; therefore, the muscle cannot develop much tension
  c. An overstretched muscle cannot develop much tension because the thick myofilaments are too far from the thin myofilaments
  d. Strongest maximal contraction is possible only when the skeletal muscle has been stretched to its optimal length
 6. Stretch reflex (**Figure 17-25**)
  a. The load imposed on a muscle influences the strength of a skeletal contraction
  b. Stretch reflex—the body tries to maintain constancy of muscle length in response to increased load
  c. Maintains a relatively constant length as load is increased up to a maximum sustainable level

C. Mobilizing and stabilizing contractions (**Figure 17-27**)
 1. Isotonic contraction (mobilizing contraction)
  a. Contraction in which the tone or tension within a muscle remains the same as the length of the muscle changes
   (1) Concentric—muscle shortens as it contracts
   (2) Eccentric—muscle lengthens while contracting
  b. Isotonic—literally means "same tension"
  c. All of the energy of contraction is used to pull on thin myofilaments and thereby change the length of a fibre's sarcomeres
 2. Isometric contraction (stabilizing contraction)
  a. Contraction in which muscle length remains the same while muscle tension increases
  b. Isometric—literally means "same length"
 3. Most body movements occur as a result of both types of contractions

UNIT 2

Function of Cardiac and Smooth Muscle Tissue (Table 17-1)

A. Cardiac muscle (**Figure 17-28**)
 1. Found only in the heart; forms the bulk of the wall of each chamber
 2. Also known as *striated involuntary muscle*
 3. Contracts rhythmically and continuously to provide the pumping action needed to maintain constant blood flow
 4. Cardiac muscle resembles skeletal muscle but has unique features related to its role in continuously pumping blood
  a. Each cardiac muscle contains parallel myofibrils (**Figure 17-28**)
  b. Cardiac muscle fibres form strong, electrically coupled junctions (intercalated discs) with other fibres; individual cells also exhibit branching
  c. Syncytium—continuous, electrically coupled mass
  d. Cardiac muscle fibres form a continuous, contractile band around the heart chambers that conducts a single impulse across a virtually continuous sarcolemma
  e. T tubules are larger and form diads with a rather sparse sarcoplasmic reticulum
  f. Cardiac muscle sustains each impulse longer than in skeletal muscle; therefore, impulses cannot come rapidly enough to produce tetanus (**Figure 17-29**)
  g. Cardiac muscle does not run low on ATP and does not experience fatigue
  h. Cardiac muscle is self-stimulating

B. Smooth muscle
 1. Smooth muscle is composed of small, tapered cells with single nuclei (**Figure 17-30**)
 2. No T tubules are present, and only a loosely organized sarcoplasmic reticulum is present
 3. Ca^{++} comes from outside the cell and binds to calmodulin instead of troponin to trigger a contraction
 4. No striations because thick and thin myofilaments are arranged differently than in skeletal or cardiac muscle fibres; myofilaments are not organized into sarcomeres

5. Two types of smooth muscle tissue (**Figure 17-31**)
   a. Single-unit (visceral) smooth muscle
      (1) Gap junctions join smooth muscle fibres into large, continuous sheets
      (2) Most common type; forms a muscular layer in the walls of hollow structures such as the digestive, urinary, and reproductive tracts
      (3) Exhibits autorhythmicity and produces peristalsis
   b. Multiunit smooth muscle
      (1) Does not act as a single unit but is composed of many independent cell units
      (2) Each fibre responds only to nervous input

The Big Picture: Muscle Tissue and the Whole Body

A. Function of all three major types of muscle is integral to function of the entire body
B. All three types of muscle tissue provide the movement necessary for survival
C. Relative constancy of the body's internal temperature is maintained by "waste" heat generated by muscle tissue
D. Maintains the body in a relatively stable position

REVIEW QUESTIONS

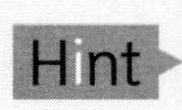

Write out the answers to these questions after reading the chapter and reviewing the Chapter Summary. Note—writing out your answers will consolidate learning and provide a valuable resource of information.

1. Define the terms *sarcolemma*, *sarcoplasm*, and *sarcoplasmic reticulum*.
2. Describe the function of the sarcoplasmic reticulum.
3. How are acetylcholine, Ca^{++}, and adenosine triphosphate (ATP) involved in the excitation and contraction of skeletal muscle?
4. Describe the general structure of ATP and tell how it relates to its function.
5. How does ATP provide energy for muscle contraction?
6. Describe the anatomical arrangement of a motor unit.
7. Compare and contrast the different types of skeletal muscle contractions.
8. Define the term *recruited* as it applies to muscles.
9. Describe rigor mortis.
10. What are the effects of *strength training* and *endurance training* on skeletal muscles?

CRITICAL THINKING QUESTIONS

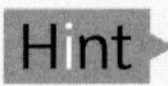

After finishing the Review Questions, write out the answers to these more in-depth questions to help you apply your new knowledge. Go back to sections of the chapter that relate to concepts that you find difficult.

1. Explain how skeletal muscles provide movement, heat, and posture. Are all of these functions unique to muscles? Explain your answer.
2. The characteristic of excitability is shared by what other system? What differentiates the two systems? Relate contractility and extensibility to the concept of agonist and antagonist discussed in Chapter 15.
3. Explain how cardiac muscle fibres avoid fatigue and what functional advantage this might have for the body.
4. Explain how the structure of myofilaments is related to their function.
5. Explain how the sliding filament theory allows for the shortening of a muscle fibre.
6. Compare and contrast the role of Ca^{++} in excitation, contraction, and relaxation of skeletal muscle.
7. Using fibre types, design a muscle for a marathon runner and a different muscle for a 100 metre sprinter. Explain your choice.
8. Explain the meaning of a "unit of combined cells" as it relates to cardiac muscle. How does this structural arrangement affect its function?
9. Which of the two smooth muscle types would be most affected by damage to the nerves that stimulate them?
10. Outline the route a calcium ion would travel from the blood in an arteriole supplying a bundle of muscle fibres to its use in contraction of a myofilament.

UNIT 3

Communication, Control, and Integration

The anatomical structures and functional mechanisms that permit communication, control, and integration of body functions are discussed in the chapters of Unit 3. To maintain homeostasis, the body must have the ability to monitor and then respond appropriately to changes that may occur in either the internal or external environment. The nervous and endocrine systems provide this capability. Information originating in sensory nerve endings found in complex special sense organs such as the eye and in simple receptors located in skin or other body tissues provides the body with the necessary input. Nervous signals travelling rapidly from the brain and spinal cord over nerves to muscles and glands initiate immediate coordinating and regulating responses. Slower acting chemical messengers, hormones produced by endocrine glands, serve to effect more long-term changes in physiological activities to maintain homeostasis. •

18 Nervous System Cells

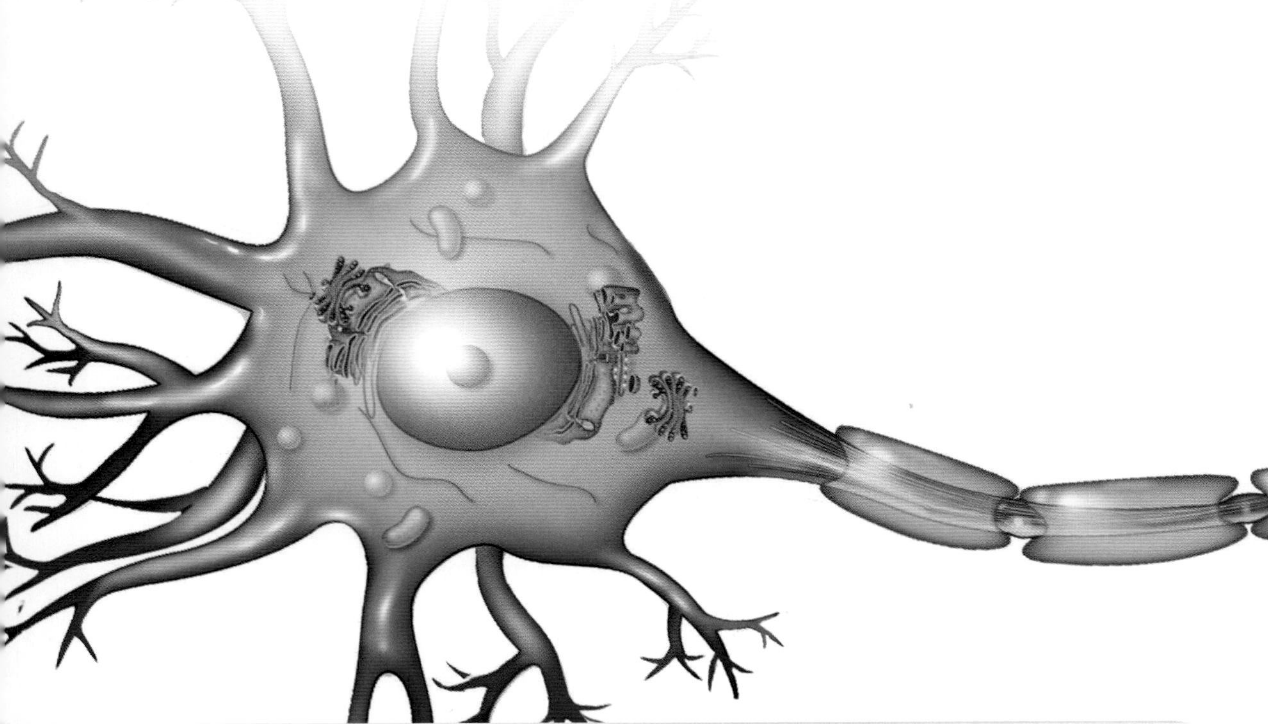

CHAPTER OUTLINE

Hint: *Scan this outline before you begin to read the chapter, as a preview of how the concepts are organized.*

LANGUAGE OF SCIENCE

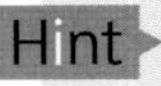
Hint: *Use this list to aid your pronunciation of unfamiliar words.*

afferent division (AF-fer-ent)
[*a-* **toward,** *-fer-* **carry,** *-ent* **relating to**]

afferent (sensory) neuron (AF-fer-ent NYOO-ron)
[*ad-* **toward,** *-fer-* **carry,** *-ent* **relating to**]

astrocyte (ASS-troh-syte)
[*astro-* **star shaped,** *-cyte* **cell**]

autonomic nervous system (ANS) (aw-toh-NOM-ik)
[*auto-* **self,** *-nom-* **rule,** *-ic* **relating to,** *nerv-* **nerves,** *-ous* **relating to**]

axon (AK-son)
[*axon* **axle**]

axon hillock (AK-son HILL-ok)
[*axon* **axle,** *hill-* **hill** *-ock* **little**]

axonal transport (AK-soh-nal trans-PORT)
[*axon* **axle,** *-al* **relating to,** *trans-* **across,** *-port* **carry**]

bipolar neuron (bye-POH-lar NYOO-ron)
[*bi-* **two,** *-pol-* **pole,** *-ar* **relating to,** *neuron* **string or nerve**]

dendrite (DEN-dryte)
[*dendr-* **tree,** *-ite* **part (branch) of**]

efferent division (EF-fer-ent)
[*e-* **away,** *-fer-* **carry,** *-ent* **relating to**]

efferent (motor) neuron (EF-fer-ent NYOO-ron)
[*e-* **away,** *-fer-* **carry,** *-ent* **relating to**]

endoneurium (en-doh-NYOO-ree-um)
[*endo-* **inward,** *-neuri-* **nerve,** *-um* **thing**] *pl.,* endoneuria

enteric nervous system (ENS) (en-TER-ik)
[*enter-* **intestine,** *-ic* **relating to**]

ependymal cell (eh-PEN-di-mal)
[*ep-* **over,** *-en-* **on,** *-dyma-* **put,** *-al* **relating to,** *cell* **storeroom**]

epineurium (ep-i-NYOO-ree-um)
[*epi-* **upon,** *-neuri-* **nerve,** *-um* **thing**] *pl.,* epineuria

fascicle (FAS-i-kul)
[*fasci-* **band or bundle,** *-cle* **small**]

glia (GLEE-ah)
[*glia* **glue**] *sing.,* glial cell

interneuron (in-ter-NYOO-ron)
[*inter-* **between,** *-neuron* **string or nerve**]

continued on p. 407

The nervous system and the endocrine system together perform a vital function for the body—communication. Communication provides the means to control and integrate the many different functions performed by organs, tissues, and cells. Integrating means unifying. Unifying body functions allows them to work together like a machine to maintain homeostasis and thus survival.

The nervous system—made up of the brain, spinal cord, and nerves—is probably the most intriguing body system (**Figure 18-1**). Facts, theories, and questions about this system are as fascinating as they are abundant. We shall begin our study of the nervous system in this chapter by considering the organization of the nervous system and the cells of the nervous tissue that comprises it. In Chapter 19, we explore the processes of nerve signalling. Then in Chapter 20 we discuss the brain and spinal cord. Chapter 21 presents the major peripheral nerves of the body and Chapter 22 discusses the role of the autonomic nervous system in the subconscious control of body functions. Chapters 23 and 24 continue the discussion by describing the structure and function of the sense organs. •

ORGANIZATION OF THE NERVOUS SYSTEM

The nervous system is organized to detect changes (stimuli) in the internal and external environment, evaluate that information, and possibly respond by initiating changes in muscles or glands. Recall from Chapter 2 that such sensing, integration, and control systems can act as feedback loops that help us maintain the homeostatic balance that ensures our survival.

To make the complex network of information lines and processing circuits involved in nervous control easier to understand, biologists have subdivided the nervous system into the smaller "systems" and "divisions" described in the following paragraphs and illustrated in **Figure 18-2**. Note as you read through the next several sections that the nervous system can be divided in various ways: by structure, direction of information flow, or control of effectors.

CENTRAL AND PERIPHERAL NERVOUS SYSTEMS

The classic manner of subdividing the nervous system is based on the gross dissections of early anatomists. It simply categorizes all nervous system tissues by their relative positions in the body: central or peripheral.

Central Nervous System (CNS)

The **central nervous system** (CNS) is, as its name implies, the structural and functional centre of the entire nervous system. Consisting of the brain and spinal cord, the CNS integrates incoming pieces of sensory information, evaluates the information, and initiates an outgoing response. Today, neurobiologists include only those cells that begin and end within the anatomical boundaries of the brain and spinal cord as part of the CNS. Cells that begin in the brain or cord

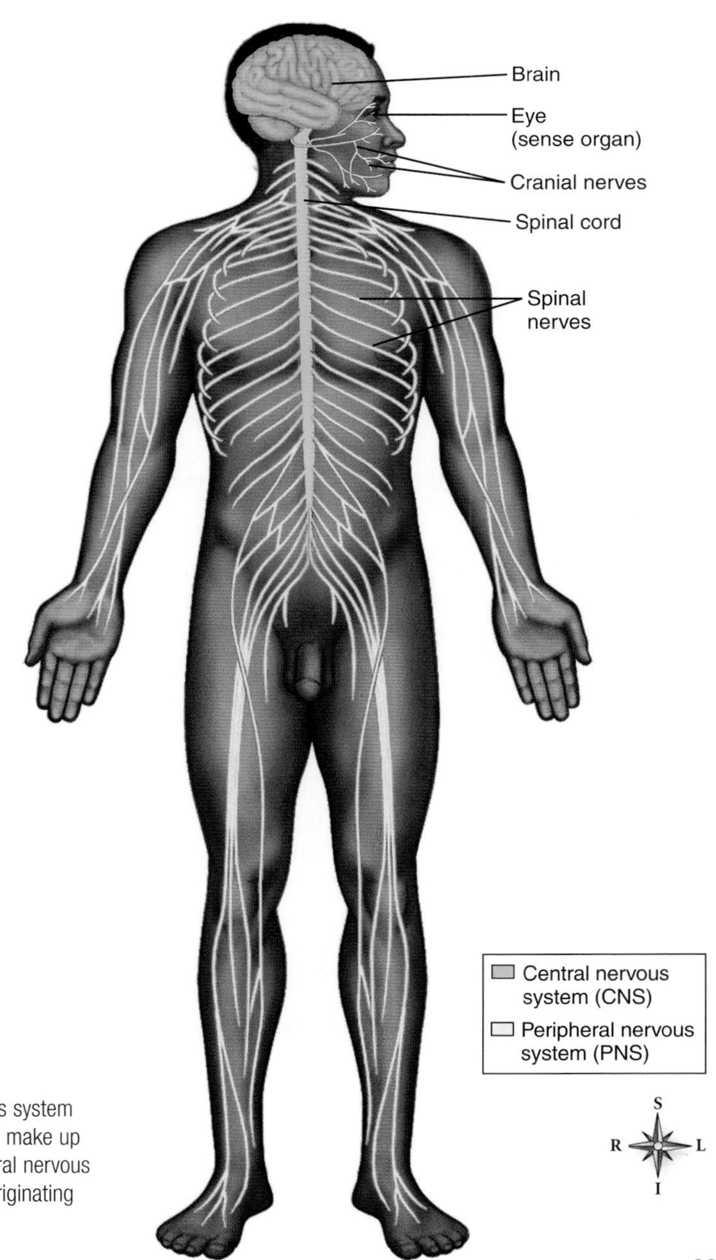

FIGURE 18-1 The nervous system. Major anatomical features of the human nervous system include the brain, the spinal cord, and each of the individual nerves. The brain and spinal cord make up the central nervous system (CNS), and all the nerves and their branches make up the peripheral nervous system (PNS). Nerves originating from the brain are classified as *cranial nerves,* and nerves originating from the spinal cord are called *spinal nerves.*

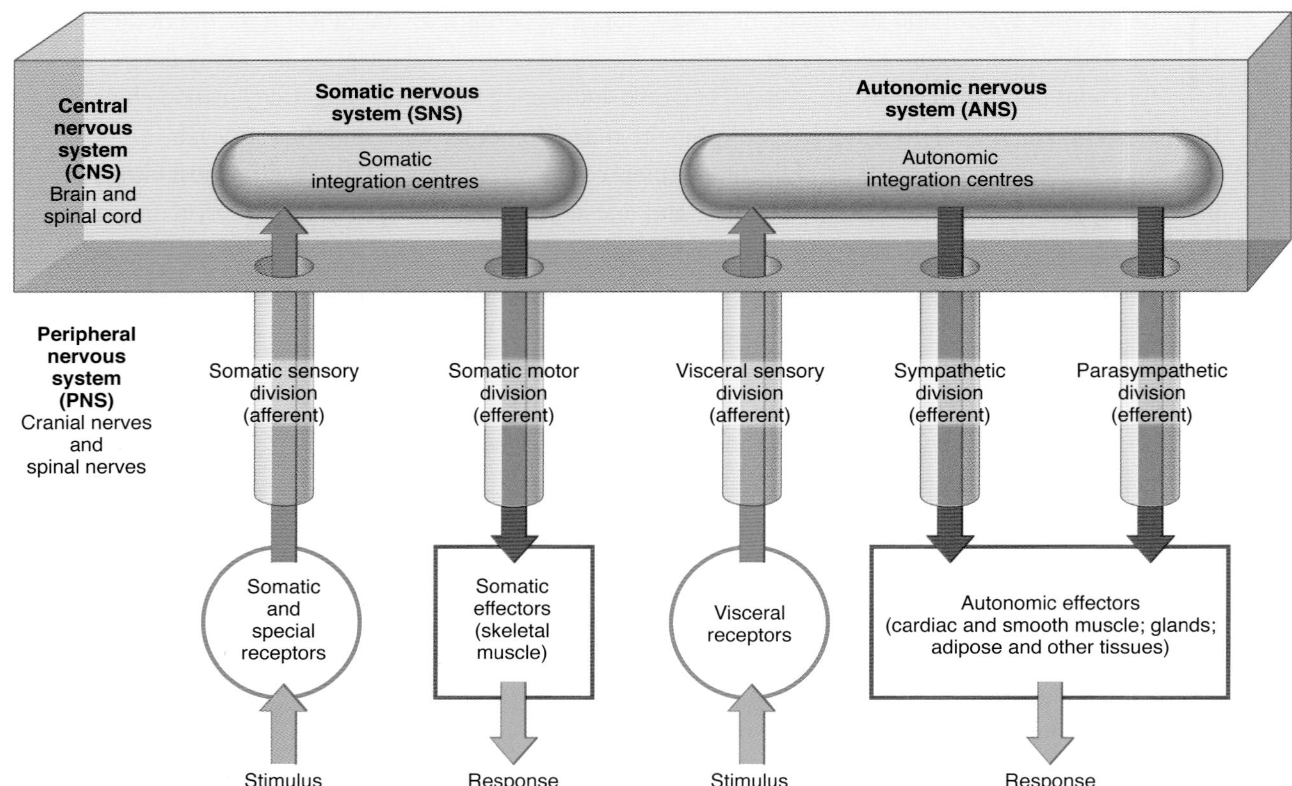

FIGURE 18-2 Organizational plan of the nervous system. Diagram summarizes the scheme used by most neurobiologists in studying the nervous system. Both the somatic nervous system (SNS) and the autonomic nervous system (ANS) include components in the central nervous system (CNS) and peripheral nervous system (PNS). Somatic sensory pathways conduct information toward integrators in the CNS, and somatic motor pathways conduct information toward somatic effectors. In the ANS, visceral sensory pathways conduct information toward CNS integrators, whereas the sympathetic and parasympathetic pathways conduct information toward autonomic effectors.

but extend out through a nerve are thus not included in the central nervous system.

Peripheral Nervous System (PNS)

The **peripheral nervous system (PNS)** consists of the nerve tissues that lie in the periphery, or "outer regions", of the nervous system. Nerves that originate from the brain or exit through the skull are called *cranial nerves*, and nerves that originate from the spinal cord and do not exit the skull are called *spinal nerves*.

The terms *central* and *peripheral* are often used as directional terms in the nervous system. For example, nerve cell extensions called *nerve fibres* may be called *central fibres* if they extend from the cell body toward the CNS. Likewise, they may be called *peripheral fibres* if they extend from the cell body away from the CNS.

Figure 18-1 represents the anatomical components of the CNS and PNS and their relative positions in the body. **Figure 18-2** represents the relationship of the CNS and PNS in diagram form.

Afferent and Efferent Divisions

The tissues of both the central and the peripheral nervous systems include nerve cells that form incoming information pathways and outgoing pathways. For this reason, it is often convenient to categorize the nervous pathways into divisions according to the direction in which they carry information. The **afferent division** of the nervous system consists of all of the incoming *sensory* or *afferent* pathways. The **efferent division** of the nervous system consists of all the outgoing *motor* or *efferent* pathways. The literal meanings of the terms *afferent* (carry toward) and *efferent* (carry away) may help you distinguish between these two divisions of the nervous system more easily.

Look at **Figure 18-2** and try to distinguish the afferent and efferent pathways represented there. Here, and throughout the rest of this book, afferent pathways are typically represented in blue and efferent pathways in red.

Somatic and Autonomic Nervous Systems

Yet another way to organize the components of the nervous system for ease of study is to categorize them according to the type of effectors they regulate. This is a functional approach.

Somatic Nervous System (SNS)

The **somatic nervous system (SNS)** regulates the *somatic effectors*, which are the skeletal muscles. The motor pathways that directly control the skeletal muscles make up the somatic motor division. As **Figure 18-2** shows, the somatic nervous system also includes the afferent pathways, making up the **somatic sensory division,** that provide feedback from the somatic effectors. The SNS also includes the integrating centres that receive the sensory information and generate the efferent response signal.

Autonomic Nervous System (ANS)

Efferent pathways of the **autonomic nervous system** (**ANS**) carry information to the *autonomic*, or *visceral*, effectors, which are mainly the smooth muscles, cardiac muscle, glands, adipose tissue, and other "involuntary" tissue. As its name implies, the autonomic nervous system seems autonomous of voluntary control—it usually appears to govern itself without our conscious knowledge. We now know that the autonomic nervous system is influenced by the conscious mind, but the historical name for this part of the nervous system has remained.

The efferent pathways of the ANS can be divided into the *sympathetic division* and the *parasympathetic division*. The sympathetic division, made up of pathways that exit the middle portions of the spinal cord, is involved in preparing the body to deal with immediate threats to the internal environment. It produces the "fight-or-flight" response. The parasympathetic pathways exit at the brain or lower portions of the spinal cord and coordinate the body's normal resting activities. The parasympathetic division is thus sometimes called the "rest-and-repair" division.

The afferent pathways of the ANS belong to the **visceral sensory division,** which carries feedback information to the autonomic integrating centres in the central nervous system.

Figure 18-2 summarizes the various ways in which the nervous system is subdivided and combines these approaches into a single "big picture".

Enteric Nervous System (ENS)

The **enteric nervous system** (**ENS**) is a so-called "second brain" in the wall of the gut. The term *enteric* means "intestinal", so you can think of this system as the "intestinal nervous system".

Because it communicates with both afferent and efferent pathways of the ANS, it was long considered to be an ordinary part of the autonomic nervous system. Experiments eventually revealed that the complex network of nerve pathways embedded in the intestinal wall has "a mind of its own"—a network of integrators and feedback loops that can act somewhat independently. Despite some "independent thinking", most physiologists still consider the ENS to be a division of the ANS.

Quick CHECK

1. List the major subdivisions of the human nervous system.
2. What two organs make up the central nervous system?
3. Contrast the somatic nervous system with the autonomic nervous system.

GLIA

Two main types of cells compose the nervous system, namely, *neurons* and *glia*. **Neurons** are excitable cells that conduct the impulses that make possible all nervous system functions. In other words, they form the "wiring" of the nervous system's information circuits. **Glia,** or *glial cells*, on the other hand, do not usually conduct information themselves but support the function of neurons in various ways. Some of the major types of glia and neurons are described in the following sections.

OVERVIEW OF GLIA

Our understanding of glia, or **neuroglia** as they are sometimes called, has been slow in coming. In the late nineteenth century the Italian cell biologist Camillo Golgi (after whom the Golgi apparatus is named) accidentally dropped a piece of brain tissue into a bath of silver nitrate. When he finally found it, Golgi could see a vast network of various kinds of darkly stained cells surrounding the neurons—proof that glia existed. However, they were almost immediately set aside as mere packing material. In fact, *glia* literally means "glue". For more than a century almost all research efforts focused on neurons. Fortunately, the tide has turned, and studies of glia and their functions are one of the hottest areas in *neurobiology*, the study of the nervous system. We are now finding that they have a major role in how the nervous system works.

For a long time, scientists thought that glia far outnumbered neurons, but research has shown that there are equally large numbers of both neurons and glia in the human nervous system. One study estimates that there are roughly 85 billion neurons and about the same number of glia in the human brain—a staggering number! However, this one-to-one ratio of neurons to glia is not uniform across the brain. Some brain regions have a four-to-one ratio and other regions have a one-to-eleven ratio of neurons to glia.

Unlike some neurons, glial cells retain their capacity for cell division throughout adulthood. Although this characteristic gives them the ability to replace themselves, it also makes them susceptible to abnormalities of cell division—such as cancer. Most benign and malignant tumours found in the nervous system originate in glial cells.

As stated earlier, glia serve various roles in supporting the function of neurons. To get a sense of this variety of functions, we shall briefly examine five major types of glia (**Figure 18-3**):

1. Astrocytes
2. Microglia
3. Ependymal cells
4. Oligodendrocytes
5. Schwann cells

The first four glial types in this list are located in the CNS. Only the Schwann cells are located in the PNS.

CENTRAL GLIA

Astrocytes

The star-shaped glia, **astrocytes** (**Figure 18-3**, A), derive their name from the Greek *astron*, "star". Found only in the central nervous system, they are the largest and most numerous type of glia. Their long, delicate "points" extend through brain tissue, attaching to both neurons and the tiny blood capillaries of the brain. Astrocytes have been called "stars of the nervous system" because of the many important functions they perform.

Astrocytes actually "feed" the neurons by picking up glucose from the blood, converting it to lactate, and passing it along to the neurons to which they are connected. (See Chapter 41 for a fuller discussion of the role of lactate in energy metabolism.) Astrocytes also help restore ion imbalances in the extracellular fluid during intense neuron activity, when excess K^+ ions may accumulate.

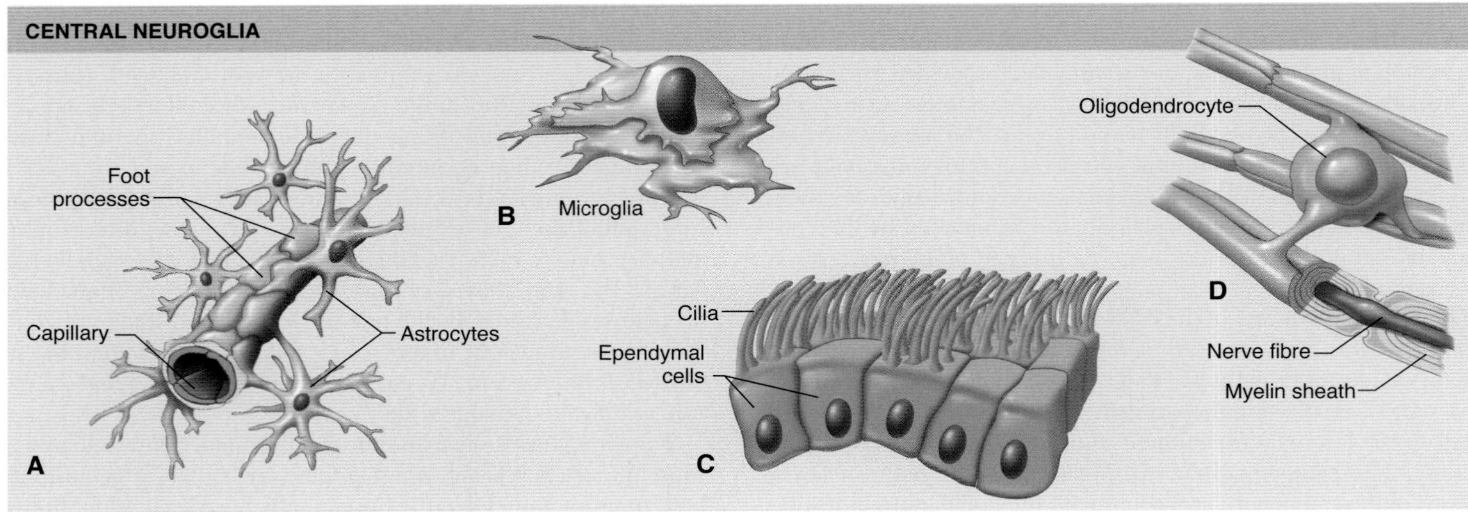

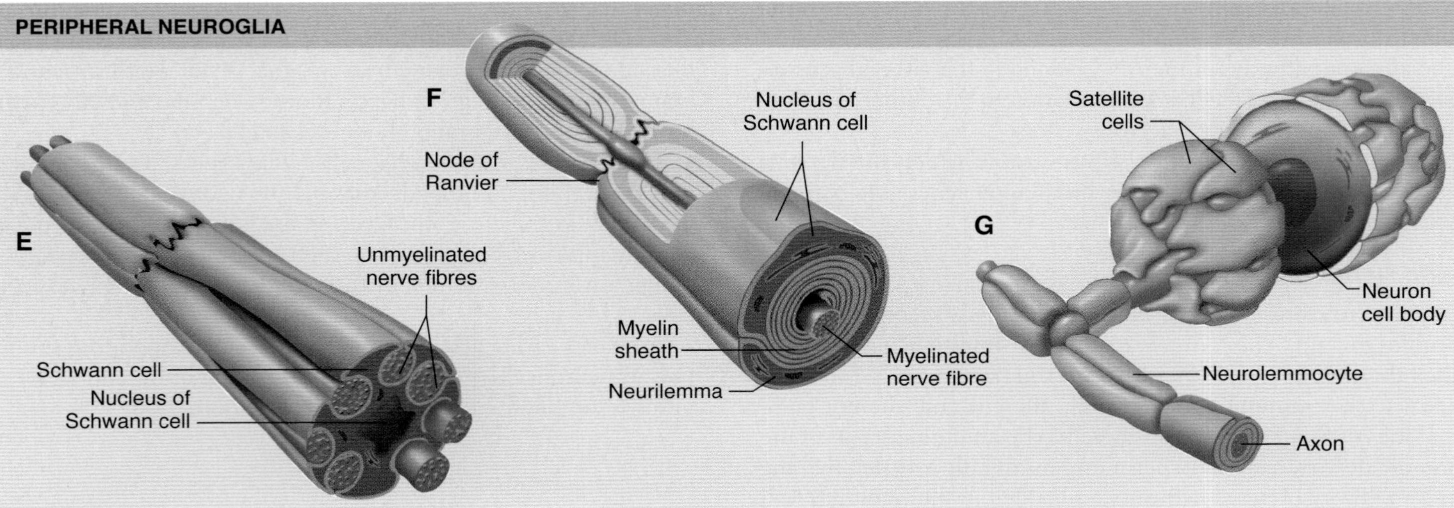

FIGURE 18-3 Types of neuroglia. Neuroglia of the central nervous system (CNS): **A,** Astrocytes attached to the outside of a capillary blood vessel in the brain. **B,** A phagocytic microglial cell. **C,** Ciliated ependymal cells forming a sheet that usually lines fluid cavities in the brain. **D,** An oligodendrocyte with processes that wrap around nerve fibres in the CNS to form myelin sheaths. Neuroglia of the peripheral nervous system (PNS): **E,** A Schwann cell supporting a bundle of nerve fibres in the PNS. **F,** Another type of Schwann cell wrapping around a peripheral nerve fibre to form a thick myelin sheath. **G,** Satellite cells, another type of Schwann cell, surround and support cell bodies of neurons in the PNS.

Astrocytes are key players in the early development of the nervous system, coordinating the production of new neurons and neural connections. Astrocytes work at nerve connections called *synapses* to recycle chemical transmitters. Astrocytes not only influence the growth of neurons and how the neurons connect to form circuits, but they may also transmit information along "astrocyte pathways" themselves.

Webs of astrocyte "feet" attach to the brain's blood capillaries, helping to form the blood–brain barrier (BBB). The BBB is an astrocyte regulated transport barrier made up of tight junctions between the endothelial cells that make up the walls of the capillaries. Small molecules (e.g., oxygen, carbon dioxide, water, alcohol) diffuse rapidly through the barrier to reach brain neurons and other glia. Larger molecules penetrate it slowly or not at all (**Box 18-1**).

Microglia

Microglia (**Figure 18-3**, *B*) are small, usually stationary cells found in the central nervous system. By contrast, all other glia and neurons in nerve tissue are called *macroglia.* In inflamed or degenerating brain tissue, however, microglia enlarge greatly, move about, and carry on phagocytosis. In other words, they engulf and destroy microorganisms and cellular debris. They may also play a role in "pruning" unneeded processes of neurons during brain development, thus increasing the efficiency of neural circuits.

Although classified as glia, microglia are functionally and developmentally unrelated to most other nervous system cells.

Ependymal Cells

Ependymal cells (**Figure 18-3**, *C*) are glia that resemble epithelial cells, forming thin sheets that line fluid-filled cavities in the brain

BOX 18-1 health matters | The Blood–Brain Barrier

The **blood–brain barrier (BBB)** helps maintain the very stable environment required for normal functioning of the brain. The BBB is formed as astrocytes wrap their "feet" around capillaries in the brain (part *A* of figure). More precisely, the covering formed by foot-like extensions of the astrocytes induces cells of the capillary wall to form tight junctions—forming a barrier that regulates the passage of most ions between the blood and the brain tissue (part *B* of figure). If they crossed to and from the brain freely, ions such as sodium (Na^+) and potassium (K^+) could disrupt the transmission of nerve impulses. Water, oxygen, carbon dioxide, and glucose can cross the barrier easily. Small, lipid-soluble molecules such as alcohol can also diffuse easily across the barrier.

The blood–brain barrier must be considered by researchers trying to develop new drug treatments for brain disorders. Many drugs and other chemicals simply will not pass through the barrier, although they might have therapeutic effects if they could get to the cells of the brain.

For example, the abnormal control of muscle movements characteristic of **Parkinson disease (PD)** can often be alleviated by the substance dopamine, which is deficient in the brains of PD patients. Because dopamine cannot cross the blood–brain barrier, dopamine injections or tablets are ineffective. Researchers found that the chemical used by brain cells to make dopamine, **levodopa (L-dopa),** can cross the barrier. Part *C* of the figure shows how L-dopa is used in brain cells to form dopamine. Levodopa administered to patients with Parkinson disease crosses the barrier and converts to dopamine, and the effects of the condition are thereby reduced.

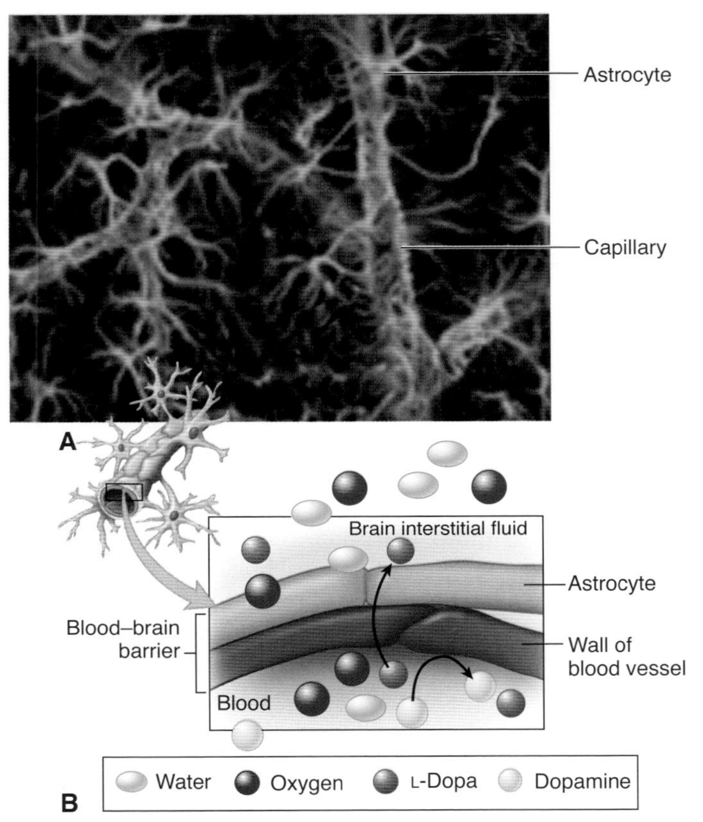

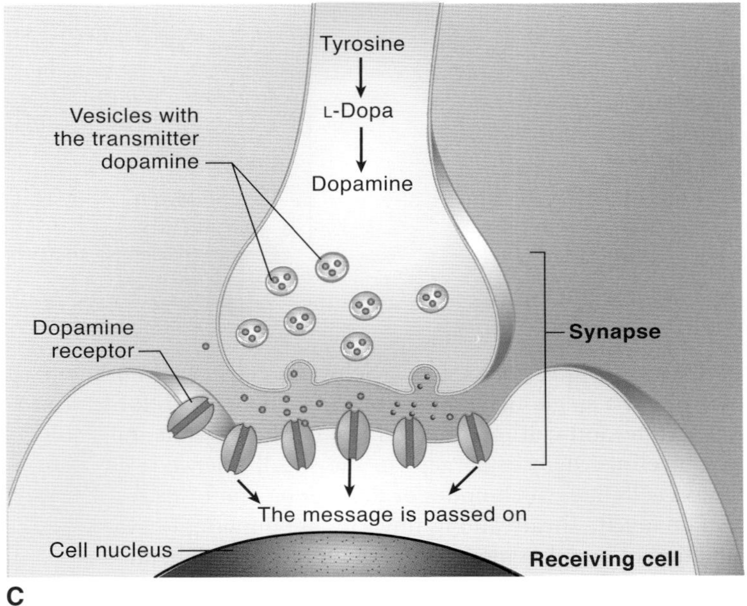

Blood–brain barrier. A, Micrograph of fluorescent-stained astrocytes shows how they attach to capillaries, forming a coating around these tiny blood vessels. **B,** Diagram showing a cross-section of the blood–brain barrier, made up of the foot processes of astrocytes and the wall of the blood capillary. **C,** Diagram showing how dopamine is formed from L-dopa before being released as a neurotransmitter. See **Figure 19-18** for a more detailed look at the formation of dopamine.

and spinal cord. Some ependymal cells take part in producing the fluid that fills these spaces. Other ependymal cells have motile cilia that help keep the fluid circulating within the cavities.

Oligodendrocytes

Oligodendrocytes (**Figure 18-3**, *D*) are smaller than astrocytes and have fewer processes. The name *oligodendrocytes* literally means "cell with few branches" (*oligo-* few, *-dendro-* branch, *-cyte* cell). Some oligodendrocytes lie clustered around nerve cell bodies; and some are arranged in rows between nerve fibres in the brain and cord. Oligodendrocytes help hold nerve fibres together and also serve another and probably more important function—they produce the fatty **myelin sheath** around the long fibres formed by some neurons in the central nervous system (**Box 18-2**). A myelin sheath permits rapid conduction of nerve impulses.

Note in **Figure 18-3**, *D*, how their processes wrap around surrounding nerve fibres to form this sheath.

Peripheral Glia

Schwann cells (**Figure 18-3**, *E* to *G*) are found only in the peripheral nervous system. Here they serve as the functional equivalent of the oligodendrocytes, supporting nerve fibres and sometimes forming a myelin sheath around them.

BOX 18-2 *health matters* | Multiple Sclerosis (MS)

Several diseases are associated with disorders of the oligodendrocytes. Because these glial cells are involved in myelin formation, the diseases are called **myelin disorders.** The most common primary disease of the central nervous system is a myelin disorder called **multiple sclerosis (MS).** It is characterized by myelin loss and destruction accompanied by varying degrees of oligodendrocyte injury and death. The result is *demyelination* throughout the white matter of the central nervous system. Hard plaquelike lesions replace the destroyed myelin, and affected areas are invaded by inflammatory cells. As the myelin surrounding nerve fibres is lost, nerve conduction is impaired, and weakness, loss of coordination, visual impairment, and speech disturbances occur. Although the disease occurs in both sexes and among all age groups, it is most common in women between 20 and 40 years of age.

The cause of MS is thought to be related to autoimmunity and to viral infections in some individuals. Susceptibility to MS is inherited in some individuals. MS is characteristically relapsing and chronic in nature, but some cases of acute and unremitting disease have been reported. In most instances, the disease is prolonged, with remissions and relapses occurring over a period of many years. There is no known cure.

Effects of multiple sclerosis (MS). **A,** A normal myelin sheath allows rapid conduction. **B,** In MS, the myelin sheath is damaged, disrupting nerve conduction.

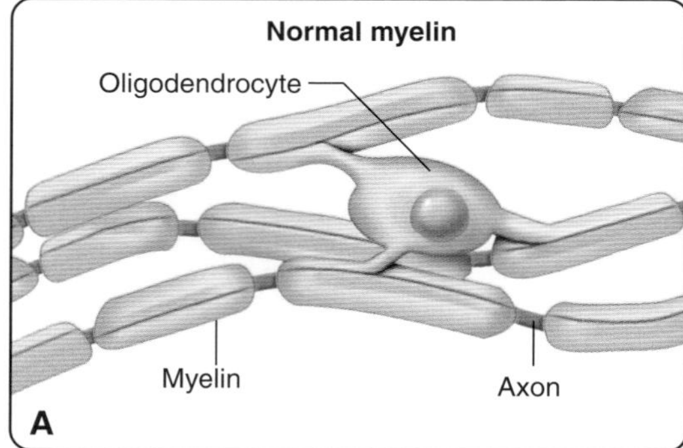

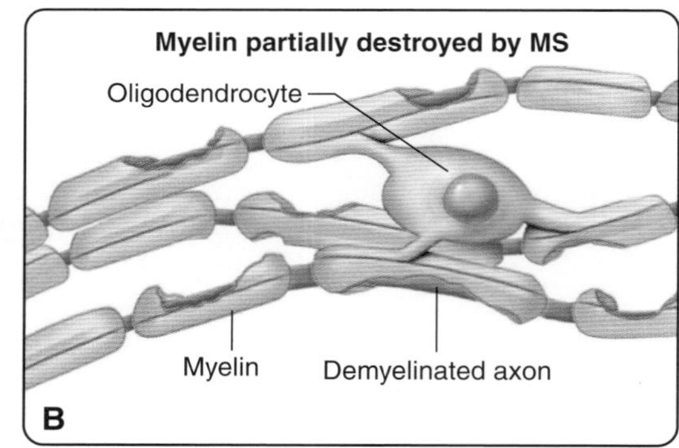

UNIT 3

As **Figure 18-3**, *F*, shows, many Schwann cells can wrap themselves around a single nerve fibre. The myelin sheath is formed by layers of Schwann cell membrane containing the white, fatty substance **myelin.** Microscopic gaps in the sheath, between adjacent Schwann cells, are called **nodes of Ranvier** or simply *myelin sheath gaps*. The myelin sheath and its tiny gaps are important in the rapid conduction of impulses along nerve fibres in the peripheral nervous system.

As you can see in **Figure 18-4**, the developing Schwann cell wraps around the nerve fibre in a way that forms an inner core of many layers of plasma membrane, made up mostly of the myelin (a type of phospholipid). Note that the Schwann cell's nucleus and cytoplasm are squeezed to the perimeter to form the **neurilemma.** The neurilemma is essential to normal nerve growth and the regeneration of injured nerve fibres. Schwann cells are also called *neurolemmocytes*. The myelin sheath along with the neurilemma is sometimes called the *neuronal sheath*.

Figure 18-3, *E*, shows that some Schwann cells do not wrap around nerve fibres to form a thick myelin sheath but simply hold fibres together in a bundle. Nerve fibres with many Schwann cells forming a thick myelin sheath are called **myelinated fibres,** or *white fibres*. When several nerve fibres are held by a single Schwann cell that does not wrap around them to form a thick myelin sheath, the fibres are called *unmyelinated fibres*, or *grey fibres*.

Figure 18-3, *G*, shows a type of Schwann cell often called a **satellite cell.** Like satellites positioned around a planet, these special Schwann cells surround the cell body of

FIGURE 18-4 Development of the myelin sheath. A Schwann cell (neurolemmocyte) migrates to a neuron and wraps around an axon. The Schwann cell's cytoplasm is pushed to the outer layer, leaving a dense multilayered covering of plasma membrane around the axon. Because the plasma membrane of the Schwann cell is mostly the phospholipid myelin, the dense wrapping around the axon is called a *myelin sheath*. The outer layer of cytoplasm is called the *neurilemma*. The extensions of oligodendrocytes also wrap around axons to form a myelin sheath.

TABLE 18-1 Major Types of Nervous System Cells

CELL TYPE	LOCATION	DESCRIPTION	FUNCTION
Glia	Brain, spinal cord, nerves	Support cells; far outnumber neurons	Structural and functional support of neurons
Astrocytes	CNS	Central body with many radiating processes	Promote nervous tissue development; provide nutrients to neurons, restore ion balance; help form and regulate synapses; part of blood–brain barrier
Microglia	CNS	Very small and stationary but can enlarge and move when stimulated	Engulf microbes and debris; prune neural circuits
Ependymal cells	CNS	Form sheets with motile cilia	Line fluid space; propel fluid
Oligodendrocytes	CNS	Central body with processes that wrap around neuron processes	Form insulating myelin sheath around CNS nerve fibres, which promotes rapid conduction along neurons
Schwann cells	PNS	Entire cell wraps around neuron processes; outer portion called neurilemma	Form insulating myelin sheath around PNS nerve fibres, which promotes rapid conduction along neurons; promotes regeneration of damaged nerve fibres
Neurons	Brain, spinal cord, nerves	Central body with fibre-like processes	Detect stimuli; conduct impulses; signal other cells
Multipolar neurons	Brain and spinal cord	Single axon, multiple dendrites	Process (integrate) information, conduct impulses along motor pathways
Bipolar neurons	Retina of eye, inner ear, olfactory pathway	Single axon; single highly branched dendrite	Conduct information along sensory pathways
Unipolar neurons (pseudounipolar)	Sensory pathways	Single process branches to form a central and a peripheral process	Conduct information along sensory pathways

a neuron. Satellite cells support neuronal cell bodies in regions called *ganglia* in the peripheral nervous system.

Table 18-1 summarizes important cells of the nervous system, including major types of glia.

Quick **CHECK**

4. What are the five main types of glia?
5. Describe the myelin sheath found on some nerve fibres.
6. What is a neurilemma?
7. Describe the three different forms of Schwann cells.

NEURONS

STRUCTURE AND FUNCTION OF NEURONS

The human brain is estimated to contain almost 85 billion neurons, or about half of the total number of nervous system cells in the brain. All neurons consist of a **cell body** (also called the **perikaryon,** or *soma*) and at least two processes: one **axon** and one or more **dendrites** (**Figure 18-5**). Because dendrites and axons are thread-like extensions from a neuron's cell body, they are often called **nerve fibres.**

In many respects the cell body, the largest part of a nerve cell, resembles other cells. It contains a nucleus, cytoplasm, and various organelles found in other cells, for example, mitochondria and a Golgi apparatus. The location of the nucleus in the cell body not only makes it easy to find in a microscopic specimen but also provides the name *perikaryon* (literally, "surrounding the nucleus"). A neuron's cytoplasm extends through its cell body and its processes. A plasma membrane encloses the entire neuron.

In the cell body, rough endoplasmic reticulum (ER) and its attached ribosomes provide protein molecules for the neuron. In neurons, the ER and ribsomes are sometimes called the **Nissl substance** or *chromatophilic substance*. Some of the proteins made here are then processed and packaged into vesicles by the Golgi apparatus. Some protein molecules in these vesicles are needed for the transmission of nerve signals from one neuron to another. Such proteins are called **neurotransmitters.** Other proteins are used in the maintenance and repair of the neuron.

The cell body also contains many mitochondria, which replicate themselves in the cell body. Some of the resulting mitochondria are transported to the end of the axon to provide energy (adenosine triphosphate [ATP]) for nerve signalling there. **Box 18-3** describes how neurons provide a back-up supply of oxygen for ATP production.

Dendrites usually branch extensively from the cell body—like tiny trees. In fact, their name derives from the Greek word for *tree*. The distal ends of dendrites of sensory neurons may be called *receptors* because they receive the stimuli that initiate nerve signals. Some dendrites in the brain have small knoblike *dendritic spines*, which serve as connection points for other neurons. Dendrites receive stimuli and conduct electrical signals toward the cell body and axon of the neuron.

BOX 18-3 ***neuroglobin***

Neuroglobin (Ngb) is a protein molecule very similar to the oxygen-binding proteins *haemoglobin (Hb)* in red blood cells (see Chapters 27 and 37) and *myoglobin* in muscle fibres (see Chapter 17). As the myoglobin in muscle fibres, neuroglobin temporarily stores a "backup" supply of oxygen for times when oxygen availability is low. In brain tissues, such a circumstance may occur during a stroke *(cerebrovascular accident [CVA])* or mini-stroke *(transient ischaemic attack [TIA])*, when the blood supply to the brain is disrupted. It could also occur during respiratory accidents, such as suffocation. Until normal blood flow is restored, neuroglobin can supply oxygen to the cell for a short time. •

The axon of a neuron is a single process that usually extends from a tapered portion of the cell body called the **axon hillock.** Axons conduct impulses away from the cell body. Although a neuron has only one axon, that axon often has one or more side branches, called *axon collaterals.* Moreover, the distal tips of axons form branches called **telodendria** that each terminate in a **synaptic knob** (see **Figure 18-5**). Each synaptic knob contains mitochondria and numerous vesicles.

Some axons have *varicosities,* or swellings, which act as points of contact with other cells such as smooth muscle fibres (see **Figure 17-31** on p. 383). Axons vary in both length and diameter. Some are a metre long. Some, however, measure only a few millimetres. Axon diameters also vary considerably, from about 20 μm down to about 1 μm—a point of interest because axon diameter relates to velocity of impulse conduction. In general, the larger the diameter, the more rapid the conduction.

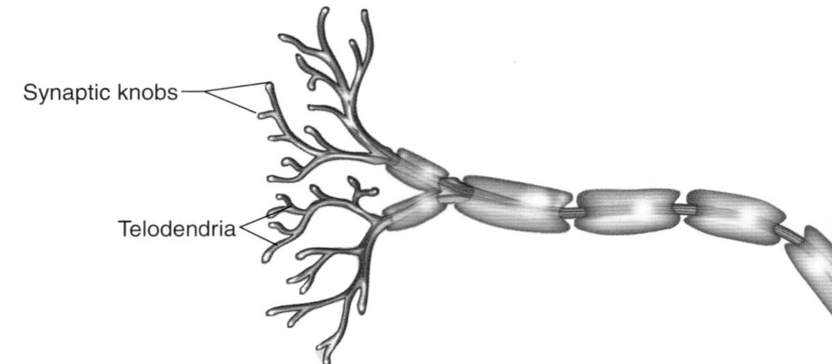

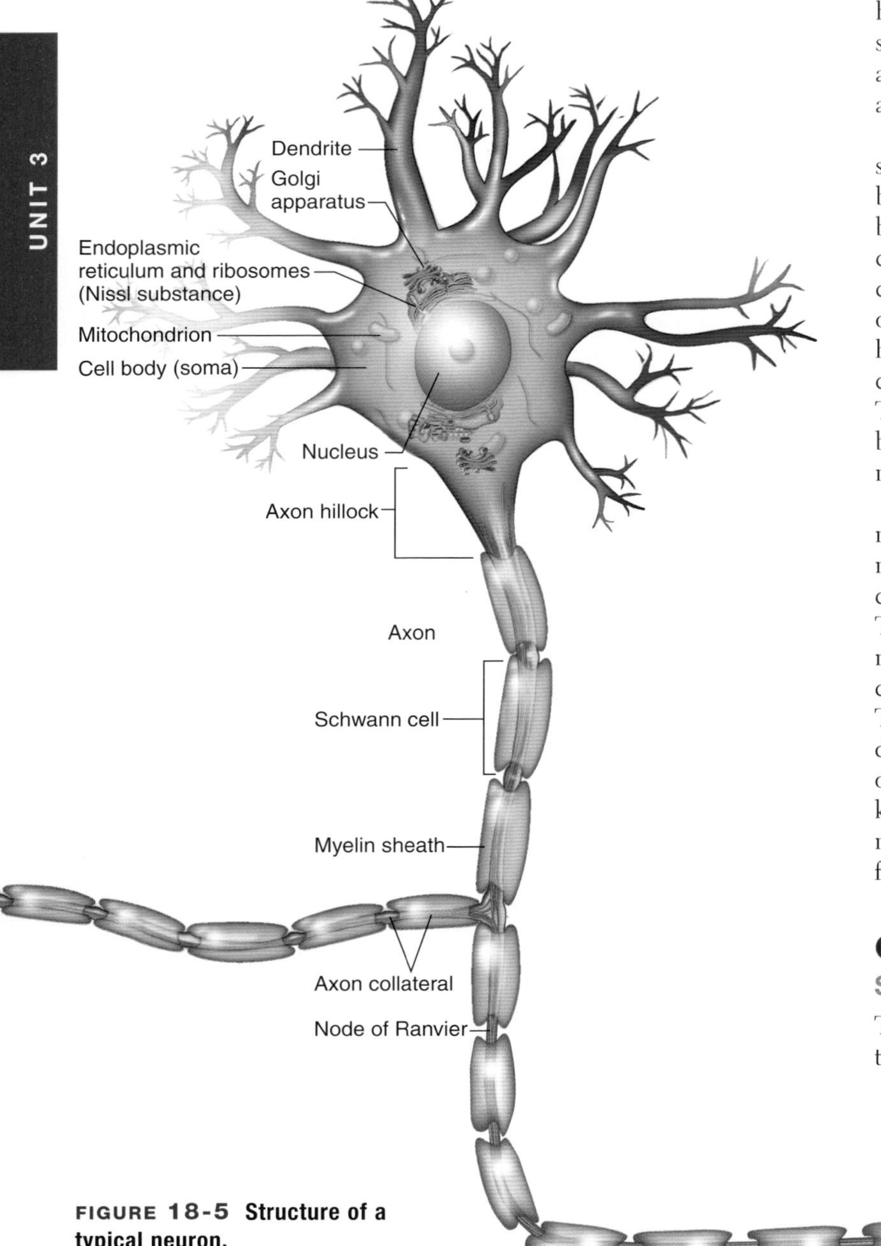

FIGURE 18-5 Structure of a typical neuron.

Whether an axon is myelinated or not also affects the speed of impulse conduction. **Figure 18-6** shows a cross-section of a typical myelinated axon. Note in the figure how a series of Schwann cells have grown over the axon in a spiral fashion to form the myelin sheath and neurilemma (see also **Figure 18-4**). Only axons may have a myelin sheath—dendrites do not. The role of the myelin sheath and nodes of Ranvier in impulse conduction is discussed later.

Extending through the cytoplasm of each neuron are fine strands sometimes called **neurofibrils** (see **Figure 18-6**). Neurofibrils are bundles of intermediate filaments called *neurofilaments.* Microtubules and microfilaments are additional components of the neuron's cytoskeleton. Along with providing structural support, a neuron's cytoskeleton forms a sort of "railway" for the rapid transport of small organelles to and from the far ends of a neuron. **Figure 18-7** shows how small "motor molecules" attach to mitochondria and vesicles containing neurotransmitters and carry them to the end of the axon. The "used" vesicles and transmitters are then returned to the cell body by the same process, but in reverse, for recycling. This type of movement is called **axonal transport.**

Figure 18-8 summarizes the different functional regions of the neurons, based on their role in receiving and conducting nerve signals. The dendrites and cell body act primarily as an *input zone,* receiving nerve stimulation and initiating nerve impulses in response. The axon hillock acts as a *summation zone* by adding together all the nerve impulses arriving from the cell body and dendrites—and deciding whether to send the impulse any farther along the neuron. The axon is the *conduction zone* because its primary job is to conduct the nerve impulse from the axon hillock all the way to the end of the neuron. The telodendria of the axon, along with their synaptic knobs, together act as an *output zone* where vesicles of neurotransmitter are released for possible reception by a nearby neuron or effector cell (muscle or gland cell).

Classification of Neurons

Structural Classification

The three types of neurons classified according to the number of their extensions from the cell body (**Figure 18-9**) are as follows:

1. Multipolar
2. Bipolar
3. Unipolar

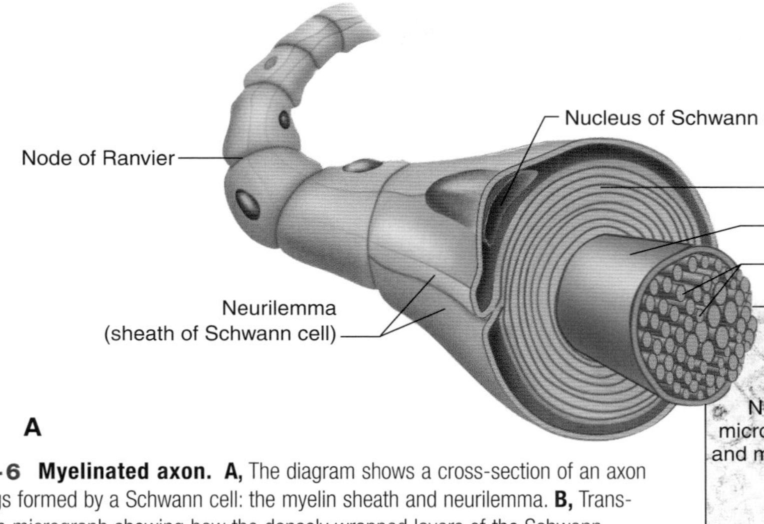

FIGURE 18-6 Myelinated axon. A, The diagram shows a cross-section of an axon and its coverings formed by a Schwann cell: the myelin sheath and neurilemma. **B,** Transmission electron micrograph showing how the densely wrapped layers of the Schwann cell's plasma membrane form the fatty myelin sheath.

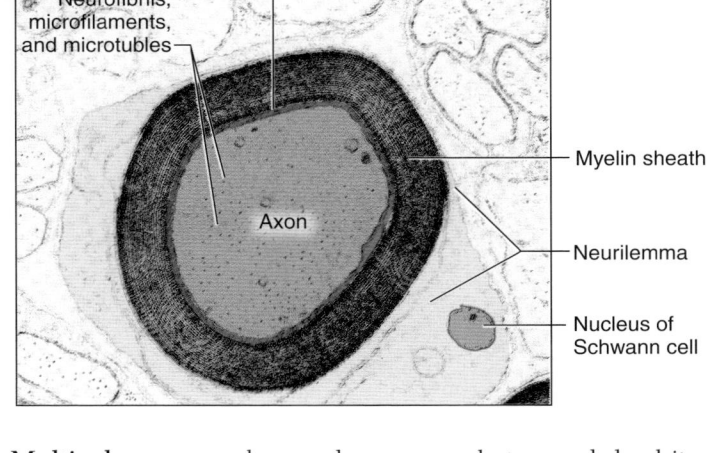

Multipolar neurons have only one axon but several dendrites. Most of the neurons in the brain and spinal cord are multipolar. In the brain, many subtypes of multipolar neurons are named for their appearance when stained, such as *basket cells*, *pyramidal cells*, and *spiny neurons*. Neurons in motor pathways are typically multipolar.

Bipolar neurons have only one axon and also only one highly branched dendrite. Bipolar neurons are the least numerous kind of neuron. They are found in the retina of the eye, in the inner ear, and in the olfactory pathway.

Unipolar neurons, also called **pseudounipolar neurons,** have a single process extending from the cell body. This single process branches to form a central process (toward the CNS) and a peripheral process (away from the CNS). These two processes together form an axon, conducting impulses away from the dendrites found at the distal end of the peripheral process. Unipolar neurons are always sensory neurons, conducting information toward the central nervous system.

Functional Classification

The three types of neurons classified according to the direction in which they conduct impulses are as follows:

1. Afferent neurons
2. Efferent neurons
3. Interneurons

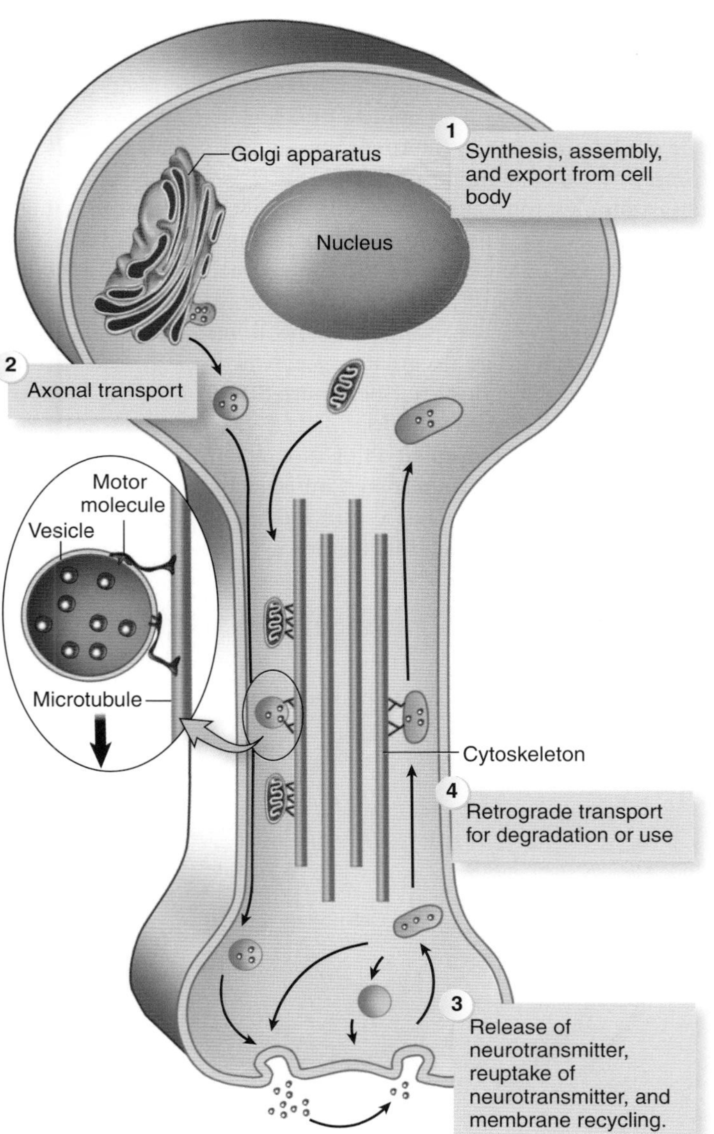

FIGURE 18-7 Axonal transport. Various cellular materials such as mitochondria and vesicles containing neurotransmitter can be shuttled quickly and efficiently from their point of origin *(1)* in the soma (perikaryon) all the way to the end of the axon *(2)* by using the neuron's cytoskeleton as a kind of railway system. The inset shows how motor molecules "walk" the material along a microtubule in the axon. The system also permits reverse transport, such as bringing the membranes of spent neurotransmitter vesicles *(3)* back up to the soma *(4)*.

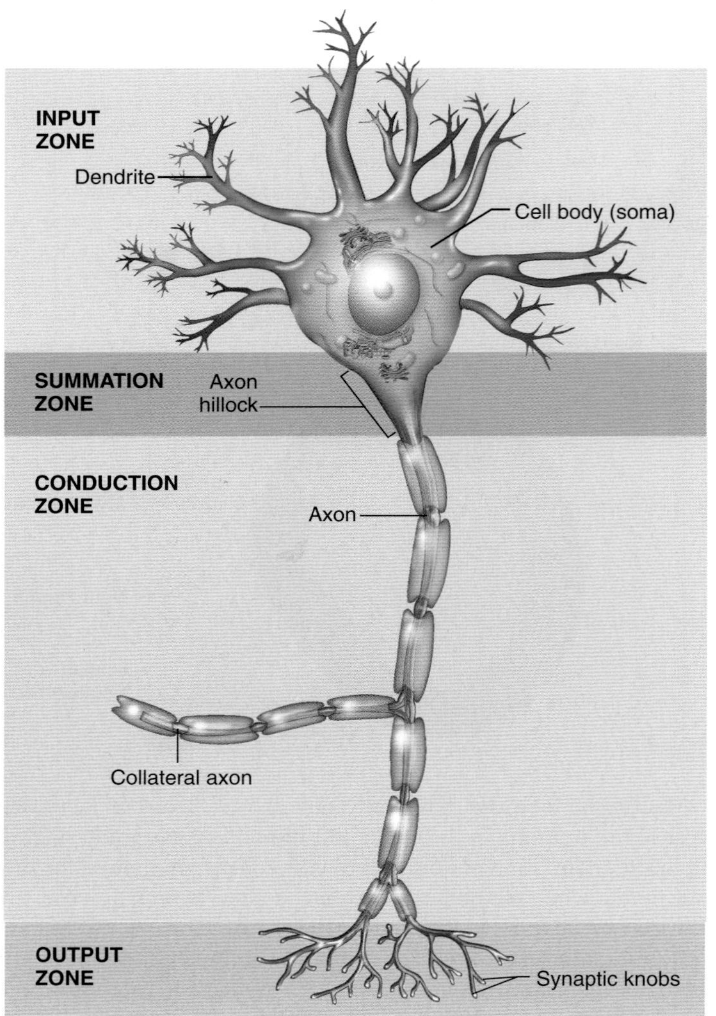

FIGURE 18-8 Functional regions of the neuron's plasma membrane. The *input zone* (dendrites and soma) receives input from other neurons or from sensory stimuli (stimulus-gated ion channels present). The *summation zone* (axon hillock) serves as the site where the nerve impulses combine and possibly trigger an impulse that will be conducted along the axon—or *conduction zone.* Both the summation (trigger) zone and conduction zone have many voltage-gated Na^+ channels and K^+ channels imbedded in the plasma membrane. The *output zone* (distal end of axon) is where the nerve impulse triggers the release of neurotransmitters. The output zone includes many voltage-gated Ca^{++} channels in the membrane.

Figure 18-10 shows one neuron of each of these types. **Afferent neurons**, also called **sensory neurons**, transmit nerve impulses to the spinal cord or brain. **Efferent neurons**, also called **motor neurons**, transmit nerve impulses away from the brain or spinal cord to or toward muscles or glands. **Interneurons** conduct impulses from afferent neurons to or toward motor neurons. Interneurons lie entirely within the central nervous system (brain and spinal cord).

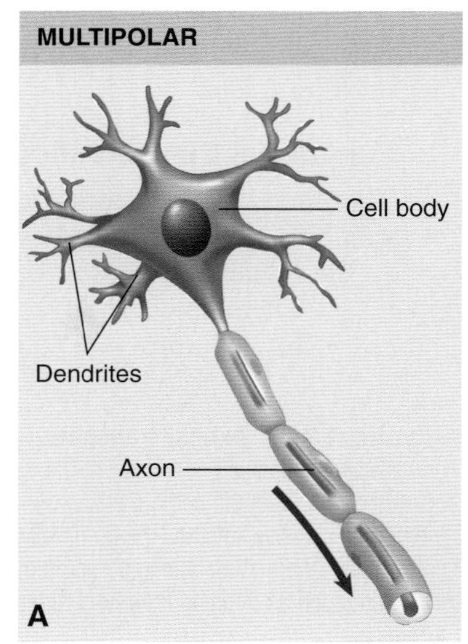

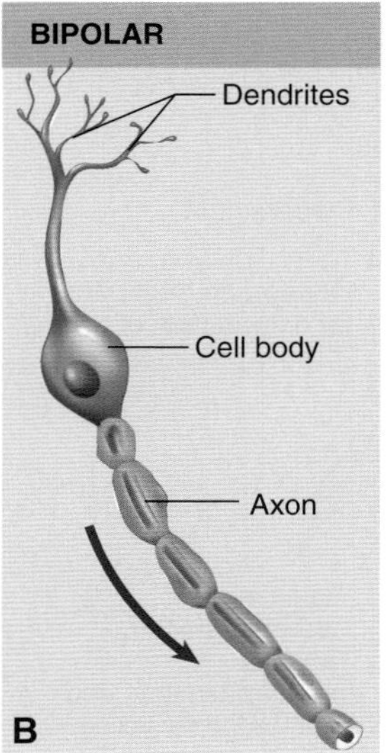

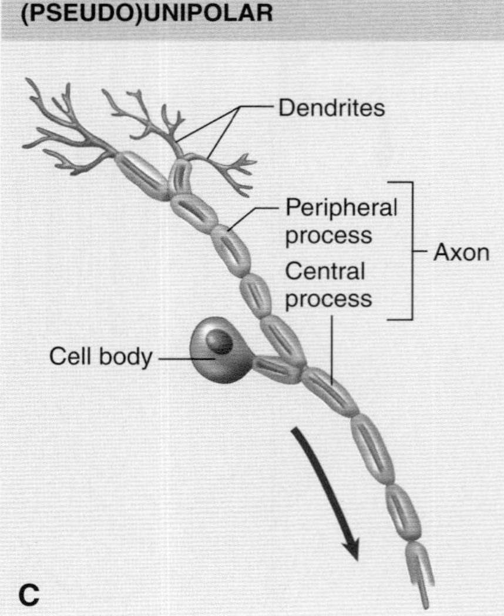

FIGURE 18-9 Structural classification of neurons. A, Multipolar neuron: neuron with multiple extensions from the cell body. **B,** Bipolar neuron: neuron with exactly two extensions from the cell body. **C,** (Pseudo) unipolar neuron: neuron with only one extension from the cell body. The central process is an axon; the peripheral process is a modified axon with branched dendrites at its extremity. (The *red arrows* show the direction of impulse travel.)

Table 18-1 summarizes important cells of the nervous system, including neurons.

REFLEX ARC

Note in **Figure 18-10** that neurons are often arranged in a pattern called a **reflex arc.** Basically, a reflex arc is a signal conduction route to and from the central nervous system (the brain and spinal cord).

The most common form of reflex arc is the three-neuron arc (**Figure 18-11**, A). It consists of an afferent neuron, an interneuron, and an efferent neuron. Afferent, or sensory, neurons conduct signals to the central nervous system from *sensory receptors* in the peripheral nervous system. Efferent neurons, or *motor neurons,* conduct signals from the central nervous system to effectors. An effector is muscle tissue or glandular tissue. Interneurons conduct signals from afferent neurons toward or to motor neurons.

In its simplest form, a reflex arc consists of an afferent neuron and an efferent neuron; this is called a *two-neuron arc.* In essence, a reflex arc is a signal conduction route from receptors to the central nervous system and out to effectors. By now you should recognize that the reflex arc is an example of the information pathway described in Chapter 2 as a regulatory *feedback loop.* To confirm this point, compare the reflex arc (see **Figure 18-10**) with the feedback loop illustrated in **Figure 2-3**, *B*, p. 27.

Now look again at **Figure 18-11**, *A*. Note the two labels for synapse. A **synapse** is the place where nerve information is transmitted from one neuron to another. Synapses are located between the synaptic knobs on one neuron and the dendrites or cell body of another

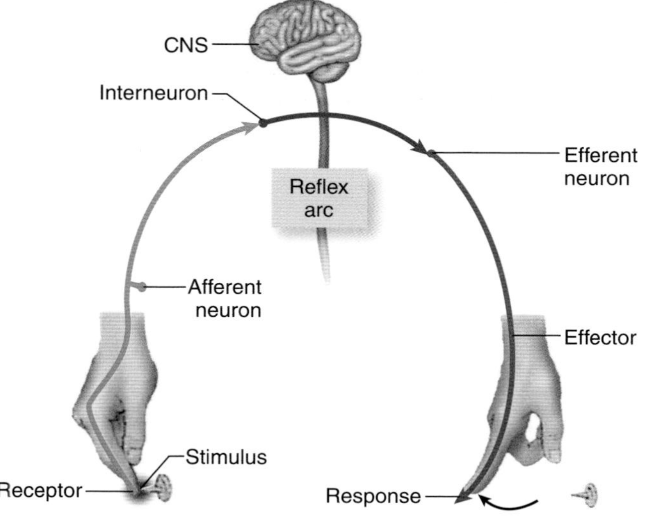

FIGURE 18-10 Functional classification of neurons in a reflex arc. Neurons can be classified according to the direction in which they conduct impulses. The most basic route of signal conduction follows a pattern called the *reflex arc.*

neuron. For example, in **Figure 18-11**, *A*, the first synapse lies between the sensory neuron's synaptic knobs and the interneuron's dendrites. The second synapse lies between the interneuron's synaptic knobs and the motor neuron's dendrites. This reflex arc is called an *ipsilateral reflex arc* because the receptors and effectors are located on the same side of the body. **Figure 18-11**, *B*, shows a *contralateral reflex arc*, one whose receptors and effectors are located on opposite sides of the body.

Besides simple two-neuron and three-neuron arcs, *intersegmental arcs* (**Figure 18-11**, *C*)—even more complex multineuron, multisynaptic arcs—also exist. An important principle is this: all electrical signals that start in receptors do not invariably travel over a complete reflex arc and terminate in effectors. Many signals fail to be conducted across synapses. Moreover, all signals that terminate in effectors do not invariably start in receptors. Many of them, for example, are thought to originate in the brain.

Quick CHECK

8. What is the difference between an axon and a dendrite?
9. What are the three structural categories of neurons?
10. What are the three main functional categories of neurons?
11. What are the essential components of a reflex arc?

NERVES AND TRACTS

Nerves and tracts are bundles of nerve fibres that connect different regions of the nervous system, much like the cables found in wired telephone and computer networks in a building.

NERVES

Nerves are bundles of peripheral nerve fibres held together by several layers of connective tissues that together form a multilayered sheath (**Figure 18-12**).

Surrounding the Schwann cell of each nerve fibre is a delicate layer of reticular fibrous connective tissue called the **endoneurium.**

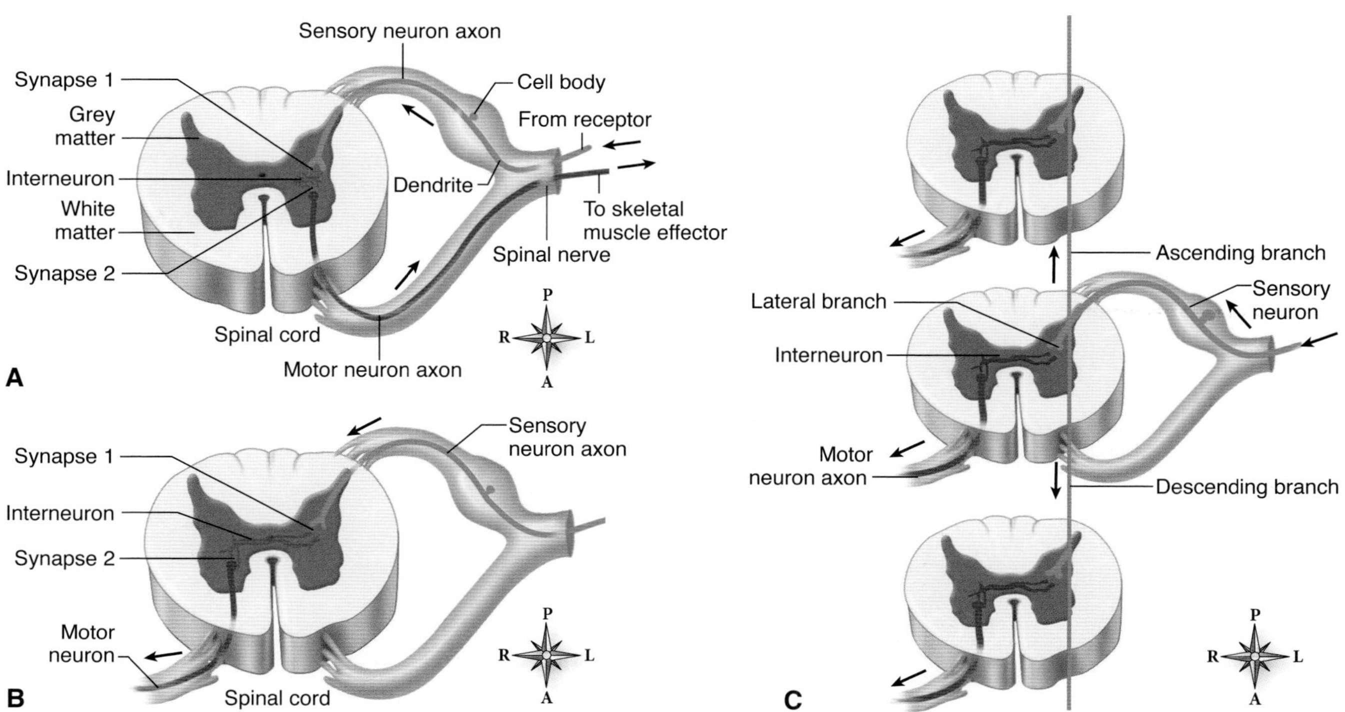

FIGURE 18-11 Examples of reflex arcs. A, Three-neuron ipsilateral reflex arc. Sensory information enters the central nervous system (CNS) and motor information leaves the CNS on the same side. **B,** Three-neuron contralateral reflex arc. Sensory information enters on the side of the CNS that is opposite from the side where motor information exits the CNS. **C,** Intersegmental contralateral reflex arc. Divergent branches of a sensory neuron bring information to several segments of the CNS at the same time. Motor information leaves each segment on the opposite side of the CNS.

Bundles of nerve fibres (each with its own endoneurium) are called **fascicles.** Each fascicle is bound together as a bundle by a connective tissue layer called the **perineurium.** The perineurium is sheet made up of several layers of flattened fibroblasts held together by tight junctions. The perineurium acts as a **blood–nerve barrier (BNB)**, regulating movement of substances between nerve tissue and the surround blood supply—much as the *blood–brain barrier* does in the brain (see **Box 18-1** on p. 397).

Numerous fascicles, along with the blood vessels that supply them, are held together to form a complete nerve by a fibrous coat called the **epineurium.** As you can see in **Figure 18-12**, the epineurium has a superficial part that surrounds the whole nerve and a deep part that extends between the fascicles. The superficial epineurium is dense, irregular fibrous connective tissue that forms a tough, flexible outer jacket of the nerve. The deep epineurium is made up of loose collagen bundles along with adipose tissue and blood vessels.

Most nerves in the human nervous system are *mixed nerves*. That is, they contain both sensory (afferent) fibres and motor (efferent) fibres. Nerves that contain predominantly afferent fibres are often called *sensory nerves*. Likewise, nerves that contain mostly efferent fibres are called *motor nerves*.

TRACTS

Within the central nervous system, however, bundles of nerve fibres are called **tracts** rather than nerves. Unlike nerves, tracts do not have connective tissue coverings. Individual nerve fibres that originate in the peripheral nervous system and pass through a nerve may continue into the spinal cord or brain as part of a tract. Likewise, an individual nerve fibre that originates in the brain or spinal cord and passes through a tract may continue into the peripheral nervous system within a nerve.

WHITE AND GREY MATTER

The creamy white colour of myelin distinguishes bundles of myelinated fibres from surrounding unmyelinated tissues, which appear darker in comparison. Bundles of myelinated fibres make up the so-called **white matter,** or *white substance*, of the nervous system. In the peripheral nervous system, white matter consists of myelinated nerves; in the central nervous system, white matter consists of myelinated tracts.

Cell bodies and unmyelinated fibres make up the darker **grey matter,** or *grey substance*, of the nervous system. Small, distinct regions of grey matter within the central nervous system are usually called *nuclei*. In peripheral nerves, similar regions of grey matter are more often called *ganglia*.

REPAIR OF NERVE FIBRES

For a long time, neuroscientists believed that mature neurons could not be replaced—and therefore nervous tissue had severe limitations to self-healing of damage. Evidence now clearly shows that neurons are in fact replaced. In fact, fresh new neurons are often added to the existing network. As we learn more about this process, neuroscientists hope to understand the details of these mechanisms and develop therapies to prevent and treat nerve damage or degeneration.

Another option in the body for healing injured or diseased nervous tissue is repairing the neurons that are already present. Unfortunately, neurons have a somewhat limited capacity to repair themselves. Nerve fibres can sometimes be repaired if the damage is not extensive, when the cell body and neurilemma (Schwann cells) remain intact, and when scarring has not occurred. **Figure 18-13** shows the stages of the healing process in the axon of a peripheral motor neuron.

Immediately after the injury occurs, the distal portion of the axon degenerates, as does its myelin sheath. Macrophages then move into the area and remove the debris. The remaining neurilemma (Schwann

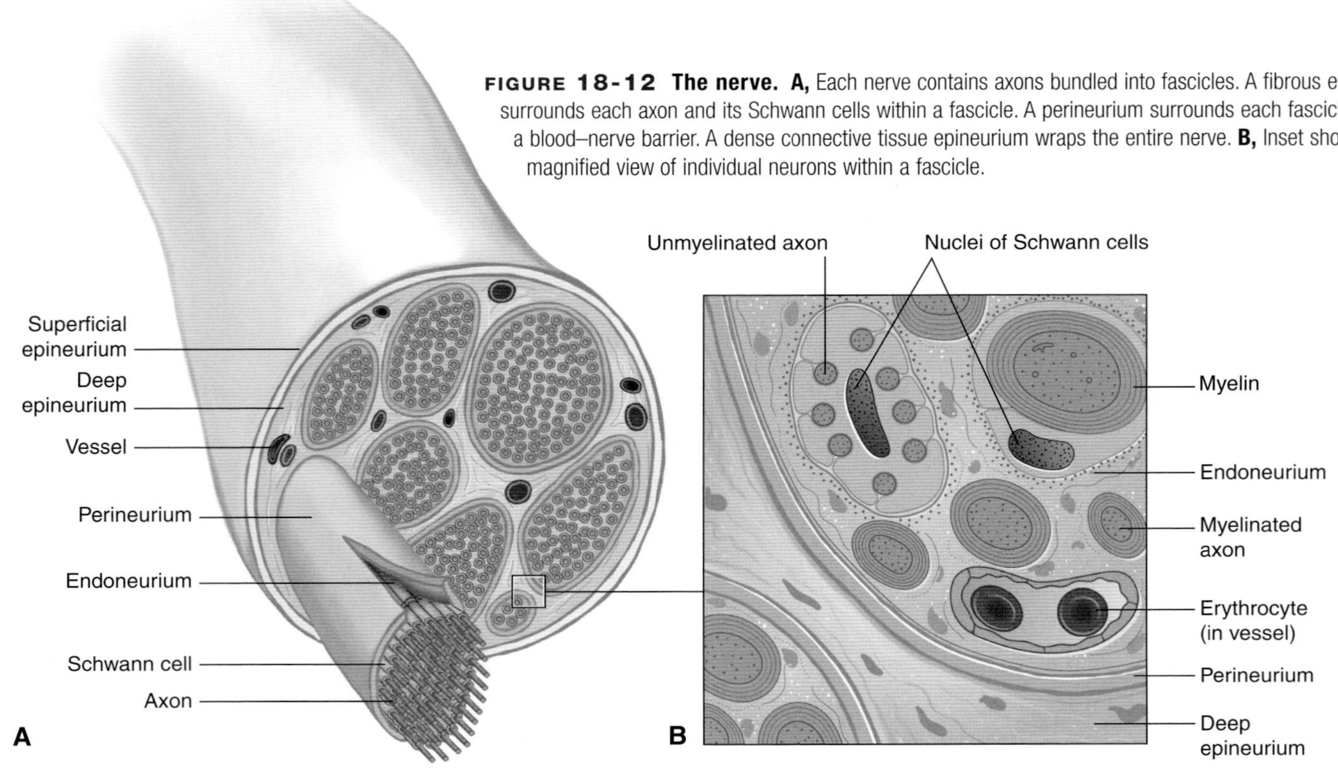

FIGURE 18-12 The nerve. A, Each nerve contains axons bundled into fascicles. A fibrous endoneurium surrounds each axon and its Schwann cells within a fascicle. A perineurium surrounds each fascicle, forming a blood–nerve barrier. A dense connective tissue epineurium wraps the entire nerve. **B,** Inset showing magnified view of individual neurons within a fascicle.

UNIT 3

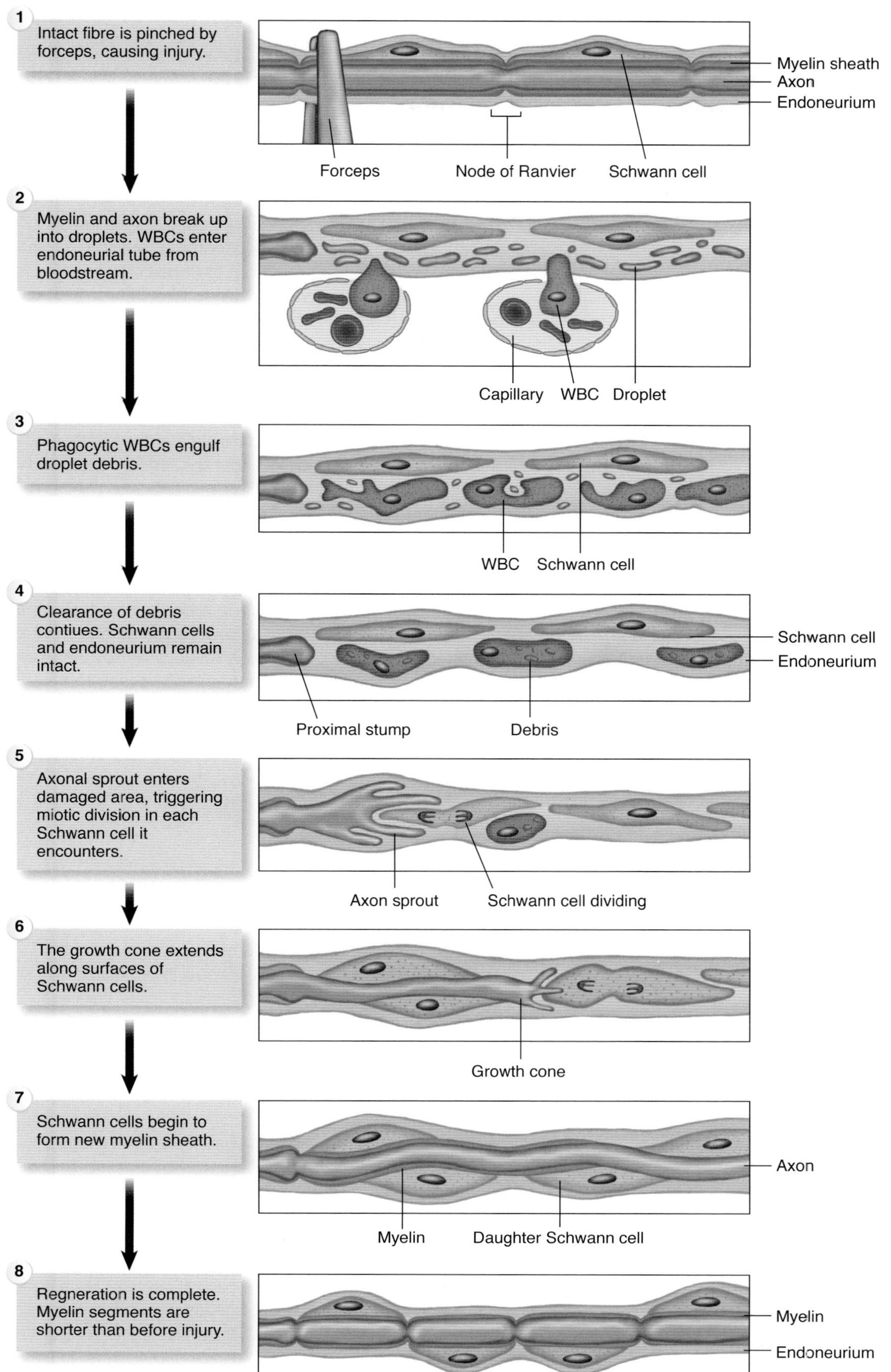
1
Intact fibre is pinched by forceps, causing injury.
Myelin sheath
Axon
Endoneurium
Forceps
Node of Ranvier
Schwann cell
2
Myelin and axon break up into droplets. WBCs enter endoneurial tube from bloodstream.
Capillary
WBC
Droplet
3
Phagocytic WBCs engulf droplet debris.
WBC
Schwann cell
4
Clearance of debris contiues. Schwann cells and endoneurium remain intact.
Schwann cell
Endoneurium
Proximal stump
Debris
5
Axonal sprout enters damaged area, triggering miotic division in each Schwann cell it encounters.
Axon sprout
Schwann cell dividing
6
The growth cone extends along surfaces of Schwann cells.
Growth cone
7
Schwann cells begin to form new myelin sheath.
Axon
Myelin
Daughter Schwann cell
8
Regneration is complete. Myelin segments are shorter than before injury.
Myelin
Endoneurium

FIGURE 18-13 Repair of a peripheral nerve fibre. *WBC*, white blood cell.

BOX 18-4 *health matters*

Reducing Damage to Nerve Fibres

Crushing and bruising cause most injuries to the spinal cord—often damaging nerve fibres irreparably. This usually results in **paralysis** or loss of function in the muscles normally supplied by the damaged fibres. Unfortunately, the inflammation of the injury site usually damages even more fibres and thus increases the extent of the paralysis. People with high-risk factor cervical spinal injuries such as those sustained in car accidents will require full in-line immobilization of their spines to prevent further damage to nerve fibres. The initial assessment and management of their injuries can have major implications for future quality of life. It is estimated that 1200 people in the UK are paralysed from spinal cord injury every year.

cells) and endoneurium form a pathway or tunnel from the point of injury to the effector. New Schwann cells are produced by mitotic division within this tunnel, maintaining a path for regrowth of the axon.

Meanwhile, the cell body of the damaged neuron has reorganized its ER and ribosomes (*Nissl substance*) to provide the proteins necessary to extend the remaining healthy portion of the axon. One or more growing axon "sprouts" appear. When one of these growing fibres reaches the tunnel (if there was a break in the fibre), it increases its growth rate—growing as much as 3 to 5 mm per day. If all goes well, the neuron's connection with the effector is quickly reestablished.

In a motor neuron, skeletal muscle cell supplied by the damaged neuron atrophies during the absence of nervous input. Only after the nervous connection is reestablished and stimulation resumed does the muscle cell grow back to its original size. If the damaged axon fails to repair itself, a nearby, undamaged axon from an adjacent neuron may form a sprout that reaches the effector cell and thus reestablishes a connection with the nervous system.

If the damaged nerve is connected to another nerve, the receiving nerve may also wither and die. In fact, because the preceding neuron may now have no functioning neuron to send a signal to, it may wither as well. In short, damage to a single axon can shut down an entire nerve pathway if not repaired—and repaired quickly.

In the central nervous system, similar repair of damaged nerve fibres is very unlikely. First of all, neurons in the central nervous system lack the neurilemma needed to form the guiding tunnel from the point of injury to the distal connection. Second, astrocytes quickly fill damaged areas and thus block regrowth of the axon with scar tissue. Despite great strides made by researchers looking for ways to stimulate the repair of neurons in the central nervous system, most injuries to the brain and spinal cord cause permanent damage (**Box 18-4**).

Quick CHECK

12. What are the three layers of connective tissues that hold the fibres of a nerve together?
13. What is the difference between a nerve and a tract?
14. How does white matter differ from grey matter?
15. In what circumstances can a nerve fibre be repaired?

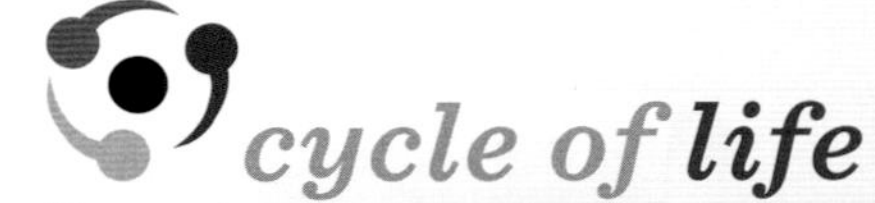

Nervous System Cells The development of nerve tissue begins from the *ectoderm* during the first weeks after conception and exhibits many complicated stages before the nervous system becomes mature by early adulthood. The most rapid and obvious development of nervous tissue occurs in the womb and for several years shortly after birth.

One of the most remarkable aspects of neural development involves the way in which nervous cells become organized to form a coordinated network spread throughout the body. Although we know very little about these processes, we do know that neurons require the coordinated actions of several agents to promote proper "wiring" of the nervous system. For example, we know that *nerve growth factors* released by effector cells stimulate the growth of neuron processes and help direct them to the proper destination.

During the first years of neural development, synapses are made, broken, and reformed until the basic organization of the nervous system is intact. Neurobiologists believe that the sensory stimulation that serves as the essence of early learning in infants and children has a critical role in directing the formation of synapses in the nervous system. The formation of new synapses, selective strengthening of existing synapses, and selective removal of synapses are thought to be primary physiological mechanisms of learning and memory.

In older adulthood, our brain processing may slow a bit. But that often allows us to make better use of stored memories and learned problem-solving skills to exhibit enhanced wisdom. In advanced old age, degeneration of neurons, glia, and the blood vessels that supply them may destroy certain portions of nervous tissue. This, coupled with age-related syndromes such as *Alzheimer disease (AD),* may produce a loss of memory, coordination, and other neural functions sometimes referred to as *senility.*

the big picture

Nervous System Cells and the Whole Body

Neurons, the conducting cells of the nervous system, act as the "wiring" that connects the structures needed to maintain the internal constancy that is so vital to our survival. They also form processing "circuits" that make decisions regarding appropriate responses to stimuli that threaten our internal constancy. Sensory neurons act as sensors or receptors that detect changes in our external and internal environment that may be potentially threatening. Sensory neurons then relay this information to integrator mechanisms in the central nervous system. There, the information is processed—often by one or more interneurons—and an outgoing response signal is relayed to effectors by way of motor neurons. At the effector, a chemical messenger or neurotransmitter triggers a response that tends to restore homeostatic balance. Neurotransmitters released into the bloodstream, where they are called *hormones,* can enhance and prolong such homeostatic responses.

Of course, neurons do much more than simply respond to stimuli in a preprogrammed manner. Circuits of interneurons are capable of remembering, learning new responses, generating rational and creative thought, and implementing other complex processes. The exact mechanisms of many of these complex integrative functions are yet to be discovered, but you will learn some of what we already know in the next few chapters.

mechanisms of disease

Disorders of Nervous System Cells

Most disorders of nervous system cells involve glia rather than neurons. *Multiple sclerosis (MS),* one of the myelin disorders discussed in **Box 18-2** (p. 398), is a good example of this principle. A few other important disorders involving glia are described in the following paragraphs.

The general name for tumours arising in nervous system structures is **neuroma.** Tumours do not usually develop directly from neurons but from glia, membrane tissues, and blood vessels. A common type of brain tumour—**glioma**—occurs in glia. Gliomas are usually benign but may still be life threatening. Because they often develop in deep areas of the brain, they are difficult to treat. Untreated gliomas may grow to a size that disrupts normal brain function—perhaps leading to death. Most malignant tumours of glia and other tissues in the nervous system do not originate there but are secondary tumours resulting from metastasis of cancer cells from the breast, lung, or other organs.

Tumours in the Central Nervous System

Astrocytoma is a type of glioma that originates from astrocytes. It is a slow-growing, infiltrating tumour of the brain that usually appears during the fourth decade of life. Seizures, headaches, or neurological deficits indicative of the area of the brain involved are usual presenting symptoms. **Glioblastoma multiforme,** a highly malignant form of astrocytic tumour, spreads throughout the white matter of the brain. Because of its invasive nature, surgical removal is difficult and the average survival is less than 1 year. **Ependymoma** is a glial tumour arising from ependymal cells, which line the fluid-filled cavities *(ventricles)* of the brain and spinal cord. This is the most common glioma in children but can occur in adults. Because of its location, fluid pathways are obstructed, causing increased pressure in the brain, which in turn causes neurological damage. Surgical correction is possible, and the average postoperative survival is roughly 5 years. Glioma of oligodendrocytes is called **oligodendroglioma.** This tumour commonly occurs in the anterior portion of the brain and has a peak incidence at 40 years of age. In Europe, more than 40% of patients survive for 5 years or more.

Tumours in the Peripheral Nervous System

Glial tumours can also develop in or on the cranial nerves. **Acoustic neuroma** is a lesion of the sheath of Schwann cells surrounding the eighth cranial nerve, responsible for hearing and balance. The tumour may be only the size of a pea or walnut, but the person with this tumour typically experiences difficulty deciphering speech through the affected ear, dizziness, tinnitus (ringing in the ear), and a slow, progressive hearing loss. With the use of microsurgical techniques, the tumour can be removed, but some nerve damage caused by the surgical procedure is common.

Glial tumours can also appear in other regions of the peripheral nervous system. **Neurofibromatosis** is a group of genetic diseases often characterized by numerous fibrous neuromas and skin spots throughout the body (**Figure 18-14**). Although usually inherited, many cases occur from spontaneous mutations of the genetic code in an individual—who can then pass along the disease to offspring. The tumours are benign, appearing first as small nodules in the Schwann cells of nerve fibres in the skin. In some cases, involvement spreads in the form of large, disfiguring fibrous tumours that develop in many areas of the body, including muscles, bones, and internal organs.

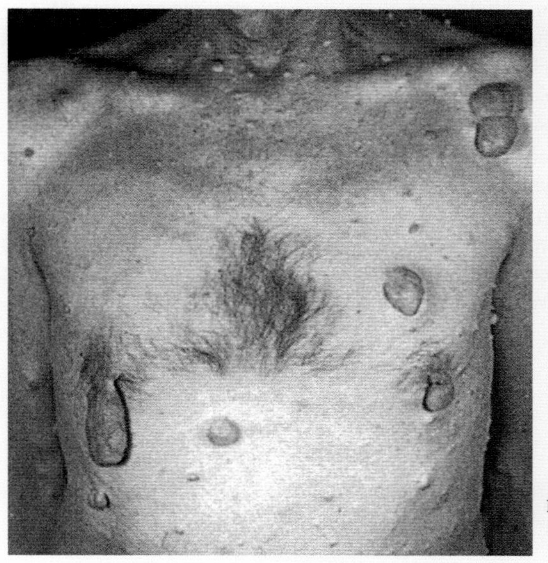

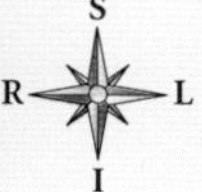

FIGURE 18-14 Neurofibromatosis. Multiple tumours of supportive cells in nerves of the skin that are characteristic of this group of genetic conditions.

UNIT 3

LANGUAGE OF SCIENCE *(continued from p. 392)*

microglia (my-KROG-lee-ah)
[*micro-* **small** *-glia* **glue**] *sing.*, microglial cell

motor neuron (MOH-ter NYOO-ron)
[*mot-* **move,** *-or* **agent,** *neuron* **string or nerve**]

multipolar neuron (mul-ti-POL-ar NYOO-ron)
[*multi-* **many,** *-pol-* **pole,** *-ar* **relating to,** *neuron* **string or nerve**]

myelin (MY-eh-lin)
[*myel-* **marrow,** *-in* **substance**]

myelin sheath (MY-eh-lin sheeth)
[*myel-* **marrow,** *-in* **substance**]

myelinated fibre (MY-eh-li-nay-ted)
[*myel-* **marrow,** *-in-* **substance,** *-ate* **act of**]

neurilemma (nyoo-ri-LEM-mah)
[*neuri-* **neuron,** *-lemma* **sheath**] *pl.*, neurilemmae

neurofibril (nyoo-roh-FYE-bril)
[*neuro-* **nerve,** *-fibr-* **thread or fibre,** *-il* **small**]

neuroglia (nyoo-ROG-lee-ah)
[*neuro-* **nerve,** *-glia* **glue**] *sing.*, neuroglial cell

neuroglobin (Ngb) (NYOO-roh-gloh-bin)
[*neuro-* **nerve,** *-glob-* **ball,** *-in* **substance**]

neuron (NYOO-ron)
[*neuron* **string or nerve**]

neurotransmitter (nyoo-roh-tranz-MIT-ter)
[*neuro-* **nerve,** *-trans-* **across,** *-mitt-* **send,** *-er* **agent**]

LANGUAGE OF SCIENCE *(continued from p. 392)*

Nissl substance (NISS-ul SUB-stans)
[*Franz Nissl* **German neurologist**]

node of Ranvier (rahn-vee-AY)
[*nod-* **knot,** *Louis A. Ranvier* **French pathologist**]

oligodendrocyte (ohl-i-go-DEN-droh-syte)
[*oligo-* **few,** *-dendr-* **part (branch) of,** *-cyte* **cell**]

perikaryon (pair-i-KAR-ee-on)
[*peri-* **around,** *-karyon* **nut or kernel**]

perineurium (pair-i-NYOO-ree-um)
[*peri-* **around,** *-neuri-* **nerve,** *-um* **thing**]
pl., perineuria

peripheral nervous system (PNS) (peh-RIF-er-al)
[*peri-* **around,** *-phera-* **boundary,** *-al* **relating to,** *nerv-* **nerve,** *-ous* **relating to**]

reflex arc
[*re-* **back or again,** *-flex* **bend,** *arc* **curve**]

satellite cell (SAT-i-lyte)
[*satell-* **attendant,** *-ite* **relating to,** *cell* **storeroom**]

Schwann cell (shwon or shvon)
[*Theodor Schwann* **German anatomist**]

sensory neuron (SEN-sor-ee NYOO-ron)
[*sens-* **feel,** *-ory* **relating to,** *neuron* **string or nerve**]

somatic nervous system (SNS) (so-MAH-tik)
[*soma-* **body,** *-ic* **relating to,** *nerv-* **nerve,** *-ous* **relating to**]

somatic sensory division (so-MAH-tik)
[*soma-* **body,** *-ic* **relating to,** *sens-* **feel,** *-ory* **relating to**]

synapse (SIN-aps)
[*syn-* **together,** *-aps-* **join**]

synaptic knob (si-NAP-tik nob)
[*syn-* **together,** *-apt-* **join,** *-ic* **relating to**]

telodendrion (tel-oh-DEN-dree-on)
[*telo-* **end,** *-dendr-* **part (branch) of**]
pl., telodendria

tract (trakt)
[*trac-* **course**]

unipolar (pseudounipolar) neuron (yoo-nee-POH-lar [SOO-doh-yoo-nee-POH-lar] NYOO-ron)
[*uni-* **single,** *-pol-* **pole,** *-ar* **relating to,** *pseudo-* **false,** *neuron* **string or nerve**]

visceral sensory division (VISS-er-al)
[*viscer-* **internal organs,** *-al* **relating to,** *sens-* **feel,** *-ory* **relating to**]

LANGUAGE OF MEDICINE

acoustic neuroma (ah-KOOS-tik nyoo-ROH-mah)
[*acoust-* **hear,** *-ic* **relating to,** *neuro-* **nerve,** *-oma* **tumour**]

astrocytoma (ass-troh-sye-TOH-mah)
[*astro-* **star,** *-cyt-* **cell,** *-oma* **tumour**]

ependymoma (eh-pen-di-MOH-mah)
[*ep-* **over,** *-en-* **on,** *-dyma-* **put,** *-oma* **tumour**]

glioblastoma multiforme (glye-oh-blas-TOH-ma mul-ti-FOR-mee)
[*glio-* **glue,** *-blasto-* **bud,** *-oma* **tumour,** *multi-* **many,** *-form-* **shape**]

glioma (glee-OH-mah)
[*glio-* **neuroglia,** *-oma* **tumour**]

levodopa (L-dopa) (LEEV-oh-doh-pah)
[*levo-* **left (form of molecule),** *-dopa* **acronym denoting 3,4-*d*ihydr*o*xy-*p*henyl*a*lanine**]

multiple sclerosis (MS) (MUL-ti-pul skleh-ROH-sis)
[*multi-* **many,** *-pl-* **fold,** *sclera-* **hard,** *-osis* **condition**]

myelin disorder (MY-eh-lin)
[*myel-* **marrow,** *-in* **substance**]

neurofibromatosis (nyoo-roh-fye-broh-mah-TOH-sis)
[*neuro-* **nerve,** *-fibr-* **thread or fibre,** *-oma-* **tumour,** *-osis* **condition**]

neuroma (nyoo-ROH-mah)
[*neur-* **nerve,** *-oma* **tumour**]

oligodendroglioma (ohl-i-go-DEN-droh-glye-OH-mah)
[*oligo-* **few,** *-dendro-* **part (branch) of,** *-glio-* **glue,** *-oma* **tumour**]

Parkinson disease (PD) (PARK-in-son)
[*James Parkinson* **English physician**]

paralysis (pah-RAL-i-sis)
[*para-* **beside,** *-lysis* **loosening**]

case study

Rachel, a 37-year-old woman, consulted her optometrist complaining of double vision (diplopia) and pain when moving her eyes. She was also experiencing dizziness, fatigue and co-ordination problems whilst walking. The optometrist noticed Rachel's right optic nerve was inflamed and she informed Rachel's GP. Following examination at the surgery, an urgent appointment was made for her with a neurology consultant.

After a series of tests and scans the neurologist confirmed that Rachel was developing multiple sclerosis (MS), a serious condition for which there is currently no cure. The neurologist instigated treatment with disease-modifying drugs (DMDs) to try and reduce the number and severity of relapses that characterize this condition.

1. Multiple sclerosis is a neurological disease associated with glial cells that behave in an abnormal way and die. Which type of glial cell is involved in the development of MS?
   a. The ependymal cell
   b. The oligodendrocyte
   c. The astrocyte
   d. The microglial cell
2. What is thought to be the cause of multiple sclerosis (MS)?
   a. MS is related to autoimmunity and to viral infections in some individuals.
   b. MS is related to an imbalance of hormones secreted by the pituitary gland.
   c. Dietary deficiencies have been thought to be the underlying cause of MS.
   d. Overexposure to certain antibiotics may initiate the onset of MS.
3. Which of the following characterizes multiple sclerosis?
   a. Demyelination throughout the white matter of the central nervous system
   b. Presence of hard plaque-like lesions replacing the myelin
   c. Impairment of nerve conduction with occurrence of weakness, loss of coordination, visual impairment, and speech disturbances
   d. All of the above characterize multiple sclerosis

Hint To solve a case study, you may have to refer to the glossary or index, other chapters in this textbook, ***Connect It!,*** and other resources.

CHAPTER SUMMARY

To download an MP3 version of the chapter summary for use with your mobile device, access the ***Audio Chapter Summaries*** *online at evolve.elsevier.com.*

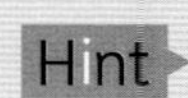

Scan this summary after reading the chapter to help you reinforce the key concepts. Later, use the summary as a quick review before your class or before a test.

Introduction

A. Function of nervous system, along with the endocrine system, is to communicate
B. Nervous system made up of the brain, spinal cord, and nerves (**Figure 18-1**)

Organization of the Nervous System

A. Organized to detect changes in internal and external environments, evaluate the information, and initiate an appropriate response
B. Subdivided into smaller "systems" by location (**Figure 18-2**)
  1. Central nervous system (CNS)
    a. Structural and functional centre of the entire nervous system
    b. Consists of the brain and spinal cord
    c. Integrates sensory information, evaluates it, and initiates an outgoing response
  2. Peripheral nervous system (PNS)
    a. Nerves that lie in the "outer regions" of the nervous system
    b. Cranial nerves—originate from the brain
    c. Spinal nerves—originate from the spinal cord
C. Afferent and efferent divisions
  1. Afferent division—consists of all incoming sensory pathways
  2. Efferent division—consists of all outgoing motor pathways
D. "Systems" categorized according to types of organs they innervate (**Figure 18-2**)
  1. Somatic nervous system (SNS)
    a. Somatic motor division carries information to the somatic effectors (skeletal muscles)
    b. Somatic sensory division carries feedback information to somatic integration centres in the CNS
  2. Autonomic nervous system (ANS)
    a. Efferent division of ANS carries information to the autonomic or visceral effectors (smooth and cardiac muscles, glands, and adipose and other tissues)
      (1) Sympathetic division—prepares the body to deal with immediate threats to the internal environment; produces "fight-or-flight" response
      (2) Parasympathetic division—coordinates the body's normal resting activities; sometimes called the "rest-and-repair" division
    b. Visceral sensory division carries feedback information to autonomic integrating centres in the CNS
    c. Enteric nervous system (ENS)
      (1) Located within intestinal wall, the ENS regulates digestive function
      (2) Has some independent integration abilities, so is considered to be a special division of the ANS

Cells of the Nervous System

A. Glia (neuroglia; **Table 18-1**)
  1. Glial cells support the neurons
  2. Five major types of glia (**Figure 18-3**)
    a. Central glia
      (1) Astrocytes (in CNS)
        (a) Star-shaped, largest, and most numerous type of glia
        (b) Cell extensions connect to both neurons and capillaries
        (c) Astrocytes transfer nutrients from the blood to the neurons
        (d) Form sheaths around brain capillaries, and induce formation of tight junctions between capillary endothelial cells, thus forming a blood–brain barrier (BBB)
      (2) Microglia (in CNS)
        (a) Small, usually stationary cells
        (b) In inflamed brain tissue, they enlarge, move about, and carry on phagocytosis
      (3) Ependymal cells (in CNS)
        (a) Resemble epithelial cells and form thin sheets that line fluid-filled cavities in the CNS
        (b) Some produce fluid; others aid in circulation of fluid
      (4) Oligodendrocytes (in CNS)
        (a) Smaller than astrocytes with fewer processes
        (b) Hold nerve fibres together and produce the myelin sheath
    b. Peripheral glia
      (1) Schwann cells (in PNS)
        (a) Found only in peripheral neurons
        (b) Support nerve fibres and form myelin sheaths (**Figure 18-4**)
        (c) Myelin sheath gaps are often called *nodes of Ranvier*
        (d) Neurilemma is formed by cytoplasm of Schwann cell (neurolemmocyte) wrapped around the myelin sheath; essential for nerve regrowth
        (e) Neuronal sheath is the myelin sheath plus the neurilemma (that is, the whole Schwann wrapping around the axon)
      (2) Satellite cells are Schwann cells that cover and support cell bodies in the PNS
B. Neurons (**Table 18-1**)
  1. Excitable cells that initiate and conduct impulses that make possible all nervous system functions
  2. Components of neurons (**Figure 18-5**)
    a. Cell body (perikaryon)
      (1) Ribosomes, rough endoplasmic reticulum (ER), Golgi apparatus
        (a) Provide protein molecules (neurotransmitters) needed for transmission of nerve signals from one neuron to another

(b) Neurotransmitters are packaged into vesicles
(c) Provide proteins for maintaining and regenerating nerve fibres
(2) Mitochondria provide energy (ATP) for neuron; some are transported to end of axon

b. Dendrites
(1) Each neuron has one or more dendrites, which branch from the cell body
(2) Conduct nerve signals to the cell body of the neuron
(3) Distal ends of dendrites of sensory neurons are receptors
(4) Dendritic spines—small knoblike protrusions on dendrites of some brain neurons; serve as connection points for axons of other neurons

c. Axon
(1) A single process extending from the axon hillock, sometimes covered by a fatty layer called a *myelin sheath* (**Figure 18-6**)
(2) Conducts nerve impulses away from the cell body of the neuron
(3) Distal tips of axons are telodendria, each of which terminates in a synaptic knob
(4) Axon varicosities—swellings that make contact (synapse) with other cells

d. Cytoskeleton
(1) Microtubules and microfilaments, as well as neurofibrils (bundles of neurofilaments)
(2) Allow the rapid transport of small organelles (**Figure 18-7**)
(a) Vesicles (some containing neurotransmitters), mitochondria
(b) Motor molecules shuttle organelles to and from the far ends of a neuron

e. Functional regions of the neuron (**Figure 18-8**)
(1) Input zone—dendrites and cell body
(2) Summation zone—axon hillock
(3) Conduction zone—axon
(4) Output zone—telodendria and synaptic knobs of axon

C. Classification of neurons
1. Structural classification—classified according to number of processes extending from cell body (**Figure 18-9**)
a. Multipolar—one axon and several dendrites
b. Bipolar—only one axon and one dendrite; least numerous kind of neuron
c. Unipolar (pseudounipolar)—one process comes off neuron cell body but divides almost immediately into two fibres: central fibre and peripheral fibre
2. Functional classification (**Figure 18-10**)
a. Afferent (sensory) neurons—conduct impulses to spinal cord or brain
b. Efferent (motor) neurons—conduct impulses away from spinal cord or brain toward muscles or glandular tissue
c. Interneurons

D. Reflex arc
1. A signal conduction route to and from the CNS, with the electrical signal beginning in receptors and ending in effectors
2. Three-neuron arc—most common; consists of afferent neurons, interneurons, and efferent neurons (**Figure 18-11**)
a. Afferent neurons—conduct impulses to the CNS from the receptors
b. Efferent neurons—conduct impulses from the CNS to effectors (muscle or glandular tissue)
3. Two-neuron arc—simplest form; consists of afferent and efferent neurons
4. Synapse
a. Where nerve signals are transmitted from one neuron to another

Nerves and Tracts

A. Nerves—bundles of peripheral nerve fibres held together by several layers of connective tissue (**Figure 18-12**)
1. Endoneurium—delicate layer of fibrous connective tissue surrounding each nerve fibre
2. Perineurium—connective tissue holding together fascicles (bundles of fibres)
3. Epineurium—fibrous coat surrounding numerous fascicles and blood vessels to form a complete nerve

B. Tracts—bundles of nerve fibres within the CNS
1. Unlike nerves, tracts do not have connective tissue coverings
2. Individual fibres may extend through both a nerve and a tract as it passes into or out of the CNS

C. White matter
1. PNS—myelinated nerves
2. CNS—myelinated tracts

D. Grey matter
1. Made up of cell bodies and unmyelinated fibres
2. CNS—referred to as *nuclei*
3. PNS—referred to as *ganglia*

E. Mixed nerves
1. Contain sensory and motor neurons
2. Sensory nerves—nerves with predominantly sensory neurons
3. Motor nerves—nerves with predominantly motor neurons

Repair of Nerve Fibres

A. Mature neurons are incapable of cell division; therefore damage to nervous tissue can be permanent

B. Neurons have limited capacity to repair themselves

C. If the damage is not extensive, the cell body and neurilemma (Schwann cells) are intact, and scarring has not occurred, nerve fibres can be repaired

D. Stages of repair of an axon in a peripheral motor neuron (**Figure 18-13**)
1. Following injury, distal portion of axon and myelin sheath degenerates
2. Macrophages remove the debris
3. Remaining neurilemma and endoneurium form a tunnel from the point of injury to the effector

4. New Schwann cells grow in the tunnel to maintain a path for regrowth of the axon
5. Cell body reorganizes its Nissl bodies to provide the needed proteins to extend the remaining healthy portion of the axon
6. Axon "sprouts" appear
7. When "sprout" reaches tunnel, its growth rate increases
8. The skeletal muscle cell atrophies until the nervous connection is reestablished

E. In CNS, similar repair of damaged nerve fibres is unlikely

Cycle of Life: Nervous System Cells

A. Nerve tissue development
   1. Begins in ectoderm
   2. Occurs most rapidly in womb and in first 2 years

B. Nervous cells organize into body network

C. Synapses
   1. Form and re-form until nervous system is intact
   2. Formation of new synapses and strengthening or elimination of old synapses stimulate learning and memory

D. Ageing causes degeneration of the nervous system, which may lead to senility

The Big Picture: Nervous System Cells and the Whole Body

A. Neurons act as the "wiring" that connects structures needed to maintain homeostasis

B. Sensory neurons—act as receptors to detect changes in the internal and external environment; relay information to integrator mechanisms in the CNS

C. Information is processed, and a response is relayed to the appropriate effectors through the motor neurons

D. At the effector, neurotransmitter triggers a response to restore homeostasis

E. Neurotransmitters released into the bloodstream are called *hormones*

F. Neurons are responsible for more than just responding to stimuli; circuits are capable of remembering or learning new responses, generation of thought, and so on

REVIEW QUESTIONS

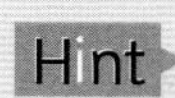

Write out the answers to these questions after reading the chapter and reviewing the Chapter Summary. Note—writing out your answers will consolidate learning and provide a valuable resource of information.

1. Briefly explain the general function the nervous system performs for the body.
2. Identify the other body system that performs the same general function.
3. Which glial cell helps form the *blood–brain barrier* (BBB)?
4. What is the difference between an ipsilateral reflex arc and a contralateral reflex arc.
5. List and describe disorders of the nervous system cells.

CRITICAL THINKING QUESTIONS

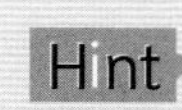

After finishing the Review Questions, write out the answers to these more in-depth questions to help you apply your new knowledge. Go back to sections of the chapter that relate to concepts that you find difficult.

1. Compare and contrast the characteristics of the central nervous system and the peripheral nervous system. Also, explain how the somatic and autonomic nervous systems could be included in the afferent and efferent divisions.
2. There are relatively few neurons in the brain. Describe the characteristics and roles of neuroglia and indicate whether they could be classified as tissue other than nervous tissue.
3. All neurons have axons and dendrites. Explain where these parts of the neuron are located in multipolar, bipolar, and unipolar neurons.
4. Compare and contrast white and grey matter. What would result if there were a loss of myelination?
5. Explain why high risk cervical spine injury requires immobilization. Give one possible consequence of failing to immobilize the spine following an accident.
6. Nerve fibres in the peripheral nervous system are much more successful than nerve fibres in the central nervous system in repairing themselves. How would you explain this difference?
7. Many antibiotics that should kill the causative agents of meningitis are ineffective if given orally. Explain the anatomical mechanism that could cause this ineffectiveness.

19 Nerve Signalling

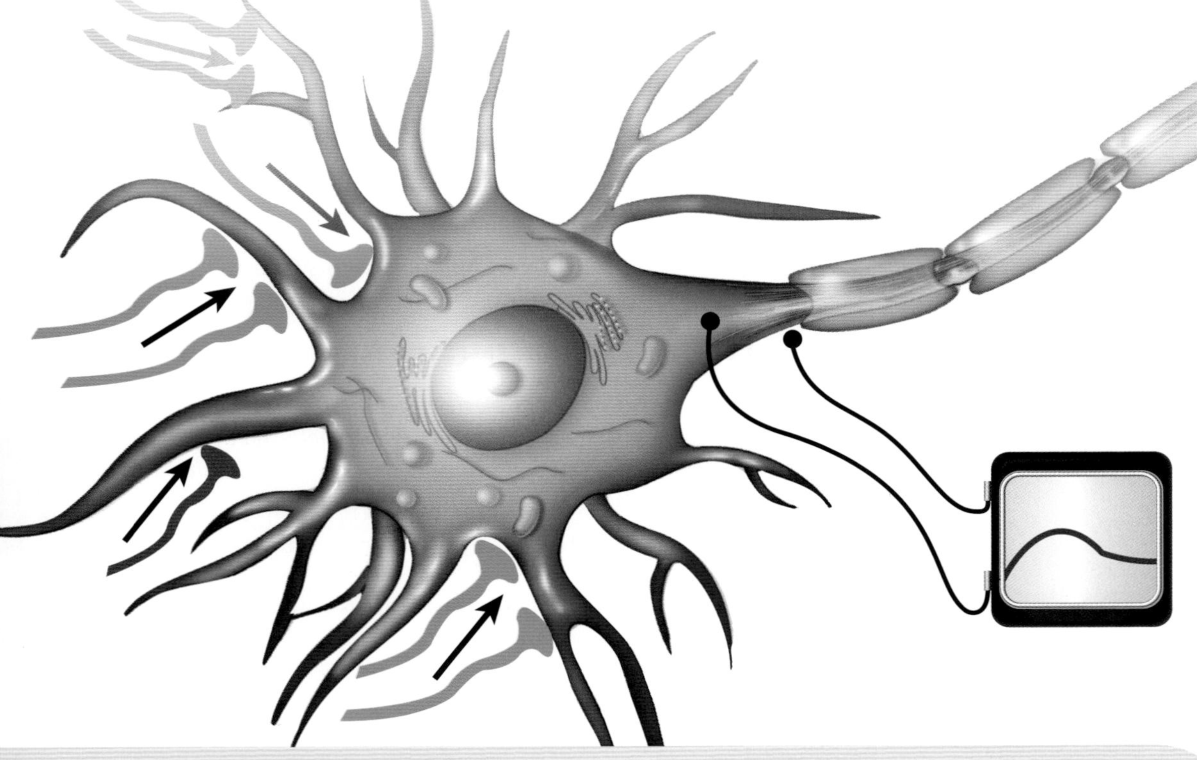

CHAPTER OUTLINE

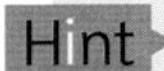

Hint ▸ *Scan this outline before you begin to read the chapter, as a preview of how the concepts are organized.*

LANGUAGE OF SCIENCE

Hint ▸ *Use this list to aid your pronunciation of unfamiliar words.*

absolute refractory period (AB-so-loot ree-FRAK-toh-ree) [*absolut-* **unrestricted,** *re-* **back or again,** *-fract-* **break,** *-ory* **relating to,** *period* **circuit**]

acetylcholine (ACh) (ass-ee-til-KOH-leen) [*acetyl-* **vinegar,** *-chole-* **bile,** *-ine* **made of**]

action potential (AK-shun poh-TEN-shal) [*potent-* **power,** *-ial* **relating to**]

amine (AM-een) [*amine* **ammonia compound**]

catecholamine (kat-eh-KOHL-ah-meen) [*catech-* **melt,** *-ol-* **alcohol,** *-amine* **ammonia compound**]

convergence (kon-VER-jens) [*con-* **together,** *-verg-* **incline,** *-ence* **state**]

depolarization (dee-poh-lar-i-ZAY-shun) [*de-* **opposite,** *-pol-* **pole,** *-ar-* **relating to,** *-ization* **process**]

divergence (dye-VER-jens) [*di-* **separate,** *-verg-* **incline,** *-ence* **state**]

excitatory postsynaptic potential (EPSP) (ek-SYE-tah-toh-ree post-si-NAP-tik poh-TEN-shal) [*excita-* **arouse,** *-ory* **relating to,** *post-* **after,** *-syn-* **together,** *-apt-* **join,** *-ic* **relating to,** *potent-* **power,** *-ial* **relating to**]

G-protein–coupled receptor (GPCR) (jee-PROH-teen-kup-eld ree-SEP-ter) [*G* **for guanine-nucleotide-binding,** *-prote-* **first rank,** *-in* **substance,** *recept-* **receive,** *-or* **agent**]

hyperpolarization (hye-per-pol-ar-i-ZAY-shun) [*hyper-* **excessive,** *-pol-* **pole,** *-ar-* **relating to,** *-ization* **process**]

inhibitory postsynaptic potential (IPSP) (in-HIB-i-tor-ee post-si-NAP-tik poh-TEN-shal) [*inhib-* **restrain,** *-ory* **relating to,** *post-* **after,** *-syn-* **together,** *-apt-* **join,** *-ic* **relating to,** *potent-* **power,** *-ial* **relating to**]

continued on p. 432

At the beginning of our study of anatomy and physiology, we learned that regulatory feedback loops that detect changes and respond to them are necessary for homeostasis—for health and survival. In the previous chapter, we learned that neurons working together in reflex arcs can operate as these needed regulatory feedback loops. We learned that neurons can detect sensory stimuli, can conduct impulses, and can pass information to other cells by using neurotransmitters. But how do nerve cells do this? How is a neuron triggered to produce a nerve impulse? What is an impulse? How do neurotransmitters work? We find answers to these questions in this chapter, which sets the stage for later studies of the nervous system and how nerve regulation works in other systems. •

ELECTRICAL NATURE OF NEURONS

Neurons are remarkable among cells because they initiate and conduct electrical signals called *nerve impulses.* Expressed differently, neurons exhibit both *excitability* and *conductivity.* What exactly is a nerve impulse? How is a neuron able to conduct this electrical signal along its entire length—sometimes a full metre? These questions, and more, are answered in the paragraphs that follow.

MEMBRANE POTENTIALS

One way to describe a nerve impulse is as a wave of electrical fluctuation that travels along the plasma membrane. To understand this phenomenon more fully, however, requires some familiarity with the electrical nature of the plasma membrane.

All living cells, including neurons, maintain a difference in the concentration of ions across their membranes. There is a slight excess of positive ions on the outside of the membrane and a slight excess of negative ions on the inside of the membrane. This, of course, results in a difference in electrical charge across their plasma membranes called the **membrane potential.**

This difference in electrical charge is called a *potential* because it is a type of stored energy called *potential energy.* Whenever opposite electrical charges (in this case, opposite ions) are thus separated by a membrane, they have the potential to move toward one another if they are allowed to cross the membrane. When a membrane potential is maintained by a cell, opposite ions are held on opposite sides of the membrane like water behind a dam—ready to rush through with force when the proper membrane channels open.

A membrane that exhibits a membrane potential is said to be *polarized.* That is, its membrane has a negative pole (the side on which there is an excess of negative ions) and a positive pole (the side on which there is an excess of positive ions). The magnitude of potential difference between the two sides of a polarized membrane is measured in volts (V) or millivolts (mV).

The voltage across a membrane can be measured by a device called a *voltmeter,* which is shown in **Figure 19-1**. The sign of a membrane's voltage indicates the charge on the inside surface of a polarized membrane. For example, the value −70 mV indicates that the potential difference has a magnitude of 70 mV and that the inside of the membrane is negative with respect to the outside surface (see **Figure 19-1**). A value of +30 mV indicates a potential difference of 30 mV and that the inside of the membrane is positive (and thus the outside of the membrane is negative).

To understand the electrical activity of the neuron—which is an essential concept of neurobiology—we will need to understand the different membrane potentials that occur in different circumstances in the plasma membrane of a neuron.

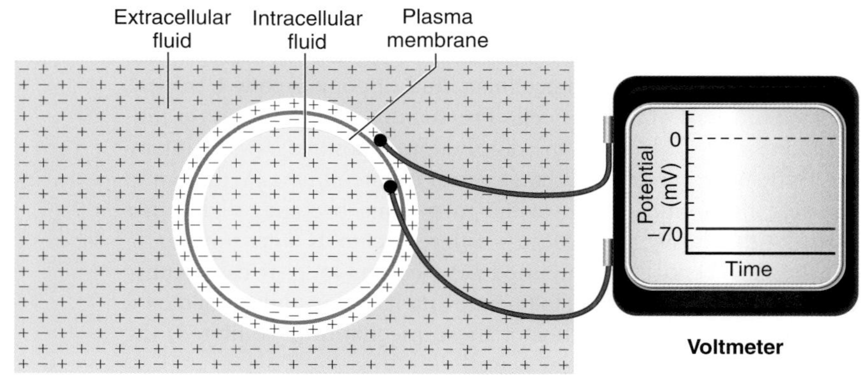

FIGURE 19-1 Membrane potential. The diagram on the left represents a cell maintaining a very slight difference in the concentration of oppositely charged ions across its plasma membrane. The voltmeter records the magnitude of electrical difference over time, which, in this case, does not fluctuate from −70 mV (voltage recorded over time as a red line).

RESTING MEMBRANE POTENTIALS

When a neuron is not conducting electrical signals, it is said to be "resting". At rest, a neuron's membrane potential is typically maintained at about −70 mV (see **Figure 19-1**). The membrane potential maintained by a nonconducting neuron's plasma membrane is called the **resting membrane potential (RMP).** Although the RMP can vary somewhat, we will use −70 mV as our typical value for the sake of discussion.

The mechanisms that produce and maintain the RMP do so by promoting a slight ionic imbalance across the neuron's plasma membrane. Specifically, these mechanisms produce a slight excess of positive ions on its outer surface. This imbalance of ion concentrations is produced primarily by ion transport mechanisms in the neuron's plasma membrane.

Recall from Chapters 5 and 6 that the permeability characteristics of each cell's plasma membrane are determined in part by the presence of specific membrane transport channels. Some ion channels, often called *leak channels,* are always open. Many of the membrane's ion channels are instead *gated channels,* allowing specific molecules to diffuse across the membrane only when the "gate" of each channel is open (see **Figure 6-6** on p. 103).

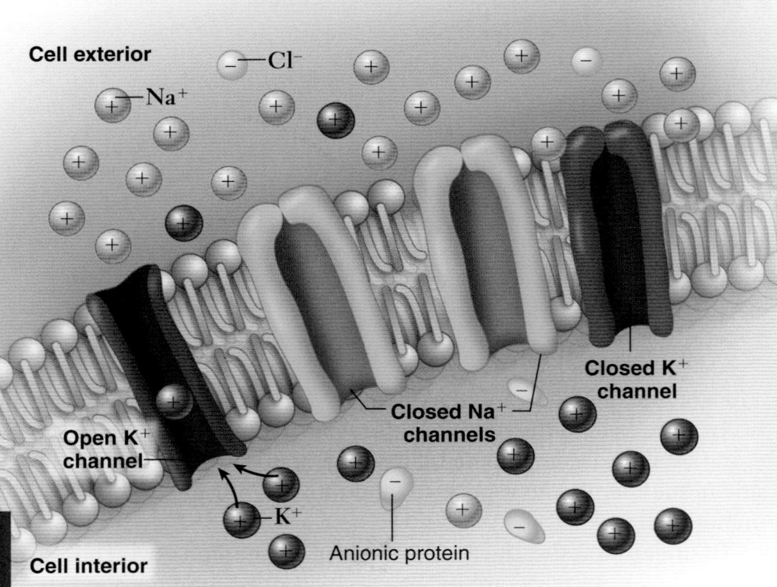

FIGURE 19-2 Role of ion channels in maintaining the resting membrane potential (RMP). Some K^+ channels are open in a "resting" membrane, allowing K^+ to diffuse down its concentration gradient (out of the cell) and thus add to the excess of positive ions on the outer surface of the plasma membrane. Diffusion of Na^+ in the opposite direction would counteract this effect but is prevented from doing so by closed Na^+ channels. Compare this figure with **Figure 19-3**.

In the neuron's plasma membrane, channels for the transport of the major anions (negative particles) are either nonexistent or mostly closed. For example, there are no channels to allow the exit of the large anionic protein molecules that dominate the intracellular fluid. Chloride ions (Cl^-), the dominant extracellular anions, are likewise "trapped" on one side of the membrane because chloride ions are repelled by the protein anions inside the cell. This means that the only ions that can move efficiently across a neuron's membrane are the positive ions sodium and potassium.

In a resting neuron, some of the potassium channels are open leak channels, but most of the sodium channels are closed gated channels (**Figure 19-2**). This means that potassium ions pumped into the neuron can diffuse or leak back out of the cell in an attempt to equalize its concentration gradient, but very little of the sodium pumped out of the cell can diffuse (leak) back into the neuron (**Figure 19-3**). Thus the membrane's selective permeability characteristics create and maintain a slight excess of positive ions on the outer surface of the membrane.

Another mechanism also operates to maintain the RMP. The sodium–potassium pump is an active transport mechanism in the plasma membrane that transports sodium ions (Na^+) and potassium ions (K^+) in opposite directions and at different rates (see **Figure 19-3**). It moves three sodium ions out of a neuron for every two potassium ions it moves into it. If, for instance, the pump transports 100 potassium ions into a neuron from the extracellular fluid, it concurrently transports 150 sodium ions out of the cell. The sodium–potassium pump thus maintains an imbalance in the distribution of positive ions, maintaining a difference in electrical charge across the membrane. As this pump operates, the inside surface of the membrane becomes slightly *less positive*—that is, slightly *negative*—with respect to its outer surface.

The RMP can be maintained by a cell as long as its sodium–potassium pumps continue to operate and its permeability characteristics remain stable. If either of these mechanisms is altered, the membrane potential changes as well.

Local Potentials

In neurons, membrane potentials can fluctuate above or below the resting membrane potential in response to certain stimuli (**Figure 19-4**). A slight shift away from the RMP in a specific region of the plasma membrane is often called a **local potential.**

Excitation of a neuron occurs when a stimulus triggers the opening of stimulus-gated Na^+ channels. **Stimulus-gated channels** are ion channels that open in response to chemicals produced by a sensory stimulus or by a chemical stimulus received from another neuron. Stimulus-gated channels are often called ligand-gated channels because they are triggered by ligands, which are signal molecules that bind to a receptor. Many stimulus-gated channels are located in the membrane of the neuron's input zone—the dendrites and soma (see **Figure 18-8** on p. 402).

The opening of stimulus-gated Na^+ channels in response to a stimulus permits more Na^+ to enter the cell. As the excess of positive ions

FIGURE 19-3 Sodium–potassium pump. This mechanism in the plasma membrane actively pumps sodium ions (Na^+) out of the neuron and potassium ions (K^+) into the neuron—at an unequal (3 : 2) rate. Because very little sodium reenters the cell via diffusion, this maintains an imbalance in the distribution of ions and thus maintains the resting potential. (See **Figure 19-2** for the role of ion channels in the diffusion of ions.)

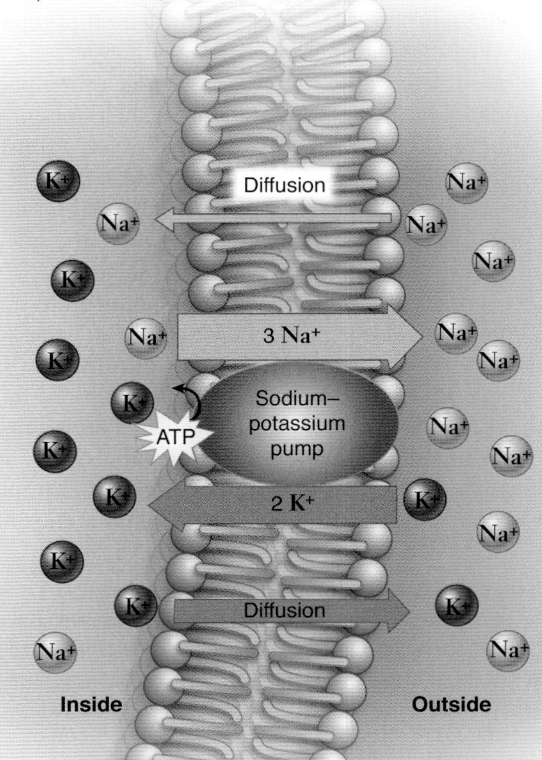

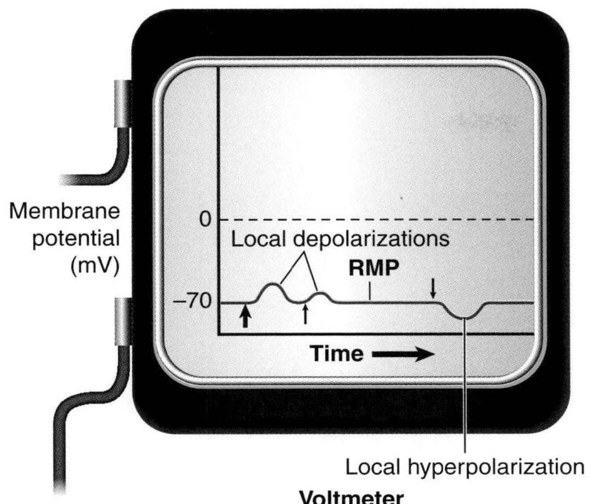

FIGURE 19-4 Local potentials. Recording voltmeter shows that excitatory stimuli (↑) cause depolarizations (movements toward 0 mV) in proportion to the strength of the stimuli. Inhibitory stimuli (↓) cause hyperpolarizations, local deviations away from 0 mV that cause the membrane potential to dip below the level of the resting membrane potential (RMP). Voltage is recorded as a red line on the screen of the voltmeter. Upward deviations of the red line are depolarizations; downward deviations of the red line are hyperpolarizations.

outside the plasma membrane decreases, the magnitude of the membrane potential is reduced. Such movement of the membrane potential toward zero is called **depolarization.** In *inhibition*, a stimulus triggers the opening of stimulus-gated K^+ channels. As more K^+ diffuses out of the cell, the excess of positive ions outside the plasma membranes increases—increasing the magnitude of the membrane potential.

Movement of the membrane potential away from zero (thus below the usual RMP) is called **hyperpolarization.**

Local potentials are called *graded potentials* because the magnitude of deviation from the RMP is proportional to the magnitude of the stimulus. In short, local potentials can be large or small—they are not all-or-none events. Local potentials exhibit *decremental* conduction, which means that their magnitude decreases as they travel along a membrane. Local potentials are called "local" nerve signals because they are more or less isolated to a particular region of the plasma membrane. That is, local potentials do not spread all the way to the end of a neuron's axon.

Quick CHECK

1. What mechanisms are involved in producing the resting membrane potential?
2. In a resting neuron, what positive ion is most abundant outside the plasma membrane? What positive ion is most abundant inside the plasma membrane?
3. How does depolarization of a membrane differ from hyperpolarization?

ACTION POTENTIALS

An **action potential** is, as the term suggests, the membrane potential of an active neuron—that is, one that is conducting an impulse. A synonym commonly used for action potential is *nerve impulse*. The action potential is an electrical fluctuation that travels along the surface of a neuron's plasma membrane.

MECHANISM OF THE ACTION POTENTIAL

As with local potentials, understanding how action potentials are generated requires familiarity with gated ion channels. **Table 19-1** summarizes the types and functions of gated channels for sodium and potassium that are important for understanding changes in membrane potential.

A step-by-step description of the mechanism that produces the action potential is given in the following paragraphs and in **Table 19-2**. Refer to **Figure 19-5** and **Figure 19-6** as you read each step.

1. When an adequate stimulus is applied to a neuron, the stimulus-gated Na^+ channels at the point of stimulation open. Na^+ diffuses rapidly into the cell because of the concentration gradient and electrical gradient, producing a local depolarization (see **Figure 19-5**, *B*).
2. If the magnitude of the local depolarization surpasses a limit called the **threshold potential** (for example, −59 mV), voltage-gated Na^+ channels are stimulated to open. **Voltage-gated channels** are ion channels that open in response to voltage fluctuations, usually at least −50 mV to −60 mV. There are many voltage-gated Na^+ channels and K^+ channels in the membrane of the neuron's summation zone (axon hillock) and conduction zone (axon) (see **Figure 18-8** on p. 402). The threshold potential is the minimum magnitude a voltage fluctuation in the summation or conduction zone must have to trigger the opening of a voltage-gated ion channel.

TABLE 19-1 Sodium and Potassium Channel Types and Functions

CHANNEL	EFFECT ON ION TRANSPORT*	EFFECT ON MEMBRANE POTENTIAL	TYPES	TRIGGER	RESPONSE
Sodium (Na^+) channels	Na^+ ions diffuse into cell	Increase (more positive)	Stimulus-gated	Sensory stimulus	Rapid response
				Chemical stimulus (neurotransmitter)	Rapid response
			Voltage-gated	Increase in membrane potential (to threshold potential [−59 mV] or beyond)	Rapid response
Potassium (K^+) channels	K^+ ions diffuse out of cell	Decrease (more negative)	Stimulus-gated	Sensory stimulus	Rapid response
				Chemical stimulus (neurotransmitter)	Rapid response
			Voltage-gated	Increase in membrane potential (to threshold potential [−59 mV] or beyond)	Slow response

*Net diffusion of ions down their respective concentration gradients.

TABLE 19-2 Steps of the Mechanism That Produces an Action Potential

STEP	DESCRIPTION
1	A stimulus triggers stimulus-gated Na^+ channels to open and allow inward Na^+ diffusion. This causes the membrane to depolarize.
2	As the threshold potential is reached, voltage-gated Na^+ channels open.
3	As more Na^+ enters the cell through voltage-gated Na^+ channels, the membrane depolarizes even further.
4	The magnitude of the action potential peaks (at +30 mV) when voltage-gated Na^+ channels close.
5	Repolarization begins when voltage-gated K^+ channels open, allowing outward diffusion of K^+.
6	After a brief period of hyperpolarization, the resting potential is restored by the sodium-potassium pump and the return of ion channels to their resting state.

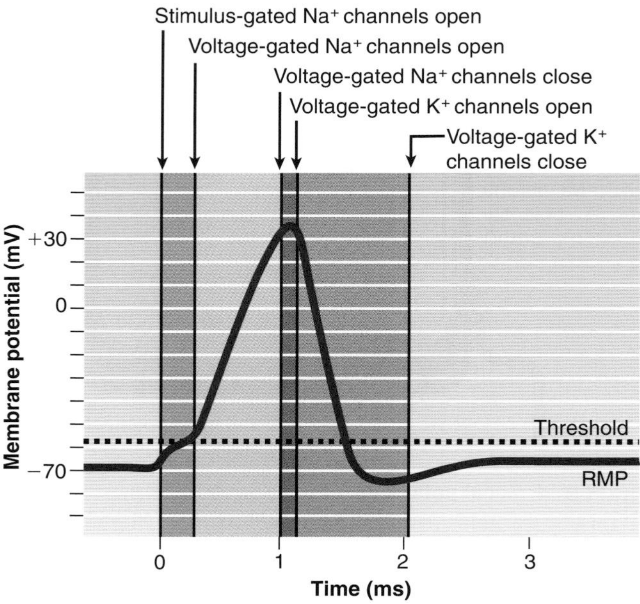

FIGURE 19-6 The action potential. Changes in membrane potential in a local area of a neuron's membrane result from changes in membrane permeability.

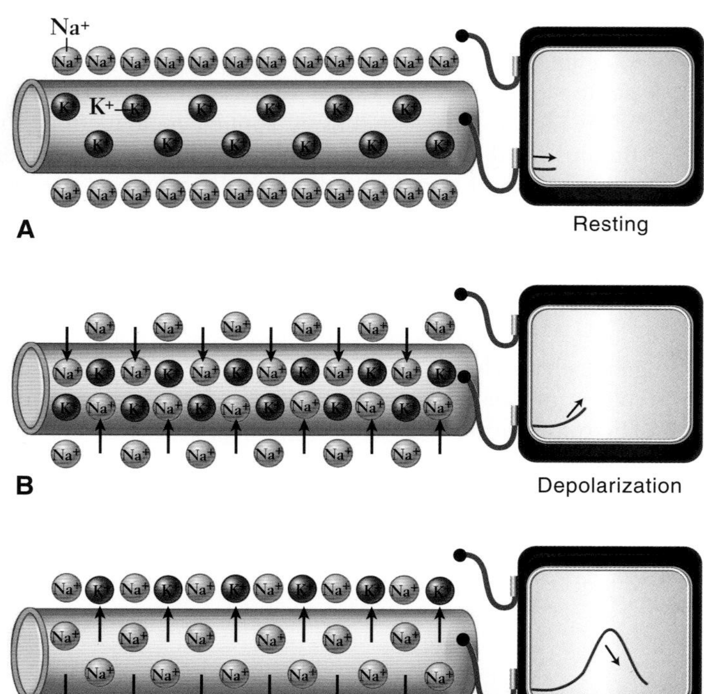

FIGURE 19-5 Depolarization and repolarization. A, Resting membrane potential (RMP) results from an excess of positive ions on the outer surface of the plasma membrane. More Na^+ ions are on the outside of the membrane than K^+ ions are on the inside of the membrane. **B,** Depolarization of a membrane occurs when Na^+ channels open, allowing Na^+ to move to an area of lower concentration (and more negative charge) *inside* the cell—reversing the polarity to an inside-positive state. **C,** Repolarization of a membrane occurs when K^+ channels then open, allowing K^+ to move to an area of lower concentration (and more negative charge) *outside* the cell—reversing the polarity back to an inside-negative state. Each voltmeter records the changing membrane potential as a red line.

3. As more Na^+ rushes into the cell, the membrane moves rapidly toward 0 mV and then continues in a positive direction to a peak of +30 mV (see **Figure 19-6**). The positive value at the peak of the action potential indicates that there is an excess of positive ions *inside* the membrane. If the local depolarization fails to cross the threshold of −59 mV, the voltage-gated Na^+ channels do not open, and the membrane simply recovers back to the resting potential of −70 mV without producing an action potential.
4. Voltage-gated Na^+ channels stay open for only about 1 millisecond (ms) before they automatically close. This means that once they are stimulated, the Na^+ channels always allow sodium to rush in for the same amount of time, which in turn produces the same magnitude of action potential. In other words, the action potential is an *all-or-none* response. If the threshold potential is surpassed, the full peak of the action potential is always reached; if the threshold potential is not surpassed, no action potential will occur at all.
5. Once the peak of the action potential is reached, the membrane potential begins to move back toward the resting potential (−70 mV) in a process called **repolarization.** Surpassing the threshold potential triggers the opening of not only voltage-gated Na^+ channels but also voltage-gated K^+ channels. The voltage-gated K^+ channels are slow to respond, however, and thus do not begin opening until the inward diffusion of Na^+ ions has caused the membrane potential to reach +30 mV. Once the K^+ channels open, K^+ rapidly diffuses out of the cell because of the concentration gradient and because it is repulsed by the now-positive interior of the cell. The outward rush of K^+ restores the original excess of positive ions on the outside surface of the membrane—thus repolarizing the membrane (see **Figure 19-5**).

TABLE 19-3 Types of Membrane Potentials

MEMBRANE POTENTIAL	POLARIZATION	TYPICAL VOLTAGE*	SUMMATION	CONDUCTION	DESCRIPTION
Resting membrane potential (RMP)	Polarized	−70 mV	Not applicable	Not applicable	Membrane voltage when the neuron is not excited and not conducting an impulse
Local potential	Depolarized (excitatory; EPSP)	Graded; varies higher than −70 mV	Yes	Decremental	Temporary fluctuation in a local region of the membrane in response to a sensory or nerve stimulus; may be an upward or downward fluctuation in voltage; loses amplitude as it spreads along membrane
	Hyperpolarized (inhibitory; IPSP)	Graded; varies lower than −70 mV	Yes	Decremental	
Threshold potential	Depolarized	−59 mV	Yes	Triggers action potential	Minimum local depolarization needed to trigger voltage-gated channels that produce the action potential
Action potential	Depolarized	+30 mV	No	Nondecremental	Temporary maximum depolarization of membrane voltage that travels to end of axon without losing amplitude

*Example used in this chapter; actual values in body vary depending on many diverse factors.
EPSP, Excitatory postsynaptic potential; *IPSP,* inhibitory postsynaptic potential.

6. Because the K^+ channels often remain open as the membrane reaches its resting potential, too much K^+ may rush out of the cell. This causes a brief period of *after-hyperpolarization* before the resting potential is restored when K^+ channels return to their resting state.

Table 19-3 summarizes essential characteristics of the action potential along with other important types of membrane potentials discussed so far in this chapter.

Note that when the threshold potential is reached, a *positive feedback* event occurs to produce the action potential. The influx of Na^+ produces just enough depolarization to trigger some voltage-gated Na^+ channels to open, which causes more depolarization, which opens more Na^+ channels, which causes more membrane depolarization, which opens more channels—until finally the amplification stops when all the available channels have opened.

Refractory Period

The refractory period is a brief period during which a local area of an axon's membrane resists restimulation (**Figure 19-7**, A). For about 0.5 ms after the membrane surpasses the threshold potential, it will not respond to any stimulus, no matter how strong. This is called the **absolute refractory period.** The **relative refractory period** is the few milliseconds after the absolute refractory period—the time during which the membrane is repolarizing and restoring the resting membrane potential. During the relative refractory period the membrane will respond only to very strong stimuli.

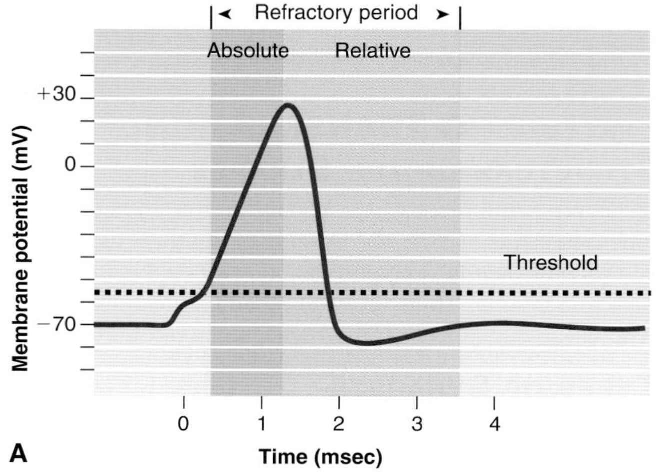

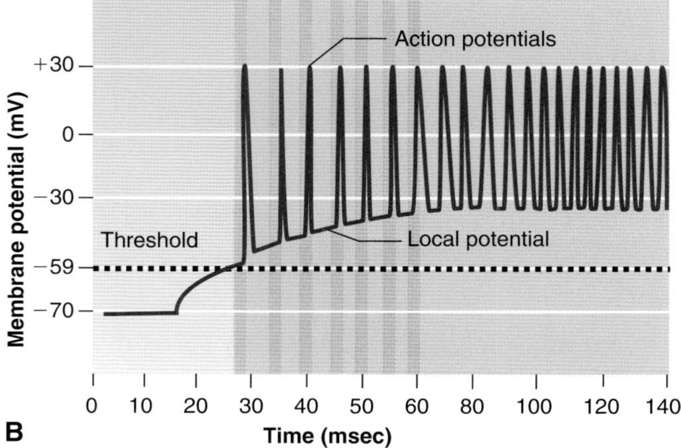

FIGURE 19-7 Refractory period. A, During the absolute refractory period, the membrane will not respond to any stimulus. During the relative refractory period, however, a very strong stimulus may elicit a response in the membrane. **B,** As the local potential increases, a new action potential may begin during the relative refractory period. The higher the local potential, the sooner a new action potential can be generated. As the graph shows, high local potentials produce a higher frequency of action potentials than lower local potentials.

Because only very strong stimuli can produce an action potential during the relative refractory period, a series of closely spaced action potentials can occur only when the magnitude of the stimulus is great. The greater the magnitude of the stimulus, the earlier a new action potential can be produced, and thus the greater the frequency of action potentials (**Figure 19-7**, *B*). This means that although the magnitude of the stimulus does not affect the magnitude of the action potential, which is an all-or-none response, it does cause a proportional increase in the frequency of impulses. Thus the nervous system uses the frequency of nerve impulses to code for the strength of a stimulus—not changes in the magnitude of the action potential.

Conduction of the Action Potential

At the peak of the action potential, the inside of the axon's plasma membrane is positive relative to the outside. That is, its polarity is now the reverse of that of the resting membrane potential. Such reversal in polarity causes electrical current to flow between the site of the action potential and the adjacent regions of membrane. This local current flow triggers voltage-gated Na^+ channels in the next segment of membrane to open. As Na^+ rushes inward, this next segment exhibits an action potential. The action potential thus has moved from one point to the next continuously along the axon's membrane (**Figure 19-8**).

This cycle repeats itself because each action potential always causes enough local current flow to surpass the threshold potential for the next region of membrane. Because each action potential is an all-or-none phenomenon, the fluctuation in membrane potential moves along the membrane without any decrement, or decrease, in magnitude.

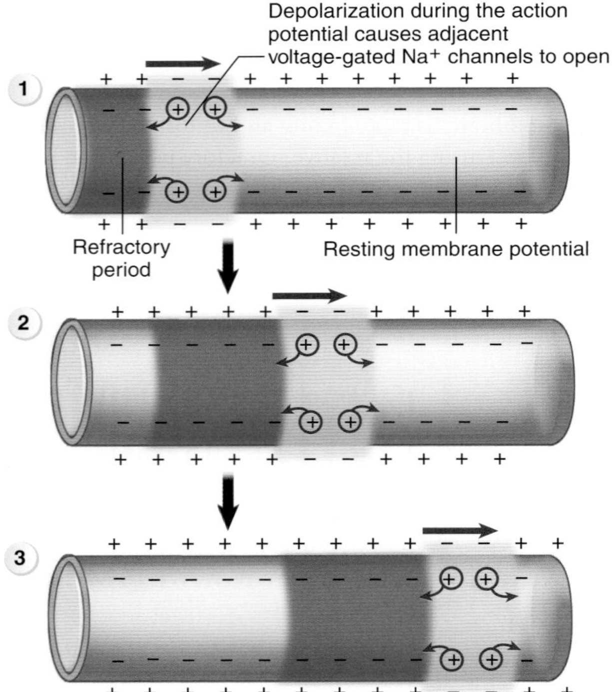

FIGURE 19-8 Continuous conduction of the action potential. The reverse polarity characteristic of the peak of the action potential causes local current flow to adjacent regions of the membrane *(small arrows)*. This stimulates voltage-gated Na^+ channels to open and thus create a new action potential. This cycle continues, producing wavelike conduction of the action potential from point to point along a nerve fibre. Adjacent regions of membrane behind the action potential do not depolarize again because they are still in their refractory period.

The action potential never moves backward, restimulating the region from which it just came. It is prevented from doing so because the previous segment of membrane remains in a refractory period too long to allow such restimulation. This is the mechanism responsible for the one-way movement of action potentials along axons.

In myelinated fibres, the insulating properties of the thick myelin sheath resist ion movement and the resulting local flow of current. Electrical changes in the membrane can only occur at gaps in the myelin sheath—that is, at the nodes of Ranvier. **Figure 19-9** shows that when an action potential occurs at one node, most of the current flows *under* the insulating myelin sheath to the next node. This stimulates regeneration of an action potential at that node by opening voltage-gated channels, which in turn stimulates the next node. Thus the action potential seems to "leap" from node to node along the myelinated fibre. This type of impulse regeneration is called **saltatory conduction** (from the Latin verb *saltare*, "to leap").

How fast does a nerve fibre conduct impulses? It depends on its diameter and on the presence or absence of a myelin sheath. The speed of conduction of a nerve fibre is proportional to its diameter: the larger the diameter, the faster it conducts impulses. Myelinated fibres conduct impulses more rapidly than unmyelinated fibres. This is because saltatory conduction is more rapid than point-to-point, continuous conduction.

The fastest fibres, such as those that innervate the skeletal muscles, can conduct impulses up to about 130 metres per second (468 km per hour). The slowest fibres, such as those from sensory receptors in the skin, may conduct impulses at only about 0.5 metre per second (1.8 km per hour).

Box 19-1 outlines how disrupting conduction of nerve impulses can be used to block pain signals.

Quick CHECK

4. List the events that lead to the initiation of an action potential.
5. What is meant by the term *threshold potential*?
6. How does impulse conduction in an unmyelinated fibre differ from impulse conduction in a myelinated fibre?

SYNAPTIC TRANSMISSION

Structure of the Synapse

A **synapse** is the place where signals are transmitted from one neuron, called the *presynaptic neuron*, to another neuron, called the *postsynaptic neuron*. The postsynaptic cell could also be an effector, such as a muscle. There are many such connections in our nervous system—more than 100 trillion synapses in our brain alone!

Types of Synapses

There are two types of synapses: electrical synapses and chemical synapses.

Electrical Synapse

Electrical synapses occur where two cells are joined end-to-end by gap junctions (**Figure 19-10**, A). Because the plasma membranes and cytoplasm are functionally continuous in this type of junction, an action

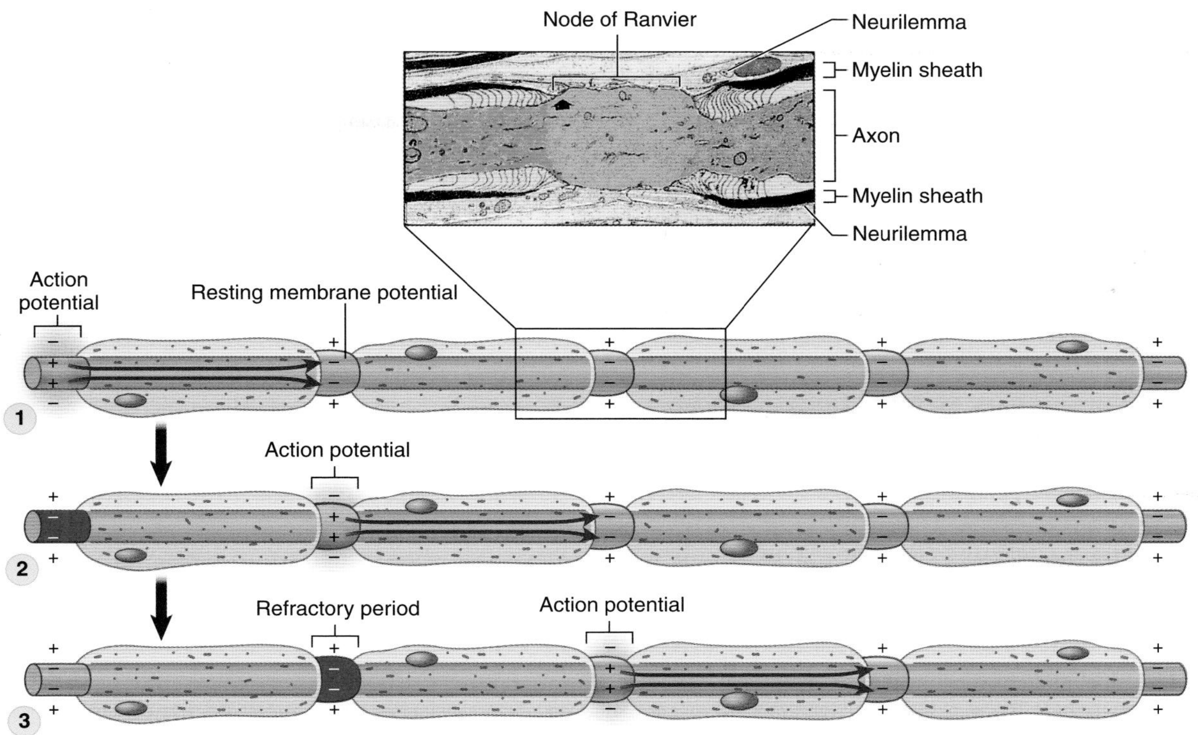

FIGURE 19–9 Saltatory conduction. This series of diagrams shows that the insulating nature of the myelin sheath prevents ion movement everywhere but at the nodes of Ranvier. The action potential at one node triggers current flow *(arrows)* across the myelin sheath to the next node—producing an action potential there. The action potential thus seems to "leap" rapidly from node to node. The inset is a transmission electron micrograph showing a node of Ranvier in a myelinated fibre.

potential can simply continue along the postsynaptic plasma membrane as if it belonged to the same cell. Electrical synapses occur between cardiac muscle cells and between some types of smooth muscle cells. Electrical synapses are found throughout the nervous system early in development. These early electrical synapses are thought to be eventually replaced by the more complex chemical synapses. However, evidence suggests that electrical synapses may be more abundant, and more critical to certain functions, in adults than previously thought.

Chemical synapses are called that because they use a chemical transmitter called a *neurotransmitter* to send a signal from the **presynaptic** cell to the **postsynaptic** cell (**Figure 19-10**, *B*). Because of its importance and complexity, it is the chemical synapse that we will consider carefully in the following paragraphs.

Chemical Synapse

Three structures make up a chemical synapse:

1. A synaptic knob
2. A synaptic cleft
3. The plasma membrane of a postsynaptic neuron

BOX 19-1 *health matters* | Anaesthetics

Anaesthetics are substances or procedures that are administered to reduce or eliminate the sensation of pain—thus producing a state called **anaesthesia.**

Many anaesthetics produce their effects by inhibiting the opening of sodium channels and thus blocking the initiation and conduction of nerve impulses. For example, electrical stimulation that disrupts nerve conduction along sensory neurons has been used in some dental procedures (see figure). Hypnosis and other mind-based methods can block awareness of pain sensations in dentistry, in childbirth, and in managing chronic pain.

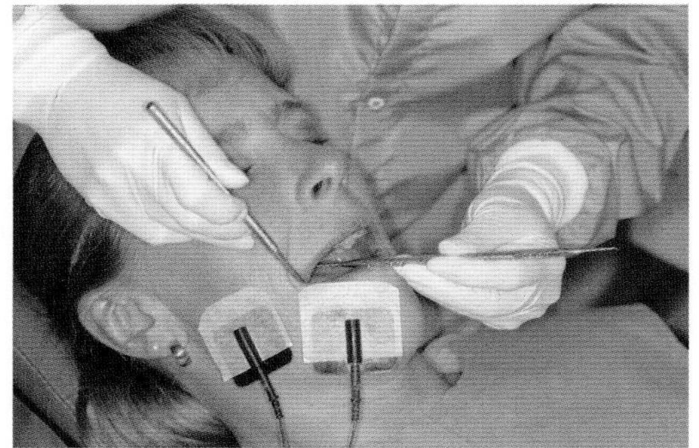

The anaesthetic drug lidocaine, in combination with epinephrine, is widely used in dentistry to minimize the pain involved in tooth extractions and other dental procedures.

Bupivacaine has likewise been used to block the transmission of electrical signals in the spinal cord and is used in a range of procedures including caesarean sections and orthopaedic surgery. Benzocaine, a local anaesthetic found in several over-the-counter products, helps relieve pain associated with sore throat, teething and aphthous ulcers. Benzocaine blocks the initiation and conduction of nerve impulses by inhibiting voltage-dependent sodium channels found on the membranes of sensory neurons.

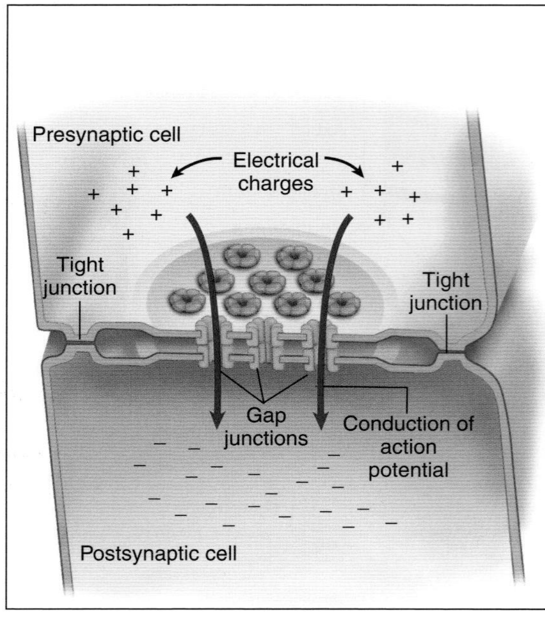

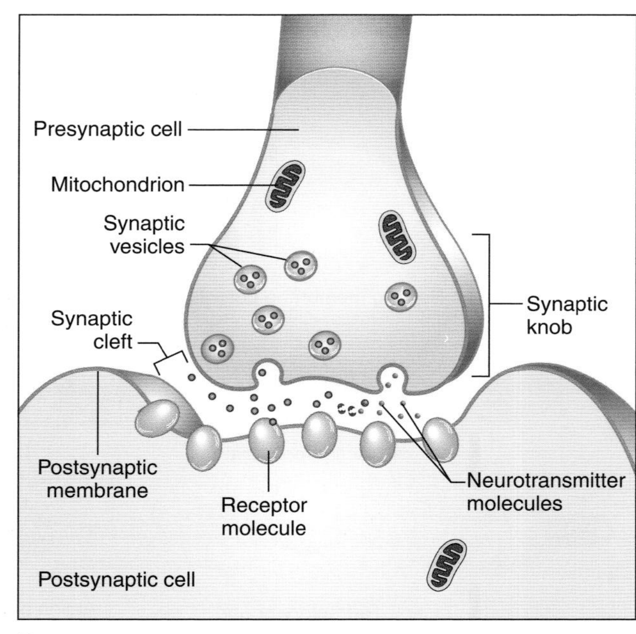

FIGURE 19-10 Electrical and chemical synapses. A, Electrical synapses involve gap junctions that allow action potentials to move from cell to cell directly by allowing electrical current to flow between cells. **B,** Chemical synapses involve transmitter chemicals (neurotransmitters) that signal postsynaptic cells, possibly inducing an action potential.

A *synaptic knob* is a tiny bulge at the end of a terminal branch of a presynaptic neuron's axon (see **Figure 19-10**). Each synaptic knob, or synaptic terminal, contains numerous small sacs or vesicles. Each vesicle contains about 10,000 neurotransmitter molecules. Some of these are released from the presynaptic neuron into a **synaptic cleft**—the space between a synaptic knob and the plasma membrane of a postsynaptic neuron.

FIGURE 19-11 Arrangements of synapses. The axon of a presynaptic neuron may form a synapse at the dendrite, soma, or axon of another neuron.

The synaptic cleft is an incredibly narrow space—only 20 to 30 nanometres (nm) in width. Identify the synaptic cleft in **Figure 19-10**. The synaptic cleft is not an empty space—it contains fluid, enzymes, adhesion molecules, and other substances.

Figure 19-11 shows that an axon may form a synapse at any of several points along a postsynaptic neuron:

- At the dendrite (axodendritic synapses)
- At the soma (axosomatic synapses)
- At the axon (axoaxonic synapses)

Synapses at the dendrite or soma are the most common arrangements in many areas of the nervous system. Synapses of an axon with the axon of another neuron are less common but offer a way for one neuron to inhibit or facilitate synaptic transmission by another neuron.

The plasma membrane of a postsynaptic neuron has protein molecules embedded in it, each facing toward the synaptic knob (see **Figure 19-10**). These membrane molecules serve as receptors to which neurotransmitter molecules bind and trigger responses in the postsynaptic cell.

Mechanisms of Synaptic Transmission

An action potential that has travelled the length of a neuron stops at its axon terminals. Action potentials cannot cross synaptic clefts, minuscule barriers though they are. Instead, neurotransmitters are released from the synaptic knob, cross the synaptic cleft, and bring about a response by the postsynaptic neuron. *Excitatory* neurotransmitters cause depolarization of the postsynaptic membrane, whereas *inhibitory* neurotransmitters cause hyperpolarization of the postsynaptic membrane (see **Figure 19-4**).

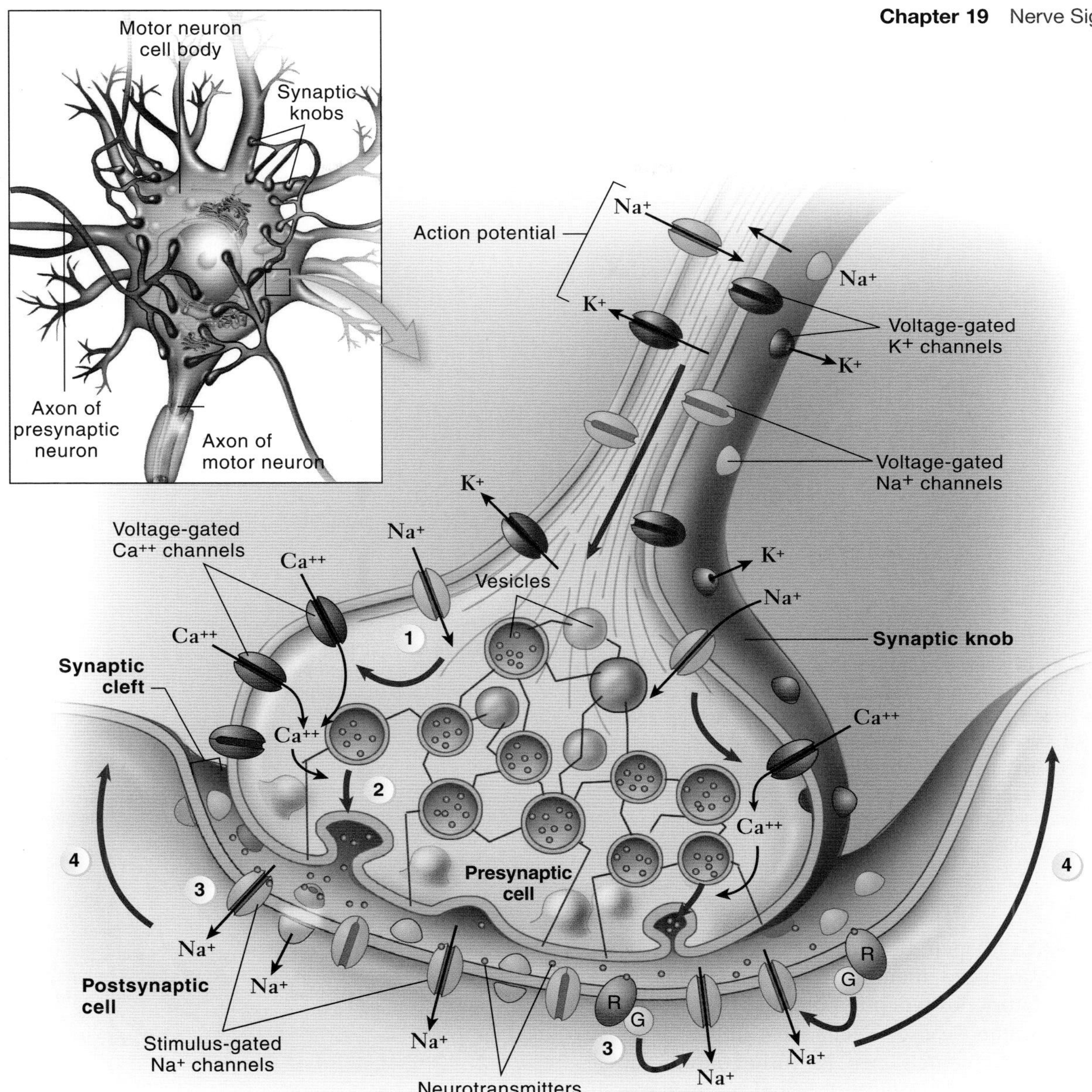

FIGURE 19-12 The chemical synapse. Diagram shows detail of synaptic knob, or axon terminal, of presynaptic neuron, the plasma membrane of a postsynaptic neuron, and a synaptic cleft. On the arrival of an action potential at a synaptic knob, voltage-gated Ca^{++} channels open and allow extracellular Ca^{++} to diffuse into the presynaptic cell *(step 1)*. In step 2, the Ca^{++} signals molecular motors in the cytoskeleton and thereby triggers the rapid exocytosis of neurotransmitter molecules from vesicles in the knob. In step 3, neurotransmitter diffuses into the synaptic cleft and binds to receptor molecules in the plasma membrane of the postsynaptic neuron. The postsynaptic receptors directly or indirectly trigger the opening of stimulus-gated ion channels, initiating a local potential in the postsynaptic neuron. In step 4, the local potential may move toward the axon, where an action potential may begin.

The mechanism of synaptic transmission, summarized in **Figure 19-10** and **Figure 19-12**, consists of the following sequence of events:

1. When an action potential reaches a synaptic knob, voltage-gated calcium channels in its membrane open and allow calcium ions (Ca^{++}) to diffuse into the knob rapidly. Many voltage-gated Ca^{++} channels are present in the membrane of the neuron's output zone (see **Figure 18-8**).
2. The increase in intracellular Ca^{++} concentration triggers molecular motors to pull neurotransmitter vesicles to the plasma membrane of the synaptic knob. Once there, the vesicles fuse with the membrane and release their neurotransmitter via exocytosis. Thousands of neurotransmitter molecules spurt out of the open vesicles into the synaptic cleft.
3. The released neurotransmitter molecules almost instantaneously diffuse across the narrow synaptic cleft and contact the postsynaptic neuron's plasma membrane. Here, neurotransmitters briefly bind to receptor molecules that are also gated channels or that are coupled to gated channels. Binding of neurotransmitters triggers the channels to open.
4. The opening of ion channels in the postsynaptic membrane may produce a local potential called a **postsynaptic potential.** Excitatory neurotransmitters cause both Na^{+} channels

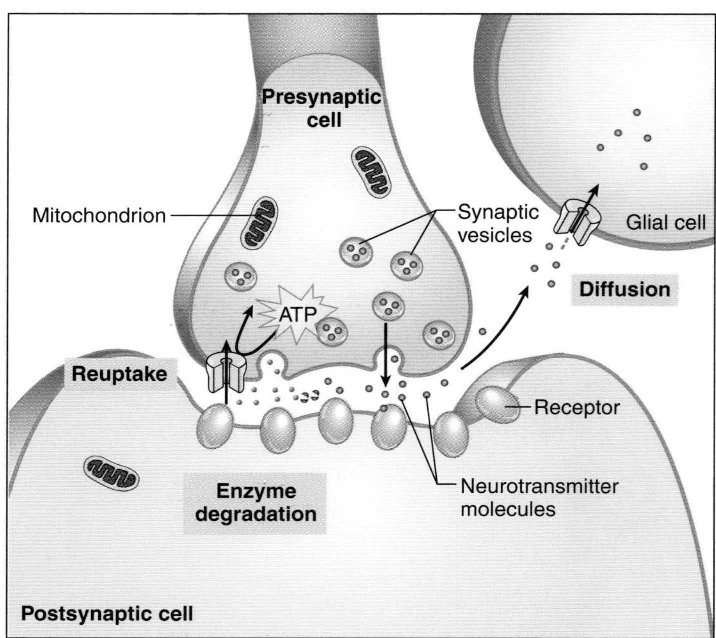

FIGURE 19-13 Fate of neurotransmitters. After synaptic transmission, the signal must be stopped by removing neurotransmitters from the synaptic cleft. Many neurotransmitters are immediately transported back into the presynaptic neuron in a process called *reuptake.* Some neurotransmitters are broken down by enzymes in the synaptic cleft, and the resulting molecules are transported back into the presynaptic neuron for recycling. Some neurotransmitter molecules may diffuse out of the synapse and be transported into a nearby glial cell (which may return an altered form of the molecule to the presynaptic neuron).

and K^+ channels to open. Because Na^+ rushes inward faster than K^+ rushes outward, there is a temporary depolarization called an **excitatory postsynaptic potential (EPSP).** Inhibitory neurotransmitters cause K^+ channels and/or Cl^- channels to open. If K^+ channels open, K^+ rushes outward; if Cl^- channels open, Cl^- rushes inward. Either event makes the inside of the membrane even more negative than at the resting potential. This temporary hyperpolarization is called an **inhibitory postsynaptic potential (IPSP).**

5. Once a neurotransmitter binds to its postsynaptic receptors, its action is quickly terminated (**Figure 19-13**). Several mechanisms bring this about. Some neurotransmitter molecules are transported back into the synaptic knobs, where they can be repacked into vesicles and used again. Some neurotransmitter molecules are metabolized into inactive compounds by synaptic enzymes. Other neurotransmitter molecules simply diffuse out of the synaptic cleft and are transported into nearby glial cells. The glial cells may release them again for reuptake by the presynaptic neuron, sometimes after breaking them down into another form.

Some mechanisms of synaptic transmission are illustrated in **Figures 19-12** and **19-13**. The diagram in **Figure 19-14** summarizes all the main events of synaptic transmission.

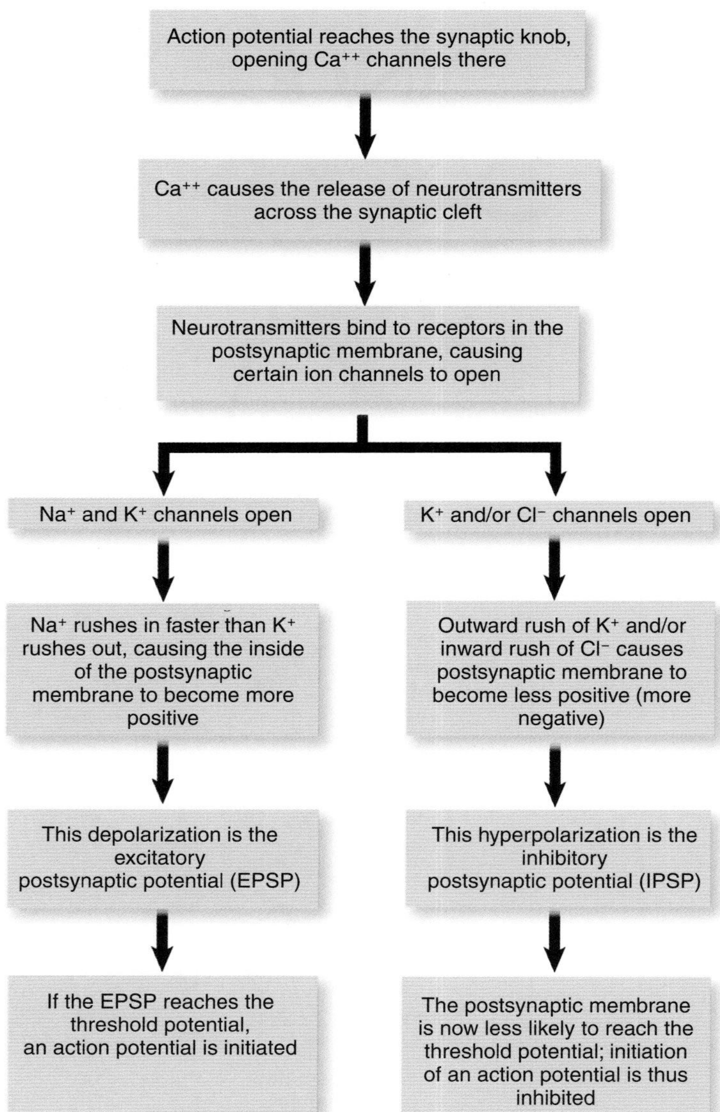

FIGURE 19-14 Summary of synaptic transmission.

SUMMATION

At least several, usually thousands, and in some cases more than 100,000 knobs synapse with a single postsynaptic neuron. The amount of excitatory neurotransmitter released by one knob is not enough to trigger an action potential. It may, however, *facilitate* initiation of an action potential by producing a local depolarization of the synaptic membrane—an EPSP. When several knobs are activated simultaneously, neurotransmitters stimulate different locations on the postsynaptic membrane. These local potentials may spread far enough to reach the axon hillock, where they may add together, or *summate*. If the sum of the local potentials reaches the threshold potential, voltage-gated channels in the axon membrane open, producing an action potential (**Figure 19-15**, A). This phenomenon is called **spatial summation.**

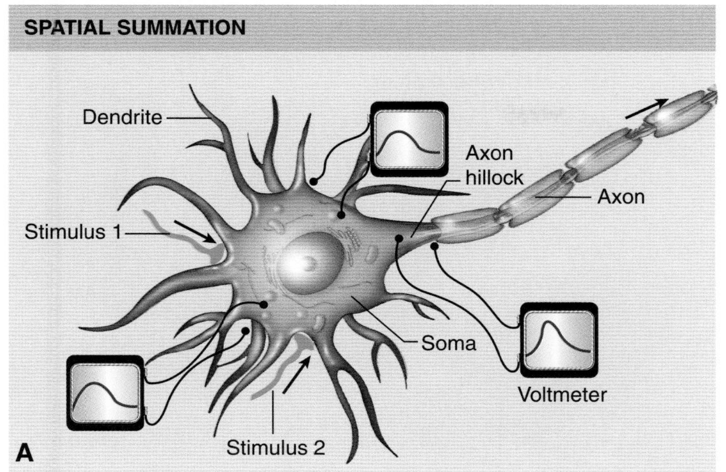

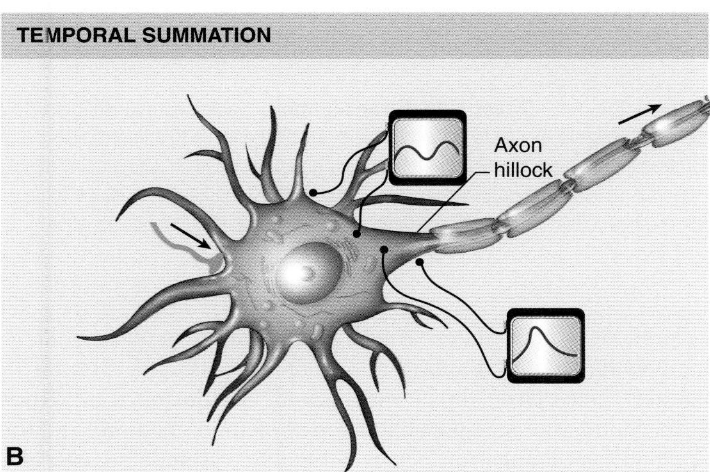

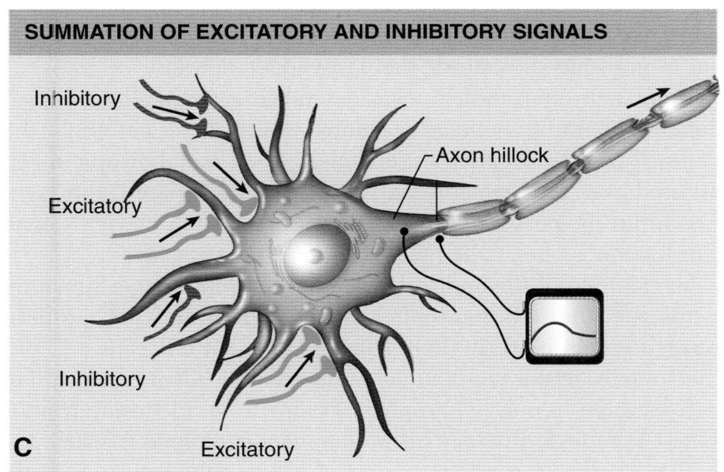

FIGURE 19-15 Summation. A, Spatial summation is the effect produced by simultaneous stimulation by a number of synaptic knobs on the same postsynaptic neuron. Voltmeters placed near the site of stimulation show small depolarizations, and a voltmeter at the axon hillock shows the large depolarization resulting from the combined effect of both smaller depolarizations. **B,** Temporal summation is the effect produced by a rapid succession of stimuli on a single postsynaptic neuron. The figure shows two stimuli in a short burst that produce two small depolarizations that combine at the axon hillock to produce a large depolarization. **C,** Summation of many excitatory and inhibitory effects produces the potential at the axon hillock. Here, depolarizations triggered by five excitatory presynaptic neurons *(green)* are partially offset by hyperpolarizations triggered by three inhibitory presynaptic neurons *(red)* to produce only a small depolarization at the axon hillock. This will occur only if there is sufficient depolarization to surpass the threshold potential.

Likewise, when synaptic knobs stimulate a postsynaptic neuron in rapid succession, their effects can add up over a brief period to produce an action potential (**Figure 19-15**, *B*). This type of summation is called **temporal summation.**

Usually both excitatory and inhibitory transmitters are released at the same postsynaptic neuron. The excitatory neurotransmitters produce local EPSPs, and the inhibitory neurotransmitters produce local IPSPs. Summation of these opposing local potentials occurs at the axon hillock, where many voltage-gated ion channels are located. If the EPSPs predominate over the IPSPs enough to depolarize the membrane to the threshold potential, the voltage-gated channels will respond and produce an action potential (**Figure 19-15**, *C*). The action potential is then conducted without decrement along the axon's membrane.

On the other hand, if the IPSPs predominate over the EPSPs, the membrane will not reach the threshold potential. The voltage-gated channels at the axon hillock will not respond, and no action potential will be conducted along the axon.

One reason summation is important for our understanding of the nervous system is that it helps explain how information can be processed as it moves through a network of neurons. For example, not all of the sensory information your sensory neurons are receiving right now is actually getting to the conscious part of your brain.

Of course, it would be overwhelming if all that information did get into your consciousness. Much of it would have been stopped at synapses where threshold was not reached, as described in the preceding paragraphs. Thus summation is a mechanism for *making decisions* about what information should continue onward in the neural network.

Synapses and Memory

Current theories of memory state that synapses play a key role in how memories are stored in the nervous system. The most widely held idea is that information is stored in the form of an increased flow of information at synapses in particular pathways (depending on the memory stored). In other words, memories form when the flow of information is facilitated at synapses.

Short-term memories, lasting only a few seconds or minutes, may result from presynaptic facilitation or inhibition at particular synapses. Go back to **Figure 19-11** on p. 420 to see how an axoaxonic synapse would permit one neuron to influence the presynaptic events of another neuron.

Intermediate long-term memory lasts from minutes to weeks. To get these memories to remain that long, facilitation of presynaptic activity has to last longer. One way that the nervous system does this involves the neurotransmitter *serotonin.* Serotonin is released at an axoaxonal synapse and triggers the axon terminal of a presynaptic neuron to block its potassium channels for up to several weeks. Thus whenever there is an action potential arriving at that presynaptic neuron, it lasts longer (because potassium fails to rapidly repolarize the membrane, as shown in **Figure 19-6** on p. 416). A prolonged action potential means that the presynaptic calcium channels stay open longer and trigger the release of more neurotransmitter than usual—thus facilitating synaptic transmission.

Long-term memories, the kind of memories needed for learning anatomy and physiology, last for months or years. Such long-term facilitation of synaptic transmission requires longer-lasting structural changes in the synapses. These changes may involve just one element or be a combination of the following: an increase in the number of vesicles stored, an increase in membrane locations from which the vesicles can release their neurotransmitters, an increase in the number of presynaptic axon terminals, or changes in the dendrites that permit postsynaptic facilitation.

Because nearby astrocytes can enhance or alter synaptic transmission by releasing transmitters of their own, they may also play a role in storing memories. Prion proteins (PrP), which can change shape and then cause other proteins in a neuron to change shape, have also been suggested as a memory mechanism.

Quick **CHECK**

7. What are the three structural components of a synapse?
8. List the steps of synaptic transmission.
9. What is an EPSP? What is an IPSP?
10. How does temporal summation differ from spatial summation?
11. How are memories formed?

NEUROTRANSMITTERS

Neurotransmitters are the means by which neurons talk to one another. The presynaptic neurons at the trillions of synapses located throughout the body release neurotransmitters that act to facilitate, stimulate, or inhibit postsynaptic neurons and effector cells. More than 50 compounds are known to be neurotransmitters. At least 50 other compounds are suspected of being neurotransmitters. For the most part, they are not distributed diffusely or at random throughout the nervous system. Instead, specific neurotransmitters are localized in discrete groups of neurons and thus released in specific nerve pathways.

Neurotransmitters are commonly classified by their function or by their chemical structure, depending on the context in which they are discussed.

FUNCTIONAL CLASSIFICATION OF NEUROTRANSMITTERS

You are already familiar with two major functional classifications: *excitatory neurotransmitters* and *inhibitory neurotransmitters.* Some neurotransmitters can have inhibitory effects at some synapses and excitatory effects at other synapses. For example, the neurotransmitter *acetylcholine,* discussed in Chapter 17, excites skeletal muscle cells but inhibits cardiac muscle cells. This illustrates an important point about the action of neurotransmitters: their function is determined by the postsynaptic receptors, not by the neurotransmitters themselves.

Another way to classify neurotransmitters by the function of their receptors is to identify the mechanism by which they cause a change in the postsynaptic neuron or effector cell—or *signal transduction.*

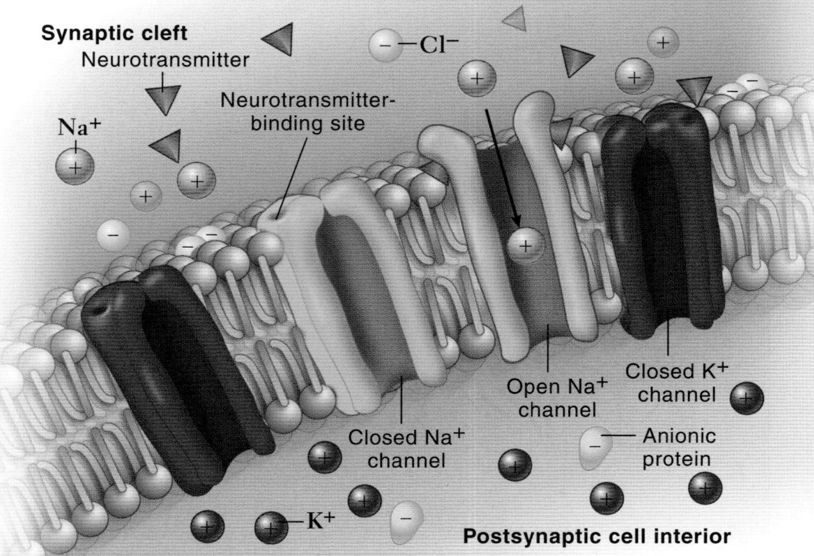

FIGURE 19-16 Direct signal transduction. Some neurotransmitters, such as acetylcholine, initiate nerve signals by binding directly to one or both neurotransmitter-binding sites on the stimulus-gated ion channel acting as a "direct" or *ionotropic* receptor. Such binding causes the channel to change its shape to an open position. When the neurotransmitter is removed, the channel again closes.

Some neurotransmitters trigger the opening or closing of ion channels directly, by binding to one or both receptor sites on the channel itself. This "direct mechanism" is illustrated in **Figure 19-16**. Membrane receptors that are part of an ion channel and thus act directly to change ion permeability when stimulated are called **ionotropic receptors.** Recent evidence shows that ionotropic resonses can be regulated by a complex variety of subtle chemical signals from inside and outside the postsynpatic neuron.

Other neurotransmitters instead bind to a receptor that sets in motion a chain of chemical reactions—a metabolic pathway—that eventually opens or closes ion channels. Such **metabotropic receptors** are linked to G *proteins* that, in turn, activate chemical messengers within the postsynaptic cell. For this reason, this style of signal transduction is often called the *second messenger model.*

An example of this indirect type of second-messenger signalling occurs when the neurotransmitter *norepinephrine* binds to **G protein–coupled receptors (GPCRs).** Triggering the GPCR causes G proteins to activate the membrane-bound enzyme *adenyl cyclase*. The adenyl cyclase removes phosphate groups from adenosine triphosphate (ATP) to form *cyclic adenosine monophosphate (cAMP)*. Cyclic AMP is the "second messenger", triggering the activation of the *protein kinase* A enzyme that eventually causes Na^+ channels in the postsynaptic membrane to open (**Figure 19-17**).

The metabotropic second-messenger mechanism is usually slower and longer lasting than the more direct ionotropic mechanism. And because the second messenger mechanism involves intracellular messengers, it can regulate other cellular processes, such as cytoskeleton movement, gene expression, and shuttling of proteins along the axonal transport system.

Mapping out these mechanisms of neurotransmitter signalling has revolutionized our understanding of neurobiology—and thus

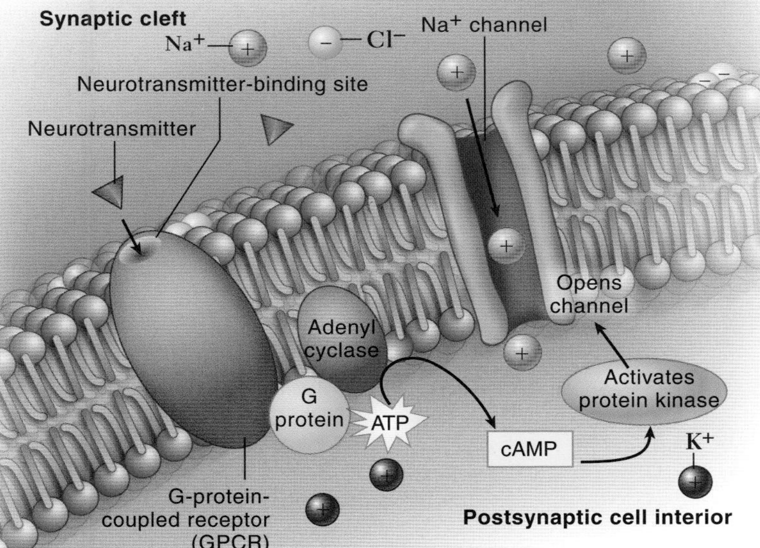

FIGURE 19-17 Indirect signal transduction. Norepinephrine and many other neurotransmitters initiate nerve signals indirectly by binding to a *metabotropic* G-protein–coupled receptor (GPCR) that changes shape to activate the enzyme *adenylate cyclase,* which in turn catalyzes the conversion of ATP to cyclic AMP (cAMP). cAMP is a "second messenger" that induces a change in the shape of a stimulus-gated channel. (Compare with **Figure 19-16**.)

our ability to prevent and treat illnesses. Many drugs and herbal supplements used in prevention and therapy today either enhance or inhibit particular steps of the mechanisms just described.

You may now more clearly see why classifying neurotransmitters by function is really just a way of classifying them by how their receptors translate their signal. It is useful to know that there are several types of receptor that can respond to any one neurotransmitter. That explains how acetylcholine can produce different responses in skeletal muscle than in cardiac muscle—different types of acetylcholine receptors are found in these two tissues.

Structural Classification of Neurotransmitters

Because the functions of specific neurotransmitters vary by location where different types of receptors may exist, it is often most useful to classify them according to their chemical structure. Neurotransmitters can thus be grouped into two main groupings: *small-molecule transmitters* and *large-molecule transmitters.*

Small-molecule neurotransmitters are, as their name implies, molecules of a smaller size than those in the large-molecule category. Small-molecule neurotransmitters are amino acids or are derived from individual amino acids. Large-molecule neurotransmitters, on the other hand, are made up of more than one amino acid—usually chains of 2 to 40 amino acids.

Small-molecule transmitters are subdivided into four main chemical classes:

Class I Acetylcholine
Class II Amines
Class III Amino acids
Class IV Other small molecules

Large-molecule neurotransmitters are all neuropeptides—chains of several amino acids strung together by peptide bonds. Examples of neurotransmitters in each of these groupings are given in the following sections, in **Figure 19-18** and **Figure 19-19**, and in **Table 19-4**.

Acetylcholine

The neurotransmitter **acetylcholine (ACh)** is in a class of its own because it has a chemical structure unique among neurotransmitters. It is synthesized in neurons by combining an acetate (acetyl coenzyme A) with choline (sometimes listed as a B vitamin)—as you can see in **Figure 19-18**.

Postsynaptic membranes contain the enzyme *acetylcholinesterase,* which rapidly inactivates the acetylcholine bound to postsynaptic receptors. Choline molecules released by this reaction are transported back into the presynaptic neuron, where they are combined with acetate to form more acetylcholine.

As **Table 19-4** shows, acetylcholine is found in various locations in the nervous system. In many of these locations, it has an excitatory effect (for example, at the neuromuscular junctions of skeletal muscles). In others, it has an inhibitory effect (for example, at the neuromuscular junctions of cardiac muscle tissue).

Amines

Amine neurotransmitters are synthesized from amino acid molecules, such as tyrosine, tryptophan, or histidine. Amines include the neurotransmitters of the **monoamine** subclass: *serotonin* and *histamine.* Monoamines have a single amine (NH_2) group, as their name implies. Also included are neurotransmitters of the **catecholamine** subclass: *dopamine, epinephrine,* and *norepinephrine.* Catecholamines, which are all derived from the amino acid tyrosine, also have only one amine group, but unlike monoamines they have a catechol ring.

Figure 19-18 shows how these subclasses of neurotransmitters are derived from different amino acids. It is not important to focus on the detailed chemical structures shown in the diagram. However, seeing that these neurotransmitters are chemically related to amino acids—and to each other—will help you better understand concepts in nutrition, pharmacology, and other health science applications.

The amine neurotransmitters are found in various regions of the brain, where they affect learning, emotions, motor control, and other activities (**Box 19-2**). In a previous section, we discussed the role of serotonin in forming memories. Dopamine, another amine, is also found in some of the mood pathways. Dopamine also has an inhibitory effect on certain somatic motor pathways. When dopamine is deficient, the tremors and general overstimulation of muscles characteristic of *parkinsonism* occur. This effect will be discussed further in Chapter 20.

Epinephrine and norepinephrine, like serotonin and dopamine, are also involved in mood. They are also involved in motor control, specifically in the sympathetic pathways of the autonomic nervous system. Some autonomic neurons in the adrenal gland do not terminate at a postsynaptic effector cell but instead release their neurotransmitters directly into the bloodstream. When this occurs, epinephrine and norepinephrine are called *hormones* instead of neurotransmitters.

ACETYLCHOLINE

$H_3C-\overset{O}{\overset{||}{C}}-O-CoA + HO-\underset{H_2}{C}-\underset{H_2}{C}-\overset{\oplus}{N}-(CH_3)_3$

Acetyl CoA

Choline

Choline acetyltransferase

$H_3C-\overset{O}{\overset{||}{C}}-O-\underset{H_2}{C}-\underset{H_2}{C}-\overset{\oplus}{N}-(CH_3)_3$

Acetylcholine

AMINO ACIDS

$HOOC-\underset{H_2}{C}-\underset{H_2}{C}-\underset{H}{\overset{NH_2}{C}}-COOH$

Glutamic acid (Glu)

Glutamic acid decarboxylase (GAD)

$HOOC-\underset{H_2}{C}-\underset{H_2}{C}-\underset{H}{\overset{NH_2}{C}}-H$

γ-Aminobutyric acid (GABA)

$H_2\overset{NH_2}{C}-COOH$

Glycine (Gly)

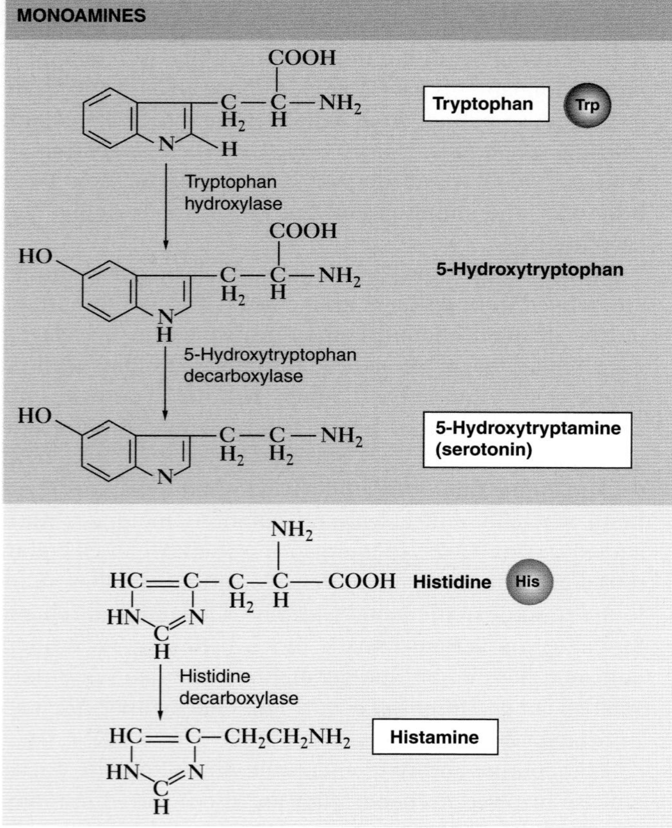

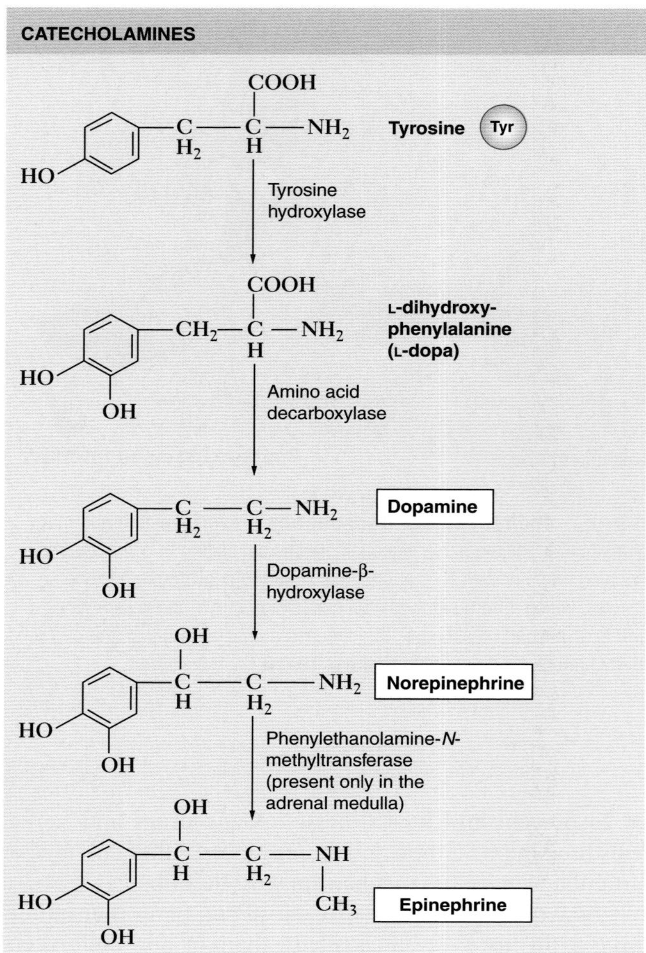

FIGURE 19-18 Examples of small-molecule neurotransmitters. Many of the small-molecule transmitters are amino acid molecules or are derived from the amino acids tryptophan, histidine, or tyrosine.

Vasoactive intestinal peptide (VIP)

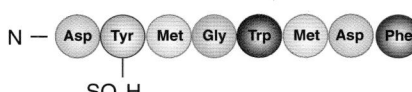

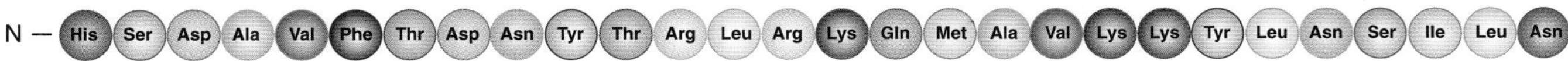

Cholecystokinin-like peptide (CCK8)

N — Asp Tyr Met Gly Trp Met Asp Phe

SO_3H

Met-enkephalin

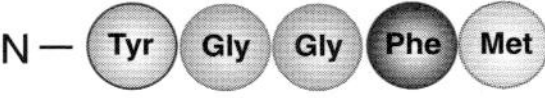

Substance P

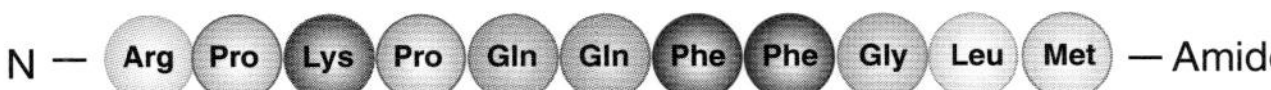

Leu-enkephalin

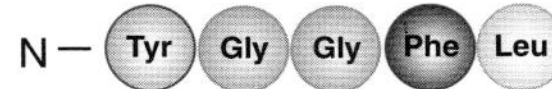

β-Endorphin

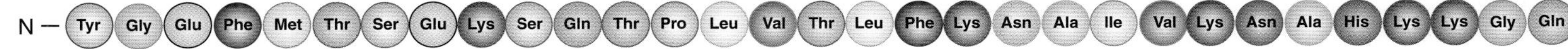

FIGURE 19-19 Examples of neuropeptides. Large-molecule transmitters are made up of more than one amino acid.

TABLE 19-4 Examples of Neurotransmitters

NEUROTRANSMITTER	LOCATION*	FUNCTION*
Small-Molecule Transmitters		
Class I		
Acetylcholine (ACh)	Junctions with motor effectors (muscles, glands); many parts of brain	Excitatory or inhibitory; involved in memory
Class II: Amines (derived from amino acids)		
Monoamines (contain one amino group)		
Serotonin (5-HT†)	Several regions of the CNS	Mostly inhibitory; involved in moods and emotions, sleep
Histamine	Brain	Mostly excitatory; involved in emotions and regulation of body temperature and water balance
Catecholamines (contain a catechol ring and one amino group)		
Dopamine (DA)	Brain; autonomic system	Mostly inhibitory; involved in emotions and moods and in regulating motor control
Epinephrine (Epi)	Several areas of the CNS and in the sympathetic division of the ANS	Excitatory or inhibitory; acts as a hormone when secreted by sympathetic neurosecretory cells of the adrenal gland
Norepinephrine (NE)	Several areas of the CNS and in the sympathetic division of the ANS	Excitatory or inhibitory; regulates sympathetic effectors; in brain, involved in emotional responses
Class III: Amino Acids (contain an amine group, carboxylic acid group, and a specific R group)		
Glutamate (glutamic acid, Glu)	CNS	Excitatory; most common excitatory neurotransmitter in CNS
Gamma-aminobutyric acid (GABA)	Brain	Inhibitory; common inhibitory neurotransmitter in brain
Glycine (Gly)	Spinal cord	Inhibitory; common inhibitory neurotransmitter in spinal cord
Class IV: Other Small Molecules		
Nitric oxide (NO)	Several regions of the nervous system	May be a signal from postsynaptic to presynaptic neuron
Purines (contain adenine, a double-ring purine structure)		
Adenosine triphosphate (ATP)	Autonomic ganglia, brain	Regulation of autonomic signalling; regulates nerve repair; glia-neuron communication
Adenosine (ADO)	Brain	May be involved in regulating sleep

*These are examples only; most of these neurotransmitters are also found in other locations, and many have additional functions.

†5-hydroxytryptamine (synonym for serotonin).

CNS, Central nervous system; *ANS,* autonomic nervous system.

(continued)

TABLE 19-4 Examples of Neurotransmitters—cont'd

NEUROTRANSMITTER	LOCATION*	FUNCTION*
Large-Molecule Transmitters		
Neuropeptides (chains of amino acids)		
Vasoactive intestinal peptide (VIP)	Brain; some ANS and sensory fibres; retina; gastrointestinal tract	Function in nervous system uncertain
Cholecystokinin (CCK)	Brain; retina	May be involved in memory, learning, mood
Substance P	Brain, spinal cord, sensory pain pathways; gastrointestinal tract	Mostly excitatory; transmits pain information
Enkephalins	Several regions of CNS; retina; intestinal tract	Mostly inhibitory; opioids that modulate pain
Endorphins	Several regions of CNS; retina; intestinal tract	Mostly inhibitory; opioids that modulate pain
Dynorphin	Several CNS locations	Mostly inhibitory; opioids that modulate pain
Neuropeptide Y (NPY)	Brain, some ANS fibres	Variety of functions including enhancing blood vessel constriction by ANS, regulation of energy balance, learning, and memory

Amino Acids

Many biologists now believe that amino acids are among the most common neurotransmitters in the central nervous system. For example, it is thought that the amino acid *glutamate (glutamic acid)* is responsible for up to 75% of the excitatory signals in the brain. *Gamma-aminobutyric acid (GABA)*, which is derived from glutamate, is the most common inhibitory neurotransmitter in the brain. In the spinal cord, the most widely distributed inhibitory neurotransmitter is the simple amino acid *glycine*. These three neurotransmitters are shown in **Figure 19-18**.

Amino acids are found in all cells of the body, where they are used to synthesize various structural and functional proteins. In the nervous system, however, they are also stored in synaptic vesicles and used as neurotransmitters. Certain membrane receptors in the postsynaptic membrane are sensitive to high quantities of certain amino acids and thus trigger specific responses in the postsynaptic cell. It is believed that an imbalance of certain amino acids in the body could produce similar effects and thus alter the function of the nervous system.

Other Small-Molecule Transmitters

The term *other* is not a very descriptive name for a category of compounds, but the discovery of a new group of small neurotransmitter molecules is so recent that a standard name for class IV neurotransmitters has not been adopted.

The prime example of this group is **nitric oxide (NO)**. Nitric oxide is a small gas molecule that the cell makes from the amino acid arginine. NO was the first gas to be identified as a transmitter,

BOX 19-2 *health matters* | Antidepressants

Antidepressants are prescribed widely for outpatients suffering from depression associated with their ongoing illness. Depression also can be a distinct mental illness that can be caused by a variety of factors. The exact mechanisms of severe depression remain incompletely explained. A classic explanation states that a deficit of *serotonin, dopamine, norepinephrine,* or other amine neurotransmitters exists at synapses along particular pathways of the brain that affect one's mood. More recent explanations theorize that it is a lack of sufficient synaptic connections in the mood pathways of the brain that are to blame.

One class of antidepressant drugs inhibit *catechol-O-methyl transferase* (COMT), the enzyme that inactivates norepinephrine. When COMT is inhibited by an antidepressant drug, the amount of active norepinephrine in brain synapses increases—relieving the symptoms of depression. Antidepressants such as phenelzine block the action of *monoamine oxidase (MAO),* the enzyme that inactivates dopamine and serotonin. Such drugs are in a class called *monoamine oxidase inhibitors (MAOIs).*

Antidepressants such as imipramine and amitriptyline increase amine neurotransmitter levels at brain synapses by blocking their uptake into the axon terminals. The popular drugs fluoxetine, citalopram, and related drugs called *selective serotonin reuptake inhibitors (SSRIs)* produce antidepressant effects by inhibiting the uptake of serotonin. *Norepinephrine reuptake inhibitors (NRIs)* such as atomoxetine selectively reduce the reuptake of noradrenaline. *Serotonin and norepinephrine reuptake inhibitors (SNRIs)* such as venlafaxine and duloxetine are also used to treat depression.

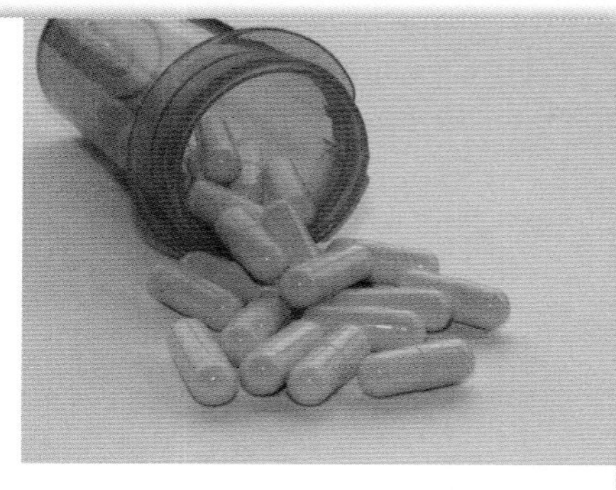

Amine-uptake inhibition with SSRIs and SNRIs is thought to cause an increase in the amount of serotonin in the synapse, thereby reversing the serotonin deficit that may contribute to feelings of depression. However, it may be these drugs' ability to produce new neurons that produces most of the antidepressant effect. This may explain why such drugs take days or weeks to alleviate symptoms of depression.

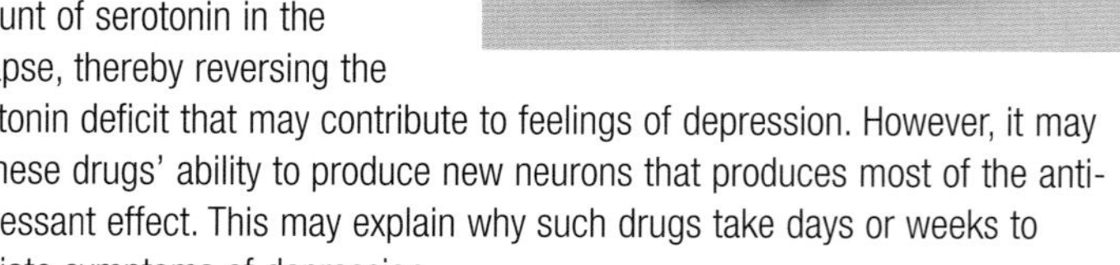

Cocaine, which is rarely used in medical practice as a local anaesthetic, produces a temporary feeling of well-being in cocaine abusers by similarly blocking the uptake of dopamine. Unfortunately, cocaine and similar drugs can also adversely affect blood flow and heart function when taken inappropriately—leading to death in some individuals.

Researchers continue to study other drugs, such as the anaesthetic *ketamine,* that more rapidly erase depression by increasing synaptic communication among existing neurons in the brain's mood pathways.

but *carbon monoxide (CO)* may be another. Nitric acid is released from postsynaptic neurons and *diffuses backward* toward the presynaptic neuron, where it has its biochemical effects. This gives postsynaptic neurons a mechanism by which they can "talk back" to the presynaptic neuron, establishing the opportunity for feedback.

Several other small molecules have been identified as acting as neurotransmitters, including *adenosine triphosphate (ATP)* and *adenosine (ADO)* (see **Figure 4-19** on p. 68). These two molecules are chemically classified as *purine neurotransmitters* because they contain the adenosine group—a type of purine structure.

Neuropeptides

The **neuropeptide** neurotransmitters are short strands of amino acids called *polypeptides* or, more simply, *peptides.* Neuropeptide neurotransmitters are often called *neuroactive peptides.* Because they are made up of chains of amino acids, peptides are very large molecules compared with the neurotransmitters previously discussed, most of which are derived from a single amino acid (see **Figure 19-19**).

Peptides were first discovered to have regulatory effects in the digestive tract, where they act as hormones and regulate digestive function. In the 1970s some of these "gut" polypeptides, such as *vasoactive intestinal peptide (VIP), cholecystokinin (CCK),* and *substance P,* were also found to be acting as neurotransmitters in the brain. In addition, researchers found that receptors of many of the gut–brain peptides also bind morphine and other opium derivatives. For example, two subclasses of peptides—*enkephalins* and *endorphins*—that bind to the opiate receptors serve as the body's own supply of opiates. Enkephalins and endorphins have important pain-relieving effects in the body.

Although neuropeptides may be secreted by a synaptic knob by themselves, some may be secreted along with a second, or even third, neurotransmitter. In such cases, the neuropeptide is thought to act as a **neuromodulator.** A neuromodulator is a "co-transmitter" that regulates or modulates the effects of the neurotransmitter(s) released along with it.

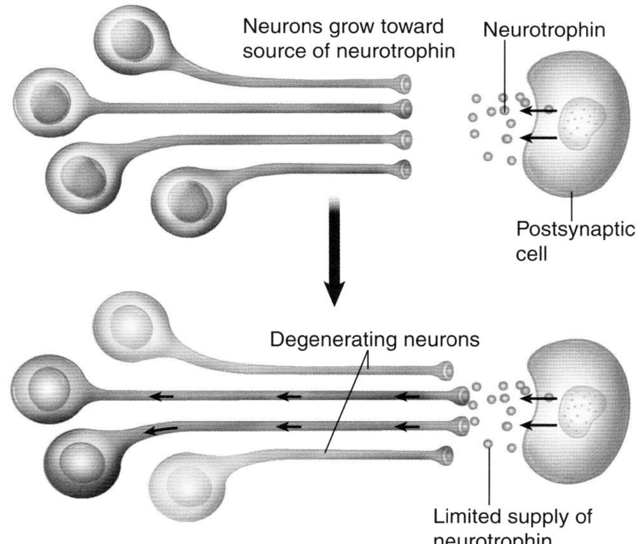

FIGURE 19-20 Development of neural networks. Neurotrophins help form synaptic connections as nerve tissue develops.

An important class of neuropeptides in the nervous system is the **neurotrophins,** or *neurotrophic factors.* When these were first discovered, researchers found that they stimulate neuron development, hence the name neurotrophin (literally, "nerve growth factor"). **Figure 19-20** shows how neurotrophins help regulate neuron growth. More recently, we have discovered that neurotrophins also participate in synaptic transmission and neuromodulation. In fact, one type of neurotrophin released by neurons is required to form any memory lasting more than a day.

NEURAL NETWORKS

The Network Model

Nervous pathways, or **neural networks,** conduct information along complex series of neurons joined together by synapses. The model of nerves forming a network has developed slowly over time using the methods of science.

From the very birth of neuroscience, biologists have argued about which metaphor is best to describe the role of cells in the nervous system. One camp has argued on behalf of the *neuron doctrine,* which states that the neuron is the basic structural and functional unit of the nervous system and that neurons are independent units connected by chemical synapses. The competing *reticular theory* stated that the nervous system is best understood as a large integrated network—one endless piece. Once the presence of chemical synapses separating independent neurons was confirmed, it seemed as if the neuron doctrine was proved true and the reticular theory proved wrong.

However, today neuroscience has advanced to a point at which the neuron doctrine has been expanded to include concepts of the reticular theory. For example, we now know that along with chemical synapses, there are many electrical synapses that functionally unite neurons into large information-processing networks. We also know that signals can be sent both forward and backward in the chemical synapses of the neural network. We know that the concentration of neurotransmitters at synapses in certain neural pathways can affect health (see **Box 19-2**). And today, we are learning more about how neuroglia communicate with each other and regulate the information-carrying functions of neurons. In fact, a very active area of neuroscience research relates to studying the integrated behaviour of large neural networks. Our understanding of the role of nervous system cells is growing rapidly.

Development of Neural Networks

Research shows that such networks develop during a person's early life and are influenced by the various sensory learning experiences that we have as our nerve tissue develops. One process that facilitates the formation of connections involves the *neurotrophins* mentioned earlier in this chapter—nerve growth factors that are released by various cells of the body.

As **Figure 19-20** shows, the axons of several developing neurons grow toward the cell that releases neurotrophins. However, only those axons that can be supported by the amount of available neurotrophin will remain—the rest of the neurons will degenerate. Many other factors, such as repeated stimulation of a pathway, influence this process. Recall from the previous chapter that microglia are involved in pruning unneeded connections from neural networks as they develop.

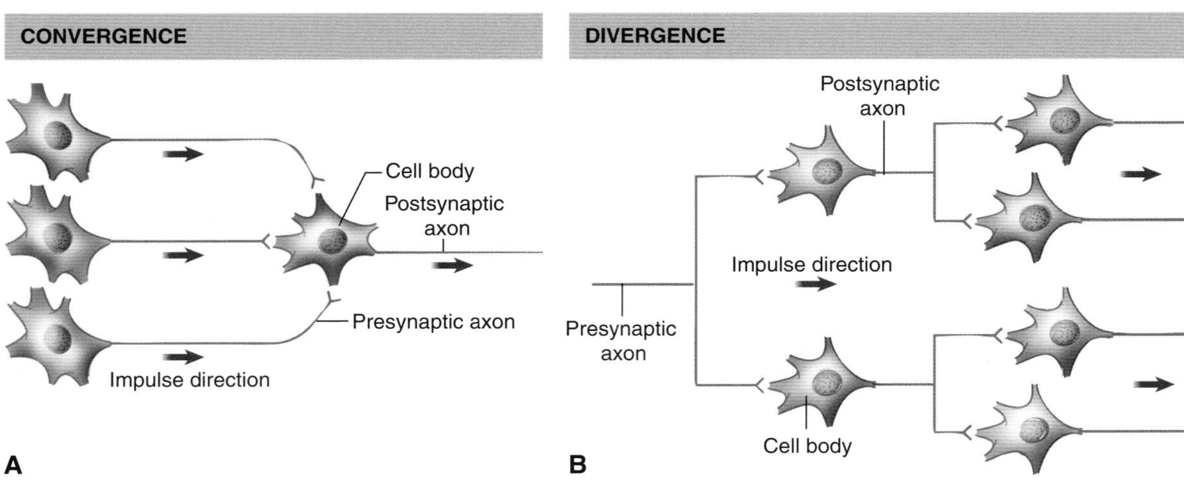

FIGURE 19-21 Complexity in neural networks. A, Convergence occurs when several nerve pathways come together. **B,** Divergence occurs when a single pathway splits into several pathways.

BOX 19-3 *fyi* | Visualizing Neural Networks

In 1837, Italian scientist Camillo Golgi (discoverer of the Golgi apparatus) introduced a staining method in which one could see entire neurons and their surrounding glia—a breakthrough for studying neural networks. Since that time, many advances in visualizing neural networks have set the stage for the current worldwide effort to map the entire human neural network—the *Human Connectome Project.*

One of the tools used in this effort is the "brainbow" technique developed at Harvard's Center for Brain Science. Using genetic engineering methods, researchers insert a set of genes into lab animals (usually mice) that randomly produce fluorescent proteins in different individual neurons. With use of a light microscope equipped with an ultraviolet light, glia without the fluorescent proteins are invisible and different individual neurons fluoresce with different colour combinations. This produces images like that seen here, which help scientists determine the pattern of neural networks. •

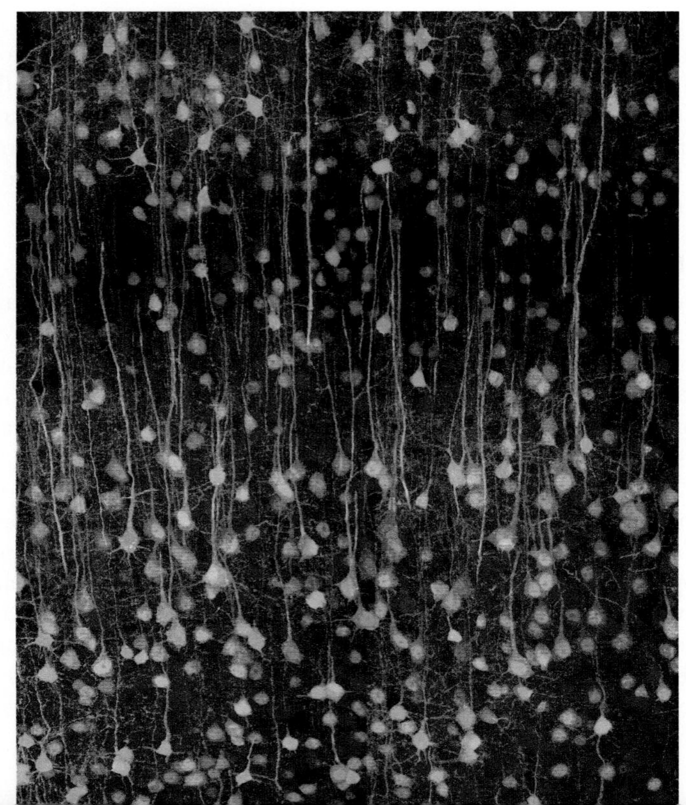

Once neural networks become mature in adulthood, they are less likely to accept the addition of new neurons—even though neural stem cells do exist in the adult nervous system.

Complexity in Neural Networks

Something that makes the pathways of neural networks structurally complex—thus allowing complexity of function—is that they often *converge* and *diverge.*

Convergence occurs when more than one presynaptic axon synapses with a single postsynaptic neuron (**Figure 19-21**, *A*). Convergence allows information from several different pathways to be funneled into a single pathway. For example, the pathways that innervate the skeletal muscles may originate in several different areas of the central nervous system. Because pathways from each of these motor control areas converge on a single motor neuron, each area has an opportunity to control the same muscle.

Divergence occurs when a single presynaptic axon synapses with many different postsynaptic neurons (**Figure 19-21**, *B*). Divergence allows information from one pathway to be "split" or "copied" and sent to different destinations in the nervous system. For example, a single bit of visual information may be sent to many different areas of the brain for processing.

Box 19-3 discusses some techniques used to visualize the complex structure of neural networks.

Besides complexity of structure, neural networks exhibit complexity of function when using summation, neuromodulation, synaptic regulation by glia, and other functional mechanisms to filter information.

CONNECT IT! 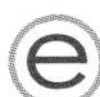

The concept that signals can be sent "backward" at a synapse is called **retrograde signalling.** See how this works at ***Retrograde Signalling*** online at ***Connect It!***

Quick CHECK

12. How do excitatory neurotransmitters differ from inhibitory neurotransmitters?
13. What are the four chemical classes of neurotransmitters?
14. What are neuromodulators?

the big picture | Nerve Signalling and the Whole Body

In the previous chapter, we first encountered the idea that neurons act as the "wiring" that forms the "circuits" of the nervous system. In this chapter, we looked more closely at how this wiring actually works. Nerve impulses are not exactly like electrical current flowing through house wiring or a telephone landline. Instead, they are temporary disturbances to the ion balances along a neuron's membrane—which briefly change the membrane's voltage. These disturbances can be triggered by sensory stimuli or chemical signals from other neurons. And these disturbances can trigger events that lead to similar disturbances in adjacent neurons, perhaps even triggering a change in an effector cell such as a muscle or gland.

Such nerve signalling serves as an important mechanism in operating the homeostatic feedback loops that maintain a healthy internal environment. Nerve signalling therefore affects every part of the body. But nerve signalling can operate properly only if there are sufficient fatty acids available to build myelin sheaths and amino acids available to produce neurotransmitters. Ion balances in the internal environment must be kept constant or membrane potentials would not be generated properly. Neurons and glia must have oxygen available to do the work of maintaining ion gradients and synthesizing and recycling neurotransmitters.

mechanisms of disease

Disorders of Nerve Signalling

Many diverse disorders of the body result from malfunctions of nerve signalling. Some of these disorders have been discussed in previous chapters and many more will be discussed in later chapters. Here, we briefly review a few examples of disorders that result from faulty nerve signalling.

Disorders of Nerve Conduction

Any of the *myelin disorders*, such as *multiple sclerosis (MS),* discussed in **Box 18-2** (p. 398) can be considered to be disorders of nerve conduction. Because myelin is necessary for efficient saltatory conduction in many nerve pathways, many diverse dysfunctions of the body may result.

Nerve damage, which can result from many different mechanisms, can also produce a wide array of dysfunctions in the body. For example, physical injury can cause either local or widespread loss of sensation or motor control. In some spinal cord injuries, *paralysis* may occur (see p. 406). Viral infections can also cause damage to nerves, as can *autoimmune* reactions triggered by viral infections (see p. 398).

In *cerebrovascular accidents (CVAs),* or strokes, and *transient ischaemic attacks (TIAs),* or mini-strokes, reduction of blood flow from blockage or leakage can reduce glucose and oxygen delivery and damage nerve fibres (see Chapter 20, p. 469). In a CVA, prolonged oxygen starvation can kill neurons, which then release stored excitatory neurotransmitters such as glutamate. These transmitters flood nearby cells, acting as **excitotoxins** that harm nearby neurons—thus spreading the loss of function caused by the CVA.

Nerve conduction problems also occur when the internal environment's concentration of ions such as K^+, Na^+, and Ca^{++} get too far above or below the set point. Such homeostatic imbalances, even temporary, can disrupt not only nerve conduction but also synaptic function.

Synaptic Disorders

Myasthenia gravis, discussed in Chapter 17 (p. 385), is an autoimmune disorder in which antibodies bind to acetylcholine receptors at neuromuscular junctions of skeletal muscles (**Figure 19-22**). This causes mild to severe muscle weakness.

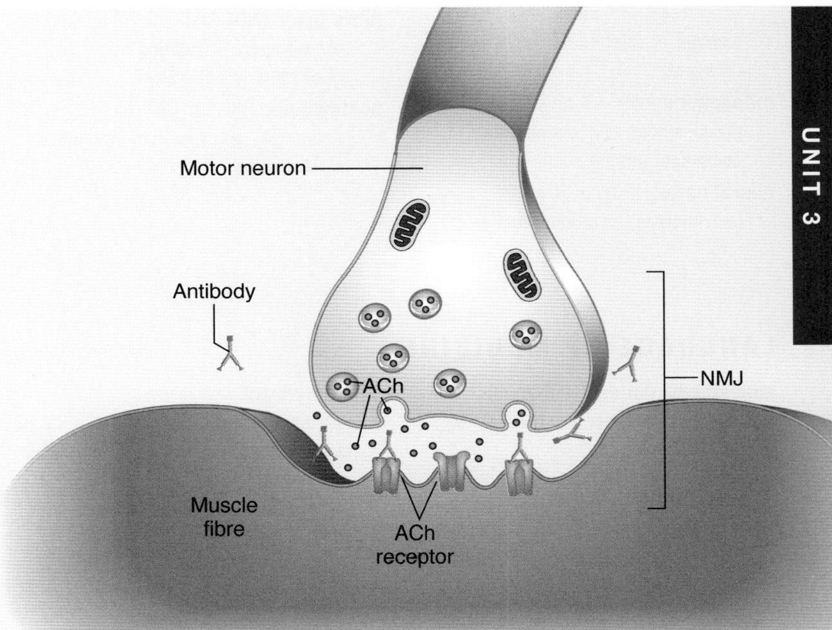

FIGURE 19-22 Myasthenia gravis. Simplified diagram showing *antibodies* (proteins produced by immune cells) binding to acetylcholine (ACh) receptors in the neuromuscular junction (NMJ). This reduces transmission of information at the NMJ and thus weakens muscle response.

Parkinson disease, discussed in **Box 18-1** (p. 397), produces malfunctions of muscle control when certain motor pathways fail to release enough dopamine at their synapses for normal muscle control.

Depression, anxiety, and many other disorders of mood and mental function are thought to have synaptic dysfunctions at their roots (see **Box 19-2** on p. 428). Even disorders with a wide range of symptoms such as **autism spectrum disorder (ASD)** may involve synaptic malfunctions. ASD, also called *autism,* is a group of neurological disorders characterized by various combinations and severity of difficulties in social interactions, verbal and nonverbal communication, and repetitive behaviours. ASD is often understood as a developmental problem involving "mistakes in wiring" of the synapses of the brain's neural network.

LANGUAGE OF SCIENCE *(continued from p. 412)*

ionotropic receptor (eye-on-eh-TROH-pik ree-SEP-tor) [*ion-* **to go (ion),** *-trop-* **turn or change,** *-ic* **relating to,** *recept-* **receive,** *-or* **agent**]

ligand-gated channel (LYE-gund or LIG-und GAY-ted CHAN-el) [*liga-* **bind,** *-and* **agent**]

membrane potential [*membran-* **thin skin,** *potent-* **power,** *-ial* **relating to**]

metabotropic receptor (meh-TAB-eh-TROH-pik ree-SEP-tor) [*meta-* **over,** *-bo-* **throw,** *-trop-* **turn or change,** *-ic* **relating to,** *recept-* **receive,** *-or* **agent**]

monoamine (mon-oh-ah-MEEN) [*mono-* **single,** *-amine* **ammonia compound (amino acid)**]

neural network (NYOOR-al) [*neur-* **nerves,** *-al* **relating to**]

neuromodulator (nyoo-roh-MOD-yoo-lay-tor) [*neuro-* **nerve,** *-modul-* **regulate,** *-at(e)-* **act of,** *-or* **agent**]

neuropeptide (nyoo-roh-PEP-tyde) [*neuro-* **nerves,** *-pept-* **digest,** *-ide* **chemical**]

neurotransmitter (nyoo-roh-tranz-MIT-ter) [*neuro-* **nerves,** *-trans-* **across,** *-mitt-* **send,** *-er* **agent**]

neurotrophin (nyoo-roh-TROF-in) [*neuro-* **nerve,** *-troph-* **nutrition,** *-in* **substance**]

nitric oxide (NO) (NYE-trik AWK-side) [*nitr-* **nitrogen,** *-ic* **relating to,** *ox-* **oxygen,** *-ide* **chemical**]

postsynaptic (post-si-NAP-tik) [*post-* **after,** *-syn-* **together,** *-apt-* **join,** *-ic* **relating to**]

postsynaptic potential (post-sih-NAP-tik poh-TEN-shal) [*post-* **after,** *-syn-* **together,** *-apt-* **join,** *-ic* **relating to,** *potent-* **power,** *-ial* **relating to**]

presynaptic (pree-sih-NAP-tik) [*pre-* **before,** *-syn-* **together,** *-apt-* **join,** *-ic* **relating to**]

relative refractory period (ree-FRAK-tor-ee) [*re-* **back or again,** *-fract-* **break,** *-ory* **relating to,** *period* **circuit**]

repolarization (ree-poh-lah-rih-ZAY-shun) [*re-* **back or again,** *-pol-* **pole,** *-ar-* **relating to,** *-ization* **process**]

resting membrane potential (RMP) [*membran-* **thin skin,** *potent-* **power,** *-ial* **relating to**]

retrograde signalling (RET-roh-grayd SIG-nah-ling) [*retro-* **backward,** *-grad-* **step,** *sign-* **mark,** *-al* **relating to**]

saltatory conduction (SAL-tah-tor-ee) [*salta-* **leap,** *-ory* **relating to**]

spatial summation (SPAY-shal sum-MAY-shun) [*spati-* **space,** *-al* **relating to,** *summa-* **total,** *-tion* **process**]

stimulus-gated channel (STIM-yoo-lus GAY-ted) [*stimulus* **incitement**]

synapse (SIN-aps) [*syn-* **together,** *-aps-* **join**]

synaptic cleft (si-NAP-tik kleft) [*syn-* **together,** *-apt-* **join,** *-ic* **relating to**]

temporal summation (TEM-poh-ral sum-MAY-shun) [*tempor-* **time,** *-al* **relating to**]

threshold potential (THRESH-hold poh-TEN-shal) [*potent-* **power,** *-ial* **relating to**]

voltage-gated channel (VOL-tij GAY-ted) [*volt-* **unit of electrical force (after** *Alessandro Volta* **Italian physicist),** *-age* **amount**]

LANGUAGE OF MEDICINE

anaesthesia (an-es-THEE-zhah) [*an-* **absence,** *-aesthesi-* **feeling,** *-ia* **condition**]

antidepressant (an-tee-deh-PRESS-ant) [*anti-* **against,** *-de-* **down,** *-press-* **press,** *-ant* **agent**]

autism spectrum disorder (ASD) (AWT-izem SPEK-trum dis-OR-der) [*aut-* **self,** *-ism* **condition,** *spectrum* **appearance (range),** *dis-* **opposite of,** *-order* **order**]

excitotoxin (ek-SYE-toh-TAWK-sin) [*excit-* **arouse,** *-tox-* **poison,** *-in* **substance**]

case study

Kelly had been having difficulty focusing her eyes for a couple of weeks. She assumed her recent lack of sleep was the cause. However, when she started dropping her keys and feeling unsteady when walking down the stairs, she became worried enough to go to the doctor. After the results of several tests were known, the doctor told her she had myasthenia gravis. This is an autoimmune, neuromuscular disease in which the body's white blood cells start attacking acetylcholine receptors.

1. What is the connection between acetylcholine and Kelly's symptoms?
   a. Acetylcholine is a hormone released during stress.
   b. Acetylcholine is found primarily in sensory neuron connections.
   c. Acetylcholine is found primarily in motor neuron connections.
   d. Acetylcholine affects communication primarily with smooth muscles.

2. Select an answer that best fits the missing words. If the binding of acetylcholine to receptors opened sodium channels on the postsynaptic membrane, this would cause a temporary ________, called an ________.
   a. depolarization; excitatory postsynaptic potential
   b. hyperpolarization; excitatory postsynaptic potential
   c. depolarization; inhibitory postsynaptic potential
   d. hyperpolarization; inhibitory postsynaptic potential

Some muscle relaxants used during surgery bind to acetylcholine receptors, effectively blocking the action of acetylcholine—just as in myasthenia gravis. The drugs (anticholinesterases) used after surgery to reverse the effect of relaxants are the same as those used to treat myasthenia gravis.

3. What is the action of this type of drug?
   a. Blocks the release of acetylcholine
   b. Blocks the action of acetylcholinesterase
   c. Increases the production of choline
   d. Increases the action of acetylcholinesterase

Hint To solve a case study, you may have to refer to the glossary or index, other chapters in this textbook, ***Connect It!,*** and other resources.

CHAPTER SUMMARY

To download an MP3 version of the chapter summary for use with your mobile device, access the ***Audio Chapter Summaries*** *online at evolve.elsevier.com.*

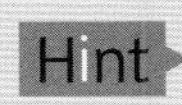

Scan this summary after reading the chapter to help you reinforce the key concepts. Later, use the summary as a quick review before your class or before a test.

Electrical Nature of Neurons

A. Membrane potentials
  1. All living cells maintain a difference in the concentration of ions across their membranes
  2. Membrane potential—slight excess of positively charged ions on the outside of the membrane and slight deficiency of positively charged ions on the inside of the membrane (**Figure 19-1**)
  3. Difference in electrical charge is called *potential* because it is a type of stored energy
  4. Polarized membrane—a membrane that exhibits a membrane potential
  5. Magnitude of potential difference between the two sides of a polarized membrane is measured in volts (V) or millivolts (mV); the sign of a membrane's voltage indicates the charge on the inside surface of a polarized membrane

B. Resting membrane potential (RMP)
  1. Membrane potential maintained by a nonconducting neuron's plasma membrane; typically −70 mV
  2. The slight excess of positive ions on a membrane's outer surface is produced by ion transport mechanisms and the membrane's permeability characteristics
  3. The membrane's selective permeability characteristics help maintain a slight excess of positive ions on the outer surface of the membrane (**Figure 19-2**)
  4. Sodium–potassium pump (**Figure 19-3**)
     a. Active transport mechanism in plasma membrane that transports Na^+ and K^+ in opposite directions and at different rates
     b. Maintains an imbalance in the distribution of positive ions, resulting in the inside surface becoming slightly negative with respect to its outer surface

C. Local potentials
  1. Local potentials—slight shift away from the resting membrane in a specific region of the plasma membrane (**Figure 19-4**)
  2. Excitation—when a stimulus triggers the opening of additional Na^+ channels, allowing the membrane potential to move toward zero (depolarization)
  3. Inhibition—when a stimulus triggers the opening of additional K^+ channels, increasing the membrane potential (hyperpolarization)
  4. Local potentials are called *graded potentials* because the magnitude of deviation from the resting membrane potential is proportional to the magnitude of the stimulus

Action Potentials

A. Action potential—the membrane potential of a neuron that is conducting an impulse; also known as a *nerve impulse*

B. Mechanism that produces the action potential (**Figures 19-5** and **19-6**)
  1. When an adequate stimulus triggers stimulus-gated Na^+ channels to open, allowing Na^+ to diffuse rapidly into the cell, a local depolarization is produced
  2. As threshold potential is reached, voltage-gated Na^+ channels open and more Na^+ enters the cell, causing further depolarization
  3. As more Na^+ rushes into cell, the membrane moves rapidly toward and continues in a positive direction to the peak of the action potential
  4. Voltage-gated Na^+ channels stay open for only about 1 ms before they automatically close; action potential is an all-or-none response
  5. After action potential peaks, membrane begins to move back toward the resting membrane potential when K^+ channels open, allowing outward diffusion of K^+; process is known as *repolarization*
  6. Brief period of after-hyperpolarization occurs, and then the resting membrane potential is restored when K^+ channels close

C. Refractory period (**Figure 19-7**)
  1. Absolute refractory period—brief period (lasting approximately 0.5 ms) during which a local area of a neuron's membrane resists restimulation and will not respond to a stimulus, no matter how strong
  2. Relative refractory period—time during which the membrane is repolarized and restoring the resting membrane potential; the few milliseconds after the absolute refractory period; will respond only to a very strong stimulus

D. Conduction of the action potential
  1. At the peak of the action potential, the plasma membrane's polarity is now the reverse of the RMP
  2. The reversal in polarity causes electrical current to flow between the site of the action potential and the adjacent regions of membrane and triggers voltage-gated Na^+ channels in the next segment to open; this next segment exhibits an action potential (**Figure 19-8**)
  3. This cycle continues to repeat, producing continuous conduction
  4. The action potential never moves backward because of the refractory period
  5. In myelinated fibres, action potentials in the membrane only occur at the nodes of Ranvier; this type of impulse conduction is called *saltatory conduction* (**Figure 19-9**)
  6. Speed of nerve conduction depends on diameter and on the presence or absence of a myelin sheath

Synaptic Transmission

A. Two types of synapses (junctions) (**Figure 19-10**)
  1. Electrical synapses occur where cells joined by gap junctions allow an action potential to simply continue along postsynaptic membrane

2. Chemical synapses occur where presynaptic cells release chemical transmitters (neurotransmitters) across a tiny gap to the postsynaptic cell, possibly inducing an action potential there

B. Structure of the chemical synapse (**Figure 19-12**)
1. Synaptic knob—tiny bulge at the end of a terminal branch of a presynaptic neuron's axon that contains vesicles housing neurotransmitters
2. Synaptic cleft—space between a synaptic knob and the plasma membrane of a postsynaptic neuron
3. Arrangements of synapses
   a. Axodendritic—axon signals postsynaptic dendrite; common
   b. Axosomatic—axon signals postsynaptic soma; common
   c. Axoaxonic—axon signals postsynaptic axon; may regulate action potential of postsynaptic axon
4. Plasma membrane of a postsynaptic neuron—has protein molecules that serve as receptors for the neurotransmitters

C. Mechanism of synaptic transmission (**Figure 19-12**)—sequence of events is as follows:
1. Action potential reaches a synaptic knob, causing calcium ions to diffuse into the knob rapidly
2. Increased calcium concentration triggers the release of neurotransmitter by way of exocytosis
3. Neurotransmitter molecules diffuse across the synaptic cleft and bind to receptor molecules, causing ion channels to open
4. Opening of ion channels produces a postsynaptic potential, either an excitatory postsynaptic potential (EPSP) or an inhibitory postsynaptic potential (IPSP)
5. The neurotransmitter's action is quickly terminated by neurotransmitter molecules being transported back into the synaptic knob (reuptake) and/or metabolized into inactive compounds by enzymes and/or diffused and taken up by nearby glia (**Figure 19-13**)

D. Summation (**Figure 19-15**)
1. Spatial summation—adding together the effects of several knobs being activated simultaneously and stimulating different locations on the postsynaptic membrane, producing an action potential
2. Temporal summation—when synaptic knobs stimulate a postsynaptic neuron in rapid succession, their effects can summate over a brief period to produce an action potential

E. Synapses and memory
1. Memories are stored by facilitating (or inhibiting) synaptic transmission
2. Short-term memories (seconds or minutes) may result from axoaxonic facilitation or inhibition of the presynaptic axon terminal
3. Intermediate long-term memory (minutes to weeks) happens when serotonin blocks potassium channels in the presynaptic terminal—thus prolonging the action potential and increasing the amount of neurotransmitter released
4. Long-term memories (months or years) require structural changes at the synapse—for example, more vesicles, more vesicle release sites, more presynaptic terminals, more sensitive postsynaptic membranes

Neurotransmitters

A. Neurotransmitters—means by which neurons communicate with one another; there are more than 50 compounds known to be neurotransmitters, and dozens of others are suspected

B. Classification of neurotransmitters—commonly classified by the following:
1. Function
   a. Function of a neurotransmitter is determined by the postsynaptic receptor
   b. Two major functional classifications are excitatory neurotransmitters and inhibitory neurotransmitters
   c. Can also be classified according to whether the receptor directly opens a channel (ionotropic) or instead uses an indirect second-messenger mechanism (metabotropic) involving G protein–coupled receptors (GPCRs) and intracellular signals (**Figures 19-16** and **19-17**)
2. Chemical structure
   a. Because functions of specific neurotransmitters vary by location, they are often instead classified according to chemical structure
   b. Small-molecule neurotransmitters comprise four main classes
   c. Large-molecule neurotransmitters are polypeptides called neuropeptides

C. Small-molecule neurotransmitters (**Figure 19-18**)
1. Acetylcholine
   a. Unique chemical structure; acetate (acetyl coenzyme A) with choline
   b. Acetylcholine is deactivated by acetylcholinesterase, with the choline molecules being released and transported back to the presynaptic neuron to combine with acetate
   c. Present at various locations, sometimes in an excitatory role; other times, inhibitory
2. Amines
   a. Synthesized from amino acid molecules
   b. Two categories: monoamines and catecholamines
   c. Found in various regions of the brain, affecting learning, emotions, motor control, and so on
3. Amino acids
   a. Believed to be among the most common neurotransmitters of the central nervous system
   b. In the peripheral nervous system, amino acids are stored in synaptic vesicles and used as neurotransmitters
4. Other small-molecule transmitters
   a. Nitric oxide (NO) derived from the amino acid arginine
   b. NO from a postsynaptic cell signals the presynaptic neuron, providing feedback in a neural pathway

D. Neuropeptides—large-molecule neurotransmitters
1. Neuropeptides are short strands of amino acids called polypeptides or peptides (**Figure 19-19**)
2. Peptides first discovered to have regulatory effects in the digestive tract; also act as neurotransmitters in the brain
3. May be secreted by themselves or in conjunction with a second or third neurotransmitter; in this case, neuropeptides act as a neuromodulator, a "co-transmitter" that regulates the effects of the neurotransmitter released along with it

4. Neurotrophins (neurotrophic [nerve growth] factors) stimulate neuron development but also can act as neurotransmitters or neuromodulators

Neural Networks

A. The "network model" of the nervous system as evolved over time:
   1. Neuron doctrine—proposes neuron is basic structural and functional unit of the nervous system and neurons are independent units connected by chemical synapses
   2. Reticular theory—proposes nervous system is best understood as a large integrated network
   3. Today, the dominant neuron doctrine has expanded to include concepts of the reticular theory—neurons are distinct units but also participate in a network; some neurons are functionally connected by electrical synapses, and chemical signals can move in two directions at the same synapse
   4. Because neuroglia also participate in the neural network, the whole concept of nervous system cell function is rapidly expanding

B. Development of neural networks involves the action of neurotrophins (nerve growth factors) and pruning away of unused connections (**Figure 19-20**)

C. Complexity in neural networks (**Figure 19-21**)
   1. Convergence—more than one presynaptic axon synapses with a single postsynaptic neuron
   2. Divergence—a single presynaptic axon synapses with many different postsynaptic neurons

The Big Picture: Nerve Signalling and the Whole Body

A. Neurons act as the "wiring" that forms the "circuits" of the nervous system

B. Nerve impulses are temporary disturbances to the ion balances along a neuron's membrane which can be triggered by sensory stimuli or chemical signals from other neurons

C. Nerve signalling serves as an important mechanism in operating the feedback loops that maintain homeostasis

D. Nerve signalling affects every part of the body but can only operate properly if there are sufficient fatty acids available to build myelin sheaths and amino acids available to produce neurotransmitters

E. Neurons and glia must have oxygen available to maintain ion gradients and synthesize and recycle neurotransmitters

REVIEW QUESTIONS

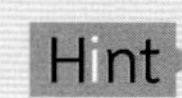

Write out the answers to these questions after reading the chapter and reviewing the Chapter Summary. Note—writing out your answers will consolidate learning and provide a valuable resource of information.

1. Describe the function of sodium and potassium in the generation of an action potential.
2. Why is an action potential an all-or-none response?
3. How does the myelin sheath affect the speed of an action potential? What about the diameter of the nerve fibre?
4. Describe the structure of a synapse.
5. Describe the series of events that mediate conduction across synapses.
6. List and describe the four main chemical classes of transmitters.
7. Describe the actions of acetylcholine.
8. Put the terms in order of their occurrence in a neuron plasma membrane: hyperpolarization, depolarization, polarization and repolarization.

CRITICAL THINKING QUESTIONS

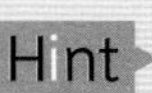

After finishing the Review Questions, write out the answers to these more in-depth questions to help you apply your new knowledge. Go back to sections of the chapter that relate to concepts that you find difficult.

1. Define *potential*. The following is a list of times and charges taken during a nerve impulse. Identify them as being either an action potential or not and as occurring either during the absolute or relative refractory period. (Assume the stimulus starts at 0 ms.)
   0 mV at 1 ms
   −50 mV at 0.5 ms
   +25 mV at 1.5 ms
   +25 mV at 3 ms
2. Describe the mechanisms that allow subthreshold stimuli to generate an action potential.
3. Explain one of the ways an anaesthetic may relieve the sensation of pain.
4. Referred pain is a condition in which the pain is not felt where the injury is actually occurring but rather is felt over a wider area or in some other part of the body. What structural aspect of the nervous system might explain referred pain?
5. Following the conduction of an action potential, an axon's membrane will not respond immediately to a second stimulus. Explain why there is a delay of about 0.5 ms before another action potential can be generated.
6. We often read in the media that common salt is bad for us. Using your knowledge of neuron physiology, explain why this statement cannot be justified.

20 Central Nervous System

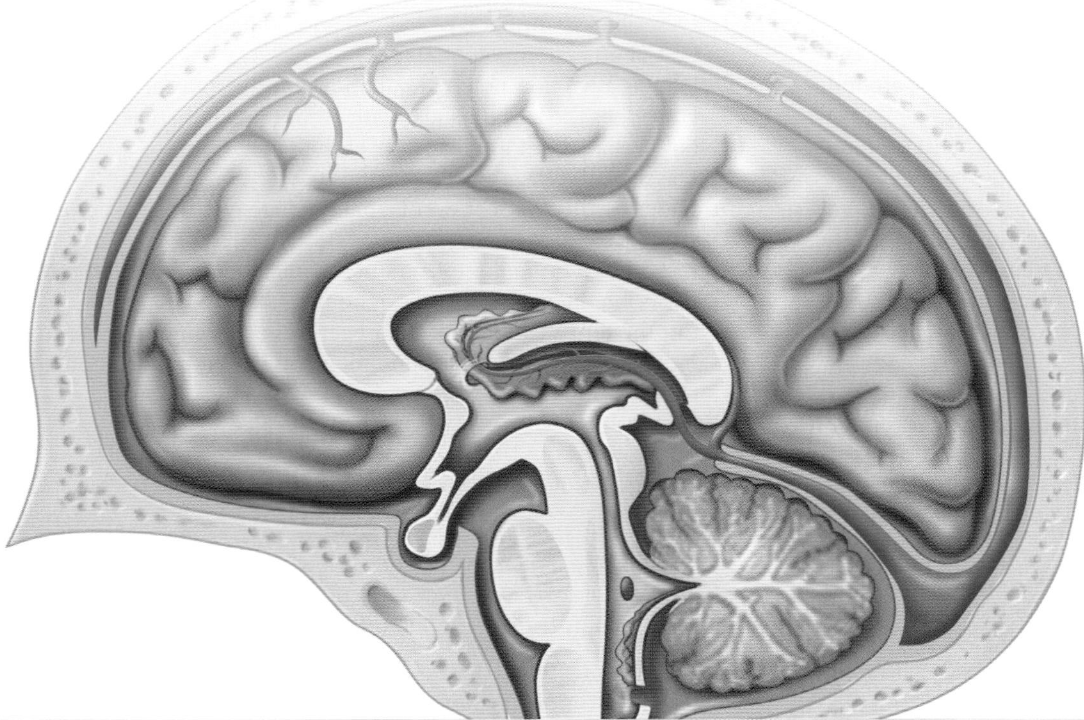

CHAPTER OUTLINE

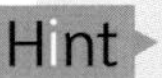 Scan this outline before you begin to read the chapter, as a preview of how the concepts are organized.

Recall from Chapter 18 that the nervous system is said to be composed of two major divisions: the central nervous system (CNS) and the peripheral nervous system (PNS). The reason for designating two distinct divisions is to make the study of the nervous system easier. In this chapter, we discuss the part of the nervous system that lies at the centre of the regulatory process: the central nervous system. Comprising both the brain and the spinal cord, the central nervous system is the principal integrator of sensory input and motor output. Thus the central nervous

LANGUAGE OF SCIENCE

Hint *Use this list to aid your pronunciation of unfamiliar words.*

amygdaloid nucleus (ah-MIG-dah-loyd NYOO-klee-us) [*amygdal-* **almond,** *-oid* **like**] *pl.*, nuclei

anterior corticospinal tract (an-TEER-ee-or KOR-ti-koh-spy-nal trakt) [*ante-* **front,** *-er-* **more,** *-or* **quality,** *cortic-* **cortex (bark),** *-spin-* **backbone,** *-al* **relating to,** *tract-* **trail**]

anterior spinothalamic tract (an-TEER-ee-or SPY-no-tha-lam-ik trakt) [*ante-* **front,** *-er-* **more,** *-or* **quality,** *spino-* **backbone,** *-thalam-* **inner chamber,** *-ic* **relating to**]

arbor vitae (AR-bor VI-tay) [*arbor* **tree,** *vitae* **of life**] *pl.*, arbores vitae

ascending tract (ah-SEND-ing trakt) [*ascend-* **climb,** *tract-* **trail**]

basal nuclei (BAY-sal NYOO-klee-eye) [*bas-* **foundation,** *-al* **relating to,** *nucle-* **nut or kernel**] *sing.*, nucleus

biological clock (bye-oh-LOJ-i-kal) [*bio-* **life,** *-o-* **combining form,** *-log-* **words (study of),** *-ical* **relating to**]

brainstem (BRAYN-stem)

cauda equina (KAW-da eh-KWY-nah) [*caud-* **tail,** *equina* **of a horse**] *pl.*, caudae equinae

caudate nucleus (KAW-dayt NYOO-klee-us) [*caud-* **tail,** *-ate* **of or like,** *nucleus* **nut or kernel**] *pl.*, nuclei

central sulcus (Rolando fissure) (SUL-kus [roh-LAHN-doh FISH-ur]) [*sulcus* **trench,** *Luigi Rolando* **Italian physician**] *pl.*, sulci

cerebellum (sair-eh-BELL-um) [*cereb-* **brain,** *-ellum* **small thing**] *pl.*, cerebella or cerebellums

cerebral hemisphere (seh-REE-bral HEM-i-sfeer) [*cerebr-* **brain,** *-al* **relating to,** *hemi-* **half,** *-sphere* **globe**]

cerebral peduncle (seh-REE-bral peh-DUNG-kul) [*cerebr-* **brain,** *-al* **relating to,** *ped-* **foot,** *-uncl-* **little**]

continued on p. 470

system is capable of evaluating incoming information and formulating responses to changes that threaten our homeostatic balance.

This chapter begins with a description of the protective coverings of the brain and spinal cord. After that, we briefly discuss the watery *cerebrospinal fluid (CSF)* and the spaces in which it is found. We then outline the overall structure and function of the major organs of the central nervous system, beginning at the bottom with the spinal cord—the simplest and least complex part of the CNS.

Then our focus moves upward to the more complex brain, beginning first with the narrow brainstem (**Figure 20-1**) and the roughly spherical cerebellum attached to its dorsal surface. Again shifting our attention upward, we describe the structure and function of the diencephalon and then move on to a discussion of the cerebrum.

As we move up the central nervous system, the complexity of both structure and function increases. The spinal cord mediates simple reflexes, whereas the brainstem and diencephalon are involved in the regulation of the more complex maintenance functions, such as regulation of heart rate and breathing. The cerebral hemispheres, which together form the largest part of the brain, perform complex integrative functions such as conscious thought, learning, memory, language, and problem solving.

We end the chapter with a discussion of the somatic sensory pathways and the somatic motor pathways. This prepares us for Chapter 21, which covers the structures of the peripheral nervous system, Chapter 22, which covers autonomic regulation of vital functions, and Chapters 23 and 24, which cover the senses. •

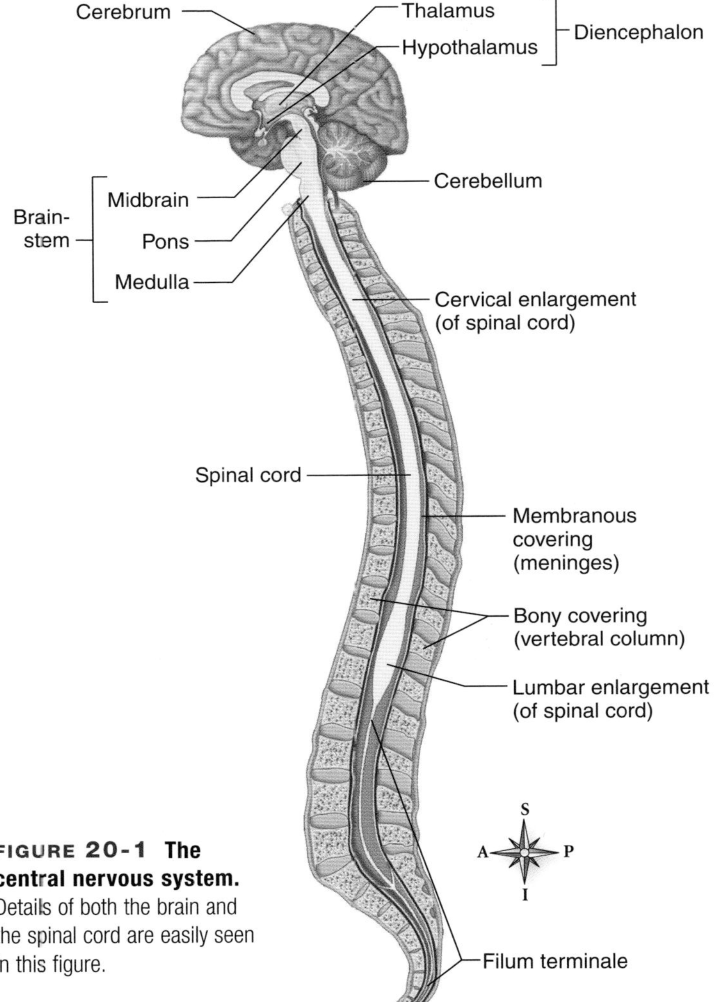

FIGURE 20-1 The central nervous system. Details of both the brain and the spinal cord are easily seen in this figure.

COVERINGS OF THE BRAIN AND SPINAL CORD

Because the brain and spinal cord are both delicate and vital, nature has provided them with two protective coverings. The outer covering consists of bone: cranial bones encase the brain; vertebrae encase the spinal cord. The inner covering consists of membranes known as **meninges.** Three distinct layers compose the meninges:

1. Dura mater
2. Arachnoid mater
3. Pia mater

Observe their respective locations in **Figure 20-2** and **Figure 20-3**. The dura mater, made of strong white fibrous tissue, serves as the outer layer of the meninges and also as the inner periosteum of the cranial bones. The arachnoid mater, a delicate, spiderweb-like layer, lies between the dura mater and the pia mater, or innermost layer of the meninges. The transparent pia mater adheres to the outer surface of the brain and spinal cord and contains blood vessels.

The dura mater has three important inward extensions:

1. **Falx cerebri.** The falx cerebri projects downward into the longitudinal fissure to form a kind of partition between the two cerebral hemispheres. The Latin word *falx* means "sickle" and refers to the curving sickle shape of this partition as it extends from the roof of the cranial cavity (see **Figure 20-2**, *B*).
2. **Falx cerebelli.** The falx cerebelli is a sickle-shaped extension that separates the two halves, or hemispheres, of the cerebellum.
3. **Tentorium cerebelli.** The tentorium cerebelli separates the cerebellum from the cerebrum. It is called a *tentorium* (meaning "tent") because it forms a tentlike covering over the cerebellum.

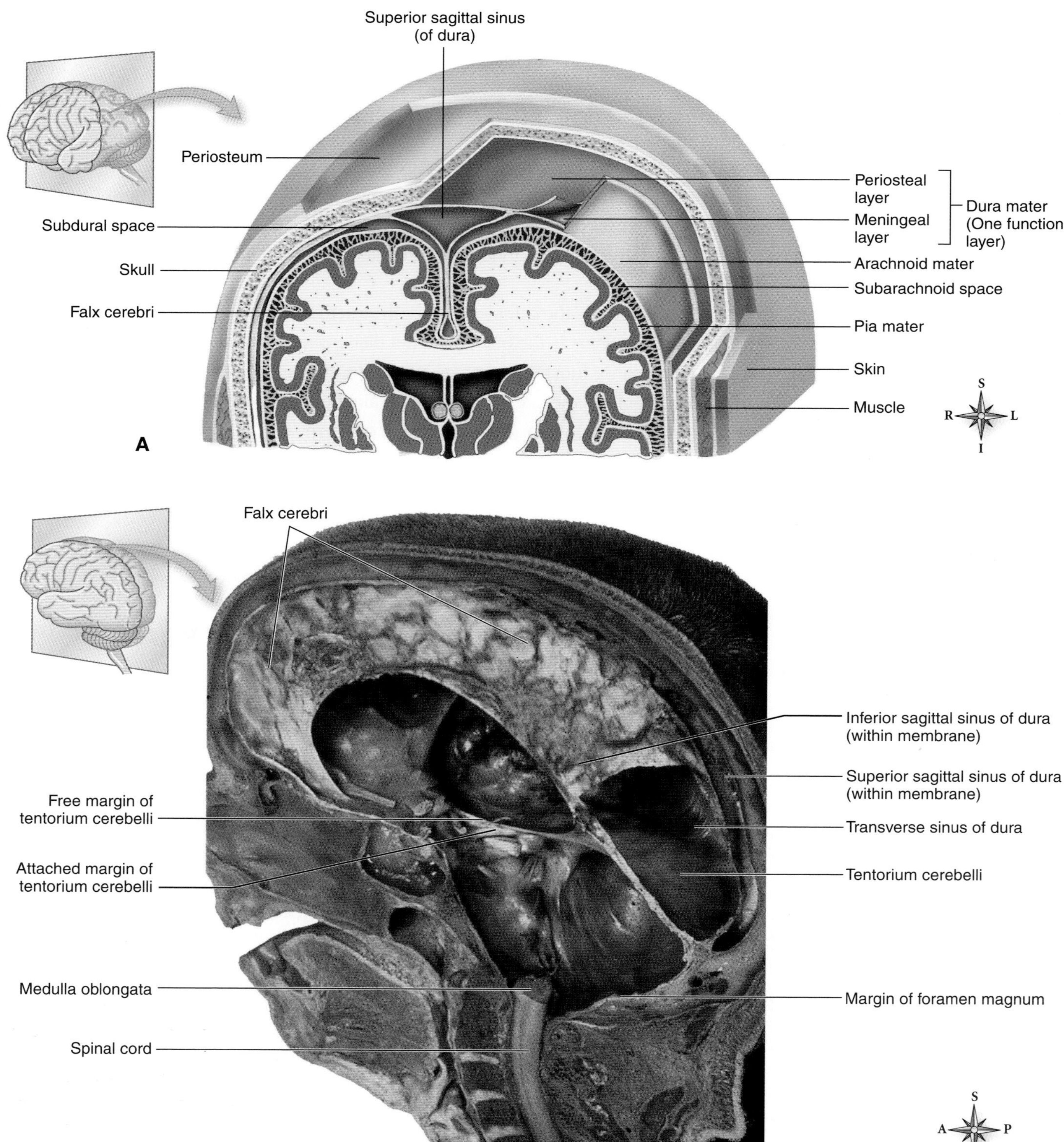

FIGURE 20-2 Coverings of the brain. **A,** Coronal (frontal) section of the superior portion of the head, as viewed from the front. Both the bony and the membranous coverings of the brain can be seen. **B,** Sagittal section of the skull, viewed from the left. The dura mater has been retained in this specimen to show how it lines the inner roof of the cranium and the falx cerebri extending inward.

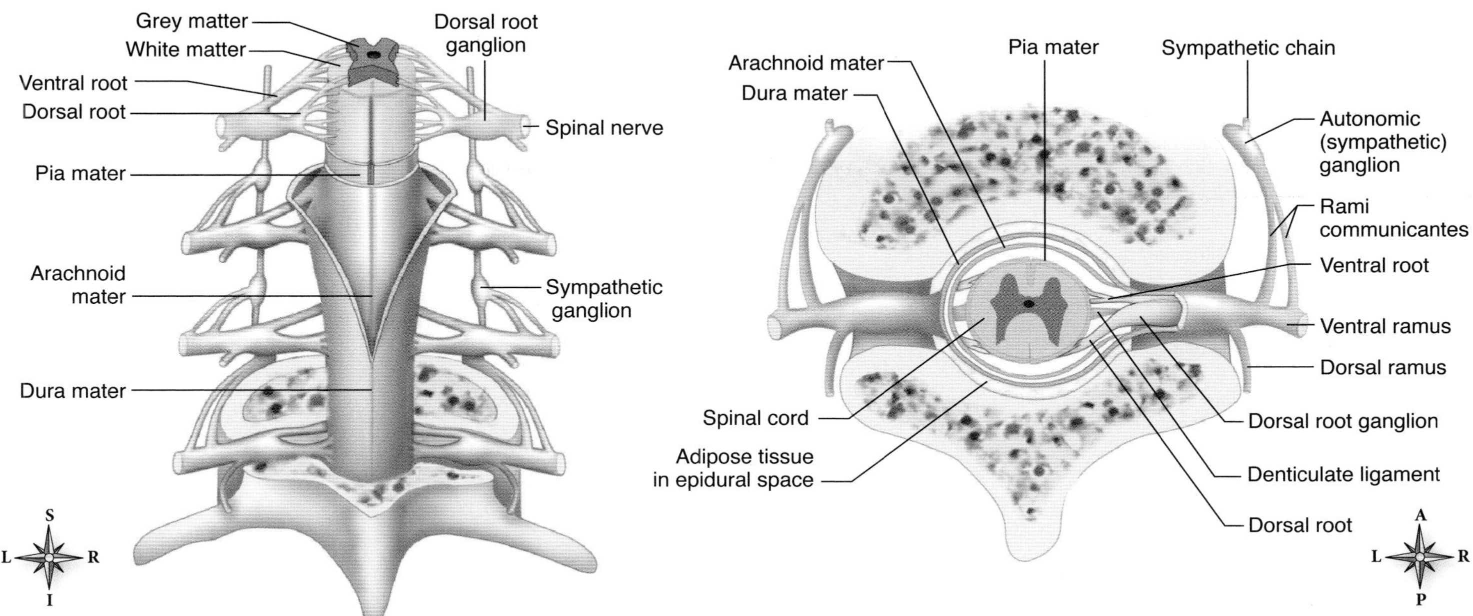

FIGURE 20-3 Coverings of the spinal cord. The dura mater is shown in purple. Note how it extends to cover the spinal nerve roots and nerves. The arachnoid mater is highlighted in pink and the pia mater in orange.

Figure 20-2 shows a large space within the dura, where the falx cerebri begins to descend between the left and right cerebral hemispheres. This space, called the *superior sagittal sinus,* is one of several dural sinuses. Dural sinuses function as venous reservoirs, collecting blood from brain tissues for the return trip to the heart.

A number of spaces lie between and around the meninges (see **Figure 20-2**). Three of these spaces are the following:

1. **Epidural space.** The epidural ("on the dura") space is immediately outside the dura mater but inside the bony coverings of the spinal cord. It contains a supporting cushion of fat and other connective tissues. Around the brain, because the dura mater is continuous with the periosteum on the inside face of the cranial bones, no epidural space is normally present.
2. **Subdural space.** The subdural ("under the dura") space is between the dura mater and arachnoid mater. The subdural space is only a potential space, but it can become a real space if blood leaks into it, forming a subdural haematoma. Normally it contains a small amount of lubricating serous fluid.
3. **Subarachnoid space.** As its name suggests, the *subarachnoid space* is under the arachnoid and outside the pia mater. This space contains a significant amount of cerebrospinal fluid.

The meninges of the cord (see **Figure 20-3**) continue on down inside the spinal cavity for some distance below the end of the spinal cord. The pia mater forms a slender filament known as the **filum terminale** (see **Figure 20-1**). At the level of the third segment of the sacrum, the filum terminale blends with the dura mater to form a fibrous cord that disappears in the periosteum of the coccyx.

CONNECT IT! 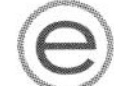

Infection or inflammation of the meninges is termed **meningitis.** Learn more about this condition and check out some medical images at ***Meningitis*** online at ***Connect It!***

CEREBROSPINAL FLUID

In addition to its bony and membranous coverings, nature has further protected the brain and spinal cord against injury by providing a cushion of fluid both around the organs and within them. This fluid is the **cerebrospinal fluid (CSF).**

The CSF does more than simply provide a supportive, protective cushion, however. It is also a reservoir of circulating fluid that, along with blood, the brain monitors for changes in the internal environment. For example, changes in the carbon dioxide (CO_2) content of CSF trigger homeostatic responses in the respiratory control centres of the brainstem that help regulate the overall CO_2 content and pH of the body.

Fluid Spaces

Cerebrospinal fluid is found in the subarachnoid space around the brain and spinal cord and within the cavities and canals of the brain and spinal cord.

The four large, fluid-filled spaces within the brain are called **ventricles.** Two of them, the lateral (or first and second) ventricles, are located one in each hemisphere of the cerebrum. As you can see in **Figure 20-4**, the third ventricle is little more than a thin, vertical pocket of fluid below and medial to the lateral ventricles. The fourth ventricle is a tiny, diamond-shaped space where the cerebellum attaches to the back of the brainstem. Actually, the fourth ventricle is simply a slight expansion of the central canal extending up from the spinal cord.

Formation and Circulation of Cerebrospinal Fluid

Formation of CSF occurs mainly by separation of fluid from blood in the **choroid plexuses.** Choroid plexuses are networks of capillaries that project from the pia mater into the lateral ventricles and into the roofs of the third and fourth ventricles. Each choroid plexus is

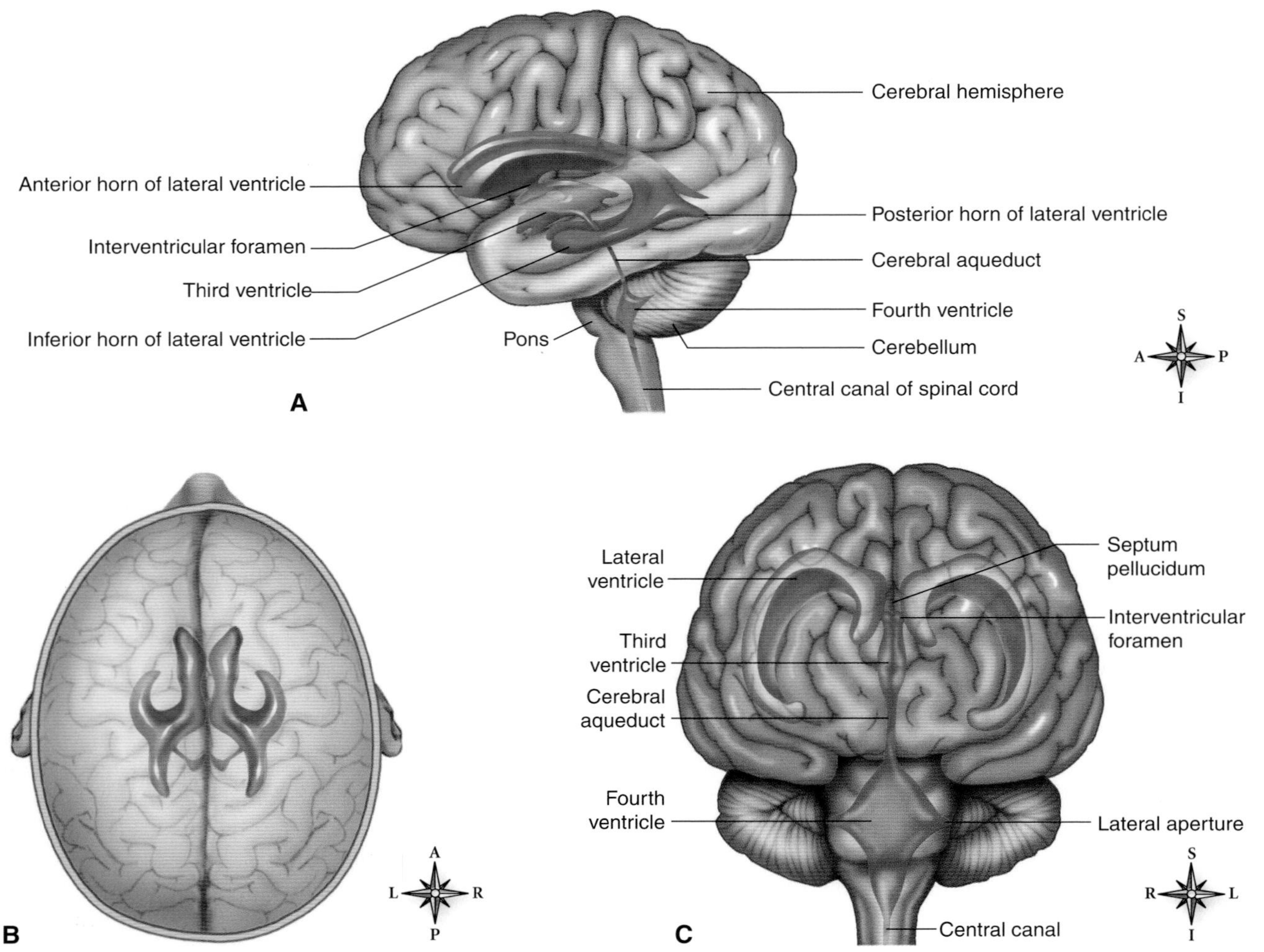

Cerebral hemisphere
Anterior horn of lateral ventricle
Interventricular foramen
Third ventricle
Inferior horn of lateral ventricle
Pons
Posterior horn of lateral ventricle
Cerebral aqueduct
Fourth ventricle
Cerebellum
Central canal of spinal cord
A

B

Lateral ventricle
Third ventricle
Cerebral aqueduct
Fourth ventricle
Septum pellucidum
Interventricular foramen
Lateral aperture
Central canal
C

FIGURE 20-4 Fluid spaces of the brain. A, Ventricles highlighted in blue within a translucent brain in a left lateral view. **B,** Ventricles as seen from above. **C,** Ventricles as seen from the front.

covered with a sheet of a special type of ependymal (glial) cell that releases the CSF into the fluid spaces.

From each lateral ventricle the fluid seeps through an opening, the *interventricular foramen (Monro foramen)*, into the third ventricle, then through a narrow channel, the *cerebral aqueduct (Sylvius aqueduct)*, into the fourth ventricle (**Figure 20-5**). Some of the fluid moves from the fourth ventricle directly into the central canal of the cord. Some of it moves out of the fourth ventricle through openings in its roof, two *lateral foramina (Luschka foramina)* and one *median foramen (Magendie foramina)*. These openings allow CSF to move into the *cisterna magna*, a space behind the medulla that is continuous with the subarachnoid space around the brain and cord.

The fluid circulates in the subarachnoid space and then is absorbed into venous blood through the *arachnoid villi*. These villi are tiny fingerlike projections of the arachnoid mater into the brain's venous sinuses.

Briefly, here is the circulation route of cerebrospinal fluid: it is formed as fluid is separated from blood in the choroid plexuses, then flows into the ventricles of the brain, circulates through the ventricles and into the central canal and subarachnoid spaces, and is then absorbed back into blood.

The amount of CSF in the average adult is about 140 mL (about 23 mL in the ventricles and 117 mL in the subarachnoid space of the brain and cord). But it is continually refreshed as new CSF is formed and older CSF is reabsorbed. **Box 20-1** explains the diagnostic value of testing a patient's cerebrospinal fluid.

CONNECT IT! 

When the circulation of cerebrospinal fluid (CSF) is blocked, there can be dramatic effects on the structure of the brain. An example is **hydrocephalus,** a condition in which the CSF produces abnormal fluid pressure in the brain, sometimes causing tremendous swelling of the head. A brief description of hydrocephalus and how it can be treated, along with some dramatic clinical images, can be found in ***Hydrocephalus*** online at ***Connect It!***

Quick CHECK

1. Name the three membranous coverings of the central nervous system in order, beginning with the outermost layer.
2. Trace the path of cerebrospinal fluid from its formation by a choroid plexus to its reabsorption into the blood.

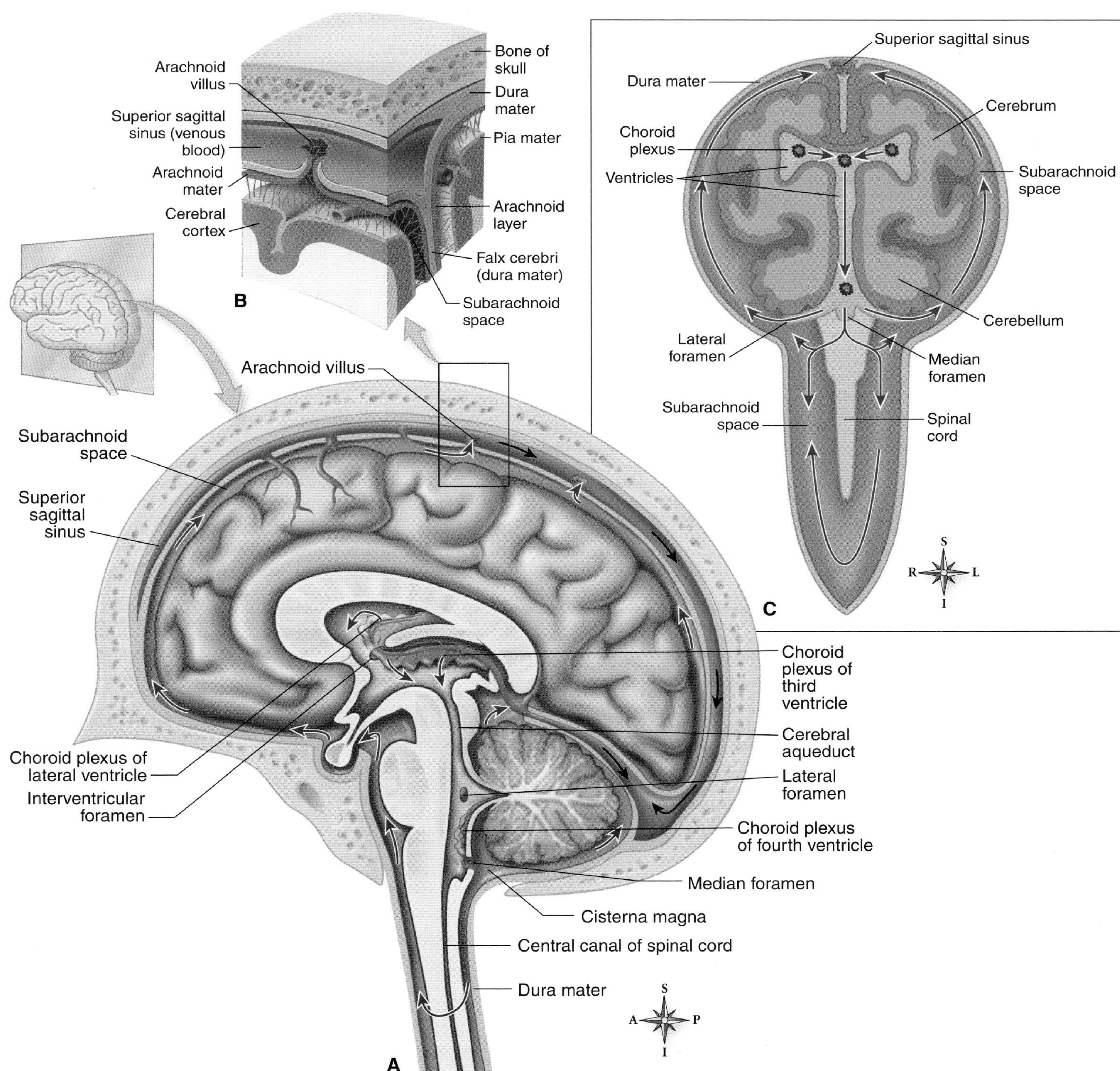

FIGURE 20-5 Flow of cerebrospinal fluid (CSF). A, The CSF produced by filtration of blood by the choroid plexus of each ventricle flows inferiorly through the lateral ventricles, interventricular foramen, third ventricle, cerebral aqueduct, fourth ventricle, and subarachnoid space and to the blood. **B,** Inset showing arachnoid villus, where CSF is reabsorbed into the blood of the superior sagittal sinus. **C,** Simplified diagram showing flow of CSF.

BOX 20-1 *diagnostic study* | Lumbar Puncture

The meninges extends beyond the cord, which provides a convenient location for performing lumbar punctures without danger of injuring the spinal cord. A **lumbar puncture** is a withdrawal of some of the cerebrospinal fluid (CSF) from the subarachnoid space in the lumbar region of the vertebral column. The physician inserts a needle just above or below the fourth lumbar vertebra, knowing that the spinal cord ends 2 or more centimetres above that level (Figure 1). The fourth lumbar vertebra can be easily located because it lies on a line with the iliac crest. Placing a patient on his or her side with the knees and chest drawn together to arch the back separates the vertebrae sufficiently to create a space in which the needle can be inserted. As the needle enters the CSF, the thin nerve roots roll off the tip of the needle—thus allowing collection of CSF without damaging nerve tissue.

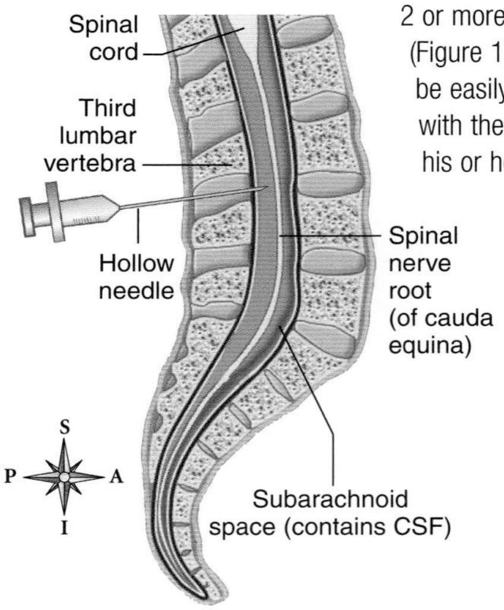

FIGURE 1 Location of lumbar puncture. The needle is inserted a few centimetres below the spinal cord.

Cerebrospinal fluid removed through a lumbar puncture can be tested for the presence of blood cells, bacteria, or other abnormal characteristics that may indicate an injury or infection, such as meningitis (Figure 2). A sensor called a *manometer* is sometimes attached to the needle to determine the pressure of the CSF within the subarachnoid space. The lumbar puncture can also be used to introduce diagnostic agents, such as radiopaque dyes for **x-ray photography,** into the subarachnoid space. •

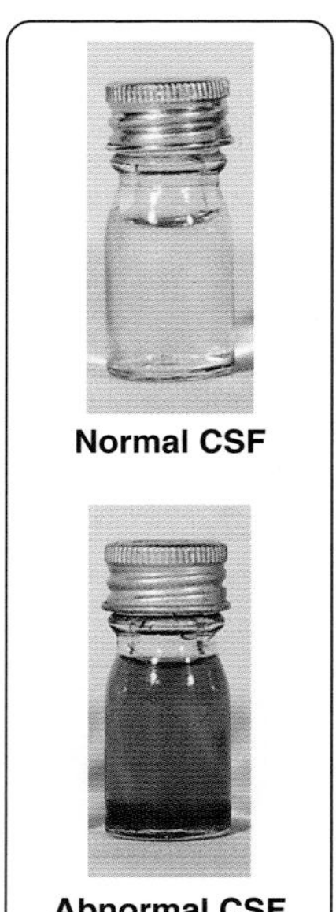

FIGURE 2 Cerebrospinal fluid (CSF) examination. These samples were taken by a lumbar puncture or "spinal tap". The top sample shows the normal, clear appearance of CSF. The bottom sample was taken from a patient with haemorrhage in the subarachnoid space. Blood is seen settling to the bottom of the sample. The yellowish tinge of the fluid is from the breakdown of blood cells before the fluid was removed from the body.

SPINAL CORD

STRUCTURE OF THE SPINAL CORD

The spinal cord lies within the spinal cavity, extending from the foramen magnum to the lower border of the first lumbar vertebra (**Figure 20-6**), a distance of about 45 cm in the average body. The spinal cord does not completely fill the spinal cavity—which also contains the meninges, CSF, a cushion of adipose tissue, and blood vessels.

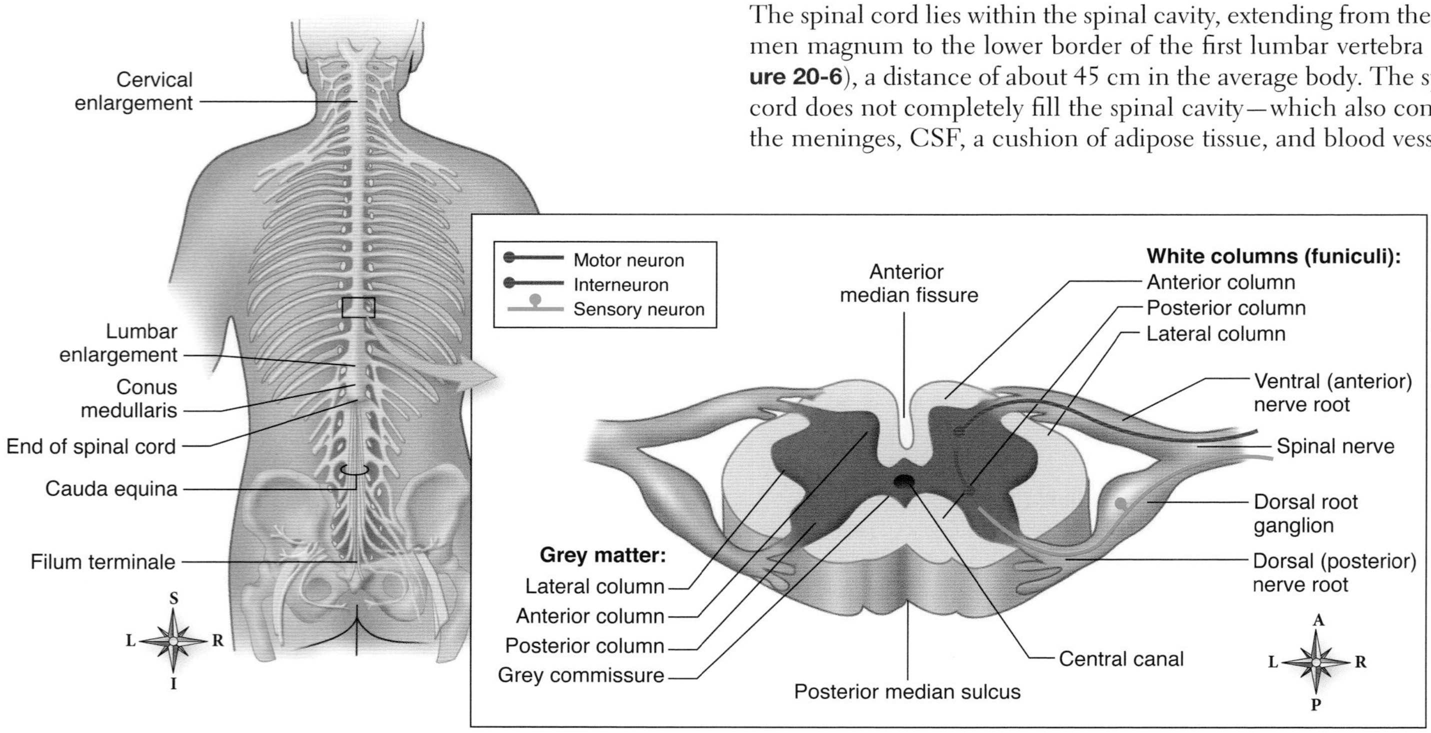

FIGURE 20-6 Spinal cord. The inset illustrates a transverse section of the spinal cord shown in the broader view.

The spinal cord is an oval cylinder that tapers slightly as it descends and has two bulges, one in the cervical region and the other in the lumbar region (see **Figure 20-6**). Two deep grooves, the *anterior median fissure* and the *posterior median sulcus,* just miss dividing the cord into separate symmetrical halves. The anterior fissure is the deeper and the wider of the two grooves—a useful fact to remember when you examine spinal cord diagrams. It enables you to tell at a glance which part of the cord is anterior and which is posterior.

Two bundles of nerve fibres called *nerve roots* project from each side of the spinal cord (see **Figure 20-6**). Fibres comprising the **dorsal nerve root,** also called **posterior nerve root,** carry sensory information into the spinal cord. Cell bodies of these unipolar, sensory neurons make up a small region of grey matter in the dorsal nerve root called the *dorsal (posterior) root ganglion.* Fibres of the **ventral nerve root,** also called **anterior nerve root,** carry motor information out of the spinal cord. Cell bodies of these multipolar, motor neurons are in the grey matter that composes the inner core of the spinal cord. Numerous interneurons are also located in the grey matter core of the spinal cord.

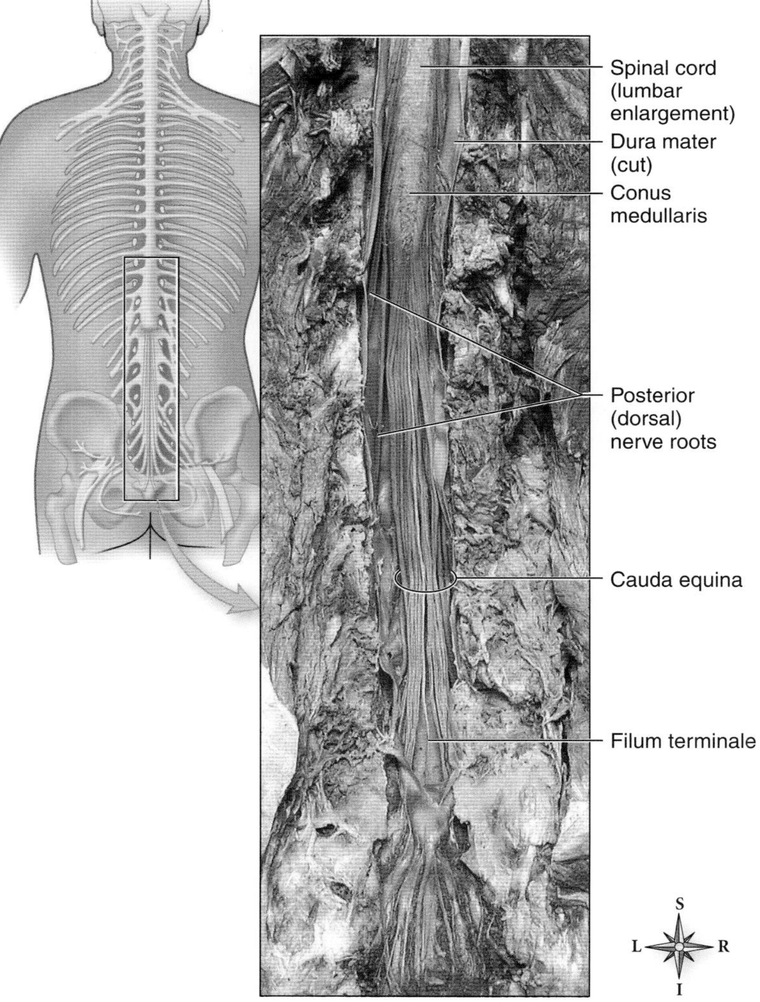

FIGURE 20-7 Cauda equina. Photograph shows the inferior portion of the dura mater dissected posteriorly, revealing the cauda equina and nearby structures.

On each side of the spinal cord, the dorsal and ventral nerve roots join together to form a single mixed nerve called, simply, a **spinal nerve.** Spinal nerves, components of the peripheral nervous system, are considered in more detail in the next chapter.

The spinal cord ends at vertebra L1 in a tapered cone called the **conus medullaris.** As you can see in **Figure 20-7**, many nerve roots extending from the conus medullaris form a sort of "horse tail" of spinal nerve roots called the **cauda equina.** Within the cauda equina the long cordlike *filum terminale* is formed from the spinal meninges.

Although the grey matter core of the spinal cord looks like a flat letter H in transverse sections of the cord, it actually has three dimensions, because the grey matter extends the length of the cord. The H-shaped rod of grey matter is made up of anterior, lateral, and posterior **grey columns.** When viewed in a cross-section, as in **Figure 20-6**, the columns forming the H appear to spread out like animal horns—and thus are also called *anterior, posterior,* and *lateral grey horns.* The left and right grey columns are joined in the middle by a band called the **grey commissure.** It is through the grey commissure that the central canal carries CSF through the spinal cord. The grey columns consist predominantly of cell bodies of interneurons and motor neurons.

White matter surrounding the grey matter is subdivided in each half of the cord into three white columns or **funiculi:** the anterior, posterior, and lateral white columns. Each white column, or funiculus, consists of a large bundle of nerve fibres (axons) divided into smaller bundles called **spinal tracts,** shown in **Figure 20-8**.

The names of most spinal cord tracts indicate the white column in which the tract is located, the structure in which the axons that make up the tract originate, and the structure in which they terminate. For example, the lateral corticospinal tract is located in the lateral white column of the cord. The axons that compose it originate from neuron cell bodies in the spinal cortex (of the cerebrum) and terminate in the spinal cord. The anterior spinothalamic tract lies in the anterior white column. The axons that compose it originate from neuron cell bodies in the spinal cord and terminate in a portion of the brain called the *thalamus.*

You may wish to refer to Part 3 of the BRIEF ATLAS OF THE HUMAN BODY, where you will find detailed photographs of a human spinal cord. How many structures can you identify in the atlas by sight?

FUNCTIONS OF THE SPINAL CORD

The spinal cord performs two general functions. Briefly, it provides conduction routes to and from the brain and serves as the integrator, or reflex centre, for all spinal reflexes.

Spinal cord tracts provide conduction paths to and from the brain. **Ascending tracts** conduct sensory impulses up the cord to the brain. **Descending tracts** conduct motor impulses down the cord from the brain. Bundles of axons compose all tracts.

Tracts are both structural and functional organizations of the nerve fibres of the spinal cord. They are *structural* organizations in that all the axons of any one tract originate from neuron cell bodies located in the same area of the central nervous system, and all the axons terminate in a single structure elsewhere in the central nervous system. For example, all the fibres of the spinothalamic tract are axons originating from neuron cell bodies located in the spinal cord and terminating in the thalamus. Tracts are *functional* organizations

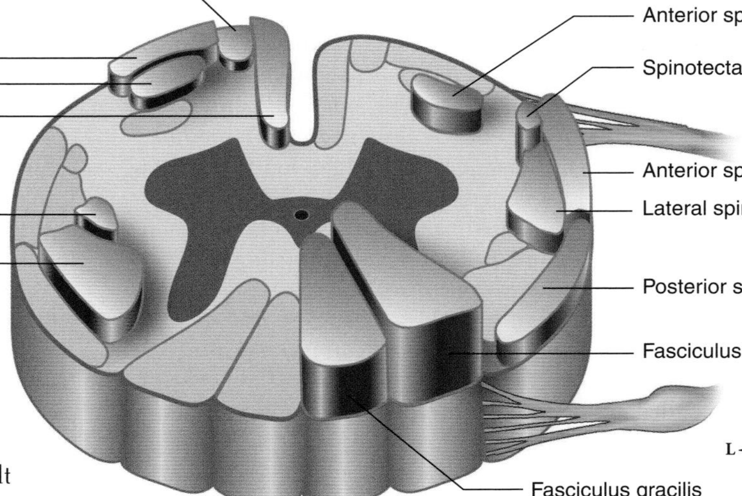

FIGURE 20-8 Major tracts of the spinal cord. The major ascending (sensory) tracts are highlighted in blue. The major descending (motor) tracts are highlighted in red.

in that all the axons that compose one tract serve one general function. For instance, fibres of the spinothalamic tracts serve a sensory function. They transmit impulses that produce the sensations of crude touch, pain, and temperature.

Because so many different tracts make up the white columns of the cord, we mention only a few of the more important ones. Locate each tract in **Figure 20-8**. Consult **Table 20-1** and **Table 20-2** for a brief summary of these tracts.

Five important ascending, or sensory, tracts and their functions, stated very briefly, are as follows:

1. **Lateral spinothalamic tracts:** crude touch, pain, and temperature
2. **Anterior spinothalamic tracts:** crude touch and pressure
3. **Fasciculi gracilis** and **cuneatus tracts:** discriminating touch and conscious sensation of position and movement of body parts (kinaesthesia)
4. **Spinocerebellar tracts:** subconscious kinaesthesia
5. **Spinotectal tracts:** touch that triggers visual reflexes

Further discussion of the sensory neural pathways may be found on pp. 464–465.

Six important descending, or motor, tracts and their functions described in brief are as follows:

1. **Lateral corticospinal tracts:** voluntary movement; contraction of individual or small groups of muscles, particularly those moving hands, fingers, feet, and toes on opposite side of body
2. **Anterior corticospinal tracts:** same as preceding except mainly muscles of same side of body
3. **Reticulospinal tracts:** help maintain posture during skeletal muscle movements
4. **Rubrospinal tracts:** transmit impulses that coordinate body movements and maintenance of posture
5. **Tectospinal tracts:** head and neck movement related to visual reflexes
6. **Vestibulospinal tracts:** coordination of posture and balance

Further discussion of motor neural pathways may be found on pp. 466–468.

The spinal cord also serves as the reflex centre for all spinal reflexes. The term *reflex centre* means the centre of a reflex arc or the place in the arc where incoming sensory impulses become outgoing motor impulses. They are structures that switch impulses from afferent to efferent neurons. In two-neuron arcs, reflex centres are merely synapses between neurons. In all other arcs, reflex centres consist of interneurons interposed between afferent and efferent neurons. Spinal reflex centres are located in the grey matter of the cord.

TABLE 20-1 Major Ascending Tracts of Spinal Cord

NAME	FUNCTION	LOCATION	ORIGIN*	TERMINATION†
Lateral spinothalamic	Pain, temperature, and crude touch on opposite side	Lateral white columns	Posterior grey column on opposite side	Thalamus
Anterior spinothalamic	Crude touch and pressure	Anterior white columns	Posterior grey column on opposite side	Thalamus
Fasciculi gracilis and cuneatus	Discriminating touch and pressure sensations, including vibration, stereognosis, and two-point discrimination; also conscious kinaesthesia	Posterior white columns	Spinal ganglia on same side	Medulla
Anterior and posterior spinocerebellar	Unconscious kinaesthesia	Lateral white columns	Anterior or posterior grey column	Cerebellum
Spinotectal	Touch related to visual reflexes	Lateral white columns	Posterior grey columns	Superior colliculus (midbrain)

*Location of cell bodies of neurons from which axons of tract arise.

†Structure in which axons of tract terminate.

TABLE 20-2 Major Descending Tracts of Spinal Cord

NAME	FUNCTION	LOCATION	ORIGIN*	TERMINATION†
Lateral corticospinal (or crossed pyramidal)	Voluntary movement, contraction of individual or small groups of muscles, particularly those moving hands, fingers, feet, and toes of opposite side	Lateral white columns	Motor areas or cerebral cortex of opposite side from tract location in cord	Lateral or anterior grey columns
Anterior corticospinal (direct pyramidal)	Same as lateral corticospinal except mainly muscles of same side	Anterior white columns	Motor cortex but on same side as location in cord	Lateral or anterior grey columns
Reticulospinal	Maintain posture during movement	Anterior white columns	Reticular formation (midbrain, pons, medulla)	Anterior grey columns
Rubrospinal	Coordination of body movement and posture	Lateral white columns	Red nucleus (of midbrain)	Anterior grey columns
Tectospinal	Head and neck movement during visual reflexes	Anterior white columns	Superior colliculus (midbrain)	Medulla and anterior grey columns
Vestibulospinal	Coordination of posture/balance	Anterior white columns	Vestibular nucleus (pons, medulla)	Anterior grey columns

*Location of cell bodies of neurons from which axons of tract arise.

†Structure in which axons of tract terminate.

CONNECT IT! 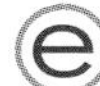

Reflex centres can act as **pain control areas.** Pain control areas can inhibit the pain information heading toward the conscious processing centres of the brain. Identifying pain control areas and how they work has led to the development of **transcutaneous electrical nerve stimulation (TENS)** units and other therapies to reduce pain. To learn more about this check out ***Pain Control Areas*** online at ***Connect It!***

Quick CHECK

3. What are spinal nerve roots? How does the dorsal root differ from the ventral root?
4. Name the regions of the white and grey matter seen in a horizontal section of the spinal cord.
5. Contrast ascending tracts and descending tracts of the spinal cord. Can you give an example of each?

BRAIN

The brain is one of the largest organs in adults. It consists, in round numbers, of almost 85 billion neurons and roughly the same number of glia. In most adults, it weighs about 1.4 kg. Large, detailed photographs of the brain are found in Part 3 of the BRIEF ATLAS OF THE HUMAN BODY.

REGIONS OF THE BRAIN

Six major divisions of the brain, named from below, upward, are as follows: *medulla oblongata, pons, midbrain, cerebellum, diencephalon*, and *cerebrum*. Very often the medulla oblongata, pons, and midbrain are referred to collectively as the *brainstem*. Look at these three structures in **Figure 20-9**. Do you agree that they seem to form a stem for the rest of the brain?

BRAIN DEVELOPMENT

Most of the production of new neurons in the brain occurs during prenatal development and during the first few months of postnatal life. Malnutrition during the crucial prenatal months of neuron multiplication can result in fewer brain cells. After birth, the neurons grow mainly in size rather than in number. The brain attains full size by about the eighteenth year but grows rapidly only during the first 9 years or so. However, some regions of the brain retain *neural stem cells (NSCs)* that can continue to add small numbers of new neurons to the brain throughout adulthood. Throughout life many new synapses form and others are broken, making the brain a very dynamic and adaptive structure.

The processes of prenatal development—or **embryology**—of the brain are worth noting here. As you learned in **Figure 8-1** (p. 140), the brain develops from the *ectododerm*, which is the outermost of three *primary germ layers* of the growing embryo. As that illustration shows, along the dorsal surface of the embryo, the ectoderm folds in on itself to form a hollow tube. This **neural tube** eventually forms a series of connected vesicles of fluid that develop into the brain and spinal cord. **Table 20-3** shows how each of the major regions of the brain develop from these vesicles. Note also that the fluid inside the neural tube eventually forms the fluid spaces that we explored earlier in this chapter.

Knowing the basics of brain embryology is helpful in several ways. Envisioning the brain and spinal cord as sections of a long tube makes it easier for some students to learn the basic anatomy of the CNS. In fact, the vesicle names are often used as synonyms for the adult brain regions. Neurological assessments, for example, often report dysfunctions related to the cerebellum as "hindbrain" disorders. Embryology often explains important concepts about pathology. *Spina bifida*, a developmental disorder of the spine, is best understood in terms of errors in neural tube development. A sonographer or obstetrician may use the names of the primary or secondary vesicles of the embryonic brain in reporting key developmental stages.

As you continue your study of the brain, you may want to become familiar with these embryological terms as you study each region of the adult.

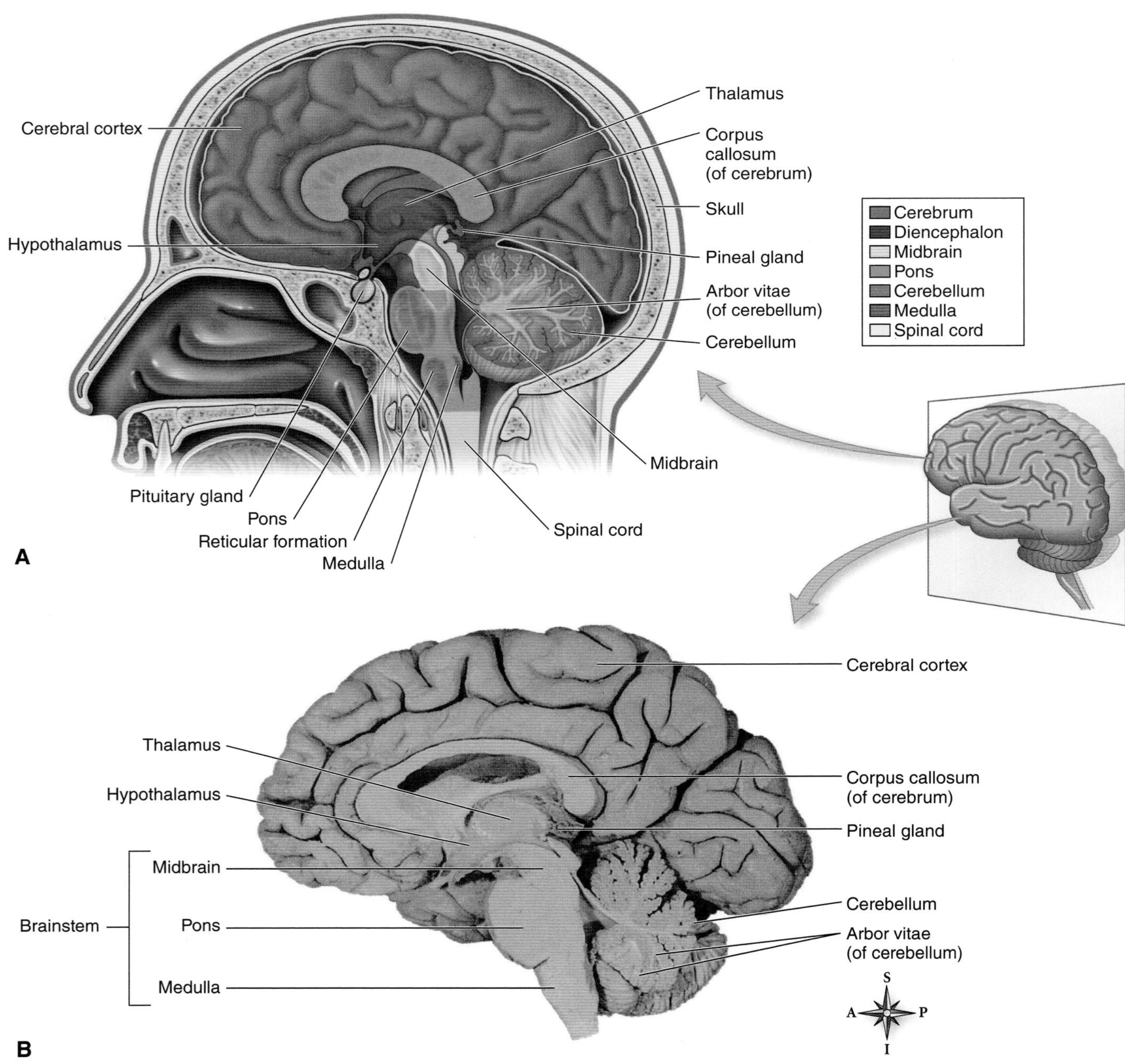

FIGURE 20-9 Divisions of the brain. A midsagittal section of the brain reveals features of its major divisions.

> **CONNECT IT!**
>
> Review the diagrams in the ***Connect It!*** article ***Embryonic Development of Tissues*** to see now the neural tube folds inward to form a fluid-filled canal that forms the series of vesicles, which in turn develops into the brain and spinal cord.

Structure of the Brainstem

Three divisions of the brain make up the **brainstem.** The **medulla oblongata** forms the lowest part of the brainstem, the **midbrain** forms the uppermost part, and the **pons** lies between them—that is, above the medulla and below the midbrain. Ten of the twelve pairs of cranial nerves arise from the brainstem.

Medulla Oblongata

The medulla oblongata is the part of the brain that attaches to the spinal cord. It is, in fact, an enlarged extension of the spinal cord located just above the foramen magnum. It measures only a few centimetres in length and is separated from the pons above by a horizontal groove. It is composed of white matter (projection tracts) and a network of grey and white matter called the **reticular formation** (look ahead to **Figure 20-20** on p. 460).

TABLE 20-3 Embryology of the Brain

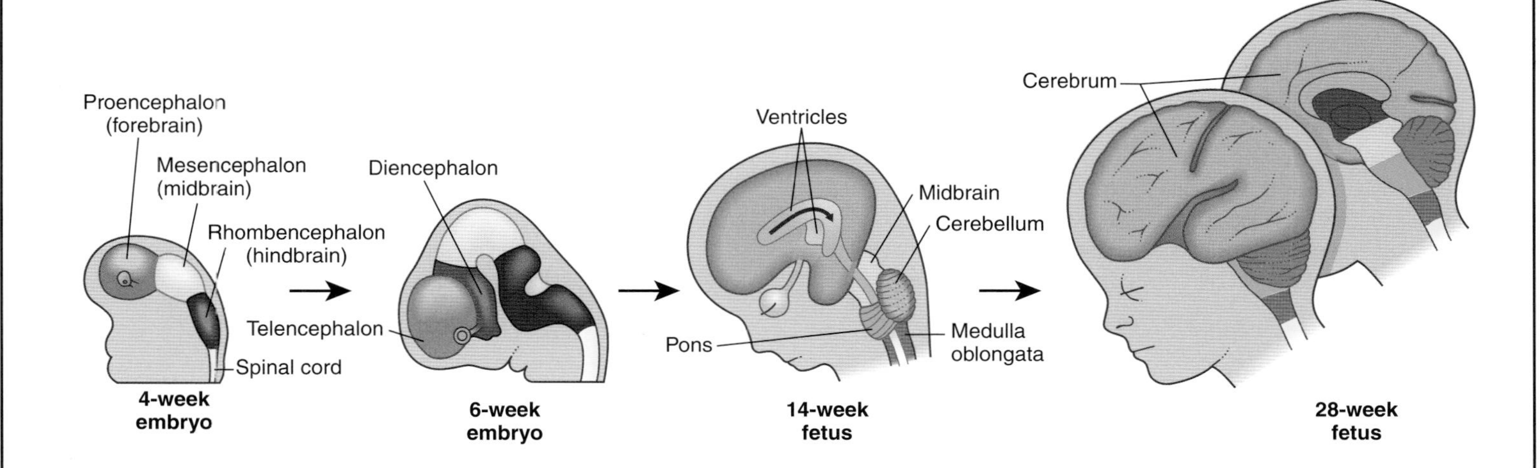

PRIMARY BRAIN VESICLES*	SECONDARY BRAIN VESICLES*	AT BIRTH: BRAIN REGIONS	AT BIRTH: FLUID SPACES
Proencephalon (forebrain)	Telencephalon	Cerebrum	Lateral ventricles
	Diencephalon	Diencephalon	Third ventricle
Mesencephalon (midbrain)	Mesencephalon	Midbrain	Cerebral aqueduct (of Sylvius)
Rhombencephalon (hindbrain)	Metencephalon	Pons	Fourth ventricle
		Cerebellum	
	Myelencephalon	Medulla oblongata	

*Pronunciations and translations of new terms are found in the glossary starting on p. 1151.

UNIT 3

The **pyramids** (**Figure 20-10**) are two bulges of white matter located on the ventral surface of the medulla. Fibres of the so-called pyramidal tracts form the pyramids.

The **olive** (see **Figure 20-10**) of the medulla is an oval projection appearing one on each side of the ventral surface of the medulla, lateral to the pyramids. See **Box 20-2** for another view of pyramids and olives.

Located in the medulla's reticular formation are various *nuclei*, or clusters of neuron cell bodies. Some nuclei are called *control centres*—for example, the cardiac, respiratory, and vasomotor control centres (**Box 20-3**).

Pons

Just above the medulla lies the pons, composed, like the medulla, of white matter and reticular formation. Fibres that run transversely across the pons and through the middle cerebellar peduncles into the cerebellum make up the external white matter of the pons and give it its arching, bridgelike appearance.

Midbrain

The midbrain *(mesencephalon)* is appropriately named. It forms the midsection of the brain, because it lies above the pons and below the cerebrum.

Both white matter (tracts) and reticular formation compose the midbrain. Extending divergently through it are two ropelike masses of white matter named **cerebral peduncles** (see **Figure 20-10**). Tracts in the peduncles conduct impulses between the midbrain and cerebrum.

In addition to the cerebral peduncles, another landmark of the midbrain is the **corpora quadrigemina** (literally, "body of fourfold twins"). The corpora quadrigemina are two **inferior colliculi** and two **superior colliculi.** Note the location of the two sets of twin colliculi, or the corpora quadrigemina, in **Figure 20-10**, *B*. They form the posterior, upper part of the midbrain, the part that lies just above the cerebellum. Certain auditory centres are located in the inferior colliculus. The superior colliculus contains visual centres.

Two other midbrain structures are the *red nucleus* and the *substantia nigra*. Each of these consists of clusters of cell bodies of neurons involved in muscular control. The substantia nigra (literally, "black matter") gets its name from the dark pigment in some of its cells.

Functions of the Brainstem

The brainstem, like the spinal cord, performs sensory, motor, and reflex functions. The spinothalamic tracts are important sensory tracts that pass through the brainstem on their way to the thalamus in the diencephalon. The fasciculi cuneatus and gracilis and the spinoreticular tracts are sensory tracts whose axons terminate in the grey matter of the brainstem. Corticospinal and reticulospinal tracts

BOX 20-2 *fyi* | Studying Human Brains

As with any part of the body, the best way to learn the anatomy of the brain is to look at actual specimens. Recall from Chapter 1 (see **Figure 1-1**, p. 4) that this is the traditional method of learning human anatomy. When cadavers are not available for this purpose, one useful alternative is photographs of well-dissected cadavers.

Part *A* of the figure below is an oblique coronal (frontal) section of the human brain, as seen from the front of the subject. This photograph shows details of the internal features of all the major brain divisions. Compare this view of the brain with part *B,* which shows the brain cut on horizontal (transverse) planes at two slightly different levels, as seen from above. Then compare these photographs with those shown in the small atlas that accompanies this book. How does viewing sections in different planes of the brain benefit your understanding of the three-dimensional aspects of brain anatomy? What benefits are there to studying the brains of human cadavers, rather than relying solely on artists' renderings of the brain? Are there any advantages to using artists' renderings of brain anatomy?

Refer to these photographs—and those in the atlas that accompanies this book—often as you study the details of brain anatomy. •

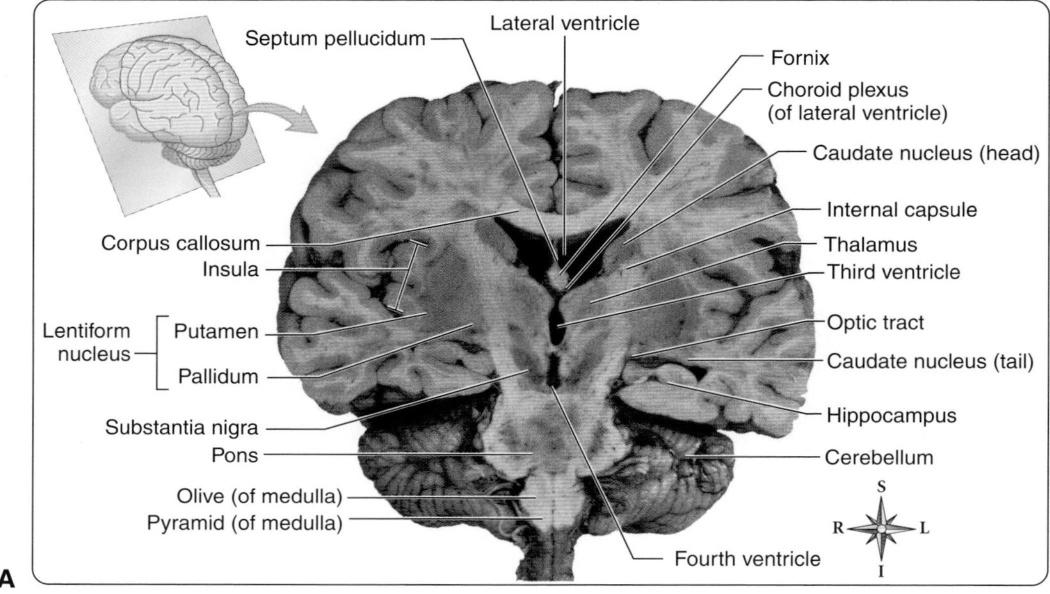

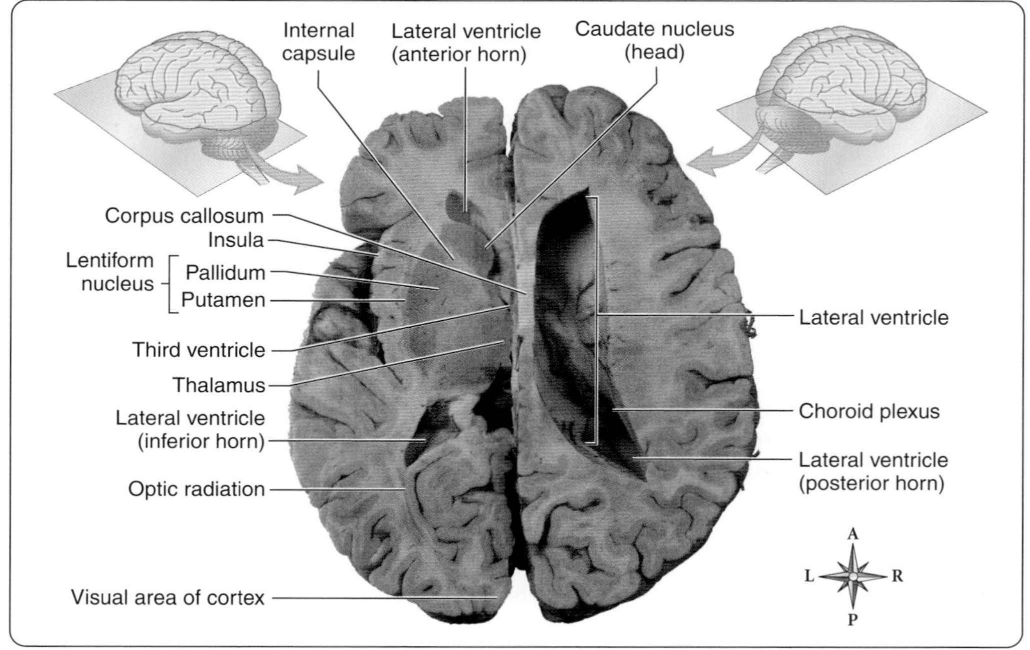

Human brain specimens. A, Oblique coronal (frontal) section. **B,** Horizontal sections (left section is slightly inferior to right section).

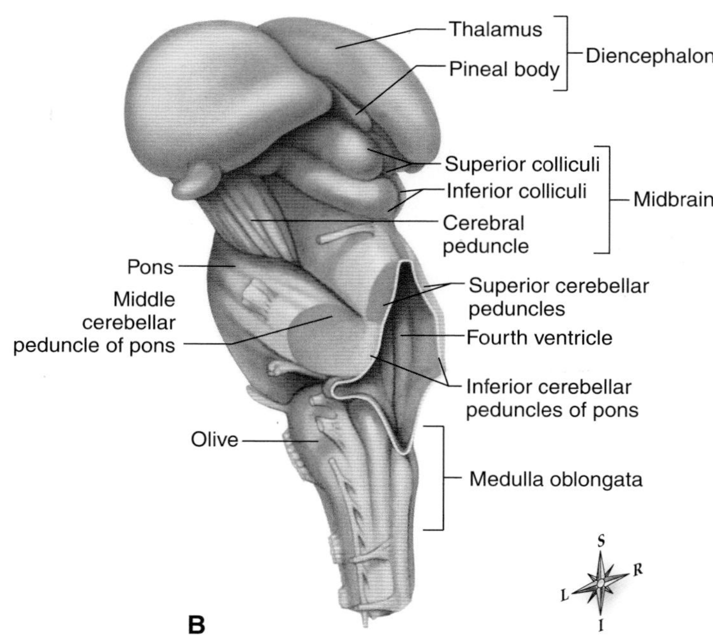

FIGURE 20-10 The brainstem and diencephalon. A, Anterior aspect. **B,** Posterior aspect (shifted slightly to lateral).

are two of the major tracts present in the white matter of the brainstem.

Nuclei in the medulla contain a number of reflex centres. Of first importance are the cardiac, vasomotor (vessel muscle), and respiratory centres. Other centres present in the medulla are for various nonvital reflexes such as vomiting, coughing, sneezing, hiccupping, and swallowing.

The pons contains centres for reflexes mediated by the fifth, sixth, seventh, and eighth cranial nerves. The locations and functions of these peripheral nerves are discussed in Chapter 21. In addition, the pons contains the pneumotaxic centres that help regulate respiration.

The midbrain, like the pons, contains reflex centres for certain cranial nerve reflexes, for example, pupillary reflexes and eye movements, mediated by the third and fourth cranial nerves, respectively.

BOX 20-3 *health matters* | **Vital Centres**

Because the cardiac, vasomotor, and respiratory control centres are essential for survival, they are called the *vital centres.* They serve as the centres for various reflexes controlling heart action, blood vessel diameter, and respiration. Because the medulla contains these centres, it is the most vital part of the entire brain—so vital that injury or disease of the medulla often proves fatal. Blows at the base of the skull and bulbar poliomyelitis, for example, cause death if they interrupt impulse conduction in the vital respiratory centres.

Structure of the Cerebellum

The **cerebellum** (literally "little brain") is located just below the posterior portion of the cerebrum and is partially covered by it (**Figure 20-11**). A transverse fissure separates the cerebellum from the cerebrum.

The cerebellum is the second largest part of the brain (after the cerebrum) but has more neurons than all the other parts of the nervous system combined! Thus the cerebellum has a lot of "computing power" compared with other parts of the brain.

The cerebrum and cerebellum have several structural characteristics in common. For instance, grey matter makes up the outer portion, or *cortex*, of each. White matter predominates in the interior of each. Look at **Figure 20-11**, *C*, and find the internal white matter of the cerebellum called the **arbor vitae** (literally "tree of life"). Note the arbor vitae's distinctive pattern, similar to the branches of a tree. Note, too, that the surfaces of both the cerebellum and the cerebrum have numerous grooves *(sulci)* and raised areas *(gyri)*. The gyri of the cerebellum, however, are much more slender and less prominent than those of the cerebrum. These delicate, roughly parallel gyri are also called **folia** (literally "leaves").

Like the cerebrum, the cerebellum consists of two large lateral masses, the left and right *cerebellar hemispheres*, and a central section called the **vermis.**

The internal white matter of the cerebellum is composed of some short and some long tracts. The shorter tracts conduct impulses from neuron cell bodies located in the cerebellar cortex to neurons whose dendrites and cell bodies compose nuclei located in the interior of the cerebellum. The longer tracts conduct impulses to and from the

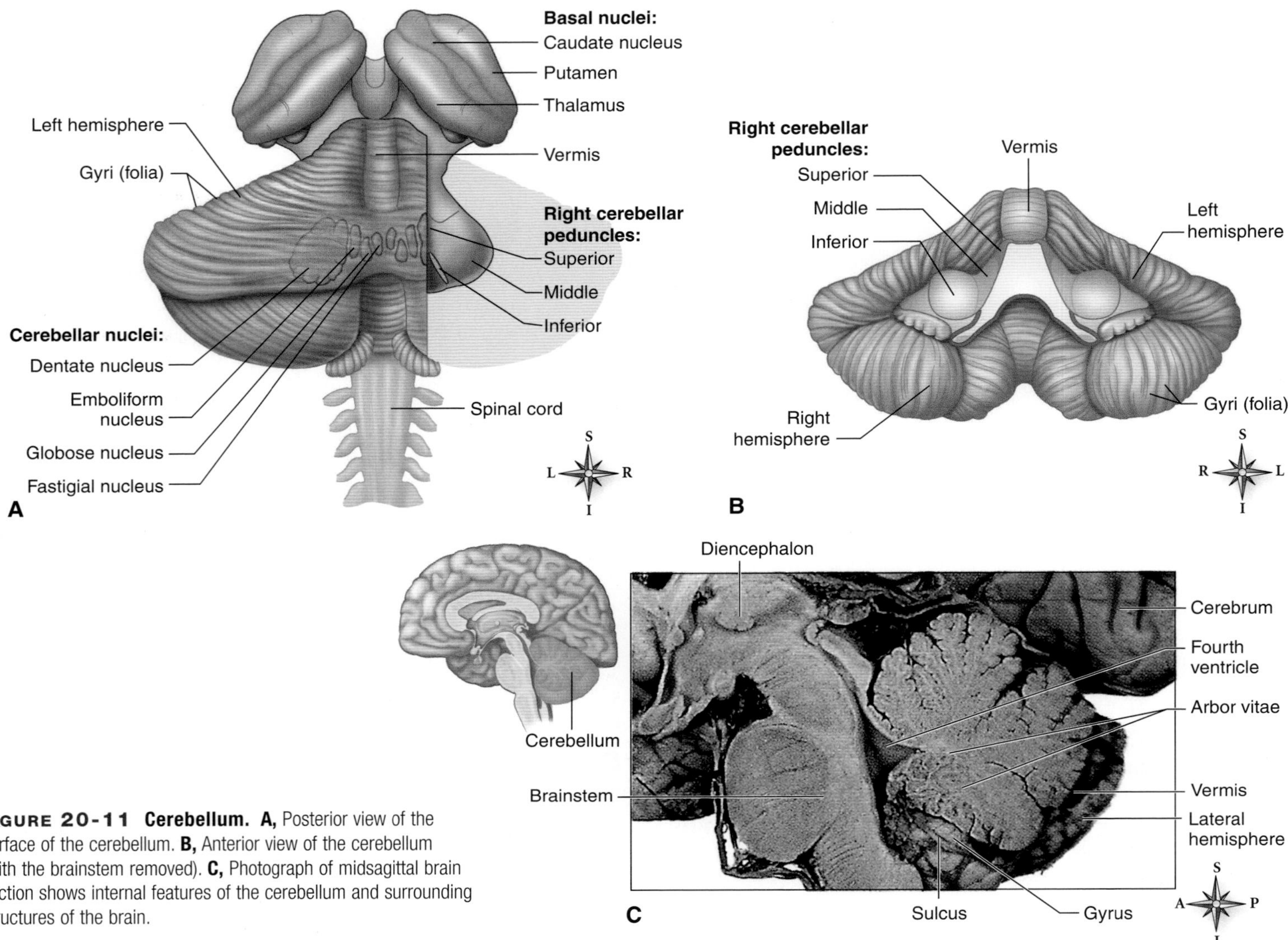

FIGURE 20-11 Cerebellum. A, Posterior view of the surface of the cerebellum. **B,** Anterior view of the cerebellum (with the brainstem removed). **C,** Photograph of midsagittal brain section shows internal features of the cerebellum and surrounding structures of the brain.

cerebellum. Fibres of the longer tracts enter or leave the cerebellum by way of its three pairs of peduncles (see **Figure 20-11**, *B*), as follows:

1. **Inferior cerebellar peduncles:** composed chiefly of tracts into the cerebellum from the medulla and cord (notably spinocerebellar, vestibulocerebellar, and reticulocerebellar tracts)
2. **Middle cerebellar peduncles:** composed almost entirely of tracts into the cerebellum from the pons—that is, pontocerebellar tracts
3. **Superior cerebellar peduncles:** composed principally of tracts from dentate nuclei in the cerebellum through the red nucleus of the midbrain to the thalamus

An important pair of cerebellar nuclei is the **dentate nuclei,** one of which lies in each hemisphere. Tracts connect these nuclei with the thalamus and with motor areas of the cerebral cortex. By means of these tracts, cerebellar impulses influence the motor cortex. Impulses in other tracts enable the motor cortex to influence the cerebellum.

Functions of the Cerebellum

The cerebellum shares similarities with the cerebrum, functionally as well as structurally. The current view of cerebellar function states that the cerebellum performs a variety of different functions that complement or assist the cerebrum, many of which involve the planning and coordination of skeletal muscle activity and maintaining balance in the body.

Coordinated control of muscle action is a function of the upper part of the cerebellum working with the motor control areas of the cerebrum. Normal muscle action involves groups of muscles, the various members of which function together as a unit. In any given action, for example, the prime mover contracts and the antagonist relaxes but then contracts weakly at the proper moment to act as a brake, checking the action of the prime mover. Also, the synergists contract to assist the prime mover, and the fixation muscles of the neighboring joint contract. Through such harmonious, coordinated patterns and group action, normal movements are smooth, steady, and precise as to force, rate, and extent. These patterns, such as the sequence of leg movements needed for walking, are learned and stored in the cerebellum.

Achievement of coordinated movements results from the combined efforts of the cerebrum and cerebellum. Impulses from the cerebrum may trigger the action, but those from the cerebellum plan and coordinate the contractions and relaxations of the various muscles once they have begun.

Figure 20-12 shows how the cerebrum and cerebellum work together. Impulses from the motor control areas of the cerebrum travel down the corticospinal tract and, through peripheral nerves, to skeletal muscle tissue. At the same time, the impulses go to the cerebellum. The cerebellum compares the motor commands of the cerebrum with information coming in from sensory receptors in the muscles (proprioception). Using "sensory maps" of the body, the cerebellum compares the intended movement with the actual state of the body and its current position or movement. Impulses then travel from the cerebellum to both the cerebrum and the muscle tissue to adjust or coordinate the movements to produce the intended action.

Interestingly, the cerebellum becomes involved when a person is just thinking about doing some activity, thus "getting ready" for possible later movement. Some physiologists consider the planning and coordination of movement to be the main functions of the cerebellum.

The cerebellum is also thought to be concerned with both exciting and inhibiting the postural reflexes that help us maintain a stable body position. Sensory impulses from equilibrium (balance) receptors in the ear reach the cerebellum. Using this information, the cerebellum then stimulates or inhibits various muscles to maintain stability of the body.

Not only does the cerebellum work with the cerebrum as a sort of "executive assistant" to coordinate and plan movement and maintain balance—evidence suggests that the cerebellum is an all-around assistant or planner of a variety of functions normally associated with the cerebrum. In fact, it is becoming clear that the cerebellum coordinates incoming sensory information as much or more than it coordinates outgoing motor information.

Cerebellar disease (e.g., abscess, haemorrhage, tumours, trauma) produces certain characteristic symptoms. Predominant among them are ataxia (muscle incoordination), hypotonia, tremors, and disturbances of gait and balance. One example of ataxia is overshooting a mark or stopping before reaching it when trying to touch a given point on the body (finger-to-nose test). Drawling, scanning, and singsong speech are also examples of ataxia. Tremors are particularly pronounced toward the end of the movements and with the exertion of effort. Disturbances of gait and balance vary, depending on the muscle groups involved. The walk, for instance, is often characterized by staggering or lurching and by a clumsy manner of raising the foot too high and bringing it down with a clap. Paralysis does not result from loss of cerebellar function.

To briefly summarize its general functions, the cerebellum:

- Acts with the cerebral cortex to produce skilled movements by planning and coordinating the activities of groups of muscles
- Helps control posture: functions below the level of consciousness to make movements smooth instead of jerky, steady instead of trembling, and efficient and coordinated instead of ineffective, awkward, and uncoordinated
- Controls skeletal muscles to maintain balance
- Coordinates incoming sensory information and acts in other ways to complement and assist various functions of the cerebrum

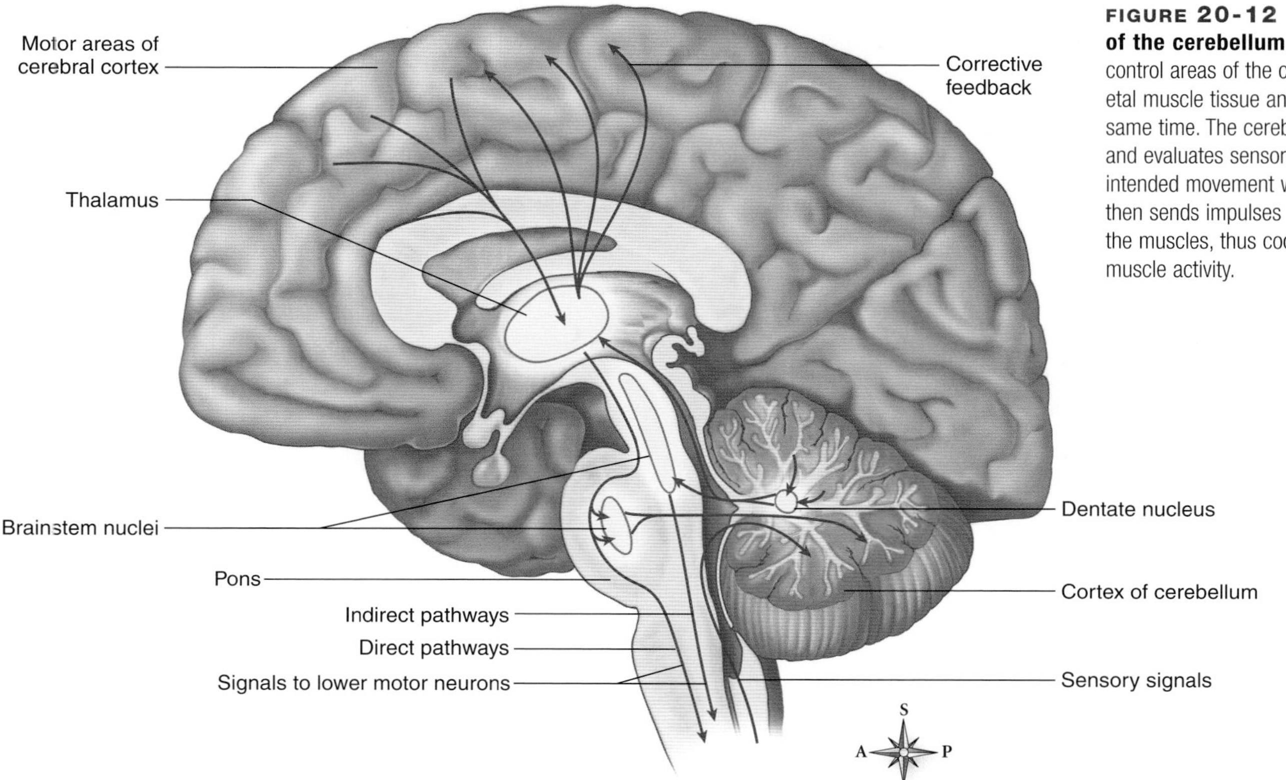

FIGURE 20-12 Coordinating function of the cerebellum. Impulses from the motor control areas of the cerebrum travel down to skeletal muscle tissue and to the cerebellum at the same time. The cerebellum, which also receives and evaluates sensory information, compares the intended movement with the actual movement. It then sends impulses to both the cerebrum and the muscles, thus coordinating and "smoothing" muscle activity.

Quick CHECK

6. Name the three major divisions of the brainstem, and briefly describe the function of each.
7. What are gyri or folia? What are sulci?
8. How does the cerebellum work with the cerebrum to coordinate muscle activity?

DIENCEPHALON

The **diencephalon** (literally, "between brain") is the part of the brain located between the cerebrum and the midbrain (mesencephalon). Although the diencephalon consists of several structures located around the third ventricle, the main ones are the *thalamus* and *hypothalamus*. The diencephalon also includes the **optic chiasma,** the **pineal gland,** and several other small but important structures.

Thalamus

The **thalamus** is a dumbbell-shaped mass of grey matter made up of many nuclei. As **Figure 20-10** and **Figure 20-13** show, each *lateral mass* of the thalamus forms one lateral wall of the third ventricle. Extending through the third ventricle, and thus joining the two lateral masses of the thalamus, is the *intermediate mass*. Two important groups of nuclei that make up the thalamus are the *geniculate bodies*, located in the posterior region of each lateral mass. The geniculate bodies play a role in processing auditory and visual input.

Large numbers of axons conduct impulses into the thalamus from the spinal cord, brainstem, cerebellum, basal nuclei, and various parts of the cerebrum. These axons terminate in thalamic nuclei, where they synapse with neurons whose axons conduct impulses out of the thalamus to virtually all areas of the cerebral cortex. Thus the

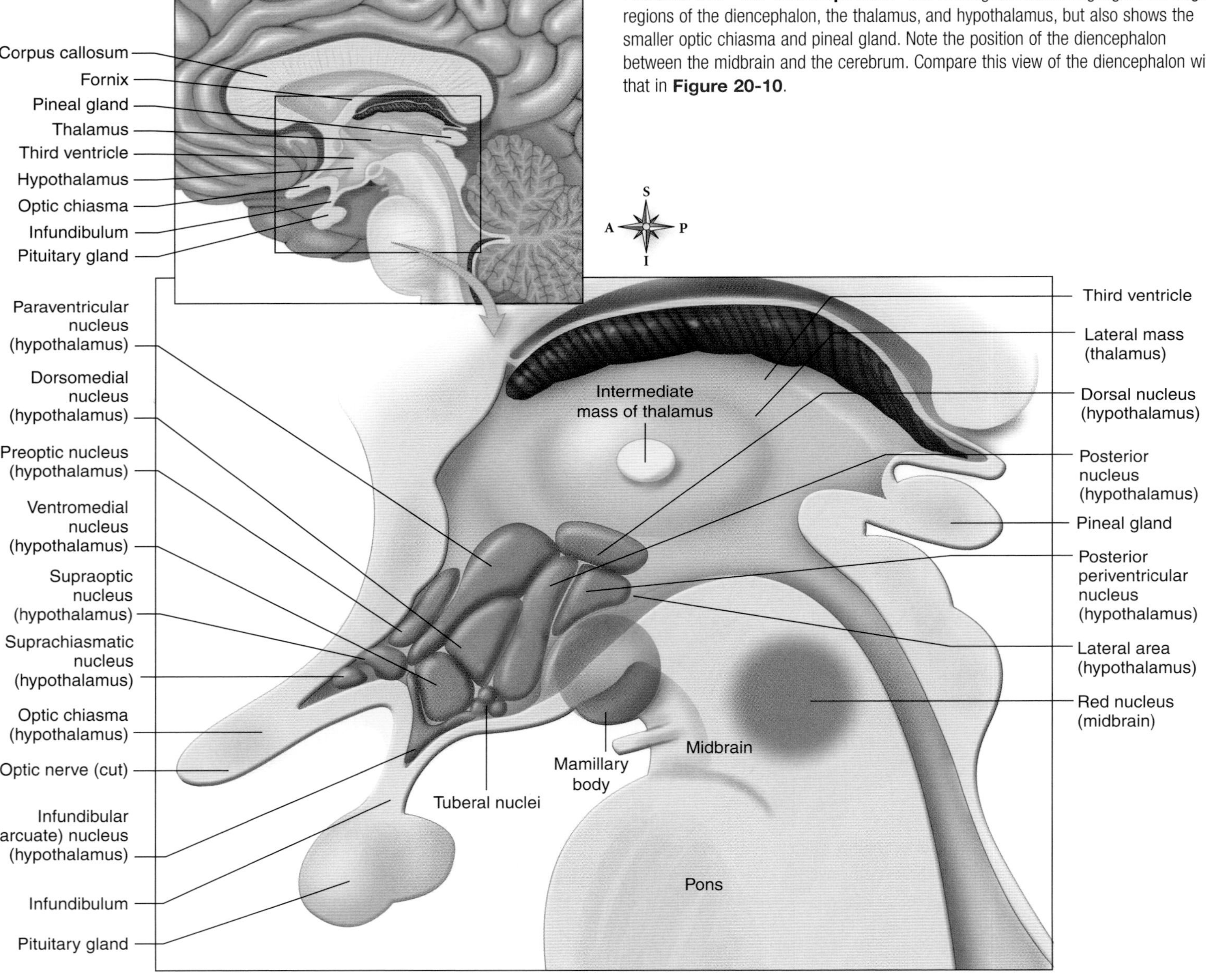

FIGURE 20-13 Diencephalon. This midsagittal section highlights the largest regions of the diencephalon, the thalamus, and hypothalamus, but also shows the smaller optic chiasma and pineal gland. Note the position of the diencephalon between the midbrain and the cerebrum. Compare this view of the diencephalon with that in **Figure 20-10**.

thalamus serves as the major relay station for sensory impulses on their way to the cerebral cortex.

The thalamus performs the following primary functions:

- Plays two parts in the mechanism responsible for sensations
  1. Impulses from appropriate receptors, on reaching the thalamus, produce conscious recognition of the crude, less critical sensations of pain, temperature, and touch
  2. Neurons whose dendrites and cell bodies lie in certain nuclei of the thalamus relay all kinds of sensory impulses, except possibly olfactory, to the cerebrum
- Plays a part in the mechanism responsible for emotions by associating sensory impulses with feelings of pleasantness and unpleasantness
- Plays a part in the arousal or alerting mechanism
- Plays a part in mechanisms that produce complex reflex movements.

Hypothalamus

The **hypothalamus** consists of several structures that lie beneath the thalamus and form the floor of the third ventricle and the lower part of its lateral walls.

Prominent among the structures composing the hypothalamus are the *supraoptic nuclei*, the *paraventricular nuclei*, and the *mamillary bodies*. The supraoptic nuclei consist of grey matter located just above and on either side of the *optic chiasma*. The optic chiasma is the X-shaped junction of the optic tracts and optic nerves. The paraventricular nuclei of the hypothalamus are named for their location, which is close to the wall of the third ventricle. The midportion of the hypothalamus gives rise to the **infundibulum,** the stalk leading to the posterior lobe of the *pituitary gland (neurohypophysis)*. The posterior part of the hypothalamus consists mainly of the mamillary bodies (see **Figure 20-13**, *inset*), which are involved with the olfactory sense (smell).

The hypothalamus is a small but functionally important area of the brain. It weighs little more than 7 grams, yet it performs many functions of the greatest importance both for survival and for the enjoyment of life.

The hypothalamus is widely known as a link between the psyche (mind) and the soma (body). It also links the nervous system to the endocrine system. Certain areas of the hypothalamus function as pleasure centres or reward centres for the primary drives such as eating, drinking, and sex. The following list briefly summarizes hypothalamic functions.

- The hypothalamus functions as a higher autonomic centre or, rather, as several higher autonomic centres. By this we mean that axons of neurons whose dendrites and cell bodies lie in nuclei of the hypothalamus extend in tracts from the hypothalamus to both parasympathetic and sympathetic centres in the brainstem and cord. Thus impulses from the hypothalamus can simultaneously or successively stimulate or inhibit few or many lower autonomic centres. In other words, the hypothalamus serves as a regulator and coordinator of autonomic activities. It helps control and integrate the responses made by autonomic (visceral) effectors all over the body.
- The hypothalamus functions as the major relay station between the cerebral cortex and lower autonomic centres. Tracts conduct impulses from various centres in the cortex to the hypothalamus. Then, by way of numerous synapses in the hypothalamus, these impulses are relayed to other tracts that conduct them on down to autonomic centres in the brainstem and cord and also to spinal cord somatic centres (lower motor neurons). Thus the hypothalamus functions as the link between the cerebral cortex and lower centres—hence between the psyche and the soma. It provides a crucial part of the route by which emotions can express themselves in changed body functions. It is the all-important relay station in the neural pathways that makes possible the mind's influence over the body—sometimes, unfortunately, even to the profound degree of producing psychosomatic disease. The positive benefits of this mind–body link are the dramatic influences our conscious mind can have in healing the body of various illnesses.
- Neurons in the supraoptic and paraventricular nuclei of the hypothalamus synthesize the hormones released by the posterior pituitary gland (neurohypophysis). Because one of these hormones affects the volume of urine excreted, the hypothalamus plays an indirect but essential role in maintaining water balance (see Chapters 42 and 43).
- Some neurons in the hypothalamus have endocrine functions. Their axons secrete chemicals, *releasing hormones*, into blood, which circulate to the anterior pituitary gland. Releasing hormones control the release of certain anterior pituitary hormones—specifically growth hormone and hormones that control hormone secretion by sex glands, the thyroid gland, and the adrenal cortex (discussed in Chapter 26). Thus indirectly the hypothalamus helps control the functioning of every cell in the body.
- The hypothalamus plays an essential role in maintaining the waking state. Presumably it functions as part of an arousal or alerting mechanism. Clinical evidence of this is that somnolence (sleepiness) characterizes some hypothalamic disorders.
- The hypothalamus functions as a crucial part of the mechanism for regulating appetite and therefore the amount of food intake. Experimental and clinical findings indicate the presence of an "appetite centre" in the lateral part of the hypothalamus and a "satiety centre" located medially. For example, an animal with an experimental lesion in the ventromedial nucleus of the hypothalamus consumes tremendous amounts of food. Similarly, a human with a tumour in this region of the hypothalamus may eat insatiably and gain an enormous amount of weight.
- The hypothalamus functions as a crucial part of the mechanism for maintaining normal body temperature. Hypothalamus neurons whose fibres connect with autonomic centres for vasoconstriction, dilation, and sweating and with somatic centres for shivering constitute heat-regulating centres. Marked elevation of body temperature often characterizes injuries or other abnormalities of the hypothalamus.

Pineal Gland

Although the thalamus and hypothalamus account for most of the tissue that makes up the diencephalon, there are several smaller structures of importance.

For example, the *optic chiasma* is a region where the right and left *optic nerves* cross each other before entering the brain—exchanging fibres as they do so. The resulting bundles of fibres are called the *optic tracts.*

Various small nuclei just outside the thalamus and hypothalamus, collectively referred to as the **epithalamus,** are also included among the structures of the diencephalon. One of the most intriguing of the epithalamic structures is the *pineal gland* or *pineal body* (formerly known as the *epiphysis*).

As **Figures 20-10** and **20-13** show, the pineal gland is located just above the corpora quadrigemina of the midbrain. Its name comes from the fact that it resembles a pine nut.

The functions of the pineal gland are still not completely understood. However, we do know that the tiny pineal gland is an important part of the body's biological clock mechanism. The function of the body's internal **biological clock** depends partly on the pineal gland varying its secretion of the hormone **melatonin.** Melatonin is a *hormone* because it is a molecule released into the blood to regulate functions elsewhere in the body—a concept we will explore further in Chapters 25 and 26. However, melatonin is in fact simply an altered form of the neurotransmitter serotonin.

Changing light levels of the sun and moon throughout the day–night cycle trigger changes in the rate of melatonin secretion. When sunlight levels are high, melatonin secretion decreases (**Figure 20-14** and **Figure 2-6**, *E*, on p. 30). When light levels are low, melatonin levels increase proportionally. The changing levels of blood melatonin exhibit a *circadian* cycle that synchronizes the body's internal biological clock mechanisms with the day–night cycle of the external environment.

If we lived in a cave, with no exposure to the sun and moon, our internal clock would still keep our body on a 24- to 25-hour circadian rhythm—but it would not match the external day–night cycle because the pineal gland would not be receiving natural light stimuli from the external environment. Melatonin is thus often called the "timekeeping hormone"—but because high blood levels of melatonin signal the body that it is time to sleep, it is also called the "sleep hormone".

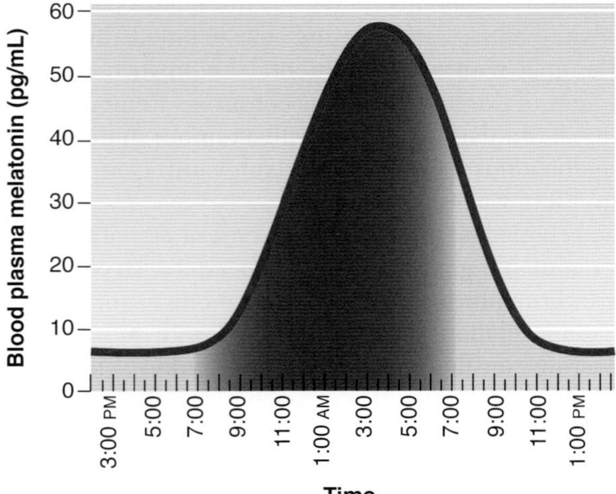

FIGURE 20-14 Melatonin. Graph comparing typical blood melatonin levels throughout the day. Sunlight suppresses melatonin secretion during the day. As the sun goes down, however, melatonin levels begin to rise—dropping again sharply when the sun comes up.

When a person travels to another time zone, or when the seasons change, the altered sunlight patterns cause corresponding time shifts to the melatonin cycle. Likewise, often subtle changes occur in each melatonin cycle depending on how much moonlight (reflected sunlight) is present each evening. Thus the body can sometimes tell what time of the (lunar) month it is—a mechanism that may help regulate the female reproductive cycle.

CONNECT IT! 

To see diagrams that clarify the pineal mechanism of timekeeping in the body, review ***The Timekeeping Hormone*** online at ***Connect It!***

Quick **CHECK**

9. What are the two main components of the diencephalon? Where are they located?
10. Name three general functions of the thalamus.
11. Name three general functions of the hypothalamus.
12. What is the pineal gland's primary function?

STRUCTURE OF THE CEREBRUM

Cerebral Cortex

The **cerebrum,** the largest and uppermost division of the brain, consists of two halves, the right and left **cerebral hemispheres.** The surface of the cerebrum—called the *cerebral cortex*—is made up of grey matter only 2 to 4 mm thick. But despite its thinness, the cortex has six layers, each composed of millions of axon terminals synapsing with millions of dendrites and cell bodies of other neurons.

If one uses a little imagination, the surface of the cerebral cortex looks like a group of small sausages. Each "sausage" is actually a **convolution,** or gyrus. Names of some of these are the *precentral gyrus, postcentral gyrus, cingulate gyrus,* and *hippocampal gyrus (hippocampus).*

Between adjacent gyri lie either shallow grooves called *sulci* or deeper grooves called *fissures* (**Box 20-4**). Fissures, as well as a few, largely imaginary boundaries, divide each cerebral hemisphere into five *lobes.* Four of the lobes are named for the bones that lie over them: **frontal lobe, parietal lobe, temporal lobe,** and **occipital lobe** (**Figure 20-15**). A fifth lobe, the **insula** *(Reil island),* lies hidden from view in the lateral fissure. The lobes are highlighted in **Figure 20-15**. The insula can also be seen in the photographs in **Box 20-2** (p. 448).

Names and locations of prominent cerebral fissures are as follows (see **Figure 20-15**):

- **Longitudinal fissure:** the deepest groove in the cerebrum; divides the cerebrum into two hemispheres
- **Central sulcus (Rolando fissure):** groove between the frontal and parietal lobes
- **Lateral fissure (Sylvius fissure):** a deep groove between the temporal lobe below and the frontal and parietal lobes above; island of Reil lies deep in the lateral fissure
- **Parietooccipital sulcus:** groove that separates the occipital lobe from the parietal lobe

BOX 20-4 *fyi* | Brain Wrinkles

One of the first things that people notice about the brain is the very wrinkled appearance of the two largest regions of the brain: the cerebellum and cerebrum. Wrinkling of the skin is associated with ageing and degeneration, but the wrinkles in the surfaces of these two brain regions provide great advantages. Such folding increases the total amount of grey-matter surface area and thereby increases the processing power of the cerebrum and cerebellum. See a diagram of how this works in ***Brain Wrinkles*** online at ***Connect It!*** •

Fissure
Gyrus
Sulcus
Sulcus
Grey matter
White matter

Wrinkles and grooves of the brain. Grey matter on the surface of the cerebrum is folded to form bumps or gyri. The valleys between the bumps are called *sulci*. Larger sulci are often called *fissures*.

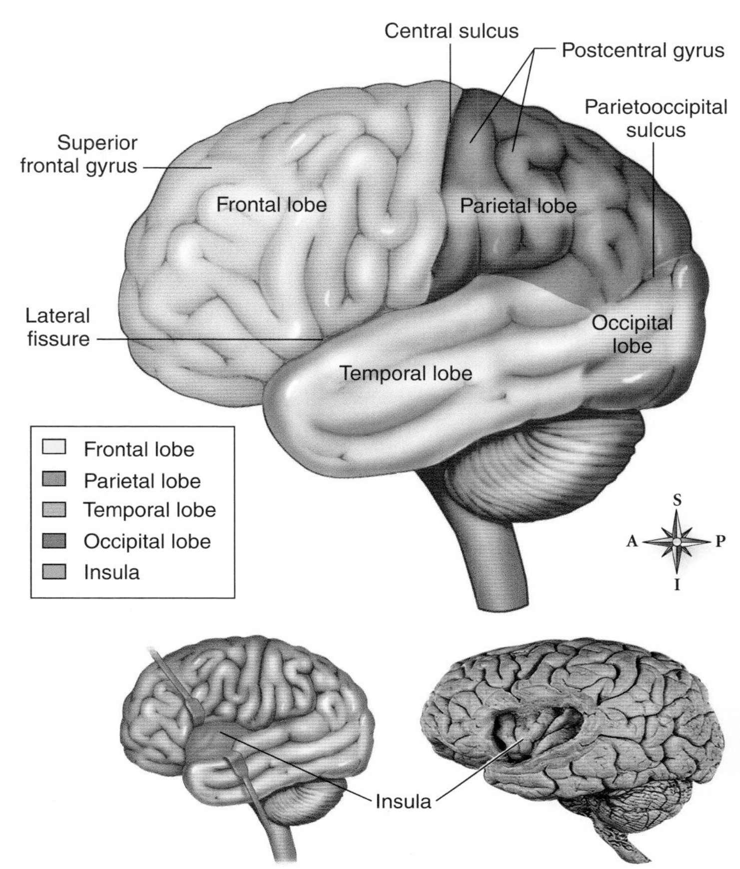

FIGURE 20-15 Left hemisphere of cerebrum, lateral surface. Note the highlighted lobes of the cerebrum.

Cerebral Tracts and Basal Nuclei

Beneath the cerebral cortex lies the large interior of the cerebrum. It is mostly white matter made up of numerous tracts. Tracts that make up the cerebrum's internal white matter are of three types: projection tracts, association tracts, and commissural tracts (**Figure 20-16**).

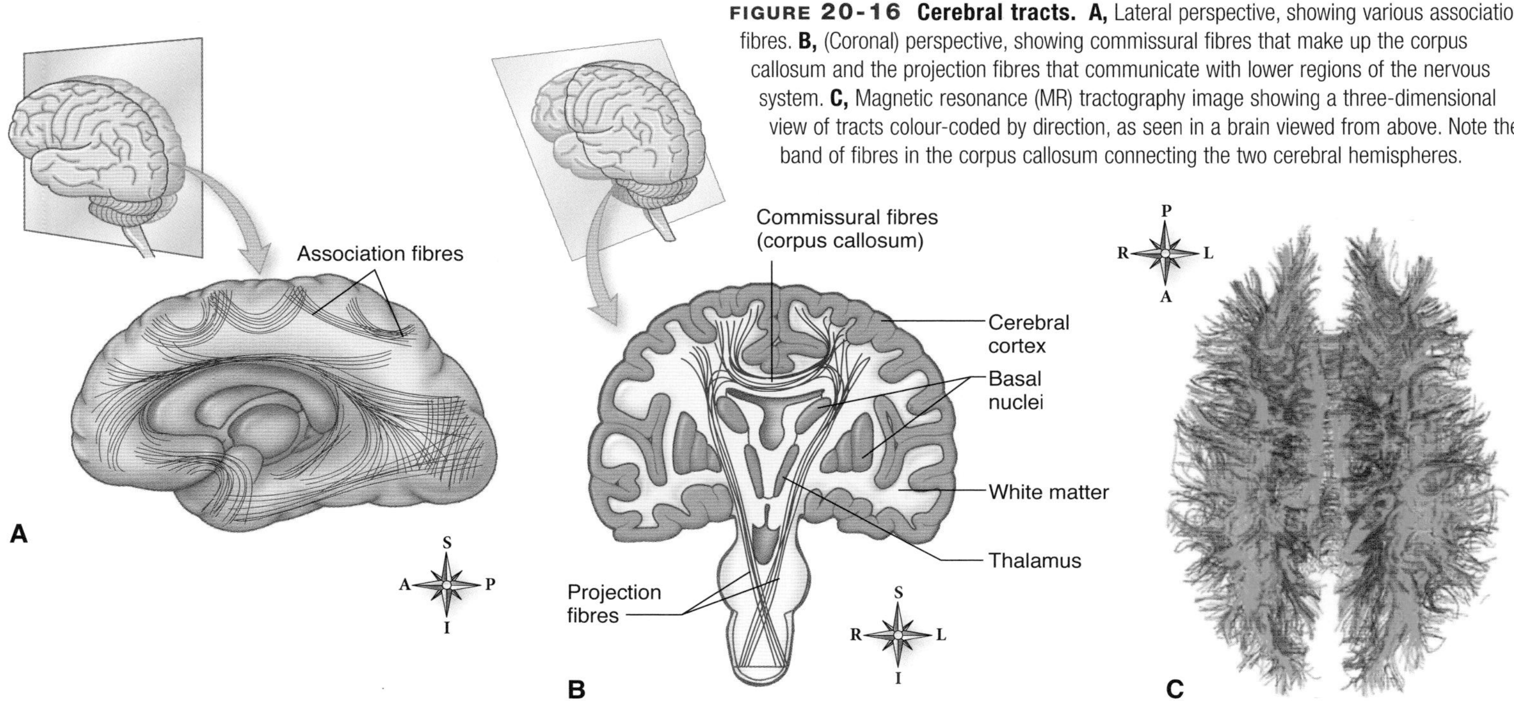

FIGURE 20-16 Cerebral tracts. A, Lateral perspective, showing various association fibres. **B,** (Coronal) perspective, showing commissural fibres that make up the corpus callosum and the projection fibres that communicate with lower regions of the nervous system. **C,** Magnetic resonance (MR) tractography image showing a three-dimensional view of tracts colour-coded by direction, as seen in a brain viewed from above. Note the band of fibres in the corpus callosum connecting the two cerebral hemispheres.

Projection tracts are extensions of the ascending, or sensory, spinothalamic tracts and descending, or motor, corticospinal tracts. *Association tracts* are the most numerous of cerebral tracts; they extend from one convolution to another in the same hemisphere. *Commissural tracts*, in contrast, extend from a point in one hemisphere to a point in the other hemisphere. Commissural tracts compose the **corpus callosum** (prominent white curved structure seen in **Figure 20-9**) and the anterior and posterior commissures.

All of the connections within the human cortex to the rest of the brain—the human **connectome**—are currently being mapped out. This massive, international effort hopes to generate better understanding of the complex functions of the human brain. **Figure 20-16**, *C*, shows an example of a type of magnetic resonance imaging (MRI) technology used in this effort.

A few islands of grey matter lie deep inside the white matter of each hemisphere. Collectively these are called **basal nuclei** (or historically, *basal ganglia*). Basal nuclei, seen in **Figure 20-17**, include the following masses of grey matter in the interior of each cerebral hemisphere:

- **Caudate nucleus:** observe the curving "tail" shape of this basal nucleus
- **Lentiform nucleus:** so named because of its lenslike shape; note in **Figure 20-17** that the lentiform nucleus consists of two structures, the putamen and the pallidum; the putamen lies lateral to the pallidum (also called the *globus pallidus*)
- **Amygdaloid nucleus:** observe the location of this almond-shaped structure at the tip of the caudate nucleus (also called the *amygdala*, literally "almond")

A structure associated with the basal nuclei is the **internal capsule.** It is a large mass of white matter located, as **Figure 20-17** shows, between the caudate and lentiform nuclei and between the lentiform nucleus and thalamus. The caudate nucleus, internal capsule, and lentiform nucleus constitute the *corpus striatum*, a term that means "striped body".

Researchers are still investigating the exact functions of the basal nuclei, but we already know that this part of the cerebrum plays an important role in regulating voluntary motor functions. For example, most of the muscle contractions involved in maintaining posture, walking, and performing other gross or repetitive movements seem to be initiated or modulated in the basal nuclei (**Box 20-5**). The basal nuclei may also play a role in thinking and learning.

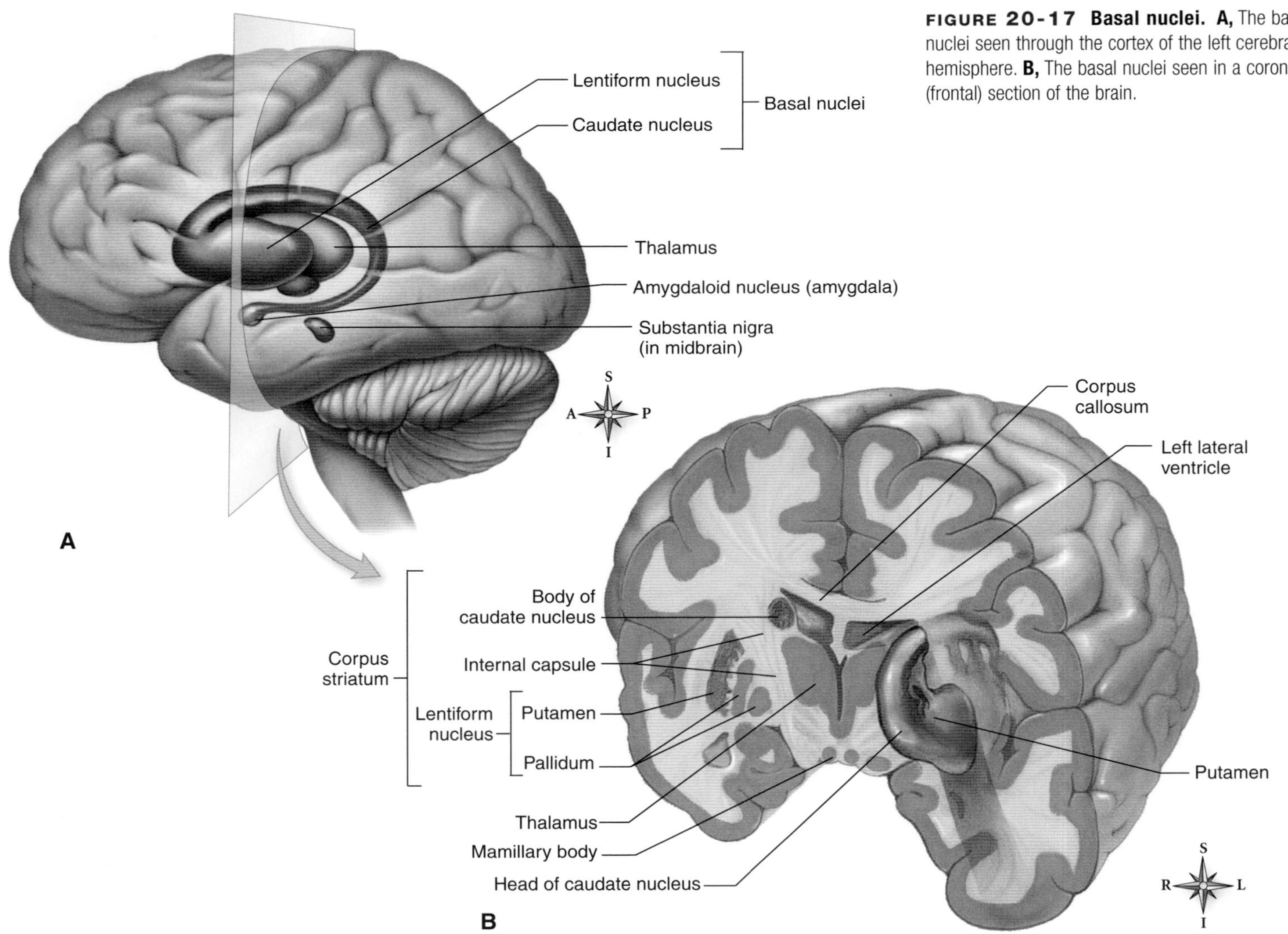

FIGURE 20-17 Basal nuclei. A, The basal nuclei seen through the cortex of the left cerebral hemisphere. **B,** The basal nuclei seen in a coronal (frontal) section of the brain.

BOX 20-5 *health matters* | Parkinson Disease

The importance of the basal nuclei in regulating voluntary motor functions is made clear in cases of **Parkinson disease (PD).** Normally, neurons that lead from the substantia nigra to the basal nuclei secrete dopamine. Dopamine inhibits the excitatory effects of acetylcholine produced by other neurons in the basal nuclei. Such inhibition by *dopaminergic* (dopamine-producing) neurons produces a balanced, restrained output of muscle-regulating signals from the basal nuclei. In PD, however, neurons leading from the substantia nigra degenerate and thus do not release normal amounts of dopamine. Without dopamine, the excitatory effects of acetylcholine are not restrained, and the basal nuclei produce an excess of signals that affect voluntary muscles in several areas of the body. Overstimulation of postural muscles in the neck, trunk, and upper limbs produces the syndrome of effects that typify this disease: rigidity and tremors of the head and limbs; an abnormal, shuffling gait; absence of relaxed arm-swinging while walking; and a forward tilting of the trunk.

Frontal lobe
Basal nuclei
Dopamine pathways
A
Forward tilt of trunk
Rigidity and trembling of head
Reduced arm-swinging
Rigidity and trembling of extremities
Shuffling gait with short steps
B

A, Dopaminergic pathways of the brain. **B,** Signs of Parkinson disease (PD).

Quick CHECK

13. Name the five lobes that make up each cerebral hemisphere. Where is each located?
14. Name the basal nuclei, and describe where they are located within the cerebrum.

Functions of the Cerebral Cortex

Functional Areas of the Cortex

During the past few decades, research scientists in various fields—neurophysiology, neurosurgery, neuropsychiatry, and others—have added mountains of information to our knowledge about the brain. However, new questions come faster than answers, and a clear, complete understanding of the brain's mechanisms still eludes us. Perhaps it always will. Perhaps the capacity of the human brain falls short of the ability to fully understand its own complexity.

We do know that certain areas of the cortex in each hemisphere of the cerebrum engage predominantly in one particular function—at least on the average. Differences between genders and among individuals of both genders are not uncommon. The fact that many cerebral functions have a typical location is known as the concept of cerebral localization. The concept that localization of function varies from person to person, and even at different times in an individual's life when the brain has sustained damage, is called **cerebral plasticity.**

The function of each region of the cerebral cortex depends on the structures with which it communicates. For example, the postcentral gyrus (**Figure 20-18** and **Figure 20-19**) functions mainly as a general somatic sensory area. It receives impulses from receptors activated by heat, cold, and touch stimuli. The precentral gyrus, on the other hand, functions chiefly as the somatic motor area (see **Figures 20-18** and **20-19**). Impulses from neurons in this area descend over motor tracts and eventually stimulate somatic effectors, the skeletal muscles. The transverse gyrus of the temporal lobe serves as the primary auditory area. The primary visual areas are in the occipital lobe. It is important to remember that no part of the brain functions alone. Many structures of the central nervous system must function together for any one part of the brain to function normally.

CONNECT IT!

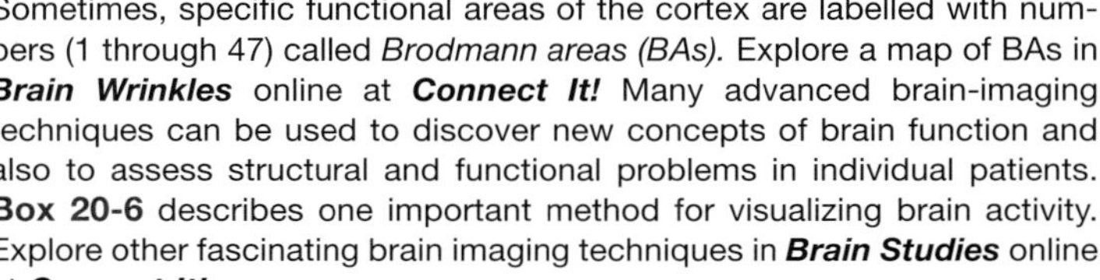
Sometimes, specific functional areas of the cortex are labelled with numbers (1 through 47) called *Brodmann areas (BAs).* Explore a map of BAs in ***Brain Wrinkles*** online at ***Connect It!*** Many advanced brain-imaging techniques can be used to discover new concepts of brain function and also to assess structural and functional problems in individual patients. **Box 20-6** describes one important method for visualizing brain activity. Explore other fascinating brain imaging techniques in ***Brain Studies*** online at ***Connect It!***

UNIT 3

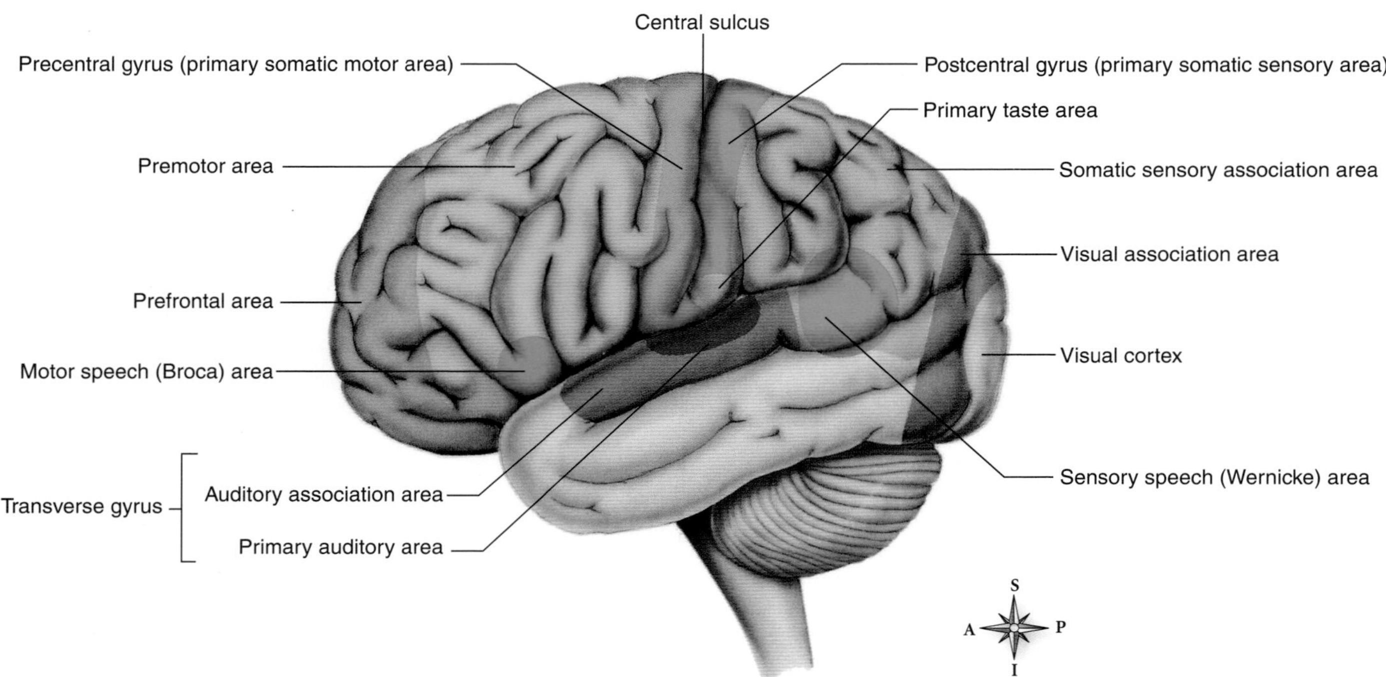

FIGURE 20-18 Functional areas of the cerebral cortex.

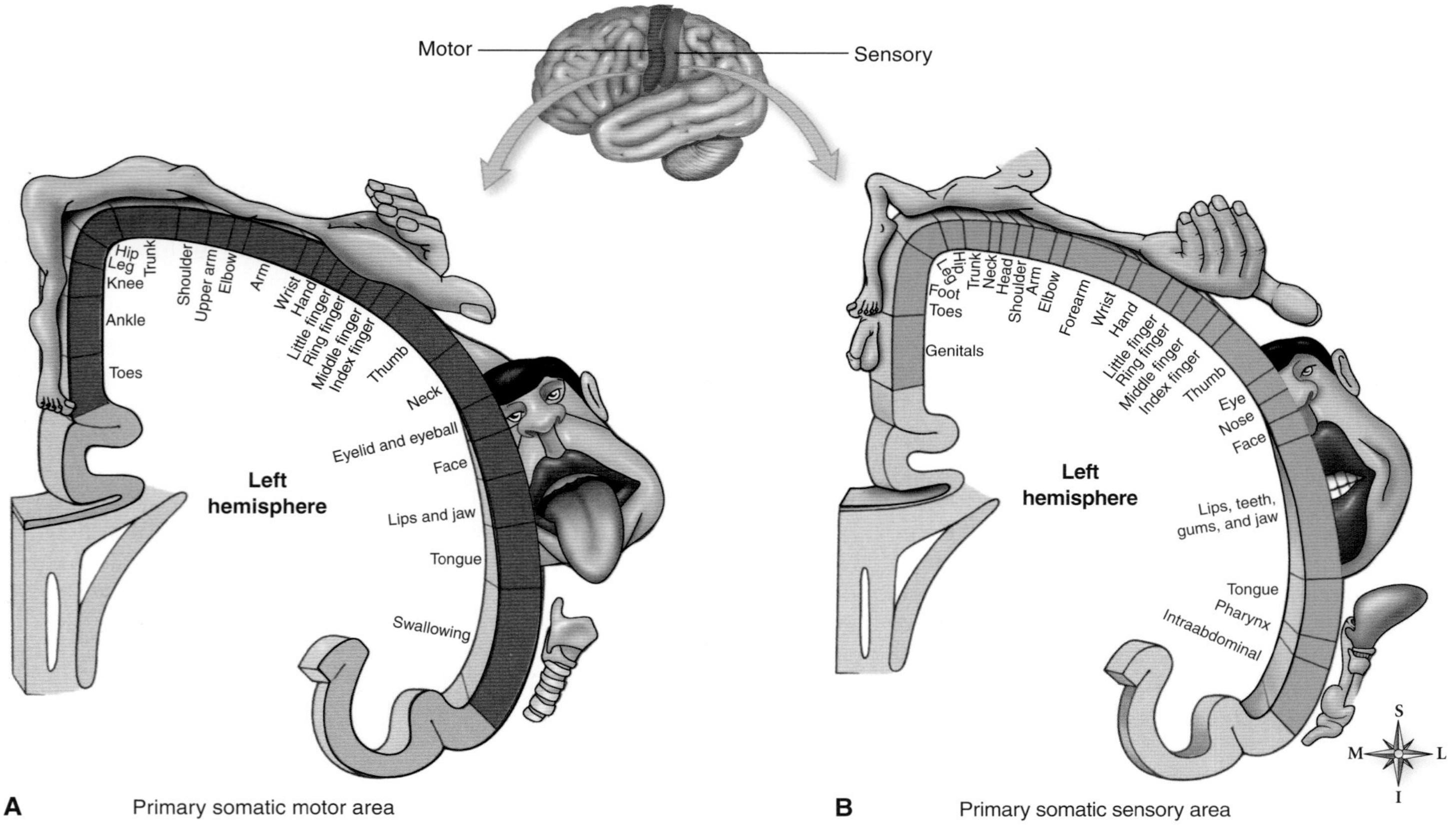

FIGURE 20-19 Primary somatic motor (A) and sensory (B) areas of the cortex. The body parts illustrated here show which parts of the body are "mapped" to specific areas of each cortical area. The exaggerated face indicates that more cortical area is devoted to processing information to and from the many receptors and motor units of the face than for the leg or arm, for example.

BOX 20-6 *diagnostic study* | The Electroencephalogram (EEG)

Cerebral activity goes on as long as life itself. Only when life ceases (or moments before) does the cerebrum cease its functioning. Only then do all its neurons stop conducting impulses. Proof of this has come from records of brain electrical potentials known as **electroencephalograms,** or **EEGs.** These records are usually made from data detected by a number of electrodes placed on different regions of the scalp; they are records of wave activity—*brainwaves* (parts *A* and *B* of the figure).

Four types of brainwaves are recognized based on frequency and amplitude of the waves. Frequency, or the number of wave cycles per second, is usually expressed in *hertz* (Hz, from Hertz, a German physicist). Amplitude means voltage. Listed in order of frequency from fastest to slowest, brainwaves are designated as *beta, alpha, theta,* and *delta. Beta waves* have a frequency of more than 13 Hz and a relatively low voltage. *Alpha waves* have a frequency of 8 to 13 Hz and a relatively high voltage. *Theta waves* have both a relatively low frequency—4 to 7 Hz—and a low voltage. *Delta waves* have the slowest frequency—less than 4 Hz—but a high voltage. Brainwaves vary in different regions of the brain, in different states of awareness, and in abnormal conditions of the cerebrum.

Fast, low-voltage beta waves characterize EEGs recorded from the frontal and central regions of the cerebrum when an individual is awake, alert, and attentive, with eyes open. Beta waves predominate when the cerebrum is busiest, that is, when it is engaged with sensory stimulation or mental activities. In short, beta waves are "busy waves". Alpha waves, in contrast, are "relaxed waves". They are moderately fast, relatively high-voltage waves that dominate EEGs recorded from the parietal lobe, occipital lobe, and posterior parts of the temporal lobes when the cerebrum is idling, so to speak. The individual is awake but has eyes closed and is in a relaxed, nonattentive state. This state is sometimes called the "alpha state". When drowsiness descends, moderately slow, low-voltage theta waves appear. Theta waves are "drowsy waves". "Deep sleep waves", on the other hand, are known as delta waves. These slowest brainwaves characterize the deep sleep from which one is not easily aroused. For this reason, deep sleep is referred to as slow-wave sleep.

Physicians use EEGs to help localize areas of brain dysfunction, to identify altered states of consciousness, and often to establish death. Two flat EEG recordings (no brainwaves) taken 24 hours apart in conjunction with no spontaneous respiration and total absence of somatic reflexes are criteria accepted as evidence of brain death. •

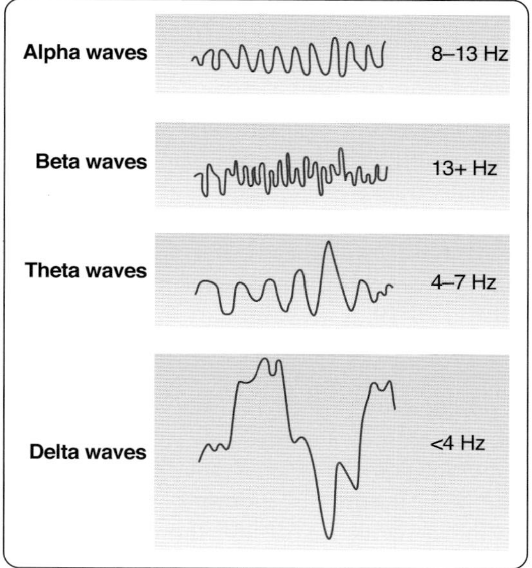

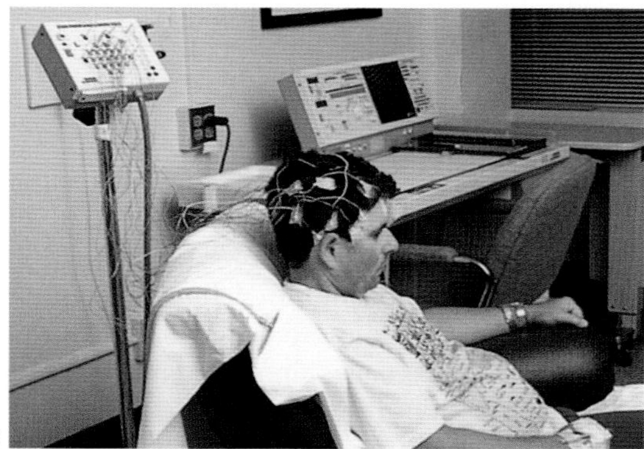

The electroencephalogram (EEG). A, Examples of alpha, beta, theta, and delta waves seen on an EEG. **B,** Photograph showing a person undergoing an EEG test. Notice the scalp electrodes that detect voltage fluctuations within the cranium.

Sensory Functions of the Cortex

Various areas of the cerebral cortex are essential for normal functioning of the somatic, or "general", senses, as well as the so-called special senses. The somatic senses include sensations of touch, pressure, temperature, body position (proprioception), and similar perceptions that do not require complex sensory organs. The special senses include vision, hearing, and other types of perception that require complex sensory organs, such as the eye and the ear.

As stated earlier, the postcentral gyrus serves as a primary area for the general somatic senses. As **Figure 20-19**, *B*, shows, sensory fibres carrying information from receptors in specific parts of the body terminate in specific regions of the somatic sensory area. In other words, the cortex contains a sort of "somatic sensory map" of the body. Areas such as the face and hand have a proportionally larger number of sensory receptors, so their part of the somatic sensory map is larger. Likewise, information regarding vision is mapped in the visual cortex, and auditory information is mapped in the primary auditory area (see **Figure 20-18**).

The cortex does more than just register separate and simple sensations, however. Information sent to the primary sensory areas is in turn relayed to the various sensory association areas, as well as to other parts of the brain. There the sensory information is compared and evaluated. Eventually, the cortex integrates separate bits of information into whole perceptions.

Suppose, for example, that someone put an ice cube in your hand. You would, of course, see it and sense something cold touching your hand. But also you would probably know that it was an ice cube because you would perceive a total impression compounded of many sensations such as temperature, shape, size, colour, weight, texture, and movement and position of your hand and arm.

Discussion of somatic sensory pathways begins on p. 464. The special senses are discussed in Chapter 24.

Motor Functions of the Cortex

Mechanisms that control voluntary movements are extremely complex and imperfectly understood. It is known, however, that for normal movements to take place, many parts of the nervous system—including certain areas of the cerebral cortex—must function.

The precentral gyrus—that is, the most posterior gyrus of the frontal lobe—constitutes the primary somatic motor area (see **Figures 20-18** and **20-19**, A). A secondary motor area lies in the gyrus immediately anterior to the precentral gyrus. Neurons in the precentral gyrus are said to control individual muscles, especially those that produce movements of distal joints (wrist, hand, finger, ankle, foot, and toe movements). Notice in **Figure 20-19** that the primary somatic motor area is mapped according to the specific areas of the body it controls. Neurons in the premotor area just anterior to the precentral gyrus are thought to activate groups of muscles simultaneously.

Motor pathways descending from the cerebrum through the brainstem and spinal cord are discussed on pp. 466–468. Autonomic motor pathways are discussed in Chapter 22.

Integrative Functions of the Cortex

Integrative functions is a murky term. Even more obscure, however, are the neural processes it designates. They consist of all events that take place in the cerebrum between its reception of sensory impulses and its sending out of motor impulses. Integrative functions of the cerebrum include consciousness and mental activities of all kinds. Consciousness, use of language, emotions, and memory are the integrative cerebral functions that we shall discuss—but only briefly.

Consciousness

Consciousness may be defined as a state of awareness of oneself, one's environment, and other humans. Very little is known about the neural mechanisms that produce consciousness. We do know, however, that consciousness depends on excitation of cortical neurons by impulses conducted to them by a network of neurons known as the *reticular activating system*.

The **reticular activating system** (**RAS**) consists of centres in the brainstem's *reticular formation* that receive impulses from the spinal cord and relay them to the thalamus and from the thalamus to all parts of the cerebral cortex (**Figure 20-20**). Both direct spinal reticular tracts and collateral fibres from the sensory tracts (spinothalamic, lemniscal, auditory, and visual) relay impulses over the reticular activating system to the cortex. Without continual excitation of cortical neurons by reticular activating impulses, an individual is unconscious and cannot be aroused. Here, then, are two current concepts about the reticular activating system: (1) It functions as the arousal or alerting system for the cerebral cortex, and (2) its functioning is crucial for maintaining consciousness. Drugs known to depress the reticular activating system decrease alertness and induce sleep.

Barbiturates, for example, produce these effects. On the other hand, amphetamine, a drug known to stimulate the cerebrum and to enhance alertness and produce wakefulness, probably acts by stimulating the reticular activating system.

Certain variations in the levels or state of consciousness are normal. All of us, for example, experience different levels of wakefulness. At times, we are highly alert and attentive. At other times, we are relaxed and nonattentive. All of us also experience different levels of sleep.

In addition to the various normal states of consciousness, altered states of consciousness also occur in certain conditions. Anaesthetic drugs produce an altered state of consciousness, namely, *anaesthesia*. Disease or injury of the brain may produce an altered state called **coma.**

Peoples of various cultures have long been familiar with an altered state called *meditation*. Meditation is a waking state but differs markedly in certain respects from the usual waking state. According to some, meditation is a "higher" or "expanded" level of consciousness. This higher consciousness is accompanied, almost paradoxically, by a high degree of both relaxation and alertness. With training in meditation techniques and practice, an individual can enter the meditative state at will and remain in it for an extended period.

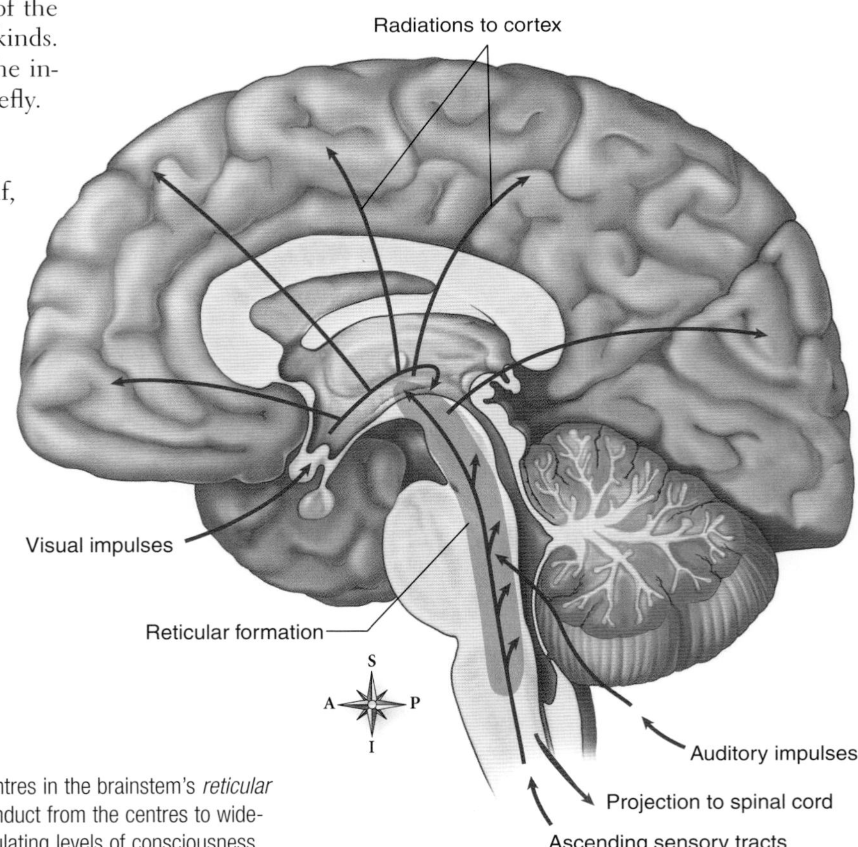

FIGURE 20-20 Reticular activating system (RAS). Consists of centres in the brainstem's *reticular formation* plus fibres that conduct to the centres from below and fibres that conduct from the centres to widespread areas of the cerebral cortex. Functioning of the RAS is essential for regulating levels of consciousness.

CONNECT IT! 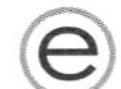

Sleep is a fascinating and mysterious process that we are just beginning to understand. What we do understand is that sleep involves changes in the level of brain activity, as seen in the figure. Shortly after falling asleep, we fall into a deep **slow-wave sleep (SWS)** characterized by slow electroencephalogram (EEG) waves. Approximately every 90 minutes or so, brain activity increases during a dream stage called **rapid eye movement (REM) sleep.** Learn more about the sleep cycle in ***Sleep*** online at ***Connect It!***

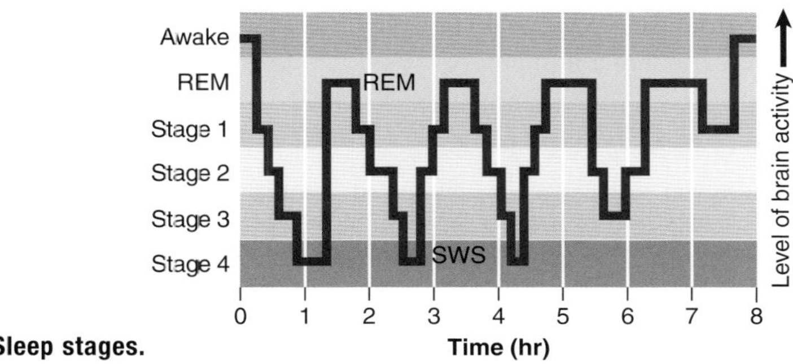

Sleep stages.

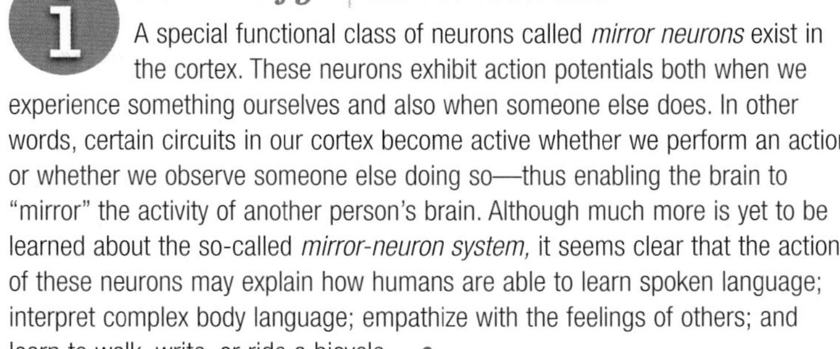

BOX 20-7 *fyi* **Mirror Neurons**

A special functional class of neurons called *mirror neurons* exist in the cortex. These neurons exhibit action potentials both when we experience something ourselves and also when someone else does. In other words, certain circuits in our cortex become active whether we perform an action or whether we observe someone else doing so—thus enabling the brain to "mirror" the activity of another person's brain. Although much more is yet to be learned about the so-called *mirror-neuron system,* it seems clear that the action of these neurons may explain how humans are able to learn spoken language; interpret complex body language; empathize with the feelings of others; and learn to walk, write, or ride a bicycle. •

Language

Language functions consist of the ability to speak and write words and the ability to understand spoken and written words. Certain areas in the frontal, parietal, and temporal lobes serve as speech centres—as crucial areas, that is, for language functions. The left cerebral hemisphere contains these areas in about 90% of the population; in the remaining 10%, either the right hemisphere or both hemispheres contain them.

Lesions in speech centres give rise to language defects called *aphasias*. For example, with damage to an area in the inferior gyrus of the frontal lobe (motor speech area, see **Figure 20-18**), a person becomes unable to articulate words but can still make vocal sounds and understand words heard and read.

Box 20-7 discusses a newly discovered class of neurons that may help us learn and use language.

Emotions

Emotions—both the subjective experiencing of them and the objective expression of them—involve functioning of the cerebrum's **limbic system.** The name *limbic* (Latin for "border or fringe") suggests the shape of the cortical structures that make up the system. They form a curving border around the corpus callosum, the structure that connects the two cerebral hemispheres.

Look now at **Figure 20-21**. Here on the medial surface of the cerebrum lie most of the structures of the limbic system. They are the cingulate gyrus and the hippocampus (the extension of the hippocampal gyrus that protrudes into the floor of the inferior horn of the lateral ventricle). These limbic system structures have primary connections with various other parts of the brain, notably the thalamus, fornix, septal nucleus, amygdaloid nucleus (the tip of the caudate nucleus, one of the basal nuclei), and the hypothalamus. Some physiologists therefore include these connected structures as parts of the limbic system.

The limbic system (or to use its more descriptive name, the *emotional brain*) functions in some way to make us experience many kinds of emotions—anger, fear, joy, sadness, surprise, and disgust, for example. To bring about the normal expression of emotions, parts of the cerebral cortex other than the limbic system must also function. Considerable evidence exists to indicate that limbic activity without the modulating influence of the other cortical areas may bring on the attacks of abnormal, uncontrollable rage suffered periodically by some unfortunate individuals.

Memory

Memory is one of our major mental activities. The cortex is capable of storing and retrieving both *short-term memory* and *long-term memory*. Short-term memory involves the storage of information over a few seconds or minutes. Short-term memories can be somehow

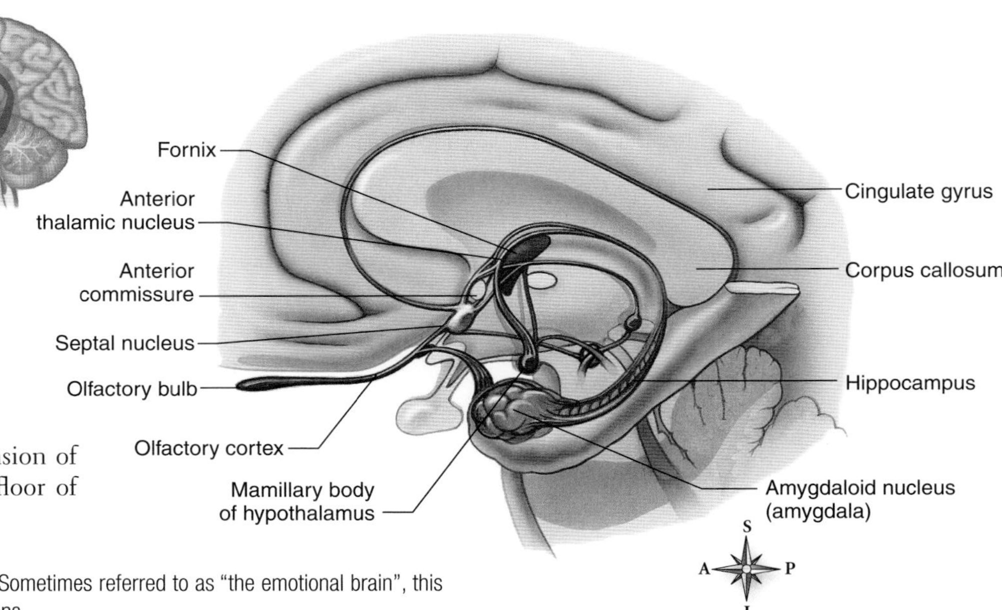

FIGURE 20-21 Structures of the limbic system. Sometimes referred to as "the emotional brain", this network of brain structures functions as we experience emotions.

consolidated by the brain and stored as long-term memories that can be retrieved days—or even years—later.

Both short-term memory and long-term memory are functions of many parts of the cerebral cortex, especially of the temporal, parietal, and occipital lobes. Findings by Dr. Wilder Penfield, a noted Canadian neurosurgeon, first gave evidence of this almost 100 years ago. He electrically stimulated the temporal lobes of epileptic patients undergoing brain surgery. They responded, much to his surprise, by recalling in the most minute detail songs and events from their past.

Such long-term memories are believed to consist of some kind of structural changes in the synapses of the cerebral cortex, as you learned in Chapter 19 (see pp. 423–424). Repeated impulse conduction over a given neuronal circuit produces the synaptic change. Two possible changes are an increase in the number of presynaptic axon terminals or an increase in the number of receptor proteins in the postsynaptic neuron's membrane. Other possible changes involve changes in the average concentrations of neurotransmitters at certain synapses or changes in the functions of astrocytes. All of these changes somehow facilitate impulse transmission at the synapses.

More recent data suggest that different kinds of memories may be stored in different ways. Some memories are perhaps stored by way of changes at synapses and some by changes in the neurons themselves. For example, some neurons have been shown to react only when a specific person is seen or mentioned—thus somehow acting as a "recognition neuron" for the particular individual who is recognized.

Many research findings indicate that the cerebrum's limbic system—the "emotional brain"—plays a key role in memory. To mention one role, when the hippocampus (part of the limbic system) is removed, the patient loses the ability to recall new information. Your own personal experience substantiates a relationship between emotion and memory.

CONNECT IT!

Have you ever heard someone called "left-brained" or "right-brained" in their approach to work or learning? What does that mean? Find out in ***Specialization of Cerebral Hemispheres*** online at ***Connect It!***

Table 20-4 briefly summarizes the major structures and functions of the central nervous system. Take a moment now to review it. This will help you reinforce what you have just learned about the CNS before moving on to the last topics of the chapter.

TABLE 20-4 Summary of CNS Structures and Functions

REGION	STRUCTURE*	FUNCTION*
Spinal cord 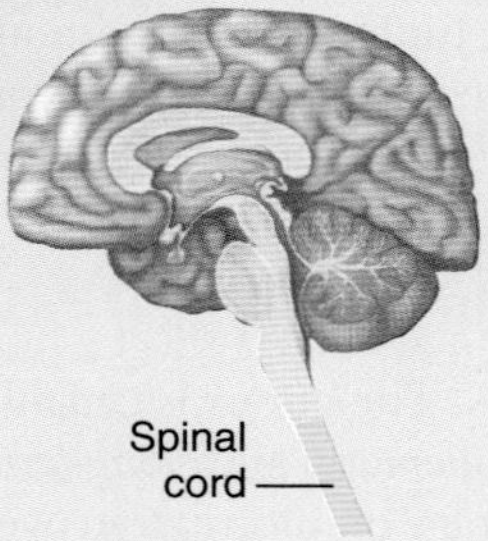	Elongated cylinder extending from the brainstem through the foramen magnum of the skull; grey matter interior surrounded by white matter; 31 pairs of spinal nerves attached by dorsal and ventral nerve roots	Integration of simple, subconscious spinal reflexes; conduction of nerve impulses
Grey matter	Numerous synapses and interneurons arranged into anterior, lateral, and posterior grey columns linked by a grey commissure	Integration of spinal reflexes and filtering of information going to higher centres (as in gated pain control)
White matter	Myelinated nerve tracts arranged into anterior, lateral, and posterior white columns (funiculi)	Ascending tracts conduct sensory information to higher CNS centres; descending tracts conduct motor information from higher CNS centres
Brainstem	Extends inferiorly from diencephalon to foramen magnum of skull, where it meets the spinal cord; central grey matter nuclei surrounded and connected by white matter tracts; 10 of the 12 pairs of cranial nerves attached here	Subconscious integration of basic vital functions
Medulla oblongata 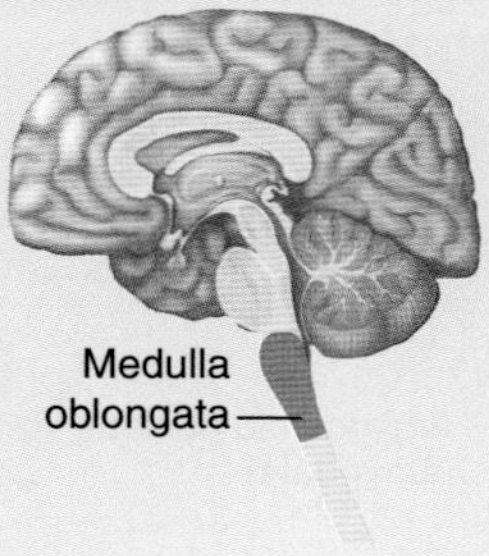	Inferior region of brainstem between the spinal cord and the pons	Integration of cardiac, vasomotor (vessel muscle), respiratory, digestive and other reflexes

*Summary only; see chapter text and figures for detailed descriptions of structure and function.

CNS, Central nervous system.

TABLE 20-4 Summary of CNS Structures and Functions—cont'd

REGION	STRUCTURE*	FUNCTION*
Pons 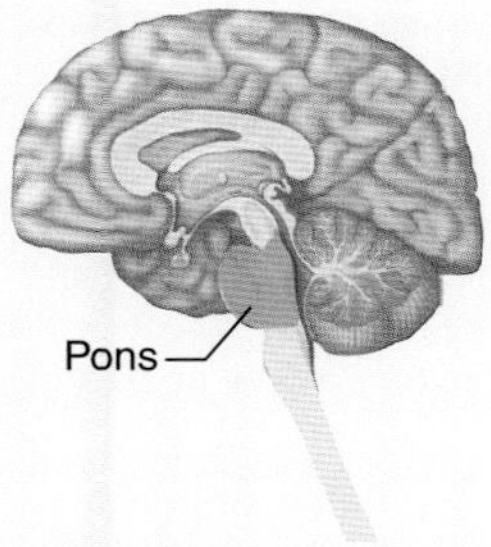	Intermediate region of brainstem between the medulla and the midbrain	Integration of numerous autonomic reflexes mediated by cranial nerves V, VI, VII, and VIII (see Chapters 21 and 22) and respiration
Midbrain 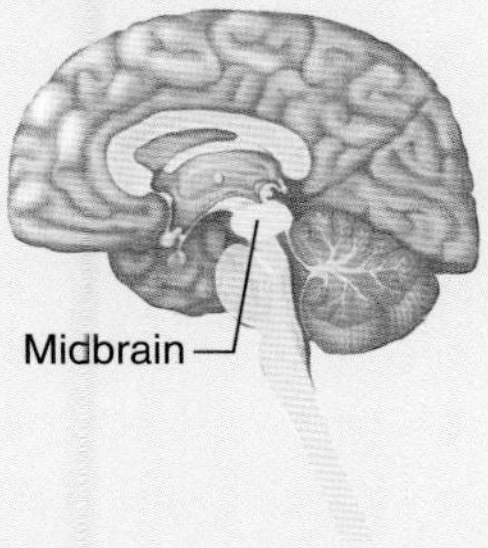	Superior region of the brainstem between the pons and the diencephalon	Integration of numerous cranial nerve reflexes, such as eye movements, pupillary reflex, ear (sound muffling) reflexes
Reticular formation 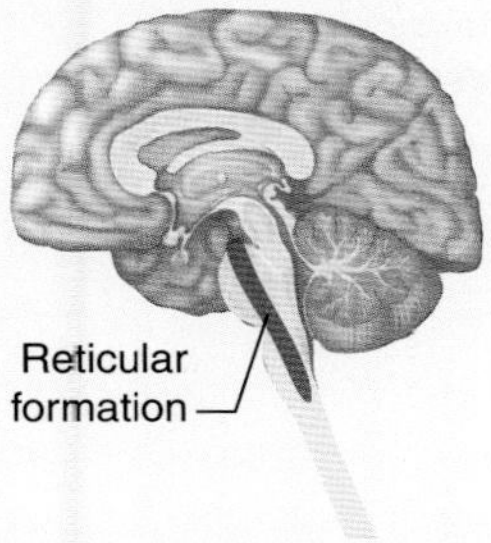	Roughly cylindrical network of nerve pathways and centres extending through the brainstem and into the diencephalon	Operates the reticular activating system (RAS) that regulates state of consciousness
Cerebellum 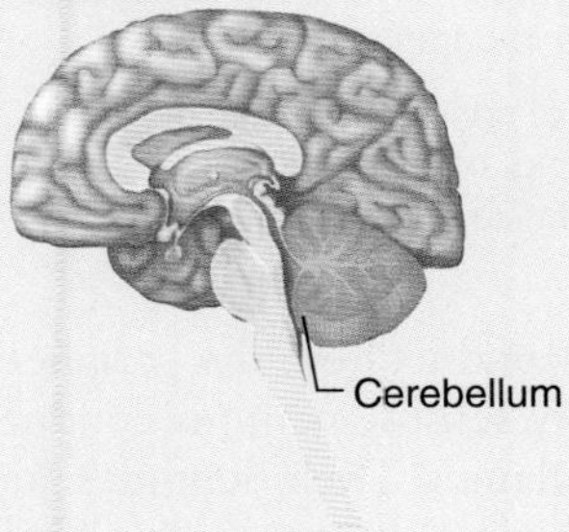	Roughly spherical structure attached at the posterior of the brainstem; wrinkled grey matter cortex, branched network of white fibres inside (arbor vitae), and several small grey nuclei	Coordinates many functions of cerebrum, including planning and control of skilled movements, posture, balance, coordination of sensory information relating to body position and movement
Diencephalon 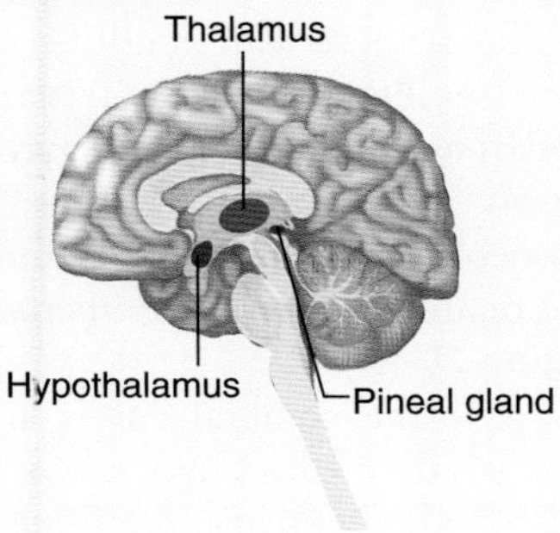	Brain region in the central part of the brain, between the cerebrum and brainstem (midbrain); made up of various grey-matter nuclei	Numerous coordinating and integrating functions

(continued)

TABLE 20-4 Summary of CNS Structures and Functions—cont'd

REGION	STRUCTURE*	FUNCTION*
Thalamus	Large ovoid of grey matter, divided into two large lateral masses connected by an intermediate mass	Crude sensations, coordination of sensory information relayed to cerebrum; involved in emotional response to sensory information; involved in arousal; general processing of information to/from cerebrum
Hypothalamus	Numerous grey-matter nuclei clustered below the thalamus	Integration/coordination of many autonomic reflexes, hormonal functions; involved in arousal, appetite, thermoregulation
Pineal gland	Single nucleus of neuroendocrine tissue posterior to the thalamus	Produces melatonin, a timekeeping hormone, as part of the body's biological clock
Cerebrum 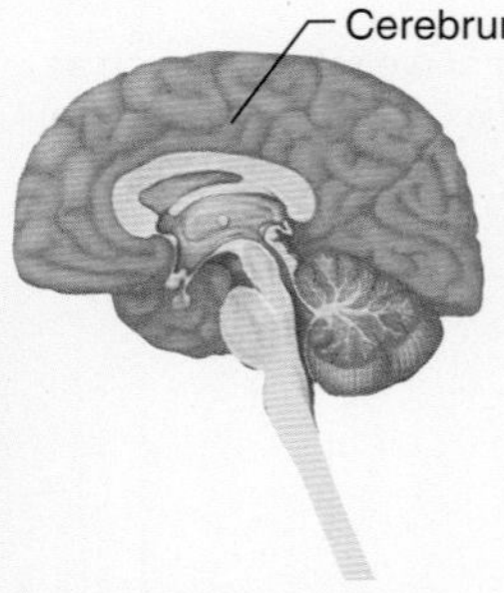	Largest, most superior region of brain; divided into right and left hemispheres, connected by the corpus callosum	Complex processing of sensory and motor information; complex integrative functions
Cerebral cortex 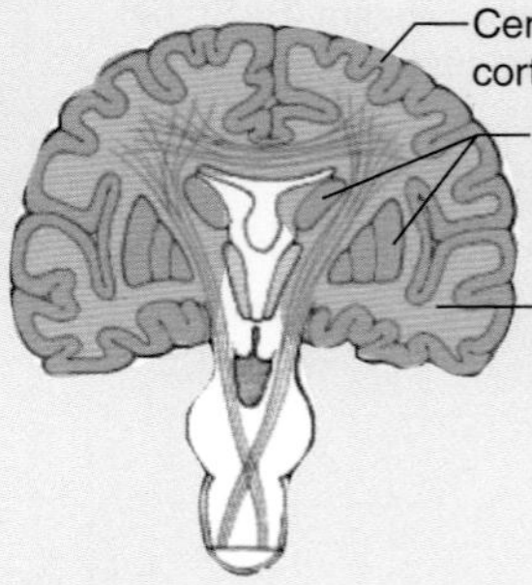	Highly wrinkled grey-matter surface of the cerebrum; divided into five major lobes per hemisphere; functionally mapped based on concept of localization	Higher-level processing of sensory and motor information, including conscious sensation and motor control; complex integrative functions such as consciousness, language, memory, emotions
Cerebral tracts	White-matter tracts connect various regions of the cortex with each other and with inferior CNS structures	Conduction information between CNS areas to facilitate complex processing and integration
Basal nuclei	Grey-matter nuclei deep in the cerebrum	Integration and regulation of conscious motor control, especially posture, walking, other repetitive movements; possible roles in thinking and learning

***Quick* CHECK**

15. Where is the primary somatic motor area of the cerebral cortex? Where is the primary somatic sensory area?
16. What does the reticular activating system have to do with alertness?
17. What is the function of the limbic system?

SOMATIC SENSORY PATHWAYS IN THE CENTRAL NERVOUS SYSTEM

For the cerebral cortex to perform its *sensory* functions, impulses must first be conducted to its sensory areas by way of relays of neurons referred to as *sensory pathways*. Most impulses that reach the sensory areas of the cerebral cortex have travelled over at least three pools of sensory neurons. We shall designate these as *primary sensory neurons*, *secondary sensory neurons*, and *tertiary sensory neurons* (**Figure 20-22**).

Primary sensory neurons of the relay conduct from the periphery to the central nervous system. Secondary sensory neurons conduct from the cord or brainstem up to the thalamus. Their dendrites and cell bodies are located in spinal cord or brainstem grey matter. Their axons ascend in ascending tracts up the cord, through the brainstem, and terminate in the thalamus. Here they synapse with dendrites or cell bodies of tertiary sensory neurons (see **Figure 20-22**). Tertiary sensory neurons conduct from the thalamus to the postcentral gyrus of the parietal lobe, the somaticosensory area. Bundles of axons of tertiary sensory neurons form thalamocortical tracts. They extend through the portion of cerebral white matter known as the *internal capsule* to the cerebral cortex (see **Figure 20-22**).

For the most part, sensory pathways to the cerebral cortex are crossed pathways. This means that each side of the brain registers sensations from the opposite side of the body. Look again at **Figure 20-22**. The axons that *decussate* (cross from one side to the other) in

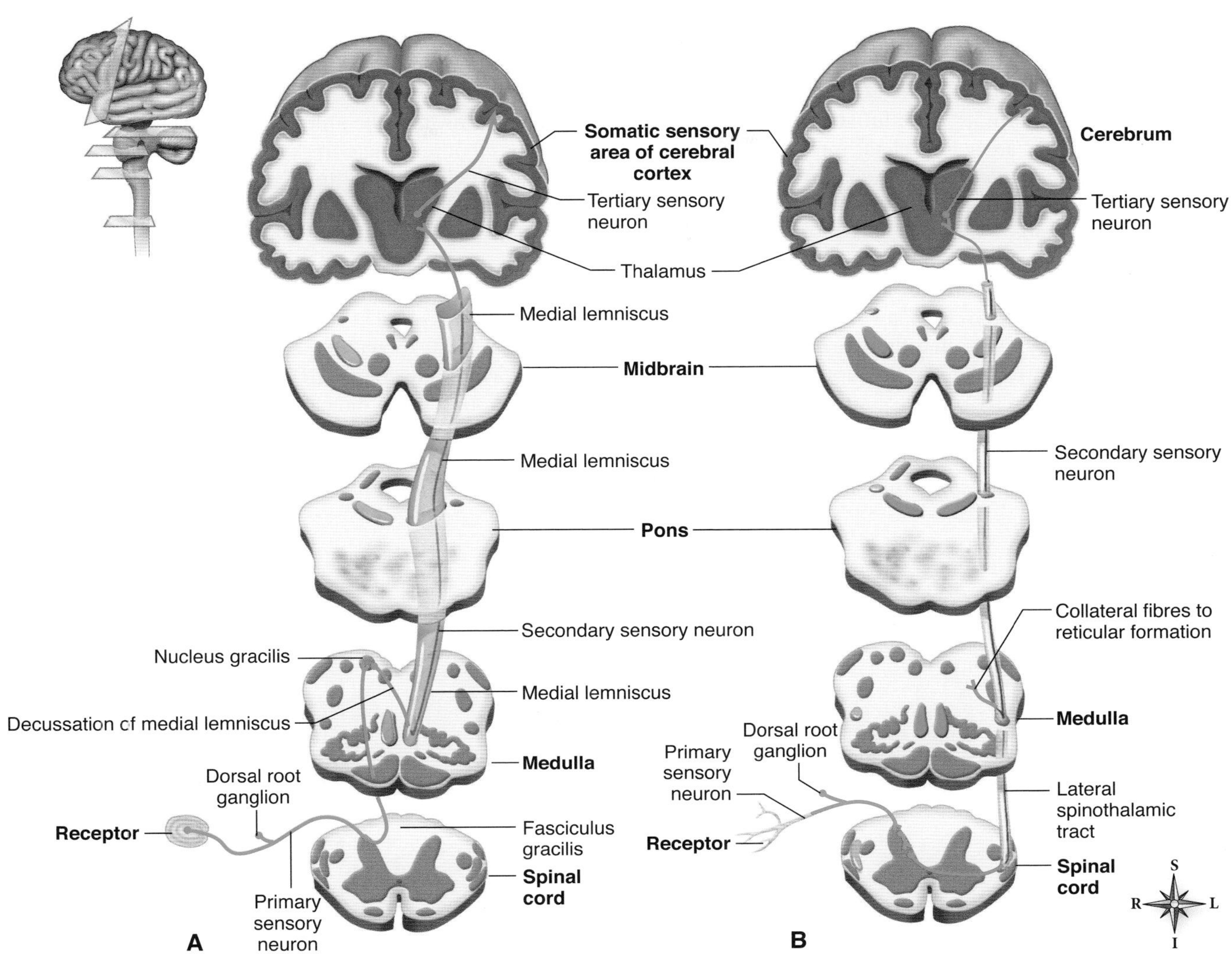

FIGURE 20-22 Examples of somatic sensory pathways. A, A pathway of the medial lemniscal system that conducts information about discriminating touch and kinaesthesia. **B,** A spinothalamic pathway that conducts information about pain and temperature.

these sensory pathways are which sensory neurons: primary, secondary, or tertiary? Usually it is the axon of a secondary sensory neuron that decussates at some level in its ascent to the thalamus. Thus general sensations of the right side of the body are predominantly experienced by the left somatic sensory area. General sensations of the left side of the body are predominantly experienced by the right somatic sensory area.

Two sensory pathways conduct impulses that produce sensations of touch and pressure, namely, the *medial lemniscal system* and the *spinothalamic pathway* (see **Figure 20-22**). The medial lemniscal system consists of the tracts that make up the posterior white columns of the cord (the fasciculi cuneatus and gracilis) plus the *medial lemniscus*, a flat band of white fibres extending through the medulla, pons, and midbrain. (The term *lemniscus* literally means "ribbon", referring to this tract's flattened shape.)

The fibres of the medial lemniscus, like those of the spinothalamic tracts, are axons of secondary sensory neurons. They originate from cell bodies in the medulla, decussate, and then extend upward to terminate in the thalamus on the opposite side. The function of the medial lemniscal system is to transmit impulses that produce our more discriminating touch and pressure sensations, including *stereognosis* (awareness of an object's size, shape, and texture), precise localization, two-point discrimination, weight discrimination, and sense of vibrations. The sensory pathway for kinaesthesia (sense of movement and position of body parts) is also part of the medial lemniscal system.

Crude touch and pressure sensations are functions of the **spinothalamic pathway.** Knowing that something is touching the skin is a crude touch sensation, whereas knowing its precise location, size, shape, or texture involves the discriminating touch sensations of the medial lemniscal system.

Quick CHECK

18. Over how many afferent neurons does somatic sensory information usually pass?
19. Explain why stimuli on the left side of the body are perceived by the right side of the cerebral cortex.

SOMATIC MOTOR PATHWAYS IN THE CENTRAL NERVOUS SYSTEM

For the cerebral cortex to perform its *motor* functions, impulses must be conducted from its motor areas to skeletal muscles by relays of neurons referred to as *somatic motor pathways*. Somatic motor pathways consist of motor neurons that conduct impulses from the central nervous system to somatic effectors—that is, skeletal muscles. Some motor pathways are extremely complex and not at all clearly defined. Others, notably spinal cord reflex arcs, are simple and well established. You read about those in Chapter 18.

Look now at **Figure 20-23**. Note that there are at least two neurons along any motor pathway. One is the upper motor neuron (UMN), which carries impulses from the brain. The other is the lower motor neuron (LMN), which carries impulses from the anterior grey horn of the spinal cord to skeletal muscle fibres. From this pattern you can derive a cardinal principle about somatic motor pathways—the *principle of the final common path*. It is this: only one final common path (the LMN of the anterior grey horn of the spinal cord) conducts *impulses* to a specific motor unit within a skeletal muscle. Axons from the anterior grey horn of the spinal cord are the only ones that terminate in skeletal muscle cells.

This principle of the final common path to skeletal muscles has important practical implications. For example, it means that any condition that makes lower motor neurons unable to conduct impulses also makes skeletal muscle cells supplied by these neurons unable to contract. They cannot be willed to contract nor can they contract reflexively. They are, in short, so flaccid that they are paralyzed. Most well known of the diseases that produce flaccid paralysis by destroying lower motor neurons is *poliomyelitis*.

Numerous somatic motor paths conduct impulses from motor areas of the cerebrum down to lower motor neurons at all levels of the cord.

Two methods are used to classify somatic motor pathways—one based on the location of their fibres in the medulla and the other on

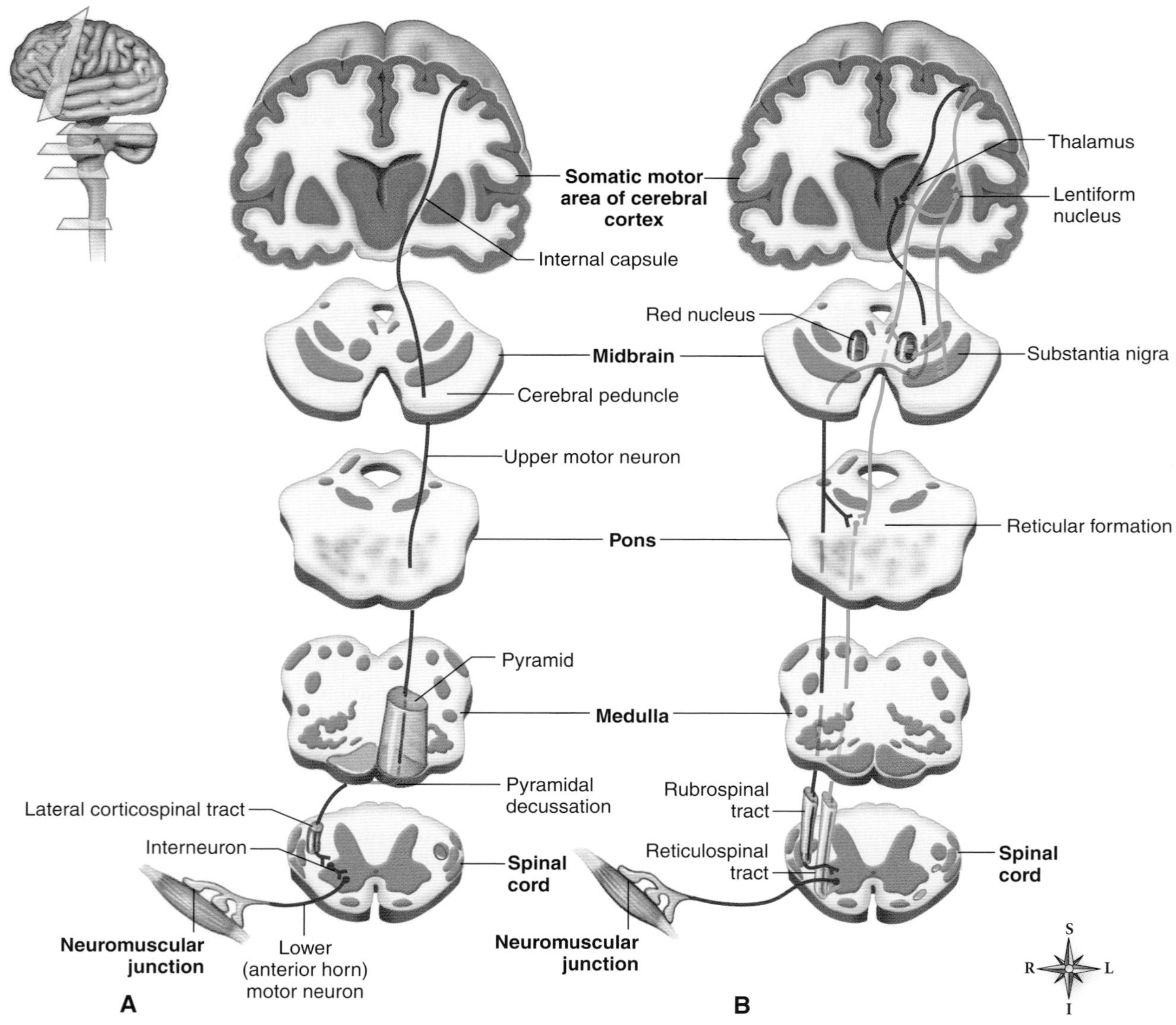

FIGURE 20-23 Examples of somatic motor pathways. A, A pyramidal pathway, through the lateral corticospinal tract. **B,** Extrapyramidal pathways, through the rubrospinal and reticulospinal tracts.

their influence on the lower motor neurons. The first method divides them into pyramidal and extrapyramidal tracts. The second classifies them as facilitatory and inhibitory tracts.

Pyramidal Tracts

Pyramidal tracts are those whose fibres come together in the medulla to form the pyramids, hence their name (see **Figure 20-23**, A). Because axons composing the pyramidal tracts originate from neuron cell bodies located in the cerebral cortex, they also bear another name—*corticospinal tracts.* About three quarters of their fibres decussate (cross over from one side to the other) in the medulla. After decussating, they extend down the spinal cord in the crossed corticospinal tract located on the opposite side of the spinal cord in the lateral white column.

About one quarter of the corticospinal fibres do not decussate. Instead, they extend down the same side of the spinal cord as the cerebral area from which they came. One pair of uncrossed tracts lies in the anterior white columns of the cord, namely, the anterior corticospinal tracts. The other uncrossed corticospinal tracts form part of the lateral corticospinal tracts.

About 60% of corticospinal fibres are axons that arise from neuron cell bodies in the precentral (frontal lobe) region of the cortex. About 40% of corticospinal fibres originate from neuron cell bodies located in postcentral areas of the cortex, areas classified as sensory; now, more accurately, they are often called *sensorimotor areas.*

Relatively few corticospinal tract fibres synapse directly with lower motor neurons. Most of them synapse with interneurons, which in turn synapse with lower motor neurons. All corticospinal fibres conduct impulses that depolarize resting lower motor neurons. The effects of depolarizations occurring rapidly in any one neuron add up, or summate. Each impulse, in other words, depolarizes a lower motor neuron's resting potential a little bit more. If sufficient numbers of impulses impinge rapidly enough on a neuron, its potential reaches the threshold level. At that moment the neuron starts conducting impulses—it is stimulated.

Stimulation of lower motor neurons by corticospinal tract impulses results in stimulation of individual muscle groups (mainly of the hands and feet). Precise control of their contractions is, in short, the function of the corticospinal tracts. Without stimulation of lower motor neurons by impulses over corticospinal fibres, willed movements cannot occur. This means that paralysis results whenever pyramidal corticospinal tract conduction is interrupted. For instance, the paralysis that so often follows **cerebrovascular accidents** (CVAs, or *strokes*) comes from pyramidal neuron injury—sometimes of their cell bodies in the motor areas, sometimes of their axons in the internal capsule (see **Figure 20-23**).

Extrapyramidal Tracts

Extrapyramidal tracts are much more complex than pyramidal tracts. They consist of all motor tracts from the brain to the spinal cord lower motor neurons except the corticospinal (pyramidal) tracts. Within the brain, extrapyramidal tracts consist of numerous relays of motor neurons between motor areas of the cortex, basal nuclei, thalamus, cerebellum, and brainstem. In the cord, some of the most important extrapyramidal tracts are the reticulospinal tracts.

Fibres of the *reticulospinal tracts* originate from cell bodies in the reticular formation of the brainstem and terminate in grey matter of the spinal cord, where they synapse with interneurons that synapse with lower (anterior horn) motor neurons. Some reticulospinal tracts function as facilitatory tracts and others as inhibitory tracts. Summation of these opposing influences determines the lower motor neuron's response. It initiates impulse conduction only when facilitatory impulses exceed inhibitory impulses sufficiently to decrease the lower motor neuron's negativity to its threshold level.

Conduction by extrapyramidal tracts plays a crucial part in producing our larger, more automatic movements because extrapyramidal impulses bring about contractions of groups of muscles in sequence or simultaneously. Such muscle action occurs, for example, in swimming and walking and, in fact, in all normal voluntary movements.

Conduction by extrapyramidal tracts plays an important part in our emotional expressions. For instance, most of us smile automatically at things that amuse us and frown at things that irritate us. It is extrapyramidal, not pyramidal, impulses that produce the smiles or frowns.

Axons of many different neurons converge on—that is, synapse with—each lower motor neuron (see **Figure 20-23**). Hence many impulses from diverse sources—some facilitatory and some inhibitory—continually bombard this final common path to skeletal muscles. Together the added, or summated, effect of these opposing influences determines lower motor neuron functioning.

Facilitatory impulses reach the lower motor neurons by way of sensory neurons (whose axons, you will recall, lie in the posterior roots of spinal nerves), pyramidal (corticospinal) tracts, and extrapyramidal facilitatory reticulospinal tracts. Impulses over facilitatory reticulospinal fibres facilitate the lower motor neurons that supply extensor muscles. At the same time, they reciprocally inhibit the lower motor neurons that supply flexor muscles. Hence facilitatory reticulospinal impulses tend to increase the tone of extensor muscles and decrease the tone of flexor muscles.

Inhibitory impulses reach lower motor neurons mainly by way of inhibitory reticulospinal fibres that originate from cell bodies located in the *bulbar inhibitory area* in the medulla. They inhibit the lower motor neurons to extensor muscles (and reciprocally stimulate those to flexor muscles). Hence inhibitory reticulospinal impulses tend to decrease extensor muscle tone and increase flexor muscle tone; note that these effects are opposite from those of facilitatory reticulospinal impulses.

The set of coordinated commands that control the programmed muscle activity mediated by extrapyramidal pathways is often called a **motor program.** Traditionally, the primary somatic motor areas of the cerebral cortex were thought to be the principal organizer of motor programs sent along the extrapyramidal pathway. That view has been replaced by the concept illustrated in **Figure 20-24**. This newer concept holds that motor programs result from the interaction of several different centres in the brain. Apparently, many voluntary motor programs are organized in the basal nuclei and cerebellum—perhaps in response to a willed command by the cerebral cortex. Impulses that constitute the motor program are then channelled through the thalamus and back to the cortex, specifically to the primary motor area. From there, the motor program is sent down to the inhibitory and facilitatory regions of the brainstem. Signals from the brainstem then continue on down one or more spinal tracts and out

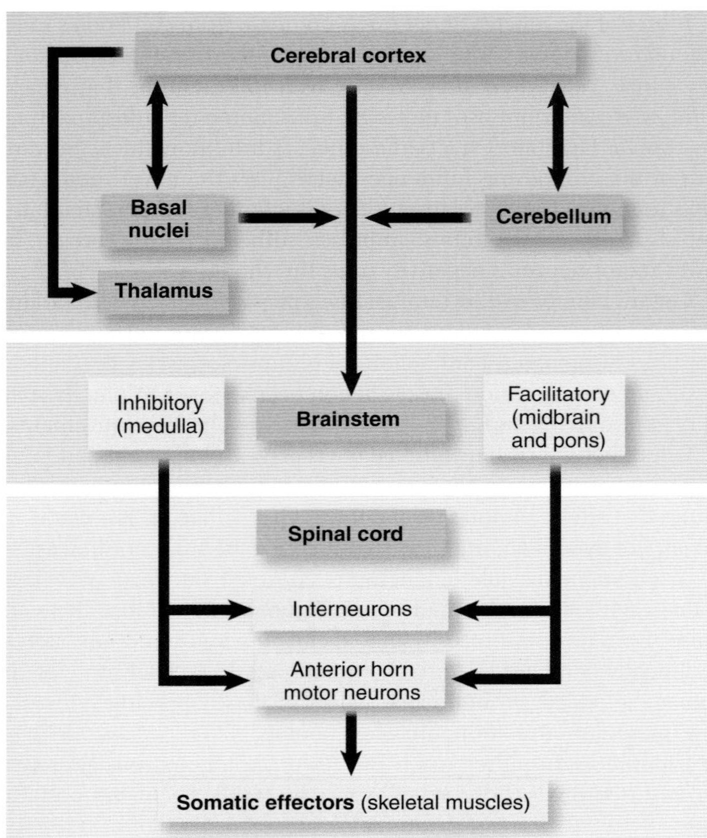

FIGURE 20-24 Concept of extrapyramidal motor control. Programmed movements result from a set of impulses called a *motor program.* The motor program organized in the basal nuclei and cerebellum in response to a command from the cortex is sent back to the primary motor control area of the cortex. From there, it is sent to the brainstem and then on through the spinal cord to the skeletal muscles. All along the motor pathway, the motor program can be refined by various components of this complex pathway.

to the muscles by way of the lower (anterior horn) motor neurons. All along the way, neural connections among the various motor control centres allow refinement and adjustment of the motor program.

If all this sounds complicated and confusing, imagine what it must be like to be a neurobiologist trying to figure out how all this works! In fact, scientists working in this field admit that they have not worked out all the details of the extrapyramidal circuits—or exactly how they control muscle activity. However, the model shown in **Figure 20-24** summarizes the current notion that it is a complex, interactive process.

Knowing about all these motor pathways helps us understand and treat injuries and disorders that affect motor functions. **Box 20-8** discusses some of the clinical signs of motor pathway injury.

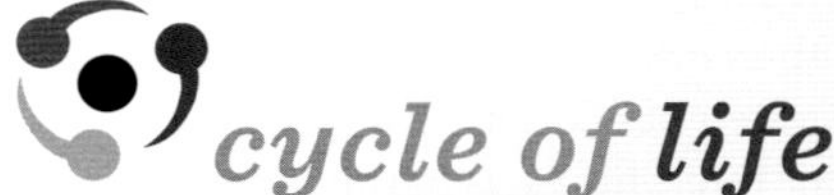

Quick CHECK

20. What is the "principle of final common path" as it pertains to somatic motor pathways?
21. Distinguish between pyramidal and extrapyramidal pathways.

BOX 20-8 *health matters* | Signs of Motor Pathway Injury

Injury of upper motor neurons (those whose axons lie in either pyramidal or extrapyramidal tracts) produces symptoms frequently referred to as "pyramidal signs", notably a spastic type of paralysis, exaggerated deep reflexes, and a positive Babinski reflex (see p. 497). Actually, pyramidal signs result from interruption of both pyramidal and extrapyramidal pathways. The paralysis stems from interruption of pyramidal tracts, whereas the spasticity (rigidity) and exaggerated reflexes come from interruption of inhibitory extrapyramidal pathways.

Injury to lower motor neurons produces symptoms different from those of upper motor neuron injury. Anterior horn cells or lower motor neurons, you will recall, constitute the final common path by which impulses reach skeletal muscles. This means that if they are injured, impulses can no longer reach the skeletal muscles they supply. This, in turn, results in the absence of all reflexes and willed movements produced by contraction of the muscles involved. Unused, the muscles soon lose their normal tone and become soft and flabby (flaccid). In short, absence of reflexes and flaccid paralysis are the chief "lower" motor neuron signs. •

cycle of life

Central Nervous System If the most obvious *structural* changes over the life span are the overall growth and then degeneration of the skeleton and other body parts, then the most obvious *functional* changes are the development and then degeneration of the complex integrative capacity of the central nervous system.

Although the development of the brain and spinal cord begins in the womb, further development beyond the time of birth is required. The lack of development of the CNS in a newborn is evidenced by lack of the more complex integrative functions, such as language, complex memory, comprehension of spatial relationships, and complex motor skills such as walking.

As childhood proceeds, one can easily see evidence of the increasing capacity of the CNS for complex function. A child learns to use language, to remember both concrete and abstract ideas, to walk, and even to behave in ways that conform to the norms of society. By the time a person reaches adulthood, most, if not all, of these complex functions have become fully developed. We use them throughout adult life to help us maintain internal stability in an unstable external world.

As we enter very late adulthood, the tissues of the brain and spinal cord may degenerate. If they do degenerate—and they may not—the degree of change varies from one individual to the next. In some cases, the degeneration is profound—or it occurs in a critical part of the brain—and an older person becomes unable to communicate, to walk, or to perform some other complex functions. In many cases, however, the degeneration produces milder effects, such as temporary lapses in memory or fumbling with certain very complex motor tasks. As our understanding of this process increases, we are finding ways to avoid entirely such changes associated with ageing. •

the big picture | The Central Nervous System and the Whole Body

The central nervous system is the ultimate regulator of the entire body. It serves as the anatomical and functional centre of the countless feedback loops that maintain the relative constancy of the internal environment. The CNS directly or indirectly regulates, or at least influences, nearly every organ in the body.

The intriguing thing about the way in which the CNS regulates the whole body is that it is able to integrate, or bring together, literally billions of bits of information from all over the body and make sense of it all. The CNS not only makes sense of all this information but also compares it with previously stored memories and makes decisions based on its own conclusions about the data. The complex integrative functions of human language, consciousness, learning, and memory enable us to adapt to situations that less complex organisms could not. Thus our wonderfully complex CNS is essential to our survival.

mechanisms of disease

Disorders of the Central Nervous System

Destruction of Brain Tissue

Injury or disease can damage or destroy neurons in the brain or spinal cord. Several examples follow.

Stroke

A common example is the destruction of neurons of the motor area of the cerebrum that results from a *cerebrovascular accident (CVA)*. A CVA, or *stroke,* is a haemorrhage from or cessation of blood flow through cerebral blood vessels. When this happens, the oxygen supply to portions of the brain is disrupted and neurons cease functioning. If the lack of oxygen is prolonged, the neurons die. If the damage from a CVA occurs in a motor control area of the brain (see **Figures 20-18** and **20-19**), a person can no longer voluntarily move the parts of the body controlled by the affected area or areas. Because motor neurons cross over from side to side in the brainstem (see **Figure 20-23**), flaccid paralysis appears on the side of the body opposite the side of the brain on which the CVA occurred. The term *hemiplegia* refers to paralysis (loss of voluntary muscle control) of one whole side of the body.

A temporary episode of blood disruption of brain is often called a **transient ischaemic attack (TIA)** or *mini-stroke.*

Cerebral Palsy

One of the most common crippling diseases that appears during childhood, **cerebral palsy,** also results from damage to brain tissue. Cerebral palsy involves permanent, nonprogressive damage to motor control areas of the brain. Such damage is present at birth or occurs shortly after birth and remains throughout life. Possible causes of brain damage include prenatal infections or diseases of the mother; mechanical trauma to the head before, during, or after birth; nerve-damaging poisons; reduced oxygen supply to the brain; and other factors. The resulting impairment to voluntary muscle control can manifest in various ways. Many people with cerebral palsy exhibit **spastic paralysis,** a type of paralysis characterized by involuntary contractions of affected muscles. In cerebral palsy, spastic paralysis often affects one entire side of the body **(hemiplegia),** both legs **(paraplegia),** both legs and one arm **(triplegia),** or all four extremities **(quadriplegia).**

Physical Injury

A **traumatic brain injury (TBI)** occurs when an outside force causes brain dysfunction. An *open (or penetrating) TBI* involves a break in the skull and dura matter, exposing the brain tissue. *Closed (or blunt) TBIs* are more common and involve a hard bump to the head or violent shaking, which causes disruption of brain function—often caused by torn nerve fibres, accompanied by bleeding, swelling, and other internal damage to the brain. **Figure 20-25** shows nerve fibre damage resulting from a closed TBI.

A *mild TBI (MTBI)*, or **concussion,** is sometimes characterized by temporary loss of consciousness—but not always, so some people have concussions and are not aware of it. A person with a concussion may also experience temporary disorientation, amnesia, or other symptoms. Any concussion requires time to repair damaged nerve fibres and thus repeated concussions, which may occur in some sports, tend to disrupt healing and often lead to long-term brain damage.

Chronic traumatic encephalopathy (CTE) results from repeated trauma to the brain, including TBIs, as occurs in some sports, physical abuse, seizure disorders or head-banging behaviour. CTE involves accumulation of abnormal proteins in the brain and memory loss and is also characterized by parkinsonism, disordered thinking and other neurological symptoms.

Dementia

Various degenerative diseases can result in destruction of neurons in the brain. This degeneration can progress to adversely affect memory, attention span, intellectual capacity, personality, and motor control. The general term for this syndrome is **dementia.**

Alzheimer disease (AD) is characterized by dementia. Its characteristic lesions develop in the cortex during the middle to late adult years. Exactly what causes dementia-producing lesions to develop in the brains of individuals with

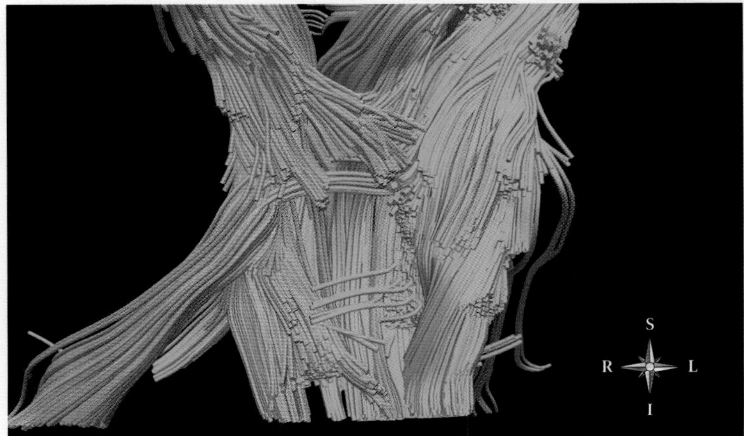

FIGURE 20-25 Traumatic brain injury (TBI). A magnetic resonance (MR) tractography image shows damage to nerve fibres in the brain resulting from a head injury in an all-terrain vehicle (ATV) accident. The right side *(yellow)* is damaged and produced paralysis in the patient's left leg, arm, and hand. The normal left side in *green* shows undamaged neural pathways.

Alzheimer disease is not known. There is strong evidence that this disease has a genetic basis—at least in some families. A current theory is that more than one of the handful of different genes associated with AD has to be abnormal before AD occurs. Other evidence indicates that environmental factors may have a role. Because the exact cause of Alzheimer disease is still not precisely known, development of an effective treatment has proven difficult. People diagnosed with AD are often treated by helping them maintain their remaining mental abilities and looking after their hygiene, nutrition, and other aspects of personal health management. Drugs such as memantine and donepezil are available to slow down the progression of AD or lessen the severity of some of the symptoms.

Huntington disease (HD) is an inherited disease characterized by chorea (involuntary, purposeless movements) that progresses to severe dementia and death. The initial symptoms of this disease first appear between ages 30 and 40 years, with death generally occurring by age 55 years. The gene responsible for Huntington disease causes the body to make the protein *huntingtin* incorrectly. In brain cells, the abnormal form of huntingtin apparently clings to molecules too tightly and thus prevents normal function.

Acquired immunodeficiency syndrome (AIDS), caused by human immunodeficiency virus (HIV) infection, can also cause dementia. The immune deficiency characteristic of AIDS results from HIV infection of white blood cells that are critical to the proper function of the immune system (see Chapter 33). However, HIV also infects neurons and can cause progressive degeneration of the brain—resulting in dementia.

Diseases caused by prions, pathogenic protein molecules, can also cause dementia. For example, *bovine spongiform encephalopathy,* also known as BSE or "mad cow disease", is a degenerative disease of the central nervous system caused by prions that convert normal proteins of the nervous system into abnormal proteins, causing loss of nervous system function, including dementia. **Variant Creutzfeldt–Jakob disease (vCJD)** is another prion disease that similarly reduces brain function, causing dementia. These diseases have caused alarm occasionally when animal brains (the tissue that carries prions to other organisms) were fed to other animals in the human food chain, increasing the risk of infecting large numbers of humans. The mechanism of prion disease was outlined in Chapter 2, p. 32.

Seizure Disorders

Some of the most common nervous system abnormalities belong to the group of conditions called *seizure disorders.* These disorders are characterized by **seizures**—sudden bursts of abnormal neuron activity that result in temporary changes in brain function. Seizures may be very mild, causing subtle changes in the level of consciousness, motor control, or sensory perception. On the other hand, seizures may be quite severe—resulting in jerky, involuntary muscle contractions called *convulsions* or even unconsciousness.

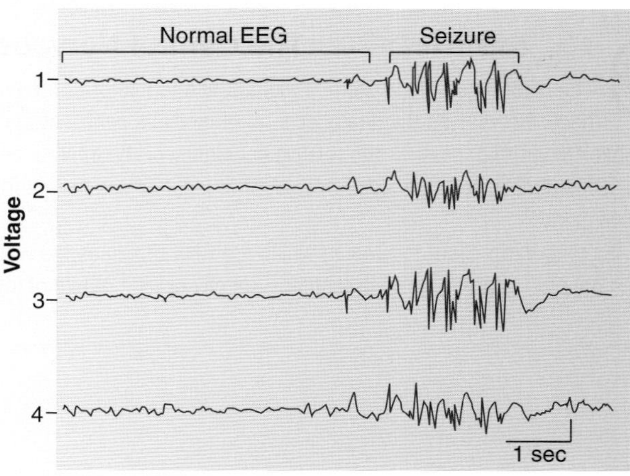

FIGURE 20-26 Electroencephalogram (EEG).

Recurring or chronic seizure episodes constitute a condition called **epilepsy.** Although some cases of epilepsy can be traced to specific causes such as tumours or chemical imbalances, most epilepsy is idiopathic (of unknown cause). Epilepsy is often treated with anticonvulsive drugs such as *phenytoin* or *valproic acid* that block neurotransmitters in affected areas of the brain. By thus blocking synaptic transmission, such drugs inhibit the explosive bursts of neuron activity associated with seizures. With proper medication, many people with epilepsy lead normal lives without the fear of experiencing uncontrollable seizures. Even those who have not responded well to drug therapies often have gained some relief from surgeries that cut or destroy areas of the brain prone to severe seizures.

Diagnosis and evaluation of epilepsy or any seizure disorder often rely on **electroencephalography** (see **Box 20-6**, p. 459). As **Figure 20-26** illustrates, a normal EEG shows the moderate rise and fall of voltage in various parts of the brain, but a seizure manifests as an explosive increase in the size and frequency of voltage fluctuations. Different classifications of epilepsy are based on the location, duration, and severity of these changes in brain activity.

LANGUAGE OF SCIENCE *(continued from p. 436)*

cerebrospinal fluid (CSF) (seh-ree-broh-SPY-nal FLOO-id) [*cerebr-* **brain,** *-spin-* **backbone,** *-al* **relating to**]

cerebrum (SAIR-eh-brum) [*cerebrum* **brain**] *pl.,* cerebra or cerebrums

choroid plexus (KOH-royd PLEK-sus) [*chorio-* **skin,** *-oid* **like,** *plexus* **braid or network**] *pl.,* plexi or plexuses

connectome (kon-NEK-tohm) [*con-* **together,** *-nect-* **bind,** *-ome* **complete set**]

conus medullaris (KOH-nus MED-yoo-lair-is) [*conus* **cone,** *medulla* **marrow or pith (middle)**] *pl.,* coni medullares

convolution (kon-voh-LOO-shun) [*con-* **together,** *-volut-* **roll,** *-tion* **process**]

corpora quadrigemina (KOHR-pohr-ah kwod-rih-JEM-ih-nah) [*corpora* **bodies,** *quadri-* **fourfold,** *-gemina* **twin**]

corpus callosum (KOHR-pus kah-LOH-sum) [*corpus* **body,** *callosum* **callous or tough**] *pl.,* corpora callosa

dentate nucleus (DEN-tayt NYOO-klee-us) [*dent-* **tooth,** *-ate* **of or like,** *nucleus* **nut or kernel**] *pl.,* nuclei

descending tract (dih-SEND-ing trakt) [*de-* **down,** *-scend-* **climb,** *tract* **trail**]

diencephalon (dye-en-SEF-ah-lon) [*di-* **between,** *-en-* **within,** *-cephalon* **head**] *pl.,* diencephala or diencephalons

dorsal (posterior) nerve root (DOR-sal) [*dors-* **back,** *-al* **relating to**]

embryology (em-bree-OL-oh-gee) [*em-* **in,** *-bryo-* **fill to bursting,** *-log-* **words (study of),** *-y* **activity**]

epidural space (ep-ih-DYOO-ral)
[*epi-* **upon,** *-dura-* **hard,** *-al* **relating to**]

epithalamus (ep-ih-THAL-ah-mus)
[*epi-* **upon,** *-thalamus* **inner chamber**] *pl.,* epithalami

extrapyramidal tract (eks-trah-pih-RAH-mih-dal)
[*extra-* **outside,** *-pyramid-* **pyramid,** *-al* **relating to,** *tract* **trail**]

falx cerebelli (falks ser-eh-BEL-lee)
[*falx* **sickle,** *cerebelli* **of the cerebellum (small brain)**] *pl.,* falces cerebelli

falx cerebri (falks SER-eh-bree)
[*falx* **sickle,** *cerebri* **of the cerebrum**] *pl.,* falces cerebri

fasciculus cuneatus (fah-SIK-yoo-lus KYOO-nee-ay-tus)
[*fasci-* **bundles,** *-iculus* **little,** *cuneatus* **wedgelike**] *pl.,* fasciculi

fasciculus gracilis (fah-SIK-yoo-lus GRAH-sil-iss)
[*fasci-* **bundles,** *-iculus* **little,** *gracilis* **thin**] *pl.,* fasciculi

filum terminale (FYE-lum ter-mih-NAL-ee)
[*filum* **thread,** *termin-* **boundary,** *-al* **relating to**] *pl.,* fila terminales

folia (FOH-lee-ah)
[*folia* **leaves**] *sing.,* folium

frontal lobe (FRON-tal)
[*front-* **forehead,** *-al* **relating to**]

funiculus (fuh-NIK-yoo-lus)
[*funi-* **rope,** *-icul-* **little**] *pl.,* funiculi

grey column (grey KOL-umm)

grey commissure (KOHM-is-shoor)
[*commissur-* **a joining**]

hypothalamus (hye-poh-THAL-ah-muss)
[*hypo-* **under or below,** *-thalamus* **inner chamber**] *pl.,* hypothalami

inferior cerebellar peduncle (SAIR-eh-bell-ar peh-DUNG-kul)
[*infer-* **lower,** *-or* **quality,** *cerebell-* **cerebellum (small brain),** *-ar* **relating to,** *ped-* **foot,** *-uncl-* **little**]

inferior colliculi (koh-LIK-yoo-lee)
[*infer-* **lower,** *-or* **quality,** *colli-* **hill,** *-iculus* **small**] *sing.,* colliculus

infundibulum (in-fun-DIB-yoo-lum)
[*infundibulum* **funnel**] *pl.,* infundibula

insula (IN-soo-lah)
[*insula* **island**] *pl.,* insulae

internal capsule
[*intern-* **inside,** *-al* **relating to,** *caps-* **box,** *-ula* **little**]

lateral corticospinal tract (LAT-er-al kohr-tih-koh-SPY-nal trakt)
[*later-* **side,** *-al* **relating to,** *cortico-* **cortex (bark),** *-spin-* **backbone,** *-al* **relating to,** *tract* **trail**]

lateral fissure (Sylvius fissure) (LAT-er-al FISH-ur [SIL-vee-us FISH-ur])
[*later-* **side,** *-al* **relating to,** *Franciscus Sylvius* **German medical professor**]

lateral spinothalamic tract (LAT-er-al spy-no-tha-LAM-ik trakt)
[*later-* **side,** *-al* **relating to,** *spino-* **backbone,** *-thalam-* **inner chamber,** *-ic* **relating to,** *tract* **trail**]

lentiform nucleus (LEN-tih-form NYOO-klee-us)
[*lent-* **lentil (lens),** *-form* **shape,** *nucleus* **nut or kernel**] *pl.,* nuclei

limbic system (LIM-bik)
[*limb-* **edge,** *-ic* **relating to**]

longitudinal fissure (lon-ji-TOO-dih-nal FISH-ur)
[*longitud-* **length,** *-al* **relating to**]

medulla oblongata (meh-DUL-ah ob-long-GAH-tah)
[*medulla* **marrow or pith (middle),** *oblongata* **oblong**] *pl.,* medullae oblongatae

melatonin (mel-ah-TOH-nin)
[*mela-* **black,** *-ton-* **tone,** *-in* **substance**]

meninges (meh-NIN-jeez)
[*meninx* **membrane**] *sing.,* meninx

midbrain (MID-brayn)
[*mid-* **middle**]

middle cerebellar peduncle (SAIR-eh-bell-ar peh-DUNG-kul)
[*cerebell-* **cerebellum (small brain),** *-ar* **relating to,** *ped-* **foot,** *-uncl* **little**]

motor program
[*mot-* **move,** *-or* **agent**]

occipital lobe (ok-SIP-it-al)
[*occipit-* **back of head,** *-al* **relating to**]

olive (OL-iv)

optic chiasma (OP-tik kye-AS-mah)
[*opti-* **vision,** *-ic* **relating to,** *chiasma* **crossed lines**] *pl.,* chiasmata, chiasms, or chiasmas

parietal lobe (pah-RYE-eh-tal)
[*parie-* **wall,** *-al* **relating to**]

parietooccipital sulcus (pah-RYE-eh-toh-ok-SIP-ih-tal SUL-kus)
[*parieto-* **wall,** *-occipit-* **back of head,** *-al* **relating to,** *sulcus* **trench**] *pl.,* sulci

pineal gland (PIN-ee-al)
[*pine-* **pine,** *-al* **relating to,** *gland* **acorn**]

pons (ponz)
[*pons* **bridge**] *pl.,* pontes

pyramid (PEER-ah-mid)

pyramidal tract (pi-RAM-ih-dal trakt)
[*pyrami-* **pyramid,** *-al* **relating to,** *tract* **trail**]

reticular activating system (RAS) (reh-TIK-yoo-lar)
[*ret-* **net,** *-ic-* **relating to,** *-ul-* **little,** *-ar* **characterized by**]

reticular formation (reh-TIK-yoo-lar)
[*ret-* **net,** *-ic-* **relating to,** *-ul-* **little,** *-ar* **characterized by**]

reticulospinal tract (reh-TIK-yoo-loh-SPY-nal trakt)
[*ret-* **net,** *-ic-* **relating to,** *-ul-* **little,** *-spin-* **backbone,** *-al* **relating to,** *tract* **trail**]

rubrospinal tract (roo-broh-SPY-nal trakt)
[*rubro-* **red,** *-spin-* **backbone,** *-al* **relating to,** *tract* **trail**]

spinal nerve (SPY-nal nerv)
[*spin-* **backbone,** *-al* **relating to**]

spinal tract (SPY-nal trakt)
[*spin-* **backbone,** *-al* **relating to,** *tract* **trail**]

spinocerebellar tract (SPY-no-sair-eh-BELL-ar trakt)
[*spino-* **backbone,** *-cerebell-* **cerebellum (small brain),** *-ar* **relating to,** *tract* **trail**]

spinotectal tract (SPY-no-TEK-tal trakt)
[*spino-* **backbone,** *-tect-* **roof,** *-al* **relating to,** *tract* **trail**]

spinothalamic pathway (spy-no-thah-LAM-ik)
[*spino-* **backbone,** *-thalam-* **inner chamber,** *-ic* **relating to**]

subarachnoid space (sub-ah-RAK-noyd)
[*sub-* **beneath,** *-arachn-* **spider,** *-oid* **like**]

subdural space (sub-DOO-ral)
[*sub-* **beneath,** *-dura-* **hard or tough,** *-al* **relating to**]

superior cerebellar peduncle (SAIR-eh-bell-ar peh-DUNG-kul)
[*super-* **over or above,** *-or* **quality,** *cerebell-* **cerebellum (small brain),** *-ar* **relating to,** *ped-* **foot,** *-uncl* **little**]

superior colliculi (koh-LIK-yoo-lee)
[*super-* **over or above,** *-or* **quality,** *colli-* **hill,** *-iculus* **small**] *sing.,* colliculus

tectospinal tract (tek-toh-SPY-nal trakt)
[*tecto-* **roof,** *-spin-* **backbone,** *-al* **relating to,** *tract* **trail**]

temporal lobe (TEM-poh-ral)
[*tempor-* **temple of head,** *-al* **relating to**]

tentorium cerebelli (ten-TOR-ee-um sair-eh-BEL-lee)
[*tentorium* **tent,** *cerebelli* **of the cerebellum (small brain)**] *pl.,* tentoria cerebelli

thalamus (THAL-ah-muss)
[*thalamus* **inner chamber**] *pl.,* thalami

ventral (anterior) nerve root (VEN-tral)
[*ventr-* **belly,** *-al* **relating to**]

ventricle (VEN-trih-kul)
[*ventr-* **belly,** *-icle* **little**]

vermis (VER-mis)
[*vermis* **worm**] *pl.,* vermes

vestibulospinal tract (ves-TIB-yoo-loh-SPY-nal trakt)
[*vestibul-* **entrance hall,** *-spino-* **backbone,** *-al* **relating to,** *tract* **trail**]

UNIT 3

LANGUAGE OF MEDICINE

acquired immunodeficiency syndrome (AIDS) (ah-KWY-erd IM-yoon deh-FISH-en-see SIN-drohm)
[*syn-* **together,** *-drome* **running or (race)course**]

Alzheimer disease (AD) (AHLZ-hye-mer)
[*Alois Alzheimer* **German neurologist**]

cerebral palsy (seh-REE-bral PAWL-zee)
[*cerebr-* **brain,** *-al* **relating to,** *palsy* **paralysis** (*para-* **beyond,** *-lysis* **loosening**)]

cerebral plasticity (seh-REE-bral plas-TIS-ih-tee)
[*cerebr-* **brain,** *-al* **relating to,** *plastic-* **mouldable,** *-ity* **state**]

cerebrovascular accident (CVA) (SAIR-eh-broh-VAS-kyoo-lar)
[*cerebr-* **brain,** *-vas-* **vessel,** *cul-* **little,** *-ar* **relating to**]

coma (KOH-mah)
[*coma* **deep sleep**]

concussion (kon-KUSH-un)
[*con-* **with,** *-cuss-* **shake,** *-ion* **condition**]

dementia (de-MEN-shah)
[*de-* **off,** *-mens-* **mind,** *-ia* **condition of**]

electroencephalogram (EEG) (eh-lek-troh-en-SEF-ah-loh-gram) [*electro-* **electricity,** *-en-* **within,** *-cephal-* **head,** *-gram* **drawing**]

electroencephalography (eh-lek-troh-en-SEF-ah-lo-grah-fee) [*electro-* **electricity,** *-en-* **inside,** *-cephal* **head,** *-graph-* **draw,** *-y* **activity**]

epilepsy (EP-ih-lep-see) [*epi-* **upon,** *-lep(t)-* **seize,** *-sy* **state or condition**]

hemiplegia (hem-ee-PLEE-jee-ah) [*hemi-* **half,** *-pleg-* **stricken,** *-ia* **condition**]

Huntington disease (HD) (HUN-ting-ton) [*George S. Huntington* **American physician**]

hydrocephalus (hye-droh-SEF-ah-lus) [*hydro-* **water,** *-cephalus* **head**]

lumbar puncture (LUM-bar) [*lumb-* **loin,** *-ar* **relating to**]

meningitis (men-in-JYE-tis) [*mening-* **membrane,** *-itis* **inflammation**]

paraplegia (pair-ah-PLEE-jee-ah) [*para-* **beside,** *-pleg-* **stricken,** *-ia* **condition**]

Parkinson disease (PD) (PAR-kin-son) [*James Parkinson* **English physician**]

quadriplegia (kwod-rih-PLEE-jee-ah) [*quadri-* **fourfold,** *-pleg-* **stricken,** *-ia* **condition**]

spastic paralysis (SPAS-tik pah-RAL-ih-sis) [*spast-* **pull,** *-ic* **relating to,** *para-* **beyond,** *-lysis* **loosening**]

transcutaneous electrical nerve stimulation (TENS) unit (tranz-kyoo-TAY-nee-us) [*trans-* **across,** *-cutan-* **skin,** *-ous* **relating to**]

traumatic brain injury (TBI) (truh-MAT-ik brayn IN-jur-ee) [*trauma-* **wound,** *-atic* **relating to**]

transient ischaemic attack [TIA] (is-KEE-mik) [*trans-* **across,** *-ent* **state,** *isch-* **hold back,** *-aem-* **blood,** *-ic* **relating to**]

triplegia (try-PLEE-jee-ah) [*tri-* **three,** *-pleg-* **stricken,** *-ia* **condition**]

variant Creutzfeldt-Jakob disease (vCJD) (KROYTS-felt YAH-kobe) [*Hans G. Creutzfeldt* **German neurologist,** *Alfons M. Jakob* **German neurologist**]

UNIT 3

case study

Paula finally went to the university clinic hoping to get some analgesics for a severe headache that had been troubling her for several days. Upon examination she also revealed that she had other symptoms: a stiff neck, sore muscles, and some red blotches on her skin. Instead of being sent home with analgesics, she was immediately sent to the hospital for a lumbar puncture (also called a spinal tap) to determine whether she had contracted meningitis. To perform a lumbar puncture and obtain a sample of cerebrospinal fluid, a needle is inserted into the meninges in the lumbar region above or below the fourth lumbar vertebra.

1. In what order will the needle pierce the meninges?
   a. Pia mater, arachnoid mater, dura mater
   b. Arachnoid mater, pia mater, dura mater
   c. Dura mater, arachnoid mater, pia mater
   d. Dura mater, pia mater, arachnoid mater
2. Where exactly will the cerebrospinal fluid be drawn from?
   a. Epidural space
   b. Subdural space
   c. Epiarachnoid space
   d. Subarachnoid space

Anyone performing a spinal tap must be extremely careful. If the needle goes past its mark, it could puncture the posterior portion of the spinal cord. One of the tracts in this region is the fasciculus gracilis.

3. The transmission of what type of information would be affected if the fasciculus gracilis were damaged?
   a. Discriminating touch
   b. Crude touch
   c. Voluntary movement
   d. Coordination of posture and balance

One possible (though rare) complication of meningitis (inflammation of the meninges) could be spread of the bacterial infection to the cerebellum.

4. Which of the following is NOT a function of the cerebellum?
   a. Coordinates skilled movement
   b. Controls language
   c. Helps control posture
   d. Controls balance

Hint To solve a case study, you may have to refer to the glossary or index, other chapters in this textbook, ***Connect It!,*** and other resources.

CHAPTER SUMMARY

To download an MP3 version of the chapter summary for use with your mobile device, access the **Audio Chapter Summaries** *online at evolve.elsevier.com.*

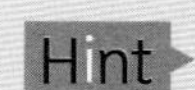

Scan this summary after reading the chapter to help you reinforce the key concepts. Later, use the summary as a quick review before your class or before a test.

Coverings of the Brain and Spinal Cord

A. Two protective coverings (**Figure 20-2**)
   1. Outer covering is bone; cranial bones encase the brain, and vertebrae encase the spinal cord (**Figure 20-1**)
   2. Inner covering is the meninges; the meninges of the cord continue inside the spinal cavity beyond the end of the spinal cord
B. Meninges—three membranous layers (**Figure 20-3**)
   1. Dura mater—strong, white fibrous tissue; outer layer of meninges and inner periosteum of the cranial bones; has three important extensions
      a. Falx cerebri
         (1) Projects downward into the longitudinal fissure between the two cerebral hemispheres
         (2) Dural sinuses—function as veins, collecting blood from brain tissues for return to the heart
         (3) Superior sagittal sinus—one of several dural sinuses

b. Falx cerebelli—separates the two hemispheres of the cerebellum
c. Tentorium cerebelli—separates the cerebellum from the cerebrum
2. Arachnoid mater—delicate, spiderweb-like layer between the dura mater and pia mater
3. Pia mater—innermost, transparent layer; adheres to the outer surface of the brain and spinal cord; contains blood vessels; beyond the spinal cord, forms a slender filament called *filum terminale*, at level of sacrum, blends with dura mater to form a fibrous cord that disappears into the periosteum of the coccyx
4. Several spaces exist between and around the meninges
    a. Epidural space—located between the dura mater and inside the bony covering of the spinal cord; contains a supporting cushion of fat and other connective tissues (virtually absent around brain because dura is continuous with periosteum of bone)
    b. Subdural space—located between the dura mater and arachnoid mater; contains lubricating serous fluid
    c. Subarachnoid space—located between the arachnoid and pia mater; contains a significant amount of cerebrospinal fluid (CSF)

Cerebrospinal Fluid

A. Functions
1. Provides a supportive, protective cushion
2. Reservoir of circulating fluid, which is monitored by the brain to detect changes in the internal environment

B. Fluid spaces
1. Cerebrospinal fluid—found within the subarachnoid space around the brain and spinal cord and within the cavities and canals of the brain and spinal cord
2. Ventricles—fluid-filled spaces within the brain; four ventricles within the brain (**Figure 20-4**)
    a. First and second ventricles (lateral)—one located in each hemisphere of the cerebrum
    b. Third ventricle—thin, vertical pocket of fluid below and medial to the lateral ventricles
    c. Fourth ventricle—tiny, diamond-shaped space where the cerebellum attaches to the back of the brainstem

C. Formation and circulation of cerebrospinal fluid (**Figure 20-5**)
1. Occurs by separation of fluid from blood in the choroid plexuses
    a. Fluid from the lateral ventricles seeps through the interventricular foramen into the third ventricle
    b. From the third ventricle, fluid goes through the cerebral aqueduct into the fourth ventricle
    c. From the fourth ventricle, fluid goes to two different areas
        (1) Some fluid flows directly into the central canal of the spinal cord
        (2) Some fluid leaves the fourth ventricle through openings in its roof and goes into the cisterna magna, a space that is continuous with the subarachnoid space
    d. Fluid circulates in the subarachnoid space and then is absorbed into venous blood through the arachnoid villi

Spinal Cord

A. Structure of the spinal cord (**Figure 20-6**)
1. Lies within the spinal cavity and extends from the foramen magnum to the lower border of the first lumbar vertebra
2. Oval-shaped cylinder that tapers slightly from above downward
3. Two bulges, one in the cervical region and one in the lumbar region
4. Anterior median fissure and posterior median sulcus are two deep grooves; anterior fissure is deeper and wider
5. Nerve roots
    a. Fibres of dorsal nerve root
        (1) Carry sensory information into the spinal canal
        (2) Dorsal root ganglion—cell bodies of unipolar, sensory neurons make up a small region of grey matter in the dorsal nerve root
    b. Fibres of ventral nerve root
        (1) Carry motor information out of the spinal cord
        (2) Cell bodies of multipolar, motor neurons are in the grey matter of the spinal cord
6. Interneurons are located in the spinal cord's grey matter core
7. Spinal nerve—a single mixed nerve on each side of the spinal cord where the dorsal and ventral nerve roots join together
8. Cauda equina—bundle of nerve roots extending (along with the filum terminale) from the conus medullaris (inferior end of spinal cord) (**Figure 20-7**)
9. Grey matter
    a. Columns of grey matter extend the length of the cord
    b. Consists predominantly of cell bodies of interneurons and motor neurons
    c. In transverse section, looks like an H with the limbs being called the *anterior, posterior,* and *lateral horns of grey matter;* crossbar of H is the *grey commissure*
10. White matter
    a. Surrounds the grey matter and is subdivided in each half on the cord into three funiculi: anterior, posterior, and lateral white columns
    b. Each funiculus consists of a large bundle of axons divided into tracts
    c. Names of spinal tracts indicate the location of the tract, the structure in which the axons originate, and the structure in which they terminate

B. Functions of the spinal cord
1. Provides conduction routes to and from the brain
    a. Ascending tracts—conduct impulses up the cord to the brain
    b. Descending tracts—conduct impulses down the cord from the brain
    c. Bundles of axons compose all tracts
    d. Tracts are both structural and functional organizations of nerve fibres
        (1) Structural—all axons of any one tract originate in the same structure and terminate in the same structure

(2) Functional—all axons that compose one tract serve one general function

e. Important ascending (sensory) tracts (**Figure 20-8**)
   (1) Lateral spinothalamic tracts—crude touch, pain, and temperature
   (2) Anterior spinothalamic tracts—crude touch, pressure
   (3) Fasciculi gracilis and cuneatus—discriminating touch and conscious kinaesthesia
   (4) Spinocerebellar tracts—subconscious kinaesthesia
   (5) Spinotectal—touch related to visual reflexes

f. Important descending (motor) tracts (**Figure 20-8**)
   (1) Lateral corticospinal tracts—voluntary movements on opposite side of the body
   (2) Anterior corticospinal tracts—voluntary movements on same side of body
   (3) Reticulospinal tracts—maintain posture during movement
   (4) Rubrospinal tracts—transmit impulses that coordinate body movements and maintenance of posture
   (5) Tectospinal tracts—head and neck movements during visual reflexes
   (6) Vestibulospinal tracts—coordination of posture and balance

g. Spinal cord—reflex centre for all spinal reflexes; spinal reflex centres are located in the grey matter of the cord

Brain

A. Size and regions
   1. One of the largest organs in the adult body (1.4 kg) having almost 85 billion neurons and as many glia
   2. Regions (**Table 20-4**)
      a. Brainstem—medulla oblongata, pons, midbrain
      b. Cerebellum
      c. Diencephalon
      d. Cerebrum

B. Brain development
   1. Most new neurons are produced before and shortly after birth; synapses are made and broken throughout life
   2. Embryology—study of processes of prenatal development
   3. Neural tube forms along dorsum of embryo by inward folding of ectoderm (primary germ layer)
      a. Forms series of connected primary, then secondary, vesicles (**Table 20-3**)
      b. Vesicles develop into adult brain regions and spinal cord
      c. Fluid canal forms fluid spaces of brain and spinal cord

C. Structure of the brainstem (**Figures 20-9** and **20-10**)
   1. Medulla oblongata
      a. Lowest part of the brainstem
      b. Part of the brain that attaches to spinal cord, located just above the foramen magnum
      c. A few centimetres in length and separated from the pons above by a horizontal groove
      d. Composed of white matter and a network of grey and white matter called the *reticular formation network*
      e. Pyramids—two bulges of white matter located on the ventral side of the medulla; formed by fibres of the pyramidal tracts
      f. Olive—oval projection located lateral to the pyramids
      g. Nuclei—clusters of neuron cell bodies located in the reticular formation
   2. Pons
      a. Located above the medulla and below the midbrain
      b. Composed of white matter and reticular formation
   3. Midbrain
      a. Located above the pons and below the cerebrum; forms the midsection of the brain
      b. Composed of white tracts and reticular formation
      c. Extending divergently through the midbrain are cerebral peduncles; conduct impulses between the midbrain and cerebrum
      d. Corpora quadrigemina—landmark in midbrain
         (1) Made up of two inferior colliculi and two superior colliculi
         (2) Forms the posterior, upper part of the midbrain that lies just above the cerebellum
         (3) Inferior colliculus—contains auditory centres
         (4) Superior colliculus—contains visual centres
      e. Red nucleus and substantia nigra—clusters of cell bodies of neurons involved in muscular control

D. Functions of the brainstem
   1. Performs sensory, motor, and reflex functions
   2. Spinothalamic tracts—important sensory tracts that pass through the brainstem
   3. Fasciculi cuneatus and gracilis and spinoreticular tracts—sensory tracts whose axons terminate in the grey matter of the brainstem
   4. Corticospinal and reticulospinal tracts—two of the major tracts present in the white matter of the brainstem
   5. Nuclei in medulla—contain reflex centres
      a. Of primary importance—cardiac, vasomotor, and respiratory centres
      b. Nonvital reflexes—vomiting, coughing, sneezing, and so on
   6. Pons—contains reflexes mediated by fifth, sixth, seventh, and eighth cranial nerves and pneumotaxic centres that help regulate respiration
   7. Midbrain—contains centres for certain cranial nerve reflexes

E. Structure of the cerebellum (**Figure 20-11**)
   1. Second largest part of the brain—contains more neurons than the rest of the nervous system
   2. Located just below the posterior portion of the cerebrum; transverse fissure separates these two parts of the brain
   3. Grey matter makes up the cortex, and white matter predominates in the interior
   4. Arbor vitae—internal white matter of the cerebellum; distinctive pattern similar to the veins of a leaf
   5. Cerebellum has numerous sulci and delicate, parallel gyri (folia)
   6. Consists of the cerebellar hemispheres and the vermis
   7. Internal white matter—composed of short and long tracts
      a. Shorter tracts—conduct impulses from neuron cell bodies located in the cerebellar cortex to neurons whose

dendrites and cell bodies compose nuclei located in the interior of the cerebellum
   b. Longer tracts—conduct impulses to and from the cerebellum; fibres enter or leave by way of three pairs of peduncles
      (1) Inferior cerebellar peduncles—composed chiefly of tracts into the cerebellum from the medulla and cord
      (2) Middle cerebellar peduncles—composed almost entirely of tracts into the cerebellum from the pons
      (3) Superior cerebellar peduncles—composed principally of tracts from dentate nuclei in the cerebellum through the red nucleus of the midbrain to the thalamus
8. Dentate nuclei
   a. Important pair of cerebellar nuclei, one of which is located in each hemisphere
   b. Nuclei connected with thalamus and with motor areas of the cerebral cortex by tracts
   c. By means of the tracts, cerebellar impulses influence the motor cortex, and the motor cortex influences the cerebellum

F. Functions of the cerebellum
1. Cerebellum compares the motor commands of the cerebrum with the information coming from proprioceptors in the muscle; impulses travel from the cerebellum to both the cerebrum and muscles to coordinate movements to produce the intended action (**Figure 20-12**)
2. General functions
   a. Acts with cerebral cortex to produce skilled movements by coordinating the activities of groups of muscles
   b. Controls skeletal muscles to maintain balance
   c. Controls posture; operates at subconscious level to smooth movements and make movements efficient and coordinated
   d. Processes sensory information; complements and assists various functions of the cerebrum

G. Diencephalon (**Figure 20-13**)
1. Located between the cerebrum and the midbrain
2. Consists of several structures located around the third ventricle: thalamus, hypothalamus, optic chiasma, pineal gland, and several others
3. Thalamus
   a. Dumbbell-shaped mass of grey matter made up of many nuclei
   b. Each lateral mass forms one lateral wall of the third ventricle
   c. Intermediate mass—extends through the third ventricle and joins the two lateral masses
   d. Geniculate bodies—two of the most important groups of nuclei comprising the thalamus; located in posterior region of each lateral mass; play role in processing auditory and visual input
   e. Serves as a major relay station for sensory impulses on their way to the cerebral cortex
   f. Performs the following primary functions:
      (1) Plays two parts in mechanism responsible for sensations
         (a) Impulses produce conscious recognition of the crude, less critical sensations of pain, temperature, and touch
         (b) Neurons relay all kinds of sensory impulses, except possibly olfactory, to the cerebrum
      (2) Plays part in the mechanism responsible for emotions by associating sensory impulses with feelings of pleasantness and unpleasantness
      (3) Plays part in arousal mechanism
      (4) Plays part in mechanisms that produce complex reflex movements
4. Hypothalamus
   a. Consists of several structures that lie beneath the thalamus
   b. Forms floor of the third ventricle and lower part of lateral walls
   c. Prominent structures found in the hypothalamus
      (1) Supraoptic nuclei—grey matter located just above and on either side of the optic chiasma
      (2) Paraventricular nuclei—located close to the wall of the third ventricle
      (3) Mamillary bodies—posterior part of hypothalamus, involved with olfactory sense
   d. Infundibulum—the stalk leading to the posterior lobe of the pituitary gland
   e. Small but functionally important area of the brain, performs many functions of greatest importance for survival and enjoyment
   f. Links mind and body
   g. Links nervous system to endocrine system
   h. Summary of hypothalamic functions
      (1) Regulator and coordinator of autonomic activities
      (2) Major relay station between the cerebral cortex and lower autonomic centres; crucial part of the route by which emotions can express themselves in changed bodily functions
      (3) Synthesizes hormones secreted by posterior pituitary and plays an essential role in maintaining water balance
      (4) Some neurons function as endocrine glands
      (5) Plays crucial role in arousal mechanism
      (6) Crucial part of mechanism regulating appetite
      (7) Crucial part of mechanism maintaining normal body temperature
5. Pineal gland
   a. Located just above the corpora quadrigemina of the midbrain
   b. Involved in regulating the body's biological clock (**Figure 20-14**)
   c. Produces melatonin as a "timekeeping hormone"
      (1) Melatonin is made from the neurotransmitter serotonin

(2) Melatonin levels increase when sunlight is absent; decrease when sunlight is present, thus regulating the circadian (daily) biological clock (**Figure 20-14**)

(3) Melatonin is the "sleep hormone"

H. Structure of the cerebrum

1. Cerebral cortex

a. Largest and uppermost division of the brain; consists of right and left cerebral hemispheres; each hemisphere is divided into five lobes (**Figure 20-15**)

(1) Frontal lobe

(2) Parietal lobe

(3) Temporal lobe

(4) Occipital lobe

(5) Insula (island of Reil)

b. Cerebral cortex—outer surface made up of six layers of grey matter

c. Gyri—convolutions; some are named: precentral gyrus, postcentral gyrus, cingulate gyrus, and hippocampal gyrus

d. Sulci—shallow grooves

e. Fissures—deeper grooves, divide each cerebral hemisphere into lobes; four prominent cerebral fissures

(1) Longitudinal fissure—deepest fissure; divides cerebrum into two hemispheres

(2) Central sulcus (fissure of Rolando)—groove between frontal and parietal lobes

(3) Lateral fissure (fissure of Sylvius)—groove between temporal lobe below and parietal lobes above; Reil island lies deep in lateral fissure

(4) Parietooccipital sulcus—groove that separates occipital lobe from parietal lobes

2. Cerebral tracts and basal nuclei

a. Cerebral tracts make up cerebrum's white matter; there are three types (**Figure 20-16**)

(1) Projection tracts—extensions of the sensory spinothalamic tracts and motor corticospinal tracts

(2) Association tracts—most numerous cerebral tracts; extend from one convolution to another in the same hemisphere

(3) Commissural tracts—extend from one convolution to a corresponding convolution in the other hemisphere; compose the corpus callosum and anterior and posterior commissures

b. Connectome—entire network of neural connections in the brain

c. Basal nuclei

(1) Structure—islands of grey matter located deep inside the white matter of each hemisphere (**Figure 20-17**); include the following:

(a) Caudate nucleus

(b) Lentiform nucleus—consists of putamen and pallidum

(c) Amygdaloid nucleus

(2) Function—regulation of voluntary (conscious) motor control related to posture, walking, and other repetitive movements; possible roles in thinking and learning

d. Corpus striatum—composed of caudate nucleus, internal capsule, and lentiform nucleus

I. Functions of the cerebral cortex

1. Functional areas of the cortex—certain areas of the cerebral cortex engage in predominantly one particular function (**Figures 20-18** and **20-19**)

a. Postcentral gyrus—mainly general somatic sensory area; receives impulses from receptors activated by heat, cold, and touch stimuli

b. Precentral gyrus—chiefly somatic motor area; impulses from neurons in this area descend over motor tracts and stimulate skeletal muscles

c. Transverse gyrus—primary auditory area

d. Occipital lobe—primary visual areas

2. Sensory functions of the cortex

a. Somatic senses—sensations of touch, pressure, temperature, proprioception, and similar perceptions that require complex sensory organs

b. Cortex contains a "somatic sensory map" of the body

c. Information sent to primary sensory areas is relayed to sensory association areas, as well as to other parts of the brain

d. The sensory information is compared and evaluated, and the cortex integrates separate bits of information into whole perceptions

3. Motor functions of the cortex

a. For normal movements to occur, many parts of the nervous system must function

b. Precentral gyrus—primary somatic motor area; controls individual muscles

c. Secondary motor area—in the gyrus immediately anterior to the precentral gyrus; activates groups of muscles simultaneously

4. Integrative functions of the cortex

J. Consciousness (**Figure 20-20**)

1. State of awareness of oneself, one's environment, and other humans

2. Depends on excitation of cortical neurons by impulses conducted to them by the reticular activating system

3. Two current concepts about the reticular activating system

a. Functions as the arousal system for the cerebral cortex

b. Its functioning is crucial for maintaining consciousness

K. Language

1. Ability to speak and write words and ability to understand spoken and written words

2. Speech centres—areas in the frontal, parietal, and temporal lobes

3. Left cerebral hemisphere contains speech centres in approximately 90% of the population; in the remaining 10%, contained in either the right hemisphere or both

4. Aphasias—lesions in speech centres

L. Emotions (**Figure 20-21**)

1. Subjective experiencing and objective expressing of emotions involve functioning of the limbic system

2. Limbic system—also known as the "emotional brain"
   a. Most structures of limbic system lie on the medial surface of the cerebrum; they are the cingulate gyrus and hippocampus
   b. Have primary connections with other parts of the brain, such as the thalamus, fornix, septal nuclei, amygdaloid nucleus, and hypothalamus

M. Memory
   1. One of our major mental activities
   2. Cortex is capable of storing and retrieving both short- and long-term memory
   3. Temporal, parietal, and occipital lobes are among the areas responsible for short- and long-term memory
   4. Structural changes in the neural pathways of the cerebral cortex store long-term memories
   5. Limbic system plays a key role in memory

Somatic Sensory Pathways in the Central Nervous System

A. For the cerebral cortex to perform its sensory functions, impulses must first be conducted to the sensory areas by sensory pathways (**Figure 20-22**)

B. Three main pools of sensory neurons
   1. Primary sensory neurons—conduct impulses from the periphery to the central nervous system
   2. Secondary sensory neurons
      a. Conduct impulses from the cord or brainstem to the thalamus
      b. Dendrites and cell bodies are located in the grey matter of the cord and brainstem
      c. Axons ascend in ascending tracts up the cord and through the brainstem, terminating in the thalamus, where they synapse with dendrites or cell bodies of tertiary sensory neurons
   3. Tertiary sensory neurons
      a. Conduct impulses from thalamus to the postcentral gyrus of the parietal lobe
      b. Bundle of axons of tertiary sensory neurons form the thalamocortical tracts
      c. Extend through the internal capsule to the cerebral cortex

C. Sensory pathways to the cerebral cortex are crossed

D. Two sensory pathways conduct impulses that produce sensations of touch and pressure
   1. Medial lemniscal system
      a. Consists of tracts that make up the fasciculi cuneatus and gracilis, and the medial lemniscus
      b. Axons of secondary sensory neurons make up medial lemniscus
      c. Functions—transmit impulses that produce discriminating touch and pressure sensations and kinaesthesia
   2. Spinothalamic pathway—functions are crude touch and pressure sensations

Somatic Motor Pathways in the Central Nervous System

A. Final common path
   1. For the cerebral cortex to perform its motor functions, impulses are conducted from its motor areas to skeletal muscles by somatic motor pathways
   2. Pathways consist of motor neurons that conduct impulses from the central nervous system to skeletal muscles
      a. Some motor pathways are extremely complex, and others are very simple
      b. At least two neurons: upper motor neuron (UMN) from the brain and lower motor neuron (LMN) from the anterior grey horn of the spinal cord to muscle fibres
   3. Principle of the final common path—cardinal principle about somatic motor pathways; only one final common path, the lower motor neuron from the anterior grey horn of the spinal cord, conducts impulses to skeletal muscles
   4. Two methods used to classify somatic motor pathways: pyramidal and extrapyramidal tracts (**Figure 20-24**)

B. Pyramidal tracts—also known as *corticospinal tracts*
   1. Approximately three quarters of the fibres decussate in the medulla and extend down the cord in the crossed corticospinal tract located on the opposite side of the spinal cord in the lateral white column
   2. Approximately one quarter of the fibres do not decussate but extend down the same side of the spinal cord as the cerebral area from which they came

C. Extrapyramidal tracts—much more complex than pyramidal tracts
   1. Consist of all motor tracts from the brain to the spinal cord lower motor neurons except the corticospinal tracts
   2. Within the brain, consist of numerous relays of motor neurons between motor areas of the cortex, basal nuclei, thalamus, cerebellum, and brainstem
   3. Within the spinal cord, some important tracts are the reticulospinal tracts
   4. Conduction by extrapyramidal tracts plays a crucial part in producing large, automatic movements
   5. Conduction by extrapyramidal tracts plays an important part in emotional expressions

D. Facilitatory and inhibitory tracts
   1. Facilitatory impulses increase tone of extensor muscles and decrease tone of flexor muscles
   2. Inhibitory impulses decrease tone of extensor muscles and increase tone of flexor muscles

E. Motor program—set of coordinated commands that control the programmed motor activity mediated by extra-pyramidal pathways (**Figure 20-24**)

Cycle of Life: Central Nervous System

A. Development and degeneration of CNS—most obvious functional change over the life span

B. Development of brain and spinal cord begins in the womb

UNIT 3

C. Lack of development in the newborn is evidenced by lack of complex integrative functions
   1. Language
   2. Complex memory
   3. Comprehension of spatial relationships
   4. Complex motor skills
D. Complex functions develop by adulthood
E. Late adulthood—tissues degenerate
   1. Profound degeneration—unable to perform complex functions
   2. Milder degeneration—temporary memory lapse or difficulty with complex motor tasks

The Big Picture: The Central Nervous System and the Whole Body

A. Central nervous system—ultimate regulator of the body; essential to survival
B. Able to integrate bits of information from all over the body, make sense of it, and make decisions

UNIT 3

REVIEW QUESTIONS

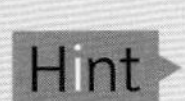

Write out the answers to these questions after reading the chapter and reviewing the Chapter Summary. Note—writing out your answers will consolidate learning and provide a valuable resource of information.

1. What term refers to the membranous covering of the brain and cord? What three layers compose this covering? Which layer could be described as lacy?
2. What are the large fluid-filled spaces within the brain called? How many are there? What do they contain?
3. Describe the formation and circulation of cerebrospinal fluid.
4. Describe the structure and general functions of the spinal cord.
5. List the major components of the brainstem, and identify their general functions.
6. Describe the general functions of the cerebellum.
7. Describe the general functions of the thalamus.
8. Describe the general functions of the hypothalamus.
9. Describe the general functions of the cerebrum.
10. What general functions does the cerebral cortex perform? Why do scientists consider that it is the cerebral cortex that makes us human?
11. Define *consciousness.* Name the normal states, or levels, of consciousness.
12. Name some altered states of consciousness.
13. Identify the following kinds of brainwaves according to their frequency, voltage, and the level of consciousness in which they predominate: alpha, beta, delta, theta.
14. Locate the dendrite, cell body, and axon of primary, secondary, and tertiary sensory neurons.
15. Compare and contrast the general structure of the cerebrum and cerebellum.

CRITICAL THINKING QUESTIONS

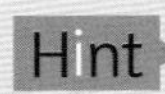

After finishing the Review Questions, write out the answers to these more in-depth questions to help you apply your new knowledge. Go back to sections of the chapter that relate to concepts that you find difficult.

1. Explain what the term *reflex centre* means. Is an interneuron necessary for a reflex centre? Explain your answer.
2. Explain briefly what is meant by the arousal or alerting mechanism.
3. Some people claim meditation has a wide range of benefits. What benefits can be supported by scientific evidence?
4. If a researcher discovered that a substantial reduction in neurotransmitter concentration caused difficulty in forming memory, what theory of memory formation would be refuted?
5. In Chapter 19, an action potential was explained in terms of electrical activity. Explain the process of measuring that activity to differentiate the types of brainwaves.
6. A person exhibiting an absence of any reflex and a person having exaggerated deep tendon reflexes both show signs of different motor pathway injuries. Using these symptoms as the basis, explain the motor pathway that was damaged and what other symptoms each person might have.
7. Compare pyramidal tract and extrapyramidal tract functions.
8. A patient with a brain infection can be diagnosed by culturing cerebrospinal fluid. The greatest concentration of the disease-causing organism can be drawn from the fluid as soon as it leaves the brain at the level of the third or fourth vertebra. Why would this be an unwise place to take the sample? Where would a better location be? Explain your answer.
9. Discuss the pattern of naming the system of the brain's ventricles. Give the location of the ventricles.
10. A young driver at a roadside police checkpoint is suspected of driving under the influence of drink or drugs. The alcohol and drug tests are negative, but the driver has an uncoordinated gait, cannot touch her nose with both index fingers, jerky eye movements and slurred speech. Suggest a neurological cause of this behaviour.

21 Peripheral Nervous System

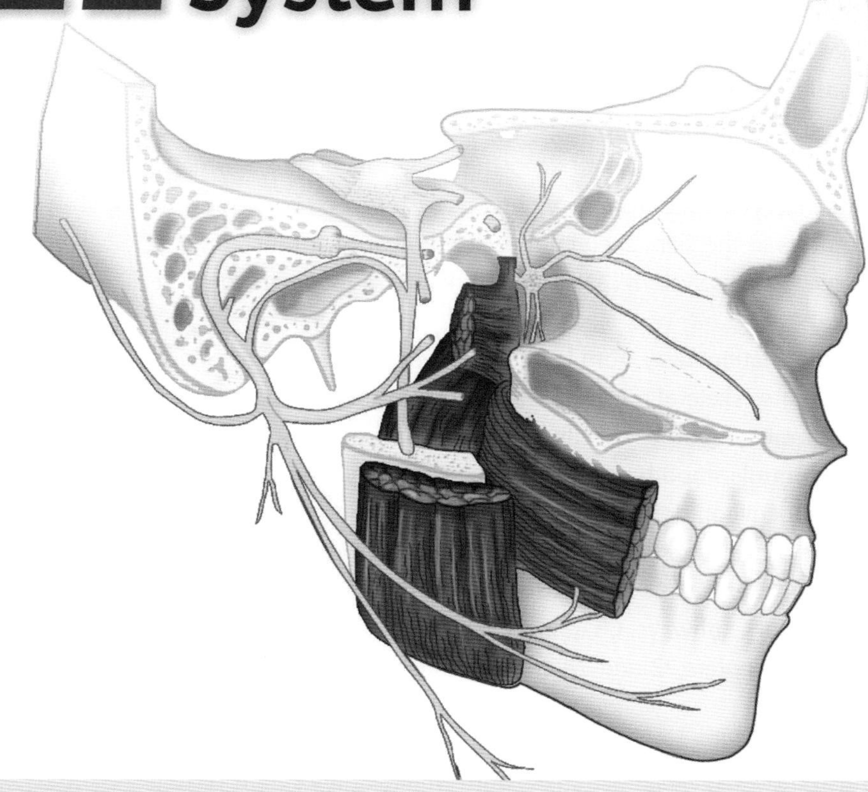

CHAPTER OUTLINE

Hint *Scan this outline before you begin to read the chapter, as a preview of how the concepts are organized.*

LANGUAGE OF SCIENCE

Hint *Use this list to aid your pronunciation of unfamiliar words.*

abdominal reflex (ab-DOM-i-nal REE-fleks) [*abdomin-* **belly,** *-al* **relating to,** *re-* **again,** *-flex* **bend**]

abducens nerve (ab-DYOO-sens nerv) [*ab-* **away,** *-duc-* **lead,** *-ens* **process**]

accessory nerve (ak-SES-oh-ree)

acetylcholine (ACh) (ass-ee-til-KOH-leen) [*acetyl-* **vinegar,** *-chole-* **bile,** *-ine* **made of**]

ankle jerk reflex [*re-* **again,** *-flex* **bend**]

autonomic (visceral) reflex (aw-toh-NOM-ik [VISS-er-al] REE-fleks) [*auto-* **self,** *-nomo-* **law,** *-ic* **relating to,** *viscer-* **internal organ,** *-al* **relating to,** *re-* **again,** *-flex* **bend**]

brachial plexus (BRAY-kee-al PLEK-sus) [*brachi-* **arm,** *-al* **relating to,** *plexus* **braid or network**] *pl.,* plexi or plexuses

cauda equina (KAW-dah eh-KWY-nah) [*cauda* **tail,** *equina* **of a horse**] *pl.,* caudae equinae

cervical plexus (SER-vih-kal PLEK-sus) [*cervic-* **neck,** *-al* **relating to,** *plexus* **braid or network**] *pl.,* plexi or plexuses

corneal reflex (KOR-nee-al REE-fleks) [*corn-* **horn,** *-al* **relating to,** *re-* **again,** *-flex* **bend**]

cranial nerve (KRAY-nee-al nerv) [*crani-* **skull,** *-al* **relating to**]

cranial reflex (KRAY-nee-al REE-fleks) [*crani-* **skull,** *-al* **relating to,** *re-* **again,** *-flex* **bend**]

dermatome (DER-mah-tohm) [*derma-* **skin,** *-tome* **cut segment or region**]

dorsal ramus (DOR-sal RAY-mus) [*dors-* **the back,** *-al* **relating to,** *ramus* **branch**] *pl.,* rami

dorsal root (DOR-sal) [*dors-* **the back,** *-al* **relating to**]

facial nerve (FAY-shal nerv) [*faci-* **face,** *-al* **relating to**]

ganglion (GANG-lee-on) [*gangli-* **knot,** *-on* **unit**] *pl.,* ganglia

continued on p. 498

In Chapter 20, you learned about the structure and function of the central nervous system (CNS). In this chapter we explore the nerve pathways that lead to and from the CNS, which together make up the peripheral nervous system (PNS). The PNS is made up of the 31 pairs of spinal nerves that emerge from the spinal cord, the 12 pairs of cranial nerves that emerge from the brain, and all the smaller nerves that branch from these "main" nerves. **Figure 21-1** shows an overview of the PNS.

Recall from earlier discussions that afferent fibres carry information into the CNS. Afferent fibres, part of the sensory nervous system, help us maintain homeostasis by sensing changes in our internal or external environment—providing the feedback necessary to keep the body functioning normally. Afferent fibres belonging to the somatic sensory or special sensory nervous system feed back information regarding changes detected by receptors in the skin, skeletal muscles, and special sense organs. Afferent fibres belonging to the autonomic nervous system (ANS) feed back information regarding the effects of autonomic control of the viscera.

Recall also that efferent fibres carry information away from the CNS. Efferent fibres may belong to the somatic nervous system (SNS) that regulates skeletal muscles, allowing us to survive by defending ourselves, getting food, or performing other essential tasks. Efferent fibres may, on the other hand, belong to the ANS. Autonomic regulation controls smooth and cardiac muscle and glands in ways that help us maintain homeostasis of the internal environment.

The first sections of this chapter explore concepts regarding the structure and function of the spinal and cranial nerves. The last portion of the chapter is devoted to discussion of the peripheral elements of the SNS, with an emphasis on efferent (motor) pathways. Chapter 22 then picks up the story, emphasizing efferent pathways of the ANS. Finally, Chapters 23 and 24 explore major concepts of sensation via the afferent pathways.

This study of peripheral nerve pathways clarifies and expands the understanding of the nervous system gained in previous chapters. It also serves as a foundation for understanding important clinical applications (**Box 21-1**). •

BOX 21-1 *health matters*

Peripheral Neuropathy

The term **peripheral neuropathy** tells you exactly what it signifies: disease of the peripheral nerves. The term is used to designate many different diseases with many different causes—but all involve damage to peripheral nerves. These disorders can also be called *peripheral neuritis.* If many nerves are involved, peripheral neuropathy can also be called *polyneuropathy* or *polyneuritis.* The most common cause of peripheral nerve damage in the UK is ***diabetes mellitus.*** There are estimated to be 4.5 million people with diabetes, and up to 50% have some form of peripheral neuropathy. See ***Diabetes Mellitus*** online at ***Connect It!*** Other causes include: metabolic problems such as kidney disease, injuries such as sports mishaps, poisoning as in drug neurotoxicity and alcohol abuse, infections such as in *leprosy (Hansen disease; Mycobacterium leprae)* or shingles (see **Box 21-3**, p. 488), and genetic mutations such as *Leber hereditary optic neuropathy* (see Chapter 48, p. 1137). •

SPINAL NERVES

Thirty-one pairs of **spinal nerves** are connected to the spinal cord. They have no special names but are merely numbered according to the level of the vertebral column at which they emerge from the spinal cavity (**Figure 21-2**). Although there are only seven cervical vertebrae, there are eight cervical nerve pairs (C1 through C8), twelve thoracic nerve pairs (T1 through T12), five lumbar nerve pairs (L1 through L5), five sacral nerve pairs (S1 through S5), and one coccygeal pair of spinal nerves. The first pair of cervical nerves emerges from the cord in the space above the first cervical vertebra, and the eighth cervical nerve emerges between the last cervical vertebra and the first thoracic vertebra. Thus nerve pair C1 passes between the skull and vertebra C1, nerve pair C2 passes between vertebrae C1 and C2, nerve pair C3 passes between vertebrae C2 and C3, and so on. All the thoracic nerves pass out of the spinal cavity horizontally through the intervertebral foramina below their respective vertebrae.

Lumbar, sacral, and coccygeal nerve roots, on the other hand, descend from their point of origin at the lower end of the spinal cord (which terminates at the level of the first lumbar vertebra) before reaching the intervertebral foramina of their respective vertebrae,

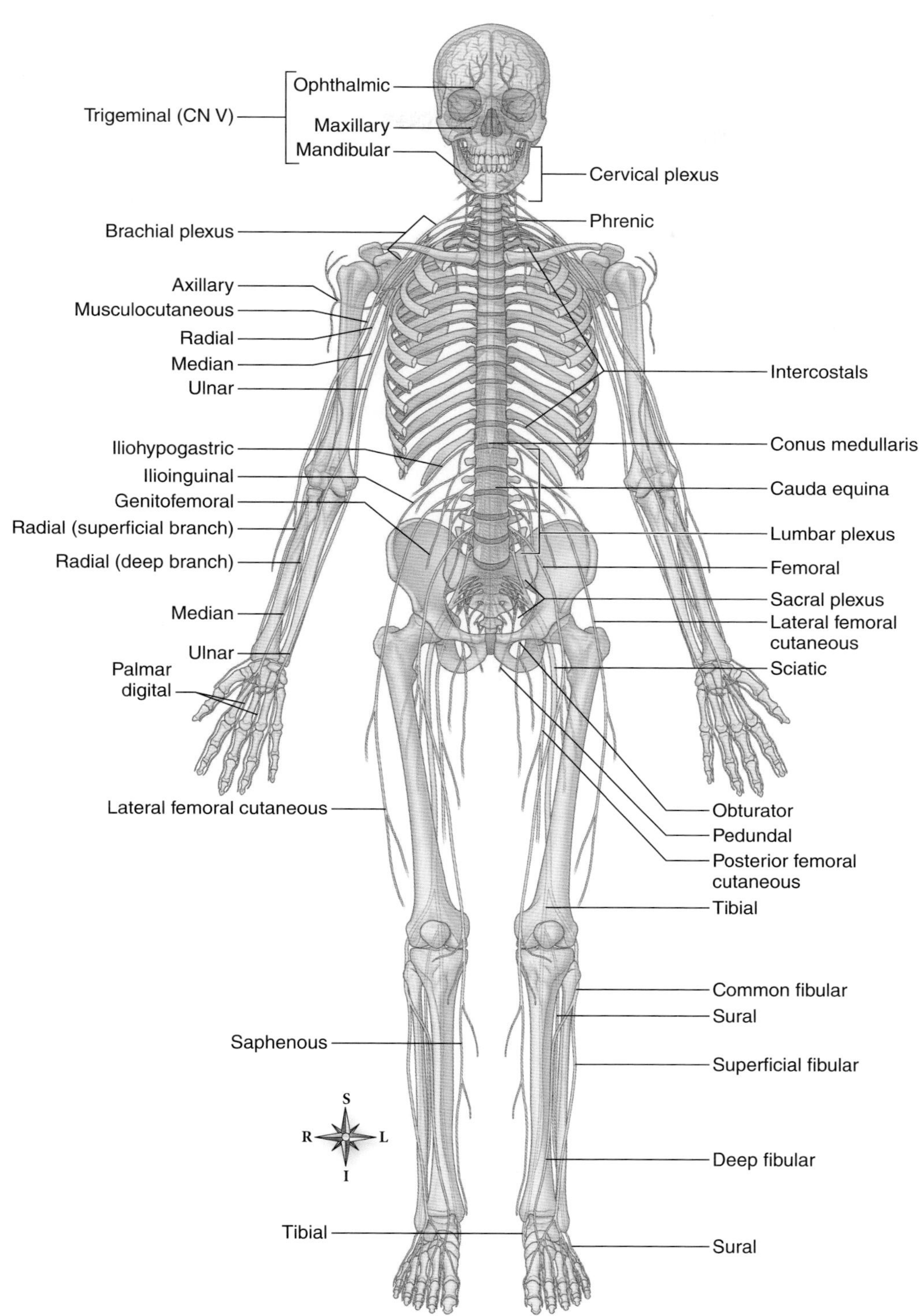

FIGURE 21-1 Overview of major peripheral nerves.

UNIT 3

through which the nerves then emerge. This gives the lower end of the cord, with its attached spinal nerve roots, the appearance of a horse's tail. In fact, it bears the name **cauda equina,** which is the Latin equivalent for "horse's tail" (see **Figure 21-2**).

Structure of Spinal Nerves

Each spinal nerve attaches to the spinal cord by means of two short roots, a **ventral** (anterior) **root** (*anterior root*) and a **dorsal root** (*posterior root*). The dorsal root of each spinal nerve is easily recognized by a swelling called the dorsal root **ganglion,** or *spinal ganglion* (**Figure 21-3**). The roots and dorsal ganglia lie within the spinal cavity, as **Figure 21-3** shows.

As described in Chapter 20, the ventral root includes motor neurons that carry information from the CNS and toward effectors (muscles and glands). Recall that in each somatic motor pathway, a single motor fibre stretches from the anterior grey horn of the spinal cord, through the ventral root, and on through the spinal nerve toward a skeletal muscle. Autonomic fibres, which also carry motor

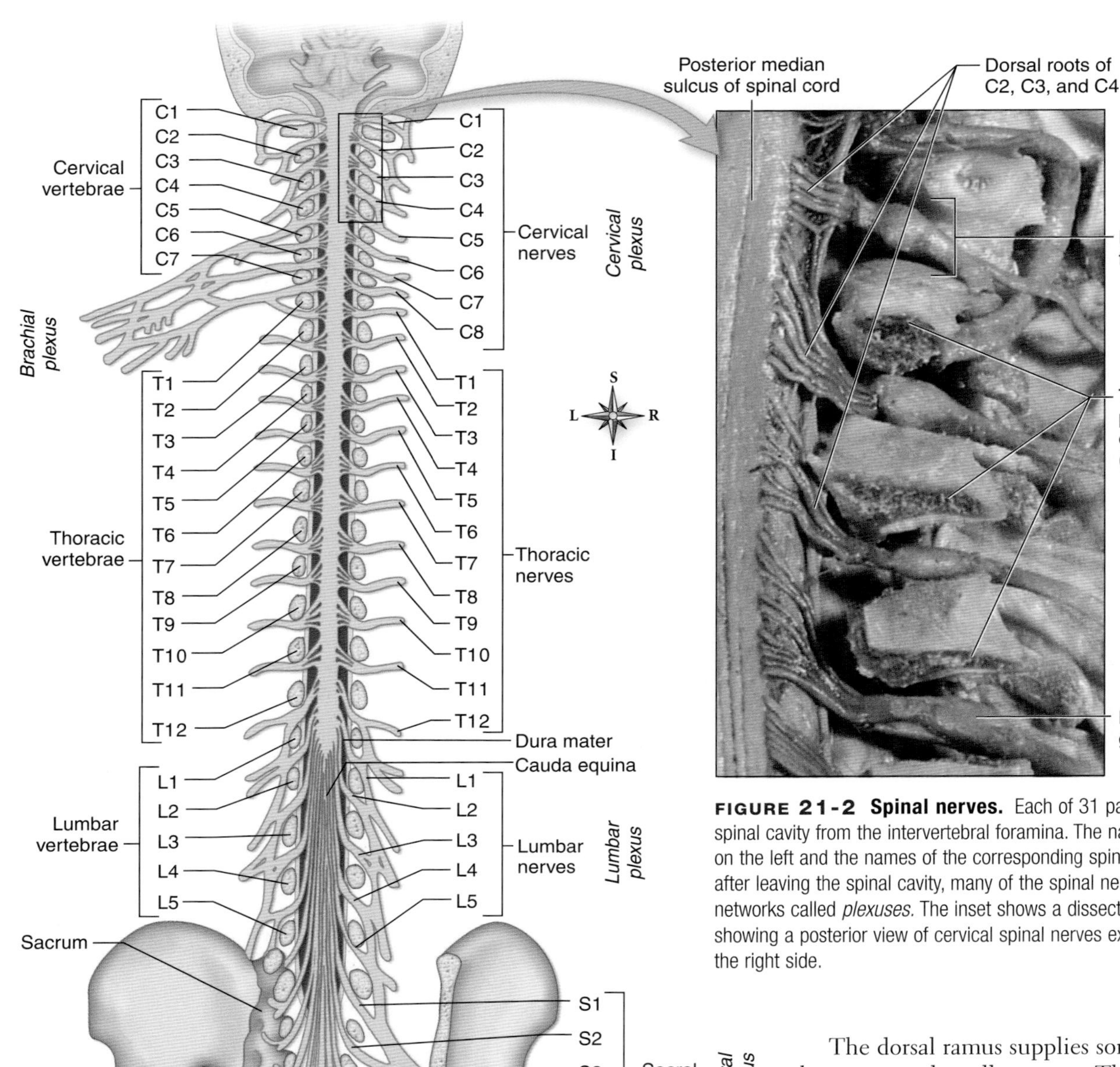

FIGURE 21-2 Spinal nerves. Each of 31 pairs of spinal nerves exits the spinal cavity from the intervertebral foramina. The names of the vertebrae are given on the left and the names of the corresponding spinal nerves on the right. Note that after leaving the spinal cavity, many of the spinal nerves interconnect to form networks called *plexuses.* The inset shows a dissection of the cervical region, showing a posterior view of cervical spinal nerves exiting intervertebral foramina on the right side.

information toward effectors, may also pass through the ventral root to become part of a spinal nerve. The dorsal root of each spinal nerve includes sensory fibres that carry information from receptors in the peripheral nerves. The dorsal root ganglion contains the cell bodies of the sensory neurons. Because all spinal nerves contain both motor and sensory fibres, they are designated as **mixed nerves.**

Soon after each spinal nerve emerges from the spinal cavity, it forms several large branches, each of which is called a **ramus** (*plural,* rami). As **Figure 21-3** shows, each spinal nerve splits into a distinct **dorsal ramus** and **ventral ramus.**

The dorsal ramus supplies somatic motor and sensory fibres to several smaller nerves. These smaller nerves, in turn, innervate the muscles and skin of the posterior surface of the head, neck, and trunk.

The structure of the ventral ramus is a little more complex. Autonomic motor fibres split away from the ventral ramus, heading toward a ganglion of the *sympathetic chain.* There, some of the autonomic fibres synapse with autonomic neurons that eventually continue on to autonomic effectors by way of *splanchnic nerves* (see **Figure 21-3**). However, some fibres synapse with autonomic neurons whose fibres rejoin the ventral ramus. The two thin rami formed by this splitting away, then rejoining, of autonomic fibres are together called the *sympathetic rami.* Motor (autonomic and somatic) and sensory fibres of the ventral rami innervate muscles and glands in the upper and lower extremities and in the lateral and ventral portions of the neck and trunk.

Nerve Plexuses

The ventral rami of most spinal nerves—all but nerves T2 through T12—subdivide to form complex networks called **plexuses.** As **Figure 21-2** shows, there are four major pairs of plexuses: the cervical

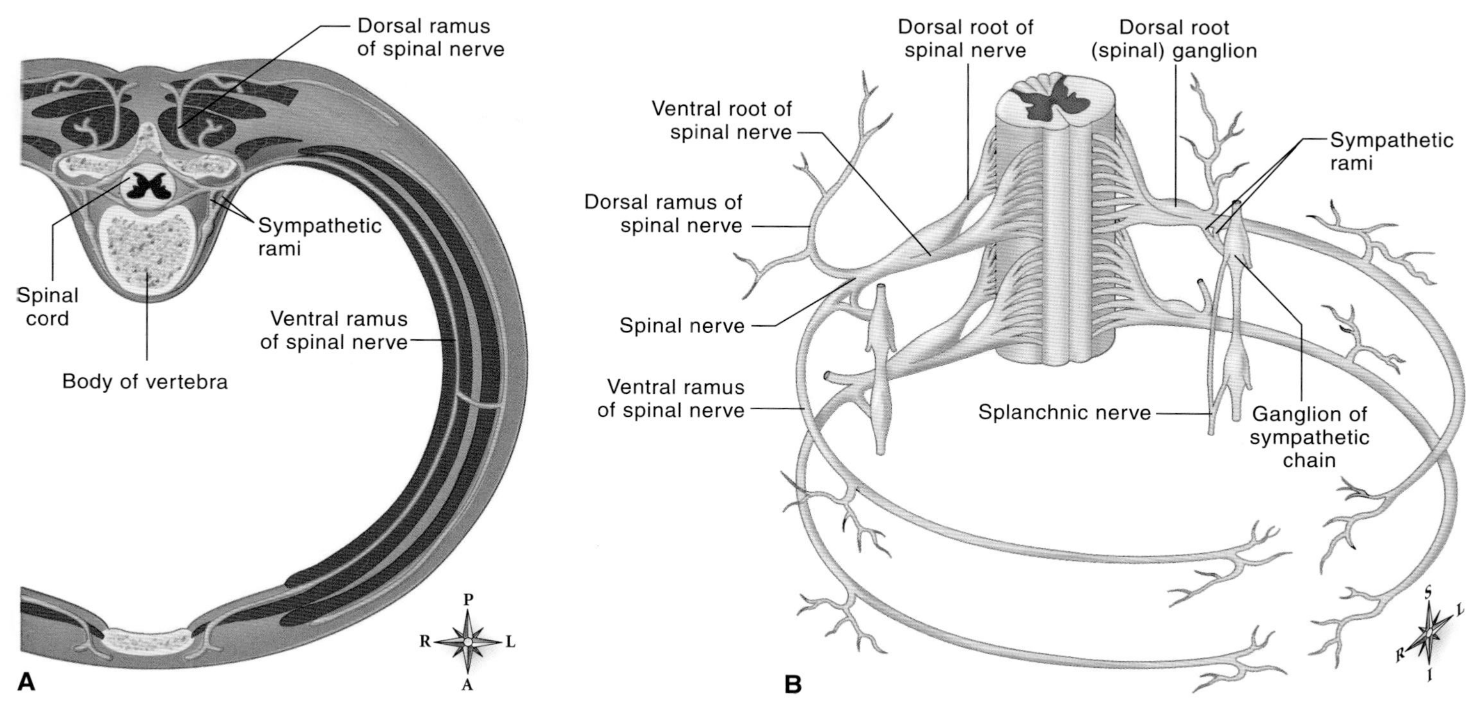

FIGURE 21-3 Rami of the spinal nerves. Note that ventral and dorsal roots join to form a spinal nerve. The spinal nerve then splits into a *dorsal ramus* (plural, *rami*) and *ventral ramus*. The ventral ramus communicates with a chain of sympathetic (autonomic) ganglia by way of a pair of thin sympathetic rami. **A,** Superior view of a pair of thoracic spinal nerves. **B,** Anterior view of several pairs of thoracic spinal nerves.

plexus, the brachial plexus, the lumbar plexus, and the sacral plexus. **Table 21-1** summarizes important information about these major plexuses.

The term *plexus* is the Latin word for "braid". This is an apt name for a structure in which fibres of several different rami join together to form individual nerves. Each individual nerve that emerges from a plexus contains all the fibres that innervate a particular region of the body. In fact, the destination of each nerve serves as a basis for its name (see **Table 21-1**). Because spinal nerve fibres are thus rearranged according to their ultimate destination, the plexus reduces the number of nerves needed to supply each body part. And because each body region is innervated by fibres that originate from several adjacent spinal nerves, damage to one spinal nerve does not mean a complete loss of function in any one region.

Cervical Plexus

The **cervical plexus**, shown in **Figure 21-4**, is found deep within the neck. Ventral rami of the first four cervical spinal nerves (C1 through C4), along with a branch of the ventral ramus of C5, exchange fibres in the cervical plexus. Individual nerves emerging from this plexus innervate the muscles and skin of the neck, upper shoulders, and part of the head. Also exiting this plexus is the **phrenic nerve,** which

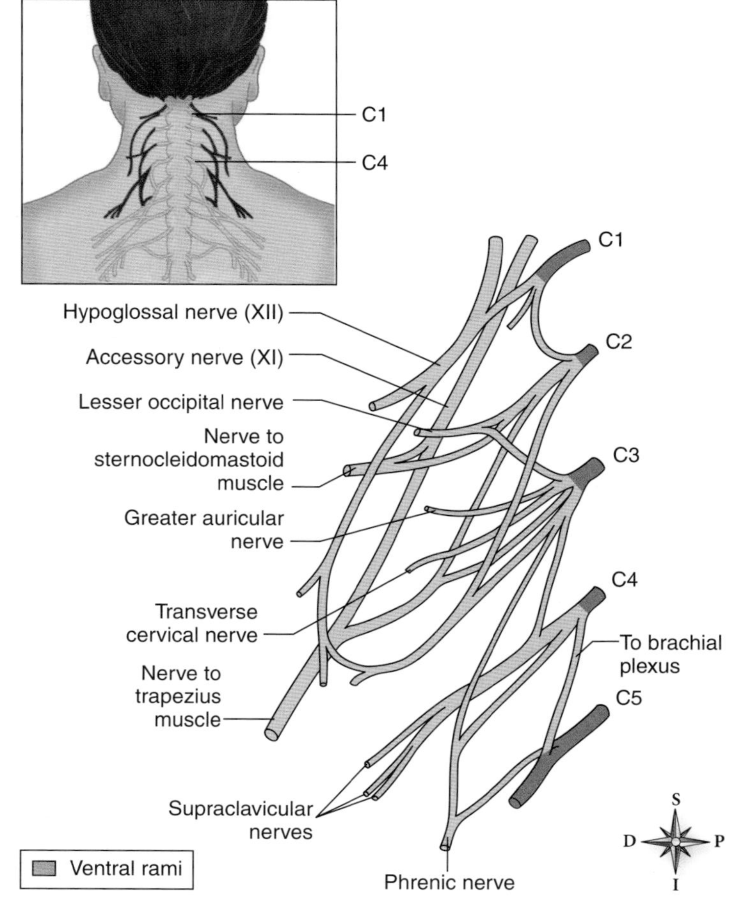

FIGURE 21-4 Cervical plexus. Ventral rami of the first four cervical spinal nerves (C1 through C4) exchange fibres in this plexus found deep within the neck. Notice that some fibres from C5 also enter this plexus to form a portion of the phrenic nerve.

TABLE 21-1 Spinal Nerves and Peripheral Branches

SPINAL NERVES	PLEXUSES FORMED FROM ANTERIOR RAMI	SPINAL NERVE BRANCHES FROM PLEXUSES	PARTS SUPPLIED
Cervical 1, 2, 3, 4	Cervical plexus	Lesser occipital Greater auricular Cutaneous nerve of neck Supraclavicular nerves Branches to muscles	Sensory to back of head, front of neck, and upper part of shoulder; motor to numerous neck muscles
		Phrenic nerve[†]	Diaphragm
Cervical 5, 6, 7, 8 ***Thoracic (or Dorsal)*** 1	Brachial plexus	Suprascapular and dorsoscapular	Superficial muscles* of scapula
		Thoracic nerves, medial and lateral branches	Pectoralis major and minor
		Long thoracic nerve	Serratus anterior
		Thoracodorsal	Latissimus dorsi
		Subscapular	Subscapular and teres major muscles
		Axillary (circumflex)	Deltoid and teres minor muscles and skin over deltoid
		Musculocutaneous	Muscles of front of arm (biceps brachii, coracobrachialis, brachialis) and skin on outer side of forearm
		Ulnar	Flexor carpi ulnaris and part of flexor digitorum profundus; some muscles of hand; sensory to medial side of hand, little finger, and medial half of fourth finger
		Median	Rest of muscles of front of forearm and hand; sensory to skin of palmar surface of thumb, index, and middle fingers
		Radial	Triceps muscle and muscles of back of forearm; sensory to skin of back of forearm and hand
		Medial cutaneous	Sensory to inner surface of arm and forearm
2, 3, 4, 5, 6, 7, 8, 9, 10, 11, 12	No plexus formed; branches run directly to intercostal muscles and skin of thorax		
Lumbar 1, 2, 3, 4, 5 ***Sacral*** 1, 2, 3, 4, 5	Lumbosacral plexus	Iliohypogastric (Sometimes fused)	Sensory to anterior abdominal wall
		Ilioinguinal (Sometimes fused)	Sensory to anterior abdominal wall and external genitalia; motor to muscles of abdominal wall
		Genitofemoral	Sensory to skin of external genitalia and inguinal region
		Lateral femoral cutaneous	Sensory to outer side of thigh
		Femoral	Motor to quadriceps, sartorius, and iliacus muscles; sensory to front of thigh and medial side of leg (saphenous nerve)
		Obturator	Motor to adductor muscles of thigh
		Tibial[‡] (medial popliteal)	Motor to muscles of calf of leg; sensory to skin of calf of leg and sole of foot
		Common peroneal (lateral popliteal)	Motor to evertors and dorsiflexors of foot; sensory to lateral surface of leg and dorsal surface of foot
		Nerves to hamstring muscles	Motor to muscles of back of thigh
		Gluteal nerves	Motor to buttock muscles and tensor fasciae latae
		Posterior femoral cutaneous	Sensory to skin of buttocks, posterior surface of thigh, and leg
		Pudendal nerve	Motor to perineal muscles; sensory to skin of perineum
Coccygeal 1	Coccygeal plexus	Anococcygeal nerves	Sensory to skin overlying coccyx

*Although nerves to muscles are considered motor, they do contain some sensory fibres that transmit proprioceptive impulses.

†Most fibres in the phrenic nerve originate in C4, but a few fibres originate in C3 and C5; thus, this nerve originates in both the cervical and brachial plexuses; some remember this with the phrase *3, 4, and 5 keep the diaphragm alive.*

‡Sensory fibres from the tibial and peroneal nerves unite to form the medial cutaneous (or sural) nerve that supplies the calf of the leg and the lateral surface of the foot. In the thigh the tibial and common peroneal nerves are usually enclosed in a single sheath to form the *sciatic nerve,* the largest nerve in the body with a width of approximately 2 cm. About two thirds of the way down the posterior part of the thigh, it divides into its component parts. Branches of the sciatic nerve extend into the hamstring muscles.

BOX 21-2 *health matters* | **Phrenic Nerves**

The right and left phrenic nerves, whose fibres come from the cervical plexus, are of considerable clinical interest because they supply the diaphragm muscle. Contraction of the diaphragm permits inspiration, and relaxation of the diaphragm permits expiration. If the neck is broken in a way that severs or crushes the spinal cord above this level, nerve impulses from the brain can no longer reach the phrenic nerves and therefore the diaphragm stops contracting. Unless artificial respiration of some kind is provided, the patient dies of respiratory paralysis as a result of the broken neck. Any disease or injury that damages the spinal cord between the third and fifth cervical segments may paralyze the phrenic nerve and, therefore, the diaphragm.

Brachial plexus

C5
T1
A
S
D P
I
C4
C5
C6
C7
C8
T1
Dorsoscapular nerve
Suprascapular nerve
Subclavian nerve
Axillary nerve
Radial nerve
Musculocutaneous nerve
Medial and lateral pectoral nerves
Median nerve
Ulnar nerve
Long thoracic nerve
Medial brachial cutaneous nerve

Ventral rami
Trunks
Cords
Anterior divisions
Posterior divisions
Nerves

Dorsal scapular nerve
Suprascapular nerve
Superior trunk
Middle trunk
Inferior trunk
C4
C5
C6
C7
C8
T1
Musculocutaneous nerve
Median nerve
Radial nerve
Ulnar nerve
Lateral antebrachial cutaneous nerve
Superficial branch of radial nerve
Deep radial nerve
S
D P
I
Ulnar nerve
Median nerve
Palmar digital nerves
B

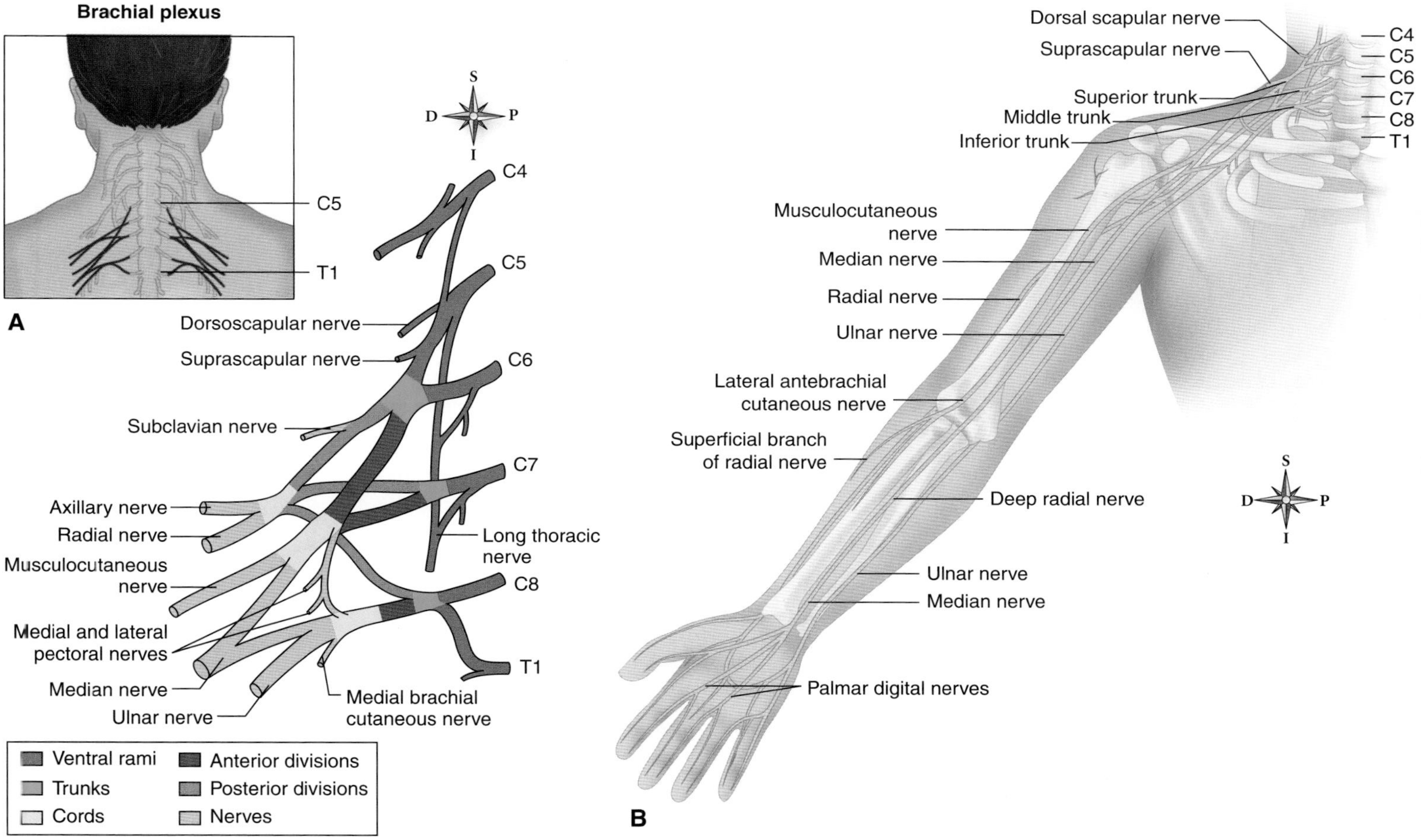

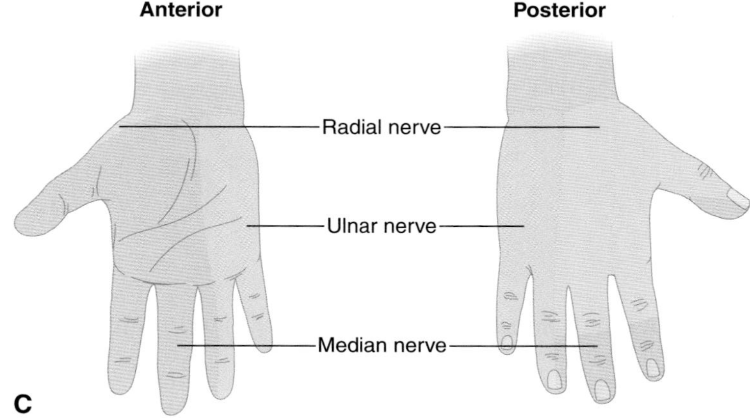

FIGURE 21-5 Brachial plexus. A, From the five rami, C5 through T1, the plexus forms three "trunks". Each trunk in turn subdivides into an anterior and posterior "division". The divisional branches then reorganize into three "cords". The cords then give rise to the individual nerves that exit this plexus. **B,** Nerves of the brachial plexus. **C,** Innervation of the hand.

innervates the diaphragm (**Box 21-2**). Two cranial nerves, the accessory nerve (XI) and the hypoglossal nerve (XII), receive small branches that emerge from the cervical plexus.

Brachial Plexus

The **brachial plexus,** shown in **Figure 21-5**, is found deep within the shoulder. It passes from the ventral rami of spinal nerves C5 through T1, beneath the clavicle (collarbone), and toward the arm. Individual nerves that emerge from the brachial plexus innervate the lower part of the shoulder and the entire upper extremity.

UNIT 3

Lumbar Plexus

Another spinal nerve plexus is the **lumbar plexus,** which is formed by the intermingling of fibres from the first four lumbar nerves (**Figure 21-6**). This network of nerves is located in the lumbar region of the back near the psoas muscle. The large femoral nerve is one of several nerves emerging from the lumbar plexus. It divides into many branches supplying the thigh and leg.

Sacral Plexus and Coccygeal Plexus

Fibres from the fourth and fifth lumbar nerves (L4 and L5) and the first four sacral nerves (S1 through S4) form the **sacral plexus.** It lies in the pelvic cavity on the anterior surface of the piriformis muscle. Because of their close proximity and overlap of fibres, the lumbar and sacral plexuses are often considered together as the *lumbosacral* plexus (see **Figure 21-6**). Among other nerves that emerge from the sacral plexus are the tibial and common fibular nerves. In the thigh, they form the largest nerve in the body, the great **sciatic nerve.** It pierces the buttocks and runs down the back of the thigh. Its many branches supply nearly all the skin of the leg, the posterior thigh muscles, and the leg and foot muscles. *Sciatica,* or neuralgia of the sciatic nerve, is a fairly common and very painful condition.

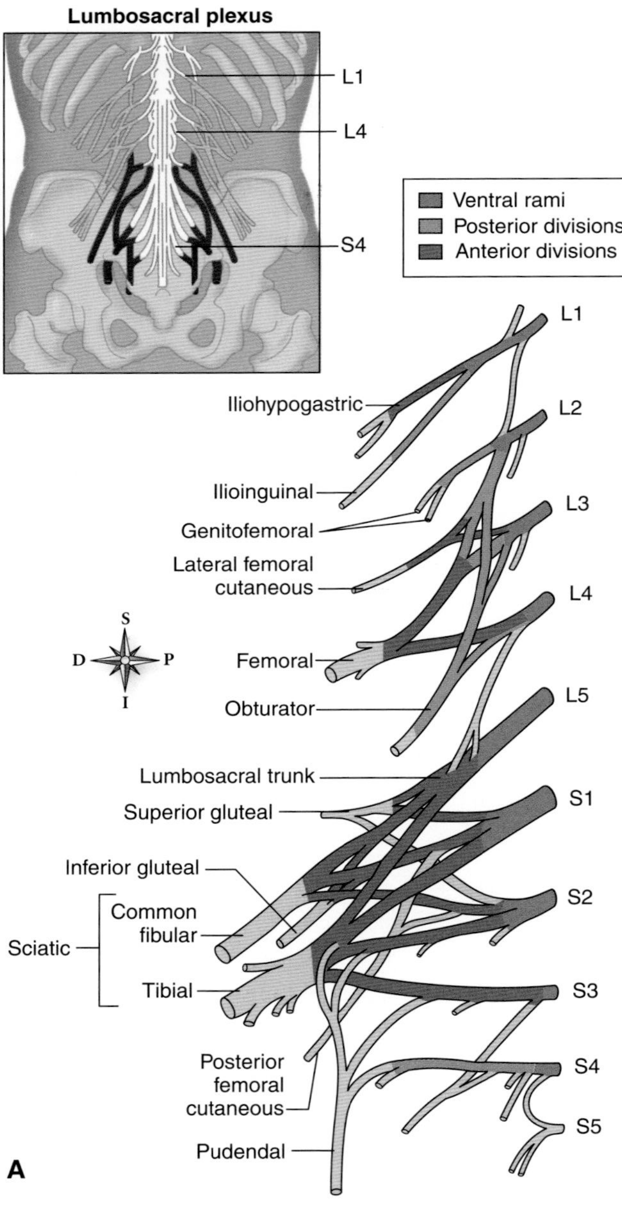

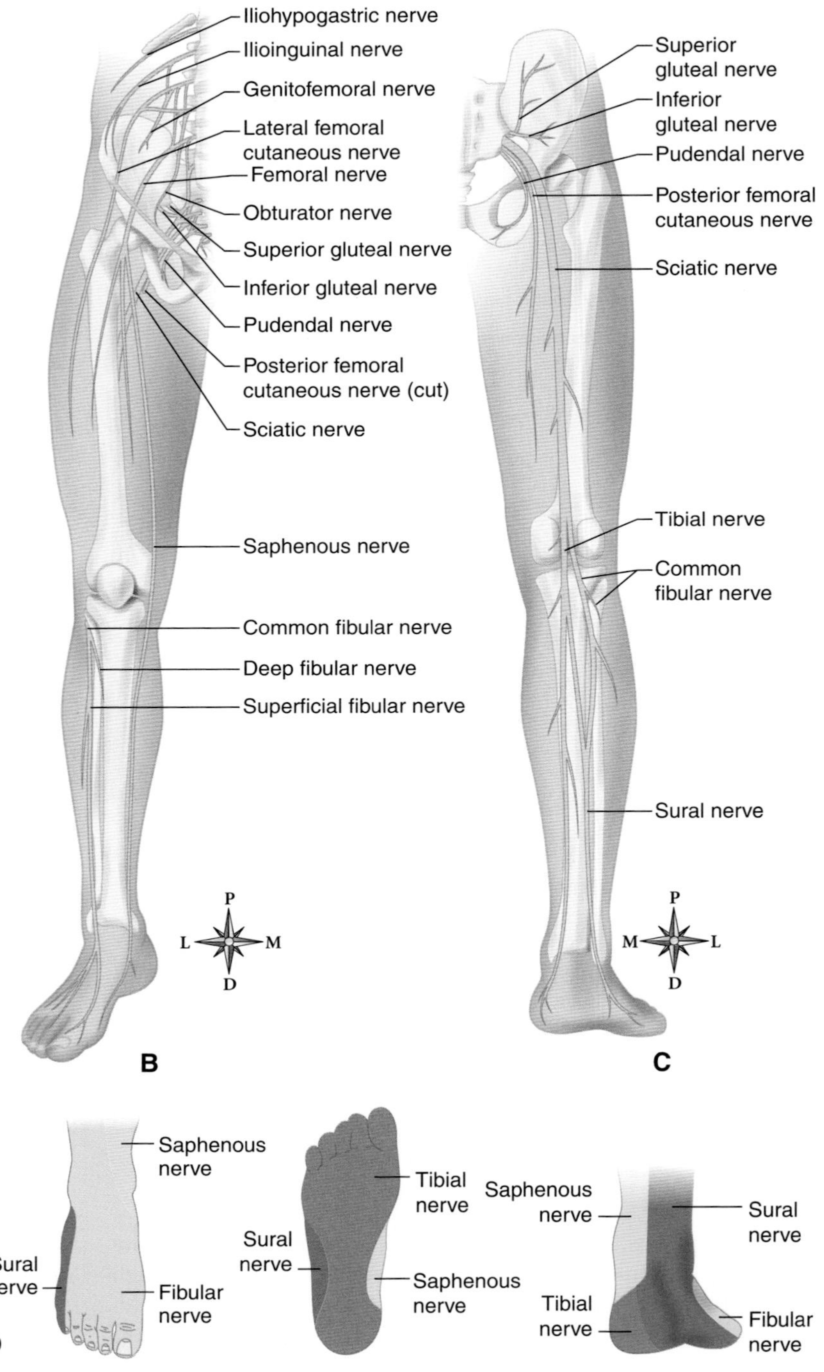

FIGURE 21-6 Lumbosacral plexus. A, This plexus is formed by the combination of the lumbar plexus with the sacral plexus, as shown in the inset. Note that the ventral rami split into anterior and posterior "divisions" before reorganizing into the various individual nerves that exit this plexus. **B,** Anterior view of lumbosacral plexus nerves. **C,** Posterior view of lumbosacral plexus nerves. **D,** Innervation of the foot and ankle.

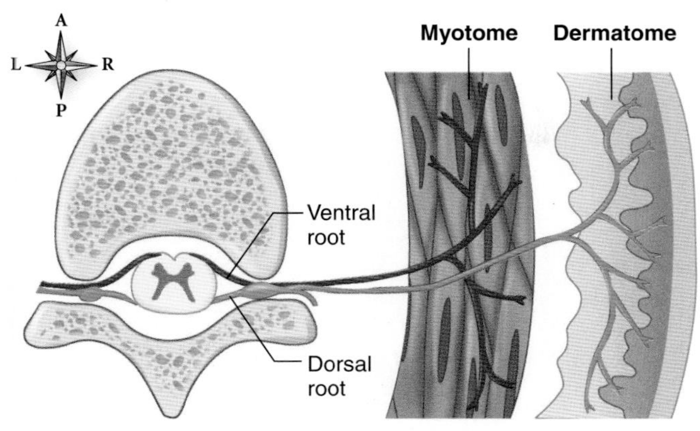

FIGURE 21-7 Segmental distribution of spinal nerves. A dermatome is a region of skin supplied by afferent (sensory) fibres of a given spinal nerve. A myotome is a region of skeletal muscle innervated by efferent (motor) fibres of a given spinal nerve. Spinal nerves at different segments of the spinal cord innervate different sets of dermatomes and myotomes.

The last sacral spinal nerve (S5), along with a few fibres from S4, joins with the coccygeal nerve to form a small *coccygeal plexus*. Thin anococcygeal nerves arising from this plexus supply the skin that lies over the coccyx bone.

Dermatomes and Myotomes

At first glance the distribution of spinal nerves does not appear to follow an ordered arrangement, but detailed mapping of the skin surface has revealed a close relationship between the spinal origin of each spinal nerve and the region of the body it innervates. Knowledge of the segmental arrangement of spinal nerves and the region of the body innervated by each segment has proved useful to health professionals. For instance, one can identify the site of spinal cord or nerve abnormality by locating the corresponding area of the body insensitive to a pinprick. Each skin surface area supplied by sensory fibres of a given spinal nerve is called a **dermatome,** a name that means "skin section" (**Figure 21-7** and **Figure 21-8**).

The body maps in **Figure 21-8** show sharp boundaries between sensory dermatomes, but there is actually quite a bit of overlap between adjacent dermatomes. Overlap of dermatomes results from

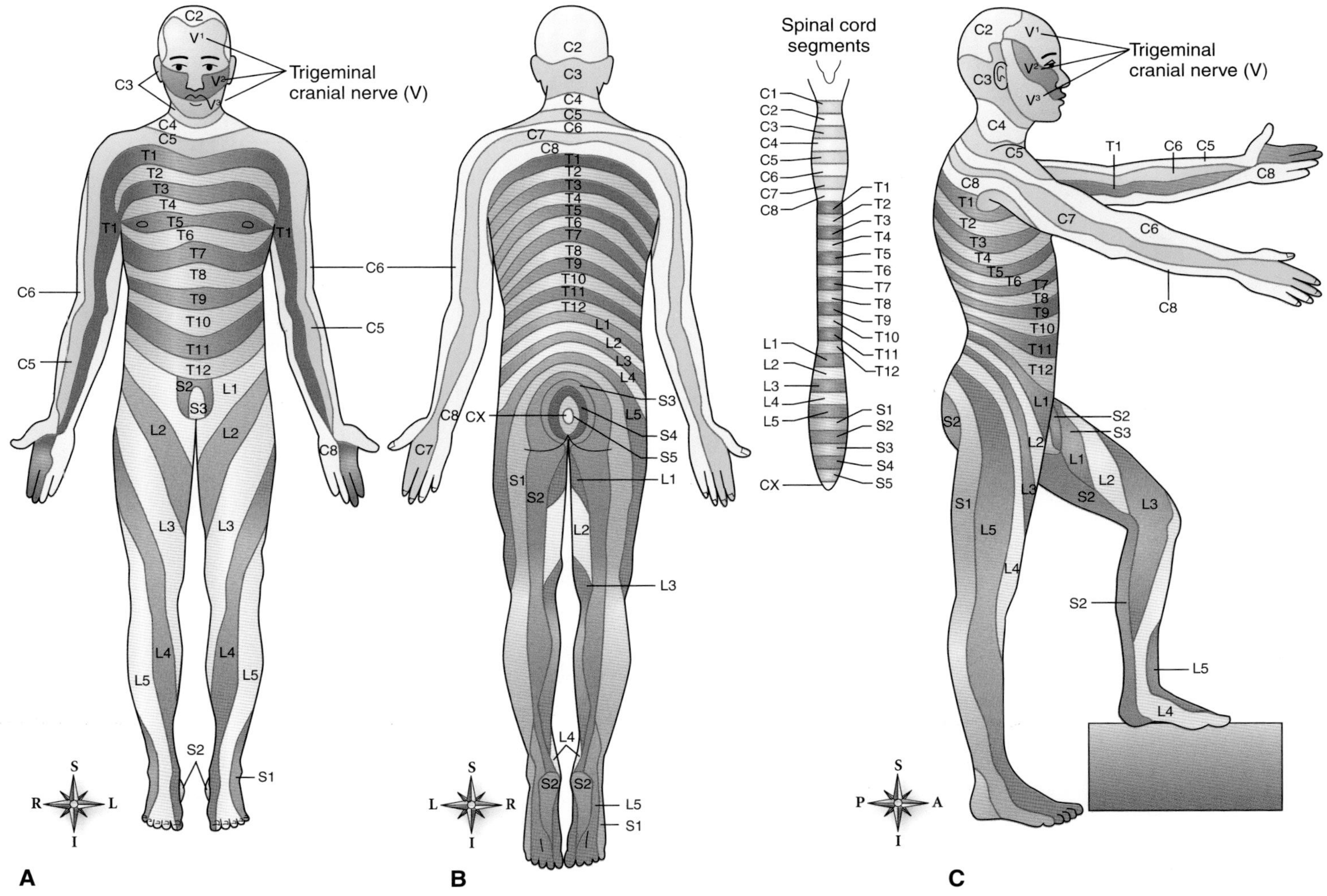

FIGURE 21-8 Dermatome distribution of spinal nerves. A, The front of the body's surface. **B,** The back of the body's surface. **C,** The side of the body's surface. The inset shows the segments of the spinal cord connected with each of the spinal nerves associated with the sensory dermatomes shown. *T,* thoracic segments and spinal nerves; *L,* lumbar segments and spinal nerves; *S,* sacral segments and spinal nerves.

BOX 21-3 *health matters* | Herpes Zoster

Herpes zoster, or **shingles,** is a unique viral infection that almost always affects the skin of a single dermatome. It is caused by the *varicella zoster virus (VZV)* of chickenpox. About 3% of the population will develop shingles at some time in their lives. In most cases the disease results from reactivation of the varicella virus. The virus most likely travels through a cutaneous nerve and remains dormant in a dorsal root ganglion for years after an initial episode of chickenpox. If the body's immunological protective mechanism becomes diminished, as in the elderly or as a result of stress, or because of radiation therapy or immunosuppressive drugs, the virus may reactivate. If this occurs, the virus will travel over the sensory nerve to the skin of a single dermatome.

The figure shows involvement of dermatome T4 in a 13-year-old boy. The result is a painful eruption of red swollen plaques or vesicles that eventually rupture and crust before clearing in 2 to 3 weeks. In severe cases, extensive inflammation, haemorrhagic blisters, and secondary bacterial infection may lead to permanent scarring. In most cases of shingles, the eruption of vesicles is preceded by 4 to 5 days of preeruptive pain, burning, and itching in the affected dermatome. *Postherpetic neuralgia*—pain that lingers long after the outbreak has cleared up—is most likely to occur in older adults.

Unfortunately, an attack of herpes zoster does not confer lasting immunity, but an effective vaccine is available and recommended for people 60 years old and older. Unvaccinated individuals sometimes have three or more episodes in a lifetime.

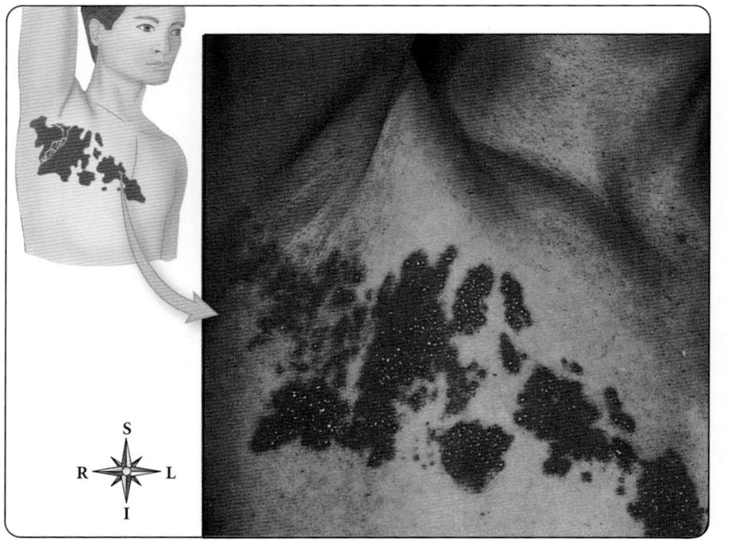

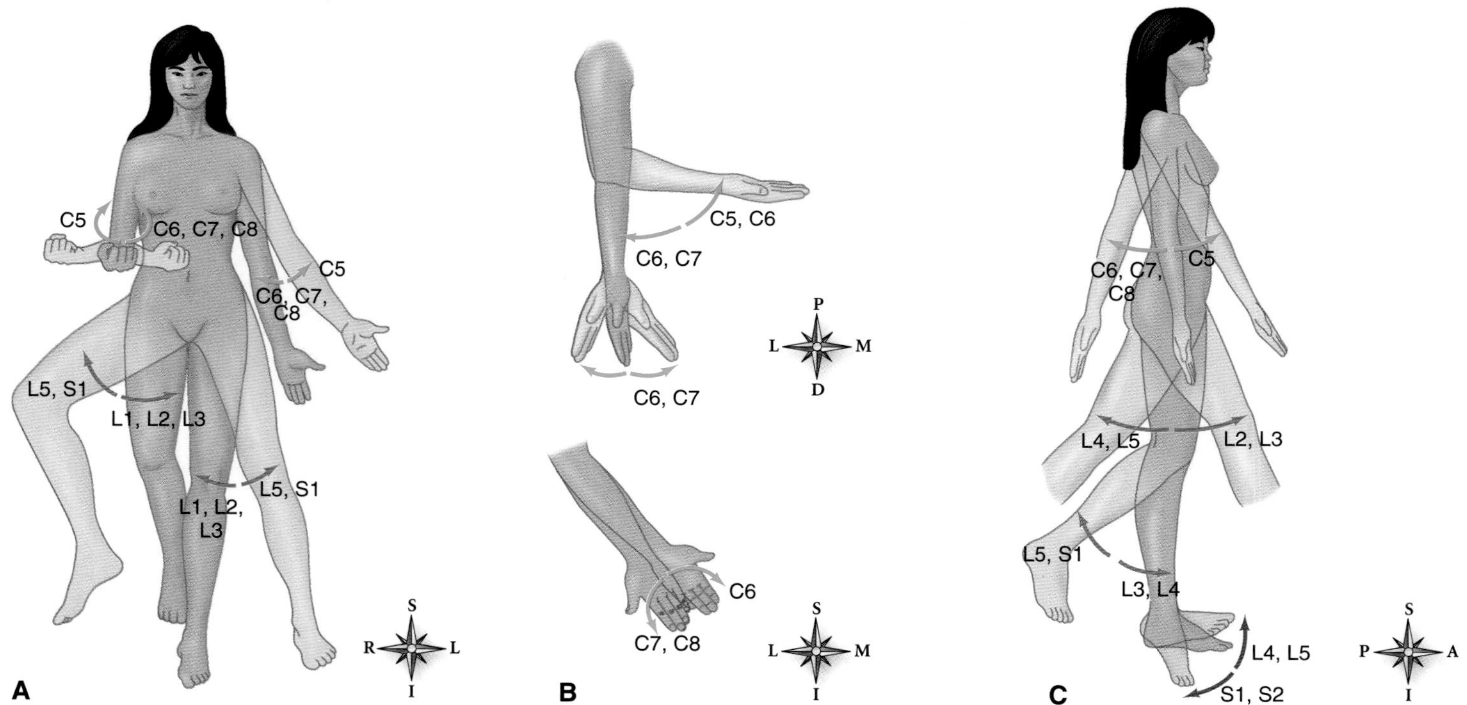

FIGURE 21-9 Myotomes and body movement. Myotomes are skeletal muscles innervated by one or more given spinal nerves. These examples show which spinal nerves innervate the skeletal muscles that produce the movements indicated by the arrows. **A,** Rotation and abduction/adduction of arm and hip. **B,** Flexion/extension of hand and wrist; pronation/supination of hand. **C,** Flexion/extension/hyperextension of arm, hip, knee; dorsiflexion and plantar flexion of foot. *C,* Cervical spinal nerves; *L,* lumbar spinal nerves; *S,* sacral spinal nerves.

differences in the way various types of sensory receptors are distributed in the skin. Dermatome maps help us to better understand cutaneous sensation, discussed later in Chapter 23, and also certain conditions that appear on the skin, such as shingles (**Box 21-3**).

A **myotome** is a skeletal muscle or group of muscles that receives motor axons from a given spinal nerve. There is some overlap among myotomes also. Thus some skeletal muscle organs may be innervated by motor axons from more than one spinal nerve. **Figure 21-9** shows examples of how myotomes relate to specific movements of the body.

CRANIAL NERVES

Twelve pairs of **cranial nerves** connect to the undersurface of the brain (**Figure 21-10**), mostly on the brainstem. Cranial nerves pass through small foramina (holes) in the cranial cavity of the skull, allowing them to extend to or from their peripheral destinations.

Both names and numbers identify the cranial nerves. Their names suggest either their distribution—where they extend to (or from). For example, the optic nerve extends from the eye, carrying visual information. Their numbers indicate the order in which they connect to the brain from anterior to posterior. Roman numerals are most often used for cranial nerves (review Roman numerals in the Quick Guide to the Language of Science and Medicine). Numerals are sometimes used with the acronym CN (for "cranial nerve"). For example, the optic nerve is also known as *cranial nerve II* or *CN II*. Less commonly, Arabic numerals are used, as in CN 2.

As with all nerves, cranial nerves are made up of bundles of axons. **Mixed cranial nerves** contain axons of sensory and motor neurons. **Sensory cranial nerves** consist of sensory axons only, and **motor cranial nerves** consist mainly of motor axons. Cranial nerves classified as "motor nerves" contain a small number of sensory fibres. These sensory fibres are *proprioceptive* fibres that carry information regarding tension in the muscles controlled by the motor fibres of the same motor nerve. **Table 21-2** lists the name, number, and functional

TABLE 21-2 Names, Numbers, and Functional Classifications of Cranial Nerves

NAME*	NUMBER	FUNCTIONAL CLASSIFICATION†
Olfactory	I	Sensory
Optic	II	Sensory
Oculomotor	III	Motor
Trochlear	IV	Motor
Trigeminal	V	Mixed
Abducens	VI	Motor
Facial	VII	Mixed
Vestibulocochlear	VIII	Sensory
Glossopharyngeal	IX	Mixed
Vagus	X	Mixed
Accessory	XI	Motor
Hypoglossal	XII	Motor

*The first letter of each word in the following sentence correlates with the first letter of the name of each of the cranial nerves, in the correct order, I to XII: **O**n **O**ld **O**lympus' **T**iny **T**ops, **A F**riendly **V**iking **G**rew **V**ines **A**nd **H**ops. Many anatomy students find that using this sentence, or one like it, helps in memorizing the names and numbers of the cranial nerves.

†The following sentence is a memory aid for learning the functional classification of each cranial nerve: ***S**ome **S**ay "**M**arry **M**oney," **B**ut **M**y **B**rothers **S**ay "**B**ad **B**usiness, **M**arry **M**oney."* In this sentence, **S** indicates *sensory,* **M** indicates *motor,* and **B** indicates *both* sensory and motor (mixed).

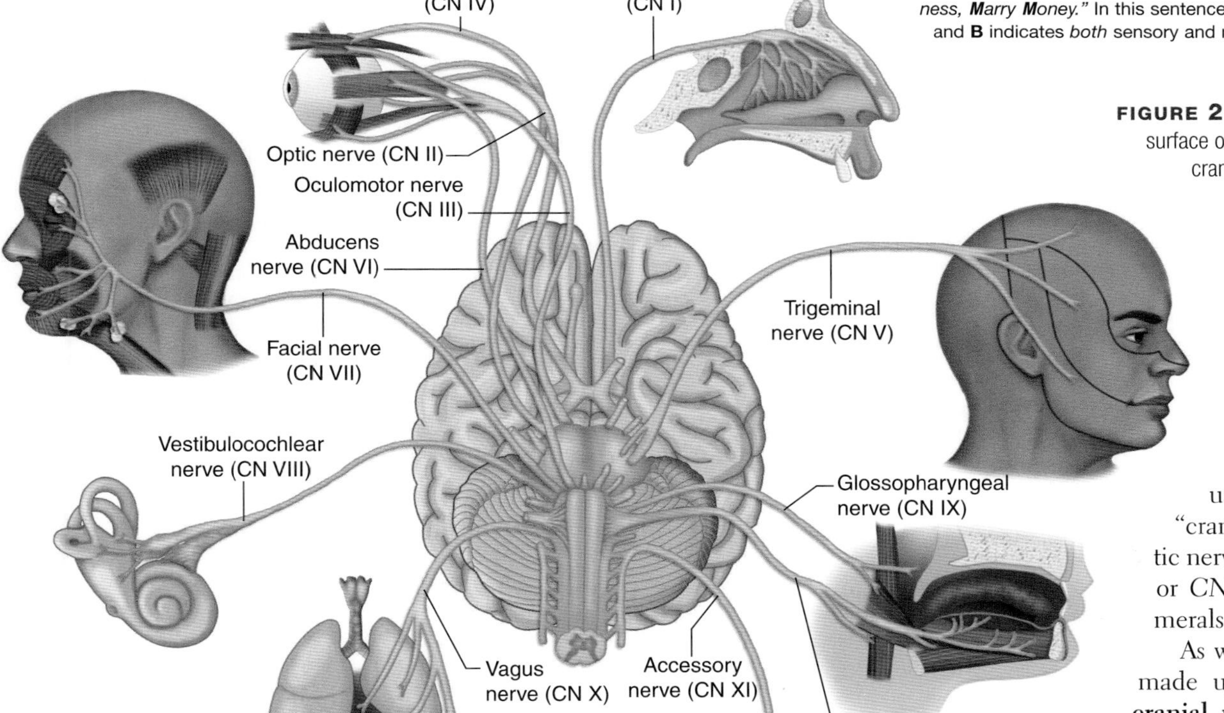

FIGURE 21-10 Cranial nerves. Ventral surface of the brain showing attachment of the cranial nerves.

UNIT 3

TABLE 21-3 Structure and Function of the Cranial Nerves

■ sensory (afferent) ■ motor (efferent)

	SENSORY FIBRES			MOTOR FIBRES		
NERVE	RECEPTORS	CELL BODIES	TERMINATION	CELL BODIES	TERMINATION	FUNCTIONS
CN I Olfactory	Nasal mucosa	Nasal mucosa	Olfactory bulbs (new relay of neurons to olfactory cortex)	—	—	Sense of smell
CN II Optic	Retina (proprioceptive)	Retina	Nucleus in thalamus (lateral geniculate); some fibres terminate in superior colliculus of midbrain	—	—	Vision
CN III Oculomotor	External eye muscles except superior oblique and lateral rectus	Trigeminal ganglion	Midbrain (oculomotor nucleus)	Midbrain (oculomotor nucleus)	External eye muscles except superior oblique and lateral rectus; autonomic fibres terminate in ciliary ganglion and then to ciliary and iris muscles	Eye movements, regulation of size of pupil, accommodation (for near vision), proprioception (muscle sense)
CN IV Trochlear	Superior oblique (proprioceptive)	Trigeminal ganglion	Midbrain	Midbrain	Superior oblique muscle of eye	Eye movements, proprioception
CN V Trigeminal	Skin and mucosa of head, teeth	Trigeminal ganglion	Pons (sensory nucleus)	Pons (motor nucleus)	Muscles of mastication	Sensations of head and face, chewing movements, proprioception
CN VI Abducens	Lateral rectus (proprioceptive)	Trigeminal ganglion	Pons	Pons	Lateral rectus muscle of eye	Abduction of eye, proprioception
CN VII Facial	Taste buds of anterior two thirds of tongue	Geniculate ganglion	Medulla (nucleus solitarius)	Pons	Superficial muscles of face and scalp; autonomic fibres to salivary and lacrimal glands	Facial expressions, secretion of saliva and tears, taste

(continued on page 493)

classification of each of the 12 pairs of cranial nerves. Details of the structure and function of each cranial nerve are described in **Table 21-3** and in the paragraphs that follow.

CONNECT IT! 

For more tips on learning cranial nerves, check out ***Learning Cranial Nerves*** online at ***Connect It!***

***Quick* CHECK**

1. How many pairs of spinal nerves are there? Name them.
2. What is a plexus? Name the four major pairs of plexuses.
3. What is a dermatome? A myotome?

Olfactory Nerve (CN I)

The **olfactory nerves** are composed of axons of neurons whose dendrites and cell bodies lie in the nasal mucosa, high up along the septum and superior conchae (turbinates). Axons of these neurons form about 20 small bundles of fibres that pierce each cribriform plate and terminate in the olfactory bulbs (see **Figure 24-1**, p. 533). Here they synapse with the second pool of olfactory neurons, whose axons compose the olfactory tracts. The olfactory nerves carry information about the sense of smell.

CONNECT IT! 

Although you will not find it in most introductory anatomy texts, there is an additional pair of cranial nerves not found in the classic list of 12. The **terminal nerve,** or cranial *nerve zero (CN 0),* is a very thin nerve located near each olfactory nerve. Why is it often missing from the list? Why is it called nerve "zero"? And why are some scientists calling it the "sex nerve"? Check out ***Nerve Zero*** online at ***Connect It!*** to find out!

Optic Nerve (CN II)

Axons from the innermost layer of sensory neurons of the retina compose the second pair of cranial nerves. They are called **optic nerves** because they carry visual information from the eyes to the brain. After entering the cranial cavity through the optic foramina, the two optic nerves unite to form the x-shaped *optic chiasma* of the diencephalon, in which some of the fibres of each nerve cross to the opposite side and continue inward through the *optic tract* of that side (see **Figure 24-26**, p. 552). Thus each optic nerve contains fibres only from the retina of the same side, whereas each optic tract of the brain has fibres in it from both retinas, an important fact in interpreting certain visual disorders.

Most of the optic tract fibres terminate in the thalamus (in the portion known as the *lateral geniculate nucleus*). From here a new relay of fibres runs to the visual area of the occipital lobe cortex. A few optic tract fibres terminate in the superior colliculi of the midbrain, where they synapse with motor fibres to the external eye muscles (CN III, CN IV, CN VI).

Oculomotor Nerve (CN III)

Fibres of each **oculomotor nerve** originate from cells in the oculomotor nucleus in the ventral part of the midbrain and extend to the various external eye muscles, with the exception of the superior oblique and the lateral rectus. Autonomic fibres are also present in the oculomotor nerves. They extend to the intrinsic muscles of the eye, which regulate the amount of light entering the eye and aid in focusing on near objects.

Yet a third group of fibres is found in the third cranial nerves. These are sensory fibres from proprioceptors in the eye muscles.

Trochlear Nerve (CN IV)

Motor fibres of each **trochlear nerve** have their origin in cells in the midbrain, from which they extend to the superior oblique muscles of the eye. The name *trochlear*, from a Greek word meaning "pulley", refers to the fact that the superior oblique muscles of the eye pass through a pulleylike ligament (see **Figure 24-15**, p. 544). Afferent fibres from proprioceptors in these muscles are also contained in the trochlear nerves.

Trigeminal Nerve (CN V)

The fifth pair of cranial nerves is called **trigeminal nerves** because they each split into three large branches. The name trigeminal means "three pairs". The three branches of each pair are the *ophthalmic nerve, maxillary nerve*, and *mandibular nerve* (**Figure 21-11**).

Sensory neurons in all three branches of the trigeminal nerve carry afferent impulses from the skin and mucosa of the head and from the teeth to cell bodies in the trigeminal ganglion (lodged in the petrous part of the temporal bone). Fibres extend from the ganglion to the main sensory nucleus of the fifth cranial nerve situated in the pons. Some of the sensory pathways carry information from the mouth about the texture and temperature of food. The so-called *trigeminal senses* that contribute to the flavours of foods are discussed further in Chapter 24. Damage to some of the sensory pathways of the trigeminal nerve could lead to trigeminal neuralgia (**Box 21-4**).

Motor fibres of the trigeminal nerve originate in the trifacial motor nucleus located in the pons just medial to the sensory nucleus. These motor fibres run to the muscles of mastication by way of the mandibular nerve.

CONNECT IT! ⓔ

Review ***Sensing Food*** online at ***Connect It!*** to see how sensory information from the trigeminal nerve helps us analyze the food we eat.

Abducens Nerve (CN VI)

Each **abducens nerve** is a motor nerve with fibres originating from a nucleus in the pons in the floor of the fourth ventricle and extending to the lateral rectus muscles of the eyes (see **Figure 24-15**, p. 544). The lateral rectus muscle *abducts* the eye to which it is attached, hence the name *abducens* for this nerve. The sixth cranial nerve also contains some afferent fibres from proprioceptors in the lateral rectus muscles.

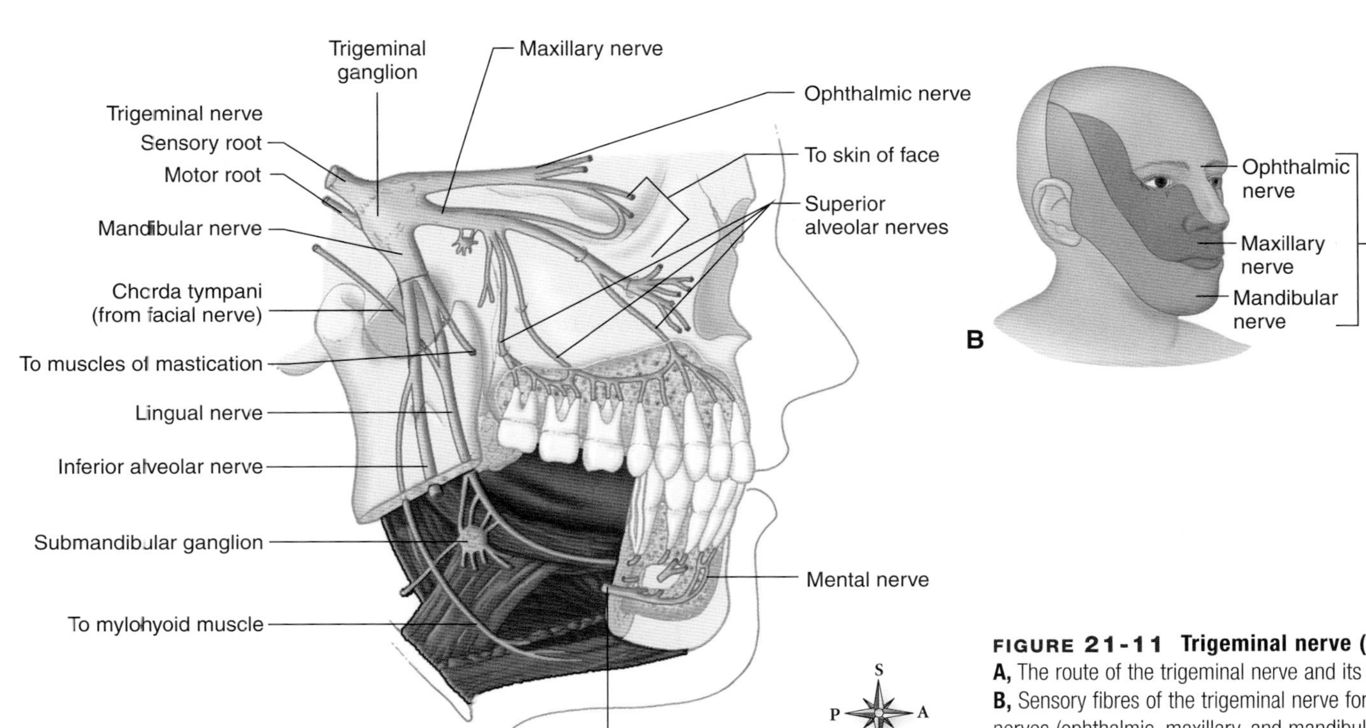

FIGURE 21-11 Trigeminal nerve (CN V). **A,** The route of the trigeminal nerve and its major branches. **B,** Sensory fibres of the trigeminal nerve form three branch nerves (ophthalmic, maxillary, and mandibular nerves), each of which conducts information from a different region of the face.

BOX 21-4 *health matters* | **Trigeminal Neuralgia**

Compression, inflammation, or degeneration of the fifth cranial nerve, the trigeminal nerve, may result in a condition called **trigeminal neuralgia** or **tic douloureux**. This condition is characterized by recurring episodes of intense stabbing pain, or *neuralgia,* radiating from the angle of the jaw along a branch of the trigeminal nerve on one side of the face (see the figure).

Treatment with the drug carbamazepine provides relief in most cases. If drugs do not provide relief, surgical methods may be used. The most drastic method of pain reduction is removal of the trigeminal ganglion on the posterior portion of the nerve (see **Figure 21-11**). This large ganglion contains the cell bodies of the nerve's afferent fibres. After such an operation, the patient's face, scalp, teeth, and conjunctiva on the side treated show anaesthesia (loss of sensation). Therefore, special care, such as wearing protective goggles and irrigating the eye frequently, is prescribed. The patient is also instructed to visit the dentist regularly because he or she can no longer experience a toothache—a warning of diseased teeth.

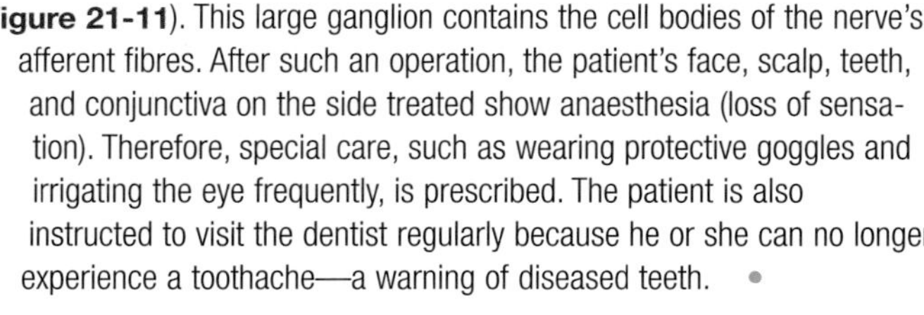

Pain zones in trigeminal neuralgia.

Facial Nerve (CN VII)

Motor fibres of the **facial nerves,** medial root (or motor root) arise from a nucleus in the lower part of the pons, from which they extend by way of several branches to the superficial muscles of the face and scalp (**Figure 21-12**). The smaller root, or intermediate nerve, carries efferent autonomic fibres of the facial nerve that extend to the submaxillary and sublingual salivary glands, as well as to the lacrimal (tear) glands. Sensory fibres from the taste buds of the anterior two thirds of the tongue run in the intermediate nerve to cell bodies in the geniculate ganglion, a small swelling on the facial nerve, where it passes through a canal in the temporal bone. From the ganglion, fibres extend to a nucleus in the medulla.

Vestibulocochlear Nerve (CN VIII)

The **vestibulocochlear nerve** has two distinct divisions: the *vestibular nerve* and the *cochlear nerve* (see **Figure 24-7**, p. 538). Both are sensory.

Fibres from the semicircular canals in the inner ear run to the vestibular ganglion (in the internal acoustic meatus). Here, the neurons' cell bodies are located, and from them, fibres extend to the vestibular nuclei in the pons and medulla. Together, these fibres constitute the *vestibular nerve*. Some of its fibres run to the cerebellum. The vestibular nerve transmits impulses that result in sensations of equilibrium.

The *cochlear nerve* consists of peripheral axon fibres starting in the organ of Corti in the cochlea of the inner ear. They have their cell bodies in the spiral ganglion in the cochlea, and their central axon fibres terminate in the cochlear nuclei located between the medulla and pons. Conduction by the cochlear nerve results in sensations of hearing. Damage to this nerve can cause deafness (**Box 21-5**). Because of its role in hearing, the eighth cranial nerve is sometimes still called the *auditory* or *acoustic* nerve.

Glossopharyngeal Nerve (CN IX)

Both sensory and motor fibres compose the **glossopharyngeal nerve.** This nerve supplies fibres not only to the tongue and pharynx (throat), as its name implies, but also to other structures (**Figure 21-13**). One is the carotid sinus. The carotid sinus plays an important part in the control of blood pressure. Sensory fibres, with their receptors in the pharynx and posterior one third of the tongue, have their cell bodies in the jugular (superior) and petrous (inferior) ganglia. These are located, respectively, in the jugular foramen

FIGURE 21-12 Facial nerve (CN VII). Artist's interpretation of the location of the various branches of the facial nerve.

TABLE 21-3 Structure and Function of the Cranial Nerves—cont'd

■ sensory (afferent) ■ motor (efferent)

	SENSORY FIBRES			MOTOR FIBRES		
NERVE	**RECEPTORS**	**CELL BODIES**	**TERMINATION**	**CELL BODIES**	**TERMINATION**	**FUNCTIONS**
CN VIII Vestibulo-cochlear	*Vestibular branch* Semicircular canals and vestibule (utricle and saccule)	Vestibular ganglion	Pons and medulla (vestibular nuclei)	—	—	Balance or equilibrium sense
	Cochlear (auditory) branch Spiral (Corti) organ in cochlear duct	Spiral ganglion	Pons and medulla (cochlear nuclei)	—	—	Hearing
CN IX Glossopharyngeal	Pharynx; taste buds and other receptors of posterior one third of tongue	Jugular and petrous ganglia	Medulla (nucleus solitarius)	Medulla (nucleus ambiguus)	Muscles of pharynx	Sensations of tongue, swallowing movements, secretion of saliva, aid in reflex control of blood pressure and respiration
	Carotid sinus and carotid body	Jugular and petrous ganglia	Medulla (respiratory and vasomotor centres)	Medulla at junction of pons (nucleus salivatorius)	Otic ganglion and then to parotid salivary gland	
CN X Vagus	Pharynx, larynx, carotid body, thoracic and abdominal viscera	Jugular and nodose ganglia	Medulla (nucleus solitarius), pons (nucleus of fifth cranial nerve)	Medulla (dorsal motor nucleus)	Ganglia of vagal plexus and then to muscles of pharynx, larynx, and autonomic fibres to thoracic and abdominal viscera	Sensations and movements of organs supplied; e.g., slows heart, increases peristalsis, contracts muscles for voice production
CN XI Accessory	Trapezius and sternocleidomastoid (proprioceptive)	Upper, cervical ganglia	Spinal cord	Anterior grey column of first five or six cervical segments of spinal cord	Trapezius and sternocleidomastoid muscle	Shoulder movements, turning movements of head, proprioception
CN XII Hypoglossal	Tongue muscles (proprioceptive)	Trigeminal ganglion	Medulla (hypoglossal nucleus)	Medulla (hypoglossal nucleus)	Muscles of tongue and throat	Tongue movements, proprioception

UNIT 3

BOX 21-5 *health matters* | Cranial Nerve Damage

Severe head injuries often damage one or more of the cranial nerves, producing symptoms that reflect loss of the functions mediated by the affected nerve or nerves. For example, injury of the sixth cranial nerve causes the eye to turn in because of paralysis of the abducting muscle of the eye. Injury of the eighth cranial nerve, on the other hand, produces deafness. Injury to the facial nerve results in a pokerfaced expression and a drooping of the corner of the mouth from paralysis of the facial muscles. •

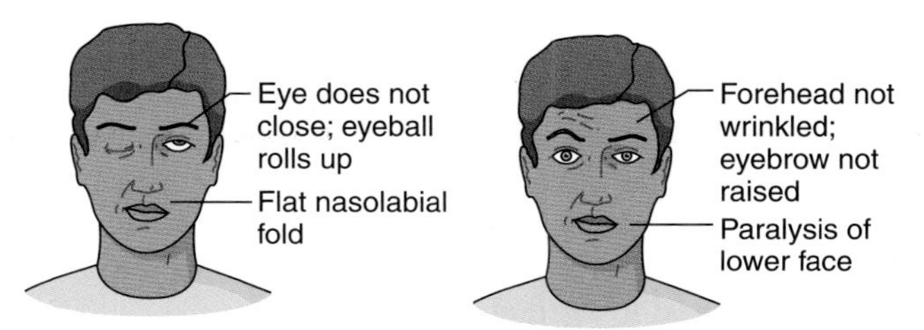

Signs of damage to the facial nerve (CN VII).

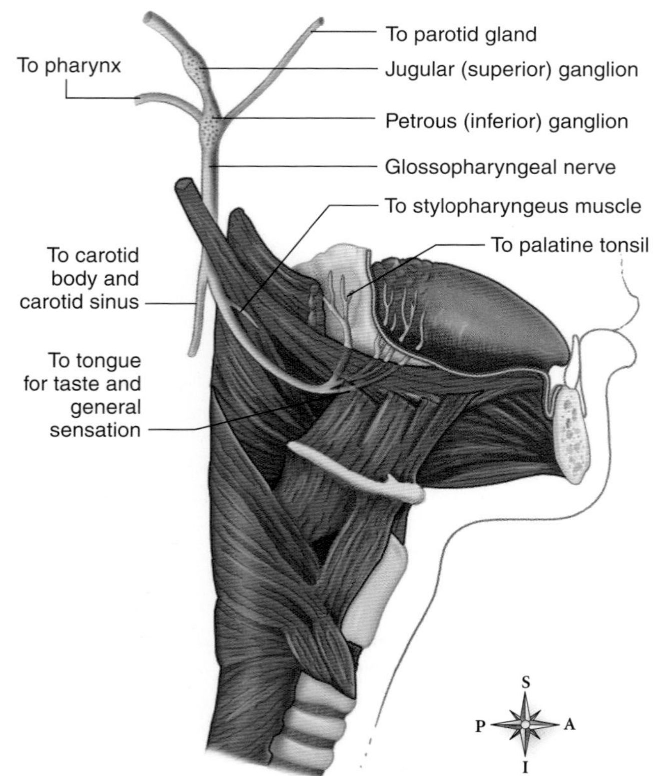

FIGURE 21-13 Glossopharyngeal nerve (CN IX). As its name implies (*glosso-*, "tongue"; *-pharyng-*, "throat"), the ninth cranial nerve supplies fibres to the tongue and throat. It is a mixed nerve that carries both sensory and motor fibres.

and the petrous part of the temporal bone. The ganglia fibres extend to a nucleus in the medulla.

The motor fibres of the ninth cranial nerve originate in another medullary nucleus and run to muscles of the pharynx. Also present in this nerve are autonomic fibres that originate in a nucleus at the junction of the pons and medulla. These fibres run to the otic ganglion, from which postganglionic fibres extend to the parotid gland.

Vagus Nerve (CN X)

The **vagus nerve** contains both sensory and motor fibres. The name *vagus* means "wanderer" and aptly describes this nerve with many widely distributed branches. Its sensory fibres supply the pharynx, larynx, trachea, heart, carotid body, lungs, bronchi, oesophagus, stomach, small intestine, and gallbladder (**Figure 21-14**). Cell bodies attached to these sensory fibres lie in the jugular and nodose ganglia, which are located, respectively, in the jugular foramen and just inferior to it on the trunk of the nerve. The sensory axons terminate in the medulla and in the pons. Somatic motor fibres of the vagus travel to the pharynx and larynx (voice box), where they control muscles involved in swallowing.

Most motor fibres of the vagus nerve are autonomic (parasympathetic) fibres. They originate in cells in the medulla and extend to various autonomic ganglia. From there, the fibres run to muscles of the pharynx, larynx, and thoracic and abdominal organs, where they control heart rate and other "visceral" activities.

Accessory Nerve (CN XI)

The **accessory nerve** is a motor nerve historically considered to be an "accessory" to the vagus nerve. In most individuals, fibres forming the cranial division originate in cells of the medulla, join the fibres of the vagus nerve and then travel as motor nerves to muscles of the abdomen, pharynx and larynx. Fibres of the spinal division of this nerve originate in the upper cervical region (C1–C5) of the spinal cord—and none of the fibres originate in the brain. From there, they extend to the trapezius and sternocleidomastoid muscles (**Figure 21-15**).

The accessory nerve is still classified as a cranial nerve because some of its fibres originate in the brainstem. Even fibres in the spinal cord pass into the foramen magnum and then out of the cranial cavity by way of the jugular foramen, thus also meeting the criterion for "cranial nerves".

Because of its spinal roots, the eleventh cranial nerve was formerly called the *spinal accessory nerve.*

Hypoglossal Nerve (CN XII)

Motor fibres with cell bodies in the hypoglossal nucleus of the medulla compose the twelfth cranial nerve. They supply the muscles of the tongue (see **Figure 21-10**). The **hypoglossal nerve** also contains

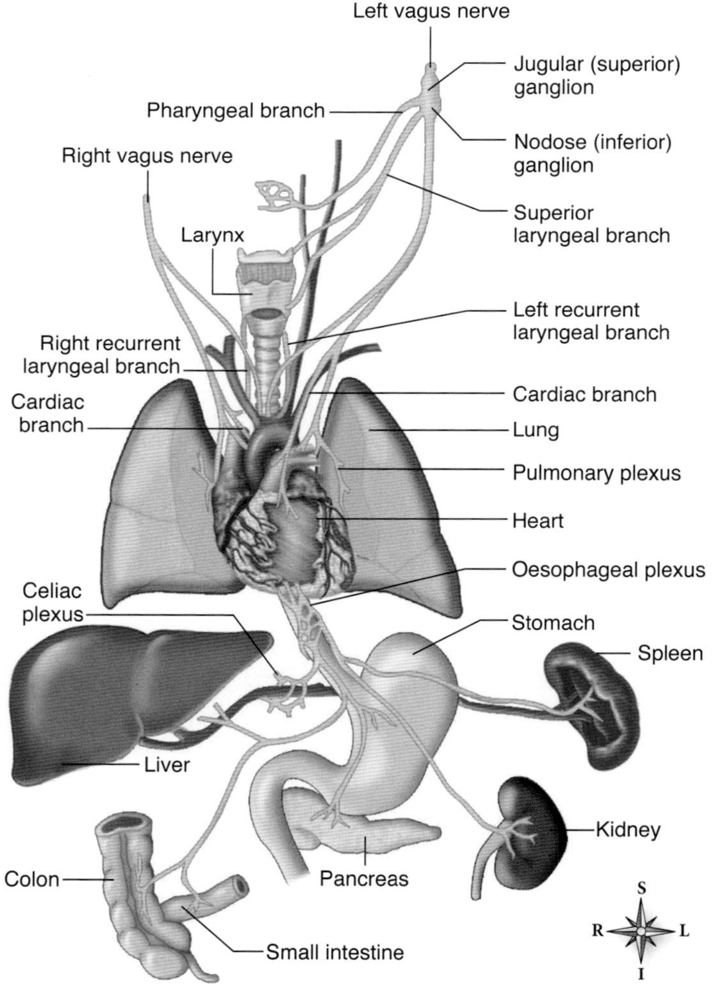

FIGURE 21-14 Vagus nerve (CN X). The vagus nerve is a mixed cranial nerve with many widely distributed branches—hence the name *vagus*, which is the Latin word for "wanderer".

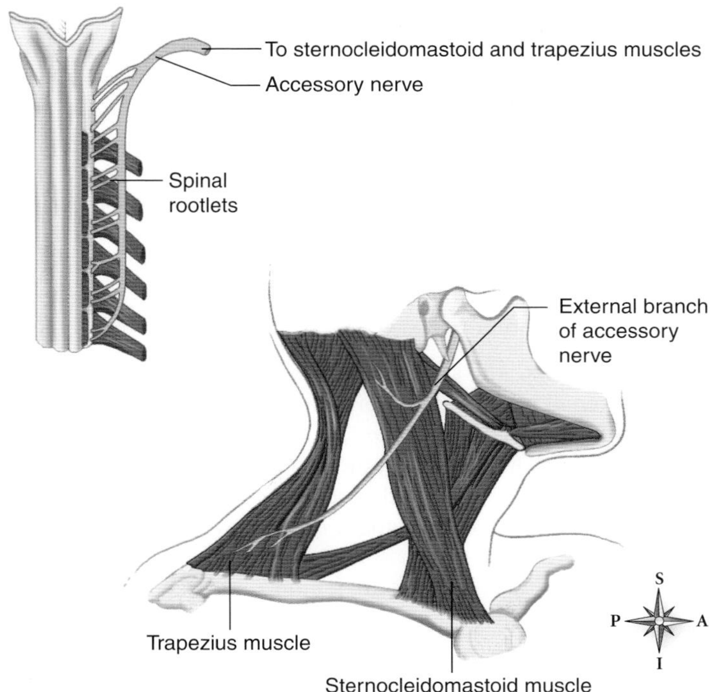

FIGURE 21-15 Accessory nerve (CN XI). Originally thought to be an "accessory" to the vagus nerve by contributing a few nerve fibres, this cranial nerve usually includes only fibres that originate in the cervical spinal segments and travel through an external nerve branch to the trapezius and sternocleidomastoid muscles of the neck. The medulla also contributes fibres to the vagus nerve. Because all the fibres leave the cranial cavity, this nerve is defined as a cranial nerve.

sensory fibres from proprioceptors in muscles of the tongue. The name *hypoglossal* means "under the tongue".

Table 21-3 summarizes the main facts about the distribution and function of each of the cranial nerve pairs.

Quick **CHECK**

4. List the names and numbers of the 12 pairs of cranial nerves.
5. Identify the primary function of each pair of cranial nerves.
6. Distinguish between a motor nerve, sensory nerve, and mixed nerve.

SOMATIC MOTOR NERVOUS SYSTEM

Divisions of the Peripheral Nervous System

Recall from Chapter 18 that the PNS includes all the nervous pathways *outside* the brain and spinal cord (see **Figure 18-2**, p.394). Thus the entire PNS includes the fibres present in the cranial nerves, the spinal nerves, and all their individual branches. Although many of these nerves are *mixed nerves*—containing both sensory and motor fibres—it is often convenient to consider the PNS as having two functional divisions: the sensory (afferent) division and the motor (efferent) division. In this chapter, we concentrate on some essential details of the somatic motor division of the PNS—the *somatic motor nervous system*. Then in Chapter 22 we move on to discuss the efferent pathways of the *autonomic nervous system*. Details of the sensory division of the PNS are discussed in Chapters 23 and 24.

Basic Principles of Somatic Motor Pathways

The somatic motor nervous system includes all the voluntary motor pathways outside the CNS. That is, it involves the peripheral pathways to the skeletal muscles, which are the *somatic effectors*. Recall from Chapter 20 that all these pathways operate according to the principle of *final common path*. This means that all the somatic motor pathways involve a single motor neuron whose axon stretches from the cell body in the CNS all the way to the effector innervated by that neuron. For fibres that originate in the spinal cord, this means that the axon extends from the anterior grey horn, through the ventral nerve root, and out to a skeletal muscle.

Another important principle of somatic motor pathways was mentioned in Chapter 17, when we were discussing skeletal muscle contraction. This principle states that the axon of the last somatic motor neuron—also called the *anterior horn neuron* or *lower motor neuron*—stimulates effector cells by means of the neurotransmitter **acetylcholine.**

This fact will have added importance later when we compare the somatic motor nervous system with the ANS.

Because the basic plan of the somatic motor pathways was discussed in Chapter 20, and the effect of acetylcholine on the somatic effectors (skeletal muscles) has already been outlined in Chapter 17, we will end our discussion of the somatic motor division of the PNS with a brief review of the concept of the reflex arc and how it relates to peripheral motor pathways.

Somatic Reflexes

Nature of a Reflex

The action that results from a nerve impulse passing over a reflex arc is called a **reflex** (see **Figure 18-10**, p. 403). In other words, a reflex is a predictable response to a stimulus. It may or may not be conscious. Usually the term is used to mean only involuntary responses rather than those directly willed. If the centre of a reflex arc is in the brain, the response it mediates is called a **cranial reflex.** If the centre of a reflex arc is in the spinal cord, the response is called a **spinal reflex.**

A reflex consists of either muscle contraction or glandular secretion.

Somatic reflexes are contractions of skeletal muscles. Impulse conduction over somatic reflex arcs—arcs whose motor neurons are somatic motor neurons (i.e., anterior horn neurons or lower motor neurons)—produces somatic reflexes.

Autonomic reflexes, or **visceral reflexes,** consist of contractions of smooth or cardiac muscle or secretion by glands. Visceral reflexes are mediated by impulse conduction over autonomic reflex arcs, the motor neurons of which are autonomic neurons (discussed later).

The following paragraphs describe only somatic reflexes.

Withdrawal Reflexes

One of the most obvious experiences of a spinal reflex occurs when you are injured—or are about to become injured. When you accidentally touch a very hot surface such as a heated pan, for example, you reflexively withdraw from it to avoid further injury. This type of reflex is therefore called a **withdrawal reflex.** The withdrawal reflex in which you pull away from a painful stimulus just described is also a *flexor reflex* because you use flexor muscles of the upper extremity to flex the elbow and pull away.

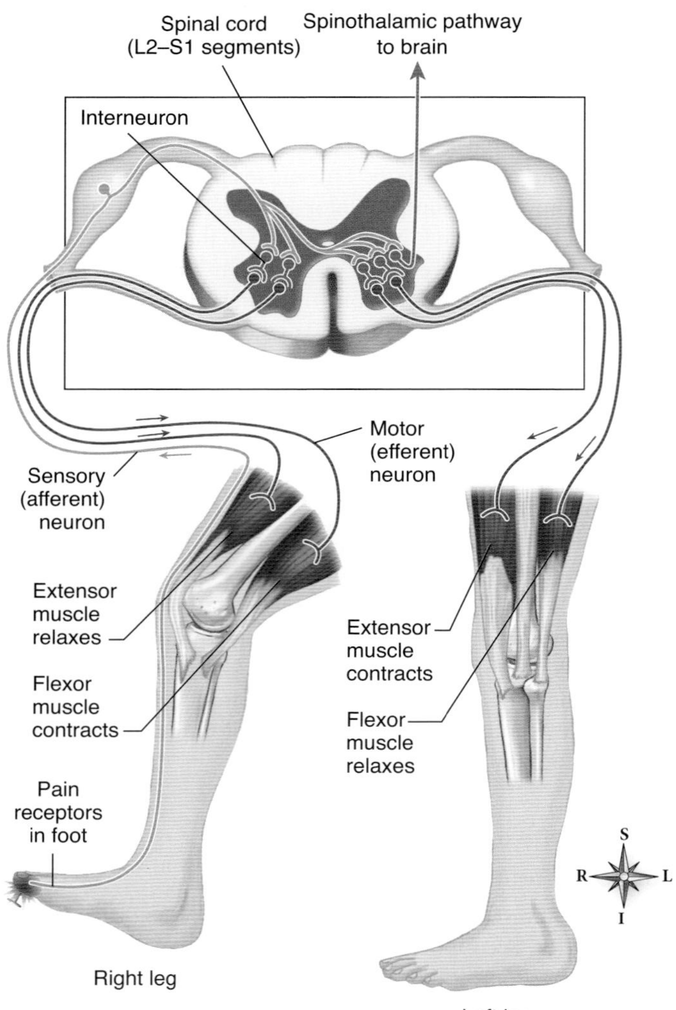

FIGURE 21-16 Flexor reflex and crossed-extensor reflex. A painful stimulus can trigger both an ipsilateral (same side) *flexor reflex* to withdraw from the stimulus and a contralateral (other side) *extensor reflex* to stabilize the body as weight shifts. This reflex involves several lower spinal segments (not shown) and may also trigger cranial reflexes involving the cerebrum and cerebellum. Note that as prime mover muscles contract, their antagonists relax.

If you had instead stepped on a hot pan or a sharp object, then your response would have been a bit more complex. You may experience a flexor reflex along with a *crossed-extensor reflex*. **Figure 21-16** shows how the painful stimulus detected in the skin receptors of the foot would cause an ipsilateral (same side) flexion of the knee to pull away from it—an ordinary flexor reflex. At the same time, however, impulses would move intersegmentally (through several segments) and across the spinal cord to trigger contralateral (other side) extension of the opposite knee. Extension of the opposite knee stabilizes it so that you can shift your weight away from the injured extremity. This crossed-extensor reflex that extends the opposite extremity helps prevent a fall and thus perhaps an even more serious injury.

Review diagrams of ipsilateral versus contralateral reflex arcs and intersegmental reflex arcs in **Figure 18-11** on p. 403.

This example is even more complex, however, because sensory information also travels up the *lateral spinothalamic tract* to the brain. The cerebrum and cerebellum may then become involved in *cranial reflexes* that help you maintain your posture and perhaps move farther away from the danger. Some of these cranial reflexes may be *learned reflexes*—reflexes that develop through prior experience—rather than *instrinsic reflexes* that are inborn and need not be learned.

Somatic Reflexes of Clinical Importance

Clinical interest in reflexes stems from the fact that they deviate from normal in certain diseases. Therefore the testing of reflexes is a valuable diagnostic aid. The following reflexes are commonly tested: knee jerk, ankle jerk, plantar reflex, corneal reflex, and abdominal reflex.

Knee Jerk Reflex. The **knee jerk reflex,** or *patellar reflex,* is an extension of the leg in response to tapping of the patellar ligament (**Figure 21-17** and **Figure 21-18**, *A*). The tap stretches the ligament, pulling on the patella and the tendon of the quadriceps femoris muscles and thereby stimulates muscle spindles (receptors) in the muscle and initiates conduction over the following two-neuron reflex arc:

- Sensory neurons
  Peripheral axon fibres—in femoral and second, third, and fourth lumbar nerves
  Cell bodies—second, third, and fourth lumbar ganglia
  Central axon fibres—in posterior roots of second, third, and fourth lumbar nerves; terminate in these segments of the spinal cord; synapse directly with lower motor neurons
- Reflex centre—synapses in anterior grey column between axons of sensory neurons and dendrites and cell bodies of lower motor neurons
- Motor neurons
  Dendrites and cell bodies—in spinal cord anterior grey column
  Axons—in anterior roots of second, third, and fourth lumbar spinal nerves and femoral nerves; terminate in quadriceps femoris muscle

The knee jerk can be classified in various ways as follows:

- As a *spinal cord reflex*—because the centre of the reflex arc (which transmits the impulses that activate the muscles producing the knee jerk) lies in the spinal cord grey matter
- As a *segmental reflex*—because impulses that mediate it enter and leave the same segment of the cord
- As a *monosynaptic reflex*—because impulses travel through only one synapse; in *polysynaptic reflexes*, however, impulses travel through more than one synapse (see **Figure 21-16**)
- As an *ipsilateral reflex*—because the impulses that mediate it come from and go to the same side of the body (a *contralateral reflex*, on the other hand, would trigger a response on the opposite side of the body)
- As a *stretch reflex* or *myotatic reflex* (from *myo-*, "muscle", *-tactic*, "stretch")—because of the kind of stimulation used to evoke it
- As an *extensor reflex*—because it is produced by extensors of the leg (muscles located on the anterior surface of the thigh, which extend the leg)
- As a *deep reflex*—because of the deep location (in muscle) of the receptors stimulated to produce this reflex (as opposed to *superficial reflexes*—those elicited by stimulation of receptors located in the skin or mucosa)

When testing a patient's reflexes, a physician interprets the test results on the basis of what is known about the reflex arcs that must function to produce normal reflexes.

To illustrate, suppose that a patient has been diagnosed as having poliomyelitis. During the examination the physician finds that she cannot elicit the knee jerk when she taps the patient's patellar tendon. She knows that the poliomyelitis virus attacks anterior horn motor neurons. She also knows the information previously related about which spinal cord segments contain the reflex centres for the knee jerk. On the basis of this knowledge, therefore, she deduces that in this patient the poliomyelitis virus has damaged the second, third, and fourth lumbar segments of the spinal cord. Do you think that this patient's leg would be paralyzed, that he would be unable to move it voluntarily? What neurons would not be able to function that must function to produce voluntary contractions?

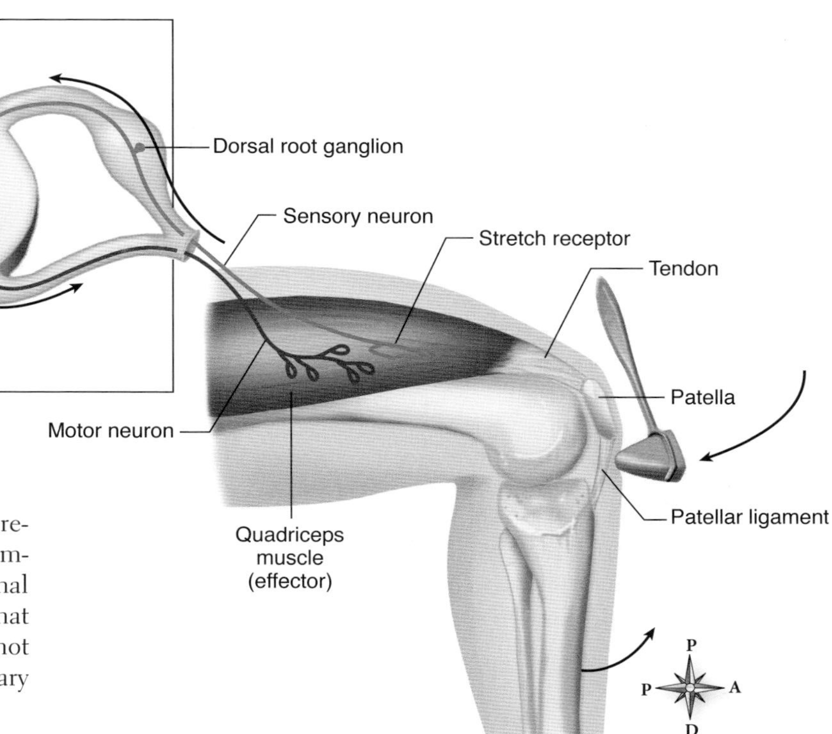

FIGURE 21-17 Patellar reflex. Neural pathway involved in the patellar (knee jerk) reflex.

Ankle Jerk Reflex. **Ankle jerk reflex,** or *Achilles reflex*, is an extension (plantar flexion) of the foot in response to tapping of the Achilles tendon (**Figure 21-18**, *B*). As with the knee jerk, it is a tendon reflex and a deep reflex mediated by two-neuron spinal arcs. The centres for the ankle jerk lie in the first and second sacral segments of the cord.

Plantar Reflex. The **plantar reflex** consists of a curling under of all the toes (plantar flexion) plus a slight turning in and flexion of the anterior part of the foot in response to stimulation of the outer edge of the sole.

The **Babinski sign,** however, is an extension of the great toe, with or without fanning of the other toes, in response to stimulation of the outer margin of the sole of the foot (**Figure 21-18**, *C*). Normal infants, up until they are about 1½ years old, exhibit this Babinski sign. At about 18 months, corticospinal fibres have become fully myelinated and the Babinski sign becomes suppressed. A Babinski sign after this age is abnormal and is one of the pyramidal signs (see **Box 20-8**, p. 468). It is interpreted to mean destruction of pyramidal tract (corticospinal) fibres.

Corneal Reflex. The **corneal reflex** is blinking in response to the cornea being touched. It is mediated by reflex arcs with sensory fibres in the ophthalmic branch of the fifth cranial nerve, centres in the pons, and motor fibres in the seventh cranial nerve.

Abdominal Reflex. The **abdominal reflex** occurs when the umbilicus moves in response to stroking the side of the abdomen

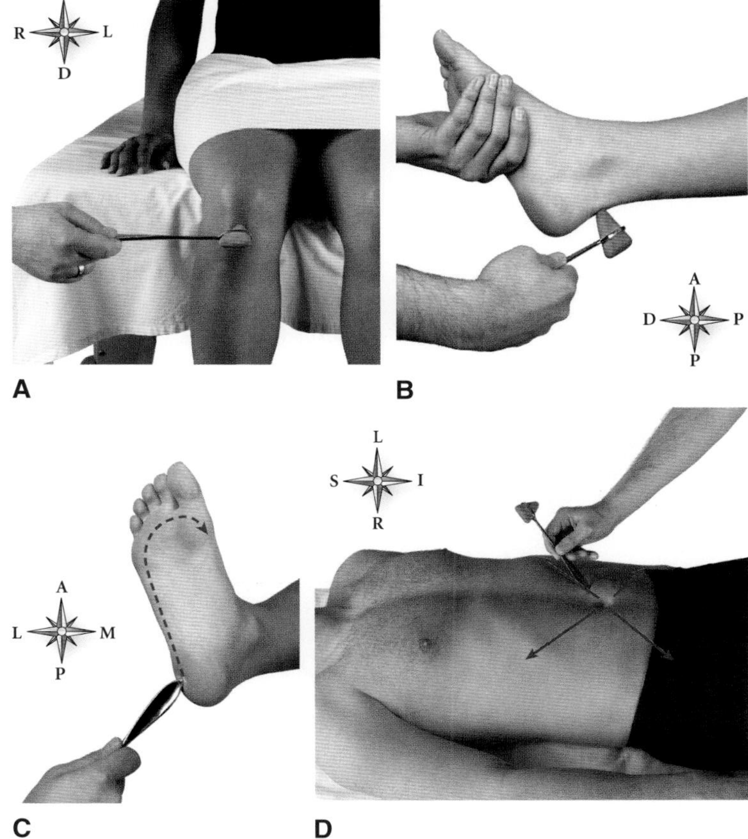

FIGURE 21-18 Common clinical reflex tests. A, Knee jerk reflex. **B,** Ankle jerk reflex. **C,** Plantar reflex showing the Babinski sign (*arrow* shows path of stimulation along plantar surface). **D,** Abdominal reflexes (one of several ways to test this type of reflex). As an object is moved away from the umbilicus and toward the side, the rectus abdominis muscles pull the umbilicus toward the stroked side.

(**Figure 21-18**, *D*). It is mediated by arcs with sensory and motor fibres in the ninth to twelfth thoracic spinal nerves and centres in these segments of the cord. It is classified as a superficial reflex. A decrease in this reflex or its absence occurs in lesions involving pyramidal tract upper motor neurons. It can, however, be absent without any pathological condition—in pregnancy, for example.

Quick CHECK

7. What are the somatic effectors?
8. State the principle of final common path as it applies to the somatic motor nervous system.
9. Explain how the knee jerk reflex can be both a stretch reflex and a spinal reflex.

the big picture | Peripheral Nervous System and the Whole Body

The peripheral nervous system is made up of all the afferent nervous pathways coming into the CNS and all the efferent pathways going out of the CNS. After reviewing all the major spinal and cranial nerves, including their major branches, we turned our attention to the efferent somatic pathways. The next chapter (22) will continue the story by picking up with the efferent autonomic pathways. We will finally finish the story of the nervous system with the peripheral afferent (sensory) pathways in Chapters 23 and 24.

The peripheral motor pathways are simply those nervous pathways that lead from the integrator (CNS) to the effectors. The somatic motor pathways lead to skeletal muscle effectors, allowing them to carry information that regulates how and when our voluntary muscles contract. This allows us to move our skeleton and accomplish many of the tasks that promote survival and make life productive and enjoyable. Somatic motor pathways also control our breathing—a topic we will explore in later chapters. Less obviously—but just as importantly—somatic motor pathways are directly involved in producing heat with our skeletal muscles.

LANGUAGE OF SCIENCE *(continued from p. 479)*

glossopharyngeal nerve (glos-oh-fah-RIN-jee-al nerv) [*glosso-* **tongue,** *-pharyng-* **throat,** *-al* **relating to**]

hypoglossal nerve (hye-poh-GLOS-al nerv) [*hypo-* **under or below,** *-gloss-* **tongue,** *-al* **relating to**]

lumbar plexus (LUM-bar PLEK-sus) [*lumb-* **loin,** *-ar* **relating to,** *plexus* **braid or network**] *pl.,* plexi or plexuses

mixed cranial nerve (KRAY-nee-al nerv) [*crani-* **skull,** *-al* **relating to**]

motor cranial nerve (MOH-tor KRAY-nee-al nerv) [*mot-* **move,** *-or* **agent,** *crani-* **skull,** *-al* **relating to**]

myotome (MY-oh-tohm) [*myo-* **muscle,** *-tome* **cut segment or region**]

oculomotor nerve (awk-yoo-loh-MOH-tor nerv) [*oculo-* **eye,** *-mot-* **move,** *-or* **agent**]

olfactory nerve (ol-FAK-tor-ee nerv) [*olfact-* **smell,** *-ory* **relating to**]

optic nerve (OP-tik nerv) [*opt-* **vision,** *-ic* **relating to**]

phrenic nerve (FREN-ik nerv) [*phren-* **mind,** *-ic* **relating to**]

plantar reflex (PLAN-tar REE-fleks) [*planta-* **sole,** *-ar* **relating to,** *re-* **again,** *-flex* **bend**]

plexus (PLEK-sus) [*plexus* **braid or network**] *pl.,* plexi or plexuses

ramus (RAY-mus) [*ramus* **branch**] *pl.,* rami

reflex (REE-fleks) [*re-* **again,** *-flex* **bend**]

sacral plexus (SAY-kral PLEK-sus) [*sacr-* **sacred,** *-al* **relating to,** *plexus* **braid or network**] *pl.,* plexi or plexuses

sciatic nerve (sye-AT-ik nerv) [*(i)sci-* **hip joint,** *-atic* **relating to**]

sensory cranial nerve (SEN-sor-ee KRAY-nee-al nerv) [*sens-* **feel,** *-ory* **relating to,** *crani-* **skull,** *-al* **relating to**]

somatic reflex (so-MAH-tik REE-fleks) [*soma-* **body,** *-ic* **relating to,** *re-* **again,** *-flex* **bend**]

spinal nerve (SPY-nal nerv) [*spine-* **backbone,** *-al* **relating to**]

spinal reflex (SPY-nal REE-fleks) [*spine-* **backbone,** *-al* **relating to,** *re-* **again,** *-flex* **bend**]

terminal nerve (TER-mih-nal nerv) [*termin-* **boundary,** *-al* **relating to**]

trigeminal nerve (try-JEM-i-nal nerv) [*tri-* **three,** *-gemina-* **twin or pair,** *-al* **relating to**]

trochlear nerve (TROK-lee-ar nerv) [*trochlea-* **pulley,** *-al* **relating to**]

vagus nerve (VAY-gus nerv) [*vagus* **wanderer**]

ventral ramus (VEN-tral RAY-mus) [*ventr-* **belly,** *-al* **relating to** *ramus* **branch**] *pl.,* rami

ventral root (VEN-tral root) [*ventr-* **belly,** *-al* **relating to**]

vestibulocochlear nerve (ves-TIB-yoo-loh-kok-lee-ar nerv) [*vestibulo-* **entrance hall,** *-cochle-* **sea shell,** *-ar* **relating to**]

withdrawal reflex [*with-* **away,** *-draw* **to draw,** *-al* **relating to,** *re-* **again,** *-flex* **bend**]

LANGUAGE OF MEDICINE

Babinski sign (bah-BIN-skee) [*Joseph F.F. Babinski* **French neurologist**]

herpes zoster (HER-peez ZOS-ter) [*herpe* **creep,** *zoster* **girdle**]

peripheral neuropathy (peh-RIF-er-al nyoo-ROP-ahthee) [*peri-* **around,** *-phera-* **boundary,** *-al* **relating to,** *neuro-* **nerves,** *-path-* **disease,** *-y* **state**]

shingles (SHING-guls) [**from** *cingul-* **girdle**]

tic douloureux (tik doo-loo-ROO) [*tic* **spasm,** *douloureux* **painful** (French)]

trigeminal neuralgia (try-JEM-i-nal nyoo-RAL-jee-ah) [*tri-* **three,** *-gemina-* **twins or pair,** *-al* **relating to,** *neur-* **nerves,** *-algia* **pain**]

case study

The supermarket was only two blocks away. Tomasina was in such a hurry and the store was so close, she didn't bother to look in the garage for her helmet. She jumped on her bike and peddled quickly toward the store. From out of nowhere, a car sped by too close to the side of the road and clipped Tomasina with the side mirror, knocking her to the ground. Unfortunately, Tomasina sustained a brain injury, and when she regained consciousness she was in hospital. Tomasina was told some tests would be conducted to see whether her cranial nerves had been affected by the trauma.

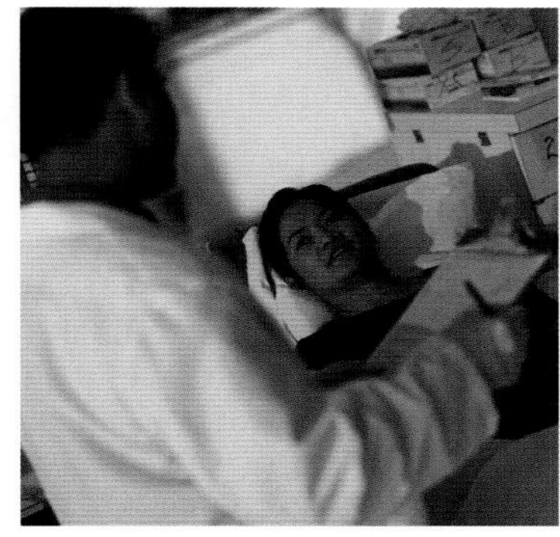

1. In one of the tests, Tomasina was asked to stick out her tongue. Which cranial nerve was being tested?
   a. Glossopharyngeal
   b. Hypoglossal
   c. Vagus
   d. Trigeminal
2. In a second test, Tomasina's hearing was evaluated. What cranial nerve is involved in the sense of hearing?
   a. Accessory
   b. Vagus
   c. Vestibulocochlear
   d. Trochlear
3. Tomasina was having difficulty focusing her eyes and following the doctor's finger on command. Which of the following cranial nerves does not control eye movement?
   a. Optic
   b. Oculomotor
   c. Trochlear
   d. Abducens
4. The nurse touched a series of swabs with different tastes to the front portion of Tomasina's tongue—sugar, salt, lemon juice, and dissolved aspirin. Which cranial nerve was the nurse testing?
   a. Glossopharyngeal
   b. Olfactory
   c. Trigeminal
   d. Facial
5. Tomasina was later discharged from the hospital and her GP was informed of her accident. Which condition on her discharge letter refers to her head injury?
   a. CVA
   b. TIA
   c. TBI
   d. VZV

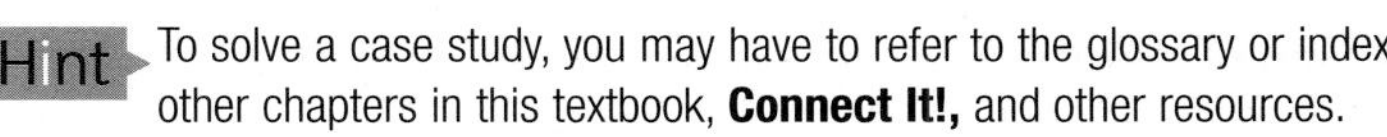

Hint To solve a case study, you may have to refer to the glossary or index, other chapters in this textbook, **Connect It!,** and other resources.

UNIT 3

CHAPTER SUMMARY

To download an MP3 version of the chapter summary for use with your mobile device, access the ***Audio Chapter Summaries*** *online at evolve.elsevier.com.*

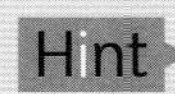

Scan this summary after reading the chapter to help you reinforce the key concepts. Later, use the summary as a quick review before your class or before a test.

Overview

A. Peripheral nervous system (PNS) (**Figure 21-1**)
   1. Thirty-one pairs of spinal nerves
   2. Twelve pairs of cranial nerves

Spinal Nerves

A. Overview (**Figure 21-2**)
   1. Thirty-one pairs of spinal nerves are connected to the spinal cord (**Figure 21-3**)
   2. No special names; numbered by level of vertebral column at which they emerge from the spinal cavity
      a. Eight cervical nerve pairs (C1 through C8)
      b. Twelve thoracic nerve pairs (T1 through T12)
      c. Five lumbar nerve pairs (L1 through L5)
      d. Five sacral nerve pairs (S1 through S5)
      e. One coccygeal nerve pair
   3. Lumbar, sacral, and coccygeal nerve roots descend from point of origin to the lower end of the spinal cord (level of first lumbar vertebra) before reaching the intervertebral foramina of the respective vertebrae, through which the nerves emerge
   4. Cauda equina—describes the appearance of the lower end of the spinal cord and its spinal nerves as a horse's tail

B. Structure of spinal nerves
   1. Each spinal nerve attaches to spinal cord by a ventral (anterior) root and a dorsal (posterior) root
   2. Dorsal root ganglion—swelling in the dorsal root of each spinal nerve
   3. All spinal nerves are mixed nerves
   4. Ramus
      a. One of several large branches formed after each spinal nerve emerges from the spinal cavity (**Figure 21-3**)
      b. Dorsal ramus—supplies somatic motor and sensory fibres to smaller nerves that innervate the muscles and skin of the posterior surface of the head, neck, and trunk

c. Ventral ramus
(1) Structure is more complex than that of dorsal ramus
(2) Autonomic motor fibres split from the ventral ramus and head toward a ganglion of the sympathetic chain
(3) Some autonomic fibres synapse with neurons that continue on to autonomic effectors through splanchnic nerves; others synapse with neurons whose fibres rejoin the ventral ramus
(4) Sympathetic rami—splitting and rejoining of autonomic fibres
(5) Motor and sensory fibres innervate muscles and glands in the extremities and lateral and ventral portions of neck and trunk

C. Nerve plexuses
1. Plexuses—complex networks formed by the ventral rami of most spinal nerves (not T2 through T12) subdividing and then joining together to form individual nerves
2. Each individual nerve that emerges contains all the fibres that innervate a particular region of the body
3. In plexuses, spinal nerve fibres are rearranged according to their ultimate destination, reducing the number of nerves needed to supply each body part
4. Four major pairs of plexuses
a. Cervical plexus (**Figure 21-4**)
(1) Located deep within the neck
(2) Made up of ventral rami of C1 through C4 and a branch of the ventral ramus of C5
(3) Individual nerves emerging from cervical plexus innervate the muscles and skin of the neck, upper shoulders, and part of the head
(4) Phrenic nerve exits the cervical plexus and innervates the diaphragm
b. Brachial plexus (**Figure 21-5**)
(1) Located deep within the shoulder
(2) Made up of ventral rami of C5 through T1
(3) Individual nerves emerging from brachial plexus innervate the lower part of the shoulder and the entire arm
c. Lumbar plexus (**Figure 21-6**)
(1) Located in the lumbar region of the back in the psoas muscle
(2) Formed by intermingling fibres of L1 through L4
(3) Femoral nerve exits the lumbar plexus, divides into many branches, and supplies the thigh and leg
d. Sacral plexus and coccygeal plexus (**Figure 21-6**)
(1) Located in the pelvic cavity in the anterior surface of the piriformis muscle
(2) Formed by intermingling of fibres from L4 through S4
(3) Tibial, common fibular, and sciatic nerves exit the sacral plexus and supply nearly all the skin of the leg, posterior thigh muscles, and leg and foot muscles

D. Dermatomes and myotomes (**Figure 21-7**)
1. Dermatome—region of skin surface area supplied by afferent (sensory) fibres of a given spinal nerve (**Figure 21-8**)
2. Myotome—skeletal muscle or muscles supplied by efferent (motor) fibres of a given spinal nerve (**Figure 21-9**)

UNIT 3

Cranial Nerves

A. Overview (**Tables 21-2** and **21-3**)
1. Twelve pairs of cranial nerves connect to the brain, mostly the brainstem (**Figure 21-10**)
2. Identified by name (determined by either distribution or function) or number (order in which they emerge, anterior to posterior) or both
3. Made up of bundles of axons
a. Mixed cranial nerve—axons of sensory and motor neurons
b. Sensory cranial nerve—axons of sensory neurons only
c. Motor cranial nerve—mainly axons of motor neurons and a small number of sensory fibres (proprioceptors)

B. Olfactory nerve (CN I)
1. Composed of axons of neurons whose dendrites and cell bodies lie in nasal mucosa and terminate in olfactory bulbs
2. Carries information about sense of smell

C. Optic nerve (CN II)
1. Composed of axons from the innermost layer of sensory neurons of the retina
2. Carries visual information from the eyes to the brain

D. Oculomotor nerve (CN III)
1. Fibres originate from cells in the oculomotor nucleus and extend to some of the external eye muscles
2. Efferent autonomic fibres are also present, which extend to the intrinsic muscles of the eye to regulate amount of light entering eye and aid focusing on near objects
3. Sensory fibres from proprioceptors in the eye muscles are also present

E. Trochlear nerve (CN IV)
1. Motor fibres originate in cells of the midbrain and extend to the superior oblique muscles of the eye
2. Also contains afferent fibres from proprioceptors in the superior oblique muscles of the eye

F. Trigeminal nerve (CN V) (**Figure 21-11**)
1. Has three branches: ophthalmic nerve, maxillary nerve, and mandibular nerve
2. Sensory neurons carry afferent impulses from skin and mucosa of head and teeth to cell bodies in the trigeminal ganglion
3. Motor fibres originate in trifacial motor nucleus and extend to the muscles of mastication through the mandibular nerve

G. Abducens nerve (CN VI)
1. Motor nerve with fibres originating from a nucleus in the pons on the floor of the fourth ventricle and extending to the lateral rectus muscles of the eye
2. Contains afferent fibres from proprioceptors in the lateral rectus muscles

H. Facial nerve (VII)
1. Motor root fibres originate from a nucleus in lower part of pons and extend to superficial muscles of the face and scalp (**Figure 21-12**)
2. Intermediate nerve—the smaller of two facial nerve roots
a. Autonomic fibres extend to submaxillary and sublingual salivary glands
b. Also contains sensory fibres from taste buds of anterior two thirds of the tongue

I. Vestibulocochlear nerve (CN VIII)
  1. Two distinct divisions that are both sensory: vestibular nerve and cochlear nerve
  2. Vestibular nerve fibres originate in the semicircular canals in inner ear and transmit impulses that result in sensations of equilibrium
  3. Cochlear nerve fibres originate in the organ of Corti in the cochlea of the inner ear and transmit impulses that result in sensations of hearing

J. Glossopharyngeal nerve (CN IX)
  1. Composed of sensory, motor, and autonomic nerve fibres
  2. Supplies fibres to tongue, pharynx, and carotid sinus (**Figure 21-13**)

K. Vagus nerve (CN X)
  1. Composed of sensory and motor fibres with many widely distributed branches
  2. Sensory fibres supply pharynx, larynx, trachea, heart, carotid body, lungs, bronchi, oesophagus, stomach, small intestine, and gallbladder (**Figure 21-14**)
  3. Somatic motor fibres innervate the pharynx and larynx and are mostly autonomic fibres

L. Accessory nerve (CN XI)
  1. Motor nerve that was once thought to be an "accessory" to the vagus nerve
  2. Fibres of the cranial division innervate muscles of the abdomen, pharynx and larynx
  3. Fibres of the spinal division innervate the trapezius and sternocleidomastoid muscles (**Figure 21-15**)

M. Hypoglossal nerve (CN XII)
  1. Composed of motor and sensory fibres
  2. Motor fibres innervate the muscles of the tongue
  3. Contains sensory fibres from proprioceptors in muscles of the tongue

Somatic Motor Nervous System

A. Two functional divisions of the peripheral nervous system (PNS)
  1. Afferent (sensory) division
  2. Efferent (motor) division
    a. Somatic motor nervous system (SNS)
    b. Autonomic nervous system (ANS) efferent pathways; ANS is discussed in Chapter 22

B. Basic principles of somatic motor pathways
  1. Somatic nervous system—includes all voluntary motor pathways outside the central nervous system
  2. Somatic effectors—skeletal muscles

C. Somatic reflexes
  1. Nature of a reflex
    a. Reflex—action that results from a nerve impulse passing over a reflex arc; predictable response to a stimulus
      (1) Cranial reflex—centre of reflex arc is in the brain
      (2) Spinal reflex—centre of reflex arc is in the spinal cord
    b. Reflex consists of either muscle contraction or glandular secretion
      (1) Somatic reflex—contraction of skeletal muscles
      (2) Autonomic (visceral) reflex—either contraction of smooth or cardiac muscle or secretion by glands
  2. Withdrawal reflexes—cause the body to withdraw from irritating stimuli (**Figure 21-16**)
    a. Flexor reflex—response in which flexors in an extremity contract
    b. Extensor reflex—response in which extensors in an extremity contract
    c. Crossed-extensor reflex—response in which extensor contralateral to the stimulus contracts
    d. Learned reflexes develop through prior experience but instrinsic reflexes are inborn
  3. Somatic reflexes of clinical importance—reflexes deviate from normal in certain diseases, and reflex testing is a valuable diagnostic aid (**Figure 21-18**)
    a. Knee jerk reflex (also known as *patellar reflex*)—extension of the leg in response to tapping the patellar ligament; tendon and muscles are stretched, stimulating muscle spindles and initiating conduction over a two-neuron reflex arc (**Figure 21-17**); may be classified in several different ways
      (1) Spinal cord reflex—centre of reflex arc located in spinal cord grey matter
      (2) Segmental reflex—mediating impulses enter and leave at same cord segment
      (3) Ipsilateral reflex—mediating impulses come from and go to the same side of the body
      (4) Stretch or myotatic reflex—result of type of stimulation used to evoke reflex
      (5) Extensor reflex—produced by extensors of the leg
      (6) Deep reflex—result of deep location of receptors stimulated to produce reflex
    b. Ankle jerk reflex (also known as *Achilles reflex*)—extension of the foot in response to tapping the Achilles tendon
      (1) Tendon reflex and deep reflex mediated by two-neuron spinal arcs
      (2) Centres lie in first and second sacral segments of the cord
    c. Plantar reflex—plantar flexion of all toes and a slight turning in and flexion of the anterior part of the foot in response to stimulation of the outer edge of the sole; compare to Babinski sign (below)
      (1) Babinski sign—extension of great toe, with or without fanning of other toes, in response to stimulation of outer margin of sole of foot
      (2) Present in normal infants until approximately 1½ years of age and then becomes suppressed when corticospinal fibres become fully myelinated
      (3) In humans older than 1½ years of age, a positive Babinski reflex is one of the pyramidal signs indicating destruction of corticospinal (pyramidal tract) fibres; compare to the normal adult plantar reflex (above)

d. Corneal reflex—winking in response to the cornea being touched; mediated by reflex arcs with sensory fibres in the ophthalmic branch of the fifth cranial nerve, centres in the pons, and motor fibres in the seventh cranial nerve
e. Abdominal reflex—drawing in of the abdominal wall in response to stroking the side of the abdomen; superficial reflex; mediated by arcs with sensory and motor fibres in T9 through T12 and centres in these segments of the cord; decreased or absent reflex may involve lesions of pyramidal tract upper motor neurons

The Big Picture: The Peripheral Nervous System and the Whole Body

A. The peripheral nervous system is made of all the afferent nervous pathways coming into the CNS and all the efferent pathways going out of the central nervous system
B. Peripheral efferent (motor) pathways are pathways that lead from the integrator central nervous system to the effectors; allow the central nervous system to communicate regulatory information to the nervous effectors in the body
C. Somatic motor pathways regulate skeletal movements needed for survival, breathing, and heat production

REVIEW QUESTIONS

Hint

Write out the answers to these questions after reading the chapter and reviewing the Chapter Summary. Note—writing out your answers will consolidate learning and provide a valuable resource of information.

1. Identify the direction of the information carried by the ventral root of a spinal nerve.
2. Define *mixed nerves.*
3. Identify the areas innervated by the individual nerves emerging from the cervical plexus.
4. Explain the concept of a dermatome.
5. Explain the correlation between a myotome and a specific movement of the body.
6. Which cranial nerves transmit impulses that result in vision? In eye movement?
7. Which cranial nerves transmit impulses that result in hearing? In taste sensations?
8. What pathways are found in the somatic motor nervous system?
9. Describe what happens when the fifth cranial nerve is compressed.
10. Describe the condition of shingles. Who can be affected by this disease?

CRITICAL THINKING QUESTIONS

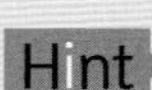

After finishing the Review Questions, write out the answers to these more in-depth questions to help you apply your new knowledge. Go back to sections of the chapter that relate to concepts that you find difficult.

1. Distinguish between the reflexes that cause cardiac muscle to react and those that cause skeletal muscles to react.
2. An adult has an extension of the great toe and the fanning of the other toes in response to stimulation of the outer margin of the sole of the foot. Why is this a concern, and where would the problem most likely be?
3. A single reflex can be classified in several ways. What example can you find that would show this? In what ways can this reflex be classified?
4. Predict the respiratory consequences of an injury that damaged the spinal cord between the third and fifth cervical segments. What specific mechanism would cause these consequences?
5. Contrast the difference between the CNS and the PNS.

22 Autonomic Nervous System

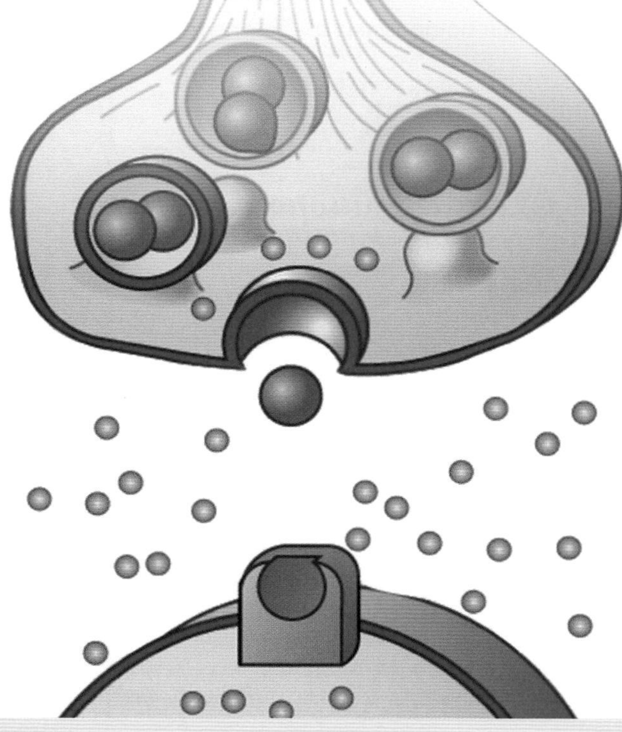

CHAPTER OUTLINE

Hint *Scan this outline before you begin to read the chapter, as a preview of how the concepts are organized.*

LANGUAGE OF SCIENCE

Hint *Use this list to aid your pronunciation of unfamiliar words.*

acetylcholine (ACh) (ass-ee-til-KOH-leen) [*acetyl-* **vinegar,** *-chole-* **bile,** *-ine* **made of**]

adrenergic (ad-ren-ER-jik) [*ad-* **toward,** *-ren-* **kidney,** *-erg-* **work,** *-ic* **relating to**]

alpha (α) receptor (AL-fah ree-SEP-tor) [*alpha* **first letter of Greek alphabet,** *recept-* **receive,** *-or* **agent**]

autonomic nervous system (ANS) (aw-toh-NOM-ik) [*auto-* **self,** *-nomo-* **law,** *-ic* **relating to**]

autonomic (visceral) reflex (aw-toh-NOM-ik REE-fleks) [*auto-* **self,** *-nomo-* **law,** *-ic* **relating to,** *re-* **again,** *-flex* **bend**]

beta (β) receptor (BAY-tah ree-SEP-tor) [*beta* **second letter of Greek alphabet,** *recept-* **receive,** *-or* **agent**]

cholinergic (koh-lin-ER-jik) [*chole-* **bile,** *-erg-* **work,** *-ic* **relating to**]

collateral ganglion (koh-LAT-er-al GANG-glee-on) [*co-* **together,** *-later-* **side,** *-al* **relating to,** *gangli-* **knot,** *-on* **unit**] *pl.,* ganglia

co-transmission (koh-tranz-MISH-un) [*co-* **together,** *-trans-* **across,** *-miss-* **send,** *-ion* **process**]

enteric nervous system (ENS) (en-TER-ik) [*enter-* **intestine,** *-ic* **relating to**]

"fight-or-flight" reaction (fyte or flyte ree-AK-shun) [*re-* **again,** *-action* **action**]

ganglion (GANG-lee-on) [*gangli-* **knot,** *-on* **unit**] *pl.,* ganglia

muscarinic (M) receptor (mus-kah-RIN-ik ree-SEP-tor) [*musca-* **fly,** *-in-* **substance,** *-ic* **relating to (after the toxic mushroom** *A. muscaria*)**,** *recept-* **receive,** *-or* **agent**]

nicotinic (N) receptor (NIK-oh-tin-ik ree-SEP-tor) [*Jean Nicot Villemain* **French diplomat (brought tobacco to France),** *-in-* **substance,** *-ic* **relating to (after plant genus** *Nicotiana*)**,** *recept-* **receive,** *-or* **agent**]

continued on p. 516

In Chapter 21, we explored the efferent (motor) pathways of the somatic nervous system (SNS) that regulates skeletal muscles, allowing us to survive by defending ourselves, getting food, or performing other essential tasks. This chapter continues the story by exploring the efferent pathways of the autonomic nervous system (ANS).

Autonomic regulation operates below the conscious level to control smooth and cardiac muscle, glands, and other tissues. Such regulation helps us maintain homeostasis of the internal environment and deal with threats to that stability. •

OVERVIEW OF THE AUTONOMIC NERVOUS SYSTEM

Role of the Autonomic Nervous System

The **autonomic nervous system (ANS)** is a subdivision of the nervous system that regulates involuntary effectors (**Figure 22-1**). Because it controls involuntary effectors, we can think of the autonomic system as our system of subconscious regulation of body functions.

It is the ANS that carries efferent signals to the autonomic, or *visceral*, effectors—cardiac muscle, smooth muscle, glandular epithelia, and adipose and other tissues (**Box 22-1**). Some autonomic pathways connect to the skeletal muscles, which are ordinarily considered somatic effectors. In skeletal muscles, subconscious autonomic stimulation helps prevent fatigue during intense exercise—it does not directly control muscle contractions.

The major functions of the ANS are heartbeat regulation, smooth muscle contraction, glandular secretion, and metabolism regulation in ways that maintain homeostatic balance or respond to threats to that balance. Recall from the previous chapter that **autonomic reflexes,** or **visceral reflexes,** can produce these effects over a visceral reflex pathway, which you can see illustrated as a simple reflex arc in **Figure 22-1**.

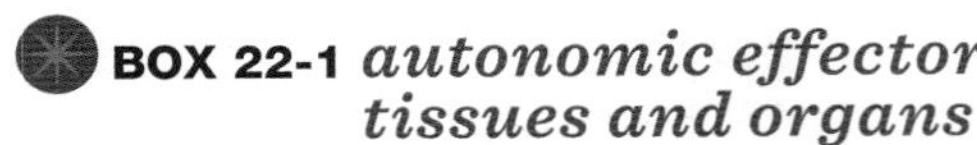

BOX 22-1 *autonomic effector tissues and organs*

Smooth Muscle
- Blood vessels
- Bronchial tubes
- Stomach
- Gallbladder
- Intestines
- Urinary bladder
- Spleen
- Eye (iris, ciliary muscles)
- Hair follicles

Cardiac Muscle
- Heart

Glandular Epithelium
- Sweat glands
- Lacrimal glands
- Digestive glands (salivary, gastric, pancreas, liver)
- Adrenal medulla

Other Tissues
- Adipose tissue
- Kidneys
- Skeletal muscle*

*Skeletal muscle is primarily a somatic effector, but sympathetic fibres help regulate contractility of skeletal muscle during intense exercise to avoid fatigue.

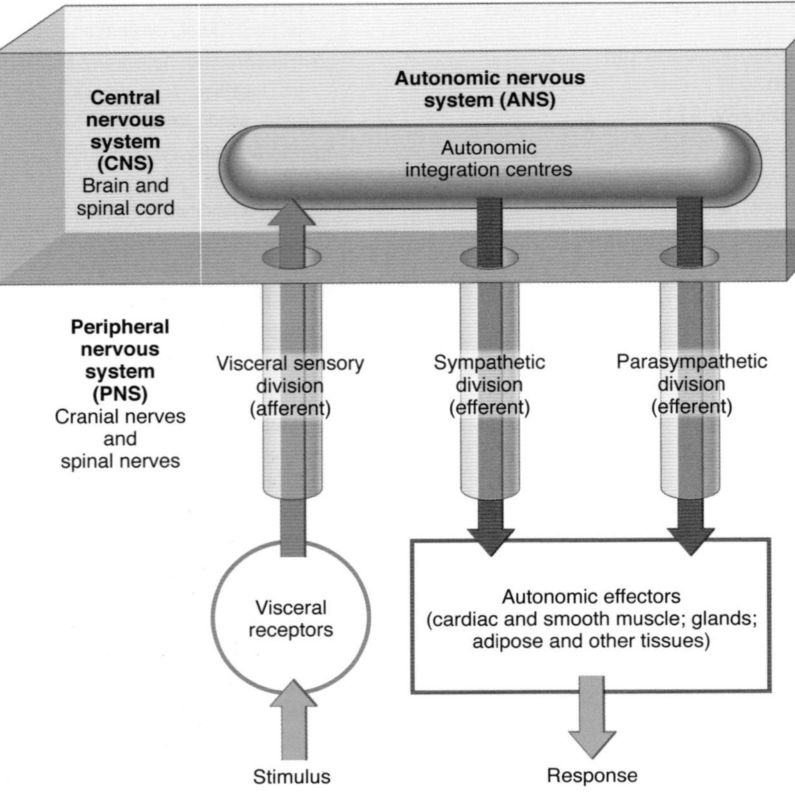

FIGURE 22-1 Organization of the autonomic nervous system. Note the simple arc pattern to information flow in the diagram. Compare to **Figure 18-2** on p. 394 to see how this part of the nervous system fits into the big picture of nervous regulation.

Divisions of the Autonomic Nervous System

Sympathetic and Parasympathetic Divisions

Although the ANS also includes sensory pathways (afferent pathways) that provide the feedback necessary to regulate effectors, we will emphasize the motor pathways (efferent pathways) in this chapter. Sensory functions as a whole are discussed in the next two chapters.

The ANS has two efferent divisions: the **sympathetic division** and the **parasympathetic division.** The sympathetic division consists of neural pathways that are separate from the parasympathetic pathways.

As you can see in **Figure 22-2**, however, even though the two divisions follow separate pathways, many autonomic effectors are *dually* *innervated.* That is, many autonomic effectors receive input from both sympathetic and parasympathetic pathways.

In dually innervated effectors, the effects of the two systems are often antagonistic: one inhibits the effector and the other stimulates the effector. This is similar to the antagonistic effects of an accelerator and brake in a vehicle. The opposing influences allow a dually innervated effector to be controlled with remarkable precision. Such antagonism also allows a dually innervated effector to participate in timed events, such as the sexual response, in which effectors must be stimulated and then rapidly inhibited (or vice versa) in a specific timed sequence.

Some autonomic effectors are *singly innervated,* receiving input from only the sympathetic division.

Enteric Nervous System

As first mentioned in Chapter 18 (see p. 395), the **enteric nervous system (ENS)** is a special part of the ANS. The ENS is the "intestinal nervous system" that is made up of a complex network of nerve plexuses buried between layers of the intestinal (gut) wall. The ENS controls visceral effectors in the gut wall, including endocrine cells, exocrine cells, and smooth muscles. Even though the various enteric nerve cells can regulate digestive function in the gut independently, efficiency is maximized when extrinsic sympathetic and parasympathetic stimuli are able to modulate ENS function.

A simple way to think of the ENS is that it is a regional part of the ANS that controls its own region but is in turn managed by the ANS. We explore the ENS in more detail in Chapter 40 when we discuss digestive function in the intestine.

STRUCTURE OF THE AUTONOMIC NERVOUS SYSTEM

Basic Plan of Autonomic Pathways

Each efferent autonomic pathway, whether sympathetic or parasympathetic, is made up of autonomic nerves, ganglia, and plexuses. These structures, in turn, are made up of efferent autonomic neurons. They conduct impulses away from the brainstem or spinal cord to autonomic effectors. As with all efferent neurons, efferent autonomic neurons function in reflex arcs. Thus, as with somatic motor regulation, efferent autonomic regulation ultimately depends on feedback from the sensory pathways.

A relay of two autonomic neurons conducts information from the central nervous system (CNS) to the autonomic effectors. The first is called a **preganglionic neuron**—an awkward name but a descriptive one. Preganglionic neurons conduct impulses from the brainstem or spinal cord to an autonomic **ganglion,** locating them *before* the ganglion—thus *pre*ganglionic. Within an autonomic ganglion, the preganglionic neuron synapses with a second efferent neuron. Because this second neuron conducts impulses away from the ganglion and to the effector, it is called the **postganglionic neuron.**

As you can see in **Figure 22-3**, A, this plan fundamentally differs from the efferent pathways of the somatic motor nervous system. Conduction to somatic effectors requires only one efferent neuron, the somatic motor neuron that originates in the anterior grey horn of the spinal cord. Conduction to autonomic effectors, however, requires a sequence of two efferent neurons from the CNS to the effector. Essential features of the somatic motor pathways and autonomic efferent pathways are further compared and contrasted in **Table 22-1**.

Structure of the Sympathetic Pathways

Sympathetic Preganglionic Neurons

Sympathetic preganglionic neurons begin within the spinal cord. Specifically, they have their dendrites and cell bodies within the lateral grey horns of the thoracic and lumbar segments of the spinal cord (see **Figure 22-3**, A). For this

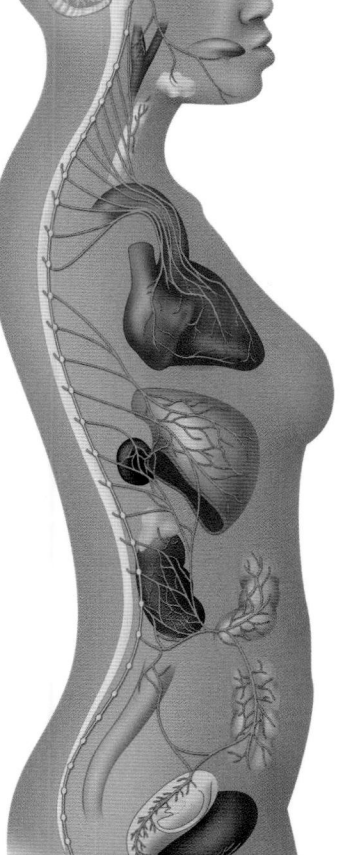

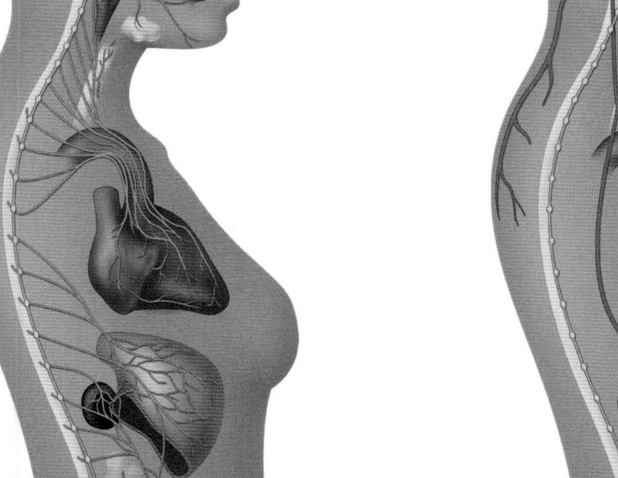

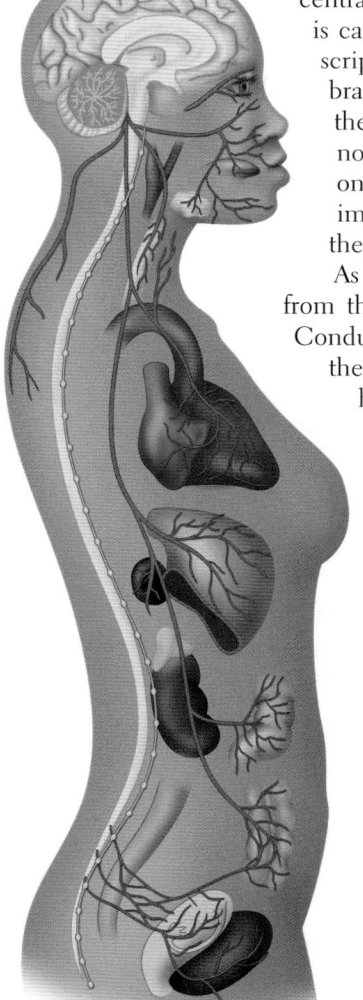

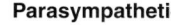

FIGURE 22-2 Divisions of the autonomic nervous system. Note that although the sympathetic pathways are separate from the parasympathetic pathways, most autonomic effectors are innervated by both pathways.

UNIT 3

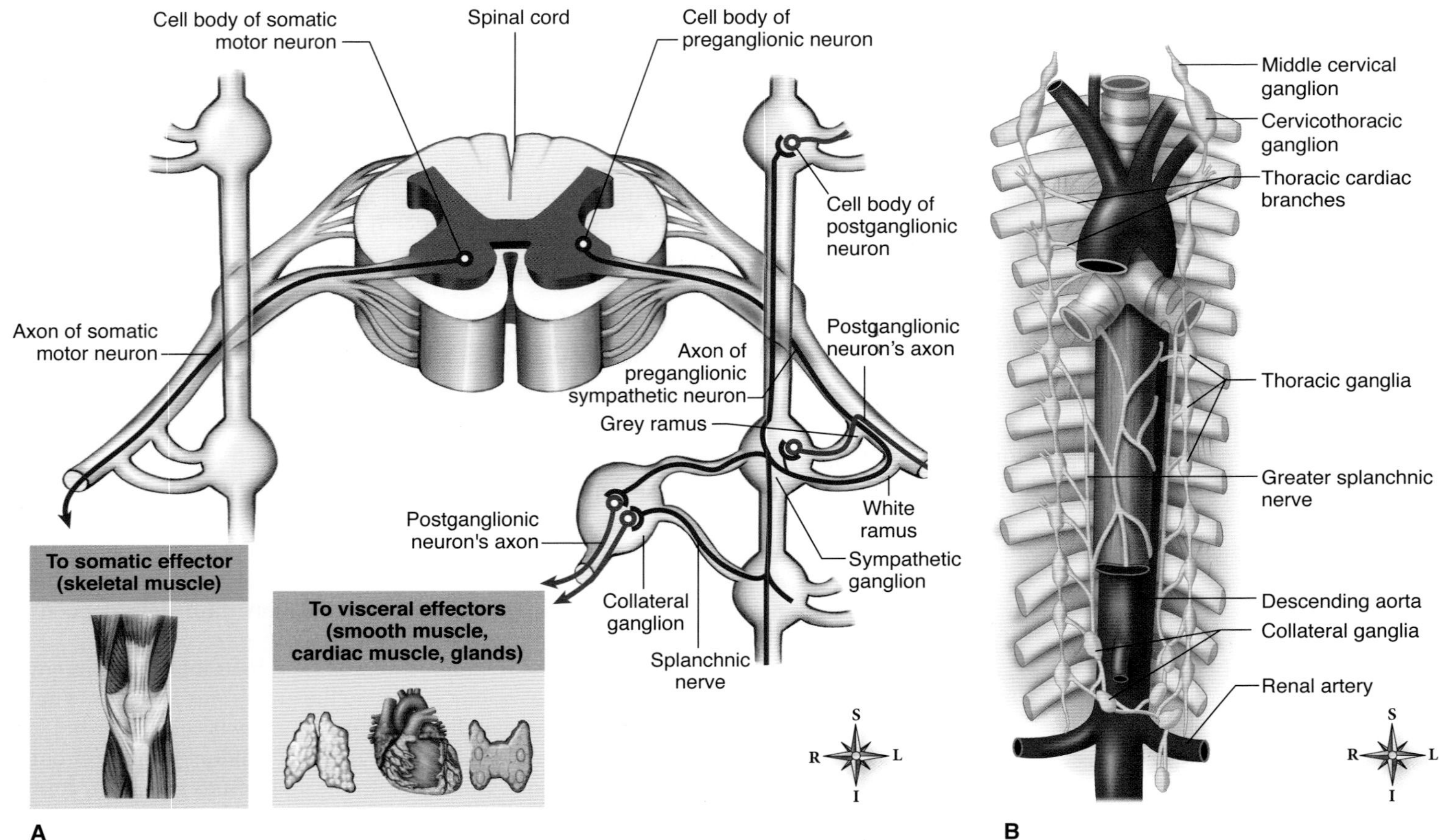

FIGURE 22-3 Diagram of autonomic conduction paths. A, The left side of the diagram shows that one somatic motor neuron conducts impulses all the way from the spinal cord to a somatic effector. Conduction from the spinal cord to any visceral effector, however, requires a relay of at least two autonomic motor neurons—a preganglionic and a postganglionic neuron, shown on the right side of the diagram. **B,** Sketch showing a portion of the left and right sympathetic chain or trunk.

reason, the sympathetic division has also been called the *thoracolumbar division.*

Most of the ganglia of the sympathetic division lie along either side of the anterior surface of the vertebral column (see **Figure 21-3**, p. 483). Both grey rami and white rami are sympathetic rami. Sympathetic axon collaterals bridge the gap between adjacent ganglia that lie on the same side of the vertebral column. This arrangement forms a structure that resembles a chain of beads (see **Figure 22-3**, *B*). Thus the linked ganglia are often referred to as the *sympathetic chain ganglia*, or the **sympathetic trunk.**

Each chain runs from the second cervical vertebra in the neck all the way down to the level of the coccyx. There are usually

TABLE 22-1 Comparison of Somatic Motor and Autonomic Pathways

FEATURE	SOMATIC MOTOR PATHWAYS	AUTONOMIC EFFERENT PATHWAYS
Direction of information flow	Efferent	Efferent
Number of neurons between CNS and effector	One (somatic motor neuron)	Two (preganglionic and postganglionic)
Myelin sheath present	Yes	Preganglionic: yes Postganglionic: no
Location of peripheral fibres	Most cranial nerves and all spinal nerves	Most cranial nerves and all spinal nerves
Effector innervated	Skeletal muscle (voluntary)	Smooth and cardiac muscle, glands, and adipose and other tissues (involuntary)
Neurotransmitter	Acetylcholine	Acetylcholine or norepinephrine

CNS, Central nervous system.

22 sympathetic chain ganglia on each side of the vertebral column: three cervical, eleven thoracic, four lumbar, and four sacral. Axons of sympathetic preganglionic neurons leave the cord by way of the ventral roots of the thoracic and first four lumbar spinal nerves. From there, they split away from other spinal nerve fibres by means of a small branch called the *white ramus*. The white ramus gets its name from the fact that most of the sympathetic preganglionic fibres within it are myelinated axons. Note in **Figure 22-3** that the sympathetic preganglionic axon extends through the white ramus to a sympathetic chain ganglion.

If we trace the axon inside the sympathetic chain ganglion, we see that the preganglionic fibre may branch along any of three paths:

1. It can synapse with a sympathetic postganglionic neuron.
2. It can send ascending or descending branches through the sympathetic trunk to synapse with postganglionic neurons in other chain ganglia.
3. It can pass through one or more ganglia without synapsing.

Preganglionic neurons that pass through chain ganglia without synapsing continue on through **splanchnic nerves** to other sympathetic ganglia (see **Figures 22-3** and **22-4**). These **collateral ganglia**, or *prevertebral ganglia*, are pairs of sympathetic ganglia located a short distance from the spinal cord. The collateral ganglia are named for nearby blood vessels. For example, the *coeliac ganglion* (also called the *solar plexus*) is a large ganglion that lies next to the coeliac artery just below the diaphragm. Other examples include the *superior mesenteric ganglion* and the *inferior mesenteric ganglion*, each located close to the beginning of an artery of the same name.

Some of the preganglionic fibres that enter the coeliac ganglion do not synapse there but continue on to the central portion (medulla) of the *adrenal gland*. Within the adrenal medulla, they synapse with modified postganglionic neurons. These modified postganglionic cells are actually endocrine cells that release hormones (mostly epinephrine) into the bloodstream. These chemical messengers may reach the various sympathetic effectors, where they enhance and prolong the effects of sympathetic stimulation.

Sympathetic Postganglionic Neurons

Most of the sympathetic postganglionic neurons have their dendrites and cell bodies in the sympathetic chain ganglia or collateral ganglia.

Some postganglionic axons return to a spinal nerve by way of a short branch called the *grey ramus*, so named because most postganglionic fibres are unmyelinated (see **Figure 22-3**). Once in the spinal nerve, the postganglionic fibres are distributed with other nerve fibres to the various sympathetic effectors. On the other hand, some postganglionic fibres are distributed to sympathetic effectors by way of separate autonomic nerves. The course of postganglionic fibres through these autonomic nerves is complex, involving the redistribution of fibres in autonomic plexuses before they reach their respective destinations.

In the sympathetic division, preganglionic neurons are relatively short and postganglionic neurons are relatively long.

The axon of any one sympathetic preganglionic neuron synapses with many postganglionic neurons, and these often terminate in widely separated organs. This anatomical fact partially explains a well-known physiological principle: Sympathetic responses are usually widespread, involving many organs—not just one.

Quick CHECK

1. Do autonomic pathways follow the principle of final common path?
2. Why is the sympathetic division of the ANS also known as the *thoracolumbar division*?
3. Describe the path generally taken by an impulse along a sympathetic pathway from the CNS to an autonomic effector.

Structure of the Parasympathetic Pathways

Parasympathetic Preganglionic Neurons

Parasympathetic preganglionic neurons have their cell bodies in nuclei in the brainstem or in the lateral grey columns of the sacral cord. For this reason, the parasympathetic division has also been called the *craniosacral division*.

Axons of parasympathetic preganglionic neurons are contained in cranial nerves III, VII, IX, and X and in some pelvic nerves. They extend a considerable distance before synapsing with postganglionic neurons. For example, at least 75% of all parasympathetic preganglionic fibres travel in the *vagus nerve* (CN X) for a distance of 30 cm or more before synapsing with postganglionic fibres in **terminal ganglia** near effectors in the chest and abdomen (**Figure 22-4** and **Table 22-2**).

Parasympathetic Postganglionic Neurons

Parasympathetic postganglionic neurons have their dendrites and cell bodies in parasympathetic ganglia. Unlike sympathetic ganglia that lie near the spinal column, parasympathetic ganglia lie near or embedded in autonomic effectors.

For example, note the ciliary ganglion in **Figure 22-4**. This and the other ganglia shown near it are parasympathetic ganglia located in the skull.

In a parasympathetic ganglion, preganglionic axons synapse with postganglionic neurons that send their short axons into the nearby autonomic effector. A parasympathetic preganglionic neuron therefore usually synapses with postganglionic neurons to a single effector. For this reason, parasympathetic stimulation often involves response by only one organ. Sympathetic stimulation, on the other hand, usually evokes responses by numerous organs.

CONNECT IT! 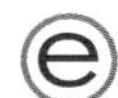

Recent evidence suggests that the sacral portion of the autonomic pathways may be sympathetic—not parasympathetic as first described over a century ago. Find out more at ***New Model of ANS Pathways*** online at ***Connect It!***

UNIT 3

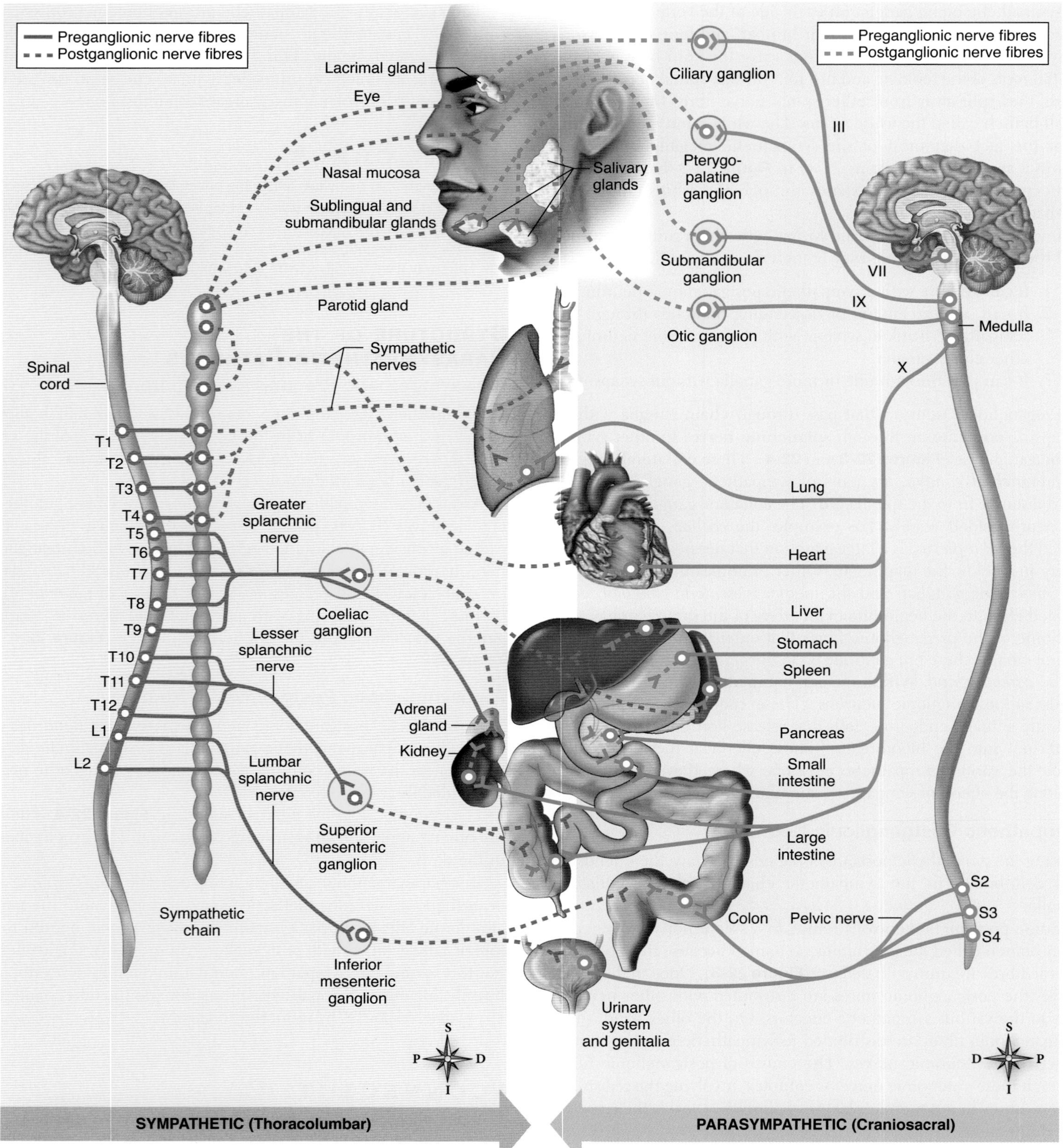

FIGURE 22-4 Major autonomic pathways.

TABLE 22-2 Comparison of Structural Features of the Sympathetic and Parasympathetic Pathways

NEURONS	SYMPATHETIC PATHWAYS	PARASYMPATHETIC PATHWAYS
Preganglionic Neurons		
Dendrites and cell bodies	In lateral grey columns of thoracic and first two or three lumbar segments of spinal cord	In nuclei of brainstem and in lateral grey columns of sacral segments of cord
Axons	In anterior roots of spinal nerves to spinal nerves (thoracic and first four lumbar), to and through white rami to terminate in sympathetic ganglia at various levels or to extend through sympathetic ganglia, to and through splanchnic nerves to terminate in collateral ganglia	From brainstem nuclei through cranial nerve III to ciliary ganglion From nuclei in pons through cranial nerve VII to sphenopalatine or submaxillary ganglion From nuclei in medulla through cranial nerve IX to otic ganglion or through cranial nerves X and XI to cardiac and coeliac ganglia, respectively
Distribution	Short fibres from CNS to ganglion	Long fibres from CNS to ganglion
Neurotransmitter	Acetylcholine	Acetylcholine
Ganglia	Sympathetic chain ganglia (22 pairs); collateral ganglia (coeliac, superior, inferior mesenteric)	Terminal ganglia (in or near effector)
Postganglionic Neurons		
Dendrites and cell bodies	In sympathetic and collateral ganglia	In parasympathetic ganglia (e.g., ciliary, sphenopalatine, submaxillary, otic, cardiac, coeliac) located in or near visceral effector organs
Receptors	Cholinergic (nicotinic)	Cholinergic (nicotinic)
Axons	In autonomic nerves and plexuses that innervate thoracic and abdominal viscera and blood vessels in these cavities In grey rami to spinal nerves, to smooth muscle of skin, blood vessels, and hair follicles, and to sweat glands	In short nerves to various visceral effector organs
Distribution	Long fibres from ganglion to widespread effectors	Short fibres from ganglion to single effector
Neurotransmitter	Norepinephrine (many); acetylcholine (few)	Acetylcholine

CNS, Central nervous system.

UNIT 3

AUTONOMIC NEUROTRANSMITTERS AND RECEPTORS

Axon terminals of autonomic neurons release either of two neurotransmitters: **norepinephrine** (NE) or **acetylcholine** (ACh). Axons that release norepinephrine are known as **adrenergic** fibres. Axons that release acetylcholine are called **cholinergic** fibres. Autonomic cholinergic fibres are the axons of preganglionic sympathetic neurons and of both preganglionic and postganglionic parasympathetic neurons. This leaves the axons of postganglionic sympathetic neurons as the only autonomic adrenergic fibres, and as you can see in **Figure 22-5**, *B*, not all of these are adrenergic. Sympathetic postganglionic axons to sweat glands and some blood vessels are instead cholinergic fibres.

Norepinephrine and Its Receptors

Norepinephrine affects visceral effectors by first binding to *adrenergic receptors* in their plasma membranes. The adrenergic receptors are of two main types, one named **alpha (α) receptors** and the other named **beta (β) receptors** (**Figure 22-6**, A). Different subtypes of alpha and beta receptors, such as alpha-1 (α_1), alpha-2 (α_2), beta-1 (β_1), beta-2 (β_2), and beta-3 (β_3), exist among cells that have adrenergic receptors.

The binding of norepinephrine to alpha receptors in the smooth muscle of blood vessels has a stimulating effect on the muscle that causes the vessel to constrict. The binding of norepinephrine to beta receptors in smooth muscle of a different blood vessel produces opposite effects. It inhibits the muscle, causing the vessel to dilate. But the binding of norepinephrine to beta receptors in cardiac muscle has a stimulating effect that results in a faster and stronger heartbeat.

Epinephrine released by the sympathetic postganglionic cells in the adrenal medulla also stimulates the adrenergic receptors, enhancing and prolonging the effects of sympathetic stimulation. Because epinephrine has a greater effect on some beta receptors than norepinephrine, effectors with a large proportion of these beta receptors are more sensitive to epinephrine.

All these facts point to an important principle about nervous regulation: the effect of a neurotransmitter on any postsynaptic cell is determined by the characteristics of the receptor and not by the neurotransmitter itself. This principle has been given due consideration in development of therapies that affect autonomic functions (**Box 22-2**).

The actions of norepinephrine and epinephrine are terminated in two ways. Most of the neurotransmitter molecules are taken back up by the synaptic knobs of postganglionic neurons, where they are broken down by the enzyme *monoamine oxidase (MAO)*. The remaining neurotransmitter molecules are eventually broken down by another enzyme, *catechol-O-methyl transferase (COMT)*. Both of these mechanisms are very slow compared with the rapid deactivation of acetylcholine by acetylcholinesterase. This fact partly

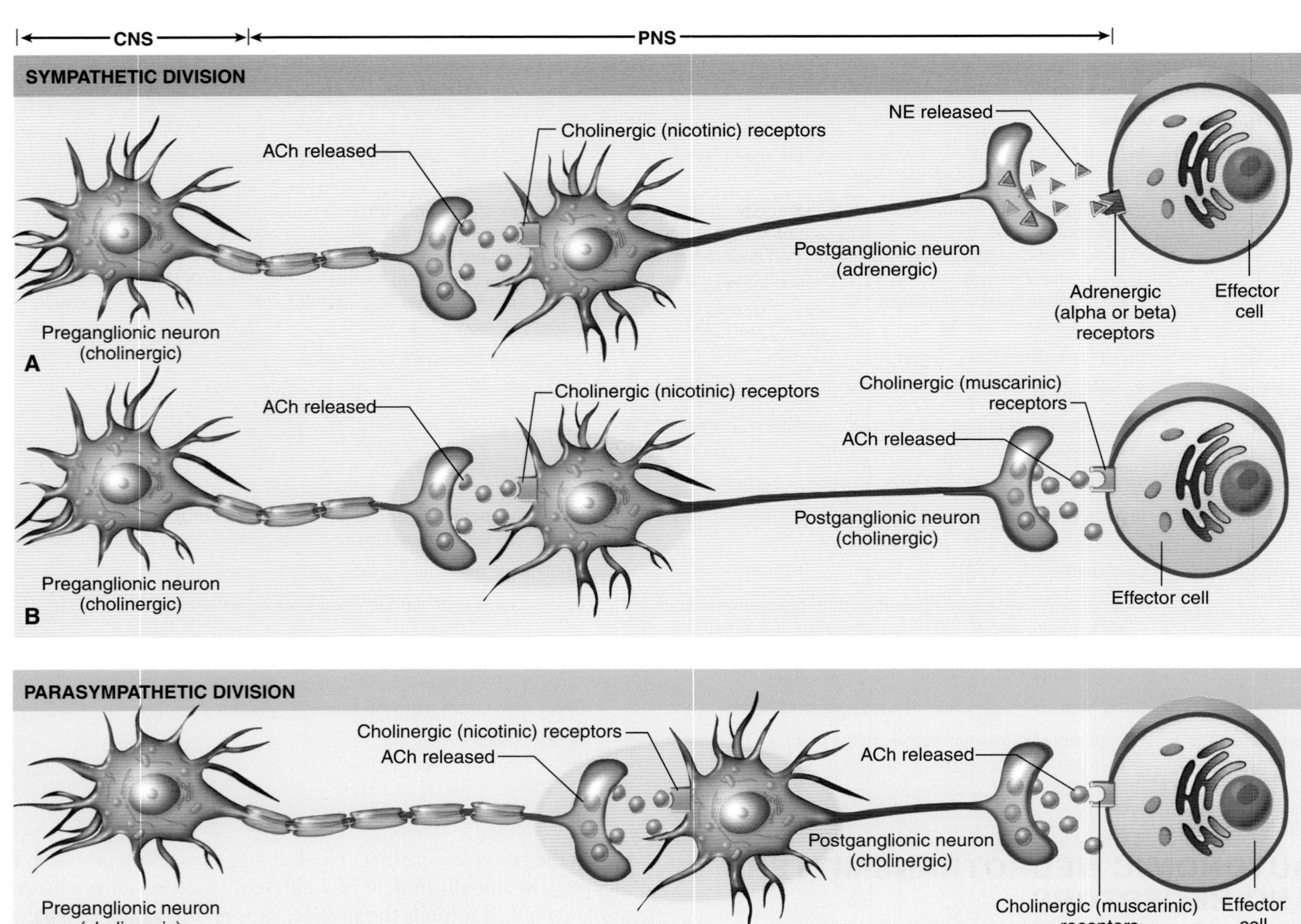

FIGURE 22-5 Locations of neurotransmitters and receptors of the autonomic nervous system. In all pathways, preganglionic fibres are cholinergic, secreting acetylcholine *(ACh),* which stimulates nicotinic receptors in the postganglionic neuron. Most sympathetic postganglionic fibres are adrenergic **(A),** secreting norepinephrine *(NE),* thus stimulating alpha or beta adrenergic receptors. A few sympathetic postganglionic fibres are cholinergic, stimulating muscarinic receptors in effector cells **(B).** All parasympathetic postganglionic fibres are cholinergic **(C),** stimulating muscarinic receptors in effector cells.

explains why adrenergic effects often linger for some time after stimulation has ceased.

Acetylcholine and Its Receptors

Acetylcholine binds to cholinergic receptors. The two main types of cholinergic receptors are **nicotinic (N) receptors** and **muscarinic (M) receptors** (**Figure 22-6**, *B*). Nicotinic receptors derive their name from the fact that they were first discovered when nicotine, a drug, was shown to bind to them. Muscarinic receptors are named for the fact that their discovery came about when it was shown that muscarine, a toxin from mushrooms, binds to them. Like the adrenergic receptors, cholinergic receptors have subtypes such as nicotinic-1 (N_1), nicotinic-2 (N_2), muscarinic-1 (M_1), muscarinic-2 (M_2), and muscarinic-3 (M_3).

In the ganglia of both autonomic divisions, acetylcholine binds to nicotinic receptors in the membranes of postganglionic cells.

BOX 22-2 *health matters* | **Beta Blockers**

Drugs that bind to beta receptors, and thus block the binding of norepinephrine and epinephrine, are informally called **beta blockers.** Beta-1 receptor blocking agents such as atenolol prevent stimulation of the beta-1 adrenergic receptors at the nerve endings of the sympathetic nervous system in the heart and blood vessels. The action of atenolol reduces systolic pressure, heart rate, cardiac contractility and cardiac output, which together decrease the demand of the heart for oxygen. Beta-blockers have therapeutic benefits for the treatment of hypertension, angina pectoris, arrhythmias (e.g. tachycardia) and myocardial infarction (heart attack).

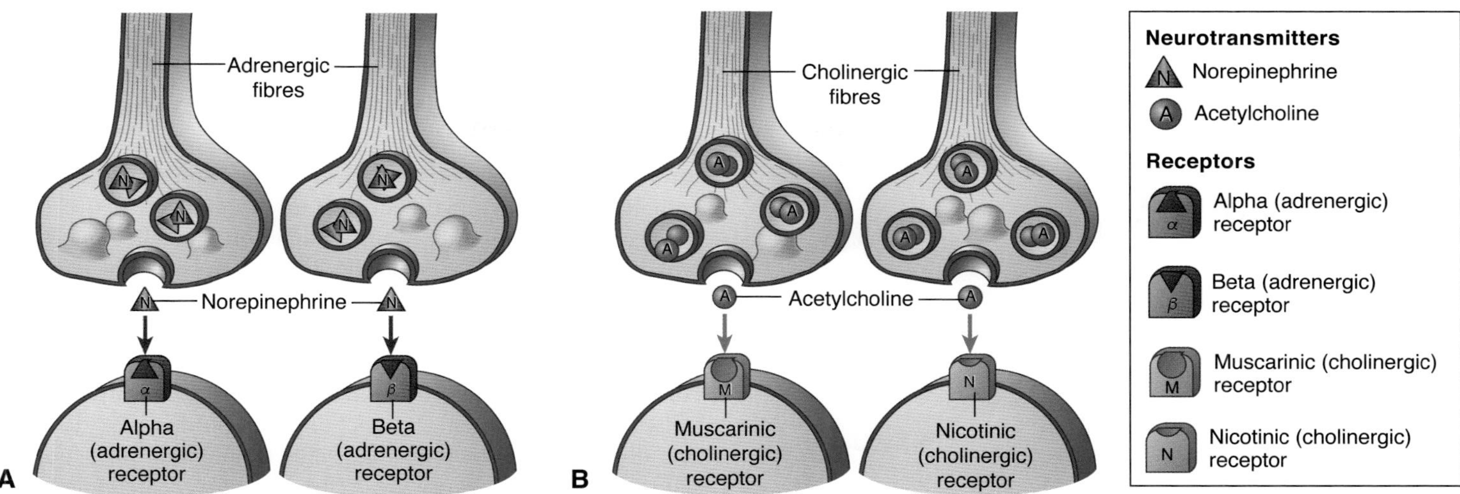

FIGURE 22-6 Functions of autonomic neurotransmitters and receptors. A, Norepinephrine released from adrenergic fibres binds to alpha or beta adrenergic receptors according to the lock-and-key model to produce regulatory effects in the postsynaptic cell. **B,** Acetylcholine released from cholinergic fibres similarly binds to muscarinic or nicotinic cholinergic receptors to produce postsynaptic regulatory effects.

Acetylcholine, released by all parasympathetic postganglionic cells and the few sympathetic postganglionic cells that are cholinergic, binds to muscarinic receptors in the membranes of effector cells. As mentioned previously, the action of acetylcholine is quickly terminated by its being hydrolyzed by the enzyme *acetylcholinesterase*.

Nonadrenergic-Noncholinergic Transmission

Research clearly shows that many neurotransmitters besides norepinephrine and acetylcholine bind to autonomic receptors. Thus a concept of **nonadrenergic-noncholinergic (NANC) transmission** has evolved.

Substances that research shows to be involved in NANC transmission across peripheral autonomic synapses include small-molecule neutrotransmitters such as nitric oxide (NO), gamma-aminobutyric acid (GABA), and the purine neurotransmitters adenosine (ADO) and adenosine triphosphate (ATP). Also involved in NANC transmission are neuropeptides such as neuropeptide Y, vasoactive intestinal peptide (VIP), luteinizing hormone–releasing hormone (LHRH), and others.

A theory of autonomic transmission called **co-transmission** states that all or most postganglionic fibres release either norepinephrine or acetylcholine along with NANC transmitters or modulators and that each substance combines with postsynaptic or presynaptic receptors to produce regulatory effects. **Figure 22-7** illustrates this concept.

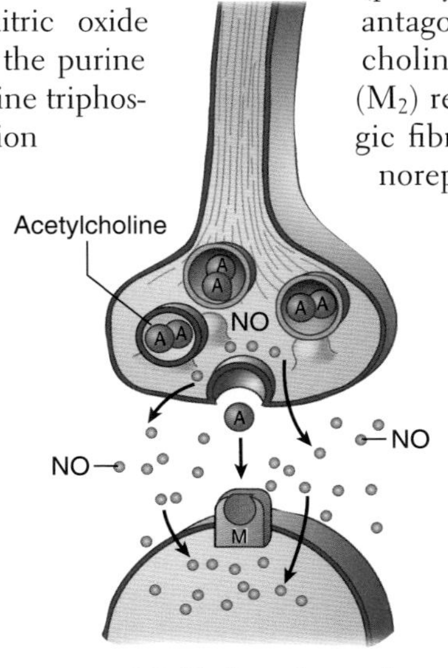

FIGURE 22-7 Nonadrenergic-noncholinergic (NANC) transmission. In this example, nitric oxide *(NO)* is released from a cholinergic fibre along with acetylcholine *(A)*.

Discoveries in autonomic co-transmission have led to a number of therapeutic breakthroughs. One of the better known of these discoveries is the drug sildenafil citrate, used to treat **erectile dysfunction** (ED) in males. During the male sexual response, co-transmission of NO in the parasympathetic nerves helps relax smooth muscles in the blood vessels—thus increasing blood flow to the penis. This class of drugs enhances that effect by reducing the natural breakdown of NO in blood vessels of the penis.

Synaptic Complexity

Figure 22-8 shows the complex manner in which neurotransmitters and receptors may function at a synapse with a dually innervated autonomic effector cell. Norepinephrine released from a sympathetic adrenergic fibre binds to alpha (or beta) receptors of the effector cell, producing adrenergic (sympathetic) effects. As the figure also shows, norepinephrine may also bind to alpha (α_2) receptors in the presynaptic membrane of a nearby cholinergic (parasympathetic) fibre. This inhibits that fibre's release of the antagonistic neurotransmitter, acetylcholine. Likewise, acetylcholine released from cholinergic fibres may bind to muscarinic (M_2) receptors in the presynaptic membranes of nearby adrenergic fibre. This inhibits the release of acetylcholine's antagonist, norepinephrine.

Autonomic pathways also co-transmit additional neurotransmitters to supplement norepinephrine and acetylcholine, further enhancing the complexity of autonomic regulation.

Because of this complexity of function, the effector cell can be controlled with great precision by balancing the effects of sympathetic and parasympathetic stimulation in various ways.

Pharmacology

The interest in autonomic transmitters and receptors is not simply theoretical. Knowledge of specific transmitter-receptor locations and types, their various interactions, and how they are modulated in co-transmission is important for understanding how many common drugs work. **Pharmacology**, the study of drug actions, has used such knowledge to determine how known drugs—and even

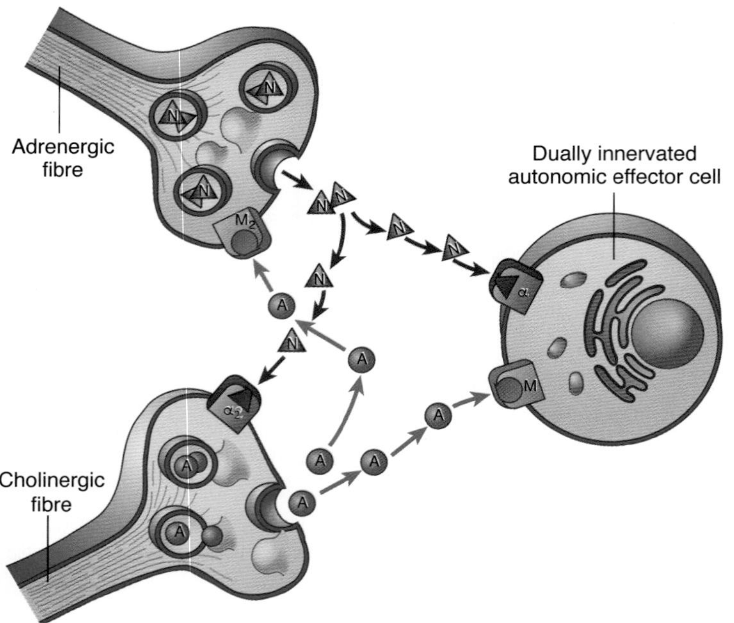

FIGURE 22-8 Complexity at autonomic synapses. The complex manner in which neurotransmitters and receptors regulate dually innervated effector cells shows that a summation of effects on receptors at both presynaptic and postsynaptic locations may occur. For example, norepinephrine released by an adrenergic fibre may bind to postsynaptic alpha (or beta) receptors to influence the effector cell and may also bind to presynaptic alpha (α_2) receptors in a cholinergic fibre to inhibit the release of acetylcholine, a possible antagonist to norepinephrine.

traditional therapies—work in the body. Pharmacology also uses this knowledge to develop newer and better drug therapies.

Take a look at **Table 22-3**. It seems overwhelming at first glance, but the purpose of this table is not for your memorization of every fact. Instead, this table gives you a set of facts organized to reveal helpful patterns if you take a moment to study it. For example, the table's information gives you a glimpse of how pharmacologists apply principles of ANS transmission in developing and classifying drugs. It gives concrete examples of drugs that act at particular receptors—and how they act. By comparing the desired drug action with possible side effects, you can more clearly see the overall strategy of autonomic regulation of body functions.

The table also compares how receptor *agonists*—drugs that mimic the neurotransmitter—differ in their actions from receptor *antagonists*—drugs that block the neurotransmitter's usual effects.

Taking a few minutes now to review these applications of autonomic concepts will help you later as you encounter adrenomimetics, beta blockers, anticholinergics, and many other drug therapies classified and understood by their autonomic effects.

Quick CHECK

4. Describe the pathway taken by an impulse travelling along a parasympathetic pathway.
5. What is the difference between a cholinergic fibre and an adrenergic fibre? Between a cholinergic receptor and an adrenergic receptor?
6. Name the two major types of cholinergic receptors and the two major types of adrenergic receptors.

FUNCTIONS OF THE AUTONOMIC NERVOUS SYSTEM

Overview of Autonomic Function

The ANS as a whole functions to regulate autonomic effectors in ways that tend to maintain or quickly restore homeostasis. Both sympathetic and parasympathetic divisions are *tonically active*. That is, they continually conduct impulses to autonomic effectors. They often exert opposite, or antagonistic, influences on them. We can call this concept the *principle of autonomic antagonism*.

If sympathetic impulses tend to stimulate an effector, parasympathetic impulses tend to inhibit it. Dually innervated effectors continually receive both sympathetic and parasympathetic impulses. Summation of the two opposing influences determines the dominating or controlling effect. For example, continual sympathetic impulses to the heart tend to accelerate the heart rate, whereas continual parasympathetic impulses tend to slow it. The actual heart rate is determined by whichever influence dominates. To find other examples of autonomic antagonism, examine **Table 22-4**.

An emerging concept in autonomic physiology holds that some sympathetic–parasympathetic regulation exhibits a synergistic or cooperative effect rather than antagonistic effects. Such cooperation is most clearly seen in autonomic regulation of urinary and reproductive reflexes, where the two divisions seem to operate more as a team than as opponents.

The ANS does not function autonomously as its name suggests. It is continually influenced by impulses from the so-called autonomic centres. These are clusters of neurons located at various levels in the brain whose axons conduct impulses directly or indirectly to autonomic preganglionic neurons. Autonomic centres function as a hierarchy in their control of the ANS (**Figure 22-9**). Highest ranking in the hierarchy are the autonomic centres in the cerebral cortex—for example, in the frontal lobe and limbic system (structures near the medial surface of the cerebrum that form a border around the corpus callosum). Neurons in these centres send impulses to other autonomic centres in the brain, notably in the hypothalamus. Then neurons in the hypothalamus send either stimulating or inhibiting impulses to parasympathetic and sympathetic preganglionic neurons located in the lower autonomic centres of the brainstem and cord.

You may be wondering why the name *autonomic system* was ever chosen if the system is really not autonomous. Originally the term seemed appropriate. The autonomic system seemed to be self-regulating and independent of the rest of the nervous system. Common observations furnished abundant evidence of its independence from cerebral control—from direct control by the will, that is. Later, however, even this was found to be not entirely true. Some rare and startling exceptions were discovered. For example, a man in a brightly lighted amphitheater can learn to change the size of his pupils from small, constricted dots (normal response to bright lights) to widely dilated circles. It is also possible to will the smooth muscle of the hairs on the arms to contract, producing gooseflesh. **Box 22-3** discusses how this knowledge can be used in therapy.

TABLE 22-3 Autonomic Receptors

RECEPTOR TYPE	LOCATION (FUNCTION)*	DRUG (ACTION)†	CONDITION TREATED BY DRUG	SIDE EFFECTS‡
Adrenergic				
alpha-1 (α_1)	Smooth muscle in blood vessels, urogenital tract, sphincters (excitatory)	Phenylephrine (agonist)	Decongestant	Hypertension (high blood pressure)
		Prazosin (antagonist)	Hypertension	Orthostatic hypotension (low blood pressure on standing); nasal congestion
alpha-2 (α_2)	Presynaptic ANS terminals (inhibitory)	Clonidine (agonist)	Hypertension	Dizziness, orthostatic hypertension
beta-1 (β_1)	Cardiac muscle (excitatory)	Dobutamine (agonist)	Heart failure	Hypertension
		Atenolol (antagonist)	Hypertension	Sleep disturbance
beta-2 (β_2)	Smooth muscles of airways, gut, vessels (inhibitory)	Salbutamol (agonist)	Asthma, COPD	Tremor, anxiety, headache, muscle cramps
beta-3 (β_3)	Smooth muscle in urinary bladder (inhibitory), adipose cells (release of FFAs)	Mirabegron (agonist)	Overactive bladder	Hypertension
Cholinergic				
nicotinic-1 (N_1)	Skeletal muscle (excitatory)	Atracurium (antagonist)	Muscle relaxant (during surgery)	Bronchospasm
nicotinic-2 (N_2)	Postganglionic ANS cells; adrenal medulla (excitatory)	Nicotine patch (agonist)	Smoking cessation	Addiction, hypertension, elevated heart rate
muscarinic-1 (M_1)	Smooth muscle (mixed)	Pilocarpine drops (agonist)	Glaucoma	Blurred vision, eye discomfort, sweating
		Dicycloverine (antagonist)	Irritable bowel syndrome	Dry mouth
muscarinic-2 (M_2)	Heart, smooth muscle (inhibitory)	Bethanechol (agonist)	Difficult urination	Nausea, vomiting, dizziness
		Atropine (antagonist)	Bradycardia (low heart rate)	Elevated heart rate, heart fibrillation
muscarinic-3 (M_3)	Glands (excitatory)	Pilocarpine (agonist)	Dry mouth (Sjögren syndrome)	Excessive sweating, nausea
		Atropine (antagonist)	Hyperhydrosis (excessive sweating)	Dry mouth
Nonadrenergic-Noncholinergic (NANC)				
Purinergic P_1 (ADO receptor)	Autonomic effectors (neuromodulator)	Adenosine (agonist)	Tachycardia	Chest discomfort, breathing problems
		Caffeine (antagonist)	Migraine and other headaches	Insomnia, restlessness
Purinergic P2Y (ADP receptor)	Platelets	Clopidogrel ADP (antagonist)	Heart attack, stroke	Haemorrhage
Nitric oxide (NO receptor)	Smooth muscle in vessels (inhibitory)	Glyceryl trinitrate (GTN, promotes synthesis)	Angina (heart pain)	Headache, dizziness

*Examples of several possible locations.

†Examples of drugs that act on each receptor type; agonists stimulate receptor action, and antagonists block receptor action.

‡Example of side effect to illustrate possible action at receptors in unintended targets.

ADO, adenosine; *ADP,* adenosine diphosphate; *ANS,* autonomic nervous system; *COPD,* chronic obstructive pulmonary disease; *FFA,* free fatty acid.

FUNCTIONS OF THE SYMPATHETIC DIVISION

In ordinary, resting conditions the sympathetic division can act to maintain the normal functioning of dually innervated autonomic effectors. It does this by opposing the effects of parasympathetic impulses to these structures. For example, by counteracting parasympathetic impulses that tend to slow the heart and weaken its beat, sympathetic impulses function to maintain the heartbeat's normal rate and strength.

TABLE 22-4 Autonomic Functions

AUTONOMIC EFFECTOR	EFFECT OF SYMPATHETIC STIMULATION (NEUROTRANSMITTER: NOREPINEPHRINE UNLESS OTHERWISE STATED)	EFFECT OF PARASYMPATHETIC STIMULATION (NEUROTRANSMITTER: ACETYLCHOLINE)
Cardiac Muscle	Increased rate and strength of contraction (beta receptors)	Decreased rate and strength of contraction
Smooth Muscle of Blood Vessels		
Skin blood vessels	Constriction (alpha receptors)	No effect
Skeletal muscle blood vessels	Dilation (beta receptors)	No effect
Coronary blood vessels	Constriction (alpha receptors) Dilation (beta receptors)	Dilation
Abdominal blood vessels	Constriction (alpha receptors)	No effect
Blood vessels of external genitalia	Constriction (alpha receptors)	Dilation of blood vessels causing erection
Smooth Muscle of Hollow Organs and Sphincters		
Bronchioles	Relaxation (dilation)	Constriction
Digestive tract, except sphincters	Decreased peristalsis	Increased peristalsis
Sphincters of digestive tract	Contraction	Relaxation
Urinary bladder	Relaxation	Contraction
Urinary sphincters	Contraction	Relaxation
Reproductive ducts	Constriction	Relaxation
Eye		
Iris	Contraction of radial muscle; dilated pupil	Contraction of circular muscle; constricted pupil
Ciliary	Relaxation; accommodates for far vision	Contraction; accommodates for near vision
Hairs (arrector pili muscles)	Contraction produces goose pimples, or piloerection (alpha receptors)	No effect
Skeletal Muscle*	During intense exercise, regulates contractility to prevent fatigue (beta receptors)	No effect
Glands		
Sweat	Increased sweat (neurotransmitter, acetylcholine)	No effect
Lacrimal	No effect	Increased secretion of tears
Digestive (salivary, gastric, etc.)	Decreased secretion of saliva; not known for others	Increased secretion of saliva
Pancreas, including islets	Decreased secretion	Increased secretion of pancreatic juice and insulin
Liver	Increased glycogenolysis (beta receptors); increased blood sugar level	No effect
Adrenal medulla†	Increased epinephrine secretion	No effect
Adipose	Increased lipolysis	No effect

*Skeletal muscle is primarily a somatic effector, but during intense exercise subconscious autonomic stimulation also occurs.

†Sympathetic preganglionic axons terminate in contact with secreting cells of the adrenal medulla. Thus the adrenal medulla functions, to quote someone's descriptive phrase, as a "giant sympathetic postganglionic neuron".

BOX 22-3 *fyi* | Biofeedback

We now know that individuals can learn to control specific autonomic effectors if two conditions are fulfilled. First, they must be informed that they are achieving the desired response, and second, they must be rewarded for it. Various kinds of **biofeedback** instruments have been developed to provide these conditions. For example, a biofeedback instrument that detects slight temperature changes has been used with patients who experience migraine headaches. (Migraine headaches initially involve distention of blood vessels in the head.) The instrument is attached to the hands and emits a high sound each time the blood vessels in the hand dilate. The reward for these patients is a lessening of the migraine pain—presumably because of the shunting of blood away from the head to the hands.

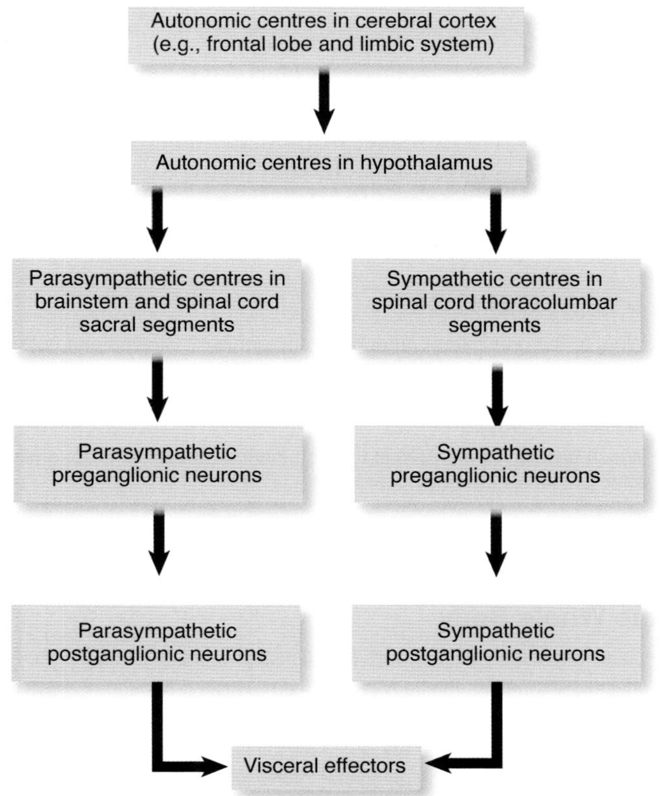

FIGURE 22-9 Central nervous system hierarchy that regulates autonomic functions.

The sympathetic division also serves another important function in usual conditions. Because only sympathetic fibres innervate the smooth muscle in blood vessel walls, sympathetic impulses function to maintain the normal tone of this muscle. By so doing, the sympathetic system plays a crucial role in maintaining blood pressure in usual conditions.

The major function of the sympathetic division, however, is that it serves as an "emergency" system. When we perceive that the homeostasis of the body might be threatened—that is, when we are under physical or psychological stress—outgoing sympathetic signals increase greatly. In fact, one of the very first steps in the body's complex defence mechanism against stress is a sudden and marked increase in sympathetic activity. This brings about a group of responses that all go on at the same time. Together they make the body ready to expend maximum energy and thus to engage in the maximum muscular exertion needed to deal with the perceived threat—as, for example, in running or fighting. Walter B. Cannon coined the descriptive and now-famous phrase **"fight-or-flight" reaction** as his name for this group of sympathetic responses.

Read **Table 22-5** to find many of the fight-or-flight physiological changes. Some particularly important changes for maximum energy expenditure by skeletal muscles are faster, stronger heartbeat, dilated blood vessels in skeletal muscles, and dilated bronchi. Stimulation of glycogenolysis (breakdown of stored glycogen) and lipolysis (breakdown of stored fat) increases available blood levels of glucose, fatty acids, and related nutrients that can be used for energy in muscle cells. Stimulation of the medulla of each adrenal gland triggers its secretion of epinephrine and some norepinephrine. These hormones reinforce and prolong effects of the norepinephrine released by sympathetic postganglionic fibres.

The fight-or-flight reaction is a normal response in times of stress. Without such a response, we might not be able to resist or retreat from something that actually threatens our well-being. However, chronic exposure to stress can lead to dysfunction of sympathetic effectors—and perhaps even to the dysfunction of the ANS itself. Some concepts regarding the effects of chronic stress are discussed in Chapter 34.

TABLE 22-5 Summary of the Sympathetic "Fight-or-Flight" Reaction

RESPONSE	ROLE IN PROMOTING ENERGY USE BY SKELETAL MUSCLES
Increased heart rate	Increased rate of blood flow, thus increased delivery of oxygen and glucose to skeletal muscles
Increased strength of cardiac muscle contraction	Increased rate of blood flow, thus increased delivery of oxygen and glucose to skeletal muscles
Dilation of coronary vessels of the heart	Increased delivery of oxygen and nutrients to cardiac muscle to sustain increased rate and strength of heart contractions
Dilation of blood vessels in skeletal muscles	Increased delivery of oxygen and nutrients to skeletal muscles
Increased stimulation at neuromuscular junctions and increased ion pump activity in skeletal muscles	Increased availability of ACh at the neuromuscular junction and more efficient restoration of resting ion balance in muscle fibres both reduce fatigue in skeletal muscles
Constriction of blood vessels in digestive and other organs	Shunting of blood to skeletal muscles to increase oxygen and glucose delivery
Contraction of spleen and other blood reservoirs	More blood discharged into general circulation, causing increased delivery of oxygen and glucose to skeletal muscles
Dilation of respiratory airways	Increased loading of oxygen into blood
Increased rate and depth of breathing	Increased loading of oxygen into blood (indirect effect)
Increased sweating	Increased dissipation of heat generated by skeletal muscle activity
Increased conversion of glycogen into glucose	Increased amount of glucose available to skeletal muscles
Increased breakdown of stored fats	Increased amount of fatty acids and glycerol available to skeletal muscles

ACh, acetylcholine.

CONNECT IT! 

The sympathetic system can also directly affect skeletal muscle function in ways that avoid fatigue during intense activity. To learn more, check out ***Sympathetic Stimulation of Skeletal Muscle*** online at ***Connect It!***

Functions of the Parasympathetic Division

The parasympathetic division is the dominant controller of most autonomic effectors most of the time. In quiet, nonstressful conditions, more impulses reach autonomic effectors by cholinergic parasympathetic fibres than by adrenergic sympathetic fibres. If the sympathetic division dominates during times that require fight-or-flight, then the parasympathetic division dominates during the in-between times of "rest and repair".

Acetylcholine, the neurotransmitter of the parasympathetic system, tends to slow the heartbeat but acts to promote digestion and elimination. For example, it stimulates digestive gland secretion. It also increases peristalsis by stimulating the smooth muscle of the digestive tract. Identify other parasympathetic effects in **Table 22-4**.

Quick CHECK

7. What is the principle of autonomic antagonism? Give an example.
8. Name the responses that occur in the fight-or-flight reaction. How does each of these prepare the body to expend a maximum amount of muscular energy?
9. Which division of the ANS is the dominant controller of autonomic effectors when the body is at rest?

UNIT 3

the big picture | Autonomic Nervous System and the Whole Body

As you know, the main role of the nervous system as a whole is to detect changes in the internal and external environment, to evaluate those changes in terms of their effect on homeostatic balance, and to regulate effectors accordingly. The autonomic efferent pathways lead to the cardiac muscle effectors, smooth muscle effectors, glandular effectors, and other effectors. Such regulation not only helps us maintain our homeostatic balance, it can also react rapidly when that balance is threatened.

Because the autonomic pathways communicate with endocrine glands, endocrine effectors throughout the body can also be regulated through nervous mechanisms. Every major organ of the body is thus influenced, directly or indirectly, by autonomic output. Although the CNS is an overall controller of the major homeostatic functions of the body, the autonomic pathways are the means to exert that control. •

LANGUAGE OF SCIENCE *(continued from p. 503)*

nonadrenergic-noncholinergic (NANC) transmission (non-AD-ren-er-jik non-KOHL-in-er-jik tranz-MISH-un) [*non-* **not,** *-ad-* **toward,** *-ren-* **kidney,** *-erg-* **work,** *-ic* **relating to,** *non-* **not,** *-chole-* **bile,** *-erg-* **work,** *-ic* **relating to**]

norepinephrine (NE) (nor-ep-ih-NEF-rin) [*nor-* **chemical prefix (unbranched C chain),** *-epi-* **upon,** *-nephr-* **kidney,** *-ine* **substance**]

parasympathetic division (pair-ah-sim-pah-THET-ik) [*para-* **beside,** *-sym-* **together,** *-pathe-* **feel,** *-ic* **relating to**]

postganglionic neuron (post-gang-glee-ON-ik NYOO-ron) [*post-* **after,** *-ganglion-* **knot,** *-ic* **relating to,** *neuron* **string or nerve**]

preganglionic neuron (pree-gang-glee-ON-ik NYOO-ron) [*pre-* **before,** *-ganglion-* **knot,** *-ic* **relating to,** *neuron* **string or nerve**]

splanchnic nerve (SPLANK-nik nerv) [*splanchn-* **internal organ,** *ic* **relating to**]

sympathetic division (sim-pah-THET-ik) [*sym-* **together,** *-pathe-* **feel,** *-ic* **relating to**]

sympathetic trunk (sim-pah-THET-ik) [*sym-* **together,** *-pathe-* **feel,** *-ic* **relating to**]

terminal ganglion (TER-mih-nal GANG-glee-on) [*termin-* **boundary,** *-al* **relating to,** *gangli-* **knot,** *-on* **unit**] *pl.,* ganglia

LANGUAGE OF MEDICINE

beta blocker (BAY-tah) [*beta* **second letter of Greek alphabet**]

biofeedback (bye-oh-FEED-bak) [*bio-* **life**]

erectile dysfunction (ED) (eh-REK-tyle dis-FUNK-shun) [*erect-* **upright,** *-ile* **relating to,** *dys-* **bad or painful,** *-func-* **perform,** *-tion* **process**]

pharmacology (far-mah-KOL-oh-jee) [*pharmaco-* **drug,** *-log-* **words (study of),** *-y* **activity**]

case study

After an exhausting day mountain biking, Tim awoke at 1:00 AM to the sound of sirens, breaking glass and a strong smell of smoke. He grabbed his dressing gown and left his fourth floor flat via the stairs and fire door. Tim noticed his heart was now racing! He was very relieved to enter the street and was thankful to see the fire brigade extinguishing a blaze in his neighbour's flat and that everyone seemed to be safe.

1. Which statement is true given the circumstances in which Tim found himself?
   a. The racing heart resulted from a tiring day mountain biking.
   b. Increased heart rate is abnormal, given that Tim was rested.
   c. Tim experienced a normal reaction to a threat.
   d. Tim experienced the rest and repair response.
2. What triggered Tim's physiological reaction to the smell of smoke and the noisy commotion in the street?
   a. Sympathetic stimulation of the heart
   b. Parasympathetic stimulation of the heart
   c. Somatic motor stimulation of the heart
   d. Both sympathetic and parasympathetic stimulation of the heart
3. What other effect(s) did Tim likely experience besides a rapid heart rate? Choose all that apply.
   a. Increased rate of breathing
   b. Increased sweating
   c. Dilation of pupils
   d. Increased digestive activity
4. Which neurotransmitter produced the effects Tim experienced?
   a. Serotonin
   b. Dopamine
   c. Acetylcholine
   d. Norepinephrine
5. Which type of tissue was primed for maximum efficiency by Tim's physiological response?
   a. Smooth muscle
   b. Skeletal muscle
   c. Connective tissue in joints
   d. Smooth muscle in the digestive system mucosa
6. Which type of effect did Tim's body experience?
   a. Adrenergic
   b. Dopaminergic
   c. Cholinergic
   d. Anaphylactic

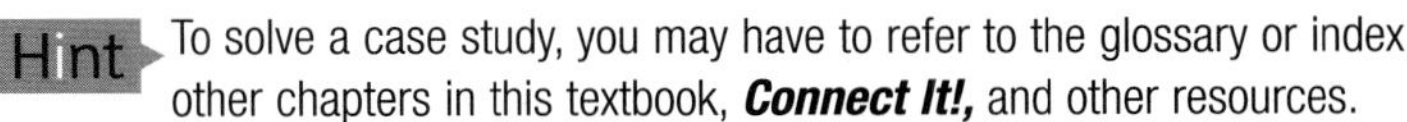

Hint To solve a case study, you may have to refer to the glossary or index, other chapters in this textbook, ***Connect It!,*** and other resources.

UNIT 3

CHAPTER SUMMARY

To download an MP3 version of the chapter summary for use with your mobile device, access the ***Audio Chapter Summaries*** *online at evolve.elsevier.com.*

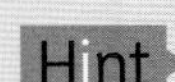

Scan this summary after reading the chapter to help you reinforce the key concepts. Later, use the summary as a quick review before your class or before a test.

Overview of the Autonomic Nervous System

A. Role of the autonomic nervous system (ANS)
   1. Contains afferent (sensory) and efferent (motor) components (**Figure 22-1**)
      a. Efferent components of ANS are emphasized in this chapter
      b. Sensory concepts of the ANS are discussed in Chapter 23
   2. Carries fibres to and from the autonomic effectors (**Box 22-1**)
   3. Major function—to regulate heartbeat, smooth muscle contraction, glandular secretions, and metabolic functions to maintain homeostatic balance and react to threats to that balance

B. Divisions of the autonomic nervous system
   1. Sympathetic and parasympathetic divisions
      a. Two efferent divisions—sympathetic division and parasympathetic division
      b. Sympathetic division consists of neural pathways that are separate from parasympathetic pathways (**Figure 22-2**)
      c. Many autonomic effectors are dually innervated, which allows remarkably precise control of an effector
   2. Enteric nervous system (ENS)—regional part of ANS in the intestinal wall regulates gut function with input from the sympathetic and parasympathetic divisions

Structure of the Autonomic Nervous System

A. Basic plan of efferent autonomic pathways (**Figure 22-3**)
   1. Each pathway is made up of autonomic nerves, ganglia, and plexuses, which are made of efferent autonomic neurons
   2. All autonomic neurons function in reflex arcs called *autonomic reflexes* or *visceral reflexes*
   3. Efferent autonomic regulation ultimately depends on feedback from sensory receptors
   4. Relay of two efferent autonomic neurons conducts information from the central nervous system to autonomic effectors
      a. Preganglionic neuron—conducts impulses from the central nervous system to an autonomic ganglion

b. Postganglionic neuron—efferent neuron with which a preganglionic neuron synapses within an autonomic ganglion

B. Structure of the sympathetic pathways
1. Sympathetic chain ganglia (sympathetic trunk)
a. Most sympathetic division ganglia lie along either side of the anterior surface of the vertebral column; joined with the other ganglia located on the same side
b. Each chain runs from the second cervical vertebra to the level of the coccyx
c. Usually 22 sympathetic chain ganglia on each side of vertebral column: three cervical, eleven thoracic, four lumbar, and four sacral
2. Thoracolumbar division
a. Sympathetic preganglionic neurons have dendrite and cell bodies in lateral grey horns of the thoracic and lumbar segments of the spinal cord
b. Axons leave the cord by way of the ventral roots of the thoracic and first four lumbar spinal nerves; split away from other spinal nerve fibres by means of the white ramus; extend to a sympathetic chain ganglion
3. Preganglionic fibres may take one of three paths once inside the sympathetic chain ganglion
a. Synapse with sympathetic postganglionic neuron
b. Send ascending or descending branches through the sympathetic trunk to synapse with postganglionic neurons in other chain ganglia
c. Pass through one or more chain ganglia without synapsing
4. Sympathetic postganglionic neurons
a. Dendrites and cell bodies are mostly in sympathetic chain ganglia or collateral ganglia
b. Grey ramus—short branch by which some postganglionic axons return to a spinal nerve
5. In the sympathetic division, preganglionic neurons are relatively short, and postganglionic neurons are relatively long
6. Axon of one sympathetic preganglionic neuron synapses with many postganglionic neurons, terminating in widely spread organs (**Figure 22-4**)

C. Structure of the parasympathetic pathways
1. Parasympathetic preganglionic neurons—cell bodies are located in nuclei in the brainstem or lateral grey columns of the sacral cord; extend a considerable distance before synapsing with postganglionic neurons
2. Parasympathetic postganglionic neurons—dendrites and cell bodies are located in parasympathetic ganglia, which are embedded in or near autonomic effectors
3. Parasympathetic preganglionic neurons synapse with postganglionic neurons that each lead to a single effector (**Figure 22-4**)

Autonomic Neurotransmitters and Receptors

A. Axon terminal of autonomic neurons releases either of two neurotransmitters: norepinephrine or acetylcholine (**Figure 22-5**)
1. Adrenergic fibres—release norepinephrine; axons of postganglionic sympathetic neurons
2. Cholinergic fibres—release acetylcholine; axons of preganglionic sympathetic neurons and of preganglionic and postganglionic parasympathetic neurons

B. Norepinephrine and its receptors (**Figure 22-6**)
1. Norepinephrine affects visceral effectors by first binding to one of two types of adrenergic receptors in plasma membranes: alpha receptors or beta receptors
a. Binding of norepinephrine to alpha receptors in smooth muscle of blood vessels is stimulating, causing the vessels to constrict
b. Binding of norepinephrine to beta receptors in smooth muscle of blood vessels is inhibitory, causing blood vessels to dilate; in cardiac muscle, has stimulating effect
2. Epinephrine also stimulates adrenergic receptors, enhancing and prolonging effects of sympathetic stimulation
3. Effect of a neurotransmitter on any postsynaptic cell is determined by characteristics of the receptors, not by the neurotransmitter
4. Termination of actions of norepinephrine and epinephrine
a. Monoamine oxidase (MAO)—enzyme that breaks up neurotransmitter molecules taken back up by the synaptic knobs
b. Catechol-O-methyl transferase (COMT)—enzyme that breaks down the remaining neurotransmitter

C. Acetylcholine and its receptors (**Figure 22-6**)
1. Acetylcholine binds to two types of cholinergic receptors: nicotinic receptors and muscarinic receptors
2. Termination of action of acetylcholine is by the enzyme acetylcholinesterase

D. Nonadrenergic-noncholinergic (NANC) transmission (**Figure 22-7**)
1. Co-transmission occurs when other neurotransmitters are released along with ACh or NE at autonomic synapses
2. Allows modulation of effects

E. Synaptic complexity (**Figure 22-8**)
1. Autonomic neurotransmitters and receptors may influence different types of presynaptic and postsynaptic receptors at synapses with dually innervated effectors
2. Co-transmission adds yet more complexity of function
3. Summation of effects increases precision of control

F. Pharmacology—study of drug actions (**Table 22-3**)
1. Concepts of autonomic transmission important in understanding how drugs work
2. Autonomic concepts used in development of new drug therapies

Functions of the Autonomic Nervous System

A. Overview of autonomic function (**Figure 22-9**)
1. Autonomic antagonism
a. Autonomic nervous system functions to regulate visceral effectors in ways that tend to maintain or quickly restore homeostasis
b. Sympathetic and parasympathetic divisions are tonically active, often exerting antagonistic influences on visceral effectors

c. Dually innervated effectors continually receive both sympathetic and parasympathetic impulses, and the summation of the two determines the controlling effect
d. Sometimes cooperation is the effect of sympathetic–parasympathetic interaction (rather than antagonism)

2. Hierarchy of autonomic regulation
   a. Autonomic centres in the brain regulate both divisions
   b. Autonomic centres are arranged in a hierarchy, or levels of control
   c. The term autonomic is not accurate because this system is not autonomous

B. Functions of the sympathetic division
   1. In resting conditions it can act to maintain the normal functioning of dually innervated autonomic effectors
   2. Sympathetic impulses function to maintain normal tone of the smooth muscle in blood vessel walls
   3. Major function of sympathetic division is that it serves as an "emergency" system—the "fight-or-flight" reaction (review **Table 22-5**)

C. Functions of the parasympathetic division (review **Table 22-4**)
   1. Dominant controller of most autonomic effectors most of the time
   2. Acetylcholine—slows heartbeat and acts to promote digestion and elimination

The Big Picture: Autonomic Nervous System and the Whole Body

A. The autonomic nervous system maintains homeostatic balance and can react rapidly to threats to that balance
B. Every major organ is influenced, directly or indirectly, by autonomic nervous system output

REVIEW QUESTIONS

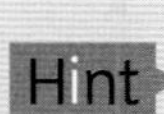

Write out the answers to these questions after reading the chapter and reviewing the Chapter Summary. Note—writing out your answers will consolidate learning and provide a valuable resource of information.

1. Describe an autonomic preganglionic neuron.
2. Identify the paths that a nerve signal may take once it is inside the sympathetic chain ganglion.
3. Differentiate between the sympathetic preganglionic and postganglionic neurons in terms of length.
4. Describe the actions of norepinephrine. How are these actions terminated? Explain what survival advantages norepinephrine gives the body in the fight or flight reaction.
5. Describe the responses caused by acetylcholine release. How are these actions terminated?

CRITICAL THINKING QUESTIONS

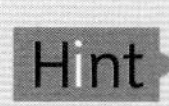

After finishing the Review Questions, write out the answers to these more in-depth questions to help you apply your new knowledge. Go back to sections of the chapter that relate to concepts that you find difficult.

1. What is the distinction between the reflexes that cause cardiac muscle to react and those that cause skeletal muscles to react?
2. Using the control of the speed of a car as an example, explain dual innervation in the autonomic nervous system.
3. What distinguishes the function of autonomic transmitters from that of receptors? How do they regulate dually innervated effector cells?
4. Based on what you know, explain why the autonomic nervous system is not an "automatic" nervous system with little control from the higher brain centres.
5. There are reports of people performing almost superhuman feats of strength when under great stress. Specifically, what is happening in the body that would allow this to happen?
6. The drug atenolol blocks the effect of a portion of the sympathetic nervous system. To what class of drugs does atenolol belong, and what are its therapeutic effects?
7. Identify substances (other than acetylcholine and norepinephrine) that respond to receptors for the autonomic nervous system. What name is given to this group of substances, and what is their most likely role?
8. The muscles of the bladder neck that keep the bladder closed contain mainly alpha adrenergic receptors. The detrusor muscles (that contract to empty the bladder) contain mainly beta receptors. What is the effect of increased secretion of norepinephrine on the bladder?
9. A patient having a heart attack has cold and clammy (moist) skin. What division of the ANS is being strongly stimulated?
10. How do parasympathetic ganglia differ from sympathetic ganglia in terms of location?

23 General Senses

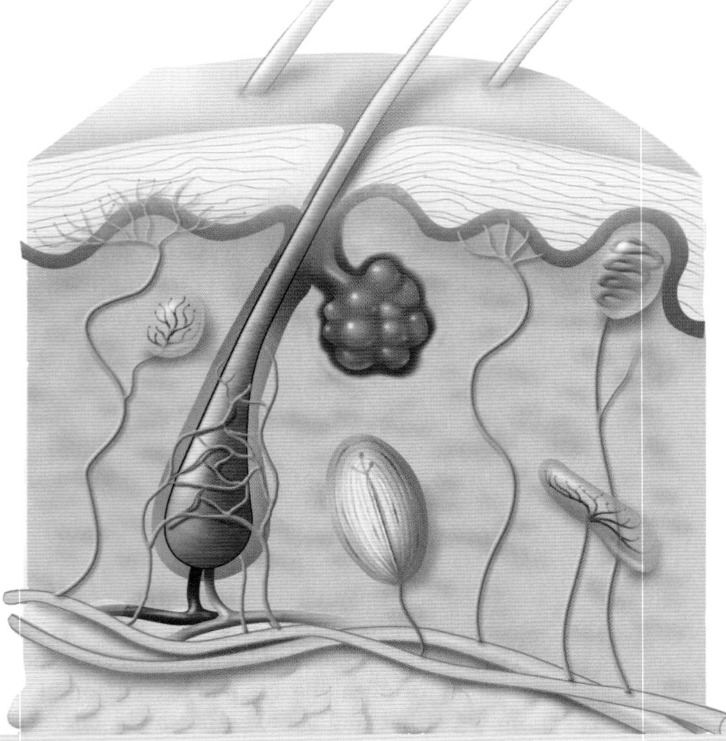

CHAPTER OUTLINE

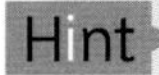 Scan this outline before you begin to read the chapter, as a preview of how the concepts are organized.

The body has millions of sense organs that contain sensory receptors, which detect changes in our internal and external environments. Sense organs fall into two main categories: *general sense organs* and *special sense organs*. Of these, by far the most numerous are the microscopic general sense receptors buried within the skin, muscles, and other organs. These tiny general sense organs—often called *somatic sense organs*—function to mediate general body senses such as touch, temperature, and pain. This sensory information may then initiate various reflexes necessary for maintaining homeostasis. Special sense organs are complex structures dedicated to mediating the special senses: vision, hearing, balance, taste, smell. They too initiate reflexes important for homeostasis.

LANGUAGE OF SCIENCE

Hint *Use this list to aid your pronunciation of unfamiliar words.*

adaptation (ad-ap-TAY-shun)
[*adapt-* **adjust,** *-tion* **process**]

alpha motor neuron
(AL-fah MOH-tor NYOO-ron)
[*alpha* (α) **first letter of Greek alphabet,** *mot-* **move,** *-or* **agent,** *neuron* **string or nerve**]

bulboid corpuscle
(BUL-boyd KOR-pus-ul)
[*bulb-* **swollen root,** *-oid* **like,** *corpus-* **body,** *-cle* **little**]

bulbous corpuscle
(BUL-bus KOR-pus-ul)
[*bulb-* **swollen root,** *-ous* **relating to,** *corpus-* **body,** *-cle* **little**]

chemoreceptor (kee-moh-ree-SEP-tor)
[*chemo-* **chemical,** *-recept-* **receive,** *-or* **agent**]

exteroceptor (eks-ter-oh-SEP-tor)
[*exter-* **outside,** *-cept-* **receive,** *-or* **agent**]

gamma motor neuron
(GAM-mah MOH-tor NYOO-roon)
[*gamma* (γ) **third letter of Greek alphabet,** *mot-* **move,** *-or* **agent,** *neuron* **string or nerve**]

Golgi tendon organ
(GOL-jee TEN-don OR-gan)
[*Camillo Golgi* **Italian histologist,** *tend-* **pulled tight,** *-on* **unit**]

Golgi tendon receptor
(GOL-jee TEN-don ree-SEP-tor)
[*Camillo Golgi* **Italian histologist,** *-cept-* **receive,** *-or* **agent**]

interoceptor (in-ter-oh-SEP-tor)
[*inter-* **inward,** *-cept-* **receive,** *-or* **agent**]

lamellar corpuscle
(lah-MEL-ar KOR-pus-ul)
[*lam-* **plate,** *-ella-* **little,** *-ar* **relating to,** *corpus-* **body,** *-cle* **little**]

mechanoreceptor
(mek-an-oh-ree-SEP-tor)
[*mechano-* **machine (mechanical),** *-cept-* **receive,** *-or* **agent**]

muscle spindle
[*mus-* **mouse,** *-cle* **small**]

nociceptor (noh-see-SEP-tor)
[*noci-* **to harm,** *-cept-* **receive,** *-or* **agent**]

continued on p. 528

In this chapter we begin with a brief overview of how all sensory receptors function, then follow that with discussion of some of the major general senses. We continue our exploration of senses in Chapter 24 with a survey of the special senses.

SENSORY RECEPTORS

Sense organs called **sensory receptors** make it possible for the body to respond to stimuli caused by changes occurring in our external or internal environment. This function is crucial to survival. The abilities to see and hear, for example, may provide the necessary warning to help us avoid injury from dangers in our external environment. Internal sensations ranging from pain and pressure to hunger and thirst help us maintain homeostasis of our internal environment.

RECEPTOR RESPONSE

The general function of receptors is to respond to stimuli by converting them to nerve impulses. Receptors are often described as the sensitive dendritic endings or "end organs" of sensory neurons. As a rule, different types of receptors respond to different types of stimuli. Heat receptors, for example, do not respond to light or stretch stimuli.

When an adequate stimulus acts on a receptor, a local potential develops in the receptor's membrane. This **receptor potential** is a graded response, graded to the strength of the stimulus (see Chapter 19, pp. 414–415). When a receptor potential reaches a certain threshold, it triggers an action potential in the sensory neuron's axon. These impulses then travel over sensory pathways to the brain and spinal cord, where they are interpreted as a particular **sensation,** such as heat or cold, or they initiate some type of reflex action, such as withdrawal of a limb from a painful stimulus.

Certain sensory impulses terminating in the brainstem may affect so-called vital sign reflexes that help regulate heart or respiratory rate. Others may end in the thalamus or cerebral cortex, where they trigger imprecise or "crude" sensation awareness (thalamus) or very precise and specific awareness of not only a specific type of sensation but also its exact location and level of intensity (cerebral cortex).

Receptors often exhibit a functional characteristic known as adaptation. **Adaptation** refers to the process by which the magnitude of the receptor potential decreases over time in response to a continuous stimulus (**Figure 23-1**). As a result, the rate of impulse conduction by the sensory neuron's axon also decreases. So too does the intensity of the resulting sensation. A familiar example of adaptation is feeling the touch of your clothing when you first put it on and then soon not sensing it at all. Touch receptors adapt rapidly. In contrast, the proprioceptors in our muscles, tendons, and joints adapt slowly. As long as stimulation of them continues, they continue sending impulses to the brain.

If we not only remain aware of a particular sensation over time but also interpret what that sensation means in a larger context, the process is called **perception.** Although we may have no conscious perception of certain sensory inputs, they often play a critical role in maintaining homeostasis. Examples might include our ability to sense and respond to changing levels of blood glucose and carbon dioxide—but not at a conscious level.

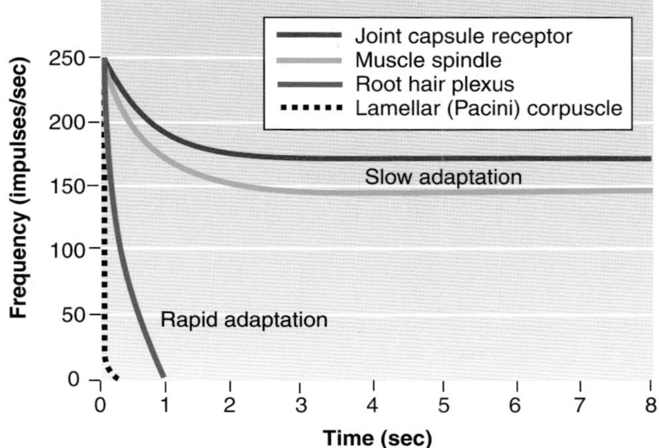

FIGURE 23-1 Adaptation of sensory receptors. In the presence of a continuous stimulus, the rate (frequency) of impulses declines quickly in rapidly adapting receptors of the skin. Here the initial stimulus, representing a *change,* is valuable information. However, continued sensation from the skin may be distracting. In slow-adapting joint and muscle receptors, the rate of impulses instead declines gradually and levels off to a constant, moderately high level. Thus information about body position is continually sent to the central nervous system. (Specific receptor types are discussed later in this chapter.)

DISTRIBUTION OF RECEPTORS

Receptors responsible for the **special senses** of smell, taste, vision, hearing, and equilibrium are grouped into localized areas (such as nasal mucosa or the tongue) or into complex organs such as the eye and ear. The **general sense organs,** on the other hand, consist of microscopic receptors widely distributed throughout the body in the skin, mucosa, connective tissues, muscles, tendons, joints, and viscera. **Figure 23-2** shows a variety of general sense organs in the skin.

Sensations produced by the receptors of general sense organs are often called the *somatic senses.* The distribution of general sense receptors is not uniform in all areas. In some, it is very dense; in others, it is sparse. The skin covering the fingertips, for instance, contains many more receptors to touch than does the skin on the back.

A simple procedure, the **two-point discrimination test,** demonstrates this fact. A subject reports the number of touch points felt when an investigator touches the skin simultaneously with two points of a compass or caliper. If the skin on the fingertip is touched with the compass points barely 3 mm apart, the subject senses them as two points. If the skin on the back is touched with the compass points this close together, they will be felt as only one point. Unless they are 25 mm or more apart, they cannot be discriminated as two points. Why this difference? Because touch receptors are so densely distributed in the fingertips that two points very close to each other still stimulate two different receptors—they are sensed as two points.

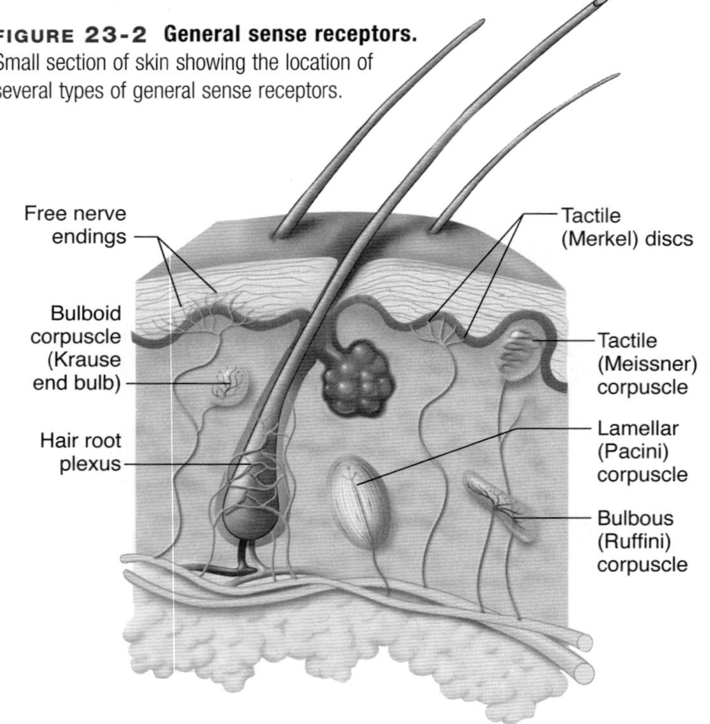

FIGURE 23-2 General sense receptors. Small section of skin showing the location of several types of general sense receptors.

The situation is quite different in the skin on the back. There, touch receptors are so widely scattered that two points have to be at least 25 mm apart to stimulate two receptors and be felt as two points.

CLASSIFICATION OF RECEPTORS

Receptors can be classified in four ways:

Classification by Sensory Pathway

Somatic sensory pathways are those that bring information about the **somatic senses,** which are the senses of which we are usually consciously aware. *Somatic sensory receptors* are found in the skin, muscles, ligaments, eyes, and ears, for example, and mediate a wide variety of sensory information such as touch, pain, body position, vision, and hearing.

The autonomic (visceral) sensory pathways carry information about the visceral senses. We are not consciously aware of our **visceral senses,** which rely on *visceral receptors* embedded in the walls of our internal organs, such as the digestive tract, urinary tract, blood vessels, and other internal organs. The visceral receptors detect changes in pH, chemical concentration, temperature, pressure, and other variables that are important in maintaining internal stability, or homeostasis.

Classification by Location

Three groups or classes of receptors can be identified by their location:

1. **Exteroceptors,** as the name implies, are located on or very near the body surface and respond most frequently to stimuli that arise external to the body itself. Receptors in this group are sometimes called *cutaneous receptors* because of their placement in the skin. However, the special sense organs, which are described later in the chapter, are also classified as exteroceptors. Examples of exteroceptors include those that detect pressure, touch, pain, and temperature.

2. **Visceroceptors (interoceptors)** are located internally, often within the substance of body organs (viscera), and when stimulated provide information about the internal environment. They are activated by stimuli such as pressure, stretching, and chemical changes that may originate in diverse internal organs, such as the major blood vessels, intestines, and urinary bladder. Visceroceptors are also involved in mediating sensations such as hunger and thirst.

3. **Proprioceptors** are a special type of visceroceptor. They are less numerous and generally more specialized than other internally placed receptors, and their location is limited to skeletal muscle, joint capsules, and tendons. Proprioceptors provide us with information about body movement, orientation in space, and muscle stretch.

Activation of two types of proprioceptors, called *tonic* and *phasic* proprioceptors, allows us to orient our body in space and provides us with positional information about specific body parts while at rest or during movement. The firing of the nonadapting tonic proprioceptors allows us to locate, for example, our arm, hand, or foot at rest without having to look. Phasic proprioceptors are rapidly adapting receptors, so they are triggered only when there is a change in position. Phasic proprioceptors therefore permit us to feel the changing position of our body parts during continuous movement.

Classification by Stimulus Detected

Receptors are often classified into six categories based on the types of stimuli that activate them:

1. **Mechanoreceptors**—activated by mechanical stimuli that in some way "deform" or change the position of the receptor, resulting in the generation of a receptor potential. Examples include pressure applied to the skin or to blood vessels or pressure caused by stretch or pressure in muscle, tendon, or lung tissue.
2. **Chemoreceptors**—activated by either the amount or the changing concentration of certain chemicals. Our senses of taste and smell depend on chemoreceptors. Some chemoreceptors in the body also detect the concentration of specific chemicals such as carbon dioxide (CO_2) and blood glucose.
3. **Thermoreceptors**—activated by changes in temperature.
4. **Nociceptors**—activated by intense stimuli of any type that results in tissue damage. The cause may be a toxic chemical, intense light, sound, pressure, or heat. The sensation produced is one of pain.
5. **Photoreceptors**—found only in the eye. Photoreceptors respond to light stimuli if the intensity is great enough to generate a receptor potential.
6. **Osmoreceptors**—concentrated in the hypothalamus and sense levels of osmotic pressure in body fluids. They are important in detecting changes in concentration of electrolytes in extracellular fluids and in stimulating the hypothalamic thirst centre.

Classification by Structure

Regardless of their location or how they are activated, the general (somatic) sensory receptors may be classified anatomically as either of the following:

- Free nerve endings
- Encapsulated nerve endings

Free nerve endings are the simplest, most common, and most widely distributed sensory receptors. They are located both on the surface of the body (exteroceptors) and in the deep visceral organs (visceroceptors). These slender sensory fibres often terminate in small swellings called *dendritic knobs*.

TABLE 23-1 Classification of Somatic Sensory Receptors

BY STRUCTURE	BY LOCATION AND TYPE	BY ACTIVATION STIMULUS	BY SENSATION OR FUNCTION
Free Nerve Endings			
Nociceptor (Dendritic knobs)	Either exteroceptor or visceroceptor—most body tissues	Almost any noxious stimulus; temperature change; mechanical	Pain; temperature; itch; tickle
Tactile (Merkel) disc (meniscus) (Tactile epithelial cell; Tactile disc)	Exteroceptor	Light pressure; mechanical	Discriminative touch
Root hair plexus	Exteroceptor	Hair movement; mechanical	Sense of "deflection" type of movement of hair

(continued on page 527)

The six types of encapsulated nerve endings have in common some type of connective tissue capsule that surrounds their terminal or dendritic end. In addition, most of the encapsulated receptors are primary mechanoreceptors. Thus they are most often activated by a mechanical or "deforming" type of stimulus. Encapsulated receptors vary in size and anatomical characteristics, as well as in numbers and distribution throughout the body.

Table 23-1 organizes some of the major receptors for the general senses by structure.

SENSE OF PAIN

We begin with what many have called our most important sense for health and survival: pain.

The term **nociceptor** is used to describe the free nerve endings that serve as the primary sensory receptors for pain. Nerve fibres that carry pain impulses from nociceptors to the brain can be divided into two types—**acute** or **fast (A) pain** fibres and **chronic** or **slow (B) pain** fibres.

A fibres are concentrated in the skin, mucous membranes, and other superficial areas. Fast pain is sometimes described as a sharp, "take your breath away" type of pain associated with superficial injury or trauma. If you have ever slammed your finger while closing a car door, you have experienced this type of fast or **somatic pain.**

The type of deep or **visceral pain** that develops more slowly over time and travels over B fibres is often described as dull or aching. It originates in deeper body (visceral) structures and can be severe if caused by conditions such as intestinal obstruction or passage of a kidney stone or gallstone.

It is important to stress that in responding to powerful stimuli of any kind, including chemical or thermal burns, intense light, sound, or pressure, the generation of a receptor potential in free nerve endings most often results in the sensation of pain—often the first indication of injury or disease.

Brain tissue is unique in that it lacks the type of nociceptors that transmit sensations of pain and is therefore incapable of sensing painful stimuli. Just the opposite is true of many deep visceral organs, in which the presence of free nerve endings makes pain one of the few sensations that can be evoked.

Pain is experienced differently by different people. Many factors cause this—many of which are unknown. Certainly the brain's filtering and processing of sensory information plays a large part. **Box 23-1** describes a common phenomenon in which visceral pain is perceived as external pain.

Pain is a "bad news/good news" type of sensation. The bad news, of course, is its relationship to disease and injury. The good news is the important role pain plays in alerting us to threats in our environment. Pain expert Paul Brand often called pain "the gift that nobody

BOX 23-1 *fyi* | Referred Pain

The stimulation of pain receptors in deep structures may be felt as pain in the skin that lies over the affected organ or in an area of skin on the body surface far removed from the site of disease or injury. **Referred pain** is the term for this phenomenon.

The cause of referred pain is related to a convergence of sensory nerve impulses from both the diseased organ and the skin in the area of referred pain. For example, pain originating in an organ deep in the abdominal cavity is often interpreted as coming from an area of skin whose sensory fibres enter the same segment of the spinal cord as the sensory fibres from the deep structure. A classic example is the referred pain often associated with a heart attack. Sensory fibres from the skin on the chest over the heart and from the tissue of the heart itself enter the first to the fifth thoracic spinal cord segments and so do sensory fibres from the skin areas over the left shoulder and inner surface of the left arm. Part *A* of the figure shows the primary sensory fibres from both the skin and heart converging in the spinal cord. Sensory impulses from both these areas travel to the brain over a common pathway—the secondary sensory fibre. Thus the brain may feel the pain of a heart attack in the shoulder or arm (part *B* of the figure).

Misinterpretation in the brain with regard to the true location of sensory neurons being stimulated causes referred pain. In clinical medicine, an understanding of referred pain is often an important determinant of whether the correct diagnosis of disease is made (see figure). Review ***Pain Control Areas*** at ***Connect It!*** to see how such understanding can also be used to therapeutically control unwanted pain.

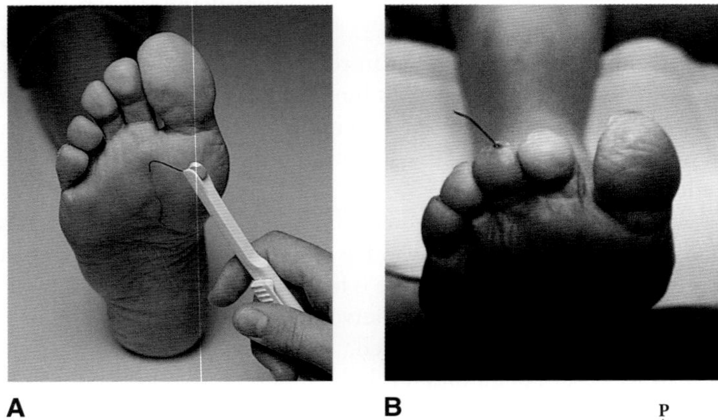

FIGURE 23-3 The importance of cutaneous sensation. **A,** Using a monofilament to check for sensation on the bottom of the foot. **B,** Foreign body (wire) in the toe of a diabetic patient may not trigger appropriate sensations of pain because of nerve damage (diabetic neuropathy).

wants". Individuals who are unable to adequately sense pain on the body surface tend to have other types of sensory loss as well. They are very much at risk for injury because they lack the ability to sense the "warning signs" that a normally functioning sensory system can provide.

Individuals with uncontrolled or poorly controlled diabetes often lose their ability to sense pain on certain areas of the body surface—especially on the skin of the feet. Other sensations are also commonly diminished or lost over time in diabetics because of nerve damage called **diabetic neuropathy.** For this reason physicians closely monitor the adequacy of cutaneous sensation on the bottom of the foot (**Figure 23-3**, A). Recognizing early signs of diabetic neuropathy can help prevent later injury. **Figure 23-3**, *B*, shows a foreign body (a piece of wire) protruding from the tip of the third toe in a diabetic patient. The individual lacked sensation in the feet and only after visually noticing it sought medical attention. This is just one example, but a common one, of a failure of "the gift of pain" to give an appropriate warning of an injury.

In a syndrome called **fibromyalgia (FM)**, chronic and widespread musculoskeletal pain is usually accompanied by distress and a variety of other symptoms. The primary mechanism of FM seems to be an abnormal amplification of pain information processed in the central nervous system. However, other mechanisms are also being investigated as contributing factors. The drug *pregabalin* reduces the pain of FM mainly by blocking calcium channels in the pain-pathway neurons of the spinal cord. Reducing calcium influx, as you probably recall (see **Figure 19-14** on p. 422), inhibits the release of pain neurotransmitters.

CONNECT IT! 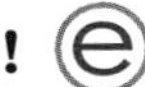

Next time you have some hot chicken wings or a spicy jalapeño pepper on your pizza, think about how mild pain actually adds to your food experience. How can that be? Check out how pain and other general senses combine with taste (a special sense) to produce a complete food sensation at ***Sensing Food*** online at ***Connect It!***

SENSE OF TEMPERATURE

We have multiple senses of temperature that can detect changes in various ranges of heat and cold. Our brain integrates all these senses into a single feeling of either localized or general temperature.

Free nerve endings called **thermoreceptors** mediate sensations of heat and cold. When small cold or warm probes are used to "map" the skin's sensitivity to temperature, small areas called "receptive fields" about 1 mm across can be identified on the skin surface as being sensitive to *either* cold or warmth but not both. Research has shown that these receptive fields represent separate *warm receptors* and *cold receptors* that respond to different thermal sensations and are sensitive to a range of relatively hot or cold temperatures. Thermal maps have also shown that thermoreceptors, like other types of cutaneous receptors, are not spread uniformly across the skin surface.

Both types of thermoreceptors undergo rapid adaptation. As a result, the intensity of the warm or cold sensations they initially produce when activated soon fade. We adapt to the heat of a sauna or a cool shower in a short time.

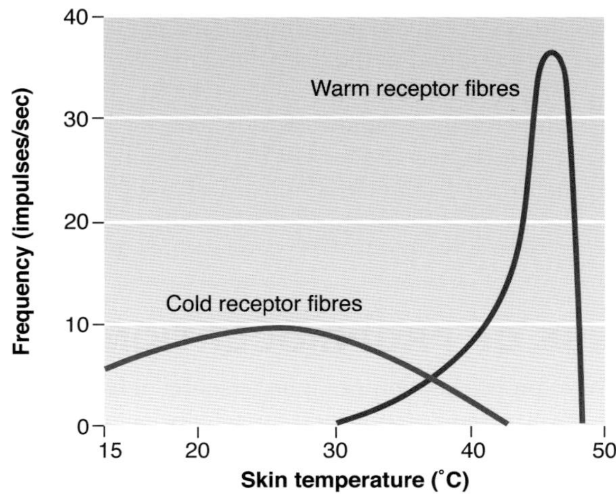

FIGURE 23-4 Range of temperature receptor sensitivity.

Warm receptors, which are located in the dermis, are activated above about 25°C and increase their firing rate until the temperature reaches about 46°C. **Figure 23-4** shows the range of temperature receptor sensitivity. Beyond a temperature of about 48°C a sensation of burning pain begins.

Cold receptors, which are located in the deepest layer of the epidermis, have a broader temperature response than warm receptors (see **Figure 23-4**). They are most active between about 10°C and 40°C. Below 10°C the firing of cold receptors decreases dramatically. The falling temperature first acts as a local anaesthetic and then activates nociceptors, resulting in a sensation of freezing pain. Between temperature extremes the brain senses a particular temperature sensation by integrating sensory inputs from both receptor types.

SENSE OF TOUCH

Like many of the senses, touch is really more than one sense because it includes the ability to detect many different types of changes in or on our skin. Some of these tactile sensations are mediated by free nerve endings and others by encapsulated nerve endings (see **Table 23-1**).

Skin Movement

Root hair plexuses are rapidly adapting free nerve endings that are activated when very slight movement on or in the skin bends or deforms a hair shaft or follicle surrounded by the receptor. When you feel a mosquito "bite", it may not be caused by the piercing of the skin by the mouth of the insect. Instead, it may be the movement of your own hair or skin caused by the mosquito's activity that triggers or stimulates a root hair plexus. In any event, it's a good idea to swat the mosquito, which is a known vector for several human diseases!

Itch

The term *itch* is used to describe several different tactile sensations mediated by free nerve endings. Most people would describe it as a sensation that makes you want to scratch. It can vary in intensity from almost imperceptible to intense and disabling. The cause is generally chemical irritation of free nerve endings by inflammatory chemicals, such as bradykinin or histamine. These types of chemicals are often released by injured tissue after insect bites or during allergic reactions.

Itches can also be induced by suggestion, like a yawn. Scientists are just now working out the types of itch that occur in humans and how these itch mechanisms work.

Tickle

Tickle is a unique sensation in that it most often results from tactile stimulation of the skin, not by you, but by someone else. It is mediated by free nerve endings and is a good but somewhat baffling example of how perception can alter the conscious interpretation of a nervous impulse when it reaches the brain.

We know that neural pathways in tickle involve both the thalamus and cerebellum before the impulses reach the cerebral cortex. However, the circuits involved in the cerebral cortex and how these circuits interact with neurons in other areas of the brain are not well

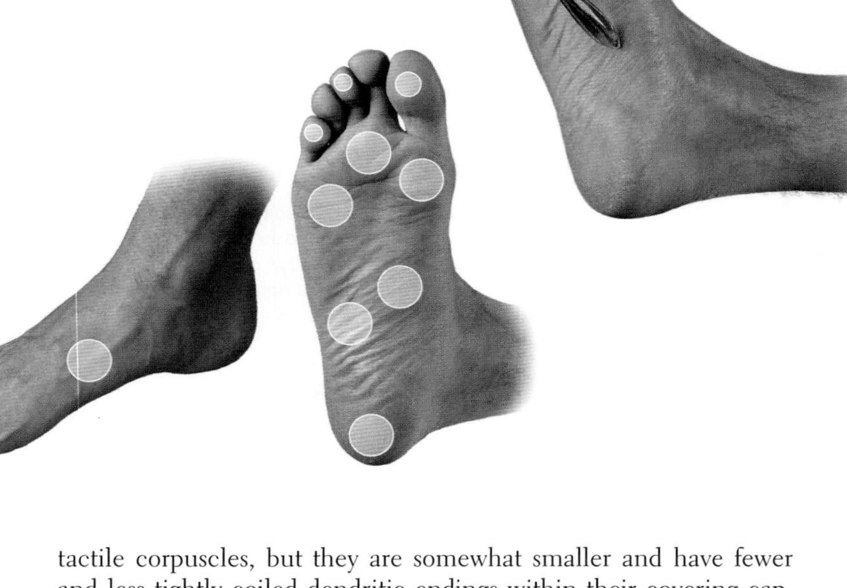

FIGURE 23-5 Discriminative "light" touch. A, Normally, sensation can be elicited by a light stroke to the skin. **B,** Examples of specific sites used to verify sensation of discriminative touch.

understood. Obviously, knowing consciously that a particular tactile sensation generally occurs only when you are touched by someone else requires complex nervous system involvement. What begins as a simple receptor potential in a free nerve ending ends in a complex, consciously interpreted tactile sensation.

Light Touch

Discriminative touch, or "light touch", refers to an often very subtle sensation that can be located exactly in certain areas of the skin (**Figure 23-5**).

Light touch is mediated by a flattened or disc-shaped variation of a free nerve ending called a **tactile disc** or *Merkel disc.* It may also be called a *tactile meniscus.* This structure was first described by the German anatomist Friedrich Merkel (1885–1919) when he studied delicate nervous elements near the skin surface.

Structurally, the tactile receptor unit is made up of two cells. One is an epithelial cell called the *tactile epithelial cell,* located in the epidermis of the skin (see **Figure 10-4**, p. 183). The other cell is a sensory neuron called the *tactile disc.* The tactile epithelial cell is rather stiff and transmits compression of the outer layer of the skin to the tactile disc neuron. The tactile disc is a delicate mechanoreceptor that is not encapsulated and has a superficial placement in the epidermis of the skin (see **Figure 23-2**). It is therefore easily "deformed" when pressed by the stiff tactile cell and capable of generating an action potential when exposed to very minimal stimulation. Tactile discs adapt slowly, thus maintaining information flow to the central nervous system for some time.

In addition to discriminative or light touch, the tactile receptor unit is also capable of detecting subtle changes in surface form and contours.

Deep Touch

Deep touch, which is mediated by several different types of encapsulated receptors, is a little more complex than light touch, which is mediated by free nerve endings.

Tactile corpuscles are encapsulated tactile end organs, also called *Meissner corpuscles,* first described by the German physiologist Georg Meissner (1829–1905). Note in **Figure 23-2** and **Table 23-1** that they are superficially placed ovoid or egg-shaped mechanoreceptors that are larger than tactile discs. The encapsulated receptor fibres are coiled and enmeshed in connective tissue. They are located in or very close to the dermal papillae in hairless skin areas such as the fingertips, lips, nipples, and genitals. Although their covering capsule requires slightly more of a "deforming" stimulus to generate an action potential than a tactile (Merkel) disc, they do mediate light touch in addition to textural sensations and low-frequency vibration.

Two important anatomical variants of tactile (Meissner) corpuscles also act as mechanoreceptors. One is called the **bulboid corpuscle** or *Krause end bulb.* Bulboid corpuscles are egg shaped, like tactile corpuscles, but they are somewhat smaller and have fewer and less tightly coiled dendritic endings within their covering capsule. These receptors are more numerous in mucous membranes than in skin and are sometimes called *mucocutaneous corpuscles.* They are involved in touch and low-frequency vibration.

The other variant of the tactile (Meissner) corpuscle is the **bulbous corpuscle,** also known as the *Ruffini corpuscle* (see **Figure 23-2**). Although considered to be a variant of the tactile corpuscle, it has a more flattened capsule and is more deeply located in the dermis of the skin. These receptors mediate sensations of crude, heavy, and persistent touch. Because they are slow adapting, they permit the skin of the fingers to remain sensitive to deep pressure for long periods. The ability to grasp an object, such as the steering wheel of a car, for long periods and still be able to "sense" its presence between the fingers depends on these receptors.

Lamellar corpuscles (*Pacini corpuscles*) are large mechanoreceptors, which, when sectioned, show thick laminated connective tissue capsules. They are found in the deep dermis of the skin—especially in the hands and feet—and are also numerous in joint capsules throughout the body (see **Figure 23-2**). Pacini, or lamellar, corpuscles respond quickly to sensations of deep pressure, high-frequency vibration, and stretch. Although sensitive and quick to respond, these receptors adapt quickly, and the sensations they evoke seldom last for long.

SENSE OF PROPRIOCEPTION

Our sense of proprioception or "muscle sense" tells us at each moment the level of contraction and stretch in each of our skeletal muscles. Thus, even with our eyes closed, we can tell where our body parts are located—even if we move them. For example, if you close your eyes and then adduct your fingers you will know where your fingers are even though you cannot see them.

TABLE 23-1 Classification of Somatic Sensory Receptors—cont'd

BY STRUCTURE	BY LOCATION AND TYPE	BY ACTIVATION STIMULUS	BY SENSATION OR FUNCTION
Encapsulated Nerve Endings			
Touch and Pressure Receptors			
Tactile (Meissner) corpuscle 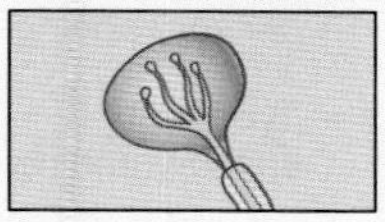	Exteroceptor; epidermis, hairless skin	Light pressure, mechanical	Touch; low-frequency vibration
Bulboid (Krause) corpuscle 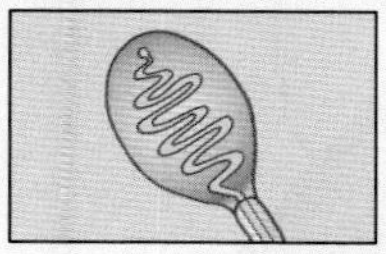	Exteroceptor; mucous membranes	Mechanical	Touch; low-frequency vibration; textural sensation
Bulbous (Ruffini) corpuscle 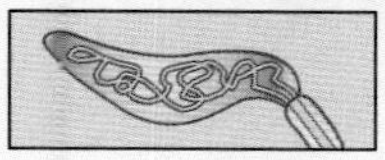	Exteroceptor; dermis of skin	Mechanical	Crude and persistent touch
Lamellar (Pacini) corpuscle 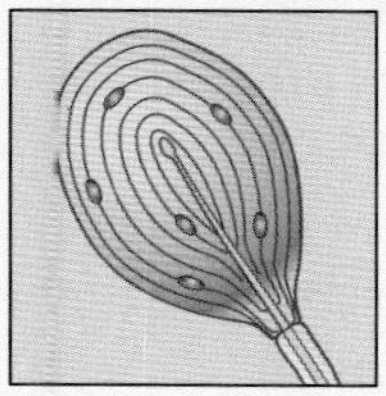	Exteroceptor; dermis of skin, joint capsules	Deep pressure, mechanical	Deep pressure; high-frequency vibration; stretch
Stretch Receptors			
Muscle spindles 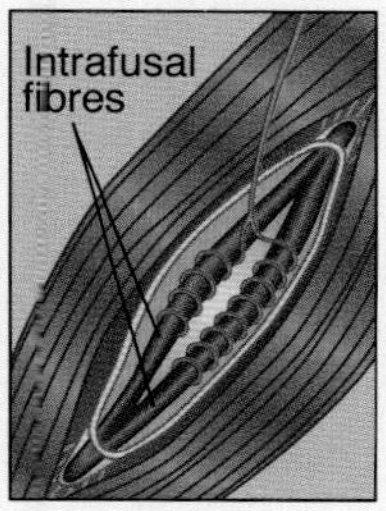	Interoceptor; skeletal muscle	Stretch; mechanical	Sense of muscle length (proprioception)
Golgi tendon receptors 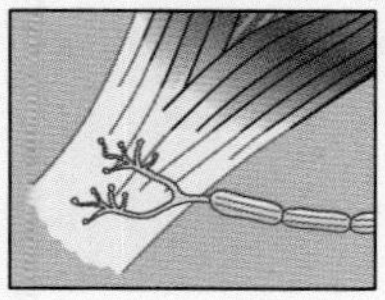	Interoceptor; tendon (near muscle tissue)	Force of contraction and tendon stretch; mechanical	Sense of muscle tension (proprioception)

The most important stretch receptors are associated with muscles and tendons and are classified as proprioceptors. Two types of stretch receptors, called **muscle spindles** and **Golgi tendon receptors**, operate to provide the body with information concerning muscle length and the strength of muscle contraction (**Figure 23-6**).

Anatomically, each muscle spindle consists of a discrete grouping of about 5 to 10 modified muscle fibres called *intrafusal fibres*, which are surrounded by a delicate capsule. These fibres have striated ends that are capable of contraction but are devoid of contractile filaments in their central areas where, instead, there are several nuclei surrounded by clear cytoplasm and two types of sensory nerve fibres that are described later. The muscle spindles can be found lying between and parallel to the regular muscle fibres called *extrafusal fibres*. Both ends of each spindle are connected or anchored to connective tissue elements within the muscle mass.

Two types of sensory (afferent) nerve fibres are found encircling the central area of each spindle. Both large-diameter and rapidly conducting type Ia and slower-conducting, small-diameter type II fibres encircle the clear central area of each spindle. When stretching occurs, afferent impulses from these sensory neurons pass to the spinal cord and are relayed to the brain, providing a mechanism to monitor changes in muscle length.

The striated ends of the muscle spindle fibres (intrafusal fibres) are capable of contraction when stimulated by efferent impulses generated in **gamma motor neurons,** whereas regular muscle fibres (extrafusal fibres) are stimulated to contract by efferent impulses generated in **alpha motor neurons.** Both types of neurons are located in the anterior grey horn of the spinal cord.

Muscle spindles are stimulated if the length of a muscle is stretched and exceeds a certain limit. The result of stimulation is a **stretch reflex** that shortens a muscle or muscle group, thus aiding in the maintenance of posture or the positioning of the body or one of its extremities in a way that may be opposed by the force of gravity (see **Figure 17-25**, p. 379). We do this unconsciously, even though these receptors do contribute to conscious proprioception.

Golgi tendon organs, often called simply *tendon organs,* like muscle spindles, are proprioceptors. They are located at the point of junction between muscle tissue and tendon. Each Golgi tendon organ consists of dendrites *(Golgi tendon receptors)* of afferent (sensory) nerves called *type Ib nerve fibres,* which are associated with bundles of collagen fibres from the tendon and surrounded by a capsule. These sensory organs act in a way opposite that of muscle spindles. Golgi tendon organs are stimulated by excessive stretch of a tendon—as when pulling too great a load for the muscle to bear safely. When the Golgi tendon organ is activated, the skeletal muscle relaxes. This response, called a *Golgi tendon reflex,* protects muscles from tearing internally or pulling away from their tendinous points of attachment to bone because of excessive contractile force.

Table 23-1 summarizes the different types of somatic sense receptors, their locations, and their functions.

Quick CHECK

1. Classify receptors into six groups based on the type of stimuli that activate them.
2. Distinguish between the special and the general, or somatic, senses.
3. Name the three types of sense receptors classified according to location in the body.
4. Name the receptors associated with pain, touch, pressure, and stretch responses.

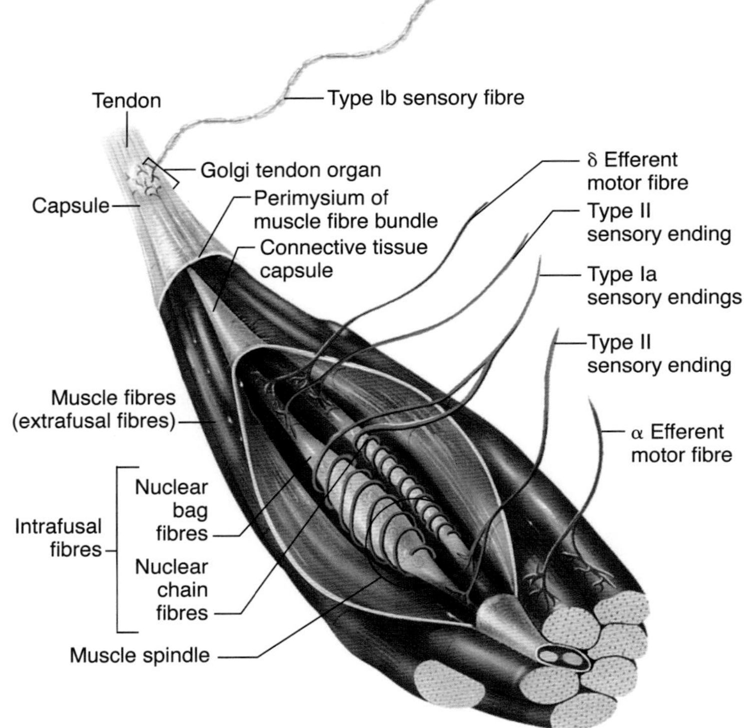

FIGURE 23-6 Proprioceptors. General sense organs for proprioception or "muscle sense" are found in muscle organs, including the tendon.

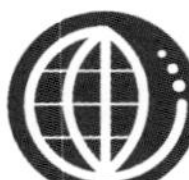

the big picture | General Senses

Almost invariably, as you study the various organ systems of the body, seeing the "big picture" involves an understanding of how that organ system affects homeostasis. Both the structure and function of the body sense organs illustrate this relationship.

The somatic sense organs are widely distributed throughout the body, and they serve to provide the body with vital information related to both external and internal conditions that affect homeostasis. For example, pain—regardless of cause—is very often the first indicator of homeostatic imbalance. Furthermore, the ability to sense touch, pressure, vibration, stretch, or temperature changes on or in the body before these stimuli reach levels that may cause injury is vital to survival.

LANGUAGE OF SCIENCE *(continued from p. 520)*

osmoreceptor (os-moh-ree-SEP-tor)
[*osmo-* **push (osmosis),** *-cept-* **receive,** *-or* **agent**]

perception (per-SEP-shun)

photoreceptor (FOH-toh-ree-sep-tor)
[*photo-* **light,** *-cept-* **receive,** *-or* **agent**]

proprioceptor (proh-pree-oh-SEP-tor)
[*propri-* **one's own,** *-cept-* **receive,** *-or* **agent**]

receptor potential (ree-SEP-tor poh-TEN-shal)
[*recept-* **receive,** *-or* **agent,** *potent-* **power,** *-ial* **relating to**]

sensory receptor (SEN-soh-ree ree-SEP-tor)
[*sens-* **feel,** *-ory* **relating to,** *recept-* **receive,** *-or* **agent**]

somatic pain (so-MAH-tik)
[*soma-* **body,** *-ic* **relating to**]

stretch reflex
[*re-* **again,** *-flex* **bend**]

tactile corpuscle (TAK-tyle KOR-pus-ul)
[*tact-* **touch,** *-ile* **relating to,** *corpus-* **body,** *-cle* **little**]

tactile disc (TAK-tyle)
[*tact-* **touch,** *-ile* **relating to**]

thermoreceptor (ther-moh-ree-SEP-tor)
[*thermo-* **heat,** *-cept-* **receive,** *-or* **agent**]

visceral pain (VISS-er-al)
[*viscera* **internal organs**]

visceroceptor (viss-er-oh-SEP-tor)
[*viscero-* **internal organs,** *-cept-* **receive,** *-or* **agent**]

LANGUAGE OF MEDICINE

diabetic neuropathy
(dye-ah-BET-ik nyoo-ROP-ah-thee)
[*diabet-* **pass-through or siphon (diabetes mellitus),** *-ic* **relating to,** *neuro-* **nerve,** *-path-* **disease,** *-y* **state**]

fibromyalgia (FM)
(fye-broh-my-AL-jah)
[*fibr-* **thread or fibre,** *-my-* **muscle,** *-algia* **pain**]

case study

As an active 40-year-old man, Donald had enjoyed playing recreational rugby for several years. Recently he began to experience dull, aching lower back pain. He complained to his doctor that the constant lower back pain was coupled with a shooting pain into the left leg from his buttock to his foot. Donald explained that there was nothing he could do to ease his discomfort and that he had difficulty sleeping. The symptoms had been present for almost two months, and he was anxious to resume his active lifestyle.

Neurological tests and magnetic resonance imaging (MRI) indicated evidence of significant sciatic nerve irritation. Donald's doctor referred him to an orthopaedic surgeon, who performed a surgical procedure called a microdiscectomy to remove part of a herniated disc. After a brief stay in the hospital, Donald received post-operative care that included physiotherapy exercises to help restore his full range of movement.

1. Receptors are often classified into categories based on the type of stimuli that activate them. Which receptors were activated when Donald experienced his lower back pain?
   a. Osmoreceptors
   b. Thermoreceptors
   c. Nociceptors
   d. Photoreceptors
2. Which type of nerve fibre carries impulses from pain receptors to the brain?
   a. Acute fibres
   b. Fast (A) pain fibres
   c. Slow (B) pain fibres
   d. Fast (B) pain fibres
3. The pain that Donald experienced can best be described as:
   a. Somatic pain
   b. Acute pain
   c. Visceral pain
   d. Referred pain
4. What would best explain why the pain in Donald's lower back radiated downwards from his left buttock to his foot?
   a. When a herniated disc ruptures, it pinches out and compresses the nerves that lead down the leg, leading to nerve irritation.
   b. A mixing or converging of sensory neurons from the lower back to the foot
   c. A phantom pain phenomenon radiating from the lower back to the foot
   d. A misinterpretation by the brain with regard to the true location of sensory neurons

Hint To solve a case study, you may have to refer to the glossary or index, other chapters in this textbook, ***Connect It!,*** and other resources.

CHAPTER SUMMARY

*To download an MP3 version of the chapter summary for use with your mobile device, access the **Audio Chapter Summaries** online at evolve.elsevier.com.*

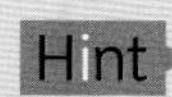

Scan this summary after reading the chapter to help you reinforce the key concepts. Later, use the summary as a quick review before your class or before a test.

Introduction

A. Sense organs have sensory receptors that detect changes in the internal and external environment
B. Two categories of sense organs or senses
   1. General (somatic) senses—have receptors buried in many different organs throughout the body to detect touch, temperature, pain, etc.
   2. Special senses—complex organs to detect vision, hearing, balance, taste, smell

Sensory Receptors

A. Sensory receptors make it possible for the body to respond to stimuli caused by changes occurring in our internal or external environment
B. Receptor response
   1. General function—responds to stimuli by converting them to nerve impulses
   2. Different types of receptors respond to different stimuli
   3. Receptor potential
      a. The potential that develops when an adequate stimulus acts on a receptor; it is a graded response
      b. When a threshold is reached, an action potential in the sensory neuron's axon is triggered

c. Impulses travel over sensory pathways to the brain and spinal cord where either they are interpreted as a particular sensation or they initiate a reflex action

4. Adaptation—a functional characteristic of receptors; receptor potential decreases over time in response to a continuous stimulus, which leads to a decreased rate of impulse conduction and a decreased intensity of sensation (**Figure 23-1**)

C. Distribution of receptors
   1. Receptors for special senses of smell, taste, vision, hearing, and equilibrium are grouped into localized areas or into complex organs
   2. General sense organs of somatic senses are microscopic receptors widely distributed throughout the body in the skin, mucosa, connective tissue, muscles, tendons, joints, and viscera (**Figure 23-2**)

Classification of Receptors

A. Classification by sensory pathway
   1. Somatic sensory receptors—found in skin, muscles, ligaments, eyes, ears and mediate our conscious somatic senses such as touch, pain, body position, special senses, etc.
   2. Autonomic (visceral) sensory receptor—found in internal organs and mediate our subconscious visceral senses (e.g., pH, chemical concentrations, temperature, pressure)

B. Classification by location
   1. Exteroceptors
      a. On or near body surface
      b. Often called *cutaneous receptors;* examples: pressure, touch, pain, temperature
   2. Visceroceptors (interoceptors)
      a. Located internally—often within body organs, or viscera
      b. Provide body with information about internal environment; examples: pressure, stretch, chemical changes, hunger, thirst
   3. Proprioceptors—special type of visceroceptor
      a. Location limited to skeletal muscle, joint capsules, and tendons
      b. Provide information on body movement, orientation in space, and muscle stretch
      c. Two types—tonic and phasic proprioceptors provide positional information on body or body parts while at rest or during movement

C. Classification by stimulus detected
   1. Mechanoreceptors—activated when “deformed” to generate receptor potential
   2. Chemoreceptors—activated by amount or changing concentration of certain chemicals, for example, taste and smell
   3. Thermoreceptors—activated by changes in temperature
   4. Nociceptors—activated by intense stimuli that may damage tissue; sensation produced in pain
   5. Photoreceptors—found only in the eye; respond to light stimuli if the intensity is great enough to generate a receptor potential
   6. Osmoreceptors—concentrated in the hypothalamus; activated by changes in concentration of electrolytes (osmolarity) in extracellular fluids.

D. Classification by structure
   1. Free nerve endings
   2. Encapsulated nerve endings (**Table 23-1**)

Sense of Pain

A. Nociceptor—describes the free nerve endings that serve as the primary sensory receptors for pain

B. Pain sensations (**Figure 23-3**)
   1. Acute or fast (A) pain fibres—mediate sharp, intense, localized pain
   2. Chronic or slow (B) pain fibres—mediate less intense but more persistent dull or aching pain

C. Somatic pain—fast, “take your breath away” pain associated with superficial injury or trauma

D. Visceral pain—dull or aching pain that develops more slowly over time and travels over B fibres

Sense of Temperature

A. Multiple senses of temperature can detect changes in various ranges of heat and cold

B. Thermoreceptors—mediate sensations of heat and cold
   1. Warm receptors and cold receptors (**Figure 23-4**)
   2. Thermal maps—indicate thermoreceptors are not spread uniformly across skin surface
   3. Warm receptors located in dermis
   4. Cold receptors located in deepest layer of epidermis

Sense of Touch

A. Sense of touch includes the ability to detect many different changes in or on our skin

B. Tactile sensations are mediated by free nerve endings or encapsulated nerve endings (**Table 23-1**)

C. Skin movement
   1. Root hair plexuses

D. Itch
   1. Mediated by free nerve endings

E. Tickle
   1. Mediated by free nerve endings
   2. Involves both the thalamus and cerebellum before impulses reach cerebral cortex

F. Light touch (**Figure 23-5**)
   1. Tactile (Merkel) discs (**Figure 23-2**)
      a. Tactile receptor unit is made up of two cells: tactile epithelial cell and tactile disc
      b. Capable of detecting subtle changes in surface form and contours

G. Deep touch
   1. Tactile corpuscle (Meissner corpuscle), relatively large and superficial in placement; mediates touch and low-frequency vibration; large numbers in hairless skin areas, such as nipples, fingertips, and lips; two anatomical variations of tactile (Meissner) corpuscle
      a. Bulboid corpuscles (Krause end bulbs)—small, with less tightly coiled dendritic endings within their capsule; involved in touch, low-frequency vibrations

b. Bulbous (Ruffini) corpuscles—have a flattened capsule and are deeply located in the dermis; mediate crude and persistent touch

2. Lamellar (Pacini) corpuscles—large mechanoreceptors that respond quickly to sensations of deep pressure, high-frequency vibration, and stretch; found in deep dermis and in joint capsules—they adapt quickly, and sensations they evoke seldom last for long periods

Sense of Proprioception

A. Proprioception or "muscle sense" tells at each moment the level of contraction and stretch in each of our skeletal muscles

B. Stretch receptors—two types; operate to provide body with information concerning muscle length and strength of muscle contraction

1. Muscle spindle—composed of 5 to 10 intrafusal fibres lying between and parallel to regular (extrafusal) muscle fibres (**Figure 23-6**)
   a. Large-diameter and rapid-conducting type Ia and smaller-diameter and slower-conducting type II afferent fibres carry messages to brain concerning changes in muscle length
   b. If the length of a muscle exceeds a certain limit, a stretch reflex is initiated to shorten the muscle, thus helping to maintain posture
2. Golgi tendon organs—located at junction between muscle tissue and tendon; made up of encapsulated neuron endings associated with collagen bundles (**Figure 23-6**)
   a. Type Ib sensory neurons (Golgi tendon receptors) are stimulated by excessive contraction—when stimulated, they cause muscle to *relax*
   b. Golgi tendon reflex protects muscle from tearing internally because of excessive contractile force

The Big Picture: General Senses

A. Somatic sense organs are widely distributed throughout the body

B. Somatic sense organs provide the body with vital information related to both external and internal conditions that affect homeostasis

REVIEW QUESTIONS

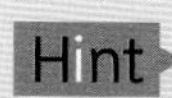

Write out the answers to these questions after reading the chapter and reviewing the Chapter Summary. Note—writing out your answers will consolidate learning and provide a valuable resource of information.

1. Define *general senses* and compare them to *special senses.*
2. Define *receptor potential.*
3. Define *adaptation* with reference to receptor response.
4. Distinguish *exteroceptors, visceroceptors,* and *proprioceptors.*
5. Describe the function of each of the following: mechanoreceptors, chemoreceptors, thermoreceptors, nociceptors, photoreceptors. Indicate where these receptors are likely to be located.
6. Describe the phenomenon of *referred pain.*
7. List and describe the different types of touch.
8. Describe *proprioception.*

CRITICAL THINKING QUESTIONS

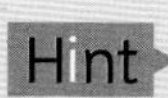

After finishing the Review Questions, write out the answers to these more in-depth questions to help you apply your new knowledge. Go back to sections of the chapter that relate to concepts that you find difficult.

1. With regard to location, explain the difference between an above-threshold receptor potential and the sensation of that stimulus.
2. Explain why the sense of pain is vital to our survival.
3. Why is it accurate to state that humans have more than one sense of temperature?
4. How does proprioception through *muscle spindles* differ from proprioception through *Golgi tendon organs?*
5. Describe the response that allows us to be aware of our clothes 100% of the time.

24 Special Senses

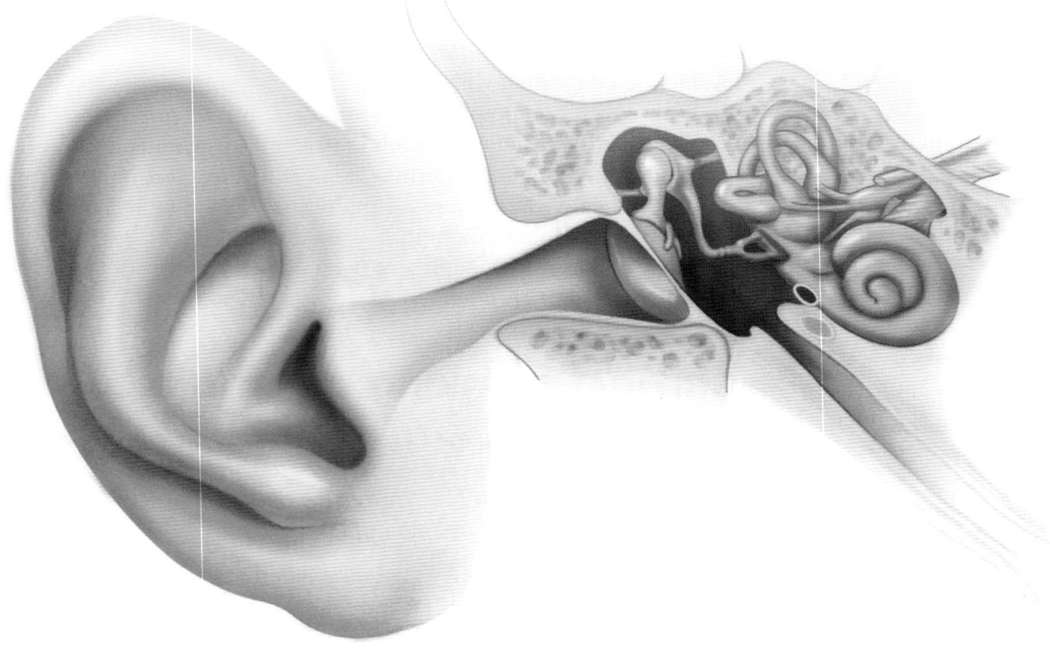

LANGUAGE OF SCIENCE

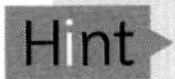

Hint *Use this list to aid your pronunciation of unfamiliar words.*

accommodation
(ah-kom-oh-DAY-shun)
[*accommoda-* **adjust,** *-ation* **process**]

anterior cavity
(an-TEER-ee-or KAV-i-tee)
[*ante-* **front,** *-er-* **more,** *-or* **quality,** *cav-* **hollow,** *-ity* **state**]

auditory ossicle
(AW-dih-toh-ree OS-ik-ul)
[*audit-* **hear,** *-ory* **relating to,** *os-* **bone,** *-icle* **little**]

auditory tube (AW-dih-toh-ree tyoob)
[*audit-* **hear,** *-ory* **relating to**]

basal cell (BAY-sal)
[*bas-* **foundation,** *-al* **relating to,** *cell* **storeroom**]

basilar membrane (BAYS-ih-lar)
[*bas-* **foundation,** *-ar* **relating to,** *membran-* **thin skin**]

ciliary body (SIL-ee-air-ee)
[*ciliary* **eyelids or eyelashes**]

circumvallate papillae
(sir-kum-VAL-ayt pah-PIL-ah)
[*circum-* **around,** *-vall-* **post or stake,** *-ate* **relating to,** *papilla* **nipple**]
pl., papillae

cornea (KOR-nee-ah)
[*corn-* **horn,** *-a* **thing**]

crista ampullaris
(KRIS-tah am-pyoo-LAIR-iss)
[*crista* **ridge,** *ampu-* **flask,** *-ulla-* **little,** *-ar-* **relating to**, *-is* **thing**] *pl.*, cristae ampulares

cupula (KYOO-pyoo-lah)
[*cup-* **tub,** *-ula* **little**] *pl.*, cupulae

dynamic equilibrium
(dye-NAM-ik ee-kwih-LIB-ree-um)
[*dynam-* **moving force,** *-ic* **relating to,** *equi-* **equal,** *-libr-* **balance**]

endolymph (EN-doh-limf)
[*endo-* **within,** *-lymph* **water**]

epithelial support cell
(ep-ih-THEE-lee-al)
[*epi-* **upon,** *-theli* **nipple,** *-al* **relating to**]

equilibrium (e-kwih-LIB-ree-um)
[*equi-* **equal,** *-libr-* **balance**]
pl., equilibria

eustachian tube (yoo-STAY-shun tyoob)
[*Bartolomeo Eustachio* **Italian anatomist,** *-an* **relating to**]

continued on p. 556

CHAPTER OUTLINE

Hint *Scan this outline before you begin to read the chapter, as a preview of how the concepts are organized.*

The previous chapter outlined the basic structure and function of sensory receptors and discussed the body's general senses. We learned that sensory information may initiate reflexes that help us maintain homeostatic balance by reacting to disturbances—or potential disturbances—to our body's internal stability.

In this chapter, we turn our attention to the special senses: smell, taste, hearing, balance, and vision. Special senses provide feedback about both internal and external environments of the body. This information tells us about actual or potential disturbances to our stability. As you progress through this chapter, try to focus on two main themes: how the structure of special sense organs determines their functions and what roles each special sense may play in maintaining a stable internal environment. •

SENSE OF SMELL

We begin our study of the special senses with olfaction. Olfaction is our sense of smell. It helps us interpret our environment by detecting molecules, called odourants, given off by organisms and substances around us.

OLFACTORY RECEPTORS

The **olfactory** epithelium consists of yellow-coloured **epithelial support cells, basal cells,** and bipolar-type **olfactory sensory neurons.** The olfactory sensory neurons, also called *olfactory receptor neurons,* have unique *olfactory cilia,* that populate the surface of the olfactory epithelium lining the upper surface of the nasal cavity. The olfactory sensory neurons are *chemoreceptors.* They are unique because they are replaced on a regular basis by **basal cells** in the olfactory epithelium.

The olfactory cilia have membrane receptors embedded in them that bind to odourants. These odourant receptors generate receptor potentials in olfactory sensory neurons when gas molecules or chemicals dissolved in the mucus covering the olfactory epithelium (**Figure 24-1**) bind to them. Gentle, random movement of the cilia helps "mix" the covering mucus and increases its efficiency as a solvent.

The olfactory epithelium is located in the most superior portion of the nasal cavity (see **Figure 24-1**). Functionally, this is a poor location because a great deal of inspired air flows around and down the nasal passageways without contacting the protein odourant receptors located in the cell membranes of the olfactory receptor cells. The location of these receptor neurons explains the necessity for sniffing, or drawing air forcefully up into the nose, to smell delicate odours.

The olfactory receptors are extremely sensitive—that is, capable of being stimulated by even very slight odours caused by just a few molecules of a particular chemical. However, rapid adaptation of olfactory sensations in the face of continuous stimulation occurs. It is due to both the inhibition of action potentials by **granule cells** in the olfactory bulbs and to fatigue of odourant receptor function caused by ongoing stimulation of the olfactory sensory neurons.

Although humans have a sense of smell far less keen than many animals, some individuals can distinguish several thousand different odours, and most of us can easily identify at least several hundred. Examples of well-known primary scents include putrid, floral, peppermint, and musky odours. Many odours are combinations of primary scents.

In 2004 U.S. researchers Drs. Linda Buck and Richard Axel received the Nobel prize in Physiology or Medicine for their pioneering work that explained for the first time how the sense of smell or olfaction in humans actually "works". Their research identified almost 1000 different types of odourant receptors in the cell membranes of human olfactory sensory neurons. All of them are G protein–coupled receptors (GPCRs), which we encountered in an earlier chapter (see **Figure 19-17** on p. 425).

In a series of sophisticated experiments, they were able to show that by stimulating the entire olfactory epithelium—or specific odourant

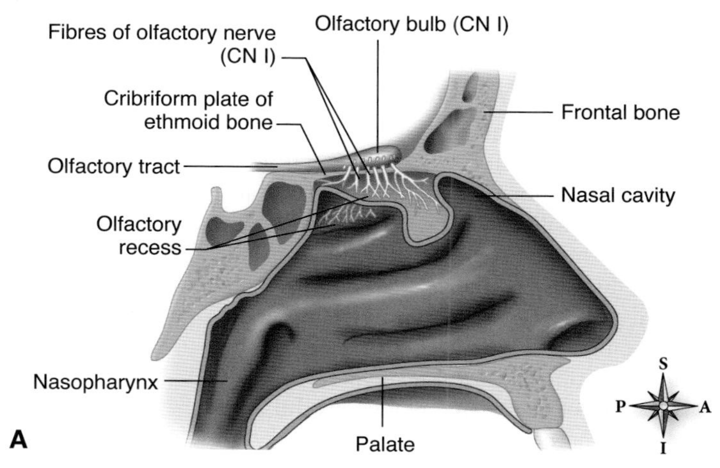

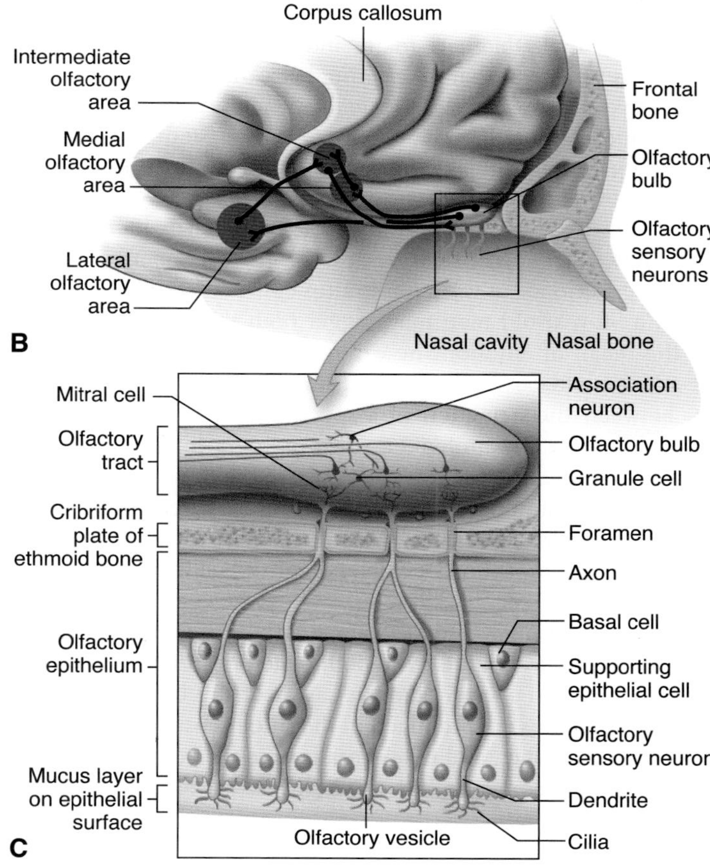

FIGURE 24-1 Olfaction. Location of olfactory epithelium, olfactory bulb, and neural pathways involved in olfaction. **A,** Midsagittal section of the nasal area shows the locations of major olfactory sensory structures. **B,** Major olfactory integration centres of the brain. **C,** Details of the olfactory bulb and olfactory epithelium.

receptors, or combinations or sequences of these receptor proteins—different odours could be identified. If the membrane receptor proteins are compared with the letters of the alphabet, activation of specific letters, formation of different "words", or word sequences, will cause differing olfactory sensory neurons or groups of neurons to transmit impulses to the brain that are perceived as unique odours. More recent research shows that this system allows the average person to discriminate more than a *trillion* different odours!

Olfactory Pathway

If the level of odourants dissolved in the mucus surrounding the olfactory cilia reaches a threshold level, a receptor potential and then an action potential will be generated and passed to the olfactory nerves in the olfactory bulb. From there, the impulse passes through the olfactory tract and into the thalamic and olfactory centres of the brain for interpretation, integration, and memory storage.

The sense of smell can create powerful and long-lasting memories. Memories coupled with unique sensory inputs, especially distinctive odours, often persist from early childhood to death. Dental office smells, baby smells, kitchen smells, and new car smells are examples of olfactory "triggers" that often bring back memories of events that occurred years earlier. In addition to the olfactory cortex and thalamic areas of the brain, components of the limbic system, including the cingulate gyrus and hippocampus, play a key role in coupling olfactory sense inputs to both short- and long-term memory.

Not only can specific odours trigger long-term memory, they often allow the individual to recall emotions associated with the recalled experience as well. For example, the smell of an evergreen tree by a 90-year-old man may trigger both the memory of events and the recall of emotions he experienced at Christmas when he was a 9-year-old boy. The mechanism of such a complex association between the detection of a specific odour and recall of the actual emotions and ambiance surrounding a long-term memory remains unknown.

People who suffer from permanent **anosmia,** complete lack of smell, can develop serious depression. Apparently, the loss of smell can have more impact on our psychological health than the loss of any other sense.

Our senses of smell and taste are closely related. Note in **Figure 24-2** that the neural inputs from both olfactory and gustatory (taste) receptors travel in several common areas of the brain. Ultimately, olfactory sensations are produced in the smell sensory cortex located in the temporal lobes, and taste sensations result from stimulation of the taste sensory cortex in the parietal lobes.

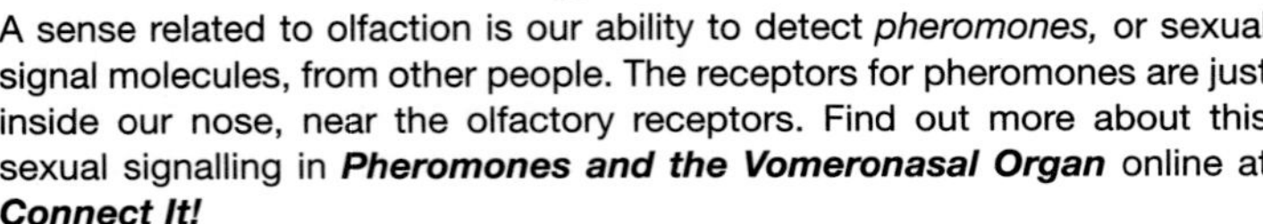

CONNECT IT!

A sense related to olfaction is our ability to detect *pheromones,* or sexual signal molecules, from other people. The receptors for pheromones are just inside our nose, near the olfactory receptors. Find out more about this sexual signalling in ***Pheromones and the Vomeronasal Organ*** online at ***Connect It!***

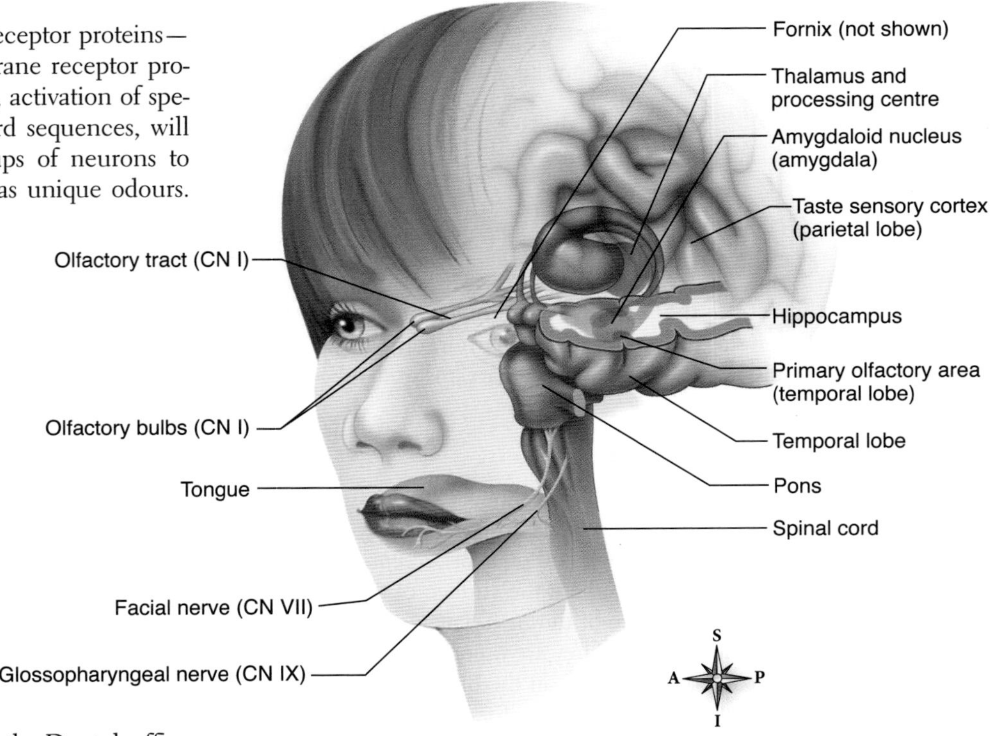

FIGURE 24-2 Relationship of olfactory and gustatory pathways.

SENSE OF TASTE

Taste Buds

The **taste buds** are the sense organs that respond to **gustatory** stimuli, or taste stimuli. Although a few taste buds are located in the lining of the mouth and on the soft palate, most are associated with small, elevated projections on the tongue, called **papillae** (**Figure 24-3**, *A* and *B*).

Tongue papillae are classified by their structure:

Fungiform papillae—large, mushroom-shaped bumps found in the anterior two thirds of the tongue surface; each one contains one or a few taste buds

Circumvallate papillae—huge, dome-shaped bumps that form a transverse row near the back of the tongue surface; each one contains thousands of taste buds

Foliate papillae—red, leaflike ridges of mucosa on the lateral edges of the posterior tongue surface; each contains about a hundred or so taste buds

Filiform papillae—bumps with tiny, threadlike projections; these papillae are scattered among the fungiform papillae; they do not contain taste buds but allow us to experience food texture and "feel"

Although the different varieties of papillae are distributed differently across the tongue surface, no regional difference exists regarding where a particular taste can be detected. For example, the long-held belief that bitter taste was localized at the back of the tongue with its high concentration of circumvallate papillae (see **Figure 24-3**, *A*) or that sweet taste is detected best at the tip of the tongue is simply not true. No tongue or taste "map" accurately indicates

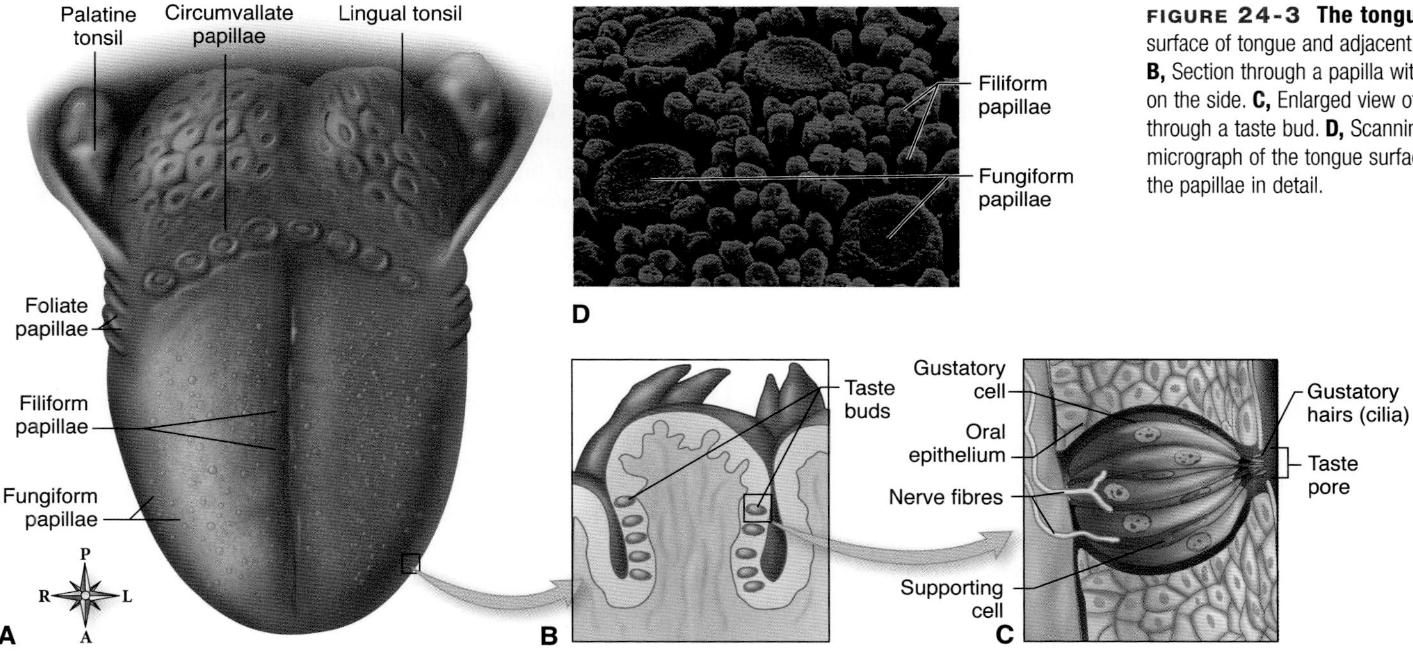

FIGURE 24-3 The tongue. A, Dorsal surface of tongue and adjacent structures. **B,** Section through a papilla with taste buds on the side. **C,** Enlarged view of a section through a taste bud. **D,** Scanning electron micrograph of the tongue surface showing the papillae in detail.

regional areas of particular sensitivity to different tastes. All tastes can be detected in all areas of the tongue that contain taste buds.

Taste buds house the chemoreceptors responsible for taste. They are stimulated by chemicals, called *tastants,* dissolved in the saliva. Each taste bud is like a banana cluster that contains 50 to 125 of these chemoreceptors, called **gustatory cells,** which are surrounded by a supportive epithelial cell capsule. Cilia, here called *gustatory hairs,* extend from each of the gustatory cells and project into an opening called the *taste pore,* which is bathed in saliva (see **Figure 24-3**, C).

The sense of taste depends on the creation of a receptor potential in gustatory cells. Only then can an action potential be generated and a nerve impulse relayed to the brain for interpretation. Generation of a receptor potential begins when G-protein–coupled receptors (GPCRs) or ion channels in the plasma membranes of gustatory hairs bind to taste-producing chemicals (tastants) dissolved or suspended in the saliva. See **Figure 19-17** (p. 425) to review GPCRs and **Figure 19-16** (p. 424) to review ion channels acting as receptors. The nature and concentration of the tastants that bind to either the receptor sites or ion channels determine how fast the receptor potential is generated.

Taste cells appear similar structurally, and all of them can respond at least in some degree to most tastants. Each taste receptor cell, however, responds most effectively to only one of five "primary" taste sensations: sour, sweet, bitter, umami (savoury), and salty. The *labelled-line model,* shown in **Figure 24-4**, holds that our brain can determine which taste we are detecting by the fact that signals from different types of receptors are conducted along different lines or neural pathways. Our ability to experience a larger variety of tastes results from combinations of the five primary sensations.

The exact mechanism by which a chemical tastant binds to a particular receptor site or ion channel on a gustatory hair is unknown. Chemical structure plays a part but is not the only factor involved, because substances that are very different chemically, such as artificial sweeteners, chloroform, and table sugar, produce a sweet taste. Some chemical compounds and specific ions, however, are definitely associated with specific tastes. Sour (H^+) and salty (Na^+) tastes activate ion channels, whereas sweet, umami, and bitter tastes result from stimulation of receptor sites. As chemoreceptors, the taste buds, like olfactory receptors, tend to be quite sensitive initially but fatigue easily. Very low levels of taste-producing chemicals are required to generate a receptor potential. However, adaptation often begins within a few seconds after a taste sensation is first noticed and is generally complete in a few minutes.

The adaptive value of our sense of taste is obvious: Taste allows us to chemically test our food before swallowing it. We can then selectively eat salty foods when our body is low in sodium, or avoid foods that contain too much sodium. We can determine which foods are high in sugars when they taste sweet. Foods with a savoury, or umami, taste are likely to be high in amino acids. Umami receptors detect *L-glutamate,* a form of the common amino acid

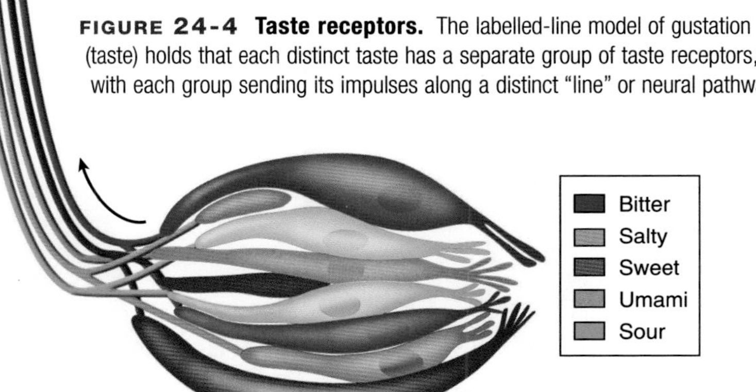

FIGURE 24-4 Taste receptors. The labelled-line model of gustation (taste) holds that each distinct taste has a separate group of taste receptors, with each group sending its impulses along a distinct "line" or neural pathway.

glutamic acid released from proteins in cooked, fermented, and ripened foods. Bitter tastes, to which we have a natural aversion if strong, signal a variety of toxins and other druglike chemicals such as caffeine that are sometimes present in plants. Research shows that there may be additional taste modalities such as "metallic" taste, or even "water" taste.

CONNECT IT!

We experience food by more sensations than just taste—review how other senses combine to give us a complete experience of food in ***Sensing Food*** online at ***Connect It!***

NEURAL PATHWAY FOR TASTE

The taste sensation begins with creation of a receptor potential in the gustatory cells of a taste bud. The generation and propagation of an action potential, or nerve impulse, then transmits the sensory input to the brain.

Nerve impulses generated in the anterior two thirds of the tongue travel over the facial nerve (cranial nerve [CN] VII), whereas those generated from the posterior one third are conducted by fibres of the glossopharyngeal nerve (CN IX). A third cranial nerve, the vagus nerve (CN X), plays a minor role in taste. It contains a few fibres that carry taste sensation from a limited number of taste buds located in the walls of the pharynx and on the epiglottis.

All three cranial nerves carry impulses into the medulla oblongata. The fact that, unlike any other special sense, taste has several different pathways to the brain is evidence that taste information is very important for survival. Once taste information is processed in the medulla, relays then carry the impulses into the thalamus and then into the taste, or gustatory, area of the cerebral cortex in the parietal lobe of the brain (see **Figure 24-2**).

We generally think of taste in terms of the "primary" sensations of sour, sweet, bitter, umami, and salty (and perhaps metallic). However, touch, texture, and temperature are also involved in taste and whether we sense it as pleasant, neutral, or unpleasant. Take the sensation of *flavour* as an example. Flavour, as the term is normally used, is a combined sense of smell, taste, and the so-called *trigeminal senses* (mediated by CN V) that detect irritants, textures, and other characteristics present in spices and most other foods. When we breathe out as we are chewing or savouring food in the mouth, olfactory receptors are triggered at the same time as receptors in taste buds and the rest of the oral mucosa. This information is integrated in the brain, and we sense the combination of smells, tastes, heat (as in pepper), cold (as in mint), and texture as a single, complex flavour experience.

***Quick* CHECK**

1. List the special senses.
2. Discuss how a receptor potential is generated in olfactory cells.
3. Discuss how a receptor potential is generated in gustatory cells.
4. Trace the path of a nervous impulse carrying (1) olfactory and (2) gustatory sense information from its point of origin to that area of the brain where interpretation occurs.
5. List the five "primary" taste sensations.
6. Locate on the tongue where taste buds are detected.

SENSES OF HEARING AND BALANCE

The ear has dual sensory functions. In addition to its role in hearing, it also functions as the sense organ of balance, or equilibrium. The stimulation, or "trigger", responsible for hearing and balance involves activation of mechanoreceptors called *hair cells.* Sound waves and fluid movement are the physical forces that act on hair cells to generate receptor potentials and then nerve impulses, which are eventually perceived in the brain as sound or balance. The ear is divided into three anatomical parts: **external ear, middle ear,** and **inner ear** (**Figure 24-5** and **Figure 24-6**).

STRUCTURE OF THE EAR

The structures illustrated in **Figure 24-6** are not drawn to scale. Instead, the smaller components of the middle and inner ear are enlarged so that they can be more easily identified. In addition, this

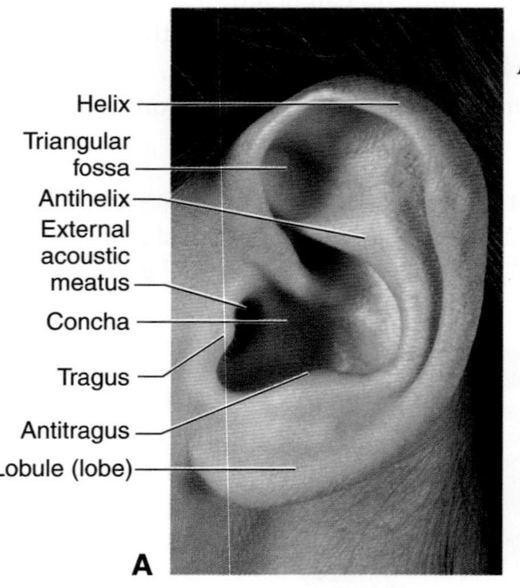

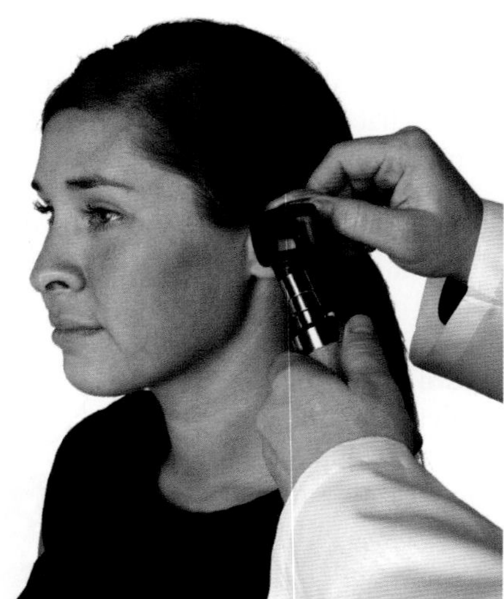

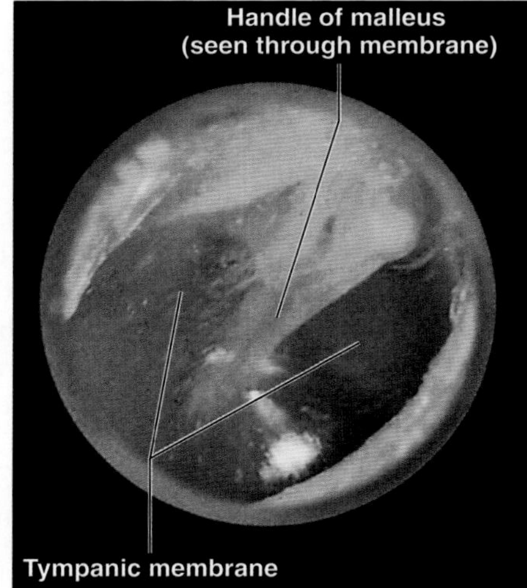

FIGURE 24-5 Examining the external ear. A, Anatomical structures of the auricle (external ear). **B,** Using a lighted otoscope to view the external ear canal and tympanic membrane. **C,** Note the translucent, pearly-grey appearance of a normal tympanic membrane (with a bit of white glare from the otoscope light in the lower right). The "handle" of the malleus can be seen attaching near the centre of the inner surface of the membrane.

type of artistic rendering makes it easier to see the anatomical relationships of these tiny elements to one another and to adjacent structures.

External Ear

The external ear has two divisions: the *auricle* or *pinna* and the *external acoustic meatus* (ear canal). The auricle is the visible appendage on the side of the head surrounding the opening of the external acoustic meatus. A number of anatomical components of the auricle are identified in **Figure 24-5**.

Because it lies exposed against the bony surface of the skull, the auricle is often injured by blunt trauma. Bruising may then cause an accumulation of blood and tissue fluid between the skin and underlying cartilage. If bruising is left untreated, the dramatic swelling of "cauliflower ear" may develop and become permanent. The sun-exposed auricle, especially the tops of the helix, is also a common site for development of skin cancer, often squamous cell carcinoma (see Chapter 10).

The *lobule* or lobe of the auricle is a common site of piercing for cosmetic reasons. Piercings of the cartilage in other areas of the auricle carry a higher risk of infection and slower healing because the blood supply is far less than in the lobule.

Note in **Figure 24-5** that the *tragus* of the auricle is located just in front of the opening to the ear in adults. This external acoustic meatus is a canal about 3 cm long. Initially this canal slants upward a bit and then curves downward before travelling into the temporal bone in an inward and forward direction. It ends at the **tympanic membrane,** or **eardrum,** which stretches across the inner end of the canal, separating it from the middle ear.

A lighted instrument called an **otoscope** is used to examine the external ear canal and outer surface of the tympanic membrane (see **Figure 24-5**, *B*). Changes in the appearance of the ear canal and tympanic membrane can provide a skilled observer with a great deal of information. For example, middle ear infection, called **otitis media,** will cause the eardrum to become red and inflamed and to bulge outward into the ear canal as pus and other fluids accumulate in the middle ear (see Mechanisms of Disease, p. 553). Accumulation of the waxlike substance *cerumen* (see **Figure 24-27** on p. 554), which is secreted by modified sweat glands in the auditory canal, may cause pain and temporary deafness. It is easily identified during otoscopic examination of the ear canal.

Middle Ear

The middle ear (tympanic cavity), a tiny epithelial-lined cavity hollowed out of the temporal bone, contains the three **auditory ossicles:** the *malleus, incus,* and *stapes* (see **Figure 24-6**). The names of these very small bones describe their shapes (hammer, anvil, stirrup). The "handle" of the malleus is attached to the inner surface of the tympanic membrane, whereas the "head" attaches to the incus, which in turn attaches to the stapes. Note in **Figure 24-6** that tiny ligaments and muscles connect to the ossicles to help stabilize them and reflexively dampen vibrations when sounds are dangerously loud.

There are several openings into the middle ear cavity: one from the external acoustic meatus, covered with the tympanic membrane; two into the internal ear, the **oval window** (into which the stapes fits) and the **round window,** which is covered by a membrane; and one into the auditory (eustachian) tube.

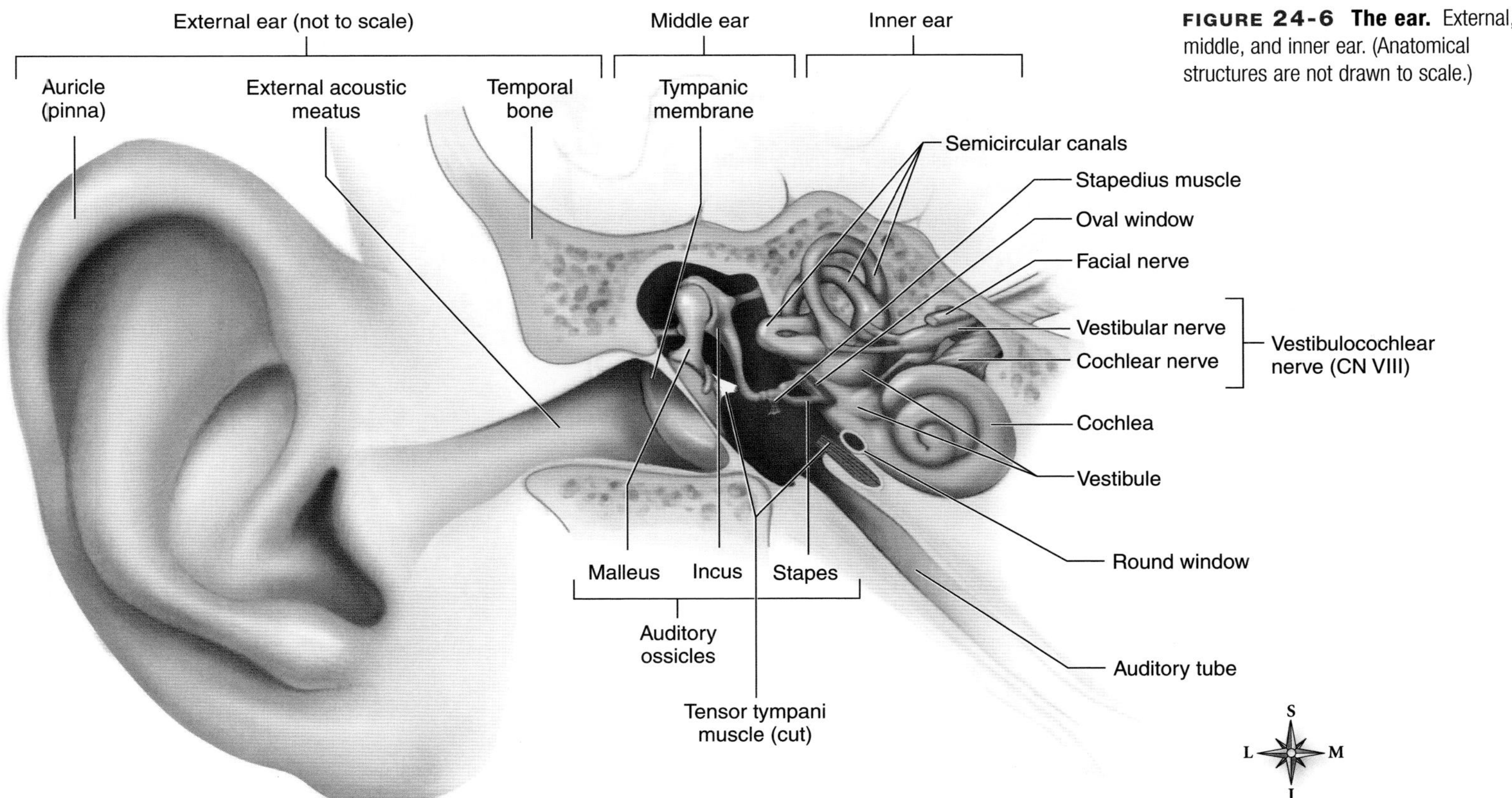

FIGURE 24-6 The ear. External, middle, and inner ear. (Anatomical structures are not drawn to scale.)

Posteriorly the middle ear cavity is continuous with numerous mastoid air spaces in the temporal bone. The clinical importance of these middle ear openings is that they provide routes through which infection can travel. Head colds, for example, especially in children, may lead to middle ear or mastoid infections by way of the nasopharynx–auditory tube, middle ear–mastoid path.

The **auditory tube,** or **eustachian tube,** is composed partly of bone and partly of cartilage and fibrous tissue and is lined with mucosa. It extends downward, forward, and inward from the middle ear cavity to the nasopharynx, or pharyngotympanic tube (the part of the throat behind the nose).

The auditory tube serves a useful function: It makes possible equalization of pressure against inner and outer surfaces of the tympanic membrane and therefore prevents membrane rupture and the discomfort that marked pressure differences produce. The way the auditory tube equalizes tympanic membrane pressure is this: When you swallow or yawn, air spreads rapidly through the open tube. Atmospheric pressure then presses against the inner surface of the tympanic membrane. Because atmospheric pressure is continually exerted against its outer surface, the pressures are equal.

In a variation of a procedure called the *Valsalva manoeuvre*, one can close the mouth, pinch the nose shut, and exhale moderately to push air into the auditory tube if needed to equalize pressure on the tympanic membrane. This move is done as a last resort if swallowing or yawning fails to equalize pressures.

Inner Ear

The inner ear is also called the **labyrinth** because of its complicated shape. It consists of two main parts, a bony labyrinth and, inside this, a membranous labyrinth. The bony labyrinth consists of three parts: the *vestibule, cochlea,* and *semicircular canals* (**Figure 24-7**). The membranous labyrinth consists of the *utricle* and *saccule* inside the vestibule, the *cochlear duct* inside the cochlea, and the membranous *semicircular ducts* inside the bony ones. The vestibule (containing the membranous utricle and saccule) and the semicircular canals (and membranous ducts) are involved in balance; the cochlea (and membranous cochlear duct) is involved in hearing.

The term **endolymph** is used to describe the clear and potassium-rich fluid that fills the membranous labyrinth. **Perilymph,** a fluid similar to cerebrospinal fluid, surrounds the membranous labyrinth and therefore fills the space between this membranous tunnel and its contents and the bony walls that surround it (see **Figure 24-7**).

The Process of Hearing

Now that we have outlined the basic organization of the ear, we are ready to explore the first of the senses mediated by the ear: hearing. The sensors for sound are within the cochlea, so we begin there.

Cochlea and Cochlear Duct

The word *cochlea,* which means "snail", describes the outer appearance of this part of the bony labyrinth. When sectioned, the cochlea resembles a tube wound spirally around a cone-shaped core of bone, the *modiolus.* The modiolus houses the spiral ganglion, which consists of cell bodies of the first sensory neurons in the auditory relay.

Inside the cochlea lies the membranous *cochlear duct*—the only part of the internal ear concerned with hearing. This structure is shaped like a somewhat triangular tube. It forms a shelf across the inside of the bony cochlea, dividing it into upper and lower sections all along its winding course (see **Figure 24-7**). The upper section (above the cochlear duct) is called the *scala vestibuli* (vestibular duct), whereas the lower section below the cochlear duct is called the *scala tympani* (tympanic duct). The roof of the cochlear duct is

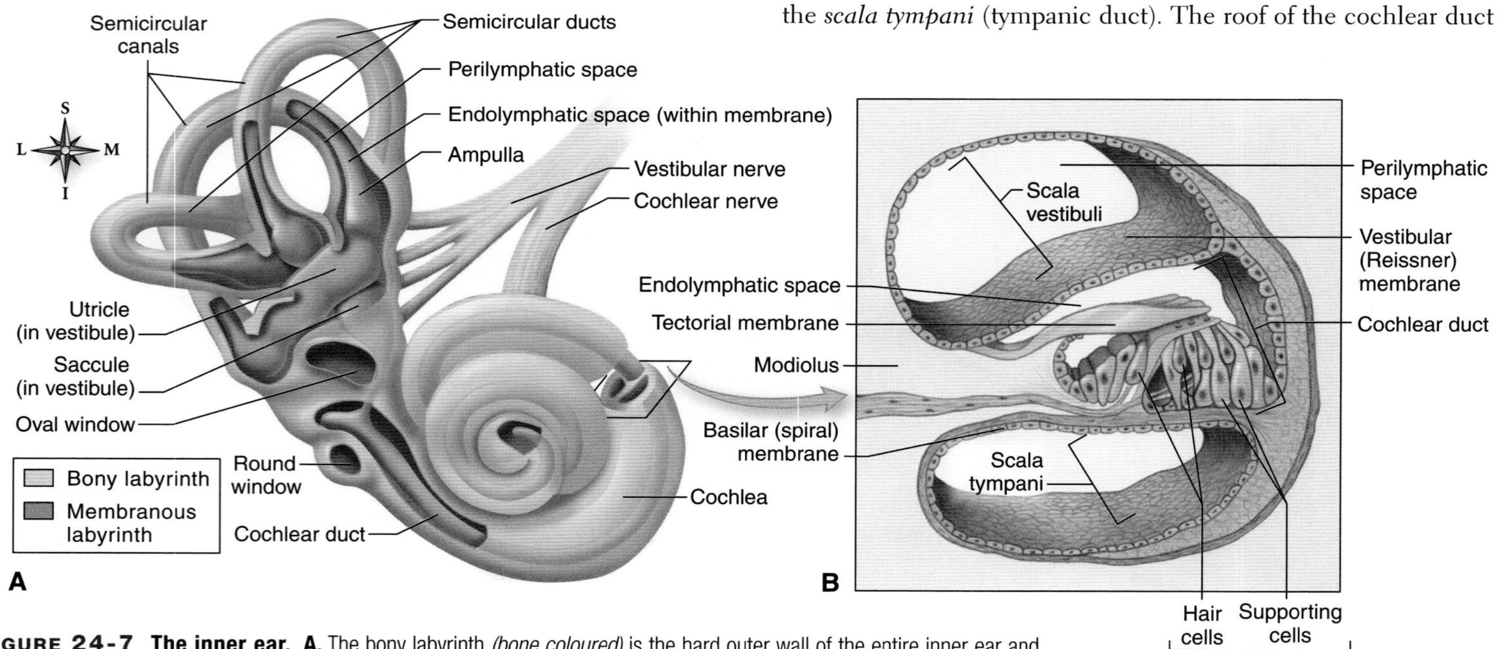

FIGURE 24-7 The inner ear. A, The bony labyrinth *(bone coloured)* is the hard outer wall of the entire inner ear and includes semicircular canals, vestibule, and cochlea. Within the bony labyrinth is the membranous labyrinth *(purple),* which is surrounded by perilymph and filled with endolymph. Each ampulla in the vestibule contains a crista ampullaris that detects changes in head position and sends sensory impulses through the vestibular nerve to the brain. **B,** The inset shows a section of the membranous cochlea. Hair cells in the organ of Corti (spiral organ) detect sound and send the information through the cochlear nerve. The vestibular and cochlear nerves join to form the eighth cranial nerve.

known as the **vestibular membrane** *(Reissner membrane)*. The **basilar membrane** is located on the floor of the cochlear duct. It is also called the *spiral membrane* and is supported by bony and fibrous projections from the wall of the cochlea.

Perilymph fills the scala vestibuli and scala tympani, and endolymph fills the cochlear duct.

The hearing sense organ, named the **organ of Corti,** rests on the basilar membrane throughout the entire length of the cochlear duct. The organ of Corti is also called the *spiral organ* because of its spiraling curl within the cochlea. The structure of the organ of Corti consists of supporting cells, as well as important hair cells that project into the endolymph and are topped by an adherent gelatinous membrane called the **tectorial membrane.**

Dendrites of the sensory neurons, whose cell bodies lie in the spiral ganglion in the modiolus, have their beginnings around the bases of the inner row of ciliated hair cells of the organ of Corti. Sound vibrations bend the cilia, which causes the membrane potential to change—thus transducing sound into a neural signal. Axons of these neurons extend to form the cochlear nerve (a branch of the eighth cranial nerve) to the brain. They conduct impulses that produce the sensation of hearing.

The outer rows of hair cells respond to vibrations by shortening or elongating in ways that amplify the vibrations—making the ear more sensitive. When sounds are dangerously loud, reflexive neural signals to the outer hair cells cause them to reduce their amplification activity to protect the delicate inner hair cells.

Perceiving Sound

Sound is created by vibrations that may occur in air, fluid, or solid material. When we speak, for example, the vibrating vocal cords create sound waves by producing vibrations in air passing over them.

Numerous terms are used to describe sound waves. The number of sound waves that occur during a specific time unit (frequency) determines the tone or pitch. Pitch is measured in waves per second, a unit called hertz (Hz). High frequencies may be expressed in thousands of waves per second, or kilohertz (kHz). Human hearing ranges between 20 Hz–20 kHz, but is most sensitive between 1–4 kHz. The height, or amplitude, of a sound wave determines its perceived loudness, or volume. Volume is measured in logarithmic units called decibels (dB). Many humans can hear pitches around 3 kHz as low as 0 dB, but pitches above and below 3 kHz require volumes that range up to 60 dB or higher. Sounds louder than 85 dB, if sustained, can cause permanent hearing damage. Our ability to hear sound waves depends in part on volume, pitch, and other acoustic properties. Sound waves must be of sufficient amplitude to initiate movement of the tympanic membrane and have a frequency that is capable of stimulating the hair cells in the organ of Corti at some point along the basilar membrane.

The basilar membrane is not the same width and thickness throughout its length. Because of this, different frequencies of sound will cause the basilar membrane to vibrate and bulge upward at different places along its length. Two bulges are shown in **Figure 24-8**, A.

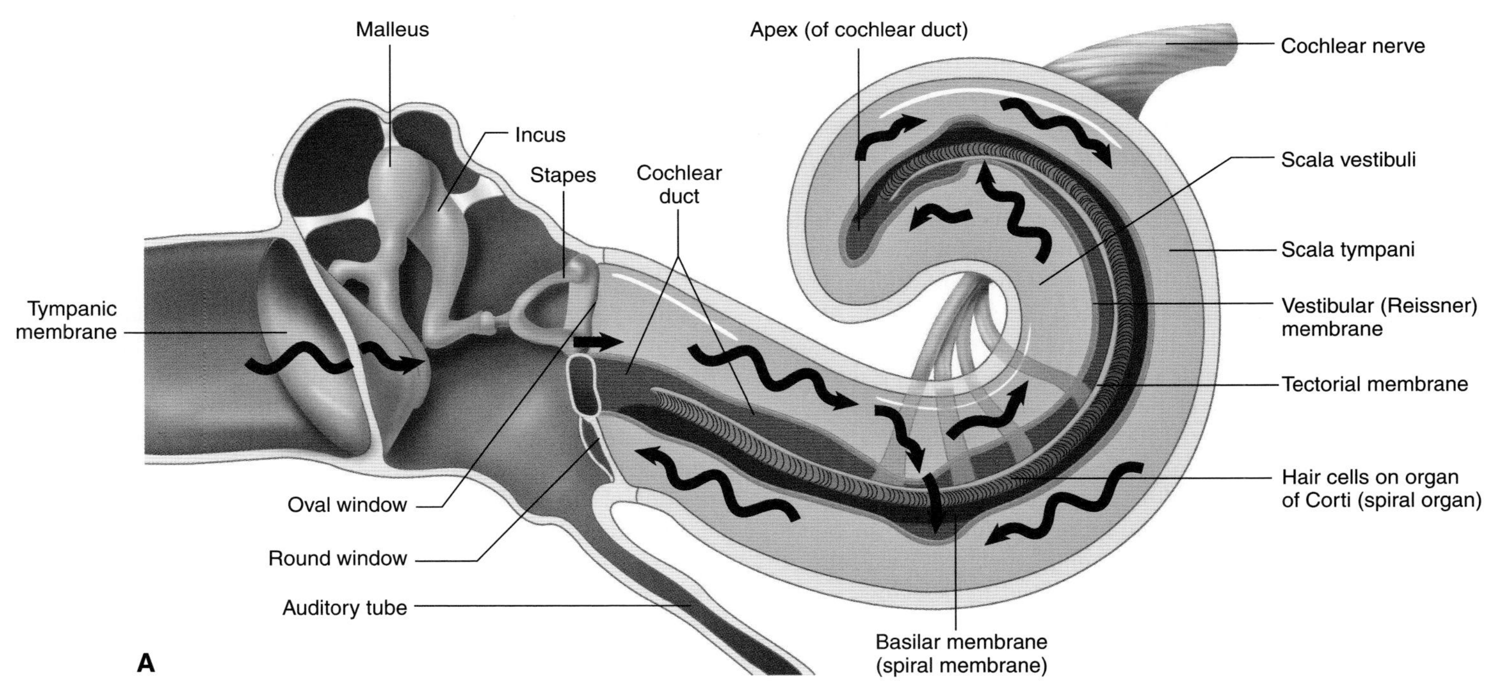

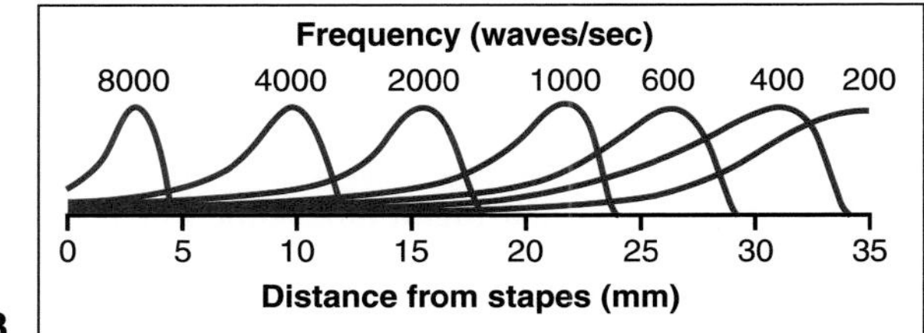

FIGURE 24-8 Effect of sound waves on cochlear structures. A, Sound waves strike the tympanic membrane and cause it to vibrate. This causes the membrane of the oval window to vibrate, which causes the perilymph in the bony labyrinth of the cochlea and the endolymph in the membranous labyrinth of the cochlea, or cochlear duct, to move. This movement of endolymph causes the basilar membrane (spiral membrane) to vibrate, which in turn stimulates hair cells on the organ of Corti (spiral organ) to transmit nerve impulses along the cochlear nerve. Eventually, nerve impulses reach the auditory cortex and are interpreted as sound. **B,** High-frequency (high-pitch) waves stimulate hair cells nearer the stapes (oval window) and low-frequency (low-pitch) waves stimulate hair cells nearer the distal end of the cochlea. The location of peak stimulation of the hair cells allows the brain to interpret the pitch of the sound.

High-frequency sound waves cause the narrow portion of the basilar membrane near the oval window to vibrate, whereas low frequencies vibrate the membrane near the apex of the cochlea, where it is considerably wider and thicker (**Figure 24-8**, *B*). This ability of sound waves of differing frequency to vibrate and cause a bulge, or displacement, of the basilar membrane at differing points along its length explains how specific groups of hair cells respond to specific frequencies of sound. When a particular portion of the basilar membrane bulges upward, the cilia on hair cells attached to that particular area are stimulated, and ultimately, sound of a particular pitch is perceived.

Our perception of different degrees of loudness of the same sound is determined by the amplitude, or movement, of the basilar membrane at any particular point along its length. The higher the upward bulge, the more the cilia on the attached hair cells are bent or stimulated. This causes an increase in perceived loudness. The moving wave of perilymph caused by upward displacement of the basilar membrane is soon dampened as it moves through the cochlea.

Hearing results from stimulation of the auditory area of the cerebral cortex. First, however, sound waves must be projected through air, bone, and fluid to stimulate nerve endings and set up impulse conduction over nerve fibres.

CONNECT IT!

Check out ***Cochlear Implants*** online at ***Connect It!***

Pathway of Sound Waves

Sound waves in the air enter the external auditory canal with aid from the pinna. At the inner end of the canal, they strike against the tympanic membrane, causing it to vibrate. Vibrations of the tympanic membrane move the malleus, whose handle attaches to the membrane. The head of the malleus attaches to the incus, and the incus attaches to the stapes. So when the malleus vibrates, it moves the incus, which moves the stapes against the oval window into which it fits so precisely. At this point, fluid conduction of sound waves begins. When the stapes moves against the oval window, pressure is exerted inward into the perilymph in the scala vestibuli of the cochlea. This starts a "ripple" in the perilymph that is transmitted through the vestibular membrane (the roof of the cochlear duct) to endolymph inside the duct and then to the organ of Corti and to the basilar membrane that supports the organ of Corti and forms the floor of the cochlear duct. From the basilar membrane the ripple is next transmitted to and through the perilymph in the scala tympani and finally expends itself against the round window—like an ocean wave as it breaks against the shore, but on a much reduced scale.

Figure 24-8 summarizes the steps involved in detecting sound stimuli in the ear.

Neural Pathway of Hearing

Dendrites of neurons whose cell bodies lie in the spiral ganglion and whose axons make up the cochlear nerve terminate around the bases of the hair cells of the organ of Corti, and the tectorial membrane adheres to their upper surfaces. The movement of the hair cells against the adherent tectorial membrane somehow stimulates these dendrites and initiates impulse conduction by the cochlear nerve to the brainstem. Before reaching the auditory area of the temporal lobe, impulses pass through "relay stations" in nuclei in the medulla, pons, midbrain, and thalamus.

Quick **CHECK**

7. List the three anatomical divisions of the ear.
8. Identify the three auditory ossicles.
9. Name the divisions of both the membranous and bony labyrinths.
10. Name the specific sense organ responsible for hearing.

BALANCE

The sense organs involved in the sense of balance, or **equilibrium,** are found in the vestibule and semicircular canals. The sense organs located in the utricle and saccule function in **static equilibrium**—a function needed to sense the position of the head relative to gravity or to sense acceleration or deceleration of the body, such as would occur when seated motionless in a vehicle that was increasing or decreasing in speed. The sense organs associated with the semicircular ducts function in **dynamic equilibrium**—a function needed to maintain balance when the head or body itself is rotated or suddenly moved.

Vestibule and Semicircular Canals

The vestibule constitutes the central section of the bony labyrinth. Look again at **Figure 24-7**, *A*. Note that the bony labyrinth opens into the oval and round windows from the middle ear, as well as the three semicircular canals of the internal ear. The utricle and saccule are the membranous structures within the vestibule. Both have walls of simple cuboidal epithelium and are filled with endolymph.

Three semicircular canals, each in a plane approximately at right angles to the others, are found in each temporal bone (see **Figure 24-7**, *A*). Within the bony semicircular canals and separated from them by perilymph are the membranous semicircular ducts. Each contains endolymph and connects with the utricle inside the bony vestibule. Near its junction with the utricle each canal enlarges into an *ampulla*.

Static Equilibrium

A small patchlike strip of epithelium called the **macula** is found within both the utricle and saccule (**Figure 24-9**, *A*). It is sensory epithelium containing receptor hair cells and supporting cells covered with a gelatinous matrix. Movements of the macula provide information related to head position or acceleration. Action potentials are generated by movement of the hair cells, which occurs when the position of the head relative to gravity changes.

Otoliths—tiny "ear stones" composed of protein and calcium carbonate—are located within the matrix of the macula (**Figure 24-9**, *B*). Now note the relative positions of the utricular and saccular maculae in **Figure 24-9**, *A*. The two maculae are oriented almost at right angles to each other: the one in the utricle is parallel to the base of the skull, and the one in the saccule is perpendicular.

Changing the position of the head produces a change in the amount of pressure on the otolith-weighted matrix, which, in turn, stimulates the hair cells (**Figure 24-9**, *C* and *D*). This stimulates the adjacent receptors of the vestibular nerve. Its fibres conduct impulses to the brain that produce a sense of the position of the head and also a sensation of a change in the pull of gravity—for example, a sensation of acceleration.

In addition, stimulation of the macula evokes *righting reflexes*, muscular responses to restore the body and its parts to their normal

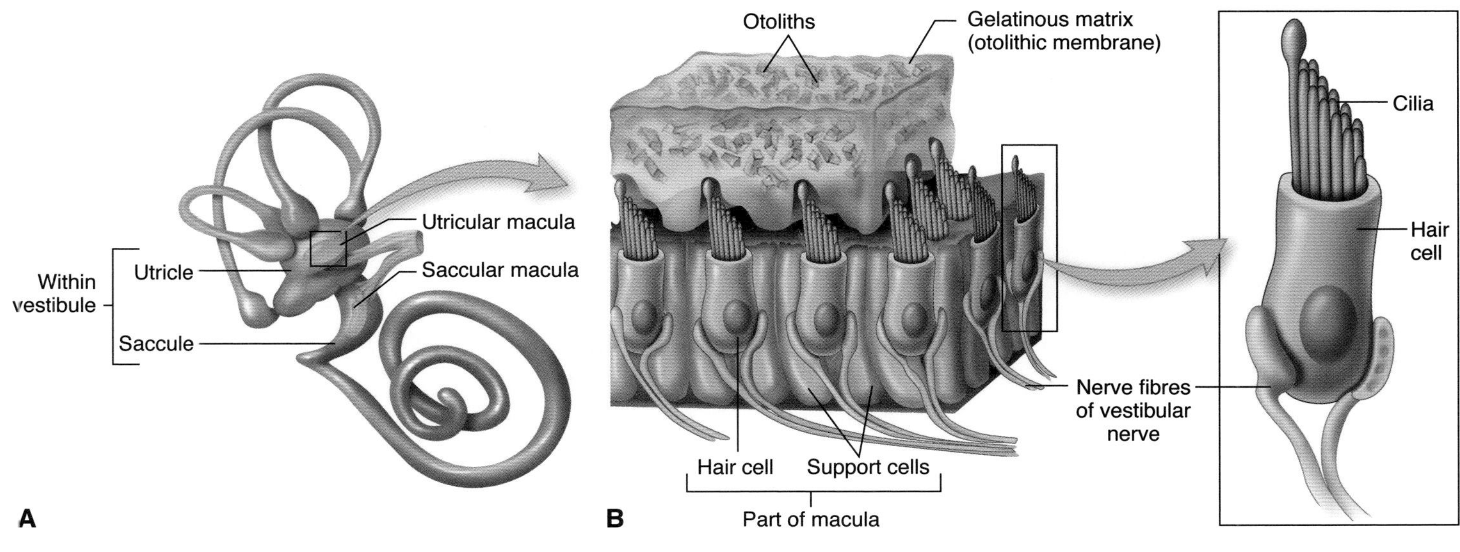

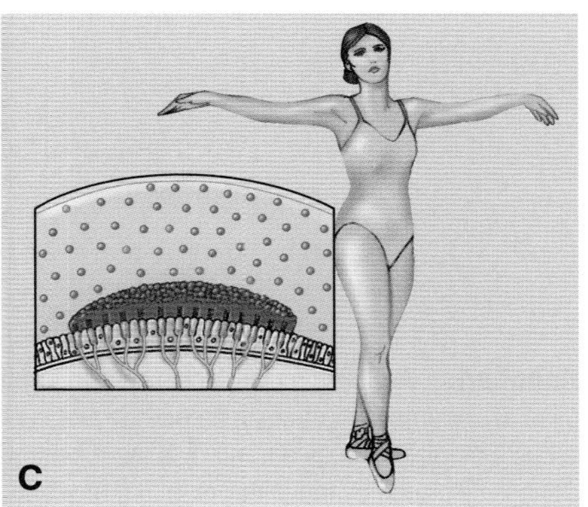

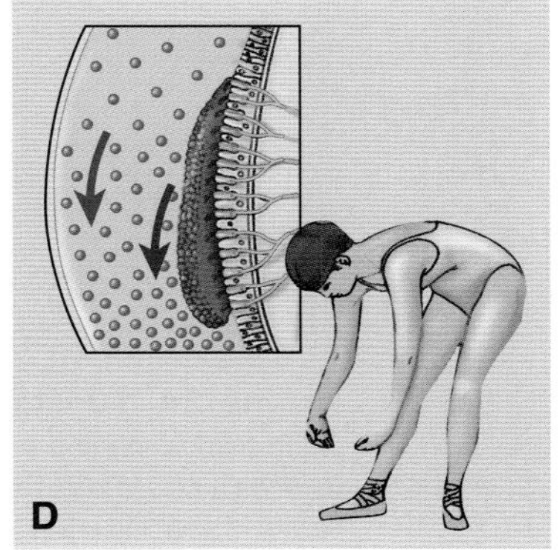

FIGURE 24-9 The macula. A, Structure of vestibule showing placement of utricular and saccular maculae. **B,** Section of macula showing otoliths. **C,** Macula stationary in upright position. **D,** Macula displaced by gravity as person bends over.

position when they have been displaced. Impulses from proprioceptors and from the eyes also activate righting reflexes. Interruption of the vestibular, visual, or proprioceptive impulses that initiate these reflexes may cause disturbances of equilibrium, nausea, vomiting, and other symptoms.

Dynamic Equilibrium

Dynamic equilibrium depends on the functioning of the **crista ampullaris,** located in the ampulla of each semicircular duct. It is also called the *ampullary crest.* This unique structure is a form of sensory epithelium that is similar in many ways to the maculae. Each ridgelike crista is dotted with many hair cells, each with its processes embedded in a gelatinous flap called the **cupula** (**Figure 24-10**, *A* and *B*).

The cupula is not weighted with otoliths and does not respond to the pull of gravity. It serves, instead, much like a float that moves with the flow of endolymph in the semicircular ducts. Like the maculae, the semicircular ducts are placed nearly at right angles to each other. This arrangement enables detection of movement in all directions. As the cupula moves, it bends the hairs embedded in it, producing first a receptor and then an action potential that passes through the vestibular portion of the eighth cranial nerve to the medulla oblongata and, from there, to other areas of the brain and spinal cord for interpretation, integration, and response.

When a person spins (**Figure 24-10**, *C* and *D*), the semicircular ducts move with the body, but inertia keeps the endolymph in them from moving at the same rate. The cupula therefore moves in a direction opposite to head movement until after the initial movement stops. Dynamic equilibrium is thus able to detect changes in both the direction and the rate at which movement occurs.

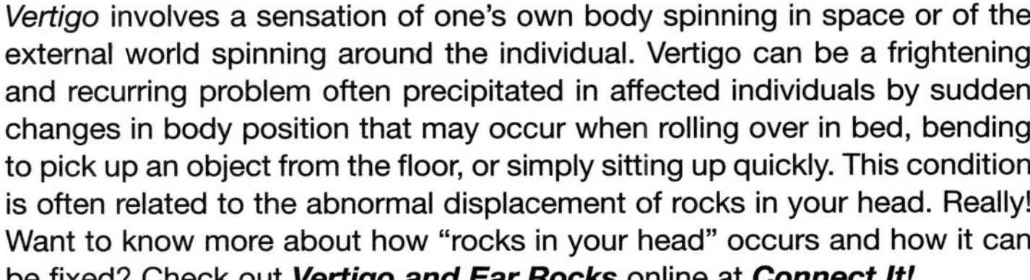

CONNECT IT!

Vertigo involves a sensation of one's own body spinning in space or of the external world spinning around the individual. Vertigo can be a frightening and recurring problem often precipitated in affected individuals by sudden changes in body position that may occur when rolling over in bed, bending to pick up an object from the floor, or simply sitting up quickly. This condition is often related to the abnormal displacement of rocks in your head. Really! Want to know more about how "rocks in your head" occurs and how it can be fixed? Check out ***Vertigo and Ear Rocks*** online at ***Connect It!***

SENSE OF VISION

One of the most important sensations involved in maintaining homeostasis is vision, and the eye is the body's sense organ for this important function. Vision is a truly remarkable sensory ability and is used to guide almost all that we do. It allows us to activate and respond to a multitude of warning systems and provides us with almost

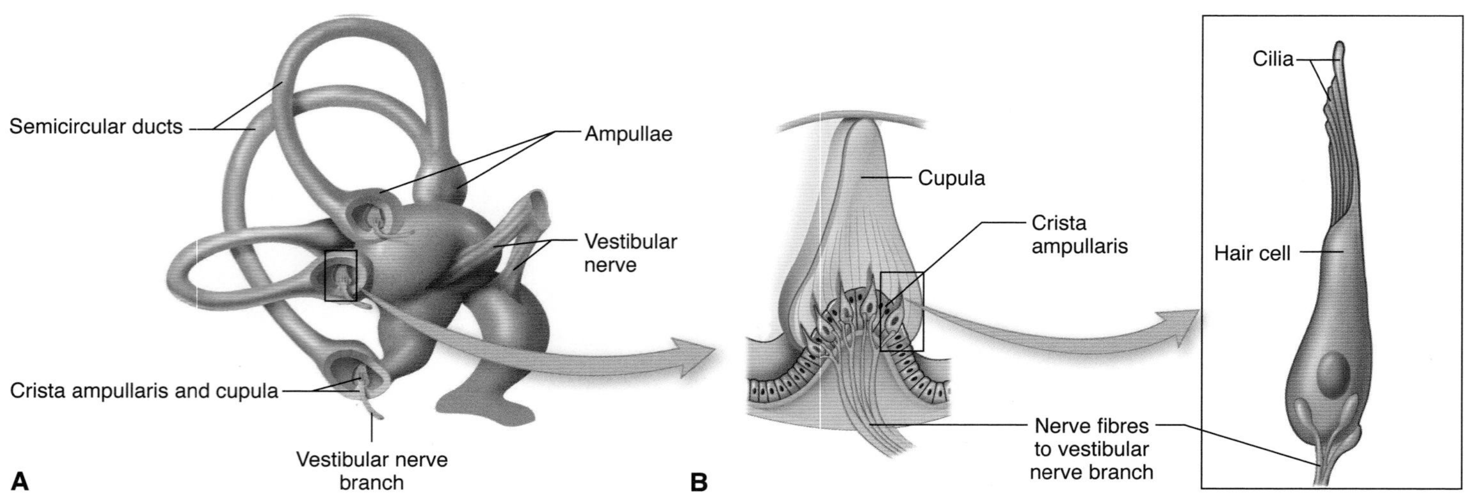

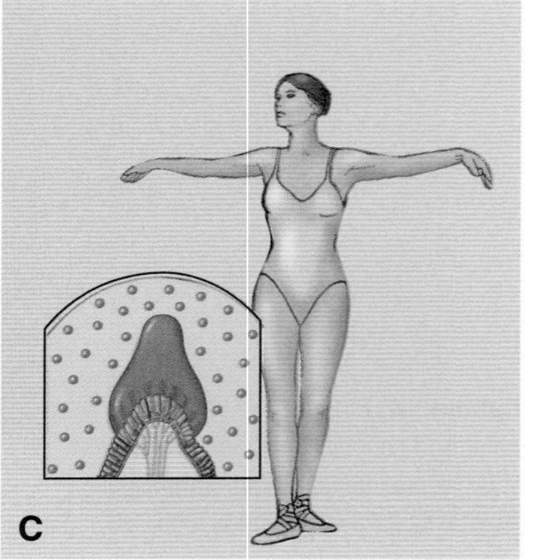

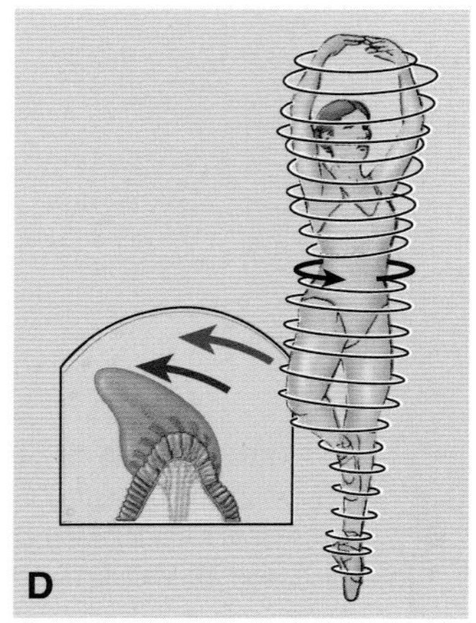

FIGURE 24-10 Crista ampullaris. A, Semicircular ducts showing location of the crista ampullaris in ampullae. **B,** Enlargement of crista ampullaris and cupula. **C,** When a person is at rest, the crista ampullaris does not move. **D,** As a person begins to spin, the crista ampullaris is displaced by the endolymph in a direction opposite to the direction of spin.

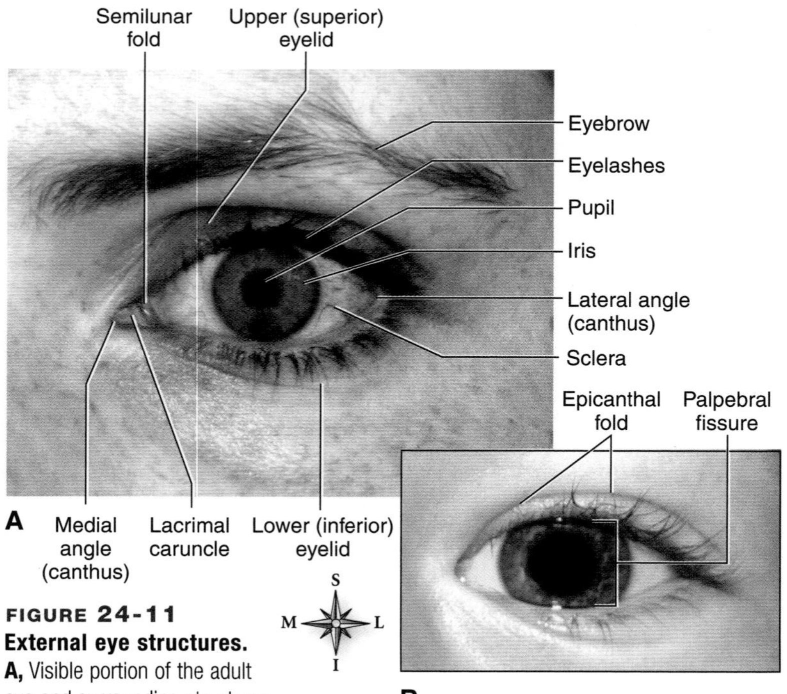

FIGURE 24-11 External eye structures. **A,** Visible portion of the adult eye and surrounding structures. **B,** Eye structures in a toddler.

constant feedback on various types of form and movement in an ever-changing environment. It is the eye that uses as a stimulus the pervasive nature of light to convert stored photochemical energy into nervous impulses that are ultimately interpreted by the brain as sight.

The study of vision and the visual apparatus is an important area of ongoing research and clinical interest. Clinical **ophthalmology** is a medical practice specialty concerned with pathological conditions of the eye and the diagnosis and treatment of eye disorders. A number of allied health professionals, including optometrists, optical assistants, laboratory technicians, and dispensing opticians, work closely with ophthalmologists in administrative, research, and clinical environments.

We will first discuss the various structures of the eye and then move on to the ways in which these structures enable the eye to control the amount of light entering it and how the conversion to electrical stimuli actually occurs.

Structure of the Eye

External Structures

A number of the anatomical structures of the external eye are visible in **Figure 24-11** and discussed in the sections that follow. Some of these structures, such as the sclera, iris, and pupil, are structures of the eye itself. Accessory structures of the eye discussed here include the eyebrows, eyelashes, eyelids, and lacrimal apparatus.

Eyebrows and Eyelashes

The eyebrows and eyelashes serve a cosmetic purpose and give some protection against foreign objects entering the eyes. They also help shade the eyes and provide at least minimal protection from direct light. Small glands located at the base of the lashes secrete a lubricating fluid. They often become infected, forming a *sty*.

Eyelids

The eyelids, or *palpebrae* (sing., *palpebra*), consist mainly of voluntary muscle and skin, with a border of thick connective tissue at the free edge of each lid, known as the *tarsal plate*. One can feel the tarsal plate as a ridge when turning back the eyelid to remove a foreign object. A lateral and medial angle or *canthus* forms where the superior and inferior eyelids meet. An additional fold of skin over the upper eyelid and medial angle of most infants and toddlers, and many adults, is called an epicanthal fold (**Figure 24-11**, *B*). The epicanthal fold is especially prominent in many people of Asian descent.

Mucous membrane, called *conjunctiva*, lines each lid (**Figure 24-12**). It continues over the surface of the eyeball, where it is modified to give transparency. Inflammation of the conjunctiva (conjunctivitis) is a fairly common infection. Because it produces a pinkish discolouration of the eye's surface, it is called *pink eye* (**Figure 24-13**).

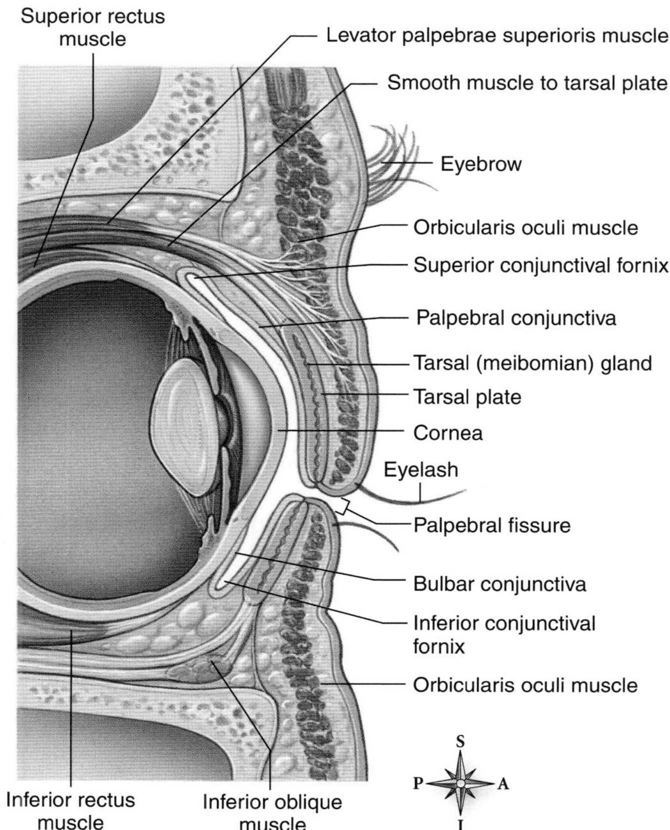

FIGURE 24-12 Accessory structures of the eye. Lateral view with eyelids closed.

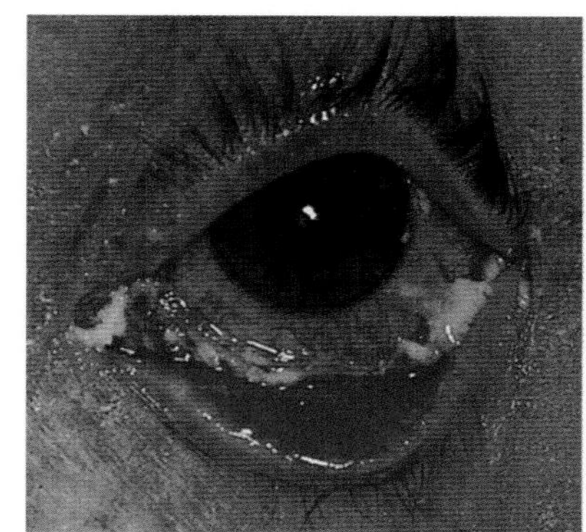

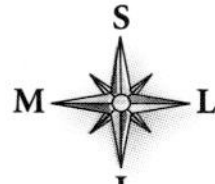

FIGURE 24-13 Acute bacterial conjunctivitis. Note the discharge of pus characteristic of this highly contagious infection of the conjunctiva.

Tiny exocrine glands, called tarsal glands or meibomian glands, at the edge (tarsus) of the eyelid secrete a lipid layer over the mucus of the conjunctiva. This oily coat helps prevent rapid drying of the eye's surface. Degeneration of or damage to the tarsal glands can contribute to "dry eye" conditions.

The opening between the eyelids bears the technical name of *palpebral fissure*. The height of the fissure determines the apparent size of the eyes. If the eyelids are habitually held wide open, the eyes appear large, although the difference in eyeball size among most adults is not significant. Eyes appear small if the upper eyelids droop. Plastic surgeons can correct this common ageing change with an operation called **blepharoplasty.**

Lacrimal Apparatus

The *lacrimal apparatus* consists of the structures that secrete tears and drain them from the surface of the eyeball. They are the lacrimal glands, lacrimal ducts, lacrimal sacs, and nasolacrimal ducts (**Figure 24-14**).

The *lacrimal glands*, comparable in size and shape to a small almond, are located in a depression of the frontal bone at the upper

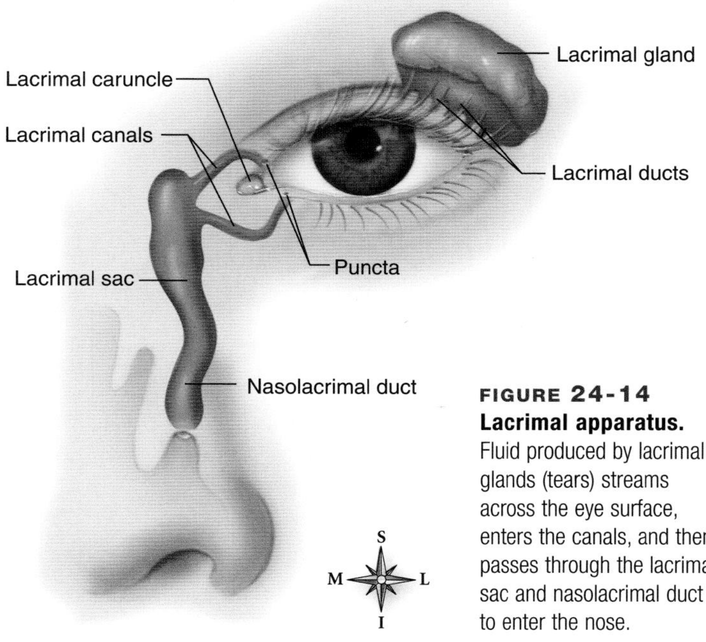

FIGURE 24-14 Lacrimal apparatus. Fluid produced by lacrimal glands (tears) streams across the eye surface, enters the canals, and then passes through the lacrimal sac and nasolacrimal duct to enter the nose.

outer margin of each orbit. Approximately a dozen small ducts lead from each gland, draining the tears onto the conjunctiva at the upper outer corner of the eye.

The *lacrimal canals* are small channels, one above and the other below each *caruncle* (small red body at the inner canthus). They empty into the lacrimal sacs. The openings into the canals are called *puncta* (*sing.*, punctum) and can be seen as two small dots at the medial angle (inner canthus) of the eye. The *lacrimal sacs* are located in a groove in the lacrimal bone. The *nasolacrimal ducts* are small tubes that extend from the lacrimal sac into the inferior meatus of the nose.

All the tear ducts are lined with mucous membrane, an extension of the mucosa that lines the nose. When this membrane becomes inflamed and swollen, the nasolacrimal ducts become plugged, causing the tears to overflow from the eyes instead of draining into the nose as they do normally. Hence when we have a common cold, "watery" eyes add to our discomfort.

Muscles of the Eye

Eye muscles are of two types: *extrinsic* and *intrinsic*.

Extrinsic eye muscles are skeletal muscles that attach to the outside of the eyeball and to the bones of the orbit. They move the eyeball in any desired direction and are, of course, voluntary muscles. Four of them are straight muscles, and two are oblique. Their names describe their positions on the eyeball. They are the superior, inferior, medial, and lateral rectus muscles and superior and inferior oblique muscles (**Figure 24-15**).

Intrinsic eye muscles are smooth, or involuntary, muscles located within the eye. These are called the *iris* and the *ciliary muscle*. Incidentally, the eye is one of only a few organs in the body in which both voluntary and involuntary muscles are found. The iris regulates the size of the pupil. The ciliary muscle controls the shape of the lens. As the ciliary muscle contracts, it releases the suspensory ligament from the backward pull usually exerted on it, and this allows the elastic lens, suspended in the ligament, to bulge, or become more convex. The role of both these muscles in vision is discussed later in this chapter.

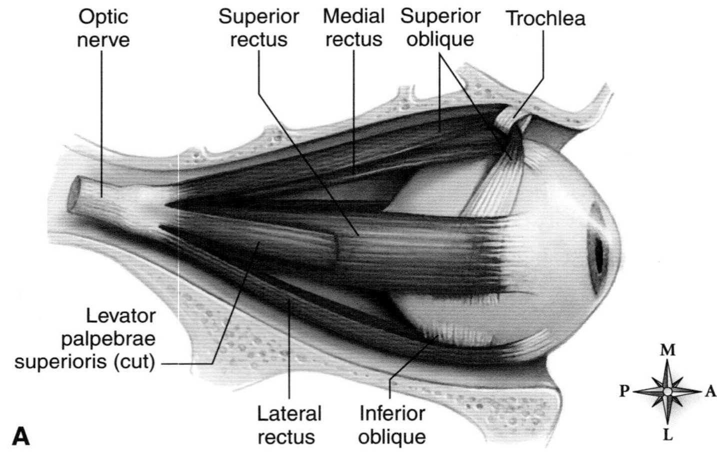

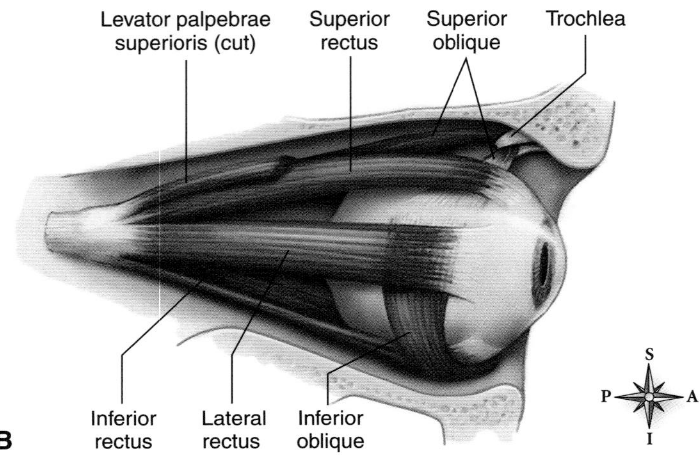

FIGURE 24-15 Extrinsic muscles of the right eye. A, Superior view. **B,** Lateral view.

Layers of the Eyeball

Approximately five sixths of the eyeball, a spherelike globe about 22 to 25 mm in diameter, lies recessed in and is protected by the bony orbit or eye socket. Only the small anterior surface of the eyeball is exposed. Three layers of tissues compose the eyeball. From the outside in, the following three layers of tissues and their component parts or regions form the eyeball.

1. Fibrous layer
   - Sclera
   - Cornea
2. Vascular layer
   - Choroid
   - Ciliary body
   - Iris
3. Inner layer
   - Retina
   - Optic nerve
   - Retinal blood vessels

Refer to **Figure 24-16** as you explore the following sections.

Fibrous Layer

The outer coat of the eyeball is the *fibrous layer*. The anterior portion of the fibrous layer is called the **cornea** and lies over the coloured part of the eye, the *iris* (see **Figures 24-11** and **24-16**). The cornea is transparent, whereas the rest of the fibrous coat—or **sclera**—is white and opaque. This fact explains why the sclera is usually spoken of as the "white" of the eye. The white colour comes from dense arrangements of collagen bundles alternating with thin elastin layers.

No blood vessels are found in the cornea or in the lens. The sclera has almost no blood vessels, but deep within the anterior part of the sclera, at its junction with the cornea, is a ring-shaped *scleral venous sinus*, formerly called the *canal of Schlemm*. The tiny blood vessels visible on the surface of the anterior sclera are in the conjunctiva, not the sclera itself.

CONNECT IT!

Corneas that have lost their transparency are often replaced with clear corneas from a donor—check out photos of transplanted corneas at ***Corneal Transplants*** online at ***Connect It!***

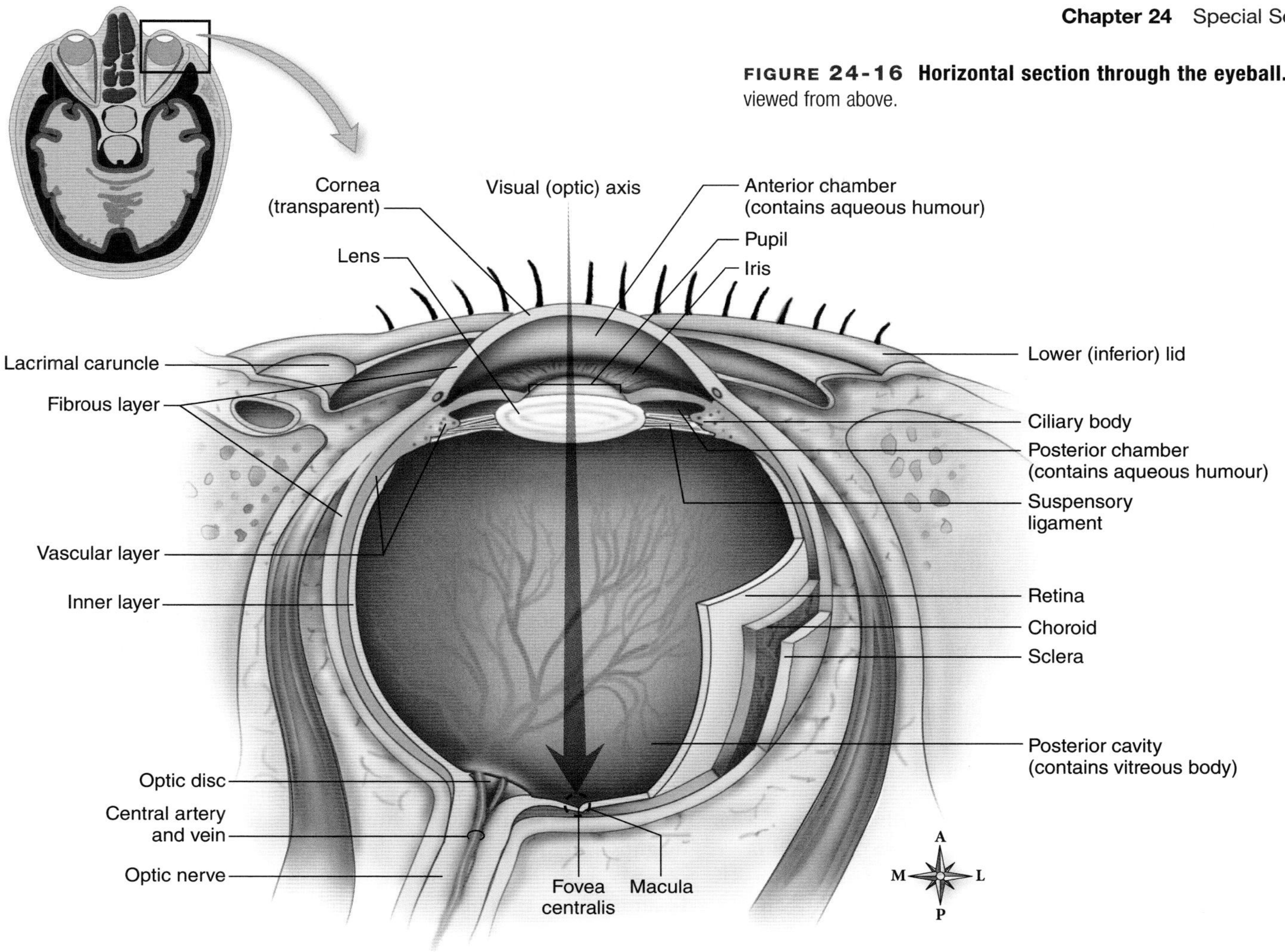

FIGURE 24-16 Horizontal section through the eyeball. The eye is viewed from above.

Vascular Layer

As noted earlier, the middle coat of the eyeball is the *vascular layer*. It consists of three component parts or regions—the choroid, ciliary body, and iris. This layer is characterized by many blood vessels and a large amount of melanin pigment. Most of this layer, forming the middle and posterior coating just inside the fibrous coat, is the highly pigmented choroid.

The **ciliary body** is formed by a thickening of the choroid and fits like a collar into the area between the anterior margin of the retina and the posterior margin of the iris (**Figure 24-17**). The small *ciliary muscle*, composed of both radial and circular smooth muscle fibres, lies in the anterior part of the ciliary body. Folds in the ciliary body are called *ciliary processes*, and attached to these are the *suspensory ligaments*, which blend with the elastic capsule of the *lens* and hold it suspended in place.

The **iris,** or the coloured part of the eye, consists of circular and radial smooth muscle fibres arranged to form a doughnut-shaped structure. It attaches to the ciliary body. The hole-shaped opening in the middle of the iris is the **pupil.** By adjusting the diameter of the opening, the iris acts like the diaphragm of a camera. It controls the amount of light that enters the eye by adjusting the size of the pupil. Eye colour is determined by the amount, placement, and type of melanin in the iris—and the reflection of light bouncing off the iris.

In *ocular albinism*, a genetic disorder, there is little or no pigmentation of the vascular layer, and thus light entering the eye passes

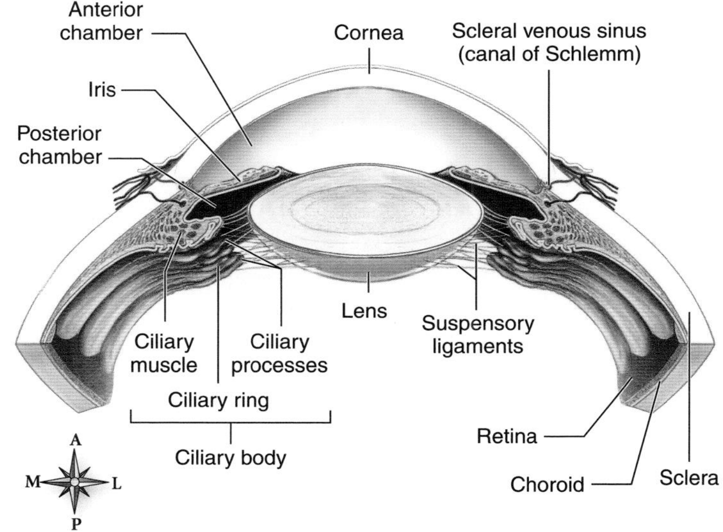

FIGURE 24-17 Lens, cornea, iris, and ciliary body. Note the suspensory ligaments that attach the lens to the ciliary body.

through this layer and reflects off of the white fibrous coat. This both amplifies the light inside the eye and disrupts the formation of a clear image—often leading to full or partial blindness.

Inner Layer

The **retina** is the incomplete innermost coat of the eyeball—incomplete in that it has no anterior portion. Melanin-containing epithelial cells form the layer of the retina next to the choroid coat. This part of the retina is called the *pigmented retina.*

Most of the retina, however, is made up of nervous tissue and is called the *sensory retina*. Three layers of neurons form the basic structure of the sensory retina. Named in the order in which they conduct impulses, these neurons are the main *photoreceptor cells, bipolar cells,* and *ganglion cells.* Identify each of these in **Figure 24-18**, *A*. Note that the main photoreceptor cells are the deepest, then the bipolar cells, then the ganglion cells.

The distal ends of the dendrites of the main photoreceptor neurons have names that describe their shapes. Because some look like tiny rods and others look like cones, they are called **rods** and **cones,** respectively (**Figure 24-18**, *B* and *C*). Because they are sensitive to light rays, they act as our principal visual receptors. Their light-sensitive outer (distal) segments are continuously regenerated, with the older sections at their tips sloughing off and then phagocytosed by the nearby pigmented epithelial cells.

Rods and cones differ in numbers, distribution, and function. Cones are less numerous than rods and are most densely concentrated in the **fovea centralis,** a small depression in the centre of a yellowish area, the **macula lutea,** found near the centre of the retina (see **Figures 24-16** and **24-19**). The macula lutea (the Latin name) is called simply the *macula* in English. The cones become less and less dense from the fovea outward. Rods, on the other hand, are absent entirely from the fovea and macula and increase in density toward the periphery of the retina. How these anatomical facts relate to rod and cone functions is discussed on pp. 550–552.

The bipolar cells are neurons that receive impulses from the rods and cones and pass these impulses to the ganglion neurons. Note in **Figure 24-18** that a bipolar neuron connects either to one cone or to many rods.

The ganglion neurons collect information from the primary photoreceptor neurons—the rods and cones. But they also act as photoreceptors themselves. Additional sets of neurons allow lateral connections among rods and cones (*horizontal cells*) and among bipolar and ganglion cells (*amacrine cells*). The lateral connecting cells are thought to help us detect patterns of movement.

All the axons of ganglion neurons extend back to a small circular area in the posterior part of the eyeball known as the **optic disc.** This part of the sclera contains perforations through which the fibres emerge from the eyeball as the **optic nerve** (second cranial nerve). The optic disc is also called the **blind spot** because light rays striking this area cannot be seen. Why? Because it contains no rods or cones, only nerve fibres. **Box 24-1** shows you how to locate the blind spots in your own eyes.

Just as an otoscope is used to view the external auditory canal and surface of the tympanic membrane, a lighted **ophthalmoscope** can be used to examine the retinal surface, called the *fundus*, and internal eye structures by viewing them through the pupil (see **Figure 24-19**). This noninvasive technique is a safe and effective aid in the diagnosis of many types of disease (see Mechanisms of Disease, p. 554). Locate the branching network of retinal blood vessels in **Figure 24-19**, *B*. These vessels supply the retinal tissues and are

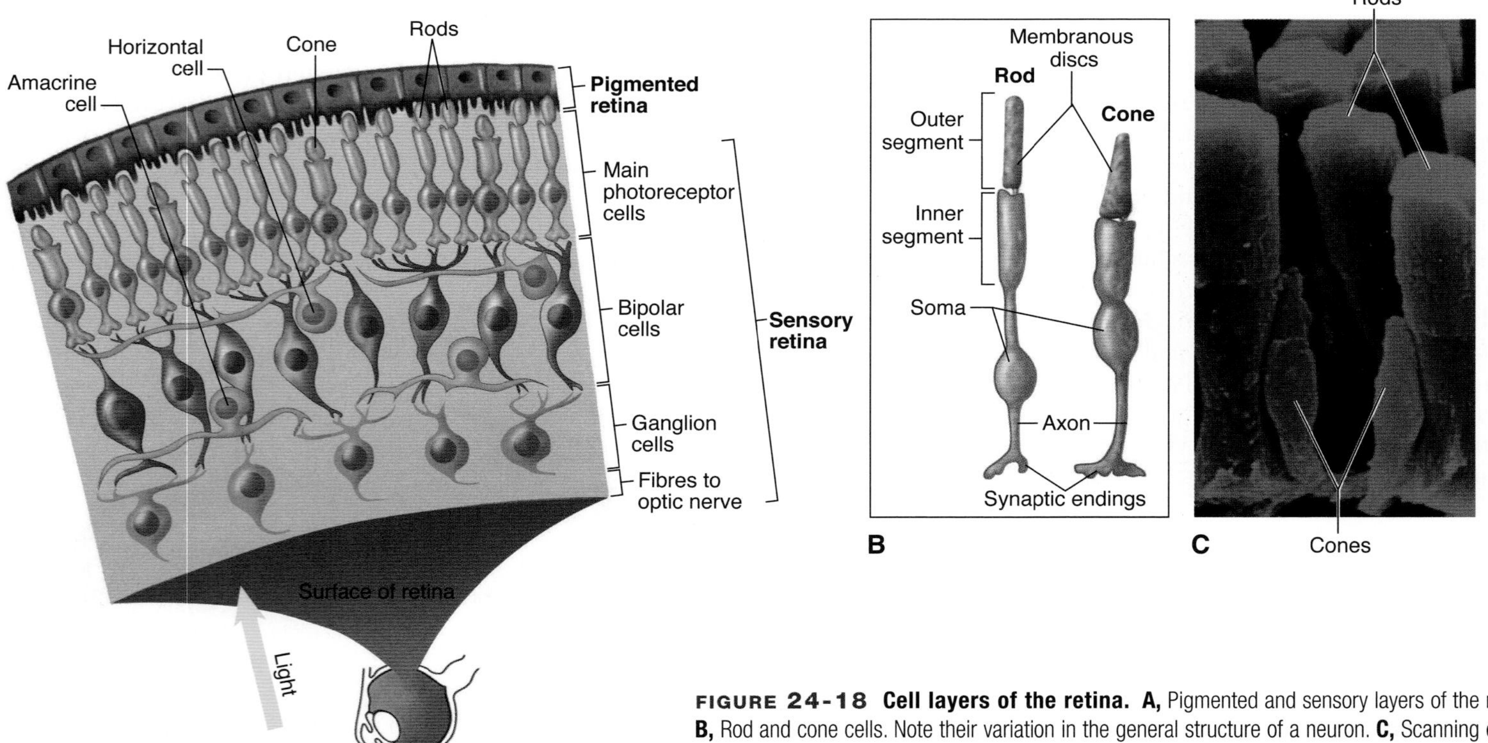

FIGURE 24-18 Cell layers of the retina. A, Pigmented and sensory layers of the retina. **B,** Rod and cone cells. Note their variation in the general structure of a neuron. **C,** Scanning electron micrograph of rod and cone cells.

UNIT 3

BOX 24-1 *fyi* | **Finding Your Blind Spot**

Demonstrate the location of the blind spot in your visual field by covering your left eye and looking at the objects below. While staring at the square, begin about 30 cm from objects and slowly bring the figures closer to your eye. At one point, the circle will seem to disappear because its image has fallen on the blind spot.

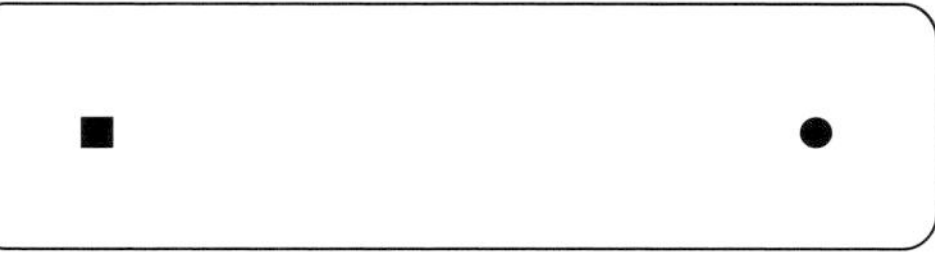

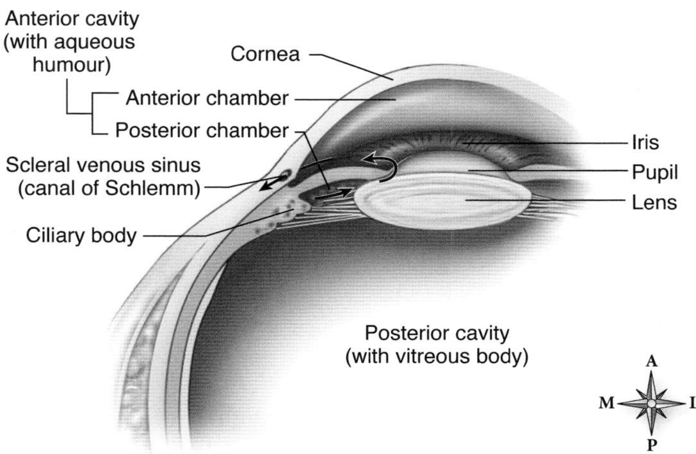

FIGURE 24-20 Formation of aqueous humour. Aqueous humour *(arrows)* is believed to be formed mainly by secretion by the ciliary body into the posterior chamber. It passes into the anterior chamber through the pupil, from which it is drained away by the ring-shaped scleral venous sinus (canal of Schlemm), and finally into the anterior ciliary veins.

critical for normal visual function. Diseases such as diabetes mellitus and atherosclerosis can reduce blood flow to these vessels, causing loss of vision.

Cavities and Humours

The eyeball is not a solid sphere; rather it contains a large interior space that is divided into two cavities: anterior and posterior.

The **anterior cavity** has two subdivisions, known as the *anterior* and *posterior chambers.* As **Figure 24-16** shows, the entire anterior cavity lies in front of the **lens.** The posterior chamber of the anterior cavity consists of the small space directly posterior to the iris but anterior to the lens. And the anterior chamber of the anterior cavity is the space anterior to the iris but posterior to the cornea. *Aqueous humour* fills both chambers of the anterior cavity. This substance is clear and watery and often leaks out when the eye is injured.

The **posterior cavity** of the eyeball is considerably larger than the anterior, because it occupies the entire space posterior to the lens, suspensory ligament, and ciliary body (see **Figure 24-16**). It contains the *vitreous body,* which is a sac filled with a soft, watery gel. Microscopically, the vitreous body is composed of a *stroma*—a fine meshwork of fibres—filled with a thick *vitreous humour.* The firm gel of the vitreous body, along with the watery aqueous humour, helps maintain sufficient intraocular pressure to prevent the eyeball from collapsing.

Aqueous humour forms from blood in capillaries (located mainly in the ciliary body). The ciliary body actively secretes aqueous humour into the posterior chamber, but passive filtration from capillary blood contributes also to aqueous humour formation. From the posterior chamber, aqueous humour moves from the area between the iris and the lens through the pupil into the anterior chamber. From here, it drains into the scleral venous sinus and moves into small veins (**Figure 24-20**).

Normally, aqueous humour drains out of the anterior chamber at the same rate at which it enters the posterior chamber, so the amount of aqueous humour in the eye remains relatively constant—and so, too, does intraocular pressure. But sometimes something happens to upset this balance, and intraocular pressure increases above the normal level of about 12 to 22 mm Hg (1.6–2.9 kPa). The individual may then develop the eye disease known as *glaucoma,* which, if untreated, can lead to retinal damage and blindness. Either excess formation or, more often, decreased drainage is seen as an immediate cause of this condition, but underlying causes are unknown (see Mechanisms of Disease, p. 555).

An outline summary of the cavities of the eye appears in **Table 24-1**. The cavities and lens are not part of the layers of the eyeball.

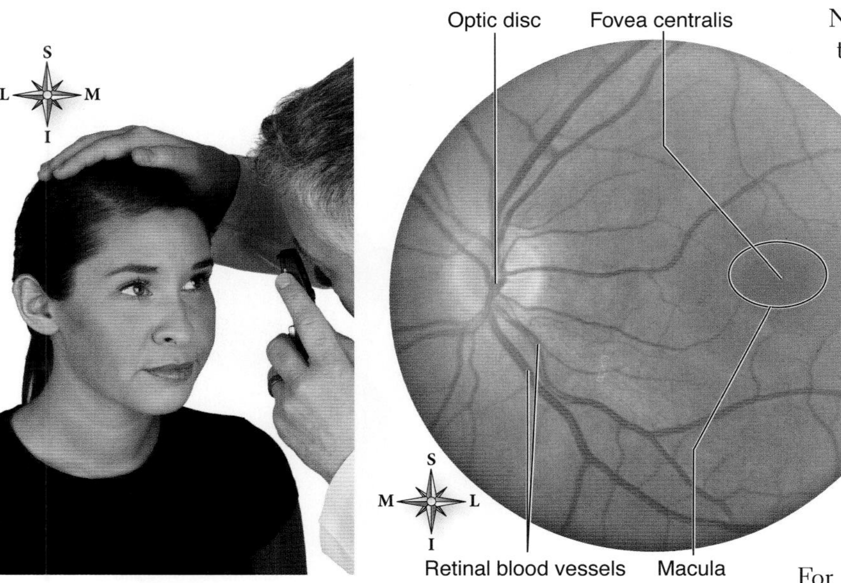

FIGURE 24-19 Examining the eye. A, Using the ophthalmoscope to view the retina. **B,** Ophthalmoscopic view of the retina as seen through the pupil.

The Process of Seeing

For vision to occur, the following conditions must be fulfilled: An image must be formed on the retina to stimulate its receptors (rods and cones), and the resulting nerve impulses must be conducted to the visual areas of the cerebral cortex for interpretation.

TABLE 24-1 Cavities of the Eye

CAVITY	DIVISIONS	LOCATION	CONTENTS
Anterior	Anterior chamber	Anterior to iris and posterior to cornea	Aqueous humour
	Posterior chamber	Posterior to iris and anterior to lens	Aqueous humour
Posterior	None	Posterior to lens	Vitreous body (stroma and vitreous humour)

Formation of Retinal Image

Four processes focus light rays so that they form a clear image on the retina: *refraction* of the light rays, *accommodation* of the lens, *constriction* of the pupil, and *convergence* of the eyes.

Refraction of Light Rays

Refraction is the deflection, or bending, of light rays. It is produced by light rays passing obliquely from one transparent medium into another of different optical density; the more convex the surface of the medium, the greater its refractive power. The refracting media of the eye are the cornea, aqueous humour, lens, and vitreous body. Light rays are bent, or refracted, at the anterior surface of the cornea as they pass from the air into the denser cornea, at the anterior surface of the lens as they pass from the aqueous humour into the denser lens, and at the posterior surface of the lens as they pass from the lens into the less dense gel of the vitreous body.

When an individual goes to an optometrist or ophthalmologist for an eye examination, the doctor performs a "refraction". In other words, by various specially designed methods, the refractory, or light-bending, power of that person's eyes is determined. Tests of visual acuity also rely on a person's ability to refract light properly (**Box 24-2**).

In a relaxed normal eye, the four refracting media together bend light rays sufficiently to bring to a focus on the retina the parallel rays reflected from an object 6 m or more away. Of course a normal eye can also focus on objects located much nearer than 6 m from the eye. This is accomplished by a mechanism known as *accommodation* (discussed next).

Many eyes, however, show errors of refraction; that is, they are not able to focus the rays on the retina in the stated conditions. Some common errors of refraction that are discussed later in the chapter are nearsightedness (myopia), farsightedness (hyperopia), and astigmatism.

Accommodation for Near Vision

Accommodation for near vision necessitates three changes: (1) increase in the curvature of the lens, (2) constriction of the pupils, and (3) convergence of the two eyes.

Light rays from objects 6 m or more away are practically parallel. The normal eye, as previously noted, refracts such rays sufficiently to focus them clearly on the retina. However, light rays from nearer objects are divergent rather than parallel. So obviously they must be bent more acutely to bring them to a focus on the retina. Accommodation of the lens or, in other words, an increase in its curvature takes place to achieve this greater refraction.

Change in Lens Shape. Contraction of the ciliary muscle pulls the choroid layer closer to the lens (see **Figure 24-17**). This, in turn,

BOX 24-2 *fyi* | Visual Acuity

Visual acuity is the clearness or sharpness of visual perception. Acuity is affected by our focusing ability, the efficiency of the retina, and the proper function of the visual pathway and processing centres in the brain.

Visual acuity is measured using the Snellen scale. A Snellen test usually consists of a number of rows of letters that get smaller as you read down the chart. The subject is asked to identify the smallest letter that he or she can see from a distance of 6 m. The resulting determination of visual acuity is expressed as a double number such as 6/6. The first number represents the distance in metres between the subject and the test chart; the standard is 6. The second number represents the number of metres a person with normal acuity would stand to see the same objects clearly. Thus a finding of 6/6 is normal because the subject can see at 6 metres what a person with normal acuity can see at 6 metres. A person with 6/30 vision can see objects at 6 metres that a person with normal vision can see at 30 metres.

People whose distant-vision acuity is worse than 6/60 with a very reduced field of vision are considered to be severely sight impaired and are certified as blind. Other criteria for registration include a visual acuity of less than 3/60 with a full visual field or between 3/60 and 6/60 with a severe reduction of field vision.

Certification is used to identify the severity of a wide variety of visual disorders so that laws that involve visual acuity can be enforced. For example, laws that govern the awarding of driving licenses require that drivers have a minimum level of visual acuity.

The image shows a common test for near-vision acuity. A chart or sample of print of different sized fonts is held at a distance of 30 to 50 cm and the subject is asked to read it. In both near-vision and distant-vision acuity tests, the subject attempts the test with each eye separately, then both eyes together. •

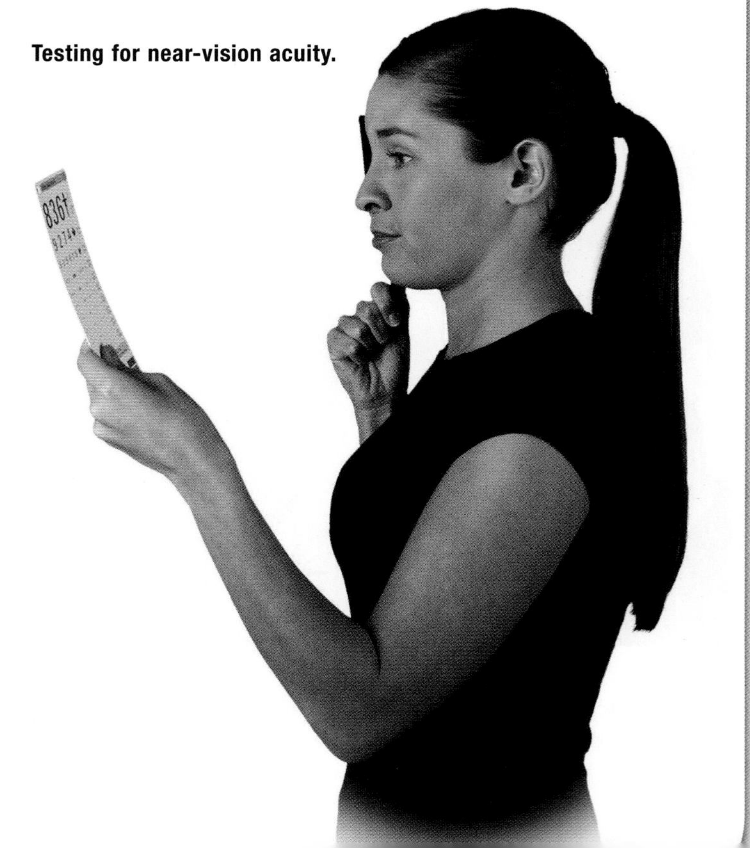

Testing for near-vision acuity.

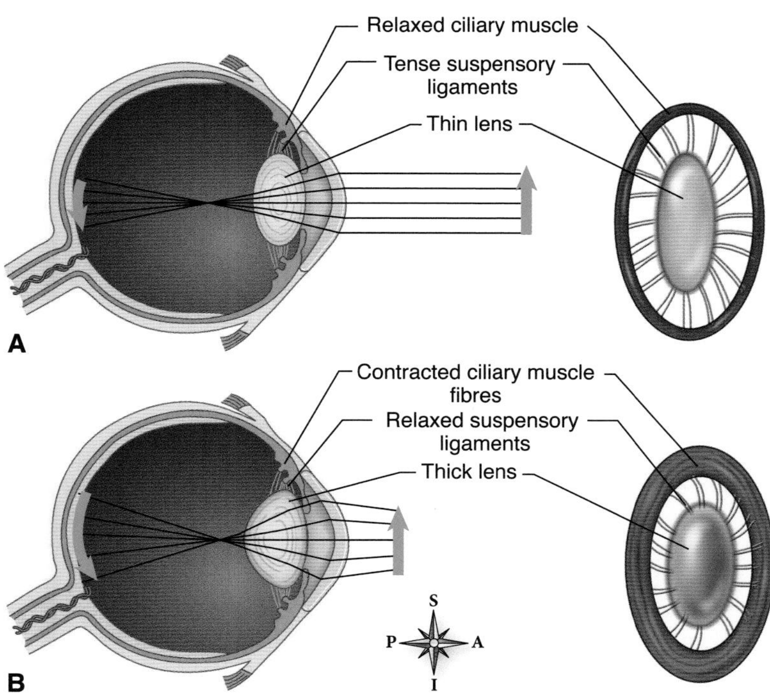

FIGURE 24-21 Accommodation of lens. A, Distant image: the lens is flattened (ciliary muscle relaxed), and the image is focused on the retina. **B,** Close image: the lens is rounded (ciliary muscle contracted), and the image is focused on the retina.

loosens the tension of the suspensory ligaments, allowing the lens to bulge. For near vision, the ciliary muscle is contracted and the lens is bulging. For far vision, however, the ciliary muscle is relaxed and the lens is comparatively flat (**Figure 24-21**). Continual use of the eyes for near work produces eyestrain because of the prolonged contraction of the ciliary muscle. Some of the strain can be avoided by looking into the distance at intervals while doing close work.

As people grow older, they tend to become farsighted because lenses lose their elasticity and therefore lose their ability to bulge and to accommodate for near vision. This condition is called *presbyopia*.

Constriction of Pupil. The muscles of the iris play an important part in the formation of clear retinal images (**Figure 24-22**). Part of the accommodation mechanism consists of contraction of the inner circular smooth muscle fibres of the iris as the outer radial fibres relax, which constricts the pupil. Such constriction prevents divergent rays from the object from entering the eye through the periphery of the cornea and lens. Such peripheral rays could not be refracted sufficiently to be brought to a focus on the retina and therefore would cause a blurred image. Constriction of the pupil for near vision is called the *near reflex* of the pupil and occurs simultaneously with accommodation of the lens in near vision.

As **Figure 24-22** shows, the pupil constricts in bright light (*photopupil reflex* or *pupillary light reflex*) to protect the retina from stimulation that is too intense or too sudden. As the same figure also shows, relaxation of inner circular fibres and contraction of the outer radial fibres cause dilation of the pupil in dim light. Pupil dilation allows more light to enter and form a more intense image in low-light environments.

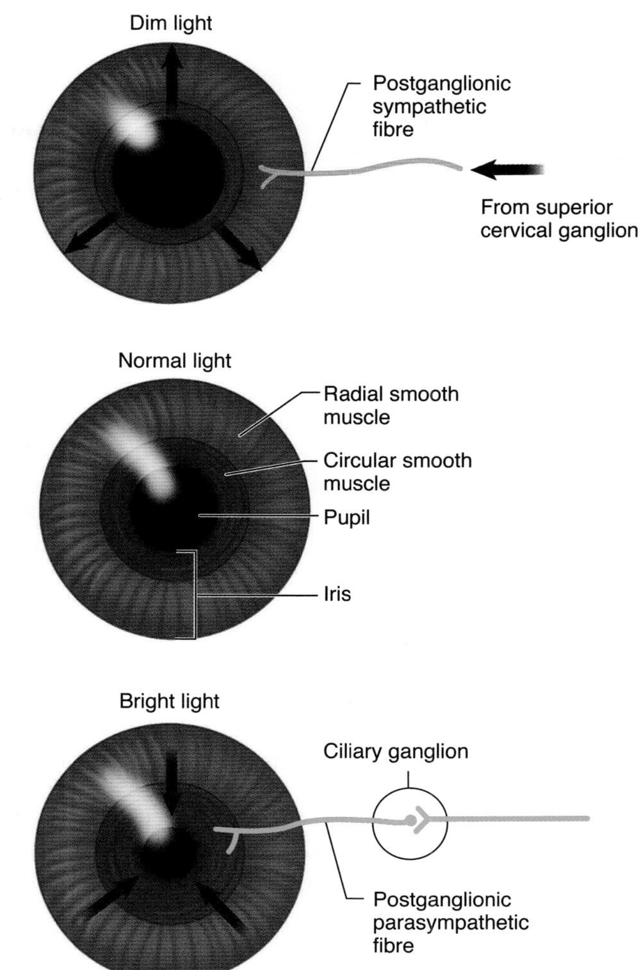

FIGURE 24-22 Constriction and dilation of pupil. Only the muscular part of the iris is shown.

Convergence of Eyes. Single binocular vision (seeing only one object instead of two when both eyes are used) occurs when light rays from an object fall on corresponding points of the two retinas. The foveae and all points lying equidistant and in the same direction from the foveae are corresponding points. Whenever the eyeballs move in unison, either with the visual axes parallel (for far objects) or converging on a common point (for near objects), light rays strike corresponding points of the two retinas.

Convergence is the movement of the two eyeballs inward so that their visual axes come together, or converge, at the object viewed. The nearer the object is, the greater the degree of convergence necessary to maintain single vision. A simple procedure demonstrates the fact that single binocular vision results from stimulation of corresponding points on two retinas. Gently press one eyeball out of line while viewing an object. Instead of one object, you will see two. To achieve unified movement of the two eyeballs, a functional balance between the antagonistic extrinsic muscles must exist.

For clear distant vision, the muscles must hold the visual axes of the two eyes parallel. For clear near vision, the muscles must converge the eyes. These conditions cannot be met if, for example, the medial rectus muscle of one eye contracts more forcefully than its

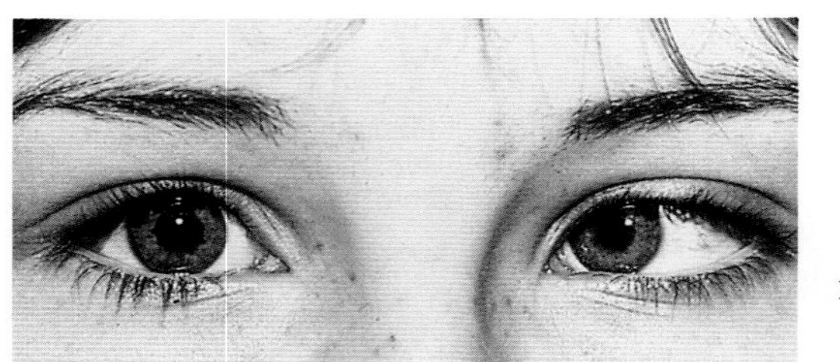

FIGURE 24-23 Strabismus. This child exhibits convergent left eye strabismus.

antagonist, the lateral rectus muscle. That eye is then pulled in toward the nose. The movement of its visual (optic) axis does not coordinate with that of the other eye. Light rays from an object then fall on noncorresponding points of the two retinas, and the object is seen double **(diplopia). Strabismus** (cross-eye or squint) is an exaggerated condition that cannot be overcome by neuromuscular effort (**Figure 24-23**). However, an individual with strabismus usually does not have double vision, as you might expect, because he or she learns to suppress one of the images.

The Role of Photopigments

Rods and cones are our main photoreceptor cells. Both rods and cones contain *photopigments*, or light-sensitive pigmented compounds that are found in the numerous membranes stacked in the outer (distal) area of both types of photoreceptors near the pigmented retina (see **Figure 24-18**). Chemically, all photopigments can be broken down into a glycoprotein called **opsin** and a vitamin A (retinol) derivative called **retinal,** which acts as the light-absorbing portion of all photopigments.

Rods

The single photopigment found in rods is named **rhodopsin.** Rhodopsin is so highly light sensitive that even dim light causes retinal to change its shape and leave the opsin molecule—a process called **bleaching.** This activity triggers a second-messenger mechanism involving G proteins that causes the rod cell's membrane potential to hyperpolarize (**Figure 24-24**). The neural signal then travels along the neural pathway until it is finally interpreted by the visual centres of the brain.

Meanwhile, ATP generated by the mitochondria in the inner segment of the rod cell is used to restore retinal's shape. Retinal again attaches to opsin to form rhodopsin, restoring its sensitivity to light. Light can almost instantly trigger a neural signal, but it takes several minutes to restore retinal. In dim light, the system can keep enough rhodopsins ready to continuously sense light. But in bright light, all of the rhodopsin is bleached and the retinal cannot be restored quickly enough to maintain continuous light sensitivity. This is why it takes a few moments to regain dim light vision after having been in bright light.

The colour of light is determined by its wavelength measured in nanometres (nm). We perceive different wavelengths of radiant energy (light) as different colours. **Figure 24-25** shows that rods are most sensitive to light in the green range of wavelengths, peaking at about 500 nm. However, the brain perceives information from the rods only as intensity of light, not as a colour. Thus the rods produce a kind of *monochrome,* or "black-and-white", vision.

Because rods are very sensitive to light and thus not only become bleached easily but also remain bleached in bright light, they are used only for "dim light" vision.

Cones

Three types of cones are present in the retina. Each contains its own version of the rhodopsin photopigment, different from the rhodopsin found in rod cells. Blue-sensitive cones are sensitive in the blue range of wavelengths (see **Figure 24-25**) and are often called *S cones* (for "short" wavelengths). Green-sensitive cones are often called *M cones* for "medium" wavelengths. Red-sensitive cones are called *L cones* for "long" wavelengths.

Our perception of a range of colours results from the combined neural input from varying numbers of the three different cone types. Abnormal function in any of the cones disrupts the normal perception of colours—a condition called *colour blindness* (**Box 24-3**).

Because cone photopigments are less sensitive to light than the rhodopsin in rods, brighter light is necessary for their breakdown. Cones therefore function to produce vision only in bright light.

In addition, cones contribute more than rods to the perception of sharp images. The reason for this difference involves the way in which information generated by the stimulation of rods and cones is "processed" before it reaches the brain. Look again at **Figure 24-18.** Note that information obtained by the bipolar cells is collated from many rods, whereas bipolar cells tend to synapse with only a single cone receptor. Recall that this property of combining input from several receptors is called *convergence.* The result of convergence is that, although the rods combine their input to make a bipolar cell fire in dimmer light, the brain is unable to determine exactly which rod was stimulated when a given bipolar or ganglion cell fires.

BOX 24-3 *fyi* | **Colour Blindness**

Colour blindness, usually an inherited condition, is caused by mistakes in the functioning of the three *photopigments* in the cones. Each photopigment is sensitive to one of the three primary colours of light: green, blue, and red (see **Figure 24-25**). In many cases, the green-sensitive photopigment is missing or deficient; other times, the red-sensitive photopigment is abnormal. (Dysfunction of the blue-sensitive cone is rare.) Colour-blind individuals see colours, but they cannot distinguish between them normally.

Figures such as parts *A* and *B* shown here are often used to screen individuals for colour blindness. A person with red-green colour blindness cannot see the *74* in part *A* of the figure, whereas a person with normal vision can. To determine which photopigment is deficient, a colour-blind person may try a figure similar to part *B.* Persons with a deficiency of red-sensitive photopigment can distinguish only the *2;* those deficient in green-sensitive photopigment can only see the *4.*

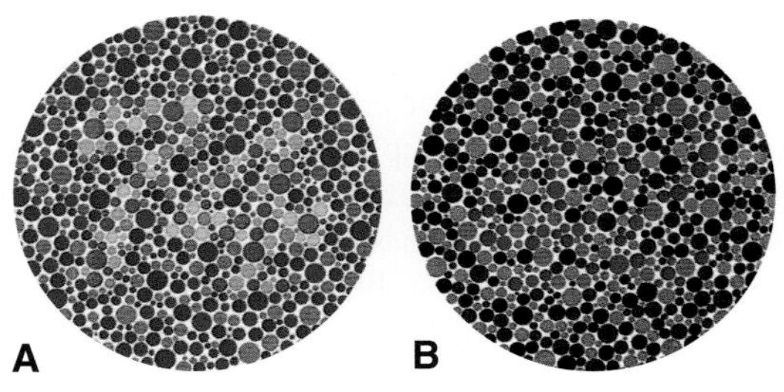

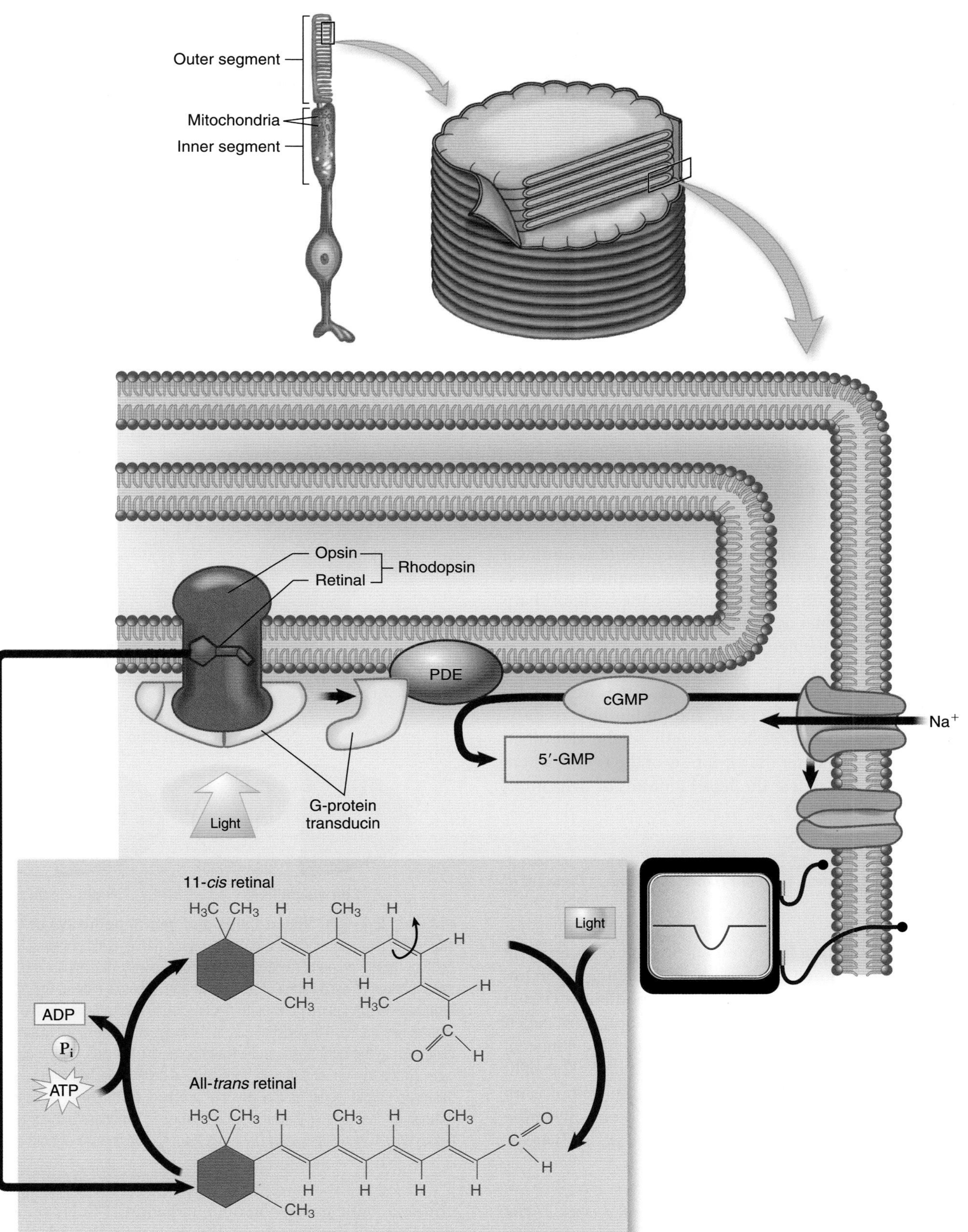

FIGURE 24-24 Rhodopsin cycle. Rhodopsin (*retinal* + *opsin*) embedded in the membranes stacked inside the rod's outer segment is hit by light, which changes retinal's shape from bent to straight. As the retinal leaves the opsin to be regenerated by ATP from mitochondria in the rod's inner segment, *G-protein transducin* is triggered to activate the membrane enzyme *phosphodiesterase (PDE)*. PDE breaks down *cyclic guanosine monophosphate (cGMP)* into 5′-GMP. Reduced availability of cGMP causes cGMP-gated sodium (Na^+) channels to close and thus hyperpolarize the membrane—resulting in neural signalling.

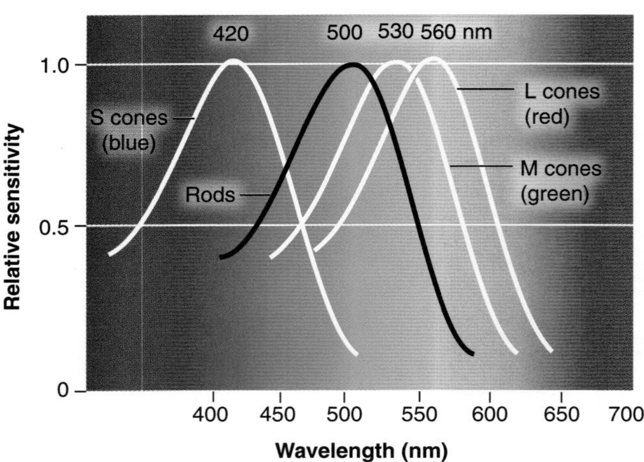

FIGURE 24-25 Colour sensitivity of rods and cones. Rods *(black line)* are sensitive only in dim-light conditions in the range of greenish wavelengths—but their information is perceived only as light and dark, not green. Three types of cones *(white lines)* perceive colours in bright-light conditions. Blue (*S*, short-wave) cones are sensitive in the blue range, green (*M*, medium-wave) cones in the green range, and red (*L*, long-wave) cones in the red range. Information from all three cone types is combined to produce a large palette of colour perception in the brain.

Convergence of impulses from cones is rare. There is almost a one-to-one relationship between cones and the ganglion cells that carry impulses toward the brain. Interpretation by the brain of sharp images is therefore much better as a result of cone stimulation.

The fovea contains the greatest concentration of cones and is therefore the point of clearest vision in good light. For this reason, when we want to see an object clearly in the daytime, we look directly at it to focus the image on the fovea. But in dim light or darkness, we see an object better if we look slightly to the side of it, thereby focusing the image nearer the periphery of the retina, where the more plentiful rods can detect the lesser amount of light information and generate an image.

CONNECT IT! ⓔ

Learn more about colour blindness in ***Colour Blindness*** online at ***Connect It!***

Ganglion Cells

Although the rods and cones are the dominant form of photoreceptor cell in the retina, and are entirely responsible for detecting visual images, some ganglion cells are now known to act in an additional visual system. The ganglion photoreceptors contain a photopigment called *melanopsin*. Melanopsin is sensitive to light in the blue range of wavelengths that seem to predominate at dawn and dusk. The light information from this system is not used to form an image but is instead needed to adjust our biological clock—a function involving the pineal body of the brain discussed in Chapter 20 (see pp. 453–454).

CONNECT IT! 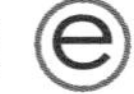

Review the role of ganglion cells in maintaining the body's clock in ***The Timekeeping Hormone*** online at ***Connect It!***

Neural Pathway of Vision

Fibres that conduct impulses from the rods and cones reach the visual cortex in the occipital lobes by way of the optic nerves, optic chiasma, optic tracts, and optic radiations. "Relay stations" along the way include the superior colliculi and the lateral geniculate nuclei of the thalamus. Look closely at **Figure 24-26**. Note that each optic nerve contains fibres from only one retina but that the optic chiasma contains fibres from the nasal portions of both retinas. Each optic tract also contains fibres from both retinas.

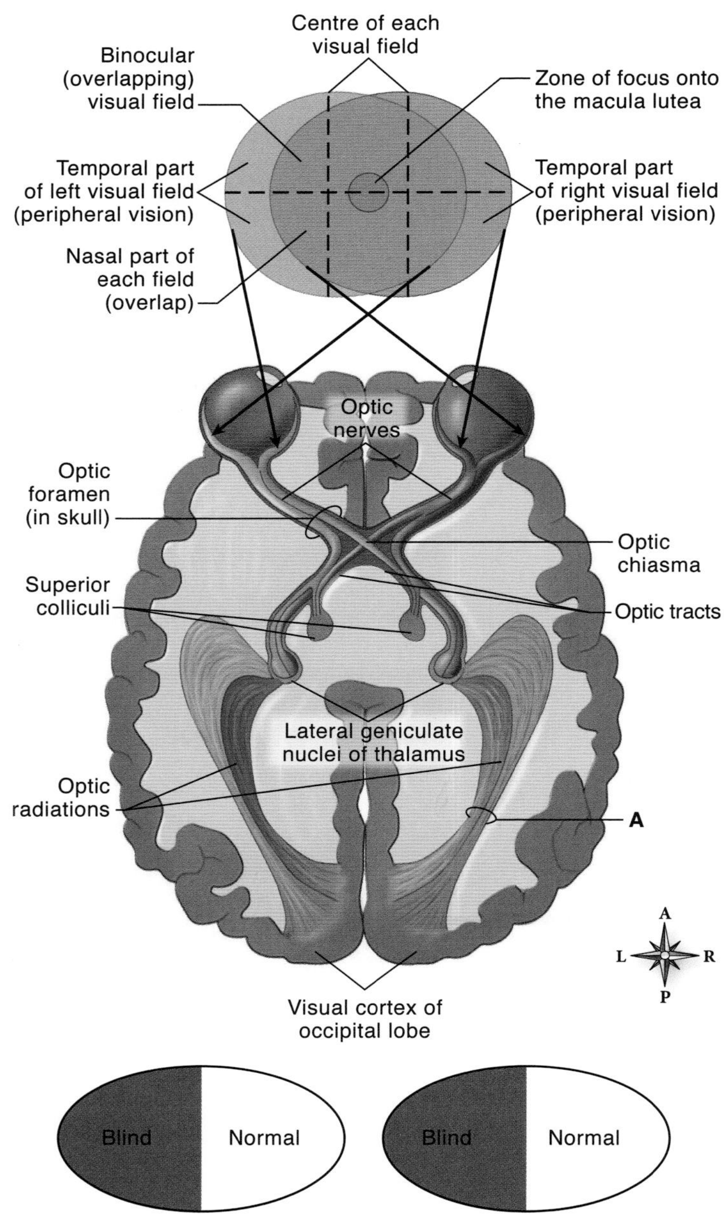

FIGURE 24-26 Visual fields and neural pathways of the eye. Note the structures that make up each pathway: optic nerve, optic chiasma, lateral geniculate body of thalamus, optic radiations, and visual cortex of occipital lobe. Fibres from the nasal portion of each retina cross over to the opposite side at the optic chiasma and terminate in the lateral geniculate nuclei. Location of a lesion in the visual pathway determines the resulting visual defect. Damage at point *A*, for example, would cause blindness in the right nasal and left temporal visual fields, as the ovals beneath indicate. (Trace the visual pathway from point *A* back to the visual field map to see why this is so.) What would be the effect of pressure on the optic chiasma—by a pituitary tumour, for instance? (*Answer:* It would produce blindness in both temporal visual fields. Why? Because it destroys fibres from the nasal side of both retinas.)

These anatomical facts explain certain peculiar visual abnormalities that sometimes occur. Suppose a person's right optic tract were injured so that it could not conduct impulses—say, at point A in **Figure 24-26**. This person would be totally blind in neither eye but partially blind in both eyes. Specifically, this person would be blind in the right nasal and left temporal visual fields. Here are the reasons: the right optic tract contains fibres from the right retina's temporal area, the area that sees the right nasal visual field. In addition, the right optic tract contains fibres from the left retina's nasal area, the area that sees the left temporal visual field.

CONNECT IT! 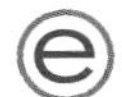

To learn about visual phenomena where one sense leads to the experience of a second sensory pathway, such as numbers associated with colours, go to the online ***Connect It!*** article ***Synaesthesia.***

Quick CHECK

11. Name the layers, or coats, of the eyeball.
12. Identify the layers of the retina.
13. Name the four processes that function to focus a clear image on the retina.
14. Outline the steps of the rhodopsin cycle.

cycle of **life**

Special Senses The ability of the sense organs to respond to stimuli caused by changes in the body's internal or external environment varies during life. Ultimately, all sensory information is acquired through depolarization of sensory nerve endings. Anything that interferes with the generation of a receptor potential or its transmission to and interpretation by areas of the central nervous system influences sensory acuity. Age, disease, structural defects, and lack of maturation all affect our ability to identify and respond to sensory input.

Structure and function response capabilities of the sense organs are related to developmental factors associated with age. For example, a newborn baby has limited sight, hearing, and tactile identification capabilities. As maturation occurs and normal development progresses, the senses become more acute. By late adulthood, presbyopia, progressive hearing loss, and a reduced sense of taste and smell are common.

Some loss of sensory capability in old age is directly related to structural change in receptor cells or other necessary sense organ structures. The lens of the eye becomes harder and less able to change shape, taste buds become less functional, and exteroceptors of all types become less responsive to stimuli because of structural deterioration. •

the big picture | Special Senses

As with the general senses, all the special senses play important homeostatic roles by acting as *sensors* in various feedback loops that maintain a stable internal environment in the body. Classic examples include vision and hearing that help us monitor our often hostile external environment and avoid or respond to dangers that might otherwise be life-threatening. Also, consider the sensation of thirst. It helps us to regulate our water intake and thus avoid dehydration or the sensation or "craving" for salt, which may signal a dangerous loss of sodium from the body. Other examples include a bitter taste or offensive odour, which are sensations often associated with poisonous materials or toxic fumes and thus serve as important defence mechanisms. Take a few minutes to review each of the special senses by integrating their structure and functions with the "big picture" of homeostasis and survival. •

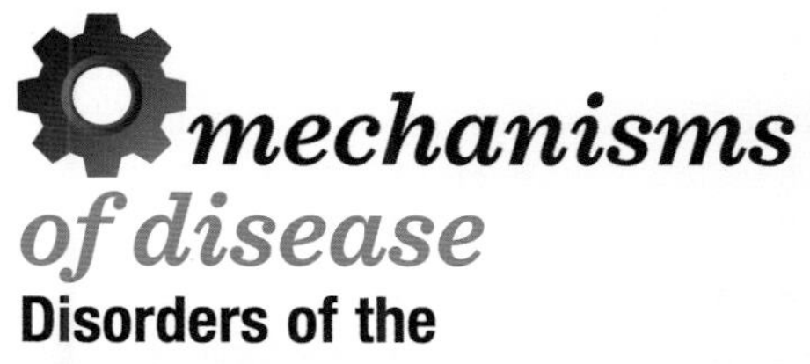

mechanisms of disease

Disorders of the Special Senses

Disorders of the Ear

Hearing problems can be divided into two basic categories: *conduction impairment* and *nerve impairment.* Conduction impairment refers to the blocking of sound waves as they are conducted through the external and middle ear to the sensory receptors of the inner ear (the conduction pathway). Nerve impairment results in insensitivity to sound because of inherited or acquired nerve damage.

The most obvious cause of conduction impairment is blockage of the external auditory canal. Waxy buildup of cerumen (**Figure 24-27**, *C*) commonly blocks conduction of sound toward the tympanic membrane. Foreign objects, tumours, and other matter can block conduction in the external or middle ear. An inherited bone disorder called **otosclerosis** impairs conduction by causing structural irregularities in the stapes. Otosclerosis usually first appears during childhood or early adulthood as **tinnitus,** or "ringing in the ear".

Temporary conduction impairment often results from ear infection, or **otitis.** The structure of the auditory tube, especially its connection with the nasopharynx, makes the middle ear prone to bacterial or viral *otitis media* (**Figure 24-27**, *A*). Otitis media often produces swelling and pus formation that block the conduction of sound through the middle ear. Surgical insertion of a grommet, also called a *ventilation* or **tympanotomy tube** (**Figure 24-27**, *B*) is sometimes employed to relieve pressure and permit drainage. Permanent damage to structures of the middle ear occasionally occurs in severe cases.

Hearing loss because of nerve impairment is common in the elderly. Called **presbycusis,** this progressive hearing loss associated with ageing results from degeneration of nerve tissue in the ear and the vestibulocochlear nerve. A similar type of hearing loss occurs after chronic exposure to loud noises that damages receptors in the organ of Corti. Because different sound *frequencies* (tones) stimulate different regions of the organ of Corti, hearing impairment is limited to only those frequencies associated with the portion of the organ of Corti that is damaged. For example, the portion of the organ of Corti that degenerates first in presbycusis is normally stimulated by high-frequency sounds. Thus the inability to hear high-pitched sounds is common among older adults.

Two small muscles, the *tensor tympani* and *stapedius,* help prevent damage to hearing caused by prolonged loud noise. The tensor tympani attaches to and limits movement of the eardrum, thus preventing excess displacement caused by prolonged loud sounds.

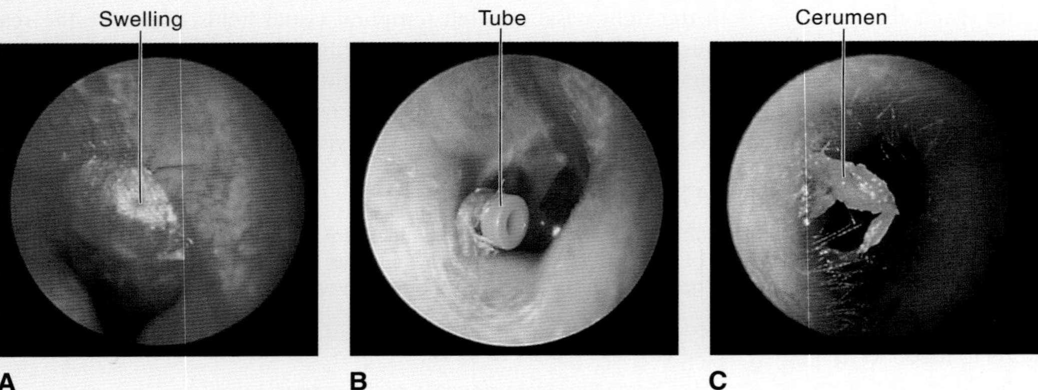

FIGURE 24-27 Disorders of the ear. **A,** Acute otitis media. Note the red, thickened, and bulging tympanic membrane. **B,** A grommet or tympanotomy tube. Inserted to relieve pressure and permit drainage in otitis media. **C,** Cerumen (earwax) in ear canal.

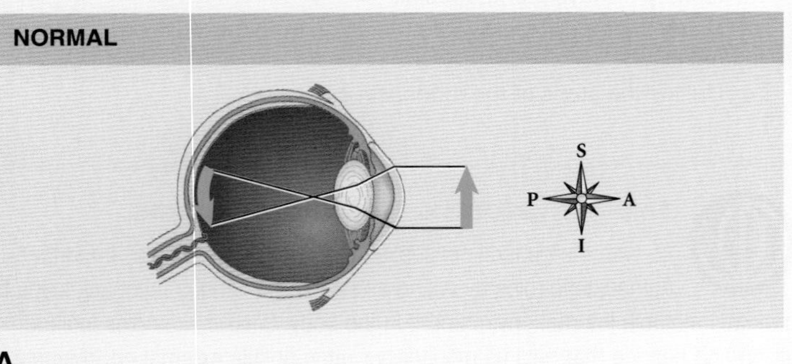

MYOPIA

Uncorrected

Corrected

B

C

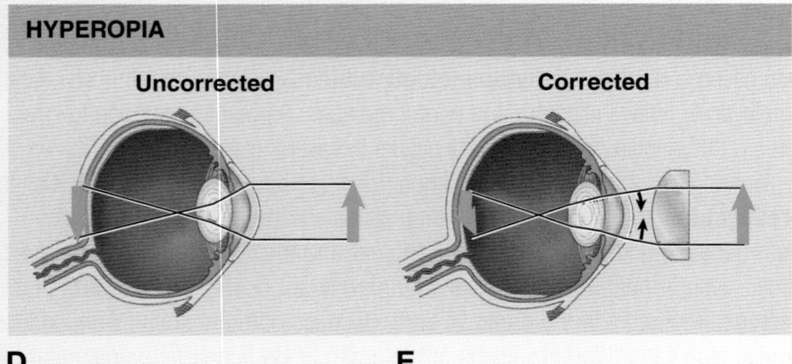

FIGURE 24-28 Correcting refraction disorders. **A,** Normal eye structure results in a well-focused retinal image. **B,** In myopia, an elongated eyeball causes the image to focus in front of the retina. **C,** An external lens can refocus the image on the retina, correcting the effects of myopia. **D,** In hyperopia, a flattened eyeball causes the image to focus behind the retina. **E,** An external lens can refocus the image on the retina.

In addition, the smallest of all body muscles, the tiny stapedius, limits excess movement of the stapes and thus protects the oval window from prolonged noise-related damage. Only protective devices, such as earplugs, can protect hearing from damage caused by very sudden loud noises, such as a gunshot.

Nerve damage can also occur in **Ménière disease,** a chronic inner ear disease of unknown cause. Ménière disease is characterized by tinnitus, progressive nerve deafness, and **vertigo** (sensation of spinning).

Disorders of the Eye

Healthy vision requires three basic processes: formation of an image on the retina (refraction), stimulation of rods and cones, and conduction of nerve impulses to the brain. Malfunction of any of these processes can disrupt normal vision.

Refraction Disorders

Focusing a clear image on the retina is essential for good vision. In the normal eye, light rays enter the eye and are focused into a clear, upside-down image on the retina (**Figure 24-28**, *A*). The brain can easily right the upside-down image in our conscious perception but cannot correct an image that is not sharply focused. If our eyes are elongated, the image focuses in front of the retina rather than on it. The retina receives only a fuzzy image. This condition, called **myopia** or *nearsightedness,* can be corrected by use of concave contact lenses or glasses or by performing refractive eye surgery (**Figure 24-28**, *B* and *C*). If our eyes are shorter than normal, the image focuses behind the retina, also producing a fuzzy image. This condition, called **hyperopia** or *farsightedness,* can also be corrected by convex lenses or refractive eye surgery (**Figure 24-28**, *D* and *E*).

CONNECT IT! 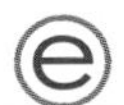

You have probably heard of eye surgeries such as RK, CK, PRK, or LASIK. But you may have wondered, *what is* a LASIK? Check out ***Refractive Eye Surgery*** online at ***Connect It!*** to explore the common refractive eye surgeries and how they are done.

Various other conditions can prevent the formation of a clear image on the retina. For example, the inability to focus the lens properly as we age, or **presbyopia,** has already been mentioned. Older individuals can compensate for presbyopia by using reading glasses when near vision is needed. An irregularity in the curvature of the cornea or lens, a condition called **astigmatism,** can also be corrected with glasses or contact lenses that are formed with the opposite curvature. **Cataracts,** cloudy spots in the eye's lens that develop as we age, may also interfere with focusing (**Figure 24-29**). Cataracts are especially troublesome in dim light because weak beams of light cannot pass through the cloudy spots the way some brighter light can. This fact accounts for the trouble many older adults have with their night vision.

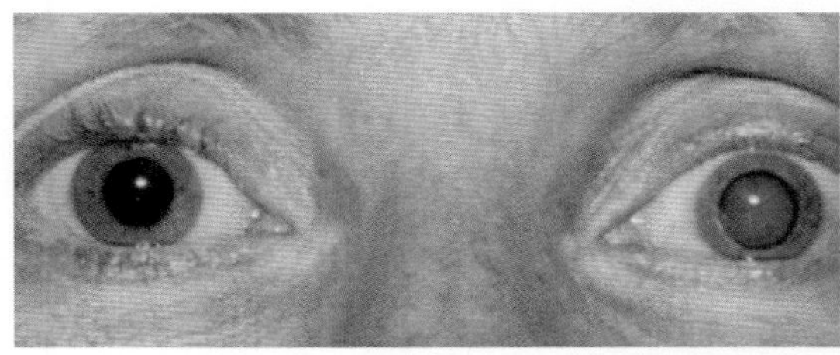

FIGURE 24-29 Cataract. Note the prominent cataract of the left eye.

Infections of the eye also have the potential to impair vision, sometimes permanently. Most eye infections begin in the conjunctiva, producing an inflammation response known as "pink-eye", or **conjunctivitis.** Various pathogens can cause conjunctivitis. For example, the bacterium *Chlamydia trachomatis* that commonly infects the reproductive tract can cause a chronic infection called *chlamydial conjunctivitis,* or **trachoma.** Because *Chlamydia* and other pathogens often inhabit the birth canal, antibiotics are routinely applied to the eyes of newborns to prevent conjunctivitis. Highly contagious *acute bacterial conjunctivitis,* characterized by drainage of a mucous pus, is most commonly caused by bacteria such as *Staphylococcus* and *Haemophilus* (see **Figure 24-13**, p. 543).

Conjunctivitis may produce lesions on the inside of the eyelid that can damage the cornea and thus impair vision. Occasionally infections of the conjunctiva spread to the tissues of the eye proper and cause permanent injury—even total blindness. Besides infection, conjunctivitis may also be caused by allergies. The red, itchy, watery eyes commonly associated with allergic reactions to pollen and other substances result from an allergic inflammatory response of the conjunctiva.

Disorders of the Retina

Damage to the retina impairs vision because even a well-focused image cannot be perceived if some or all of the light receptors do not function properly. For example, in a condition called **retinal detachment,** part of the retina falls away from the tissue supporting it (**Figure 24-30**, *A*). This condition may result from ageing, eye tumours, or blows to the head—as in a sporting injury. Common warning signs include the sudden appearance of floating spots that may decrease over a period of weeks and odd "flashes of light" that appear when the eye moves. If left untreated, the retina may detach completely and cause total blindness in the affected eye.

Diabetes mellitus, a disorder involving the hormone insulin, may cause a condition known as **diabetic retinopathy**. In this disorder the diabetes causes small haemorrhages in retinal blood vessels that disrupt the oxygen supply to the photoreceptors (**Figure 24-30**, *B*). The eye responds by building new, but abnormal, vessels that block vision and may cause detachment of the retina. Diabetic retinopathy is one of the leading causes of blindness in the United Kingdom. Diabetic retinopathy and other complications of diabetes are often associated with high blood pressure, or *hypertension*, which also causes retinal haemorrhages (**Figure 24-30**, *C*).

Another condition that can damage the retina is **glaucoma.** Recall that glaucoma is excessive *intraocular pressure* caused by abnormal accumulation of aqueous humour. As fluid pressure against the retina increases above normal, blood flow through the retina slows. Reduced blood flow causes degeneration of the retina and thus leads to loss of vision. Although acute forms of glaucoma can occur, most cases of glaucoma develop slowly over a period of years. This chronic form may not produce any symptoms, especially in its early stages. For this reason, routine eye examinations typically include a screening test for glaucoma. As chronic glaucoma progresses, damage first appears at the edges of the retina—causing a gradual loss of peripheral vision. Blurred vision and headaches may also occur. As the damage becomes more extensive, "halos" are seen around bright lights. If untreated, glaucoma eventually produces total, permanent blindness. One of the most common characteristic early retinal changes associated with glaucoma is swelling or "cupping" of the optic disc (**Figure 24-30**, *D*).

Degeneration of the retina can cause difficulty seeing at night or in dim light. This condition, called **nyctalopia,** or "night blindness", can also be caused by a deficiency of vitamin A. Recall that vitamin A is needed to make retinal, a component of rhodopsin. A deficiency of rhodopsin impairs the function of rod cells, which are needed for dim light vision.

Disorders of the Visual Pathway

Damage or degeneration in the optic nerve, the brain, or any part of the visual pathway between them, can impair vision. For example, the pressure associated with glaucoma can also damage the optic nerve. Diabetes, already cited as a cause of retina damage, can also cause degeneration of the optic nerve.

Damage to the visual pathway does not always result in total loss of sight. Depending on where the damage occurs, only a part of the visual field may be affected. For example, a certain form of neuritis (nerve inflammation), often associated with multiple sclerosis, can cause loss of only the centre of the visual field—a condition called **scotoma.**

A stroke can cause vision impairment when the resulting tissue damage occurs in one of the regions of the brain that processes visual information. For example, damage to an area that processes information about colours may result in a rare condition called **acquired cortical colour blindness.** This condition is characterized by difficulty in distinguishing any colour—not just one or two colours as in the more common inherited forms of colour blindness.

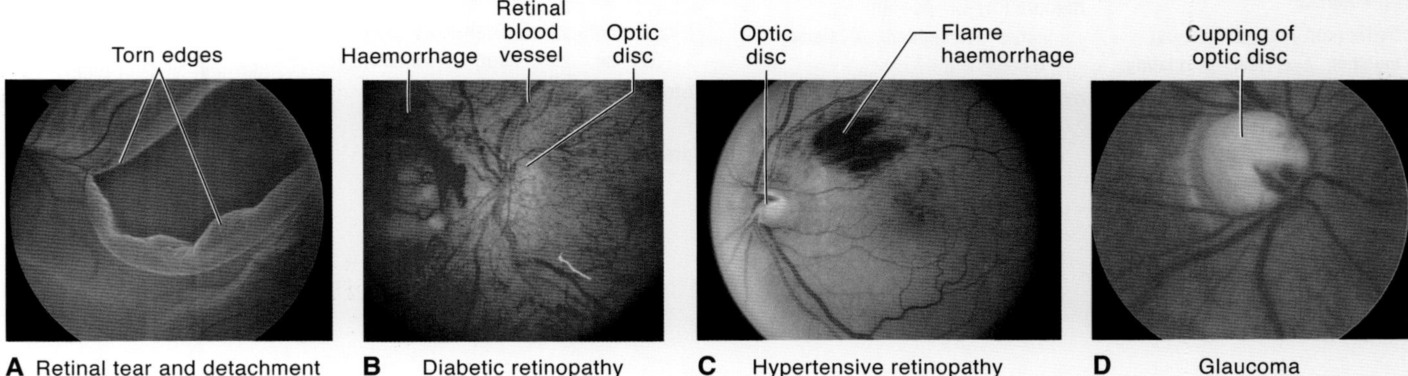

FIGURE 24-30 Retinal pathological conditions. A, Retina tear and detachment. **B,** Diabetic retinopathy. Note the abnormal blood vessels and haemorrhages in the retina caused by diabetes. **C,** Hypertensive retinopathy. Large "flame haemorrhages" in the retina are associated with high blood pressure. **D,** Glaucoma. Note "cupping" of the optic disc caused by increased intraocular pressure. (Compare to normal retina in **Figure 24-19** on p. 547.)

LANGUAGE OF SCIENCE *(continued from p. 532)*

extrinsic eye muscle (eks-TRIN-sik)
[*extr-* **outside,** *-sic* **beside,** *mus-* **mouse,** *-cle* **small**]

filiform papilla (FIL-ih-form pah-PIL-ah)
[*fili-* **thread,** *-form* **shape,** *papilla* **nipple**] *pl.*, papillae

foliate papilla (FOL-ee-ayt pah-PIL-ah)
[*foli-* **leaf,** *-ate* **relating to,** *papilla* **nipple**] *pl.*, papillae

fovea centralis (FOH-vee-ah sen-TRAL-is)
[*fovea* **pit,** *centralis* **centre**] *pl.*, foveae centrales

fungiform papilla (FUN-jih-form pah-PIL-ah)
[*fungi-* **mushroom,** *-form* **shape,** *papilla* **nipple**] *pl.*, papillae

granule cell (GRAN-yool)
[*gran-* **grain,** *-ule* **little**]

gustatory (GUS-tah-tor-ee)
[*gusta-* **taste,** *-ory* **relating to**]

gustatory cell (GUS-tah-tor-ee sell)
[*gusta-* **taste,** *-ory* **relating to,** *cell* **storeroom**]

intrinsic eye muscle (in-TRIN-sik)
[*intr-* **within,** *-sic* **beside,** *mus-* **mouse,** *-cle* **small**]

iris
[*iris* **rainbow**]

labyrinth (LAB-ih-rinth)
[*labyrinth* **maze**]

lens (lenz)
[*lens* **lentil**]

macula (MAK-yoo-lah)
[*macula* **spot**] *pl.*, maculae or maculas

macula lutea (MAK-yoo-lah LOO-tee-ah)
[*macula* **spot,** *lutea* **yellow**] *pl.*, maculae luteae

olfactory (ohl-FAK-tor-ee)
[*olfact-* **smell,** *-ory* **relating to**]

olfactory sensory neuron (ol-FAK-tor-ee SEN-sor-ee NYOO-ron)
[*olfact-* **smell,** *-ory* **relating to,** *neuron* **string or nerve**]

opsin (OP-sin)
[*ops-* **vision,** *-in* **substance**]

optic disc (OP-tik disk)
[*opti-* **vision,** *-ic* **relating to**]

optic nerve (OP-tik)
[*opt-* **vision,** *-ic* **relating to**]

organ of Corti (OR-gan of KOR-tee)
[*Alfonso Corti* **Italian anatomist**]

otolith (O-toh-lith)
[*oto-* **ear,** *-lith* **stone**]

papilla (pah-PIL-ah)
[*papilla* **nipple**] *pl.*, papillae

perilymph (PAIR-ih-limf)
[*peri-* **around,** *-lymph* **water**]

posterior cavity (pohs-TEER-ee-or KAV-i-tee)
[*poster-* **behind,** *-or* **quality,** *cav-* **hollow,** *-ity* **state**]

pupil (PYOO-pill)
[*pup-* **doll,** *-il* **little**]

refraction (ree-FRAK-shun)
[*re-* **back or again,** *-fract-* **break,** *-tion* **process**]

retina (RET-ih-nah)
[*ret-* **net,** *-in-* **relating to,** *-a* **thing**]

retinal (RET-ih-nal)
[*ret-* **net,** *-in-* **relating to,** *-al* **relating to**]

rhodopsin (roh-DOP-sin)
[*rhodo-* **red,** *-ops-* **vision,** *-in* **substance**]

sclera (SKLEH-rah)
[*scler-* **hard,** *-a* **thing or substance**]

static equilibrium (STAT-ik ee-kwih-LIB-ree-um)
[*stat-* **stand,** *-ic* **relating to,** *equi-* **equal,** *-libr-* **balance**]

tectorial membrane (tek-TOH-ree-al)
[*tect-* **roof,** *-or-* **quality,** *-al* **relating to,** *membran-* **thin skin**]

tympanic membrane (tim-PAN-ik)
[*tympan-* **drum,** *-ic* **relating to,** *membran-* **thin skin**]

vestibular membrane (ves-TIB-yoo-lar)
[*vestibul-* **entrance hall,** *-ar* **relating to,** *membran-* **thin skin**]

LANGUAGE OF MEDICINE

acquired cortical colour blindness (ah-KWY-erd KOHR-tih-kahl)
[*cortic-* **cortex (bark),** *-al* **relating to**]

anosmia (an-OZ-mee-ah)
[*an-* **without,** *-osm-* **smell,** *-ia* **condition**]

astigmatism (ah-STIG-mah-tiz-em)
[*a-* **not,** *-stigma-* **point,** *-ism* **condition**]

blepharoplasty (blef-ar-oh-PLAS-tee)
[*blepharo-* **eyelid or eyelash,** *-plasty* **surgical repair**]

cataracts (KAT-ah-rakts)
[*cataract* **waterfall**]

conjunctivitis (kon-junk-tih-VYE-tis)
[*con-* **together,** *-junct-* **join,** *-iv-* **relating to,** *-itis* **inflammation**]

diabetic retinopathy (dye-ah-BET-ik ret-in-OP-ath-ee)
[*diabet-* **pass-through or siphon (diabetes mellitus),** *-ic* **relating to,** *ret-* **net,** *-in-* **relating to,** *-path-* **disease,** *-y* **state**]

diplopia (dih-PLOH-pee-ah)
[*di-* **double,** *-op-* **vision,** *-ia* **condition**]

glaucoma (glaw-KOH-mah)
[*glauco-* **grey or silver,** *-oma* **tumour (growth)**]

hyperopia (hye-per-OH-pee-ah)
[*hyper-* **excessive or above,** *-op-* **vision,** *-ia* **condition**]

Ménière disease (men-ee-AIR)
[*Prosper Ménière* **French physician**]

myopia (my-OH-pee-ah)
[*myops-* **nearsighted,** *-op-* **vision,** *-ia* **condition**]

nyctalopia (nik-tah-LOH-pee-ah)
[*nyct-* **night,** *-op-* **vision,** *-ia* **condition**]

ophthalmology (off-thal-MOL-eh-jee)
[*oph-* **eye or vision,** *-thalm-* **inner chamber,** *-o-* **combining form,** *-log-* **words (study of),** *-y* **activity**]

ophthalmoscope (off-THAL-mah-skohp)
[*oph-* **eye or vision,** *-thalmo-* **inner chamber,** *-scop-* **see**]

otitis (o-TYE-tis)
[*ot-* **ear,** *-itis* **inflammation**]

otitis media (o-TYE-tis MEE-dee-ah)
[*ot-* **ear,** *-itis* **inflammation,** *medi-* **middle,** *-al* **relating to**]

otosclerosis (o-toh-skleh-ROH-sis)
[*oto-* **ear,** *-sclero-* **hard,** *-sis* **condition**]

otoscope (O-toh-skohp)
[*oto-* **ear,** *-scop-* **see**]

presbycusis (pres-bih-KYOO-sis)
[*presby-* **elderly,** *-cusis* **hearing**]

presbyopia (pres-bee-OH-pee-ah)
[*presby-* **elderly,** *-op-* **vision,** *-ia* **condition**]

retinal detachment (RET-ih-nal)
[*ret-* **net,** *-in-* **relating to,** *-al* **relating to**]

scotoma (skoh-TOH-mah)
[*scoto-* **darkness,** *-oma* **tumour**]

strabismus (strah-BIS-mus)
[*strab-* **squinting,** *-ismus* **condition**]

tinnitus (tih-NYE-tus or TIN-nit-us)
[*tinnitis* **a ringing or tinkling**]

trachoma (trah-KOH-mah)
[*trach-* **rough,** *-oma* **tumour**]

tympanotomy tube (tim-pah-NOT-eh-mee)
[*tympan-* **drum,** *-tom-* **cut,** *-y* **action**]

vertigo (VER-ti-go)
[*vertigo* **turning**]

case study

Why were the headlights of the oncoming cars so bright? Rita flashed her car lights as the next car approached, but when the driver flashed his lights in return, she saw his lights had been on the low setting all along. She also noticed the street signs were difficult to read in dim light. When she got to her daughter's house, Rita was quite relieved to be off the road! Over the years, her vision had always been excellent; not being able to see well was a new experience for her. Her daughter suggested she should have her eyes checked as soon as possible.

The following week Rita tried to read one of the magazines in the optometrist's waiting room and realized she could not get the letters to come into focus unless she held the magazine at arm's length; yet another sign of trouble with her eyesight.

1. What could be causing Rita's inability to focus on close objects?
   a. Myopia
   b. Presbyopia
   c. Conjunctivitis
   d. Scotoma

A few minutes later she heard the secretary calling her name for her appointment with the optometrist.

2. What type of receptor in Rita's ear responded to the secretary's voice?
   a. A mechanoreceptor
   b. A photoreceptor
   c. A thermoreceptor
   d. A chemoreceptor

As the optometrist leaned closer to get a better look at her eyes, Rita could smell her perfume.

3. What type of receptor in Rita's nose responded to the perfume?
   a. A mechanoreceptor
   b. A photoreceptor
   c. A thermoreceptor
   d. A chemoreceptor

When the examination was complete, the optometrist told Rita that the lenses of her eyes had cloudy spots in them, and this would account for the vision problems she experienced when driving at night.

4. What condition could the cloudy spots indicate?
   a. Presbyopia
   b. Glaucoma
   c. Cataracts
   d. Myopia

Hint: To solve a case study, you may have to refer to the glossary or index, other chapters in this textbook, ***Connect It!,*** and other resources.

UNIT 3

CHAPTER SUMMARY

*To download an MP3 version of the chapter summary for use with your mobile device, access the **Audio Chapter Summaries** online at evolve.elsevier.com.*

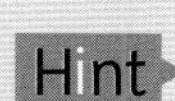

Scan this summary after reading the chapter to help you reinforce the key concepts. Later, use the summary as a quick review before your class or before a test.

Introduction

A. Special senses include smell, taste, hearing, balance, and vision
B. Special senses provide feedback about both the internal and external environments, possibly initiating reflexes that maintain homeostasis

Sense of Smell

A. Olfactory receptors
   1. Olfactory sense organs consist of epithelial support cells and olfactory sensory neurons (**Figure 24-1**)
      a. Olfactory cilia—located on olfactory sensory neurons that touch the olfactory epithelium lining the upper surface of the nasal cavity
      b. Olfactory cells—chemoreceptors—gas molecules or odourants dissolved in the mucus covering the nasal epithelium stimulate the olfactory cells
      c. Olfactory epithelium—located in most superior portion of the nasal cavity
      d. Olfactory receptors—extremely sensitive and easily fatigued
B. Olfactory pathway—when the level of odourants reaches a threshold level, the following occurs (**Figure 24-2**):
   1. Receptor potential and then action potential are generated and passed to the olfactory nerves in the olfactory bulb
   2. The impulse then passes through the olfactory tract and into the thalamic and olfactory centres of the brain for interpretation, integration, and memory storage

Sense of Taste

A. Taste buds—sense organs that respond to gustatory, or taste, stimuli
   1. Associated with papillae
      a. Fungiform—large, mushroom-shaped; anterior two thirds of tongue
      b. Circumvallate—huge, dome-shaped; form row near back of tongue
      c. Foliate—leaflike; lateral edges of posterior tongue
      d. Filiform—threadlike; scattered among fungiform papillae
   2. Chemoreceptors that are stimulated by chemicals dissolved in the saliva

3. Gustatory cells—sensory cells in taste buds; gustatory hairs extend from each gustatory cell into the taste pore
4. Sense of taste depends on the creation of a receptor potential in gustatory cells because of taste-producing chemicals (tastants) in the saliva
5. Taste buds are similar structurally; functionally, each taste bud responds most effectively to one of five primary taste sensations: sour, sweet, bitter, umami, and salty (and perhaps others, such as metallic or water) (**Figures 24-3** and **24-4**)
6. Adaptation and sensitivity thresholds differ for each of the primary taste sensations

B. Neural pathway for taste
1. Taste sensation begins with a receptor potential in the gustatory cells of a taste bud; generation and propagation of an action potential then transmits the sensory input to the brain
2. Nerve impulses from the anterior two thirds of the tongue travel over the facial nerve; those from the posterior one third of the tongue travel over the glossopharyngeal nerve; the vagus nerve plays a minor role in taste
3. Nerve impulses are carried to the medulla oblongata, relayed into the thalamus, and then relayed into the gustatory area of the cerebral cortex in the parietal lobe of the brain
4. Flavour results from integration of taste, smell, and the trigeminal senses (textures and irritants)

Senses of Hearing and Balance

A. Structure of the ear
1. External ear—two divisions (**Figures 24-5** and **24-6**)
   a. Auricle, or pinna—the visible portion of the ear
   b. External acoustic meatus—tube leading from the auricle into the temporal bone and ending at the tympanic membrane
2. Middle ear (**Figure 24-6**)
   a. Tiny, epithelium-lined cavity hollowed out of the temporal bone
   b. Contains three auditory ossicles
      (1) Malleus (hammer)—attached to the inner surface of the tympanic membrane
      (2) Incus (anvil)—attached to the malleus and stapes
      (3) Stapes (stirrup)—attached to the incus
   c. Openings into the middle ear cavity
      (1) Opening from the external acoustic meatus covered with tympanic membrane
      (2) Oval window—opening into inner ear; stapes fits here
      (3) Round window—opening into inner ear; covered by a membrane
      (4) Opening into the auditory (eustachian) tube
3. Inner ear (**Figure 24-7**, *A*)
   a. Structure of the inner ear (labyrinth)
      (1) Bony labyrinth—made up of the vestibule, cochlea, and semicircular canals
      (2) Membranous labyrinth—made up of utricle and saccule inside the vestibule, cochlear duct inside the cochlea, and membranous semicircular ducts inside the bony semicircular canals
      (3) Vestibule and semicircular canal organs are involved with balance
      (4) Cochlea—involved with hearing
      (5) Endolymph—clear, potassium-rich fluid filling the membranous labyrinth
      (6) Perilymph—similar to cerebrospinal fluid, surrounds the membranous labyrinth, filling the space between the membranous tunnel and its contents and the bony walls that surround it

B. The process of hearing
1. Cochlea and cochlear duct (**Figure 24-7**, *B*)
   a. Cochlea—bony labyrinth
   b. Modiolus—cone-shaped core of bone that houses the spiral ganglion, which consists of cell bodies of the first sensory neurons in the auditory relay
   c. Cochlear duct
      (1) Lies inside the cochlea; only part of the internal ear concerned with hearing; contains endolymph
      (2) Shaped like a triangular tube
      (3) Divides the cochlea into the scala vestibuli, the upper section, and the scala tympani, the lower section; both sections filled with perilymph
      (4) Vestibular membrane—the roof of the cochlear duct
      (5) Basilar (spiral) membrane—floor of the cochlear duct
      (6) Organ of Corti—rests on the basilar membrane; consists of supporting cells and hair cells; also called *spiral organ*
      (7) Axons of the neurons that begin around the organ of Corti, extend in the cochlear nerve to the brain to produce the sensation of hearing
      (8) Outer rows of hair cells respond to vibrations by shortening or elongating in ways that amplify the vibrations—making ear more sensitive
2. Perceiving sound
   a. Sound is created by vibrations
   b. Ability to hear sound waves depends on volume, pitch, and other acoustic properties
   c. Sound waves must be of sufficient amplitude to move the tympanic membrane and have a frequency capable of stimulating the hair cells in the organ of Corti (spiral organ) (**Figure 24-8**, *A*)
   d. Basilar membrane width and thickness varies throughout its length
      (1) High-frequency sound waves vibrate the narrow portion near the oval window
      (2) Low frequencies vibrate the wider, thicker portion near the apex of the cochlea
      (3) Each frequency stimulates different hair cells and facilitates perception of different pitches (**Figure 24-8**, *B*)
      (4) Perception of loudness is determined by movement amplitude; the greater the movement, the louder the perceived sound
      (5) Hearing results from stimulation of the auditory area of the cerebral cortex

3. Pathway of sound waves (**Figure 24-8**)
   a. Enter external auditory canal
   b. Strike tympanic membrane, causing vibrations
   c. Tympanic vibrations move the malleus, which in turn moves the incus and then the stapes
   d. The stapes moves against the oval window, which begins the fluid conduction of sound waves
   e. The perilymph in the scala vestibuli of the cochlea begins a "ripple" that is transmitted through the vestibular membrane to the endolymph inside the duct, to the basilar membrane, and then to the organ of Corti
   f. From the basilar membrane, the ripple is transmitted through the perilymph in the scala tympani and then expends itself against the round window
4. Neural pathway of hearing
   a. A movement of hair cells against the tectorial membrane stimulates the dendrites that terminate around the base of the hair cells and initiates impulse conduction by the cochlear nerve to the brainstem
   b. Impulses pass through "relay stations" in the nuclei in the medulla, pons, midbrain, and thalamus before reaching the auditory area of the temporal lobe

C. Balance
1. Vestibule and semicircular canals (**Figure 24-7**, *A*)
   a. Vestibule—the central section of the bony labyrinth; the utricle and saccule are the membranous structures within the vestibule
   b. Three semicircular canals—found in each temporal bone
      (1) Each canal is at a right angle to the other
      (2) Membranous semicircular ducts, within the canals; each contains endolymph and connects with the utricle
      (3) Each canal enlarges into an ampulla near junction with utricle
2. Static equilibrium—ability to sense the position of the head relative to gravity or to sense acceleration or deceleration (**Figure 24-9**)
   a. Movements of the maculae, located in both the utricle and saccule almost at right angles to each other, provide information related to head position or acceleration
   b. Otoliths are located within the matrix of the macula
   c. Changing head position produces a change of pressure on the otolith-weighted matrix, which stimulates the hair cells that in turn stimulate the receptors of the vestibular nerve
   d. Vestibular nerve fibres conduct impulses to the brain and produce a sensation of the position of the head and also a sensation of a change in the pull of gravity
   e. Righting reflexes—muscular responses to restore the body and its parts to their normal position when they have been displaced; caused by stimuli of the macula and impulses from proprioceptors and from the eyes
3. Dynamic equilibrium—needed to maintain balance when the head or body is rotated or suddenly moved; able to detect changes both in direction and rate at which movement occurs (**Figure 24-10**)
   a. Depends on the functioning of the cristae ampullare, which are located in the ampulla of each semicircular duct
   b. Cupula—gelatinous cap in which the hair cells of each crista are embedded
      (1) Does not respond to gravity
      (2) Moves with the flow of endolymph in the semicircular ducts
   c. Semicircular ducts are arranged at nearly right angles to each other to detect movement in all directions
   d. Hair cells bend as cupula moves, producing a receptor potential followed by an action potential
      (1) Action potential passes through the vestibular portion of the eighth cranial nerve to the medulla oblongata
      (2) Sent next to other areas of the brain and spinal cord for interpretation, integration, and response

Vision

A. Structure of the eye (**Figures 24-11** through **24-20**)
1. External structures (**Figures 24-11** through **24-15**)
   a. Eyebrows and eyelashes—give some protection against foreign objects entering the eye; cosmetic purposes
   b. Eyelids—consist of voluntary muscle and skin with a tarsal plate
      (1) Lined with conjunctiva, a mucous membrane
      (2) Palpebral fissure—opening between the eyelids
      (3) Angle or canthus—where the upper and lower eyelids join
   c. Lacrimal apparatus—structures that secrete tears and drain them from the surface of the eyeball (**Figure 24-14**)
      (1) Lacrimal glands—size and shape of a small almond
         (a) Located at the upper, outer margin of each orbit
         (b) Approximately a dozen small ducts lead from each gland
         (c) Drain tears onto the conjunctiva
      (2) Lacrimal canals—small channels that empty into lacrimal sacs
      (3) Lacrimal sacs—located in a groove in the lacrimal bone
      (4) Nasolacrimal ducts—small tubes that extend from the lacrimal sac into the inferior meatus of the nose
   d. Muscles of the eye
      (1) Extrinsic eye muscles (**Figure 24-15**)—skeletal muscles that attach to the outside of the eyeball and to the bones of the orbit
         (a) Named according to their position on the eyeball
         (b) Include the superior, inferior, medial, and lateral rectus muscles and superior and inferior oblique muscles
      (2) Intrinsic eye muscles—smooth muscles located within the eye
         (a) Iris—regulates size of pupil
         (b) Ciliary muscle—controls shape of lens

2. Layers of the eyeball—three coats of tissues compose the eyeball (**Figure 24-16**)
   a. Fibrous layer—outer coat
      (1) Sclera—tough, white, fibrous tissue
      (2) Cornea—the transparent anterior portion that lies over the iris; no blood vessels found in the cornea or in the lens
      (3) Scleral venous sinus (canal of Schlemm)—ring-shaped venous sinus found deep within the anterior portion of the sclera at its junction with the cornea
   b. Vascular layer—middle coat
      (1) Contains many blood vessels and a large amount of pigment
      (2) Choroid—pigmented membrane lining more than two thirds of the posterior fibrous outer coat
      (3) Anterior portion has three different structures (**Figure 24-16**)
         (a) Ciliary body—thickening of choroid, fits between anterior margin of retina and posterior margin of iris; ciliary muscle lies in anterior part of ciliary body; ciliary processes—fold in the ciliary body
         (b) Suspensory ligament—attached to the ciliary processes and blends with the elastic capsule of the lens, to hold it in place
         (c) Iris—coloured part of the eye; consists of circular and radial smooth muscle fibres that form a doughnut-shaped structure; attaches to the ciliary body
   c. Inner layer—incomplete innermost coat of the eyeball
      (1) Retina—made up of an outer layer of pigmented epithelium (pigmented retina) and an inner layer of nervous tissue (sensory retina) (**Figure 24-18**)
      (2) Three layers of neurons make up the sensory retina
         (a) Photoreceptor cells—visual receptors, sensitive to light rays
            (i) Rods—absent from the fovea and macula; increased in density toward the periphery of the retina
            (ii) Cones—less numerous than rods; most densely concentrated in the fovea centralis in the macula lutea
         (b) Bipolar cells
         (c) Ganglionic cells—all axons of these neurons extend back to the optic disc; part of the sclera, which contains perforations through which the fibres emerge from the eyeball as the optic nerve
         (d) Horizontal and amacrine cells allow lateral connections within the sensory retina
      (3) Optic nerve—second cranial nerve (CN II) extends from the eyeball to the brain
      (4) Retinal blood vessels—critical to normal visual function (**Figure 24-19**)
3. Cavities and humours
   a. Cavities—eyeball has a large interior space divided into two cavities
      (1) Anterior cavity—lies in front of the lens; has two subdivisions
         (a) Anterior chamber—space anterior to the iris and posterior to the cornea
         (b) Posterior chamber—small space posterior to the iris and anterior to the lens
      (2) Posterior cavity—larger than the anterior cavity; occupies all the space posterior to the lens, suspensory ligament, and ciliary body
   b. Humours
      (1) Aqueous humour—fills both chambers of the anterior cavity; clear, watery fluid that often leaks out when the eye is injured; formed from blood in capillaries located in the ciliary body (**Figure 24-20**)
      (2) Vitreous body—gel-filled sac fills the posterior cavity; fibrous meshwork (stroma) filled with thick vitreous humour
      (3) Humours help to maintain sufficient intraocular pressure to give the eyeball its shape

B. The process of seeing
1. Formation of retinal image
   a. Refraction of light rays—deflection, or bending, of light rays produced by light rays passing obliquely from one transparent medium into another of different optical density; cornea, aqueous humour, lens, and vitreous body are the refracting media of the eye
   b. Accommodation for near vision requires three changes:
      (1) Change of lens shape (**Figure 24-21**)
         (a) Increase in curvature of the lens to achieve the greater refraction needed for near vision
         (b) Contraction of ciliary muscle reduces tension in suspensory ligaments, allowing lens to bulge to better see near objects
         (c) Relaxation of ciliary muscle increases tension in suspensory ligaments, flattening lens for distant vision
      (2) Constriction of pupil—muscles of iris are important to formation of a clear retinal image (**Figure 24-22**)
         (a) Pupil constriction prevents divergent rays from object from entering eye through periphery of the cornea and lens
         (b) Near reflex—constriction of pupil that occurs with accommodation of the lens in near vision
         (c) Photopupil reflex—pupil constricts in bright light
      (3) Convergence of eyes—movement of the two eyeballs inward so that their visual axes come together at the object viewed
         (a) The closer the object, the greater the degree of convergence necessary to maintain single vision
         (b) For convergence to occur, a functional balance between antagonistic extrinsic muscles must exist
         (c) Strabismus (crossed eyes) is abnormal convergence (**Figure 24-23**)

2. The role of photopigments—light-sensitive pigmented compounds undergo structural changes that result in generation of nerve impulses, which are interpreted by the brain as sight
   a. Rods—photopigment in rods is rhodopsin
      (1) Rhodopsin (retinal + opsin) is found in membranes stacked in the rod cell's outer segment
      (2) Retinal changes shape quickly when light strikes it and rhodopsin breaks down into opsin and retinal
      (3) A second-messenger system involving G proteins then triggers hyperpolarization of the rod cell, resulting in neural signalling
      (4) ATP from mitochondria in the rod cell's inner segment is needed to re-form rhodopsin (**Figure 24-24**)
   b. Cones—three types of cones are present in the retina, with each having a different variation of the rhodopsin photopigment: blue (S) cones, green (M) cones, and red (L) cones
      (1) Perception of a large variety of colours results from the combination of signals from different cone types
      (2) Cone pigments are less light-sensitive than rhodopsin and need brighter light to break down (**Figure 24-25**)
      (3) Cones are densely distributed at the fovea (centre of the visual field), in contrast to rods, which are densest outside the fovea
   c. Ganglion cells—relay information from rods and cones (by way of bipolar cells) but also relay non-image light information to the body's biological clock; photopigment is melanopsin
3. Neural pathway of vision (**Figure 24-26**)
   a. Fibres that conduct impulses from the rods and cones reach the visual cortex in the occipital lobes by way of the optic nerves, optic chiasma, optic tracts, and optic radiations
   b. Optic nerve contains fibres from only one retina, but optic chiasma contains fibres from the nasal portion of both retinas; these anatomical facts explain peculiar visual abnormalities that sometimes occur

Cycle of Life: Special Senses

A. Sensory information is acquired through depolarization of sensory nerve endings
   1. Age, disease, structural defects, or lack of maturation affects ability to identify and respond
B. Structure and function response capabilities are related to developmental factors associated with age
C. Senses become more acute with maturation
D. Sensory capability loss in old age related to structural change in receptor cells or other sense organ structures

The Big Picture: Special Senses

A. Special senses act as sensors in homeostatic feedback loops
B. Many special senses help us monitor our external environment for dangers or help us find essential nutrients such as water or salt

REVIEW QUESTIONS

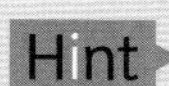

Write out the answers to these questions after reading the chapter and reviewing the Chapter Summary. Note—writing out your answers will consolidate learning and provide a valuable resource of information.

1. Identify the pathway involved for the production of the sense of smell.
2. What are G-protein–mediated receptor sites?
3. Describe the main features of the middle ear.
4. Name the parts of the bony and membranous labyrinths and describe the relationship of those parts.
5. In what ear structure or structures is the hearing sense organ located? In which main ear structures are the sense organs associated with equilibrium of the body located?
6. What is the name of the hearing sense organ? Name the sense organs of equilibrium.
7. Describe the path of sound waves as they enter the ear.
8. Define *vertigo*. How is vertigo treated?
9. Describe the role of the basilar (spiral) membrane in hearing.
10. What is the difference between static and dynamic equilibrium? Describe the general mechanisms by which each is maintained.
11. Name two involuntary muscles in the eye. Explain their functions.
12. Define the term *refraction*. Name the refractory media of the eye.
13. Explain briefly the mechanism for accommodation for near vision.
14. Name the photopigments present in rods and in cones. Explain their role in vision.
15. Explain why "night blindness" may occur in marked vitamin A deficiency.

CRITICAL THINKING QUESTIONS

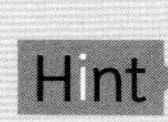

After finishing the Review Questions, write out the answers to these more in-depth questions to help you apply your new knowledge. Go back to sections of the chapter that relate to concepts that you find difficult.

1. Describe the neural pathways for taste and smell. What would be most likely to stimulate a memory: the taste of apple pie or the smell of apple pie? Explain your answer.
2. Describe the various ways that the body protects the sensory structures of the ears when external sounds are dangerously loud.
3. Compare and contrast the three coats of the eye. Include the specific functions of each within your answer.
4. Describe how the receptors for vision in dim light and those for vision in bright light are different.
5. How is sensory response related to age?
6. If you were told you had to lose a special sense but could pick which one, which would it be? Indicate which sensory pathway would no longer be in use and how it would affect your quality of life.

25 Endocrine Regulation

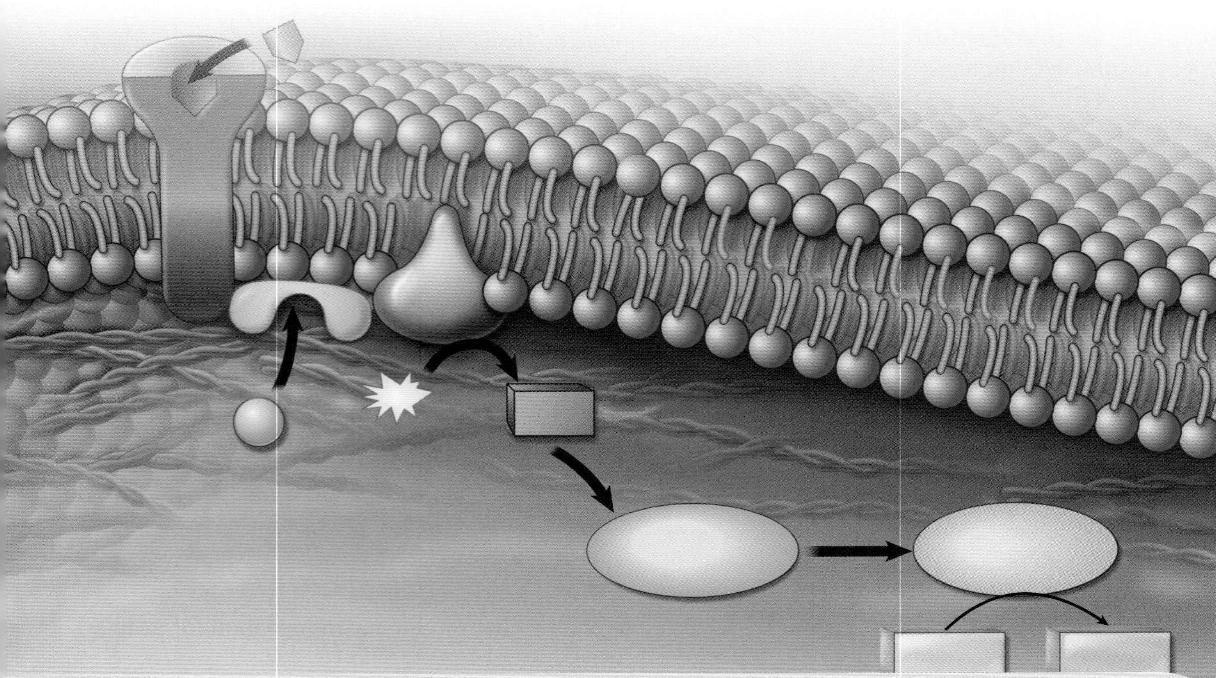

CHAPTER OUTLINE

Hint *Scan this outline before you begin to read the chapter, as a preview of how the concepts are organized.*

In the previous chapters we explored important sensory and regulatory mechanisms involving the nervous system. Our study of the regulation of body function continues in this chapter, in which we discuss the regulatory function of the endocrine system. The endocrine system uses signalling molecules called hormones, which are released by glands into the bloodstream and sent throughout the body. These hormones can thus affect any or all tissues of the body. As you learn concepts of hormone function, try to see them as part of an overall system of regulating the body's functions. In the next chapter, we continue the story of endocrine regulation by exploring specific endocrine glands and the hormones they produce. •

LANGUAGE OF SCIENCE

Hint *Use this list to aid your pronunciation of unfamiliar words.*

amino acid derivative hormone (ah-MEE-no ASS-id deh-RIV-i-tiv HOR-mohn)
[*amino* **NH_2,** *acid* **sour,** *hormon-* **excite**]

anabolic hormone (an-ah-BOL-ik HOR-mohn)
[*anabol-* **build up,** *-ic* **relating to,** *hormon-* **excite**]

antagonism (an-TAG-oh-niz-em)
[*ant-* **against,** *-agon-* **struggle,** *-ism* **condition**]

autocrine hormone (AW-toh-krin HOR-mohn)
[*auto-* **self,** *-crin-* **secrete,** *hormon-* **excite**]

down-regulation (down reg-yuh-LAY-shun)
[*regula-* **rule,** *-tion* **process**]

eicosanoid (eye-KOH-sah-noyd)
[*eicosa-* **twenty,** *-an(e)-* **chemical,** *-oid* **of or like**]

endocrine hormone (EN-doh-krin HOR-mohn)
[*endo-* **within,** *-crin-* **secrete,** *hormon-* **excite**]

G protein-coupled receptor (GPCR) (jee-PROH-teen-kup-eld ree-SEP-ter)
[*G* **for guanine-nucleotide-binding,** *prote-* **first rank,** *-in* **substance,** *recept-* **receive,** *-or* **agent**]

glycoprotein hormone (glye-koh-PRO-teen HOR-mohn)
[*glyco-* **sweet (glucose),** *-prote-* **first rank,** *-in* **substance,** *hormon-* **excite**]

hormone (HOR-mohn)
[*hormon-* **excite**]

leukotriene (loo-koh-TRY-een)
[*leuko-* **white,** *-tri-* **three,** *-ene* **chemical**]

mobile-receptor model (MO-bil-ree-SEP-tor)
[*recept-* **receive,** *-or* **agent**]

neuroendocrine system (nyoo-roh-EN-doh-krin)
[*neuro-* **nerve,** *-endo-* **within,** *-crin-* **secrete**]

neurosecretory tissue (nyoo-roh-sek-REE-tor-ee TISH-yoo)
[*neuro-* **nerve,** *-secret-* **separate,** *-ory* **relating to,** *tissu-* **fabric**]

continued on p. 575

ORGANIZATION OF THE ENDOCRINE SYSTEM

The endocrine system and the nervous system both function to achieve and maintain stability of the internal environment. Each system may work alone or in concert with each other as a single **neuroendocrine system,** performing the same general functions within the body: communication, integration, and control.

Both the endocrine system and the nervous system perform their regulatory functions by means of chemical messengers sent to specific cells. In the nervous system, neurons secrete neurotransmitter molecules to signal nearby cells that have the appropriate receptor molecules. In the endocrine system, secreting cells send **hormone** (from the Greek *hormaein,* "to excite") molecules by way of the bloodstream to signal specific **target cells** throughout the body. Tissues and organs that contain endocrine target cells are called *target tissues* and *target organs,* respectively. As with postsynaptic cells, endocrine target cells must have the appropriate receptor to be influenced by the signalling chemical—a process called *signal transduction.* Many cells have receptors for both neurotransmitters and hormones, so they can be influenced by both types of chemicals.

Whereas neurotransmitters are sent over very short distances across a synapse, hormones diffuse into the blood to be carried to nearly every point in the body. The nervous system can directly control only muscles and glands that are innervated with efferent fibres, whereas the endocrine system can regulate most cells in the body. The effects of neurotransmitters are rapid and short-lived compared with the effects of hormones, which appear more slowly and last longer. **Table 25-1** compares endocrine structure and function with nervous structure and function (**Figure 25-1**).

Endocrine glands secrete their products, hormones, directly into the blood. Because they do not have ducts, they are often called "ductless glands". This characteristic distinguishes *endocrine glands* from *exocrine glands,* which secrete their products into ducts (see Chapter 9, p. 161). Many endocrine glands are made of glandular epithelium, whose cells manufacture and secrete hormones. However, a few endocrine glands are made of **neurosecretory tissue.** Neurosecretory cells are simply modified neurons that secrete chemical messengers that diffuse into the bloodstream rather than across a synapse. In such cases, the chemical messenger is called a *hormone* rather than a *neurotransmitter.* For example, when norepinephrine is released by neurons, diffuses across a synapse, and binds to an adrenergic receptor in a postsynaptic neuron, we call norepinephrine a *neurotransmitter.* On the other hand, we call norepinephrine a *hormone* when it diffuses into the blood (because no postsynaptic cell is present) and then binds to an adrenergic receptor in a distant target cell.

Glands of the endocrine system are widely scattered throughout the body. New discoveries in *endocrinology* continue to add to the long list of hormone-secreting tissues. However, even the most newly

TABLE 25-1 Comparison of the Endocrine System and the Nervous System

FEATURE	ENDOCRINE SYSTEM	NERVOUS SYSTEM
Overall Function	Regulation of effectors to maintain homeostasis	Regulation of effectors to maintain homeostasis
Control by regulatory feedback loops	Yes (endocrine reflexes)	Yes (nervous reflexes)
Effector tissues	Endocrine effectors: virtually all tissues	Nervous effectors: muscle and glandular tissue
Effector cells	Target cells (throughout the body)	Postsynaptic cells (in muscle and glandular tissue)
Chemical Messenger	Hormone	Neurotransmitter
Cells that secrete the chemical messenger	Glandular epithelial cells or neurosecretory cells (modified neurons)	Neurons
Distance travelled (and method of travel) by chemical messenger	Long (by way of circulating blood)	Short (across a microscopic synapse)
Location of receptor in effector cell	On the plasma membrane or within the cell	On the plasma membrane
Characteristics of regulatory effects	Slow to appear, long-lasting	Appear rapidly, short-lived

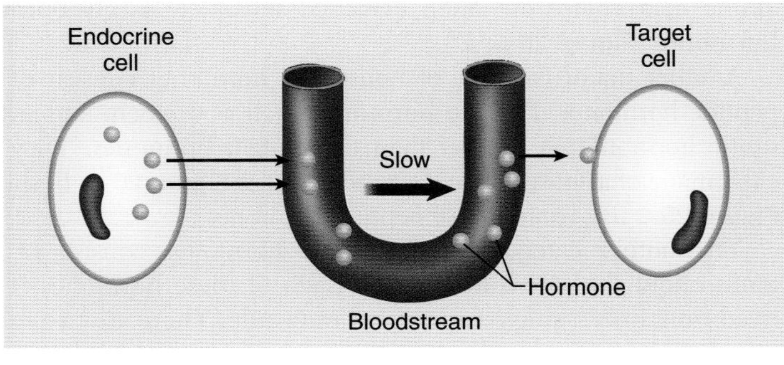

A

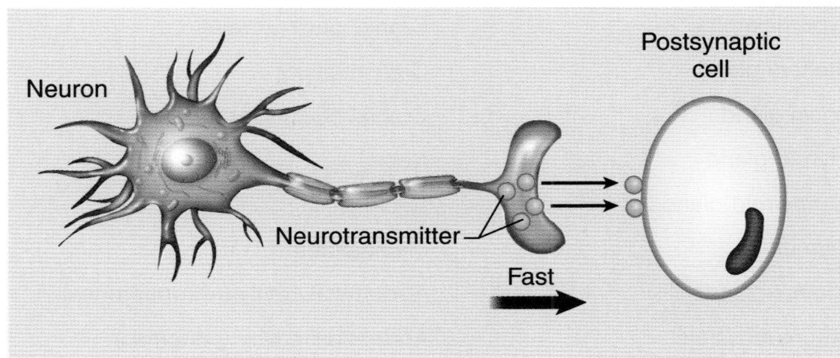

B

FIGURE 25-1 Mechanisms of endocrine (A) and nervous (B) signals.

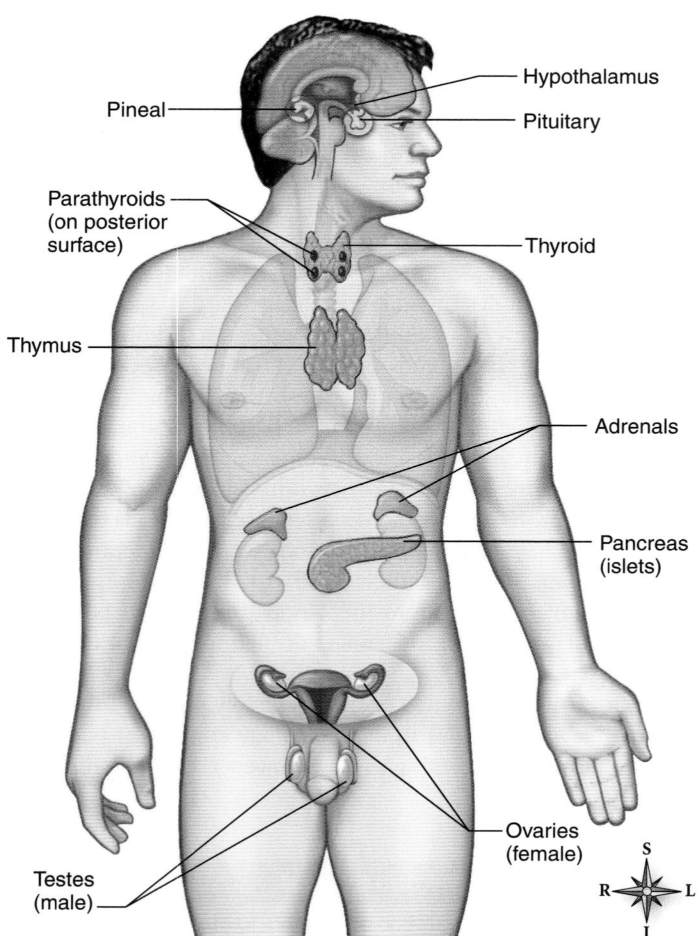

FIGURE 25-2 Locations of some major endocrine glands.

discovered endocrine tissues and their hormones operate according to some basic physiological principles.

In this chapter, we focus our discussion primarily on a few major endocrine glands and their principal hormones. **Figure 25-2** and **Table 25-2** summarize the names and locations of these representative endocrine glands. After you are familiar with the basic principles of endocrinology and the major examples of glands and their hormones, you will be prepared for additional examples that you will encounter as you continue your study of the human body.

TABLE 25-2 Some of the Major Endocrine Glands

NAME	LOCATION
Hypothalamus	Cranial cavity (brain)
Pituitary gland	Cranial cavity
Pineal gland	Cranial cavity (brain)
Thyroid gland	Neck
Parathyroid glands	Neck
Thymus	Mediastinum
Adrenal glands	Abdominal cavity (retroperitoneal)
Pancreatic islets	Abdominal cavity (pancreas)
Ovaries	Pelvic cavity
Testes	Scrotum
Placenta	Pregnant uterus

Quick CHECK

1. What is meant by the term *target cell*?
2. Describe how the nervous system and the endocrine system differ in the way they control effectors.

CLASSIFICATION OF HORMONES

Hormone molecules can be classified in various useful ways. For example, when classified by general function, hormones can be identified as **tropic hormones** (hormones that target other endocrine glands and stimulate their growth and secretion), **sex hormones** (hormones that target reproductive tissues), **anabolic hormones** (hormones that stimulate anabolism in their target cells), and many other functional names. Another useful way to classify hormones is by their chemical structure. Because this method of classifying hormones is so widely used, we will briefly describe it in the following paragraphs.

STEROID HORMONES

All of the many hormones secreted by endocrine tissues can be classified simply as **steroid** or **nonsteroid** (**Figure 25-3**). Steroid hormone molecules are manufactured by endocrine cells from cholesterol, an important type of lipid in the human body (see Chapter 4, p. 60). As **Figure 25-4** shows, because all steroid hormones are derived from a common molecule, cholesterol, they have a characteristic chemical group at the core of each molecule. Because steroids are lipid-soluble, they can easily pass through the phospholipid plasma membrane of target cells. **Figure 25-5** outlines the metabolic pathways used by endocrine cells to convert cholesterol into steroid hormones. Examples of important steroid hormones include cortisol, aldosterone, oestrogen, progesterone, and testosterone.

NONSTEROID HORMONES

Most nonsteroid hormones are synthesized primarily from amino acids rather than from cholesterol (**Figure 25-6**). Some nonsteroid hormones are **protein hormones.** These hormones are long, folded chains of amino acids, a structure typical of protein molecules of any sort (see Chapter 4, p. 64). Included among the protein hormones are insulin, parathyroid hormone, and others listed in **Figure 25-3**. Protein hormones that have carbohydrate groups attached to their amino acid chains are often classified separately as **glycoprotein hormones** (**Figure 25-6**, *D*).

Another major category of nonsteroid hormones consists of the peptide hormones. **Peptide hormones** such as oxytocin and antidiuretic hormone are smaller than the protein hormones. They are each made of a short chain of amino acids, as **Figure 25-6**, *B*, shows. **Figure 25-3** lists examples of peptide hormones.

Yet another category of nonsteroid hormones consists of the **amino acid derivative hormones.** Each of these hormones is derived from only a single amino acid molecule. There are two major subgroups within this category. One subgroup, the *amine hormones*, is synthesized by modifying a single molecule of an amino acid—either tyrosine or tryptophan. Amine hormones such as epinephrine and norepinephrine are produced by neurosecretory cells (secreted

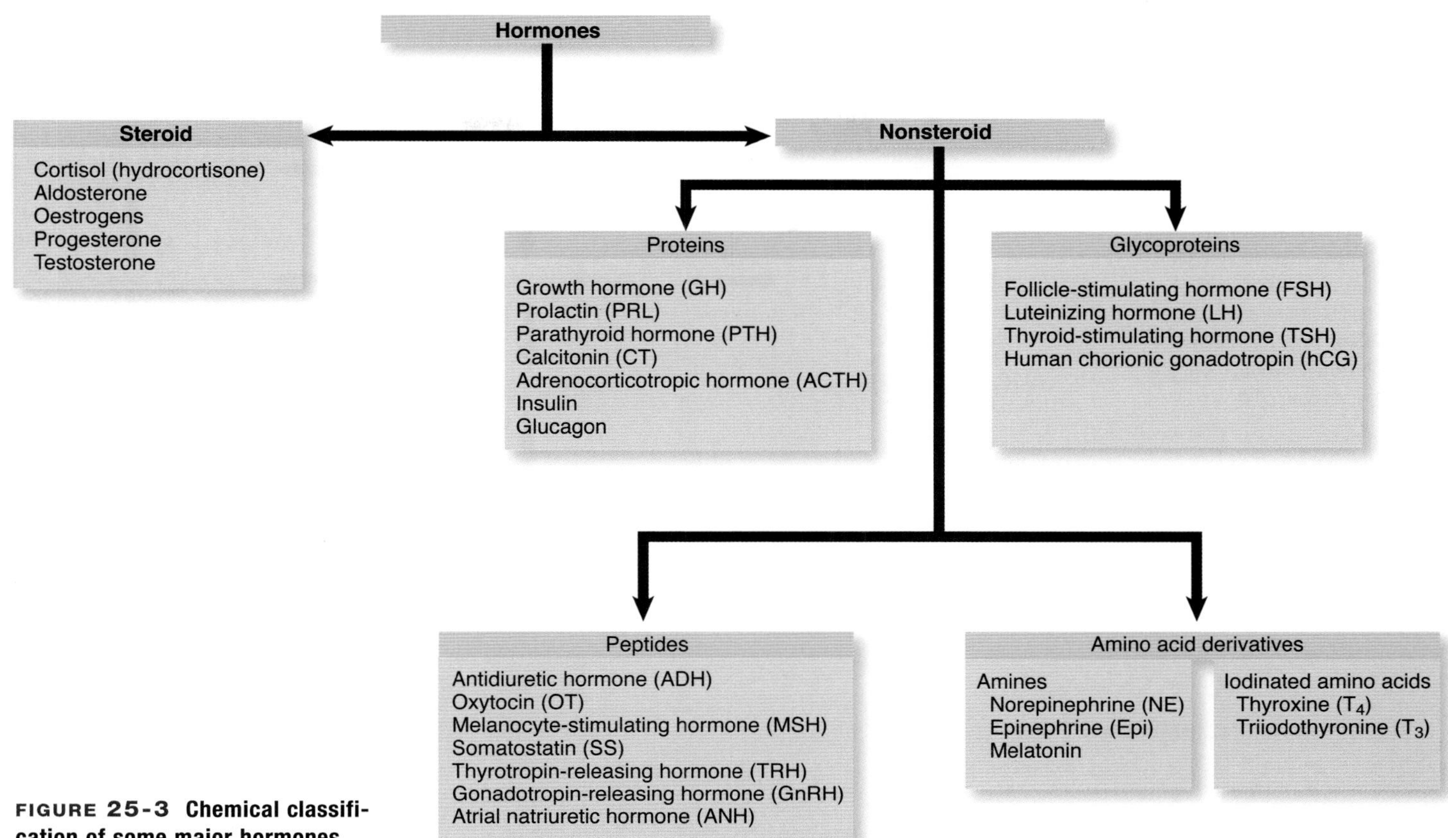

FIGURE 25-3 Chemical classification of some major hormones.

as hormones) and by neurons (secreted as neurotransmitters). Another subgroup of amino acid derivatives produced by the thyroid gland are all synthesized by adding iodine (I) atoms to a tyrosine molecule (**Figure 25-6**, *C*). **Figure 25-3** lists examples of hormones derived from single amino acids.

Quick CHECK

3. How are steroid hormones able to pass through a cell's plasma membrane easily?
4. Name some of the different general types of nonsteroid hormones. Give an example of each.

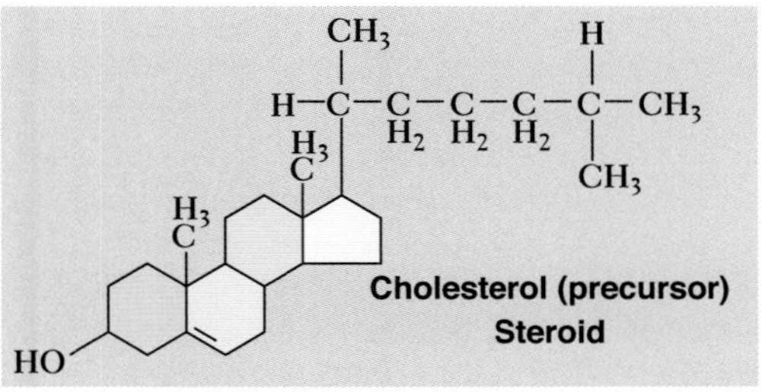

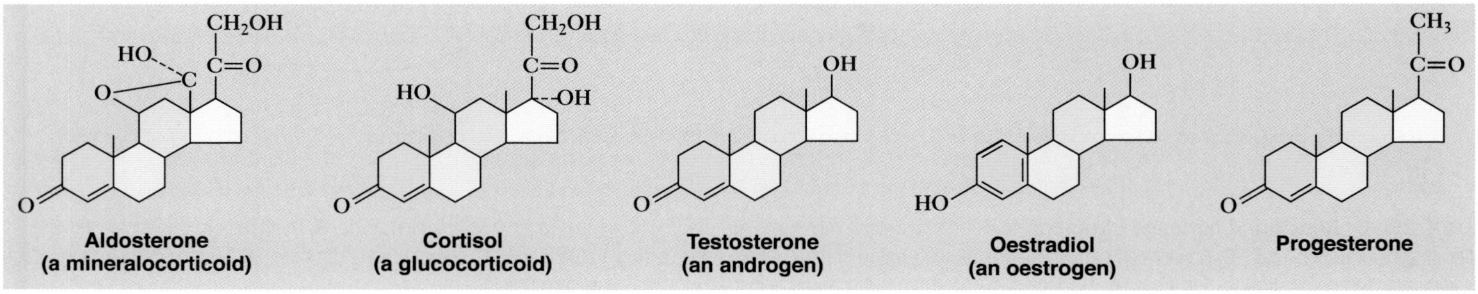

FIGURE 25-4 Steroid hormone structure. As these examples show, steroid hormone molecules are very similar in structure to cholesterol *(top left),* particularly in having a four-ring steroid nucleus at their core. Cholesterol is the precursor molecule from which the steroid hormones are all derived.

Cholesterol (precursor) Steroid

Aldosterone (a mineralocorticoid)

Cortisol (a glucocorticoid)

Testosterone (an androgen)

Oestradiol (an oestrogen)

Progesterone

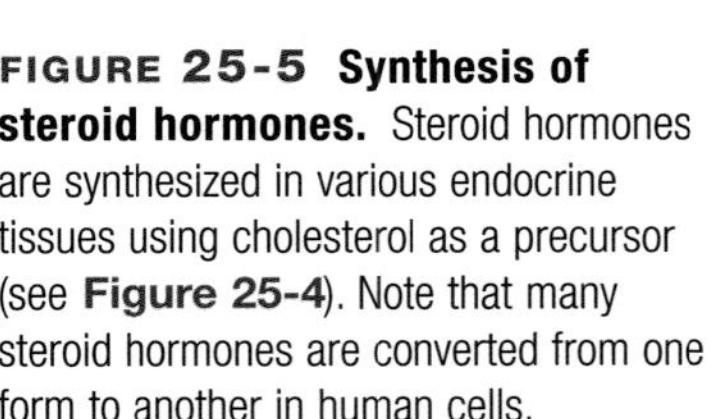

FIGURE 25-5 Synthesis of steroid hormones. Steroid hormones are synthesized in various endocrine tissues using cholesterol as a precursor (see **Figure 25-4**). Note that many steroid hormones are converted from one form to another in human cells.

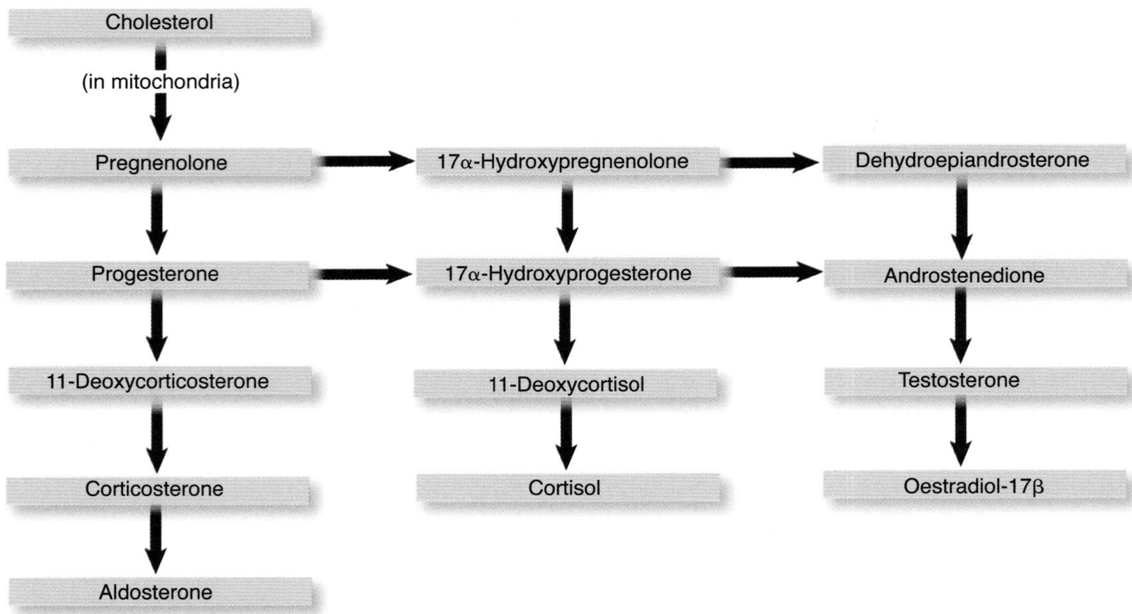

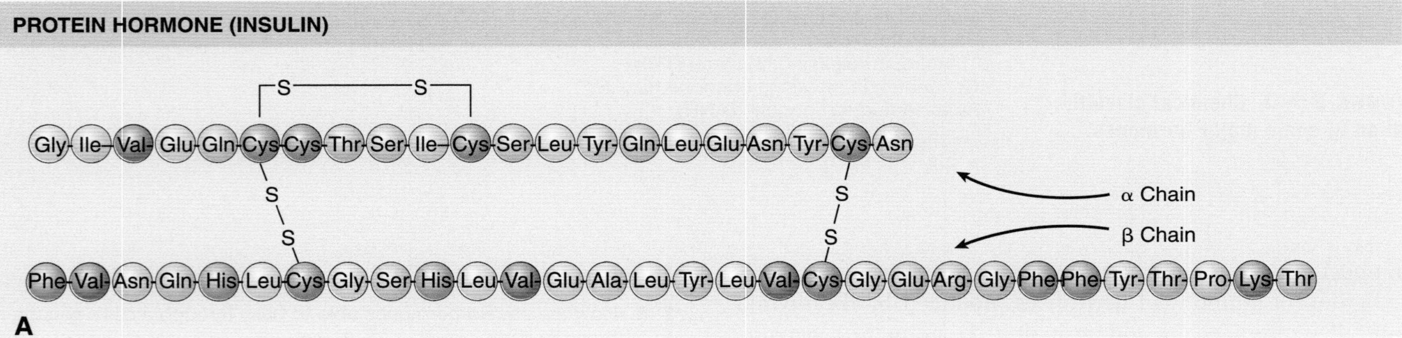

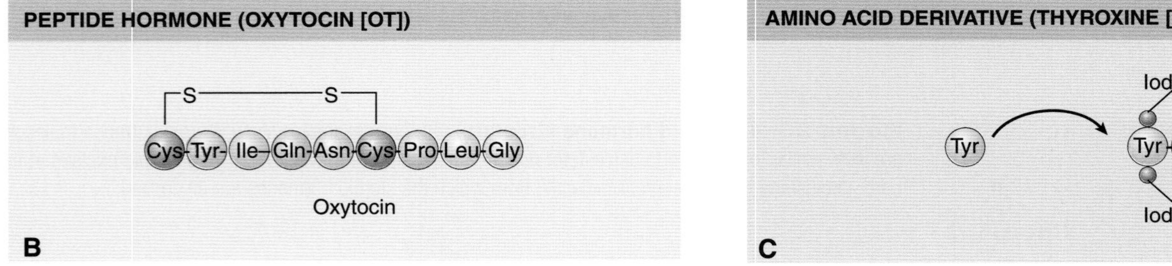

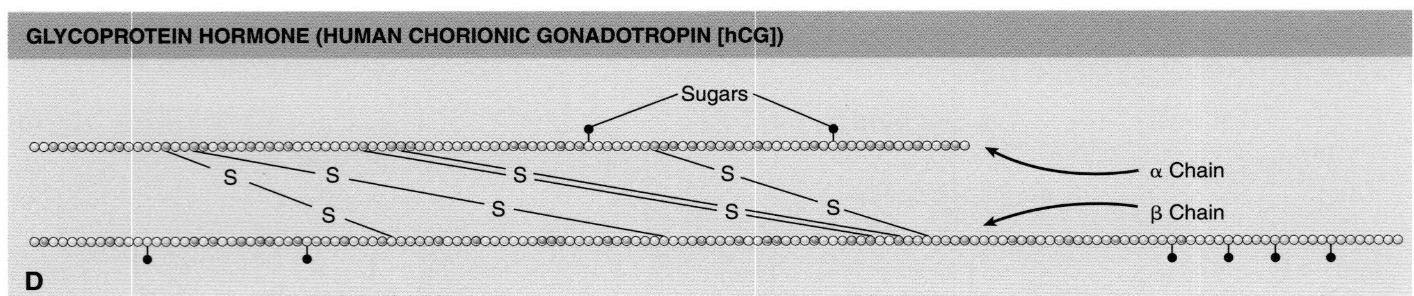

FIGURE 25-6 Nonsteroid hormone structure. A, Protein hormone molecules are made of long, folded strands of amino acids. **B,** Peptide hormone molecules are smaller strands of amino acids. **C,** Amino acid derivatives are, as their name implies, derived from a single amino acid. **D,** Glycoprotein hormones are long, folded strands of amino acids with attached sugar groups. See **Figure 4-12** on p. 62 for abbreviations and colour key for individual amino acids.

HOW HORMONES WORK

GENERAL PRINCIPLES OF HORMONE ACTION

As previously stated, hormones signal a cell by binding to specific receptors on or in the cell. In a "lock-and-key" mechanism, hormones will bind only to receptor molecules that "fit" them exactly. Any cell with one or more receptors for a particular hormone is said to be a *target* of that hormone (**Figure 25-7**). Cells usually have many different types of receptors; therefore they are *target cells* of many different hormones.

In a complex process called *signal transduction*, each different hormone-receptor interaction produces different regulatory changes within the target cell. These cellular changes are usually accomplished by altering the chemical reactions within the target cell. For example, some hormone-receptor interactions initiate synthesis of new proteins. Other hormone-receptor interactions trigger the activation or inactivation of certain enzymes and thus affect the metabolic reactions regulated by those enzymes. Still other hormone-receptor interactions regulate cells by opening or closing specific ion channels in the plasma membrane. Specific mechanisms of signal transduction and endocrine effects in target cells are outlined in the next section.

Different hormones may work together to enhance each other's influence on a target cell. In a phenomenon called **synergism,** combinations of hormones have a greater effect on a target cell than the sum of the effects that each would have if acting alone. Combined hormone actions may exhibit instead the phenomenon of **permissiveness.** Permissiveness occurs when a small amount of one hormone allows a second hormone to have its full effect on a target cell; the first hormone "permits" the full action of the second hormone. A common type of combined action of hormones is seen in the phenomenon of **antagonism.** In antagonism, one hormone produces the opposite effect of another hormone. Antagonism between hormones can be used to "fine tune" the activity of target cells with great accuracy, signalling the cell exactly when (and by how much) to increase or decrease a certain cellular process.

Although our discussion is focused on the primary actions of only a few selected hormones, ongoing studies make it clear that hormones usually have many diverse secondary functions in the body. For example, prolactin (PRL) is a hormone with primary actions that regulate milk production (lactation) and reproduction, but it also has about 300 secondary actions in the body. Most secondary effects of hormones modulate, or influence, the activity of other regulatory mechanisms. The primary effect of a hormone, on the other hand, is a more direct regulatory mechanism.

As previously stated, hormones travel to their target cells by way of the circulating bloodstream. This means that all hormones travel throughout the body. Because they affect only their target cells, however, the effects of a particular hormone may be limited to specific tissues in the body. Some hormone molecules are attached to plasma proteins while they are carried along in the bloodstream. Such hormones must free themselves from the plasma protein to leave the blood and combine with their receptors. Because blood carries hormones nearly everywhere in the body, even where there are no target cells, not all hormone molecules produced by endocrine glands actually hit their target. Unused hormones usually are quickly excreted by the kidneys or broken down by metabolic processes.

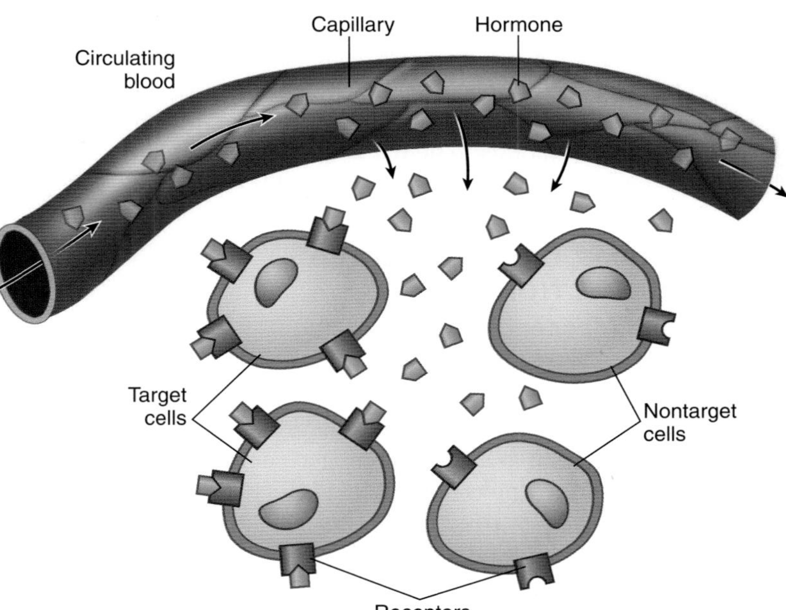

FIGURE 25-7 The target cell concept. A hormone acts only on cells that have receptors specific to that hormone because the shape of the receptor determines which hormone can react with it. This is an example of the lock-and-key model of biochemical reactions.

MECHANISM OF STEROID HORMONE ACTION

Steroid hormones are lipids and thus are not very soluble in blood plasma, which is mostly water. Instead of travelling in the plasma as free molecules, they attach to soluble plasma proteins. As you can see in **Figure 25-8**, a steroid hormone molecule dissociates from its carrier before approaching the target cell.

Because steroid hormones are lipid-soluble and thus can pass into cells easily, it is not surprising that many of their receptors are found inside the cell rather than on the surface of the plasma membrane. After a steroid hormone molecule has diffused into its target cell, it passes into the nucleus, where it binds to a mobile-receptor molecule to form a *hormone-receptor complex.* Some hormones must be activated by enzymes before they can bind to their receptors. Because steroid hormone receptors are not attached to the plasma membrane, but seem to move freely in the nucleoplasm, this model of hormone action has been called the **mobile-receptor model,** or the *nuclear-receptor model.*

Once formed, the hormone-receptor complex activates a certain gene sequence to begin transcription of messenger RNA (mRNA) molecules. The newly formed mRNA molecules then move out of the nucleus into the cytosol, where they associate with ribosomes and begin synthesizing protein molecules.

The new protein molecules synthesized by the target cell would not have been made if not for the arrival of the steroid hormone molecule. Steroid hormones regulate cells by regulating their production of certain critical proteins, such as enzymes that control intracellular reactions or integral membrane proteins that alter the permeability of a cell.

This mechanism of steroid hormone action implies several things about the effects of these hormones. For one thing, the more hormone-receptor complexes are formed, the more mRNA molecules are transcribed, the more new protein molecules are formed, and thus the greater the magnitude of the regulatory effect. In short, the *amount* of steroid hormone present determines the magnitude of a target cell's response. Also, because transcription and protein synthesis take some time, responses to steroid hormones can be slow—from 45 minutes to several days before the full effect is seen.

Mechanisms of Nonsteroid Hormone Action

The Second Messenger Mechanism

Nonsteroid hormones typically operate according to a mechanism originally called the **second messenger model.**

According to this concept of signal transduction, a nonsteroid hormone molecule acts as a "first messenger", delivering its chemical message to fixed receptors in the target cell's plasma membrane. The "message" is then passed into the cell where a "second messenger" triggers the appropriate cellular changes. This concept of nonsteroid hormone action is also called the *fixed-membrane-receptor model.*

In the example illustrated in **Figure 25-9**, a nonsteroid hormone can trigger a **G-protein–coupled receptor (GPCR)** embedded in the membrane of a target cell. The activated GPCR causes an integral membrane protein, called the *G protein,* to bind to a nucleotide called *guanosine triphosphate (GTP).* This in turn activates another membrane protein, *adenyl cyclase.* Adenyl cyclase is an enzyme that promotes the removal of two phosphate groups from adenosine triphosphate (ATP) molecules in the cytosol. The product thus formed is cyclic adenosine monophosphate *(cAMP).* The cAMP molecule acts as a second messenger within the cell. cAMP activates *protein kinases,* a set of enzymes that activate other types of enzymes. It is this final set of specific enzymes, which are now activated, that catalyze the cellular reactions that characterize the target cell's response. In short, the hormone first messenger binds to a membrane receptor, triggering formation of an intracellular second messenger, which activates a cascade of chemical reactions that produces the target cell's response.

Since the time Sutherland first began his pioneering work, other second messenger systems for signal transduction have been discovered. As a matter of fact, the study of second messenger mechanisms remains a central area of physiology research. Although many nonsteroid hormones seem to use cAMP as the second messenger, we now know that some hormones use nucleotides such as inositol triphosphate (IP_3) and cyclic guanosine monophosphate (cGMP) as the second messenger.

FIGURE 25-8 Steroid hormone mechanism. According to the mobile-receptor model, lipid-soluble steroid hormone molecules detach from a carrier protein **(1)** and pass through the plasma membrane **(2)**. The hormone molecules then pass into the nucleus where they bind with a mobile receptor to form a hormone-receptor complex **(3)**. This complex then binds to a specific site on a DNA molecule **(4)**, triggering transcription of the genetic information encoded there **(5)**. The resulting mRNA molecule moves to the cytosol, where it associates with a ribosome, initiating synthesis of a new protein **(6)**. This new protein—usually an enzyme or channel protein—produces specific effects in the target cell **(7)**. Some steroid hormones also have additional secondary effects such as influencing signal transduction pathways at the plasma membrane.

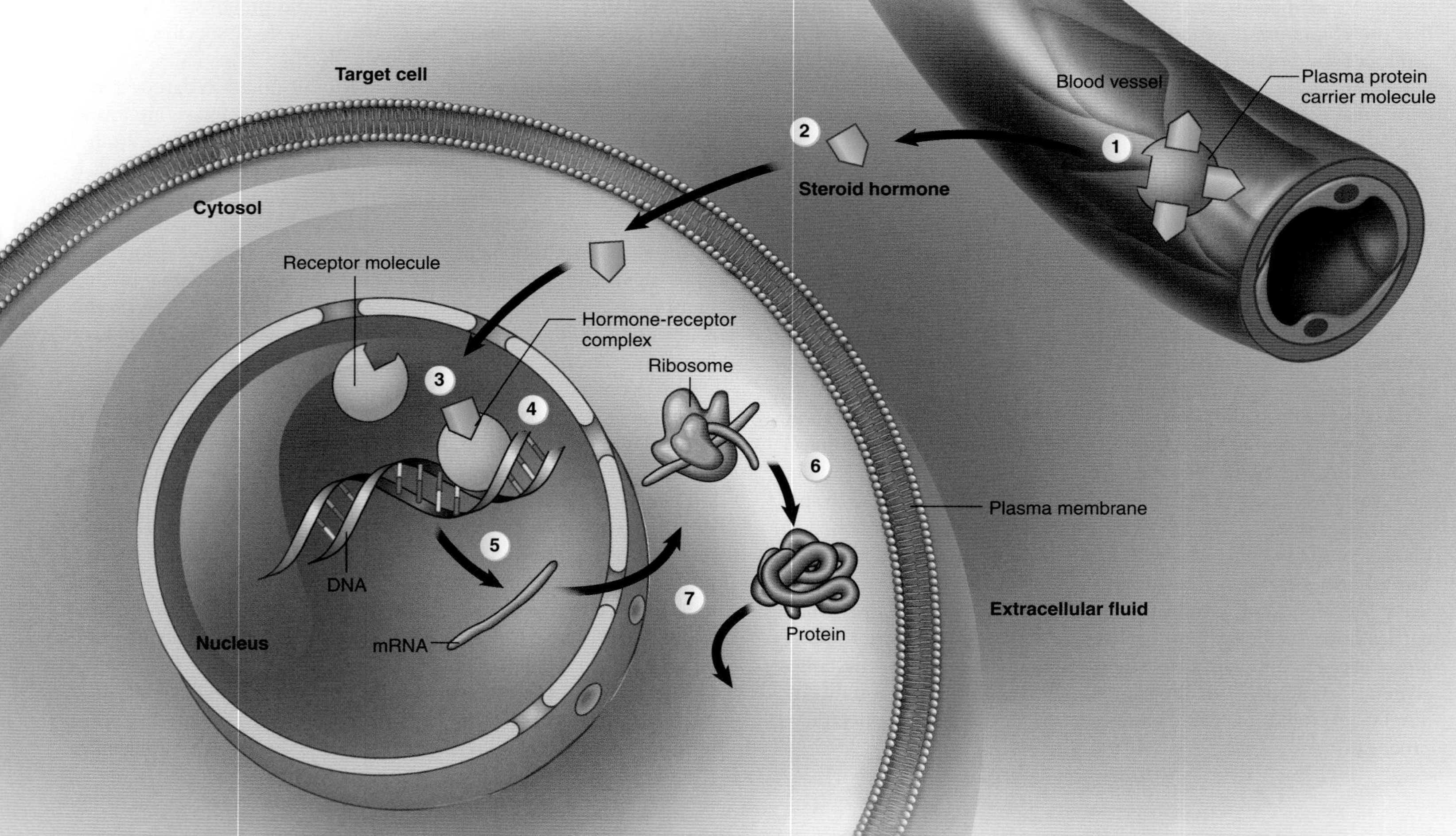

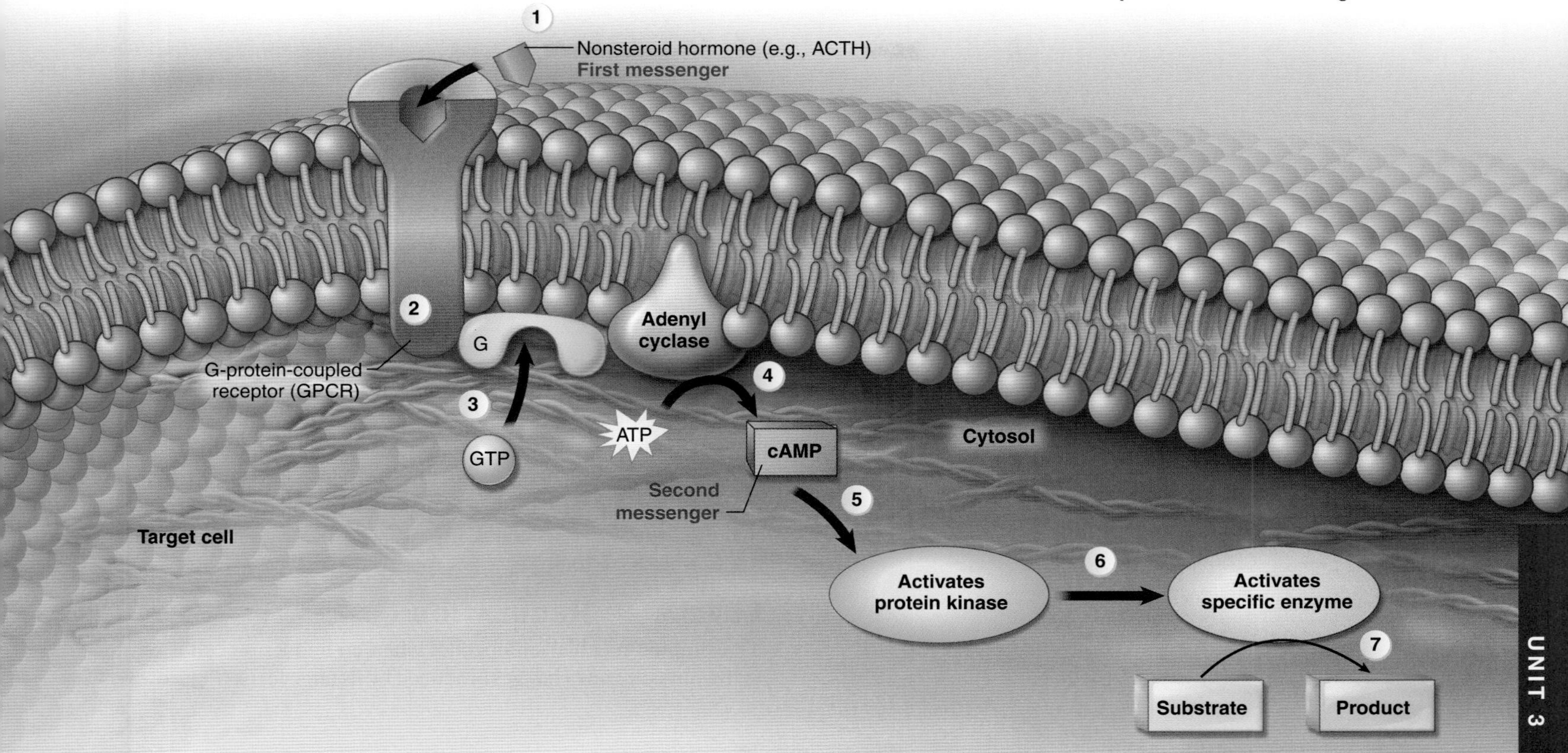

FIGURE 25-9 Example of a second messenger mechanism. A nonsteroid hormone (first messenger) binds to a fixed G-protein–coupled receptor (GPCR) in the plasma membrane of the target cell **(1)**. The hormone-receptor complex activates the G protein **(2)**. The activated G protein reacts with GTP, which in turn activates the membrane-bound enzyme adenyl cyclase **(3)**. Adenyl cyclase removes phosphates from ATP, converting it to cAMP (second messenger) **(4)**. cAMP activates or inactivates protein kinases **(5)**. Protein kinases activate specific intracellular enzymes **(6)**. These activated enzymes then influence specific cellular reactions, thus producing the target cell's response to the hormone **(7)**. *GTP,* Guanosine triphosphate; *ATP,* adenosine triphosphate; *cAMP,* cyclic adenosine monophosphate.

UNIT 3

Still other hormones produce their effects by triggering the opening of calcium (Ca^{++}) channels in the target cell's membranes, as you can see in **Figure 25-10**. Binding of a hormone to a fixed membrane receptor (GPCR) activates a chain of integral membrane proteins (G protein and phosphatidylinositol 4,5-biphosphate, PIP_2) that in turn trigger the opening of calcium channels in the plasma membrane. Ca^{++} ions that enter the cytosol when the channels open bind to an intracellular molecule called *calmodulin.* The Ca^{++}–calmodulin complex thus formed acts as a second messenger, influencing the enzymes that produce the target cell's response.

Research findings also show that in second messenger systems, the hormone-receptor complexes may be taken into the cell by means of endocytosis. Although the purpose of this may be primarily to break down the complexes and recycle the receptors, the hormone-receptor complex may continue to have physiological effects after it is taken into the cell.

The second messenger mechanism of signal transduction produces target cell effects that differ from steroid hormone effects in several important ways (**Table 25-3**). First, the cascade of reactions produced in the second messenger mechanism greatly amplifies the effects of the hormone. Thus the effects of many nonsteroid hormones are disproportionately great when compared with the amount of hormone present. Recall that steroid hormones produce effects in proportion to the amount of hormone present. Also, the second messenger mechanism operates much more quickly than the steroid mechanism. Many nonsteroid hormones produce their full effects within seconds or minutes of initial binding to the target cell receptors—not the hours or days sometimes seen with steroid hormones.

The Nuclear-Receptor Mechanism

Not all nonsteroid hormones operate according to the second messenger model. The notable exception is the pair of thyroid hormones, thyroxine (T_4) and triiodothyronine (T_3). These small iodinated amino acids apparently enter their target cells and bind to receptors already associated with a DNA molecule within the nucleus of the target cell. Formation of a hormone-receptor complex triggers transcription of mRNA and the synthesis of new enzymes in a signal transduction system similar to the steroid mechanism.

Regulation of Hormone Secretion

Hormonal secretion is usually controlled by negative and positive feedback loops. Responses that result from the operation of these loops within the endocrine system are called *endocrine reflexes,* just as responses to nervous feedback loops (reflex arcs) are called *nervous reflexes.*

Negative Feedback

The principle of negative feedback can be illustrated by using the hormone insulin as an example. Normally, elevated blood glucose occurs after a meal, after the absorption of glucose from the digestive

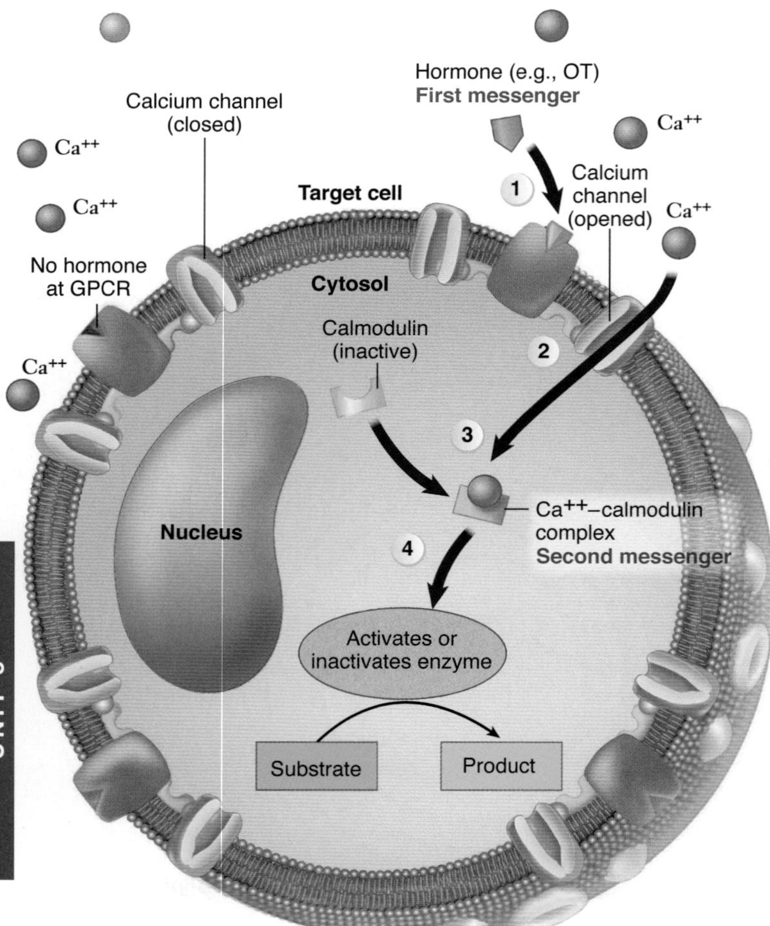

FIGURE 25-10 Calcium–calmodulin as a second messenger. In this example of a second messenger mechanism, a nonsteroid hormone (first messenger) first binds to a fixed receptor (G-protein–coupled receptor, GPCR) in the plasma membrane **(1)**, which activates membrane-bound proteins (G protein and PIP_2) that trigger the opening of calcium channels **(2)**. Calcium ions, which are normally at a higher concentration in the extracellular fluid, diffuse into the cell and bind to a calmodulin molecule **(3)**. The Ca^{++}–calmodulin complex thus formed is a second messenger that binds to an enzyme to produce an allosteric effect that promotes or inhibits the enzyme's regulatory effect in the target cell **(4)**. *PIP_2*, Phosphatidylinositol 4,5-biphosphate.

tract takes place. The elevated blood glucose stimulates the release of insulin from the pancreas. Insulin then assists in the transfer of glucose from the blood into cells, causing blood glucose to drop back toward the normal set point.

As blood glucose concentration drops, the endocrine cells in the pancreas slow their production and release of insulin. These responses are negative because they reverse the direction of a disturbance to the stability of the internal environment. This homeostatic mechanism is called a negative feedback control mechanism because it reverses the change in blood glucose.

Positive Feedback

Positive feedback mechanisms amplify changes rather than reverse them. Usually such amplification threatens homeostasis, but in some situations it can help the body maintain its stability.

For example, during labour, the muscle contractions that push the fetus through the birth canal become stronger and stronger by means of a positive feedback mechanism that regulates secretion of the hormone oxytocin.

Levels of Regulation

The simplest mechanism operates when an endocrine cell is sensitive to the physiological changes produced by its target cells (**Figure 25-11**).

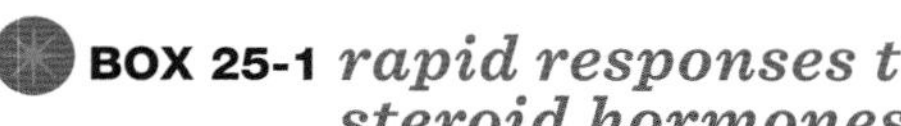

BOX 25-1 *rapid responses to steroid hormones*

The conventional view of steroid hormone regulation of gene activity states that 1 or more hours pass before the effects of the hormone reach their peak. Steroid hormones, however, can also produce some rapid effects in target cells—in just seconds or minutes. How is this possible? We now know that additional steroid hormone receptors at the plasma membrane enable many steroid hormones to regulate signal transduction in target cells. That is, steroid hormones have a secondary effect that can change the messages sent by other regulatory molecules, such as other hormones or neurotransmitters.

The emerging view therefore is that steroid hormones produce both slow and rapid effects in target cells. Slow effects result from stimulating the transcription of specific genes in the target cell's nucleus, thus producing new proteins. Rapid effects result from altering signal transduction mechanisms in the plasma membrane of the target cell. •

TABLE 25-3 Comparison of Steroid and Nonsteroid Hormones

CHARACTERISTIC	STEROID HORMONES*	NONSTEROID HORMONES†
Chemical structure	Lipid	One or more amino acids, sometimes with added sugar groups
Stored in secretory cell	No	Yes; stored in secretory vesicles before release
Interaction with plasma membrane	No; simple diffusion through plasma membrane and into target cell	Yes; binds to specific plasma membrane receptor
Receptor	Mobile receptor in cytoplasm or nucleus	Embedded in plasma membrane
Action	Regulates gene activity (transcription of new proteins that eventually produce effects in the cell)	Triggers signal transduction cascade, producing internal "second messengers" that trigger rapid effects in the target cell
Response time	1 hour to several days	Several seconds to a few minutes

*See **Box 25-1** above for additional emerging concepts of steroid hormone characteristics.

†Some nonsteroid hormones derived from amino acids (e.g., thyroid hormones T_3 and T_4) have gene-activating actions similar to steroid hormones.

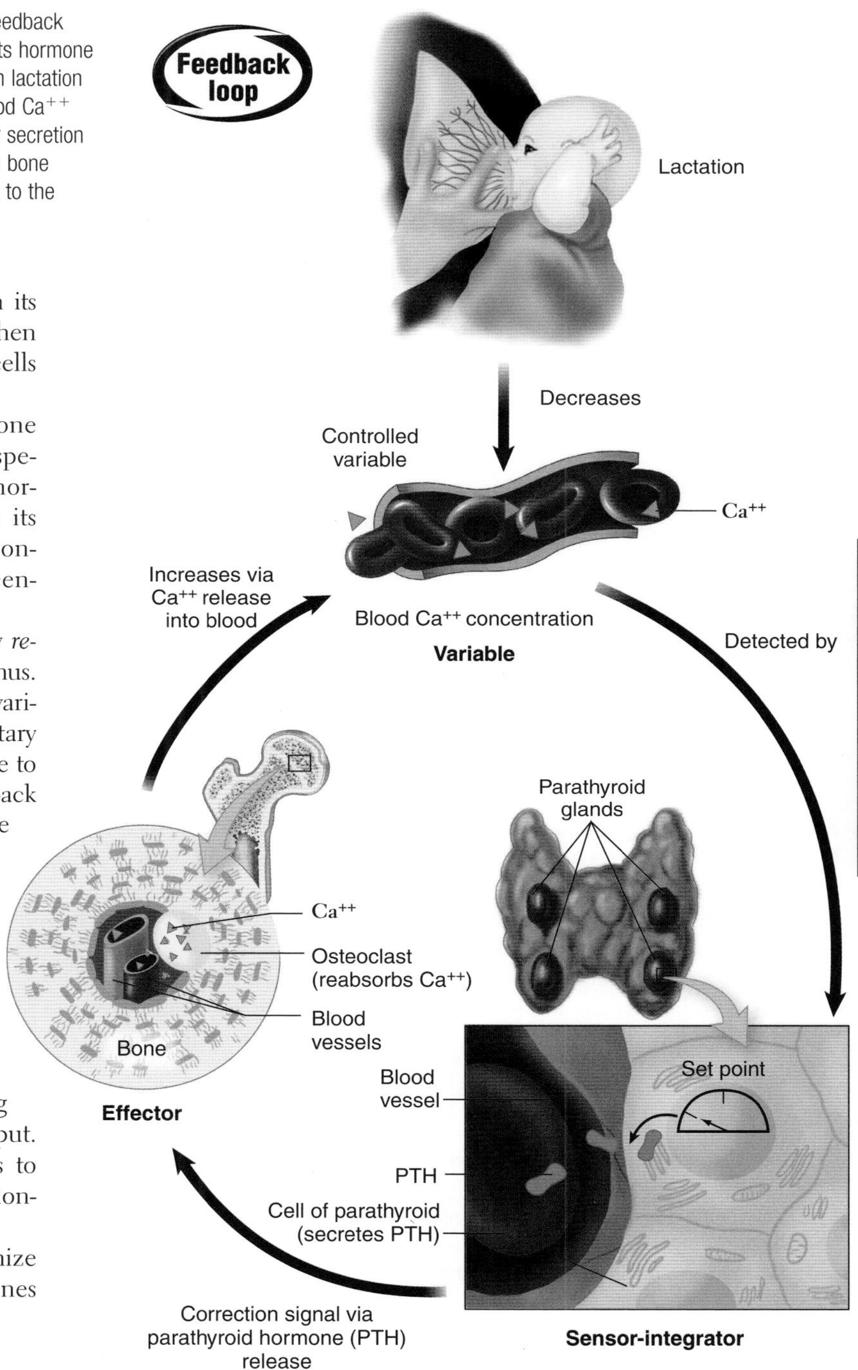

FIGURE 25-11 Endocrine feedback loop. In this example of a short feedback loop, each parathyroid gland is sensitive to changes in the physiological variable its hormone (parathyroid hormone [PTH]) controls—blood calcium (Ca^{++}) concentration. When lactation (milk production) in a breastfeeding woman consumes Ca^{++} and thus lowers blood Ca^{++} concentration, the parathyroids sense the change and respond by increasing their secretion of PTH. PTH stimulates osteoclasts in bone to release more Ca^{++} from storage in bone tissue (among other effects), which increases maternal blood Ca^{++} concentration to the setpoint level.

For example, parathyroid hormone (PTH) produces responses in its target cells that increase Ca^{++} concentration in the blood. When blood Ca^{++} concentration exceeds the setpoint value, parathyroid cells sense it and reflexively reduce their output of PTH.

Secretion by many endocrine glands is regulated by a hormone produced by another gland. For example, the pituitary gland (specifically, the anterior portion) produces thyroid-stimulating hormone (TSH), which stimulates the thyroid gland to release its hormones. The anterior pituitary responds to changes in the controlled physiological variable and to changes in the blood concentration of hormones secreted by its target gland.

Secretion by the anterior pituitary can in turn be regulated by *releasing hormones* or *inhibiting hormones* secreted by the hypothalamus. Hypothalamic secretion is responsive to changes in the controlled variable, as well as changes in the blood concentration of anterior pituitary and target gland hormones. Although the target gland may be able to adjust its own output, the additional controls exerted by long feedback loops involving the anterior pituitary and hypothalamus allow more precise regulation of hormone secretion—and thus more precise regulation of the internal environment.

Another mechanism that may influence the secretion of hormones by a gland is input from the nervous system. For example, secretion by the posterior pituitary is not regulated by releasing hormones but by direct nervous input from the hypothalamus. Likewise, sympathetic nerve impulses that reach the medulla of the adrenal glands trigger the secretion of epinephrine and norepinephrine. Many other glands, including the pancreas, are also influenced to some degree by nervous input. That the nervous system operates with hormonal mechanisms to produce endocrine reflexes emphasizes the close functional relationship between these two systems.

Although the operation of long feedback loops tends to minimize wide fluctuations in secretion rates, the output of several hormones typically rises and falls dramatically within a short period.

Regulation of Target Cell Sensitivity

The sensitivity of a target cell to any particular hormone partly depends on how many receptors for that hormone it has. The more receptors there are, the more sensitive is the target cell. Hormone receptors, as with other cell components, are constantly broken down by the cell and replaced with newly synthesized receptors. This mechanism not only ensures that all cell parts are "new" and working properly but also provides a method by which the number of receptors can be changed from time to time.

If synthesis of new receptors occurs faster than degradation of old receptors, the target cell will have more receptors and thus be more sensitive to the hormone. This phenomenon, illustrated in **Figure 25-12**, *A*, is often called **up-regulation** because the number of receptors goes up. If, on the other hand, the rate of receptor degradation exceeds the rate of receptor synthesis, the target cell's number of receptors will decrease (**Figure 25-12**, *B*). Because the number of receptors, and thus the sensitivity of the target cell, go down, this phenomenon is often called **down-regulation.**

Of course, regulation of signal transduction mechanisms and gene transcription triggered by various hormones can also play a role in adjusting the sensitivity of target cells to a particular hormone at a particular time. For example, one hormone may affect the signal transduction of another hormone, thus inhibiting or enhancing the second hormone's effects (**Box 25-2**).

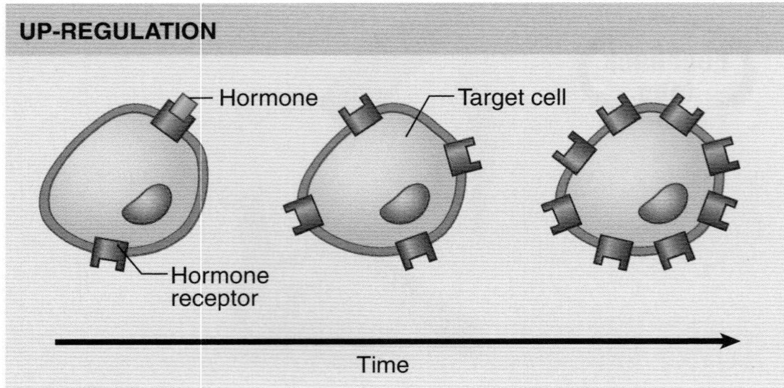

A

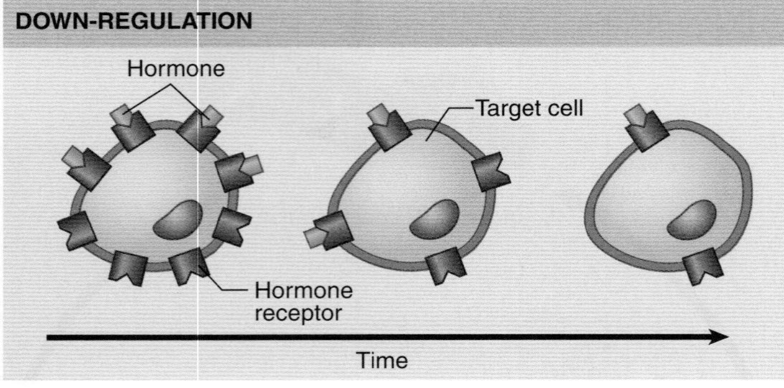

B

FIGURE 25-12 Regulation of target cell sensitivity. A, Up-regulation. **B,** Down-regulation.

Endocrinologists are just now learning the mechanisms that control the process of receptor turnover and signal transduction in the cell and how this affects the functions of the target cell. Information uncovered so far has already led to a better understanding of important and widespread endocrine disorders such as diabetes mellitus.

Quick CHECK

5. Name some ways in which hormones can work together to regulate a tissue.
6. Why is the concept of steroid hormone action called the *mobile-receptor model*?
7. Why is the concept of nonsteroid hormone action often called the *second messenger model*? Why is it known as the *fixed-membrane-receptor model*?
8. Name some ways that the secretion of an endocrine cell can be controlled.

BOX 25-2 health matters | "Too Much or Too Little"

Diseases of the endocrine system are numerous, varied, and sometimes spectacular. Tumours or other abnormalities commonly cause the glands to secrete too much or too little of their hormones. Production of too much hormone by a diseased gland is called **hypersecretion.** If too little hormone is produced, the condition is called **hyposecretion.**

Various endocrine disorders that appear to result from hyposecretion are actually caused by a problem in the target cells. If the usual target cells of a particular hormone have damaged receptors, too few receptors, or some other abnormality, they will not respond to that hormone properly. In other words, lack of target cell response could be a sign of hyposecretion or a sign of target cell insensitivity. *Diabetes mellitus (DM),* for example, can result from insulin hyposecretion or from the target cells' insensitivity to insulin.

Polyendocrine disorders are caused by hypersecretion and/or hyposecretion of more than one hormone. Often, an imbalance of one hormone will lead to an imbalance of other hormones as well.

EICOSANOIDS

Tissue Hormones

Before continuing our discussion of endocrine glands and hormones, let us pause for a moment to consider the **eicosanoid** compounds (**Table 25-4**). Sometimes called *icosanoids*, these compounds are a unique group of lipid molecules that serve important and widespread integrative functions in the body but do not meet the usual definition of a hormone (**Box 25-3**). Eicosanoids include *prostaglandins*, *thromboxanes*, and *leukotrienes*.

Eicosanoids are 20-carbon unsaturated fatty acids and contain a 5-carbon ring (**Figure 25-13**). The word part *eicosa-* means "twenty". Eicosanoids are made by cells throughout the body by breaking apart membrane phospholipids and using their fatty acid "tails" (specifically, *arachidonic acid*). **Box 4-2** on p. 61 discusses one of the enzymes (*cyclooxygenase* or COX) used to convert arachidonic acid to prostaglandin.

Although eicosanoids may be secreted directly into the bloodstream, they are rapidly metabolized, so that circulating levels are extremely low. The term *tissue hormone* is appropriate because the secretion is produced in a tissue and diffuses only a short distance to other cells within the same tissue. Whereas typical hormones integrate activities of widely separated organs, eicosanoids tend to integrate activities of neighbouring cells.

TABLE 25-4 Eicosanoids

HORMONE	SOURCE	TARGET	PRINCIPAL ACTION
Prostaglandins (PGs)	Many diverse tissues of the body	Local cells within the source tissue	Diverse local (paracrine/autocrine) effects such as regulation of inflammation, muscle contraction in blood vessels
Thromboxanes (TXs)	Platelets	Other platelets; muscles in blood vessel walls	Increase stickiness of platelets; promote blood clotting; cause constriction of blood vessels
Leukotrienes	Several types of white blood cells (leucocytes)	Local cells of various types	Produce local inflammatory responses triggered by allergens, including constriction of airways (as in asthma) and other inflammatory responses

BOX 25-3 *local hormones*

The classical view of hormones is that they are secreted from a tissue into the bloodstream and have their effects in target cells at some distance from their source. This is the standard definition of an **endocrine hormone** (part *A* of figure). That is, hormones have "global" effects in the body.

However, some hormones and related agents have primarily local effects—that is, effects *within* the source tissue. To distinguish classical endocrine hormones from local regulators such as prostaglandins and related compounds, scientists often use more precise terms for "local" hormones. Here are examples of terms used to designate local regulators:

Paracrine hormones—hormones that regulate activity in nearby cells within the same tissue as their source (part *B* of figure)

Autocrine hormones—hormones that regulate activity in the secreting cell itself (part *C* of figure)

To avoid confusion, scientists most often refer only to endocrine hormones simply as *hormones.* For local regulators, scientists use general terms such as *tissue hormone* or *local regulator*—or more specific terms such as *paracrine* or *autocrine* factor. •

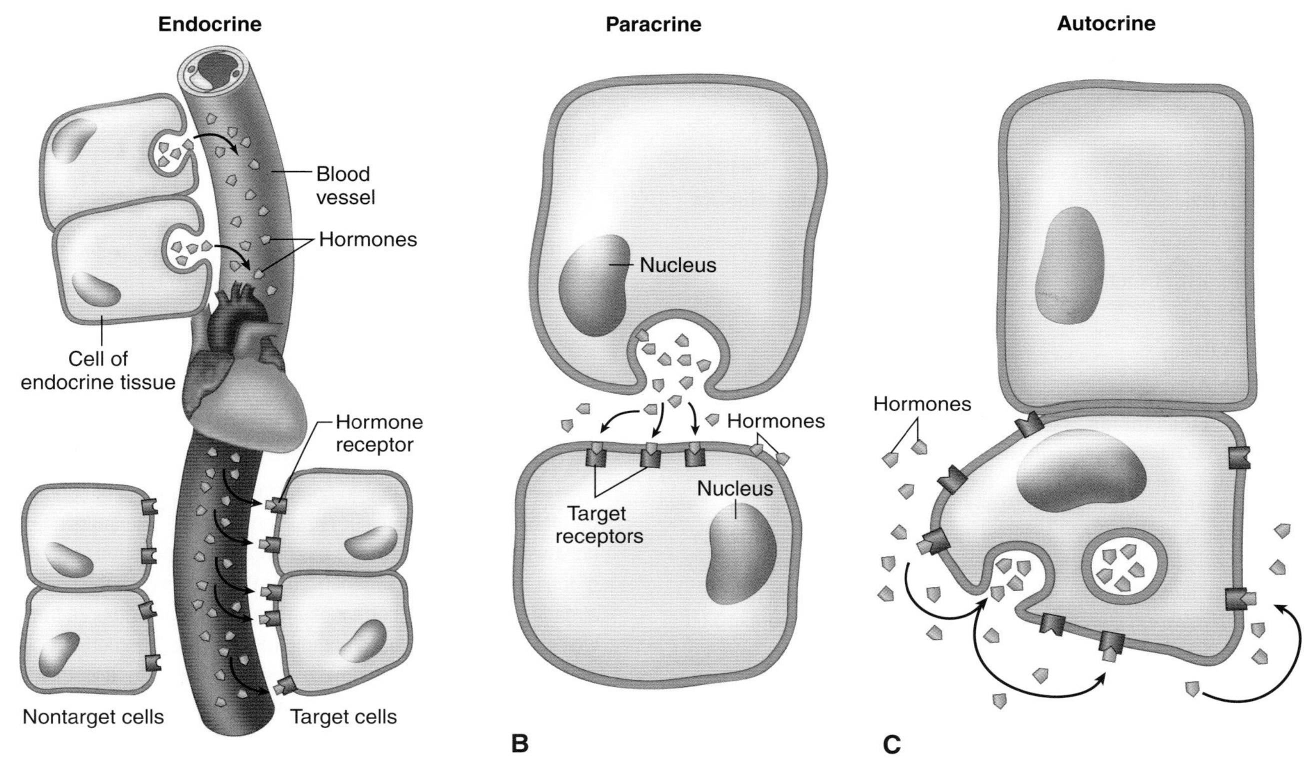

PROSTAGLANDINS

There are at least 16 different **prostaglandins (PGs)**, falling into nine structural classes—prostaglandin A (PGA) through prostaglandin I (PGI). Prostaglandins have been isolated and identified from a variety of tissues. The first prostaglandin was discovered in semen, so it was attributed to the prostate gland (hence the name, prostaglandin). Later, researchers found that the seminal vesicles, not the prostate, secreted the prostaglandin that they had found. Many other tissues are now known to secrete prostaglandins.

As a group, the prostaglandins have diverse physiological effects and are among the most varied and potent of any naturally occurring biological compounds. They are intimately involved in overall endocrine regulation by influencing adenyl cyclase–cAMP interaction within the cell's plasma membrane (see **Figure 25-9**). Specific biological effects depend on the class of prostaglandin.

Intraarterial infusion of prostaglandins A (PGAs) results in an immediate fall in blood pressure accompanied by an increase in regional blood flow to several areas, including the coronary and renal systems. PGAs apparently produce this effect by causing relaxation of smooth muscle fibres in the walls of certain arteries and arterioles.

Prostaglandins E (PGEs) have an important role in various vascular, metabolic, and gastrointestinal functions. Vascular effects include regulation of red blood cell deformability and platelet aggregation (see Chapter 27). PGEs also have a role in systemic inflammations, such as fever. Common antiinflammatory agents such as aspirin and ibuprofen produce some of their effects by inhibiting PGE synthesis. These drugs act by blocking one or more of the prostaglandin-producing *cyclooxygenase* enzymes such as *COX-1* and COX-2, as you may recall from **Box 4-2** on p. 61. PGE also regulates hydrochloric acid secretion in the stomach, helping to prevent gastric ulcers.

Prostaglandins F (PGFs) have an especially important role in the reproductive system. They cause uterine muscle contractions, so

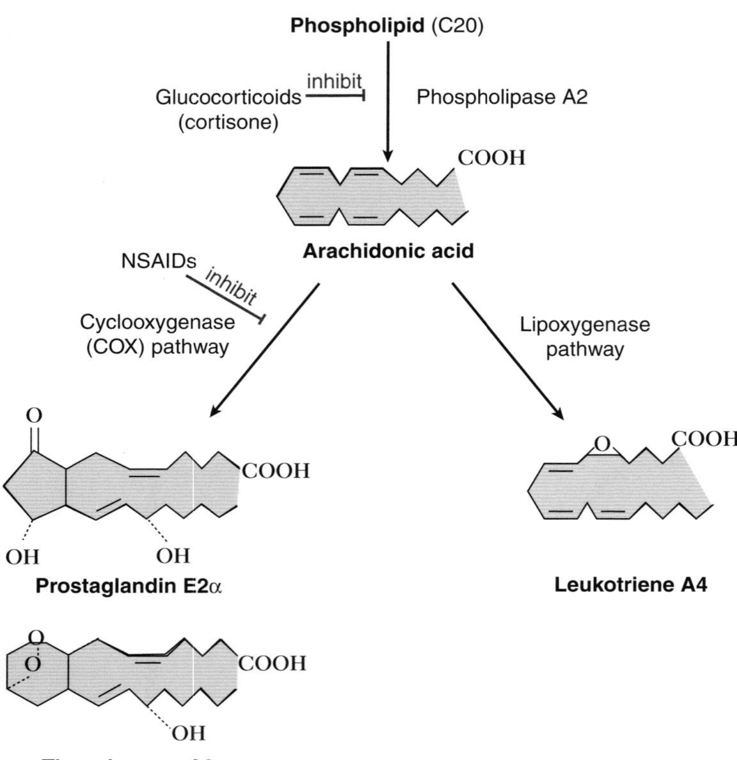

FIGURE 25-13 Eicosanoids. Membrane phospholipids containing the 20-carbon fatty acid arachidonic acid are enzymatically broken apart (C20, 20-carbon). Therapeutic use of glucocorticoids such as cortisone can inhibit this pathway, thus reducing the amount (and effects) of any of the resulting regulator molecules. Arachidonic acid is then converted by the COX pathway to either prostaglandins or thromboxanes (*left*). This step can be therapeutically inhibited by nonsteroidal antiinflammatory drugs (NSAIDs). Arachidonic acid may alternatively be converted by the lipoxygenase pathway to a leukotriene. See also **Figure 4-10** on p. 60. *COX,* Cyclooxygenase.

they have been used to induce labour and thus accelerate delivery of a baby. PGFs also affect intestinal motility and are required for normal peristalsis.

Thromboxanes and Leukotrienes

In addition to prostaglandins, various tissues also synthesize other eicosanoid compounds that are structurally and functionally similar to prostaglandins (see **Figure 25-13**).

One example is the **thromboxanes.** *Thromboxane* A2 is a regulator synthesized by blood platelets and is important in blood clotting. Aspirin targets thromboxane A2 synthesis, thereby reducing the blood's ability to clot. We will discuss thromboxane in Chapter 27, when we study blood clotting.

Another important example of eicosanoids is a group called the **leukotrienes,** which are regulators of immunity (discussed in Chapter 32). As with any of the eicosanoids, these compounds may also be referred to as "tissue hormones" because of their local, yet potent, regulatory effects.

The potential therapeutic use of eicosanoid compounds, which are found in almost every body tissue and are capable of regulating hormone activity on the cellular level, has been described as the most revolutionary development in medicine since the advent of antibiotics. They are likely to play increasingly important roles in the treatment of diverse conditions such as hypertension, coronary thrombosis, asthma, and ulcers.

Quick CHECK

9. Why are prostaglandins sometimes called *tissue hormones*?
10. Why are prostaglandins considered to be important in clinical applications?

the big picture | Endocrine Regulation and the Whole Body

It is important to appreciate the precision of control afforded by the partnership of the two major regulatory systems: the endocrine system and the nervous system. Some of the more important endocrine glands and the actions of their hormones are summarized in the following chapter. However, we have already seen how the hormones interact with each other in functional teams, as well as how their functions complement those of the nervous system. Although there is still much to be learned, we can see that a basic understanding of hormonal regulatory mechanisms is required to fully appreciate the nature of homeostasis in the human organism. As we continue our study of human anatomy and physiology, we will often encounter the critical integrative role played by the endocrine system. Having explored the basic principles of hormonal regulation, we are now ready for the specific examples of important glands and hormones outlined in the next chapter.

mechanisms of disease: Endocrine Disorders

As we have stated throughout this chapter, endocrine disorders typically result from either elevated or depressed hormone levels (hypersecretion or hyposecretion). At first thought, this may seem very simple and straightforward. In reality, however, nothing could be further from the truth. A variety of specific mechanisms may produce hypersecretion or hyposecretion of hormones. A few of the more well-known mechanisms are briefly explained here.

Mechanisms of Hypersecretion

Excessively high blood concentration of a hormone—or any condition that mimics high hormone levels—is called *hypersecretion.* Specific types of hypersecretion are usually named by placing the prefix *hyper-* in front of the name of the source gland and the suffix *-ism* at the end. For example, hypersecretion of thyroid hormone—no matter what the specific cause—is called **hyperthyroidism.** Hyperthyroidism is not a disease itself but a condition that characterizes several different diseases (e.g., Graves disease, toxic nodular goitre).

Any of several different mechanisms may be responsible for a particular case of hypersecretion. For example, tumours are often responsible for an abnormal proliferation of endocrine cells and the resulting increase in hormone secretion. Pituitary adenomas, for example, are benign tumours that may cause **hyperpituitarism.** As many as one in five people may have pituitary adenomas, but the majority of tumours are microscopic and asymptomatic. Larger tumours may, however, cause hyperpituitarism with possible outcomes of **gigantism** or **acromegaly.**

Another cause of hypersecretion is a phenomenon called **autoimmunity.** In autoimmunity the immune system functions abnormally. In **Graves disease,** for example, autoimmune antibodies against the thyroid-stimulating hormone (TSH) receptor actually stimulate the receptor and mimic the activity of TSH. As a result, the thyroid gland hypertrophies and excess thyroid hormone is produced.

Another possible cause of hypersecretion of a hormone is a failure of the feedback mechanisms that regulate secretion of a particular hormone. For example, a condition called **primary hyperparathyroidism** is characterized by a failure of the parathyroid gland to adjust its output to compensate for changes in blood calcium levels. Instead, the parathyroid gland seems to operate independently of the normal feedback loop and thus overproduces parathyroid hormone.

Mechanisms of Hyposecretion

Depressed blood hormone levels—or any condition that mimics low hormone levels—is termed *hyposecretion.* Specific types of hyposecretion are named in a manner similar to that in which hypersecretion disorders are named: by the addition of the *hypo-* prefix and the *-ism* suffix. For example, hyposecretion of thyroid hormone is called *hypothyroidism.*

Various different mechanisms have been shown to cause hyposecretion of hormones. For example, although most tumours cause oversecretion of a hormone, they may instead cause a gland to undersecrete its hormone or hormones. Tissue death, perhaps caused by a blockage or other failure of the blood supply, can also cause a gland to reduce its hormonal output. Hypopituitarism (hyposecretion by the anterior pituitary) can occur this way. Still another way in which a gland may reduce its secretion below normal levels is through abnormal operation of regulatory feedback loops.

An example of this is in the case of hyposecretion of testosterone and gonadotropic hormones in males who abuse **anabolic steroids.** Men who take testosterone steroids increase their blood concentration of this hormone above setpoint levels. The desired effect is to promote muscle growth and increased strength. However, the body responds to this overabundance by reducing its own output of testosterone (i.e., gonadotropins). This may lead to sterility and other complications.

Abnormalities of immune function may also cause hyposecretion. For example, an autoimmune attack on glandular tissue sometimes has the effect of reducing hormone output. Some endocrinologists theorize that autoimmune destruction of pancreatic islet cells, perhaps in combination with viral and genetic mechanisms, is a culprit in many cases of *type 1 (insulin-dependent) diabetes mellitus (DM).*

Many types of hyposecretion disorders have been shown to be caused by insensitivity of the target cells to tropic hormones rather than from actual hyposecretion. A few major types of abnormal responses in target cells are as follows:

- An abnormal decrease in the number of hormone receptors
- Abnormal function of hormone receptors, resulting in failure to bind to hormones properly
- Antibodies bind to hormone receptors, thus blocking binding of hormone molecules
- Abnormal metabolic response to the hormone-receptor complex by the target cell
- Failure of the target cell to produce enough second messenger molecules

For example, type 2 (non–insulin-dependent) diabetes mellitus is thought to be caused by target cell abnormalities that render the cells insensitive to insulin.

The next chapter will give several examples of many specific endocrine disorders. Apply the principles you have learned here to determine whether each primarily involves functional hyposecretion or functional hypersecretion of the hormones involved.

UNIT 3

LANGUAGE OF SCIENCE *(continued from p. 562)*

nonsteroid (nahn-STAYR-oyd)
[*non-* **not,** *-stero-* **solid,** *-oid* **like**]

paracrine hormone
(PAIR-ah-krin HOR-mohn)
[*para-* **beside,** *-crin-* **secrete,** *hormon-* **excite**]

peptide hormone
(PEP-tyde HOR-mohn)
[*pept-* **to digest,** *-ide* **chemical,** *hormon-* **excite**]

permissiveness (per-MISS-iv-ness)

prostaglandin (PG)
(pross-tah-GLAN-din)
[*pro-* **before,** *-stat-* **set or place (prostate),** *-gland-* **acorn (gland),** *-in* **substance**]

protein hormone
(PRO-teen HOR-mohn)
[*prote-* **first rank,** *-in* **substance,** *hormon-* **excite**]

second messenger model
(SEK-und MESS-en-jer MOD-el)

sex hormone (seks HOR-mohn)
[*hormon-* **excite**]

steroid (STAYR-oyd)
[*stero-* **solid,** *-oid* **like**]

synergism (SIN-er-jiz-em)
[*syn-* **together,** *-erg-* **work,** *-ism* **condition**]

target cell
[*cell* **storeroom**]

thromboxane (throm-BOKS-ayne)
[*thrombo-* **clot,** *-oxa-* **oxygen,** *-ane* **chemical**]

tropic hormone (TROH-pik HOR-mohn)
[*trop-* **turn or change,** *-ic* **relating to,** *hormon-* **excite**]

up-regulation (uhp reg-yuh-LAY-shun)
[*regula-* **rule,** *-tion* **process**]

LANGUAGE OF MEDICINE

acromegaly (ak-roh-MEG-ah-lee)
[*acro-* **extremities,** *-mega-* **great,** *-aly* **state**]

anabolic steroid
(an-ah-BOL-ik STAYR-oyd)
[*anabol-* **build up,** *-ic* **relating to,** *stero-* **solid,** *-oid* **like**]

autoimmunity
(aw-toh-ih-MYOO-nih-tee)
[*auto-* **self,** *-immun-* **free,** *-ity* **state**]

gigantism (jye-GAN-tiz-em)
[*gigant-* **great,** *-ism* **condition**]

Graves disease (grayvz)
[*Robert J. Graves* **Irish physician**]

hyperpituitarism
(hye-per-pih-TYOO-i-tar-iz-em)
[*hyper-* **excessive,** *-pituitar-* **phlegm (pituitary gland),** *-ism* **condition**]

hypersecretion
(hye-per-seh-KREE-shun)
[*hyper-* **excessive,** *-secret-* **separate,** *-tion* **process**]

hyperthyroidism
(hye-per-THY-royd-iz-em)
[*hyper-* **excessive,** *-thyr-* **shield (thyroid gland),** *-oid* **like,** *-ism* **condition**]

hyposecretion
(hye-poh-seh-KREE-shun)
[*hypo-* **under or below,** *-secret-* **separate,** *-tion* **process**]

primary hyperparathyroidism
(hye-per-pair-ah-THY-royd-iz-em)
[*prim-* **first,** *-ary* **relating to,** *hyper-* **excessive,** *-para-* **beside,** *-thyr-* **shield (thyroid),** *-oid* **like,** *-ism* **condition**]

CHAPTER SUMMARY

To download an MP3 version of the chapter summary for use with your mobile device, access the **Audio Chapter Summaries** *online at evolve.elsevier.com.*

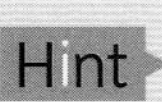

Scan this summary after reading the chapter to help you reinforce the key concepts. Later, use the summary as a quick review before your class or before a test.

Organization of the Endocrine System

A. The endocrine and nervous systems function to achieve and maintain homeostasis (**Figure 25-1**, **Table 25-1**)
B. When the two systems work together, referred to as the *neuroendocrine system,* they perform the same general functions: communication, integration, and control
C. In the endocrine system, secreting cells send hormone molecules by way of the blood to specific target cells contained in target tissues or target organs
D. Hormones—carried to almost every point in the body; can regulate most cells; effects work more slowly and last longer than those of neurotransmitters
E. Endocrine glands are "ductless glands"; many are made of glandular epithelium whose cells manufacture and secrete hormones; a few endocrine glands are made of neurosecretory tissue
F. Glands of the endocrine system are widely scattered throughout the body (**Figure 25-2**; **Table 25-2**)

Classification of Hormones

A. Classification by general function
  1. Tropic hormones—hormones that target other endocrine glands and stimulate their growth and secretion
  2. Sex hormones—hormones that target reproductive tissues
  3. Anabolic hormones—hormones that stimulate anabolism in target cells
B. Classification by chemical structure (**Figure 25-3**; **Table 25-3**)
  1. Steroid hormones
  2. Nonsteroid hormones
C. Steroid hormones (**Figure 25-4**)
  1. Synthesized from cholesterol (**Figure 25-5**)
  2. Lipid-soluble and can easily pass through the phospholipid plasma membrane of target cells
  3. Examples of steroid hormones: cortisol, aldosterone, oestrogen, progesterone, and testosterone
D. Nonsteroid hormones (**Figure 25-6**)
  1. Synthesized primarily from amino acids
  2. Protein hormones—long, folded chains of amino acids; e.g., insulin, parathyroid hormone
  3. Glycoprotein hormones—protein hormones with carbohydrate groups attached to the amino acid chain
  4. Peptide hormones—smaller than protein hormones; short chain of amino acids; e.g., oxytocin, antidiuretic hormone (ADH)
  5. Amino acid derivative hormones—each is derived from a single amino acid molecule
    a. Amine hormones—synthesized by modifying a single molecule of tyrosine or tryptophan; produced by neurosecretory cells and by neurons; e.g., epinephrine, norepinephrine
    b. Amino acid derivatives produced by the thyroid gland; synthesized by adding iodine to tyrosine

How Hormones Work

A. General principles of hormone action
  1. Target cells—hormones signal a cell by binding to the target cell's specific receptors in a "lock-and-key" mechanism (**Figure 25-7**)
  2. Signal transduction—different hormone-receptor interactions produce different regulatory changes within the target cell through chemical reactions
  3. Combined hormone actions
    a. Synergism—combinations of hormones acting together have a greater effect on a target cell than the sum of the effects that each would have if acting alone
    b. Permissiveness—when a small amount of one hormone allows a second one to have its full effects on a target cell
    c. Antagonism—one hormone produces the opposite effects of another hormone; used to "fine tune" the activity of target cells with great accuracy
  4. Primary and secondary actions—most hormones have primary effects that directly regulate target cells and many secondary effects that influence or modulate other regulatory mechanisms in target cells
  5. High blood concentration of hormones—endocrine glands produce more hormone molecules than actually are needed; the unused hormones are quickly excreted by the kidneys or broken down by metabolic processes

B. Mechanisms of steroid hormone action (**Figure 25-8**)
   1. Steroid hormones are lipid-soluble, and their receptors are normally found in the target cell's cytosol
   2. After a steroid hormone molecule has diffused into the target cell, it binds to a receptor molecule to form a hormone-receptor complex
   3. Mobile-receptor model—the hormone passes into the nucleus, where it binds to a mobile receptor and activates a certain gene sequence to begin transcription of mRNA; newly formed mRNA molecules move into the cytosol, associate with ribosomes, and begin synthesizing protein molecules that produce the effects of the hormone
   4. Steroid hormones regulate cells by regulating production of certain critical proteins
   5. The amount of steroid hormone present determines the magnitude of a target cell's response
   6. Because transcription and protein synthesis take time, responses to steroid hormones are often slow

C. Mechanisms of nonsteroid hormone action
   1. The second messenger mechanism—also known as the *fixed-membrane-receptor model* (**Figure 25-9**)
      a. A nonsteroid hormone molecule acts as a "first messenger" and delivers its chemical message to fixed receptors in the target cell's plasma membrane
      b. The "message" is then passed by way of a G-protein–coupled receptor (GPCR) into the cell where a "second messenger" triggers a G protein, which leads to the appropriate cellular changes
      c. Second messenger mechanism—produces target cell effects that differ from steroid hormone effects in several important ways
         (1) The effects of the hormone are amplified by the cascade of reactions
         (2) There are a variety of second messenger mechanisms—e.g., IP_3, cGMP, calcium–calmodulin mechanisms (**Figure 25-10**)
         (3) The second messenger mechanism operates much more quickly than the steroid mechanism
   2. The nuclear-receptor mechanism—small iodinated amino acids (T_4 and T_3) enter the target cell and bind to receptors associated with a DNA molecule in the nucleus; this binding triggers transcription of mRNA and synthesis of new enzymes

D. Regulation of hormone secretion
   1. Control of hormonal secretion is usually part of a negative feedback loop called an endocrine reflex (**Figure 25-11**)
   2. Negative feedback—mechanisms that reverse the direction of a change in a physiological system
   3. Positive feedback—(uncommon) mechanisms that amplify physiological changes
   4. Levels of regulation—different levels of homeostatic control
      a. Simplest mechanism—when an endocrine gland is sensitive to the physiological changes produced by its target cells
      b. Endocrine gland secretions may also be regulated by a hormone produced by another gland
      c. Endocrine gland secretions may be influenced by nervous system input; this fact emphasizes the close functional relationship between the two systems

E. Regulation of target cell sensitivity
   1. Sensitivity of target cell depends in part on number of receptors (**Figure 25-12**)
      a. Up-regulation—increased number of hormone receptors increases sensitivity
      b. Down-regulation—decreased number of hormone receptors decreases sensitivity
   2. Sensitivity of target cell may also be regulated by factors that affect signal transcription or gene transcription

Eicosanoids

A. Tissue hormones
   1. Unique group of lipid hormones (20-carbon fatty acid with 5-carbon ring) that serve important and widespread integrative functions in the body but do not meet the usual definition of a hormone (**Figure 25-13**; **Table 25-4**)
   2. Called *tissue hormones* because the secretion is produced in a tissue and diffuses only a short distance to other cells within the same tissue; PGs tend to integrate activities of neighbouring cells

B. Prostaglandins
   1. Many structural classes of prostaglandins have been isolated and identified
      a. Prostaglandin A (PGA)—intraarterial infusion resulting in an immediate fall in blood pressure accompanied by an increase in regional blood flow to several areas
      b. Prostaglandin E (PGE)—vascular effects: regulation of red blood cell deformability and platelet aggregation; inflammation (which can be blocked with drugs that inhibit PG-producing enzymes such as COX-1 and COX-2); gastrointestinal effects: regulates hydrochloric acid secretion
      c. Prostaglandin F (PGF)—especially important in reproductive system, causing uterine contractions; also affects intestinal motility and is required for normal peristalsis
   2. Many tissues are known to secrete PGs
   3. PGs have diverse physiological effects

C. Thromboxanes and leukotrienes
   1. Thromboxane A2 involved in blood clotting; aspirin inhibits thromboxane A2 synthesis and thus inhibits blood clotting; discussed in Chapter 27
   2. Leukotrienes regulate immunity; discussed in Chapters 32 and 33

The Big Picture: Endocrine Regulation and the Whole Body

A. Nearly every process in the human organism is kept in balance by the intricate interaction of different nervous and endocrine regulatory chemicals

B. The endocrine system operates with the nervous system to finely adjust the many processes they regulate

REVIEW QUESTIONS

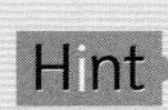

Write out the answers to these questions after reading the chapter and reviewing the Chapter Summary. Note—writing out your answers will consolidate learning and provide a valuable resource of information.

1. Define the terms *hormone* and *target organ.*
2. Describe the characteristic chemical structure found at the core of each steroid hormone.
3. Identify the major categories of nonsteroid hormones.
4. Identify the sequence of events involved in a second messenger mechanism.
5. What is the function of calmodulin?
6. List the classes of prostaglandins. Identify the functions of three of these classes.

CRITICAL THINKING QUESTIONS

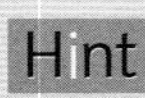

After finishing the Review Questions, write out the answers to these more in-depth questions to help you apply your new knowledge. Go back to sections of the chapter that relate to concepts that you find difficult.

1. Driving a car requires rapid response of selected muscles. The regulation of blood sugar level requires regulating almost every cell in the body. Based on the characteristics of each system, explain why driving would be a nervous system function and blood sugar regulation would be an endocrine function.
2. Explain the ways in which one hormone interacts with another and its effect on the cell.
3. Compare and contrast the action mechanisms of steroid and nonsteroid hormones.
4. Why are thyroid hormones exceptions to the usual mode of nonsteroid hormone functioning?
5. Using the parathyroid gland as an example, explain the concept of a negative feedback loop in the regulation of blood calcium (Ca^{++}) levels. Outline how the parathyroid is involved in bone-forming activity.

26 Endocrine Glands

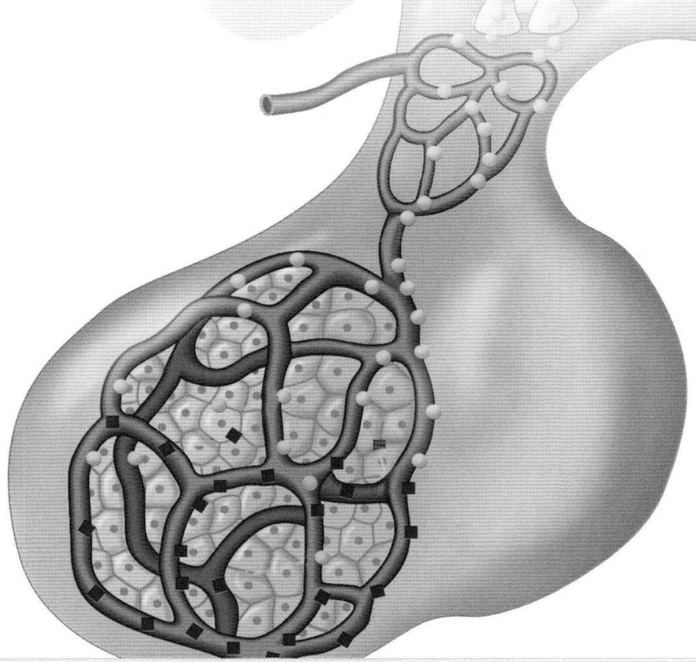

CHAPTER OUTLINE

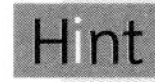

Hint *Scan this outline before you begin to read the chapter, as a preview of how the concepts are organized.*

LANGUAGE OF SCIENCE

Hint *Use this list to aid your pronunciation of unfamiliar words.*

adenohypophysis
(ad-eh-no-hye-POF-ih-sis)
[*adeno-* **gland,** *-hypo-* **under or below,** *-physis* **growth**] *pl.,* adenohypophyses

adrenal cortex
(ah-DREE-nal KOR-teks)
[*ad-* **toward,** *-ren-* **kidney,** *-al* **relating to,** *cortex* **bark**] *pl.,* cortices

adrenal gland (ah-DREE-nal)
[*ad-* **toward,** *-ren-* **kidney,** *-al* **relating to,** *gland* **acorn**]

adrenal medulla
(ah-DREE-nal meh-DUL-eh)
[*ad-* **toward,** *-ren-* **kidney,** *-al* **relating to,** *medulla* **marrow or pith (middle)**] *pl.,* medullae or medullas

adrenocorticotropic hormone (ACTH)
(ah-dree-no-kor-teh-koh-TROH-pik HOR-mohn)
[*adreno-* **gland,** *-cortic-* **cortex (bark),** *-trop-* **nourish,** *-ic* **relating to,** *hormon-* **excite**]

aldosterone
(AL-doh-steh-rohn or al-DOS-tair-ohn)
[*aldo-* **aldehyde,** *-stero-* **solid or steroid derivative,** *-one* **chemical**]

alpha cell (AL-fah)
[*alpha (α)* **first letter of Greek alphabet,** *cell* **storeroom**]

angiotensin I (an-jee-oh-TEN-sin)
[*angio-* **vessel,** *-tens-* **pressure or stretch,** *-in* **substance,** *I* **Roman numeral one**]

angiotensin II (an-jee-oh-TEN-sin)
[*angio-* **vessel,** *-tens-* **pressure or stretch,** *-in* **substance,** *II* **Roman numeral two**]

angiotensinogen
(an-jee-oh-TEN-sin-oh-jen)
[*angio-* **vessel,** *-tens-* **pressure or stretch,** *-in-* **substance,** *-gen* **produce**]

antidiuretic hormone (ADH)
(an-tee-dye-yoo-RET-ik HOR-mohn)
[*anti-* **against,** *-dia-* **through,** *-uret-* **urination,** *-ic* **relating to,** *hormon-* **excite**]

arginine vasopressin (AVP)
(AHR-jih-neen vas-oh-PRES-in)
[*arginine* **type of amino acid,** *vaso-* **vessel,** *-press-* **pressure,** *-in* **substance**]

continued on p. 602

In the previous chapter we outlined the basic mechanisms of endocrine regulation and its partnership with nervous regulation. We learned how hormones released from endocrine glands into the bloodstream can signal target tissues to alter their functions in ways that promote homeostasis. Our study of neuroendocrine regulation of body function continues in this chapter, in which we explore the structure and function of some of the major endocrine glands. By looking at a few of the important glands and their hormones, a clear picture emerges of how endocrine regulation works. As you learn the specific actions of the major hormones, think of them as part of an overall system of regulating the body's functions. In later chapters, we will encounter many of these hormones again as we explore the various body functions they regulate. •

PITUITARY GLAND

STRUCTURE OF THE PITUITARY GLAND

The **pituitary gland** (also called the *hypophysis cerebri*) is a small but mighty structure. It measures only 1.2 to 1.5 cm across. By weight, it is even less impressive—only about 0.5 gram! And yet so crucial are the functions of the anterior lobe of the pituitary gland that, in past centuries, it was referred to as the "master gland".

The pituitary gland has a well-protected location within the skull on the ventral surface of the brain (**Figure 26-1**). It lies in the *pituitary fossa* of the sella turcica and is covered by a portion of the dura mater called the *pituitary diaphragm.* The gland has a stemlike stalk, the **infundibulum,** which connects it to the hypothalamus of the brain.

Although the pituitary looks like one gland, it actually consists of two separate glands—the *adenohypophysis*, or anterior pituitary gland, and the *neurohypophysis*, or posterior pituitary gland. In the embryo, the adenohypophysis develops from an upward projection of the pharynx and is composed of regular endocrine tissue. The neurohypophysis, on the other hand, develops from a downward projection of the brain and is composed of neurosecretory tissue. These histological differences are incorporated into their names—*adeno* means "gland", and *neuro* means "nervous". As you may suspect, the hormones secreted by the adenohypophysis serve very different functions from those released by the neurohypophysis.

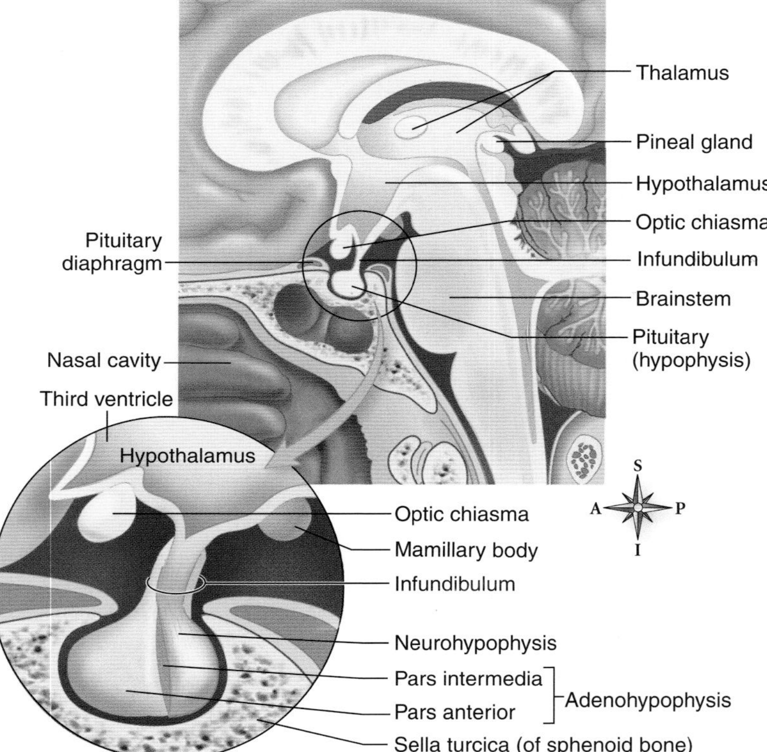

FIGURE 26-1 Location and structure of the pituitary gland. The pituitary gland is located within the sella turcica of the skull's sphenoid bone and is connected to the hypothalamus by a stalklike infundibulum. The infundibulum passes through a gap in the portion of the dura mater that covers the pituitary (the pituitary diaphragm). The inset shows that the pituitary is divided into an anterior portion, the adenohypophysis, and a posterior portion, the neurohypophysis. The adenohypophysis is further subdivided into the pars anterior and pars intermedia. The pars intermedia is almost absent in the adult pituitary.

ADENOHYPOPHYSIS (ANTERIOR LOBE OF PITUITARY)

The **adenohypophysis,** the anterior portion of the pituitary gland, is divided into two parts—the *pars anterior* and the *pars intermedia.* The pars anterior forms the major portion of the adenohypophysis and is divided from the tiny pars intermedia by a narrow cleft and some connective tissue (see **Figure 26-1**).

The tissue of the adenohypophysis is composed of irregular clumps of secretory cells supported by fine connective tissue fibres and surrounded by a rich vascular network.

Traditionally, histologists have identified three types of cells according to their affinity for certain types of stains: *chromophobes* (literally "afraid of colour"), *acidophils* ("acid [stain] lovers"), and *basophils* ("base [stain] lovers"). All three types are visible in the photomicrograph shown in **Figure 26-2**. Currently, however, cells of the adenohypophysis are more often classified by their secretions into five types:

1. **Somatotrophs**—secrete growth hormone (GH)
2. **Corticotrophs**—secrete adrenocorticotropic hormone (ACTH)
3. **Thyrotrophs**—secrete thyroid-stimulating hormone (TSH)
4. **Lactotrophs**—secrete prolactin (PRL)
5. **Gonadotrophs**—secrete luteinizing hormone (LH) and follicle-stimulating hormone (FSH)

Figure 26-3 summarizes the hormones of the adenohypophysis and shows the primary locations of their target cells.

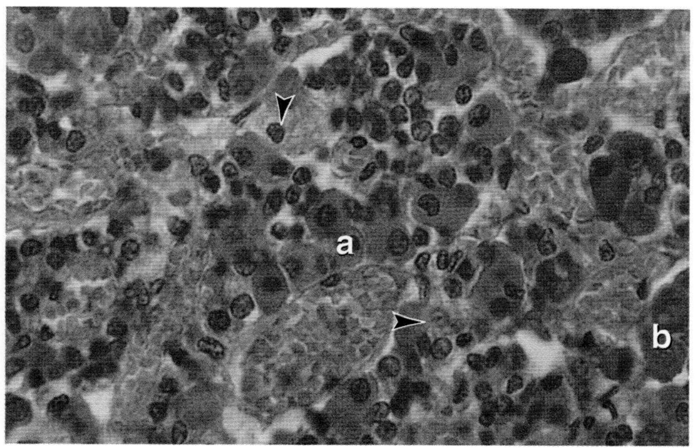

FIGURE 26-2 Histology of the adenohypophysis. In this light micrograph, nonstaining chromophobes are indicated by arrowheads. Examples of hormone-secreting cells are labelled *a* (acidophil) and *b* (basophil).

Growth Hormone

Growth hormone (GH), or **somatotropin (STH)**, promotes bodily growth indirectly by stimulating the liver and other tissues to produce another hormone called *insulin-like growth factor 1 (IGF-1)*, which, in turn, produces most of the effects attributed to GH.

One of the functions of GH, by way of IGF-1, is to accelerate amino acid transport into cells. Rapid entrance of amino acids from the blood into the cells allows protein anabolism within the cells to accelerate. Increased protein anabolism allows an increased rate of growth. GH promotes the growth of bone, muscle, and other tissues (**Box 26-1**).

In addition to stimulating protein anabolism, GH also stimulates fat metabolism. GH accelerates mobilization of lipids from storage in adipose cells and also speeds up the catabolism of those lipids after they have entered another cell. In this way, GH tends to shift a cell's use of nutrients away from carbohydrate (glucose) catabolism and toward lipid catabolism as an energy source. Because less glucose is then removed from the blood by cells, the blood glucose levels tend to rise. Thus GH is said to have a *hyperglycemic effect*. Insulin (from

FIGURE 26-3 Pituitary hormones. Some of the major hormones of the adenohypophysis and neurohypophysis and their principal target organs.

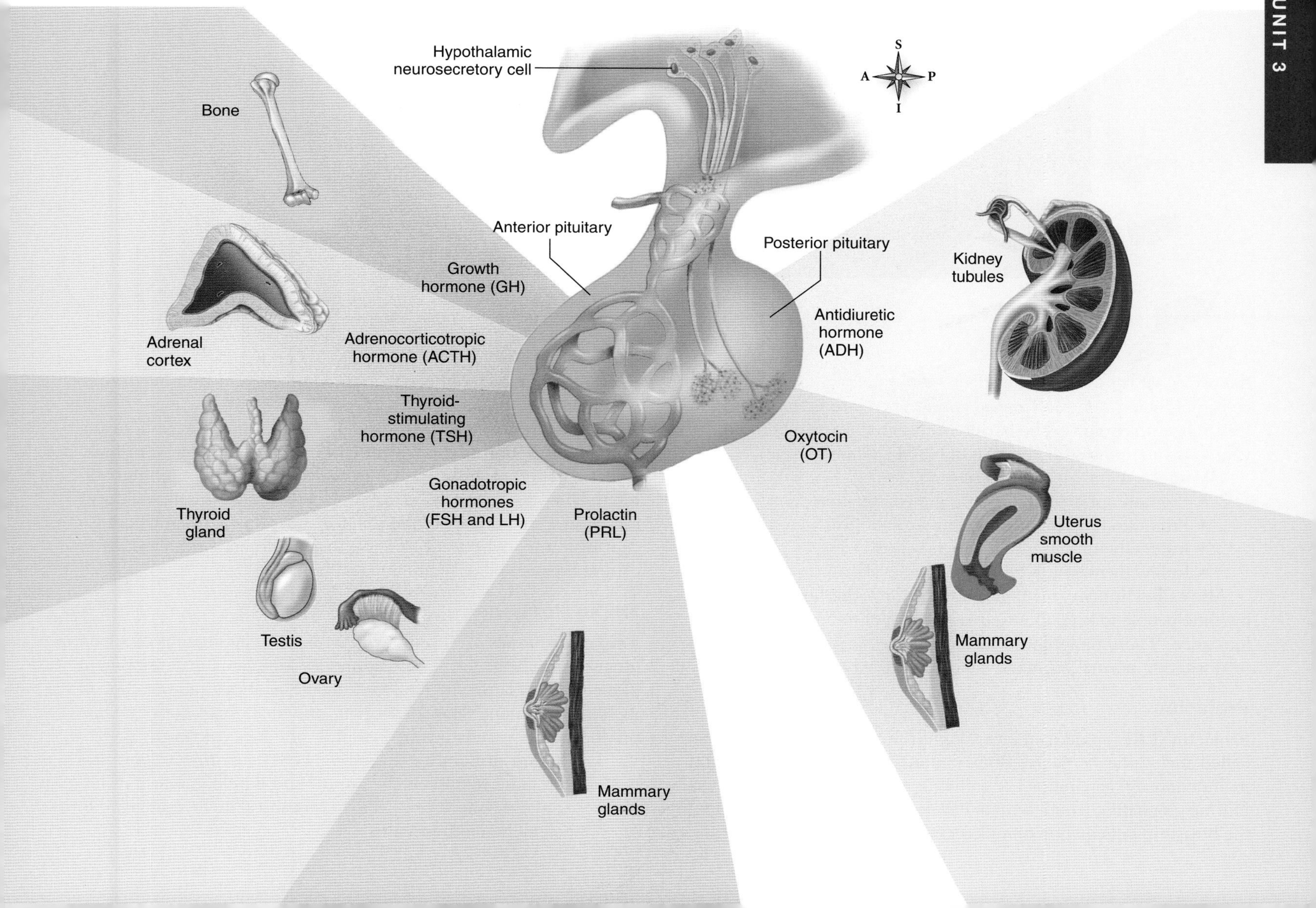

BOX 26-1 *health matters* | Growth Hormone Abnormalities

Hypersecretion of growth hormone (GH) during the growth years (before ossification of the epiphyseal plates) causes an abnormally rapid rate of skeletal growth. This condition is known as **gigantism** (see *A, left*). Hypersecretion after skeletal fusion has occurred can result in **acromegaly,** a condition in which cartilage still left in the skeleton continues to form new bone (see *B*). This abnormal growth may result in a distorted appearance because of the enlargement of the hands, feet, face, jaw (causing separation of the teeth), and other body parts. Overlying soft tissue may also be affected—for instance, the skin often thickens and the pores become more pronounced.

Hyposecretion of GH during growth years may result in stunted body growth, known as **pituitary dwarfism**. Formerly, patients were treated only with GH extracted from human tissues. Since 1987, the availability of human GH produced by genetically engineered bacteria has made the treatment obtainable for many more patients.

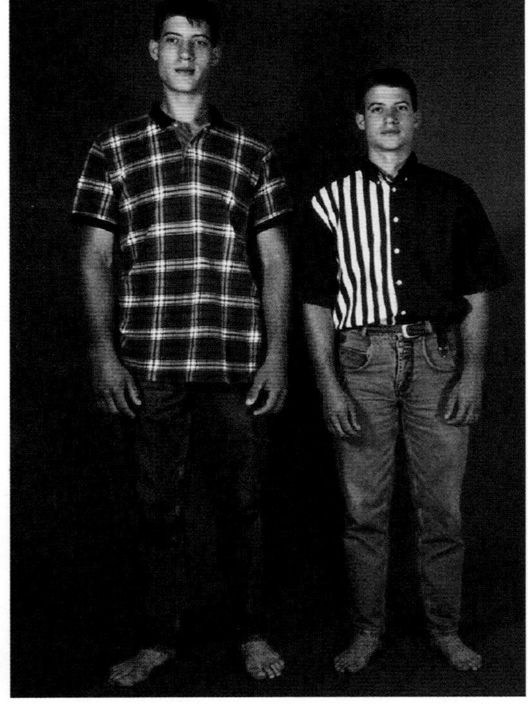

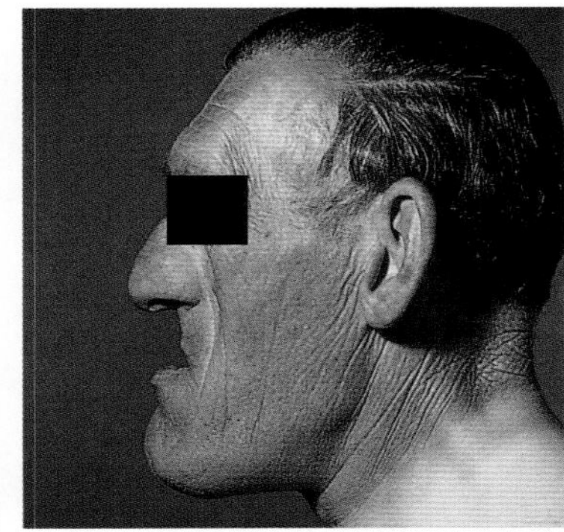

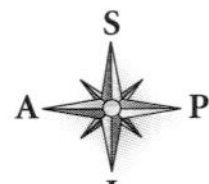

Growth hormone abnormalities. A, The 22-year-old man on the left with gigantism is much taller than his identical twin on the right. **B,** Acromegaly. Notice the large head, exaggerated projection of the lower jaw, and protrusion of the ridge above the eye orbits.

the pancreas) has the opposite effect—it promotes glucose entry into cells, producing a *hypoglycaemic effect.* Therefore GH and insulin function as antagonists. The balance between these two hormones is vital to maintaining a homeostasis of blood glucose levels.

GH affects metabolism in these ways:

- Promotes protein anabolism (growth, tissue repair)
- Promotes lipid mobilization and catabolism
- Indirectly inhibits glucose metabolism
- Indirectly increases blood glucose levels

Also called human growth hormone (hGH), this hormone is used by some people to keep themselves youthful or to boost athletic performance. These unapproved uses can have dangerous side effects by disrupting normal hormone balances in the body.

Prolactin

Prolactin (PRL), produced by acidophils in the pars anterior, is also called *lactogenic hormone.* Both names of this hormone suggest its function in "generating" or initiating milk secretion (lactation). During pregnancy, a high level of PRL promotes the development of the breasts in anticipation of milk secretion. At the birth of an infant, PRL in the mother stimulates the mammary glands to begin milk secretion.

Hypersecretion of PRL may cause lactation in nonnursing women, disruption of the menstrual cycle, and impotence in men. Hypersecretion of prolactin can be caused by a benign pituitary tumour called prolactinoma. Most prolactinomas are small and occur mostly in women. **Hyposecretion** of PRL is usually insignificant except in women who want to nurse their children. Milk production cannot be initiated or maintained without PRL.

Tropic Hormones

Tropic hormones are hormones that have a stimulating effect on other endocrine glands. These hormones stimulate the development of their target glands and tend to stimulate synthesis and secretion of the target hormone (**Box 26-2**). Four principal tropic hormones are produced and secreted by the basophils of the pars anterior:

1. **Thyroid-stimulating hormone (TSH),** or *thyrotropin,* promotes and maintains the growth and development of its target gland—the thyroid. TSH also causes the thyroid gland to secrete thyroid hormone.

BOX 26-2 *health matters*

Tropic Hormone Abnormalities

Hypersecretion of the tropic hormones may result from a pituitary tumour. The tropic hormones, produced at higher than normal levels, cause hypersecretion in their target glands. This may result in various effects throughout the body. Early hypersecretion of gonadotropins, for example, may lead to an abnormally early onset of puberty.

Hyposecretion of tropic hormones often causes their target glands to secrete less than a normal amount of their hormones. This may disrupt reproduction, kidney function, overall metabolism, and other processes.

2. **Adrenocorticotropic hormone (ACTH),** or *adrenocorticotropin,* promotes and maintains normal growth and development of the cortex of the adrenal gland. ACTH also stimulates the adrenal cortex to synthesize and secrete some of its hormones.
3. **Follicle-stimulating hormone (FSH)** stimulates structures within the ovaries, primary follicles, to grow toward maturity. Each follicle contains a developing egg cell (ovum), which is released from the ovary during ovulation. FSH also stimulates the follicle cells to synthesize and secrete oestrogens (female sex hormones). In the male, FSH stimulates the development of the seminiferous tubules of the testes and maintains spermatogenesis (sperm production) by them.
4. **Luteinizing hormone (LH)** stimulates the formation and activity of the corpus luteum of the ovary. The corpus luteum (meaning "yellow body") is the tissue left behind when a follicle ruptures to release its egg during ovulation. The corpus luteum secretes progesterone and oestrogens when stimulated by LH. LH also supports FSH in stimulating the maturation of follicles. In males, LH stimulates interstitial cells in the testes to develop and then synthesize and secrete testosterone (the male sex hormone).

FSH and LH are called **gonadotropins** because they stimulate the growth and maintenance of the gonads (ovaries and testes). During childhood the adenohypophysis secretes insignificant amounts of the gonadotropins. A few years before puberty, gonadotropin secretion is gradually increased. Then, suddenly, their secretion spurts, and the gonads are stimulated to develop and begin their normal functions.

In addition to those listed, the adenohypophysis produces many other hormones in small amounts. Many of these are also produced elsewhere in the body. For example, *alpha melanocyte-stimulating hormone (α-MSH)* and other melanocortins discussed in Chapter 10 (see p. 189) are produced in the skin and other tissues, with a relatively insignificant amount also produced in the adenohypophysis.

Control of Secretion in the Adenohypophysis

The cell bodies of neurons in certain parts of the hypothalamus synthesize chemicals that their axons then secrete into the blood. These chemicals, generally called **releasing hormones,** travel through a complex of small blood vessels called the **hypophyseal portal system** (**Figure 26-4**). A *portal system* is an arrangement of blood vessels in which blood exiting one tissue is immediately carried to a second tissue before being returned to the heart and lungs for oxygenation and redistribution. The hypophyseal portal system carries blood from the hypothalamus directly to the adenohypophysis, where the target cells of the releasing hormones are located. The advantage of a portal system in the hypophysis is that a small amount of hormone can be delivered directly to its target tissue without the great dilution that would occur in the general circulation. The releasing hormones that arrive in the adenohypophysis by means of this portal system influence the secretion of hormones by acidophils and basophils. In this manner, the hypothalamus directly regulates the secretion of the adenohypophysis. You can see that the supposed "master gland" really has a master of its own—the hypothalamus.

The following is a list of some of the important hormones secreted by the hypothalamus into the hypophyseal portal system:

- Growth hormone–releasing hormone (GHRH)
- Growth hormone–inhibiting hormone (GHIH) (also called somatostatin [SS])
- Corticotropin-releasing hormone (CRH)
- Thyrotropin-releasing hormone (TRH)
- Gonadotropin-releasing hormone (GnRH)
- Prolactin-releasing hormone (PRH)
- Prolactin-inhibiting hormone (PIH)

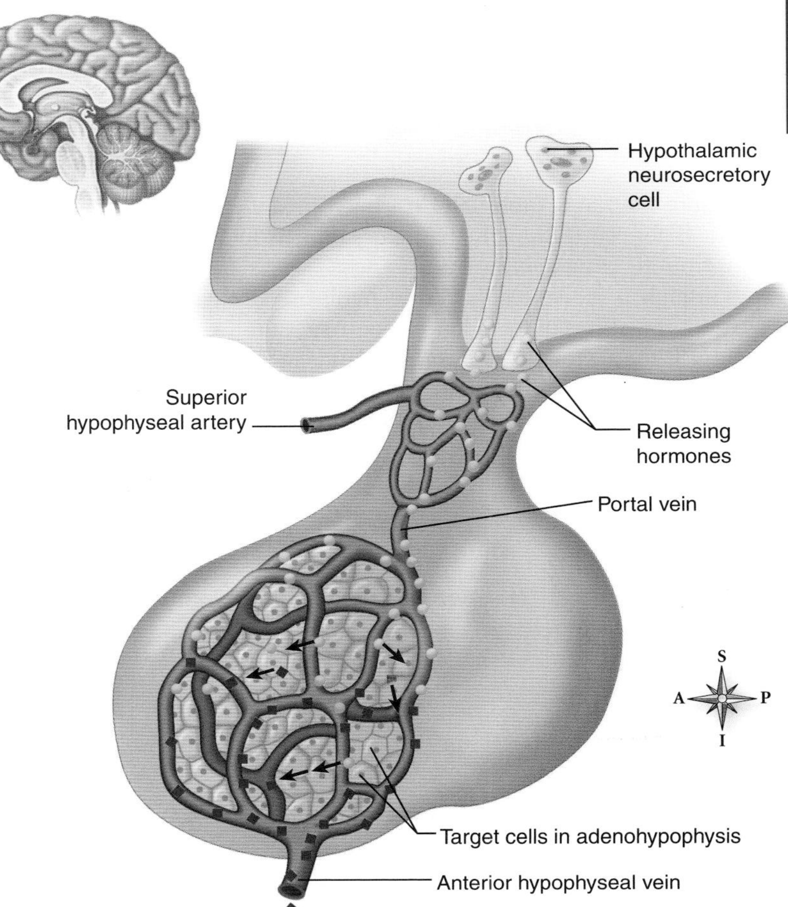

FIGURE 26-4 Hypophyseal portal system. Neurons in the hypothalamus secrete releasing hormones into vessels that carry the releasing hormones directly to the vessels of the adenohypophysis, thus bypassing the normal circulatory route.

UNIT 3

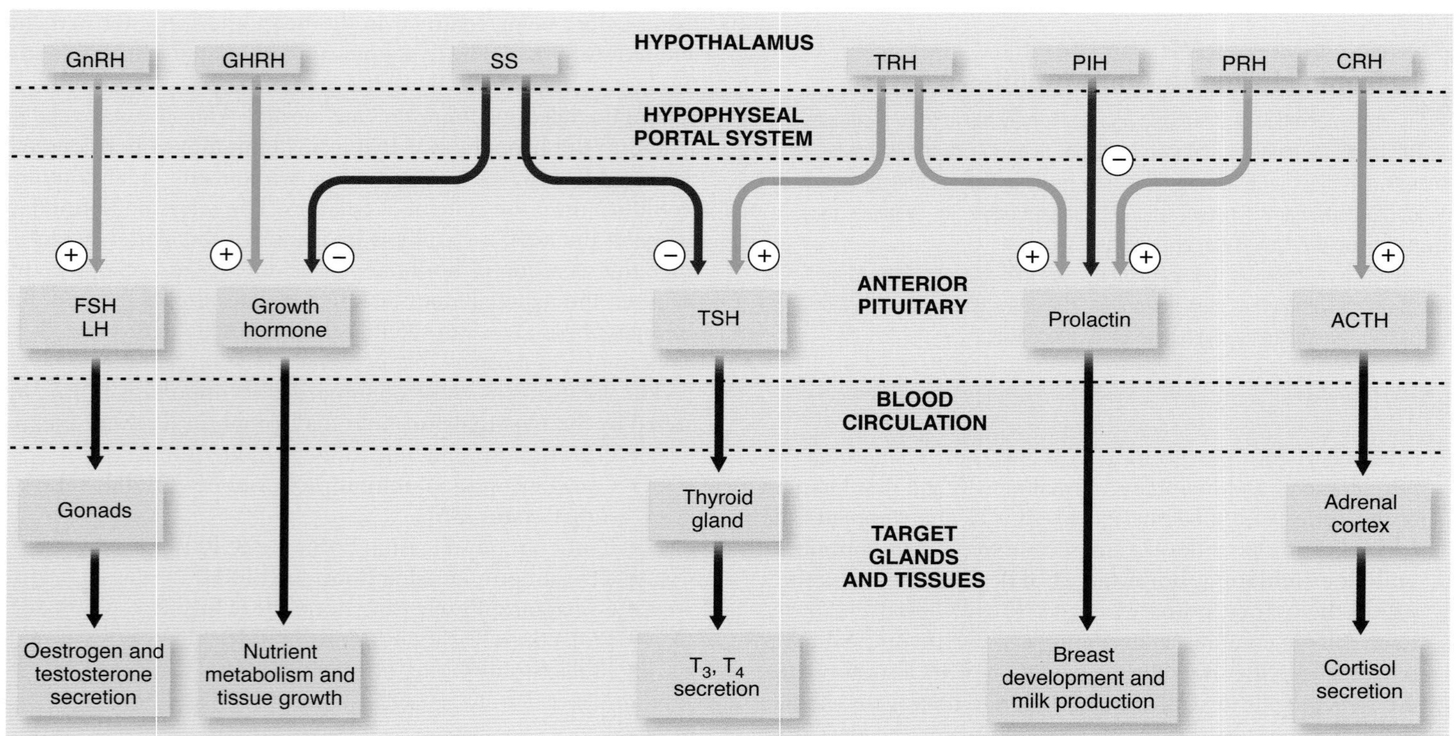

FIGURE 26-5 Action of hypothalamic hormones. Hypothalamic hormones have releasing or inhibiting effects on the various cells of the anterior pituitary, thus regulating anterior pituitary secretion—and thus ultimately regulating the effects of anterior pituitary hormones throughout the body. *ACTH,* Adrenocorticotropic hormone; *CRH,* corticotropin-releasing hormone; *FSH,* follicle-stimulating hormone; *GHRH,* growth hormone–releasing hormone; *GnRH,* gonadotropin-releasing hormone; *LH,* luteinizing hormone; *PIH,* prolactin-inhibiting hormone; *PRH,* prolactin-releasing hormone; *SS,* somatostatin; *TRH,* thyroid-releasing hormone; *TSH,* thyroid-stimulating hormone; T_3, triiodothyronine; T_4, thyroxine.

Figure 26-5 and **Table 26-1** list functions of each releasing hormone. Before consulting the figure or table, try to deduce their functions from their names.

Through negative feedback mechanisms, the hypothalamus adjusts the secretions of the adenohypophysis, and the adenohypophysis adjusts the secretions of its target glands, which in turn adjust the activity of their target tissues. For example, **Figure 26-6** shows the negative feedback control of the secretion of TSH and thyroid hormone (T_3 and T_4).

Hormone secretion can occur in pulses or peaks, as we see in a graph of minute-by-minute variations in GH secretion (**Figure 26-7**). The peaks result from many somatotroph cells in the pituitary collectively increasing their rate of secretion of GH. Such increases result from pulses in GHRH secretion by the hypothalamus (see **Figure 26-5**), which are especially large during sleep. Exercise, stress, and high-protein meals can cause an increase in the frequency of these peaks.

Before leaving the subject of control of pituitary secretion, we call your attention to another concept involving the hypothalamus. It functions as an important part of the body's complex machinery for responding to stress situations. For example, in severe pain or intense emotions, the cerebral cortex—especially the limbic area—sends

TABLE 26-1 Hormones of the Hypothalamus

HORMONE	SOURCE	TARGET	PRINCIPAL ACTION
Growth hormone–releasing hormone (GHRH)	Hypothalamus	Adenohypophysis (somatotrophs)	Stimulates secretion (release) of growth hormone
Growth hormone–inhibiting hormone (GHIH), or somatostatin	Hypothalamus	Adenohypophysis (somatotrophs)	Inhibits secretion of growth hormone
Corticotropin-releasing hormone (CRH)	Hypothalamus	Adenohypophysis (corticotrophs)	Stimulates release of adrenocorticotropic hormone (ACTH)
Thyrotropin-releasing hormone (TRH)	Hypothalamus	Adenohypophysis (thyrotrophs)	Stimulates release of thyroid-stimulating hormone (TSH)
Gonadotropin-releasing hormone (GnRH)	Hypothalamus	Adenohypophysis (gonadotrophs)	Stimulates release of gonadotropins (FSH and LH)
Prolactin-releasing hormone (PRH)	Hypothalamus	Adenohypophysis (corticotrophs)	Stimulates secretion of prolactin
Prolactin-inhibiting hormone (PIH)	Hypothalamus	Adenohypophysis (corticotrophs)	Inhibits secretion of prolactin

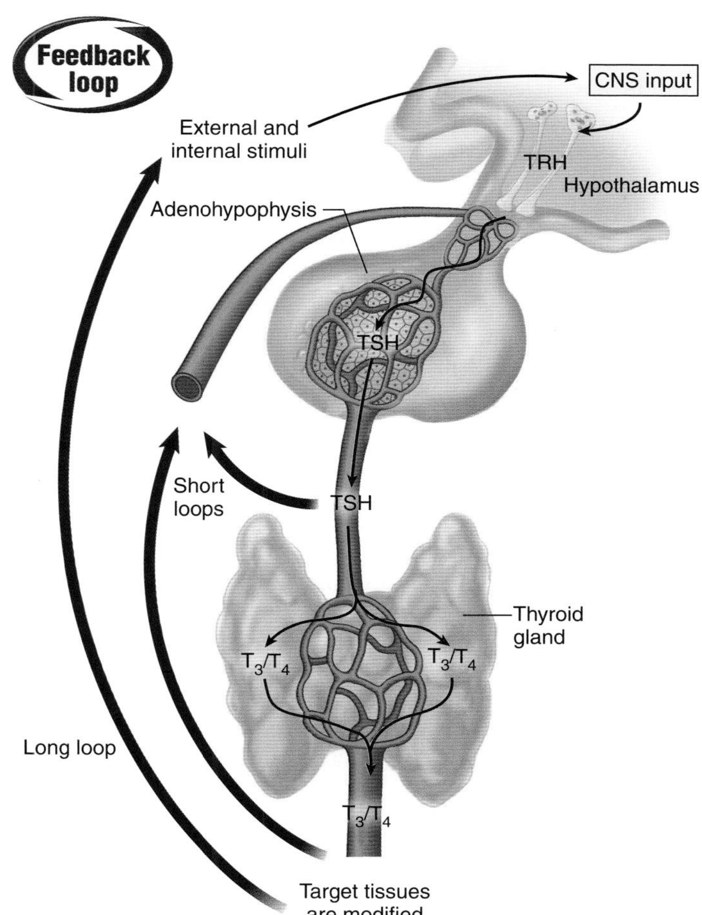

FIGURE 26-6 Negative feedback control by the hypothalamus. In this example, the secretion of thyroid hormone (T_3 and T_4) is regulated by a number of negative feedback loops. A long negative feedback loop *(long red arrow)* allows the central nervous system (CNS) to influence hypothalamic secretion of thyrotropin-releasing hormone (TRH) by nervous feedback from the targets of T_3/T_4 (and from other nerve inputs). The secretion of TRH by the hypothalamus and thyroid-stimulating hormone (TSH) by the adenohypophysis is also influenced by shorter feedback loops *(shorter red arrows),* allowing great precision in the control of this system.

impulses to the hypothalamus. The impulses stimulate the hypothalamus to secrete its releasing hormones into the hypophyseal portal veins. Circulating quickly to the adenohypophysis, they stimulate it to secrete more of its hormones. These in turn stimulate increased activity by the pituitary's target structures. In essence, what the hypothalamus does through its releasing of hormones is to translate nerve impulses into hormone secretion by endocrine glands. Thus the hypothalamus links the nervous system to the endocrine system. It integrates the activities of these two great integrating systems—particularly, it seems, in times of stress. When survival is threatened, the hypothalamus can take over the adenohypophysis and thus gain control of literally every cell in the body. We discuss stress in more detail in Chapter 34.

The mind–body link provided by the hypothalamus has tremendous implications. It means that the cerebrum can do more than just receive sensory impulses and send out impulses to muscles and glands. It means that our thoughts and emotions—our minds—can, by way of the hypothalamus, influence the functions of all of our trillions of cells. In short, the brain has two-way contact with every

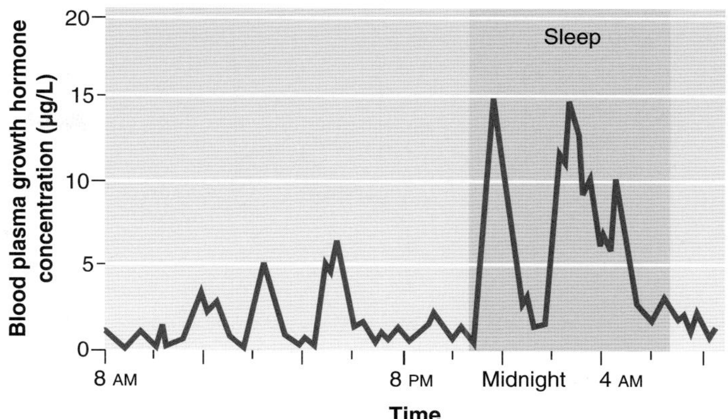

FIGURE 26-7 Secretion of growth hormone (GH). The amount of GH in the blood plasma of a 23-year-old woman was plotted on a graph every 5 minutes over the course of 24 hours. Note that GH fluctuates chaotically minute by minute, with occasional peaks that get larger after she falls asleep. The surges of GH result in part from pulses of GHRH (GH-releasing hormone) from the hypothalamus.

tissue of the body. Thus the state of the body can influence mental processes, and the state of the mind can affect the functioning of the body. Therefore both psychosomatic (mind influencing the body) and somatopsychic (body influencing the mind) relationships exist between human body systems and the brain.

Quick **CHECK**

1. What are the two main divisions of the pituitary called? How are they distinguished by location and histology?
2. Name three hormones produced by the adenohypophysis, and give their main functions.
3. What is a tropic hormone? A releasing hormone?

Neurohypophysis (Posterior Lobe of Pituitary)

The **neurohypophysis** serves as a storage and release site for two hormones: **antidiuretic hormone (ADH)** and **oxytocin (OT).** The cells of the neurohypophysis do not themselves make these hormones. Instead, neurons whose bodies are in either the *supraoptic* or the *paraventricular nuclei* of the hypothalamus synthesize them (**Figure 26-8**).

From the cell bodies of these neurons in the hypothalamus, the hormones pass down along axons (in the hypothalamohypophyseal tract) into the neurohypophysis. Instead of the chemical-releasing factors that trigger secretion of hormones from the adenohypophysis, release of ADH and OT into the blood is controlled by nervous stimulation.

Antidiuretic Hormone

The term *antidiuresis* literally means "opposing the production of a large urine volume". And this is exactly what ADH does—it prevents the formation of a large volume of urine. In preventing large losses of fluid through the excretion of dilute urine, ADH helps the body conserve water. In other words, ADH maintains water balance in the body. When the body dehydrates, the increased osmotic pressure of the blood is detected by special *osmoreceptors* near the supraoptic

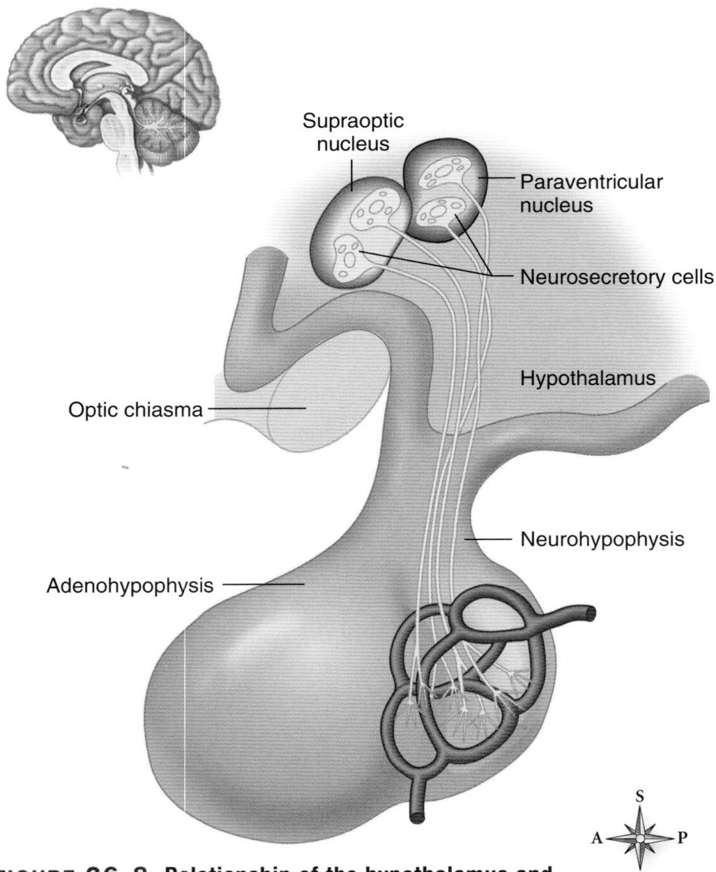

FIGURE 26-8 Relationship of the hypothalamus and neurohypophysis. Neurosecretory cells have their cell bodies in the hypothalamus and their axon terminals in the neurohypophysis. Thus hormones synthesized in the hypothalamus are actually released from the neurohypophysis.

nucleus. This triggers the release of ADH from the neurohypophysis. ADH causes water to be reabsorbed from the tubules of the kidney and returned to the blood (see Chapter 42). This increases the water content of the blood, restoring the osmotic pressure to its normal lower level. Thus, ADH is a major regulator of fluid balance in the body.

ADH has many other effects in the body as well. One of the most well known is that ADH stimulates contraction of muscles in the walls of small arteries (blood vessels that supply tissues), thus increasing blood pressure. For that reason, ADH is also known as *vasopressin* (literally, "vessel pressure substance"). Human vasopressin contains the amino acid arginine, unlike the vasopressin of some other organisms, so it is called **arginine vasopressin (AVP).**

Box 26-3 discusses some abnormalities associated with ADH.

BOX 26-3 *health matters*

Antidiuretic Hormone Abnormalities

Hyposecretion of antidiuretic hormone (ADH) can lead to **diabetes insipidus,** a condition in which the patient produces abnormally large amounts of urine. Drugs such as desmopressin, which mimic ADH, can alleviate this symptom. Studies have shown that ADH may be involved in learning and memory, so investigators are looking into the possibility of administering ADH to reverse the memory loss associated with senility.

Oxytocin

Oxytocin has at least two primary actions: It stimulates rhythmic contraction of smooth muscles in the uterus, and it causes milk ejection from the breasts of lactating women.

Under the influence of OT, muscle-like *myoepithelial* cells surrounding the milk-storing *alveoli* of the mammary glands squeeze milk into the ducts of the breast. **Figure 46-17** on p. 1077 clearly shows the structures involved. This action is very important because milk cannot be removed by suckling unless it has first been ejected into the ducts. Throughout nursing, the mechanical and psychological stimulation of the baby's suckling action triggers the release of more OT. In other words, OT secretion is regulated by a *positive feedback* mechanism: the baby suckles, which increases OT levels, which provides more milk, so the baby continues to suckle, which increases OT levels, and so on.

OT, together with prolactin, ensures successful nursing. Prolactin prepares the breast for milk production and stimulates cells to produce milk. The milk is not released, however, until OT stimulates its release.

The other major action of OT—its stimulation of uterine contractions—is the source of its name: oxytocin (literally "swift childbirth"). OT stimulates the uterus to strengthen the strong, muscular labour contractions that occur during childbirth. OT secretion is regulated here again by means of a positive feedback mechanism. After they have begun, uterine contractions stimulate stretch receptors in the pelvis, which triggers the release of more OT, which again stretches the pelvic receptors, and so on. Review the diagram in **Figure 2-4** (p. 29) outlining this positive feedback loop.

The wavelike contractions continue to some degree after childbirth, which helps the uterus expel the placenta and then return to its unstretched shape. Commercial preparations of synthetic OT have been given to stimulate contractions after childbirth to lessen the danger of uterine haemorrhage.

OT rises during sexual arousal in both males and females. The increased OT is related to rhythmic smooth muscle contractions associated with sexual arousal and orgasm.

OT's effect on muscle tissue also extends to skeletal muscle by supporting muscle regeneration. Some of the loss of skeletal muscle mass in ageing may be due, in part, to reduced secretion of OT as we age.

Interestingly, recent research shows that the smell of OT can increase the feeling of social connection to the person releasing it (perhaps in sweat). This may enhance a strong feeling of trust the newborn has for its mother. The role of oxytocin as a pheromone in social recognition and bonding is still being investigated—possibly leading to a better understanding of autism and other disorders that involve disruptions of social bonding.

Important characteristics of the hormones secreted by the pituitary—both the adenohypophysis and the neurohypophysis—are summarized in **Table 26-2**.

PINEAL GLAND

The **pineal gland,** or *pineal body,* is a tiny 1 cm structure resembling a pine nut (or a large kernel of corn) located on the dorsal aspect of the brain's diencephalon region (see **Figure 26-1**). It is a member of two body systems because it acts as a part of the nervous system (because it receives and processes nerve stimuli relayed from other parts

TABLE 26-2 Hormones of the Pituitary Gland

HORMONE	SOURCE	TARGET	PRINCIPAL ACTION
Growth hormone (GH) (somatotropin [STH])	Adenohypophysis (somatotrophs)	General	Promotes growth by stimulating protein anabolism and fat mobilization
Prolactin (PRL) (lactogenic hormone)	Adenohypophysis (lactotrophs)	Mammary glands (alveolar secretory cells)	Promotes milk secretion
Thyroid-stimulating hormone (TSH)*	Adenohypophysis (thyrotrophs)	Thyroid gland	Stimulates development and secretion in the thyroid gland
Adrenocorticotropic hormone (ACTH)*	Adenohypophysis (corticotrophs)	Adrenal cortex	Promotes development and secretion in the adrenal cortex
Follicle-stimulating hormone (FSH)*	Adenohypophysis (gonadotrophs)	Gonads (primary sex organs)	*Female:* promotes development of ovarian follicle; stimulates oestrogen secretion *Male:* promotes development of testes; stimulates sperm production
Luteinizing hormone (LH)*	Adenohypophysis (gonadotrophs)	Gonads	*Female:* triggers ovulation; promotes development of corpus luteum *Male:* stimulates production of testosterone
Antidiuretic hormone (ADH), or arginine vasopressin (AVP)	Neurohypophysis	Kidney	Promotes water retention by kidney tubules; raises blood pressure by stimulating muscles in walls of small arteries
Oxytocin (OT)	Neurohypophysis	Uterus and mammary glands	Stimulates uterine contractions; stimulates ejection of milk into ducts of mammary glands; involved in social bonding

*Tropic hormones.

of the nervous system) and as a part of the endocrine system (because it secretes hormones).

The pineal gland produces small amounts of many different hormones, but the principal hormone is melatonin. Recall from Chapter 20 that melatonin is an altered form of serotonin that acts as a hormone because it is released by neurosecretory cells of the pineal gland into the blood to regulate functions throughout the body. Recall also that melatonin levels rise and fall in a cycle related to the changing levels of sunlight throughout the day—melatonin levels rise when sunlight is absent, triggering sleepiness. Thus the pineal gland and melatonin act as important parts of a person's *biological clock*—the timekeeping mechanism of the body.

Melatonin, whose secretion is inhibited by the presence of sunlight, may also affect a person's mood. This is not surprising, given melatonin's relationship to another mood-altering molecule—serotonin. Serotonin is a precursor of melatonin, making both molecules structurally similar.

A mental disorder called *seasonal affective disorder (SAD)*, in which a patient suffers severe depression only in winter (when there are fewer hours of daylight), has been linked to the pineal gland. Patients who experience this "winter depression" are often advised to expose themselves to special high-intensity lights for several hours each evening during the winter months. Apparently, light stimulates the pineal gland for a longer period, which shifts the phase of melatonin peaks in the bloodstream. For reasons not fully understood, this phase shift often reduces or eliminates symptoms of depression. Apparently, keeping the body's clock well timed is important for maintaining a healthy mood.

CONNECT IT! 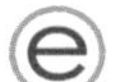

To see diagrams that clarify the pineal mechanism of timekeeping in the body, review ***The Timekeeping Hormone*** online at ***Connect It!***

***Quick* CHECK**

4. Where are the hormones of the neurohypophysis manufactured? From which location in the body are they released into the bloodstream?
5. Name the two hormones of the neurohypophysis.
6. How does the pineal gland adjust the body's biological clock?

THYROID GLAND

STRUCTURE OF THE THYROID GLAND

Two large **lateral lobes** and a narrow connecting isthmus make up the **thyroid gland** (**Figure 26-9**). Often a thin wormlike piece of thyroid tissue, called the *pyramidal lobe,* extends upward from the isthmus. The weight of the gland in the adult is variable, but it is around 30 grams. The thyroid is located in the neck, on the anterior and lateral surfaces of the trachea, just below the larynx. Figure 3-8 in the BRIEF ATLAS OF THE HUMAN BODY shows the position of the thyroid gland in the neck.

Thyroid tissue is composed of tiny structural units called **follicles,** the site of thyroid hormone synthesis. Each follicle is a small hollow sphere with a wall of simple cuboidal glandular epithelium (**Figure 26-10**). The interior is filled with a thick fluid called **thyroid colloid.** The colloid is produced by the cuboidal cells of the follicle wall (**follicular cells**) and contains protein–iodine complexes known as **thyroglobulins**—the precursors of thyroid hormones. Scattered around the outside of the follicles are *parafollicular cells,* which produce a hormone called calcitonin (CT).

THYROID HORMONE

The substance that is often called *thyroid hormone* (TH) is actually two different hormones. The most abundant TH is **tetraiodothyronine** (T_4), or **thyroxine.** The other is called **triiodothyronine** (T_3).

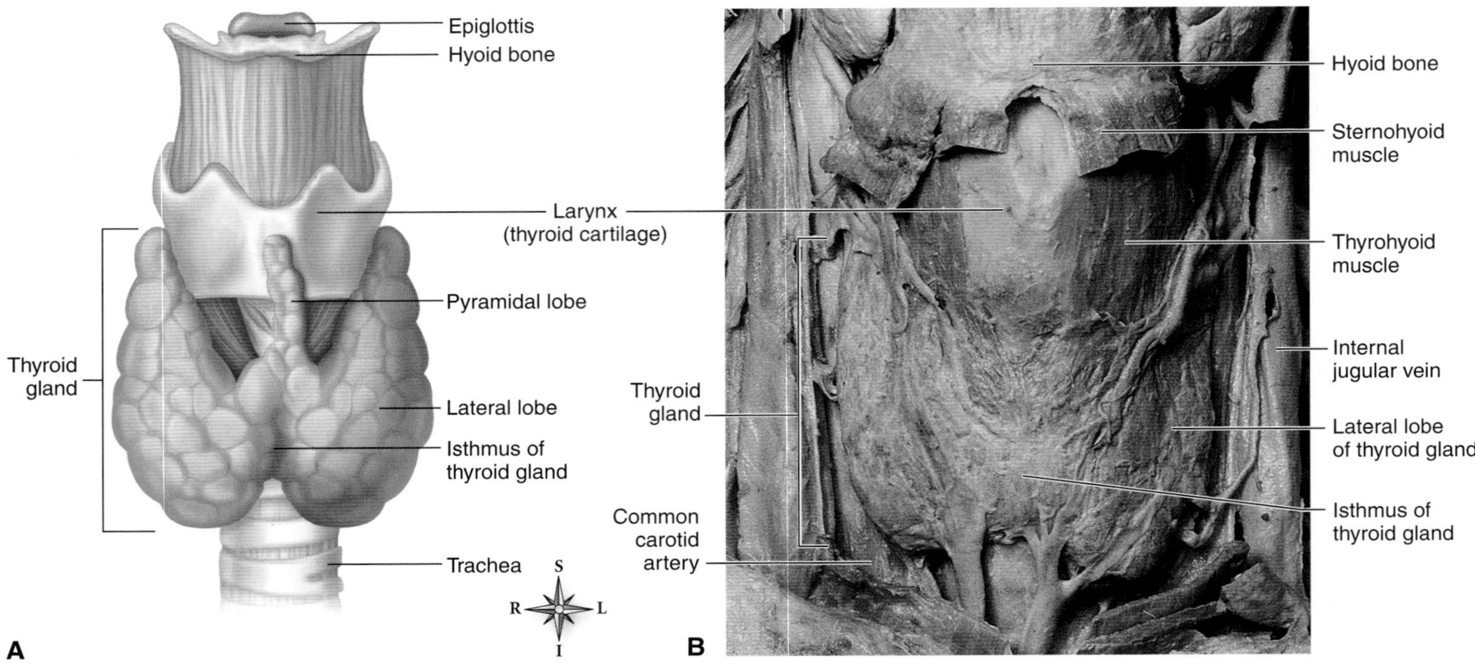

FIGURE 26-9 Thyroid gland. A, In this drawing, the relationship of the thyroid to the larynx (voice box) and to the trachea is easily seen. **B,** In this photo of a dissected cadaver, the location of the thyroid relative to the carotid arteries and jugular veins is seen.

One molecule of T_4 contains four iodine atoms, and one molecule of T_3 contains three iodine atoms. After synthesizing a preliminary form of its hormones, the thyroid gland stores considerable amounts of them before secreting them (**Figure 26-11**). This is unusual because none of the other endocrine glands stores its hormones in another form for later release.

T_3 and T_4 form in the colloid of the follicles on globulin molecules, forming thyroglobulin complexes. When they are to be released, T_3 and T_4 detach from the globulin and enter the blood. Once in the bloodstream, however, they attach to plasma proteins, principally a globulin called *thyroid-binding globulin (TBG)* and albumin, and circulate as a hormone–globulin complex. When they near their target cells, T_3 and T_4 detach from the plasma globulin.

Although the thyroid gland releases about 20 times more T_4 than T_3, T_3 is much more potent than T_4 and is considered by physiologists to be the principal thyroid hormone. Why is this? T_4 binds more strongly to plasma globulins than T_3, so T_4 is not removed from the blood by target cells as quickly as T_3. The small amount of T_4 that enters target tissues is usually converted to T_3. Add this to the fact that experiments have shown that T_3 binds more efficiently than T_4 to nuclear receptors in target cells, and the evidence is overwhelming that T_3 is the principal thyroid hormone. Although T_4 may influ-

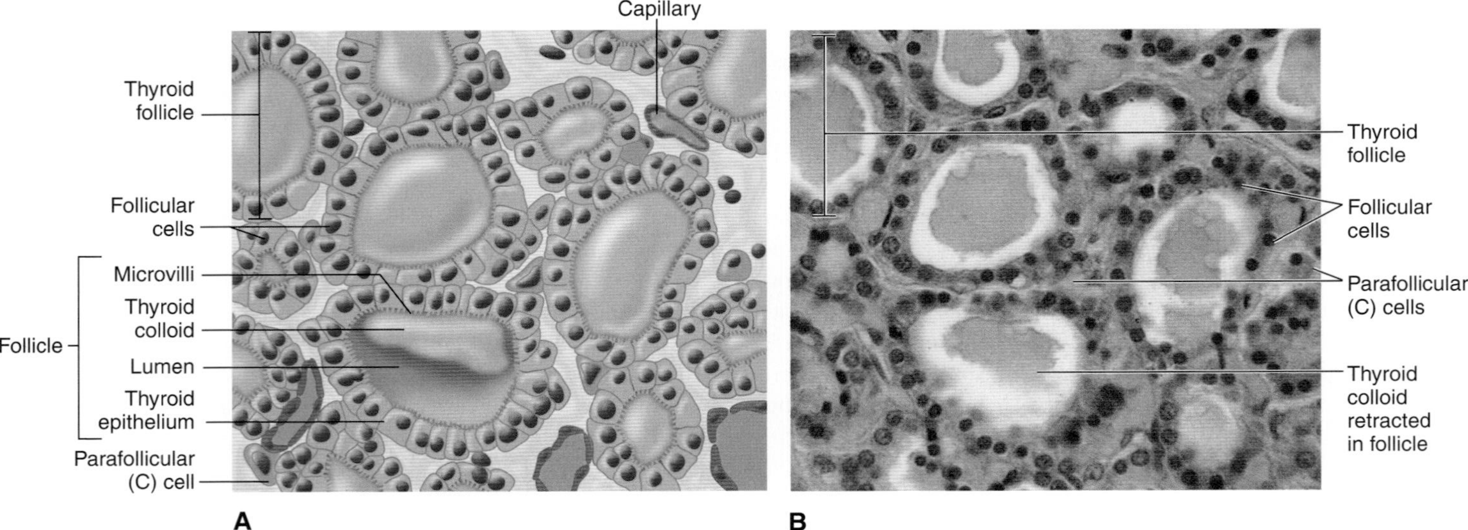

FIGURE 26-10 Thyroid gland tissue. In the drawing **(A)** and the photomicrograph **(B)** note that each of the thyroid follicles is filled with colloid. In the micrograph (×140), the thyroid colloid has separated from the follicular cells during preparation of the specimen.

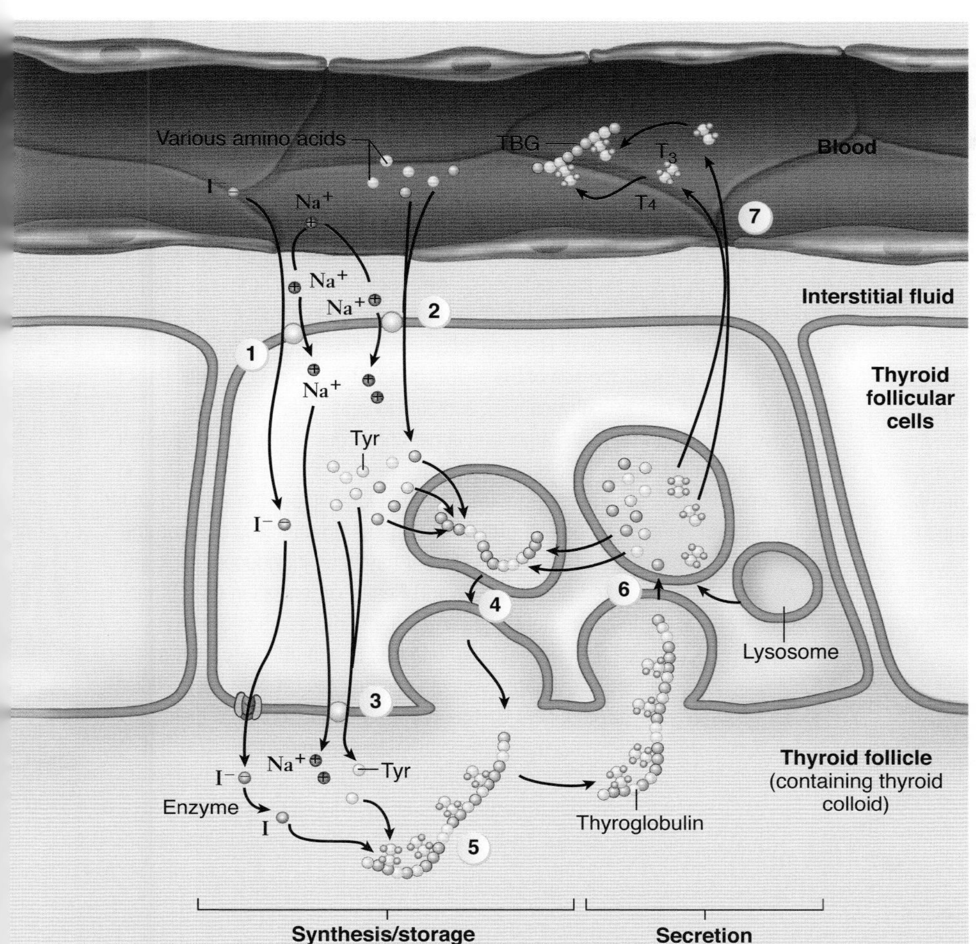

1 **Step 1.** Iodide ions (I^-) present in the blood enter follicular cells in the thyroid by sodium cotransport (see Box 6-3, p. 105). I^- then moves into the thyroid follicle through an ion channel, after which it is converted to iodine (I).

2 **Step 2.** At the same time, various amino acids (including tyrosine) enter follicular cells by sodium cotransport.

3 **Step 3.** Tyrosine amino acids move into the follicle.

4 **Step 4.** Some of the amino acids form a polypeptide, which is released into the follicle to be used as a structural "backbone" for thyroglobulin.

5 **Step 5.** The iodine (I) and tyrosine (Tyr) molecules are added to the polypeptide backbone to form thyroglobulin.

6 **Step 6.** When needed, thyroglobulin molecules move into follicular cells by endocytosis, where they are digested and thus release "free" T_3 and T_4 molecules.

7 **Step 7.** Thyroid hormones (T_3 and T_4) are secreted into the bloodstream, where they bind to plasma proteins called *thyroid-binding globulins (TBGs)* and travel to other parts of the body.

FIGURE 26-11 Synthesis, storage, and release of thyroid hormone (T_3 and T_4).

ence target cells to some extent, its major importance is as a precursor to T_3. Such hormone precursors are often called *prohormones*.

Thyroid hormone helps regulate the metabolic rate of all cells, as well as the processes of cell growth and tissue differentiation (**Box 26-4**). Because thyroid hormone can potentially interact with any cell in the body, it is said to have a "general" target.

Calcitonin

Besides thyroid hormone (T_3 and T_4), the thyroid gland also produces a hormone called **calcitonin (CT).** You might wonder why some hormones of the thyroid qualify for the name "thyroid hormone", whereas calcitonin does not. The answer lies in the simple fact that for many years, we had no idea that a hormone other than thyroid hormone was produced by the thyroid gland. By the time calcitonin was discovered, and later shown to be made in the thyroid gland, the term *thyroid hormone* was too well established to change it easily.

Produced by *parafollicular cells* (cells associated with the thyroid follicles) called **C cells,** calcitonin influences the processing of calcium by bone cells. Calcitonin apparently controls calcium content of the blood by increasing bone formation by osteoblasts and inhibiting bone breakdown by osteoclasts. This means more calcium is removed from the blood by the osteoblasts, and less calcium is released into the blood by osteoclasts.

Calcitonin in humans does not seem to have a great effect—but it may slightly decrease blood calcium levels and promote conservation of hard bone matrix. Calcitonin contained in nasal spray has been used for the treatment of bone loss in *osteoporosis*.

Parathyroid hormone, discussed later, is an antagonist to calcitonin, because it has the opposite effect. Together, calcitonin and parathyroid hormone help maintain calcium homeostasis (look ahead to **Figure 26-14** on p. 591).

Table 26-3 summarizes hormones of the thyroid gland.

PARATHYROID GLANDS

Structure of the Parathyroid Glands

There are usually four or five **parathyroid glands** embedded in the posterior surface of the thyroid's lateral lobes (**Figure 26-12**). They appear as tiny rounded bodies within thyroid tissue formed by compact, irregular rows of cells (**Figure 26-13** and Figure 5-44 in the Brief Atlas of the Human Body).

Parathyroid Hormone

The parathyroid glands secrete **parathyroid hormone (PTH),** or *parathormone* (see **Table 26-3**). PTH is the main hormone the body uses to maintain calcium homeostasis. PTH acts on bone and kidney cells by increasing the release of calcium into the blood. The bone

BOX 26-4 *health matters* | Thyroid Hormone Abnormalities

Hypersecretion of thyroid hormone occurs in **Graves disease,** which is thought to be an autoimmune condition. Graves disease patients may suffer from unexplained weight loss, nervousness, increased heart rate, and **exophthalmos** (protrusion of the eyeballs resulting, in part, from oedema of tissue at the back of the eye socket; see part *B* of the figure).

Hyposecretion of thyroid hormone during growth years may lead to **congenital hypothyroidism,** a condition characterized by a low metabolic rate, retarded growth and sexual development, and possibly mental retardation. People with profound manifestations of this condition are said to have deformed *dwarfism* (as opposed to the proportional dwarfism caused by hyposecretion of growth hormone). Hyposecretion later in life produces a condition characterized by decreased metabolic rate, loss of mental and physical vigour, gain in weight, loss of hair, yellow dullness of the skin, and myxoedema. **Myxoedema** is a swelling (oedema) and firmness of the skin caused by accumulation of mucopolysaccharides in the skin.

In the condition called **simple goitre,** the thyroid enlarges when there is a lack of iodine in the diet (part *A* of figure). This condition is an interesting example of how the feedback control mechanisms illustrated in **Figure 26-6** operate.

Because iodine is required for the synthesis of T_3 and T_4, lack of iodine in the diet results in a drop in the production of these hormones. When the reserve (in thyroid colloid) is exhausted, feedback informs the hypothalamus and adenohypophysis of the deficiency. In response, the secretion of thyrotropin-releasing hormone (TRH) and thyroid-stimulating hormone (TSH) increases in an attempt to stimulate the thyroid to produce more thyroid hormone. Because there is no iodine available to do this, the only effect is to increase the size of the thyroid gland. This information feeds back to the hypothalamus and adenohypophysis, and both increase their secretions in response. Thus the thyroid gets larger and larger and larger—all in a futile attempt to increase thyroid hormone secretion to normal levels.

This condition is still common in areas of the world where the soil and water contain little or no iodine. The use of iodized salt has dramatically reduced the incidence of simple goitre in countries where it has been introduced, such as the United States. The World Health Organization (WHO) has made iodine deficiency a global priority and has been campaigning for at-risk countries to add iodine to their salt. Recent investigations have indicated the UK is iodine-deficient, as salt producers are not required to add iodine to their salt. Young women of child-bearing age are most at risk as they now drink less milk, which is an important dietary source of iodine in the UK. Iodine deficiency may also have an impact on the developing brain of a fetus, as well as causing goitre in the mother.

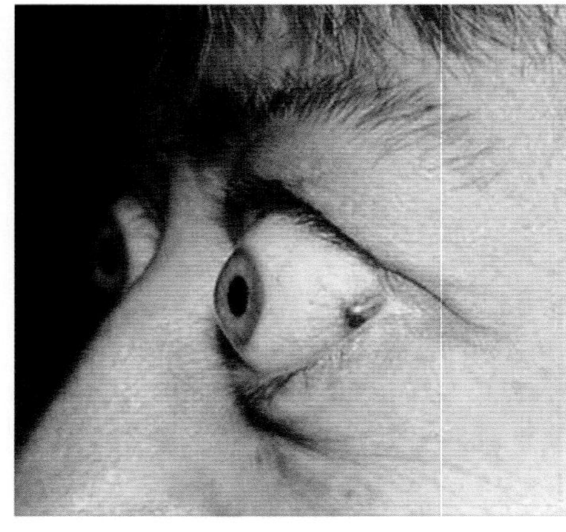

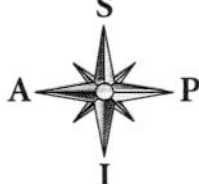

Thyroid hormone abnormalities. A, Simple goitre. **B,** Exophthalmos goitre (anterior view).

cells are especially affected, causing less new bone to be formed and more old bone to be dissolved, yielding calcium and phosphate. These minerals are then free to move into the blood, elevating blood levels of calcium and phosphate. In the kidney, however, only calcium is reabsorbed from urine into the blood. Under the influence of PTH, phosphate is secreted by kidney cells *out* of the blood and into the urine to be excreted.

PTH also increases the body's absorption of calcium from food by activating **vitamin D** *(cholecalciferol)*. If you go back to **Figure 10-14** (p. 192), you can see that vitamin D is converted to the active hormone *calcitriol* in the kidney, which then permits Ca^{++} to be transported through intestinal cells and into the blood.

The maintenance of calcium homeostasis, achieved through the interaction of PTH and calcitonin, is very important for healthy survival

TABLE 26-3 Hormones of the Thyroid and Parathyroid Glands

HORMONE	SOURCE	TARGET	PRINCIPAL ACTION
Triiodothyronine (T_3)	Thyroid gland (follicular cells)	General	Increases rate of metabolism
Tetraiodothyronine (T_4), or thyroxine	Thyroid gland (follicular cells)	General	Increases rate of metabolism (usually converted to T_3 first)
Calcitonin (CT)	Thyroid gland (parafollicular cells)	Bone tissue	Increases calcium storage in bone, lowering blood Ca^{++} levels
Parathyroid hormone (PTH), or parathormone	Parathyroid glands	Bone tissue and kidney	Increases calcium removal from storage in bone and produces the active form of vitamin D in the kidneys, increasing absorption of calcium by intestines and increasing blood Ca^{++} levels

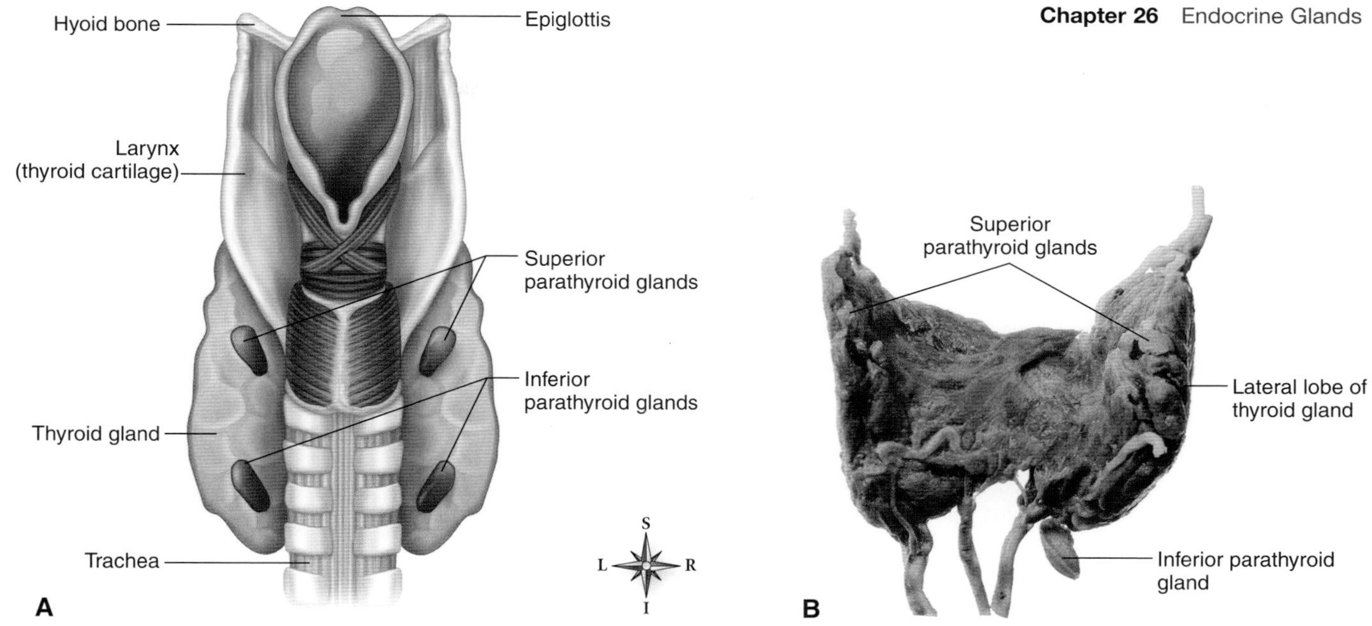

FIGURE 26-12 Parathyroid gland. A, In this drawing from a posterior view, note the relationship of the parathyroid glands to each other, to the thyroid gland, to the larynx (voice box), and to the trachea. **B,** Photo of a cadaver dissection (also from a posterior view) showing several parathyroid glands on the posterior surface of the lateral lobes of an isolated thyroid gland.

(**Figure 26-14**). You learned in Chapter 11 that adequate calcium in the blood is needed to build and maintain a healthy skeleton. Normal neuromuscular excitability, blood clotting, cell membrane permeability, and normal functioning of certain enzymes all depend on the maintenance of normal levels of calcium in the blood. For example, hyposecretion of PTH can lead to hypocalcaemia (**Box 26-5**). Hypocalcaemia increases neuromuscular irritability—sometimes so much that it produces muscle spasms and convulsions. Conversely, high blood calcium levels decrease the irritability of muscle and nerve tissue so that constipation, lethargy, and even coma can result.

Quick CHECK

7. Where is the thyroid located? What does it look like?
8. Thyroid hormone is really two distinct compounds—what are they? Which of the two is considered more physiologically active?
9. How do calcitonin and parathyroid hormone act together to regulate homeostasis of blood calcium concentration?

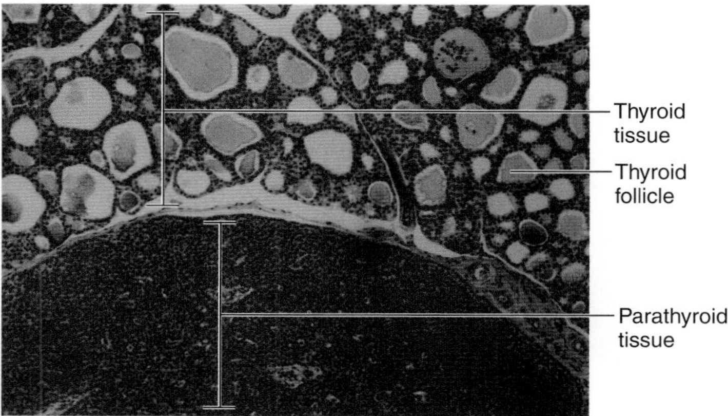

FIGURE 26-13 Parathyroid tissue. This microscopic specimen shows a portion of a parathyroid gland bordered by the surrounding thyroid tissue.

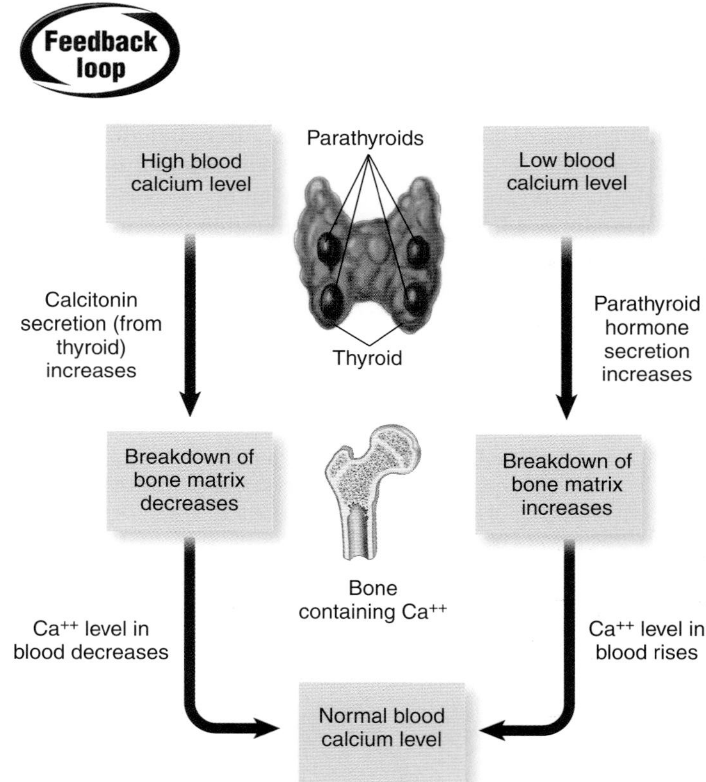

FIGURE 26-14 Regulation of blood calcium levels. Calcitonin and parathyroid hormones have antagonistic (opposite) effects on calcium concentration in the blood. (Also see **Figure 25-11**.)

BOX 26-5 *health matters*

Parathyroid Treatments

In cases of hyperparathyroidism, elevated parathyroid hormone (PTH) levels cause increases in blood calcium levels and possible development of osteoporosis and kidney stones. Treatment often involves surgical removal of one or more of the parathyroid glands.

However, knowing just how much parathyroid tissue to remove is a problem for the surgeon. If too much tissue is removed, the resulting drop in PTH below normal limits can result in **hypocalcaemia** that requires a lifetime of *PTH replacement therapy.*

A special deep freezing technique permits **cryopreservation,** or frozen storage, of the removed parathyroid tissue for up to 1 year. If too much tissue was removed at the time of surgery, a "banked" portion can be reimplanted (generally below the skin in the forearm) and will function to restore normal blood PTH levels.

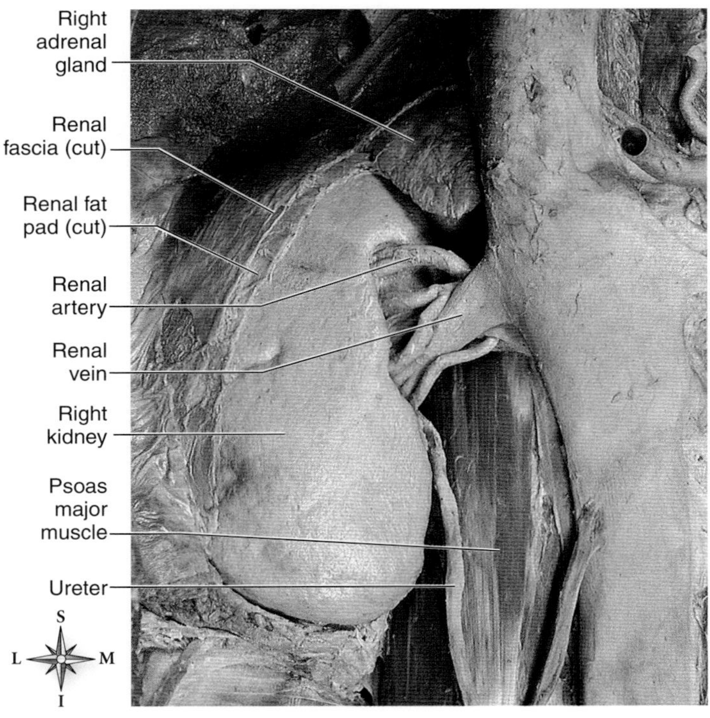

FIGURE 26-15 Location of the adrenal gland. Photograph of a cadaver dissection showing the location of the adrenal gland just superior to the kidney. Note that the adrenal glands are covered by the renal fascia but not the renal fat pad, both of which cover the kidney.

ADRENAL GLANDS

Structure of the Adrenal Glands

The **adrenal glands,** or *suprarenal glands,* are located atop the kidneys, fitting like a cap over these organs. **Figure 26-15** in this book and Figure 3-13 in the Brief Atlas of the Human Body show the position of the adrenal gland in relation to the kidney.

The outer portion of the gland is called the **adrenal cortex,** and the inner portion of the gland is called the **adrenal medulla** (**Figure 26-16**). Even though the adrenal cortex and adrenal medulla are part of the same organ, they have different embryological origins and are structurally and functionally so different that they are often spoken of as if they were separate glands. The adrenal cortex is composed of regular endocrine tissue, but the adrenal medulla is made of neurosecretory tissue (**Figure 26-17**). As you might guess, each of these tissues synthesizes and secretes a different set of hormones (**Figure 26-18** and **Table 26-4**).

Adrenal Cortex

The adrenal cortex is composed of three distinct layers, or zones, of secreting cells (see **Figures 26-16** to **26-18**). Starting with the zone directly under the outer connective tissue capsule of the gland, they are the **zona glomerulosa, zona fasciculata,** and **zona reticularis.** Cells of the outer zone secrete a class of hormones called *mineralocorticoids.* Cells of the middle zone secrete *glucocorticoids.* The

FIGURE 26-16 Structure of the adrenal gland. The zona glomerulosa of the cortex secretes aldosterone. The zona fasciculata secretes abundant amounts of glucocorticoids, chiefly cortisol. The zona reticularis secretes minute amounts of sex hormones and glucocorticoids. A portion of the medulla is visible at lower right at the bottom of the drawing.

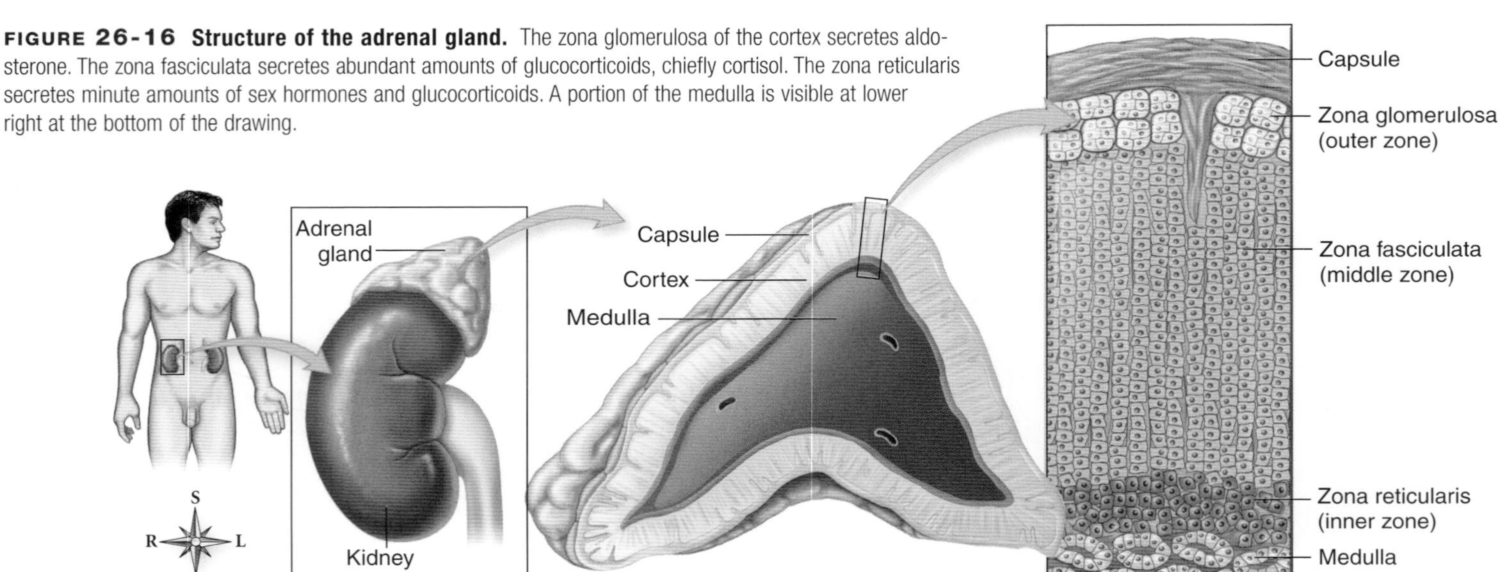

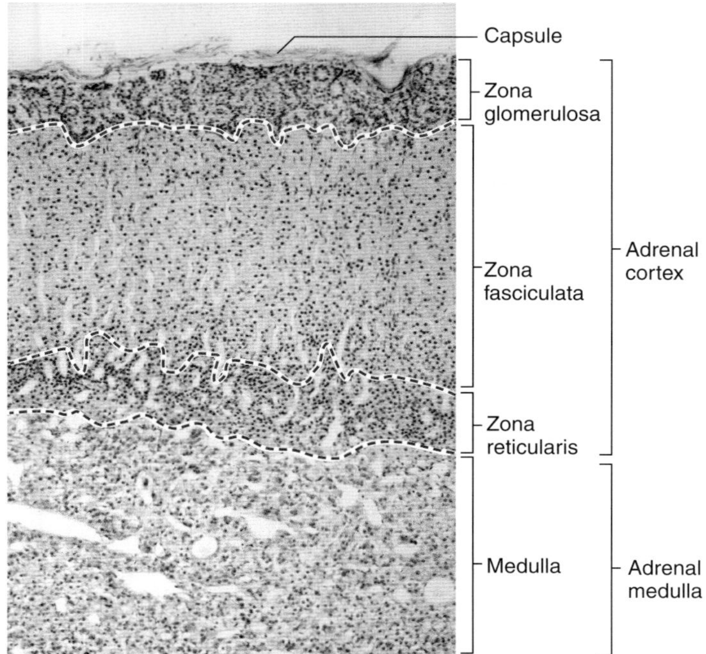

FIGURE 26-17 Adrenal tissue. The major regions of the adrenal gland are shown in a light micrograph of a stained specimen. The cortex is made up of epithelial endocrine tissue, and the medulla is instead made up of neurosecretory tissue. Compare with drawing in **Figure 26-16**.

inner zone secretes small amounts of *glucocorticoids* and *gonadocorticoids* (**sex hormones**). All these cortical hormones are steroids, so together they are known as *corticosteroids*.

Mineralocorticoids

Mineralocorticoids, as their name suggests, have an important role in regulating how mineral salts (electrolytes) are processed in the body. In the human, **aldosterone** is the only physiologically important mineralocorticoid. Its primary function is the maintenance of sodium homeostasis in the blood. Aldosterone accomplishes this by increasing sodium reabsorption in the kidneys. Sodium ions are reabsorbed from the urine back into the blood in exchange for potassium or hydrogen ions. In this way, aldosterone not only adjusts blood sodium levels but also can influence potassium and pH levels in the blood.

Zona glomerulosa
Zona fasciculata
Zona reticularis
Medulla
Mineralocorticoids
Glucocorticoids
Gonadocorticoids
Cortex
Catecholamines

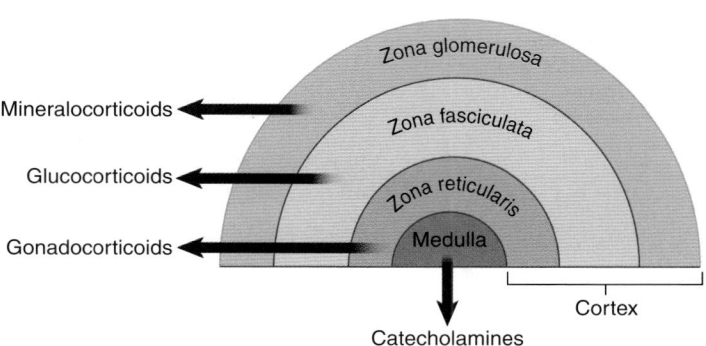

FIGURE 26-18 Adrenal hormones.

Because the reabsorption of sodium ions causes water to also be reabsorbed (partly by triggering the secretion of ADH), aldosterone promotes water retention by the body. Altogether, aldosterone can increase sodium and water retention and promote the loss of potassium and hydrogen ions.

Aldosterone secretion is controlled mainly by the **renin–angiotensin–aldosterone system (RAAS)** and by blood potassium concentration. The RAAS (**Figure 26-19**) operates as indicated in this sequence of steps:

1. When the incoming blood pressure in the kidneys drops below a certain level, a piece of tissue near the vessels (the *juxtaglomerular apparatus*) secretes *renin* into the blood.
2. **Renin,** an enzyme, causes **angiotensinogen** (a normal constituent of blood) to be converted to *angiotensin I.*
3. **Angiotensin I** circulates through the bloodstream, where *angiotensin-converting enzyme (ACE)* in blood capillaries (mostly in the lungs) splits the molecule, forming *angiotensin II.*
4. **Angiotensin II** circulates to the adrenal cortex, where it stimulates the secretion of aldosterone. (Some aldosterone is also synthesized in the heart and blood vessels.)
5. **Aldosterone** causes increased reabsorption of sodium, which causes increased water retention. As water is retained, the volume of blood increases. The increased volume of blood creates higher blood pressure—which then causes the renin–angiotensin–aldosterone system to stop.

TABLE 26-4 Hormones of the Adrenal Glands

HORMONE	SOURCE	TARGET	PRINCIPAL ACTION
Aldosterone	Adrenal cortex (zona glomerulosa)	Kidney	Stimulates kidney tubules to conserve sodium, which in turn triggers the release of ADH and the resulting conservation of water by the kidney
Cortisol (hydrocortisone)	Adrenal cortex (zona fasciculata)	General	Influences metabolism of food molecules; in large amounts, it has an antiinflammatory effect
Adrenal androgens	Adrenal cortex (zona reticularis)	Sex organs, other effectors	Exact role uncertain but may support sexual function
Adrenal oestrogens	Adrenal cortex (zona reticularis)	Sex organs	Thought to be physiologically insignificant
Epinephrine (Epi) (adrenaline)	Adrenal medulla	Sympathetic effectors	Enhances and prolongs the effects of the sympathetic division of the autonomic nervous system
Norepinephrine (NE)	Adrenal medulla	Sympathetic effectors	Enhances and prolongs the effects of the sympathetic division of the autonomic nervous system

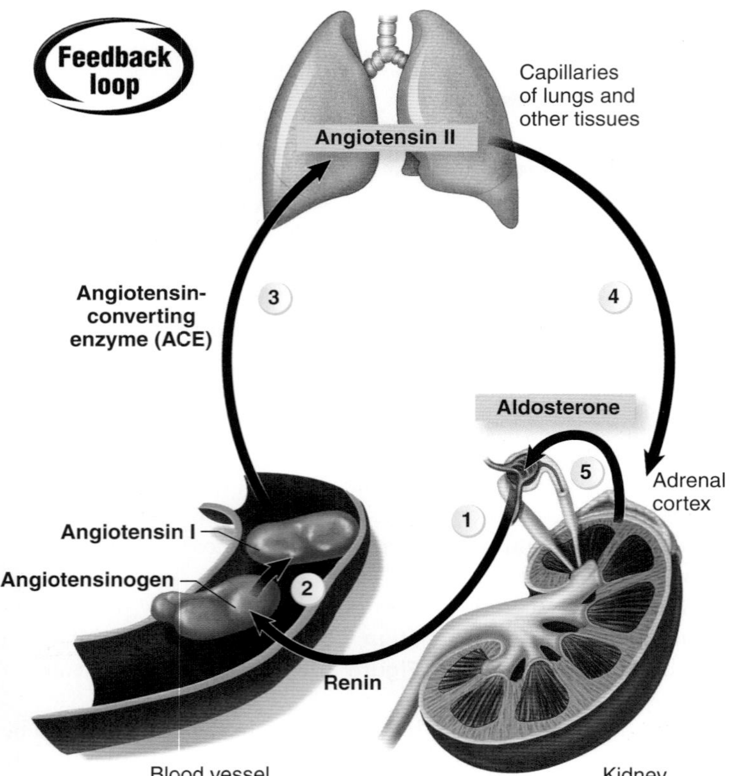

FIGURE 26-19 Renin–angiotensin–aldosterone system (RAAS) for regulating aldosterone secretion. The numbers correspond to the steps outlined in the text. Angiotensin-converting enzyme (ACE) is produced by capillaries throughout the body but is most concentrated in the lung capillaries.

The renin–angiotensin–aldosterone system is a negative feedback mechanism that helps maintain homeostasis of blood pressure. One way is to increase the overall volume of blood, a function of aldosterone. Another way is by the action of angiotensin II, which increases the tone of smooth muscle in the walls of arteries—thus increasing arterial blood pressure. A type of drug called an *ACE inhibitor* reduces abnormally high blood pressure by blocking the formation of angiotensin II (see step 3 earlier) and thus reducing both of these blood-pressure enhancing effects.

Glucocorticoids

The chief glucocorticoids secreted by the zona fasciculata of the adrenal cortex are **cortisol** (also called *hydrocortisone*), *cortisone*, and *corticosterone*. Of these, only cortisol is secreted in significant quantities in the human. Glucocorticoids affect every cell in the body. Although much remains to be discovered about their precise mechanisms of action, we do know enough to make some generalizations:

- Glucocorticoids accelerate the breakdown of proteins into amino acids (except in liver cells). These "mobilized" amino acids move out of the tissue cells and into the blood. From there, they circulate to the liver cells, where they are changed to glucose in a process called *gluconeogenesis*. A prolonged high blood concentration of glucocorticoids in the blood therefore results in a net loss of tissue proteins ("tissue wasting") and hyperglycaemia (high blood glucose). Glucocorticoids are protein-mobilizing, gluconeogenic, and hyperglycaemic.
- Glucocorticoids tend to accelerate mobilization of both lipids from adipose cells and lipid catabolism by nearly every cell in the body. In other words, glucocorticoids tend to cause a shift from carbohydrate catabolism to lipid catabolism as an energy source. The mobilized lipids may also be used in the liver for gluconeogenesis. This effect contributes to the hyperglycaemic effect already observed.
- Glucocorticoids are essential for maintaining a normal blood pressure. Without adequate amounts of glucocorticoids in the blood, the hormones norepinephrine and epinephrine cannot produce their vasoconstricting effect on blood vessels, and blood pressure falls. In other words, glucocorticoids exhibit *permissiveness* in that they permit norepinephrine and epinephrine to have their full effects. When glucocorticoids are present in high concentrations for a prolonged time, they may elevate blood pressure beyond normal (hypertension).
- A high blood concentration of glucocorticoids rather quickly causes a marked decrease in the number of white blood cells called *eosinophils* in the blood (eosinopenia) and marked atrophy of lymphatic tissues. The thymus gland and lymph nodes are particularly affected. This in turn leads to a decrease in the number of lymphocytes and plasma cells in the blood. Because of the decreased number of lymphocytes and plasma cells (antibody-processing cells), antibody formation decreases. Antibody formation is an important part of immunity—the body's defence against infection.
- Normal amounts of glucocorticoids act with epinephrine, a hormone secreted by the adrenal medulla, to bring about normal recovery from injury produced by inflammatory agents. How they act together to bring about this antiinflammatory effect is still uncertain.
- Glucocorticoid secretion increases as part of the stress response. One advantage gained by increased secretion may be the increase in glucose available for skeletal muscles needed in fight-or-flight responses. However, prolonged stress can lead to immune dysfunction, probably as a result of prolonged exposure to high levels of glucocorticoids (see Chapter 34).
- Except during the stress response, glucocorticoid secretion is controlled mainly by means of a negative feedback mechanism that involves ACTH from the adenohypophysis.
- As with many hormones, including all the adrenal cortical hormones, glucocorticoid secretion occurs in pulses and also shows a daily pattern of pulses of different amounts of hormone secretion (**Figure 26-20**).

Gonadocorticoids

The term *gonadocorticoid* refers to sex hormones that are released from the zona fasciculata and zona reticularis of the adrenal cortex rather than the gonads. The normal adrenal cortex secretes small amounts of male hormones (androgens). Normally, not enough androgen is produced to give women masculine characteristics, but it is sufficient to influence the appearance of pubic and axillary hair in both boys and girls.

Box 26-6 discusses some adrenal cortical hormone disorders.

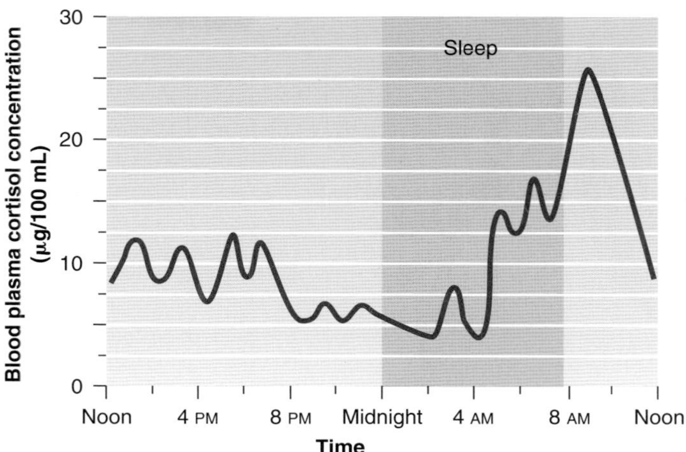

FIGURE 26-20 Secretion of cortisol. As with many hormones, the amount of cortisol secreted into the blood varies chaotically throughout the day. However, pulses of increased hormone secretion occur occasionally, with the highest peaks shortly before and after waking. Pulsing secretion (in response to specific conditions in the body) with a daily, or *diurnal,* pattern is seen in many hormones—including all of the adrenal cortical hormones.

Adrenal Medulla

The adrenal medulla is composed of neurosecretory tissue—that is, tissue composed of neurons adapted to secrete their products into the blood rather than across a synapse. Actually, the medullary cells are modified versions of sympathetic postganglionic fibres of the autonomic nervous system. They are innervated by sympathetic preganglionic fibres, so that when the sympathetic nervous system is activated (as in the stress response), the medullary cells secrete their hormones directly into the blood.

The adrenal medulla secretes two important hormones, both of which are in the class of nonsteroid hormones called catecholamines. **Epinephrine (Epi),** or *adrenaline,* accounts for about 80% of the medulla's secretion. The other 20% is **norepinephrine** (**NE** or **NR**). You may recall that norepinephrine is also the neurotransmitter produced by postganglionic sympathetic fibres. Sympathetic effectors such as the heart, smooth muscle, and glands have receptors for norepinephrine. Both epinephrine and norepinephrine produced by the adrenal medulla can bind to the receptors of sympathetic effectors to prolong and enhance the effects of sympathetic stimulation by the autonomic nervous system (**Figure 26-21**).

Quick CHECK

10. Distinguish between the histology of the adrenal cortex and the adrenal medulla.
11. Name some effects of cortisol in the body.
12. How does the function of the adrenal medulla overlap with the function of the autonomic nervous system?

PANCREATIC ISLETS

Structure of the Pancreatic Islets

The pancreas is an elongated gland (12 to 15 cm long) weighing up to 100 grams (**Figure 26-22**). The "head" of the gland lies in the C-shaped beginning of the small intestine (duodenum), with its body extending horizontally behind the stomach and its tail touching the spleen.

The tissue of the pancreas is composed of both endocrine and exocrine tissues. The endocrine portion is made up of scattered, tiny islands of cells, called **pancreatic islets** *(islets of Langerhans)* that account for only about 2% or 3% of the total mass of the pancreas. These hormone-producing islets are surrounded by cells called

UNIT 3

BOX 26-6 *health matters* | Adrenal Cortical Hormone Abnormalities

Hypersecretion of cortisol from the adrenal cortex often produces a collection of symptoms called **Cushing syndrome.** Hypersecretion of glucocorticoids results in a redistribution of body fat. The fatty "moon face" and thin, reddened skin characteristic of Cushing syndrome are shown in part *A* of the figure. Part *B* shows the face of the same boy 4 months after treatment. Hypersecretion of aldosterone, *aldosteronism,* leads to increased water retention and muscle weakness resulting from potassium loss. Hypersecretion of androgens can result from tumours of the adrenal cortex, called *virilizing tumours.* They are so called because the increased blood level of male hormones in women can cause them to acquire male characteristics, such as facial hair. People with Cushing syndrome may suffer from all the symptoms just described.

Hyposecretion of mineralocorticoids and glucocorticoids, as in **Addison disease,** may lead to a drop in blood sodium and blood glucose, an increase in blood potassium levels, dehydration, and weight loss.

Pharmacological preparations of glucocorticoids have been used for many years to temporarily relieve the symptoms of severe inflammatory conditions such as rheumatoid arthritis. Over-the-counter creams and ointments containing hydrocortisone are widely available for use in treating the pain, itching, swelling, and redness of skin rashes. •

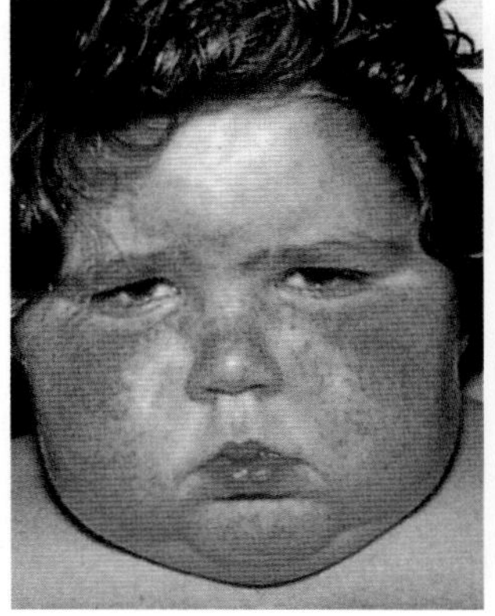

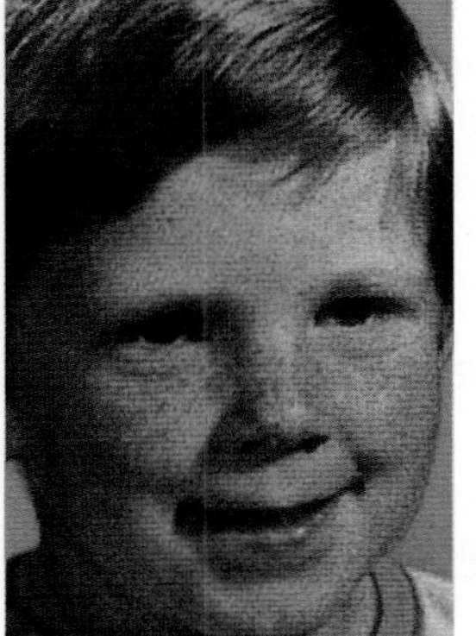

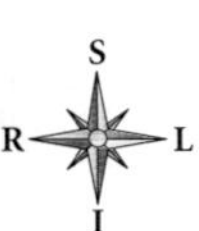

Cushing syndrome. A, Fatty "moon face" in a boy with Cushing syndrome. **B,** The face of the same boy 4 months after treatment.

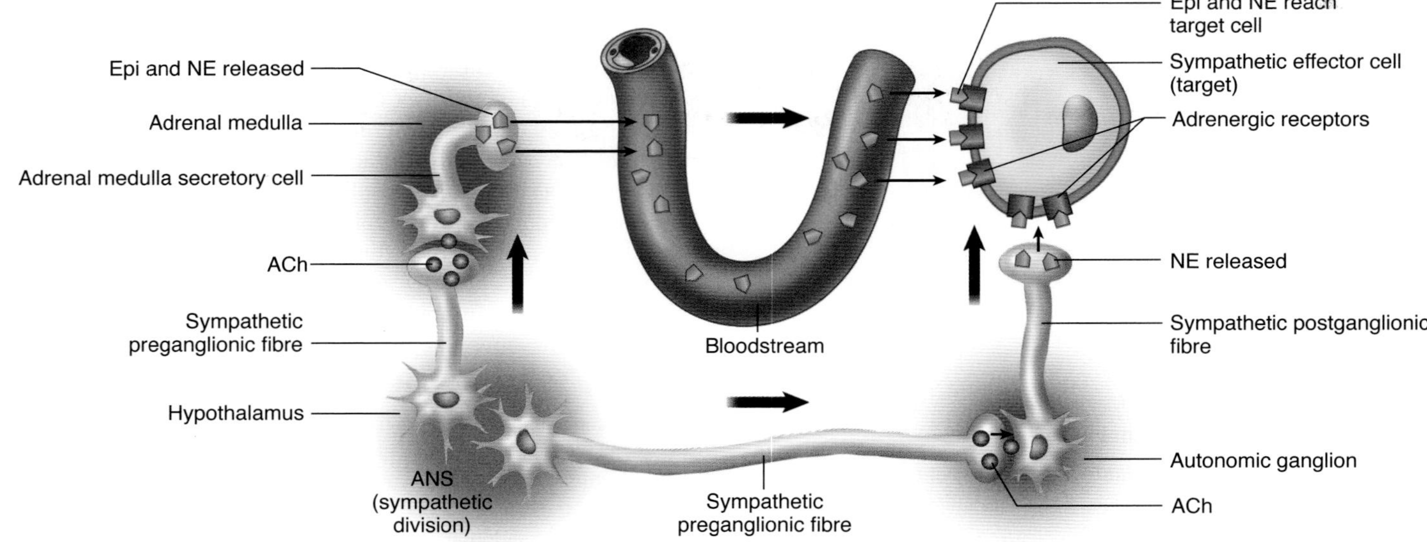

FIGURE 26-21 Combined nervous and endocrine influence on sympathetic effectors. A sympathetic centre in the hypothalamus sends efferent impulses through preganglionic fibres. Some preganglionic fibres synapse with postganglionic fibres that deliver norepinephrine *(NE)* across a synapse with the effector cell. Other preganglionic fibres synapse with postganglionic neurosecretory cells in the adrenal medulla. These neurosecretory cells secrete epinephrine *(Epi)* and norepinephrine into the bloodstream, where they travel to the target cells (sympathetic effectors). Compare this figure with **Figure 25-1**. *ACh,* Acetylcholine; *ANS,* autonomic nervous system.

acini, which secrete a serous fluid containing digestive enzymes into ducts that drain into the small intestine (see **Figure 26-22**). The digestive roles of the pancreas are discussed in Chapters 39 and 40. For the moment, we will concentrate on the endocrine part of this gland, the pancreatic islets.

Each of the 1 to 2 million pancreatic islets in the pancreas contains a combination of four primary types of endocrine cells, all joined to each other by gap junctions. Each type of cell secretes a different hormone, but the gap junctions may allow for some coordination of these functions as a single secretory unit. One type of pancreatic islet cell is the **alpha cell** (α or *A cell*), which secretes the hormone glucagon. **Beta cells** (β or *B cells*) secrete the hormone insulin; **delta cells** (δ or *D cells*) secrete the hormone somatostatin; **pancreatic polypeptide cells** (*F,* or *PP, cells*) secrete pancreatic polypeptide; and **epsilon cells** (ϵ *cells*) secrete the hormone ghrelin. Beta cells, which account for about three quarters of all the pancreatic islet cells, are usually found near the centre of each islet, whereas cells of the other three types are more often found in the outer portion.

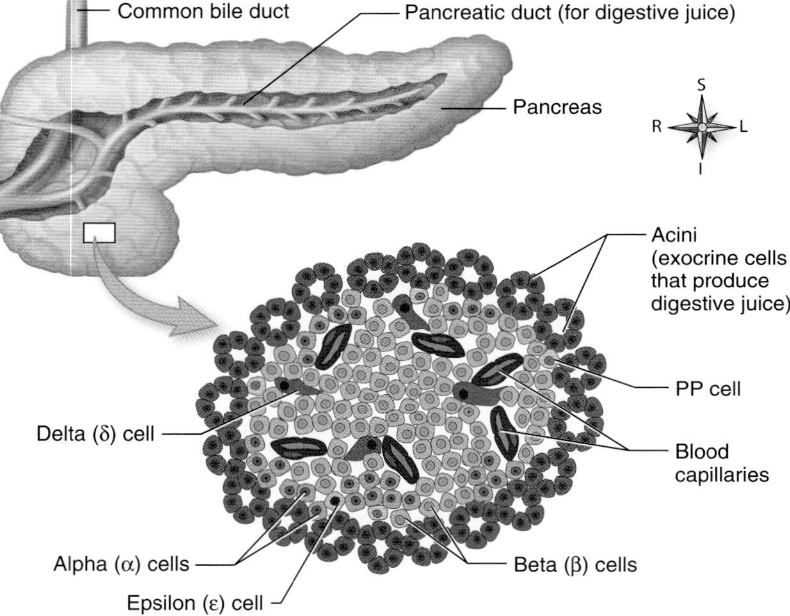

FIGURE 26-22 Pancreas. A pancreatic islet, or hormone-producing area, is evident among the pancreatic cells that produce the pancreatic digestive juice. The pancreatic islets are more abundant in the tail of the pancreas than in the body or head.

Pancreatic Hormones

The pancreatic islets produce several hormones, the most important of which are described in **Table 26-5** and in the following list:

- **Glucagon,** produced by alpha cells, tends to increase blood glucose levels by stimulating the conversion of glycogen to glucose in liver cells. It also stimulates gluconeogenesis (transformation of fatty acids and amino acids into glucose) in liver cells. The glucose produced by way of the breakdown of glycogen and by gluconeogenesis is released into the bloodstream, producing a hyperglycaemic effect.
- **Insulin,** produced by beta cells, tends to promote the movement of glucose, amino acids, and fatty acids out of the blood and into tissue cells. Hence insulin tends to lower the blood concentrations of these food molecules and to promote their metabolism by tissue cells. The antagonistic effects that glucagon and insulin have on blood glucose levels are summarized in **Figure 26-23** and discussed further in Chapter 41.
- **Somatostatin,** produced by delta cells, may affect many different tissues in the body, but its primary role seems to be in regulating the other endocrine cells of the pancreatic islets. Somatostatin inhibits the secretion of glucagon, insulin, and

TABLE 26-5 Hormones of the Pancreatic Islets

HORMONE	SOURCE	TARGET	PRINCIPAL ACTION
Glucagon	Pancreatic islets (alpha [α] cells, or A cells)	General	Promotes movement of glucose from storage and into the blood
Insulin	Pancreatic islets (beta [β] cells, or B cells)	General	Promotes movement of glucose out of the blood and into cells
Somatostatin (SS)	Pancreatic islets (delta [δ] cells, or D cells)	Pancreatic cells and other effectors	Can have general effects in the body, but primary role seems to be regulation of secretion of other pancreatic hormones
Pancreatic polypeptide (PP)	Pancreatic islets (pancreatic polypeptide [PP] or F cells)	Intestinal cells and other effectors	Exact function uncertain but seems to influence absorption in the digestive tract
Ghrelin (GHRL)	Stomach mucosa, pancreatic islets (epsilon [ϵ] cells)	Hypothalamus; other diverse tissues	Stimulates hypothalamus to boost appetite; affects energy balance in various tissues

pancreatic polypeptide. It also inhibits the secretion of growth hormone (somatotropin) from the anterior pituitary.

- **Pancreatic polypeptide** is produced by PP (or F) cells in the periphery of pancreatic islets. Although much is yet to be learned about pancreatic polypeptide, we do know that it influences gastrointestinal (GI) motility, secretion by the exocrine pancreas and feelings of hunger or fullness (satiety).
- **Ghrelin (GHRL)** is produced in tiny amounts by epsilon cells near the outer boundary of pancreatic islets. It acts by stimulating the hypothalamus to boost appetite. Because it also acts on other body tissues to slow metabolism and reduce fat burning, it may play an important role in contributing to obesity. GHRL is also secreted by the gastric mucosa.

UNIT 3

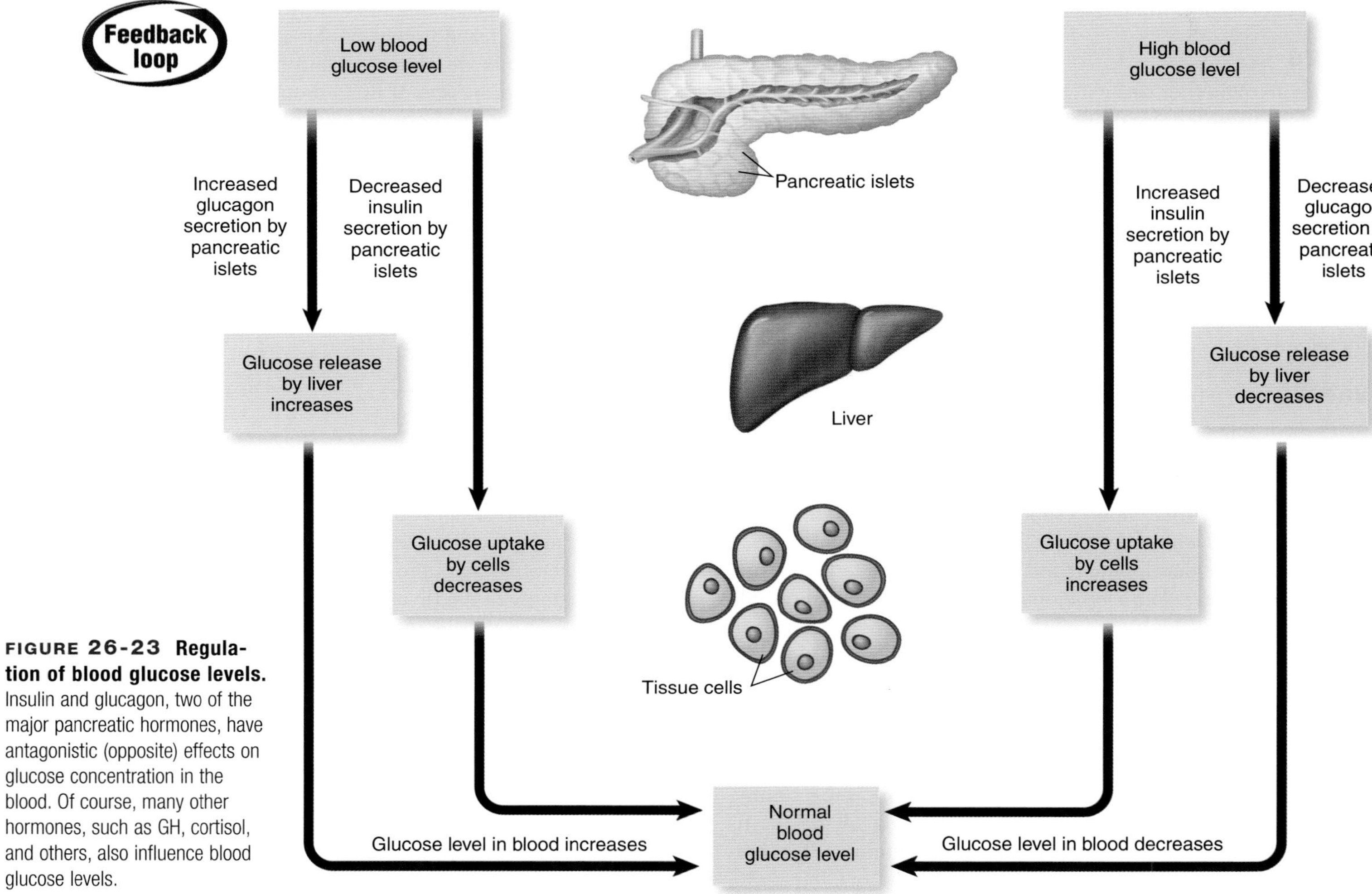

FIGURE 26-23 Regulation of blood glucose levels. Insulin and glucagon, two of the major pancreatic hormones, have antagonistic (opposite) effects on glucose concentration in the blood. Of course, many other hormones, such as GH, cortisol, and others, also influence blood glucose levels.

All of the pancreatic hormones work together as a team to maintain a homeostasis of nutrient molecules (glucose, fatty acids, and amino acids). More about their respective roles in overall nutrient metabolism is discussed in Chapter 41.

CONNECT IT!

Diabetes mellitus (DM) is one of the most common endocrine disorders. It involves a variety of abnormal effects in the body, all related to either hyposecretion of insulin or a reduction of insulin effects in target cells (or both). For a brief discussion of this disorder, and a chart showing the causes of the common symptoms of DM, check out ***Diabetes Mellitus*** online at ***Connect It!***

***Quick* CHECK**

13. Name two of the four principal hormones secreted by the pancreatic islets.
14. In what way do insulin and glucagon exert antagonistic influences on the concentration of glucose in the blood?

GONADS

Gonads are the primary sex organs in the male (*testes*; singular, *testis*) and in the female *(ovaries)*. Each is structured differently, and each produces its own unique set of hormones (**Table 26-6**).

Testes

The testes are paired organs within a sac of skin called the *scrotum*, which hangs from the groin area of the trunk (see **Figure 25-2** on p. 564). They are composed mainly of coils of sperm-producing *seminiferous tubules* with a scattering of endocrine *interstitial cells* found in areas between the tubules. These interstitial cells produce androgens (male sex hormones); the principal androgen is **testosterone.** Testosterone is responsible for the growth and maintenance of male sexual characteristics and for sperm production. Testosterone secretion is regulated principally by gonadotropin (especially LH) levels in the blood.

Ovaries

Ovaries are a set of paired glands in the pelvis (see **Figure 25-2** on p. 564) that produce several types of sex hormones, including those described briefly in the following list:

- **Oestrogens,** including oestradiol and oestrone, are steroid hormones secreted by the cells of the ovarian follicles that promote the development and maintenance of female sexual characteristics. With other hormones, they are responsible for breast development and the proper sequence of events in the female reproductive cycle (menstrual cycle). More details of their function are discussed in Chapter 46.
- **Progesterone** is a hormone whose name, which means "pregnancy-promoting steroid", indicates its chief function. Secreted by the corpus luteum (the tissue left behind after the rupture of a follicle during ovulation), progesterone (along with oestrogen) maintains the lining of the uterus necessary for successful pregnancy (gestation). This hormone, along with others, is discussed in detail in Chapter 46.

Regulation of ovarian hormone secretion is complex, to say the least, but basically depends on the changing levels of follicle-stimulating hormone (FSH) and LH (gonadotropins) from the adenohypophysis.

PLACENTA

Another reproductive tissue that functions as an important endocrine gland is the placenta. The **placenta,** the tissue that forms on the lining of the uterus as an interface between the circulatory systems of the mother and developing child, serves as a temporary endocrine gland.

The placenta produces **human chorionic gonadotropin (hCG).** This hormone is called *chorionic* because it is secreted by the chorion, a fetal tissue component of the placenta. It is called *gonadotropin* because, as with the gonadotropins of the adenohypophysis, it stimulates development and hormone secretion by maternal ovarian tissues. Chorionic gonadotropin secretion is high during the early part of pregnancy and serves as a signal to the mother's gonads to maintain the uterine lining rather than allow it to degenerate and fall away (as in menstruation).

The discovery of hCG many years ago led to the development of early pregnancy tests. The high levels of hCG in the urine of women who are in the early part of their pregnancies can be detected through several means. The most familiar test involves the use of an over-the-counter kit that tests for hCG in urine by means of an antigen-antibody reaction that can be easily interpreted.

As the placenta develops past the first trimester (3 months) of pregnancy, its production of hCG drops as its production of oestrogens and progesterone increases. The placenta therefore more or less takes over the job of ovaries in producing these hormones necessary for a successful pregnancy.

The placenta also produces additional oestrogen and progesterone during pregnancy, as well as several other hormones (see **Table 26-6**). These include **human placental lactogen (hPL)** and **relaxin.**

More about how placental hormones work is discussed in Chapter 47.

THYMUS

The **thymus** is a gland in the mediastinum, just beneath the sternum (see **Figure 25-2** on p. 564). It is large in children until puberty, when it begins to atrophy. It continues to atrophy throughout adulthood, so that by the time an individual reaches old age, the gland is but a vestige of fat and fibrous tissue.

The anatomy of the thymus is described in Chapter 31.

Although it is considered to be primarily a lymphatic organ (see Chapter 31), the hormones **thymosin** and **thymopoietin** have been isolated from thymus tissue and are considered to be largely responsible for its endocrine activity (see **Table 26-6**). *Thymosin* and *thymopoietin* actually refer to two entire families of peptides that together have a critical role in the development of the immune system. Specifically, thymosin and thymopoietin are thought to stimulate the production of special lymphocytes involved in the immune response called *T cells.* The role of T cells in the immune system is discussed in Chapter 33.

TABLE 26-6 Examples of Additional Hormones of the Body

HORMONE	SOURCE	TARGET	PRINCIPAL ACTION
Cholecalciferol (vitamin D_3)	Skin, liver, kidney (in progressive steps)	Intestines, bones, most other tissues	Promotes calcium absorption from food, regulates mineral balance in bones, regulates growth and differentiation of many cell types
Dehydroepiandrosterone (DHEA)	Adrenal gland, testis, ovary, other tissues	Converted to other hormones	Eventually converted to oestrogens, testosterone, or both (see **Figure 25-5**), has a role in stress as functional antagonist to cortisol
Melatonin	Pineal gland	Timekeeping tissues of the nervous system	Helps "set" the biological clock mechanisms of the body by signalling light changes during the day, month, and seasons; may help induce sleep
Testosterone	Testis (small amounts in adrenal and ovary)	Sperm-producing tissues of testis, muscles, other tissues	Stimulates sperm production, stimulates growth and maintenance of male sexual characteristics, promotes muscle growth
Oestrogen, including oestradiol (E_2) and oestrone	Ovary and placenta (small amounts in adrenal and testis)	Uterus, breasts, other tissues	Stimulates development of female sexual characteristics, breast development, bone and nervous system maintenance
Progesterone	Ovary and placenta	Uterus, mammary glands, other tissues	Helps maintain proper conditions for pregnancy
Human chorionic gonadotropin (hCG)	Placenta	Ovary	Stimulates secretion of oestrogen and progesterone during pregnancy
Human placental lactogens (hPLs)	Placenta	Mammary glands; pancreas and other tissues	Promote development of mammary glands during pregnancy; help regulate energy balance in fetus
Relaxin	Placenta	Uterus and joints	Inhibits uterine contractions during pregnancy and softens pelvic joints to facilitate childbirth
Thymosins and thymopoietins	Thymus gland	Certain lymphocytes (type of white blood cell)	Stimulate development of T lymphocytes, which are involved in immunity
Gastrin	Stomach mucosa	Exocrine glands of stomach	Triggers increased gastric juice secretion
Secretin	Intestinal mucosa	Stomach and pancreas	Increases alkaline secretions of the pancreas and slows emptying of stomach; helps regulate water homeostasis
Cholecystokinin (CCK)	Intestinal mucosa	Gallbladder and pancreas	Triggers the release of bile from gallbladder and enzymes from the pancreas
Atrial natriuretic hormone (ANH) and other atrial natriuretic peptides (ANPs)	Heart muscle	Kidney	Promote loss of sodium from body into urine, thus promoting water loss from the body and a resulting decrease in blood volume and pressure
Inhibins	Ovary and testis	Hypothalamus Adenohypophysis (anterior pituitary)	Inhibit secretion of GnRH by hypothalamus and FSH by the anterior pituitary, thus helping to regulate the female reproductive cycle
Erythropoietin (EPO)	Kidneys, liver	Red marrow	Promotes increased production of red blood cells
Irisin	Skeletal muscle	Adipose, other tissues	Promotes conversion of white fat to brown fat
Interleukin-6 (IL-6)	Skeletal muscle	Liver	Promotes release of glucose into blood during prolonged exercise
Leptin	Adipose tissue	Hypothalamus; other diverse tissues	Affects energy balance, perhaps as a signal of how much fat is stored; affects various immune, neuroendocrine, reproductive, and developmental functions throughout body
Resistin	Adipose tissue and macrophages	Liver and other tissues	Reduces sensitivity to insulin (a pancreatic islet hormone), thus increasing blood glucose levels
Palmitoleate	Adipose tissue (thighs)	Muscle, liver, other tissues	Increases insulin sensitivity
Insulin-like growth factor 1 (IGF-1)	Liver, kidney, and other tissues	Bone, muscle, and other tissues	Secreted in response to growth hormone (GH) IGF-1 carries out many functions attributed to GH

UNIT 3

GASTRIC AND INTESTINAL MUCOSA

The mucous lining of the gastrointestinal (GI) tract, like the pancreas, contains cells that produce both endocrine and exocrine secretions (see **Table 26-6**).

GI hormones such as **gastrin**, **secretin**, and **cholecystokinin (CCK)** have important regulatory roles in coordinating the secretory and motor activities involved in the digestive process. For example, secretin is released when acids make contact with the intestinal mucosa. Secretin carried by the blood triggers its target cells in the stomach to reduce acid secretion. Secretin also triggers its target cells in the pancreas to release an alkaline fluid, and it acts with CCK to trigger the pancreas to release digestive enzymes. CCK triggers the gallbladder to release more bile, which helps break up fat droplets. In effect, secretin and CCK are signals from the intestine to other parts of the digestive system that promote an effective coordination of GI functions.

The appetite-boosting hormone *ghrelin (GHRL)* is secreted by endocrine cells in the gastric mucosa as well as in the pancreatic islets.

Chapter 40 describes the hormonal control of digestion in the stomach and small intestine in more detail (see **Table 40-5**, p. 918).

HEART

The heart is another organ with a secondary endocrine role. Although the heart's main function is to pump blood, a specific area in its wall contains some hormone-producing cells. These cells produce several peptide hormones (see **Table 26-6**). This group of hormones is collectively called *atrial natriuretic peptide (ANP)*, and the principal hormone of the group is called **atrial natriuretic hormone (ANH).**

The name atrial natriuretic hormone reveals much about its role in the body. The term *atrial* refers to the fact that ANH is secreted by cells in an upper chamber of the heart called an *atrium*. Atrial cells increase their secretion of ANH in response to an increase in the stretch of the atrial wall caused by abnormally high blood volume or blood pressure. The term *natriuretic* refers to the fact that its principal effect is to promote the loss of sodium (Latin, *natrium*) from the body by means of the urine. When sodium is thus lost from the internal environment, water follows. Water loss results in a decrease in blood volume (and thus a decrease in blood pressure). We can then state that the primary effect of ANH is to oppose increases in blood volume or blood pressure. We can also state that ANH is an antagonist to ADH and aldosterone.

ANH is also known by several other names, including *atrial natriuretic factor (ANF), atrial natriuretic peptide,* and simply, *atrial peptide.*

ADIPOSE TISSUE

Adipose tissue serves many functions in the body, including endocrine regulation. Adipose tissue secretes **leptin,** a protein hormone that plays a role in energy balance, regulation of immunity and neuroendocrine function, and development. Leptin has some subtle effects on reproductive function in humans by stimulating GnRH release from the hypothalamus. Leptin may reduce or stop menstruation in women who are starving or overexercising, and it may promote early onset of menstruation (menarche) in obese girls.

Another hormone secreted by adipose tissue and macrophages—**resistin**—reduces sensitivity to insulin and thus raises blood glucose levels.

Adipose tissue also produces a recently discovered type of lipid hormone called a **lipokine**. The primary example is the lipokine *palmiteolate,* derived from the fatty acid palmitoleic acid. Secreted primarily from adipose tissue in the thighs, palmiteolate increases insulin sensitivity in other tissues.

CONNECT IT! 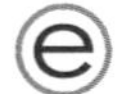

People with body shapes with fatty thighs (pear-shaped body type) tend to have reduced risk for cardiovascular disease and diabetes. Lipokines from adipose tissue in the thighs may play a role in reducing health risks. Review ***Body Types and Disease*** online at ***Connect It!***

OTHER ENDOCRINE GLANDS AND HORMONES

In this chapter, we have outlined the structure and function of only a few of the more central endocrine glands. And we have discussed only a few of their principal hormones. Many of the glands we have discussed in this chapter produce many more hormones, all of which are important to normal body function.

For example, the ovaries produce the hormone **inhibin**—a glycoprotein hormone that helps to regulate FSH levels in women. Hormones produced by muscle tissues are called myokines. An example is the hormone irisin, which helps to convert white fat into brown fat. Another of the myokines is interleukin-6 (IL-6), which signals the liver to release glucose during prolonged exercise. *Erythropoietin (EPO)* is a hormone produced by the kidneys that promotes red blood cell production—a topic to be discussed in our next chapter.

In addition to the primary effects described in this book, many hormones have additional effects—including some yet to be discovered.

Many other tissues throughout the body produce hormones—perhaps all tissues in the body produce hormones. **Table 26-6** summarizes a few additional examples of hormones that you are likely to encounter in your studies.

It is neither within the scope of this chapter—nor within the scope of this book—to discuss every known human hormone. Such a discussion would be longer than this *whole* book is now! Having had this brief preview, however, you will now be prepared for additional examples that you will encounter as you continue your study of the human body.

***Quick* CHECK**

15. What are the major hormones secreted by reproductive tissues (gonads and the placenta)?
16. Which gland produces a hormone that regulates the development of cells important to the immune system?
17. Secretin was the first substance in the body to be identified as a hormone. What structure produces secretin?
18. Which type of body tissue produces the hormone *leptin*?

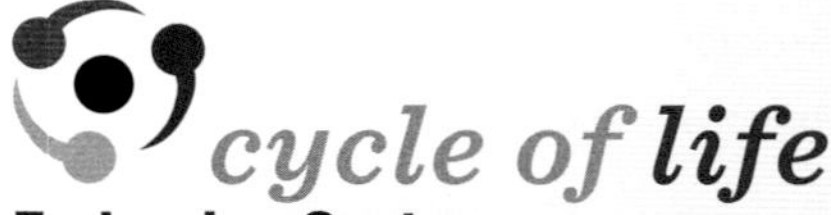

Endocrine System Endocrine regulation of body processes first begins during early development in the womb. By the time a baby is born, many of the hormones are already at work influencing the activity of target cells throughout the body. As a matter of fact, it is a hormonal signal from the fetus to the mother that signals the onset of labour and delivery. Many of the basic hormones are active from birth, but most of the hormones related to reproductive functions are not produced or secreted until puberty. Secretion of male reproductive hormones follows the same pattern as most nonreproductive hormones: continuous secretion from puberty until a slight tapering off occurs in late adulthood. The secretion of female reproductive hormones such as oestrogens also declines late in life, but more suddenly and completely—often during or just at the end of middle adulthood. •

the big picture

The Endocrine System and the Whole Body

In the previous chapter we identified the precision of control afforded by the partnership of the two major regulatory systems: the endocrine system and the nervous system. In this chapter we have encountered many examples of this partnership.

The neuroendocrine system is able to finely adjust the availability and processing of nutrients through a diverse array of mechanisms: growth hormone, thyroid hormone, cortisol, epinephrine, somatostatin, autonomic nervous regulation, and so on. The absorption, storage, and transport of calcium ions are kept in balance by the antagonistic actions of calcitonin and parathyroid hormone (and its effects on vitamin D). Reproductive ability is triggered, developed, maintained, and timed by the complex interaction of the nervous system with follicle-stimulating hormone, luteinizing hormone, oestrogen, progesterone, testosterone, chorionic gonadotropin, prolactin, oxytocin, and melatonin. Nearly every process in the human organism is kept in balance by the incredibly complex, but precise, interaction of all these different nervous and endocrine regulatory chemicals.

In this chapter, we have also seen the many different structures and regulatory mechanisms that make up the endocrine system. Some of the more important hormones and their characteristics are summarized in tables throughout the chapter. As we continue our study of human anatomy and physiology, we will often encounter these hormones and the critical integrative role played by the endocrine system.

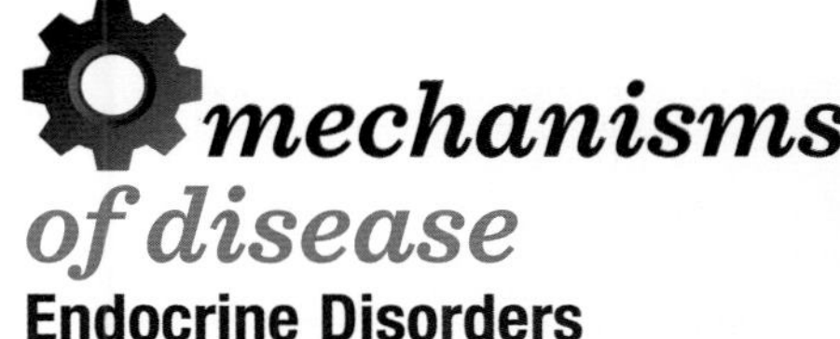

Endocrine Disorders

In Chapter 25 (see p. 572, **Box 25-2**) we stated that nearly all endocrine disorders are caused by abnormal hormonal effects in target tissues. This could result from hypersecretion or hyposecretion of hormones. Or it could result from oversensitivity or undersensitivity in the target tissues, which can produce effects similar to hypersecretion or hyposecretion of hormones. Throughout this chapter, we have seen examples of many such disorders. **Table 26-7** summarizes some important examples of endocrine disorders.

UNIT 3

TABLE 26-7 Examples of Endocrine Conditions

CONDITION	MECHANISM	DESCRIPTION
Acromegaly	Hypersecretion of growth hormone (GH) during adulthood	Chronic metabolic disorder characterized by gradual enlargement or elongation of facial bones and extremities
Addison disease	Hyposecretion of adrenal cortical hormones (adrenal cortical insufficiency)	Caused by tuberculosis, autoimmunity, or other factors, this life-threatening condition is characterized by weakness, anorexia, weight loss, nausea, irritability, decreased cold tolerance, dehydration, increased skin pigmentation, and emotional disturbance; it may lead to an acute phase (adrenal crisis) characterized by circulatory shock
Aldosteronism	Hypersecretion of aldosterone	Often caused by adrenal hyperplasia, this condition is characterized by sodium retention and potassium loss—producing Conn syndrome: severe muscle weakness, hypertension (high blood pressure), kidney dysfunction, cardiac problems
Congenital hypothyroidism (formerly cretinism, a term now deemed inappropriate by healthcare workers)	Hyposecretion of thyroid hormone during early development	Congenital condition characterized by dwarfism, retarded mental development, facial puffiness, dry skin, umbilical hernia, lack of muscle coordination
Cushing disease	Hypersecretion of adrenocorticotropic hormone (ACTH)	Caused by adenoma of the anterior pituitary; increased ACTH causes hypersecretion of adrenal cortical hormones, producing *Cushing syndrome*
Cushing syndrome	Hypersecretion (or injection) of glucocorticoids	Metabolic disorder characterized by fat deposits on upper back, striated pad of fat on chest and abdomen, rounded "moon" face, muscular atrophy, oedema, hypokalaemia (low blood potassium level), possible abnormal skin pigmentation; occurs in Cushing disease
Diabetes insipidus	Hyposecretion of (or insensitivity to) antidiuretic hormone (ADH)	Metabolic disorder characterized by extreme polyuria (excessive urination) and polydipsia (excessive thirst) because of a decrease in the kidney's retention of water
Gestational diabetes mellitus (GDM)	Temporary decrease in blood levels of insulin during pregnancy	Carbohydrate-metabolism disorder occurring in some pregnant women; characterized by polydipsia, polyuria, overeating, weight loss, fatigue, irritability
Gigantism	Hypersecretion of GH before age 25 years	Condition characterized by extreme skeletal size caused by excess protein anabolism during skeletal development
Graves disease	Hypersecretion of thyroid hormone	Inherited, possibly autoimmune disease characterized by hyperthyroidism, exophthalmos (protruding eyes)

(continued)

TABLE 26-7 Examples of Endocrine Conditions—cont'd

CONDITION	MECHANISM	DESCRIPTION
Hashimoto disease	Autoimmune damage to thyroid causing hyposecretion of thyroid hormone	Enlargement of thyroid (goitre) is sometimes accompanied by hypothyroidism, typically occurring between ages 30 and 50 years; 20 times more common in females than males
Hyperparathyroidism	Hypersecretion of parathyroid hormone (PTH)	Condition characterized by increased reabsorption of calcium from bone tissue and kidneys and increased absorption by the gastrointestinal tract; produces hypercalcaemia, resulting in confusion, anorexia, abdominal pain, muscle pain, and fatigue, possibly progressing to circulatory shock, kidney failure, death
Hyperthyroidism (adult)	Hypersecretion of thyroid hormone	Condition characterized by nervousness, tremor, weight loss, excessive hunger, fatigue, heat intolerance, heart arrhythmia, and diarrhoea; caused by a general acceleration of body function
Hypothyroidism (adult)	Hyposecretion of thyroid hormone	Condition characterized by sluggishness, weight gain, skin dryness, constipation, arthritis, and general slowing of body function; may lead to myxoedema, coma, or death if untreated
Insulin shock	Hypersecretion (or overdose injection) of insulin, decreased food intake, excessive exercise	Hypoglycaemic (low blood glucose) shock characterized by nervousness, sweating and chills, irritability, hunger, and pallor—progressing to convulsion, coma, and death if untreated
Myxoedema	Extreme hyposecretion of thyroid hormone during adulthood	Severe form of adult hypothyroidism characterized by oedema of the face and extremities; often progressing to coma and death
Osteoporosis	Hyposecretion of oestrogen in postmenopausal women	Bone disorder characterized by loss of minerals and collagen from bone matrix, producing holes or porosities that weaken the skeleton
Pituitary dwarfism	Hyposecretion of GH before age 25 years	Condition characterized by reduced skeletal size caused by decreased protein anabolism during skeletal development
Simple goitre	Lack of iodine in diet	Enlargement of thyroid tissue results from the inability of the thyroid to make thyroid hormone because of a lack of iodine; a positive feedback situation develops in which low thyroid hormone levels trigger hypersecretion of thyroid-stimulating hormone (TSH) by pituitary—which stimulates thyroid growth
Sterility	Hyposecretion of sex hormones	Loss of reproductive function
Type 1 diabetes mellitus	Hyposecretion of insulin	Inherited condition with sudden childhood onset characterized by polydipsia, polyuria, overeating, weight loss, fatigue, and irritability, resulting from the inability of cells to secure and metabolize carbohydrates
Type 2 diabetes mellitus	Insensitivity of target cells to insulin	Carbohydrate-metabolism disorder with slow adulthood onset thought to be caused by a combination of genetic and environmental factors and characterized by polydipsia, polyuria, overeating, weight loss, fatigue, irritability
Winter (seasonal) depression	Hypersecretion of (or hypersensitivity to) melatonin	Abnormal emotional state characterized by sadness and melancholy resulting from exaggerated melatonin effects; melatonin levels are inhibited by sunlight so they increase when day length decreases during winter

LANGUAGE OF SCIENCE *(continued from p. 579)*

atrial natriuretic hormone (ANH) (AY-tree-al nay-tree-yoo-RET-ik HOR-mohn)
[*atria-* **entrance courtyard (atrium of heart),** *-al* **relating to,** *natri-* **natrium (sodium),** *-uret-* **urination,** *-ic* **relating to,** *hormon-* **excite**]

beta cell (BAY-tah)
[*beta (β)* **second letter of Greek alphabet,** *cell* **storeroom**]

C cell
[*C* **for calcitonin,** *cell* **storeroom**]

calcitonin (CT) (kal-sih-TOH-nin)
[*calci-* **lime (calcium),** *-ton-* **tone,** *-in* **substance**]

cholecystokinin (CCK) (koh-lee-sis-toh-KYE-nin)
[*chole-* **bile,** *-cyst-* **bag,** *-kin-* **movement,** *-in* **substance**]

corticotroph (kohr-tih-koh-TROHF)
[*cortic-* **cortex (bark),** *-troph* **nourish**]

cortisol (KOHR-tih-sol)
[*cortis-* **cortex (bark),** *-ol* **alcohol**]

delta cell
[*delta (δ)* **fourth letter of Greek alphabet,** *cell* **storeroom**]

epinephrine (Epi) (ep-ih-NEF-rin)
[*epi-* **upon,** *-nephr-* **kidney,** *-ine* **substance**]

epsilon cell (EP-sih-lon)
[*epsilon (ϵ)* **fifth letter of Greek alphabet,** *cell* **storeroom**]

follicle (FOL-lih-kul)
[*foll-* **bag,** *-icle* **little**]

follicle-stimulating hormone (FSH) (FOL-lih-kul-STIM-yoo-lay-ting HOR-mohn)
[*foll-* **bag,** *-icle-* **little,** *hormon-* **excite**]

follicular cell (foh-LIK-yoo-lar)
[*foll-* **bag,** *-icul-* **small,** *-ar* **relating to,** *cell* **storeroom**]

gastrin (GAS-trin)
[*gastr-* **stomach,** *-in* **substance**]

ghrelin (GHRL) (GRAY-lin)
[*ghrel-* **grow (also acronym for growth hormone–releasing peptide),** *-in* **substance**]

glucagon (GLOO-kah-gon)
[*gluc-* **glucose,** *-agon* **drive**]

gonad (GO-nad)
[*gon-* **offspring,** *-ad* **relating to**]

gonadotroph (go-NAD-oh-trohf)
[*gon-* **offspring,** *-ad-* **relating to,** *-troph* **nourish**]

gonadotropin (go-nah-doh-TROH-pin)
[*gon-* **offspring,** *-ad-* **relating to,** *-trop-* **turn or change,** *-in* **substance**]

human chorionic gonadotropin (hCG) (koh-ree-ON-ik go-nah-doh-TROH-pin)
[*chorion-* **skin,** *-ic* **relating to,** *gon-* **offspring,** *-ad-* **relating to,** *-trop-* **nourish,** *-in* **substance**]

human placental lactogen (hPL) (plah-SEN-tal lak-TOH-jen)
[*placenta* **flat cake,** *-al* **relating to,** *lacto-* **milk,** *-gen* **produce**]

hypophyseal portal system (hye-poh-FIZ-ee-al POR-tal)
[*hypo-* **under or below,** *-physis-* **growth,** *-al* **relating to,** *portal* **doorway**]

infundibulum (in-fun-DIB-yoo-lum)
[*infundibulum* **funnel**]

inhibin (in-HIB-in)
[*inhib-* **inhibit,** *-in* **substance**]

insulin (IN-suh-lin)
[*insul-* **island,** *-in* **substance**]

lactotroph (lak-toh-TROHF)
[*lacto-* **milk,** *-troph* **nourish**]

lateral lobe (LAT-er-all)
[*later-* **side,** *-al* **relating to**]

leptin (LEP-tin)
[*lept-* **thin,** *-in* **substance**]

lipokine (LIP-oh-kyne)
[*lipo-* **fat,** *-kine* **motion**]

luteinizing hormone (LH) (loo-tee-in-EYE-zing HOR-mohn)
[*lute-* **yellow,** *-in-* **substance,** *-iz-* **to cause,** *hormon-* **excite**]

neurohypophysis (nyoo-roh-hye-POF-ih-sis)
[*neuro-* **nerve,** *-hypo-* **under or below,** *-physis* **growth**] *pl.,* neurohypophyses

norepinephrine (NE or NR) (nor-ep-ih-NEF-rin)
[*nor-* **chemical prefix (unbranched C chain),** *-epi-* **upon,** *-nephr-* **kidney,** *-ine* **substance**]

oxytocin (OT) (ock-see-TOH-sin)
[*oxy-* **sharp (oxygen),** *-toc-* **birth,** *-in* **substance**]

pancreatic islet (pan-kree-AT-ik eye-let)
[*pan-* **all,** *-creat-* **flesh,** *-ic* **relating to,** *isl-* **island,** *-et* **little**]

pancreatic polypeptide cell (pan-kree-AT-ik pol-ee-PEP-tyde)
[*pan-* **all,** *-creat-* **flesh,** *-ic* **relating to,** *poly-* **many,** *-pept-* **to digest,** *-ide* **chemical,** *cell* **storeroom**]

parathyroid gland (pair-ah-THYE-royd)
[*para-* **beside,** *-thyr-* **shield,** *-oid* **like,** *gland* **acorn**]

parathyroid hormone (PTH) (pair-ah-THYE-royd HOR-mohn)
[*para-* **besides,** *-thyr-* **shield,** *-oid* **like,** *hormon-* **excite**]

pineal gland (PIN-ee-al)
[*pine-* **pine,** *-al* **relating to,** *gland* **acorn**]

pituitary gland (pih-TYOO-ih-tair-ee)
[*pituit-* **phlegm,** *-ary* **relating to,** *gland* **acorn**]

placenta (plah-SEN-tah)
[*placenta* **flat cake**] *pl.,* placentae or placentas

progesterone (proh-JES-ter-ohn)
[*pro-* **before,** *-gester-* **bearing (pregnancy),** *-stero-* **solid or steroid derivative,** *-one* **chemical**]

prolactin (PRL) (proh-LAK-tin)
[*pro-* **before,** *-lact-* **milk,** *-in* **substance**]

relaxin (reh-LAK-sin)
[*relax-* **relaxation,** *-in* **substance**]

releasing hormone (ree-LEE-sing HOR-mohn)
[*hormon-* **excite**]

renin (REE-nin)
[*ren-* **kidney,** *-in* **substance**]

renin–angiotensin–aldosterone system (RAAS) (REE-nin-an-jee-oh-TEN-sin-al-DOS-tair-ohn)
[*ren-* **kidney,** *-in* **substance,** *angio-* **vessel,** *-tens-* **pressure or stretch,** *-in* **substance,** *aldo-* **aldehyde,** *-stero-* **solid or steroid derivative,** *-one* **chemical**]

resistin (reh-SIS-tin)
[*resist-* **withstand,** *-in* **substance**]

secretin (seh-KREE-tin)
[*secret-* **separate,** *-in* **substance**]

somatostatin (soh-mah-toh-STAT-in)
[*soma-* **body,** *-stat-* **stand,** *-in* **substance**]

somatotroph (soh-mah-toh-TROHF)
[*soma-* **body,** *-troph* **nourish**]

somatotropin (STH) (soh-mah-toh-TROH-pin)
[*soma-* **body,** *-trop-* **turn or change,** *-in* **substance**]

testosterone (tes-TOS-teh-rohn)
[*testo-* **witness (testis),** *-stero-***solid or steroid derivative,** *-one* **chemical**]

tetraiodothyronine (T4) (tet-rah-eye-oh-doh-THY-roh-neen)
[*tetra-* **four,** *-iodo-* **violet (iodine),** *-thyro-* **shield (thyroid gland),** *-ine* **chemical**]

thymopoietin (thy-moh-POY-eh-tin)
[*thymo-* **thymus gland,** *-poiet-* **make,** *-in* **substance**]

thymosin (THY-moh-sin)
[*thymos-* **thyme flower (thymus gland),** *-in* **substance**]

thymus (THY-mus)
[*thymus* **thyme flower**]

thyroglobulin (thy-roh-GLOB-yoo-lin)
[*thyro-* **shield (thyroid gland),** *-glob-* **ball,** *-ul-* **small,** *-in* **substance**]

thyroid colloid (THY-royd KOL-oyd)
[*thyro-* **shield (thyroid gland),** *-oid* **like,** *coll-* **glue,** *-oid* **like**]

thyroid gland (THY-royd)
[*thyro-* **shield,** *-oid* **like,** *gland* **acorn**]

thyroid-stimulating hormone (TSH) (THY-royd STIM-yoo-lay-ting HOR-mohn)
[*thyro-* **shield,** *-oid* **like,** *hormon-* **excite**]

thyrotroph (thy-roh-TROHF)
[*thyro-* **shield (thyroid gland),** *-troph* **nourish**]

thyroxine (thy-ROK-sin)
[*thyro-* **shield (thyroid gland),** *-ox-* **oxygen,** *-ine* **chemical**]

triiodothyronine (T_3) (try-eye-oh-doh-THY-roh-neen)
[*tri-* **three,** *-iodo-* **violet (iodine),** *-thyro-* **shield (thyroid gland),** *-nine* **chemical**]

tropic hormone (TROH-pik HOR-mohn)
[*trop-* **turn or change,** *-ic* **relating to,** *hormon-* **excite**]

vitamin D (VYE-tah-min D)
[*vit-* **life,** *-amin(e)* **ammonia compound**]

zona fasciculata (ZOH-nah fas-sic-yoo-LAY-tah)
[*zona* **belt,** *fasci-* **bundle,** *-cul-* **little,** *-ata* **characterized by**] *pl.,* zonae fasciculatae

zona glomerulosa (ZOH-nah gloh-mair-yoo-LOH-sah)
[*zona* **belt,** *glomerulosa* **having small balls**] *pl.,* zonae glomerulosae

zona reticularis (ZOH-nah reh-tik-yoo-LAIR-is)
[*zona* **belt,** *reticularis* **having little nets**] *pl.,* zonae reticulares

UNIT 3

LANGUAGE OF MEDICINE

acromegaly (ak-roh-MEG-ah-lee)
[*acro-* **extremities,** *-mega-* **great,** *-aly* **state**]

Addison disease (AD-ih-son)
[*Thomas Addison* **English physician**]

cryopreservation (krye-oh-prez-er-VAY-shun)
[*cryo-* **cold,** *-preserv-* **to keep,** *-tion* **process**]

Cushing syndrome (KOOSH-ing SIN-drohm)
[*Harvey W. Cushing* **American neurosurgeon,** *syn-* **together,** *-drome* **running or (race) course**]

diabetes insipidus (dye-ah-BEE-teez in-SIP-ih-dus)
[*diabetes* **pass-through or siphon,** *insipidus* **without zest**]

diabetes mellitus (dye-ah-BEE-teez mell-EYE-tus)
[*diabetes* **pass-through or siphon,** *mellitus* **honey sweet**]

exophthalmos (ek-soff-THAL-mus)
[*ex-* **outside,** *-oph-* **eye,** *-thalm-* **inner chamber,** *-ic* **relating to**]

gigantism (jye-GAN-tiz-em)
[*gigant-* **great,** *-ism* **condition**]

Graves disease (grayvz)
[*Robert J. Graves* **Irish physician**]

hypersecretion (hy-per-seh-KREE-shun)
[*hyper-* **excessive,** *-secret-* **separate,** *-tion* **process**]

(continued)

hypocalcaemia
(hye-poh-kal-SEE-mee-ah)
[*hypo-* **under or below,** *-calc-* **lime (calcium),** *-aem-* **blood,** *-ia* **condition**]

hyposecretion
(hye-poh-seh-KREE-shun)
[*hypo-* **under or below,** *-secret-* **separate,** *-tion* **process**]

myxoedema (mik-seh-DEE-mah)
[*myx-* **mucus,** *-oedema* **swelling**]

pituitary dwarfism
(pih-TYOO-ih-tair-ee DWARF-iz-em)
[*pituita-* **phlegm,** *dwar-* **tiny,** *-ism* **condition**]

simple goitre (GOY-ter)
[**from** *gutter* **throat**]

case study

"Why are you so grumpy lately?" Sharon was the third person to ask that in the past week. When she stopped to think about it, Cara realized that she had been getting angry over minor issues. "Perhaps I just need more sleep," she thought. But that didn't really make sense, either. She'd been getting about 9 hours of sleep each night, but could barely keep her eyes open during dinner. She made a routine appointment to see her GP the following week.

Cara informed her doctor that she was experiencing severe fatigue, irritability, increased urination and back-ache.

1. Increased urination is a symptom associated with which endocrine disorder?
   a. Diabetes mellitus
   b. Acromegaly
   c. Hyperthyroidism
   d. Hypothyroidism

The practice nurse called Cara in to take her vital signs and weight. Cara was surprised to see that she had gained more than a kilo because her arms felt so thin. Her blood pressure was much higher than usual, too. Cara also told the nurse she was concerned that a cut on her hand wasn't healing after three days, as it should.

2. Changes in the secretion of which hormone could account for Cara's increase in weight (in the trunk area), high BP and slow healing of her wound?
   a. Insulin
   b. Cortisol
   c. Thyroid hormone
   d. Testosterone

3. Which condition would you choose as a diagnosis?
   a. Addison disease
   b. Graves disease
   c. Hashimoto disease
   d. Cushing disease

4. One of the most common causes of Cara's condition is a tumour in the anterior pituitary gland. If this is the case for Cara, what will her blood levels show?
   a. Increased CRH; increased ACTH; increased cortisol
   b. Increased CRH; decreased ACTH; increased cortisol
   c. Decreased CRH; increased ACTH; increased cortisol
   d. Decreased CRH; decreased ACTH; increased cortisol

Hint To solve a case study, you may have to refer to the glossary or index, other chapters in this textbook, ***Connect It!,*** and other resources.

CHAPTER SUMMARY

*To download an MP3 version of the chapter summary for use with your mobile device, access the **Audio Chapter Summaries** online at evolve.elsevier.com.*

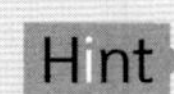

Scan this summary after reading the chapter to help you reinforce the key concepts. Later, use the summary as a quick review before your class or before a test.

Pituitary Gland

A. Structure of the pituitary gland
   1. Formerly known as *hypophysis*
   2. Size: 1.2 to 1.5 cm across; weight: 0.5 gram
   3. Located on the ventral surface of the brain within the skull (**Figure 26-1**)
   4. Infundibulum—stemlike stalk that connects pituitary to the hypothalamus
   5. Made up of two separate glands, the adenohypophysis (anterior pituitary gland) and the neurohypophysis (posterior pituitary gland)

B. Adenohypophysis (anterior lobe of pituitary)
   1. Divided into two parts
      a. Pars anterior—forms the major portion of the adenohypophysis
      b. Pars intermedia
   2. Tissue composed of irregular clumps of secretory cells supported by fine connective tissue fibres and surrounded by a rich vascular network
   3. Three types of cells can be identified according to their affinity for certain stains (**Figure 26-2**)
      a. Chromophobes—do not stain
      b. Acidophils—stain with acid stains
      c. Basophils—stain with basic stains
   4. Five functional types of secretory cells exist
      a. Somatotrophs—secrete GH
      b. Corticotrophs—secrete ACTH
      c. Thyrotrophs—secrete TSH
      d. Lactotrophs—secrete prolactin (PRL)
      e. Gonadotrophs—secrete LH and FSH
   5. Growth hormone (GH) (**Figure 26-3**; **Table 26-2**)
      a. Also known as somatotropin (STH)
      b. Promotes growth of bone, muscle, and other tissues by accelerating amino acid transport into the cells
      c. Stimulates fat metabolism by mobilizing lipids from storage in adipose cells and speeding up catabolism of the lipids after they have entered another cell
      d. GH tends to shift cell chemistry away from glucose catabolism and toward lipid catabolism as an energy source; this leads to increased blood glucose levels
      e. GH functions as an insulin antagonist and is vital to maintaining homeostasis of blood glucose levels
   6. Prolactin (PRL; **Table 26-2**)
      a. Produced by acidophils in the pars anterior
      b. Also known as *lactogenic hormone*
      c. During pregnancy, PRL promotes development of the breasts, anticipating milk secretion; after the baby is born, PRL stimulates the mother's mammary glands to produce milk
   7. Tropic hormones—hormones that have a stimulating effect on other endocrine glands; four principal tropic hormones are produced and secreted by the basophils of the pars anterior (**Table 26-2**)
      a. Thyroid-stimulating hormone (TSH), or thyrotropin—promotes and maintains the growth and development of the thyroid; also causes the thyroid to secrete its hormones
      b. Adrenocorticotropic hormone (ACTH), or adrenocorticotropin—promotes and maintains normal growth and development of the cortex of the adrenal gland; also stimulates the adrenal cortex to secrete some of its hormones
      c. Follicle-stimulating hormone (FSH)—in the female, stimulates primary follicles to grow toward maturity; also stimulates the follicle cells to secrete oestrogens; in the male, FSH stimulates the development of the seminiferous tubules of the testes and maintains spermatogenesis
      d. Luteinizing hormone (LH)—in the female, stimulates the formation and activity of the corpus luteum of the ovary; corpus luteum secretes progesterone and oestrogens when stimulated by LH; LH also supports FSH in stimulating maturation of follicles; in the male, LH stimulates interstitial cells in the testes to develop and secrete testosterone; FSH and LH are called *gonadotropins* because they stimulate the growth and maintenance of the gonads
   8. Control of secretion in the adenohypophysis
      a. Hypothalamus secretes releasing hormones into the blood, which are then carried to the hypophyseal portal system (**Figure 26-5**; **Table 26-1**)
      b. Hypophyseal portal system carries blood from the hypothalamus directly to the adenohypophysis, where the target cells of the releasing hormones are located (**Figure 26-4**)
      c. Releasing hormones influence the secretion of hormones by acidophils and basophils
      d. Through negative feedback, the hypothalamus adjusts the secretions of the adenohypophysis, which then adjusts the secretions of the target glands that in turn adjust the activity of their target tissues (**Figure 26-6**)
      e. Minute-by-minute variations in hormone secretion can exhibit occasional large peaks, caused by pulses in releasing hormone secretion by the hypothalamus (**Figure 26-7**)
      f. In stress, the hypothalamus translates nerve impulses into hormone secretions by endocrine glands, basically creating a mind–body link

C. Neurohypophysis (posterior lobe of pituitary)
   1. Serves as storage and release site for antidiuretic hormone (ADH) and oxytocin (OT), which are synthesized in the hypothalamus (**Figure 26-8**; **Table 26-2**)
   2. Release of ADH and OT into the blood is controlled by nervous stimulation
   3. Antidiuretic hormone (ADH)
      a. Prevents the formation of a large volume of urine, thereby helping the body conserve water

b. Causes a portion of each tubule in the kidney to reabsorb water from the urine it is forming
c. Dehydration triggers the release of ADH
d. Also called arginine vasopressin (AVP) because it stimulates a rise in blood pressure, partly by increasing contraction in small arteries
4. Oxytocin (OT)—has at least two primary actions
a. Causes milk ejection from the lactating breast; regulated by positive feedback mechanism; PRL cooperates with oxytocin
b. Stimulates contraction of uterine muscles that occurs during and after childbirth; regulated by positive feedback mechanism
c. Involved in sexual arousal and social bonding
d. Helps maintain normal skeletal muscle regeneration

Pineal Gland

A. Tiny, pine cone–shaped structure located on the dorsal aspect of the brain's diencephalons
B. Member of the nervous system because it receives visual stimuli and also a member of the endocrine system because it secretes hormones
C. Pineal gland supports the body's biological clock
D. Principal pineal secretion is melatonin (**Table 26-6**)

Thyroid Gland

A. Structure of the thyroid gland
1. Made up of two large lateral lobes and a narrow connecting isthmus (**Figure 26-9**)
2. A thin, wormlike projection of thyroid tissue often extends upward from the isthmus
3. Weight of the thyroid in an adult is approximately 30 grams
4. Located in the neck, on the anterior and lateral surfaces of the trachea, just below the larynx
5. Composed of follicles (**Figure 26-10**)
a. Small, hollow spheres
b. Filled with thyroid colloid that contains thyroglobulins
B. Thyroid hormone (**Figure 26-11**; **Table 26-3**)
1. Actually two different hormones
a. Tetraiodothyronine (T_4), or thyroxine—contains four iodine atoms; approximately 20 times more abundant than T_3; major importance is as a precursor to T_3
b. Triiodothyronine (T_3)—contains three iodine atoms; considered to be the principal thyroid hormone; T_3 binds efficiently to nuclear receptors in target cells
2. Thyroid gland stores considerable amounts of a preliminary form of its hormones *before* secreting them
3. Before being stored in the colloid of follicles, T_3 and T_4 are attached to globulin molecules, forming thyroglobin complexes
4. Before release, T_3 and T_4 detach from globulin and enter the bloodstream
5. Once in the blood, T_3 and T_4 attach to a plasma protein called *thyroid-binding globulins (TBGs)* and travel as a hormone-globulin complex
6. T_3 and, to a lesser extent, T_4 detach from plasma globulin as they near the target cells
7. Thyroid hormone—helps regulate the metabolic rate of all cells and cell growth and tissue differentiation; it is said to have a "general" target
C. Calcitonin (CT) (**Table 26-3**)
1. Produced by thyroid gland in the parafollicular cells
2. In humans, CT may subtly influence the processing of calcium by bone cells by decreasing blood calcium levels and promoting conservation of hard bone matrix
3. Parathyroid hormone acts as antagonist to calcitonin to maintain calcium homeostasis

Parathyroid Glands

A. Structure of the parathyroid glands
1. Four or five parathyroid glands embedded in the posterior surface of the thyroid's lateral lobes (**Figure 26-12**)
2. Tiny, rounded bodies within thyroid tissue formed by compact, irregular rows of cells (**Figure 26-13**)
B. Parathyroid hormone (PTH) (**Table 26-3**)
1. PTH is an antagonist to calcitonin and is the primary hormone to maintain calcium homeostasis (**Figure 26-14**)
2. PTH acts on bone and kidney
a. Causes more bone to be dissolved, yielding calcium and phosphate, which enters the bloodstream
b. Causes phosphate to be secreted by the kidney cells into the urine to be excreted
c. Causes increased intestinal absorption of calcium by stimulating the kidney to produce active vitamin D (the hormone calcitriol), which increases calcium absorption in gut

Adrenal Glands

A. Structure of the adrenal glands
1. Located on top of the kidneys, fitting like caps (**Figure 26-15**)
2. Made up of two portions (**Figure 26-16**; **Table 26-4**)
a. Adrenal cortex—composed of endocrine tissue (**Figure 26-17**)
b. Adrenal medulla—composed of neurosecretory tissue
B. Adrenal cortex—all cortical hormones are steroids and known as *corticosteroids* (**Figure 26-18**)
1. Composed of three distinct layers of secreting cells
a. Zona glomerulosa—outermost layer, directly under the outer connective tissue capsule of the adrenal gland; secretes mineralocorticoids
b. Zona fasciculata—middle layer; secretes glucocorticoids
c. Zona reticularis—inner layer; secretes small amounts of glucocorticoids and gonadocorticoids
2. Mineralocorticoids
a. Have an important role in the regulatory process of sodium in the body
b. Aldosterone
(1) Only physiologically important mineralocorticoid in the human; primary function is maintenance of sodium homeostasis in the blood by increasing sodium reabsorption in the kidneys
(2) Aldosterone also increases water retention and promotes the loss of potassium and hydrogen ions
(3) Aldosterone secretion is controlled by the renin–angiotensin–aldosterone system (RAAS) and by blood potassium concentration (**Figure 26-19**)

3. Glucocorticoids
   a. Main glucocorticoids secreted by the zona fasciculata are cortisol, cortisone, and corticosterone, with cortisol the only one secreted in significant quantities
   b. Affect every cell in the body
   c. Are protein mobilizing, gluconeogenic, and hyperglycaemic
   d. Tend to cause a shift from carbohydrate catabolism to lipid catabolism as an energy source
   e. Essential for maintaining normal blood pressure by aiding norepinephrine and epinephrine to have their full effect, causing vasoconstriction
   f. High blood concentration causes eosinopenia and marked atrophy of lymphatic tissues
   g. Act with epinephrine to bring about normal recovery from injury produced by inflammatory agents
   h. Secretion increases in response to stress
   i. Except during stress response, secretion is mainly controlled by a negative feedback mechanism involving ACTH from the adenohypophysis
   j. Secretion is characterized by several large pulses of increased hormone levels throughout the day—the largest occurring just before waking (**Figure 26-20**)
4. Gonadocorticoids—sex hormones (androgens) that are released from the adrenal cortex

C. Adrenal medulla
1. Neurosecretory tissue—tissue composed of neurons that secrete their products into the blood
2. Adrenal medulla secretes two important hormones—epinephrine and norepinephrine; they are part of the class of nonsteroid hormones called *catecholamines*
3. Both hormones bind to the receptors of sympathetic effectors to prolong and enhance the effects of sympathetic stimulation by the ANS (**Figure 26-21**)

Pancreatic Islets

A. Structure of the pancreatic islets (**Figure 26-22**)
1. Elongated gland, weighing approximately 100 grams; its head lies in the duodenum, extends horizontally behind the stomach and, then, touches the spleen
2. Composed of endocrine and exocrine tissues
   a. Pancreatic islets (islets of Langerhans)—endocrine portion
   b. Acini—exocrine portion—secretes a serous fluid containing digestive enzymes into ducts draining into the small intestine
3. Pancreatic islets—each islet contains five primary types of endocrine cells joined by gap junctions
   a. Alpha cells (A cells)—secrete glucagon
   b. Beta cells (B cells)—secrete insulin; account for up to 75% of all pancreatic islet cells
   c. Delta cells (D cells)—secrete somatostatin
   d. Pancreatic polypeptide cells (F cells, or PP cells)—secrete pancreatic polypeptide
   e. Epsilon cells (ϵ cells)—secrete ghrelin

B. Pancreatic hormones (**Table 26-5**)—work as a team to maintain homeostasis of food molecules (**Figure 26-23**)
1. Glucagon—produced by alpha cells; tends to increase blood glucose levels; stimulates gluconeogenesis in liver cells
2. Insulin—produced by beta cells; lowers blood concentration of glucose, amino acids, and fatty acids and promotes their metabolism by tissue cells
3. Somatostatin—produced by delta cells; primary role is regulating the other endocrine cells of the pancreatic islets
4. Pancreatic polypeptide—produced by F (or PP) cells; functions uncertain but probably influences GI motility, secretion by exocrine pancreas and satiety
5. Ghrelin (GHRL)—hormone secreted by epsilon cells at periphery of pancreatic islets; stimulates hypothalamus to boost appetite; slows metabolism and fat burning; may contribute to obesity

Gonads

A. Testes (**Figure 25-2**; **Table 26-6**)
1. Paired organs within the scrotum in the male
2. Composed of seminiferous tubules and a scattering of interstitial cells
3. Testosterone is produced by the interstitial cells and is responsible for the growth and maintenance of male sexual characteristics
4. Testosterone secretion is mainly regulated by gonadotropin levels in the blood

B. Ovaries (**Figure 25-2**; **Table 26-6**)
1. Primary sex organs in the female
2. Set of paired glands in the pelvis that produce several types of sex hormones
   a. Oestrogens—steroid hormones secreted by ovarian follicles; promote development and maintenance of female sexual characteristics
   b. Progesterone—secreted by corpus luteum; maintains the lining of the uterus necessary for successful pregnancy
   c. Ovarian hormone secretion depends on the changing levels of FSH and LH from the adenohypophysis

Placenta

A. Tissues that form on the lining of the uterus as a connection between the circulatory systems of the mother and developing fetus

B. Serves as a temporary endocrine gland that produces human chorionic gonadotropin, oestrogens, and progesterone (**Table 26-6**)

Thymus

A. Gland located in the mediastinum just beneath the sternum (**Figure 25-2**)

B. Thymus is large in children, begins to atrophy at puberty, and, by old age, is a vestige of fat and fibrous tissue

C. Considered to be primarily a lymphatic organ, but the hormone thymosin has been isolated from thymus tissue (**Table 26-6**)

D. Thymosin—stimulates development of T cells

Gastric and Intestinal Mucosa

A. The mucous lining of the GI tract contains cells that produce both endocrine and exocrine secretions (**Table 26-6**)

B. GI hormones, such as gastrin, secretin, and cholecystokinin (CCK), play regulatory roles in coordinating the secretory and motor activities involved in the digestive process
C. Ghrelin (GHRL)—appetite-boosting hormone secreted by endocrine cells in gastric mucosa as well as in pancreatic islets

Heart

A. The heart has a secondary endocrine role
B. Hormone-producing cells produce several atrial natriuretic peptides (ANPs), including atrial natriuretic hormone (ANH) (**Table 26-6**)
C. ANH's primary effect is to oppose increases in blood volume or blood pressure; also an antagonist to ADH and aldosterone

Adipose Tissue

A. Leptin plays a role in energy balance, immunity, neuroendocrine, reproductive functions
B. Resistin reduces insulin sensitivity
C. Lipokines (palmiteolate) increase insulin sensitivity

Other Endocrine Glands and Organs

A. Major endocrine glands produce more hormones than are outlined in this book (e.g., inhibin secreted by the ovaries, irisin and interleukin-6 (IL-6) secreted by muscle, erythropoietin secreted by kidneys) (**Table 26-6**)
B. Many tissues (perhaps all tissues) produce hormones

Cycle of Life: Endocrine System

A. Endocrine regulation begins in the womb
B. Many active hormones are active from birth—evidence that a hormonal signal from fetus to mother signals the onset of labour
C. Hormones related to reproduction begin at puberty
D. Secretion of male reproductive hormones—continuous production from puberty, slight decline in late adulthood
E. Secretion of female reproductive hormones declines suddenly and completely in middle adulthood

The Big Picture: The Endocrine System and the Whole Body

A. The endocrine system operates with the nervous system to finely adjust the many processes they regulate
B. Neuroendocrine system adjusts nutrient supply
C. Calcitonin, parathyroid hormone, and vitamin D balance calcium ion use
D. The nervous system and hormones regulate reproduction

REVIEW QUESTIONS

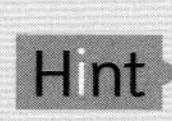

Write out the answers to these questions after reading the chapter and reviewing the Chapter Summary. Note—writing out your answers will consolidate learning and provide a valuable resource of information.

1. Name the two subdivisions of the adenohypophysis.
2. Discuss and identify, by staining tendency and relative percentages, the cell types present in the anterior pituitary gland.
3. Discuss the functions of growth hormone.
4. How does growth hormone affect metabolism?
5. List the four tropic hormones secreted by the basophils of the anterior pituitary gland. Which of the tropic hormones are also called *gonadotropins*?
6. How does antidiuretic hormone act to alter urine volume?
7. Describe the feedback associated with oxytocin. Identify the mechanism as positive or negative.
8. Discuss the synthesis and storage of thyroxine and triiodothyronine. How are they transported in the blood?
9. Describe the functions of parathyroid hormone.
10. List the hormones produced by each "zone" of the adrenal cortex, and describe the actions of these hormones.
11. Discuss the normal function of hormones produced by the adrenal medulla.
12. Identify the hormones produced by each of the cell types in the pancreatic islets.
13. Identify the "pregnancy-promoting" hormone.
14. Where is human chorionic gonadotropin produced? What is its function?
15. Describe the role of atrial natriuretic hormone.
16. Identify the conditions resulting from both hypersecretion and hyposecretion of growth hormone during growth years.
17. Describe the face of a patient with Cushing syndrome.
18. How does exercise affect diabetes mellitus?

CRITICAL THINKING QUESTIONS

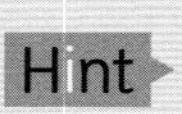

After finishing the Review Questions, write out the answers to these more in-depth questions to help you apply your new knowledge. Go back to sections of the chapter that relate to concepts that you find difficult.

1. What examples can you find that apply the concept of a negative feedback loop to the regulation of hormone secretion?
2. A hyposecretion of which hormone would make it difficult for a mother to nurse her child? How would you summarize the effects of this hormone?
3. Why can the hypothalamus be called the "mind–body link"?
4. Explain the hormonal interaction that helps maintain the setpoint value for the glucose in the blood.
5. Explain how the cell is able to become more or less sensitive to a specific hormone.
6. What is the relationship between increased blood level concentrations of FSH and menopause?
7. A lack of iodine in the diet will cause a simple goitre. Describe the feedback loop that will cause its formation.
8. A friend of yours is considering the use of anabolic steroids. Based on what you know of their effects, how would you explain why using these steroids could be harmful?
9. Describe the role of a tropic hormone. Explain why the pituitary gland was originally referred to as a "master gland".
10. If you were to eat a large slice of cake and drink a glass of sugary fruit juice, which pancreatic hormone would be released at a higher level, insulin or glucagon? Outline the response of these hormones to the intake of cake and juice.

UNIT 4

Transportation and Defence

The chapters in Unit 4 are concerned with transportation, how the body defends itself, and stress. Blood (Chapter 27), a complex fluid tissue, is discussed, and the text explains how blood serves to transport respiratory gases and key nutrients to cells and carry away wastes. The body's blood is pumped by the heart (Chapter 28) through the blood vessels (Chapter 29) by way of a complex set of circulatory mechanisms (Chapter 30).

The elements of the lymphatic system (Chapter 31) provide an open pathway for return of fluid and proteins from the interstitial spaces and for fats, which are absorbed from the intestine into the general circulation. The lymphatic system is also involved in immunity, or resistance to disease, and in the removal and destruction of old red blood cells. The immune system is more fully discussed in Chapters 32 and 33. Elements of the immune system provide a multilayered defence mechanism involving both phagocytic cells and defensive proteins called *antibodies*. Stress—and the body's often maladaptive response to it—is discussed in Chapter 34. •

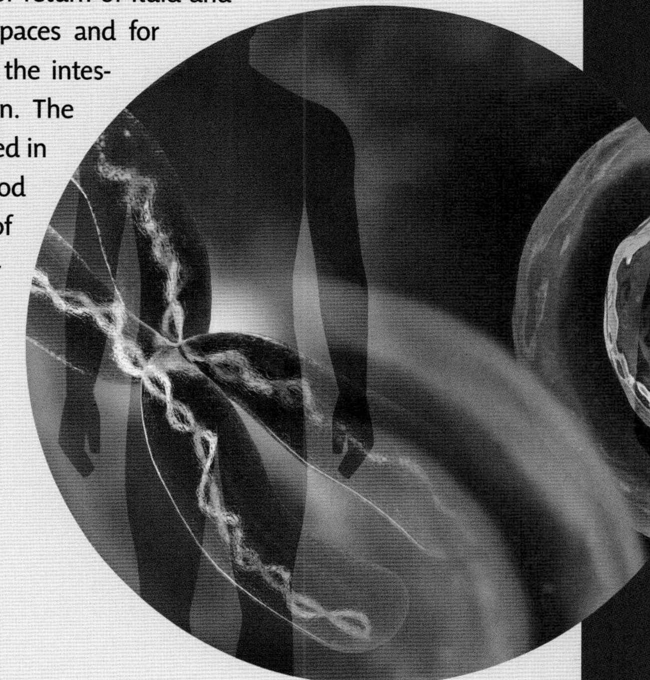

27 Blood

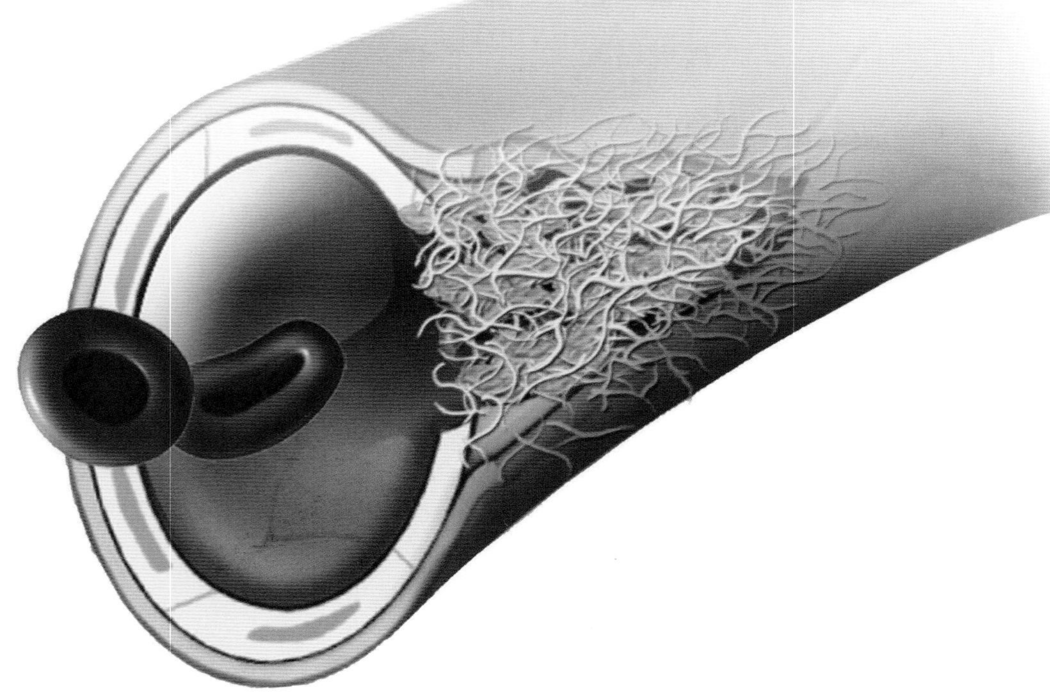

CHAPTER OUTLINE

Hint Scan this outline before you begin to read the chapter, as a preview of how the concepts are organized.

LANGUAGE OF SCIENCE

Hint *Use this list to aid your pronunciation of unfamiliar words.*

agranulocyte (ah-GRAN-yoo-loh-syte)
[*a-* **without,** *-gran-* **grain,** *-ul-* **little**]

antibody (AN-tih-bod-ee)
[*anti-* **against**]

antigen (AN-tih-jen)
[*anti-* **against,** *-gen* **produce**]

basophil (BAY-so-fil)
[*bas-* **foundation,** *-phil* **love**]

basophilic erythroblast (BAY-so-fil-ik eh-RITH-roh-blast)
[*bas-* **foundation,** *-phil-* **love,** *-ic* **relating to,** *erythro-* **red,** *-blast* **bud**]

bicarbonate ion (bye-KAR-boh-nayte EYE-on)
[*bi-* **twice,** *-carbo-* **coal,** *-ate* **oxygen**]

blood serum (SEER-um)
[*serum* **watery fluid**] *pl.,* sera

buffy coat (BUHF-ee koht)

carbonic anhydrase (CA) (kar-BON-ik an-HYE-drays)
[*carbo-* **coal,** *-ic* **relating to,** *a-* **without,** *-hydr-* **water,** *-ase* **enzyme**]

chemotaxis (kee-moh-TAK-sis)
[*chemo-* **chemical,** *-taxis* **movement or reaction**]

diapedesis (dye-ah-peh-DEE-sis)
[*dia-* **apart or through,** *-pedesis* **oozing**]

electrolyte (eh-LEK-troh-lyte)
[*electro-* **electricity,** *-lyt-* **loosening**]

embryonic stem cell (em-bree-ON-ik)
[*em-* **in,** *-bryo-* **fill to bursting,** *-ic* **relating to**]

eosinophil (ee-oh-SIN-oh-fil)
[*eosin-* **reddish colour,** *-phil* **love**]

erythrocyte (eh-RITH-roh-syte)
[*erythro-* **red,** *-cyte* **cell**]

erythropoiesis (eh-rith-roh-poy-EE-sis)
[*erythro-* **red,** *-poiesis* **making**]

erythropoietin (EPO) (eh-RITH-roh-POY-eh-tin)
[*erythro-* **red,** *-poiet-* **make,** *-in* **substance**]

extrinsic clotting pathway (eks-TRIN-sik)
[*extr-* **outside,** *-sic* **beside**]

extrinsic factor (eks-TRIN-sik)
[*extr-* **outside,** *-sic* **beside**]

fibrinolysis (fye-brin-OL-ih-sis)
[*fibr-* **thread or fibre,** *-lysis* **loosening**]

continued on p. 632

Five chapters in this unit deal with transportation, one of the body's vital functions. Homeostasis of the internal environment—and therefore survival itself—depends on continual transportation to and from body cells. This chapter discusses the major transportation fluid, blood. Chapters 28 through 30 consider the major transportation system, the cardiovascular system, and Chapter 31 explains a supplementary drainage system, the lymphatic system. •

COMPOSITION OF BLOOD

STRUCTURE AND FUNCTION OF BLOOD

Blood is much more than the simple liquid it seems to be. It consists of not only a fluid but also cells and cell fragments.

The watery fluid portion of blood is the extracellular matrix of blood tissue, a type of connective tissue. Usually called **plasma,** it is one of the three major body fluids (interstitial and intracellular fluids are the other two). Plasma, when separated from "whole blood", is a clear straw-coloured fluid that consists of about 90% water and 10% solutes.

The term **formed elements** is used to designate the various kinds of blood cells and cell fragments (*platelets*) that are normally present in blood (**Table 27-1**). The formed elements of blood are as follows:

- Red blood cells (RBCs) or erythrocytes
- White blood cells (WBCs) or leucocytes
- Platelets or thrombocytes

TABLE 27-1 Classes of Blood Cells

CELL TYPE	DESCRIPTION	FUNCTION	LIFE SPAN
Erythrocyte	7 μm in diameter; concave disc shape; entire cell stains pale pink; no nucleus	Transportation of respiratory gases (O_2 and CO_2)	105–120 days
Neutrophil	12–15 μm in diameter; spherical shape; multilobed nucleus; small, pink-purple–staining cytoplasmic granules	Cellular defence—phagocytosis of small pathogenic microorganisms	Hours to 3 days
Basophil	11–14 μm in diameter; spherical shape; generally two-lobed nucleus; large purple-staining cytoplasmic granules	Secretes heparin (anticoagulant) and histamine (important in inflammatory response)	Hours to 3 days
Eosinophil	10–12 μm in diameter; spherical shape; generally two-lobed nucleus; large, orange-red–staining cytoplasmic granule	Cellular defence—some phagocytosis; chemical attack of large pathogenic microorganisms (such as protozoa) and parasitic worms; helps regulate allergic reactions and other inflammatory responses	10–12 days
Lymphocyte	6–9 μm in diameter; spherical shape; round (single-lobed) nucleus; small lymphocytes have scant cytoplasm	Humoral defence—secretes antibodies; involved in immune system response and regulation	Days to years
Monocyte	12–17 μm in diameter; spherical shape; nucleus generally kidney-bean or horseshoe shaped with convoluted surface; ample cytoplasm often "steel blue" in colour	Capable of migrating out of the blood to enter tissue spaces as a macrophage—an aggressive phagocytic cell capable of ingesting bacteria, cellular debris, and cancerous cells	Months
Platelet	2–5 μm in diameter; irregularly shaped fragments; cytoplasm contains very small, pink-staining granules	Releases clot-activating substances and helps in formation of actual blood clot by forming platelet "plugs"	7–10 days

Blood transfusions most often involve all major blood components—plasma, platelets, and red blood cells. In the UK, approximately 1.7 million red blood cell transfusion units are used each year. In addition, 250,000 units of platelets, 215,000 units of fresh frozen plasma and 165,000 units of cryoprecipitate are distributed by the blood transfusion service. (Cryoprecipitate contains frozen blood clotting factors and fibrinogen.)

CONNECT IT! 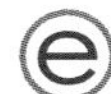

Blood transfusions are an important therapeutic tool. Learn more about blood transfusions, blood banking, and even artificial blood in ***Blood Transfusions*** online at ***Connect It!***

As explained later, the quantity of whole blood found in the body (blood volume) is often expressed as a percent of total body weight. However, the measurement of the plasma and formed elements is generally expressed as a percent of the *whole blood volume.* Using these measurement criteria, whole blood constitutes about 8% of total body weight, plasma accounts for 55%, and the formed elements account for about 45% of the total blood volume (**Figure 27-1**).

Blood is a complex transport medium that performs vital pickup and delivery services for the body. It picks up food and oxygen from the digestive and respiratory systems and delivers them to cells while also picking up wastes from cells for delivery to excretory organs. Blood also transports hormones, enzymes, buffers, and various other biochemical substances that serve important functions.

Blood serves another critical function. It is the keystone of the body's heat-regulating mechanism. Certain physical properties of blood make it especially effective in this role. Its high specific heat and conductivity enable this unique fluid to absorb large quantities of heat without an appreciable increase in its own temperature and to transfer this absorbed heat from the core of the body to its surface, where the heat can be more readily dissipated (see **Figure 10-15**, p. 193).

Blood Volume

How much blood does the body contain? The answer is about 8% of total body weight in average-sized adults. In a healthy young female, that amounts to about 4 to 5 litres and in a male about 5 to 6 litres. In addition to gender differences, blood volume varies with age, body composition, and method of measurement. A *unit* of blood is 0.45 of a litre that is collected from a blood donor for transfusion purposes. It constitutes about 10% of total blood volume in many adults.

Blood volume can be determined using direct methods or indirect methods of measurement. *Direct* measurement of total blood volume can be accomplished only by complete removal of all blood from an experimental animal. In humans, *indirect* methods of measurement that employ "tagging" of red blood cells or plasma components with radioisotopes are used. The principle is simply to introduce a known amount of radioisotope into the circulation, allow the material to be distributed uniformly throughout the blood, and then analyze its concentration in a representative blood sample. Having an accurate measurement is important in replacing blood lost because of haemorrhage or in treating other serious conditions such as shock.

One of the chief variables influencing normal blood volume is the amount of body fat. Blood volume per kilogram of body weight varies inversely with the amount of excess body fat. This means that the less fat there is in your body, the more blood you have per kilogram of your body weight. Because females normally have a higher

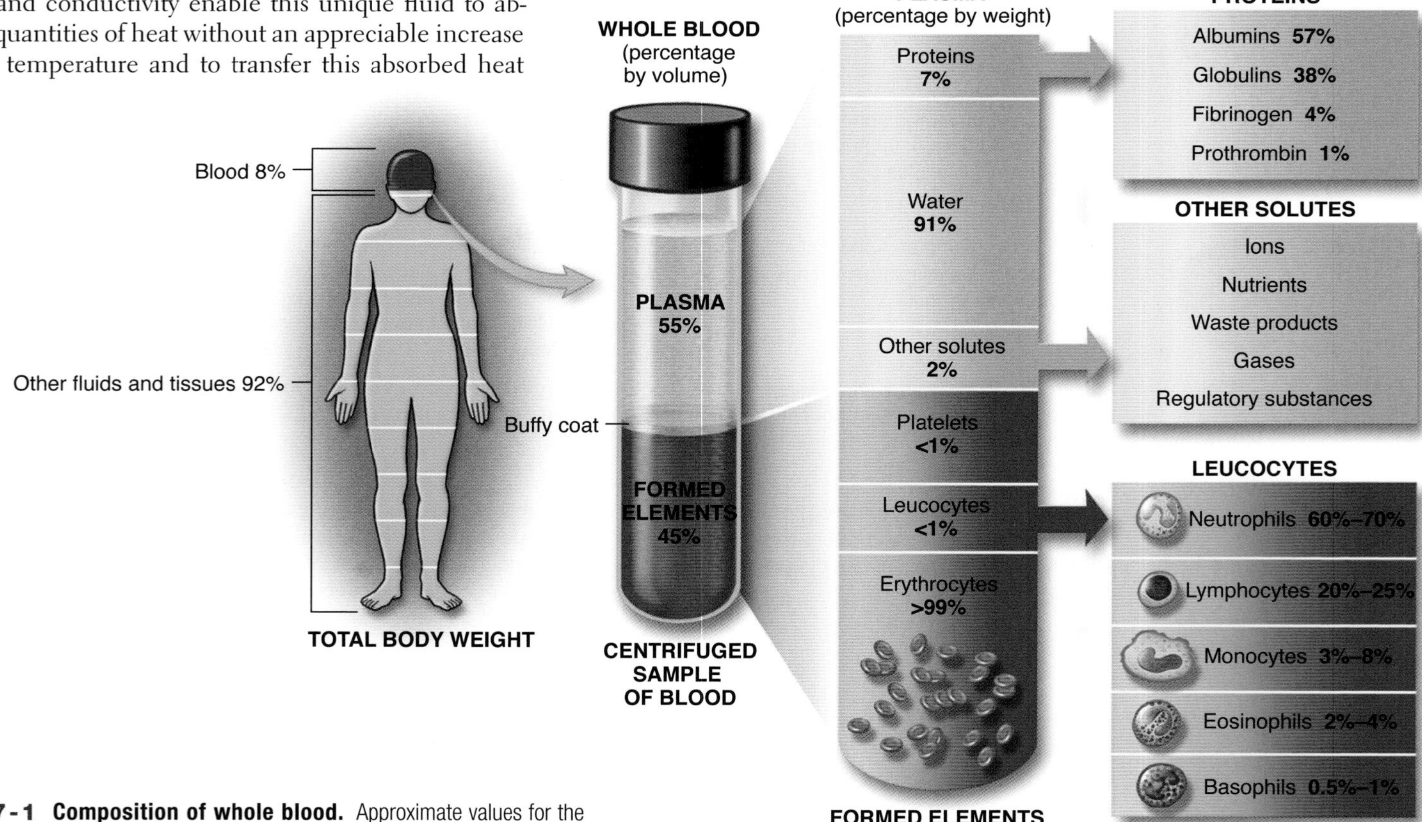

FIGURE 27-1 Composition of whole blood. Approximate values for the components of blood in a normal adult.

percent of body fat than males, they have less blood per kilogram of body weight and therefore a lower blood volume.

HAEMATOCRIT

If a tube of whole blood—that is, plasma and formed elements—is allowed to stand or is spun in a centrifuge, separation will occur. The term **haematocrit (Hct)** or **packed cell volume (PCV)** is used to describe the volume percent of red blood cells (RBCs) in whole blood.

In **Figure 27-2**, *A*, a sample of normal whole blood has been separated by spinning in a centrifuge so that the formed elements are forced to the bottom. The percentage of plasma is about 55% of the total sample, whereas the packed cell volume, or haematocrit, is 45%. An Hct of 45% means that in every 100 mL of whole blood there are 45 mL of RBCs and 55 mL of fluid plasma.

Normally the average Hct for a man is about 45% (40% to 54%, normal range) and for a woman about 42% (38% to 47%, normal range). Conditions that result in decreased RBC numbers (**Figure 27-2**, *B*) are called **anaemias** and are characterized by a reduced Hct value. Healthy individuals who live and work in high altitudes often have elevated RBC numbers and haematocrit values (**Figure 27-2**, *C*). The condition is called **physiological polycythaemia** (from word parts meaning "condition of many blood cells").

Changes in plasma volume can also affect the Hct value. In dehydration, the Hct may be high because the plasma volume is low, not because there are more red blood cells.

White blood cells (WBCs), or leucocytes, and platelets make up less than 1% of blood volume. Note in **Figure 27-2** that a thin white layer of leucocytes and platelets, called the **buffy coat,** is present at the interface between the packed red cells and plasma.

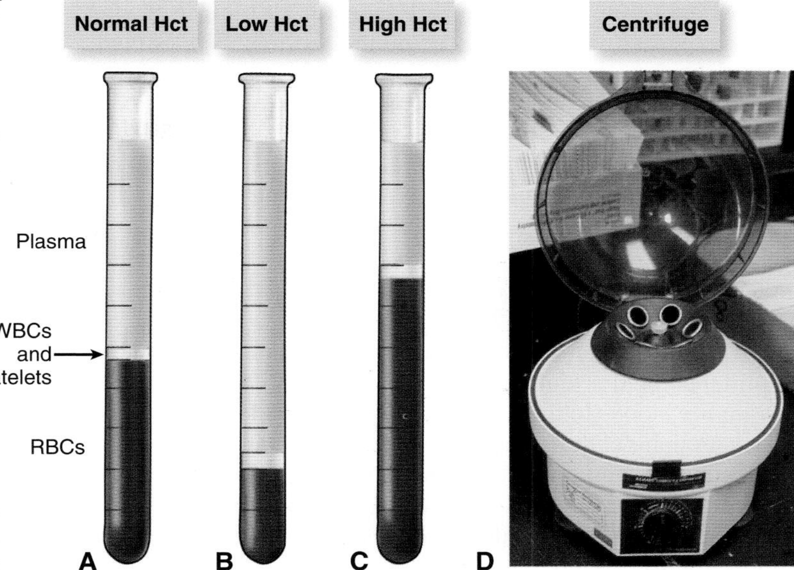

FIGURE 27-2 Haematocrit (Hct) test. Note the buffy coat located between the packed RBCs and the plasma. **A,** Normal blood with the typical percent of RBCs. **B,** Anaemia (a low percent of RBCs). **C,** Polycythaemia (a high percent of RBCs). **D,** Centrifuge that spins tubes of blood, causing RBCs to become densely packed into the bottom of the tubes.

CONNECT IT!

Another commonly done clinical blood test that involves separating RBCs from plasma is called the **erythrocyte sedimentation rate,** or **ESR.** To learn more about this procedure, check out the illustrated article ***Erythrocyte Sedimentation Rate*** online at ***Connect It!***

Quick CHECK

1. Name the fluid portion of whole blood.
2. What constitutes the formed elements of blood?
3. What factors influence blood volume?
4. Identify the component percentages of the normal haematocrit.

BLOOD PLASMA

Plasma is the liquid part of blood—whole blood minus formed elements (**Figure 27-3**). In the laboratory, whole blood that has not clotted is centrifuged to form plasma. This consists of a rapid whirling process that hurls the blood cells to the bottom of the centrifuge tube. A clear, straw-coloured fluid—blood plasma—lies above the cells.

Plasma consists of 90% water and 10% solutes. By far the largest quantity of these solutes is proteins; normally, they constitute about 6% to 8% of the plasma. Proteins such as factor VIII regulate blood clotting; and others such as gamma globulins, which are important in treating weakened immune systems, and albumin, a blood volume expander, are common transfusion products. Other solutes present in much smaller amounts in plasma are nutrient substances (principally glucose, amino acids, and lipids), compounds formed by metabolism (e.g., urea, uric acid, creatinine, and lactate), respiratory gases (oxygen and carbon dioxide), and regulatory substances (hormones, enzymes, and certain other substances).

Some solutes present in blood plasma are true solutes, or crystalloids. Others are colloids. *Crystalloids* are solute particles less than 1 nm in diameter (e.g., ions, glucose, and other small molecules).

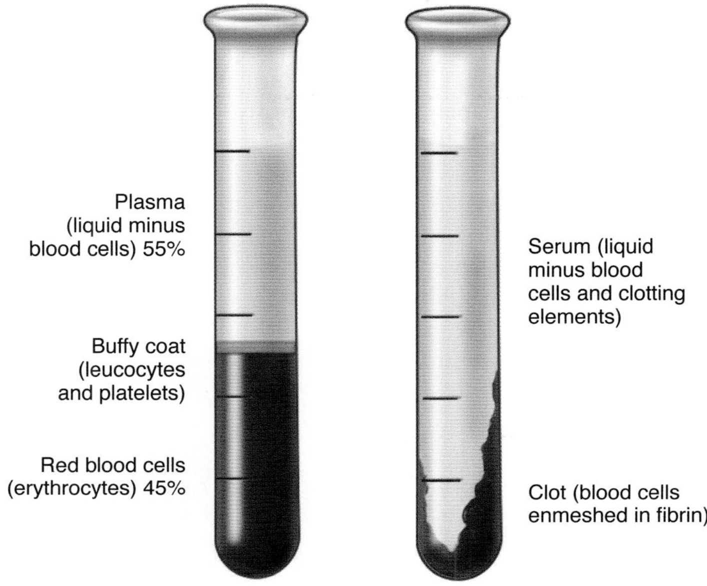

FIGURE 27-3 Difference between blood plasma and blood serum. Plasma is whole blood minus cells. Serum is whole blood minus the clotting elements. Plasma is prepared by centrifuging anticoagulated blood. Serum is prepared by allowing blood to clot.

Colloids are solute particles from 1 to about 100 nm in diameter (e.g., proteins of all types). Blood solutes also may be classified as **electrolytes** (molecules that ionize in solution) or **nonelectrolytes**—for example, proteins and inorganic salts are electrolytes; glucose and lipids are nonelectrolytes.

The proteins in blood plasma consist of three main kinds of compounds: *albumins*, *globulins*, and clotting proteins, principally *fibrinogen*. Measuring the amounts of these compounds reveals that 100 mL of plasma contains a total of approximately 6 to 8 grams of protein. Albumins constitute about 55% of this total, globulins about 38%, and fibrinogen about 7%.

Plasma proteins are crucially important substances. Fibrinogen, for instance, and a clotting protein named prothrombin have key roles in the blood-clotting mechanism. Globulins function as essential components of the immunity mechanism. Many modified globulins, called gamma globulins, serve important roles as circulating antibodies (see also immunoglobulins, Chapter 33). All plasma proteins contribute to the maintenance of normal blood viscosity, blood osmotic pressure, and blood volume. Therefore plasma proteins have an essential part in maintaining normal circulation.

Synthesis of plasma proteins occurs in liver cells. They form all kinds of plasma proteins, except some of the gamma globulin antibodies synthesized by plasma cells. Plasma cells are a type of lymphocyte (WBC). Cancer of plasma cells, called *multiple myeloma*, causes production of an abnormal myeloma antibody—a gamma globulin—that results in numerous and very serious disease symptoms (see Mechanisms of Disease, p. 629).

The pale yellowish liquid left after a clot forms is **blood serum.** How do you think serum differs from plasma? To check your answers, see **Figure 27-3**.

RED BLOOD CELLS

STRUCTURE OF RED BLOOD CELLS

A normal, mature RBC has no nucleus and is only about 7.5 μm in diameter. More than 1300 of them could be placed side by side in a 1 cm space. Before the cell reaches maturity and enters the bloodstream from the bone marrow, the nucleus is extruded. As you can see in **Figure 27-4**, normal, mature RBCs are shaped like tiny biconcave discs.

The mature **erythrocyte** is also unique in that it does not contain ribosomes, mitochondria, and other organelles typical of most body cells. Instead, the primary component of each RBC is the red protein pigment, **haemoglobin (Hb).** It accounts for more than one third of the cell volume and is critically important to its primary function.

The depression on each flat surface of the cell results in a thin centre and thicker edges. This unique shape of the RBC gives it a large surface area relative to its volume compared with a sphere. A flattened shape also permits interior haemoglobin to be close to the plasma membrane where gas exchange occurs. Perhaps most importantly, the biconcave disc shape of RBCs reduces cell spinning and thus minimizes turbulence as blood flows through large vessels. The disc shape of erythrocytes can passively change as they forcibly pass through blood capillaries that often are smaller than the typical 7.5 μm diameter of an erythrocyte.

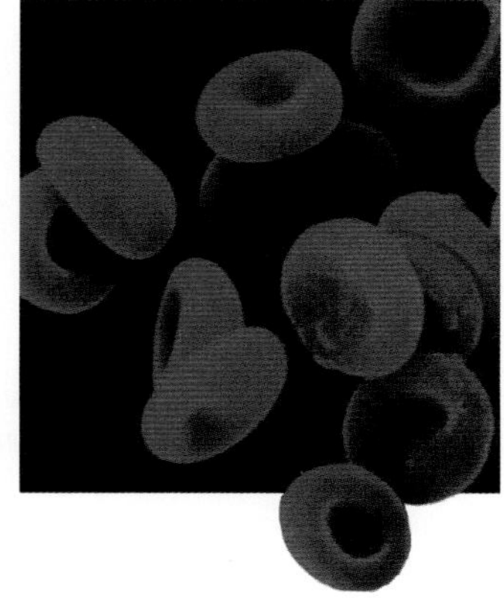

FIGURE 27-4 Erythrocytes. Colour-enhanced scanning electron micrograph shows normal erythrocytes.

The flexibility of RBC shape is possible because of the presence of stretchable fibres composed of a unique protein called *spectrin*. These fibres, which are part of the cytoskeleton, adhere to the inside of the erythrocyte plasma membrane. It is the presence of flexible spectrin fibres that permits the plasma membrane surrounding the RBC to accommodate change from a more typical biconcave shape to a smaller cup-shaped cell size and then back to its normal size and appearance when deforming pressures are no longer being applied to the surface of the plasma membrane.

This ability to change shape is necessary for the survival of RBCs, which are under almost constant mechanical shearing and bursting strains as they pass through the capillary system. In addition, the degree of cell deformity that is possible influences the speed of blood flow in the microcirculation.

RBCs are the most numerous of the formed elements in the blood. In men, RBC counts average about 5,500,000 per cubic millimeter (mm^3) of blood (5.5×10^{12}/L); in women, 4,800,000/mm^3 (4.8×10^{12}/L). Gender differences in RBC numbers may be influenced by the stimulating effect of the male sex hormone testosterone on RBC production. RBC numbers in females are normally lower than those in males.

CONNECT IT! 

To explore the normal values for a variety of blood constituents, including RBC values, scan the list in ***Clinical and Laboratory Values*** online at ***Connect It!***

FUNCTION OF RED BLOOD CELLS

RBCs play a critical role in the transport of oxygen and carbon dioxide in the body. Chapter 37 includes a detailed discussion of how oxygen is transported from air in the lungs to the body cells and how carbon dioxide moves from body cells to the lungs for removal. Both of these functions depend on haemoglobin.

In addition to haemoglobin, the presence of an enzyme, **carbonic anhydrase (CA)**, in RBCs catalyzes a reaction that joins carbon dioxide and water to form carbonic acid. Dissociation of the acid then generates **bicarbonate ions** (HCO_3^-) and hydrogen ions (H^+), which diffuse out of the RBCs. Because carbon dioxide (CO_2) is chemically incorporated into the newly formed bicarbonate ions, it can be transported in this new form in the blood plasma until it is excreted from the body. Bicarbonate ions also have an important role in maintaining normal blood pH levels (see Chapter 44).

Considered together, the total surface area of all the RBCs in an adult is enormous. It provides an area larger than a football field for the exchange of respiratory gases between haemoglobin found in circulating erythrocytes and interstitial fluid that bathes the body cells. This is an excellent example of the relationship between form and function.

UNIT 4

HAEMOGLOBIN

Packed within each RBC are an estimated 200 to 300 million molecules of haemoglobin, which make up about 95% of the dry weight of each cell. Each haemoglobin molecule is composed of four protein chains. Each chain, called a **globin,** is bound to a red pigment, identified in **Figure 27-5**, as a **haem** group. Each haem group contains one iron atom. Therefore one haemoglobin molecule contains four iron atoms. This structural fact enables one haemoglobin molecule to unite with four oxygen molecules to form *oxyhaemoglobin* (a reversible reaction). Haemoglobin can also combine with carbon dioxide to form *carbaminohaemoglobin* (also reversible). But in this reaction the structure of the globin part of the haemoglobin molecule, rather than its haem part, makes the combining possible.

CONNECT IT! 

Learn more about oxygen saturation of haemoglobin (%SO_2) in ***Measuring Oxygen Saturation*** online at ***Connect It!***

A man's blood usually contains more haemoglobin than a woman's. In most normal men, 100 mL of blood contains 14 to 16 grams of haemoglobin. The normal haemoglobin content of a woman's blood is a little less—specifically, in the range of 12 to 14 grams/100 mL. Recall that testosterone in the male tends to stimulate erythrocyte production and cause an increase in RBC numbers. Increased levels of haemoglobin in males are directly related to increased erythrocyte numbers.

An adult who has a haemoglobin content of less than 10 grams/100 mL of blood is diagnosed as having **anaemia.** The term *anaemia* also may be used to describe a reduction in the number or volume of functional RBCs in a given unit of whole blood. Anaemias are classified according to the size and haemoglobin content of RBCs.

CONNECT IT! 

Sickle cell anaemia is a condition in which haemoglobin is present in a normal amount, but is defective. This causes distortion of RBC shape, which causes many different problems to occur. Check out ***Sickle Cell Anaemia*** online at ***Connect It!*** for more.

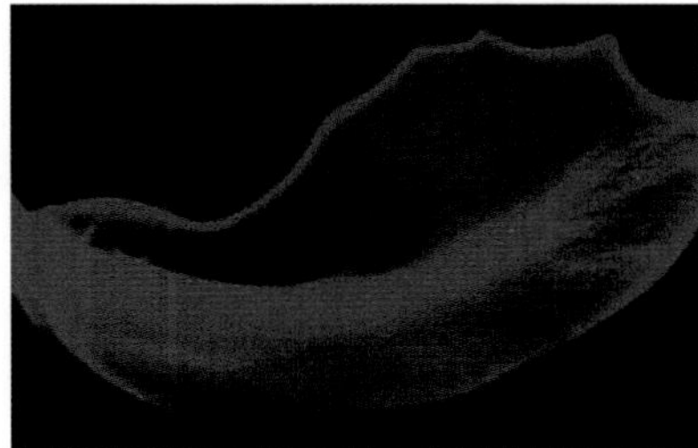

FORMATION OF RED BLOOD CELLS

The entire process of RBC formation is a type of haematopoiesis called **erythropoiesis.** In the adult, erythrocytes begin their maturation sequence in the red bone marrow from nucleated cells known as **haematopoietic stem cells (HSCs),** or adult blood-forming stem cells. *Adult stem cells* are cells that have the ability to maintain a constant population of newly differentiating cells of a specific type. These adult blood-forming stem cells divide by mitosis; some of the daughter cells remain as undifferentiated adult stem cells, whereas others go through several stages of development to become erythrocytes.

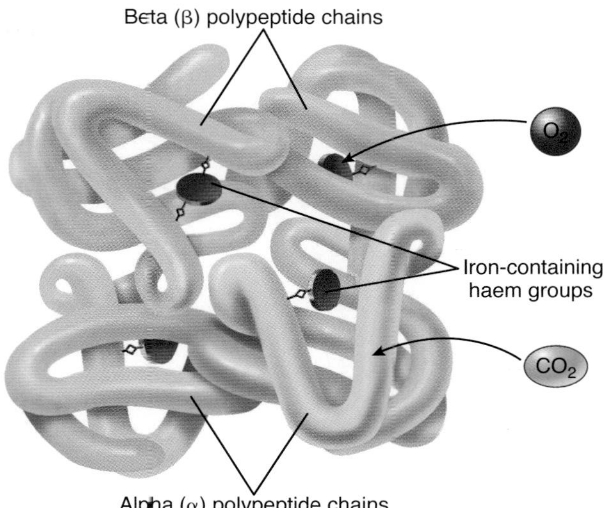

FIGURE 27-5 Haemoglobin. Four protein chains (globins), each with a haem group, form a haemoglobin molecule. Each haem contains one iron atom. Carbon dioxide (CO_2) can bind to amino acids in the globin part or oxygen (O_2) may bind to the haem groups.

Figure 27-6 shows the classic model of developmental stages that can be identified as transformation from the immature form to the mature red blood cell occurs. The entire maturation process requires about 4 days and proceeds from step to step by gradual transition. Just what influences direct **embryonic stem cells** (found in the embryo and in umbilical cord blood) to develop into a specific type of **adult stem cell** (e.g., haematopoietic stem cells) and then eventually differentiate into a specific cell type, such as an RBC, is a topic of intense research.

As you can see in **Figure 27-6**, all blood cells are derived from haematopoietic stem cells. In RBCs, differentiation begins with the appearance of **proerythroblasts.** Mitotic divisions then produce **basophilic erythroblasts.** The next maturation division produces **polychromatic erythroblasts,** which produce haemoglobin. These cells subsequently lose their nuclei and become **reticulocytes.** Once released into the circulating blood, reticulocytes lose their delicate reticulum and become mature erythrocytes in about 24 to 36 hours. Note in **Figure 27-6** that overall cell size decreases as the maturation sequence progresses

Every day of our adult lives we produce more than 200 billion RBCs to replace an equal number destroyed during that brief time. Because in health the number of RBCs remains relatively constant, efficient homeostatic mechanisms must operate to balance the number of cells formed against the number destroyed.

The rate of RBC production soon speeds up if blood oxygen levels reaching the tissues decrease. Oxygen deficiency increases RBC numbers by increasing the secretion of a glycoprotein hormone named **erythropoietin (EPO).** An inactive form of this hormone, called an *erythropoietinogen*, is released into the blood primarily from the liver on an ongoing basis. If oxygen levels decrease, the kidneys release increasing amounts of erythropoietin, which in turn stimulates bone marrow to accelerate its production of red blood cells. With increasing numbers of RBCs, oxygen delivery to tissues increases, less erythropoietin is produced, and consequently less is available to stimulate RBC production in the red bone marrow.

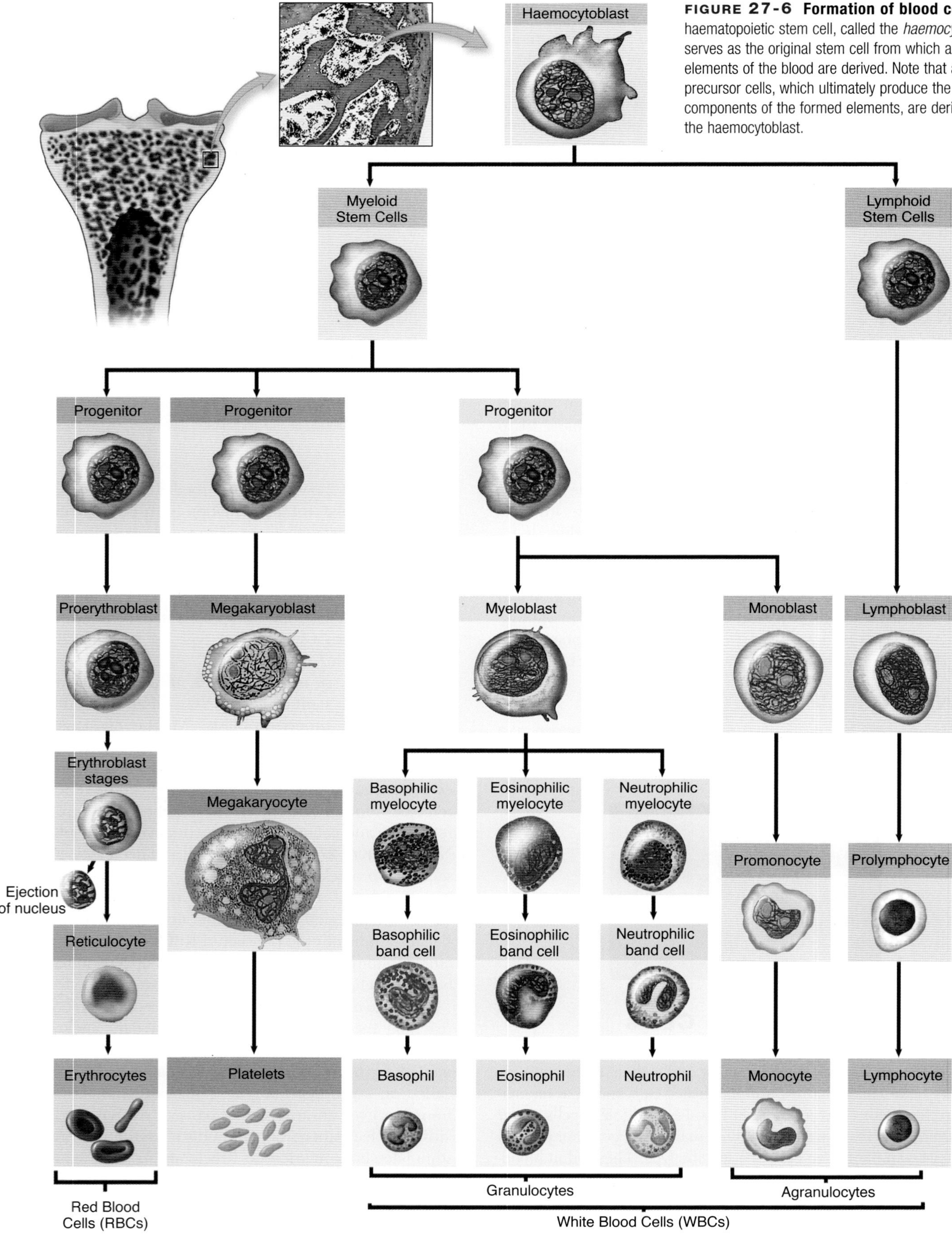

FIGURE 27-6 Formation of blood cells. The haematopoietic stem cell, called the *haemocytoblast,* serves as the original stem cell from which all formed elements of the blood are derived. Note that all five precursor cells, which ultimately produce the different components of the formed elements, are derived from the haemocytoblast.

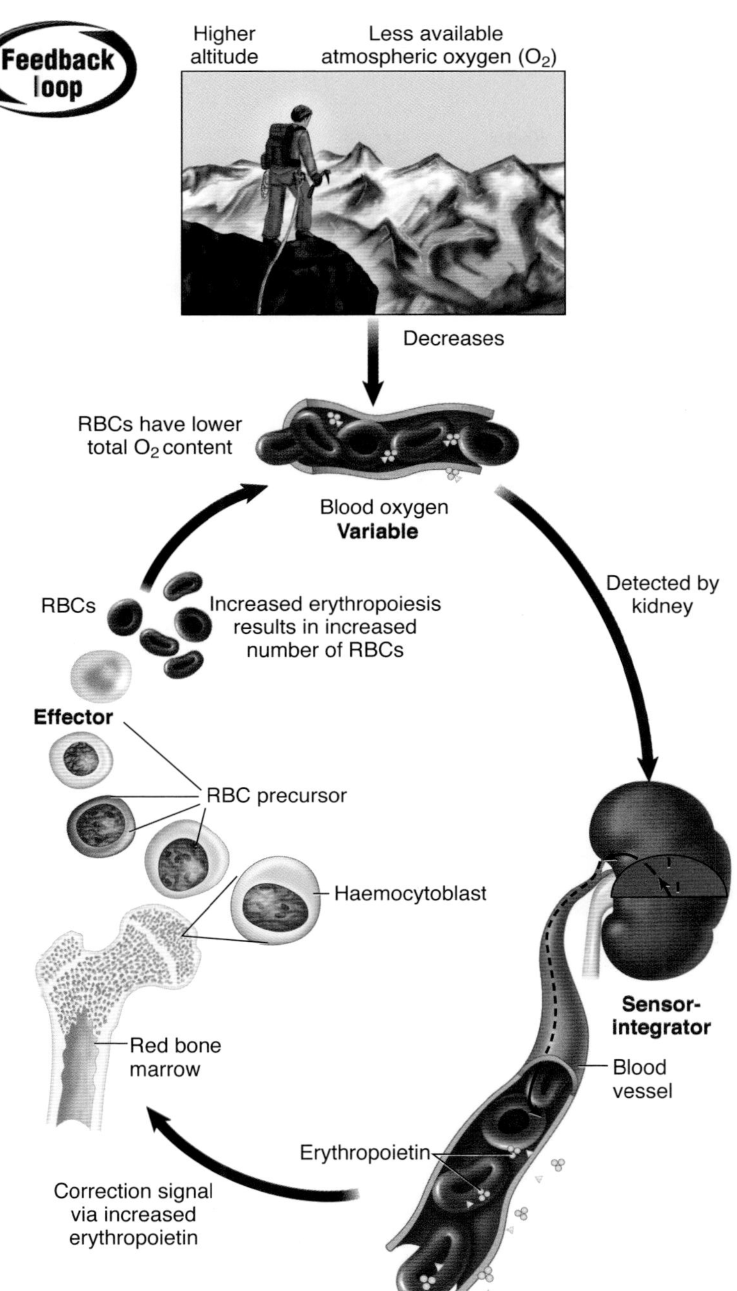

FIGURE 27-7 Erythropoiesis. In response to decreased blood oxygen, the kidneys release erythropoietin, which stimulates erythrocyte production in the red bone marrow.

Figure 27-7 shows how erythropoietin production is controlled by a negative feedback loop that is activated by decreasing oxygen concentration in the tissues.

CONNECT IT! 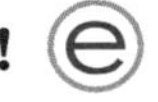

The practice among elite athletes of boosting RBC numbers artificially has been in the news for decades. To find out more about **blood doping** or **blood boosting** check out ***Blood Doping*** online at ***Connect It!*** Also review ***Sites of Haematopoiesis*** online at ***Connect It!***

Life Cycle of Red Blood Cells

The life span of RBCs circulating in the bloodstream averages about 105 to 120 days. They often break apart, or fragment, in the capillaries as they age. Macrophage cells in the lining of blood vessels, particularly in the liver and spleen, phagocytose (ingest and destroy) the aged, abnormal, or fragmented red blood cells (**Figure 27-8**).

The RBC dismantling process results in breakdown of haemoglobin, with the release of amino acids, iron, and the pigment bilirubin. Iron is returned to the bone marrow for use in synthesis of new haemoglobin, and bilirubin is transported to the liver, where it is excreted into the intestine as part of bile. Amino acids, released from the globin portion of the degraded haemoglobin molecule, are used by the body for energy or for synthesis of new proteins.

For the RBC homeostatic mechanism to succeed in maintaining a normal number of RBCs, the bone marrow must function adequately. To do this the blood must supply it with adequate amounts of several substances with which to form the new red blood cells—vitamin B_{12}, iron, and amino acids, for example, and also copper and cobalt to serve as catalysts. In addition, the gastric mucosa must provide some unidentified intrinsic factor necessary for absorption of vitamin B_{12} (also called **extrinsic factor** because it derives from external sources in foods and is not synthesized by the body; vitamin B_{12} is also called the **antianaemic principle**).

Blood Types

In 1902, the Austrian pathologist Karl Landsteiner announced his discovery of blood types, one of the most important medical discoveries of the time. The term *blood type* refers to the type of cell markers or antigens present on RBC membranes. Landsteiner discovered the most important blood antigens: A and B. The presence or absence of these antigens determines a person's blood type in the ABO system. In 1940, Landsteiner found that a group of six Rh (or D) antigens previously found in rhesus monkeys was also found in humans. Continuing research by Landsteiner and others revealed nearly two dozen additional blood antigens that vary from person to person.

The fact that not everyone has the same blood antigens is very important. This means that our immune system may "attack" donated blood cells (from a transfusion) if they have antigens different from our own. Antigens A, B, and Rh are the most important blood antigens as far as transfusions and newborn survival are concerned. The other blood antigens are less important clinically but may still cause occasional problems.

Why do different people have different antigens on their RBCs? We do not have a complete answer to that question, but their presence or absence probably gives some biological advantage related to conditions within different human populations. For example, an antigen called *Duffy* (after the patient in whom it was first discovered) is often missing in populations that have lived with the threat of malaria for many generations. The Duffy antigen is used by the malaria parasite to enter RBCs, so its absence protects a person against developing malaria. However, we know very little about functions of the other antigens.

The term *agglutinins* is often used to describe the antibodies dissolved in plasma that react with specific blood group antigens or *agglutinogens*. We use the terms *agglutinin* and *agglutinogen* because when they combine and react, they cause the RBCs to clump together, or agglutinate. It is the specific agglutinogens or antigens

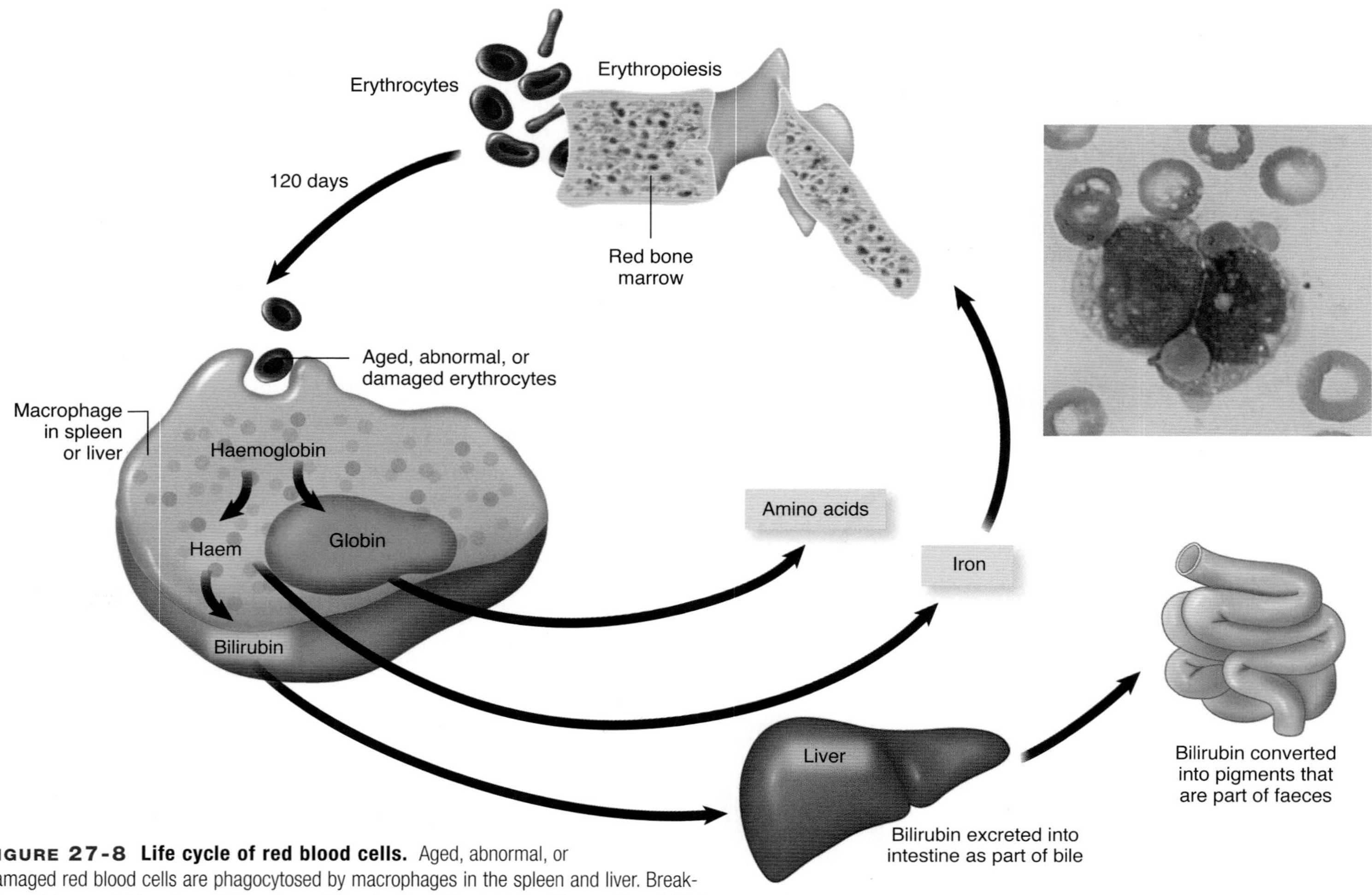

FIGURE 27-8 Life cycle of red blood cells. Aged, abnormal, or damaged red blood cells are phagocytosed by macrophages in the spleen and liver. Breakdown of haemoglobin released from the red blood cells yields globin and haem. The globin is converted to amino acids and used as an energy source or for protein synthesis. Note that the released haem is further degraded into iron, which may be stored or used immediately to produce both new haemoglobin and bilirubin; the bilirubin is ultimately excreted in the bile. Photo inset shows phagocytosis of erythrocytes by macrophages in the liver.

on red cell membranes that characterize the different ABO blood groups, which are described in the following paragraphs.

When a blood transfusion is performed, great care must be taken to prevent a mixture of agglutinogens (antigens) and agglutinins (antibodies) that would result in the agglutination of the donor and recipient blood—a potentially fatal event known as a **transfusion reaction.** Clinical laboratory tests, called *blood typing* and *cross-matching*, ensure the proper identification of blood group antigens and antibodies in both donor and recipient blood and demonstrate the lack of an agglutination reaction when they are mixed together.

The ABO System

Every person's blood belongs to one of the four ABO blood types (or groups). Blood types are named according to the antigens present (agglutinogens) on RBC membranes. Here, then, are the four ABO blood types:

1. Type A—antigen A on RBCs
2. Type B—antigen B on RBCs
3. Type AB—both antigen A and antigen B on RBCs
4. Type O—neither antigen A nor antigen B on RBCs

Blood plasma may or may not contain antibodies (agglutinins) that can react with red blood cell antigens A or B. An important principle related to this is that plasma never contains antibodies against the antigens present on its own red blood cells—for obvious reasons. If it did, the antibody would react with the antigen and thereby destroy the RBCs. However (and this is an equally important principle), plasma does contain antibodies against antigen A or antigen B if they are *not* present on its RBCs. So by applying these two principles, we can deduce the following: In type A blood, antigen A is present on its RBCs; therefore its plasma contains no anti-A antibodies but does contain anti-B antibodies. In type B blood, antigen-B is present on its RBCs; therefore its plasma contains no anti-B antibodies but does contain anti-A antibodies (**Figure 27-9**).

Note in **Figure 27-10**, A, that type A blood donated to a type A recipient does not cause an agglutination transfusion reaction because the anti-B antibodies in the recipient do not combine with the A antigens in the donated blood. However, type A blood donated to a type B recipient causes an agglutination reaction because the anti-A antibodies in the recipient combine with the A antigens in the

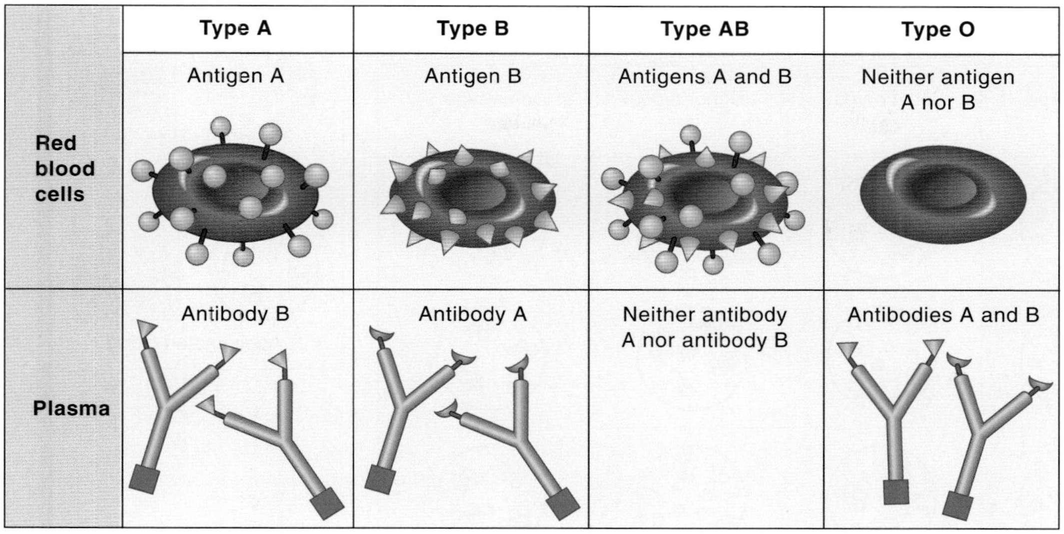

	Type A	Type B	Type AB	Type O
Red blood cells	Antigen A	Antigen B	Antigens A and B	Neither antigen A nor B
Plasma	Antibody B	Antibody A	Neither antibody A nor antibody B	Antibodies A and B

FIGURE 27-9 ABO blood types. Note that antigens characteristic of each blood type are bound to the surface of RBCs. The antibodies of each blood type are found in the plasma and exhibit unique structural features that permit agglutination to occur if exposure to the appropriate antigen occurs.

donated blood (**Figure 27-10**, *B*). **Figure 27-11** shows the results of different combinations of donor and recipient blood.

Because type O blood does not contain either antigen A or B, it has been referred to as *universal donor* blood, a term that implies that it can safely be given to any recipient. This, however, is not true because the recipient's plasma may contain agglutinins other than anti-A or anti-B antibodies. For this reason the recipient's and the donor's blood—even if it is type O—should be cross-matched; that is, mixed and observed for agglutination of the donor's red blood cells.

Universal recipient (type AB) blood contains neither anti-A nor anti-B antibodies, so it cannot agglutinate type A or type B donor red

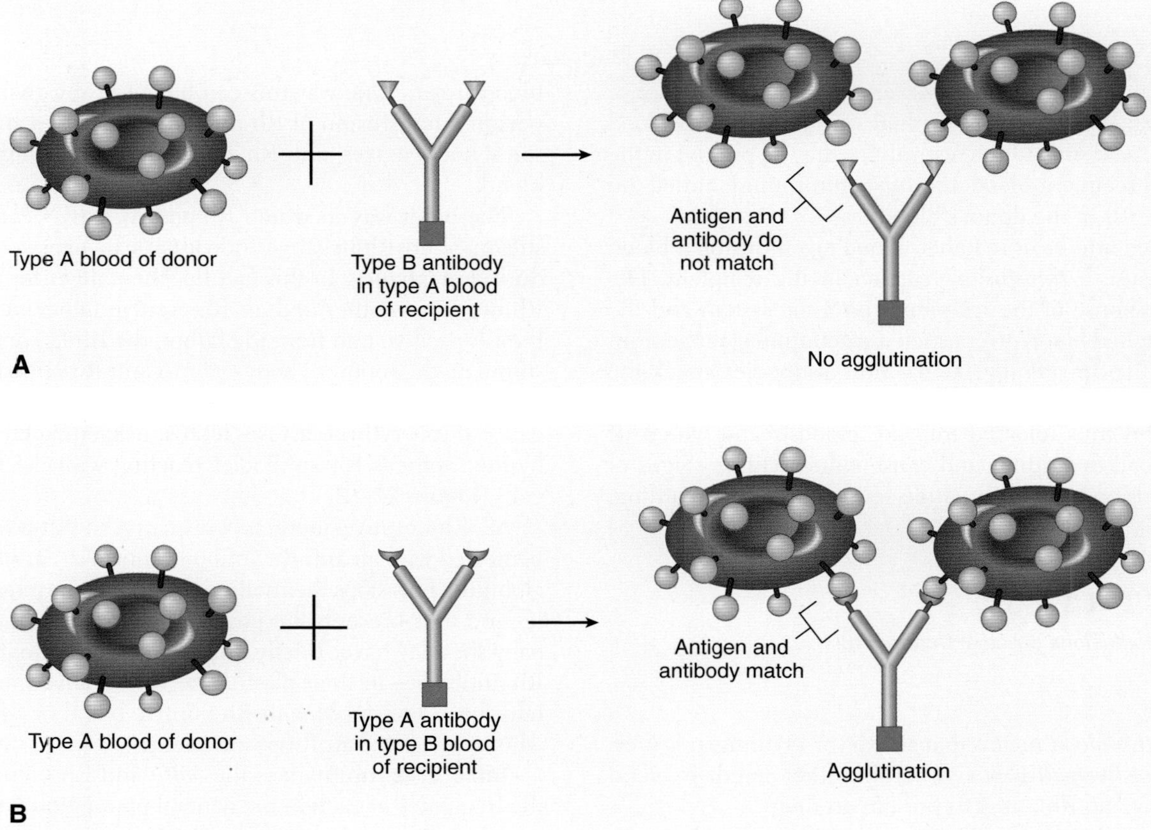

FIGURE 27-10 Agglutination. A, When mixing of donor and recipient blood of the same type *(A)* occurs, there is no agglutination because only anti-B antibodies are present. **B,** If type A donor blood is mixed with type B recipient blood, agglutination will occur because of the presence of anti-A antibodies in the type B recipient blood.

Recipient's blood		Reactions with donor's blood			
RBC antigens	Plasma antibodies	Donor type O	Donor type A	Donor type B	Donor type AB
None (Type O)	Anti-A Anti-B				
A (Type A)	Anti-B				
B (Type B)	Anti-A				
AB (Type AB)	(None)				

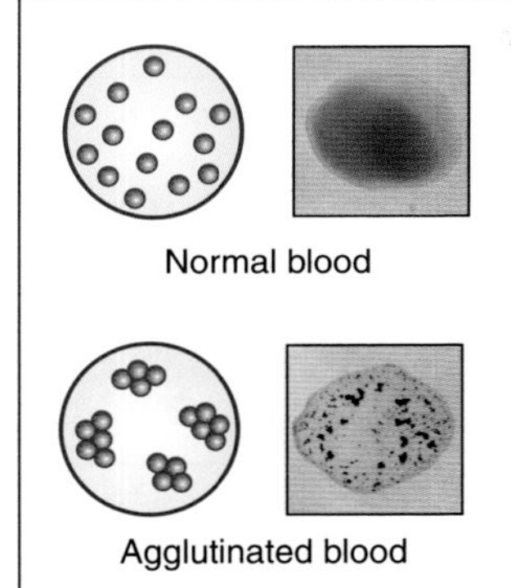

FIGURE 27-11 Results of (cross-matching) different combinations (types) of donor and recipient blood. The left columns show the antigen and antibody characteristics that define the recipient's blood type, and the top row shows the donor's blood type. Cross-matching identifies either a compatible combination of donor-recipient blood (no agglutination) or an incompatible combination (agglutinated blood). Photo inset shows drops of blood showing appearance of agglutinated and nonagglutinated red blood cells.

blood cells. This does not mean, however, that any type of donor blood may be safely given to an individual who has type AB blood without first cross-matching. Other agglutinins may be present in the so-called universal recipient blood and may clump unidentified antigens (agglutinogens) in the donor's blood.

Improperly typed and cross-matched blood given during a blood transfusion can cause a *transfusion reaction* in the recipient. Depending on the response of the recipient's immune system and the amount of mismatched blood given, such a reaction may range from mild to severe to life-threatening. As the host antibodies attack the donor RBCs, the RBCs are broken apart—a process called *haemolysis*. Haemoglobin is thus released into the bloodstream, which (if severe) may overload the kidney and cause kidney failure. Signs of this type of transfusion reaction include fever, difficulty breathing, and pink urine.

CONNECT IT! ⓔ

Review ***Blood Transfusions*** online at ***Connect It!***

The Rh System

The term *Rh-positive blood* means that an Rh (or D) antigen is present on its RBCs. *Rh-negative blood,* on the other hand, is blood whose red cells have no Rh antigens present on them.

Blood does not normally contain anti-Rh antibodies. However, anti-Rh antibodies can appear in the blood of an Rh-negative person, provided Rh-positive RBCs have at some time entered the bloodstream. One way this can happen is by giving an Rh-negative person a transfusion of Rh-positive blood. In a short time, the person's body makes anti-Rh antibodies, and these remain in the blood.

The other way in which Rh-positive RBCs can enter the bloodstream of an Rh-negative individual can happen only to a woman during pregnancy. In this fact lies the danger for a baby born to an Rh-negative mother and an Rh-positive father. If the baby inherits the Rh-positive trait from the father, the Rh factor on the RBCs may stimulate the mother's body to form anti-Rh antibodies. Then, if she later carries another Rh-positive fetus, the fetus may develop a disease called **erythroblastosis fetalis,** a haemolytic condition caused by the mother's Rh antibodies reacting with the baby's Rh-positive cells (**Figure 27-12**).

All Rh-negative mothers who carry an Rh-positive fetus should be treated with an anti-Rh antibody known as Anti-D (RH$_o$) immunoglobulin. This stops the mother's body from forming anti-Rh antibodies and thus prevents the possibility of harm to the next Rh-positive baby she may have. Briefly, the only people who can ever have anti-Rh antibodies in their plasma are Rh-negative men or women who have been transfused with Rh-positive blood or Rh-negative women who have carried an Rh-positive fetus.

Table 27-2 summarizes the ABO and Rh blood types, including the frequency of each in the general population—that is, the human population as a whole. Of course the frequency of these and other blood types may be different within a family or ethnic group based on regional differences in the human gene pool.

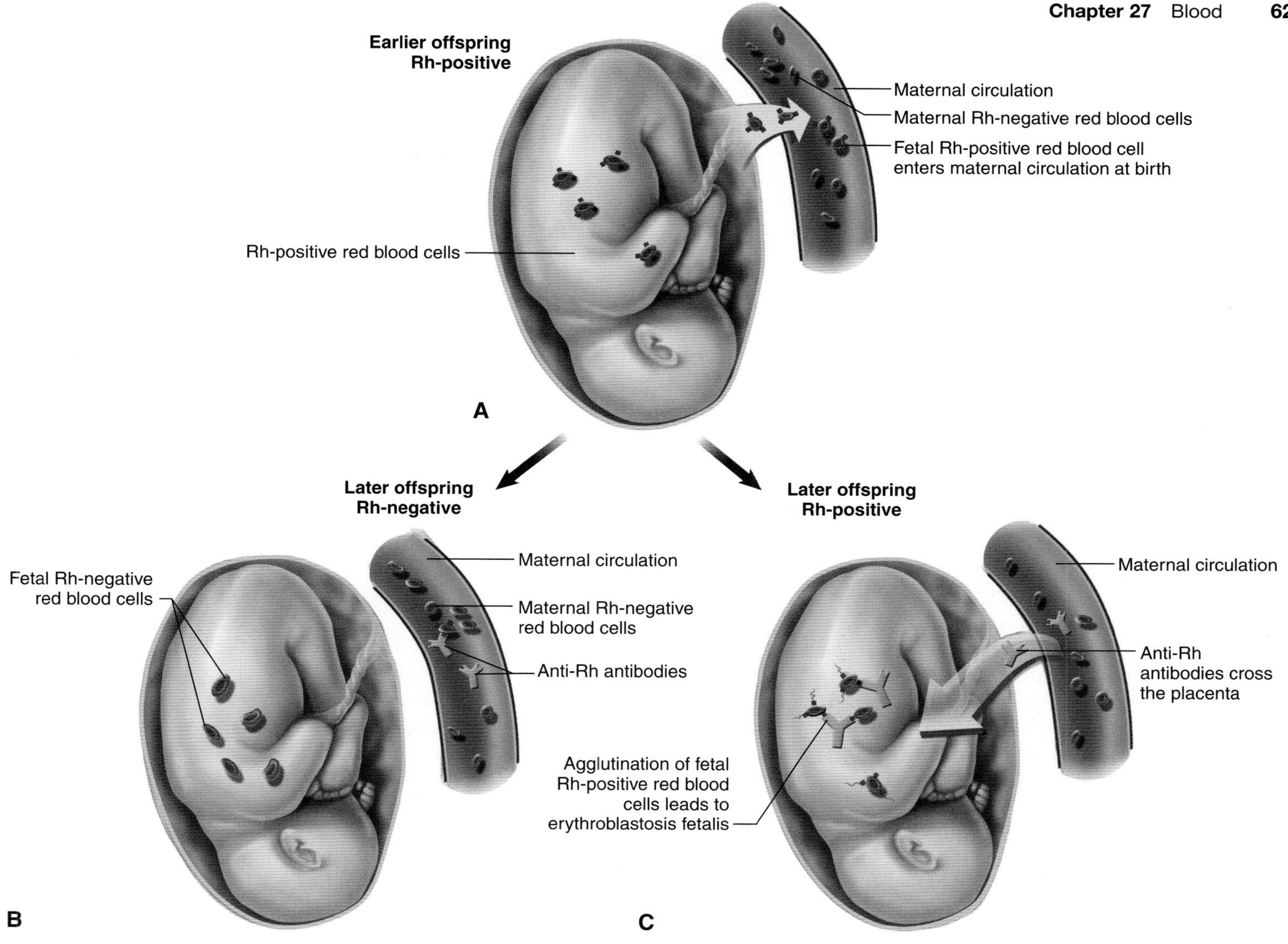

FIGURE 27-12 Erythroblastosis fetalis. A, Rh-positive blood cells enter the mother's bloodstream during delivery of an Rh-positive baby. If not treated, the mother's body will produce anti-Rh antibodies. **B,** A later pregnancy involving an Rh-negative baby is normal because there are no Rh antigens in the baby's blood. **C,** A later pregnancy involving an Rh-positive baby may result in erythroblastosis fetalis. Anti-Rh antibodies enter the baby's blood supply and cause agglutination of RBCs with the Rh antigen.

Quick CHECK

5. Name the red pigment found in RBCs, and list the normal range (in grams per 100 mL of blood) for women and men.
6. Trace the formation of an erythrocyte from stem cell precursor to a mature and circulating RBC.
7. Explain the negative feedback loop that controls erythropoiesis.
8. Discuss the destruction of RBCs in the body.

WHITE BLOOD CELLS

White blood cells, or **leucocytes,** do not contain pigments; but these transparent cells appear white when collected together—just like clear snowflakes that appear white when grouped together. Because they are colourless, WBCs can be seen easily under a microscope only when stained. Five general types of WBCS can be classified according to their staining characteristics, including the presence or absence of stained granules in their cytoplasm.

TABLE 27-2 Blood Typing

BLOOD TYPE (ABO AND Rh)	ANTIGENS PRESENT*	ANTIBODIES PRESENT*	PERCENT OF GENERAL POPULATION
O+	Rh	anti-A, anti-B	35%
O− §	None	anti-A, anti-B, anti-Rh?	7%
A+	A, Rh	anti-B	35%
A−	A	anti-B, anti-Rh?	7%
B+	B, Rh	anti-A	8%
B−	B	anti-A, anti-Rh?	2%
AB+ ǁ	A, B, Rh	None	4%
AB−	A, B	anti-Rh?	2%

Adapted from Pagana KD, Pagana TJ: *Mosby's manual of diagnostic and laboratory tests,* ed 5, St Louis, 2013, Mosby.

*Anti-Rh antibodies *may* be present, depending on exposure to Rh antigens.

§Universal donor.

ǁUniversal recipient.

Granulocytes, or granular leucocytes include the three WBCs that have large granules in their cytoplasm. They are named according to their cytoplasmic staining properties:

1. Neutrophils
2. Eosinophils
3. Basophils

Agranulocytes, or agranular leucocytes (WBCs without stained cytoplasmic granules) include the following:

1. Lymphocytes
2. Monocytes

WBCs have nuclei and are generally larger than RBCs, as you can see in **Table 27-1** (p. 611). The table, and the sections that follow, briefly outline the main functions of each type of WBC. In Chapters 32 and 33 we more fully explore many of these defensive functions of leucocytes.

Granulocytes

Neutrophils

Neutrophils (**Figure 27-13**) take their name from the fact that their cytoplasmic granules stain a very light purple with neutral dyes. The granules in these cells are small and numerous and tend to give the cytoplasm a coarse appearance. Because their nuclei have two, three, or more lobes, neutrophils are also called **polymorphonuclear leucocytes** or, to avoid that tongue twister, simply *polys.*

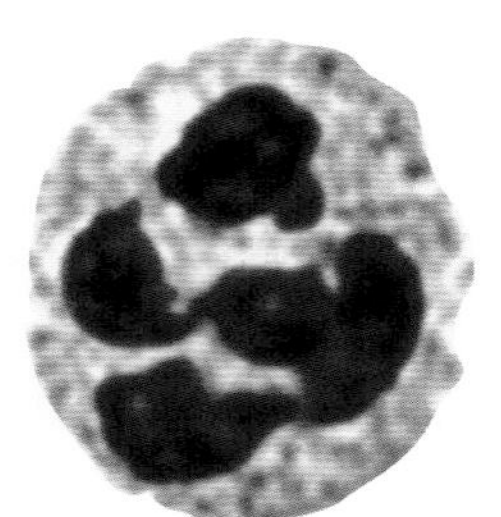

FIGURE 27-13 Neutrophil.

Neutrophil numbers average about 65% of the total WBC count in a normal blood sample. These leucocytes are highly mobile, active phagocytic cells that can migrate out of blood vessels and enter the tissue spaces. The process is called **diapedesis.** The cytoplasmic granules in neutrophils contain powerful lysosomes, the organelles with digestive-like enzymes that are capable of destroying bacterial cells.

Bacterial infections that produce an inflammatory response cause the release of chemicals from damaged cells that attract neutrophils and other phagocytic WBCs to the infection site. The process, called **chemotaxis,** helps the body concentrate phagocytic cells at focal points of infection.

Eosinophils

Eosinophils (**Figure 27-14**) contain cytoplasmic granules that are large, numerous, and stain orange with acid dyes such as eosin. Their nuclei generally have two lobes. Normally, eosinophils account for about 2% to 5% of circulating WBCs. They are also numerous in mucous membranes such as the lining of the respiratory and digestive tracts.

Although eosinophils are weak phagocytes, their major role is the release of chemicals from their granules. These immune chemicals include cell toxins and many regulators of the body's immune response. Perhaps their most important overall functions involve protection against infections caused by parasitic worms and involvement in regulating allergic reactions such as asthma.

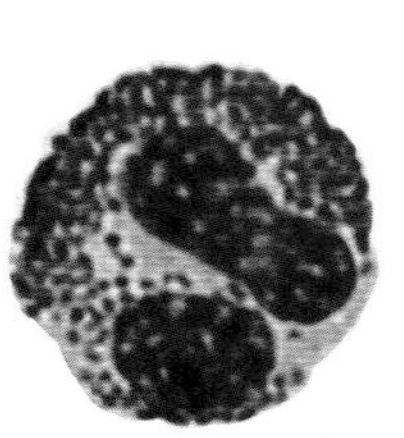

FIGURE 27-14 Eosinophil.

Basophils

Basophils (**Figure 27-15**) have relatively large, but sparse, cytoplasmic granules that stain a dark purple with basic dyes. They are the least numerous of the WBCs, numbering only 0.5% to 1% of the total leucocyte count. Basophils are both motile and capable of diapedesis. They exhibit S-shaped, but indistinct, nuclei. The cytoplasmic granules of these WBCs contain *histamine* (an inflammatory chemical) and *heparin* (an anticoagulant).

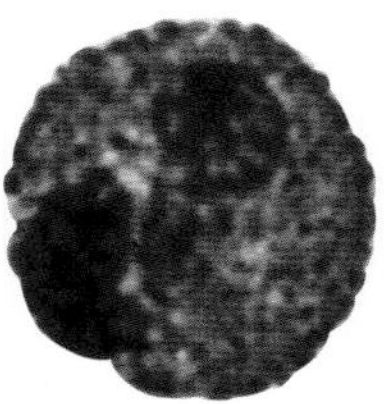

FIGURE 27-15 Basophil.

Agranulocytes

Although all agranulocytes share the characteristic that their cytoplasmic particles do not stain with typical haematological stains, lymphocytes and monocytes are very different from one another in both size and function.

Lymphocytes

Lymphocytes (**Figure 27-16**) found in the blood are the smallest of the leucocytes, averaging about 6 to 9 μm in diameter. They have large, spherical nuclei surrounded by a very limited amount of pale blue–staining cytoplasm. Next to neutrophils, lymphocytes are the most numerous WBCs. They account for about 25% of all the leucocyte population. Two types of lymphocytes, called *T lymphocytes* and *B lymphocytes*, have important roles in immunity. T lymphocytes function by directly attacking an infected or cancerous cell, whereas B lymphocytes produce antibodies against specific antigens. Activated B lymphocytes are also called *plasma cells.* The functions of both types of lymphocytes are fully discussed in Chapter 33.

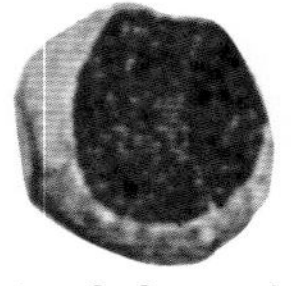

FIGURE 27-16 Lymphocyte.

Monocytes

Monocytes (**Figure 27-17**) are the largest of the leucocytes. They have dark, kidney bean–shaped nuclei surrounded by large quantities of distinctive blue-grey cytoplasm. Monocytes are motile and highly phagocytic cells capable of engulfing large bacterial organisms and viral-infected cells.

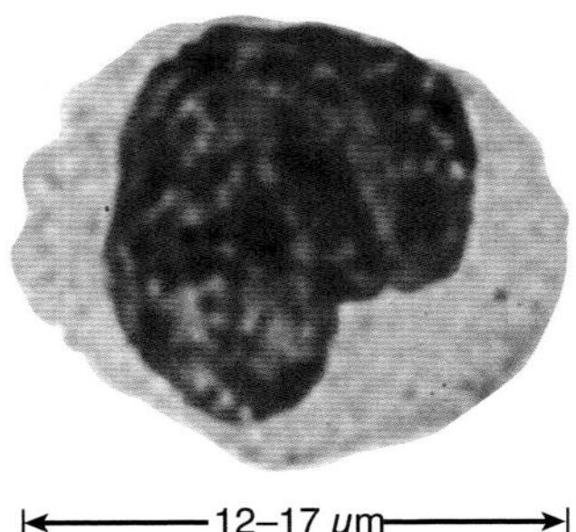

FIGURE 27-17 Monocyte.

White Blood Cell Numbers

One cubic millimetre of normal blood usually contains about 4000 to 11,000 leucocytes (4.0–11.0 × 10^9/L), with different percentages of each type. Because these numbers change in certain abnormal conditions, they have clinical significance. In acute appendicitis, for example, the percentage of neutrophils increases and so, too, does the total WBC count. In fact, these characteristic changes may be the deciding points for surgery.

BOX 27-1 *diagnostic study*
Complete Blood Cell Count

One of the most useful and commonly performed clinical blood tests is called the **complete blood cell count** or simply the **CBC.** The CBC is a collection of tests whose results, when interpreted as a whole, can yield an enormous amount of information regarding a person's health. Standard red blood cell, white blood cell, and thrombocyte counts; the differential white blood cell count; haematocrit; haemoglobin content; and other characteristics of the formed elements are usually included in this battery of tests. The CBC is also known as a full blood count (FBC). •

An overall decrease in the number of WBCs is called **leucopenia.** An increase in the number of WBCs is **leucocytosis.**

A special type of white blood cell count called a **differential WBC count** reveals more information than simply the total number of all of the different types of WBCs in a blood sample. In a differential WBC count, a component test in the *complete blood cell count*, or CBC (**Box 27-1**), the *proportions* of each type of white blood cell are reported as percentages of the total WBC count. Normal percentages are shown in **Table 27-3**. A lab technician may count the first 100 WBCs seen in a blood smear under a microscope to estimate the percentage of each type of WBC, but often this is done using advanced image-recognition computer technology (**Figure 27-18**).

Because all disorders do not affect each WBC type the same way, the differential WBC count is a valuable diagnostic tool. For example, although some parasite infestations do not cause an increase in the total WBC count, they often do cause an increase in the proportion of eosinophils that are present. The reason? This type of WBC specializes in defending against parasites (see **Table 27-1**).

Formation of White Blood Cells

The haematopoietic stem cell serves as the precursor of not only the erythrocytes but also the leucocytes and platelets in blood. **Figure 27-6**, p. 616, shows the sequence of **leucopoiesis** that results in formation of the various types of leucocytes from the undifferentiated haematopoietic stem cell (HSC or haemocytoblast).

TABLE 27-3 Differential Count of White Blood Cells

CLASS	DIFFERENTIAL COUNT*	
	NORMAL RANGE (%)	TYPICAL VALUE (%)†
Neutrophils	65–75	65
Lymphocytes (large and small)	20–25	25
Monocytes	3–8	6
Eosinophils	2–5	3
Basophils	½–1	1
TOTAL	100	100

*In any differential count the sum of the percentages of the different kinds of white blood cells (WBCs) must, of course, total 100%.

†The following mnemonic phrase may help you remember percent values in decreasing order by class of WBC: "**N**ever **L**et **M**onkeys **E**at **B**ananas."

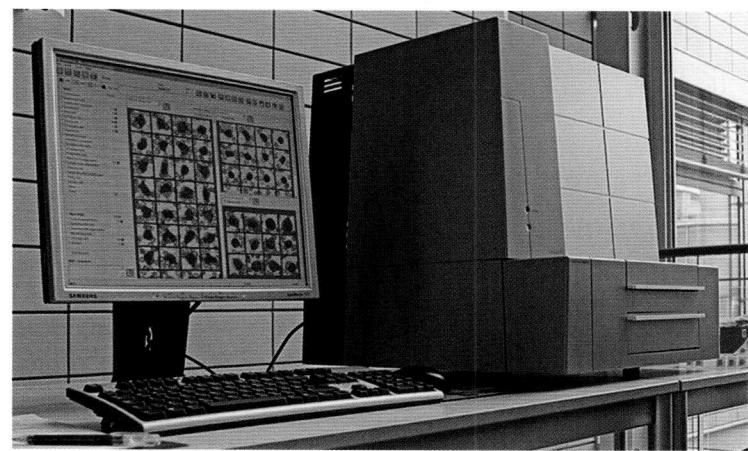

FIGURE 27-18 Differential WBC count. Automated microscope systems use advanced image-recognition technology to identify and count different WBC types in blood smear samples and produce the differential WBC count.

In the classic model of blood cell development, two lines of blood stem cells emerge early in the process of leucopoiesis: the *myeloid* stem cell line and the *lymphoid* stem cell line.

The myeloid line, or "marrow line", diverges into lines of development that produce the granular leucocytes (neutrophils, eosinophils, and basophils) and monocytes. The myeloid line also produces the erythrocyte and thrombocyte lines. As the name implies, the blood cells produced by the myeloid lines develop within the red bone marrow. However, when white blood cells leave the marrow, they may take up temporary residence in other tissues, including the lymphoid tissue found with lymphatic organs such as the spleen and lymph nodes.

The lymphoid line, on the other hand, produces only lymphocytes. The term *lymphocyte* is generic and often refers to a stem cell in the lymphoid line that leaves the bone marrow and migrates to lymphoid tissue, where it differentiates into a specific type of lymphocyte. For example, lymphocytes that migrate to the lymphoid tissue of the thymus gland differentiate into *T lymphocytes* or simply T cells. Lymphocytes that migrate to lymph nodes may differentiate into *B lymphocytes* or B cells. *Natural killer (NK) lymphocytes* may differentiate in the bone marrow or lymphoid tissue in the thymus.

Myeloid tissue (bone marrow) and lymphoid tissue together constitute the haematopoietic, or blood cell–forming, tissues of the body. Red bone marrow is myeloid tissue and gets its red colour from the red blood cells it contains. Yellow marrow, on the other hand, is yellow because it has been converted to mostly adipose tissue. It is not active in the business of blood cell formation as long as it remains yellow. Sometimes, however, it becomes active and turns red in colour when an extreme and prolonged need for red blood cell production occurs.

We have learned that EPO regulates erythropoiesis. Is there an equivalent regulator of leucopoiesis? Given the various types and subtypes that are produced, leucopoiesis is more complex. So it is not surprising that there are dozens of intrinsic and extrinsic regulators that have been identified. Among them are various *colony-stimulating factors (CSFs)*, **interleukins (ILs)**, and other regulator molecules. However, they all operate on the same principle as EPO does—adjustment of blood cell production to maintain homeostatic balance in the body.

CONNECT IT!

Where in the body are the sources of new blood cells? The illustrations in ***Sites of Haematopoiesis*** online at ***Connect It!*** will help you visualize the many locations of blood cell production.

PLATELETS

STRUCTURE AND FUNCTION OF PLATELETS

To compare **platelets** with other blood cells in terms of appearance and size, see **Table 27-1**. In circulating blood, platelets are small, nearly colourless bodies that usually appear as irregular spindles or oval discs about 2 to 4 μm in diameter.

Three important physical properties of platelets—namely, agglutination, adhesiveness, and aggregation—make attempts at classification on the basis of size or shape in dry blood smears all but impossible. As soon as blood is removed from a vessel, the platelets adhere to each other and to every surface they contact; in so doing, they assume various shapes and irregular forms.

Platelet counts in adults average about 250,000/mm^3 of blood (250×10^9/L). A range of 150,000 to 400,000/mm^3 ($150–400 \times 10^9$/L) is considered normal. Newborn infants often show reduced counts, but these rise gradually to reach normal adult values at about 3 months of age. There are no differences between the sexes in platelet count.

Platelets play an important role in **haemostasis** (from the Greek *stasis*, "a standing"), the process of reducing bleeding from injured blood vessels. This is a complex process that deserves its own discussion, which follows later in this chapter.

FORMATION AND LIFE SPAN OF PLATELETS

Formation of platelets, often called thrombocytes, is referred to as **thrombopoiesis.** It begins with stimulation of precursor cells called megakaryoblasts (see **Figure 27-6**) and is controlled by the hormone *thrombopoietin.*

Mature megakaryocytes are huge cells (20 to 100 μm) with large nuclei containing as many as 20 lobes (**Figure 27-19**). They often have a bizarre shape. The cytoplasm of a stained specimen is blue to pink in colour, is abundant, and contains a variable number of very fine granules. Mature megakaryocytes are largely confined to red bone marrow, although some are located in the lungs and, to a lesser extent, the spleen.

Between 2000 and more than 3000 platelets are released when the irregular cytoplasmic membrane surrounding the mature megakaryocyte ruptures. The resulting platelets have a limiting plasma membrane but, like RBCs, no nucleus. Platelets have a short life span, an average of about 7 days.

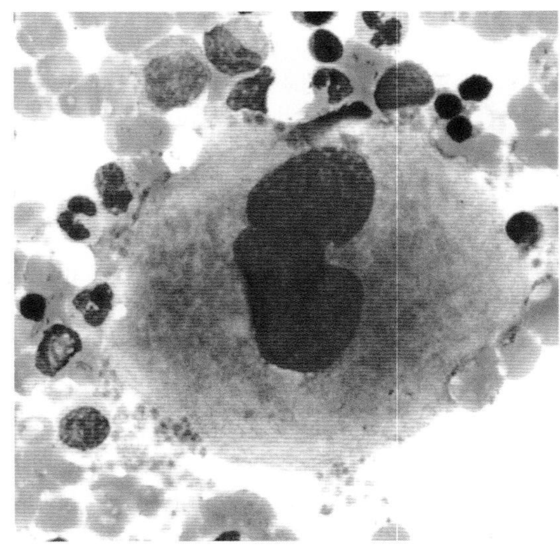

FIGURE 27-19 Megakaryocyte. Note the large size of the cell and multinucleated nucleus. This bone marrow smear also shows a number of WBCs scattered among more numerous RBCs.

HAEMOSTASIS

Recall that haemostasis is the process that slows and stops bleeding when a vessel is injured. A secondary and less well known function of the haemostasis mechanism is to help in defending us against infection. In an injury, bacteria may find an opportunity to invade our tissues. However, a blood clot will hopefully trap and bind enough of them to prevent such an invasion.

Haemostasis is an interrelated set of complex mechanisms that can adapt to many different scenarios involving bleeding. Put simply, there are three major phases to haemostasis:

1. Vasoconstriction
2. Platelet plug formation
3. Blood clotting (coagulation)

VASOCONSTRICTION

Injury to a blood vessel is usually followed by spasms of smooth muscle fibres in the wall of damaged blood vessels, which causes **vasoconstriction.** Vasoconstriction applies pressure that causes temporary closure of a damaged vessel and lessens blood loss until a platelet plug and subsequent coagulation effectively stop the haemorrhage.

Physical injury is the stimulus that causes smooth muscle fibres to reflexively constrict. Vasoconstriction after an injury is enhanced by *thromboxane* A2 released from platelets. Damaged endothelial cells lining the vessel release potent local regulators, such as *endothelin-1*, that promote vasoconstriction.

Collapse of injured vessels is further enhanced by factors outside the blood vessel. For example, external pressure from reflexive contraction of nearby skeletal muscles in response to pain can help collapse a vessel to stop bleeding. Similarly, pressure applied to a wound by a first responder may have the same effect.

PLATELET PLUG FORMATION

Within 1 to 5 seconds after injury to a blood capillary, platelets will adhere to the damaged lining of the vessel and to each other to form a haemostatic **platelet plug** that helps stop the flow of blood into the tissues.

The formation of a temporary platelet plug is an important step in haemostasis. The formation of a platelet plug results when platelets undergo a change caused by an encounter with a damaged capillary wall, or with underlying connective tissue fibres. This transformation in platelets results in the creation of *sticky platelets,* which bind to underlying tissues and each other.

In addition to adhesion of platelets to form a physical plug at the site of injury, platelets are activated to secrete several chemical signals. These chemical signals include adenosine diphosphate (ADP), thromboxane A2, and a fatty acid (arachidonic acid). When released, these substances affect both local blood flow (by vasoconstriction) and increased platelet aggregation at the site of injury.

Vasoconstriction and platelet plug formation are short-lived and cannot stop the bleeding if an injury is extensive. In the case of an

BOX 27-2 *health matters* | Anticoagulant and Antiplatelet Drug Treatments

Many types of drugs are now available to physicians that help prevent thrombosis and embolism. If an individual is at risk for thrombus formation, the selection of a so-called targeted or rational drug treatment may depend on the location in the vascular system in which the clots may form. Research has shown that venous thrombi consist mainly of fibrin and red blood cells, whereas arterial thrombi consist mainly of platelet aggregates. This information provides a theoretical basis for selecting different types of drug treatment for conditions caused by either venous or arterial thrombi.

For example, **anticoagulant drugs** such as aspirin, heparin, and warfarin should be more effective in prevention of venous thrombi, and drugs that decrease the tendency for platelets to become sticky and form aggregates **(antiplatelet drugs)** should be more effective in preventing arterial thrombi.

A daily low dose of aspirin inhibits the cyclooxygenase-1 (COX-1) enzyme, thus blocking production of the platelet inhibitor thromboxane (see **Figure 25-13** on p. 574). Daily low-dose (81 mg) aspirin therapy prevents thrombosis that can trigger a myocardial infarction (MI). A larger dose of aspirin taken during an MI can lessen its severity (see figure).

Heparin is a naturally occurring "blood thinner" that can be used to prevent excessive clotting. Heparin inhibits the conversion of prothrombin to thrombin, preventing the formation of a thrombus. Warfarin, an oral anticoagulant, is also commonly used to prevent excessive clotting. It blocks the stimulating effect of vitamin K on the liver, and consequently the liver cells make less prothrombin. The prothrombin content soon falls low enough to prevent abnormal clotting.

Despite anticoagulant drugs being called "blood thinners", they do not really dilute the blood. They instead make blood less likely to clot and more likely to flow easily, just as adding "paint thinner" to paint prevents clumping and promotes the smooth flow of paint.

The antiplatelet drug cilostazol inhibits an enzyme called phosphodiesterase, which is involved in platelet aggregation activity. The mechanism of action of this type of drug may explain why a condition such as **intermittent claudication,** which involves cramplike pain in the calves after walking that is caused by occasional arterial microvascular blockages by platelet plugs, often responds well to antiplatelet but not to anticoagulant drug therapy.

Another popular antiplatelet drug is clopidogrel, which exerts its antiplatelet action by blocking adenosine diphosphate (ADP) receptors on the platelet membranes. This drug is used to prevent arterial clots that may cause an MI or stroke. •

Aspirin. Acetylsalicylic acid (aspirin) is a commonly used cyclooxygenase (COX) inhibitor that reduces prostaglandin effects in the body, including blood clotting.

extensive injury, the blood-clotting mechanism is activated to assist in haemostasis.

Platelet plugs are extremely important in controlling so-called microhaemorrhages, which may involve a break in a single capillary. Failure to arrest haemorrhage from these very minor but numerous and widespread capillary breaks can result in life-threatening blood loss.

Platelet plugs are also believed to be involved in causing intermittent arterial microvascular occlusion in certain types of peripheral vascular disease (**Box 27-2**).

Blood Clotting (Coagulation)

The **blood-clotting—or coagulation—**mechanism involves a series of chemical reactions that takes place in a definite and rapid sequence resulting in a net of fibres that traps red blood cells (**Figure 27-20**).

Because of the function of coagulation, the mechanism for producing it must be swift and sure when needed, such as when a vessel is cut or ruptured. Equally important, however, coagulation needs to be prevented from happening when it is not needed because clots can plug up vessels that need to stay open if cells are to receive blood's life-sustaining cargo of oxygen.

The three stages of coagulation described in the following paragraphs are illustrated in **Figure 27-21** and summarized on the right.

These stages of coagulation occur by the action of a host of *coagulation factors* (clotting factors), each of which is essential to normal haemostasis (**Table 27-4**).

Stage 1: Activation pathways
- Intrinsic pathway
- Extrinsic pathway

Stage 2: Thrombin formation

$$\text{Prothrombin} \xrightarrow[\text{Ca}^{++}]{\text{Prothrombin activator}} \text{Thrombin}$$

Stage 3: Fibrin clot formation

$$\text{Fibrinogen} \xrightarrow[\text{Ca}^{++}]{\text{Thrombin}} \text{Fibrin}$$

Activation Pathways

Stage 1 of the clotting mechanism—or *activation*—can be divided into two separate mechanisms called the **extrinsic clotting pathways** and **intrinsic clotting pathways.**

In both pathways a sequential series of chemical reactions called a *clotting cascade* precedes the formation of prothrombin activator. This substance is the catalyst needed for conversion of prothrombin to thrombin in stage 2 of the clotting process (see **Figure 27-21**).

In the extrinsic pathway, chemicals released from damaged tissues that are outside or extrinsic to the blood trigger the cascade of events that ultimately result in formation of prothrombin activator. Initially, tissue damage results in release of a mixture of lipoproteins and phospholipids called *tissue factor* or *factor III*. In the coordinated series of chemical reactions that follow, this factor, in the presence

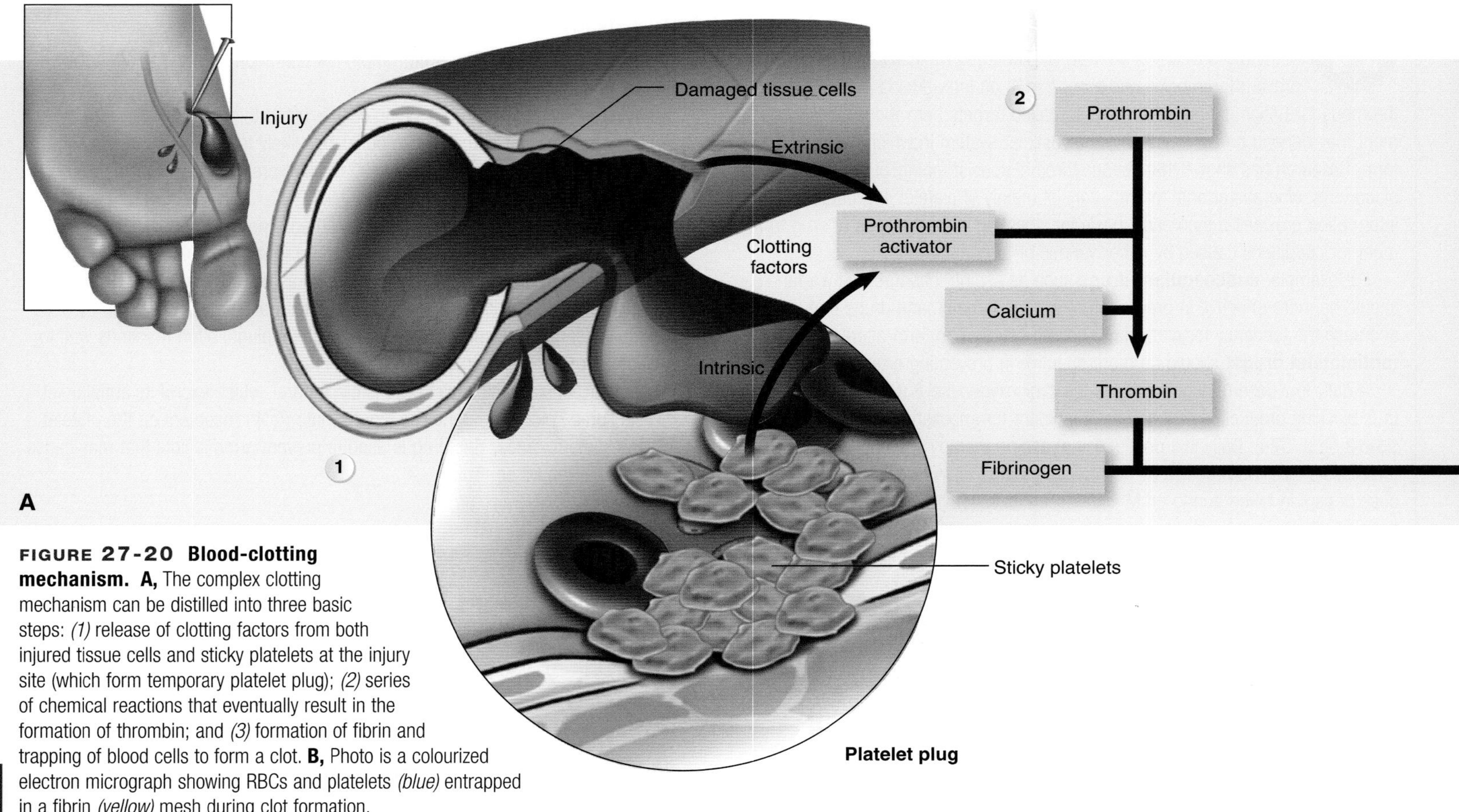

FIGURE 27-20 Blood-clotting mechanism. A, The complex clotting mechanism can be distilled into three basic steps: *(1)* release of clotting factors from both injured tissue cells and sticky platelets at the injury site (which form temporary platelet plug); *(2)* series of chemical reactions that eventually result in the formation of thrombin; and *(3)* formation of fibrin and trapping of blood cells to form a clot. **B,** Photo is a colourized electron micrograph showing RBCs and platelets *(blue)* entrapped in a fibrin *(yellow)* mesh during clot formation.

TABLE 27-4 Coagulation Factors—Standard Nomenclature and Synonyms

FACTOR	COMMON SYNONYM(S)
Factor I	Fibrinogen
Factor II	Prothrombin
Factor III	Thromboplastin Thrombokinase
Factor IV (now obsolete)	Calcium
Factor V	Proaccelerin Labile factor
Factor VI (now obsolete)	Activated factor V (Va)
Factor VII	Serum prothrombin conversion accelerator (SPCA)
Factor VIII	Antihaemophilic globulin (AHG) Antihaemophilic factor (AHF)
Factor IX	Plasma thromboplastin component (PTC), Christmas factor
Factor X	Stuart factor
Factor XI	Plasma thromboplastin antecedent (PTA)
Factor XII	Hageman factor
Factor XIII	Fibrin-stabilizing factor

of calcium ions, factor V, and factor VII, forms a complex that in turn activates factor X and produces prothrombin activator (see **Figure 27-21**, *A*).

The intrinsic pathway involves a series of reactions that begin with factors normally present in, or intrinsic to, the blood. Damage to the endothelial lining of blood vessels exposes collagen fibres, which in turn causes the activation of a number of coagulation factors present in plasma. When activated in this manner, factor XII (Hageman factor) then causes factor XI to activate factor IX. Sticky platelets participate in the intrinsic pathway by releasing a phospholipid called *platelet factor VIII.* This substance activates factor X, which then produces the prothrombin activator (prothrombinase) (see **Figure 27-21**, *B*).

Common Pathway

Regardless of the activation pathway involved, after prothrombin activator is produced, stages 2 and 3 of the blood-clotting mechanism are initiated and a clot will form. Thrombin formed in stage 2 accelerates in stage 3 conversion of the soluble plasma protein fibrinogen to insoluble fibrin. The stage 3 polymerization of fibrin strands into a fibrin clot is accelerated by the presence of activated factor XIII.

Fibrin appears in blood as fine threads all tangled together. Blood cells catch in the entanglement, and because most of the cells are

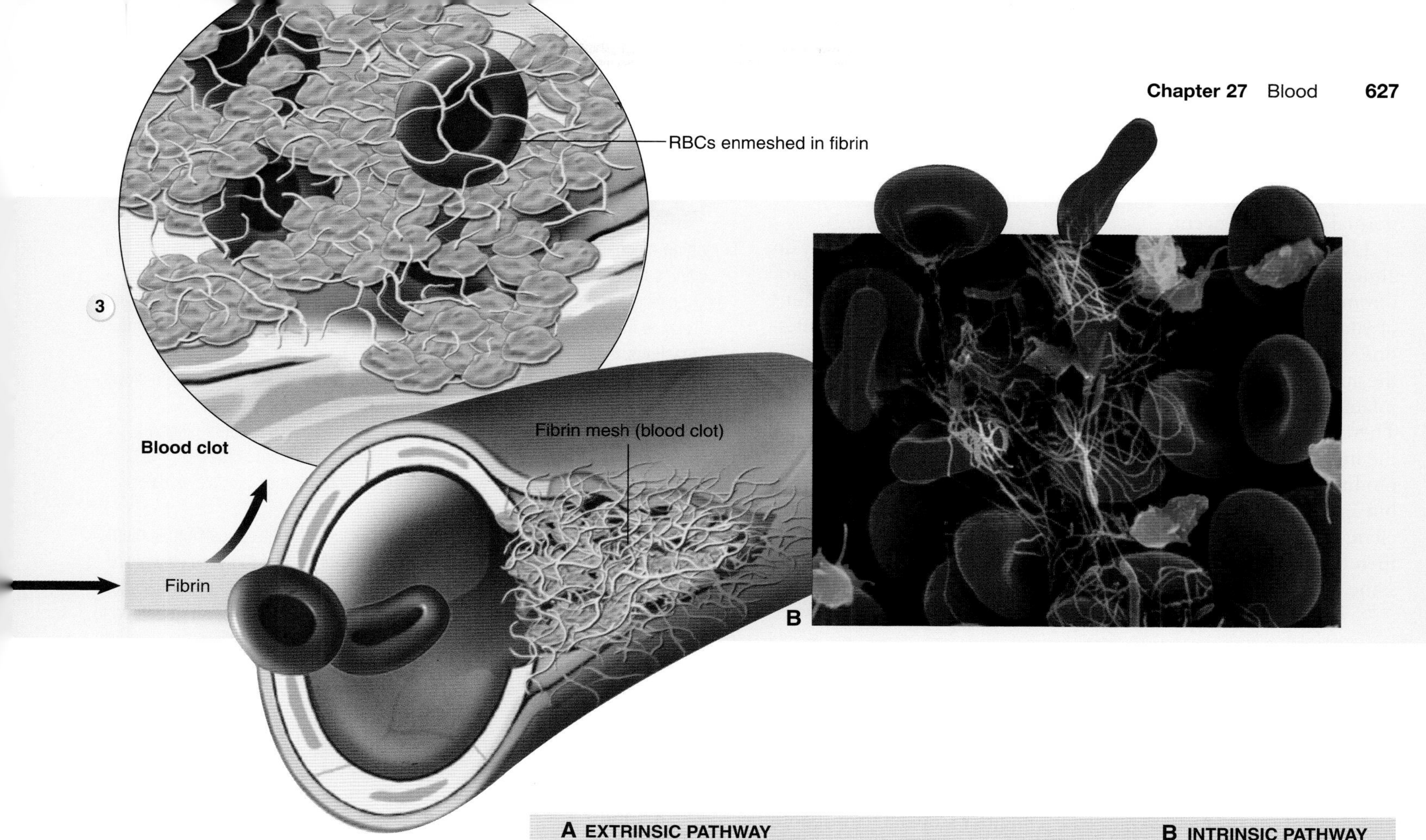

RBCs enmeshed in fibrin

3

Blood clot

Fibrin

Fibrin mesh (blood clot)

B

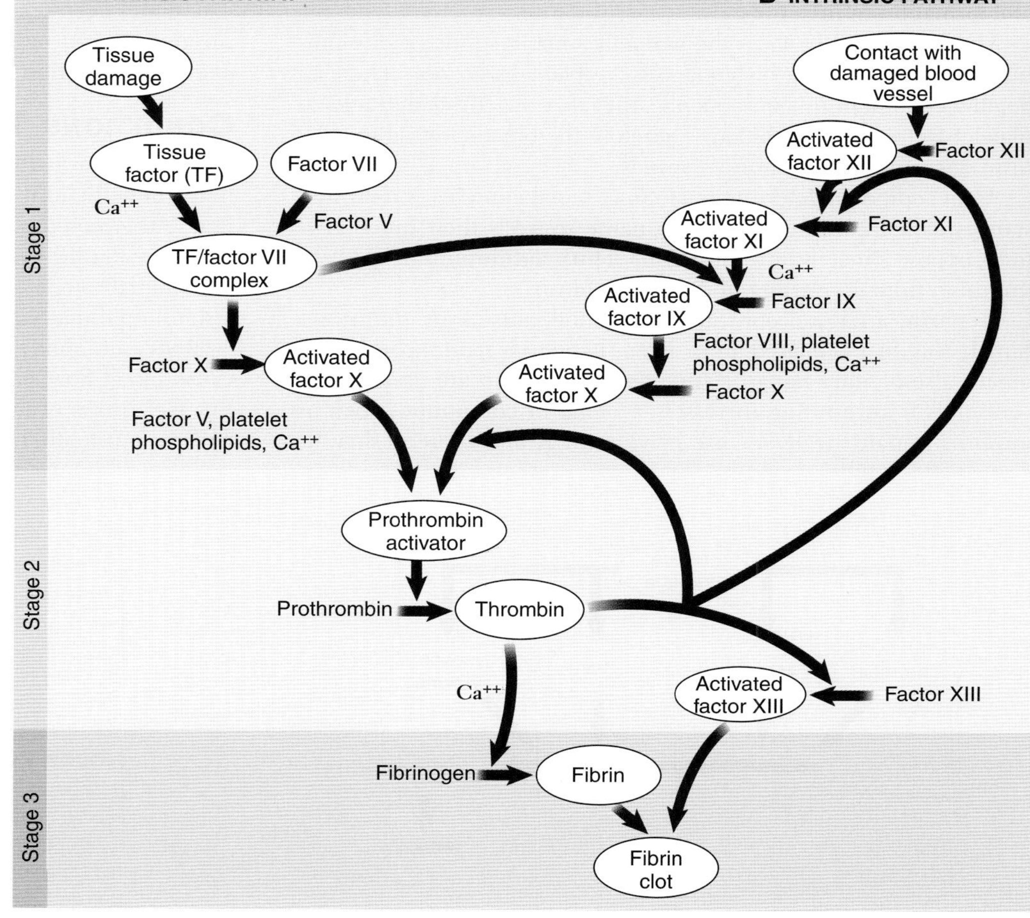

FIGURE 27-21 Clot formation. A, *Extrinsic clotting pathway. Stage 1:* Damaged tissue releases tissue factor, which with factor VII and calcium ions activates factor X. Activated factor X, factor V, phospholipids, and calcium ions form prothrombin activator (prothrombinase). *Stage 2:* Prothrombin is converted to thrombin by prothrombin activator. *Stage 3:* Fibrinogen is converted to fibrin by thrombin. Fibrin forms a clot. **B,** *Intrinsic clotting pathway. Stage 1:* Damaged vessels cause activation of factor XII. Activated factor XII activates factor XI, which activates factor IX. Factor IX, along with factor VIII and platelet phospholipids, activates factor X. Activated factor X, factor V, phospholipids, and calcium ions form prothrombin activator. Stages 2 and 3 constitute the *common pathway* and thus take the same course as after extrinsic activation.

RBCs, clotted blood has a red colour. Note that several of the clotting factors require calcium ions as a co-factor. This explains the need for the presence of adequate calcium levels in the blood for normal clotting to occur.

Liver cells synthesize both prothrombin and fibrinogen as they do almost all other plasma proteins. For the liver to synthesize prothrombin at a normal rate, blood must contain an adequate amount of vitamin K. Vitamin K is absorbed into the blood from the intestine. Some foods contain this vitamin, but it is also synthesized in the intestine by certain bacteria (not fully developed in newborn infants). Because vitamin K is fat soluble, its absorption requires bile. Therefore if the bile ducts become obstructed and bile cannot enter the intestine, a vitamin K deficiency develops. The liver cannot then produce prothrombin at its normal rate, and the blood's prothrombin concentration soon falls below normal. A prothrombin deficiency gives rise to a bleeding tendency. As a preoperative safeguard, therefore, patients with obstructive jaundice are generally given some kind of vitamin K preparation.

CONNECT IT! 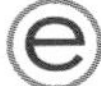

The role of gut microorganisms in producing the vitamin K needed for blood clotting is found in ***The Human Microbiome*** at ***Connect It!***

Conditions That Oppose Clotting

Although blood clotting goes on continuously and concurrently with clot dissolution (*fibrinolysis*), several conditions operate to oppose clot formation in intact vessels.

Most important by far is the perfectly smooth surface of the normal endothelial lining of blood vessels. Platelets do not adhere to healthy endothelium; consequently, they do not activate and release platelet factors into the blood. Therefore the blood-clotting mechanism does not begin in normal vessels.

As an additional deterrent to clotting, blood contains certain substances called *antithrombins*. The name suggests their function—they oppose (inactivate) thrombin. Thus antithrombins prevent thrombin from converting fibrinogen to fibrin.

Heparin, a natural constituent of blood, acts as an antithrombin. It was first prepared from liver (hence its name), but other organs also contain heparin. Injections of heparin are used to prevent clots from forming in vessels. *Coumarin* compounds such as *warfarin* impair the liver's use of vitamin K and thereby slow its synthesis of prothrombin and factors VII, IX, and X. Indirectly, therefore, coumarin compounds retard coagulation. Direct thrombin inhibitors such as dabigatran can be administered orally to prevent clotting.

Citrates keep donor blood from clotting before transfusion. Aspirin and other drugs, such as clopidogrel or cilostazol, that inhibit platelet aggregation also inhibit coagulation (see **Box 27-2**).

Conditions That Hasten Clotting

Two conditions particularly favour thrombus formation: a rough spot in the endothelium (blood vessel lining) and abnormally slow blood flow. Atherosclerosis, for example, is associated with an increased tendency toward **thrombosis,** the abnormal formation of clots. It is endothelial rough spots in the form of plaques of accumulated cholesterol lipid material that could trigger abnormal clot formation.

Body immobility, on the other hand, may lead to thrombosis because blood flow slows down as movements decrease. Incidentally, this fact is one of the major reasons why physicians insist that bed patients must either move or be moved frequently.

Once started, a clot tends to grow. Platelets enmeshed in the fibrin threads activate, releasing more thromboplastin, which, in turn, causes more clotting, which enmeshes more platelets, and so on, in a positive-feedback loop. Normally, this is desirable because it quickly builds a large clot to stop bleeding when the need arises. However, it can be harmful when a clot forms inappropriately. Clot-retarding substances

BOX 27-3 *health matters*

Clinical Methods of Hastening Clotting

One way of treating excessive bleeding is to speed up the blood-clotting mechanism. This can be accomplished by increasing any of the *procoagulation* substances essential for clotting, for example:

- Applying a rough surface such as gauze causes more platelets to activate and release more platelet factors. This in turn accelerates the first of the clotting reactions.
- Gently squeezing the tissues around a cut vessel constricts vessels and slows bleeding, which helps the coagulation process.
- Applying purified thrombin (in the form of sprays or impregnated gelatin sponges that can be left in a wound) accelerates the third stage.
- Applying cold compresses, which causes vasoconstriction and slows blood flow, can stop some superficial bleeding.
- Applying an alginate dressing made from calcium alginate or calcium sodium alginate derived from brown seaweed. Alginate dressings form a highly absorbent gel suitable for use on exuding wounds. They also act as a haemostatic, but caution is needed because blood clots can cause the dressing to adhere to the wound surface.

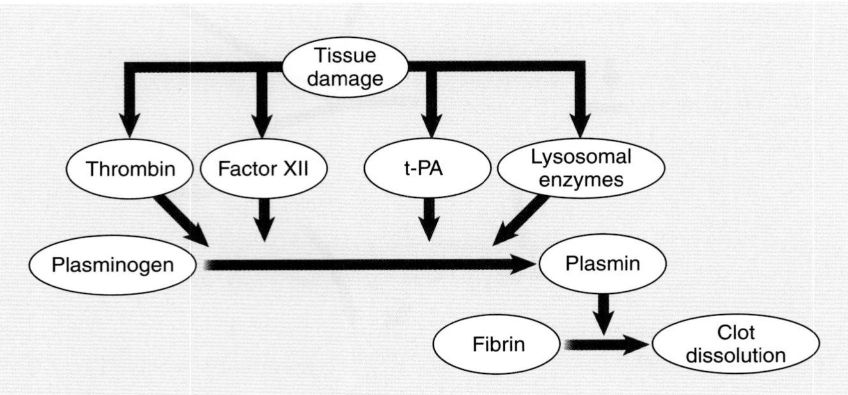

FIGURE 27-22 Fibrinolysis. Dissolution of a clot by fibrinolysis is triggered by the same events as those producing the clot but operates at a slower rate. Plasminogen is converted into the active enzyme plasmin by thrombin, factor XII, tissue plasminogen activator *(t-PA),* and lysosomal enzymes. Plasmin hydrolyzes fibrin strands and dissolves the clot.

have proved valuable for retarding this process. **Box 27-3** discusses some methods for therapeutically hastening clotting to stop bleeding.

Clot Dissolution

The physiological mechanism that dissolves clots is known as **fibrinolysis** (**Figure 27-22**). Evidence indicates that the two opposing processes of clot formation and fibrinolysis go on continuously. Normal blood contains an inactive plasma protein called *plasminogen* that can be activated by several substances released from damaged cells. These converting substances include thrombin, factor XII, tissue plasminogen activator (t-PA), and lysosomal enzymes. Plasmin hydrolyzes fibrin strands and dissolves the clot (see **Figure 27-22**).

In today's clinical practice, several different kinds of proteins are used to dissolve blood clots that are causing an acute medical crisis. These are enzymes that generate plasmin when injected into patients. Streptokinase (SK) is a plasminogen-activating factor made by certain *Streptococci* bacteria. It and recombinant t-PA can be used to dissolve clots in the large arteries of the heart, which, when blocked, can result in myocardial infarction (heart attack). In addition, t-PA has been recognized as a promising drug for the early treatment of strokes. If given within the first 6 hours after a clot forms in a cerebral vessel, it can often improve blood flow and greatly reduce the serious aftereffects of a stroke.

The fact that streptococcal bacteria can form blood-dissolving factors such as SK is an important one. Recall that a secondary function of blood clotting is to trap bacteria that attempt to enter our tissues. To make their attack more effective, many bacteria, such as *Streptococcus* "strep" species, *Staphylococcus* "staph" species, *Escherichia coli* (*E. coli*), and others, release anticlotting agents to overcome our defences. Such agents often activate plasminogen and thus disrupt formation of the initial blood clot. Some bacterial agents instead bind fibrinogen to disrupt normal clotting.

Quick CHECK

9. List the granulocytic and agranulocytic leucocytes.
10. List the normal percentages of the different WBCs in a differential count.
11. List the four ABO blood groups, and identify the antigens and antibodies (if any) associated with each.
12. Identify the two basic coagulation steps.

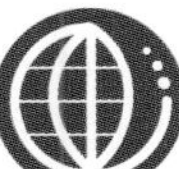

the big picture | Blood and the Whole Body

In every chapter of this book we have referred to the notion that the whole body's function is geared toward maintaining stability of the internal fluid environment—that is, *homeostasis.* The fluid that makes up the internal environment in which cells are bathed—the fluid that must be kept stable—includes the plasma of the blood. As a matter of fact, it is the blood plasma that transports substances, and even heat, around the internal environment so that all body tissues are linked together. The various tissues of the body are linked by the plasma, which circulates between any two points served by blood vessels. This, of course, means that substances such as nutrients, wastes, dissolved gases, water, antibodies, and hormones can be transported between almost any two points in the body.

Blood tissue is not just plasma, however. It contains the *formed elements*—the blood cells and platelets. The RBCs participate in the mechanisms that permit the efficient transport of the gases oxygen and carbon dioxide. WBCs are important in the defence mechanisms of the whole body. Their presence in blood ensures that they are available to all parts of the body, all of the time, to fight cancer, resist infectious agents, and clean up injured tissues. Platelets provide mechanisms for preventing loss of the fluid that constitutes our internal environment.

All other organs and systems of the body rely on blood to perform their many functions. No organ or system can maintain proper levels of nutrients, dissolved gases, or water without direct or indirect help from the blood. On the other hand, many other systems help blood do its job. For example, the respiratory system excretes carbon dioxide from the blood and picks up oxygen. Organs of the digestive system pick up nutrients, remove some toxins, and dispose of old blood cells. The endocrine system regulates the production of blood cells and the water content of the plasma. Besides removing toxic wastes such as urea, the urinary system has a vital role in maintaining homeostasis of plasma water concentration and pH.

Of course, blood is useless unless it continually and rapidly flows around the whole body—and continues to transport, defend, and maintain balance. The next several chapters outline the structures and functions that make this possible. Chapters 28 through 30 discuss the plan of the blood circulation and how adequate blood flow is maintained. Chapter 31 discusses the role of the lymphatic system in maintaining the fluid balance of the blood. Chapters 32 through 34 deal with the defensive mechanisms of blood and related tissues. As a matter of fact, most of the remaining chapters feature the role of blood in maintaining stability of the whole body.

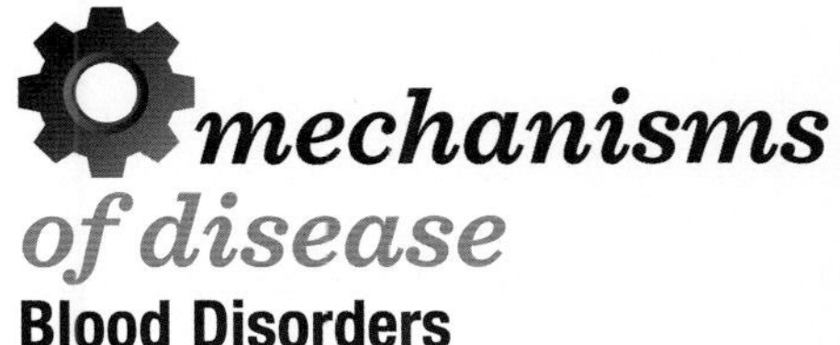

Blood Disorders

Most blood diseases are disorders of the formed elements. Thus it is not surprising that the basic mechanism of many blood diseases is the failure of the blood-producing myeloid and lymphatic tissues to properly form blood cells. In many cases, this failure is the result of damage by drugs, toxic chemicals, or radiation. In other cases, it results from an inherited defect or even cancer.

If bone marrow failure is the suspected cause of a particular blood disorder, a sample of myeloid tissue may be drawn into a syringe. The bone marrow is obtained from inside the pelvic bone (iliac crest) or the sternum. This procedure, called **aspiration biopsy cytology** (ABC), allows examination of the tissue that may help confirm or reject a tentative diagnosis. If the bone marrow is severely damaged, the choice of a **bone marrow transplant** may be offered to the patient. In this procedure, myeloid tissue from a compatible donor is introduced into the recipient intravenously. If the recipient's immune system does not reject the new tissue, which is always a danger in this type of tissue transplant, the donor cells may establish a colony of new, healthy tissue in the bone marrow. In some cases, infusion of healthy marrow follows total body irradiation. This treatment destroys the diseased marrow, permitting the new tissue to grow.

Red Blood Cell Disorders

Anaemia

The term *anaemia* is used to describe different disease conditions caused by an inability of the blood to carry sufficient oxygen to the body cells. Anaemias can result from inadequate numbers of RBCs or a deficiency of oxygen-carrying haemoglobin. Thus anaemia can occur if the haemoglobin in RBCs is inadequate, even if normal numbers of RBCs are present.

Anaemia Resulting from Changes in RBC Number

Anaemias caused by an actual change in the number of RBCs can occur if blood is lost by haemorrhage, as with accidents or bleeding ulcers or if the blood-forming tissues cannot maintain normal numbers of blood cells. Such failures occur because of cancer, chemotherapy treatment, radiation (x-ray) damage, and certain types of infections. If bone marrow produces an excess of RBCs, the result is a condition called **polycythaemia.** The blood in individuals suffering from this condition may contain so many RBCs that it may become too thick to flow properly.

One type of anaemia characterized by an abnormally low number of red blood cells is **aplastic anaemia.** Although idiopathic forms of this disease occur, most cases result from destruction of bone marrow by drugs, toxic chemicals, or radiation. Less commonly, aplastic anaemia results from bone marrow destruction by cancer. Because tissues that produce other formed elements are also affected, aplastic anaemia is usually accompanied by a decreased number of WBCs and platelets. Bone marrow transplants have been successful in treating some cases of aplastic anaemia.

Pernicious anaemia is another disorder characterized by a low number of RBCs. Pernicious anaemia sometimes results from a dietary deficiency of vitamin B_{12}. Vitamin B_{12} is used in the formation of new RBCs in the bone marrow. In many cases, pernicious anaemia results from the failure of the stomach lining to produce *intrinsic factor*—the substance that allows vitamin B_{12} to be absorbed. Pernicious anaemia can be fatal if not successfully treated. One method of treatment involves intramuscular injections of vitamin B_{12}.

Folate deficiency anaemia is similar to pernicious anaemia because it also causes a decrease in the RBC count resulting from a vitamin deficiency. In this condition, it is *folic acid* (vitamin B_9) that is deficient. Folic acid deficiencies are common among individuals with alcoholism and other malnourished individuals. Treatment for folate deficiency **acute anaemia** involves taking vitamin supplements until a balanced diet can be restored.

Of course, a significant reduction in the number of RBCs can occur as a result of blood loss. **Blood loss anaemia** often occurs after haemorrhages associated with trauma, extensive surgeries, or other situations involving a sudden loss of blood. **Anaemia of chronic disease** can be a serious complication of chronic inflammatory diseases and cancer; the cause is often unknown.

Changes in Haemoglobin

The amount and quality of haemoglobin within RBCs are just as important as the number of RBCs. In haemoglobin disorders, RBCs are sometimes classified as **hyperchromic** (abnormally high haemoglobin content) or **hypochromic** (abnormally low haemoglobin content).

Iron (Fe) is a critical component of the haemoglobin molecule, forming the central core of each haem group (see **Figure 27-5** on p. 615). Without adequate iron in the diet, the body cannot manufacture enough haemoglobin. The result is **iron deficiency anaemia**—a worldwide medical problem. Although the body carefully protects its iron reserves, they may be depleted through haemorrhage, increased requirements such as wound healing or pregnancy, or low intake. Unfortunately, iron deficiency is the most common nutritional deficiency in the world. The tragic result is that an estimated 10% of the population in some developed countries and up to 50% in developing countries suffers from iron deficiency anaemia. Oral administration of iron-containing compounds, such as ferrous sulfate or ferrous gluconate, is very effective in treating the basic iron deficiency seen in the disease. **Figure 27-23** shows a peripheral blood smear from an individual with iron deficiency anaemia. The numbers of RBCs are only slightly below normal. Note, however, that the cells are small (microcytic) and appear pale (hypochromic) because of the reduction in haemoglobin content.

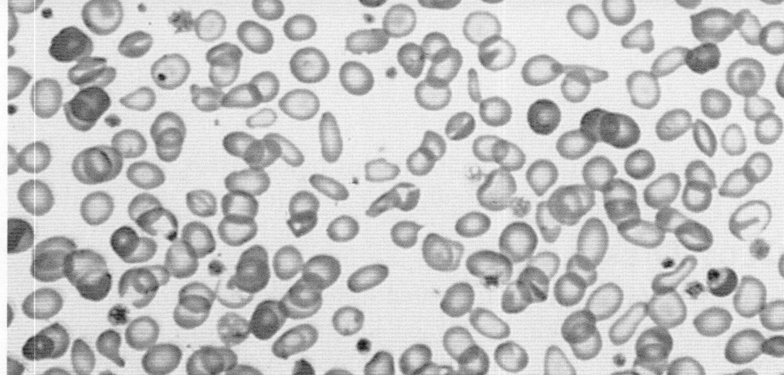

FIGURE 27-23 Iron deficiency anaemia. Note the small (microcytic), pale (hypochromic) red blood cells (RBCs). Lack of adequate colour in the RBCs is due to reduced haemoglobin content.

The term **haemolytic anaemia** applies to any of a variety of inherited blood disorders characterized by abnormal types of haemoglobin. The term *haemolytic* means "relating to blood breakage" and emphasizes the fact that abnormal haemoglobin often causes red blood cells to become distorted and easily broken. An example of a haemolytic anaemia is **sickle cell anaemia.** Another type of haemolytic anaemia is **thalassaemia**. As with sickle cell anaemia, thalassaemia is an inherited disorder, with both a mild and a severe form (*thalassaemia minor* and *thalassaemia major*).

White Blood Cell Disorders

The term *leucopenia* refers to an abnormally low WBC count (less than 4000 cells/mm^3 [4.0×10^9/L] of blood). Various disease conditions may affect the immune system and decrease the amount of circulating WBCs. Acquired immunodeficiency syndrome, or AIDS, results in marked leucopenia. *Leucocytosis* refers to an abnormally high WBC count. It is a much more common problem than leucopenia, is seen in most types of leukaemia, and almost always accompanies bacterial infections.

Two major groups of disease conditions constitute a majority of WBC and blood-related cancers, or malignant neoplasms. **Lymphoid neoplasms** arise from lymphoid precursor cells that normally produce B lymphocytes, T lymphocytes, or their descendent cell types. **Myeloid neoplasms** appear as a result of malignant transformation of myeloid stem or precursor cells that normally produce granulocytic WBCs, monocytes, RBCs, and platelets.

Multiple Myeloma

Multiple myeloma is cancer of antibody-secreting B lymphocytes called *plasma cells* (**Figure 27-24**, *B*). It is one of the most common and one of the most deadly forms of blood-related cancers in people older than 65 years of age. The cancerous transformation of plasma cells results in impairment of bone marrow function, production of defective antibodies, recurrent infections (from neutropenia), anaemia, and the painful destruction and fracture of bones in the skull and throughout the skeletal system. The x-ray photo in **Figure 27-24**, *A,* shows the typical "honeycomb" or "punched-out" defects in skull bones caused by the defective myeloma antibody.

Leukaemia

Leukaemia is the term used to describe a number of blood cancers affecting the WBCs. In almost every form of leukaemia, marked leucocytosis occurs. Leucocyte counts in excess of 100,000/mm^3 (100×10^9/L) in circulating blood are common. The different types of leukaemia are identified as either *acute* or

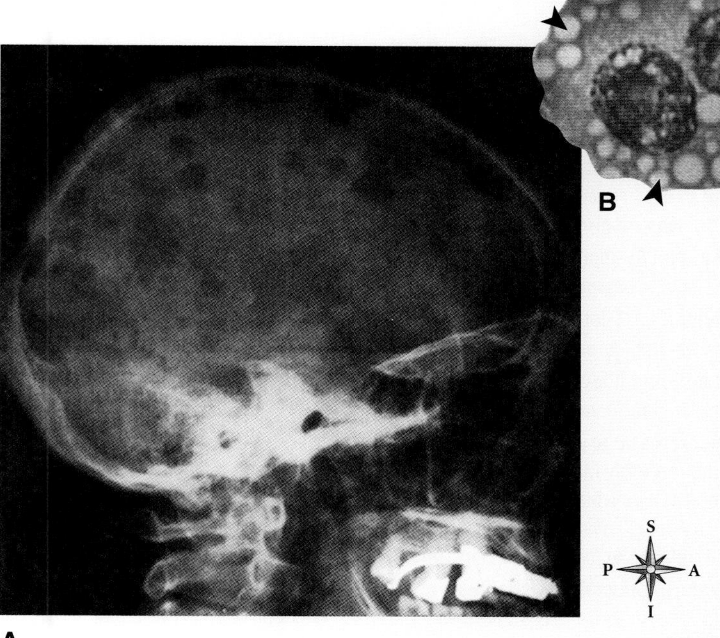

FIGURE 27-24 Multiple myeloma. A, Radiograph of skull showing "honeycomb" or "punched-out" appearance of bones caused by defective antibodies from plasma cells. Normal skull bones would instead have a more uniform (less mottled) appearance in a radiograph. **B,** Malignant plasma cell. Vesicles *(arrowheads)* contain defective antibodies.

chronic, based on how quickly symptoms appear after the disease begins, and as *lymphocytic* or *myeloid,* depending on the cell type involved.

CONNECT IT! 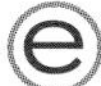

Four of the most common leukaemias are briefly described and illustrated in ***Types of Leukaemia*** online at ***Connect It!***

Infectious Mononucleosis

Infectious mononucleosis is a common noncancerous WBC disorder appearing most often in adolescents and young adults between 15 and 25 years of age. It is caused by a virus found in the saliva of infected individuals. Leucocytosis is common early in the disease, with total WBC counts averaging between 12,000 and 18,000/mm^3 (12.0–18.0 $\times$ 10^9/L). More than 60% of the leucocytes can be identified in a differential WBC count as large, *atypical* (abnormal) lymphocytes that have abundant cytoplasm and a large nucleus (**Figure 27-25**). Symptoms vary greatly, but, in addition to the leucocytosis and atypical lymphocytes seen in peripheral blood, fever, sore throat, rash, severe fatigue, and enlargement of lymph nodes and the spleen are common findings. Infectious "mono" is generally self-limited and resolves without complications in about 4 to 6 weeks, although fatigue may last for longer periods.

Clotting Disorders

Unfortunately, clots sometimes form in unbroken blood vessels of the heart, brain, lungs, or other organs—a dreaded thing because clots may produce sudden death by shutting off the blood supply to a vital organ. When a clot stays in the place where it formed, it is called a **thrombus,** and the condition itself is spoken of as *thrombosis.* If all or part of a clot dislodges and circulates through the bloodstream, it is called an **embolus,** and the condition is called an **embolism.**

Thrombosis and embolism cause most myocardial infarctions (MIs or "heart attacks") and cerebrovascular accidents (CVAs or "strokes"), making them the leading cause of death in developed countries. **Box 27-2** on p. 625 discusses various therapies to prevent the dangers of thrombus formation.

Haemophilia is an X-linked inherited disorder that affects 1 in every 10,000 males worldwide. It results from a failure to produce one or more plasma proteins responsible for blood clotting—a process illustrated in **Figure 27-20**. Thus haemophilia is characterized by a relative inability to form blood clots. Because minor blood vessel injuries are common in ordinary life, haemophilia can be a life-threatening condition. The most common form is called *haemophilia A.* It is caused by absence of factor VIII protein and affects more than 300,000 people around the world.

CONNECT IT! 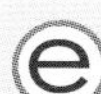

Crushing injuries of skeletal muscle can cause widespread abnormal clotting. Review the article ***Rhabdomyolysis*** online at ***Connect It!***

Historically, factor VIII was obtained by plasma fractionation. This method cannot meet demand given the shortage of available donated blood. Currently, recombinant methods are used to produce enough recombinant antihaemophilic factor VIII (rAHF) to meet the therapeutic needs of the world's haemophiliac population. Increasing amounts are needed to meet the larger quantities required as adolescent patients mature and as physicians prescribe more factor VIII to prevent as well as to treat bleeding episodes. A more common type of clotting disorder results from a decrease in the platelet count—a condition called **thrombocytopenia.** This condition is characterized by bleeding from many small blood vessels throughout the body, most visibly in the skin and mucous membranes. If the number of thrombocytes falls to 20,000/mm^3 (20 $\times$ 10^9/L) or less (normal range is 150,000 to 400,000/mm^3 [150–400 $\times$ 10^9/L]), catastrophic bleeding may occur. Although a number of different mechanisms can result in thrombocytopenia, the usual cause is bone marrow destruction by drugs or an immune system disease, chemicals, radiation, or cancer. Drugs may cause thrombocytopenia as a side effect. In such cases, stopping the drug usually solves the problem.

CONNECT IT! 

The blood's ability to clot can be determined by tests such as *prothrombin time (PT),* which help monitor the success of therapies for clotting disorders. For a brief synopsis of this clinical lab test, check out ***Prothrombin Time*** online at ***Connect It!***

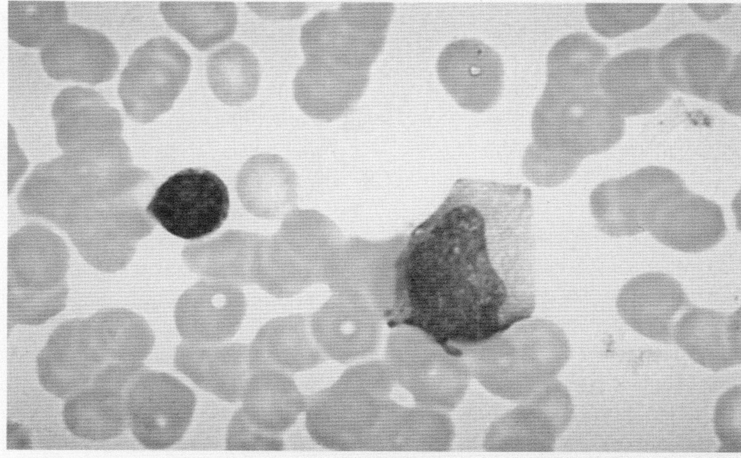

FIGURE 27-25 Infectious mononucleosis. The cell on the left is a typical small lymphocyte with the nucleus almost filling the cell. The larger atypical lymphocyte on the right has much more cytoplasm and a larger nucleus.

LANGUAGE OF SCIENCE *(continued from p. 610)*

formed element (formd EL-eh-ment)
[*element* **first principle**]

globin (GLOH-bin)
[*glob-* **ball,** *-in* **substance**]

granulocyte (GRAN-yoo-loh-syte)
[*gran-* **grain,** *-ul-* **little,** *-cyte* **cell**]

haematopoietic stem cell (hee-mah-toh-poy-ET-ik)
[*haemato-* **blood,** *-poietic* **referring to making**]

haem (heem)
[*haem-* **blood**]

haemoglobin (Hb) (hee-moh-GLOH-bin)
[*haemo-* **blood,** *-globus* **ball**]

heparin (HEP-ah-rin)
[*hepar-* **liver,** *-in* **substance**]

interleukin (IL) (in-ter-LOO-kin)
[*inter-* **between,** *-leuco-* **white (blood cell),** *-in* **substance**]

intrinsic clotting pathway (in-TRIN-sik)
[*intr-* **within,** *-sic* **beside**]

leucocyte (LOO-koh-syte)
[*leuco-* **white,** *-cyte* **cell**]

leucopoiesis (loo-koh-poy-EE-sis)
[*leuco-* **white,** *-poiesis* **making**]

lymphocyte (LIM-foh-syte)
[*lymph-* **water (lymphatic system),** *-cyte* **cell**]

monocyte (MON-oh-syte)
[*mono-* **single,** *-cyte* **cell**]

neutrophil (NYOO-troh-fil)
[*neutr-* **neither,** *-phil* **love**]

nonelectrolyte (non-ee-LEK-troh-lyte)
[*non-* **not,** *-electro-* **electricity,** *-lyt-* **loosening**]

plasma (PLAZ-mah)
[*plasma* **substance**]

platelet (PLAYT-let)
[*plate-* **flat,** *-let* **small**]

platelet plug (PLAYT-let)
[*plate-* **flat,** *-let* **small**]

polychromatic erythroblast (pol-ee-kroh-MAT-ik ee-RITH-roh-blast)
[*poly-* **many,** *-chromat-* **colour,** *-ic* **relating to,** *erythro-* **red,** *-blast* **bud**]

polymorphonuclear leucocyte (pol-ee-mohr-foh-NYOO-klee-er LOO-koh-syte)
[*poly-* **many,** *-morph-* **form,** *-nucle-* **nut or kernel,** *-ar* **relating to,** *leuco-* **white,** *-cyte* **cell**]

proerythroblast (proh-eh-rith-roh-BLAST)
[*pro-* **first,** *-erythro-* **red,** *-blast* **bud**]

reticulocyte (reh-TIK-yoo-loh-syte)
[*ret-* **net,** *-ic-* **relating to,** *-ul-* **little,** *-cyte* **cell**]

thrombopoiesis (throm-boh-poy-EE-sis)
[*thromb-* **clot,** *-poiesis* **making**]

thrombus (THROM-bus)
[*thrombus* **clot**] *pl.,* thrombi

vasoconstriction (vay-soh-kon-STRIK-shun)
[*vas-* **vessel,** *-constrict-* **draw tight,** *-tion* **state**]

LANGUAGE OF MEDICINE

acute anaemia (ah-KYOOT ah-NEE-mee-ah)
[*acu-* **sharp,** *an-* **without,** *-aem-* **blood,** *-ia* **condition**]

acute lymphocytic leukaemia (ALL) (ah-KYOOT LIM-foh-sit-ik loo-KEE-mee-ah)
[*acu-* **sharp,** *lymph-* **water (lymphatic system),** *-cyt-* **cell,** *-ic* **relating to,** *leuk-* **white,** *-aem-* **blood,** *-ia* **condition**]

acute myeloid leukaemia (AML) (ah-KYOOT MY-eh-loyd loo-KEE-mee-ah)
[*acu-* **sharp,** *myel-* **marrow,** *-oid* **like,** *leuk-* **white,** *-aem-* **blood,** *-ia* **condition**]

anaemia (ah-NEE-mee-ah)
[*an-* **without,** *-aem-* **blood,** *-ia* **condition**]

anaemia of chronic disease (ah-NEE-mee-ah KRON-ik)
[*an-* **without,** *-aem-* **blood,** *-ia* **condition,** *chron-* **time,** *-ic* **relating to**]

antianaemic principle (an-tee-ah-NEE-mik)
[*anti-* **against,** *-an-* **without,** *-aem-* **blood,** *-ia* **condition,** *-ic* **relating to**]

anticoagulant drug (an-tee-koh-AG-yoo-lant)
[*anti-* **against,** *-coagul-* **curdle,** *-ant* **agent**]

antiplatelet drug (an-tee-PLAYT-let)
[*anti-* **against,** *-plate-* **flat,** *-let* **small**]

aplastic anaemia (a-PLAS-tik ah-NEE-mee-ah)
[*a-* **without,** *-plast-* **form,** *-ic* **relating to,** *an-* **without,** *-aemia-* **condition of blood**]

aspiration biopsy cytology (ass-pih-RAY-shen BYE-op-see sye-TOL-oh-jee)
[*a-* **act of,** *-spir-* **breathe,** *-ation* **process,** *bio-* **life,** *-ops-* **view,** *-y* **act of,** *cyt-* **cell,** *-o-* **combining form,** *-log-* **words (study of),** *-y* **activity**]

blood loss anaemia (ah-NEE-mee-ah)
[*an-* **without,** *-aem-* **blood,** *-ia* **condition**]

bone marrow transplant (bohn MAIR-oh TRANZ-plant)

chronic lymphocytic leukaemia (CLL) (KRON-ik LIM-foh-sit-ik loo-KEE-mee-ah)
[*chron-* **time,** *-ic* **relating to,** *lymph-* **water (lymphatic system),** *-cyte* **cell,** *leuk-* **white,** *-aem-* **blood,** *-ia* **condition**]

chronic myeloid leukaemia (CML) (KRON-ik MY-eh-loyd loo-KEE-mee-ah)
[*chron-* **time,** *-ic* **relating to,** *myel-* **bone marrow,** *leuk-* **white,** *-aem-* **blood,** *-ia* **condition**]

coagulation (koh-ag-yoo-LAY-shen)
[*coagul-* **curdle,** *-ation* **process**]

complete blood cell count (CBC) (kom-PLEET blud sel kownt)

differential white blood cell count (dif-er-EN-shal)
[*different-* **difference,** *-al* **relating to,** *cell-* **storeroom**]

embolism (EM-boh-liz-em)
[*embol-* **plug,** *-ism* **condition**]

embolus (EM-boh-lus)
[*embolus* **plug**]

erythroblastosis fetalis (eh-rith-roh-blas-TOH-sis feh-TAL-is)
[*erythro-* **red,** *-blast-* **bud,** *-osis* **condition,** *fet-* **offspring**, *-al-* **relating to,** *-is* **thing**]

erythrocyte sedimentation rate (ESR) (eh-RITH-roh-syte sed-i-men-TAY-shen)
[*erythro-* **red,** *-cyte* **cell**]

folate deficiency anaemia (FOH-layt deh-FISH-en-see ah-NEE-mee-ah)
[*fol-* **leaf,** *-ate* **relating to,** *an-* **without,** *-aem-* **blood,** *-ia* **condition**]

haematocrit (Hct) (hee-MAT-oh-krit)
[*haemato-* **blood,** *-crit* **separate**]

haemolytic anaemia (hee-moh-LIT-ik ah-NEE-mee-ah)
[*haemo-* **blood,** *-lyt-* **loosen,** *-ic* **relating to,** *an-* **without,** *-aem-* **blood,** *-ia* **condition**]

haemophilia (hee-moh-FIL-ee-ah)
[*haemo-* **blood,** *-phil-* **love,** *-ia* **condition**]

haemostasis (hee-moh-STAY-sis)
[*haemo-* **blood,** *-stasis* **standing**]

hyperchromic (hye-per-KROH-mik)
[*hyper-* **excessive,** *-chrom-* **colour,** *-ic* **relating to**]

hypochromic (hye-poh-KROH-mik)
[*hypo-* **under or below,** *-chrom-* **colour,** *-ic* **relating to**]

infectious mononucleosis (in-FEK-shuss mon-oh-nyoo-klee-OH-sis)
[*infect-* **stain,** *-ous* **relating to,** *mono-* **single,** *-nucle-* **nut,** *-osis* **condition**]

intermittent claudication (in-ter-MIT-tent klaw-dih-KAY-shun)
[*inter-* **between,** *-mitt-* **send,** *claudica-* **limping,** *-ation* **process**]

iron deficiency anaemia (EYE-ern deh-FISH-en-see ah-NEE-mee-ah)
[*iron* **strong metal,** *de-* **down,** *-fic-* **perform,** *-ency* **state,** *an-* **without,** *-aem-* **blood,** *-ia* **condition**]

leukaemia (loo-KEE-mee-ah)
[*leuk-* **white,** *-aem-* **blood**, *-ia* **condition**]

leucocytosis (loo-koh-sye-TOH-sis)
[*leuco-* **white,** *-cyt-* **cell,** *-osis* **condition**]

leucopenia (loo-koh-PEE-nee-ah)
[*leuco-* **white,** *-penia* **lack**]

lymphoid neoplasm (LIM-foyd NEE-oh-plaz-em)
[*lymph-* **water (lymphatic system),** *-oid* **like,** *neo-* **new,** *-plasm* **substance**]

multiple myeloma (my-eh-LOH-mah)
[*myel-* **marrow,** *-oma* **tumour**]

myeloid neoplasm
(MY-eh-loyd NEE-oh-plaz-em)
[*myel-* **marrow,** *-oid* **like,** *neo-* **new,** *-plasm* **substance**]

packed cell volume (PCV)
(pakt sell VOL-yoom)

pernicious anaemia
(per-NISH-us ah-NEE-mee-ah)
[*pernici-* **destruction,** *-ous* **relating to,** *an-* **without,** *-aem-* **blood,** *-ia* **condition**]

physiological polycythaemia
(fiz-ee-oh-LOJ-ih-kal pol-ee-sye-THEE-mee-ah)
[*physi-* **nature,** *-o-* **combining form,** *-log-* **words (study of),** *-y* **activity,** *poly-* **many,** *-cyt-* **cell,** *-(h)aem-* **blood,** *-ia* **condition**]

polycythaemia
(pahl-ee-sye-THEE-mee-ah)
[*poly-* **many,** *-cyt-* **cell,** *-(h)aem-* **blood,** *-ia* **condition**]

sickle cell anaemia
(SIK-ul sell ah-NEE-mee-ah)
[*sickle* **crescent,** *cell* **storeroom,** *an-* **without,** *-aem-* **blood,** *-ia* **condition**]

thalassaemia (thal-ah-SEE-mee-ah)
[*thalass-* **sea,** *-aem-* **blood,** *-ia* **condition**]

thrombocytopenia
(throm-boh-sye-toh-PEE-nee-ah)
[*thrombo-* **clot,** *-cyto-* **cell,** *-penia* **lack**]

thrombosis (throm-BOH-sis)
[*thrombo-* **clot,** *-osis* **condition**]

transfusion reaction
(tranz-FYOO-zhun ree-AK-shun)
[*trans-* **across,** *-fus-* **pour,** *-sion* **process,** *re-* **again,** *-action* **action**]

case study

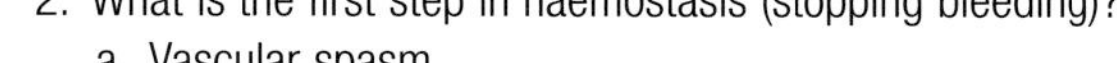

Duncan is slicing a bagel to put in the toaster. When the microwave beeps, he glances in that direction, taking his eyes off the bagel for a split second. In that split second, the knife slips and cuts deeply into his finger. Immediately, blood starts spurting out of the damaged blood vessels.

Duncan grabs a towel and wraps it tightly around the cut, while holding his hand above his heart.

1. What is the main component of the blood by volume coming out of Duncan's finger?
   a. Erythrocytes
   b. Leucocytes
   c. Plasma
   d. Thrombocytes

Because of the damage to his blood vessels, Duncan's body will immediately start the blood-clotting process.

2. What is the first step in haemostasis (stopping bleeding)?
   a. Vascular spasm
   b. Platelet plug formation
   c. Coagulation
   d. Leucocytic plug formation
3. What is the last step in clot formation?
   a. Fibrinogen converted to fibrin
   b. Prothrombin converted to thrombin
   c. Profibrin converted to fibrin
   d. Factor VIII converted to factor IX
4. If Duncan were missing factor VIII, what condition would he have?
   a. Thrombocytopenia
   b. Pernicious anaemia
   c. Polycythaemia
   d. Haemophilia

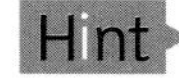
To solve a case study, you may have to refer to the glossary or index, other chapters in this textbook, ***Connect It!,*** and other resources.

UNIT 4

CHAPTER SUMMARY

To download an MP3 version of the chapter summary for use with your mobile device, access the ***Audio Chapter Summaries*** *online at evolve.elsevier.com.*

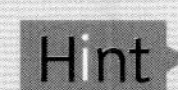
Scan this summary after reading the chapter to help you reinforce the key concepts. Later, use the summary as a quick review before your class or before a test.

Composition of Blood

A. Structure and function of blood (**Figure 27-1**)
   1. Blood—made up of plasma and formed elements
   2. Blood—complex transport medium that performs vital pickup and delivery services for the body
   3. Blood—keystone of body's heat-regulating mechanism

B. Blood volume
   1. Young adult male has approximately 5 litres of blood
   2. Blood volume varies according to age, body type, sex, and method of measurement

C. Haematocrit (Hct)—volume percent of whole blood that is red blood cells

Blood Plasma

A. Plasma—liquid part of blood; clear, straw-coloured fluid; made up of 90% water and 10% solutes (**Figure 27-3**)

B. Solutes—6% to 8% of plasma solutes are proteins, consisting of three main compounds:
   1. Albumins—help maintain osmotic balance of the blood
   2. Globulins—essential component of the immunity mechanism
   3. Fibrinogen—key role in blood clotting

C. Plasma proteins have an essential role in maintaining normal blood circulation

Red Blood Cells

A. Structure of RBCs (**Figure 27-4**)
   1. Mature RBCs (erythrocytes) have no nucleus and are shaped like tiny biconcave discs
   2. Do not contain ribosomes, mitochondria, and other organelles typical of most body cells
   3. Primary component is haemoglobin
   4. Most numerous of the formed elements

B. Function of RBCs
   1. RBCs' critical role in the transport of oxygen and carbon dioxide depends on haemoglobin
   2. Carbonic anhydrase (CA)—enzyme in RBCs that catalyzes a reaction that joins carbon dioxide and water to form carbonic acid
   3. Carbonic acid—dissociates and generates bicarbonate ions, which diffuse out of the RBC and serve to transport carbon dioxide in the blood plasma

C. Haemoglobin (**Figure 27-5**)
   1. Within each RBC are approximately 200 to 300 million molecules of haemoglobin
   2. Haemoglobin is made up of four globin chains, with each attached to a haem group
   3. Haemoglobin is able to unite with four oxygen molecules to form oxyhaemoglobin to allow RBCs to transport oxygen where it is needed
   4. A male has a greater amount of haemoglobin than a female
   5. Anaemia—a decrease in number or volume of functional RBCs in a given unit of whole blood

D. Formation of RBCs (review **Figures 27-6** and **27-7**)
   1. Erythropoiesis—entire process of RBC formation
   2. RBC formation begins in the red bone marrow as haematopoietic stem cells and goes through several stages of development to become erythrocytes; entire maturation process requires approximately 4 days
   3. RBCs are created and destroyed at approximately 200 billion per day in an adult; homeostatic mechanisms operate to balance the number of cells formed against the number of cells destroyed

E. Life cycle of RBCs (**Figure 27-8**)
   1. Life span of a circulating RBC averages 105 to 120 days
   2. Macrophage cells phagocytose the aged, abnormal, or fragmented RBCs
   3. Haemoglobin is broken down, and amino acids, iron, and bilirubin are released

F. Blood types (blood groups)
   1. The ABO system (**Figures 27-9** to **27-11**)
      a. Every person's blood belongs to one of four ABO blood groups
      b. Named according to antigens present on RBC membranes
         (1) Type A—antigen A on RBCs
         (2) Type B—antigen B on RBCs
         (3) Type AB—both antigen A and antigen B on RBCs; known as universal recipient
         (4) Type O—neither antigen A nor antigen B on RBCs; known as universal donor
   2. The Rh system (**Figure 27-12**)
      a. Rh-positive blood—Rh antigen is present on the RBCs
      b. Rh-negative—RBCs have no Rh antigen present
      c. Anti-Rh antibodies are not normally present in blood; anti-Rh antibodies can appear in Rh-negative blood if it has come in contact with Rh-positive RBCs

White Blood Cells

A. White blood cells also called leucocytes or WBCs (review **Table 27-1**)

B. Transparent cells with nuclei; generally larger than RBCs

C. Classified by their staining properties
   1. Granulocytes—large granules in cytoplasm stain with different stains
      a. Neutrophils
      b. Eosinophils
      c. Basophils
   2. Agranulocytes—no stained granules in cytoplasm
      a. Lymphcytes
      b. Monocytes

D. Have defensive functions outlined below and in later chapters

E. Granulocytes
   1. Neutrophils (review **Figure 27-13**)—make up approximately 65% of total WBC count in a normal blood sample; highly mobile and very active phagocytic cells; capable of diapedesis; cytoplasmic granules contain lysosomes
   2. Eosinophils (review **Figure 27-14**)—account for 2% to 5% of circulating WBCs; numerous in mucous lining of respiratory and digestive tracts; weak phagocytes; release chemicals of immunity; provide protection against infections caused by parasitic worms, and help regulate allergic reactions
   3. Basophils (review **Figure 27-15**)—account for only 0.5% to 1% of circulating WBCs; motile and capable of diapedesis; cytoplasmic granules contain histamine and heparin

F. Agranulocytes (**Figures 27-16** and **27-17**)
   1. Lymphocytes—smallest of the WBCs; second most numerous WBC; account for approximately 25% of circulating WBCs; NK cells, T lymphocytes and B lymphocytes have an important role in immunity—T lymphocytes directly attack an infected or cancerous cell, and B lymphocytes produce antibodies against specific antigens
   2. Monocytes—largest leucocytes; mobile and highly phagocytic cells

G. WBC numbers—1 mm^3 of normal blood usually contains 4000 to 11000 leucocytes ($4\text{-}11 \times 10^9$/L), with different percentages for each type; WBC numbers have clinical significance because they change with certain abnormal conditions (**Figure 27-18**)

H. Formation of WBCs (review **Figure 27-6**)
  1. Granular and agranular leucocytes mature from the undifferentiated haematopoietic stem cell
  2. Neutrophils, eosinophils, basophils, and a few lymphocytes and monocytes originate in red bone marrow; most lymphocytes and monocytes develop from haematopoietic stem cells in lymphatic tissue

Platelets (review **Figure 27-6**)

A. Structure and function of platelets
  1. In circulating blood, platelets are small, pale bodies that appear as irregular spindles or oval discs
  2. Three important properties are agglutination, adhesiveness, and aggregation
  3. Platelet counts in adults average 250,000/mm^3 (250 $\times$ 10^9/L) of blood; normal range is 150,000 to 400,000/mm^3 (150–400 $\times$ 10^9/L)
  4. Important role in haemostasis (stoppage of bleeding)

B. Formation and life span of platelets (average of 7 days)—formed in red bone marrow, lungs, and spleen by fragmentation of megakaryocytes

Haemostasis

A. Haemostasis
  1. Stops bleeding and prevents loss of vital body fluid
  2. Secondary role in defending against bacterial attacks

B. Vasoconstriction
  1. Smooth muscle spasms in vessel wall collapse vessel and slow bleeding
  2. Can be enhanced by
    a. Chemical regulators such as thromboxane A2 from platelets or endothelin-1 from endothelium
    b. Application of external pressure to constrict vessels

C. Platelet plug formation
  1. Platelets adhere to damaged endothelial lining and to each other 1 to 5 seconds after injury to vessel wall, forming a platelet plug
  2. Temporary platelet plug is an important step in haemostasis—but if injury is extensive, the blood-clotting mechanism is activated to assist
  3. "Sticky platelets" form physical plug and activate to secrete several chemicals involved in the coagulation process; chemicals also stimulate more platelet aggregation, which releases even more chemicals (positive feedback)

D. Blood clotting (coagulation) (**Figure 27-20**)
  1. Stages
    a. Stage I—production of thromboplastin activator by *either* of the following:
      (1) Chemicals released from damaged tissues (extrinsic pathway)
      (2) Chemicals present in the blood (intrinsic pathway)
    b. Stage II—conversion of prothrombin to thrombin
    c. Stage III—conversion of fibrinogen to fibrin and production of fibrin clot
  2. Activation pathways (**Figure 27-21**)
    a. Extrinsic clotting pathways; chemicals released from damaged tissues that are outside or extrinsic to the blood trigger cascade of events that result in the formation of prothrombin activator
    b. Intrinsic clotting pathways; involves a series of reactions that begin with factors normally present, or intrinsic to, the blood
  3. Common pathway
    a. After prothrombin activator is produced, stages 2 and 3 of the blood-clotting mechanism are initiated and a clot will form
    b. Fibrin appears in blood as fine threads all tangled together

E. Conditions that oppose clotting
  1. Clot formation in intact vessels is opposed
  2. Several factors oppose clotting
    a. Perfectly smooth surface of the normal endothelial lining of blood vessels does not allow platelets to adhere
    b. Antithrombins—substances in the blood that oppose or inactivate thrombin; prevent thrombin from converting fibrinogen to fibrin; for example, heparin

F. Conditions that hasten clotting
  1. Rough spot in the endothelium
  2. Abnormally slow blood flow

G. Clot dissolution (**Figure 27-22**)
  1. Fibrinolysis—physiological mechanism that dissolves the clot once it has formed
  2. Plasmin—enzyme in the blood that catalyzes the hydrolysis of fibrin, causing it to dissolve; it is activated by chemicals released from damaged cells and acts slowly to dissolve the clot
  3. Substances that generate plasmin can be used as a therapy to dissolve blood clots

The Big Picture: Blood and the Whole Body

A. Blood plasma transports substances, including heat, around the body, linking all body tissues together

B. Blood tissue contains formed elements—blood cells and platelets
  1. RBCs assist in the transport of oxygen and carbon dioxide
  2. WBCs assist in the defence mechanisms of the whole body
  3. Platelets prevent loss of the fluid that constitutes the internal environment

C. Blood is needed by all organs and body systems to function properly, just as many body systems aid the functions of blood

D. Blood is useless to the body unless it continues to flow around the body and performs its functions of transport, defence, and balance (or homeostasis)

REVIEW QUESTIONS

Hint

Write out the answers to these questions after reading the chapter and reviewing the Chapter Summary. Note—writing out your answers will consolidate learning and provide a valuable resource of information.

1. What are the formed elements of blood?
2. What is the function of carbonic anhydrase?
3. Describe the structure of haemoglobin.
4. How does the structure of haemoglobin allow it to combine with oxygen?
5. Discuss the steps involved in erythropoiesis.
6. What is the average life span of a circulating red blood cell?
7. Compare and contrast granulocytes and agranulocytes.
8. Define the term *chemotaxis.*
9. List the important physical properties of platelets.
10. Explain what is meant by *type AB blood.* Explain Rh-negative blood.
11. Which organ is responsible for the synthesis of most plasma proteins?
12. What is the normal plasma protein concentration?
13. What are some functions served by plasma proteins?
14. Describe the role of platelets in haemostasis and blood clotting.
15. What triggers blood clotting?
16. Identify factors that oppose blood clotting. Do the same for factors that hasten blood clotting.
17. Describe the physiological mechanism that dissolves clots.
18. Describe the haemoglobin in a person with sickle cell trait.
19. List and describe three blood disorders.
20. What is the functional advantage of erythrocytes containing no nucleus?

CRITICAL THINKING QUESTIONS

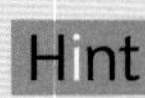

After finishing the Review Questions, write out the answers to these more in-depth questions to help you apply your new knowledge. Go back to sections of the chapter that relate to concepts that you find difficult.

1. A modern hospital laboratory has machines that can automatically do blood cell counts based on the size of cells. If the lab technician did not want to count erythrocytes, for what size range would the machine be set? What white blood cells would be missed? What would be the classes, functions, and life spans of the white blood cells that were counted?
2. A friend received a report detailing the laboratory results related to his recent physical examination and noted that his haematocrit (Hct) was below normal. Because he knows you are taking anatomy and physiology, he has come to you for an explanation. Based on what you know, explain to him what a haematocrit value is, how it is determined, and what value would put him below normal.
3. You are a medical examiner and are asked to determine the cause of death of a body brought to the mortuary. You find a very large agglutination (not a clot) in a major vein. Based on this, what judgment would you make regarding the cause of death?
4. Suppose a person had a thyroid disorder that caused the production of calcitonin to be many times higher than it should be. Elaborate on why a possible side effect of this condition might be a very slow blood-clotting time.
5. A patient comes into accident and emergency with severe bleeding. What can be done to speed the formation of a clot?
6. Some athletes, seeking a competitive edge, may resort to blood doping. How would you explain blood doping? What information would you use to discourage athletes from participating in the practice of blood doping?
7. Summarize the condition *erythroblastosis fetalis.*
8. A friend who has haemophilia has a headache and wants to take an aspirin. What would you advise him to do?

28 Heart

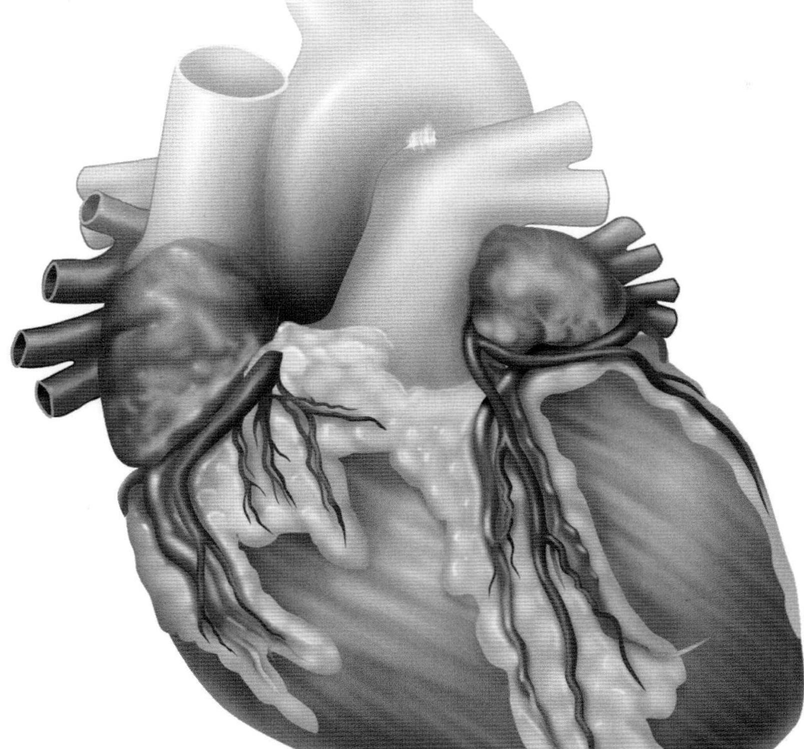

CHAPTER OUTLINE

Hint *Scan this outline before you begin to read the chapter, as a preview of how the concepts are organized.*

The cardiovascular system is sometimes called simply the circulatory system. It consists of the heart, which is a muscular pumping device, and a closed system of vessels called arteries, capillaries, and veins. As the name implies, blood contained in the circulatory system is pumped by the heart around a closed circle or circuit of vessels as it passes again and again through the various circulations of the body (see **Figure 29-5** on p. 671).

As in the adult, survival of the developing embryo depends on the circulation of blood to maintain homeostasis and a favourable cellular environment. In response to this need, the cardiovascular system makes its appearance early in development and reaches a functional state long before any other major organ system. Incredible as it seems, the heart begins to beat regularly early in the fourth week after fertilization.

LANGUAGE OF SCIENCE

Hint *Use this list to aid your pronunciation of unfamiliar words.*

anastomosis (ah-nas-toh-MOH-sis)
[*ana-* **again or anew,** *-stomo-* **mouth,** *-osis* **condition**] *pl.,* anastomoses

aorta (ay-OR-tah)
[*aort-* **lifted,** *-a* **thing**] *pl.,* aortae or aortas

artery (AR-ter-ee)
[*arteri-* **vessel**]

atrioventricular (AV) bundle (ay-tree-oh-ven-TRIK-yoo-lar BUN-del)
[*atrio-* **entrance courtyard,** *-ventr-* **belly,** *-icul-* **little,** *-ar* **relating to**]

atrioventricular (AV) node (ay-tree-oh-ven-TRIK-yoo-lar)
[*atrio-* **entrance courtyard,** *-ventr-* **belly,** *-icul-* **little,** *-ar* **relating to,** *-ar* **relating to,** *nod-* **knot**]

atrioventricular (AV) valve (ay-tree-oh-ven-TRIK-yoo-lar)
[*atrio-* **entrance courtyard,** *-ventr-* **belly,** *-icul-* **little,** *-ar* **relating to**]

atrium (AY-tree-um)
[*atrium* **entrance courtyard**] *pl.,* atria

bicuspid valve (bye-KUS-pid)
[*bi-* **double,** *-cusp-* **point,** *-id* **characterized by**]

capillary (kah-PILL-er-ee)
[*capill-* **hair,** *-ary* **relating to**]

cardiac cycle (KAR-dee-ak)
[*cardi-* **heart,** *-ac* **relating to,** *cycle* **circle**]

chordae tendineae (KOR-dee ten-DIN-ee-ee)
[*chorda* **string or cord,** *tendinea* **pulled tight**] *sing.,* chorda tendinea

coronary artery (KOHR-oh-nair-ee AR-ter-ee)
[*corona-* **crown,** *-ary* **relating to,** *arteri-* **vessel**]

cuspid valve (KUS-pid)
[*cusp-* **point,** *-id* **characterized by**]

diastole (dye-ASS-toh-lee)
[*dia-* **through,** *-stole* **position**]

endocardium (en-doh-KAR-dee-um)
[*endo-* **within,** *-cardi-* **heart,** *-um* **thing**]

endothelium (en-doh-THEE-lee-um)
[*endo-* **within,** *-theli-* **nipple,** *-um* **thing**]

epicardium (ep-ih-KAR-dee-um)
[*epi-* **on or upon,** *-cardi-* **heart,** *-um* **thing**]

continued on p. 660

This chapter explores the structure and function of the heart as a pump. Chapter 29 continues the story of circulation by describing the blood vessel types and outlining the various circulatory routes of the body. Chapter 30 then integrates all of these concepts by discussing the coordinated processes that keep blood flowing. •

HEART STRUCTURE

Location of the Heart

The human heart is a four-chambered muscular organ, shaped and sized roughly like a person's closed fist (**Figure 28-1**). It lies in the mediastinum, or middle region of the thorax, just behind the body of the sternum between the points of attachment of the second through the sixth ribs. Approximately two thirds of the heart's mass is to the left of the midline of the body, and one third is to the right (**Figure 28-2**).

Posteriorly the heart rests against the bodies of the fifth to the eighth thoracic vertebrae. Because of its placement between the sternum in front and the bodies of the thoracic vertebrae behind, it can be compressed by application of pressure to the lower portion of the body of the sternum using the heel of the hand (**Figure 28-2**, *E*). Rhythmic compression of the heart in this way can maintain blood flow in cases of cardiac arrest and, if combined with effective artificial respiration, the resulting procedure, called *cardiopulmonary resuscitation* (CPR), can be life-saving.

The anatomical position of the heart in the thoracic cavity is shown in **Figure 28-2**. The lower border of the heart, which forms a blunt point known as the *apex*, lies on the diaphragm, pointing toward the left. To count the apical beat, one must place a stethoscope directly over the apex—that is, in the space between the fifth and sixth ribs (fifth intercostal space) on a line with the midpoint of the left clavicle.

The upper border of the heart—that is, its base—lies just below the second rib. The boundaries, which indicate its size, have considerable clinical importance, because a marked increase in heart size accompanies certain types of heart disease. Therefore, when diagnosing heart disorders, the physician charts the boundaries of the heart. The "normal" boundaries of the heart are, however, influenced by factors such as age, body build, and state of contraction.

Size and Shape of the Heart

At birth the heart is said to be transverse (wide) in type and appears large in proportion to the diameter of the chest cavity. In the infant, it is 1⁄130 of the total body weight compared with about 1⁄300 in the adult. Between puberty and 25 years of age the heart attains its adult shape and weight—about 310 grams is average for the male and 225 grams for the female.

In the adult the shape of the heart tends to resemble that of the chest. In tall, thin individuals the heart is often described as elongated, whereas in short, stocky individuals it has greater width and is described as transverse. In individuals of average height and weight it is neither long nor transverse but somewhat intermediate between the two. Its approximate dimensions are 12 cm long, 9 cm wide, and 6 cm deep.

Figure 28-3 in this book and Figure 3-7 in the Brief Atlas of the Human Body show details of the heart and great vessels in external views.

Quick CHECK

1. In anatomical terms, where is the heart located?
2. Describe the shape of the heart.
3. When does the heart attain its adult shape and weight?

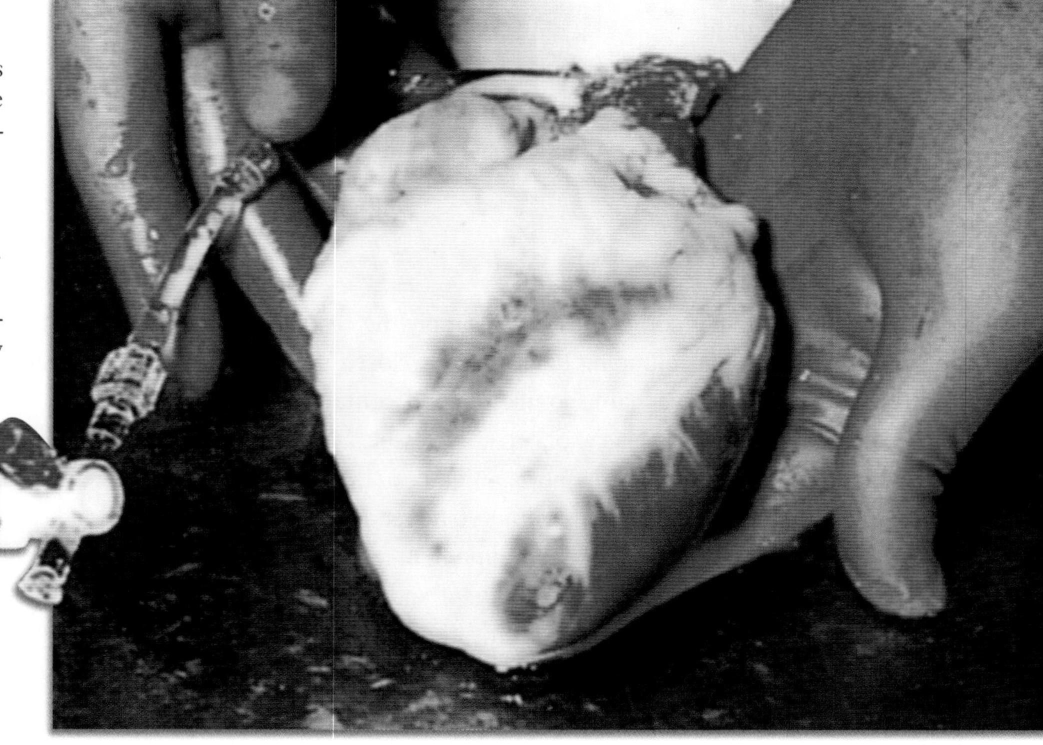

FIGURE 28-1 Appearance of the heart. This photograph shows a living human heart prepared for transplantation into a patient. Note its size relative to the hands that are holding it.

UNIT 4

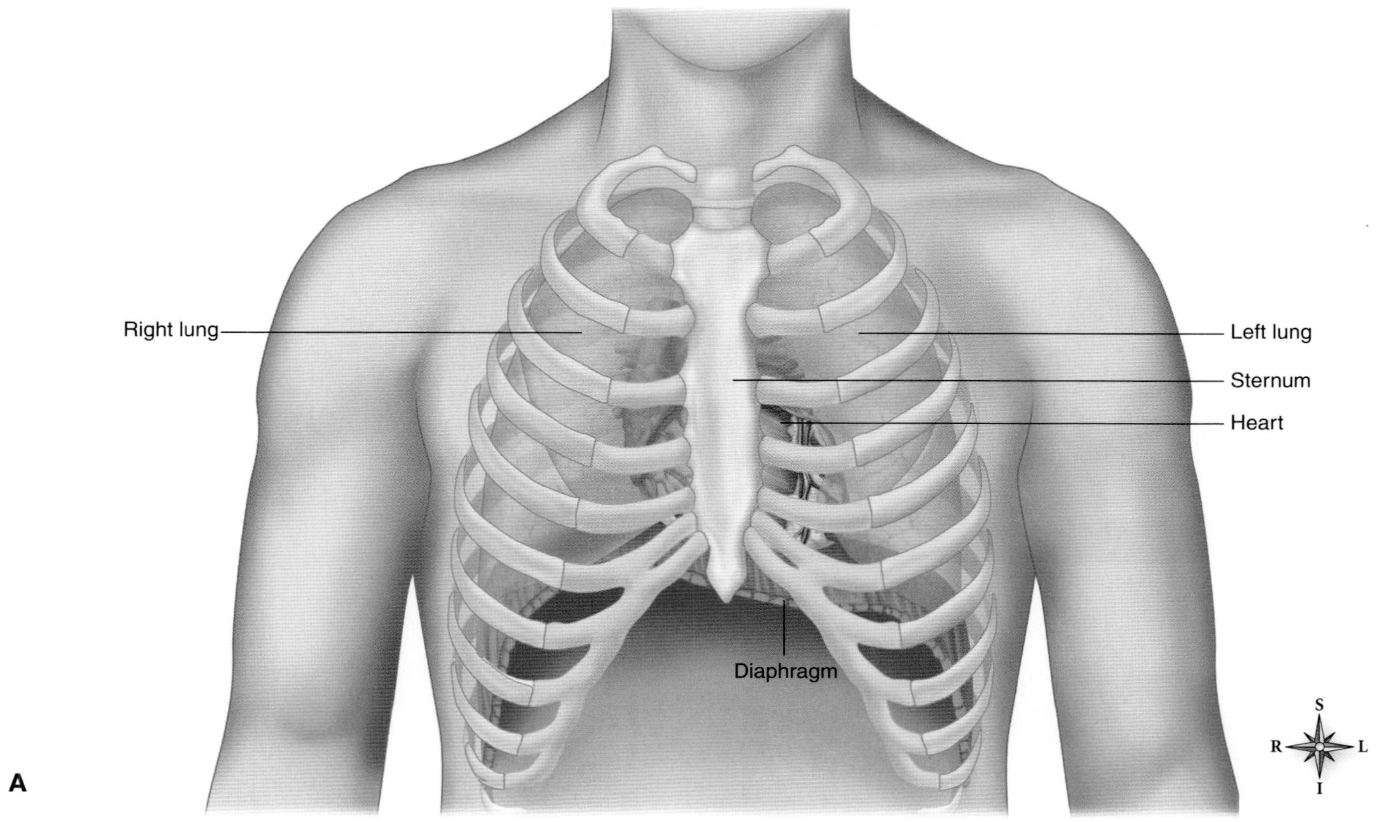

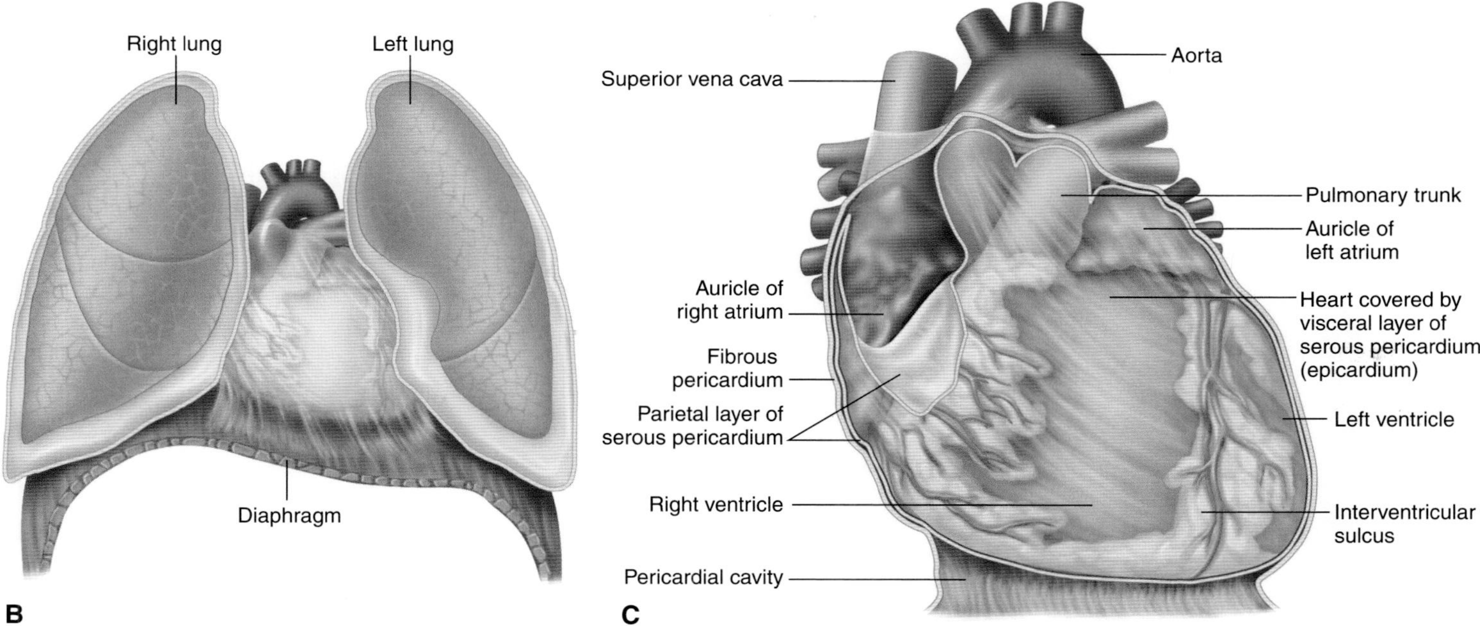

FIGURE 28-2 Location of the heart. **A,** Heart in mediastinum showing relationship to lungs and other anterior thoracic structures. **B,** Anterior view of isolated heart and lungs. Portions of the parietal pleura and pericardium have been removed. **C,** Detail of heart resting on diaphragm with pericardial sac opened. *(continued)*

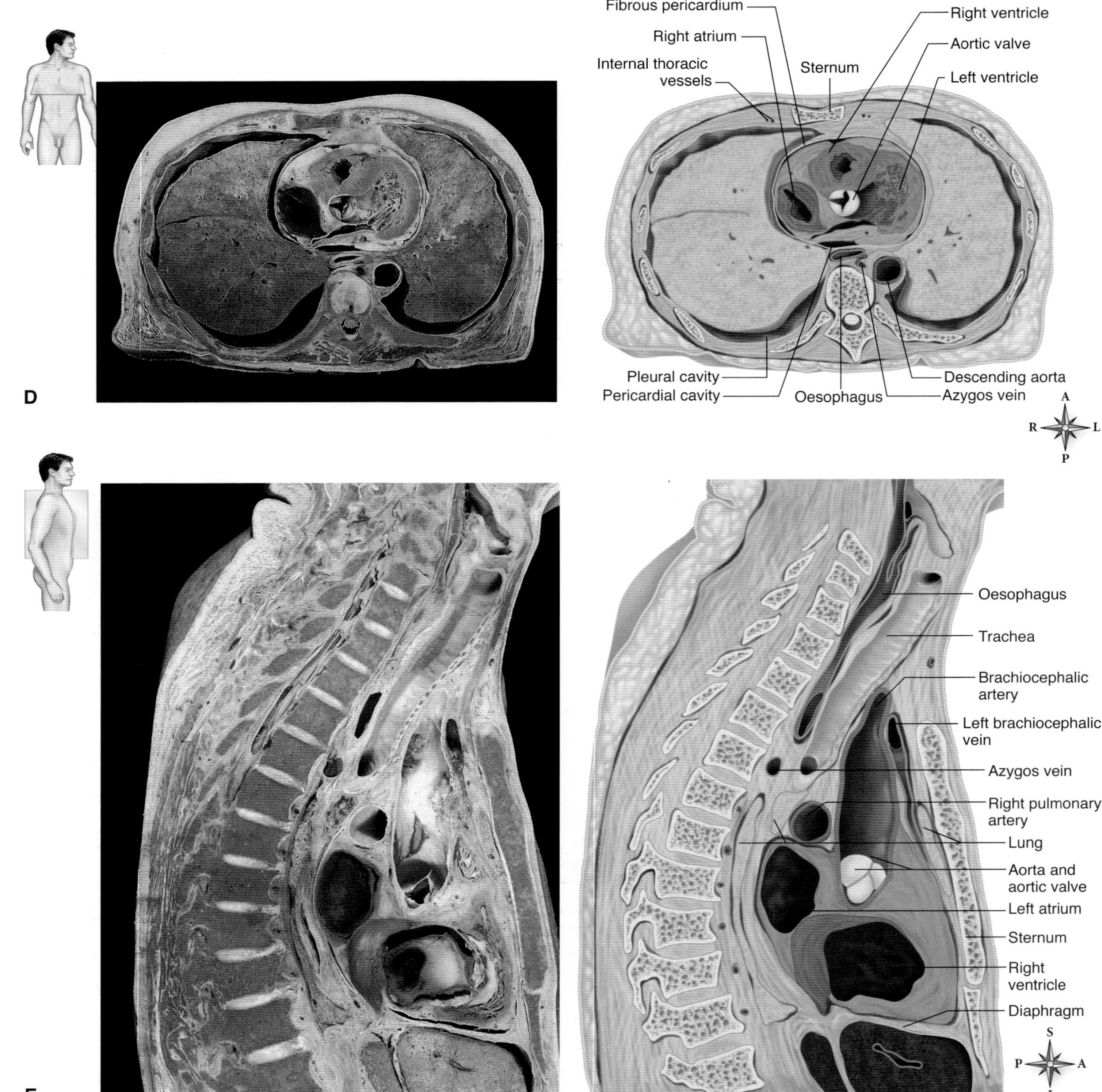

FIGURE 28-2 Location of the heart *(continued).* **D,** Transverse section of cadaver specimen and colour drawing of thoracic structures at the level of the sixth thoracic vertebra (inferior aspect). **E,** Midline sagittal section of cadaver specimen and colour drawing showing thorax structures. Note the placement of the heart between the sternum in front and thoracic vertebrae behind—a fact that explains how CPR compressions can squeeze the heart to keep blood flowing.

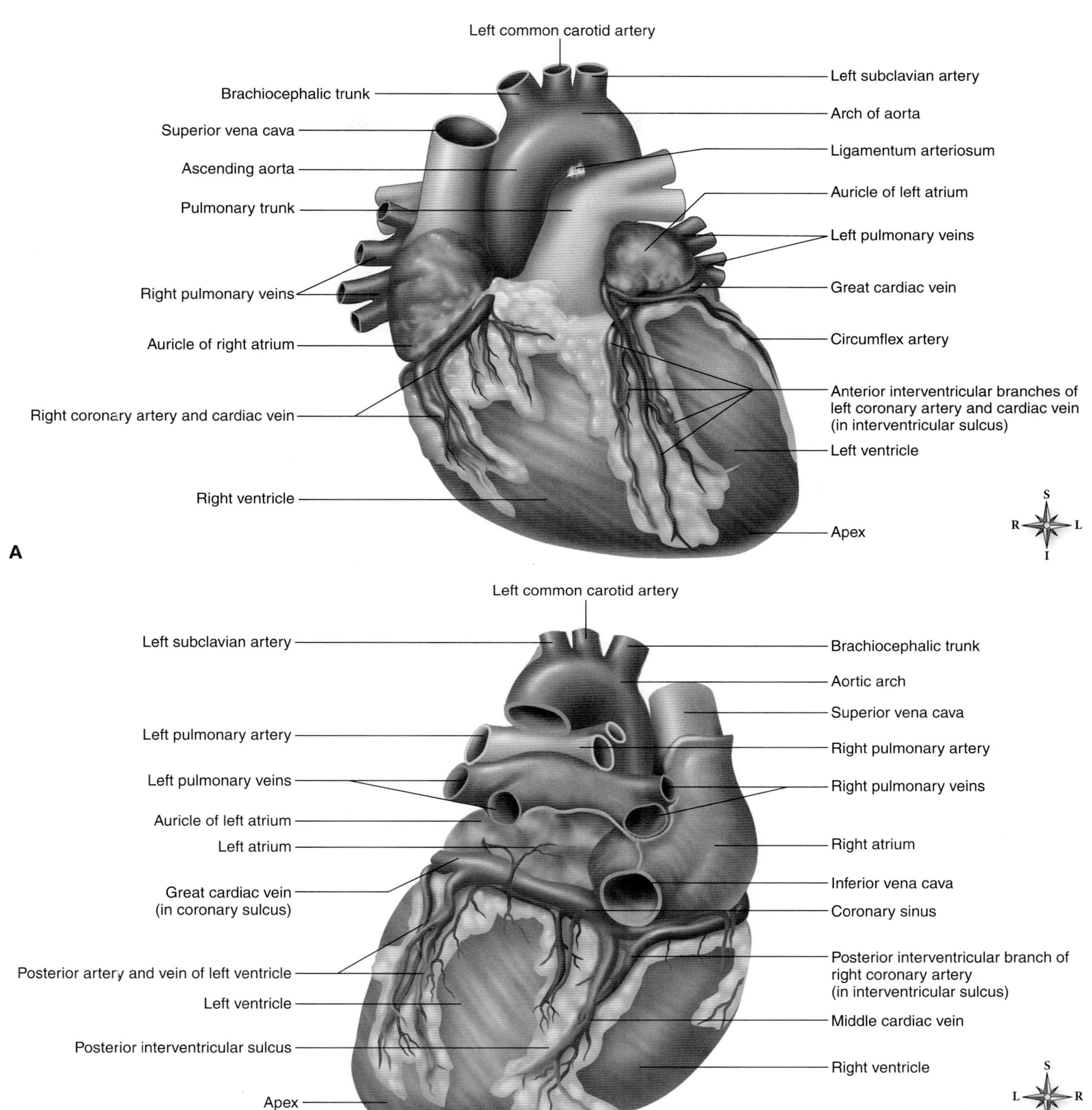

FIGURE 28-3 The heart and great vessels. A, Anterior view. **B,** Posterior view. A shallow depression called the *coronary sulcus* encircles the heart, marking the boundary between atria above and ventricles below. Similar depressions, an *anterior* and *posterior interventricular sulcus*, mark the boundary between left and right ventricles. Coronary blood vessels lie along these sulci.

UNIT 4

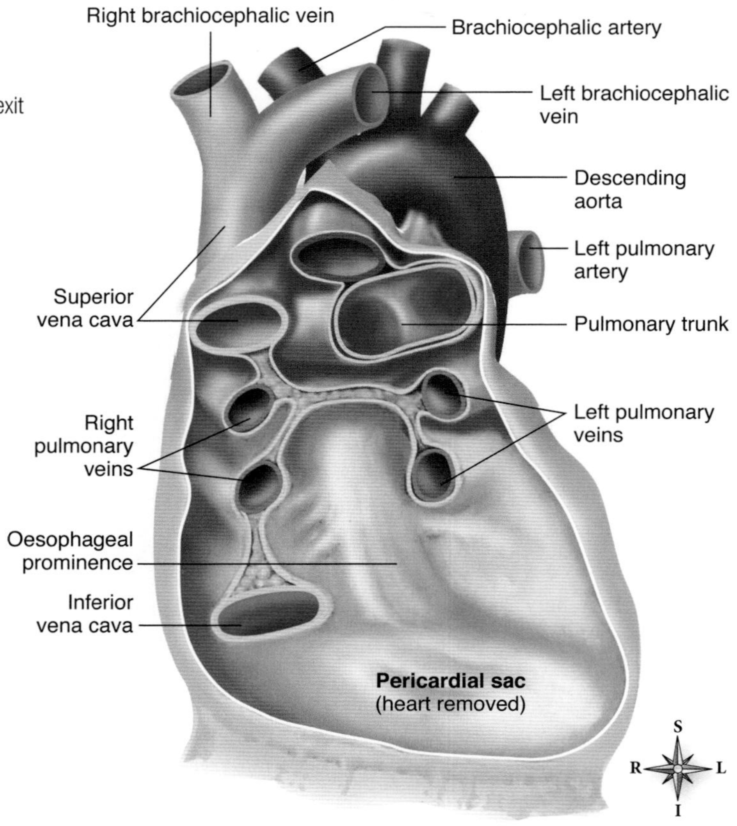

FIGURE 28-4 Pericardium. Coronal (frontal) view diagram showing cut pericardial sac with heart removed. Note that the pericardial sac attaches to the great vessels that enter and exit the heart, not to the heart itself. For a different view of the pericardium, see **Figure 28-2**, *C*.

Coverings of the Heart

Structure of the Heart Coverings

The heart has its own special covering, a loose-fitting inextensible sac called the **pericardium.** The pericardial sac, with the heart removed, can be seen in **Figure 28-4**.

The pericardium consists of two parts: a fibrous portion and a serous portion (**Figure 28-5**). The sac itself is made of tough white fibrous tissue but is lined with smooth, moist serous membrane—the parietal layer of the serous pericardium. The same kind of membrane covers the entire outer surface of the heart. This covering layer is known as the *visceral layer* of the serous pericardium or the **epicardium.**

The fibrous sac attaches to the large blood vessels emerging from the top of the heart but not to the heart itself (see **Figure 28-4**). Therefore it fits loosely around the heart, with a slight space between the visceral layer adhering to the heart and the parietal layer adhering to the inside of the fibrous sac. This space is called the **pericardial space.** It contains 10 to 15 mL of **pericardial fluid**, a lubricating fluid secreted by the serous membrane. **Figure 1-6** on p. 11 illustrates the basic concept of serous membrane anatomy.

To summarize, the layers of the pericardium from superficial to deep are as follows:

Fibrous pericardium—tough, loose-fitting, and inelastic sac around the heart

Serous pericardium—consisting of two layers:

1. *Parietal layer*—lining inside the fibrous pericardium
2. *Visceral layer (epicardium)*—adhering to the outside of the heart; between visceral and parietal layers is a space, the pericardial space, that contains a few drops of pericardial fluid

Function of the Heart Coverings

The fibrous pericardial sac with its smooth, well-lubricated serous lining provides protection against friction. The heart moves easily in this loose-fitting jacket with no danger of irritation from friction between the two surfaces, as long as the serous pericardium remains normal and continues to produce lubricating serous fluid.

Structure of the Heart

Vessels of the Heart

Looking at **Figure 28-3**, one cannot help but notice the great vessels of the heart that connect it to the rest of the cardiovascular system. These include the sup.vena cava, inf.vena cava, pulmonary arteries, pulmonary veins and the aorta.

Wall of the Heart

Three distinct layers of tissue make up the heart wall (see **Figure 28-5**) in both the atria and the ventricles: the epicardium, myocardium, and endocardium.

Epicardium

The outer layer of the heart wall is called the **epicardium,** a name that literally means "on the heart". The epicardium is actually the visceral layer of the serous pericardium already described. In other words, the same structure has two different names: epicardium and serous pericardium.

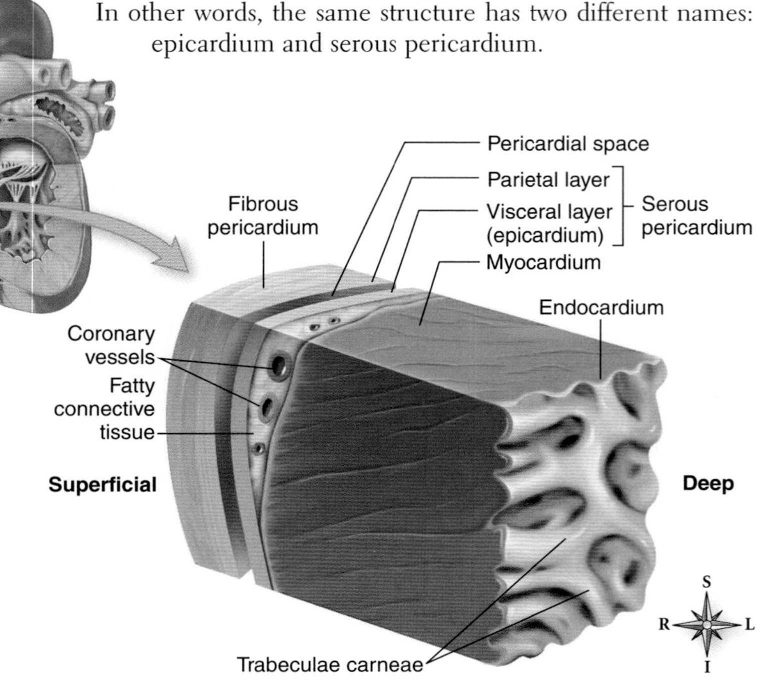

FIGURE 28-5 Wall of the heart. The cutout section of the heart wall shows the outer fibrous pericardium and the parietal and visceral layers of the serous pericardium (with the pericardial space between them). Note that a layer of fatty connective tissue is located between the visceral layer of the serous pericardium (epicardium) and the myocardium. Note also that the endocardium covers beamlike projections of myocardial muscle tissue, called *trabeculae carneae.*

Myocardium

The bulk of the heart wall is the thick, contractile, middle layer of specially constructed and arranged cardiac muscle cells called the **myocardium.** The minute structure of cardiac muscle has been described in Chapters 9 and 17. Review **Table 17-1** on p. 381 for a brief overview of cardiac muscle.

Recall that cardiac muscle tissue is composed of many branching cells that are joined into a continuous mass by end-to-end junctions called *intercalated discs* (see **Figure 9-32** on p. 172). Because each intercalated disc includes many gap junctions, large areas of cardiac muscle are electrically coupled into a single functional unit called a *syncytium* (meaning "joined cells"). **Figure 19-10** on p. 420 shows how such electrical connections work. Because they form an electrically coupled syncytium, cardiac muscle cells can pass an action potential from fibre to fibre along a large area of the heart wall—thus stimulating contraction in each muscle fibre of the syncytium.

Another advantage of the linked structure of myocardial cells is that the cardiac fibres form a continuous sheet of muscle that wraps entirely around the cavities within the heart. Thus the encircling myocardium can compress the heart cavities, and the blood within them, with great force.

Recall also that cardiac muscles are *autorhythmic,* meaning that they can contract on their own in a slow, steady rhythm. As we explained in Chapter 17, cardiac muscle cells cannot summate contractions to produce tetanus and thus do not fatigue—a useful characteristic for muscle tissue that must maintain a continuous cycle of alternating contraction and relaxation for the entire span of life. Because the muscular myocardium can contract powerfully and rhythmically, without fatigue, the heart is an efficient and dependable pump for blood.

If the myocardium is damaged, as it may be in a "heart attack" or myocardial infarction (MI), then it will not pump as efficiently—which may quickly lead to death if the damage is severe.

CONNECT IT! 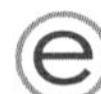

Blood tests can be used to detect **C-reactive protein (CRP)** associated with inflammation that may lead to an MI. The cardiac marker detected by the **troponins test** may help diagnose an MI by revealing the presence of molecules released into the bloodstream by damaged myocardial fibres. To learn more, check out ***Cardiac Marker Studies*** online at ***Connect It!***

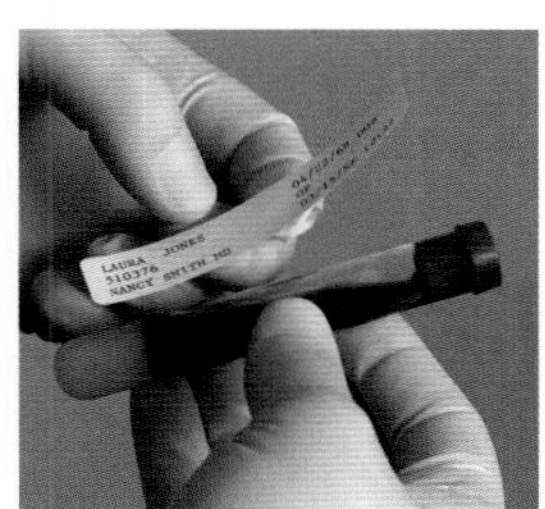

Endocardium

The lining of the interior of the myocardial wall is a delicate layer known as the **endocardium.** The endocardium is made of a type of tissue called endothelial tissue, or simply **endothelium.** Endothelium lines the heart (where it is called the *endocardium*) and continues on to line all of the blood vessels. Endothelium is a specialized type of simple squamous epithelium.

Note in **Figure 28-5** that the endocardium covers beamlike projections of myocardial tissue. These muscular projections are called *trabeculae carneae* (meaning "fleshy beams") and help to add force to the inward contraction of the heart wall.

Inward folds or pockets formed by the endocardium and supporting connective tissue make up the flaps or cusps of the major heart valves. These valves ensure the one-way flow of blood through the chambers of the heart, thus enabling the heart to act as a pump.

Chambers of the Heart

The interior of the heart is divided into four cavities, or heart chambers (**Figure 28-6**). The two upper chambers are called *atria* (singular, *atrium*), and the two lower chambers are called *ventricles.* The left chambers are separated from the right chambers by an extension of the heart wall called the *septum.*

Atria

The two superior chambers of the heart—the **atria**—are separated into left and right chambers by the *interatrial septum.* Atria are often called the "receiving chambers" because they receive blood from vessels called *veins.* **Veins** are the large blood vessels that return blood from various tissues to the heart so that the blood can be pumped out to tissues again.

Figure 28-7 shows how the atria alternately relax and contract to receive blood, then push it into the lower chambers. Because the atria need not generate great pressure to move blood such a small distance, the myocardial wall of each atrium is not very thick.

If you look at **Figures 28-2**, *C*, and **28-3**, *A*, you will see that part of each atrium is labelled as an *auricle.* The term *auricle* (meaning "little ear") refers to the earlike flap protruding from each atrium. Thus the auricles are *part of* the atria. The terms *auricles* and *atria* should not be used synonymously.

Ventricles

The **ventricles** are the two lower chambers of the heart. The ventricles are separated into left and right chambers by the *interventricular septum.* Because the ventricles receive blood from the atria and pump blood out of the heart into arteries, the ventricles are considered to be the primary "pumping chambers" of the heart.

Because more force is needed to pump blood a farther distance from the ventricles than from the atria, the myocardium of each ventricle is thicker than the myocardium of either atrium. The myocardium of the left ventricle is thicker than that of the right ventricle because the left ventricle pushes blood through most vessels of the body, whereas the right ventricle pushes blood only through the nearby pulmonary vessels that serve the gas exchange tissues of the lungs.

The pumping action of the heart chambers is summarized in **Figure 28-7** and described more fully later in this chapter.

Valves of the Heart

The heart valves are structures that permit the flow of blood in one direction only—allowing the heart to act as a pump that forces the continuous flow of blood in one direction.

Four valves are of importance to the normal functioning of the heart (**Figure 28-8**; see **Figure 28-7**). Because they guard the openings between the atria and the ventricles, two of the valves are called the **atrioventricular (AV) valves.** The atrioventricular valves have pointed leaflets or flaps called *cusps* and are therefore also called **cuspid valves.** The other two heart valves, the heart's **semilunar (SL) valves,** are located where the trunk of the pulmonary artery joins the right ventricle (pulmonary valve) and where the aorta joins the left ventricle (aortic valve).

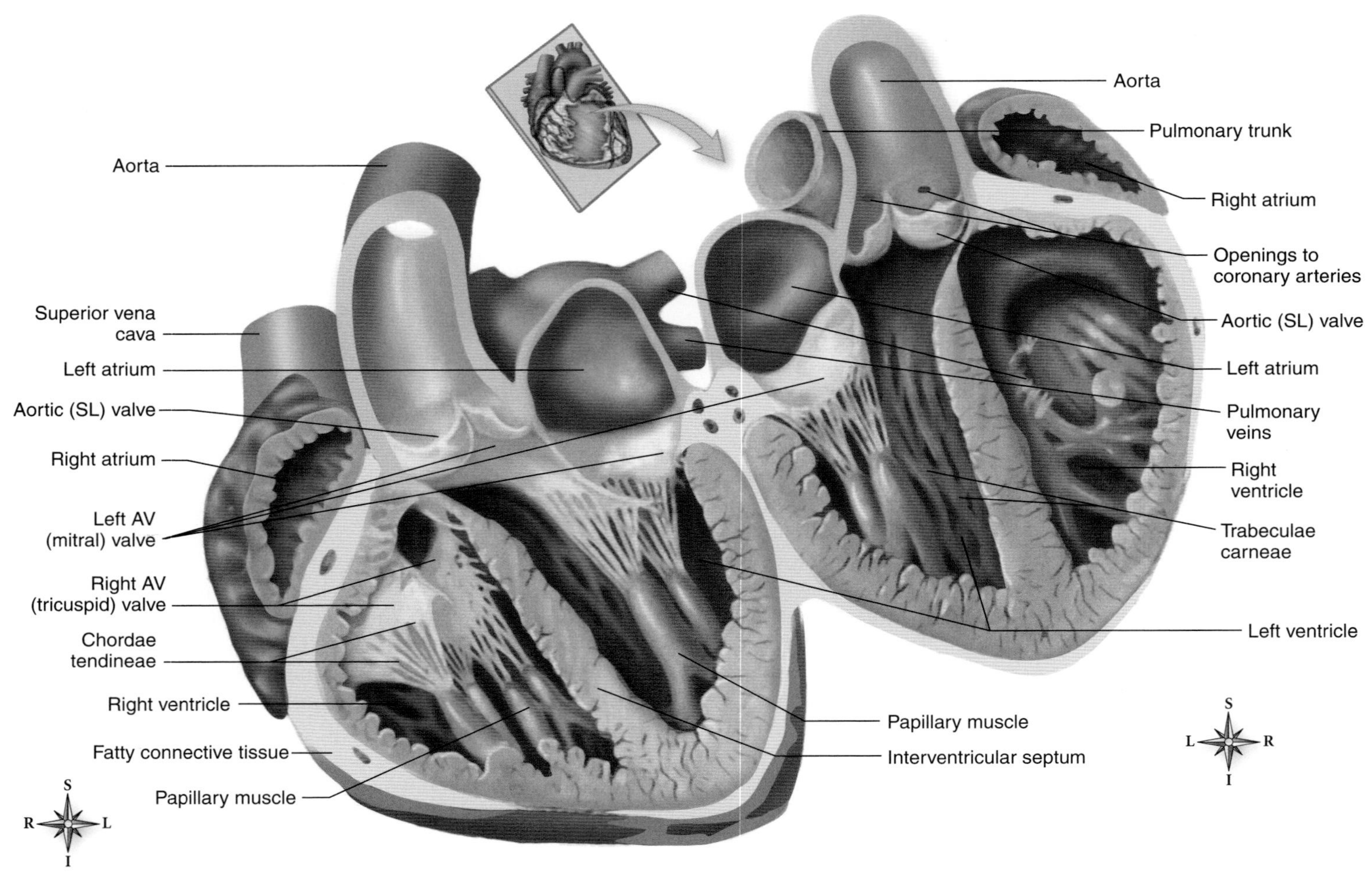

FIGURE 28-6 Interior of the heart. This illustration shows the heart as it would appear if it were cut along a coronal (frontal) plane and opened like a book. The front portion of the heart lies to the reader's right; the back portion of the heart lies to the reader's left. (Note each portion has a separate anatomical compass rosette to facilitate orientation.) The four chambers of the heart—two atria and two ventricles—are easily seen. *AV,* Atrioventricular; *SL,* semilunar.

Atrioventricular Valves

The atrioventricular valve regulating flow through the right atrioventricular opening consists of three flaps (cusps) of endocardium. The free edge of each flap is anchored to the *papillary muscles* of the right ventricle by several *tendinous cords* that are more often called **chordae tendineae.**

Because the right atrioventricular valve has three flaps or cusps, it is also called the **tricuspid valve.** The valve that guards the left atrioventricular opening is similar in structure to the right atrioventricular valve, except that it has only two flaps and is therefore also called the **bicuspid valve.** Most commonly, however, the left AV valve is called the **mitral valve**—a name it gets from its resemblance to the miter, a double-cusped hat worn by bishops.

The construction of both atrioventricular valves allows blood to flow from the atria into the ventricles but prevents it from flowing back up into the atria from the ventricles. When ventricles are relaxed, blood can flow through the AV valve from the atrium by simply pushing the flimsy valve cusps aside, into the ventricle.

Ventricular contraction, also called ventricular systole, forces the blood in the ventricles hard against the valve flaps, closing the valves. The papillary muscles contract along with the rest of the ventricular myocardium, thus pulling on the edges of the cusps by way of the chordae tendineae. By holding the edges of the cusps firmly during ventricular systole, the chordae tendineae prevent the edges of the flaps from bending backward and allowing blood to flow back into the atria. The harder the ventricular myocardium contracts, the more strongly it pushes against the AV valve—and the more strongly the papillary muscles pull on the chordae tendineae to hold the AV valves shut. This mechanism thus prevents backflow, no matter how strongly the heart ventricles contract. Keeping the AV valves closed during ventricular systole ensures the movement of the blood upward into the pulmonary trunk and aorta as the ventricles contract (see **Figure 28-7**).

Semilunar Valves

The *semilunar (SL) valves* of the heart consist of pocketlike flaps (leaflets) extending inward from the lining of the trunk of the pulmonary artery and aorta. *Semilunar,* which literally means "half moon", refers to the crescent shape of the valve cusps visible in a coronal (frontal) section of the heart.

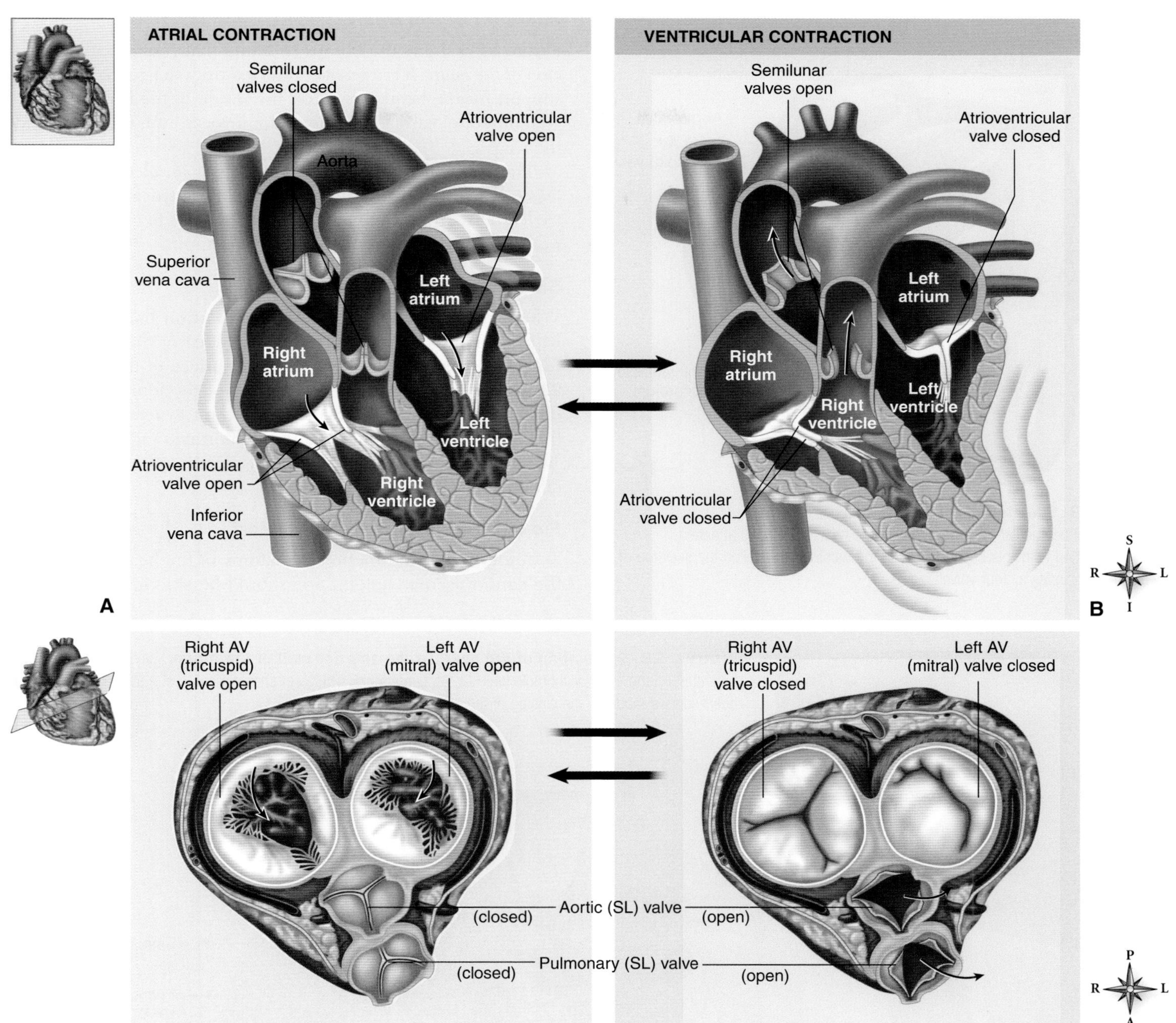

FIGURE 28-7 Chambers and valves of the heart. A, During atrial contraction cardiac muscle in the atrial wall contracts, forcing blood through the atrioventricular (AV) valves and into the ventricles. Bottom illustration shows superior view of all four valves, with semilunar (SL) valves closed and AV valves open. **B,** During ventricular contraction that follows, the AV valves close and the blood is forced out of the ventricles through the SL valves and into the arteries. Bottom illustration shows superior view of SL valves open and AV valves closed.

The semilunar valve at the entrance of the pulmonary trunk is called the *pulmonary valve*. The semilunar valve at the entrance of the aorta is called the *aortic valve*. When the pulmonary and aortic valves are closed, as in **Figure 28-7**, *A*, blood fills the spaces between the leaflets and the vessel wall. Each leaflet then looks like a tiny, filled bucket. Inflowing blood smoothes the leaflets against the blood vessel walls, collapsing the buckets and thereby opening the valves (see **Figure 28-7**, *B*). Closure of the semilunar valves, as of the atrioventricular valves, simultaneously prevents backflow and ensures forward flow of blood in places where there would otherwise be considerable backflow.

Whereas the atrioventricular valves prevent blood from flowing back up into the atria from the ventricles, the semilunar valves prevent it from flowing back down into the ventricles from the aorta and pulmonary trunk.

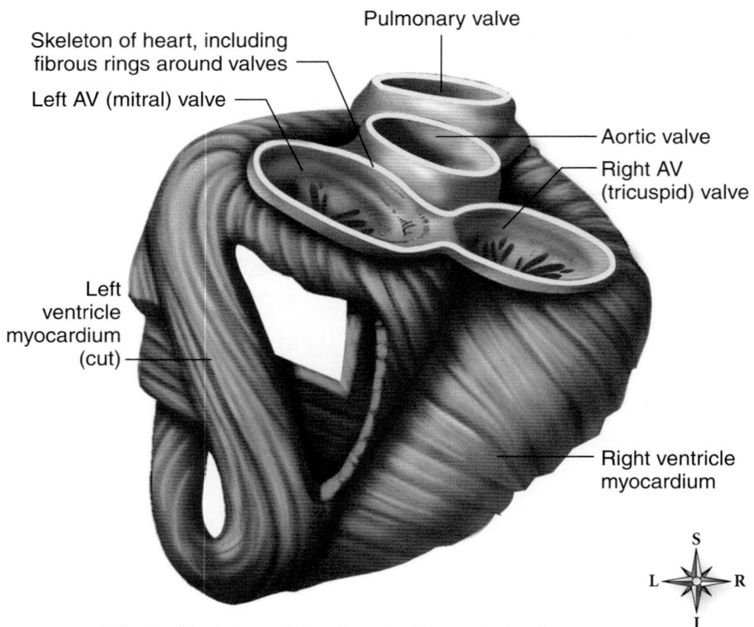

FIGURE 28-8 Skeleton of the heart. This posterior view shows part of the ventricular myocardium with the heart valves still attached. The rim of each heart valve is supported by a fibrous structure, called the skeleton of the heart, that encircles all four valves.

Skeleton of the Heart

Figure 28-8 shows the fibrous structure that is often called the *skeleton of the heart.* It is a set of connected rings that serve as a semirigid support for the heart valves (on the inside of the rings) and for the attachment of cardiac muscle of the myocardium (on the outside of the rings).

The skeleton of the heart also serves as an electrical barrier between the myocardium of the atria and the myocardium of the ventricles. This arrangement allows the ventricles to contract separately from the atria, thus ensuring effective pumping of blood.

Surface Projection

When listening to the sounds of the heart on the body surface, as with a stethoscope, one must have an idea of the relationship between the valves of the heart and the surface of the thorax. **Figure 28-9** indicates the surface relationship of the four heart valves and other features of the heart. It is important to remember, however, that considerable variation within the normal range makes a precise "surface projection" outline of the heart's structure on the chest wall difficult.

Flow of Blood Through the Heart

To understand the functional anatomy of the heart and the rest of the cardiovascular system, one should be able to trace the flow of

FIGURE 28-9 Relation of the heart to the anterior wall of the thorax. Valves of the heart are projected on the anterior thoracic wall. *AV,* Atrioventricular. The inset shows the use of a stethoscope to listen to heart sounds made by the closing of the valves.

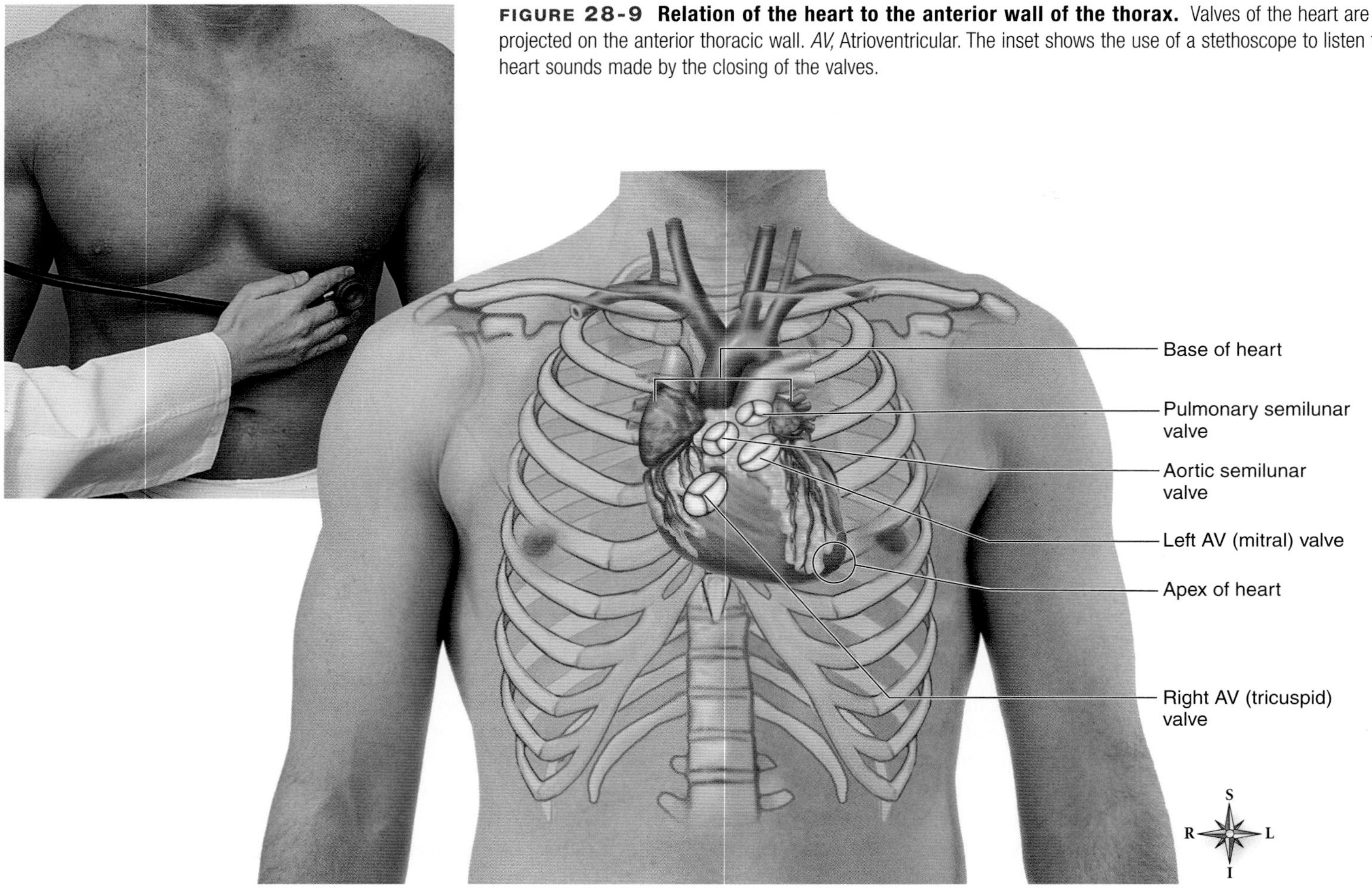

blood through the heart. As we take you through one complete pass through the right side of the heart, then the left side of the heart, trace the path of blood flow with your finger, using **Figure 28-7**.

We can trace the path of blood flow through the right side of the heart by beginning in the right atrium. From the right atrium, blood flows through the right atrioventricular (tricuspid) valve into the right ventricle. From the right ventricle, blood flows through the pulmonary semilunar valve into the first portion of the pulmonary artery, the pulmonary trunk. The pulmonary trunk branches to form the left and right pulmonary arteries, which conduct blood to the gas exchange tissues of the lung. From there, blood flows through pulmonary veins into the left atrium.

We can begin to trace the path of blood flow through the left side of the heart from the left atrium. From the left atrium, blood flows through the left atrioventricular (mitral) valve into the left ventricle. From the left ventricle, blood flows through the aortic semilunar valve into the aorta. Branches of the aorta supply all the tissues of the body except the gas-exchange tissues of the lungs. Blood leaving the head, neck, and upper extremities empties into the superior vena cava. Blood leaving the lower body empties into the inferior vena cava. Both large vessels conduct blood into the right atrium, bringing us back to the point where we began.

CONNECT IT!

Modern sound-wave technology such as **echocardiography** allows us to visualize the action of the heart valves and the flow of blood through the chambers and great vessels of the heart using sound waves—the same technology often used to visualize fetuses developing within the womb. Learn how this technology is used and see the images it produces in ***Echocardiography*** online at ***Connect It!***

Quick CHECK

4. Name the layers of tissues that make up the pericardium.
5. What is the function of the pericardium?
6. Name the three layers of tissue that make up the wall of the heart. What is the function of each layer?
7. Name the four chambers of the heart and the valves associated with them.
8. How do atrioventricular valves differ from semilunar valves?

Blood Supply of Heart Tissue

Coronary Arteries

Myocardial cells receive blood by way of two small vessels, the right and left **coronary arteries.** *Coronary* means "crown"—an apt name when you visualize the position of the left and right coronary arteries encircling the myocardium along a *coronary sulcus*, much as a crown encircles the head (**Figure 28-10**, *A*). Because the openings into these vitally important vessels lie behind leaflets of the aortic semilunar valve, they come off the aorta at its very beginning and are its first branches.

Figure 28-10, *B*, shows that the placement of the openings of the coronary arteries behind the leaflets or flaps of the aortic valve permits an unusual and necessary method of arterial filling. Ordinarily, arteries that branch from the aorta fill during ventricular systole when the great force of ventricular pressure pushes blood into the arteries. However, the coronary arteries are squeezed during ventricular systole and could not fill during this time. Because the coronary artery openings are placed behind the leaflets of the aortic valve, blood flow is diverted from these openings during ventricular contraction when the valve leaflets are against the wall of the aorta. During ventricular relaxation, also called ventricular diastole, when the coronary arteries expand somewhat, blood flow is diverted into the coronary artery openings by the closing of the aortic valve—allowing the coronary arteries to fill.

Both right and left coronary arteries have two main branches, as shown in **Figure 28-10** and **Figure 28-11**.

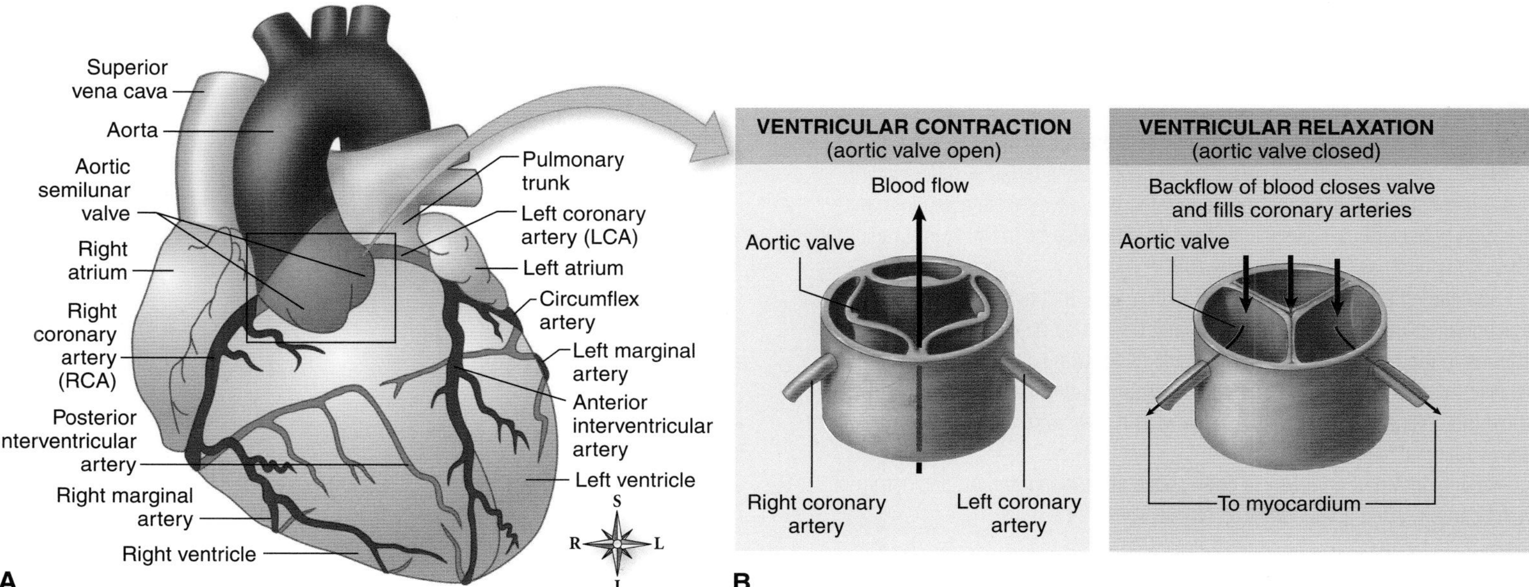

FIGURE 28-10 Coronary arteries. A, Diagram showing the major coronary arteries (anterior view). Clinicians often refer to the interventricular arteries as *descending* arteries. Thus a cardiologist would refer to the *left anterior descending (LAD) artery* and an anatomist would refer to the same vessel as the *anterior interventricular artery.* **B,** The unusual placement of the coronary artery opening behind the leaflets of the aortic valve allows the coronary arteries to fill during ventricular relaxation.

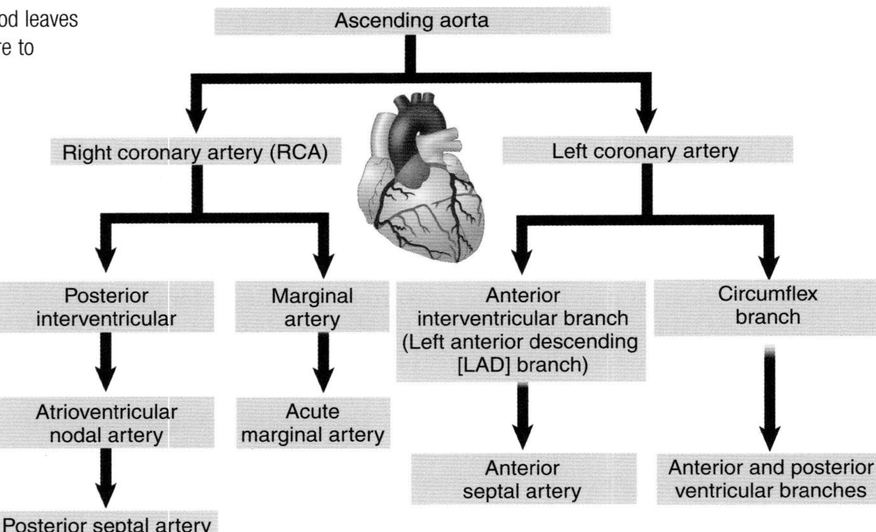

FIGURE 28-11 Blood flow through the coronary arteries. Blood leaves the ascending aorta and flows through the myocardium of the heart. Compare to **Figure 28-10**.

Approximately 70,000 people die every year from coronary artery disease (CAD) in the UK, and over 2 million men and women are living with some narrowing of their coronary arteries. Obstruction of these vessels may cause chest pain (**angina pectoris**). Knowledge about the distribution of coronary artery branches therefore has great practical importance. Here, then, are some principles related to the heart's own blood supply that are worth noting:

- Both ventricles receive their blood supply from branches of the right and left coronary arteries.
- Each atrium, in contrast, receives blood only from a small branch of the corresponding coronary artery.
- The most abundant blood supply goes to the myocardium of the left ventricle—an appropriate amount—because the left ventricle does the most work and so needs the most oxygen and nutrients delivered to it.
- The right coronary artery is dominant in the hearts of about 50% of all people; the left coronary artery is dominant in about 20%; and in about 30%, neither right nor left coronary artery dominates.

Another fact about the heart's own blood supply—one of life-and-death importance—is that only a few connections, or anastomoses, exist between the larger branches of the coronary arteries. An **anastomosis** consists of one or more branches from the proximal part of an artery to a more distal part of itself or of another artery. Thus anastomoses provide detours in which arterial blood can travel if the main route becomes obstructed. In short, they provide collateral circulation to a part. This explains why the scarcity of anastomoses between larger coronary arteries looms so large as a threat to life.

If, for example, a blood clot plugs one of the larger coronary artery branches, as it often does in coronary thrombosis or embolism, too little or possibly no blood at all can reach some of the heart muscle cells. They become ischaemic, in other words. Deprived of oxygen, metabolic function is impaired and cell survival is threatened. **Myocardial infarction (MI)**—death of ischaemic heart muscle cells—soon results.

Another anatomical fact, however, brightens the picture somewhat: although few anastomoses exist between the larger coronary arteries, many anastomoses do exist between the very small arterial vessels in the heart. Given time, new anastomoses between the very small coronary arteries develop and provide collateral circulation to ischaemic areas. Several surgical procedures have been devised to aid this process (see Mechanisms of Disease, p. 656).

Box 28-1 discusses a method for visualizing blood channels through the coronary arteries.

BOX 28-1 *diagnostic study* | Angiography of the Heart

A special type of radiography called **angiography** is often used to visualize arteries, including the coronary arteries. A radiopaque dye—a substance that cannot be penetrated by x-rays—is injected into an artery to better visualize vessels that would otherwise be invisible in a radiograph. This dye is often called *contrast medium.*

Sometimes the dye is released through a long, thin tube called a catheter—a procedure called *catheterization.* The catheter can be pushed through peripheral arteries to the heart or another organ until its tip is in just the right location to release the dye. As the dye begins to circulate, an *angiogram* (radiograph) will show the outline of the arteries as clearly as if they were made of bone or other dense material (see figure).

An angiogram of an artery is often called an *arteriogram.* An angiogram of veins can be called a *venogram* or *phlebogram.* •

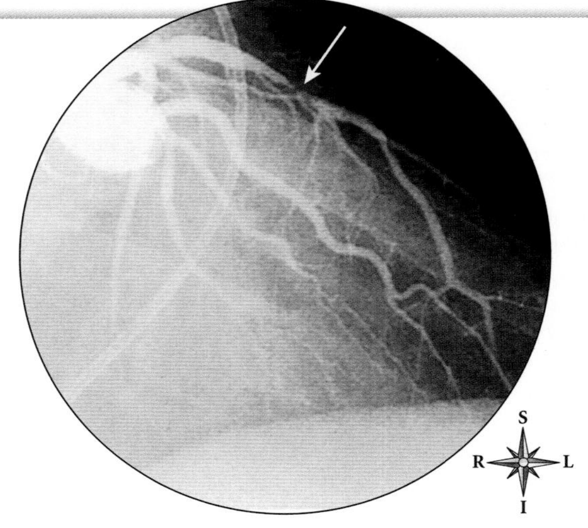

Widow maker. Coronary arteriogram of the coronary arteries shows a narrowing *(arrow)* of the channel in the left anterior descending (LAD) artery of the heart. Partial or complete occlusion of the LAD coronary artery is sometimes called the "widow maker" because complete occlusion of this artery results in a massive heart attack and sudden death—often occurring in men in their 50s.

CONNECT IT!

To learn more about radiography, check out ***Medical Imaging of the Body*** online at ***Connect It! Cardiac Nuclear Scanning*** is also used to assess blood flow in coronary vessels. Read all about it at ***Connect It!***

UNIT 4

Cardiac Veins

After blood has passed through **capillary** networks in the myocardium, it enters a series of cardiac veins before draining into the right atrium through a common venous channel called the *coronary sinus.* Several veins that collect blood from a small area of the right ventricle do not end in the coronary sinus but instead drain directly into the right atrium. As a rule, the cardiac veins (**Figure 28-12**) follow a course that closely parallels that of the coronary arteries.

Figures 3-18 and 3-19 in the BRIEF ATLAS OF THE HUMAN BODY show detailed, three-dimensional casts of the blood supply of the heart.

Nerve Supply of the Heart

The myocardium is autorhythmic and can thus produce its own action potentials without the influence of afferent nerve signals. To coordinate effective self-activation, the heart has a system of myocardial fibres specialized for rapid electrical conduction along a pathway extending from the top to the bottom of the heart. The myocardial structures that generate and conduct action potentials are called the *conduction system of the heart.* The structure and function of this important system are discussed later in this chapter.

Although the heart can generate its own rhythm of impulses (action potentials) and thus generate its own pumping contractions, the body sometimes has need to increase or decrease that rhythm. For example, when you increase the use of skeletal muscles and thus use oxygen more rapidly, your heart must increase its rate of pumping to keep the blood oxygen level near the set point. So it is no surprise that the heart receives efferent (motor) nerves that permit such regulation of the contractions of the heart.

Both divisions of the autonomic nervous system send fibres to the heart. Sympathetic fibres (contained in the middle, superior, and inferior cardiac nerves) and parasympathetic fibres (in branches of the vagus nerve) combine to form cardiac plexuses located close to the arch of the aorta. From the cardiac plexuses, fibres accompany the right and left coronary arteries to enter the heart. Here most of the fibres terminate in the *sinoatrial (SA) node* near the junction of the superior vena cava and right atrial wall. The SA node acts as the heart's *pacemaker* and is part of the heart's own conduction system, a concept we explore in the next section of this chapter.

However, some of the fibres end in the *atrioventricular (AV) node* (another part of the heart's conduction system) and in the atrial myocardium. A few parasympathetic fibres extend to the ventricular part of the heart's conduction system.

Because they increase the heart rate by stimulating the heart's built-in pacemaker, sympathetic nerves to the heart are also called *accelerator nerves.* Vagus fibres to the heart instead serve as *inhibitory* or *depressor nerves.*

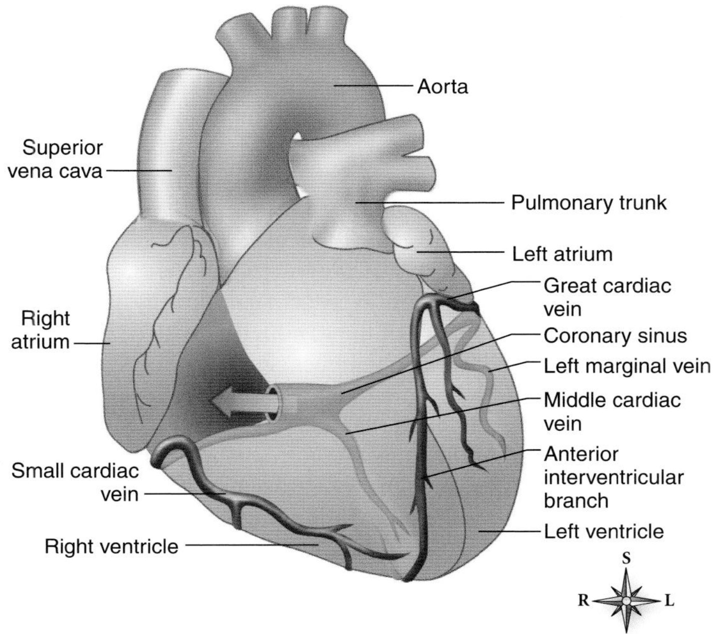

FIGURE 28-12 Coronary veins. Diagram showing the major veins of the coronary circulation (anterior view). Vessels near the anterior surface are more darkly coloured than vessels of the posterior surface seen through the heart.

Quick CHECK

9. Briefly describe the general structure and the function of the coronary circulation.
10. Why is an understanding of the coronary circulation so critical to understanding major types of heart disease?
11. What is meant by the term *conduction system of the heart*?
12. What is a myocardial infarction?

THE HEART AS A PUMP

Earlier in this chapter, we discussed the functional anatomy of the heart. Its four chambers and their valves make up two pumps: a left pump and a right pump. The left pump (left side of the heart) helps move blood through the systemic circulation, and the right pump (right side of the heart) helps move blood through the pulmonary circulation. We will now step back from our previous discussion of the valves and chambers of the heart to look at the bigger picture and see how these two linked pumps function together as a single unit. First, we will discuss the role of the electrical conduction system of the heart in coordinating heart contractions. Then we will discuss how these coordinated contractions produce the pumping cycle of the heart.

CONDUCTION SYSTEM OF THE HEART

For the heart to pump effectively, the impulses (action potentials) that trigger myocardial contraction must be coordinated carefully. This requires a system for generating rhythmic impulses and distributing them quickly to the different regions of the myocardium along impulse-conducting pathways. Without such a system, different regions of the myocardium would be contracting too slowly and at slightly different rates.

Four structures make up the core of the electrical conduction system of the heart:

1. **Sinoatrial (SA) node**
2. **Atrioventricular (AV) node**
3. **Atrioventricular (AV) bundle** (bundle of His)
4. **Subendocardial branches** (Purkinje fibres)

These structures are represented in **Figure 28-13** and described in the following paragraphs.

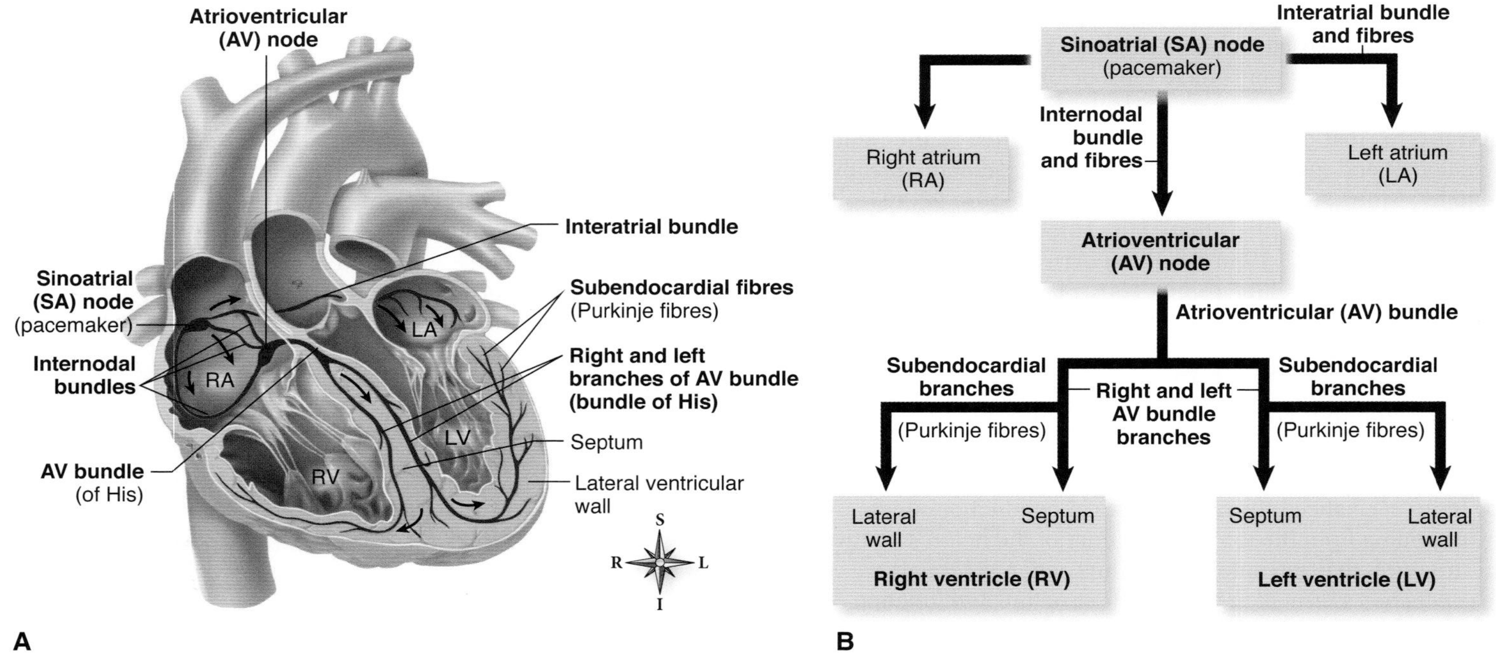

FIGURE 28-13 Conduction system of the heart. Specialized cardiac muscle cells *(boldface type)* in the wall of the heart rapidly initiate or conduct an electrical impulse throughout the myocardium. Both the sketch of the conduction system **(A)** and the flowchart **(B)** show the origin and path of conduction. The signal is initiated by the SA node (pacemaker) and spreads to the rest of the right atrial myocardium directly, to the left atrial myocardium by way of a bundle of interatrial conducting fibres, and to the AV node by way of three internodal bundles. The AV node then initiates a signal that is conducted through the ventricular myocardium by way of the AV bundle (of His) and subendocardial branches (Purkinje fibres).

Each of the structures of the heart's conduction system consists of cardiac muscle modified enough in structure to differ in function from ordinary cardiac muscle. The specialty of ordinary cardiac muscle is contraction. In this, it is like all muscle, and like all muscle, ordinary cardiac muscle can also conduct impulses. However, the myocardial fibres of the conduction system are more highly specialized, both structurally and functionally, than ordinary cardiac muscle tissue. They are not contractile. Instead, they permit only generation or rapid conduction of an action potential through the heart.

Fibres that initiate signals are called *pacemaker fibres*. During the resting membrane potential of a pacemaker fibre, there is leakage of K^+ ions out of the cell and an increasing flow of Na^+ and Ca^{++} ions inward. This slowly depolarizes the membrane, eventually reaching the threshold potential and triggering an action potential. Because this happens continuously, it produces an *intrinsic rhythm* of action potentials—setting the pace for other fibres in the syncytium connected together by gap junctions.

Conduction fibres are specially adapted for rapid conduction through the syncytium of connected cardiac fibres. These are the "high speed" fibres that quickly carry the action potential from pacemaker fibres out to more distant areas of the syncytium.

The normal cardiac impulse that initiates mechanical contraction of the heart arises in the SA node (or **pacemaker**), located just beneath the right atrial epicardium at its junction with the superior vena cava (**Figure 28-13**, A).

Each impulse generated at the SA node travels swiftly throughout the muscle fibres of both atria. An **interatrial bundle** of conduction fibres facilitates rapid conduction to the left atrium. Thus stimulated, the atria begin to contract. As the action potential enters the AV node by way of three **internodal bundles** of conduction fibres, its conduction slows markedly, thus allowing for complete contraction of both atrial chambers before the impulse reaches the ventricles.

After passing slowly through the AV node, conduction velocity increases as the impulse is relayed through the AV bundle (bundle of His) into the ventricles. Here, right and left *bundle branches* and the subendocardial branches (Purkinje fibres) in which they terminate conduct the impulses throughout the muscle of both ventricles, stimulating them to contract almost simultaneously.

Thus the SA node initiates each heartbeat and sets its pace—it is the heart's own natural *pacemaker*. Under the influence of autonomic and endocrine control, the SA node will normally "discharge", or "fire", at an intrinsic rhythmical rate of 70 to 75 beats/min in resting conditions. However, if for any reason the SA node loses its ability to generate an impulse, pacemaker activity will shift to another excitable component of the conduction system, such as the AV node or the subendocardial branches (Purkinje fibres). Pacemakers other than the SA node are abnormal and are usually **ectopic pacemakers.** Ectopic is a word that means "out of place". Although ectopic pacemakers fire rhythmically, their rate of discharge is generally much slower than that of the SA node. For example, a pulse of 40 to 60 beats/min would result if the AV node were forced to assume pacemaker activity.

CONNECT IT! 

If the heart's own pacemaker fails to maintain a healthy heart rhythm, an artificial pacemaker can be implanted to restore normal function. Check out ***Artificial Cardiac Pacemakers*** online at ***Connect It!*** to see how this is done.

ELECTROCARDIOGRAM (ECG)

Electrocardiography

Impulse conduction generates tiny electrical currents in the heart that spread through surrounding tissues to the surface of the body. This fact has great clinical importance. Why? Because from the skin, visible records of the heart's electrical activity can be made with an instrument called an *electrocardiograph*. Skilled interpretation of these records may sometimes make the difference between life and death.

The **electrocardiogram** (ECG) is a graphic record of the heart's electrical activity, its conduction of impulses. It is not a record of the heart's contractions but of the *electrical events* that precede them. To produce an electrocardiogram, electrodes of a recording voltmeter (electrocardiograph) are attached to the limbs and/or chest of the subject (**Figure 28-14**, A). Changes in voltage, which represent changes in the heart's electrical activity, are observed as deflections of a line drawn on paper or traced on a video monitor.

Figure 28-15 explains the basic theory behind **electrocardiography.** To keep things simple, a single cardiac muscle fibre is shown with the two electrodes of a recording voltmeter nearby. Before the action potential reaches either electrode, there is no difference in charge between the electrodes, and thus no change in voltage is recorded on the voltmeter graph (**Figure 28-15**, step *1*). As an action potential reaches the first electrode, the external surface of the sarcolemma becomes relatively negative and so the voltmeter records a difference in charge between the two electrodes as an upward deflection of the pen on the recording chart (**Figure 28-15**, step *2*). When the action potential also reaches the second electrode, the pen returns to the zero baseline because there is no difference in charge between the two electrodes (**Figure 28-15**, step *3*). As the end of the action potential passes the first electrode, the sarcolemma is again relatively positive on its outer surface, causing the pen to again deflect away from the baseline. This time, because the direction of the negative and positive electrodes is reversed, the pen deflects downward rather than upward (**Figure 28-15**, step *4*). After the end of the action potential also passes the second electrode, the pen again returns to the zero baseline (**Figure 28-15**, step *5*). In short, depolarization of cardiac muscle causes a deflection of the graphed line; repolarization causes a deflection in the opposite direction.

Electrocardiography electrodes are normally quite some distance from myocardial tissue, but, given the massive size of the myocardial syncytium, it should not be surprising that even cutaneous electrodes can detect changes in the heart's polarity.

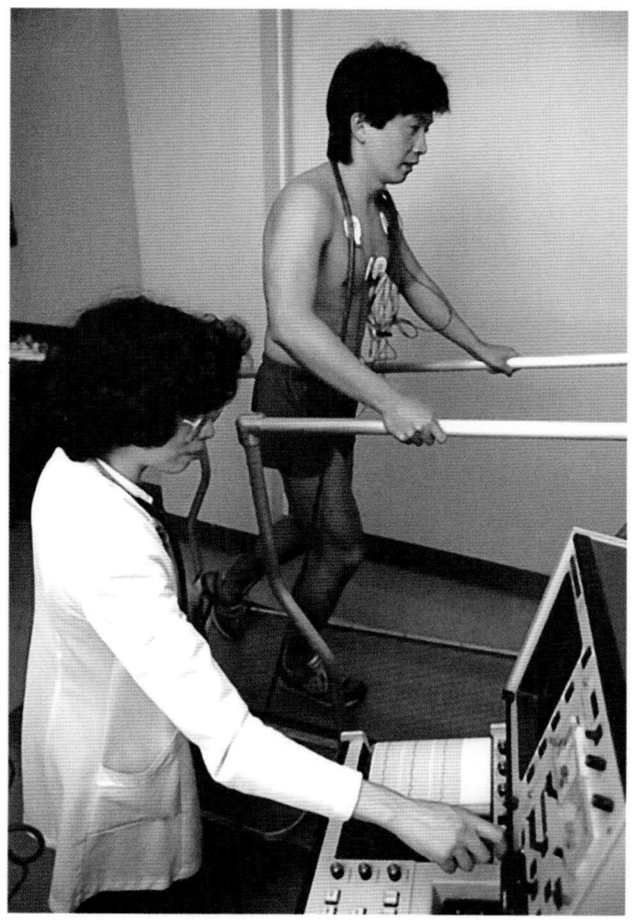

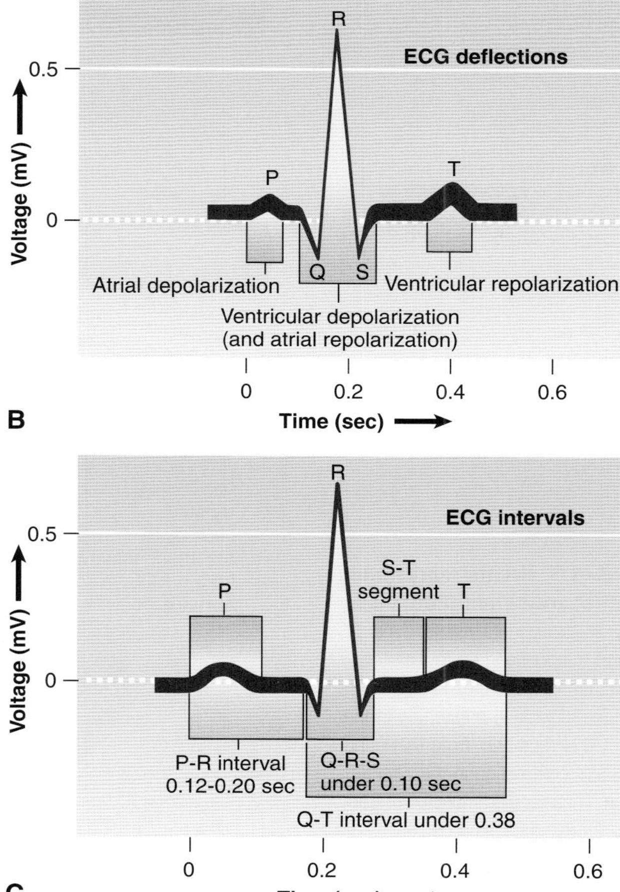

FIGURE 28-14 Electrocardiogram (ECG). A, A nurse monitors a patient's ECG as he exercises on a treadmill. **B,** Idealized ECG deflections represent depolarization and repolarization of cardiac muscle tissue. **C,** Principal ECG intervals between P, QRS, and T waves. Note that the P–R interval is measured from the start of the P wave to the start of the Q wave. The fact that ECG tracings in **B** and **C** are not exactly identical reflects normal variations in the heart's electrical activity.

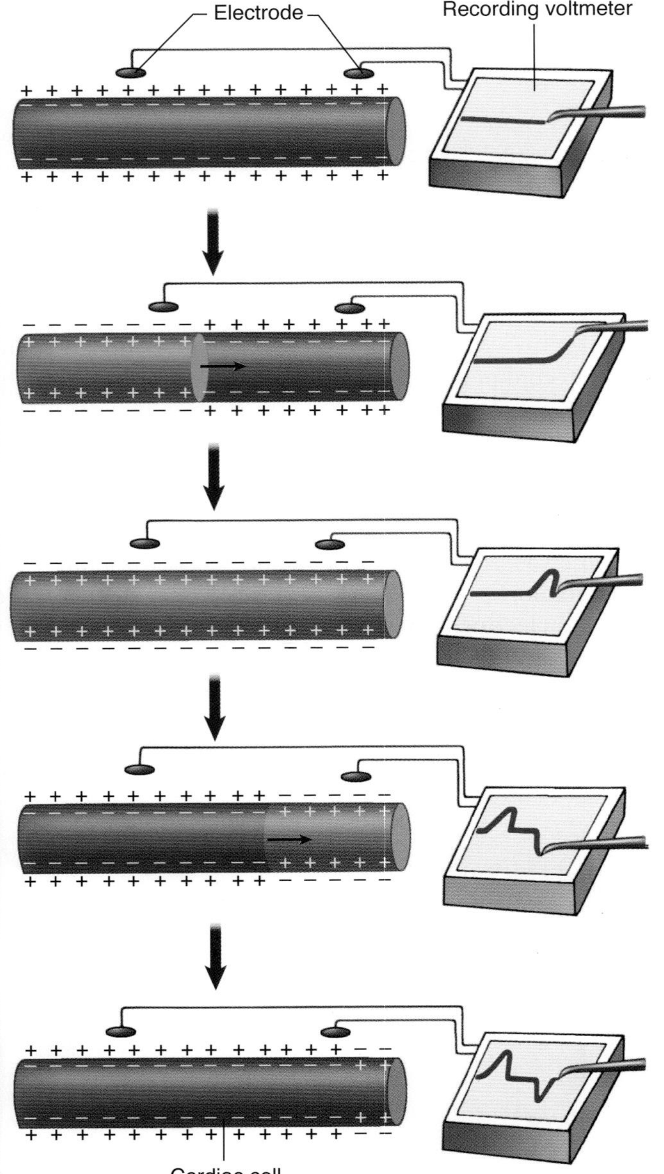

FIGURE 28-15 The basic theory of electrocardiography.

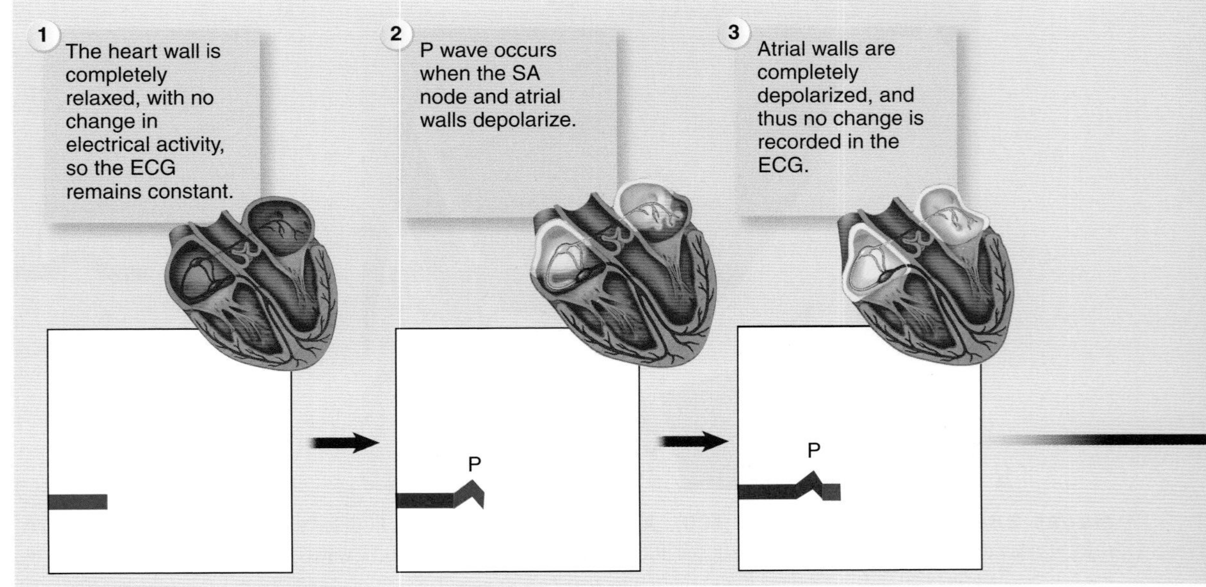

1
The heart wall is completely relaxed, with no change in electrical activity, so the ECG remains constant.
2
P wave occurs when the SA node and atrial walls depolarize.
P
3
Atrial walls are completely depolarized, and thus no change is recorded in the ECG.
P

FIGURE 28-16 Events represented by the electrocardiogram (ECG). It is impossible to illustrate the invisible, dynamic events of heart conduction in a few cartoon panels or "snapshots", but the sketches here give you an idea of what is happening in the heart as an ECG is recorded. Note that depolarization triggers contraction in the affected muscle tissue. Thus cardiac muscle contraction occurs *after* depolarization begins.

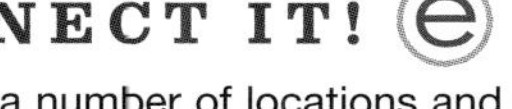

There are a number of locations and patterns of attaching ECG leads. Different ECG setups produce different results—thus allowing physicians to "see" the electrical activity of the heart from different angles. See how this is done in ***Electrocardiography*** online at ***Connect It!***

ECG Waves

Because electrocardiography is far too complex a subject to explain fully here, normal ECG *deflection waves* and the *ECG intervals* between them will be discussed only briefly. As shown in **Figure 28-14**, *B*, and **Figure 28-16**, the normal ECG is composed of deflection waves called the *P wave*, *QRS complex*, and *T wave*. (The letters do not represent any words; they are simply an arbitrarily chosen sequence of letters of the alphabet.)

P Wave

The **P wave** represents depolarization of the atria. That is, the P wave is the deflection caused by the passage of an electrical impulse from the SA node through the musculature of both atria. P wave abnormalities often reflect atrial enlargement.

QRS Complex

The **QRS complex** represents depolarization of the ventricles. Depolarization of the ventricles is a complex process, involving depolarization of the interventricular septum and the subsequent spread of depolarization by the subendocardial branches (Purkinje fibres) through the lateral ventricular walls. Rather than getting mired in a detailed explanation, let us simplify matters by stating that the combined duration of all three deflections of the QRS complex (Q, R, and S) represents the time required (0.07–0.11 second) for ventricular depolarization. (See **Figure 28-14**, *C*.)

At the same time that the ventricles are depolarizing, the atria are repolarizing. As we explained earlier, we should expect to see a deflection that is opposite in direction to the P wave that represented depolarization. However, the massive ventricular depolarization that is occurring at the same time overshadows the voltage fluctuation produced by atrial repolarization. Thus we can say that the QRS complex represents both ventricular depolarization and atrial repolarization. If the QRS duration is prolonged, ventricular conduction delay is probably occurring.

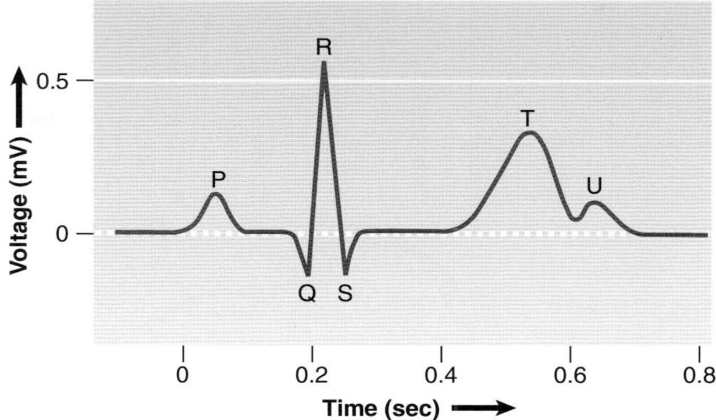
Voltage (mV)
0.5
0
R
P
T
U
Q S
0
0.2
0.4
0.6
0.8
Time (sec)

FIGURE 28-17 The U wave. This electrocardiogram (ECG) recording shows the presence of a U wave, which follows the T wave—or appears as a "hump" on the back of the T wave. The U wave represents a sudden, late repolarization of subendocardial branches (Purkinje fibres) in the papillary muscle.

T Wave

The **T wave** reflects repolarization of the ventricles. In atria, the first part of the myocardium to depolarize is the first to repolarize. In ventricles, on the other hand, the first part of the myocardium to depolarize is the last to repolarize. Thus ECG deflections for both depolarization and repolarization are in the same direction. An inverted T wave is often seen after myocardial muscle damage.

Sometimes, an additional **U wave** may be seen in the electrocardiogram (**Figure 28-17**). The U wave, when visible, appears as a tiny "hump" at the end of the T wave. The U wave is thought to represent late repolarization of subendocardial branches (Purkinje fibres) in the papillary muscle of the ventricular myocardium. However, some cardiologists believe it is simply a two-part T wave resulting from

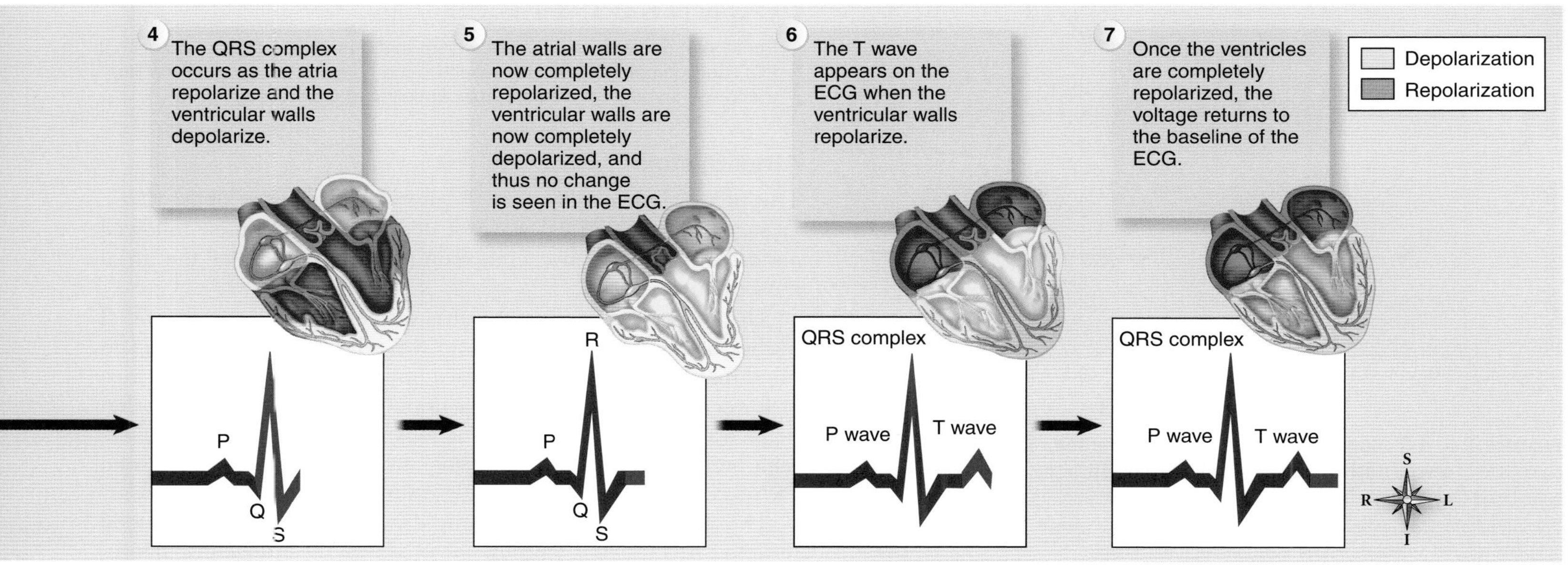
4 The QRS complex occurs as the atria repolarize and the ventricular walls depolarize.
5 The atrial walls are now completely repolarized, the ventricular walls are now completely depolarized, and thus no change is seen in the ECG.
6 The T wave appears on the ECG when the ventricular walls repolarize.
7 Once the ventricles are completely repolarized, the voltage returns to the baseline of the ECG.
Depolarization
Repolarization
P
Q
S
R
P
Q
S
QRS complex
P wave
T wave
QRS complex
P wave
T wave
S
R
L
I

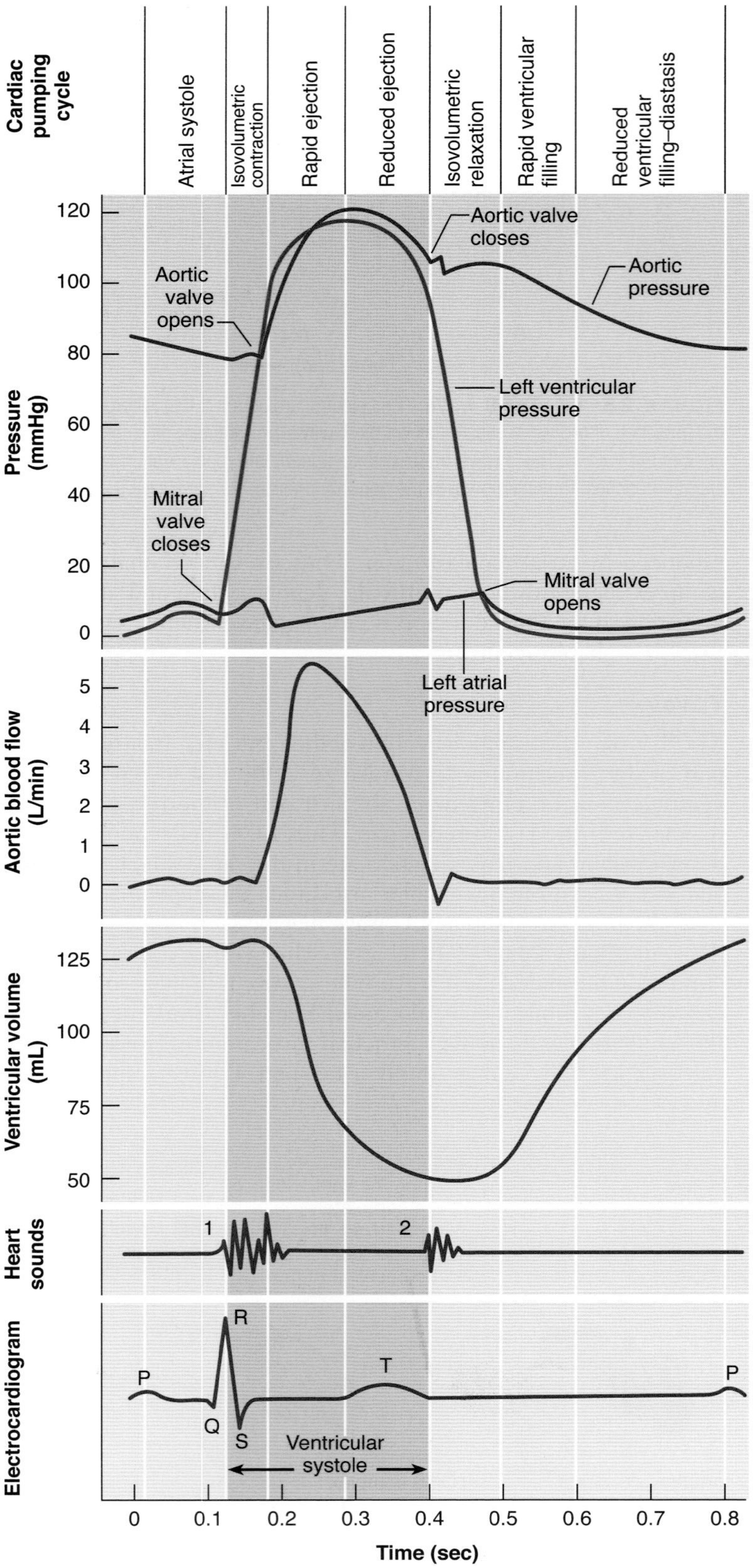

FIGURE 28-18 Composite chart of heart function. This chart is a composite of several diagrams of heart function (cardiac pumping cycle, blood pressure, blood flow, volume, heart sounds, and electrocardiogram [ECG]), all adjusted to the same time scale. Although it appears daunting at first glance, you will find it a valuable reference tool as you proceed through this chapter.

longer duration of the action potential in some ventricular myocardial cells. If not too big, U waves are usually considered to be normal. Sometimes, however, U waves can be a sign of **hypokalaemia** (low blood potassium) or too much **digoxin** (a heart medication).

ECG Intervals

The principal ECG intervals between P, QRS, and T waves are shown in **Figure 28-14**, C. Measurement of these intervals can provide valuable information concerning the rate of conduction of an action potential through the heart, as we shall see later in this chapter. **Figure 28-16** summarizes the relationship between the electrical events of the myocardium and the ECG recordings.

Quick CHECK

13. List the principal structures of the heart's conduction system.
14. What are the three deflection waves seen in a typical ECG?
15. What event does each ECG wave represent?

Cardiac Cycle

The term **cardiac cycle** means a complete heartbeat, or pumping cycle, consisting of contraction (**systole**) and relaxation (**diastole**) of both atria and both ventricles. The two atria contract simultaneously. Then, as the atria relax, the two ventricles contract and relax, instead of the entire heart contracting as a unit. This gives a kind of pumping action to the movements of the heart. The atria remain relaxed during part of the ventricular relaxation and then start the cycle over again. The cycle as a whole is often divided into time intervals for discussion and study. The following sections describe several of the important events of the cardiac cycle. As you read through these sections, refer frequently to **Figure 28-18**, which is a composite chart that graphically illustrates and integrates changes in pressure gradients in the left atrium, left ventricle, and aorta with ECG and heart sound recordings. Aortic blood flow and changes in ventricular volume are also shown. Refer also to **Figure 28-19**, which shows the major phases of the cardiac cycle.

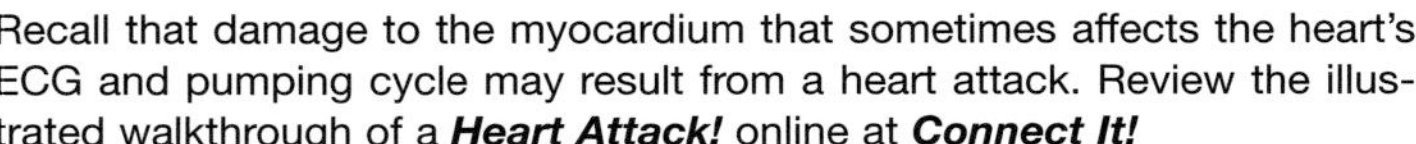

CONNECT IT!

Recall that damage to the myocardium that sometimes affects the heart's ECG and pumping cycle may result from a heart attack. Review the illustrated walkthrough of a ***Heart Attack!*** online at ***Connect It!***

Atrial Systole

This phase of the cardiac cycle begins with the P wave of the ECG. Passage of the electrical wave of depolarization is then followed almost immediately by actual contraction (systole) of the atrial musculature.

The contracting force of the atria creates a pressure gradient that pushes blood out of the atria into the relaxed ventricles. Keep in mind that fluid moves from an area of high pressure toward an area of lower pressure—an important principle of haemodynamics that helps explain how the heart functions as a pump. Because of the high pressure of atrial blood during atrial systole, blood moves into the relaxed ventricles, where the pressure is lower.

The pressure gradient not only drives the movement of blood from the atria into the ventricles, it also keeps the atrioventricular (or

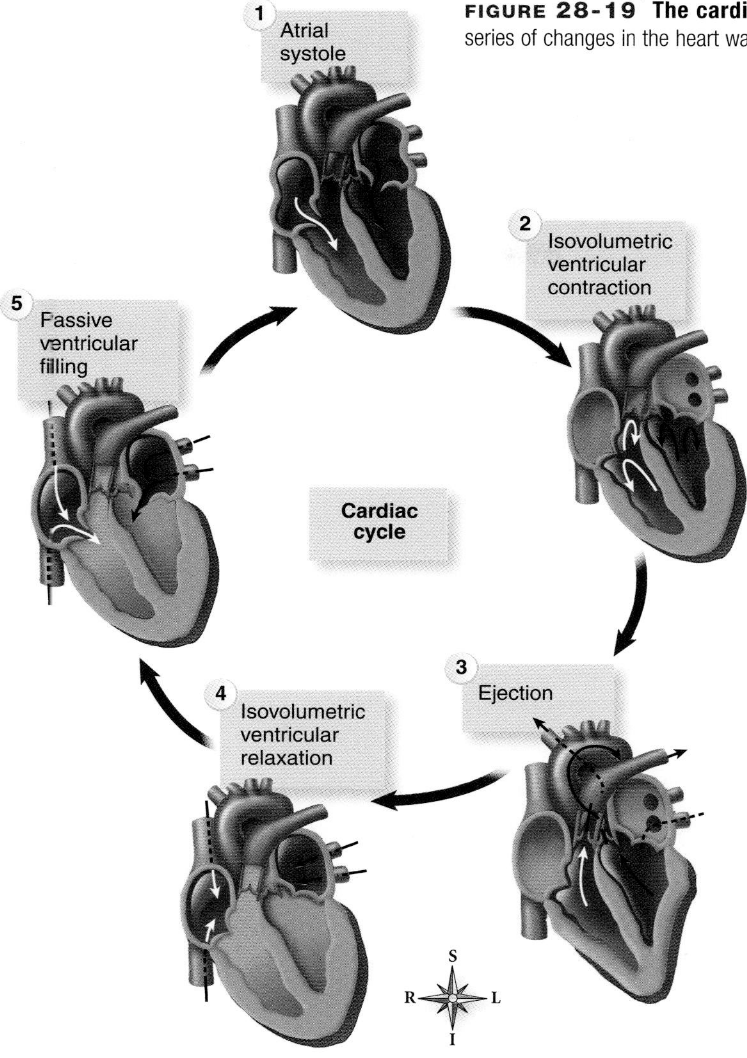

FIGURE 28-19 The cardiac cycle. The five steps of the heart's pumping cycle described in the text are shown as a series of changes in the heart wall and valves.

cuspid) valves open during this phase. The ventricles are relaxed and rapidly filling with blood. The semilunar valves are closed because during this phase the arterial pressure is higher than pressure in the relaxed ventricles. This pressure gradient pushes blood against the semilunar valves and thereby prevents reentry of blood from the pulmonary artery or aorta.

Isovolumetric Ventricular Contraction

The onset of ventricular systole coincides with the R wave of the ECG and the appearance of the first heart sound.

Iso- is a combining form denoting equality or uniformity, and *volumetric* denotes measurement of volume. Thus *isovolumetric* is a term that means "having the same measured volume". During the brief period of isovolumetric ventricular contraction, the intraventricular pressure begins to increase. This is enough of a pressure increase in the ventricles to overcome atrial pressure and close the atrioventricular valves—producing the first heart sound—but not enough to overcome arterial pressure and open the semilunar valves. This phase occurs between the start of ventricular systole and the opening of the semilunar valves, during which ventricular volume remains constant as the pressure increases rapidly.

Ejection

The semilunar valves open and blood is ejected from the heart when the pressure in the ventricles exceeds the pressure in the pulmonary artery and aorta. An initial, shorter phase, called *rapid ejection*, is characterized by a marked increase in ventricular and aortic pressure and in aortic blood flow. The T wave of the ECG appears during the later, longer phase of *reduced ejection* (characterized by a less abrupt decrease in ventricular volume). A considerable quantity of blood, called the **residual volume,** normally remains in the ventricles at the end of the ejection period. In heart failure the residual volume remaining in the ventricles may greatly exceed that ejected during systole.

Isovolumetric Ventricular Relaxation

Ventricular diastole, or relaxation, begins with the isovolumetric ventricular relaxation period of the cardiac cycle. It is the period between closure of the semilunar valves and opening of the atrioventricular valves. At the end of ventricular ejection, the semilunar valves close when the ventricular pressure drops below arterial pressure and pushes the valve flaps closed. As the valves snap shut, they produce the second heart sound. Closure of the semilunar valves prevents blood from reentering the ventricular chambers from the pulmonary trunk and aorta. Both sets of valves are closed, and the ventricles are relaxing.

Ventricular relaxation causes a dramatic fall in intraventricular pressure but not enough to open the atrioventricular valves. Because the valves are closed, there is no change in volume. The atrioventricular valves do not open until the pressure in the atrial chambers increases above that in the relaxing ventricles.

Passive Ventricular Filling

As the ventricles continue to relax, the intraventricular pressure continues to drop. That, along with rising intraatrial pressure produced by return of venous blood, produces a pressure gradient sufficient to force open the atrioventricular valves. Blood then rushes into the relaxing ventricles.

The rapid influx of blood into the ventricles lasts about 0.1 second and results in a dramatic increase in ventricular volume. The term *diastasis* is often used to describe a later, longer period of slow ventricular filling as ventricular diastole ends. The abrupt inflow of blood that occurred immediately after opening of the atrioventricular valves is followed by a slow but continuous flow of venous blood into the atria and then through the open atrioventricular valves into the ventricles. Diastasis lasts about 0.2 second and is characterized by a gradual increase in ventricular pressure and volume.

At the end of this phase of the cardiac cycle, a new P wave triggers the contraction of atria that marks the beginning of another *atrial systole* phase—and new cardiac cycle.

CONNECT IT! 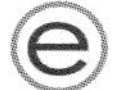

Review ***Echocardiography*** online at ***Connect It!*** to learn how sound waves are used to visualize the events of the cardiac cycle.

Heart Sounds

The heart makes certain typical sounds during each cardiac cycle that are described as sounding like "lubb-dupp" when heard through a stethoscope.

The first heart sound (S1) is caused primarily by the contraction (systole) of the ventricles and also by vibrations of the closing AV, or cuspid, valves. It is longer and lower than the second heart sound (S2), which is short and sharp and is caused by vibrations of the closing SL valves as the ventricles relax (diastole) (see **Figure 28-18**). S1 and S2 are sometimes called the systolic and diastolic sounds, respectively.

Heart sounds have clinical significance because they provide information about the valves of the heart. Any variation from normal in the sounds indicates imperfect functioning of the valves. For example, a third heart sound (S3), producing a "lubb-dupp-up" pattern, may be produced by a sudden myocardial stretching during rapid ventricular filling (atrial systole). S3 is normal in children and thin, young adults. However, S3 may indicate pericarditis or ventricular failure in older adults.

A fourth heart sound (S4) may occur just before S1, producing a "la-lubb-dupp" pattern. S4 may be found in healthy older adults, but may also indicate a stiff ventricular wall or abnormally increased pressure at the end of ventricular diastole, which may occur in a variety of cardiac disorders.

If S3 is also present, the pattern is more like "la-lubb-dupp-up". Because they make the heartbeat somewhat resemble the sound of hoofbeats, S3 and/or S4 patterns are sometimes called heart gallop patterns.

Heart murmur is one type of commonly heard abnormal heart sound. It is sometimes described as a "swishing" sound that may signify incomplete closing of the valves (valvular insufficiency) or stenosis (constriction, or narrowing) of them.

cycle of life

Heart At the beginning of this chapter, we mentioned that the heart is one of the first organs to begin functioning during embryonic development. Throughout childhood, adolescence, and adulthood, the heart normally maintains its basic structure and function—pumping continuously and thus permitting continued survival of the individual. Perhaps the only apparent normal changes in these structures occur as a result of regular exercise. The myocardium thickens and the supply of blood vessels in skeletal muscle tissues increases in response to increased oxygen and glucose use during prolonged exercise.

As we pass through adulthood, especially later adulthood, various degenerative changes can occur in the heart. For example, a type of "hardening of the arteries", called **atherosclerosis,** can result in blockage or weakening of critical coronary arteries—perhaps causing a myocardial infarction or stroke. The heart valves and myocardial tissues often degenerate with age, becoming hardened or fibrotic and less able to perform their functions properly. This reduces the heart's pumping efficiency and therefore threatens homeostasis of the entire internal environment. •

Quick CHECK

16. Using **Figure 28-19** as a guide, describe the major events of the cardiac cycle.
17. As the ventricles contract, their volume remains constant for a time. Explain why the volume does not begin to decrease immediately.

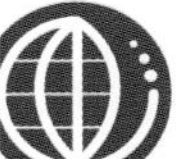

the big picture | Heart

You have just explored the complex structures of the heart and how they allow it to act as a pump to keep blood circulating through the vast network of vessels that reach nearly every part of your body. Without the pumping of the heart, blood could not transport substances quickly around the body's internal environment. Cells of the brain would starve for oxygen. Every organ would soon run out of the water that is essential to life. Mitochondria would have no nutrients to "recharge" the ATP that provides energy for life. Wastes could not be removed from tissues and excreted from the body. Not a single organ in the body could do its job of maintaining the relative constancy of the internal environment. It is no wonder, then, that the heart has often been considered the most vital of all of our organs—the most necessary for life. We are learning that there is no "one" organ that supports life, but we can now better appreciate why the heart plays this metaphorical role in our thinking. •

mechanisms of disease

Disorders of the Heart

Disorders of Heart Structure

Disorders Involving the Pericardium

If the pericardium becomes inflamed, a condition called **pericarditis** results. Pericarditis may be caused by various factors: trauma, viral or bacterial infection, tumours, and other factors. The pericardial oedema that characterizes this condition often causes the visceral and parietal layers of the serous pericardium to rub together—causing severe chest pain. Pericardial fluid, pus, or blood (in the case of an injury) may accumulate in the space between the two pericardial layers and impair the pumping action of the heart. This is termed **pericardial effusion** and may develop into a serious compression of the heart called **cardiac tamponade.**

Pericarditis may be acute or chronic, depending on the rate, severity, and duration of symptoms. Clinical manifestations include pericardial pain that increases with respirations or coughing, a "friction rub" (a grating, scratching sound heard over the left sternal border and upper ribs) resulting from the swollen pericardial layers rubbing against each other, difficulty breathing, restlessness, and an accumulation of pericardial fluid. Cardiac tamponade requires immediate pericardial drainage **(pericardiocentesis).** Antibiotics are usually prescribed to treat the causative organism, and nonsteroidal antiinflammatory agents such as aspirin are prescribed to reduce the inflammation and thus control the symptoms.

Disorders Involving Heart Valves

Disorders of the cardiac valves can have several effects. For example, a congenital defect in valve structure can result in mild to severe pumping inefficiency. Incompetent valves leak, allowing some blood to flow back into the chamber from

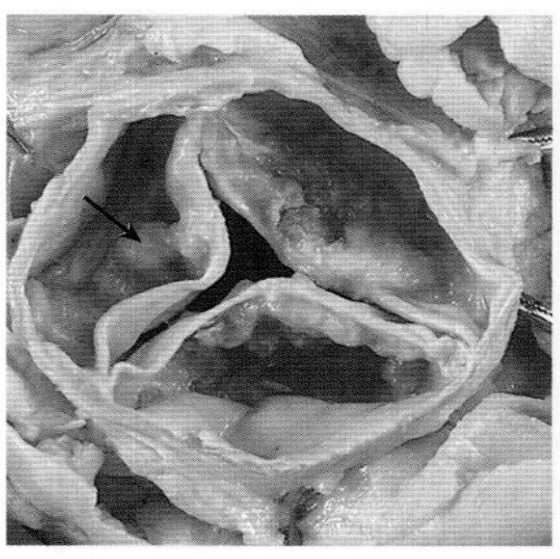

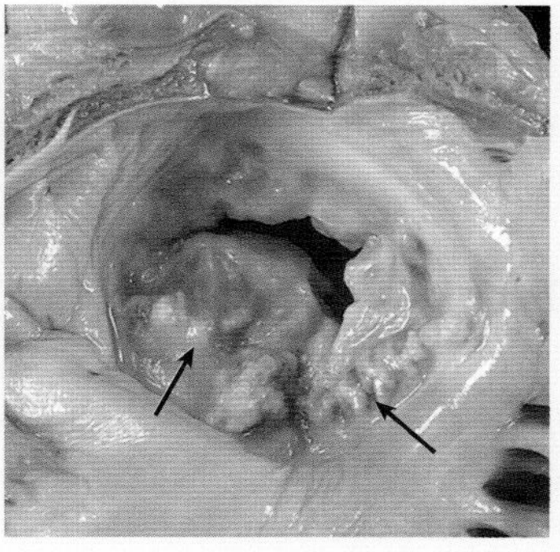

FIGURE 28-20 Stenosed valves. *Left,* Aortic valve; *right,* mitral valve. Note the calcific nodules *(arrows)* attached to the cusps, thus narrowing the opening and slowing blood flow.

which it came. **Stenosed valves** are valves that are narrower than normal, slowing blood flow from a heart chamber (**Figure 28-20**).

Rheumatic heart disease results from a delayed inflammatory response to streptococcal infection that occurs most often in children. A few weeks after an improperly treated streptococcal infection, the cardiac valves and other tissues in the body may become inflamed—a condition called **rheumatic fever.** If severe, the inflammation can result in stenosis or other deformities of the valves, chordae tendineae, or myocardium.

Mitral valve prolapse (MVP), a condition affecting the bicuspid or mitral valve has a genetic basis in some cases but can result from rheumatic fever or other factors. A prolapsed mitral valve is one whose flaps extend back into the left atrium, causing incompetence (leaking) of the valve (**Figure 28-21**). Although this condition is common, occurring in up to 1 in every 20 people, most cases are asymptomatic. In severe cases, patients experience chest pain and fatigue.

Aortic regurgitation is a condition in which blood not only ejects forward into the aorta but also regurgitates back into the left ventricle because of a leaky aortic semilunar valve. This causes a volume overload on the left ventricle, with subsequent hypertrophy and dilation of the left ventricle. The left ventricle attempts to compensate for the increased load by increasing its strength of contraction. Such a heavy load may eventually stress the heart to the point of causing myocardial **ischaemia** (decreased blood flow causing muscle cell impairment).

Damaged or defective cardiac valves can often be replaced surgically—a procedure called **valvuloplasty.** Artificial valves made from synthetic materials, as well as valves taken from other mammals such as swine, are often used in these valve replacement procedures.

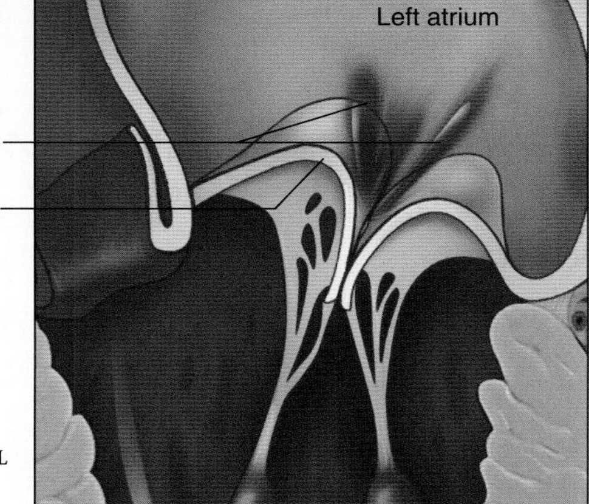

FIGURE 28-21 Mitral valve prolapse. The normal mitral valve *(left)* prevents backflow of blood from the left ventricle into the left atrium during ventricular systole (contraction). The prolapsed mitral valve *(inset)* permits leakage because the valve flaps billow backward, parting slightly.

Disorders Involving the Myocardium

One of the leading causes of death in the UK is **coronary artery disease (CAD).** This condition can result from many causes, all of which somehow reduce the flow of blood to the vital myocardial tissue. For example, in both coronary thrombosis and coronary embolism, a blood clot occludes, or plugs, some part of a coronary artery. Blood cannot pass through the occluded vessel and so cannot reach the heart muscle cells it normally supplies. Deprived of oxygen, these cells soon die or are damaged. In medical terms, a **myocardial infarction (MI),** or tissue death, occurs.

A myocardial infarction (heart attack) is a common cause of death during middle and late adulthood. Recovery from a myocardial infarction is possible if the amount of heart tissue damaged is small enough that the remaining undamaged heart muscle can pump blood effectively enough to supply the needs of the rest of the heart, as well as the body.

CONNECT IT! ⓔ

How does a heart attack develop? Take a tour through an illustrated description of the process of an MI in ***Heart Attack!*** online at ***Connect It!*** At the same time check out Heart Sounds online at ***Connect It!***

Coronary arteries may also become blocked as a result of *atherosclerosis,* a type of "hardening of the arteries" in which lipids and other substances build up within the wall of blood vessels and eventually calcify, making the vessel wall hard and brittle. Mechanisms of atherosclerosis are discussed elsewhere in this chapter. Coronary atherosclerosis has increased dramatically over the last half century to become the leading cause of death in western countries. Many pathophysiologists believe this increase results from a change in lifestyle. They cite several important risk factors associated with coronary atherosclerosis: cigarette smoking, high-fat and high-cholesterol blood plasma, diabetes, and hypertension (high blood pressure).

The term **angina pectoris** is used to describe the severe chest pain that occurs when the myocardium is deprived of adequate oxygen. It is often a warning that the coronary arteries are no longer able to supply enough blood and oxygen to the heart muscle. **Coronary bypass surgery** is a common treatment for those with severely restricted coronary artery blood flow. In this procedure, veins and sometimes arteries are "harvested" from other areas of the body and used to bypass partial blockages in coronary arteries (**Figure 28-22**).

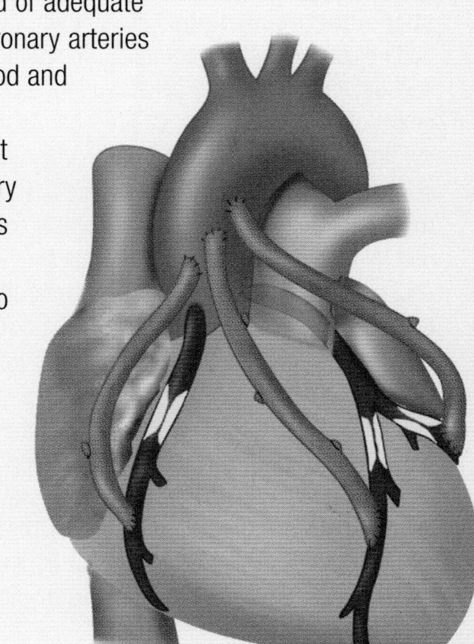

FIGURE 28-22 Coronary bypass. In coronary bypass surgery, blood vessels are "harvested" or "rerouted" from other parts of the body and used to construct detours around blocked coronary arteries. Artificial vessels can also be used.

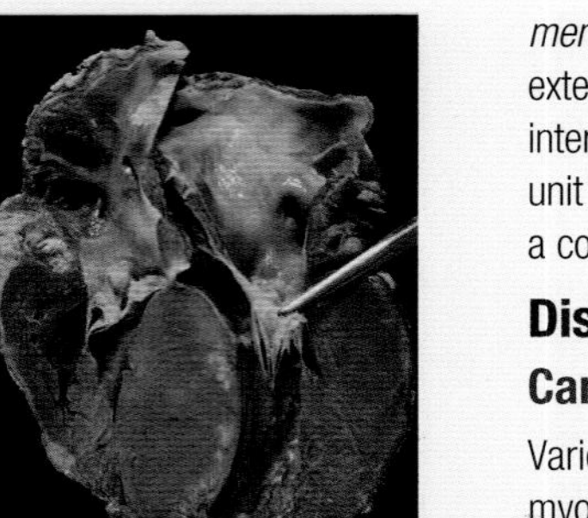

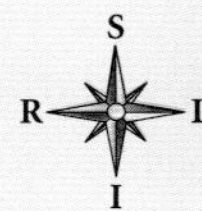
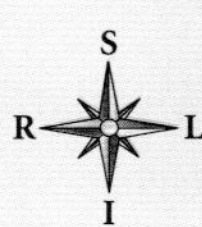

FIGURE 28-23 Hypertrophic cardiomyopathy. Note the dramatic increase of myocardial tissue. This genetic condition may cause sudden heart failure in the apparent absence of warning symptoms.

The term **cardiomyopathy** is used to describe a number of different types of heart diseases that result in abnormal enlargement. In addition to left and right ventricular hypertrophy, another form of enlargement is called **hypertrophic cardiomyopathy** and is caused by a genetic defect. **Figure 28-23** shows the appearance of the heart in this condition. It is one of the most common causes of sudden unexplained death in young athletes.

CONNECT IT! 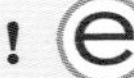

Have you ever heard of broken heart syndrome? Also called stress cardiomyopathy, this is a temporary condition induced by intense physical or emotional stress—but can mimic serious cardiac conditions. Find out more in ***Broken Heart*** online at ***Connect It!***

Patients in danger of death because of heart failure may be candidates for heart *transplants* or heart *implants.* Heart transplants are surgical procedures in which healthy hearts from recently deceased donors replace the hearts of patients with heart disease. Unfortunately, a continuing problem with this procedure is the tendency of the body's immune system to reject the new heart—perceiving it as a foreign tissue. More details about the rejection of transplanted tissues are found in later chapters.

Heart implants are artificial hearts that are made of biologically inert synthetic materials. On July 3, 2001, the first artificial heart was successfully implanted into Robert Tools by University of Louisville researchers. The 1-kg *AbioCor Implantable Replacement Heart* ("artificial heart") allowed the patient to move about freely without any external pumps. Portable external battery packs are used to recharge the small internal battery that powers the internal pumping unit. The success of the AbioCor unit and other artificial heart models gives hope that artificial hearts will one day be a commonplace and effective treatment for patients with severe heart disease.

Disorders of Heart Function

Cardiac Dysrhythmia

Various conditions such as inflammation of the endocardium (endocarditis) or myocardial infarction (heart attack) can damage the heart's conduction system and thereby disturb the normal rhythmical beating of the heart (**Figure 28-24**, *A*). The term **dysrhythmia** refers to an abnormality of heart rhythm. Dysrhythmia may also be called *arrhythmia.*

One kind of dysrhythmia is called a **heart block.** In AV node block, impulses are blocked from getting through to the ventricular myocardium, resulting in the ventricles contracting at a much slower rate than normal. On an ECG, there may be a large interval between the P wave and the R peak of the QRS complex (**Figure 28-24**, *B*). *Complete heart block* occurs when the P waves do not

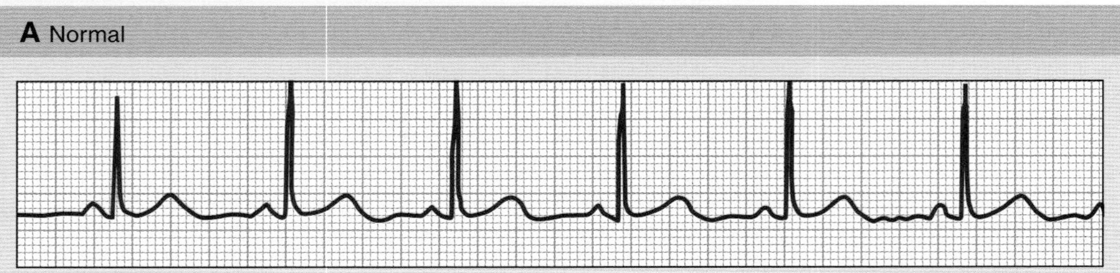

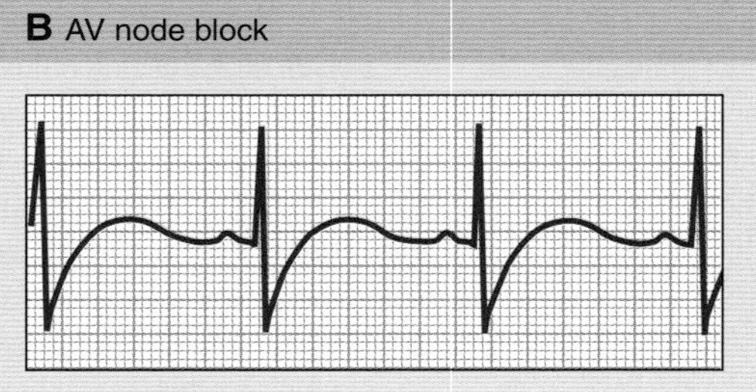

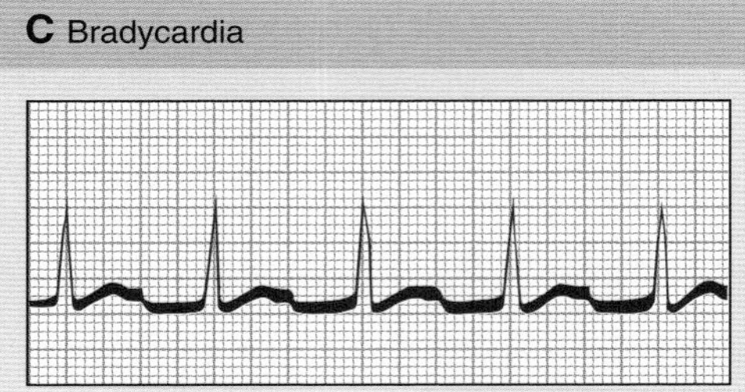

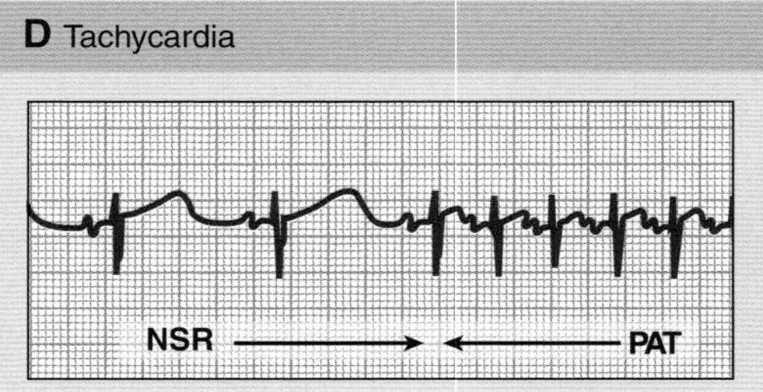

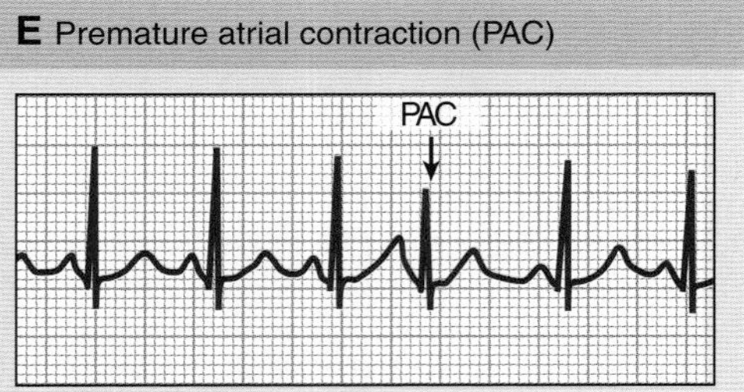

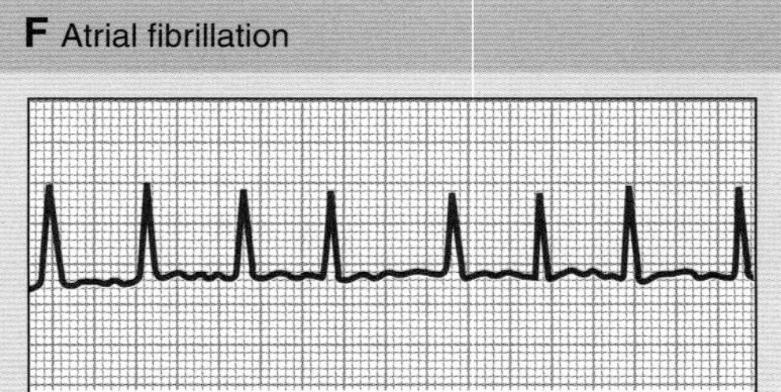

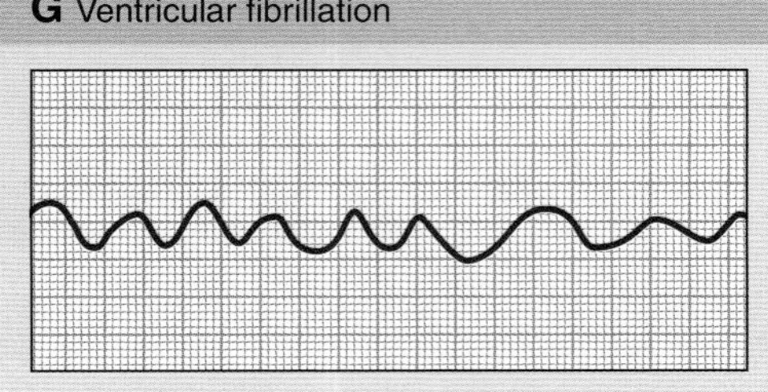

FIGURE 28-24 Electrocardiogram (ECG) strip chart recordings. A, Normal ECG. **B,** AV node block. Very slow ventricular contraction (25 to 45 beats/min at rest); P waves widely separated from peaks of QRS complexes. **C,** Bradycardia. Slow heart rhythm (less than 60 beats/min); no disruption of normal rhythm pattern. **D,** Tachycardia. Rapid heart rhythm (greater than 100 beats/min); no disruption of normal rhythm pattern. *NSR,* Normal sinus rhythm; *PAT,* paroxysmal (sudden) atrial tachycardia. **E,** Premature atrial contraction (PAC). Unexpected, early P wave that differs from normal P waves; PR interval may be shorter or longer than normal; normal QRS complex; more than 6 PACs per minute may precede atrial fibrillation. **F,** Atrial fibrillation. Irregular, rapid atrial depolarizations; P wave rapid (greater than 300/min) with irregular QRS complexes (110–180 beats/min). **G,** Ventricular fibrillation. Complete disruption of normal heart rhythm.

match up at all with the QRS complexes—as in an ECG that shows two or more P waves for every QRS complex. A physician may treat heart block by implanting in the heart an *artificial pacemaker.*

Bradycardia is a slow heart rhythm—below 60 beats/min (**Figure 28-24**, *C*). Slight bradycardia is normal during sleep and in conditioned athletes while they are awake (but at rest). Abnormal bradycardia can result from improper autonomic nervous control of the heart or from a damaged SA node. If the problem is severe, artificial pacemakers can be used to increase the heart rate by taking the place of the SA node.

Tachycardia is a very rapid heart rhythm—more than 100 beats/min (**Figure 28-24**, *D*). Tachycardia is normal during and just after exercise and during the stress response. Abnormal tachycardia can result from improper autonomic control of the heart, blood loss or shock, the action of drugs and toxins, fever, and other factors.

Sinus dysrhythmia is a variation in heart rate during the breathing cycle. Typically, the rate increases during inspiration and decreases during expiration. The causes of sinus dysrhythmia are not clear. This phenomenon is common in young people and usually does not require treatment.

Premature contractions, or *extrasystoles,* are contractions that occur before the next expected contraction in a series of cardiac cycles. For example, *premature atrial contractions (PACs)* may occur shortly after the ventricles contract—seen as early P waves on the ECG (**Figure 28-24**, *E*). Premature atrial contractions often occur with lack of sleep, too much caffeine or nicotine, alcoholism, or heart damage. Ventricular depolarizations that appear earlier than expected are called *premature ventricular contractions (PVCs).* PVCs appear on the ECG as early, wide QRS complexes without a preceding related P wave. PVCs are caused by a variety of circumstances that include stress, electrolyte imbalance, acidosis, hypoxaemia, ventricular enlargement, or drug reactions. Occasional PVCs are not clinically significant in otherwise healthy individuals. However, in people with heart disease they may reduce cardiac output.

Frequent premature contractions can lead to fibrillation, a condition in which cardiac muscle fibres contract out of step with each other. This event can be seen in an ECG as the absence of regular P waves or abnormal QRS and T waves. In fibrillation, the affected heart chambers do not effectively pump blood.

Atrial fibrillation (A-fib or AF) occurs commonly in mitral stenosis, rheumatic heart disease, and infarction of the atrial myocardium (**Figure 28-24**, *F*). This condition can be treated with drugs such as digoxin (a digitalis preparation) or by *cardioversion*—the application of carefully timed electrical shocks to restore the normal myocardial rhythm. Sometimes chronic AF is triggered by "extra beats" originating in the pulmonary veins. This can be treated by AF *ablation therapy* in which the myocardium near each pulmonary vein is cauterized to electrically "disconnect" the veins from the atrial myocardium.

Ventricular fibrillation (V-fib or VF) is an immediately life-threatening condition in which the lack of ventricular pumping suddenly stops the flow of blood to vital tissues (**Figure 28-24**, *G*). Ventricular fibrillation is often treated by *defibrillation*—application of electrical shock to force cardiac muscle fibres to contract in unison (**Figure 28-25**). Unless ventricular fibrillation is corrected immediately by defibrillation or some other method, death may occur within minutes.

Other types of defibrillators, besides those used by health professionals in emergency situations, also save lives. For example, *automatic internal cardiac defibrillators (AICDs)* are preprogrammed devices placed inside the body of a patient who is at a high risk for fibrillation. An AICD will automatically fire a defibrillating shock as needed. Increasingly, *automatic external defibrillators (AEDs)* that can be used by nearly anyone have become available in public areas or for private use (see **Figure 28-25**).

Heart Failure

Heart failure is the inability of the heart to pump enough blood to sustain life. Heart failure is often measured as a decline in the *ejection fraction (EF)* below normal. The lower the EF, the more severe the heart failure.

Heart failure can result from many different heart diseases. Valve disorders can reduce the pumping efficiency of the heart enough to cause heart failure. Cardiomyopathy, or disease of the myocardial tissue, may reduce pumping effectiveness. A specific event such as myocardial infarction can result in myocardial damage that causes heart failure. Dysrhythmias such as complete heart block or ventricular fibrillation can also impair the pumping effectiveness of the heart and thus cause heart failure.

Congestive heart failure (CHF), or simply *left-sided heart failure,* is the inability of the left ventricle to pump blood effectively. Most often, such failure results from chronic systemic hypertension (high blood pressure) or from myocardial infarction caused by coronary artery disease (**Figure 28-26**, *A*). It is called *congestive heart failure* because it decreases pumping pressure in the systemic circulation, which in turn causes the body to retain fluids. Portions of the systemic circulation thus become congested with extra fluid. Left-sided heart failure also causes congestion of blood in the pulmonary circulation, termed

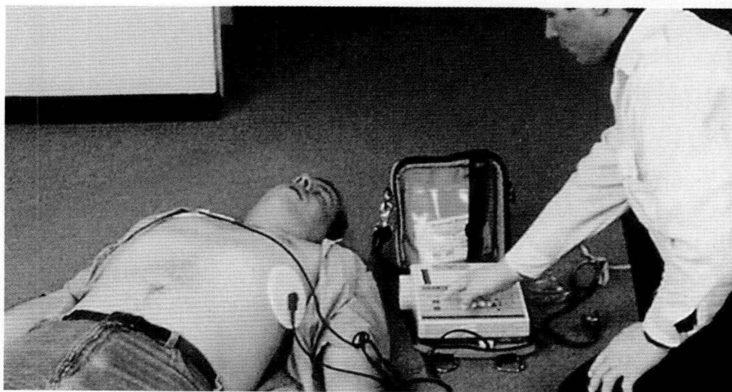

FIGURE 28-25 Defibrillation. Application of an electrical shock (a countershock) depolarizes some of the heart muscle allowing the SAN (pacemaker) to reestablish a normal sinus rhythm. The automatic external defibrillator (AED) shown above has saved many lives by correcting ventricular fibrillation.

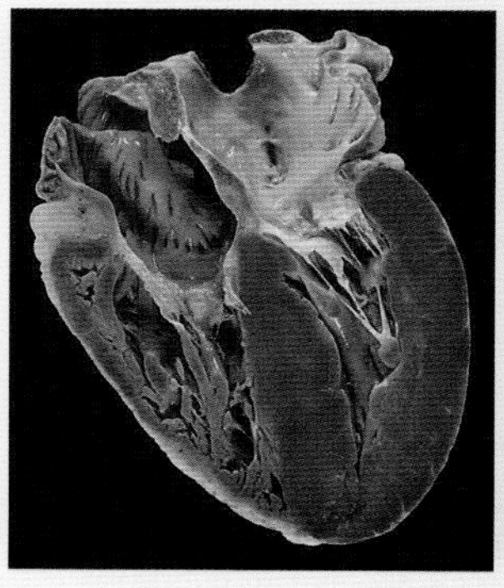

A

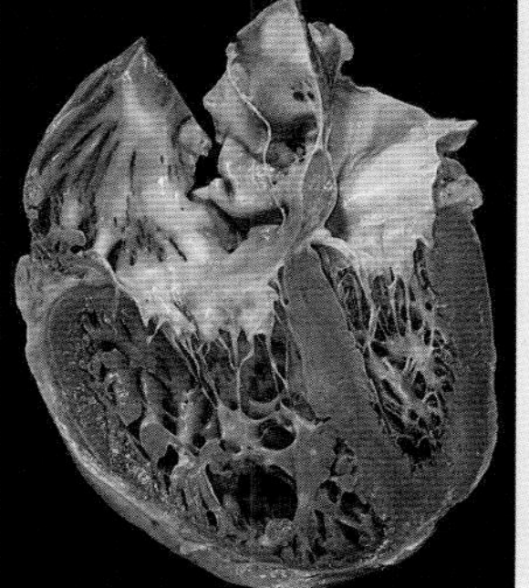

B

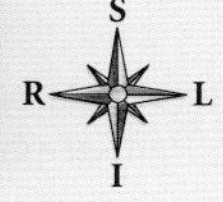

FIGURE 28-26 Congestive heart failure. A, Left ventricle hypertrophy (left-sided heart failure). Note the hypertrophy of the left ventricle, often caused by chronic systemic hypertension. **B,** Right ventricular hypertrophy (right-sided heart failure or *cor pulmonale*). Note the right ventricular hypertrophy and dilation caused by pulmonary hypertension.

pulmonary oedema—possibly leading to right-sided heart failure and pulmonary hypertension (**Figure 28-26**, *B*).

Right-sided heart failure often results from the progression of disease that begins in the left side of the heart. Failure of the left side of the heart results in reduced pumping of blood returning from the lungs. Blood backs up into the pulmonary circulation and then into the right side of the heart—causing an increase in pressure that the right side of the heart simply cannot overcome. Right-sided heart failure can also be caused by lung disorders that obstruct normal pulmonary blood flow and thus overload the right side of the heart—a condition called **cor pulmonale**.

Heart Medication

Although numerous drugs are used in the treatment of heart disease, the following have proven to be basic tools of the cardiologist**: anticoagulants** prevent clot formation; **beta-adrenergic blockers** block norepinephrine receptors and thus reduce the strength and rate of heart beats; **calcium channel blockers** reduce heart contractions by preventing the flow of Ca^{++} into cardiac muscle cells; **digitalis** slows and increases the strength of cardiac contractions; **nitroglycerin** dilates coronary blood vessels and thus improves O_2 supply to myocardium; and **tissue plasminogen activator (t-PA)** helps dissolve clots.

LANGUAGE OF SCIENCE *(continued from p. 637)*

fibrous pericardium (FYE-brus pair-i-KAR-dee-um) [*fibr-* **thread or fibre,** *-ous* **relating to,** *peri-* **around,** *-cardi-* **heart,** *-um* **thing**]

inferior vena cava (in-FEER-ee-or VEE-nah KAY-vah) [*infer-* **lower,** *-or* **quality,** *vena* **vein,** *cava* **hollow**] *pl.*, venae cavae

interatrial bundle (in-ter-AT-tree-al) [*inter-* **between,** *-atri-* **entrance courtyard,** *-al* **relating to**]

internodal bundle (in-ter-NOH-dal) [*inter-* **between,** *-nod-* **knot,** *-al* **relating to**]

mitral valve (MY-tral) [*mitr-* **bishop's hat,** *-al* **relating to**]

myocardium (my-oh-KAR-dee-um) [*myo-* **muscle,** *-cardi-* **heart,** *-um* **thing**] *pl.*, myocardia

pacemaker (PAYS-may-ker)

pericardial fluid (pair-i-KAR-dee-al) [*peri-* **around,** *-cardi-* **heart,** *-al* **relating to**]

pericardial space (pair-i-KAR-dee-al) [*peri-* **around,** *-cardi-* **heart,** *-al* **relating to**]

pericardium (pair-i-KAR-dee-um) [*peri-* **around,** *-cardi-* **heart,** *-um* **thing**] *pl.*, pericardia

residual volume (ree-ZID-yoo-al) [*residu-* **remainder,** *-al* **relating to**]

semilunar (SL) valve (sem-i-LOO-nar) [*semi-* **half,** *-luna* **moon**]

serous pericardium (SEER-us pair-i-KAR-dee-um) [*sero-* **watery fluid,** *-ous* **relating to,** *peri-* **around,** *-cardi-* **heart,** *-um* **thing**] *pl.*, pericardia

sinoatrial (SA) node (sye-no-AY-tree-al) [*sin-* **hollow (sinus),** *atri-* **entrance courtyard,** *-al* **relating to,** *nod-* **knot**]

subendocardial branch (sub-en-doh-KAR-dee-al) [*sub-* **under,** *-endo-* **within,** *-cardi-* **heart,** *-al* **relating to**]

superior vena cava (soo-PEER-ee-or VEE-nah KAY-vah) [*super-* **over or above,** *-or* **quality,** *vena* **vein,** *cava* **hollow**] *pl.*, venae cavae

systole (SIS-toh-lee) [*sy(n)-* **together**, *-stol-* **position**]

tricuspid valve (try-KUS-pid) [*tri-* **three,** *-cusp-* **point,** *-id* **characterized by**]

vein (vayn) [*vena* **blood vessel**]

ventricle (VEN-trih-kul) [*ventr-* **belly,** *-icle* **little**]

LANGUAGE OF MEDICINE

angina pectoris (an-JYE-nah PEK-tor-is) [*angina* **strangling,** *pector-* **breast,** *-is* **relating to**]

angiography (an-jee-OG-rah-fee) [*angi-* **vessel,** *-graph-* **draw,** *-y* **process**]

anticoagulant (an-tee-koh-AG-yoo-lant) [*anti-* **against,** *-coagul-* **curdle,** *-ant* **agent**]

aortic regurgitation (ay-OR-tik ree-gur-jih-TAY-shun) [*aort-* **lifted,** *-ic* **relating to,** *re-* **again,** *-gurgit-* **flow,** *-ation* **process**]

atherosclerosis (ath-er-oh-skleh-ROH-sis) [*athero-* **porridge,** *-scler-* **hardening,** *-osis* **condition**]

atrial fibrillation (A-fib or AF) (AY-tree-al fih-bril-LAY-shun) [*atri-* **entrance courtyard,** *-al* **relating to,** *fibr-* **thread or fibre,** *-illa-* **little,** *-ation* **process**]

beta-adrenergic blocker (BAY-tah-ad-ren-ER-jik) [*beta (β)* **second letter of Greek alphabet,** *ad-* **toward,** *-ren-* **kidney,** *-erg-* **work,** *-ic* **relating to**]

bradycardia (bray-dee-KAR-dee-ah) [*brady-* **slow,** *-cardi-* **heart,** *-ia* **condition**]

C-reactive protein (CRP) (see re-AK-tiv PRO-teen) [*C* **C-polysaccharide,** *re-* **again,** *-act-* **act,** *-ive* **characterized by,** *prote-* **first rank,** *-in* **substance**]

calcium channel blocker (KAL-see-um CHAN-al)

cardiac tamponade (KAR-dee-ak tam-puh-NOD) [*cardi-* **heart,** *-ac* **relating to,** *tampon-* **plug,** *-ade* **process**]

cardiomyopathy (kar-dee-oh-my-OP-ah-thee) [*cardio-* **heart,** *-myo-* **muscle,** *-path-* **disease,** *-y* **state**]

congestive heart failure (CHF) (kon-JES-tive) [*congest-* **crowd together,** *-ive* **relating to**]

coronary artery disease (CAD) (KOR-oh-nair-ee AR-ter-ee) [*corona-* **crown,** *-ary* **relating to,** *arteri-* **vessel**]

coronary bypass surgery (KOR-oh-nair-ee) [*corona-* **crown,** *-ary* **relating to**]

cor pulmonale (kohr pul-mah-NAL-ee) [*cor* **heart,** *pulmon-* **lung,** *-ale* **relating to**]

digitalis (dij-i-TAL-is) [*digit-* **finger,** *-al-* **relating to,** *-is* **thing (from finger-shaped flower of foxglove)**]

digoxin (di-JOK-sin) [*dig-* **finger (from digitalis or finger-like foxglove),** *-oxin* **poison or toxin**]

dysrhythmia (dis-RITH-mee-ah) [*dys-* **disordered,** *-rhythm-* **movement in time,** *-ia* **condition**]

echocardiography (ek-oh-kar-dee-OG-rah-fee) [*echo-* **reflect sound,** *-cardi-* **heart,** *-graph-* **draw,** *-y* **activity**]

ectopic pacemaker (ek-TOP-ik PAYS-may-ker) [*ec-* **out of,** *-top-* **place,** *-ic* **relating to**]

electrocardiogram (ECG) (eh-lek-troh-KAR-dee-oh-gram) [*electro-* **electricity,** *-cardio-* **heart,** *-gram* **drawing**]

electrocardiography (eh-lek-troh-kar-dee-OG-rah-fee) [*electro-* **electricity,** *-cardio-* **heart,** *-graph-* **draw,** *-y* **process**]

heart block (hart blok)

heart failure (hart FALE-yer)

heart murmur [*murmur* **mutter**]

hypertrophic cardiomyopathy (hye-PER-troh-fik kar-dee-oh-my-OP-ah-thee) [*hyper-* **excessive,** *-troph-* **nourishment,** *-ic* **relating to,** *cardi-* **heart,** *-myo-* **muscle,** *-path-* **disease,** *-y* **state**]

hypokalaemia (hye-poh-kal-EE-mee-ah) [*hypo-* **under or below,** *-kal-* **potassium,** *-aem-* **blood,** *-ia* **condition**]

ischaemia (is-KEE-mee-ah) [*isch-* **hold back,** *-aem-* **blood,** *-ia* **condition**]

mitral valve prolapse (MVP) (MY-tral valv PROH-laps) [*mitr-* **bishop's hat,** *-al* **relating to,** *pro-* **forward,** *-laps-* **fall**]

myocardial infarction (MI) (my-oh-KAR-dee-al in-FARK-shun) [*myo-* **muscle,** *-cardi-* **heart,** *-al* **relating to,** *in-* **in,** *-farc-* **stuff or block**]

nitroglycerin (nye-troh-GLIS-eh-rin) [*nitro-* **nitrogen,** *-glyc-* **sweet (sugar),** *-in* **substance**]

pericardial effusion (pair-i-KAR-dee-all ef-FYOO-shen) [*peri-* **around,** *-cardi-* **heart,** *-al* **relating to,** *e(x)-* **outside,** *-fus-* **pour,** *-sion* **process**]

pericardiocentesis (pair-ee-KAR-dee-oh-sen-TEE-sis) [*peri-* **around,** *-cardi-* **heart,** *-centesis* **pricking**]

pericarditis (pair-i-kar-DYE-tis) [*peri-* **around,** *-cardi-* **heart,** *-itis* **inflammation**]

premature contraction (pree-mah-TUR kon-TRAK-shun)

P wave [**named for 16th letter of Roman alphabet**]

pulmonary oedema (PUL-moh-nair-ee eh-DEE-mah) [*pulmon-* **lung,** *-ary* **relating to,** *oedema* **swelling**]

QRS complex (Q R S KOM-pleks) [**named for 17th-19th letters of Roman alphabet**]

rheumatic fever (roo-MAT-ik FEE-ver) [*rheuma-* **flow,** *-ic* **relating to**]

rheumatic heart disease (roo-MAT-ik) [*rheuma-* **flow,** *-ic* **relating to,** *dis-* **opposite of,** *-ease* **comfort**]

sinus dysrhythmia (SYE-nus dis-RITH-mee-ah) [*sinus* **hollow,** *dys-* **disordered,** *-rhythm-* **movement in time,** *-ia* **condition**]

stenosed valve (steh-NOSD) [*stenos-* **narrow,** *-osis* **condition**]

tachycardia (tak-ih-KAR-dee-ah) [*tachy-* **rapid,** *-cardi-* **heart,** *-ia* **condition**]

tissue plasminogen activator (t-PA) (TISH-yoo plaz-MIN-oh-jen AK-tih-vay-tor) [*tissue-* **fabric,** *plasm-* **substance (plasma),** *-in-* **substance,** *-gen* **produce**]

troponins test (TROH-poh-ninz) [*tropo-* **turn,** *-in* **substance**]

T wave [**named for 20th letter of Roman alphabet**]

U wave [**named for 21st letter of Roman alphabet**]

valvuloplasty (VAL-vyoo-loh-plas-tee) [*valv-* **valve,** *-plasty* **surgical repair**]

ventricular fibrillation (V-fib or VF) (ven-TRIK-yoo-lar fib-ril-LAY-shun) [*ventr-* **belly,** *-icul-* **little,** *-ar* **relating to,** *fibr-* **thread or fibre,** *-illa-* **little,** *-ation* **process**]

case study

Bobby was in a hurry to finish the last job of the day. Being an electrician, he had been called in to help complete and inspect the wiring in a museum that was due to open the next week. Bobby called to his co-worker Jerry to confirm the current was off to the electrical box on which he was working. When he heard a positive response, he climbed the ladder and reached up to tighten a few loose screws. As he was tightening the screws with his right hand, he lost his balance and reached up with his left hand to catch hold of the ladder but instead caught a live wire that sent a jolt of electricity through his body. Jerry came running and knocked the ladder out from under Bobby so he would fall to the floor, breaking the connection to earth. "Are you okay?" he asked Bobby, who appeared dazed but was conscious. "I don't feel so great," he replied, smiling weakly; then he collapsed.

Jerry yelled at the other workers in the room to call 999, checked Bobby's pulse and started CPR. The foreman rushed in with an automatic external defibrillator (AED) and attached the electrodes to Bobby's chest. The AED's mechanical voice said, "V-fib. Recommend shock. Press button when clear."

1. What is V-fib that the AED registered?
   a. Ventricular fibrosis
   b. Venous fibrillation
   c. Ventricular fibrillation
   d. Vasomotor fibrosis

When activated, the AED delivers a dose of electric current to the heart (a countershock). This depolarizes the heart muscle, removes the dysrhythmia and allows the body's natural pacemaker to re-establish its normal sinus rhythm.

2. What bundle of cells in Bobby's heart (and yours) is known as the pacemaker?
   a. SV node
   b. SA node
   c. AV node
   d. AV bundle

When the paramedics arrived, they rushed Bobby to the hospital. "Get an ECG!" the attending specialty registrar called out immediately.

3. What is an ECG?
   a. Electrocardiogram
   b. Electrocirculogram
   c. Encephalocardiogram
   d. Emergencycardiogram

4. Ventricular depolarization is shown as which part of the ECG?
   a. V wave
   b. P wave
   c. T wave
   d. QRS complex

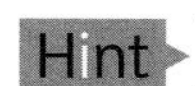

To solve a case study, you may have to refer to the glossary or index, other chapters in this textbook, ***Connect It!,*** and other resources.

CHAPTER SUMMARY

*To download an MP3 version of the chapter summary for use with your mobile device, access the **Audio Chapter Summaries** online at evolve.elsevier.com.*

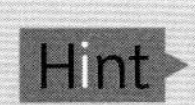

Scan this summary after reading the chapter to help you reinforce the key concepts. Later, use the summary as a quick review before your class or before a test.

Heart Structure

A. Location of the heart (**Figure 28-2**)
1. Lies in the mediastinum, behind the body of the sternum between the points of attachment of ribs two through six; approximately two thirds of its mass is to the left of the midline of the body, and one third is to the right
2. Posteriorly the heart rests on the bodies of thoracic vertebrae five through eight
3. Apex lies on the diaphragm, pointing to the left
4. Base lies just below the second rib
5. Boundaries of the heart are clinically important as an aid in diagnosing heart disorders

B. Size and shape of the heart (**Figures 28-1** and **28-2**)
1. At birth, the heart is transverse and appears large in proportion to the diameter of the chest cavity
2. Between puberty and 25 years of age, the heart attains its adult shape and weight
3. In adults, the shape of the heart tends to resemble that of the chest

C. Coverings of the heart
1. Structure of the heart coverings
   a. Pericardium (**Figure 28-4**)
      (1) Fibrous pericardium—tough, loose-fitting inextensible sac
      (2) Serous pericardium—parietal layer lies inside the fibrous pericardium, and visceral layer (epicardium) adheres to the outside of the heart
      (3) Pericardial space—lies between visceral and parietal layers and contains 10 to 15 mL of pericardial fluid
2. Function of the heart coverings—provides protection against friction

D. Structure of the heart
1. Vessels of the heart
   a. The large vessels to and from the heart are called great vessels of the heart. These include the sup.vena cava, inf.vena cava, pulmonary arteries, pulmonary veins and the aorta.
   b. Smaller coronary vessels serve the cardiac muscle tissue within the heart wall
2. Wall of the heart—made up of three distinct layers (**Figure 28-5**)
   a. Epicardium—outer layer of heart wall
   b. Myocardium—thick, contractile middle layer of heart wall; compresses the heart cavities, and the blood within them, with great force
   c. Endocardium—delicate inner layer of endothelial tissue
3. Chambers of the heart—divided into four cavities with the right and left chambers separated by the septum (**Figures 28-6** and **28-7**)
   a. Atria
      (1) Two superior chambers known as "receiving chambers" because they receive blood from veins
      (2) Atria alternately relax to receive blood and then contract to push blood into ventricles
      (3) Myocardial wall of each atrium is not very thick, because little pressure is needed to move blood such a small distance
      (4) Auricle—earlike flap protruding from each atrium
   b. Ventricles
      (1) Two lower chambers known as "pumping chambers" because they push blood into the large network of vessels
      (2) Ventricular myocardium is thicker than the myocardium of the atria because great force must be generated to pump the blood a large distance; myocardium of left ventricle is thicker than the right, because it must push blood much farther
4. Valves of the heart—mechanical devices that permit the flow of blood in one direction only (**Figure 28-8**)
   a. Atrioventricular (AV) valves—prevent blood from flowing back into the atria from the ventricles when the ventricles contract
      (1) Tricuspid valve (right AV valve)—guards the right atrioventricular orifice; free edges of three flaps of endocardium are attached to papillary muscles by chordae tendineae
      (2) Bicuspid, or mitral, valve (left AV valve)—similar in structure to tricuspid valve except has only two flaps
   b. Semilunar (SL) valves—half-moon–shaped flaps growing out from the lining of the pulmonary trunk and aorta; prevent blood from flowing back into the ventricles from the aorta and pulmonary trunk
      (1) Pulmonary valve—valve at entrance of the pulmonary trunk
      (2) Aortic valve—valve at entrance of the aorta
   c. Skeleton of the heart
      (1) Set of connected rings that serve as a semirigid support for the heart valves and for the attachment of cardiac muscle of the myocardium
      (2) Serves as an electrical barrier between the myocardium of the atria and that of the ventricles
   d. Surface projection (review **Figure 28-9**)
   e. Flow of blood through heart (review **Figure 28-7**)
5. Coronary circulation—blood supply of heart tissue (**Figures 28-10**, **28-11**, and **28-12**)
   a. Coronary arteries—myocardial cells receive blood from the right and left coronary arteries
      (1) First branches to come off the aorta
      (2) Ventricles receive blood from branches of both right and left coronary arteries
      (3) Each ventricle receives blood only from a small branch of the corresponding coronary artery

(4) Most abundant blood supply goes to the myocardium of the left ventricle

(5) Right coronary artery is dominant in approximately 50% of all hearts and the left in about 20%; in approximately 30%, neither coronary artery is dominant

(6) Few anastomoses exist between the larger branches of the coronary arteries

b. Cardiac veins

(1) As a rule, veins follow a course that closely parallels that of coronary arteries

(2) After going through cardiac veins, blood enters the coronary sinus to drain into the right atrium

(3) Several veins drain directly into the right atrium

6. Nerve supply of the heart

a. Conduction system of the heart—made up of modified cardiac muscle, it generates and distributes the heart's own rhythmic contractions; can be regulated by afferent nerves

b. Cardiac plexuses—located near the arch of the aorta, made up of the combination of sympathetic and parasympathetic fibres

c. Fibres from the cardiac plexus accompany the right and left coronary arteries to enter the heart

d. Most fibres end in the SA node, but some end in the AV node and in the atrial myocardium; the SA node acts as the heart's pacemaker

e. Sympathetic nerves—accelerator nerves

f. Vagus fibres—inhibitory, or depressor, nerves

The Heart as a Pump

A. Conduction system of the heart (**Figure 28-13**)

1. Composed of four major structures

a. Sinoatrial (SA) node

b. Atrioventricular (AV) node

c. AV bundle (bundle of His)

d. Subendocardial branches (Purkinje fibres)

2. Conduction system structures are more highly specialized than ordinary cardiac muscle tissue and permit rapid conduction of an action potential through the heart

3. SA node (pacemaker)

a. Initiates each heartbeat and sets its pace

b. Specialized pacemaker cells in the node possess an intrinsic rhythm

4. Sequence of cardiac stimulation

a. After being generated by the SA node, each impulse travels throughout the muscle fibres of both atria and the atria begin to contract

b. As the action potential enters the AV node from the right atrium, its conduction slows to allow complete contraction of both atrial chambers before the impulse reaches the ventricles

c. After the AV node, conduction velocity increases as the impulse is relayed through the AV bundle into the ventricles

d. Right and left branches of the bundle fibres and subendocardial branches (Purkinje fibres) conduct the impulses throughout the muscles of both ventricles, stimulating them to contract almost simultaneously

B. Electrocardiogram (ECG)

1. Graphic record of the heart's electrical activity, its conduction of impulses; a record of the electrical events that precede the contractions of the heart

2. Production of an ECG (**Figure 28-14**)

a. Electrodes are attached to the subject

b. Voltage changes that represent the heart's electrical activity are sensed by electrodes and recorded on paper (**Figure 28-15**)

3. Composition (ECG waves) of normal ECG recording (**Figures 28-14** and **28-16**) is composed of:

a. P wave—represents depolarization of the atria

b. QRS complex—represents depolarization of the ventricles and repolarization of the atria

c. T wave—represents repolarization of the ventricles

d. U wave—tiny "hump" at end of T wave—represents repolarization of the papillary muscle (or a two-part T wave) and may appear on ECG as well (**Figure 28-17**)

(1) Absent or small U waves usually considered normal

(2) U waves may be a sign of hypokalaemia or too much digoxin

e. ECG intervals between P, QRS, and T waves can provide information about rate of conduction of an action potential through the heart

C. Cardiac cycle—a complete heartbeat

1. Consists of contraction (systole) and relaxation (diastole) of both atria and both ventricles

2. Cycle is often divided into time intervals (**Figures 28-18** and **28-19**)

3. Atrial systole

a. This cycle begins with the P wave of the ECG, which triggers atrial contraction

b. Contraction of atria creates a pressure gradient that pushes blood out of the atria into the relaxed ventricles

c. Because of pressure gradients, AV valves are open; SL valves are closed

d. Ventricles are relaxed and filling with blood from atria

4. Isovolumetric ventricular contraction

a. Onset of ventricular systole coincides with the R wave of the ECG and the appearance of the first heart sound

b. Occurs between the start of ventricular systole and the opening of the SL valves

c. Ventricular volume remains constant as the pressure increases rapidly

(1) Intraventricular pressure rises enough to close AV valves, producing the first heart sound

(2) Intraventricular pressure is not yet high enough to open the SL valves

5. Ejection

a. SL valves open and blood is ejected from the ventricles when the intraventricular pressure exceeds the pressure in the pulmonary artery and aorta

b. Rapid ejection—initial short phase characterized by a marked increase in ventricular and aortic pressure and in aortic blood flow
c. Reduced ejection—characterized by a less abrupt decrease in ventricular volume; coincides with the T wave of the ECG

6. Isovolumetric ventricular relaxation
   a. Ventricular diastole begins with this phase
   b. Occurs between closure of the SL valves and opening of the AV valves
   c. A dramatic fall in intraventricular pressure but not enough to open the AV valves, thus no change in volume
   d. Second heart sound is heard during this period
7. Passive ventricular filling
   a. Continued ventricular relaxation reduces intraventricular pressure and returning venous blood increases intraatrial pressure, producing enough of a pressure gradient to push open the AV valves
   b. Blood rushes into the relaxing ventricles; influx lasts approximately 0.1 second and results in a dramatic increase in ventricular volume
   c. Diastasis—later longer period of slow ventricular filling near end of ventricular diastole lasting approximately 0.2 second; characterized by a gradual increase in ventricular pressure and volume
   d. The cardiac cycle then begins again with a new atrial systole

D. Heart sounds
   1. Systolic sound—first sound, believed to be caused primarily by contraction of the ventricles and by vibrations of the closing AV valves
   2. Diastolic sound—short, sharp sound; thought to be caused by vibrations of the closing of SL valves
   3. Heart sounds have clinical significance because they provide information about the functioning of the valves of the heart

Cycle of Life: Heart

A. Heart and blood vessels maintain basic structure and function from childhood through adulthood
B. Only apparent normal changes occur as a result of exercise
   1. Exercise thickens myocardium
   2. Exercise increases the supply of blood vessels in skeletal muscle tissue
C. Adulthood through later adulthood—degenerative changes
   1. Atherosclerosis—blockage or weakening of critical arteries
   2. Heart valves and myocardial tissue degenerate—reduces pumping efficiency

The Big Picture: Heart

A. The heart acts as a pump to circulate blood to every part of the body
B. Pumping of blood quickly transports essential oxygen, water, wastes, and other substances throughout the body to maintain overall internal stability

REVIEW QUESTIONS

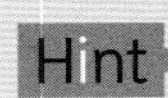

Write out the answers to these questions after reading the chapter and reviewing the Chapter Summary. Note—writing out your answers will consolidate learning and provide a valuable resource of information.

1. Discuss the size, position, and location of the heart in the thoracic cavity.
2. Describe the pericardium, differentiating between the fibrous and serous portions.
3. Exactly where is pericardial fluid found? Explain its function.
4. Define the following terms: *intercalated discs*, *syncytium*, *autorhythmic*.
5. Name and locate the chambers and valves of the heart.
6. Trace the flow of blood through the heart.
7. Identify, locate, and describe the function of each of the following structures: SA node, AV node, AV bundle, and subendocardial branches (Purkinje fibres).
8. What does an electrocardiogram measure and record? List the normal ECG deflection waves and intervals. What do the various ECG waves represent?
9. What is meant by the term *cardiac cycle*?
10. List the “phases” of the cardiac cycle and briefly describe the events that occur in each.
11. What is meant by the term *residual volume* as it applies to the heart?
12. Describe and explain the origin of the heart sounds.
13. Explain the purpose of echocardiography.
14. Identify the clinical significance of cardiac markers.
15. Identify possible causes of coronary artery disease. What are the first symptoms to appear in a patient developing coronary artery disease?
16. Define congestive heart failure.
17. Describe the various types of cardiac dysrhythmias.
18. Put these structures in order of their electrical conduction beginning with the “pacemaker”: AV node, bundle of His, Purkinje fibres and SA node.

CRITICAL THINKING QUESTIONS

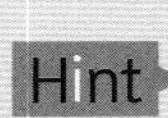

After finishing the Review Questions, write out the answers to these more in-depth questions to help you apply your new knowledge. Go back to sections of the chapter that relate to concepts that you find difficult.

1. How is CPR accomplished? What is the significance of the placement of the heart in the thoracic cavity and successful CPR?
2. What would result if there were a lack of anastomosis in the arteries of the heart?
3. What is an ectopic pacemaker? What would be the effect on the heart rate if an ectopic pacemaker took over for the SA node?
4. Explain the functional importance of the valve cusps (leaflets) that extend into the lumen of the aorta near its origin in the heart.
5. Briefly describe the coronary artery system and explain why one specific artery is known as the “widow maker”.

29 Blood Vessels

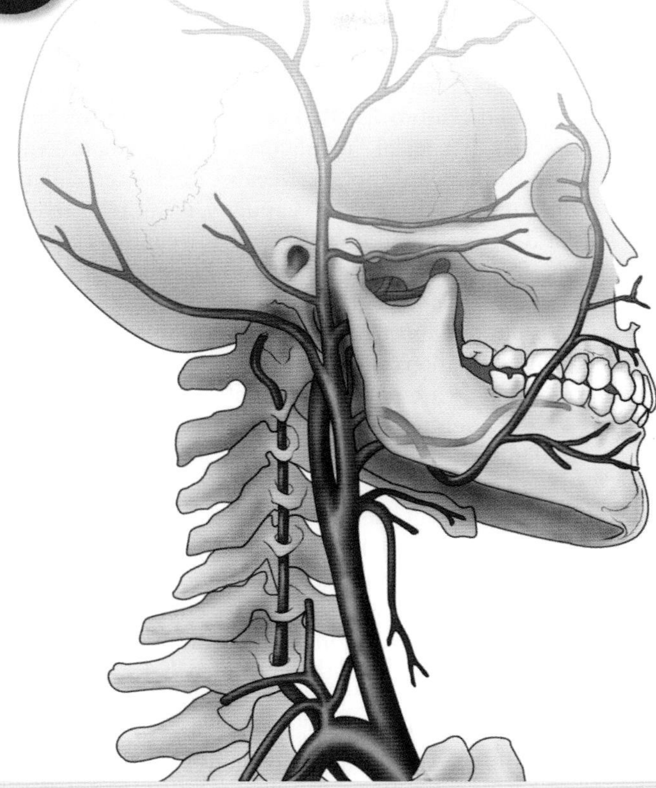

CHAPTER OUTLINE

Hint Scan this outline before you begin to read the chapter, as a preview of how the concepts are organized.

The name *cardiovascular system* implies this system's two major structural components: the heart *(cardio-)* and the vessels *(-vas-)*. In the previous chapter, we explored the heart's functional anatomy and its role in pumping blood. Now we turn our attention to the vast network of blood vessels that carry life-sustaining blood to nearly every corner of our body.

First, we describe the various types of vessels that carry our blood and their roles in the cardiovascular system. Then we outline the major circulatory routes taken by these vessels, including some "special" cases that don't follow the usual pattern of circulation. Chapter 30 continues our story by bringing together and applying all of the concepts of the last few chapters in an overview of the interrelated mechanisms that keep blood flowing. •

LANGUAGE OF SCIENCE

Hint Use this list to aid your pronunciation of unfamiliar words.

abdominal aorta
(ab-DOM-i-nal ay-OR-tah)
[*abdomin-* **belly,** *-al* **relating to,** *aort-* **lifted,** *-a* **thing**] *pl.,* aortae or aortas

accessory hemiazygos vein
(ak-SES-oh-ree hem-ee-ah-ZYE-gos vayn)
[*hemi-* **half,** *-a-* **without,** *-zygo-* **union or yoke,** *vena* **blood vessel**]

angiogenesis (an-jee-oh-JEN-eh-sis)
[*angi-* **vessel,** *-gen-* **produce,** *-esis* **process**]

anterior tibial vein
(an-TEER-ee-or TIB-ee-al vayn)
[*ante-* **front,** *-er-* **more,** *-or* **quality,** *tibia* **shin bone,** *-al* **relating to,** *vena* **blood vessel**]

aorta (ay-OR-tah)
[*aort-* **lifted,** *-a* **thing**] *pl.,* aortae or aortas

aortic arch (ay-OR-tik)
[*aort-* **lifted,** *-ic* **relating to**]

arterial anastomosis (ar-TEER-ee-al ah-nas-tuh-MOH-sis)
[*arteria-* **vessel,** *-al* **relating to,** *ana-* **anew,** *-stomo-* **mouth,** *-osis* **condition**] *pl.,* anastomoses

arteriole (ar-TEER-ee-ohl)
[*arteri-* **vessel,** *-ole* **little**]

arteriovenous anastomosis
(ar-teer-ee-oh-VEE-nus ah-nas-tuh-MOH-sis)
[*arteri-* **vessel,** *-ven-* **vein,** *-ous* **relating to,** *ana-* **again or anew,** *-stomo-* **mouth,** *-osis* **condition**] *pl.,* anastomoses

artery (AR-ter-ee)
[*arteri-* **vessel**]

ascending aorta
(ah-SEND-ing ay-OR-tah)
[*ascend-* **climb,** *aort-* **lifted,** *-a* **thing**] *pl.,* aortae or aortas

axillary vein (AK-sih-lair-ee vayn)
[*axilla* **wing,** *-ary* **relating to,** *vena* **blood vessel**]

azygos vein (AZ-ih-gohs vayn)
[*a-* **without,** *-zygo-* **union or yoke,** *vena* **blood vessel**]

basilic vein (bah-SIL-ik vayn)
[*bas-* **foundation,** *-ic* **relating to,** *vena* **blood vessel**]

continued on p. 694

BLOOD VESSEL TYPES

There are nearly 100,000 km of vessels carrying blood through your body right now. These vessels developed through the complex process of **angiogenesis** (*angi-* means "vessel") that begins during embryonic development and continues through the life span. As scientists work out how angiogenesis is guided by chemical signals, they also develop new therapies to promote angiogenesis after tissue injury and to inhibit the accelerated angiogenesis in tumours that allows them to spread as cancer.

You have already been introduced to the different roles that blood vessels play in the body: *arteries* conduct blood away from the heart, *capillaries* conduct blood through tissues and permit exchange of materials, and *veins* conduct blood back toward the heart. In the following sections, we explore a few important details of blood vessel anatomy.

ARTERIES

An **artery** is a vessel that carries blood away from the heart. There are several types of arteries in the cardiovascular system.

Elastic arteries (also called *conducting arteries*) are the largest in the body and include the aorta and some of its major branches. As the name implies, elastic arteries can stretch without causing injury to accommodate the surge of blood that is forced into them when the ventricles contract and then can recoil as the ventricles relax.

Muscular arteries (also called *distributing arteries*) carry blood farther away from the heart to specific organs and areas of the body. They are smaller in diameter than elastic arteries. However, the muscular layer in the wall of these vessels is proportionately thicker. Because of the thick muscle layer, muscular arteries have a thicker vessel wall than similar-sized veins (**Figure 29-1**). Like elastic arteries, muscular arteries are given names. Examples are the brachial, gastric, and superior mesenteric arteries.

Arterioles, also called *resistance vessels,* are the smallest arteries. **Figure 29-2** shows the structure of arterioles in comparison to muscular and elastic arteries. Arterioles are not named individually, but as a group they are critically important in regulating blood flow throughout the body. They function in this way by variable contraction of smooth muscle in their walls, which in turn increases resistance to blood flow and helps regulate blood pressure as well as determining the quantity of blood that enters a particular organ. The concept of flow resistance and its relationship to blood vessel diameter are discussed further in Chapter 30.

Metarteriole is the term used to describe the short connecting vessel that connects a true arteriole with the proximal end of between 20 and 100 capillaries and then extends through the capillary bed (**Figure 29-3**). The proximal ends of metarterioles are encircled by special "regulatory valves"—smooth muscle cells called **precapillary sphincters.** Because each precapillary sphincter wraps around the entrance to a capillary, it can relax or contract to increase or decrease blood flow into specific capillary networks.

The distal end of a metarteriole is devoid of precapillary sphincters and is called a *thoroughfare channel.* It is possible for blood passing directly through a metarteriole into a thoroughfare channel to bypass the intervening capillary bed. After birth all arteries except the pulmonary artery and its branches carry oxygenated blood.

Research has confirmed the existence of the scheme of microcirculation in **Figure 29-3** in only a few human structures, primarily the *mesenteries*—the folds of serous membrane between the digestive organs and the wall of the abdomen. Specific schemes of microcirculation vary widely among different tissues and organs, confirming the principle of structure fits function. A current theory holds that in most tissues, the same regulatory effects are achieved in roughly the same manner by altering the overall **precapillary tone** in the smooth muscles that encircle the arterioles that supply the capillaries.

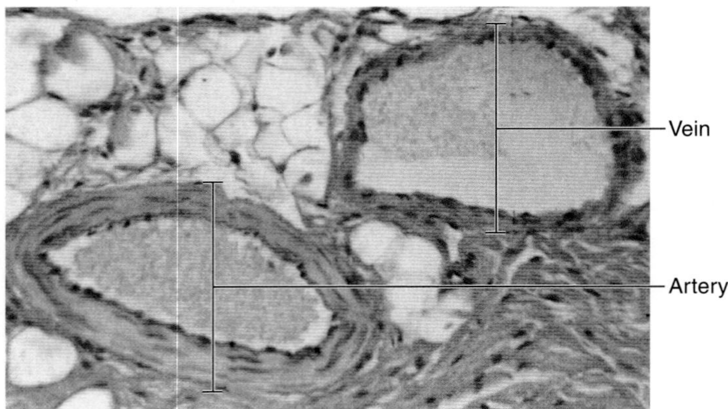

FIGURE 29-1 Artery and vein. Light micrograph of a cross-section of similar-sized artery *(left)* and vein *(right).* Notice the thick muscular wall of the artery as compared to the thin-walled vein.

CAPILLARIES

Capillaries are the microscopic vessels that carry blood from arterioles to venules. Blood flow through the arterioles, venules, and capillaries is called the *microcirculation* (see **Figure 29-3**). Transfer of nutrients and other vital substances between blood and tissue cells occurs at or very near a capillary—in so-called capillary beds or networks. It is for this reason that capillaries are sometimes known as the *primary exchange vessels* of the cardiovascular system. So vital is this function that no cell in the body is far removed from a capillary.

Although capillaries are small in size, the number of them in the body is estimated to be in excess of 1 billion. They are not, however, uniformly distributed. Some body tissues, such as liver or cardiac muscle, have high metabolic rates and require large numbers of capillary vessels. Other tissues, such as cartilage and epithelium, are avascular and lack capillary networks altogether.

True capillaries receive blood flowing out of small arterioles. If the precapillary tone in arteriolar smooth muscle is low (relaxed), blood flows into the capillaries. However, if the precapillary tone is high, very little blood flows into the local capillaries. Capillaries are often categorized into three groups by the ease of passage of substances through their walls or by structural differences that affect their permeability.

Continuous capillaries have a continuous lining of endothelial cells with only small openings called *intercellular clefts* between them (**Figure 29-4**). This type of capillary is typically found in skeletal muscle, lung, and many types of connective tissue. **Fenestrated capillaries** also have intercellular clefts between their lining endothelial cells. But, in addition, they also have small "holes" or fenestrations through the plasma membrane of the endothelial cell itself. This unique structural adaptation allows for special function. Under-

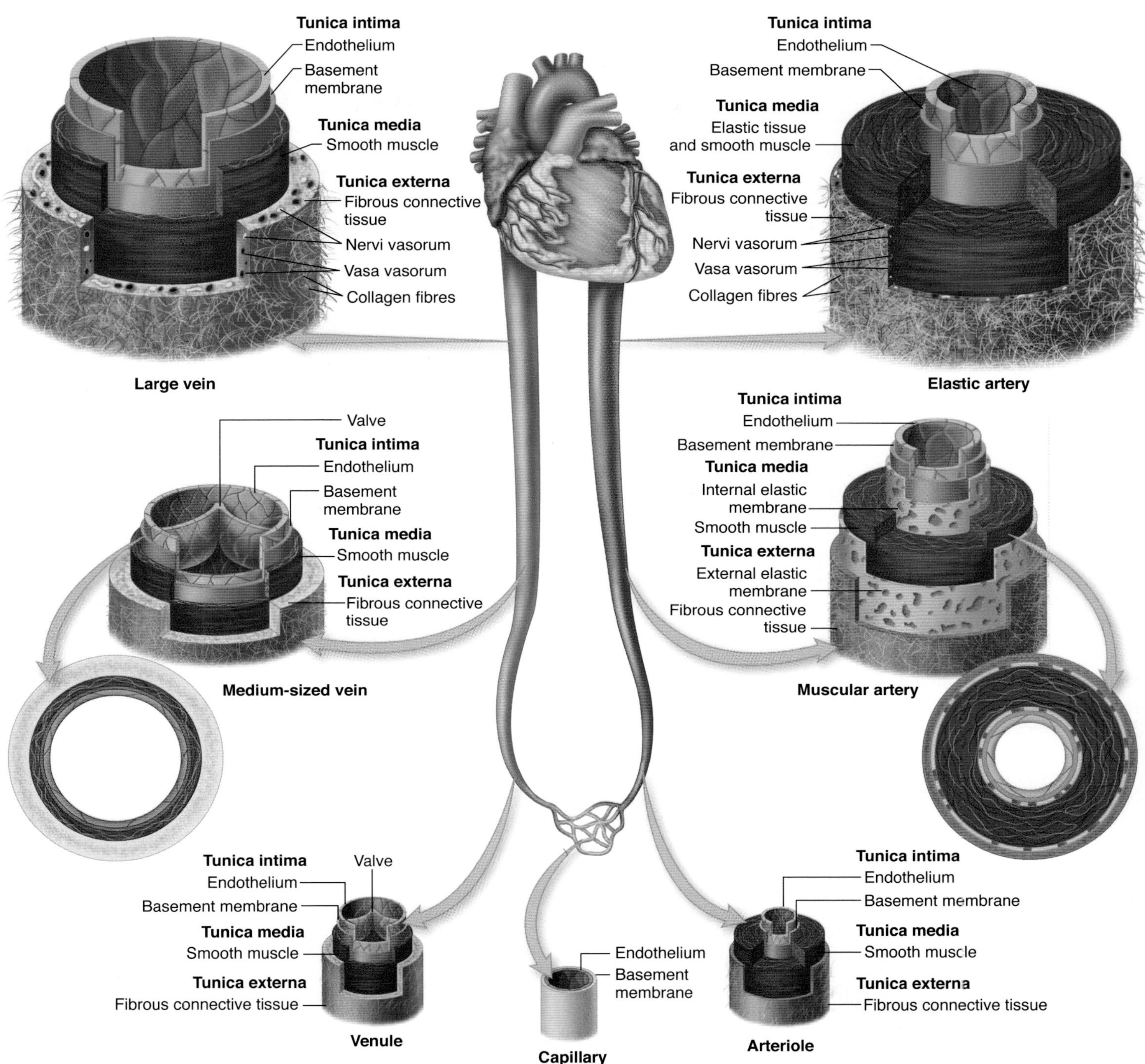

FIGURE 29-2 Structure of blood vessels. The tunica externa of the veins are colour-coded blue and the arteries red.

standing the anatomy of these tiny vessels will be helpful in understanding the function of a number of major organs, such as the kidneys and small intestines, discussed later in the text.

Sinusoid is the term used to describe a type of capillary that has a much larger lumen and more winding or tortuous course than other capillary vessels. The basement membrane that completely covers other capillaries is either absent or incomplete in sinusoids. In addition, the fenestrations present both between and within the endothelial lining cells are much larger than in other capillary types. The result is great porosity. Because of this structural adaptation, sinusoids in the bone marrow and liver, for example, are able to permit migration of blood cells from the intravascular space into surrounding tissues.

VEINS

A **vein** is a vessel that carries blood toward the heart. After passing through the complex capillary network of vessels, blood from several capillaries flows into the distal end of the metarteriole, the

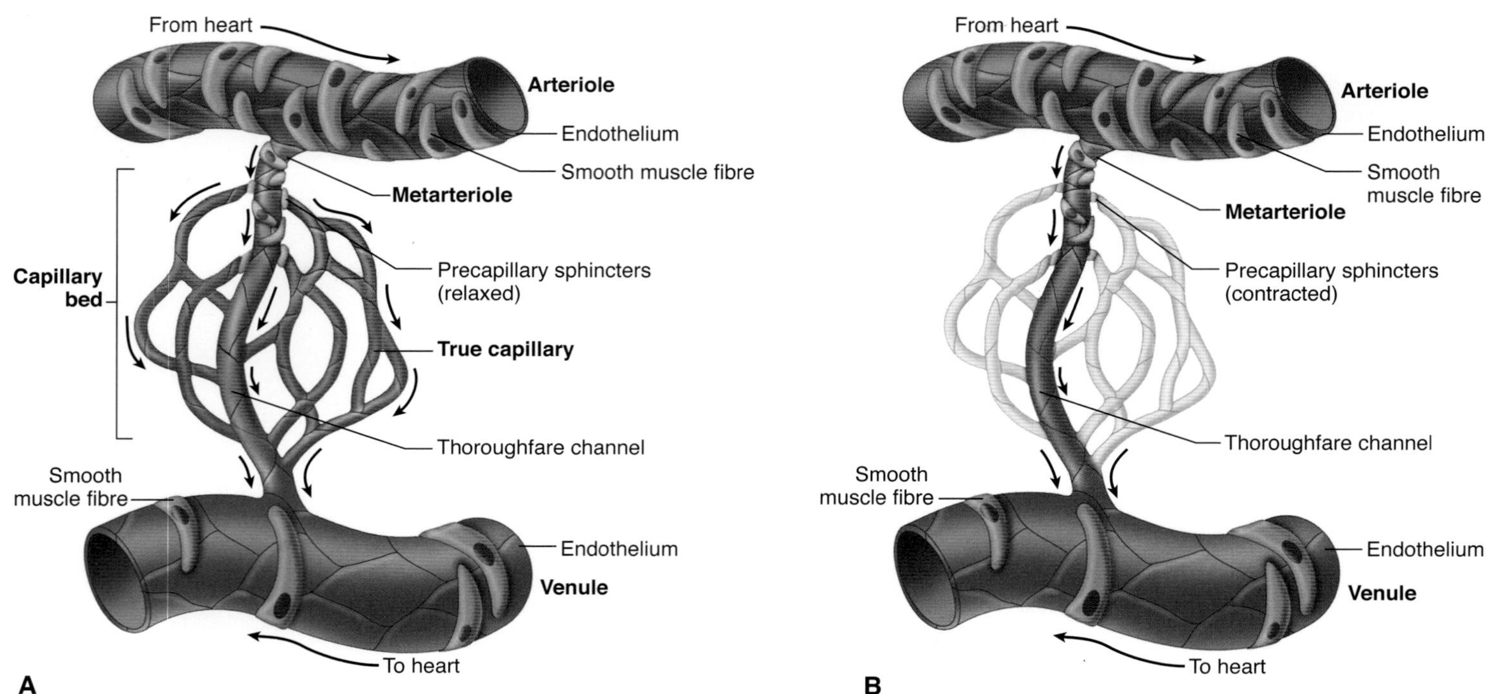

FIGURE 29-3 Microcirculation. Classic model of control of local blood flow through a capillary network is regulated by altering the tone of precapillary sphincters surrounding arterioles and metarterioles. Recent models recognize that in most tissues, it is the overall tone in arteriolar smooth muscle that regulates blood flow into capillary networks. **A,** Sphincters are relaxed, permitting blood flow to enter the capillary bed. **B,** With sphincters contracted, blood flows from metarteriole directly into thoroughfare channel, bypassing the capillary bed.

thoroughfare channel, or directly enters the first of a series of vessels that will eventually return it to the heart.

The first venous structures are small-diameter vessels called **venules.** Initially, these tiny veins, especially those closest to the capillary bed, have very narrow lumens and porous, thin walls. As in capillaries, fluid can be exchanged between blood in the smallest venules and the tissue spaces. Their walls consist of little more than endothelial cells, a few smooth muscle cells and an occasional fibroblast. In addition to movement of fluid through the wall of the venule, phagocytic white blood cells (WBCs) also move out of the cardiovascular system and into areas of inflamed tissue by passing through the pores in walls of venules (see discussion of diapedesis on pp. 622 and 756).

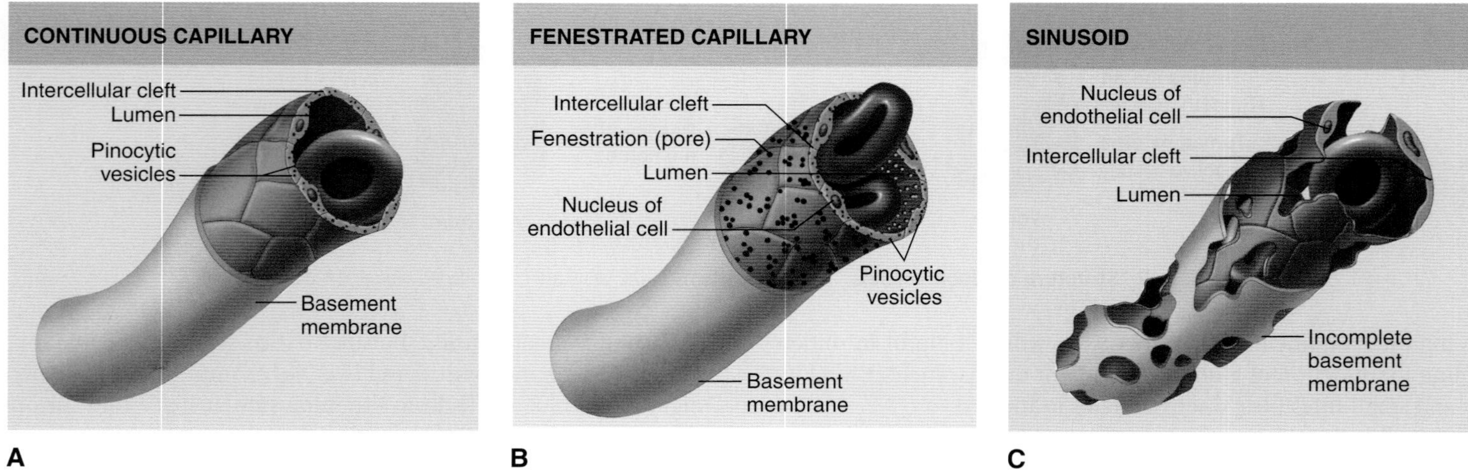

FIGURE 29-4 Types of capillaries. **A,** Continuous capillary. Note the presence of clefts only between adjacent endothelial cells. **B,** Fenestrated capillary. In addition to intercellular clefts, fenestrations (pores) exist in the plasma membranes of endothelial cells. **C,** Sinusoid. In addition to large intercellular clefts and cellular fenestrations, the basement membrane is incomplete or absent.

As blood exits the smaller venules it enters progressively larger venous channels—the veins. Their names correspond to their arterial counterparts. However, whereas arteries become progressively smaller as blood flows away from the heart and into branches feeding other areas of the body, named veins become progressively larger as additional blood flows into them as they approach the heart. Structural changes occur in the walls of veins as they grow in size to accommodate and regulate additional blood volume and flow.

Veins can accommodate varying amounts of blood with almost no change in blood pressure. This results from their great ability to stretch. Ease of stretch is also called *capacitance*. Therefore, the veins are often referred to as the *capacitance vessels* of the cardiovascular system. High capacitance permits veins to serve as reservoirs for blood as well as conduits for its passage back to the heart.

Another structural adaptation in veins that has an important functional significance is the presence of one-way valves similar to the heart's semilunar valves. These valves develop from the thin membrane (**endothelium**) that lines the lumen of these vessels. The peripheral veins in the extremities have more valves than other veins of the body. Valves keep blood moving toward the heart and prevent its potential backflow.

The term **venous sinus** is used to describe large venous structures that have very thin endothelial walls. Since no smooth muscle cells or other support tissues found in the outer layers of typical large veins are located in the walls of venous sinuses, they cannot change their shape and thus depend on surrounding structures for support. Examples of venous sinuses include the dural venous sinuses of the brain (look ahead to **Figure 29-16** on p. 684) and the coronary sinus of the heart (see **Figure 28-12** on p. 649). After birth, all the veins except the pulmonary veins contain deoxygenated blood.

Structure of Blood Vessels

Components of the Blood Vessel Wall

Differences in the amounts of the tissue components present in blood vessel walls occur in different types of arteries and veins (see **Figure 29-2**). Regardless of how thick a vessel wall might be, four types of "fabrics" that make up a vessel wall are commonly present: (1) lining *endothelial tissue*, (2) *collagen fibres*, (3) *elastic fibres*, and (4) *smooth muscle tissue*.

Endothelial Tissue

Endothelial tissue or *endothelium* is a specific type of simple squamous epithelium. Recall from Chapter 9 (see **Figure 9-1** on p. 157) that this tissue forms a thin, smooth membrane made up of flattened cells. The endothelial membrane that lines the entire vascular tree exhibits specific features and performs a number of different functions in different regions of the vascular system. By providing a smooth luminal surface, endothelium influences blood flow and inhibits intravascular coagulation.

Intercellular clefts between adjacent endothelial cells and the presence, size, and number of pores or fenestrations in their cytoplasmic membranes influence diffusion and movement of substances or cells out of and into the circulating blood (see **Figure 29-4**). Endothelial cells are also capable of transporting substances rapidly across their boundaries by using pinocytic vesicles (see **Box 5-1**, p. 80).

Cellular reproduction provides new cells to increase blood vessel size, replace damaged cells, and provide growing cords of cells that are forerunners of new blood vessels. Besides producing several important growth factors, endothelium releases a variety of signalling molecules that play important roles in maintaining cardiovascular health.

Collagen Fibres

Collagen fibres in the vascular wall are woven together much like the reinforcing strands found in the wall of a tyre or hose. They form from fibrous protein molecules that aggregate into fibres several micrometres in diameter and are clearly visible with a light microscope (see **Figure 8-3** on p. 142 and **Figure 9-12** on p. 163).

In physiological conditions, collagen fibres are very flexible—but far less extensible than the elastic fibres described later. They do not stretch more than 2% to 3%. The collagen fibres function more to keep the lumen of the vessel open and strengthen the wall than to contribute to overall tension or recoil ability.

Elastic Fibres

Individual elastic fibres are composed largely of an insoluble protein polymer called *elastin* and are quite small (0.1 to 1 μm in diameter). Once secreted into the extracellular matrix, they form into a rubberlike network that is highly elastic and capable of stretching more than 100% in physiological conditions (see **Figure 8-5** on p. 144).

In large elastic arteries, especially, wavy elastic fibres are organized or arranged in concentric, almost circular patterns. Elastic fibres allow for recoil after distention. This property of elastic fibres plays an important role in maintaining *passive tension* in the vessels of the cardiovascular system. This type of tension is required to maintain normal blood pressure levels throughout the cardiac cycle—a process that is discussed in Chapter 30.

Smooth Muscle Tissue

Smooth muscle cells are found in the wall of all segments of the vascular system except capillaries. Recall from Chapters 9 and 17 that smooth muscle is an involuntary muscle found in the wall of most hollow organs of the body.

Smooth muscle cells are most numerous in elastic and muscular arteries and exert *active tension* in these vessels when contracting.

Layers of the Blood Vessel Wall

The walls of arteries and veins consist of three separate layers or "coats" called the *tunica externa*, *tunica media*, and *tunica intima*. These layers are arranged in sequence from the outside, to the middle, and then to the interior, or luminal, surface of the vessel. As blood vessels decrease in diameter, the relative thickness of their walls also decreases.

When considering the general structure of the walls of vessels in the circulatory system, capillaries are the exception. They consist of only a single layer of endothelial cells (tunica intima) surrounded by a basement membrane (see **Figure 29-4**).

TABLE 29-1 Structure of Blood Vessels

	TYPICAL DIAMETER	TYPICAL WALL THICKNESS	TUNICA INTIMA	TUNICA MEDIA	TUNICA EXTERNA
Typical histology		Endothelium	Smooth muscle; elastic fibres	Collagen fibres	
Arteries	Aorta: 25 mm Small artery: 4 mm Arteriole: 30 μm	Aorta: 2 mm Small artery: 1 mm Arteriole: 8 μm	Smooth lining	Allows constriction and dilation of vessels; thicker than in veins; muscle innervated by autonomic fibres	Provides flexible support that resists collapse or injury; thicker than in veins; thinner than tunica media
Veins	Vena cava: 30 mm Vein: 5 mm Venule: 20 μm	Vena cava: 1.5 mm Vein: 0.5 mm Venule: 1 μm	Smooth lining with valves to ensure one-way flow	Allows constriction and dilation of vessels; thinner than in arteries; muscle innervated by autonomic fibres	Provides flexible support that resists collapse or injury; thinner than in arteries; thicker than tunica media
Capillaries	5 μm	0.5 μm	Makes up entire wall of capillary; thinness permits ease of transport across vessel wall	(Absent)	(Absent)

Outer Layer

The walls of the larger blood vessels, the arteries and veins, have three layers (see **Figure 29-2** and **Table 29-1**). The outermost layer is called the **tunica externa.** This Latin name literally means "outside coat". The tunica externa, also called *tunica adventitia,* is made of strong, flexible fibrous connective tissue. This layer prevents tearing of the vessel walls during body movements. Collagen fibres extend outward from this layer to connect to nearby structures—anchoring the vessel and helping to hold it open. In veins, the tunica externa is the thickest of the three layers of the venous wall. In arteries, it is usually a little thinner than the middle layer of the arterial wall.

Middle Layer

The middle layer, or **tunica media** (Latin for "middle coat"), is made of a layer of smooth muscle tissue sandwiched together with a layer of elastic connective tissue. Some anatomists consider the elastic portion of the tunica media to be distinct enough to call it a separate *external elastic membrane* of the wall. The encircling smooth muscles of the tunica media permit changes in blood vessel diameter. The smooth muscle tissue of the tunica media is innervated by autonomic nerves called *nervi vasorum* ("nerves of the vessel") and supplied with blood by tiny *vasa vasorum* ("vessels of the vessel") that extend inward from the tunica externa. As a rule, arteries have a thicker layer of smooth muscle than do veins.

Inner Layer

The innermost layer of a blood vessel is called the **tunica intima**—Latin for "inside coat". The tunica intima is made up of endothelium that is continuous with the endothelium that lines the heart. The endothelium has a basement membrane to support it. Elastic arteries also have an *internal elastic membrane.*

In arteries, the endothelium provides a completely smooth lining. In veins, however, the endothelium also forms valves that help maintain the one-way flow of blood. The smallest of the vessels, the capillaries, have only one thin coat: the endothelium. This structural feature is important because the thinness of the capillary wall allows for efficient exchange of materials between the blood plasma and the interstitial fluid of the surrounding tissues.

Quick CHECK

1. Name the three major types of blood vessels.
2. How does the structure of each major type of vessel differ from the other types?
3. How does the function of capillaries relate to the structure of their walls?

CIRCULATORY ROUTES

The term *circulation of blood* suggests its meaning—namely, blood flow through vessels arranged to form a circuit or circular pattern.

The **systemic circulation** route conducts blood flow from the heart (left ventricle) through blood vessels to all parts of the body (except the gas-exchange tissues in the lungs) and back to the heart (to the right atrium) (**Figure 29-5**). The left ventricle pumps blood into the ascending aorta. From here it flows into arteries that carry it into the various tissues and organs of the body. Within each organ or structure, blood moves, as indicated in **Figure 29-5**, from arteries to arterioles to capillaries. Here the vital two-way exchange of substances occurs between the blood and cells. Blood flows next out of each organ by way of its venules and then its veins to drain eventually into the inferior or superior vena cava. These two great veins of the body return venous blood to the right atrium of the heart to complete the systemic circulation. But the blood does not quite come full circle back to its starting point, the left ventricle.

To start on its way again, blood must first flow through another circuit, the **pulmonary circulation** route. Observe in **Figure 29-5** that deoxygenated blood moves from the right atrium to the right ventricle to the pulmonary artery to lung arterioles and capillaries. Here, exchange of gases between blood and air takes place, converting deoxygenated blood to oxygenated blood. This oxygenated blood then flows on through lung venules into four pulmonary veins and returns to the left atrium of the heart. From the left atrium it enters the left ventricle to be pumped again through the systemic circulation.

Movement of blood as shown in **Figure 29-5** follows a general rule of thumb often used when studying the circulatory system—namely, that blood passes through only one capillary network in the systemic circulation from the time it leaves the heart until it returns. Although this is certainly true in most instances, two important exceptions to the rule do occur. In a **portal system,** blood flowing through the systemic circulation passes through two consecutive capillary beds rather than one. For example, note in **Figure 29-5** that blood coming from the digestive organs passes through a second capillary network in the liver before returning to the heart. The liver's portal circulation is discussed later in this chapter.

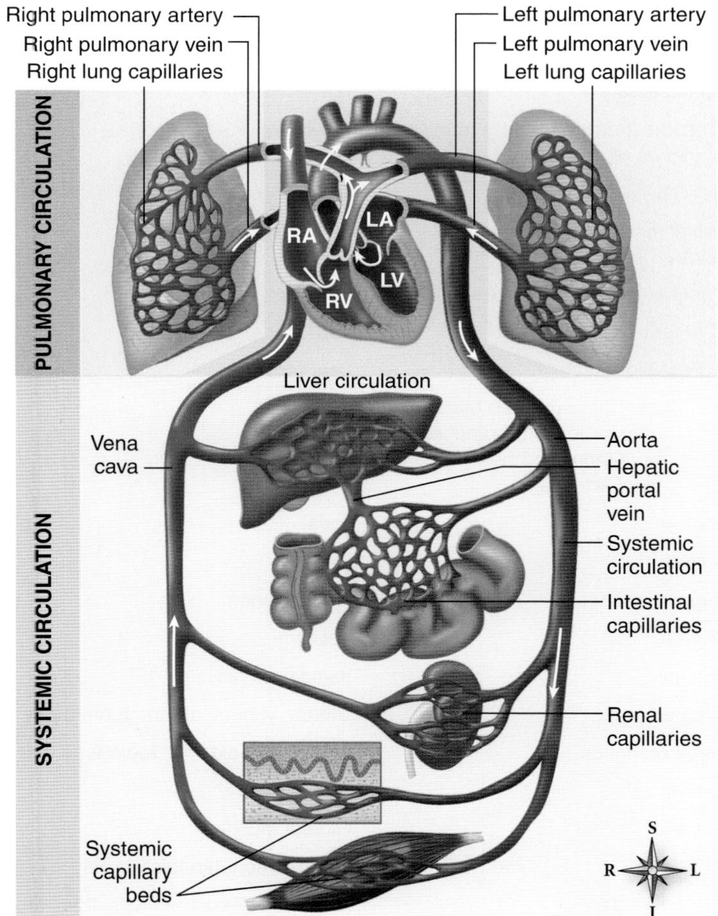

FIGURE 29-5 Circulatory routes. The pulmonary circulation routes blood flow to and from the gas-exchange tissues of the lungs. The systemic circulation, on the other hand, routes blood flow to and from the oxygen-consuming tissues of the body.

The term **vascular anastomosis** is used to describe a second type of exception. It involves the direct connection or merger of blood vessels to one another. In vascular anastomoses, blood moves from veins to other veins or arteries to other arteries without passing through an intervening capillary network.

Arterial anastomoses involve the merger of one artery directly into another artery and may develop in response to disease. Such an anastomosis may permit "bypass" of a partially blocked artery, thus allowing blood to flow into a capillary network and an area of tissue that would otherwise be deprived of an adequate supply of oxygen and nutrients. As stated earlier, arterial anastomoses between the smaller **coronary arteries** may permit development of "collateral circulation" and movement of blood into areas of ischaemic cardiac muscle tissue. However, because very few natural arterial anastomoses exist between the larger coronary arteries, surgical arterial bypass procedures are often required to correct inadequate blood flow to heart muscle (see discussion of myocardial infarction in Mechanisms of Disease, p. 657).

Venous anastomoses, which are much more common, involve direct linkage between different veins. Multiple venous drainage routes from an organ or body area provide a safety mechanism if occlusion of one venous return route should occur. This is especially true of the deep veins. Catastrophic consequences from a so-called *deep vein thrombosis (DVT)* may be prevented or lessened because of these anastomoses.

Arteriovenous anastomoses, or **shunts,** occur when blood flows from an artery directly into a vein without passing through a capillary bed. Heat loss occurs when blood passes through capillary beds in the skin. In cases of hypothermia, heat loss can be avoided by shunting of blood directly from skin arteries to veins without permitting it to pass through capillary beds near the skin surface (see **Figure 10-15** on p. 193).

SYSTEMIC CIRCULATION

The systemic circulatory route includes most of the vessels of the body. The following paragraphs, tables, and illustrations outline some of the major vessels of the systemic circulation and give tips for understanding this circulatory route.

Systemic Arteries

Locate the arteries listed in **Table 29-2** (see also **Figures 29-6** to **29-14**). You may find it easier to learn the names of blood vessels and the relation of the vessels to each other from diagrams and tables than from narrative descriptions.

General Principles Concerning Arteries

As you learn the names of the main arteries, keep in mind that these are only the major pipelines distributing blood from the heart to the

TABLE 29-2 Major Systemic Arteries

ARTERY*	REGION SUPPLIED
Ascending Aorta	
Coronary arteries	Myocardium
Arch of Aorta	
Brachiocephalic (Innominate)	Head, upper extremity
Right common carotid	Head, neck
Right internal carotid[†]	Brain, eye, forehead, nose
Right external carotid[†]	Thyroid, tongue, tonsils, ear, etc.
Right subclavian	Head, upper extremity
Right vertebral[†]	Spinal cord, brain
Right axillary (continuation of subclavian)	Shoulder, chest, axillary region
Right brachial (continuation of axillary)	Arm, hand
Right radial	Forearm, hand (lateral)
Right ulnar	Forearm, hand (medial)
Superficial and deep palmar arches (formed by anastomosis of branches of radial and ulnar)	Hand, fingers
Digital	Fingers
Left Common Carotid	Head, neck
Left internal carotid[†]	Brain, eye, forehead, nose
Left external carotid[†]	Thyroid, tongue, tonsils, ear, etc.
Left Subclavian	Head, upper extremity
Left vertebral[†]	Spinal cord, brain
Left axillary (continuation of subclavian)	Shoulder, chest, axillary region
Left brachial (continuation of axillary)	Arm, hand
Left radial	Forearm, hand (lateral)
Left ulnar	Forearm, hand (medial)
Superficial and deep palmar arches (formed by anastomosis of branches of radial and ulnar)	Hand, fingers
Digital	Fingers
Descending Thoracic Aorta	
Visceral Branches	Thoracic viscera
Bronchial	Lungs, bronchi
Oesophageal	Oesophagus
Parietal Branches	Thoracic walls
Intercostal	Lateral thoracic walls (rib cage)
Superior phrenic	Superior surface of diaphragm

ARTERY*	REGION SUPPLIED
Descending Abdominal Aorta	
Visceral Branches	Abdominal viscera
Coeliac artery (trunk)	Abdominal viscera
Left gastric	Stomach, oesophagus
Common hepatic	Liver
Splenic	Spleen, pancreas, stomach
Superior mesenteric	Pancreas, small intestine, colon
Inferior mesenteric	Descending colon, rectum
Suprarenal	Adrenal (suprarenal) gland
Renal	Kidney
Ovarian	Ovary, uterine tube, ureter
Testicular	Testis, ureter
Parietal Branches	Walls of abdomen
Inferior phrenic	Inferior surface of diaphragm, adrenal gland
Lumbar	Lumbar vertebrae, muscles of back
Median sacral	Lower vertebrae
Common Iliac (formed by terminal branches of aorta)	Pelvis, lower extremity
External Iliac	Thigh, leg, foot
Femoral (continuation of external iliac)	Thigh, leg, foot
Popliteal (continuation of femoral)	Leg, foot
Anterior tibial	Leg, foot
Posterior tibial	Leg, foot
Plantar arch (formed by anastomosis of branches of anterior and posterior tibial arteries)	Foot, toes
Digital	Toes
Internal Iliac	Pelvis
Visceral branches	Pelvic viscera
Middle rectal	Rectum
Vaginal	Vagina, uterus
Uterine	Uterus, vagina, uterine tube, ovary
Parietal branches	Pelvic wall, external regions
Lateral sacral	Sacrum
Superior gluteal	Gluteal muscles
Obturator	Pubic region, hip joint, groin
Internal pudendal	Rectum, external genitals, floor of pelvis
Inferior gluteal	Lower gluteal region, coccyx, upper thigh

*Branches of each artery are indented below its name.

†See text and/or figures for branches of the artery.

various organs and that, in each organ, the main artery resembles a tree trunk in that it gives off numerous branches that continue to branch and rebranch, forming ever-smaller vessels (arterioles), which also branch, forming microscopic vessels, the capillaries. In other words, most arteries eventually diverge into smaller arterioles, then into capillaries. An artery that provides the only supply of oxygen and nutrients to a particular tissue is called a terminal artery or end artery. Important organs or areas of the body supplied by end arteries are subject to serious damage or death in occlusive arterial disease. As an example, permanent blindness results when the central artery of the retina, an end artery, is occluded. Therefore arterial disease that occludes (blocks) blood flow, such as **atherosclerosis,** is of clinical concern when it affects important organs having an end-arterial blood supply.

FIGURE 29-6 Principal arteries of the body.

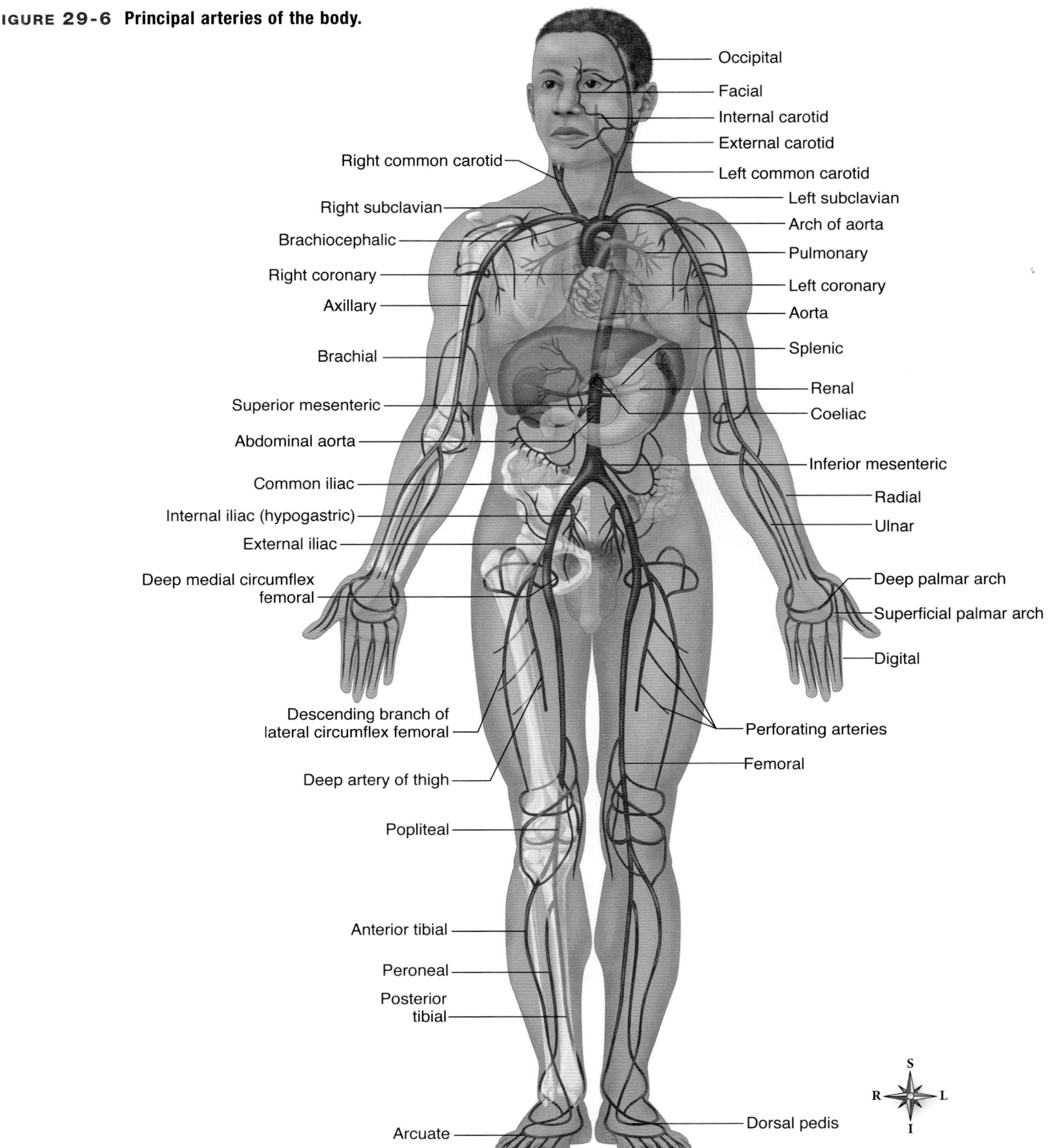

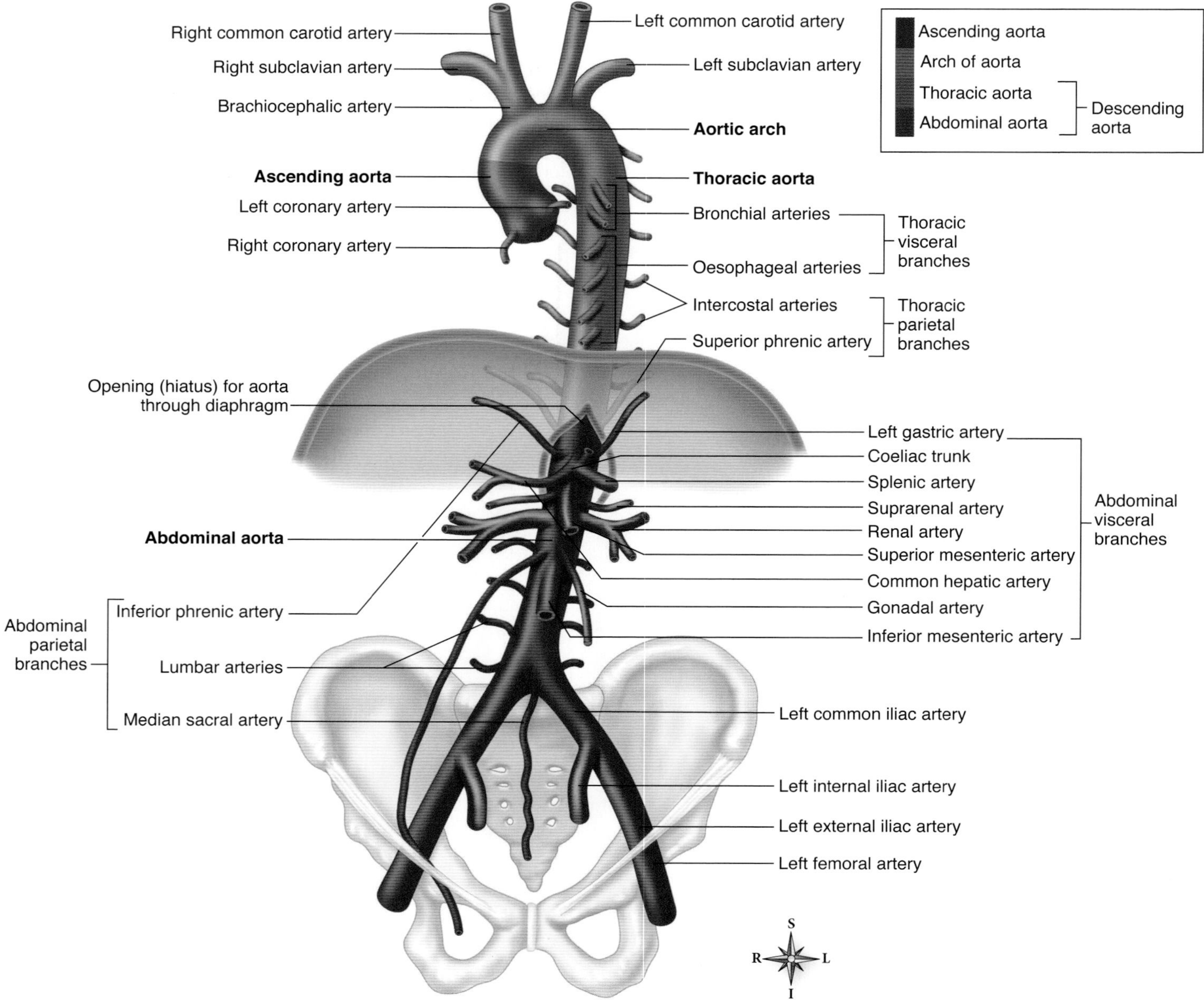

FIGURE 29-7 Divisions and primary branches of the aorta (anterior view). The aorta is the main systemic artery, serving as a trunk from which other arteries branch. Blood is conducted from the heart first through the ascending aorta, then through the arch of the aorta, and then through the thoracic and abdominal segments of the descending aorta. Note the designation of visceral and parietal branches in the thoracic and abdominal aortic divisions. **Table 29-2** and the flow charts showing branches of the aortic divisions in **Figure 29-10**, **Figure 29-12**, and **Figure 29-14** are intended to assist you in interpreting the artist's depiction of arterial vessels.

A few arteries open into other branches of the same or other arteries. Such a communication was described earlier as an **arterial anastomosis.** Anastomoses, we have already noted, fulfil an important protective function in that they provide detour routes for blood to travel through in the event of obstruction of a main artery. The incidence of arterial anastomoses increases as distance from the heart increases, and smaller arterial branches tend to anastomose more often than larger vessels. Examples of arterial anastomoses are the palmar and plantar arches and the cerebral arterial circle (of Willis) at the base of the brain (look ahead to **Figure 29-9** on p. 676). Other examples are found around several joints, as well as in other locations.

Another general principle to remember as you study the systemic arteries is that the **aorta** is the major artery that serves as the main trunk of the entire systemic arterial system. Notice in **Figures 29-6** and **29-7** that different segments of the aorta are known by different names. Because the first few centimetres of the aorta conduct blood upward out of the left ventricle, this region is known as the **ascending aorta.** The coronary arteries are branches of the ascending aorta (look back to **Figures 28-10** and **28-11** on pp. 647–648). The aorta then turns 180 degrees, forming a curved segment called the *arch of the aorta* or simply **aortic arch.** Arterial blood is conducted downward from the arch of the aorta through the **descending aorta.** The descending aorta passes through the thoracic cavity, where it is known as the **thoracic aorta,** to the abdominal cavity, where it is known as the **abdominal aorta.**

If you check **Table 29-2** or **Figure 29-6**, you will see that all systemic arteries branch from the aorta or one of its branches.

Look again at **Figures 29-6** and **29-7**. Note how the main branches from the arch of the aorta are different on the right compared with the left. The right side of the head and neck are supplied by the **brachiocephalic artery,** which branches to become the right **subclavian artery** and right **common carotid artery.** On the left, however, the left subclavian artery and the left common carotid artery branch directly from the arch of the aorta—without an intervening brachiocephalic artery.

Arteries of the Head and Neck

Figure 29-8 shows the major arteries of the head, neck, and face. Trace the branching of arteries in the figure with your finger as you read through **Table 29-2**. Note in this figure how the right and left vertebral arteries extend from their origin as branches of the subclavian arteries up the neck, through foramina in the transverse processes of the cervical vertebrae, through the foramen magnum, and into the cranial cavity.

Next, take a look at **Figure 29-9**, which shows the arteries at the base of the brain. Note how the vertebral arteries unite on the undersurface of the brainstem to form the *basilar artery*, which shortly branches into the right and left *posterior cerebral arteries* (see **Figure 29-9**). The basilar artery also branches to the pons and cerebellum (see **Table 29-2**). The internal carotid arteries enter the cranial cavity in the midpart of the cranial floor, where they become known as the *anterior cerebral arteries.* Small vessels, the *communicating arteries,* join the anterior and posterior cerebral arteries in such a way as to form the **cerebral arterial circle** *(of Willis)* at the base of the brain, a good example of arterial anastomosis (see **Figure 29-9**).

Typical of vascular anastomoses, the exact structure of the cerebral arterial circle varies somewhat among individuals. Recent studies suggest that missing components of the circle may increase the risk of *migraine headaches.*

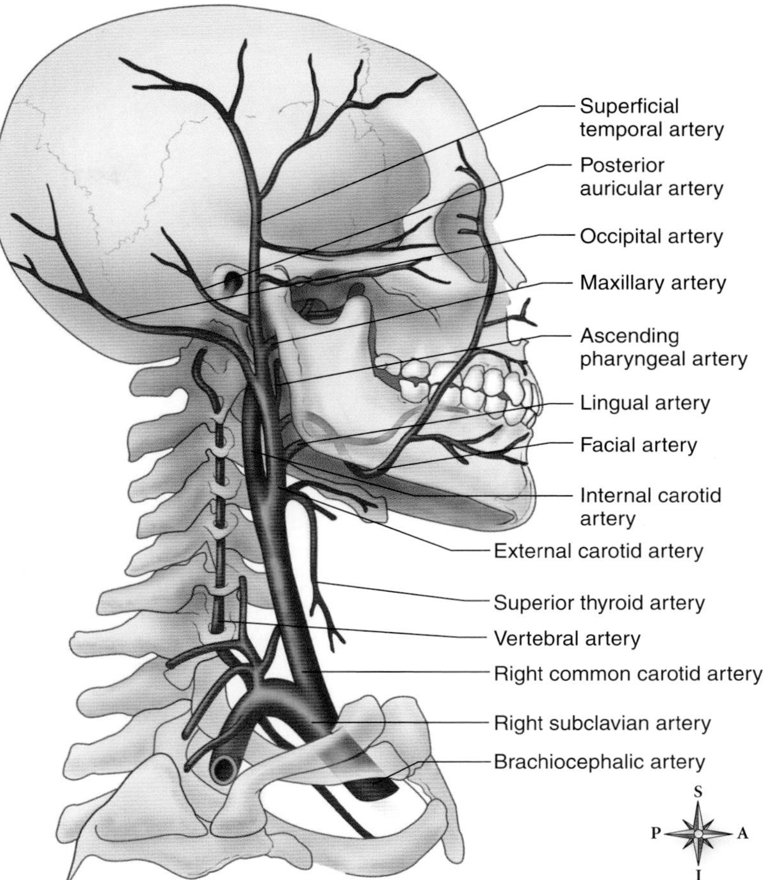

FIGURE 29-8 Major arteries of the head and neck. See **Figure 29-9** for arteries at the base of the brain.

Arteries of the Trunk

The arch of the aorta continues downward as the **thoracic aorta.** It begins at the level of the fifth thoracic vertebra and ends at the diaphragm. *Parietal* branches of the thoracic aorta (posterior intercostal, superior phrenic, and subcostal arteries) supply blood to the body wall. Four *visceral* branches (mediastinal, bronchial, oesophageal, and pericardial) provide arterial blood to internal thoracic structures.

Just as the thoracic aorta is a downward continuation of the aortic arch so, too, is the **abdominal aorta** a downward continuation of the thoracic portion above it. It extends from the diaphragm above to the point where it divides into the right and left common iliac arteries at the level of the fourth lumbar vertebra. Note in **Figure 29-7** that this

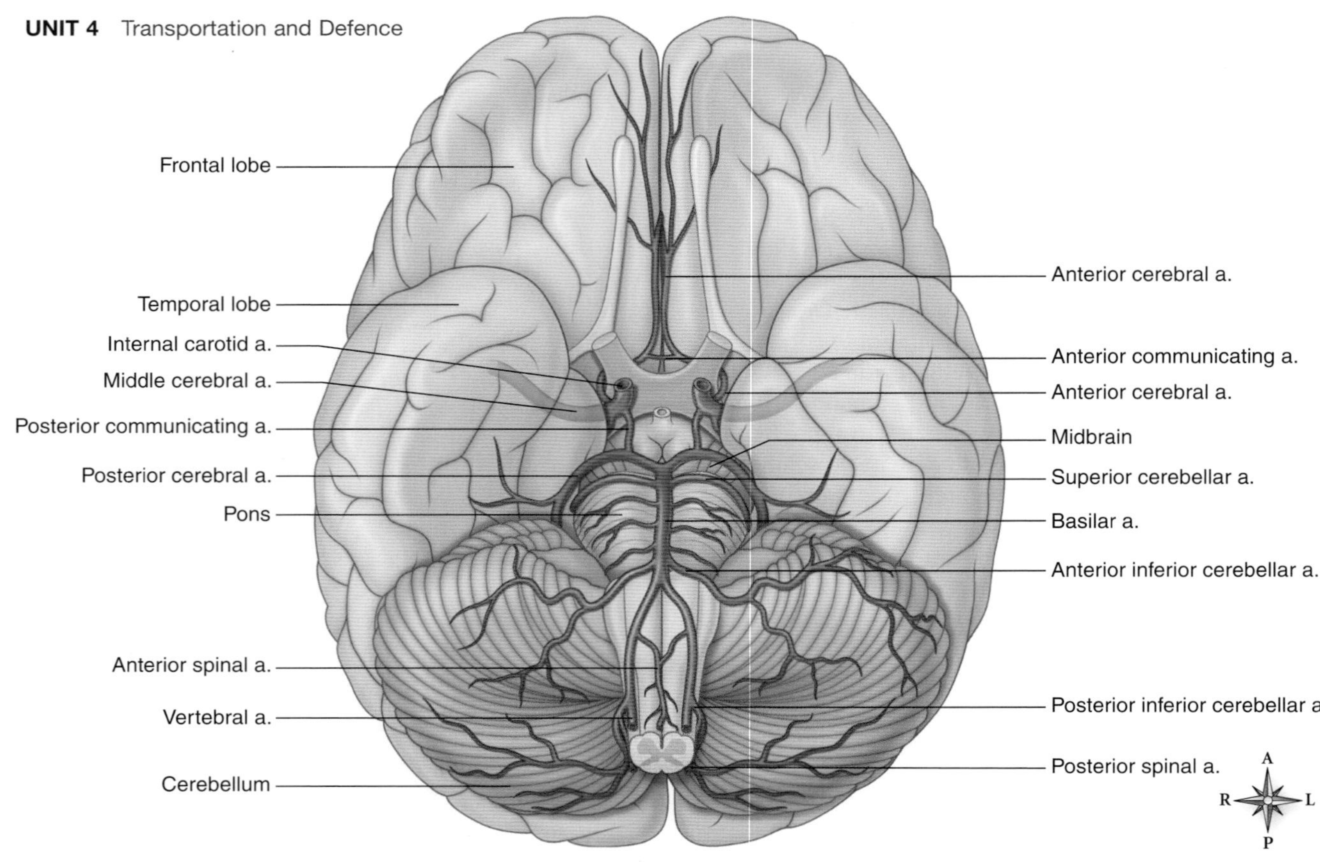

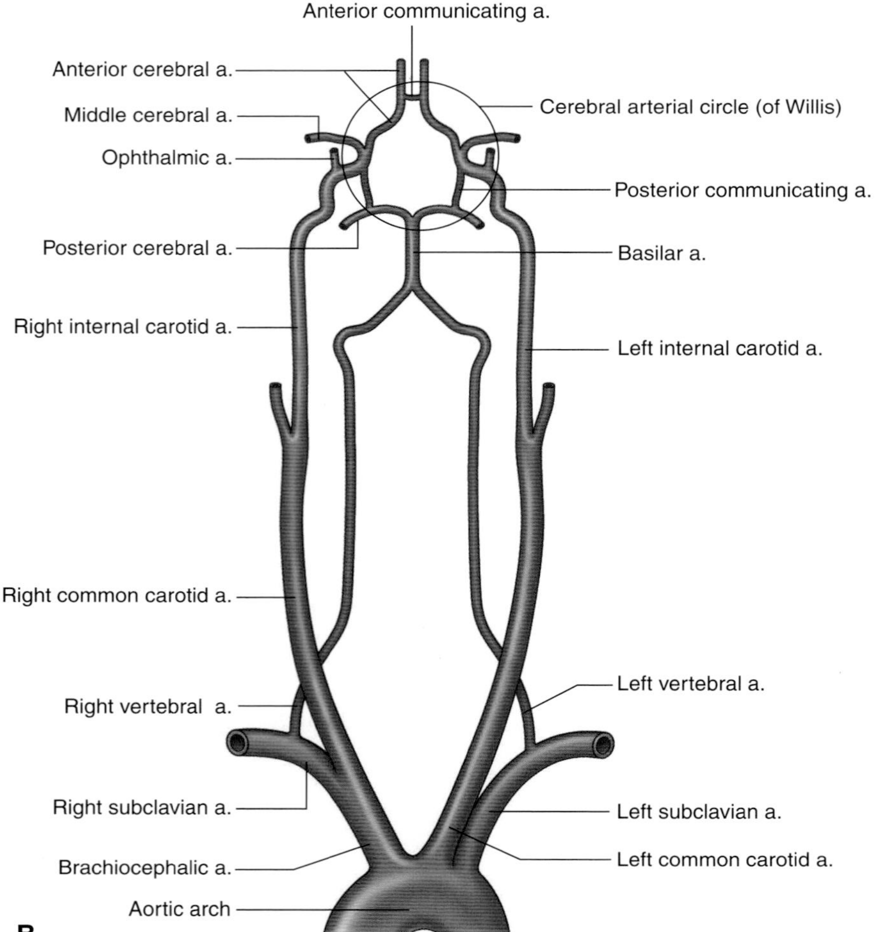

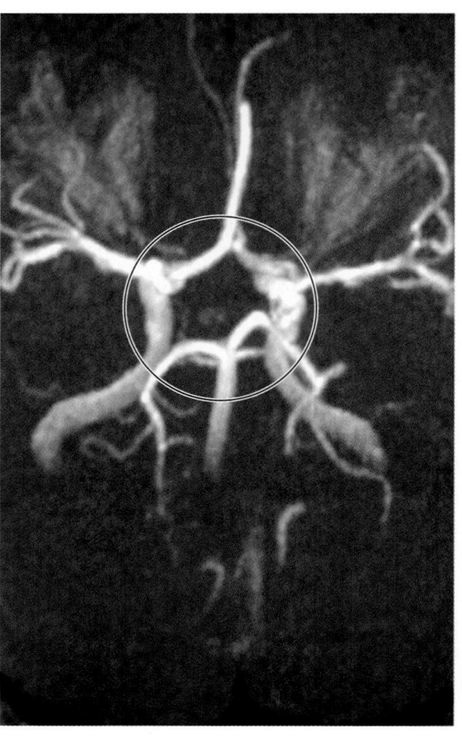

FIGURE 29-9 Arteries at the base of the brain. A, Diagram shows the cerebral arterial circle (of Willis) and related structures on the base of the brain. Note the arterial anastomoses. **B,** Origins of blood vessels that form the cerebral arterial circle. **C,** Magnetic resonance image of the cerebral arterial circle.

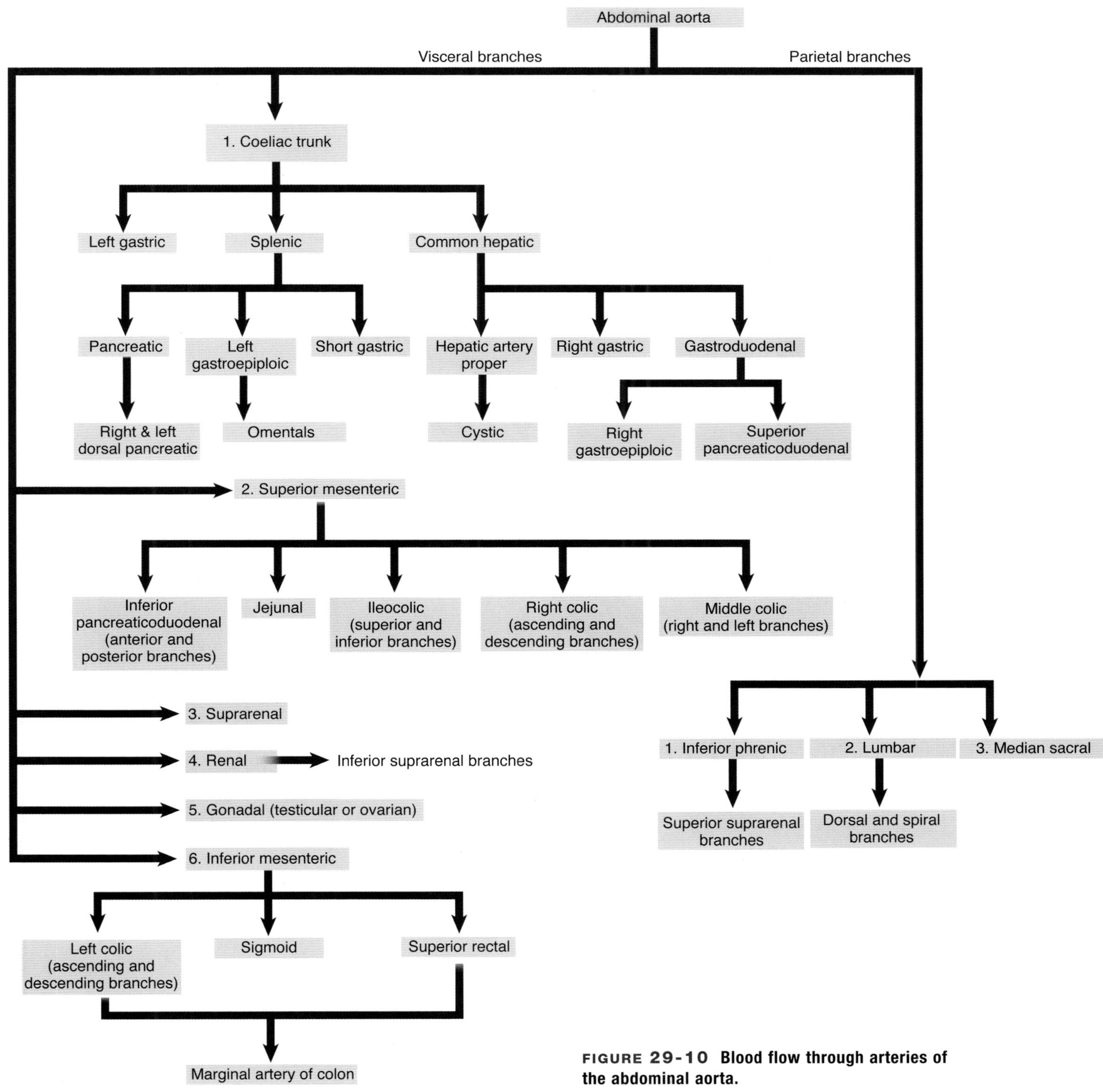

FIGURE 29-10 Blood flow through arteries of the abdominal aorta.

UNIT 4

segment of the aorta lies just anterior to the vertebral bodies. As a result, a physician can feel the aortic pulse during deep palpation of the abdomen when the vessel is compressed against the underlying vertebrae. The presence of a pulsating swelling along the aorta—an aortic aneurysm—is often diagnosed in this way.

Major abdominal and pelvic branches of the abdominal aorta may also be described as parietal or visceral depending on the location of the end organ or structures they supply with blood. Branches of this segment of the aorta are illustrated in **Figures 29-6** and **29-7** and shown in schematic form in **Figure 29-10**.

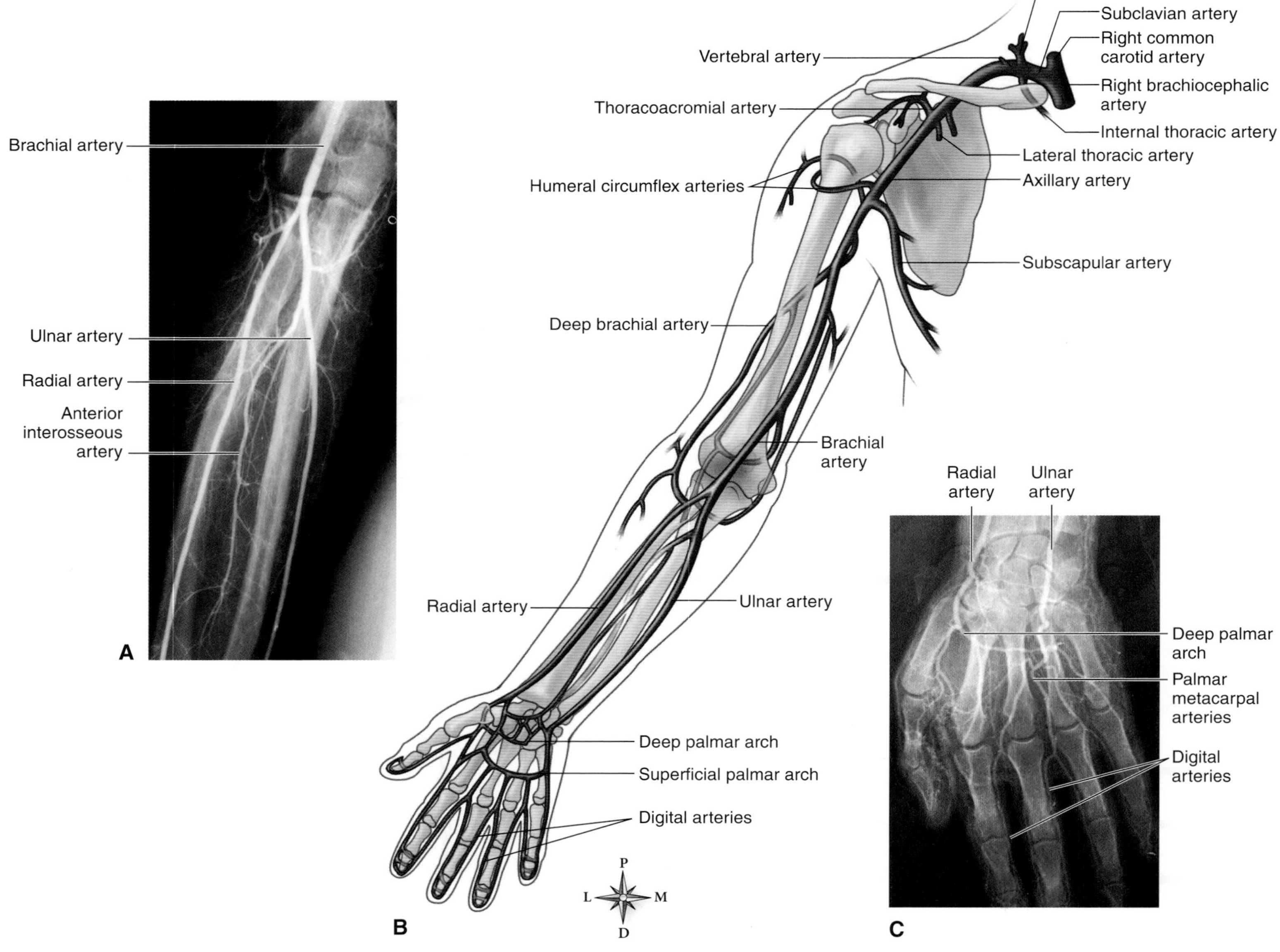

FIGURE 29-11 Major arteries of the upper extremity. A, Arteriogram of brachial and upper forearm arteries. **B,** Diagram of major arteries of upper extremity (anterior view). **C,** Arteriogram of hand arteries.

Arteries of the Extremities

Next, take a look at **Figures 29-11** and **29-12**, which outline the arteries of the upper extremity. Then take a look at **Figures 29-13** and **29-14**, which outline the arteries of the lower extremity. Trace these arteries with your finger as you compare each figure to **Table 29-2**. Because of differences in orientation, not every artery listed in the table appears in every illustration.

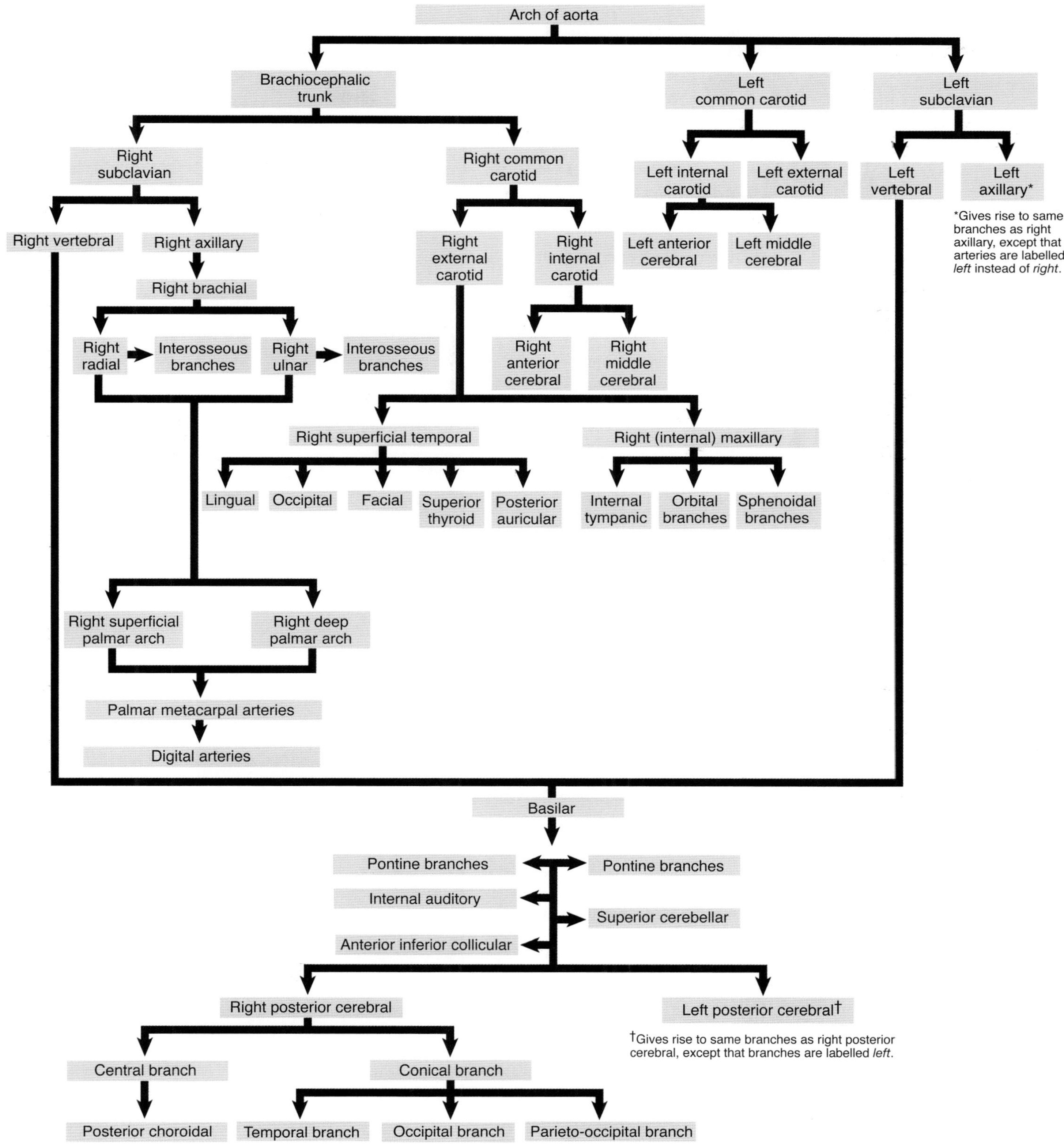

FIGURE 29-12 **Blood flow through arteries of the aortic arch.**

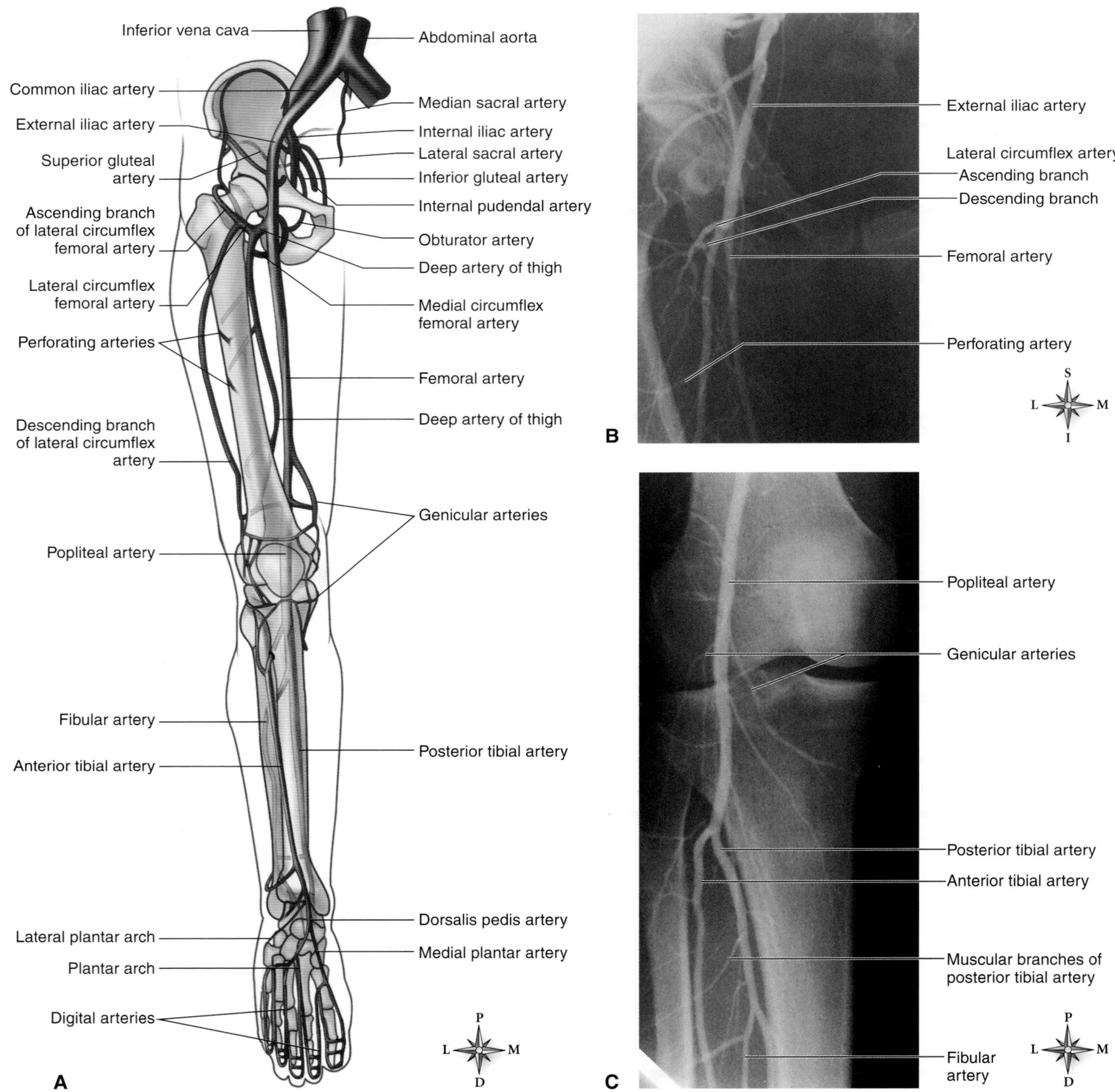

FIGURE 29-13 Major arteries of the lower extremity. A, Diagram of major arteries of lower extremity. Anterior view of the right hip and leg. **B,** Femoral arteriogram. Contrast material passing through the external iliac artery in the abdomen has entered the femoral artery and its branches in the thigh. **C,** Popliteal arteriogram.

FIGURE 29-14 Blood flow through arteries of the lower extremity.

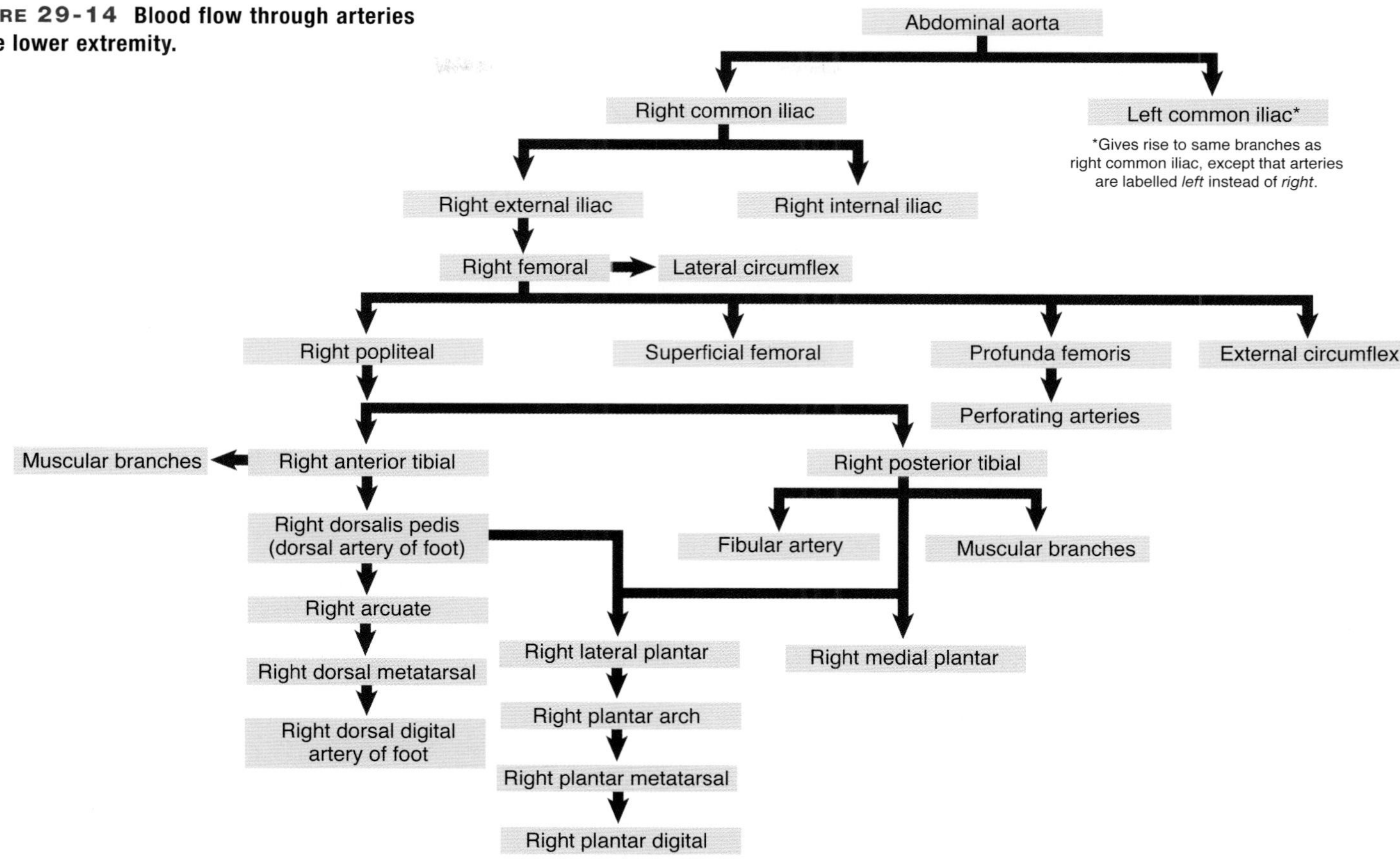

Systemic Veins

Locate the veins listed in **Table 29-3** (see also **Figures 29-15** to **29-22**). As with the arteries, you may find it easier to learn the names of veins and their anatomical relation to each other from diagrams and tables than from narrative descriptions.

General Principles Concerning Veins

The following facts should be borne in mind while learning the names and locations of veins:

- Veins are the ultimate extensions of capillaries, just as capillaries are the eventual extensions of arteries. Whereas arteries branch into vessels of decreasing size to form arterioles and eventually capillaries, capillaries unite into vessels of increasing size to form venules and, eventually, veins.
- Although all vessels vary considerably in location and branches—and whether or not they are even present—the veins are especially variable. For example, the **median cubital vein** in the forearm is absent in many individuals.
- Many of the main arteries have corresponding veins bearing the same name and are located alongside or near the arteries. These veins, like the arteries, lie in deep, well-protected areas, for the most part, close along the bones. Examples are the femoral artery and femoral vein, both located along the femur bone.
- Veins found in the deep parts of the body are called **deep veins,** in contrast to **superficial veins,** which lie near the surface. The latter are the veins that can be seen through the skin.
- The large veins of the cranial cavity, formed by the dura mater, are not usually called veins but are instead called *dural sinuses*, or, simply, **sinuses.** They should not be confused with the bony, air-filled sinuses of the skull.
- Veins communicate (anastomose) with each other in the same way as arteries. In fact, the venous portion of the systemic circulation has even more anastomoses than the arterial portion. Such venous anastomoses provide for collateral return blood flow in cases of venous obstruction.
- Venous blood from the head, neck, upper extremities, and thoracic cavity, with the exception of the lungs, drains into the superior vena cava. Blood from the lower extremities and abdomen enters the inferior vena cava.

Table 29-3 identifies the major systemic veins. Locate each one as you read the table and trace them with your finger on **Figures 29-15** to **29-22**.

TABLE 29-3 Major Systemic Veins

VEIN*	REGION DRAINED	VEIN*	REGION DRAINED
Superior Vena Cava	Head, neck, thorax, upper extremity	***Inferior Vena Cava***	Lower trunk and extremity
Brachiocephalic (Innominate)	Head, neck, upper extremity	**Phrenic**	Diaphragm
Internal jugular (continuation of sigmoid sinus)	Brain	**Hepatic Portal System**	Upper abdominal viscera
Lingual	Tongue, mouth	Hepatic veins (continuations of liver venules and sinusoids and ultimately the hepatic portal vein)	Liver
Superior thyroid	Thyroid, deep face	Hepatic portal vein	Gastrointestinal organs, pancreas, spleen, gallbladder
Facial	Superficial face	Cystic	Gallbladder
Sigmoid sinus (continuation of transverse sinus; direct tributary of internal jugular)	Brain, meninges, skull	Gastric	Stomach
Superior and inferior petrosal sinuses	Anterior brain, skull	Splenic	Spleen
Cavernous sinus	Anterior brain, skull	Inferior mesenteric	Descending colon, rectum
Ophthalmic veins	Eye, orbit	Pancreatic	Pancreas
Transverse sinus (direct tributary of sigmoid sinus)	Brain, meninges, skull	Superior mesenteric	Small intestine, most of colon
Occipital sinus	Inferior, central region of cranial cavity	Gastroepiploic	Stomach
Straight sinus	Central region of brain, meninges	**Renal**	Kidneys
Inferior sagittal sinus	Central region of brain, meninges	Suprarenal	Adrenal (suprarenal) gland
Superior sagittal (longitudinal) sinus	Superior region of cranial cavity	Left ovarian	Left ovary
External jugular	Superficial, posterior head, neck	Left testicular	Left testis
Subclavian (continuation of axillary; direct tributary of brachiocephalic)	Axilla, lower extremity	Left ascending lumbar (anastomoses with hemiazygos)	Left lumbar region
Cephalic	Lateral arm and forearm, hand	**Right Ovarian (Gonadal)**	Right ovary
Axillary (continuation of basilic; direct tributary of subclavian)	Axilla, lower extremity	**Right Testicular (Gonadal)**	Right testis
Brachial	Deep arm	**Right Ascending Lumbar** (anastomoses with azygos)	Right lumbar region
Radial	Deep lateral forearm	**Common Iliac** (continuation of external iliac; common iliacs unite to form inferior vena cava)	Lower extremity
Ulnar	Deep medial forearm	External iliac (continuation of femoral direct tributary of common iliac)	Thigh, leg, foot
Basilic (direct tributary of axillary)	Medial arm and forearm, hand	Femoral (continuation of popliteal direct tributary of external iliac)	Thigh, leg, foot
Median cubital (formed by anastomosis of cephalic and basilic)	Forearm, hand	Popliteal	Leg, foot
Deep and superficial palmar venous arches (formed by anastomosis of cephalic and basilic)	Hand	Small (external, short) saphenous	Superficial posterior leg, lateral foot
Digital	Fingers	Dorsal veins of foot (also drain into great saphenous)	Anterior (dorsal) foot, toes
Azygos (anastomoses with right ascending lumbar)	Right posterior wall of thorax and abdomen, oesophagus, bronchi, pericardium, mediastinum	Medial and lateral plantar	Sole of foot
Hemiazygos (anastomoses with left renal)	Left inferior posterior wall of thorax and abdomen, oesophagus, mediastinum	Anterior tibial	Anterior leg, foot
Accessory hemiazygos	Left superior posterior wall of thorax	Fibular (peroneal)	Lateral and anterior leg, foot
		Posterior tibial	Deep posterior leg
		Great (internal, long) saphenous	Superficial medial and anterior thigh, leg, foot
		Dorsal veins of foot	Anterior (dorsal) foot, toes
		Dorsal venous arch	Anterior (dorsal) foot, toes
		Digital	Toes
		Internal iliac (unites with external iliac to form common iliac)	Pelvic region

*Tributaries of each vein are identified below its name; deep veins are printed in dark blue, and superficial veins are printed in light blue.

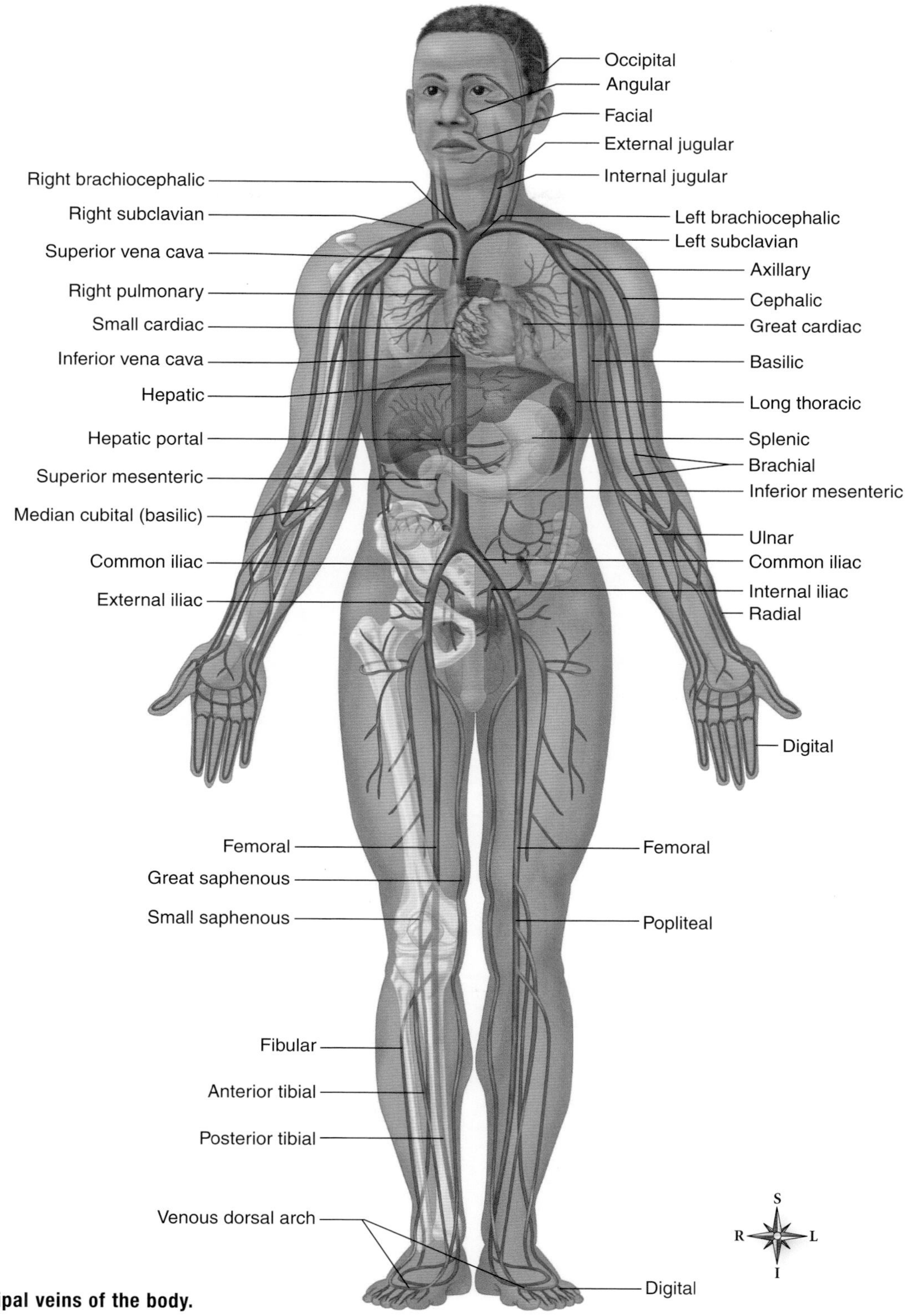

FIGURE 29-15 Principal veins of the body.

Veins of the Head and Neck

The deep veins of the head and neck lie mostly within the cranial cavity (see **Figure 29-16**). These are mainly dural sinuses and other veins that drain into the **internal jugular vein.** The internal jugular vein also receives blood from superficial veins of the face and neck.

The superficial veins that lie over the cranium drain into the right and left **external jugular veins** in the neck. The external jugular veins also receive blood from deep veins of the face. Each external jugular vein terminates in a *subclavian vein.* Small emissary veins connect veins of the scalp and face with blood sinuses of the cranial

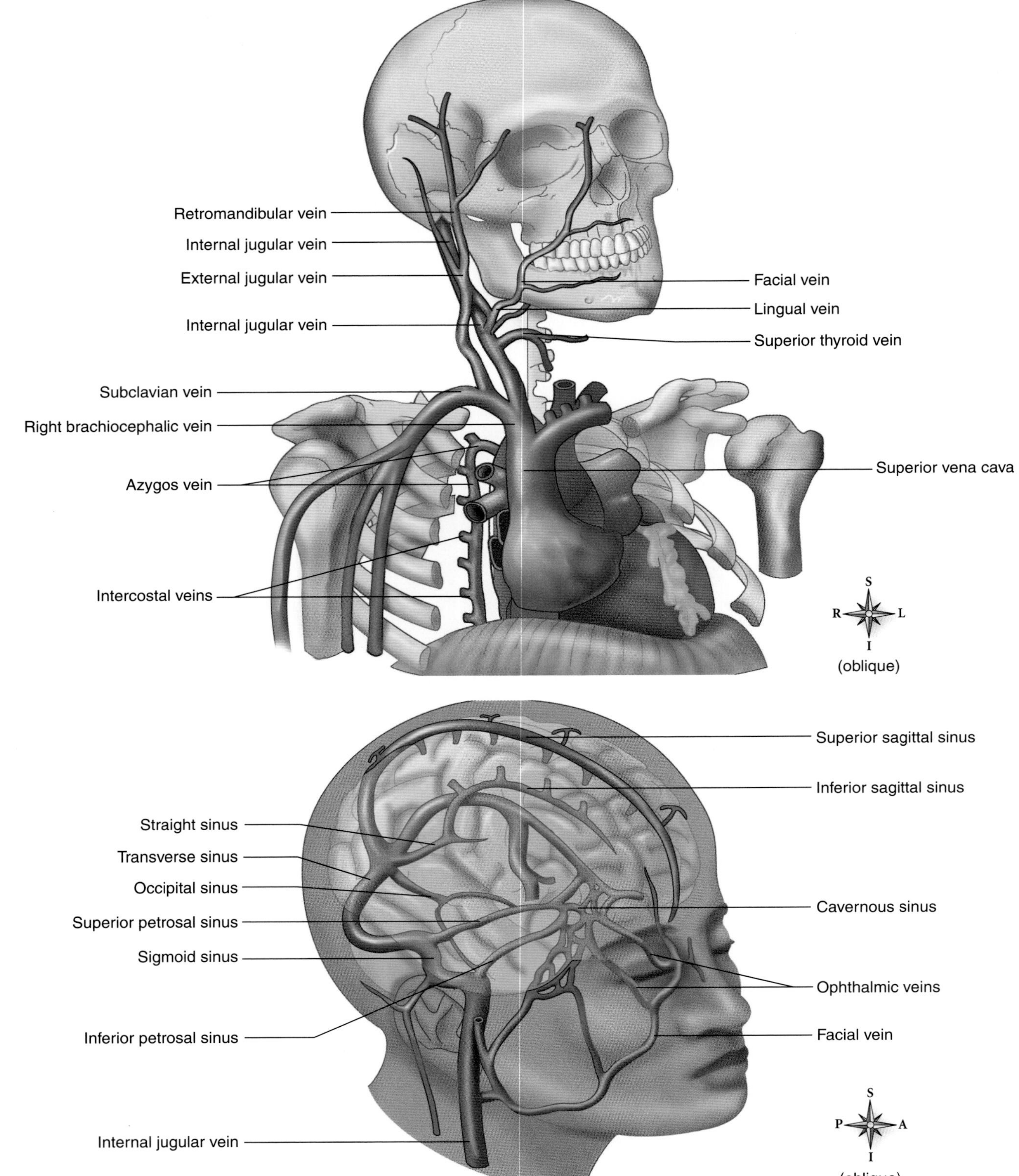

FIGURE 29-16 Major veins of the head and neck. A, Anterior view showing veins on the right side of the head and neck. **B,** Lateral, superior view showing the position of major veins relative to the brain. The venous sinuses shown here are within the dura mater and are thus called *dural sinuses.*

cavity, a fact of clinical interest as a possible avenue for infections to enter the cranial cavity.

Veins of the Upper Extremity

Deep veins of the upper extremity drain into the **brachial vein,** which in turn drains into the **axillary vein** and then the **subclavian vein** before joining the **brachiocephalic vein,** a major tributary of the **superior vena cava.** The major veins of the upper extremity are shown in **Figures 29-17** and **29-18**. At this point, it is interesting to note that the tributaries of the superior vena cava are more symmetrical from left to right than the nearby branches of the aorta. Compare **Figures 29-6** and **29-15** to verify this point.

Superficial veins of the hand form the **palmar venous arches,** which, together with a complicated network of superficial veins of the forearm, finally pour their blood into two large veins: the **cephalic vein** (thumb side) and **basilic vein** (little finger side). These two veins empty into the deep **axillary vein.**

Veins of the Thorax

Several small veins—such as the **bronchial vein, oesophageal vein,** and **pericardial vein**—return blood from thoracic organs (except gas exchange tissues in the lungs) directly into the **superior vena cava** or **azygos vein.** Refer to **Figure 29-19** to see how these veins are arranged. The azygos vein lies to the right of the spinal column and extends from the inferior vena cava (at the level of the first or second lumbar vertebra) through the diaphragm to the terminal part of the superior vena cava. The **hemiazygos vein** lies to the left of the spinal column, extending from the lumbar level of the inferior vena cava through the diaphragm to terminate in the azygos vein. The **accessory hemiazygos vein** connects some of the **superior intercostal veins** with the azygos or hemiazygos vein.

Veins of the Abdomen

The abdominal tributaries offer another opportunity to see a slight difference between the left and right portions of the systemic venous circulation. For example, **Figure 29-19** shows that the gonadal veins—*ovarian vein* or *testicular (spermatic) vein*—and left **suprarenal vein** usually drain into the left **renal vein** instead of into the **inferior vena cava.** This is the opposite of the arrangement of these veins on the right. For a description of the return of blood from the abdominal digestive organs, see the subsequent discussion of the **hepatic portal circulation.**

Hepatic Portal Circulation

Veins from the spleen, stomach, pancreas, gallbladder, and intestines do not pour their blood directly into the inferior vena cava, as do the veins from other abdominal organs. They send their blood to the liver by means of the hepatic portal vein. Here the blood mingles with the arterial blood in the capillaries and is eventually drained from the liver by the hepatic veins that join the inferior vena cava. Any arrangement in which venous blood flows through a second capillary network before returning to the heart is called a *portal* circulatory route. Portal comes from the Latin *porta,* meaning "gateway", and is used here because the hepatic portal vein to the liver is a gateway through which blood returning from the digestive tract must pass before it returns to the heart.

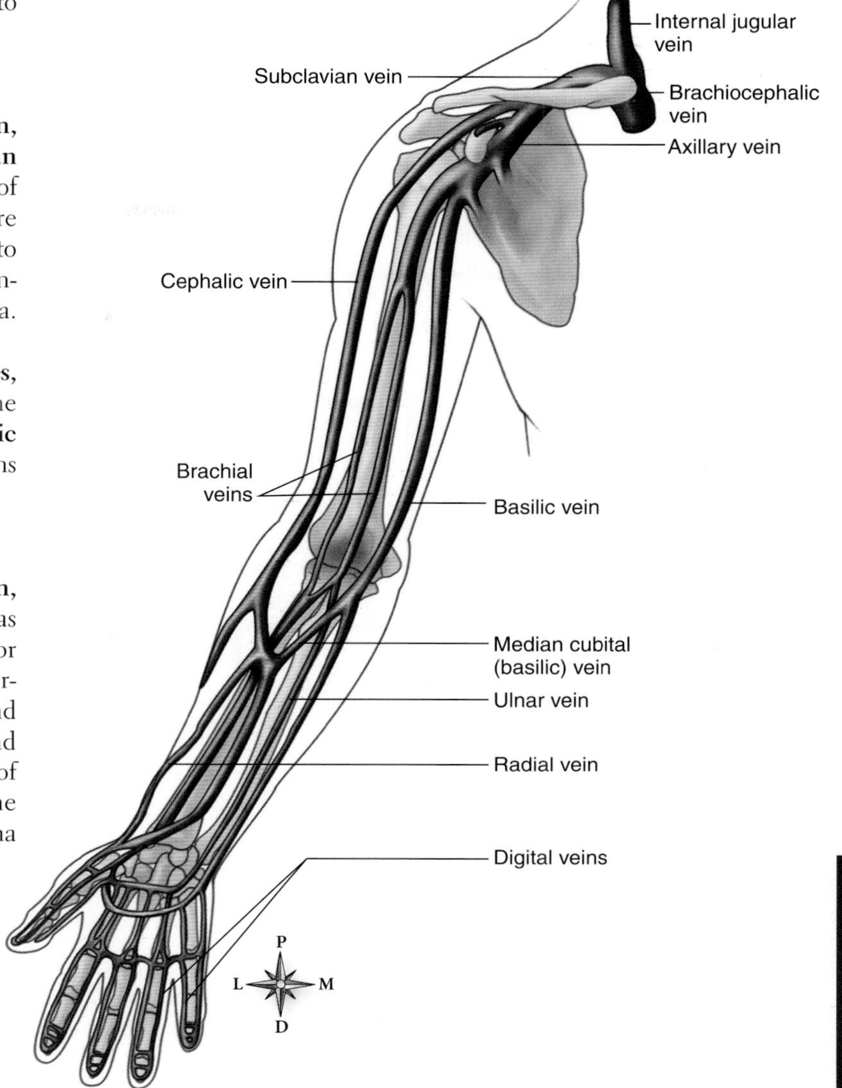

FIGURE 29-17 Major veins of the upper extremity. The median cubital (basilic) vein is commonly used for removing blood from the body as when obtaining blood specimens or adding blood as when giving intravenous infusions (anterior view).

There are several advantages to detouring blood from the digestive tract through the liver before it returns to the heart. Shortly after a meal, blood flowing through digestive organs begins absorbing glucose and other simple nutrients. The result is a tremendous increase in the blood glucose level. As the blood travels through the liver, however, excess glucose is removed from the blood and stored in liver cells as glycogen. Thus blood returned to the heart carries only a moderate level of glucose. Many hours after food has yielded its nutrients, low-glucose blood coming from the digestive organs can pick up glucose released from the glycogen stores held in the liver cells before returning to the heart.

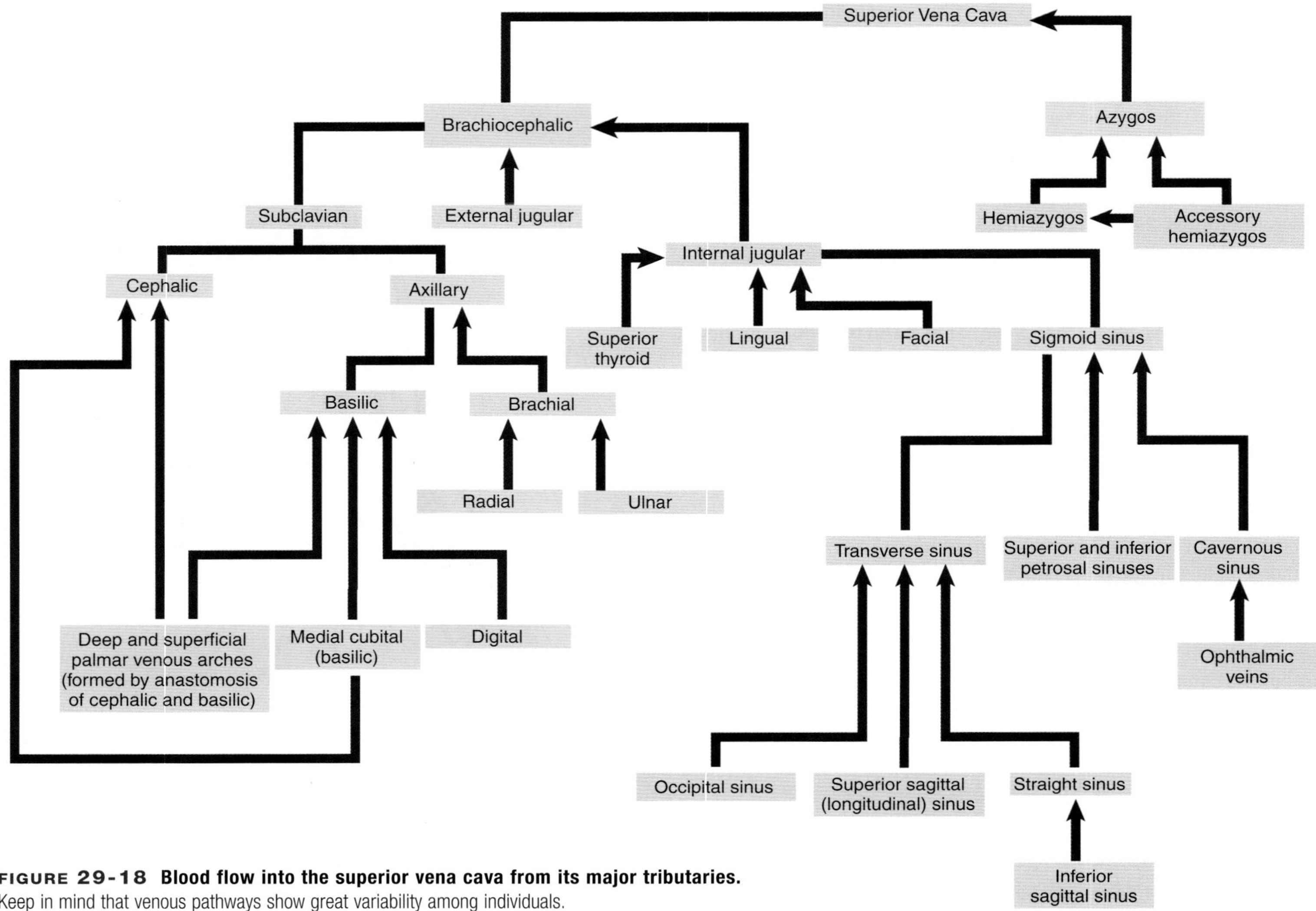

FIGURE 29-18 Blood flow into the superior vena cava from its major tributaries. Keep in mind that venous pathways show great variability among individuals.

Another advantage of the hepatic portal scheme is that toxic molecules such as alcohol can be partially removed or detoxified before the blood is distributed to the rest of the body. Additional information regarding the role of the liver, and the advantages of the portal circulation through the liver, are discussed in Chapters 39 and 40.

Figure 29-5 (p. 671) shows the plan of the hepatic portal system in relation to the overall scheme of circulation. **Figure 29-20** shows the details of the veins involved in the hepatic portal circulation. In most individuals the hepatic portal vein is formed by the union of the splenic and superior mesenteric veins, but blood from the gastric, pancreatic, and inferior mesenteric veins drains into the splenic vein before it merges with the superior mesenteric vein.

If either hepatic portal circulation or venous return from the liver is interfered with (as often occurs in certain types of liver disease or heart disease), venous drainage from most of the other abdominal organs is necessarily obstructed also. The accompanying increased capillary pressure accounts, at least in part, for the occurrence of abdominal bloating, or **ascites,** in these conditions.

Veins of the Lower Extremity

As **Figure 29-21** shows, deep veins of the leg drain from the **anterior tibial vein,** the **fibular vein (peroneal vein),** and the **posterior tibial vein.** These veins join the **popliteal vein,** which runs behind the knee joint and continues up along the femur as the deep femoral vein. The

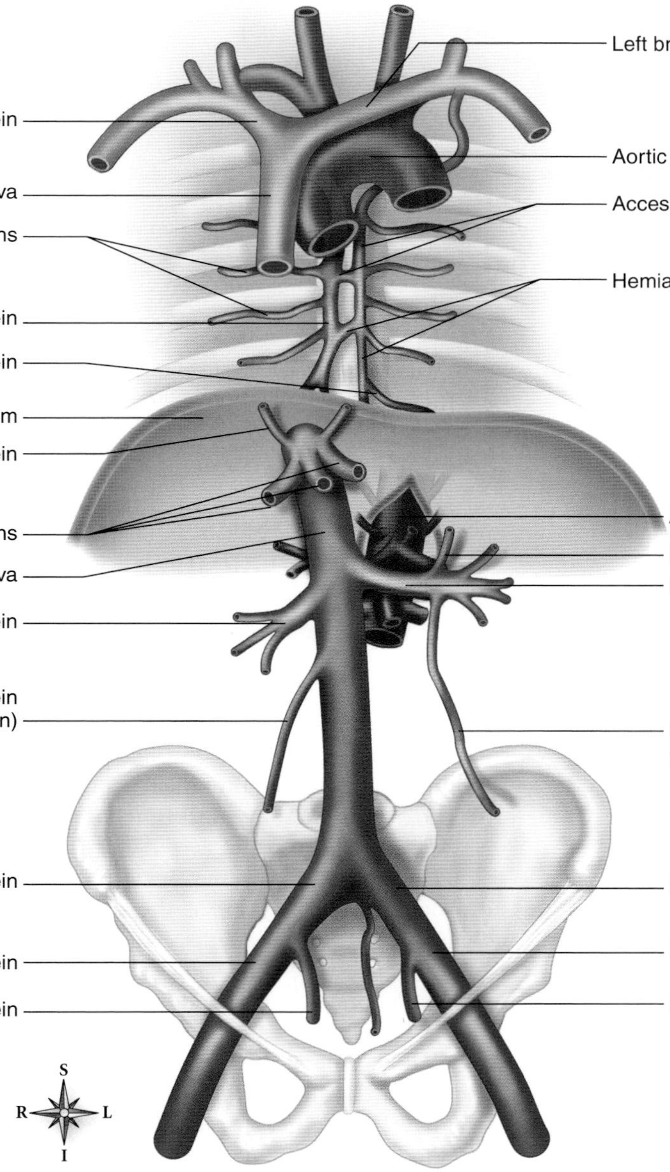

Left brachiocephalic vein
Right brachiocephalic vein
Aortic arch
Superior vena cava
Accessory hemiazygos vein
Intercostal veins
Hemiazygos vein
Azygos vein
Ascending lumbar vein
Diaphragm
Phrenic vein
Aorta
Hepatic veins
Inferior vena cava
Left suprarenal vein
Left renal vein
Right renal vein
Right ovarian or testicular vein (gonadal vein)
Left ovarian or testicular vein (gonadal vein)
Right common iliac vein
Left common iliac vein
Right external iliac vein
Left external iliac vein
Right internal iliac vein
Left internal iliac vein
S
R
L
I

FIGURE 29-19 Inferior vena cava and its abdominopelvic tributaries. Anterior view of ventral body cavity with many of the viscera removed. Note the close anatomical relationship between the inferior vena cava and the descending aorta. Smaller veins of the thorax drain blood into the inferior vena cava or into the azygos vein—both are shown here. The hemiazygos vein and accessory hemiazygos vein on the left drain into the azygos vein on the right.

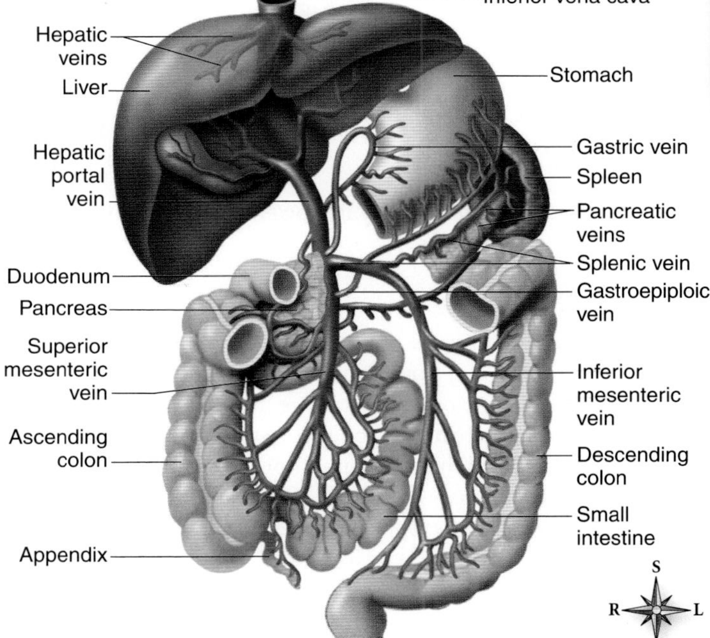

FIGURE 29-20 Hepatic portal circulation. In this unusual circulatory route, a vein is located between two capillary beds (see **Figure 29-3**). The hepatic portal vein collects blood from capillaries in visceral structures located in the abdomen and empties it into the liver. Hepatic veins return blood to the inferior vena cava.

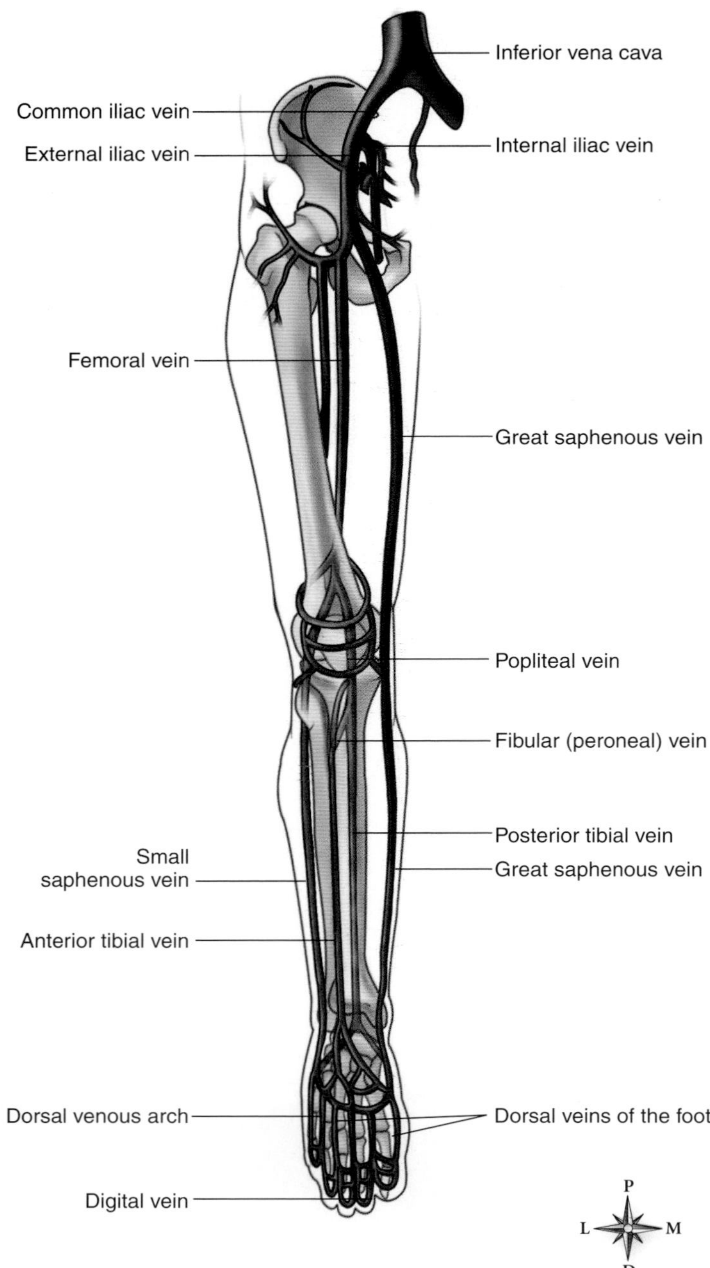

FIGURE 29-21 Major veins of the lower extremity (anterior view).

femoral vein continues as the **external iliac vein,** draining into the common iliac vein and from there into the **inferior vena cava.**

Superficial veins of the lower extremity include the **small saphenous vein,** a tributary of the popliteal vein, and the **great saphenous vein,** which drains much of the superficial leg and foot. The name *saphenous* is from the Greek *saphenes,* a word that means "apparent"—an appropriate name for these visible, superficial veins.

Figure 29-22 summarizes blood flow from the abdomen and lower extremities into the inferior vena cava.

Quick CHECK

4. What is the difference between the pulmonary circulation and the systemic circulation?
5. What is the function of arterial anastomoses? What is the function of venous anastomoses?
6. How are systemic arteries and veins usually named?
7. What are the advantages of a portal circulation through the liver?

CONNECT IT! 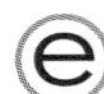

A valuable skill is the ability to trace the flow of blood completely through the normal adult circulatory route. Check out ***How to Trace the Flow of Blood*** online at ***Connect It!*** for some tips and a handy diagram of the route of blood flow through the body.

FETAL CIRCULATION

THE BASIC PLAN OF FETAL CIRCULATION

Circulation in the body before birth necessarily differs from circulation after birth for one main reason—fetal blood secures oxygen and nutrients from maternal blood instead of from fetal lungs and digestive organs. Obviously, then, there must be additional blood vessels in the fetus to carry the fetal blood into close approximation with the maternal blood and to return it to the fetal body. These structures are the two **umbilical arteries,** the **umbilical vein,** and the **ductus venosus.**

Also, some structure must function as the lungs and digestive organs do after birth—that is, provide a place where an exchange of gases, nutrients, and wastes between the fetal and maternal blood can occur. This structure is the *placenta* (**Figure 29-23**). The exchange of substances occurs without any actual mixing of maternal and fetal blood, because each flows in its own separate space.

In addition to the placenta and umbilical vessels, three structures located within the fetus's own body play an important part in fetal circulation. One of them (the ductus venosus) serves as a detour by which most of the blood returning from the placenta bypasses the fetal liver. The other two (the foramen ovale and ductus arteriosus) provide detours by which blood bypasses the lungs. A brief description of each of the six structures necessary for fetal circulation follows (**Figure 29-24**):

1. The two **umbilical arteries** are branches of the internal iliac (hypogastric) arteries and carry fetal blood to the placenta.
2. The **placenta** is a structure attached to the uterine wall. Exchange of oxygen and other substances between maternal and fetal blood takes place in the placenta, although no mixing of maternal and fetal blood occurs. **Box 29-1** discusses how alcohol from the maternal blood can damage developing fetal tissues.
3. The **umbilical vein** returns oxygenated blood from the placenta, enters the fetal body through the umbilicus, extends up to the undersurface of the liver where it gives off two or three branches to the liver, and then continues on as the ductus venosus. Two umbilical arteries and the umbilical vein together constitute the umbilical cord; these are shed at birth along with the placenta.
4. The **ductus venosus** is a continuation of the umbilical vein along the undersurface of the liver that drains into the inferior vena cava. Most of the blood returning from the placenta

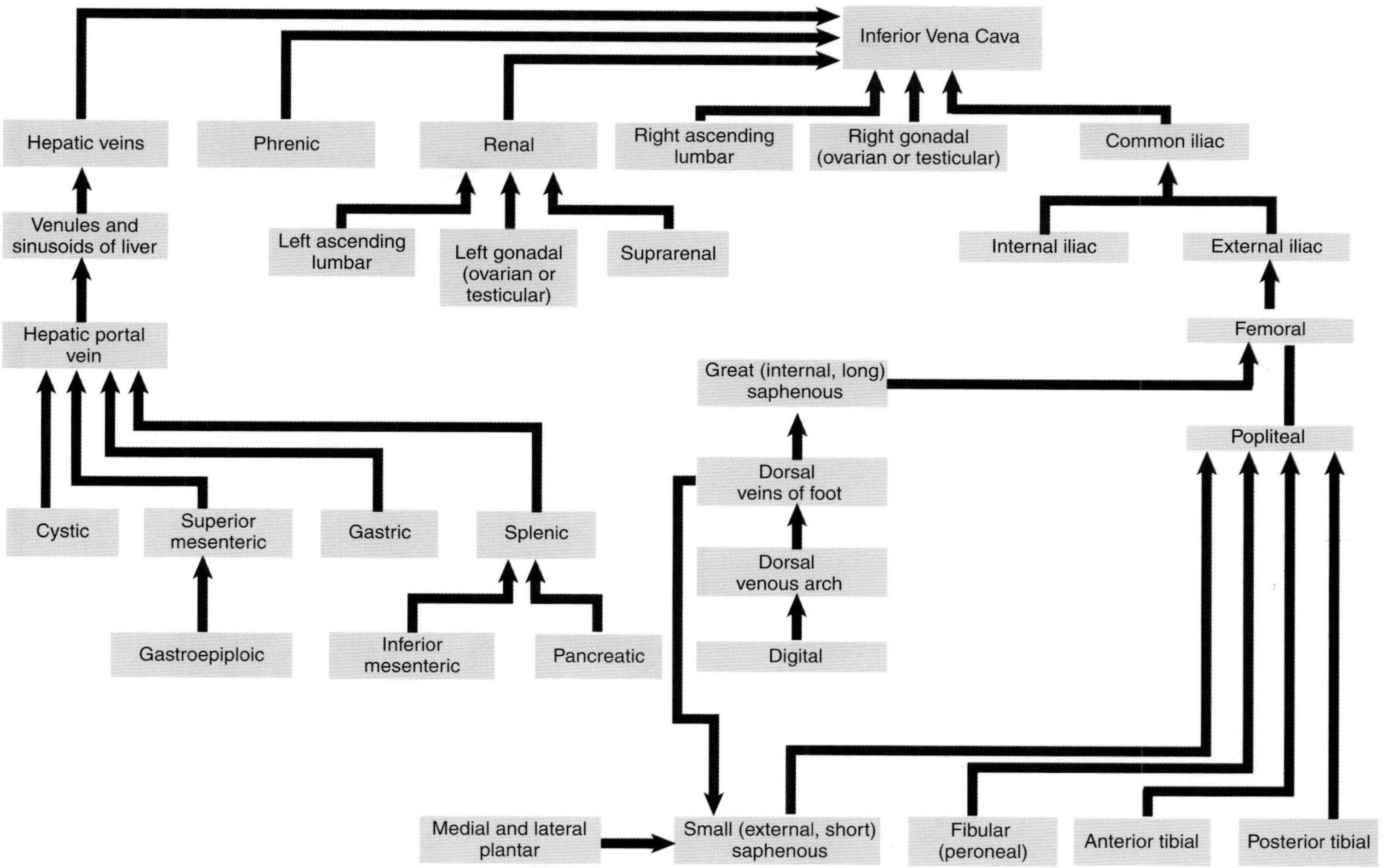

Inferior Vena Cava
Hepatic veins
Phrenic
Renal
Right ascending lumbar
Right gonadal (ovarian or testicular)
Common iliac
Venules and sinusoids of liver
Left ascending lumbar
Left gonadal (ovarian or testicular)
Suprarenal
Internal iliac
External iliac
Hepatic portal vein
Femoral
Great (internal, long) saphenous
Popliteal
Dorsal veins of foot
Cystic
Superior mesenteric
Gastric
Splenic
Dorsal venous arch
Gastroepiploic
Inferior mesenteric
Pancreatic
Digital
Medial and lateral plantar
Small (external, short) saphenous
Fibular (peroneal)
Anterior tibial
Posterior tibial

FIGURE 29-22 Blood flow into the inferior vena cava from its major tributaries. Keep in mind that venous pathways show great variability among individuals.

UNIT 4

Maternal arteriole
Endometrium
Maternal venule
Chorionic villi
Maternal blood
Fetal arteriole
Fetal venule
Placenta
Umbilical vein
Umbilical arteries
Umbilical cord

FIGURE 29-23 Placental circulation. The placenta is an organ that permits exchange of blood gases (O_2 and CO_2), nutrients, and wastes between fetal blood and maternal blood. Fetal capillaries found within branched villi are bathed in maternal blood. Note that fetal and maternal blood is separated by a membranous barrier. Other special features of fetal circulation are shown in **Figure 29-24** and **Figure 29-25**.

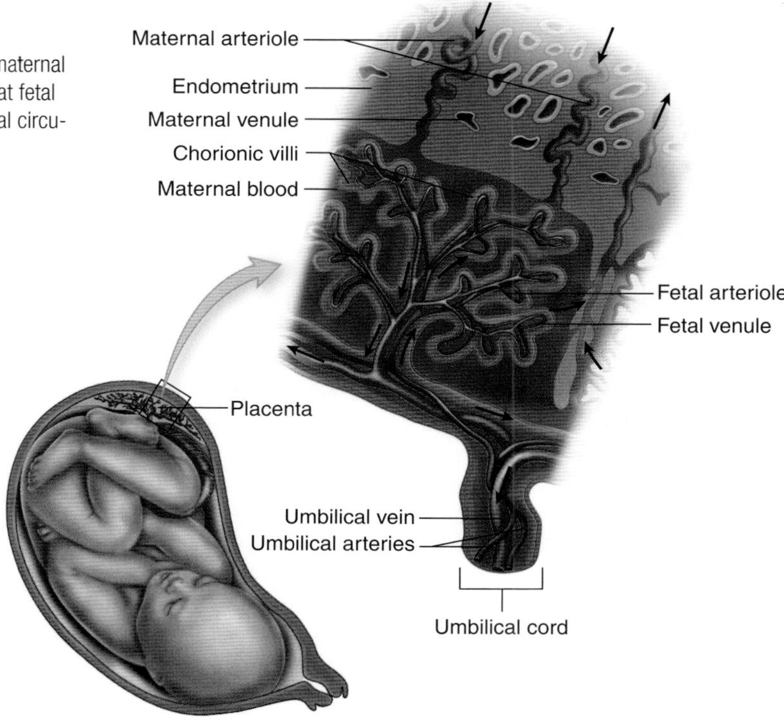

bypasses the liver. Only a relatively small amount of blood enters the liver by way of the branches from the umbilical vein into the liver.

5. The **foramen ovale** is an opening in the septum between the right and left atria. A valve at the opening of the inferior vena cava into the right atrium directs most of the blood through the foramen ovale into the left atrium so that it bypasses the fetal lungs. A small percentage of the blood leaves the right atrium for the right ventricle and pulmonary trunk. But most of this blood does not flow on into the lungs. Still another detour, the ductus arteriosus, diverts it.
6. The **ductus arteriosus** is a small vessel connecting the pulmonary trunk with the aortic arch. It therefore enables another portion of the blood to detour into the systemic circulation without going through the lungs.

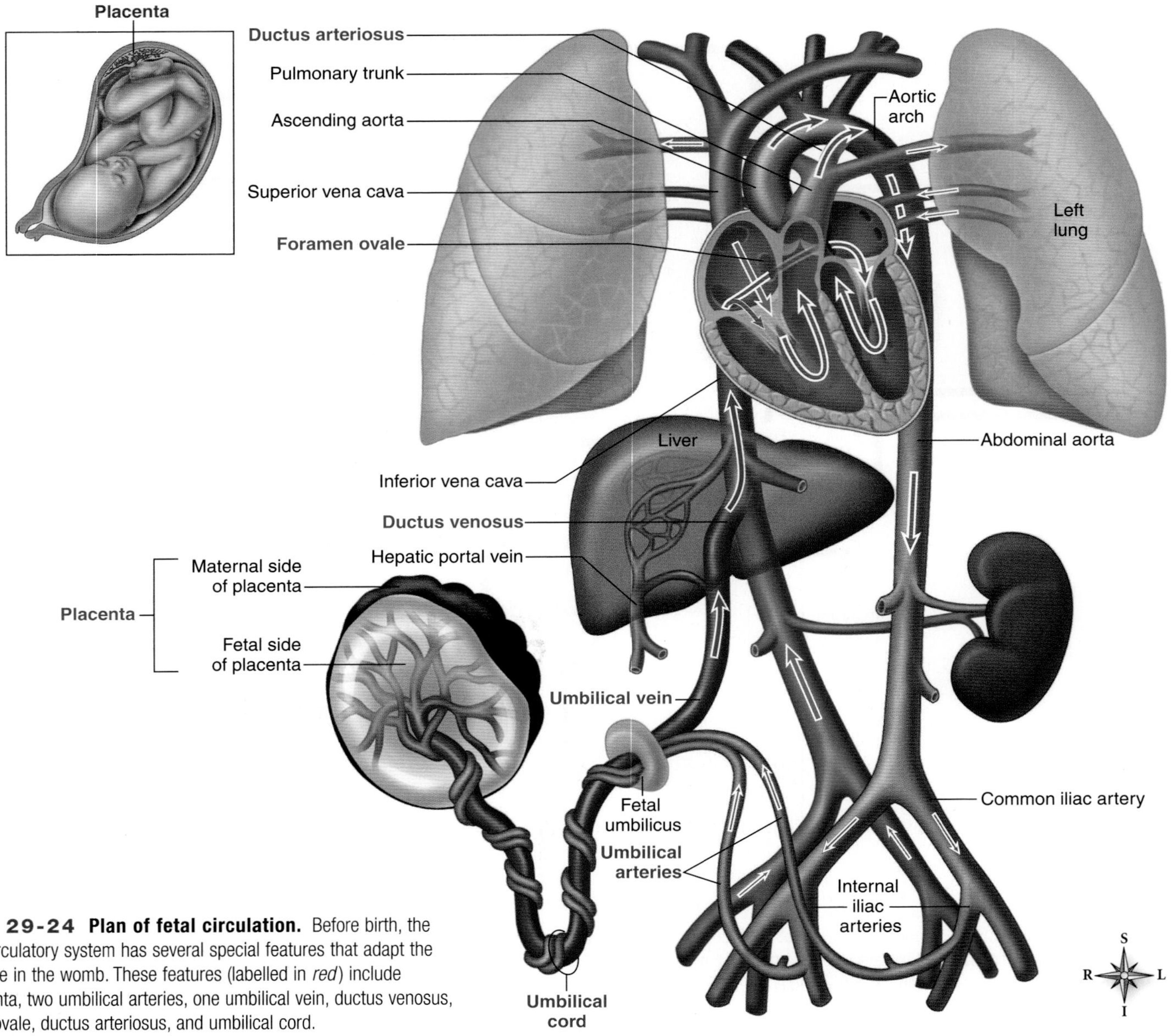

FIGURE 29-24 Plan of fetal circulation. Before birth, the human circulatory system has several special features that adapt the body to life in the womb. These features (labelled in *red*) include the placenta, two umbilical arteries, one umbilical vein, ductus venosus, foramen ovale, ductus arteriosus, and umbilical cord.

BOX 29-1 *health matters* | Fetal Alcohol Syndrome

Consumption of alcohol by a woman during her pregnancy can have tragic effects on the developing fetus. Educational efforts to inform pregnant women about the dangers of alcohol are now receiving national attention. Even very limited consumption of alcohol during pregnancy poses significant hazards to the developing fetus because alcohol can easily cross the placental barrier and enter the fetal bloodstream.

When alcohol enters the fetal blood, the potential result, called **fetal alcohol syndrome (FAS),** can include tragic congenital abnormalities such as "small head", or **microcephaly**; low birth weight; cardiovascular defects; developmental disabilities such as physical and intellectual disability; and even fetal death.

The photograph shows the small head, thinned upper lip, horizontally narrow eye openings *(palpebral fissures),* epicanthal folds, and receded upper jaw *(retrognathia)* typical of infants born with fetal alcohol syndrome.

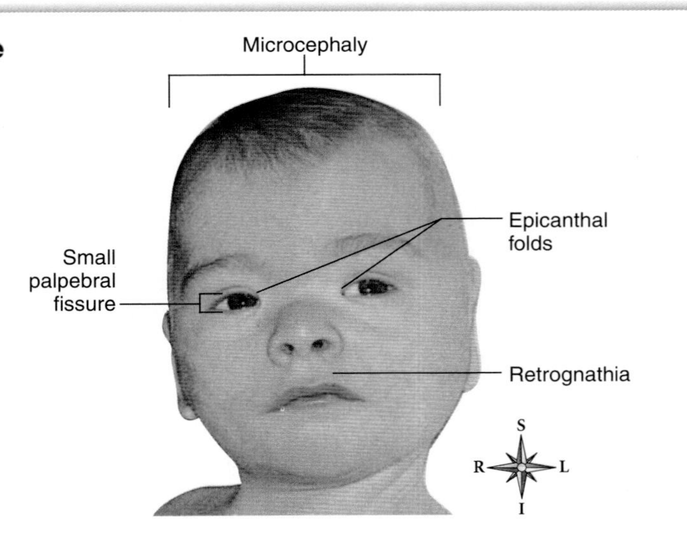

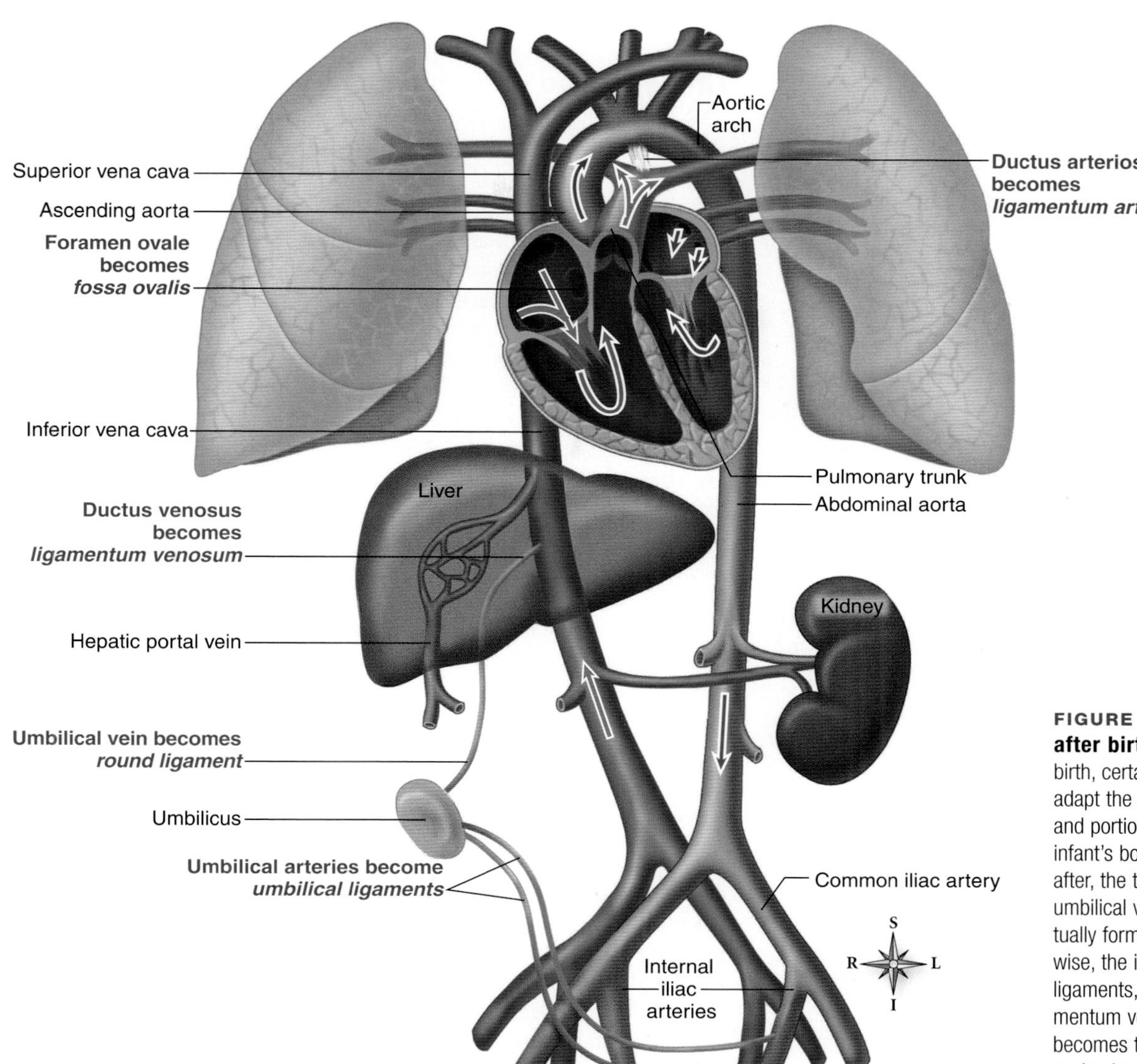

FIGURE 29-25 Changes in circulation after birth. Within the first year after the time of birth, certain changes in the circulatory plan occur to adapt the body to life outside the womb. The placenta and portions of the umbilical vessels outside the infant's body are removed or fall off at, or shortly after, the time of birth. The internal portion of the umbilical vein constricts and becomes fibrous, eventually forming the round ligament of the liver. Likewise, the internal umbilical arteries become umbilical ligaments, the ductus venosus becomes the ligamentum venosum, and the ductus arteriosus becomes the ligamentum arteriosum. The foramen ovale closes, forming a thin region of the atrial wall called the *fossa ovalis*.

Almost all fetal blood is a mixture of oxygenated and deoxygenated blood. Examine **Figure 29-24** carefully to determine why this is so. What happens to the oxygenated blood returned from the placenta by way of the umbilical vein? Note that it flows into the inferior vena cava.

Changes in Circulation at Birth

Because the six structures that serve fetal circulation are no longer needed after birth, several changes take place (**Figure 29-25**). As soon as the umbilical cord is cut, the two umbilical arteries, the placenta, and the umbilical vein obviously no longer function. The placenta is shed from the mother's body as the *afterbirth* with part of the umbilical vessels attached. The sections of these vessels remaining in the infant's body eventually become fibrous cords, which remain throughout life (the umbilical vein becomes the *round ligament* of the liver).

The ductus venosus, no longer needed to bypass blood around the liver, eventually becomes the *ligamentum venosum* of the liver.

The foramen ovale normally becomes functionally closed soon after a newborn takes the first breath and full circulation through the lungs becomes established. Complete structural closure, however, usually requires 9 months or more. Eventually, the foramen ovale becomes a mere depression *(fossa ovalis)* in the wall of the right atrial septum.

The ductus arteriosus contracts as soon as respiration is established. Eventually, it also turns into a fibrous cord, the *ligamentum arteriosum*. Compare the blood flow in **Figures 29-24** and **29-25**. Notice how separation of oxygenated and deoxygenated blood occurs *after* birth.

Quick CHECK

8. Name some structures of the fetal circulation that are not part of the adult circulation.
9. What is the function of the placenta and umbilical vessels?
10. What changes in the circulatory system occur at the time of birth?

cycle of life

Blood Vessels As with all body structures, the blood vessels undergo profound anatomical changes during early development in the womb. At birth, the switch from a placenta-dependent system causes another set of profound anatomical changes. As with the heart, throughout childhood, adolescence, and adulthood, the blood vessels normally maintain their basic structure and function—permitting continued survival of the individual. Normal changes include regrowth of vessels in damaged areas of the body and an increased number of blood vessels in skeletal muscles and the heart when we stay active.

In middle and late adulthood, our vessels often become less elastic, which can cause an overall increase in blood pressure. In the last chapter, we mentioned the risk of *atherosclerosis* in coronary arteries in adulthood—a risk that applies to all the arteries of the body—which can contribute to reduced elasticity of vessels. Although the risk of abnormal bulges, or *aneurysms*, is always present, such risk increases as we get older when the thinned vessel walls in an aneurysm may get closer to bursting if our resting blood pressure increases. •

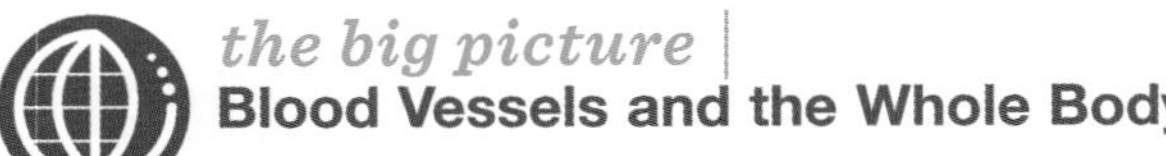

the big picture | Blood Vessels and the Whole Body

In this chapter, we have briefly outlined the functional anatomy of many different structures: the major arteries and veins, as well as the tiny arterioles, venules, and capillaries.

In essence, we have described a complex, interconnected network of flexible transport pipes for blood. Part of what you learned from this description is how each component of this blood-transporting network is constructed and just a little bit about how each works as an individual unit. Step back from this collection of facts for a moment, and think about how each component of the heart works with the other components to keep blood flowing continuously through the heart. Broaden the picture now in your mind's eye to include each of the other components of the network: the arteries, the veins, and the capillaries. As you continue to study this chapter, keep this "big picture" in mind and add to it your deepening understanding of where each vessel gets its blood and where it delivers the blood. Before long, you will have a useful understanding of how the entire network functions as a system.

In the next chapter, we build on your understanding of the functional anatomy of the cardiovascular system by discussing mechanisms of blood flow. In other words, all of the next chapter deals with issues relating to the big picture of cardiovascular function and its importance to survival. •

mechanisms of disease

Disorders of the Blood Vessels

Disorders of Arteries

As mentioned earlier in this chapter, arteries contain blood that is maintained at a relatively high pressure. This means the arterial walls must be able to withstand a great deal of force or they will burst. The arteries must also stay free of obstruction; otherwise they cannot deliver their blood to the capillary beds (and thus the tissues they serve).

A common type of vascular disease that occludes (blocks) arteries and weakens arterial walls is called **arteriosclerosis,** or *hardening of the arteries.* Arteriosclerosis is characterized by thickening of arterial walls that eventually progresses to hardening as calcium deposits form. The thickening and calcification reduce the flow of blood to the tissues. If blood slows in peripheral tissues such as the hands, legs, or feet, the condition is often referred to as **peripheral vascular disease (PVD)** or **peripheral arterial disease (PAD)** and the result is ischaemia.

Ischaemia, or decreased blood supply to a tissue, involves the gradual death of cells and may lead to complete tissue death— a condition called **necrosis.** If a large section of tissue becomes necrotic, it may begin to decay because of bacterial action. Necrosis that has progressed this far is called **gangrene.** Gangrene is a very serious consequence of ischaemia or blocked blood flow in PVD and is, unfortunately, a common problem in uncontrolled diabetes (**Figure 29-26**). PVD may also cause occasional pain, cramping, or weakness in the extremities—a condition called *intermittent claudication* (see **Box 27-2** on p. 625).

Because of the tissue damage involved, arteriosclerosis is not only painful—it is life-threatening. As we have previously stated, ischaemia of heart muscle can lead to *myocardial infarction* and death.

There are several types of arteriosclerosis, but perhaps the most well known is *atherosclerosis*—described earlier as the blockage of arteries by lipids and other matter (see **Figure 29-26**). Eventually, the fatty deposits in the arterial walls become fibrous and perhaps calcified—resulting in sclerosis (hardening). High blood levels of triglycerides and cholesterol, which may be caused by a high-fat and high-cholesterol diet, smoking, and a genetic predisposition, are associated with atherosclerosis.

In general, arteriosclerosis develops with advanced age, diabetes, high-fat and high-cholesterol diets, hypertension (high blood pressure), and smoking. Arteriosclerosis can be treated by drugs, called **vasodilators,** that trigger the smooth muscles of the arterial walls to relax, thus causing the arteries to dilate (widen).

Some cases of atherosclerosis are treated by mechanically opening the affected area of an artery in a type of procedure called **percutaneous coronary intervention (PCI).** In one PCI procedure called **angioplasty,** a deflated balloon attached to a long, thin tube called a **catheter** is inserted into a partially blocked artery and then inflated (**Figure 29-27**). As the balloon inflates, the *atherosclerotic plaque* (fatty deposits and tissue) is pushed outward, and the artery widens to allow near-normal blood flow. In a similar procedure, metal springs or mesh tubes, called **stents**, are inserted in affected arteries to hold them open.

Similar types of PCIs called **atherectomies** use lasers, drills, or spinning loops of wire to clear the way for normal blood flow. Severely affected arteries can also be surgically bypassed or replaced.

Damage to arterial walls caused by arteriosclerosis or other factors may lead to the formation of an **aneurysm.** An aneurysm is a section of an artery that has become abnormally widened because of a weakening of the arterial wall. Aneurysms sometimes form a saclike extension of the arterial wall. One reason aneurysms are dangerous is because they, like atherosclerotic plaques, promote the formation of thrombi (abnormal clots). A thrombus may cause an embolism

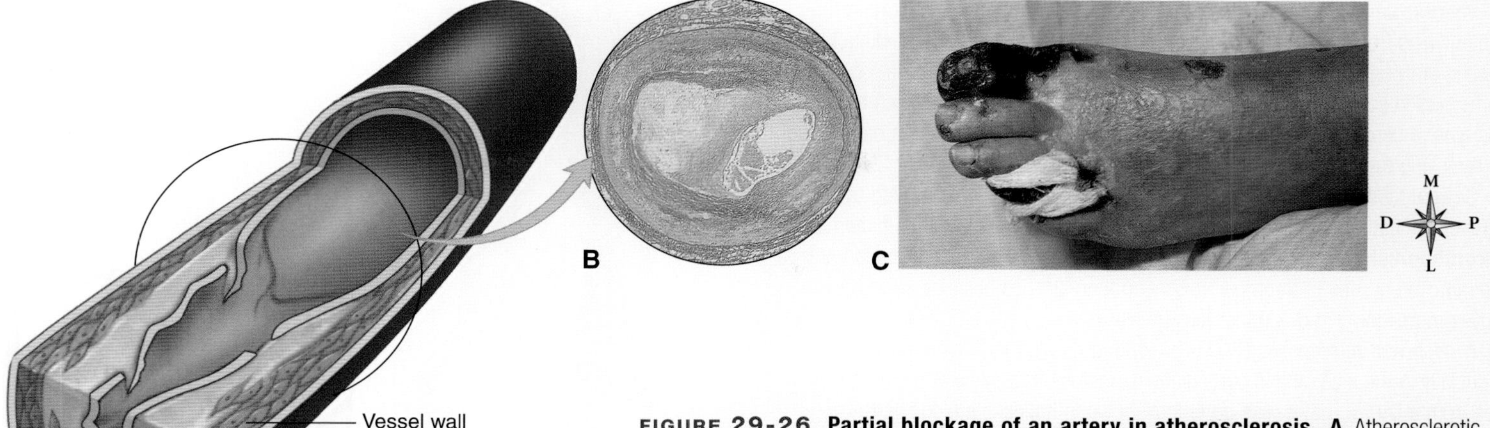

FIGURE 29-26 Partial blockage of an artery in atherosclerosis. A, Atherosclerotic plaque develops from the deposition of fats and other substances in the wall of the artery—a classic symptom of peripheral vascular disease. **B,** Photograph of a cross-section of an artery showing partial blockage of lumen by atherosclerotic plaque. **C,** Photograph showing diabetic gangrene that results from decreased peripheral blood flow.

(blockage) in the heart or some other vital tissue. Another reason aneurysms are dangerous is their tendency to burst, causing severe haemorrhaging that may result in death.

A brain aneurysm may lead to a **stroke,** or **cerebrovascular accident (CVA).** A stroke results from ischaemia of brain tissue caused by an embolism or ruptured aneurysm. Depending on the amount of tissue affected and the place in the brain the CVA occurs, effects of a stroke may range from hardly noticeable to crippling to fatal.

Disorders of Veins

Varicose veins are enlarged veins in which blood tends to pool rather than continue on toward the heart. Varicose veins, also called *varices* (*singular,* **varix**), commonly occur in *superficial veins* near the surface of the body. The *great saphenous vein,* the largest superficial vein of the leg (see **Figure 29-21**), often becomes varicose in people who stand for long periods. The force of gravity slows the return of venous blood to the heart in such cases, causing blood-engorged veins to dilate. As the veins dilate, the distance between the flaps of venous valves widens—eventually making them incompetent (leaky) (**Figure 29-28**). Incompetence of valves causes even more pooling in affected veins—a positive feedback phenomenon.

Haemorrhoids, or *piles,* are varicose veins in the anal canal (look ahead to **Figure 39-19** on p. 896). Excessive straining during defaecation can create pressures that cause haemorrhoids. The unusual pressures of carrying a child during pregnancy predispose expectant mothers to haemorrhoids and other varicosities.

UNIT 4

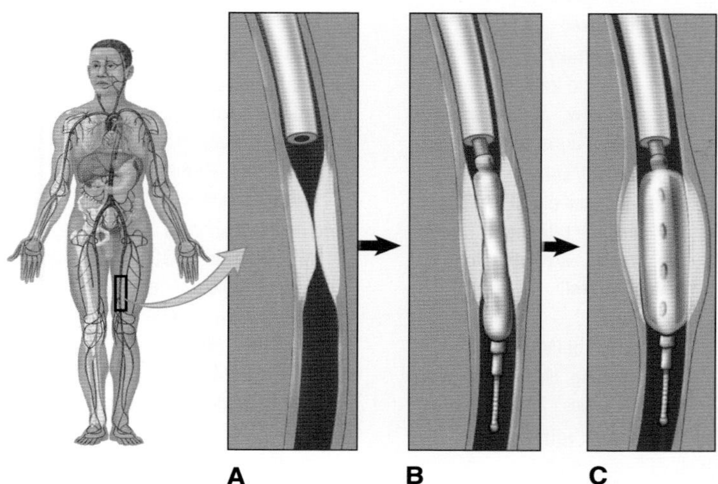

FIGURE 29-27 Balloon angioplasty. A, A catheter is inserted into the vessel until it reaches the affected region. **B,** A probe with a metal tip is pushed out the end of the catheter into the blocked region of the vessel. **C,** The balloon is inflated, pushing the walls of the vessel outward. Sometimes metal coils or tubes, called "stents", are inserted to keep the vessel open. Drug-coated stents may further reduce delayed scarring and reclogging of arteries following angioplasty in many patients.

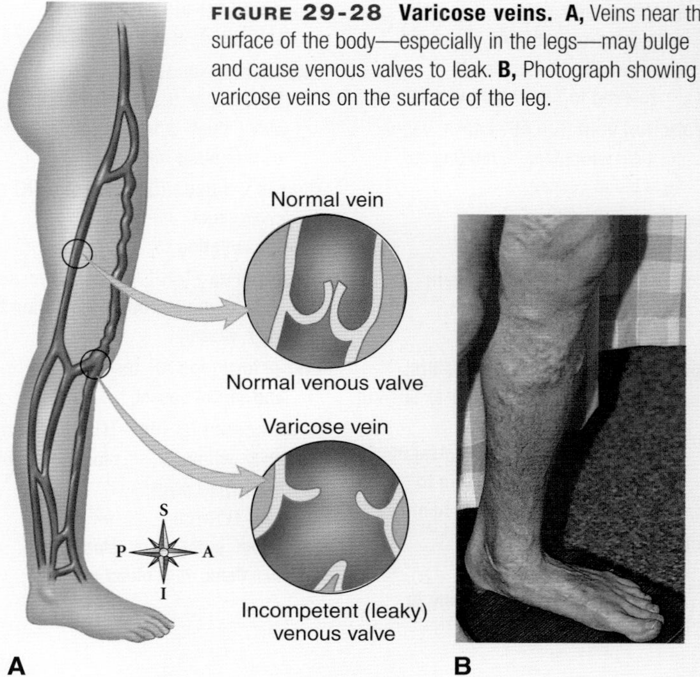

FIGURE 29-28 Varicose veins. A, Veins near the surface of the body—especially in the legs—may bulge and cause venous valves to leak. **B,** Photograph showing varicose veins on the surface of the leg.

Varicose veins in some parts of the body can be treated by supporting the dilated veins from the outside. For instance, support stockings can reduce blood pooling in the great saphenous vein. Surgical removal of varicose veins can be performed in severe cases. Advanced cases of haemorrhoids are often treated by this type of surgery. Symptoms of milder cases of varicose veins can be relieved by removing the pressure that caused the condition.

Several factors can cause **phlebitis,** or vein inflammation. Irritation by an intravenous catheter, for example, is a common cause of vein inflammation. **Thrombophlebitis** is acute phlebitis caused by clot (thrombus) formation. Veins are more likely sites of thrombus formation than arteries because venous blood moves more slowly and is under less pressure.

A *deep vein thrombosis (DVT)* is a clot that has formed in a deep vein, especially in the legs, and is particularly dangerous. If a piece of a clot breaks free from a DVT, it may cause an embolism when it blocks a blood vessel. **Pulmonary embolism,** for example, could result when an embolus lodges in the circulation of the lung (**Figure 29-29**). Pulmonary embolism can lead to death quickly if too much blood flow is blocked.

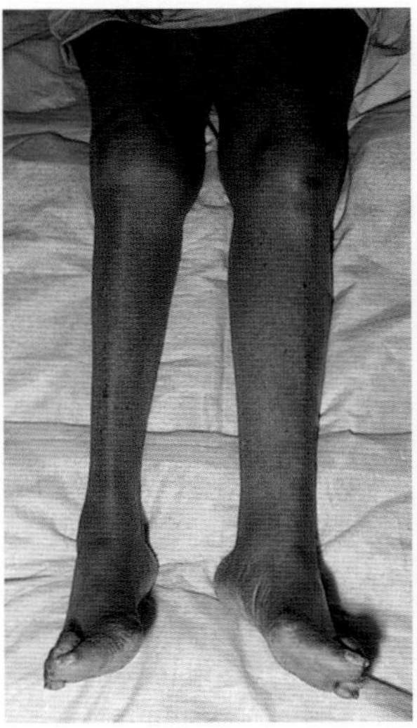

A

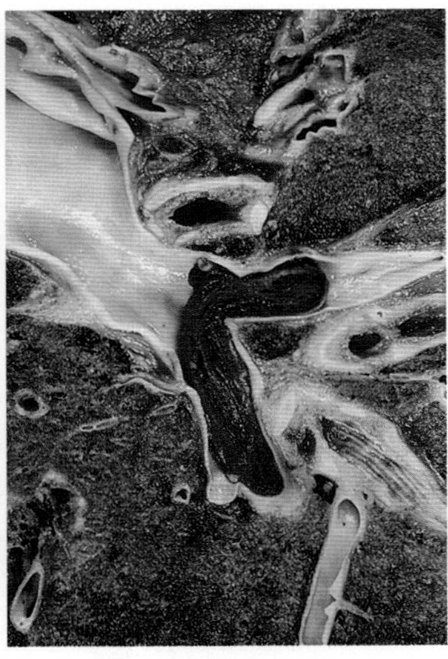

B

FIGURE 29-29 Deep vein thrombosis (DVT). A, Note the swelling in the left leg of this patient caused by a deep femoral vein thrombosis secondary to cancer. **B,** Large embolus derived from a lower extremity DVT and now located in a pulmonary artery branch. This type of blood clot is sometimes called a "saddle" or "straddling embolism" because it straddles a dividing blood vessel.

LANGUAGE OF SCIENCE *(continued from p. 665)*

brachial vein (BRAY-kee-al vayn)
[*brachi-* **arm,** *-al* **relating to,** *vena* **blood vessel**]

brachiocephalic artery
(brayk-ee-oh-seh-FAL-ik AR-ter-ee)
[*brachi-* **arm,** *-cephal-* **head,** *-ic* **relating to,** *arteri-* **vessel**]

brachiocephalic vein
(brayk-ee-oh-seh-FAL-ik vayn)
[*brachi-* **arm,** *-cephal-* **head,** *-ic* **relating to,** *vena* **blood vessel**]

bronchial vein (BRONK-kee-al vayn)
[*bronch-* **windpipe,** *-al* **relating to,** *vena* **blood vessel**]

capillary (kah-PILL-er-ee)
[*capill-* **hair,** *-ary* **relating to**]

cephalic vein (seh-FAL-ik vayn)
[*cephal-* **head,** *-ic* **relating to,** *vena* **blood vessel**]

cerebral arterial circle (of Willis)
(seh-REE-bral ar-TEER-ee-al SIR-kul [ov WILL-is])
[*cerebr-* **brain (cerebrum),** *-al* **relating to,** *arteria-* **vessel,** *-al* relating to (*Thomas Willis* **English physician**)]

common carotid artery
(kah-ROT-id AR-ter-ee)
[*caro-* **heavy sleep,** *-id* **relating to,** *arteri-* **vessel**]

continuous capillary (kah-PILL-er-ee)
[*capill-* **hair,** *-ary* **relating to**]

coronary artery
(KOHR-oh-nair-ee AR-ter-ee)
[*corona-* **crown,** *-ary* **relating to,** *arteri-* **vessel**]

descending aorta
(dih-SEND-ing ay-OR-tah)
[*aort-* **lifted,** *-a* **thing**] *pl.,* aortae or aortas

ductus arteriosus
(DUK-tus ar-teer-ee-OH-sus)
[*ductus* **duct,** *arteri-* **vessel,** *-osus* **relating to**]

ductus venosus (DUK-tus veh-NO-sus)
[*ductus* **duct,** *ven-* **vein,** *-osus* **relating to**]

elastic artery (eh-LAS-tik AR-ter-ee)
[*elast-* **to drive propel,** *-ic* **relating to,** *arteri-* **vessel**]

end artery (end AR-ter-ee)
[**end** *-arteri-* **vessel**]

endothelium (en-doh-THEE-lee-um)
[*endo-* **within,** *-theli-* **nipple,** *-um* **thing**]

external iliac vein
(eks-TER-nal IL-ee-ak vayn)
[*extern-* **outside,** *-al* **relating to,** *ilium* **flank,** *vena* **blood vessel**]

external jugular vein
(eks-TER-nal JUG-yoo-lar vayn)
[*extern-* **outside,** *-al* **relating to,** *jugul-* **neck,** *-ar* **relating to,** *vena* **blood vessel**]

femoral vein (FEM-or-al vayn)
[*femor-* **thigh,** *-al* **relating to,** *vena* **blood vessel**]

fenestrated capillary
(fen-es-TRAY-tid kah-PILL-er-ee)
[*fenestra-* **window,** *-ate* **characterized by,** *capill-* **hair,** *-ary* **relating to**]

fibular (peroneal) vein
(FIB-yoo-lar [per-oh-NEE-al] vayn)
[*fibula-* **clasp,** *-ar* **relating to,** *perone-* **brooch,** *-al* **relating to,** *vena* **blood vessel**]

foramen ovale
(foh-RAY-men oh-VAL-ee)
[*foramen* **opening,** *ovale* **egg shaped**] *pl.,* foramina ovales

great saphenous vein
(sah-FEE-nus vayn)
[*saphen-* **manifest,** *-ous* **relating to,** *vena* **blood vessel**]

hemiazygos vein
(hem-ee-AZ-ih-gohs vayn)
[*hemi-* **half,** *-a-* **without,** *-zygo-* **union or yoke,** *vena* **blood vessel**]

hepatic portal circulation
(heh-PAT-ik POR-tal)
[*hepa-* **liver,** *-ic* **relating to,** *port-* **doorway,** *-al* **relating to,** *circulat-* **go around,** *-tion* **process**]

inferior vena cava
(in-FEER-ee-or VEE-nah KAY-vah)
[*infer-* **lower,** *-or* **quality,** *vena* **vein,** *cava* **hollow**] *pl.,* venae cavae

internal jugular vein
(JUG-yoo-lar vayn)
[*intern-* **inside,** *-al* **relating to,** *jugul-* **neck,** *-ar* **relating to,** *vena* **blood vessel**]

median cubital vein
(MEE-dee-an KYOO-bih-tal vayn)
[*medi-* **middle,** *-an* **relating to,** *cubit-* **elbow,** *-al* **relating to,** *vena* **blood vessel**]

metarteriole (met-ar-TEER-ee-ohl)
[*meta-* **middle,** *arteri-* **vessel,** *-ole* **little**]

palmar venous arch
(PAHL-mar VEE-nus)
[*palm-* **palm of hand,** *-ar* **relating to,** *ven-* **vein,** *-ous* **relating to**]

pericardial vein
(pair-ih-KAR-dee-al vayn)
[*peri-* **around,** *-cardi-* **heart,** *-al* **relating to,** *vena* **blood vessel**]

placenta (plah-SEN-tah)
[*placenta* **flat cake**] *pl.,* placentae or placentas

popliteal vein (pop-lih-TEE-al vayn)
[*poplit-* **back of knee,** *-al* **relating to,** *vena* **blood vessel**]

portal system (POR-tal)
[*port-* **doorway,** *-al* **relating to**]

posterior tibial vein
(pohs-TEER-ee-or TIB-ee-al vayn)
[*poster-* **behind,** *-or* **quality,** *tibia* **shin bone,** *-al* **relating to,** *vena* **blood vessel**]

precapillary sphincter
(pree-kah-PILL-er-ee SFINGK-ter)
[*pre-* **before,** *-capill-* **hair,** *-ary* **relating to,** *sphinc-* **bind tight,** *-er* **agent**]

precapillary tone
(pree-kah-PILL-er-ee tohn)
[*pre-* **before,** *-capill-* **hair,** *-ary* **relating to,** *tone* **tension**]

pulmonary circulation
(PUL-moh-nair-ee sur-kyoo-LAY-shun)
[*pulmon-* **lung,** *-ary* **relating to,** *circulat-* **go around,** *-tion* **process**]

renal vein (REE-nal vayn)
[*ren-* **kidney,** *-al* **relating to,** *vena* **blood vessel**]

sinus (SYE-nus)
[*sinus* **hollow**]

sinusoid (SYE-nah-soyd)
[*sinus-* **hollow,** *-oid* **like**]

small saphenous vein
(sah-FEE-nus vayn)
[*saphen-* **manifest,** *-ous* **relating to,** *vena* **blood vessel**]

subclavian artery
(sub-KLAY-vee-an AR-ter-ee)
[*sub-* **below,** *-clavi-* **key,** *-ula* **little,** *arteri-* **vessel**]

subclavian vein
(sub-KLAY-vee-an vayn)
[*sub-* **below,** *-clavi-* **key (clavicle bone),** *-an* **relating to,** *vena* **blood vessel**]

superficial vein (soo-per-FISH-al vein)
[*super-* **over or above,** *-fici-* **face,** *-al* **relating to,** *vena* **blood vessel**]

superior intercostal vein
(soo-PEER-ee-or inter-KOS-tal vayn)
[*super-* **over or above,** *-or* **quality,** *inter-* **between,** *-costa-* **rib,** *-al* **relating to,** *vena* **blood vessel**]

superior vena cava
(soo-PEER-ee-or VEE-nah KAY-vah)
[*super-* **over or above,** *-or* **quality,** *vena* **vein,** *cava* **hollow**] *pl.,* venae cavae

suprarenal vein
(soo-prah-REE-nal vayn)
[*supra-* **above or over,** *-ren-* **kidney,** *-al* **relating to,** *vena* **blood vessel**]

systemic circulation
(sis-TEM-ik sur-kyoo-LAY-shun)
[*system-* **organized whole,** *-ic* **relating to,** *circulat-* **go around,** *-tion* **process**]

thoracic aorta (tho-RASS-ik ay-OR-tah)
[*thorac-* **chest,** *-ic* **relating to,** *aort-* **lifted,** *-a* **thing**] *pl.,* aortae or aortas

tunica externa
(TYOO-nih-kah ex-TER-nah)
[*tunica* **tunic or coat,** *extern-* **outside**] *pl.,* tunicae externae

tunica intima (TYOO-nih-kah IN-tih-mah)
[*tunica* **tunic or coat,** *intima* **innermost**] *pl.,* tunicae intimae

tunica media
(TYOO-nih-kah MEE-dee-ah)
[*tunica* **tunic or coat,** *media* **middle**] *pl.,* tunicae mediae

umbilical artery
(um-BIL-ih-kul AR-ter-ee)
[*umbilic-* **navel,** *-al* **relating to,** *arteri-* **vessel**]

umbilical vein (um-BIL-ih-kul vayn)
[*umbilic-* **navel,** *-al* **relating to,** *vena* **blood vessel**]

vascular anastomosis
(VAS-kyoo-lar ah-nas-toh-MOH-sis)
[*vas-* **vessel,** *-ular* **relating to,** *ana-* **again or anew,** *-stomo-* **mouth,** *-osis* **condition**] *pl.,* anatomoses

venous sinus (VEE-nus SYE-nus)
[*ven-* **vein,** *-ous* **relating to,** *sinus* **hollow**]

venule (VEN-yool)
[*ven-* **vein,** *-ule* **little**]

LANGUAGE OF MEDICINE

aneurysm (AN-yoo-riz-em)
[*aneurysm* **widening**]

angioplasty (AN-jee-oh-plass-tee)
[*angio-* **vessel,** *-plasty* **surgical repair**]

arteriosclerosis
(ar-teer-ee-oh-skleh-ROH-sis)
[*arteri-* **vessel,** *-scler-* **hardening,** *-osis* **condition**]

ascites (ah-SYE-tees)
[*asc-* **belly,** *-ites* **swelling**]

atherectomy (ath-er-EK-to-mee)
[*ather-* **porridge,** *-ec-* **out,** *-tom-* **cut,** *-y* **action**]

atherosclerosis
(ath-er-oh-skleh-ROH-sis)
[*athero-* **porridge,** *-scler-* **hardening,** *-osis* **condition**]

catheter (KATH-eh-ter)
[*cathe-* **send down,** *-er* **agent**]

cerebrovascular accident (CVA)
(SAIR-eh-broh-VAS-kyoo-lar)
[*cerebr-* **brain,** *-vas-* **vessel,** *-ular* **relating to**]

fetal alcohol syndrome (FAS)
(FEE-tal AL-koh-hol SIN-drohm)
[*fet-* **offspring,** *-al* **relating to,** *syn-* **together,** *-drome* **running or (race) course**]

gangrene (GANG-green)
[*gangren-* **gnawing sore**]

haemorrhoid (HEM-uh-royd)
[*haemo-* **blood,** *-rrhoid-* **flow**]

ischaemia (is-KEE-mee-ah)
[*ische-* **hold back,** *-aem-* **blood,** *-ia* **condition**]

microcephaly (my-kroh-SEF-ah-lee)
[*micro-* **small,** *-ceph-* **head,** *-aly* **relating to**]

necrosis (neh-KROH-sis)
[*necr-* **death,** *-osis* **condition**]

percutaneous coronary intervention (PCI) (per-kyoo-TAYN-ee-us KOR-oh-nair-ee in-ter-VEN-shun)
[*per-* **through,** *cut-* **skin,** *-aneous* **relating to,** *corona-* **crown,** *-ary* **relating to,** *inter-* **between,** *-ven-* **go,** *-tion* **process**]

peripheral arterial disease (PAD)
(peh-RIF-er-al ar-TEER-ee-al)
[*peri-* **around,** *-pher-* **boundary,** *-al* **relating to,** *-arteri-* **vessel,** *-al* **relating to,** *dis-* **opposite of,** *-ease* **comfort**]

peripheral vascular disease (PVD)
(peh-RIF-er-al VAS-kyoo-lar)
[*peri-* **around,** *-pher-* **boundary,** *-al* **relating to,** *-vas-* **vessel,** *-ular* **relating to,** *dis-* **opposite of,** *-ease* **comfort**]

phlebitis (fleh-BYE-tis)
[*phleb-* **vein,** *-itis* **inflammation**]

pulmonary embolism
(PUL-moh-nair-ee EM-boh-liz-em)
[*pulmon-* **lung,** *-ary* **relating to,** *embol-* **plug,** *-ism* **condition**]

shunt (shuhnt)

stent (stent)
[*Charles Stent* **English dentist**]

stroke (strohk)

thrombophlebitis
(throm-boh-fleh-BYE-tis)
[*thrombo-* **clot,** *-phleb-* **vein,** *-itis* **inflammation**]

varicose vein (VAIR-ih-kohs vayn)
[*varic-* **swollen vein,** *-ose* **characterized by,** *vena* **blood vessel**]

varix (VAIR-iks)
[*varix* **swollen vein**] *pl.,* varices

vasodilator (vay-so-DYE-lay-tor)
[*vas-* **vessel or duct,** *-dilat-* **widen,** *-or* **agent**]

case study

John, a 45-year-old builder, finally gave into his wife's insistence that he should pay a visit to his GP; he'd been sweating, feeling nauseous and experiencing minor chest pain for a couple of days. John had convinced himself the pain was from strained muscles caused by his recent weight lifting. The doctor measured John's blood pressure and recorded his heart rate and ECG using a portable electrocardiograph.

Following his initial examination, the doctor made an emergency appointment for John to have an angiogram and consultation with a cardiologist at the main hospital.

1. The GP suspected a blockage in which part of John's body?
   a. The cerebral arteries
   b. The hepatic artery
   c. The common carotid artery in the neck
   d. The coronary arteries

2. At the main hospital John was taken to the cardiac catheterization laboratory (Cath Lab) and a catheter was inserted into his thigh. Through which vessel did the surgeon thread the catheter?
   a. Brachial artery
   b. Popliteal artery
   c. Femoral artery
   d. Tibial artery

3. Once inserted, through which pathway was the catheter moved?
   a. External iliac artery, abdominal aorta, descending aorta, aortic arch, ascending aorta
   b. Internal iliac artery, abdominal aorta, ascending aorta, aortic arch, descending aorta
   c. Abdominal aorta, descending aorta, aortic arch, ascending aorta
   d. Popliteal artery, external iliac artery, abdominal aorta, thoracic aorta, aortic arch

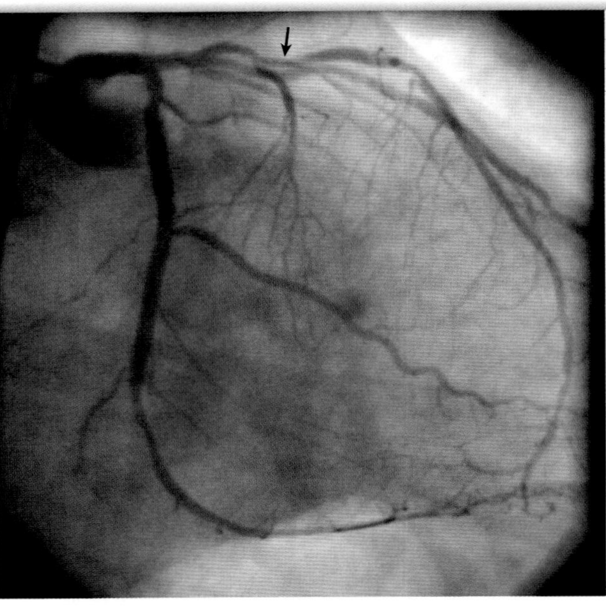

During the procedure, dye was injected through the catheter to enhance the view of the coronary vessels. John's right coronary artery appeared to be partially occluded. The surgeon inserted a balloon through the catheter that was then inflated to press against the sides of the artery and enlarge its diameter. Next she inserted a metal stent to keep the lumen of the artery open and restore the supply of blood to the myocardium.

4. The myocardium of which heart chamber receives the most abundant blood supply from the coronary arteries?
   a. Left atrium
   b. Left ventricle
   c. Right atrium
   d. Right ventricle

Hint To solve a case study, you may have to refer to the glossary or index, other chapters in this textbook, ***Connect It!,*** and other resources.

UNIT 4

CHAPTER SUMMARY

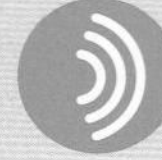

To download an MP3 version of the chapter summary for use with your mobile device, access the ***Audio Chapter Summaries*** *online at evolve.elsevier.com.*

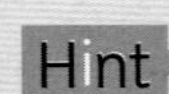

Scan this summary after reading the chapter to help you reinforce the key concepts. Later, use the summary as a quick review before your class or before a test.

Blood Vessel Types

A. Types of blood vessels (**Figures 29-1** and **29-2**)
   1. Angiogenesis—formation of new blood vessels
   2. Arteries
      a. Carry blood away from heart—all arteries except pulmonary artery carry oxygenated blood
      b. Elastic (conducting) arteries—largest in body
         (1) Examples: aorta and its major branches
         (2) Able to stretch without injury
         (3) Accommodate surge of blood when heart contracts and able to recoil when ventricles relax
      c. Muscular (distributing) arteries
         (1) Smaller in diameter than elastic arteries
         (2) Muscular layer is thick
         (3) Examples: brachial, gastric, superior mesenteric

d. Arterioles (resistance vessels)
 (1) Smallest arteries
 (2) Important in regulating blood flow to end organs (precapillary tone)
e. Metarterioles (exist in some tissues)
 (1) Each is a short connecting vessel between true arteriole and 20 to 100 capillaries
 (2) Encircled by precapillary sphincters in some tissues
 (3) Distal end called *thoroughfare channel*, which is free of precapillary sphincters

3. Capillaries—primary exchange vessels
 a. Microscopic vessels
 b. Carry blood from arterioles to venules—together, arterioles, capillaries, and venules constitute the microcirculation (**Figure 29-3**)
 c. Not evenly distributed—highest numbers in tissues with high metabolic rate; may be absent in some "avascular" tissues, such as cartilage
 d. Types of capillaries (**Figure 29-4**)
  (1) True capillaries—receive blood flowing from metarteriole with input regulated by precapillary tone (in arteriolar smooth muscle)
  (2) Continuous capillaries
   (a) Continuous lining of endothelial cells
   (b) Openings called *intercellular clefts* exist between adjacent endothelial cells
  (3) Fenestrated capillaries
   (a) Have both intercellular clefts and "holes" or fenestrations through plasma membrane to facilitate exchange functions
  (4) Sinusoids
   (a) Large lumen and tortuous course
   (b) Absent or incomplete basement membrane
   (c) Very porous—permit migration of cells into or out of vessel lumen
4. Veins
 a. Carry blood toward the heart
 b. Act as collectors and as reservoir vessels; called *capacitance vessels*

B. Structure of blood vessels (**Figure 29-1** and **29-2**)
 1. Components or "building blocks" commonly present
  a. Lining endothelial tissue—one layer of squamous endothelial cells
   (1) Only lining found in capillary
   (2) Lines entire vascular tree
   (3) Provides a smooth luminal surface—protects against intravascular coagulation
   (4) Intercellular clefts, cytoplasmic pores, and fenestrations in cells allow exchange to occur between blood and tissue fluid
   (5) Capable of secreting a number of substances
   (6) Capable of reproduction
  b. Collagen fibres
   (1) Exhibit woven appearance
   (2) Formed from protein molecules that aggregate into fibres
   (3) Visible with light microscope
   (4) Have only a limited ability to stretch (2% to 3%) in physiological conditions
   (5) Function to strengthen and keep lumen of vessel open
  c. Elastic fibres
   (1) Composed of insoluble protein called *elastin*
   (2) Form highly elastic networks
   (3) Wavy fibres can stretch more than 100% in physiological conditions
   (4) Play important role in creating passive tension to help regulate blood pressure throughout the cardiac cycle
  d. Smooth muscle tissue
   (1) Present in all segments of vascular system except capillaries
   (2) Most abundant in elastic and muscular arteries
   (3) Exerts active tension in vessels when contracting
 2. Layers
  a. Tunica externa—found in arteries and veins (tunica adventitia)
  b. Tunica media—found in arteries and veins
  c. Tunica intima—found in all blood vessels; only layer present in capillaries

Circulatory Routes (Figure 29-5)

A. Systemic circulation—blood flows from the left ventricle of the heart through blood vessels to all parts of the body (except gas exchange tissues of lungs) and back to the right atrium
B. Pulmonary circulation—deoxygenated blood moves from right atrium to right ventricle to pulmonary artery to lung arterioles and capillaries, where gases are exchanged; oxygenated blood returns to left atrium by way of pulmonary veins; from left atrium, blood enters the left ventricle

Systemic Circulation

A. Systemic arteries (review **Table 29-2** and **Figures 29-6** to **29-14**)
 1. Main arteries give off branches, which continue to rebranch, forming arterioles and then capillaries
 2. End arteries—terminal arteries that are the only blood supply to a particular tissue
 3. Arterial anastomosis—arteries that open into other branches of the same or other arteries; incidence of arterial anastomoses increases as distance from the heart increases
 4. Arteriovenous anastomoses or shunts occur when blood flows from an artery directly into a vein
B. Systemic veins (review **Table 29-3** and **Figures 29-15** to **29-22**)
 1. Veins are the ultimate extensions of capillaries; unite into vessels of increasing size to form venules and then veins
 2. Large veins of the cranial cavity are called *dural sinuses*
 3. Veins anastomose the same as arteries
 4. Venous blood from the head, neck, upper extremities, and thoracic cavity (except lungs) drains into superior vena cava
 5. Venous blood from thoracic organs drains directly into superior vena cava or azygos vein
 6. Hepatic portal circulation (**Table 29-3** and **Figures 29-5** and **29-20**)
  a. Veins from the spleen, stomach, pancreas, gallbladder, and intestines send their blood to the liver by way of the hepatic portal vein

b. In the liver the venous blood mingles with arterial blood in the sinusoids and is eventually drained from the liver by hepatic veins that join the inferior vena cava
7. Venous blood from the lower extremities and abdomen drains into the inferior vena cava

Fetal Circulation

A. Basic plan of fetal circulation—additional vessels needed to allow fetal blood to secure oxygen and nutrients from maternal blood at the placenta (**Figure 29-24**)
   1. Two umbilical arteries—extensions of the internal iliac arteries; carry fetal blood to the placenta
   2. Placenta—attached to uterine wall; where exchange of oxygen and other substances between the separated maternal and fetal blood occurs (**Figure 29-23**)
   3. Umbilical vein—returns oxygenated blood from the placenta to the fetus; enters body through the umbilicus and goes to the undersurface of the liver where it gives off two or three branches and then continues as the ductus venosus
   4. Ductus venosus—continuation of the umbilical vein; drains into inferior vena cava
   5. Foramen ovale—opening in septum between the right and left atria
   6. Ductus arteriosus—small vessel connecting the pulmonary trunk with the aortic arch

B. Changes in circulation at birth (compare **Figures 29-24** and **29-25**)
   1. When umbilical cord is cut, the two umbilical arteries, the placenta and umbilical vein, no longer function
   2. Umbilical vein within the baby's body becomes the round ligament of the liver
   3. Ductus venosus becomes the ligamentum venosum of the liver
   4. Foramen ovale—functionally closed shortly after a newborn's first breath and pulmonary circulation is established; structural closure takes approximately 9 months
   5. Ductus arteriosus—contracts with establishment of respiration, becomes ligamentum arteriosum

UNIT 4

Cycle of Life: Blood Vessels

A. Birth—change from placenta-dependent system
B. Heart and blood vessels maintain basic structure and function from childhood through adulthood
C. Only normal changes occur as a result of exercise
   1. Exercise thickens myocardium
   2. Exercise increases the supply of blood vessels in skeletal muscle tissue
D. Adulthood through later adulthood—degenerative changes
   1. Atherosclerosis—blockage or weakening of critical arteries (**Figure 29-26**)
   2. Heart valves and myocardial tissue degenerate—reduces pumping efficiency

The Big Picture: Blood Vessels and the Whole Body

A. Blood vessels act as transport pipes for blood
B. Blood vessels each act as a component of a complex, interconnected network

REVIEW QUESTIONS

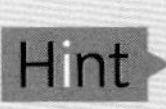

Write out the answers to these questions after reading the chapter and reviewing the Chapter Summary. Note—writing out your answers will consolidate learning and provide a valuable resource of information.

1. Identify the vessels that join to form the hepatic portal vein.
2. Describe the six unique structures necessary for fetal circulation.
3. Explain how the separation of oxygenated and deoxygenated blood occurs after birth.
4. How might a jugular vein spread infection?
5. Briefly define the following terms: *aneurysm, atherosclerosis, phlebitis.*
6. Explain how haemorrhoids develop.
7. Describe the structures in veins that ensure a one-way circulation. Explain the mechanisms involved in ensuring blood also flows in one direction in the arterial system.

CRITICAL THINKING QUESTIONS

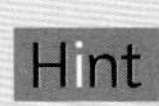

After finishing the Review Questions, write out the answers to these more in-depth questions to help you apply your new knowledge. Go back to sections of the chapter that relate to concepts that you find difficult.

1. The general public thinks the most important structure in the cardiovascular system is the heart. Anatomists know it is the capillary. What information would you use to support this view?
2. Compare and contrast arterial blood in systemic circulation and arterial blood in pulmonary circulation.
3. Explain the distinction between an occlusion of an end artery and an occlusion of other small arteries?
4. Determine which of the following veins drain into the superior vena cava and which drain into the inferior vena cava: longitudinal sinus, great saphenous, basilic, internal jugular, azygos, popliteal, and hepatic portal.
5. Describe the functional advantage of a portal system.
6. Naming the vessels and organs involved, trace the path taken by a single RBC. Begin at the right atrium, proceed to the left great toe, and return to the right atrium.
7. Explain the changes that occur in the cardiovascular system during the normal cycle of one's life.
8. Suggest which cardiovascular system disorder may produce dementia, and give reasons for your answer.

30 Circulation of Blood

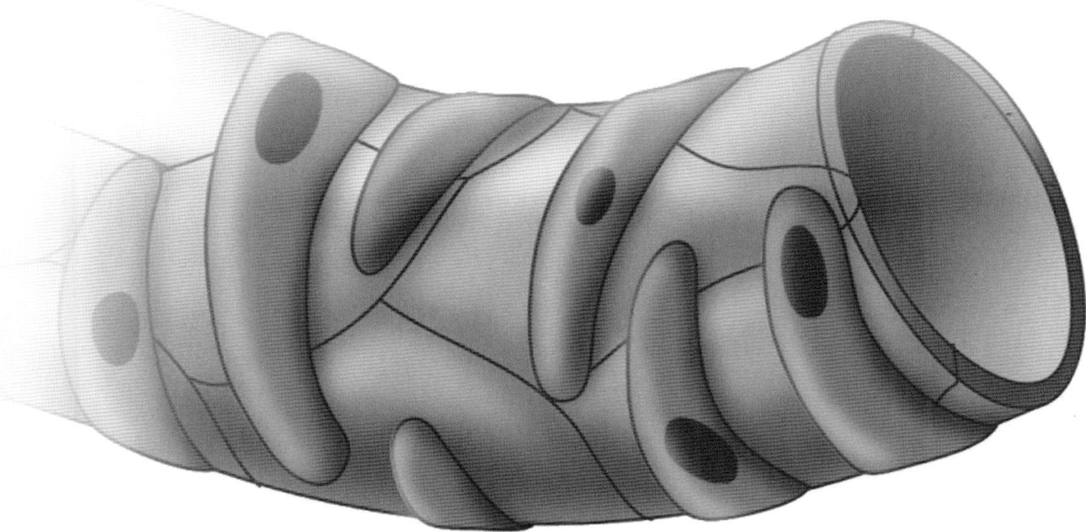

LANGUAGE OF SCIENCE

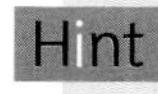

Use this list to aid your pronunciation of unfamiliar words.

aortic reflex (ay-OR-tik REE-fleks) [*aort-* **lifted,** *-ic* **relating to,** *re-* **back or again,** *-flex* **bend**]

baroreceptor (bar-oh-ree-SEP-tor) [*baro-* **pressure,** *-recept-* **receive,** *-or* **agent**]

capillary exchange (kah-PILL-er-ee) [*capill-* **hair,** *-ary* **relating to**]

cardiac reserve (KAR-dee-ak ree-ZERV) [*cardi-* **heart,** *-ic* **relating to**]

cardiac output (CO) (KAR-dee-ak) [*cardi-* **heart,** *-ac* **relating to**]

carotid sinus reflex (kah-ROT-id SYE-nus REE-fleks) [*caro-* **heavy sleep,** *-id* **relating to,** *sinus* **hollow,** *re-* **back or again,** *-flex* **bend**]

chemoreceptor reflex (kee-moh-ree-SEP-tor REE-fleks)

chronotropic (kroh-noh-TROH-pik) [*chron-* **time,** *-trop-* **turn or change,** *-ic* **relating to**]

ejection fraction (EF) (ee-JEK-shun FRAK-shun)

end-diastolic volume (EDV) (end-dye-ah-STOL-lik) [*dia-* **through,** *-stol-* **position,** *-ic* **relating to**]

haemodynamics (hee-moh-dye-NAM-iks) [*haemo-* **blood,** *-dynam-* **moving force,** *-ic* **relating to**]

inotropic (ee-noh-TROH-pik) [*in-* **sinew,** *-trop-* **turn or change,** *-ic* **relating to**]

ischaemic (is-KEE-mik) [*isch-* **hold back,** *aem-* **blood,** *-ic* **relating to**]

mean arterial pressure (MAP) (meen ar-TEER-ee-al PRESH-er) [*mean* **average,** *arteri-* **vessel,** *-al* **relating to**]

medullary ischaemic reflex (med-ULL-air-ee is-KEE-mik REE-fleks) [*medulla-* **marrow or pith (middle),** *-ary* **relating to,** *isch-* **hold back,** *-aem-* **blood** *-ic* **relating to,** *re-* **back or again,** *-flex* **bend**]

minute volume (MI-nit VOL-yoom)

continued on p. 722

CHAPTER OUTLINE

Hint *Scan this outline before you begin to read the chapter, as a preview of how the concepts are organized.*

The vital role of the cardiovascular system in maintaining homeostasis depends on the continuous and controlled movement of blood through the thousands of kilometres of capillaries that permeate every tissue and reach every cell in the body. Blood must not only be kept moving through its closed circuit of vessels by the pumping activity of the heart, but also must be directed and delivered to those capillary beds surrounding cells that need it most. Because variations in cellular activity require uneven distribution of blood, regulation of blood pressure and flow must change in response to cellular activity.

Numerous control mechanisms help regulate and integrate the diverse functions and component parts of the cardiovascular system to supply blood to specific body areas according to need. These mechanisms ensure a constant *milieu intérieur*—that is, a constant internal environment surrounding each body cell regardless of differing demands for nutrients or production of waste products. This chapter explores the control mechanisms that regulate the pumping activity of the heart and the smooth and directed flow of blood through the complex channels of the circulation. •

HAEMODYNAMICS

Haemodynamics is a term used to describe a collection of mechanisms that influence the active and changing—or dynamic—circulation of blood (**Figure 30-1**).

Circulation is, of course, a vital function. It constitutes the only means by which cells can receive materials needed for their survival and can have their wastes removed. Circulation is necessary, and circulation of different volumes of blood per minute at different times is also essential for healthy survival. For example, more active cells need more blood per minute than less active cells. The reason underlying this principle is obvious. The more work cells do, the more energy they use, and the more oxygen and nutrients they remove from the blood. Because blood circulates, it can continually bring in more oxygen and nutrients to replace what is consumed.

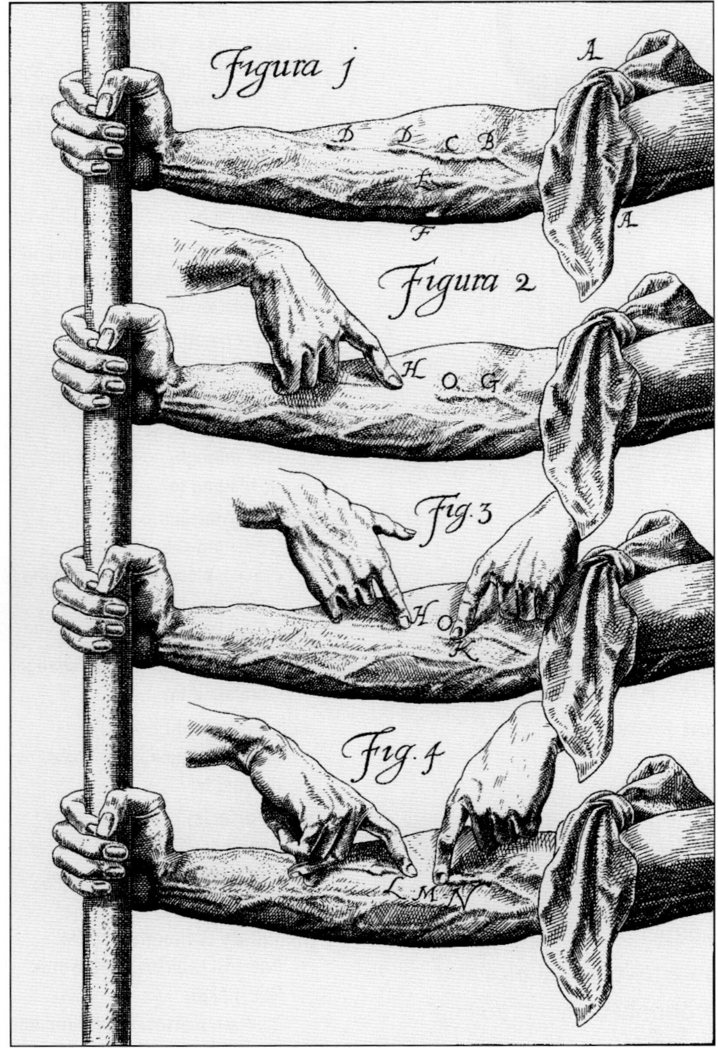

FIGURE 30-1 Haemodynamics. An illustration of a famous experiment in haemodynamics conducted by English scientist William Harvey in the early seventeenth century. Through a series of such experiments, this one showing how valves ensure one-way flow of blood through veins, Harvey finally proved that blood flows in a circuit out through the arteries and back through the veins—a concept on which most other haemodynamic concepts are based.

The greater the activity of any part of the body, the greater the volume of blood circulating through it. This requires that circulation control mechanisms accomplish two functions: maintain circulation (keep blood flowing) and vary the volume and distribution of the blood circulated. Therefore as any structure increases its activity, an increased volume of blood must be distributed to it; that is, blood must be shifted from the less active tissues to the more active tissues.

To achieve these two ends, a great many factors must operate together as one smooth-running, although complex, machine. Incidentally, this is an important physiological principle that you have no doubt observed by now—that every body function depends on many other functions. A constellation of separate processes or mechanisms acts as a single integrated mechanism. Together, these separate mechanisms perform one large function. For example, many mechanisms together accomplish the large function we call *circulation*.

This chapter is about haemodynamics—the mechanisms that keep blood flowing in ways that maintain relative constancy of the body's internal environment.

PRIMARY PRINCIPLE OF CIRCULATION

Blood circulates for the same reason that any fluid flows—whether it is water in a river, water in a garden hose, fluid in hospital tubing, or blood in vessels. A fluid flows because a pressure gradient exists between different parts of its volume (**Figure 30-2**).

This primary fluid flow principle derives from Newton's first and second laws of motion. In essence, these laws state the following principles:

1. A fluid does not flow when the pressure is the same throughout.
2. A fluid flows only when its pressure is higher in one area than in another, and it flows always from its higher pressure area toward its lower pressure area.

Thus the primary principle about circulation is this: Blood flows because of a pressure gradient. We have already seen this principle

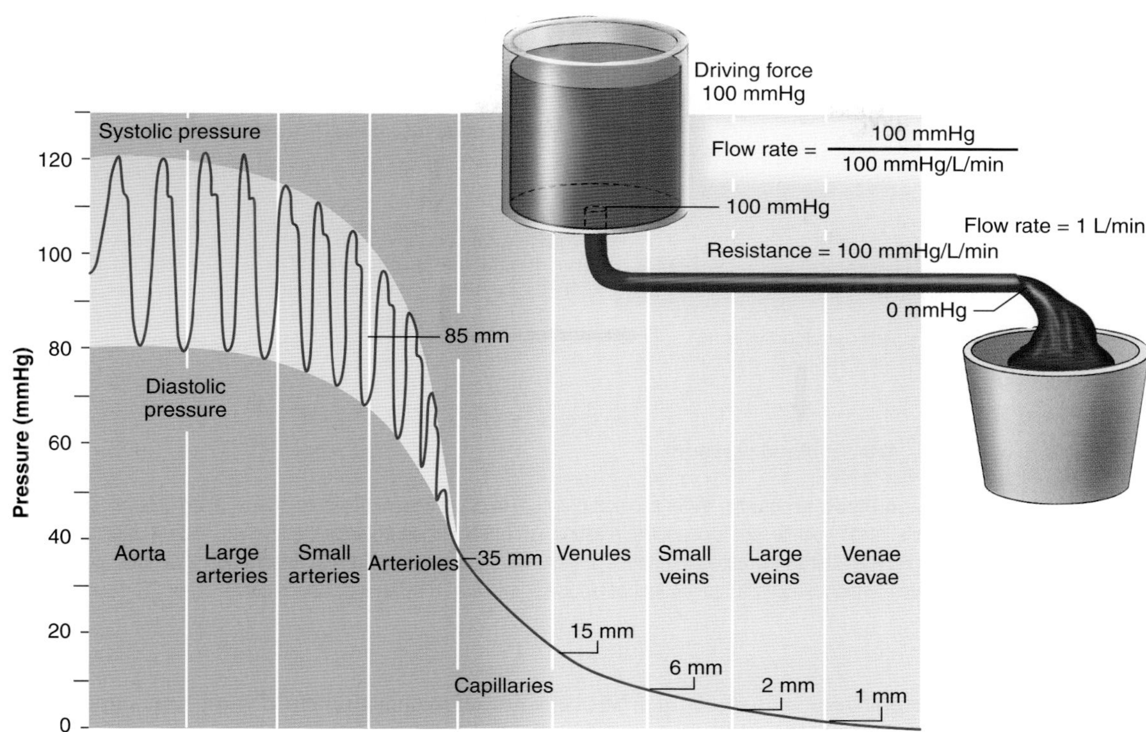

FIGURE 30-2 The primary principle of circulation. Fluid always travels from an area of high pressure to an area of low pressure. Fluid flows from an area of high pressure in the tank (100 mmHg) toward the area of low pressure above the bucket (0 mmHg). Blood likewise tends to move from an area of high pressure at the beginning of the aorta (100 mmHg) toward the area of lowest pressure at the end of the venae cavae (0 mmHg). Blood flow between any two points in the circulatory system can always be predicted by the pressure gradient.

operate to drive the flow of blood through the heart during the cardiac cycle (see pp. 654–655). It also applies to a whole circulatory loop—blood circulates from the left ventricle and returns to the right atrium of the heart because a blood pressure gradient exists between these two structures. Likewise, blood circulates from the right ventricle and returns to the left atrium because of a pressure gradient. By blood pressure gradient, we mean the difference between the blood pressure in one structure and the blood pressure in another.

An example of a normal blood pressure measurement in the aorta, as the left ventricle contracts and thereby pumps blood into it, is 120 mmHg. As the left ventricle relaxes, blood pressure decreases to 80 mmHg. The midpoint of aortic pressure in this instance is 100 mmHg.

Figure 30-2 shows the systolic and diastolic pressures in the arterial system and illustrates the progressive fall in pressure from a midpoint of 100 mmHg in the aorta down to 0 mmHg by the time blood reaches the venae cavae and right atrium. The progressive fall in pressure as blood passes through the circulatory system is directly related to flow resistance. Resistance to blood flow in the aorta is almost zero. Although the pumping action of the heart causes fluctuations in aortic blood pressure (systolic 120 mmHg; diastolic 80 mmHg), the midpoint of pressure remains almost constant, dropping perhaps only 1 or 2 mmHg.

The greatest drop in pressure (about 50 mmHg) occurs as blood goes through the arterioles because they present the greatest resistance to blood flow. The importance of flow resistance to maintaining a healthy pressure gradient is explored further in the next part of the chapter.

P_1–P_2 is often used to represent a pressure gradient, with P_1 the symbol for the higher pressure and P_2 the symbol for the lower pressure. For example, blood enters the arterioles at 85 mmHg and leaves at 35 mmHg. Which measurement is P_1? P_2? What is the blood pressure gradient? It would cause blood to flow through the arterioles toward the capillaries.

Of course, this principle applies to local blood flow as well as an entire circulatory loop. For example, pressure in the arteries and arterioles of the kidney must be higher than the blood pressure in the capillaries and veins of the kidney in order for blood to flow through the tissues of the kidney. This local pressure gradient needed to maintain blood flow in a tissue is called **perfusion pressure** (*perfusion* means "flow through").

ARTERIAL BLOOD PRESSURE

According to the primary principle of circulation, high pressure in the arteries must be maintained to keep blood flowing through the cardiovascular system. The chief determinant of arterial blood pressure is the volume of blood in the arteries. Arterial blood pressure is directly proportional to arterial blood volume. This means that an increase in arterial blood volume tends to increase arterial pressure, and conversely, a decrease in arterial volume tends to decrease arterial pressure.

Many factors determine arterial pressure through their influence on arterial volume. Two of the most important—*cardiac output* and *peripheral resistance*—are directly proportional to blood volume (**Figure 30-3**).

Cardiac Output

Cardiac output (**CO**) is the amount of blood that flows out of a ventricle of the heart per unit of time. The resting cardiac output from the left ventricle into the systemic arteries is roughly 5000 mL/min, for example. As **Figure 30-4** shows, the cardiac output influences the flow rate to the various organs of the body. For the sake of discussion, we focus mainly on cardiac output from the left ventricle into the

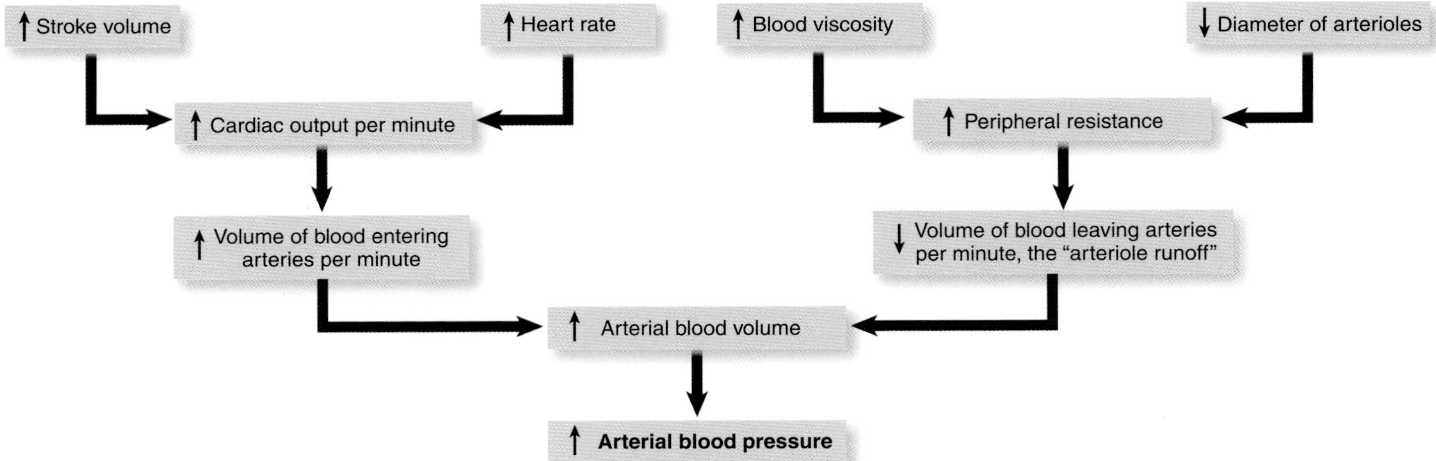

FIGURE 30-3 Relationship between arterial blood volume and blood pressure. Arterial blood pressure is directly proportional to arterial blood volume. Cardiac output (CO) and peripheral resistance (PR) are directly proportional to arterial blood volume, but for opposite reasons: CO affects blood *entering* the arteries, and PR affects blood *leaving* the arteries. If cardiac output increases, the amount of blood entering the arteries increases and tends to increase the volume of blood in the arteries. If peripheral resistance increases, it decreases the amount of blood leaving the arteries, which tends to increase the amount of blood left in them. Thus an increase in either CO or PR results in an increase in arterial blood volume, which increases arterial blood pressure.

systemic loop—but the same principles apply to cardiac output from either the left or the right ventricle.

Cardiac output is determined by the volume of blood pumped out of a ventricle by each beat (**stroke volume,** or **SV**) and by heart rate (HR). Because contraction of the heart is called *systole,* the volume of blood pumped by one contraction is known as *systolic discharge.* Stroke volume means the same thing, the amount of blood pumped by one stroke (contraction) of the ventricle.

Stroke volume, or volume pumped per heartbeat, is one of two major factors that determine CO. CO can be computed by the following simple equation:

$$\text{SV (volume/beat)} \times \text{HR (beat/min)} = \text{CO (volume/min)}$$

Thus the greater the stroke volume, the greater the CO (but only if the heart rate remains constant). In practice, computing the CO is far from simple. It requires introducing a catheter into the right side of the heart (cardiac catheterization) and solving a computation known as *Fick's formula.*

Because the heart's rate and stroke volume determine its output, anything that changes the rate of the heartbeat or its stroke volume tends to change CO, arterial blood volume, and blood pressure in the same direction. In other words, anything that makes the heart beat faster or anything that makes it beat stronger (increases its stroke volume) *tends* to increase CO and therefore arterial blood volume and pressure. Conversely, anything that causes the heart to beat more slowly or more weakly tends to decrease CO, arterial volume, and blood pressure.

Do not overlook the word *tends* in the preceding sentences. A change in heart rate or stroke volume does not *always* change the heart's output, or the amount of blood in the arteries, or the blood pressure. To see whether this is true, do the following arithmetic calculation, using the simple formula for computing CO. Assume a normal rate of 72 beats/min and a normal stroke volume of 70 mL.

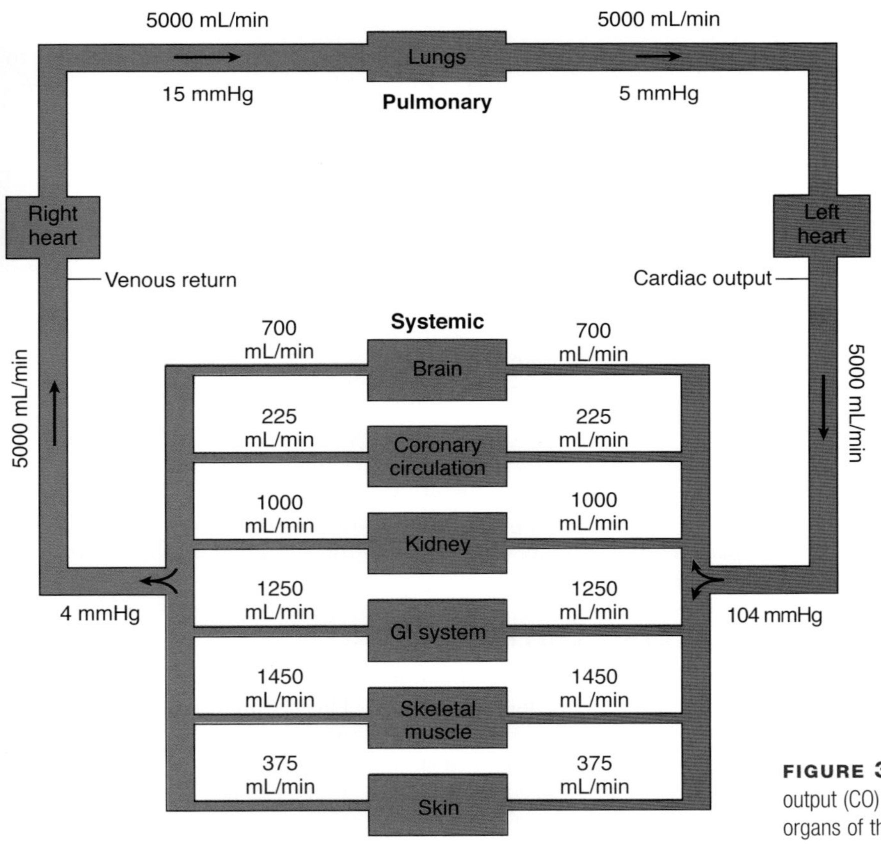

FIGURE 30-4 Cardiac output. This diagram shows that a typical resting cardiac output (CO) of 5000 mL/min (or 5 L/min) is distributed among the various systems and organs of the body. *GI,* Gastrointestinal.

Next, suppose the rate drops to 60 and the stroke volume increases to 100 mL. Does the decrease in heart rate actually cause a decrease in CO in this case? Clearly not—the CO increases. Do you think it is valid, however, to say that a slower rate tends to decrease the heart's output? By itself, without any change in any other factor, would not a slowing of the heartbeat cause CO volume, arterial volume, and blood pressure to fall?

The amount that the CO can increase above the resting value is called the **cardiac reserve.** In other words, it is pumping capacity that is held "in reserve" until needed—perhaps for increased physical activity. Cardiac reserve is often expressed in percent above resting CO. In a healthy young adult it may be 300% to 400% and in some athletes twice that.

Factors That Affect Stroke Volume

Factors that affect the strength of myocardial contraction—and therefore the stroke volume—are called **inotropic** factors. These include mechanical, neural, and chemical factors. One mechanical factor that helps determine stroke volume is the length of myocardial fibres at the beginning of ventricular contraction.

Many years ago, an English physiologist named Ernest Starling described a principle that later became known as **Starling's law of the heart.** Because the principle was partly based on the earlier work of Otto Frank, it is sometimes called the *Frank–Starling mechanism.* In this principle, Starling stated the factor he had observed as the main regulator of heartbeat strength in experiments performed on denervated animal hearts. Starling's law of the heart is this: within limits, the longer, or more stretched, the heart fibres at the beginning of contraction, the stronger is their contraction. Compare this concept with the length–tension relationship in skeletal muscle described in Chapter 17 (p. 378).

The factor determining how stretched the animal hearts were at the beginning of contractions was, as you might deduce, the amount of blood in the hearts at the end of diastole—the **end-diastolic volume (EDV).** The more blood returned to the heart per minute, the more stretched were their fibres, the stronger were their contractions, and the larger was the volume of blood they ejected with each contraction. If, however, too much blood stretched the hearts beyond a certain critical point, they seemed to lose their elasticity. They then contracted less vigorously, similar to how a band of elastic, stretched too much, rebounds with less force (**Figure 30-5**).

Thus, according to Starling's law of the heart, the heart pumps out what it receives. That is, within certain limits, the strength of myocardial contraction matches the pumping load or *preload*—unlike mechanical pumps that do not adjust themselves to their input with every stroke.

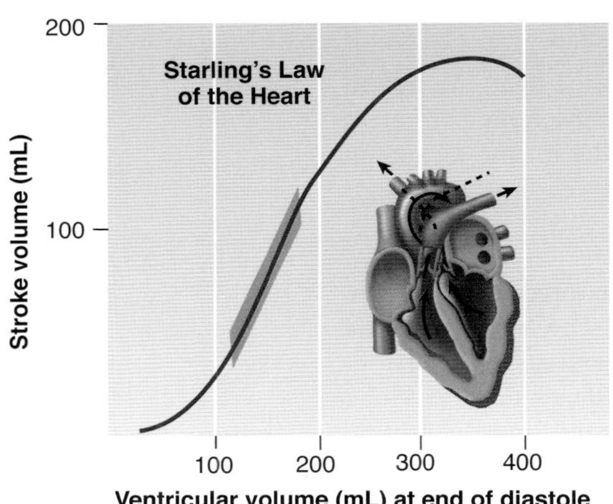

FIGURE 30-5 Starling's law of the heart. This curve represents the relationship between the stroke volume and the ventricular volume at the end of diastole. The range of values observed in a typical heart is shaded. Note that if the ventricle has an abnormally large volume at the end of diastole *(far right portion of the curve)*, the stroke volume cannot compensate.

Although Starling's law of the heart was first described in animal experiments, most physiologists agree that it operates in humans as a major regulator of stroke volume in ordinary conditions. Operation of Starling's law of the heart ensures that increased amounts of blood returned to the heart will be pumped out of it. It automatically adjusts CO to venous return in usual conditions. Factors that influence the amount of blood returned to the heart—venous return—are discussed in a later section.

Other factors that influence stroke volume are neural and endocrine chemical factors. You already know from our discussions in earlier chapters that norepinephrine (NE) released by sympathetic fibres in the cardiac nerve and epinephrine released into the blood by the adrenal medulla can both increase the strength of contraction, or *contractility*, of the myocardium. This increased contractility of heart muscle pushes more blood out of the heart per cardiac stroke—thus increasing the stroke volume. As **Figure 30-6** shows, both the increased contractility from these chemical factors and the effects of Starling's law of the heart can change the stroke volume—and therefore also cardiac output. Factors such as the stress of exercise can trigger these neural and endocrine responses.

The **ejection fraction (EF)** is related to the stroke volume. The ejection fraction is the ratio of the stroke volume (SV) to the end-diastolic volume (EDV), often expressed as a percentage. Expressed as a formula, EF = (SV/EDV) × 100. Thus as SV goes up, EF goes up—and as SV goes down, EF also goes down. An EF of 55% or higher is typical in healthy adults. The EF declines when the myocardium fails to function properly and cannot contract strongly enough to eject a normal amount of blood—as sometimes happens after a myocardial infarction (MI).

CONNECT IT! 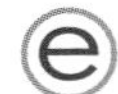

The ejection fraction is usually measured by echocardiography, a procedure described in ***Echocardiography*** online at ***Connect It!***

Another factor to consider is the cardiac *afterload*—the pumping work that the heart must do to push blood into the arteries. The harder it is to push blood out of the ventricles, the lower the stroke volume will be. For example, if pulmonary blood flow "backs up" in the pulmonary arteries because of obstructions in pulmonary blood flow, the stroke volume can be reduced below normal—causing a type of *heart failure* (see p. 659).

Factors That Affect Heart Rate

Although the sinoatrial node normally initiates each heartbeat, the rate it sets is not an unalterable one. Various factors—often called **chronotropic** factors—can and do change the rate of the heartbeat.

One major modifier of sinoatrial node activity—and therefore of the heart rate—is the ratio of sympathetic and parasympathetic impulses conducted to the node per minute. Autonomic control of heart rate is the result of opposing influences between parasympathetic (chiefly vagus nerve) and sympathetic (cardiac nerve) stimulation.

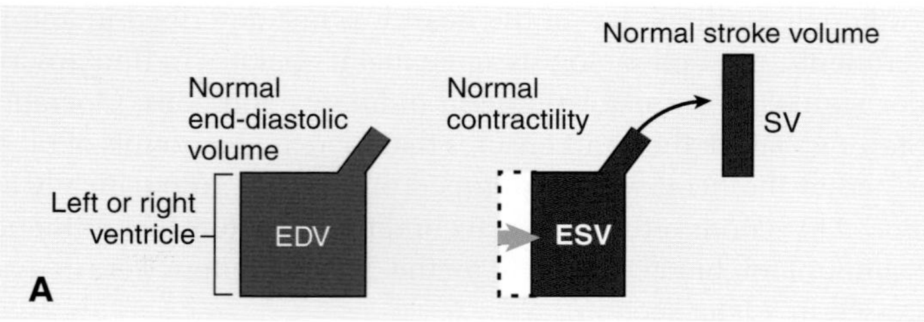

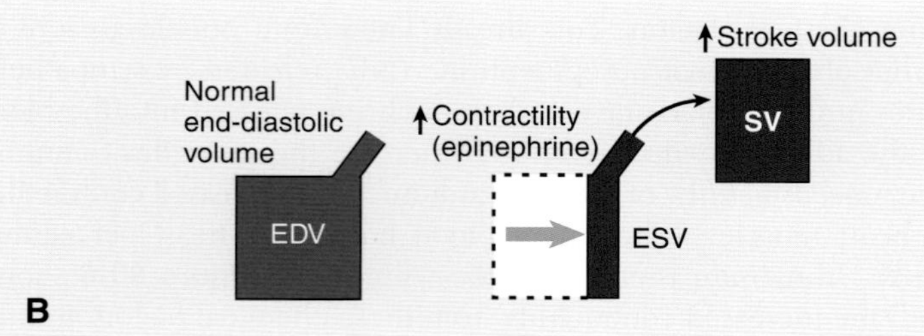

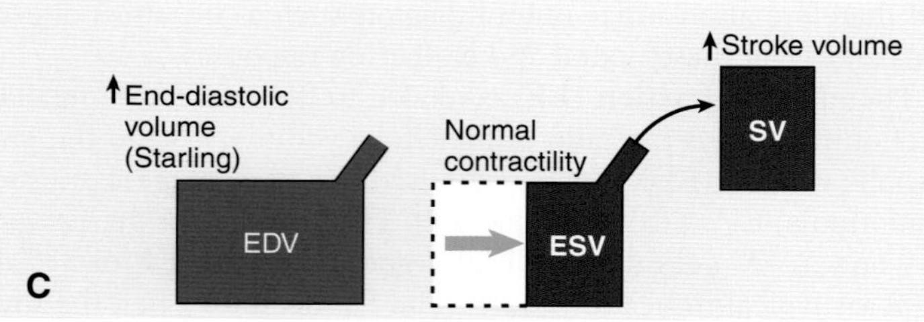

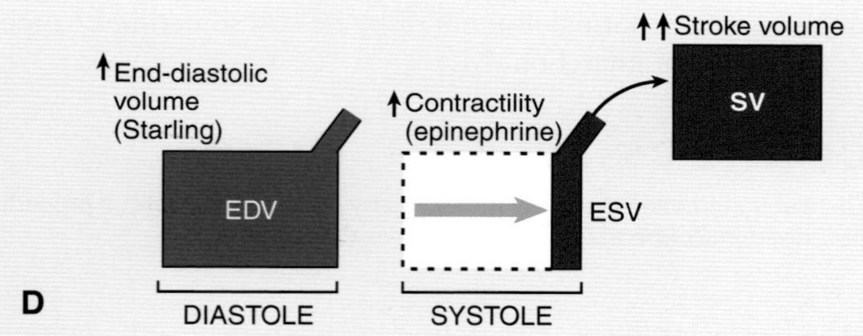

FIGURE 30-6 Stroke volume. Changes in stroke volume caused by increasing the end-diastolic volume (EDV) or contractility. **A,** Normal stroke volume (no external influences). **B,** When EDV remains constant and contractility increases (from epinephrine), stroke volume increases. **C,** When contractility remains constant and EDV increases, stroke volume increases (Starling's law of the heart). **D,** When both EDV and contractility increase, a combined effect increases the stroke volume even more. *EDV,* End-diastolic volume; *ESV,* end-systolic volume; *SV,* stroke volume.

The results of parasympathetic stimulation on the heart are inhibitory and are mediated by vagal release of acetylcholine, whereas sympathetic (stimulatory) effects result from the release of norepinephrine at the distal end of the cardiac nerve.

Cardiac Pressoreflexes

Receptors sensitive to changes in pressure (**baroreceptors**) are located in two places near the heart (**Figure 30-7**). Called the *aortic baroreceptors* and *carotid baroreceptors,* they send afferent nerve fibres to cardiac control centres in the medulla oblongata. These stretch receptors, located in the aorta and carotid sinus, constitute a very important heart rate control mechanism because of their effect on the autonomic cardiac control centres—and therefore on parasympathetic and sympathetic outflow. Baroreceptors operate with integrators in the cardiac control centres in negative feedback loops called **pressoreflexes** or *baroreflexes* that oppose changes in pressure by adjusting heart rate.

Carotid Sinus Reflex

The carotid sinus is a small dilation at the beginning of the internal carotid artery just above the branching of the common carotid artery to form the internal and external carotid arteries (see **Figure 30-7**).

The sinus lies just under the sternocleidomastoid muscle at the level of the upper margin of the thyroid cartilage. Sensory (afferent) fibres from carotid sinus baroreceptors (pressure sensors) run through the carotid sinus nerve (of Hering) and on through the glossopharyngeal (or ninth cranial) nerve. These nerves relay feedback information to an integrator area of the medulla called the *cardiac control centre.* If the integrators in the cardiac control centre detect an increase in blood pressure above the set point, then a correction signal is sent to the SA node by way of efferent parasympathetic fibres in the vagus (tenth cranial) nerve. Acetylcholine released by vagal fibres decreases the rate of SA node firing, thus decreasing the heart rate back toward the set point. The vagus

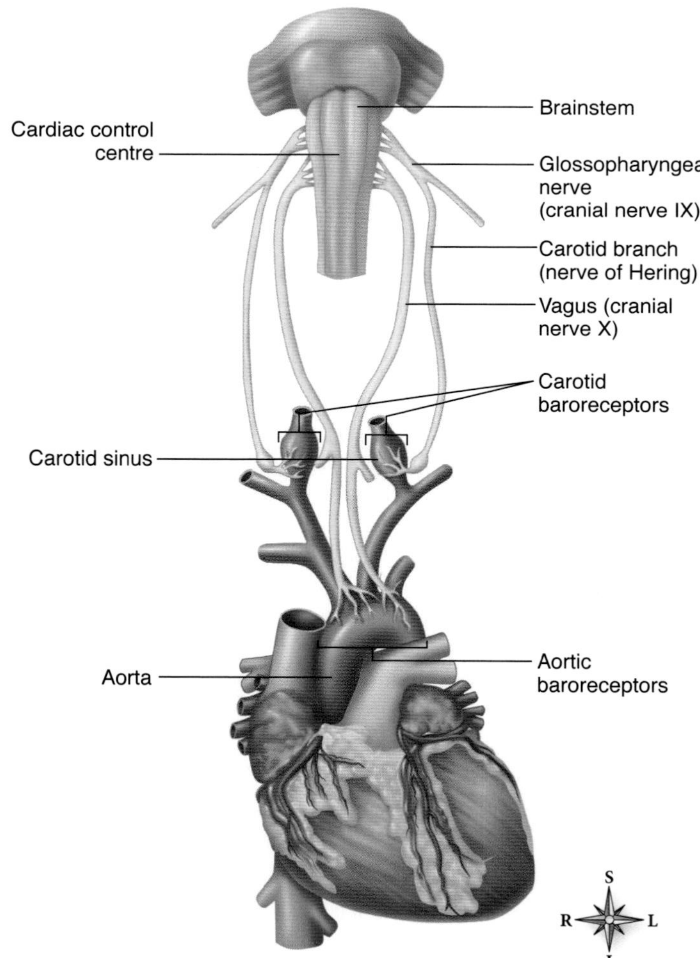

FIGURE 30-7 Cardiac baroreceptors. Location of aortic and carotid baroreceptors and the sensory nerves that carry feedback information about blood pressure back to the central nervous system.

is said to act as a "brake" on the heart—a situation called *vagal inhibition*. **Figure 30-8** summarizes this negative feedback loop, which is often called the **carotid sinus reflex.**

Aortic Reflex

Sensory (afferent) nerve fibres also extend from baroreceptors located in the wall of the arch of the aorta through the aortic nerve and then through the vagus (tenth cranial) nerve to terminate in the cardiac control centre of the medulla (see **Figure 30-7**).

If blood pressure within the aorta or carotid sinus suddenly increases beyond the set point, it stimulates the aortic or carotid baroreceptors, as shown in **Figure 30-8**. Stimulation of these stretch receptors causes the cardiac control centre to increase vagal inhibition, thus slowing the heart and returning blood pressure back toward the normal set point. A decrease in aortic or carotid blood pressure usually allows some acceleration of the heart by way of correction signals through the cardiac nerve. Because it involves receptors located in the wall of the aorta, this feedback loop is called the **aortic reflex.**

More details of pressoreflex activity are included later in the chapter as part of a mechanism that tends to maintain or restore homeostasis of arterial blood pressure.

Other Reflexes That Influence Heart Rate

Reflexes involving important factors such as emotions, exercise, hormones, blood temperature, pain, and stimulation of various exteroceptors also influence heart rate. Anxiety, fear, and anger often make the heart beat faster. Grief, in contrast, tends to slow it. Emotions produce changes in the heart rate through the influence of impulses from the "higher centres" in the cerebrum by way of the hypothalamus. Such impulses can influence activity of the cardiac control centres.

During exercise the heart normally accelerates. The mechanism for this acceleration is not definitely known, but it is thought to include impulses from the cerebrum through the hypothalamus to the cardiac centre. Epinephrine is the hormone most noted as a cardiac accelerator.

Increased blood temperature or stimulation of skin heat receptors tends to increase the heart rate, and decreased blood temperature or stimulation of skin cold receptors tends to slow it. Sudden, intense stimulation of pain receptors in visceral structures such as the gallbladder, ureters, or intestines can result in such slowing of the heart that fainting may result.

FIGURE 30-8 Aortic and carotid sinus pressoreflexes. These pressoreflexes operate in a feedback loop that maintains the homeostasis of blood pressure by decreasing the heart rate when the blood pressure surpasses the set point—as when recovering from a stress event after being startled.

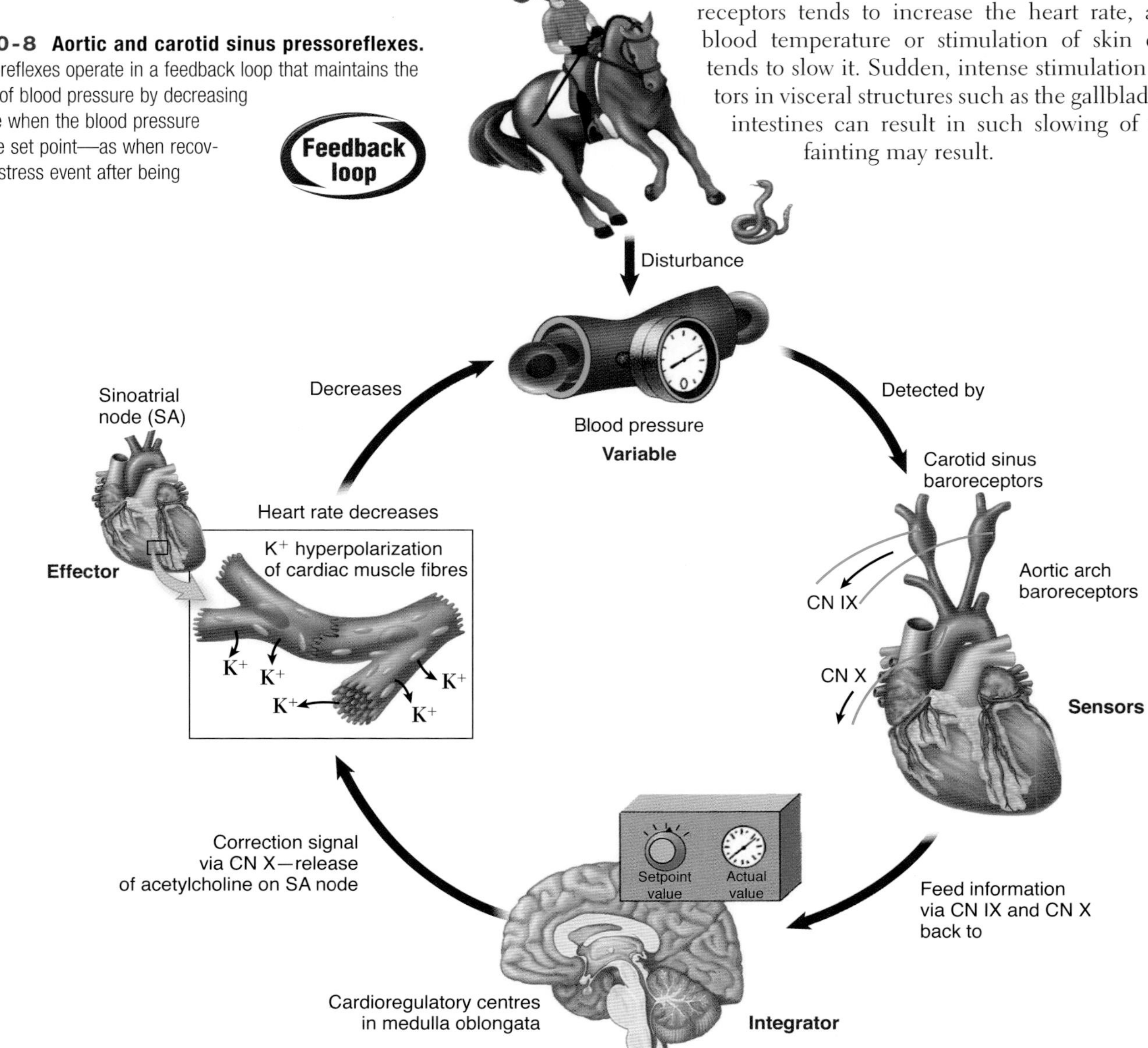

Reflexive increases in heart rate often result from an increase in sympathetic stimulation of the heart. Sympathetic impulses originate in the cardiac control centre of the medulla and reach the heart by way of sympathetic fibres (contained in the middle, superior, and inferior cardiac nerves). Norepinephrine released as a result of sympathetic stimulation increases heart rate and strength of cardiac muscle contraction.

Quick CHECK

1. State the primary principle of circulation.
2. Relate stroke volume and heart rate to cardiac output.
3. If the amount of blood returned to the heart increases, what happens to the stroke volume? What principle explains this?
4. How does the body use a pressoreflex to counteract an abnormal increase in heart rate? An abnormal decrease in heart rate?

PERIPHERAL RESISTANCE

How Resistance Influences Blood Pressure

Peripheral resistance means the resistance to blood flow imposed by the force of friction between blood and the walls of its vessels. Friction develops partly because of a characteristic of blood—its **viscosity**, or thickness—and partly from the small diameter of arterioles and capillaries. The resistance offered by arterioles, in particular, accounts for almost one half of the total resistance in systemic circulation.

Peripheral resistance in arterioles helps determine arterial blood pressure because the more resistance there is in the arterioles, the more blood "backs up" in the arteries to increase fluid pressure. This mechanism can help maintain the pressure gradient needed to keep blood flowing (review again **Figure 30-2** on p. 701). Think of what happens when you pinch off the end of a garden hose. The water backs up in the hose and the increased pressure gradient gives more force to the water flowing out of the hose.

Blood viscosity stems mainly from the proportion of red blood cells (haematocrit) but also partly from the protein molecules present in blood. An increase in either blood protein concentration or haematocrit tends to increase viscosity, and a decrease in either tends to decrease it (**Figure 30-9**). In normal circumstances, blood viscosity changes very little. But in certain abnormal conditions, such as marked anaemia or haemorrhage, a decrease in blood viscosity may be the crucial factor lowering peripheral resistance and arterial pressure, even to the point of circulatory failure.

The muscular coat of the arterioles allows them to constrict or dilate and thus change the amount of resistance to blood flow. This muscular mechanism in the vessels is called the **vasomotor mechanism.** Reduction in vessel diameter caused by increased contraction of the muscular coat, or **vasoconstriction,** increases resistance to blood flow, and thus blood flow into the tissue decreases. **Vasodilation,** the increase in vessel diameter caused by relaxation of vascular muscles, decreases resistance to blood flow, and thus blood flow into the tissue increases.

As **Figure 30-10** shows, small changes in diameter can cause proportionally large changes in resistance—and therefore large changes in local blood flow. This makes the vasomotor mechanism well suited for quickly and dramatically changing blood flow in varying conditions in the body, as we shall see.

Peripheral resistance helps determine arterial pressure by controlling the rate of "arteriole runoff", the amount of blood that runs out of the arteries into the arterioles (**Figure 30-11**). The greater the resistance, the less the arteriole runoff, or outflow, tends to be—and therefore the more blood left in the arteries, the higher the arterial pressure tends to be. This can occur locally, within a particular tissue or organ, or it can occur throughout the systemic loop when enough arterioles constrict and increase the **total peripheral resistance (TPR).**

Vasomotor Control Mechanism

Blood distribution patterns, as well as blood pressure, can be influenced by factors that control changes in the diameter of arterioles. Such factors might be said to constitute the vasomotor control mechanism. Like most physiological control mechanisms, it consists of many parts. An area in the medulla called the *vasomotor centre,* or *vasoconstrictor centre,* will, when stimulated, initiate an impulse outflow by way of sympathetic fibres that ends in the smooth muscle surrounding resistance vessels, arterioles, venules, and veins of the "blood reservoirs", causing their constriction. Thus the vasomotor control mechanism plays a role both in the maintenance of the general blood pressure and in the distribution of blood to areas of special need.

The main blood reservoirs are the venous plexuses and sinuses in the skin and abdominal organs (especially in the liver and spleen). In other words, blood reservoirs are the venous networks in most parts of the body—all but those in the skeletal muscles, heart, and brain. **Figure 30-12** shows that the volume of blood in the systemic veins and venules in a resting adult is extremely large compared with the volume in other vessels of the body. The term *reservoir* is apt, because the systemic veins and venules serve as a kind of slowly moving stockpile or reserve of blood. Blood can quickly be moved out of blood reservoirs by **venoconstriction** that squeezes the vein walls and thereby "shifts" blood toward arteries that supply heart and skeletal muscles when increased activity demands (**Figure 30-13**).

A change in either arterial blood's oxygen or carbon dioxide content sets a chemical vasomotor control mechanism in operation. A change in arterial blood pressure initiates a **vasomotor pressoreflex.**

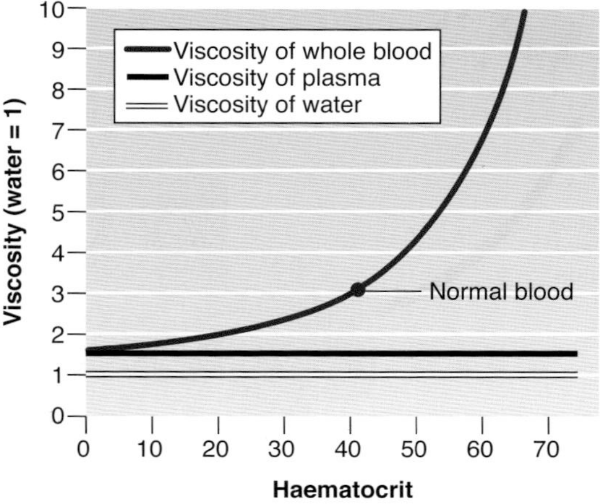

FIGURE 30-9 Blood viscosity. The effect of a changing haematocrit (percentage of red blood cells in blood) on blood viscosity is shown here. As haematocrit increases (horizontal axis of graph), the viscosity increases. Water is the reference value at viscosity = 1. Plasma is slightly more viscous than water—at approximately 1.5. As the total viscosity of blood increases, the resistance to blood flow increases.

UNIT 4

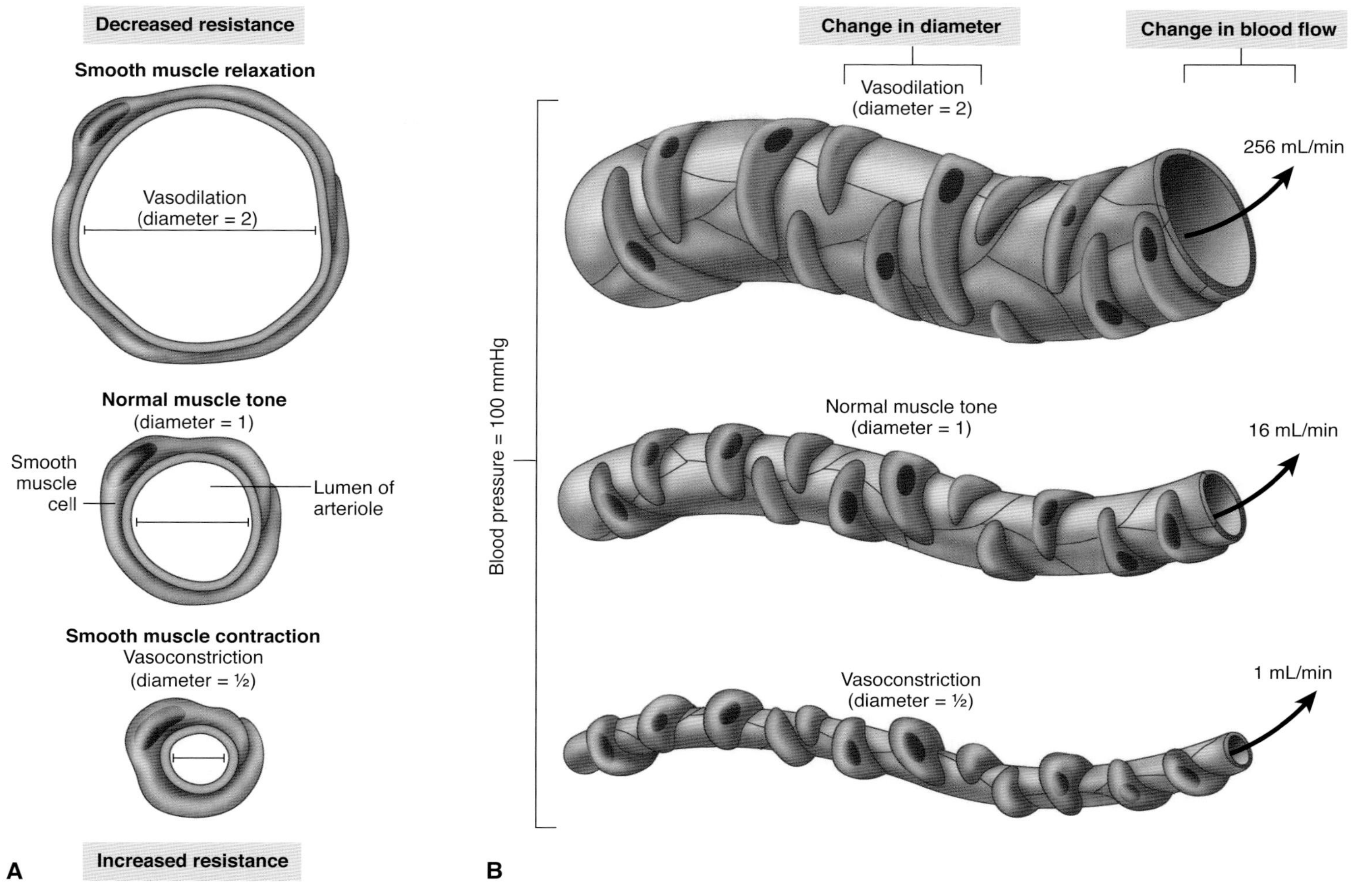

A

Decreased resistance

Smooth muscle relaxation

Vasodilation (diameter = 2)

Normal muscle tone (diameter = 1)

Smooth muscle cell

Lumen of arteriole

Smooth muscle contraction

Vasoconstriction (diameter = ½)

Increased resistance

B

Change in diameter

Change in blood flow

Blood pressure = 100 mmHg

Vasodilation (diameter = 2)

256 mL/min

Normal muscle tone (diameter = 1)

16 mL/min

Vasoconstriction (diameter = ½)

1 mL/min

FIGURE 30-10 Vessel diameter. The effect of changing diameter of arterioles on peripheral resistance and blood flow. **A,** Cross-sections of an arteriole showing vasodilation *(top),* normal diameter *(centre),* and vasoconstriction *(bottom)* as tension in smooth muscle fibres changes. **B,** Diagram showing that relatively small changes from the normal diameter of an arteriole (normal = 1) cause very large changes in peripheral resistance to blood flow. For example, reducing diameter to one half of normal reduces blood flow to 1/16 of normal. Likewise, doubling the vessel diameter does not double the blood flow—it increases blood flow 16 times the normal flow!

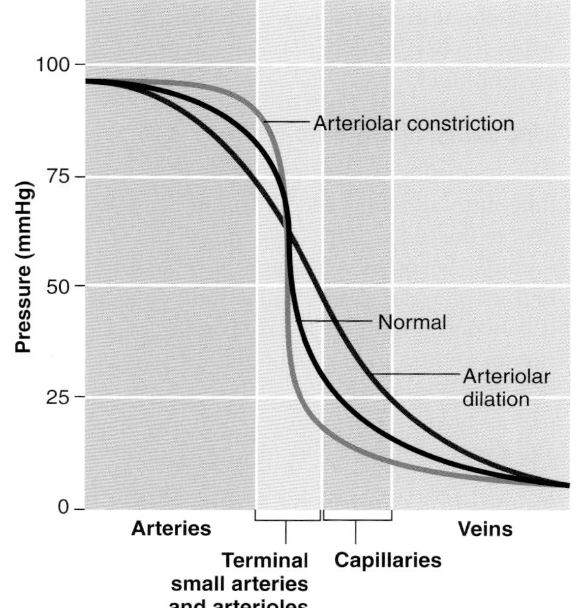

FIGURE 30-11 Vasomotor effects on blood pressure. The normal blood pressures in various vessels are shown by the *black line.* The *green line* shows a shift in blood pressures during vasoconstriction of the arterioles. Note that because there is more resistance in the arterioles, blood flow in the arteries backs up and thus increases arterial blood pressure. The *purple line* shows that vasodilation of the arterioles increases blood flow from the arteries and therefore reduces arterial blood pressure.

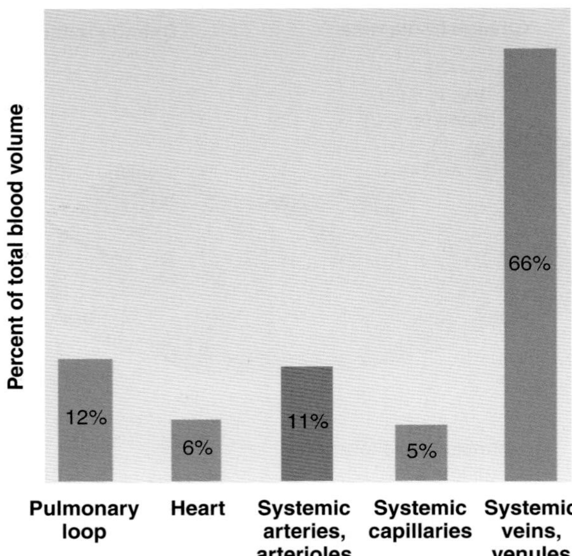

FIGURE 30-12 Relative blood volumes. The relative volumes of blood at rest in different parts of the adult cardiovascular system expressed as percentages of total blood volume. Note that at rest most of the body's blood supply is in the systemic veins and venules.

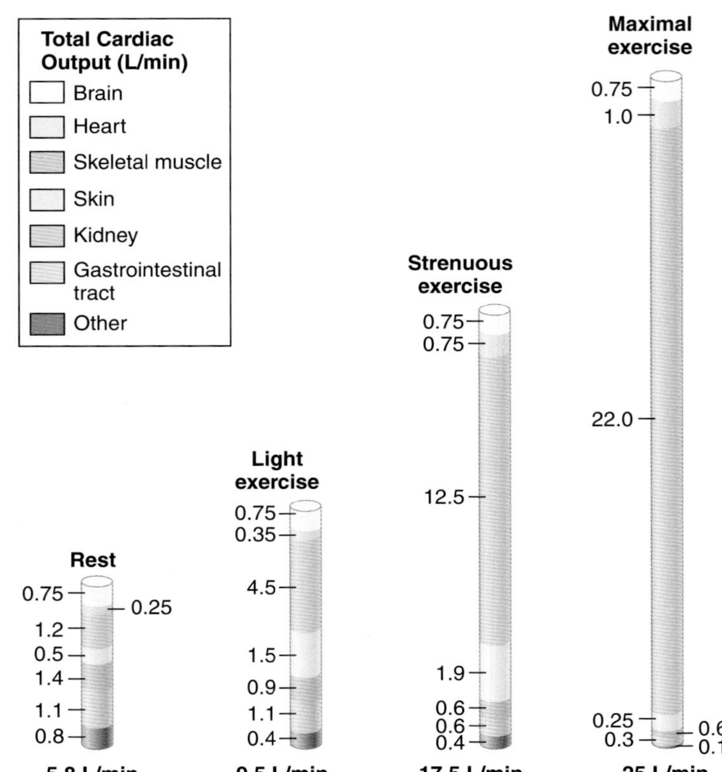

FIGURE 30-13 Changes in local blood flow during exercise. Graphic representation of blood flow (L/min) in an individual in various circumstances: at rest and during light, strenuous, and maximal exercise. During exercise, the vasomotor centre of the medulla sends sympathetic signals to certain blood vessels to change diameter and thus shunt blood away from "maintenance" organs, such as the digestive organs in the abdomen, and toward the skeletal muscles. Local regulators of blood flow add to this effect. Note that blood flow in the brain is held constant. Note also that the total blood flow (cardiac output) in this individual increases from 5.8 L/min (rest) to 25 L/min—a fivefold increase in cardiac output—as the intensity of exercise increases. This increase in cardiac output represents use of the cardiac reserve.

Vasomotor Pressoreflexes

A sudden increase in arterial blood pressure stimulates aortic and carotid baroreceptors—the same ones that initiate cardiac reflexes. Not only does this stimulate the cardiac control centre to reduce heart rate (see **Figure 30-8**), but also it inhibits the vasoconstrictor centre. More impulses per second go out over parasympathetic fibres to the heart. As a result, the heartbeat slows. Because sympathetic vasoconstrictor impulses predominate at normal arterial pressures, inhibition of these is considered the major mechanism of vasodilation. The nervous pathways involved in this mechanism are illustrated in **Figure 30-14**.

A decrease in arterial pressure causes the aortic and carotid baroreceptors to send fewer impulses to the medulla's vasoconstrictor centres, signalling the change in blood pressure. These centres then send more impulses by way of the sympathetic fibres to stimulate vascular smooth muscle and cause vasoconstriction. When arterioles constrict, it "backs up" arterial blood and increases arterial blood pressure. Vasoconstriction also squeezes more blood out of the blood reservoirs, increasing the amount of venous blood return to the heart.

During exercise, blood from reservoirs is redistributed to more active structures such as skeletal muscles and heart because their arterioles become dilated largely from the operation of a local mechanism (discussed later). Thus the vasoconstrictor pressoreflex and the local vasodilating mechanism together serve as an important device for shifting blood from reservoirs to tissues that need it during exercise (**Box 30-1**; also see **Figure 30-13**).

Vasomotor Chemoreflexes

Chemoreceptors located in the aortic and carotid bodies are particularly sensitive to excess blood carbon dioxide (**hypercapnia**) and somewhat less sensitive to a deficiency of blood oxygen (**hypoxia**) and to decreased arterial blood pH. When one or more of these conditions stimulates the chemoreceptors, their fibres transmit more impulses to the medulla's vasoconstrictor centres, and vasoconstriction of arterioles and venous reservoirs soon follows (**Figure 30-15**). This **chemoreceptor reflex** functions as an emergency mechanism when hypoxia or hypercapnia endangers the stability of the internal environment.

Medullary Ischaemic Reflex

The **medullary ischaemic reflex** mechanism is said to exert powerful control of blood vessels during emergency situations when blood flow to the brain drops below normal. When the blood supply to the medulla becomes inadequate (**ischaemic**), its neurons suffer from both oxygen deficiency and carbon dioxide excess. But, presumably, it is hypercapnia that intensely and directly stimulates the vasoconstrictor centres to bring about marked arteriole and venous constriction (see **Figure 30-15**). If the oxygen supply to the medulla decreases below a certain level, its neurons, of course, cannot function and the medullary ischaemic reflex cannot operate.

Vasomotor Control by Higher Brain Centres

Impulses from centres in the cerebral cortex and in the hypothalamus are believed to be transmitted to the vasomotor centres in the medulla and to thereby help control vasoconstriction and dilation.

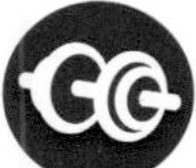

BOX 30-1 *sports and fitness* | The Cardiovascular System and Exercise

Exercise produces short-term and long-term changes in the cardiovascular system.

Short-term changes involve negative feedback mechanisms that maintain setpoint levels of blood oxygen and glucose, as well as other physiological variables. Because moderate to strenuous use of skeletal muscles greatly increases the body's overall rate of metabolism, oxygen and glucose are used up at a faster rate. This requires an increase in transport of oxygen and glucose by the cardiovascular system to maintain normal setpoint levels of these substances. One response by the cardiovascular system is to increase the cardiac output (CO) from 5 to 6 L/min at rest to up to 30 to 40 L/min during strenuous exercise. This represents a fivefold to eightfold increase in the blood output of the heart! Such an increase is accomplished by a reflexive increase in heart rate (see **Figure 30-8**) coupled with an increase in stroke volume (see **Figures 30-5** and **30-6**). Exercise can also trigger a reflexive change in local distribution of blood flow to various tissues, shown in **Figure 30-13**, that results in a larger share of blood flow going to the skeletal muscles than to some other tissues. A number of central and local regulatory effects that operate during exercise are summarized in the figure.

Long-term changes in the cardiovascular system come only when moderate to strenuous exercise occurs regularly over a long period. •

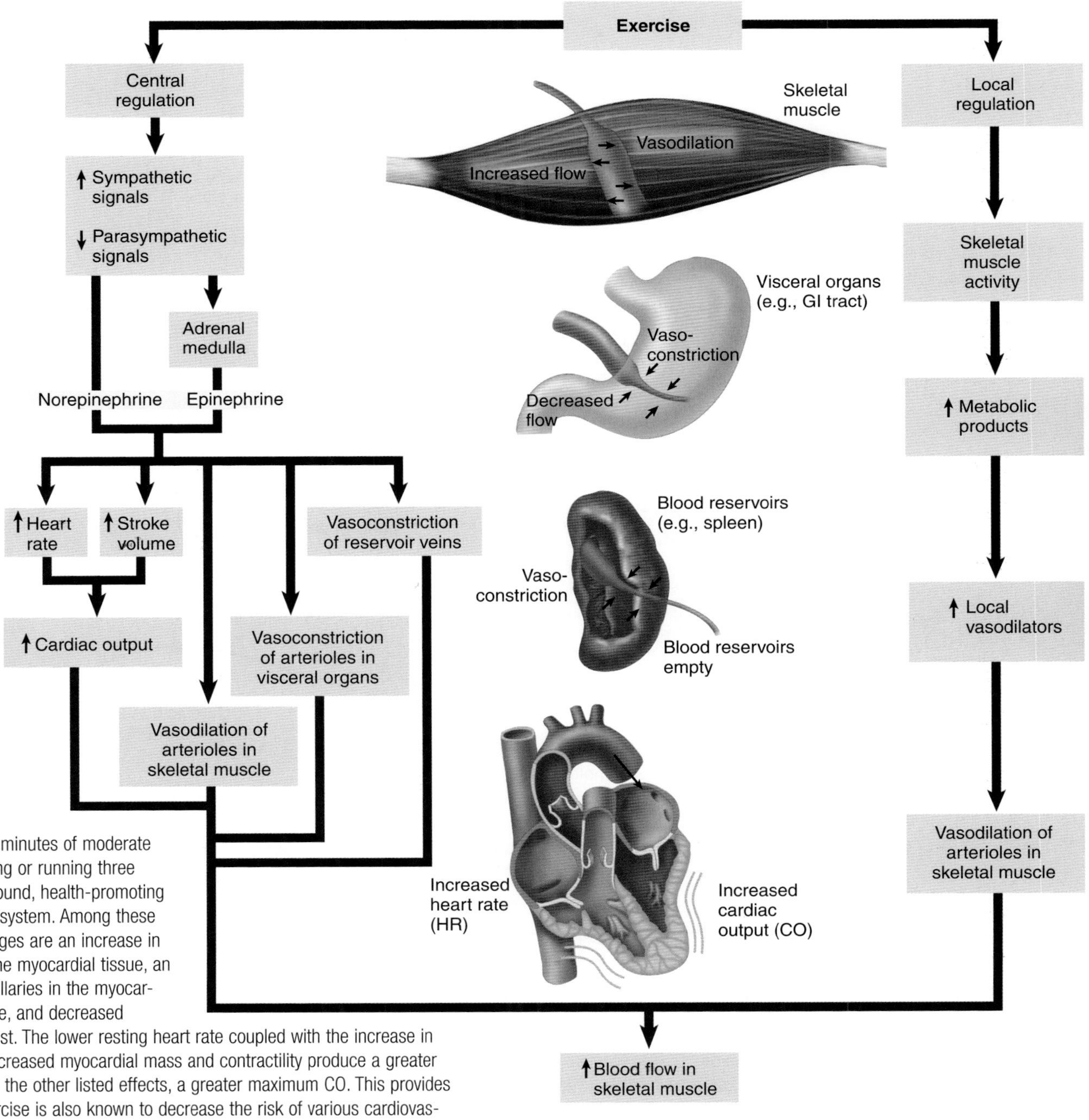

Exercise

Central regulation

↑ Sympathetic signals

↓ Parasympathetic signals

Adrenal medulla

Norepinephrine Epinephrine

↑ Heart rate

↑ Stroke volume

↑ Cardiac output

Vasoconstriction of reservoir veins

Vasoconstriction of arterioles in visceral organs

Vasodilation of arterioles in skeletal muscle

Skeletal muscle

Vasodilation

Increased flow

Visceral organs (e.g., GI tract)

Vaso-constriction

Decreased flow

Blood reservoirs (e.g., spleen)

Vaso-constriction

Blood reservoirs empty

Increased heart rate (HR)

Increased cardiac output (CO)

Local regulation

Skeletal muscle activity

↑ Metabolic products

↑ Local vasodilators

Vasodilation of arterioles in skeletal muscle

↑ Blood flow in skeletal muscle

Evidence shows that 20 to 30 minutes of moderate aerobic exercise such as cycling or running three times per week produces profound, health-promoting changes in the cardiovascular system. Among these long-term cardiovascular changes are an increase in the mass and contractility of the myocardial tissue, an increase in the number of capillaries in the myocardium, a lower resting heart rate, and decreased peripheral resistance during rest. The lower resting heart rate coupled with the increase in stroke volume possible with increased myocardial mass and contractility produce a greater range of CO, and coupled with the other listed effects, a greater maximum CO. This provides a greater cardiac reserve. Exercise is also known to decrease the risk of various cardiovascular disorders, including arteriosclerosis, hypertension, and heart failure.

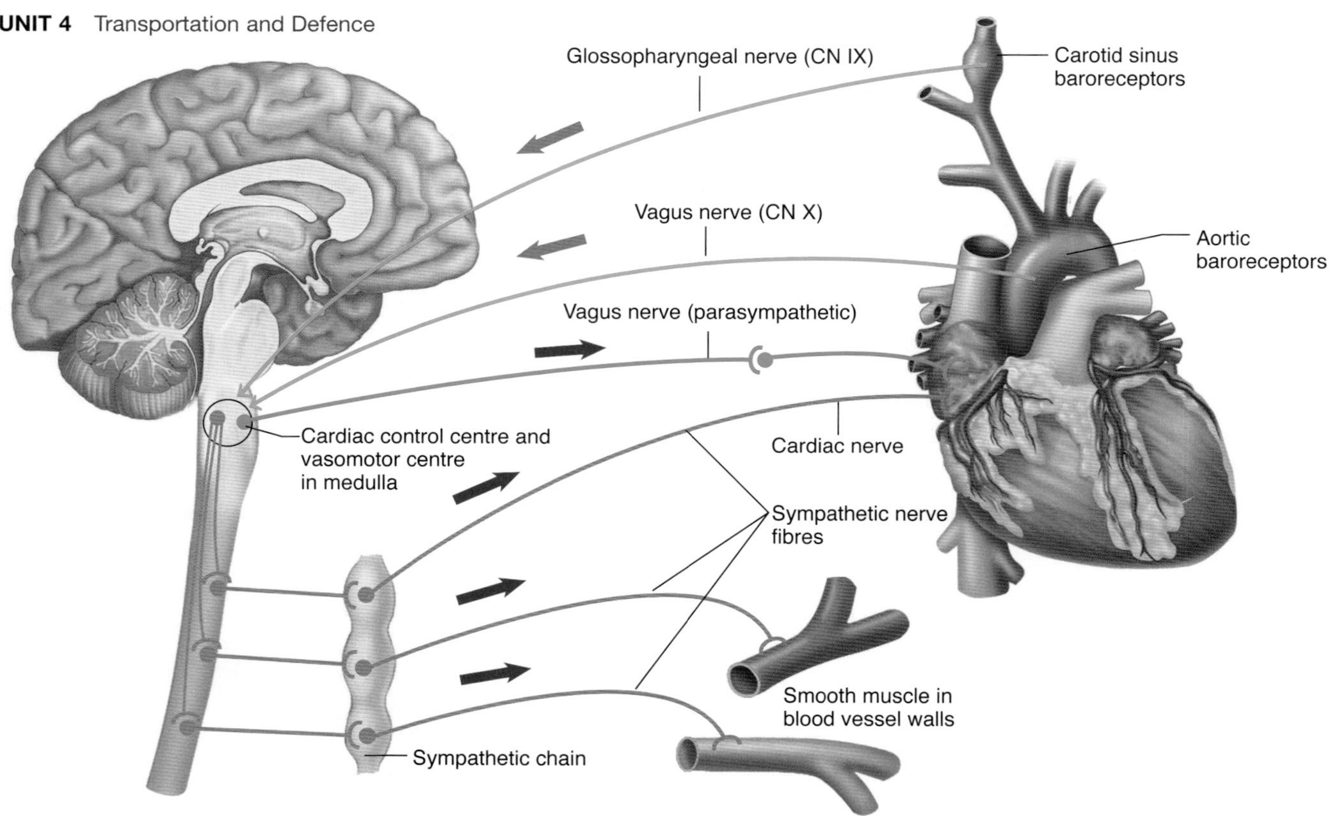

FIGURE 30-14 Vasomotor pressoreflexes. Carotid sinus and aortic baroreceptors detect changes in blood pressure and feed the information back to the cardiac control centre and the vasomotor centre in the medulla. In response, these control centres alter the ratio between sympathetic and parasympathetic output. If the pressure is too high, increased parasympathetic impulses and reduced sympathetic impulses will reduce it by slowing heart rate, reducing stroke volume, and dilating blood "reservoir" vessels. If the pressure is too low, an increase in sympathetic impulses will increase it by increasing heart rate and stroke volume and constricting arterioles and reservoir vessels.

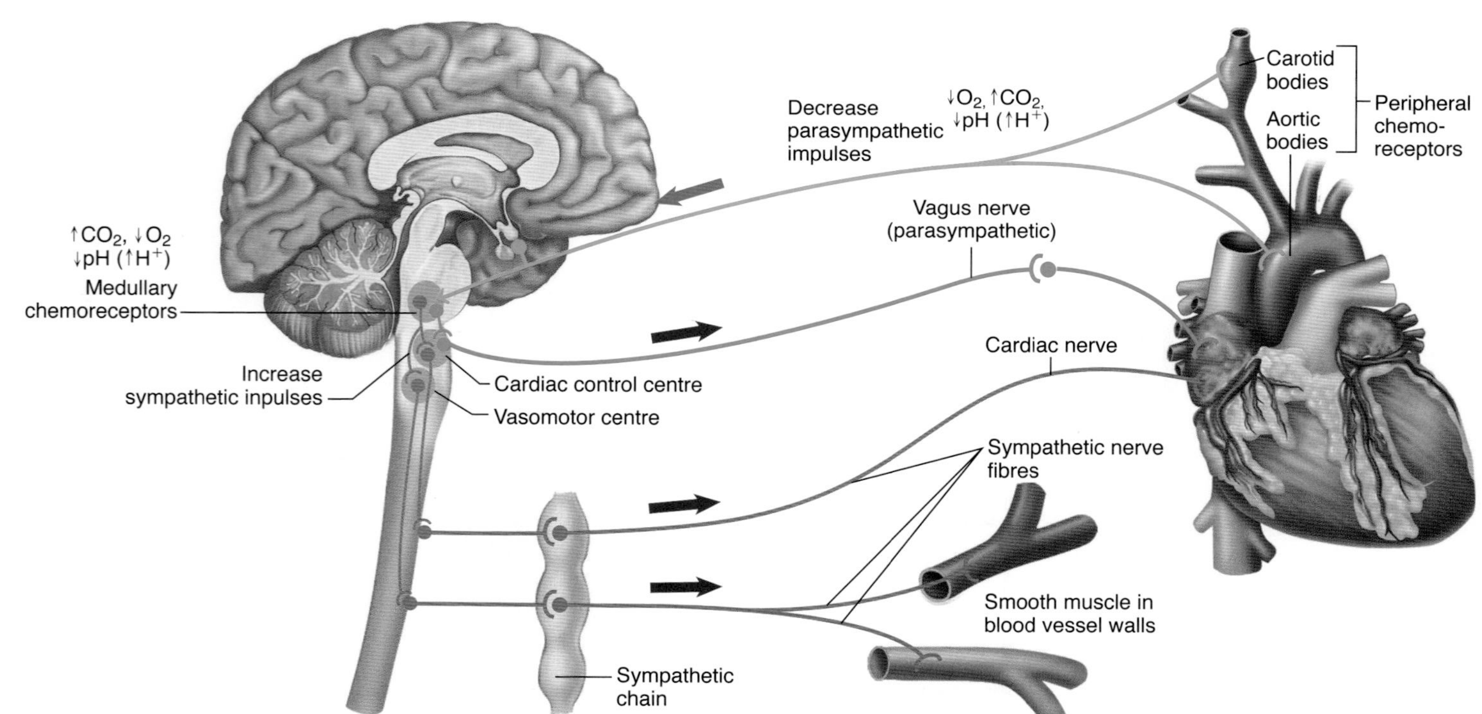

FIGURE 30-15 Vasomotor chemoreflexes. Chemoreceptors in the carotid and aortic bodies, as well as chemoreceptive neurons in the vasomotor centre of the medulla itself, detect increases in carbon dioxide (CO_2), decreases in blood oxygen (O_2), and/or decreases in pH (which is really an increase in H^+). This information feeds back to the cardiac control centre and the vasomotor control centre of the medulla, which in turn alter the ratio of parasympathetic and sympathetic output. When O_2 drops, CO_2 increases and/or pH drops, a dominance of sympathetic impulses increases heart rate and stroke volume and constricts reservoir vessels in response.

Evidence supporting this view is that vasoconstriction and a rise in arterial blood pressure characteristically accompany emotions of intense fear or anger. Also, laboratory experiments on animals in which stimulation of the posterior or lateral parts of the hypothalamus leads to vasoconstriction support the belief that higher brain centres influence the vasomotor centres in the medulla.

Local Control of Arterioles

Several kinds of local mechanisms operate to produce vasodilation in localized areas. Although not all these mechanisms are clearly understood, they are known to function in times of increased tissue activity. For example, they probably account for the increased blood flow into skeletal muscles during exercise. They also operate in ischaemic tissues, serving as a homeostatic mechanism that tends to restore normal blood flow. Some locally produced substances, such as nitric oxide, activate the local vasodilator mechanism, whereas others, such as *endothelin*, constrict the arterioles. Local vasodilation is also referred to as *active hyperaemia*.

Quick CHECK

5. Peripheral resistance is affected by two major factors: blood viscosity and what else?
6. If the diameter of the arteries decreases, what effect does it have on peripheral resistance?
7. In general, how do vasomotor pressoreflexes affect the flow of blood?
8. What is a chemoreflex? How do chemoreflexes affect the flow of blood?

VENOUS RETURN TO THE HEART

Venous return refers to the amount of blood that is returned to the heart by way of the veins. Various factors influence venous return, including the reservoir function of veins, which occurs whenever blood pressure drops and the elasticity of the venous walls adapts the diameter of veins to the lower pressure, thus maintaining blood flow and venous return to the heart. Likewise, when overall blood pressure rises, the elastic nature of blood vessels allows them to expand and adapt to the higher pressure to maintain normal blood flow. This effect, which occurs in all blood vessels to some degree (with certain limitations to its adaptability), is often called the **stress-relaxation effect.**

Another factor that influences venous return is gravity. **Figure 30-16** shows that when a person is reclining, the force of gravity is not pulling blood downward toward the legs. However, when a person is sitting or standing, the blood *is* pulled by gravity toward the legs. Because the venous blood is already at a low blood pressure and because the venous walls are compliant (easily stretched), it is easy for the force of gravity to work against venous return back to the heart and cause some blood to remain in the veins of the limbs. The shift of the blood reservoir to the veins in the legs when standing is often called the **orthostatic effect** because *orthostasis* means "standing upright".

A factor that can help to overcome the influence of gravity is the operation of **venous pumps** that maintain the pressure gradients necessary to keep blood moving into the central veins (e.g., venae cavae) and from there into the atria of the heart.

Changes in the total volume of blood in the vessels can also alter venous return. Venous return and total blood volume are discussed in the paragraphs that follow.

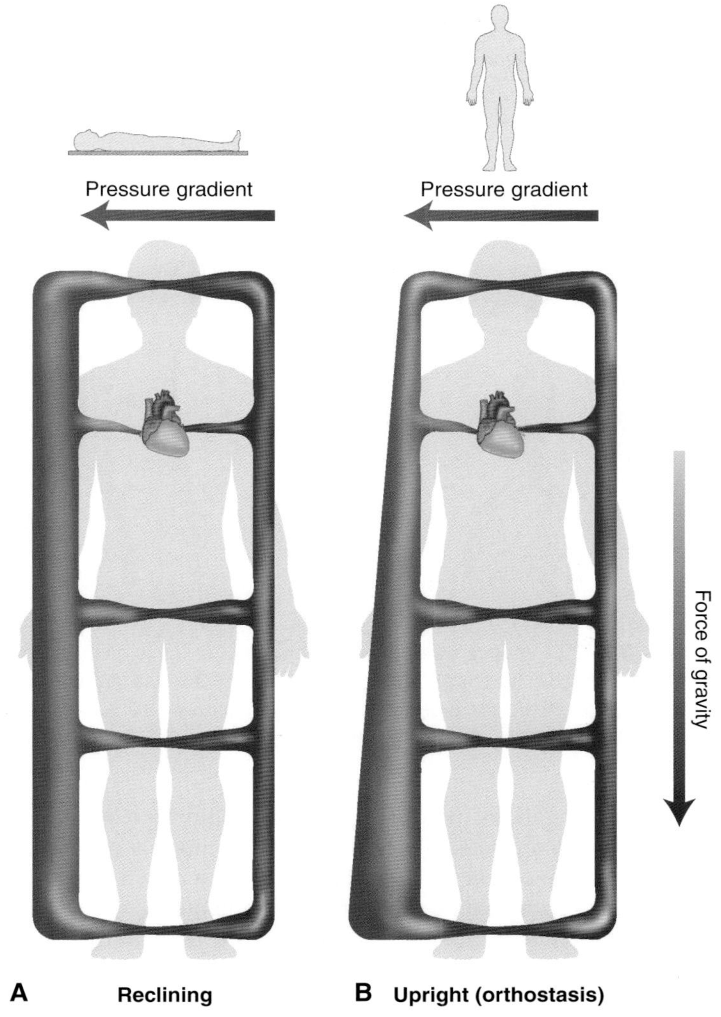

FIGURE 30-16 Influence of gravity on blood distribution in veins. **A,** When a person is lying flat, the pull of gravity is equal above and below the heart. **B,** When a person stands upright (orthostasis), the pull of gravity combined with the compliance (ease of stretch) of the veins causes a redistribution of venous blood to the lower limbs. This *orthostatic effect* can reduce venous return to the heart if not counteracted by other forces.

Venous Pumps

One important factor that promotes the return of venous blood to the heart is the blood-pumping action of respirations and skeletal muscle contractions. Both actions produce their facilitating effect on venous return by increasing the pressure gradient between the peripheral veins and the venae cavae (central veins).

The process of inspiration increases the pressure gradient between peripheral and central veins by decreasing central venous pressure and also by increasing peripheral venous pressure. Each time the diaphragm contracts, the thoracic cavity necessarily becomes larger and the abdominal cavity smaller. Therefore the pressures in the thoracic cavity, in the thoracic portion of the vena cava, and in the atria decrease, and those in the abdominal cavity and the abdominal veins increase. As **Figure 30-17**, A, shows, this change in pressure between expiration and inspiration acts as a "respiratory pump" that moves blood along the venous route.

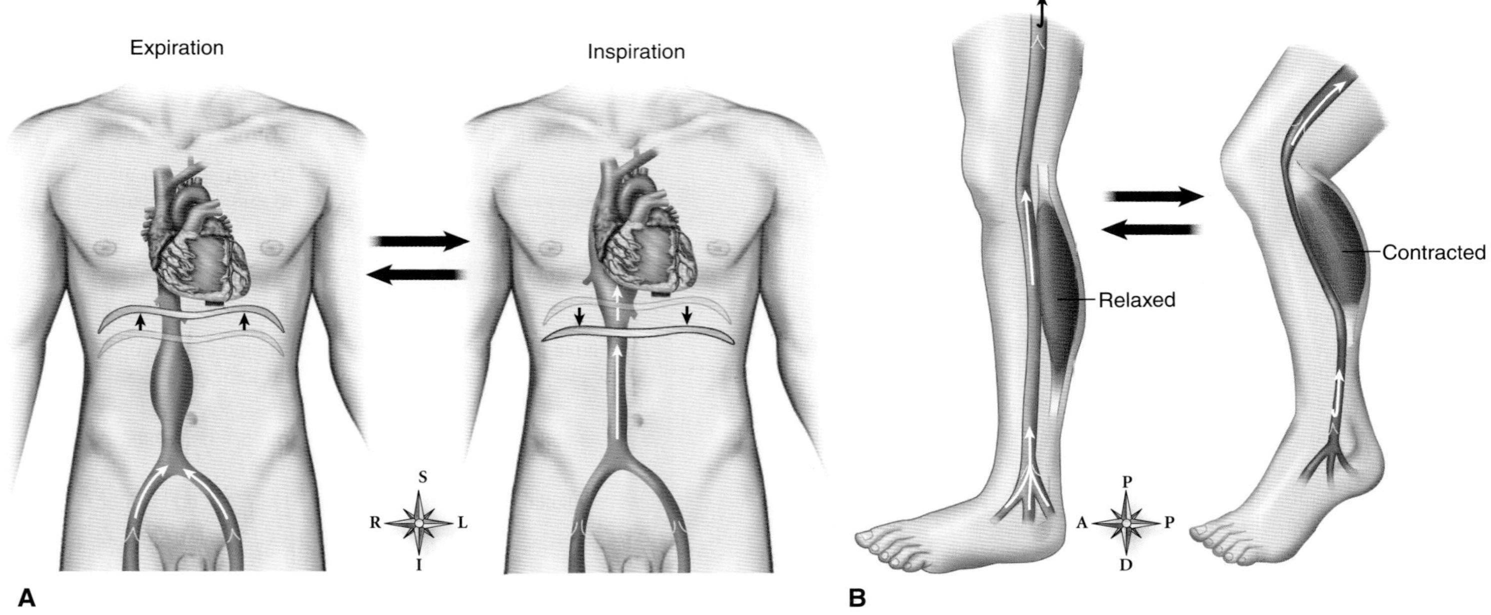

FIGURE 30-17 Venous pumping mechanisms. A, The respiratory pump operates by alternately increasing pressure in the thorax during expiration (thus pushing central venous blood into the heart) and decreasing thoracic pressure during inspiration (thus pulling venous blood into the central veins). **B,** The skeletal muscle pump operates by the alternate increase and decrease in peripheral venous pressure that normally occurs when the skeletal muscles are used for the activities of daily living. Both pumping mechanisms rely on the presence of one-way valves in the veins to prevent backflow during the low-pressure points in the pumping cycle (see **Figure 30-18**).

Deeper respirations intensify these effects and therefore tend to increase venous return to the heart more than normal respirations. This is part of the reason the principle is true—increased respirations and increased circulation tend to go hand in hand.

Skeletal muscle contractions serve as "booster pumps" for the heart. The skeletal muscle pump promotes venous return in the following way. As each skeletal muscle contracts, it squeezes the soft veins scattered through its interior, thereby "milking" the blood in them upward, or toward the heart (**Figure 30-17**, *B*). The closing of the one-way valves present in veins prevents blood from falling back as the muscle relaxes. Their flaps catch the blood as gravity pulls backward on it (**Figure 30-18**). The net effect of skeletal muscle contraction plus venous valvular action therefore is to move venous blood toward the heart, to increase the venous return.

The value of skeletal muscle contractions in moving blood through veins is illustrated by a common experience. Who has not noticed how much more uncomfortable and tiring standing still is than walking? After several minutes of standing quietly, the feet and legs feel "full" and swollen. Blood has accumulated in the veins because the skeletal muscles are not contracting and squeezing it upward. The repeated contractions of the muscles when walking naturally in comfortable shoes, on the other hand, keep the blood moving in the veins and prevent the discomfort of distended veins.

Total Blood Volume

The return of venous blood to the heart can be influenced by factors that change the total volume of blood in the closed circulatory pathway. Stated simply, the greater the total volume of blood, the greater the volume of blood returned to the heart. What mechanisms can increase or decrease the total volume of blood? The mechanisms that change total blood volume most quickly, making them most useful in maintaining constancy of blood flow, are those that cause water to quickly move into the plasma (increasing total blood volume) or out of the plasma (decreasing total blood volume). Most mechanisms that accomplish such changes in plasma volume operate by altering the body's retention of water.

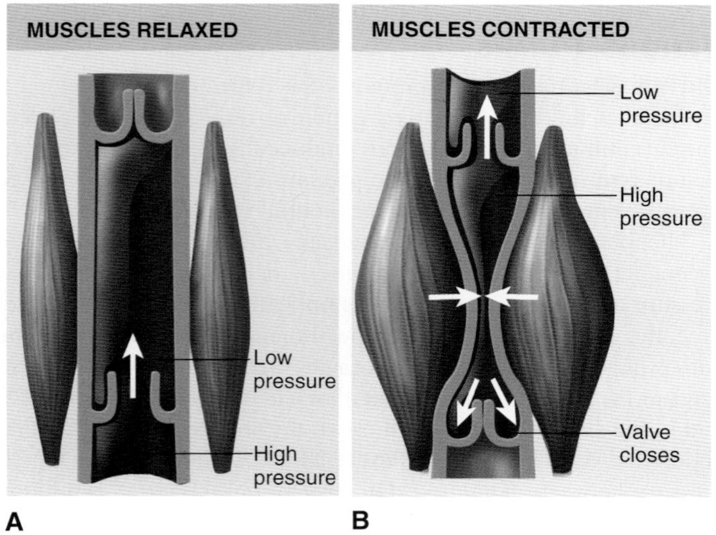

MUSCLES RELAXED
Low pressure
High pressure
A

MUSCLES CONTRACTED
Low pressure
High pressure
Valve closes
B

FIGURE 30-18 Venous valves. In veins, one-way valves aid circulation by preventing backflow of venous blood when pressure in a local area is low. **A,** Local high blood pressure pushes the flaps of the valve to the side of the vessel, allowing easy flow. **B,** When pressure below the valve drops, blood begins to flow backward but fills the "pockets" formed by the valve flaps, pushing the flaps together and thus blocking further backward flow.

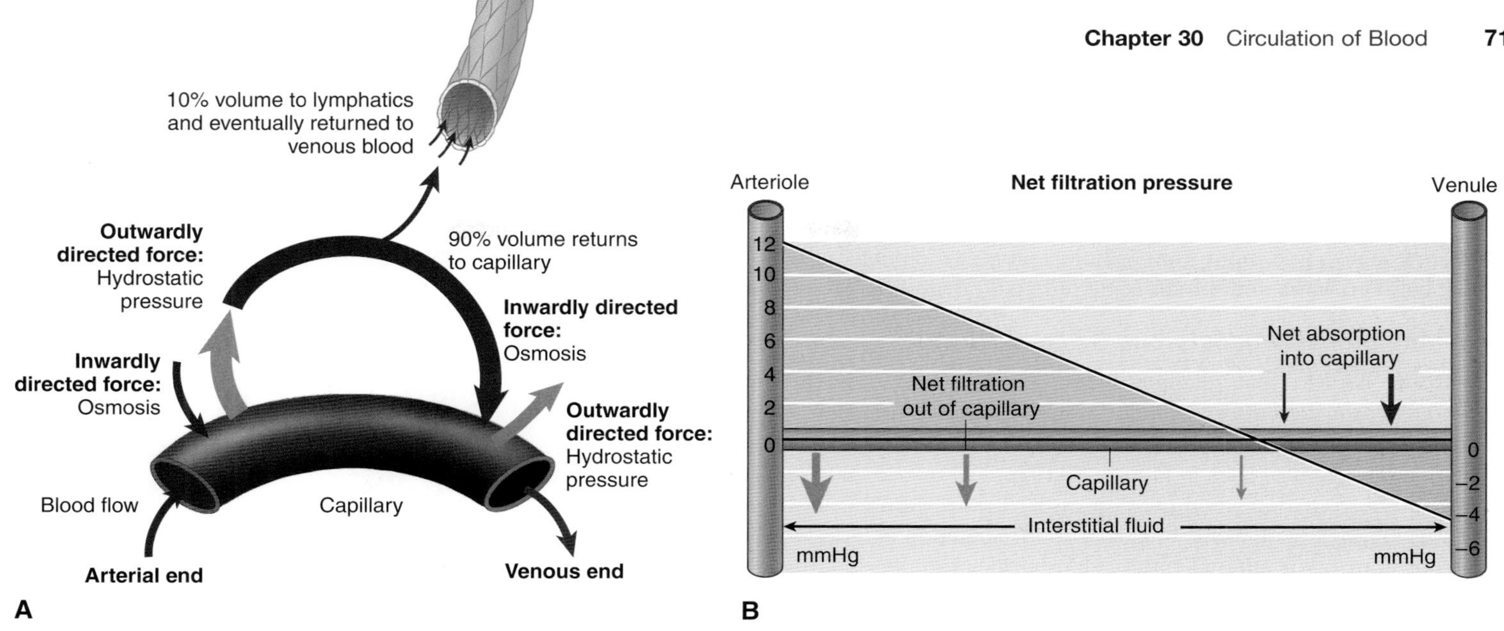

FIGURE 30-19 Starling's law of the capillaries. A, At the arterial end of a capillary the outward driving force of blood pressure (hydrostatic pressure of blood) is larger than the inwardly directed force of osmosis—thus fluid moves out of the vessel. At the venous end of a capillary the inward driving force of osmosis is greater than the outwardly directed force of hydrostatic pressure—thus fluid enters the vessel. About 90% of the fluid leaving the capillary at the arterial end is recovered by the blood before it leaves the venous end. The remaining 10% is recovered by the venous blood eventually, by way of the lymphatic vessels (see Chapter 31). **B,** Graph showing the shift in net filtration force along the length of a capillary, according to Starling's law of the capillaries. At the arterial end, net movement of fluid is *out of* the capillary; at the venous end, net movement of fluid shifts *into* the capillary.

Capillary Exchange and Total Blood Volume

We begin our discussion of fluid movement into and out of the blood plasma with a brief overview of **capillary exchange**—the exchange of materials between plasma in the capillaries and the surrounding interstitial fluid of the systemic tissues.

According to a principle first proposed by Ernest Starling, several factors govern the movement of fluid (and solutes contained in the fluid) back and forth across a capillary wall—a principle now known as **Starling's law of the capillaries.** These factors, illustrated in **Figure 30-19**, include inwardly directed forces and outwardly directed forces. It is the balance between these forces that determines whether fluids will move into or out of the plasma at any particular point.

One type of force, osmotic pressure, tends to promote diffusion of fluid into the plasma. Osmotic pressure generated by blood colloids (large solute particles such as plasma proteins) in the plasma that cannot cross the vessel wall tends to draw water osmotically into the plasma. At the arterial end of a capillary (and in some thin-walled arterioles) the potential osmotic pressure is small and thus generates only a small, inwardly directed force. However, a much larger, outwardly directed force is operating at the arterial end of a capillary, namely, a hydrostatic pressure gradient. Recall from Chapter 6 that hydrostatic pressure gradients promote filtration across a barrier with filtration pores, such as the capillary wall. At the arterial end of a capillary, the blood pressure in the vessel is much greater than the hydrostatic pressure of the interstitial fluid (IF), thus generating a very large, outwardly directed force. In short, the stronger, outwardly directed forces at the arterial end of a capillary drive fluids out of the blood vessel and into the surrounding IF—producing a net loss of blood volume.

At the venous end of the capillary, however, the loss of water has increased the blood colloid osmotic pressure—promoting osmosis of water back into the plasma. This inwardly directed force is much larger than the hydrostatic pressure gradient, which has dissipated somewhat with the loss of water at the arterial end of the vessel. In short, the capillary recovers much of the fluid it lost—recovering some of the previously lost blood volume.

If you look carefully at **Figure 30-19**, A, you will see that about 90% of the fluid lost at the arterial end of a capillary is recovered at the venous end by the forces operating in Starling's law of the capillaries. Does that mean that there is a constant loss of blood volume? No. Note that 10% of the fluid loss is recovered by the lymphatic system and returned to the venous blood before it reaches the heart. Details of how the lymphatic system accomplishes this fluid recovery are discussed in the next chapter. For now, we will simply state that if the lymphatic system operates normally and the osmotic and hydrostatic pressure gradients remain relatively constant, there is no net loss of blood volume resulting from capillary exchange. If any of these factors change, however, fluid retention by the blood and tissue fluids will be affected.

UNIT 4

CONNECT IT! ⓔ

For a quick refresher on the principle of osmosis and related terminology, check out the illustrated article ***Osmotic Pressure of a Solution*** online at ***Connect It!***

Changes in Total Blood Volume

You have already studied the primary mechanisms for altering water retention in the body—they are the endocrine reflexes previewed in Chapter 26.

ADH Mechanism

One endocrine reflex that regulates total blood volume is the *antidiuretic hormone (ADH) mechanism*. Recall that ADH is released by the neurohypophysis (posterior pituitary) and acts on the kidneys in a way that reduces the amount of water lost by the body. ADH does this by increasing the amount of water that the kidneys reabsorb from urine before the urine is excreted from the body. The more ADH is secreted, the more water will be reabsorbed into the blood from the urine, and the greater the blood plasma volume will become. The ADH mechanism can be triggered by various factors, such as input from baroreceptors and input from osmoreceptors (which detect the balance between water and solutes in the internal environment).

Renin–Angiotensin–Aldosterone System (RAAS)

Another mechanism that changes blood plasma volume is the *renin–angiotensin mechanism* of aldosterone secretion—the **renin–angiotensin–aldosterone system (RAAS).**

You may want to turn back to **Figure 26-19** (p. 594) to see that the enzyme renin is released when blood pressure in the kidney is low. Renin triggers a series of events that leads to the secretion of aldosterone, a hormone of the adrenal cortex. Aldosterone promotes sodium retention by the kidney, which in turn stimulates the osmotic flow of water from kidney tubules back into the blood plasma—but only when ADH is present to permit the movement of water. Thus low blood pressure increases the secretion of aldosterone, which in turn stimulates retention of water and thus an increase in blood volume.

Another effect of the renin–angiotensin mechanism is the vasoconstriction of blood vessels caused by an intermediate compound called *angiotensin II*. This complements the volume-increasing effects of the mechanism and thus also promotes an increase in overall blood flow. Because angiotensin-converting enzyme (ACE) regulates the amount of available angiotensin II, drugs that act as ACE inhibitors can reduce angiotensin II and thus block vasoconstriction—an effect that is useful in reducing abnormally high blood pressure (hypertension).

ANH Mechanism

Yet another mechanism that can change blood plasma volume and thus venous return of blood to the heart is the *atrial natriuretic hormone (ANH) mechanism*. Recall that ANH is secreted by specialized cells in the atrial wall in response to overstretching. Overstretching of the atrial wall, of course, occurs when venous return to the heart is abnormally high. ANH adjusts venous return back down to its setpoint value by promoting the loss of water from the plasma and the resulting decrease in blood volume. ANH accomplishes this feat by increasing urine sodium loss, which causes water to follow osmotically. Sodium loss also inhibits the secretion of ADH. ANH may also have other complementary effects, such as promoting vasodilation of blood reservoirs.

Balance of Regulation

Thus various mechanisms influence blood volume and therefore venous return. These primary mechanisms are summarized in **Figure 30-20**. The ANH mechanism opposes ADH and RAAS mechanisms to produce a balanced, precise control of blood volume. Precision of blood volume control contributes to precision in controlling venous return, which in turn contributes to precision in the overall control of blood circulation.

In summary, many different factors help regulate blood pressure and therefore regulate blood flow. **Figure 30-21** summarizes some of the rapidly acting, intermediate, and long-term responses that can return blood pressure and blood flow back to normal after a sudden change. Most of these responses have been discussed in this chapter and previous chapters, but some will be explored further in later chapters.

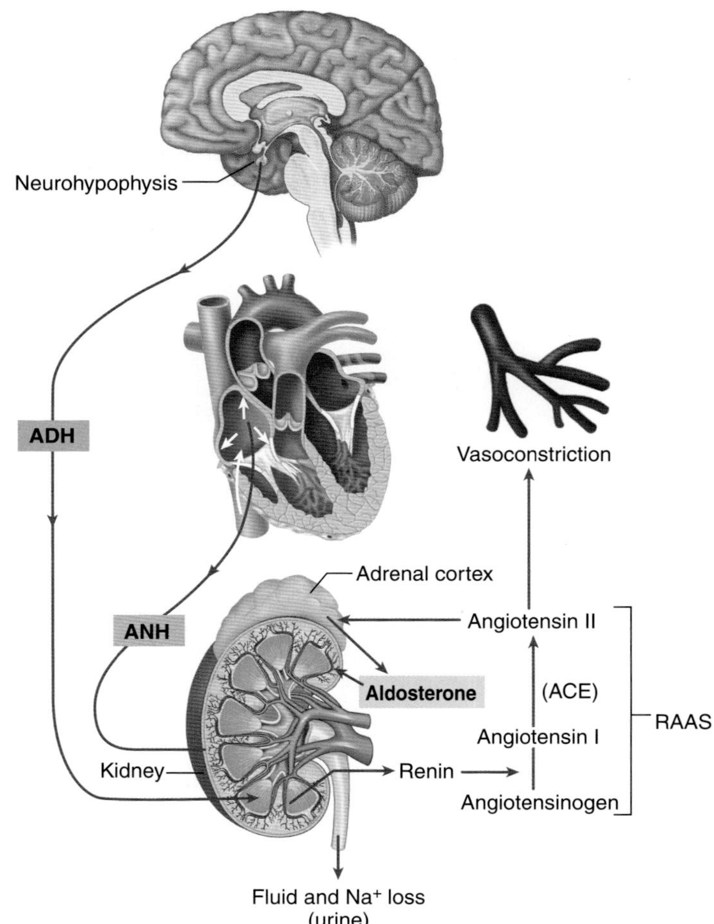

FIGURE 30-20 Three mechanisms that influence total plasma volume. The antidiuretic hormone (ADH) mechanism and renin–angiotensin–aldosterone system (RAAS) tend to increase water retention and thus increase total plasma volume. The atrial natriuretic hormone (ANH) mechanism antagonizes these mechanisms by promoting water loss and thus promoting a decrease in total plasma volume. *ACE,* Angiotensin-converting enzyme.

Quick **CHECK**

9. What is meant by the term *venous return*?
10. Briefly describe how the respiratory pump and skeletal muscle pump work.
11. How does Starling's law of the capillaries explain capillary exchange?
12. What three hormonal mechanisms work together to regulate blood volume?

MEASURING BLOOD PRESSURE

ARTERIAL BLOOD PRESSURE

Blood pressure is measured with the aid of an apparatus known as a **sphygmomanometer,** which makes it possible to measure the amount of air pressure equal to the blood pressure in an artery. The measurement is made in terms of how many millimetres (mm) high the air pressure raises a column of mercury (Hg) in a glass tube.

Sphygmomanometers originally consisted of a rubber cuff attached by a rubber tube to a compressible bulb and by another tube to a column of mercury that was marked off in millimetres

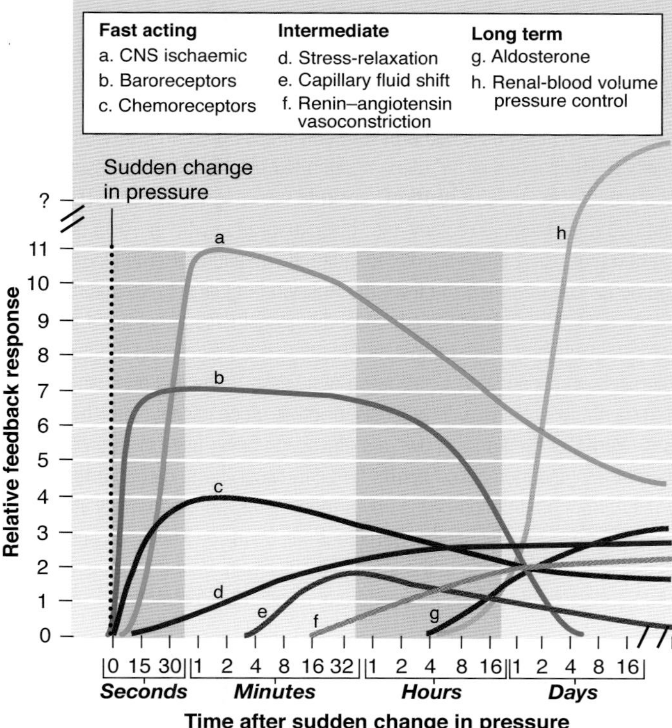

FIGURE 30-21 Feedback responses of various arterial pressure mechanisms. This composite graph shows the relative regulatory shifts that can be carried out by different regulatory mechanisms in response to a sudden shift in blood pressure—all with the outcome of moving arterial blood pressure back to its setpoint value. Note that some responses have their maximum effect within a few seconds or minutes. Other responses take longer to reach their maximum effect. *CNS,* Central nervous system.

(**Figure 30-22**). Pressure in the cuff and rubber tube pushes the column of mercury to a new height. Therefore, pressure can be expressed as *millimetres of mercury (mmHg).* Because of the hazardous nature of mercury, many sphygmomanometers in use today have mercury-free mechanical or electronic pressure sensors that are calibrated to the mercury scale.

The cuff of the sphygmomanometer is wrapped around the arm over the brachial artery, and air is pumped into the cuff by means of the bulb. In this way, air pressure is exerted against the outside of the artery. Air is added until the air pressure exceeds the blood pressure within the artery or, in other words, until it compresses the artery. At this time, no pulse can be heard through a stethoscope placed over the brachial artery at the bend of the elbow along the inner margin of the biceps muscle.

By slowly releasing the air in the cuff, the air pressure is decreased until it approximately equals the blood pressure within the artery. At this point, the vessel opens slightly and a small spurt of blood comes through, producing sharp "tapping" sounds. This is followed by increasingly louder sounds that change suddenly. They become more muffled, then disappear altogether. These sounds are often called *Korotkoff sounds* (**Box 30-2**).

Health professionals train themselves to hear the Korotkoff sounds and simultaneously read the column of mercury, because the first tapping sound appears when the column of mercury indicates the **systolic blood pressure.** Systolic pressure is the force with which the blood is pushing against the artery walls at its highest pressure—during the ejection phase of the cardiac cycle when the ventricles are contracting. The lowest point at which the sounds can be heard, just before they disappear, is approximately equal to the **diastolic blood pressure,** or the force of the blood against the arterial walls when the ventricles are relaxed. Diastolic pressure is observed at the end of ventricular relaxation and as isovolumetric contraction of the ventricle occurs, as you can see near the top of the diagram in **Figure 28-18** (p. 654).

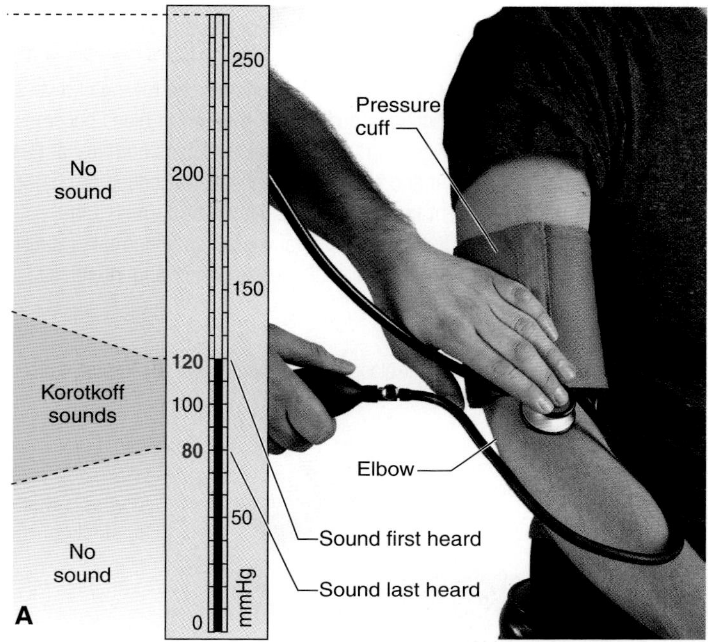

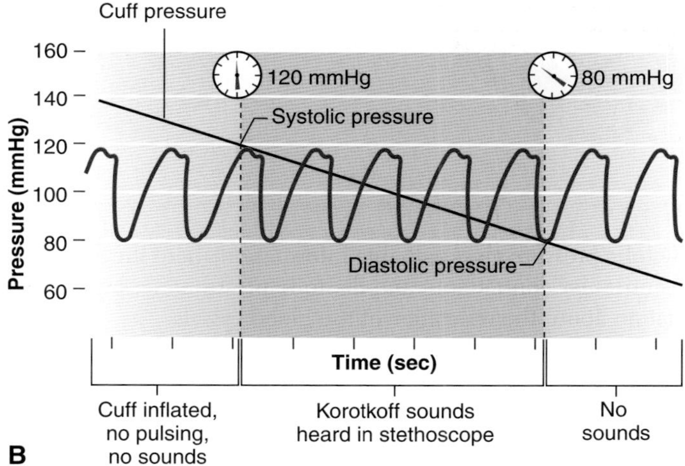

FIGURE 30-22 Sphygmomanometer. This mercury-filled pressure sensor is used in clinical and research settings to quickly and accurately measure arterial blood pressure. **A,** The pressure cuff is pumped with air until the pressure inside the cuff exceeds the expected systolic pressure of the large arteries of the arm. No sound caused by pulsing of blood in the arteries can then be heard with a stethoscope. As the pressure inside the cuff is slowly released from a valve, the air pressure equals the maximum pressure of the pulse waves in the artery—thus the pulsing sounds can then be heard. **B,** The sounds of pulsing (Korotkoff sounds) continue as long as the cuff pressure is equal to pressures of the pulse wave. The sounds disappear at the point that cuff pressure drops below the minimum pulse pressure in the arteries.

BOX 30-2 *diagnostic study* | Focus on Turbulent Blood Flow

Understanding the mechanics of fluid flow through blood vessels facilitates comprehension of the bigger picture of haemodynamics.

Normally, blood flows through vessels with smooth walls that taper or enlarge only slightly, if at all. The manner in which a fluid, in this case blood, flows through a smooth vessel is termed **laminar flow.** The Latin word *lamina* means layer, an apt description of the way fluids flow through tubes in concentric, cylindrical layers—as you can see in part *A* of the figure. Because of friction against the inner face of the vessel wall, the outer layers of blood flow more slowly than the inner layers. Laminar flow is the normal pattern of blood flow in most healthy vessels.

When smooth, laminar flow is disrupted by branching or narrowing of a vessel, a sharp turn, or a sudden constriction or obstruction, the flow of blood becomes turbulent. **Turbulent flow,** shown in part *B* of the figure, occurs normally at heart valves and contributes to the first and second heart sounds described on p. 656.

However, significant turbulent flow in most vessels is not normal. If the sounds of turbulence are detected in a peripheral vessel, an abnormal or unusual constriction may exist. Such constrictions could be temporary and intentional, as in the case of an inflated blood pressure cuff pressing on an artery and creating turbulence. The sounds of turbulence generated by such blood pressure measurements are called **Korotkoff sounds** (see **Figure 30-22**). These sounds are named after Nicolai Korotkov, the Russian surgeon who in 1905 developed the method for using these sounds to indirectly measure arterial blood pressure. His name has been romanized from the Russian language to Korotkoff.

Some sounds of turbulence are caused by constrictions that are a serious threat to one's health. For example, in Chapter 29 we discussed the fact that arteriosclerosis can cause such a narrowing of a vessel's channel and can ultimately lead to death by ischaemia, thrombosis, or other mechanisms (see **Figure 29-26**). Part *C* of the figure shows a stethoscope being used to listen for low-pitched blowing sounds called **bruits** that can occur in the carotid arteries. Bruits may result from obstruction caused by arteriosclerosis or abnormally increased pulse pressure. A usually benign, but abnormal, condition known as venous hum produces a humming noise in the internal jugular vein. Venous hum is common in children and probably results from vigorous myocardial contraction. •

Turbulent blood flow. A, Laminar blood flow (no turbulence). **B,** Turbulent blood flow. **C,** Listening for bruits.

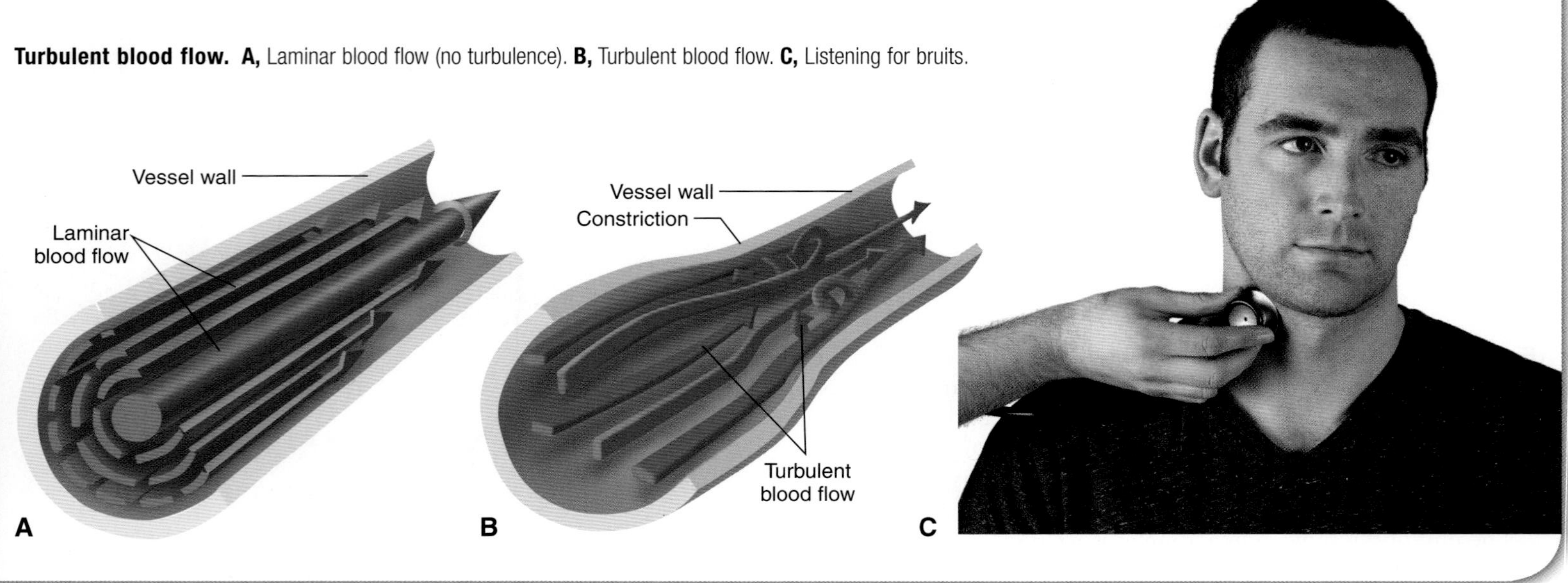

Systolic pressure gives valuable information about the force of the left ventricular contraction, and diastolic pressure gives valuable information about the resistance of the blood vessels.

Blood in the arteries of an adult with a blood pressure reading at the high end of the normal range exerts a pressure equal to that required to raise a column of mercury about 120 mm high in a glass tube during systole of the ventricles and 80 mm high during diastole. For the sake of brevity, this is expressed as a blood pressure of "120 over 80" or 120/80. The first, or upper, figure represents systolic pressure, and the second represents diastolic pressure. Note, the SI unit for pressure the pascal (Pa) has not been adopted in clinical practice for measuring blood pressure.

From the figures just given, we can see that blood pressure fluctuates considerably during each heartbeat. During ventricular systole, the force is great enough to raise the mercury column 40 mm higher than during ventricular diastole. This difference between systolic and diastolic pressure is called **pulse pressure (PP).** It characteristically increases in arteriosclerosis, mainly because systolic pressure increases more than diastolic pressure. Pulse pressure increases even more markedly in aortic valve insufficiency because of both a rise in systolic pressure and a fall in diastolic pressure.

The **mean arterial pressure (MAP)** is an average blood pressure in the arteries often calculated by this equation:

$$\text{MAP} = \frac{(2 \times \text{diastolic BP}) + \text{systolic BP}}{3}$$

For a BP of 120/80, the MAP would be 93 mmHg using this equation. Diastolic pressure is weighted more heavily to calculate the average because about two thirds of the cardiac cycle is spent in ventricular diastole. A MAP of at least 60 mmHg is enough perfusion pressure to sufficiently supply the coronary arteries, brain, kidneys, and other vital organs. If the MAP drops below this number, vital tissues may become ischaemic and cease to function. MAP normally ranges between 70 mmHg to 110 mmHg at rest.

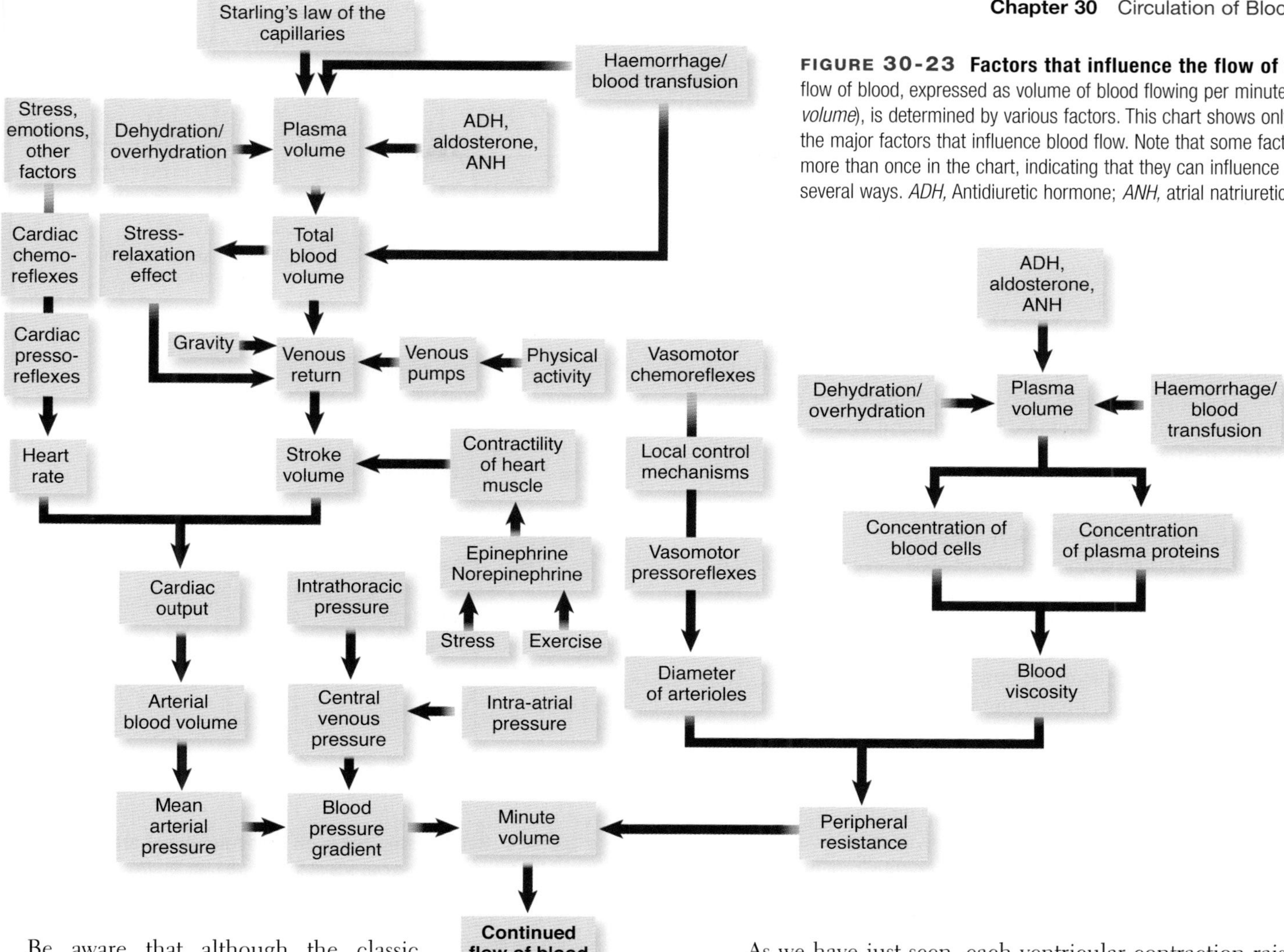

FIGURE 30-23 Factors that influence the flow of blood. The flow of blood, expressed as volume of blood flowing per minute (or *minute volume*), is determined by various factors. This chart shows only some of the major factors that influence blood flow. Note that some factors appear more than once in the chart, indicating that they can influence blood flow in several ways. *ADH,* Antidiuretic hormone; *ANH,* atrial natriuretic hormone.

Be aware that although the classic method of indirect arterial blood pressure assessment involves a column of mercury, and the units in which blood pressure is expressed are based on the height of a mercury column, very few modern sphygmomanometers actually use mercury. The reason is twofold. First, mercury is a very hazardous substance. Should the mercury column break, an environmental health hazard would be created. Second, it is much more cost-effective to use inexpensive and durable mechanical or electronic pressure sensors that are calibrated to the mercury scale than to construct fragile columns of mercury in glass.

Blood pressure can also be measured directly in various ways. For example, a small tube called a *cannula* with a removable pointed insert can be pushed directly into a vessel, the insert withdrawn, and the cannula connected to a manometer or electronic pressure sensor. A long, flexible tube called a *catheter* can likewise be placed in a blood vessel or even into a chamber of the heart. These techniques can be used in critical care, but the more indirect methods described previously are more practical for routine screening and clinical evaluation.

Blood Pressure and Bleeding

Because blood exerts a comparatively high pressure in arteries and a very low pressure in veins, it gushes forth with considerable force from a cut artery but seeps in a slow, steady stream from a vein.

As we have just seen, each ventricular contraction raises arterial blood pressure to the systolic level, and each ventricular relaxation lowers it to the diastolic level. As the ventricles contract, the blood spurts forth forcefully because of the increased pressure in the artery, but as the ventricles relax, the flow ebbs to almost nothing because of the fall in pressure. In other words, blood escapes from an artery in spurts because of the alternate raising and lowering of arterial blood pressure but flows slowly and steadily from a vein because of the low, practically constant pressure.

A uniform, instead of a pulsating, pressure exists in the capillaries and veins. Why? Because the arterial walls, being elastic, continue to squeeze the blood forward while the ventricles are in diastole. Therefore blood enters capillaries and veins under a relatively steady pressure (see **Figure 30-2**).

MINUTE VOLUME OF BLOOD

The volume of blood circulating through the body per minute (**minute volume**) is determined by the magnitude of the blood pressure gradient and the peripheral resistance (**Figure 30-23**).

A nineteenth-century physiologist and physicist, Jean Poiseuille, described the relation between these three factors—pressure gradient, resistance, and minute volume—with a mathematical equation known as **Poiseuille's law.** In general, but with certain modifications, it applies to blood circulation. We can state the law in a simplified form as follows: the volume of blood circulated per minute is directly related to mean arterial pressure minus central venous pressure and is inversely related to resistance:

$$\text{Volume of blood circulated per minute} = \frac{\text{Mean arterial pressure} - \text{Central venous pressure}}{\text{Resistance}}$$

$$\text{Minute volume} = \frac{\text{Pressure gradient}}{\text{Resistance}}$$

This mathematical relationship needs qualifying with regard to the influence of peripheral resistance on circulation. For instance, according to the equation, an increase in peripheral resistance tends to decrease blood flow. (Why? Increasing peripheral resistance increases the denominator of the fraction in the preceding equation. Increasing the denominator of any fraction necessarily does what to its value? It decreases the value of the fraction.)

Increased peripheral resistance, however, has a secondary action that opposes its primary tendency to decrease blood flow. An increase in peripheral resistance hinders or decreases arteriole runoff. This, of course, tends to increase the volume of blood left in the arteries and so tends to increase arterial pressure.

Note also that increasing arterial pressure tends to increase the value of the fraction in Poiseuille's equation. Therefore it tends to increase circulation. In short, to say unequivocally what the effect of an increased peripheral resistance will be on circulation is impossible. It depends also on arterial blood pressure—whether it increases, decreases, or stays the same when peripheral resistance increases. The clinical condition *arteriosclerosis with hypertension* (high blood pressure) illustrates this point. Both peripheral resistance and arterial pressure are increased in this condition. If resistance were to increase more than arterial pressure, circulation (i.e., volume of blood flow per minute) would decrease. But if arterial pressure increases proportionately to resistance, circulation remains normal.

Quick CHECK

13. What is meant by the term *minute volume*?
14. How is minute volume related to peripheral resistance?

VELOCITY OF BLOOD FLOW

The speed with which the blood flows—that is, distance per minute—through its vessels is governed in part by the physical principle that when a liquid flows from an area of one cross-sectional size to an area of larger size, its velocity slows in the area with the larger cross-section (**Figure 30-24**). For example, a narrow river whose bed widens flows more slowly through the wide section than through the narrow section.

In terms of the blood vascular system, the total cross-sectional area of all arterioles together is greater than that of the arteries. Therefore blood flows more slowly through arterioles than through arteries. Likewise, the total cross-sectional area of all capillaries together is greater than that of all arterioles, and therefore capillary flow is slower than arteriole flow. The venule cross-sectional area, on the other hand, is smaller than the capillary cross-sectional area.

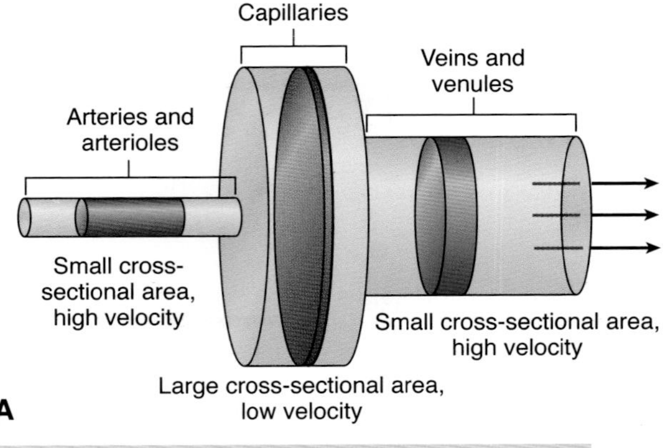

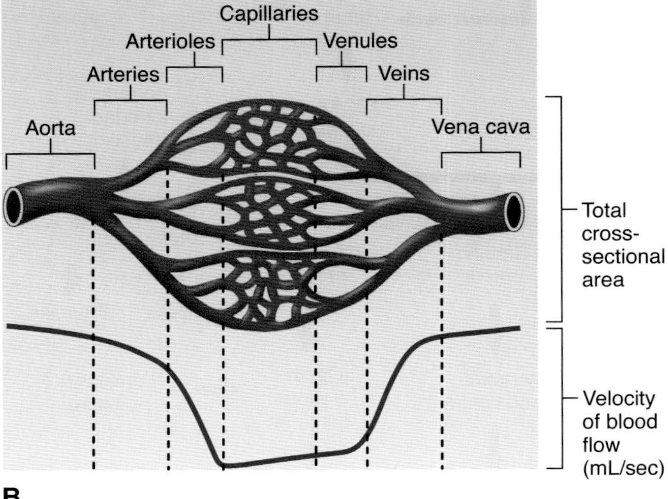

FIGURE 30-24 Relationship between cross-sectional area and velocity of blood flow. As you can see in the simple diagram **(A)** and the blood vessel chart **(B),** blood flows with great speed in the large arteries. However, branching of arterial vessels increases the total cross-sectional area of the arterioles and capillaries, reducing the flow rate. When capillaries merge into venules and venules merge into veins, the total cross-sectional area decreases, causing the flow rate to increase.

Therefore blood velocity increases in venules and again in veins, which have a still smaller cross-sectional area.

In short, the most rapid blood flow takes place in arteries and the slowest in capillaries. Can you think of a valuable effect stemming from the fact that blood flows most slowly through the capillaries?

PULSE

MECHANISM

Pulse is defined as the alternate expansion and recoil of an artery. Two factors are responsible for the existence of a pulse that can be felt:

1. Intermittent injections of blood from the heart into the aorta, which alternately increase and decrease the pressure in that vessel. If blood poured steadily out of the heart into the aorta, the pressure there would remain constant and there would be no pulse.
2. The elasticity of the arterial walls, which allows them to expand with each injection of blood and then recoil. If the vessels were fashioned from rigid material such as glass, there would still be an alternate raising and lowering of pressure within them with each systole and diastole of the ventricles, but the walls could not expand and recoil and therefore no pulse could be felt.

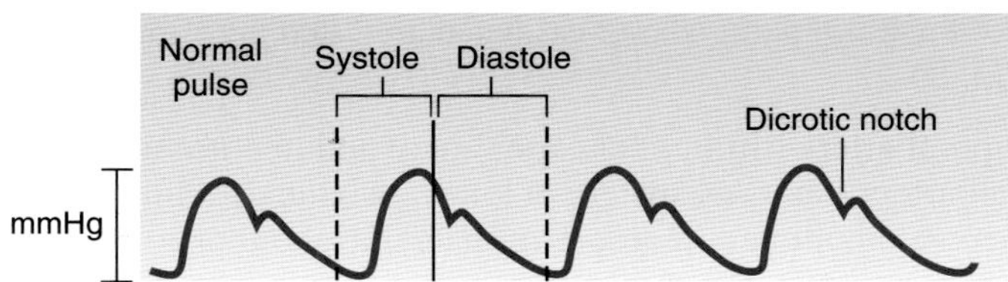

FIGURE 30-25 Normal carotid pulse wave. This series of pulse waves shows rhythmic increases and decreases in pressure as measured at the common carotid artery in the neck. The dicrotic notch represents the pressure fluctuation generated by closure of the aortic valve.

Pulse Wave

Each ventricular systole starts a new pulse that proceeds as a wave of expansion throughout the arteries and is known as the pulse wave. It gradually dissipates as it travels, disappearing entirely in the capillaries.

The pulse wave felt at the common carotid artery in the neck is large and powerful, rapidly following the first heart sound. **Figure 30-25** shows that the carotid pulse wave begins during ventricular systole. Note that the closure of the aortic valve produces a detectable *dicrotic notch* in the pulse wave. However, the pulse felt in the radial artery at the wrist does not coincide with the contraction of the ventricles. It follows each contraction by an appreciable interval (the length of time required for the pulse wave to travel from the aorta to the radial artery). The farther from the heart the pulse is taken, therefore, the longer that interval is.

Almost everyone is aware of the diagnostic importance of the pulse. It reveals important information about the cardiovascular system, heart action, blood vessels, and circulation.

Not everyone is aware of the basic functional role of the pulse wave, however. The pulse wave actually conserves energy produced by the pumping action of the heart (**Figure 30-26**). The great force of pressure with which blood is ejected from the heart during ventricular systole expands the wall of the aorta. At that point, the stretched aortic wall has potential energy stored in it—just as a stretched rubber band has potential energy. During ventricular diastole, the elastic nature of the aortic wall allows it to recoil. This recoil exerts pressure on the blood and thus keeps it moving. If the wall of the aorta were inelastic, it would not alternately expand and recoil—and would thus not keep blood moving continuously. Instead, arterial blood would simply spurt, then stop, then spurt, then stop, and so on.

Where the Pulse Can Be Felt

The pulse can be felt wherever an artery lies near the surface and over a bone or other firm background. Some specific locations

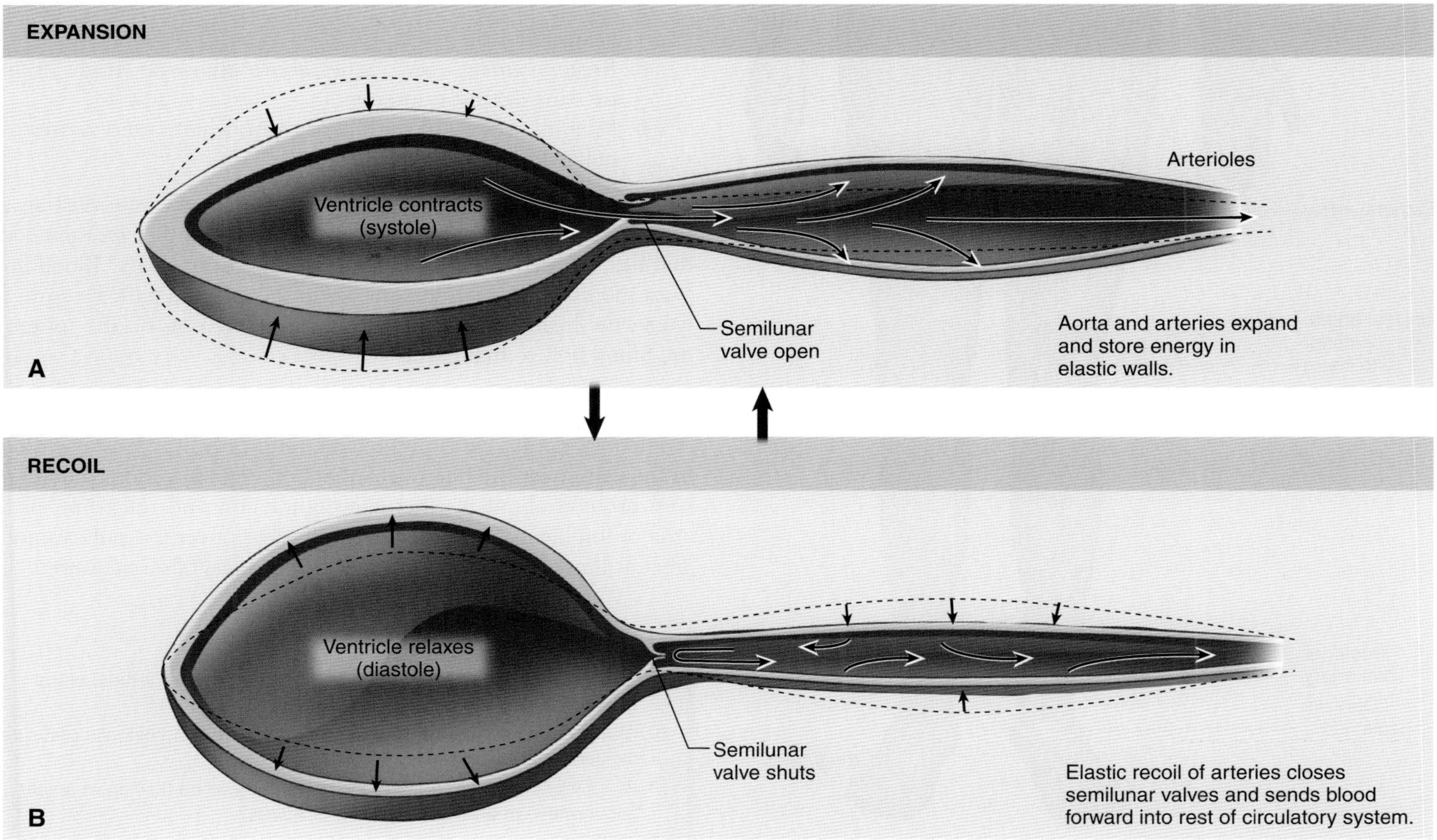

EXPANSION
Ventricle contracts (systole)
Arterioles
Semilunar valve open
Aorta and arteries expand and store energy in elastic walls.
A

RECOIL
Ventricle relaxes (diastole)
Semilunar valve shuts
Elastic recoil of arteries closes semilunar valves and sends blood forward into rest of circulatory system.
B

FIGURE 30-26 Functional role of the pulse wave. The arterial pulse conserves energy by absorbing and storing force from the ventricular contraction by causing elastic expansion of the arterial wall. The energy is used to maintain continued blood flow during ventricular relaxation by elastic recoil of the arterial wall—thus producing enough arterial pressure to keep blood flowing.

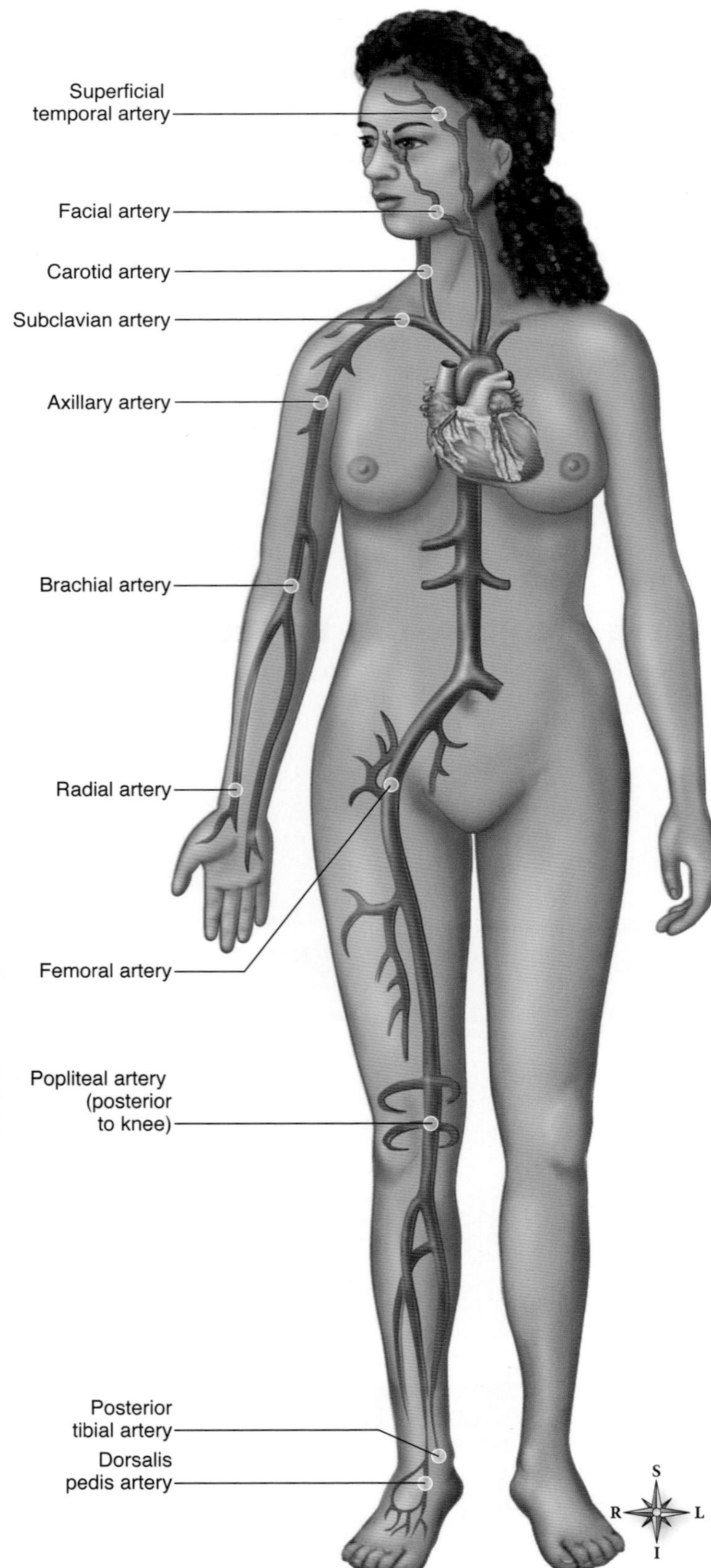

FIGURE 30-27 Pulse points. Each pulse point is named after the artery with which it is associated. (Some arteries in the figure have been enlarged to clarify the location of pulse points.)

where the pulse point is most easily felt are listed here and shown in **Figure 30-27**:

Temporal artery—in front of ear or above and to outer side of eye
Facial artery—at lower margin of lower jawbone on a line with corners of mouth and in groove in mandible about one third of the way forward from angle
Common carotid artery—along anterior edge of sternocleidomastoid muscle at level of lower margin of thyroid cartilage
Subclavian artery—deep to superior margin of the clavicle
Axillary artery—in armpit
Brachial artery—at bend of elbow along inner margin of biceps muscle
Radial artery—at wrist
Femoral artery—in middle of groin, where artery passes over pelvic bone
Popliteal artery—behind the knee
Posterior tibial artery—behind the medial malleolus (inner "ankle bone")
Dorsalis pedis artery—on dorsum (upper surface) of foot

Six important pressure points can be used to stop arterial bleeding:

1. *Temporal artery*—in front of ear
2. *Facial artery*—same place at which pulse is taken
3. *Common carotid artery*—point where pulse is taken, with pressure back against spinal column
4. *Subclavian artery*—behind medial third of clavicle, pressing against first rib
5. *Brachial artery*—few inches above elbow on inside of arm, pressing against humerus
6. *Femoral artery*—in middle of groin, where artery passes over pelvic bone (where pulse is felt)

In trying to stop arterial bleeding by pressure, one must always remember to apply the pressure at the pulse point, or *pressure point*, that lies between the bleeding part and the heart. Why? Blood flows from the heart through the arteries to the affected part. Pressure between the heart and bleeding point therefore cuts off the source of the blood flow to that point.

Venous Pulse

A detectable pulse exists in the large veins only. It is most prominent in the veins near the heart because of changes in venous blood pressure brought about by alternate contraction and relaxation of the atria of the heart. The clinical significance of venous pulse is not as great as that of arterial pulse, and thus it is less often measured.

Quick CHECK

15. What device is used in clinical settings to measure arterial blood pressure?
16. Which is more important for assessing health—the systolic pressure or the diastolic pressure?
17. In which type of vessel is blood most likely to be flowing at a very slow rate—an artery, a capillary, or a vein?
18. Without being specific, where are pulse points normally located in the body?

cycle of life

Cardiovascular Physiology Changes in the function of the heart and blood vessels usually parallel the structural changes in these organs over the life span. For example, changes at the time of birth that adapt the circulatory system to life outside the womb cause changes in the blood pressure gradients that alter the flow of blood in many parts of the body. Likewise, the degenerative changes associated with ageing reduce the heart's ability to maintain cardiac output and the ability of arteries to withstand high pressure.

Changes in arterial blood pressure are among the most apparent changes in the function of the cardiovascular system associated with the progression through the life cycle. In a newborn, normal arterial blood pressure is only about 90/55 mmHg—much lower than the arterial pressure of just under 120/80 mmHg in most healthy young adults. In older adults hypertension can develop—with arterial blood pressures commonly reaching 150/90 mmHg.

Another commonly observed change in cardiovascular function relates to heart rate. The heart rates of infants and children typically vary more than those in adults. Compared with adults, children often exhibit very large increases in heart rate in response to stressors such as illness, pain, tension, and exercise. Whereas a typical resting heart rate for adults is about 72 beats/min, the resting heart rate of a newborn can range from 120 to 170 beats/min, and the resting heart rate of a preschooler can range from 80 to 160 beats/min. In older adults, resting heart rates range from lows of around 40 beats/min to 100 beats/min. •

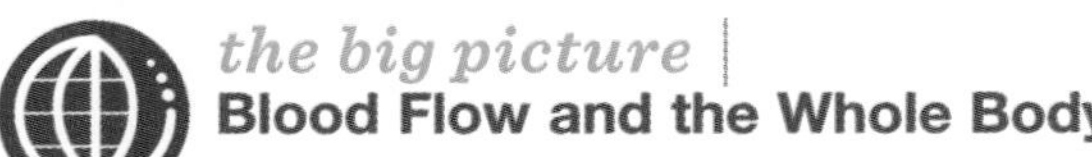

the big picture | Blood Flow and the Whole Body

As stated in this chapter and many times throughout this book, one of the essential concepts of homeostasis is the renewable fluid that makes up our internal environment. If we were not able to maintain the chemical nature and other physical characteristics of our internal fluid environment, we would not survive.

To maintain the constancy of the internal fluid, we must be able to shift nutrients, gases, hormones, waste products, agents of immunity, and other materials around in the body. As certain materials are depleted in one tissue and new materials enter the internal environment in another tissue, redistribution must occur. What better way than through a system of circulating fluid? This fluid shifts materials from place to place and also redistributes heat and pressure. Recall from your study of the integumentary and muscular systems that shifting the flow of blood to or away from warm tissues at the proper time is essential to maintaining the homeostasis of body temperature. As we will learn in Chapter 42, the ability of our blood to increase or decrease blood pressure in the kidney has a great impact on that organ's vital function of filtering the internal environment. Understanding the basic mechanisms of almost any system in the body requires an understanding of the dynamics of blood flow.

What we have seen in this chapter is a wonderfully complex array of mechanisms that work together in concert with the actions of other systems to maintain the constancy of the *milieu intérieur*—the internal environment. •

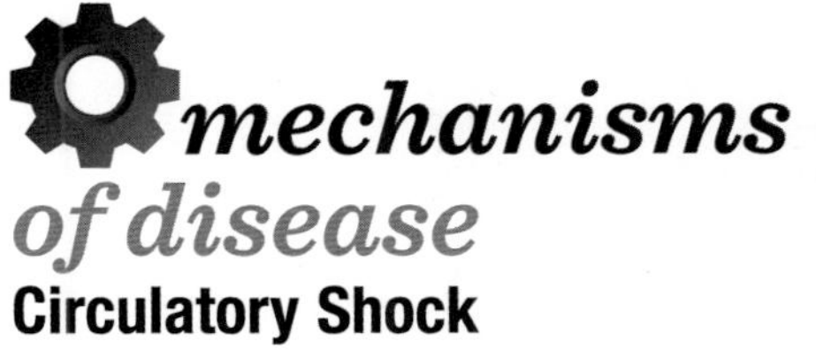

mechanisms of disease
Circulatory Shock

The term **circulatory shock** refers to the failure of the circulatory system to adequately deliver oxygen to the tissues, resulting in the impairment of cell function throughout the body. If left untreated, circulatory shock may lead to death. Circulatory failure has many causes, all of which somehow reduce the flow of blood through the blood vessels of the body. Because of the variety of causes, circulatory shock is often classified into the following types:

Cardiogenic shock results from any type of heart failure, such as that after severe myocardial infarction (heart attack), heart infections, and other heart conditions. Because the heart can no longer pump blood effectively, blood flow to the tissues of the body decreases or stops.

Hypovolaemic shock results from the loss of blood volume in the blood vessels (hypovolaemia means "low blood volume"). Reduced blood volume results in low blood pressure and reduced flow of blood to tissues. Haemorrhage is a common cause of blood volume loss leading to hypovolemic shock. Hypovolaemia can also be caused by loss of interstitial fluid, causing a drain of blood plasma out of the vessels and into the tissue spaces. Loss of interstitial fluid is common in chronic diarrhoea or vomiting, dehydration, intestinal blockage, severe or extensive burns, and other conditions.

Neurogenic shock results from widespread dilation of blood vessels caused by an imbalance in autonomic stimulation of smooth muscle in vessel walls. It is also sometimes called **vasodilatory shock.** You may recall from Chapter 22 that autonomic effectors such as smooth muscle tissues are controlled by a balance of stimulation from the sympathetic and parasympathetic divisions of the autonomic nervous system. Normally, sympathetic stimulation maintains the muscle tone that keeps blood vessels at their usual diameter. If sympathetic stimulation is disrupted by an injury to the spinal cord or medulla, depressive drugs, emotional stress, or some other factor, blood vessels dilate significantly. Widespread vasodilation reduces blood pressure, thus reducing blood flow.

Anaphylactic shock results from an acute allergic reaction called *anaphylaxis.* Anaphylaxis causes the same kind of blood vessel dilation characteristic of neurogenic shock.

Septic shock results from complications of septicaemia, a condition in which infectious agents release toxins into the blood. The toxins often dilate blood vessels, thereby causing shock. The situation is usually made worse by the damaging effects of the toxins on tissues combined with the increased cell activity caused by the accompanying fever. One type of septic shock is *toxic shock syndrome (TSS),* which usually results from staphylococcal infections that begin in the vagina of menstruating women and spread to the blood.

The body has numerous mechanisms that compensate for the changes that occur during shock. However, these mechanisms may fail to compensate for changes that occur in severe cases, and this failure often results in death.

Hypertension

One of the most frequent reasons for a patient visiting their doctor is a condition called **hypertension (HTN).** In the UK it accounts for approximately 12% of all consultations, and it is estimated that more than 24% of the population have GP recorded or undiagnosed hypertension. This condition occurs when the force of blood exerted by the arterial blood vessel exceeds a blood pressure of 140/90 mmHg. Ninety percent of HTN cases are classified as *primary-essential,* or idiopathic, with no single known causative etiology. Another classification, *secondary HTN,* is caused by kidney disease or hormonal problems or induced by oral contraceptives, pregnancy, or other causes.

The chart in **Figure 30-28** shows the range of blood pressures used to aid the diagnosis of hypertension and grade the condition according to severity.

Blood Pressure (BP) Classification

Category	Systolic		Diastolic
Optimal	<120	and	<80
Normal	120–129	and/or	80–84
High normal	130–139	and/or	85–89
Grade 1 hypertension	140–159	and/or	90–99
Grade 2 hypertension	160–179	and/or	100–109
Grade 3 hypertension	≥180	and/or	≥110
Isolated systolic hypertension	≥140	and	<90

140/90

FIGURE 30-28 Classification of hypertension.

Many risk factors have been identified in the development of HTN. Genetic factors play a large role. There is an increased susceptibility or predisposition with a family history of HTN. Up to the age of 64, men in the UK experience more HTN than women. Studies have also shown that people of recent African origin have rates of HTN that exceed those of European descent. There is also a direct relationship between age and high blood pressure. This is because as age advances, the blood vessels become less compliant and there is a higher incidence of atherosclerotic plaque buildup. HTN can also be fatal if undetected in women taking oral contraceptives. Risk factors include high stress levels, obesity, calcium deficiencies, high levels of alcohol and caffeine intake, smoking, and lack of exercise.

Untreated HTN has many potential complications. Ischaemic heart disease and heart failure, kidney failure, and stroke are some examples. As many as 152,000 people per year experience a stroke. Because HTN manifests minimal or no overt signs, it is known as the "silent killer". Headaches, dizziness, and fainting have been reported but are not always symptomatic of HTN. Regular screenings at workplaces, health centres and hospitals often help to identify asymptomatic HTN.

Hypotension

Blood pressure that is lower than normal is called **hypotension,** or low blood pressure. Hypotension may be temporary, as in *orthostatic hypotension* when a person stands up suddenly (see **Figure 30-16** on p. 711) or when blood pressure drops because of a sudden loss of blood. Unexplained or *essential* hypotension is generally chronic and may result from heart disease or genetic influences. Whether acute or chronic, hypotension may cause rapid heart rate and pulse as the body attempts to maintain constant blood pressure for good circulation. Rapid heart rate may, in turn, lead to dysrhythmias or other cardiac problems. If normal circulation cannot be maintained, reduced blood flow in local areas may cause damage or dysfunction in the affected areas. For example, hypotension in the elderly may cause cognitive impairment when proper blood flow to the brain cannot be maintained.

LANGUAGE OF SCIENCE *(continued from p. 699)*

orthostatic effect (or-thoh-STAT-ik ef-FEKT) [*ortho-* **upright,** *-stat-* **standing,** *-ic* **relating to,** *effect* **accomplishment**]

perfusion pressure (per-FYOO-shun) [*per-* **through,** *-fus-* **pour,** *-sion* **process**]

peripheral resistance (peh-RIF-er-al ree-ZIS-tens) [*peri-* **around,** *-phera-* **boundary,** *-al* **relating to,** *resist-* **withstand,** *-ance* **act of**]

Poiseuille's law (pwah-ZWEE-ez) [*Jean L.M. Poiseuille* **French physiologist**]

pressoreflex (pres-oh-REE-fleks) [*press-* **pressure,** *-re-* **back or again,** *-flex* **bend**]

renin–angiotensin–aldosterone system (RAAS) (REE-nin-an-jee-oh-TEN-sin-al-DOS-tair-ohn) [*ren-* **kidney,** *-in* **substance,** *angio-* **vessel,** *-tens-* **pressure or stretch,** *-in* **substance,** *aldo-* **aldehyde,** *-stero-* **solid or steroid derivative,** *-one* **chemical**]

Starling's law of the capillaries (STAR-lingz) [*Ernest H. Starling* **English physiologist,** *capill-* **hair,** *-ary* **relating to**]

Starling's law of the heart (STAR-lingz) [*Ernest H. Starling* **English physiologist**]

stress-relaxation effect (stres-ree-laks-AY-shun ef-FEKT) [*stress-* **tighten,** *relax-* **loosen,** *-ation* **process,** *effect* **accomplishment**]

stroke volume (SV) (strohk VOL-yoom)

total peripheral resistance (TPR) (peh-RIF-er-al ree-ZIS-tens) [*peri-* **around,** *-phera-* **boundary,** *-al* **relating to,** *resist-* **withstand,** *-ance* **act of**]

vasoconstriction (vay-soh-kon-STRIK-shun) [*vas-* **vessel,** *-constrict-* **draw tight,** *-tion* **state**]

vasodilation (vay-soh-dye-LAY-shun) [*vas-* **vessel,** *-dilat-* **widen,** *-tion* **state**]

vasomotor mechanism (vay-so-MOH-tor) [*vas-* **vessel,** *-motor* **move,** *mechan-* **machine,** *-ism* **state**]

vasomotor pressoreflex (vay-so-MOH-tor press-oh-REE-fleks) [*vas-* **vessel,** *-motor* **move,** *press-* **pressure,** *-re-* **back or again,** *-flex* **bend**]

venoconstriction (vee-noh-kon-STRIK-shun) [*ven-* **vein,** *-constrict-* **draw tight,** *-tion* **state**]

viscosity (vis-KOS-ih-tee)
[*viscos-* **sticky,** *-ity* **state**]

LANGUAGE OF MEDICINE

anaphylactic shock (an-ah-fih-LAK-tik)
[*ana-* **without,** *-phylact-* **protection,** *-ic* **relating to**]

bruits (BROO-eez)
[*bruits* **noise**]

cardiogenic shock (kar-dee-oh-JEN-ik)
[*cardi-* **heart,** *-gen-* **produce,** *-ic* **relating to**]

circulatory shock (SUR-kyoo-lah-tor-ee)
[*circulat-* **go around,** *-ory* **relating to**]

diastolic blood pressure (dye-ah-STOL-ik blud PRESH-ur)
[*dia-* **apart or through,** *-stol-* **position,** *-ic* **relating to**]

hypercapnia (hye-per-KAP-nee-ah)
[*hyper-* **excessive,** *-capn-* **vapour (CO_2),** *-ia* **condition**]

hypertension (HTN) (hye-per-TEN-shun)
[*hyper-* **excessive,** *-tens-* **stretch or pull tight,** *-sion* **state**]

hypotension (hye-poh-TEN-shun)
[*hypo-* **under or below,** *-tens-* **stretch or pull tight,** *-sion* **state**]

hypovolaemic shock (hye-poh-voh-LEE-mik)
[*hypo-* **under or below,** *-vol-* **whirl,** *-aem-* **blood,** *-ic* **relating to**]

hypoxia (hye-POK-see-ah)
[*hypo-* **under or below,** *-ox-* **oxygen,** *-ia* **condition**]

Korotkoff sound (kor-ROT-koff)
[*Nicolai Korotkoff* **Russian physician**]

laminar flow (LAM-ih-nar)
[*lamina-* **plate,** *-ar* **relating to**]

neurogenic shock (nyoo-roh-JEN-ik)
[*neuro-* **nerve,** *-gen-* **produce,** *-ic* **relating to**]

pulse pressure (PP)
[*pulse* **beat**]

septic shock (SEP-tik shok)
[*septi-* **putrid,** *-ic* **relating to**]

sphygmomanometer (sfig-moh-mah-NOM-eh-ter)
[*sphygmo-* **pulse,** *-mano-* **pressure,** *-meter* **measure**]

systolic blood pressure (sis-TOL-ik blud PRESH-ur)
[*sy(n)-* **together,** *-stol-* **position,** *-ic* **relating to**]

turbulent flow (TUR-byoo-lent flo)

vasodilatory shock (vay-soh-DYE-lah-tor-ee)
[*vas-* **vessel,** *-dilat-* **widen,** *-ory* **relating to**]

case study

Over the past few weeks, Luke experienced headaches and dizziness. During a routine physical examination, Luke's doctor informed him that his blood pressure was 150/90. As a result of this reading, Luke was diagnosed with hypertension (HTN). Luke's doctor encouraged him to watch his diet and begin exercising on a regular basis.

1. Luke's doctor used a sphygmomanometer and stethoscope to measure his blood pressure. After releasing the air in the cuff, the doctor listened for sounds of turbulence generated by the blood pressure changes in the brachial artery. What are these sounds called?
   a. Turbulent sounds
   b. Laminar sounds
   c. Korotkoff sounds
   d. Bruit sounds
2. Blood pressure fluctuates considerably during each heartbeat. This difference between systolic pressure and diastolic pressure is called pulse pressure (PP). Based on Luke's blood pressure reading, calculate his pulse pressure.
   a. 40
   b. 50
   c. 60
   d. 70
3. The mean arterial pressure (MAP) is an average blood pressure in the arteries. Calculate Luke's MAP.
   a. 110 mmHg
   b. 140 mmHg
   c. 210 mmHg
   d. 270 mmHg

Hint To solve a case study, you may have to refer to the glossary or index, other chapters in this textbook, ***Connect It!,*** and other resources.

UNIT 4

CHAPTER SUMMARY

To download an MP3 version of the chapter summary for use with your mobile device, access the ***Audio Chapter Summaries*** *online at evolve.elsevier.com.*

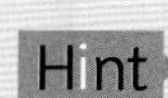

Scan this summary after reading the chapter to help you reinforce the key concepts. Later, use the summary as a quick review before your class or before a test.

Introduction

A. Vital role of the cardiovascular system in maintaining homeostasis depends on the continuous and controlled movement of blood through the capillaries

B. Numerous control mechanisms help regulate and integrate the diverse functions and component parts of the cardiovascular system to supply blood in response to specific body area needs

Haemodynamics

A. Haemodynamics—collection of mechanisms that influence the dynamic (active and changing) circulation of blood (**Figure 30-1**)

B. Circulation of different volumes of blood per minute is essential for healthy survival

C. Circulation control mechanisms must accomplish two functions:
   1. Maintain circulation
   2. Vary volume and distribution of the blood circulated

Primary Principle of Circulation

A. Blood flows because a pressure gradient exists between different parts of its volume; this is based on Newton's first and second laws of motion (**Figure 30-2**)

B. For example, blood circulates from the left ventricle to the right atrium of the heart because a blood pressure gradient exists between these two structures; likewise, a blood pressure gradient drives blood flow from the right ventricle to the left atrium

C. P_1–P_2 is the symbol used to represent a pressure gradient, with P_1 representing the higher pressure and P_2 the lower pressure

D. Perfusion pressure—the pressure gradient needed to maintain blood flow through a local tissue

Arterial Blood Pressure

A. Primary determinant of arterial blood pressure is the volume of blood in the arteries; a direct relationship exists between arterial blood pressure and arterial blood volume (**Figure 30-3**)

B. Cardiac output (CO)—volume of blood pumped out of the heart per unit of time (mL/min or L/min) (**Figure 30-4**)
   1. General principles and definitions
      a. Cardiac output (CO)—determined by stroke volume and heart rate
      b. Stroke volume (SV)—volume pumped per heartbeat
      c. CO (volume/min) = SV (volume/beat) × HR (beats/min)
      d. In practice, CO is computed by Fick's formula
      e. Heart rate and stroke volume determine CO, so anything that changes either also tends to change CO, arterial blood volume, and blood pressure in the same direction
      f. Cardiac reserve—amount the CO can increase above resting CO, usually expressed in percent above resting value
   2. Factors that affect stroke volume
      a. Starling's law of the heart (Frank–Starling mechanism) (**Figure 30-5**)
         (1) Within limits, the longer, or more stretched, the heart fibres at the beginning of contraction, the stronger the contraction
         (2) The amount of blood in the heart at the end of diastole determines the amount of stretch or preload placed on the heart fibres
         (3) The myocardium contracts with enough strength to match its pumping load (within certain limits) with each stroke—unlike mechanical pumps
      b. Contractility (strength of contraction) can also be influenced by chemical factors (**Figure 30-6**)
         (1) Neural—norepinephrine; endocrine—epinephrine
         (2) Triggered by stress, exercise
      c. Ejection fraction (EF)—the ratio of stroke volume (SV) to end-diastolic volume (EDV)
         (1) Usually expressed as a percentage: EF = (SV/EDV) × 100
         (2) Healthy adults have EFs of at least 55%
         (3) EF goes down as the myocardium fails
      d. Afterload—the pumping work that the heart must do to push blood into the arteries
         (1) The harder it is to push blood out of the ventricles, the lower the stroke volume will be
         (2) Abnormally high afterload from flow resistance in arteries can cause heart failure
   3. Factors that affect heart rate—SA node normally initiates each heartbeat; however, various factors can and do change the rate of the heartbeat
      a. Cardiac pressoreflexes
         (1) Aortic baroreceptors and carotid baroreceptors, located in the aorta and carotid sinus
         (2) Extremely important because they affect the autonomic cardiac control centre, and therefore parasympathetic and sympathetic outflow, to aid in control of blood pressure (**Figures 30-7** and **30-8**)
      b. Carotid sinus reflex
         (1) Located at the beginning of the internal carotid artery
         (2) Sensory fibres from carotid sinus baroreceptors run through the carotid sinus nerve and the glossopharyngeal nerve to the cardiac control centre
         (3) Parasympathetic impulses leave the cardiac control centre, travel through the vagus nerve to reach the SA node
      c. Aortic reflex
         (1) Sensory fibres extend from baroreceptors located in the wall of the arch of the aorta through the aortic nerve and through the vagus nerve to terminate in the cardiac control centre
         (2) Stimulation causes cardiac control centre to increase vagal inhibition, thus slowing the heart
      d. Other reflexes that influence heart rate
         (1) Anxiety, fear, and anger often increase heart rate
         (2) Grief tends to decrease heart rate
         (3) Emotions produce changes in heart rate through the influence of impulses from the cerebrum by way of the hypothalamus
         (4) Exercise normally increases heart rate
         (5) Increased blood temperature or stimulation of skin heat receptors increases heart rate
         (6) Decreased blood temperature or stimulation of skin cold receptors decreases heart rate

C. Peripheral resistance—resistance to blood flow imposed by the force of friction between blood and the walls of its vessels
   1. Factors that influence peripheral resistance
      a. Blood viscosity—the thickness of blood as a fluid (**Figure 30-9**)
         (1) High plasma protein concentration can slightly increase blood viscosity
         (2) High haematocrit (% RBC) can increase blood viscosity
         (3) Anaemia, haemorrhage, or other abnormal conditions may also affect blood viscosity

b. Diameter of arterioles (**Figure 30-10**)
   (1) Vasomotor mechanism—muscles in walls of arteriole may constrict vessel (vasoconstriction) or dilate vessel (vasodilation), thus changing diameter of arteriole
   (2) Small changes in blood vessel diameter cause large changes in resistance, making the vasomotor mechanism ideal for regulating blood pressure and blood flow

2. How resistance influences blood pressure
   a. Arterial blood pressure tends to vary directly with peripheral resistance
   b. Friction caused by viscosity and small diameter of arterioles and capillaries
   c. Muscular coat of arterioles allows them to constrict or dilate and change the amount of resistance to blood flow
   d. Peripheral resistance helps determine arterial pressure by controlling the amount of blood that runs from the arteries to the arterioles (**Figure 30-11**)
      (1) Increased resistance and decreased arteriole runoff lead to higher arterial pressure
      (2) Can occur locally (in one organ), or the total peripheral resistance (TPR) may increase, thus generally raising systemic arterial pressure
3. Vasomotor control mechanism—controls changes in the diameter of arterioles; plays role in maintenance of the general blood pressure and in distribution of blood to areas of special need (**Figures 30-12** and **30-13**)
   a. Vasomotor pressoreflexes (**Figure 30-14**)
      (1) Sudden increase in arterial blood pressure stimulates aortic and carotid baroreceptors; results in arterioles and venules of the blood reservoirs dilating
      (2) Decrease in arterial blood pressure results in stimulation of vasoconstrictor centres, causing vascular smooth muscle to constrict
   b. Vasomotor chemoreflexes (**Figure 30-15**)—chemoreceptors located in aortic and carotid bodies are sensitive to hypercapnia, hypoxia, and decreased arterial blood pH
   c. Medullary ischaemic reflex—acts during emergency situation when there is decreased blood flow to the medulla; causes marked arteriole and venous constriction
   d. Vasomotor control by higher brain centres—impulses from centres in cerebral cortex and hypothalamus are transmitted to vasomotor centres in medulla to help control vasoconstriction and dilation
4. Local control of arterioles—several local mechanisms produce vasodilation in localized areas; referred to as *active hyperaemia*

Venous Return to the Heart

A. Venous return—amount of blood returned to the heart by the veins

B. Stress-relaxation effect—occurs when a change in blood pressure causes a change in vessel diameter (because of elasticity) that accommodates the new pressure and thereby keeps blood flowing (works only within certain limits)

C. Gravity—the pull of gravity on venous blood while sitting or standing tends to cause a decrease in venous return (orthostatic effect) (**Figure 30-16**)

D. Venous pumps—blood-pumping action of respirations and skeletal muscle contractions facilitate venous return by increasing pressure gradient between peripheral veins and venae cavae (**Figure 30-17**)
   1. Respirations—inspiration increases the pressure gradient between peripheral and central veins by decreasing central venous pressure and also by increasing peripheral venous pressure
   2. Skeletal muscle contractions—promote venous return by squeezing veins through a contracting muscle and milking the blood toward the heart
   3. One-way valves in veins prevent backflow (**Figure 30-18**)

E. Total blood volume—changes in total blood volume change the amount of blood returned to the heart
   1. Capillary exchange—governed by Starling's law of the capillaries (**Figure 30-19**)
      a. At arterial end of capillary, outward hydrostatic pressure is strongest force; moves fluid out of plasma and into interstitial fluid (IF)
      b. At venous end of capillary, inward osmotic pressure is strongest force; moves fluid into plasma from IF; 90% of fluid lost by plasma at arterial end is recovered
      c. Lymphatic system recovers fluid not recovered by capillary and returns it to the venous blood before it is returned to the heart
   2. Changes in total blood volume—mechanisms that change total blood volume most quickly are those that cause water to quickly move into or out of the plasma (**Figure 30-20**)
      a. ADH mechanism—decreases the amount of water lost by the body by increasing the amount of water that kidneys resorb from urine before the urine is excreted from the body; triggered by input from baroreceptors and osmoreceptors
      b. Renin–angiotensin–aldosterone system (RAAS)—decreases water loss
         (1) Renin—released when blood pressure in kidney is low; leads to increased secretion of aldosterone, which stimulates retention of sodium, causing increased retention of water and an increase in blood volume
         (2) Angiotensin II—intermediate compound that causes vasoconstriction, which complements the volume-increasing effects of renin and promotes an increase in overall blood flow
      c. ANH mechanism—adjusts venous return from an abnormally high level by promoting the loss of water from plasma, causing a decrease in blood volume; increases urine sodium loss, which causes water to follow osmotically

F. A variety of feedback responses restore normal blood pressure after a sudden change in pressure (**Figure 30-21**)

Measuring Blood Pressure

A. Arterial blood pressure
   1. Measured with the aid of a sphygmomanometer and stethoscope; listen for Korotkoff sounds as the pressure in the cuff is gradually decreased (**Figure 30-22**)
   2. Systolic blood pressure—force of the blood pushing against the artery walls while ventricles are contracting
   3. Diastolic blood pressure—force of the blood pushing against the artery walls when ventricles are relaxed and during isovolumetric ventricular contraction
   4. Pulse pressure (PP)—difference between systolic and diastolic blood pressure
   5. Mean arterial pressure (MAP)—average blood pressure in arteries for perfusion of tissues

B. Relation to arterial and venous bleeding
   1. Arterial bleeding—blood escapes from artery in spurts because of alternating increase and decrease of arterial blood pressure
   2. Venous bleeding—blood flows slowly and steadily because of low, practically constant pressure

Minute Volume of Blood (Figure 30-23)

A. Minute volume—determined by the magnitude of the blood pressure gradient and peripheral resistance

B. Poiseuille's law—Minute volume = Pressure gradient ÷ Resistance

Velocity of Blood Flow

A. Governed by the physical principle that when a liquid flows from an area of one cross-sectional size to an area of larger size, its velocity decreases in the area with the larger cross-section (**Figure 30-24**)

B. Blood flows more slowly through arterioles than arteries because total cross-sectional area of arterioles is greater than that of arteries, and capillary blood flow is slower than arteriole blood flow

C. Venule cross-sectional area is smaller than capillary cross-sectional area, causing blood velocity to increase in venules and then veins with a still smaller cross-sectional area

Pulse

A. Mechanism
   1. Pulse—alternate expansion and recoil of an artery (**Figure 30-25**)
      a. Clinical significance: reveals important information regarding the cardiovascular system, blood vessels, and circulation
      b. Physiological significance: expansion stores energy released during recoil, conserving energy generated by the heart and maintaining relatively constant blood flow (**Figure 30-26**)
   2. Existence of pulse is due to two factors
      a. Alternating increase and decrease of pressure in the vessel
      b. Elasticity of arterial walls allows walls to expand with increased pressure and recoil with decreased pressure

B. Pulse wave
   1. Each pulse starts with ventricular contraction and proceeds as a wave of expansion throughout the arteries
   2. Gradually dissipates as it travels, disappearing in the capillaries

C. Where the pulse can be felt—wherever an artery lies near the surface and over a bone or other firm background (**Figure 30-27**)

D. Venous pulse—detectable pulse exists only in large veins; most prominent near the heart; not of clinical importance

Cycle of Life: Cardiovascular Physiology

A. Changes in the function of the heart and blood vessels usually parallel the structural changes in these organs over the life span

B. Changes in arterial blood pressure are among the most apparent changes in function of the cardiovascular system associated with the progression through the life cycle

C. Heart rates of infants and children typically vary more than those in adults

The Big Picture: Blood Flow and the Whole Body

A. Blood flow shifts materials from place to place and redistributes heat and pressure

B. Vital to maintaining homeostasis of internal environment

REVIEW QUESTIONS

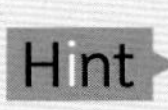

Write out the answers to these questions after reading the chapter and reviewing the Chapter Summary. Note—writing out your answers will consolidate learning and provide a valuable resource of information.

1. Which blood vessels present the greatest resistance to blood flow?
2. What is the primary determinant of arterial blood pressure?
3. List the two most important factors that indirectly determine arterial pressure by their influence on arterial volume.
4. How is cardiac output determined?
5. List the effect of the following factors on heart rate: exercise, blood temperature, pain, anxiety and grief. Suggest why the response to grief may be different.
6. What mechanisms control peripheral resistance? Cite an example of the operation of one or more parts of this mechanism to increase resistance and to decrease it.
7. What are the components of the vasomotor control mechanism?
8. Explain how antidiuretic hormone can change the total blood volume.
9. What is the effect of low blood pressure in relation to aldosterone and antidiuretic hormone secretion?
10. Describe the measurement of arterial blood pressure.
11. Identify the eight locations where the pulse point is most easily felt. List the six pressure points at which pressure can be applied to stop arterial bleeding distal to that point.

CRITICAL THINKING QUESTIONS

Hint *After finishing the Review Questions, write out the answers to these more in-depth questions to help you apply your new knowledge. Go back to sections of the chapter that relate to concepts that you find difficult.*

1. State in your own words the primary principle of circulation. How does it govern the various mechanisms involved in blood flow?
2. What is Starling's law of the heart? What role does *venous return* play in Starling's law?
3. Explain how the heart rate is a good example of dual innervation in the autonomic nervous system. Include the nerves and neurotransmitters involved.
4. Explain how blood pressure in the brain is prevented from getting too high.
5. What is arterial runoff? What is the relationship of arteriole runoff and peripheral resistance?
6. Explain what occurs when the carbon dioxide level in the medulla rises above the set point. What emergency mechanism operates when hypoxia (low O_2) or hypercapnia (high CO_2) in the internal environment endangers homeostasis?
7. By the time blood gets to the veins, almost all the pressure from the contracting ventricles has been lost. What mechanisms does the body use to assist in returning blood to the heart?
8. Explain the forces that act on capillary exchange on both the arterial and venous ends of the capillary. Is the recovery of fluid at the venous end 100% effective?
9. State in your own words Poiseuille's law. What equation expresses this law? According to the equation, an increase in resistance would lower the minute volume. Give an example of where this would not be the case.
10. What two factors determine blood viscosity? What does viscosity mean? Give an example of a condition in which blood viscosity decreases. Explain its effects on resistance, arterial pressure, and circulation.

31 Lymphatic System

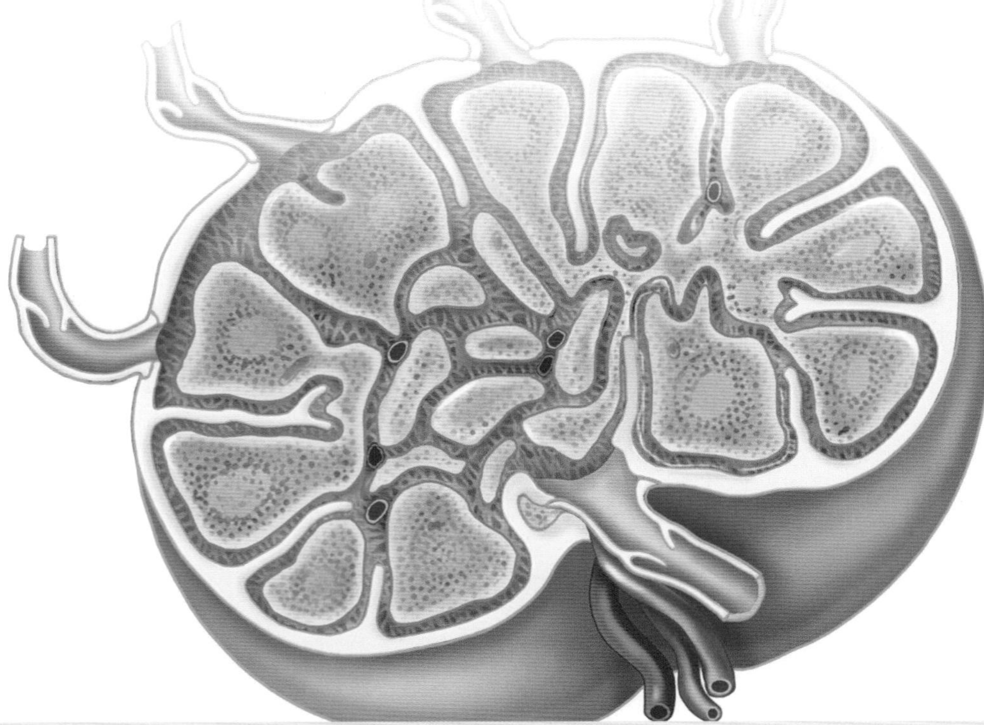

CHAPTER OUTLINE

Hint ▸ *Scan this outline before you begin to read the chapter, as a preview of how the concepts are organized.*

LANGUAGE OF SCIENCE

Hint ▸ *Use this list to aid your pronunciation of unfamiliar words.*

aggregated lymphoid nodules (ag-rah-GAYT-ed LIM-foyd NOD-yoolz)
[*a[d]-* **to,** *-grega-* **collect,** *lymph-* **water,** *-oid* **like,** *nod-* **knot,** *-ule* **small**]

anastomosis (ah-nas-tuh-MOH-sis)
[*ana-* **again or anew,** *-stomo-* **mouth,** *-osis* **conditions of**] *pl.,* anastomoses

axillary lymph node (AK-sih-lair-ee limf nohd)
[*axilla-* **wing,** *-ary* **relating to,** *lymph* **water,** *nod-* **knot**]

chyle (kile)
[*chyl-* **juice**]

cisterna chyli (sis-TER-nah KYE-lye)
[*cisterna* **vessel,** *chyli* **of juice**]

cortical nodule (KOHR-tih-kal NOD-yool)
[*cortic-* **cortex (bark),** *-al* **relating to,** *nod-* **knot,** *-ule* **small**]

iliac lymph node (ILL-ee-ak limf nohd)
[*ilia-* **loin or gut [ileum],** *-ac* **relating to,** *lymph* **water,** *nod-* **knot**]

inguinal lymph node (ING-gwih-nal limf nohd)
[*inguin-* **groin,** *-al* **relating to,** *lymph* **water,** *-atic* **relating to,** *nod-* **knot**]

interstitial fluid (IF) (in-ter-STISH-al)
[*inter-* **between,** *-stit-* **stand,** *-al* **relating to**]

involution (in-voh-LOO-shun)
[*in-* **in,** *-volu-* **roll,** *-tion* **state**]

lacteal (LAK-tee-al)
[*lact-* **milk,** *-al* **relating to**]

lingual tonsil (LING-gwal TON-sil)
[*lingua-* **tongue,** *-al* **relating to,** *tons-* **goitre,** *-il* **little**]

lymph (limf)
[*lymph* **water**]

lymph node (limf nohd)
[*lymph* **water,** *nod-* **knot**]

lymphatic capillary (lim-FAT-ik kah-PILL-air-ee)
[*lymph-* **water,** *-atic* **relating to,** *capill-* **hair,** *-ary* **relating to**]

lymphatic vessel (lim-FAT-ik)
[*lymph-* **water,** *-atic* **relating to**]

lymphoid tissue (LIM-foyd)
[*lymph-* **water (lymphatic system),** *-oid* **like,** *tissu-* **fabric**]

continued on p. 745

The lymphatic system serves various functions in the body. The two most important functions of this system are maintenance of fluid balance in the internal environment and immunity. Although both of these important functions are discussed in this chapter, details of immunity are discussed more fully in Chapters 32 and 33. A third, somewhat less important, function of the lymphatic system is the absorption of lipids from digested food in the small intestine and its transport to the large systemic veins. This fat-transport function of the lymphatic system is discussed in Chapter 40.

OVERVIEW OF THE LYMPHATIC SYSTEM

The importance of the lymphatic system in maintaining a balance of fluid in the internal environment is best explained by the diagram in **Figure 31-1**. As this figure shows, plasma filters into interstitial spaces from blood flowing through capillaries. Most of this interstitial fluid (IF) is absorbed by tissue cells or reabsorbed by the blood before it flows out of the tissue. However, a small percentage of the interstitial fluid remains behind (review **Figure 30-19**, A, on p. 713). If this continued for even a brief period, the increased interstitial fluid would cause massive oedema (swelling) of the tissue. The high fluid pressure from this oedema could cause tissue destruction or perhaps even death as normal functions became disrupted. Such a problem is avoided by the presence of lymphatic vessels that act as "drains" to collect the excess tissue fluid and return it to the venous blood just before it reaches the heart.

The lymphatic system is a component of the circulatory system because it consists of a moving fluid (lymph) derived from the blood and tissue fluid and a group of vessels (lymphatics) that return the lymph to the blood. In general, the lymphatic vessels that drain the peripheral areas of the body parallel the venous return.

In addition to lymph and the lymphatic vessels, the system includes various structures that contain **lymphoid tissue**—a type of reticular tissue (see Chapter 9) that contains lymphocytes and other defensive cells. For example, lymph nodes are located along the paths of the collecting lymphatic vessels. Isolated nodules of lymphatic tissue, such as the **aggregated lymphoid nodules** called *Peyer patches* in the intestinal wall or the nodules of the vermiform appendix of the large intestine, are other examples. Additional lymphoid structures include the tonsils, thymus, spleen, and bone marrow (**Figure 31-2**).

Although it serves a unique transport function by returning tissue fluid, proteins, fats, and other substances to the general circulation, lymph flow differs from the true "circulation" of blood seen in the cardiovascular system. Unlike vessels in the blood vascular system, lymphatic vessels do not form a closed ring, or circuit, but instead

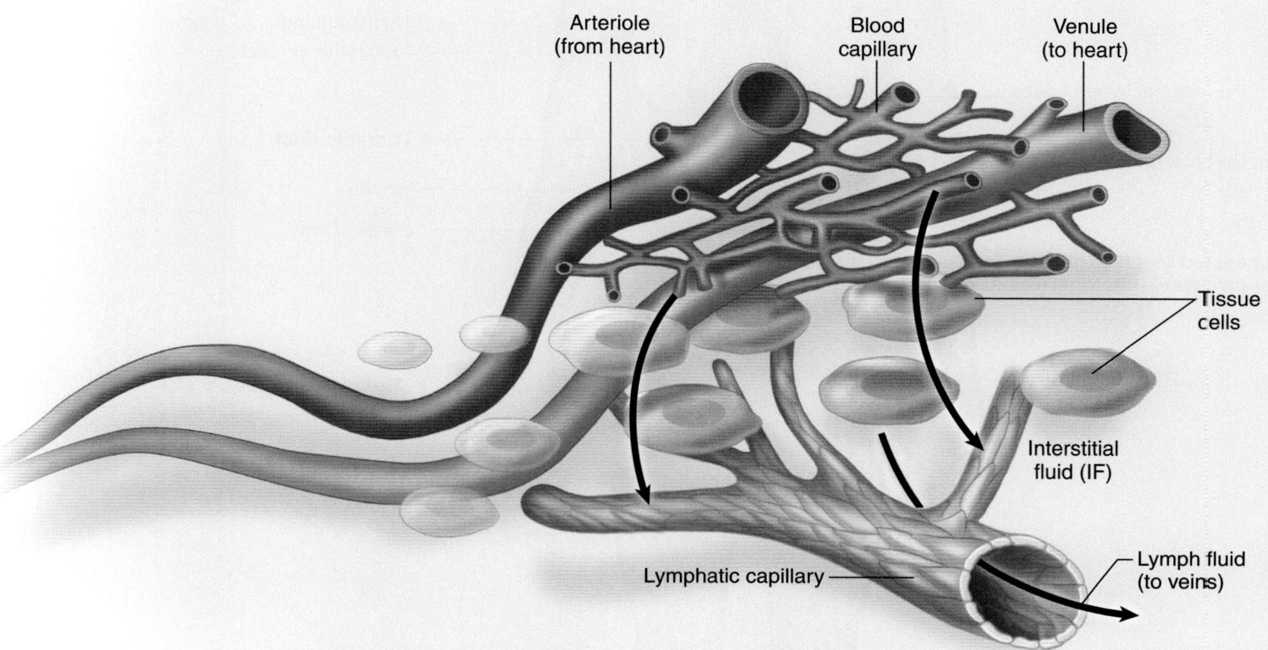

FIGURE 31-1 Role of the lymphatic system in fluid balance. Fluid from plasma flowing through the capillaries moves into interstitial spaces. Although *most* of this interstitial fluid is either absorbed by tissue cells or resorbed by blood capillaries, *some* of the fluid tends to accumulate in the interstitial spaces. As this fluid builds up, it tends to drain into lymphatic vessels *(green)* that eventually return the fluid to the venous blood. Lymphatic structures are not actually green. Green is used in diagrams to contrast lymphatic structures with nearby blood vessels *(red, blue)* or nerves *(yellow)*.

begin blindly in the intercellular spaces of the soft tissues of the body (see **Figure 31-1**).

LYMPH AND INTERSTITIAL FLUID

Lymph (or *lymphatic fluid*) is the clear, watery-appearing fluid found in the lymphatic vessels. **Interstitial fluid (IF),** which fills the spaces between the cells, is not the simple fluid it seems to be. Studies show that it is an important and complex part of the *ECM (extracellular matrix)*. Interstitial fluid and blood plasma together constitute the extracellular fluid compartment of the body, or in the words of Claude Bernard, the "internal environment of the body"—the fluid environment of cells in contrast to the atmosphere, or external environment, of the body.

Both lymph and interstitial fluid closely resemble blood plasma in composition. The main difference is that they contain a lower percentage of proteins than does plasma. Lymph is isotonic and almost identical in chemical composition to interstitial fluid when comparisons are made between the two fluids taken from the same area of the body. However, the average concentration of protein (4 grams/100 mL) in lymph taken from the thoracic duct (see **Figure 31-2**) is about twice that found in most interstitial fluid samples.

The elevated protein level of thoracic duct lymph (a mixture of lymph from all areas of the body) results from protein-rich lymph flowing into the duct from the liver and small intestine. A little more than one half of the 2800 to 3000 mL total daily lymph flowing through the thoracic duct is derived from these two organs.

Box 31-1 discusses the effects of abnormal loss of lymphatic fluid.

> **BOX 31-1** *health matters*
>
> **Loss of Lymphatic Fluid**
>
> Lymph does not clot. Therefore, if damage to the main lymphatic trunks in the thorax occurs as a result of penetrating injury, the flow of lymph must be stopped surgically or death ensues. It is impossible to maintain adequate plasma protein concentration by dietary means if significant loss of lymph continues over time. As lymph is lost, rapid emaciation occurs, with a progressive and eventually fatal decrease in total blood fat and protein concentration.

LYMPHATIC VESSELS

Distribution of Lymphatic Vessels

Lymphatic vessels—often simply called *lymphatics*—originate as microscopic blind-end vessels called *lymphatic capillaries*. (Those originating in the villi of the small intestine are called *lacteals*; see Chapter 40.) The wall of each **lymphatic capillary** consists of a single layer of flattened endothelial cells.

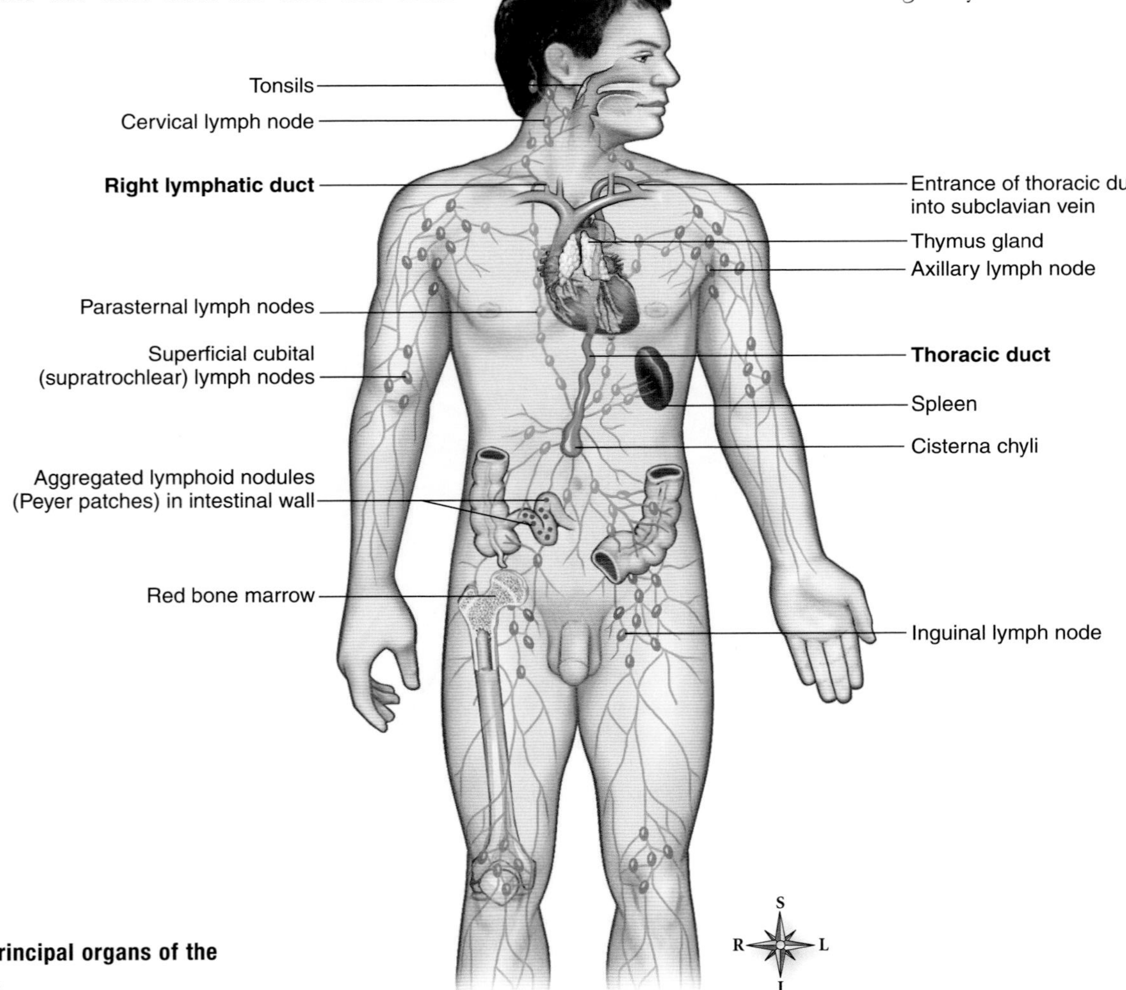

FIGURE 31-2 Principal organs of the lymphatic system.

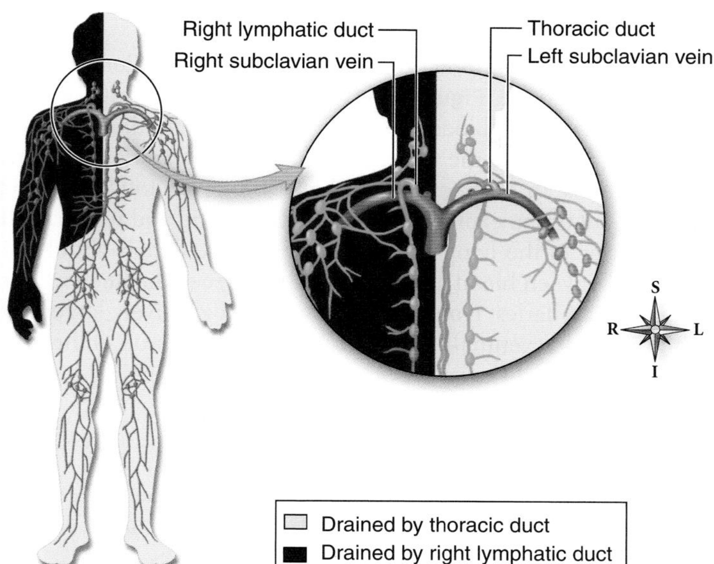

FIGURE 31-3 Lymphatic drainage. The right lymphatic duct drains lymph from the upper right quadrant *(dark blue)* of the body into the right subclavian vein. The thoracic duct drains lymph from the rest of the body *(green)* into the left subclavian vein. The lymphatic fluid is thus returned to the systemic blood just before entering the heart.

Each blindly ending capillary is attached, or fixed, to surrounding cells by tiny connective tissue filaments. Networks of lymphatic capillaries branch and anastomose extensively. Lymphatic networks are located in the intercellular (interstitial) spaces and are widely distributed throughout the body. As a rule, lymphatic and blood capillary networks lie side by side but are always independent of each other.

As twigs of a tree join to form branches, branches join to form larger branches, and larger branches join to form the tree trunk, so do lymphatic capillaries merge, forming slightly larger lymphatics that join other lymphatics to form still larger vessels, which merge to form the main lymphatic trunks: the **right lymphatic duct** and the **thoracic duct** (see **Figure 31-2**).

Lymph from the entire body, except for the upper right quadrant, drains eventually into the thoracic duct, which drains into the left subclavian vein at the point where it joins the left internal jugular vein (**Figure 31-3**). Lymph from the upper right quadrant of the body empties into the right lymphatic duct and then into the right subclavian vein. However, this structure can vary among individuals. For example, in most people there are three separate lymphatic ducts that drain into the right subclavian vein rather than a single right lymphatic duct.

Because most of the lymph of the body returns to the bloodstream by way of the thoracic duct, this vessel is considerably larger than the other main lymph channels, the right lymphatic ducts, but is much smaller than the large veins, which it resembles in structure. The thoracic duct has an average diameter of about 5 mm and a length of about 40 cm. It originates as a dilated structure, the **cisterna chyli** or *chyle cistern,* in the lumbar region of the abdominal cavity—where fatty lymph called *chyle* from the intestinal tract collects. The cisterna chyli can be up to 15 mm in diameter. The thoracic duct then ascends a curving pathway to the root of the neck, where it joins the subclavian vein as just described (see **Figures 31-2** and **31-3**).

Structure of Lymphatic Vessels

Lymphatics resemble veins in structure with these exceptions:

- Lymphatics have thinner walls.
- Lymphatics contain more valves.
- Lymphatics contain lymph nodes located at certain intervals along their course.

The lymphatic capillary wall is formed by a single layer of large but very thin and flat endothelial cells (**Figure 31-4**). Although the openings (clefts) between endothelial cells of lymphatic capillary walls are small, they are larger than those found in blood capillaries—a fact that explains the remarkable permeability of this system.

As lymph flows from the thin-walled capillaries into vessels with a larger diameter (0.2 to 0.3 mm), the walls become thicker and exhibit the three coats, or layers, typical of arteries and veins (see **Table 29-1**, p. 670). Interlacing elastic fibres and several strata of circular smooth muscle bundles are found in both the tunica media and the tunica externa of the large lymphatic vessel wall. Boundaries between layers are less distinct in the thinner lymphatic vessel walls than in arteries or veins.

One-way valves are extremely numerous in lymphatics of all sizes and give the vessels a somewhat varicose and beaded appearance. Valves are present every few millimetres in large lymphatics and are even more numerous in the smaller vessels. Formed from folds of the tunica intima, each valve projects into the vessel lumen in a slightly expanded area circled by bundles of smooth muscle fibres.

Experimental evidence suggests that most lymph vessels have the capacity for repair or regeneration when damaged. Formation of new lymphatic vessels occurs by extension of solid cellular cores, or sprouts, formed by mitotic division of endothelial cells in existing vessels, which later become "canalized".

Functions of Lymphatic Vessels

The lymphatics play a critical role in numerous interrelated homeostatic mechanisms. The high degree of permeability of the lymphatic capillary wall permits very large molecules and even particulate

FIGURE 31-4 Structure of a typical lymphatic capillary. Note that interstitial fluid enters through clefts between overlapping endothelial cells that form the wall of the vessel. Valves ensure one-way flow of lymph out of the tissue. Small fibres anchor the wall of the lymphatic capillary to the surrounding extracellular matrix (ECM) and cells, thus holding it open to allow entry of fluids and small particles.

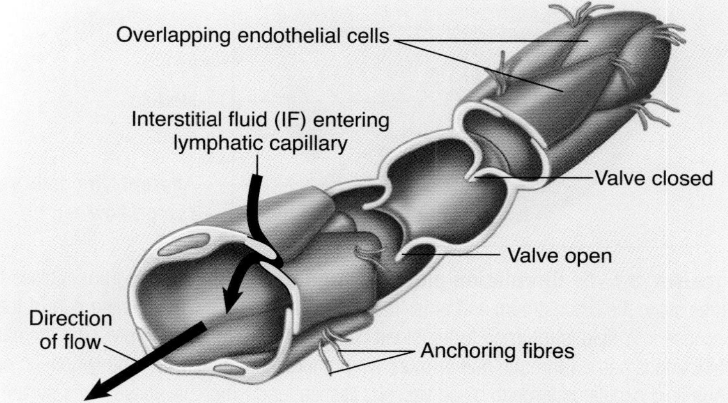

matter, which cannot be absorbed into a blood capillary, to be removed from the interstitial spaces. Proteins that accumulate in the tissue spaces can return to blood only by way of lymphatics. This fact has great clinical importance. For instance, if anything blocks lymphatic return, blood protein concentration and blood osmotic pressure soon fall below normal, and fluid imbalance and death will result (discussed in Chapter 43).

Lacteals (lymphatic capillaries in the villi of the small intestine) serve an important function in the absorption of fats and other nutrients. The milky lymph found in lacteals after digestion contains 1% to 2% fat and is called **chyle.** Interstitial fluid has a much lower lipid content than chyle (see Chapter 40).

CIRCULATION OF LYMPH

Water and solutes continually filter out of capillary blood into the interstitial fluid (see **Figure 31-1**). To balance this outflow, fluid continually reenters blood from the interstitial fluid. Newer evidence has disproved the old idea that healthy capillaries do not "leak" proteins. In truth, each day about 50% of the total blood proteins leak out of the capillaries into the tissue fluid and return to the blood by way of the lymphatic vessels. For more details about fluid exchange between blood and interstitial fluid, see Chapter 43. From lymphatic capillaries, lymph flows through progressively larger lymphatic vessels to eventually reenter blood at the junction of the internal jugular and subclavian veins (**Figure 31-5**).

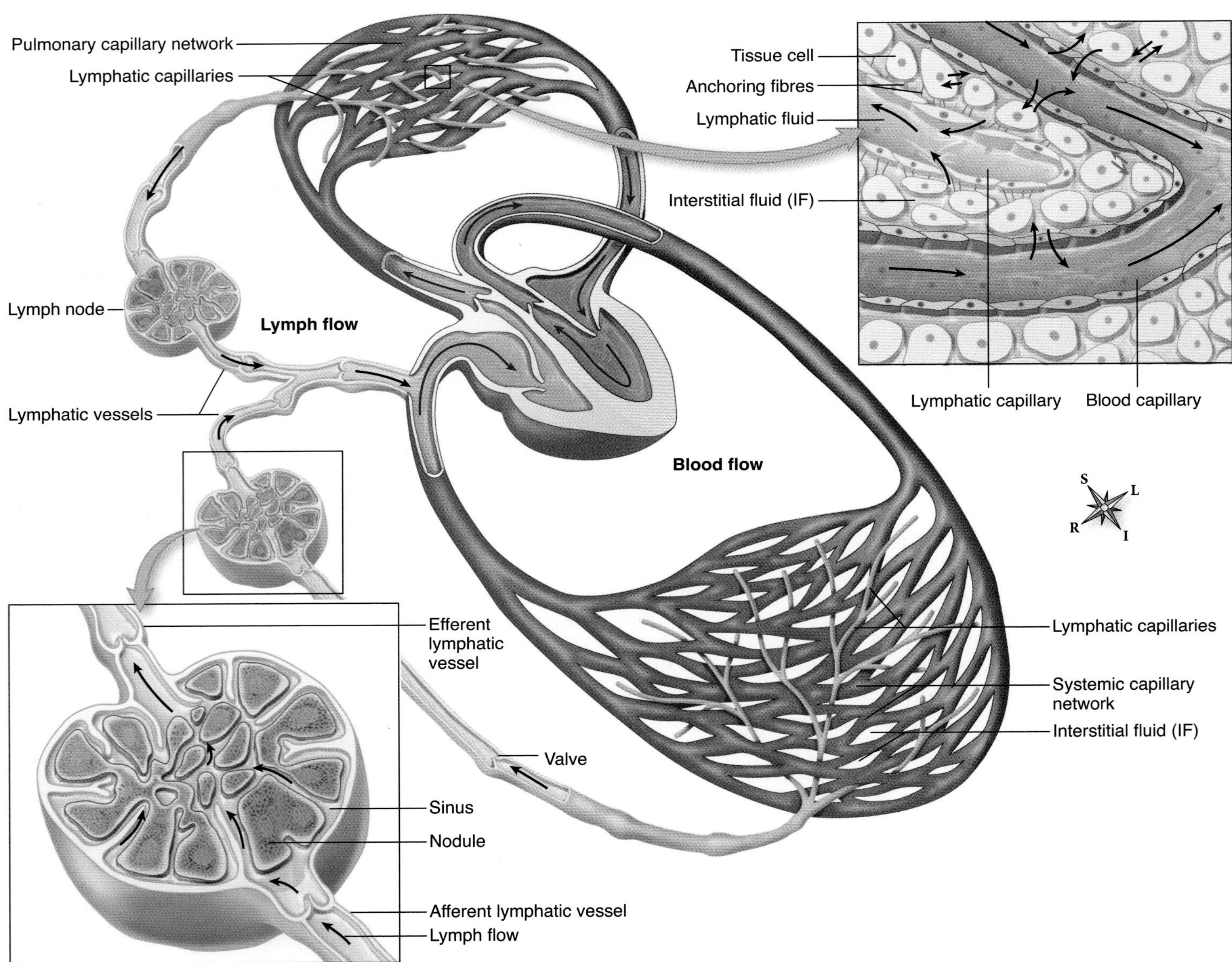

FIGURE 31-5 Circulation plan of lymphatic fluid. This diagram outlines the general scheme for lymphatic circulation. Fluids from the systemic and pulmonary capillaries leave the bloodstream and enter the interstitial space, thus becoming part of the interstitial fluid (IF). The IF also exchanges materials with the surrounding tissues. Often, because less fluid is returned to the blood capillary than had left it, IF pressure increases—causing IF to flow into the lymphatic capillary. The fluid is then called *lymph* (lymphatic fluid) and is carried through one or more lymph nodes and finally to large lymphatic ducts. The lymph enters a subclavian vein, where it is returned to the systemic blood plasma. Thus fluid circulates through blood vessels, tissues, and lymphatic vessels in a sort of "open circulation".

BOX 31-2 *health matters*

Lymphatic Drainage and Artificial Limbs

An understanding of the anatomy of lymphatic drainage of the skin is critically important in surgical amputation of an extremity. A majority of the lymphatics draining the skin are located in plexus-like networks lying on the deep fascia. To prevent stasis of lymph in the stump after amputation, the surgeon retains the deep fascia and its lymphatic vessels with the skin flaps that are used to cover the cut end of the extremity. This procedure results in minimal oedema and swelling—a matter of obvious importance to the patient and artificial-limb fitter.

The Lymphatic Pump

Although there is no muscular pumping organ connected with the lymphatic vessels to force lymph onward as the heart forces blood, lymph still moves slowly and steadily along in its vessels. Lymph flows through the thoracic duct and reenters the general circulation at the rate of about 3 litres per day. This occurs despite the fact that most of the flow is against gravity, or "uphill". It moves through the system in the right direction because of the large number of valves that permit fluid flow only in the central direction.

What mechanisms establish the pressure gradient required by the basic law of fluid flow? Two of the same mechanisms that contribute to the blood pressure gradient in veins also establish a lymph pressure gradient. These are breathing movements and skeletal muscle contractions (see **Figure 30-17**, p. 712). **Box 31-2** explains one of many reasons a working knowledge of lymphatic flow is important.

Activities that result in central movement, or flow, of lymph are called *lymphokinetic* actions (*-kinet-* "move"). Thus the flow of lymph may be called **lymphokinesis.** X-ray films taken after radiopaque material is injected into the lymphatics show that lymph pours into the central veins most rapidly at the peak of inspiration. This method of visualizing lymphatic vessels is called **lymphangiography** (**Figure 31-6**).

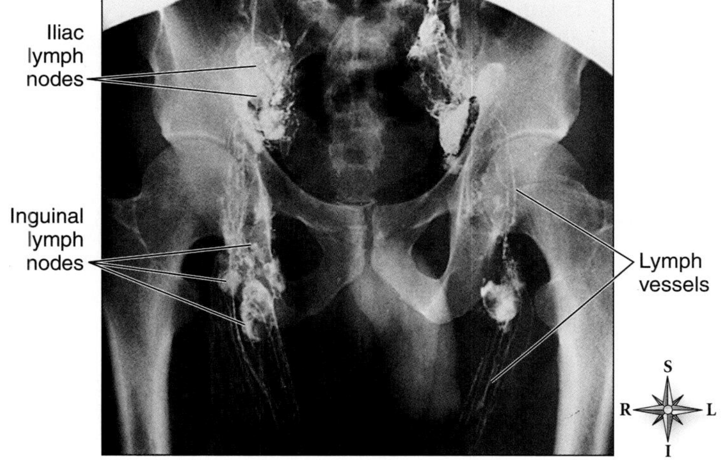

FIGURE 31-6 Lymphangiogram. A dye that is radiopaque (blocks x-rays) is injected into the interstitial fluid that eventually drains into nearby lymphatic pathways. There the dye is seen as bright areas outlining the location of pelvic (iliac) and inguinal lymphatic vessels and lymph nodes.

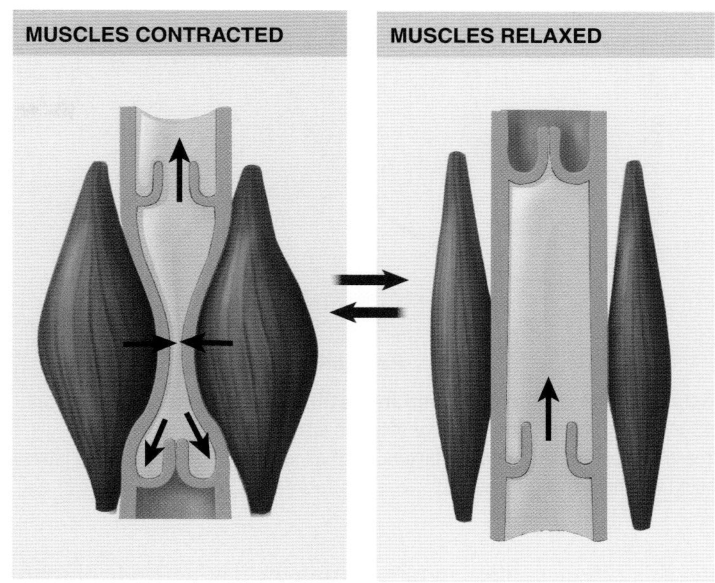

FIGURE 31-7 Lymphatic pump. The diagram shows a "muscle pump" in a lymphatic vessel similar to that which moves blood through the veins. Increased external pressure from muscle contraction also increases lymphatic pressure, pushing it past one-way lymphatic valves. Because the valves prevent backflow, the system becomes a pump that keeps lymph moving in one direction (toward a subclavian vein).

The mechanism of inspiration, resulting from the descent of the diaphragm, causes intraabdominal pressure to increase as intrathoracic pressure decreases. This simultaneously causes pressure to increase in the abdominal portion of the thoracic duct and to decrease in the thoracic portion. In other words, the process of inspiring establishes a pressure gradient in the thoracic duct that causes lymph to flow upward through it.

Research studies have shown that thoracic duct lymph is literally "pumped" into the venous system during the inspiration phase of pulmonary ventilation. The rate of flow, or ejection, of lymph into the venous circulation is proportional to the depth of inspiration. The total volume of lymph that enters the central veins during a given period depends on the depth of the inspiration phase and the overall breathing rate.

Most lymph flow in the body is the result of contracting skeletal muscles. As muscles contract, they "milk" the lymphatic vessels and push the lymph forward (**Figure 31-7**). The actual pressure generated in the system remains very low, and movement of lymph proceeds quite slowly when compared with the circulation of blood. During exercise, lymph flow may increase as much as 10 to 15 times. In addition to lymph flow caused by skeletal muscle contractions, a very limited amount of smooth muscle exists in the walls of the large lymphatic trunks. Contraction of the smooth muscle in the thoracic vessel walls permits lymphatic vessels to pulse rhythmically and thus help move lymph from one valved segment to the next.

Other pressure-generating factors that can compress the lymphatics also contribute to the effectiveness of the "lymphatic pump". Examples of such lymphokinetic factors include interstitial fluid pressure (**Figure 31-8**), arterial pulsations, postural changes, and passive compression (massage) of the body soft tissues.

Although the overall volume of lymph that enters the bloodstream during each 24-hour period averages about 3 litres, it may

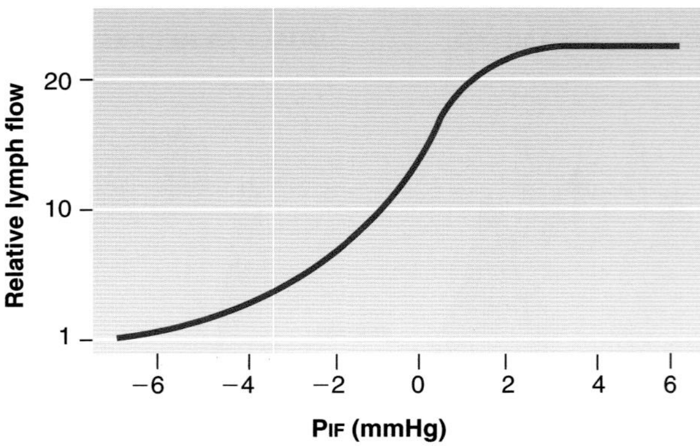

FIGURE 31-8 Lymph flow and interstitial fluid (IF) pressure. As the pressure of IF (PIF) increases, the flow of lymph increases. Muscle pumps can increase IF pressure, as can other factors, such as accumulation of additional interstitial fluid volume within a tissue.

enter the system at different rates during the day. The rate of return varies, depending on the level of generalized physical activity and other factors, including changes in the interstitial fluid pressure and the rate and depth of respiration. As physical activity increases, so does the outflow of fluid from blood capillaries into the tissue spaces of the body. The increased flow of lymph that occurs with increased physical activity helps return this fluid to the cardiovascular system and thus serves as an important balancing or homeostatic mechanism.

Quick CHECK

1. What is the overall function of the lymphatic system?
2. What is the origin of lymph?
3. Compare lymphatic vessels with blood vessels.

LYMPH NODES

Structure of Lymph Nodes

Lymph nodes are oval-shaped or bean-shaped structures (**Figure 31-9**). Some are as small as a pinhead, and others are as large as a butter bean. Each lymph node (from 1 mm to more than 20 mm in diameter) is enclosed by a fibrous capsule. Note in **Figure 31-10** that lymph moves into a node by way of numerous *afferent* lymphatic vessels and emerges at the notch or hilum by one or more *efferent* vessels.

Think of a lymph node as a biological filter placed in the channel of several afferent lymph vessels (as you saw in **Figure 31-5**). Once lymph enters the node, it "percolates" slowly through the spaces known as sinuses before draining into the single efferent exit vessel. One-way valves in both the afferent and efferent vessels keep lymph flowing in one direction.

Fibrous septa, or *trabeculae*, extend from the covering capsule toward the centre of the node. **Cortical nodules** within sinuses along the periphery, or cortex, of the node are separated from each other by these connective tissue trabeculae. Each cortical nodule is composed of packed lymphocytes that surround a less dense area called a *germinal centre* (see **Figure 31-10**).

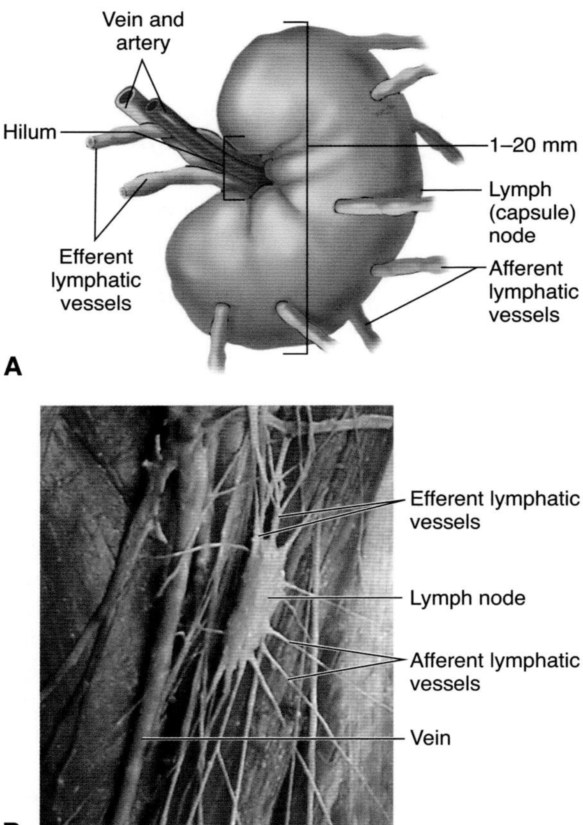

FIGURE 31-9 External structure of a lymph node. A, A lymph node is typically a small structure into which afferent lymphatic ducts empty their lymph and out of which efferent lymphatic ducts drain the lymph. An outer fibrous capsule maintains the structural integrity of the node. **B,** Photograph of a dissected cadaver shows a lymph node and its associated lymphatic vessels, along with nearby muscles, nerves, and blood vessels.

Figure 31-10, *B*, is a low-power (×35) light micrograph of a portion of a typical lymph node. When an infection is present, germinal centres form and the node begins to release lymphocytes. B lymphocytes (B cells) begin their final stages of maturation within the less dense germinal centre of the nodule and then are pushed to the more densely packed outer layers as they mature to become antibody-producing plasma cells. The centre, or medulla, of a lymph node is composed of sinuses and medullary cords (see **Figure 31-10**). Both the cortical and medullary sinuses are lined with reticuloendothelial cells (macrophages) capable of phagocytosis.

Locations of Lymph Nodes

With the exception of comparatively few single nodes, most lymph nodes occur in groups, or clusters, in certain areas. The group locations of greatest clinical importance are as follows:

Preauricular lymph nodes—located just in front of the ear; these nodes drain the superficial tissues and skin on the lateral side of the head and face (**Figure 31-11**).

Submental group and **submandibular group** *(submaxillary)*—in the floor of the mouth; lymph from the nose, lips, and teeth drains through these nodes (see **Figure 31-11**).

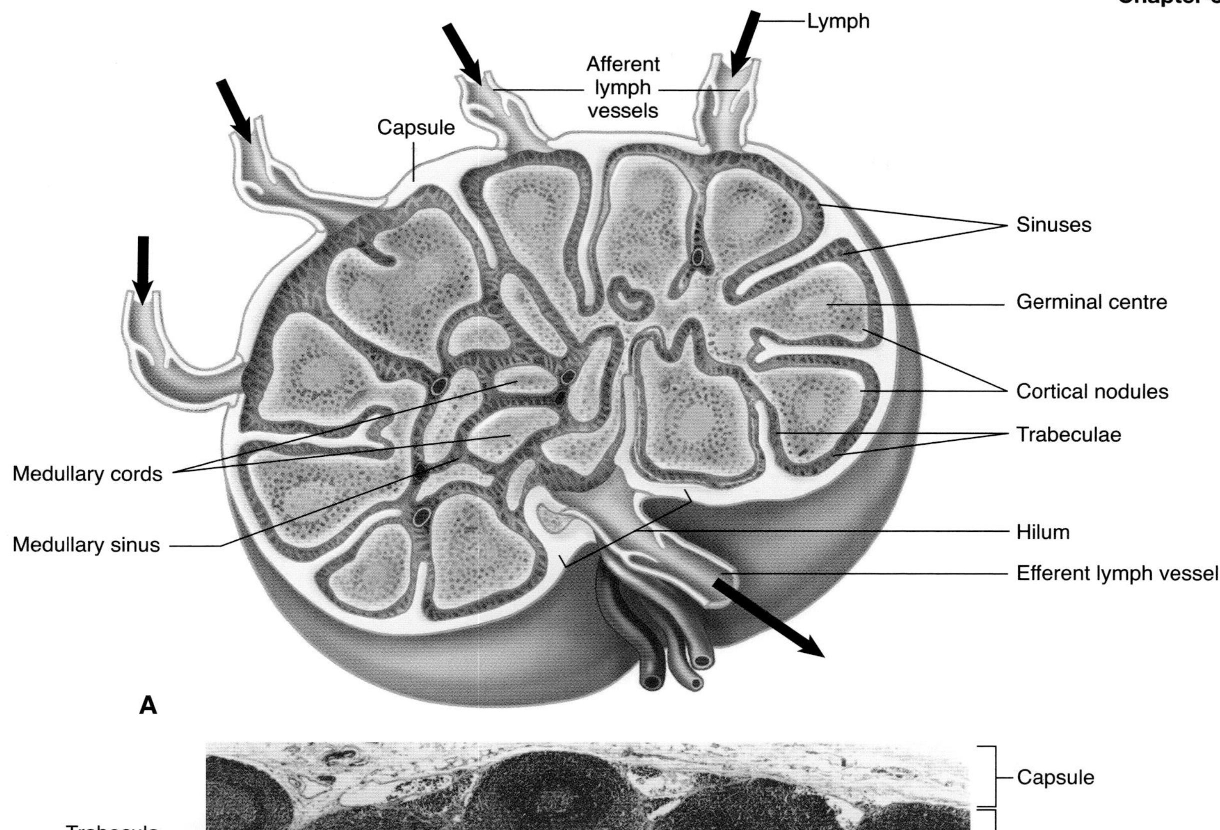

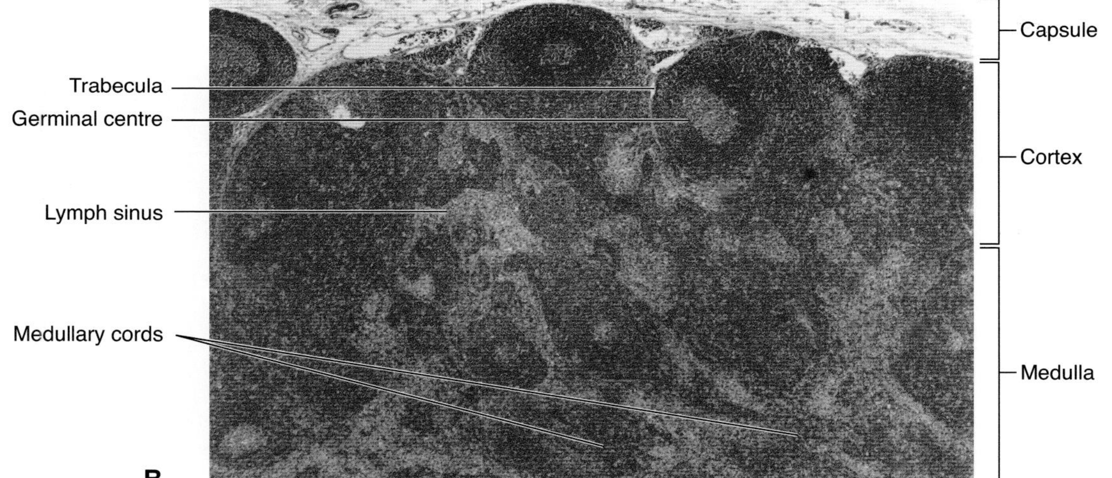

FIGURE 31-10 Internal structure of a lymph node. **A,** Several afferent valved lymphatics bring lymph to the node. In this example, a single efferent lymphatic leaves the node at a concave area called the *hilum.* Note that the artery and vein also enter and leave at the hilum. Arrows show direction of lymph flow. **B,** Photomicrograph showing a portion of the cortex and medulla of a lymph node.

Superficial cervical lymph nodes—in the neck along the sternocleidomastoid muscle, these nodes drain lymph (which has already passed through other nodes) from the head and neck (**Figure 31-12**; see also **Figure 31-11**).

Superficial cubital lymph nodes (supratrochlear lymph nodes)—located just above the bend of the elbow; lymph from the forearm passes through these nodes (see **Figure 31-2**).

Axillary lymph nodes—20 to 30 large nodes clustered deep within the underarm and upper chest regions; lymph from the arm and upper part of the thoracic wall, including the breast, drains through these nodes (see **Figure 31-2**).

Iliac lymph nodes and **inguinal lymph nodes**—in the pelvis and groin; lymph from the pelvic organs, legs, and external genitals drains through these nodes (**Figure 31-13**; see **Figure 31-6**).

Functions of Lymph Nodes

Lymph nodes perform at least two distinct functions: defence and haematopoiesis.

Defence Functions: Filtration and Phagocytosis

The structure of the sinus channels within lymph nodes slows the lymph flow through them. This gives the reticuloendothelial cells that line the channels time to remove the microorganisms and other injurious particles—soot, for example—from the lymph and phagocytose them (**Figure 31-14**). Lymph nodes physically stop particles from progressing farther in the body—a process called *mechanical filtration*. Because lymph nodes also make use of biological processes such as phagocytosis to destroy particles, *biological filtration* also occurs here.

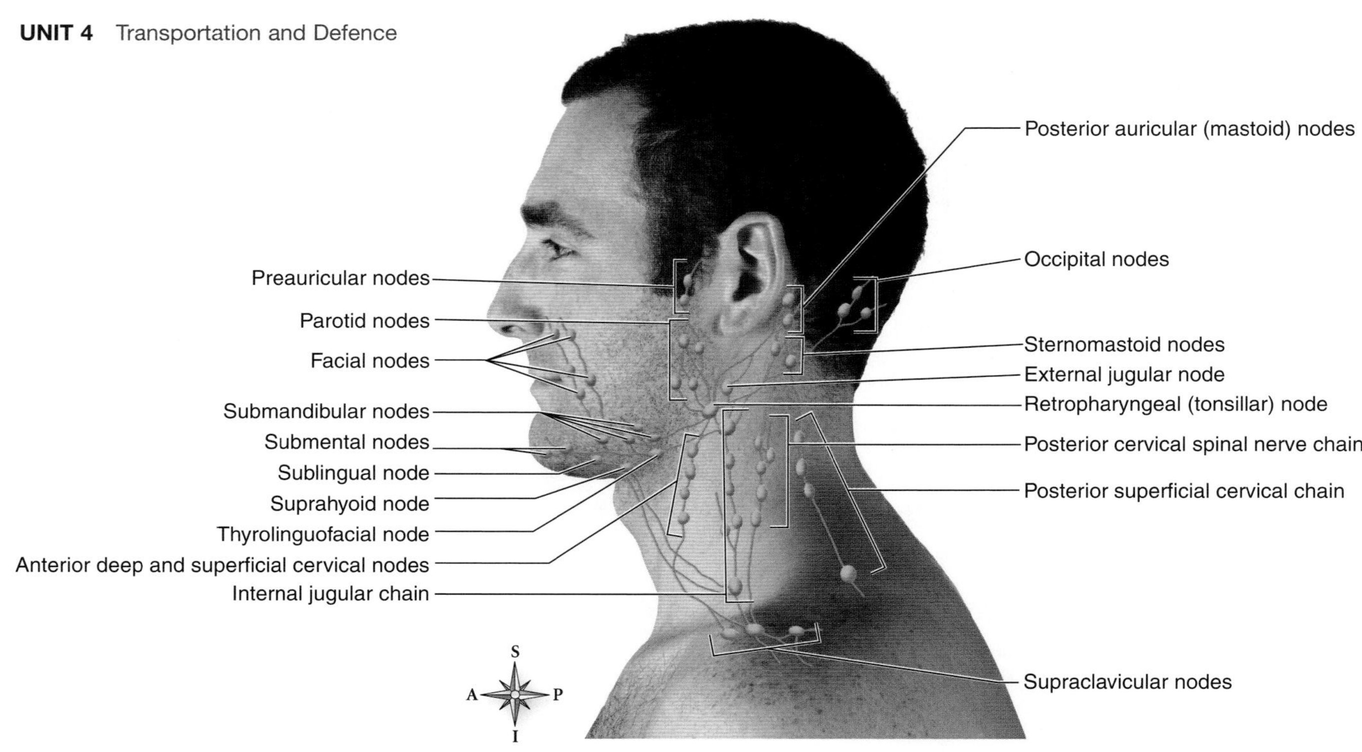

FIGURE 31-11 Lymphatic drainage of the head and neck. The head and neck contain many lymph nodes (and associated lymphatic vessels) that are often of clinical significance in certain infections and cancers.

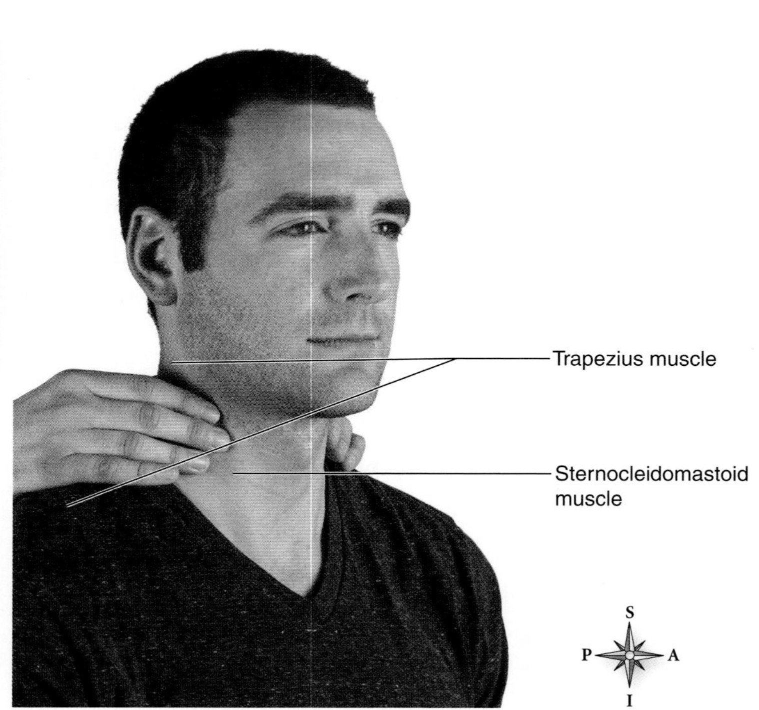

FIGURE 31-12 Palpation of the posterior cervical lymph nodes. The pads of the fingertips are used to palpate (feel) along the anterior surface of the trapezius muscle and then moved slowly in a circular motion to the posterior surface of the sternocleidomastoid muscle. Swollen lymph nodes may be a sign of infection, cancer, blocked lymphatic drainage, or some other abnormal condition.

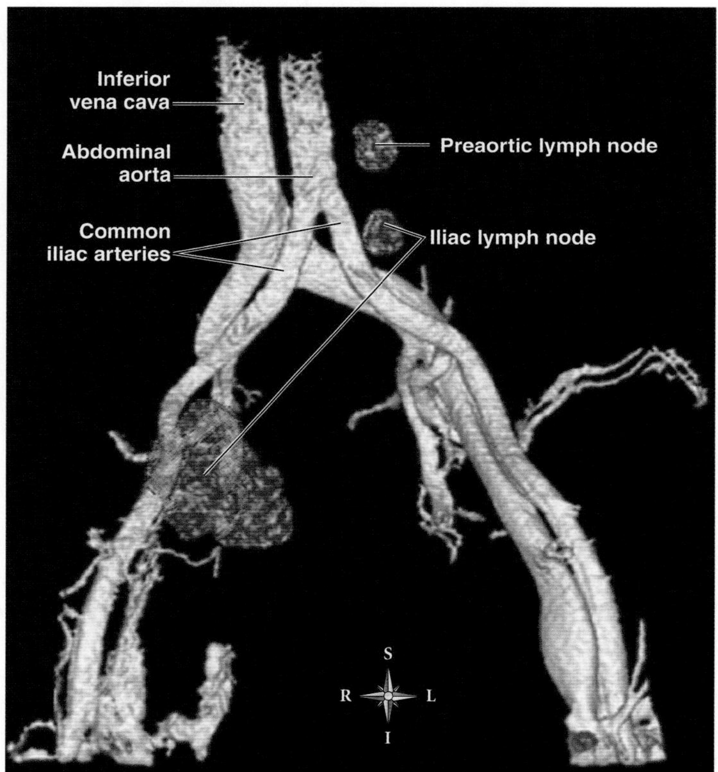

FIGURE 31-13 MRI of lymph nodes. This three-dimensional magnetic resonance image (MRI) has been enhanced by the use of specially engineered nanoparticles that are injected into the blood and then later ingested by macrophages in the lymphoid tissue of the lymph nodes. In lymphoid tissue containing metastasized cancer cells, there is a recognizable, abnormal pattern calculated in the MRI software (colour-coded *red* in this image). Thus cancerous lymph nodes can be identified and accurately located for surgical removal or other therapy.

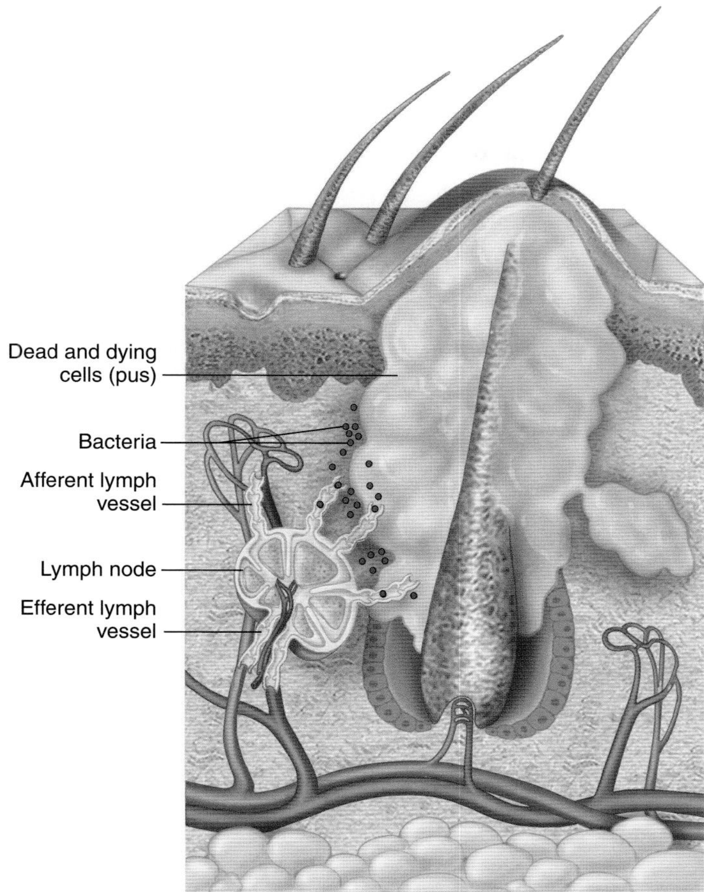

FIGURE 31-14 Role of a lymph node in a skin infection. Leucocytes phagocytose many bacteria in tissue spaces. Others may enter the lymph nodes by way of afferent lymphatics. The nodes filter out these bacteria; reticuloendothelial cells within the nodes usually destroy all the bacteria by phagocytosis. (Lymph node is shown smaller than actual size.)

Sometimes, however, such hordes of microorganisms enter the nodes that the phagocytes cannot destroy enough of them to prevent injury to the node. An infection of the node, *adenitis*, then results. Also, because cancer cells often break away from a malignant tumour and enter lymphatics, they travel to the lymph nodes, where they may set up new growths and block flow of lymph. This may leave too few channels for lymph to return to the blood. For example, if tumours block axillary node channels, fluid accumulates in the interstitial spaces of the arm, causing the arm to become markedly swollen. Even viruses such as human immunodeficiency virus (HIV) and other types of pathogens can infect or infest lymph nodes, as seen in **Figure 31-15**.

Haematopoiesis

The lymphoid tissue of lymph nodes serves as the site of the final stages of maturation for some types of lymphocytes and monocytes that have migrated from the bone marrow. In addition to lymph nodes and the major lymphatic organs described later in the chapter, small aggregates of diffuse lymphoid tissue and other lymphatic cell types are found throughout the body—especially in connective tissues and under mucous membranes.

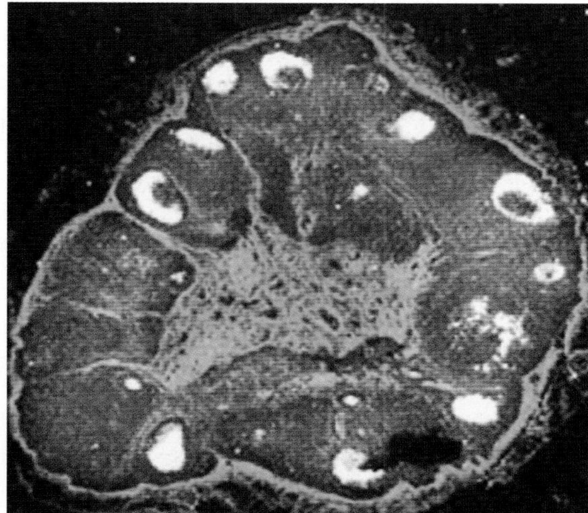

FIGURE 31-15 Infected lymph node. This lymph node is infected with human immunodeficiency virus (HIV), seen in this specially stained micrograph as *white areas.* Researchers at the National Institute of Allergy and Infectious Disease (NIAID) found that lymphoid tissue is a major reservoir for HIV, thus providing a sanctuary for viral replication while the virus is being cleared from the bloodstream by the immune system.

CONNECT IT!

See a micrograph of the blood-forming lymphoid tissue of a lymph node in ***Sites of Haematopoiesis*** online at ***Connect It!***

LYMPHATIC DRAINAGE OF THE BREAST

Cancer of the breast is one of the most common forms of malignancy in women. Unfortunately, cancerous cells from a single "primary" tumour in the breast often spread to other areas of the body through the lymphatic system. An understanding of the lymphatic drainage of the breast is therefore of particular importance in the diagnosis and treatment of this type of malignancy (**Box 31-3**).

Breast infections (**mastitis**) are also a serious health concern, especially among women who are nursing infants. Breast infections, like cancer, can also spread easily through lymphatic pathways

BOX 31-3 *health matters*
Lymphoedema After Breast Surgery

Surgical procedures called *mastectomies,* in which some or all of the breast tissue is removed, are sometimes performed to treat breast cancer. Because cancer cells can spread so easily through the extensive network of lymphatic vessels associated with the breast (see **Figure 31-16**), the lymphatic vessels and their nodes are sometimes also removed. Occasionally, such procedures interfere with the normal flow of lymph fluid from the arm. When this happens, tissue fluid may accumulate in the arm—resulting in swelling, or *lymphoedema.* Fortunately, adequate lymph drainage is almost always restored by the reestablishment of new lymphatic vessels, which grow back into the area.

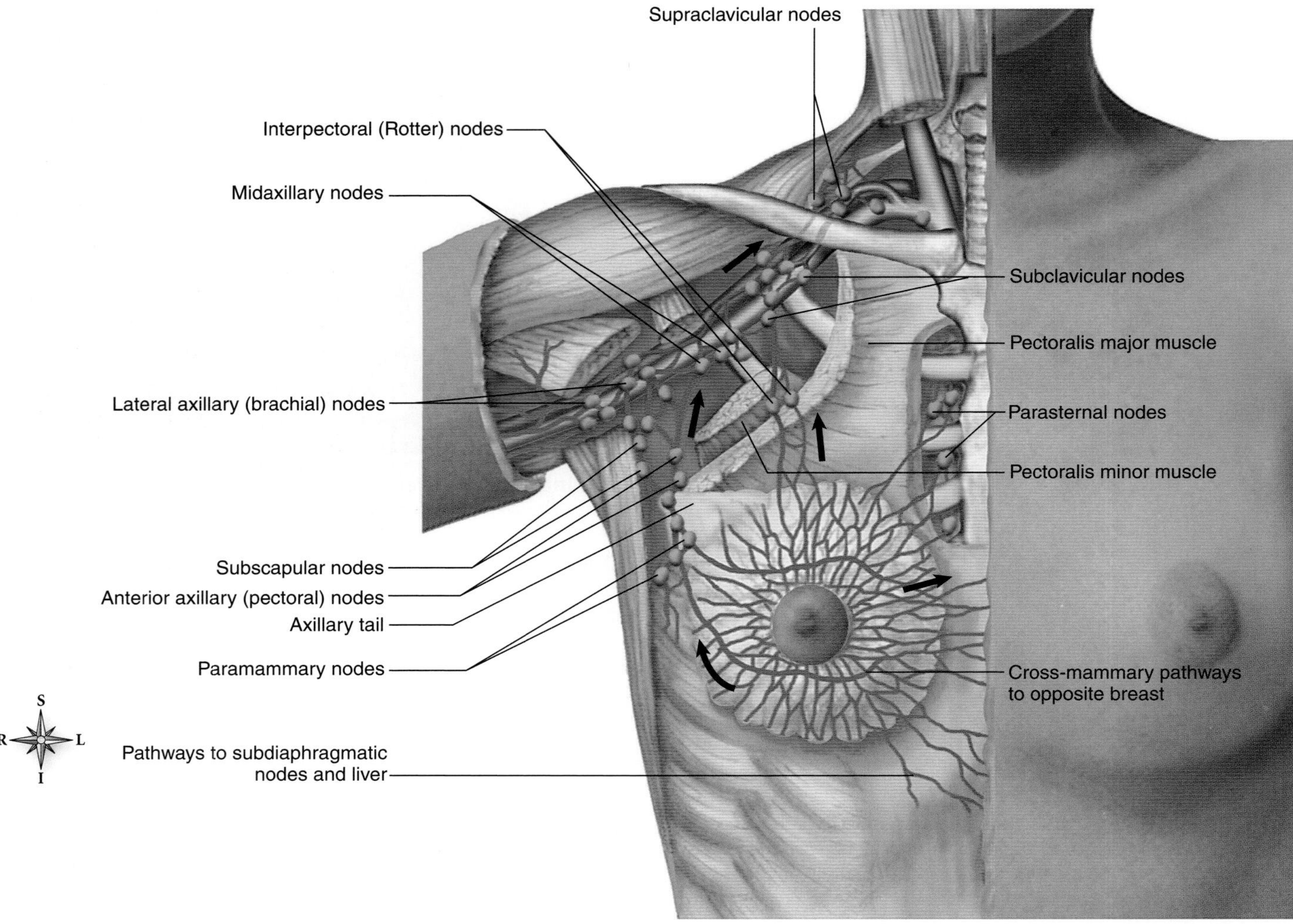

FIGURE 31-16 Lymphatic drainage of the breast. Note the extensive network of lymphatic vessels and nodes that receive lymph from the breast.

BOX 31-4 *health matters* | **Lymphatic Anastomoses and Breast Cancer**

Anastomoses (connections) occur between superficial lymphatics from both breasts across the middle line. Such communication can result in the spread of cancerous cells in one breast to previously healthy tissue in the other breast.

Both superficial and deep lymphatic vessels also communicate with lymphatics in the fascia of the pectoralis major muscle. Removal of a wide area of deep fascia is therefore required in surgical treatment of advanced or diffuse breast malignancy (radical mastectomy). In addition, cancer cells from a breast tumour sometimes reach the abdominal cavity because of lymphatic communication through the upper part of the linea alba.

A more thorough discussion of breast cancer is found in Chapter 46 on p. 1083.

associated with the breast. Refer to **Figure 31-16** as you study the lymphatic drainage of the breast.

Distribution of Lymphatics in the Breast

The breast—mammary gland and surrounding tissues—is drained by the following two sets of lymphatic vessels:

1. Lymphatics that originate in and drain the skin over the breast, with the exception of the areola and nipple
2. Lymphatics that originate in and drain the underlying substance of the breast itself, as well as the skin of the areola and nipple

Superficial vessels that drain lymph from the skin and surface areas of the breast converge to form a diffuse *cutaneous lymphatic plexus*. Communication between the cutaneous plexus and large lymphatics that drain the secretory tissue and ducts of the breast occurs in the *subareolar plexus (plexus of Sappey)* located under the areola surrounding the nipple.

Box 31-4 discusses the numerous connections of the breast lymphatic pathways.

Lymph Nodes Associated with the Breast

More than 85% of the lymph from the breast enters the lymph nodes of the axillary region (see **Figure 31-16**). Most of the remainder enters lymph nodes along the lateral edges of the sternum.

Several very large nodes in the axillary region are in actual physical contact with an extension of breast tissue called the *axillary tail (tail of Spence)*. Because of the physical contact between these nodes and breast tissue, cancerous and infectious cells may spread by both lymphatic extension and contiguity of tissue. Other nodes in the axilla or chest wall will enlarge and swell after being "seeded" with malignant cells or bacteria as lymph from a cancerous or infected breast flows through them. For example, interpectoral nodes (Rotter nodes) found between the pectoralis major and minor muscles often contain metastases from mammary cancer.

A **sentinel lymph node (SLN)** is the first lymph node to which a cancerous tumour can spread. When a tumour is detected, the nearby SLN may be identified and examined in a biopsy to determine whether cancer cells are present—showing that the cancer has metastasized.

Quick CHECK

4. Describe the overall structure of a typical lymph node.
5. Where are lymph nodes usually found?
6. What functions are carried out by lymph nodes?
7. How do the lymphatic structures of the breast relate to breast cancer?

TONSILS

Masses of lymphoid tissue, called **tonsils,** are located in a protective ring under the mucous membranes in the mouth and back of the throat (**Figure 31-17**, A). This ring is called the *pharyngeal lymphoid ring*. The ring of tonsils helps protect against bacteria that may invade tissues in the area around the openings between the nasal and oral cavities.

The **palatine tonsils** are located on each side of the throat. The **pharyngeal tonsils,** known as *adenoids* when they become swollen, are near the posterior opening of the nasal cavity. A third type of tonsil, the **lingual tonsils,** is near the base of the tongue. A fourth type of tonsil, the *tubal tonsils*, is located near the opening of the auditory (eustachian) tube. Each of the tonsils has deep recesses called *tonsillar crypts* that trap bacteria and put them in close contact with cells of the immune system.

The tonsils serve as the first line of defence from the exterior and as such are subject to chronic infection, or **tonsillitis** (**Figure 31-17**, B). They are sometimes removed surgically if antibiotic therapy is not successful or if swelling impairs breathing. This procedure, called **tonsillectomy,** is no longer a routine treatment because of the critical immunological role played by the lymphoid tissue.

CONNECT IT! 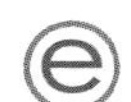

Because it is exposed to the external environment, the respiratory tract could be extremely vulnerable. Look at the structure of a tonsil and learn about its defensive role in ***Protective Strategies of the Respiratory Tract*** online at ***Connect It!***

THYMUS

Location and Appearance of the Thymus

Intensive study and experimentation have identified the **thymus** as a primary organ of the lymphatic system. It is an unpaired organ consisting of two pyramidal lobes with delicate and finely lobulated surfaces. The thymus is located in the mediastinum, extending up into the neck as far as the lower edge of the thyroid gland and inferiorly as far as the fourth costal cartilage (**Figure 31-18**, A). Its size relative to the rest of the body is largest in a child about 2 years old. Its absolute size is largest at puberty, when its weight ranges between 35 and 40 grams. From then on, it gradually atrophies until, in advanced old age, it may be largely replaced by fat, weigh less than 10 grams, and be barely recognizable. By age 60, the lymphoid tissue is about half its maximum size and is virtually gone by age 80 or so. The process of shrinkage of an organ in this manner is called **involution.** The thymus is pinkish grey in early childhood but, with advancing age, becomes yellowish as lymphoid tissue is replaced by fat.

UNIT 4

FIGURE 31-17 Location of the tonsils. A, Small segments of the roof and floor of the mouth have been removed to show the protective ring of tonsils (pharyngeal lymphoid ring) around the internal openings of the nose and throat. Tubal tonsils are not visible in this view. **B,** Tonsillitis. Note the swelling and presence of a white coating (exudate) indicating an infection.

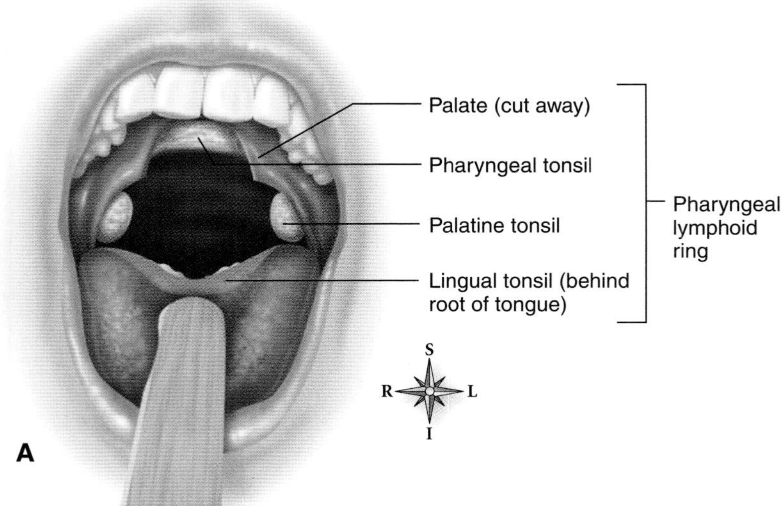

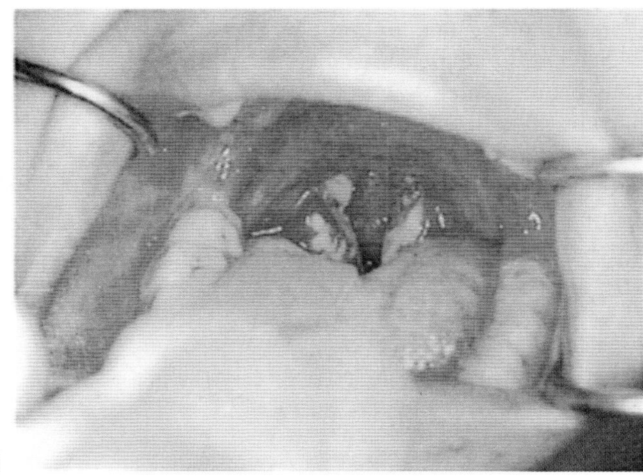

Structure of the Thymus

The lobes of the thymus are subdivided into small (1- to 2-mm) lobules by connective tissue septa that extend inward from a fibrous covering capsule. Each lobule is composed of a dense cellular cortex and an inner, less dense medulla (**Figure 31-18**, *B*). Both cortex and medulla are composed of lymphocytes in an epithelial framework quite different from the supporting connective tissue seen in other lymphoid organs.

In stained histological sections of thymus, medullary tissue can be identified by the presence of rather large (30- to 150-mm) laminated spherical structures called **thymic corpuscles,** or *Hassall corpuscles.* Composed of concentric layers of keratinized epithelial cells, thymic corpuscles have a unique onionlike appearance. These corpuscles may serve as a place to break down dead, keratinized epithelial cells migrating inward from the outer parts of each lobule. They also secrete some of the regulatory molecules that affect white blood cell (WBC) development described in the next section.

Function of the Thymus

One of the body's best-kept secrets has been the function of the thymus. Before 1961 there were no significant clues as to its role. Then a young Briton, Dr. Jacques F.A.P. Miller, removed the thymus glands from newborn mice. His findings proved startling and crucial. Almost like a chain reaction, further investigations followed, leading to the gradual uncovering of the thymus's long-held secrets. It is now clear that this small structure plays a critical part in the body's defences against infections—in its vital immunity mechanism (see Chapter 33).

The thymus performs at least two important functions. First, it serves as the final site of lymphocyte development before birth. (The fetal bone marrow forms immature lymphocytes, which then move to the thymus.) Many lymphocytes leave the thymus and circulate to the spleen, lymph nodes, and other lymphoid tissues. Second, soon after birth the thymus begins secreting a group of hormones (collectively called *thymosin*) and other regulators that enable lymphocytes to develop into mature T cells. Only T cells (T lymphocytes) that pass immunological testing by lymphoid cells such as *macrophages* and *dendritic cells*—only about 5% of the cells that mature each day—are released into the bloodstream. **Figure 31-19** outlines some essential steps in T-cell development within the thymus.

Because T cells attack foreign or abnormal cells and also serve as regulators of immune function, the thymus functions as an important part of the immune mechanism. It is most active in childhood. Beginning at puberty, involution of the thymus reduces its function gradually through adulthood. By the time a person is 50, only 10% of functional thymus tissue remains. Elderly people have virtually no functional thymus tissue left, a factor that contributes to reduced immune function associated with ageing.

SPLEEN

Location of the Spleen

The **spleen** is located in the left hypochondrium of the abdominopelvic cavity, directly below the diaphragm. The spleen is just above most of the left kidney and the descending colon and behind the fundus of the stomach (**Figure 31-2** and **Figure 31-20**). In addition, it is common to find small *accessory spleens* embedded in the double fold of serous membrane that connects the spleen and stomach. Accessory spleens often form from splenic cells released from the spleen during even minor injuries to its structure.

Structure of the Spleen

As **Figure 31-20** and **Figure 31-21** show, the spleen is roughly ovoid in shape. Its size varies in different individuals and in the same individual at different times (**Box 31-5**). For example, it hypertrophies during infectious diseases and atrophies in old age.

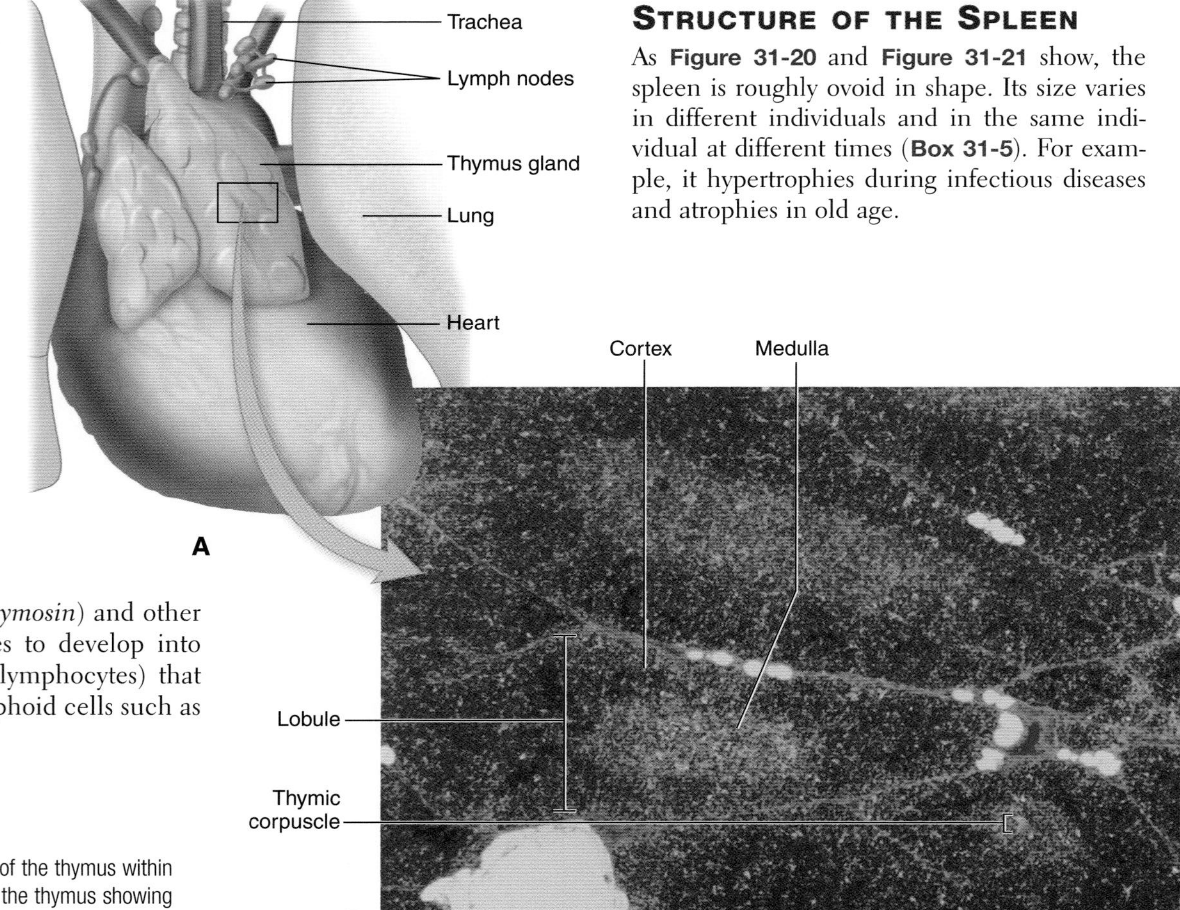

FIGURE 31-18 Thymus. A, Location of the thymus within the mediastinum. **B,** Microscopic structure of the thymus showing several lobules, each with a cortex and a medulla.

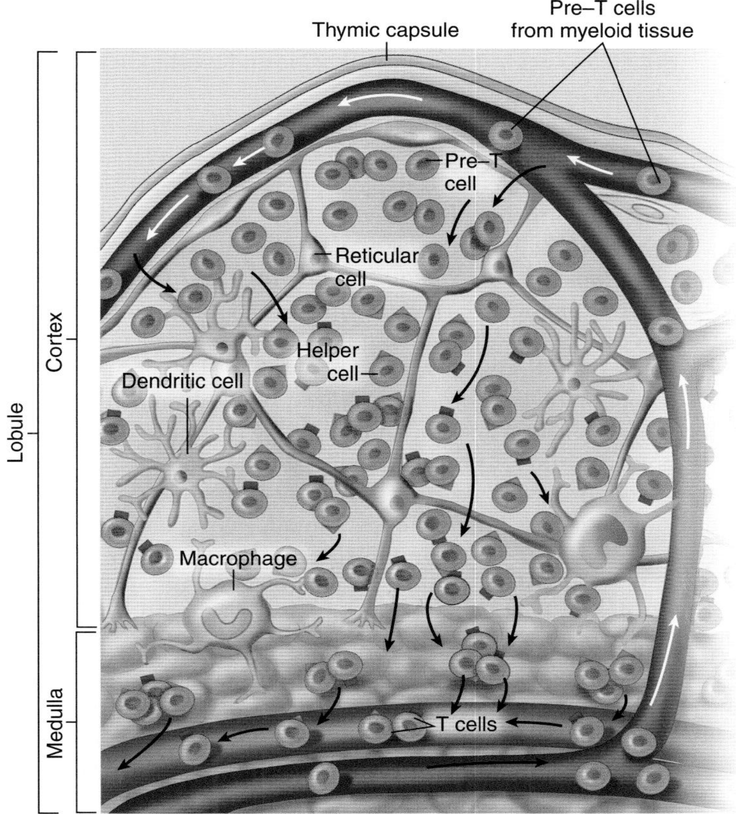

FIGURE 31-19 T-cell development in the thymus. This diagram shows part of a lobule, with the cortex at the top and the medulla at the bottom. Pre–T cells derived from haematopoietic stem cells in red bone marrow (myeloid tissue) travel through the bloodstream to the cortex of the thymus. Under the influence of thymosin and other regulators, the pre–T cells divide and mature as they migrate toward the medulla. Along the way, the developing T cells (T lymphocytes) are tested for immune capability against various lymphoid immune cells, such as dendritic cells and macrophages. Only about 5% of the cells pass these tests and are released into the bloodstream to defend the body.

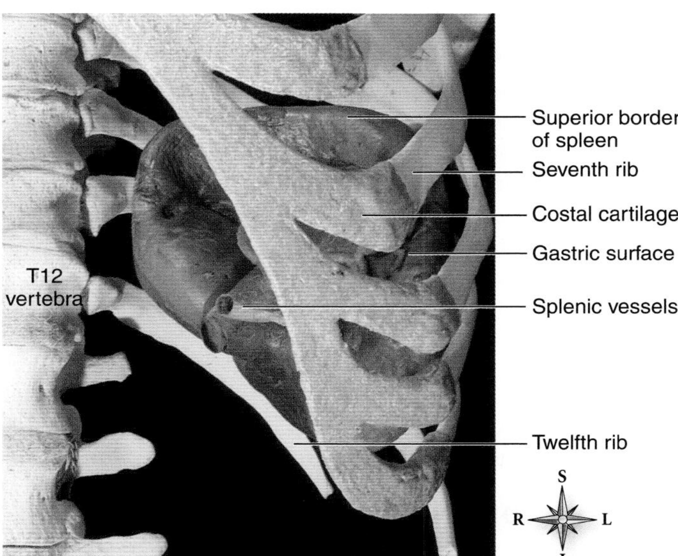

FIGURE 31-20 Location of the spleen. The spleen is located in the left hypochondrium of the abdominopelvic cavity, just inferior to the diaphragm and just deep to the lower portion of the rib cage.

Like other lymphoid organs, the spleen is surrounded by a fibrous capsule with inward extensions that roughly divide the organ into compartments. One such compartment is shown in **Figure 31-21**, *B*. Arteries leading into each compartment are surrounded by dense masses (nodules) of developing lymphocytes. Because of its whitish appearance, this tissue is called *white pulp*.

Near the outer regions of each compartment is tissue called *red pulp*, made up of a network of fine reticular fibres submerged in blood that comes from the nearby arterioles. The red pulp network supports cords of WBCs and related cells surrounded by blood-filled

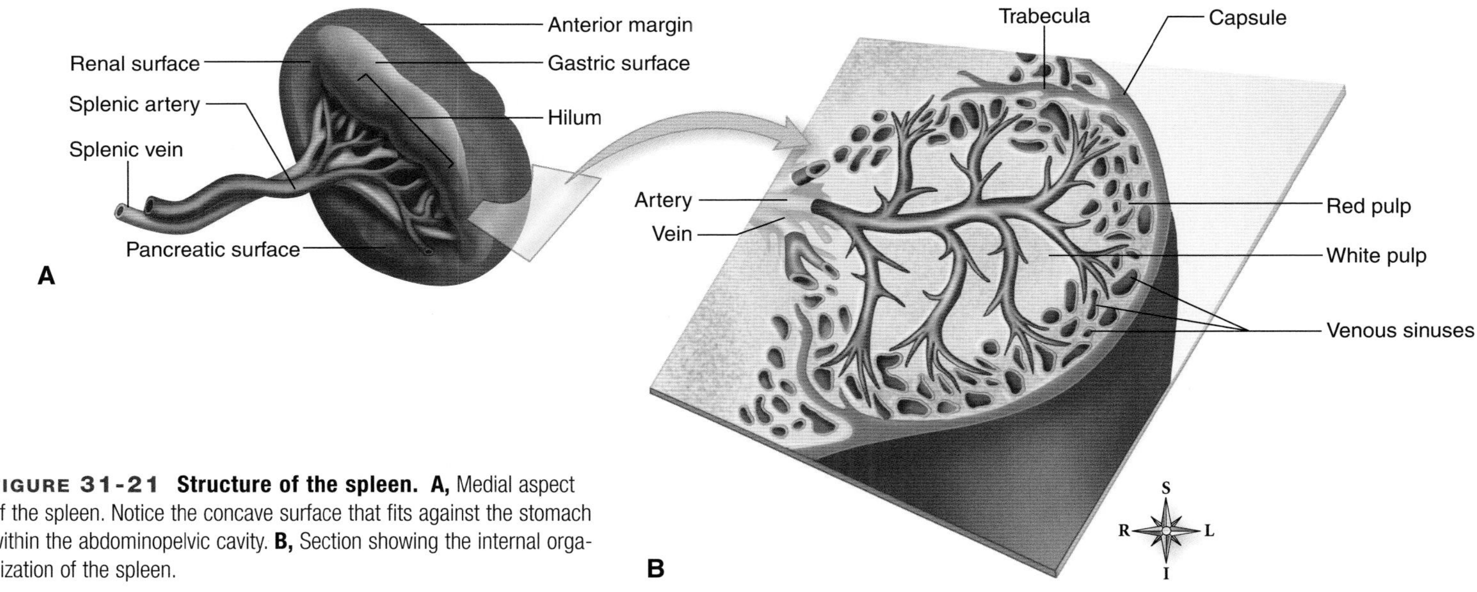

FIGURE 31-21 Structure of the spleen. A, Medial aspect of the spleen. Notice the concave surface that fits against the stomach within the abdominopelvic cavity. **B,** Section showing the internal organization of the spleen.

BOX 31-5 *health matters* | Splenomegaly

Splenomegaly, or abnormal spleen enlargement, is observed in various disorders. For example, infectious conditions such as scarlet fever, syphilis, and typhoid fever may be characterized by splenomegaly. Spleen enlargement sometimes accompanies hypertension. Splenomegaly also accompanies some forms of haemolytic anaemia in which red blood cells appear to be broken apart at an abnormally fast rate. Surgical removal of the spleen often prevents death in such cases.

sinusoids. After passing through the reticular meshwork, blood collects in venous sinuses and then returns to the heart through veins.

Functions of the Spleen

The spleen has many and sundry functions, including defence, haematopoiesis, and red blood cell and platelet destruction; it also serves as a reservoir for blood.

- ***Defence.*** As blood passes through the sinusoids of the spleen, reticuloendothelial cells (macrophages) lining these venous spaces remove microorganisms from the blood and destroy them by phagocytosis. Therefore the spleen plays a part in the body's defence against microorganisms.
- ***Tissue repair.*** Monocytes found in the cords of WBCs in red pulp just under the spleen's outer capsule are mobilized when significant tissue damage occurs, such as in heart attack (MI) or stroke (CVA). A large number of monocytes migrate quickly to the injured tissue and assist in healing and repair.
- ***Haematopoiesis.*** Nongranular leucocytes—that is, monocytes and lymphocytes—complete their development and become activated in the spleen. Before birth, red blood cells are also formed in the spleen, but after birth, the spleen forms red blood cells only in cases of extreme haemolytic anaemia.
- ***Red blood cell destruction** and **platelet destruction.*** Macrophages lining the spleen's sinusoids remove worn-out red blood cells and imperfect platelets from the blood and destroy them by phagocytosis. They also break apart the haemoglobin molecules from the destroyed red blood cells and salvage their iron and globin content by returning them to the bloodstream for storage in bone marrow and liver.
- ***Blood reservoir.*** At any given point in time the pulp of the spleen and its venous sinuses contain a considerable amount of blood. Although continually moving slowly through the spleen, blood can rapidly be added back into the circulatory system from this functional reservoir if needed. Its normal volume of about 350 mL is said to decrease by about 200 mL in less than 1 minute after sympathetic stimulation that produces marked constriction of its smooth-muscle capsule. This "self-transfusion" occurs, for example, as a response to the stress imposed by haemorrhage.

Although the spleen's functions make it a most useful organ, it is not a vital one. Dr. Charles Austin Doan in 1933 took the daring step of performing the first **splenectomy.** He removed the spleen from a 4-year-old girl who was dying of haemolytic anaemia. Presumably,

TABLE 31-1 Major Lymphatic Organs

ORGAN	STRUCTURE	FUNCTION
Lymphatic vessels	Thin-walled vessels with numerous valves that ensure one-way flow of lymphatic fluid (lymph); larger vessels have three layers (similar to veins)	Collect fluids draining from tissues of the body (lymph) and return it to the blood circulation
Lymphatic capillaries	Microscopic, blind-end vessels, made up of single endothelial layer having many gaps	Collect tissue fluid (forming lymph) Transport lymph to larger lymphatic vessels
Lymphatic ducts	Large lymphatic vessels formed by many tributaries throughout the body; connect to the subclavian veins	Collect lymph from network of lymphatic vessels and drain it into the blood circulation
Lymphoid organs	Have a significant component of lymphoid tissue (developing white blood cells)	Haematopoiesis (WBCs) Immunity Filter body fluids
Lymph nodes	Fibrous capsule surrounding a maze of sinuses, each with lymphoid tissue nodule suspended by reticular fibres	Filtration of lymph before it enters bloodstream Mechanical filtration: removing particles Biological filtration: cells destroy and remove particles
Aggregated lymph nodules (tonsils, Peyer patches)	Groupings of nodules (lumps of lymphoid tissue) embedded in mucous membranes	Immunity at common points of entry for pathogenic microbes
Thymus	Two pyramid-shaped lobes subdivided into smaller lobules containing lymphoid tissue	Haematopoiesis—site of T-lymphocyte (T-cell) development Hormone production—thymosin regulates T-cell development
Spleen	Ovoid fibrous capsule with internal maze of sinuses containing dense lymphoid tissue (white pulp) surrounded by blood sinusoids having cords of lymphoid tissue (red pulp)	Haematopoiesis (WBCs) Immunity Filtration of blood Tissue repair Destruction of old RBCs, platelets Blood reservoir

RBC, Red blood cell; *WBC,* white blood cell.

UNIT 4

he justified his radical treatment on the basis of what was then merely conjecture—that is, that the spleen destroys red blood cells. The child recovered, and Dr. Doan's operation proved to be a landmark. It created a great upsurge of interest in the spleen and led to many investigations of this organ.

Because of its role as a blood reservoir, the spleen contains a high volume of blood at any one time—especially during rest. If the spleen is accidentally ruptured, as it might be when the ribs are broken and pushed into the spleen, significant internal bleeding could occur. If the blood loss is rapid and is not stopped in time, death could result. Surgical repair or removal of the spleen can stop the blood loss and save a life.

Table 31-1 summarizes the essential characteristics of the major types of lymphatic organs.

Quick CHECK

8. Where are the major tonsils located? What is their role?
9. What major role does the thymus play in immunity?
10. What are the major functions of the spleen?

cycle of life

Lymphatic System Many of the structural features of the lymphatic system exhibit dramatic changes as a person progresses through a life span. Most of the organs containing masses of developing lymphocytes appear before birth and continue growing through most of childhood until just before puberty. After puberty, these lymphoid organs typically begin to slowly atrophy until they reach much smaller size by late adulthood. These organs—including the thymus, lymph nodes, tonsils, and other lymphoid structures—shrink and become fatty or fibrous. The notable exception to this principle is the spleen, which develops early in life and remains intact until very late adulthood.

Despite the fact that lymphocyte-producing lymphoid tissues decline after puberty, the overall function of the immune system is maintained until late adulthood. During the late adult years, deficiency of the immune system permits a greater risk of infections and cancer, and hypersensitivity of the immune system may make autoimmune conditions more likely to occur. •

the big picture | Lymphatic System and the Whole Body

One way to imagine the role of the lymphatic system in the "society of cells" that makes up the human body is as a sort of wastewater system. Like wastewater systems used in the cities of human society, the lymphatic system drains away excess, or "runoff", water from large areas. After collecting the body's runoff, or lymph, the lymphatic system conducts it through a network of lymphatic vessels, or "drainpipes", to miniature "treatment facilities" called *lymph nodes.* Contaminants are there removed from lymph, just as contaminants are removed in a wastewater treatment plant. The "clean" fluid is then returned to the bloodstream much as clean wastewater is returned to a nearby river or lake. Like municipal wastewater systems, the lymphatic system not only prevents dangerous fluid buildups, or "floods", but also prevents the spread of disease.

All systems of the body benefit from the fluid-balancing and immune functions of the lymphatic system. Some parts of the body, such as the digestive and respiratory tracts, make special use of the defensive capacities of lymphatic organs such as aggregated lymph nodules (Peyer patches) and tonsils. Likewise, body structures such as the breasts and limbs make more use of the fluid-draining capacities of the lymphatic system than do other regions of the body. Overall, however, the entire body benefits from the fluid balance and freedom from disease conferred by the proper functioning of this important body system. •

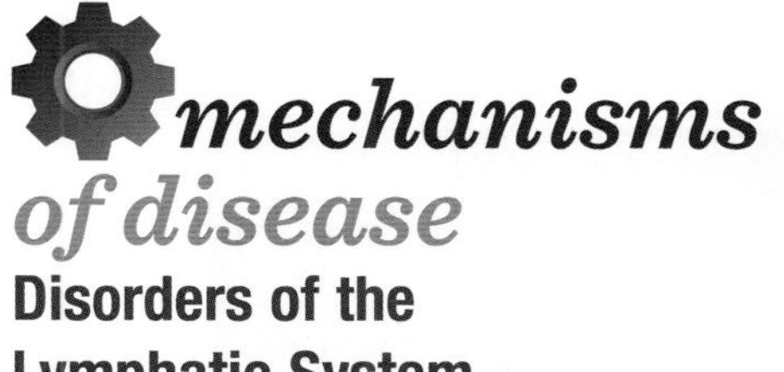

mechanisms of disease

Disorders of the Lymphatic System

Disorders Associated with Lymphatic Vessels

Lymphoedema is an abnormal condition in which swelling of tissues in the extremities occurs because of an obstruction of the lymphatics and accumulation of lymph (**Figure 31-22**). The most common type of lymphoedema is *congenital lymphoedema* (lymphoedema praecox), more often seen in females between the ages of 15 and 25 years. The obstruction in lymphoedema can be in both the lymphatic vessels and lymph nodes themselves. Initially, the swelling, or oedema, in the extremity will be soft, but as the condition progresses, it becomes firm, painful, and unresponsive to treatment. Frequent infections, involving high fever and chills, may occur with chronic lymphoedema. Diuretics (agents that cause water loss) to reduce the swelling have been shown to be effective, along with strict bed rest, massage, and elevation of the involved extremities. If the oedema is severe and unresponsive to these measures, or infection has occurred, or the person's mobility is severely compromised, surgical removal of the involved subcutaneous tissue and fascia may be required. Other procedures involving surgical "shunting" of superficial lymphatic drainage into the deep lymphatic system have been tried.

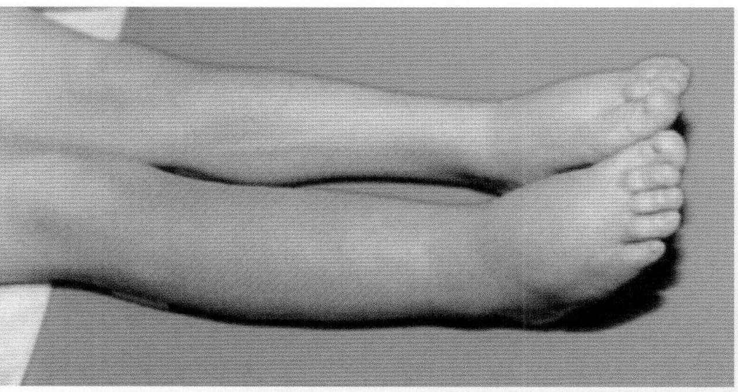

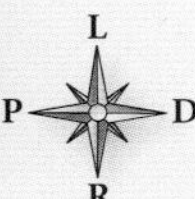

FIGURE 31-22 Lymphoedema. Notice the significant swelling in the subject's right leg and foot.

Lymphoedema may be caused by small parasitic worms (nematodes) called **filaria** that infest the lymph vessels. The condition is endemic in the tropical and

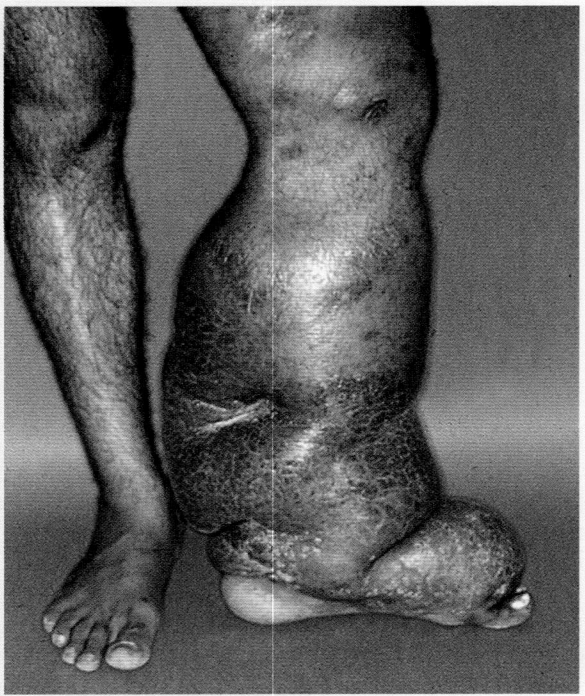
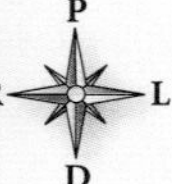

FIGURE 31-23 Elephantiasis. Prolonged infestation of the lymphatic system by *Filaria* worms produces so much swelling (lymphoedema) that the affected limbs begin to resemble those of an elephant!

subtropical parts of Africa, Asia, South and Central America, and the Pacific Island nations. The flow of lymph is blocked, causing oedema in the affected extremities that, in severe cases, become so swollen that they resemble an elephant's limbs (**Figure 31-23**). For this reason, the condition is referred to as **elephantiasis**—literally "condition of being an elephant". Chronic swelling, thickening of the subcutaneous tissue, and frequent bouts of infections are common in this condition.

Lymphangitis, an acute inflammation of the lymphatic vessels, stems from invasion of an infectious organism. This condition is characterized by thin, red streaks extending from an infected region up the arm or leg (**Figure 31-24**). The lymph nodes also become enlarged, tender, and reddened. Necrosis, or tissue death, along with development of an abscess (collection of fluid and pus) can occur, leading to a condition known as *suppurative lymphadenitis.* The lymph nodes commonly involved are in the groin, axilla, and cervical regions. The infectious agents that cause lymphangitis may eventually spread into the bloodstream, causing *septicaemia* (blood poisoning) and possible death from septic shock, but this is rare if the proper antibiotic therapy is initiated.

Disorders Associated with Lymph Nodes and Other Lymphatic Organs

Tonsillitis

The tonsils, composed of lymphoid tissue, serve as the first line of defence from the exterior and also are subject to acute or chronic infection, known as tonsillitis. Fever, sore throat, and difficulty swallowing are common signs and symptoms. Enlarged pharyngeal tonsils (adenoids) may cause nasal obstruction. The infection may extend to the middle ear by way of the auditory (eustachian) tubes, causing *acute otitis media* (middle ear infection) and possible deafness if left untreated. Antibiotics are usually initiated after diagnosis of tonsillitis. If these are unsuccessful, and swelling has endangered the airway and breathing, a *tonsillectomy,* or surgical removal of the tonsils, may be performed.

Lymphoma

Lymphoma is a term that refers to a tumour of the cells of lymphoid tissue. Lymphomas are often malignant but, in rare cases, can be benign. They usually originate in isolated lymph nodes but can involve lymphoid tissue in the liver, spleen, and gastrointestinal tract. Widespread involvement is common because the disease spreads from node to node through the many anastomoses of the lymphatic vessels throughout the body. The exact cause of these neoplasms is unknown.

Two principal categories of lymphomas are *Hodgkin lymphoma (HL)* and *non-Hodgkin lymphoma (NHL).* Hodgkin lymphoma (or **Hodgkin disease**) is a malignancy with an uncertain aetiology. Some pathophysiologists believe that it originates as a pathogen-induced tumour of T cells, although there is currently no evidence to support this conclusively. Other factors such as exposure to chemicals or other environmental hazards may also be involved. This condition usually begins as painless, nontender, enlarged lymph nodes in the neck or axilla (**Figure 31-25**). Soon, lymph nodes in other regions enlarge in the same manner. If they involve the trachea or oesophagus, pressure results in difficulty breathing or swallowing. HL is considered to be one of the most curable forms of cancer if detected early.

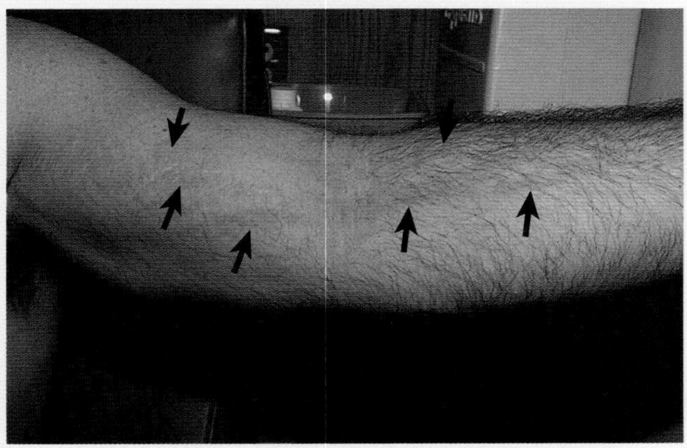
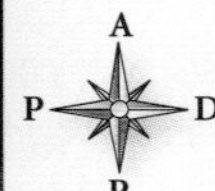

FIGURE 31-24 Lymphangitis. Black arrows mark the location of red streaks that result from inflamed lymphatic vessels in this arm.

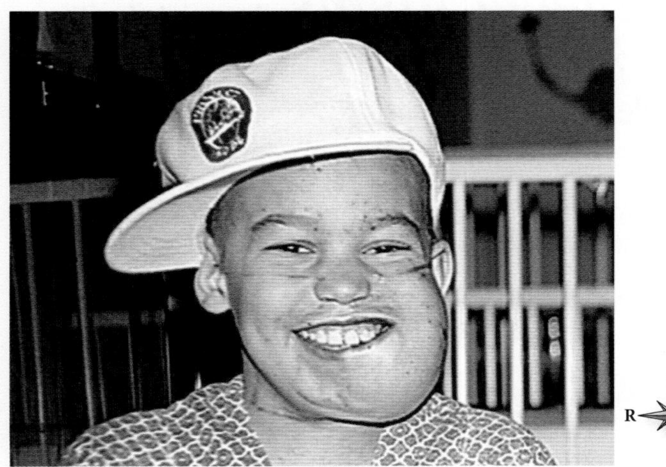

FIGURE 31-25 Hodgkin lymphoma. Enlarged lymph nodes in the neck or axilla characterize this condition.

Lymphoedema caused by blockage of lymph nodes may cause enlargement of the extremities. Occasionally the disease may obstruct flow into or out of the liver, leading to liver enlargement and failure. Anaemia, leucocytosis, fever, and weight loss occur as the condition progresses. Hodgkin lymphoma is potentially curable with radiation therapy, provided it has not spread beyond the lymphatic system. Chemotherapy is used in addition to radiation therapy in more advanced cases. Infection, from both the disease and the treatments, is a common complication.

Non-Hodgkin lymphoma is the name given to a malignancy of lymphoid tissue other than Hodgkin lymphoma. Again, the aetiology is uncertain but the disease has been hypothesized to be caused by a virus. Patients with immunodeficiencies such as AIDS often develop this condition. Manifestations are similar to those of Hodgkin lymphoma, but there is usually a more generalized involvement of lymph nodes. The central nervous system is also often involved. Radiation and chemotherapy are treatments of choice.

LANGUAGE OF SCIENCE *(continued from p. 728)*

lymphokinesis (lim-foh-kih-NEE-sis)
[*lymph-* **water,** *-kinesis* **activation**]

palatine tonsil (PAL-ah-tyne TON-sil)
[*palat-* **palate,** *-ine* **relating to,** *tons-* **goitre,** *-il* **little**]

pharyngeal tonsil (fair-IN-jee-al TON-sil)
[*pharyng-* **throat,** *-al* **relating to,** *tons-* **goitre,** *-il* **little**]

preauricular lymph node (pree-ah-RIK-yoo-lar limf nohd)
[*pre-* **before,** *-auri-* **ear,** *-cula-* **little,** *-ar* **relating to,** *lymph* **water,** *nod-* **knot**]

right lymphatic duct (lim-FAT-ik)
[*lymph-* **water,** *-atic* **relating to**]

submandibular group (sub-man-DIB-yoo-lar)
[*sub-* **beneath,** *-mandibul-* **chew (mandible or jawbone),** *-ar* **relating to**]

submental group (sub-MEN-tal)
[*sub-* **beneath,** *-ment-* **chin,** *-al* **relating to**]

superficial cervical lymph node (soo-per-FISH-al SER-vih-kal limf nohd)
[*super-* **over or above,** *-fici-* **face,** *-al* **relating to,** *cervic-* **neck,** *-al* **relating to,** *lymph* **water,** *nod-* **knot**]

superficial cubital lymph node (soo-per-FISH-al KYOO-bih-tal limf nohd)
[*super-* **over or above,** *-fici-* **face,** *-al* **relating to,** *cubit-* **elbow,** *-al* **relating to,** *lymph* **water,** *nod-* **knot**]

supratrochlear lymph node (soo-prah-TROHK-lee-ar limf nohd)
[*supra-* **above,** *-trochlea-* **pulley,** *-ar* **relating to,** *lymph* **water,** *nod-* **knot**]

thoracic duct (thoh-RAS-ik)
[*thorac-* **chest (thorax),** *-ic* **relating to**]

thymic corpuscle (THYE-mik KOR-pus-ul)
[*thym-* **thyme flower (thymus gland),** *-ic* **relating to,** *corpus-* **body,** *-cle* **little**]

thymus (THY-mus)
[*thymus* **thyme flower**] *pl.,* thymuses

tonsil (TON-sil)
[*tons-* **goitre,** *-il* **little**]

LANGUAGE OF MEDICINE

elephantiasis (el-eh-fan-TYE-ah-sis)
[*elephant-* **elephant,** *-iasis* **condition**]

filaria (fih-LAR-ee-a)
[*fila-* **thread,** *-ar-* **like,** *-ia* **things**]
pl., filariae

Hodgkin disease (HOJ-kin)
[*Thomas Hodgkin* **English physician**]

lymphangiography (lim-fan-jee-OG-reh-fee)
[*lymph-* **water,** *-angi-* **vessel,** *-graph-* **draw,** *-y* **process**]

lymphangitis (lim-fan-JYE-tis)
[*lymph-* **water,** *-angi-* **vessel,** *-itis* **inflammation**]

lymphoedema (lim-fah-DEE-mah)
[*lymph-* **water,** *-oedema* **swelling**]

lymphoma (lim-FOH-mah)
[*lymph-* **water (lymphatic system),** *-oma* **tumour**]

mastitis (mass-TYE-tis)
[*mast-* **breast,** *-itis* **inflammation**]

sentinel lymph node (SLN) (SEN-tin-el limf nohd)
[*sentinel* **lookout,** *lymph* **water,** *nod-* **knot**]

splenectomy (spleh-NEK-toh-mee)
[*splen-* **spleen,** *-ec-* **out,** *-tom-* **cut,** *-y* **action**]

tonsillectomy (ton-sih-LEK-toh-mee)
[*tons-* **goitre,** *-il* **little,** *-ec-* **out,** *-tom-* **cut,** *-y* **action**]

tonsillitis (ton-sih-LYE-tis)
[*tons-* **goitre,** *-il* **little,** *-itis* **inflammation**]

case study

Karen, a dental student, was in Ghana with several of her classmates. Each summer, the students had an opportunity to combine study abroad with volunteering at a dental clinic in Accra. On their second day at the clinic, Karen met Juba, a local farmer's daughter. Juba's right foot and leg below the knee were extremely swollen, seemingly blown up like a balloon. In contrast, Juba's left leg had no swelling at all and appeared quite normal. One of the local dentists told Karen that Juba had elephantiasis, a type of lymphoedema caused by a blockage.

1. What caused Juba's right leg to swell?
   a. Blocked arteries
   b. Blocked veins
   c. Blocked capillaries
   d. Blocked lymphatic vessels
2. Which of the following is NOT a function of the lymphatic system?
   a. Removing excess fluid from the blood
   b. Absorbing lipids from the small intestines
   c. Returning fluid from the interstitial areas back to the bloodstream
   d. Filtering lymph to remove foreign organisms and particulates

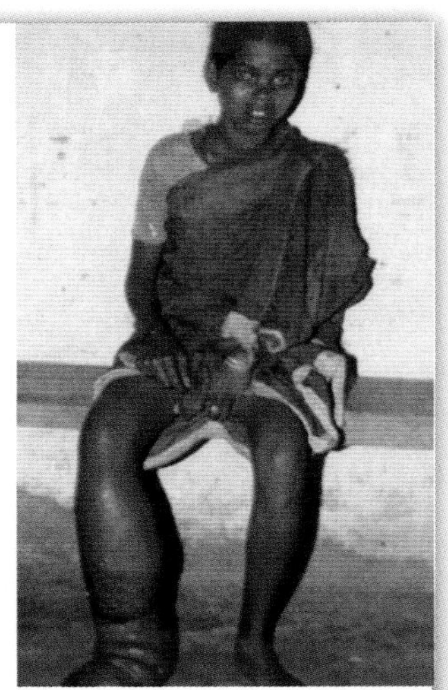

3. What helps circulate the lymph (fluid) through the lymph vessels?
   a. Ventricular contraction
   b. Skeletal muscle contractions
   c. Exhalation
   d. Lymphatic vessel contraction

4. Before Juba's leg became affected by this disorder, the lymph would have passed first through which nodes?
   a. Cervical
   b. Axillary
   c. Inguinal
   d. Mediastinal

Hint To solve a case study, you may have to refer to the glossary or index, other chapters in this textbook, ***Connect It!,*** and other resources.

CHAPTER SUMMARY

To download an MP3 version of the chapter summary for use with your mobile device, access the ***Audio Chapter Summaries*** *online at evolve.elsevier.com.*

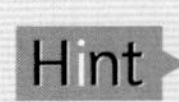

Scan this summary after reading the chapter to help you reinforce the key concepts. Later, use the summary as a quick review before your class or before a test.

Overview of the Lymphatic System

A. Two most important functions—maintain fluid balance in the internal environment and immunity; a third function is to collect absorbed fat from the intestines and transport it to the systemic veins
B. Lymph vessels act as "drains" to collect excess tissue fluid and return it to the venous blood just before it returns to the heart (**Figure 31-1**)
C. Lymphatic system—component of the circulatory system; made up of lymph, lymphatic vessels, and isolated structures containing lymphoid tissue: lymph nodes, aggregated lymphoid nodules, tonsils, thymus, spleen, and bone marrow (**Figure 31-2**)
D. Transports tissue fluid, proteins, fats, and other substances to the general circulation
E. Lymphatic vessels begin blindly in the intercellular spaces of the soft tissues; do not form a closed circuit

Lymph and Interstitial Fluid

A. Lymph (lymphatic fluid)
   1. Clear, watery-appearing fluid found in the lymphatic vessels
   2. Closely resembles blood plasma in composition but has a lower percentage of protein; isotonic
   3. Elevated protein concentration in thoracic duct lymph because of protein-rich lymph from the liver and small intestine
B. Interstitial fluid (IF)
   1. Complex, organized fluid that fills the spaces between the cells and is part of the ECM (extracellular matrix)
   2. Resembles blood plasma in composition with a lower percentage of protein
   3. Along with blood plasma, constitutes the extracellular fluid

Lymphatic Vessels

A. Distribution of lymphatic vessels (lymphatics) (**Figures 31-2** and **31-3**)
   1. Lymphatic capillaries—microscopic blind-end vessels where lymphatic vessels originate; wall consists of a single layer of flattened endothelial cells; networks branch and anastomose freely
   2. Lymphatic capillaries merge to form larger lymphatics and eventually form the main lymphatic trunks, the right lymphatic ducts, and the thoracic duct
   3. Lymph from upper right quadrant empties into right lymphatic duct and then into right subclavian vein
   4. Lymph from rest of the body empties into the thoracic duct, which then drains into the left subclavian vein; thoracic duct originates as the cisterna chyli (chyle cistern)
B. Structure of lymphatic vessels (**Figure 31-4**)
   1. Similar to veins except lymphatic vessels have thinner walls, have more valves, and contain lymph nodes
   2. Lymphatic capillary wall is formed by a single layer of thin, flat endothelial cells
   3. As the diameter of lymphatic vessels increases from capillary size, the walls become thicker and have three layers
   4. One-way valves are present every few millimetres in large lymphatics and even more frequently in smaller lymphatics
C. Functions of the lymphatic vessels
   1. Remove high-molecular-weight substances and even particulate matter from interstitial spaces
   2. Lacteals absorb fats and other nutrients from the small intestine

Circulation of Lymph

A. From lymphatic capillaries, lymph flows through progressively larger lymphatic vessels to eventually reenter blood at the junction of the internal jugular and subclavian veins (**Figure 31-5**)
B. The lymphatic pump
   1. Lymphokinesis—the movement (flow) of lymph; can be visualized in a lymphangiogram (**Figure 31-6**)
   2. Lymph moves through the system in the right direction because of the large number of valves
   3. Breathing movements and skeletal muscle contractions (**Figure 31-7**) establish a fluid pressure gradient, as they do with venous blood

4. Other factors, such as IF pressure, also drive lymphokinesis (**Figure 31-8**)
5. Lymphokinetic actions—activities that result in a central flow of lymph

Lymph Nodes

A. Structure of lymph nodes
   1. Lymph nodes are oval-shaped structures enclosed by a fibrous capsule (**Figure 31-9**)
   2. Nodes are a type of biological filter
   3. Once lymph enters a node, it moves slowly through sinuses to drain into the efferent exit vessel (**Figure 31-10**)
   4. Trabeculae extend from the covering capsule toward the centre of the node
   5. Cortical and medullary sinuses are lined with reticuloendothelial cells capable of phagocytosis

B. Locations of lymph nodes
   1. Most lymph nodes occur in groups
   2. Groups with greatest clinical importance are preauricular lymph nodes, submental and submaxillary groups, and superficial cervical, superficial cubital, axillary, iliac, and inguinal lymph nodes (**Figures 31-11** through **31-13**)

C. Functions of lymph nodes—perform two distinct functions
   1. Defence functions
      a. Filtration
         (1) Mechanical filtration—physically stopping particles from progressing further in the body
         (2) Biological filtration—biological activity of cells destroys and removes particles
      b. Phagocytosis—reticuloendothelial cells remove micro-organisms and other injurious particles from lymph and phagocytose them (biological filtration)
      c. If overwhelmed, lymph nodes can become infected or damaged (**Figures 31-14** and **31-15**)
   2. Haematopoiesis—lymphoid tissue is the site for the final stages of maturation of some lymphocytes and monocytes

Lymphatic Drainage of the Breast

A. Clinically important because cancer cells and infections can spread along lymphatic pathways to lymph nodes and other organs of the body

B. Distribution of lymphatics in the breast (**Figure 31-16**)
   1. Drained by two sets of lymphatic vessels
      a. Lymphatics that drain the skin over the breast with the exception of the areola and nipple
      b. Lymphatics that drain the underlying substance of the breast, as well as the skin of the areola and nipple
   2. Superficial vessels converge to form a diffuse, cutaneous lymphatic plexus
   3. Subareolar plexus—located under the areola surrounding the nipple; where communication between the cutaneous plexus and large lymphatics that drain the secretory tissue and ducts of the breast occurs

C. Lymph nodes associated with the breast
   1. More than 85% of the lymph from the breast enters the lymph nodes of the axillary region
   2. Remainder of lymph enters lymph nodes along the lateral edges of the sternum

Tonsils

A. Form a broken ring under the mucous membranes in the mouth and back of the throat—the pharyngeal lymphoid ring (**Figure 31-17**)
   1. Palatine tonsils—located on each side of the throat
   2. Pharyngeal tonsils—located near the posterior opening of the nasal cavity
   3. Lingual tonsils—located near the base of the tongue
   4. Tubal tonsils—located near the openings of the auditory (eustachian) tubes

B. Protect against bacteria that may invade tissues around the openings between the nasal and oral cavities; bacteria are trapped in tonsillar crypts and put in close contact with immune system cells

Thymus

A. Location and appearance of the thymus (**Figure 31-18**)
   1. Primary organ of lymphatic system
   2. Single, unpaired organ located in the mediastinum, extending upward to the lower edge of the thyroid and inferiorly as far as the fourth costal cartilage
   3. Thymus is pinkish grey in childhood; with advancing age, becomes yellowish as lymphoid tissue is replaced by fat

B. Structure of the thymus
   1. Two pyramid-shaped lobes are subdivided into small lobules
   2. Each lobule is composed of a dense cellular cortex and an inner, less dense medulla
   3. Medullary tissue can be identified by presence of thymic corpuscles

C. Function of the thymus
   1. Plays vital role in immunity mechanism
   2. Source of lymphocytes before birth
   3. Shortly after birth, thymus secretes thymosin and other regulators, which enables lymphocytes to develop into T cells (**Figure 31-19**)

Spleen

A. Location of the spleen—in the left hypochondrium, directly below the diaphragm, above the left kidney and descending colon, and behind the fundus of the stomach (**Figures 31-2** and **31-20**)

B. Structure of the spleen (**Figure 31-21**)
   1. Ovoid in shape
   2. Surrounded by fibrous capsule with inward extensions that divide the organ into compartments
   3. White pulp—dense masses of developing lymphocytes

4. Red pulp—near outer regions, made up of a network of fine reticular fibres submerged in blood that comes from nearby arterioles; made up of cords of WBCs and related cells surrounded by sinusoids

C. Functions of the spleen
  1. Defence—macrophages lining the sinusoids of the spleen remove microorganisms from the blood and phagocytose them
  2. Tissue repair—the spleen holds a reservoir of monocytes that migrate in a large mass to sites of injury to help with tissue healing and repair
  3. Haematopoiesis—monocytes and lymphocytes complete their development in the spleen
  4. Red blood cell and platelet destruction—macrophages remove worn-out RBCs and imperfect platelets and destroy them by phagocytosis; also salvage iron and globin from destroyed RBCs
  5. Blood reservoir—pulp of spleen and its sinuses store blood

Cycle of Life: Lymphatic System

A. Dramatic changes throughout life
B. Organs with lymphocytes appear before birth and grow until puberty
C. Postpuberty
  1. Organs atrophy through late adulthood
    a. Shrink in size
    b. Become fatty or fibrous
  2. Spleen—develops early, remains intact
D. Overall function maintained until late adulthood
E. Later adulthood
  1. Deficiency permits risk of infection and cancer
  2. Hypersensitivity—likelihood of autoimmune conditions

The Big Picture: The Lymphatic System and the Whole Body

A. Lymphatic system drains away excess water from large areas
B. Lymph is conducted through lymphatic vessels to nodes, where contaminants are removed
C. Lymphatic system benefits the whole body by maintaining fluid balance and freedom from disease

REVIEW QUESTIONS

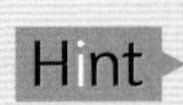

Write out the answers to these questions after reading the chapter and reviewing the Chapter Summary. Note—writing out your answers will consolidate learning and provide a valuable resource of information.

1. List the anatomical components of the lymphatic system.
2. How do interstitial fluid and lymph differ from blood plasma?
3. How do lymphatic vessels originate?
4. Briefly describe the anatomy of the lymphatic capillary wall.
5. Lymph from what body areas enters the general circulation by way of the thoracic duct? By way of the right lymphatic ducts?
6. What is the cisterna chyli?
7. Where does lymph enter the blood vascular system?
8. In general, lymphatics resemble veins in structure. List three exceptions to this general rule.
9. What are the unique lymphatic vessels that originate in the villi of the small intestine called?
10. What is chyle? Where is it formed?
11. Give examples of lymphokinetic factors and explain how they contribute to the "lymphatic pump".
12. List several important groups, or clusters, of lymph nodes.
13. Explain how lymph nodes function in body defence and haematopoiesis.
14. If cancer cells from breast cancer enter the lymphatics of the breast, where are they likely to lodge and start new growths? Explain why, using your knowledge of the anatomy of the lymphatic and circulatory systems.
15. Locate the thymus, and describe its appearance and size at birth, at maturity, and in old age.
16. Explain the function of the thymus.
17. Describe the location and functions of the spleen.
18. What happens when there is a loss of lymphatic fluid?
19. Explain why lymphoedema may occur after breast surgery.

CRITICAL THINKING QUESTIONS

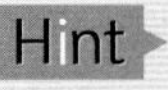

After finishing the Review Questions, write out the answers to these more in-depth questions to help you apply your new knowledge. Go back to sections of the chapter that relate to concepts that you find difficult.

1. Even though the lymphatic system is a component of the circulatory system, why is the term *circulation* not the most appropriate term to describe the flow of lymph?
2. Explain how lymph is formed. What would be the impact on lymph formation if the osmotic force at the venous end of the capillary was more successful at recovering fluid lost at the arterial end?
3. Discuss the importance of valves in the lymphatic system.
4. Explain the role of the lymphatic system in the spread of breast cancer and its surgical treatment.
5. The spleen can be removed if diseased or injured. Explain how this organ with several important functions can be removed without harming or killing the patient.

32 Innate Immunity

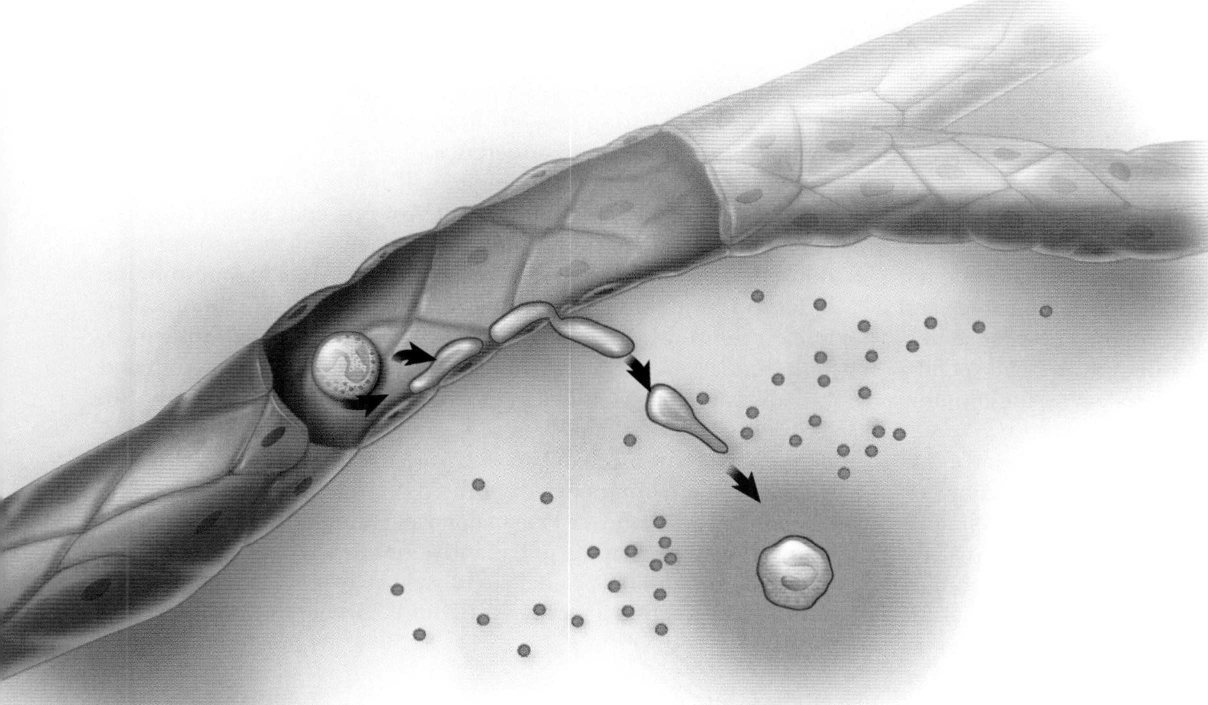

CHAPTER OUTLINE

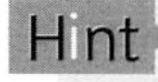 Scan this outline before you begin to read the chapter, as a preview of how the concepts are organized.

Enemies of many kinds and in great numbers assault the body during a lifetime. Among the most threatening are hordes of microorganisms. We live our lives in a virtual sea of protozoa, fungi, bacteria, viruses, and other pathogens. So ever-present and potentially lethal are these small but formidable foes that no newborn could live through infancy, much less survive to adulthood or old age, without effective defences against them. We also are threatened by enemies from within. Inside the body, abnormal body cells appear on an irregular but continual basis. If allowed to survive, these abnormal cells reproduce and form a tumour. At the very least, a tumour alone can damage surrounding tissues and can be life-threatening as it continues to enlarge, and there is always the possibility that a tumour could become cancerous and spread (metastasize) to many

LANGUAGE OF SCIENCE

Hint *Use this list to aid your pronunciation of unfamiliar words.*

adaptive immunity (ah-DAP-tiv ih-MYOO-nih-tee) [*adapt-* **adjust,** *-ive* **relating to,** *immun-* **free,** *-ity* **state**]

antigen (AN-tih-jen) [*anti-* **against,** *-gen* **produce**]

antigen-presenting cell (APC) (AN-tih-jen) [*anti-* **against,** *-gen* **produce, presenting,** *cell* **storeroom**]

chemotactic factor (kee-moh-TAK-tik) [*chemo-* **chemical,** *-tact-* **movement,** *-ic* **relating to**]

chemotaxis (kee-moh-TAK-sis) [*chemo-* **chemical,** *-taxis* **movement**]

complement (KOM-pleh-ment) [*comple-* **complete,** *-ment* **result of action**]

cytokine (SYE-toh-kyne) [*cyto-* **cell,** *-kine* **movement**]

dendritic cell (DC) (den-DRIH-tik) [*dendr-* **tree,** *-it-* **(branch) of,** *-ic* **relating to,** *cell* **storeroom**]

diapedesis (dye-ah-peh-DEE-sis) [*dia-* **through,** *-pedesis* **an oozing**]

immunocompetence (ih-myoo-noh-KOM-peh-tens) [*immuno-* **free (immunity),** *-competence* **capability**]

inflammatory response (in-FLAM-ah-toh-ree) [*inflamm-* **set afire,** *-ory* **relating to**]

innate immunity (IN-ayt ih-MYOO-nih-tee) [*innat-* **inborn,** *immun-* **free,** *-ity* **state**]

interferon (IFN) (in-ter-FEER-on) [*inter-* **between,** *-fer-* **strike,** *-on* **substance**]

macrophage (MAK-roh-fayj) [*macro-* **large,** *-phage* **eat**]

major histocompatibility complex (MHC) (MAY-jer HIST-oh-kom-pat-ib-IL-it-ee KOM-pleks) [*histo-* **tissue,** *-compatibil-* **agreeable,** *-ity* **state,** *com-* **together,** *-plex* **weave or braid**]

membrane attack complex (MAC) (MEM-brayn at-TAK KOM-pleks) [*com-* **together,** *-plex* **weave or braid**]

natural killer (NK) cell (NACH-ur-ul KIL-er sell)

nonself (NON-self)

continued on p. 760

other locations within the body. Without an internal "security force" to deal with such abnormal cells when they first appear, we would live very short lives.

This chapter and the next present a brief overview of the system that provides defences against both external and internal enemies—the immune system. •

ORGANIZATION OF THE IMMUNE SYSTEM

DEFENCE OF THE BODY

Like any security force, the components and mechanisms of the immune system are organized in an efficient—almost military-like—manner. They are not just ready at a moment's notice; they are *continually* patrolling the body for foreign or internal enemies and shoring up the various lines of defence to fend off a possible attack. Before we begin studying the specifics of immunity, we will spend a moment mapping out the overall defensive strategy of the immune system.

First, it is important to recognize that cells, viruses, and other particles have unique molecules and groups of molecules on their surfaces that can be used to identify them. These molecular markers visible to the immune system are called **antigens.** This is similar to military operations in which enemy aircraft, vehicles, or soldiers can be identified by their distinctive insignia that are different from the insignia seen on "our side". This ability to activate an effective response to an antigen is called *immunologic competence* or **immunocompetence.**

Our own cells also have unique cell markers embedded in our plasma membranes that identify each of our cells as **self**—that is, belonging to us as an individual. And foreign cells or particles have **nonself** molecules that serve as recognition markers for our immune system. The ability of our immune system to attack abnormal or foreign cells but spare our own normal cells is called **self-tolerance.**

In human society, any good security force employs numerous and varied strategies to guard its territory and take action if necessary. So, too, does the body's "society of cells" employ a system that uses many different kinds of mechanisms to ensure the integrity and survival of the internal environment. All of these defence mechanisms can be categorized into one of two major categories of immune mechanisms: **innate immunity** and **adaptive immunity.**

Innate immunity is called such because it is "in place" before a person is exposed to a particular harmful particle or condition. The

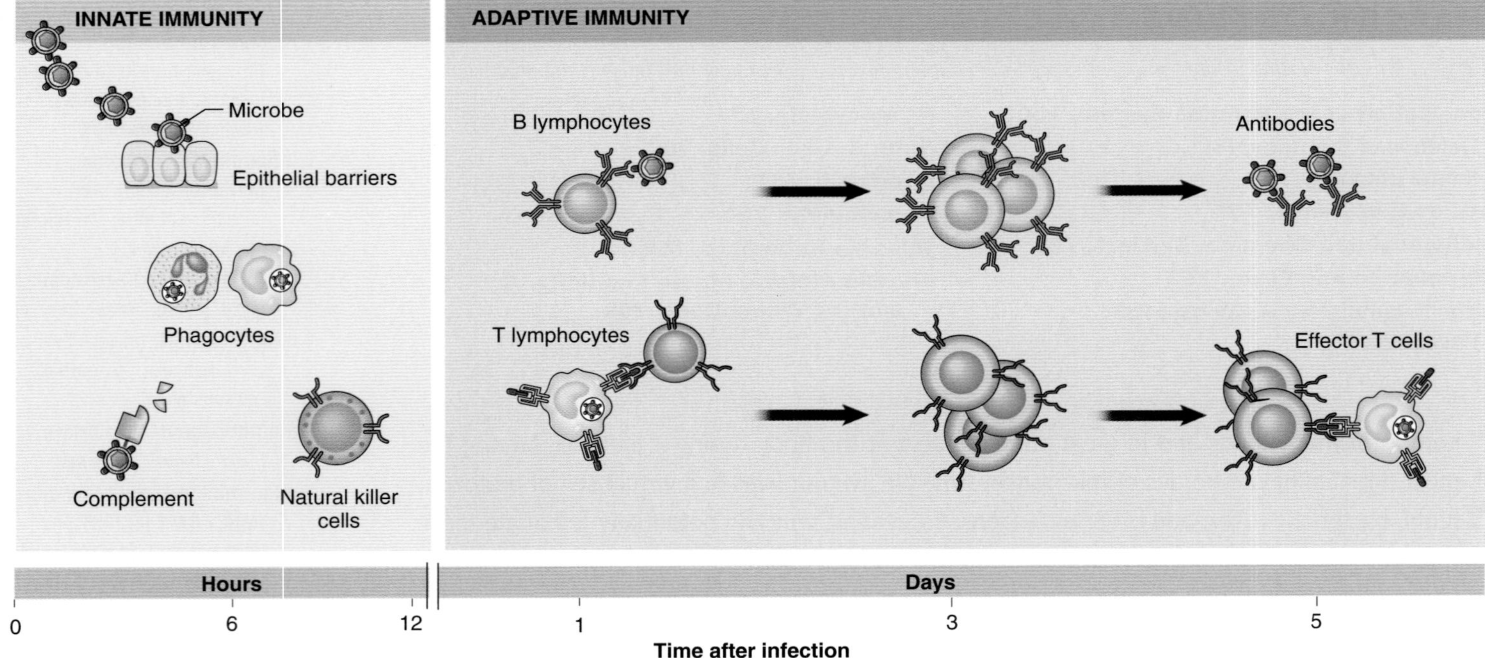

FIGURE 32-1 Innate and adaptive immunity. Innate (nonspecific) immune mechanisms are "built in" and ready for action—thus providing the initial defence against infections and other assaults on the body. Adaptive (specific) immune mechanisms develop later, as lymphocytes are activated to work against specific foreign or abnormal cells and particles. The timeframes are generalizations.

UNIT 4

TABLE 32-1 **Innate and Adaptive Immunity**

		INNATE IMMUNITY	ADAPTIVE IMMUNITY
Synonyms	Commonly used alternate terminology	Nonspecific immunity, native immunity, genetic immunity	Specific immunity, acquired immunity
Characteristics			
Specificity	Unique antigens produce unique responses of the immune system	Not specific—recognizes variety of different groups of foreign cells or particles	Specific—recognizes specific antigens on specific cells or particles
Speed of reaction	Reaction time of the immune responses	Rapid: immediate up to several hours	Slower: several hours to several days
Memory	Enhanced responses to repeated exposures to the same antigen	None	Yes
Does not react to self	Prevents injury to the individual's own cells*	Yes	Yes
Components			
Barriers	Prevent entry of harmful particles	Skin, mucosa, antimicrobial chemicals	Lymphocytes in epithelia; antibodies released at epithelial surfaces
Blood proteins	Circulate throughout body, providing wide area of protection	Complement, interferon (IFN), others	Antibodies
Cells	Types of leucocytes involved in immunity	Phagocytes (macrophages, neutrophils), natural killer (NK) cells	Lymphocytes (B cells and T cells)

*Assumes healthy function. Anti-self immunity (autoimmunity) is a characteristic of many disorders.

word *innate* refers to something that is already present naturally at birth. Because it includes mechanisms that resist a wide variety of threatening agents or conditions, innate immunity is also called **nonspecific immunity.** The term *nonspecific* implies that these immune mechanisms do not act on only one or two specific invaders but rather provide a more general defence by simply acting against a wide variety of particles recognized as *nonself.*

Adaptive immunity, on the other hand, involves mechanisms that recognize *specific* threatening agents and then *adapt,* or respond, by targeting their activity against these agents—and these agents only. Because it targets only specific harmful particles, adaptive immunity is also called **specific immunity.** Adaptive immune mechanisms often take some time to recognize their targets and react with sufficient force to overcome the threat, at least on their first exposure to a specific kind of threatening agent. Innate mechanisms, because they are already in place, have the advantage of being able to meet an enemy as soon as it presents itself. As we discuss examples of each major type of immunity, you will come to understand how each type works and appreciate the distinction between them. You will also come to appreciate the value in having two complementary strategies for defending the body.

As in any body system, the work of the immune system is done by cells or substances made by cells. The primary types of cells involved in innate immunity are these: epithelial barrier cells, phagocytic cells (neutrophils, macrophages), and aptly named *natural killer (NK) cells.* The primary types of cells involved in adaptive immunity are two types of lymphocytes called *T cells* and *B cells.*

Cytokines, which are chemicals released from cells to trigger or regulate innate and adaptive immune responses, also participate in innate immunity. Examples of cytokines include *interleukins (ILs), leukotrienes,* and *interferons (IFNs)*—all of which are described later in this chapter. Other chemicals, in addition to cytokines, play a regulatory role in immunity—these include *complements,* other enzymes, and the amine *histamine.*

Awesome indeed is the army of cells and molecules that make up the immune system. More than 1 trillion lymphocytes, for example, and 100 million trillion (10^{20}) plasma protein molecules (antibodies) are a few of the many agents that help your body resist damage and disease. **Figure 32-1** and **Table 32-1** summarize some of the essential characteristics of innate and adaptive immunity that we discuss in this chapter.

UNIT 4

Quick CHECK

1. What is the difference between *self* and *nonself*?
2. What is the difference between *adaptive* and *innate* immunity?
3. What is a *cytokine*? What are some examples of cytokines?

INNATE IMMUNITY

The general, innate defensive mechanisms of the body are many and varied (**Table 32-2**). Only the major types of innate immune mechanisms are listed here; many other examples appear in other chapters throughout this book. You will probably recognize examples in this chapter that you have encountered already in previous chapters. Phagocytes are a good example. They are often referred to by different names when identified in specific body areas. For example, phagocytic cells in the skin were identified as *dendritic cells (DCs)* of the epidermis (Langerhans cells; Chapter 10, p. 182).

TABLE 32-2 Mechanisms of Innate Defence

MECHANISM	DESCRIPTION
Species Resistance	Genetic characteristics of the human species protect the body from certain pathogens
Mechanical and Chemical Barriers	Physical impediments to the entry of foreign cells or substances
Skin and mucosa	Forms a continuous wall that separates the internal environment from the external environment, preventing the entry of pathogens
Secretions	Secretions such as sebum, mucus, acids, and enzymes chemically inhibit the activity of pathogens
Inflammation	The inflammatory response isolates the pathogens and stimulates the speedy arrival of large numbers of immune cells
Fever	Fever may enhance immune reactions and inhibit pathogens
Phagocytosis	Ingestion and destruction of pathogens by phagocytic cells
Neutrophils	Granular leucocytes that are usually the first phagocytic cell to arrive at the scene of an inflammatory response
Macrophages	Monocytes that have enlarged to become giant phagocytic cells capable of consuming many pathogens; often called by other, more specific names when found in specific tissues of the body
Natural Killer (NK) Cells	Group of lymphocytes that kill many different types of cancer cells and virus-infected cells
Interferon	Protein produced by cells after they become infected by a virus; inhibits the spread or further development of a viral infection
Complement	Group of plasma proteins (inactive enzymes) that produce a cascade of chemical reactions that ultimately causes lysis (rupture) of a foreign cell; the complement cascade can be triggered by adaptive or innate immune mechanisms
Toll-Like Receptors (TLRs)	Membrane receptors that recognize nonspecific patterns in microbial molecules (not human molecules) and trigger a variety of innate immune responses (many of those listed in this table)

SPECIES RESISTANCE

Species resistance refers to a phenomenon in which the genetic characteristics common to a particular kind of organism, or *species*, provide defence against certain *pathogens* (disease-causing agents). The human species *(Homo sapiens)*, for example, is resistant to many life-threatening infections and infestations that often spread easily among plants and other animals. For example, humans do not have to worry about getting Dutch elm disease, a fungal infection that nearly eradicated the English elm tree, or becoming infected with canine viral distemper, a virus to which young dogs are susceptible. Usually, species resistance in humans results from the fact that our internal environment is not suitable for certain pathogens. We may also have resistance because a particular microbe may not be biochemically compatible with the various molecules on our cell membranes that the microbes would need to gain entry into a host cell.

MECHANICAL AND CHEMICAL BARRIERS

The internal environment of the human body is protected by a continuous mechanical barrier formed by the cutaneous membrane (skin) and mucous membranes (see **Figure 8-9**, p. 146). Often called the *first line of defence*, these membranes provide several layers of densely packed cells and other materials— forming a sort of "castle wall"—that protects the internal environment from invasion by foreign cells (**Figure 32-2**).

Besides forming a protective wall, the skin and mucous membranes operate various additional immune mechanisms. For example, substances such as *sebum* (which contains pathogen-inhibiting agents), *mucus* (in which pathogens become stuck and are then swept away), enzymes (which may hydrolyze pathogens), and hydrochloric acid in gastric mucosa (which may destroy pathogens) also may be present to act as innate defence mechanisms. These chemical barriers act as a sort of moat around the castle wall formed by the membranes.

The epithelial barriers of the body are essentially innate, nonspecific defences. However, the protective epithelial membranes also have adaptive (specific) defences that reinforce them. The combined innate and adaptive immune functions of protective mucous membranes are discussed in the next chapter (see **Box 33-6** on p. 777).

CONNECT IT! 

The beneficial bacteria that live on our skin and mucous membranes themselves form a defensive line that protects us from attacks by pathogens. Review the various roles of the human *microbiome* in ***The Human Microbiome*** at ***Connect It!***

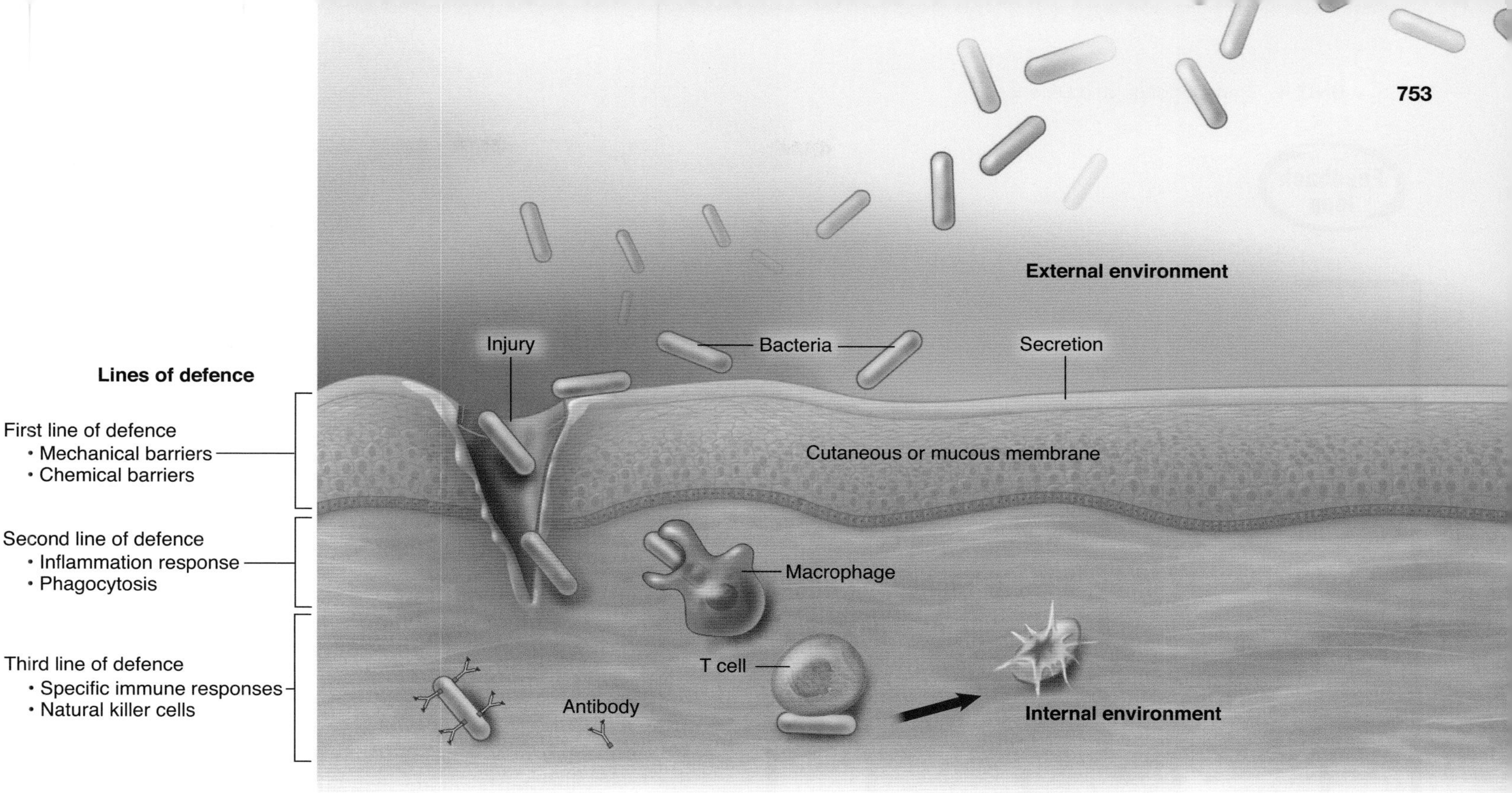

FIGURE 32-2 Lines of defence. Immune function—that is, defence of the internal environment against foreign cells, proteins, and viruses—includes three layers of protection. The first line of defence is a set of barriers between the internal and external environments, the second involves the innate inflammatory response (including phagocytosis), and the third includes the adaptive immune responses and the innate defence offered by natural killer cells. Of course, tumour cells that arise within the body are not affected by the first two lines of defence and must be attacked by the third line of defence. This diagram is a simplification of the complex function of the immune system; in reality, a great deal of crossover of mechanisms occurs between these "lines of defence".

INFLAMMATION AND FEVER

THE INFLAMMATORY RESPONSE

If bacteria or other invaders break through the chemical and mechanical barriers formed by the membranes and their secretions, the body has a *second line of defence* at the ready: the inflammatory response (see **Figure 32-2**). The **inflammatory response** has already been discussed in some detail in previous chapters and ***Connect It!: Inflammation*** online). For the purpose of a quick review, recall that tissue damage elicits a host of responses that counteract the injury and promote a return to normal. An example of how local inflammation works is illustrated in **Figure 32-3**. In the example, bacteria cause tissue damage that, in turn, triggers the release of various inflammation mediators from cells such as the *mast cells* found in connective tissues (**Figure 32-4**). These inflammation mediators include *histamine, kinins, prostaglandins, leukotrienes, interleukins (ILs),* and related compounds. Many of these mediators are chemotactic factors—that is, substances that attract white blood cells to the area in a process called **chemotaxis.** As **Figure 32-5** shows, chemotaxis is the process by which a cell navigates toward the source of the **chemotactic factor** *(chemotaxin)* by way of detecting and then moving toward higher concentrations of the factor.

In addition, many of the factors released from tissue cells and phagocytes, such as the peptide fragment called *C5a* from complement, produce the mechanisms that cause characteristic signs of inflammation: heat, redness, pain, and swelling (**Figure 32-6**). These signs result from increased blood flow and vascular permeability in the affected region, which help phagocytic white blood cells reach the general area and then enter the affected tissue. Also, some inflammation mediators trigger fibroblasts to grow and produce more collagen fibres to promote repair and regeneration.

CONNECT IT! 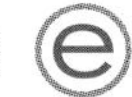

Inflammation is an important defensive reaction in the body's tissues. Check out ***Inflammation*** online at ***Connect It!*** for a brief review of the inflammatory response and its effects on the tissues of your body.

FEVER

Besides local inflammation, systemic inflammation may occur when the inflammation mediators trigger responses that occur on a body-wide basis. A body-wide inflammatory response may be manifested by a **fever**—a state of abnormally high body temperature. For example, bacterial infections that spread widely throughout the body

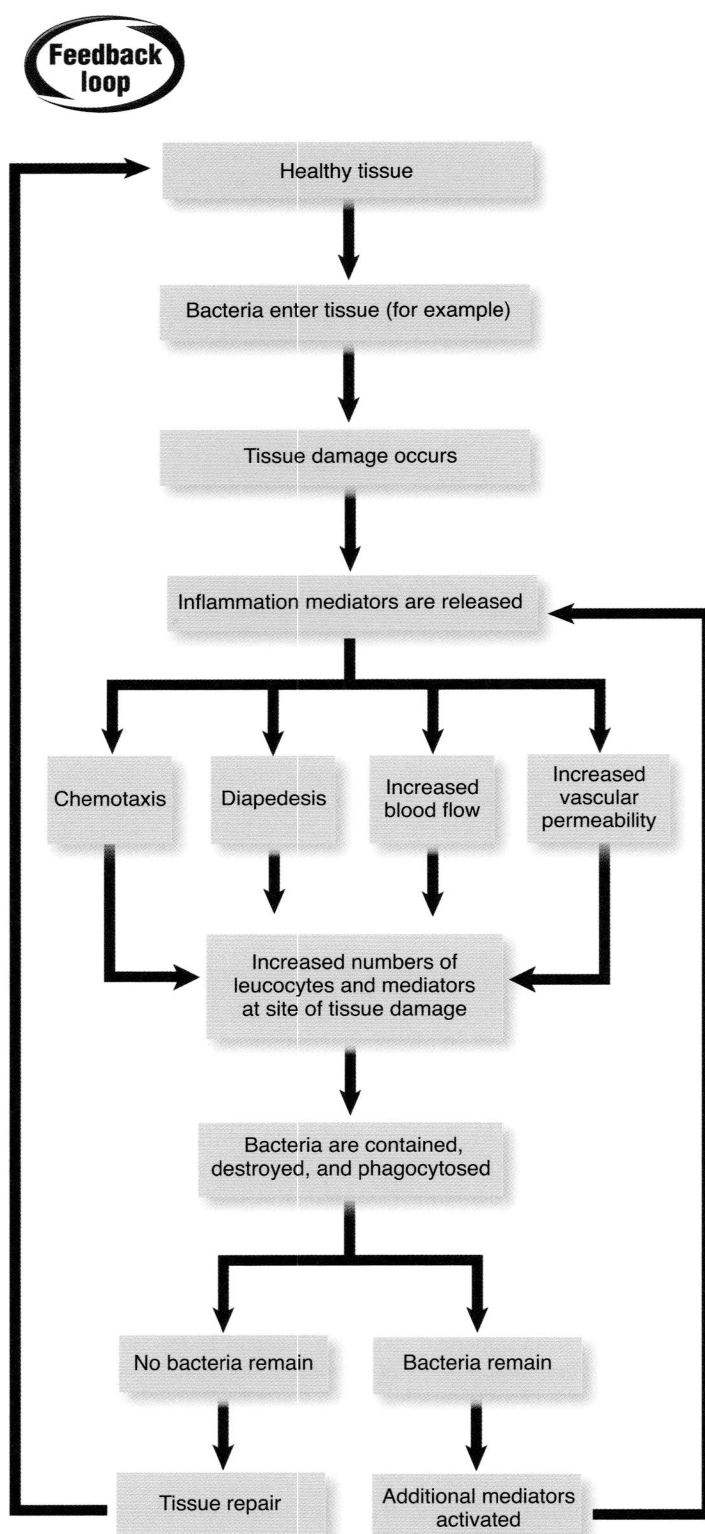
Feedback loop
Healthy tissue
Bacteria enter tissue (for example)
Tissue damage occurs
Inflammation mediators are released
Chemotaxis
Diapedesis
Increased blood flow
Increased vascular permeability
Increased numbers of leucocytes and mediators at site of tissue damage
Bacteria are contained, destroyed, and phagocytosed
No bacteria remain
Bacteria remain
Tissue repair
Additional mediators activated

FIGURE 32-3 Example of the inflammatory response. Tissue damage caused by bacteria triggers a series of events that produces the inflammatory response and promotes phagocytosis at the site of injury. These responses tend to inhibit or destroy the bacteria, eventually bringing the tissue back to its healthy state. Similar reactions will occur in the presence of other abnormal or injurious particles or conditions.

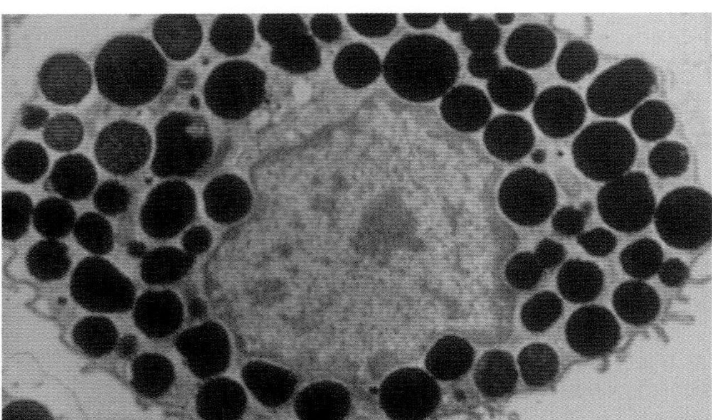

FIGURE 32-4 Mast cell. This colourized micrograph shows a mast cell filled with dense red granules of the inflammation mediator called *histamine.*

may produce *systemic inflammatory response syndrome (SIRS)*. SIRS involves an abnormally high neutrophil (phagocytic white blood cell [WBC]) count and fever. Viral infections, tumours, allergies, and other abnormal conditions also can cause fevers.

Recall from Chapter 2, p. 29, that fevers result from a "reset" of the body's thermostat in the hypothalamus, which temporarily increases the set point or target temperature to a higher-than-normal value. The body then shivers or we cover ourselves and otherwise seek heat until the new setpoint temperature—a fever—is reached.

As we have already learned in earlier chapters, *pyrogen* molecules trigger the fever response by promoting production of prostaglandins (PGs), which then reset the body's thermostat in the hypothalamus. Aspirin and other cyclooxygenase (COX) inhibitors reduce the activity of the COX enzymes (COX-1 and COX-2) that produce these prostaglandins—thus having a fever-reducing effect (see **Figure 25-13** on p. 574). Pyrogens can be released from damaged cells (endogenous pyrogens) or could be introduced from outside the body (exogenous pyrogens).

The elevated temperature of a fever may facilitate some immune reactions and may also inhibit the reproduction of some microbial pathogens. However, immunologists still debate the role of fever in protecting the body.

PHAGOCYTOSIS

A major component of the body's second line of defence is the mechanism of **phagocytosis**—the ingestion and destruction of microorganisms or other small particles. There are many types of *phagocytes*—that is, cells capable of phagocytosis, in the body. As **Figure 32-7** shows, when phagocytes approach a microorganism, they extend footlike projections (pseudopods) toward it. Soon the pseudopods encircle the organism and form a complete sac, called a *phagosome*, around it. The phagosome then moves into the interior of the cell, where a lysosome fuses with it. The contents of the lysosome, chiefly digestive enzymes and hydrogen peroxide, drain into the phagosome and destroy the microorganisms within it.

Because phagocytosis defends us against various kinds of agents, it is classified as an *innate defence*. However, phagocytes also "cross

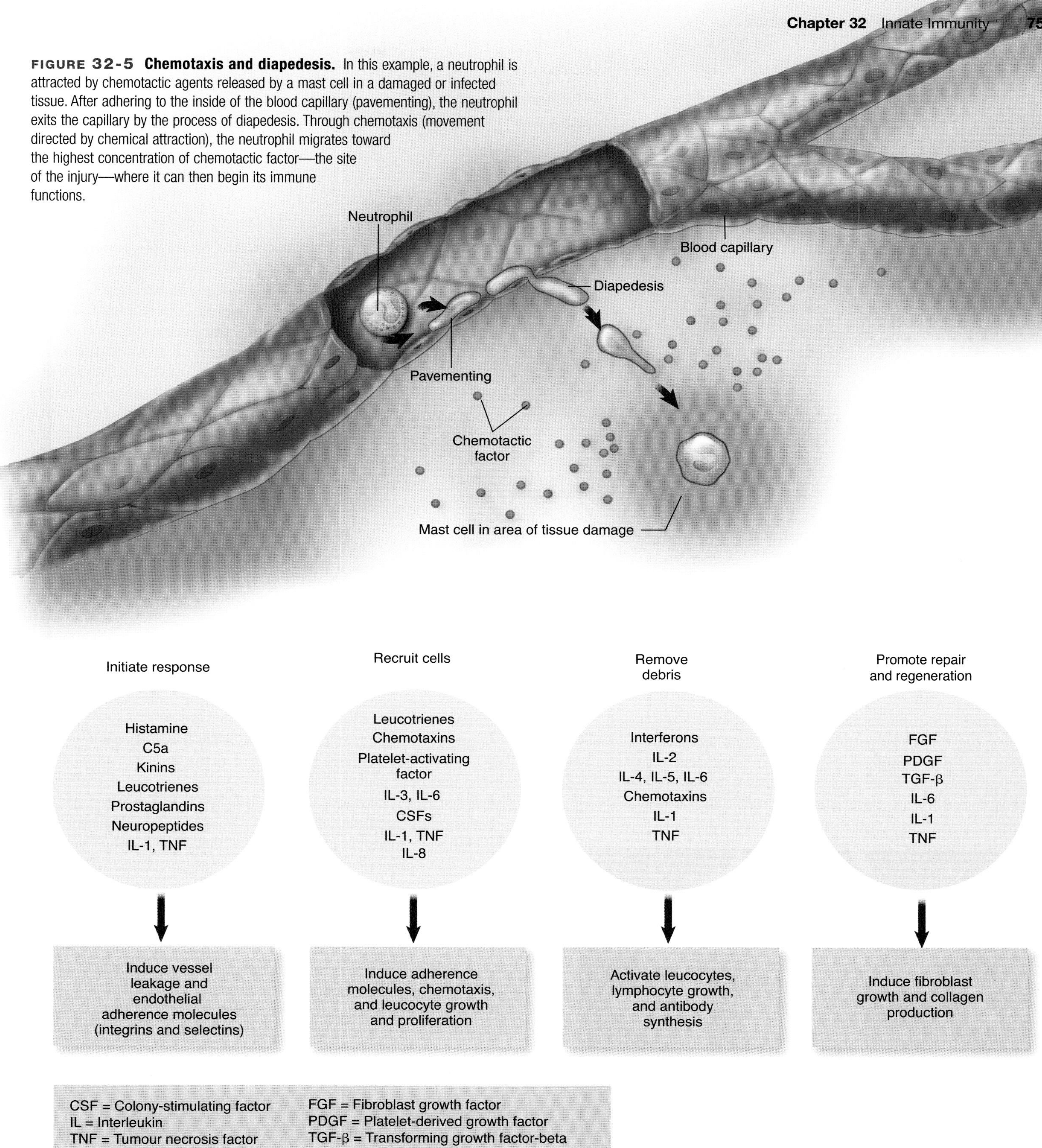

FIGURE 32-5 Chemotaxis and diapedesis. In this example, a neutrophil is attracted by chemotactic agents released by a mast cell in a damaged or infected tissue. After adhering to the inside of the blood capillary (pavementing), the neutrophil exits the capillary by the process of diapedesis. Through chemotaxis (movement directed by chemical attraction), the neutrophil migrates toward the highest concentration of chemotactic factor—the site of the injury—where it can then begin its immune functions.

FIGURE 32-6 Inflammation mediators. A wide variety of chemical mediators help regulate the immune response, as this generalized chart shows. Some of the processes shown overlap in time and are thus sometimes concurrent.

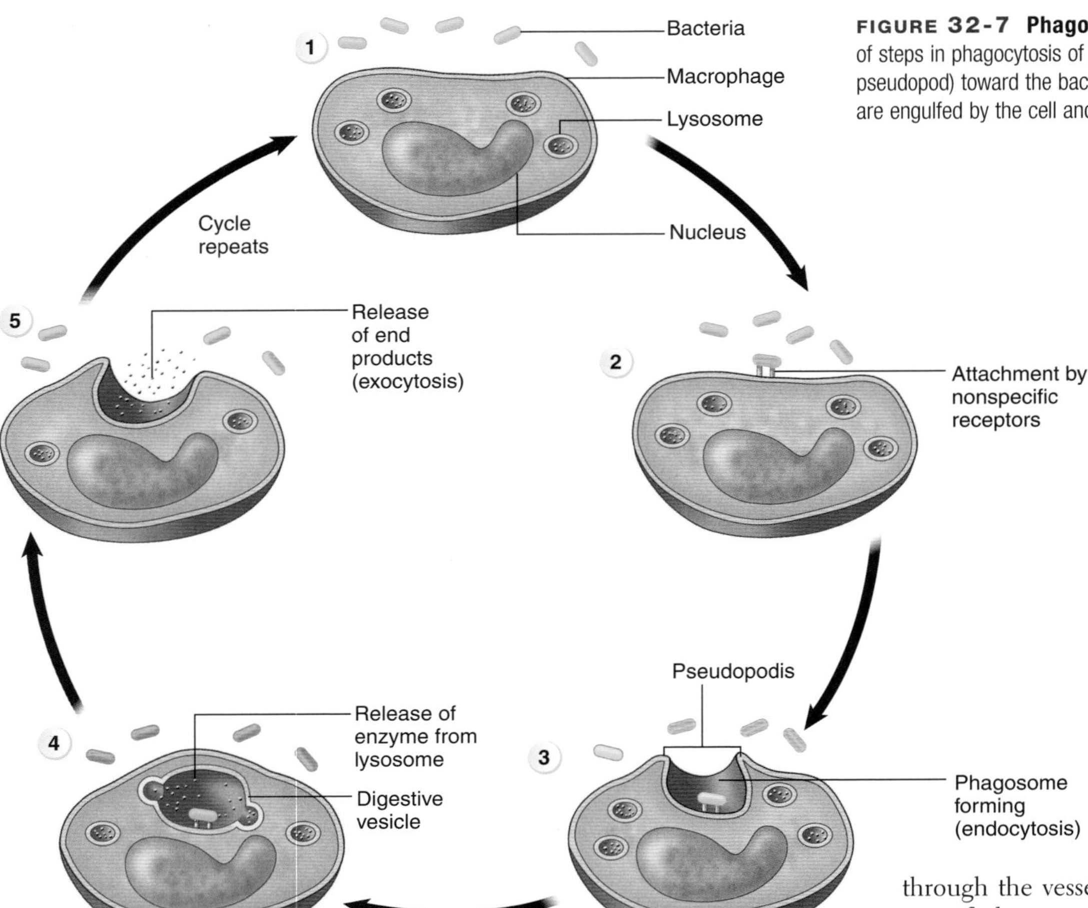

FIGURE 32-7 Phagocytosis of bacteria. Drawing shows sequence of steps in phagocytosis of bacteria. The plasma membrane extends (as a pseudopod) toward the bacterial cells, then envelops them. Once trapped, they are engulfed by the cell and destroyed by lysosomal enzymes.

over" to play an important role in adaptive immunity as well. After digesting the offending particle, a phagocyte will often process the proteins and display bits of the protein—peptides—on the surface of the phagocyte. These peptides are then recognized by cells of the adaptive immune system as antigens, thus possibly triggering an adaptive immune response. Cells that perform this function are called *antigen-presenting cells (APCs)*.

You learned in Chapter 27 that the most numerous type of phagocyte is the *neutrophil*, a granular, neutral-staining type of WBC. After being released at a site of inflammation or tissue damage, chemotactic factors diffuse into adjoining capillaries. Once in the bloodstream, they cause neutrophils and other phagocytes to adhere to the vessel's endothelial lining in a process called **pavementing** (see **Figure 32-5**). Numbers of these adherent phagocytes pass between the endothelial cells that form the capillary wall, dissolve the underlying basement membrane, and then exit through the vessel wall in the inflamed area. The movement of phagocytes from blood vessel to inflammation site is called **diapedesis.** Phagocytes have a very short life span, and thus dead cells tend to "pile up" at the inflammation site—forming most of the white substance called **pus.**

Another common type of phagocyte is the **macrophage** (meaning "large eater"). Macrophages are phagocytic monocytes (nongranular WBCs) that have grown to several times their original size after migrating out of the bloodstream. Macrophages are important APCs.

Yet another important type of phagocyte is the **dendritic cell (DC)** found in many tissues of the body that are in contact with the external environment, such as the skin and mucous membranes (**Figure 32-8**). This type of phagocytic APC is called *dendritic* because of its many branches (*dendr-*, branch). Dendritic cells are also sometimes called *stellate* ("star shaped") *cells.*

Phagocytic APCs of various types are present in many areas of the body, even on the outside surface of some mucous membranes (e.g., in the respiratory tract). Phagocyte types are often known by specific names that designate their location (**Table 32-3**). The importance of phagocytes to our overall defence of the body is made clear by the

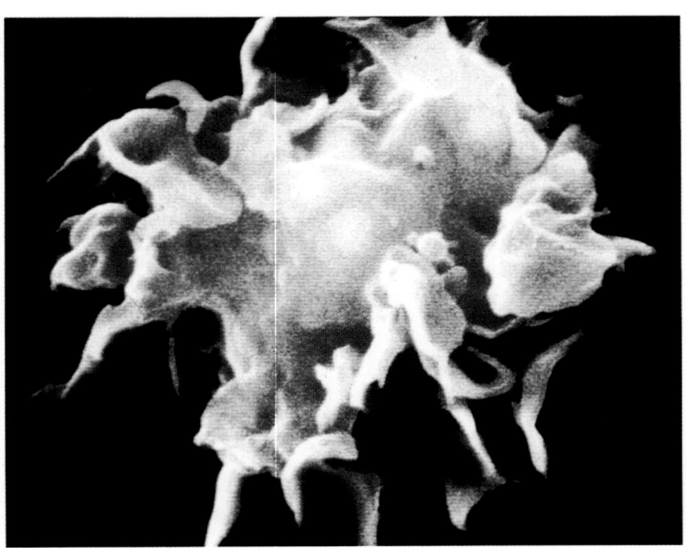

FIGURE 32-8 Dendritic cell (DC). Scanning electron micrograph showing the detail of projections of the plasma membrane in DCs. Also called *stellate (star-shaped) cells,* DCs are phagocytic antigen-presenting cells (APCs) that are found in many areas of the body (see also **Figure 33-15** on p. 771).

TABLE 32-3 Examples of Phagocyte Locations

PHAGOCYTES	LOCATION
Circulating phagocytes	Bloodstream
Osteoclasts; bone marrow (fixed) phagocytes	Bone and bone marrow
Microglia	Central nervous system
Histiocytes	Connective tissues
Epidermal dendritic cells (Langerhans cells)	Epidermis
Stellate macrophages (Kupffer cells)	Liver
Alveolar macrophages (dust cells); dendritic cells	Lung
Fixed and free lymphoid macrophages; dendritic cells	Lymph nodes
Pleural macrophages; peritoneal macrophages	Serous fluids
Splenic macrophages	Spleen

fact that 10% to 15% (by number) of all cells in any organ of the body are phagocytic cells!

NATURAL KILLER CELLS

Besides phagocytes, the body has another important set of cells that provides innate defence of the body. These are the **natural killer (NK) cells.** NK cells are a group of lymphocytes that kill many types of tumour cells and cells infected by different kinds of viruses. As a group they are produced in the red bone marrow and constitute about 15% of the total lymphocyte cell numbers. NK cells are neither T cells nor B cells, as described later under the topic of adaptive immunity. Because they have such a broad action and do not have to be activated by a specific foreign antigen to become active, they are usually included among the innate immune strategies. However, they can also participate in adaptive immunity.

In innate immune responses, NK cells recognize abnormal cells by using two different recognition receptors: a killer-activating receptor and a killer-inhibiting receptor (**Figure 32-9**). The killer-activating receptor binds to any of several common surface molecules found in cells. Thus the NK cell can bind to any cell of the body as well as any foreign cells. However, if the killer-inhibiting receptor happens to bind to an MHC (major histocompatibility complex) protein also, then the killing action is stopped. **Box 32-1** explains that MHCs are surface proteins on all normal cells and are unique to each individual person. Thus only abnormal and foreign cells fail to bind to the killer-inhibitor centres—and therefore are killed by the NK cell.

The NK cells use several different methods for killing cells, most of which involve chemically triggering apoptosis (programmed cell death) that progresses to lysis (breaking apart). NK cells must engage their target cells by direct contact (binding of receptors) to cause cell destruction.

INTERFERON

Several types of cells, if invaded by viruses, respond rapidly by synthesizing the protein **interferon (IFN)** and releasing some of it into the circulation. As the name suggests, interferon proteins interfere with the ability of viruses to cause disease. One way that they do this is by preventing viruses from multiplying in cells. IFN production is triggered by viral infection in a cell, probably by the presence of viral dsRNA (double-strand RNA). The IFN is then released to nearby cells, where it triggers signal transduction that activates antiviral genes in the neighbouring cells. These genes produce an "antiviral state" by producing several enzymes that block viral replication if the cell becomes infected. Thus IFN acts as a paracrine (local) hormone that allows virus-infected cells to send an "alarm" to nearby cells that protects the uninfected cells.

Some interferons also promote synthesis of more MHC proteins, thus allowing them to present viral antigens and promote immune destruction of infected cells (see **Box 32-1**). By promoting the destruction of cells that are already infected, the chance of the virus spreading to other cells is reduced.

Interferon comes in several varieties, each with somewhat different antiviral actions. Leucocyte interferon (β), fibroblast interferon (α), and immune interferon (γ) are the three major types of interferon proteins. All three have now been produced by using gene-splicing techniques.

CONNECT IT!

Studies exploring antiviral and anticancer activities of interferons are currently under way. To learn more, check out ***Interferon Therapy*** online at ***Connect It!***

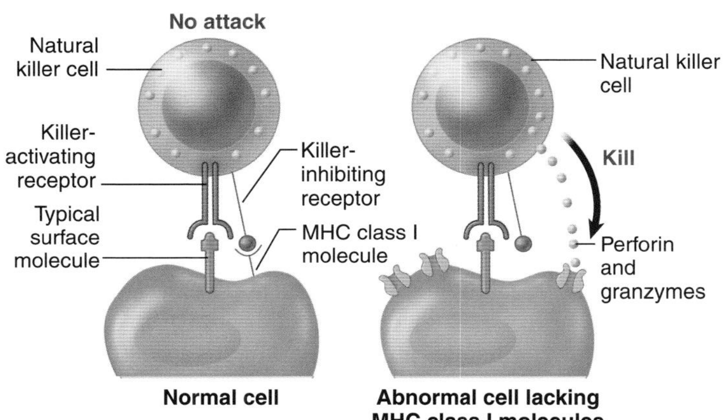

FIGURE 32-9 Natural killer (NK) cells. NK cells are a type of lymphocyte distinct from B cells and T cells. NK cells have killer-activating receptors that recognize any of several molecules commonly found in plasma membranes. NK cells also have killer-inhibiting receptors that recognize major histocompatibility complex (MHC) class I surface molecules, which act as "self" markers (see **Box 32-1** on p. 758). If both the NK receptors bind, as they would in a normal cell with the proper MHC class I surface molecule, then the killing action of the cell is inhibited and the target cell remains alive. However, if the MHC class I marker is absent—as would happen with a foreign cell or a virus-infected cell—then the killer-inhibiting receptor has nothing to bind. Thus the killing action of the NK cell is not inhibited and the target cell is destroyed by chemicals released from the NK cell.

BOX 32-1 *fyi* | Major Histocompatibility Complex

The **major histocompatibility complex (MHC)** is a set of genes in chromosome 6 that all code for antigen-presenting proteins and other immune system proteins (part *A* of figure). Antigens are proteins that potentially trigger a specific immune response. The MHC proteins produced by MHC genes in class I and class II also are called *human leucocyte antigens (HLAs).* Their function is to present different protein fragments (peptides) at the surface of the cell for possible recognition as either self- or nonself-antigens by immune system cells.

The MHC class I proteins, or HLAs, are present in every nucleated cell of the body. Their function is to present protein fragments from within the cell at the surface as antigens. An immune cell will then recognize the presented antigen as a *self-antigen* or as a *nonself-antigen* (part *B* of figure). Self-antigens are normally ignored by the immune cell. Nonself-antigens are instead recognized as abnormal and attacked by the mechanisms described later in this chapter. If a normal cell becomes infected with a virus or becomes cancerous, it may present some abnormal antigens on the surface and thus be identified by the immune system.

MHC class I proteins are also involved in the mechanism by which natural killer (NK) cells recognize abnormal cells. As **Figure 32-9** shows, the absence of MHC class I proteins fails to inhibit the killing action of the NK cell. Cells from outside the body are likely to have no MHC class I proteins or have a different version of the MHC class I proteins. Infected or damaged cells are also likely to have missing or damaged MHC class I surface proteins.

MHC class II proteins are expressed in immune cells that specialize in presenting antigens. These "professional" **antigen-presenting cells (APCs)** include macrophages, dendritic cells (DCs), and B cells, for example. The APCs use their MHC class II proteins to present fragments of proteins that they've brought in from outside the cell— perhaps from a bacterial cell. Thus they alert the immune system to the presence of these invaders and trigger certain adaptive (specific) immune responses.

MHC class III proteins include a wide variety of different immune-related proteins such as complement components, some cytokines, and a number of immune and nonimmune proteins.

The MHC first came to the attention of researchers trying to find out why transplants and tissue grafts were often rejected by the recipient. They found that individuals with different MHC genes rejected tissues transplanted from one to the other. Thus they coined the term *histocompatibility* for this set of genes because the genes seemed to regulate the compatibility of transplants and grafts.

There are hundreds of different versions or alleles of the principal MHC genes—far more genetic variability than in any other group of genes in the human genome! Scientists are still trying to find a satisfactory explanation for this tremendous variation.

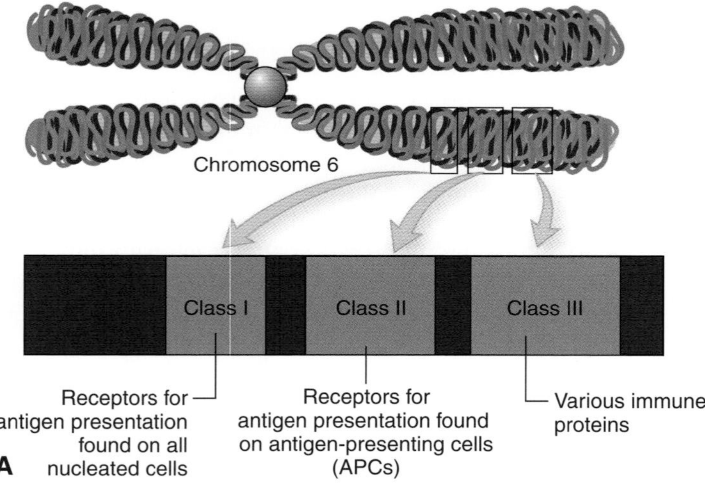

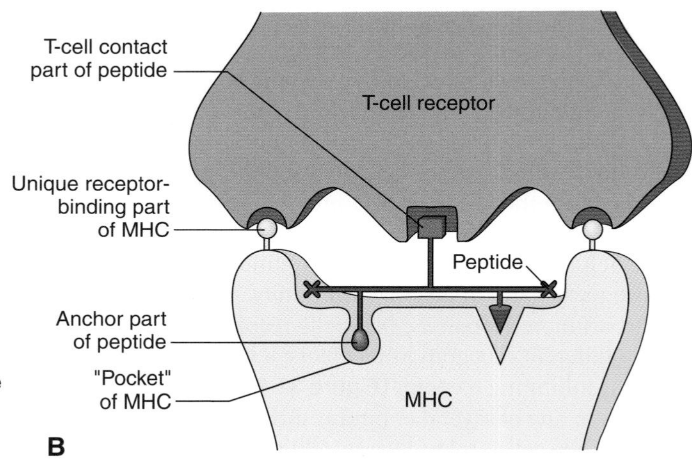

A, Major histocompatibility complex (MHC). The MHC is a region of chromosome 6 that codes for proteins important in immune system function. MHC class I proteins present antigens on the surfaces of all cells of the body that possess a nucleus—which is most cells. MHC class II proteins present antigens on the surfaces of cells that specialize in presenting antigens—the antigen-presenting cells (APCs). MHC class III proteins include complement, cytokines, and other proteins of the immune system. **B, MHC function.** This simplified diagram shows that the MHC protein displays an antigen (protein fragment or peptide) on the surface of the cell. A receptor on the surface of a T cell may then bind to the unique receptor-binding part of the MHC and to a complementary part of the T cell. Antigens (peptides) presented this way can then be recognized by immune cells as being "self" or "nonself".

COMPLEMENT

Complement is the name given to each of a group of about 20 inactive enzymes in the plasma and on cell surfaces. Individual complement proteins are often designated by C (for complement) followed by a number, such as C1, C2, C3, and so on. Subtypes of each complement are usually identified by a lower-case letter, such as C4b or C5a—or by Greek letters, as in C5bα or C8β.

Complement molecules are activated in a cascade of chemical reactions triggered by either adaptive or innate mechanisms. There are several pathways of activating the *complement cascade*

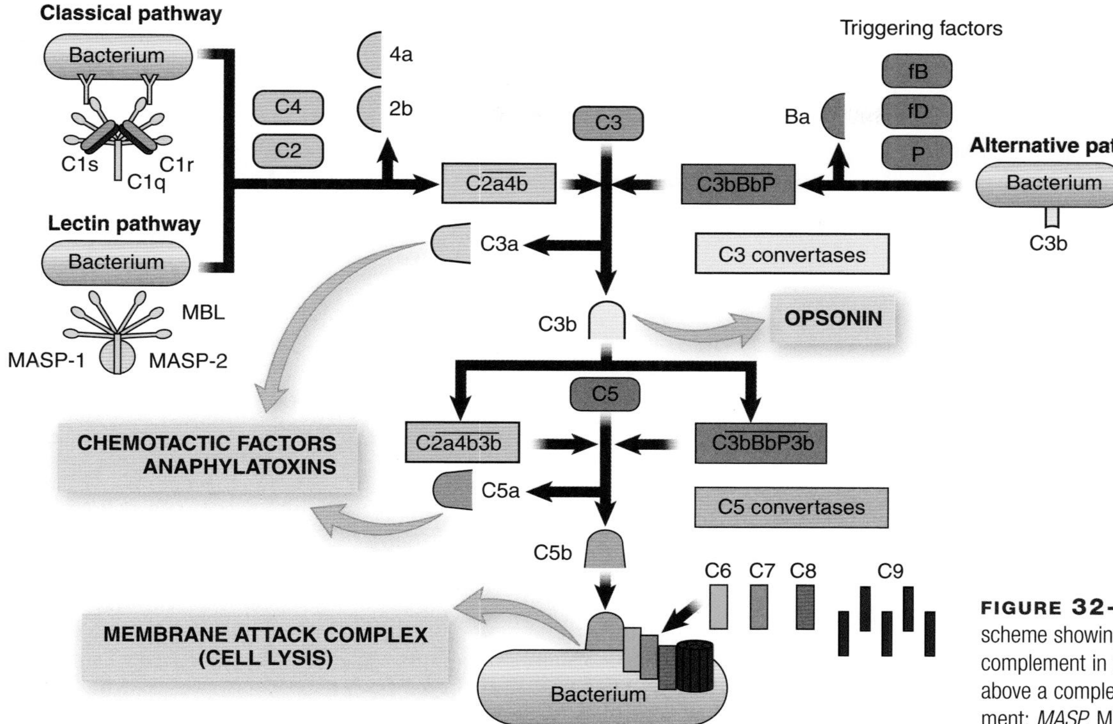

FIGURE 32-10 Complement cascade. Simplified scheme showing three possible pathways showing activation of complement in response to the presence of pathogens. A bar above a complement name indicates an enzyme. *C,* Complement; *MASP,* MBL-related enzyme; *MBL,* mannose-binding lectin.

(**Figure 32-10**). The *classical pathway* is usually activated by antigen–antibody reactions. The *lectin pathway* is triggered when mannose-binding lectin (MBL) attaches to mannose-rich surface structures on pathogenic bacteria. The *alternative pathway* can be triggered by different factors, such as polysaccharides on bacteria.

Ultimately, the *complement cascade* causes lysis (rupture) of the foreign cell that triggered the response by producing an ominous-sounding structure called the **membrane attack complex (MAC).** The MAC will be discussed more fully in the next chapter.

Complements may act as chemotactic factors or act as *anaphylatoxins* to trigger inflammatory responses. Complement can also act as an *opsonin* to mark microbes for destruction by phagocytic cells—a process called **opsonization.** Some of these functions of complement are discussed in more detail later in the next chapter.

TOLL-LIKE RECEPTORS

Triggering of many of the innate responses already mentioned requires action by **Toll-like receptors (TLRs)** in the membranes of host cells. They get their odd name from *Toll* (German for "weird"), the name of a gene for this receptor family that was first discovered to cause strange body shapes in fruit flies when damaged. Later, the proteins produced by the gene were also found to have a primitive immune function.

Each of the many types of TLRs present in membranes of human cells can recognize the general pattern of a whole group of molecules that originate in microbes (but not in human cells). That is, they are **pattern-recognition receptors (PRRs)** and thus do not identify specific antigens. Instead, they have a *nonspecific* ability to identify a large variety of different bacterial molecules such as toxins and flagella proteins, viral RNA and glycoproteins, and fungal molecules.

When triggered, TLRs facilitate many of the nonspecific immune mechanisms described earlier. For example, they help initiate the inflammatory response, antigen presentation to immune cells, phagocytosis, release of cytokines and interferon—and even apoptosis of an infected host cell. TLRs are key facilitators of the overall innate immune response of the body.

Quick CHECK

4. Why are the skin and mucous membranes together called the body's first line of defence?
5. Name some of the events of the inflammatory response. How does each help protect the body?
6. What is the role of macrophages in the defence of the body?
7. How do interferons and complement protect the body?

the big picture | Innate Immunity and the Whole Body

Because we have only just begun our story of the immune system, we are not quite ready for "the" big picture. However, taking a step back to look at the broader view will help us orient ourselves before moving on. We now have a general idea of how the immune system works using the analogy of a military defence force. In this chapter, we focused on the rapid first responses that our immune system stands ready to mount at any time. Such "early defences" are vitally important in any military strategy. Now that we have completed our "basic training" on immunity and know the standard responses against threats, we are ready to move on to "advanced training" in the special "military" skills brought into play in adaptive immunity.

LANGUAGE OF SCIENCE *(continued from p. 749)*

nonspecific immunity (non-speh-SIF-ik ih-MYOO-nih-tee) [*non-* **not,** *-spec-* **form or kind,** *-ific* **relating to,** *immun-* **free,** *-ity* **state**]

opsonization (OP-so-nih-ZAY-shen) [*opsoni-* **supply food,** *-ation* **process**]

pattern-recognition receptor (PRR) (PAT-urn rek-ug-NISH-un ree-SEP-tor)

pavementing (PAYV-ment-ing) [*pave-* **cover with stones,** *-ment-* **process**]

phagocytosis (fag-oh-sye-TOH-sis) [*phago-* **eating,** *-cyt-* **cell,** *-osis* **condition**]

species resistance (SPEE-sheez ree-ZIS-tens) [*species* **form or kind,** *resist-* **withstand,** *-ance* **act of**]

specific immunity (ih-MYOO-nih-tee) [*spec-* **form or kind,** *-ific* **relating to,** *immun-* **free,** *-ity* **state**]

Toll-like receptor (TLR) [*Toll-* **weird or amazing,** *-like,* *recept-* **receive,** *-or* **agent**]

LANGUAGE OF MEDICINE

fever (FEE-ver)

pus (puhs)

CHAPTER SUMMARY

To download an MP3 version of the chapter summary for use with your mobile device, access the ***Audio Chapter Summaries*** *online at evolve.elsevier.com.*

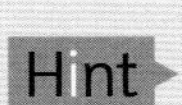

Scan this summary after reading the chapter to help you reinforce the key concepts. Later, use the summary as a quick review before your class or before a test.

Introduction

A. The immune system protects against assaults on the body
   1. External assaults include microorganisms—protozoans, bacteria, and viruses
   2. Internal assaults—abnormal cells reproduce and form tumours that may become cancerous and spread

Organization of the Immune System

A. Immune system continually patrols and protects the body
B. Identification of cells and other particles
   1. Markers, or antigens, are unique molecules recognized by the immune system
   2. Self markers—molecules on the surface of our cells that are unique to an individual, thus identifying the cell as "self" to the immune system
   3. Nonself markers—molecules on the surface of foreign or abnormal cells or particles that identify the particle as "nonself" to the immune system
   4. Self-tolerance—the ability of our immune system to attack abnormal or foreign cells but spare our own normal cells
C. Two major categories of immune mechanisms—innate immunity and adaptive immunity (**Figure 32-1**; **Table 32-1**)
   1. Innate immunity provides a general, nonspecific defence against anything that is not "self"
   2. Adaptive immunity acts as a specific defence against specific threatening agents
   3. Primary cells of innate immunity—epithelial barrier cells, phagocytes (neutrophils, macrophages, dendritic cells), and natural killer cells; chemicals used in innate immunity—complement and interferon
   4. Primary cells of adaptive immunity—lymphocytes called T cells and B cells
   5. Cytokines—chemicals released from cells to promote or trigger innate and adaptive immune responses (e.g., interleukin, interferon, leukotriene)
   6. Other chemicals (e.g., complement, other enzymes, histamine) also play regulatory roles in immunity

Species Resistance (Table 32-2)

A. Genetic characteristics of an organism or species defend against pathogens

Mechanical and Chemical Barriers

A. First line of defence (**Figure 32-2**)
   1. Internal environment of the body is protected by a barrier formed by the skin and the mucous membranes
   2. Skin and mucous membranes provide additional immune mechanisms—sebum, mucus, enzymes, and hydrochloric acid in the stomach

Inflammation and Fever

A. Second line of defence (**Figure 32-3**)
   1. Inflammatory response—tissue damage elicits responses to counteract injury and promote normality
      a. Inflammation mediators include histamine, kinins, prostaglandins, and related compounds (**Figure 32-4**)
      b. Chemotactic factors—substances that attract white blood cells to area of injury in a process called *chemotaxis* (**Figure 32-6**)
      c. Characteristic signs of inflammation—heat, redness, pain, and swelling
      d. Systemic inflammation—occurs from a body-wide inflammatory response
   2. Fever—abnormally high body temperature triggered by inflammation mediators
      a. Triggered in SIRS (systemic inflammatory response syndrome) and other events such as viral infections, tumours, allergies

b. Pyrogens released from damaged tissues (endogenous) or introduced into the body (exogenous)
   (1) Promote prostaglandin (PG) production
   (2) PGs reset the hypothalamic "thermostat" to a higher temperature
   (3) Aspirin and other COX inhibitors interfere with COX enzymes necessary for PG production
c. Fever is thought to increase immune function and inhibit pathogens

Phagocytosis

A. Ingestion and destruction of microorganisms or other small particles by phagocytes (**Figure 32-7**)
   1. Phagocytes—many types capable of phagocytosis (**Table 32-3**)
   2. Antigen-presenting cells (APCs)—phagocytes that ingest foreign particles, isolate protein segments (peptides), and display them as antigens on their surface to trigger an immune response when recognized by a specific (adaptive) immune cell
      a. Neutrophil—most numerous phagocyte; usually first to arrive at site of injury; migrates out of bloodstream during diapedesis; forms pus
      b. Diapedesis—process by which immune cells squeeze through the wall of a blood vessel to get to the site of injury or infection (**Figure 32-5**)
      c. Macrophage—large phagocytic monocyte cells that grow to several times original size after migrating out of bloodstream; important APCs
      d. Dendritic cell (DC)—type of APC with long branches or extensions (**Figure 32-8**)
      e. Phagocytes often identified by location—histiocytes in connective tissue, microglia in nervous system, and Kupffer cells (stellate macrophages) in liver

Natural Killer (NK) Cells

A. Lymphocytes that kill tumour cells and cells infected by viruses (**Figure 32-9**)
   1. Method of recognizing abnormal or nonself cells—target cell is killed if killer-inhibiting receptor on NK cell does not bind to a proper MHC surface protein
   2. Method of killing cells—lysing cells by damaging plasma membranes

Interferon (IFN)

A. Protein synthesized and released into circulation by certain cells if invaded by viruses to signal other nearby cells to enter a protective antiviral state

Complement

A. Group of enzymes that produce a cascade of reactions resulting in a variety of immune responses (**Figure 32-10**)
   1. Cascade may be triggered through multiple pathways
   2. Lyse cells when activated by either adaptive or innate mechanisms
      a. Membrane attack complex (MAC) discussed in next chapter
   3. Anaphylatoxins trigger inflammatory responses
   4. Opsonization—process that marks cells for destruction by phagocytes by complements acting as opsonins
   5. Variety of other immune responses (**Figure 32-10**)

Toll-Like Receptors (TLRs)

A. Pattern-recognition receptors in the membranes of host cells
B. When triggered, TLRs stimulate many different kinds of innate immune responses

The Big Picture: Innate Immunity and the Whole Body

A. Rapid first responses of our immune system are ready to mount at any time

REVIEW QUESTIONS

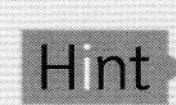

Write out the answers to these questions after reading the chapter and reviewing the Chapter Summary. Note—writing out your answers will consolidate learning and provide a valuable resource of information.

1. Define the term *innate immunity.*
2. List several mechanisms of innate defence, and give a brief description of each one.
3. Identify the body's first line of defence. Why is it inadequate at times?
4. What changes occur in a local area during the inflammatory response?
5. Describe chemotactic factors released from the mast cell.
6. Describe the function of an NK cell.
7. What is the function of interferon?
8. What are complements and what is their role in innate immunity?

CRITICAL THINKING QUESTIONS

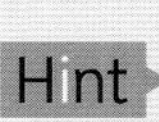

After finishing the Review Questions, write out the answers to these more in-depth questions to help you apply your new knowledge. Go back to sections of the chapter that relate to concepts that you find difficult.

1. The causative organism of tuberculosis has a coat around it that makes it much more resistant than other bacteria to digestive enzymes and hydrogen peroxide. What can you say about this characteristic, and why is it more difficult for the body to fight off these bacteria?
2. If a person had a mutation that prevented the formation of the complement proteins, what capabilities would be lessened in the immune system?
3. How does having a fever help your body recover from injury or infection?
4. How does phagocytosis help protect the internal environment of the body?
5. If the genes that produce Toll-like receptors (TLRs) were abnormal, what effect might that have on a person's immunity?
6. What characteristics of innate immunity make it well suited as an early defence system?
7. Explain the importance to the body of immune system cells that can recognize cells and antigens as self or non-self.

33 Adaptive Immunity

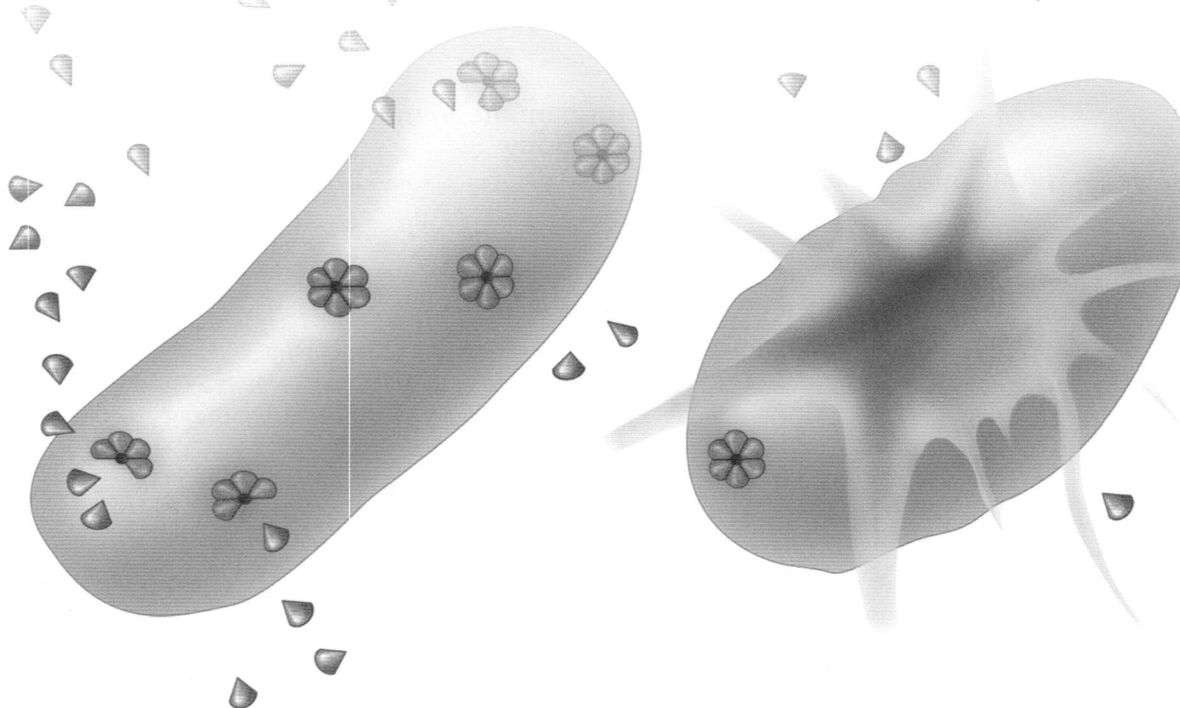

CHAPTER OUTLINE

Hint Scan this outline before you begin to read the chapter, as a preview of how the concepts are organized.

The previous chapter introduced the immune system and the military model of an "internal defence force"—the *immune system.* Beginning with innate immunity, we learned that the body has agents "on duty" and ready to mount a rapid first response to injuries, infections, and other problems. But the innate immune responses are not sufficient for all attacks on the relative constancy of our internal environment. Sometimes, pathogens and tumours cannot be stopped easily and we need more specific defences to provide stronger resistance. This is where our *adaptive* immune responses come into play. Adaptive immunity works in close coordination with our innate defences to protect and preserve our "home territory"—our internal fluid environment and all the cells that live there. This chapter finishes the story of immunity begun in the previous chapters. •

LANGUAGE OF SCIENCE

Hint *Use this list to aid your pronunciation of unfamiliar words.*

antibody (AN-tih-bod-ee)
[*anti-* **against**]

antibody-mediated immunity (AN-tih-bod-ee-MEE-dee-ayt-ed ih-MYOO-nih-tee)
[*anti-* **against,** *medi-* **middle,** *-ate* **process,** *immun-* **free,** *-ity* **state**]

antigen (AN-tih-jen)
[*anti-* **against,** *-gen* **produce**]

antigen–antibody complex (AN-tih-jen-AN-tih-bod-ee KOM-pleks)
[*anti-* **against,** *-gen* **produce,** *anti-* **against,** *body, com-* **together,** *-plex* **weave or braid**]

antigenic determinant (AN-tih-jen-ik deh-TUR-mih-nant)
[*anti-* **against,** *-gen* **produce,** *-ic* **relating to,** *determin-* **limit,** *-ant* **agent of**]

antigen-presenting cell (APC) (AN-tih-jen)
[*anti-* **against,** *-gen* **produce, presenting,** *cell* **storeroom**]

autoimmunity (aw-toh-ih-MYOO-nih-tee)
[*auto-* **self,** *-immun-* **free,** *-ity* **state**]

B cell
[*B* **bursa-equivalent tissue,** *cell* **storeroom**]

cell-mediated immunity (sell-MEE-dee-ayt-ed ih-MYOO-nih-tee)
[*cell* **storeroom,** *medi-* **middle,** *-ate* **process,** *immun-* **free,** *-ity* **state**]

cellular immunity (SELL-yoo-lar ih-MYOO-nih-tee)
[*cell* **storeroom,** *-ular* **relating to,** *immun-* **free,** *-ity* **state**]

chemotactic factor (kee-moh-TAK-tik)
[*chemo-* **chemical,** *-tact-* **movement,** *-ic* **relating to**]

clone (klohn)
[*clon* **a plant cutting**]

combining site (kom-BYNE-ing syte)
[*com-* **together,** *-bine* **two at a time**]

complement (KOM-pluh-munt)
[*comple-* **complete,** *-ment* **result of action**]

cytokine (SYE-toh-kyne)
[*cyto-* **cell,** *-kine* **movement**]

continued on p. 781

OVERVIEW OF ADAPTIVE IMMUNITY

Unlike the innate, nonspecific mechanisms of immunity, the various types of adaptive immune mechanisms attack *specific* agents that the body recognizes as abnormal or nonself. Adaptive immunity, part of the body's *third line of defence*, is orchestrated by two different classes of a type of white blood cell called the *lymphocyte* (**Figure 33-1**).

Originally, lymphocytes are formed in the red bone marrow of the fetus. They, like all blood cells, derive from primitive cells known as *haematopoietic stem cells (HSCs)* (see Chapter 27). The stem cells destined to become lymphocytes of the adaptive immune system follow two developmental paths and differentiate into two major classes of lymphocytes—*B lymphocytes* and *T lymphocytes*, or simply **B cells** and **T cells** (**Figure 33-2**).

CONNECT IT!

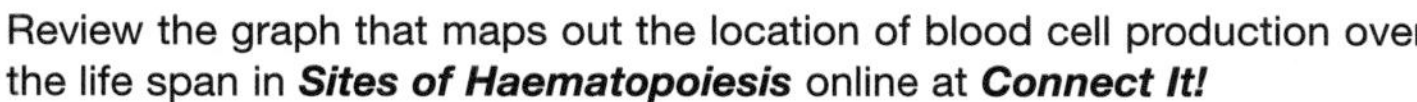

Review the graph that maps out the location of blood cell production over the life span in ***Sites of Haematopoiesis*** online at ***Connect It!***

B cells do not attack pathogens themselves but instead produce molecules called **antibodies** that attack the pathogens or direct other cells, such as phagocytes, to attack them. B cell mechanisms are therefore often classified as **antibody-mediated immunity.** Because antibodies disperse freely in the blood plasma, where they accomplish their immune functions, this type of immunity is sometimes also called **humoral immunity.** The word *humoral* refers to body fluids, especially blood plasma. (Note: In ancient Greek times, the body was thought to contain four fluids, called humours. Derived from the original word, the use of humor is preferred in immunology rather than humour). Many of these terms are further explained in **Box 33-1**.

Because T cells attack pathogens more directly, T cell immune mechanisms are classified as **cell-mediated immunity** or, more simply, **cellular immunity** (**Figure 33-3**).

Lymphocytes express proteins on their surfaces known as *surface markers.* Some of these proteins are unique to lymphocytes; some are shared by other types of cells. B cells and T cells each have some unique surface markers that not only distinguish B cells from T cells but also subdivide these categories into *subsets.* Lymphocyte subsets are clinically meaningful. For example, the condition of a patient's T-cell subsets is very important in understanding AIDS. The international system for naming surface markers on blood cells is the **CD system** (CD stands for *cluster of differentiation*; the number after "CD" refers to a single, defined surface marker protein). For example, the T-cell subsets that are clinically important in diagnosing and assessing AIDS or other immune deficiencies are the $CD4^+$ and $CD8^+$ T-cell subsets. These T-cell types are noted with + because they are "positive" for their respective CD markers.

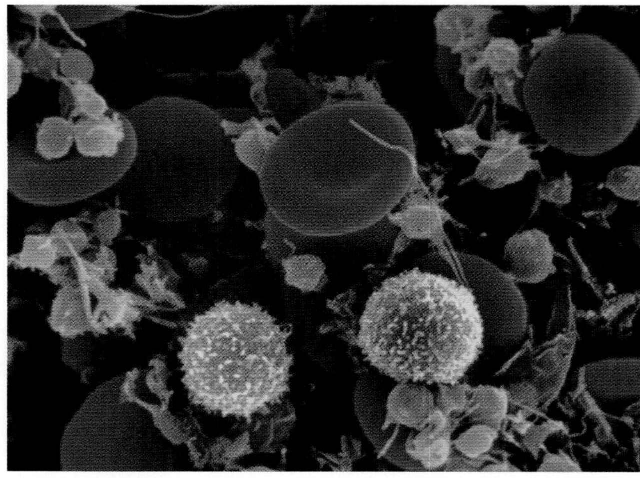

FIGURE 33-1 Lymphocytes. Colour-enhanced scanning electron micrograph showing lymphocytes in yellow, red blood cells in red, and platelets in green.

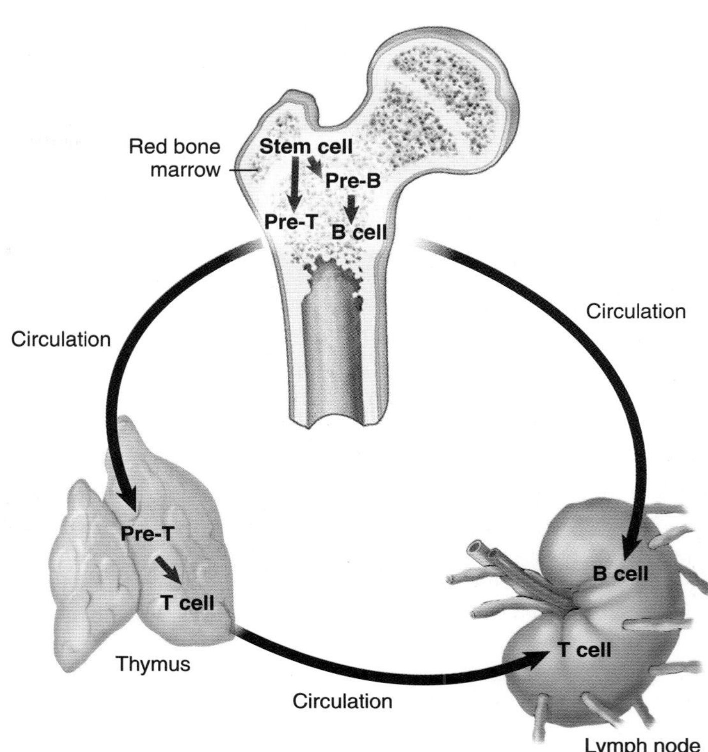

FIGURE 33-2 Development of B cells and T cells. Both types of lymphocytes originate from stem cells in the red bone marrow. Pre–B cells that are formed by dividing stem cells develop in the "bursa-equivalent" tissues in the yolk sac, fetal liver, and bone marrow. Likewise, pre–T cells migrate to the thymus, where they continue developing. Once they are formed, B cells and T cells circulate to the lymph nodes and spleen.

Adaptive immunity requires activation of lymphocyte populations, which then begin their immune attack of specific antigens (or cells or viruses bearing those antigens). Such activation requires two activating signals: a specific antigen and a chemical signal (**Figure 33-4**). Each lymphocyte has receptors both for antigens and for signalling chemicals. Both receptors must be activated for the lymphocyte to begin its active immune function. Chemicals required to stimulate immune function may come from injured or infected cells or from microbes themselves.

The densest populations of lymphocytes—the cells directly involved in adaptive immunity—occur in the bone marrow, thymus gland, lymph nodes, and spleen (**Figure 33-5**). From these structures, lymphocytes pour into the blood and then distribute themselves throughout the tissues of the body. After wandering through the tissue spaces, they eventually find their way into lymphatic capillaries. Lymph flow transports the lymphocytes through a succession

BOX 33-1 *fyi* | The Language of Adaptive Immunity

Learning the mechanisms of adaptive (specific) immunity will be easier if you first become familiar with the following terms:

Antigens—macromolecules (large molecules) that induce the immune system to make certain responses. Most antigens are foreign proteins. Some, however, are polysaccharides, and some are nucleic acids. *Haptens,* sometimes called "incomplete antigens", are very small molecules that must first bind to a protein before they can induce an immune response. Many antigens that enter the body are macromolecules located in the walls or outer membranes of microorganisms or the outer coats of viruses. Of course, antigens on the surfaces of some tumour cells (tumour markers) are not really from outside the body but are "foreign" in the sense that they are recognized as "not belonging". The membrane molecules that identify all the normal cells of the body are called *self-antigens* or *major histocompatibility complex (MHC) antigens* (see **Box 32-1** on p. 758). Foreign and tumour cell antigens can be called *nonself-antigens.*

Antigenic determinants—variously shaped, small regions on the surface of an antigen molecule; a less cumbersome name is *epitopes.* In a protein molecule, for instance, an epitope consists of a sequence of only about 10 amino acids that are part of a much longer, folded chain of amino acids. The sequence of the amino acids in an epitope determines its shape. Because the sequence differs in different kinds of antigens, each kind of antigen usually has specific and uniquely shaped epitopes.

Antibodies—plasma proteins of the class called *immunoglobulins.* Unlike most antigens, all antibodies are native molecules—that is, they are normally present in the body.

Combining sites—two small concave regions on the surface of an antibody molecule. Like epitopes, combining sites have specific and unique shapes. An antibody's combining sites are shaped so that an antigen's epitope that has a complementary shape can fit into the combining site and thereby bind the antigen to the antibody to form an **antigen–antibody complex.** Because combining sites receive and bind antigens, they are also called *antigen receptors* and *antigen-binding sites.*

Clone—family of cells, all of which have descended from one cell.

Complement—a group of proteins that, when activated, work together to destroy foreign cells.

Effector cell—a B cell or T cell that is actively producing an immune response, such as secreting antibodies (effector B cells) or directly attacking other cells (effector T cells); effector cells usually die during or just after their immune response; effector B cells are also called *plasma cells.*

Memory cell—a B or T cell that has been activated (no longer naïve) but is not an effector cell producing an active response; rather, a memory cell survives for a long period in the lymph nodes and if later exposed to the same specific antigen, forms a clone of cells that rapidly produce a specific immune response.

Naïve—refers to a B or T cell that is inactive, meaning it has not yet been exposed to (or had an opportunity to react with) a specific antigen; synonymous with "inactive" or "virgin".

	Antibody-mediated (humoral) immunity	Cell-mediated immunity	
Microbe	Extracellular microbes	Phagocytosed microbes in macrophage	Intracellular microbes (e.g., viruses) replicating within infected cell
Responding lymphocytes	B lymphocyte	Helper T lymphocyte	Cytotoxic T lymphocyte
Effector mechanism	Secreted antibody		
Distributed by	Blood plasma (antibodies)	Cells (T lymphocytes)	Cells (T lymphocytes)
Main functions	**Block infections and eliminate extracellular microbes**	**Activate macrophages to kill phagocytosed microbes**	**Kill infected cells and eliminate reservoirs of infection**

FIGURE 33-3 Two strategies of adaptive immunity. Simplified summary of antibody-mediated (humoral) immunity and cell-mediated (cellular) immunity.

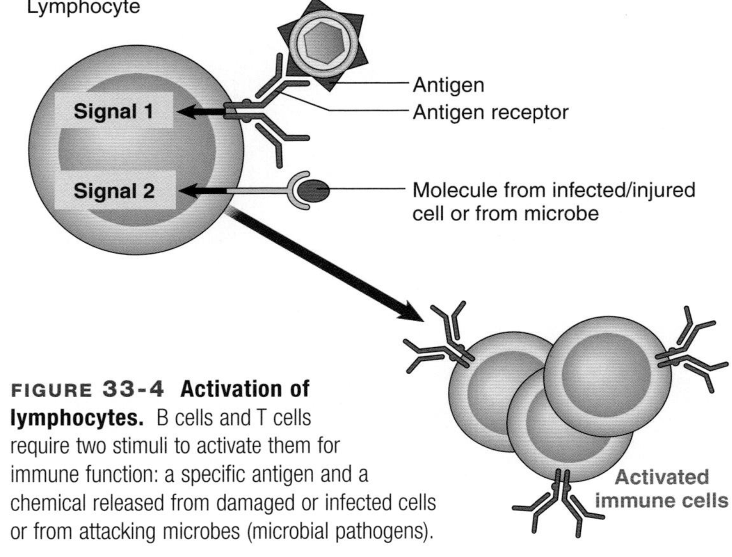

FIGURE 33-4 Activation of lymphocytes. B cells and T cells require two stimuli to activate them for immune function: a specific antigen and a chemical released from damaged or infected cells or from attacking microbes (microbial pathogens).

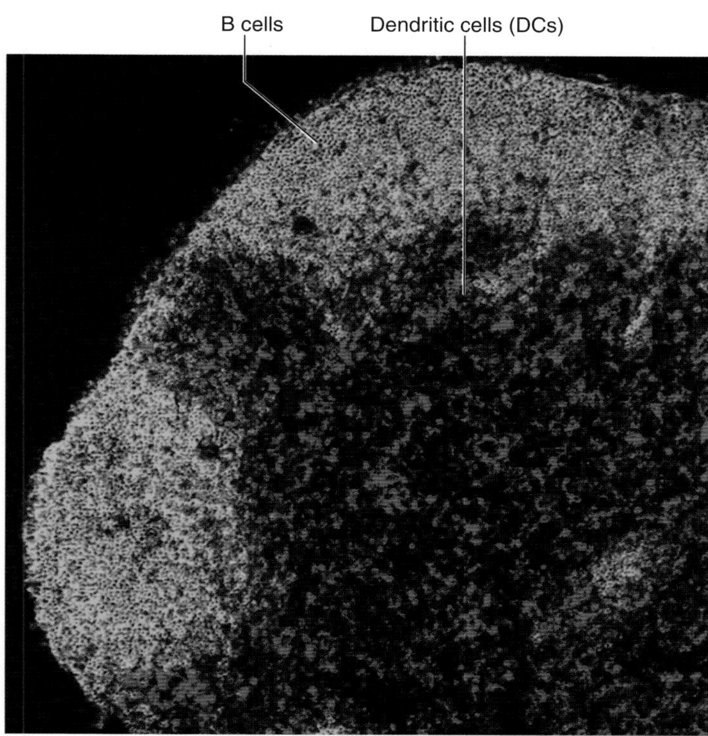

B cells
Dendritic cells (DCs)

FIGURE 33-5 B cells in a lymph node. This micrograph of a lymph node shows fluorescent green stain in B cells, which are densely packed in the nodules of the lymph node. The cells marked by the red stain are a type of macrophage called *dendritic cells* (see **Figure 32-8** on p. 756).

of lymph nodes and lymphatic vessels and empties them by way of the thoracic and right lymphatic ducts into the subclavian veins. Thus returned to the blood, the lymphocytes embark on still another long journey—through blood, tissue spaces, and lymph and then back to blood. The survival value of the continued recirculation of lymphocytes and of their widespread distribution throughout body tissues seems apparent. It provides these major cells of the immune system ample opportunity to perform their functions of searching out, recognizing, and destroying foreign invaders.

Before reading further, please review the basic terminology used to explain adaptive immunity, which is presented in **Box 33-1**.

Quick **CHECK**

1. What is an antigen? What is the difference between a *self-antigen* and a *nonself-antigen*?
2. What is meant by the term *clone*?

B CELLS AND ANTIBODY-MEDIATED IMMUNITY

Development and Activation of B Cells

The development of the lymphocytes called *B cells* occurs in two stages (**Figure 33-6**). In chickens the first stage of B-cell development occurs in the *bursa of Fabricius*—hence the name *B cells*. Because humans do not have a bursa of Fabricius, another organ must serve as the site for the first stage of B-cell development. The bursa-equivalent tissue in humans is the yolk sac and fetal liver during

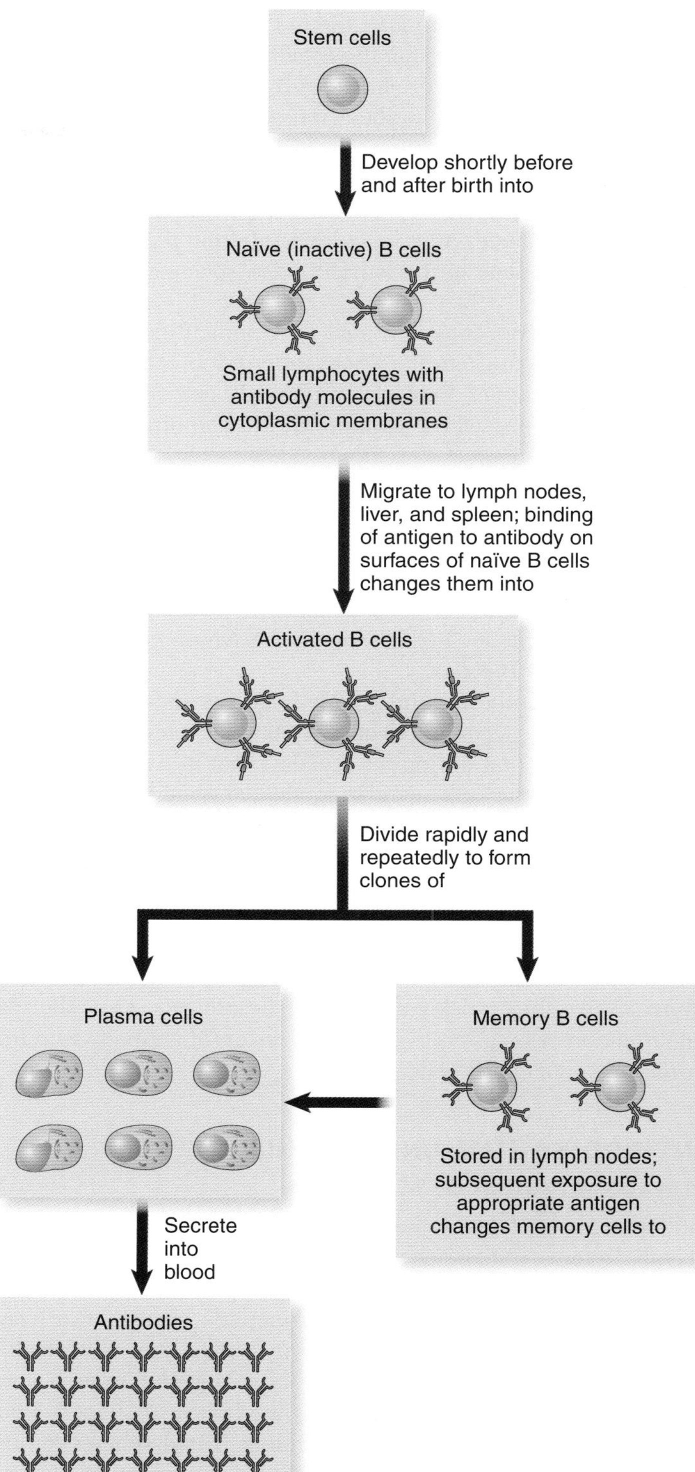

Stem cells
Develop shortly before and after birth into
Naïve (inactive) B cells
Small lymphocytes with antibody molecules in cytoplasmic membranes
Migrate to lymph nodes, liver, and spleen; binding of antigen to antibody on surfaces of naïve B cells changes them into
Activated B cells
Divide rapidly and repeatedly to form clones of
Plasma cells
Memory B cells
Stored in lymph nodes; subsequent exposure to appropriate antigen changes memory cells to
Secrete into blood
Antibodies

FIGURE 33-6 B-cell development. B-cell development takes place in two stages. *First stage:* Shortly before and after birth, stem cells develop into naïve B cells. *Second stage* (occurs only if naïve B cell contacts its specific antigen): Naïve B cell develops into activated B cell, which divides rapidly and repeatedly to form a clone of plasma cells and a clone of memory cells. Plasma cells secrete antibodies capable of combining with specific antigens that cause naïve B cell to develop into active B cell. Stem cells maintain a constant population of newly differentiating cells.

early development and then later the red marrow. After completing their first developmental stage, the B cells are then known as **naïve B cells,** or sometimes *inactive* or *virgin* B cells.

Naïve B cells synthesize antibody molecules but secrete few if any of them. Instead, they insert on the surface of their plasma membranes perhaps 100,000 antibody molecules. The combining sites of these surface antibody molecules serve as receptors for a specific antigen if encountered. After being released from the bone marrow, naïve B cells circulate to the lymph nodes, spleen, and other lymphoid structures.

The second major stage of B-cell development occurs when the naïve B cells become activated. Activation of a B cell must be initiated by an encounter between a naïve B cell and its specific antigen—that is, one whose epitopes fit the combining sites of the B cell's surface antibodies (see **Figure 33-6**).

The antigen binds to these antibodies on the B cell's surface. Antigen–antibody binding activates the B cell, triggering a rapid series of mitotic divisions. By dividing repeatedly, a single B cell produces a clone, or family, of identical B cells. Some of them differentiate to form **effector B cells** or **plasma cells.** Others do not differentiate completely but remain in the lymphatic tissue as the so-called **memory B cells.**

Plasma cells synthesize and secrete huge amounts of antibody. A single plasma cell, according to one estimate, secretes 2000 antibody molecules per second during the few days that it lives. All the cells in a clone of plasma cells secrete identical antibodies because they have all descended from the same B cell.

Memory B cells do not themselves secrete antibodies, but if they are later exposed to the antigen that triggered their formation, memory B cells then rapidly divide to produce more plasma cells and memory cells. The newly formed plasma cells then quickly secrete antibodies that can combine with the initiating antigen (see **Figure 33-6**)—thus quickly combating the antigen. Thus the ultimate function of B cells is to serve as ancestors of antibody-secreting plasma cells (effector B cells).

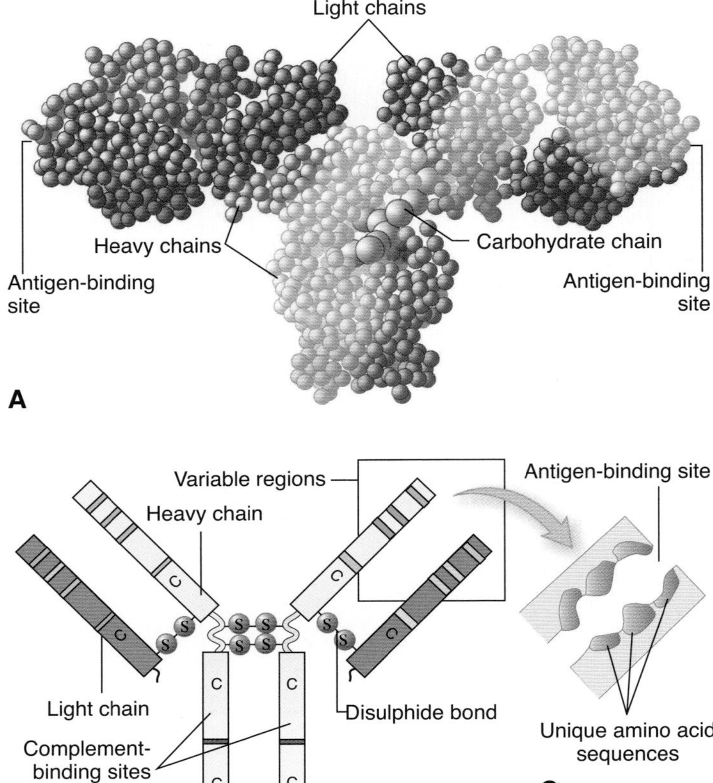

FIGURE 33-7 Structure of the antibody molecule. A, In this molecular model of a typical antibody molecule, the light chains are represented by strands of red spheres (each represents an individual amino acid). Heavy chains are represented by strands of blue spheres. Notice that the heavy chains can complex with a carbohydrate chain. **B,** This simplified diagram shows the variable regions, highlighted by coloured bars, that represent amino acid sequences unique to that molecule. Constant regions of the heavy and light chains are marked. **C,** The variable regions at the end of each arm of the molecule form a cleft that serves as an antigen-binding site.

ANTIBODIES (IMMUNOGLOBULINS)

Structure of Antibody Molecules

Antibodies are proteins of the family called **immunoglobulin (Ig).** Like all proteins, antibodies are very large molecules and are composed of long chains of amino acids (polypeptides). Each immunoglobulin molecule consists of four polypeptide chains—two heavy chains and two light chains. Each polypeptide chain is intricately folded to form globular regions that are joined together in such a way that the immunoglobulin molecule as a whole is Y-shaped. Look now at **Figure 33-7**, A. The twisted strands of red spheres (amino acids) in the diagram represent the light chains, and the two twisted strands of blue spheres represent the heavy chains. Each heavy chain consists of 446 amino acids. Heavy chains therefore are about twice as long and weigh about twice as much as light chains.

The regions with coloured bars seen in **Figure 33-7**, *B*, represent *variable regions*—that is, regions in which the sequence of amino acids varies in different antibody molecules. Note the relative positions of the variable regions of the light and heavy chains; they lie directly opposite each other. Because the amino acid sequence determines conformation or shape, and because different sequences of amino acids occur in the variable regions of different antibodies, the shapes of the sites between the variable regions also differ. At the end of each "arm" of the Y-shaped antibody molecule, the unique shapes of the variable regions form a cleft that serves as the antibody's combining sites, or antigen-binding sites. It is this structural feature that enables antibodies to recognize and combine with specific antigens, both of which are crucial first steps in the body's defence against invading microorganisms and other foreign cells.

In addition to its variable region, each light chain in an antibody molecule also has a constant region. The constant region consists of 106 amino acids whose sequence is identical in all antibody molecules. Each heavy chain of an antibody molecule consists of three constant regions in addition to its one variable region. Identify the constant and variable regions of the light and heavy chains in **Figure 33-7**. Note the location of two *complement-binding sites* on the antibody molecule (one on each heavy chain).

In summary, an immunoglobulin, or antibody molecule, consists of two heavy and two light polypeptide chains. Each light chain consists of one variable region and one constant region. Each heavy chain consists of one variable region and three constant regions. Disulphide bonds join the two heavy chains to each other; they also bind each heavy chain to its adjacent light chain. An antibody has two antigen-binding sites—one at the top of each pair of variable regions—and two complement-binding sites located as shown in **Figure 33-7**.

Diversity of Antibodies

Every normal baby is born with an enormous number of different clones of B cells populating his or her bone marrow, lymph nodes, and spleen. All the cells of each clone are committed to synthesizing a specific antibody with a sequence of amino acids in its variable regions that is different from the sequence synthesized by any other of the innumerable clones of B cells.

How does this astounding diversity originate? One suggested answer is called the *somatic recombination hypothesis*. According to this explanation, our chromosomes do not contain whole genes for producing the heavy and light polypeptide chains that make up each antibody molecule. Instead, the genetic code is a set of separate sequences that are assembled into whole genes as a B cell develops. Because the separate sequences can be assembled in an astounding number of different combinations to form each whole gene, and because several different polypeptides are needed to make one antibody, any particular B cell is not likely to synthesize *exactly* the same antibody as any other B cell. Thus somatic recombination is a sort of "genetic lottery" that produces millions of unique genes by combining different gene segments and millions of unique antibodies by combining different polypeptides.

Antibody diversity may also be influenced by occasional mutations in the gene segments used to form the genes needed to produce antibodies. Evidence from several different studies shows that random genetic mutations—slight changes in the master DNA code—result in slight differences in the variable regions of antibodies.

If these hypotheses about antibody diversity are correct, it is possible to produce B cells that make antibodies against self-antigens. It is thought that although most such B cells are eliminated early in their development, before they produce antibodies that would attack a person's own cells, all humans have some "anti-self" B cells in their bodies.

Classes of Antibodies

There are five classes of antibodies, identified by letter names as immunoglobulins M, G, A, E, and D (**Figure 33-8**). *Immunoglobulin M (IgM)* is the antibody that immature B cells synthesize and insert into their plasma membranes. It is also the predominant class of antibody produced after initial contact with an antigen. The most abundant circulating antibody, the one that normally makes up about 75% of all the antibodies in the blood, is *IgG*. It is the predominant antibody of the secondary antibody response—that is, after subsequent contacts with a given antigen. The IgG antibodies are those that cross the placental barrier during pregnancy to impart natural passive immunity to the offspring (**Table 33-1**; see **Box 33-5**). *IgA* is the major class of antibody present in the mucous membranes of the body, in saliva, and in tears (see **Box 33-6**). *IgE*, although minor in amount, can produce major harmful effects, such as those associated with allergies. *IgD* is present in the blood in very small amounts, and its precise function is as yet unknown. As **Figure 33-8** shows, some immunoglobulin molecules are formed by the joining of several basic antibody units.

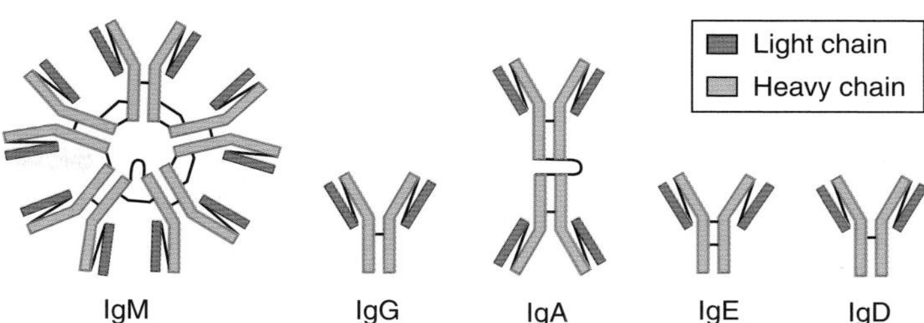

FIGURE 33-8 Classes of antibodies. Antibodies are classified into five major groups: immunoglobulin M (IgM), immunoglobulin G (IgG), immunoglobulin A (IgA), immunoglobulin E (IgE), and immunoglobulin D (IgD). Notice that each IgM molecule has five Y-shaped basic antibody units and most of the others have a single basic antibody unit. IgA is shown here with two antibody units, which is the form found in mucous secretions. But IgA also has a single-unit form found in the blood plasma.

Functions of Antibodies

The function of antibody molecules—some 100 million trillion of them—is to produce antibody-mediated immunity. As we stated earlier, this type of immunity is also called *humoral immunity* because it occurs within plasma, which is one of the humors, or fluids, of the body.

Antigen-Antibody Reactions

Antibodies fight disease first by recognizing substances that are foreign or abnormal. In other words, they distinguish nonself-antigens from self-antigens. Recognition occurs when an antigen's epitopes (small regions on its surface) fit into and bind to an antibody molecule's antigen-binding sites (**Figure 33-9**). The binding of the antigen to antibody forms an antigen–antibody complex that may produce one or more effects. For example, it transforms antigens that are toxins (chemicals poisonous to cells) into harmless substances. It agglutinates antigens that are molecules on the surface of microorganisms. In other words, it makes them stick together in clumps, and this in turn makes it possible for macrophages and other phagocytes to dispose of them more rapidly by ingesting and digesting large

TABLE 33-1 Types of Adaptive Immunity

TYPE	DESCRIPTION OR EXAMPLE
Natural Immunity	Exposure to the causative agent is not deliberate
Active (exposure)	A child develops measles and acquires an immunity to a subsequent infection
Passive (exposure)	A fetus receives protection from the mother through the placenta, or an infant receives protection through the mother's milk
Artificial Immunity	Exposure to the causative agent is deliberate
Active (exposure)	Injection of the causative agent, such as a vaccination against polio, confers immunity
Passive (exposure)	Injection of protective material (antibodies) that was developed by another individual's immune system

UNIT 4

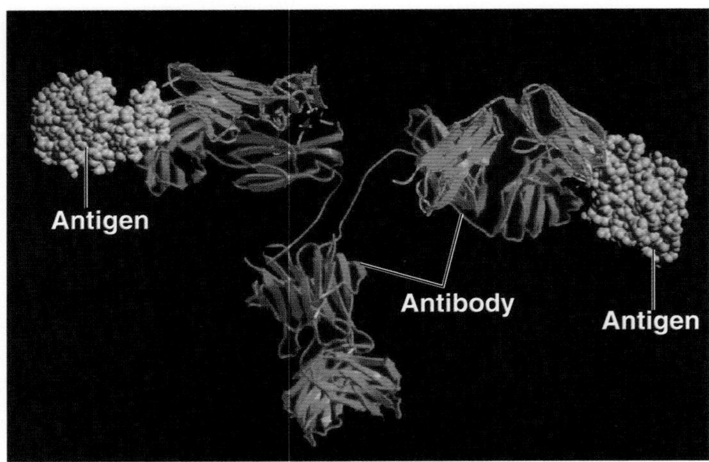

FIGURE 33-9 Binding of antigen by an antibody. This ribbon model of an antibody shows the heavy chains in blue and the light chains in red. Note the green antigen molecules bound to each antigen-binding site.

numbers of them at one time. The binding of antigens to antibodies often produces still another effect: it alters the shape of the antibody molecule—not very much, but enough to expose the molecule's previously hidden complement-binding sites. This seems a trivial enough change, but it is not so. It initiates an astonishing series of reactions that culminate in the destruction of microorganisms and other foreign cells (**Figure 33-10**).

CONNECT IT!

Techniques that permit biologists to produce and isolate large quantities of pure and very specific antibodies called **monoclonal antibodies (MAbs)** and tiny antibody fragments called **nanobodies** have resulted in dramatic advances in medicine. Learn how this works in ***Monoclonal Antibodies and Nanobodies*** online at ***Connect It!***

Complement

Complement is a component of blood plasma that consists of about 20 protein compounds. They are inactive enzymes that become activated in a definite sequence to catalyze a series of intricately linked reactions. The binding of an antibody to an antigen located on the surface of a cell alters the shape of the antibody molecule in a way that exposes its complement-binding sites. By binding to these sites, complement protein 1 becomes activated and touches off the catalytic activity of the next complement protein in the series. A rapid sequence, or cascade, of activity by the next protein, then the next, and the next, follows until the entire series of enzymes has functioned. The end result of this rapid-fire activity challenges the imagination. Some of the resulting reactions were summarized in **Figure 32-10** (p. 759).

One of the more spectacular results of the complement cascade is the formation of **membrane attack complexes (MACs).** Molecules formed by the reactions of the complement cascade assemble themselves on the enemy cell's surface in such a way as to form a doughnut-shaped structure—complete with a hole in the middle (**Figure 33-11**). In effect, the complement has drilled a hole through the foreign cell's surface membrane. Ions and water rush into the cell through the MAC; consequently, it swells and bursts (**Figure 33-12**). **Cytolysis** is the technical name for this process. Nucleated cells usually resist cytolysis, but the influx of ions triggers apoptosis and thus kills the target cell another way.

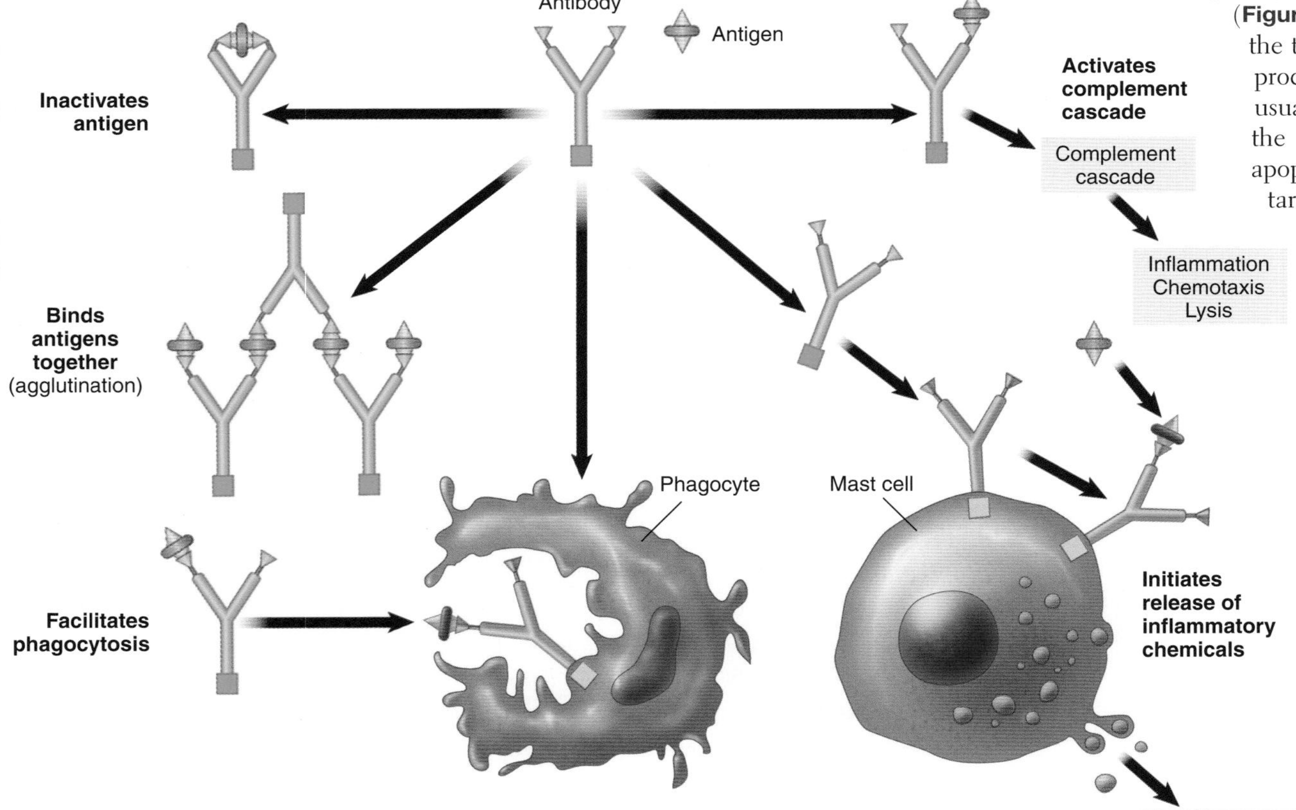

FIGURE 33-10 Actions of antibodies. Antibodies act on antigens by inactivating and bending them together to facilitate phagocytosis and by initiating inflammation and activating the complement cascade.

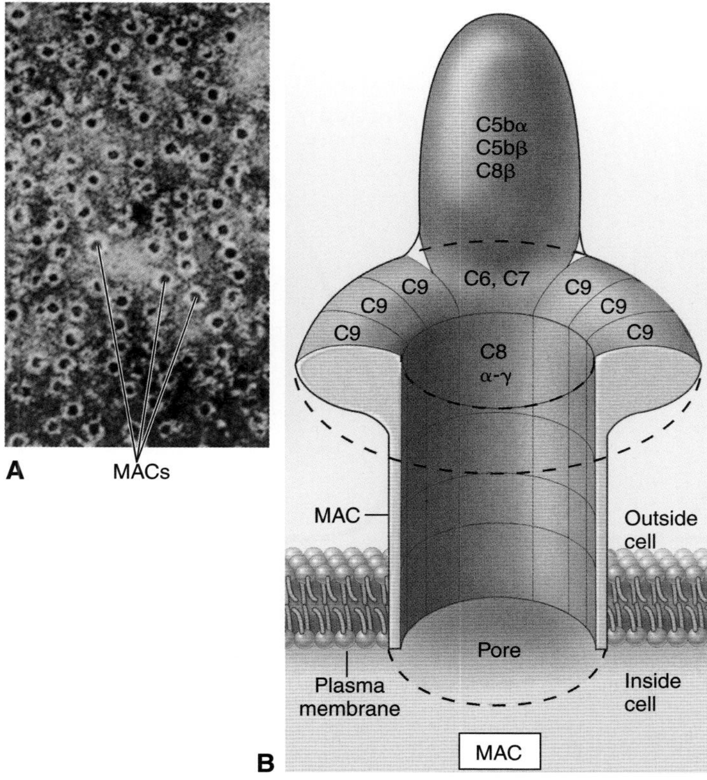

FIGURE 33-11 Membrane attack complex (MAC). Complement components assemble to form a ringlike complex that forms a pore in the membrane of a cell. **A,** Electron micrograph showing numerous MAC pores, each about 10 nm in diameter. **B,** Diagram of the structure of a MAC embedded in a plasma membrane.

Briefly, then, complement functions to kill foreign cells by cytolysis. In addition, various complement proteins serve other functions. Some, for example, cause vasodilation in the invaded area, and some attract neutrophils to the site and enhance phagocytosis.

The complement cascade can also be initiated by innate immune mechanisms. Complement protein 3 (C3) can become activated without any stimulation by an antigen. C3 is normally inactivated by enzymes, but it can produce the full complement effect if it binds to bacteria or viruses in the presence of a protein called *properdin.* Thus lysis of various foreign cells and viruses by complement can occur even when antibodies are not involved. This method of activating the complement cascade is often called the "alternate pathway" to distinguish it from the "classical pathway" involving antibodies.

FIGURE 33-12 Cytolysis of a bacterial cell. A, Complement molecules activated by antibodies form doughnut-shaped membrane attack complexes (MACs) in a bacterium's plasma membrane. **B,** Holes in the complement complex allow sodium (Na^+) and then water (H_2O) to diffuse into the bacterium. **C,** After enough water has entered, the swollen bacterium bursts. In nucleated cells that resist cytolysis, the influx of calcium ions triggers apoptosis and thus kills the target cell another way.

Primary and Secondary Responses

As **Figure 33-13** shows, an initial encounter with a specific antigen produces a *primary response* of increased antibody production in a few days. As the antigen is dealt with, the antibody levels decrease to their normal baseline levels. However, memory B cells that can respond to the triggering antigen have also been produced and wait for another encounter with the antigen. A later encounter with the same antigen triggers the waiting memory B cells and thus produces a secondary response in much less time. The memory B cells quickly divide to form more memory cells and a large number of plasma cells that produce antibodies against the known antigen. Thus the secondary response can be quicker and thus more effective. The strength of the secondary response can be used to boost the effectiveness of immunizations (**Box 33-2**).

CONNECT IT!

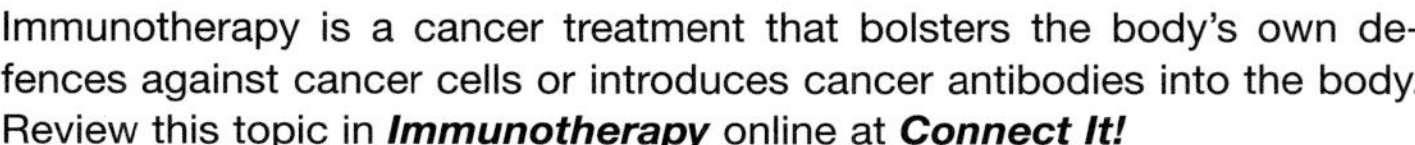

Immunotherapy is a cancer treatment that bolsters the body's own defences against cancer cells or introduces cancer antibodies into the body. Review this topic in ***Immunotherapy*** online at ***Connect It!***

Clonal Selection Theory

The *clonal selection theory,* which deals with antigen destruction, was first proposed in 1959 by Sir Macfarlane Burnet (**Figure 33-14**). It has two basic tenets. First, it holds that the body contains an enormous number of diverse clones of cells, each committed by certain of its genes to synthesize a different antibody. Second, the clonal selection theory postulates that when an antigen enters the body, it selects the clone whose cells are committed to synthesizing its specific antibody and stimulates these cells to proliferate and to thereby produce more antibodies.

We now know that the clones selected by antigens consist of lymphocytes. We also know how antigens select lymphocytes—by the shape of antigen receptors on the lymphocyte's plasma membrane. An antigen recognizes receptors that fit its epitopes and combines with them. By thus selecting the precise clone committed to making its specific antibody, each antigen provokes its own destruction.

It has also been demonstrated that clones with antigen receptors against self-antigens are normally deleted, rather than

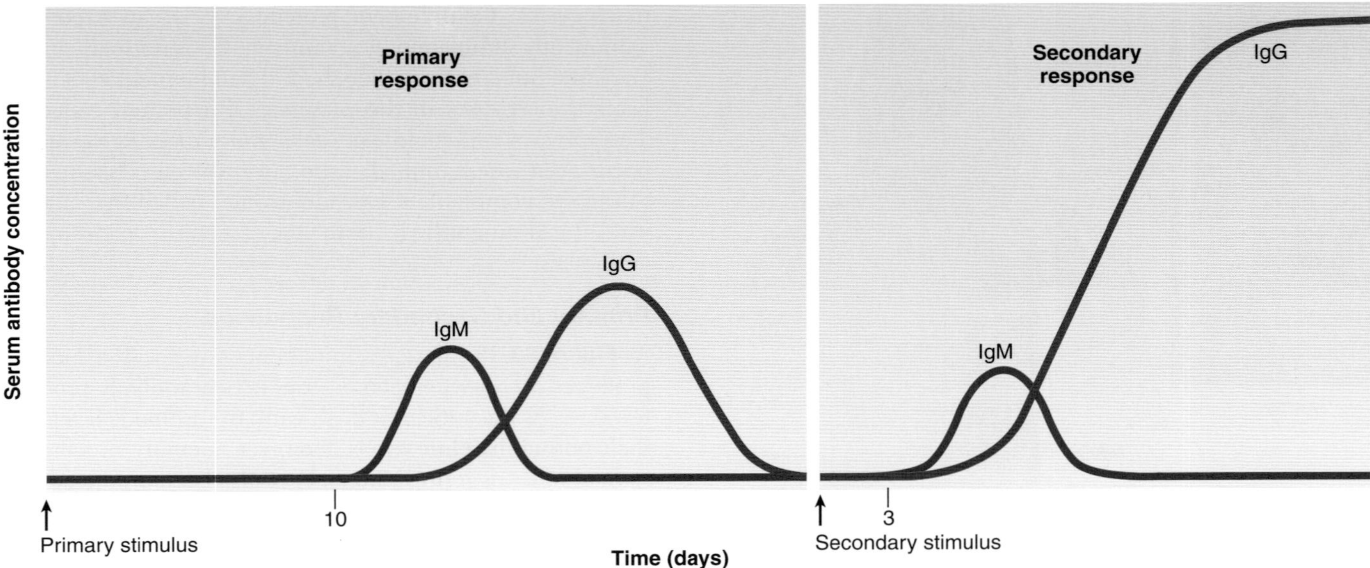

FIGURE 33-13 Antibody response times. The initial encounter with a specific antigen (primary stimulus) produces a primary response (increased production of IgM and IgG) in a few days. A later encounter (secondary stimulus) produces a secondary response in much less time. Note that both IgM production and IgG production occur more quickly in the secondary response—and IgG production also increases in the total amount of antibody produced.

selected. This *clonal deletion* is necessary to maintain self-tolerance. But in autoimmune disorders, clonal deletion may fail and our immune system attacks our own normal cells.

Clonal selection and deletion also occurs in T lymphocytes, whose role in immunity we explore next.

Quick CHECK

3. From what structure was the term *B cell* originally derived?
4. How do B cells help defend the body against pathogens?
5. How does the structure of an antibody relate to its function?
6. Describe the mechanism by which complement destroys foreign cells.

BOX 33-2 *health matters* | Immunization

Active immunity can be established artificially by using a technique called **vaccination.** The first vaccine was a live cowpox virus that was injected into healthy people to cause a mild cowpox infection. The term *vaccine* literally means "cow substance". Because the cowpox virus is similar to the deadly *smallpox virus,* vaccinated individuals developed antibodies that imparted immunity against both cowpox and smallpox viruses.

Modern vaccines work on a similar principle; substances that trigger the formation of antibodies against specific pathogens are introduced orally or by injection. Some of these vaccines are killed pathogens or live, *attenuated* (weakened) pathogens. Such pathogens still have their specific antigens intact, so they can trigger formation of the proper antibodies, but they are no longer *virulent* (able to cause disease). Although rare, these vaccines sometimes backfire and actually cause an infection. Many of the newer vaccines avoid this potential problem by using only the part of the pathogen that contains antigens. Because the disease-causing portion is missing, such vaccines cannot cause infection.

The amount of antibodies in a person's blood produced in response to vaccination or an actual infection is called the **antibody titre.** As you can see in the figure, the initial injection of vaccine triggers a rise in the antibody titre that gradually diminishes. Often, a **booster shot,** or second injection, is given to keep the antibody titre high or to raise it to a level that is more likely to prevent infection. The secondary response is more intense than the primary response because memory B cells are ready to produce a large number of antibodies at a moment's notice. A later accidental exposure to the pathogen will trigger an even more intense response—thus preventing infection.

Rigorous studies have shown that vaccines are generally safe and effective. A complete immunization schedule is available from Public Health England on the GOV.UK website every year.

Toxoids are similar to vaccines but use an altered form of a bacterial toxin to stimulate production of antibodies. Injection of toxoids imparts protection against toxins, whereas administration of vaccines imparts protection against pathogenic organisms and viruses.

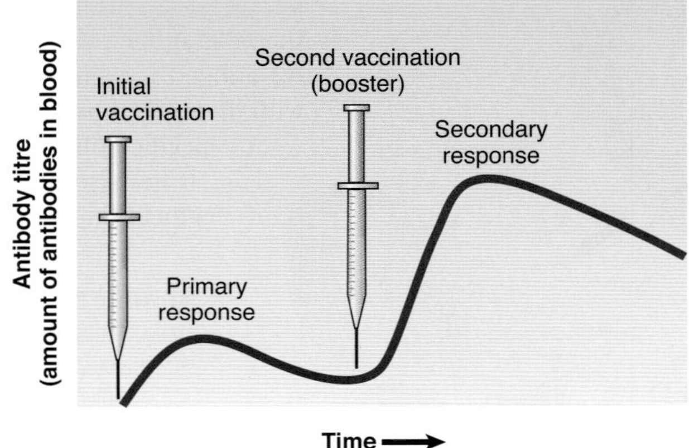

Changes in blood antibody titres after primary and secondary (booster) vaccinations.

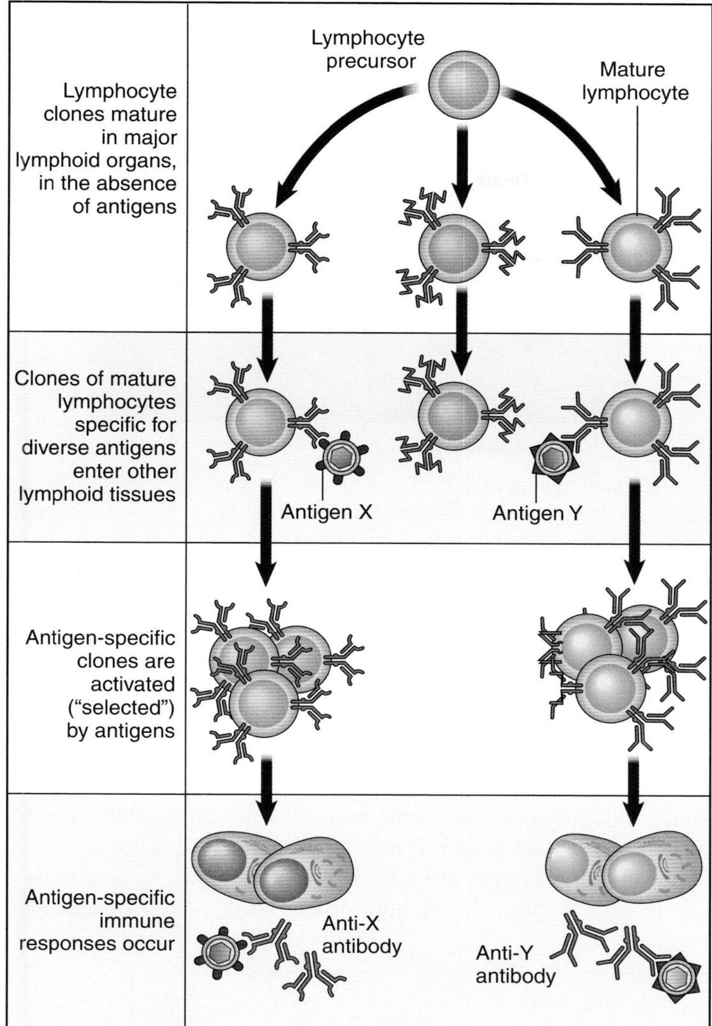

FIGURE 33-14 The clonal selection theory. This theory of immunity states that each specific antigen (here shown as X and Y) activates—selects—a previously produced clone of lymphocytes. The clone is "selected" because it is specifically targeted at the selecting antigen. The clone, when thus activated, produces effector cells that attack the antigen. B cells are shown here, but the same principle also applies to T cells.

T CELLS AND CELL-MEDIATED IMMUNITY

DEVELOPMENT OF T CELLS

T cells, by definition, are lymphocytes that have made a detour through the thymus gland before migrating to the lymph nodes and spleen (see **Figure 33-2**). During their residence in the thymus, pre–T cells develop into **thymocytes,** cells that proliferate as rapidly as any in the body. Thymocytes divide up to three times each day, and, as a result, their numbers increase enormously in a relatively short time. They stream out of the thymus into the blood and find their way to a new home in areas of the lymph nodes and spleen called *T-dependent zones.* From this time on, they are known as T cells.

ACTIVATION AND FUNCTIONS OF T CELLS

Each T cell, like each B cell, displays antigen receptors on its surface membrane. They are not immunoglobulins as are B-cell receptor molecules but are proteins similar to them. When an antigen (preprocessed and presented by phagocytes) encounters a naïve T cell whose surface receptors fit the antigen's epitopes, the antigen binds to the T cell's receptors. Here is where we see one of several differences between antibody-mediated immunity and cell-mediated immunity: antibodies can react to soluble antigens dissolved in the plasma, but T cells can only react to protein fragments presented on the surfaces of **antigen-presenting cells (APCs)** or infected cells. Thus T cells react to cells that are already infected—or have otherwise engulfed the antigen. B cells, on the other hand, react mainly to antigens that are in the plasma.

The presentation of an antigen by an antigen-presenting cell activates or sensitizes the T cell. The T cell then divides repeatedly to form a clone of identical *sensitized T cells* that form **effector T cells** and **memory T cells.** Effector T cells include **cytotoxic T cells,** which cause contact killing of a target cell. Cytotoxic T cells are also called *cytolytic T lymphocytes (CTLs)* or *killer T cells.* Memory T cells remain in red bone marrow until they ultimately produce additional active T cells when needed. The process of T-cell development and activation is summarized in **Figure 33-15**.

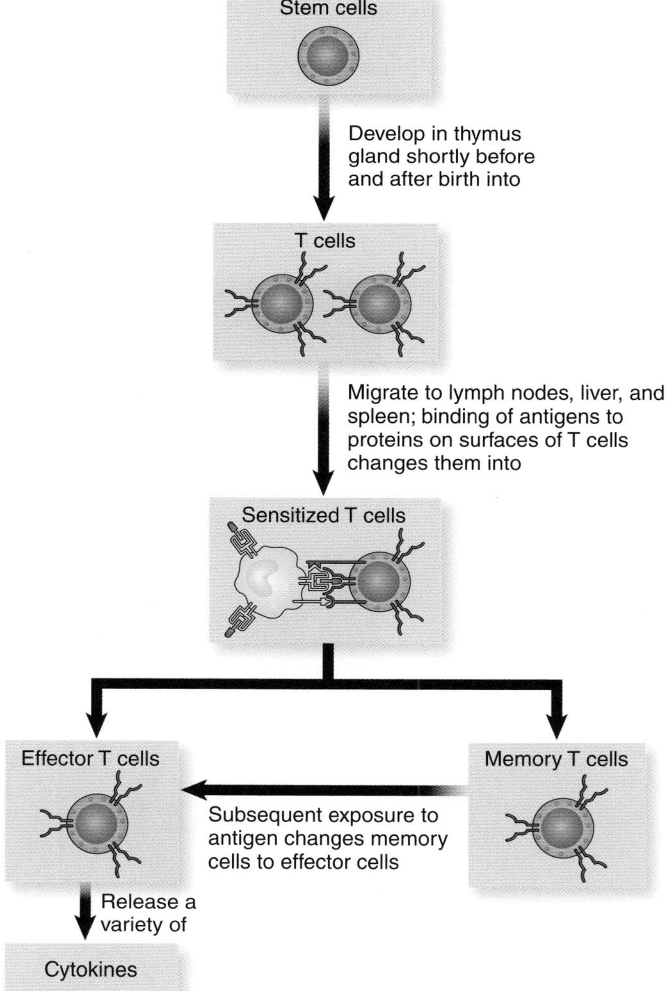

FIGURE 33-15 T-cell development. The *first stage* occurs in the thymus gland shortly before and after birth. Stem cells maintain a constant population of newly differentiating cells as they are needed. The *second stage* occurs only if a T cell is presented an antigen, which combines with certain proteins on the T cell's surface.

UNIT 4

BOX 33-3 *fyi* | Immunological Synapses

Immune cells often make contact with other immune cells or their target cells so that they can carry out their various functions. Their contact points are similar in many ways to the neurological synapse that you learned about in Chapter 19 (see **Figure 19-10**, *B*, on p. 420). Therefore, these contact points made by immune cells are called *immunological synapses (ISs).*

Some ISs are temporary junctions formed when an antigen-presenting cell (APC) connects to an effector cell, such as a cytotoxic T cell. For example, see the effector mechanisms for cell-mediated immunity in **Figure 33-13**. ISs also form when natural killer (NK) cells or cytotoxic T cells temporarily attach to a target cell to destroy it (see the figure). The junctions seen in **Figures 32-9** and **33-16** are examples. ISs also form a temporary junction between immune cells to allow cytokines to pass efficiently from one cell to another. The junctions seen in the effector functions of helper T cells are shown in **Figure 33-17**. •

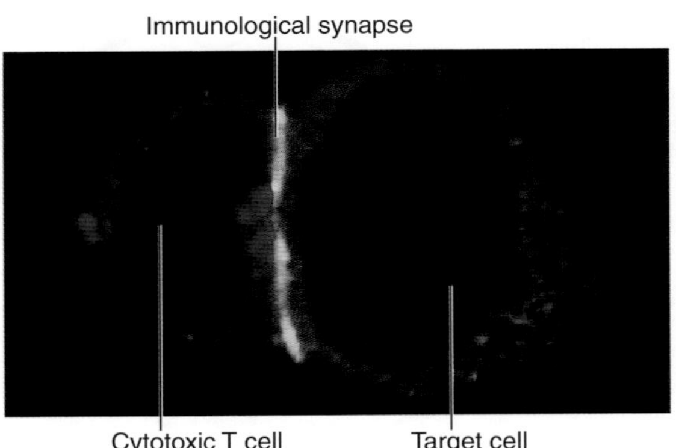

Immunological synapses (IS). Fluorescence micrograph that highlights integral membrane proteins involved in the formation of a temporary junction—immunological synapse—between a cytotoxic T cell and the target cell it is about to destroy. Other types of ISs permit efficient communication between two or more immune cells.

The effector T cells then travel to the site where the antigens originally entered the body. There, in the inflamed tissue, the sensitized T cells bind to antigens of the same kind that led to their formation. However, T cells bind to their specific antigen only if the antigen is presented by an APC such as a macrophage or dendritic cell. The T cell and APC form a temporary junction called an **immunological synapse (IS)**, as explained in **Box 33-3**. The antigen-bound sensitized T cells then release chemical messengers into the inflamed tissues.

The chemical messengers released by T cells are called **cytokines**—a term we first encountered in the previous chapter. Because some cytokines are secreted mainly by lymphocytes, such cytokines are sometimes called *lymphokines*. Names of a few individual cytokines are chemotactic factor, migration inhibition factor, macrophage activating factor, interleukin, and lymphotoxin.

Chemotactic factors attract macrophages, causing hundreds of them to migrate into the vicinity of the antigen-bound, sensitized

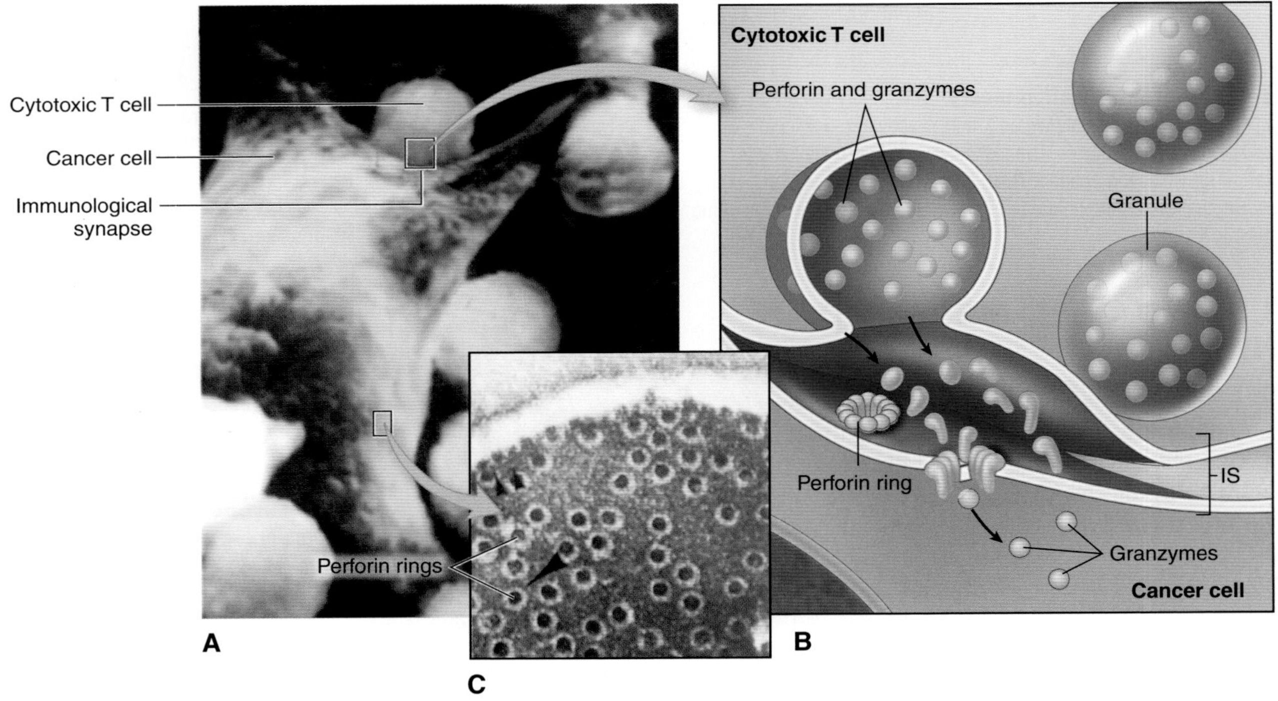

FIGURE 33-16 Killing by cytotoxic T cells. A, The blue spheres seen in this scanning electron microscope view are cytotoxic T cells attacking a much larger cancer cell. T cells are a significant part of our defence against cancer and other abnormal or foreign cells. **B,** After forming an immunological synapse (IS) with the tumour cell, the cytotoxic T cell releases perforin, which forms ringlike holes in the tumour cell's membrane, and granzymes, which pass through the perforin rings to trigger apoptosis (programmed cell death) in the tumour cell. **C,** Electron micrograph showing perforin rings with an average diameter of about 160 Å, which is much larger than the major histocompatibility complex (MHC) rings formed by complement (compare with **Figure 33-11**).

T cell. *Migration inhibition factor* halts macrophage migration. *Macrophage activating factor* prods the assembled macrophages to destroy antigens by phagocytosing them at a rapid rate. **Interleukins (ILs)** are a class of about a dozen different cytokines that are involved in regulating a wide variety of immune functions in different cell types. **Lymphotoxin** is a powerful poison that acts more directly, quickly killing any cell it attacks.

Effector T cells that release lymphotoxin are the *cytotoxic T cells.* **Figure 33-16** shows how lymphotoxins work in killing a cell—a cancer cell in this case. After having been activated by the presentation of tumour cell antigens by an APC such as a dendritic cell, the cytotoxic T cell then becomes active and finds a tumour cell bearing that antigen. The cytotoxic T cell binds directly to the surface of the tumour cell and releases two kinds of molecules: perforin and granzymes. The lymphotoxins called *perforin* produce a ringlike hole in the plasma membrane of the target cell, similar to the one produced by the MAC formed by complement (see **Figure 33-16**). The *granzymes* enter the target cell through the perforin-ring hole and trigger apoptosis of the cell—thus killing it.

Besides cytotoxic T cells, at least two other populations of effector T cells are found in the body: **helper T cells (T_H cells)** and **suppressor T cells.** Both types of cells help regulate adaptive immune function by regulating B-cell and T-cell function. Helper T cells help other lymphocytes by secreting cytokines that stimulate B cells and cytotoxic T cells. T_H cytokines also stimulate phagocytes and other leucocytes (**Figure 33-17**). These cytokines include *interleukin-2 (IL-2)* and *interleukin-4* (IL-4 or B-cell differentiating factor). Like other effector T cells, naïve T_H cells are activated by antigens presented on the surfaces of APCs and form a clone that differentiates into *effector T_H cells* and *memory T_H cells.*

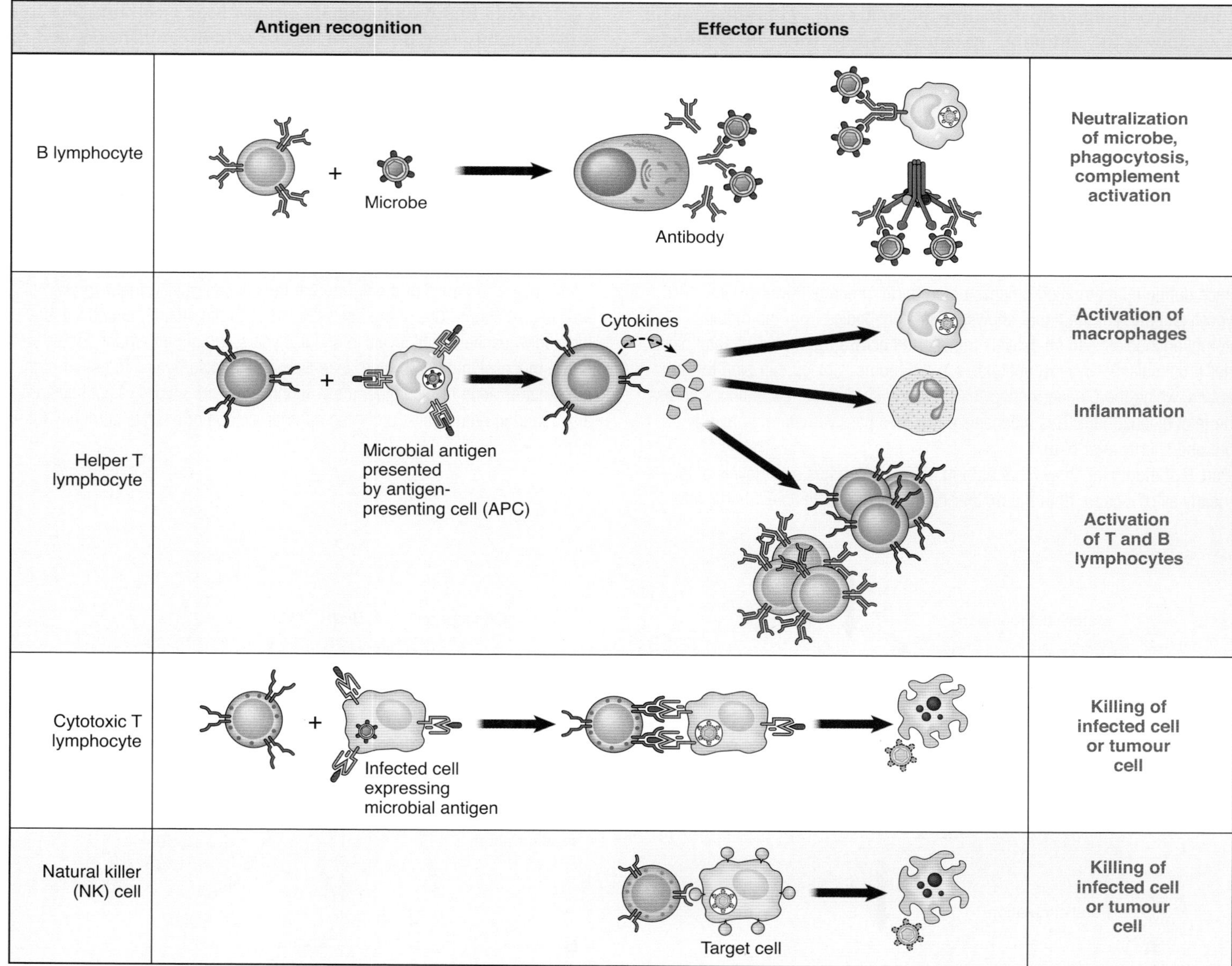

FIGURE 33-17 Lymphocyte functions. This diagram summarizes, in a simplified way, the main functions of the major classes of lymphocytes. B and T lymphocytes participate in adaptive immunity and NK cells participate in innate immunity.

BOX 33-4 *health matters* | Immunity and Cancer

One of the many functions of the immune system is to constantly guard against the development of cancer. Cell mutations occur frequently in the normal body, and many of the mutated cells formed are cancer cells. Cancer cells, you may recall, are cells capable of forming tumours in many different parts of the body—unless they are destroyed before this can happen. Abnormal antigens presented on cancer cells, called **tumour-specific antigens,** are present in the plasma membranes of some cancer cells in addition to self-antigens. Lymphocytes, in their continual wanderings through body tissues, are almost sure to come in contact with newly formed cancer cells. Hopefully, the lymphocytes recognize these cells by their abnormal antigens and quickly initiate reactions that kill the cancer cells. Abnormal antigens on cancer cells, called tumour-specific antigens or **tumour markers,** are present in the plasma membranes of some cancer cells in addition to self-antigens or major histocompatibility complex (MHC) antigens. Examples of cancer markers include (1) **carcinoembryonic antigen (CEA)**—found normally in the fetus and elevated in colorectal and other adult cancers; (2) **alpha-fetoprotein (AFP)**—normal fetal protein, whose presence in the adult strongly suggests liver or germ cell cancer; (3) **CA-125**—tumour antigen associated with ovarian cancer; and (4) **prostate-specific antigen (PSA),** which is elevated in both benign and malignant prostate disease. The relationship between cancer and the immune system continues to be an area of intense research by scientists looking for effective cancer treatments. •

Suppressor T cells, often called *regulator T cells (T-regs)*, act to suppress B-cell differentiation into plasma cells. The antagonistic action allows the immune system to finely tune its antibody-mediated response. Suppressor T cells also regulate other T cells, helping "turn off" an immune response to restore homeostasis, for example. Suppressor T cells help maintain self-tolerance by reducing T-cell reactions to self-antigens. For this reason, researchers are trying to find ways to enhance suppressor T-cell function to treat autoimmunity (see p. 778) or in organ transplants to prevent rejection of donor tissue.

Summarizing briefly, the function of T cells is to produce cell-mediated immunity. They search out, recognize, and bind to

BOX 33-5 *fyi* | Prenatal Immunity

Without direct access to external antigens, it is no wonder that the immune system is not very capable (on its own) of a vigorous defence during its maturation process before birth (prenatal development). However, as part *A* of the figure shows, certain antibodies from the mother (maternal antibodies) can be actively transported across the maternal–fetal blood barrier (trophoblast). Only IgG antibodies in the mother's blood can bind to the receptors, which then trigger endocytosis and transport each IgG antibody across to the fetal bloodstream. This mechanism provides passive natural immunity before and shortly after birth.

Part *B* of the figure shows that at birth, the newborn has adult levels of IgG—but nearly all of it came from the mother (maternal IgG, *blue line*). Shortly after birth, the maternal IgG is broken down *(blue line)* and replaced with new IgG made by the newborn's own immune system *(red line)*.

Note also in part *B* of the figure that the concentration of IgM *(broken blue line)* is only about 20% of the adult level at birth but steadily increases after birth. IgM reaches adult levels in about 2 years. IgA, an important component of the mucosal immune system (see **Box 33-6**), also begins to rise at birth. IgA reaches adult levels in just a few months. All three types of antibody are also found in breast milk, providing another avenue of passive immunity after birth. •

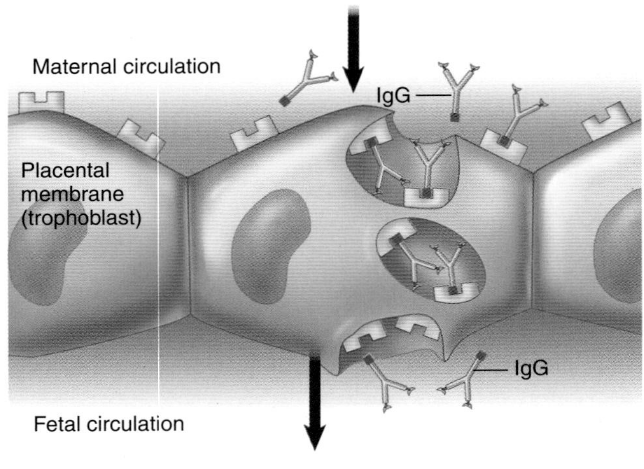

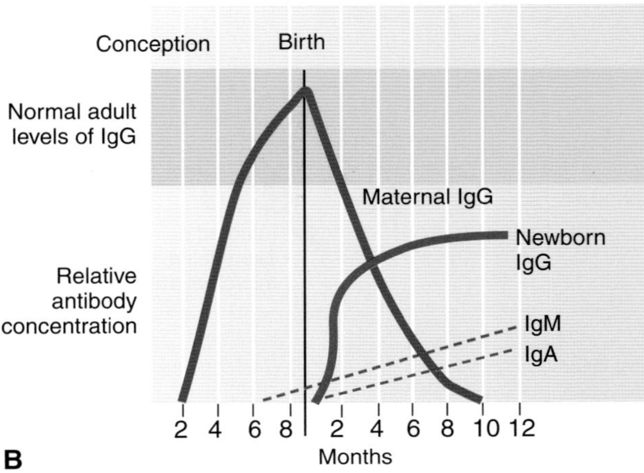

A, Transport of antibodies across the placenta. **B,** Antibody concentrations before and after birth.

UNIT 4

appropriate antigens located on the surfaces of cells. This kills the cells—the ultimate function of killer T cells. Usually these are not the body's own normal cells but are cells that have been invaded by viruses, that have become malignant (**Box 33-4**), or that have been transplanted into the body. Killer T cells therefore function to defend us from viral diseases and cancer, but they also bring about rejection of transplanted tissues or organs. T cells also serve as overall regulators of adaptive immune mechanisms.

***Quick* CHECK**

7. From what structure is the term *T cell* derived?
8. What causes a T cell to become sensitized or activated?
9. How do cytotoxic T cells destroy pathogens?

TYPES OF ADAPTIVE IMMUNITY

B-cell immunity and T-cell immunity, the two major types of adaptive immunity, can be further classified according to the manner in which they develop.

Recall that innate immunity, also called *inborn* or *inherited immunity*, occurs when nonspecific immune mechanisms are put in place by genetic mechanisms during the early stages of human development in the womb (see **Table 33-1**).

Adaptive immunity, our focus here, is instead a specific kind of resistance that develops after we are born. Acquired immunity may be further classified as either *natural immunity* or *artificial immunity*, depending on how the body is exposed to the antigen.

Natural exposure is not deliberate and occurs in the course of everyday living. We are naturally exposed to many disease-causing agents on a regular basis. Artificial, or deliberate, exposure to potentially harmful antigens is called *immunization*.

Natural and artificial immunity may be "active" or "passive". Active immunity occurs when an individual's own immune system responds to a harmful agent, regardless of whether that agent was naturally or artificially encountered. Passive immunity results when immunity to a disease that has developed in another individual or animal is transferred to an individual who was not previously immune. For example, antibodies in a mother's milk confer passive immunity to her nursing infant (see **Box 33-5**). Active immunity generally lasts longer than passive immunity. Passive immunity, although temporary, provides immediate protection.

Table 33-1 lists the various forms of adaptive immunity.

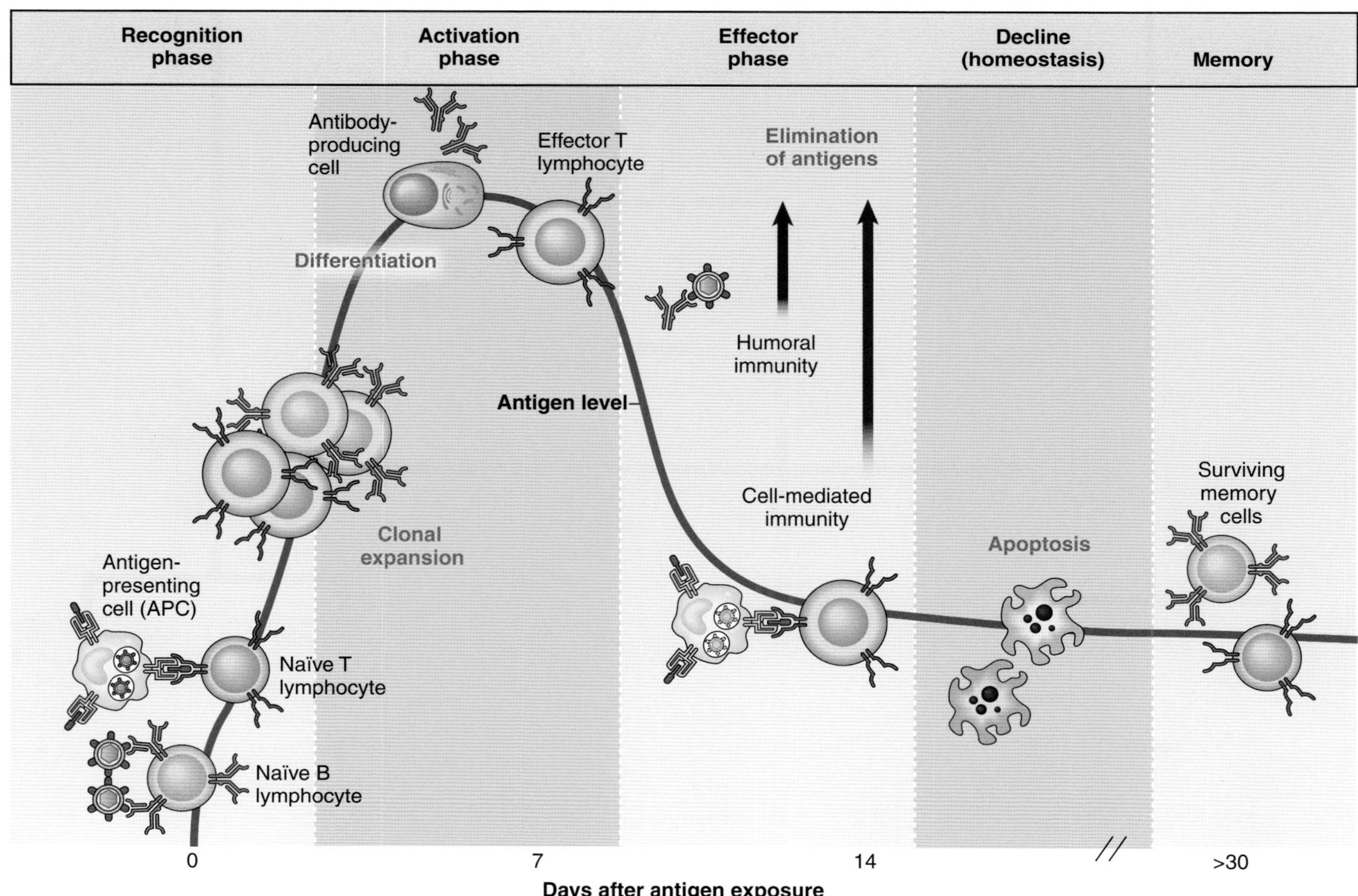

FIGURE 33-18 Stages of adaptive immune response. First, B cells and T cells recognize a specific antigen. Next, the B and T cells are activated—expanding their population (clonal expansion) while differentiating into effector cells and memory cells. Then the effector cells get to work attacking the source or sources of the antigen—humoral (antibody-mediated) immunity and cell-mediated immunity. As antigen levels decline, effector cells die off (apoptosis). Memory cells then remain—ready to quickly engage the antigen again later.

SUMMARY OF ADAPTIVE IMMUNITY

Adaptive immunity is specific immunity—that is, it targets specific antigens. Two special types of lymphocytes play a major role in immunity: B cells and T cells. As **Figure 33-17** shows, B cells recognize specific antigens and produce specific antibodies (immunoglobulins) to destroy the antigen—antibody-mediated or humoral immunity. T cells recognize antigens presented on cell surfaces to attack infected and abnormal cells in several ways—cell-mediated or cellular immunity.

Adaptive immunity progresses along a pathway of stages outlined in **Figure 33-18**. First, B cells and T cells recognize a specific antigen. Next, the B and T cells are activated—expanding their population (a clone) and thus producing effector cells and memory cells. Then, the effector cells get to work attacking the source or sources of the antigen. When there are no longer enough antigens to continue stimulating these immune responses, the effector B and effector T cells die off through the process of apoptosis. This represents a return to a homeostatic balance after the immune response. However, a number of memory cells remain—ready to quickly engage the antigen again should it reappear later.

Figure 33-19 summarizes the activity of the adaptive immune system in a different way. This figure shows the

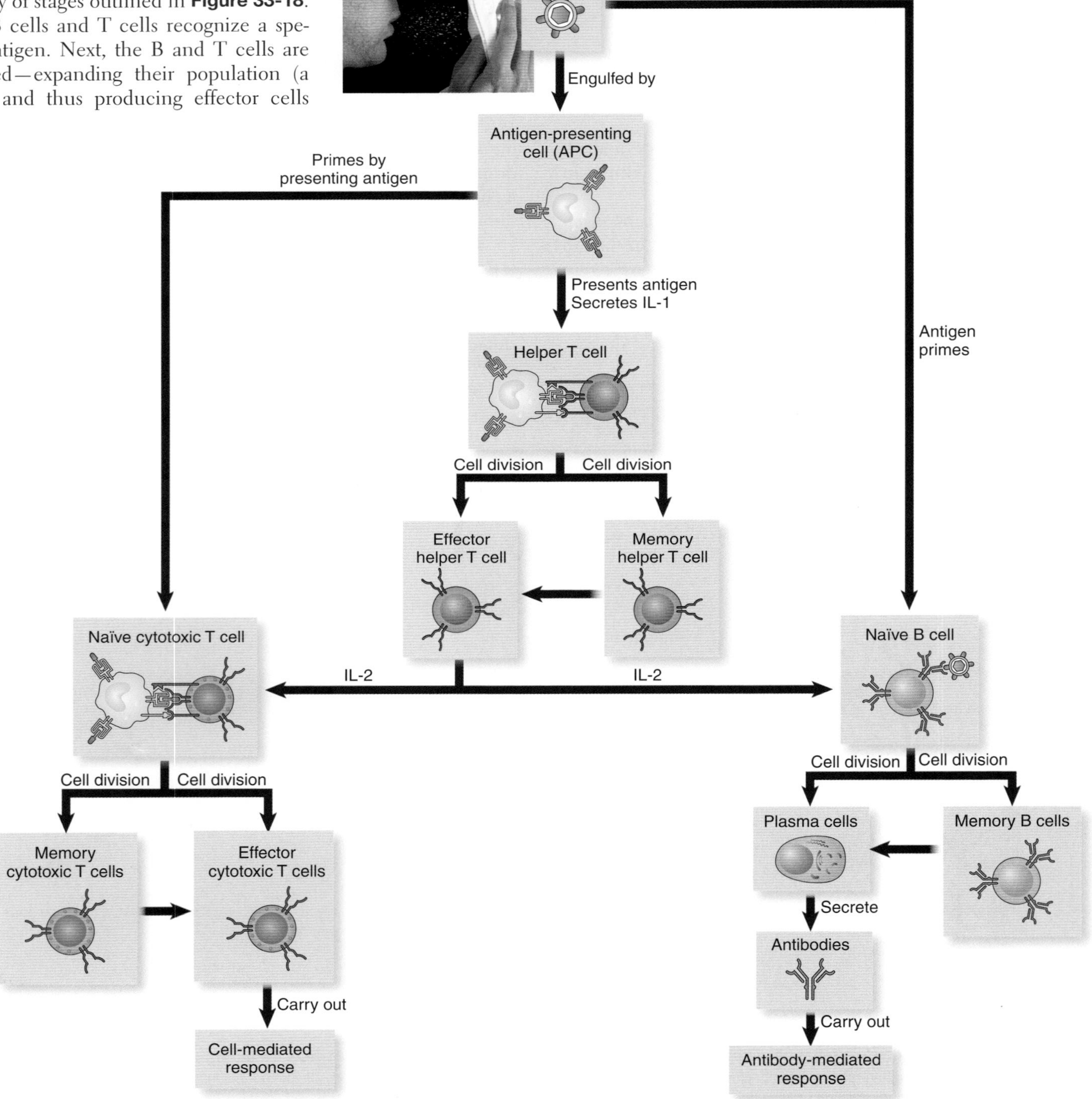

FIGURE 33-19 Summary of adaptive immunity. Flowchart summarizing an example of adaptive immune response when exposed to a microbial pathogen.

interaction of different cells and cytokines (in this case, interleukins) in a simplified model of the cooperative nature of the adaptive immune responses.

Box 33-6 explores an additional immune system of the body found in the mucosa.

Quick CHECK

10. What is the difference between inherited and acquired immunity?
11. What is the difference between natural and artificial immunity?
12. What is the difference between active and passive immunity?

BOX 33-6 *fyi* | Mucosal Immunity

The **mucosal immune system** is a complex system of defence distinct from the systemic (internal) immune system that we have been discussing in these last two chapters. It is an innate and adaptive system that is localized to the mucous barriers of the body: digestive tract, urinary/reproductive tracts, respiratory tract, exocrine ducts, conjunctiva, middle ear, and so on. The immune cells that make up the mucosal immune system are located mainly in or near **mucosa-associated lymphoid tissue (MALT).**

The main functions of the mucosal immune system involve preventing pathogens from colonizing the mucous surfaces of the body, preventing the accidental absorption of antigens from outside the body, and preventing inappropriate or intense responses of the systemic immune system to these external antigens.

As the figure shows, there are several components of the mucosal immune system. Large numbers of IgA antibodies are secreted by effector B cells (plasma cells) into the mucous layer lining the mucosal surfaces of the body. These secretory IgA molecules are dimers (double molecules) that resist being broken down by digestive and other enzymes (see **Figure 33-8**). Secretory IgA protects against a diverse group of pathogens such as viruses, bacteria, fungi, and animal parasites, thus forming an effective first line of defence.

Besides B cells, T cells also make up part of the mucosal immune system. T cells are located in both the epithelial layer and connective layer (lamina propria) of the mucous membrane, as well as in organized *regional lymphoid nodules* such as the aggregated lymphoid nodules (Peyer patches) of the intestines, the appendix, and the tonsils. Most of these T cells have distinctive structural and functional characteristics that distinguish them from the T cells of the systemic immune system. The mucosal T cells may be activated by antigens presented by APCs such as dendritic cells (DCs) present in the mucous membrane. Some antigens are processed by special *M (membrane) cells* in the surface of the epithelial layer and sent to lymphoid nodules, where APCs can present them to T cells. Interestingly, T cells activated in one mucosal membrane can migrate directly to mucous membranes in other parts of the body. They accomplish this through special "homing" receptors on the surface of each mucosal T cell.

Understanding the mucosal immune system and its cooperation with the systemic (internal) immune system promises to reveal new strategies of immunization. For example, researchers have found that immunizing through the bloodstream activates only the internal (systemic) B cells and T cells. Thus a pathogen would have to actually enter the internal environment before this type of specific immunity could protect us. Immunization of the mucosal lymphocytes, however, can activate both mucosal and systemic lymphocytes—providing a more thorough type of protection. Another advantage of mucosal immunization is that it is easier to administer to patients than immunizations injected under the skin or into the bloodstream. For example, immunization can be delivered by nasal sprays or drops instead of "shots". •

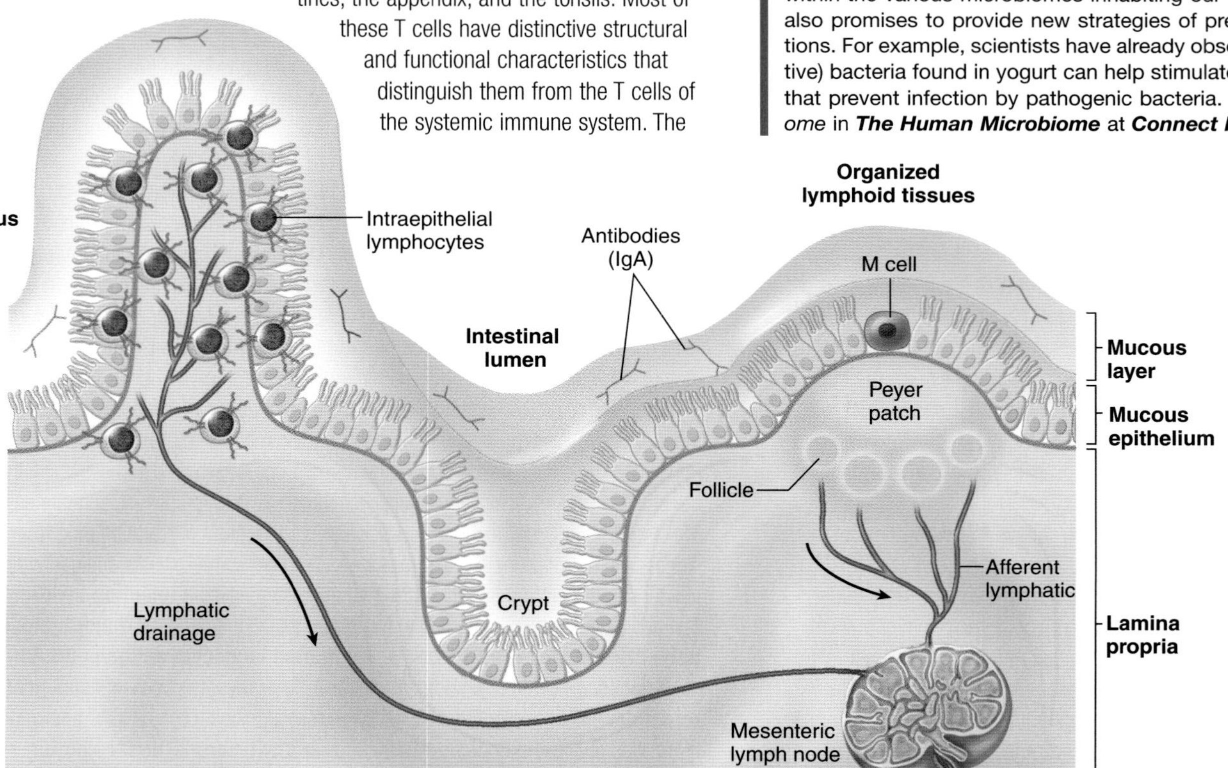

Diagram of the mucosal immune system. Lymphoid tissue associated with mucous membranes is called mucosa-associated lymphoid tissue (MALT).

CONNECT IT! 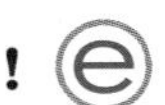

Understanding how the mucosal immune system cooperates with microbes within the various microbiomes inhabiting our body's mucous membranes also promises to provide new strategies of preventing or managing infections. For example, scientists have already observed how *probiotic* (protective) bacteria found in yogurt can help stimulate mucosal immunity in ways that prevent infection by pathogenic bacteria. Review the human *microbiome* in ***The Human Microbiome*** at **Connect It!**

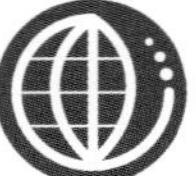

the big picture | Immune System and the Whole Body

The "big picture" of the immune system's role in maintaining the relative constancy of the internal environment is probably easier to "see" than any other system. After all, its agents—antibodies, lymphocytes, and other substances and cells—are everywhere in the body. They even stand guard on the outside surface of the body. Without the defensive activity of the immune system, our internal constancy would be decimated by cancer, infections, and even minor injuries.

In describing the various mechanisms of the immune system, we have used the analogy of a militaristic-style security force. As useful as this analogy might be, it may mislead us into believing that the immune system is a completely independent group of defensive agents. Nothing could be further from the truth.

First of all, evidence shows that the immune system is regulated to some degree by the nervous and endocrine systems—triggering the development of the emerging field of *neuroimmunology.* These systems, as you already know, are in turn influenced by feedback from all parts of the body.

Second, the agents of the immune system are not a separate, distinct group of cells and substances. They include blood cells, skin cells, mucosal cells, brain cells, liver cells, and many other types of cells and their secretions. Thus the immune system is more like a self-defence force made up of ordinary citizens who work shoulder-to-shoulder with military specialists.

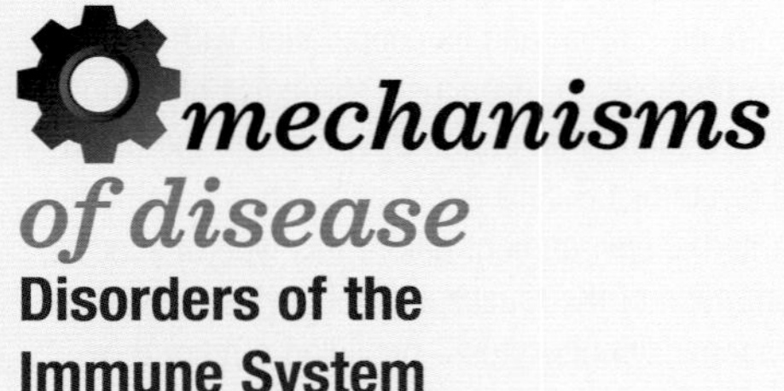

Disorders of the Immune System

There are two basic mechanisms for disorders of immunity. The immune defences can either overreact to antigens or fail to react to an antigen and thus produce disease. A few examples of each of these mechanisms are briefly described in the paragraphs that follow.

Hypersensitivity of the Immune System

Hypersensitivity is a type of inappropriate or excessive response of the immune system. The three major types of immune hypersensitivity discussed in the following sections are allergy, autoimmunity, and alloimmunity.

Allergy

The term **allergy** is used to describe hypersensitivity of the immune system to relatively harmless environmental antigens. Antigens that trigger an allergic response are often called **allergens.** The UK has some of the highest prevalence rates of allergic conditions in the world, with over 20% affected by one or more allergic disorders. Both genetic predisposition and environmental factors are known to be involved in the formation of an allergy.

Immediate allergic responses involve antigen–antibody reactions, mainly IgE. Before such a reaction occurs, a susceptible person must be exposed repeatedly to an **allergen**—triggering the production of antibodies. After a person is thus *sensitized,* exposure to an allergen causes antigen–antibody reactions that trigger the release of histamine, kinins, and other inflammatory substances. These responses usually cause typical allergy symptoms such as runny nose, conjunctivitis, and *urticaria* (hives). In some cases, however, these substances may cause constriction of the airways, relaxation of blood vessels, and irregular heart rhythms that can progress to a life-threatening condition called **anaphylactic shock** (see Chapter 30, p. 721). Drugs called **antihistamines** are sometimes used to relieve the symptoms of this type of allergy.

Delayed allergic responses, on the other hand, involve cell-mediated immunity. In **contact dermatitis,** for example, T cells trigger events that lead to local skin inflammation a few hours or days after initial exposure to an antigen. Exposure to poison ivy, soaps, and certain cosmetics may cause contact dermatitis in this manner. Hypersensitive individuals may use **hypoallergenic** products (products without common allergens) to avoid such allergic reactions.

Autoimmunity

Autoimmunity is an inappropriate and excessive response to self-antigens. Disorders that result from autoimmune responses are called **autoimmune diseases. Table 33-2** gives examples of autoimmune diseases. Self-antigens are molecules that are native to a person's body and that are used by the immune system to identify components of "self". In autoimmunity, the immune system inappropriately attacks these antigens.

A common autoimmune disease is **systemic lupus erythematosus (SLE),** or simply *lupus.* Lupus is a chronic inflammatory disease that affects many tissues in the body: joints, blood vessels, kidney, nervous system, and skin. The name *lupus erythematosus* refers to the red rash that often develops on the faces of those afflicted with SLE. The "systemic" part of the name comes from the fact that the disease affects many systems throughout the body. The systemic nature of SLE results from the production of IgG antibodies against a person's own DNA.

Alloimmunity

Alloimmunity is a normal but often undesirable reaction of the immune system to antigens from a different individual of the same species. Alloimmunity is important in two situations: pregnancy and tissue transplants. Alloimmunity is also called isoimmunity.

During pregnancy, antigens from the fetus may enter the mother's blood supply and sensitize her immune system. Antibodies that are formed as a result of this sensitization may enter the fetal circulation and cause an inappropriate immune reaction. One example, erythroblastosis fetalis, was discussed in Chapter 27. Other pathological conditions may also be caused by damage to developing fetal tissues resulting from attack by the mother's immune system. Examples include congenital heart defects, Graves disease, and myasthenia gravis.

Tissue or organ **transplants** are medical procedures in which tissue from a donor is surgically *grafted* into the body. For example, skin grafts are often performed to repair damage caused by burns. Donated whole blood tissue is often transfused into a recipient after massive haemorrhaging. A kidney is sometimes removed from a living donor or cadaver and grafted into a person suffering from kidney failure. Unfortunately, the immune system sometimes reacts against foreign antigens in the grafted tissue, causing what is often called a **rejection syndrome.** The antigens commonly involved in transplant rejection are called **major histocompatibility complex (MHC)** proteins—or **human leucocyte antigens (HLAs).**

Rejection of grafted tissues can occur in two ways: (1) **host-versus-graft rejection**—the recipient's immune system recognizes foreign HLAs and attacks them, destroying the donated tissue, and (2) **graft-versus-host rejection**—the donated tissue (e.g., bone marrow) attacks the recipient's HLAs, destroying tissue throughout the recipient's body. Graft-versus-host rejection may lead to death.

There are two ways to prevent rejection syndrome. One strategy is called *tissue typing,* in which HLAs and other antigens of a potential donor and recipient are identified. If they match, tissue rejection is unlikely to occur. Another strategy is the use of **immunosuppressive drugs** in the recipient. Immunosuppressive drugs such as *cyclosporine* and *prednisone* suppress the immune system's ability to attack the foreign antigens in the donated tissue.

Deficiency of the Immune System

Immunodeficiency, or immune deficiency, is the failure of immune system mechanisms to defend against pathogens. Immune system failure usually results from disruption of lymphocyte (B cell or T cell) function. The chief characteristic of immunodeficiency is the development of unusual or recurring severe infections or cancer. Although immunodeficiency by itself does not cause death, the resulting infections or cancer can.

The two broad categories of immune deficiencies, based on the mechanism of lymphocyte dysfunction, are *congenital* and *acquired.* Each of these types is outlined in the following discussion.

Congenital Immunodeficiency

Congenital immunodeficiency, which is rare, results from improper lymphocyte development before birth. Depending on which stage of the development of stem cells, B cells, or T cells the defect occurs, different diseases can result. For example, improper B-cell development can cause insufficiency or absence of antibodies in the blood. If stem cells are missing or are unable to grow properly, a condition called **severe combined immunodeficiency (SCID)** occurs. In most forms of SCID, both humoral immunity and cell-mediated immunity are defective. Temporary immunity can be imparted to children with SCID by injecting them with a preparation of antibodies (gamma globulin). Bone marrow transplants, which replace the defective stem cells with healthy donor cells, have proven effective in treating some cases of SCID.

Acquired Immunodeficiency

Acquired immune deficiency develops after birth (and is not related to genetic defects). Many factors can contribute to acquired immunodeficiency: nutritional deficiencies, immunosuppressive drugs or other medical treatments, trauma, stress, and viral infection.

One of the best known examples of acquired immunodeficiency is **acquired immunodeficiency syndrome (AIDS).** AIDS affects millions of people worldwide. This syndrome is caused by the **human immunodeficiency virus,** or **HIV.** HIV, a retrovirus, contains RNA that produces its own DNA inside infected cells. The viral DNA often becomes part of the cell's DNA (**Figure 33-20**). When the viral DNA is activated by cytokines, it directs the cell to synthesize viral RNA

TABLE 33-2 Examples of Autoimmune Diseases

DISEASE	POSSIBLE SELF-ANTIGEN	DESCRIPTION
Addison disease	Surface antigens on adrenal cells	Hyposecretion of adrenal hormones, resulting in weakness, reduced blood glucose, nausea, loss of appetite, and weight loss
Cardiomyopathy	Cardiac muscle	Disease of cardiac muscle (i.e., the myocardium), resulting in loss of pumping efficiency (heart failure)
Diabetes mellitus (type 1)	Pancreatic islet cells, insulin, insulin receptors	Hyposecretion of insulin by the pancreas, resulting in extremely elevated blood glucose levels (in turn causing a host of metabolic problems, even death if untreated)
Glomerulonephritis	Blood antigens that form immune complexes that deposit in kidney	Disease of the filtration apparatus of the kidney (renal corpuscle), resulting in fluid and electrolyte imbalance and possibly total kidney failure and death
Graves disease (type of hyperthyroidism)	TSH receptors on thyroid cells	Hypersecretion of thyroid hormone and resulting increase in metabolic rate
Haemolytic anaemia	Surface antigens on RBCs	Condition of low RBC count in the blood resulting from excessive destruction of mature RBCs (haemolysis)
Hypothyroidism	Antigens in thyroid cells	Hyposecretion of thyroid hormone in adulthood, causing decreased metabolic rate and characterized by reduced mental and physical vigour, weight gain, hair loss, and oedema
Multiple sclerosis (MS)	Antigens in myelin sheaths of nervous tissue	Progressive degeneration of myelin sheaths, resulting in widespread impairment of nerve function (especially muscle control)
Myasthenia gravis	Antigens at neuromuscular junction	Muscle disorder characterized by progressive weakness and chronic fatigue
Pernicious anaemia	Antigens on parietal cells, intrinsic factor	Abnormally low RBC count resulting from the inability to absorb vitamin B_{12}, a substance critical to RBC production
Reproductive infertility	Antigens on sperm or tissue surrounding ovum (egg)	Inability to produce offspring (in this case, resulting from destruction of gametes)
Rheumatic fever	Cardiac cell membranes (cross reaction with group A streptococcal antigen)	Rheumatic heart disease; inflammatory cardiac damage (especially to the endocardium and valves)
Rheumatoid arthritis (RA)	Collagen	Inflammatory joint disease characterized by synovial inflammation that spreads to other fibrous tissues
Systemic lupus erythematosus (SLE)	Numerous	Chronic inflammatory disease with widespread effects and characterized by arthritis, a red rash on the face, and other signs
Ulcerative colitis	Mucous cells of colon	Chronic inflammatory disease of the colon characterized by watery diarrhoea containing blood, mucus, and pus

RBC, Red blood cell; *TSH,* thyroid-stimulating hormone.

and viral proteins—producing new retroviruses. HIV thus "steals" raw materials from the cell. When this occurs in the $CD4^+$ subset of T cells (helper T cells), the cell is destroyed and immunity is seriously impaired.

As the T cell dies, it releases new retroviruses that can spread the HIV infection. As the HIV infection progresses, more and more $CD4^+$ lymphocytes are lost. This change in $CD4^+$ lymphocyte number is one of the principal clinical methods for monitoring AIDS (**Figure 33-21**, *A*).

HIV can invade several types of human cells, including brain cells. However, when $CD4^+$ T-cell (helper T-cell) function is impaired, infectious organisms and cancer cells can grow and spread much more easily than normal. Infections and tumours that rarely occur in healthy people, such as *Pneumocystis jiroveci pneumonia* (a protozoal infection) and *Kaposi sarcoma* (*KS*) (a type of skin cancer), commonly are seen in people with AIDS. Because their immune system is deficient, people with AIDS usually die from one of these infections or cancers.

After they are infected with HIV, T cells may not show signs of AIDS for years. This is because the immune system can hold the infection at bay for a long time before finally succumbing to it. **Figure 33-21**, *B*, shows the progression of HIV infection to AIDS.

There are several strategies for controlling AIDS and related conditions. Many agencies are trying to slow the spread of AIDS by educating people about how to avoid contact with the HIV retrovirus. HIV is spread by direct contact with body fluids, so preventing such contact reduces HIV transmission. Sexual relations, blood transfusions, breastfeeding, and intravenous use of contaminated needles are the usual modes of HIV transmission.

Most patients with AIDS have an abundance of antibodies against the HIV in their blood. This is another important clinical test for diagnosing and monitoring AIDS patients (often referred to as a *Western blot*). Unfortunately, for the majority of patients, the antibody response to HIV is not sufficient to suppress the disease. However, a few patients who demonstrated a strong antibody response were able to shed the virus completely. Studies of these few cases are fuelling an intensive, worldwide research effort to develop a vaccine for treating AIDS. The fast rate at which these viruses mutate (change their protein structure), however, is making vaccine development an extremely difficult challenge.

A drug called enfuvirtide can disrupt the HIV particle's ability to fuse with a host cell—the first drug in a class called *fusion inhibitors.* Inhibition of fusion can stop HIV from infecting cells that are not yet infected.

A way to inhibit symptoms of the disease is by means of chemicals such as zidovudine (also called azidothymidine [AZT]) and ritonavir that block HIV's ability to reproduce within infected cells.

A breakthrough in the treatment of HIV occurred when it was discovered that a "cocktail" of several antiviral drugs working together greatly reduces the number of virus particles in a patient's blood. More than 100 such compounds in various combinations are being evaluated for use in halting the progress of HIV infections. Currently, the recommended treatment for HIV infection is a combination of at least three medications in an individually tailored regimen called *highly active antiretroviral therapy (HAART).*

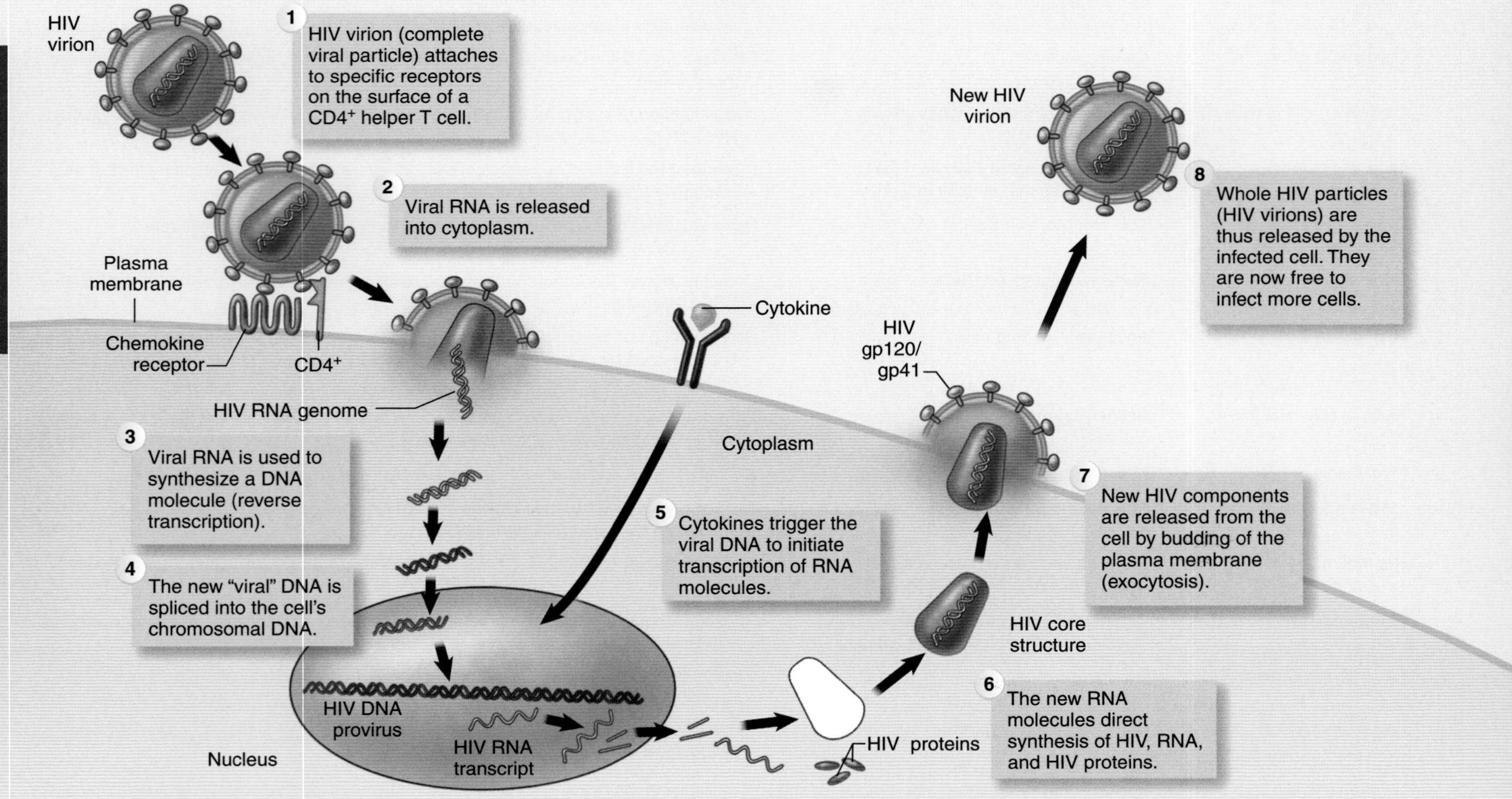

FIGURE 33-20 Mechanisms of HIV infection. HIV is an RNA-containing virus *(retrovirus)* that appears to infect T cells by way of the mechanism described in the diagram and simplified into 8 steps.

UNIT 4

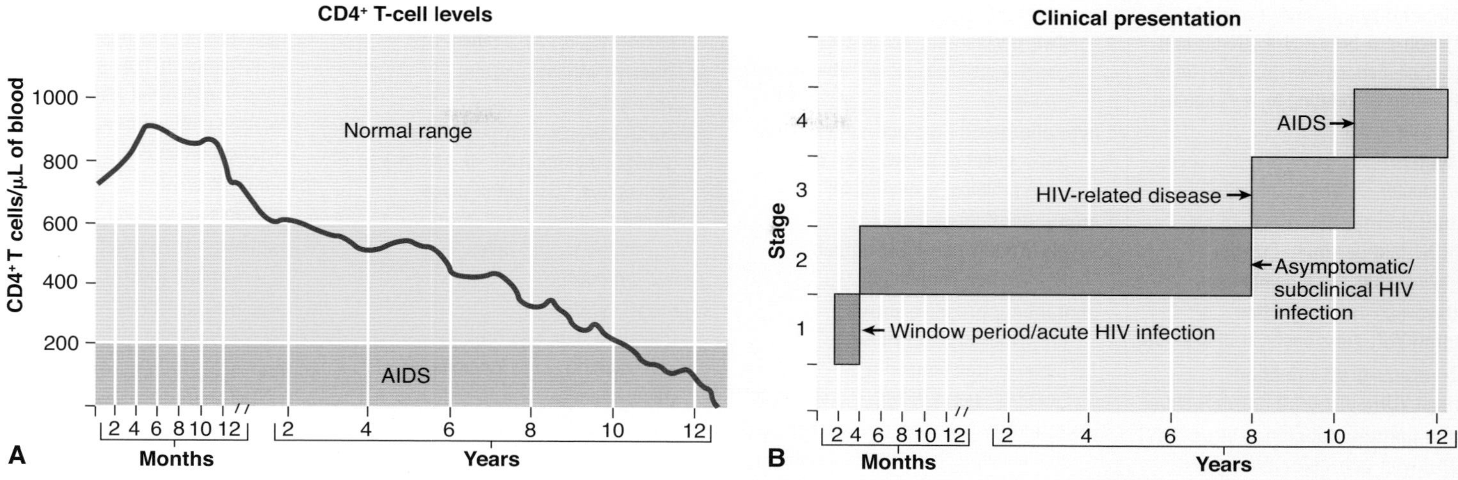

FIGURE 33-21 **Clinical progression of HIV/AIDS. A,** Changing numbers of $CD4^+$ T cells as an HIV infection progresses to AIDS. **B,** Progression from initial HIV infection to full-blown AIDS is usually described in four stages: (1) Acute viral infection with common viral symptoms; called "window period" because anti-HIV antibodies are not yet detectable by laboratory tests. (2) Subclinical stage in which there are often no (or minor) symptoms, but the virus is replicating. (3) HIV-related disease, with symptoms of acute viral infection and high levels of anti-HIV antibodies found in laboratory tests. (4) AIDS, including opportunistic infections and cancers.

LANGUAGE OF SCIENCE *(continued from p. 762)*

cytolysis (sye-TOL-ih-sis)
[*cyto-* **cell,** *-lysis* **loosening**]

cytotoxic T cell
(sye-toh-TOK-sik tee sel)
[*cyto-* **cell,** *-toxic* **poison,** *T* **thymus gland,** *cell* **storeroom**]

effector B cell (ef-FEK-tor bee sel)
[*effect-* **accomplish,** *-or* **agent,** *B* **bursa-equivalent tissue,** *cell* **storeroom**]

effector cell (ef-FEK-tor sel)

effector T cell (ef-FEK-tor tee sel)
[*effect-* **accomplish,** *-or* **agent,** *T* **thymus gland,** *cell* **storeroom**]

helper T cell (T_H cell)
[*T* **thymus gland**, *cell* **storeroom**]

human leucocyte antigen (HLA)
(LOO-koh-syte AN-tih-jen)
[*leuco-* **white,** *-cyte* **cell,** *anti-* **against,** *-gen* **produce**]

humoral immunity
(HYOO-mor-al ih-MYOO-nih-tee)
[*humor-* **liquid,** *-al* **relating to,** *immun-* **free,** *-ity* **state**]

immunoglobulin (Ig)
(ih-myoo-noh-GLOB-yoo-lin)
[*immuno-* **free (immunity),** *-glob-* **ball,** *-ul-* **small,** *-in* **substance**]

immunological synapse (IS)
(ih-myoo-noh-LOJ-ih-kal SIN-aps)
[*immuno-* **free (immunity),** *-log-* **words (study of),** *-ical* **relating to,** *syn-* **together,** *-aps-* **join**]

interleukin (IL) (in-ter-LOO-kin)
[*inter-* **between,** *-leuk-* **white (blood cell),** *-in* **substance**]

lymphotoxin (lim-foh-TOK-sin)
[*lympho-* **water (lymphocyte),** *-tox-* **poison,** *-in* **substance**]

major histocompatibility complex (MHC) (MAY-jer HIST-oh-kom-pat-ib-IL-it-ee KOM-pleks)
[*histo-* **tissue,** *-compatibil-* **agreeable,** *-ity* **state,** *com-* **together,** *-plex* **weave or braid**]

membrane attack complex (MAC)
(MEM-brayn at-TAK KOM-pleks)
[*com-* **together,** *-plex* **weave or braid**]

memory B cell (MEM-oh-ree bee sel)
[*B* **bursa-equivalent tissue,** *cell* **storeroom**]

memory cell (MEM-oh-ree sel)

memory T cell (MEM-oh-ree tee sel)
[*T* **thymus gland,** *cell* **storeroom**]

mucosal-associated lymphoid tissue (MALT) (myoo-KOH-sal-ah-soh-she-AYT-ed LIM-foyd)
[*muc-* **slime or mucus,** *-osal* **relating to,** *associa-* **unite,** *-ate* **process,** *lymph-* **water (lymphatic system),** *-oid* **like,** *tissue-* **fabric**]

mucosal immune system
(myoo-KOH-sal ih-MYOON)
[*muc-* **slime or mucus,** *-osal* **relating to,** *immun-* **free**]

naïve (nye-EEV)
[*naïve* **natural**]

naïve B cell (nye-EEV bee sel)
[*naïve* **natural,** *B* **bursa-equivalent tissue,** *cell* **storeroom**]

plasma cell (PLAZ-mah sel)
[*plasma* **something moulded (blood plasma),** *cell* **storeroom**]

suppressor T cell
(suh-PRESS-er tee sel)
[*suppress-* **press down,** *-or* **agent,** *T* **thymus gland,** *cell* **storeroom**]

T cell
[*T* **thymus gland,** *cell* **storeroom**]

thymocyte (THY-moh-syte)
[*thymo-* **thyme flower (thymus gland),** *-cyte* **cell**]

LANGUAGE OF MEDICINE

acquired immunodeficiency syndrome (AIDS) (ah-KWYRD ih-MYOON deh-FISH-en-see)
[*acquire* **obtain,** *immun-* **free,** *syn-* **together,** *-drome* **running or (race) course**]

allergen (AL-er-jen)
[*all-* **other,** *-erg-* **work,** *-gen* **produce**]

allergy (AL-er-jee)
[*all-* **other,** *-erg-* **work,** *-y* **state**]

alpha-fetoprotein (AFP)
(al-fah-fee-toh-PRO-teen)
[*alpha-* **first letter of Greek alphabet (α),** *feto-* **offspring (fetus)**]

anaphylactic shock (an-ah-fih-LAK-tik)
[*ana-* **without,** *-phylact-* **protection,** *-ic* **relating to**]

antibody titre (AN-tih-bod-ee TYE-ter)
[*anti-* **against,** *titre* **proportion (in a solution)**]

antihistamine (an-tih-HIS-tah-meen)
[*anti-* **against,** *-histo-* **tissue,** *-amine* **ammonia compound**]

autoimmune diseases
(aw-toh-ih-MYOON)
[*auto-* **self,** *-immun-* **free (immunity)**]

CA-125
[*C* **cancer,** *A* **antigen**]

UNIT 4

carcinoembryonic antigen (CEA) (kar-sin-oh-em-bree-ON-ik AN-tih-jen)
[*carcino-* **cancer,** *-em-* **in,** *-bryo-* **fill to bursting,** *-ic* **relating to,** *anti-* **against,** *-gen* **produce**]

CD system
[*C* **cluster,** *D* **differentiation**]

contact dermatitis
(KON-takt der-mah-TYE-tis)
[*derma-* **skin,** *-itis* **inflammation**]

graft-versus-host rejection
(graft VUR-suhz host reh-JEK-shun)

host-versus-graft rejection
(host VUR-suhz graft reh-JEK-shun)

human immunodeficiency virus (HIV)
(ih-myoo-noh-deh-FISH-en-see VYE-rus)
[*immuno-* **free (immunity),** *-de-* **down,** *-fic-* **perform,** *-ency* **state,** *virus* **poison**]

hypersensitivity
(hye-per-sen-sih-TIV-ih-tee)
[*hyper-* **excessive,** *sensitiv-* **able to feel,** *-ity* **state**]

hypoallergenic (hye-poh-al-er-JEN-ik)
[*hypo-* **under or below,** *-aller-* **other,** *-gen-* **produce,** *-ic* **relating to**]

immunodeficiency
(ih-MYOON deh-FISH-en-see)
[*immun-* **free (immunity)**]

immunosuppressive drugs
(ih-myoo-no-soo-PRES-iv)
[*immuno-* **free (immunity),** *-suppress-* **press down,** *-ive* **relating to**]

isoimmunity (eye-soh-ih-MYOO-ni-tee)
[*iso-* **equal,** *-immun-* **free,** *-ity* **state**]

monoclonal antibody (MAb)
(mon-oh-KLONE-al AN-tih-bod-ee)
[*mono-* **single,** *-clon-* **(plant) cutting,** *-al* **relating to,** *anti-* **against**]

nanobody (NAN-oh-bod-ee)
[*nano* **small**]

prostate-specific antigen (PSA)
(PROSS-tayt speh-SIF-ik AN-tih-jen)
[*pro-* **before,** *-stat-* **set or place (prostate gland),** *specif-* **form,** *-ic* **relating to,** *anti-* **against,** *-gen* **produce**]

rejection syndrome
(reh-JEK-shun SIN-drohm)
[*syn-* **together,** *-drome* **running or (race) course**]

severe combined immunodeficiency (SCID)
(ih-myoo-no-deh-FISH-en-see)
[*immun-* **free**]

systemic lupus erythematosus (SLE)
(sis-TEM-ik LOO-pus er-ih-them-ah-TOH-sus)
[*system-* **organized whole,** *-ic* **relating to,** *lupus* **wolf,** *erythema-* **redness,** *-osus* **condition**]

toxoid (TOK-soyd)
[*tox-* **poison,** *-oid* **like**]

transplant (tranz-PLANT [verb] or TRANZ-plant [noun])

tumour marker (TYOO-mer)
[*tumour* **swelling**]

tumour-specific antigen
(TYOO-mer-speh-SIF-ik AN-tih-jen)
[*tumour* **swelling,** *specif-* **form,** *-ic* **relating to,** *anti-* **against,** *-gen* **produce**]

vaccination (vak-sih-NAY-shun)
[*vaccin-* **cow (cowpox),** *-ation* **process**]

case study

George remembered getting the flu (influenza) last winter: coughing, fever, achiness all over his body, watery eyes, and fatigue. He felt awful! This year he argued, "What's the point of a flu vaccination, when all it does is give you the flu?" George did not understand that the flu vaccine is a combination of several inactivated (killed) viruses; no live viruses are injected into the body. So, as for the injected vaccine "causing" the flu—people who claim that could already have been exposed to a flu virus before the vaccination or could have been exposed to one of the strains not included in that year's vaccine. Some people produce a mild immune reaction that can be mistaken for the flu. In the end, George relented and got his flu vaccine!

1. Which of George's cells will respond to the flu antigens introduced in the vaccine?
   a. Erythrocytes
   b. Thrombocytes
   c. Lymphocytes
   d. Platelets

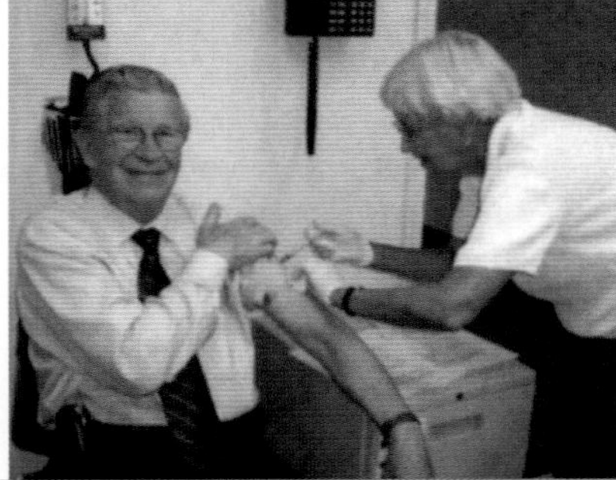

2. Which specific cell types will begin producing antibodies to the antigens?
   a. Z cells
   b. T cells
   c. A cells
   d. B cells
3. Which antibody is primarily involved in this response to vaccine?
   a. IgM
   b. IgE
   c. IgG
   d. IgD
4. The release of which type of molecule helped to stimulate an increase in George's body temperature and bring on a fever in his previous influenza infection? (Note: The molecules trigger an increase in the thermoregulatory set point controlled by the hypothalamus.)
   a. A vulcanogen
   b. Histamine
   c. A pyrogen
   d. An antibody
5. What would you call the specific type of immunity George developed as a result of the vaccination?
   a. Natural active immunity
   b. Artificial active immunity
   c. Natural passive immunity
   d. Artificial passive immunity

Hint To solve a case study, you may have to refer to the glossary or index, other chapters in this textbook, ***Connect It!,*** and other resources.

CHAPTER SUMMARY

To download an MP3 version of the chapter summary for use with your mobile device, access the ***Audio Chapter Summaries*** *online at evolve.elsevier.com.*

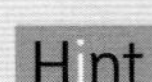

Scan this summary after reading the chapter to help you reinforce the key concepts. Later, use the summary as a quick review before your class or before a test.

Overview of Adaptive Immunity

A. Adaptive immunity
   1. Part of the third line of defence consisting of lymphocytes
   2. Two different classes of a white blood cell (lymphocyte) involved (**Figure 33-1**)

UNIT 4

B. Classes of lymphocytes (**Figure 33-2**)—B lymphocytes (B cells) and T lymphocytes (T cells)
   1. B-cell mechanisms—antibody-mediated immunity (humoral immunity); produce antibodies that attack pathogens (**Figure 33-3**)
   2. T-cell mechanisms—attack pathogens more directly—classified as cell-mediated immunity (cellular immunity)
   3. Lymphocytes have protein markers on their surfaces
      a. Surface markers named using the CD (cluster of differentiation) system
      b. Examples are $CD4^+$ and $CD8^+$ cells, clinically important in diagnosing AIDS
   4. Activation of lymphocytes require two stimuli: a specific antigen and activating chemicals (**Figure 33-4**)
   5. Lymphocytes are densest where they develop—in bone marrow, thymus gland, lymph nodes, and spleen (**Figure 33-5**)
   6. Lymphocytes flow through the bloodstream, become distributed in tissues, and return to the bloodstream in a continuous recirculation

B Cells and Antibody-Mediated Immunity

A. Development and activation of B cells
   1. Development occurs in two stages (**Figure 33-6**)
      a. Pre–B cells develop in red bone marrow (prenatal, in the yolk sac and fetal liver)
      b. Second stage occurs in lymph nodes and spleen—activation of a naïve B cell after it binds to a specific antigen
      c. B cells divide repeatedly—serve as ancestors to antibody-secreting plasma cells
         (1) Some of the clone cells differentiate to form B cells or plasma cells
         (2) Others remain in lymphatic tissue and become memory B cells

B. Antibodies—proteins (immunoglobulins) secreted by activated B cell (**Figure 33-6**)
   1. Structure of antibody molecules
      a. An antibody molecule consists of two heavy and two light polypeptide chains
      b. Each molecule has two antigen-binding sites and two complement-binding sites (**Figure 33-7**)
   2. Diversity of antibodies
      a. Babies are born with different clones of B cells in bone marrow, lymph nodes, and spleen
      b. Cells of the clone synthesize a specific antibody with a sequence of amino acids in its variable region that differs from the sequence synthesized by other clones
   3. Classes of antibodies (**Figure 33-8**)—immunoglobulins M, G, A, E, and D
      a. IgM—antibody that naïve B cells synthesize and insert into their own plasma membranes; the predominant class produced after initial contact with an antigen
      b. IgG—makes up 75% of antibodies in the blood; predominant antibody of the secondary antibody response
      c. IgA—major class of antibody in the mucous membranes, in saliva and tears (also found in plasma)
      d. IgE—small amount; produces harmful effects such as allergies
      e. IgD—small amount in blood; precise function unknown
   4. Functions of antibodies (**Figure 33-9**)
      a. Antigen-antibody reactions
         (1) Transform toxic antigens into harmless substances
         (2) Agglutinate antigens to make disposal by phagocytes more rapid
         (3) Alter the shape of antigen molecule to expose complement-binding sites (**Figure 33-10**)
      b. Complement—a component of blood plasma consisting of several protein compounds (inactive enzymes)
         (1) Antibodies can activate complement after binding to an antigen by exposing complement-binding sites that trigger a cascade of linked chemical reactions to produce a variety of immune effects
            (a) Membrane attack complex (MAC)—complement cascade can form doughnut-shaped structures that produce a hole in a foreign cell's membrane, causing cytolysis (cell rupture) (**Figures 33-11** and **33-12**)
            (b) Complement can also cause vasodilation, enhance phagocytosis, and have other effects
         (2) Complement activity can also be initiated by innate immune mechanisms
            (a) Complement protein 3 (C3)—activated without antigen stimulation—produces full complement effect by binding to bacteria or viruses in presence of properdin
            (b) Complement activation by innate immunity is called the alternate pathway
      c. Primary and secondary responses (**Figure 33-13**)
         (1) Primary response—initial encounter with a specific antigen triggers the formation and release of specific antibodies that reaches its peak in a few days
         (2) Secondary response—a later encounter with the same antigen triggers a much quicker response; B memory cells rapidly divide, producing more plasma cells and thus more antibodies

C. Clonal selection theory (**Figure 33-14**)
   1. Two basic tenets
      a. Body contains many diverse clones of cells, each committed by its genes to synthesize a different antibody
      b. When an antigen enters the body, it selects the clone whose cells are synthesizing its antibody and stimulates them to proliferate and create more antibody
   2. The clones selected by antigens consist of lymphocytes and are selected by the shape of antigen receptors on the lymphocyte's plasma membrane

T Cells and Cell-Mediated Immunity

A. Development of T cells
   1. T cells are lymphocytes that go through the thymus gland before migrating to the lymph nodes and spleen
   2. Pre–T cells develop into thymocytes while in the thymus
   3. Thymocytes stream into the blood and are carried to the T-dependent zones in the spleen and the lymph nodes

B. Activation of T cells
   1. T cells display antigen receptors on their surface membranes that are similar to antibodies

2. A T cell is activated when an antigen (in an infected cell or presented by an APC) binds to its receptors (at an IS), causing the T cell to divide repeatedly to form a clone of identical T cells (**Figure 33-15**)
   a. Cells of the clone differentiate into effector T cells and memory T cells
   b. Effector T cells go to the site where the antigen entered, bind to antigens, and begin their attack
   c. Memory T cells remain in bone marrow until needed later to produce more effector T cells and memory T cells

C. Functions of T cells
1. Cytotoxic T cells—T cells release lymphotoxin to kill cells (**Figure 33-16**)
2. Helper T cells (T_H cells)—regulate the function of B cells, T cells, phagocytes, and other leucocytes (**Figure 33-17**)
3. Suppressor T cells—regulatory T cells that suppress lymphocyte function, thus regulating immunity and promoting self-tolerance
4. T cells function to produce cell-mediated immunity and help to regulate adaptive immunity in general

Types of Adaptive Immunity (Table 33-1)

A. Innate immunity (inborn or inherited immunity)—genetic mechanisms put innate immune mechanisms in place during development in the womb
B. Adaptive or acquired immunity; resistance developed after birth; two types:
1. Natural immunity results from nondeliberate exposure to antigens
2. Artificial immunity results from deliberate exposure to antigens, called *immunization*

C. Natural and artificial immunity may be active or passive
1. Active immunity—when the immune system responds to a harmful agent regardless of whether it was natural or artificial; lasts longer than passive
2. Passive immunity—immunity developed in another individual is transferred to an individual who was not previously immune; it is temporary but provides immediate protection

Summary of Adaptive Immunity

A. Adaptive immunity is specific immunity—targeting specific antigens
B. Adaptive immunity involves two classes of lymphocyte: B cells and T cells (**Figure 33-17**)
1. B cells—antibody-mediated (humoral) immunity
2. T cells—cell-mediated (cellular) immunity

C. Adaptive immunity occurs in a series of stages (**Figure 33-18**)
1. Recognition of antigen
2. Activation of lymphocytes
3. Effector phase (immune attack)
4. Decline of antigen causes lymphocyte death (homeostatic balance)
5. Memory cells remain for later response if needed

D. B cells and T cells work together in a coordinated system of adaptive immunity (**Figure 33-19**)

The Big Picture: Immune System and the Whole Body

A. Immune system regulated to some degree by nervous and endocrine systems
B. Agents of the immune system include blood cells, skin cells, mucosal cells, brain cells, liver cells, and other types of cells and their secretions

REVIEW QUESTIONS

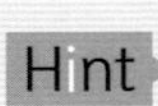

Write out the answers to these questions after reading the chapter and reviewing the Chapter Summary. Note—writing out your answers will consolidate learning and provide a valuable resource of information.

1. Define the following terms: antigens, antibodies, antigenic determinants, combining sites, clone.
2. What two terms are synonyms for combining sites?
3. When an antigen–antibody complex is formed, what region on the antigen molecule fits into what region on the antibody molecule?
4. Activated B cells develop into clones of what two kinds of cells?
5. What cells synthesize and secrete copious amounts of antibodies?
6. Explain the function of memory cells.
7. Antibodies belong to what class of compounds? With the aid of a diagram describe the structure of an antibody.
8. Explain the two basic tenets of Burnet's clonal selection theory.
9. What are cytokines? Lymphotoxins?
10. Differentiate between the classifications of natural and artificial immunity.
11. Describe the process behind the functioning of modern vaccines.
12. What are monoclonal antibodies, and how do they function?

CRITICAL THINKING QUESTIONS

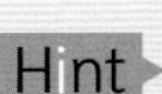

After finishing the Review Questions, write out the answers to these more in-depth questions to help you apply your new knowledge. Go back to sections of the chapter that relate to concepts that you find difficult.

1. Explain how the various types of T cells can fine-tune the immune system.
2. Why do you think the development of cancer can be seen as a failure of the immune system?
3. For each pair of characteristics, determine which one best fits innate immunity and which one best fits adaptive immunity.
   a. Specific threats, general threats
   b. Rapid response, slow response
   c. Various targets, specific targets
   d. Memory of antigens, no memory of antigens
4. One of the best-known examples of acquired immunodeficiency is acquired immunodeficiency syndrome (AIDS). The human immunodeficiency virus (HIV) causes this syndrome. Summarize the mechanism of HIV infection.
5. Some parents believe deliberately exposing a child to chickenpox by allowing contact with other infected children is a good way to develop immunity to this condition. What dangers does this practice pose?

34 Stress

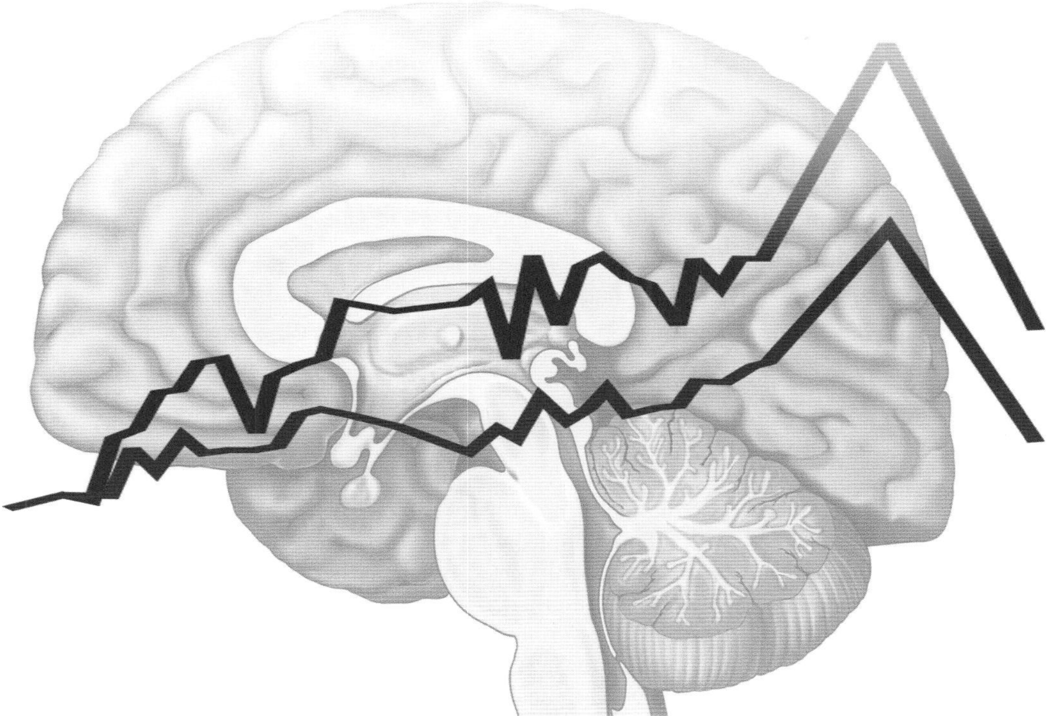

CHAPTER OUTLINE

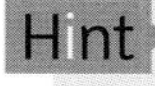 Scan this outline before you begin to read the chapter, as a preview of how the concepts are organized.

Stress affects people of all ages and in all walks of life. Children at play, students preparing for an examination, college graduates on their first day of work, and even a fetus before birth are all subjected to stress. Although some stress can be beneficial, excessive or prolonged stress can often negatively affect health and quality of life.

People experiencing severe stress are often overwhelmed by tension, anger, fear, and frustration. As a result, blood epinephrine (Epi or adrenaline) levels rise, blood pressure and heart rate increase, breathing patterns change, and blood levels of nutrients such as glucose and fatty acids deviate from their normal set points. The immune system even becomes less effective, so people under severe, long-term stress are more susceptible to infection and commonly develop stress-related illnesses. Because no two people experience the same stress-related symptoms, diagnosis

LANGUAGE OF SCIENCE

Hint: *Use this list to aid your pronunciation of unfamiliar words.*

adaptation (ad-ap-TAY-shun)
[*adapt-* **adjust,** *-ation* **process**]

alarm reaction (uh-LARM ree-AK-shun)
[*al-* **toward,** *-arm* **weapon,** *re-* **again,** *-action*]

allostasis (al-lo-STAY-sis)
[*allo-* **different,** *-stasis* **standing still**]

corticoid (KOHR-tih-koyd)
[*cortic-* **cortex (bark),** *-oid* **like**]

fetal programming (FEE-tal)
[*fet-* **offspring,** *-al* **relating to**]

fight-or-flight reaction (fyte or flyte ree-AK-shun)
[*re-* **again,** *-action*]

hypothalamic–pituitary–adrenal (HPA) axis (hye-poh-THAL-ah-mik pih-TYOO-it-air-ee ah-DREE-nal AK-sis)
[*hypo-* **under or below,** *-thalam-* **inner chamber,** *-ic* **relating to,** *pituit-* **phlegm,** *-ary* **relating to,** *ad-* **toward,** *-ren-* **kidney,** *-al* **relating to,** *axis* **axle**]

neuropeptide Y (NYOOR-oh-pep-tyde)
[*neuro-* **nerve,** *-pept-* **digest,** *-ide* **chemical**]

psychological stressor (sye-koh-LOJ-ih-kal STRESS-or)
[*psycho-* **the mind,** *-log-* **words (study),** *-ical* **relating to,** *stress-* **tighten,** *-or* **agent**]

stage of exhaustion (stayj ov eg-ZAWS-chun)
[*exhaust-* **drain away,** *-ion* **process**]

stage of resistance (stayj ov ree-ZIS-tens)
[*resist-* **withstand,** *-ance* **act of**]

stress
[*stress-* **tighten**]

stress response (stres ree-SPONS)
[*stress-* **tighten**]

stress triad (stres TRYE-ad)
[*stress-* **tighten,** *triad* **group of three**]

stressor (STRESS-or)
[*stress-* **tighten,** *-or* **agent**]

continued on p. 796

and treatment are difficult. Quite often, though, stress makes it difficult to focus on tasks—which then interferes with problem-solving skills, whether at school or at work. Stress is also associated with sleep disorders, depression, and complaints of stomach pain, heart palpitations, fatigue, and muscle aches.

Contemporary medicine now acknowledges that excessive, long-term stress is a critically important and widespread risk factor for disease. It disrupts homeostasis of numerous physiological control systems in the body and must be controlled to ensure good health.

Insight and research data from diverse disciplines such as molecular genetics, neurobiology, psychology, endocrinology, immunology, and sociology are necessary when trying to understand the physiological impact of stress. The result is a holistic model of stress that affirms the importance of mind–body interactions in both health and disease.

For decades, most of what we knew about stress came from the pioneering and classic research done by Hans Selye. Though our current understanding of stress extends beyond the nonspecific physiological responses suggested over 80 years ago, Selye's work had a dramatic and critical impact on stress research. Because his work provided a scientific basis for ongoing research in this complex area, we begin the chapter by summarizing Selye's concept of stress. •

SELYE'S CONCEPT OF STRESS

In 1935, Hans Selye of McGill University in Montreal made an accidental discovery that launched him on a lifelong career and led him to conceive the idea of stress. This chapter tells briefly the story of how Selye developed his stress concept and also describes the mechanism of stress that he postulated. It then presents some current ideas about stress.

Development of the Stress Concept

Selye made his accidental discovery when he was trying to determine whether there was another sex hormone besides those already known. He injected rats with various extracts derived from ovaries and placenta, expecting to find different changes had occurred in animals injected with different hormonal preparations. But to his surprise and puzzlement, he found the same three changes in all the animals. The cortices of their adrenal glands were enlarged, but their lymphatic organs—thymus glands, spleens, and lymph nodes—were atrophied, and bleeding ulcers of the stomach and duodenum had developed in every animal. Next he injected many other substances—for example, extracts from pituitary glands, kidneys, and spleens and even a poison, formaldehyde. Every time he found the same three changes in the animal subjects: enlarged adrenals, shrunken lymphatic organs, and bleeding gastrointestinal ulcers. Selye believed that these symptoms were a specific syndrome.

A syndrome, according to the classical definition, is a set of signs and symptoms that occur together and that characterize one particular disease. The three changes, or "stress triad", Selye had observed occurred together, but they seemed to characterize not any one particular kind of injury but instead all kinds of harmful stimuli. More experiments using various chemicals and injurious agents confirmed for him that the three changes truly were a syndrome of injury. His first publication on the subject was a short paper titled "A Syndrome Produced by Diverse Nocuous Agents"; it appeared in the July 1936 issue of the British journal *Nature*. Years later, in 1956, he published his monumental technical treatise, *The Stress of Life*.

Although a majority of the current literature credits Hans Selye with the first published reports on stress, Walter B. Cannon used the term "emotional stress" much earlier (1914) when discussing his theory of homeostasis. It seems Cannon was also convinced stress had both a psychological (emotional) and a physiological origin. It was Selye, however, who brought our knowledge of stress and its importance in health and disease into the forefront of modern medicine.

Definitions

Stress, according to Selye's use of the word, is a state, or condition, of the body produced by "diverse nocuous agents" and manifested by a syndrome of changes. We know as well that stress and its negative effects can also be caused by a wide variety of mental, emotional, and other psychological events that an individual may perceive as threatening or undesirable. Selye named the agents that produce stress *stressors* and coined a name—*general adaptation syndrome (GAS)*—for the syndrome or group of changes that make the presence of stress in the body known.

Stressors

A **stressor** is any agent or stimulus that produces stress. However, just how an individual interacts with or relates to a particular type of physiological or cognitive situation may well determine whether that particular event is stressful or not. Even the same intensity of a particular physiological stressor, such as temperature change, may be perceived as a threat and activate a stress response in one individual and not another.

In addition to variances in ability to handle physiological stress, some people have the ability to cope better than others when faced with difficult events in life, such as divorce or bereavement. As a result, they suffer less from negative stress-related symptoms or illness.

Clearly, a precise classification of stimuli as stressors or nonstressors is not possible. We can, however, make these five generalizations about the character of stressors.

1. Stressors are extreme stimuli—too much or too little of almost anything. The *perception* of the individual is critical. A particular event or circumstance that is viewed as undesirable or goes beyond what the individual is capable of coping with may be viewed as "extreme" and cause one or more of the psychological or physiological responses associated with stress. In contrast, almost anything in moderation or that engenders only mild stimuli are nonstressors. Thus coolness, warmth, and soft sounds are nonstressors, whereas extreme cold, extreme heat, and extremely loud sounds almost always act as stressors. Not only extreme excesses but also extreme deficiencies may be perceived as stressors. One example of this kind of stressor is an extreme lack of social contact stimuli. Solitary confinement in a prison, space travel, social isolation because of blindness or deafness, and in some cases, old age have all been identified as stressors. But the opposite extreme, an excess of social contact stimuli (e.g., caused by overcrowding) also acts as a stressor (**Figure 34-1**). We now know that various types of stress in young children and even prenatal infants may occur as a result of negative stimuli that are experienced by a parent. For example, severe psychological or physical trauma, environmental hazards, and nutri-

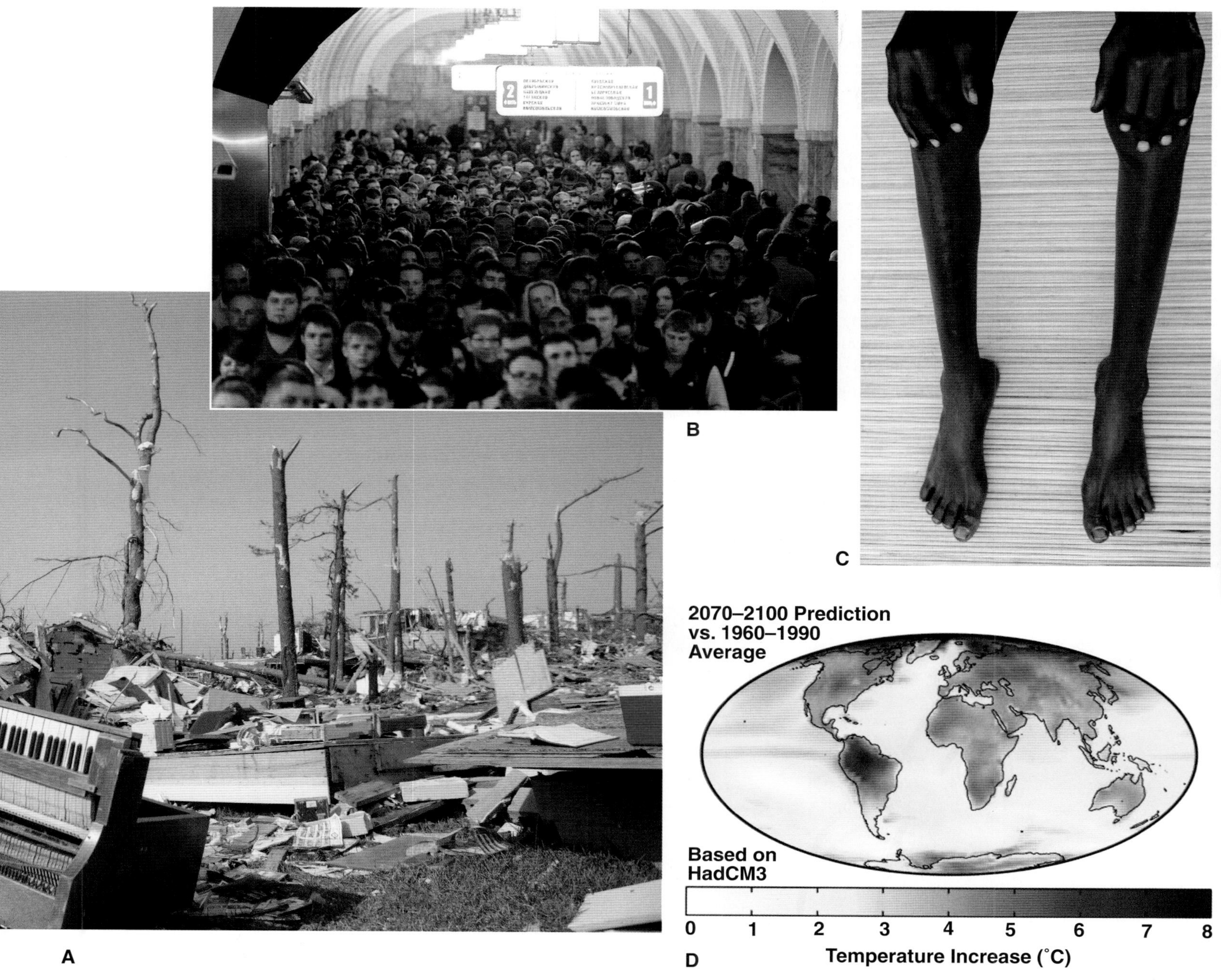

FIGURE 34-1 Causes of stress. A, Natural disaster, such as a tornado. **B,** Overcrowding. **C,** Malnutrition. **D,** Environmental dangers (climate change). *HadCM3,* Hadley Centre Coupled Model version 3.

tional deficiencies or abuses, when encountered by a pregnant or nursing woman, can all have a stress-related impact on her child that may result in immediate or delayed behavioural, physiological, or anatomical anomalies. Intrauterine stress is discussed in detail later in the chapter. Poverty and illness, typically associated with stress, are often coupled with alcoholism, drug abuse, and malnutrition. These conditions often result either directly or indirectly in premature births, developmental anomalies, increased susceptibility to many types of mental and physical diseases, and myriad other physical defects that may occur immediately in the children involved, or they may develop later in life.
2. Stressors very often are injurious, unpleasant, or painful stimuli—but not always. "A painful blow and a passionate kiss," Selye wrote, "can be equally stressful."
3. Anything that an individual perceives as a threat, whether real or imagined, arouses fear or anxiety. These emotions act as stressors. So, too, does the emotion of grief.
4. The reaction to stressors differs in different individuals and in one individual at different times. A stimulus that is a stressor for you may not be a stressor for me. A stimulus that is a stressor for you today may not be a stressor for you tomorrow and might not have been a stressor for you yesterday. Many factors—including one's physical and mental health, heredity, past experiences, coping habits, and even diet—determine which stimuli are stressors for each individual.
5. Stress can occur even in a developing fetus—a circumstance called *prenatal stress.* In many instances prenatal stress will result from a physical or nutritional stressor experienced by the mother. For example, in England in 2014, there were 272 hospital admissions for fetal alcohol syndrome (FAS). Studies suggest significant underreporting, and the condition may be as high as 2–5% in school-aged children. FAS involves signs ranging from poor prenatal and infant growth to mental retardation. In this context, alcohol consumed during pregnancy is a dangerous stressor. Even in small amounts it can produce prenatal brain damage that may permanently affect the ability of the child to concentrate, think abstractly, use appropriate judgment, or learn effectively. When a woman consumes alcohol during pregnancy, real or perceived stress is often the impetus for such behaviour. Education that promotes healthy habits and teaches coping strategies must be a part of any social programs intended to eliminate alcohol consumption during pregnancy and the incidence of FAS.

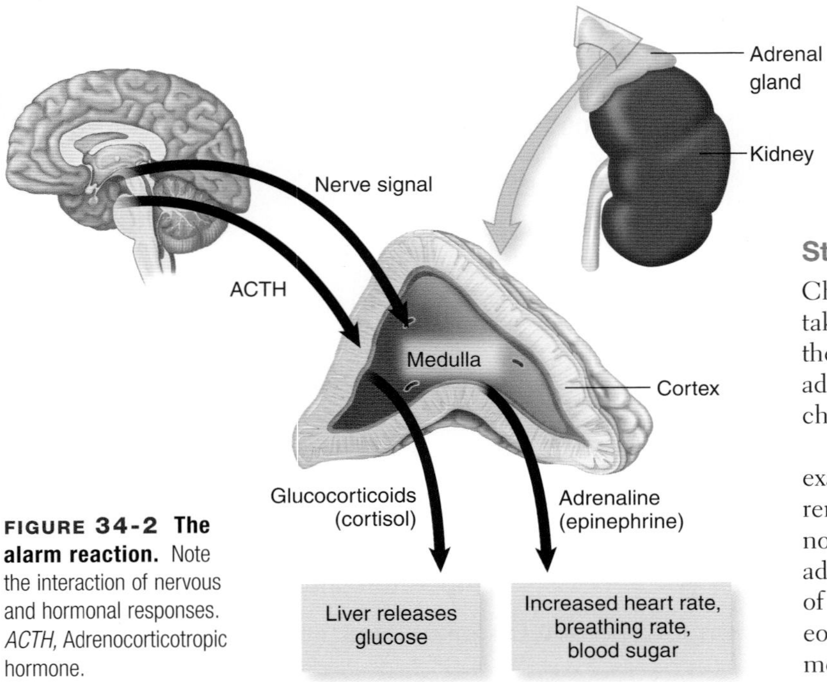

Quick CHECK

1. Define the term *stress.*
2. Identify the three changes Hans Selye called the "stress triad".
3. List four characteristics of stressors.

General Adaptation Syndrome

Manifestations

Stress, like health or any other state or condition, is an intangible phenomenon. It cannot be seen, heard, tasted, smelled, felt, or measured directly. How, then, can we know that stress exists? It can be inferred to exist when certain visible, tangible, and measurable responses occur. Selye, for example, inferred that the animals on which he experimented were in a state of stress when he found the syndrome of the three changes previously noted—hypertrophied adrenals, atrophied lymphatic organs, and bleeding gastrointestinal ulcers. Because this syndrome indicated the presence of stress and consisted of three changes, he called them the **"stress triad"**.

Eventually he found that many other changes also took place as a result of stress. He named the entire group of changes or responses the **general adaptation syndrome (GAS).** In coining this term, he reasoned that the word *general* suggested that the syndrome was "produced only by agents that have a general effect on large portions of the body". The word **adaptation** was meant to imply that the syndrome of changes made it possible for the body to adapt, to cope successfully with stress. Selye thought that these responses seemed to protect the animals from serious damage by extreme stimuli and to promote their healthy survival. He looked on the general adaptation syndrome as a crucial part of the body's complex defence mechanism.

Stages

Changes that make up the general adaptation syndrome do not all take place simultaneously but over time in three stages. Selye named these stages: (1) the alarm reaction, (2) the stage of resistance or adaptation, and (3) the stage of exhaustion. A different syndrome of changes, he noted, characterized each stage.

Among the responses characteristic of the **alarm reaction,** for example, were the stress triad already described—hypertrophied adrenal cortex, atrophied lymphatic organs (thymus, spleen, lymph nodes), and bleeding gastric and duodenal ulcers. In addition, the adrenal cortex increased its secretion of glucocorticoids, the number of lymphocytes decreased markedly, and so, too, did the number of eosinophils. Also, the sympathetic nervous system and the adrenal medulla greatly increased their activity (**Figure 34-2**). Each of these

FIGURE 34-2 The alarm reaction. Note the interaction of nervous and hormonal responses. *ACTH,* Adrenocorticotropic hormone.

UNIT 4

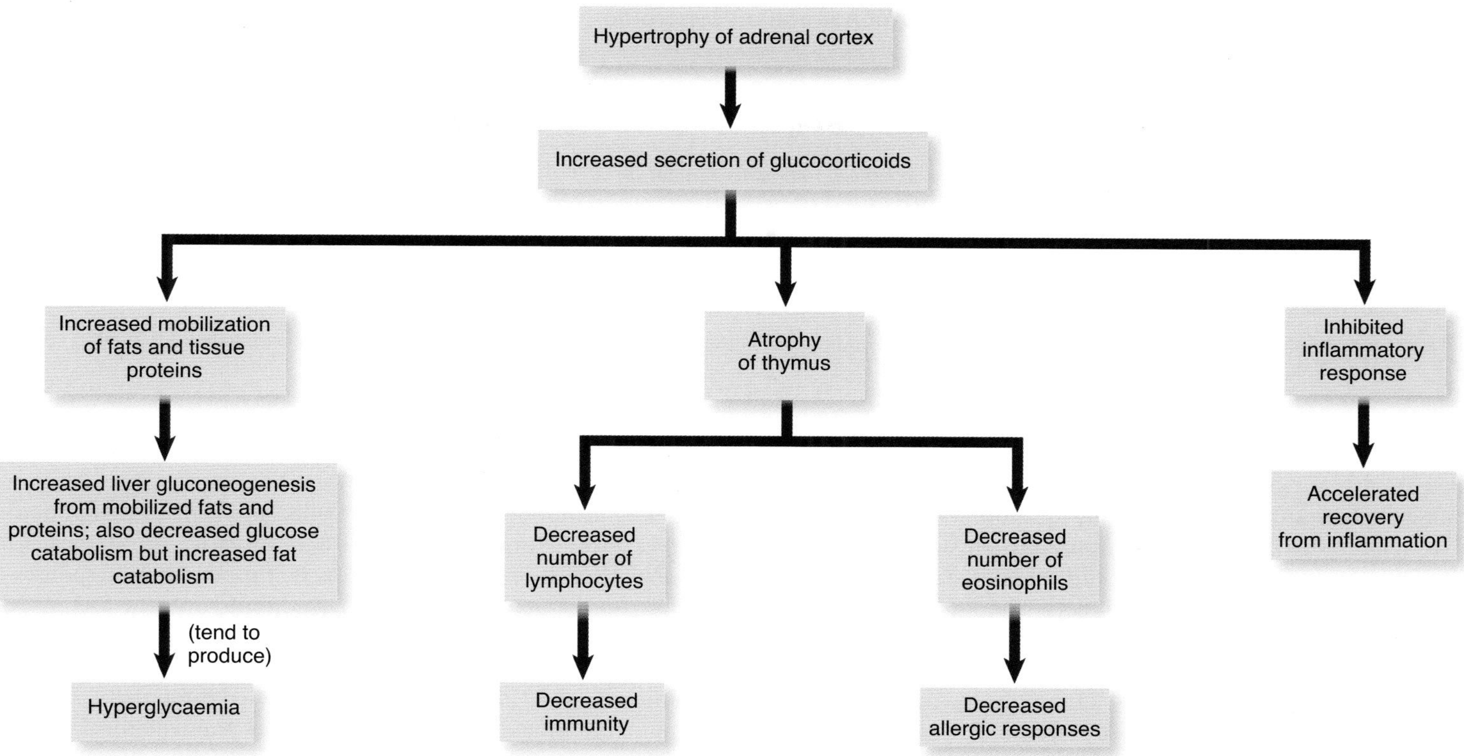

FIGURE 34-3 Alarm reaction responses resulting from hypertrophy of adrenal cortex.

changes, in turn, produced other widespread changes. **Figure 34-3** indicates some of the changes stemming from adrenal cortical hypertrophy. **Figure 34-4** shows responses produced by increased sympathetic activity and increased secretion by the adrenal medulla of its hormone, epinephrine (adrenaline).

Quite different responses characterize the **stage of resistance.** For instance, the adrenal cortex and medulla return to their normal rates of hormone secretion. The changes that take place during the alarm stage as a result of increased corticoid secretion disappear during the stage of resistance. All of us go through the first and second stages of

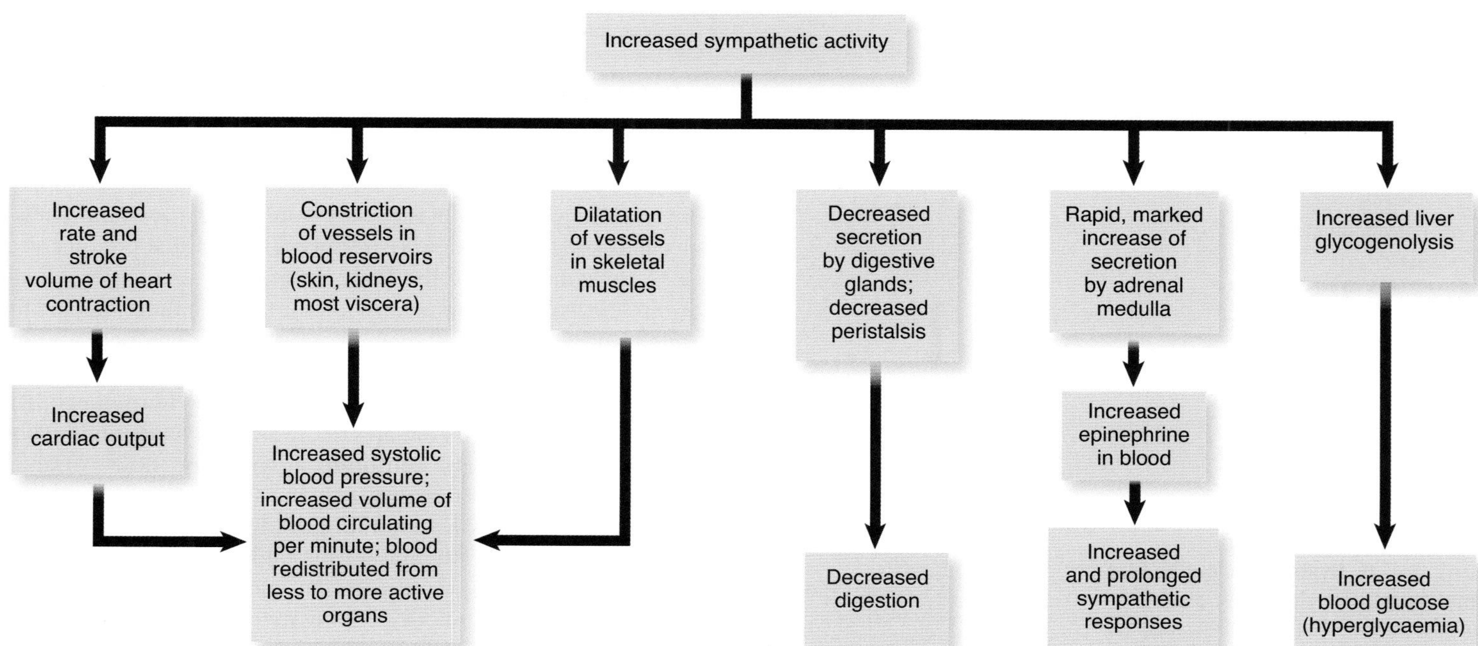

FIGURE 34-4 Alarm reaction responses resulting from increased sympathetic activity. Note that these are the responses commonly referred to as the "fight-or-flight" reaction.

TABLE 34-1 The Three Stages of the General Adaptation Syndrome

ALARM	RESISTANCE	EXHAUSTION
Increased secretion of glucocorticoids and resultant changes (see **Figure 34-2**)	Glucocorticoid secretion returns to normal	Initially increased glucocorticoid secretion but eventually markedly decreased secretion
Increased activity of sympathetic nervous system	Sympathetic activity returns to normal	Stress triad (hypertrophied adrenals, atrophied thymus and lymph nodes, bleeding ulcers in stomach and duodenum)
Increased norepinephrine secretion by adrenal medulla	Norepinephrine secretion returns to normal	—
Fight-or-flight reaction (see **Figure 34-4**)	Fight-or-flight reaction disappears	—
Low resistance to stressors	High resistance (adaptation) to stressor	Loss of resistance to stressor; may lead to death

the stress syndrome many times in our lifetimes. Stressors of one kind or another act on most of us every day. They may upset or alarm us, but we soon resist them successfully. In short, we adapt; we cope.

The **stage of exhaustion** develops only when stress is extremely severe or when it continues over long periods. Otherwise, when stress is mild and of short duration, it ends with a successful stage of resistance and adaptation to the stressor. If stress continues until the body reaches the stage of exhaustion, corticoid secretion and adaptation eventually decrease markedly. The body can no longer cope successfully with the stressor and death may ensue as a result. For a brief summary of the changes characteristic of the three stages of the general adaptation syndrome, see **Table 34-1**.

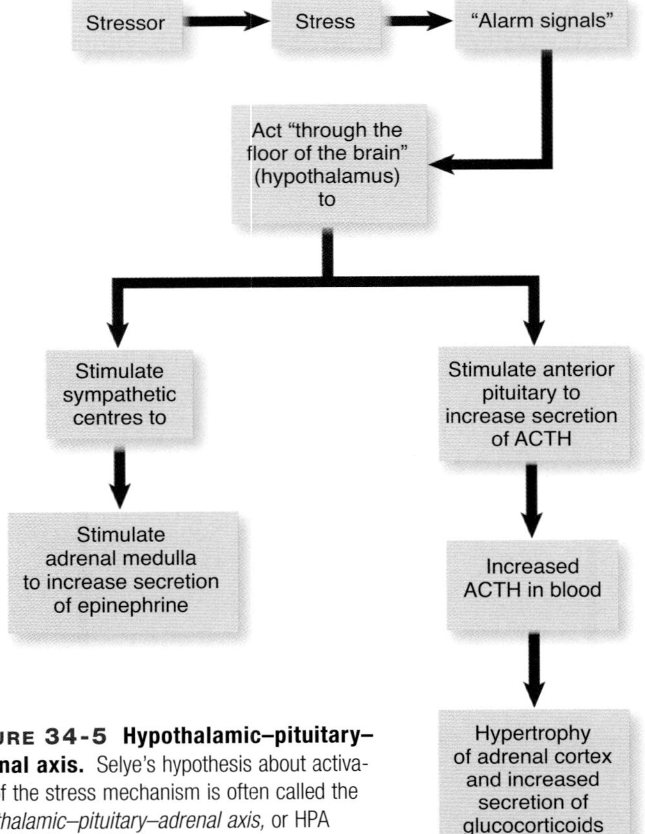

FIGURE 34-5 Hypothalamic–pituitary–adrenal axis. Selye's hypothesis about activation of the stress mechanism is often called the *hypothalamic–pituitary–adrenal axis,* or HPA mechanism. *ACTH,* Adrenocorticotropic hormone.

Mechanism of Stress

Stressors produce a state of stress. A state of stress in turn inaugurates a series of responses that Selye called the *general adaptation syndrome.* More simply, a state of stress turns on the stress response mechanism. It activates the organs that produce the responses that make up the general adaptation syndrome; but just how stress—a state of the body—does this is not clear. Selye could only guess about it, and his terms were vague. For instance, he postulated that, by some unknown "alarm signals", stress "acted through the floor of the brain" (presumably the hypothalamus) to stimulate the sympathetic nervous system and the pituitary gland.

In **Figure 34-5** you can see Selye's hypothesis in diagram form. Because it involves the **hypothalamic–pituitary–adrenal (HPA) axis**, many scientists refer to this process as the *HPA mechanism.*

Quick CHECK

4. What is the general adaptation syndrome?
5. Identify the three stages of the general adaptation syndrome. How do they differ?
6. Discuss the types of responses produced in the body by increased sympathetic activity.

SOME CURRENT CONCEPTS ABOUT STRESS

Definitions

Some of today's physiologists use the terms *stressors* and *stress* as Selye did—that is, they define stressors as stimuli that produce stress, a state (or condition) of the body. In contrast, many physiologists now use the word *stress* to mean something much more specific than a state of the body. **Stress,** according to their operational definition, is any stimulus that directly or indirectly stimulates neurons of the hypothalamus to release corticotropin-releasing hormone (CRH). CRH acts as a trigger that initiates many diverse changes in the body. Together, these changes constitute a syndrome now commonly called the **stress syndrome,** or simply the **stress response.**

The term **allostasis** is sometimes used to refer to the stress syndrome, or the body's attempts to reestablish homeostatic balance while under stress. The word part *allo-* means "different". One can think of allostasis as the body's coping mechanisms when things are different. *Allostatic load* refers to the broad effects of allostasis on the body, such as increased energy expenditure, alterations of neural and endocrine mechanisms, and changes in behaviour. One can think of allostatic load as the physiological load placed on the body by stress.

Stress Syndrome

Look now at **Figure 34-6**. It summarizes some current major ideas about the syndrome of stress responses. Beginning at the top of the diagram, note that the initiator of the stress syndrome is stress—any factor that stimulates the hypothalamus to release CRH. Most often, stress consists of injurious or extreme stimuli. These may act directly on the hypothalamus to stimulate it. Instead, or in addition, they may act indirectly on the hypothalamus.

An example of stress that stimulates the hypothalamus directly is hypoglycaemia. A lower than normal concentration of glucose in the blood circulating to the hypothalamus stimulates it to release CRH.

Indirect stimulation of the hypothalamus occurs in this way: Stress stimulates the cerebral part of the brain's limbic system—the so-called *emotional brain*—and other parts of the cerebral cortex, and these regions then send stimulating impulses to the hypothalamus (also part of the limbic system). The hypothalamus releases CRH in response.

In addition to releasing CRH, note in **Figure 34-6** that the stress-stimulated hypothalamus sends stimulating impulses to sympathetic centres and to the posterior pituitary gland.

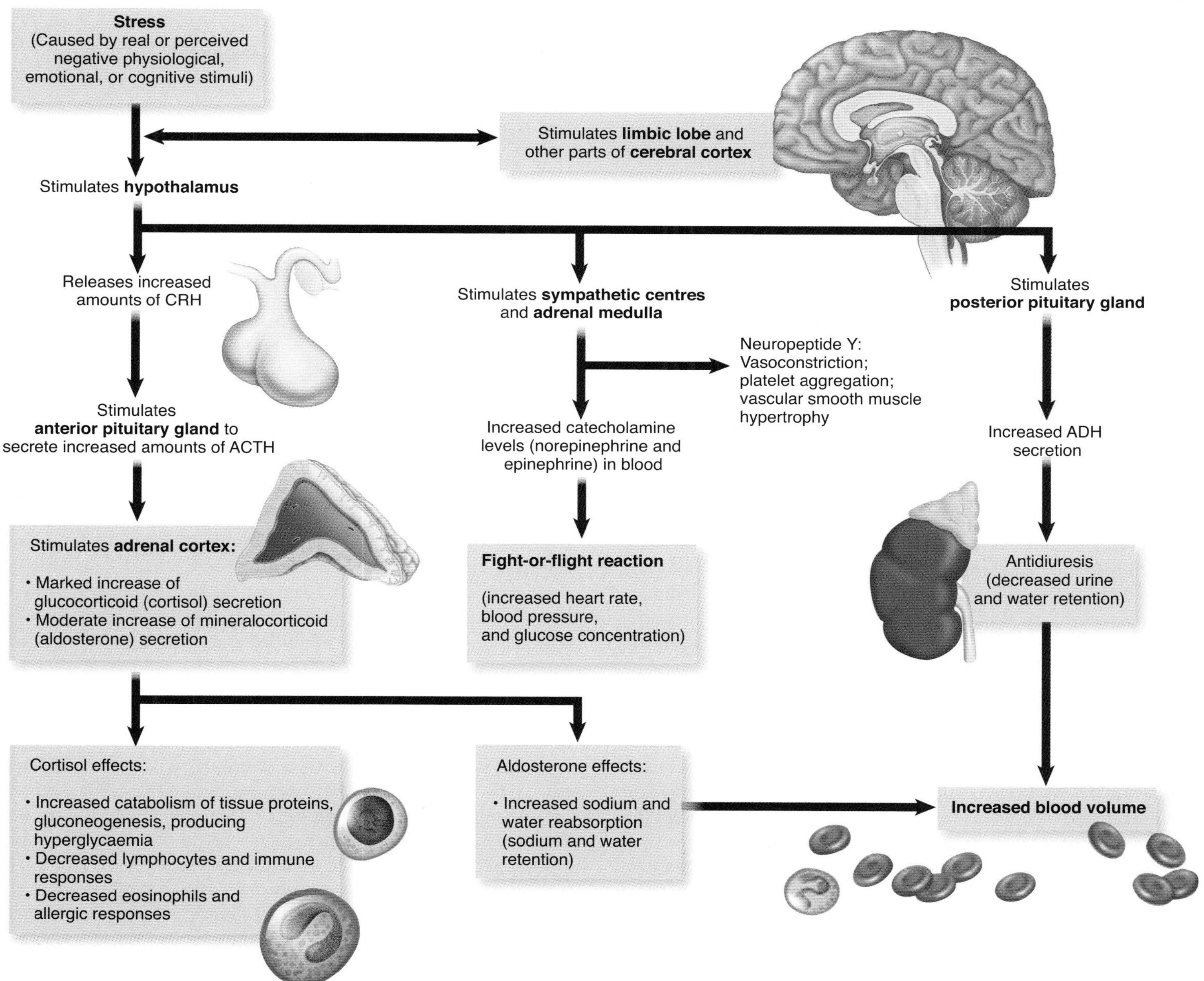

FIGURE 34-6 Current concepts of the stress syndrome. Some effects are immediate, such as the sympathetic fight-or-flight reaction, and some effects are longer-term, such as the hormonal effects. *ACTH,* Adrenocorticotropic hormone; *ADH,* antidiuretic hormone; *CRH,* corticotropin-releasing hormone.

UNIT 4

CRH stimulates the anterior pituitary gland to secrete increased amounts of adrenocorticotropic hormone (ACTH). ACTH stimulates the adrenal cortex to secrete greatly increased amounts of cortisol and more moderately increased amounts of aldosterone. These two hormones induce various stress responses. Some important ones worth remembering are listed in **Figure 34-6** under cortisol effects and aldosterone effects.

Recall from Chapter 22 that stimulation of sympathetic centres by impulses from the stress-stimulated hypothalamus leads to many stress responses, known collectively as the **fight-or-flight reaction.** These *adrenergic responses* include important changes such as an increase in the rate and strength of the heartbeat, a rise in blood pressure, and hyperglycaemia. Other sympathetic stress responses are pallor and coolness of the skin, sweaty palms, and dry mouth. Review **Table 22-5** on p. 515 for a listing of the adrenergic effects observed in the fight-or-flight reaction.

Water retention and an increase in blood volume are common stress responses. They stem, as you can see in **Figure 34-6**, from increased ADH and increased aldosterone secretion.

Evidence also suggests that prolonged stress produces yet another hormone, called **neuropeptide Y,** that is secreted from the sympathetic nerves and adrenal medulla. This stress-related hormone causes vasoconstriction, platelet aggregation, and, over time, hypertrophy of vascular smooth muscle.

Stress and Disease

Stress, as we have observed several times, produces different results in different individuals and different results in the same individual at different times. In one person, a certain amount of stress may induce responses that maintain or even enhance health. But in another person the same amount of stress appears to cause sickness. Whether stress is "good" or "bad" for you seems to depend more on your own body's responses to it than on the severity of the stressors inducing it.

You may recall that Selye emphasized the adaptive nature of stress responses. He coined the term *general adaptation syndrome* because he believed that stress responses usually enable the body to adapt successfully to the many stressors that assail it. He held that the state of stress activates physiological mechanisms to meet the challenge imposed by stressors. But a challenge issued does not necessarily mean a challenge successfully met. Selye proposed that sometimes the body's adaptive mechanisms fail to meet the challenge issued by stressors and that when they fail, disease results—diseases of adaptation, he called them. In today's terms, we might say that when the allostatic load becomes high, fatigue or disease may result.

Around the middle of the last century, one of the problems studied was the relationship of blood glucocorticoid concentration to disease. If stress is adaptive, the investigators reasoned, and helps the body combat the effects of many kinds of stressors (e.g., infection, injury, and burns), then possibly various diseases might be treated by adding to the body's natural output of glucocorticoids (cortisone).

Indicators of Stress

Whether an individual's body is responding to stress stimuli can be determined by certain measurements and observations (**Figure 34-7**). Some examples follow: an increase in the rate and force of heartbeat, a rise in systolic blood pressure, an increase in blood and urine concentration of epinephrine and norepinephrine, sweating of the

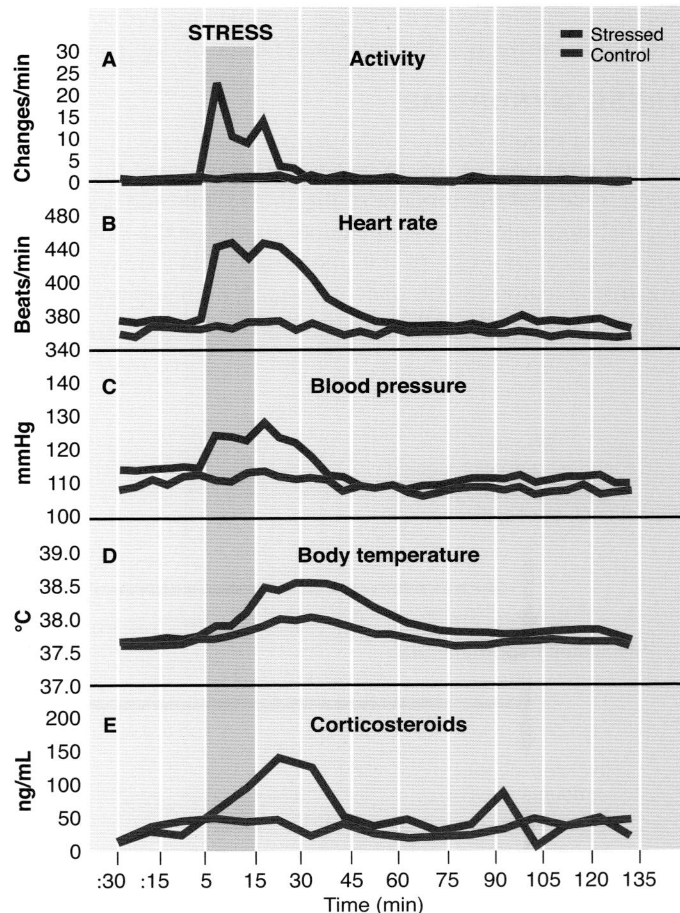

FIGURE 34-7 Stress indicators. Graphs showing a variety of physiological changes in mice when presented with a stressor: increased movements **(A)**, elevated heart rate **(B)**, elevated blood pressure **(C)**, elevated body temperature **(D)**, and increased plasma corticosteroids **(E)**. Similar stress responses occur in all mammals.

palms of the hands, and dilation of pupils. The heart rate has been shown to increase in response to varied stress stimuli, such as anaesthesia and annoying sounds. Even anticipation by patients in a coronary care unit of their upcoming transfer to a less closely supervised convalescent unit has been identified as a stress stimulus that causes the heart rate to speed up.

A decrease in the number of eosinophils and lymphocytes in the blood indicates that the individual is responding to stress stimuli. Soldiers stressed by prolonged marching, for example, have been found to have fewer circulating eosinophils than normal. This same stress indicator has been observed in college athletes when they were anticipating performing in an important event. It has also been observed in heart patients when they were anticipating the various types of procedures required to treat their illness.

The amount of urinary adrenocorticoids is often used as a measure of stress. It has been found to increase in depressed persons feeling hopeless and doomed, in test pilots anticipating a scheduled flight, and in college students taking examinations or watching exciting movies. In contrast, urinary corticoids were found to drop markedly in persons watching boring films.

The level of adrenocorticoids in the blood plasma of disturbed patients having acute psychotic episodes has been found to be 70%

higher than that in normal individuals or in calm patients. Another study showed that the plasma corticoid levels of chronically depressed patients were significantly lower than those of acutely anxious patients. Smoking and exposure to nicotine have also been shown to be stressors that caused a marked rise in plasma adrenocorticoids—by as much as 77% in humans and in experimental animals.

CONNECT IT! 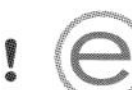

Stress cardiomyopathy, or broken heart syndrome, is a temporary condition induced by physical or emotional stress but can mimic serious cardiac conditions. Review this condition in ***Broken Heart*** online at ***Connect It!***

Corticoids and Resistance to Stress

Selye thought that the increase in **corticoids** that occurred in his stressed animals enabled them to adapt to and resist stress. Today many physiologists doubt this. No one questions that adrenal cortical hormones increase during stress. That fact has been clearly established. But what many question is how essential this increase is for *resisting stress.*

No one has proved by an unequivocal experiment that a higher than normal blood level of corticoids increases an animal's ability to adapt to stress, and increasing corticoid levels may in themselves be problematic—especially in the developing fetus. Some clinical evidence, however, seems to indicate that it does increase a human's coping ability. For instance, patients who have been taking cortisol for some time are known to require increased doses of this hormone to successfully resist stresses such as surgery or severe injury.

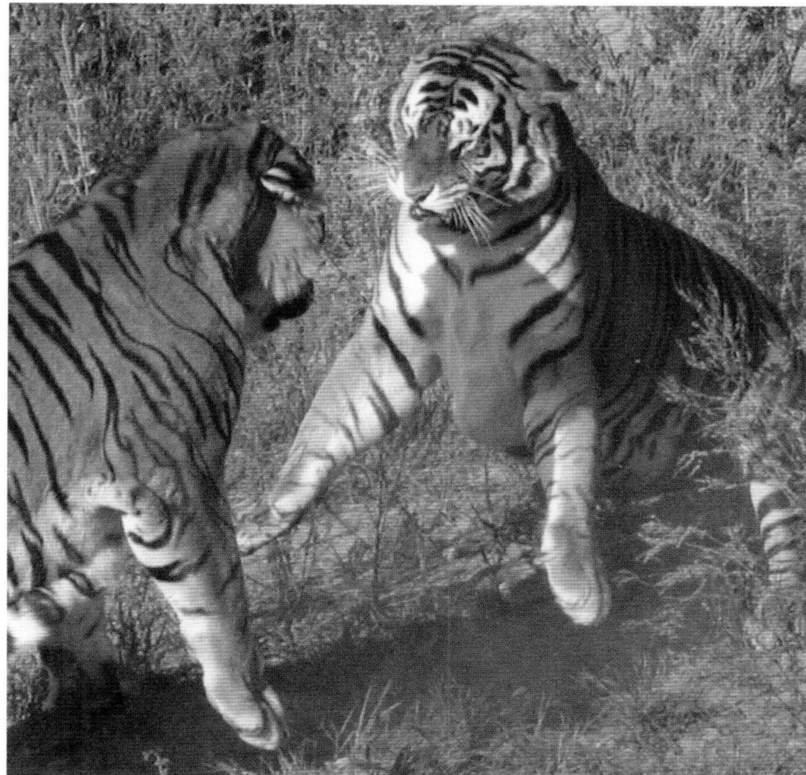

FIGURE 34-8 Psychological stress. For any animal, a stressor is a perceived threat to survival. The threat may be real (pictured) or imagined. Regardless, it will produce protective stress responses in the body.

Psychological Stress

Stress as defined by Selye is physiological stress—that is, a state of the body. Psychological stress, in contrast, might be defined as a state of the mind. It is caused by psychological stressors and manifested by a syndrome.

A **psychological stressor** is anything that an individual perceives as a threat—a threat to survival or to self-image. Moreover, the threat does not need to be real—it needs only to be real to the individual, who must see it as a threat, although in truth, it may not be so. The ability to recognize threats is vital to the survival of any animal, including humans (**Figure 34-8**). But perceiving nonharmful stimuli as stressors will also produce stress effects in the body.

Psychological stressors produce a syndrome of subjective and objective responses. Dominant among the subjective reactions is a feeling of anxiety. Other emotional reactions, such as anger, hate, depression, fear, and guilt, are also common subjective responses to psychological stressors.

Some characteristic objective responses are restlessness, fidgeting, criticizing, quarrelling, lying, and crying. Another objective indicator of psychological stress is that the concentration of lactate in the blood increases. Lactate, a molecule related to glucose, is released by glia to nourish nearby neurons. Increased blood lactate is an indicator of tissue hypoxia. Hypoxia may result from changes in breathing patterns.

Does psychological stress relate to physiological stress? The answer is clearly "yes". Physiological stress usually is accompanied by some degree of psychological stress. And conversely, in most people, psychological stress produces some physiological stress responses. Ancient peoples intuitively recognized this fact. For example, it is said that in ancient times when the Chinese suspected a person of lying, they made that person chew rice powder and then spit it out. If the powder came out dry, not moistened by saliva, they judged the suspect guilty. They seemed to know that lying makes a person nervous—and that nervousness makes a person's mouth dry. We "moderns" also know these facts, but we describe them with more technical language. Lying, we might say, induces psychological stress, and psychological stress acts in some way to cause the physiological stress response of decreased salivation.

Within recent decades, a scientific discipline called *psychophysiology* has come into being. Psychophysiologists, using accepted research methods, blood analyses, and sophisticated instruments—including polygraphs designed especially for this type of research—have investigated various physiological responses made by individuals subjected to psychological stressors. Their findings amply confirm the principle that psychological stressors often produce physiological stress responses in all age groups.

Especially apparent are the links among the immune, nervous, and endocrine systems. **Table 34-2** lists a number of stress-related diseases and conditions. Psychophysiologists have found, however, that identical psychological stressors do not necessarily induce identical physiological responses in different individuals. For example, stress may result in heart rate and blood pressure changes in one individual and changes in breathing patterns in another. Another of their interesting discoveries is that some organ systems become less responsive after they have been stimulated a number of times. We now know that infancy and early childhood, once overlooked as

TABLE 34-2 Stress-Related Diseases and Conditions

TARGET ORGAN OR SYSTEM	DISEASE OR CONDITION
Cardiovascular system	Coronary artery disease Hypertension Stroke Disturbances of heart rhythm
Muscles	Tension headaches Muscle contraction backache
Connective tissues	Rheumatoid arthritis (autoimmune disease) Related inflammatory diseases of connective tissue
Pulmonary system	Asthma (hypersensitivity reaction) Hay fever (hypersensitivity reaction) Changes in breathing patterns
Immune system	Immunosuppression or immune deficiency Autoimmune diseases
Gastrointestinal system	Ulcer Irritable bowel syndrome Diarrhoea Nausea and vomiting Ulcerative colitis
Genitourinary system	Diuresis Impotence (erectile dysfunction) Loss of libido (sexual desire)
Skin	Eczema Neurodermatitis Acne
Endocrine system	Diabetes mellitus Amenorrhoea
Central nervous system	Fatigue and lethargy Type A behaviour Overeating Depression Insomnia

potentially stressful periods in life, do indeed present youngsters with challenges that result in stress. The result is often manifested by physical or behavioural adaptations intended to assist in coping. As young children mature, they continue to face multiple periods of often stressful transition to new roles in social relationships, self-concept, personal identity, and, later, sexual identity and behaviour. These challenges are highly individualistic and often temporary—existing for only short periods during childhood and adolescence.

In the adult years, the types of stressors characteristic of earlier periods of development, such as the transition from childhood to sexual maturity, will often change and maladaptive responses will vary. Adults often face higher levels of ongoing stress than do children because of the many complex social interactions they must deal with day in and day out, including the need to make ethical judgments and decisions related to standards of conduct.

Maladaptive responses to chronic stress in adults often affect not only their physical health but also the emotional, social, and intellectual aspects of their lives. Living with chronic stress as an adult often leads to a decreased quality of life. Ulcers, hypertension, chemical dependency, impaired relationships, and even loss of contact with reality may occur. Adults struggling with unhealthy levels of stress over time often develop multiple problems that limit their ability to function in society as their general level of both physical and psychological health deteriorates.

Teaching these individuals how to manage stress is an important component of holistic treatment programs designed to improve both their physical and psychological health. In addition to specific drugs and counselling, such programs may include use of relaxation techniques, such as massage, meditation, and positive imagery, and educational components that focus on development of coping strategies.

Elderly people are at high risk for stress-related illness (**Box 34-1**). It is estimated that the UK population of very elderly individuals (85 years or older) will double to reach 3.6 million by 2039. These individuals must deal with unique and very significant stressors during their later years. Unfortunately, loss of health and general well-being, fear of death or dying, a sense of abandonment and social isolation, poverty, and often the death of a spouse result in frequent maladaptive responses to stress in this age group. Family support and societal support are particularly important for elderly individuals struggling with stress.

In summary, here are some principles to remember about psychological stress:

- Physiological stress almost always is accompanied by some degree of psychological stress.
- In most people, psychological stress leads to some physiological stress responses. Many of these are measurable autonomic responses, such as accelerated heart rate and increased systolic blood pressure (**Box 34-2**).
- Identical psychological stressors do not always induce identical physiological responses in different individuals.
- In any one individual, certain autonomic responses are better indicators of psychological stress than others.

BOX 34-1 *fyi* | **The Stress–Age Syndrome**

The **stress–age syndrome** refers to a group of anatomical, neurohormonal, and immune system changes related to ageing that influence both physiological and psychological stress responses. The syndrome includes a wide array of changes, including:

- Decrease in coping skills
  - Alteration of limbic system and hypothalamus excitability
  - Increases in catecholamines, adrenocorticotropic hormone (ACTH), and cortisol
  - Decreases in testosterone, oestrogen, thyroxine, and other hormones
  - Immunodepression
  - Decreases in neuromuscular transmitter chemicals resulting in chronic fatigue and reduced physical strength
  - Changes in blood lipid profile
  - Increased potential for hypercoagulation of the blood
- Disturbances of the sleep/wake cycle and other circadian rhythms

Although not all age-related changes connected with stress are damaging, a majority result in a lower potential for positive adaptation to change.

> **BOX 34-2 *fyi* | Type A Behaviour and Stress**
>
> Hard-driving, competitive type A individuals who put themselves in high-stress situations have been found to be at a somewhat greater risk of elevated systolic blood pressure and coronary disease than individuals with the more relaxed and less impatient type B personality. Studies show that type A behaviour patterns can be reduced by psychological guidance. Counselling of type A individuals helps them reduce stress and may cut in half their chances of suffering a heart attack (myocardial infarction, or MI) because of stress. •

Effects of Intrauterine Stress

We now know that a fetus develops both short-term and long-term responses to stress experienced during intrauterine development.

Maternal malnutrition is one of the most common stressors experienced by a pregnant woman and her unborn child. In malnourished women who smoke, oxygen delivery to the fetus will also decrease. The result is hypoxic as well as nutritional stress. Physicians have known for years that when a fetus is stressed by toxins such as alcohol (see generalization number 5 on p. 788) or by a lack of necessary nutrients or oxygen during development, the immediate outcome for the fetus is often preterm delivery and low birth weight. Both of these outcomes are associated with potential problems, including developmental delays, anatomical (congenital) anomalies, functional deficits, and overt disease.

The fetus is not simply a passive recipient of the negative results of maternal stress during pregnancy. And early delivery, low birth weight, or both are not the only outcomes related to fetal stress. Stress-related changes in the intrauterine environment may also trigger numerous development problems that may become apparent during gestation or at the time of delivery. Many are related to oversecretion of endocrine secretions, especially cortisol, by both mother and developing fetus (**Figure 34-9**). Intrauterine levels of cortisol are influenced by the maternal–fetoplacental unit and by the shared maternal–fetal HPA axis (review **Figure 34-5**).

Not only do abnormal increases in the intrauterine level of cortisol have an immediate impact on the fetus or newborn baby, they also produce intermediate and long-term effects on the individual over a lifetime. The process is now called **fetal programming.** It refers to the relationship between events occurring during the course of fetal development and the appearance of specific anatomical, physiological, or disease states that develop later in life. Early research in the area of fetal programming focused on trying to explain the relationship known to exist between the stress of inadequate fetal nutrition, low birth weight, and subsequent adult rates of cardiovascular disease and its precursors—including elevated cholesterol levels, high blood pressure, and diabetes.

Fetal programming is strongly influenced by elevated intrauterine levels of cortisol and other stress hormones, and it affects not only the cardiovascular system but also many other body systems and physiological variables over a lifetime. Cortisol-induced fetal programming changes are known to influence body composition; growth rates; age at maturity; the functioning of the adult immune, endocrine, renal, and reproductive systems; the ageing process; and even life expectancy.

Although sophisticated experimental work has shown that fetal programming does indeed occur and that it is often influenced by stress before birth, the mechanism that would explain exactly how it works has yet to be discovered. Fully understanding the role of cortisol in regulating the "partitioning" or allocation of energy (nutrients) available for use by different organ systems during intrauterine development will most certainly be important in solving the puzzle.

Many scientists believe the answer will be related to what are described as *biological tradeoffs*. For example, for a developing fetus, the "tradeoff" of simply surviving a dangerous pregnancy caused by the stress of maternal malnutrition might be to "accept" the dangers associated with preterm delivery and low birth weight. Diverting very limited nutrients to support central nervous system development required to sustain life at birth rather than using the same amount of energy resource to protect future reproductive system function might be another "acceptable" biological tradeoff. In a biological sense, in the cycle of life, the "big picture" focuses on survival. It is therefore appropriate to state that stress plays an important role in the health of an individual in every stage of the cycle of life from conception to death.

New research data related to fetal programming and its relationship to stress experienced by the fetus during development have dramatically increased interest in this area in both the scientific and medical communities. For example, knowing that a particular disease or condition is caused by prenatal stress related to a nutritional deficiency in the maternal diet, and not by genetic susceptibility, will drastically change public health and disease prevention strategies intended to reduce the incidence of that disease or condition in the

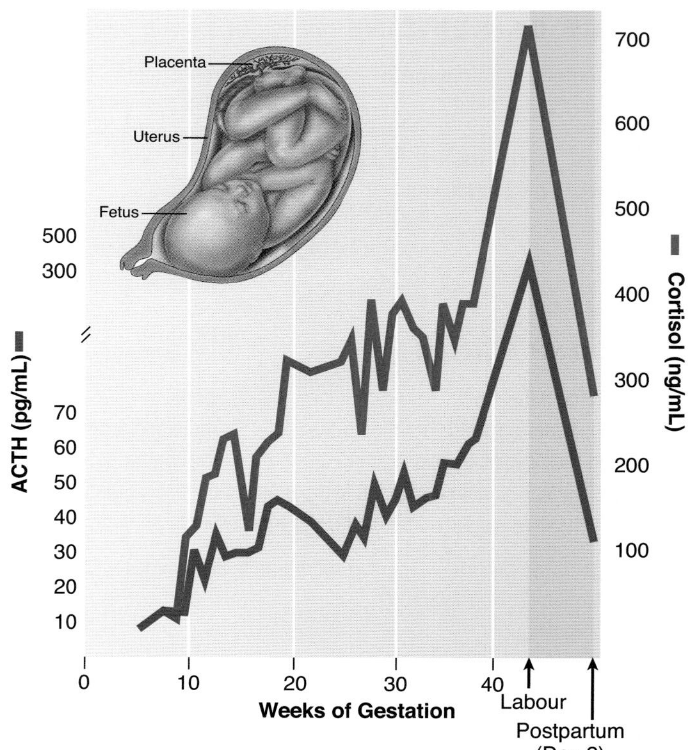

FIGURE 34-9 Stress hormones during pregnancy. The graph shows increasing levels of the maternal stress hormones cortisol and ACTH during pregnancy. Notice that they decrease dramatically after birth *(shaded area)*.

population. A good example is prevention of certain congenital defects in the central nervous system by addition of an important micronutrient, folic acid, to the diet of pregnant women.

Expanding our knowledge about prenatal stress has resulted in new commitments being made to improve nutrition for women during pregnancy and to increase access to educational programs intended to decrease smoking and alcohol consumption.

Quick CHECK

7. What is meant by the phrase *diseases of adaptation*?
8. What is the fight-or-flight reaction?
9. List four indicators of stress.
10. What is the difference between physiological and psychological stress?

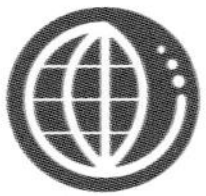

the big picture | Stress and the Whole Body

Although our understanding of physiological and psychological stress is still evolving, we are certain of this: stress affects the entire body. Stress responses involve numerous physiological mechanisms, many of which are suspected to occur but are as yet unproven.

So far, we understand that stress responses involve nearly every system of the body. The nervous system detects and integrates the factors, or stressors, that trigger the stress responses. Physiological stress responses result from signals sent from the nervous system directly—or by way of the endocrine system. Many of these "stress signals" have been discovered in recent decades. Many different kinds of neurotransmitters, hormones, and perhaps other regulatory chemicals influence the function of the skeletal muscles, the digestive system, the urinary system, the reproductive system, the respiratory system, the cardiovascular system, the integumentary system—perhaps every system, organ, and tissue in the body.

Because the regulatory agents associated with stress influence the function of blood cells, stress can have a profound effect on the function of the immune system. Although the fact that stress inhibits immune function has been known for some time, many of the exact mechanisms that accomplish this have been discovered only in the past few decades. Biologists now better appreciate the link between the mind and the immune system and thus are better able to explain how stress causes disease—and even death. In fact, an emerging field within human biology is devoted to studying the mind–immunity link—the field of *neuroimmunology*. Some researchers in this field have found their studies tend to incorporate diverse fields such as endocrinology, psychology, and haematology.

Considering the effect that stress can have on the entire internal environment—the whole body—and the high levels of stress that characterize the modern cultures in which many of us live and work, advancements in stress research hold the promise of improving the length and quality of our lives.

LANGUAGE OF MEDICINE *(continued from p. 785)*

general adaptation syndrome (GAS) (JEN-er-al ad-ap-TAY-shun SIN-drohm) [*adapt-* **adjust,** *-tion* **process,** *syn-* **together,** *-drome* **running or (race) course**]

stress syndrome (stres SIN-drohm) [*stress* **tighten,** *syn-* **together,** *-drome* **running or (race) course**]

stress–age syndrome (stres-AYJ SIN-drohm) [*stress-* **tighten,** *syn-* **together,** *-drome* **running or (race) course**]

case study

"What's the matter with me?" Jane thinks. Her palms are sweaty; her heart is racing; her mouth feels dry. She's finding it difficult to concentrate on the physiology exam sitting on her desk. No matter how many times she tells herself to calm down, the symptoms continue. She glances over at her friend, who is taking the same exam. Her friend seems perfectly calm!

1. Which stage of the general adaptation syndrome is Jane experiencing?
   a. Alert reaction
   b. Stage of resistance
   c. Stage of exhaustion
   d. Alarm reaction
2. If we were to do a blood test on Jane at this moment, the levels of which hormone would be elevated?
   a. TRH
   b. CRH
   c. TSH
   d. Melatonin
3. Which of the following is NOT included in the "stress triad"?
   a. Enlarged lymphatic organs
   b. Increased size of adrenal glands
   c. Gastrointestinal ulcers
   d. Decreased size of lymphatic organs
4. All of the following statements are FALSE, except which one?
   a. Stressors are perceived in an infant before and after birth.
   b. All stressors have the same effect on all people.
   c. Stressors are always intensely negative experiences.
   d. Stressors cannot be an imagined threat; they must be a real, physical threat.

Hint To solve a case study, you may have to refer to the glossary or index, other chapters in this textbook, ***Connect It!,*** and other resources.

CHAPTER SUMMARY

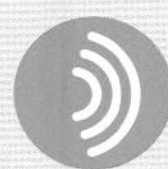

To download an MP3 version of the chapter summary for use with your mobile device, access the ***Audio Chapter Summaries*** *online at evolve.elsevier.com.*

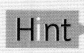

Scan this summary after reading the chapter to help you reinforce the key concepts. Later, use the summary as a quick review before your class or before a test.

Selye's Concept of Stress

A. Development of the stress concept
   1. Selye found that animals exposed to noxious agents all responded with the same syndrome of changes, or "stress triad"
   2. Changes included enlarged adrenal glands, atrophied lymphatic organs, and bleeding ulcers of the stomach and duodenum

B. Definitions
   1. Stress—a state, or condition, of the body produced by "diverse nocuous agents" and manifested by a syndrome of changes (**Figure 34-1**)
   2. Stressors—agents that produce stress
   3. General adaptation syndrome—group of changes that manifest the presence of stress

C. Stressors
   1. Stressors are extreme stimuli—too much or too little of almost anything
   2. Stressors are very often injurious or painful stimuli
   3. Anything an individual perceives as a threat is a stressor for that individual
   4. Reaction to stressors differs for different individuals and for one individual at different times
   5. Physical or nutritional stressors experienced by a pregnant woman can cause her fetus to develop prenatal stress

D. General adaptation syndrome
   1. Manifestations
      a. Stress is intangible but can be inferred by physiological changes
      b. Three changes initially noted by Selye named *stress triad;* subsequently, many other changes were noted
      c. Entire group of changes or responses were named *general adaptation syndrome (GAS)*
   2. Stages
      a. Changes occur in stages over time, not simultaneously
      b. Three successive stages: alarm reaction, stage of resistance, stage of exhaustion (**Figures 34-2**, **34-3**, and **34-4**)
      c. Each stage characterized by different syndrome of changes (**Table 34-1**)

E. Mechanism of stress
   1. State of stress turns on stress response mechanism—general adaptation syndrome
   2. Stimulus that produces stress and thereby activates stress mechanism is nonspecific or variable
   3. Stress mechanism often referred to as hypothalamic–pituitary–adrenal (HPA) axis or HPA mechanism (**Figure 34-5**)

Some Current Concepts about Stress

A. Definitions
   1. Stress—any stimulus that directly or indirectly stimulates the hypothalamus to release corticotropin-releasing hormone (CRH)
   2. Stress syndrome—also called the *stress response;* many diverse changes initiated by stress
   3. Allostasis—term sometimes used instead of stress syndrome to describe the body's attempts to restore homeostasis during stress
   4. Allostatic load—the effect of allostasis on the body (stress effects)

B. Stress syndrome—see **Figure 34-6**
   1. Direct or indirect stress stimulation of hypothalamus triggers release of CRH and stimulation of sympathetic centres and posterior pituitary gland
      a. CRH triggers release of adrenocorticotropic hormone (ACTH), which in turn triggers release of cortisol and aldosterone from adrenal cortex
      b. Sympathetic activation produces collection of adrenergic effects called the fight-or-flight reaction (e.g., increased heart rate and blood pressure); review **Table 22-5** on p. 515
   2. Additional hormones such as neuropeptide Y may produce additional stress responses

C. Stress and disease—Selye held that stress could result in disease instead of adaptation; in today's terms: high allostatic load can produce fatigue or disease

D. Indicators of stress (**Figure 34-7**)
   1. Stress response determined by physiological measurements and observations—faster, stronger heartbeat; higher blood pressure; sweaty palms; dilated pupils
   2. Laboratory tests reveal decreased eosinophils and lymphocytes; increased level of adrenocorticoids

E. Corticoids and resistance to stress
   1. Increase in corticoids when experiencing stress is proved reaction to stress
   2. Role of higher levels of corticoids in helping body resist stress not yet proven

F. Psychological stress
   1. Psychological stressors—anything that an individual perceives as a threat to survival or self-image (**Figure 34-8**)
   2. A syndrome of subjective and objective responses characterizes the mental state of psychological stress including anxiety (dominant subjective response), restlessness, irritability, lying, crying
   3. Psychological stressors produce physiological stress (see summary of principles on p. 793)

G. Effects of intrauterine stress
   1. Fetus develops short- and long-term responses to stress experienced during intrauterine development (**Figure 34-9**)
      a. Common stressors include maternal malnutrition, hypoxia, and exposure to toxins such as alcohol
      b. Low birth weight and preterm delivery are common immediate responses to intrauterine stress

2. Maternal–fetal blood levels of cortisol, important mediators of stress, are influenced by endocrine secretory activity of maternal–fetoplacental unit and the shared maternal–fetal hypothalamic–pituitary–adrenal (HPA) mechanism
3. Fetal programming responses to stress often result in negative outcomes later in life and affect many organ systems and even life expectancy
4. Concept of *biological tradeoffs* may be involved in fetal programming outcomes; for example, low birth weight and preterm delivery may be tradeoffs for stress of maternal malnutrition by the fetus to ensure survival

The Big Picture: Stress and the Whole Body

A. Stress affects the entire body
B. Nervous system detects and integrates stressors that trigger stress responses
C. Stress can have profound effect on immune system
D. Emerging field of neuroimmunology studies mind–immunity link

REVIEW QUESTIONS

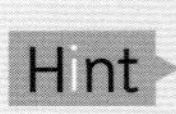

Write out the answers to these questions after reading the chapter and reviewing the Chapter Summary. Note—writing out your answers will consolidate learning and provide a valuable resource of information.

1. Define the terms *stress, stressor,* and *general adaptation syndrome*.
2. Describe a few generalizations about the kinds of stimuli that constitute stressors.
3. What three stages make up the general adaptation syndrome? What changes characterize each stage?
4. What changes constitute the "stress triad"?
5. An increase in what three hormones brought about the changes that Selye named the general adaptation syndrome?
6. What function, according to Selye, does the general adaptation syndrome serve?
7. Stress, according to Selye, is a state, or condition, of the body. What is a more specific definition of stress?
8. What part of the brain, according to current ideas, plays the key role in initiating stress syndrome responses?
9. What parts of the nervous system other than that named in question 8 are involved in inducing the stress syndrome?
10. Briefly, what role, if any, does each of the following hormones play when the body is subjected to stress: ACTH, ADH, aldosterone, cortisol, CRH, epinephrine, and norepinephrine?
11. What has been proven about corticoids in relation to stress?
12. What issue is considered controversial regarding corticoids as they relate to stress?
13. Cite several examples of psychological stressors.
14. Are psychological stressors the same for all individuals? Give an example.
15. Give some examples of subjective indicators of psychological stress.
16. Give some examples of objective responses that are part of psychological stress.

CRITICAL THINKING QUESTIONS

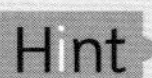

After finishing the Review Questions, write out the answers to these more in-depth questions to help you apply your new knowledge. Go back to sections of the chapter that relate to concepts that you find difficult.

1. Based on what you know regarding Selye's experimental results, explain why stress could be described as a nonspecific response.
2. What is the relationship between stress and disease? If stress levels were high in a person, how might age and personality type affect the risk for specific diseases?
3. What observations and clinical test results would indicate an individual was under stress?
4. Use your knowledge of psychophysiology to explain the Chinese rice powder test.
5. Compare and contrast psychological stress and physiological stress. What is the relationship between physiological stress and psychological stress?

UNIT 5

Respiration, Nutrition, and Excretion

The chapters in Unit 5 provide a discussion of respiration, digestion, processing of nutrients, and excretion of wastes by the urinary system. The concluding chapters of this unit discuss fluid and electrolyte balance and acid–base balance. Ultimately, all homeostatic mechanisms function to maintain what can best be described as a "dynamic constancy" at the cellular level. For example, although in normal conditions the oxygen (O_2) and carbon dioxide (CO_2) content of blood does not change much over time, the quantity of O_2 and CO_2 that enters and exits the blood can vary widely with exercise. Delivery of oxygen and elimination of carbon dioxide and other wastes resulting from the metabolism of nutrients must be regulated within narrow limits so that cellular function remains normal. Maintaining the dynamic constancy of fluid and electrolyte balance and acid–base balance at the cellular level is also required for survival. The anatomical structures and functional control mechanisms discussed in this unit all relate, in the last analysis, to cellular homeostasis.

35 Respiratory Tract

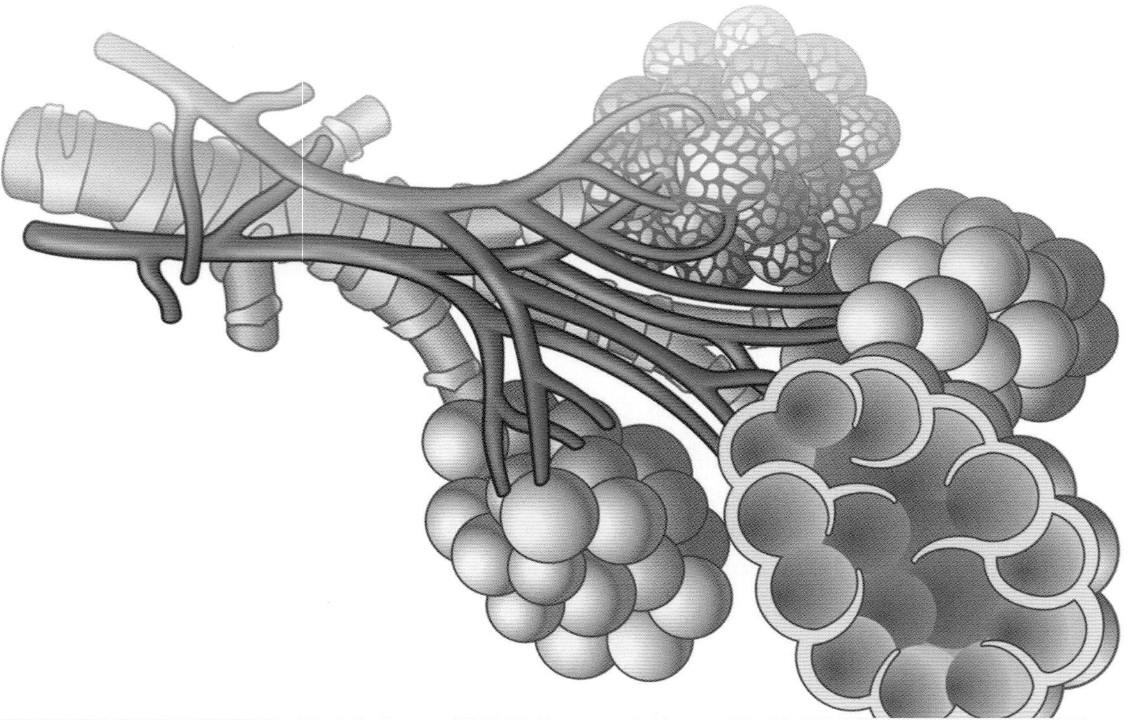

CHAPTER OUTLINE

Hint *Scan this outline before you begin to read the chapter, as a preview of how the concepts are organized.*

The respiratory system functions as an air distributor and a gas exchanger so that oxygen can be supplied to and carbon dioxide removed from the body's cells. Because most of our trillions of cells lie too far from air to exchange gases directly with it, air must first exchange gases with blood, blood must circulate, and finally, blood and cells must exchange gases. These events require the functioning of two systems—namely, the respiratory system and the circulatory system. All parts of the respiratory system—except its microscopic-sized sacs called alveoli—function as air distributors. Only the alveoli and the tiny alveolar ducts that open into them serve as gas exchangers.

In addition to air distribution and gas exchange, the respiratory system effectively filters, warms, and humidifies the air we breathe. Respiratory organs also help produce sounds, including

LANGUAGE OF SCIENCE

Hint *Use this list to aid your pronunciation of unfamiliar words.*

alveolar duct (al-VEE-oh-lar)
[*alve-* **hollow,** *-ol-* **little,** *-ar* **relating to**]

alveolus (al-VEE-oh-lus)
[*alve-* **hollow,** *-olus* **little**] *pl.,* alveoli

apex (AY-peks)
[*apex* **tip**] *pl.,* apices

arytenoid cartilage (ah-RIT-en-oyd or ar-ih-TEE-noyd KAR-ti-lij)
[*aryten-* **ladle,** *-oid* **like**]

bronchial tree (BRONG-kee-al)
[*bronch-* **windpipe,** *-al* **relating to**]

bronchiole (BRONG-kee-ohl)
[*bronch-* **windpipe,** *-ol-* **little**]

bronchopulmonary segment (brong-koh-PUL-moh-nair-ee)
[*bronch-* **windpipe,** *-pulmon-* **lung,** *-ary* **relating to**]

concha (KONG-kah)
[*concha* **sea shell**] *pl.,* conchae

costal surface (KOS-tal)
[*costa-* **rib,** *-al* **relating to**]

cribriform plate (KRIB-rih-form)
[*cribr-* **sieve,** *-form* **shape**]

epiglottis (ep-ih-GLOT-is)
[*epi-* **upon,** *-glottis* **mouth of windpipe**] *pl.,* epiglottides or epiglottises

glottis (GLOT-is)
[*glottis* **mouth of windpipe**] *pl.,* glottides or glottises

hilum (HYE-lum)
[*hilum* **least bit**] *pl.,* hila

horizontal fissure (hor-ih-ZON-tal FISH-ur)
[*fissur-* **cleft**]

laryngopharynx (lah-ring-go-FAIR-inks)
[*laryng-* **voicebox (larynx),** *-pharynx* **throat**] *pl.,* laryngopharynges or laryngopharynxes

larynx (LAIR-inks)
[*larynx* **voicebox**] *pl.,* larynges or larynxes

lingual tonsil (LING-gwal TON-sil)
[*ling-* **tongue,** *-al* **relating to,** *tons-* **goitre,** *-il* **little**]

nasal mucosa (NAY-zal myoo-KOH-sah)
[*nas-* **nose,** *-al* **relating to,** *mucus* **slime**] *pl.,* mucosae

nasopharynx (nay-zoh-FAIR-inks)
[*naso-* **nose,** *-pharynx* **throat**] *pl.,* nasopharynges or nasopharynxes

continued on p. 820

speech used in communicating oral language. Special sensory epithelium in the respiratory tract makes the sense of smell (olfaction) possible. The respiratory system also plays an important role in the regulation, or homeostasis, of pH in the body.

In this chapter, we explore the structural aspects of the respiratory system and in Chapters 36 and 37 we explore the functional aspects.

STRUCTURAL PLAN OF THE RESPIRATORY TRACT

For purposes of study, the respiratory system may be divided into upper and lower tracts, or structural divisions. The organs of the upper respiratory tract are located outside the thorax, or chest cavity, whereas those in the lower tract, or division, are located almost entirely within it (**Figure 35-1**).

The **upper respiratory tract** is composed of the nose, nasopharynx, oropharynx, laryngopharynx, and larynx. The **lower respiratory tract,** or division, consists of the trachea, all segments of the bronchial tree, and the lungs. Functionally, the respiratory system also

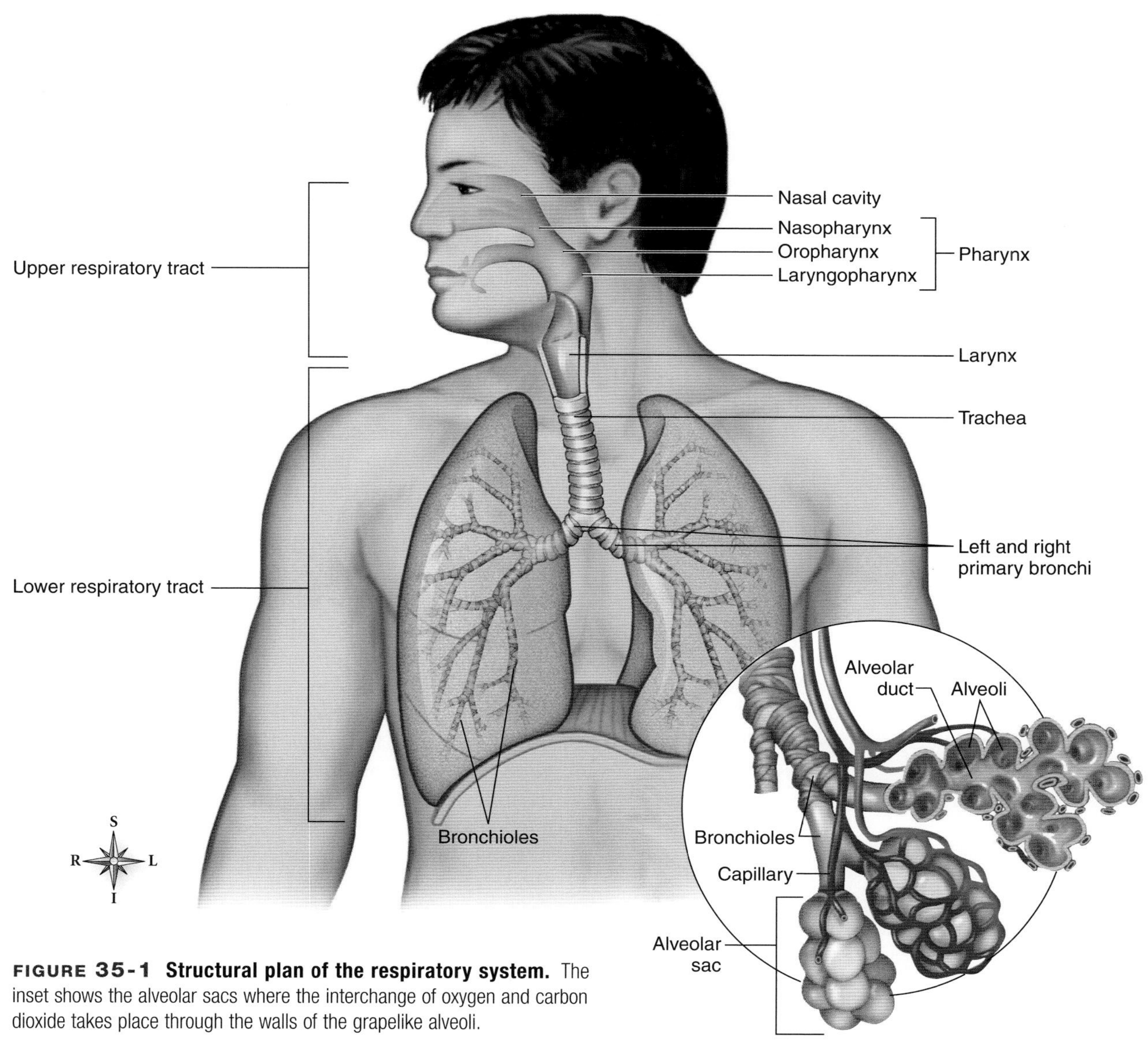

FIGURE 35-1 Structural plan of the respiratory system. The inset shows the alveolar sacs where the interchange of oxygen and carbon dioxide takes place through the walls of the grapelike alveoli.

UNIT 5

includes several accessory structures, such as the oral cavity, ribcage, and respiratory muscles including the diaphragm. Together, these structures constitute the lifeline, the air supply line of the body. This chapter describes the functional anatomy of these organs. The functional aspects of respiration are discussed in Chapters 36 and 37. Cells require a constant supply of oxygen for the vital energy conversion process carried out within each cell's mitochondria—a process called *cellular respiration* (Chapter 41). Cellular respiration produces carbon dioxide (CO_2) as a waste product, which must be removed before it accumulates to dangerously high levels.

CONNECT IT! 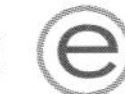

The ecology of the respiratory tract's microbiome, which varies by location in the upper and lower portions, affects our ability to resist respiratory infections and other disorders. Review the human *microbiome* in ***The Human Microbiome*** at ***Connect It!***

UPPER RESPIRATORY TRACT

NOSE

Structure of the Nose

The nose has external and internal structures. The external portion—that is, the part that protrudes from the face—consists of a bony and cartilaginous framework overlaid by skin containing many sebaceous glands. The two nasal bones meet in the centre of the face just below the forehead, where they are surrounded by the frontal bone to form the root of the nose. The nose is surrounded by the maxilla laterally and inferiorly at its base. The flaring cartilaginous expansion forming and supporting the outer side of each oval nostril opening is called the *ala*.

The internal portion of the nose, or nasal cavity, lies over the roof of the mouth where the palatine bones, which form the floor of the nose and the roof of the mouth, separate the nasal cavities from the mouth cavity. Sometimes the palatine bones fail to unite completely and produce a condition known as **cleft palate.** When this abnormality exists, the mouth is only partially separated from the nasal cavity, and consequently difficulties arise in swallowing and speaking.

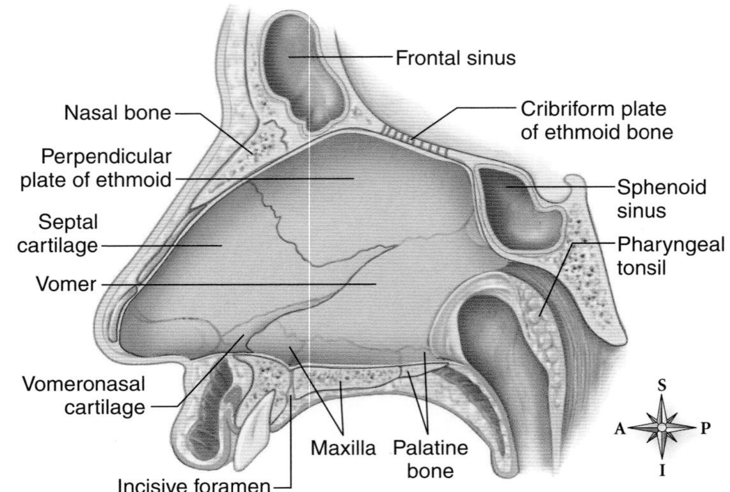

FIGURE 35-2 Nasal septum. The nasal septum consists of the perpendicular plate of the ethmoid bone, the vomer, and the septal and vomeronasal cartilages.

The roof of the nose is separated from the cranial cavity by a portion of the ethmoid bone called the **cribriform plate** (**Figure 35-2** and **Figure 35-3**). The cribriform plate is perforated by many small openings that permit branches of the olfactory nerve responsible for the special sense of smell to enter the cranial cavity and reach the brain.

Separation of the nasal and cranial cavities by a thin, perforated plate of bone presents real hazards. If the cribriform plate is damaged as a result of trauma to the nose, it is possible for potentially infectious material to pass directly from the nasal cavity into the cranial fossa and infect the brain and its covering membranes.

The hollow nasal cavity is separated by a midline partition, the **septum** (see **Figure 35-2**), into right and left cavities. Note in **Figure 35-2** that the nasal septum is made up of four main structures: the perpendicular plate of the ethmoid bone above, the vomer bone, and the septal nasal and vomeronasal cartilages below. In the adult the nasal septum is often deviated to one side or the other, interfering with respiration and with drainage of the nose and sinuses. The nasal septum has a rich blood supply. Nosebleeds, or *epistaxis*, often occur as a result of septal contusions caused by a direct blow to the nose. Epistaxis may also result from weak blood vessels combined with high blood pressure. Though seemingly dramatic, nosebleeds are seldom a serious health problem.

Each nasal cavity is divided into three passageways named the *superior, middle,* and *inferior meatuses.* These incomplete tubes are formed by the projection of the **conchae,** or **turbinates,** curving from the lateral walls of the internal portion of the nose (see **Figure 35-3**). The superior and middle conchae are processes of the ethmoid bone, whereas the inferior conchae are separate bones.

The external openings into the nasal cavities, commonly referred to as nostrils, have the technical name of *anterior nares* (singular, *naris*). They are sometimes called *external nares.* The anterior nares open into an area covered by skin that is reflected from the wings (ala) of the nose. This area, called the **vestibule,** is located just inside the nasal cavity below the inferior meatus. The vestibule is lined with skin. Coarse hairs called **vibrissae,** sebaceous glands, and numerous sweat glands are found in the skin of the vestibule. Once air has passed over the skin of the vestibule, it enters the **respiratory portion** of each nasal passage. This area extends from the inferior meatus to the small funnel-shaped orifices of the *posterior (internal) nares.* The posterior nares are openings that allow air to pass from the nasal cavity into the next major segment of the upper respiratory tract—the pharynx.

If one were to trace the movement of air through the nose into the pharynx, it would be found that air passes through several structures on the way. The sequence is as follows:

1. Anterior (external) nares
2. Vestibule
3. Inferior, middle, and superior meatuses, simultaneously
4. Posterior (internal) nares

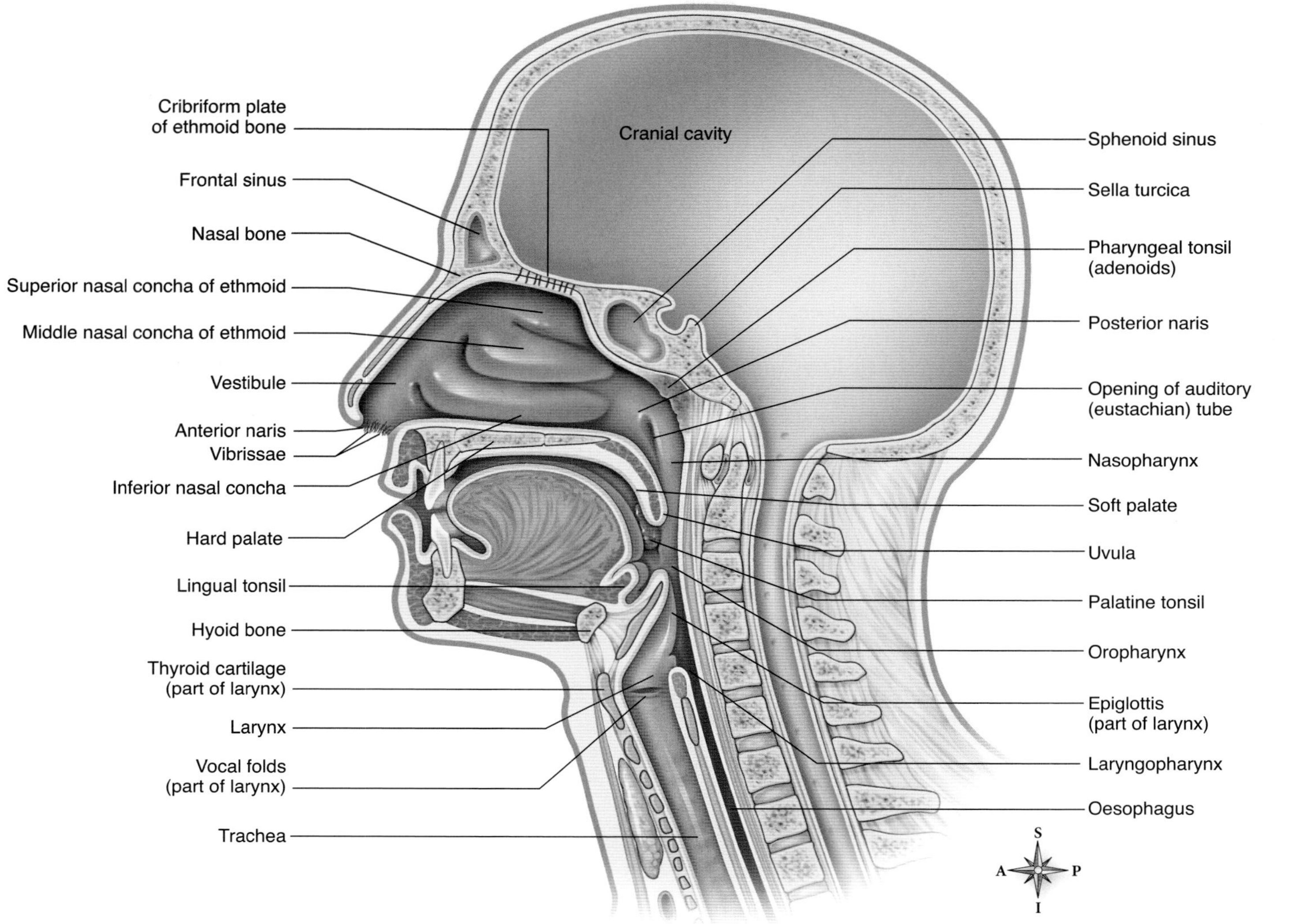

Cribriform plate of ethmoid bone
Frontal sinus
Nasal bone
Superior nasal concha of ethmoid
Middle nasal concha of ethmoid
Vestibule
Anterior naris
Vibrissae
Inferior nasal concha
Hard palate
Lingual tonsil
Hyoid bone
Thyroid cartilage (part of larynx)
Larynx
Vocal folds (part of larynx)
Trachea
Cranial cavity
Sphenoid sinus
Sella turcica
Pharyngeal tonsil (adenoids)
Posterior naris
Opening of auditory (eustachian) tube
Nasopharynx
Soft palate
Uvula
Palatine tonsil
Oropharynx
Epiglottis (part of larynx)
Laryngopharynx
Oesophagus
S
A
P
I

FIGURE 35-3 Upper respiratory tract. In this midsagittal section through the upper respiratory tract, the nasal septum has been removed to reveal the turbinates (nasal conchae) of the lateral wall of the nasal cavity. The three divisions of the pharynx (nasopharynx, oropharynx, and laryngopharynx) are also visible.

Nasal Mucosa

Once air has passed over the skin of the vestibule and enters the respiratory portion of the nasal passage, it passes over the **respiratory mucosa.** This mucous membrane has a pseudostratified ciliated columnar epithelium rich in goblet cells (**Figure 35-4**). The respiratory mucosa possesses a rich blood supply, especially over the inferior turbinate, and is bright pink or red. Near the roof of the nasal cavity and over the superior turbinate and opposing portion of the septum, the mucosa turns pale and has a yellowish tint. In this area it is referred to as the **olfactory epithelium.** This membrane contains many olfactory nerve cells and has a rich lymphatic plexus. Ciliated mucous membrane lines the rest of the respiratory tract down as far as the smaller bronchioles.

Goblet cell
Cilia
Pseudostratified ciliated columnar epithelium
Connective tissue

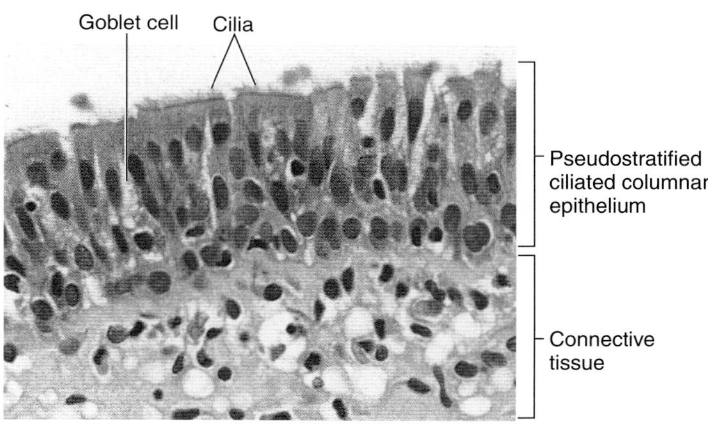

FIGURE 35-4 Respiratory mucosa. This epithelium is typically ciliated and exhibits numerous goblet cells that produce and release mucus.

CONNECT IT! 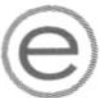

Besides the olfactory sensory neurons imbedded in the nasal mucosa, a structure called the **vomeronasal organ (VNO)** is located in the mucosa of the inferior nasal septum. The VNO is thought to be involved in sensing pheromones, which are sex-signalling chemicals. Want to know more? Check out ***Pheromones and the Vomeronasal Organ*** and ***Nerve Zero*** online at ***Connect It!***

Paranasal Sinuses

The four pairs of **paranasal sinuses** are air-containing spaces that lighten the weight of the skull and open, or drain, into the nasal cavity. They take their names from the skull bones in which they are located (see Chapter 12). These paranasal sinuses are the frontal, maxillary, ethmoid, and sphenoid sinuses (**Figure 35-5**). Like the nasal cavity, each paranasal sinus is lined by respiratory mucosa. The mucous secretions produced in the sinuses are continually being swept into the nose by the ciliated surface of the respiratory membrane. The exact size and shape of the paranasal sinuses varies among individuals.

The right and left frontal sinuses are located just above the corresponding orbit, whereas the maxillary, the largest of the sinuses, extends into the maxilla on either side of the nose. The sphenoid sinuses lie in the body of the sphenoid bone on either side of the midline in close proximity to the optic nerves and pituitary gland.

Note in **Figure 35-5** that the ethmoid sinuses are not single large cavities but a collection of small air cells divided into anterior, middle, and posterior groups that open independently into the upper part of the nasal cavity.

The paranasal sinuses drain as follows:

- Into the middle meatus (passageway below the middle concha)—frontal, maxillary, anterior, and middle ethmoidal sinuses
- Into the superior meatus—posterior ethmoidal sinuses
- Into the space above the superior conchae (sphenoethmoidal recess)—sphenoid sinuses

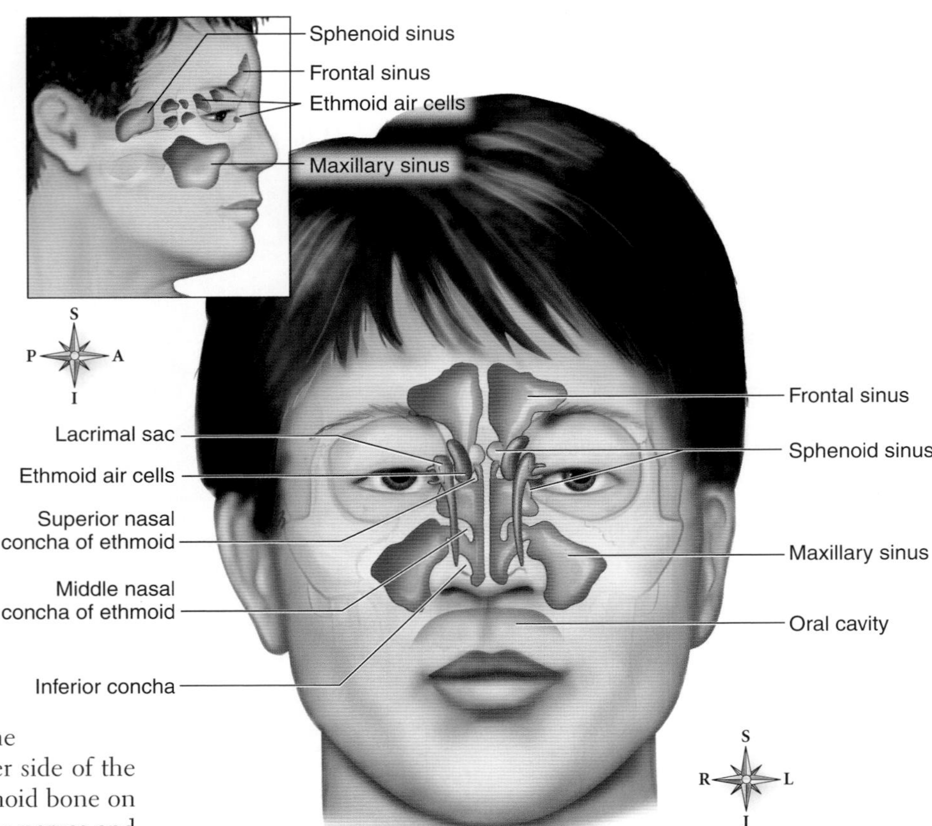

FIGURE 35-5 The paranasal sinuses. The anterior view shows the anatomical relationship of the paranasal sinuses to each other and to the nasal cavity. The inset is a lateral view of the position of the sinuses.

Functions of the Nose

The nose serves as a passageway for air going to and from the lungs. However, if the nasal passages are obstructed, it is possible for air to bypass the nose and enter the respiratory tract directly through the mouth.

Air that enters the system through the nasal cavity is filtered of impurities, warmed, moistened, and chemically examined (by olfaction) to detect substances that might prove irritating to the delicate lining of the respiratory tract. The vibrissae, or *nasal hairs*, in the vestibule serve as an initial "filter" that screens particulate matter from air that is entering the system. The conchae, or turbinates, then serve as baffles to slow and stir the air—as well as provide a large mucus-covered surface area over which air must pass before reaching the pharynx. The respiratory membrane produces copious quantities of mucus and possesses a rich blood supply, especially over the inferior conchae, which permits rapid warming and moistening of the dry inspired air. Mucous secretions provide the final "trap" where some of the remaining particulate matter from air is removed as it travels through the nasal passages. Fluid from the lacrimal glands (see **Figure 24-14** on p. 543) and additional mucus produced in the paranasal sinuses also help trap particulate matter and moisten air passing through the nose.

In addition, the hollow sinuses act to lighten the bones of the skull and serve as resonating chambers for speech. Swirling of air by the middle and superior conchae over the olfactory epithelium makes the special sense of olfaction possible.

***Quick* CHECK**

1. What are the overall functions of the respiratory system? Which other body system is involved in accomplishing these functions?
2. Name the principal organs of the upper respiratory tract. Name the principal organs of the lower respiratory tract.
3. Describe the paranasal sinuses. What is their anatomical relationship to the nose?

PHARYNX

Structure of the Pharynx

Another name for the **pharynx** is the throat. It is a tubelike structure about 12.5 cm long that extends from the base of the skull to the oesophagus and lies just anterior to the cervical vertebrae. It is made of muscle and is lined with mucous membrane.

The pharynx has three anatomical divisions. The **nasopharynx** is located behind the nose and extends from the posterior nares to the level of the soft palate. The **oropharynx** is located behind the mouth from the soft palate above to the level of the hyoid bone below. Finally, the **laryngopharynx** extends from the hyoid bone to the oesophagus. **Figure 35-3** shows the divisions of the pharynx.

Seven openings are found in the pharynx (see **Figure 35-3**):

- Right and left auditory (eustachian) tubes opening into the nasopharynx
- Two posterior nares opening into the nasopharynx
- The opening from the mouth, known as the fauces, into the oropharynx
- The opening into the larynx from the laryngopharynx
- The opening into the oesophagus from the laryngopharynx

The **pharyngeal tonsils** are located in the nasopharynx on its posterior wall opposite the posterior nares. The pharyngeal tonsils are referred to as *adenoids* when they are enlarged. Although the cavity of the nasopharynx differs from the oral and laryngeal divisions in that it does not collapse, it still may become obstructed. If these tonsils enlarge to become adenoids, they may fill the space behind the posterior nares and make it difficult or even impossible for air to travel from the nose into the throat. Small *tubal tonsils* are located in the nasopharynx near the opening of the auditory (eustachian) tube.

Two pairs of organs are found in the oropharynx: the **palatine tonsils,** located behind and below the pillars of the fauces, and the **lingual tonsils,** located at the base of the tongue. The palatine tonsils are the ones most commonly removed in the procedure referred to as a tonsillectomy. Only rarely are the lingual tonsils also removed.

You may want to review details of the structure and function of tonsils in Chapter 31.

Functions of the Pharynx

The pharynx serves as a common pathway for the respiratory and digestive tracts, because both air and food must pass through this structure before reaching the appropriate tubes—the trachea (air) and oesophagus (food). It also affects phonation (speech production). For example, only by changing the shape of the pharynx can the different vowel sounds of speech be formed.

LARYNX

Location of the Larynx

The **larynx,** or voice box, lies between the root of the tongue and the upper end of the trachea just below and in front of the lowest part of the pharynx (see **Figure 35-1**). It might be described as a vestibule opening into the trachea from the pharynx. It normally extends between the third, fourth, fifth, and sixth cervical vertebrae but is often positioned somewhat higher in females and during childhood for both genders. The lateral lobes of the thyroid gland and the carotid artery within its covering sheath touch the sides of the larynx.

Structure of the Larynx

The triangle-shaped larynx consists largely of cartilages that are attached to one another and to surrounding structures by muscles or by fibrous and elastic tissue components (**Figure 35-6**). It is lined by a ciliated mucous membrane. The cavity of the larynx extends from

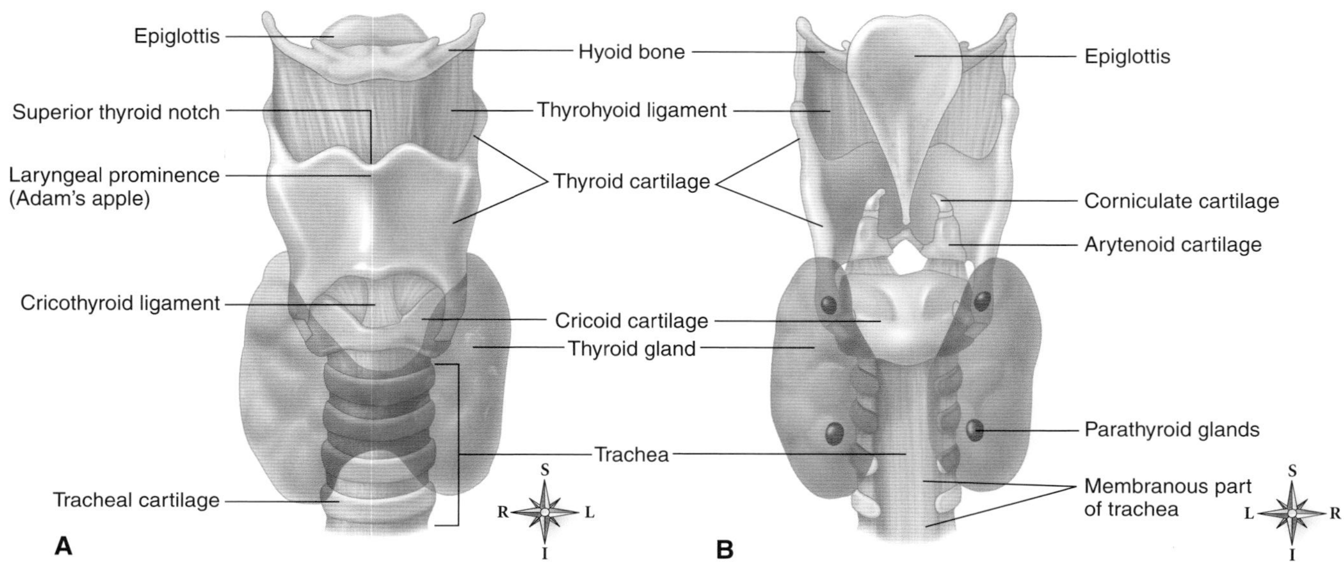

FIGURE 35-6 Laryngeal cartilages. Some softer tissues of the larynx and surrounding structures have been removed to make it possible to see the cartilages of the larynx. Note the position of the nearby thyroid gland. **A,** Anterior view. **B,** Posterior view.

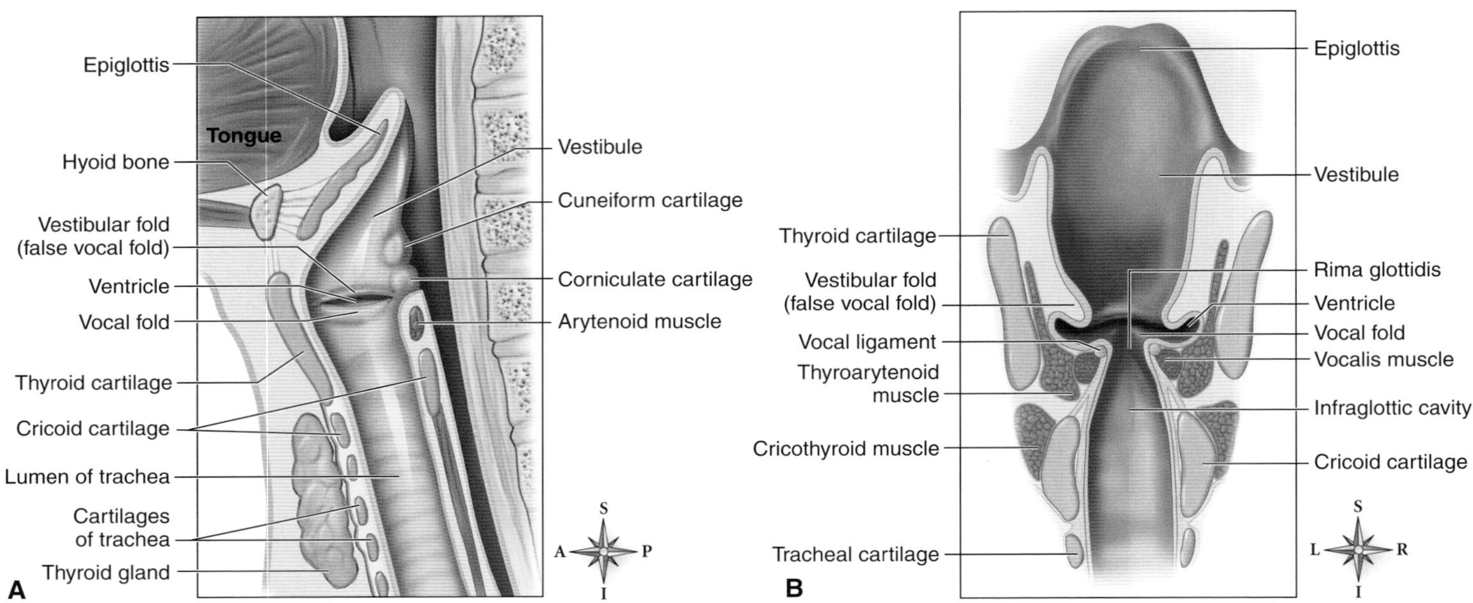

FIGURE 35-7 Larynx. These illustrations depict the mucosal lining of the larynx, with its folds and underlying muscles and ligaments visible. **A,** Sagittal section. **B,** Coronal (frontal) section, viewed from behind.

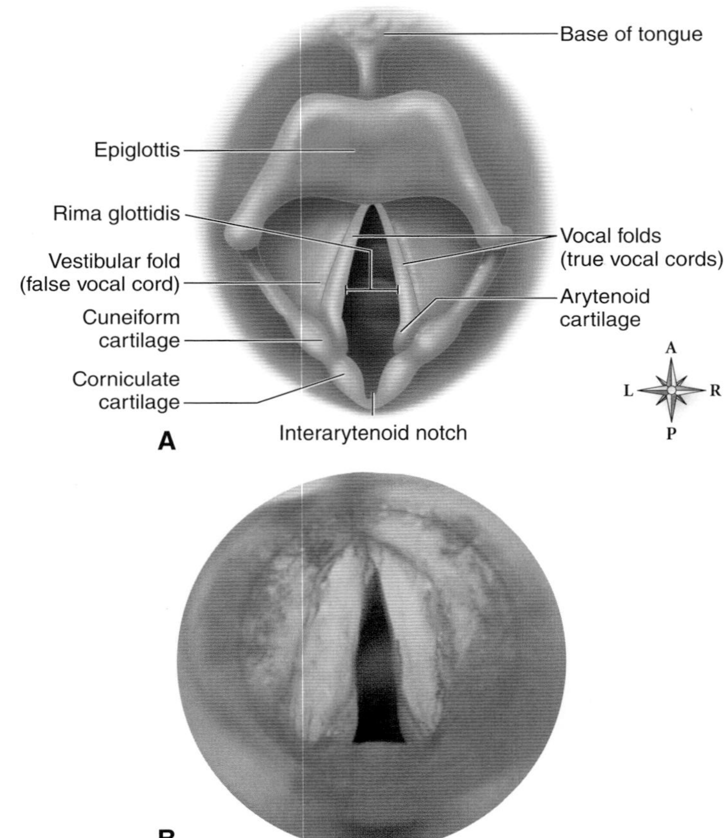

FIGURE 35-8 Vocal folds. **A,** Vocal folds viewed from above. **B,** Photograph taken with an endoscope showing the vocal folds in the open position.

its triangle-shaped inlet at the epiglottis to the circular outlet at the lower border of the cricoid cartilage, where it is continuous with the lumen of the trachea (**Figure 35-7**).

The larynx is lined primarily with respiratory mucosa—pseudostratified ciliated columnar epithelium. The mucous membrane lining the larynx forms two pairs of lateral folds that jut inward into its cavity. The upper folds are called the **vestibular folds.** They are also sometimes called the *false vocal folds* for the rather obvious reason that they play no part in vocalization. The lower pair serves as the **vocal folds,** which produce sounds needed for speech and other vocalizations. The vocal folds are sometimes called the *true vocal folds* or simply *vocal cords.* Each vocal fold is covered with nonkeratinized stratified squamous epithelium and supported at its medial edge by a strong *vocal ligament.* The slitlike space between the left and right vocal folds, called the *rima glottidis,* is the narrowest part of the larynx.

The vocal folds and the space between them (rima glottidis) are together designated as the **glottis.** An endoscopic view of the vocal folds and related structures is shown in **Figure 35-8**, *B.*

The laryngeal cavity above the vestibular folds is called the **vestibule**. The very short middle portion of the cavity between the vestibular and vocal folds is the **ventricle** of the larynx, or *laryngeal ventricle.* The *infraglottic cavity* is the open space below the glottis.

Cartilages of the Larynx

Nine cartilages form the framework of the larynx. The three largest—the thyroid cartilage, the epiglottis, and the cricoid cartilage—are single structures. The other six are three pairs of smaller accessory cartilages—namely, the arytenoid, corniculate, and cuneiform cartilages.

- The **thyroid cartilage** is the largest cartilage of the larynx and is the one that gives the characteristic triangular shape to its anterior wall. An anterior laryngeal eminence is often called the Adam's apple. It is usually larger in men than in women and has less of a fat pad lying over it—two reasons that a man's thyroid cartilage protrudes more than a woman's.
- The **epiglottis** is a small leaf-shaped cartilage that projects upward behind the tongue and hyoid bone. It is attached below to the thyroid cartilage, but its free superior border can flex to move up and down during swallowing to prevent food or liquids from entering the trachea (see **Figures 35-6** and **35-7**). The epiglottis is covered with nonkeratinized stratified squamous epithelium.
- The pyramid-shaped **arytenoid cartilages** are the most important of the paired laryngeal cartilages. The base of each cartilage articulates with the superior border of the cricoid cartilage (see **Figure 35-6**). The anterior angles of these cartilages serve as points of attachment for the vocal folds.

Muscles of the Larynx

The muscles of the larynx are often divided into intrinsic and extrinsic groups. Intrinsic muscles have both their origin and insertion on the larynx. They are important in controlling vocal fold length and tension and in regulating the shape of the laryngeal inlet. Extrinsic muscles insert on the larynx but have their origin on some other structure—such as the hyoid bone. Therefore, contraction of the extrinsic muscles actually moves or displaces the larynx as a whole. Muscles in both groups play important roles in respiration, vocalization, and swallowing. During swallowing, for example, contraction of the intrinsic aryepiglottic muscles (those that connect the arytenoid cartilages with the epiglottis) prevents entry of food or fluid into the trachea by squeezing the laryngeal inlet shut.

Two other pairs of intrinsic laryngeal muscles function to open and close the glottis by adducting or abducting the vocal folds. These events are crucial to both respiration and voice production. Certain other intrinsic muscles of the larynx function to influence the pitch of the voice by either lengthening and tensing or shortening and relaxing the vocal folds.

Functions of the Larynx

The larynx functions in respiration because it constitutes part of the vital airway to the lungs. This unique passageway, like the other components of the upper respiratory tract, is lined with a ciliated mucous membrane that helps in removal of dust particles and in warming and humidification of inspired air. In addition, it protects the airway against the entrance of solids or liquids during swallowing.

It also serves as the organ of voice production—hence its popular name, the *voice box.* Air being expired through the glottis, narrowed by partial adduction of the vocal folds, causes them to vibrate. Their vibration produces the voice. Several other structures besides the larynx contribute to the sound of the voice by acting as sounding boards or resonating chambers. Thus the size and shape of the nose, mouth, pharynx, and bony sinuses help determine the quality of the voice.

CONNECT IT! 

Oedema (swelling) of the mucosa covering the vocal folds and other laryngeal tissues can be a potentially lethal condition. Even a moderate amount of swelling can obstruct the glottis so much that air cannot get through and asphyxiation results. To find out more, check out ***Swollen Larynx*** online at ***Connect It!***

***Quick* CHECK**

4. What are the three main divisions of the pharynx?
5. Describe where the tonsils are located.
6. Distinguish between true and false vocal folds.

LOWER RESPIRATORY TRACT

Trachea

Structure of the Trachea

The **trachea,** or windpipe, is a tube about 11 cm long that extends from the larynx in the neck to the primary bronchi in the thoracic cavity (**Figure 35-9**). Its diameter measures about 2.5 cm.

The outside of the tracheal wall is covered in a fibrous *adventitia.* Smooth muscle, in which are embedded C-shaped rings of cartilage at regular intervals, makes up most of the wall of the trachea (**Figure 35-10**, *A*). The posterior wall also contains many elastic fibres.

The cartilaginous rings are incomplete on the posterior surface (look back at **Figure 35-6**, *B*). They give firmness to the wall and tend to prevent it from collapsing and shutting off the vital airway. The fact that the rings are incomplete allows the oesophagus, which runs just posterior to the trachea, to expand as food moves toward the stomach during swallowing (**Figure 35-10**, *B*).

The trachea is lined with *respiratory mucosa.* This type of mucosa is characterized by pseudostratified ciliated columnar epithelium and is typical of the respiratory tract as a whole (**Figure 35-11**). Goblet cells in the epithelium produce the blanket of mucus that continually moves upward towards the pharynx.

Function of the Trachea

The trachea performs a simple, but vital function—it furnishes part of the open passageway through which air can reach the lungs from the outside. Obstruction of this airway for even a few minutes causes death from asphyxiation (**Box 35-1**).

Bronchi and Alveoli

Structure of the Bronchi

The trachea divides at its lower end into two **primary bronchi,** the right bronchus being slightly larger and more vertical than the left. This anatomical fact helps explain why aspirated foreign objects often lodge in the right bronchus.

In structure the bronchi resemble the trachea. The bronchi walls have incomplete cartilaginous rings in the sections superior to the

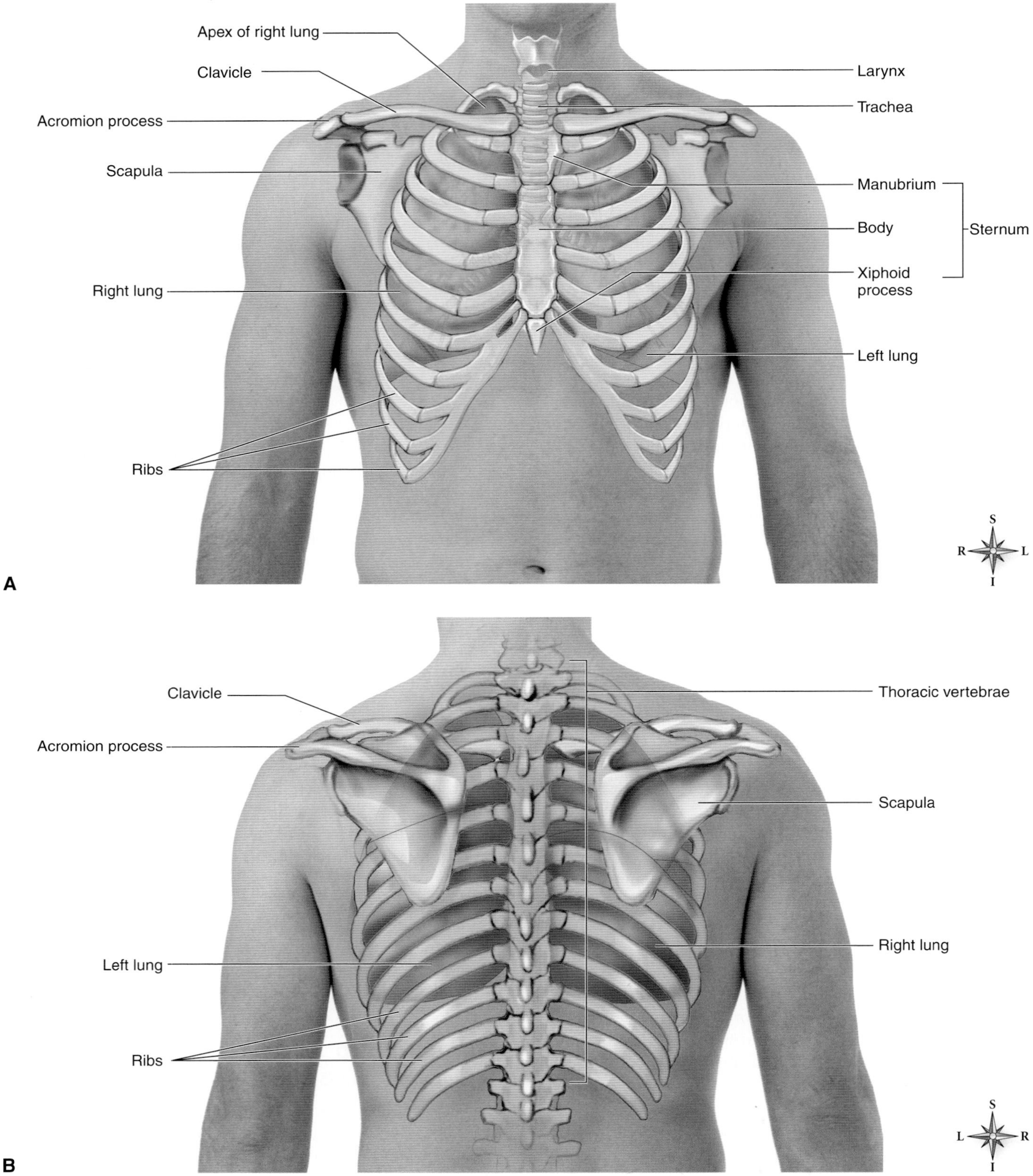

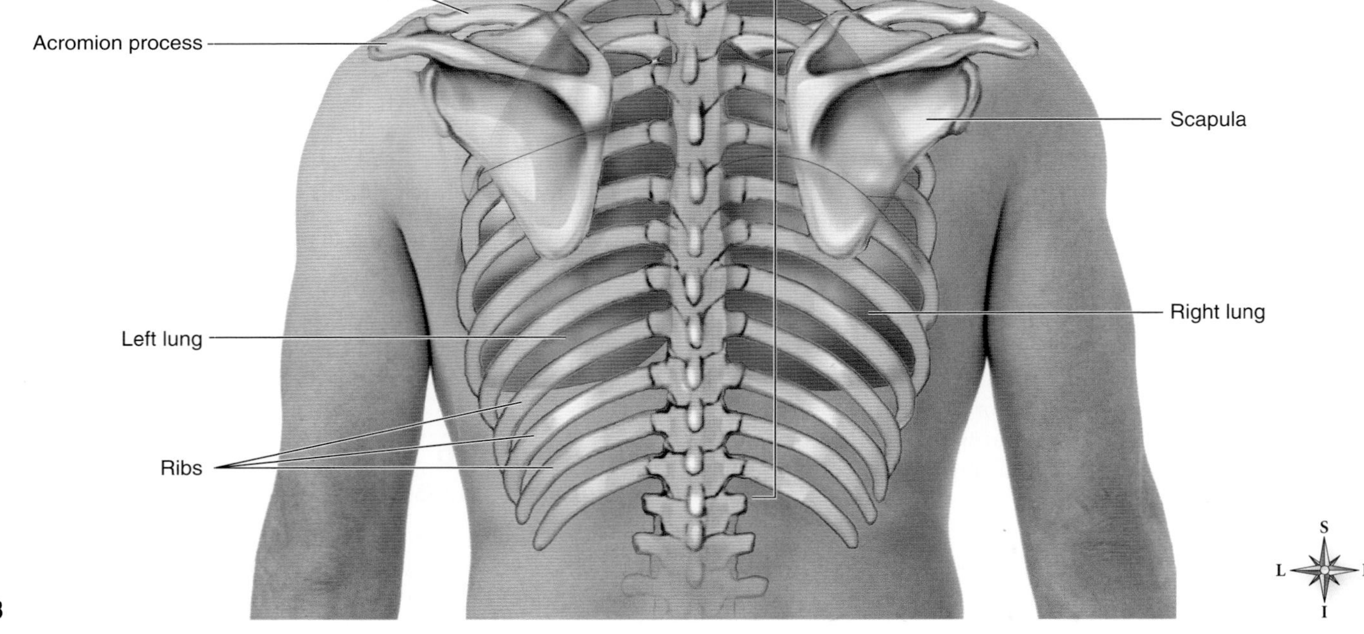

FIGURE 35-9 Bony structures of the chest. These structures form a protective and expandable cage around the lungs and heart. **A,** Anterior view. **B,** Posterior view.

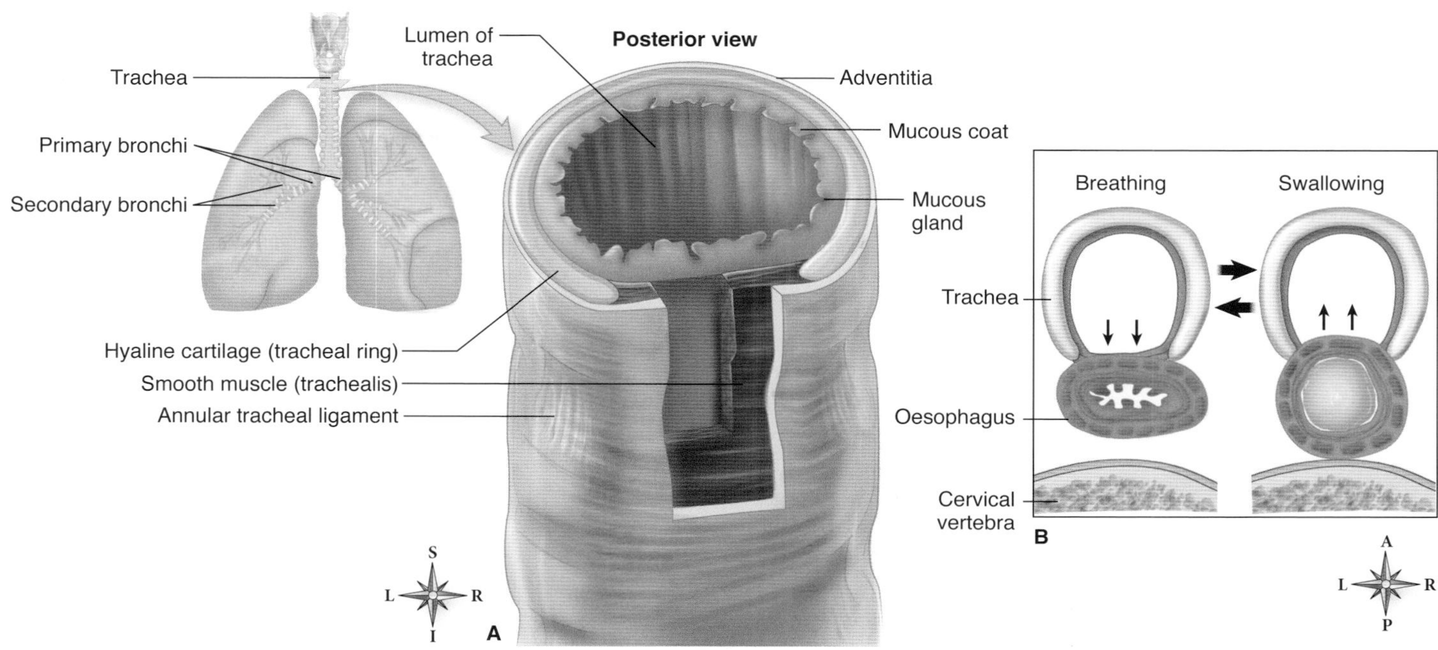

FIGURE 35-10 Cross-section of the trachea. The inset at the top shows where the section was cut. **A,** Structure of the trachea. **B,** Incomplete tracheal rings and elasticity of posterior tracheal wall allow the oesophagus to expand during swallowing.

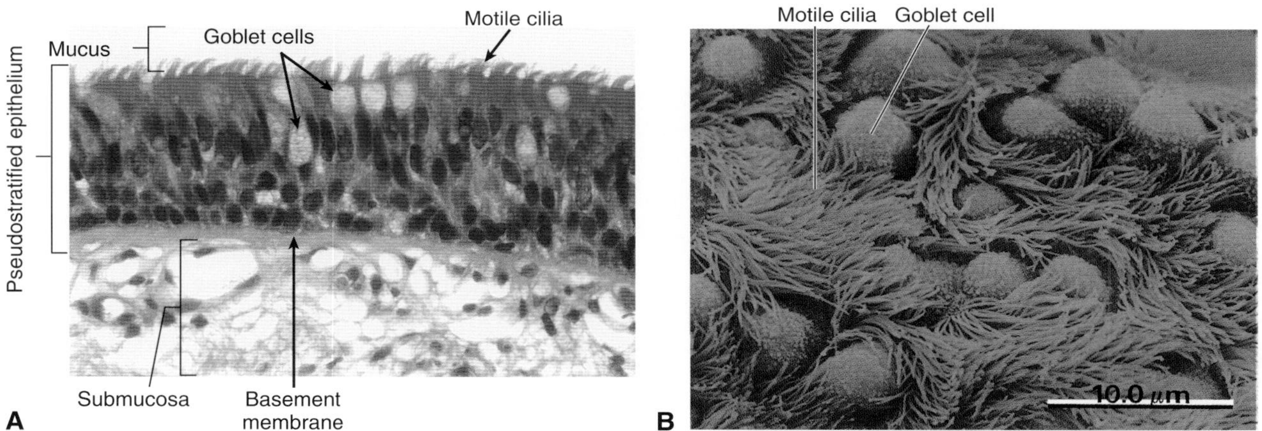

FIGURE 35-11 Respiratory mucosa. A, Light micrograph (×200) and **B,** Scanning electron micrograph (×2000) of respiratory mucosa. Note the numerous motile (moving) cilia and mucus-producing goblet cells.

lungs, but have complete rings in the sections within the lungs. Ciliated mucosa lines the bronchi, as it does the trachea.

Each primary bronchus enters the lung on its respective side and there immediately divides into smaller branches called **secondary bronchi.** The secondary bronchi continue to branch and form tertiary bronchi and then small **bronchioles.** The trachea and the two primary bronchi and their many branches resemble an inverted tree trunk with its branches and are therefore spoken of as the **bronchial tree** (**Figure 35-12**).

There are 23 levels of branching in the bronchial tree, producing a huge number of tiny bronchioles. As these bronchioles subdivide into smaller and smaller tubes, they eventually terminate in microscopic branches sometimes called *terminal bronchioles*. The terminal bronchioles are the last branches that serve solely to conduct air.

The terminal bronchioles divide into *respiratory bronchioles* that have thin, gas-exchanging walls. The respiratory bronchioles proceed onward into **alveolar ducts,** which end in one or more alveolar

BOX 35-1 *health matters* | Keeping the Trachea Open

Often a tube is placed through the mouth, pharynx, and larynx into the trachea before patients leave the operating room, especially if they have been given a muscle relaxant. This procedure is called **endotracheal intubation.** The purpose of the tube is to ensure an open airway (see parts *A* and *B* of the figure). To ensure that the tube enters the trachea rather than the nearby oesophagus (which leads to the stomach), anatomical landmarks such as the vocal folds are visualized. Likewise, the distinct feel of the V-shaped groove called the *interarytenoid notch* (see **Figure 35-8**, *A*) can help guide the proper insertion of the tube.

Another procedure done commonly in today's modern hospitals is a **tracheostomy—**that is, the cutting of an opening into the trachea (part *C* of the figure). A surgeon may perform this procedure so that a suction device can be inserted to remove secretions from the bronchial tree or so that mechanical ventilation can be used to improve ventilation of the lungs.

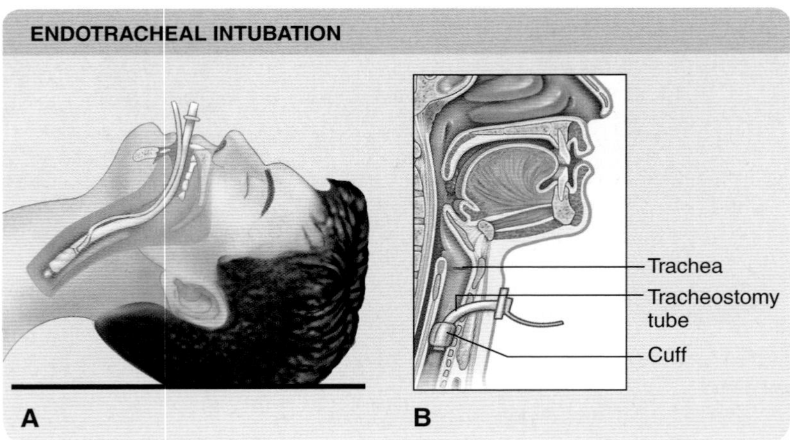

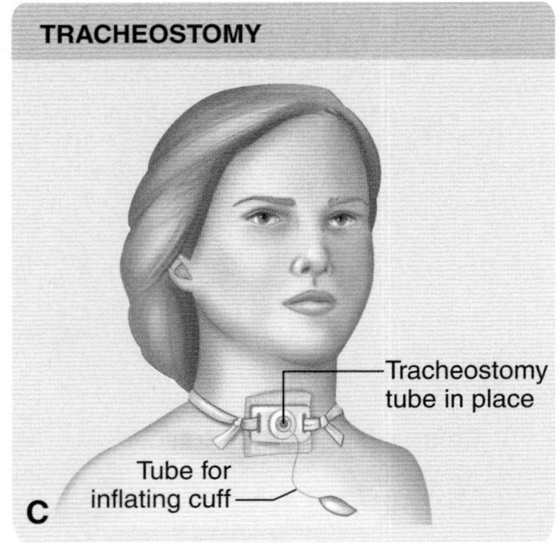

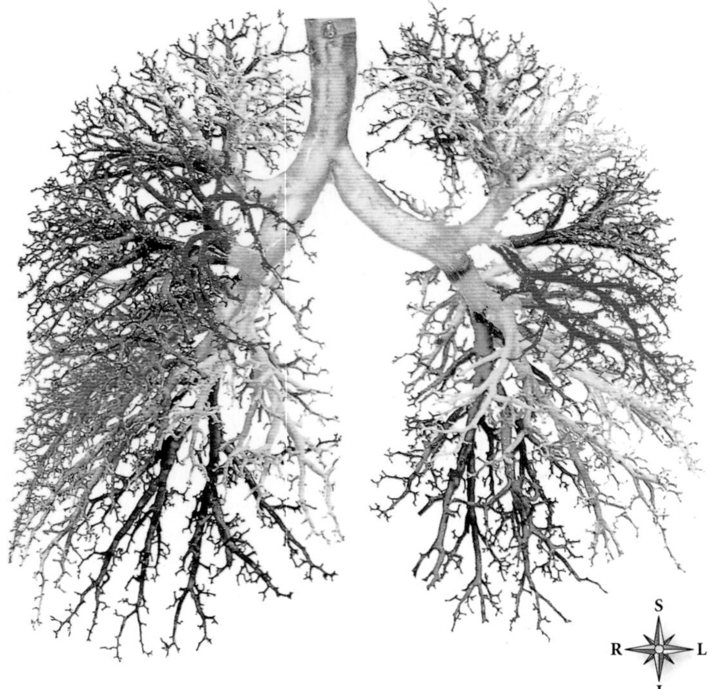

FIGURE 35-12 Plastic cast of air spaces of the lungs. The cast was prepared by pouring liquid plastic into the airways of a cadaver lung—a different colour for each bronchopulmonary segment supplied by its own tertiary bronchus. After the plastic hardened, the soft tissue was removed, leaving the branched form of the lower respiratory tract that is pictured here (compare with **Figure 35-17**).

sacs, the walls of which consist of numerous **alveoli** (**Figure 35-13**; see also **Figure 35-1**). Some 300 million alveoli are estimated to be present in our two lungs.

The structure of the secondary and tertiary bronchi and bronchioles shows some modification of the primary bronchial structure. The cartilaginous rings become irregular and disappear entirely into the smaller bronchioles. By the time the branches of the bronchial tree dwindle to form the respiratory bronchioles, alveolar ducts and sacs, and the alveoli, only the internal surface layer of cells remains. In other words, the walls of these microscopic structures consist of a single layer of simple, squamous epithelial tissue (**Figure 35-14**; see **Figure 35-13**). As we shall see, this structural fact makes it possible for them to perform their functions.

Figure 3-20 in the Brief Atlas of the Human Body shows a detailed, three-dimensional cast of the entire bronchial tree of both lungs.

Structure of the Alveoli

Note the spongelike structure of the alveoli in **Figure 35-13**, *B*, and **35-14**. Besides the bronchiolar pathways leading to and from the alveoli, alveolar pores through the septa separating adjacent alveoli also permit air movement. It may be helpful to imagine the lung as a moist sponge that draws air into and out of numerous tiny, wet air spaces as the sponge is squeezed and released.

The alveoli are the primary gas exchange structures of the respiratory tract (**Figure 35-15**; see **Figure 35-14**). Alveoli are very effective in exchanging carbon dioxide (CO_2) and oxygen (O_2) because each alveolus is extremely thin-walled, each alveolus lies in contact with blood capillaries, and there are millions of alveoli in each lung.

The barrier across which gases are exchanged between alveolar air and blood is called the **respiratory membrane** (see **Figure 35-15**, *inset*). The respiratory membrane consists of the alveolar epithelium, the capillary endothelium, and their joined basement membranes.

The surface of the respiratory membrane inside each alveolus is coated with a fluid containing **surfactant** produced by *type II cells* of the alveolar wall. Surfactant helps reduce surface tension—the force of attraction between water molecules—of the fluid. Thus it helps prevent each alveolus from collapsing and "sticking shut" as air moves in and out during respiration. In the next chapter, we explore this important role of surfactant further.

Another factor that helps prevent alveolar collapse is the structural interdependence of all the connected alveoli. Looking at the sponge-like structure of lung tissue in **Figure 35-13**, *B*, and **Figure 35-14**, you can see that alveoli are connected to one another and exert a pull on each other to help keep them all open—just as in a sponge.

Functions of the Bronchi and Alveoli

The tubes composing the bronchial tree perform the same function as the trachea—that of distributing air to the lung's interior. Calculations show that 23 levels of branching produce the optimum ability

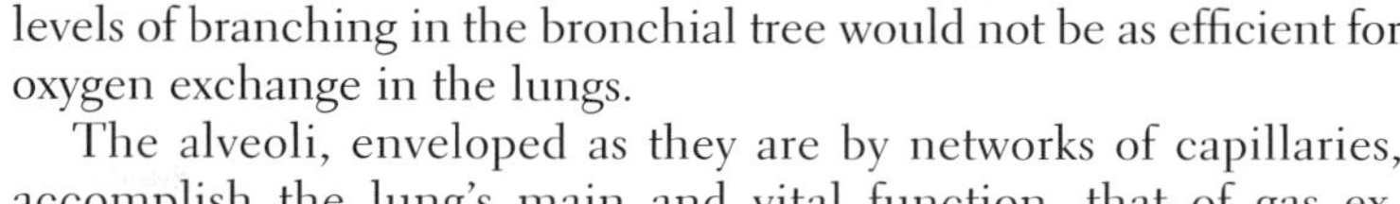

to transfer oxygen to the pulmonary blood. Any more or any fewer levels of branching in the bronchial tree would not be as efficient for oxygen exchange in the lungs.

The alveoli, enveloped as they are by networks of capillaries, accomplish the lung's main and vital function, that of gas exchange between air and blood. It has been observed that "the lung passages all serve the alveoli" just as "the circulatory system serves the capillaries".

Recall that in addition to serving as air distribution passageways or gas exchange surfaces, the anatomical components of the respiratory tract and lungs cleanse, warm, and humidify inspired air. Air entering the nose is generally contaminated with one or more common irritants; examples include insects, dust, pollen, and bacterial organisms. A remarkably effective air purification mechanism removes almost every form of contaminant before inspired air reaches the alveoli or terminal air sacs in the lungs.

The layer of protective mucus that covers a large portion of the membrane that lines the respiratory tree serves as the most important air purification mechanism. More than 125 mL of respiratory mucus is produced daily. It forms a continuous sheet, called a *mucus blanket*, that covers the lining of the air distribution tubes in the respiratory tree. This layer of cleansing mucus moves upward to the pharynx from the lower portions of the bronchial tree on millions of hairlike cilia that cover the epithelial cells in the respiratory mucosa (see **Figure 35-11**). The microscopic cilia that cover epithelial cells in the respiratory mucosa are motile, beating or moving in only one direction. The result is movement of mucus toward the pharynx—a mechanism sometimes called the *ciliary escalator*.

Respiratory cilia can "taste" bitter toxins and respond by moving more rapidly in an effort to clear the toxin molecules from the airway. Prolonged exposure to toxins, as with cigarette smoke, can paralyze the cilia. Eventually, the ciliary escalator begins to fail and accumulations of mucus trigger the typical smoker's cough, an effort to clear the secretions.

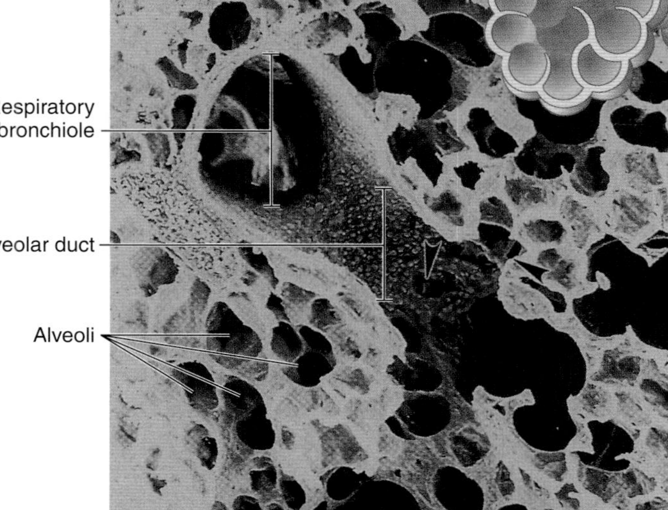

FIGURE 35-13 Alveoli. A, Respiratory bronchioles subdivide to form tiny tubes called *alveolar ducts*, which end in clusters of alveoli called *alveolar sacs*. **B,** Scanning electron micrograph of a bronchiole, alveolar ducts, and surrounding alveoli. The *arrowhead* indicates the opening of alveoli into the alveolar duct.

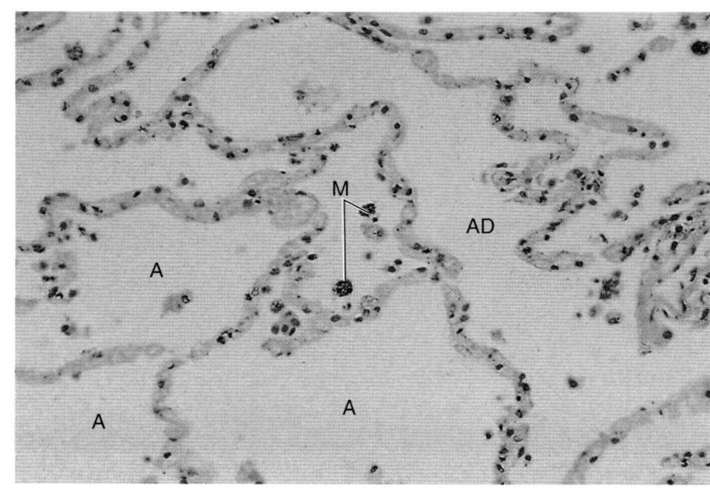

FIGURE 35-14 Micrograph of alveoli. Note the thin alveolar walls and open alveolar spaces *(A)*. An occasional macrophage *(M)*, which provides immune defence, can be seen in several of the alveolar spaces. *AD,* Alveolar duct.

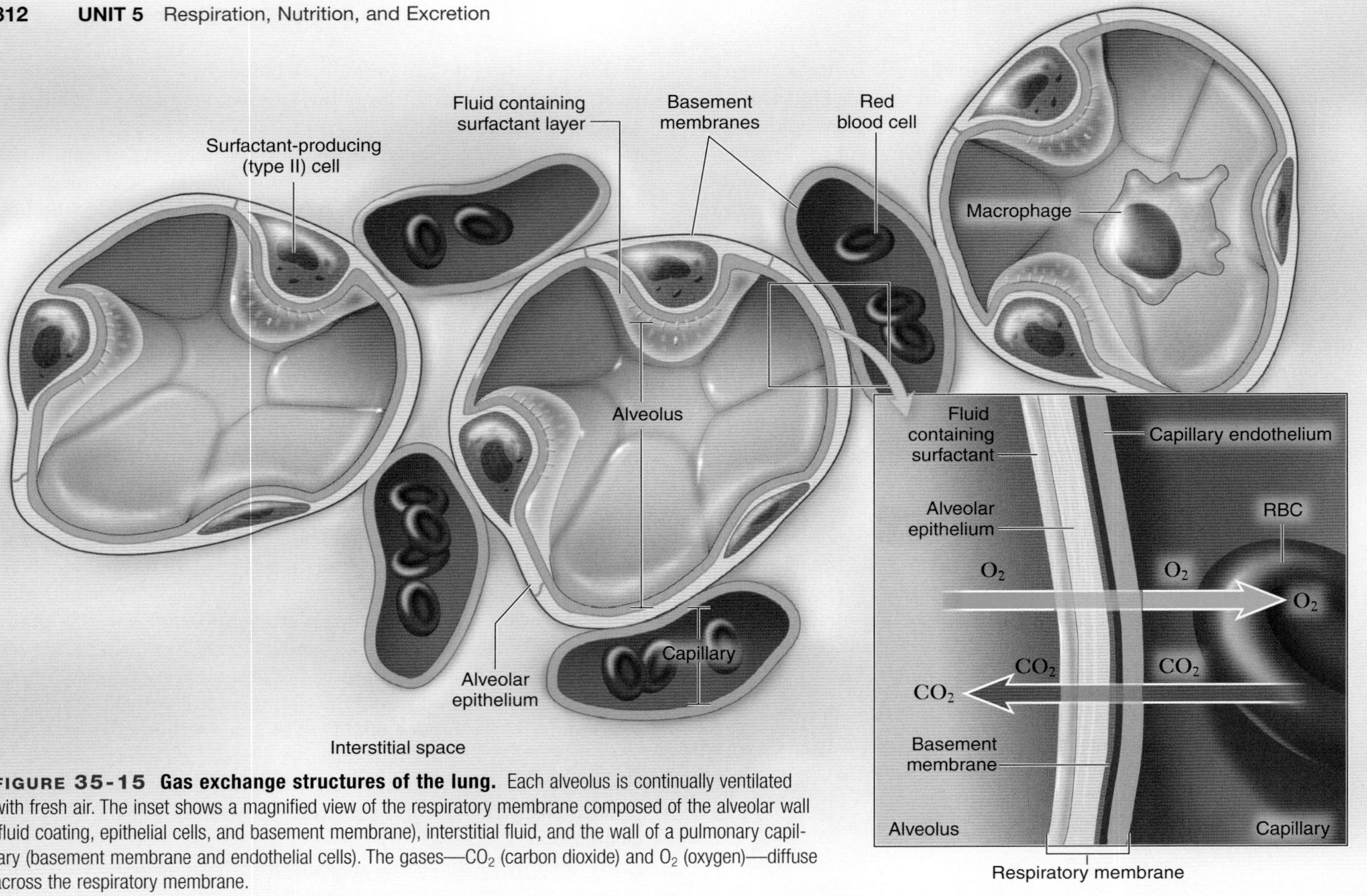

FIGURE 35-15 Gas exchange structures of the lung. Each alveolus is continually ventilated with fresh air. The inset shows a magnified view of the respiratory membrane composed of the alveolar wall (fluid coating, epithelial cells, and basement membrane), interstitial fluid, and the wall of a pulmonary capillary (basement membrane and endothelial cells). The gases—CO_2 (carbon dioxide) and O_2 (oxygen)—diffuse across the respiratory membrane.

Additional information about the functional anatomy of each section of the respiratory tract can be found in **Table 35-1**.

CONNECT IT! 

Because it is exposed to the external environment, the respiratory tract could be extremely vulnerable. Visualize how the respiratory tract defends itself in ***Protective Strategies of the Respiratory Tract*** online at ***Connect It!***

Quick CHECK

7. How are the trachea and primary bronchi held open so that they do not collapse during inspiration?
8. What is meant by the term *bronchial tree*?
9. What characteristics of alveoli enable them to efficiently exchange gases with blood?

LUNGS

Structure of the Lungs

The lungs are cone-shaped organs, large enough to fill the pleural portion of the thoracic cavity completely (see **Figure 35-9**). They extend from the diaphragm to a point slightly above the clavicles and lie against the ribs both anteriorly and posteriorly. The medial surface of each lung is roughly concave to allow room for the mediastinal structures and for the heart, but the concavity is greater on the left than on the right because of the position of the heart. The primary bronchi and pulmonary blood vessels (bound together by connective tissue to form what is known as the **root** of the lung) enter each lung through a slit on its medial surface called the **hilum.**

The broad inferior surface of the lung, which rests on the diaphragm, constitutes the **base,** whereas the pointed upper margin is the **apex** (**Figure 35-16**). Each apex projects above a clavicle (see **Figure 35-9**, A). The **costal surface** of each lung lies against the ribs and is rounded to match the contours of the thoracic cavity.

Each lung is divided into lobes by fissures. The left lung is partially divided into two lobes (superior and inferior) and the right lung into three lobes (superior, middle, and inferior). Note in **Figure 35-17**, A, that an **oblique fissure** is present in both lungs. In the right lung a **horizontal fissure** is also present that separates the superior from the middle lobe. After the primary bronchi enter the lungs, they branch into *secondary*, or *lobar*, bronchi that enter each lobe. Thus, in the right lung, three secondary bronchi are formed that enter the superior, middle, and inferior lobes. Each secondary

TABLE 35-1 Summary of Respiratory Tract Structures*

STRUCTURE	DESCRIPTION	FUNCTION
Upper Respiratory Tract	Portion of the respiratory tract outside the thoracic cavity	Processing of incoming air Conducts air to/from lungs Vocalization and phonation Olfaction
Nasal cavity	Lumen of nose, separated into left and right portions by nasal septum supported by cartilage, vomer, and perpendicular plate of ethmoid; supported laterally by nasal conchae	Conducts air between atmosphere (external environment) and pharynx Warms, humidifies, cleans inspired air
Anterior nares (external nares)	Nostrils External openings of nasal cavity	Boundary between external environment and nasal cavity
Vestibule	Extends from the anterior nares to the inferior meatus Supported by cartilage of septum and ala Lined with skin epidermis (keratinized stratified squamous epithelium) with vibrissae (hairs)	Conducts air between external environment and respiratory portion of nasal cavity Vibrissae prevent entry of large contaminants
Respiratory portion	Extends from vestibule to posterior nares Supported by bones of septum and nasal conchae, which curve to form meatuses Lined with highly vascular respiratory mucosa (pseudostratified ciliated columnar epithelium) Olfactory epithelium in superior lining contains numerous sensory receptors	Conducts air between vestibule and pharynx Meatuses create turbulence to assist processing of inspired air Mucosa warms, humidifies, and cleans inspired air Olfaction
Paranasal sinuses	Four pairs of air-filled spaces within frontal, maxillary, ethmoid, and sphenoid bones of skull Lined with pseudostratified ciliated columnar epithelium Drain into the nasal cavity	Reduce weight of skull Help warm and humidify air
Posterior nares (internal nares)	Openings from the nasal cavity into the pharynx	Boundary between nasal cavity and pharynx
Pharynx	Throat Extends from posterior nares to the oesophagus Supported by occipital bone and skeletal muscle Lined with mucous membrane (nonkeratinized stratified squamous epithelium)	Conducts air between nasal cavity and larynx
Nasopharynx	Segment of pharynx posterior to nasal cavity Pharyngeal tonsils in posterior wall	Conducts air between posterior nares and oropharynx
Oropharynx	Segment of pharynx posterior to oral cavity Pair of palatine tonsils in lateral walls Lingual tonsils in anterior wall, at base of tongue	Conducts air between nasopharynx and/or oral cavity and laryngopharynx
Laryngopharynx	Segment of pharynx posterior to opening of larynx and superior to opening of oesophagus	Conducts air between oropharynx and larynx
Tonsils	Ring of individual aggregations of lymphoid nodules	Immune protection of respiratory and digestive mucosa (see Chapter 31)
Larynx	Voicebox Extends from laryngopharynx to trachea Supported by nine cartilages connected by muscle and ligaments Lined with mucosa (pseudostratified ciliated columnar epithelium, except epiglottis and vocal folds)	Conducts air between the pharynx and trachea Prevents food from entering lower airways Vocalization Ciliary escalator removes contaminants
Epiglottis	Flexible "lid" of larynx Covered/lined with nonkeratinized stratified squamous, transitioning through simple columnar to pseudostratified ciliated columnar epithelium at border with vestibule	Flexes during swallowing to cover larynx and prevent food from entering lower airways (see Chapter 40)
Vestibule	Extends from base of epiglottis to vestibular folds	Conducts air between pharynx and vestibular folds
Vestibular folds (false vocal folds)	Superior pair of lateral mucosal folds	Slow contaminants dripping toward lower airways
Ventricle (laryngeal ventricle)	Space between the vestibular folds and vocal folds	Conducts air between mucosal folds of larynx

*Listed in order of air flow during inspiration.

(continued)

TABLE 35-1 Summary of Respiratory Tract Structures—cont'd

STRUCTURE	DESCRIPTION	FUNCTION
Upper Respiratory Tract—cont'd		
Larynx—cont'd		
Vocal folds (true vocal folds or vocal cords)	Inferior pair of lateral mucosal folds Each fold supported by skeletal muscle and strong vocal ligament at medial edge Covered with nonkeratinized stratified squamous epithelium Glottis: vocal folds and space between them (rima glottidis)	Prevent contaminants from entering lower airways Produce vibrations when pulled together during expiration (vocalization)
Infraglottic cavity	Segment below glottis, between vocal folds and trachea	Conducts air between vocal folds and trachea
Lower Respiratory Tract	Portion of respiratory tract within the thoracic cavity Also called bronchial tree	Conducts air to/from gas-exchange tissues of lungs
Trachea	Windpipe Extends from larynx to primary bronchi Supported by C-shaped cartilage rings Lined with respiratory mucosa (pseudostratified ciliated columnar epithelium)	Conducts air between the larynx and bronchi Ciliary escalator removes contaminants
Bronchi	Treelike branching of airways 23 levels of branching, producing a huge number of individual airways Supported by cartilage rings (incomplete outside lungs; complete inside lungs) Lined with respiratory mucosa (pseudostratified ciliated columnar epithelium)	Conduct air between trachea and lungs Ciliary escalator removes contaminants
Primary bronchi	Left and right branch from trachea, one to each lung	Conduct air to/from the lungs
Secondary bronchi (lobar bronchi)	Branches of the primary bronchi; three from the right, two from the left	Conduct air to/from the lobes of lungs
Tertiary bronchi (segmental bronchi)	Branches of the secondary bronchi	Conduct air to/from the various bronchopulmonary segments of lungs
Bronchioles	Smallest branches (20 levels of branching)	Conduct air to/from alveoli
Alveoli	Microscopic air spaces at terminals of bronchial tree Lined with simple squamous epithelium that joins with pulmonary capillary endothelium to form the respiratory membrane	Exchange of gases (CO_2, O_2) between air and pulmonary blood Surfactant lining alveoli prevents collapse of air spaces

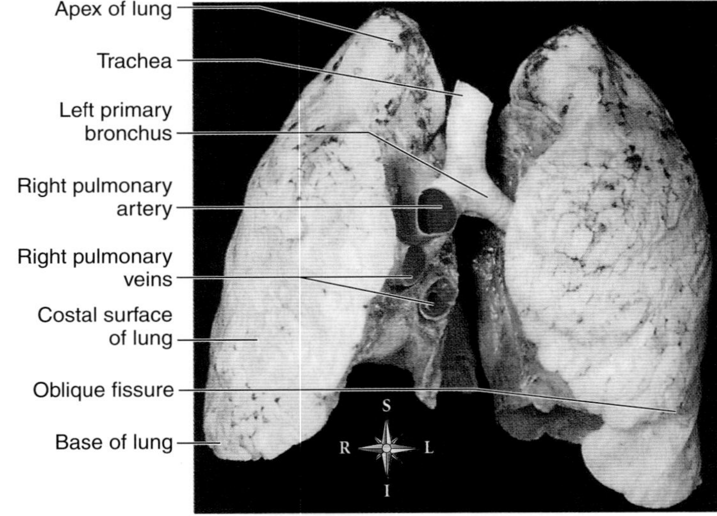

FIGURE 35-16 Anterior view of trachea, bronchi, and lungs. The lower respiratory tract has been dissected from a cadaver and its organs separated to show them clearly.

bronchus is named for the lung lobe that it enters; for example, the superior secondary bronchus enters the superior lobe. The left primary bronchus divides into two secondary bronchi entering the superior and inferior lobes of that lung.

The lobes of the lung can be further subdivided into functional units called **bronchopulmonary segments** (see **Figure 35-17**, *B*). These segments may be called by their anatomically descriptive names (for example, *anterior segment of superior lobe*) or by Roman numerals. Both systems of naming the segments are shown in **Figure 35-17**, *B*.

Each bronchopulmonary segment is served by a separate *tertiary*, or *segmental*, bronchus. The interior of each bronchopulmonary segment consists of almost innumerable tubes of dwindling diameter that make up the bronchial tree and serve as air distributors. The smallest tubes terminate in the smallest, but functionally most important, structures of the lung—the alveoli, or "gas exchangers".

Visceral pleura covers the outer surfaces of the lungs and adheres to them much as the skin of an apple adheres to the apple (**Figure 35-18**).

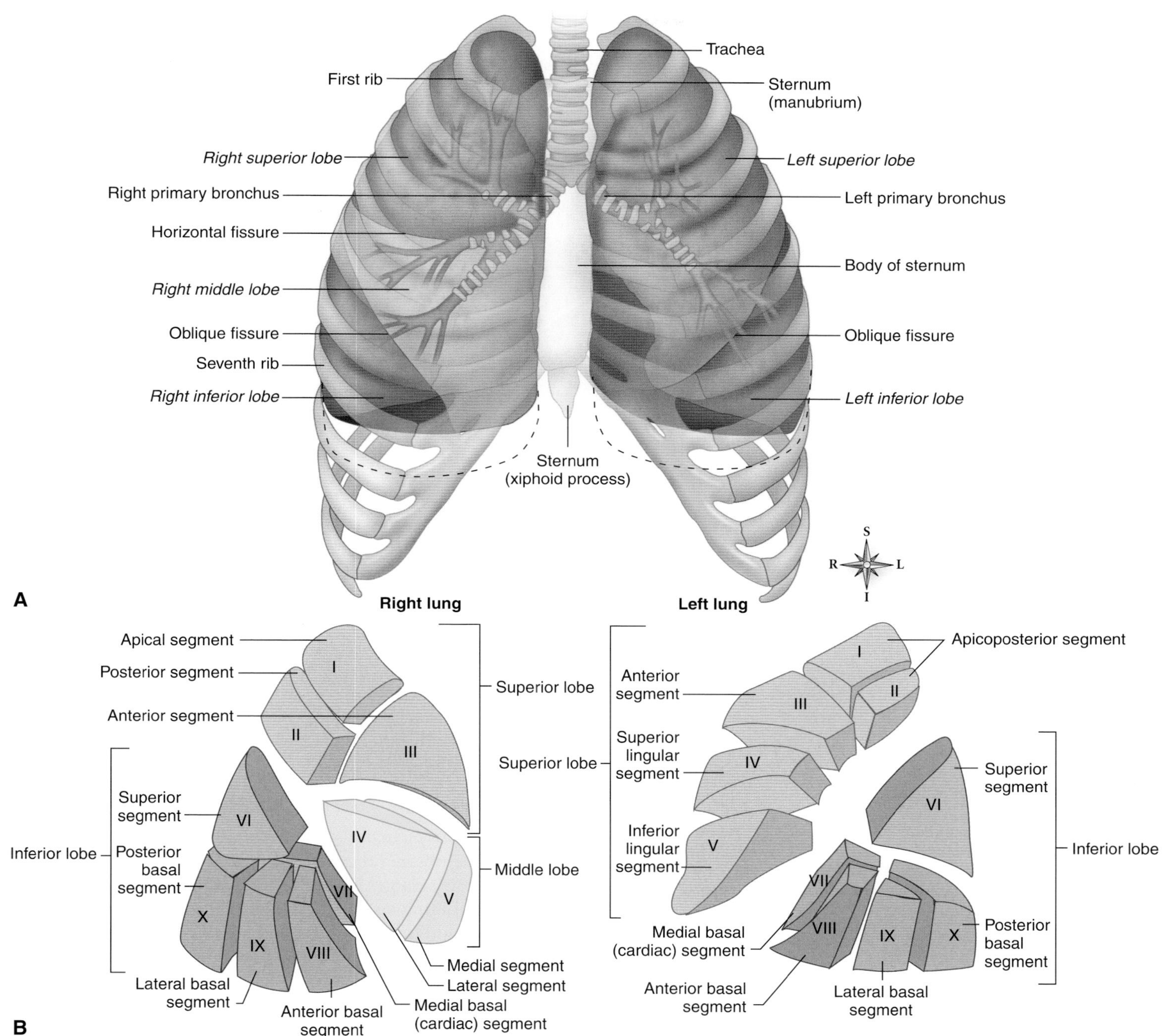

FIGURE 35-17 Lobes and segments of the lungs. A, Anterior view of the lungs, bronchi, and trachea. **B,** Expanded diagram showing the bronchopulmonary segments. Note—the left lung is divided into ten bronchopulmonary segments. Often a pair of segments fuse in the superior lobe and a pair fuse in the inferior lobe, resulting in a total of eight segments in the left lung.

Functions of the Lungs

The lungs perform two functions—air distribution and gas exchange. Air distribution to the alveoli is the function of the tubes of the bronchial tree. Gas exchange between air and blood is the joint function of the alveoli and the networks of blood capillaries that envelop them. These two structures—one part of the respiratory system and the other part of the circulatory system—together serve as highly efficient gas exchangers. Why? Because together they provide an enormous surface area, the **respiratory membrane,** where the very thin-walled alveoli and equally thin-walled pulmonary capillaries come in contact (see **Figures 35-14** and **35-15**). This makes possible extremely rapid diffusion of gases between alveolar air and pulmonary capillary blood. It has been estimated that if the lungs' 300 million or so alveoli could be opened up flat, they would form a surface about the size of a small home's floor plan—that is, about 85 square metres, more than 40 times the surface area of the entire

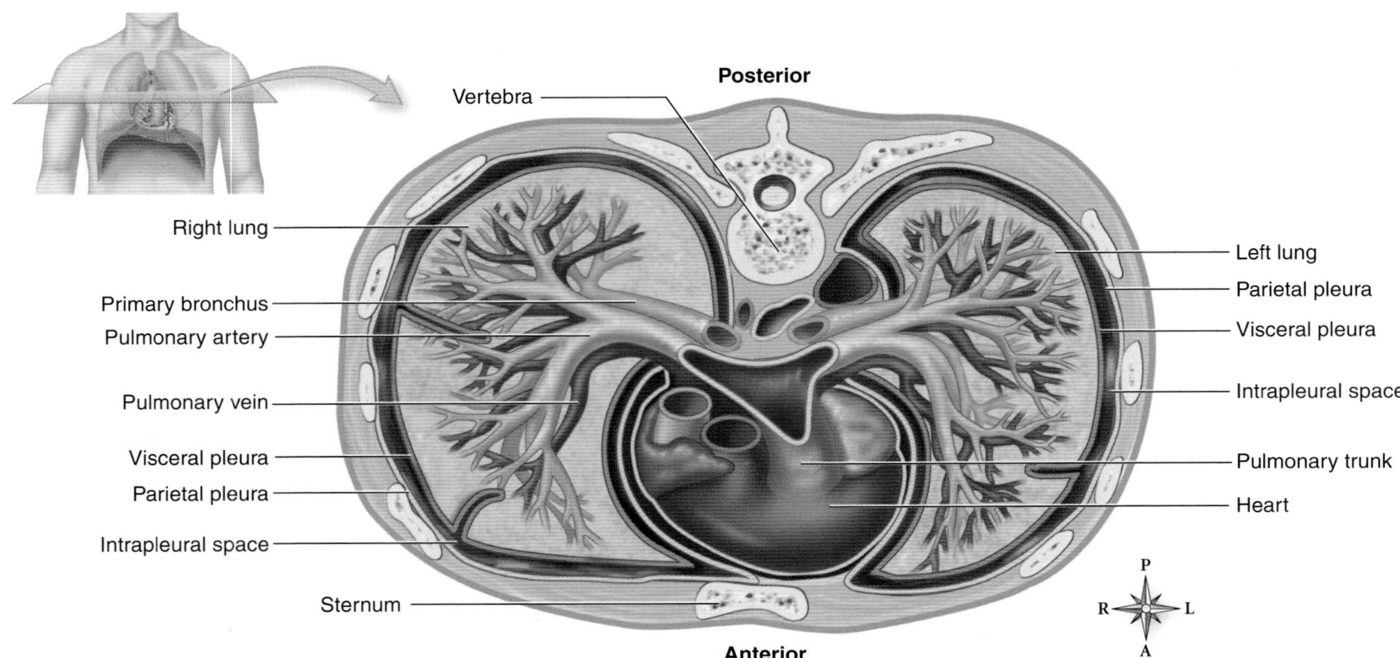

FIGURE 35-18 Lungs and pleura (transverse section). Note the parietal pleura lining the right and left pleural divisions of the thoracic cavity before folding inward near the bronchi to cover the lungs as the visceral pleura. The intrapleural space separates the parietal and visceral pleura. The heart, oesophagus, and aorta are shown in the central mediastinum.

body! No wonder such large amounts of oxygen can be so quickly loaded into the blood while large amounts of carbon dioxide are rapidly unloaded from it.

CONNECT IT! 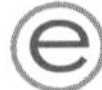

The surgical removal of portions of the lung is a "treatment of last resort" for severe cases of emphysema, which is classified as a **chronic obstructive pulmonary disease,** or **COPD.** For more information and photographs, check out ***Lung Volume Reduction Surgery*** online at ***Connect It!***

THORAX

Structure of the Thoracic Cavity

As described in Chapter 1, the thoracic cavity has three divisions, separated from each other by partitions of **pleura.** The parts of the cavity occupied by the lungs are the *pleural divisions.* The space between the lungs occupied mainly by the oesophagus, trachea, large blood vessels, and heart is the *mediastinum* (see **Figure 35-18**).

The **parietal pleura** lines the entire thoracic cavity. It adheres to the internal surface of the ribs and the superior surface of the diaphragm, and it partitions off the mediastinum. A separate pleural sac thus encases each lung. Because the outer surface of each lung is covered by the visceral layer of the pleura, the visceral pleura lies against the parietal pleura, separated only by a potential space (pleural space) that contains just enough pleural fluid for lubrication (see **Figure 35-18**). Thus, when the lungs inflate with air, the smooth, moist visceral pleura coheres to the smooth, moist parietal pleura. Friction is thereby avoided, and respirations are painless. In *pleurisy* (pleuritis), on the other hand, the pleura is inflamed and respirations become painful.

Functions of the Thoracic Cavity

The thorax plays a major role in respiration. Because of the elliptical shape of the ribs and the angle of their attachment to the spine, the thorax becomes larger when the chest is raised and smaller when it is lowered. Lifting up the chest raises the ribs so that they no longer slant downward from the spine, and because of their elliptical shape, both the depth (from front to back) and the width of the thorax are enlarged. (If this does not sound convincing to you, examine a skeleton to see why it is so.) An even greater change in thoracic volume occurs when the diaphragm contracts and relaxes. When the diaphragm contracts, it flattens out and thus pulls the floor of the thoracic cavity downward—thereby enlarging the volume of the thorax. When the diaphragm relaxes, it returns to its resting, domelike shape—thus reducing the volume of the thoracic cavity. It is these changes in thorax size that bring about inspiration and expiration (discussed on pp. 828–830 in Chapter 36).

Quick CHECK

10. What is meant by the term *lobe of the lung*? What is a bronchopulmonary segment?
11. How does the structure of the diaphragm enable it to participate in breathing movements?

cycle of life

Respiratory Tract Respiration involves the exchange of O_2 and CO_2 between the organism and its environment. The exchange must occur between air in the lungs and blood and then between blood and every body cell. In addition to the structural components of the body through which the respiratory gases must pass, haemoglobin plays a vital role in the respiration process. Each component of the system may be affected by developmental defects, by age-related structural changes, pulmonary disease, or by loss of function during the life cycle.

Premature birth can cause potentially fatal respiratory problems. A very low birth weight baby may have inadequate blood flow to the lungs, an inability to ventilate properly, and inadequate quantities of surfactant. Other diseases that cause serious respiratory problems are also associated with specific age groups. Examples are cystic fibrosis and asthma in children and certain types of obstructive pulmonary disease and emphysema in older adults. Pneumothorax occurs more often in young adult females.

Numerous age-related changes affect lung capacity, make ventilation difficult, or reduce the oxygen- or carbon dioxide–carrying capacity of blood. For example, in older adulthood the ribs and sternum tend to become more fixed and less able to expand during inspiration, the respiratory muscles are less effective, and haemoglobin levels are often reduced. The result is a general reduction in respiratory efficiency in old age. •

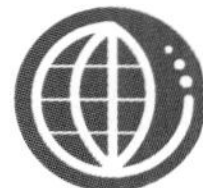

the big picture | Respiratory Tract

Understanding the relationship of structure to function is critical to an understanding of homeostasis in all body organ systems. The anatomy of the respiratory system components permits the distribution of air and the exchange of respiratory gases. This dual function ultimately allows for both exchange of gases between environmental air and blood in the lungs and, finally, gas exchange between blood and individual body cells. In addition to delivery of air to the tiny terminal air passageways and alveoli for gas exchange with blood, components of the upper respiratory tract effectively filter, warm, and humidify the air we breathe.

Respiratory functions are dependent on the structural organization of the system parts and on the interrelationship of those components with other body systems, including the nervous, cardiovascular, muscular, and immune systems. For example, nerves regulate the thoracic and abdominal muscles that drive breathing, as well as the smooth muscles that regulate airflow through the bronchial tree. The immune system guards against airborne pathogens and irritants. Understanding the proper functioning and regulation of the physiology of the respiratory system, discussed in Chapters 36 and 37, depends on your understanding of its structural components and their relationships to one another and to other body organ systems—the "big picture" of total-body homeostasis. •

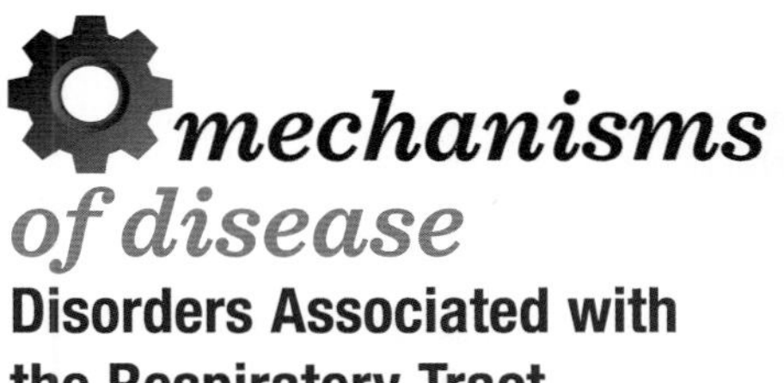

Disorders Associated with the Respiratory Tract

Disorders of the Upper Respiratory Tract

Inflammation and Infection

Any infection localized in the mucosa of the upper respiratory tract (nose, pharynx, and larynx) can be called an **upper respiratory infection (URI)** and is often named for the specific structure involved.

Rhinitis (from the Greek *rhinos,* "nose") is an inflammation of the mucosa of the nasal cavity. It is commonly caused by a viral infection, as in the common cold (caused by rhinoviruses) or flu (caused by influenza viruses). The colder temperatures in the nasal cavity during the winter allow rhinoviruses to replicate more rapidly, contributing to the higher rates and severity of the common cold during cold weather. Rhinitis can also be caused by nasal irritants or an allergic reaction to airborne allergens. Allergic rhinitis, or "hay fever", occurs in sensitive people in a seasonal pattern, depending on the allergens involved (e.g., pollen). The excessive mucus production that results from the inflammatory response involved in rhinitis can cause fluid to drip down the pharynx and into the oesophagus and lower respiratory tract. This dripping may cause sore throat, coughing, and upset stomach. Irritation of the **nasal mucosa** itself often triggers the sneeze reflex. Elimination of the causative factor, rest, and the use of antihistamines and decongestants usually relieve these symptoms.

Pharyngitis is inflammation or infection of the pharynx. Commonly referred to as a "sore throat", it is often due to viral invasion. Bacterial infection by *Streptococcus* bacteria is termed "strep throat". The common complaint is a sore throat, but redness and difficulty swallowing (dysphagia) often accompany it. Throat lozenges, rest, and fluid intake are encouraged, and antibiotics are prescribed for severe infections.

Laryngitis, or inflammation of the mucous lining of the larynx, is characterized by oedema of the vocal folds, resulting in hoarseness (dysphonia) or loss of voice. Besides infections, inhalation of toxic or irritating fumes (i.e., smoking), endotracheal intubation, vocal abuse (i.e., public speaking), and alcohol ingestion can precipitate laryngitis. In children younger than 5 years, it may cause difficulty breathing, a condition often called **croup.** Conservative treatment, including limiting speech, is usually effective. A rare but much more severe and rapidly progressing viral form of laryngeal oedema called **epiglottitis** is always treated as a medical emergency because of the potential for airway obstruction (see ***Swollen Larynx*** online at ***Connect It!***).

Tonsillitis is inflammation of one or more of the masses of lymphatic tissue embedded in the mucous membrane of the pharynx (see p. 739). Most cases of tonsillitis result in inflammation and swelling of the palatine tonsils in the oropharynx and the pharyngeal tonsils or adenoids in the nasopharynx. Repeated episodes of infection and chronic swelling of these tonsillar tissues require aggressive antibiotic therapy and, in severe cases, even surgical removal.

However, **tonsillectomy,** the surgical procedure used to remove inflamed or enlarged tonsillar tissue, is no longer considered a "first-choice" treatment option in routine cases of tonsillitis. As a result, the number of tonsillectomies performed each year continues to decrease. Physicians now recognize the value of lymphatic tissue in the body's defence mechanism and delay tonsillectomy with its rare but potentially serious complications—including severe haemorrhage—until more conservative treatment options have proved ineffective.

Occasionally, surgical removal may be required, especially in children, if adenoidal and tonsillar infection and hypertrophy do not respond to antibiotic therapy. In these cases, sleep disturbance, fatigue, and other potentially serious complications involving the heart and lungs can result from progressive upper

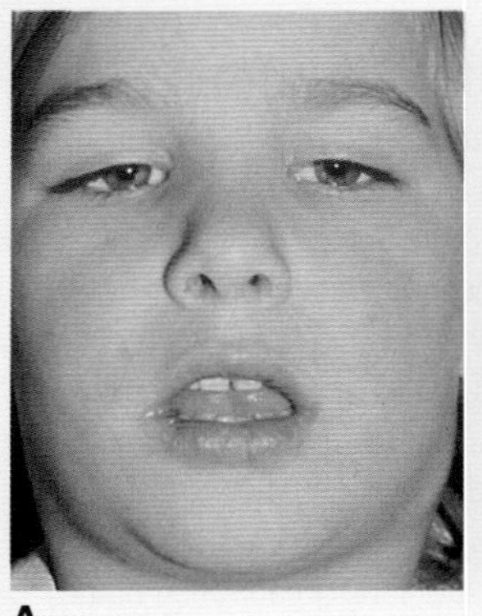
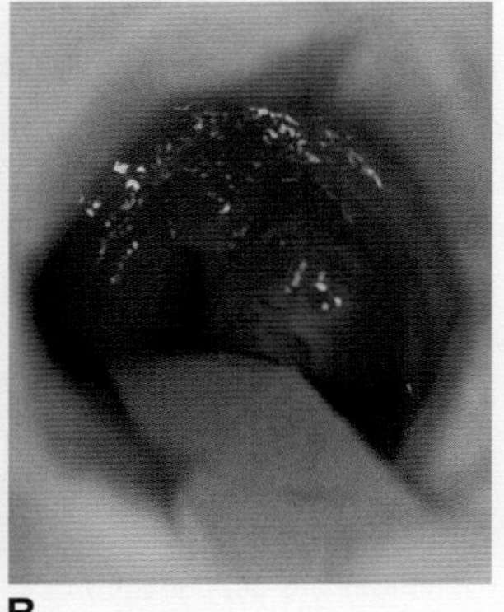
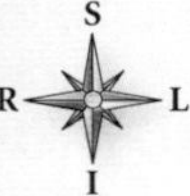

FIGURE 35-19 Tonsillitis. A, Facial appearance of a child with marked enlargement of the tonsils and adenoids. He must keep his mouth open to breathe and shows signs of fatigue. **B,** Enlarged tonsils can be seen meeting in the midline of the pharynx.

airway obstruction over time. **Figure 35-19**, *A,* shows the fatigued facial appearance of a child with severely enlarged tonsils who must keep his mouth open to breathe. In **Figure 35-19**, *B,* note how the enlarged tonsils in this child have all but filled the pharynx and are nearly meeting in the midline, thus seriously limiting airflow.

Because the upper respiratory mucosa is continuous with the mucous lining of the sinuses, auditory tube (eustachian tube), middle ear, and lower respiratory tract, URIs have the unfortunate tendency to spread. It is not unusual to see a common cold progress to **sinusitis** (sinus infection) or **otitis media** (middle ear infection).

Anatomical Disorders

Nasal obstruction can be caused by displacement of the nasal septum from the midline of the nasal cavity, called a **deviated septum.** Most individuals have a small amount of septal cartilage protruding into one nasal passage; however, some are born with a congenital defect that results in various degrees of blockage on one or both sides of the nasal cavity. Damage from injury or infection may also cause a deviated septum. If breathing is impaired, surgical intervention is required to correct the deformity.

A common problem associated with a deviated septum is snoring. Pronounced snoring may be a symptom of **sleep apnoea.** In these individuals there is a transition during sleep from loud snoring to variable periods of complete cessation of breathing. These periods of apnoea are characterized by restlessness and often end in a loud "snort" before a normal breathing pattern resumes. Sleep apnoea may be repeated many times each night and cause excessive daytime sleepiness and other symptoms related to chronic lack of oxygen.

Trauma to the nose can occur because the nose projects some distance from the front of the face. Usually, however, common bumps and other injuries cause little, if any, serious damage. **Epistaxis,** or nosebleed, can be caused by violent sneezing or nose blowing, chronic infection or inflammation (as in rhinitis), hypertension, or a strong bump or blow to the nose. Immediate direct pressure with an ice pack will often slow or stop the bleeding.

Disorders of the Lower Respiratory Tract

A range of conditions can interfere with the lower respiratory tract functions of gas exchange and ventilation. Some of these disorders, such as restrictive and obstructive conditions, are discussed in Chapter 36. For now, we concentrate on infections and lung cancer.

CONNECT IT! 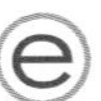

Bronchial and lung disorders are often detected and monitored by chest x-ray imaging. Find out more in ***Pulmonary Radiology*** online at ***Connect It!***

Lower Respiratory Infection

Acute bronchitis is a common condition characterized by acute inflammation of the tracheobronchial tree, most commonly caused by infection. Part of or preceded by an acute URI, it is most prevalent in winter. Predisposing factors include chilling, fatigue, malnutrition, and exposure to air pollutants. The protective functions of the bronchial epithelium are disturbed and excessive fluid accumulates in the bronchi. Acute bronchitis often begins with a nonproductive cough, but malaise, slight fever, back and muscle pain, and a sore throat occur if a URI is present. Rest is indicated until the fever subsides, and cough suppressants may be used if the cough is troublesome.

Pneumonia is a common condition characterized by acute inflammation of the lungs. Depending on the cause, the alveoli and bronchi become swollen and plugged with mucous secretions. In bacterial pneumonia, a thick fibrin and neutrophil (pus)-containing exudate forms (**Figure 35-20**).

The vast majority of pneumonia cases result from infection by *Streptococcus pneumoniae* bacteria (see **Figure 35-20**), but pneumonia can also be caused by several other bacteria, viruses, and fungi. For example, **legionnaires' disease** is a form of bacterial pneumonia caused by infection with the *Legionella pneumophila* organism. Contaminated air conditioning cooling towers and whirlpool spas are sources of infection.

Viral infections can produce pneumonia as well. A dramatic example is the 2003 outbreak of *severe acute respiratory syndrome (SARS)* caused by the SARS-associated coronavirus (SARS-CoV). Unless treated very early, most SARS cases progress to pneumonia. SARS, like most viral infections responsible for pneumonia, is transmitted by close contact of individuals.

The term *aspiration pneumonia* is used to describe lung infections caused by the inhalation of vomit or other infective material. It is common in acute alcohol intoxication and as a complication of anaesthesia.

Pneumonia is often associated with a high fever, chills, headache, cough, and chest pain. Increases in white blood cell (WBC) numbers (leucocytosis) and depressed blood oxygen levels (hypoxia) are common findings. The fact that each day more than 10,000 litres of potentially contaminated air enters the respiratory

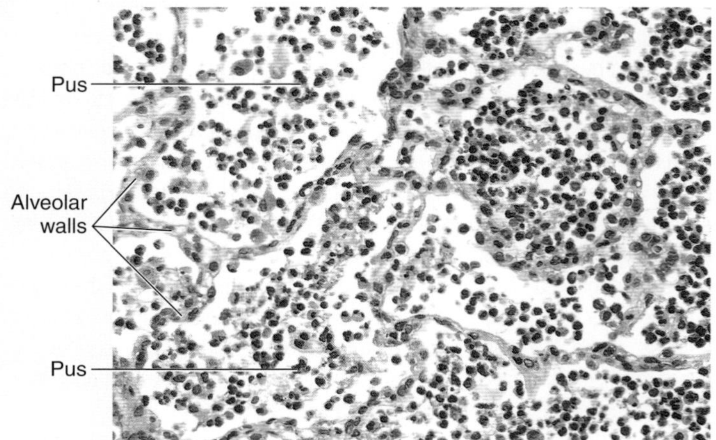

FIGURE 35-20 Acute bacterial pneumonia. The alveolar walls are thickened and the spaces filled with a fibrin exudate and neutrophils (pus)—a classic finding in acute pneumonia caused by bacterial infection.

system helps explain why pneumonia is such a common illness—especially in individuals with lowered resistance or impaired immune systems.

Types include *lobar pneumonia,* which typically affects an entire lobe of the lung (**Figure 35-21**), and *bronchopneumonia,* in which patches of infection are scattered along portions of the bronchial tree and generally involve more than one lobe. Treatment involves antimicrobial drugs to control the infection and supportive therapy, including the administration of supplemental oxygen. Removal of tracheobronchial secretions may be necessary to maintain airway integrity.

Tuberculosis (TB) is a chronic bacillus infection caused by *Mycobacterium tuberculosis.* It is a highly contagious disease, transmitted by airborne mechanisms (i.e., inhalation of infectious droplets). Inflammatory lesions called "tubercles" form around colonies of TB bacilli in the lung and produce the characteristic symptoms of cough, fatigue, chest pain, weight loss, and fever. As TB progresses, lung haemorrhage and dyspnoea (laboured breathing) may develop. If large areas of the lung are infected and tissue is destroyed, scar tissue may develop and cause reduced lung volume and restrictive lung disease. TB can invade other tissues or organs such as the lymphatic system, genitourinary system, and bone tissue. Because of the advancement of modern antimicrobial agents, the incidence of TB in the United Kingdom dropped dramatically in the last century. However, various factors have allowed multi-drug resistant tuberculosis (MDR-TB) to emerge in groups of drug users, prisoners, and specific ethnic groups born outside the UK. The incidence of TB has not reached epidemic proportions, but it continues to disproportionately affect hard-to-reach groups of people in society. The health authorities in many large cities have prioritized the delivery of appropriate clinical and public health services with the aim of achieving a year-on-year decrease in the number of cases.

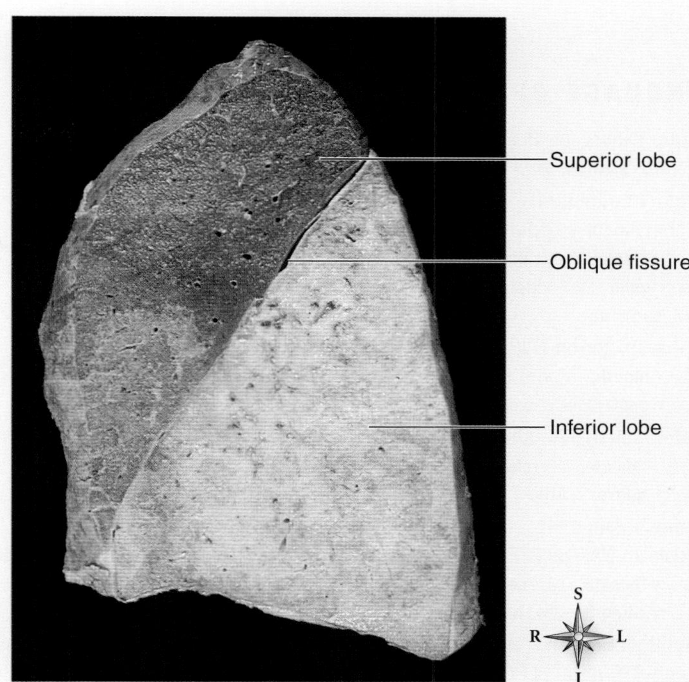

FIGURE 35-21 Lobar pneumonia. Exudate fills many of the alveoli and ducts of a single lobe of the left lung. Note the difference in texture and colour of the affected inferior lobe. (See **Figure 35-20**.)

Lung Cancer

Lung cancer is a malignancy of pulmonary tissue that not only destroys the vital gas exchange tissues of the lungs but, like other cancers, may also invade other parts of the body (metastasis). Lung cancer most often develops in damaged or diseased lungs (see **Figure 35-21**). The most common predisposing condition associated with lung cancer is cigarette smoking (accounting for about 75% of lung cancer cases). In 1950, British epidemiologist Sir Richard Doll published the results of a groundbreaking scientific study that established for the first time the deadly link between smoking and lung cancer. His pioneering research was uniquely important in medical history. At the time of his death in 2005 at age 92, Doll was regarded as one of the most eminent scientists of his generation and one whose work will ultimately prevent tens of millions of premature tobacco-related deaths around the world. Other factors thought to cause lung cancer include exposure to "secondhand" cigarette smoke, asbestos, chromium, coal products, petroleum products, rust, and ionizing radiation (as in radon gas).

Lung cancer may be arrested if detected early on routine chest x-ray films or by other diagnostic procedures such as bronchoscopy. Depending on the size, location, and exact type of malignancy involved, several strategies are available for treatment. Surgery is perhaps the most effective single treatment for most localized lung cancers. In a lobectomy, only the affected lobe of a lung is removed. **Pneumonectomy** is the surgical removal of an entire lung. Chemotherapy can also cause a cure or remission in selected cases, as can radiation therapy or concurrent (combination) chemotherapy and radiation treatment.

Unfortunately, in a high proportion of patients diagnosed with the most common type of lung cancer, called non–small cell lung cancer, the disease has already spread, or metastasized, to lymph nodes and other organs by the time a diagnosis is made. Non–small cell lung cancer (NSCLC) accounts for approximately 87% of all cancers of the lung diagnosed in the UK. Non–small cell lung cancer patients are treated with a combination of lobectomy, chemotherapy, and radiation therapy. Recently the National Institute for Health and Care Excellence (NICE) has also approved the use of an immunotherapeutic agent (pembrolizumab) for untreated, PD-L1-positive metastatic NSCLC in adults. Pembrolizumab can be used as the first-line treatment in some patients or following chemotherapy.

The 5-year survival rate for patients with NSCLC depends on their grading and stage at diagnosis. The 5-year survival rate for patients with stage 1A is about 49%, but if the cancer has spread to other parts of the body and the patient is at stage IV it falls to 1%.

So-called small cell lung cancers usually appear first in the lining of the respiratory passageways. Curable if detected very early, this type of cancerous lesion is often treated by surgical removal, with **photodynamic therapy (PDT),** or both. This deadly form of the disease spreads very rapidly and is usually not effectively treated in its later stages with either standard concurrent radiation plus chemotherapy or by the standard treatment options followed by operation.

CONNECT IT! 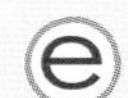

Learn how light can be used to treat lung cancer! Check out ***Photodynamic Therapy*** online at ***Connect It!***

LANGUAGE OF SCIENCE *(continued from p. 800)*

oblique fissure (oh-BLEEK FISH-ur)
[*obliqu-* **slanted,** *fissur-* **cleft**]

olfactory epithelium (ohl-FAK-tor-ee ep-ih-THEE-lee-um)
[*olfact-* **smell,** *-ory* **relating to,** *epi-* **upon,** *-theli-* **nipple,** *-um* **thing**] *pl.,* epithelia

oropharynx (or-oh-FAIR-inks)
[*oro-* **mouth,** *-pharynx* **throat**] *pl.,* oropharynges or oropharynxes

palatine tonsil (PAL-ah-tyne TON-sil)
[*palat-* **palate,** *-ine* **relating to,** *tons-* **goitre,** *-il* **little**]

paranasal sinus (pair-ah-NAY-zal SYE-nus)
[*para-* **beside,** *-nas-* **nose,** *-al* **relating to,** *sinus* **hollow**]

parietal pleura (pah-RYE-ih-tal PLOO-rah)
[*parie-* **wall,** *-al* **relating to,** *pleura* **side of body**] *pl.,* pleurae

pharyngeal tonsil (fah-RIN-jee-al TON-sil)
[*pharyng-* **throat,** *-al* **relating to,** *tons-* **goitre,** *-il* **little**]

pharynx (FAIR-inks)
[*pharynx* **throat**] *pl.,* pharynges or pharynxes

pleura (PLOO-rah)
[*pleura* **side of body**] *pl.,* pleurae

primary bronchus (BRONG-kus)
[*prim-* **first,** *-ary* **relating to,** *bronchus* **windpipe**] *pl.,* bronchi

respiratory membrane (RES-pih-rah-tor-ee)
[*re-* **again,** *-spir-* **breathe,** *-tory* **relating to,** *membran-* **thin skin**]

respiratory mucosa (RES-pih-rah-tor-ee myoo-KOH-sah)
[*re-* **again,** *-spir-* **breathe,** *-tory* **relating to,** *muc-* **slime,** *-os-* **characterized by,** *-a* **thing**]

respiratory portion (RES-pih-rah-tor-ee POR-shun)
[*re-* **again,** *-spir-* **breathe,** *-tory* **relating to**]

secondary bronchus (BRONG-kus)
[*second-* **second,** *bronchus* **windpipe**] *pl.,* bronchi

septum (SEP-tum) pl., septa

surfactant (sur-FAK-tant)
[**combination of** *surf*(ace) *act*(ive) *a*(ge)*nt*]

thyroid cartilage (THY-royd KAR-tih-lij)
[*thyr-* **shield,** *-oid* **like**]

trachea (TRAY-kee-ah)
[*trachea* **rough duct**] *pl.,* tracheae or tracheas

turbinate (TUR-bih-nayt)
[*turbin-* **top (spinning toy),** *-ate* **of or like**]

upper respiratory tract (RES-pih-rah-tor-ee trakt)
[*re-* **again,** *-spir-* **breathe,** *-tory* **relating to,** *tract* **trail**]

ventricle (VEN-trih-kul)
[*ventr-* **belly,** *-icle* **little**]

vestibular fold (ves-TIB-yoo-lar)
[*vestibul-* **entrance hall,** *-ar* **relating to**]

vestibule (VES-tih-byool)
[*vestibul-* **entrance hall**]

vibrissa (vye-BRISS-ah)
[*vibrissa* **nostril hair**] *pl.,* vibrissae

visceral pleura (VISS-er-al PLOO-rah)
[*viscer-* **internal organ,** *-al* **relating to,** *pleura* **side of body**] *pl.,* pleurae

vocal fold
[*voca-* **voice,** *-al* **relating to**]

vomeronasal organ (VNO) (voh-mer-oh-NAY-sal)
[*vomer-* **plowshare (vomer bone),** *nas-* **nose,** *-al* **relating to**]

LANGUAGE OF MEDICINE

acute bronchitis (ah-KYOOT brong-KYE-tis)
[*acut-* **sharp,** *bronch-* **windpipe,** *-itis* **inflammation**]

chronic obstructive pulmonary disease (COPD) (KRON-ik ob-STRUK-tiv PUL-moh-nair-ee)
[*chron-* **time,** *-ic* **relating to,** *pulmon-* **lung,** *-ary* **relating to**]

cleft palate (kleft PAL-ett)

croup (kroop)
[*croup* **croak**]

deviated septum (DEE-vee-ay-ted SEP-tum)
[*devia-* **turn aside,** *-ate* **process,** *septum* **partition**] *pl.,* septa

endotracheal intubation (en-doh-TRAY-kee-al in-tyoo-BAY-shun)
[*endo-* **within,** *-trache-* **rough duct,** *-al* **relating to,** *in-* **within,** *-tub-* **tube,** *-ation* **process**]

epiglottitis (epp-ih-glaw-TYE-tis)
[*epi-* **upon,** *-glotti-* **mouth of windpipe (glottis),** *-itis* **inflammation**]

epistaxis (ep-ih-STAK-sis)
[*epi-* **upon,** *-staxis* **drip**]

laryngitis (lar-in-JYE-tis)
[*laryng-* **voice box (larynx),** *-itis* **inflammation**]

legionnaires' disease (LEE-jen-airz)
[**named for American Legion convention, location of first diagnosed case**]

otitis media (oh-TYE-tis MEE-dee-ah)
[*oti-* **ear,** *-itis* **inflammation,** *media* **middle**]

pharyngitis (fair-in-JYE-tis)
[*pharyng-* **throat (pharynx),** *-itis* **inflammation**]

photodynamic therapy (PDT) (foh-toh-dye-NAM-ik)
[*photo-* **light,** *-dynam-* **moving force,** *-ic* **relating to**]

pneumonectomy (nyoo-moh-NEK-toh-mee)
[*pneumon-* **lung,** *-ec-* **out,** *-tom-* **cut,** *-y* **action**]

pneumonia (nyoo-MOH-nee-ah)
[*pneumon-* **lung,** *-ia* **condition**]

rhinitis (rye-NYE-tis)
[*rhin-* **nose,** *-itis* **inflammation**]

sinusitis (sye-nyoo-SYE-tis)
[*sinus-* **hollow,** *-itis* **inflammation**]

sleep apnoea (APP-nee-ah)
[*a-* **not,** *-pnoea* **breathe**]

tonsillectomy (ton-sih-LEK-toh-mee)
[*tons-* **goitre,** *-il* **little,** *-ec-* **out,** *-tom-* **cut,** *-y* **action**]

tonsillitis (ton-sih-LYE-tis)
[*tons-* **goitre,** *-il-* **little,** *-itis* **inflammation**]

tracheostomy (tray-kee-OS-toh-mee)
[*trache-* **rough duct,** *-os-* **mouth or opening,** *-tom-* **cut,** *-y* **action**]

tuberculosis (TB) (too-ber-kyoo-LOH-sis)
[*tuber-* **swelling,** *-cul-* **little,** *-osis* **condition**]

upper respiratory infection (URI) (RES-pih-rah-tor-ee)
[*re-* **again,** *-spir-* **breathe,** *-tory* **relating to,** *infec-* **stain,** *-tion* **process**]

case study

Sharon looked away from her toddler for just a second. Her 2-year-old daughter, Zoe, was playing on the floor next to her desk. When Sharon glanced down again, Zoe was squirming, holding her throat and making little squeaking sounds. Zoe looked up at her mother with scared eyes. *She's choking!* Sharon's voice screamed in her head. She first thought about performing abdominal thrusts on Zoe but then remembered that was not the correct action because the child was still able to breathe a little (as evidenced by the squeaking sound). She didn't want to cause whatever had been swallowed to block Zoe's airway completely. Sharon grabbed the phone and dialled the emergency service. The paramedics were there in minutes, but it seemed like hours; they took Zoe to the hospital. Based on Zoe's signs and symptoms, the doctors immediately scheduled a bronchoscopy. In this procedure, a thin tube (with a camera) is inserted through the mouth and down the throat.

1. What is the correct sequence of structures through which the bronchoscope passed into Zoe's throat?
   a. Nasopharynx, laryngopharynx, trachea, larynx
   b. Oropharynx, laryngopharynx, larynx, trachea
   c. Laryngopharynx, oropharynx, larynx, trachea
   d. Trachea, larynx, oropharynx, laryngopharynx

After finding nothing in the trachea, the doctor focused attention on the first tube to the right (after the trachea).

2. What is the name of this tube?
   a. Primary bronchiole
   b. Tracheal limb
   c. Primary bronchus
   d. Alveolar duct
3. What type of epithelium lines both this tube and the trachea?
   a. Stratified squamous
   b. Simple cuboidal
   c. Simple columnar
   d. Ciliated pseudostratified columnar

And there it was! Zoe had attempted to swallow a small magnetic ball, one of her older brother's toys. The toy had gone into her respiratory tract instead of her oesophagus. The doctor inserted forceps through the bronchoscope, clamped onto the ball, and pulled it out.

4. What structure usually directs material into the oesophagus instead of the trachea when we swallow?
   a. Epiglottis
   b. Glottis
   c. Concha
   d. Vocal fold

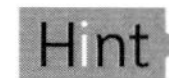
To solve a case study, you may have to refer to the glossary or index, other chapters in this textbook, ***Connect It!,*** and other resources.

CHAPTER SUMMARY

To download an MP3 version of the chapter summary for use with your mobile device, access the ***Audio Chapter Summaries*** *online at evolve.elsevier.com.*

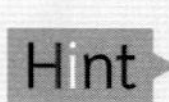
Scan this summary after reading the chapter to help you reinforce the key concepts. Later, use the summary as a quick review before your class or before a test.

Structural Plan of the Respiratory Tract

A. Structure determined by respiratory system functions of air distributor and gas exchanger—supplying oxygen and removing carbon dioxide from cells (**Figure 35-1**)
   1. Alveoli—sacs that serve as gas exchangers; all other parts of respiratory system serve as air distributors
   2. The respiratory system also warms, filters, and humidifies air
   3. Respiratory organs involved in speech, homeostasis of body pH, and olfaction

B. The respiratory system is divided into two structural divisions
   1. Upper respiratory tract—the organs are located outside the thorax and consist of the nose, nasopharynx, oropharynx, laryngopharynx, and larynx
   2. Lower respiratory tract—the organs are located within the thorax and consist of the trachea, the bronchial tree, and the lungs
   3. Accessory structures include the oral cavity, rib cage, and diaphragm

Upper Respiratory Tract

A. Nose
   1. Structure of the nose—external portion consists of a bony and cartilaginous frame covered by skin containing sebaceous glands
      a. The two nasal bones meet and are surrounded by the frontal bone to form the root
      b. The nose is surrounded by the maxilla (**Figure 35-2**)
   2. Internal portion of the nose (nasal cavity) lies over the roof of the mouth, separated by the palatine bones
      a. Cleft palate—condition in which the palatine bones fail to unite completely and only partially separate the nose and the mouth, thereby producing difficulty swallowing
      b. Cribriform plate—separates the roof of the nose from the cranial cavity
      c. Septum—separates the nasal cavity into right and left cavities; it consists of four structures: the perpendicular plate of the ethmoid bone, the vomer bone, the vomeronasal cartilages, and the septal nasal cartilage
   3. Each nasal cavity is divided into three passageways: superior, middle, and inferior meatuses (**Figure 35-3**)
   4. Anterior (external) nares—external openings to the nasal cavities; open into the vestibule
   5. Sequence of airflow through the nose into the pharynx—anterior nares to the vestibule to all three meatuses simultaneously and then to the posterior (internal) nares

6. Nasal mucosa
   a. Air passes over respiratory mucosa, which contains a rich blood supply (**Figure 35-4**)
   b. Olfactory epithelium—special sensory membrane containing many olfactory nerve cells and a rich lymphatic plexus
7. Paranasal sinuses
   a. Four pairs of air-containing spaces that open or drain into the nasal cavity
   b. Each is lined with respiratory mucosa (**Figure 35-5**)
8. Functions of the nose
   a. Provides a passageway for air travelling to and from the lungs
   b. Filters the air, aids speech, and makes possible the sense of smell

B. Pharynx (throat)
1. Structure of pharynx
   a. Tubelike structure extending from the base of the skull to the oesophagus
   b. Made of muscle and divided into three parts (**Figure 35-3**)—nasopharynx, oropharynx, and laryngopharynx
2. Pharyngeal tonsils
   a. Located in the nasopharynx
   b. Called *adenoids* when they become enlarged
3. Oropharynx contains two pair of organs—the palatine tonsils (most commonly removed in tonsillectomy) and the lingual tonsils (rarely removed)
4. Functions of the pharynx—pathway for the respiratory and digestive tracts

C. Larynx (**Figures 35-6** and **35-7**)
1. Location of larynx—positioned between the root of the tongue and the upper end of the trachea
2. Structure of larynx
   a. Consists of cartilages attached to each other by muscle
   b. Lined by a ciliated mucous membrane, which forms two pairs of folds (**Figure 35-8**)—vestibular folds (false vocal folds) and vocal folds
3. Cartilages (framework) of the larynx—formed by nine cartilages
   a. Single laryngeal cartilages—the three largest cartilages: the thyroid cartilage, the epiglottis, and the cricoid cartilages
   b. Paired laryngeal cartilages—three pairs of smaller cartilages: the arytenoid, the corniculate, and the cuneiform cartilages
4. Muscles of the larynx
   a. Intrinsic muscles both insert and originate within the larynx
   b. Extrinsic muscles insert in the larynx but originate on some other structure
5. Functions of the larynx—forms part of the airway to the lungs and produces the voice

D. Additional information is found in **Table 35-1**

Lower Respiratory Tract

A. Trachea—often called “windpipe” (**Figure 35-10**)
1. Structure of trachea
   a. Extends from the larynx to the primary bronchi
   b. Wall composed of (outer) adventitia, (middle) smooth muscle and C-shaped cartilage rings, (inner) respiratory mucosa; posterior wall is very elastic (**Figure 35-11**)
   c. Incomplete rings and posterior elasticity allows oesophagus to expand into trachea during swallowing
2. Functions of trachea—furnishes part of the open airway to the lungs; obstruction causes death

B. Bronchi and alveoli
1. Structure of bronchi
   a. Lower end of the trachea divides into two primary bronchi, one on the right and one on the left; right one is larger and more vertical than left
   b. Primary bronchi enter the lung and divide into secondary bronchi, which branch into bronchioles and eventually divide into alveolar ducts and alveoli
   c. 23 levels of branching (**Figure 35-12**)
2. Structure of alveoli—the primary gas-exchange structures (**Figures 35-13** and **35-14**)
   a. Respiratory membrane—the barrier between which gases are exchanged by alveolar air and blood (**Figure 35-15**)
   b. Respiratory membrane consists of the alveolar epithelium, the capillary endothelium, and their joined basement membranes
   c. Surfactant—a component of the fluid coating the respiratory membrane that reduces surface tension; produced by type II cells
   d. Structural interdependence of connected alveoli also helps prevent alveolar collapse
3. Functions of bronchi and alveoli
   a. Distribute air to the lung's interior; 23 levels of branching are optimal for oxygen transfer to the blood
   b. Mucus blanket cleans the airways as it is moved upward by the ciliary escalator

C. Lungs
1. Structure of the lungs—cone-shaped organs extending from the diaphragm to above the clavicles (**Figures 35-16** and **35-17**)
   a. Hilum—slit on the lung's medial surface where the primary bronchi and pulmonary blood vessels enter
   b. Base—the inferior surface of the lung that rests on the diaphragm
   c. Costal surface—lies against the ribs
   d. Left lung is divided into two lobes—superior and inferior
   e. Right lung is divided into three lobes—superior, middle, and inferior
   f. Lobes are further divided into functional units—bronchopulmonary segments
      (1) Ten segments in the right lung
      (2) Ten segments in the left lung, there can be eight or nine if segments have fused
2. Functions of the lungs—air distribution and gas exchange

D. Thorax (**Figure 35-18**)
   1. Structure of the thoracic cavity—three divisions divided by the pleura
      a. Pleural divisions—the part occupied by the lungs
      b. Mediastinum—part occupied by the oesophagus, trachea, large blood vessels, and heart
   2. Functions of the thorax—brings about inspiration and expiration

E. Additional information is found in **Table 35-1**

Cycle of Life: Respiratory Tract

A. Respiration may be affected by developmental defects, age-related structural changes, or loss of function throughout the life cycle
B. Age-related changes affect lung capacity, make ventilation difficult, or reduce the oxygen- or carbon dioxide–carrying capacity of blood
C. Respiratory efficiency is reduced in old age as a result of changes in ribs, respiratory muscles, and haemoglobin levels

The Big Picture: Respiratory Tract

A. Understanding the relationship of structure and function is critical to an understanding of homeostasis in all of the body organ systems
B. Respiratory system components permit the distribution of air and the exchange of respiratory gases
C. Respiratory functions are dependent on the structural organization of the system parts and the interrelationship of those components with other body systems

REVIEW QUESTIONS

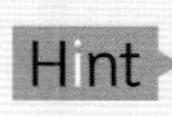

Write out the answers to these questions after reading the chapter and reviewing the Chapter Summary. Note—writing out your answers will consolidate learning and provide a valuable resource of information.

1. Identify the major anatomical structures of the nose.
2. How are the conchae arranged in the nose? What are they?
3. Describe the draining of the paranasal sinuses.
4. What organs are found in the nasopharynx?
5. What tubes open into the nasopharynx?
6. The pharynx is common to what two systems?
7. List the divisions of the larynx.
8. What is the voice box? Of what is it composed? What is the Adam's apple?
9. What is the epiglottis? What is its function?
10. What are the vocal folds? What name is given to the opening between the folds?
11. Describe the structure and function of the trachea.
12. Discuss the component parts of the bronchial tree.
13. Make a diagram showing the termination of a bronchiole in an alveolar duct with alveoli.
14. How many lobes are in the right lung? The left? What are the bronchopulmonary segments?
15. Describe the changes in thorax size during respiration.
16. List the organs that are included in the upper respiratory tract. Do the same for the lower respiratory tract.
17. What is the role of the vomeronasal organ?
18. Name the openings found in the pharynx. List the functions of the pharynx.
19. Which small, single cartilage of the larynx is associated with a life-threatening condition in children? What are the symptoms of this condition?
20. What is the function of the tracheal cartilage? What is the significance of its shape?

CRITICAL THINKING QUESTIONS

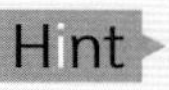

After finishing the Review Questions, write out the answers to these more in-depth questions to help you apply your new knowledge. Go back to sections of the chapter that relate to concepts that you find difficult.

1. Describe the structure and function of the respiratory mucosa. Include the types of cells it contains and where these cells are located in the respiratory system.
2. Why do you think mucus production is especially important in the olfactory epithelium?
3. Which of the paired laryngeal cartilages are the most important for vocalization? What evidence can you cite to support your answer?
4. In an earlier chapter the characteristic of water called *polarity* was described as the attraction water molecules have for each other. Why is this a problem in the respiratory system, and how is it solved?
5. Make the distinction between air distribution and gas exchange in the respiratory system. Identify the organs that serve as air distributors and gas exchangers.

36 Ventilation

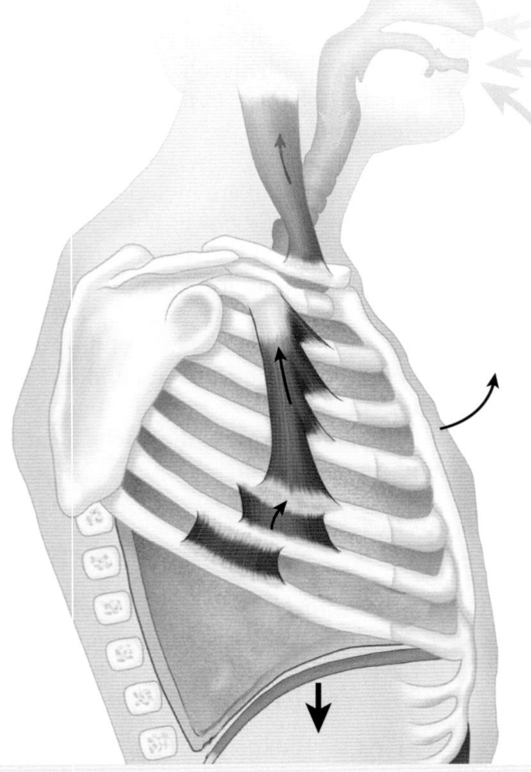

CHAPTER OUTLINE

Hint *Scan this outline before you begin to read the chapter, as a preview of how the concepts are organized.*

In Chapter 35 the anatomy of the respiratory system was presented as a basis for understanding the physiological principles that regulate air distribution and gas exchange. This chapter is the first of two chapters that deal with **respiratory physiology**—a complex series of interacting and coordinated processes that have a critical role in maintaining the stability, or constancy, of our internal environment. The proper functioning of the respiratory system ensures the tissues of an adequate oxygen supply and prompt removal of carbon dioxide. This process is complicated by the fact that control mechanisms must permit maintenance of homeostasis throughout a wide range of ever-changing environmental conditions and body demands. Adequate and efficient regulation

LANGUAGE OF SCIENCE

Hint *Use this list to aid your pronunciation of unfamiliar words.*

alveolar ventilation (al-VEE-oh-lar ven-tih-LAY-shun) [*alve-* **hollow,** *-ol-* **little,** *-ar* **relating to,** *vent-* **fan or create wind,** *-tion* **process**]

anatomical dead space (an-ah-TOM-ih-kal) [*ana-* **apart,** *-tom-* **cut,** *-ical* **relating to**]

apneustic centre (ap-NYOO-stik) [*a-* **not,** *-pneus-* **breathing,** *-ic* **relating to**]

Boyle's law (boils law) [*Robert Boyle* **English scientist**]

central chemoreceptor (SEN-tral kee-moh-ree-SEP-tor) [*centr-* **centre,** *-al* **relating to,** *chemo-* **chemical,** *-recept-* **receive,** *-or* **agent**]

Charles's law (CHARLZ-ez law)

compliance [*compli-* **fill up (complete),** *-ance* **act of**]

Dalton's law (DAL-tenz law) [*John Dalton* **English chemist and physicist**]

elastic recoil (eh-LAS-tik REE-koyl) [*elast-* **drive or propel,** *-ic* **relating to**]

expiration (eks-pih-RAY-shun) [*ex-* **out,** *-pir-* **breathe,** *-tion* **process**]

flow–volume loop (flo-VOL-yoom loop)

Henry's law [*William Henry* **English chemist**]

Hering–Breuer reflex (HER-ing BROO-er REE-fleks) [*Heinrich E. Hering* **German physiologist,** *Joseph Breuer* **Australian physician,** *re-* **back or again,** *-flex* **bend**]

ideal gas (i-DEEL gas)

inspiration (in-spih-RAY-shun) [*in-* **in,** *-spir-* **breathe,** *-ation* **process**]

law of partial pressures (PAR-shal PRESH-ur)

medullary rhythmicity area (MED-uh-lair-ee rith-MIH-sih-tee) [*medulla-* **marrow or pith (middle),** *-ary* **relating to,** *rhythm-* **rhythm,** *-ic* **relating to,** *-ity* **condition**]

continued on p. 844

of gas exchange between body cells and circulating blood in changing conditions is the essence of respiratory physiology. This complex function would not be possible without integration of numerous physiological control systems, including acid–base, water, and electrolyte balance; circulation; and metabolism.

RESPIRATORY PHYSIOLOGY

Functionally, the respiratory system is composed of an integrated set of regulated processes that include the following:

- External respiration: pulmonary ventilation (breathing) and gas exchange in the pulmonary capillaries of the lungs
- Transport of gases by the blood
- Internal respiration: gas exchange in the systemic blood capillaries and cellular respiration
- Overall regulation of respiration

Figure 36-1 summarizes the essential processes of pulmonary function. We will use this set of processes as a general framework for this and the next chapter. Cellular respiration has already been covered in Chapter 6 and will be reviewed again in greater detail in Chapter 41.

MECHANISM OF VENTILATION

PRIMARY PRINCIPLE OF VENTILATION

Pulmonary ventilation is a technical term for what most of us call breathing. One phase of it, *inspiration*, moves air into the lungs and the other phase, *expiration*, moves air out of the lungs.

Air moves in and out of the lungs for the same basic reason that any fluid (a liquid or a gas) moves from one place to another—briefly, because its pressure in one place is different from that in the other place. Or stated differently, the existence of a pressure gradient (a pressure difference) causes fluids to move. A fluid always moves *down* its pressure gradient. This means that a fluid moves from the area where its pressure is higher to the area where its pressure is lower. When applied to the flow of air in the pulmonary airways, we can call this central idea the **primary principle of ventilation.**

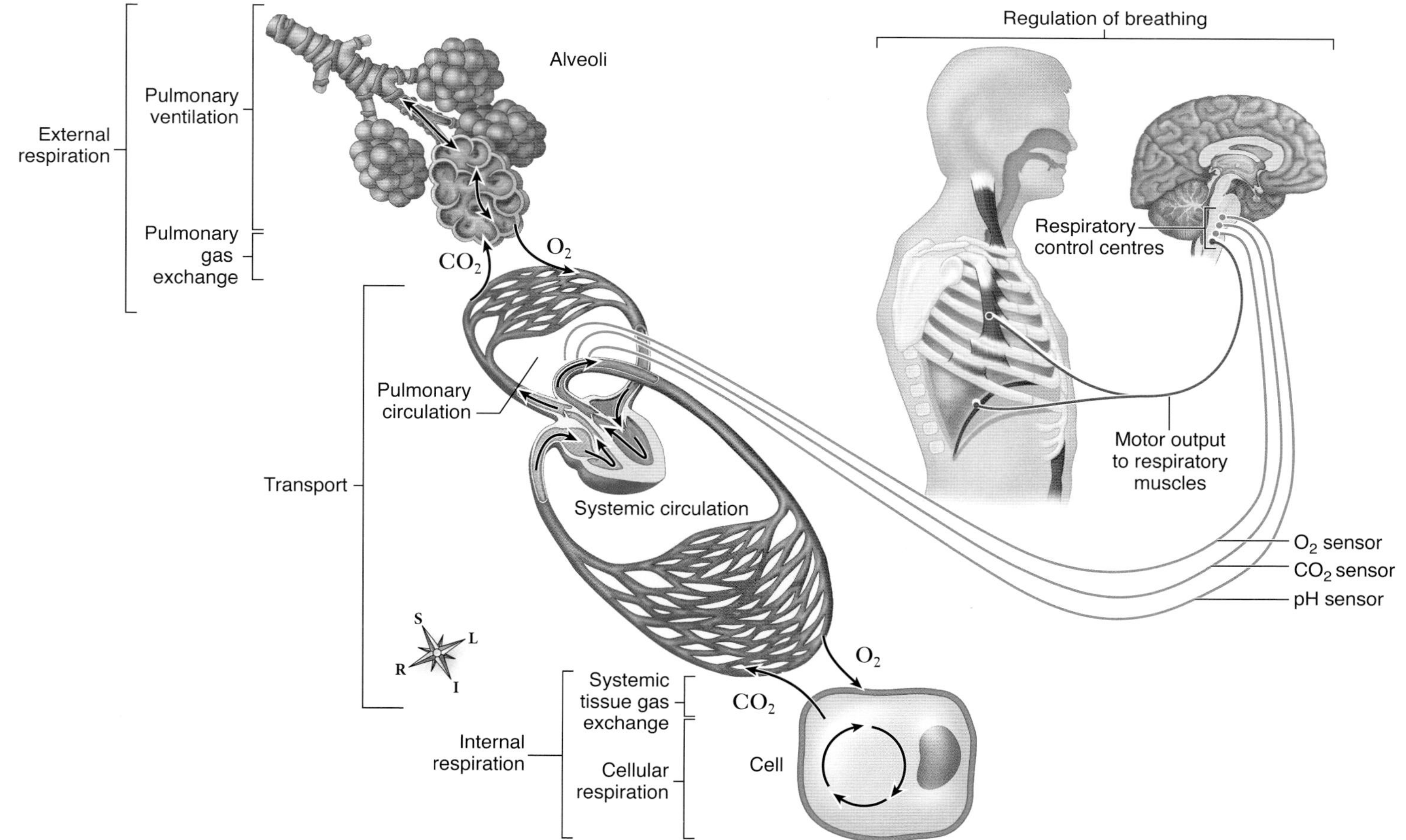

FIGURE 36-1 Overview of respiratory physiology. This chapter and the next are organized around the principle that respiratory function includes external respiration (ventilation and pulmonary gas exchange), transport of gases by blood, and internal respiration (systemic tissue gas exchange and cellular respiration). Cellular respiration is discussed separately (see Chapters 6 and 41). Regulatory mechanisms centred in the brainstem use feedback from blood gas sensors to regulate ventilation.

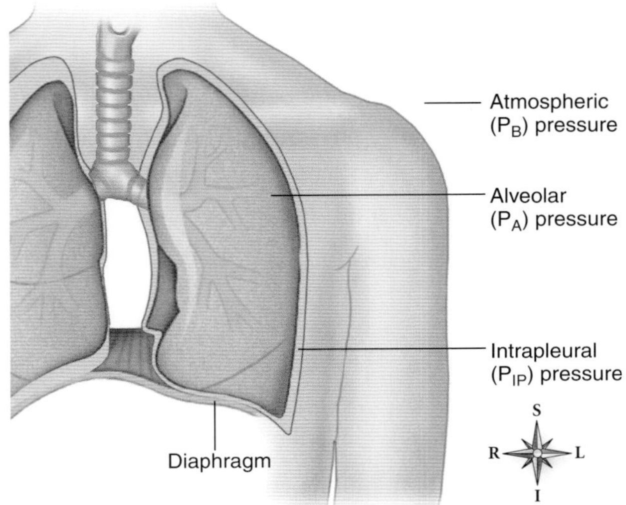

FIGURE 36-2 Pressures important in ventilation. This diagram shows the locations of pressures involved in the pressure gradients needed for ventilation (see **Figure 36-3**). Atmospheric pressure (P_B) is the air pressure of the atmosphere outside the body's airways. Alveolar pressure (P_A) is intrapulmonary pressure—the pressure at the far end of the internal airways. Intrapleural pressure (P_{IP}) is the fluid pressure of the pleural fluid between the parietal pleura and visceral pleura—or intrathoracic pressure (pressure in the thorax).

Note—The pressures of gases referred to in this chapter are given in kilopascals (kPa) and mm of mercury (mmHg). Note, 1 mmHg = 0.13 kPa.

In standard conditions, air in the atmosphere exerts a pressure of 101.3 kPa (760 mmHg). Air in the alveoli at the end of one **expiration** and before the beginning of another **inspiration** also exerts a pressure of 101.3 kPa (760 mmHg). This explains why, at that moment, air is neither entering nor leaving the lungs. The mechanism that produces pulmonary ventilation is one that establishes a gas pressure gradient between the atmosphere and the alveolar air. Keep in mind that atmospheric pressure changes with the weather and other factors—we use 101.3 kPa (760 mmHg) here as an example only.

When atmospheric pressure is greater than pressure within the lung, air flows down this gas pressure gradient. Then air moves from the atmosphere into the lungs. In other words, inspiration occurs. When pressure in the lungs becomes greater than atmospheric pressure, air again moves down a gas pressure gradient. But this time, the air moves in the opposite direction. That is, air moves out of the lungs into the atmosphere. The pulmonary ventilation mechanism, therefore, must somehow establish these two gas pressure gradients—one in which alveolar pressure (P_A, pressure within the alveoli of the lungs) is

BOX 36-1 *gas laws*

A true understanding of respiratory function requires some familiarity with some of what physical scientists call the "gas laws". The gas laws are simply statements of what we have come to understand about the physical nature of gases. The gas laws are based on the concept of an **ideal gas**—that is, a gas whose molecules are so far apart that the molecules rarely collide with one another.

The gas laws are also based on the premise that gas molecules continually collide with the walls of their container and thus produce a force against it called the *gas pressure.* Pressure exerted by a gas depends on several factors. One factor is the frequency of collisions, which is proportional to the concentration of the gas: the higher the gas concentration, the higher the number of collisions with the wall of the container and thus the higher the gas pressure. **Boyle's law** sums up this principle very neatly by stating that a gas's volume is inversely proportional to its pressure (see figure on facing page, part *A*). When the volume of a container increases, the pressure of the gas inside it decreases, and when the volume decreases, the gas pressure increases. In this chapter, Boyle's law has been applied to ventilation: when thoracic volume increases, air pressure in the airways decreases (allowing air to move inward), and when thoracic volume decreases, air pressure in the airways increases (allowing air to move outward).

Another factor that affects an ideal gas is its temperature. Temperature is really a measurement of the motion of molecules. Thus an increase in temperature signals an increase in the average velocity of gas molecules. It follows that all other things remaining the same, an increase in the temperature of a gas will increase its pressure. However, if the container is expandable, as it is in part *B* of the figure, and thus the pressure is held constant, the volume increases. This principle is summed up in **Charles's law,** which states that volume is directly proportional to temperature ($V \propto T$) when pressure is held constant (see figure, part *B*). One could extend this notion to state that pressure is proportional to temperature ($P \propto T$) when volume is held constant. One can assume, then, that during inspiration, air expands in volume as it is warmed by the respiratory mucosa.

Dalton's law takes things a step further by stating the situation when the gas in question is actually a *mixture* of different kinds of gas molecules, as in air (part *C* of the figure). Dalton's law states that the total pressure exerted by a mixture of gases is the sum of the pressure of each individual gas. That is, the collision force created by all of one type of molecule accounts for only a part of the total pressure—the collision forces of all the other types of molecules in the mixture must be included to arrive at the total gas pressure. Dalton's law, also known as the **law of partial pressures,** is used to determine the partial pressure of oxygen (Po_2) in air, for example. Because the partial pressure of a gas is determined by its relative concentration in the mixture of gases, partial pressure values can be used in much the same way as concentration values in determining the direction of net diffusion.

Another gas law, **Henry's law,** describes how the pressure of a gas relates to the concentration of that gas in a liquid solution (part *D* of the figure). If you have a beaker of water surrounded by air, which contains oxygen, the concentration of oxygen dissolved in the water will be proportional to the partial pressure of oxygen in the air. Henry's law further states that the concentration of the gas in solution is also a function of the gas's **solubility,** or its relative ability to dissolve. Thus Henry's law states that the concentration of a gas in a solution depends on the partial pressure of the gas and the solubility of the gas, as long as the temperature remains constant. This principle explains how the plasma concentration of a gas such as oxygen relates to its partial pressure.

Also see **Box 37-1** on p. 851, which discusses Fick's law. •

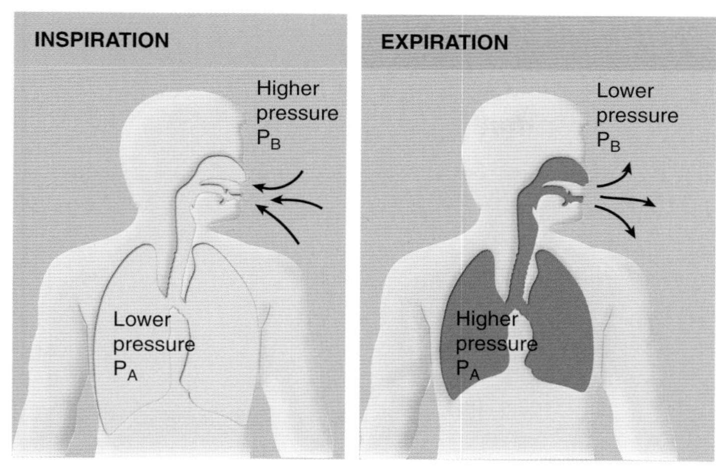

FIGURE 36-3 Primary principle of ventilation. Put simply, air moves down its pressure gradient—that is, it always moves from an area of high pressure to an area of lower pressure. To achieve inspiration, the higher pressure must be outside the body. To achieve expiration, the higher pressure must be inside the body's airways. P_A, Alveolar pressure; P_B, atmospheric [barometric] pressure. (See **Figure 36-2**.)

lower than atmospheric pressure (or barometric pressure, P_B) to produce inspiration and one in which it is higher than atmospheric pressure to produce expiration (**Figure 36-2** and **Figure 36-3**).

These pressure gradients are established by changes in the size of the thoracic cavity, which in turn are produced by contraction and relaxation of respiratory muscles. An understanding of *Boyle's law* is important for understanding the pressure changes that occur in the lungs and thorax during the breathing cycle. It is a familiar principle, stating that the volume of a gas varies inversely with pressure at a constant temperature (**Box 36-1**). One application of this principle is as follows: Expansion of the thorax (increase in volume) results in a decreased intrapleural (intrathoracic) pressure. This leads to a decreased intra-alveolar pressure, which causes air to move from the outside into the lungs.

Figure 36-4 applies the primary principle of ventilation and Boyle's law to the human airways to demonstrate the mechanics of ventilation. Because the thorax and lungs are *compliant* (stretchable), expanding the thorax and lungs by pulling the diaphragm downward increases thoracic volume—thus decreasing intrapleural pressure (P_{IP}) and alveolar pressure (P_A). This creates a pressure gradient between the atmosphere and the alveoli that results in flow of air into the airways. The opposite occurs when the elastic diaphragm recoils, decreasing internal air volumes (thus increasing internal air pressure) and forcing air out of the airways.

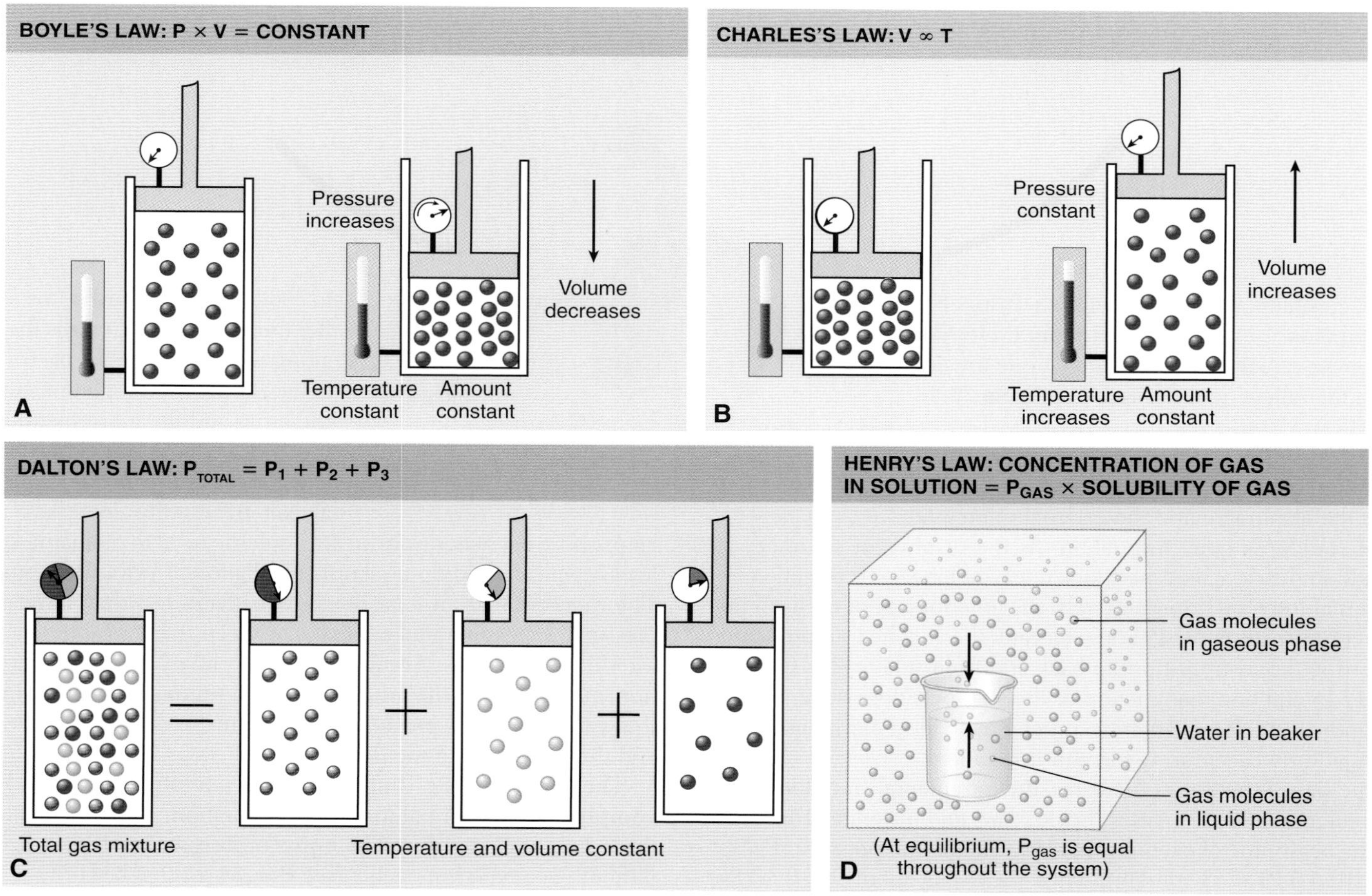

The gas laws. A, Boyle's law. **B,** Charles's law. **C,** Dalton's law. **D,** Henry's law.

UNIT 5

FIGURE 36-4 The respiratory cycle. During *inspiration,* the diaphragm contracts, increasing the volume of the thoracic cavity. This increase in volume results in a decrease in pressure, which causes air to rush into the lungs. During *expiration,* the diaphragm returns to an upward position, reducing the volume in the thoracic cavity. Air pressure thus increases, forcing air out of the lungs. See **Table 36-1** for additional details. P_A, Alveolar pressure; P_B, barometric pressure; P_{IP}, intrapleural pressure.

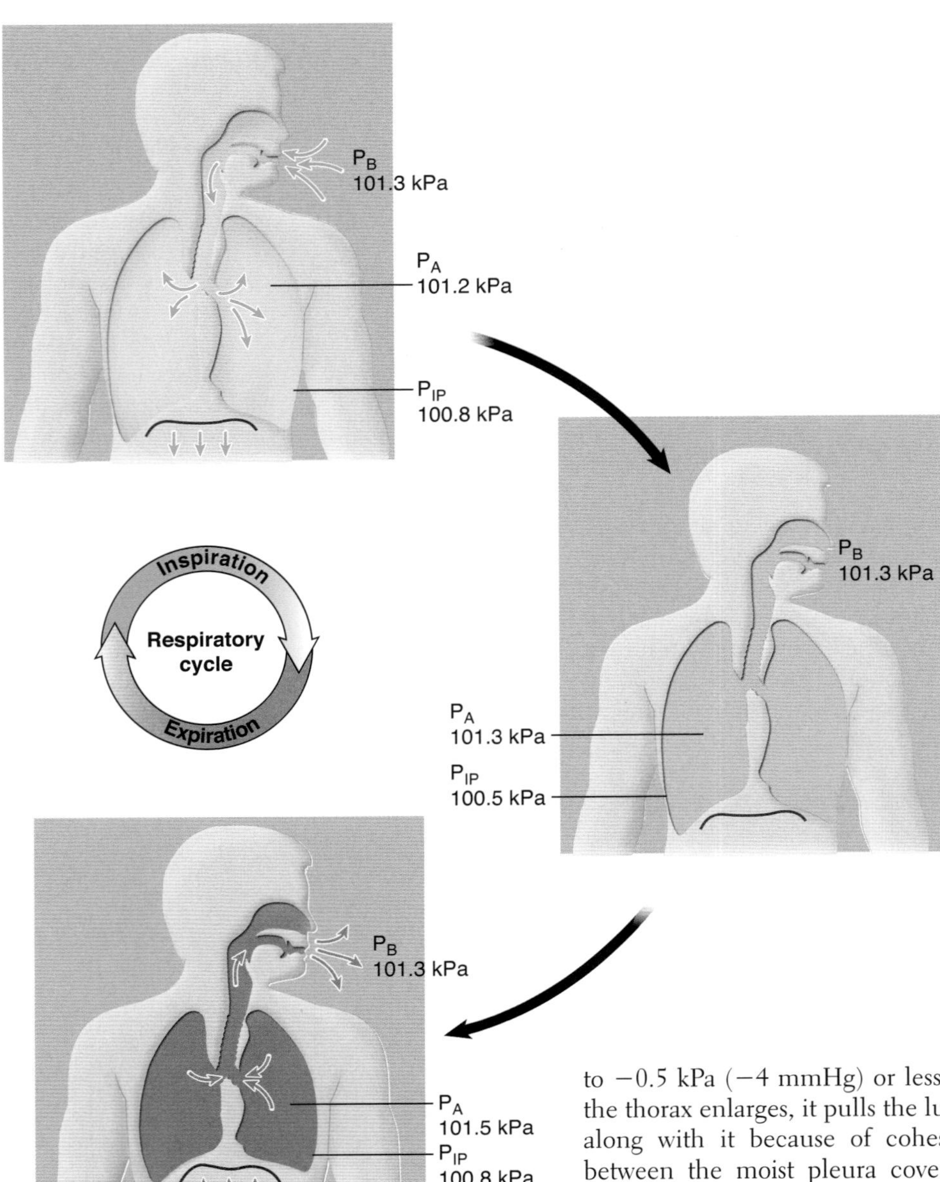

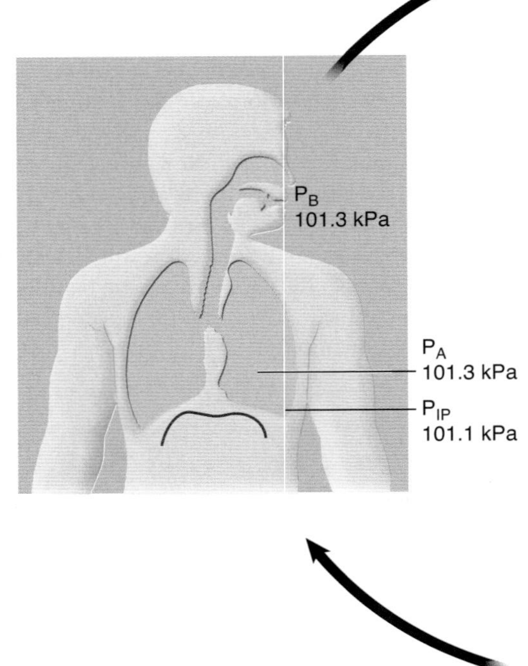

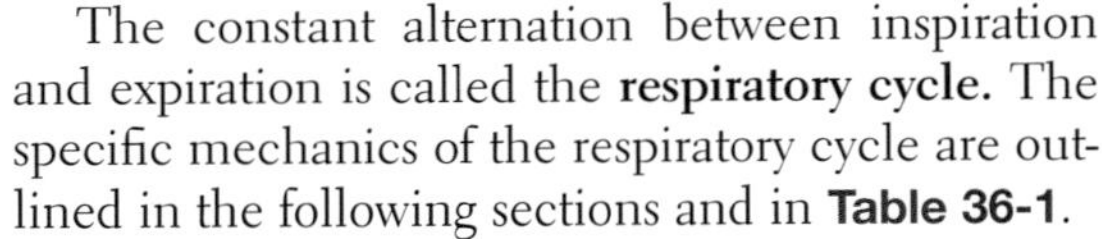

The constant alternation between inspiration and expiration is called the **respiratory cycle.** The specific mechanics of the respiratory cycle are outlined in the following sections and in **Table 36-1**.

INSPIRATION

Contraction of the diaphragm alone, or contraction of both the diaphragm and the external intercostal muscles, produces quiet inspiration. As the diaphragm contracts, it descends, and this makes the thoracic cavity longer. Contraction of the external intercostal muscles pulls the anterior end of each rib up and out (**Figure 36-5**, A). This also elevates the attached sternum and enlarges the thorax from front to back and from side to side (**Figure 36-5**, *B*). In addition, contraction of the sternocleidomastoid, pectoralis minor, and serratus anterior muscles can aid in elevation of the sternum and rib cage during forceful inspiration.

As the size of the thorax increases, the intrapleural (intrathoracic) and alveolar pressure decreases (Boyle's law) and inspiration occurs.

At the beginning of each inspiration, intrapleural pressure (P_{IP}) is about 101.1 kPa (758 mmHg). Thus the P_{IP} is about 0.2–0.3 kPa (2 mmHg) less than atmospheric pressure (often written −0.3 kPa (−2 mmHg). During normal quiet inspiration, P_{IP} decreases further to −0.5 kPa (−4 mmHg) or less. As the thorax enlarges, it pulls the lungs along with it because of cohesion between the moist pleura covering the lungs and the moist pleura lining the thorax. Thus the lungs expand and the pressure in their tubes and alveoli necessarily decreases. Alveolar pressure decreases from an atmospheric level to a subatmospheric level—typically a drop of about 0.1 kPa to 0.4 kPa (1 to 3 mmHg). The moment that alveolar pressure becomes less than atmospheric pressure, a pressure gradient exists between the atmosphere and the interior of the lungs. According to the primary principle of ventilation, air moves into the lungs. Eventually, enough air moves into the lungs to establish a pressure equilibrium between the atmosphere and the alveoli—and the flow of air then stops.

The ability of the lungs and thorax to stretch, referred to as **compliance,** is essential to normal respiration. If the compliance of these structures is reduced by injury or disease, inspiration becomes difficult—or even impossible (see **Box 36-2** on p. 832).

For a summary of the mechanism of inspiration just described, see **Figure 36-4** and **Figure 36-6**.

TABLE 36-1 The Respiratory Cycle*

P_{IP}	P_A	P_B	DESCRIPTION
Inspiration			
101.1	101.3	101.3	The diaphragm is relaxed, putting the thoracic cavity at low volume. At the beginning of inspiration $P_{IP} < P_A$, keeping alveoli open. Because $P_A = P_B$, no air is flowing yet.
100.8	101.2	101.3	The diaphragm contracts, increasing the thoracic volume and reducing P_{IP}. A decrease in P_{IP} causes a decrease in P_A. Now $P_A < P_B$, and air flows down the pressure gradient (into the lungs).
100.5	101.3	101.3	Eventually, the alveoli fill with air and P_A equilibrates with P_B. Inward airflow stops. The cycle is now ready to shift to the expiration phase. Note that P_{IP} is still dropping but P_A has not yet "caught up" with the drop.
Expiration			
100.5	101.3	101.3	As expiration is about to begin, the diaphragm is contracted maximally. Because $P_A = P_B$, there is no airflow.
100.8	101.5	101.3	The diaphragm relaxes, and elastic recoil of the thoracic walls and alveoli increases P_{IP} and P_A. Now, $P_A > P_B$. Air moves (outward) down the pressure gradient.
101.1	101.3	101.3	The diaphragm eventually relaxes fully, so the decrease in volume stops. P_A equilibrates with P_B, and airflow ceases. The system is now ready for another inspiration phase.

*All P values are expressed in *kPa* and are examples only.

P_A, Alveolar pressure (air pressure inside the alveoli); *P_B*, atmospheric (barometric) pressure (air pressure of the external environment [atmosphere]); *P_{IP}*, intrapleural pressure (air pressure in the intrapleural space).

EXPIRATION

Quiet expiration is ordinarily a passive process that begins when the pressure gradients that resulted in inspiration are reversed. The inspiratory muscles relax, causing a decrease in the size of the thorax and an increase in intrapleural pressure from about 100.5 kPa (754 mmHg) (−0.8 kPa (−6 mmHg)) before expiration to about 100.8 kPa (756 mmHg); (−0.5 kPa (−4 mmHg)) or more during expiration. It is important to understand that this pressure between the parietal and visceral pleura is always negative, that is, less than alveolar pressure. The negative intrapleural pressure is required to overcome the so-called collapse tendency of the lungs caused by surface tension of the fluid lining the alveoli and the stretch of elastic fibres that are constantly attempting to recoil.

As alveolar pressure increases, a positive-pressure gradient is established from alveoli to atmosphere—and thus expiration occurs as air flows outward through the respiratory passageways. In forced expiration, contraction of the abdominal and internal intercostal muscles can increase alveolar pressure tremendously—creating a very large air pressure gradient.

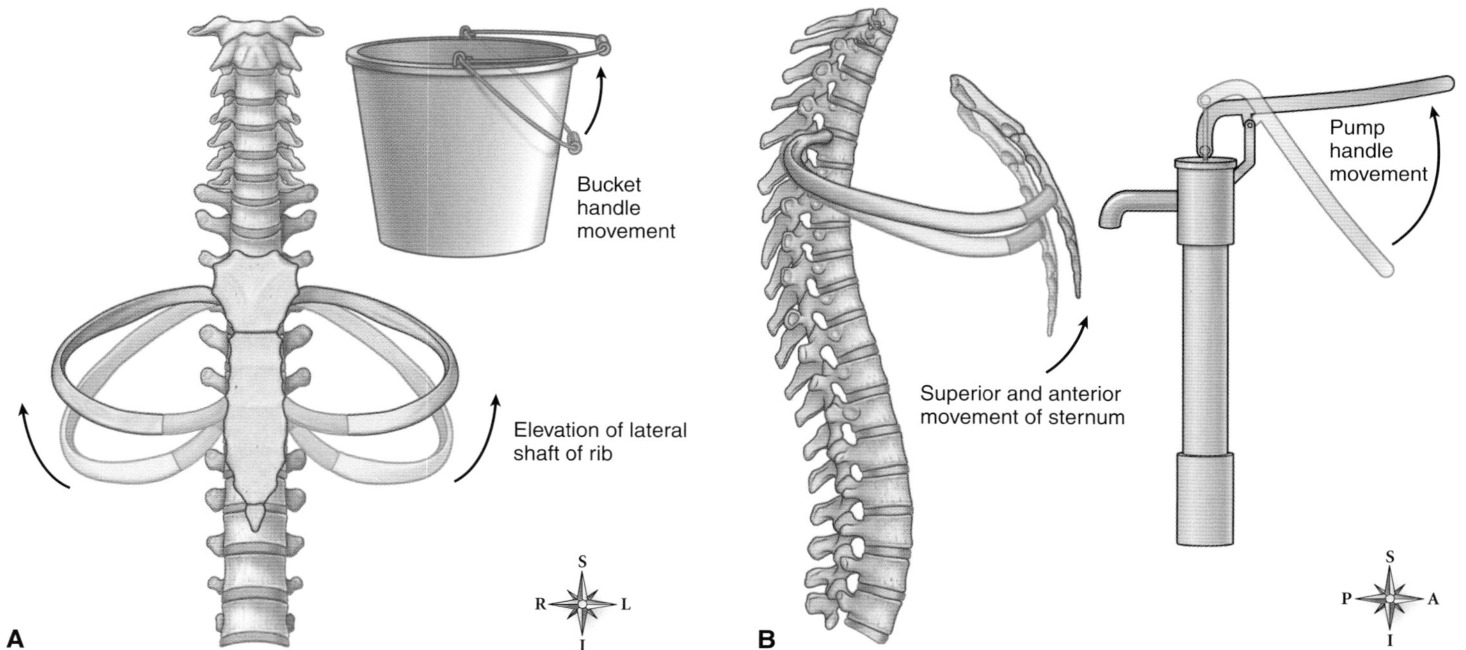

FIGURE 36-5 Movement of the rib cage during breathing. A, Inspiratory muscles pull the ribs upward and thus outward, as illustrated by lifting a bucket handle. **B,** Inspiratory muscles pull the sternum upward and thus outward, as when pulling upward on the handle of a water pump.

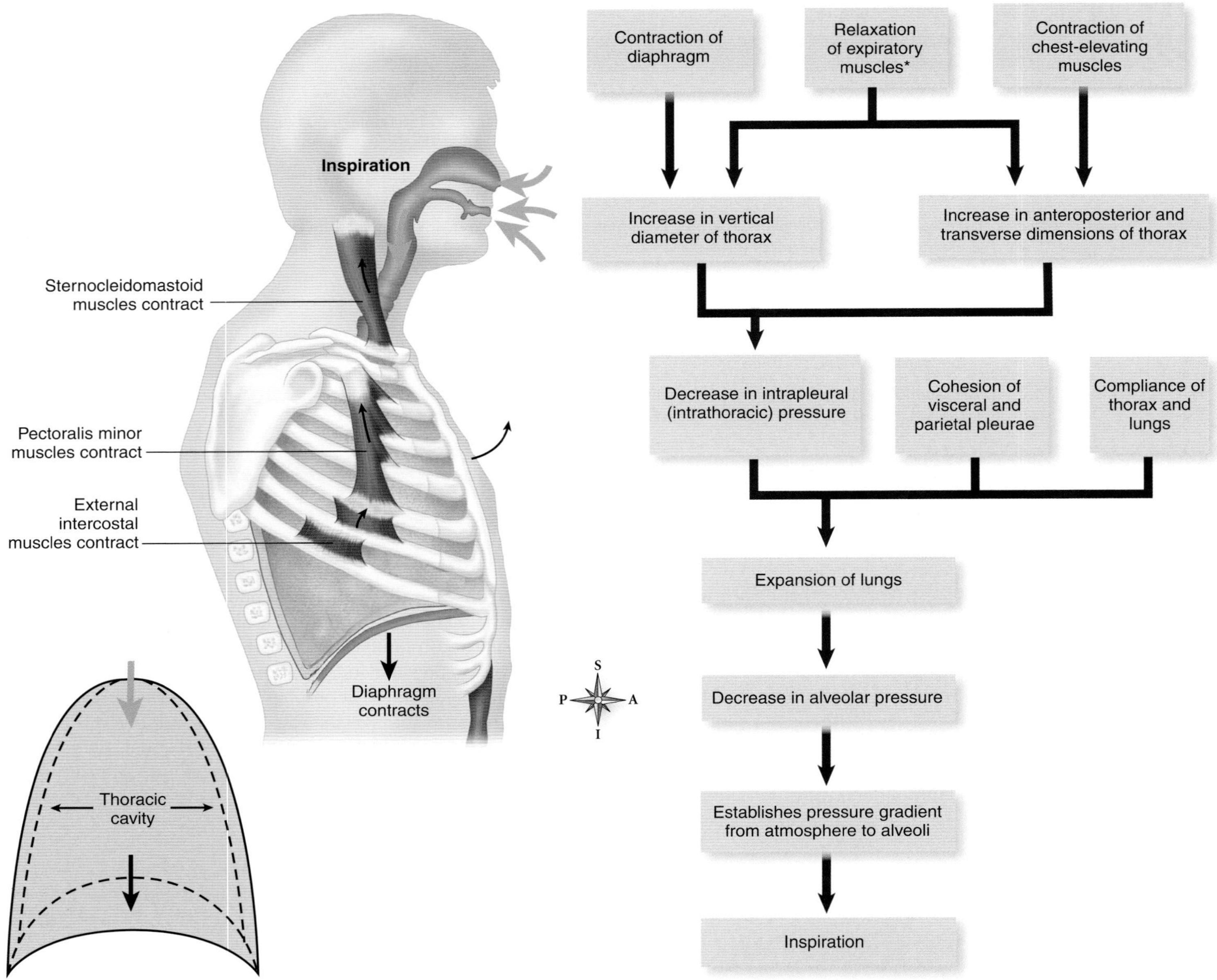

FIGURE 36-6 Mechanism of inspiration. Note the role of the diaphragm and the chest-elevating muscles (pectoralis minor and external intercostals) in increasing thoracic volume, which decreases pressure in the lungs and thus draws air inward. (*Relaxation of expiratory muscles is not needed during normal, quiet breathing.)

The tendency of the thorax and lungs to return to their preinspiration volume is a physical phenomenon called **elastic recoil.** If a disease condition reduces the elasticity of pulmonary tissues, expirations must become forced even at rest.

Figure 36-4 and **Figure 36-7** summarize the mechanism of expiration just described.

Look for a moment at **Figure 36-8**. This figure shows the repeating respiratory cycle mapped out as changes in pressures and volumes. Note that intrapleural pressure is always less than alveolar pressure. This difference ($P_{IP} - P_A$) is called the **transpulmonary pressure.** Intrapleural pressure is always "negative" with respect to alveolar pressure. Transpulmonary pressure must be negative to maintain inflation of the lungs, as stated previously.

Quick CHECK

1. What is meant by the term *pulmonary ventilation*?
2. What effect does enlargement of the thoracic cavity have on the air pressure inside the lungs?
3. Which requires more expenditure of energy during normal, quiet breathing—inspiration or expiration?

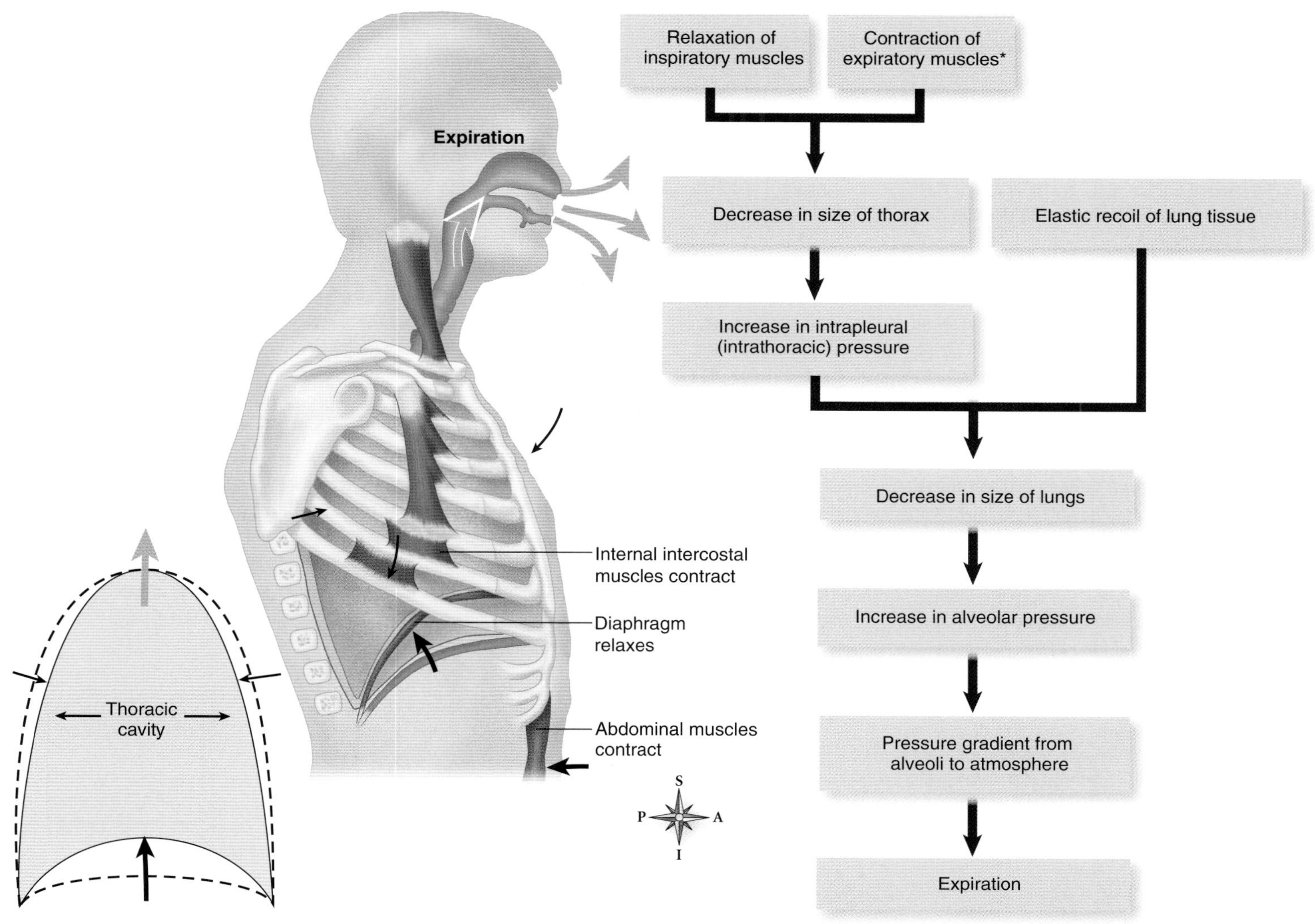

FIGURE 36-7 Mechanism of expiration. Note that relaxation of the diaphragm plus contraction of chest-depressing muscles (internal intercostals) reduces thoracic volume, which increases pressure in the lungs and thus pushes air outward. (*Contraction of expiratory muscles is not needed during normal, quiet breathing.)

PULMONARY VOLUMES AND CAPACITIES

The volumes of air moved in and out of the lungs and the volume remaining in them are matters of great importance. They must be normal so that normal exchange of oxygen and carbon dioxide can occur between alveolar air and pulmonary capillary blood.

Pulmonary Volumes

An apparatus called a **spirometer** is used to measure the volume of air exchanged in breathing (**Figure 36-9**). A graphic recording of the changing pulmonary volumes observed during breathing is called a **spirogram** (**Figure 36-10**, A). The volume of air exhaled normally after a typical inspiration is termed **tidal volume (TV).** As you can see in **Figure 36-10**, the normal volume of tidal air for an adult at rest is approximately 500 mL (or 0.5 L).

After expiration of tidal air, an individual can force still more air out of the lungs. The largest additional volume of air that one can forcibly expire after expiring tidal air is called the **expiratory reserve volume (ERV).** An adult, as **Figure 36-10** shows, normally has an ERV of between 1000 and 1200 mL (1.0 to 1.2 litres). **Inspiratory reserve volume (IRV)** is the amount of air that can be forcibly inspired over and above a normal inspiration. It is measured by having the individual exhale normally after a forced inspiration. The normal IRV is about 3300 mL (3.3 litres). No matter how forcefully one exhales, one cannot squeeze all the air out of the lungs. Some of it remains trapped in the alveoli. This amount of air that cannot be forcibly expired is known as **residual volume (RV)** and amounts to about 1200 mL (1.2 litres). Between breaths, an exchange of oxygen and carbon dioxide occurs between the trapped residual air in the alveoli and the blood. This process helps "level off" the amounts—

BOX 36-2 *surfactant and lung compliance*

As we have discussed already, inspiration cannot occur without the lungs and thorax having the ability to stretch—a characteristic called *compliance.* Of course, the natural "stretchiness" of the alveolar walls is important in determining lung compliance. Conditions that cause thickening, or fibrosis, of lung tissues reduce the ease of stretch and thus reduce lung compliance. A greater impact on lung compliance is made by **surface tension** in the fluid film that lines the alveoli.

Surface tension in an aqueous (water-based) solution results from the attractive forces between water molecules in the solution. Recall from Chapter 3 that water molecules are polar and thus are electrically attracted to one another—as though they are weak magnets. Surface tension is high as the water molecules try to move toward one another, thereby contracting the fluid. The fluid lining of each alveolus would thus tend to collapse under this contracting force. However, as we discussed in Chapter 35 (see p. 811), the presence of surfactant helps prevent such collapse of alveoli. Surfactant is formed from the protein and phospholipid secretions of **type II cells** in the wall of each alveolus. Surfactant reduces surface tension and thus prevents fluid contraction and alveolar collapse. The role of surfactant in preventing alveolar collapse is illustrated in Figure *A.*

The pressure created by the force of surface tension is greater in smaller alveoli than in larger alveoli, according to the **Young–LaPlace law**. This means that smaller alveoli would tend to have a higher pressure (P_A) than larger alveoli would. Thus air would move from the smaller alveoli into larger alveoli. However, because the surfactant on the surface of the fluid that lines the smaller alveoli is more concentrated than that on larger alveoli, surface tension is reduced proportionally. In this way, the pressure in large alveoli is equal to that in smaller alveoli. In theory, all alveoli—no matter what their size—are ventilated equally. Figure *B* summarizes the Young–LaPlace law.

Surfactant is present in most newborns. However, because surfactant formation is not fully under way until the seventh or eighth month of prenatal development, premature infants often do not have enough surfactant. The deficiency of surfactant in premature infants is called **hyaline membrane disease (HMD).** Because lack of surfactant decreases lung compliance, a premature infant will try to inflate the alveoli by increasing effort of the inspiratory muscles. Such great effort is needed to maintain normal ventilation that the baby may die of exhaustion. The effects of such alveolar collapse and ventilation difficulty are collectively called **respiratory distress syndrome (RDS).** In infants, it is more specifically called *infant respiratory distress syndrome (IRDS).*

One way to treat IRDS is to use a special type of mechanical respirator with **continuous positive airway pressure** (**CPAP,** pronounced "SEE-pap"). The respirator artificially inflates the baby's lungs and then maintains enough pressure during expiration to prevent collapse—thus relieving the baby's inspiratory muscles. Synthetic surfactants are also used commonly to prevent or treat IRDS. The surfactant is delivered through a tube directly into the airways—a method called **intratracheal injection.** •

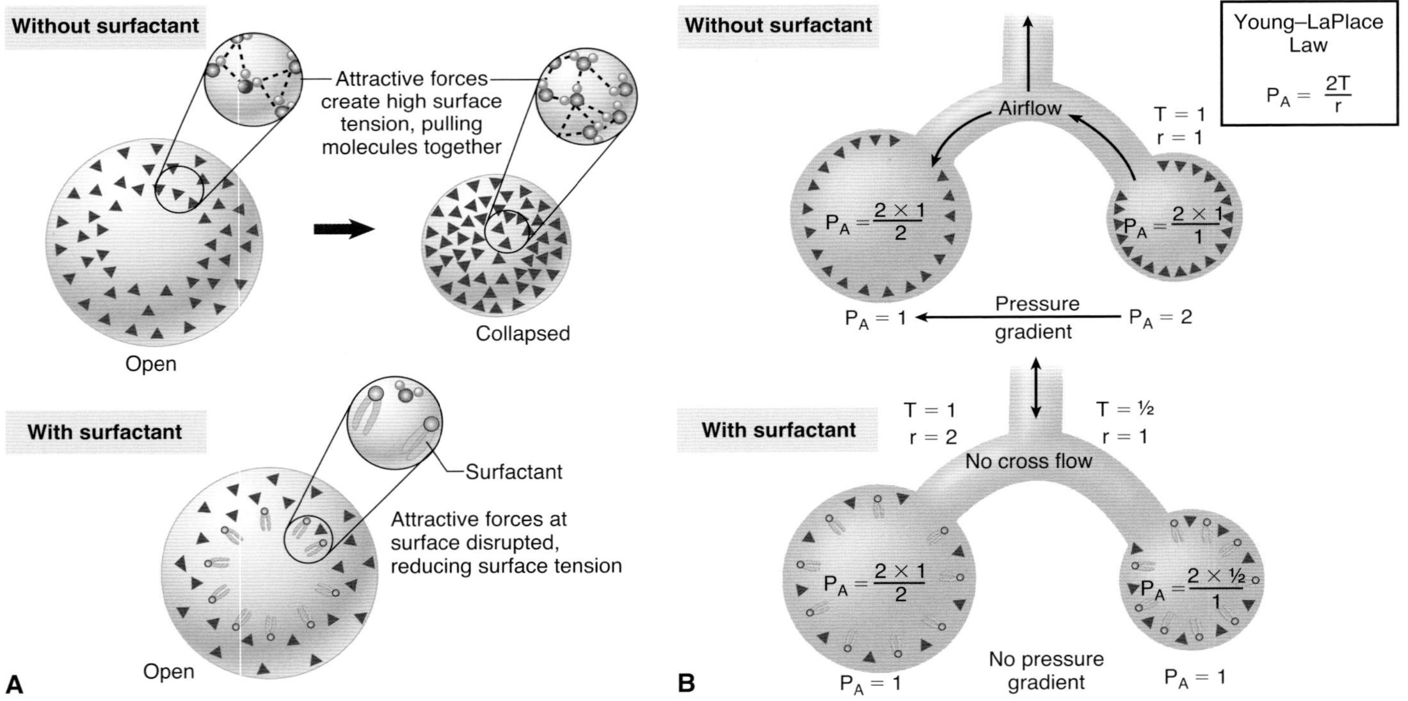

A, Role of surfactant. The surface of the water that lines the small alveoli tends to contract because of its high surface tension, thereby collapsing the entire alveolus. Surfactant disrupts some of the attractive forces and thus reduces surface tension—and the risk of alveolar collapse. **B, Young–LaPlace law.** Also called the *law of LaPlace,* this principle states that alveolar pressure (P_A) is directly proportional to surface tension (T) and inversely proportional to the radius (r) of the alveolus. Without surfactant, the pressure gradient would cause air to flow from the small alveoli to the larger alveoli—thus triggering collapse of the smaller alveoli. When surfactant is present, the concentration of the surfactant is higher as the alveolus gets smaller. Because small alveoli have less surface tension than larger alveoli do (as a result of more concentrated surfactant), the effect of the Young–LaPlace law is counterbalanced. Because P_A thus remains about the same in all alveoli, regardless of size, ventilation is not disrupted.

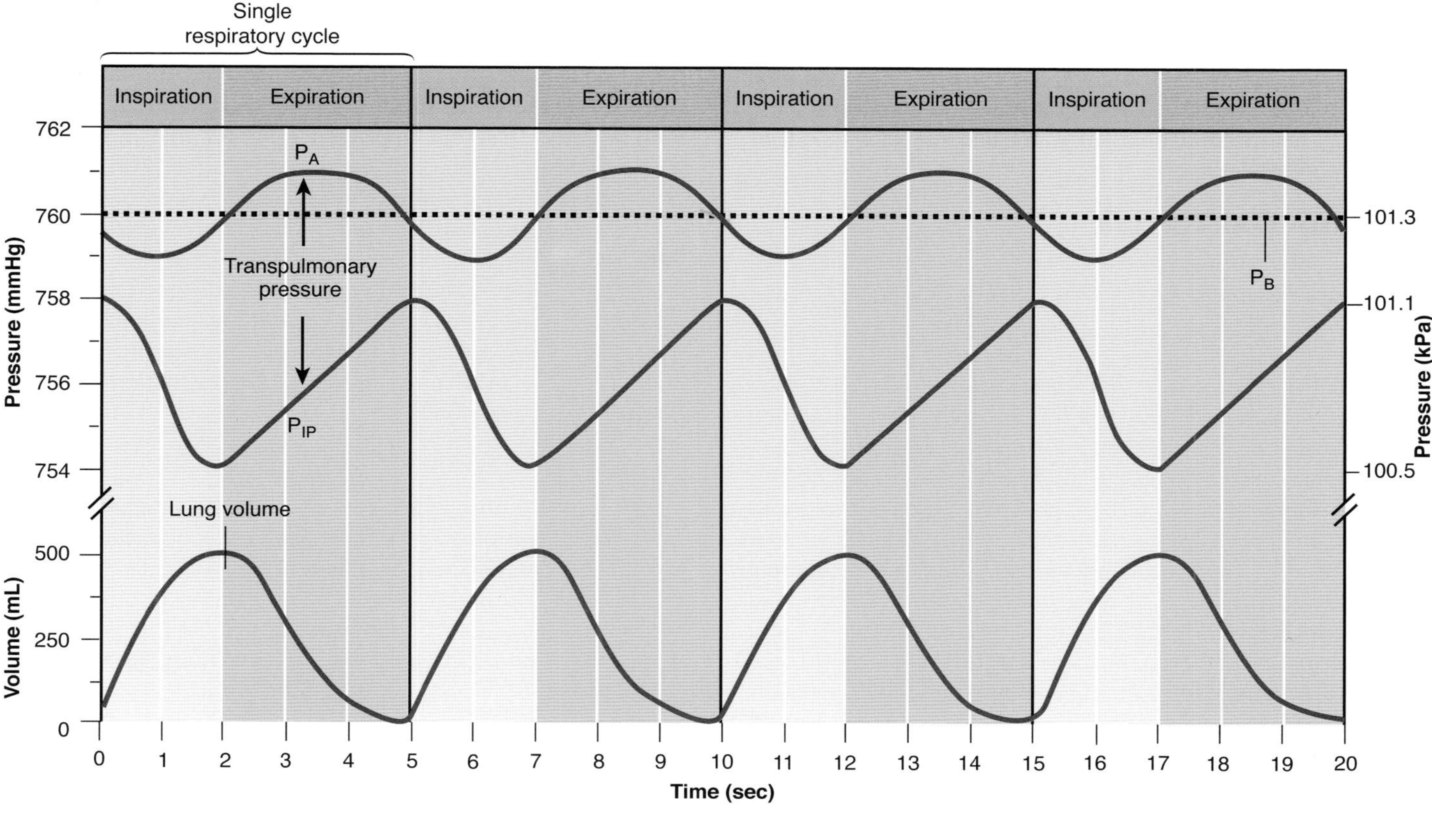

FIGURE 36-8 Rhythm of ventilation. Respiratory cycles repeat continuously in normal, quiet breathing. Notice the rhythmic rise and fall of the intrapleural pressure (P_{IP}) and alveolar pressure (P_A). You can easily see that P_{IP} is always lower than P_A (negative transpulmonary pressure), which helps keep the alveoli inflated. The lowest line shows the change in air volumes during the respiratory cycle.

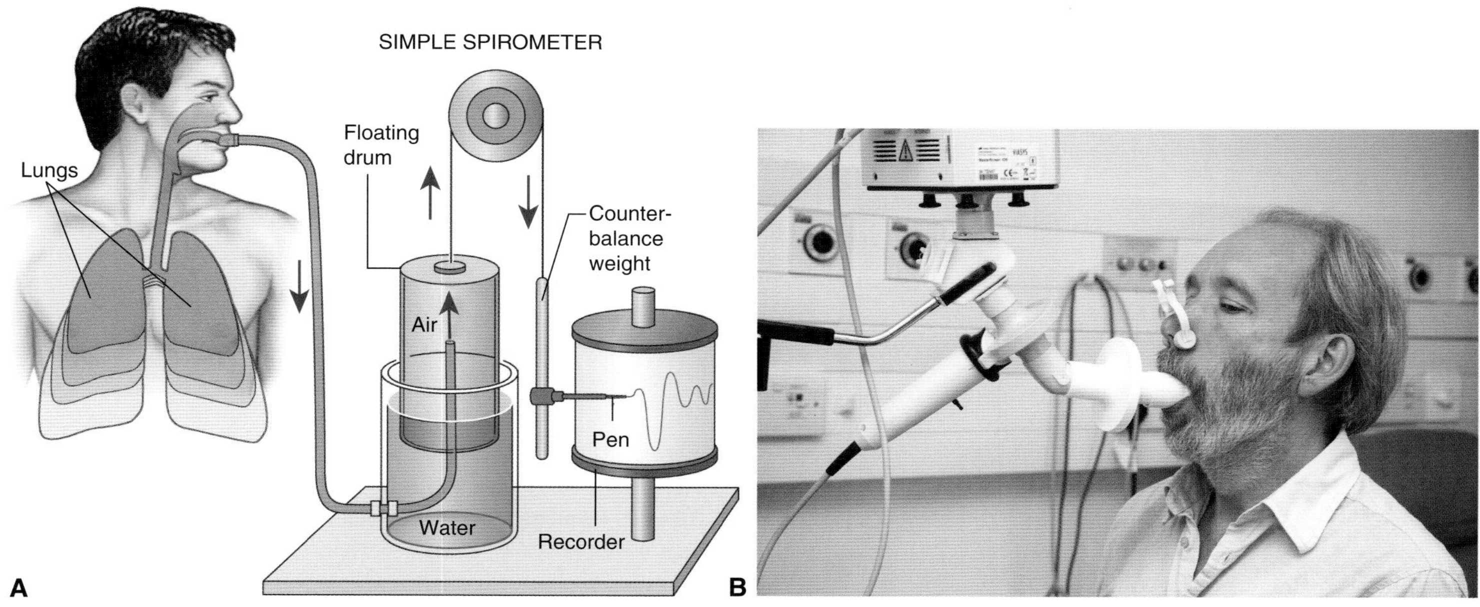

FIGURE 36-9 Spirometer. Spirometers are devices that measure the volume of gas that the lungs inhale and exhale, usually as a function of time. **A,** Diagram of a classic spirometer design showing how the volume of air exhaled and inhaled is recorded as a rising and falling line. **B,** A simple spirometer attached to a computerized recording device. This type of apparatus is used frequently for routine assessment of ventilation.

or maintain the setpoint values—of oxygen and carbon dioxide in the blood during the breathing cycle.

In *pneumothorax* (**Box 36-3**), the RV is eliminated when the lung collapses. Even after the RV is forced out, the collapsed lung has a porous, spongy texture and floats in water because of trapped air called the *minimal volume*, which is about 40% of the RV.

Pulmonary Capacities

A pulmonary "capacity" is the sum of two or more pulmonary "volumes". Notice in **Figure 36-10** that **vital capacity (VC)** is the sum of:

$$IRV + TV + ERV$$

The vital capacity represents the largest volume of air an individual can move in and out of the lungs. It is determined by measuring the largest possible expiration after the largest possible inspiration. How large a vital capacity a person has depends on many factors—the size of the thoracic cavity, posture, and various other factors. In general, a larger person has a larger vital capacity than a smaller person does. An individual has a larger vital capacity when standing erect than when stooped over or lying down. The volume of blood in the lungs also affects the vital capacity. If the lungs contain more blood than normal, the alveolar air space is encroached on and vital capacity accordingly decreases. This becomes a very important factor in congestive heart disease.

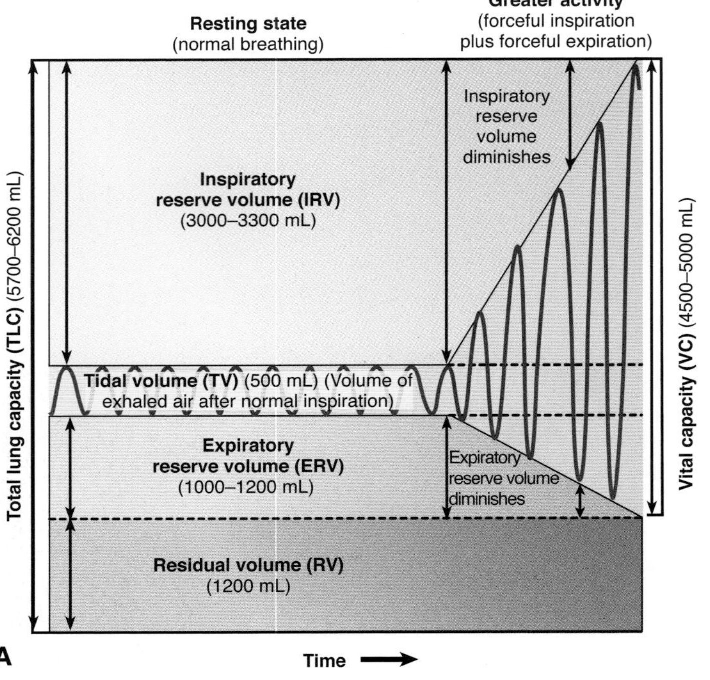

FIGURE 36-10 Pulmonary ventilation volumes and capacities. A, Spirogram. **B,** Pulmonary volumes (at rest) represented as relative proportions of an inflated balloon. During normal, quiet respirations, the atmosphere and lungs exchange about 500 mL of air (TV). With forcible inspiration, about 3300 mL more air can be inhaled (IRV). After a normal inspiration and normal expiration, approximately 1000 mL more air can be forcibly expired (ERV). Vital capacity is the amount of air that can be forcibly expired after a maximal inspiration and therefore indicates the largest amount of air that can enter and leave the lungs during respiration. Residual volume is the air that remains trapped in the alveoli.

Excess fluid in the pleural or abdominal cavities also decreases vital capacity. So, too, does the disease *emphysema*. In emphysema, the alveolar walls become stretched—that is, lose their elasticity—and are unable to recoil normally for expiration. This leads to an increased RV. In severe emphysema, the RV may increase so much that the chest occupies the inspiratory position even at rest. Excessive muscular effort is therefore necessary for inspiration, and because of the loss of elasticity of lung tissue, greater effort is required, too, for expiration.

In diagnosing lung disorders a physician may need to know the inspiratory capacity and the functional residual capacity of the patient's lungs. **Inspiratory capacity (IC)** is the maximal amount of air an individual can inspire after a normal expiration. From **Figure 36-10**, you can deduce that:

$$IC = TV + IRV$$

Using the volumes given in the figure, how many millilitres is the IC? Check your answer in **Table 36-2**, which summarizes pulmonary volumes and capacities.

Functional residual capacity (FRC) is the amount of air left in the lungs at the end of a normal expiration—that is, without contracting expiratory muscles. Therefore, as **Figure 36-10** implies,

$$FRC = ERV + RV$$

Using the volumes given, the functional residual capacity is 2200 to 2400 mL (2.2 to 2.4 litres). The total volume of air a lung can hold is called the **total lung capacity (TLC)**. It is, as **Figure 36-10** indicates, the sum of all four lung volumes.

The term **alveolar ventilation** refers to the volume of inspired air that actually reaches, or "ventilates", the alveoli. Only this volume of air takes part in the exchange of gases between air and blood. (Alveolar air exchanges some of its oxygen for some of the blood's carbon dioxide.)

With every breath we take, part of the entering air necessarily fills our air passageways—nose, pharynx, larynx, trachea, and bronchi. This portion of air does not descend into any alveoli and therefore cannot take part in gas exchange. In this sense, it is "dead air". Appropriately, the larger air passageways this air occupies are said to constitute the **anatomical dead space. Figure 36-10**, *B*, relates the volume of the anatomical dead space to the major pulmonary volumes.

In abnormal events such as a *pulmonary embolism* in which perfusion of some pulmonary blood vessels is blocked, some alveoli are not able to perform gas exchange and are therefore also "dead space". The anatomical dead space plus any alveolar dead space together make up the **physiological dead space.**

BOX 36-3 *health matters* | Pneumothorax

Air in the pleural space may accumulate when the visceral pleura ruptures and air from the lung rushes out or when atmospheric air rushes in through a wound in the chest wall and parietal pleura. In either case, the lung collapses and normal respiration is impaired. Air in the thoracic cavity is a condition known as **pneumothorax** (see figure). To apply some of the information you have learned about the respiratory mechanism, let us suppose that a surgeon makes an incision through the chest wall into the pleural space, as is done in one of the dramatic, modern open-chest operations. What change, if any, can you deduce takes place in respirations? Compare your deductions with the information in the next paragraph.

Intrapleural pressure, of course, immediately increases from its normal subatmospheric level to the atmospheric level. More pressure than normal is therefore exerted on the outer surface of the punctured lung and causes it to collapse.

Pneumothorax can also result from disruption of the visceral pleura and the resulting flow of pulmonary air into the pleural space.

Pneumothorax results in many respiratory and circulatory changes. They are of great importance in determining medical and nursing care but lie beyond the scope of this book.

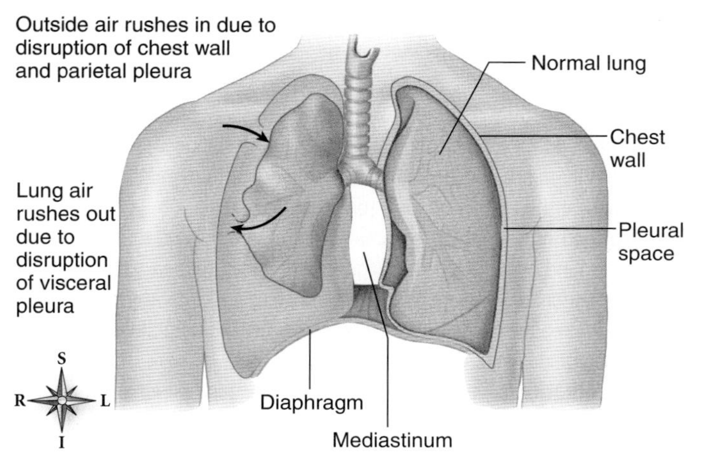

Pneumothorax. Diagram showing air entering the thoracic cavity, causing lung collapse.

One rule of thumb estimates the volume of air in the anatomical dead space to be approximately 30% of the TV (tidal volume).

$$\text{TV} - \text{dead space volume} = \text{alveolar ventilation volume}$$

Suppose you have a normal TV of 500 mL and that 30% of this, or 150 mL, fills the anatomical dead space. The amount of air reaching your alveoli—your alveolar ventilation volume—is then 350 mL per breath, or 70% of your TV.

Emphysema and certain other abnormal conditions, in effect, increase the amount of dead space air or physiological dead space. Consequently, alveolar ventilation decreases, and this in turn decreases the amount of oxygen that can enter blood and the amount of carbon dioxide that can leave it. Inadequate air–blood gas exchange, therefore, is the inevitable result of inadequate alveolar ventilation. Stated differently, the alveoli must be adequately ventilated for an adequate gas exchange to take place in the lungs.

Box 36-4 summarizes some abnormal breathing patterns seen in spirometry.

PULMONARY AIRFLOW

Various applications of spirometry can be used to generate additional information about airflow in an individual. For example, spirometry can be used to determine pulmonary airflow as the rate of pulmonary ventilation, or **total minute volume** (volume moved per minute). Tidal volume (mL/cycle) multiplied by respiration rate (cycles per minute) yields the total minute volume (mL/min). The total minute volume of a person at rest is about 6000 mL (500 mL/cycle × 12 cycles/min). **Box 36-5** discusses the concept of *maximum oxygen consumption*.

Yet another application of spirometry is the **forced expiratory volume (FEV)** test. The FEV test can determine the presence of respiratory obstruction by measuring the volume of air expired per second during forced expiration. The volume forcefully expired

TABLE 36-2 Pulmonary Volumes and Capacities

VOLUME	DESCRIPTION	TYPICAL VALUE	CAPACITY	FORMULA	TYPICAL VALUE
Tidal volume (TV)	Volume moved into or out of the respiratory tract during a normal respiratory cycle	500 mL (0.5 L)	Vital capacity (VC)	TV + IRV +ERV	4500–5000 mL (4.5–5.0 L)
Inspiratory reserve volume (IRV)	Maximum volume that can be moved into the respiratory tract after a normal inspiration	3000–3300 mL (3.0–3.3 L)	Inspiratory capacity (IC)	TV + IRV	3500–3800 mL (3.5–3.8 L)
Expiratory reserve volume (ERV)	Maximum volume that can be moved out of the respiratory tract after a normal expiration	1000–1200 mL (1.0–1.2 L)	Functional residual capacity (FRC)	ERV + RV	2200–2400 mL (2.2–2.4 L)
Residual volume (RV)	Volume remaining in the respiratory tract after maximum expiration	1200 mL (1.2 L)	Total lung capacity (TLC)	TV + IRV + ERV + RV	5700–6200 mL (5.7–6.2 L)

BOX 36-4 *types of breathing*

The alternate movement of air into and out of the lungs that we call breathing can occur in distinctive patterns that can be recognized and designated by name (see figure).

Eupnoea is the term used to describe normal quiet breathing. During eupnoea, the need for oxygen and carbon dioxide exchange is being met, and the individual is not usually conscious of the breathing pattern. Ventilation occurs spontaneously at the rate of 12 to 17 breaths per minute.

Hyperpnoea means increased breathing that is regulated to meet an increased demand by the body for oxygen. During hyperpnoea, there is always an increase in pulmonary ventilation. The hyperpnoea caused by exercise may meet the need for increased oxygen by an increase in tidal volume alone or by an increase in both tidal volume and breathing frequency.

Hyperventilation is characterized by an increase in pulmonary ventilation in excess of the need for oxygen. It sometimes results from a conscious voluntary effort preceding exertion or from psychogenic factors (hysterical hyperventilation). **Hypoventilation** is a decrease in pulmonary ventilation that results in elevated blood levels of carbon dioxide.

Dyspnoea refers to laboured or difficult breathing and is often associated with hypoventilation. A person suffering from dyspnoea is aware, or conscious, of the breathing pattern and is generally uncomfortable and in distress. **Orthopnoea** refers to dyspnoea while lying down. It is relieved by sitting or standing up. This condition is common in patients with heart disease.

Several terms are used to describe the cessation of breathing. **Apnoea** refers to the temporary cessation of breathing at the end of a normal expiration. It may occur during sleep or when swallowing. **Apneusis** is the cessation of breathing in the inspiratory position. Failure to resume breathing after a period of apnoea, or apneusis, is called **respiratory arrest.**

Cheyne–Stokes respiration is a periodic type of abnormal breathing often seen in terminally ill or brain-damaged patients. It is characterized by cycles of gradually increasing tidal volume for several breaths followed by several breaths with gradually decreasing tidal volume. These cycles repeat in a type of crescendo-decrescendo pattern.

Biot's breathing is characterized by repeated sequences of deep gasps and apnoea. This type of abnormal breathing pattern is seen in individuals suffering from increased intracranial pressure. •

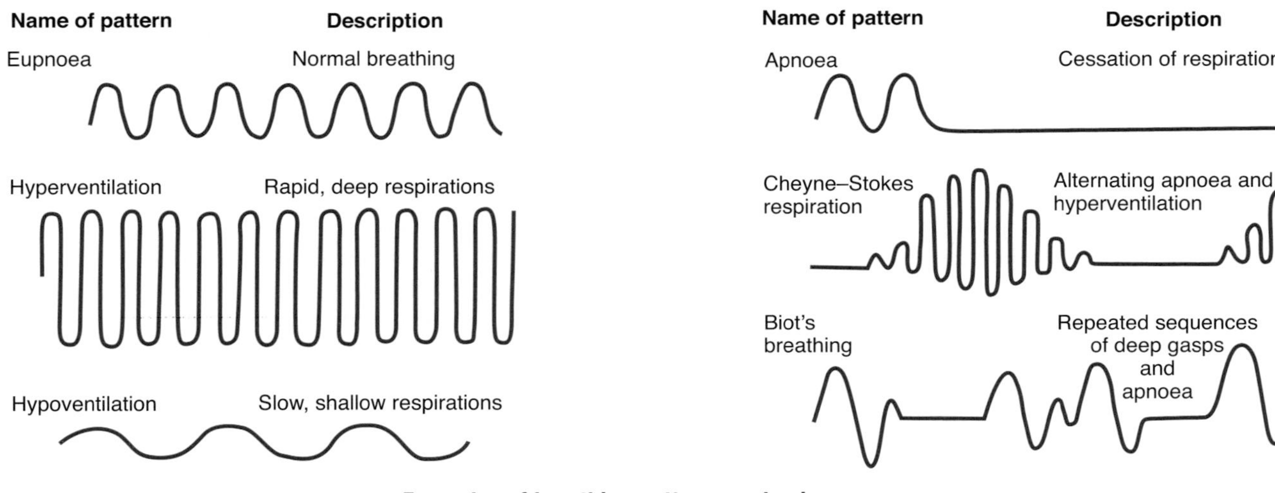

Examples of breathing patterns and spirograms.

BOX 36-5 *sports and fitness*

Maximum Oxygen Consumption

Exercise physiologists use **maximum oxygen consumption** ($VO_{2\ max}$) as a predictor of a person's capacity to do aerobic exercise. An individual's $VO_{2\ max}$ represents the amount of oxygen taken up by the lungs, transported to the tissues, and used to do work. $VO_{2\ max}$ is determined largely by hereditary factors, but aerobic (endurance) training can increase it by as much as 35%. Many endurance athletes are now using $VO_{2\ max}$ measurements to help them determine and then maintain their peak condition. •

during the first second, the FEV_1, is normally about 83% of the vital capacity (**Figure 36-11**). FEV_2, the total volume expired during the first 2 seconds, is about 94% of the VC. By the end of the third second, FEV_3, 97% of the vital capacity should have been expired. The FEV test is also sometimes called the *FVC (forced vital capacity) test.*

Some spirometers are capable of producing a graph called the **flow–volume loop.** This type of graph shows a forced expiration (forced vital capacity) as a loop rather than the peaks and valleys of the classic spirogram. In **Figure 36-12** you can see that the top portion of the loop represents expiratory airflow (litres per second) along the vertical axis and expiratory volume (litres) along the horizontal axis. The inspiratory airflow and volume are represented by the bottom portion of the loop.

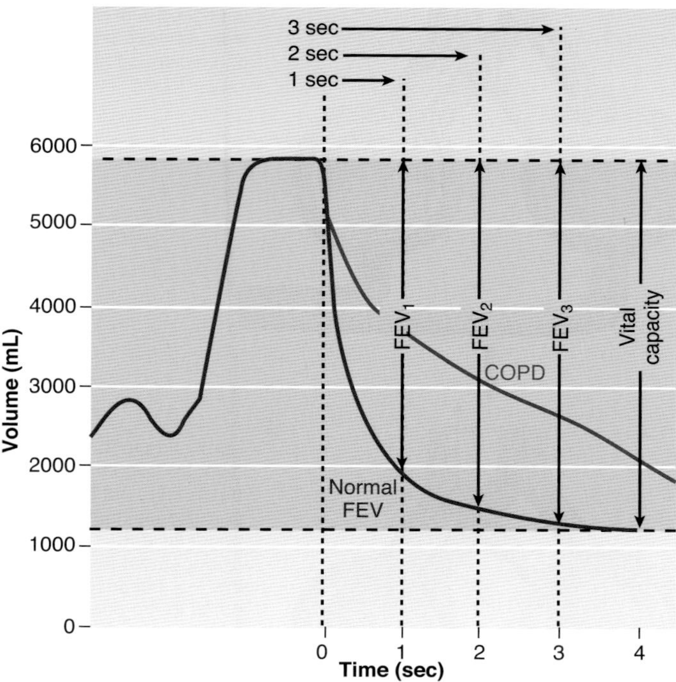

FIGURE 36-11 Forced expiratory volume (FEV). A normal individual forcefully exhales about 83% of the vital capacity (VC) during the first second (FEV_1), 94% at the end of 2 seconds (FEV_2), and 97% by the end of 3 seconds (FEV_3). The *red line* shows the results from a person with chronic obstructive pulmonary disease (COPD) who cannot forcefully exhale a large percentage of the vital capacity as quickly as a person without pulmonary obstruction *(purple line)*.

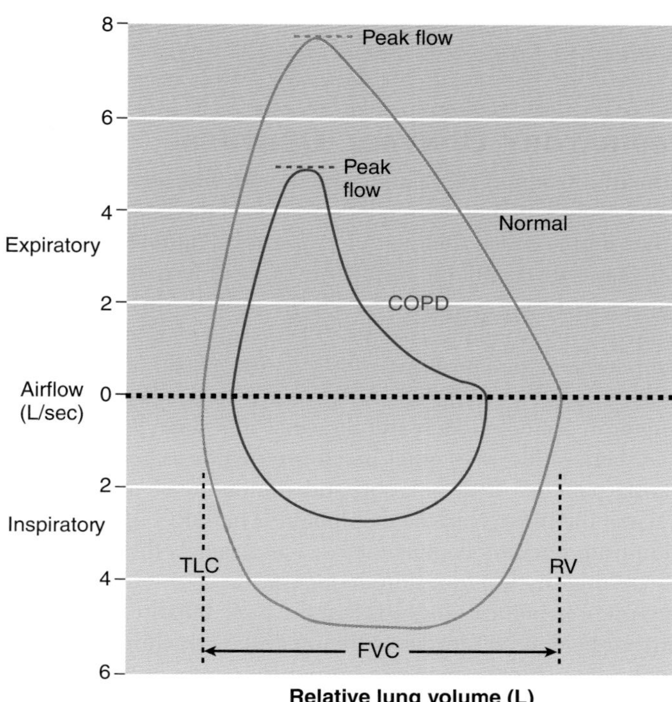

FIGURE 36-12 Flow–volume loops. The top of the loop represents expiratory flow (vertically) and volume (horizontally). The bottom of the loop represents inspiratory flow and volume. Notice that a person with chronic obstructive pulmonary disease (COPD) will produce a smaller loop with a "scooped-out" shape at the end of the expiratory curve. *FVC,* Forced vital capacity; *RV,* residual volume; *TLC,* total lung capacity.

Notice in **Figure 36-12** that the top of the flow–volume loop represents the peak expiratory flow, or more simply the *peak flow*. The peak flow is easy to measure even with simple hand-held spirometers. It is no wonder, then, that peak flow measurements are often used at home by asthma patients to keep a diary of airflow function. The flow–volume loop is especially useful in assessing such obstructive disorders because of the characteristic "scooped-out" shape of the expiratory part of the loop. In some obstructive disorders, the inspiratory portion of the loop may have a normal curve, but smaller than normal.

Quick CHECK

4. What is the difference between a pulmonary *volume* and a pulmonary *capacity*?
5. The volume of air that is expired after a normal inspiration during normal, quiet breathing is referred to by what name?
6. What is meant by the term *vital capacity*?
7. What is the *total minute volume*? How can it be calculated from a spirogram?

VENTILATION AND PERFUSION

Alveolar ventilation, as we already know, is airflow to the alveoli (see **Figure 36-1**). Alveolar perfusion is blood flow to the alveoli. Matching ventilation and perfusion is important for efficient gas exchange in the lungs.

If a poorly ventilated alveolus is well perfused, blood flow is being "wasted" on an inefficient alveolus. It is more efficient to detour some of the blood flow away from the poorly ventilated alveolus and toward a well-ventilated alveolus.

Figure 36-13 shows that perfusion can be matched—within very limited boundaries—to the ventilation status of individual groups of alveoli. As you have probably already deduced, this is accomplished through vasoconstriction (narrowing) of certain pulmonary arterioles to reduce perfusion to poorly ventilated alveoli. Such ventilation–perfusion matching in various regions of each lung can increase the overall efficiency of gas exchange.

REGULATION OF VENTILATION

HOMEOSTASIS OF BLOOD GASES AND pH

Various regulatory mechanisms operate to maintain relative constancy of the blood's oxygen and carbon dioxide levels. These blood gas concentrations are often expressed as *oxygen pressure* (PO_2) and *carbon dioxide pressure* (PCO_2) in kilopascals (kPa) or millimetres of mercury (mmHg). Because CO_2 dissolved in water produces an acid, the higher the PCO_2 of blood plasma, the lower the pH of blood plasma—a concept we explore further in the next chapter.

This homeostasis of blood gases is maintained primarily by means of changes in ventilation—the rate and depth of breathing. Changes in ventilation can also help regulate the homeostasis of pH in the body's internal environment.

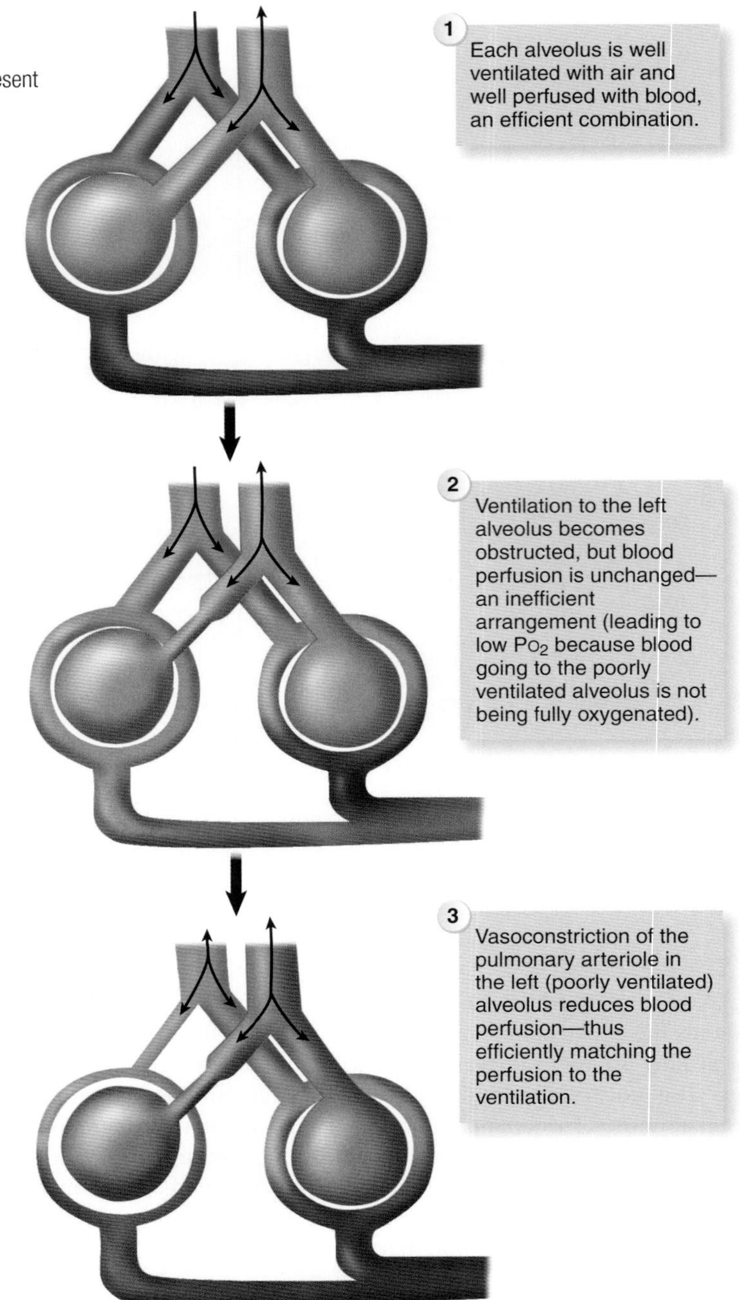

1
Each alveolus is well ventilated with air and well perfused with blood, an efficient combination.
2
Ventilation to the left alveolus becomes obstructed, but blood perfusion is unchanged—an inefficient arrangement (leading to low P_{O_2} because blood going to the poorly ventilated alveolus is not being fully oxygenated).
3
Vasoconstriction of the pulmonary arteriole in the left (poorly ventilated) alveolus reduces blood perfusion—thus efficiently matching the perfusion to the ventilation.

FIGURE 36-13 Ventilation and perfusion of the alveoli. Here, two alveoli represent typical alveoli in the lungs.

Respiratory Control Centres

The main integrators that control the nerves that affect the inspiratory and expiratory muscles are located within the brainstem and are together simply called the *respiratory centres* (**Figure 36-14**).

The basic rhythm of the respiratory cycle of inspiration and expiration seems to be generated by the **medullary rhythmicity area.** This area of the medulla consists of two regions of interconnected control centres: the *dorsal respiratory group (DRG)* and the *ventral respiratory group (VRG)*. The VRG seems to be the basic rhythm generator in animal models and thus may also serve this function in human beings. Normal, quiet breathing rhythm is generated by alternating patterns of stimulation and inhibition of motor neurons that signal the muscles of the diaphragm. The DRG integrates information from chemoreceptors for P_{CO_2} and signals the VRG to alter the breathing rhythm to restore homeostasis.

A current hypothesis suggests that the basic breathing rhythm can be altered by different inputs to the medullary rhythmicity area. For example, input from a possible **apneustic centre** in the pons may regulate the length and depth of inspiration. Damage to the nerves from the apneustic centre is thought to produce breathing characterized by abnormally long, deep inspirations, which is sometimes called "apneustic breathing".

The **pontine respiratory group** (PRG; formerly called the *pneumotaxic centre*), also in the pons, may regulate both the apneustic centre and the medullary rhythmicity area. Thus a network of interconnected centres in the brainstem regulates the rhythm of breathing. **Box 36-6** discusses some unusual breathing reflexes such as coughing and sneezing.

The *cerebral cortex* also influences breathing. Impulses to the respiratory centre from the motor area of the cerebrum may either increase or decrease the rate and strength of respirations. In other words, an individual may voluntarily speed up or slow down the breathing rate. This voluntary control of respirations, however, has certain limitations. For example, one may stop breathing and do so for a few minutes, but holding the breath results in an increase in the CO_2 content of the blood because it is not being removed by respirations. CO_2 is a powerful respiratory stimulant. So when arterial blood P_{CO_2} increases to a certain level, it stimulates the inspiratory neuron (directly and reflexively) to send motor impulses to the respiratory muscles, and breathing is resumed, even though the individual may still will contrarily.

Feedback and Responses

Feedback information to the medullary rhythmicity area comes from sensors throughout the nervous system, as well as from other control centres. The sensors that provide this feedback are primarily the **central chemoreceptors** in the brain and **peripheral chemoreceptors** in peripheral sensory nerves in the carotid bodies and aorta. These chemoreceptors are sensitive to changes in the O_2, CO_2 and hydrogen ion concentration (pH) of the fluid internal environment.

Large increases in arterial P_{CO_2} stimulate *peripheral chemoreceptors* in the carotid bodies and aorta. Stimulation of chemoreceptors by increased arterial P_{CO_2} results in faster breathing, with a greater volume of air moving in and out of the lungs per minute. **Figure 36-15** summarizes this negative feedback response.

Decreased arterial P_{CO_2} produces opposite effects—it inhibits central and peripheral chemoreceptors, which leads to inhibition of the medullary rhythmicity area and slower respirations. In fact, breathing stops entirely for a few moments (apnoea) when arterial P_{CO_2} drops moderately—to about 4.7 kPa (35 mmHg), for example.

Recall that increases in the CO_2 content of plasma are accompanied by a proportional decrease in plasma pH. A decrease in arterial blood pH (increase in acid), within certain limits, has a stimulating effect on chemoreceptors located in the carotid and aortic bodies.

Central chemoreceptors are sensitive to ongoing changes in pH in a way that differs from peripheral chemoreceptor sensitivity. This difference results from the fact that cerebrospinal fluid (CSF) and

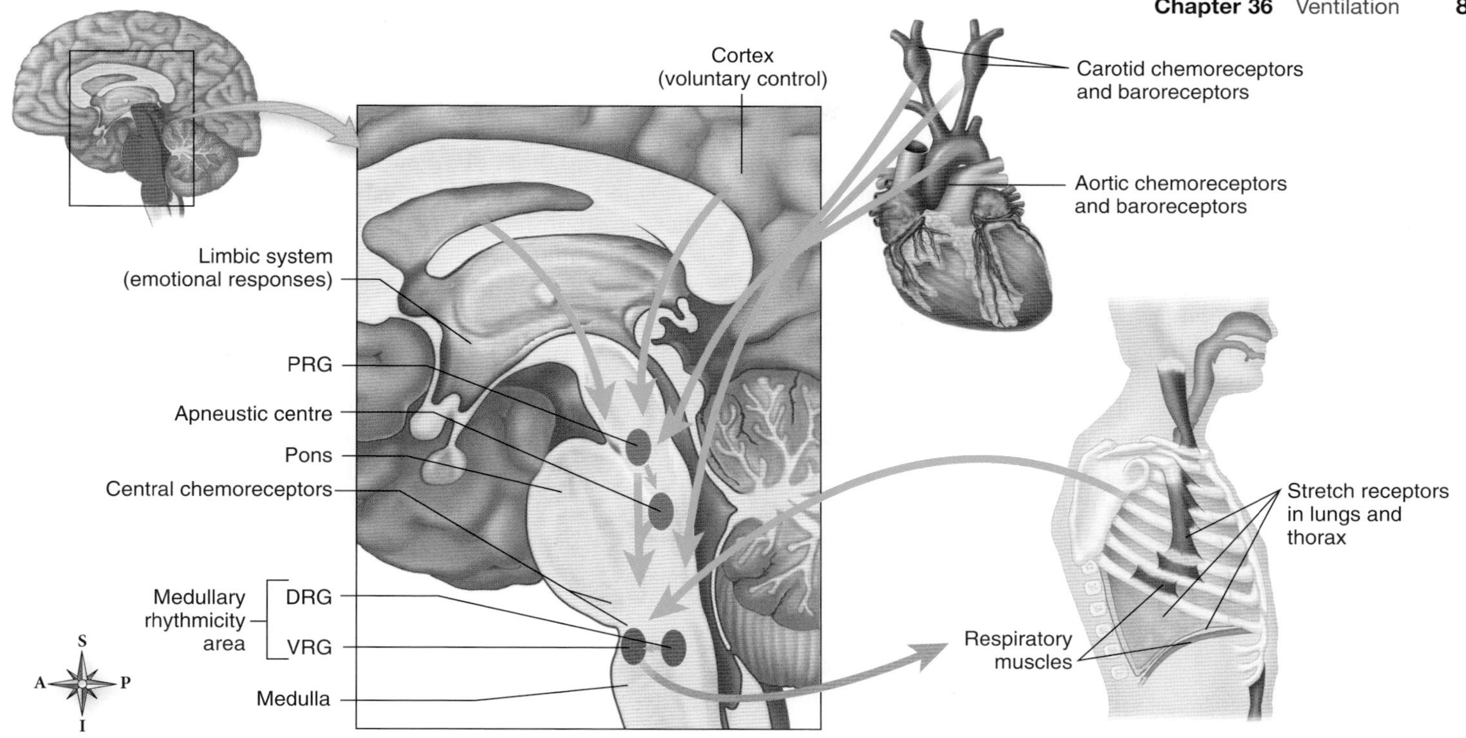

FIGURE 36-14 Regulation of breathing. The dorsal respiratory group (DRG) and ventral respiratory group (VRG) of the medulla represent the medullary rhythmicity area. The pontine respiratory group (PRG, or pneumotaxic centre) and apneustic centre of the pons influence the basic respiratory rhythm by means of neural input to the medullary rhythmicity area. The brainstem also receives input from other parts of the body; information from chemoreceptors, baroreceptors, and stretch receptors can alter the basic breathing pattern, as can emotional (limbic) and sensory input. Despite these subconscious reflexes, the cerebral cortex can override the "automatic" control of breathing to some extent to do such activities as sing or blow up a balloon. *Green arrows* show flow of information to the respiratory control centres. The *purple arrow* shows the flow of information from the control centres to the respiratory muscles that drive breathing.

BOX 36-6 *fyi* | Unusual Breathing Reflexes

The **cough reflex** is stimulated by foreign matter in the trachea or bronchi. The epiglottis and glottis reflexively close, and contraction of the expiratory muscles causes air pressure in the lungs to increase. The epiglottis and glottis then open suddenly, resulting in an upward burst of air that removes the offending contaminants—a cough.

The **sneeze reflex** is similar to the cough reflex, except that it is stimulated by contaminants in the nasal cavity. A burst of air is directed through the nose and mouth, forcing the contaminants (and mucus) out of the respiratory tract. Droplets from a sneeze can travel more than 161 km/hr and travel 3 metres. Research suggests that many pathogenic microbes produce symptoms that trigger sneezing in order to spread themselves to other people. Scientists call this *altered host behaviour* and identify it as a mechanism of microbes to efficiently spread themselves to additional human hosts.

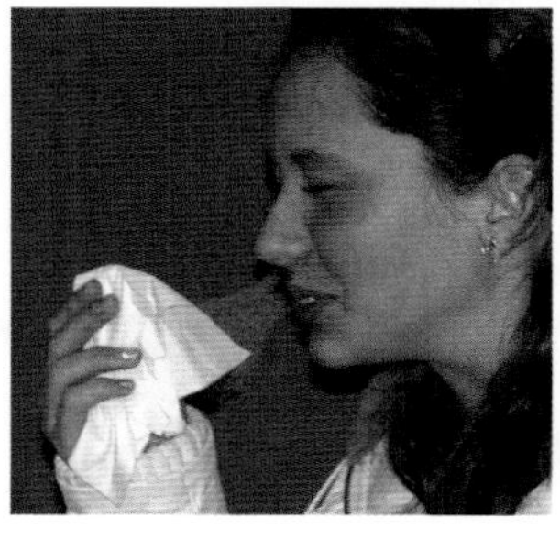

The term **hiccup** is used to describe an involuntary, spasmodic contraction of the diaphragm. When such a contraction occurs, generally at the beginning of an inspiration, the glottis suddenly closes, producing the characteristic sound. Hiccups lasting for extended periods can be disabling. They may be produced by irritation of the phrenic nerve or the sensory nerves in the stomach or by direct injury or pressure on certain areas of the brain. Fortunately, most cases of hiccups last only a few minutes and are harmless.

A **yawn** is slow, deep inspiration through an unusually widened mouth. Yawns were once thought to be reflexes that increase ventilation when blood oxygen content is low, but newer evidence suggests that this is unlikely. A current theory states that we yawn for the same reason we occasionally stretch—to prepare our muscles and our circulatory system for action. Alternate hypotheses suggest that yawning cools the brain or otherwise regulates body temperature—or that yawning is triggered by neurotransmitters related to mood. The variety of hypotheses show one thing for certain: *We do not currently understand the physiology of yawning!*

A protective physiological response called the **diving reflex** is responsible for the astonishing recovery of people in apparent drownings—including some who may have been submerged for more than 40 minutes! Survivors are most often preadolescent children who have been immersed in water below 20° C. Apparently, the colder the water, the better the chance of survival. In such cases, the person initially appears dead when pulled from the water. Breathing has stopped; the pupils are fixed and dilated; the skin is cyanotic; and the pulse has stopped.

Studies have shown that when the head and face are immersed in ice-cold water, there is immediate shunting of blood to the core body areas with peripheral vasoconstriction and slowing of the heart (bradycardia). Metabolism is slowed, and tissue requirements for oxygen and nutrients decrease. The diving reflex is a protective response of the body to cold water immersion and is a function of such physiological and environmental parameters as water temperature, age, lung volume, and posture. •

interstitial fluid (IF) of the brain is separated from the buffers present in the blood by the BBB (blood–brain barrier). Thus, when blood P_{CO_2} increases in the blood, it is partially buffered in the blood—but the CO_2 can cross the BBB and is *not* buffered in the brain's CSF and IF. The brain then senses unbuffered changes in pH (**Figure 36-16**). However, because the movement of CO_2 across the BBB is slow, the central chemoreceptors are best at detecting longer-term changes in CO_2 than rapid changes in CO_2 or pH.

The role of arterial blood P_{O_2} in controlling respirations is not entirely clear. Presumably, it has little influence as long as it stays above a certain level. But neurons of the respiratory centres, like all body cells, require adequate amounts of oxygen to function optimally. Consequently, if they become hypoxic, they become depressed and send fewer impulses to respiratory muscles. Respirations then decrease or fail entirely. This principle has important clinical significance. For example, the respiratory centres cannot respond to stimulation by an increasing blood CO_2 if, at the same time, blood P_{O_2} falls below a critical level—a fact that may become life or death important during anaesthesia.

However, a decrease in arterial blood P_{O_2} below 9.3 kPa (70 mmHg), but not so low as the critical level, stimulates chemoreceptors in the carotid and aortic bodies and causes reflex stimulation of the inspiratory neurons of the medullary rhythmicity area. This constitutes a "backup" respiratory control mechanism. It does not help regulate respirations in ordinary conditions when arterial blood P_{O_2} remains considerably higher than 9.3 kPa (70 mmHg), which is the level necessary to stimulate the chemoreceptors.

To summarize, here are a few principles of feedback and responses in regulating ventilation:

- Peripheral chemoreceptors monitor arterial blood plasma and respond to low plasma P_{O_2}, high plasma P_{CO_2}, and low plasma pH (when plasma acidity exceeds buffering capacity).

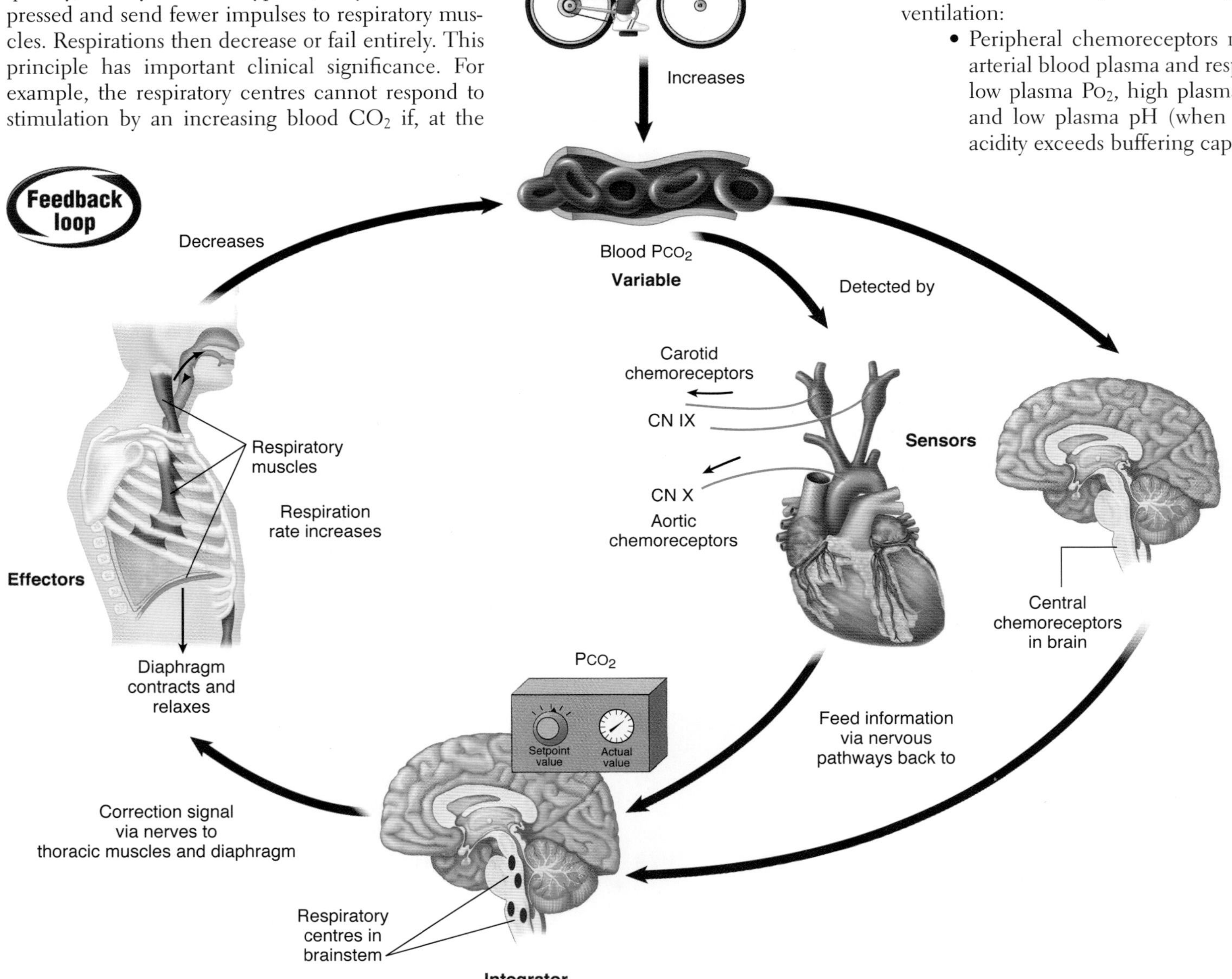

FIGURE 36-15 Negative feedback control of ventilation. This diagram summarizes the feedback loop that operates to increase the respiratory rate in response to high plasma P_{CO_2}. Increased cellular respiration during exercise causes a rise in plasma P_{CO_2}—which is detected by central chemoreceptors in the brain and perhaps peripheral chemoreceptors in the carotid sinus and aorta. Feedback information is relayed to integrators in the brainstem that respond to the increase in P_{CO_2} above the setpoint value by sending nervous correction signals to the respiratory muscles, which act as effectors. The effector muscles increase their alternate contraction and relaxation, thus increasing the rate of respiration. As the respiration rate increases, the rate of CO_2 loss from the body increases and P_{CO_2} drops accordingly. This brings the plasma P_{CO_2} back to its setpoint value.

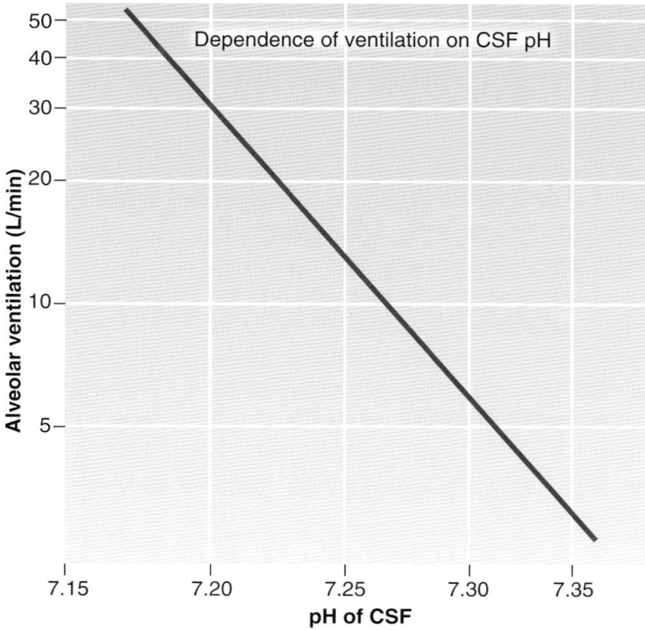

FIGURE 36-16 Regulatory effect of pH of cerebrospinal fluid. As P_{CO_2} of arterial blood increases, the pH of the cerebrospinal fluid (CSF) decreases, as does the brainstem's interstitial fluid (IF). As the graph shows, the lower the pH goes, the higher the ventilation rate rises. Higher ventilation results in increased rate of CO_2 loss from the body, eventually returning the body to a homeostatic balance.

- Central chemoreceptors respond to high CSF P_{CO_2} and/or low CSF pH.
- Peripheral chemoreceptors respond to rapid changes but chemoreceptors respond to ongoing changes.

OTHER INFLUENCES ON VENTILATION

Arterial blood pressure helps control breathing through the respiratory pressoreflex mechanism. A sudden rise in arterial pressure, by acting on aortic and carotid baroreceptors, results in reflex slowing of respirations. A sudden drop in arterial pressure brings about a reflex increase in the rate and depth of respirations. The pressoreflex mechanism is probably not of great importance in the control of respirations. It is, however, of major importance in the control of circulation.

The **Hering–Breuer reflexes** also help control respirations, particularly their depth and rhythmicity when the tidal volume is high. It is believed they regulate the depth of respirations (extent of lung expansion)—and therefore the volume of tidal air—in the following way. Presumably, when a large tidal volume of air has been inspired, the lungs are expanded enough to stimulate stretch receptors located within them. The stretch receptors then send inhibitory impulses to the inspiratory neuron, relaxation of inspiratory muscles occurs, and expiration follows the Hering–Breuer expiratory reflex. Then, when a large tidal volume of air has been expired, the lungs are sufficiently deflated to inhibit the lung stretch receptors and allow inspiration to start again—the Hering–Breuer inspiratory reflex. Evidence suggests that these reflexes do not play a significant role in resting (low tidal volume) breathing, except perhaps in newborns.

Miscellaneous factors may also influence breathing. Among these are blood temperature and sensory impulses from skin thermal receptors and from superficial or deep pain receptors:

BOX 36-7 *sports and fitness*
Control of Respirations During Exercise

Respirations increase abruptly at the beginning of exercise and decrease even more markedly as it ends. This much is known. The mechanism that accomplishes this increased breathing rate, however, is not known. It is not identical to the one that produces moderate increases in breathing. Numerous studies have shown that arterial blood P_{CO_2}, P_{O_2}, and pH do not change enough during exercise to produce the degree of hyperpnoea (faster, deeper respirations) observed. Presumably, many chemical and nervous factors and temperature changes operate as a complex, but still unknown, mechanism for regulating respirations during exercise. •

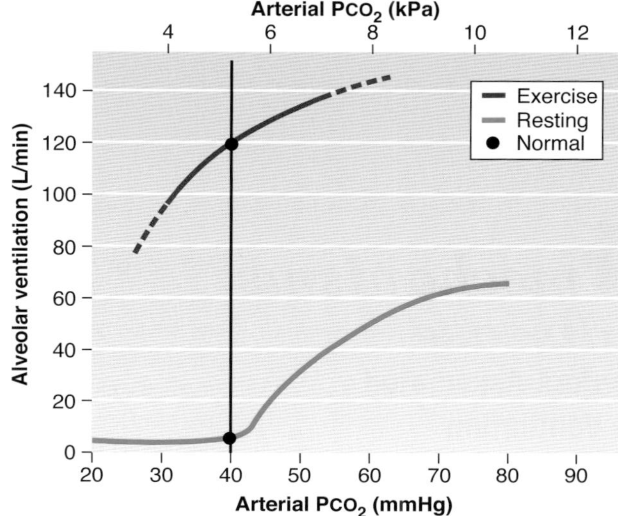

Normal effects of maximum exercise in an athlete. This graph shows that the breathing rate (vertical axis) is much higher in an athlete exercising maximally than would be expected for any given blood carbon dioxide pressure (P_{CO_2}) (horizontal axis). As you can see at the normal points of a P_{CO_2} of 40 mmHg (5.3 kPa), the exercising athlete's breathing (ventilation) rate is 120 L/min. However, at rest the athlete's breathing rate is only about 5 or 6 L/min at the same P_{CO_2}—thus showing that P_{CO_2} is not the major factor causing an increased rate of breathing during exercise.

Sudden painful stimulation produces a reflex apnoea, but continued painful stimuli cause faster and deeper respirations.

Sudden cold stimuli applied to the skin cause reflex apnoea.

Stimulation of the pharynx or larynx by irritating chemicals or by touch causes a temporary apnoea. This is the choking reflex, a valuable protective device. It operates, for example, to prevent aspiration of food or liquids during swallowing.

The major factors that influence breathing are summarized in **Figure 36-14**. Some factors that affect breathing during exercise are mentioned in **Box 36-7**.

Quick CHECK

8. Where are the chief regulatory centres of the respiratory function located?
9. Name several factors that can influence the breathing rate of an individual; tell whether each triggers an increase or a decrease in breathing rate.

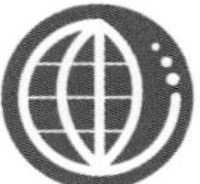

the big picture | Ventilation and the Whole Body

The homeostatic balance of the entire body, and thus the survival of each and every cell, depends on the proper functioning of the respiratory system. Because the mitochondria in each cell require oxygen for their energy conversions, and because each cell produces toxic carbon dioxide as a waste product of the very same energy conversions, the internal environment must continually acquire new oxygen and discard carbon dioxide. If each cell were immediately adjacent to the external environment—that is, atmospheric air—this would require no special system. However, because almost every one of the 37 trillion cells that make up the body are far removed from the outside air, another method of satisfying this condition must be employed—this is where the respiratory system comes in. By the process of ventilation, fresh external air continually flows less than a hair's breadth away from the circulating fluid of the body—the blood.

Specific mechanisms involved in respiratory function show the interdependence among body systems observed throughout our study of the human body. For example, without regulation by the nervous system, ventilation could not be adjusted to compensate for changes in the oxygen or carbon dioxide content of the internal environment. Without the skeletal muscles of the thorax, the airways could not maintain the flow of fresh air that is so vital to respiratory function. The skeleton itself provides a firm outer housing for the lungs and has an arrangement of bones that facilitates the expansion and recoil of the thorax, which is needed to accomplish inspiration and expiration. Without the immune system, pathogens from the external environment could easily colonize the respiratory tract and possibly cause a fatal infection.

Even more subtle interactions between the respiratory system and other body systems can be found. For example, the language function of the nervous system is limited without the speaking ability provided by the larynx and other structures of the respiratory tract.

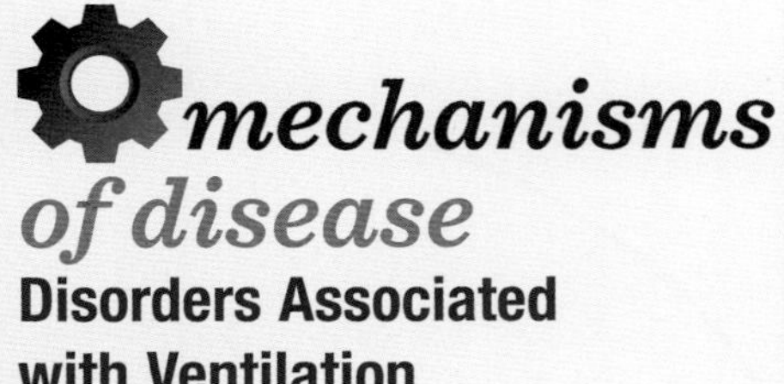

mechanisms of disease Disorders Associated with Ventilation

Many things can interfere with the functions of gas exchange and ventilation and cause respiratory failure. A few of the more important disorders are briefly described here and in **Box 36-8**.

Restrictive Pulmonary Disorders

Restrictive pulmonary disorders involve restriction of the alveoli, or reduced compliance, leading to decreased lung inflation. The hallmark of these disorders, regardless of their cause, is decreased lung volumes and capacities such as inspiratory reserve volume and vital capacity. Factors that restrict breathing can originate either within the lung or outside of it. Causes of restrictive lung disorders include alveolar fibrosis (scarring) secondary to occupational exposure to asbestos, toxic fumes, coal dust, or other contaminants; immunological diseases, as in rheumatoid lung; obesity; and metabolic disorders such as uraemia. Restriction of breathing can also be caused by pain that accompanies pleurisy (inflammation of the pleurae) or mechanical injuries (such as a fractured or bruised rib). Patients with restrictive lung disease classically experience **dyspnoea** (laboured breathing) and are not able to tolerate increased activity, which reduces their ability to work or perform normal daily activities. Therapy involves eliminating the cause of the restriction, ensuring adequate gas exchange, and improving exercise tolerance.

Obstructive Pulmonary Disorders

A variety of conditions may cause obstruction of the airways. Exposure to cigarette smoke and other common air pollutants can trigger a reflexive constriction of bronchial airways. Obstructive disorders may obstruct inspiration and expiration, whereas restrictive disorders mainly restrict inspiration.

Chronic Obstructive Pulmonary Disease

Chronic obstructive pulmonary disease (COPD) is a broad term used to describe conditions of progressive irreversible obstruction of expiratory airflow. People with COPD have chronic difficulties with breathing, mainly emptying their lungs, and have visibly hyperinflated chests. **Figures 36-11** and **36-12** (p. 837) show the effects of COPD compared with normal breathing patterns. Those with COPD often have a productive cough and intolerance of activity. The major disorders observed in people with COPD are chronic bronchitis and emphysema.

In the UK, tobacco use is the primary cause of COPD, but air pollution, asthma, and respiratory infections also play a role. COPD is a leading cause of death—one that has been *increasing* over recent years! COPD affects more men than women, but an increase in the number of women smokers has led to an increase in the incidence of this condition in women.

Acute respiratory failure can occur when any of the disorders that produce COPD become intense. Heart failure resulting from the pulmonary disease and the vascular resistance that develops with COPD is another possible outcome. Although there is no cure for chronic obstructive respiratory conditions, limiting

---

BOX 36-8 *health matters* | **Sudden Infant Death Syndrome (SIDS)**

There are between 200 and 325 unexplained infant deaths in England and Wales every year, a rate of 0.36 deaths per 1,000 live births. Almost two-thirds (65%) of these were recorded as *sudden infant death syndrome* (SIDS), commonly called "cot death", and more males are affected than females.

SIDS was first recognized in the early 1960s and is defined as "the sudden death of any infant or young child which is unexplained by history and in which a thorough post mortem examination fails to demonstrate an adequate cause of death".

Although the baby stops breathing in SIDS cases, the exact cause of this cannot be established and it remains a mystery. The main risk factors for SIDS are overheating and an unsafe sleeping environment, such as sleeping face down. More deaths occur during the winter, perhaps because of the use of extra clothing, blankets, and central heating. Other risk factors include maternal age, maternal smoking during pregnancy, and post-natal exposure to tobacco smoke. A number of other factors have also been associated with an increased risk of SIDS, for example marital status of the mother and socio-economic position of the parents.

Although the exact cause of SIDS remains unknown, genetic defects involving the structure and function of the respiratory system or unusual physiological responses to common flu or cold viruses may also play a role in this tragic problem.

symptoms can improve quality of life. Bronchodilators and corticosteroids have been used to relieve some of the airway obstruction involved in COPD.

Acute obstruction of the airways, as when a piece of food blocks airflow, requires immediate action to avoid death from suffocation.

CONNECT IT!

Knowledge of the physical principles of ventilation can have lifesaving applications in medical emergencies involving acute airway obstruction caused by foreign material. Learn about how these procedures can help people who are choking in ***Abdominal Thrusts*** online at ***Connect It!***

Bronchitis

In chronic **bronchitis,** the person produces excessive tracheobronchial secretions that obstruct airflow, and the bronchial mucous glands are enlarged (**Figure 36-17**, *B*). Risk factors include cigarette smoking (accounting for 80% to 90% of the risk of developing COPD), a normal decline in pulmonary function as a result of age, and environmental exposure to dust and chemicals. With impairment of the alveoli and loss of capillary beds, gas exchange is inefficient, which in turn produces hypoxia.

Emphysema

In **emphysema,** the air spaces distal to the terminal bronchioles are enlarged as a result of damage to lung connective tissue. As the bronchioles collapse and the alveoli enlarge, the alveolar walls rupture and fuse into large irregular spaces, and gas exchange units are destroyed (**Figure 36-17**, *D*). Although the aetiology is not fully understood, this condition is believed to be caused by proteolytic enzymes that destroy lung tissue. Hypoxia often develops in people with emphysema.

Asthma

Asthma is an obstructive lung disorder characterized by recurring inflammation of mucous membranes and spasms of the smooth muscles in the walls of the bronchial air passages. The inflammation (oedema and excessive mucus production) and contractions narrow airways, making breathing difficult (**Figure 36-17**, *C*). Initial onset of asthma can occur in children or adults. Acute episodes of asthma—so-called asthma attacks—can be triggered by stress, heavy exercise, infection, or exposure to allergens or other irritants such as dust, vapour, or fumes. Many patients with asthma have a family history of allergies.

Dyspnoea is the major symptom of asthma, but hyperventilation, headaches, numbness, and nausea can occur. One way to treat asthma is by using inhaled or systemic bronchodilators to reduce muscle spasms and thus open the airways. Other types of treatment involve the use of antiinflammatory medications including leukotriene modifiers to reduce the inflammation associated with asthma. (Recall from Chapter 32 that leukotrienes are cytokines released by immune cells to regulate the inflammation response.)

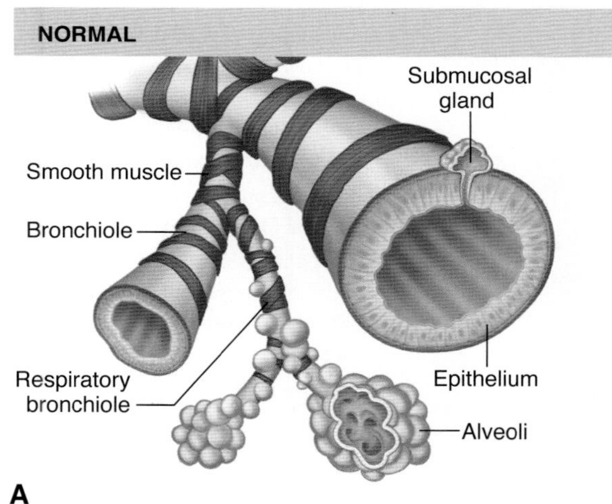

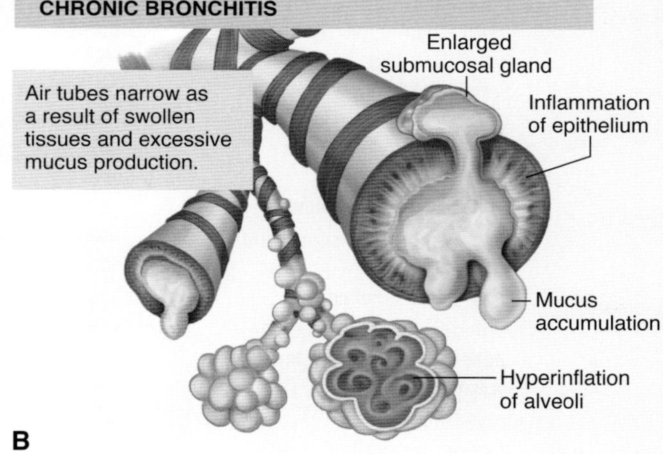

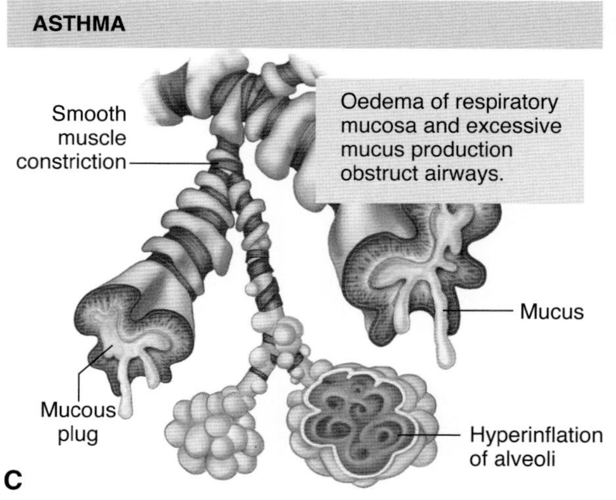

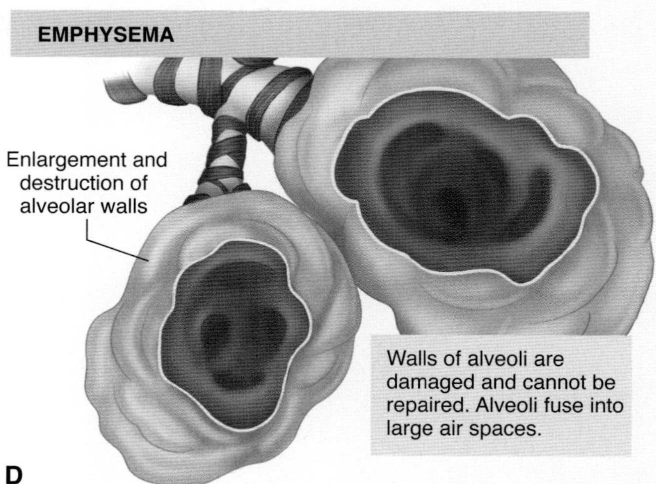

FIGURE 36-17 Obstructive pulmonary disorders. Examples of chronic disorders involving pulmonary obstruction.

LANGUAGE OF SCIENCE *(continued from p. 824)*

peripheral chemoreceptor (pe-RIF-er-al kee-moh-ree-SEP-tor) [*centr-* **centre,** *-al* **relating to,** *chemo-* **chemical,** *-recept-* **receive,** *-or* **agent**]

physiological dead space (fiz-ee-oh-LOJ-ih-kal) [*physio-* **nature,** *-log-* **words (study),** *-ical* **relating to**]

pontine respiratory group (PRG) (pon-TEEN RES-pih-rah-toh-ree groop) [*pont-* **bridge (pons),** *-ine* **relating to**]

primary principle of ventilation (ven-tih-LAY-shun) [*prim-* **first,** *-ary* **relating to,** *princip-* **foundation,** *vent-* **fan or create wind,** *-tion* **process**]

pulmonary ventilation (PUL-moh-nair-ee ven-tih-LAY-shun) [*pulmon-* **lung,** *-ary* **relating to,** *vent-* **fan or create wind,** *-tion* **process**]

solubility (sol-yoo-BIL-ih-tee) [*solu-* **dissolve,** *-bil-* **capable,** *-ity* **state**]

surface tension (SER-fes TEN-shun)

tension (TEN-shun)

transpulmonary pressure (tranz-PUHL-mohn-air-ee) [*trans-* **across,** *pulmon-* **lung,** *-ary* **relating to**]

Young–LaPlace law (law of LaPlace) (yung lah-PLAHS) [*Thomas Young* **English physician,** *Pierre Simon de LaPlace* **French physicist**]

LANGUAGE OF MEDICINE

apnoea (AP-nee-ah) [*a-* **not,** *-pnoe-* **breathe,** *-a* **condition**]

apneusis (ap-NYOO-sis) [*a-* **not,** *-pneu-* **breathe,** *-sis* **condition**]

asthma (AZ-mah) [*asthma* **panting**]

Biot's breathing (bee-OHS) [*Camille Biot* **French physician**]

bronchitis (brong-KYE-tis) [*bronch-* **windpipe,** *-itis* **inflammation**]

Cheyne–Stokes respiration (chain stokes res-pih-RAY-shun) [*John Cheyne* **Scots physician,** *William Stokes* **Irish physician,** *re-* **again,** *-spir-* **breathe,** *-ation* **process**]

chronic obstructive pulmonary disease (COPD) (KRON-ik ob-STRUK-tiv PUL-moh-nair-ee) [*chron-* **time,** *-ic* **relating to,** *pulmon-* **lung,** *-ary* **relating to**]

continuous positive airway pressure (CPAP) (CPAP)

dyspnoea (DISP-nee-ah) [*dys-* **painful,** *-pnoe-* **breathe,** *-a* **condition**]

emphysema (em-fih-SEE-mah) [*em-* **in,** *-physema* **blowing or puffing up**]

eupnoea (YOOP-nee-ah) [*eu-* **easily,** *-pnoe-* **breathe,** *-a* **condition**]

expiratory reserve volume (ERV) (eks-PYE-rah-tor-ee) [*ex-* **out of,** *-[s]pir-* **breathe,** *-tory* **relating to**]

forced expiratory volume (FEV) (eks-PYE-rah-tor-ee) [*ex-* **out of,** *-[s]pir-* **breathe,** *-tory* **relating to**]

functional residual capacity (FRC) (FUNK-shun-al reh-ZID-yoo-al kah-PAS-ih-tee) [*function-* **perform,** *-al* **relating to,** *residu-* **left over,** *-al* **relating to,** *capac-* **hold,** *-ity* **state**]

hiccup (HIK-up) [**imitation of hiccup sound**]

hyaline membrane disease (HMD) (HYE-ah-lin) [*hyal-* **glass,** *-ine* **of or like**]

hyperpnoea (hye-PERP-nee-ah) [*hyper-* **excessive,** *-pnoe-* **breathe,** *-a* **condition**]

hyperventilation (hye-per-ven-tih-LAY-shun) [*hyper-* **excessive,** *-vent-* **fan or create wind,** *-tion* **process**]

hypoventilation (hye-poh-ven-tih-LAY-shun) [*hypo-* **under or below,** *-vent-* **fan or create wind,** *-tion* **process**]

inspiratory capacity (IC) (in-SPY-rah-tor-ee kah-PASS-ih-tee) [*in-* **in,** *-spir-* **breathe,** *-tory* **relating to,** *capac-* **hold,** *-ity* **state**]

inspiratory reserve volume (IRV) (in-SPY-rah-tor-ee) [*in-* **in,** *-spir-* **breathe,** *-tory* **relating to**]

intratracheal injection (in-trah-TRAY-kee-al in-JEK-shun) [*intra-* **within,** *-trache-* **rough duct,** *-al* **relating to,** *in-* **in,** *-ject-* **throw,** *-tion* **process**]

maximum oxygen consumption ($Vo_{2\ max}$) [*maximum* **greatest,** *oxy-* **sharp,** *-gen* **produce,** *con-* **with or in,** *-sum-* **take,** *-tion* **process**]

orthopnoea (or-THOP-nee-ah) [*ortho-* **straight or upright,** *-pnoe-* **breathe,** *-a* **condition**]

pneumothorax (nyoo-moh-THOH-raks) [*pneumo-* **air or wind,** *-thorax* **chest**]

residual volume (RV) (ree-ZID-yoo-al)

respiratory distress syndrome (RDS) (RES-pih-rah-tor-ee dih-STRESS SIN-drohm) [*re-* **again,** *-spir-* **breathe,** *-tory* **relating to,** *syn-* **together,** *-drome* **running or (race)course**]

spirogram (SPY-roh-gram) [*spir-* **breathe,** *-gram* **drawing**]

spirometer (spih-ROM-eh-ter) [*spir-* **breathe,** *-meter* **measure**]

tidal volume (TV) (TYE-dal) [*tid-* **time,** *-al* **relating to**]

total lung capacity (TLC) (TOHT-il lung kah-PASS-ih-tee) [*capac-* **hold,** *-ity* **state**]

total minute volume (TOHT-il MIN-it VOL-yoom)

vital capacity (VC) (VYE-tal kah-PASS-ih-tee) [*vita-* **life,** *-al* **relating to,** *capac-* **hold,** *-ity* **state**]

case study

After having surgery to remove a stomach tumour, Robert woke up in the recovery room in extreme pain. Although it hurt to move, blink, or take even a little breath, the nurse asked him to take a deep breath and cough!

1. Which of these muscles would not contract when Robert complied with his nurse's instructions?
   a. Diaphragm
   b. Serratus anterior
   c. Rectus abdominis
   d. External intercostals

2. Which statement best describes the "mechanics" of Robert's inhalations?
   a. The thoracic cavity decreases in size, lowering the alveolar pressure, and air flows from high (atmospheric) pressure to low (alveolar) pressure.
   b. The thoracic cavity increases in size, lowering the alveolar pressure, and air flows from high (atmospheric) pressure to low (alveolar) pressure.
   c. Air flows from high (atmospheric) pressure to low (alveolar) pressure and expands the thoracic cavity.
   d. Air flows from high (intrapleural) pressure to low (alveolar) pressure and expands the thoracic cavity.

The respiratory physiotherapist measured Robert's pulmonary capacities. The results were inspiratory reserve volume: 2900 mL; tidal volume: 490 mL; and expiratory reserve volume: 1000 mL.

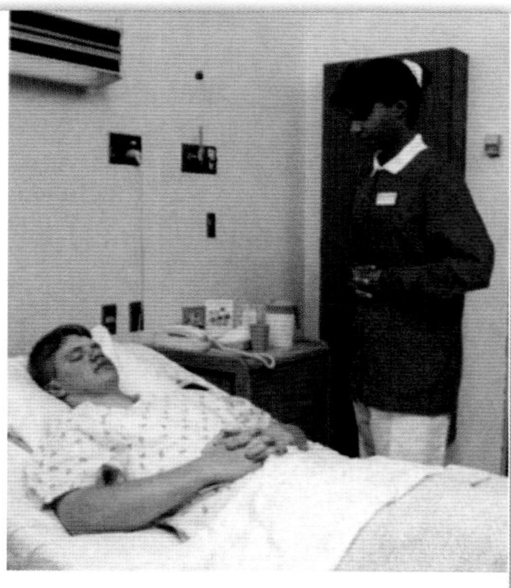

3. Using the volumes listed above, what was Robert's vital capacity following his operation?
   a. 3390 mL
   b. 4390 mL
   c. 3900 mL
   d. 1490 mL

4. The respiratory physiotherapist was concerned that air may have accumulated in the pleural space as a result of the surgery. What is the name of the condition in which air is present in the pleural space between the lung and wall of the thoracic cavity?
   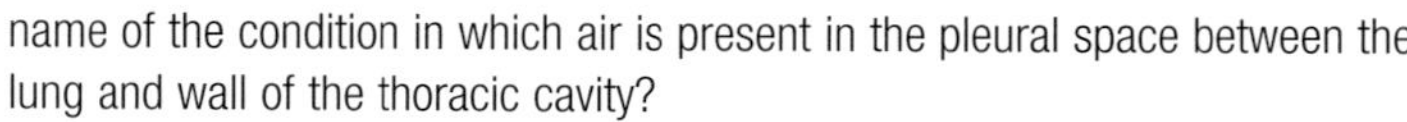
   a. Orthopnoea
   b. Eupnoea
   c. Hyperpnoea
   d. Pneumothorax

Hint To solve a case study, you may have to refer to the glossary or index, other chapters in this textbook, ***Connect It!***, and other resources.

CHAPTER SUMMARY

*To download an MP3 version of the chapter summary for use with your mobile device, access the **Audio Chapter Summaries** online at evolve.elsevier.com.*

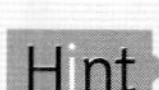

Scan this summary after reading the chapter to help you reinforce the key concepts. Later, use the summary as a quick review before your class or before a test.

Respiratory Physiology (**Figure 36-1**)

A. Definition—complex, coordinated processes that help maintain homeostasis
B. External respiration
   1. Pulmonary ventilation (breathing)
   2. Pulmonary gas exchange
C. Transport of gases by the blood
D. Internal respiration
   1. Systemic tissue gas exchange
   2. Cellular respiration
E. Regulation of respiration

Mechanism of Ventilation

A. Primary principle of ventilation (breathing)
   1. Inspiration—moves air into the lungs
   2. Expiration—moves air out of the lungs
   3. Pulmonary ventilation mechanism must establish two gas pressure gradients (**Figures 36-2** and **36-3**)
      a. One in which the pressure within the alveoli of the lungs is lower than atmospheric pressure to produce inspiration
      b. One in which the pressure in the alveoli of the lungs is higher than atmospheric pressure to produce expiration
   4. Pressure gradients are established by changes in the size of the thoracic cavity that are produced by contraction and relaxation of muscles (**Figures 36-4** and **36-5**)
   5. Boyle's law—the volume of gas varies inversely with pressure at a constant temperature
B. Inspiration—contraction of the diaphragm produces inspiration—as it contracts, it makes the thoracic cavity larger (**Figures 36-5** and **36-6**)
   1. Expansion of the thorax results in decreased intrapleural pressure (P_{IP}), leading to decreased alveolar pressure (P_A)
   2. Air moves into the lungs when alveolar pressure (P_A) drops below atmospheric pressure (P_B)
   3. Compliance—ability of pulmonary tissues to stretch, thus making inspiration possible
C. Expiration—a passive process that begins when the inspiratory muscles are relaxed, which decreases the size of the thorax (**Figure 36-7**)
   1. Decreasing thoracic volume increases the intrapleural pressure and thus increases alveolar pressure above the atmospheric pressure

UNIT 5

2. Air moves out of the lungs when alveolar pressure exceeds the atmospheric pressure
3. Pressure between parietal and visceral pleura is always less than alveolar pressure and less than atmospheric pressure; the difference between P_{IP} and P_A is called *transpulmonary pressure*
4. Elastic recoil—tendency of pulmonary tissues to return to a smaller size after having been stretched; occurs passively during expiration

D. The respiratory cycle can be imagined as rhythmic changes in pressures and volumes (**Figure 36-8**)

Pulmonary Volumes and Capacities

A. Pulmonary volumes—normal exchange of oxygen and carbon dioxide depends on the presence of normal volumes of air moving in and out and the remaining volume (**Figure 36-10**)
   1. Spirometer—instrument used to measure the volume of air (**Figure 36-9**)
   2. Tidal volume (TV)—amount of air exhaled after normal inspiration
   3. Expiratory reserve volume (ERV)—largest volume of additional air that can be forcibly exhaled (between 1.0 and 1.2 litres is normal ERV)
   4. Inspiratory reserve volume (IRV)—amount of air that can be forcibly inhaled after normal inspiration (normal IRV is 3.3 litres)
   5. Residual volume—amount of air that cannot be forcibly exhaled (1.2 litres)

B. Pulmonary capacities—the sum of two or more pulmonary volumes
   1. Vital capacity (VC)—the sum of IRV + TV + ERV
   2. Minimal volume—the amount of air remaining after RV
   3. A person's vital capacity depends on many factors, including the size of the thoracic cavity and posture
   4. Inspiratory capacity (IC)—maximal amount of air that can be inspired after a normal expiration
   5. Functional residual capacity (FRC)—the amount of air at the end of a normal respiration
   6. Total lung capacity (TLC)—the sum of all four lung volumes—the total amount of air a lung can hold
   7. Alveolar ventilation—volume of inspired air that reaches the alveoli
   8. Anatomical dead space—passageways occupied by air that does not participate in gas exchange (**Figure 36-10**, *B*)
   9. Physiological dead space—anatomical dead space plus any alveoli not able to perform gas exchange (as in pulmonary disease)
   10. Alveoli must be properly ventilated for adequate gas exchange

Pulmonary Airflow

A. Pulmonary airflow—rates of airflow into/out of the pulmonary airways
   1. Total minute volume—volume moved per minute (mL/min)
   2. Forced expiratory volume (FEV) or forced vital capacity (FVC)—volume of air expired per second during forced expiration (as a percentage of VC) (**Figure 36-11**)
   3. Flow–volume loop—graph that shows flow (vertically) and volume (horizontally), with the top of the loop representing expiratory flow–volume and the bottom of the loop representing inspiratory flow–volume relationships (**Figure 36-12**)

Ventilation and Perfusion (Figure 36-13)

A. Alveolar ventilation—airflow to the alveoli

B. Alveolar perfusion—blood flow to the alveoli

C. Efficiency of gas exchange can be maintained by limited ability to match perfusion to ventilation—for example, vasoconstricting arterioles that supply poorly ventilated alveoli and allow full blood flow to well-ventilated alveoli

Regulation of Ventilation

A. Homeostasis of blood gases and pH
   1. Various regulatory mechanisms maintain relative constancy of the blood's oxygen and carbon dioxide levels
      a. Blood gas concentrations are often expressed as *oxygen pressure* (P_{O_2}) and *carbon dioxide pressure* (P_{CO_2})

B. Respiratory control centres—the main integrators controlling the nerves that affect the inspiratory and expiratory muscles are located in the brainstem (**Figure 36-14**)
   1. Medullary rhythmicity centre—generates the basic rhythm of the respiratory cycle
      a. Consists of two interconnected control centres
         (1) Dorsal respiratory group (DRG)—integrates information from chemoreceptors to regulate the VRG pattern
         (2) Ventral respiratory group (VRG)—generates basic pattern of breathing rhythm
   2. The basic breathing rhythm can be altered by different inputs to the medullary rhythmicity centre (**Figure 36-14**)
      a. Input from the apneustic centre in the pons regulates the medullary rhythmicity area
      b. Pontine respiratory group (PRG, or pneumotaxic centre)—in the pons—inhibits the apneustic centre and medullary rhythmicity area to prevent overinflation of the lungs

C. Feedback and responses—sensors from the nervous system provide feedback to the medullary rhythmicity centre (**Figure 36-15**)
   1. Changes in the P_{O_2}, P_{CO_2}, and pH of arterial blood influence the medullary rhythmicity area
      a. P_{CO_2} acts on central chemoreceptors throughout the brainstem—if it increases, the result is faster breathing; if it decreases, the result is slower breathing
      b. A decrease in blood pH stimulates peripheral chemoreceptors in the carotid and aortic bodies and, even more so, stimulates the central chemoreceptors (because they are surrounded by unbuffered fluid) (**Figure 36-16**)
      c. Arterial blood P_{O_2} presumably has little influence if it stays above a certain level

D. Other influences on ventilation
   1. Arterial blood pressure controls breathing through the respiratory pressoreflex mechanism
   2. Hering–Breuer reflexes help control respirations by regulating depth of respirations and the volume of tidal air

3. Other miscellaneous factors may also influence breathing
    a. Blood temperature
    b. Sensory impulses from skin thermal receptors and from superficial or deep pain receptors

The Big Picture: Ventilation and the Whole Body

A. The internal system must continually acquire new oxygen and rid itself of carbon dioxide because each cell requires oxygen and produces carbon dioxide as a result of energy conversion
B. Specific mechanisms involved in respiratory function
    1. Regulation by the nervous system adjusts ventilation to compensate for changes in oxygen or carbon dioxide in the internal environment
    2. The skeletal muscles of the thorax aid the airways in maintaining the flow of fresh air
    3. The skeleton houses the lungs, and the arrangement of bones facilitates the expansion and recoil of the thorax
    4. The immune system prevents pathogens from colonizing the respiratory tract and causing infection

REVIEW QUESTIONS

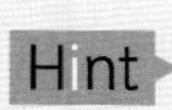

Write out the answers to these questions after reading the chapter and reviewing the Chapter Summary. Note—writing out your answers will consolidate learning and provide a valuable resource of information.

1. Define respiratory physiology.
2. What is the main inspiratory muscle?
3. Identify the separate volumes that make up the total lung capacity.
4. Normally, about what percentage of the tidal volume fills the anatomical dead space? What is the functional significance of air in this space?
5. Normally, about what percentage of the tidal volume is useful air—that is, ventilates the alveoli?
6. Identify the major factors that influence breathing.
7. Orthopnoea is a symptom of what type of disease?
8. Dyspnoea is often associated with what type of breathing?
9. Define the diving reflex and explain its physiological importance.
10. Describe four other unusual reflexes that indirectly affect breathing.
11. Describe the changes in respirations during a period of exercise.

CRITICAL THINKING QUESTIONS

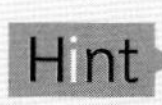

After finishing the Review Questions, write out the answers to these more in-depth questions to help you apply your new knowledge. Go back to sections of the chapter that relate to concepts that you find difficult.

1. The proper functioning of the respiratory system allows what to occur in the body? What other control system has an impact on this function?
2. Identify the various processes that allow the respiratory system to accomplish its function.
3. What is pulmonary ventilation? What evidence can you find to describe whether the lungs are active or passive during this process?
4. Compare and contrast inspiration and expiration. Include the importance of elastic recoil and compliance to these processes.
5. Compare and contrast infant and adult forms of respiratory distress syndrome.
6. After strenuous exercise, inexperienced athletes will quite often attempt to recover and resume normal breathing by bending over or sitting down. Using the mechanics of ventilation, how would you modify the recovery practices of these athletes?
7. Recall or review your knowledge of axial muscles. Name and give the actions of muscles beyond the diaphragm involved in deep breathing.
8. Patients on ventilators depend on the machine to breathe for them. An extended inhalation known as a sigh is sometimes programmed into the ventilation cycle. What is the advantage of this to the patient?

37 Gas Exchange and Transport

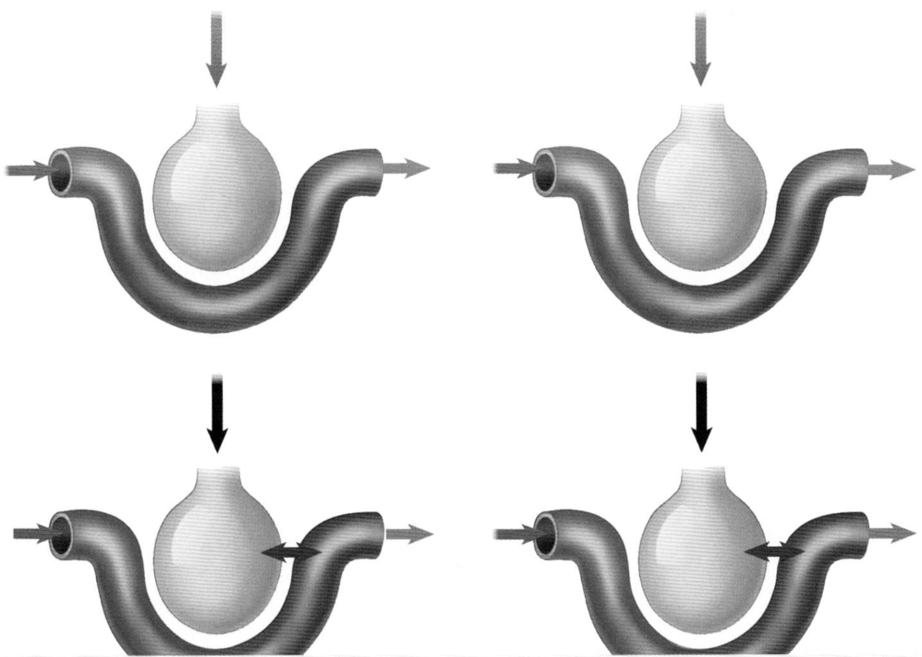

CHAPTER OUTLINE

Hint Scan this outline before you begin to read the chapter, as a preview of how the concepts are organized.

In Chapter 36 we explored the process of ventilation—how we get air to and from the lungs inside our thorax. In this chapter, we continue the story by explaining the mechanisms that move blood gases—oxygen and carbon dioxide—between the air that ventilates our lungs and the blood that perfuses our lungs. We then discuss the amazing properties of blood that allow it to efficiently load and unload these blood gases and transport them between their pickup points and drop-off points. Before beginning this chapter, we recommend going back to **Figure 36-1** on p. 825 to study the overview of respiratory function and remind yourself where the processes of gas exchange and transport fit into the big picture of respiration.

LANGUAGE OF SCIENCE

Hint Use this list to aid your pronunciation of unfamiliar words.

bicarbonate (bye-KAR-boh-nayt)
[*bi-* **two,** *-carbon* **coal (carbon),** *-ate* **oxygen compound**]

Bohr effect (bor)
[*Christian Bohr* **Danish physiologist**]

carbaminohaemoglobin (kahr-bam-ih-no-hee-moh-GLOH-bin)
[*carb-* **coal (carbon),** *-amino-* **ammonia compound (amino acid),** *-haemo-* **blood,** *-glob-* **ball,** *-in* **substance**]

chloride shift (KLOR-ide)
[*chlor-* **green,** *-ide* **chemical**]

fetal haemoglobin (FEE-tal hee-moh-GLOH-bin)
[*fet-* **offspring,** *-al* **relating to,** *haemo-* **blood,** *-glob-* **ball,** *-in* **substance**]

Fick's Law
[*Adolph Eugen Fick* **German physiologist**]

Haldane effect (HAWL-dayne)
[*John Scott Haldane* **Scots physiologist**]

haem group (heem)
[*haem* **blood**]

haemoglobin (Hb) (hee-moh-GLOH-bin)
[*haemo-* **blood,** *-glob-* **ball,** *-in* **substance**]

oxygen–haemoglobin dissociation curve (OCK-sih-jen hee-moh-GLOH-bin dih-soh-see-AY-shun)
[*oxy-* **sharp,** *-gen* **produce,** *haemo-* **blood,** *-glob-* **ball,** *-in* **substance,** *dis-* **reverse,** *-socia-* **unite,** *-ation* **process**]

oxyhaemoglobin (ock-see-hee-moh-GLOH-bin)
[*oxy-* **sharp (oxygen),** *-haemo-* **blood,** *-glob-* **ball,** *-in* **substance**]

LANGUAGE OF MEDICINE

carbon monoxide (CO) (KAR-bon mon-OKS-ide)
[*mono-* **single,** *-ox-* **sharp (oxygen),** *-ide* **chemical**]

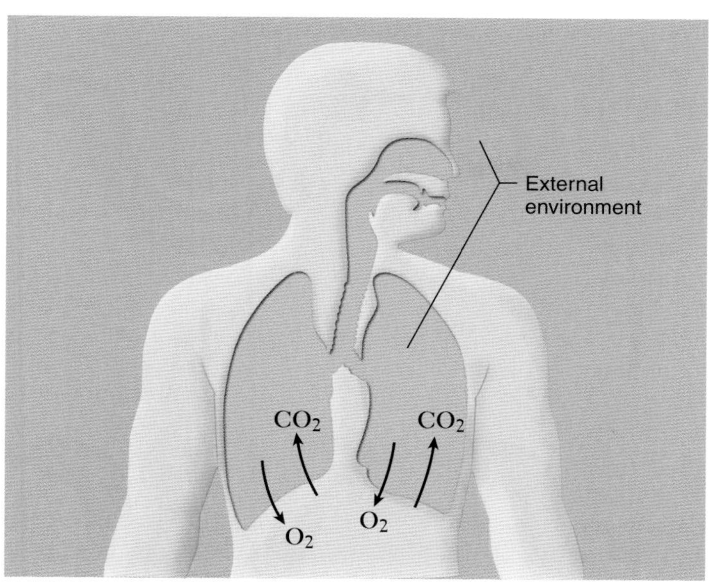

FIGURE 37-1 External–internal barrier. The respiratory membranes of the lung represent an interface or barrier that gases must cross to enter or exit the body's internal environment. The pulmonary airway is merely an extension of the external environment.

PULMONARY GAS EXCHANGE

Exchange of gases in the lungs takes place between alveolar air and blood flowing through lung capillaries. It is important to realize that physiologically speaking, air in the lung is not part of our body. That is, inspired air is not part of the internal environment. As **Figure 37-1** shows, the airways are merely inward extensions of the external environment. Before oxygen can enter our internal environment, and before carbon dioxide can leave our internal environment, these gases must cross the barrier between the external world and the internal world. Note—the pressures of gases referred to in this chapter are given in kilopascals (kPa) and millimetres of mercury (mmHg); 1 mmHg = 0.13 kPa.

PARTIAL PRESSURE

Before discussing the exchange of gases across the respiratory membranes, we need to understand the law of partial pressures (Dalton's law).

The term **partial pressure** means the pressure exerted by any one gas in a mixture of gases or in a liquid. According to the law of partial pressures, the partial pressure of a gas in a mixture of gases is directly related to the concentration of that gas in the mixture and to the total pressure of the mixture. **Figure 37-2** shows how each gas in dry atmospheric air contributes to the total atmospheric pressure. The partial pressure of each gas is directly related to its concentration in the total mixture. Suppose we apply this principle to compute the partial pressure of oxygen in a dry atmosphere. The concentration of oxygen in the atmosphere is about 21%, and the total pressure of the atmosphere is 760 mmHg (101.3 kPa) in standard conditions. Therefore:

$$\text{Atmospheric } Po_2 = 21\% \times 760 = 159.6 \text{ mmHg}$$
$$(= 21\% \times 101.3 = 21.3 \text{ kPa})$$

The symbol used to designate partial pressure is the capital letter *P* preceding the chemical symbol for the gas. Examples: alveolar air Po_2 is about 100 mmHg (13.3 kPa), arterial blood Po_2 is also about 100 mmHg (13.3 kPa), and venous blood Po_2 is about 37 mmHg (4.9 kPa). The word **tension** is often used as a synonym for the term *partial pressure*—*oxygen tension* means the same thing as Po_2.

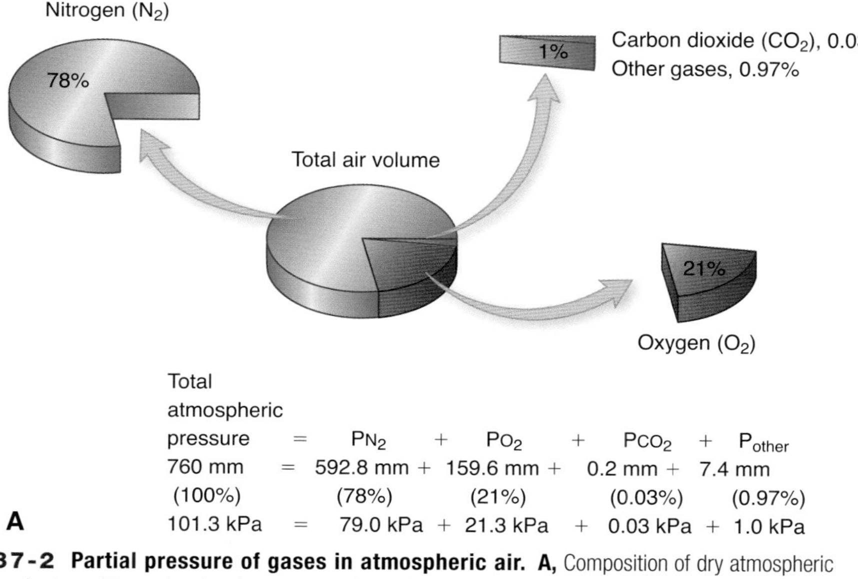

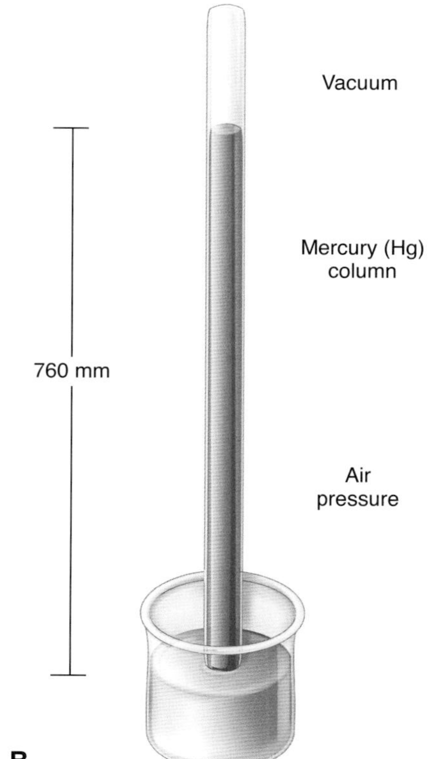

FIGURE 37-2 Partial pressure of gases in atmospheric air. A, Composition of dry atmospheric air under standard conditions showing the concentrations of nitrogen, oxygen, carbon dioxide, and other gases. **B,** A mercury barometer. The weight of air pressing down on the surface of the mercury in the open dish pushes the mercury down into the dish and up the tube. The greater the air pressure pushing down on the mercury surface, the farther up the tube the mercury will be forced. In standard conditions, air pressure causes the mercury column to rise 760 mm. A proportion of this pressure is exerted by each of the gases that make up air, according to their relative concentrations (see **A**). That is, the total atmospheric air pressure is the sum of the partial pressures of nitrogen, oxygen, carbon dioxide, water vapour, and other gases.

The partial pressure of a gas in a liquid is directly determined by the amount of that gas dissolved in the liquid, which in turn is determined by the partial pressure of the gas in the environment of the liquid. Gas molecules diffuse into a liquid from its environment and dissolve in the liquid until the partial pressure of the gas in solution becomes equal to its partial pressure in the environment of the liquid.

Alveolar air constitutes the environment surrounding blood moving through pulmonary capillaries. Standing between the blood and the air are only the very thin alveolar and capillary membranes, and both of these membranes are highly permeable to oxygen and carbon dioxide. By the time blood leaves the pulmonary capillaries as arterial blood, diffusion and approximate equilibration of oxygen and carbon dioxide across the membranes have occurred. Arterial blood Po_2 and Pco_2 therefore usually equal or very nearly equal alveolar Po_2 and Pco_2 (**Table 37-1**).

Before we begin applying the concept of partial pressures to our understanding of gas exchange, we should take a moment to emphasize that alveolar air is a bit different than dry atmospheric air. Because alveolar air has been humidified in the nose and other airways, it has gained a significant amount of water vapour. This water vapour is a gas that is added to the dry mixture of nitrogen, oxygen, carbon dioxide, and so on, as illustrated in **Figure 37-2**. The addition of gaseous water shifts the proportions of each gas in the mixture. What that means for our discussion is that you should expect to see different Po_2 and Pco_2 in alveoli than you do in dry air—as shown in **Table 37-1**. Another factor that contributes to this difference is that the alveolar air is a mix of incoming and outgoing air—so will be higher in CO_2 and lower in O_2 than the external atmosphere.

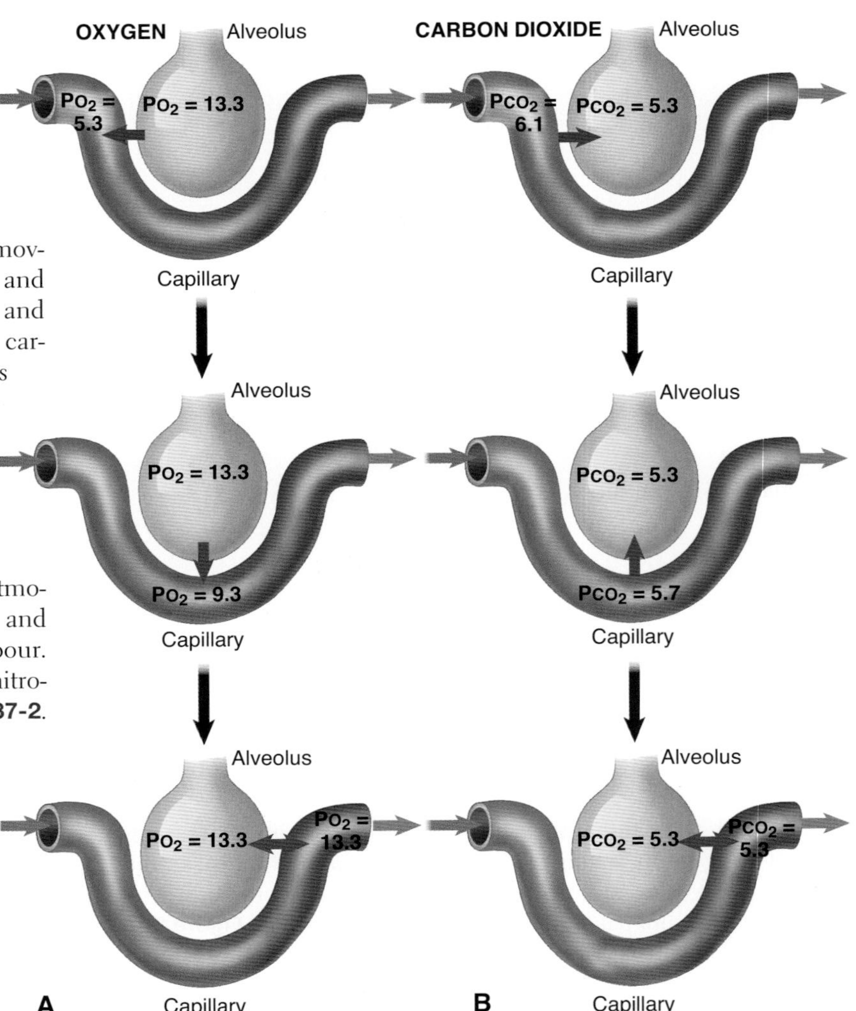

FIGURE 37-3 Pulmonary gas exchange. A, As blood enters a pulmonary capillary, oxygen diffuses down its pressure gradient (into the blood). Oxygen continues diffusing into the blood until equilibration has occurred (or until the blood leaves the capillary). **B,** As blood enters a pulmonary capillary, carbon dioxide diffuses down its pressure gradient (out of the blood). As with oxygen, carbon dioxide continues diffusing as long as there is a pressure gradient. PO_2 and PCO_2 remain relatively constant in a continually ventilated alveolus. Numbers expressed in the diagram are kPa (1 kPa = 7.5 mmHg).

EXCHANGE OF GASES IN THE LUNGS

Gases move in both directions through the respiratory membrane (see **Figure 35-15** on p. 812).

Oxygen enters blood from the alveolar air because the Po_2 of alveolar air is greater than the Po_2 of incoming blood. Another way of saying this is that oxygen diffuses “down” its pressure gradient. Simultaneously, carbon dioxide molecules exit from the blood by diffusing down the carbon dioxide pressure gradient out into the alveolar air. The Pco_2 of venous blood is a bit higher than the Pco_2 of alveolar air. This two-way exchange of gases between alveolar air and pulmonary blood converts deoxygenated blood to oxygenated blood (**Figure 37-3**).

When you look at **Figure 37-3**, you might wonder why the partial pressures of gases in the alveoli remain constant, whereas the partial pressures of gases in the blood change to equilibrate with alveolar partial pressures. The answer to this question lies in the fact that the alveoli are more or less continually ventilated. That is, there is always new air moving into the alveoli at a relatively low, stable velocity (**Figure 37-4**). Therefore, the average partial pressures of gases in the alveoli as a group are relatively constant.

TABLE 37-1 Oxygen and Carbon Dioxide*

	ATMOSPHERE	ALVEOLAR AIR	SYSTEMIC ARTERIAL BLOOD	SYSTEMIC VENOUS BLOOD
Po_2	160/21.3	100/13.3	100/13.3	40/5.3
Pco_2	0.2/0.03	40/5.3	40/5.3	46/6.1

*Values indicate approximate mmHg and kPa pressure in usual conditions.

The amount of oxygen that diffuses into blood each minute depends on several factors, notably the following four:

1. The oxygen pressure gradient between alveolar air and incoming pulmonary blood (alveolar Po_2 − blood Po_2)
2. The total functional surface area of the respiratory membrane
3. The respiratory minute volume (respiratory rate per minute times volume of air inspired per respiration)
4. Alveolar ventilation (discussed on p. 834)

All four of these factors bear a direct relation to oxygen diffusion. Anything that decreases alveolar Po_2, for instance, tends to decrease the alveolar–blood oxygen pressure gradient and therefore tends to decrease the amount of oxygen entering the blood. An application of

UNIT 5

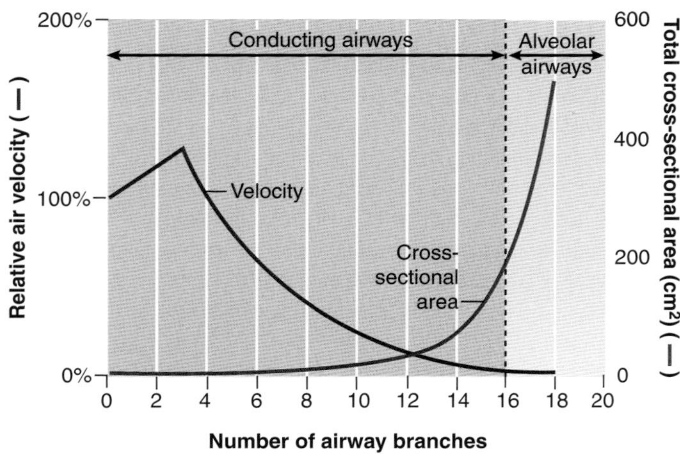

FIGURE 37-4 Airflow in airways. Air velocity (speed of flow) is high in the upper respiratory tract, where the total cross-sectional area is very low. As you can see on the left of the graph, however, the airflow slows down considerably in the alveolar airways because of the high total cross-sectional area of all of the alveoli. This accounts for the fact that ventilation of the alveoli is slow and relatively steady whereas ventilation of the upper airways is characterized by high-speed, alternating rushes of air.

this is as follows: alveolar air Po_2 decreases as altitude increases, and thus less oxygen enters the blood at high altitudes. At a certain high altitude, alveolar air Po_2 equals the Po_2 of blood entering the pulmonary capillaries. How would this affect oxygen diffusion into blood?

Anything that decreases the total functional surface area of the respiratory membrane also tends to decrease oxygen diffusion into the blood (functional surface area is meant as that which is freely permeable to oxygen). An application of this is as follows: in emphysema the total functional area decreases and is one of the factors responsible for poor blood oxygenation in this condition. Surfactant disorders (**Box 36-2** on p. 832) and pneumothorax (**Box 36-3** on p. 835) can also decrease total functional area by collapsing alveoli.

Anything that decreases the respiratory minute volume also tends to decrease blood oxygenation. For example, morphine slows respirations and therefore decreases the respiratory minute volume (volume of air inspired per minute) and tends to lessen the amount of oxygen entering the blood.

Several times we have stated the principle that structure determines function. This principle applies to gas exchange in the lungs. Several structural facts facilitate oxygen diffusion from the alveolar air into the blood in lung capillaries:

- The walls of the alveoli and the capillaries together form a very thin barrier for the gases to cross (estimated at not more than 0.004 mm thick—see **Figure 35-15**, p. 812).
- Alveolar and capillary surfaces are both extremely large (**Box 37-1**).
- Lung capillaries accommodate a large amount of blood at one time. The lung capillaries of a small individual—one who has a body surface area of 1.5 square metres—contain about 90 mL of blood at one time in resting conditions (**Figure 37-5**).
- Blood is distributed through the capillaries in a layer so thin (equal only to the diameter of one red blood cell) that each red blood cell comes close to alveolar air.

Quick CHECK

1. How does the partial pressure of a gas relate to its concentration?
2. What determines the direction in which oxygen will diffuse across the respiratory membrane?
3. List two of the four major factors that influence how much oxygen diffuses into pulmonary blood per minute.

CONNECT IT!

A variety of conditions leave us feeling like we need more oxygen—whether it is strenuous exercise or an abnormal respiratory or cardiovascular condition. Getting extra oxygen for therapeutic, sports, and even recreational use is explored in ***Oxygen Supplements*** online at ***Connect It!***

BOX 37-1 *Fick's law*

Fick's law is a principle that describes the diffusion of carbon dioxide (CO_2) and oxygen (O_2) across the respiratory membrane, including the fluid film on the surface of the alveoli. As you can see in the figure, the principle illustrates common sense: Each gas diffuses more efficiently (faster) if the surface area *(A)* is large, if the thickness of the membrane *(t)* is small, if the solubility of the gas *(S)* is high, and if the partial pressure (Po_2 or Pco_2) gradient is high. Another way of stating Fick's law is that the net gas diffusion rate across a fluid membrane is proportional to the membrane surface area *(A)*, solubility of the gas in the membrane *(S)*, and partial pressure *(P)* difference—and inversely proportional to the membrane thickness *(t)*.

The human respiratory system takes advantage of this principle by improving what it can in the equation to maximize the rate of gas diffusion. The body builds its respiratory membrane of material with as much solubility to CO_2 and O_2 as possible and makes it as thin as possible. The large number of alveoli in a fractal-like arrangement ensures a very large surface area, and a high partial pressure gradient is maintained across the respiratory membrane. •

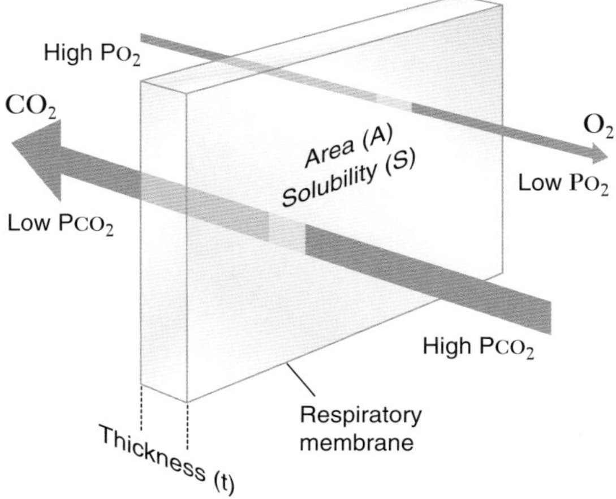

Rate of diffusion of a gas through a membrane. According to Fick's law, the membrane diffusion rate is affected by surface area *(A)*, solubility *(S)* of the gas, membrane thickness *(t)*, and the partial pressure *(P)* gradient.

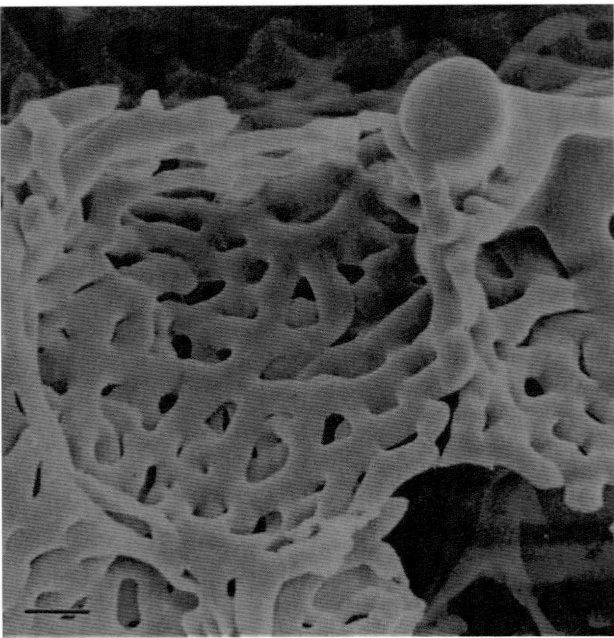

FIGURE 37-5 Alveolar blood supply. Scanning electron micrograph showing the rich blood supply to alveoli (which have been removed). The numerous, narrow branches ensure that each red blood cell is exposed to the alveolar air. (Black bar in lower left represents 10 μm.)

HOW BLOOD TRANSPORTS GASES

Blood transports oxygen and carbon dioxide either as solutes or combined with other chemicals. Immediately on entering the blood, both oxygen and carbon dioxide dissolve in the plasma, but because fluids can hold only small amounts of gas in solution, most of the oxygen and carbon dioxide rapidly form a chemical union with some other molecule—such as haemoglobin, a plasma protein, or water. Once gas molecules are bound to another molecule, their plasma concentration decreases and more gas can diffuse into the plasma. In this way, comparatively large volumes of the gases can be transported.

BOX 37-2 *carbon monoxide poisoning*

Gases other than O_2 and CO_2 can bind to the haemoglobin (Hb) molecule. **Carbon monoxide (CO)** is a molecule produced by incomplete combustion in furnaces, engines, and other circumstances. This invisible, odourless gas binds to Hb more than 200 times more strongly than O_2 does. That means that CO "knocks out" O_2 from HbO_2 and forms HbCO. As more and more HbCO is formed, less and less oxygen is being carried by your blood—a life-threatening situation. Because CO binds so strongly, it is hard to remove it from Hb. One strategy to remove CO is to place a person in a pressure chamber where the PO_2 can be driven so high that it "knocks off" the CO from the Hb, allowing O_2 to form HbO_2. •

HAEMOGLOBIN

Before we begin our discussion of transport of gases in the blood, we will pause and briefly review some facts about **haemoglobin (Hb)** (**Figure 37-6**). As we outlined in Chapter 27, haemoglobin is a reddish protein pigment found only inside red blood cells.

Haemoglobin is a quaternary protein made of four different polypeptide chains—two alpha chains and two beta chains—each associated with an iron-containing **haem group.** If you look at **Figure 37-6**, you will see that an oxygen molecule (O_2) can combine with the iron atom (Fe) in each haem group. Thus haemoglobin can act as a kind of oxygen sponge that chemically absorbs oxygen molecules from the surrounding solution. Note also in this figure that carbon dioxide (CO_2) molecules can combine with the amino acids of the alpha and beta polypeptide chains. Thus haemoglobin can also act as a carbon dioxide sponge and absorb carbon dioxide molecules from a solution. Haemoglobin, then, has exactly the chemical characteristics needed to pick up and transport gases that enter the blood. As you will learn in the following paragraphs, haemoglobin also has the chemical characteristics needed to unload these gases. **Box 37-2** explains how carbon monoxide interferes with haemoglobin's function.

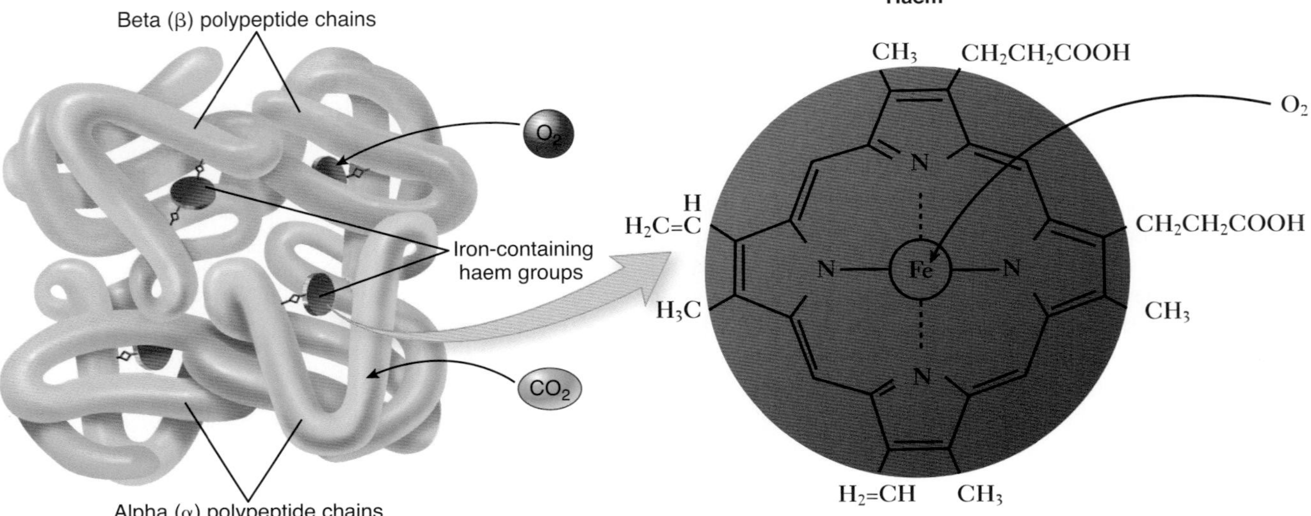

FIGURE 37-6 Haemoglobin. Sketch showing that haemoglobin is a quaternary protein consisting of four different tertiary (folded) polypeptide chains—two alpha (α) chains and two beta (β) chains. Each chain has an associated iron-containing haem group, as seen in detail in the inset. Oxygen (O_2) can bind to the iron (Fe) of the haem group, or carbon dioxide (CO_2) can bind to amine groups of the amino acids in the polypeptide chains.

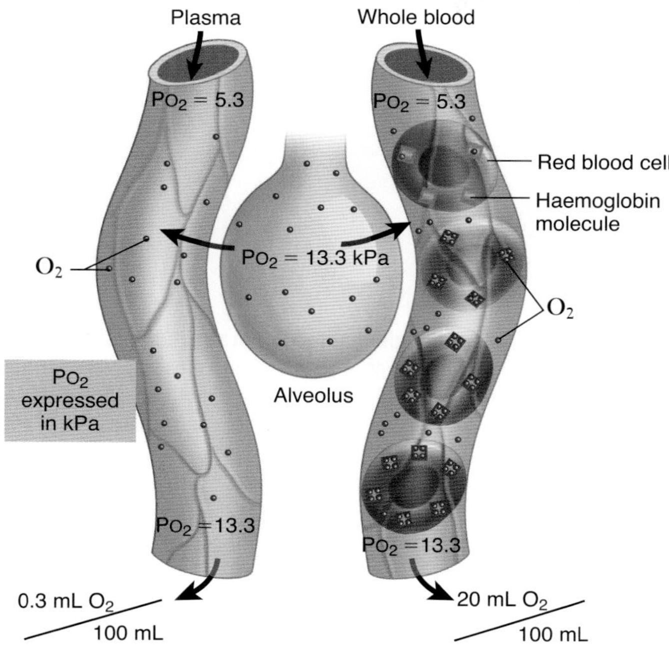

FIGURE 37-7 Oxygen-carrying capacity of blood. If blood consisted only of plasma, the maximum oxygen that could be transported would be only about 0.3 mL of O_2 per 100 mL of blood. Because the red blood cells contain haemoglobin molecules, which act as "oxygen sponges", the blood can actually carry up to 20 mL of dissolved O_2 per 100 mL of blood.

Transport of Oxygen

Because oxygenated blood has a Po_2 of 13.3 kPa (100 mmHg), it contains only about 0.3 mL of dissolved O_2 per 100 mL of blood. Many times that amount, however, combines with the haemoglobin in 100 mL of blood to form **oxyhaemoglobin.** Because each gram of haemoglobin can unite with 1.34 mL of oxygen, the exact amount of oxygen in blood depends mainly on the amount of haemoglobin present. Normally, 100 mL of blood contains about 15 grams of haemoglobin. If 100% of it combines with oxygen, 100 mL of blood will contain 15 × 1.34, or 20.1 mL, of oxygen in the form of oxyhaemoglobin. Because most (about 98.5%) of the O_2 carried by systemic arterial blood is attached to haemoglobin, only about 1.5% of the O_2 travels as dissolved O_2 in the plasma. **Figure 37-7** shows how haemoglobin increases the oxygen-carrying capacity of blood.

Another way of expressing blood oxygen content is in terms of volume percent (vol%). Normal arterial blood, with a Po_2 of 13.3 kPa (100 mmHg), contains about 20 vol% O_2 (meaning 20 mL of oxygen in each 100 mL of blood).

Blood that contains more haemoglobin can, of course, transport more oxygen. Thus blood that contains less haemoglobin can transport less oxygen. Therefore haemoglobin deficiency anaemia decreases oxygen transport and may produce marked cellular hypoxia (inadequate oxygen supply). Thus, in anaemia one may have arterial haemoglobin that is fully saturated with oxygen—perhaps exhibiting 97% oxygen saturation—but low total oxygen content because there is an abnormally low amount of haemoglobin that can become fully saturated with oxygen.

To combine with haemoglobin, oxygen must, of course, diffuse from plasma into the red blood cells where millions of haemoglobin molecules are located. Several factors influence the rate at which haemoglobin combines with oxygen in lung capillaries. For instance, as the following equation and the **oxygen–haemoglobin dissociation curve** (**Figure 37-8**) show, an increasing blood Po_2 accelerates haemoglobin association with oxygen:

$$Hb + O_2 \xrightarrow{\text{Increasing } Po_2} HbO_2$$

Decreasing Po_2, on the other hand, accelerates oxygen dissociation from oxyhaemoglobin—that is, the reverse of the preceding equation. Oxygen associates with haemoglobin rapidly—so rapidly,

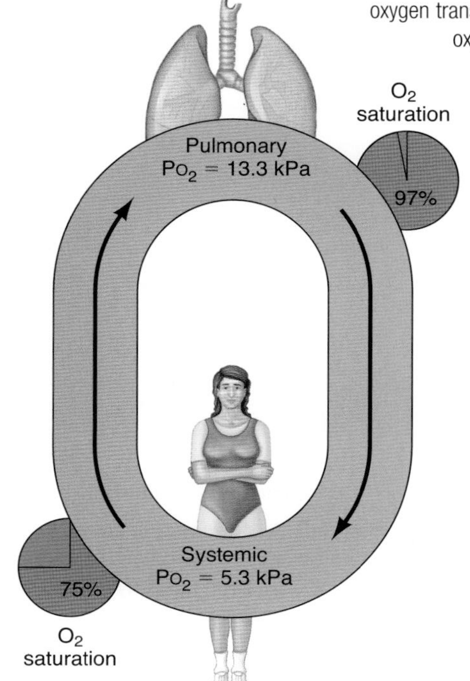

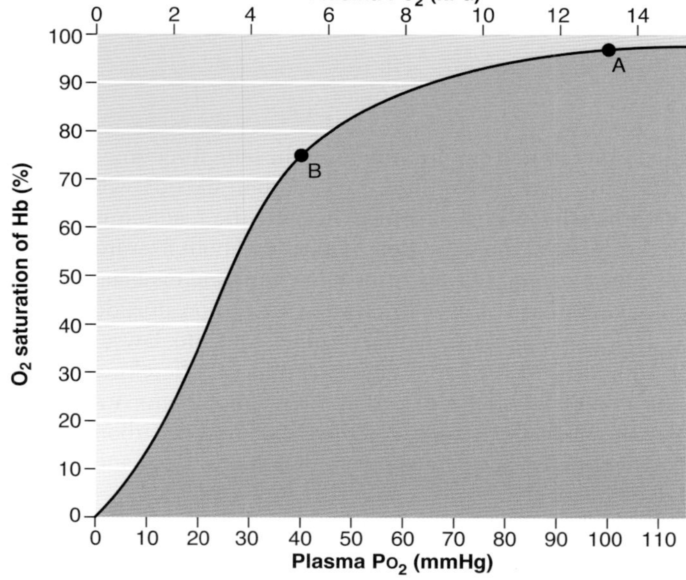

FIGURE 37-8 Oxygen–haemoglobin dissociation curve. The graph represents the relationship between Po_2 and O_2 saturation of haemoglobin (Hb-O_2 affinity). The diagram on the left shows how the graphed curve relates to oxygen transport by the blood. Notice that at high plasma Po_2 values (point *A*), haemoglobin (Hb) is fully loaded with oxygen. At low plasma Po_2 values (point *B*), Hb is only partially loaded with oxygen.

in fact, that about 97% of the blood's haemoglobin has united with oxygen by the time the blood leaves the lung capillaries to return to the heart. In other words, the average oxygen saturation of haemoglobin in oxygenated blood is about 97%.

Summing up, we can say that oxygen travels in two forms: as dissolved O_2 in the plasma and as O_2 associated with haemoglobin (oxyhaemoglobin). Of these two forms of transport, oxyhaemoglobin carries the vast majority of the total oxygen transported by the blood.

CONNECT IT!

Variations of haemoglobin exist in the body to temporarily store or carry oxygen—for example, *neuroglobin, myoglobin,* and **fetal haemoglobin.** Find out why we need more than one type of oxygen carrier in the body in ***Oxygen-binding Proteins*** online at ***Connect It!***

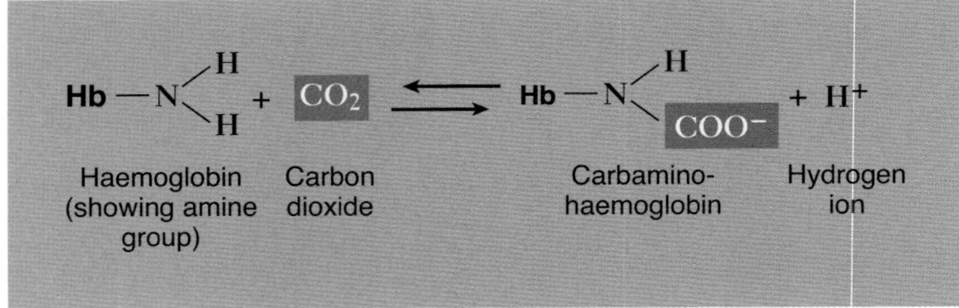

FIGURE 37-9 Carbon dioxide–haemoglobin reaction. Carbon dioxide can bind to an amine group (NH_2) in an amino acid within a haemoglobin (Hb) molecule to form carbaminohaemoglobin ($HbNCOOH^-$) and a hydrogen ion. The highlighted areas show where the original carbon dioxide molecule is in each part of the equation.

Transport of Carbon Dioxide

Carbon dioxide is carried in the blood in several ways, the most important of which are described briefly in the following paragraphs.

Dissolved Carbon Dioxide

A small amount of CO_2 dissolves in plasma and is transported as a solute. About 10% of the total amount of carbon dioxide carried by the blood is carried in the dissolved form. It is this dissolved CO_2 that produces the P_{CO_2} of blood plasma.

Carbamino Compounds

One fifth to one quarter of the carbon dioxide in blood unites with the NH_2 (amine) groups of the amino acids that make up the polypeptide chains of haemoglobin and various plasma proteins. When carbon dioxide binds to amine groups, it forms *carbamino compounds.* Because haemoglobin is the main protein that combines with carbon dioxide, most carbamino molecules are formed and transported in the red blood cells. The compound formed when carbon dioxide combines with haemoglobin has a tongue-twisting name—**carbaminohaemoglobin.** The following chemical equation, amplified in **Figure 37-9**, shows how carbon dioxide combines with amine (NH_2) in haemoglobin's polypeptide chains to produce carbaminohaemoglobin (HbNCOOH) and H^+:

$$Hb{-}NH_2 + CO_2 \rightleftharpoons Hb{-}NH{-}COO^- + H^+$$

Note that the arrows in this equilibrium point in both directions. This means that in any given conditions, some carbon dioxide will be associated with haemoglobin and some will not—the reaction is moving in both directions at the same time. The rate of both forward and reverse reactions—carbon dioxide association with and dissociation from haemoglobin—can shift with changes in carbon dioxide concentration. This principle is sometimes called the **rate law** of chemistry. The addition of more carbon dioxide to blood, therefore, will increase the rate of formation of carbaminohaemoglobin. Another way to state this principle is to say that the association of carbon dioxide with haemoglobin is accelerated by an increase in P_{CO_2} and is slowed by a decrease in P_{CO_2}.

Figure 37-10, which shows the carbon dioxide dissociation curve, illustrates that the total CO_2-carrying capacity (including plasma CO_2, carbamino compounds, and bicarbonate) of blood is affected by the rate law and thus increases as plasma P_{CO_2} increases.

Bicarbonate

More than two thirds of the CO_2 carried by blood is carried in the form of **bicarbonate** ions (HCO_3^-). When CO_2 dissolves in water (as in blood plasma), some of the CO_2 molecules associate with H_2O to form carbonic acid (H_2CO_3). Once formed, some of the H_2CO_3 molecules dissociate to form H^+ and bicarbonate (HCO_3^-) ions. This process, which is catalyzed by an enzyme present in red blood cells called *carbonic anhydrase* (CA), is summarized by the following chemical equation:

$$CO_2 + H_2O^+ \rightleftharpoons H_2CO_3 \rightleftharpoons H + HCO_3^-$$

Figure 37-11 amplifies this equation. According to the rate law of chemistry we stated earlier, as more CO_2 is added to the plasma, more will be converted to carbonic acid. Because the carbonic anhydrase enzyme in the blood is facilitating the conversion of carbon dioxide and water to carbonic acid, this reaction occurs very rapidly as CO_2 is added to the plasma. Carbonic acid concentration

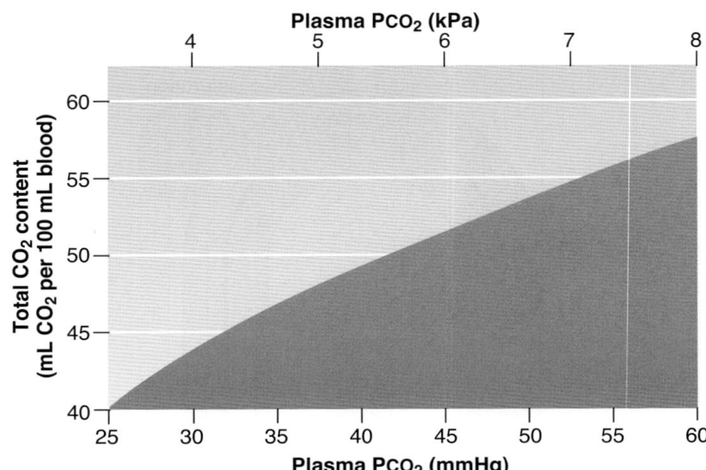

FIGURE 37-10 Carbon dioxide dissociation curve. The relationship between P_{CO_2} and total CO_2 content (mL CO_2 per 100 mL blood) is graphed as a nearly straight line. Notice that the CO_2-carrying capacity of blood increases as the plasma P_{CO_2} increases. The graph represents *total* CO_2-carrying capacity, including transport in plasma, carbaminohaemoglobin, and bicarbonate.

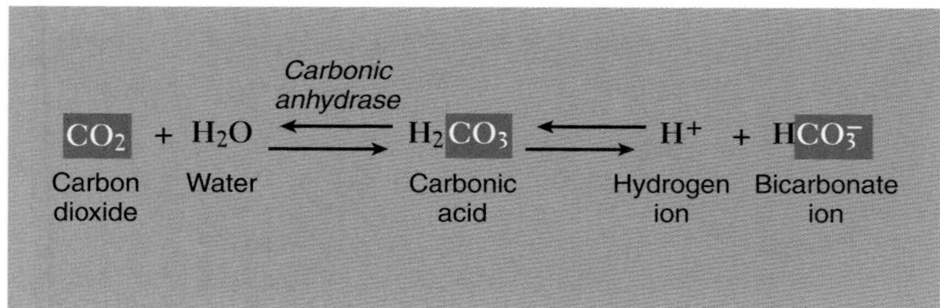

FIGURE 37-11 Formation of bicarbonate. Carbon dioxide can react with water to form carbonic acid, a reaction catalyzed by the red blood cell (RBC) enzyme carbonic anhydrase. Carbonic acid then dissociates to form bicarbonate and a hydrogen ion. The highlighted areas show where the original carbon dioxide molecule is in each part of the equation. The double arrows show that each reaction is reversible, the actual rate in each direction governed by the relative concentration of each molecule.

increases as a result, "pulling" the system toward the bicarbonate side, thus increasing the rate of bicarbonate formation. The end result is that CO_2 molecules diffusing into plasma will continually be removed from the solution and converted into bicarbonate. This allows room for even more CO_2 to dissolve in the plasma—thus increasing the CO_2-carrying capacity of the blood.

Figure 37-12, which summarizes all three forms of CO_2 transport, shows that once bicarbonate ions are formed, they diffuse down their concentration gradient into the plasma. The exit of this negative ion (HCO_3^-) from the red blood cell is balanced by the inward transport of another negative ion, chloride (Cl^-). This countertransport of negative ions is often called the **chloride shift.**

According to the rate law of chemistry described earlier, when CO_2 is removed from the plasma, the entire system, illustrated in **Figures 37-11** and **37-12**, shifts in the opposite direction. Thus the reaction that converts carbonic acid to free CO_2 becomes dominant. The declining concentration of carbonic acid then forces a shift in favour of the conversion of bicarbonate to carbonic acid. In short, CO_2 is unloaded from bicarbonate.

The relative proportions of the three different forms of carbon dioxide carried in the blood are summarized in **Figure 37-13**.

Carbon Dioxide and pH

You may have noticed by now that when carbon dioxide enters the blood, most of it is converted to carbaminohaemoglobin and hydrogen ions (H^+) or to bicarbonate and hydrogen ions. In other words, have you noticed that increasing the carbon dioxide content of the blood also increases its H^+ concentration? Thus an increase in carbon dioxide in the blood causes an increase in the acidity, or a drop in pH, in the blood. This is a very important principle in understanding how and why respiration is regulated in the manner that it is—as we learned in the previous chapter. This principle is also important to the understanding of acid–base balance in the body—a topic discussed thoroughly in Chapter 44.

Quick CHECK

4. Most oxygen carried by the blood is transported in what form?
5. Most carbon dioxide carried by the blood is transported in what form?
6. What is oxyhaemoglobin? What is carbaminohaemoglobin?
7. How does carbon dioxide affect the pH of blood?

FIGURE 37-12 Carbon dioxide transport in the blood. As the illustration shows, CO_2 dissolves in the plasma. Some of the dissolved CO_2 enters red blood cells (RBCs) and combines with haemoglobin (Hb) to form carbaminohaemoglobin ($HbCO_2$). Some of the CO_2 entering RBCs combines with H_2O to form carbonic acid (H_2CO_3), a process facilitated by the enzyme carbonic anhydrase (CA) present inside each cell. Carbonic acid then dissociates to form H^+ and bicarbonate (HCO_3^-). The H^+ combines with Hb, whereas the HCO_3^- diffuses down its concentration gradient into the plasma. As HCO_3^- leaves each RBC, Cl^- enters and prevents an imbalance in charge—a phenomenon called the *chloride shift,* which is discussed in Chapter 44.

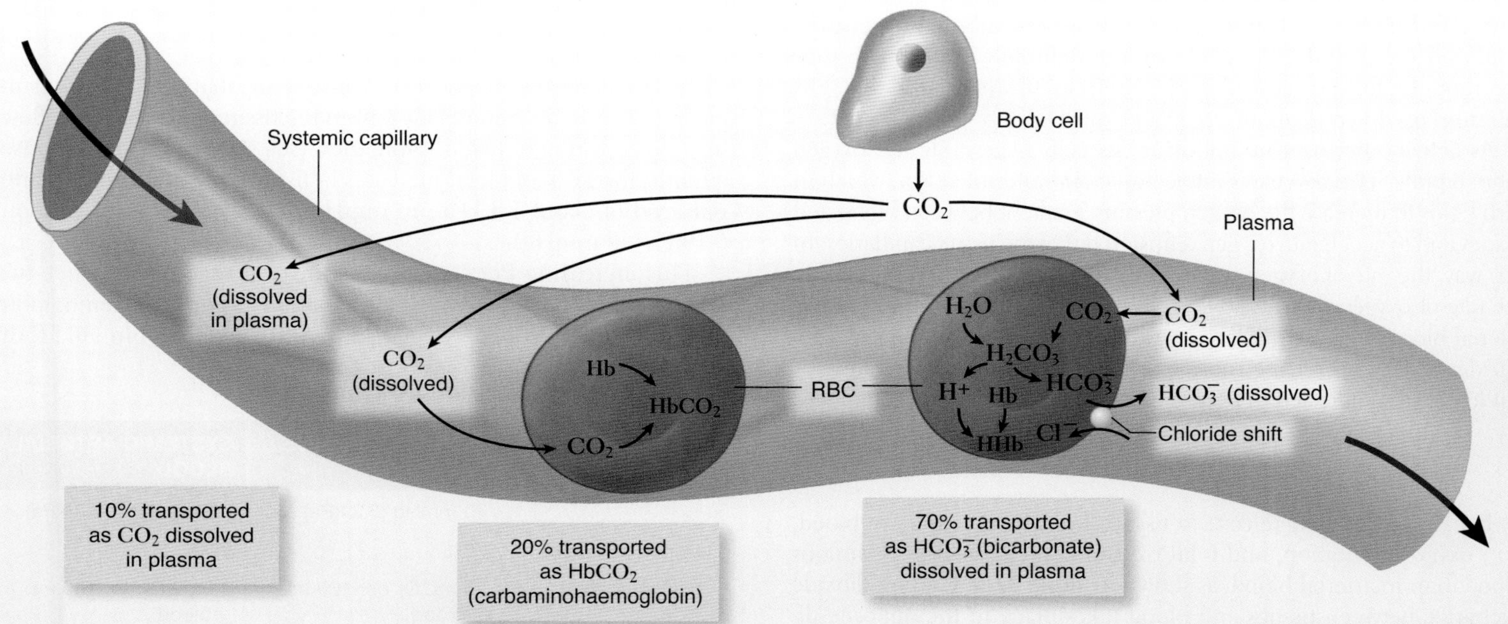

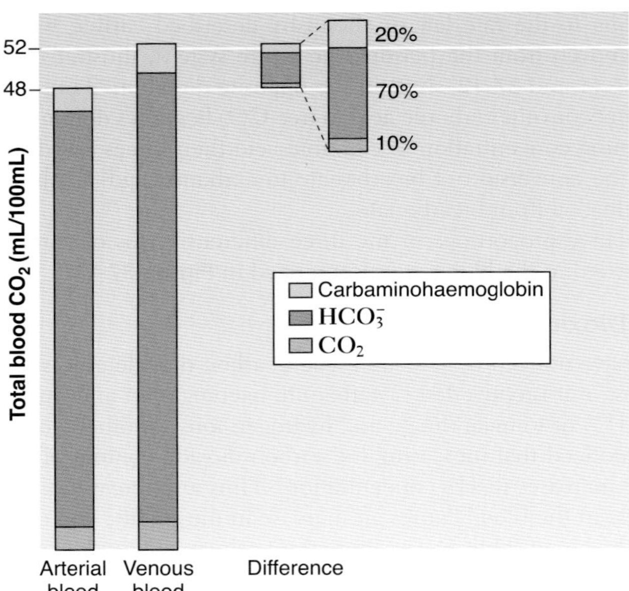

FIGURE 37-13 Proportions of carbon dioxide transported in the blood. This graph shows that systemic venous blood carries more carbon dioxide than systemic arterial blood does. The difference, shown in the upper left, represents the total amount of carbon dioxide loaded into the blood in the systemic tissues. Or it could be viewed as the total amount of carbon dioxide unloaded from the blood in the lungs. Note that most of the carbon dioxide is carried in the form of HCO_3^- (bicarbonate).

SYSTEMIC GAS EXCHANGE

Exchange of gases in tissues takes place between arterial blood flowing through tissue capillaries and cells (**Figure 37-14**). It occurs because of the principle already noted—that gases move down a gas pressure gradient. More specifically, in the tissue capillaries, oxygen diffuses out of arterial blood because the oxygen pressure gradient favours its outward diffusion (see **Figure 37-14**). Arterial blood P_{O_2} is about 13.3 kPa (100 mmHg), interstitial fluid P_{O_2} is considerably lower, and intracellular fluid P_{O_2} is still lower. Although interstitial fluid and intracellular fluid P_{O_2} are not definitely established, they are thought to vary considerably—perhaps from around 8.0 kPa (60 mmHg) down to about 0.1 kPa (1 mmHg).

As activity increases in any tissue, its cells necessarily use oxygen more rapidly. This decreases intracellular and interstitial P_{O_2}, which in turn tends to increase the oxygen pressure gradient between blood and tissues and to accelerate oxygen diffusion out of the tissue capillaries. In this way, the rate of oxygen use by cells automatically tends to regulate the rate of oxygen delivery to cells. As dissolved oxygen diffuses out of arterial blood, blood P_{O_2} decreases, and this accelerates oxyhaemoglobin dissociation to release more oxygen into the plasma for diffusion out to cells, as indicated in **Figure 37-15** and the following equation:

$$HbO_2 \xrightarrow{\text{Decreasing } P_{O_2}} Hb + O_2$$

Because of oxygen release to tissues from tissue capillary blood, P_{O_2}, oxygen saturation, and total oxygen content are less in venous blood than in arterial blood, as shown in **Table 37-2**. Carbon dioxide exchange between tissues and blood takes place in the opposite direction from oxygen exchange. Catabolism produces large amounts of CO_2 inside cells. Therefore, intracellular and interstitial P_{CO_2} are higher than arterial blood P_{CO_2}. This means that the CO_2 pressure gradient causes diffusion of CO_2 from the tissues into the blood flowing along through tissue capillaries (see **Figure 37-14**). Consequently, the P_{CO_2} of blood increases in tissue capillaries from its arterial level of about 5.3 kPa (40 mmHg) to its venous level of about 6.1 kPa (46 mmHg).

This increasing P_{CO_2} and decreasing P_{O_2} together produce two effects—they favour oxygen dissociation from oxyhaemoglobin and carbon dioxide association with haemoglobin to form

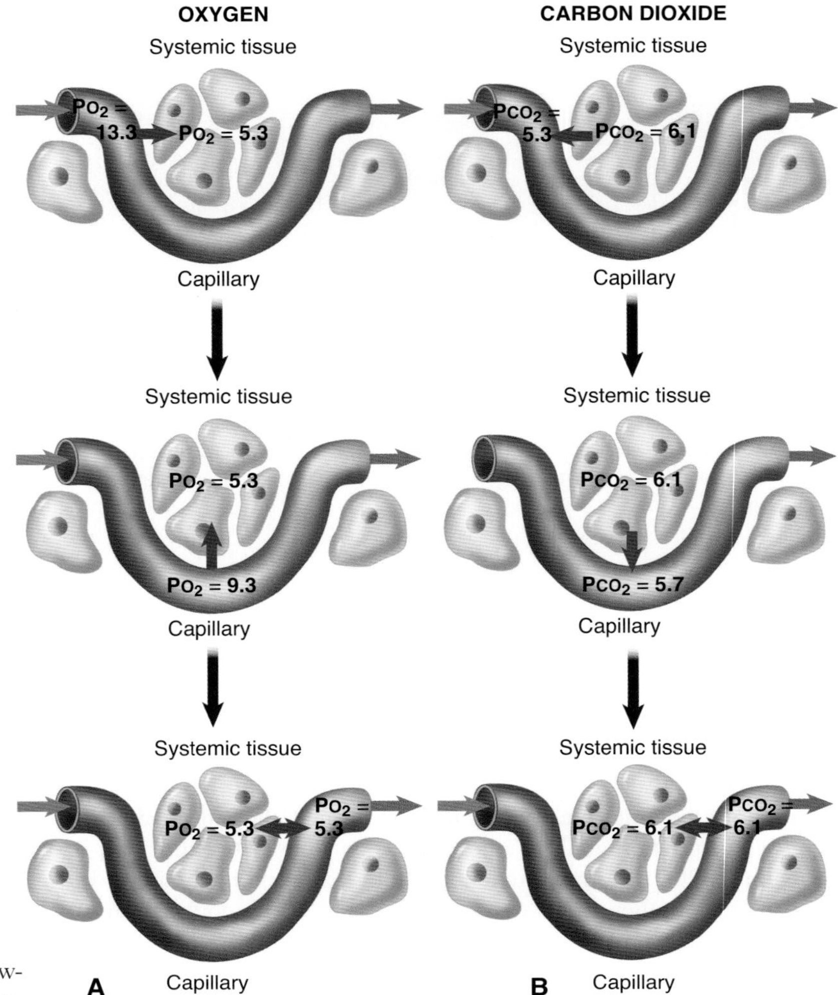

FIGURE 37-14 Systemic gas exchange. A, As blood enters a systemic capillary, O_2 diffuses down its pressure gradient (out of the blood). O_2 continues diffusing out of the blood until equilibration has occurred (or until the blood leaves the capillary). **B,** As blood enters a systemic capillary, CO_2 diffuses down its pressure gradient (into the blood). As with O_2, CO_2 continues diffusing as long as there is a pressure gradient. Numbers in the diagram are expressed as kPa (1 kPa = 7.5 mm Hg).

TABLE 37-2 Blood Oxygen

	SYSTEMIC VENOUS BLOOD	SYSTEMIC ARTERIAL BLOOD
P_{O_2}	40 mmHg (5.3 kPa)	100 mmHg (13.3 kPa)
Oxygen saturation	75%	97%
Oxygen content	15 mL O_2 per 100 mL blood	20 mL O_2 per 100 mL blood*

*Oxygen use by tissues = difference between the oxygen content of arterial and venous blood (20–15) = 5 mL O_2 per 100 mL blood circulated per minute.

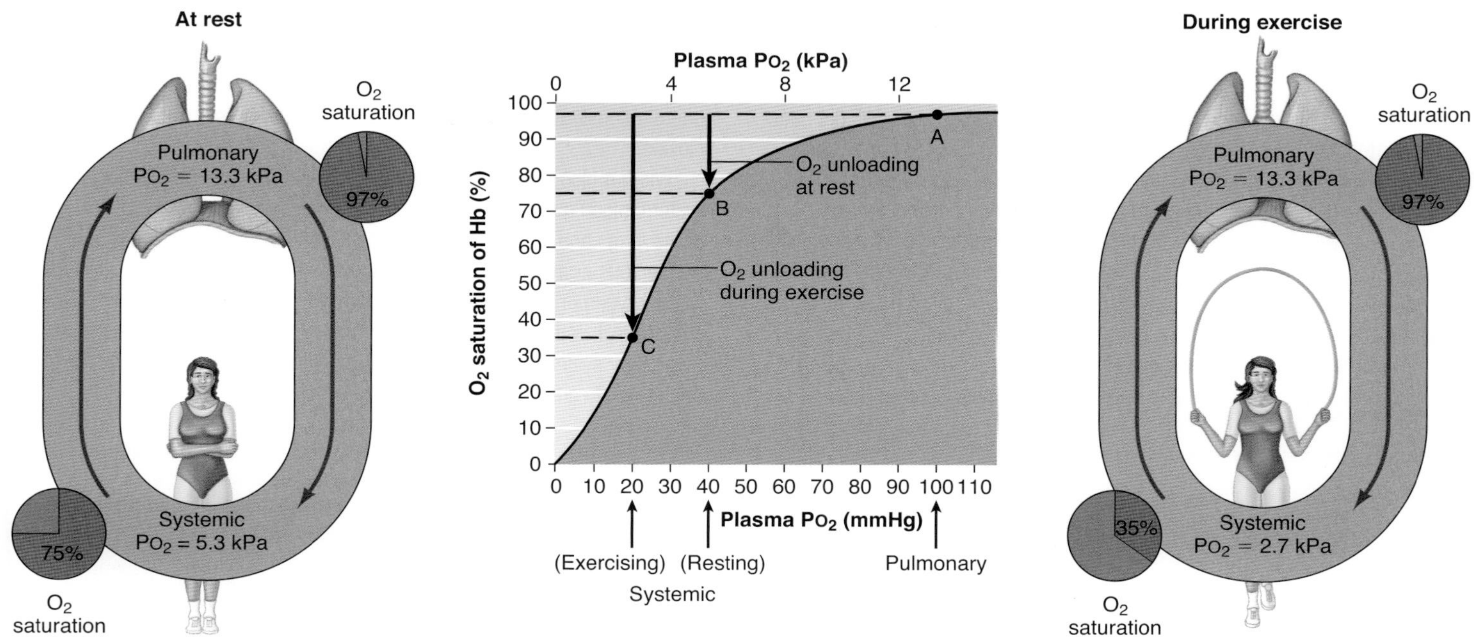

FIGURE 37-15 Oxygen unloading at rest and during exercise. At rest, fully saturated Hb unloads almost 25% of its O_2 load when it reaches the low-Po_2 (40 mmHg/ 5.3 kPa) environment in systemic tissues *(left inset)*. During exercise, the tissue Po_2 is even lower (20 mmHg/2.7 kPa)—thus causing fully saturated Hb to unload about 70% of its O_2 load *(right inset)*. As you can see in the graph, a slight drop in tissue Po_2—from point *B* to point *C*—causes a large increase in O_2 unloading.

carbaminohaemoglobin. This reciprocal interrelationship between oxygen and carbon dioxide transport mechanisms is contrasted in **Figure 37-16**. Note that increased Pco_2 decreases the affinity between haemoglobin and oxygen—this is called a "right shift". A right shift of the oxygen–haemoglobin dissociation curve resulting from increased Pco_2 is also known as the **Bohr effect,** named for Christian Bohr, who, along with other scientists, discovered this phenomenon in 1904. A drop in plasma pH, which normally accompanies an increase in blood Pco_2, also causes a right shift.

The **Haldane effect** refers to the increased total CO_2 loading caused by a decrease in Po_2. This phenomenon is named for its discoverer John Scott Haldane.

CONNECT IT!

If you are having trouble visualizing the essential process of gas exchange, check out the simplified ***Summary of Gas Exchange*** online at ***Connect It!***

Quick CHECK

8. What factors can cause the attraction between haemoglobin and oxygen to decrease?
9. What factors can cause an increase in the amount of carbon dioxide loaded into the systemic blood?

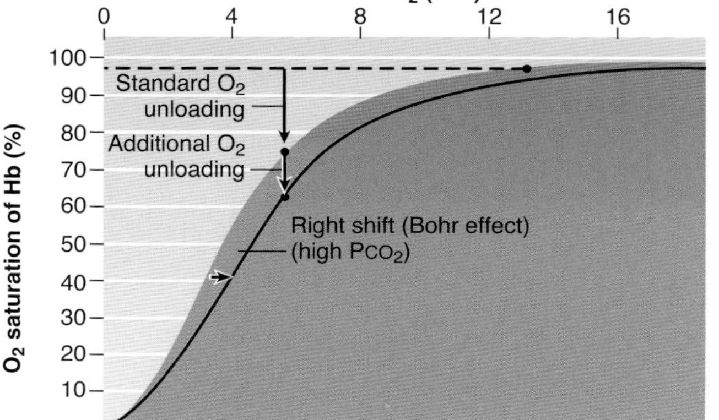

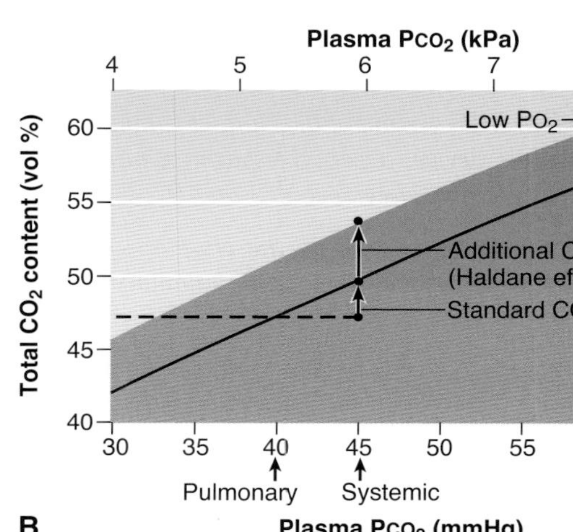

FIGURE 37-16 Effects of Po_2 and Pco_2 on gas transport by the blood. A, The increased plasma Pco_2 in systemic tissues decreases the affinity between Hb and O_2, shown as a right shift of the oxygen–haemoglobin dissociation curve. This phenomenon is known as the *Bohr effect.* A right shift can also be caused by a decrease in plasma pH. **B,** At the same time, the decreased plasma Po_2 commonly observed in systemic tissues increases the CO_2 content of the blood, shown as a left shift of the CO_2 dissociation curve. This phenomenon is known as the *Haldane effect.*

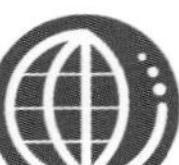

the big picture | Gas Exchange and Transport and the Whole Body

In the previous chapters, we learned that the homeostatic balance of the entire body, and thus the survival of each and every cell, depends on the proper functioning of the respiratory system. In this chapter, we focused on the ability of blood to exchange gases between the internal and external environments. By means of diffusion, oxygen enters the internal environment and carbon dioxide leaves. The efficiency of this process is enhanced by the presence of "oxygen sponges", called *haemoglobin molecules,* which immediately take oxygen molecules out of solution in the plasma so that more oxygen can rapidly diffuse into the blood. The blood, the circulating fluid tissue of the cardiovascular system, carries the blood gases throughout the body—picking up gases where there is an excess and unloading them where there is a deficiency. In this manner, each cell of the body is continually bathed in a fluid environment that offers a constant supply of oxygen and an efficient system for removing carbon dioxide.

Without blood and the maintenance of blood flow by the cardiovascular system, blood gases could not be transported between the gas exchange tissues of the lungs and the various systemic tissues of the body. Without regulation by the nervous system, ventilation could not be adjusted to compensate for changes in the oxygen or carbon dioxide content of the internal environment. The homeostasis of pH, which is regulated by a variety of systems, is influenced by the respiratory system's ability to adjust the body's carbon dioxide levels (and thus the levels of carbonic acid).

case study |

Remember Robert from the previous case study? If you recall, after Robert had surgery to remove a stomach tumour, he woke up in the recovery room in extreme pain. It hurt to move; it hurt to blink; it hurt to take even a little breath.

Robert's shallow respirations were not getting rid of as much carbon dioxide as usual. As a result, the concentration of CO_2 in his bloodstream was building to a level that would negatively affect homeostasis.

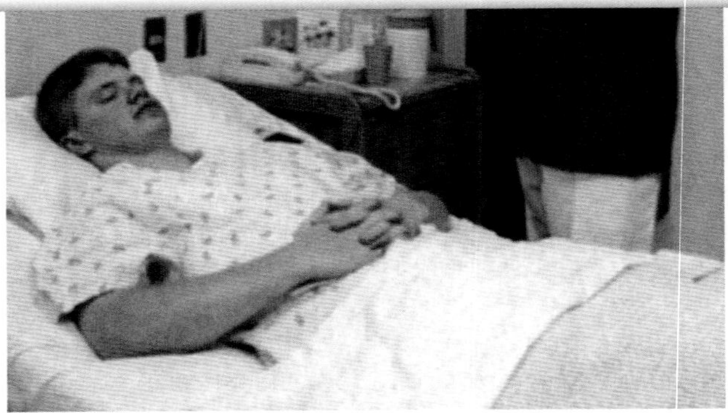

1. The increased carbon dioxide will make Robert's blood more _____?
   a. Acidic
   b. Basic
   c. Neutral
   d. None of the above
2. How is carbon dioxide transported in the blood?
   a. Dissolved in the plasma
   b. Bound to haemoglobin
   c. In the form of bicarbonate
   d. All of the above
3. How is oxygen transported in the blood?
   a. As dissolved O_2 in the plasma and as O_2 associated with haemoglobin
   b. As dissolved O_2 in the plasma and as O_2 associated with bicarbonate
   c. As O_2 associated with haemoglobin and bicarbonate
   d. As O_2 associated with haemoglobin and carbamino compounds

Hint To solve a case study, you may have to refer to the glossary or index, other chapters in this textbook, ***Connect It!,*** and other resources.

UNIT 5

CHAPTER SUMMARY

To download an MP3 version of the chapter summary for use with your mobile device, access the ***Audio Chapter Summaries*** *online at evolve.elsevier.com.*

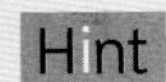

Scan this summary after reading the chapter to help you reinforce the key concepts. Later, use the summary as a quick review before your class or before a test.

Pulmonary Gas Exchange

A. Partial pressure of gases—pressure exerted by a gas in a mixture of gases or a liquid (**Figure 37-2**)
   1. Law of partial pressures (Dalton's law)—the partial pressure of a gas in a mixture of gases is directly related to the concentration of that gas in the mixture and to the total pressure of the mixture
   2. Arterial blood P_{O_2} and P_{CO_2} equal alveolar P_{O_2} and P_{CO_2}

B. Exchange of gases in the lungs—takes place between alveolar air and blood flowing through lung capillaries (**Figures 37-1, 37-3,** and **37-4**)
   1. Four factors determine the amount of oxygen that diffuses into blood
      a. The oxygen pressure gradient between alveolar air and blood
      b. The total functional surface area of the respiratory membrane
      c. The respiratory minute volume
      d. Alveolar ventilation
   2. Structural facts that facilitate oxygen diffusion from the alveolar air to the blood
      a. The walls of the alveoli and capillaries form only a very thin barrier for gases to cross
      b. The alveolar and capillary surfaces are large

c. The blood is distributed through the capillaries in a thin layer so that each red blood cell comes close to alveolar air (**Figure 37-5**)

How Blood Transports Gases

A. Oxygen and carbon dioxide are transported as solutes and as parts of molecules of certain chemical compounds
B. Haemoglobin (Hb)
   1. Made up of four polypeptide chains (two alpha chains, two beta chains), each with an iron-containing haem group
   2. Carbon dioxide can bind to amino acids in the chains and oxygen can bind to iron in the haem groups (**Figure 37-6**)
C. Transport of oxygen
   1. Oxygenated blood contains about 0.3 mL of dissolved O_2 per 100 mL of blood
   2. Haemoglobin increases the oxygen-carrying capacity of blood (**Figure 37-7**)
   3. Oxygen travels in two forms: as dissolved O_2 in plasma and as being associated with haemoglobin (oxyhaemoglobin)
      a. Increasing blood Po_2 accelerates haemoglobin association with oxygen (**Figure 37-8**)
      b. Oxyhaemoglobin carries the majority of the total oxygen transported by blood
D. Transport of carbon dioxide
   1. A small amount of CO_2 dissolves in plasma and is transported as a solute (10%)
   2. Less than one quarter of blood carbon dioxide combines with NH_2 (amine) groups of haemoglobin and other proteins to form carbaminohaemoglobin (20%) (**Figure 37-9**)
   3. Carbon dioxide's association with haemoglobin is accelerated by an increase in blood Pco_2 (**Figure 37-10**)
   4. More than two thirds of the carbon dioxide is carried in plasma as bicarbonate ions (70%) (**Figures 37-11**, **37-12**, and **37-13**)
   5. Increasing the carbon dioxide content of the blood increases its H^+ concentration, thus increasing its acidity which causes a drop in pH in the blood

Systemic Gas Exchange

A. Exchange of gases in tissues takes place between arterial blood flowing through tissue capillaries and cells (**Figure 37-14**)
   1. Oxygen diffuses out of arterial blood because the oxygen pressure gradient favours its outward diffusion
   2. As dissolved oxygen diffuses out of arterial blood, blood Po_2 decreases, which accelerates oxyhaemoglobin dissociation to release more oxygen to plasma for diffusion to cells (**Figure 37-15**)
B. Carbon dioxide exchange between tissues and blood takes place in the opposite direction from oxygen exchange
   1. Bohr effect—increased Pco_2 decreases the affinity between oxygen and haemoglobin (**Figure 37-16**, A)
   2. Haldane effect—increased carbon dioxide loading caused by a decrease in Po_2 (**Figure 37-16**, *B*)

The Big Picture: Gas Exchange and Transport and the Whole Body

A. Homeostatic balance of the entire body, and thus the survival of each and every cell, depends on the proper functioning of the respiratory system
B. Through diffusion, oxygen enters the internal environment and carbon dioxide leaves
   1. Haemoglobin molecules enhance the efficiency of this process
C. Blood and the maintenance of blood flow by the cardiovascular system allow for the transport of blood gases between the gas exchange tissues of the lungs and the various systemic tissues of the body
D. The nervous system regulates ventilation to adjust for changes in the oxygen or carbon dioxide content of the internal environment
E. Homeostasis of pH is influenced by the respiratory system's ability to adjust the body's carbon dioxide levels

REVIEW QUESTIONS

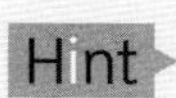

Write out the answers to these questions after reading the chapter and reviewing the Chapter Summary. Note—writing out your answers will consolidate learning and provide a valuable resource of information.

1. One gram of haemoglobin combines with how many millilitres of oxygen?
2. What factors influence the amount of oxygen that diffuses into the blood from the alveoli?
3. Increasing Pco_2 and decreasing Po_2 produce what two effects?
4. Identify the ways in which carbon dioxide is carried in the blood.
5. Identify the two ways in which oxygen travels in the blood.
6. Which form of transport carries the vast majority of the total oxygen transported in the blood?

CRITICAL THINKING QUESTIONS

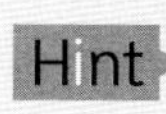

After finishing the Review Questions, write out the answers to these more in-depth questions to help you apply your new knowledge. Go back to sections of the chapter that relate to concepts that you find difficult.

1. Summarize the interaction of oxygen and carbon dioxide on gas transport in the blood. Include the Bohr and Haldane effects in your explanation.
2. Suppose your blood has a haemoglobin content of 15 grams/100 mL and an oxygen saturation of 97%. How many millilitres of oxygen would 100 mL of your arterial blood contain?
3. How does the rate of oxygen used by the cells automatically tend to regulate the rate of oxygen delivery to cells?
4. Why is the Po_2 of alveolar air significantly lower than the Po_2 of atmospheric air?

38 Upper Digestive Tract

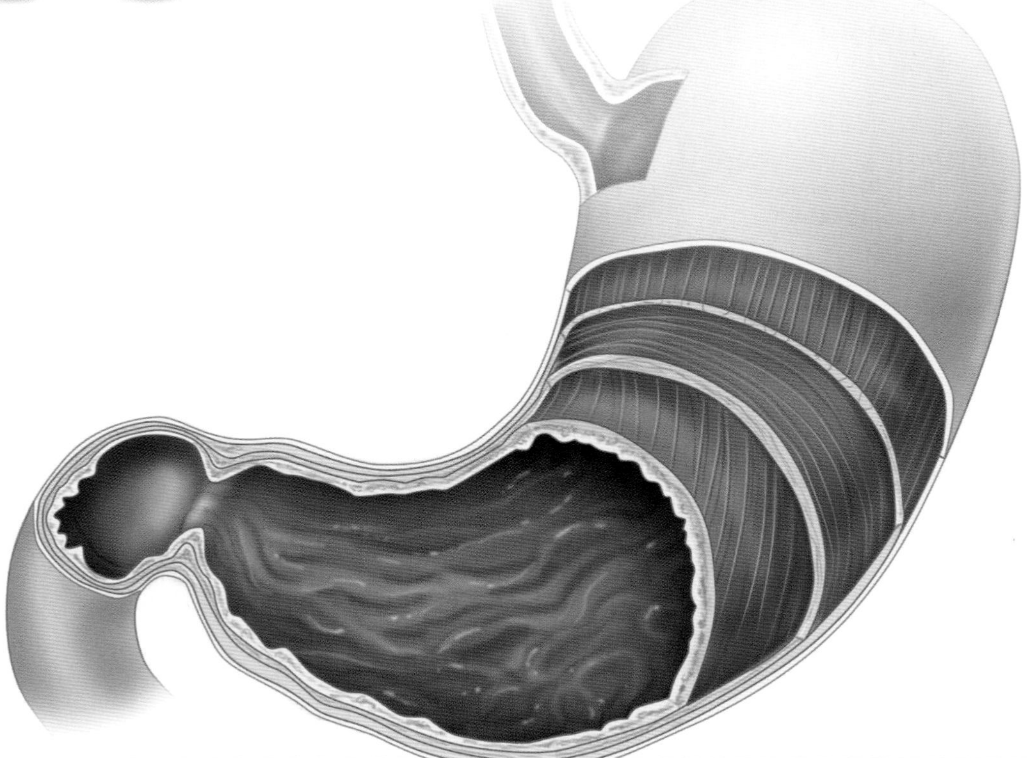

CHAPTER OUTLINE

Hint ▸ *Scan this outline before you begin to read the chapter, as a preview of how the concepts are organized.*

This chapter and the next deal with the anatomy of the digestive system. The organs of the digestive system together perform a vital function—that of preparing nutrients for absorption and for use by the millions of body cells. Most food when eaten is in a form that cannot reach the cells (because it cannot pass through the intestinal mucosa into the bloodstream), nor could it be used by the cells even if it could reach them. It must therefore be modified in both physical state and chemical composition so that nutrients can be absorbed and used by the body cells. The complete process of altering the physical and chemical composition of ingested food material so that it

LANGUAGE OF SCIENCE

Hint ▸ *Use this list to aid your pronunciation of unfamiliar words.*

alimentary canal
(al-uh-MEN-tar-ee kah-NAL)
[*aliment-* **nourishment,** *-ary* **relating to**]

cardia (KAR-dee-ah)
[*cardia* **heart**]

cementum (sih-MEN-tum)
[*cement-* **mortar,** *-um* **matter**]

deciduous teeth (deh-SID-yoo-us)
[*decid-* **fall off,** *-ous* **relating to**]

deglutition (deg-loo-TISH-un)
[*deglut-* **swallow,** *-tion* **process**]

dentin (DEN-tin)
[*dent-* **tooth,** *-in* **substance**]

enamel (i-NA-mel)
[*en-* **in,** *-amel* **melt**]

fundus (FUN-duss)
[*fundus* **bottom**] *pl.,* fundi (FUN-dye)

gastrointestinal (GI) tract
(gas-troh-in-TES-tin-ul trakt)
[*gastr-* **stomach,** *-intestin-* **intestine,** *-al* **relating to,** *tract* **trail**]

gingiva (JIN-jih-vah)
[*gingiv-* **gum,** *-a* **thing**] *pl.,* gingivae (JIN-jih-vee)

hard palate (PAL-et)

intramural plexus
(in-trah-MYOO-ral PLEK-sus)
[*intra-* **within,** *-mura-* **wall,** *-al* **relating to,** *plexus* **braid or network**] *pl.,* plexi or plexuses

lower oesophageal sphincter (LOS)
(eh-SOF-eh-JEE-ul SFINGK-ter)
[*oes-* **will carry,** *-phag-* **food (eat),** *-al* **relating to,** *sphinc-* **bind tight,** *-er* **agent**]

mastication (mas-tih-KAY-shun)
[*mastic-* **chew,** *-ation* **process**]

mesentery (MEZ-en-tair-ee)
[*mes-* **middle,** *-enter-* **intestine**]

mucosa (myoo-KOH-sah)
[*muc-* **slime,** *-os-* **relating to,** *-a* **thing**] *pl.,* mucosae

muscularis (mus-kyoo-LAIR-is)
[*mus-* **mouse,** *-cul-* **little,** *-ar-* **relating to,** *-is* **thing**] *pl.,* musculares

parietal cell (pah-RYE-ih-tal sell)
[*paires-* **wall,** *-al* **relating to,** *cell* **storeroom**]

parotid (peh-ROT-id)
[*par-* **beside,** *-ot-* **ear,** *-id* **relating to**]

continued on p. 878

can be absorbed and used by the body cells is called **digestion.** This complex process is the function of both the digestive tract and accessory organs that make up the digestive system.

This chapter begins the story of digestion with a brief survey of the upper digestive tract and Chapter 39 continues with a survey of the lower digestive tract. The physiology of digestion and absorption is discussed in Chapter 40. Assimilation and metabolism of nutrients will then be explored in Chapter 41.

ORGANIZATION OF THE DIGESTIVE SYSTEM

THE DIGESTIVE TRACT

The main organs of the digestive system (**Figure 38-1**) form a tube that goes all the way through the ventral cavities of the body. It is open at both ends. This tube is usually referred to as the **alimentary canal** or **digestive tract.** This tube can also be called the *gut*. The term **gastrointestinal (GI) tract** refers only to the stomach and intestines but is sometimes used in reference to the entire alimentary canal.

Because the digestive tract is so long—more than 10 metres in some individuals—it is often convenient to divide it into sections. There are several ways to do this. Some anatomists prefer an embryological approach, dividing the tract into the *foregut*, *midgut*, and *hindgut* based on early differentiation of the tube during embryonic development. Many clinicians prefer an upper-lower division of sections, but the boundary between them varies for several practical reasons—such as how far an endoscopy scope will reach or where certain processes take place. In this book, we designate the *upper digestive tract* as mouth through stomach and the *lower digestive tract* as small intestine to anus.

Box 38-1 lists the main organs of the digestive system—that is, the segments of the alimentary canal—and the accessory organs located in the main digestive organs or opening into them. Organs such as the larynx, trachea, diaphragm, and spleen are labelled in **Figure 38-1**, but they are not digestive organs. They are shown to assist in orienting the digestive organs to other important body structures.

BOX 38-1 ***organs of the digestive system***

Segments of the Digestive Tract

Upper Digestive Tract
- Mouth
- Pharynx
- Oesophagus
- Stomach

Lower Digestive Tract
- Small intestine
  - Duodenum
  - Jejunum
  - Ileum
- Large intestine
  - Caecum
  - Colon
    - Ascending colon
    - Transverse colon
    - Descending colon
    - Sigmoid colon
  - Rectum
- Ana canal

Accessory Organs
- Salivary glands
  - Parotid
  - Submandibular
  - Sublingual
- Tongue
- Teeth
- Liver
- Gallbladder
- Pancreas
- Vermiform appendix

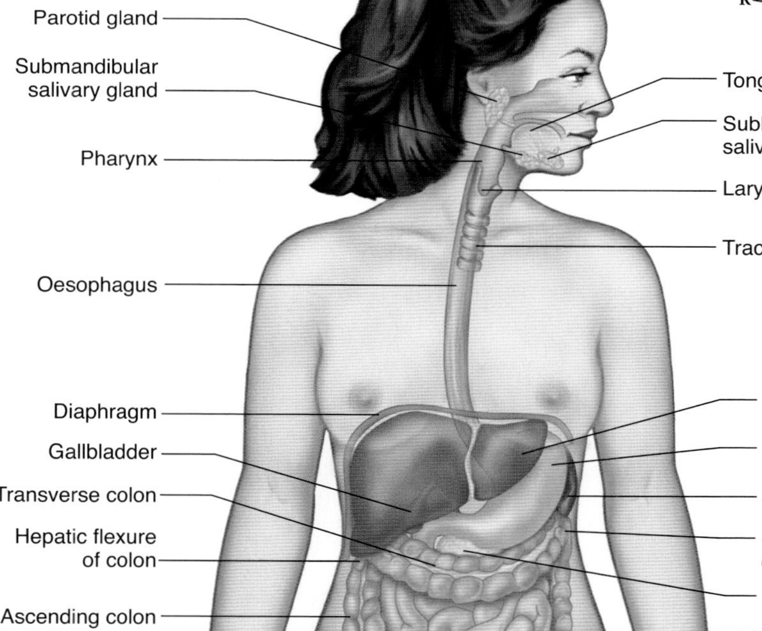

FIGURE 38-1 Location of the digestive organs and accessory organs. Note: Organs such as the larynx, trachea, diaphragm and spleen are labelled in Figure 38-1, but they are not digestive organs. They are shown to assist in orienting the digestive organs to other important body structures.

UNIT 5

It is important to realize that ingested food material passing through the lumen of the digestive tract is actually outside the internal environment of the body, even though the tube itself passes through the ventral body cavities.

Wall of the GI Tract

The GI tract is essentially a tube with walls fashioned of four layers of tissues: a mucous lining, a submucous coat of connective tissue in which are embedded the main blood vessels of the tract, a muscular layer, and a fibroserous layer (**Figure 38-2**). A large fan-like serous fold called mesentery connects the GI tract to the abdominal wall. Blood vessels and nerves travel through the mesentery to reach the GI tract throughout most of its length.

Mucosa

The innermost layer of the GI wall—the layer facing the lumen, or open space, of the tube—is called the **mucosa** or *mucous layer.* Note in **Figure 38-2** that the mucosa is made up of three layers— an inner *mucous epithelium*, a layer of loose fibrous connective tissue called the *lamina propria*, and a thin layer of smooth muscle called the *muscularis mucosae.*

Submucosa

The **submucosa** layer of the digestive tube is composed of connective tissue that is thicker than the mucosal layer. It contains numerous small glands, blood vessels, and parasympathetic nerves that form the *submucosal plexus* (Meissner plexus).

Muscularis

The **muscularis**—or *muscular layer*—is a thick layer of muscle tissue that wraps around the submucosa. This portion of the wall is characterized by an inner layer of circular and an outer layer of longitudinal smooth muscle. Like the submucosa, the muscularis contains nerves organized into a plexus called the *myenteric plexus* (Auerbach plexus). This plexus lies between the two muscle layers. Note in **Figure 38-2** that the term **intramural plexus** is used to describe both plexuses. Together they comprise the major part of the *enteric nervous system* (*ENS*) and thus play an important role in the regulation of digestive tract movement and secretion.

Serosa

The **serosa**—or *serous layer*—is the outermost layer of the GI wall. It is made up of serous membrane (see **Figures 8-8** and **8-9** on pp. 145 and 146). The serosa is actually the *visceral layer* of the **peritoneum**—the serous membrane that lines the abdominopelvic cavity and covers its organs. The lining attached to and covering the walls of the abdominopelvic cavity is called the *parietal layer* of the peritoneum.

The fold of serous membrane shown in **Figure 38-2** that connects the parietal and visceral portions is called a **mesentery.** There are similar folds described in later chapters—all of which help hold the digestive organs in place without twisting or kinking.

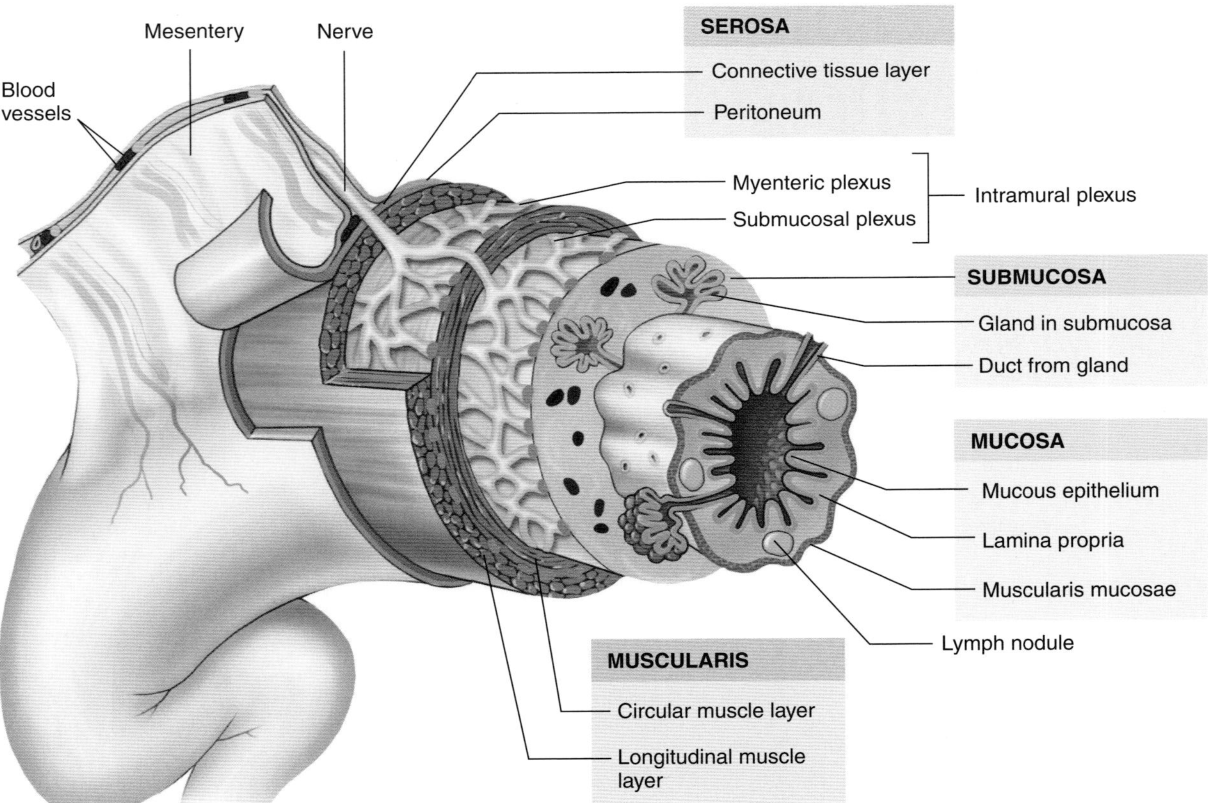

FIGURE 38-2 Wall of the GI tract. The wall of the gastrointestinal (GI) tract is made up of four layers, shown here in a generalized diagram of a segment of the GI tract. Notice that the serosa is continuous with a fold of serous membrane called a *mesentery.* Note also that digestive glands may empty their products into the lumen of the GI tract by way of ducts.

TABLE 38-1 Modifications of Layers of the Digestive Tract Wall

ORGAN	MUCOSA	MUSCULARIS	SEROSA
Oesophagus	Stratified squamous epithelium resists abrasion	Two layers—inner one of circular fibres and outer one of longitudinal fibres; striated muscle in the upper part and smooth muscle in the lower part of the oesophagus and in the rest of the tract	Outer layer, fibrous (adventitia); serous around part of the oesophagus in the thoracic cavity
Stomach	Arranged in flexible longitudinal folds called *rugae;* allow for distention; contains gastric pits with microscopic gastric glands	Has three layers instead of the usual two—circular, longitudinal, and oblique fibres; two sphincters—lower oesophageal sphincter (LOS) at the entrance of the stomach and pyloric sphincter at its exit, formed by circular fibres	Outer layer, visceral peritoneum; hangs in a double fold from the lower edge of the stomach over the intestines and forms an apronlike structure; greater omentum; lesser omentum connects the stomach to the liver
Small intestine	Contains permanent circular folds (plicae circulares) Microscopic fingerlike projections, villi with brush border Crypts (of Lieberkühn) Microscopic duodenal (Brunner) mucous glands Aggregated lymphoid nodules (Peyer patches) Numerous single lymphoid nodules called *solitary nodules*	Two layers—inner one of circular fibres and outer one of longitudinal fibres	Outer layer, visceral peritoneum, continuous with the mesentery
Large intestine	Solitary lymph nodes Intestinal mucous glands Anal columns form in the anal region	Outer longitudinal layer condensed to form three tapelike strips (taeniae coli); clumping of circular muscle produces small sacs (haustra) and give the rest of the wall of the large intestine a puckered appearance; internal anal sphincter formed by circular smooth fibres; external anal sphincter formed by striated fibres; serous membrane (visceral peritoneum) has small fatty epiploic appendages	Outer layer, visceral peritoneum, continuous with mesocolon

Modifications of Layers

Although the same four tissue layers form the various organs of the GI tract, their structures vary in different regions of the tube throughout its length. Variations in the epithelial layer of the mucosa, for example, range from stratified layers of squamous cells that provide protection from abrasion in the upper part of the oesophagus to the simple columnar epithelium, designed for absorption and secretion, which is found throughout most of the tract. Note in **Figure 38-2** that exocrine glands empty their secretions into the lumen of the GI tract through ducts. Some of these modifications are listed in **Table 38-1**; refer back to this table when each of these organs is studied in detail.

Quick CHECK

1. What is another name for the digestive tract?
2. Name the four layers of the digestive tract wall.

MOUTH

Structure of the Oral Cavity

The mouth is also called the *oral cavity.* The following structures form the oral cavity *(buccal cavity)*: the lips, which surround the orifice of the mouth and form the anterior boundary of the oral cavity; the cheeks (side walls); the tongue and its muscles (floor); and the hard palate and soft palate (roof) (**Figure 38-3**).

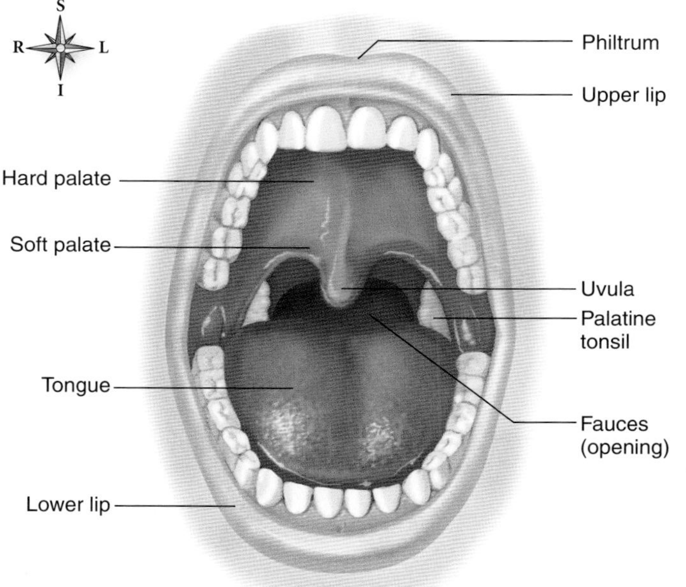

FIGURE 38-3 The oral cavity.

UNIT 5

Lips

The **lips** are covered externally by skin and internally by mucous membrane that continues into the oral cavity and lines the mouth. The junction between skin and mucous membrane is highly sensitive and easily irritated. The upper lip is marked near the midline by a shallow vertical groove called the *philtrum*, which ends at the junction between skin and mucous membrane in a slight prominence called the *tubercle*. The term *fissure* is often used to describe a cleft or groove between or separating anatomical structures. Therefore, when the lips are closed, the line of contact between them is called the *oral fissure*. Besides keeping food in the mouth while it is being chewed, the lips help sense the temperature and texture of food before it enters the mouth. The lips are also needed to form many speech sounds (syllables).

Cheeks

The **cheeks** form the lateral boundaries of the oral cavity. They are continuous with the lips in front and are lined by mucous membrane that is reflected onto the *soft palate* and the alveolar process of each jaw—forming the **gingiva,** or gums. The walls of the cheeks are formed in large part by the buccinator muscle, which is sandwiched with a considerable amount of adipose, or fat, tissue between the outer skin and mucous membrane lining. Numerous small mucus-secreting glands are located between the mucous membrane and the buccinator muscle; their ducts open opposite the last molar teeth.

Hard Palate and Soft Palate

The **hard palate** consists of portions of four bones: two maxillae and two palatines (see **Figure 12-5** on p. 240). The **soft palate,** which forms a partition between the mouth and nasopharynx (see **Figure 35-3** on p. 803), is fashioned of muscle arranged in the shape of an arch. The opening in the arch leads from the mouth into the oropharynx and is named the *fauces*. Suspended from the midpoint of the posterior border of the arch is a small cone-shaped process, the *uvula*.

Tongue

The **tongue** is a solid mass of skeletal muscle components (intrinsic muscles) covered by a mucous membrane.

Note in **Figure 38-4**, *A*, that the tongue has a blunt *root*, a *tip*, and a central *body*. The upper, or dorsal, surface of the tongue is normally moist, pink, and covered by rough elevations, called *papillae* (**Figure 38-4**, *B*). Recall from Chapter 24 that papillae possess sensory organs called *taste buds*.

The four types of papillae—circumvallate, fungiform, foliate, and filiform—are all located on the sides or upper surface (dorsum) of the tongue. Note in **Figure 38-4**, *A*, that the large circumvallate papillae form an inverted **V**-shaped row extending from a median pit named the *foramen caecum* on the posterior part of the tongue. There are 10 to 14 of these large, mushroomlike papillae. You can readily distinguish them if you look at your own tongue. **Figure 38-5** shows two micrographs of circumvallate papillae. To be tasted, a dissolved substance must enter a moatlike depression surrounding the papillae, where it contacts taste buds located on the lateral surface.

Taste buds are also located on the sides of the fungiform papillae, which are found chiefly on the sides and tip of the tongue. Foliate papillae are leaflike ridges on the posterior, lateral edges of the tongue that also possess taste buds. The numerous filiform papillae are filamentous and threadlike in appearance. They have a whitish colouration and are distributed over the anterior two thirds of the tongue. Filiform papillae do not contain taste buds. Refer back to Chapter 24, p. 534, for more discussion of papillae and taste buds.

The *lingual frenulum* (**Figure 38-6**, *A*) is a fold of mucous membrane in the midline of the undersurface of the tongue that helps anchor the tongue to the floor of the mouth. If the frenulum is too short and hinders tongue movement—a congenital condition called *ankyloglossia*—the individual is said to be tongue-tied; this causes faulty speech (**Figure 38-6**, *B*).

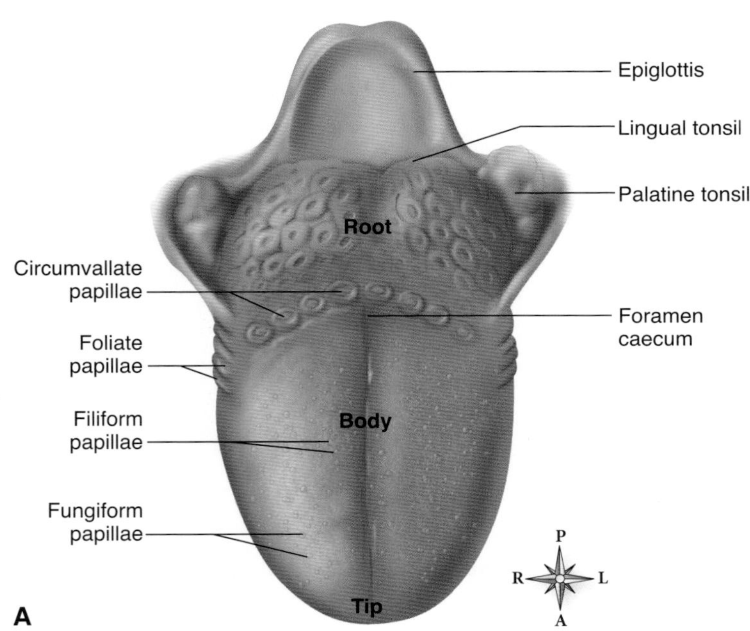

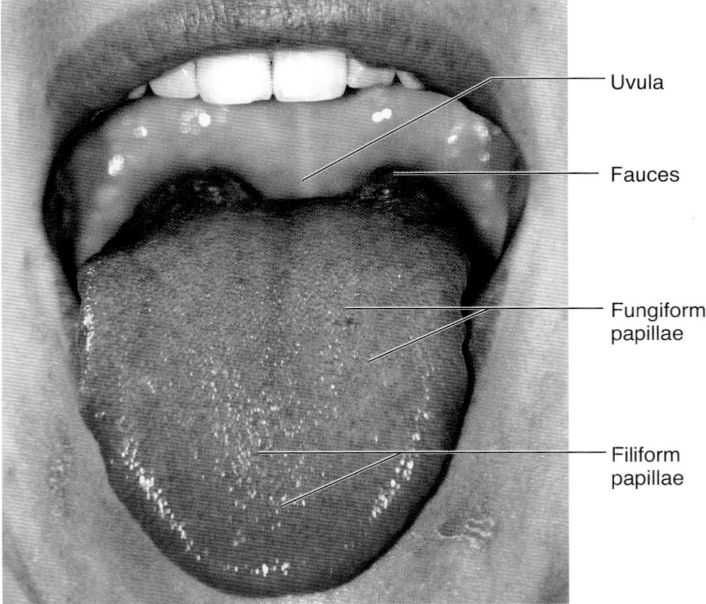

FIGURE 38-4 Dorsal surface of tongue. A, Sketch showing the three divisions of the tongue (see also **Figure 24-3** on p. 535). **B,** Photograph showing rough texture of tongue produced by papillae.

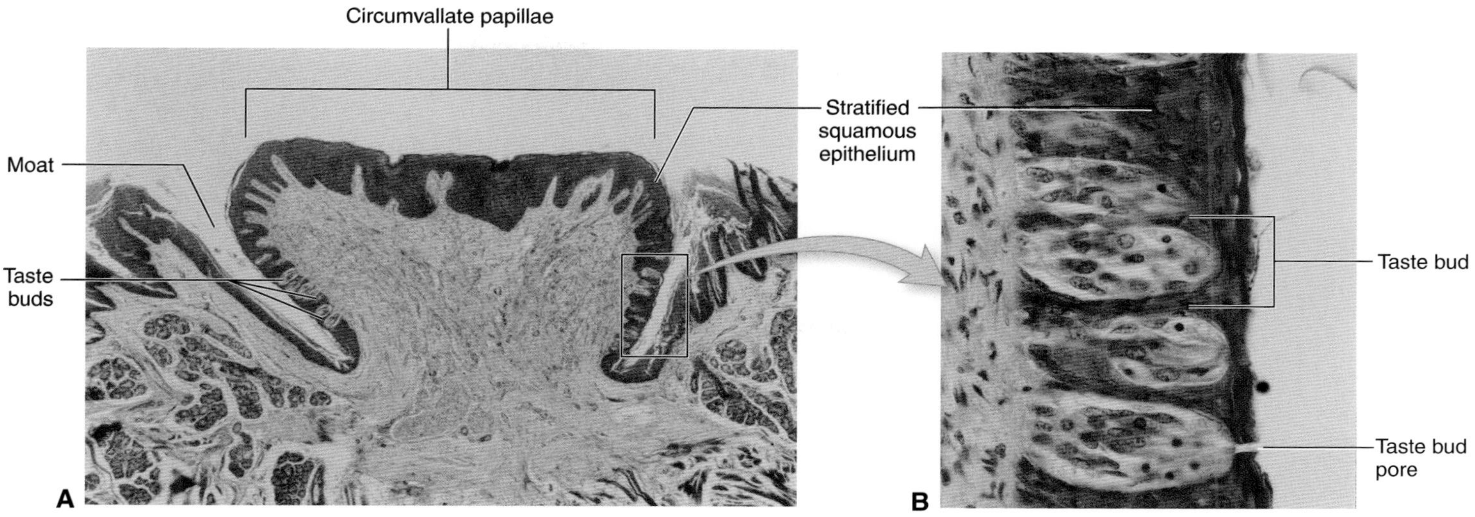

FIGURE 38-5 Circumvallate papillae on the surface of the tongue. A, Taste buds are located on the lateral surfaces of the papillae. Several taste buds can be seen opening into the moat from the sides of the papillae. (×35.) **B,** Enlargement of the photomicrograph of taste buds in **A** (×40). Compare to **Figure 24-3** on p. 535.

A fold of mucous membrane called the *fimbriated fold* (or *plica fimbriata*) (see **Figure 38-6**, *A*) extends toward the apex of the tongue on either side of the lingual frenulum. The floor of the mouth and undersurface of the tongue are richly supplied with blood vessels. The deep lingual vein can be seen (see **Figure 38-6**, *A*) shining through the mucous membrane between the lingual frenulum and fimbriated fold. In this region many vessels are extremely superficial and are covered only by a very thin layer of mucosa. Soluble drugs, such as aspirin or nitroglycerin used during a heart attack, are absorbed into the circulation rapidly if placed under the tongue.

The intrinsic muscles of the tongue have, by definition, both their origin and their insertion in the tongue itself. As you can see in **Figure 38-7**, *A*, intrinsic muscles have their fibres oriented in all directions, thus providing a basis for extreme manoeuvrability. Changes in the size and shape of the tongue caused by intrinsic muscle contraction assist in placement of food material between the teeth during **mastication** (chewing). Such movements are also necessary for forming speech syllables properly.

Extrinsic tongue muscles are those that insert into the tongue but have their origin on some other structure, such as the hyoid bone or one of the bones of the skull. Examples of extrinsic tongue muscles are the genioglossus, which protrudes the tongue, and the hyoglossus, which depresses it (see **Figure 38-7**, *B*). Contraction of the extrinsic muscles is important during **deglutition**, or swallowing, and speech.

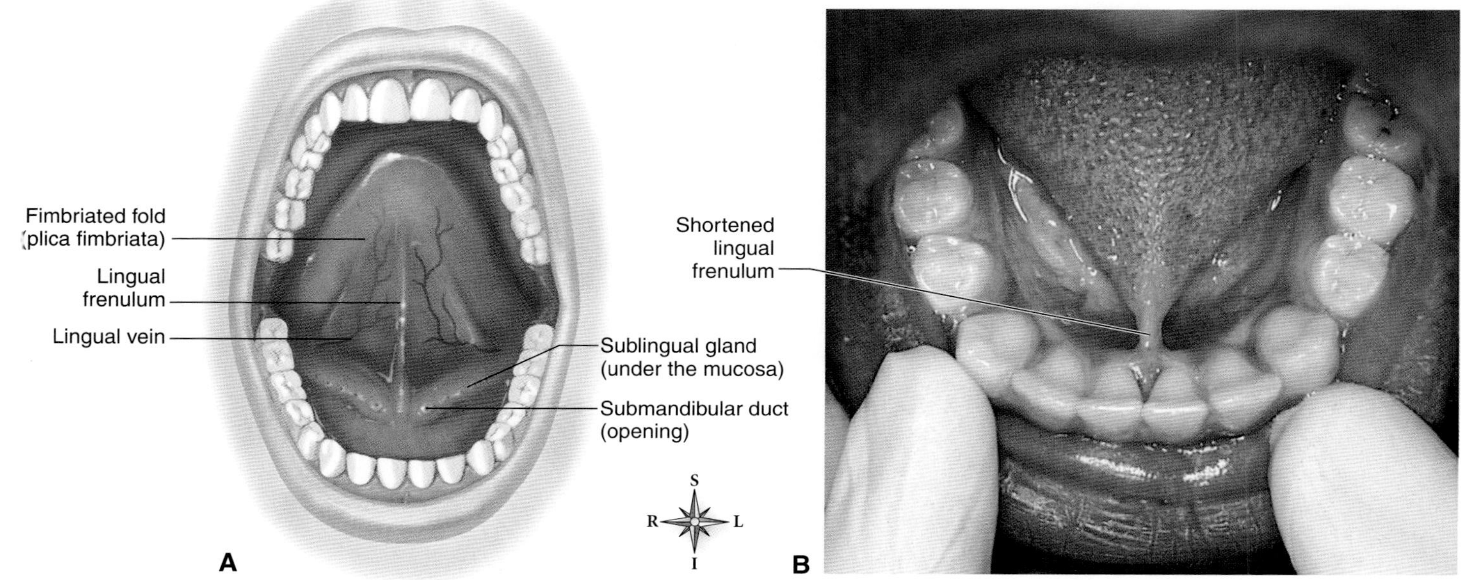

FIGURE 38-6 Floor of mouth. A, Floor of mouth and ventral surface of tongue. **B,** Photo showing ankyloglossia, characterized by an abnormally short lingual frenulum.

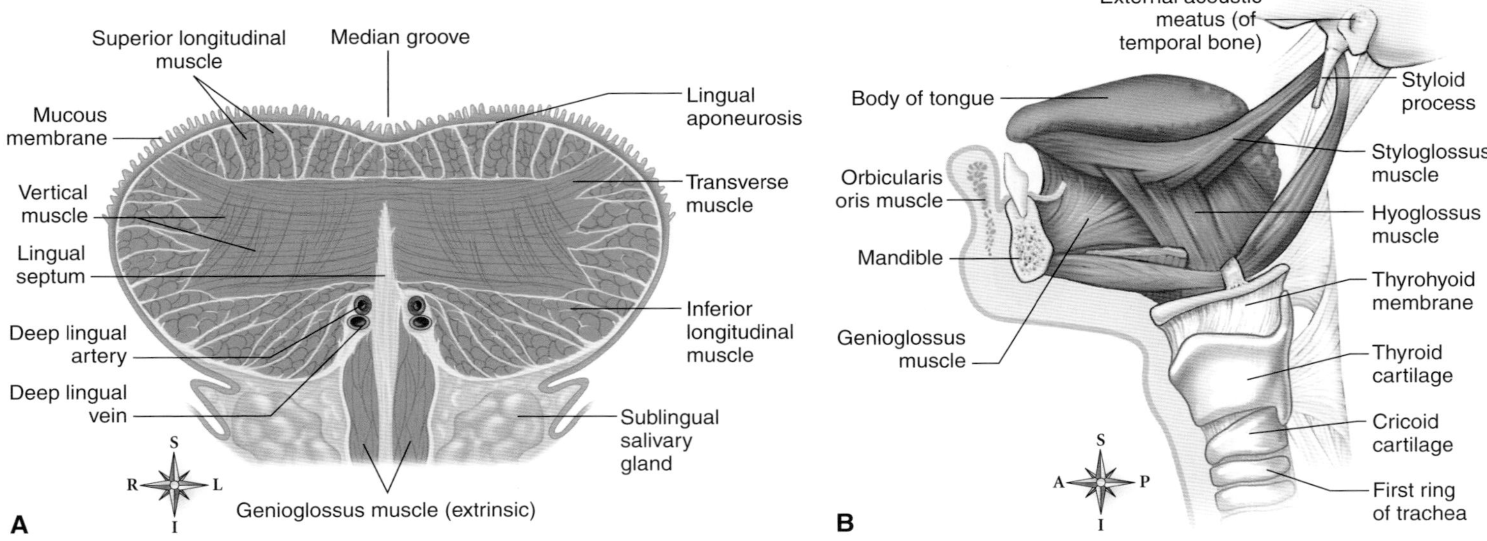

FIGURE 38-7 Muscles of the tongue. A, Intrinsic muscles of the tongue shown in a coronal (frontal) section. **B,** Extrinsic muscles of the tongue.

CONNECT IT!

Taste buds provide just one mechanism for analyzing our food before we swallow it. Review ***Sensing Food*** online at ***Connect It!*** to find out the many other ways that food is analyzed in the mouth.

SALIVARY GLANDS

The salivary glands are typical of the accessory glands associated with the digestive system. They are located outside the alimentary canal and convey their exocrine secretions by way of ducts from the glands into the lumen of the tract (**Figure 38-8**, *A*).

The mucous and serous cells seen in the compound tubuloalveolar gland pictured in **Figure 38-8**, *B*, together secrete a mixture of fluids that are then modified by the duct cells on their way out of the salivary gland. The serous cells produce a watery secretion that contains digestive enzymes. Mucous cells produce mucus. The functions of saliva and its components in the digestive process are discussed in Chapter 40.

Three pairs of major salivary glands (see **Figure 38-8**)—the parotid, submandibular, and sublingual glands—secrete a major amount (about 1 litre) of the saliva produced each day. The minor salivary glands (*buccal*, *lingual*, *palatine*, *labial*, and *molar glands*) that occur in the mucosa lining the mouth contribute less than 5% of the total salivary volume. Minor salivary gland secretion is

Parotid gland
Parotid duct
Submandibular gland
Submandibular duct
A
Sublingual gland
S
A
P
I
Duct
Mucous cells
Duct epithelium
Serous cells
B

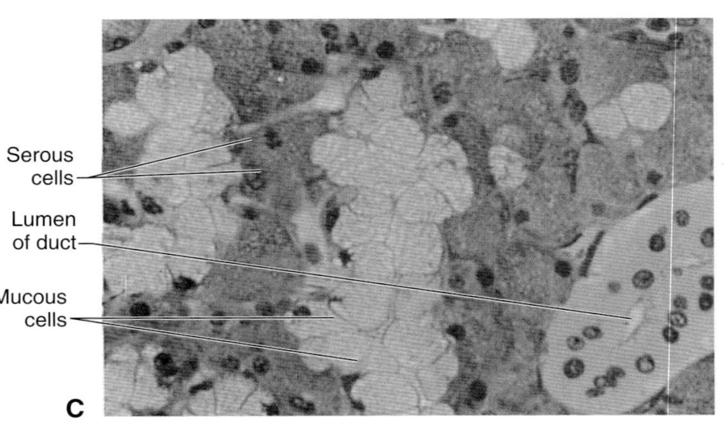

FIGURE 38-8 Salivary glands. A, Location of the salivary glands. **B** and **C,** Detail of submandibular salivary gland. This mixed- or compound-type gland produces mucus from mucous cells and enzymatic secretion from serous cells. Duct cross sections are also visible. (×140.)

UNIT 5

important, however, to the hygiene and comfort of the mouth tissues, as well as digestive enzyme production.

Parotid Glands

The pyramidal **parotids** are the largest of the paired salivary glands (see **Figure 38-8**, A). They are located between the skin and underlying masseter muscle in front of and below the external ear. The parotids produce a watery, or serous, type of saliva containing enzymes but not mucus. The *parotid ducts* (*Stensen ducts*) are about 5 cm long. They penetrate the buccinator muscle on each side and open into the mouth through the *parotid papilla* opposite the upper second molars. Inflammation of the parotids is called **mumps** or **parotitis** and is caused by *paramyxovirus* (see Mechanisms of Disease, p. 874).

Submandibular Glands

Submandibular glands (see **Figure 38-8**, A) are called *mixed* or *compound glands* because they contain both serous (enzyme) and mucus-producing elements (see **Figure 38-8**, *B* and *C*). These glands are located just below the mandibular angle. You can feel the gland by placing your index finger on the posterior part of the floor of the mouth and your thumb medial to and just in front of the angle of the mandible. The gland is irregular in form and about the size of a walnut. The ducts of the submandibular glands (*Wharton ducts*) open into the mouth on either side of the lingual frenulum.

Sublingual Glands

Sublingual glands are the smallest of the main salivary glands (see **Figure 38-8**, A). They lie in front of the submandibular glands, under the mucous membrane covering the floor of the mouth. Each sublingual gland is drained by 8 to 20 ducts (*Rivinus ducts*) that open into the floor of the mouth. Unlike the other salivary glands, the sublingual glands produce only a mucous type of saliva.

TEETH

The teeth are the organs of *mastication*, or chewing. They are designed to cut, tear, and grind ingested food so that it can be mixed with saliva and swallowed. During the process of mastication, food is ground into small bits. This increases the surface area that can be acted on by the digestive enzymes.

Typical Tooth

The tooth is made up of four special types of connective tissues called *dental tissues*:

- **Pulp**—soft, fibrous connective tissue with blood vessels and nerves at the core of each tooth
- **Dentin**—hard, mineralized connective tissue similar to bone forms the body of the tooth
- **Cementum**—hard, mineralized connective tissue similar to bone; forms a coat around the root of the tooth and helps connect to the jawbone
- **Enamel**—hard, mineralized connective tissue; harder than bone; forms hard covering of exposed tooth surfaces

A typical tooth (**Figure 38-9**) can be divided into three main parts: crown, neck, and root.

The **crown** is the exposed portion of a tooth. It is covered by enamel—the hardest and chemically most stable tissue in the body. Enamel consists of approximately 97% calcified (inorganic) material and only 3% organic material and water. Enamel develops as an interlocking set of rods that forms an incredibly strong coating over the crown. It is ideally suited to withstand the very abrasive process of mastication. Even though it no longer has any living cells by adulthood, and therefore can no longer remodel or repair itself, it is still designated as a nonliving dental "tissue" by histologists.

The *neck* of a tooth is the narrow portion shown in **Figure 38-9** that is surrounded by the gingivae, or gums. It joins the crown of the tooth to the root.

It is the **root** that fits into the socket of the alveolar process of either the upper or lower jaw. The root of a tooth may be a single peglike structure or consist of two or three separate conical projections. The root is not rigidly anchored to the alveolar process by cement but is suspended in the socket by the fibrous *periodontal membrane* (see **Figure 38-9**). This membrane is composed of many *periodontal ligaments* that intertwine with collagen fibres within both the cementum and the alveolar bone of the jaw.

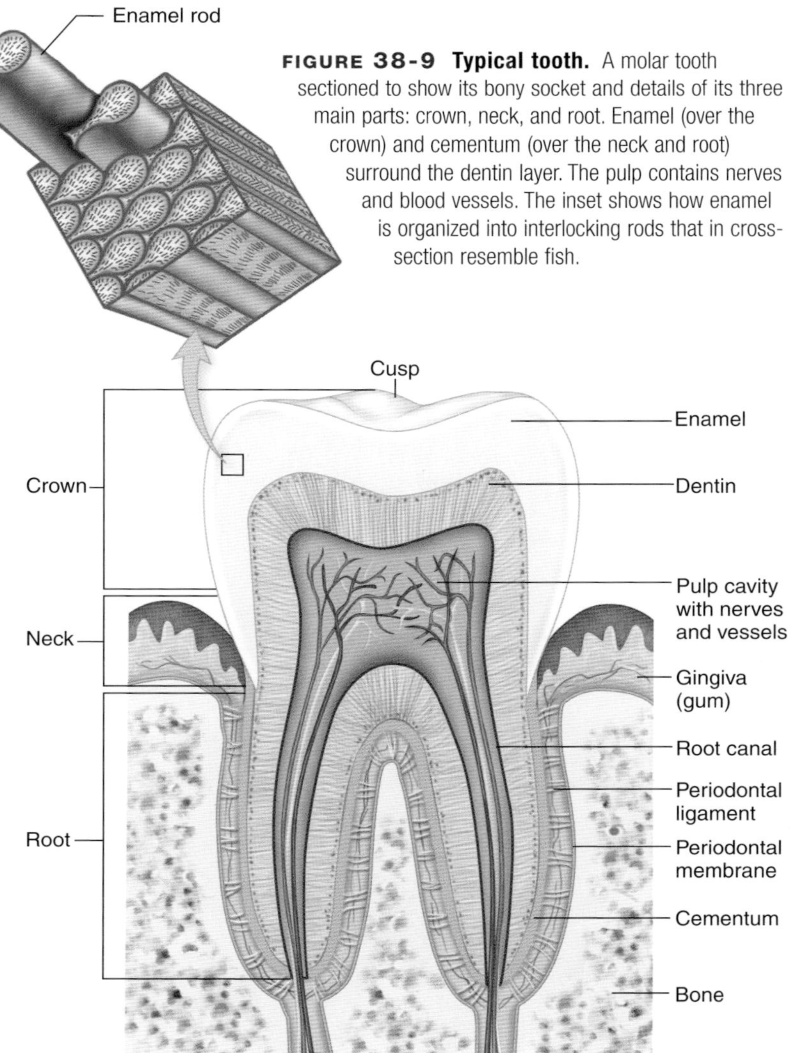

FIGURE 38-9 Typical tooth. A molar tooth sectioned to show its bony socket and details of its three main parts: crown, neck, and root. Enamel (over the crown) and cementum (over the neck and root) surround the dentin layer. The pulp contains nerves and blood vessels. The inset shows how enamel is organized into interlocking rods that in cross-section resemble fish.

TABLE 38-2 Dentition

NAME OF TOOTH	NUMBER PER JAW (UPPER OR LOWER)	
	DECIDUOUS SET	PERMANENT SET
Central incisors	2	2
Lateral incisors	2	2
Canines (cuspids)	2	2
Premolars (bicuspids)	0	4
First molars (tricuspids)	2	2
Second molars	2	2
Third molars (wisdom teeth)	0	2
TOTAL (per jaw)	10	16
TOTAL (per set)	20	32

In addition to enamel, the outer shell of each tooth is composed of two additional dental tissues—*dentin* and *cementum* (see **Figure 38-9**). Dentin makes up the greatest proportion of the tooth body. It is covered by enamel in the crown and by cementum in the neck and root area. The dentin contains a **pulp cavity** consisting of fibrous *pulp* tissue, blood and lymphatic vessels, and sensory nerves.

Types of Teeth

Dentition is the type, number, and arrangement of teeth in the jaws.

Twenty primary or **deciduous teeth,** or so-called *baby teeth*, appear early in life and are later replaced by 32 **permanent teeth** (**Figure 38-10**). The names and numbers of teeth in both sets are given in **Table 38-2**. The first deciduous tooth usually erupts at about 6 months of age. The remainder follow at the rate of one or more a month until all 20 have appeared. There is, however, great individual variation in the age at which teeth erupt. Deciduous teeth are generally shed between the ages of 6 and 13 years. The third molars (wisdom teeth) are the last to appear, and usually erupt sometime after 17 years of age.

Teeth in the upper jaw are called *maxillary teeth* because they are in the maxilla bone of the skull. Teeth in the lower jaw are called

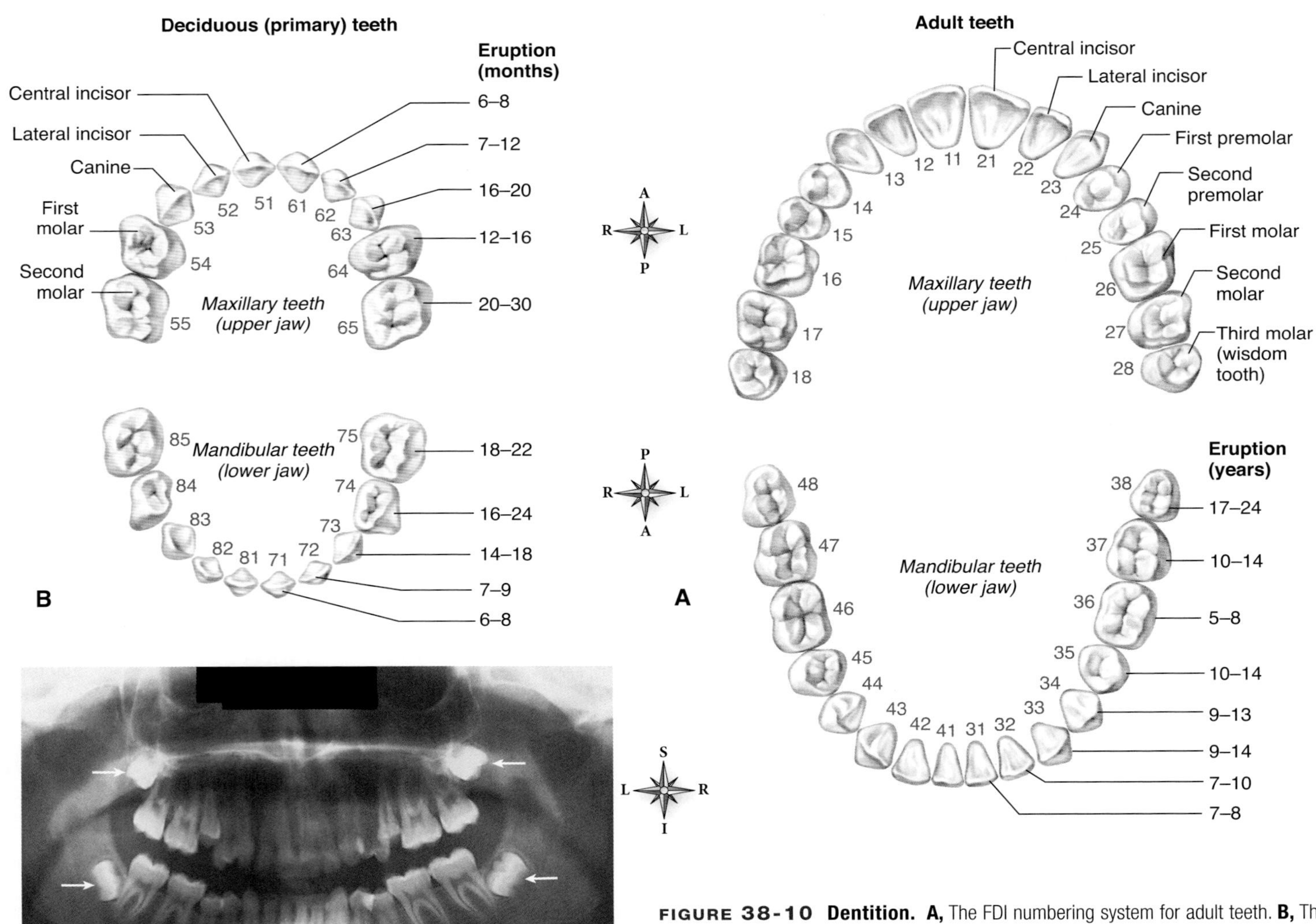

FIGURE 38-10 Dentition. A, The FDI numbering system for adult teeth. **B,** The FDI numbering system for children's teeth. In general the lower teeth erupt before the corresponding upper teeth. The photo inset is a "Panorex" dental radiograph. It displays the full dentition in a single "flattened-out" image. Arrows show the third molars or "wisdom teeth" that have not yet erupted.

mandibular teeth because they are anchored in the mandible bone. The teeth shown in **Figure 38-10** are numbered according to the internationally recognized two-digit FDI *(Fédération Dentaire Internationale)* system used by dentists.

For adults the mouth is divided into four quadrants numbered clockwise from 1 to 4, starting from the upper left of **Figure 38-10** *A*, which corresponds to the patient's upper right. The adult teeth are numbered from 1 to 8 in each quadrant going from the central incisor to the canine and premolars and then to the third molar.

For children the mouth is similarly divided into quadrants numbered clockwise from 5 to 8 starting from the upper left of **Figure 38-10** *B*. The teeth are numbered from 1 to 5 going from the central incisors to canines and molars.

CONNECT IT!

An epidemic of methamphetamine abuse has resulted in a number of health problems, including "meth mouth". See an example of this disorder and learn about its causes in ***Meth Mouth*** online at ***Connect It!***

***Quick* CHECK**

3. What are the boundaries of the oral cavity?
4. Describe the location of the taste buds in the mouth.
5. What are the names of the three types of salivary glands?
6. How do the names of the salivary glands describe their locations?
7. What are the three main parts of a typical tooth?

PHARYNX

The act of swallowing, or **deglutition,** moves a rounded mass of food, called a *bolus*, from the mouth to the stomach. As the food bolus passes from the mouth, it enters the oropharynx by passing through a constricted, archlike opening called the *fauces*. The oropharynx is the second division of the pharynx (see **Figure 35-3** on p. 803). During respiration, air passes through all three pharyngeal divisions. However, only the terminal portions of the pharynx serve the digestive system. Once a bolus has passed through the pharynx, it enters the digestive tube proper—the portion of the digestive tract that serves only the digestive system. The anatomy of the pharynx is discussed in more detail in Chapter 35 on p. 805.

CONNECT IT! 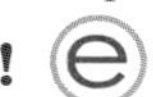

The ring of tonsils in the pharynx defends both the digestive tract and respiratory tract from infection. Visualize the tonsils and review their defensive role in ***Protective Strategies of the Respiratory Tract*** online at ***Connect It!***

OESOPHAGUS

The **oesophagus,** a collapsible, muscular, mucosa-lined tube about 25 cm long, extends from the pharynx to the stomach and pierces the diaphragm in its descent from the thoracic cavity to the abdominal cavity (**Figure 38-11**). It lies posterior to the trachea and heart and serves as a dynamic passageway for food, pushing the food toward the stomach. The short portion of the oesophagus in the neck is called the *cervical part*, the portion in the thorax is called the *thoracic part*, and the short portion in the abdomen is called the *abdominal part*.

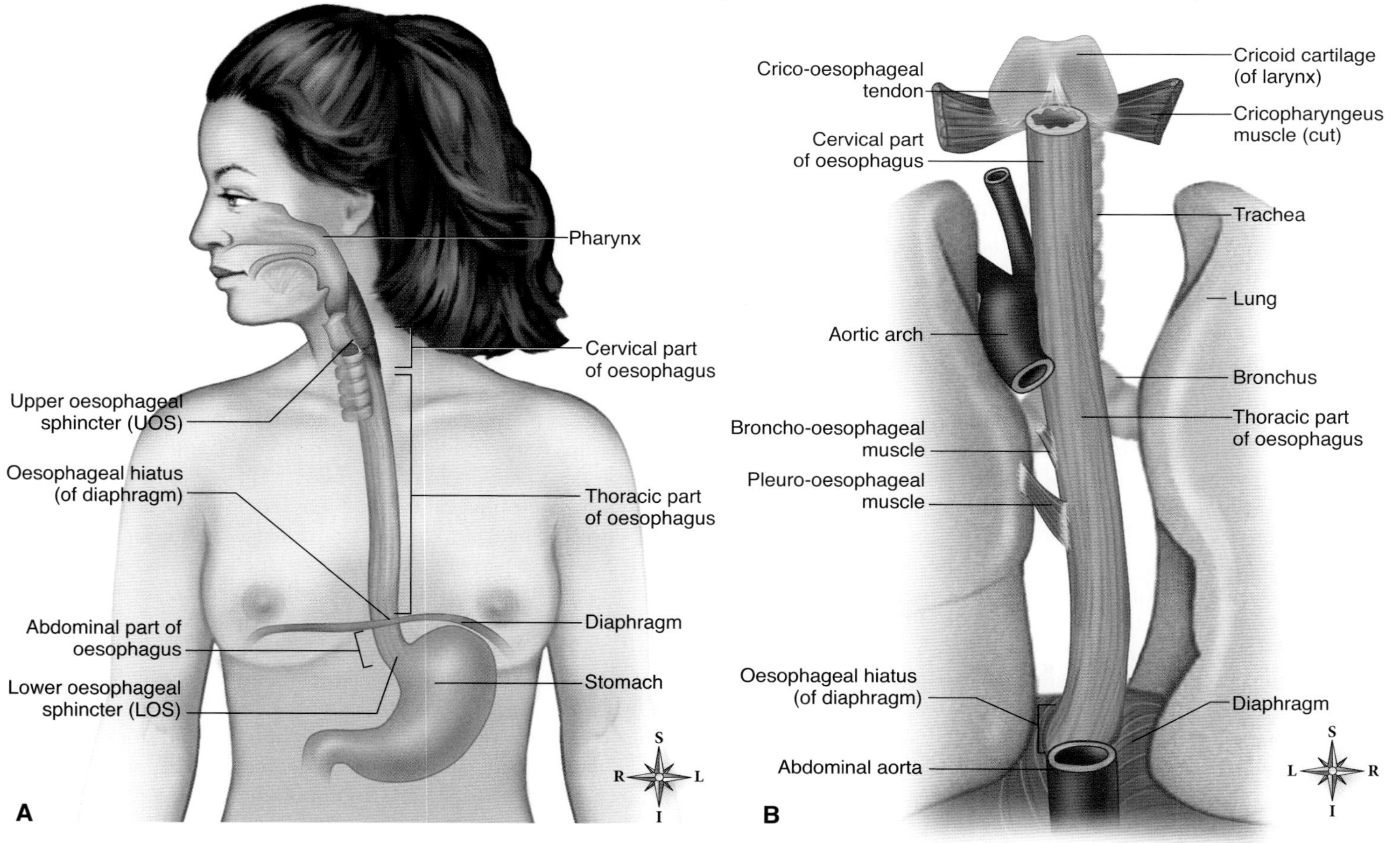

FIGURE 38-11 Oesophagus. A, Diagram showing the major features of the oesophagus. **B,** View of the muscular wall of the oesophagus from behind, showing its position relative to other structures.

UNIT 5

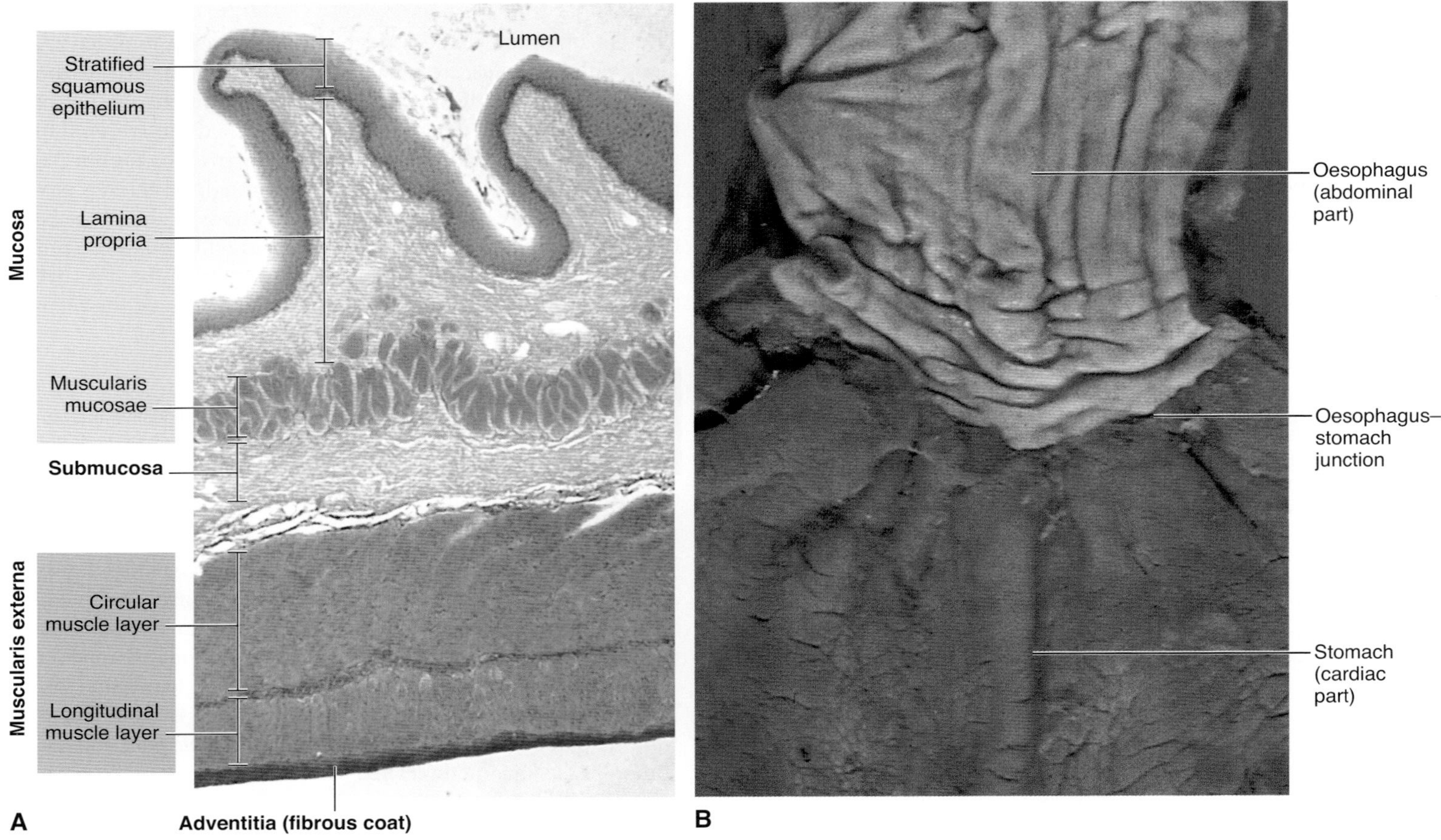

FIGURE 38-12 Wall of oesophagus. A, The four layers of the gastrointestinal (GI) wall are easily identified in this microscopic cross-section of the oesophagus (see **Table 38-1**). **B,** Cadaver dissection photograph of the mucosal lining at the junction between the lower part of the oesophagus and the stomach—a common site of irritation caused by reflux of acidic gastric secretions.

The oesophagus is the first segment of the digestive tube proper, and the four layers that form the wall of the GI tract organs can be identified there (**Figure 38-12**, *A*). The oesophagus is normally flattened, and thus the lumen is practically nonexistent in the resting state. The stratified squamous epithelium of the oesophageal mucosa seen in **Figure 38-12** provides a thick, abrasion-resistant lining that protects the oesophagus from injury. The inner circular and outer longitudinal layers of the muscular layer are striated (voluntary) in the upper third, mixed (striated and smooth) in the middle third, and smooth (involuntary) in the lower third of the tube.

Each end of the oesophagus is encircled by muscular sphincters that act as valves to regulate passage of material. The **upper oesophageal sphincter (UOS)** in the cervical part of the oesophagus helps prevent air from entering the oesophagus during respiration. The UOS is made up of several muscles, but the *cricopharyngeus muscle* (see **Figure 38-11**, *B*) that wraps around the back of the cervical oesophagus plays the primary role. Relaxation of the UOS is what permits *belching* (or *burping*), which is the sudden escape of air trapped in the stomach and oesophagus.

The **lower oesophageal sphincter (LOS)** is also called the *cardiac sphincter* or *cardial sphincter*. The intrinsic part of the LOS is located at the junction with the stomach and is made up of layers of circular muscle that are thicker than in other parts of the oesophagus. Slinglike oblique muscles from the stomach wall also form part of the LOS, adding to its strength in containing the stomach contents while the stomach is full and churning. The muscles of the diaphragm at the *oesophageal hiatus*—an opening in the diaphragm located near the junction between the terminal portion of the oesophagus and the stomach—form the extrinsic part of the LOS.

The oesophageal hiatus in the diaphragm, which permits passage of the oesophagus into the abdomen, may become stretched or otherwise enlarged. Such enlargement may permit bulging of the lower segment of the oesophagus and intrinsic LOS and part or even all of the stomach upward through the diaphragm and into the chest. The condition is called a **hiatal hernia.**

Gastro-oesophageal reflux disease, or **GORD,** is the term used to describe the backward flow of stomach acid up through the LOS and into the lower part of the oesophagus. It often causes a painful sensation called *heartburn*. Being a potentially serious medical condition, GORD is treated by elimination of the underlying causes, such as a hiatal hernia, by drugs to reduce excess stomach acid, or by surgery to reduce the lumen size or strengthen the LOS (see Mechanisms of Disease on p. 875). **Box 38-2** describes a method for imaging a hiatal hernia and other problems of the oesophagus and stomach.

The junction between the lower part of the oesophagus and stomach (see **Figure 38-12**, *B*) is an important site for a number of pathologic conditions, many associated with repeated exposure to acid gastric secretions. In the last 1- to 1.5-cm-long abdominal part of the

BOX 38-2 *diagnostic study*

Upper Gastrointestinal X-Ray Study

An upper gastrointestinal (UGI) study consists of a series of radiographs of the lower part of the oesophagus, stomach, and duodenum, usually with barium sulphate used as the contrast medium. The test is used to detect ulcerations, tumours, inflammation, or anatomical malpositions such as *hiatal hernia* (distention of the diaphragm that allows the stomach to protrude). Obstruction of the upper GI tract is also easily detected.

In this test the patient is asked to drink a flavoured liquid containing barium sulphate. As the contrast medium travels through the system, the lower portion of the oesophagus, gastric wall, pyloric channel, and duodenum are each evaluated for defects. Benign peptic ulcer is a common pathological condition affecting these areas. Tumours, cysts, or enlarged organs near the stomach can also be identified by an anatomical distortion of the outline of the upper GI tract. Identify the outline of the stomach in the figure. •

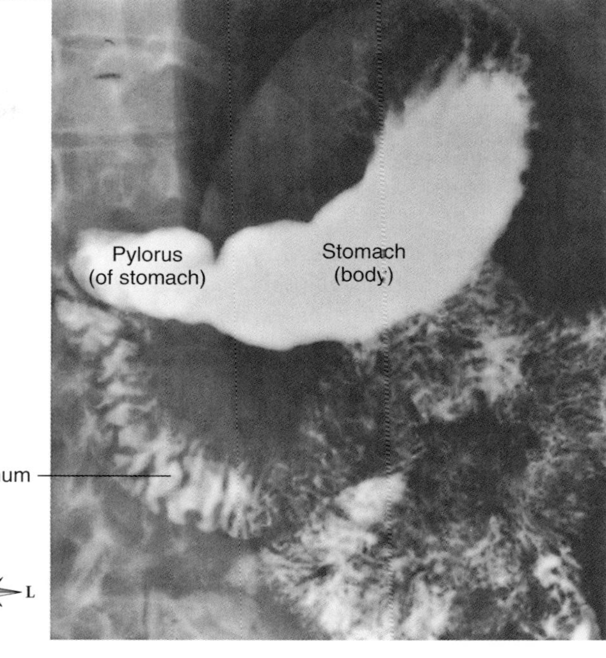

X-ray film of the lower part of the oesophagus, stomach, and duodenum.

FIGURE 38-13 Stomach. A portion of the anterior wall has been cut away to reveal the muscle layers of the stomach wall. Note that the mucosa lining the stomach forms folds called *rugae.*

oesophagus below the diaphragm, stratified squamous epithelium is replaced by columnar epithelium. It is this area of transition that is often damaged by exposure to acid and digestive enzymes from the stomach. The area of transition between the lower part of the oesophagus and stomach is clearly visible in **Figure 38-12**, *B*. The stratified squamous epithelial lining of the oesophagus appears pale, whereas the columnar gastric epithelium appears brown.

STOMACH

Size and Position of the Stomach

Just below the diaphragm, the digestive tube dilates into an elongated pouchlike structure, the stomach (**Figure 38-13**), the size of which varies according to several factors, notably the amount of distention. For some time after a meal, the stomach is enlarged because of distention of its walls, but as food passes out of the stomach, the walls partially collapse, leaving the organ about the size of a large sausage. In adults, the stomach usually holds a volume of up to 1 to 1.5 litres.

The stomach lies in the upper part of the abdominal cavity under the liver and diaphragm, with approximately five sixths of its mass to the left of the median line (see **Figure 38-1**). In other words, it is described as lying in the *epigastrium* and left *hypochondrium* (see **Figure 1-8**, p. 14, and Figure 1-18 of the BRIEF ATLAS OF THE HUMAN BODY). Its position, however, alters frequently. For example, it is pushed downward with each inspiration and upward with each expiration. When it is greatly distended from an unusually large meal, its size interferes with descent of the diaphragm on inspiration, thereby producing the familiar feeling of *dyspnoea* (breathing difficulty) that accompanies overeating. In this state, the stomach also pushes upward against the heart and may give rise to the sensation that the heart is being crowded.

Divisions of the Stomach

The **fundus, body,** and **pylorus** are the major divisions of the stomach. The fundus is the enlarged portion to the left and above the opening of the oesophagus into the stomach. The body is the central part of the stomach, and the pylorus is its lower portion (see **Figure 38-13**). The small collar or margin of the stomach at its junction with the oesophagus is often called the **cardia** or *cardiac part* (or *cardial part*).

Curves of the Stomach

The curve formed by the upper right surface of the stomach is known as the *lesser curvature*; the curve formed by the lower left surface is known as the *greater curvature* (see **Figure 38-13**).

Sphincter Muscles

Sphincter muscles regulate passage of material at both stomach openings. A sphincter muscle, as you know, consists of circular fibres arranged to form an opening in the centre of them (like the hole in a doughnut) when they are relaxed and no opening when they are fully contracted.

The *lower oesophageal sphincter* (*LOS*), or *cardiac sphincter*, controls the opening of the oesophagus into the stomach, and the **pyloric sphincter** controls the opening from the pyloric portion of the stomach into the first part of the small intestine (duodenum).

Stomach Wall

Each of the four layers of the stomach wall suits the function of this organ, as summarized in **Table 38-1** (p. 863) and shown in **Figure 38-13** and **Figure 38-14**. Of particular interest are the modifications to the stomach mucosa and muscularis, both of which are briefly described below.

Gastric Mucosa

The epithelial lining of the stomach is thrown into folds, called *rugae*, and marked by depressions called *gastric pits*. Numerous coiled tubular-type glands, *gastric glands*, are found below the level of the pits, particularly in the fundus and body of the stomach. **Figure 38-14** illustrates the anatomical relationship of the gastric pits and gastric glands. The glands secrete most of the gastric juice, a mucous fluid containing digestive enzymes and hydrochloric acid (HCl). **Figure 38-15**, *A*, a low-power micrograph of the mucosal lining in the body of the stomach, shows numerous gastric pits and a uniform underlying layer of coiled gastric glands. The mucosal lining is easily differentiated from the deeper submucosal layer in this section. **Figure 38-15**, *B*, shows an enlarged view of gastric pits and gastric glands isolated from the submucosa and surrounding tissues.

In addition to the mucus-producing cells that cover the entire surface of the stomach and line the pits, the gastric glands contain three major secretory cells—**chief cells, parietal cells,** and **endocrine cells** (see **Figure 38-14**). Chief cells (zymogenic cells) secrete the enzymes of gastric juice. Parietal cells secrete hydrochloric acid and are also thought to produce the important substance known as *intrinsic factor*. Intrinsic factor binds to vitamin B_{12} molecules to protect them from digestive juices until they reach the small intestine—and then facilitates the absorption of B_{12}. Endocrine cells secrete *ghrelin* (*GHRL*)—a

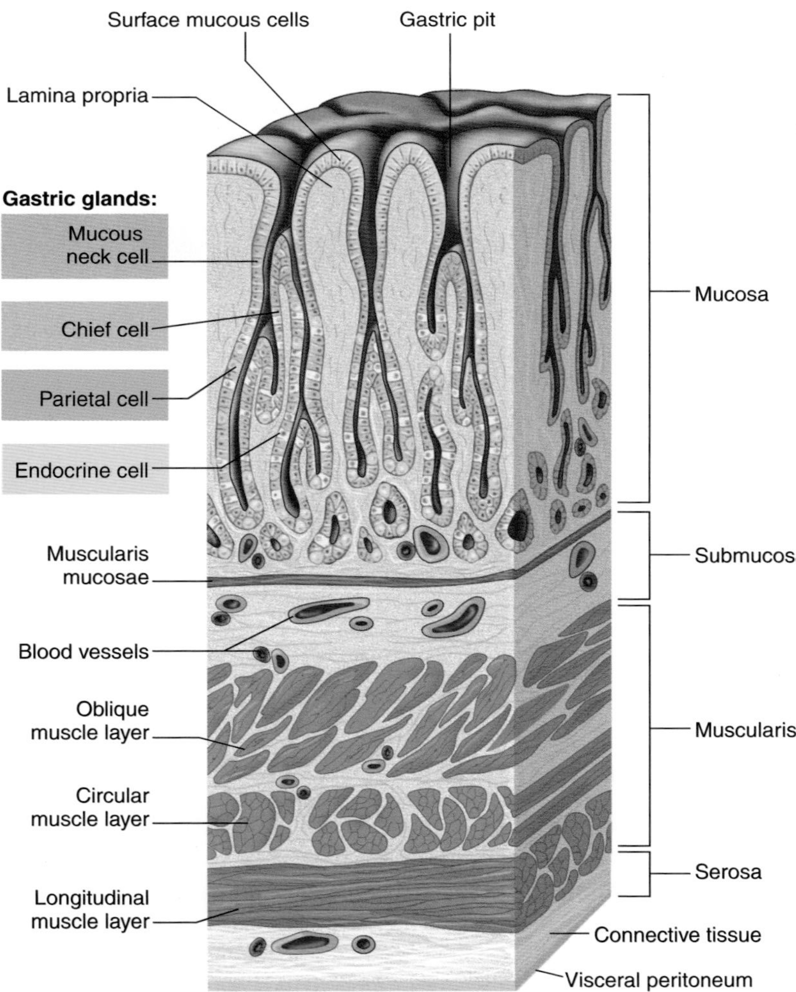

FIGURE 38-14 Gastric pits and gastric glands. Gastric pits are depressions in the epithelial lining of the stomach. At the bottom of each pit is one or more tubular *gastric glands.* Chief cells produce the enzymes of gastric juice, and parietal cells produce stomach acid. Endocrine cells secrete the appetite-boosting hormone ghrelin.

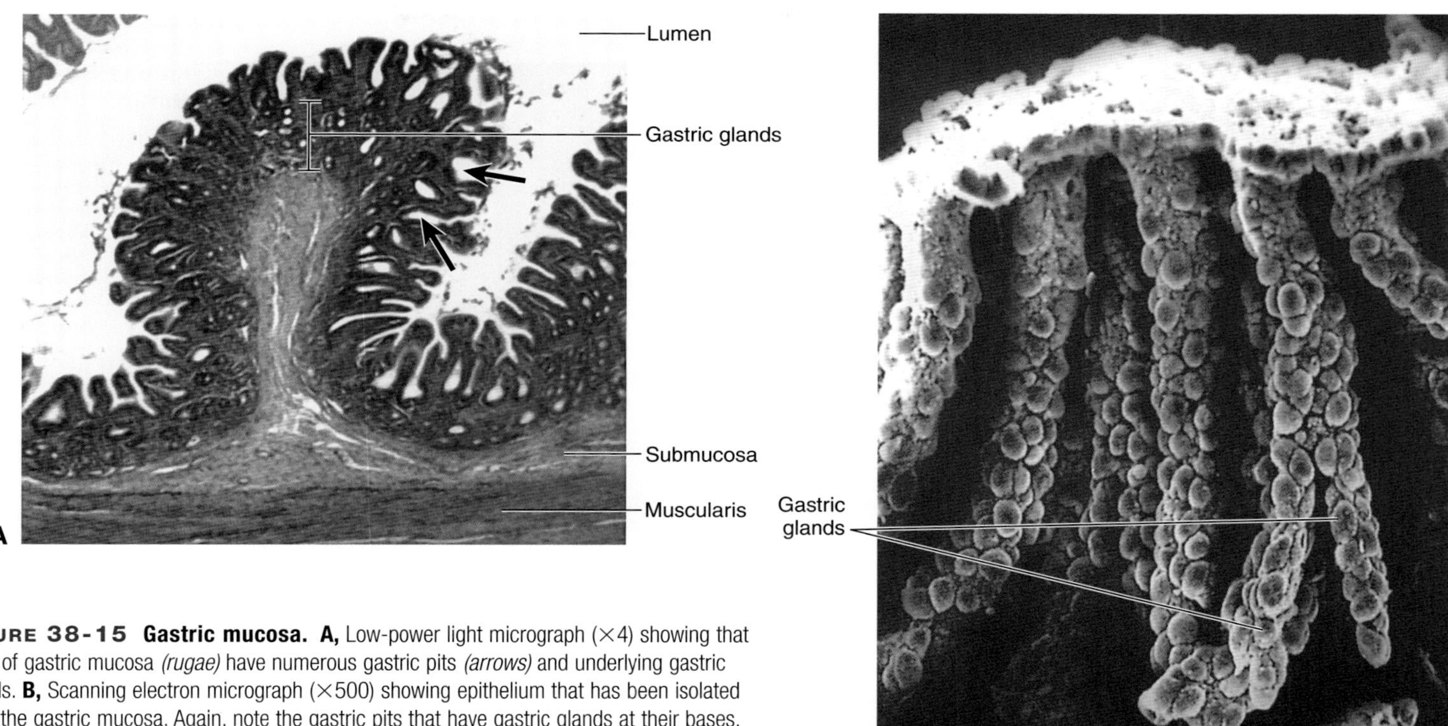

FIGURE 38-15 Gastric mucosa. A, Low-power light micrograph (×4) showing that folds of gastric mucosa *(rugae)* have numerous gastric pits *(arrows)* and underlying gastric glands. **B,** Scanning electron micrograph (×500) showing epithelium that has been isolated from the gastric mucosa. Again, note the gastric pits that have gastric glands at their bases. The outer surfaces of the parietal cells are seen as prominent dome-shaped bulges.

hormone that stimulates the hypothalamus to secrete growth hormone and increase appetite—and *gastrin,* which influences digestive functions. The roles of the gastric secretory cells are explored further in Chapter 40.

Gastric Muscle

The thick layer of muscle in the stomach wall—the **muscularis**—is made of three distinct sublayers of smooth muscle tissue. As **Figure 38-13** shows, there is the usual layer of longitudinal muscles and circular muscles, as well as an additional, underlying oblique layer. The crisscrossing pattern of smooth muscle fibres formed by this arrangement gives the stomach wall the ability to contract strongly at many angles—thus making the mixing action of this organ very efficient.

Functions of the Stomach

The stomach performs the following functions:

- Serves as a food reservoir, its main function; food is stored in the stomach until it can be partially digested and moved further along the gastrointestinal tract.
- Secretes *gastric juice,* which contains acid and enzymes that aid in the digestion of food.
- Churns the food (by contractions of its muscular coat), breaking it into small particles and mixing them well with the gastric juice; in time, gastric contents are moved along into the duodenum.
- Secretes *intrinsic factor.*
- Performs a limited amount of absorption; absorbed substances include certain drugs, some water, alcohol, and some short-chain fatty acids found in butter or milk fat.
- Produces the hormones *gastrin,* which helps regulate digestive functions, and *ghrelin (GHRL),* which increases appetite.
- Helps protect the body by destroying pathogenic bacteria swallowed with food or with mucus from the respiratory tract.

The digestive functions of the stomach are discussed further in Chapter 40.

Quick CHECK

8. What is the primary digestive function of the pharynx?
9. Describe the location of the oesophagus.
10. What are the three main divisions of the stomach?
11. What are gastric pits?

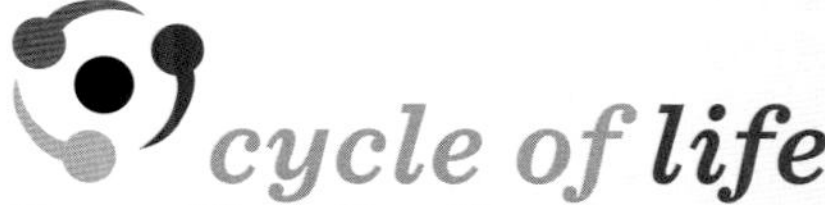

Upper Digestive Tract Significant changes in both the structure and function of the upper digestive tract can occur at different times in the human life cycle. One of the most obvious and important set of changes we observe from infancy through adulthood involves our dentition—our teeth. Necessary for survival, we are usually born without visible teeth. Gradually our deciduous dentition erupts, followed by our permanent dentition. As our jaws and permanent teeth grow, our dentition may become misaligned and require the use of retainers or braces to prevent future problems. As we age, the enamel of teeth, as hard as it is, can become worn, cracked, stained, and pitted. Periodontal ligaments may loosen, threatening loss of teeth and possible replacement with artificial dentures. Our stomach sphincter reflexes may not be mature as infants, perhaps causing regurgitation of large meals or gastric reflux. •

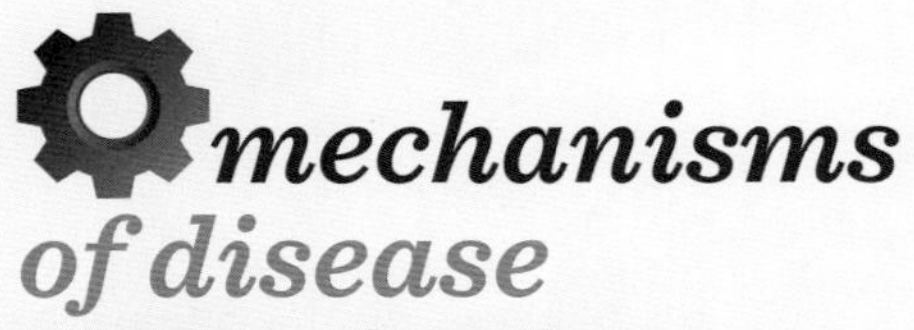

mechanisms of disease

Disorders of the Upper Digestive Tract

Disorders of the Mouth and Oesophagus

Infections, cancer, congenital defects, and other disorders of the mouth and teeth can result in a variety of serious complications. Such conditions may cause pain or damage to the mouth and teeth that makes chewing and swallowing difficult. Mouth infections or cancer may also spread to nearby tissues: the nasal cavity (then on to the sinuses, middle ear, and brain) or pharynx (and on to the oesophagus, larynx, and thoracic and other body organs).

Diseases of the salivary glands, including problems that affect their sympathetic and parasympathetic innervation, may alter both the chemical composition and the amount of saliva produced, about 1 litre per day on average. Inadequate saliva inhibits proper mixing and mastication of food, decreases production of salivary amylase (ptyalin) that initiates digestion in the mouth, and causes an imbalance in salivary pH (normally about 7.4).

Sjögren Syndrome

Sjögren syndrome is an autoimmune disease in which the body's immune system targets the salivary and tear glands for destruction. It is estimated that about half a million people in the UK are affected. The condition results in a dramatic reduction in both the production of saliva, causing dry mouth **(xerostomia),** and tears, which produces dry eyes **(xerophthalmia).** Symptoms of dry mouth and dry eyes, which cause a feeling of irritation and grittiness, become progressively worse over time. The syndrome affects many more women than men and usually begins around age 50. Among other symptoms, the lack of saliva makes chewing and swallowing difficult and contributes to a higher incidence of tooth decay. There is currently no cure for Sjögren syndrome, but for certain severely affected patients drugs such as methotrexate and azathioprine can be used to suppress the immune response. For most patients, treatment for uncomplicated Sjögren syndrome is aimed at reducing the troublesome symptoms of xerophthalmia and xerostomia.

Mumps

Mumps is an acute viral disease characterized by swelling and inflammation of the parotid gland (*parotitis*). Both parotid glands are involved in about 70% of individuals with mumps. It is caused by a paramyxovirus. Initial symptoms include fever, loss of appetite, and a generalized feeling of weakness and discomfort. Within a few hours, swelling of the parotid gland and spasm of the jaw muscles cause pain when the mouth is opened or during chewing movements. As swelling of the parotid gland becomes more pronounced, it extends over the ramus and fills the hollow behind the angle of the mandible to produce the classic "puffy" facial appearance of mumps (**Figure 38-16**). Another helpful diagnostic sign is redness of the parotid papilla on the inside of the cheek opposite the second molar tooth on one or both sides of the upper jaw.

Most of us think of mumps as a childhood disease because it most often affects children between the ages of 5 and 15 years. However, it can occur in adults—often producing a more severe infection. The mumps infection can affect other tissues in addition to the parotid gland, including the joints, pancreas, myocardium, and kidneys. In about 25% of infected men, mumps causes inflammation of the testes, or **orchitis.** Of the 25% of men in whom mumps-related orchitis develops, only about half experience atrophy of testicular tissue. Furthermore, because the problem is usually unilateral and involves only one testis, sterility rarely results, although some reduction in fertility may occur.

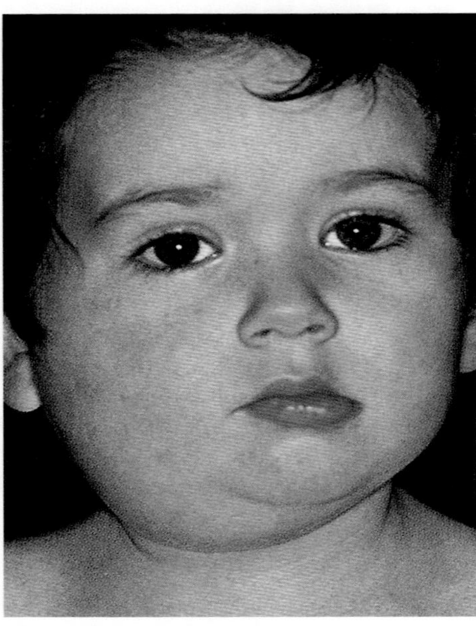

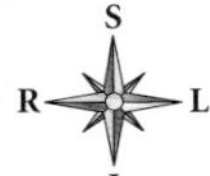

FIGURE 38-16 Mumps. This young boy with mumps has unilateral parotid swelling on the right side.

Tooth Decay

Tooth decay, or dental **caries,** is a common disease throughout the world. It is a disease of the enamel, dentin, and cementum of teeth that results in the formation of a permanent defect called a *cavity.* Most people living in the United States, Canada, and Europe are significantly affected by the disease.

Decay refers to demineralization of the hard tissues of the tooth caused by acids produced by *Streptococcus mutans* bacteria. These bacteria survive on sugars from food debris that collects around teeth, forming an acid-producing biofilm called *plaque.*

If the disease goes untreated, tooth decay results in infection, loss of teeth, and inflammation of the soft tissues in the mouth. Bacteria may also invade the paranasal sinuses or extend to the surface of the face and neck, causing even more serious complications.

Gingivitis is the general term for inflammation or infection of the gums. Most cases of gingivitis result from poor oral hygiene—inadequate brushing and no flossing. Gingivitis may also be a complication of other conditions such as diabetes mellitus, vitamin deficiency, or pregnancy.

Periodontitis is inflammation of the periodontal membrane, or *periodontal ligament,* that anchors the tooth to the bone of the jaw. Periodontitis is often a complication of advanced or untreated gingivitis and may spread to the surrounding bony tissue. Destruction of periodontal membrane and bone results in loosening and eventually complete loss of teeth. Periodontitis is the leading cause of tooth loss in adults.

Leukoplakia of the mouth is a precancerous change in the mucous membrane characterized by thickened, white, and slightly raised patches of tissue. Leukoplakia often develops in the fold "between cheek and gum" in people who chew tobacco. The condition may lead to tooth and gum disease, as well as oral cancer.

CONNECT IT! 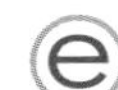

An individual's risk of dental caries and related concerns is related to the unique balance of microorganisms that live in each person's mouth. That is, some people tend to get few cavities because of the particular bacteria that live in the film on their teeth. Review the human *microbiome* in ***The Human Microbiome*** at ***Connect It!***

UNIT 5

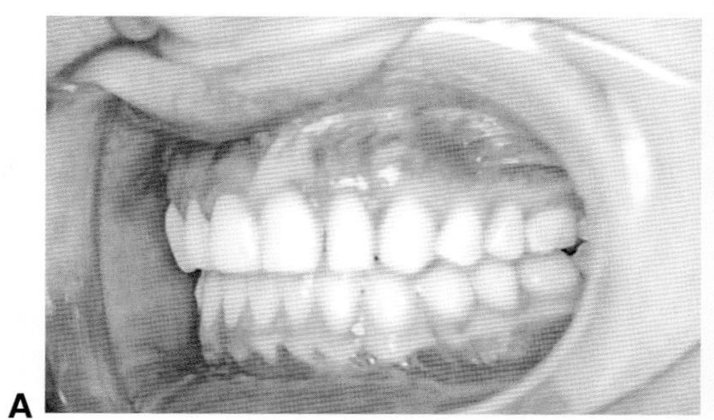

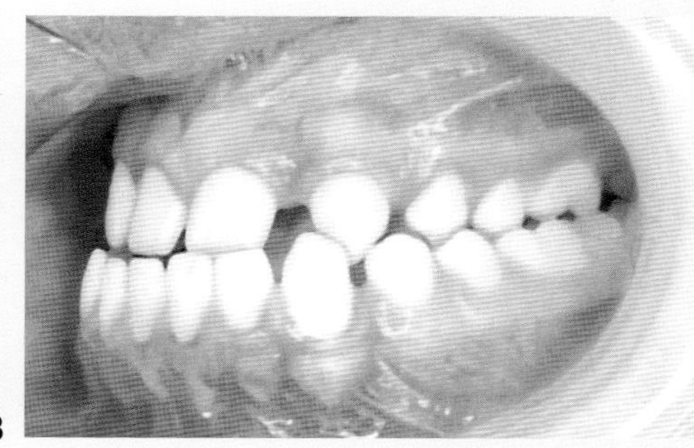

FIGURE 38-17 Malocclusion. A, Overbite. **B,** Underbite.

Malocclusion

Malocclusion of the teeth occurs when missing teeth create wide spaces in the dentition, when teeth overlap, or when malposition of one or more teeth prevents correct alignment of the maxillary and mandibular dental arches (**Figure 38-17**, *A* and *B*). Malocclusion that results in protrusion of the upper front teeth so that they hang over the lower front teeth is called *overbite (A),* whereas positioning of the lower front teeth outside the upper front teeth is called *underbite (B).*

Dental malocclusion may cause chronic pain and significant problems in functioning of the temporomandibular joint, contribute to the generation of headaches, or complicate routine mastication of food. Fortunately, even severe malocclusion problems can be corrected by the use of braces and other dental appliances. **Orthodontics** is the branch of dentistry that deals with the prevention and correction of positioning irregularities of the teeth and malocclusion.

Cleft lip and *cleft palate* (**Figure 38-18**) are the most common *congenital defects* affecting the mouth. They may occur alone or together and are caused by failure of structures in the upper lip or palate to fuse or close properly during embryonic development. Cleft lip, which may occur on one or both sides, is typically repaired soon after birth. Surgical repair of cleft palate is usually done later—but generally in the first or second year of life.

Gastro-oesophageal Reflux Disease (GORD)

The terms *heartburn* and *acid indigestion* are often used to describe a number of unpleasant symptoms experienced by more than 40% of the adult population of the UK every year. Backward flow of stomach acid into the oesophagus causes these symptoms, which typically include burning and pressure behind the breastbone. The term *gastro-oesophageal reflux disease (GORD)* is now used to better describe this common and sometimes serious medical condition.

In its simplest form, GORD symptoms are mild and occur only infrequently (twice a week or less). In these cases, avoiding problem foods or beverages, stopping smoking, or losing weight if needed may solve the problem. Additional treatment with over-the-counter antacids, non-prescription-strength proton pump inhibitors (omeprazole and others), and H_2 receptor antagonists (ranitidine and others) may also be used. More severe and frequent episodes of GORD can trigger asthma attacks, cause severe chest pain, result in bleeding, or promote a narrowing (stricture) or chronic irritation of the oesophagus, called **erosive oesophagitis** (**Figure 38-19**, *D*). In these cases, greater strength inhibitors of stomach acid such as the *proton pump inhibitor* esomeprazole may be added to the treatment prescribed. Drugs called *promotility agents,* which strengthen the lower oesophageal sphincter and thus reduce backflow of stomach acid, are also used in moderate to severe cases of GORD.

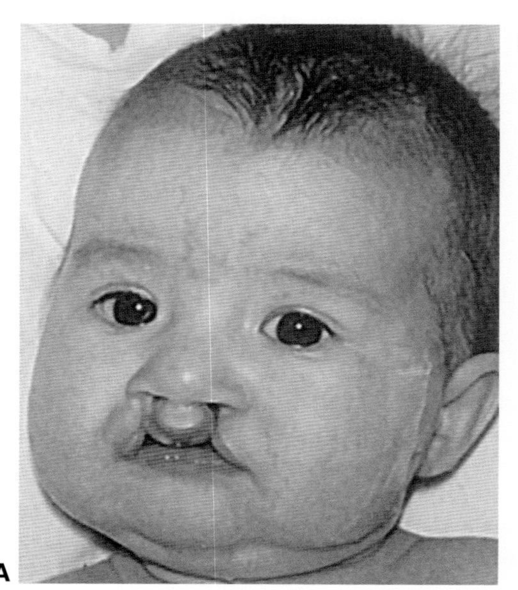

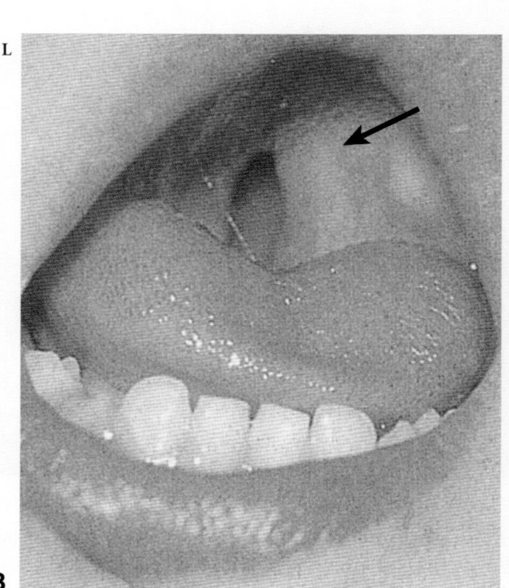

FIGURE 38-18 Congenital defects of the mouth. A, Bilateral cleft lip in an infant. **B,** Cleft palate *(arrow).* Modern reconstructive surgery techniques are extremely effective in minimizing the cosmetic, anatomical, and functional problems associated with these defects.

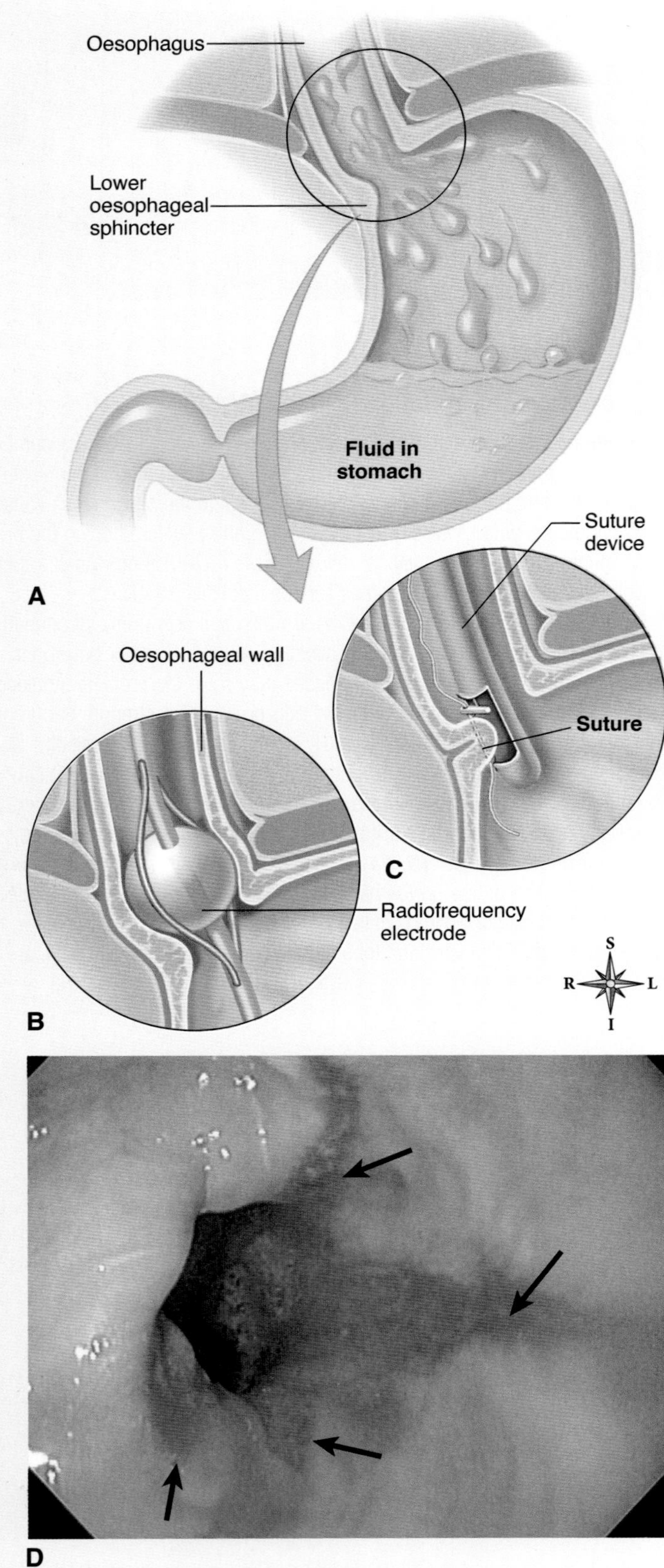

FIGURE 38-19 Gastro-oesophageal reflux disease (GORD). A, Reflux of gastric acid up into the oesophagus through the lower oesophageal sphincter. **B,** Stretta procedure. **C,** Bard endoscopic suturing system. **D,** Endoscopic view of oesophageal inflammation *(oesophagitis)* caused by "splashing back" of acids from the stomach in a patient with GORD.

Two minimally invasive procedures for treating serious cases of GORD are now available (**Figure 38-19**, *B* and *C*). One, called the *Stretta procedure,* uses radiofrequency energy emitted by a special electrode to produce small burns that tighten the muscular wall of the lower oesophageal sphincter and reduce acid reflux from the stomach. The other procedure, called the *Bard endoscopic suturing system,* uses a miniature sewing machine–like device to place two or more stitches in the muscular wall of the lower oesophageal sphincter, which are then pulled together to narrow the lumen. In both procedures, which are done on an outpatient basis, a flexible tube called an **oesophageal endoscope** is used to insert and then remove the necessary electrode or suturing device required for treatment. As a last resort, a surgical procedure called *fundoplication* may be performed to strengthen the sphincter. The procedure involves wrapping a layer of the upper stomach wall around the sphincter and terminal oesophagus to lessen the possibility of acid reflux. If GORD is left untreated, serious pathological (precancerous) changes in the oesophageal lining may develop—a condition called *Barrett oesophagus.*

Disorders of the Stomach

Gastroenterology is the study of the stomach *(gastro-)* and intestines *(-entero-)* and their diseases. The stomach is the potential site of numerous diseases and conditions, some of which are briefly described in this section. Many of these disorders are characterized by one or more of the following signs and symptoms:

Gastroenteritis—stomach inflammation (gastritis) and intestinal inflammation (enteritis)
Anorexia—chronic loss of appetite
Nausea—unpleasant feeling that often leads to vomiting
Emesis—vomiting (**Figure 38-20**)

An **ulcer** is a craterlike wound or sore in a membrane caused by tissue destruction (**Figure 38-21**). Statistics show that approximately 13% of individuals who undergo endoscopy in the UK have a gastric or duodenal ulcer. In Western populations, that is a 1 in 10 lifetime risk of developing peptic ulcer disease. Ulcers cause disintegration, loss, and death of tissue as they erode the

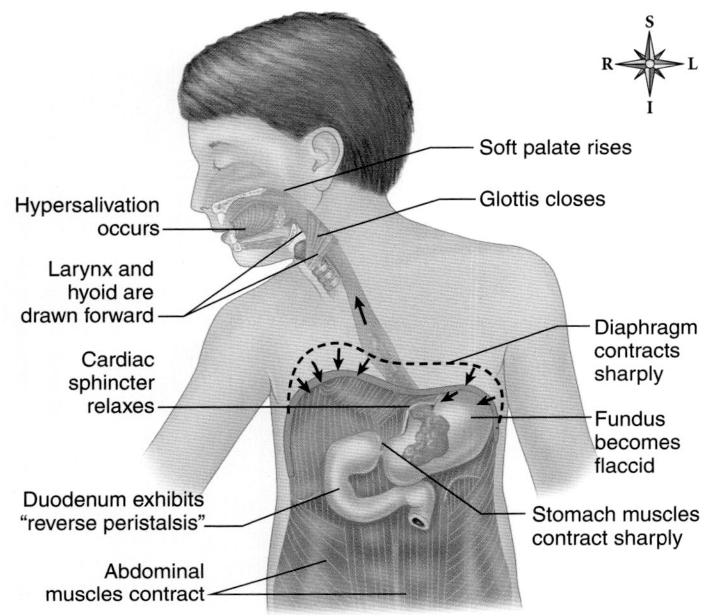

FIGURE 38-20 Emesis (vomiting). Summary of components of the vomiting reflex.

layers of the wall of the stomach or duodenum. These craterlike lesions cause gnawing or burning pain and may ultimately result in haemorrhage, perforation, widespread inflammation, scarring, and other very serious medical complications. Usually, perforation does not occur, but small, repeated haemorrhages over long periods can cause anaemia.

Two Australian scientists, Dr. Barry Marshall (a microbiologist) and Dr. J. Robin Warren (a pathologist) were awarded the 2005 Nobel Prize in Physiology or Medicine for ulcer research. In 1979 they discovered that infection with a spiral-shaped bacterium called *Helicobacter pylori (H. pylori)*—and not excessive acid secretion—was the primary cause of most ulcers. The two scientists were quick to report the relationship they observed between inflammation, lack of protective mucus, and tissue erosion around areas of bacterial colonization by *H. pylori* in tissue biopsies obtained from many ulcer patients. However, many in the medical community were initially slow to accept their research results linking *H. pylori* to ulcer development as valid. At the time, it was difficult for many clinicians to accept that ulcers were caused by a bacterium and were, therefore, more like an infectious disease than an illness caused by excess acid. Initial skepticism decreased when Marshall publicly swallowed a culture of *H. pylori* and then developed a severe case of gastritis that was successfully treated with antibiotics!

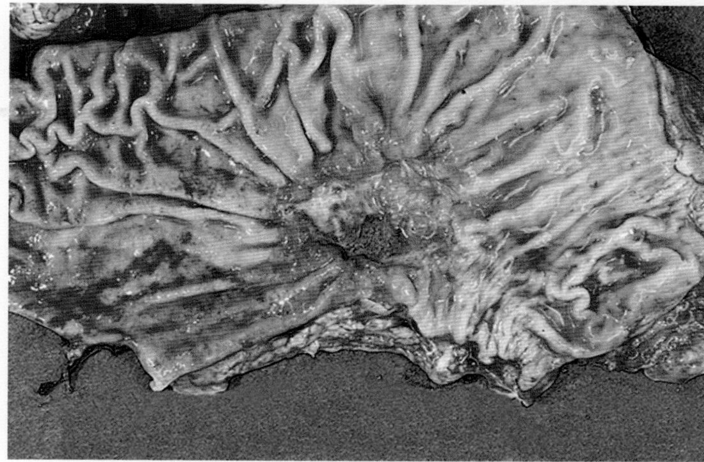

FIGURE 38-22 Stomach cancer. The abnormal tissue near the centre of this opened stomach is gastric carcinoma, or "stomach cancer". Note the distinct, normal rugae (folds) that surround the tumour tissue.

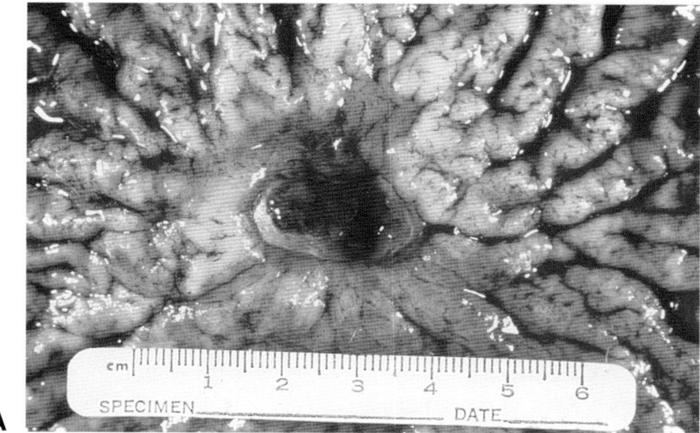

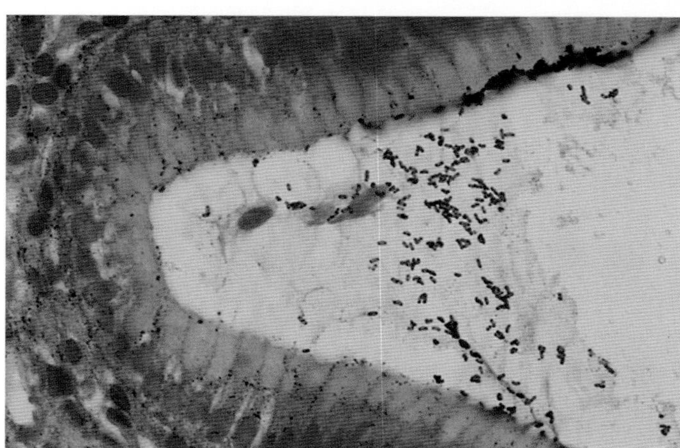

FIGURE 38-21 Ulcer. A, Gastric ulcer (actual size). **B,** Micrograph of *H. pylori (black particles)* infecting the stomach mucosa *(pink)*.

Marshall and Warren not only identified a bacterium as the cause of ulcers, their work also suggested that the time-honoured and traditional use of antacid treatment for ulcers be abandoned and replaced by antibiotic therapy. In awarding the Nobel, the committee described the research of Marshall and Warren as producing "one of the most radical and important changes in the last 50 years in the perception of a medical condition". What was once considered an unorthodox new explanation for the cause of ulcers is now a proven fact. And, antibiotic treatment is now an important part of the accepted standard of care for most ulcer patients. *H. pylori* infection in ulcer patients can be diagnosed by biopsy, breath, or blood antibody tests.

Long-term use of certain pain medications such as aspirin and ibuprofen, called *nonsteroidal antiinflammatory drugs (NSAIDs),* can also cause ulcers. These drugs interfere with prostaglandins that regulate the mucus lining of the GI tract. NSAID-induced ulcers can be treated by stopping NSAID use and taking acid-reducing drugs until the ulcer heals.

Stomach cancer (**Figure 38-22**) has been linked to *H. pylori* infection, excessive alcohol consumption, use of chewing tobacco, and eating smoked or heavily preserved food. Most stomach cancers, usually *adenocarcinomas,* have already metastasized before they are found because patients treat themselves for the early warning signs of heartburn, belching, and nausea. Later warning signs of stomach cancer include chronic indigestion, vomiting, anorexia, stomach pain, and blood in the faeces. Surgical removal of the malignant tumours has been the most successful method of treating stomach cancer. The pyloric sphincter is of clinical importance because **pylorospasm** is a fairly common condition in infants. The pyloric fibres do not relax normally to allow food to leave the stomach, and consequently, the infant vomits food instead of digesting and absorbing it. The condition is relieved by the administration of a drug that relaxes smooth muscles. Another abnormality of the pyloric sphincter is **pyloric stenosis,** an obstructive narrowing of its opening.

LANGUAGE OF SCIENCE (continued from p. 860)

peritoneum (pair-ih-toh-NEE-um)
[*peri-* **around,** *-tone-* **stretched,** *-um* **thing**] *pl.,* peritonea

pulp
[*pulp* **flesh**]

pulp cavity
[*pulp* **flesh,** *cav-* **hollow,** *-ity* **condition**]

pyloric sphincter (pye-LOR-ik SFINGK-ter)
[*pyl-* **gate,** *-or-* **to guard,** *-ic* **relating to,** *sphinc-* **bind tight,** *-er* **agent**]

pylorus (pye-LOR-us)

serosa (see-ROH-sah)
[*ser-* **watery fluid,** *-os-* **relating to,** *-a* **thing**] *pl.,* serosae

sublingual gland (sub-LING-gwall)
[*sub-* **under,** *-lingua-* **tongue,** *-al* **relating to,** *gland* **acorn**]

submandibular gland (sub-man-DIB-yoo-lar)
[*sub-* **under,** *-mandibul-* **chew (mandible or jawbone),** *-ar* **relating to,** *gland* **acorn**]

submucosa (sub-myoo-KOH-sah)
[*sub-* **under,** *-muc-* **slime,** *-os-* **relating to,** *-a* **thing**] *pl.,* submucosae

upper oesophageal sphincter (UOS) (eh-SOF-ah-JEE-ul SFINGK-ter)
[*oes-* **will carry,** *-phag-* **food (eat),** *-al* **relating to,** *sphinc-* **bind tight,** *-er* **agent**]

LANGUAGE OF MEDICINE

anorexia (an-oh-REK-see-ah)
[*an-* **without,** *-orex-* **appetite,** *-ia* **condition**]

caries (KAIR-eez)
[*caries* **decay**]

chief cell (cheef sel)
[*chief* **head,** *cell* **storeroom**]

emesis (EM-eh-sis)
[*emesis* **vomiting**]

endocrine cell (EN-doh-krin sel)
[*endo-* **within,** *-crin-* **secrete,** *cell* **storeroom**]

erosive oesophagitis (eh-ROH-siv eh-SOF-ah-jye-tis)
[*oes-* **will carry,** *-phag-* **food (eat),** *-itis* **inflammation**]

gastroenteritis (gas-troh-en-ter-EYE-tis)
[*gastr-* **stomach,** *-enter-* **intestine,** *-itis* **inflammation**]

gastroenterology (gas-troh-en-ter-OL-oh-jee)
[*gastr-* **stomach,** *-entero-* **intestine,** *-o-* **combining form,** *-log-* **words (study of),** *-y* **activity**]

gastro-oesophageal reflux disease (GORD) (gas-troh-eh-sof-eh-JEE-all REE-fluks)
[*gastro-* **stomach,** *-oes-* **will carry,** *-phag-* **food (eat),** *-al* **relating to,** *re-* **again or back,** *-flux* **flow**]

gingivitis (jin-jih-VYE-tis)
[*gingiv-* **gum,** *-itis* **inflammation**]

hiatal hernia (hye-AY-tal HER-nee-ah)
[*hiat-* **gap,** *-al* **relating to,** *hernia* **rupture**] *pl.,* herniae or hernias

leukoplakia (loo-koh-PLAY-kee-ah)
[*leuko-* **white,** *-plak-* **flat area,** *-ia* **condition**]

malocclusion (mal-oh-CLEW-zhun)
[*mal-* **bad,** *-occlu-* **close up,** *-sion* **state**]

mumps
[*mumps* **grimace**]

nausea (NAW-zee-ah)
[*nausea* **seasickness**]

oesophageal endoscope (eh-sof-ah-JEE-ul EN-doh-skohp)
[*oes-* **will carry,** *-phag-* **food (eat),** *-al* **relating to,** *endo-* **within,** *-scop-* **see**]

orchitis (or-KYE-tis)
[*orchi-* **testis,** *-itis* **inflammation**]

orthodontics (or-thoh-DON-tiks)
[*ortho-* **straight or upright,** *-odont-* **tooth,** *-ic* **relating to**]

parotitis (pair-oh-TYE-tis)
[*par-* **beside,** *-ot-* **ear (parotid salivary gland),** *-itis* **inflammation**]

periodontitis (pair-ee-oh-don-TYE-tis)
[*peri-* **around,** *-odont-* **tooth,** *-itis* **inflammation**]

pyloric stenosis (pye-LOR-ik steh-NO-sis)
[*pyl-* **gate,** *-or-* **guard,** *-ic* **relating to,** *stenos-* **narrow,** *-osis* **condition**] *pl.,* stenoses

pylorospasm (pye-LOHR-oh-spaz-um)
[*pyl-* **gate,** *-or-* **guard,** *-spasm* **twitch or involuntary contraction**]

Sjögren syndrome (SHOW-grin SIN-drohm)
[*Henrik S.C. Sjögren* **Swedish ophthalmologist,** *syn-* **together,** *-drome* **running or (race) course**]

ulcer (UL-ser)
[*ulc-* **sore**]

xerophthalmia (zee-rof-THAL-mee-ah)
[*xero-* **dryness,** *-opth-* **eye,** *-thalm-* **inner chamber,** *-ia* **condition**]

xerostomia (zee-roh-STOH-mee-ah)
[*xero-* **dryness,** *-stom-* **mouth,** *-ia* **condition**]

UNIT 5

case study

Joanne only turned away from her task of reorganizing her sewing basket for a few seconds, but it was sufficient time for her 24-month-old daughter Lucy to put a handful of buttons into her mouth. Joanne dropped down and removed the buttons from Lucy's mouth, but she had no way of knowing how many she may have ingested, and Lucy was coughing and drooling. In a panic, Joanne drove immediately to the Accident and Emergency department of the local hospital, where Lucy's neck and chest were examined and X-rayed. The radiograph showed one button lodged in Lucy's upper oesophagus.

1. With what layer of the oesophageal lining would the button be in contact?
   a. Serosa
   b. Muscularis
   c. Submucosa
   d. Mucosa
2. To enter the oesophagus the button passed through which sphincter?
   a. Upper oesophageal sphincter
   b. Lower oesophageal sphincter
   c. Cardiac sphincter
   d. Pyloric sphincter

3. What would be released from the gastric mucosa if the button entered the stomach?
   a. Mucous fluid containing digestive enzymes and sodium bicarbonate
   b. Mucous fluid containing amylase and pepsin
   c. Mucous fluid containing digestive enzymes and hydrochloric acid (HCl)
   d. Mucous fluid containing amylase, pepsin, and intrinsic factor

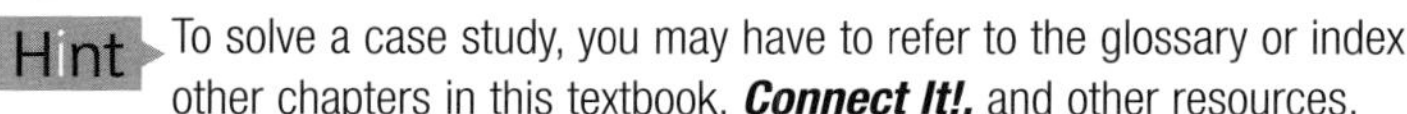

To solve a case study, you may have to refer to the glossary or index, other chapters in this textbook, ***Connect It!,*** and other resources.

CHAPTER SUMMARY

*To download an MP3 version of the chapter summary for use with your mobile device, access the **Audio Chapter Summaries** online at evolve.elsevier.com.*

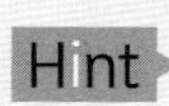

Scan this summary after reading the chapter to help you reinforce the key concepts. Later, use the summary as a quick review before your class or before a test.

Organization of the Digestive System

A. Digestive tract (**Figure 38-1**)
   1. Main organs of the digestive system form the alimentary canal (digestive tract) that extends from the mouth through the abdominopelvic cavity to the anus; gastrointestinal (GI) tract may refer to either the stomach and intestines or the entire alimentary canal
   2. This textbook divides the 10-metre-long digestive tract into two sections:
      a. Upper digestive tract—mouth through stomach
      b. Lower digestive tract—small intestine through anus
   3. Ingested food material passing through the lumen of the GI tract is outside the internal environment of the body

B. Wall of the GI tract (**Figure 38-2**)
   1. Mucosa—innermost layer
   2. Submucosa—contains numerous glands, blood vessels, and parasympathetic nerves
   3. Muscularis—thick layer of muscle tissue
   4. Serosa—outermost layer; mesentery and related structures are serous folds that connect the tract to the abdominal wall
   5. Modifications of layers—structure of layers varies in different regions throughout length of GI tract (**Table 38-1**)

Mouth

A. Structure of the oral cavity (buccal cavity) (**Figure 38-3**)
   1. Lips
      a. Covered externally by skin and internally by mucous membrane
      b. Junction between skin and mucous membrane is highly sensitive
      c. Line of contact between closed lips forms the oral fissure
   2. Cheeks
      a. Lateral boundaries of the oral cavity, continuous with the lips and lined by mucous membrane
      b. Formed in large part by the buccinator muscle covered by adipose tissue
      c. Contain mucus-secreting glands
   3. Hard palate and soft palate
      a. Hard palate consists of portions of four bones: two maxillae and two palatines
      b. Soft palate forms the partition between the mouth and nasopharynx and is made of muscle arranged in an arch
      c. Suspended from the midpoint of the posterior border of the arch is the uvula
   4. Tongue—solid mass of skeletal muscle covered by a mucous membrane; extremely maneuverable
      a. Has three parts: root, tip, and body (**Figure 38-4**)
      b. Papillae located on the dorsal and lateral surfaces of the tongue (**Figure 38-5**)
      c. Lingual frenulum anchors the tongue to the floor of the mouth (**Figure 38-6**)
      d. Intrinsic muscles important for speech and mastication; extrinsic muscles important for deglutition and speech (**Figure 38-7**)

B. Salivary glands
   1. Three main pairs of compound tubuloalveolar glands (**Figure 38-8**)
      a. Secrete approximately 1 litre of saliva each day
      b. Additional small buccal glands contribute less than 5% of the total salivary volume but provide for hygiene and comfort of oral tissues
   2. Parotid glands—largest of the paired salivary glands; produce watery saliva containing enzymes
   3. Submandibular glands—compound glands that contain enzyme- and mucus-producing elements
   4. Sublingual glands—smallest of the salivary glands; produce a mucous type of saliva

C. Teeth—organs of mastication
   1. Typical tooth (**Figure 38-9**)
      a. Four connective tissues called dental tissues:
         (1) Pulp—soft, fibrous connective tissue with blood vessels and nerves
         (2) Dentin—hard, mineralized tissue similar to bone in tooth body
         (3) Cementum—hard, mineralized tissue similar to bone around tooth roots
         (4) Enamel—hard, mineralized tissue harder than bone over crown of tooth
      b. Crown—exposed portion of a tooth, covered by enamel; ideally suited to withstand abrasion during mastication
      c. Neck—narrow portion that joins the crown to the root; surrounded by gingivae

d. Root—fits into the socket of the alveolar process; suspended by a fibrous periodontal membrane made up of periodontal ligaments
e. Outer shell contains two additional tissues: dentin and cementum
(1) Dentin—greatest portion of the tooth shell; at the crown, covered by enamel, and at the neck and root, covered by cementum
(2) Pulp cavity—located within dentin, contains loose connective pulp tissue that includes blood, lymphatic vessels, and sensory nerves
2. Types of teeth (**Figure 38-10**)
a. Deciduous teeth—20 baby teeth, which appear early in life
b. Permanent teeth—32 teeth, which replace the deciduous teeth

Pharynx

A. Tube through which a food bolus passes when moved from the mouth to the oesophagus by the process of deglutition
B. Air passes through all three divisions of the pharynx; only terminal portion involved in digestive system

Oesophagus

A. Tube that extends from the pharynx to the stomach; first segment of the digestive tube (**Figure 38-11**)
B. Lined with stratified squamous epithelium (**Figure 38-12**)
C. Each end encircled by muscular sphincters

Stomach

A. Size and position of the stomach
1. Size varies according to factors such as gender and amount of distention
a. When no food is in the stomach, it is about the size of a large sausage
b. In adults, its capacity ranges from 1.0 to 1.5 litres
2. Stomach location: upper part of the abdominal cavity under the liver and diaphragm
B. Divisions of the stomach (**Figure 38-13**)
1. Cardia—collarlike region at junction with oesophagus
2. Fundus—enlarged portion to the left and above the opening of the oesophagus into the stomach
3. Body—central portion of the stomach
4. Pylorus—lower part of the stomach
C. Curves of the stomach
1. Lesser curvature—upper right curve of the stomach
2. Greater curvature—lower left curve of the stomach
D. Sphincter muscles—circular fibres arranged so that there is an opening in the centre when relaxed and no opening when contracted
1. Lower oesophageal sphincter (LOS), or cardiac sphincter, controls the opening of the oesophagus into the stomach
2. Pyloric sphincter controls the outlet of the pyloric portion of the stomach into the duodenum
E. Stomach wall (**Figure 38-14**)
1. Gastric mucosa
a. Epithelial lining has rugae marked by gastric pits (**Figure 38-15**)
b. Gastric glands—found below the level of the pits; secrete most of the gastric juice
c. Chief cells—secretory cells found in the gastric glands; secrete the enzymes of gastric juice
d. Parietal cells—secretory cells found in the gastric glands; secrete hydrochloric acid; thought to produce intrinsic factor needed for vitamin B_{12} absorption
e. Endocrine cells—secrete gastrin and ghrelin
2. Gastric muscle
a. Thick layer of muscle with three distinct sublayers of smooth muscle tissue arranged in a crisscrossing pattern
b. This pattern allows the stomach to contract strongly at many angles
F. Functions of the stomach
1. Reservoir for food until it is partially digested and moved farther along the GI tract
2. Secretes gastric juice to aid in digestion of food
3. Breaks food into small particles and mixes them with gastric juice
4. Secretes intrinsic factor
5. Performs limited absorption
6. Produces gastrin and ghrelin
7. Helps protect the body from pathogenic bacteria swallowed with food

Cycle of Life: Upper Digestive Tract

A. Significant changes in both the structure and function of the upper digestive tract can occur at different times in the human life cycle
1. Teeth change from infancy through adulthood
2. Stomach sphincter reflexes may not be mature as infants

REVIEW QUESTIONS

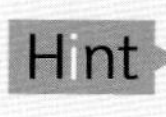

Write out the answers to these questions after reading the chapter and reviewing the Chapter Summary. Note—writing out your answers will consolidate learning and provide a valuable resource of information.

1. List the component parts or segments of the GI tract and the accessory organs of digestion.
2. Name and describe the four tissue layers that form the wall of GI tract organs.
3. Identify the structures that form the mouth.
4. Define the following terms associated with the mouth and pharynx: *philtrum, oral fissure, hard palate* and *soft palate, fauces, uvula, foramen caecum, lingual frenulum.*
5. What is ankyloglossia? How could this condition be treated surgically?
6. Identify the types of tongue papillae. What is the relationship between papillae and taste buds?
7. List and give the location of the paired salivary glands. Identify by name the ducts that drain the saliva from these glands into the mouth.
8. What type of saliva is produced by the parotid glands? What is meant by the term *mixed* or *compound salivary gland?*
9. Describe a typical tooth. Name the specific types of teeth.
10. Distinguish between deciduous and permanent teeth.
11. What is meant by the term *deglutition?*
12. Draw a labelled diagram illustrating the divisions of the stomach.
13. Identify the three major cell types of the gastric glands. What cell type produces hydrochloric acid? Gastric enzymes? Gastrin? Ghrelin?
14. Describe the seven functions of the stomach.
15. Identify the condition that can develop in men who are infected with mumps.
16. What is the difference between dental caries and periodontitis?
17. What is pyloric stenosis?

CRITICAL THINKING QUESTIONS

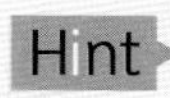

After finishing the Review Questions, write out the answers to these more in-depth questions to help you apply your new knowledge. Go back to sections of the chapter that relate to concepts that you find difficult.

1. Explain the role of the tongue's intrinsic and extrinsic muscles.
2. What property of enamel could be used to argue that it is not a type of tissue?
3. Describe the unique features of the muscular layer of the oesophagus and explain their functions.
4. What is the difference between gastric pits and gastric glands?
5. A fundus is the base of an organ. If the fundus of the stomach is its base, what forms the apex of the stomach?
6. Explain the radiography procedure used to diagnose a hiatal hernia.

39 Lower Digestive Tract

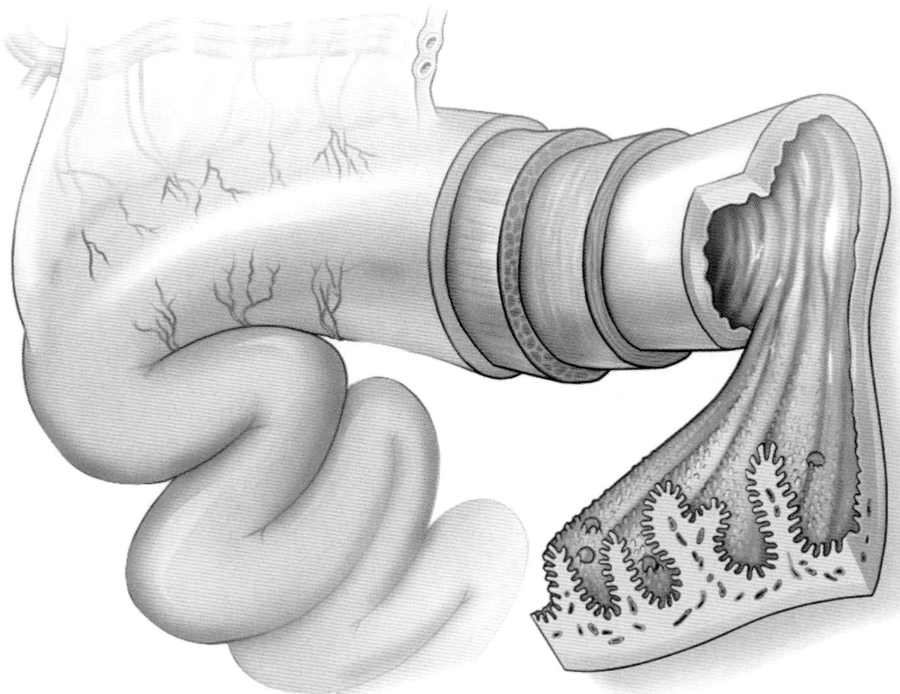

CHAPTER OUTLINE

Hint Scan this outline before you begin to read the chapter, as a preview of how the concepts are organized.

The previous chapter surveyed the upper digestive tract, from the mouth through the stomach. This chapter continues the story of digestion with an exploration of the lower digestive tract. This portion of the alimentary canal includes the small intestine and large intestine. We will also take the opportunity to discuss the large glands that open into the lower digestive tract—the liver and pancreas—and their associated structures.

LANGUAGE OF SCIENCE

Hint *Use this list to aid your pronunciation of unfamiliar words.*

anal canal (AY-nal kah-NAL)
[*an-* **ring (anus),** *-al* **relating to**]

ascending colon (ah-SEND-ing KOH-lon)
[*colon* **large intestine**]

bile (byle)

colon (KOH-lon)
[*colon* **large intestine**]

descending colon (dih-SEND-ing KOH-lon)
[*colon* **large intestine**]

duodenum (dyoo-oh-DEE-num)
[**shortened from** *intestinum duodenum digitorum* **intestine of 12 finger-widths**]
pl., duodena or duodenums

enteroendocrine cell (EN-ter-oh-EN-doh-krin cell)
[*entero-* **intestine,** *-endo-* **within,** *-crin* **secrete,** *cell* **storeroom**]

enterocyte (EN-ter-oh-syte)
[*entero-* **intestine,** *-cyte* **cell**]

epiploic appendage (eh-pih-PLOH-ik ah-PEN-daj)
[*epiplo-* **omentum,** *-ic* **relating to,** *append-* **hang upon,** *-age* **thing**]

extraperitoneal (eks-trah-pair-ih-toh-NEE-al)
[*extra-* **outside,** *peri-* **around,** *-tone-* **stretched,** *-al* **relating to**]

fractal geometry (FRAK-tal jee-OM-eh-tree)
[*fract-* **a breaking,** *-al* **relating to,** *geo-* **earth or land,** *-metr-* **measure,** *-y* **activity**]

glucagon (GLOO-kah-gon)
[*gluc-* **glucose,** *-agon* **drive**]

greater omentum (oh-MEN-tum)
[*omentum* **fatty covering of intestines**]
pl., omenta

haustra (HAW-strah)
[*haustr-* **drawer or recess**]
sing., **haustrum**

hepatic lobule (heh-PAT-ik LOB-yool))
[*hepa-* **liver,** *-ic* **relating to,** *lob-* **pod,** *-ule* **small**]

hepatocyte (heh-PAT-oh-syte)
[*hepat-* **liver,** *-cyte* **cell**]

ileum (IL-ee-um)
[*ileum* **groin or flank**] *pl.,* ilea

insulin (IN-suh-lin)
[*insul-* **island,** *-in* **substance**]

continued on p. 897

Part 3 of the BRIEF ATLAS OF THE HUMAN BODY shows detailed photographs of major structures of the lower digestive tract and accessory organs of digestion.

After we finish our tour through the digestive tract in this chapter, we move on to the overall processes of digestion and absorption in Chapter 40. Finally, in Chapter 41 we briefly discuss how the absorbed nutrients are used by the body.

SMALL INTESTINE

Size and Position of the Small Intestine

The small intestine is a tube measuring about 2.5 cm in diameter and 6 to 8 metres in length. Its coiled loops fill most of the abdominal cavity (**Figure 39-1** and **Figure 39-2**).

Divisions of the Small Intestine

The small intestine consists of three divisions: the duodenum, the jejunum, and the ileum. The **duodenum** is the uppermost division and the part to which the pyloric end of the stomach attaches. It is about 25 cm long and is shaped roughly like the letter **C**. The name *duodenum,* meaning "12 fingerbreadths", refers to the short length of this intestinal division. The duodenum becomes **jejunum** at the point where the tube turns abruptly forward and downward. The jejunal portion continues for approximately the next 2.5 metres, at the end of which it becomes the **ileum,** but without any sharp line of demarcation between the two divisions. The ileum is about 3.5 metres long.

Wall of the Small Intestine

Note in **Figure 39-3** that the intestinal lining has circular **plicae** (folds) that have many tiny projections called **villi.** Villi are important modifications of the mucosal layer of the small intestine.

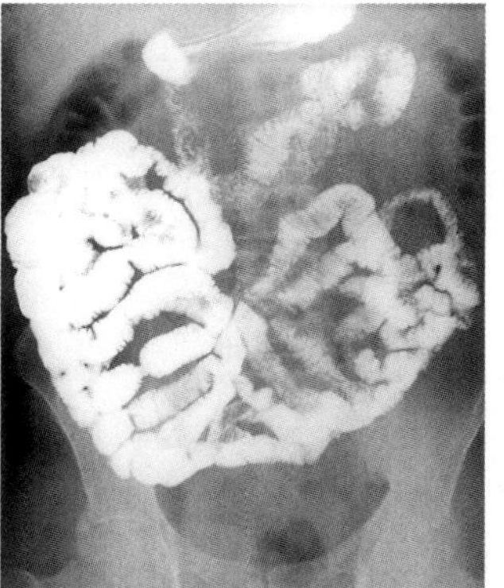

A

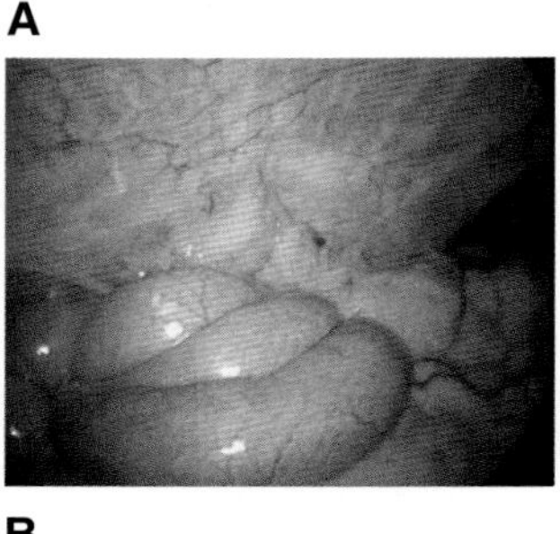

B

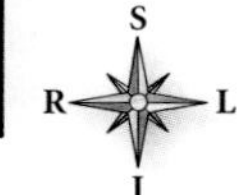

FIGURE 39-2 Viewing the small intestine. **A,** Anteroposterior (AP) x-ray image obtained during a contrast (barium-enhanced) study of the small intestine. The individual is lying supine on the x-ray table. **B,** Laparoscopic view of the small intestine.

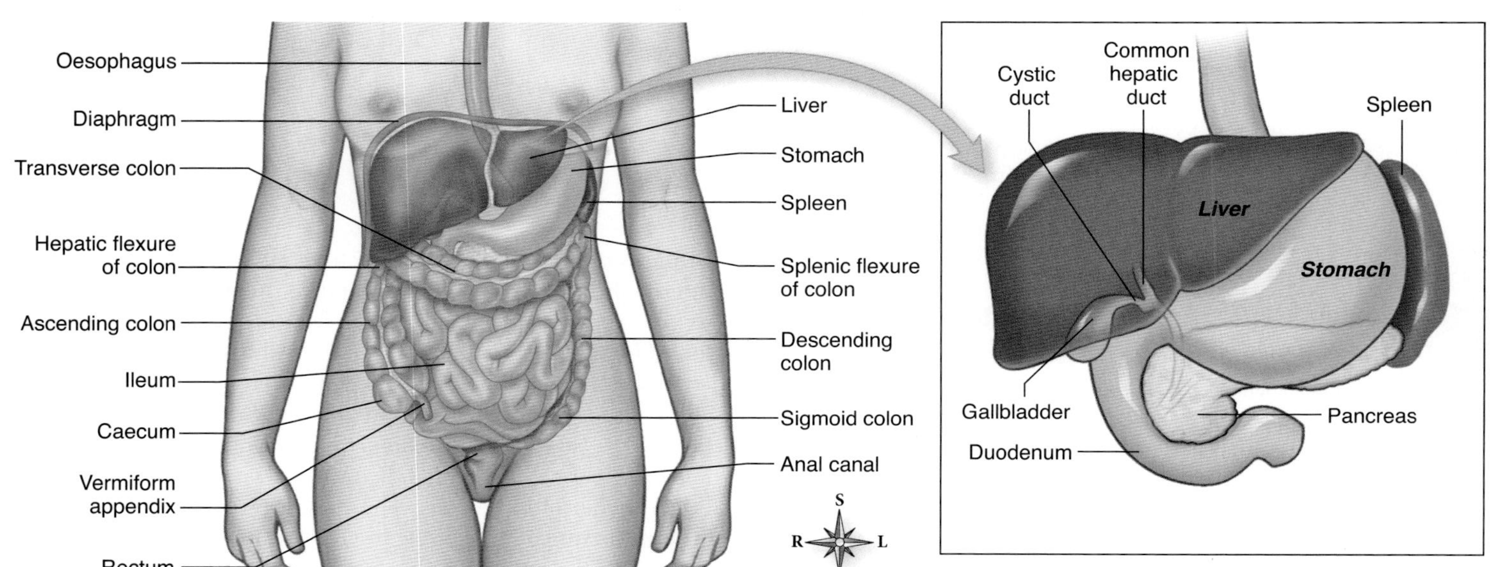

FIGURE 39-1 Location of lower digestive organs. Inset shows enlargement of liver, gallbladder, and pancreas.

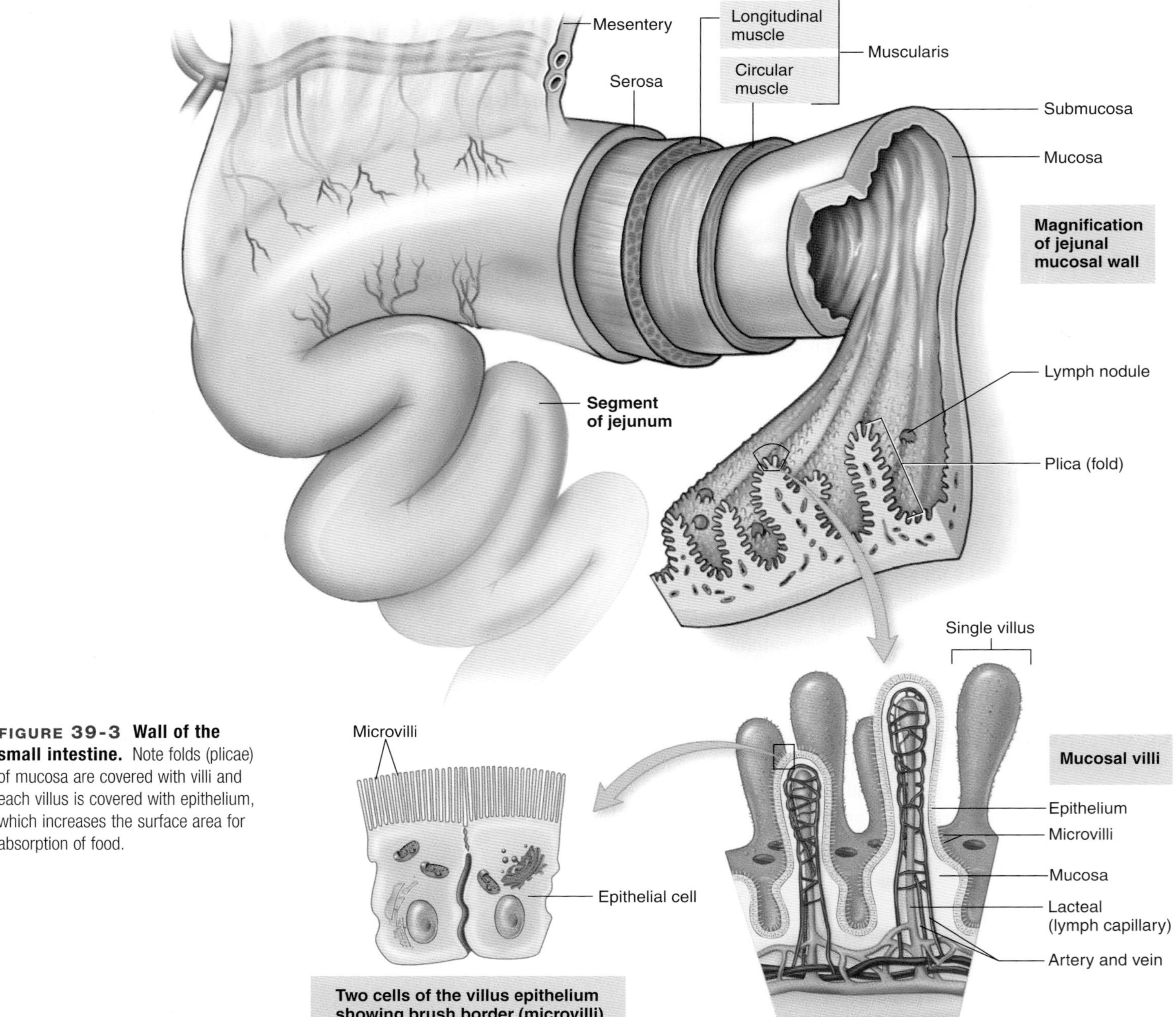

FIGURE 39-3 Wall of the small intestine. Note folds (plicae) of mucosa are covered with villi and each villus is covered with epithelium, which increases the surface area for absorption of food.

Millions of these projections, each about 1 mm in height, give the intestinal mucosa a velvety appearance. Each **villus** contains an arteriole, venule, and lymph vessel (lacteal) (see **Figure 39-3**). **Box 39-1** identifies the fractal-like structure of the intestinal lining.

Absorptive epithelial cells called **enterocytes** on the surface of villi can be seen by microscopy to have a surface resembling a fine brush. This so-called *brush border* is formed by about 1700 ultrafine *microvilli* per cell. Intestinal digestive enzymes are imbedded in the brush border of these cells. The presence of villi and microvilli increases the surface area of the small intestine hundreds of times, thus making this organ the main site of digestion and absorption. This is another example of the principle that structure fits function.

BOX 39-1 *fyi* | Fractal Geometry of the Body

Biologists are now applying the principles of the field of **fractal geometry** to human anatomy. Specialists in fractal geometry often study surfaces with a seemingly infinite area, such as the lining of the small intestine. Fractal surfaces have bumps that have bumps that have bumps, and so on. The fractal-like nature of the intestinal lining is represented in **Figure 39-3**. The plicae (folds) have villi, the villi have microvilli, and even the microvilli have bumps that cannot be seen in the figure. Thus the absorptive surface area of the small intestine is almost limitless. •

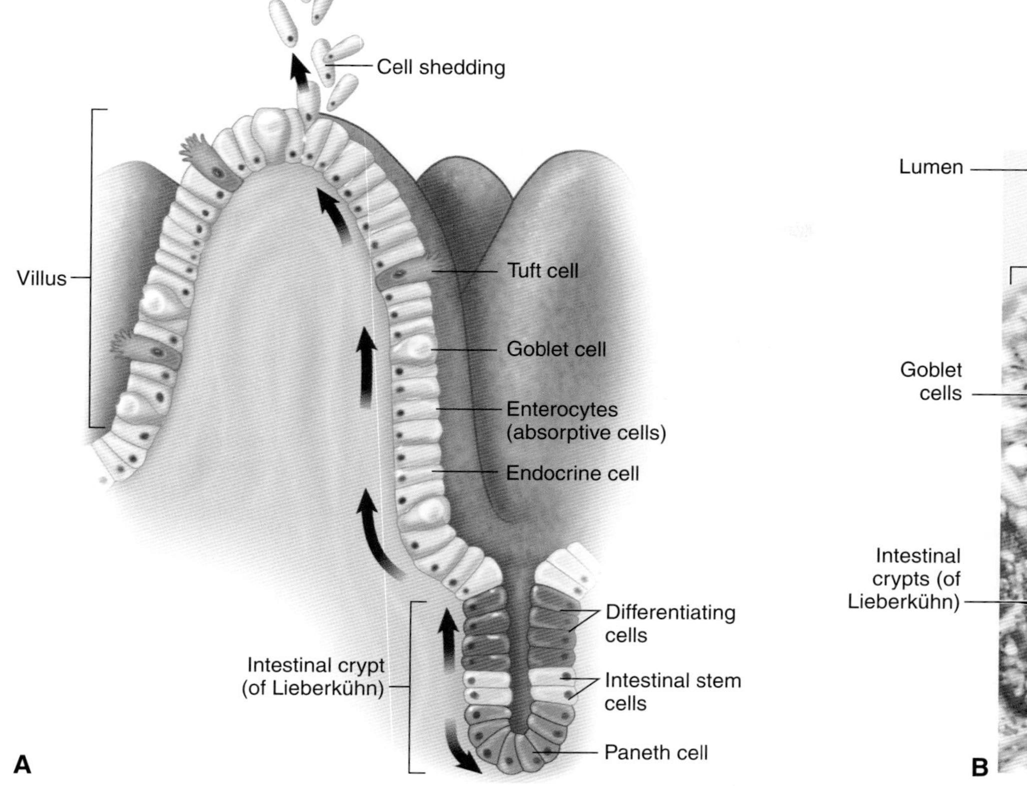

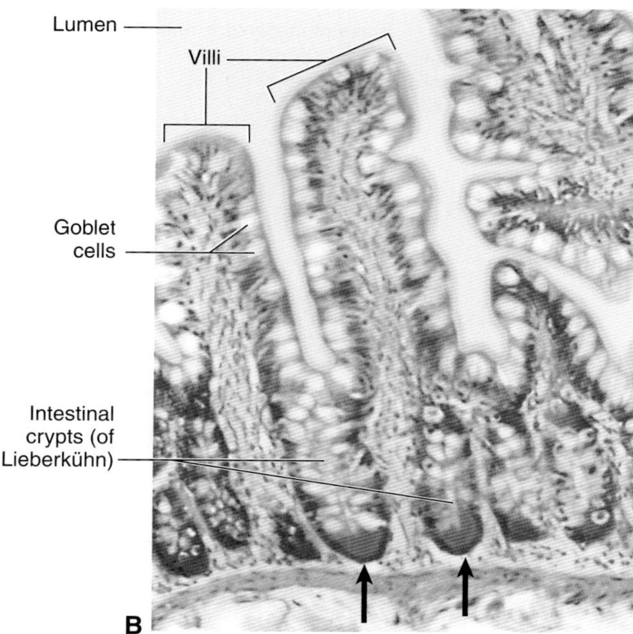

FIGURE 39-4 Intestinal villi and crypts. A, Stem cells near the bottom of each intestinal crypt divide to form daughter cells that move upward and differentiate into mucus-producing goblet cells, hormone-producing enteroendocrine cells, absorptive enterocytes, and tuft cells that secrete prostaglandins and endorphins. Eventually these cells are pushed to the top of the villus, where they are shed. Stem cells also produce Paneth cells, which move deeper into the crypt where they produce bactericidal secretions. **B,** This micrograph shows a section of the ileum wall with several villi and the intestinal crypts between them. Protective Paneth cells at the base of each crypt are marked by arrows.

Mucus-secreting goblet cells are found in large numbers on villi (**Figure 39-4**). **Enteroendocrine cells** that produce the intestinal hormones we discuss in Chapter 40 are also found in the villi. Also present are odd-looking **tuft cells** (*brush cells*) that have a dense apical tuft of long microvilli. Tuft cells secrete prostaglandins and endorphins. They can also "taste" the intestinal contents to detect the presence of amino acids and other types of nutrient.

In the valleys between villi are deep depressions called **intestinal crypts** (*of Lieberkühn*) or *intestinal glands*. Intestinal crypts serve as a site of rapid mitotic cell division. Stem cells near the bottom of each crypt keep the intestinal mucosa continuously supplied with fresh cells. New differentiating daughter cells are produced by the stem cells and pushed upward toward the mouth of the crypt. As they differentiate into enterocytes, goblet cells, tuft cells, and enteroendocrine cells, the older cells are pushed up and out of each crypt, eventually moving to the distal end of a villus, where they are shed. Thus the intestinal mucosa is continually renewed.

At the base of each crypt, protective **Paneth cells** produce enzymes and other molecules that inhibit bacterial growth in the small intestine. The location of the Paneth cells makes them especially useful in protecting the vital stem cells.

See **Table 38-1** (p. 863) and **Figure 39-3** for more information on the layers of the small intestine.

Quick CHECK

1. What are the three main divisions of the small intestine?
2. What are intestinal villi? What is their function?

LARGE INTESTINE

SIZE OF THE LARGE INTESTINE

The lower part of the alimentary canal bears the name *large intestine* because its diameter is noticeably larger than that of the small intestine. Its length, however, is much less, being about 1.5 to 1.8 metres. Its average diameter is approximately 6 cm, but the diameter decreases toward the lower end of the tube.

CONNECT IT! 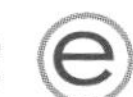

A barium enema (BE) study is a common way to produce an image of the large intestine to diagnose abnormalities. To read a description and see photographs, check out ***Barium Enema Study*** online at ***Connect It!***

DIVISIONS OF THE LARGE INTESTINE

The large intestine is divided into the caecum, colon, and rectum (**Figure 39-5**).

Caecum

The first 5 to 8 cm of the large intestine is named the *caecum.* It is a blind pouch located in the lower right quadrant of the abdomen (see **Figure 39-1**).

Colon

The **colon** is divided into the following portions: ascending, transverse, descending, and sigmoid (see **Figure 39-5**).

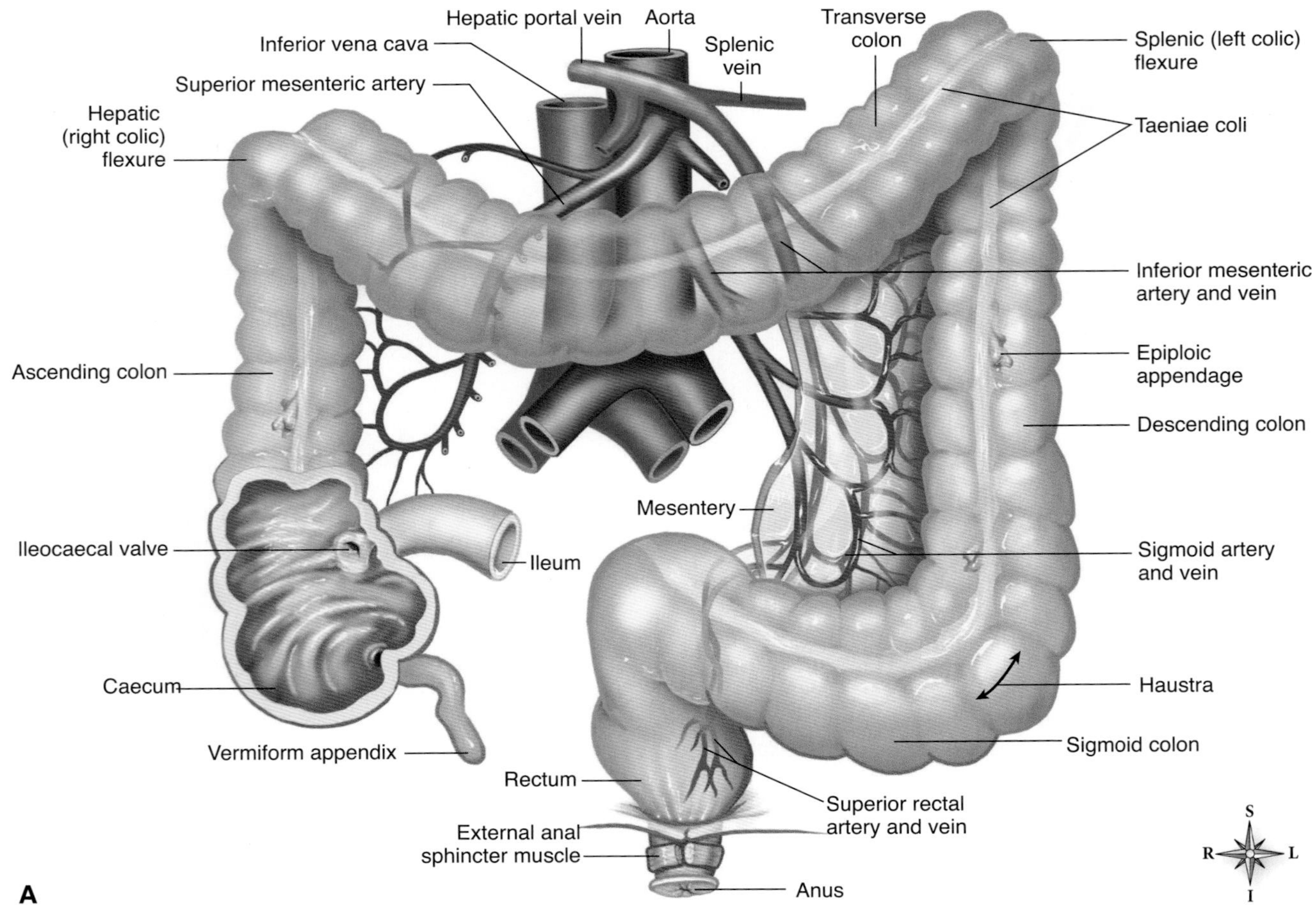

- The **ascending colon** lies in a vertical position, on the right side of the abdomen, and extends up to the lower border of the liver. The ileum joins the large intestine at the junction of the caecum and ascending colon, the place of attachment resembling the letter T (see **Figure 39-5**). The *ileocaecal valve* permits material to pass from the ileum into the large intestine, but not usually in the reverse direction.
- The **transverse colon** passes horizontally across the abdomen, below the liver, stomach, and spleen. Note that this part of the colon is above the small intestine (see **Figure 39-1**). The transverse colon extends from the *hepatic flexure* to the *splenic flexure*, the two points at which the colon bends on itself to form 90-degree angles.
- The **descending colon** lies in the vertical position, on the left side of the abdomen, and extends from a point below the stomach and spleen to the level of the iliac crest.
- The **sigmoid colon** is the portion of the large intestine that courses downward below the iliac crest. It is called *sigmoid* (meaning "S shaped") because it forms an S-shaped curve. The lower part of the curve, which joins the rectum, bends toward the left, the anatomical reason for placing a patient on the left side when giving an enema. In this position, gravity aids the flow of enema fluid from the rectum into the sigmoid flexure.

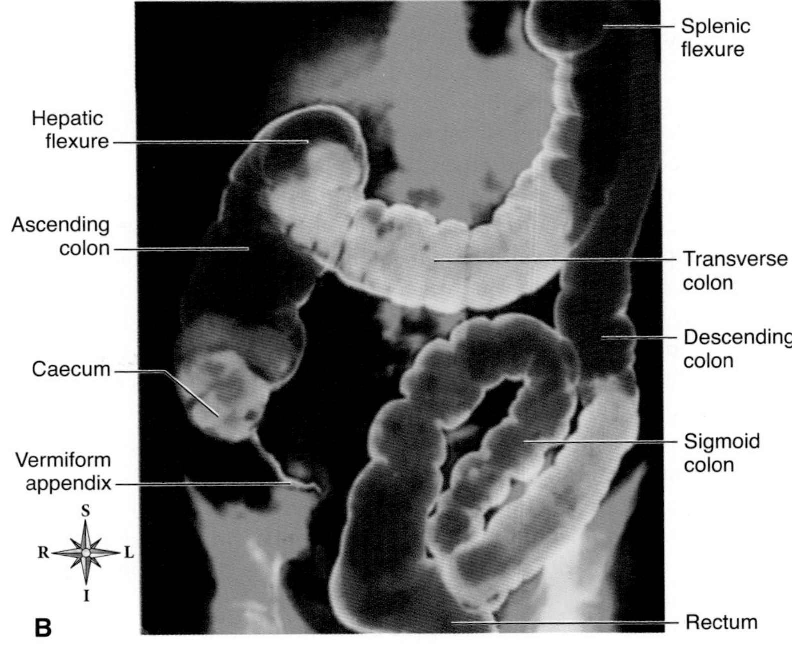

FIGURE 39-5 Divisions of the large intestine. A, Illustration showing divisions of the large intestine and adjacent vascular structures. **B,** Colourized x-ray film taken after a barium enema (see ***Barium Enema Study*** online at ***Connect It!***).

UNIT 5

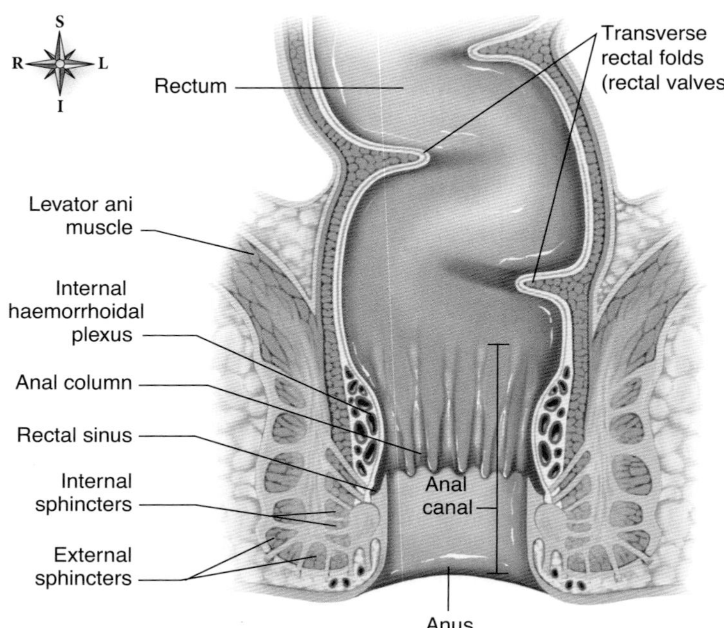

FIGURE 39-6 The rectum and anus.

Rectum

The last 17 to 20 cm of the intestinal tube is called the **rectum** (**Figure 39-6**). Crescent-shaped *transverse rectal folds,* also called *rectal valves,* help slow down the flow of faeces as it enters the rectum and hold the faeces in place until defaecation occurs. In an empty rectum, these folds may overlap and make it difficult to insert instruments during a **colonoscopy.**

The terminal 25 mm of the rectum is called the **anal canal.** Its mucous lining is arranged in numerous vertical folds known as *anal columns,* each of which contains an artery and a vein. The opening of the canal to the exterior is guarded by two sphincter muscles—an internal one of smooth muscle and an external one of striated muscle. The opening itself is called the *anus.* The anus is directed slightly posteriorly and is therefore at almost a right angle to the rectum (see **Figure 39-8**).

Wall of the Large Intestine

Table 38-1 (see p. 863) summarizes modifications of the gastrointestinal (GI) wall seen in the large intestine.

One of the most notable of these modifications is the presence of intestinal mucous glands, which produce the lubricating mucus that coats the faeces as they are formed (**Figure 39-7**). Although cells lining the large intestine have microvilli, the cells do not form villi like those that appear in the lining of the small intestine.

Another notable feature of the wall of the colon is the uneven distribution of fibres in the muscle layer. The longitudinal muscles are grouped into tapelike strips about a centimetre wide called **taeniae coli.** The circular muscles are grouped into dense rings. The presence of circular muscle rings and taeniae that are a bit shorter than the colon itself helps form pouchlike **haustra** that appear as puckered segments of the colon (see **Figure 39-5**). This arrangement promotes segmentation within the haustra.

In the rectum, rings of circular muscle form the internal rectal sphincter valves seen in **Figure 39-6**.

The outside of the colon wall is the serous membrane extension of the peritoneum, discussed further in a later section. It is often studded with pouchlike extensions filled with fat called **epiploic appendages.**

VERMIFORM APPENDIX

The **vermiform appendix** (from *vermis* "worm", *form* "shape") is, as the name implies, a wormlike tubular organ. It averages 8 to 10 cm in length and is most often found just behind the caecum or over the pelvic rim. The lumen of the appendix communicates with the caecum 3 cm below the ileocaecal valve, thus making it an accessory organ of the digestive system (see **Figure 39-5**).

The vermiform appendix serves as a sort of "breeding ground" for the nonpathogenic intestinal bacteria found throughout the colon. The normal microbiome of the colon contributes to the digestive process by digesting unused nutrients and producing essential molecules such as vitamins K and B_7 (biotin). Some bacteria also produce gases that escape from the colon through the anus—a phenomenon called flatulence or *flatus.*

Maintaining a normal intestinal microbiome also helps prevent pathogenic bacteria from becoming established. When the normal microbiome of the gut is disrupted by infection or antibiotics, for example, bacteria hidden away in the appendix can migrate into the colon to restore the normal ecological balance.

CONNECT IT!

The ecology of the human gut's microbiome is a very active field of research. Review the important role of the appendix in maintaining a healthy human *microbiome* in ***The Human Microbiome*** at ***Connect It!***

Lymph nodules appear in the wall of the appendix shortly after birth, become more prominent during the first 10 years of life, and then progressively disappear. The normal adult appendix shows only traces of lymphoid tissue. The function of lymphatic tissue present

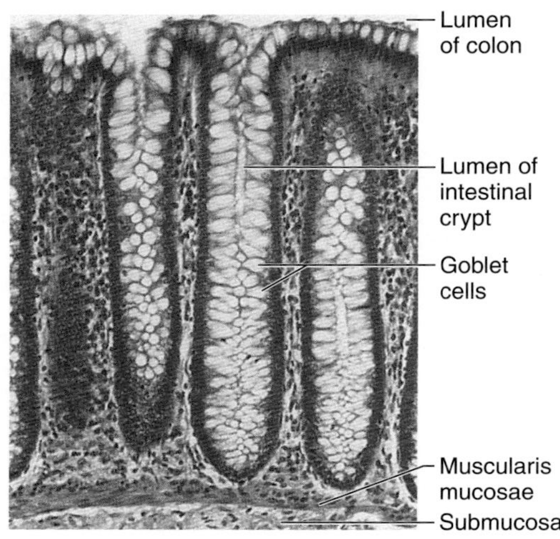

FIGURE 39-7 Wall of the colon. Note the straight nature of the intestinal glands of the colon. Many of the columnar epithelial cells are mucus-producing goblet cells.

in the appendix of young children is not fully understood but may involve regulating the gut's microbial communities.

Inflammation of the appendix, or **appendicitis,** is a common and potentially very serious medical problem (see Mechanisms of Disease, p. 895). The lifetime risk for appendicitis in the UK is 8.6% in males and 6.9% in females. A site on the surface of the anterior abdominal wall is often used to help in the diagnosis of appendicitis and to estimate the location of the appendix internally. It is called the *McBurney point* and is located in the right lower quadrant of the abdomen about a third of the way along a line from the right anterior superior iliac spine to the umbilicus. Extreme sensitivity and pain are common when the abdomen of persons with acute appendicitis is palpated over this point.

PERITONEUM

Now that we have described the entire length of the digestive tube from one end to the other, let's focus on the membrane covering most of these organs and holding them loosely in place. The **peritoneum** is a large, continuous sheet of serous membrane. It lines the walls of the entire abdominal cavity (parietal layer) and also forms the serous outer coat of the organs (visceral layer), as you can see in **Figure 39-8**.

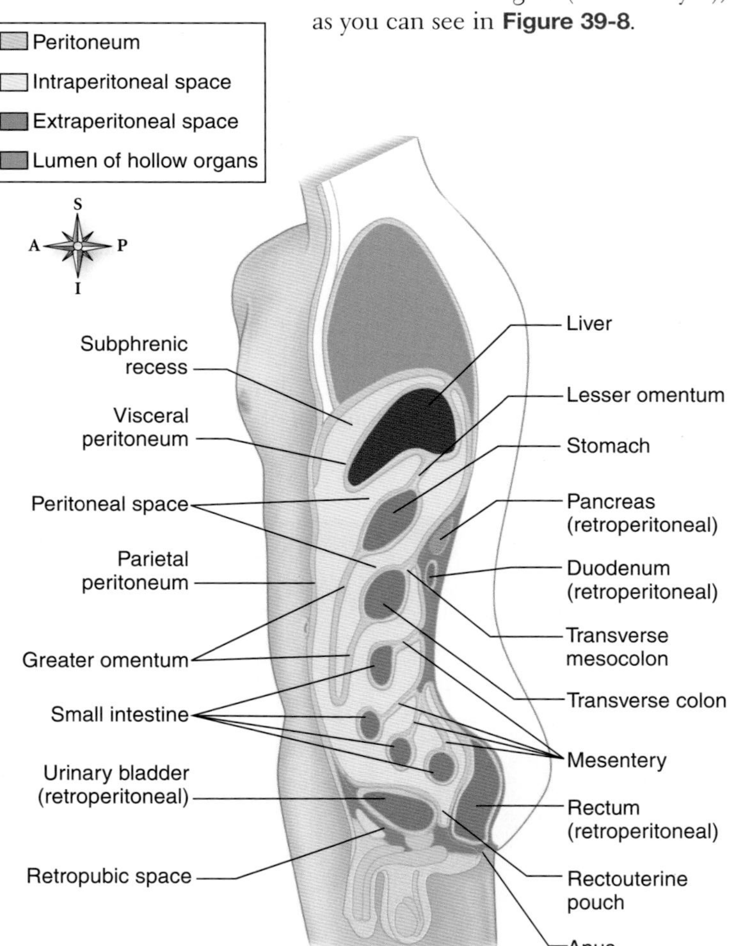

FIGURE 39-8 Peritoneum. Sagittal view of the abdomen showing a simplified scheme of the peritoneum and its reflections. *Intraperitoneal* spaces are shown in yellow and *extraperitoneal* spaces in green. The portion of the extraperitoneal space along the posterior wall of the abdomen is often called the *retroperitoneal space.*

Organs such as the stomach and most of the intestines covered with visceral peritoneum are described as being **intraperitoneal** ("within the peritoneum"). All the space outside the parietal peritoneum is called **extraperitoneal** ("outside the peritoneum") space. The extraperitoneal space along the posterior and bottom of the abdominopelvic cavity is most often identified as **retroperitoneal** ("behind the peritoneum"). Retroperitoneal organs include the pancreas (except the tail), kidneys and adrenal glands, ureters and bladder, aorta and inferior vena cava, part of the oesophagus, part of the duodenum, ascending and descending colon, and the rectum.

In several places the peritoneum forms reflections, or extensions, that bind the abdominal organs together (**Figure 39-9**; see **Figure 39-8**). The **mesentery** is a fan-shaped projection of the parietal peritoneum that extends from the lumbar region of the posterior abdominal wall. The attached posterior border of this great fan is just 15 to 20 cm long, yet the loose outer edge enclosing the jejunum and ileum is 6 metres long. The mesentery allows free movement of each coil of the intestine and helps prevent strangulation of the long tube. A similar but less extensive fold of peritoneum, called the **transverse mesocolon,** attaches the transverse colon to the posterior abdominal wall.

The **greater omentum** is a continuation of the serosa of the greater curvature of the stomach and the first part of the duodenum to the transverse colon. Spotty deposits of fat accumulate in the omentum and give it the appearance of a lace apron hanging down loosely over the intestines. In cases of localized abdominal inflammation such as appendicitis, the greater omentum envelops the inflamed area, walling it off from the rest of the abdomen.

The **lesser omentum** attaches from the liver to the lesser curvature of the stomach and the first part of the duodenum. The falciform ligament extends from the liver to the anterior abdominal wall. Examine the relationships of peritoneal extensions in **Figure 39-8**.

Quick CHECK

3. What are the four main divisions of the colon?
4. What are *haustra*?
5. Where is the vermiform appendix located?
6. Why is the greater omentum sometimes called the *lace apron*?

LIVER

LOCATION AND SIZE OF THE LIVER

The liver is the largest gland in the body. It weighs about 1.5 kg but grows and shrinks by nearly 40% in a daily cycle affected by our eating schedule. It lies immediately under the diaphragm, attached by peritoneal extensions called *coronary ligaments*. The liver occupies most of the right hypochondrium and part of the epigastrium (see **Figure 39-1**).

LIVER LOBES AND LOBULES

The liver consists of two lobes separated by the *falciform ligament* (**Figure 39-10**). The **left lobe** forms about one sixth of the liver, and the **right lobe** makes up the remainder. The right lobe has three parts, designated the *right lobe proper*, the *caudate lobe* (a small oblong area on the posterior surface), and the *quadrate lobe* (a four-sided section on the undersurface).

Each lobe is divided into numerous lobules by small blood vessels and by fibrous strands that form a supporting framework for them

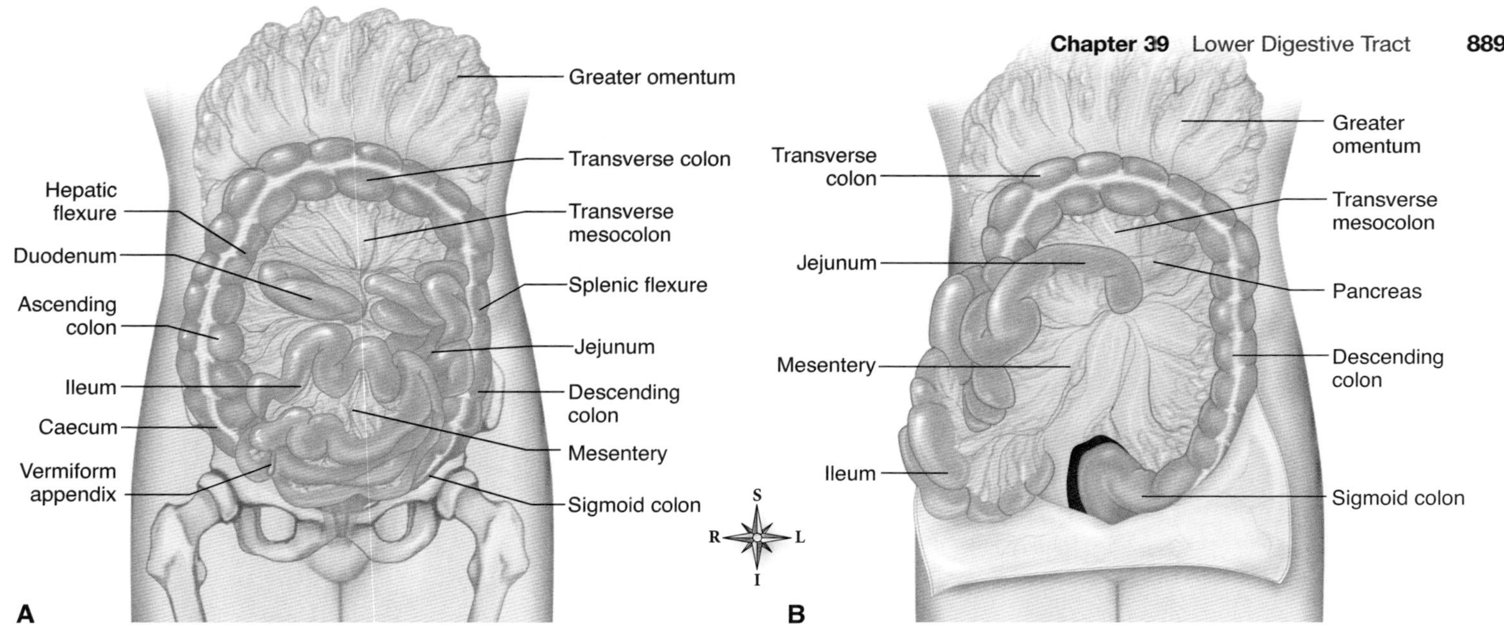

FIGURE 39-9 Projections of the peritoneum. A, Abdominal viscera from the front. The transverse colon and the greater omentum are elevated to reveal the flexures of the colon and the loops of the small intestine. **B,** The transverse colon and greater omentum are raised and the small intestine is pulled to the side to show the transverse mesocolon and mesentery.

FIGURE 39-10 Gross structure of the liver. A, Normal liver prepared for organ transplantation. Diagrams of a normal liver: **B,** anterior view; **C,** inferior view.

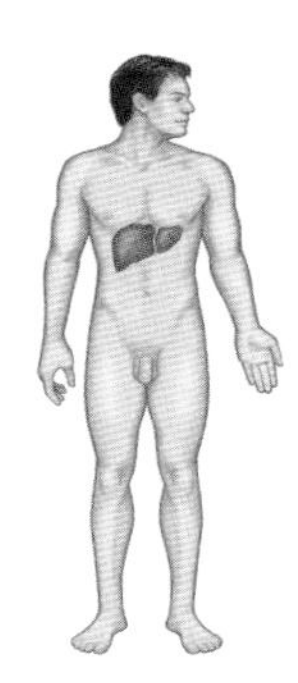

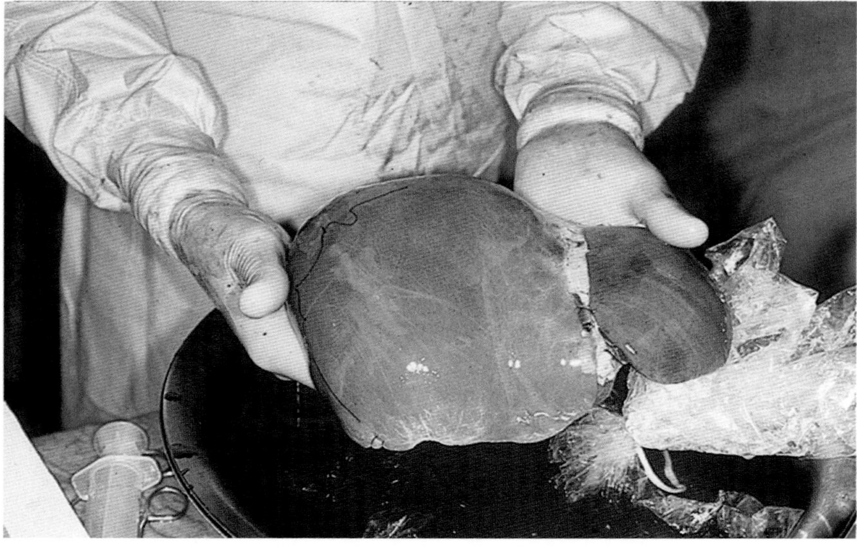

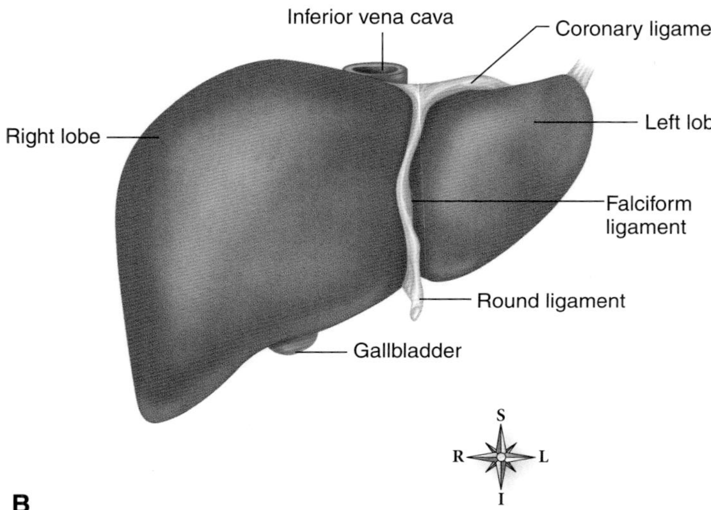

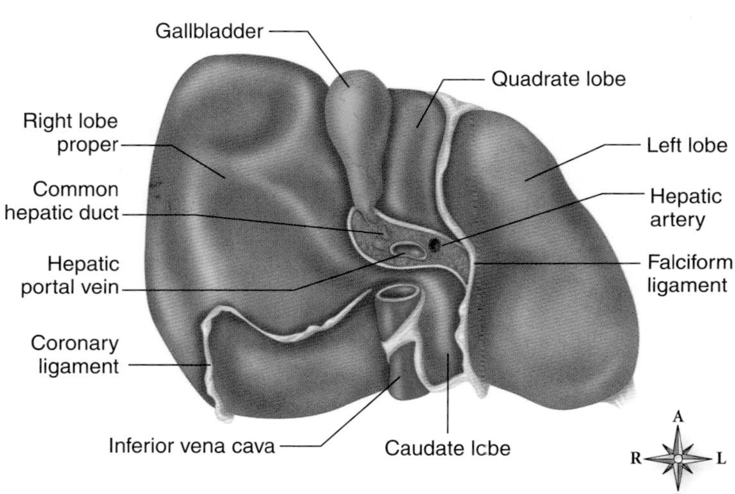

UNIT 5

FIGURE 39-11 Microscopic structure of the liver. A, This diagram shows the location of liver lobules relative to the overall circulatory scheme of the liver. **B** and **C,** Enlarged views of several lobules show how blood from the hepatic portal veins and hepatic arteries flows through sinusoids and thus past plates of hepatocytes toward a central vein in each lobule *(black arrows)*. Hepatocytes form bile, which flows through bile canaliculi toward hepatic ducts that eventually drain the bile from the liver *(yellow arrows)*.

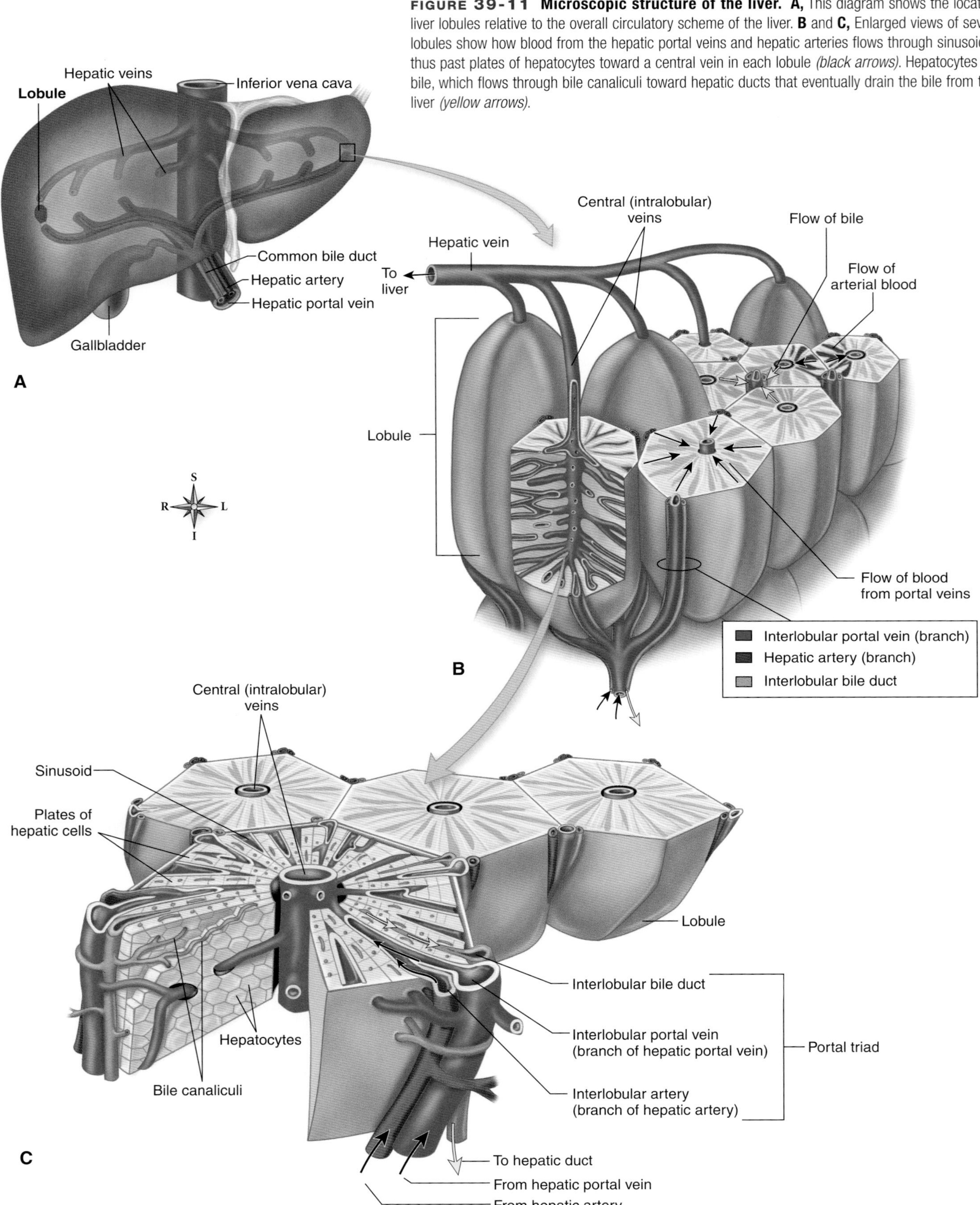

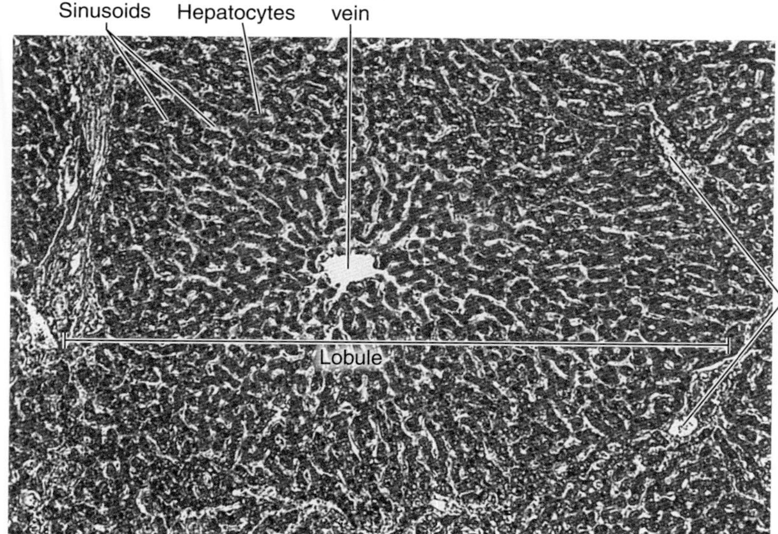

FIGURE 39-12 Liver tissue. This cross-section of a hepatic lobule shows the sinusoids that permit passage of blood from the interlobular portal veins toward the central vein. The glandular epithelium (hepatocytes) forms plates between the sinusoids.

called the *perivascular fibrous capsule*. The perivascular fibrous capsule—also called the *capsule of Glisson*—is an extension of the heavy connective tissue capsule that envelops the entire liver.

The **hepatic lobules** (**Figure 39-11**), the anatomical units of the liver, are tiny hexagonal or pentagonal cylinders about 2 mm high and 1 mm in diameter. A small branch of the hepatic vein extends through the centre of each lobule. Around this *central (intralobular) vein*, in plates or irregular walls radiating outward, are arranged the **hepatocytes** (liver cells).

On the outer corners of each lobule are several sets of tiny tubes collectively called the **portal triad** or *hepatic triad*. Each triad includes three primary structures:

1. *Interlobular artery* (branch of hepatic artery)
2. *Interlobular portal vein* (branch of hepatic portal vein)
3. *Interlobular bile duct*

Alongside these three primary structures, each portal triad also includes lymphatic vessels and branches of the vagus nerve (CN X).

From the portal triads, irregular branches (sinusoids) of the interlobular portal veins extend between the radiating plates of hepatocytes to join the central vein. Minute bile canaliculi are formed by the spaces around each cell that collect bile secreted by the hepatocytes.

Consider the function of the hepatic lobule while carefully examining **Figure 39-11** and **Figure 39-12**. Blood enters a lobule from branches of the hepatic artery and portal vein. Arterial blood oxygenates the hepatocytes, whereas blood from the portal system simply passes through the liver for "inspection".

Sinusoids in the lobule have many resident macrophages—mainly **stellate macrophages** (*Kupffer cells*)—along their lining. These phagocytic cells can remove bacteria, worn red blood cells (RBCs), and other particles from the bloodstream.

Ingested vitamins and other nutrients to be stored or metabolized by liver cells enter the hepatocytes that form radiating walls of the lobule. Dissolved toxins in the blood are also absorbed into hepatocytes, where they are detoxified (rendered harmless).

Blood continues along the sinusoids to a vein at the centre of the lobule. Such central, intralobular veins eventually lead to the main hepatic veins that drain into the inferior vena cava. **Bile** formed by hepatocytes passes through canaliculi to the periphery of the lobule to join small interlobular bile ducts in the portal triads.

Bile Ducts

The small bile ducts within the liver join to form two larger ducts that emerge from the undersurface of the organ as the *right* and *left hepatic ducts*. These ducts immediately join to form one common hepatic duct. The common hepatic duct merges with the *cystic duct* from the gallbladder to form the *common bile duct* (**Figure 39-13**), which opens into the duodenum in a small raised area called the *major duodenal papilla*. This papilla is located 7 to 10 cm below the pyloric opening from the stomach.

The inset in **Figure 39-13** shows a radiograph taken during a procedure with a long and tongue-twisting name—**endoscopic cholangiography.** During this procedure, x-ray images are taken to visualize the gallbladder and ducts that carry bile. The process begins with passage of a flexible endoscope tube surrounding a hollow catheter and other laparoscopic instruments through the mouth, oesophagus, and stomach into the duodenum. Once in the duodenum, the catheter is introduced into the major duodenal papilla, and contrast material is injected into the biliary tract. This procedure can also be used to fill the pancreatic duct and its branches with contrast material to obtain very high-quality x-ray images.

Functions of the Liver

The liver is one of the most vital organs of the body, performing more than 300 functions critical to a healthy life. Here, in brief, are its main functions:

- Liver cells detoxify various substances.
- Liver cells break down and remove old red blood cells, recycling the iron from haemoglobin.
- Liver cells secrete approximately half a litre of bile a day.
- Liver cells carry on numerous important steps in the metabolism of all three kinds of foods—proteins, fats, and carbohydrates.
- Liver cells store several substances—iron, for example, and vitamins A, B_{12}, and D.
- The liver produces important plasma proteins and serves as a site of haematopoiesis (blood cell production) during fetal development.
- The liver stores glucose in the form of glycogen, a polysaccharide.

Detoxification by Liver Cells

Numerous poisonous substances enter blood from the intestines. They circulate to the liver, where, through a series of chemical reactions, they may be changed into nontoxic compounds. Ingested substances—alcohol, paracetamol, and various other drugs, for example—and toxic substances formed in the intestines can be detoxified in the liver.

Bile Secretion by the Liver

The main components of bile are bile salts, bile pigments, and cholesterol. Bile salts (formed in the liver from cholesterol) are the most essential part of bile. They aid in the digestion and absorption of fats

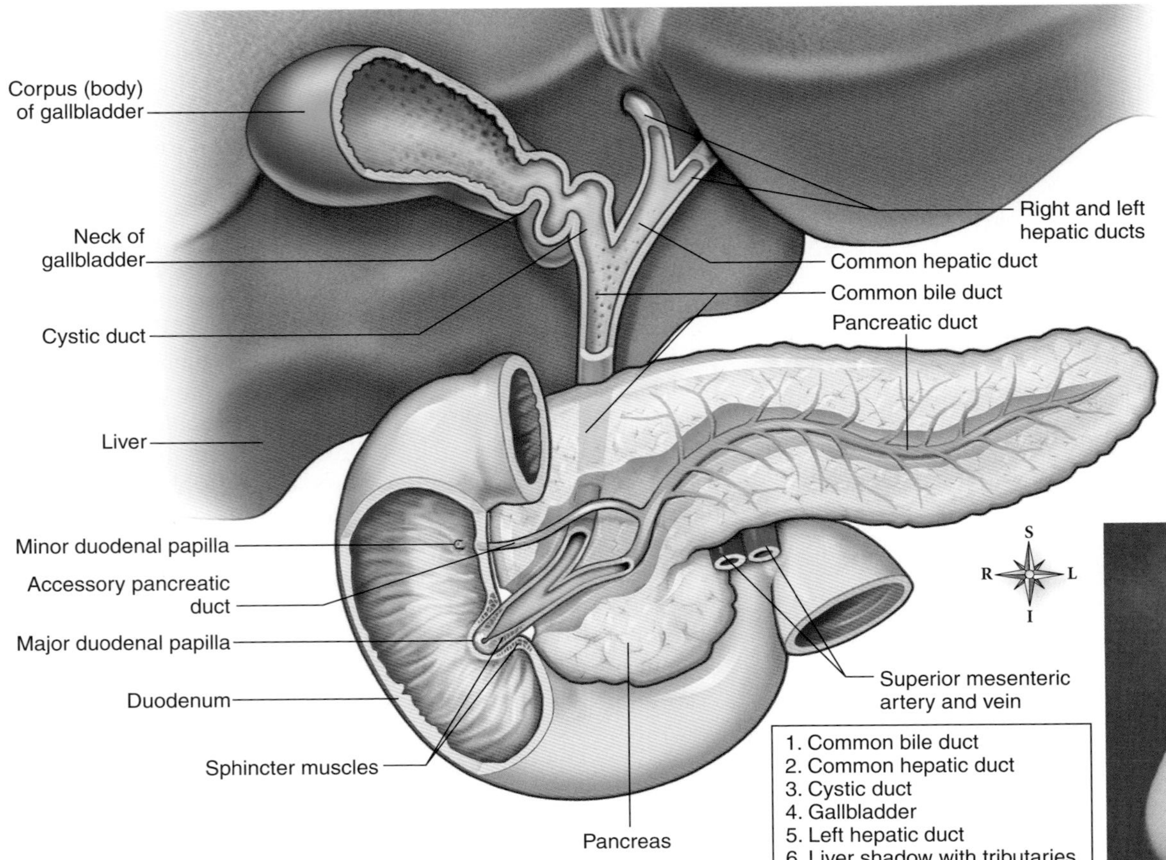

Corpus (body) of gallbladder
Neck of gallbladder
Cystic duct
Liver
Minor duodenal papilla
Accessory pancreatic duct
Major duodenal papilla
Duodenum
Sphincter muscles
Pancreas
Right and left hepatic ducts
Common hepatic duct
Common bile duct
Pancreatic duct
Superior mesenteric artery and vein
S R L I

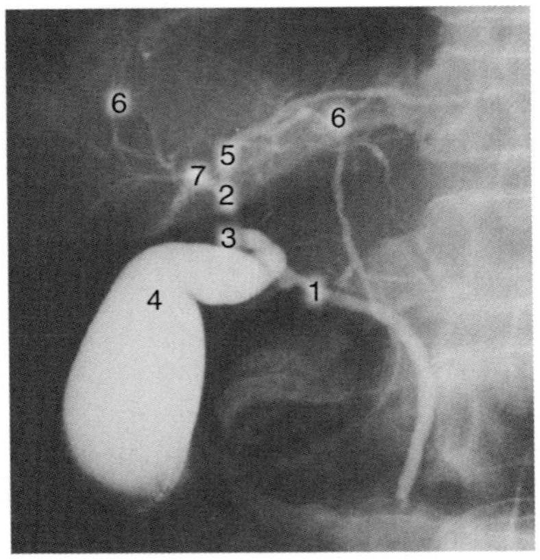

1. Common bile duct
2. Common hepatic duct
3. Cystic duct
4. Gallbladder
5. Left hepatic duct
6. Liver shadow with tributaries of hepatic ducts
7. Right hepatic duct

FIGURE 39-13 Ducts that carry bile from the liver and gallbladder. Bile exits the liver through the left and right hepatic ducts, which join to form the common hepatic duct. The common hepatic duct joins the cystic duct from the gallbladder to form the common bile duct, which enters the duodenum at the major duodenal papilla (regulated by sphincter muscles). When sphincter muscles contract, bile backs up into the gallbladder, where it is stored and concentrated. Obstruction of either the common hepatic or the common bile duct by a stone or muscle spasm prevents bile from being ejected into the duodenum. The inset shows an x-ray image of the gallbladder and the ducts that carry bile taken during a procedure called *endoscopic cholangiography.*

and then are themselves absorbed in the ileum. Eighty percent of bile salts are recycled in the liver to again become part of bile. Bile also serves as a pathway for elimination of certain breakdown products of RBCs. When aged and fragile erythrocytes are destroyed in the spleen, the haem portion of the released haemoglobin molecule is converted into bilirubin and transported by blood to the liver. Liver cells extract the bilirubin and excrete it into bile. Because it secretes bile into ducts, the liver qualifies as an exocrine gland.

A
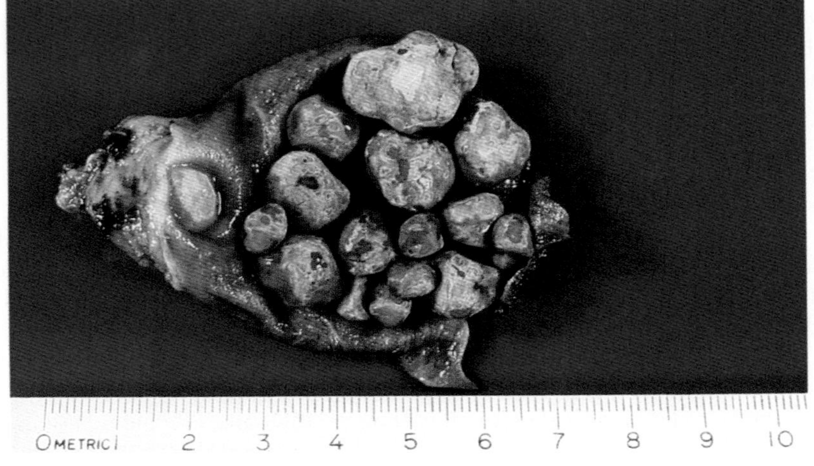

B
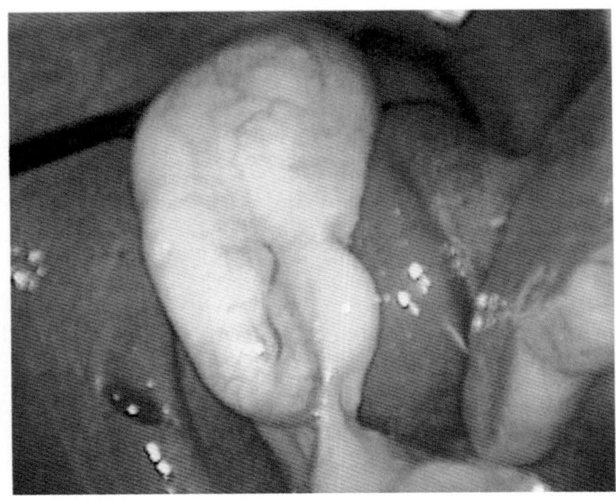

FIGURE 39-14 Gallbladder and gallstones. A, Gallbladder filled with yellow cholesterol gallstones. **B,** Laparoscopic view of the gallbladder before removal.

Liver Metabolism

Although all liver functions are important for healthy survival, some of its metabolic processes are crucial for survival itself. A fairly detailed description of the role of the liver in metabolism is given in Chapter 41.

GALLBLADDER

Size and Location of the Gallbladder

The gallbladder is a pear-shaped sac 7 to 10 cm long and 3 cm broad at its widest point (see **Figure 39-13**). The gallbladder lies on the undersurface of the liver and is attached there by areolar connective tissue.

Structure of the Gallbladder

Serous, muscular, and mucous layers compose the wall of the gallbladder. The mucosal lining is arranged in folds called *rugae*, similar in structure to those of the stomach. These rugae allow the gallbladder to expand as it receives bile that backs up into it when the sphincters of the major duodenal papilla contract. The gallbladder can hold 30 to 50 mL of bile.

Functions of the Gallbladder

The gallbladder stores bile that backs up into it. The gallbladder concentrates bile fivefold to tenfold as it is stored. When partially digested material exits the stomach, the gallbladder contracts and ejects the concentrated bile into the duodenum.

Jaundice, a yellow discolouration of the skin and mucosa, results when obstruction of bile flow into the duodenum occurs. Bile is thereby denied its normal exit from the body in faeces. Instead, it is absorbed into the blood, and an excess of bile pigments with a yellow hue enters the blood and is deposited in tissues.

Inflammation of the gallbladder is called **cholecystitis**. It is often caused by gallstone formation or **cholelithiasis** (**Figure 39-14**, *A*). Inflammation and stone formation may require surgical removal in a procedure called **cholecystectomy.** Surgical removal is now commonly performed laparoscopically, a procedure less invasive than traditional surgery (**Figure 39-14**, *B*). However, efforts to eliminate stones with drugs or nonsurgical methods, such as *ultrasound lithotripsy*, are often the treatment of choice initially.

CONNECT IT! ⓔ

Did you know that the formation of gallstones may be related to weight loss and dieting? Find out how, and see some dramatic medical images, in ***Gallstones and Weight Loss*** online at ***Connect It!***

PANCREAS

Size and Location of the Pancreas

The pancreas is a greyish pink–coloured gland about 12 to 15 cm long, weighing about 60 grams. It resembles a fish with its head and neck in the C-shaped curve of the duodenum, its body extending horizontally behind the stomach, and its tail touching the spleen (**Figure 39-15**; see **Figure 39-1** on p. 883). According to an old anatomical witticism, the "romance of the abdomen" is the pancreas lying "in the arms of the duodenum".

Structure of the Pancreas

The pancreas is composed of two different types of glandular tissue, one exocrine and one endocrine. Most of the tissue is exocrine, with a compound acinar arrangement. The word *acinar* means that the cells are in a grapelike formation and that they release their secretions into a microscopic duct within each unit (see **Figure 39-15**, *B*). The word *compound* indicates that the ducts have branches. These tiny ducts unite to form larger ducts that eventually join the main pancreatic duct, which extends throughout the length of the gland from its tail to its head.

The pancreatic duct empties into the duodenum at the same point as the common bile duct at the *major duodenal papilla.* An accessory duct is often found extending from the head of the pancreas into the duodenum, opening at the *minor duodenal papilla* about 2 cm above the major papilla (see **Figure 39-15**, *A*).

Embedded between the exocrine units of the pancreas, like so many little islands, lie clusters of endocrine cells called **pancreatic islets** (see **Figure 39-15**). Although there are about a million of these tiny islands, they constitute only about 2% of the total mass of the pancreas. Special staining techniques have revealed that several kinds of cells—mainly alpha cells and beta cells—make up the islets. They are secreting cells, but their secretion passes into blood capillaries rather than into ducts. Thus the pancreas is a dual gland—an exocrine, or duct, gland because of the acinar units and an endocrine, or ductless, gland because of the pancreatic islets.

Functions of the Pancreas

The acinar units that comprise most of the pancreatic tissue secrete pancreatic juice. This digestive juice is made up mostly of water but also contains sodium bicarbonate ($NaHCO_3$) and various digestive enzymes. Hence the exocrine part of the pancreas plays an important part in digestion (see Chapter 40).

The endocrine functions of the pancreas were introduced in Chapter 26 (see pp. 596–597) and will be discussed further in subsequent chapters. Recall that *beta cells* of the pancreatic islets secrete **insulin,** a hormone that exerts a major control over carbohydrate metabolism (see **Figure 39-15**, *B*). *Alpha cells* secrete **glucagon.** It is interesting to note that glucagon, which is produced so close to where insulin is produced, has an opposite effect on carbohydrate metabolism.

CONNECT IT! ⓔ

An abnormal decrease in insulin effects can have dramatic consequences for a person's health. To see a flowchart of how these effects create disease and possibly death, check out ***Diabetes Mellitus*** online at ***Connect It!***

***Quick* CHECK**

7. Where is the liver located?
8. Name three of the many functions of the liver.
9. Trace the route of bile from the gallbladder to the duodenum.
10. What is the function of the acinar units of the pancreas?

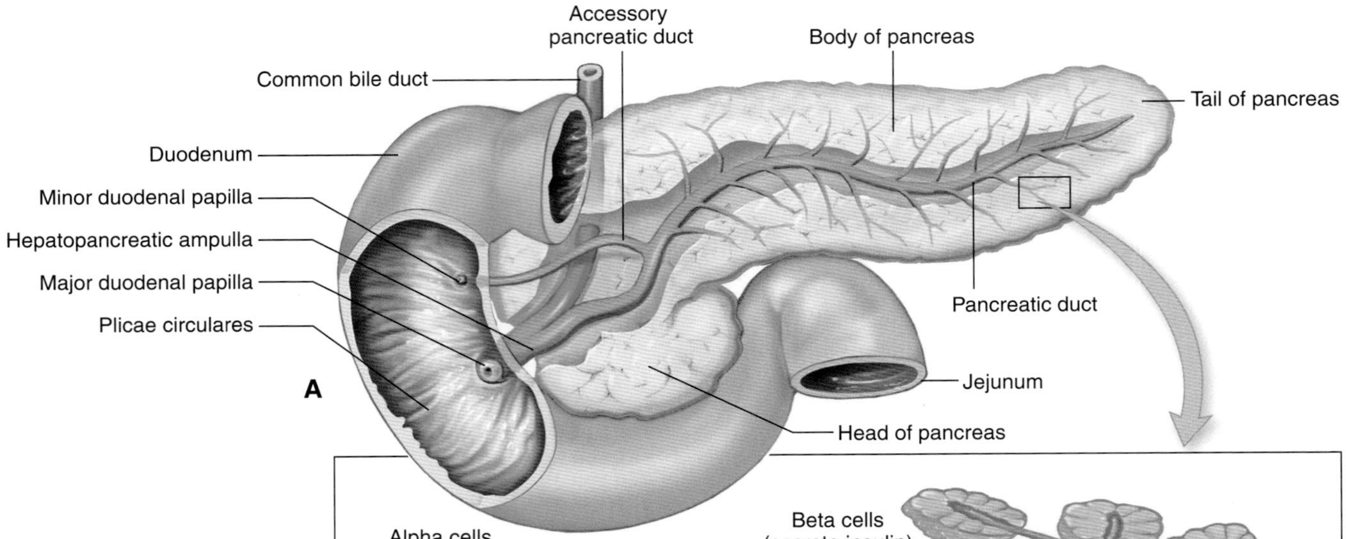

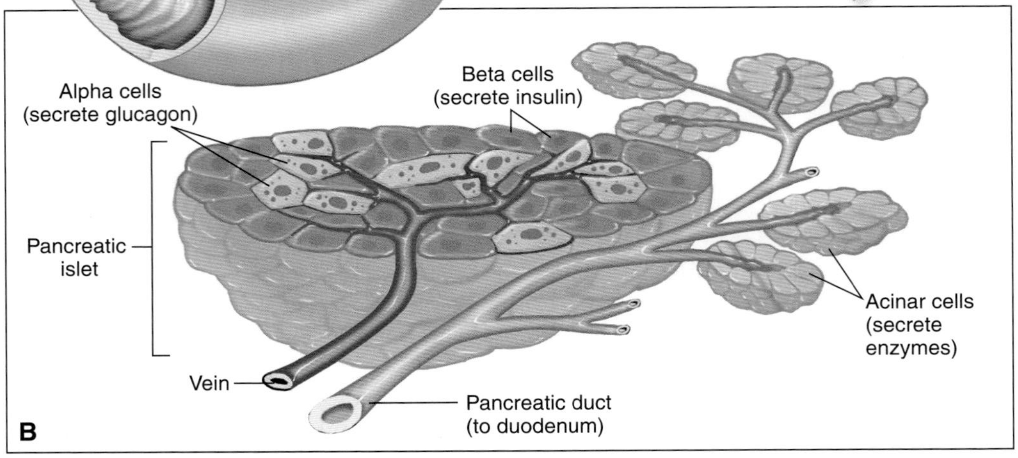

FIGURE 39-15 Pancreas. A, Pancreas dissected to show the main and accessory ducts. The main duct may join the common bile duct, as shown here, to enter the duodenum by a single opening at the major duodenal papilla (see **Figure 39-13**), or the two ducts may have separate openings. The accessory pancreatic duct is usually present and has a separate opening into the duodenum. **B,** Exocrine glandular cells (around small pancreatic ducts) and endocrine glandular cells of the pancreatic islets (adjacent to blood capillaries). Exocrine pancreatic cells secrete pancreatic juice, alpha endocrine cells secrete glucagon, and beta cells secrete insulin.

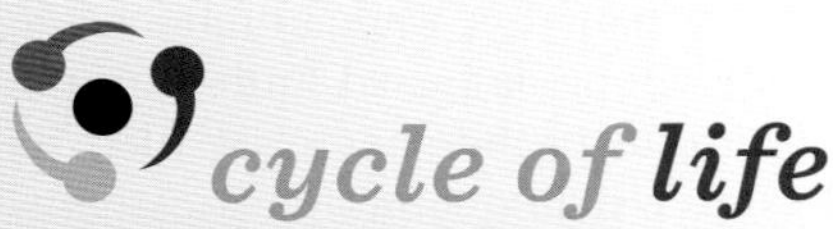

Lower Digestive Tract Various changes to the structure and function of the intestines and associated structures occur over the life span. For example, because of the immaturity of intestinal mucosa in young infants, some types of intact proteins can pass through the epithelial cells that line the tract. The result may be an early allergic response caused by the protein triggering the baby's immune system. Lactose intolerance is another age-related example of a common digestive system problem. Intestinal lactase, needed for the digestion of lactose, or milk sugar, is almost always present at the time of birth. Levels may rapidly diminish in some babies, however, and such individuals soon become unable to digest lactose.

Appendicitis occurs more commonly in adolescents. The incidence of appendicitis then decreases with age because the size of the opening between the appendix and the intestinal lumen decreases. Gallbladder disease and ulcers are primarily problems of middle age. In more elderly individuals, a decrease in volume of digestive fluids coupled with a slowing of peristalsis and reduced physical activity often results in constipation and diverticulosis. •

the big picture | **The Digestive Tract**

The process of digestion, which is discussed in the next chapter, is structure-dependent. It is the normal interrelationships of the anatomical components of the digestive system coupled with the functioning of other body organ systems that permit the highly regulated processes that result in digestion and absorption of nutrients. For example, breaking down of food involves not only the grinding action of the teeth but also the mechanical mixing of food as it passes through the GI tract. Nervous involvement in this process requires the conscious control of mastication and the parasympathetic regulation of smooth muscle contraction mediated through the intramural plexus. Endocrine cells produce hormones that also help regulate digestive tract function. A rich blood and lymphatic supply allows for efficient absorption of nutrients and transport to other parts of the body. Furthermore, the structural adaptations of the GI tract that increase the surface area for better absorption (rugae, villi, brush borders) increase overall digestive efficiency. In the next two chapters, the digestive system's role in maintaining a relatively constant supply of nutrients available to cells becomes even more clear. •

mechanisms of disease

Disorders of the Lower Digestive Tract

Disorders of the Intestines

Recall that ***gastroenterology*** is the study of the stomach *(gastro-)* and intestines *(entero-)* and their diseases. Intestinal diseases often involve these signs:

Diarrhoea—elimination of liquid faeces, perhaps accompanied by abdominal cramps

Constipation—decreased motility of colon, resulting in difficulty in defaecation

Malabsorption syndrome is a general term referring to a group of symptoms resulting from the failure of the small intestine to absorb nutrients properly. These symptoms include anorexia, abdominal bloating, cramps, anaemia, and fatigue. Numerous underlying conditions can cause malabsorption syndrome. For example, certain enzyme deficiencies can result in an absorption failure because there are no digested nutrients to absorb. Cystic fibrosis and other genetic conditions can also cause malabsorption syndrome.

Diverticulosis is the presence of abnormal saclike outpouchings of the intestinal wall called *diverticula* (**Figure 39-16**). Diverticula often develop in adults older than 50 years who eat low-fibre foods. Diverticulosis is usually asymptomatic. If the diverticula become inflamed, however, the condition is called **diverticulitis.** Diverticulitis is characterized by pain, tenderness, and fever.

Colitis refers to any inflammatory condition of the large intestine. Symptoms of colitis include diarrhoea and abdominal cramps or constipation. Some forms of colitis may also produce bleeding and intestinal ulcers. It may also result from an autoimmune disease, as in *ulcerative colitis.* Another type of colitis can occur in those with **Crohn disease.** Crohn disease results from an abnormal inflammatory response. Although it can occur in any part of the alimentary canal, it most often affects both the small intestine and the colon (**Figure 39-17**). If more conservative treatments fail, colitis may be corrected by surgical removal of the affected portions of the colon.

Irritable bowel syndrome, or *spastic colon,* is a common chronic noninflammatory condition that is often caused by stress. Irritable bowel syndrome is characterized by diarrhoea or constipation with or without pain.

Colorectal cancer is a malignancy, usually an *adenocarcinoma,* of the colon or rectum. Colorectal cancer occurs most often after the age of 50, and a low-fibre, high-fat diet and genetic predisposition are known risk factors. Early warning signs of this common type of cancer include changes in bowel habits, faecal blood, rectal bleeding, abdominal pain, unexplained anaemia or weight loss, and fatigue. Screening for colorectal cancer may be done by checking for occult (hidden) blood in the faeces or by examining the rectum and colon with a flexible scope during a *colonoscopy.*

If the mucous lining of the appendix becomes inflamed, the resulting condition is the well-known affliction **appendicitis.** As you can see in **Figure 39-5** (p. 886), the appendix is very close to the rectal wall. For patients with suspected appendicitis, a physician often evaluates the appendix by performing a digital rectal examination.

The opening between the lumen of the appendix and the caecum is quite large in children and young adults—a fact of clinical significance because food,

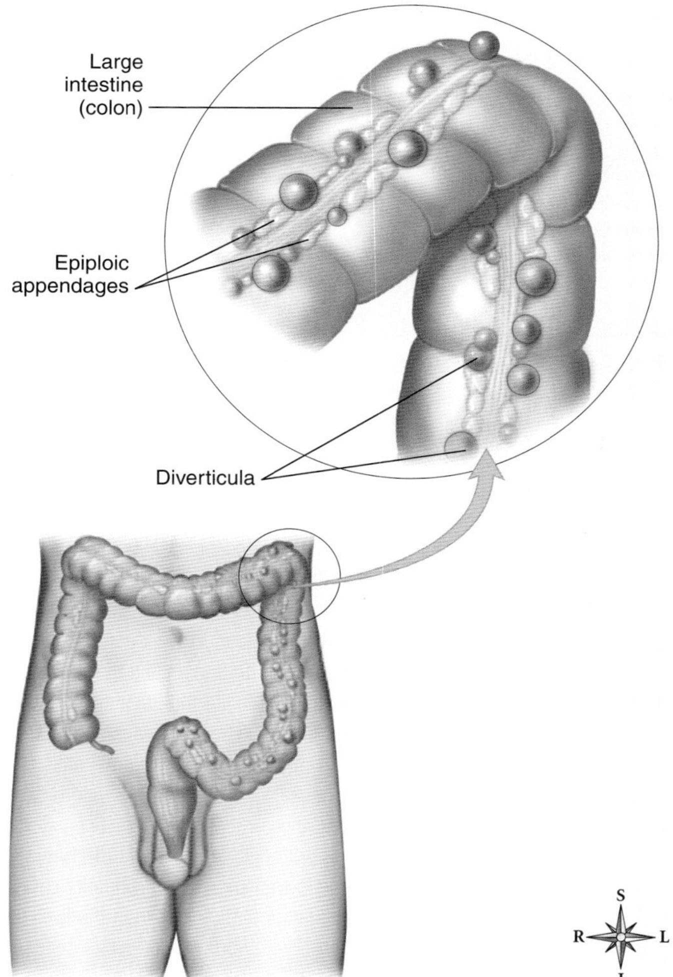

FIGURE 39-16 Diverticula. Abnormal outpouchings of the colon are called *diverticula.* When they become inflamed, the condition is called *diverticulitis.* Diverticula occur mainly in the descending colon and only very rarely in the transverse colon.

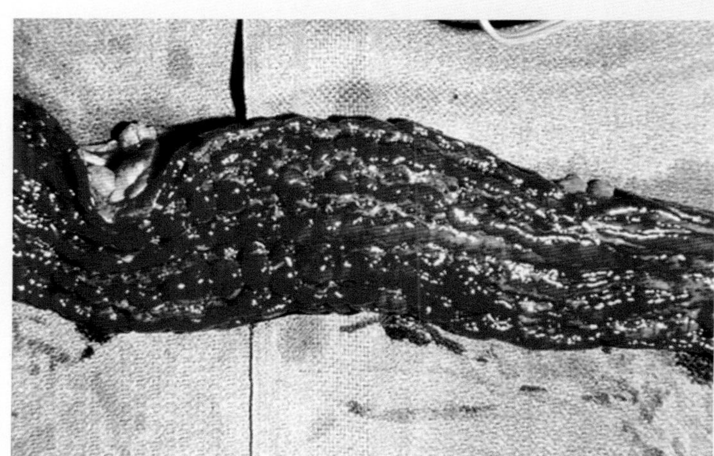

FIGURE 39-17 Crohn disease. Crohn disease, an autoimmune form of colitis, is characterized by severe inflammation that gives a sort of "cobblestone" appearance to the intestinal lining.

faecal material, or calcified, stonelike concretions called **appendicoliths** may become trapped in the opening, block the lumen, and cause irritation and inflammation resulting in appendicitis. If calcification within the appendix is visible on an x-ray image in a patient with pain in the lower right abdominal quadrant, there is an extremely high probability—physicians call it "clinical suspicion"—of acute appendicitis.

The opening between the appendix and the caecum is often completely obliterated in elderly persons, which explains the low incidence of appendicitis in this population.

If infectious material becomes trapped in an inflamed appendix (**Figure 39-18**), the appendix may rupture and release the material into the abdominal cavity. Infection of the peritoneum and other abdominal organs may result—with sometimes tragic consequences.

Rectal bleeding is a symptom that should always be investigated. Although it may signal a serious disease problem, such as cancer, most instances of this common problem are indicators of less serious and non–life-threatening conditions (**Figure 39-19**).

Haemorrhoids are dilated veins that result from direct irritation or from increases in venous pressure that often accompany pregnancy or result from constipation and the subsequent straining required to pass compact and hardened stools. Haemorrhoids most commonly develop near the anal opening or on the wall of the anal canal. Though often painful and irritating, haemorrhoids generally respond readily to treatment and are seldom a serious health concern.

Proctitis, or inflammation of the rectal mucosa, is another common cause of rectal bleeding and related symptoms such as mucus discharge or increased frequency of bowel movements. The condition may result from direct irritation or infection. In most cases, proctitis responds quickly to the administration of anti-inflammatory drugs and treatment of the underlying problem.

Anal fissures are generally minor lacerations in the lining of the anus or anal canal that result in rectal bleeding. They are caused by direct irritation—often the result of passing a hardened stool. An **anal fistula** is a more serious problem that may require surgical repair. A fistula is a passageway that often develops between the rectal wall and the skin surrounding the anus. Fistulas occur in Crohn disease, an inflammatory bowel disease.

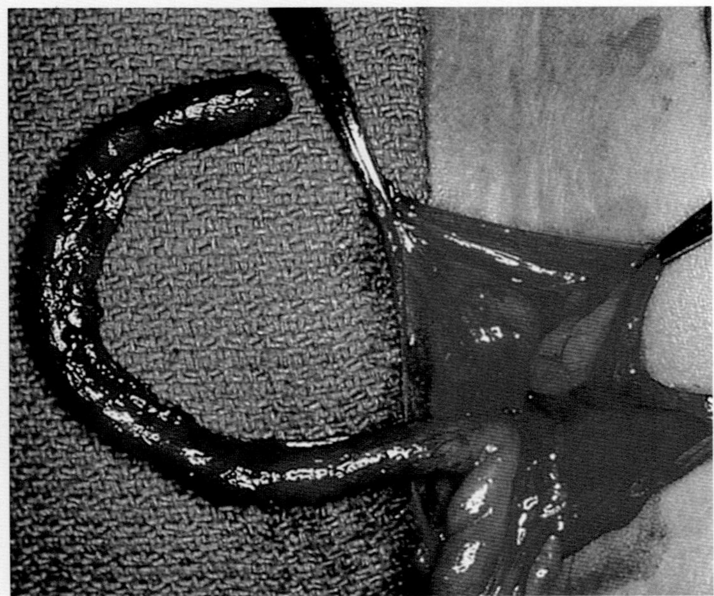

FIGURE 39-18 **Acute appendicitis.** Note the inflamed tissue surrounding the base of a gangrenous appendix.

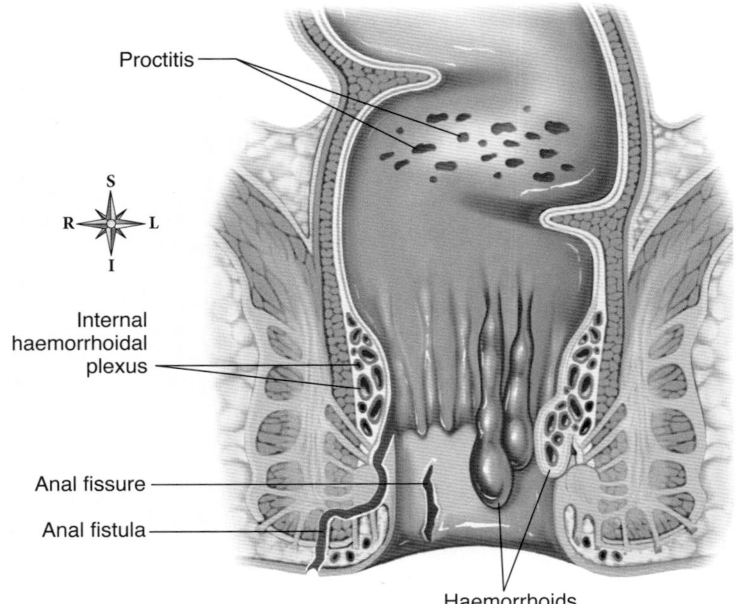

FIGURE 39-19 **Causes of rectal bleeding.**

CONNECT IT!

Monitoring for bleeding and other changes in the faeces is a way to monitor overall body health. For potential signs of health dangers in the faeces, check out ***Toilet Signs*** online at ***Connect It!***

Disorders of the Liver and Pancreas

Hepatitis is a general term referring to inflammation of the liver. Hepatitis is characterized by jaundice (yellowish discolouration of body tissues), liver enlargement, anorexia, abdominal discomfort, grey-white faeces, and dark urine. Various conditions can produce hepatitis. Alcohol, drugs, or other toxins may cause hepatitis. It may also be a complication of bacterial or viral infection or parasite infestation. *Hepatitis A,* for example, results from infection by the hepatitis A virus. Contaminated food is often a source of infection. Hepatitis A occurs commonly in young people and ranges in severity from mild to life-threatening. Another viral hepatitis, *hepatitis B,* is usually more severe. It is also called *serum hepatitis* because it is often transmitted by contaminated blood serum (plasma). The *hepatitis C virus (HCV)* causes a viral form of hepatitis that can also be transmitted by contaminated blood. The disease may become chronic and result in life-threatening liver disease many months or even years after exposure. Oral drugs are now available that have a cure rate of nearly 100% when taken for 3 months. Vaccines for hepatitis C are also being developed. Other viral forms of hepatitis include the D, E, and G types.

Hepatitis, chronic alcohol abuse, malnutrition, infection, or *nonalcoholic fatty liver disease* may lead to a degenerative liver condition known as **cirrhosis.** The liver's ability to regenerate damaged tissue is well known, but it has its limits. For example, when the toxic effects of alcohol accumulate faster than the liver can regenerate itself, damaged tissue is replaced with fibrous scar tissue instead of normal tissue (**Figure 39-20**). *Cirrhosis* is the name given to such degeneration.

Besides the endocrine disorders such as diabetes mellitus discussed in Chapter 26, the pancreas may be involved in numerous other diseases. For example, **pancreatitis,** or inflammation of the pancreas, can be caused by various factors. *Acute pancreatitis* usually results from blockage of the pancreatic duct. The blockage causes pancreatic enzymes to "back up" into the pancreas and digest it. Another condition that blocks the flow of pancreatic enzymes is *cystic fibrosis (CF)*. You may recall from Chapter 6 that this inherited disorder disrupts cell transport and causes exocrine glands to produce excessively thick secretions. Thick pancreatic secretions may build up and block pancreatic ducts, disrupting the flow of pancreatic enzymes and damaging the pancreas.

Another serious pancreatic disorder is **pancreatic cancer.** Usually a form of *adenocarcinoma,* pancreatic cancer claims the lives of nearly all its patients within 5 years after diagnosis.

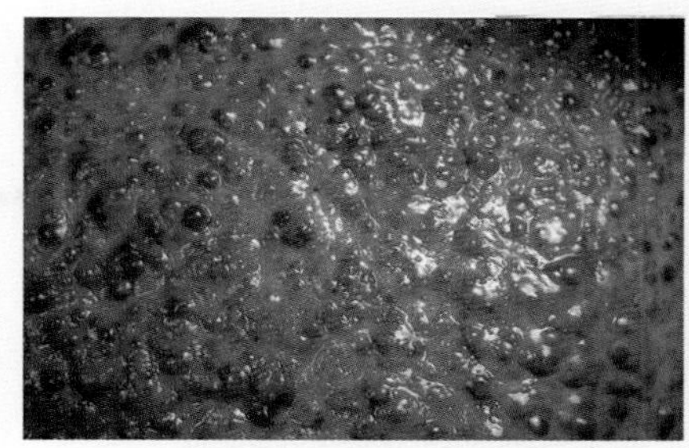

FIGURE 39-20
Cirrhosis. Alcoholic cirrhosis is characterized by hardness of the liver caused by fibrous tissue and by nodules—which can be seen clearly in this photograph of the surface of a cirrhotic liver.

LANGUAGE OF SCIENCE *(continued from p. 882)*

intestinal crypt (of Lieberkühn) (in-TES-tih-nal kript [LEE-ber-kyoon]) [*intestin-* **intestine,** *-al* **relating to,** *crypt* **hidden cave** (*Johannes Lieberkühn* **German anatomist**)]

intraperitoneal (in-trah-pair-ih-toh-NEE-al) [*intra-* **within,** *peri-* **around,** *-tone-* **stretched,** *-al* **relating to**]

jejunum (jeh-JOO-num) [*jejunus* **empty**]

left lobe (lohb)

lesser omentum (oh-MEN-tum) [*omentum* **fatty covering of intestines**]

mesentery (MEZ-en-tair-ee) [*mes-* **middle,** *-enter-* **intestine**]

pancreatic islet (pan-kree-AT-ik EYE-let) [*pan-* **all,** *-crea-* **flesh,** *-ic* **relating to,** *islet* **island**]

Paneth cell (PAH-net sel) [*Josef Paneth* **Austrian physiologist**]

peritoneum (pair-ih-toh-NEE-um) [*peri-* **around,** *-tone-* **stretched,** *-um* **thing**] *pl.,* peritonea

plica (PLYE-ka) [*plica* **fold**] *pl.,* plicae or plicas

portal triad (PORT-al TRY-ad) [*port-* **doorway,** *-al* **relating to,** *triad* **group of three**]

rectum (REK-tum) [*rect-* **straight or upright,** *-um* **thing**]

retroperitoneal (reh-troh-pair-ih-toh-NEE-al) [*retro-* **backward,** *peri-* **around,** *-tone-* **stretched,** *-al* **relating to**]

right lobe (lohb)

sigmoid colon (SIG-moyd KOH-lon) [*sigm-* **sigma (Σ or σ) 18th letter of Greek alphabet (Roman S),** *-oid* **like,** *colon* **colon**]

stellate macrophage (Kupffer cell) (STEL-ayt MAK-roh-fayj [KOOP-fer sel]) [*stell-* **star,** *-ate* **of or like,** *macro-* **large,** *-phag-* **eat** (*Karl W. von Kupffer* **German surgeon**)]

taeniae coli (TEE-nee-ee KOH-lye) [*taenia* **ribbon or tape,** *coli* **relating to the large intestine**] *sing.,* taenia coli

transverse colon (tranz-VERS KOH-lon) [*trans-* **across,** *-vers-* **turn,** *colon* **large intestine**]

transverse mesocolon (tranz-VERS MEZ-oh-koh-lon) [*trans-* **across,** *-vers-* **turn,** *meso-* **middle,** *-colon* **large intestine**]

tuft cell (tuhft sel)

vermiform appendix (VERM-ih-form ah-PEN-diks) [*vermi-* **worm,** *-form* **shape,** *append-* **hang upon,** *-ix* **thing**] *pl.,* appendices

villus (VIL-us) [*villus* **shaggy hair**] *pl.,* villi

LANGUAGE OF MEDICINE

anal fissure (AY-nal FISH-ur) [*an-* **ring (anus),** *-al* **relating to,** *fissur-* **cleft**]

anal fistula (AY-nal FISS-tyoo-lah) [*an-* **ring (anus),** *-al* **relating to,** *fistula* **pipe**] *pl.,* fistulae or fistulas

appendicitis (ah-pen-dih-SYE-tis) [*appendic-* **hang upon,** *-itis* **inflammation**]

appendicolith (ah-pen-DIK-oh-lith) [*appendic-* **hang upon,** *-lith* **stone**]

cholecystectomy (koh-leh-sis-TEK-toh-mee) [*chole-* **bile,** *-cyst-* **bag,** *-ec-* **out,** *-tom-* **cut,** *-y* **action**]

cholecystitis (koh-leh-sis-TYE-tis) [*chole-* **bile,** *-cyst-* **bag,** *-itis* **inflammation**]

cholelithiasis (koh-leh-lih-THYE-ah-sis) [*chole-* **bile,** *-lith-* **stone,** *-iasis* **condition**]

cirrhosis (sih-ROH-sis) [*cirrhos-* **yellow-orange,** *-osis* **condition**]

colitis (koh-LYE-tis) [*col-* **colon,** *-itis* **inflammation**]

colonoscopy (koh-lon-OS-kah-pee) [*colon* **large intestine,** *-scop-* **see,** *-y* **activity**]

colorectal cancer (koh-loh-REK-tal KAN-ser) [*colo-* **colon,** *-rect-* **straight or upright,** *-al* **relating to,** *cancer* **crab or malignant tumour**]

constipation (kon-sti-PAY-shun) [*constipa-* **crowd together,** *-ation* **process**]

Crohn disease (krohn) [*Burrill B. Crohn* **American physician**]

diarrhoea (dye-ah-REE-ah) [*dia-* **through,** *-rrhoea* **flow**]

diverticulitis (dye-ver-tik-yoo-LYE-tis) [*diverticul-* **turn aside,** *-itis* **inflammation**]

diverticulosis (dye-ver-tik-yoo-LOH-sis) [*diverticul-* **turn aside,** *-osis* **condition**]

endoscopic cholangiography (en-doh-SKOP-ik koh-lan-jee-OG-rah-fee) [*endo-* **within,** *-scop-* **see,** *chol-* **bile,** *angi-* **vessel,** *-graph-* **draw,** *-y* **process**]

gastroenterology (gas-troh-en-ter-OL-oh-jee) [*gastr-* **stomach,** *-entero-* **intestine,** *-o-* **combining form,** *-log-* **words (study of),** *-y* **activity**]

haemorrhoid (HEM-uh-royd) [*haemo-* **blood,** *-rrh-* **flow,** *-oid* **of or like**]

hepatitis (hep-ah-TYE-tis) [*hepat-* **liver,** *-itis* **inflammation**]

irritable bowel syndrome (IR-ih-tah-bul BOW-uhl SIN-drohm) [*irrita-* **tease,** *-ble* **capable,** *bowel* **sausage,** *syn-* **together,** *-drome* **running or (race) course**]

jaundice (JAWN-dis) [*jaun-* **yellow,** *-ice* **state**]

malabsorption syndrome (mal-ab-SORP-shun SIN-drohm) [*mal-* **bad,** *-ab-* **from,** *-sorp-* **suck,** *-tion* **process,** *syn-* **together,** *-drome* **running or (race) course**]

pancreatic cancer (pan-kree-AT-ik KAN-ser) [*pan-* **all,** *-creat-* **flesh,** *-ic* **relating to,** *cancer* **crab or malignant tumour**]

pancreatitis (pan-kree-ah-TYE-tis) [*pan-* **all,** *-creat-* **flesh,** *-itis* **inflammation**]

proctitis (prok-TYE-tis) [*proct-* **anus,** *-itis* **inflammation**]

case study

In the previous case study, remember Joanne turned away from her sewing basket to pick up her mobile phone just as her small daughter Lucy placed a handful of buttons into her mouth. Following radiography of her neck and head, medical staff at Accident and Emergency found one button in Lucy's upper oesophagus.

The button appeared to be round with no sharp points, so the decision was made to let the button "pass" through Lucy's digestive system naturally.

1. As the button makes its way through Lucy's alimentary tract, it will go through which sequence of sphincters and valves?
   a. Lower oesophageal, pyloric, ileocaecal, anal
   b. Anal, pyloric, lower oesophageal, ileocaecal
   c. Lower oesophageal, ileocaecal, pyloric, anal
   d. Pyloric, ileocaecal, anal, lower oesophageal
2. Imagine a camera is attached to the button. As the button travels through Lucy's small intestines, the viewing monitor shows many tiny projections that look like gently moving brush bristles in the lining of the small intestine. What are these projections?
   a. Plicae
   b. Rugae
   c. Villi
   d. Crowns
3. As the button enters the large intestine, the camera picks up images of longitudinal muscles grouped into three tape-like strips called:
   a. Haustra
   b. Rugae
   c. Taeniae coli
   d. Villi

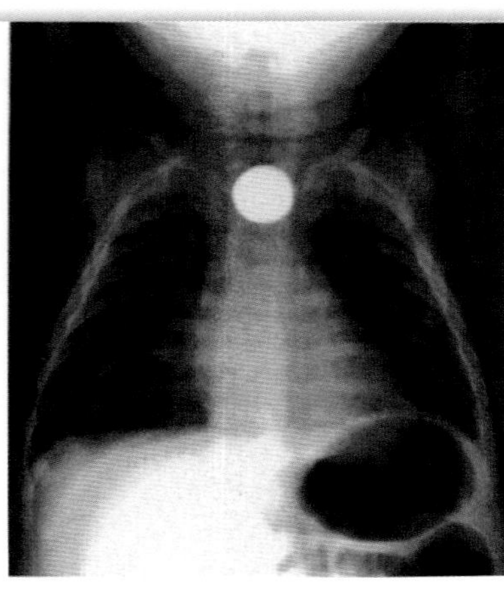

4. Identify the correct pathway the button will follow as it moves through the colon.
   a. Ascending colon, transverse colon, descending colon, sigmoid colon
   b. Sigmoid colon, ascending colon, transverse colon, descending colon
   c. Sigmoid colon, transverse colon, ascending colon, descending colon
   d. Descending colon, transverse colon, ascending colon, sigmoid colon

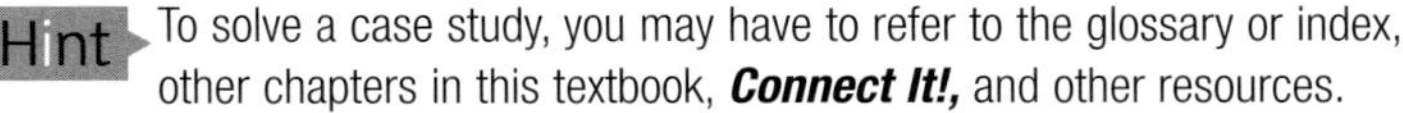
Hint To solve a case study, you may have to refer to the glossary or index, other chapters in this textbook, ***Connect It!***, and other resources.

CHAPTER SUMMARY

To download an MP3 version of the chapter summary for use with your mobile device, access the ***Audio Chapter Summaries*** *online at evolve.elsevier.com.*

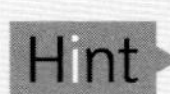

Hint *Scan this summary after reading the chapter to help you reinforce the key concepts. Later, use the summary as a quick review before your class or before a test.*

Introduction

A. Upper digestive tract—mouth through stomach
B. Lower digestive tract—small and large intestine; liver and pancreas empty secretions into lower digestive tract (**Figure 39-1**)

Small Intestine

A. Size and position of the small intestine
   1. Tube approximately 2.5 cm in diameter and 6 metres in length
   2. Coiled loops fill most of the abdominal cavity (**Figure 39-2**)
B. Divisions of the small intestine
   1. Duodenum—uppermost division; approximately 25 cm long, shaped roughly like the letter **C**
   2. Jejunum—approximately 2.5 metres long
   3. Ileum—approximately 3.5 metres long
C. Wall of the small intestine (**Figure 39-3**)
   1. Intestinal lining has plicae with villi
   2. Villi—important modifications of the mucosal layer
      a. Each villus contains an arteriole, venule, and lacteal vessel
      b. Covered by a brush border made up of 1700 ultrafine microvilli per cell
      c. Villi and microvilli increase the surface area of the small intestine hundreds of times
   3. Crypts—located between villi; contain stem cells from which other cell types are produced and then migrate upward to cover the villi, where they eventually slough off (**Figure 39-4**)

Large Intestine

A. Size of the large intestine
   1. Average diameter, 6 cm
   2. Length, approximately 1.5 to 1.8 metres
B. Divisions of the large intestine (**Figure 39-5**)
   1. Caecum—first 5 to 8 cm of the large intestine; blind pouch located in the lower right quadrant of the abdomen
   2. Colon
      a. Ascending colon—vertical position on the right side of the abdomen; the ileocaecal valve prevents material from passing from the large intestine into the ileum

b. Transverse colon—passes horizontally across the abdomen, above the small intestine; extends from the hepatic flexure to the splenic flexure
c. Descending colon—vertical position on left side of the abdomen
d. Sigmoid colon joins the descending colon to the rectum

3. Rectum
   a. Last 17 to 20 centimetres of the intestinal tube
   b. Terminal 2.5 cm is the anal canal with the opening called the *anus* (**Figure 39-6**)

C. Wall of the large intestine (**Figure 39-7**)
   1. Intestinal mucous glands produce lubricating mucus that coats faeces as they are formed
   2. Uneven distribution of fibres in the muscle coat produce tapelike taeniae coli and pouchlike haustra
   3. Fatty extensions on visceral peritoneum of the colon are called epiploic appendages

Vermiform Appendix

A. Accessory organ of digestive system
B. 8 to 10 cm in length; communicates with the caecum
C. Serves as reservoir for beneficial gut bacteria

Peritoneum

A. Large, continuous sheet of serous membrane (**Figure 39-8**)
   1. Many organs are covered with visceral peritoneum and are described as intraperitoneal; parietal peritoneum then lines the wall of the abdominopelvic cavity
   2. Extraperitoneal space is outside the parietal layer of the peritoneum; retroperitoneal identifies the extraperitoneal space along the posterior and bottom of the abdominopelvic cavity.

B. Mesentery—projection of the parietal peritoneum; allows free movement of each coil of the intestine and helps prevent strangulation of the long tube (**Figure 39-9**)
C. Transverse mesocolon—extension of the peritoneum that supports the transverse colon

Liver

A. Location and size of the liver (**Figure 39-10**)
   1. Largest gland in the body, weighs approximately 1.5 kg
   2. Lies under the diaphragm; occupies most of the right hypochondrium and part of the epigastrium

B. Liver lobes and lobules—two lobes separated by the falciform ligament
   1. Left lobe—forms about one sixth of the liver
   2. Right lobe—forms about five sixths of the liver; divides into right lobe proper, caudate lobe, and quadrate lobe
   3. Hepatic lobules (**Figures 39-11** and **39-12**)
      a. Microscopic units of the liver made up of plates of hepatocytes (liver cells) surrounded by irregular sinusoids containing stellate macrophages (Kupffer cells)
      b. A small branch of the hepatic vein extends through the centre of each lobule
      c. Portal triads (interlobular artery, portal vein, and bile duct) lie at the periphery of each lobule

C. Bile ducts (**Figure 39-13**)
   1. Small bile ducts form right and left hepatic ducts
   2. Right and left hepatic ducts immediately join to form one hepatic duct
   3. Hepatic duct merges with the cystic duct to form the common bile duct, which opens into the duodenum

D. Functions of the liver
   1. Detoxification by hepatocytes (liver cells)—ingested toxic substances and toxic substances formed in the intestines may be changed to nontoxic substances
   2. Breakdown and removal of old red blood cells, recycling the iron from haemoglobin
   3. Bile secretion by liver—bile salts are formed in the liver from cholesterol and are the most essential part of bile; liver cells secrete approximately 0.5 litres of bile per day
   4. Liver metabolism—carries out numerous important steps in metabolizing proteins, fats, and carbohydrates
   5. Storage of substances such as iron and some vitamins
   6. Production of important plasma proteins (e.g. clotting factors, albumin)
   7. A site for haematopoiesis during fetal development

Gallbladder

A. Size and location of the gallbladder
   1. Pear-shaped sac 7 to 10 cm long and 3 cm wide at its broadest point
   2. Lies on the undersurface of the liver (**Figure 39-13**)

B. Structure of the gallbladder
   1. Serous, muscular, and mucous layers compose the gallbladder wall
   2. The mucosal lining has rugae that expand to allow storage of bile; holds 30 to 50 mL of bile

C. Functions of the gallbladder
   1. Storage of bile
   2. Concentration of bile fivefold to tenfold
   3. Ejection of the concentrated bile into the duodenum

D. Gallstones—often made of cholesterol; can form when bile becomes concentrated (**Figure 39-14**)

Pancreas

A. Size and location of the pancreas
   1. Greyish pink–coloured gland; 12 to 15 cm long; weighs approximately 60 grams
   2. Runs from the duodenum, behind the stomach, to the spleen

B. Structure of the pancreas (**Figure 39-15**)—composed of endocrine and exocrine glandular tissue
   1. Exocrine portion makes up the majority of the pancreas; has a compound acinar arrangement; tiny ducts unite to form the main pancreatic duct, which empties into the duodenum
   2. Endocrine portion—embedded between exocrine units; called *pancreatic islets*; constitute only 2% of the total mass of the pancreas; made up of alpha cells and beta cells; pass secretions into capillaries

C. Functions of the pancreas
   1. Acinar units secrete digestive enzymes
   2. Beta cells secrete insulin
   3. Alpha cells secrete glucagon

Cycle of Life: Lower Digestive Tract

A. Changes in digestive function and structure are age-related
B. Infants have immature intestinal mucosa
   1. Intact proteins can pass through epithelial cells lining the tract and trigger an allergic response
   2. Lactose intolerance affects infants who lack the enzyme lactase
C. Ulcers and gallbladder disease common in middle age
D. Decreased digestive fluids, slowing of peristalsis, and reduced physical activity lead to constipation and diverticulosis in the elderly

The Big Picture: Digestive Tract

A. Specific features of structures throughout the digestive tract, such as grinding surfaces on teeth and muscles that can mix and propel nutrients, contribute to digestive function
B. External and internal nerves, along with endocrine hormones, regulate and coordinate digestive tract function
C. Blood and lymphatic tissues are available to help with nutrient absorption and transport

REVIEW QUESTIONS

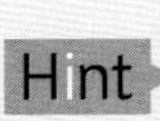

Write out the answers to these questions after reading the chapter and reviewing the Chapter Summary. Note—writing out your answers will consolidate learning and provide a valuable resource of information.

1. Draw or sketch a diagram of the divisions of the small intestine from proximal to distal.
2. In what area of the GI tract do you find villi? Haustra? Taeniae coli?
3. List the divisions of the large intestine.
4. What is believed to be the function of the vermiform appendix?
5. Discuss the general characteristics of the peritoneum and its reflections.
6. Discuss the anatomy of a typical liver lobule.
7. Identify the ducts of the liver and gallbladder.
8. Explain the functions of the gallbladder.
9. Differentiate between endocrine and exocrine functions of the pancreas.
10. Define cholelithiasis.

CRITICAL THINKING QUESTIONS

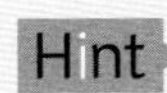

After finishing the Review Questions, write out the answers to these more in-depth questions to help you apply your new knowledge. Go back to sections of the chapter that relate to concepts that you find difficult.

1. Increasing the interior surface area of the small intestine allows it to absorb nutrients more efficiently. What structures can you identify that add to the interior surface area of the small intestine?
2. Explain the x-ray procedure used to diagnose an intestinal diverticulum.
3. If an elderly patient had abdominal pain, why would it be unlikely that it is caused by appendicitis?
4. Why is the liver considered to be a vital organ—which of the liver's functions are necessary for survival? How can a person survive after donating a lobe of their liver to another person?
5. Is the gallbladder a vital organ? Explain why or why not.
6. Which structure is responsible for preventing the intestines from becoming entangled with each other?

40 Digestion and Absorption

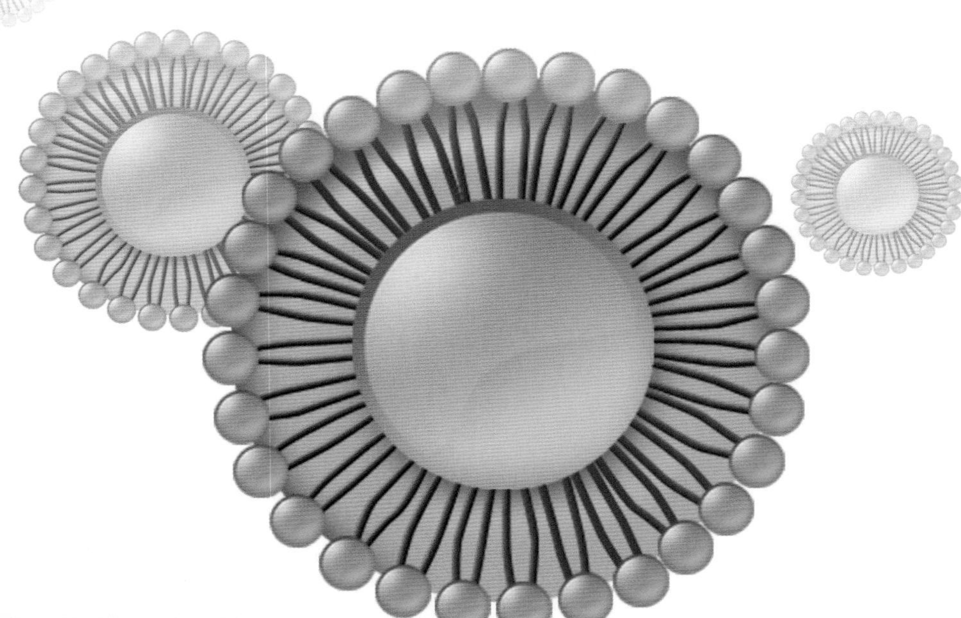

CHAPTER OUTLINE

Hint *Scan this outline before you begin to read the chapter, as a preview of how the concepts are organized.*

Now that we are familiar with the structural organization of the digestive system (Chapters 38 and 39), we are ready to understand the physiological organization of this system. The primary function of the digestive system is to bring essential nutrients into the internal environment so that they are available to each cell of the body. This chapter lays out the essential processes of digestion and absorption. Later, in Chapter 41, you will learn about how the body manages the nutrients after they have been absorbed into the internal environment.

LANGUAGE OF SCIENCE

Hint *Use this list to aid your pronunciation of unfamiliar words.*

absorption (ab-SORP-shun)
[*-ab-* **from,** *-sorp-* **suck,** *-tion* **process**]

amylase (AM-eh-layz)
[*amyl-* **starch,** *-ase* **enzyme**]

bile (byle)

bile salt (byle)

bilirubin (bil-ih-ROO-bin)
[*bili-* **bile,** *-rub-* **red,** *-in* **substance**]

cephalic phase (seh-FAL-ik fayz)
[*cephal-* **head,** *-ic* **relating to**]

cholecystokinin (CCK)
(koh-leh-sis-tuh-KYE-nin)
[*chole-* **bile,** *-cyst-* **bladder,** *-kin-* **move,** *-in* **substance**]

chylomicron (kye-loh-MY-kron)
[*chylo-* **juice (chyle),** *-micro-* **small,** *-on* **particle**]

chyme (kyme)
[*chym-* **juice**]

chymotrypsin (kye-moh-TRIP-sin)
[*chymo-* **juice,** *-tryps-* **pound,** *-in* **substance**]

colipase (koh-LYE-payz)
[*co-* **with,** *lip-* **fat,** *-ase* **enzyme**]

defaecation (def-eh-KAY-shun)
[*de-* **remove,** *-faeca-* **waste (faeces),** *-tion* **process**]

deglutition (deg-loo-TISH-un)
[*deglut-* **swallow,** *-tion* **process**]

digestion
[*digest-* **break apart,** *-tion* **process**]

elimination (ee-lim-ih-NAY-shun)
[*e-* **out,** *-limen-* **threshold,** *-ation* **process**]

emulsified (ee-MULL-seh-fyde)
[*e-* **out,** *-muls-* **milk,** *-i-* **combining form,** *-fy* **process**]

enteric nervous system (ENS)
(en-TER-ik)
[*enter-* **intestine,** *-ic* **relating to**]

enterogastric reflex
(en-ter-oh-GAS-trik)
[*entero-* **intestine,** *-gastr-* **stomach,** *-ic* **relating to,** *re-* **back or again,** *-flex* **bend**]

enterokinase (en-ter-oh-KYE-nays)
[*entero-* **intestine,** *-kin-* **movement,** *-ase* **enzyme**]

continued on p. 925

OVERVIEW OF DIGESTIVE FUNCTION

To accomplish the function of making nutrients available to each cell of the body, the digestive system uses various mechanisms (**Table 40-1**). For example, complex foods must first be taken in—a process called **ingestion.** Then, complex nutrients are broken down into simpler nutrients in the process that gives this system its name: **digestion.** To physically break large chunks of food into smaller bits and to move it along the tract, movement (or **motility**) of the gastrointestinal (GI) wall is required. Chemical digestion—that is, breakdown of large molecules into small molecules—requires **secretion** of digestive enzymes into the lumen of the GI tract. After being digested, nutrients are ready for the process of **absorption,** or movement through the GI mucosa into the internal environment. The material that is not absorbed must then be excreted to make room for more material—a process known as **elimination.** Of course, all these activities must be coordinated, which we have already learned is the process of *regulation.* Some of the major digestive processes are summarized in **Figure 40-1**. Digestive regulation is introduced in **Box 40-1**.

Note that **Figure 40-1** also illustrates that from a functional perspective, the lumen of the alimentary canal is really a tubelike extension of the external environment that goes right through the middle of the body. Thus digested materials are not truly "part of the body" until they've been absorbed into the internal environment.

After we have explored the various mechanisms of the digestive process in this chapter, we will be ready for Chapter 41, which discusses the assimilation of nutrients after they have been absorbed.

DIGESTION

After food is ingested (taken into the mouth), the process of digestion begins immediately. Digestion is the overall name for all the processes that chemically and mechanically break complex foods into simpler nutrients that can be easily absorbed. We begin our discussion with a brief overview of *mechanical digestion* and then move on to a discussion of *chemical digestion.*

TABLE 40-1 Primary Mechanisms of the Digestive System

MECHANISM	DESCRIPTION
Ingestion	Process of taking food into the mouth, starting it on its journey through the digestive tract
Digestion	A group of processes that break complex nutrients into simpler ones, thus facilitating their absorption; mechanical digestion physically breaks large chunks into small bits; chemical digestion breaks molecules apart
Motility	Movement by the muscular components of the digestive tube, including processes of mechanical digestion; examples include peristalsis and segmentation
Secretion	Release of digestive juices (containing enzymes, acids, bases, mucus, bile, or other products that facilitate digestion); some digestive organs also secrete endocrine hormones that regulate digestion or metabolism of nutrients
Absorption	Movement of digested nutrients through the gastrointestinal (GI) mucosa and into the internal environment
Elimination	Excretion of the residues of the digestive process (faeces) from the rectum, through the anus; defaecation
Regulation	Coordination of digestive activity (motility, secretion, etc.)

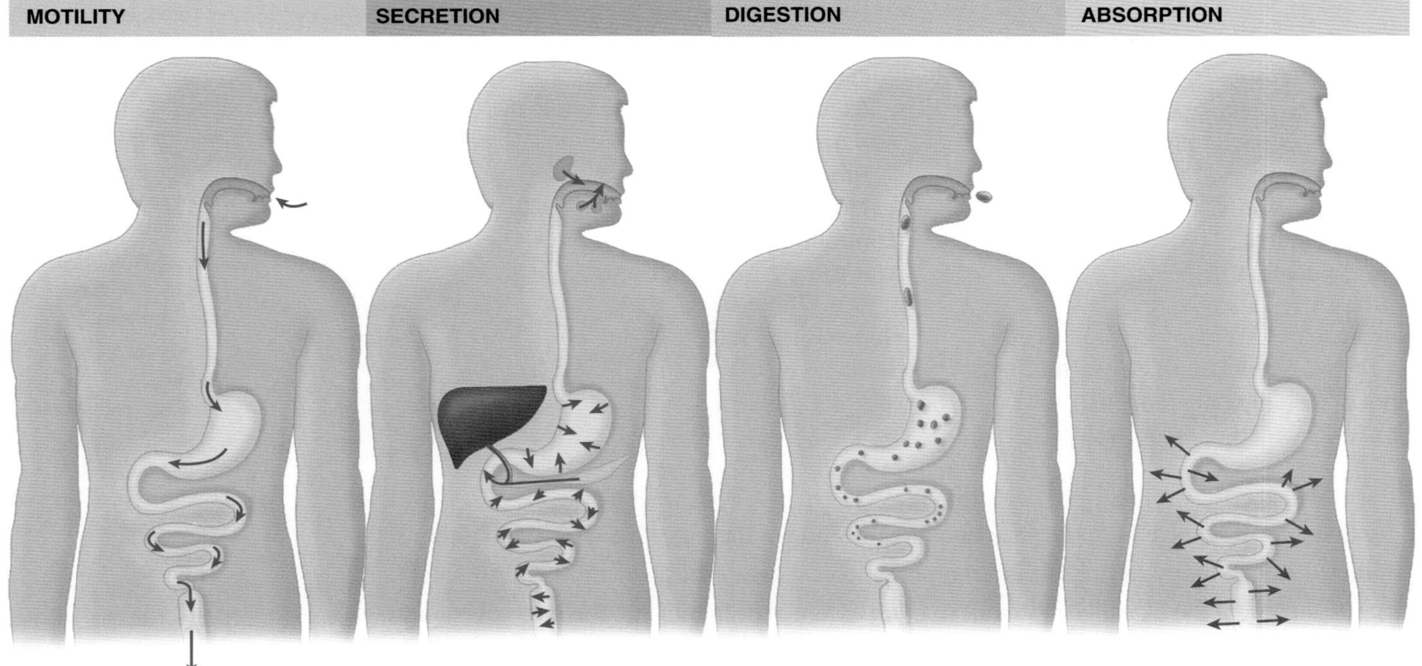

FIGURE 40-1 Overview of digestive functions. Several important digestive functions are summarized in these diagrams. Note that the digestive tract is an extension of the external environment—extending like a tunnel through the body.

BOX 40-1 *the enteric nervous system*

As we discussed in Chapter 38, the gastrointestinal (GI) wall includes an *intramural plexus* of nerve pathways. This complex arrangement of neurons is made up largely of the submucosal plexus (of Meissner) and the myenteric plexus (of Auerbach). **Figure 38-2** on p. 862 clarifies the locations of these two structures and also shows that they are connected not only to each other but also to the central nervous system (CNS) and the GI muscles and mucous membrane. All these structures work together in a coordinated system called the **enteric nervous system (ENS).**

The ENS is often called a "mini brain" or "second brain" because it includes afferent neurons, interneurons, and efferent neurons that independently operate their own nervous reflexes. Thus the ENS can act as "its own brain" in many ways. However, the ENS is certainly influenced by the CNS—as you can see in the diagram here. Because it operates as an involuntary, autonomic system, many physiologists consider the ENS to be another division of the autonomic nervous system (ANS). As the diagram shows, there is certainly communication between the ENS and the various divisions of the ANS.

Operation of the ENS, like that of the brain, seems to involve the storage and retrieval of memories and the establishment of repeating patterns of response.

Of course, this "second brain" has a complete set of different neurotransmitters that help carry out the complex functions of coordinating enteric reflexes. The list of major ENS neurotransmitters includes some familiar names: acetylcholine (ACh), enkephalins, substance P, serotonin, and nitric oxide (NO). Also on the list is an important peptide neurotransmitter, vasoactive intestinal peptide (VIP). Like other peptide neurotransmitters, VIP helps modulate neuron function—in this case, involving inhibition of intestinal smooth muscle or stimulation of intestinal secretions.

The ENS also helps establish a nervous-immune connection (*neuroimmune* function). For example, neurotransmitters from the ANS and from the ENS can stimulate mast cells in the wall of the GI tract to release histamine and other regulatory molecules. Histamine, for example, stimulates acid secretion in the stomach, besides having the immune functions previously discussed (see Chapter 32).

As we shall see throughout this chapter, the ENS works with other divisions of the nervous system, with the endocrine system, and with local regulatory mechanisms to achieve the coordination of incredibly complex, finely tuned mechanisms of motility (movement), secretion, digestion, and other functions. •

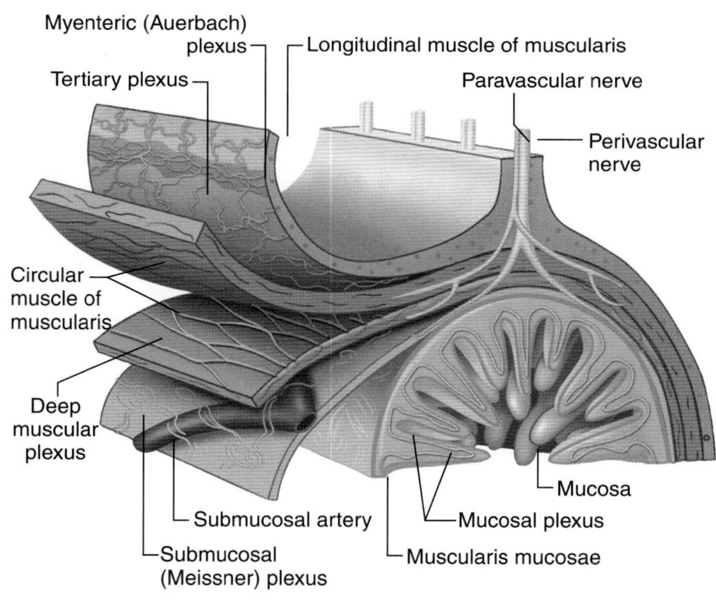

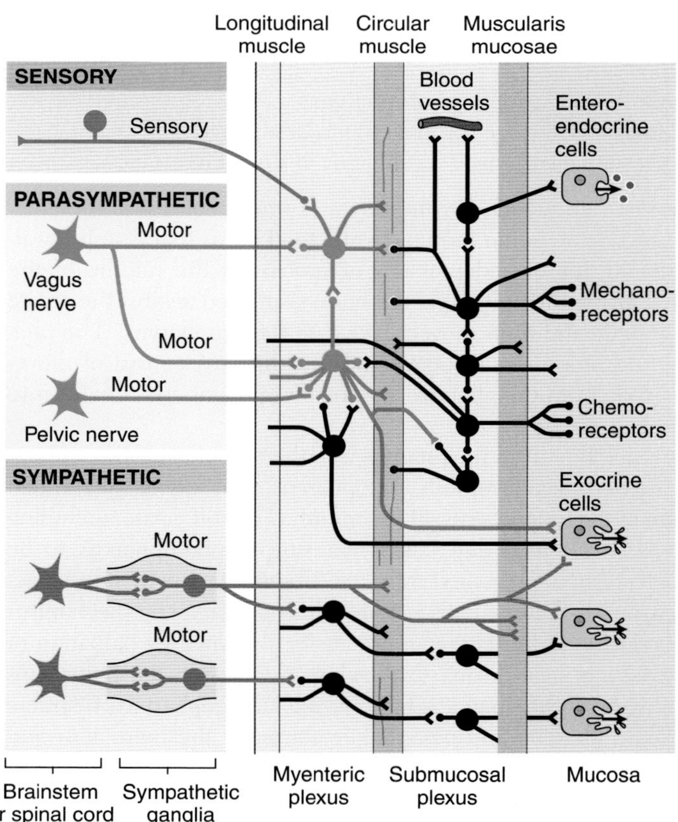

Enteric nervous system (ENS). This diagram shows some typical neural pathways involved in the ENS. Although the ENS can operate its own independent regulatory system, it is also interconnected with various divisions of the autonomic nervous system (ANS).

MECHANICAL DIGESTION

Mechanical digestion consists of all movement (motility) of the digestive tract that brings about the following:

- Change in the physical state of ingested food from comparatively large solid pieces into minute particles, thereby facilitating chemical digestion
- Churning of the contents of the GI lumen in such a way that they become well mixed with the digestive juices and all parts of them come in contact with the surface of the intestinal mucosa, thereby facilitating absorption
- Propelling the food forward along the digestive tract, and finally eliminating the digestive wastes from the body

Mastication

Mechanical digestion begins in the mouth when the particle size of ingested food material is reduced by chewing movements, or **mastication.** The tongue, cheeks, and lips play an important role in keeping food material between the cutting or grinding surfaces of the teeth when a person is biting off or chewing food. In addition to reducing particle size, chewing movements serve to mix food with saliva in preparation for swallowing.

Deglutition

The process of swallowing, or **deglutition,** involves three main steps, or stages, that may be divided into the formation and then movement of a food bolus from the mouth to the stomach (**Figure 40-2**):

1. Oral stage (mouth to oropharynx)
2. Pharyngeal stage (oropharynx to oesophagus)
3. Oesophageal stage (oesophagus to stomach)

The first step, which is voluntary and under control of the cerebral cortex, involves the formation of a food bolus that is to be swallowed by means of a depression or groove in the middle of the tongue. During the oral stage, the bolus is pressed against the palate by the tongue and then moved back into the oropharynx. The pharyngeal and oesophageal stages, both involuntary, consist of movement of food from the pharynx into the oesophagus and, finally, into the stomach.

To propel food from the pharynx into the oesophagus, three openings must be blocked: mouth, nasopharynx, and larynx. Continued elevation of the tongue seals off the mouth. The soft palate, including the uvula, is elevated and tensed, causing the nasopharynx to be closed off. Food is prevented from entering the larynx by muscle action that causes the epiglottis to block this opening. The mechanism involves raising of the larynx, a process easily noted by palpation of the thyroid cartilage during swallowing. As a result, the bolus slips over the back of the epiglottis to enter the laryngopharynx. Contractions of the pharynx and oesophagus compress the bolus into and through the oesophageal tube. These steps are involuntary and under control of the *deglutition centre* in the medulla. The presence of a bolus stimulates sensory receptors in the mouth and pharynx, thus initiating reflex pharyngeal contractions. Consequently, anaesthesia of sensory nerves from the mucosa of the mouth and pharynx by a drug such as procaine makes swallowing difficult or impossible.

Swallowing is a complex process requiring the coordination of many muscles and other structures in the head and neck. The process must not only occur smoothly but also take place rapidly because respiration is inhibited for the 1 to 3 seconds required for food to clear the pharynx during each swallow.

Peristalsis and Segmentation

After food enters the lower portion of the oesophagus, smooth muscle tissue in the wall of the GI tract takes on primary responsibility for its movement (**Box 40-2**). The motility produced by smooth muscle is of two main types: peristalsis and segmentation.

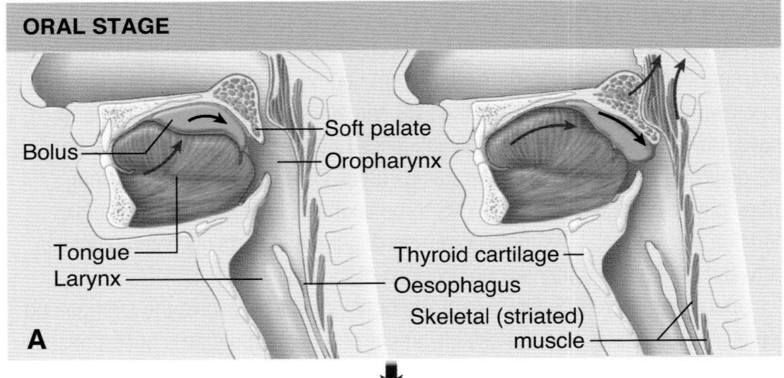

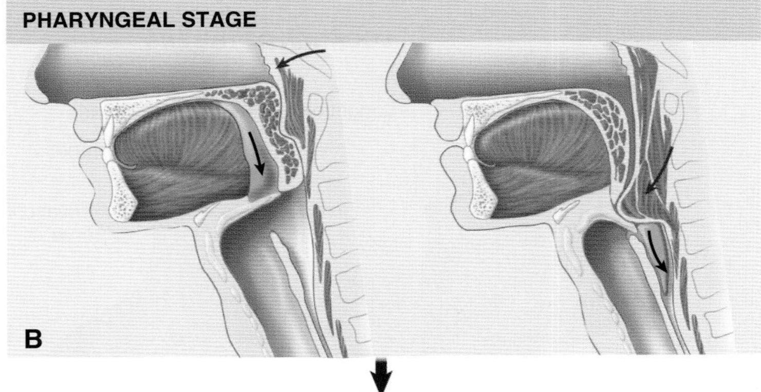

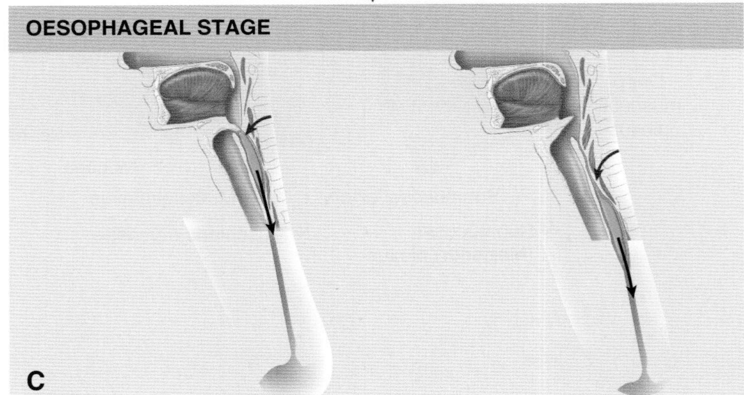

FIGURE 40-2 Deglutition. A, *Oral stage.* During this stage of deglutition (swallowing), a bolus of food is voluntarily formed on the tongue and pushed against the palate and then into the oropharynx. Notice that the soft palate acts as a valve that prevents food from entering the nasopharynx. **B,** *Pharyngeal stage.* After the bolus has entered the oropharynx, involuntary reflexes push the bolus down toward the oesophagus. Notice that upward movement of the larynx and downward movement of the bolus close the epiglottis and thus prevent food from entering the lower respiratory tract. **C,** *Oesophageal stage.* Involuntary reflexes of skeletal (striated) and smooth muscle in the wall of the oesophagus move the bolus through the oesophagus toward the stomach.

BOX 40-2 *smooth muscle function in the GI tract*

Smooth muscle tissue in the wall of the gastrointestinal (GI) tract differs from other types of muscle tissue in a number of important ways. For example, smooth muscle is slow compared with skeletal muscle. Because the sliding of myofilaments proceeds at a much slower pace than in skeletal muscle, smooth muscle often exhibits a prolonged contraction phase. Because the same amount of energy is used for slow contraction as for fast contraction, GI muscle can sustain tension for long periods without fatigue—exactly what is needed for the long process of digestion.

Another unique functional characteristic of smooth muscle is its ability to maintain *basal tone*. The basal tone is a continuous state of minimal contraction. Continuous tension is maintained in cells that have enough calcium ions free in the sarcoplasm to generate the contraction response. The force of contraction can increase above the basal tone by way of the effects of an action potential, which causes rapid influx of extracellular calcium.

Gastrointestinal *sphincter* muscles, as you recall from the previous chapter, are ringlike formations of smooth muscle in the GI wall that act as gateways or valves that regulate movement of chyme from one part of the tract to the next part. Sphincter muscles generally have a higher basal tone than does surrounding smooth muscle—thus constricting the lumen and "keeping the gate closed". Usually, stimuli in a section preceding the sphincter trigger a decrease in basal tone to allow material to pass through. Some of these reflexes are discussed later in this chapter.

Most of the smooth muscles in the GI wall are electrically coupled by gap junctions—so-called *single-unit* muscles. Such electrical coupling allows for intrinsic control of smooth muscle contraction, as in cardiac muscle. Smooth muscle fibres exhibit an intrinsic, rhythmic fluctuation in membrane voltage that is sometimes called *basic electrical rhythm (BER)*. As part *A* of the figure shows, the peaks of these slow waves sometimes reach the threshold potential—thus triggering bursts of action potentials. Because the fibres are electrically coupled, action potentials generated in one fibre spread rapidly to many surrounding fibres. This phenomenon is called *pacemaker activity* (as we have already seen in the heart with cardiac muscle fibres). Part *A* of the figure shows the effect of pacemaker activity on the force generated in a local area of the GI muscle. Between action potentials, the muscle cells exhibit the basal tone—but when stimulated by pacemaker potentials, the contractile force increases dramatically. The end result of pacemaker activity is a somewhat rhythmic increase and decrease in smooth muscle tension.

In part *B* of the figure, you can see that the small intestine shows an unusual pattern of this rhythmic pacemaker activity during the fasting state. In the fasting state, the electrical rhythm (and therefore the rhythm of contraction) is relatively quiet, except for a coordinated wave of motor activity every 1½ to 2 hours. Each wave of rhythmic contractions is called a **migrating motor complex (MMC).** One function of the MMC is thought to be that of clearing out any remaining material, such as larger, indigestible particles, bile and other secretions, bacteria, and sloughed off epithelial cells. The MMC pattern is largely triggered by the hormone **motilin** released from endocrine cells in the duodenum.

Once material enters a segment of the digestive tract, the slow basic rhythm of contraction changes to the rapid rhythms of *segmentation* (mixing actions) and *peristalsis* (progressive movement).

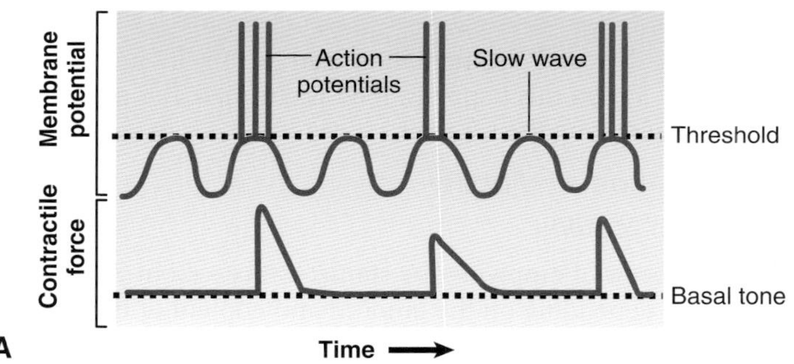

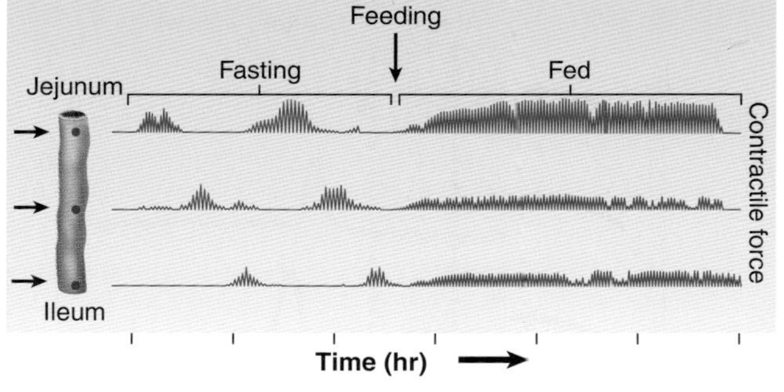

A, Pacemaker activity of smooth muscle. As the upper graph line shows, the membrane potential of smooth muscle exhibits a rhythmic fluctuation (the basic electrical rhythm). Occasionally, the fluctuating membrane potential reaches the threshold—triggering one or more action potentials that spread to surrounding muscle fibres. Smooth muscles are continually partially contracted (the basal tone), but the force of contraction increases dramatically with each burst of action potentials (bottom graph line). The more action potentials that occur in a short series, the stronger the force of contraction. **B, Migrating motor complex (MMC).** In the small intestine, the basal rhythm of smooth muscle contractions during the fasting state is characterized by occasional waves of motor activity called *migrating motor complexes (MMCs)*. These waves of contraction slowly "sweep out" the intestinal lumen between active digestive periods (fed states). During the fed state, the MMC pattern disappears and is replaced by a more rapid, active pattern that includes peristalsis and segmentation.

UNIT 5

Peristalsis is often described as a wavelike ripple of the muscle layer of a hollow organ. The diagram in **Figure 40-3** shows step by step how peristalsis occurs. A bolus stretches the GI wall, triggering a reflex contraction of circular muscle that pushes the bolus forward. This, in turn, triggers a reflex contraction in that location, pushing the bolus even further. This process continues as long as the stretch reflex is activated by the presence of food. Peristalsis is a progressive kind of motility—that is, a type of motion that produces forward movement of ingested material along the GI tract. **Figure 40-4** shows the effects of peristaltic contractions in the oesophagus during deglutition.

Segmentation can be described simply as mixing movement. Segmentation occurs when digestive reflexes cause a forward and backward movement within a single region, or segment, of the GI tract (**Figure 40-5**). Such movement helps mechanically break down food particles, mixes food and digestive juices thoroughly, and

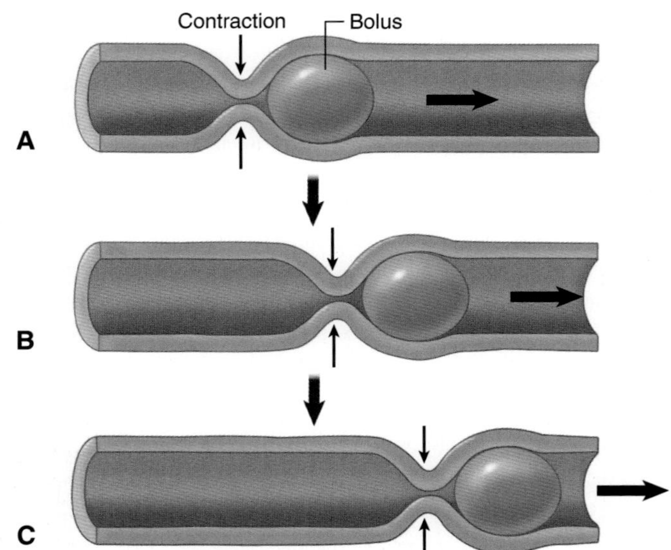

FIGURE 40-3 Peristalsis. Peristalsis is a progressive type of movement in which material is propelled from point to point along the gastrointestinal (GI) tract. **A,** A ring of contraction occurs where the GI wall is stretched, and the bolus is pushed forward. **B,** The moving bolus triggers a ring of contraction in the next region that pushes the bolus even further along. **C,** The ring of contraction moves like a wave along the GI tract to push the bolus forward.

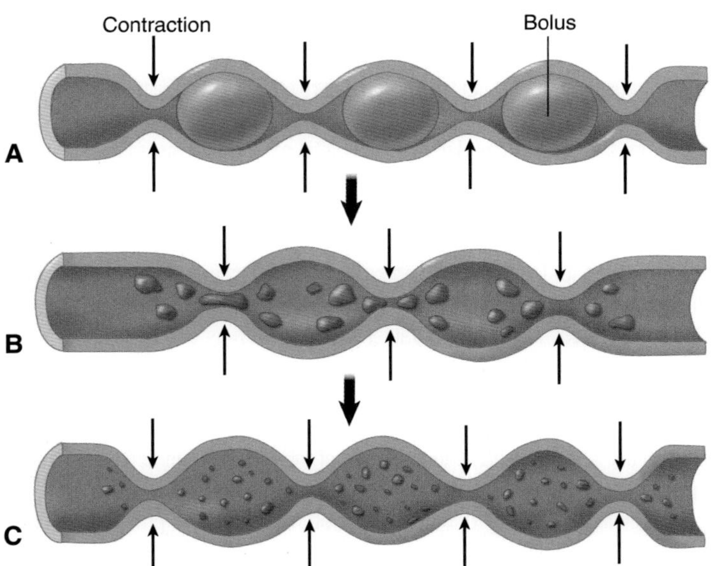

FIGURE 40-5 Segmentation. Segmentation is a back-and-forth action that breaks apart chunks of food and mixes in digestive juices. **A,** Ringlike regions of contraction occur at intervals along the gastrointestinal (GI) tract. **B,** Previously contracted regions relax and adjacent regions now contract, effectively "chopping" the contents of each segment into smaller chunks. **C,** The location of the contracted regions continues to alternate back and forth, chopping and mixing the contents of the GI lumen.

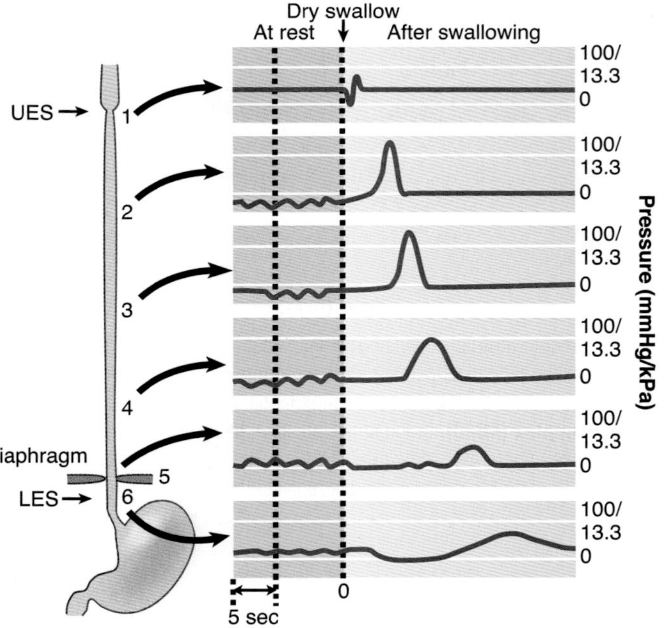

FIGURE 40-4 Pressure in the oesophagus during swallowing. This diagram shows the changing pressure (mmHg/kPa) inside the oesophagus during the oesophageal stage of deglutition (swallowing) (see **Figure 40-2**). Note that an area of high pressure moves progressively down the oesophagus—and eventually to the stomach. Note that during the rest period before swallowing, the smooth muscle exhibits a slow rhythm of weak contractions. *UES,* Upper oesophageal sphincter; *LES,* lower oesophageal [cardiac] sphincter.

brings digested food in contact with intestinal mucosa to facilitate absorption.

Peristalsis and segmentation can occur in an alternating sequence. When this happens, food is churned and mixed as it slowly progresses along the GI tract.

Regulation of Motility

Gastric Motility

The process of emptying the stomach takes about 2 to 6 hours after a meal, depending on the amount and content of the meal. During its "storage time" in the stomach, food is churned with gastric juices to form a thick, milky material known as **chyme,** which is ejected about every 20 seconds into the duodenum. As you can see in **Figure 40-6**, while chyme is in the stomach, it is continually being pushed toward the pyloric sphincter by waves of peristaltic contractions—a process called **propulsion.** Because the pyloric sphincter remains closed most of the time, the chyme is forced to move backward—a process called **retropulsion.** Thus, because the chyme is temporarily "trapped", peristalsis creates a sort of back-and-forth movement that helps mix the chyme and gastric juice. Eventually, the contraction force of the pyloric sphincter decreases, allowing a little of the chyme to pass through to the duodenum.

Because the volume of the stomach is large and that of the duodenum is small, gastric emptying must be regulated to prevent overburdening of the duodenum. Such control occurs by way of two principal mechanisms—one hormonal and one nervous. Fats and other nutrients in the duodenum stimulate the intestinal mucosa to release a hormone called **gastric inhibitory peptide (GIP)** into the

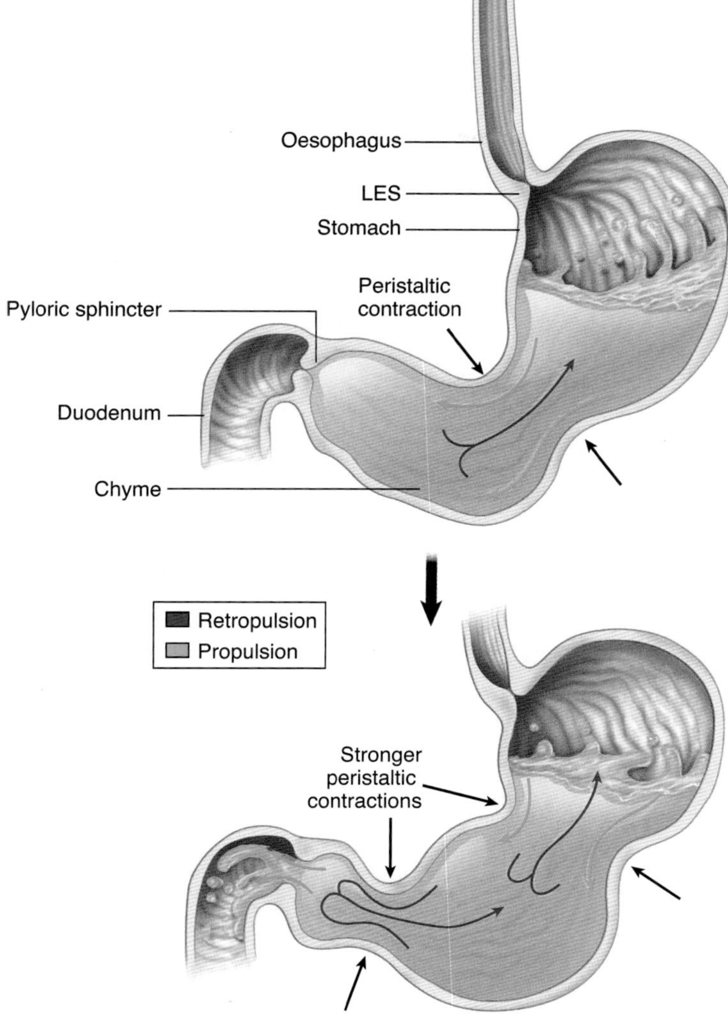

FIGURE 40-6 Gastric motility. Mixing actions in the stomach include both propulsion (forward movement) and retropulsion (backward movement). As peristaltic contractions become stronger, some of the liquid chyme squirts past the pyloric sphincter (which has decreased its muscle tone) and into the duodenum. The stomach continues to mix the chyme as it is gradually released into the duodenum.

bloodstream. GIP is also called *glucose-dependent insulinotropic polypeptide (GIP)*. When it reaches the stomach wall via the circulation, GIP has an inhibitory effect on gastric muscle, decreasing its peristalsis and thus slowing passage of food into the duodenum. Nervous control results from receptors in the duodenal mucosa that are sensitive to the presence of acid and to distention. Sensory and motor fibres in the vagus nerve then cause a reflex inhibition of gastric peristalsis. This nervous mechanism is known as the **enterogastric reflex.**

Box 40-3 discusses one important application of concepts of gastric motility.

Intestinal Motility

Intestinal motility includes both peristaltic contractions and segmentation. Segmentation in the duodenum and upper jejunum mixes the incoming chyme with digestive juices from the pancreas, liver, and intestinal mucosa. This mixing action also allows the products of digestion to contact the intestinal mucosa, where they can be absorbed into the internal environment. Peristalsis continues as the chyme nears the end of the jejunum—moving the food through the rest of the small intestine and into the large intestine. After leaving the stomach, chyme normally takes about 5 hours to pass all the way through the small intestine.

Several mechanisms are involved in the control of intestinal motility. Peristalsis is regulated in part by the intrinsic stretch reflexes already described. It is also thought to be stimulated by the hormone **cholecystokinin (CCK),** which is secreted by endocrine cells of the intestinal mucosa when chyme is present.

A list of definitions of the different processes involved in mechanical digestion, along with the organs that accomplish them, is presented in **Table 40-2**.

Quick CHECK

1. What is meant by the term *motility*?
2. Is deglutition a voluntary or involuntary process?
3. What is the purpose of peristalsis?
4. What triggers the *enterogastric reflex* to inhibit gastric emptying?

BOX 40-3 *sports and fitness* | Exercise and Fluid Uptake

Replacement of fluids lost through sweating during exercise is essential for maintaining homeostasis. Nearly everyone increases the intake of fluids during and after exercise. The main limitation to efficient fluid replacement is how quickly fluid can be absorbed rather than how much a person drinks. Very little water is absorbed until it reaches the intestines, where it is absorbed almost immediately. Thus the rate of *gastric emptying* into the intestine is critical.

Large volumes of fluid leave the stomach and enter the intestines more rapidly than small volumes do. However, having large volumes in the stomach may be uncomfortable during exercise. Cool fluids (8° to 13°C) empty more quickly than warm fluids. Fluids with a high solute concentration empty slowly and may cause nausea or stomach cramps. Thus large amounts of cool, dilute, or isotonic fluids are best for replacing fluids quickly during exercise. •

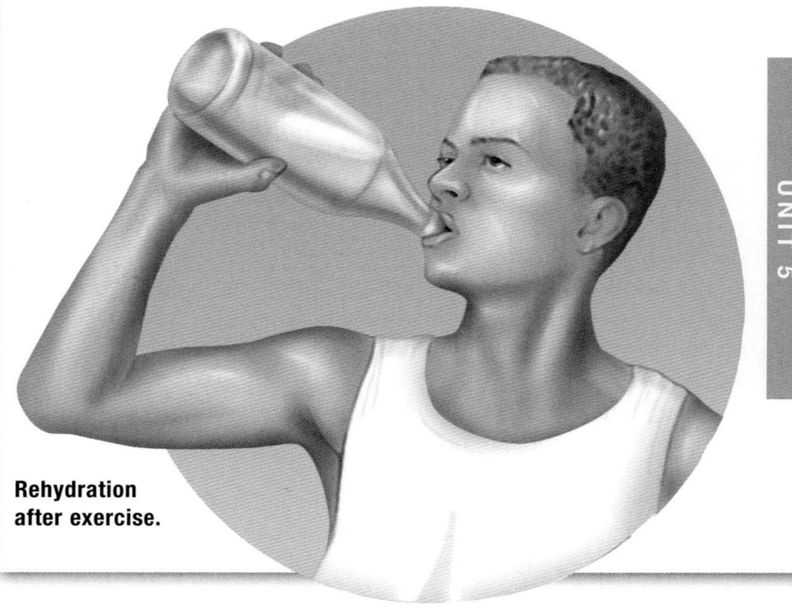

Rehydration after exercise.

UNIT 5

TABLE 40-2 Processes of Mechanical Digestion

ORGAN	MECHANICAL PROCESS	NATURE OF PROCESS
Mouth (teeth and tongue)	Mastication	Chewing movements—reduce size of food particles and mix them with saliva
	Deglutition	Swallowing—movement of food from mouth to stomach
Pharynx	Deglutition	See description above
Oesophagus	Deglutition	See description above
	Peristalsis	Rippling movements that squeeze food downward in digestive tract; a constricted ring forms first in one section, then the next, and so on, causing waves of contraction to spread along entire canal
Stomach	Churning	Forward and backward movement (propulsion/retropulsion) of gastric contents, mixing food with gastric juices to form chyme
	Peristalsis	Wave starting in body of stomach that occurs about three times per minute and sweeps toward closed pyloric sphincter; at intervals, strong peristaltic waves press chyme past sphincter into duodenum
Small intestine	Segmentation (mixing contractions)	Forward and backward movement within segment of intestine; purpose is to mix food and digestive juices thoroughly and to bring all digested food into contact with intestinal mucosa to facilitate absorption; purpose of peristalsis, on the other hand, is to propel intestinal contents along digestive tract
	Peristalsis	
Large intestine		
Colon	Segmentation	Churning movements within haustral sacs
	Peristalsis	Wavelike progressive movement of colon contents
Descending colon	Mass peristalsis	Entire contents moved into sigmoid colon and rectum; occurs three or four times a day, usually after a meal
Rectum	Defaecation	Emptying of rectum, so-called bowel movement

CHEMICAL DIGESTION

Chemical digestion consists of all the changes in chemical composition that foods undergo in their travel through the digestive tract. These changes result from the hydrolysis of foods. **Hydrolysis** is a chemical process in which a compound unites with water and then splits into simpler compounds (see Chapter 3). Numerous enzymes in the various digestive juices catalyze the hydrolysis of foods.

Digestive Enzymes

Overview of Digestive Enzymes

Enzymes were briefly introduced in Chapter 3 and their important functional roles were more fully discussed in Chapter 6 (see pp. 109–111). Although our interest until now has primarily concerned *intracellular enzymes*, our current discussion focuses on extracellular digestive enzymes. In the following paragraphs we briefly review enzymes in general and outline some characteristics of *digestive enzymes* in particular.

Recall that enzymes can be defined simply as "organic catalysts"; that is, they are organic compounds (proteins), and they accelerate chemical reactions without appearing in the final products of the reaction.

Recall the two systems used for naming enzymes: the suffix *-ase* is used with the root name of the substance whose chemical reaction is catalyzed (the substrate chemical, that is) or with the word that describes the kind of chemical reaction catalyzed. Thus, according to the first method, lipase is an enzyme that catalyzes a chemical reaction in which a lipid takes part. According to the second method, lipase might also be called a *hydrolase* because it catalyzes the hydrolysis of lipids. Enzymes investigated before these methods of nomenclature were adopted are still called by older names, such as **pepsin** and **trypsin**—both proteases (protein-digesting enzymes).

Enzymes can be classified as intracellular or extracellular, depending on whether they act within cells or outside of them in the surrounding medium. Most enzymes act intracellularly in the body; an important exception is the digestive enzymes. Digestive enzymes are classified as extracellular because they operate in the lumen of the digestive tract, outside any cells of the body. All digestive enzymes are classified chemically as hydrolases because they catalyze the hydrolysis of food molecules—the breakdown of a molecule using water.

Properties of Digestive Enzymes

As with any type of enzyme, digestive enzymes are *specific in their action*; that is, they act only on a specific substrate. This is attributed to a key-in-a-lock kind of action, the configuration of the enzyme molecule fitting the configuration of some part of the substrate molecule (**Figure 40-7**).

Digestive enzymes *function optimally at a specific pH* and become inactive if the pH deviates beyond narrow limits (**Figure 40-8**). This effect occurs because changes in the hydrogen ion (H^+) concentration influence the chemical attractions that hold all protein molecules—including enzymes—in their complex, multidimensional shapes. In short, changing the pH changes the shape of an enzyme molecule—possibly rendering it inactive.

Different digestive enzymes require different H^+ concentrations in their environment for optimal functioning. This is because the

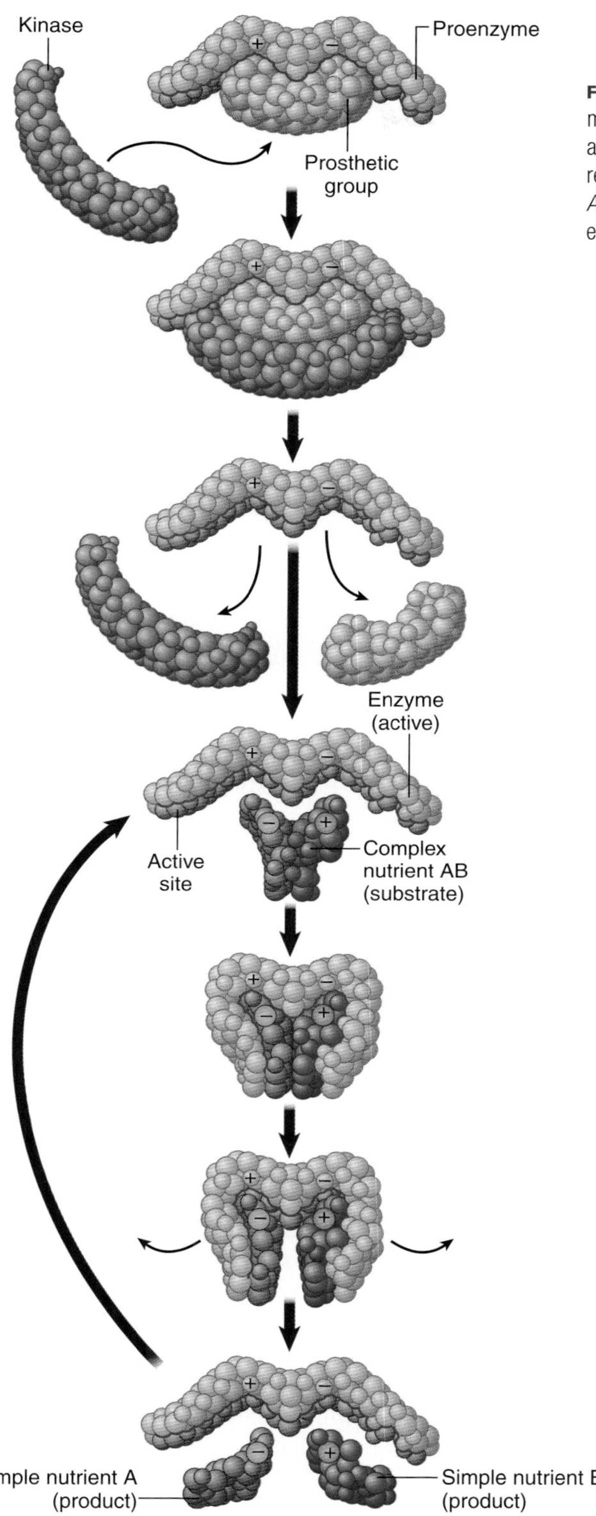

FIGURE 40-7 Model of digestive enzyme action. Enzymes are functional proteins whose molecular shape allows them to catalyze chemical reactions. First, an inactive proenzyme must be altered by an activating enzyme called a *kinase.* The kinase often accomplishes the activation by removing a prosthetic group from the proenzyme, exposing an active site. A complex nutrient molecule *AB* is acted on by the active digestive enzyme, yielding simpler nutrient molecules *A* and *B.* The active enzyme can then digest another complex nutrient molecule.

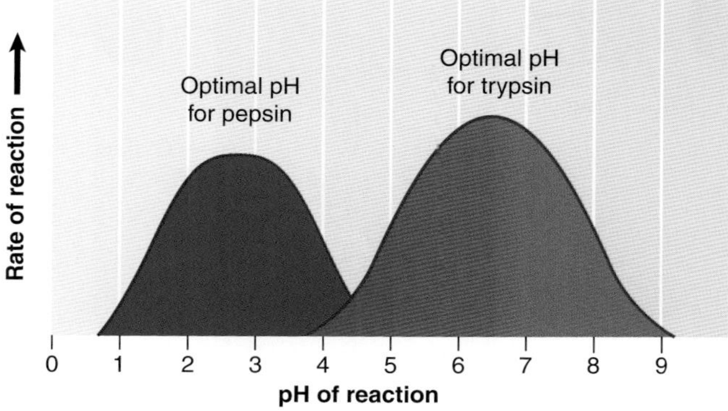

FIGURE 40-8 Effect of pH on digestive enzyme function. Digestive enzymes catalyze chemical reactions with greatest efficiency within a narrow range of pH. For example, *pepsin* (a protein-digesting enzyme in gastric juice) operates within a low pH range, whereas *trypsin* (a protein-digesting enzyme in pancreatic juice) operates within a higher pH range.

H^+ concentration influences the shape of each enzyme molecule. Amylase, the main enzyme in saliva, functions best in the neutral to slightly acid pH range characteristic of saliva. It is gradually inactivated by the marked acidity of gastric juice. In contrast, pepsin, an enzyme in gastric juice, is inactive unless sufficient hydrochloric acid is present. Therefore, in diseases characterized by gastric hypoacidity, dilute hydrochloric acid is given orally before meals.

Most enzymes catalyze a chemical reaction in both directions, the direction and rate of the reaction being governed by the rate law (law of mass action). An accumulation of a product slows the reaction and tends to reverse it. A practical application of this fact is the slowing of digestion when absorption is interfered with and the products of digestion accumulate. However, digestive enzyme reactions do not ordinarily reverse themselves in the digestive tract.

Digestive enzymes are continually being destroyed or eliminated from the body and therefore have to be continually synthesized, even though they are not used up in the reactions they catalyze.

Most digestive enzymes are synthesized and secreted as inactive **proenzymes** (see **Figure 40-7**). Enzymes that break apart proenzymes and thus convert them to active enzymes are often called *kinases.* For example, enterokinase is a kinase that changes inactive trypsinogen into active trypsin.

Although we eat six main types of chemical substances (carbohydrates, proteins, lipids, vitamins, mineral salts, and water), only the first three have to be chemically digested to be absorbed.

Carbohydrate Digestion

Carbohydrates are saccharide compounds. This means that their molecules contain one or more saccharide groups ($C_6H_{10}O_5$). Polysaccharides, notably starches and glycogen, contain many of these groups. Disaccharides (sucrose, lactose, and maltose) contain two of them, and monosaccharides (glucose, fructose, and galactose) contain only one. Polysaccharides are hydrolyzed to disaccharides by enzymes known as **amylases,** found in saliva and pancreatic juice (salivary amylase is sometimes called *ptyalin*). The enzymes that catalyze the final steps in carbohydrate digestion are *sucrase, lactase,* and *maltase* (**Figure 40-9**). These enzymes are located in the cell membrane of epithelial cells covering the villi and, therefore, lining the intestinal lumen. The substrates (disaccharides) bind onto the

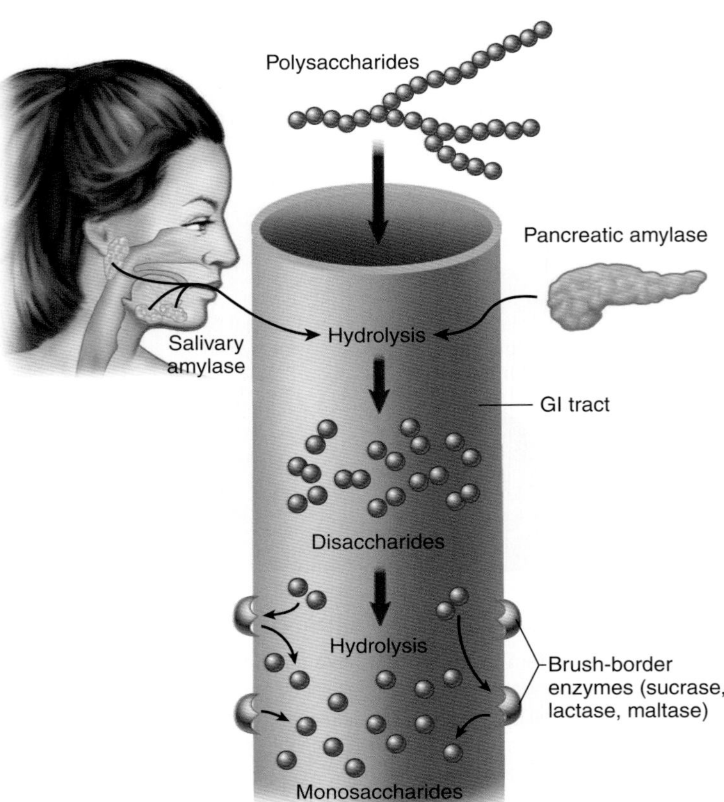

FIGURE 40-9 Carbohydrate digestion. Amylase in saliva and pancreatic juice hydrolyzes polysaccharides into disaccharides. Brush-border disaccharidases in the lining of the small intestine then promote hydrolysis of the disaccharides into monosaccharides.

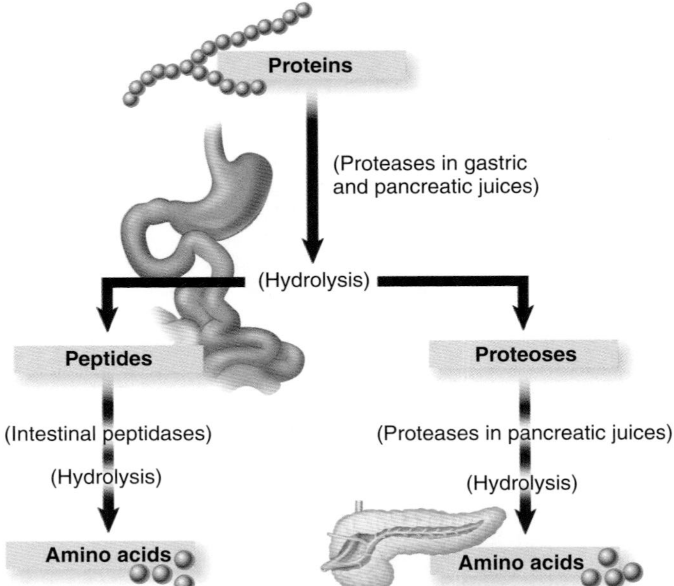

FIGURE 40-10 Protein digestion. Gastric juice protease (pepsin) and pancreatic juice proteases (trypsin and chymotrypsin) hydrolyze proteins into proteoses and peptides. Protein digestion is then completed by pancreatic proteases, which hydrolyze proteoses into amino acids, and by intestinal peptidases, which hydrolyze peptides into amino acids.

enzymes at the surface of the brush border, giving the name **contact digestion** to the process. The resulting end products of digestion, mainly glucose, are conveniently located at the site of absorption (and are not floating around somewhere in the lumen).

Protein Digestion

Protein compounds have very large molecules made up of folded or twisted chains of amino acids, often hundreds in number. Enzymes called **proteases** catalyze the hydrolysis of proteins first into a variety of intermediate compounds called proteoses and peptides, which are simply shorter strands of amino acids. Then, finally, proteases break these shorter molecules into individual amino acids (**Figure 40-10**).

The main proteases are **pepsin** in gastric juice, **trypsin** and **chymotrypsin** in pancreatic juice, and **peptidases** of the intestinal brush border (**Box 40-4**). Peptidases are also present within each intestinal cell, where they break apart dipeptides and tripeptides absorbed into these cells. Each kind of protease catalyzes the breaking apart of a specific kind of peptide bond. Because different amino acid combinations within a protein or polypeptide can have slightly different kinds of peptide bonds holding them together, a whole arsenal of different proteases is needed for efficient protein digestion.

Fat Digestion

Because fats are insoluble in water, they must be **emulsified**—that is, dispersed into very small droplets, before they can be digested. Some dietary fats such as those in dairy products may already be emulsified when ingested. Otherwise, two substances found in bile, **lecithin** and **bile salts,** will emulsify dietary oils and fats in the lumen of the small intestine. Bile is produced in the liver and stored and concentrated in the gallbladder. Bile is released into the lumen of the GI tract by way of the common bile duct.

Lecithin is a phospholipid similar to other phospholipids that make up the bulk of cellular membranes (see **Figures 4-8** on p. 60 and **5-3** on p. 79). As **Figure 40-11** shows, lecithin mixes with lipids and water, forming tiny spheres called **micelles.** In forming a micelle, lecithin molecules align to form a shell that surrounds the lipid. Alignment of lecithin molecules results from the fact that the polar heads of this molecule are attracted by polar water molecules and the nonpolar tails of lecithin are lipid-soluble. Thus the hydrophilic (polar) heads form the outer face of the shell and the hydrophobic (nonpolar) tails form the inner face of the shell. Bile salts, which are derived from the lipid cholesterol, emulsify fats by forming micelles in the same manner.

The mechanical process of emulsification facilitates chemical digestion of fats by breaking large fat drops into small droplets. This process provides a greater contact area between fat molecules and pancreatic **lipases,** the main lipid-digesting enzymes (**Figure 40-12**). Triglycerides (fats), important dietary lipids, are broken down by lipases to yield fatty acids, monoglycerides, and glycerol molecules. Other lipids are similarly broken down into their respective component chemical groups. For example, a phospholipid molecule can be

BOX 40-4 *the brush border*

The term **brush border** refers to the microvilli on the epithelial cells that line the small intestine, visible in the figures. These microvilli are on the apical surfaces of the epithelial cells—the surfaces that face the interior of the intestinal lumen. Because when viewed under high magnification the microvilli look like the bristles of a brush, the surface of the intestinal mucosa was nicknamed "brush border".

The brush border represents the boundary between the external environment (the lumen of the alimentary canal) and the internal environment of the body. It is across this border that molecules must pass if they are going to be absorbed into the body.

The brush border possesses an incredibly large surface area because the microvilli increase the apical surface area. There are usually 2000 to 3000 microvilli on each cell! Of course, the presence of intestinal villi, circular folds (plicae circulares), and numerous loops also adds to the intestinal surface area (see **Figure 39-3** on p. 884).

The large surface area of the brush border provides sites for digestive enzymes on the plasma membranes of intestinal cells—the *brush-border enzymes.* The efficiency of the last stages of digestion is thus enhanced by having more surface area for more digestive enzymes. Many of the brush border enzymes are on fine, branched filaments that extend from the surface of each microvillus and form a glycoprotein coat on the brush border called the *glycocalyx.* Because each substrate molecule must come in direct contact with a brush border enzyme before it can be digested, the process is called *contact digestion.*

The large surface area also provides more opportunities for the absorption of digested nutrients. More surface area allows for more phospholipid bilayer to absorb lipids and more carrier molecules to carry amino acids, peptides, monosaccharides, and other nutrients. •

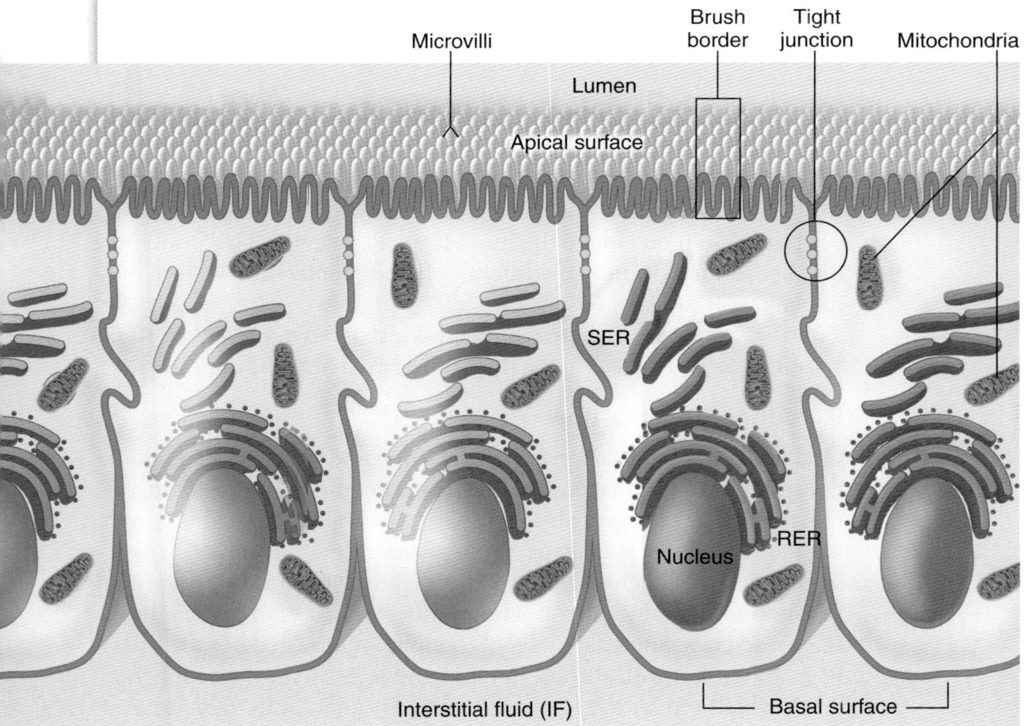

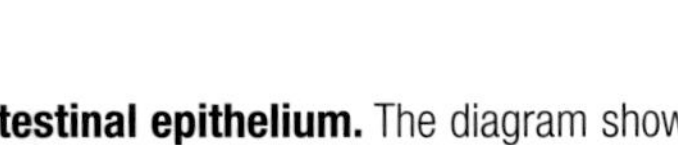

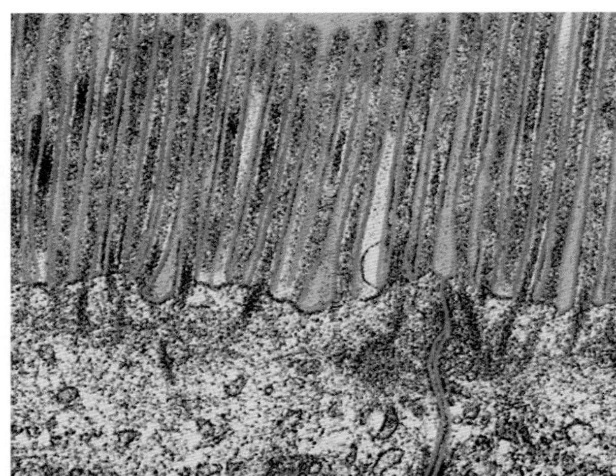

B

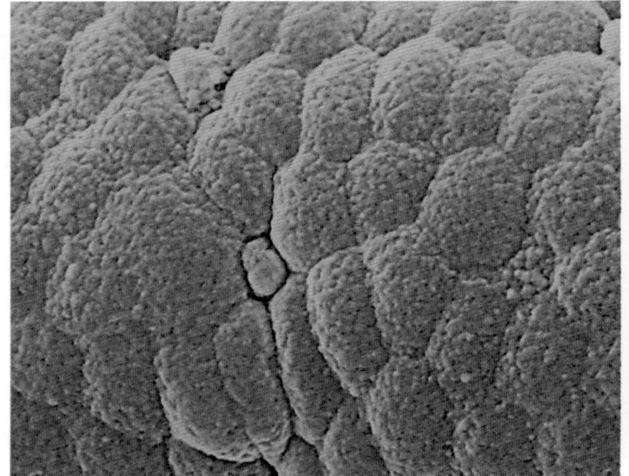

C

A, Intestinal epithelium. The diagram shows intestinal epithelial cells joined by tight junctions and covered with microvilli on their apical (lumen-facing) surfaces. *RER,* Rough endoplasmic reticulum; *SER,* smooth endoplasmic reticulum. **B, Cross-section of the brush border.** A transmission electron micrograph shows microvilli, which resemble bristles of a brush. **C, Surface view of the brush border.** A scanning electron micrograph of the surface of an intestinal villus shows the epithelial cells joined by tight junctions. Note the brushy appearance of the surface caused by the presence of microvilli.

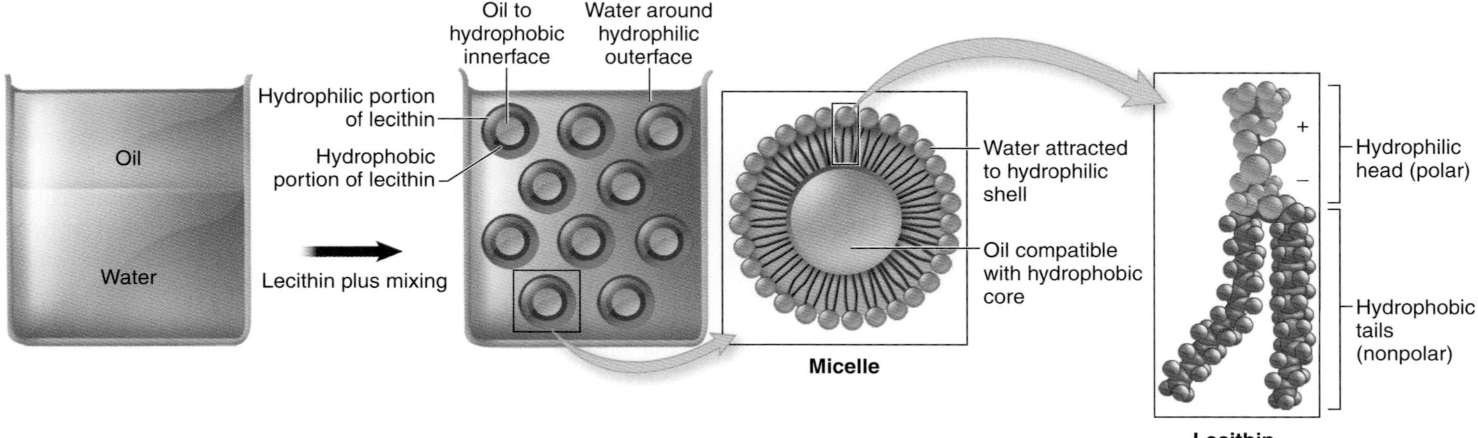

FIGURE 40-11 Formation of micelles by lecithin. Lecithin is a phospholipid in bile that mixes with oil and water to form micelles. Micelles are spherical shells formed by the orientation of lecithin molecules according to their solubility in water and lipids: the polar heads of lecithin face outward (toward water), and the nonpolar tails of lecithin face inward (toward lipid). Formation of micelles, a mechanical process called *emulsification,* breaks fat drops into small droplets and makes the droplets water-soluble.

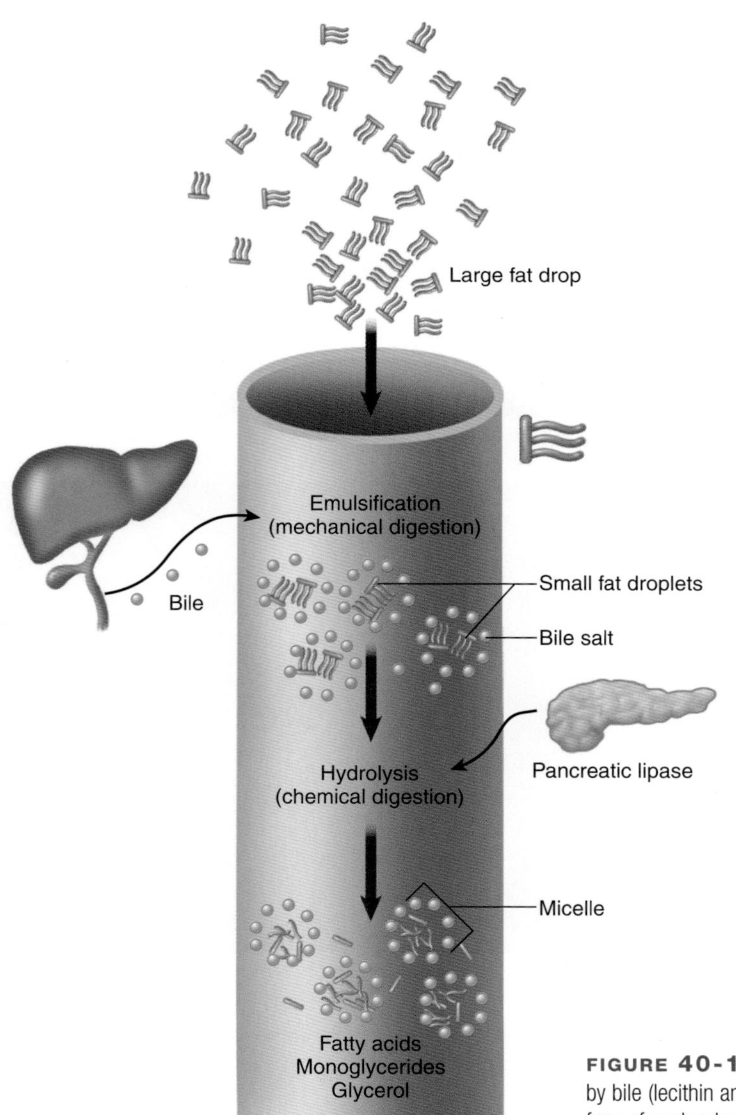

chemically broken down by a lipase called *phospholipase* to yield one free fatty acid and one lysophosphatide (a phospholipid head with a single fatty-acid tail).

The action of lipases is enhanced by a component of pancreatic juice called **colipase.** Colipase is a coenzyme molecule that anchors a lipase molecule to the inner face of a micelle. This positions the lipase for optimum hydrolysis of lipid molecules within the micelle.

For a summary of chemical digestion, see **Table 40-3**. **Box 40-5** summarizes concepts of nucleic acid digestion and absorption.

Residues of Digestion

Certain components of food resist digestion and are eliminated from the intestines in the **faeces.** Included among these *residues of digestion* are cellulose (a carbohydrate, also known as "dietary fibre") and undigested connective tissue from meat (mostly collagen). These substances remain undigested because humans lack the enzymes required to hydrolyze them. The residues of digestion also include undigested fats. Some fat molecules remain undigested because they have combined with dietary minerals such as calcium and magnesium, which render the fats indigestible. In addition to these wastes, faeces consist of bacteria, pigments, water, and mucus.

CONNECT IT!

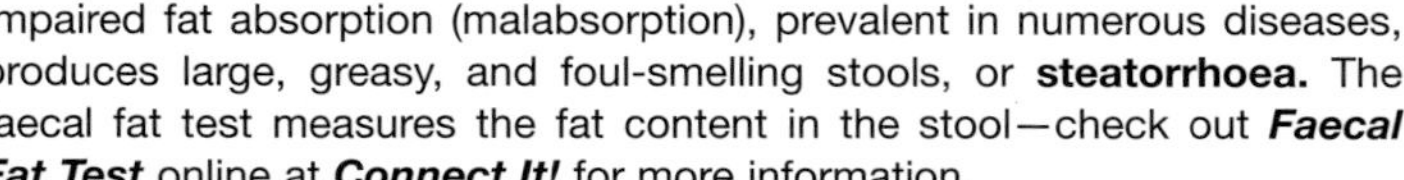

Impaired fat absorption (malabsorption), prevalent in numerous diseases, produces large, greasy, and foul-smelling stools, or **steatorrhoea.** The faecal fat test measures the fat content in the stool—check out ***Faecal Fat Test*** online at ***Connect It!*** for more information.

Monitoring for changes in the faeces is a way to monitor overall body health. For potential signs of health dangers in the faeces, review ***Toilet Signs*** online at ***Connect It!***

FIGURE 40-12 Fat digestion. Hydrolysis by the enzyme lipase is facilitated by prior emulsion of fats by bile (lecithin and bile salts). Though not pictured, colipase is needed to anchor lipase molecules to the inner face of each micelle.

TABLE 40-3 Chemical Digestion

DIGESTIVE JUICES AND ENZYMES		SUBSTANCE DIGESTED (OR HYDROLYZED)	RESULTING PRODUCT*
Saliva			
Amylase (ptyalin)		Starch (polysaccharide)	Maltose (disaccharide)
Lingual lipase		Emulsified lipids	**Fatty acids, monoglycerides,** diglycerides, and **glycerol**
Gastric Juice			
Protease (pepsin)† plus hydrochloric acid	Saliva	Proteins	Partially digested proteins
Pancreatic Juice			
Proteases (e.g., trypsin)‡	Gastric juice	Proteins (intact or partially digested)	Peptides and **amino acids**
Pancreatic lipases		Fats emulsified by bile	**Fatty acids, monoglycerides,** and **glycerol**
Amylase		Starch	Maltose
Nucleases	Pancreatic juice	Nucleic acids (DNA, RNA)	Nucleotides
Intestinal Enzymes§			
Peptidases	Intestinal enzymes	Peptides	**Amino acids**
Sucrase		Sucrose (cane sugar)	**Glucose** and **fructose¶** (monosaccharides)
Lactase		Lactose (milk sugar)	**Glucose** and **galactose** (monosaccharides)
Maltase		Maltose (malt sugar)	**Glucose**
Nucleotidases and phosphatases		Nucleotides	Nucleosides

*Substances in **boldface type** are end products of digestion (i.e., completely digested nutrients ready for absorption).

†Secreted in inactive form (pepsinogen); activated by low pH (hydrochloric acid).

‡Secreted in inactive form (trypsinogen); activated by enterokinase, an enzyme in the intestinal brush border.

§Brush-border enzymes.

¶Glucose is also called *dextrose;* fructose is also called *levulose.*

Quick CHECK

5. What type of reaction do all digestive enzymes catalyze?
6. List some factors that alter the shape of an enzyme, thus altering its function.
7. Name the final digestive products of each of the following food molecules: proteins, carbohydrates, and triclycerides.

SECRETION

Digestive secretion generally refers to the release of various substances from the exocrine glands that serve the digestive system. For example, digestive secretion includes the release of saliva, gastric juice, bile, pancreatic juice, and intestinal juice. In the paragraphs that follow, we briefly summarize the major digestive juices. Later, we discuss how secretion is regulated.

BOX 40-5 *fyi* | Nucleic Acid Digestion and Absorption

Although they are not usually considered to be essential nutrients, the nucleic acids such as DNA and RNA found in cells of food material are digested, absorbed, and used by the body.

DNA and RNA strands released during mechanical digestion are still associated with proteins and so must first be hydrolyzed by proteases to break the proteins free from the DNA or RNA strand. **Nucleases** in pancreatic juice then break down each strand into individual nucleotides. Nucleotides are simple enough to be absorbed by intestinal cells. Many of the nucleotides, however, are first stripped of their phosphate groups by intestinal *phosphatases* and *nucleotidases.* A nucleotide thus stripped of its phosphate is called a *nucleoside.*

Although nucleotides can be absorbed, most nucleic acids are absorbed in the form of nucleosides. Both nucleotides and nucleosides are absorbed through the intestinal wall by a sodium cotransport process similar to that for glucose and amino acids. After absorption, the nucleosides have phosphates added to them by cellular enzymes and are thus restored to the nucleotide form.

Although a healthy body can make its own nucleotides, nucleotides from food help the body maintain a healthy pool of nucleotides available for making DNA and RNA. This external source of nucleotides is especially useful during rapid growth and development stages (as during infancy) and during certain disease or weakened states. •

Saliva

Saliva is the secretion of the salivary glands (see **Figure 38-8** on p. 866). Saliva, as with all digestive secretions, is mostly water. Water helps mechanically digest food as it moves through the digestive tract by helping to liquefy the food. Liquefied food, called chyme after it enters the stomach, not only represents a physically broken-down form of food but also permits enzymes and other substances to mix freely with small chunks of food.

Mixed in the water is a combination of other important substances. **Mucus,** for example, is found not only in saliva but also in each of the other digestive juices. Mucus, you may recall, is a mixture of glycoproteins and related substances that is rather slippery to the touch. Mucus in intestinal juices has the primary functions of protecting the digestive mucosa and lubricating food as it passes through the alimentary canal.

Saliva, as with most other digestive juices, contains enzymes. Specifically, saliva contains **amylase**—a carbohydrate-digesting enzyme. Although salivary amylase (ptyalin) can chemically digest starches into smaller carbohydrates, the short time it has until it is destroyed by acids and enzymes in the stomach make this function relatively unimportant. Saliva also contains a small amount of **lipase,** which digests lipids. Sometimes called *lingual lipase* because it is produced by the lingual salivary glands, it functions at a low pH and thus can break down lipids as it moves into the stomach and into the upper duodenum.

Saliva also contains a small amount of sodium bicarbonate ($NaHCO_3$). Sodium bicarbonate dissociates in water to form sodium ions (Na^+) and bicarbonate ions (HCO_3^-). You may recall from Chapter 37 that bicarbonate can bind to hydrogen ions, thus taking the hydrogen ions out of solution and causing a decrease in acidity (increase in pH). This buffering mechanism keeps saliva close to neutral pH, which is optimum for amylase activity.

Gastric Juice

Gastric juice is secreted by exocrine *gastric glands,* which have ducts that lead to the gastric lumen by way of the gastric pits (see **Figure 38-14** on p. 872). Gastric juice contains not only the basic water and mucus mixture of most other digestive juices but also a unique combination of other substances.

Chief cells in the gastric glands are also called **zymogenic cells** because they secrete the enzymes in gastric juice. The prefix *zymo-* refers to enzymes and *-genic* pertains to making something. Primary among the gastric enzymes is **pepsin,** which is secreted as the inactive proenzyme **pepsinogen.**

Pepsinogen is converted to pepsin by hydrochloric acid (HCl), which is produced by **parietal cells** of the gastric glands. **Figure 40-13** shows how carbon dioxide and water form carbonic acid, which then dissociates to form the hydrogen ions needed to actively secrete hydrochloric acid. This is the very same chemical process that was outlined in Chapter 37, where we discussed carbon dioxide transport in the blood (see **Figure 37-11**, p. 855).

Note in **Figure 40-13** that there is a *chloride shift* similar to that discussed with regard to the respiratory system. In exchange for bicarbonate (also produced by dissociation of carbonic acid), chloride is shifted into the parietal cell, where it can then diffuse into the duct of the gastric gland along with hydrogen ions. The end result of this process in parietal cells is that the contents of the stomach become more acidic, or drop in pH, and the contents of the blood become more basic, or increase in pH.

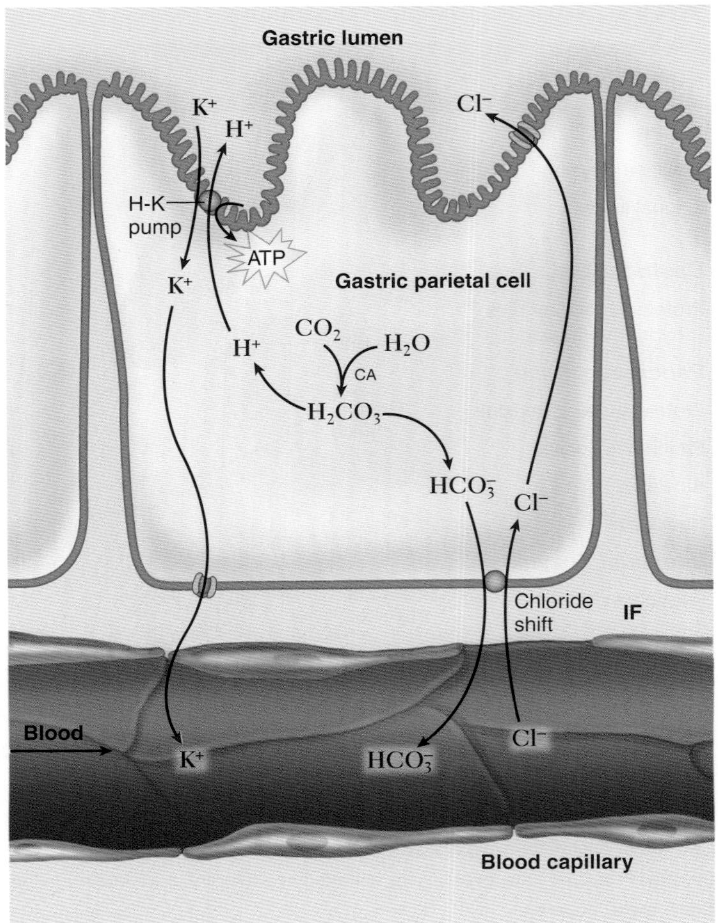

FIGURE 40-13 Acid secretion by gastric parietal cells. In this simplified diagram, you can see that hydrochloric acid (HCl) secretion by gastric parietal cells uses H^+ produced by the dissociation of carbonic acid (H_2CO_3). Recall that carbonic acid is produced by the reaction of water and carbon dioxide—a process enhanced by the enzyme carbonic anhydrase (CA). The chloride (Cl^-) of gastric HCl comes from a chloride shift into the cell in exchange for bicarbonate ions (HCO_3^-) produced by the same dissociation of carbonic acid that yielded the H^+. As Cl^- is shifted into the cell, the intracellular Cl^- concentration rises and produces a concentration gradient with the lumen of the gastric gland—forcing Cl^- to diffuse out of the parietal cell. The net effect is that active pumping of H^+ out of the cell by the H-K pump drives the concurrent shift of Cl^- into the cell from the blood and diffusion of Cl^- out of the cell and into the duct of the gastric gland. *IF,* Interstitial fluid.

The ion pump in the membrane of gastric parietal cells that pumps H^+ ions into the gastric juice is often called the **H-K pump**—or more simply, a *proton pump* (see **Figure 40-13**). It is this pump that is targeted by drugs that inhibit gastric acid secretion, such as omeprazole. By inhibiting the H-K pumps of the stomach, these drugs reduce the overall acidity of the stomach contents.

The parietal cells have an interesting and important mechanism involved with secretion of ions. As **Figure 40-14**, A, shows, when the parietal cell is not actively secreting, it has a relatively small surface area and many internal vesicles. These vesicles have H-K pumps and ion channels and carriers embedded in their membranes. When the

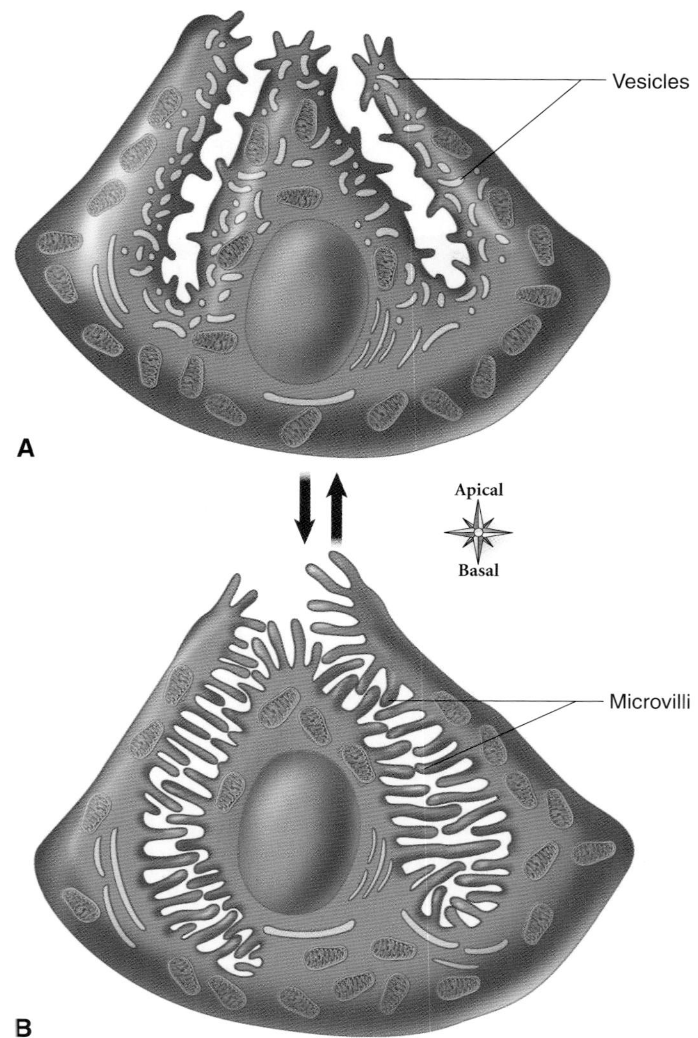

FIGURE 40-14 Parietal cell membrane surface. The surface of the resting parietal cell **(A)** can be enlarged by a factor of 100 when the cell becomes active and vesicles fuse to the apical surface of the cell **(B).** The vesicle membranes contain many ion pumps, carriers, and channels (see **Figure 40-13**) that are thus added to the additional microvilli formed by fusion of the vesicle membrane to the plasma membrane.

parietal cell becomes active, however, these vesicles move quickly to the apical surface (**Figure 40-14**, *B*). There, they fuse with the plasma membrane, forming more microvilli and increasing the overall surface area by as much as 100 times! The pumps, carriers, and channels then begin the secretion process summarized in **Figure 40-13**.

Besides secreting acid, parietal cells also produce **intrinsic factor.** Intrinsic factor binds to molecules of vitamin B_{12}, protecting them from the acids and enzymes of the stomach. Intrinsic factor remains attached to B_{12} until it reaches the lower small intestine, where it facilitates the absorption of B_{12} across the intestinal wall (**Figure 40-15**). Vitamin B_{12}, you may recall, is essential for the production of new red blood cells. In pernicious anaemia, caused by insufficient vitamin B_{12} in the body, the stomach may fail to make sufficient intrinsic factor (perhaps because of stomach cancer or ulcers). More often, however, an autoimmune mechanism produces antibodies that block the intrinsic factor from binding to vitamin B_{12}.

PANCREATIC JUICE

Pancreatic juice is secreted by the exocrine *acinar cells* of the pancreas (see **Figure 39-15** on p. 894). As with other digestive secretions, pancreatic juice is mostly water. In addition, pancreatic juice also contains various digestive enzymes. All of the pancreatic enzymes are secreted as zymogens—inactive proenzymes. For example, protein-digesting **trypsin** is released as the zymogen **trypsinogen,** which is subsequently converted to active trypsin by **enterokinase** in the intestinal lumen. Enterokinase is an activating enzyme bound to the plasma membranes of cells that line the intestinal tract. After it is activated, trypsin can then activate other enzymes such as **chymotrypsin** (and other protein-digesting enzymes), various **lipases** (lipid-digesting enzymes), **nucleases** (RNA- and DNA-digesting enzymes),

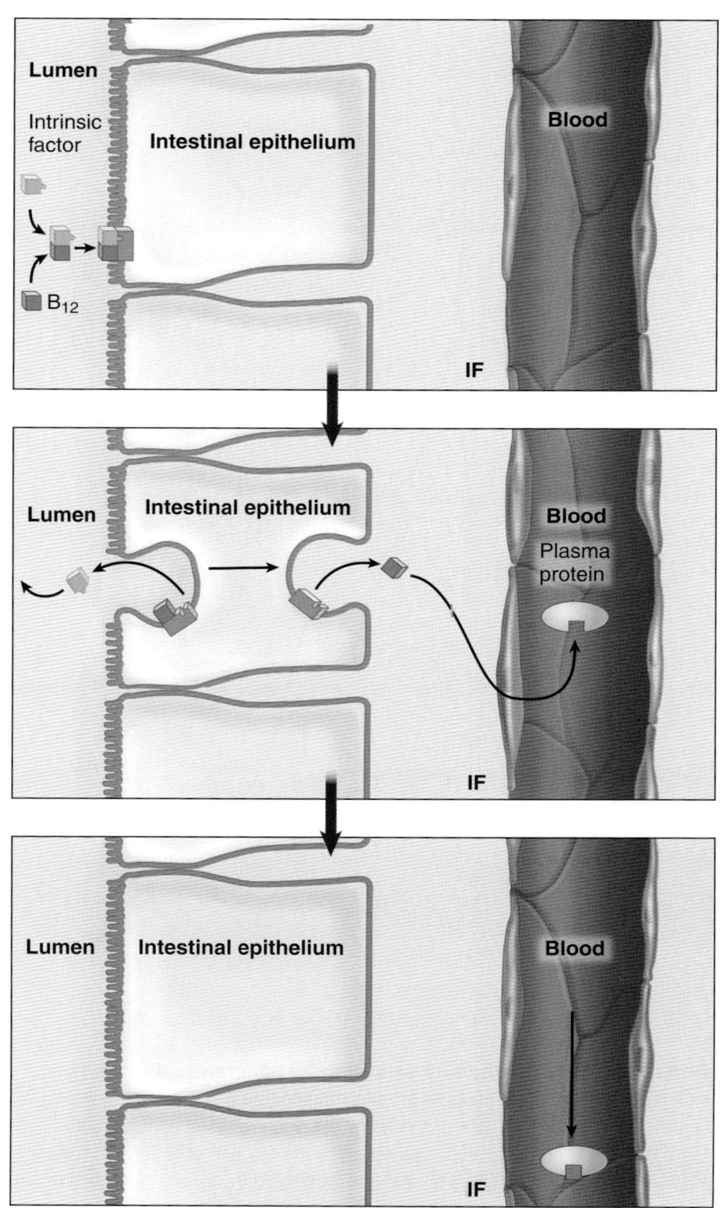

FIGURE 40-15 Role of intrinsic factor. As this series of sketches shows, intrinsic factor secreted from the stomach binds to vitamin B_{12}, which then permits the absorption of vitamin B_{12} into the bloodstream in the intestines. *IF,* Interstitial fluid.

and **amylase** (a starch-digesting enzyme). Trypsin activates these molecules by an allosteric effect: it removes a specific sequence of amino acids from the proenzyme molecule, thus changing its shape to the active enzyme form. The advantage of this system is that the enzymes will not digest the cells that make them.

Cells along the exocrine ducts of the pancreas also have a secretory function. As **Figure 40-16** shows, they produce sodium bicarbonate by more or less reversing the direction of the process described for acid secretion by gastric parietal cells and shown in **Figure 40-13**. In the pancreas, base (bicarbonate) is secreted into the GI lumen and acid is secreted into the blood—rather than the other way around, as in the stomach. This process thus provides a mechanism to neutralize the decreased pH of the chyme and the increased pH of the blood. As **Figure 40-17** shows, the pH balance of the body is preserved and loss of homeostatic stability is avoided.

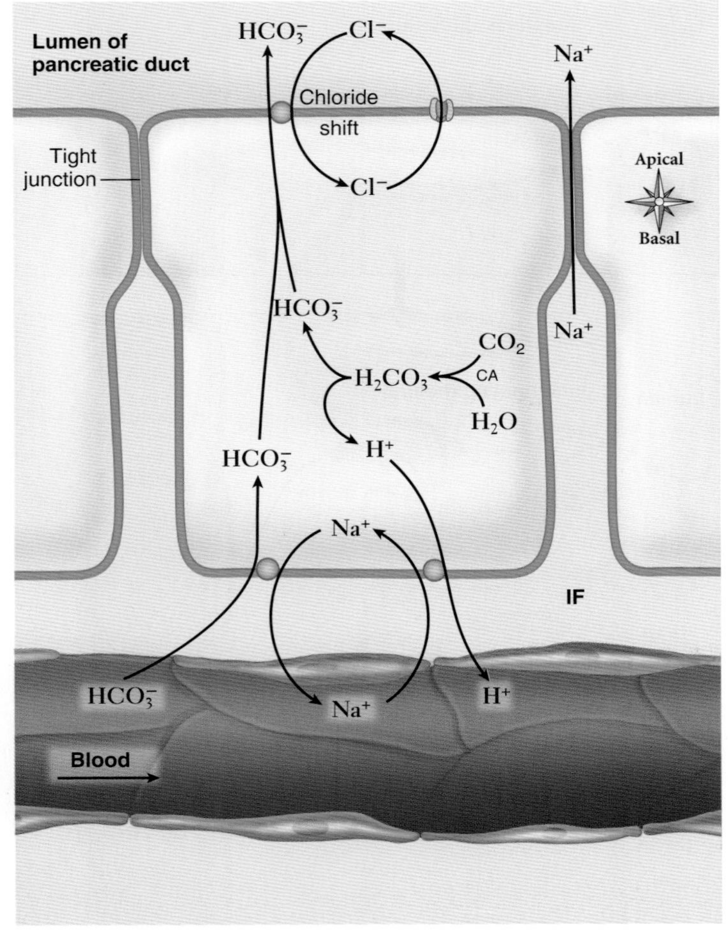

FIGURE 40-16 Bicarbonate secretion by pancreatic duct cells. In this simplified diagram, you can see that bicarbonate (HCO_3^-) secretion by cells of the pancreatic duct uses HCO_3^- produced by the dissociation of carbonic acid (H_2CO_3). Recall that carbonic acid is produced by the reaction of water and carbon dioxide—a process enhanced by the enzyme carbonic anhydrase (CA). Notice that a "reverse" chloride shift occurs as bicarbonate ions (HCO_3^-) are exchanged for Cl^- ions. The outward movement of negative bicarbonate ions into the lumen of the pancreatic ducts creates an electrical gradient that draws positive sodium ions (Na^+) from the interstitial fluid (IF), across the tight junctions, and into the pancreatic juice.

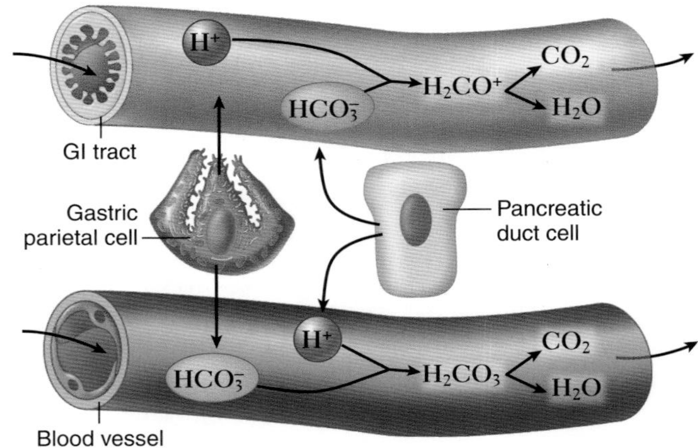

FIGURE 40-17 pH balance related to the digestive tract. Hydrochloric acid (HCl) secretion by gastric parietal cells moves H^+ into the gastrointestinal (GI) lumen, decreasing the pH of chyme. At the same time, gastric parietal cells shift bicarbonate ions (HCO_3^-) into the blood, increasing the pH of blood plasma. Eventually, this net loss of acid from the internal environment would cause alkalosis if not for the counterbalancing effects of bicarbonate secretion by the duct cells of the pancreas and other digestive glands such as the liver and intestinal glands. These cells secrete HCO_3^- into the GI lumen, increasing the pH of chyme, at the same time they move H^+ into the blood, decreasing the pH of blood back toward normal. This mechanism permits changes in the pH of chyme to facilitate the action of various enzymes without profoundly affecting the pH of the internal environment.

BILE

Bile is an interesting mixture of many different substances that is secreted by the liver and stored and concentrated by the gallbladder. As **Figure 39-13** (on p. 892) shows, bile from the liver is conducted through the right and left hepatic ducts, which merge to form a common hepatic duct. The common hepatic duct, in turn, merges with the cystic duct from the gallbladder to form the common bile duct, which delivers bile to the duodenum through the major duodenal papilla.

Bile contains several substances that aid in digestion, specifically lecithin and bile salts. As we stated previously, both of these substances break down large drops of fat into smaller droplets, thus making the fats more easily digestible. Both lecithin and bile salts wrap a hydrophilic shell around the droplets, making them water-soluble and therefore able to move freely through the watery chyme in the GI lumen. Bile also contains a small amount of sodium bicarbonate, which, as with the sodium bicarbonate secreted by pancreatic duct cells, helps neutralize chyme.

Bile also contains several substances that are ultimately destined for removal from the body by becoming part of the faeces that are eventually eliminated from the GI tract. It is therefore proper to state that these waste substances are actually *excretions*, a term that implies shedding waste, rather than *secretions*. Excreted substances in bile include cholesterol, products of detoxification, and bile pigments.

The cholesterol in bile represents excess amounts of this lipid that have been picked up from body cells by lipoproteins and delivered to the liver for disposal in bile. Products of detoxification are formed in the liver as it renders toxic molecules harmless, a process called *detoxification*. Bile pigments, chiefly **bilirubin,** are products of haemolysis (the breakdown of old red blood cells) by the liver (see **Figure 27-8** on p. 618). It is the bile pigments that are eventually eliminated from the GI tract that give faeces its characteristic brownish colour. Elimination of grey faeces, therefore, ordinarily can be interpreted as a sign that bile secretion is abnormally low.

We discuss many functions of the liver further in the next chapter.

Intestinal Juice

The term **intestinal juice** refers to the sum total of intestinal secretions rather than to a premixed combination of substances that enters the GI lumen by way of a duct. Most intestinal cells produce a water-based solution of sodium bicarbonate. This adds to the buffering effect mentioned in previous paragraphs and illustrated in **Figure 40-17**. Goblet cells of the intestinal mucosa also produce a watery solution of mucus. Thus intestinal juice is a slightly basic, mucous solution that buffers and lubricates material in the intestinal lumen.

Intestinal juice is largely a product of the small intestine, but goblet cells in the mucosa of the large intestine produce some lubricating mucus.

Table 40-4 lists various secretions of the digestive tract and their components.

Quick CHECK

8. Name the primary components of saliva.
9. Name the components of gastric juice. Which type of cell produces each component?
10. Name as many pancreatic enzymes as you can.
11. What is excretion? What components of bile are excretions?

TABLE 40-4 Digestive Secretions

DIGESTIVE JUICE	SOURCE	SUBSTANCE	FUNCTIONAL ROLE*
Saliva	Salivary glands	Mucus	*Lubricates bolus of food; facilitates mixing of food*
		Amylase (ptyalin)	**Enzyme; begins digestion of starches**
		Sodium bicarbonate	Increases pH (for optimum amylase function)
		Lingual lipase	**Enzyme; digests a third or more of fats ingested**
		Water	*Dilutes food and other substances; facilitates mixing*
Gastric juice	Gastric glands	Pepsin	**Enzyme; digests proteins**
		Hydrochloric acid	Denatures proteins; decreases pH (for optimum pepsin function)
		Intrinsic factor	**Protects and allows later absorption of vitamin B_{12}**
		Mucus	*Lubricates chyme; protects stomach lining*
		Water	*Dilutes food and other substances; facilitates mixing*
Pancreatic juice	Pancreas (exocrine portion)	Proteases (trypsin, chymotrypsin, collagenase, elastase, etc.)	**Enzymes; digest proteins and polypeptides**
		Lipases (lipase, phospholipase, etc.)	**Enzymes; digest up to two thirds of ingested lipids**
		Colipase	**Coenzyme; helps lipase digest fats**
		Nucleases	**Enzymes; digest nucleic acids (RNA and DNA)**
		Amylase	**Enzyme; digests starches**
		Water	*Dilutes food and other substances; facilitates mixing*
		Mucus	*Lubricates*
		Sodium bicarbonate	**Increases pH** (for optimum enzyme function)
Bile	Liver (stored and concentrated in gallbladder)	Lecithin and bile salts	*Emulsify lipids*
		Sodium bicarbonate	**Increases pH** (for optimum enzyme function)
		Cholesterol	Excess cholesterol from body cells, to be excreted with faeces
		Products of detoxification	From detoxification of harmful substances by hepatocytes, to be excreted with faeces
		Bile pigments (mainly bilirubin)	Products of breakdown of haem groups during haemolysis, to be excreted with faeces
		Mucus	*Lubrication*
		Water	Dilutes food and other substances; facilitates mixing
Intestinal juice	Mucosa of small and large intestine	Mucus	*Lubrication*
		Sodium bicarbonate	**Increases pH** (for optimum enzyme function)
		Water	Small amount to carry mucus and sodium bicarbonate

*__Boldface type__ indicates a chemical digestive process; *italic type* indicates a mechanical process.

UNIT 5

CONTROL OF DIGESTIVE GLAND SECRETION

Exocrine digestive glands secrete when food is present in the digestive tract or when it is seen, smelled, or imagined. Complicated nervous and hormonal reflex mechanisms control the flow of digestive juices in such a way that they appear in proper amounts when and for as long as needed.

Control of Salivary Secretion

As far as is known, only reflex mechanisms control the secretion of saliva. Chemical, mechanical, olfactory, and visual stimuli initiate afferent impulses to centres in the brainstem that send out efferent impulses to the salivary glands, stimulating them. Chemical and mechanical stimuli come from the presence of food in the mouth. Olfactory and visual stimuli come, of course, from the smell and sight of food.

Control of Gastric Secretion

Stimulation of gastric juice secretion occurs in three phases that are controlled by reflex and chemical mechanisms. Because stimuli that activate these mechanisms arise in the head, stomach, and intestines, the three phases are known as the cephalic, gastric, and intestinal phases, respectively. As you read the description of each phase, glance at the diagrams shown in **Figure 40-18**.

The **cephalic phase** is also spoken of as the "psychic phase" because psychic (mental) factors activate the mechanism. For example, the sight, smell, taste, or even thought of food that is pleasing to an individual activates control centres in the medulla oblongata from which parasympathetic fibres of the vagus nerve conduct efferent impulses to the gastric glands. Vagal nerve impulses also stimulate the production of **gastrin,** a hormone secreted by endocrine *G cells* in the gastric mucosa. Gastrin stimulates gastric secretion, thus prolonging and enhancing the response.

During the **gastric phase** of gastric secretion, the following chemical control mechanism dominates. Products of protein digestion in foods that have reached the pyloric portion of the stomach stimulate its mucosa to release *gastrin* into the blood in stomach capillaries. When it circulates to the gastric glands, gastrin greatly accelerates their secretion of gastric juice, which has a high pepsinogen and hydrochloric acid content (**Table 40-5**). Hence, this seems to be a mechanism for ensuring that when food is in the stomach, there will be enough enzymes there to digest it. Gastrin release is also stimulated by distention of the stomach (caused by the presence of food), which activates local and parasympathetic reflexes in the pylorus.

The **intestinal phase** of gastric juice secretion is less clearly understood than the other two phases. Various different mechanisms seem to adjust gastric juice secretion as chyme passes to and through the intestinal tract. Experiments show that gastric secretions are inhibited when chyme, containing fats, carbohydrates, and acid (low pH) is present in the duodenum. This probably occurs by means of endocrine reflexes that involve the hormones GIP, **secretin,** CCK, and perhaps several others. These hormones are secreted by endocrine cells in the mucosa of the duodenum. Gastric secretion may also be inhibited by the parasympathetic enterogastric reflex. We have discussed how this reflex inhibits gastric motility as food begins to fill the duodenum; now we see that it may inhibit gastric secretion as well.

In summary, we see that the rate of gastric secretion can be adjusted by nervous and endocrine reflex mechanisms in ways that improve the efficiency of the system. Anticipation of swallowing food causes the stomach to prepare itself by increasing its secretion of enzymes and acid. Thus food enters a stomach already partially filled with gastric juice. The rate of gastric secretion can then be adjusted according to the amount of food present and whether it contains proteins (the only food that can be chemically digested by gastric juice). Gastric secretion—and thus chemical digestion in the stomach—can be slowed when the duodenum becomes full. This prevents the stomach from finishing its task before the small intestine is ready to receive the chyme.

TABLE 40-5 Actions of Some Digestive Hormones Summarized

HORMONE	SOURCE	ACTION
Gastrin	Secreted by gastric mucosa in presence of partially digested proteins, when stimulated by the vagus nerve, or when the stomach is stretched	Stimulates secretion of gastric juice rich in pepsin and hydrochloric acid
Gastric inhibitory peptide (GIP)*	Secreted by intestinal mucosa in presence of glucose, fats, and perhaps other nutrients	Inhibits gastric secretion and motility; enhances insulin secretion by pancreas (see Chapter 41)
Secretin	Secreted by intestinal mucosa in presence of acid, partially digested proteins, and fats	Inhibits gastric secretion; stimulates secretion of pancreatic juice low in enzymes and high in alkalinity (bicarbonate); enhances effects of CCK
Cholecystokinin (CCK)	Secreted by intestinal mucosa in presence of fats, partially digested proteins, and acids	Stimulates ejection of bile from gallbladder and secretion of pancreatic juice high in enzymes; relaxes sphincters that regulate flow from the common bile duct; opposes the action of gastrin, raising the pH of gastric juice

*GIP is also known as *glucose-dependent insulinotropic polypeptide*.

Control of Pancreatic Secretion

Several hormones released by the intestinal mucosa are known to stimulate pancreatic secretion. One of these hormones, *secretin,* evokes the production of pancreatic fluid low in enzyme content but high in bicarbonate (HCO_3^-). This alkaline fluid acts to neutralize the acid (chyme) entering the duodenum. As you might expect, the presence of acid in the duodenum serves as the most potent stimulator of secretin. (Additional control involving the same hormone is shown by the fact that fats in the duodenum also elicit secretin,

1 **Cephalic Phase** Sensations or thoughts about food are relayed to the brainstem, where parasympathetic signals to the gastric mucosa are initiated. This directly stimulates gastric juice secretion and also stimulates the release of gastrin, which prolongs and enhances the effect.

2 **Gastric Phase** The presence of food, specifically the distention it causes, triggers local and parasympathetic nervous reflexes that increase secretion of gastric juice and gastrin (which further amplifies gastric juice secretion).

3 **Intestinal Phase** As food moves into the duodenum, the presence of fats, carbohydrates, and acid stimulates hormonal and nervous reflexes that inhibit stomach activity.

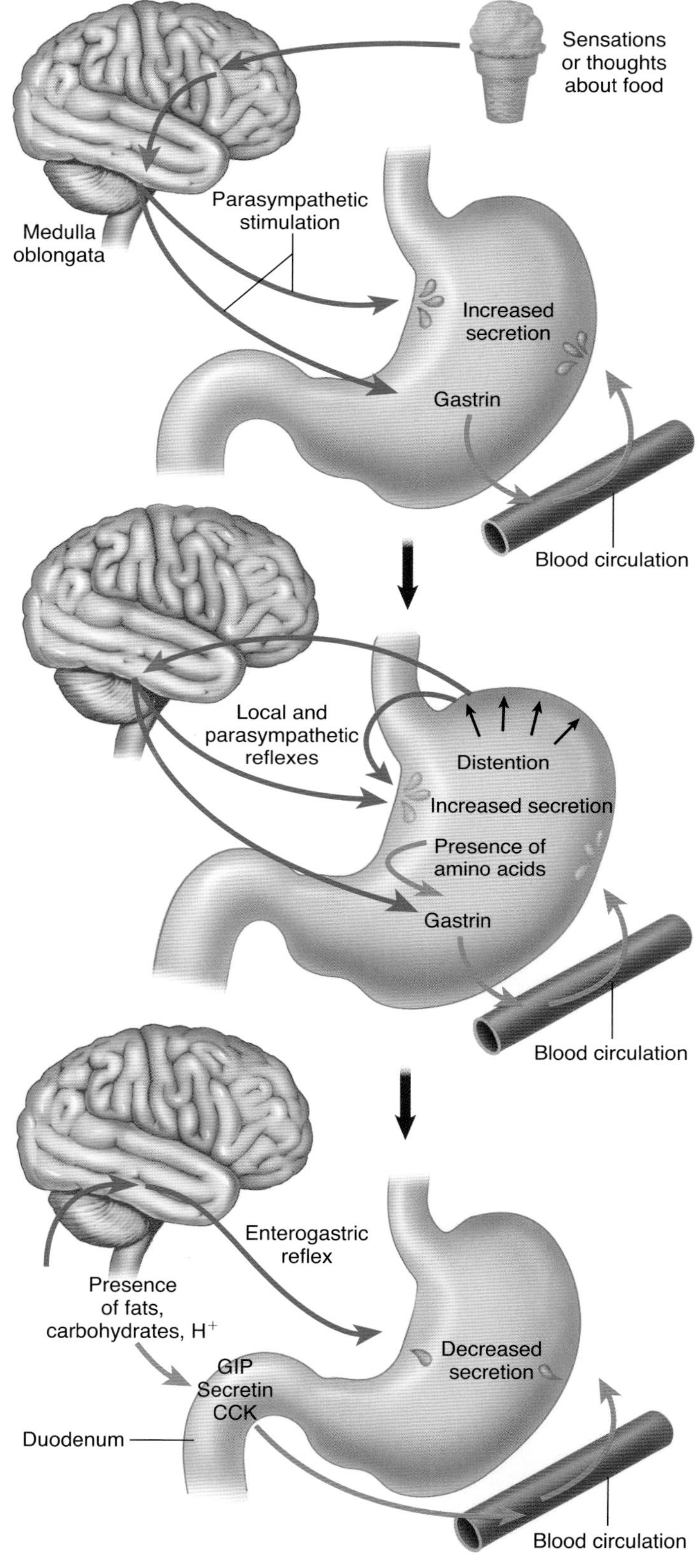

FIGURE 40-18 Phases of gastric secretion. *CCK,* Cholecystokinin, *GIP,* gastric inhibitory peptide, H^+, hydrogen ion (acid).

which then influences the gallbladder to increase its ejection of the fat emulsifier bile.)

The other intestinal hormone, known as cholecystokinin (CCK), was originally thought to be two separate substances. It has now been identified as one chemical with several important functions: (1) It causes the pancreas to increase exocrine secretions high in enzyme content; (2) it opposes the influence of gastrin on gastric parietal cells, thus inhibiting hydrochloric acid secretion by the stomach; and (3) it stimulates contraction of the gallbladder so that bile can pass into the duodenum.

Control of Bile Secretion

Bile is secreted continually by the liver and is stored in the gallbladder until needed by the duodenum. The hormones secretin and CCK, as described, stimulate ejection of bile from the gallbladder (see **Table 40-5**).

Control of Intestinal Secretion

Relatively little is known about the regulation of intestinal exocrine secretions. Some evidence suggests that the intestinal mucosa, stimulated by hydrochloric acid and food products, releases hormones into the blood, including *vasoactive intestinal peptide (VIP)*, which brings about increased production of intestinal juice. Intestinal secretions contain bicarbonate, which along with pancreatic bicarbonate, neutralizes acid from the stomach. Bicarbonate secretion is regulated by a reflex sensitive to changes in pH of the chyme. Presumably, neural mechanisms also help control the secretion of intestinal juice.

Quick CHECK

12. Name the three phases of gastric secretion.
13. What is the function of gastric inhibitory peptide?

Absorption

Process of Absorption

Absorption is the passage of substances (notably digested foods, water, salts, and vitamins) through the intestinal mucosa into the blood or lymph. As stated earlier, most absorption occurs in the small intestine, where the large surface area provided by the intestinal villi and microvilli (**Figure 40-19**) facilitates this process.

Mechanisms of Absorption

Absorption of some substances, such as mineral ions, is simple and straightforward: diffusion (or, in the case of water, osmosis). However, some substances depend on more complex mechanisms to be absorbed. Sodium is a good example. Epithelial cells that form the outer wall of the villus (see **Figure 40-19**) constantly pump sodium from the GI lumen into the internal environment through a complex process called *secondary active transport* (see **Box 6-3** on p. 105).

As **Figure 40-20**, *A*, shows, active transport carriers on the basal side, or "back side", of the cell continually pump Na^+ out of the cell. This mechanism maintains a low Na^+ concentration inside the cell. Thus it is likely that Na^+ in the GI lumen will diffuse into the low-Na^+ cell. As Na^+ diffuses in through passive carriers in the cell's luminal surface, or "lumen side", it is removed by active transport pumps in the cell's basal membrane. In short, Na^+ moves out of the GI lumen only because it is being pumped from the other side of the intestinal cells.

Another good example of a complex transport process is that involving glucose. Though considered an end product of digestion, glucose is a relatively large molecule and cannot pass freely through the brush border membrane of an intestinal mucosa cell. In addition to physical size, the lipid nature of the cell membrane (see **Figure 5-3**, p. 79) presents another barrier to glucose absorption.

Molecules the size of glucose can pass freely (passively) through the lipid cell barrier only if they are lipid-soluble (hydrophobic). Because glucose is too large physically and is hydrophilic (water soluble) in nature, it must be transported across the membrane by a carrier to enter the cell. In a process called **sodium cotransport** or coupled transport, carriers that bind both sodium ions and glucose molecules passively transport these molecules *together* out of the GI lumen (see **Figure 40-20**, *B*). However, this is another case of secondary active transport because this movement does not occur without the Na^+ concentration gradient maintained by the active transport

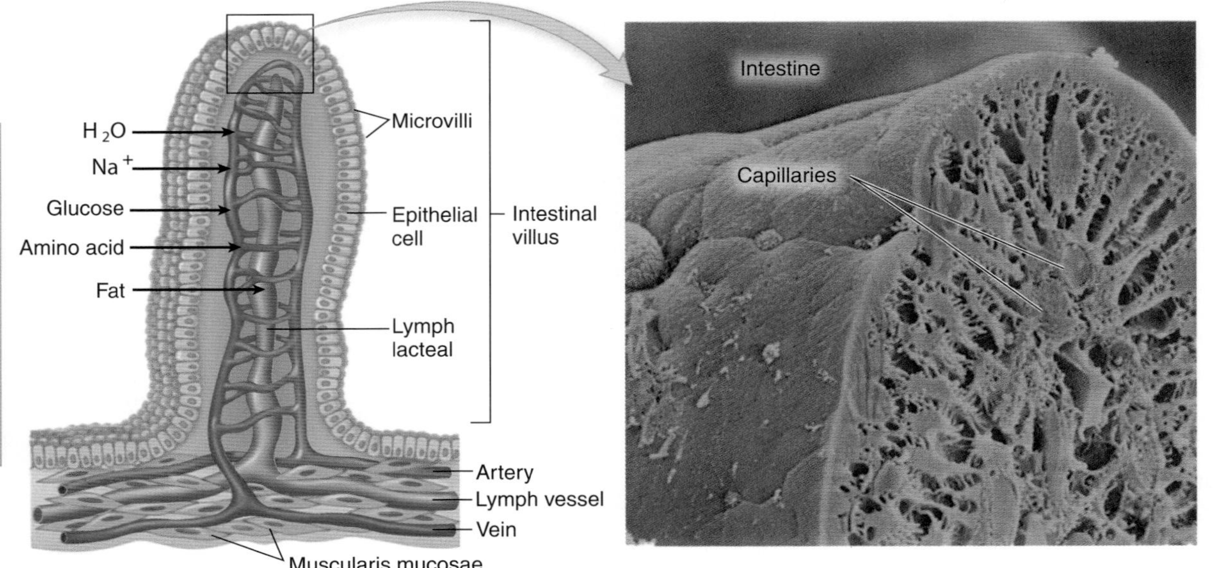

FIGURE 40-19 Intestinal villus. The presence of intestinal villi and microvilli increases the absorptive surface area of the intestinal mucosa. Most absorbed substances enter the blood in intestinal capillaries, with the exception of fat, which enters lymph by way of the intestinal lacteals. The inset is a scanning electron micrograph of the sectioned tip of a villus.

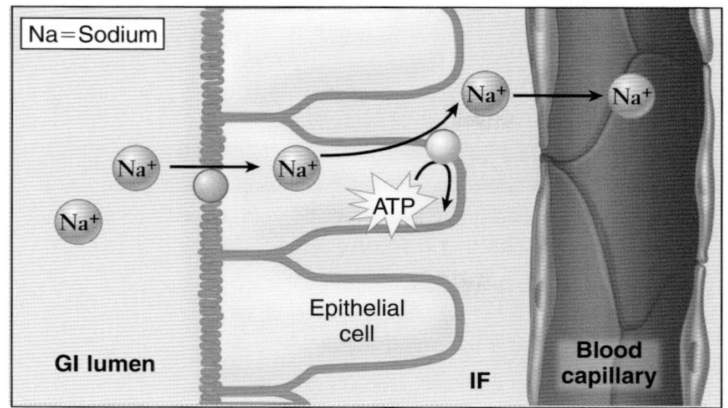

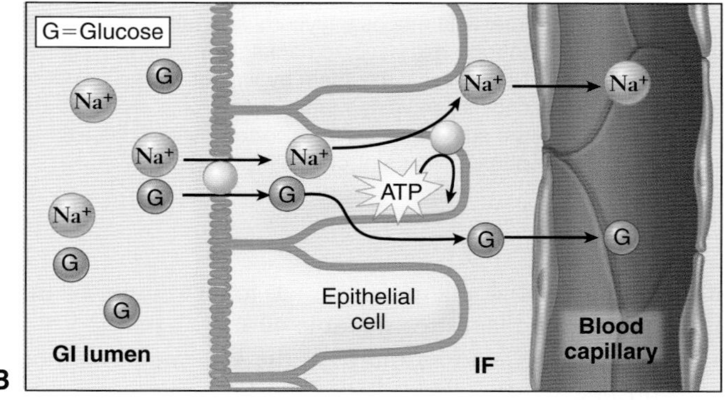

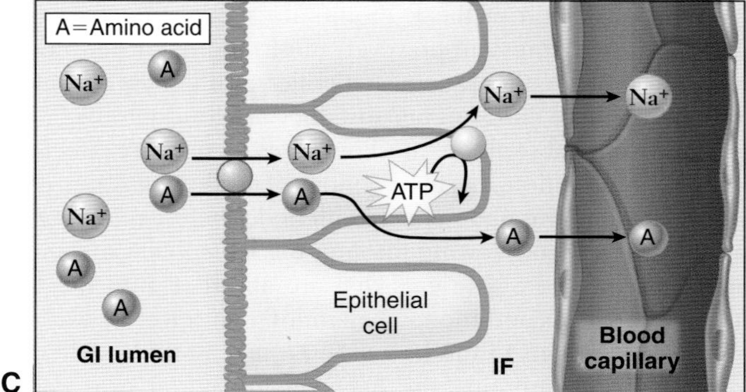

FIGURE 40-20 Absorption of sodium, glucose, and amino acids. Absorption of sodium **(A),** glucose **(B),** and amino acids **(C)** are forms of *secondary active transport* because each involves both active and passive carriers. The active carrier on the basal side of the epithelial cell maintains a sodium gradient, which facilitates passive transport of sodium, and perhaps another molecule, out of the gastrointestinal (GI) lumen via a passive carrier on the luminal side of the cell. *IF,* Interstitial fluid.

of Na^+ out of the cell's basal membrane. Amino acids and several other compounds are thought to also be absorbed by such a secondary active transport mechanism (see **Figure 40-20**, *C*).

Other mechanisms of transporting glucose and amino acids across absorptive cells have also been proposed. One hypothesis suggests that these compounds are transported by passive carriers on both the apical surfaces (lumen side) and the basal surfaces of the absorptive cells. Another hypothesis suggests that the brush border enzymes also act as carriers. It should also be noted that some short polypeptides can diffuse by way of peptide carriers into absorptive cells, where they are hydrolyzed into amino acids that can move into the blood.

Fatty acids and monoglycerides (products of fat digestion) and cholesterol are transported with the aid of lecithin and bile salts from fat droplets in the intestinal lumen to absorbing cells on villi. Lecithin and bile salts form microscopic spheres called micelles, which contain simple lipids (see **Figure 40-12** on p. 912).

As **Figure 40-21** shows, water-soluble micelles formed in the lumen of the intestine approach the brush border of absorbing cells. There, simple lipid molecules are released to pass through the plasma membrane (its phospholipid bilayer is receptive to lipids) by simple diffusion. After they are inside the cell, fatty acids are rapidly reunited with monoglycerides to form triglycerides (neutral fats).

The final step in lipid transport by the intestine is the formation of **chylomicrons,** which are simply another type of micelle. Chylomicrons are formed by the Golgi apparatus of the absorptive cell.

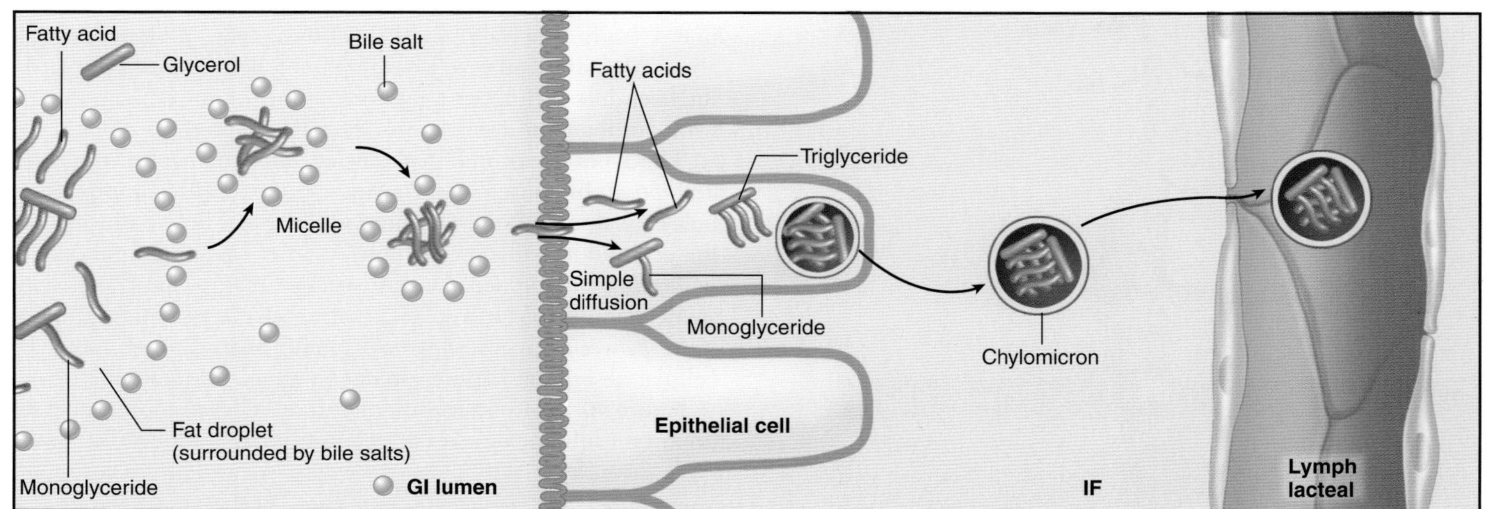

FIGURE 40-21 Absorption of lipids. Triglycerides are chemically digested within emulsified fat droplets, yielding fatty acids, monoglycerides, and glycerol *(left).* Fatty acids and other lipid-soluble compounds (such as cholesterol) leave the fat droplets in small spheres coated with bile salts (micelles). When a micelle reaches the plasma membrane of an absorptive cell, individual lipid-soluble molecules diffuse directly into the cytoplasm. The endoplasmic reticulum of the cell resynthesizes fatty acids and monoglycerides into triglycerides. A Golgi body within the cell packages the fats into water-soluble micelles called chylomicrons, which then exit the absorptive cell by exocytosis and enter a lymphatic lacteal. *IF,* Interstitial fluid.

TABLE 40-6 **Food Absorption**

FORM ABSORBED	STRUCTURES INTO WHICH ABSORBED	CIRCULATION
Protein—as amino acids Perhaps minute quantities of some short-chain polypeptides and whole proteins are absorbed; for example, some antibodies	Blood in intestinal capillaries	Portal vein, liver, hepatic vein, inferior vena cava to heart, and so on
Carbohydrates—as simple sugars	Same as amino acids	Same as amino acids
Fats		
Glycerol and monoglycerides	Lymph in intestinal lacteals	During absorption, that is, while in epithelial cells of intestinal mucosa, glycerol and fatty acids recombine to form microscopic packages of fats (chylomicrons); lymphatics carry them by way of thoracic duct to left subclavian vein, superior vena cava, heart, and so on; some fats are transported by blood in form of phospholipids or cholesterol esters
Fatty acids combine with bile salts to form water-soluble substance	Lymph in intestinal lacteals	
Some finely emulsified, undigested fats absorbed	Small fraction enters intestinal blood capillaries	

The water-soluble chylomicron allows fats to be transported through lymph and into the bloodstream (**Table 40-6**).

Vitamins A, D, E, and K, known as the *fat-soluble vitamins*, also depend on bile salts for their absorption. Some water-soluble vitamins, such as certain of the B group, are small enough to be absorbed by simple diffusion; however, most require carrier-mediated transport. Many drugs (sedatives, analgesics, antibiotics) appear to be absorbed by simple diffusion because they are lipid-soluble.

Note that after absorption, most nutrients do not pass directly into the general circulation. Lacteals conduct fats along a series of lymphatic vessels and through many lymph nodes before releasing them into the venous blood flowing through the left subclavian vein (see **Figure 31-2**, p. 730). Nutrients that are absorbed into the blood, such as amino acids and monosaccharides, first travel by way of the hepatic portal system to the liver (see **Figure 29-20**, p. 687). After absorption, blood entering the liver via the portal vein contains greater concentrations of glucose and other nutrients than does blood leaving the liver via the hepatic vein for the systemic circulation. Clearly, much of the excess of these food substances over and above normal blood levels has remained behind in the liver. What the liver does with them is part of the story of nutrition and metabolism, our topic for discussion in the next chapter.

The types of absorption discussed thus far involve *transcellular absorption*. In transcellular (meaning "across cells") absorption, particles are absorbed into the interior of the cell before moving out of the cell and into blood or lymph. Another type of absorption called *paracellular absorption* can also occur. In this type of absorption, small amounts of glucose, minerals, and even small peptides can move *between* the absorptive cells rather than through them. Paracellular absorption requires no energy expenditure by cells.

Figure 40-22 summarizes the locations where absorption of some important substances takes place. Notice that although the stomach

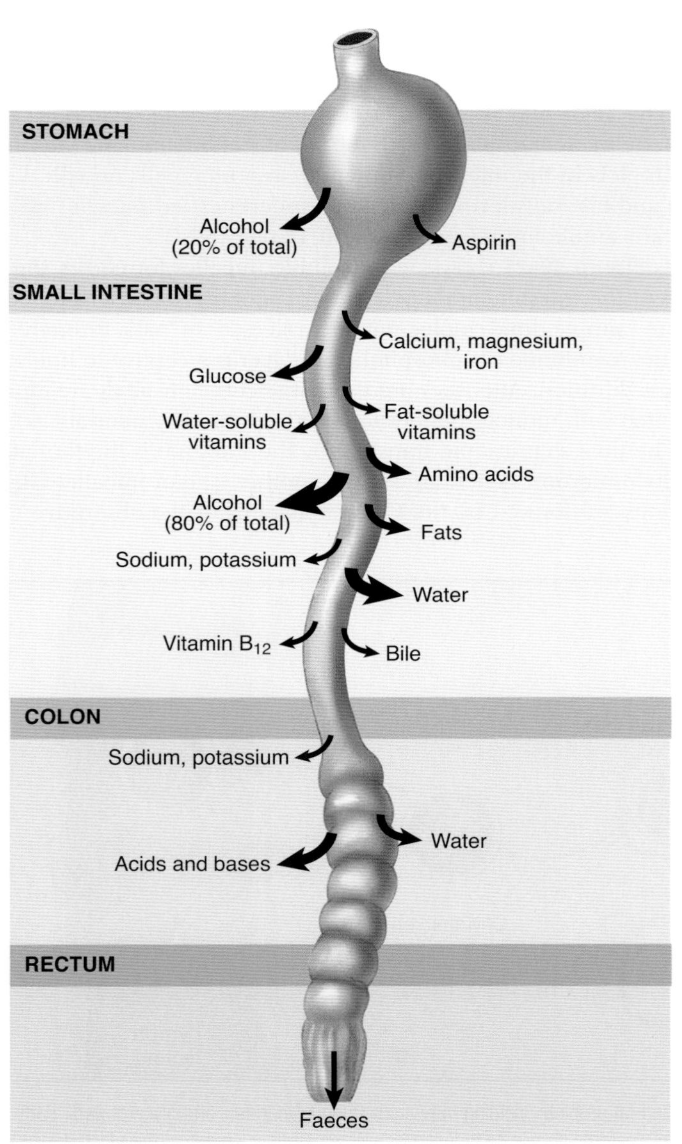

FIGURE 40-22 **Absorption sites in the digestive tract.** The size of the arrow at each site indicates the relative amount of absorption of a particular substance at that site. Note that most absorption occurs in the intestines, particularly the small intestine.

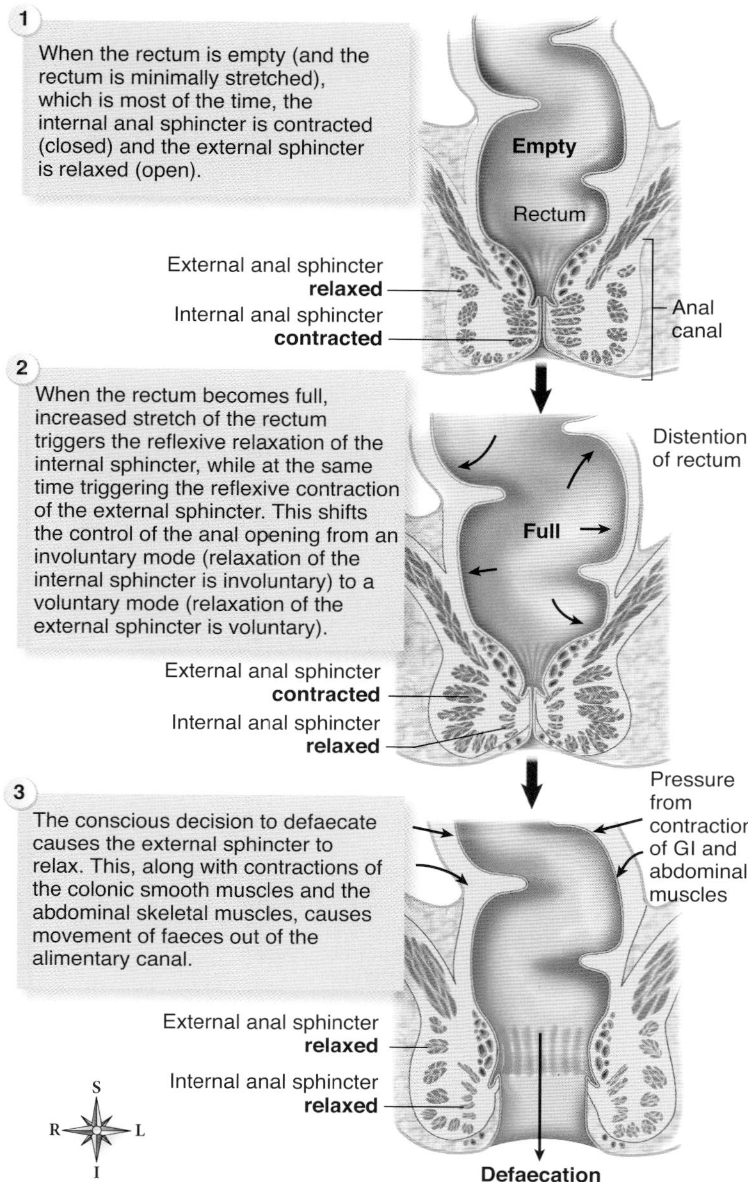
1
When the rectum is empty (and the rectum is minimally stretched), which is most of the time, the internal anal sphincter is contracted (closed) and the external sphincter is relaxed (open).
Empty
Rectum
External anal sphincter **relaxed**
Internal anal sphincter **contracted**
Anal canal
2
When the rectum becomes full, increased stretch of the rectum triggers the reflexive relaxation of the internal sphincter, while at the same time triggering the reflexive contraction of the external sphincter. This shifts the control of the anal opening from an involuntary mode (relaxation of the internal sphincter is involuntary) to a voluntary mode (relaxation of the external sphincter is voluntary).
Distention of rectum
Full
External anal sphincter **contracted**
Internal anal sphincter **relaxed**
3
The conscious decision to defaecate causes the external sphincter to relax. This, along with contractions of the colonic smooth muscles and the abdominal skeletal muscles, causes movement of faeces out of the alimentary canal.
Pressure from contraction of GI and abdominal muscles
External anal sphincter **relaxed**
Internal anal sphincter **relaxed**
S
R
L
I
Defaecation

FIGURE 40-23 Defaecation. The sketches show the role of the anal sphincters in defaecation.

can absorb a small amount of alcohol, almost all other absorption takes place in the intestines—particularly the small intestine.

ELIMINATION

The process of **elimination** is simply the expulsion of the residues of digestion—*faeces*—from the digestive tract. Formation and storage of faeces is the primary function of the colon. The act of expelling faeces is called **defaecation.**

Defaecation is a reflex brought about by stimulation of receptors in the rectal mucosa. Normally, the rectum is empty until mass peristalsis moves faecal matter out of the colon into the rectum. This distends the rectum and produces the desire to defaecate. Also, it stimulates colonic peristalsis and initiates reflex relaxation of the internal sphincter of the anus. Voluntary straining efforts and relaxation of the external anal sphincter may then follow as a result of the desire to defaecate. Together, these several responses bring about defaecation (**Figure 40-23**).

Note that the defaecation reflex is partly under voluntary control. If one voluntarily inhibits defaecation, the rectal receptors soon become depressed and the urge to defaecate does not usually recur until hours later, when mass peristalsis again takes place.

Excessive straining (sometimes referred to as modified *Valsalva manoeuvres*) to defaecate can be dangerous, especially in those with heart problems. Such straining may compress the thorax and disrupt blood flow, interrupt cardiac rhythms, or cause other serious problems.

Constipation occurs when the contents of the distal part of the colon and rectum move at a rate that is slower than normal. What is normal can range from three times a day to three times a week, depending on a variety of factors such as the amount, type, and rate of food eaten. When motility in the distal colon and rectum slows significantly, extra water is absorbed from the faecal mass, producing a hardened stool.

Diarrhoea may occur as a result of increased motility of the small intestine. Chyme moves through the small intestine too quickly, reducing the amount of absorption of water and electrolytes. Diarrhoea may also result from bacterial toxins that damage the water reabsorption mechanisms of the intestinal mucosa. The large volume of material arriving in the large intestine exceeds the limited capacity of the colon for absorption, so a watery stool results. Prolonged diarrhoea can be particularly serious, even fatal, in infants because they have a minimal reserve of water and electrolytes.

CONNECT IT! ⓔ

Intestinal disorders such as diarrhoea may sometimes be treated by restoring a healthy balance of bacteria. Review basic principles of the human *microbiome* in ***The Human Microbiome*** at ***Connect It!***

Severe diarrhoea caused by a *rotavirus,* an intestinal infection, kills more than 600,000 infants and young children worldwide each year. To learn more about how vaccines and **oral rehydration therapy (ORT)** can be used to treat infant diarrhoea, check out ***Infant Diarrhoea*** online at ***Connect It!***

Quick CHECK

14. Explain the term *secondary active transport.*
15. Describe how fatty acids are absorbed by cells of the GI mucosa.
16. What triggers the defaecation reflex?

the big picture | Digestion and the Whole Body

The process of digestion, as with any other vital function, provides a means of survival for the entire body and also requires the function of other systems. The digestive system's primary contribution to overall homeostasis is its ability to maintain a constancy of nutrient concentration in the internal environment. It accomplishes this by breaking large, complex nutrients into smaller, simpler nutrients so they can be absorbed (see figure). The digestive system also provides the means of absorption—the cellular mechanisms that operate in the absorptive cells of the intestinal mucosa. The digestive system also provides some secondary, less vital functions. For example, the teeth and tongue aid the nervous system and respiratory system in producing spoken language. Also, acid in the stomach assists the immune system by destroying potentially harmful bacteria. Some of the various vital and nonvital roles played by the different organs that make up the digestive system are summarized in the "Summary of Digestive Function" figure.

To accomplish its functions, the digestive system requires functional contributions by other systems of the body. Regulation of digestive motility and secretion requires the active participation of both the nervous system and the endocrine system. The oxygen needed for digestive activity requires the proper functioning of both the respiratory system and the circulatory system. The body's framework (integumentary and skeletal systems) is required to support and protect the digestive organs. The skeletal muscles must function if ingestion, mastication, deglutition, and defaecation are to occur normally. As you can see, the digestive system cannot operate alone—nor can any other system or organ, for that matter. The body is truly an integrated system, not a collection of independent components.

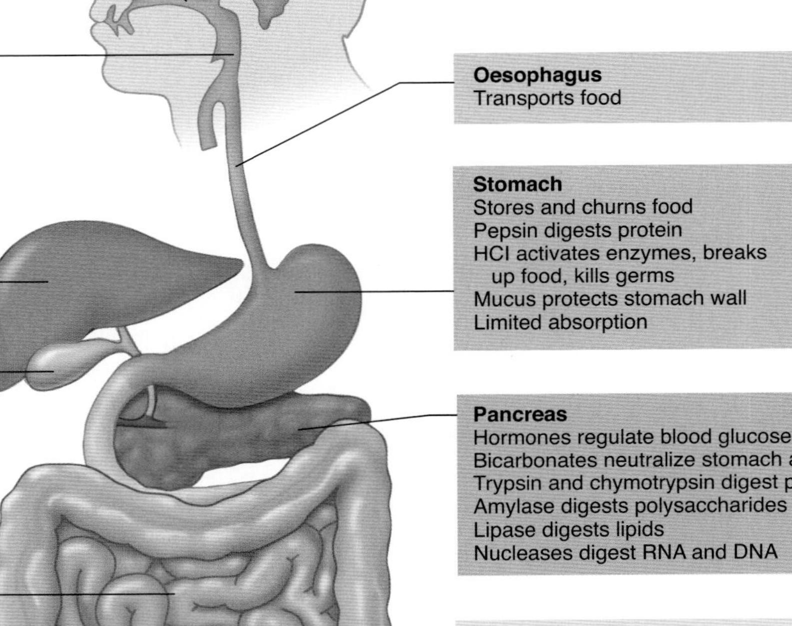
Mouth
Breaks up food particles
Assists in producing spoken language
Pharynx
Swallows
Liver
Breaks down and builds up many biological molecules
Stores vitamins and iron
Destroys old blood cells
Destroys poisons
Bile aids in digestion
Gallbladder
Stores and concentrates bile
Small intestine
Completes digestion
Mucus protects gut wall
Absorbs nutrients, most water
Peptidase digests proteins
Sucrases digest sugars
Nucleotidases and phosphatases digest nucleotides
Anus
Opening for elimination of faeces
Salivary glands
Saliva moistens and lubricates food
Amylase digests polysaccharides
Oesophagus
Transports food
Stomach
Stores and churns food
Pepsin digests protein
HCl activates enzymes, breaks up food, kills germs
Mucus protects stomach wall
Limited absorption
Pancreas
Hormones regulate blood glucose levels
Bicarbonates neutralize stomach acid
Trypsin and chymotrypsin digest proteins
Amylase digests polysaccharides
Lipase digests lipids
Nucleases digest RNA and DNA
Large intestine
Reabsorbs some water and ions
Forms and stores faeces
Rectum
Stores and expels faeces

Summary of digestive function.

LANGUAGE OF SCIENCE *(continued from p. 901)*

enzyme (EN-zyme)
[*en-* **in,** *-zyme* **ferment**]

faeces (FEE-seez)
[*faeces* **waste**]

gastric inhibitory peptide (GIP) (GAS-trik in-HIB-ih-tor-ee PEP-tyde)
[*gastr-* **stomach,** *-ic* **relating to,** *inhibit-* **restrain,** *-ory* **relating to,** *pept-* **digest,** *-ide* **chemical**]

gastric juice
[*gastr-* **stomach,** *-ic* **relating to**]

gastric phase
[*gastr-* **stomach,** *-ic* **relating to**]

gastrin (GAS-trin)
[*gastr-* **stomach,** *-in* **substance**]

H-K pump
[*H* **hydrogen,** *K* **potassium**]

hydrolysis (hye-DROHL-ih-sis)
[*hydro-* **water,** *-lysis* **loosening**]

ingestion (in-JES-chun)
[*in-* **within,** *-gest-* **carry,** *-tion* **process**]

intestinal juice (in-TES-tih-nal)
[*intestin-* **intestine,** *-al* **relating to**]

intestinal phase (in-TES-tih-nal)
[*intestin-* **intestine,** *-al* **relating to**]

intrinsic factor (in-TRIN-sik FAK-tor)
[*intr-* **inside or within,** *-insic* **beside**]

lecithin (LES-ih-thin)
[*lecith-* **yolk,** *-in* **substance**]

lipase (LYE-payz)
[*lip-* **fat,** *-ase* **enzyme**]

mastication (mas-tih-KAY-shun)
[*mastica-* **chew,** *-tion* **process**]

mechanical digestion
[*digest-* **break apart,** *-tion* **process**]

micelle (my-SELL)
[*mic-* **grain,** *-elle* **small**]

migrating motor complex (MMC)
[*migra-* **wander,** *-at-* **process,** *motor* **move,** *com-* **together,** *-plex* **weave or braid**]

motilin (moh-TIL-in)
[*mot-* **move,** *-il-* **relating to,** *-in* **substance**]

motility (moh-TIL-ih-tee)
[*mot-* **move,** *-il-* **relating to,** *-ity* **state**]

mucus (MYOO-kus)
[*mucus* **slime**]

nuclease (NYOO-klee-ayz)
[*nucle-* **nut or kernel (nucleic acid),** *-ase* **enzyme**]

pancreatic juice (pan-kree-AT-ik)
[*pan-* **all,** *-creat-* **flesh,** *-ic* **relating to**]

parietal cell (pah-RYE-ih-tal)
[*parie-* **wall,** *-al* **relating to**]

pepsin (PEP-sin)
[*peps-* **digestion,** *-in* **substance**]

pepsinogen (pep-SIN-oh-jen)
[*peps-* **digestion,** *-in* **substance,** *-o-* **combining form,** *-gen* **produce**]

peptidase (PEP-tyd-ayz)
[*pept-* **digestion,** *-ide* **chemical,** *-ase* **enzyme**]

peristalsis (pair-ih-STAL-sis)
[*peri-* **around,** *-stalsis* **contraction**]

proenzyme (pro-EN-zyme)
[*pro-* **first,** *-en-* **in,** *-zyme* **ferment**]

propulsion (proh-PUL-shun)
[*pro-* **in front,** *-pul-* **drive,** *-sion* **process**]

protease (PROH-tee-ayz)
[*prote-* **protein,** *-ase* **enzyme**]

retropulsion (ret-roh-PUL-shun)
[*retro-* **backward,** *-pul-* **drive,** *-sion* **process**]

secretin (seh-KREE-tin)
[*secret-* **separate,** *-in* **substance**]

segmentation (seg-men-TAY-shun)
[*segment-* **cut section,** *-ation* **process**]

sodium cotransport (SOH-dee-um koh-TRANS-port)
[*sod-* **soda,** *-ium* **chemical ending,** *co-* **with,** *-trans-* **across,** *-port* **carry**]

trypsin (TRIP-sin)
[*tryps-* **pound,** *-in* **substance**]

trypsinogen (trip-SIN-oh-gen)
[*tryps-* **pound,** *-in* **substance,** *-o-* **combining form,** *-gen* **produce**]

zymogenic cell (zye-moh-JEN-ik)
[*zym-* **ferment (enzyme),** *-o-* **combining form,** *-gen-* **produce,** *-ic* **relating to**]

LANGUAGE OF MEDICINE

constipation (kon-stih-PAY-shun)
[*constipa-* **crowd together,** *-tion* **process**]

diarrhoea (dye-ah-REE-ah)
[*dia-* **through,** *-rrhoea* **flow**]

oral rehydration therapy (ORT) (OR-al ree-hye-DRAY-shun THER-ah-pee)
[*or-* **mouth,** *-alis* **relating to,** *re-* **back again,** *-hydra-* **water,** *-ation* **process**]

steatorrhoea (stee-ah-toh-REE-ah)
[*steat-* **fat,** *-o-* **combining form,** *-rrhoea* **flow**]

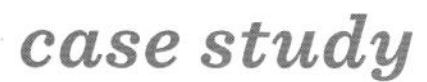

case study

Peter had been working late and picked up a takeaway meal of fish and chips to eat at home. After his meal he bent over to pick up a plate and felt a sharp, stabbing pain in his right upper back just below his shoulder blade. The pain was so intense he could hardly breathe. The discomfort lasted for about 20 minutes and then dissipated to a dull ache. Having a history of back pain he thought he had injured the same area again.

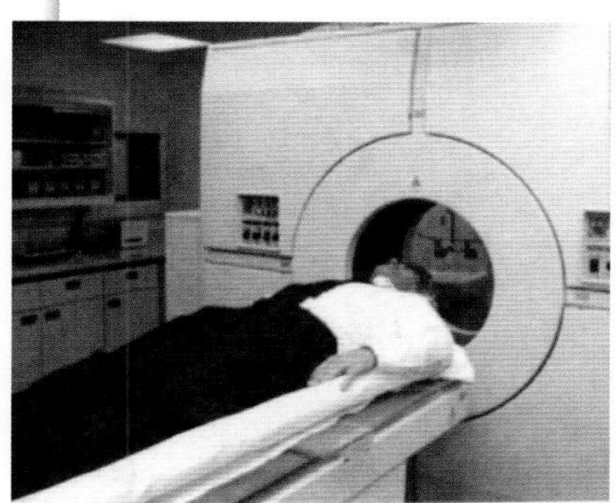

The following Monday Peter's doctor arranged a magnetic resonance imaging (MRI) scan to investigate his spine. The test results showed nothing wrong with the skeletal system and no misalignment of the spine. There was also no change in the pain with movement; the dull ache in Peter's back remained constant regardless of whether he was moving or still. A urine analysis came back normal and over the next few weeks the pain receded.

A few weeks later Peter joined some friends after work for an evening meal and within a few minutes of consuming his food the stabbing pain returned. Again Peter's late meal had a very high fat content.

1. Taking all the information into account, what system do you think may be malfunctioning to cause Peter's pain?
   a. Skeletal system
   b. Muscular system
   c. Digestive system
   d. Urinary system

2. Which of the following hormones is NOT released in response to fatty, acidic chyme entering the duodenum?
   a. Gastrin
   b. CCK
   c. Secretin
   d. GIP

3. After eating foods high in fat, Peter's body may increase the production and release of bile. Bile is stored in which organ?
   a. Liver
   b. Pancreas
   c. Stomach
   d. Gallbladder

Hint To solve a case study, you may have to refer to the glossary or index, other chapters in this textbook, ***Connect It!,*** and other resources.

CHAPTER SUMMARY

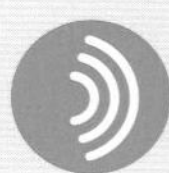

*To download an MP3 version of the chapter summary for use with your mobile device, access the **Audio Chapter Summaries** online at evolve.elsevier.com.*

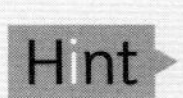

Scan this summary after reading the chapter to help you reinforce the key concepts. Later, use the summary as a quick review before your class or before a test.

Overview of Digestive Function

A. Primary function of the digestive system—to bring essential nutrients into the internal environment so that they are available to each cell of the body
B. Mechanisms used to accomplish the primary function of the digestive system (**Figure 40-1**)
   1. Ingestion—food is taken in
   2. Digestion—breakdown of complex nutrients into simple nutrients
   3. Motility of the GI wall—physically breaks down large chunks of food material and moves food along the tract
   4. Secretion—digestive enzyme secretion facilitates chemical digestion
   5. Absorption—movement of nutrients through the GI mucosa into the internal environment
   6. Elimination—excretion of material that is not absorbed
   7. Regulation—coordination of the various functions of the digestive system
C. The digestive tract is functionally an extension of the external environment—material does not truly enter the body until it is absorbed into the internal environment

Digestion

A. Mechanical digestion—movements of the digestive tract
   1. Change ingested food from large particles into minute particles, facilitating chemical digestion
   2. Churn contents of the GI lumen to mix with digestive juices and ensure contact with the surface of the intestinal mucosa, facilitating absorption
   3. Propel food along the alimentary tract, eliminating digestive waste from the body
   4. Mastication—chewing movements
      a. Reduces size of food particles
      b. Mixes food with saliva in preparation for swallowing
   5. Deglutition—process of swallowing; complex process requiring coordinated and rapid movements (**Figure 40-2**)
      a. Oral stage (mouth to oropharynx)—voluntarily controlled; formation of a food bolus in the middle of the tongue; tongue presses bolus against the palate and food is then moved into the oropharynx
      b. Pharyngeal stage (oropharynx to oesophagus)—involuntary movement; to propel bolus from the pharynx to the oesophagus, the mouth, nasopharynx, and larynx must be blocked; a combination of contractions and gravity move bolus into oesophagus
      c. Oesophageal stage (oesophagus to stomach)—involuntary movement; contractions and gravity move bolus through oesophagus and into stomach
   6. Peristalsis and segmentation—two main types of motility produced by the smooth muscle of the GI tract; can occur together, in an alternating fashion
      a. Peristalsis—wavelike ripple of the muscle layer of a hollow organ; progressive motility that produces forward movement of matter along the GI tract (**Figures 40-3** and **40-4**)
      b. Segmentation—mixing movement; digestive reflexes cause a forward-and-backward movement with a single segment of the GI tract; helps break down food particles, mixes food and digestive juices, and brings digested food in contact with intestinal mucosa to facilitate absorption (**Figure 40-5**)
   7. Regulation of motility
      a. Gastric motility
         (1) Food in the stomach is churned (propulsion and retropulsion) and mixed with gastric juices to form chyme
         (2) Chyme is ejected about every 20 seconds into the duodenum; emptying the stomach takes approximately 2 to 6 hours
      b. Gastric emptying controlled by hormonal and nervous mechanisms (**Figure 40-6**)
         (1) Hormonal mechanism—fats in duodenum stimulate the release of gastric inhibitory peptide, which acts to decrease peristalsis of gastric muscle and slows passage of chyme into duodenum
         (2) Nervous mechanism—enterogastric reflex; receptors in the duodenal mucosa are sensitive to presence of

acid and to distention; impulses over sensory and motor fibres in the vagus nerve cause a reflex inhibition of gastric peristalsis

8. Intestinal motility—includes peristalsis and segmentation
   a. Segmentation in duodenum and upper jejunum mixes chyme with digestive juices from the pancreas, liver, and intestinal mucosa
   b. Peristalsis rate picks up as chyme approaches end of jejunum, moving it through small intestine into the large intestine
   c. After leaving stomach, passage of chyme all the way through the small intestine takes approximately 5 hours
   d. Peristalsis regulated in part by intrinsic stretch reflexes; stimulated by cholecystokinin (CCK)

B. Chemical digestion—all changes in chemical composition of food as it travels through the digestive tract
   1. Chemical changes result from hydrolysis—process in which compound unites with water and breaks down further
   2. Digestive enzymes—extracellular, organic (protein) catalysts
      a. Operate in lumen of digestive tract, outside of any body cells
      b. Properties of digestive enzymes
         (1) Specific in their action (**Figure 40-7**)
         (2) Function optimally at a specific pH (**Figure 40-8**)
         (3) Most enzymes catalyze a chemical reaction in both directions
         (4) Enzymes are continually being destroyed or eliminated from the body and must continually be synthesized
         (5) Most digestive enzymes are synthesized as inactive proenzymes
   3. Carbohydrate digestion (**Figure 40-9**)
      a. Carbohydrates are saccharide compounds
      b. Polysaccharides are hydrolyzed by amylases to form disaccharides
      c. Final steps of carbohydrate digestion are catalyzed by sucrase, lactase, and maltase, found in the cell membrane of epithelial cells covering the villi that line the intestinal lumen
   4. Protein digestion (**Figure 40-10**)
      a. Protein compounds are made up of twisted chains of amino acids
      b. Proteases catalyze hydrolysis of proteins into intermediate compounds and, finally, into amino acids
      c. Main proteases: pepsin in gastric juice, trypsin in pancreatic juice, peptidases in intestinal brush border
   5. Fat digestion (**Figure 40-12**)
      a. Fats must be emulsified by bile in small intestine before being digested (**Figure 40-11**)
      b. Lipases are the main fat-digesting enzymes
   6. Residues of digestion—some compounds of food resist digestion and are eliminated as faeces

Secretion

A. Saliva—secreted by salivary glands
   1. Mucus lubricates food and, with water, facilitates mixing
   2. Amylase—an enzyme that begins digestion of starches
   3. Lingual lipase works at low pH, so can digest fats in stomach and upper duodenum
   4. Sodium bicarbonate increases the pH for optimum amylase function

B. Gastric juice—secreted by gastric glands
   1. Pepsin (secreted as inactive pepsinogen by chief cells)—a protease that begins the digestion of proteins
   2. Hydrochloric acid (HCl, secreted by parietal cells)
      a. HCl decreases the pH of chyme for activation and optimum function of pepsin (**Figure 40-13**)
      b. Released actively into the gastric juice by H-K pumps (proton pumps)
      c. Vesicles in the resting parietal cell move to the apical surface when the cell becomes active—thus increasing the surface area for the process of secretion (**Figure 40-14**)
   3. Intrinsic factor (secreted by parietal cells) protects vitamin B_{12} and later facilitates its absorption (**Figure 40-15**)
   4. Mucus and water lubricate, protect, and facilitate mixing of chyme (**Table 40-4**)

C. Pancreatic juice—secreted by acinar and duct cells of the pancreas
   1. Proteases (e.g., trypsin and chymotrypsin)—enzymes that digest proteins and polypeptides
   2. Lipases—enzymes that digest emulsified fats
   3. Nucleases—enzymes that digest nucleic acids such as DNA and RNA
   4. Amylase—an enzyme that digests starches
   5. Sodium bicarbonate increases the pH for optimum enzyme function; its manufacture also helps restore normal pH of blood (**Figures 40-16** and **40-17**)

D. Bile—secreted by the liver; stored and concentrated in the gallbladder
   1. Lecithin and bile salts emulsify fats by encasing them in shells to form tiny spheres called *micelles*
   2. Sodium bicarbonate increases pH for optimum enzyme function
   3. Cholesterol, products of detoxification, and bile pigments (e.g., bilirubin) are waste products excreted by the liver and eventually eliminated in the faeces

E. Intestinal juice—secreted by intestinal exocrine cells
   1. Mucus and water lubricate and aid in continued mixing of chyme
   2. Sodium bicarbonate increases pH for optimum enzyme function

Control of Digestive Gland Secretion

A. Control of salivary secretion
   1. Only reflex mechanisms control the secretion of saliva
   2. Chemical and mechanical stimuli come from the presence of food in the mouth
   3. Olfactory and visual stimuli come from the smell and sight of food

B. Control of gastric secretion—three phases (**Figure 40-18**)
   1. Cephalic phase—"psychic phase", because mental factors activate the mechanism; parasympathetic fibres in branches of the vagus nerve conduct stimulating efferent impulses to

the glands; stimulate production of gastrin (by G cells in the stomach)
   2. Gastric phase—when products of protein digestion reach the pyloric portion of the stomach, they stimulate release of gastrin; gastrin accelerates secretion of gastric juice, ensuring enough enzymes are present to digest food
   3. Intestinal phase—various mechanisms seem to adjust gastric secretion as chyme passes to and through the intestinal tract; endocrine reflexes involving gastric inhibitory peptide, secretin, and CCK inhibit gastric secretions

C. Control of pancreatic secretion—stimulated by several hormones released by intestinal mucosa
   1. Secretin evokes production of pancreatic fluid low in enzyme content but high in bicarbonate
   2. CCK—several functions
      a. Causes increased exocrine secretion from the pancreas
      b. Opposes gastrin, thus inhibiting gastric HCl secretion
      c. Stimulates contraction of the gallbladder so that bile is ejected into the duodenum

D. Control of bile secretion—bile secreted continually by the liver; secretin and CCK stimulate ejection of bile from the gallbladder

E. Control of intestinal secretion—little known about how intestinal secretion is regulated; suggested that the intestinal mucosa is stimulated to release hormones that increase the production of intestinal juice

Absorption

A. Process of absorption
   1. Passage of substances through the intestinal mucosa into the blood or lymph (**Figure 40-19**)
   2. Most absorption occurs in the small intestine

B. Mechanisms of absorption
   1. For some substances such as mineral ions or water, absorption occurs by simple diffusion or osmosis
   2. Other substances are absorbed through more complex mechanisms (**Figures 40-20** and **40-21**)
      a. Secondary active transport—how sodium is transported
      b. Sodium cotransport (coupled transport)—how glucose and amino acids are transported
      c. Fatty acids, monoglycerides, and cholesterol are transported with the aid of bile salts from the lumen to absorbing cells of the villi
   3. Transcellular absorption moves nutrient particle *through* cells (as described earlier) and paracellular absorption moves particles *between* cells
   4. After food is absorbed, it travels to the liver via the portal system
   5. In summary, most absorption occurs in the small intestine (**Figure 40-22**)

Elimination

A. Definition—expulsion of faeces from the digestive tract; referred to as *defaecation*

B. Defaecation—results from a reflex brought about by stimulation of receptors in the rectal mucosa that is produced when the rectum is distended (**Figure 40-23**)

C. Constipation—contents of the lower part of the colon and rectum move at a slower than normal rate; extra water is absorbed from the faeces, resulting in a hardened stool

D. Diarrhoea—result of increased motility of the small intestine, causing decreased absorption of water and electrolytes and a watery stool

The Big Picture: Digestion and the Whole Body

A. Primary contribution of the digestive system to overall homeostasis is to provide a constant nutrient concentration in the internal environment

B. Secondary roles of digestive system
   1. Absorption of nutrients
   2. Teeth and tongue, along with respiratory and nervous system, are important in producing spoken language
   3. Gastric acids aid the immune system by destroying potentially harmful bacteria

C. To accomplish its functions, digestive system needs other systems to contribute
   1. Regulation of digestive motility and secretion requires the nervous system and endocrine system
   2. Oxygen for digestive activity is dependent on proper functioning of the respiratory and circulatory systems
   3. Integumentary and skeletal systems support and protect the digestive organs
   4. Muscular system is needed for ingestion, mastication, deglutition, and defaecation to occur normally

REVIEW QUESTIONS

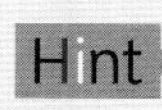

Write out the answers to these questions after reading the chapter and reviewing the Chapter Summary. Note—writing out your answers will consolidate learning and provide a valuable resource of information.

1. List four of the mechanical processes that occur during digestion.
2. List the three steps, or stages, in deglutition.
3. Discuss the function of the deglutition centre in the medulla.
4. How does gastric inhibitory peptide influence emptying of the stomach? What is the enterogastric reflex?
5. Discuss the functional roles of gastric juice.
6. What is chyme?
7. Describe the classification of digestive enzymes.
8. Discuss three important properties of digestive enzymes.
9. What substances chemically digest proteins? Carbohydrates? Fats?
10. What is meant by the term *cephalic phase* of gastric secretion? *Gastric phase? Intestinal phase?*
11. What digestive functions does the pancreas perform?
12. Describe the absorption of glucose from the lumen of the small intestine.
13. What vitamins depend on bile salts for their absorption?
14. Name each hormone that controls ejection of bile, stimulation of gastric enzymes, inhibition of gastric emptying, secretion of alkaline fluid from pancreas, and secretion of pancreatic enzymes.
15. Discuss responses that collectively result in defaecation.
16. Describe the treatment called *oral rehydration therapy*.

CRITICAL THINKING QUESTIONS

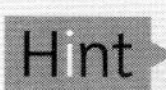

After finishing the Review Questions, write out the answers to these more in-depth questions to help you apply your new knowledge. Go back to sections of the chapter that relate to concepts that you find difficult.

1. In terms of homeostatic balance in the body, what is the function of the digestive system?
2. Explain the two types of digestive processes within the alimentary canal.
3. Describe the two types of motility within the intestine.
4. What distinction is there between trypsin and pepsin, protein and peptides, and polysaccharides and monosaccharides? Explain how one pair is different from the other two.
5. What is the relationship between hydrochloric acid production by the stomach and bicarbonate production by the pancreas?
6. Because fats are not soluble in water, what process is used by the digestive system to emulsify fats?
7. How is emulsification an example of mechanical digestion rather than chemical digestion?
8. Compare and contrast carbohydrate and protein absorption with fat absorption. Include an explanation of basal active transport.

41 Nutrition and Metabolism

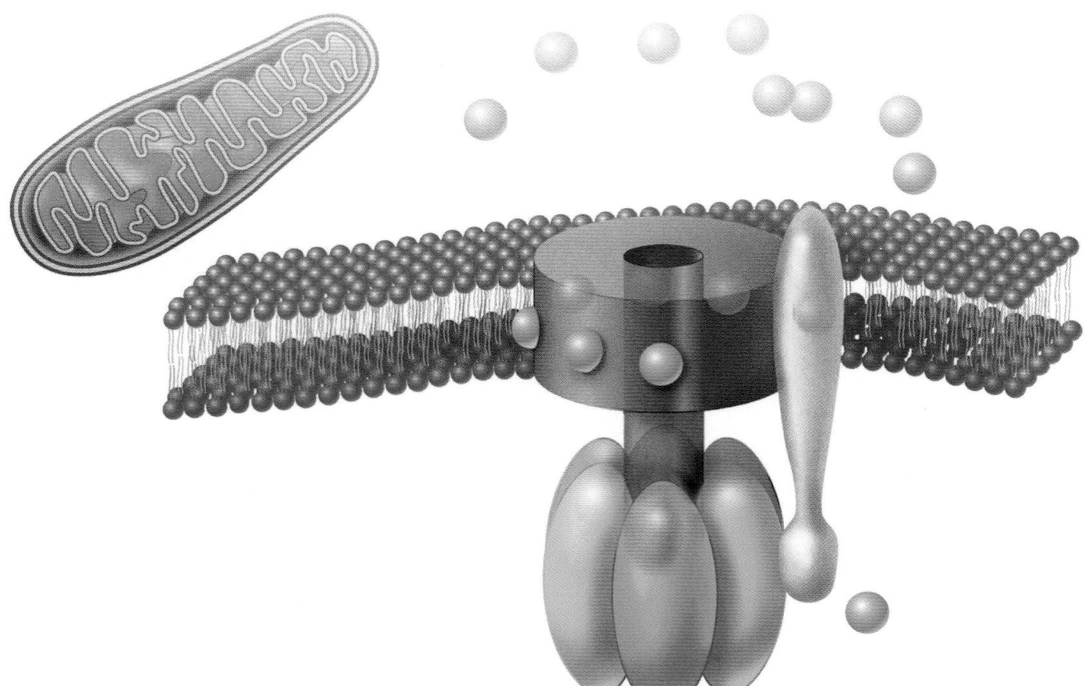

CHAPTER OUTLINE

Hint Scan this outline before you begin to read the chapter, as a preview of how the concepts are organized.

The previous chapter (Chapter 40) explains the processes of getting nutrients into the internal environment. This chapter takes the story further by discussing how the body manages the nutrients after they are absorbed—how they are stored and how they are used by the cells of the body. Before beginning this chapter, you may want to review the story of metabolism summarized in Chapters 6 and 7, beginning on p. 109.

LANGUAGE OF SCIENCE

Hint *Use this list to aid your pronunciation of unfamiliar words.*

aerobic respiration (air-OH-bik res-pih-RAY-shun) [*aero-* **air,** *-b-* **(from** *-bio-***) life,** *-ic* **relating to,** *re-* **again,** *-spir-* **breathe,** *-tion* **process**]

amino acid (ah-MEE-no ASS-id) [*amino* **NH_2,** *acid* **sour**]

anabolism (ah-NAB-oh-liz-im) [*anabol-* **build up,** *-ism* **action**]

anaerobic pathway (an-air-OH-bik) [*an-* **without,** *-aero-* **air,** *-b-* **(from** *-bio-***) life,** *-ic* **relating to**]

anorexigenic effect (an-oh-rek-sih-JEN-ik) [*an-* **without,** *-orex-* **appetite,** *-gen-* **produce,** *-ic* **relating to**]

antioxidant (an-tee-OK-sih-dent) [*anti-* **against,** *-oxi-* **sharp (oxygen),** *-ant* **agent**]

appetite centre (AP-ih-tyte) [*a(d)-* **toward,** *-pet-* **seek out,** *-ite* **relating to**]

assimilation (ah-sim-ih-LAY-shun) [*assimila-* **make alike,** *-tion* **process**]

ATP synthase (SIN-thays) [*ATP* **adenosine triphosphate,** *syn-* **together,** *-ase* **enzyme**]

basal metabolic rate (BMR) (BAY-sal met-ah-BOL-ik) [*bas-* **basis,** *-al* **relating to,** *meta-* **over,** *-bol-* **throw,** *-ic* **relating to**]

calcitriol (kal-SIT-ree-ol) [*calci-* **lime (calcium),** *-tri-* **three,** *-ol* **alcohol (after** *1,25-D_3* **or** *1,25-dihydroxycholecalciferol***)**]

catabolism (kah-TAB-oh-liz-im) [*catabol-* **break down,** *-ism* **action**]

cellulose (SEL-yoo-lohs) [*cell* **storeroom (cell),** *-ul-* **small,** *-ose* **carbohydrate**]

chylomicron (kye-loh-MY-kron) [*chylo-* **juice (chyle),** *-micro-* **small,** *-on* **particle**]

citric acid cycle (SIT-rik ASS-id SYE-kul) [*citr-* **lemony,** *-ic* **relating to,** *acid* **sour,** *cycle* **circle**]

coenzyme (koh-EN-zyme) [*co-* **together,** *-en-* **in,** *-zyme* **ferment**]

coenzyme A (CoA) (koh-EN-zyme) [*co-* **together,** *-en-* **in,** *-zyme* **ferment,** *A* **first letter of Roman alphabet**]

continued on p. 960

OVERVIEW OF NUTRITION AND METABOLISM

Nutrition and *metabolism* are words that are often used together—but what do they mean? **Nutrition** refers to the foods that we eat and the nutrients they contain. The World Health Organization (WHO) describes nutrition as the "intake of food in relation to the body's dietary needs". Good nutrition is a well-balanced diet containing all the materials required by cells to maintain homeostasis. A balanced diet is considered to be the foundation of good health when combined with regular physical activity. Poor nutrition leads to reduced immunity, increased susceptibility to disease, impaired physical and mental development, and reduced productivity.

Nutritional science includes the study of processes by which the body ingests, digests, absorbs, transports, utilizes, and excretes food substances.

Healthy nutrition requires a balance of different nutrients in healthy amounts. *Malnutrition* is a deficiency or imbalance in the consumption of food, vitamins, and minerals. As a matter of convenient communication, many nutrition experts divide the essential (required) nutrients into two major categories:

1. **Macronutrients**—usually include those nutrients that we need in large amounts, such as carbohydrates, fats, and proteins. Sometimes water is included because we need to ingest a large amount of water each day to remain healthy. Minerals that we need in large quantities to remain in good health are also often included among the macronutrients. For example, sodium, chloride, potassium, calcium, magnesium, and phosphorus are often considered to be macronutrients. This group of minerals can also be more specifically called *macrominerals*. Macronutrients are also sometimes called *bulk nutrients* because we need them in bulk quantities to survive.
2. **Micronutrients**—usually include nutrients that we need in very small amounts, such as vitamins and some minerals. Minerals in this group include iron, iodine, zinc, manganese, cobalt, and a few others. Mineral micronutrients can also be called *microminerals* or *trace elements*.

Essential nutrients (sometimes called *indispensable nutrients*) are those that are required in our diet because our bodies cannot synthesize them. *Nonessential (dispensable) nutrients* are those that our body can synthesize, given the proper raw materials (essential nutrients).

We have already stated that healthy nutrition requires a balance of nutrients in the proper amounts. What do we mean by "proper balance" of nutrients? That is a puzzle that scientists continue to work on unravelling. The answer to the puzzle will certainly be complicated because we now know that a complex interaction of slight differences in individual genetic codes and individual lifestyles and environments affect how nutrients affect our bodies. Until this puzzle is completely solved, if it ever is, we fortunately have some advice that we can rely on to help us make healthy choices. For example the UK government organization Public Health England makes use of an *Eatwell Guide* (**Figure 41-1**) to help people achieve a balance of essential nutrients in their diet.

There are numerous claims that certain types of diet encourage better eating habits, such as the so-called *Mediterranean diet*, the *5:2 diet*, and the *DASH diet*. These, along with vegetarianism and veganism, have pros and cons. However some popular diets are not always based on science and research and may be harmful, so it is probably wise for those wishing to change their diet to discuss their options with a dietitian or doctor.

As we proceed through this chapter, we will discuss most of the major nutrients in more detail and their roles in maintaining the body.

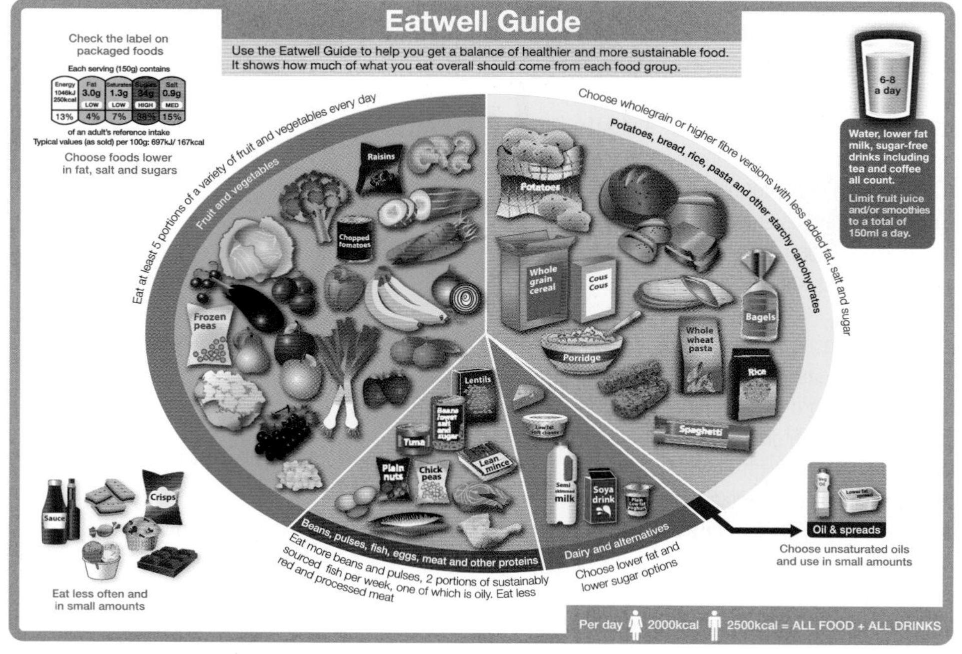

FIGURE 41-1 UK EatWell Guide.
Simple diagrams such as the Eatwell Guide help educate the public on building a diet with a balance of foods from different categories as illustrated in the diagram. The guide also shows what to eat less of or avoid.

UNIT 5

CONNECT IT! 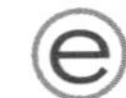

Our sense of taste provides just one mechanism for analyzing our food before we swallow it, so that we know whether our food contains the nutrients we need. Review ***Sensing Food*** online at ***Connect It!*** to find out the many other ways that food is analyzed in the mouth.

Metabolism refers to the complex, interactive set of chemical processes that make life possible. A good phrase to remember in connection with the word *metabolism* is "use of foods" because basically this is what metabolism is—the use the body makes of foods after they have been digested, absorbed, and circulated to cells.

Your body cells use nutrients from food in several ways: as fuel (energy), as material for growth and maintenance, and for regulation of body functions. Before they can be used in these different ways, nutrients have to be assimilated. **Assimilation** occurs when nutrient molecules enter cells and undergo many chemical changes.

Metabolism is a complex process made up of many other processes. Two of the major metabolic processes are **catabolism** and **anabolism.** Each of these processes, in turn, consists of a series of enzyme-catalyzed chemical reactions known as *metabolic pathways.*

Catabolism breaks food molecules down into smaller molecular compounds and, in so doing, releases energy from them. Anabolism does the opposite. It builds nutrient molecules up into larger molecular compounds and, in so doing, uses energy. Catabolism is a decomposition process. Anabolism is a synthesis process. Both catabolism and anabolism take place inside cells. Both processes go on continually and concurrently.

Catabolism releases energy in two forms: heat and chemical energy. The amount of heat generated is relatively large—so large, in fact, that it would hard-boil cells if it were released in one large burst. Fortunately, this does not happen. Catabolism releases heat in frequent, small bursts. Heat is practically useless as an energy source for cells because they cannot use it to do their work. However, this heat is important in maintaining the homeostasis of body temperature. In contrast, chemical energy released by catabolism is more obviously useful. It cannot, however, be used directly for biological reactions. First, it must be transferred to the high-energy molecule of adenosine triphosphate (ATP) (**Box 41-1**).

ATP is one of the most important compounds in the world. Why? It supplies energy directly to the energy-using reactions of all cells in all kinds of living organisms, from one-celled plants to trillion-celled humans. ATP functions as the universal biological currency. It pays the energy bills for all cells and is as important in the world of cells as money is in the world of contemporary society.

Look now at **Figure 41-2**. The structural formula at the top of the diagram shows three phosphate groups attached to the rest of the ATP molecule, two of them by high-energy bonds. Adding water to ATP yields a phosphate group (P), adenosine diphosphate (ADP), and energy, which, as the diagram indicates, is used for anabolism and other cell work. The diagram also shows that P and ADP then use energy released by catabolism to recombine and form ATP. This cycle is called the *ATP/ADP system.*

Metabolism is not identical in all cells. It differs mainly with regard to rate and the kind of products synthesized by anabolism. More

BOX 41-1 *transferring chemical energy*

The ability to transfer energy from molecule to molecule is, as you might imagine, essential to life. We have already discussed the critical role played by the nucleotide adenosine triphosphate (ATP) in transferring energy within living cells. ATP can accept energy from catabolic reactions and transfer that energy to energy-requiring anabolic reactions (see **Figure 41-2**). Although we say that ATP is an "energy storage molecule", do not suppose that the energy is stored for very long periods. In fact, an ATP molecule exists for only a brief time before its last phosphate group is broken off and its energy is transferred to another molecule in some metabolic pathway. Long-term storage of energy can be accomplished only by nutrient molecules such as glucose, glycogen, and triglycerides.

In addition to ATP, various other energy transfer molecules are essential to human life. When atoms in a molecule absorb energy, some of their electrons may move outward to a higher energy level (shell). Electrons often become so energized that they leave the atom completely. As this occurs, pairs of "high-energy" electrons can be picked up and transferred to another molecule by an electron carrier such as **flavin adenine dinucleotide (FAD)** or **nicotinamide adenine dinucleotide (NAD).** The figure shows how NAD^+ (oxidized NAD) picks up a pair of energized electrons to become NADH. It should be noted here that electrons always travel with a proton (H^+) in the metabolic pathways described in this chapter. The electrons do not stay with the electron carrier for long, however. They are immediately transferred to molecules in another metabolic pathway, as the figure shows. In the cell, pairs of electrons (and their energy) can thus be transferred from pathway to pathway by NAD and FAD.

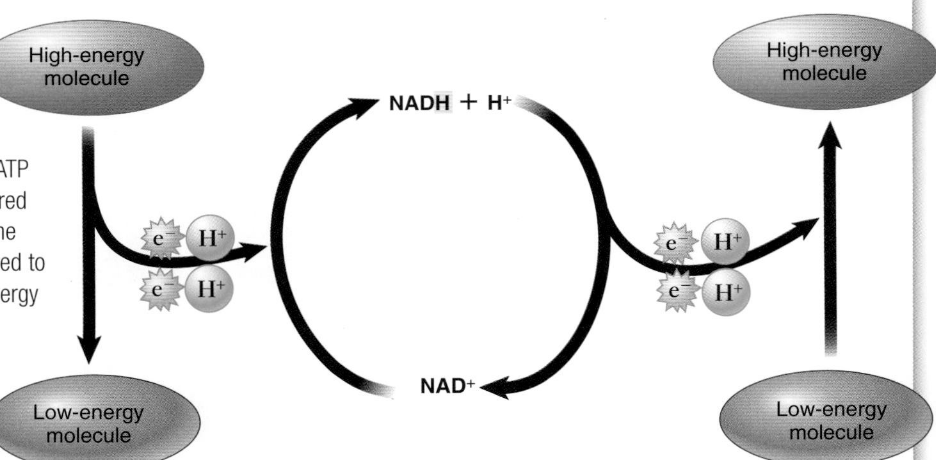

The role of coenzymes in transferring chemical energy.

NAD and FAD, though very similar in function, do have their differences. One difference is that after NAD drops off its pair of high-energy electrons, three ATP molecules are generated, and when FAD drops off its pair of electrons, only two ATP molecules are generated. •

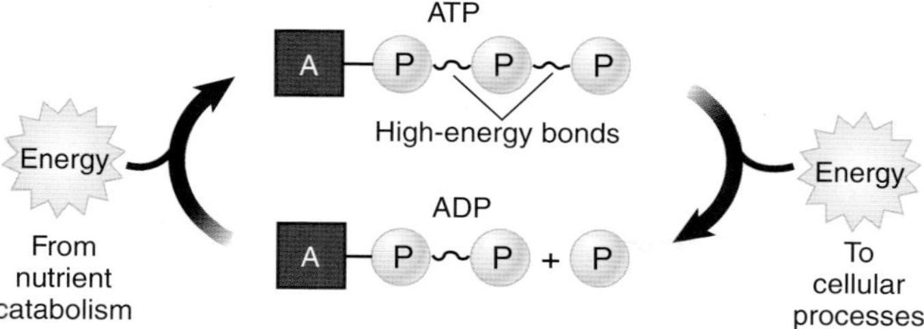

FIGURE 41-2 The role of ATP in metabolism. Adenosine triphosphate (ATP) temporarily stores energy in its last high-energy phosphate bond. When water is added and phosphate breaks free, energy is released to do cellular work. The adenosine diphosphate (ADP) and phosphate groups that result can be resynthesized into ATP, capturing additional energy from nutrient catabolism. This cycle is called the *ATP/ADP system.*

active cells have a higher metabolic rate than do less active cells. Anabolism in different kinds of cells produces different compounds. In hepatocytes (liver cells), for example, anabolism synthesizes various blood protein compounds. Not so in beta cells of the pancreas. Anabolism there produces a different compound—insulin.

The bulk of this chapter discusses concepts related to the many and varied metabolic pathways of the human body. Our attempt here is to build on what you learned in previous chapters, but not to cover the subject of metabolism in its entirety—if that is even possible. Our goal, therefore, is to underscore the *basic* concepts of nutrition and metabolism. It is important to note that our discussion, as well as the diagrams that accompany the discussion, have been simplified to facilitate understanding of these basic concepts.

CARBOHYDRATES

DIETARY SOURCES OF CARBOHYDRATES

Carbohydrates are found in most of the foods that we eat. *Complex carbohydrates*—polysaccharides such as starches in vegetables, grains, and other plant tissues—are broken down into simpler carbohydrates before they are absorbed.

Cellulose, a major component of most plant tissues, is an important exception to this principle. Because humans do not make enzymes that chemically digest this complex carbohydrate, it passes through our system without being broken down. Also called *dietary fibre* or "roughage", cellulose and other indigestible polysaccharides keep chyme thick enough for the digestive system to push it easily. They also help mix chyme, much like the ball inside a can of spray paint. Most biologists believe that a high-fibre diet reduces the risk of many forms of cancer, including colorectal cancer.

Disaccharides such as those in refined sugar must also be chemically digested before they can be absorbed. Monosaccharides in fruits and some "diet foods" are already in an absorbable form, so they can move directly into the internal environment without initially being processed. The monosaccharide *glucose* is the carbohydrate that is most useful to the typical human cell. As **Figure 41-3** shows, other important monosaccharides, *fructose* and *galactose*, are usually converted by liver cells into glucose for use by other cells of the body.

Quick CHECK

1. Name the two types of metabolism and distinguish between them.
2. Why must energy in nutrient molecules be transferred to ATP?

CARBOHYDRATE METABOLISM

The body metabolizes carbohydrates by both catabolic and anabolic processes. Because many human cells use carbohydrates—mainly glucose—as their first or preferred energy fuel, they catabolize most of the carbohydrate absorbed and anabolize a relatively small portion of it. When the amount of glucose entering cells is inadequate for their energy needs, they may make more use of an alternative pathway and catabolize fats or proteins.

We first discussed carbohydrate metabolism in Chapter 6 when we discussed basic concepts of cell metabolism (see pp. 112–115). The subject came up again in Chapter 17 when we discussed energy production in muscle tissue (see pp. 370–373). You may want to flip back to those passages and review the material before proceeding further with this chapter.

As you read through the following sections that briefly describe the process of carbohydrate metabolism, remember the ultimate result of catabolism: the transfer of energy from a nutrient molecule to ATP. It is the continued production of ATP, the energy currency of the cell, that makes nutrient catabolism so incredibly vital to the overall process of life itself.

Glucose Transport and Phosphorylation

Carbohydrate metabolism begins with the movement of glucose through cell membranes. Immediately on reaching the interior of a cell, glucose reacts with ATP to form glucose-6-phosphate (G-6-P). This step, named **glucose phosphorylation,** prepares glucose for further metabolic reactions. **Phosphorylation** is the process of adding a phosphate group to a molecule. In most cells of the body, glucose phosphorylation is an irreversible reaction. However, in a few cells—namely, those of the intestinal mucosa, liver, and renal cortex—glucose phosphorylation is reversible. These cells contain phosphatase, an enzyme that splits phosphate off from glucose-6-phosphate. This reverse glucose phosphorylation reaction forms glucose, which then moves out of the cells into the blood. (Glucose-6-phosphate cannot pass through cell membranes.) Depending on their energy needs of the moment, cells either catabolize (break apart) or anabolize (bind together) glucose-6-phosphate.

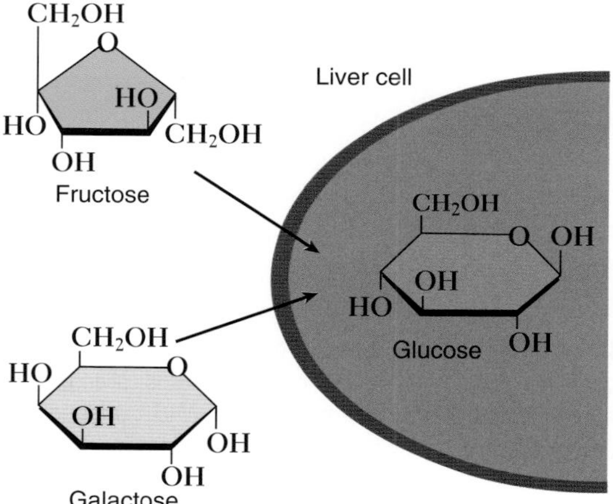

FIGURE 41-3 Conversion of monosaccharides. Monosaccharides fructose and galactose are usually converted to glucose by liver cells. Although simplified in this diagram, conversion to glucose requires several steps. Glucose is the carbohydrate used universally by all cells in the body.

UNIT 5

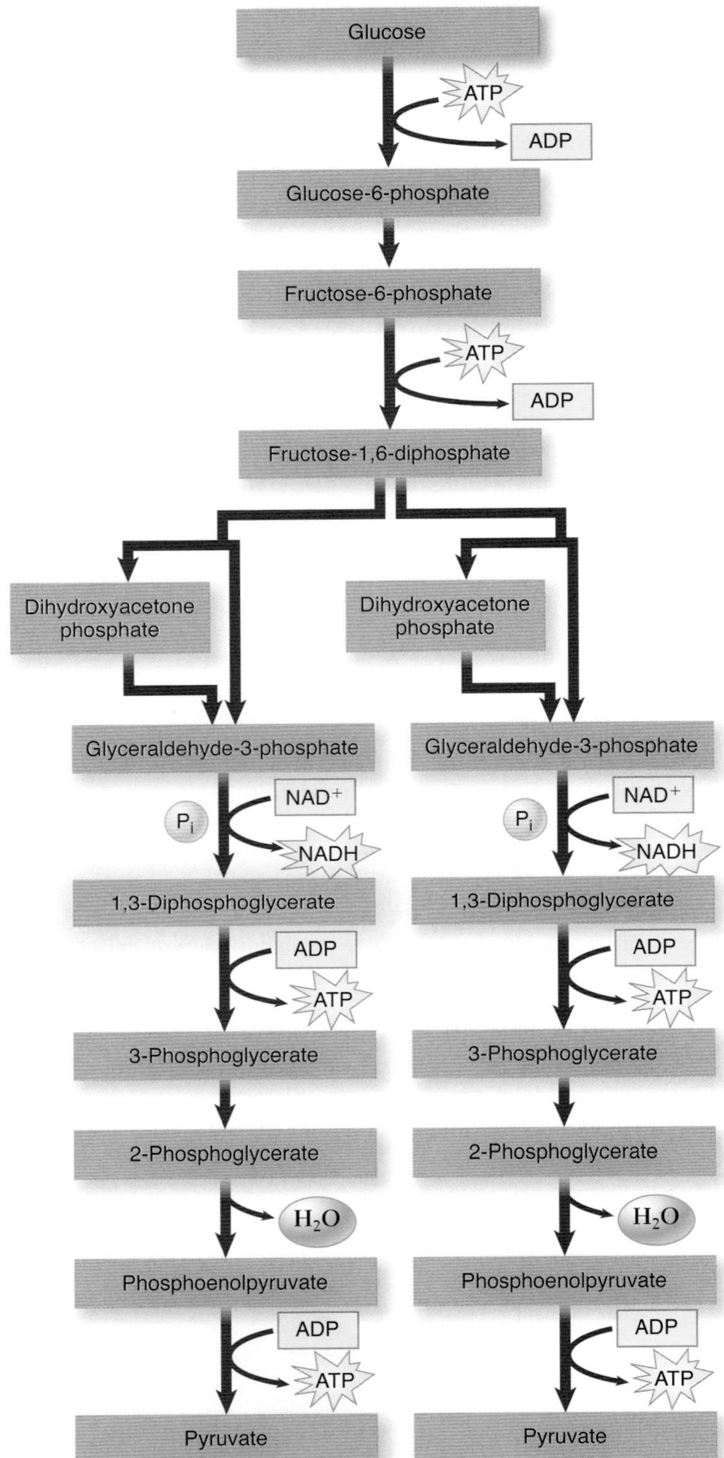

FIGURE 41-4 Glycolysis. The series of enzyme-catalyzed reactions that make up the portion of the catabolic pathway for carbohydrates is called *glycolysis. ADP,* Adenosine diphosphate; *ATP,* adenosine triphosphate; *NAD⁺*, oxidized nicotinamide adenine dinucleotide; *NADH,* reduced nicotinamide adenine dinucleotide.

CONNECT IT! 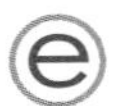

Nutritionists often talk about the "energy value" of food—that is, how much energy the body can get from that food. Do you know what it means when a label states that food energy in calories? Do you know the difference between a *calorie* and a *Calorie*? Or a calorie and a *joule* or *kilojoule*? Find answers to these questions, and also learn the energy values of major nutrients and the amount of energy expended by different physical activities in ***Measuring Energy*** online at ***Connect It!***

Glycolysis

Glycolysis is the first step in the process of carbohydrate catabolism. It breaks apart one glucose molecule to form two pyruvate molecules. (A glucose molecule contains six carbon atoms, and a pyruvate molecule contains three carbon atoms. See **Figure 41-5**.) Glycolysis consists, as **Figure 41-4** shows, of a series of chemical reactions. A specific enzyme catalyzes each of these reactions. Probably the most important facts for you to remember about glycolysis are the following:

- Glycolysis occurs in the cytoplasm of all human cells.
- Glycolysis is an *anaerobic* process; that is, it does not use oxygen. It is the only process that provides cells with energy when their oxygen supply is inadequate or even absent.
- Glycolysis breaks the chemical bonds in glucose molecules and thereby releases about 5% of the energy stored in them. Much of the released energy appears as heat, but some of it is transferred to the high-energy bonds of ATP molecules. For every molecule of glucose undergoing glycolysis, a net of two molecules of ATP is formed. About 8 kilocalories (kcal) (or 33.5 kJ) of energy (in normal physiological conditions) is stored in the high-energy bonds that bind phosphate to ADP to form 1 mole (6.02×10^{23} molecules) of ATP.
- Glycolysis is rapid (compared with the aerobic pathway). It can quickly produce ATP, which is important for the short burst of energy needed in skeletal muscle. Because of its fast rate, pyruvate that cannot enter the slower aerobic pathway converts to lactate, and this normally accumulates in the cell until it can be used. If not used in the cell, it can move through the blood to be processed in other cells, primarily the liver.
- Glycolysis is an essential process because it prepares glucose for the second step in catabolism, namely, the **citric acid cycle.** Glucose itself cannot enter the cycle but must first be converted to pyruvate, then to a compound called *acetyl CoA (coenzyme A).*

Citric Acid Cycle

Glycolysis takes place in the cytoplasm of cells, whereas the citric acid cycle occurs in their mitochondria. Some of the enzymes needed for the many steps of the citric acid cycle are dissolved in the matrix of the mitochondrion, and some are attached to the inner membrane of the mitochondrion.

As stated previously, for every glucose molecule that enters the catabolic pathway described here two pyruvate molecules are produced. Before each pyruvate molecule can proceed into the citric acid cycle, it must be converted into an acetyl group (acetate),

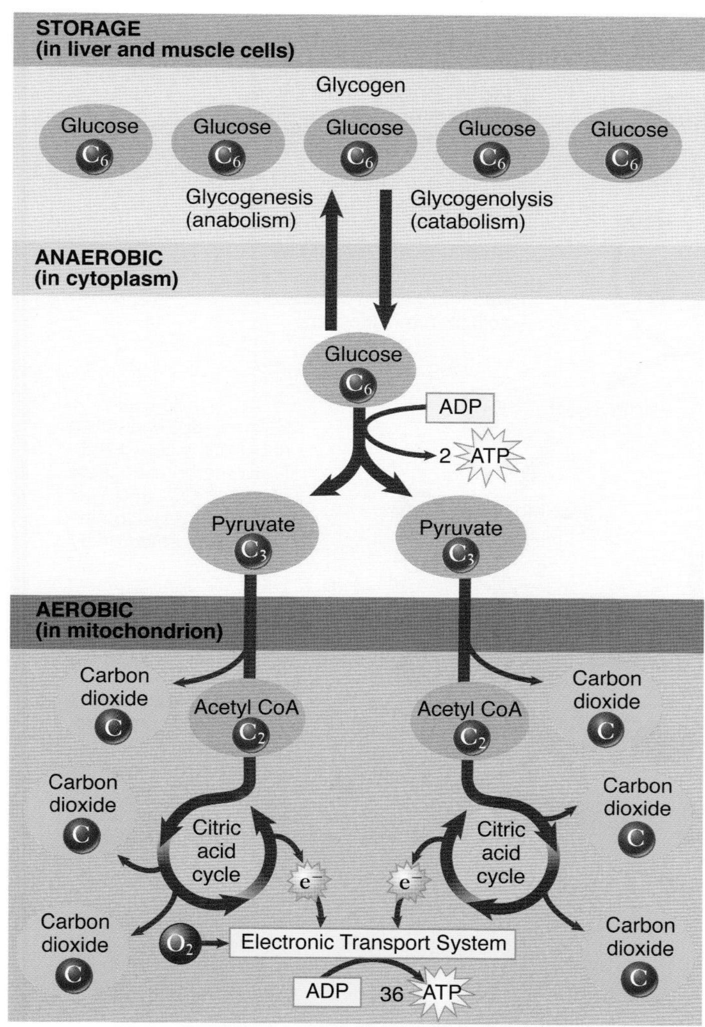

FIGURE 41-5 Catabolism of glucose. Glucose may be stored in the liver and other tissues as the polymer glycogen, which can then later be hydrolyzed to form individual glucose molecules. Glycolysis splits one molecule of glucose (six carbon atoms) into two molecules of pyruvate (three carbon atoms each). The glycolytic pathway does not require oxygen, so it is termed *anaerobic.* A transition reaction removes a carbon dioxide molecule, converting each pyruvate molecule into a two-carbon acetyl group that is escorted by coenzyme A (CoA) into the citric acid cycle. There, two more carbon dioxide molecules (one carbon atom each) are released. The carbon and oxygen atoms in the original glucose molecule are thus released as waste products. However, the real metabolic prize is energy, which is released as the molecule is broken down. Because this part of the pathway requires oxygen, it is termed *aerobic.* More detailed depictions of this process are included later in this chapter.

releasing a carbon dioxide molecule, and a pair of high-energy electrons (with their accompanying protons, H^+), as you can see near the top of **Figure 41-7**. The acetyl is then carried into the citric acid cycle by **coenzyme A (CoA).** Essentially, the citric acid cycle then converts the two acetyl molecules to four carbon dioxide and six water molecules. But many chemical reactions intervene. **Figure 41-5** shows that one glucose molecule is changed by glycolysis to two pyruvate molecules, which, by means of the citric acid cycle, yield six carbon dioxide molecules. **Figure 41-6** shows the details of the citric acid cycle.

First CoA detaches from acetyl CoA, leaving a two-carbon acetyl group, which enters the citric acid cycle by combining with oxaloacetic acid to form citric acid. This is what gives the citric acid cycle its name. The cycle is also called the **tricarboxylic acid (TCA) cycle** because citric acid is also called *tricarboxylic acid.* For many years this cycle was called the **Krebs cycle** after Sir Hans Krebs, whose brilliant work in discovering this metabolic pathway earned him the 1953 Nobel Prize.

You probably do not need to memorize the names of the intermediate products formed during the citric acid cycle, but notice that all of them are acids. You should note that a little bit of ATP is directly generated by the citric acid cycle (in step 5). In step 5, energy is transferred first to guanosine triphosphate (GTP), a nucleotide similar to ATP, and then finally to ATP.

Observe, too, that for each pyruvate molecule entering this pathway, three CO_2 molecules are formed and that certain reactions yield high-energy electrons. Most of the energy leaving the citric acid cycle is in these high-energy electrons. The next section describes how these high-energy electrons are used to generate ATP.

Electron Transport System and Oxidative Phosphorylation

High-energy electrons removed during the citric acid cycle enter a chain of carrier molecules, which is embedded in the inner membrane of mitochondria and is known as the **electron transport system (ETS). Figure 41-7** shows that high-energy electrons (along with their accompanying protons, H^+) are carried to the electron transport system by NAD and FAD. The electrons quickly move down the chain, from one membrane protein complex to the next, eventually to their final acceptor, oxygen.

As the electrons are transported, some of their energy is used to pump their accompanying protons (H^+) to the intramembrane space between the inner and outer membranes of the mitochondrion. This creates a concentration gradient of protons, and the intermembrane space thus becomes a virtual reservoir of protons. As with water behind a dam, the reservoir of protons temporarily stores energy. As in a dam possessing water wheels that convert energy, the inner membrane has "proton wheels" built into it—in the form of **ATP synthase. Figure 41-8** shows how protons move down their concentration gradient and into the ATP synthase structure, turning a molecular wheel that transfers energy by synthesizing ATP from ADP and phosphate.

At this time, the low-energy electrons (e^-) and their protons (H^+) join oxygen, forming water. As you can see, although oxygen is not needed until the very last step of aerobic respiration, its role is vital. Without oxygen to oxidize the hydrogen into water, the energy generation pathway would stop.

Oxidative phosphorylation refers to this oxygen-requiring joining of a phosphate group to ADP to form ATP—a reaction whose importance can scarcely be overemphasized.

The arrangement of catabolic "machinery" within the cell, as currently viewed, is shown in **Figure 41-9**. Glycolytic enzymes in the cytoplasm catalyze the production of pyruvate, which diffuses into

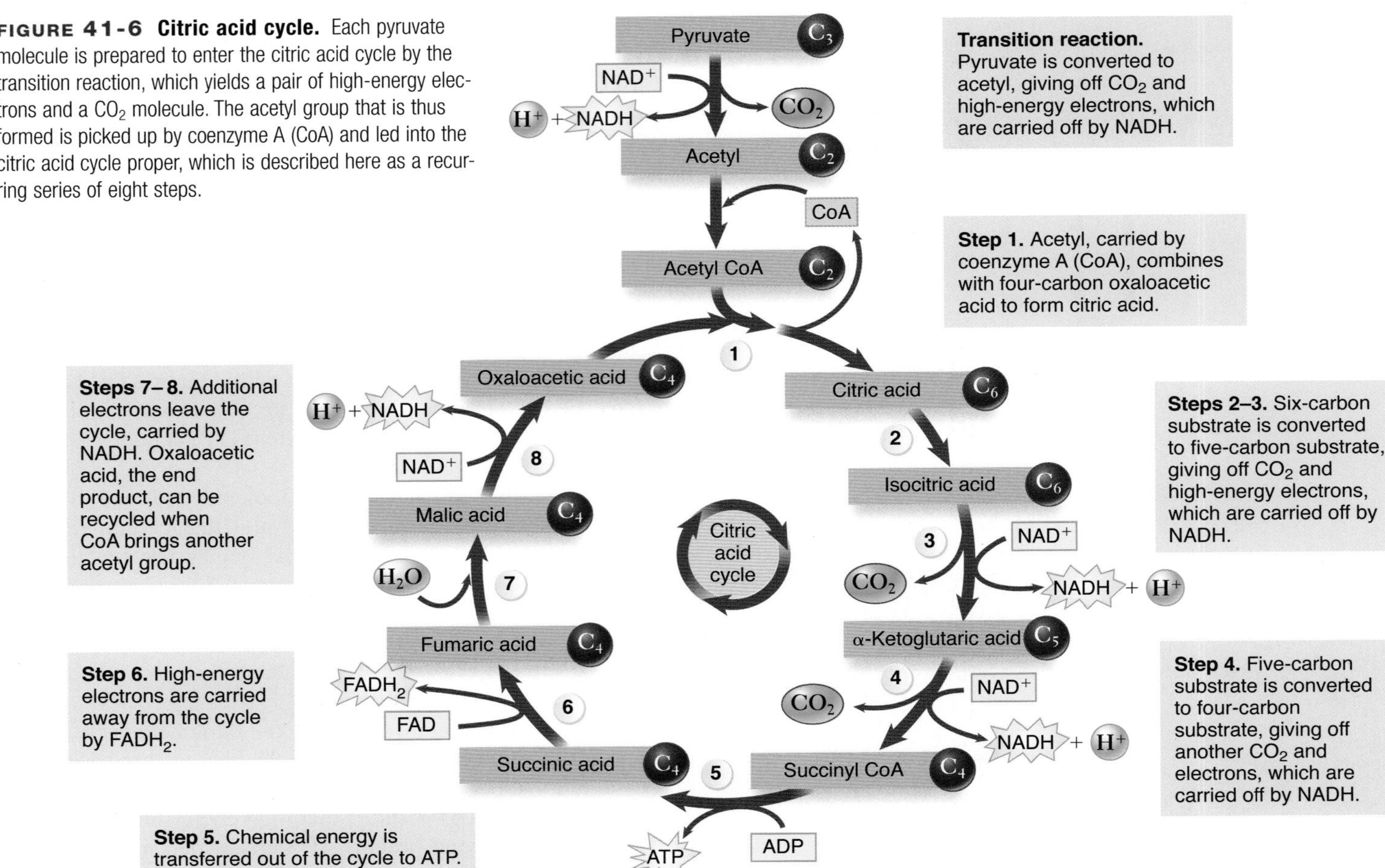

FIGURE 41-6 Citric acid cycle. Each pyruvate molecule is prepared to enter the citric acid cycle by the transition reaction, which yields a pair of high-energy electrons and a CO_2 molecule. The acetyl group that is thus formed is picked up by coenzyme A (CoA) and led into the citric acid cycle proper, which is described here as a recurring series of eight steps.

mitochondria. The enzymes of the citric acid cycle have been localized mostly to the matter (matrix) inside the inner mitochondrial membrane. The high-energy electrons and their accompanying protons are then carried to the cristae of the inner membrane, where the electron transport carriers and mechanism for phosphorylation are found. Because so many of the cell's energy-releasing enzymes are located within the mitochondria, these tiny structures are aptly described as the "power plants" or "powerhouses" of the cell.

The breakdown of ATP molecules, of course, provides virtually all the energy that does cellular work. Therefore, the process that produces some 90% of the ATP formed during carbohydrate catabolism—namely, oxidative phosphorylation—is the crucial part of catabolism (**Figure 41-10**). This vital process depends on cells receiving an adequate oxygen supply. Why? Briefly, because only when oxygen is present in cells to serve as the final acceptor of electrons and hydrogen ions can electrons then continue moving down the electron transport chain. If oxygen becomes unavailable, the movement of electrons and hydrogen ions stops. Cessation of ATP formation by oxidative phosphorylation necessarily follows. All too soon, cells have an inadequate energy supply—a lethal condition if it persists for more than a few minutes.

We can summarize the long series of chemical reactions in glucose catabolism with one short equation:

$$C_6H_{12}O_6 + 6\ O_2 \longrightarrow 6\ CO_2 + 6\ H_2O + 36\ (\text{or } 38)\ \text{ATP} + \text{Heat}$$

Quick CHECK

3. What is glycolysis? How much energy is transferred to ATP through this process?
4. What happens to a nutrient molecule as it proceeds through the citric acid cycle?
5. What is the purpose of the electron transport system?

Anaerobic Pathway

If oxygen supply is inadequate to operate the electron transport system and oxidative phosphorylation, the cell can utilize another pathway for ATP production. Recall from Chapter 17 that oxygen concentration in muscle cells can fall quickly upon beginning strenuous exercise. When this occurs the cell uses the anaerobic pathway that transfers energy to ATP using only glycolysis, a catabolic process that does not require oxygen.

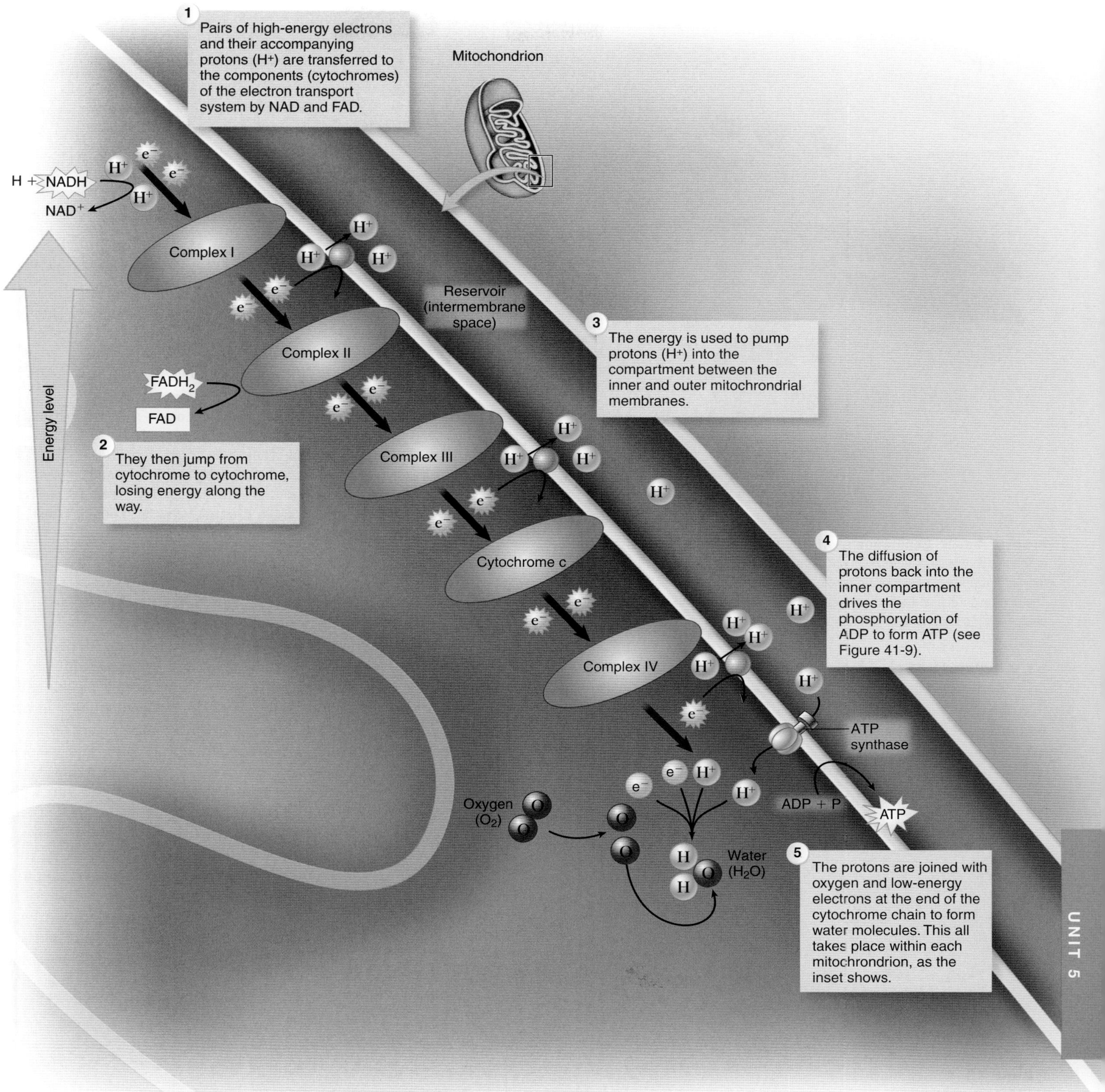

1 Pairs of high-energy electrons and their accompanying protons (H^+) are transferred to the components (cytochromes) of the electron transport system by NAD and FAD.

Mitochondrion

$H + NADH$

NAD^+

H^+

e^-

Complex I

Reservoir (intermembrane space)

Complex II

$FADH_2$

FAD

Energy level

2 They then jump from cytochrome to cytochrome, losing energy along the way.

3 The energy is used to pump protons (H^+) into the compartment between the inner and outer mitochrondrial membranes.

Complex III

Cytochrome c

Complex IV

4 The diffusion of protons back into the inner compartment drives the phosphorylation of ADP to form ATP (see Figure 41-9).

ATP synthase

ADP + P

ATP

Oxygen (O_2)

Water (H_2O)

5 The protons are joined with oxygen and low-energy electrons at the end of the cytochrome chain to form water molecules. This all takes place within each mitochrondrion, as the inset shows.

UNIT 5

FIGURE 41-7 Electron transport system (ETS). This system of energy transfer takes place entirely within each mitochondrion.

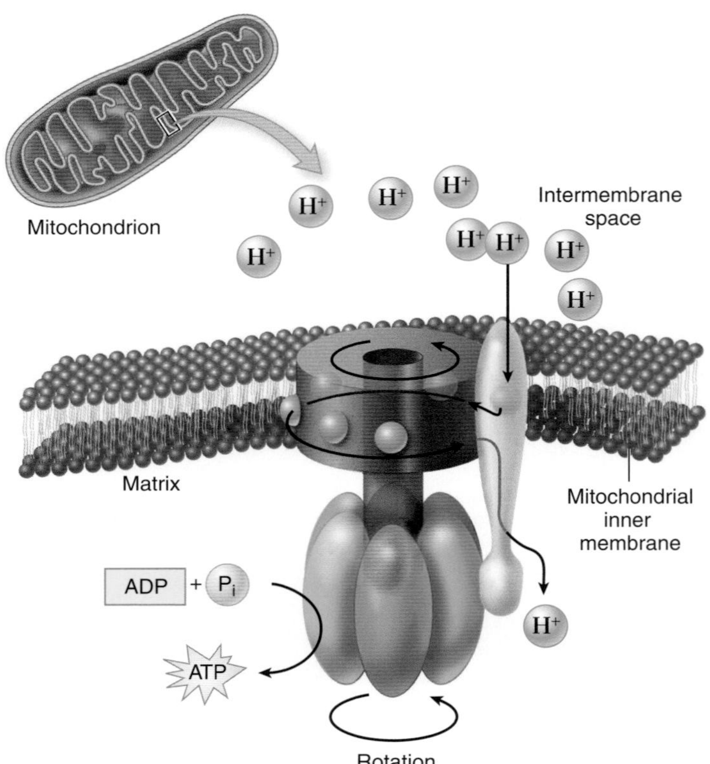

FIGURE 41-8 Generation of ATP by ATP synthase. This simplified model of the proton wheel in the mitochondrial inner membrane shows how protons (H^+) moving down their concentration gradient drive the rotation of a molecular machine. The energy of rotation then phosphorylates (adds phosphate to) adenosine diphosphate (ADP) to become adenosine triphosphate (ATP).

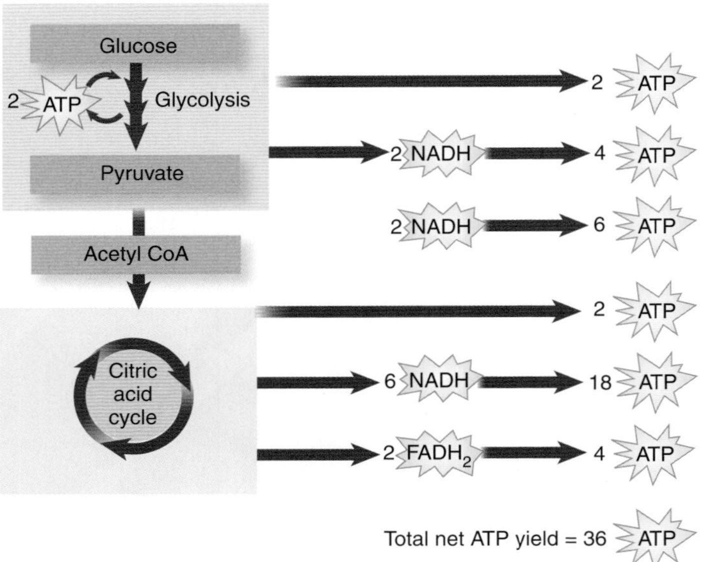

FIGURE 41-10 Energy extracted from glucose. Energy released from the breakdown of glucose is released mostly as heat, but some of it is transferred to a usable form—the high-energy bonds of adenosine triphosphate (ATP). In most human cells, one glucose molecule produces enough usable chemical energy to synthesize or "charge up" 36 ATP molecules. Some cells, such as heart and liver cells, shuttle electrons more efficiently and may be able to synthesize up to 38 ATP molecules. This represents an energy conversion efficiency of 38% to 44%, much better than the 20% to 25% typical of most machines.

As **Figure 41-11** shows, there are two main pathways that glucose or its derivatives can take. One is the pathway that ends with oxidative phosphorylation of ATP. This pathway, described in the previous sections, is called the *aerobic pathway*, or **aerobic respiration**, because it requires the presence of oxygen (**Box 41-2**). If enough oxygen is not available to operate this pathway, the cell will rely solely on glycolysis to produce ATP. Even though this process does not extract the maximum amount of energy from a glucose molecule, it is the only ATP-producing process that can operate in anaerobic conditions. Because the pyruvate molecule produced by glycolysis cannot enter the citric acid cycle, it is converted to *lactate* rather than acetyl CoA. Lactate cannot enter the citric acid cycle.

The production of lactate does something very important—it converts the NADH (reduced nicotinamide adenine dinucleotide) produced by glycolysis to NAD. As glycolysis proceeds, NAD is converted to NADH. If you look at **Figure 41-4** carefully, you will see that there is no reaction in the glycolytic pathway to turn NADH back into NAD again. This is no problem if the aerobic pathway is in operation—NADH is converted back to NAD in the electron transport system. After a short period of anaerobic activity, however, glycolysis will turn all of the cell's NAD into NADH and thus glycolysis will have to shut down because of a lack of free NAD. The production of lactate solves this biochemical dilemma because this reaction also converts NADH back to NAD.

Once oxygen becomes available again in cells that ordinarily rely on

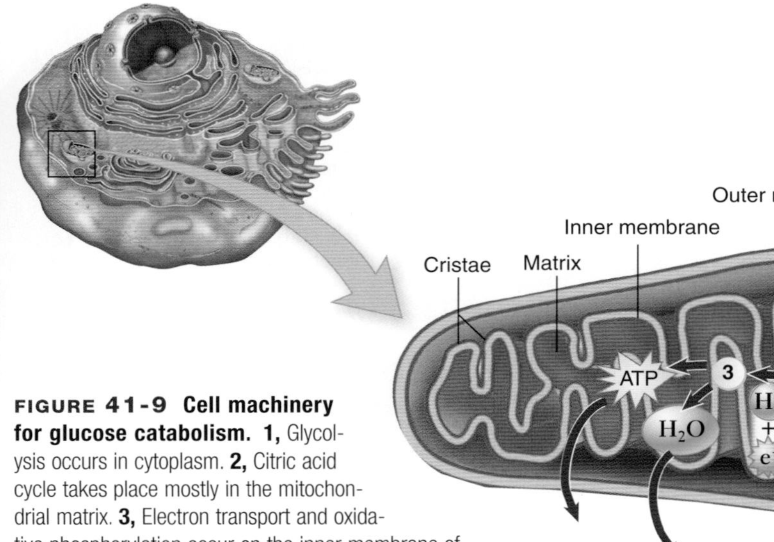

FIGURE 41-9 Cell machinery for glucose catabolism. 1, Glycolysis occurs in cytoplasm. **2,** Citric acid cycle takes place mostly in the mitochondrial matrix. **3,** Electron transport and oxidative phosphorylation occur on the inner membrane of the mitochondrion.

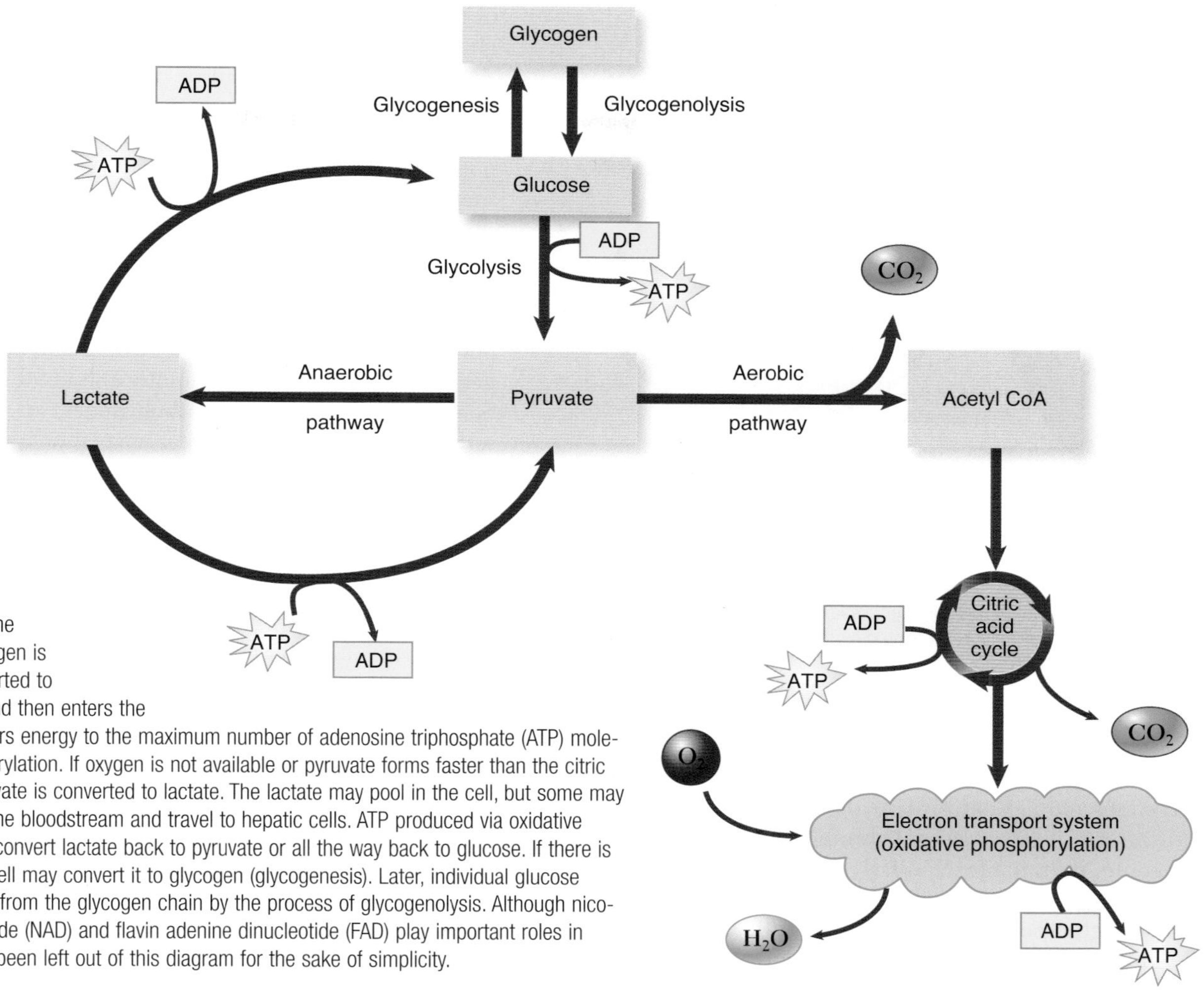

FIGURE 41-11 Summary of glucose metabolism. Glucose is catabolized to pyruvate in the process of glycolysis. If oxygen is available, pyruvate is converted to acetyl coenzyme A (CoA) and then enters the citric acid cycle and transfers energy to the maximum number of adenosine triphosphate (ATP) molecules via oxidative phosphorylation. If oxygen is not available or pyruvate forms faster than the citric acid cycle can take it, pyruvate is converted to lactate. The lactate may pool in the cell, but some may diffuse out of the cell into the bloodstream and travel to hepatic cells. ATP produced via oxidative phosphorylation is used to convert lactate back to pyruvate or all the way back to glucose. If there is an excess of glucose, the cell may convert it to glycogen (glycogenesis). Later, individual glucose molecules can be removed from the glycogen chain by the process of glycogenolysis. Although nicotinamide adenine dinucleotide (NAD) and flavin adenine dinucleotide (FAD) play important roles in these pathways, they have been left out of this diagram for the sake of simplicity.

aerobic respiration, some of the lactate is converted back to pyruvate by the cell (see **Figure 41-11**). Notice that such reconversion requires energy from ATP. Thus reconversion in muscle cells, for example, can occur only when phosphorylation has resumed and produced enough ATP to allow reconversion to occur. Once it is converted to pyruvate, the molecule can follow the aerobic pathway and become completely catabolized.

Much of the lactate produced during anaerobic glycolysis diffuses into the blood and is removed by the liver. Inside liver cells, ATP produced by oxidative phosphorylation is used to convert the lactate back into glucose. The glucose may then be stored as glycogen in the liver or be returned through the bloodstream for use by other cells. **Figure 41-12** summarizes this cycle during anaerobic glycolysis by skeletal muscles. This cycle is often called the **Cori cycle** after its discoverers, Carl and Gerty Cori.

Because anaerobic glycolysis requires the later use of ATP molecules produced by oxidative phosphorylation, more oxygen needs to be taken into the body. Historically this was called the oxygen debt, it is now referred to as excess post-exercise oxygen consumption (EPOC). When excess oxygen becomes available following exercise, the extra ATP formed is used to convert lactate to pyruvate or glucose.

BOX 41-2 *fyi* | Anaerobic Body Cells

Some body cells, specifically the red blood cells (see photo), do not have the cellular organelles and enzymes required to carry out aerobic respiration. These cells must rely solely on glycolysis for their adenosine triphosphate (ATP) production. Red blood cells produce lactate continually, which diffuses into the plasma and is carried to liver cells for conversion back to pyruvate and then to glucose and glycogen (see **Figure 41-11**). •

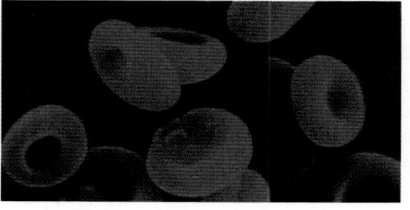

Red blood cells (RBCs). This colour-enhanced scanning electron micrograph shows several RBCs, which are unable to perform aerobic respiration because of a lack of mitochondria. They rely solely on anaerobic glycolysis for their ATP, producing lactate as a metabolic waste product.

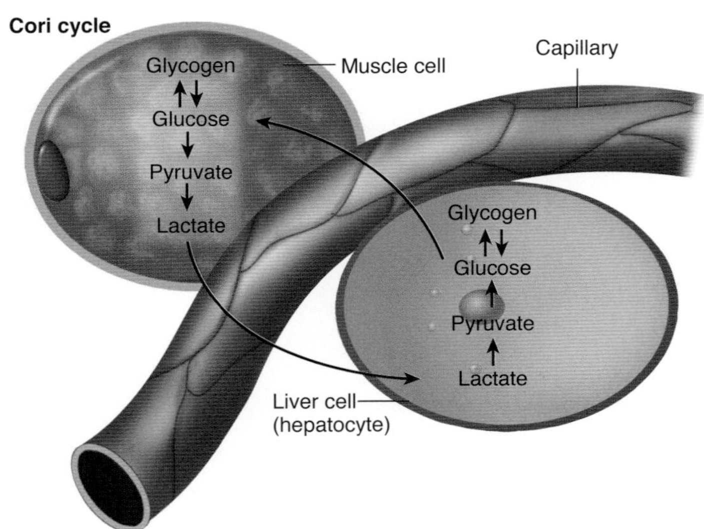

FIGURE 41-12 Cori cycle. Lactate produced by anaerobic glycolysis in skeletal muscles is carried to liver cells, where it is converted back to glucose and stored as liver glycogen or returned to the bloodstream, where the glucose may be taken up by muscle cells and used for respiration or stored as muscle glycogen.

Glycogenesis

Imagine what happens in a cell if glucose catabolism is proceeding at maximum rate. What do you do if you see a traffic jam ahead with no possible way to get through it? Probably take an alternative route, if available. Similarly, if glycolytic pathways are "saturated" because of high levels of glucose entering the cell, a "traffic jam" of glucose-6-phosphate will result. Unable to enter glycolysis, glucose-6-phosphate will begin an alternative route; that is, it will enter the anabolic pathway of glycogen formation. The process of glycogen formation, called **glycogenesis** (see **Figure 41-11**), is a series of chemical reactions in which glucose molecules are joined together to form a structure made of a branched strand of stored glucoses (**Figure 41-13**). The huge glycogen polymer molecules settle out of solution and therefore do not upset the osmotic balance of the cell—which would happen if a large quantity of individual glucose molecules is kept in the cell.

Glycogen polymers can be made by any cell, but only two types of cells store a large quantity of glycogen: muscle fibres and liver cells. Astrocytes in the brain store more glycogen than most cells, but not nearly as much as muscle fibres and liver cells. However, that small amount of glycogen may be enough to protect the brain for a short time when glucose availability is low. It is mainly the liver that acts as the glycogen reservoir for the body.

The process of glycogenesis is part of a homeostatic mechanism that operates when the blood glucose level increases above the midpoint of its normal range. The normal range of glucose in a fasting person is about 4.4 to 5.0 mmol/L (80 to 90 mg/100 mL) of blood. Soon after a meal high in carbohydrates, while glucose is being absorbed rapidly, the blood glucose may shoot up to 6.7 to 7.8 mmol/L (120 to 140 mg/100 mL) or more. Recall that blood from the digestive tract is detoured directly to the liver via the portal system before being returned to the heart (see **Figure 29-20** on p. 687). In the liver, the action of the pancreatic hormone *insulin* causes a great many glucose molecules to leave the blood for storage in hepatocytes as glycogen. As a result of glycogenesis, the blood glucose level decreases, ordinarily enough to reestablish its normal level. **Figure 41-14** summarizes this role of glycogenolysis in maintaining homeostasis of blood glucose.

Glycogenolysis

Glycogen molecules do not remain in the cell permanently but are eventually broken apart (hydrolyzed). This process of "splitting glycogen" is called **glycogenolysis** (**Figure 41-15**; see **Figure 41-11**). It is, in essence, a reversal of glycogenesis. What are the products of glycogenolysis? The answer depends on the cell. Although all cells presumably have the enzymes to break glycogen down to glucose-6-phosphate, only a few cell types (liver, kidney, intestinal mucosa)

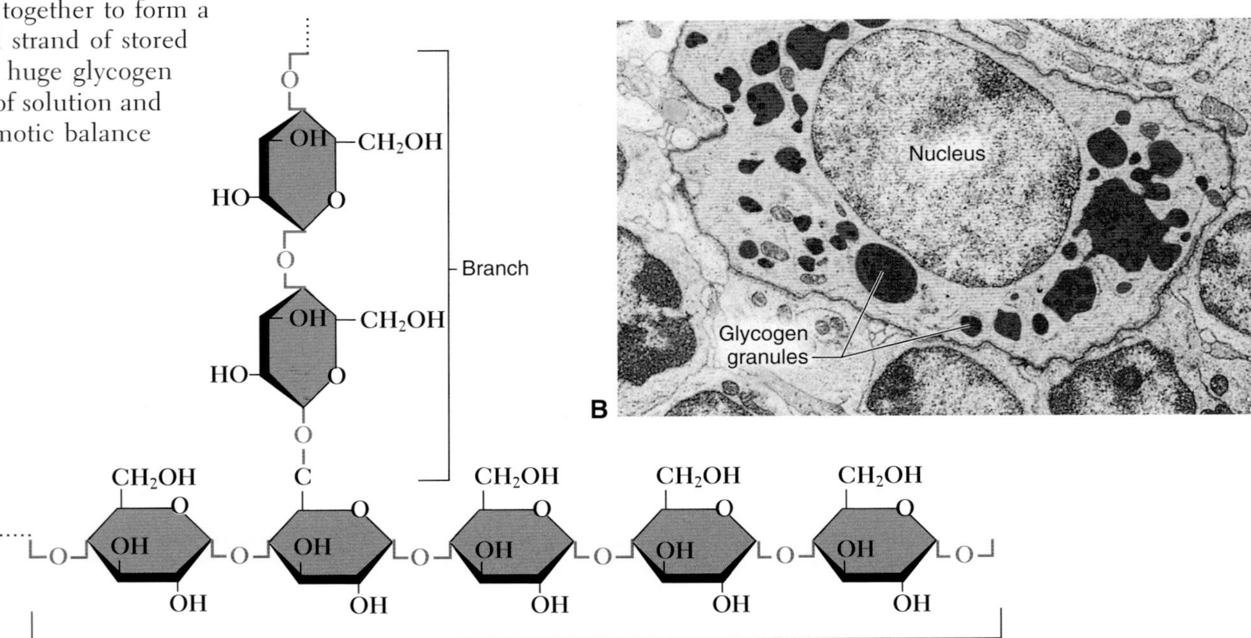

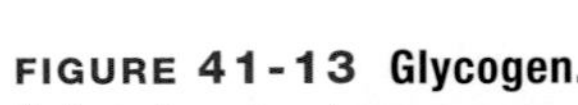

FIGURE 41-13 Glycogen. **A,** A portion of a glycogen molecule, the very large, highly branched polymer of varying numbers of glucose subunits. **B,** Transmission electron micrograph of solid glycogen granules in a liver cell. Glycogen (a polysaccharide) is the form in which human cells store glucose (a monosaccharide) without disrupting their osmotic balance.

UNIT 5

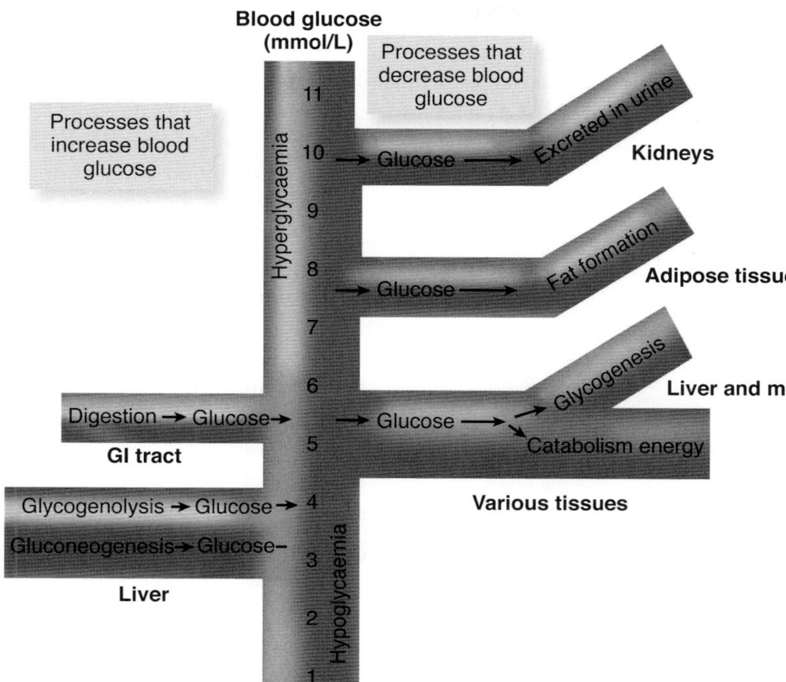

FIGURE 41-14 Homeostasis of blood glucose level. When blood glucose level starts to decrease below its normal range of about 4.4–5.0 mmol/L (80–90 mg/100 mL) (fasting), liver cells increase the rate at which they convert glycogen, amino acids, and glycerol to glucose (glycogenolysis and gluconeogenesis) and release it into blood. But when blood glucose level increases, liver cells increase the rate at which they remove glucose molecules from blood and convert them to glycogen for storage (glycogenesis). At still higher levels, glucose leaves blood for liver cells to be converted into fat and, at still higher levels, is excreted in the urine. Hormones regulate the processes shown (see **Figure 41-18**).

have the enzyme phosphatase, which allows free glucose to form and possibly leave the cell.

So the term *glycogenolysis* means different things in different cells. In muscles, glucose-6-phosphate is the product, which then undergoes glycolysis. But liver glycogenolysis (see **Figure 41-15**) results in free glucose that can leave the cell and increase the blood glucose level. Accordingly, liver glycogenolysis acts as a part of the homeostatic mechanism to maintain the blood glucose level. Example: A few hours after a meal, when the blood glucose level decreases (see **Figure 41-14**), the pancreatic hormone *glucagon* stimulates accelerated liver glycogenolysis. However, glycogenolysis alone can probably maintain homeostasis of blood glucose concentration for only 12 to 16 hours because the body can store only small amounts of glycogen.

During a stress response, elevated *epinephrine* and *cortisol* levels can stimulate glycogenolysis. This action elevates blood glucose levels, which may prove useful for the muscular activity of the "fight" or "flight" needed to resist or avoid a threat to the homeostatic balance of the body.

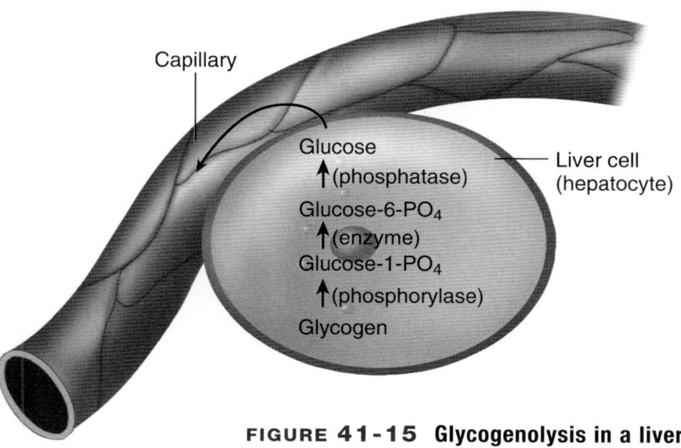

FIGURE 41-15 Glycogenolysis in a liver cell.

Gluconeogenesis

Literally, **gluconeogenesis** means the formation of "new" glucose—"new" in the sense that it is made from proteins or, less commonly, from the glycerol of fats—not from carbohydrates. The process occurs chiefly in the liver. It consists of many complex chemical reactions. The new glucose produced from proteins or lipids by gluconeogenesis (**Figure 41-16**) diffuses out of liver cells into the blood. Gluconeogenesis can therefore add glucose to the blood when needed. So, too, can the process of liver glycogenolysis. Obviously, then, the liver is a very important organ for maintaining blood glucose homeostasis.

Control of Glucose Metabolism

The complex mechanism that normally maintains homeostasis of blood glucose concentration consists of hormonal and neural devices. At least five endocrine glands—pancreatic islets, anterior pituitary gland, adrenal cortex, adrenal medulla, and thyroid gland—and at least eight hormones secreted by these glands function as key elements of the glucose homeostatic mechanism. As you read through the following paragraphs, keep in mind that each of the hormones listed has many different kinds of regulatory effects in the body—not just their effects on glucose metabolism.

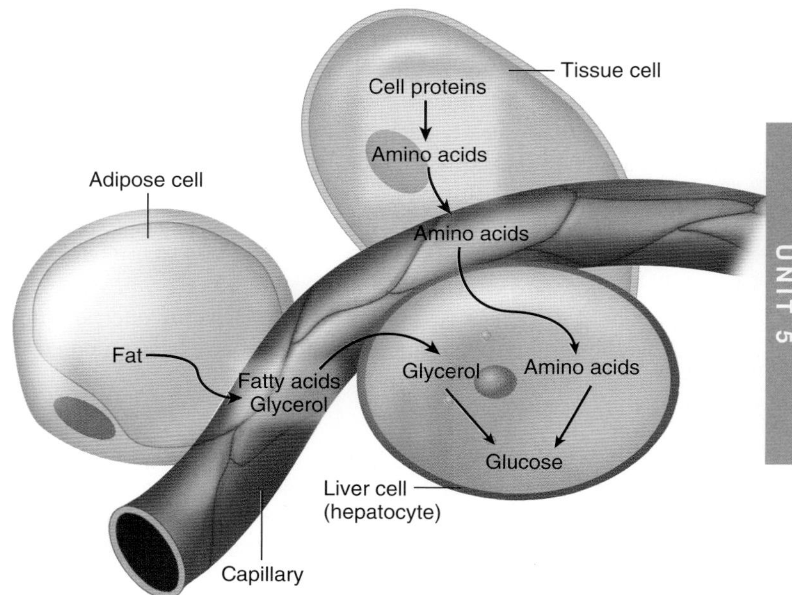

FIGURE 41-16 Gluconeogenesis. Liver cells can form glucose from mobilized tissue proteins and fats.

Beta cells of the pancreatic islets secrete the most well-known sugar-regulating hormone of all—**insulin.** Insulin decreases blood glucose level by moving glucose molecules out of the blood and into cells (**Figure 41-17**, *A*). Although the exact details of its mechanism of action are still being worked out, insulin is known to accelerate glucose transport through cell membranes. It also increases the activity of the enzyme glucokinase. Glucokinase catalyzes glucose phosphorylation, the reaction that must occur before either glycogenesis or glucose catabolism can take place. Insulin thus moves glucose into cells and increases glycogenesis and increased catabolism of glucose—all of which decrease blood glucose levels. **Figure 41-17**, *B*, demonstrates the blood glucose–lowering effects of insulin after ingestion of glucose.

CONNECT IT!

Insulin deficiency can cause slow glycogenesis and low glycogen storage, decreased glucose catabolism, and increased blood glucose, as in diabetes mellitus (DM). To learn more, visit ***Diabetes Mellitus*** online at ***Connect It!***

Alpha cells of the pancreatic islets secrete the sugar-regulating hormone **glucagon.** Whereas insulin tends to decrease the blood glucose level, glucagon tends to increase it. Glucagon increases the activity of the enzyme phosphorylase. **Figure 41-15** shows that phosphorylase promotes liver glycogenolysis, thereby causing the release of more glucose into the bloodstream.

Hormones collectively called **incretins** act to increase the amount of insulin released from the pancreatic beta cells and decrease the amount of glucagon released from pancreatic alpha cells. Thus incretins tend to decrease blood glucose levels. Incretins may also reduce the rate of gastric emptying and decrease desire for more food. Incretins are released by endocrine gastrointestinal (GI) cells in response to the presence of glucose and can increase insulin release even before blood glucose levels begin to rise after a meal. Incretins include *glucagon-like peptide 1 (GLP-1)* and *gastric inhibitory peptide (GIP)*. Because of its role as an incretin, GIP is also called *glucose-dependent insulinotropic peptide (GIP)*. Because of their insulin-elevating effects, drugs that mimic the action of incretins (incretin agonists) have emerged as possible treatments for diabetes mellitus (DM).

Epinephrine is a hormone secreted in large amounts by the adrenal medulla in times of emotional or physical stress. Like glucagon, epinephrine increases phosphorylase activity. This makes glycogenolysis occur at a faster rate. Epinephrine accelerates both liver and muscle glycogenolysis, whereas glucagon accelerates only liver glycogenolysis. Both hormones increase the blood glucose level. Epinephrine is the only hormone whose release into the systemic circulation (and therefore its effects on metabolism) is directly under the control of the nervous system.

Adrenocorticotropic hormone (ACTH) and *glucocorticoids* (e.g., cortisone) are two more hormones that increase blood glucose concentration. ACTH stimulates the adrenal cortex to increase its

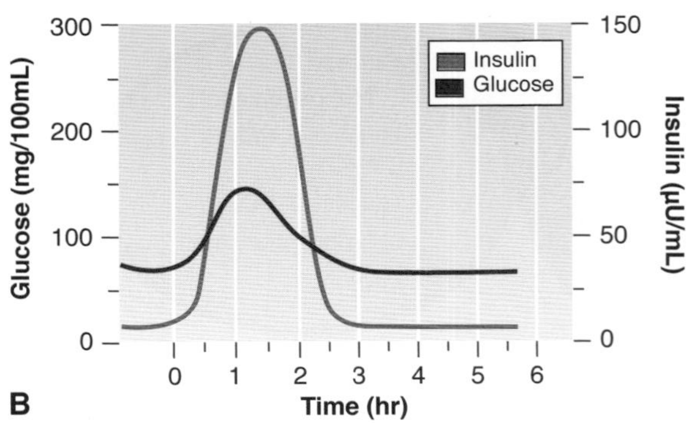

FIGURE 41-17 Role of insulin. Insulin operates in a negative feedback loop **(A)** that prevents blood glucose concentration from increasing too far above the normal range. Insulin promotes uptake of glucose by all cells of the body, enabling them to catabolize and/or store it. The liver and skeletal muscles are especially well adapted for storage of glucose as glycogen. Thus excess glucose is removed from the bloodstream, as the graph **(B)** demonstrates. If the glucose level falls below the normal range, hormones such as glucagon promote the release of glucose from storage into the bloodstream (see **Figure 41-18**). Note: mmol/L = mg/100 mL ÷ 18.

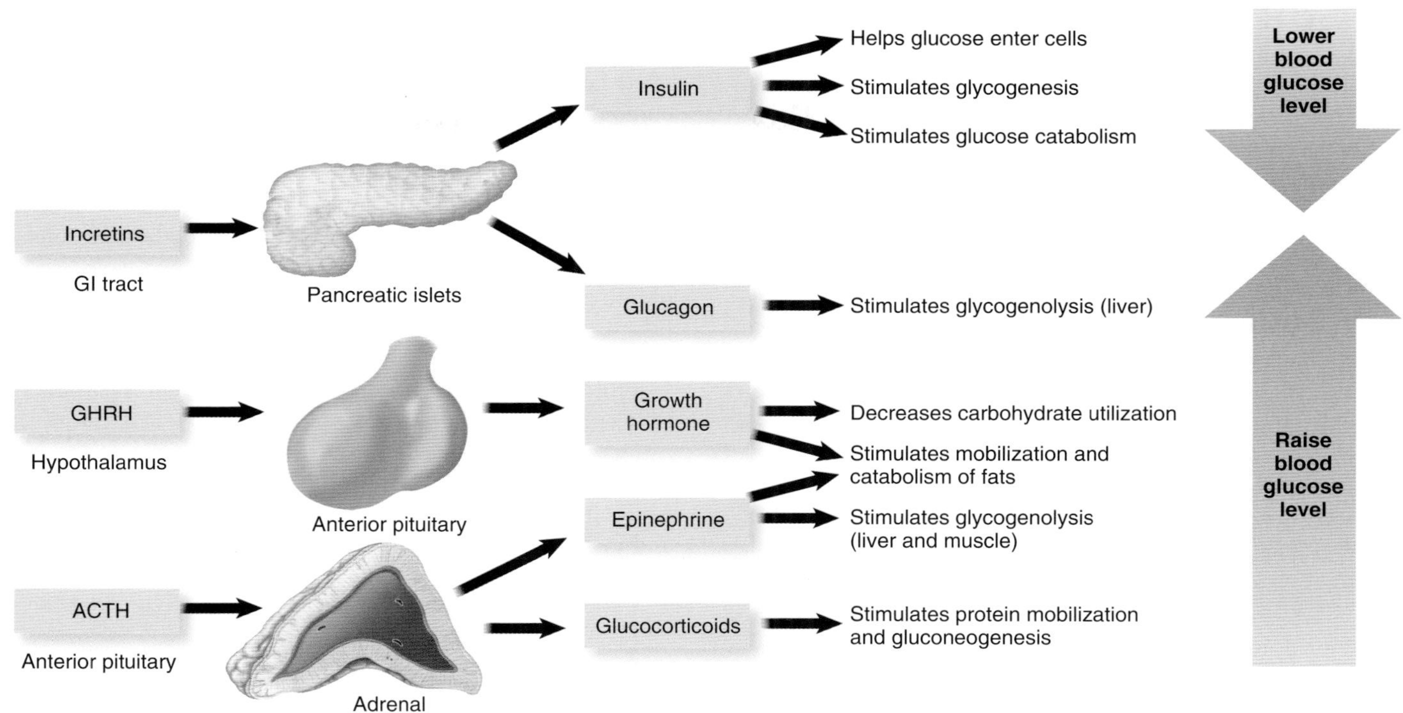

FIGURE 41-18 Hormonal control of blood glucose level. Simplified view of some of the major glucose-regulating hormones. Insulin lowers blood glucose level and is therefore hypoglycaemic. Most hormones shown here raise blood glucose level and are called *hyperglycaemic,* or *anti-insulin, hormones.* **Figure 41-14** shows how the regulated processes change blood glucose levels. *GHRH,* growth hormone–releasing hormone.

secretion of glucocorticoids. Glucocorticoids accelerate gluconeogenesis. They do this by mobilizing proteins—that is, the breakdown, or hydrolysis, of tissue proteins to amino acids. More amino acids enter the circulation and are carried to the liver. Liver cells step up their production of "new" glucose from the mobilized amino acids. Glucocorticoids help here, too, by stimulating enzymatic reversal of glycolysis and thus helping the cell in its effort to manufacture more glucose. The glucose streams out of liver cells into the blood and adds to the blood glucose level.

Growth hormone (GH), made by the anterior pituitary, also increases blood glucose level, but by a different mechanism. GH causes a shift from carbohydrate to fat catabolism. It does this by limiting the storage of fat in fat depots. Instead, more fats are mobilized and catabolized. In this way, GH "spares" carbohydrates from catabolism, and the level of glucose in the bloodstream is increased.

Thyroid-stimulating hormone (TSH) from the anterior pituitary gland and its target secretion, *thyroid hormone* (T_3 and T_4), have complex effects on metabolism. Some of these raise, and some lower, the glucose level. One of the effects of thyroid hormone is to accelerate catabolism, and because glucose is the body's "preferred fuel", the result may be a decrease in blood glucose level.

The summary of hormone control shown in **Figure 41-18** indicates that most hormones cause the glucose blood level to rise. These hormones are called *hyperglycaemic* because they tend to promote a high blood glucose concentration. The one notable exception is insulin, which is *hypoglycaemic* (tends to decrease the blood glucose level). See **Box 41-3** for more discussion of blood glucose problems.

UNIT 5

BOX 41-3 *fyi* | Abnormal Blood Glucose Concentration

The term **hyperglycaemia,** which literally means "condition of too much sugar in the blood", is used to describe any blood glucose concentration that is higher than the normal setpoint level. Hyperglycaemia is most often associated with untreated diabetes mellitus, but it can occur in newborns when too much intravenous glucose is given or in other similar situations. If untreated, the excess glucose leaves the blood in the kidney—literally "spilling over" into the urine. This increases the osmotic pressure of urine, drawing an abnormally high amount of water into the urine from the bloodstream. Thus hyperglycaemia causes loss of glucose in the urine and its accompanying loss of water—potentially threatening the fluid balance of the body. Dehydration of this sort can ultimately lead to death.

Hypoglycaemia occurs when the blood glucose concentration dips below the normal setpoint level. Hypoglycaemia can occur in various conditions, including starvation, hypersecretion of insulin by the pancreatic islets, or injection of too much insulin. Symptoms of hypoglycaemia include weakness, hunger, headache, blurry vision, anxiety, and personality changes—perhaps leading to coma and death if untreated.

Quick CHECK

6. Why might a cell switch to the anaerobic pathway as its major source of usable energy?
7. What is meant by excess post-exercise oxygen consumption (EPOC)?
8. Distinguish between glycogenesis and glycogenolysis. In what circumstances might each occur?
9. List three of the hormones that affect glucose metabolism.

LIPIDS

Dietary Sources of Lipids

Recall from Chapter 4 that **lipids** are a class of organic compounds that includes fats, oils, and related substances. The most common lipids in the diet are **triglycerides,** which are composed of a *glycerol* subunit to which are attached three *fatty acids.* Other important dietary lipids include *phospholipids* and *cholesterol.*

Dietary fats are often classified as either **saturated** or **unsaturated.** Saturated fats contain fatty acid chains in which there are no double bonds—that is, all available bonds of the hydrocarbon chain are filled (saturated) with hydrogen atoms (see **Figure 4-5**, p. 59). Saturated fats are usually solid at room temperature. Unsaturated fats contain fatty acid chains, of which there are some double bonds, meaning that not all sites for hydrogen are filled. Unsaturated fats are usually liquid at room temperature.

Triglycerides are found in nearly every food that we eat. However, the amount of triglycerides in each type of food varies considerably, as does the proportion of saturated to unsaturated types. Phospholipids are also found in nearly all foods because they make up the cellular membranes in and around each cell of all living organisms. Cholesterol, however, is found only in foods of animal origin. Cholesterol concentration also varies. For example, it is particularly high in liver and the yolks of eggs.

Transport of Lipids

Lipids are transported in blood as chylomicrons, other lipoproteins, and free fatty acids.

BOX 41-4 ***lipoproteins***

As stated in the text, high blood concentrations of low-density lipoproteins (LDLs) are associated with a high risk for atherosclerosis. Atherosclerosis is a form of "hardening of the arteries" that occurs when lipids accumulate in cells lining the blood vessels and promote the development of a plaque that eventually impedes blood flow and may trigger clot formation. Atherosclerosis may also weaken the wall of a blood vessel to the point that it ruptures. In any case, a person with atherosclerosis of the coronary arteries risks a heart attack when blood flow to cardiac muscle is impaired. If vessels in the brain are affected, there is risk of a *cerebrovascular accident (CVA),* or "stroke".

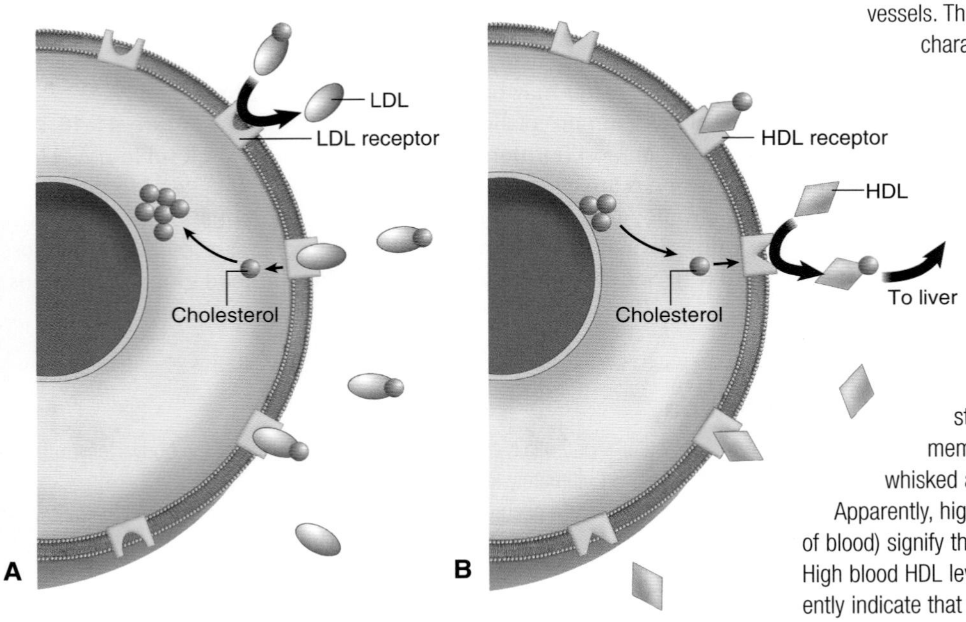

Role of blood lipoproteins. A, Simplified diagram of the role of low-density lipoprotein *(LDL)* in delivering cholesterol to cells. **B,** Proposed role of high-density lipoprotein *(HDL)* in removing cholesterol from cells.

Part *A* of the figure is a simplified version of a concept of LDL function first proposed by Nobel laureates Michael Brown and Joseph Goldstein at the University of Texas. According to their model, LDL delivers cholesterol to cells for use in synthesizing steroid hormones and stabilizing the plasma membrane. Most, if not all, cells have many LDL receptors embedded in the outer surface of their plasma membranes. These receptors attract cholesterol-bearing LDL. Once the LDL molecule binds to the receptor, specific mechanisms operate to release the cholesterol it carries into the cell. Excess cholesterol is stored in droplets near the centre of the cell. It seems that, in some individuals at least, cells have so few LDL receptors that they accumulate too much cholesterol in the blood. Some mechanism in endothelial cells moves this excess LDL into the wall of blood vessels. This has been proposed as a cause for the lipid accumulation characteristic of atherosclerosis.

High blood concentrations of high-density lipoproteins (HDLs) have been associated with a low risk of developing atherosclerosis and its many possible complications. Although the exact details of how this works have yet to be worked out or confirmed, some scientists have made some progress toward that end. Jack Oram, a cell biologist working at the University of Washington, has proposed the mechanism illustrated in part *B* of the figure. According to his model, HDL molecules are attracted to HDL receptors embedded in the plasma membranes. Once they bind to their receptors, the cell is stimulated to release some of its cholesterol from storage. The released cholesterol migrates to the plasma membrane, where it may attach to the HDL molecule and be whisked away to the liver for excretion in bile.

Apparently, high blood LDL levels (more than 180 mg/100 mL or 4.7 mmol/L of blood) signify that a large amount of cholesterol is being delivered to cells. High blood HDL levels (more than 60 mg/100 mL or 1.6 mmol/L of blood) apparently indicate that a large amount of cholesterol is being removed from cells and delivered to the liver for excretion from the body. Currently, researchers are using this information to develop treatments that may prevent—or even cure—atherosclerosis and the disorders it causes. •

UNIT 5

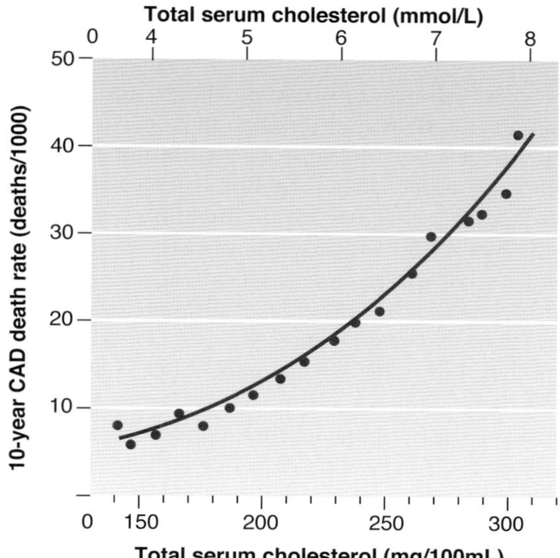

FIGURE 41-19 Cholesterol and heart disease. The graph shows a relationship between the total serum (blood plasma) cholesterol level and coronary artery disease (CAD). Note—mmol/L = mg/100 mL ÷ 38.6.

Chylomicrons are small fat droplets found in blood soon after fat absorption has occurred. Fatty acids and monoglyceride products of fat digestion combine during absorption to again form fats (triglycerides, or triacylglycerols). These triglycerides plus small amounts of cholesterol and phospholipids compose the chylomicrons. During fat absorption, the so-called *absorptive state*, blood may contain so many of these fat droplets that it appears turbid or even yellowish in colour. But during the *postabsorptive state*—usually within about 4 hours after a meal—few, if any chylomicrons remain in the blood. Their contents have moved mostly into adipose tissue cells.

In the postabsorptive state, when chylomicrons are virtually absent from the circulation, some 95% of the lipids in blood are transported in the form of other lipoproteins. **Lipoproteins** are produced mainly in the liver, and as their name suggests, they consist of lipids (triglycerides, cholesterol, and phospholipids) and protein. At all times, blood contains three types of lipoprotein, namely, very-low-density lipoprotein, low-density lipoprotein, and high-density lipoprotein. Usually, they are designated by their abbreviations: VLDL, LDL, and HDL. Diets high in saturated fats and cholesterol tend to produce an increase in blood LDL concentration, which in turn is associated with a high incidence of coronary artery disease (CAD) and atherosclerosis (**Figure 41-19** and **Box 41-4**). A high blood HDL concentration, in contrast, is associated with a low incidence of heart disease. One might therefore think of the LDLs as the "bad lipoproteins" and the HDLs as the "good lipoproteins". Considerable evidence indicates that exercise tends to elevate HDL concentration. This may partially account for the beneficial effects of exercise.

Fatty acids, on entering the blood from adipose tissue or other cells, combine with albumin to form the so-called **free fatty acids (FFAs)**. Fatty acids are transported from cells of one tissue to those of another in the form of free fatty acids. Whenever the rate of fat catabolism increases—as it does in starvation or diabetes—the free fatty acid content of blood increases markedly.

Lipid Metabolism

Lipid Catabolism

Lipid catabolism, like carbohydrate catabolism, consists of several processes. Each of these processes, in turn, consists of a series of chemical reactions. Triglycerides are first hydrolyzed to yield fatty acids and glycerol. Glycerol is then converted to glyceraldehyde-3-phosphate, which may then be converted to glucose or it may enter the glycolysis pathway directly (see **Figure 41-4**). Fatty acids, as **Figure 41-20** shows, are broken down by a process called beta-oxidation into two-carbon pieces, the familiar acetyl CoA. These molecules are then catabolized via the citric acid cycle. The final process of lipid catabolism therefore consists of the same reactions as does carbohydrate catabolism. Catabolism of lipids, however, yields considerably more energy than does catabolism of carbohydrates. Whereas catabolism of 1 gram of carbohydrates yields only 4.1 kcal (17.2 kJ) of heat, catabolism of 1 gram of fat yields 9 kcal (37.6 kJ). It is not surprising, then, that lipids are the preferred energy source for muscle tissue.

When fat catabolism occurs at an accelerated rate, as in diabetes mellitus (when glucose cannot enter cells) or fasting, excessive numbers of acetyl CoA units are formed. Liver cells then temporarily condense acetyl CoA units together to form four-carbon acetoacetic acid. Acetoacetic acid is classified as a *ketone body* and can be converted to two other types of ketone bodies, namely, acetone and beta-hydroxybutyric acid—hence the name **ketogenesis** for this process (**Box 41-5**). Liver cells oxidize a small portion of the ketone bodies for their own energy needs, but most of them are transported by the blood to other tissue cells for the change back to acetyl CoA and oxidation via the citric acid cycle (see **Figure 41-20**).

Lipid Anabolism

Lipid anabolism, also called **lipogenesis,** consists of the synthesis of various types

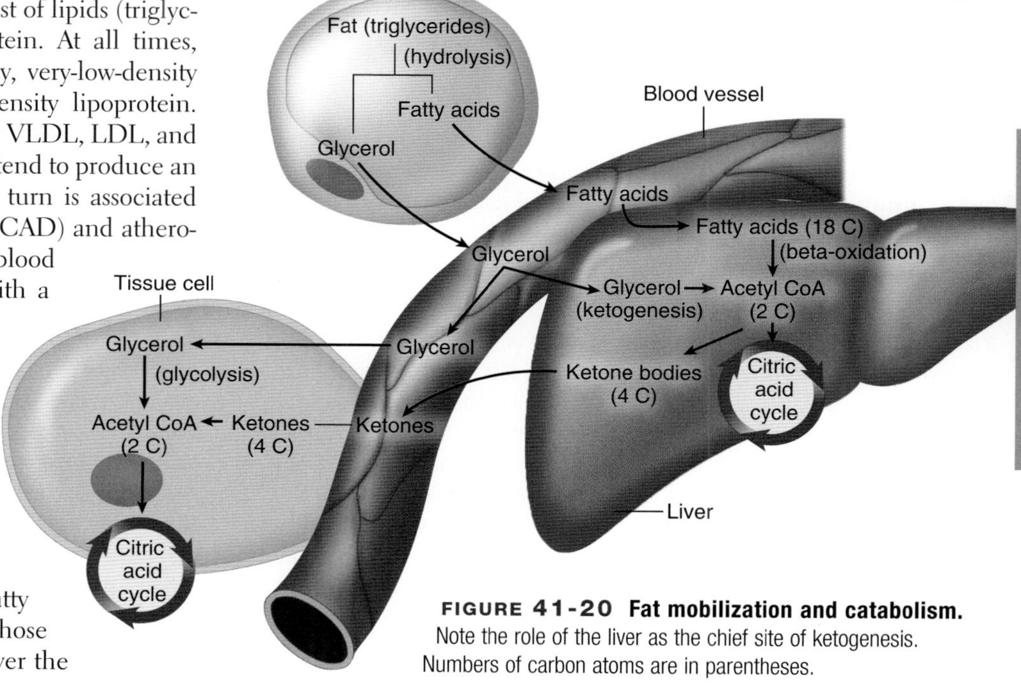

FIGURE 41-20 Fat mobilization and catabolism. Note the role of the liver as the chief site of ketogenesis. Numbers of carbon atoms are in parentheses.

UNIT 5

BOX 41-5 *health matters* | **Ketosis**

Large amounts of ketone bodies may be present in the blood of a person with uncontrolled diabetes mellitus. This condition is known as **ketosis.** Signs of it are acetone breath and *ketonuria* (high number of ketone bodies in the urine). •

of lipids, notably *triglycerides, cholesterol, phospholipids,* and *prostaglandins.* Triglycerides and structural lipids (e.g., phospholipids) are synthesized from fatty acids and glycerol or from excess glucose or amino acids. So it is possible to "get fat" from foods other than fat. Triglycerides are stored mainly in adipose tissue cells. These fat deposits constitute the body's largest reserve energy source—often too large, unfortunately. Almost limitless kilos of fat can be stored. In contrast, only a few hundred grams of carbohydrates can be stored as liver and muscle glycogen.

Most fatty acids can be synthesized by the body. A certain number of the unsaturated fatty acids must be provided by the diet and are thus called **essential fatty acids.** *Omega-3 fatty acids* found in large quantities in certain fish oils and some plant oils are examples of essential fatty acids. Some of the essential fatty acids serve as a source within the body for synthesis of an important group of lipids called *prostaglandins.* These hormone-like compounds, first discovered in the 1930s in semen, have gained increasing recognition for their occurrence in various tissues, where they support a wide spectrum of biological activity (see Chapter 25). Certain essential fatty acids are also necessary for manufacturing the phospholipids in cell membranes (see Chapter 5) and the myelin in nerve tissue (see Chapters 18 and 19).

Control of Lipid Metabolism

Lipid metabolism is controlled mainly by the following hormones:

- Insulin
- ACTH
- Growth hormone
- Glucocorticoids

You probably recall from our discussion of these hormones in connection with carbohydrate metabolism that they regulate fat metabolism in such a way that the rate of fat catabolism is inversely related to the rate of carbohydrate catabolism. If some condition such as diabetes mellitus causes carbohydrate catabolism to decrease below energy needs, increased secretion of growth hormone, ACTH, and glucocorticoids soon follows. These hormones, in turn, bring about an increase in fat catabolism. But, when carbohydrate catabolism equals energy needs, fats are not mobilized out of storage and catabolized (**Box 41-6**). Instead, they are spared and stored in adipose tissue. "Carbohydrates have a 'fat-sparing' effect", so says an old physiological maxim. Or stating this truth more descriptively: "Carbohydrates have a 'fat-storing' effect."

Research has shown that hormonal control of lipid metabolism is very complex—and still not well understood. One intriguing line of research involves the hormone **leptin.** Leptin is secreted by fat-storing cells and seems to regulate *satiety* (feeling of fullness) and how fat is metabolized. Researchers studying the complex interaction of leptin and other hormones and their receptors hope to find effective treatments for obesity, diabetes, and other fat-storage afflictions.

Quick **CHECK**

10. In what forms are lipids transported to cells?
11. How can glycerol and fatty acids enter the citric acid cycle?
12. Which fatty acids cannot be made by the body?

PROTEINS

Sources of Proteins

Recall from Chapter 4 that proteins are very large molecules composed of chemical subunits called **amino acids** (see **Figure 4-13**, p. 63). Proteins are assembled from a pool of many different kinds of amino acids. If any one type of amino acid is deficient, vital proteins cannot be synthesized—a serious health threat. One way your body maintains a constant supply of amino acids is by synthesizing them from other compounds already present in the body. Only about half of the required types of amino acids can be made by the body, however. The remaining types of amino acids must be supplied in the diet. Nutritionists often refer to the amino acids that must be in the diet as essential, or indispensable, amino acids. **Table 41-1** lists amino acids according to whether they are considered essential in the diet or nonessential (dispensable) in the diet (synthesized by the body). **Box 41-7** describes the link between blood levels of amino acids and disease.

BOX 41-6 ***PPARs and fat metabolism***

A class of proteins called *peroxisome proliferator–activated receptors,* or *PPARs,* may hold some keys as to how the body metabolizes fats. PPARs are molecules attached to the DNA molecules of cells. PPARs combine with other proteins to form a complex that regulates genes that determine how the cell takes in and breaks down fat. Initial research shows that chemicals that affect different PPARs can influence fat storage in the body. With 68% of men and 58% of women in the UK overweight and at risk for heart disease, diabetes, cancer, and other health problems, it is no wonder that scientists are scrambling to find out more about how PPARs regulate fat metabolism and how we can influence them to reduce obesity-related health risks. •

BOX 41-7 *health matters* | **Amino Acids and Disease**

The balance of amino acids circulating in the blood is associated with various diseases. High blood levels of homocysteine, one of several alternate forms of the amino acid cysteine (see **Table 41-1**), have been linked to heart disease, stroke, and dementias such as Alzheimer disease. Whether such abnormalities in homocysteine levels are the direct cause of these conditions is uncertain. Despite this uncertainty, many physicians recommend lowering abnormally high blood homocysteine levels to reduce the possible risk for these devastating conditions. Homocysteine can be reduced to normally low blood levels when there is adequate vitamin B_6, B_{12}, or B_9 (folic acid) in the diet. •

TABLE 41-1 Amino Acids

ESSENTIAL (INDISPENSABLE)	NONESSENTIAL (DISPENSABLE)
Histidine (His)*	Alanine (Ala)
Isoleucine (Ile)	Arginine (Arg)
Leucine (Leu)	Asparagine (Asn)
Lysine (Lys)	Aspartic acid (Asp)
Methionine (Met)	Cysteine (Cys)
Phenylalanine (Phe)	Glutamic acid (Glu)
Threonine (Thr)	Glutamine (Gln)
Tryptophan (Trp)	Glycine (Gly)
Valine (Val)	Proline (Pro)
	Selenocysteine (Sec)
	Serine (Ser)
	Tyrosine (Tyr)†

*Essential in infants and, perhaps, adult males.

†Can be synthesized from phenylalanine; therefore nonessential as long as phenylalanine is in the diet.

Proteins are obtained in the diet from various sources. Muscle meat and other animal tissues particularly high in proteins contain the essential amino acids. Food from a single plant or other nonanimal source does not usually contain an adequate amount of all the essential amino acids. Therefore, it is important to include meat in the diet or a mixture of different vegetables that provide all the amino acids needed by the body. Plant tissues that are particularly high in protein content include cereal grains, nuts, and legumes such as peas and beans.

Protein Metabolism

In protein metabolism, anabolism is primary and catabolism is secondary. In carbohydrate and fat metabolism, the opposite is true—catabolism is primary and anabolism is secondary. Proteins are primarily tissue-building foods. Carbohydrates and fats are primarily energy-supplying foods.

Protein Anabolism

Protein anabolism is the process by which proteins are synthesized by the ribosomes of all cells. The specific mechanisms of protein anabolism were first discussed in Chapter 4 (see pp. 61–67) and further explained in Chapter 7 (see pp. 121–127). We review the basic idea of protein anabolism here.

Every cell synthesizes its own structural proteins and its own enzymes. In addition, many cells, such as liver and glandular cells, synthesize special proteins for export. For example, liver cells manufacture the plasma proteins found in blood. The cell's genes, under the influence of signalling mechanisms, determine the specific proteins to be synthesized. Protein anabolism is truly "big business" in the body. Consider, for instance, that protein anabolism constitutes the major process of growth, reproduction, tissue repair, and the replacement of cells destroyed by daily wear and tear. Red blood cell replacement alone amounts to millions of cells per second!

Protein Catabolism

The first step in protein catabolism takes place in liver cells. Called **deamination,** it consists of the splitting off of an amino (NH_2) group from an amino acid molecule to form a molecule of ammonia and one of keto acid (e.g., alpha-ketoglutaric acid). Most of the ammonia is converted by liver cells to *urea* and later excreted in the urine. The keto acid may be oxidized via the citric acid cycle (see **Figure 41-6**) or may be converted to glucose via gluconeogenesis (**Figure 41-21**) or to fat (lipogenesis). Both protein catabolism and anabolism go on continually. Only their rates differ from time to time. With a protein-deficient diet, for example, protein catabolism exceeds protein anabolism. Various hormones, as we shall see, also influence the rates of protein catabolism and anabolism.

Protein Balance and Nitrogen Balance

Usually a state of **protein balance** exists in the normal healthy adult body; that is, the rate of protein anabolism equals or balances the rate of protein catabolism. When the body is in protein balance, it is also in a state of **nitrogen balance** because the amount of nitrogen taken into the body (in protein foods) equals the amount of nitrogen in protein catabolic waste products excreted in the urine, faeces, and sweat.

It is important to realize that there are two kinds of protein, or nitrogen, imbalance. When protein catabolism exceeds protein anabolism, the amount of nitrogen in the urine exceeds the amount of nitrogen in the protein foods ingested. The individual is then said to be in a state of **negative nitrogen balance,** or in a state of "tissue wasting"—because more of the tissue proteins are being catabolized than are being replaced by protein synthesis. Protein-poor diets, starvation, and wasting illnesses, for example, produce a negative nitrogen balance. A **positive nitrogen balance** (nitrogen intake in foods greater than nitrogen output in urine) indicates that protein anabolism is occurring at a faster rate than protein catabolism. A state of

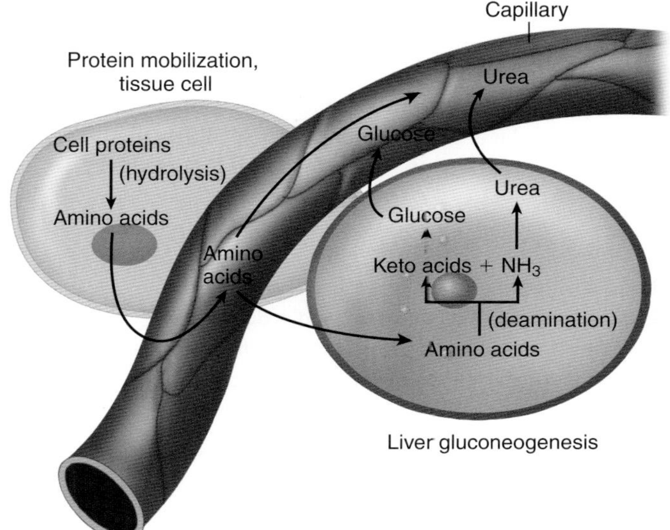

FIGURE 41-21 Protein mobilization and catabolism. Glucocorticoids tend to accelerate these processes and are therefore classified as protein catabolic hormones.

TABLE 41-2 Metabolism

NUTRIENT	ANABOLISM	CATABOLISM
Carbohydrates	Temporary excess changed into glycogen by liver cells in presence of insulin; stored in liver and skeletal muscles until needed and then changed back to glucose. True excess beyond body's energy requirements converted into adipose tissue; stored in various fat depots of body	Oxidized, in presence of insulin, to yield energy (4.1 kcal per gram) (17.2 kJ/g) and wastes (carbon dioxide and water) $C_6H_{12}O_6 + 6\ O_2 \longrightarrow \text{Energy} + 6\ CO_2 + 6\ H_2O$
Fats	Built into adipose tissue; stored in fat depots of body	Fatty acids ↓ (beta-oxidation) Acetyl CoA ⇌ Ketones ↓ (tissues; citric acid cycle) Energy (9.3 kcal/g) (38.9 kJ/g) + CO_2 + H_2O; Glycerol ↓ (glycolysis) Acetyl CoA
Proteins	Synthesized into tissue proteins, blood proteins, enzymes, hormones, etc.	Deaminated by liver, forming ammonia (which is converted to urea) and keto acids (which are either oxidized [yielding energy of 4.1 kcal/g (17.2 kJ/g)] or changed to glucose or fat)

positive nitrogen balance therefore characterizes any condition in which large amounts of tissue are being synthesized, such as during growth, pregnancy, and convalescence from an emaciating illness.

Control of Protein Metabolism

Protein metabolism, like that of carbohydrates and fats, is controlled largely by hormones rather than by the nervous system. Growth hormone and the male hormone testosterone both have a stimulating effect on protein synthesis, or anabolism. For this reason, they are referred to as *anabolic* hormones. The protein *catabolic* hormones of greatest consequence are glucocorticoids. They speed up tissue protein mobilization—that is, the hydrolysis of cell proteins to amino acids, their entry into the blood, and their subsequent catabolism (see **Figure 41-21**). ACTH functions indirectly as a protein catabolic hormone because of its stimulating effect on glucocorticoid secretion.

Thyroid hormone is necessary for and tends to promote protein anabolism and therefore growth when plenty of carbohydrates and fats are available for energy production. On the other hand, in different conditions—for example, when the amount of thyroid hormone is excessive or when the energy foods are deficient—this hormone may then promote protein mobilization and catabolism.

Some of the facts about metabolism set forth in the preceding sections are summarized in **Table 41-2** and **Figure 41-22**.

Quick CHECK

13. What is meant by the term *essential amino acid*?
14. What happens when an amino acid is deaminated?
15. What is the purpose of the process of amino acid deamination?
16. What is meant by the term *nitrogen balance*?

VITAMINS AND MINERALS

One glance at the label of any packaged food product reveals the importance we place on vitamins and minerals. We know that carbohydrates, fats, and proteins are used by our bodies to build important molecules and to provide energy. So why do we need vitamins and minerals?

VITAMINS

Vitamins are organic molecules needed in small quantities for normal metabolism throughout the body (**Box 41-8**). The first vitamins were discovered in the early twentieth century at the University of Wisconsin by Marguerite Davis and Elmer Vernon McCollum. Earlier, vitamins were hypothesized to be amines so they were originally called vitamines, later shortened to vitamins. However, Davis and McCollum discovered two lipid-soluble, nonamine substances that fit the proposed function of a vitamin and they named these factors lipid-soluble A and lipid-soluble B. This not only began a system of naming vitamins with letters but also spurred the whole science of nutrition.

Most vitamin molecules attach to enzymes or coenzymes and help them work properly. **Coenzymes** are organic, nonprotein catalysts that often act as "molecule carriers". Many enzymes or coenzymes are totally useless without the appropriate vitamins to attach to them and thus give them the shape that allows them to function properly. For example, coenzyme A (CoA), an important carrier molecule associated with the citric acid cycle, has *pantothenic acid* (vitamin B_5) as one of its major components.

Not all vitamins are involved directly with enzymes and coenzymes. Vitamins A, D, and E play a variety of different, but no less important, roles in the chemistry of the body. The form of vitamin A called *retinal*, for example, plays an important role in detecting light

BOX 41-8 *sports and fitness*
Vitamin Supplements for Athletes

Because a deficiency of vitamins *(avitaminosis)* can cause poor athletic performance, many athletes regularly consume vitamin supplements. However, research suggests that vitamin supplementation has little or no effect on a person's athletic performance. A reasonably well balanced diet supplies more than enough vitamins for even the elite athlete. The use of vitamin supplements therefore has fuelled controversy among experts. Opponents of vitamin supplements cite the cost and the possibility of liver damage associated with some forms of *hypervitaminosis,* whereas supporters cite the benefit of protecting against vitamin deficiency. •

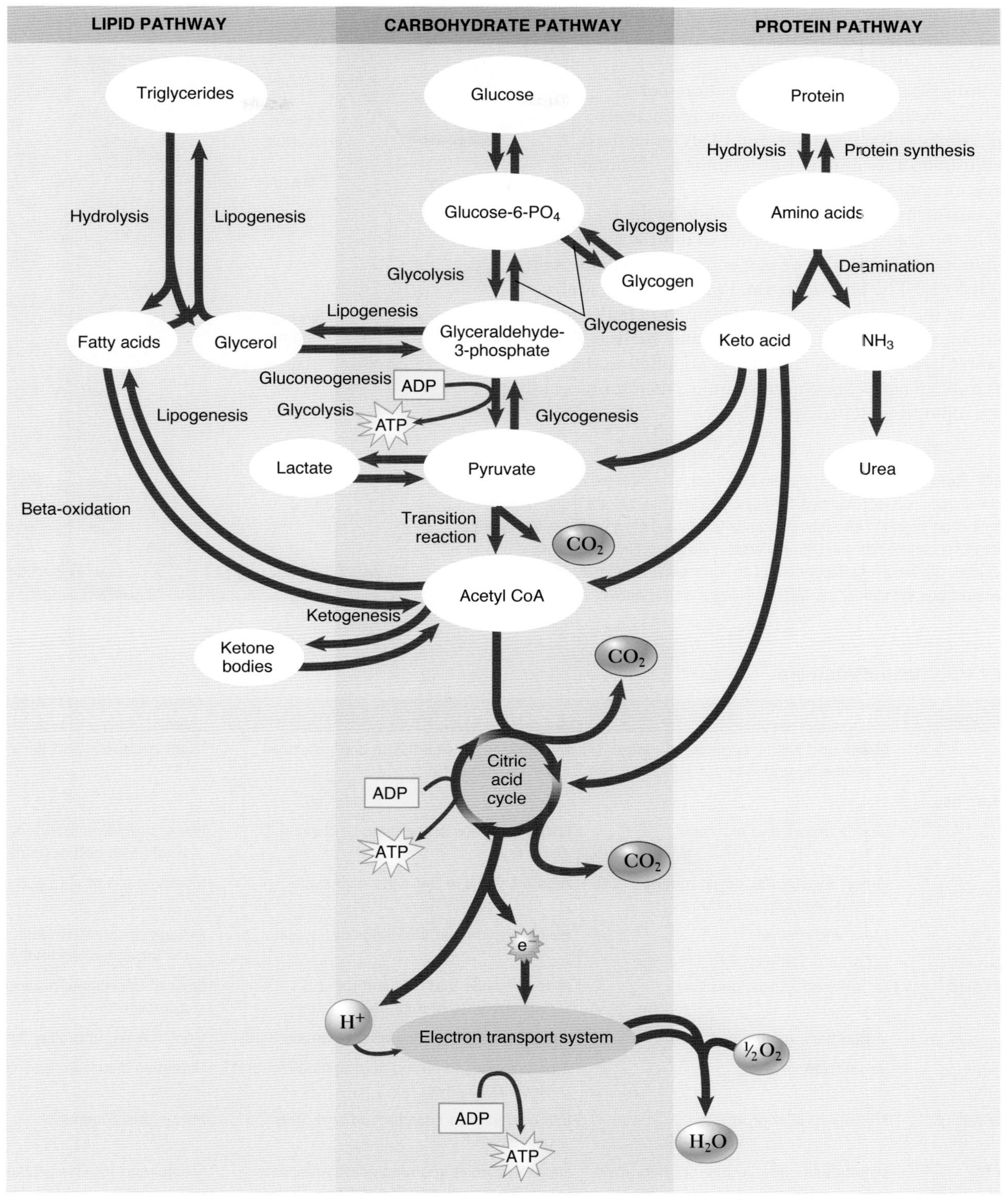

FIGURE 41-22 Summary of metabolism. Notice the central role played by the citric acid cycle and electron transport system. Notice also how different molecules can be converted to forms that may enter other pathways. *ADP,* Adenosine diphosphate; *ATP,* adenosine triphosphate; *CoA,* coenzyme A.

in sensory cells of the retina. Vitamin D acts as the hormone **calcitriol,** which plays a role in the regulation of calcium homeostasis in the body. One role of vitamin E is to serve as an **antioxidant** that prevents electron-seeking molecules such as free radicals from damaging electron-dense molecules in the cell membranes and DNA molecules. **Figure 41-23** illustrates this function of vitamin E. Vitamin C may also serve as an antioxidant.

No vitamin, except for vitamin D, can be made by the body itself. Bacteria living in the colon make two more: vitamin K and biotin. We must eat vitamins, or molecules we can convert into vitamins, in our food to get the rest. The body can store lipid-soluble vitamins—A, D, E, and K—in the liver for later use. Because the body cannot store significant amounts of water-soluble vitamins such as B vitamins and vitamin C, they must be continually supplied in the diet. **Table 41-3** lists some of the better-known vitamins, their sources and functions, and symptoms of deficiency.

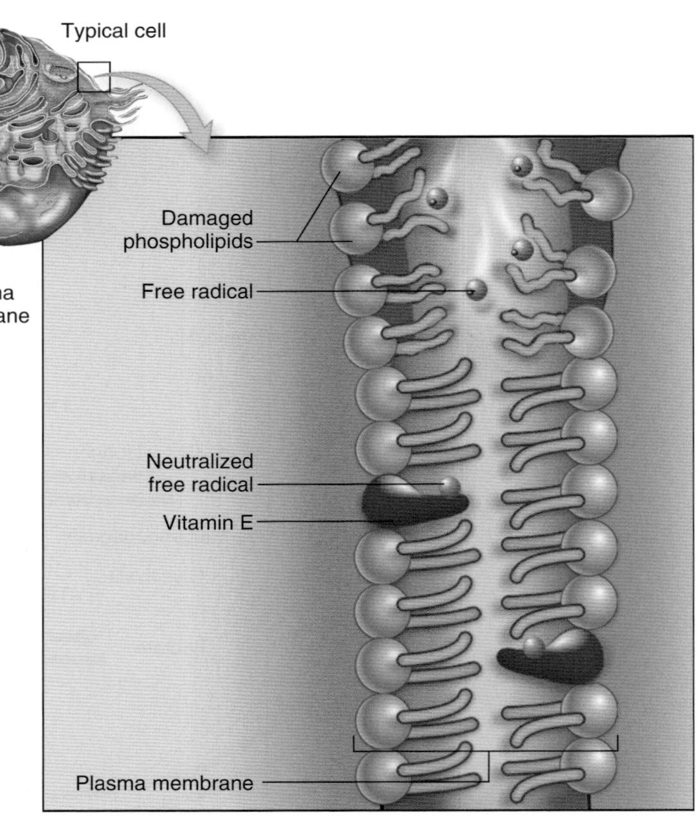

FIGURE 41-23 Role of vitamin E. Vitamin E can act as an antioxidant, attracting and neutralizing molecules with unpaired electrons. For example, free radicals are highly reactive molecules with an electron-seeking behaviour that tends to damage electron-dense areas of the cell such as membrane phospholipids and DNA molecules. Vitamin E embedded among phospholipids in cell membranes can have a protective effect as it attracts and neutralizes free radicals that would otherwise destroy the membrane. Vitamin C has a similar antioxidant effect.

TABLE 41-3 Major Vitamins

VITAMIN	DIETARY SOURCE	FUNCTIONS	SYMPTOMS OF DEFICIENCY
Vitamin A*	Green and yellow vegetables, dairy products, and liver	Maintains epithelial tissue and produces visual pigments	Night blindness and flaking skin
B-complex vitamins			
B_1 (thiamine)	Grains, meat, and legumes	Helps enzymes in the citric acid cycle	Nerve problems (beriberi), heart muscle weakness, and oedema
B_2 (riboflavin)	Green vegetables, organ meats, eggs, and dairy products	Aids enzymes in the citric acid cycle	Inflammation of skin and eyes
B_3 (niacin)	Meat and grains	Helps enzymes in the citric acid cycle	Pellagra (scaly dermatitis and mental disturbances) and nervous disorders
B_5 (pantothenic acid)	Organ meat, eggs, and liver	Aids enzymes that connect fat and carbohydrate metabolism	Loss of coordination (rare), decreased gut motility
B_6 (pyridoxine)	Vegetables, meats, and grains	Helps enzymes that catabolize amino acids	Convulsions, irritability, and anaemia
B_9 (folic acid)	Vegetables	Aids enzymes in amino acid catabolism and blood production	Digestive disorders and anaemia
B_{12} (cyanocobalamin)	Meat and dairy products	Involved in blood production and other processes	Pernicious anaemia
Biotin (vitamin H)	Vegetables, meat, eggs, gut microbes	Helps enzymes in amino acid catabolism and fat and glycogen synthesis	Mental and muscle problems (rare)
Vitamin C (ascorbic acid)	Fruits and green vegetables	Helps in manufacture of collagen fibres; antioxidant	Scurvy and degeneration of skin, bone, and blood vessels
Vitamin D* (calciferol)	Dairy products and fish liver oil	Aids in calcium absorption	Rickets and skeletal deformity
Vitamin E* (tocopherol)	Green vegetables and seeds	Protects cell membranes from being destroyed; antioxidant	Muscle and reproductive disorders (rare)
Vitamin K*	Leafy green vegetables, gut microbes	Blood coagulation, other metabolic pathways	Clotting disorders, anaemia, osteoporosis

*Lipid-soluble vitamin (all others listed are water-soluble vitamins).

CONNECT IT!

Bacteria that provide vitamin K to the body are part of a complex microbial system. Some people ingest preparations called **probiotics** that contain helpful bacteria to prevent or reverse imbalances in the gut microbiome. **Prebiotics**, which are not bacteria but have effects that alter the gut's bacterial communities, may also be used to maintain or restore normal microbial function. Review the human *microbiome* in ***The Human Microbiome*** at ***Connect It!***

Minerals

Minerals are at least as important as vitamins in our diet. Minerals are inorganic elements or salts that are found naturally in the earth. Like vitamins, mineral ions can attach to enzymes or other organic molecules and help them work. Of course, minerals such as sodium, chloride, and potassium are essential in relatively large amounts for maintaining the fluid/ion composition of the internal fluid environment (see Chapter 40).

Minerals also function in various other vital chemical reactions. For example, sodium, calcium, and other minerals are required for nerve conduction and for contraction in muscle fibres. Without these minerals, the brain, heart, and respiratory tract would cease to function. Iron is needed to manufacture haemoglobin in red blood cells, and iodine is needed to make thyroid hormones T_3 and T_4. Calcium, phosphorus, and magnesium are required to build the strong structural components of the skeleton.

Information about some of the more important minerals is summarized in **Table 41-4**. Like vitamins, minerals are beneficial only when taken in the proper amounts. Some of the minerals listed in **Table 41-4** are required in large amounts and some only in trace or ultratrace amounts. Any intake of minerals beyond or below the recommended amount may become unhealthy—perhaps even life-threatening.

Dietary **macrominerals** are those in which the adequate intakes (AIs) are at least 100 mg per day. Dietary **microminerals**—also called *trace elements*—have AIs less than 15 mg/day. Microminerals that are needed only in microgram quantities each day are called *ultratrace* minerals.

Recommended AIs of minerals can change over the life span. For example, **Figure 41-24** shows that calcium intake should increase throughout childhood and remain high throughout adulthood. However, the actual intake of calcium among females in the United Kingdom and the United States tends to fall short during adulthood—thereby increasing the risk for osteoporosis and other disorders.

Figure 41-25 shows the requirement for iron over the life span for both men and women. Although both males and females require a large amount of iron during the spurt of growth in the teenage years, the iron requirement remains high only in women during the rest of adulthood. This difference is explained by the fact that adult women must continually replace the iron lost in the menstrual flow. Note that female iron requirements drop to the level of males after menopause.

TABLE 41-4 Major Minerals

MINERAL	DIETARY SOURCE	FUNCTIONS	SYMPTOMS OF DEFICIENCY
Macrominerals			
Calcium (Ca)	Dairy products, legumes, and vegetables	Helps blood clotting, bone formation, and nerve and muscle function	Bone degeneration and nerve and muscle malfunction
Phosphorus (P)	Dairy products and meat	Aids in bone formation and is used to make ATP, DNA, RNA, and phospholipids	Bone degeneration and metabolic problems
Microminerals			
Chlorine (Cl)	Salty foods	Aids in stomach acid production and acid–base balance	Acid–base imbalance
Cobalt (Co)	Meat	Helps vitamin B_{12} in blood cell production	Pernicious anaemia
Copper (Cu)	Seafood, organ meats, and legumes	Involved in extracting energy from the citric acid cycle and in blood production	Fatigue and anaemia
Iodine (I)	Seafood and iodized salt	Required for thyroid hormone synthesis	Goitre (thyroid enlargement) and decrease in metabolic rate
Iron (Fe)	Meat, eggs, vegetables, and legumes	Involved in extracting energy from the citric acid cycle and in blood production	Fatigue and anaemia
Magnesium (Mg)	Vegetables and grains	Helps many enzymes	Nerve disorders, blood vessel dilation, and heart rhythm problems
Manganese (Mn)	Vegetables, legumes, and grains	Helps many enzymes	Muscle and nerve disorders
Potassium (K)	Seafood, milk, fruit, and meats	Helps muscle and nerve function	Muscle weakness, heart problems, and nerve problems
Selenium (Se)	Nuts, grains, meat, fish, mushrooms, eggs	Needed to make some amino acids; cofactor for enzymes	Heart muscle damage, cartilage degeneration, hypothyroidism
Sodium (Na)	Salty foods	Aids in muscle and nerve function and fluid balance	Weakness and digestive upset
Zinc (Zn)	Many foods	Helps many enzymes	Inadequate growth

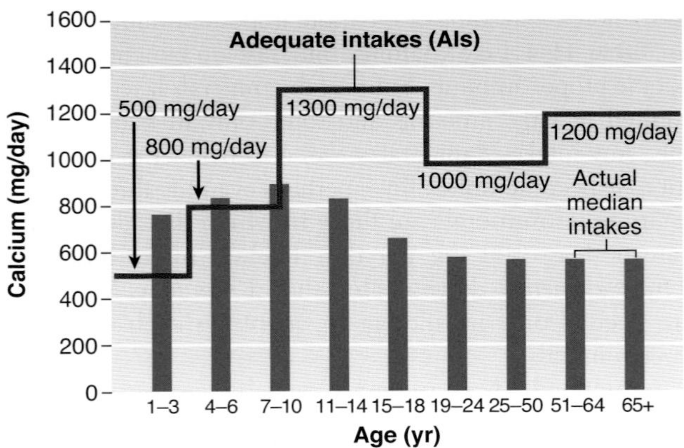

FIGURE 41-24 Calcium intake in women. The chart compares the recommended adequate intake (AIs) of calcium for women over the life span with the actual median intake of calcium among females in the United States.

Note also that the iron requirement peaks during pregnancies—when fetal blood development requires large amounts of iron.

Quick **CHECK**

17. What is a vitamin?
18. List two functions of minerals in the body.

CONNECT IT! 

One of the hottest areas in the field of nutrition today is that of *functional foods.* Find out what they are and why you may want to include them in your diet in ***Functional Foods*** online at ***Connect It!***

METABOLIC RATES

Metabolic rate refers to the amount of energy released in the body in a given time by catabolism. It is the energy that must be expended to accomplish various kinds of work. In short, metabolic rate is the catabolic rate, or the rate of energy release.

Metabolic rates are expressed in either of two ways: (1) in terms of the number of kilocalories of heat energy expended per hour or per day or (2) as normal or as a definite percentage above or below normal.

In the sections that follow, energy values are expressed in kilojoules (kJ) or megajoules (MJ) as well as in kilocalories (kcal). (Note 1 MJ = 1000 kJ.)

BASAL METABOLIC RATE

The **basal metabolic rate (BMR)** is the body's rate of energy expenditure in "basal conditions"—namely, when the individual is:

- Awake but resting—that is, lying down and, as far as possible, not moving a muscle.
- In the postabsorptive state (12 to 18 hours after the last meal).
- In a comfortably warm environment (the so-called *thermoneutral zone,* a temperature range at which metabolism is independent of ambient temperature).

Note that the BMR is not the minimum metabolic rate. It does not indicate the smallest amount of energy that must be expended to sustain life. It does, however, indicate the smallest amount of energy expenditure that can sustain life and also maintain the waking state and a normal body temperature in a comfortably warm environment.

Factors Influencing Basal Metabolic Rate

The BMR is not identical for all individuals because of the influence of various factors (**Figure 41-26** and **Figure 41-27**), some of which are described in the following paragraphs (**Box 41-9**).

Size

In computing the BMR, size is usually indicated by the amount of the body's surface area. It is computed from the individual's height and weight. A large individual has the same BMR as a small person per square metre of body surface, if other conditions are equal. However, because a large individual has more square metres of surface area, the BMR is greater than that of a small individual. For example,

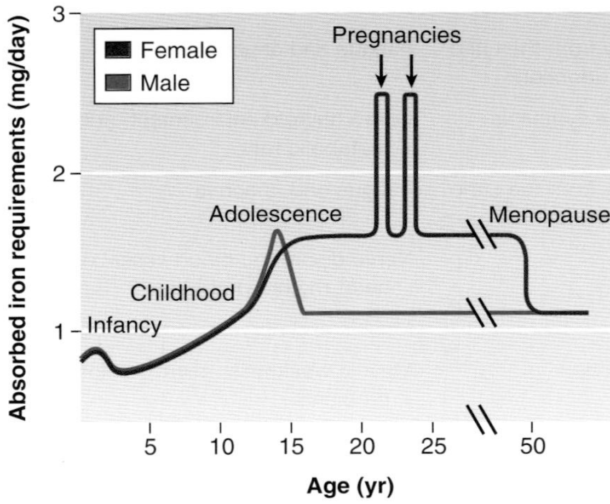

FIGURE 41-25 Iron intake requirements. The chart compares male and female absorbable iron requirements over the life span.

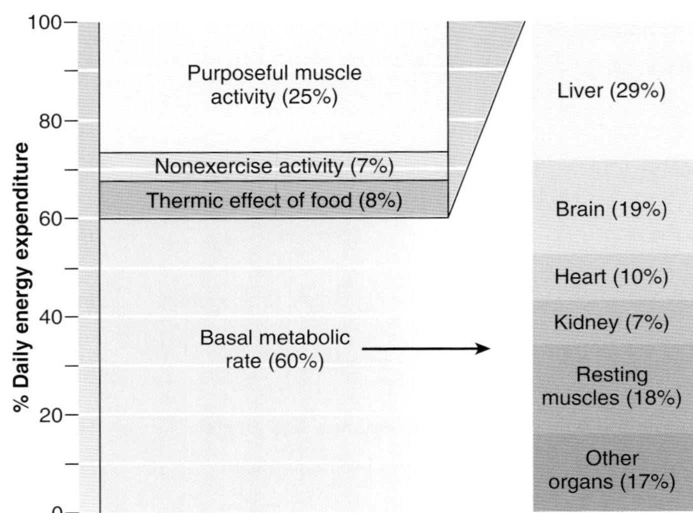

FIGURE 41-26 Daily energy expenditure. The left bar shows the total energy expenditure of the body as a combination of the basal metabolic rate (BMR), the thermic effect of food, everyday tasks, and purposeful exercise. The right bar shows the organs of the body that contribute to the basal metabolic rate.

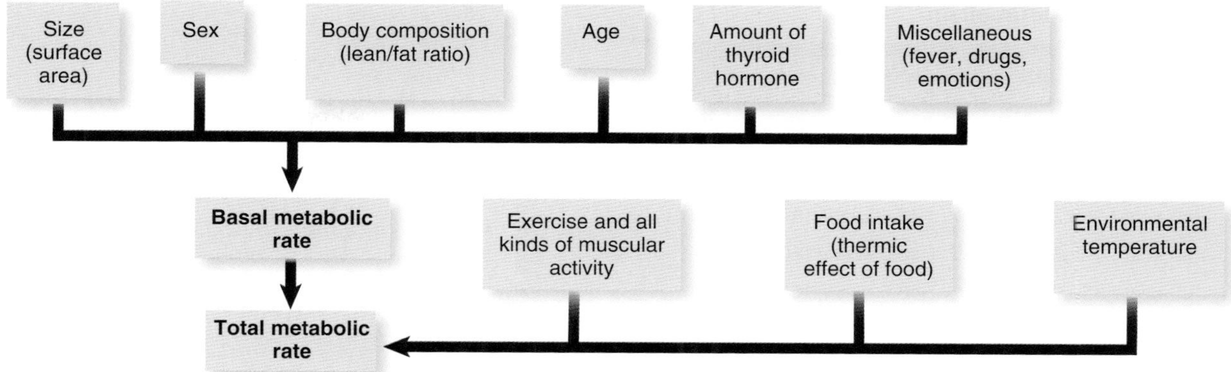

FIGURE 41-27 **Some factors that determine basal and total metabolic rates.**

BOX 41-9 *how BMR is determined*

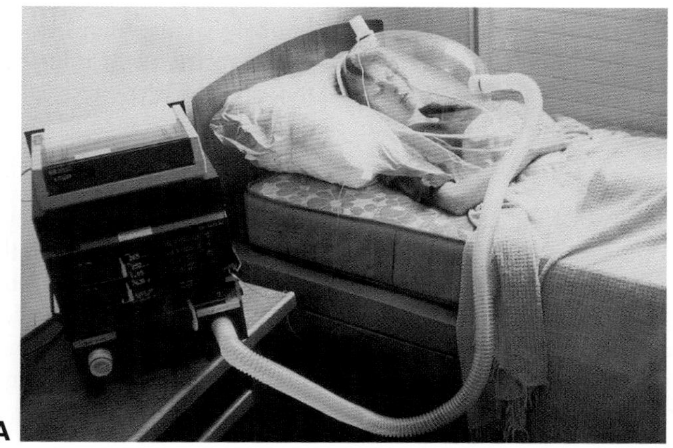

Basal metabolic rate (BMR) can be determined by a method called indirect calorimetry. The rationale underlying this method is that BMR (expressed as the number of kilocalories (or kilojoules) of heat produced per unit of time) can be calculated from the amount of oxygen consumed in a given time (part *B* of the figure). BMR can then be expressed as normal, or as a definite percentage above or below normal, by dividing the actual kilocalorie (or kilojoule) rate by the known average kilocalorie (or kilojoule) rate for normal individuals of the same size, sex, and age.

Statistical tables, based on research, list estimated normal BMRs. (If BMR was calculated to be 10% above normal, for example, it would be reported as +10.) Are you curious to know the average BMR for a person of your size, sex, and age? If so, take the following steps:

1. Start with your weight in kilograms and your height in centimetres. (Convert pounds to kilograms by dividing pounds by 2.2. Convert inches to approximate centimetres by multiplying inches by 2.5.) For example, 110 pounds = 50 kg; 5 feet, 3 inches = 158 cm.
2. Convert your weight and height to square metres by using the chart shown here (part *B* of the figure). For example, a weight of 50 kg and height of 158 cm = about 1.5 square metres of body surface area.
3. Find your age and sex in **Table 41-5** and then multiply the number of kilocalories (or kilojoules) per square metre per hour given there by your square metres of surface area and then by 24. For example, the average BMR per day for a 25-year-old woman with a weight of 50kg and height of 158cm = 1332 kcal (37 × 1.5 × 24) or 5573 kJ (154.8 x 1.5 x 24). •

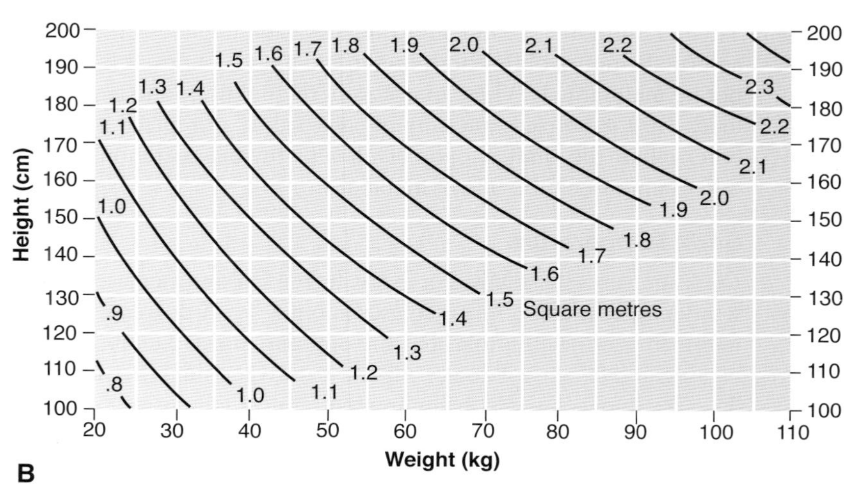

Measuring BMR. A, Indirect calorimetry calculates the rate of metabolism by measuring the rate at which oxygen is consumed. **B,** BMR estimate chart.

TABLE 41-5 Basal Metabolism

	KILOCALORIES/KILOJOULES PER HOUR PER SQUARE METRE OF BODY SURFACE	
AGE (YR)	MALE	FEMALE
10–12	51.5 kcal / 215.5 kJ	50.0 kcal / 209.2 kJ
12–14	50.0 kcal / 209.2 kJ	46.5 kcal / 194.5 kJ
14–16	46.0 kcal / 192.5 kJ	43.0 kcal / 180.0 kJ
16–18	43.0 kcal / 180.0 kJ	40.0 kcal / 167.3 kJ
18–20	41.0 kcal / 171.5 kJ	38.0 kcal / 159.0 kJ
20–30	39.5 kcal / 165.3 kJ	37.0 kcal / 154.8 kJ
30–40	39.5 kcal / 165.3 kJ	36.5 kcal / 152.7 kJ
40–50	38.5 kcal / 161.0 kJ	36.0 kcal / 150.6 kJ
50–60	37.5 kcal / 157.0 kJ	35.0 kcal / 146.4 kJ
60–70	36.5 kcal / 152.7 kJ	34.0 kcal / 142.3 kJ

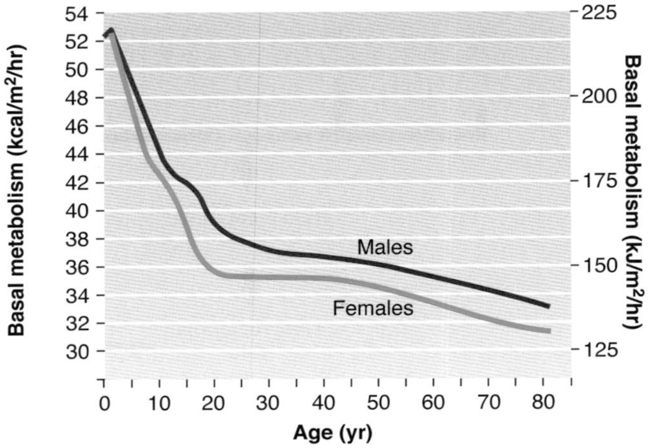

FIGURE 41-29 Basal metabolic rates over the life span. The chart shows normal basal metabolic rates (BMRs) as function of age for each sex.

the BMR for a man in his 20s is 39.5 kcal (165.3 kJ) per square metre of body surface per hour (**Table 41-5**). However, a large man with a body surface area of 1.9 square metres would have a BMR of 76 kcal (318 kJ) per hour, whereas a smaller man with a surface area of perhaps 1.6 square metres would have a BMR of only 64 kcal (268 kJ) per hour. The average surface area for UK adults is 1.7 square metres for women and 1.9 square metres for men.

Body Composition

Lean tissue is mostly "working tissue" that uses energy at a faster rate than does storage tissue or white fat tissue. Therefore, the higher the ratio of lean tissue to fat tissue in a person, the higher the BMR.

Gender

Men oxidize their food approximately 5% to 7% faster than women do. Therefore their BMRs are about 5% to 7% higher for a given size and age. A man 1.7 metres tall weighing 63.5 kg, for example, has a 5% to 7% higher BMR than a woman of the same height, weight, and age. This gender difference in BMR probably results from the difference in the proportion of body fat, which is determined by sex hormones. Women tend to have a higher percentage of body fat (and thus a lower total lean mass) than men do (**Figure 41-28**). Fat tissue is less metabolically active than lean tissues such as muscle. Differences in total lean mass not related to gender also affect the BMR. The relationship of BMR to sex and age is illustrated in **Figure 41-29**.

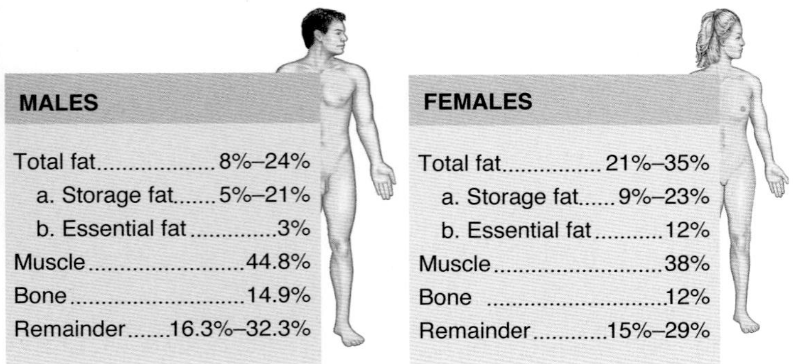

MALES
Total fat..................8%–24%
a. Storage fat.......5%–21%
b. Essential fat..............3%
Muscle..........................44.8%
Bone.............................14.9%
Remainder.......16.3%–32.3%
FEMALES
Total fat...............21%–35%
a. Storage fat......9%–23%
b. Essential fat...........12%
Muscle...........................38%
Bone 12%
Remainder............15%–29%

FIGURE 41-28 Body composition. Estimated values in healthy men and women.

Age

That the fires of youth burn more brightly than those of age is a physiological and psychological fact. In general, the younger the individual, the higher the BMR for a given size and sex (see **Table 41-5**). Exception: The BMR is slightly lower at birth than it is a few years later. That is to say, the rate increases slightly during the first 3 to 6 years, then starts to decrease and continues to do so throughout life.

Thyroid Hormone

Thyroid hormone (T_3 and T_4) stimulates basal metabolism. Without a normal amount of this hormone in the blood, a normal BMR cannot be maintained. When an excess of thyroid hormone is secreted, foods are catabolized faster, much as wood in a fireplace is burned faster when the draft is open. Deficient thyroid secretion, on the other hand, slows the rate of metabolism.

Body Temperature

Fever increases the BMR. For every degree Celsius increase in body temperature, metabolism increases about 13%. A decrease in body temperature (hypothermia) has the opposite effect. Metabolism decreases, and because it does, cells use less oxygen than they normally do. This knowledge has been applied clinically by using hypothermia in certain situations—for example, in open-heart surgery. Because circulation is reduced or interrupted during this procedure, oxygen supply necessarily decreases. Cells can tolerate this decreased oxygen supply reasonably well if their oxygen need has also decreased. Induced hypothermia decreases their rate of metabolism and thereby decreases their use of oxygen.

Drugs

Certain drugs, such as caffeine, amphetamine, and levothyroxine, increase the BMR.

Other Factors

Other factors, such as *emotions*, *pregnancy*, and *lactation* (milk production), also influence basal metabolism. All of these factors increase the BMR.

TOTAL METABOLIC RATE

Total metabolic rate is the amount of energy used or expended by the body in a given time. It is often expressed in kilocalories (or kilojoules) per hour or per day. Most of the factors that determine the total metabolic rate are shown in **Figures 41-26** and **41-27**. Of these, the main direct determinants are as follows:

Factor 1—the basal metabolic rate—that is, the energy used to do the work of maintaining life in the basal conditions previously described. Basal metabolic rate usually constitutes about 55% to 60% of the total metabolic rate.

Factor 2—the energy used to do all kinds of skeletal muscle work. This encompasses the simplest activities such as feeding oneself or sitting up in bed to the most strenuous kind of physical labour or exercise.

Factor 3—the *thermic effect* of foods. The metabolic rate increases for several hours after a meal, apparently because of the energy needed for metabolizing foods. The energy released is called the thermic effect of food (TEF). Carbohydrates and fats have a thermic effect of about 5%. Proteins have a much higher thermic effect, about 30%. This means that for every 100 kcal (418 kJ) of protein, 30 kcal (125 kJ) are used for processes such as deamination and oxidation of the protein, leaving just 70 kcal (293 kJ) available for other cell work. For this reason, proteins are "worth" fewer calories.

ENERGY BALANCE AND BODY WEIGHT

When we say that the body maintains a state of energy balance, we mean that its energy input equals its energy output. Energy input per day equals the total calories (kilocalories) in the food ingested per day. Energy output equals the total metabolic rate expressed in kilocalories. You may be wondering what energy intake, output, and balance have to do with body weight. *Everything* would be a fairly good one-word answer. Or, to be somewhat more explicit, the following basic principles describe the relationships among these factors:

- Body weight remains constant (except for possible variations in water content) when the body maintains energy balance—when the total calories in the food ingested equals the total metabolic rate. Example: If you have a total metabolic rate of 2000 kcal (8.36 MJ) per day and if the food you eat per day yields 2000 kcal (8.36 MJ), your body will be maintaining energy balance and your weight will stay constant.
- Body weight increases when energy input exceeds energy output—when the total calories of food intake per day is greater than the total calories of the metabolic rate. A small amount of the excess energy input is used to synthesize glycogen for storage in the liver and muscles. The rest is used for synthesizing fat and storing it in adipose tissue. If you were to eat 3000 kcal (12.55 MJ) each day for a week and if your total metabolic rate were 2000 kcal (8.36 MJ) per day, you would gain weight. How much you would gain you can discover by doing a little simple arithmetic:

Total energy input for week	=	21,000 kcal (87.8 MJ)
Total energy output for week	=	−14,000 kcal (−58.52 MJ)
Excess energy input for week	=	7,000 kcal (29.33 MJ)

  Approximately 3500 kcal (14.64 MJ) are used to synthesize 0.45 kg of adipose tissue. Hence, at the end of this 1 week of "overeating"—of eating 7000 kcal (29.33 MJ) over and above your total metabolic rate—you would have gained about 0.9 kg.
- Body weight decreases when energy input is less than energy output—when the total number of calories in the food eaten is less than the total metabolic rate. Suppose you were to eat only 1000 kcal (4.18 MJ) a day for a week and that you have a total metabolic rate of 2000 kcal (8.36 MJ) per day. By the end of the week, your body would have used a total of 14,000 kcal (58.52 MJ) of energy for maintaining life and doing its many kinds of work. All 14,000 kcal (58.52 MJ) of this actual energy expenditure had to come from catabolism of foods because this is the body's only source of energy. Catabolism of ingested food supplied 7000 kcal (29.28 MJ), and catabolism of stored food supplied the remaining 7000 kcal (29.28 MJ). That week your body would not have maintained energy balance, nor would it have maintained weight balance. It would have incurred an energy deficit paid out of the energy stored in approximately 0.9 kg of body fat. In short, you would have lost about 0.9 kg.

Foods are stored primarily as glycogen and fats. Many cells catabolize them preferentially in this order: carbohydrates, then fats. (Skeletal muscle cells, however, seem to put fat first in their order of preference.) If there is no food intake, almost all of the glycogen is estimated to be used up in a matter of 1 or 2 days (**Figure 41-30**). Then, with no more

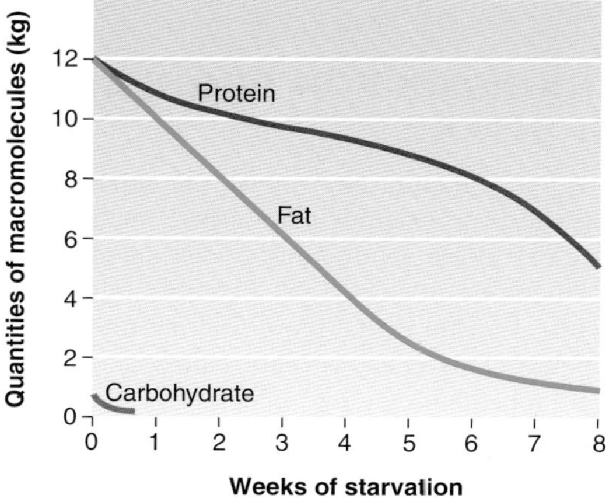

FIGURE 41-30 Effects of starvation on the body. Three major macromolecules serve as primary energy sources: carbohydrates, fats, and proteins. During starvation, the carbohydrate stores (glycogen) are rapidly depleted. However, stored lipids can mobilize and provide much of our energy needs for several weeks. Eventually, lipid stores run low and the body starts using proteins as a major source of energy—causing the breakdown of muscle and other protein-rich tissues. Muscle damage during starvation usually leads to death.

TABLE 41-6 Examples of Appetite-Regulating Factors*

OREXIGENIC FACTORS (STIMULATE APPETITE)	ANOREXIGENIC FACTORS (INHIBIT APPETITE)	SOURCE
	Leptin Interleukin 18 (IL-18)	Adipose tissue
Cortisol		Adrenal cortex
Ghrelin (GHRL)	Cholecystokinin (CCK) Glucagon-like peptide-1 (GLP-1) Oxyntomodulin (OXM) Peptide YY_{3-36} (PYY_{3-36})	GI tract
Endogenous opioid peptides (EOP) Galanin (GAL) Gamma-aminobutyric acid (GABA) Neuropeptide Y (NPY) Norepinephrine (NE) Orexins	Alpha-melanocyte–stimulating hormone (α-MSH) Cocaine- and amphetamine-regulated transcript (CART) Corticotropin-releasing hormone (CRH)	Hypothalamus
	Glucose	Liver
Emotions Environmental stimuli Food sensations Internal stimuli (e.g., blood temperature, glucose) Lifestyle choices and habits	Emotions Environmental stimuli Food sensations Internal stimuli (e.g., blood temperature, glucose) Lifestyle choices and habits	Nervous system†
	Insulin Pancreatic polypeptide (PP)	Pancreas

GI, Gastrointestinal.

*Hormones, neurotransmitters, and other factors that affect feeding centres in the hypothalamus.

†Nervous factors not specifically hypothalamic in origin.

carbohydrate to act as a fat sparer, fat is catabolized. How long it takes to deplete all of this reserve food depends, of course, on how much adipose tissue the individual has when starting the starvation diet. Finally, with no more fat available, tissue proteins are catabolized (see **Figure 41-30**). Because significant amounts of protein are not "stored" for use in catabolism, important structural and functional proteins are quickly depleted. Thus death soon ensues.

MECHANISMS FOR REGULATING FOOD INTAKE

Mechanisms for regulating food intake are still not clearly established. That the hypothalamus plays a part in these mechanisms, however, seems certain. Numerous studies seem to indicate that a cluster of neurons in the lateral hypothalamus function as an **appetite centre**—meaning that impulses from them bring about increased appetite. This effect is often called an **orexigenic effect** (meaning an "appetite-producing" effect).

Additional data suggest that a group of neurons in the ventral medial nucleus of the hypothalamus functions as a **satiety centre**—meaning that impulses from these neurons decrease appetite so that we feel sated, or satisfied. This effect is often called an **anorexigenic effect** (meaning "producing an appetite loss" effect).

What acts directly on both of these feeding centres to stimulate or depress them is still being worked out by researchers.

One factor is the temperature of the blood circulating to the hypothalamus. A moderate decrease in blood temperature stimulates the appetite centre (and inhibits the satiety centre). Result: the individual has an appetite, wants to eat, and probably does. An increase in blood temperature produces the opposite effect, a depressed appetite **(anorexia).** One well-known instance of this effect is the loss of appetite in persons who have a fever.

Another factor is blood glucose concentration and the rate of glucose use. A low blood glucose concentration or low glucose use stimulates the appetite centre, whereas a high blood glucose concentration inhibits it. This may be the action of a group of hormones called **orexins** or *hypocretins* produced in the hypothalamus in response to low blood glucose levels.

More recently, a variety of hormones and other regulators have been identified that have a profound impact on the feeding centres of the brain. The hypothalamus itself produces several hormones and neurotransmitters that affect the feeding centres, as you can see in **Table 41-6**. In addition, appetite-altering factors (hormones and neurotransmitters) are produced in many other organs such as the liver, adipose tissue, pancreas, GI tract, and autonomic nerve pathways (especially the vagal nerve). Of course, factors such as daily eating habits or patterns, emotional responses, the sensations of food, and many others must also be involved in regulating or affecting appetite.

Unquestionably, many factors operate together as a complex mechanism for regulating food intake—a mechanism that is still incompletely understood.

Quick CHECK

19. Give one of the two ways in which metabolic rates can be expressed.
20. Name three of the factors that influence basal metabolic rate.
21. Distinguish between basal metabolic rate and total metabolic rate.
22. In which division of the brain would you find the control centres for regulating food intake?

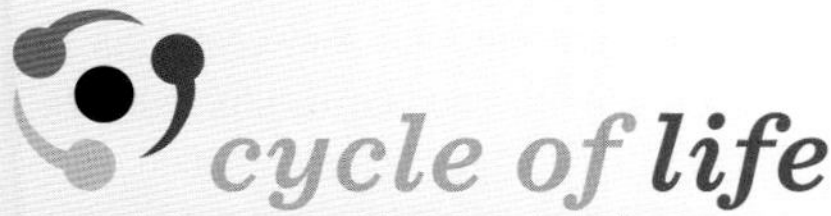

cycle of life

Nutrition and Metabolism The importance of proper nutrition to an individual's well-being begins at the moment of conception and continues until death. In the womb, various nutrients must be obtained from the mother's blood in sufficient quantity to ensure normal growth and development.

One critical nutrient during fetal development, infancy, and childhood is protein. Sufficient proteins, containing all the essential amino acids, are required to permit normal development of the nervous system, muscle tissues, and other vital structures.

Another critical nutrient during the early years of life is the mineral calcium. Large quantities of calcium are needed by a growing body to maintain normal development of the skeleton and other tissues. In the womb, a steady supply of calcium in the mother's blood is maintained by increased levels of the parathyroid hormone (PTH). Recall from Chapter 26 that PTH increases blood calcium levels by removing it from storage in the bones.

Unless a pregnant woman consumes enough calcium to replace this calcium lost from bones, she may experience the bone-softening effects of calcium deficiency. If proteins, calcium, or other necessary nutrients are in short supply anytime before the beginning of adulthood, the consequences may be permanent. For example, bone deformities resulting from a lack of calcium during childhood could become permanent if not corrected or compensated for before the skeleton ossifies completely.

In late adulthood, the number of food calories needed declines because the metabolic rate declines. This metabolic decline is thought to result largely from age-related changes in the balance of metabolic hormones such as thyroid hormones (T_3 and T_4). Even though the number of required food calories declines, the overall balance of nutrients consumed must be maintained to preserve proper metabolic function. Some nutrients, such as calcium, may be needed in greater quantity in older adults to compensate for (or avoid) age-related bone loss or other conditions. •

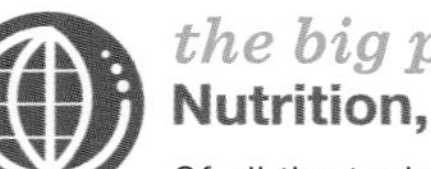

the big picture | Nutrition, Metabolism, and the Whole Body

Of all the topics we have discussed so far, the topic of nutrition and metabolism has the most easily seen role in the "big picture" of human body function. Every cell in the body must maintain the operation of its metabolic pathways to ensure its survival. Anabolic pathways are required to build the various structural and functional components of the cells. Catabolic pathways are required to convert energy to a usable form. Catabolic pathways are also needed to degrade large molecules into small subunits that can be used in anabolic pathways. Of course, the basic nutrient molecules—carbohydrates, fats, and proteins of the correct type—must be available to each cell to carry out these metabolic processes. Besides the basic nutrient molecules, cells also require small amounts of specific vitamins and minerals needed to produce the structural and functional components necessary for cellular metabolism.

Various body systems operate to make sure that essential nutrients reach the cells as needed to maintain metabolism in a manner that preserves relative constancy of the internal environment. For example, the nervous, skeletal, and muscular systems make it possible for us to take in complex foods from our external environment. The digestive system reduces these complex nutrients to simpler, more usable nutrients—then provides the mechanisms that allow us to absorb them into the internal environment. The circulatory system—both the cardiovascular and the lymphatic circulations—transports the absorbed nutrients to the individual cells for immediate use or to the liver or other organs for temporary storage. The endocrine system regulates the balance between immediate use and storage. The respiratory system, working with the cardiovascular system, provides the oxygen needed for oxidative phosphorylation—that is, using the citric acid cycle and electron transport system to transfer energy to ATP. These two systems also provide a mechanism for removing waste carbon dioxide (CO_2) generated by the catabolism of nutrient molecules. Likewise, the urinary system provides a mechanism for removing waste urea generated by protein catabolism. Even the integumentary system becomes involved, by producing vitamin D in the presence of sunlight.

Metabolism, with all the physiological mechanisms that support it, could be described as the essential process of life. It is, after all, the sum total of all the biochemical processes that distinguish a living organism from a nonliving object. •

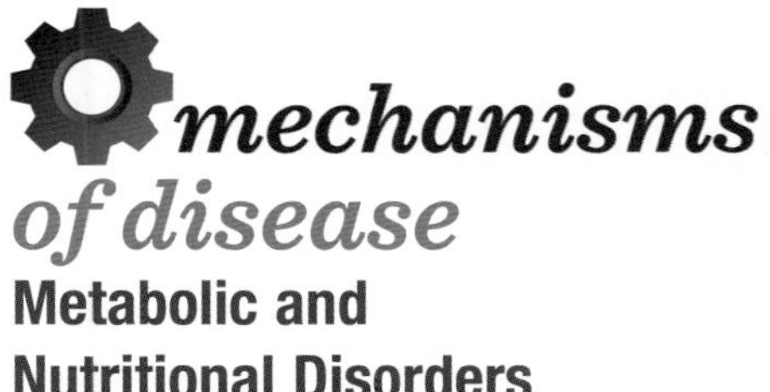

mechanisms of disease

Metabolic and Nutritional Disorders

Disorders characterized by a disruption or imbalance of normal metabolism can be caused by several different factors. For example, **inborn errors of metabolism** are a group of genetic conditions involving a deficiency or absence of a particular enzyme. Specific enzymes are required by cells to carry out each step of every metabolic reaction. Although an abnormal genetic code may affect the production of only a single enzyme, the resulting abnormal metabolism may have widespread effects. Specific diseases resulting from inborn errors of metabolism, such as **phenylketonuria,** are discussed in Chapter 48.

A number of metabolic disorders are complications of other conditions. For example, you may recall from Chapter 26 that both hyperthyroidism and hypothyroidism have profound effects on the basal metabolic rate. Diabetes mellitus affects metabolism throughout the body when an insulin deficiency limits the amount of glucose available for use by the cells.

Some metabolic disorders result from normal mechanisms in the body that maintain homeostasis. For example, the body has several mechanisms that maintain a relatively constant level of glucose in the blood—glucose required by cells for life-sustaining catabolism. As mentioned earlier in this chapter, during starvation or as a result of certain eating disorders, these mechanisms are taken to the extreme as they attempt to maintain blood glucose homeostasis. A few of the more well-known eating and nutrition disorders are briefly described in later sections.

Body Mass Index (BMI)

The **body mass index (BMI)** is a measure of a person's proportion of body weight to height. The BMI was developed in the late twentieth century as a way for researchers to easily assess body-fat percentages in large populations so they could track trends in obesity and other health conditions.

To calculate a BMI, simply divide weight (in kilograms) by the square of height (in metres): BMI $= kg/m^2$. To determine kilogram weight, divide the number of pounds by 2.2. To determine metre height, divide total inches by 39.4. Thus the BMI can quickly tell individuals whether they are above or below their ideal weight, and by approximately how much.

As discussed in the following sections and illustrated in **Figure 41-31**, a BMI that is too high or too low is associated with an increased risk of death. However, remember that BMI is most useful when looking at trends in a population as a whole and not as useful in individual risk assessments. Factors such as gender, age, and genetics play a role in such health assessments, so BMI alone is not sufficient. Measurements of waist or thigh circumference and body fat percentages (see **Box 8-1**, p. 138) are often used along with BMI to give a more complete picture.

Metabolic Syndrome

Metabolic syndrome is a collection of risk factors for coronary artery disease, stroke, and type 2 diabetes. Obesity is a risk factor in metabolic syndrome, as is *insulin resistance.* As target cells respond less efficiently to insulin, glucose cannot enter cells and the body must move triglycerides and other lipids into the blood to supply energy needs. Thus, *hyperlipidaemia* (elevated blood lipids, such as high triglyceride and LDL cholesterol) is also a risk factor included in this syndrome.

Other risk factors in this syndrome are low HDL cholesterol, hypertension, increased blood clotting, elevated inflammation mediators, and related factors. Metabolic syndrome can be treated with diet, exercise, cholesterol-lowering therapy, and other strategies to reduce central obesity.

CONNECT IT! 

A specific risk factor that usually occurs in metabolic syndrome is large waist circumference—the "apple-shaped" central obesity described in ***Body Types and Disease*** at ***Connect It!***

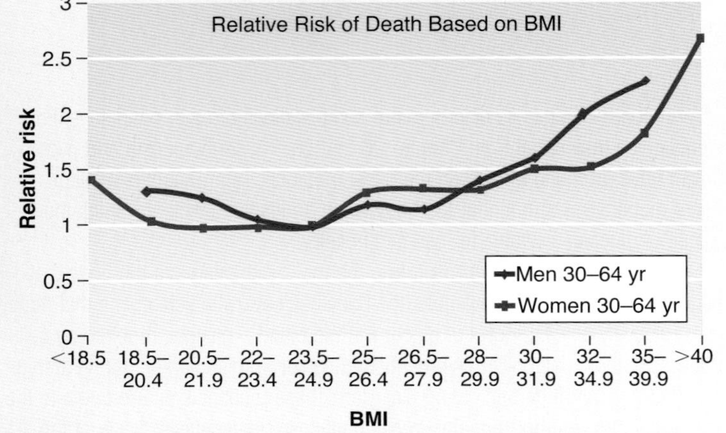

FIGURE 41-31 Body mass index (BMI) and risk of death. Mortality (death) risk is higher in individuals with a high or low BMI.

Eating Disorders

Eating disorders have been a part of the medical literature for many years, but interest and concern regarding these disorders are growing because the number of reported cases has increased dramatically. The two most common eating disorders are called *anorexia nervosa* and *bulimia.* Neither illness is completely understood, and successful treatment is often varied and sometimes controversial.

Anorexia Nervosa

Anorexia nervosa is primarily a disease of young adults. Most individuals affected are female (90% to 95%) and from 12 to 25 years of age. As many as 10% of people affected by an eating disorder are diagnosed with this condition in the UK. These individuals have a disturbed body image and an intense fear of obesity and therefore diet with a vengeance. They almost always develop unusual eating rituals and scrupulously monitor and restrict their food intake. Anorexic individuals literally starve themselves and, as a result, develop serious medical complications. The illness is characterized by a 20% to 25% loss of body mass, accompanied by slowed or impaired intellectual functioning. People affected are usually involved in excessive exercise and pursue ultimate thinness, regardless of their health. In women, menstruation ceases (amenorrhoea), and the basal metabolic rate is decreased as a result of starvation. These individuals have many skin abnormalities and an assortment of psychological, cardiovascular, and hormonal problems. They are at increased risk for sudden death from complications directly related to excessive weight loss and nutritional deficiency. Treatment is directed at resolution of both medical and psychological problems. In addition to psychotherapy and weight stabilization, pharmacological treatment with antidepressants has been used to improve mood and self-image.

Bulimia

Bulimia is an illness characterized by an eating and vomiting, or purging, cycle. It is sometimes referred to as **binge–purge syndrome.** In the UK, approximately 40% of people affected by an eating disorder have this condition. Most people who have bulimia are relatively young, single, white females. The mean age is 19, but the age of patients appears to be increasing. People with bulimia have an uncontrollable urge for food that leads to massive overeating (bingeing), which is followed by repeated forced vomiting and laxative abuse (purging). Loss of gastric and intestinal contents often leads to serious fluid and electrolyte imbalance. The result is often the development of neurological problems such as convulsions, tetany, and seizures. Vomiting may also cause aspiration pneumonia, erosion of tooth enamel, trauma of the mouth and oesophagus, and infection of the salivary glands. The longer the disease is allowed to continue without treatment, the greater the increase in mortality from medical complications. Many people who have bulimia suffer from major depression and have concomitant social problems such as alcohol abuse. About a quarter of people with bulimia are chemically dependent, and many have been sexually abused. They are especially prone to self-mutilation and suicide attempts. Nutritional counselling, psychotherapy, and treatment with antidepressants help bulimic patients cope with stress and break the binge/purge cycle.

Obesity

Obesity is not an eating disorder itself but may be a symptom of chronic overeating behaviour. Like anorexia nervosa and bulimia, eating disorders characterized by chronic overeating usually have an underlying emotional cause. Obesity may also result from metabolic disorders. Obesity is defined as an abnormal increase in the proportion of adipose tissue in the body. Usually, a person with a BMI higher than 30 is considered moderately obese. A person with a BMI higher than 40 is considered to be extremely obese. Most of the excess fat is stored in

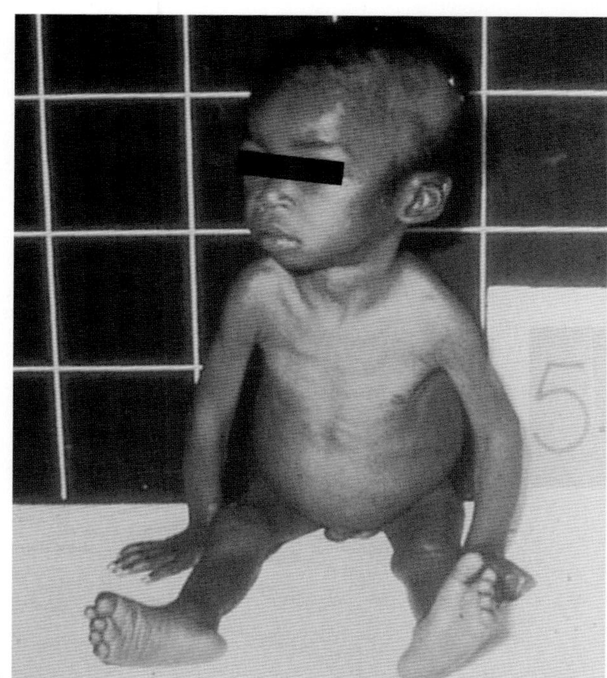

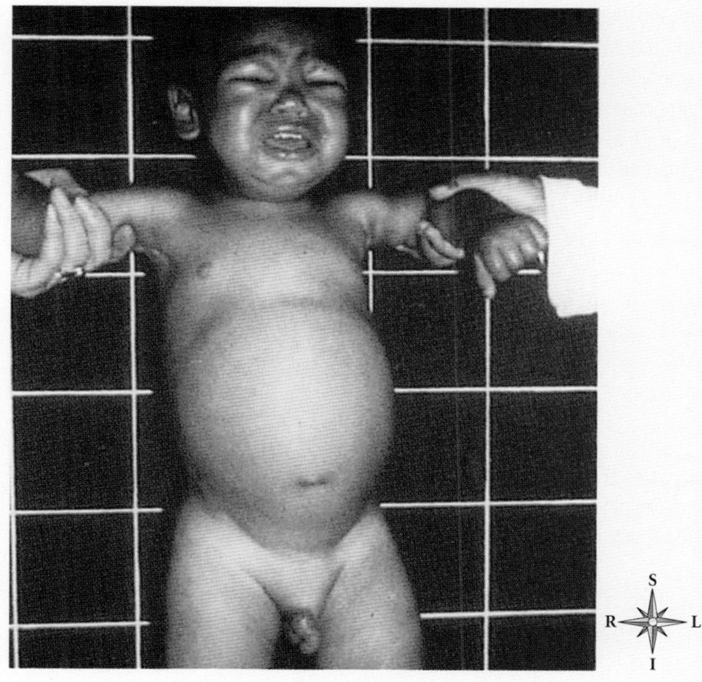

FIGURE 41-32 Protein–calorie malnutrition (PCM). PCM is an abnormal condition resulting from a deficiency of calories in general and protein in particular. Here, two forms of advanced PCM, marasmus **(A)** and kwashiorkor **(B),** are shown.

the subcutaneous tissue and around the viscera. Obesity is a risk factor in various life-threatening diseases, including many forms of cancer, diabetes, and heart disease (see **Figure 41-31**).

Nutritional Disorders

Protein–Calorie Malnutrition

Protein–calorie malnutrition (PCM) is an abnormal condition resulting from a deficiency of calories in general and protein in particular. PCM is likely to result from reduced intake of food but may also be caused by increased nutrient loss or increased use of nutrients by the body. Mild cases occur commonly in those with illness; as many as one in five patients admitted to the hospital are significantly malnourished. More severe cases of PCM are likely to occur in parts of the world where food, especially protein-rich food, is relatively unavailable. There are two forms of advanced PCM: **marasmus** and **kwashiorkor** (**Figure 41-32**). Marasmus results from an overall lack of calories and proteins, such as when sufficient quantities of food are not available. Marasmus is characterized by progressive wasting of muscle and subcutaneous tissue accompanied by fluid and electrolyte imbalances. Kwashiorkor results from a protein deficiency in the presence of sufficient calories, as when a child is weaned from milk to low-protein foods. At the same time, a child affected with kwashiorkor is also likely to have an underlying infection that further increases calorie and protein needs. Like marasmus, kwashiorkor also causes wasting of tissues, but unlike marasmus, it also causes pronounced ascites (abdominal bloating) and flaking dermatitis. The ascites results from a deficiency of plasma proteins, which changes the osmotic balance of the blood and thus promotes osmosis of water from the blood into the peritoneal space.

Vitamin Disorders

Vitamin deficiency, or **avitaminosis**, can lead to severe metabolic problems. For example, *avitaminosis C* (vitamin C deficiency) can lead to scurvy. Scurvy results from the inability of the body to manufacture and maintain collagen fibres. As you may have gathered from your studies thus far, collagen fibres compose the connective tissues that hold most of the body together. In scurvy, the body literally falls apart in the same way that a neglected house eventually falls apart (**Figure 41-33**). Other details about scurvy and other types of avitaminosis are given in **Table 41-3**.

Some forms of **hypervitaminosis**—or vitamin excess—can be just as serious as a deficiency of vitamins. For example, chronic *hypervitaminosis A* can occur if large amounts of vitamin A—more than 10 times the recommended dietary or daily allowance (RDA)—are consumed daily over a period of 3 months or more (**Figure 41-34**). This condition first manifests with dry skin, hair loss,

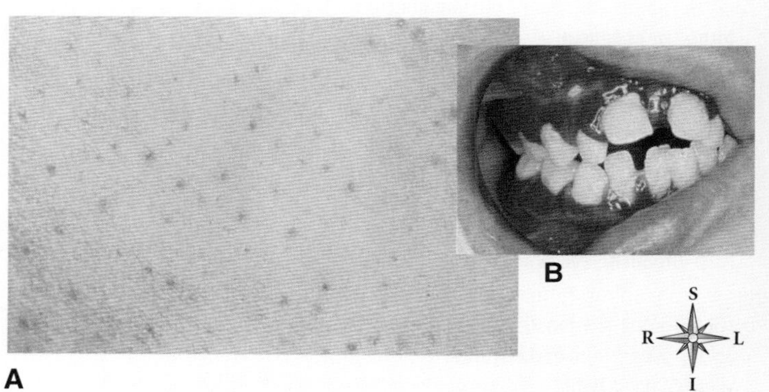

FIGURE 41-33 Scurvy. In scurvy, lack of vitamin C impairs the normal maintenance of collagen-containing connective tissues, causing bleeding and ulceration of the skin, gums, and other tissues, as these lesions on the skin **(A)** and inflamed gingiva **(B)** show.

anorexia (appetite loss), and vomiting. However, it may progress to severe headaches and mental disturbances, liver enlargement, and occasionally cirrhosis. Acute hypervitaminosis A, characterized by vomiting, abdominal pain, and headache, can occur if a massive overdose is ingested. Excesses of the lipid-soluble vitamins (A, D, E, and K) are generally more serious than excesses of the water-soluble vitamins (B complex and C), as they are stored in body tissues and accumulate to toxic levels.

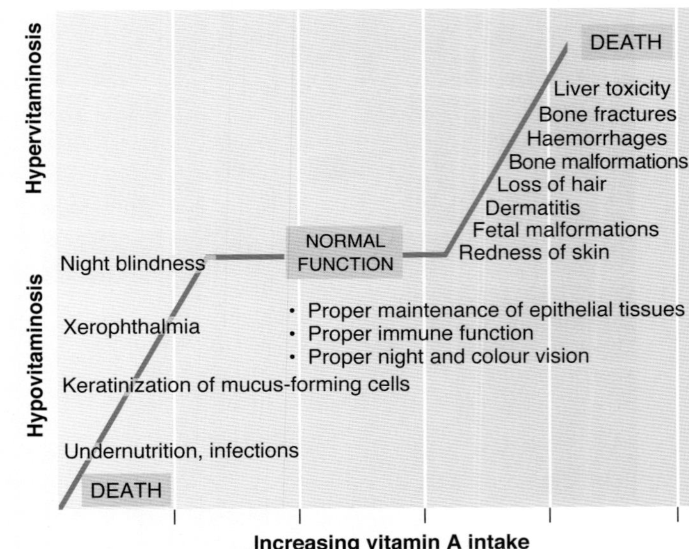

FIGURE 41-34 Vitamin A intake. This chart shows how changing the amount of vitamin A in the diet can lead to hypovitaminosis A or hypervitaminosis A. In extreme cases, either can lead to death.

LANGUAGE OF SCIENCE *(continued from p. 930)*

Cori cycle (KOR-ee SYE-kul)
[*Carl Ferdinand Cori and Gerty Theresa Radnitz Cori* **Czech-American biochemists,** *cycl-* **circle**]

deamination (dee-am-ih-NAY-shun)
[*de-* **undo,** *-amin-* **ammonia compound,** *-ation* **process**]

electron transport system (ETS)
[*electr-* **electric,** *-on* **unit,** *trans-* **across,** *-port* **carry**]

flavin adenine dinucleotide (FAD) (FLAY-vin AD-en-een dye-NYOO-klee-oh-tyde)
[*flav-* **yellow,** *-in* **substance,** *aden-* **gland,** *-ine* **chemical,** *di-* **two,** *nucleo-* **kernel (nucleus),** *-t-* **combining form,** *-ide* **chemical**]

glucagon (GLOO-kah-gon)
[*gluca-* **sweet (glucose),** *-agon* **lead or bring**]

gluconeogenesis (gloo-koh-nee-oh-JEN-eh-sis)
[*gluco-* **sweet (glucose),** *-neo-* **new,** *-gen-* **produce,** *-esis* **process**]

glucose phosphorylation (GLOO-kohs fos-for-ih-LAY-shun)
[*gluco-* **sweet,** *-ose* **carbohydrate (sugar),** *phos-* **light,** *-phor-* **carry,** *-yl-* **chemical,** *-ation* **process**]

glycogenesis (glye-koh-JEN-eh-sis)
[*glyco-* **sweet,** *-gen-* **produce,** *-esis* **process**]

glycogenolysis (glye-koh-jeh-NOL-ih-sis)
[*glyco-* **sweet (glucose),** *-gen-* **produce,** *-o-* **combining form,** *-lysis* **loosening**]

glycolysis (glye-KOHL-ih-sis)
[*glyco-* **sweet (glucose),** *-o-* **combining form,** *-lysis* **loosening**]

incretin (in-KREE-tin)
[*in-* **in,** *-cret-* **secrete,** *-in* **substance**]

insulin (IN-suh-lin)
[*insul-* **island,** *-in* **substance**]

ketogenesis (kee-toh-JEN-eh-sis)
[*keto-* **acetone,** *-gen-* **produce,** *-esis* **process**]

Krebs cycle (krebz SYE-kul)
[*Sir Hans Adolf Krebs* **British biochemist,** *cycl-* **circle**]

leptin (LEP-tin)
[*lept-* **thin,** *-in* **substance**]

lipid (LIP-id)
[*lip-* **fat,** *-id* **form**]

lipogenesis (lip-oh-JEN-eh-sis)
[*lipo-* **fat,** *-gen-* **produce,** *-esis* **process**]

lipoprotein (lip-oh-PROH-teen)
[*lipo-* **fat, protein**]

macromineral (mak-roh-MIN-er-al)
[*macro-* **large,** *-miner-* **mine,** *-al* **relating to**]

macronutrient (MAK-roh-NYOO-tree-ent)
[*macro-* **large,** *nutri-* **nourish,** *-ent* **agent**]

metabolic rate (met-ah-BOL-ik)
[*meta-* **over,** *-bol-* **throw,** *-ic* **relating to**]

metabolic syndrome (met-ah-BOL-ik SIN-drohm)
[*meta-* **over,** *-bol-* **throw,** *-ic* **relating to,** *syn-* **together,** *-drome* **running or (race)course**]

metabolism (meh-TAB-oh-liz-im)
[*meta-* **over,** *-bol-* **throw,** *-ism* **action**]

micromineral (my-kroh-MIN-er-al)
[*micro-* **small,** *-miner-* **mine,** *-al* **relating to**]

micronutrient (MY-kroh-NYOO-tree-ent)
[*micro-* **small,** *nutri-* **nourish,** *-ent* **agent**]

negative nitrogen balance (NEG-ah-tiv NYE-troh-jen)
[*negat-* **deny,** *-ive* **relating to,** *nitro-* **soda,** *-gen* **produce**]

nicotinamide adenine dinucleotide (NAD) (nik-oh-TIN-ah-myde AD-eh-neen dye-NYOO-klee-oh-tyde)
[*Jacque Nicot* **French diplomat (brought tobacco to France),** *-in-* **substance (after plant genus** *Nicotiana***),** *-am-* **ammonia,** *-ide* **chemical,** *aden-* **gland,** *-ine* **derived substance,** *di-* **two,** *nucleo-* **kernel (nucleus),** *-t-* **combining form,** *-ide* **chemical**]

nitrogen balance (NYE-troh-jen)
[*nitro-* **soda,** *-gen* **produce**]

nutrition (nyoo-TRIH-shun)
[*nutri-* **nourish,** *-tion* **process**]

orexigenic effect (oh-rek-sih-JEN-ik)
[*orex-* **appetite,** *-gen-* **produce,** *-ic* **relating to**]

orexin (oh-REK-sin)
[*orex-* **appetite,** *-in* **substance**]

oxidative phosphorylation (ock-si-DAY-tiv fos-for-ih-LAY-shun)
[*oxi-* **sharp (oxygen),** *-id-* **chemical (*-ide*),** *-at-* **action of (*-ate*),** *-ive* **relating to,** *phos-* **light,** *-phor-* **carry,** *-yl-* **chemical,** *-ation* **process**]

phosphorylation (fos-for-ih-LAY-shun)
[*phos-* **light,** *-phor-* **carry,** *-yl-* **chemical,** *-ation* **process**]

positive nitrogen balance (POZ-ih-tiv NYE-troh-jen)
[*posit-* **put or place,** *-ive* **relating to,** *nitro-* **soda,** *-gen* **produce**]

protein balance (PROH-teen)

satiety centre (sah-TYE-eh-tee)
[*sati-* **enough,** *-ety* **state**]

saturated (SACH-yoo-ray-ted)

total metabolic rate (met-ah-BOL-ik)
[*meta-* **over,** *-bol-* **throw,** *-ic* **relating to**]

tricarboxylic acid (TCA) cycle (try-kar-bok-SIL-ik ASS-id SYE-kul)
[*tri-* **three,** *-carbo-* **carbon,** *-oxy-* **sharp (oxygen),** *-yl-* **chemical,** *-ic* **relating to,** *acid* **sour,** *cyclo-* **circle**]

triglyceride (try-GLIH-ser-ide)
[*tri-* **three,** *-glycer-* **sweet,** *-ide* **chemical**]

LANGUAGE OF MEDICINE

anorexia nervosa
(an-oh-REK-see-ah ner-VOH-sah)
[*an-* **without,** *-orex-* **appetite,** *-ia* **condition,** *nerv-* **nerve,** *-os-* **relating to,** *-a* **thing**]

avitaminosis (ay-vye-tah-mih-NO-sis)
[*a-* **without,** *-vita-* **life,** *-amin-* **ammonia compound,** *-osis* **condition**]

binge–purge syndrome
[*syn-* **together,** *-drome* **running or (race)course**]

body mass index (BMI)
[*indicare-* **to make known**]

bulimia (boo-LEE-mee-ah)
[*bu-* **ox,** *-lim-* **hunger,** *-ia* **condition**]

hyperglycaemia
(hye-per-gly-SEEM-ee-ah)
[*hyper-* **above,** *-glyc-* **sweet (glucose),** *-aem-* **blood,** *-ia* **condition**]

hypervitaminosis
(hye-per-vye-tah-mih-NO-sis)
[*hyper-* **excessive,** *-vita-* **life,** *-amin-* **ammonia compound,** *osis* **condition**]

hypoglycaemia
(hye-poh-gly-SEE-mee-ah)
[*hypo-* **under or below,** *-glyc-* **sweet (glucose),** *-aem-* **blood,** *-ia* **condition**]

inborn errors of metabolism
(meh-TAB-ohl-iz-im)
[*meta-* **over,** *-bol-* **throw,** *-ism* **action**]

indirect calorimetry
(in-dir-EKT kal-oh-RIM-eh-tree)
[*in-* **not, direct,** *calor-* **heat,** *-metr-* **measuring,** *-y* **process**]

ketosis (kee-TOH-sis)
[*keto-* **acetone,** *-osis* **condition**]

kwashiorkor (kwah-shee-OR-kor)
[*kwashiorkor* **one who is displaced (from the breast)**]

marasmus (mah-RAZ-mus)
[*marasmus* **a wasting**]

phenylketonuria (PKU)
(fen-il-kee-toh-NOO-ree-ah)
[*phen-* **shining (phenol),** *-yl-* **chemical,** *-keton-* **acetone,** *-ur-* **urine,** *-ia* **condition**]

prebiotic (pree-bye-OT-ik)
[*pre-* **before,** *-bio-* **life,** *-ic* **relating to**]

probiotic (proh-bye-OT-ik)
[*pro-* **favoring,** *-bio-* **life,** *-ic* **relating to**]

protein–calorie malnutrition (PCM)
(PROH-teen KAHL-ah-ree mal-nyoo-TRISH-un)
[*mal-* **poor,** *-nutri-* **nourish,** *-tion* **process**]

case study

As part of a course investigation Karen, a nutrition and dietetics student, had to evaluate whether pizza can be regarded as a "complete meal" because it contains all the major macronutrients. Karen listed the major macronutrients: carbohydrates, lipids . . .

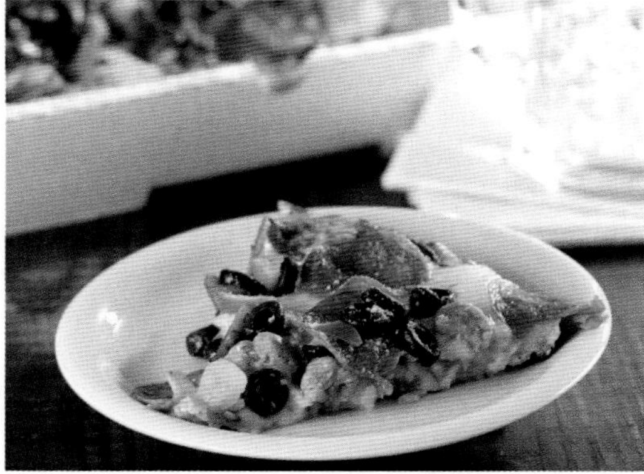

1. Which item doesn't belong to Karen's list of macronutrients?
   a. Protein
   b. Lipid
   c. Vitamin C
   d. Carbohydrate

Karen included a list of macrominerals: sodium, potassium . . .

2. Which of the minerals Karen listed is not considered a macromineral?
   a. Sodium
   b. Cobalt
   c. Potassium
   d. Calcium

3. The olive oil on pizza crust is mostly triglyceride lipids containing monounsaturated fatty acids. What is the first step in catabolizing the triglycerides in the olive oil?
   a. Hydrolysis
   b. Glycolysis
   c. Lipogenesis
   d. Deamination

4. Karen spent all day writing up her investigation and skipped lunch and dinner. By the time she had completed her investigation her blood sugar level (glucose concentration) and stored carbohydrate level were running low. Which of the following processes will restore glucose availability in her blood stream?
   a. Glycolysis
   b. Glyconeogenesis
   c. Oxidative phosphorylation
   d. Gluconeogenesis

Hint To solve a case study, you may have to refer to the glossary or index, other chapters in this textbook, ***Connect It!,*** and other resources.

CHAPTER SUMMARY

To download an MP3 version of the chapter summary for use with your mobile device, access the **Audio Chapter Summaries** *online at evolve.elsevier.com.*

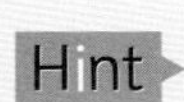

Scan this summary after reading the chapter to help you reinforce the key concepts. Later, use the summary as a quick review before your class or before a test.

Overview of Nutrition and Metabolism

A. *Nutrition* refers to the food (nutrients) we eat
 1. Malnutrition—a deficiency in the consumption of food, vitamins, and minerals
 2. Categories of nutrients
  a. Macronutrients—nutrients that the body needs in large amounts (bulk nutrients)
   (1) Macromolecules such as carbohydrates, fats (lipids), proteins
   (2) Water
   (3) Macrominerals—minerals needed in large quantities; for example, sodium, chloride, calcium
  b. Micronutrients—nutrients needed in very small amounts
   (1) Vitamins
   (2) Microminerals (trace elements)—minerals that are needed only in very small quantities, such as iron, iodine, and zinc
 3. Essential nutrients
  a. Essential (indispensable) nutrients cannot be synthesized by the body
  b. Nonessential (dispensable) nutrients can be synthesized in the body from essential nutrients
 4. Balance of nutrients is required for good health (**Figure 41-1**)

B. Metabolism—the use of nutrients—a process made up of many chemical pathways (**Figure 41-22**)
 1. Catabolism breaks food down into smaller molecular compounds and releases two forms of energy—heat and chemical energy
 2. Anabolism—a synthesis process
 3. Both catabolism and anabolism take place inside of cells continuously and concurrently
 4. Chemical energy released by catabolism must be transferred to ATP, which supplies energy directly to the energy-using reactions of all cells (**Figure 41-2**)

Carbohydrates

A. Dietary sources of carbohydrates
 1. Complex carbohydrates
  a. Polysaccharides—starches; found in vegetables and grains; glycogen is found in meat
  b. Cellulose—a component of most plant tissue; passes through the system without being broken down
  c. Disaccharides—found in refined sugar; must be broken down before they can be absorbed
  d. Monosaccharides—found in fruits; move directly into the internal environment without being processed directly
   (1) Glucose—carbohydrate most useful to the human cell
   (2) Other monosaccharides can be converted into glucose (e.g., fructose and galactose) (**Figure 41-3**)

B. Carbohydrate metabolism—human cells catabolize most of the carbohydrate absorbed and anabolize a small portion of it
 1. Glucose transport and phosphorylation—glucose reacts with ATP to form glucose-6-phosphate
  a. This step prepares glucose for further metabolic reactions
  b. This step is irreversible except in the intestinal mucosa, liver, and kidney tubules
 2. Glycolysis—the first process of carbohydrate catabolism; consists of a series of chemical reactions (**Figure 41-4**)
  a. Occurs in the cytoplasm of all human cells
  b. Only process that provides cells with energy in conditions of inadequate oxygen—an anaerobic process
  c. Breaks down chemical bonds in glucose molecules and releases about 5% of the energy stored in them
  d. Prepares glucose for the second step in catabolism—the citric acid cycle
 3. Citric acid cycle
  a. Two pyruvate molecules from glycolysis are converted to two acetyl molecules in a transition reaction, losing one carbon dioxide molecule, and two high-energy electrons (plus their protons) per pyruvate molecule converted
  b. By the end of the transition reaction and citric acid cycle, two pyruvate molecules have been broken down to six carbon dioxide and six water molecules, plus many high-energy electrons (plus their protons) (**Figures 41-5** and **41-6**)
  c. Citric acid cycle also called the *tricarboxylic acid (TCA) cycle* because citric acid is also called *tricarboxylic acid*
  d. Citric acid cycle once called Krebs cycle after Sir Hans Krebs, who discovered this process
 4. Electron transport system (**Figure 41-7**)
  a. High-energy electrons (along with their protons) removed during the citric acid cycle enter a chain of molecules embedded in the inner membrane of the mitochondria
  b. As electrons move down the chain, they release small bursts of energy to pump protons between the inner and outer membrane of the mitochondrion
  c. Protons then passively move down their concentration gradient, across the inner membrane, driving ATP synthase (**Figure 41-8**)
 5. Oxidative phosphorylation—the joining of a phosphate group to ADP to form ATP by the action of ATP synthase (**Figures 41-8** and **41-10**)
 6. Anaerobic pathway—a pathway for the catabolism of glucose; transfers energy to ATP using only glycolysis; ultimately sends pyruvates through the aerobic part of the pathway, which ends with the oxidative phosphorylation of ADP to form ATP (**Figure 41-11**)

7. Cori cycle—circular pathway in which excess lactate produced by anaerobic glycolysis in skeletal muscles is carried to liver cells, where it is converted back to glucose and stored as liver glycogen or returned to the bloodstream, where the glucose may be taken up by muscle cells and used for respiration or stored as muscle glycogen (**Figure 41-12**)
8. Glycogenesis—a series of chemical reactions in which glucose molecules are joined to form a strand of glucose beads; a process that operates when the blood glucose level increases above the midpoint of its normal range (**Figures 41-13** and **41-14**)
9. Glycogenolysis (**Figure 41-15**)—the reversal of glycogenesis; it means different things in different cells; can be stimulated by glucagon hours after a meal when blood glucose declines or by epinephrine and cortisol during a stress response to provide extra blood glucose
10. Gluconeogenesis (**Figure 41-16**)—the formation of new glucose, which occurs chiefly in the liver
11. Control of glucose metabolism—hormonal and neural devices maintain homeostasis of blood glucose concentration (**Figures 41-17** and **41-18**)
    a. Insulin—secreted by beta cells to decrease blood glucose level (**Figure 41-17**)
    b. Glucagon increases the blood glucose level by increasing the activity of the enzyme phosphorylase
    c. Incretins—GI hormones that, in the presence of glucose in the gut, stimulate insulin release from pancreas, thereby decreasing blood glucose levels; examples: GLP-1 and GIP
    d. Epinephrine—hormone secreted in times of stress; increases phosphorylase activity
    e. Adrenocorticotropic hormone stimulates the adrenal cortex to increase its secretion of glucocorticoids
    f. Glucocorticoids accelerate gluconeogenesis
    g. Growth hormone increases blood glucose level by shifting from carbohydrate to fat catabolism
    h. Thyroid-stimulating hormone has complex effects on metabolism
12. Hormones that cause the blood glucose level to rise are called *hyperglycaemic*
13. Insulin is hypoglycaemic because it causes the blood glucose level to decrease

Lipids

A. Dietary sources of lipids
  1. Triglycerides—the most common lipids—composed of a glycerol subunit that is attached to three fatty acids
  2. Phospholipids—an important lipid found in all foods
  3. Cholesterol—an important lipid found only in animal foods
  4. Dietary fats
     a. Saturated fats contain fatty acid chains in which there are no double bonds
     b. Unsaturated fats contain fatty acid chains in which there are some double bonds

B. Transport of lipids—transported in blood as chylomicrons, lipoproteins, and fatty acids
  1. In the absorptive state, many chylomicrons are present in the blood
  2. Postabsorptive state—95% of lipids are in the form of lipoproteins
     a. Consist of lipids and protein; formed in the liver
        (1) Blood contains three types of lipoproteins: very low density, low density, and high density
        (2) Cholesterol lipoproteins associated with heart disease (**Figure 41-19**)
     b. Fatty acids transported from cells of one tissue to cells of another in the form of free fatty acids

C. Lipid metabolism
  1. Lipid catabolism
     a. Triglycerides are hydrolyzed to yield fatty acids and glycerol
     b. Glycerol is converted to glyceraldehyde-3-phosphate, which enters the glycolysis pathway
     c. Fatty acids are broken down by beta-oxidation and then catabolized through the citric acid cycle (**Figure 41-20**)
  2. Lipid anabolism consists of the synthesis of triglycerides, cholesterol, phospholipids, and prostaglandins
  3. Control of lipid metabolism is through the following hormones
     a. Insulin
     b. Growth hormone
     c. ACTH
     d. Glucocorticoids

Proteins

A. Sources of proteins
  1. Proteins assembled from a pool of many different amino acids
  2. The body synthesizes amino acids from other compounds in the body
  3. Only about half the necessary types of amino acids can be produced by the body; remainder supplied through diet—found in both meat and vegetables

B. Protein metabolism—anabolism is primary and catabolism is secondary
  1. Protein anabolism—process by which proteins are synthesized by the ribosomes of the cells
  2. Protein catabolism—deamination takes place in the liver cells and forms an ammonia molecule, which is converted to urea and excreted in urine, and a keto acid molecule, which is oxidized or converted to glucose or fat (**Figure 41-21**)
  3. Protein balance—rate of protein anabolism balances rate of protein catabolism
  4. Nitrogen balance—amount of nitrogen taken in equals nitrogen in protein catabolic waste
  5. Two kinds of protein or nitrogen imbalance
     a. Negative nitrogen balance—protein catabolism exceeds protein anabolism; more tissue proteins are catabolized than are replaced by protein synthesis
     b. Positive nitrogen balance—protein anabolism exceeds protein catabolism
  6. Control of protein metabolism—achieved by hormones

Vitamins and Minerals

A. Vitamins (**Table 41-3**)—organic molecules necessary for normal metabolism; many attach to enzymes and help them work or have other important biochemical roles (**Figure 41-23**)
   1. Most of the necessary vitamins not produced by the body; must be obtained through diet
      a. The body stores lipid-soluble vitamins, but not water-soluble vitamins

B. Minerals (**Table 41-4**)—inorganic elements or salts found in the earth
   1. They attach to enzymes and help them work and function in chemical reactions
   2. Essential to the fluid/ion balance of the internal fluid environment
   3. Involved in many processes in the body such as muscle contraction, nerve function, hardening of bone, etc.
   4. Too large or too small an amount of some minerals may be harmful
   5. Recommended mineral intakes may vary over the life span (**Figures 41-24** and **41-25**)
      a. Macromineral—adequate intake (AI) is at least 100 mg/day
      b. Micromineral (trace element)—AI is less than 15 mg/day; ultratrace elements needed in microgram quantities

Metabolic Rates

A. Metabolic rate means the amount of energy released by catabolism

B. Metabolic rates expressed in two ways
   1. The number of kilocalories (or kilojoules) of heat energy expended per hour or per day
   2. As normal or as a percentage above or below normal

C. Basal metabolic rate—the rate of energy expended in basal conditions
   1. BMR not identical for all individuals because of influence of various factors
   2. Factors that influence BMR: size, body composition, gender, age, thyroid hormone, body temperature, drugs, other factors (**Figures 41-26** through **41-29**)

D. Total metabolic rate (**Figure 41-26**)
   1. Amount of energy used in a given time
   2. Main determinants
      a. Factor 1—basal metabolic rate
      b. Factor 2—energy used to do skeletal muscle work
      c. Factor 3—thermic effect of foods

E. Energy balance and body weight
   1. The body maintains a weight (state of energy balance) when the total calories in the food ingested equals the total metabolic rate
   2. Body weight increases when energy input exceeds energy output
   3. Body weight decreases when energy output exceeds energy input
   4. In starvation, the carbohydrates are used up first, then fats, then proteins (**Figure 41-30**)

Mechanisms for Regulating Food Intake (Table 41-6)

A. The hypothalamus plays a part in food intake

B. Feeding centres in the hypothalamus exert primary control over appetite
   1. Appetite centre
      a. Cluster of neurons in the lateral hypothalamus that if stimulated brings about increased appetite
      b. Orexigenic effects—factors that trigger appetite
   2. Satiety centre
      a. Group of neurons in the ventral medial nucleus of the hypothalamus that if stimulated brings about decreased appetite
      b. Anorexigenic effects—factors that suppress appetite (anorexia is loss of appetite)

Cycle of Life: Nutrition and Metabolism

A. The importance of proper nutrition to an individual's well-being begins at conception and continues until death

B. Protein is the one critical nutrient during fetal development, infancy, and childhood

C. Calcium is another critical nutrient during the early years of life
   1. Bone deformities may result from a lack of calcium during childhood

D. In late adulthood, the number of food calories needed declines because metabolic rate declines
   1. Nutrients, such as calcium, may be needed in greater quantity in older adults to compensate for age-related bone loss or other conditions

The Big Picture: Nutrition, Metabolism, and the Whole Body

A. Every cell in the body needs the maintenance of the metabolic pathways to stay alive

B. Anabolic pathways build the various structural and functional components of the cells

C. Catabolic pathways convert energy to a usable form and degrade large molecules into subunits used in anabolic pathways

D. Cells require appropriate amounts of vitamins and minerals to produce structural and functional components necessary for cellular metabolism

E. Other body mechanisms operate to ensure that nutrients reach the cells

REVIEW QUESTIONS

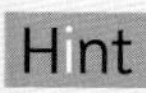

Write out the answers to these questions after reading the chapter and reviewing the Chapter Summary. Note—writing out your answers will consolidate learning and provide a valuable resource of information.

1. What is metabolism? Nutrition?
2. What two processes make up the process of metabolism?
3. Does the body digest dietary fibre? Give reasons for your answer and explain the importance of fibre in the diet.
4. Briefly describe glycolysis, the first process of carbohydrate catabolism.
5. Where in the cell does glycolysis occur?
6. Describe the process of "splitting glycogen".
7. How are dietary fats classified?
8. Explain how lipids are transported in blood.
9. List the hormones involved in the control of lipid metabolism.
10. What are the essential amino acids? Why are they called essential?
11. What does the term *metabolic rate* mean?
12. List the various factors that influence basal metabolic rate.
13. Describe various factors that influence the amount of food a person eats.
14. Define the term *calorie.*

CRITICAL THINKING QUESTIONS

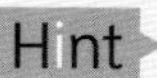

After finishing the Review Questions, write out the answers to these more in-depth questions to help you apply your new knowledge. Go back to sections of the chapter that relate to concepts that you find difficult.

1. Describe in your own words, the process of carbohydrate catabolism known as the citric acid cycle? Draw a picture to illustrate what you mean.
2. Describe the mitochondria, and explain why they are referred to as the "power plants" of the cells.
3. Compare anaerobic and aerobic pathways. What important role does lactate play in the anaerobic pathway?
4. Identify and explain the processes and hormones involved in maintaining the homeostatic level of glucose in the blood.
5. State in your own words the process of lipid catabolism. How is it similar to the carbohydrate pathway? How does this process generate ketone bodies?
6. Describe protein catabolism in your own words. How is this process related to a negative nitrogen balance?
7. Compare and contrast the functions of proteins, carbohydrates, and fats.
8. Construct a table listing the general functions of vitamins A, B-complex, C, D, E, and K. If they share a common function, include it in the table.
9. What is the difference between basal and total metabolic rates?
10. What would be the predicted basal metabolism rate in kilocalories per day of a 22-year-old man who is 1.8 m tall and weighs 80 kg?
11. A man went on a 7-day vacation. Because he planned to be more active than normal, he thought he would not have to be concerned about his diet. During the 7 days, he burned 17,500 kcal (73.22 MJ). He ate 26,500 kcal (110.87 MJ). What was the approximate difference in his body weight before and after his vacation?
12. Why do you think high blood concentrations of low-density lipoproteins may lead to atherosclerosis?

42 Urinary System

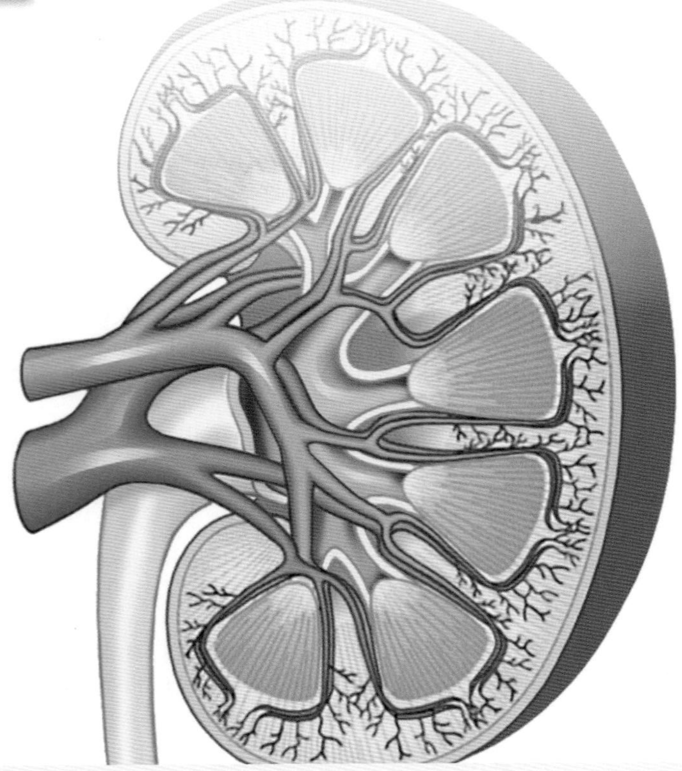

CHAPTER OUTLINE

Hint *Scan this outline before you begin to read the chapter, as a preview of how the concepts are organized.*

We often think of the urinary system primarily as a "urine producer", which it certainly is. However, a better description of the system is that of "blood plasma balancer". Each kidney processes incoming blood plasma in ways that allow it to leave the kidney in better condition. The water content is adjusted so that the body does not have too much or too little water to maintain constancy of the internal environment. Likewise, the blood content of important ions such as sodium and potassium is adjusted to match setpoint levels. Even the pH of the blood can be altered to match the setpoint level. In these ways, the urinary system regulates the content of blood plasma so that the homeostasis, or "dynamic constancy", of the entire internal fluid environment can be maintained within normal limits.

LANGUAGE OF SCIENCE

Hint *Use this list to aid your pronunciation of unfamiliar words.*

atrial natriuretic hormone (ANH) (AY-tree-al nay-tree-yoo-RET-ik HOR-mohn)
[*atrium* **entrance courtyard (atrium of heart),** *natri-* **sodium,** *-ure-* **urine,** *-ic* **relating to,** *hormon-* **excite**]

Bowman capsule (BOH-mun KAP-sul)
[*William Bowman* **English anatomist,** *caps-* **box**, *-ul-* **little**]

calyx (KAY-liks)
[*calyx* **cuplike**] *pl.*, calyces

collecting duct (CD) (koh-LEK-ting)
[*co-* **together**, *-lect-* **gather,** *duct* **path**]

cortical nephron (KOHR-tih-kal NEF-ron)
[*cortic-* **cortex (bark),** *-al* **relating to,** *nephro-* **kidney,** *-on* **unit**]

countercurrent mechanism
[*counter-* **against,** *-current* **flow**]

detrusor muscle (dee-TROO-sor)
[*detrus-* **thrust,** *-or* **agent**]

distal convoluted tubule (DCT) (DIS-tal KON-voh-LOO-ted TYOO-byool)
[*dist-* **distance,** *-al* **relating to,** *con-* **together,** *-volut-* **roll,** *tub-* **tube,** *-ul-* **little**]

filtration (fil-TRAY-shun)
[*filtr-* **strain,** *-ation* **process**]

glomerular capsular membrane (gloh-MER-yoo-lar KAP-syoo-lahr MEM-brayne)
[*glomer-* **ball,** *-ul-* **little,** *-ar* **relating to,** *caps-* **box,** *-ula-* **little,** *-ar* **relating to,** *membran-* **thin skin**]

glomerular filtration rate (GFR) (gloh-MER-yoo-lar fil-TRAY-shun)
[*glomer-* **ball,** *-ul-* **little,** *-ar* **relating to,** *filtr-* **strain,** *-ation* **process**]

glomerulus (gloh-MAIR-yoo-lus)
[*glomer-* **ball,** *-ulus* **little**] *pl.*, glomeruli

hilum (HYE-lum)
[*hilum* **least bit**] *pl.*, hila

juxtaglomerular apparatus (juks-tah-gloh-MER-yoo-lar app-ah-RAT-us)
[*juxta-* **near or adjoining,** *-glomer-* **ball,** *-ul-* **little,** *-ar* **relating to**]

continued on p. 993

This chapter explores the basic principles of urinary structure and function. The next two chapters look more closely at the role of the kidneys and other organs in fluid and ion homeostasis (Chapter 43) and pH homeostasis (Chapter 44).

ANATOMY OF THE URINARY SYSTEM

GROSS STRUCTURE

The principal organs of the urinary system are the **kidneys,** which process blood and form urine as a waste to be excreted—that is, removed from the body (**Box 42-1**). The excreted urine travels from the kidneys to the outside of the body via accessory organs: the *ureters, urinary bladder,* and *urethra.* Part 3 of the BRIEF ATLAS OF THE HUMAN BODY shows detailed photographs of the gross structures of the urinary system.

Kidney

The kidneys resemble lima beans in shape—that is, roughly oval with a medial indentation (**Figure 42-1**, A). An average-sized kidney measures approximately 11 cm by 7 cm by 3 cm. The left kidney is often slightly larger than the right. The kidneys lie in a *retroperitoneal* position, meaning posterior to the parietal peritoneum, against the posterior wall of the abdomen (**Figure 42-1**, C). They are located on either side of the vertebral column and extend from the level of the last thoracic vertebra (T12) to just above the third lumbar vertebra (L3). Note in **Figure 42-1**, *B*, that the superior or upper portions (poles) of both kidneys extend above the level of the twelfth rib and the lower edge of the thoracic parietal pleura. This anatomical relationship has important clinical implications, as when performing a

BOX 42-1 *fyi* | **Excretion**

The urinary system's chief function is to regulate the volume and composition of body fluids and excrete unwanted material, but it is not the only system in the body that is able to excrete unneeded substances.

The following table compares the excretory functions of several systems. Although all these systems contribute to the body's effort to remove wastes, only the urinary system can finely adjust the water and electrolyte balance to the degree required for normal homeostasis of body fluids.

SYSTEM	ORGAN	EXCRETION
Urinary	Kidney	Nitrogen compounds Toxins Water Electrolytes
Integumentary	Skin—sweat glands	Nitrogen compounds Electrolytes Water
Respiratory	Lung	Carbon dioxide Water
Digestive	Intestine	Digestive wastes Bile pigments Salts of heavy metals

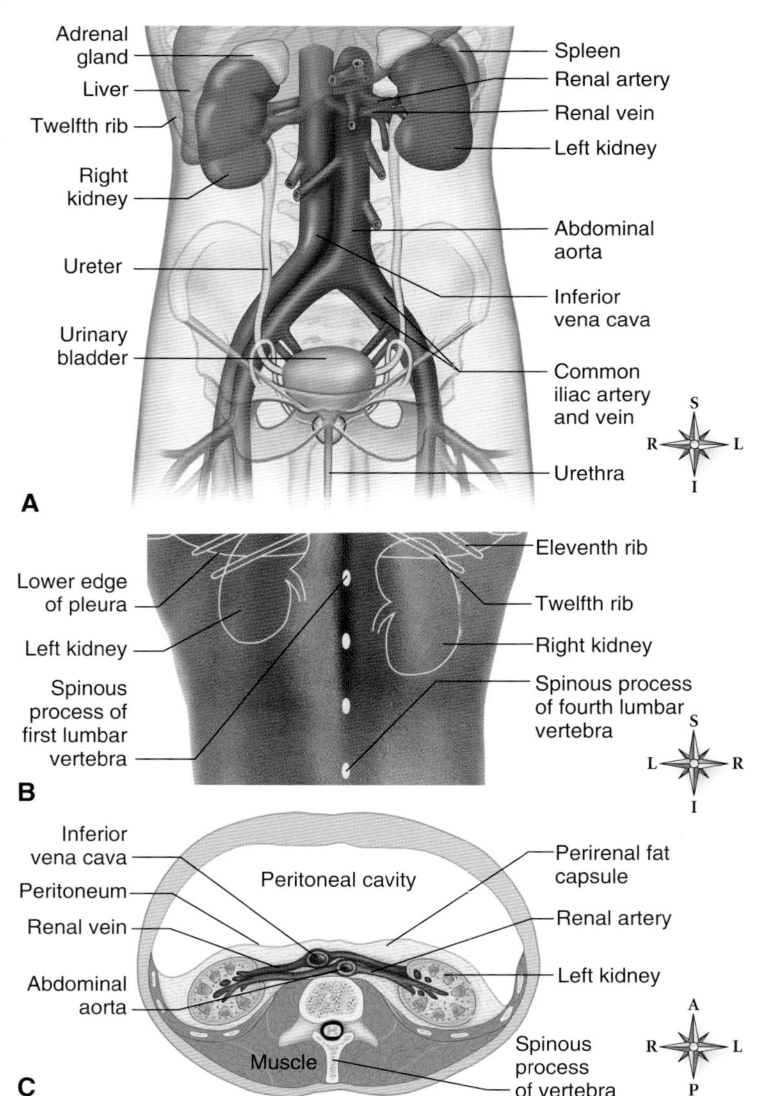

FIGURE 42-1 Location of urinary system organs. A, Anterior view of the urinary organs with the peritoneum and visceral organs removed. **B,** Surface markings of the kidneys, eleventh and twelfth ribs, spinous processes of L1 to L4, and lower edge of the pleura (posterior view). **C,** Horizontal (transverse) section of the abdomen showing the retroperitoneal position of the kidneys.

kidney biopsy. Usually the right kidney is a little lower than the left, presumably because the liver takes up some of the space above the right kidney.

A heavy cushion of fat—the **perirenal fat capsule** or *renal fat pad*—encases each kidney and holds it in position. Connective tissue, the renal fasciae, anchors the kidneys to surrounding structures and also helps maintain their normal positions.

CONNECT IT! 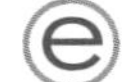

See how knowing anatomical relationships of the kidney can avoid potential dangers in ***Kidney Biopsy*** online at ***Connect It!***

The medial surface of each kidney has a concave notch called the **hilum.** Renal blood vessels and other structures enter or leave the kidney through this notch. A tough, white fibrous capsule encases each kidney (**Figure 42-2**).

The coronal section of the right kidney shown in **Figure 42-2** depicts the major internal structures of the kidney. Identify the **renal cortex,** or outer region, and the **renal medulla,** or inner region. A dozen or so distinct triangular wedges, the **renal pyramids,** make up much of the medullary tissue. The *base* of each pyramid faces outward, and the narrow *papilla* of each faces toward the hilum. Each renal papilla has multiple openings that release urine. Note that the cortical tissue dips into the medulla between the pyramids, forming areas known as **renal columns.**

Each renal papilla (point of a pyramid) juts into a cuplike structure called a **calyx.** The calyces are considered the beginnings of the "plumbing system" of the urinary system, for it is here that urine leaving the renal papilla is collected for transport out of the body. The cups that drain the renal papillae directly are called *minor calyces.* These minor calyces are stemlike branches that join together to form larger branches called *major calyces.* The major calyces join together to form a large collection basin called the **renal pelvis.** The pelvis of the kidney narrows as it exits the hilum to become the ureter. *Pelvis* is Latin for "basin", and like a lavatory basin, it collects fluid and quickly drains it away through a channel.

Blood Vessels of the Kidneys

The kidneys are highly vascular organs (**Figure 42-3**). Every minute about 1200 mL of blood flows through them. Stated another way, approximately one fifth of all the blood pumped by the heart per minute goes to the kidneys. From this fact one might guess, and correctly so, that the kidneys process the blood in important ways before returning it to the general circulation. A large branch of the abdominal aorta—the *renal artery*—brings blood into each kidney. As it nears the kidney, it divides into *segmental arteries,* which divide to become *lobar arteries.* Between the pyramids of the kidney's medulla, the lobar arteries branch to form *interlobar arteries* that extend out toward the cortex, then arch over the bases of the pyramids to form the *arcuate arteries.* From the arcuate arteries, *interlobular arteries* penetrate the cortex. Because they radiate through the cortex, the interlobular arteries are sometimes called the *cortical radiate arteries.*

Branches of the interlobular arteries called *afferent arterioles* carry blood directly to the tiny functional units of the kidney called *nephrons.* We discuss the structure and function of nephrons later in this chapter, where we will resume outlining the path of blood flow—this time at a microscopic level.

Figure 3-22 in the Brief Atlas of the Human Body shows detailed, three-dimensional casts of the blood supply of the kidneys.

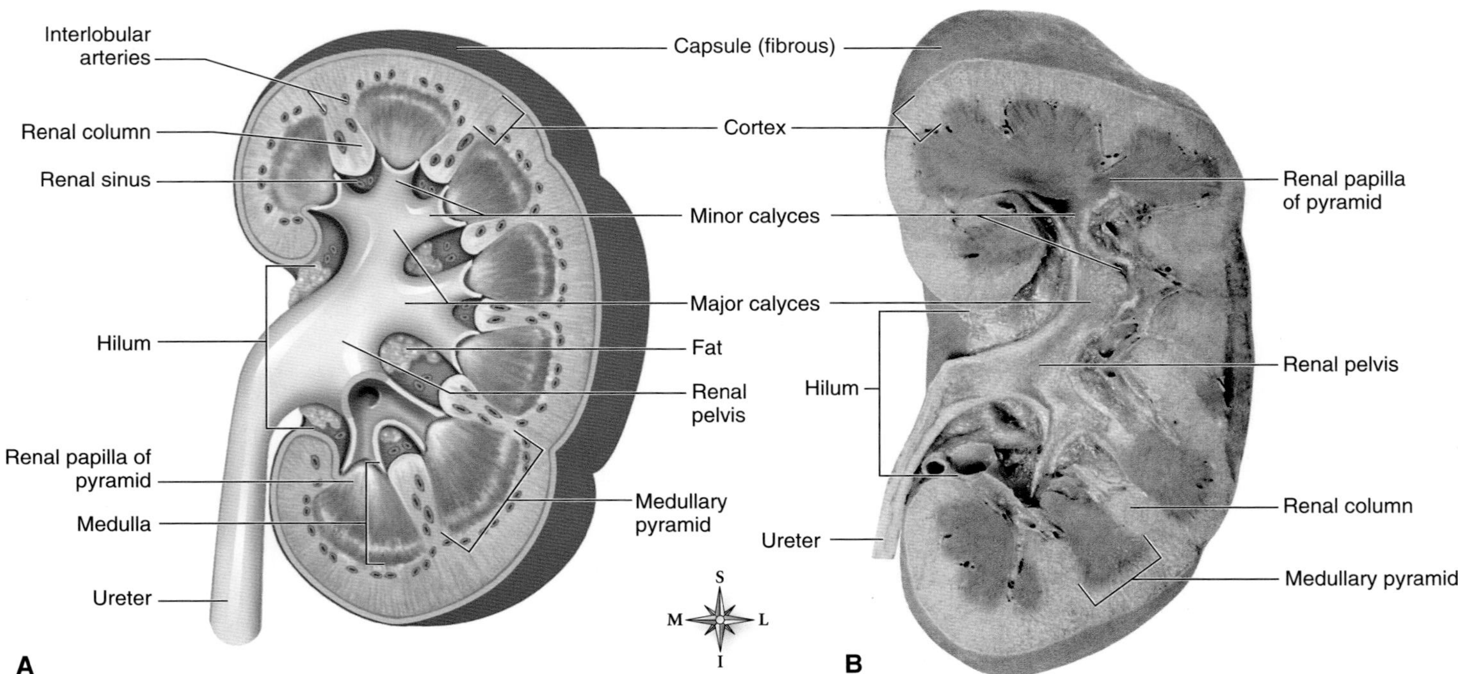

FIGURE 42-2 Internal structure of the kidney. A, Coronal section of the right kidney in an artist's rendering. **B,** Photo of a coronal section of a preserved human kidney.

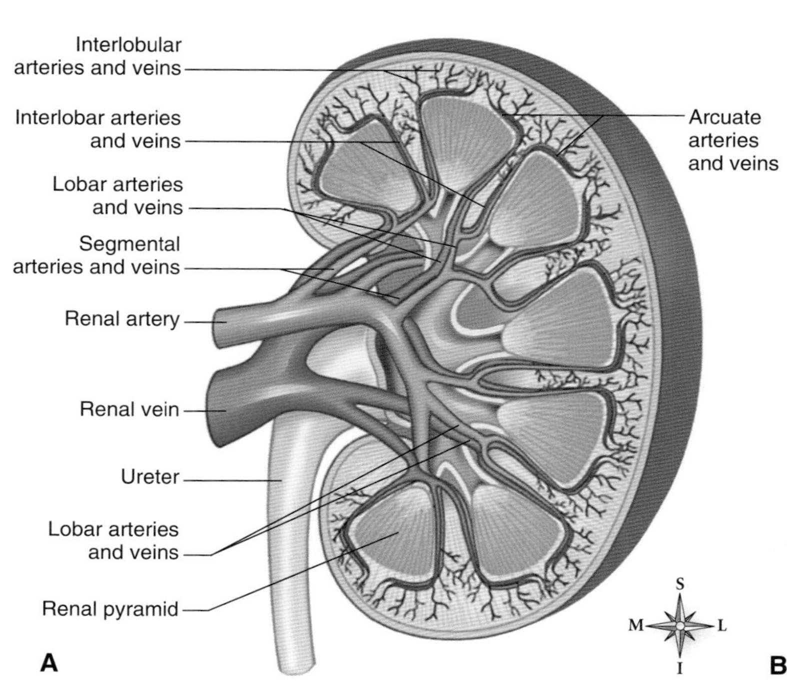

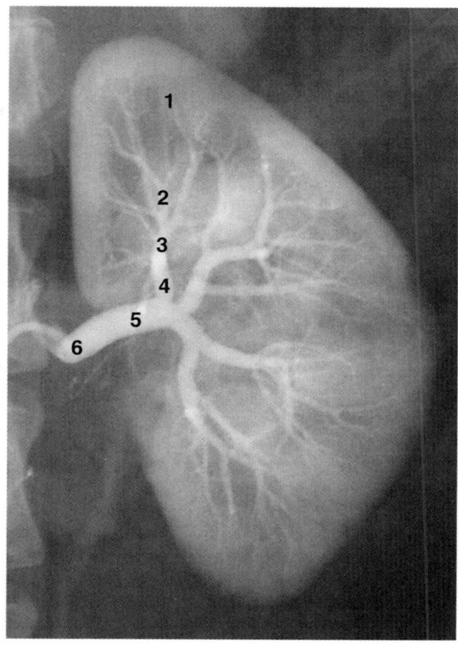

FIGURE 42-3 Circulation of blood through the kidney. A, Diagram showing the major arteries and veins of the renal circulation. **B,** Renal arteriogram. Arcuate arteries *(1)* are seen near the junction of the cortex and medulla, interlobar arteries *(2)* are present between the medullary pyramids, and lobar arteries *(3)* and segmental arteries *(4)* are seen branching from the main renal artery *(5)*. Note the tip of the catheter used to inject contrast material *(6)* into the proximal part of the main renal artery.

CONNECT IT!

Knowing the pathway of blood flow in the kidney is important for understanding how the kidney works. We continue the story later in the chapter. We put all the pieces together in an overview in ***Tracing Blood Flow in the Kidney*** online at ***Connect It!***

Quick CHECK

1. Name the accessory organs of the urinary system.
2. What is the general function of the urinary system?
3. Distinguish between the renal cortex and the renal medulla.
4. What proportion of the body's blood flow goes to the kidney?

Ureter

The **ureters,** about 28 to 34 cm in length, are the two tubes that actively convey urine from the kidneys to the urinary bladder (see **Figure 42-1**, A). They begin on each side at the narrow outlet of the renal pelvis on a level with the first lumbar vertebra (L1). Each ureter is retroperitoneal and courses into the pelvis until it reaches the bladder, where it attaches to the bottom of the bladder (**Figure 42-4**). It then runs at an angle for about 2 cm through the bladder wall and opens at the lateral angles of the trigone (floor) of the bladder (**Figure 42-5**). Because of its oblique course through the bladder wall, the ends of the tube close and act as valves when the bladder is full, thus preventing backflow of urine (**Figure 42-6**).

The ureter is lined with transitional epithelium, which is also called **urothelium** because it lines the urinary tract. Recall from Chapter 9 that this tissue is adapted to permit stretching without damage to a structure's epithelial lining. This feature permits either high or low rates of flow through the ureters.

In females, the ureters are in close proximity to the ovaries and cervix of the uterus; in males, they are in close proximity to the seminal vesicles and near the prostate gland (see **Figure 42-4**). Each ureter is composed of three layers of tissue: a mucous lining, a muscular middle layer, and a fibrous outer layer (**Figure 42-7**). The muscular layer is composed of smooth muscle, which propels the urine by peristalsis. The rate and strength of peristalsis increase with increasing urine volume.

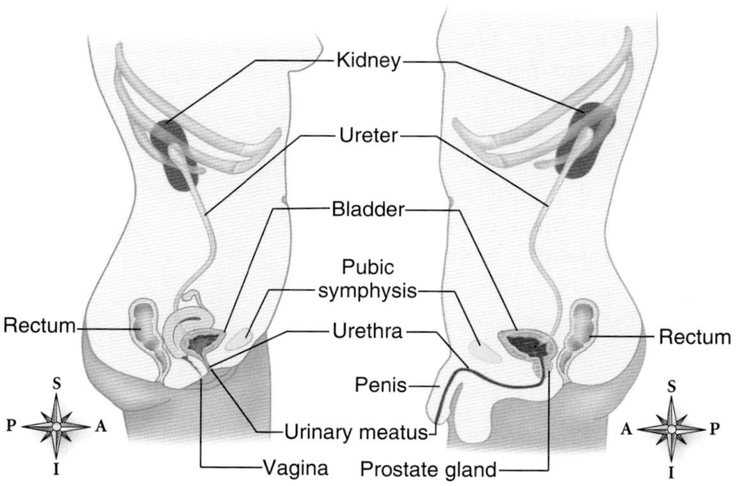

FIGURE 42-4 Sagittal view of urinary tract. The female urinary system is shown on the reader's left and the male urinary system on the reader's right, each showing a distended (stretched) bladder.

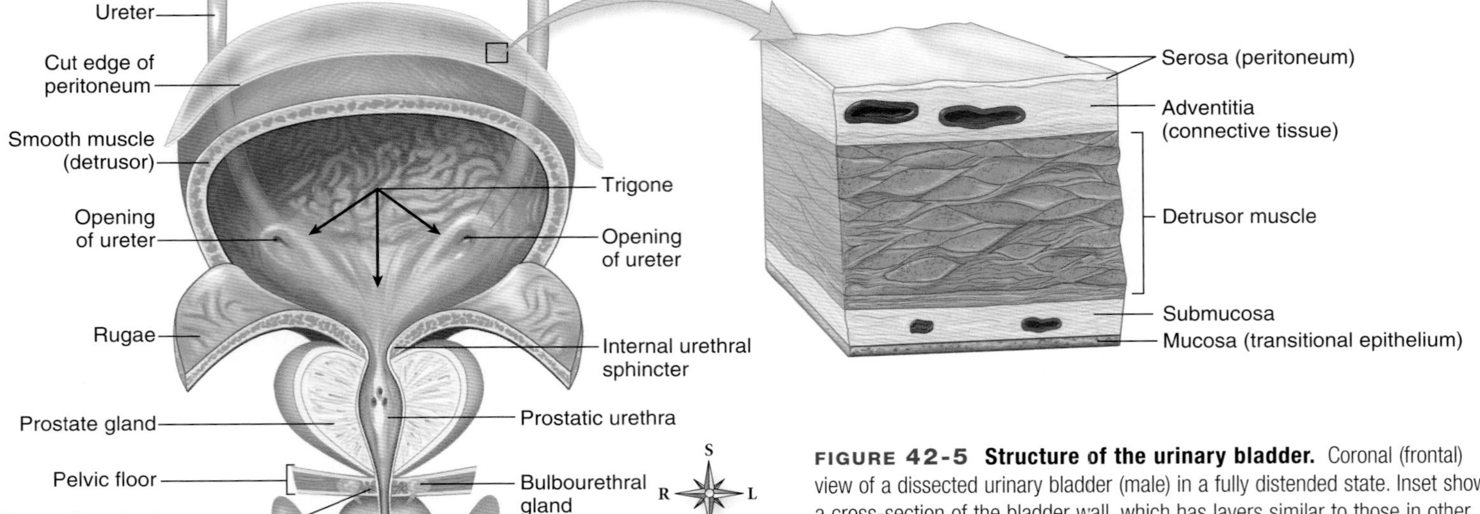

FIGURE 42-5 Structure of the urinary bladder. Coronal (frontal) view of a dissected urinary bladder (male) in a fully distended state. Inset shows a cross-section of the bladder wall, which has layers similar to those in other hollow abdominopelvic organs (compare with **Figure 38-2** on p. 862).

Urinary Bladder

The urinary bladder is a muscular, collapsible bag that is located directly behind the pubic symphysis and in front of the rectum (see **Figure 42-4**). It lies below the parietal peritoneum, which covers only its superior surface (see **Figure 42-5**). The remainder of the bladder surface is covered by a fibrous adventitia. In women it sits on the anterior of the vagina and in front of the uterus, whereas in men, it rests on the prostate.

The wall of the bladder is made mostly of smooth muscle tissue (see **Figure 42-5**). Often called the **detrusor muscle,** the muscle layer is formed by a network of crisscrossing bundles of smooth muscle fibres. The bundles run in all directions: circular, oblique, and lengthwise. The bladder is lined with mucous urothelium that forms folds called *rugae* (see **Figure 42-5**). Because of the folds and the extensibility of urothelium, the bladder can distend considerably. There are three openings in the floor of the bladder—two from the ureters and one into the **urethra.** The ureter openings lie at the posterior corners of the triangle-shaped floor—the **trigone**—and the urethral opening lies at the anterior, lower corner.

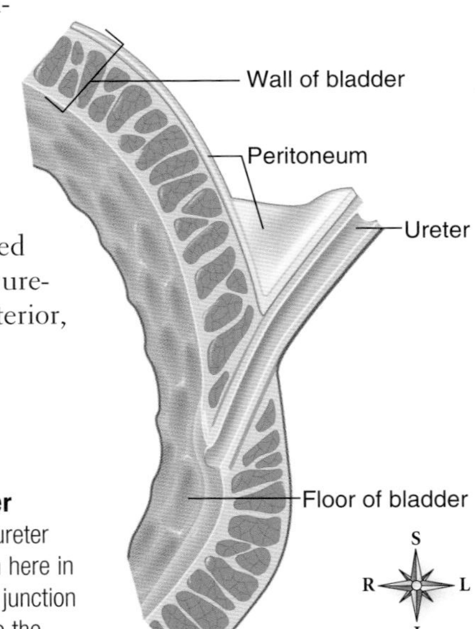

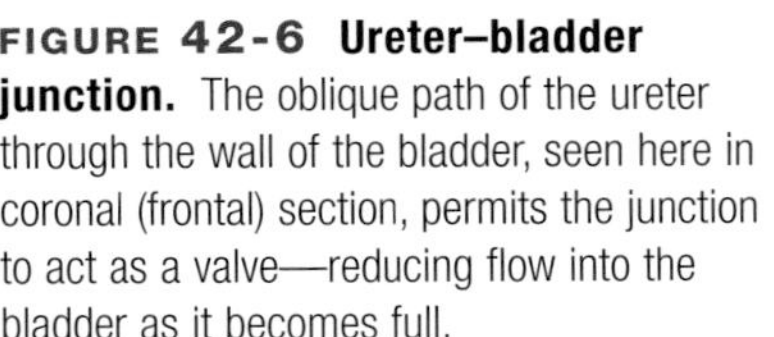
FIGURE 42-6 Ureter–bladder junction. The oblique path of the ureter through the wall of the bladder, seen here in coronal (frontal) section, permits the junction to act as a valve—reducing flow into the bladder as it becomes full.

The bladder performs two major functions:

1. It serves as a reservoir for urine before it leaves the body.
2. Aided by the urethra, it expels urine from the body.

Urethra

The urethra is a small tube lined with mucous membrane (urothelium) that leads from the floor of the bladder (*trigone*) to the exterior of the body. In females, the urethra lies directly behind the pubic symphysis and anterior to the vagina as it passes through the muscular floor of the pelvis (**Figure 42-8**). It extends down and forward from the bladder for a distance of about 3 cm and ends at the external urinary meatus (see **Figure 42-4**). The functional importance of the relationship of the urethra and vagina to the muscular pelvic floor, especially after vaginal delivery of a baby, will be discussed in Chapter 46. The male urethra, on the other hand, extends along a winding path for about 20 cm (see **Figure 42-4**). The male urethra passes through the

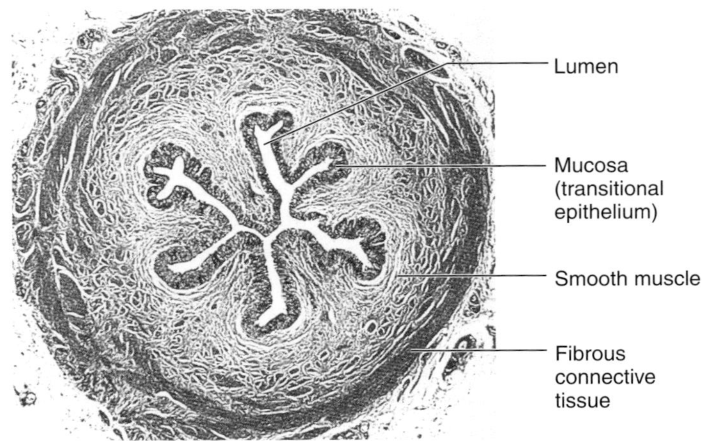

FIGURE 42-7 Ureter (cross-section). Low power micrograph. Note the convoluted folds, covered by a transitional mucous lining, that almost fill the lumen. The thick muscular layer is surrounded by a tough fibrous coat.

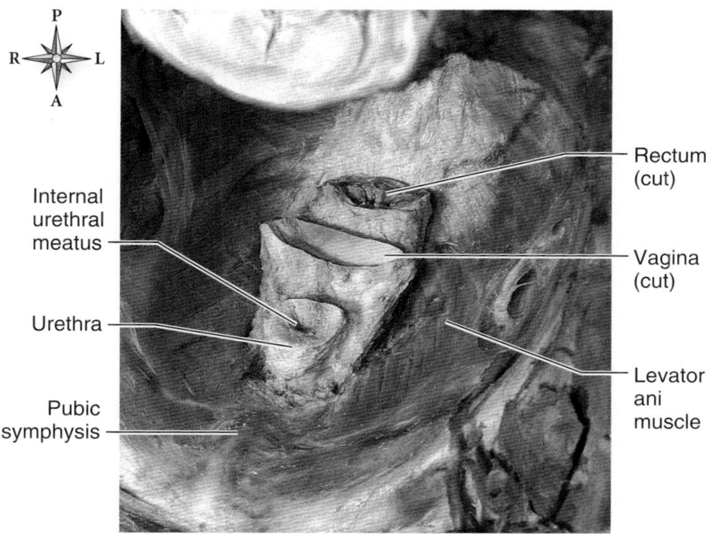

FIGURE 42-8 Female urethra piercing the muscular pelvic floor. The urethra is posterior to the pubic symphysis and anterior to the vagina. Some of the muscles of the pelvic floor act as an external urethral sphincter. (See also text discussion in Chapter 46, pp. 1059–1060.)

centre of the *prostate gland* just after leaving the bladder. Within the prostate, it is joined by two *ejaculatory ducts*. After leaving the prostate, the urethra extends down, forward, then up to enter the base of the penis. It then travels through the centre of the penis and ends as a *urinary meatus* at the tip of the penis.

Because the male urethra is joined by the ejaculatory ducts, it serves as a pathway for *semen* (fluid containing sperm) as it is ejaculated out of the body through the penis. Thus we can say that the male urethra is a part of two different systems: the urinary system (when it is used to void urine) and the reproductive system (when it is used to ejaculate semen). Urine is prevented from mixing with semen during ejaculation by a reflex closure of sphincter muscles guarding the bladder's opening. The female urethral tract, in contrast, is separate from the lower reproductive tract (vagina), which lies just behind the urethra (see **Figure 42-8**).

CONNECT IT! ⓔ

Maintaining healthy communities of microorganisms in the mucosa of the urinary and reproductive tracts helps prevent infections and other disorders. Review the human *microbiome* in ***The Human Microbiome*** at ***Connect It!***

Micturition

The mechanism for urinating begins with involuntary contractions of the detrusor muscle of the bladder wall (see **Figure 42-5**). Urination is also called *voiding* the bladder or *micturition*. **Figure 42-9** shows that as the pressure of urine against the inside of the bladder wall increases with urine volume, involuntary micturition contractions develop. This rapid succession of involuntary contractions triggered by a parasympathetic reflex get stronger and stronger as the bladder fills and the urine volume and pressure increase. The parasympathetic reflex also causes the *internal urethral sphincter* muscles to relax at the same time. The internal urethral sphincters include a ringlike part of the detrusor muscle of the bladder wall, as you can see in **Figure 42-5**. The relaxation of these internal sphincters along with the micturition contractions of the bladder wall can force urine out of the bladder and through the urethra.

Thankfully, most people learn how to consciously regulate voluntary contraction of the *external urethral sphincter* muscles to stop voiding—that is, until a suitable time. **Figure 42-5** shows that the skeletal muscles of the pelvic floor, including the *levator ani* muscle, act as external urethral sphincters (see also **Figure 15-16** on p. 333). Voluntary control of *micturition* (voiding, or urination) is possible only if the nerves supplying the pelvic floor, the projection tracts of the central nervous system (CNS), and the motor areas of the brain are all intact and functioning properly. Learning this function is not possible until the nervous system matures sufficiently—making voluntary control of urination impossible during infancy and very early childhood.

Injury to any of these parts of the nervous system, by a cerebral haemorrhage or a spinal cord injury, for example, results in involuntary emptying of the bladder at intervals. Involuntary micturition is called *incontinence* (see Mechanisms of Disease, p. 990). In the average bladder, 250 mL of urine causes a moderately distended sensation and therefore the desire to void.

***Quick* CHECK**

5. Where does the ureter enter the bladder? Why is its angle through the wall significant?
6. What type of mucous epithelium lines most of the urinary tract? What is the functional advantage of this type of epithelium?
7. What are the two major functions of the bladder?

MICROSCOPIC STRUCTURE

More than a million microscopic functional units named **nephrons** make up the bulk of each kidney. The shape of the nephron is unusual, unmistakable, and uniquely suited to its function of blood plasma processing and urine formation (**Figure 42-10**). It resembles a tiny funnel with a long, winding stem about 3 cm long.

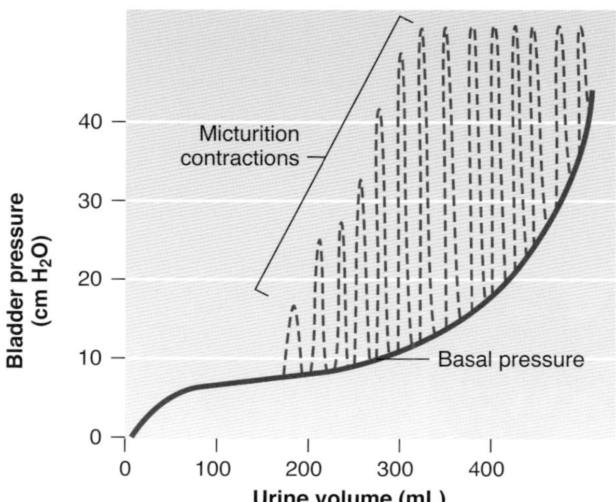

FIGURE 42-9 Micturition reflex. Increased volume of urine in the bladder causes increased internal bladder pressure. This triggers reflexive parasympathetic stimulation of micturition contractions of the detrusor muscles in the bladder wall. As these contractions get stronger, nerve signals to the internal sphincters (**Figure 42-5**) cause them to relax. *cm H_2O* - centimetres of water (a unit of pressure equal to about 0.73 mmHg (0.1 kPa)).

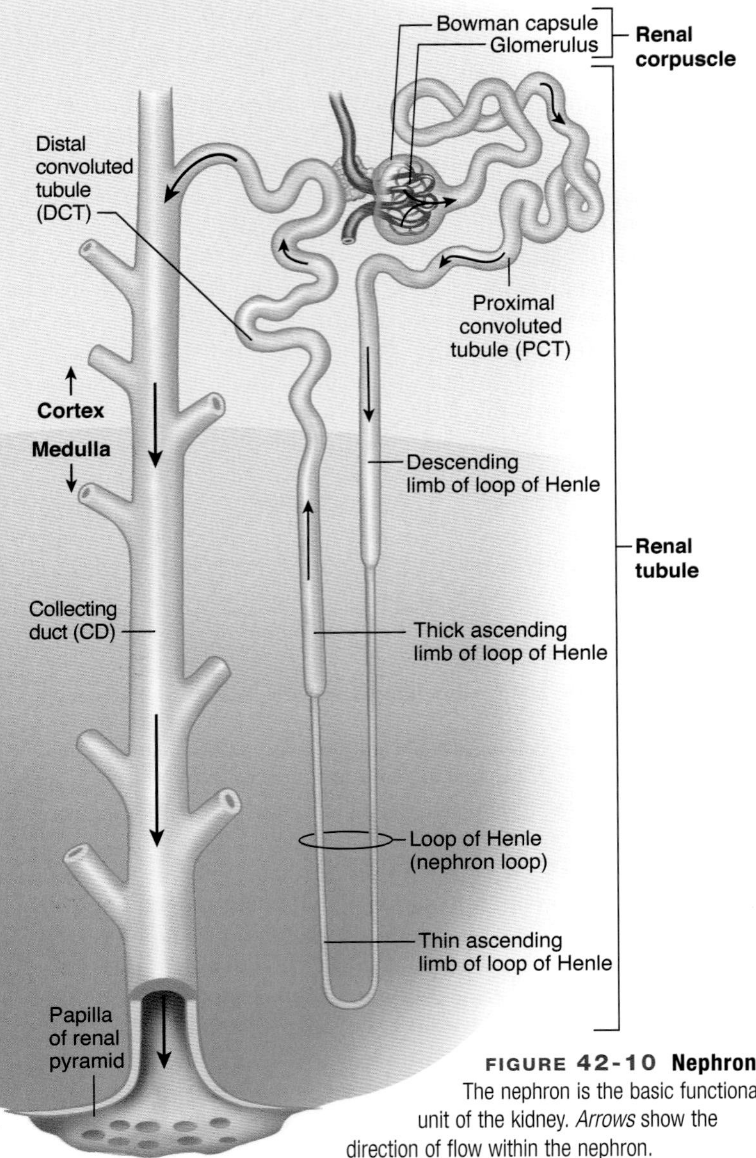

FIGURE 42-10 Nephron. The nephron is the basic functional unit of the kidney. *Arrows* show the direction of flow within the nephron.

As **Figure 42-10** shows, each nephron is made up of two main regions: the *renal corpuscle* and the *renal tubule.* Fluid is filtered out of the blood in the renal corpuscle, forming a filtrate that flows through the renal tubule and collecting duct—where much of the filtrate is returned to the blood. The remaining filtrate leaves the collecting duct as urine. We will come back to the processing of filtrate later. For now, we explore the structure of the nephron and collecting duct. Here are the main structures we explore, listed in the order in which fluid flows through them:

Nephron

- Renal corpuscle
  - Glomerulus (capillaries)
  - Bowman capsule (glomerular capsule)
- Renal tubule
  - Proximal convoluted tubule
  - Loop of Henle (nephron loop)
  - Distal convoluted tubule

Collecting duct

As you read the brief description of each of these microscopic structures, refer often to **Figure 42-10**, which shows a schematic diagram of a complete nephron.

CONNECT IT!

For our purposes, the simplified scheme of microscopic renal anatomy shown in **Figure 42-10** works well. However, some renal biologists prefer the more elaborate scheme sketched out in a ***Detailed Map of Nephron*** online at ***Connect It!***

Nephron

Renal Corpuscle

The **renal corpuscle** is the first part of the nephron and is made up of the Bowman capsule and glomerulus. Formation of a renal corpuscle is sometimes compared with pushing your fist into the end of an inflated balloon. The mechanism is shown in **Figure 42-11**. Note that as the glomerular tuft of capillaries pushes into the balloon, it becomes surrounded by a double-walled cup with parietal (outer) and visceral (inner) walls—the Bowman capsule or glomerular capsule (**Figure 42-12**).

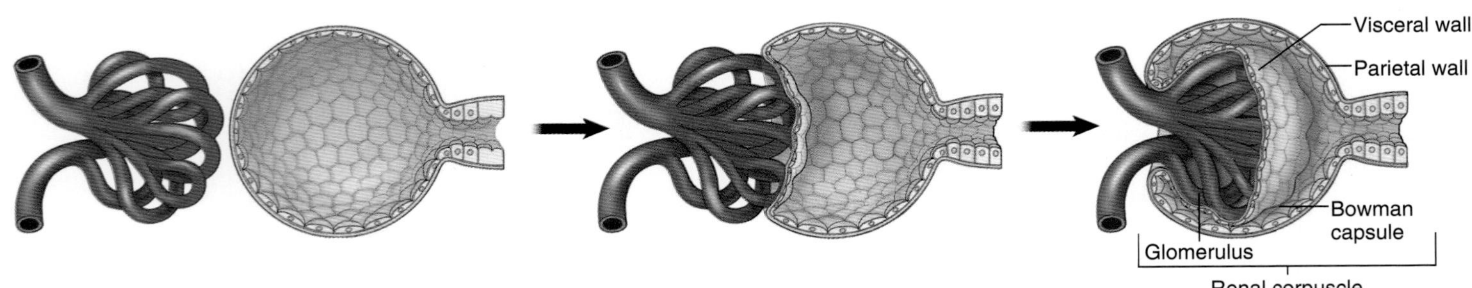

FIGURE 42-11 Overview of the renal corpuscle. Note that as the glomerular tuft of capillaries pushes into the inflated balloonlike structure representing a Bowman capsule, the visceral layer of the capsule adheres to the outer surface of the epithelial cells of the glomerular capillaries to become the visceral layer lining the capsular space. The outer layer of cells constitutes the parietal layer of a Bowman capsule. Glomerular filtrate enters the space between the parietal and visceral layers of the Bowman capsule before entering the tubular segments of the nephron.

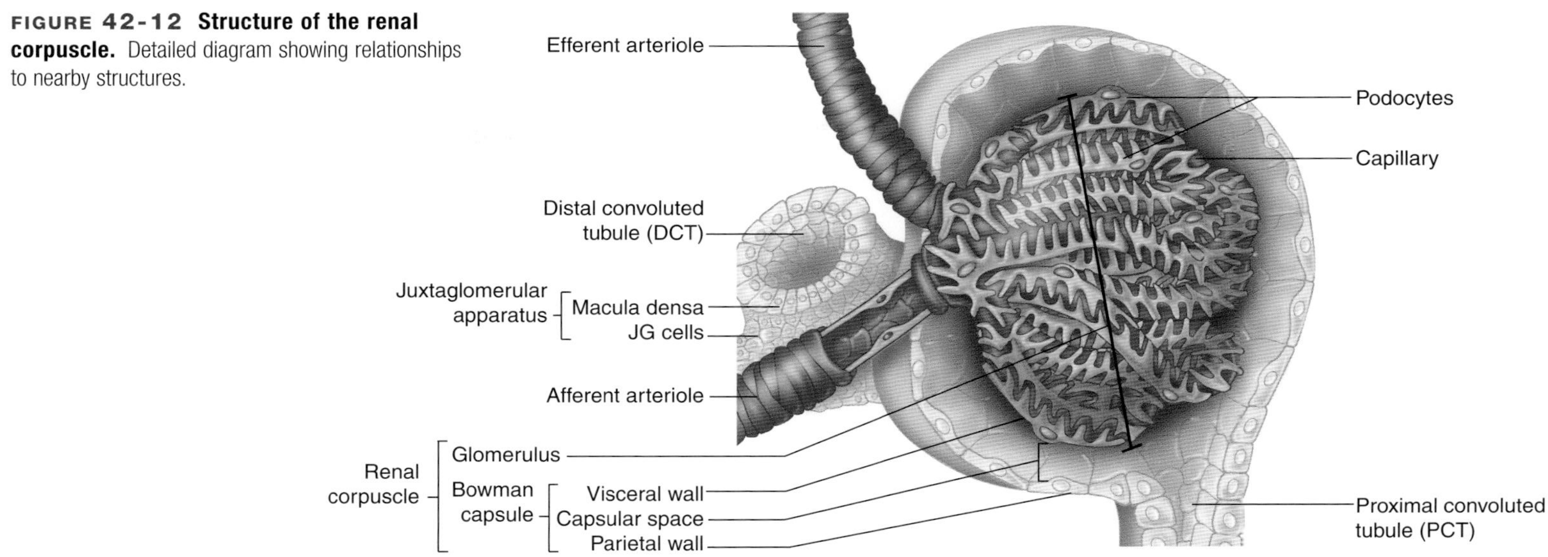

FIGURE 42-12 Structure of the renal corpuscle. Detailed diagram showing relationships to nearby structures.

Fluid from the blood first filters out of the glomerulus and then into the Bowman capsule. We begin our discussion with the Bowman capsule first, however, because it will then make it easier to understand the structure and function of the glomerulus.

Bowman Capsule. The **Bowman capsule** is the cup-shaped mouth of a nephron. It is sometimes called the *glomerular capsule*. The capsule is formed by two layers of epithelial cells with a space, called the *capsular space (Bowman space)*, between them (**Figure 42-13**). Fluids, waste products, and electrolytes that pass through the porous glomerular capillaries and enter this space constitute the *filtrate*, which will be processed in the nephron to form urine.

The parietal, or outer, wall is composed of simple squamous epithelium. It plays no role in the production of glomerular filtrate. The visceral (inner) wall, however, is quite different. It is composed of special epithelial cells called *podocytes* (meaning "cells with feet").

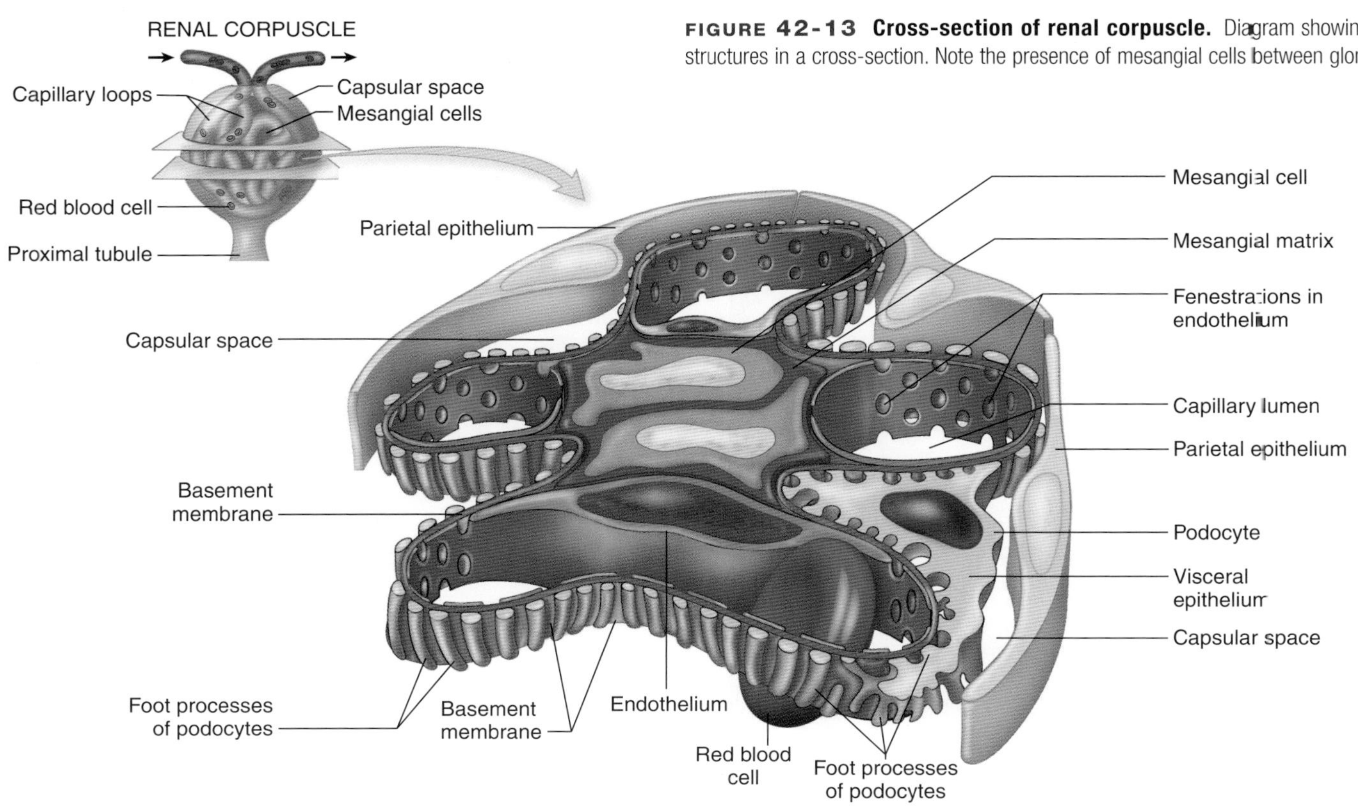

FIGURE 42-13 Cross-section of renal corpuscle. Diagram showing detail of glomerular structures in a cross-section. Note the presence of mesangial cells between glomerular capillaries.

The scanning electron micrograph in **Figure 42-14** reveals the odd shapes of podocytes. Note that the primary branches extending from the cell bodies divide into a network of branches that terminate in little "feet" called *pedicels*. The pedicels are packed so closely together that only narrow slits of space lie between them. These spaces are called *filtration slits*. The slits are not merely open spaces, however. Within them is a mesh of fine connective tissue fibres called the *slit diaphragm* that prevents the slits from enlarging under pressure while still maintaining permeability of the slit. The slit diaphragm is an important component of the filter mechanism because it prevents many large macromolecules, such as proteins, from passing through.

Glomerulus. The **glomerulus** is probably the body's most well-known capillary network and is surely one of its most important for survival. Its relationship to the Bowman capsule is clearly visible in **Figures 42-11** and **42-12**. Note in both figures that an afferent arteriole leads into the glomerular network and an efferent arteriole leads out.

Like all capillaries, glomerular capillaries have thin, membranous walls that are composed of a single layer of endothelial cells. Many pores, or *fenestrations* (meaning "windows"), are present in the glomerular endothelium (see **Figure 42-14**, *B*). These pores are not present in regular capillaries (see **Figure 29-4** on p. 668). This increased porosity is necessary for filtration to occur at the rate required for normal kidney function. The relationship between fenestration size and the rate of glomerular filtration is yet another example of the connection between form and function.

Mesangial cells (see **Figure 42-13**) are unique to renal corpuscles. They are irregular in shape, have numerous cytoplasmic processes, and are scattered in an apparently haphazard way in an extracellular matrix between the twisting glomerular capillaries. Most physiologists believe they serve a support and phagocytic function, similar in some ways to microglia and other types of glia cells found in the nervous system (see Chapter 18, p. 396). However, we now know that they also secrete paracrine regulators that play a role in various immune responses, in regulating the surface of the filtration membrane, and in control of blood flow through the glomerular loop. Mesangial cells are currently the subject of considerable research interest and may well have other important functions or play important roles in human glomerular disease.

Between a glomerulus and its Bowman capsule lies a basement membrane (basal lamina). It consists of a thin layer of fine fibrils embedded in a matrix of glycoprotein (see **Figure 8-4** on p. 143). The visceral layer of Bowman capsule contacts the basement membrane by means of countless pedicels ("feet") of the podocytes (see **Figure 42-14**, A). The glomerular endothelium, the basement membrane, and the visceral layer of Bowman capsule constitute the **glomerular capsular membrane,** a structure well suited to its function of filtration (**Figure 42-15**).

A

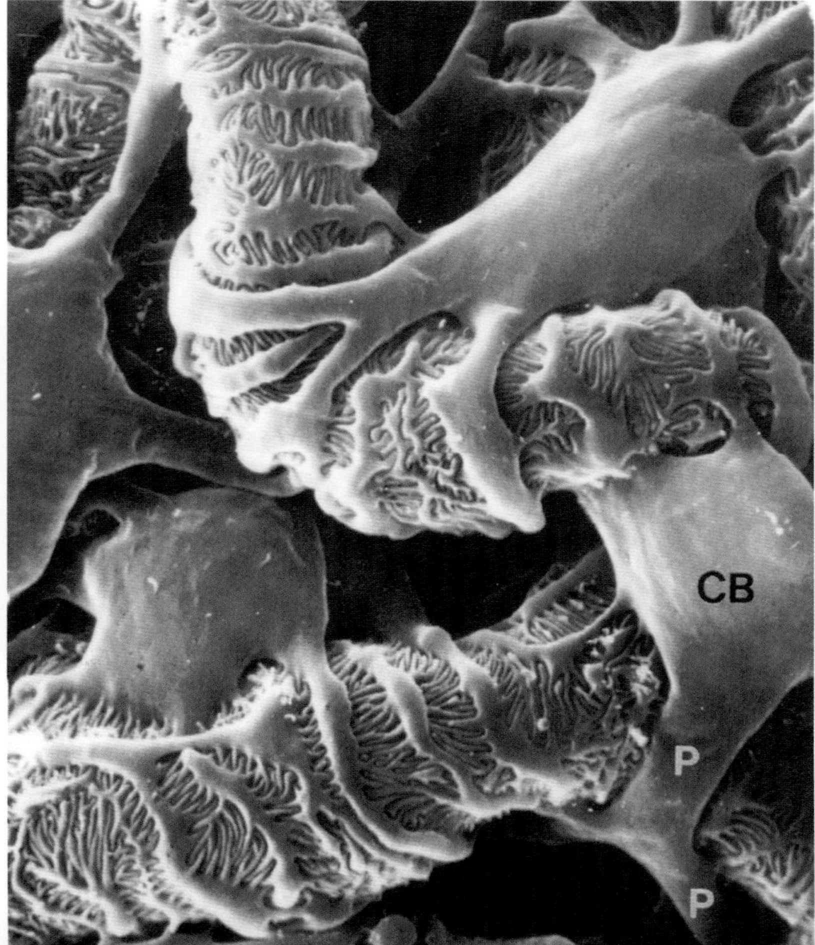

B

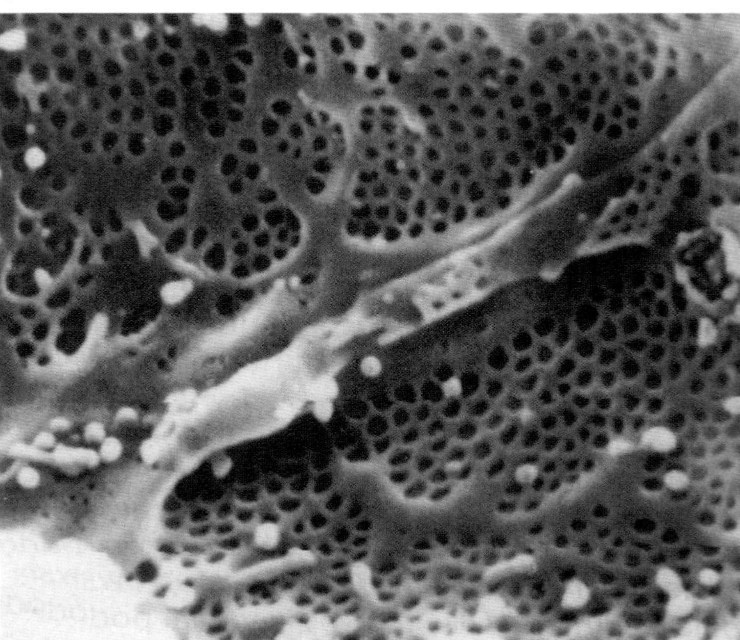

FIGURE 42-14 Glomerular capillaries. Scanning electron micrographs. **A,** View of the surface of a glomerular capillary from the vantage point of the capsular (Bowman) space. A podocyte cell body *(CB)* and podocyte foot processes *(P)* are shown on the outer surface of a capillary endothelial cell. **B,** View of the glomerular capillary wall from the vantage point of the capillary lumen. Note the multiple fenestrations that perforate the endothelial cells.

Renal Tubule

The renal tubule is a winding, hollow tube with walls largely made up of simple cuboidal and simple squamous epithelium. The epithelial cells each possess a single, *primary cilium* that acts as a sensory receptor that monitors the chemical makeup and rate of flow of the fluid flowing through the lumen of the tubule. Thus, renal tubule cells are able to respond to changes in the composition and flow of fluid to regulate the growth and functioning of the tubule. You can review the sensory role of primary cilia in the body on p. 91.

The renal tubule extends from the renal corpuscle to the end of the nephron, where it joins a collecting duct shared in common with other nearby nephrons. The renal tubule is divided into different regions: the proximal convoluted tubule, loop of Henle (nephron loop), and the distal convoluted tubule. Follow along in **Figure 42-10** (p. 972) as we briefly explore these regions.

Proximal Convoluted Tubule. The **proximal convoluted tubule (PCT)**, or more simply *proximal tubule,* is the second part of the nephron but the first part of the *renal tubule.* As its name suggests, the proximal convoluted tubule is the segment proximal, or nearest, to the Bowman capsule. Because it follows a winding, convoluted course, it is called a *convoluted* tubule. Its wall consists of one layer of epithelial cells that have a brush border facing the lumen of the tubule. Thousands of microvilli form the brush border and greatly increase its luminal surface area—a structural fact of importance to its function, as we shall see.

Loop of Henle. The **loop of Henle**, or *nephron loop,* is the segment of renal tubule just beyond the proximal tubule. It consists of a thin *descending limb,* a sharp turn, and an *ascending limb.* Note in **Figure 42-10** that the ascending limb has two regions of different wall thickness: the *thin ascending limb of (the loop of) Henle (tALH)* and the *thick ascending limb (TAL).* The length of the loop of Henle is important in the production of highly concentrated or very dilute urine.

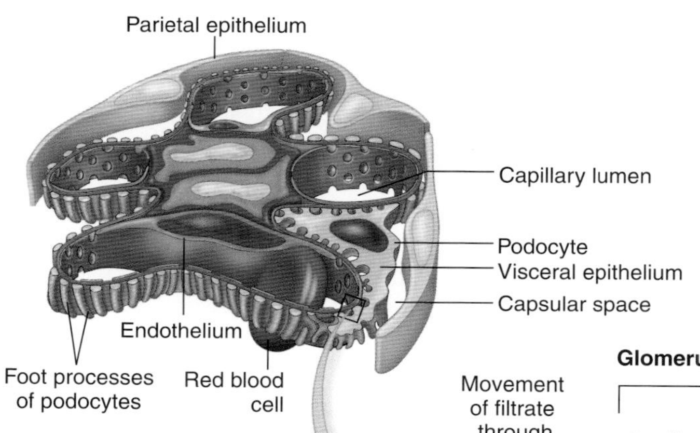

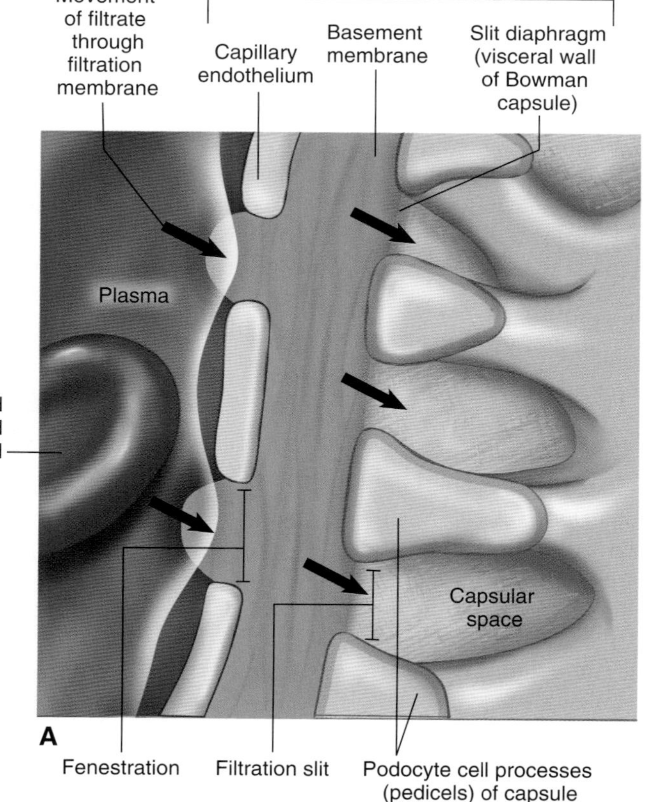

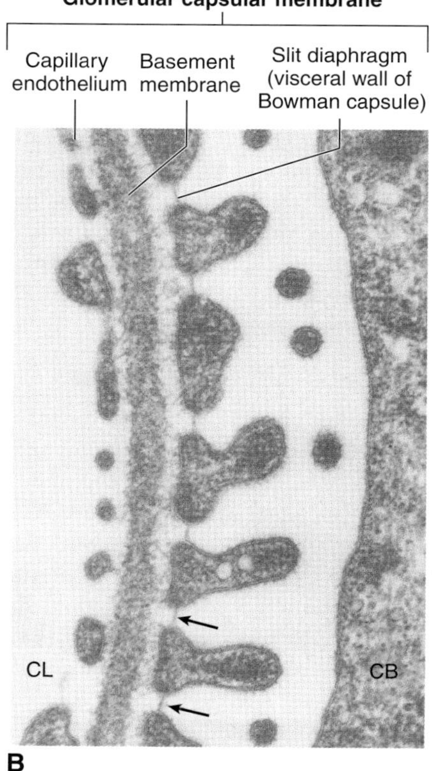

FIGURE 42-15 Glomerular capsular membrane. A, Artist's rendering of a transmission electron micrograph (TEM) showing the filtration membrane formed when footlike extensions (pedicels) of cells forming the visceral wall of the Bowman capsule share a basement membrane with the fenestrated endothelial cells that form the wall of glomerular capillaries. **B,** TEM of the glomerular capsular membrane. Note from left to right, the capillary lumen (CL), fenestrations in the capillary endothelium, and multiple podocyte foot processes separated by slit diaphragms *(arrows)* extending into the capsular (Bowman) space. A portion of an overarching podocyte cell body (CB) is visible on the right.

Distal Convoluted Tubule. The **distal convoluted tubule (DCT),** or simply *distal tubule,* is a convoluted portion of the tubule beyond (distal to) the loop of Henle. The distal convoluted tubule conducts filtrate out of the nephron and into a collecting duct.

The **juxtaglomerular apparatus** (meaning "structure near the glomerulus") is found at the point where the afferent arteriole brushes past the distal convoluted tubule (see **Figure 42-12**). Also called the *juxtaglomerular complex,* this structure is important in maintaining homeostasis of blood flow because it reflexively secretes **renin** when blood pressure in the afferent arteriole drops. Recall from Chapter 30 that renin triggers a mechanism that produces *angiotensin,* a substance that causes vasoconstriction and the resulting increase in blood pressure (see **Figure 42-27** on p. 986).

The unique cells of the juxtaglomerular apparatus represent a modification of cells in the walls of both the distal convoluted tubule and the afferent arteriole at the point where they touch one another. Large smooth muscle cells in the wall of the afferent arteriole—called **juxtaglomerular (JG) cells**—contain renin granules. These cells are sensitive to increased pressure in the arteriole and are considered functional *mechanoreceptors.* Modified distal convoluted tubule cells in the juxtaglomerular apparatus form a dense, tightly packed structure called the **macula densa.** Cells in the macula densa are *chemoreceptors* that can sense the concentration of solute materials in the fluid passing through the tubule. Acting together, both cell types in the juxtaglomerular apparatus contribute to homeostasis of renal function by influencing the ability of the kidney to produce concentrated urine.

Collecting Duct

The **collecting duct (CD)** is formed by the joining of renal tubules of several nephrons. All the collecting ducts of one renal pyramid converge at a renal papilla and release urine through their openings into one of the minor calyces (**Figure 42-16**). Bowman capsules and both convoluted tubules lie entirely within the cortex of the kidney, whereas the loops of Henle and collecting ducts extend into the medulla (see **Figure 42-10**).

Blood Supply of the Nephron

Earlier in this chapter, we traced renal blood flow through the renal artery and its branches to the afferent arteriole. Blood flows from the afferent arteriole into the glomerular capillaries and then exits through an *efferent arteriole* (**Figure 42-17**). The efferent arteriole then enters another capillary network that runs alongside the renal tubule. These capillaries are called **peritubular capillaries.** Some of the blood from the efferent arteriole flows through long hairpin-shaped loops that follow the nephron loop. These long, looping arterioles are called the **vasa recta** (*singular,* vas rectum) or *straight arterioles.* Blood flows very slowly through the vasa recta, a fact that plays an important role in the function of these vessels.

As you can see in **Figure 42-17**, blood flows through the efferent arteriole to the peritubular capillaries and vasa recta—the *peritubular blood supply*—then back toward the heart through *interlobular veins* and *arcuate veins* that head toward the large *renal veins.*

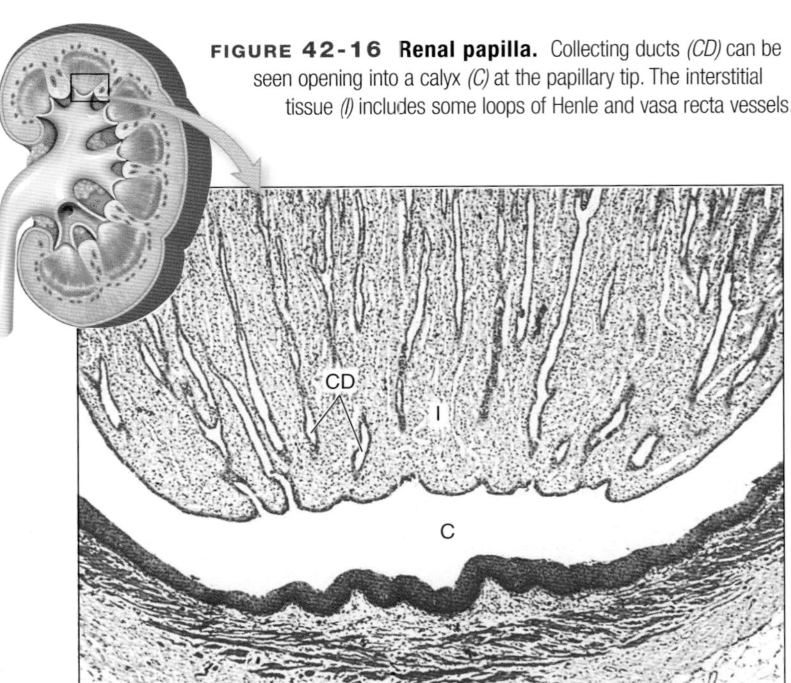

FIGURE 42-16 Renal papilla. Collecting ducts *(CD)* can be seen opening into a calyx *(C)* at the papillary tip. The interstitial tissue *(I)* includes some loops of Henle and vasa recta vessels.

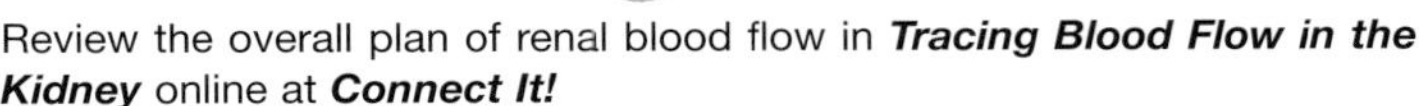

CONNECT IT!

Review the overall plan of renal blood flow in ***Tracing Blood Flow in the Kidney*** online at ***Connect It!***

Several micrographs of nephron and renal blood vessel structures are found in Part 5 of the Brief Atlas of the Human Body.

Types of Nephrons

About 85% of all nephrons are located almost entirely in the renal cortex and are called **cortical nephrons,** or short-loop nephrons. The remainder, called **juxtamedullary nephrons,** or long-loop nephrons, are found adjoining (*juxta*) the medulla. Juxtamedullary nephrons have long loops of Henle that dip far into the medulla (see **Figure 42-17**). The special role of these long loops of Henle of juxtamedullary nephrons in concentrating urine is discussed later.

Quick CHECK

8. Name the segments of the nephron in the order in which fluid flows through them.
9. What characteristics of the glomerular capsular membrane permit filtration?
10. What is the name of the blood supply that surrounds the nephron? The other name for the straight arterioles that follow the nephron loop?

PHYSIOLOGY OF THE URINARY SYSTEM

Overview of Kidney Function

The chief functions of the kidney are to process blood plasma and excrete urine. These functions are vital because they maintain the homeostatic balance of the body. For example, the kidneys are the

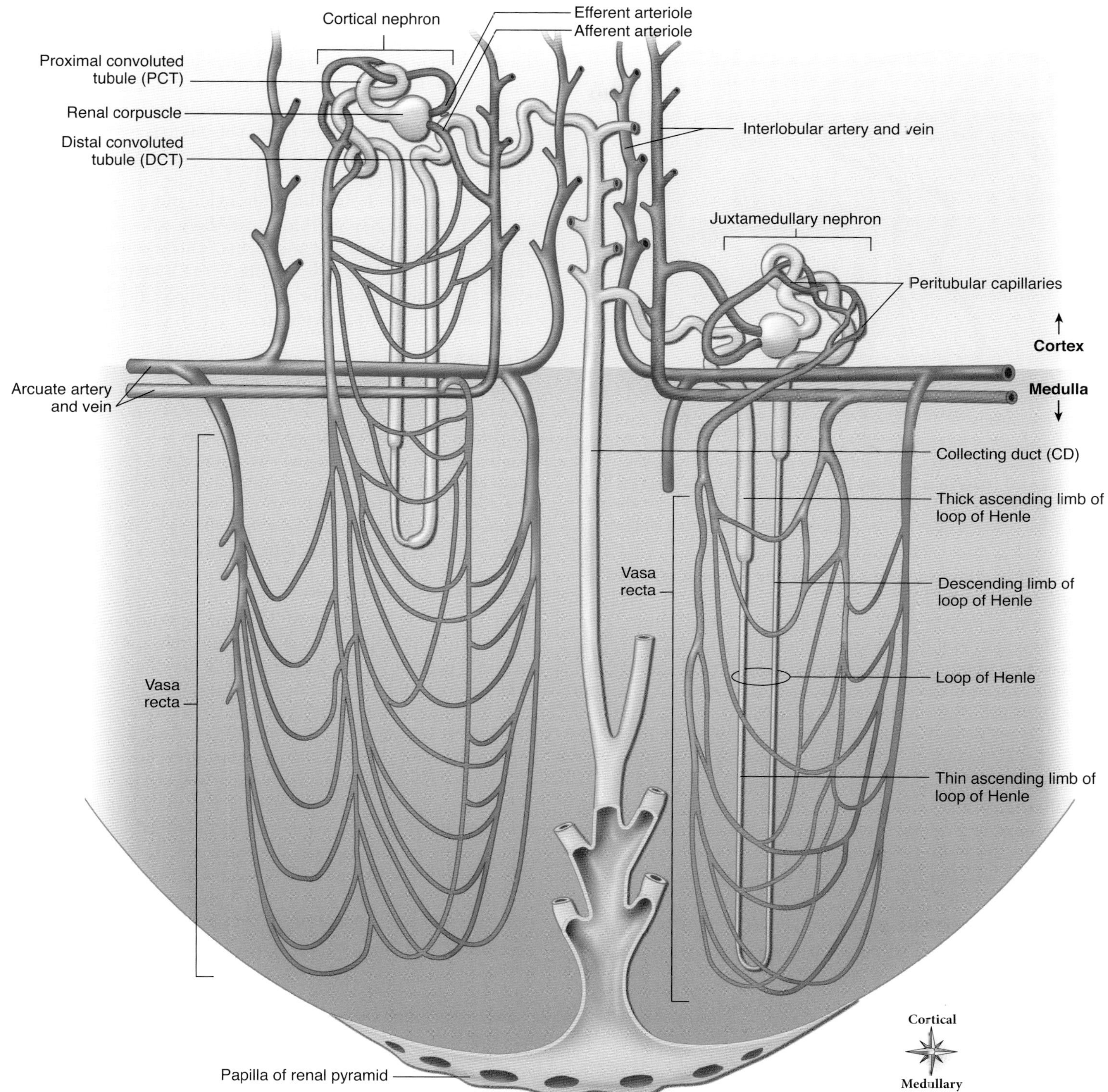

FIGURE 42-17 Blood supply of nephrons. Two types of nephrons (cortical and juxtaglomerular) are shown surrounded by the peritubular blood supply.

most important organs in the body for maintaining fluid–electrolyte and acid–base balance. The kidneys do this by varying the amount of water and electrolytes leaving the blood in the urine so that they equal the amounts of these substances entering the blood from various other avenues. Nitrogenous wastes from protein metabolism, notably *urea,* leave the blood by way of the kidneys.

Here are just a few of the blood constituents that cannot be held within their normal concentration ranges if the kidneys fail:

- Sodium
- Potassium
- Chloride
- Nitrogenous wastes (especially urea)

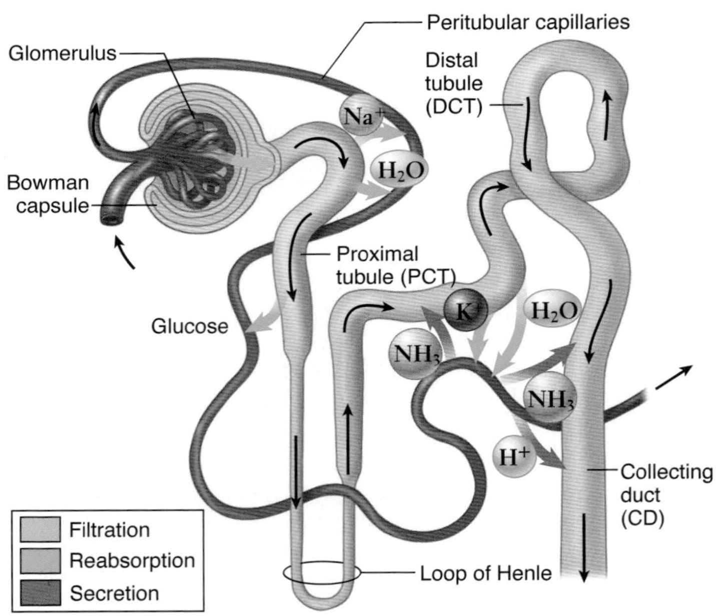

FIGURE 42-18 Overview of urine formation. The diagram shows the basic mechanisms of urine formation—filtration, reabsorption, and secretion—and where they occur in the nephron. Details of these steps are revealed later in this chapter.

In short, kidney failure means homeostatic failure and, if not relieved, inevitable death.

In addition to processing blood plasma and forming urine, the kidneys also perform other important functions. They influence the rate of secretion of the hormones antidiuretic hormone (ADH) and aldosterone and synthesize the active form of vitamin D, the hormone *erythropoietin*, and certain prostaglandins.

As you already know, the basic functional unit of the kidney is the nephron. It has two main parts—the renal corpuscle and renal tubule—that form urine by means of three processes:

1. **Filtration**—movement of water and protein-free solutes from plasma in the glomerulus, across the glomerular capsular membrane, and into the capsular space of Bowman capsule
2. **Tubular reabsorption**—movement of molecules out of the various segments of the tubule and into the peritubular blood
3. **Tubular secretion**—movement of molecules out of peritubular blood and into the tubule for excretion

These three mechanisms are used in concert to process blood plasma and form urine. First, a hydrostatic pressure gradient drives the filtration of much of the plasma into the nephron (**Figure 42-18**). Because the filtrate contains materials that the body must conserve (save), the walls of the tubules start reabsorbing these materials back into the blood. As the filtrate (urine) begins to leave the nephron, the kidney may secrete a few "last minute" items into the urine for excretion. In short, the kidney does not selectively filter out only harmful or excess material. It first filters out much of the plasma, then reabsorbs what should not be "thrown out" before the filtrate reaches the end of the tubule and becomes urine. This mechanism allows very fine adjustments to blood homeostasis, as we shall see. **Figure 42-19** shows the amounts of some important molecules that are filtered, then reabsorbed, by the nephron.

FILTRATION

Filtration, the first step in blood processing, is a physical process that occurs in the kidneys' 2.5 million renal corpuscles (see **Figures 42-10, 42-12**, and **42-15**). As blood flows through the glomerular capillaries, water and small solutes filter out of the blood into Bowman capsules. The only blood constituents that do not move out are the blood solids (cells) and most plasma proteins. The result is about 180 litres of glomerular filtrate being formed each day. This filtration takes place through the glomerular capsular membrane.

Mechanism of Filtration

Filtration from glomeruli into Bowman capsules occurs for the same reason that filtration from other capillaries into interstitial fluid occurs—because of the existence of a filtration pressure gradient. The main factor establishing the pressure gradient between the blood in the glomeruli and the filtrate in the Bowman capsule is the hydrostatic pressure of glomerular blood (**Figure 42-20**). It tends to cause filtration out of the glomerular blood plasma into Bowman capsules. The intensity of glomerular hydrostatic pressure is influenced by systemic blood pressure and the resistance to blood flow through the glomerular capillaries as described later. However, exerting force in the opposite direction are the osmotic pressure of glomerular blood plasma and the hydrostatic pressure of the capsular filtrate. The net or *effective filtration pressure (EFP)* therefore is the filtration pressure (glomerular hydrostatic pressure minus capsular hydrostatic pressure) minus the net osmotic pressure (glomerular

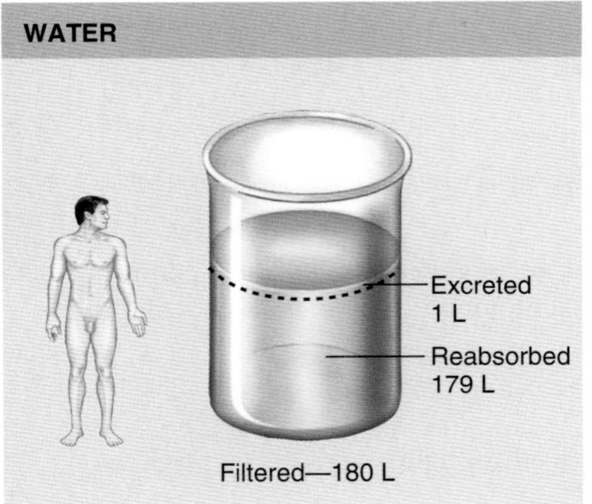

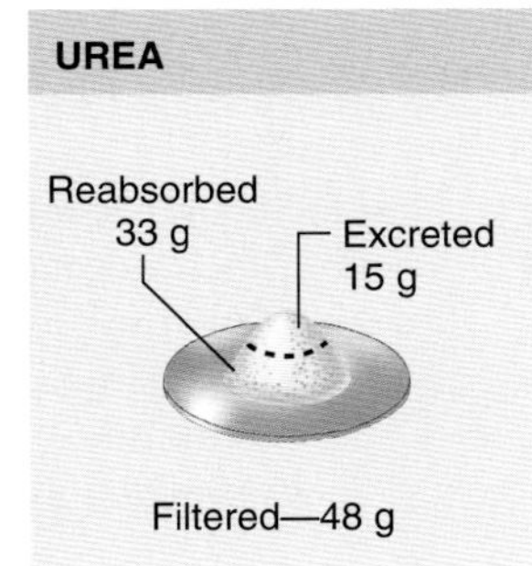

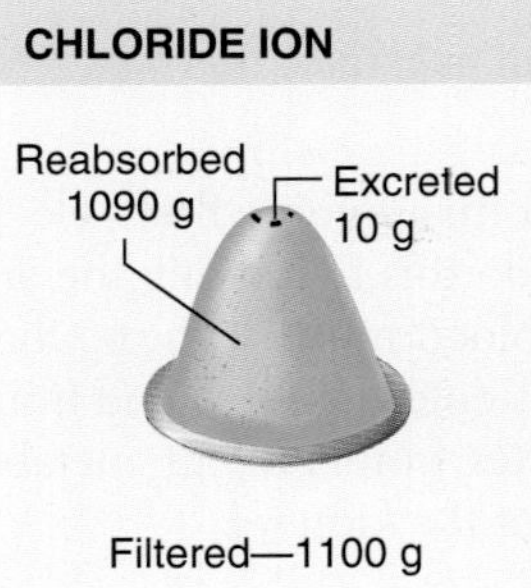

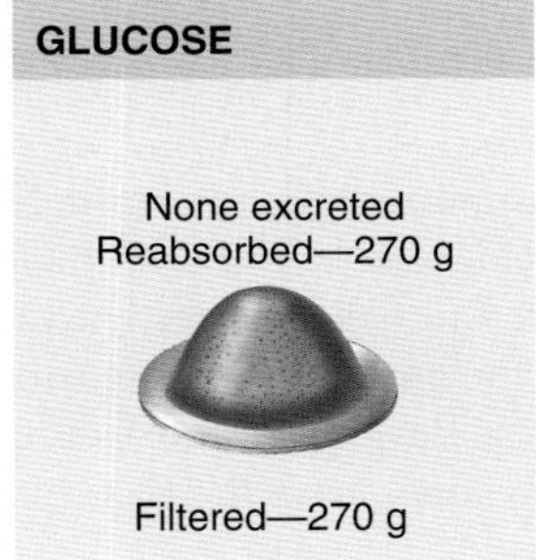

FIGURE 42-19 Filtration and reabsorption volumes. Note the enormous volume of water that is filtered out of glomerular blood per day—180 litres, or many times the total volume of blood in the body. Only a small proportion of this water, however, is excreted into urine. More than 99% of it (179 litres) is reabsorbed into tubular blood.

osmotic pressure minus capsular osmotic pressure). For example, assume the following pressures (**Figure 42-20**):

Filtration pressure
- Glomerular hydrostatic pressure = 60 mmHg (8.0 kPa)
- Capsular hydrostatic pressure = 18 mmHg (2.4 kPa)

Osmotic pressure
- Glomerular osmotic pressure = 32 mmHg (4.3 kPa)
- Capsular osmotic pressure = negligible amount (± 0 mmHg or ± 0 kPa)

The EFP, using these particular figures, equals (60 − 18) − (32 − 0), or 10 mmHg; or using kilopascals (8.0 − 2.4) − (4.3 − 0) = 1.3 kPa. An EFP of 1 mmHg (0.13 kPa), according to some investigators, produces a glomerular filtration rate (GFR) of 12.5 mL per minute (includes both kidneys).

With an EFP of 10 mmHg (1.3 kPa), the GFR would be 125 mL per minute, or about 180 litres in a 24-hour period, which is a GFR. (GFR ranges from 150 to 250 litres per day in healthy individuals.) Because only about 1.5 litres of urine is excreted each day, more than 99% of the filtrate must be reabsorbed from the tubular segments of the nephrons and collecting ducts.

Filtration occurs more rapidly out of glomeruli than out of other tissue capillaries. One reason for this is a structural difference between the endothelium of glomeruli and that of tissue capillaries. Glomerular endothelium has many more pores (fenestrations) in it, so it is more permeable than tissue capillary endothelium. Another reason for more rapid glomerular filtration than tissue capillary filtration is that glomerular hydrostatic pressure is higher than tissue capillary pressure. The reason for this, briefly, is that the efferent arteriole has a smaller diameter than the afferent arteriole does. Therefore, it offers more resistance to blood flow out of the glomerulus than venules offer to blood flow out of tissue capillaries.

Glomerular Filtration Rate

The **glomerular filtration rate (GFR)** is the rate of movement of fluid out of the glomerulus and into the capsular space.

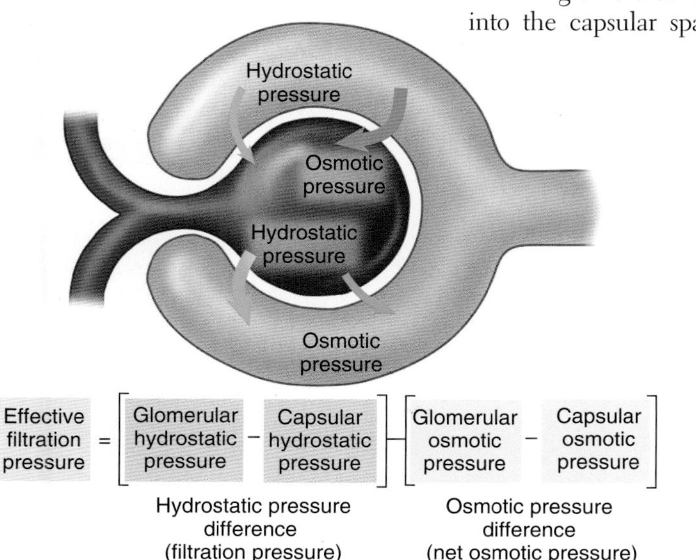

FIGURE 42-20 Forces affecting glomerular filtration. Effective filtration pressure (EFP) is determined by subtracting the forces that push fluid into the capillary from those that push it out of the capillary.

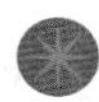

BOX 42-2 *changes in glomerular filtration rate*

In some types of kidney disease, the permeability of the glomerular endothelium increases sufficiently to allow plasma proteins to filter out into the capsule. Osmotic pressure then develops in the capsular filtrate. To determine how this affects the effective filtration pressure (EFP) in the glomeruli, first calculate the normal EFP by using the figures that the table lists as "Normal" in the formula given in **Figure 42-20**. After you have obtained your answer, apply the formula to the figures given under "Kidney Disease" in the table. You should find an EFP of 10 mmHg (1.3 kPa) with the normal figures and an EFP of 15 mmHg (2.0 kPa) with the kidney disease figures. A change in the glomerular EFP produces a similar change in the glomerular filtration rate (GFR). Therefore, loss of plasma protein into urine increases not only the EFP but also the GFR.

Intense exercise causes temporary proteinuria in many individuals. Some exercise physiologists believed that intense athletic activities cause kidney damage, but subsequent research has ruled out that explanation. One current hypothesis is that hormonal changes during strenuous exercise increase the permeability of the nephron's filtration membrane, thereby allowing more plasma proteins to enter the filtrate. Some degree of postexercise proteinuria is usually considered normal. •

Normal and Abnormal Pressure in the Renal Corpuscle

	HYDROSTATIC PRESSURE	OSMOTIC PRESSURE
Normal		
Glomerular blood	60 mmHg (8.0 kPa)	32 mmHg (4.3 kPa)
Capsular filtrate	18 mmHg (2.4 kPa)	0 mmHg (0 kPa)
Kidney Disease		
Glomerular blood	60 mmHg (8.0 kPa)	32 mmHg (4.3 kPa)
Capsular filtrate	18 mmHg (2.4 kPa)	5 mmHg (0.7 kPa)

GFR is directly proportional to the EFP and can be altered by changes in the diameter of the afferent and efferent arterioles or by changes in the systemic blood pressure (**Box 42-2**). It can also be altered indirectly by changes in the efficiency of cardiac contraction. Stress may lead to intense sympathetic stimulation of the arterioles with greater constriction of the afferent than the efferent arteriole. Consequently, glomerular hydrostatic pressure falls. In severe stress, it may even drop to a level so low that the EFP falls to zero. No glomerular filtration then occurs. The kidneys "shut down", or in technical language, *renal suppression* occurs.

Kidney disease and other factors can alter the permeability of the glomerular capsular membrane and thereby also affect GFR. Glomerular hydrostatic pressure and filtration are directly related to systemic blood pressure. That is, a decrease in systemic blood pressure tends to produce a decrease in both glomerular hydrostatic pressure and the GFR. The converse is also true. However, when systemic arterial pressure increases, a smaller increase in glomerular pressure follows because the afferent arterioles constrict. This decreases blood flow into the glomeruli and prevents a marked rise in glomerular hydrostatic pressure or glomerular filtration. For instance, when the mean arterial blood pressure doubles, glomerular filtration reportedly increases only 15% to 20%.

Clinically, the GFR can be estimated by determining the **renal clearance** of a substance—that is, the rate at which a substance is "cleared" out of the plasma and into urine by the kidney. It is expressed as a volume of plasma cleared of a particular substance by the kidney per unit of time. Renal clearance is calculated with this equation:

$$\text{Renal clearance (mL/min)} = \frac{\text{Urine concentration of substance (mg/100 mL)} \times \text{Urine flow rate (mL/min)}}{\text{Plasma concentration of substance (mg/100 mL)}}$$

For example, if the renal clearance of *creatinine* is 100 mL/min, that means that creatinine is completely cleared from 100 millilitres of plasma in 1 minute.

Creatinine is a metabolic byproduct of breaking down creatine phosphate (CP) for muscle contraction and is produced at a fairly constant rate in the body, so it is a handy substance for determining kidney function. Another substance, the fructose polysaccharide *inulin*, is not present in the body so its clearance after being injected into the blood is not subject to physiological factors that could influence the accuracy of creatinine clearance results. Creatinine clearance is used most often clinically, however, because even though it is not as accurate as inulin clearance, it is less expensive and complicated to assess.

Quick CHECK

11. What are the three basic processes a nephron uses to form urine?
12. What is the GFR? Why is a high GFR important to kidney function?
13. How does blood pressure affect filtration in the kidney?

REABSORPTION

Reabsorption takes place by means of passive and active transport mechanisms from all parts of the renal tubules. A major portion of water and electrolytes and (normally) all nutrients are, however, reabsorbed from the proximal convoluted tubules. The rest of the renal tubule reabsorbs comparatively little of the filtrate. Researchers continue to investigate the exact mechanisms of reabsorption in the various segments of the nephron. We have summarized only the essential principles of some of the current concepts in the following paragraphs.

Reabsorption in the Proximal Convoluted Tubule

Most of the 180 litres of filtrate that enters the renal tubule from Bowman capsules each day does not get very far. More than two thirds of it is reabsorbed before it reaches the end of the proximal convoluted tubule.

The process of reabsorption begins when sodium ions (Na^+) are actively transported out of the lumen of the tubule and into peritubular blood by the mechanism summarized in **Figure 42-21**. The microvilli on the luminal surface of each epithelial cell in the tubule wall form a brush border that increases the absorptive surface area of the entire inner face of the tubule. As sodium ions accumulate in the interstitial fluid, the interstitial fluid becomes temporarily positive with respect to the tubule fluid. This electrical gradient (difference in net charge) drives the diffusion of negative ions from the filtrate, into the interstitial fluid, and eventually, into the peritubular blood. In other words, the attraction between negative and positive ions is used to drive the passive transport of chloride (Cl^-), phosphate ($PO_4^{\equiv}$) and other negative ions out of the tubule.

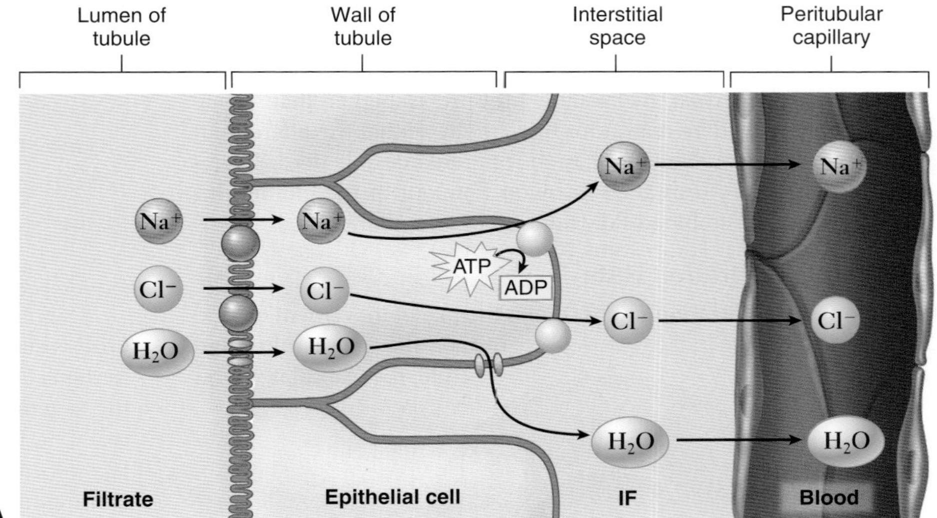

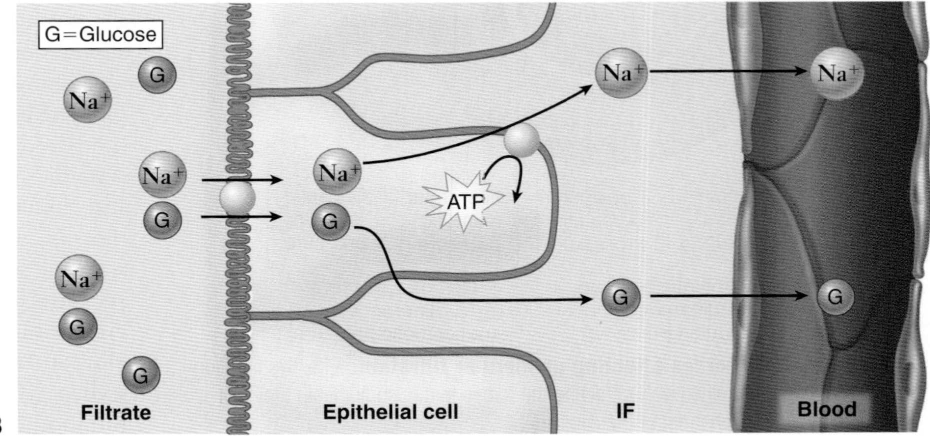

FIGURE 42-21 Mechanisms of tubular reabsorption. A, Sodium ions (Na^+) are pumped from the tubule cell to interstitial fluid (IF), thereby increasing the interstitial Na^+ concentration to a level that drives diffusion of Na^+ into blood. As Na^+ is pumped out of the cell, more Na^+ passively diffuses in from the filtrate to maintain an equilibrium of concentration. Enough Na^+ moves out of the tubule and into blood that an electrical gradient is established (blood is positive relative to the filtrate). Electrical attraction between oppositely charged particles drives diffusion of negative ions in the filtrate, such as chloride (Cl^-), into blood. As the ion concentration in blood increases, osmosis of water from the tubule occurs. Thus active transport of sodium creates a situation that promotes passive transport of negative ions and water. **B,** In sodium cotransport of glucose, a sodium–glucose carrier transports glucose (G) along with sodium in an example of secondary active transport (see **Box 6-3**, Figure *B*, on p. 105). Amino acids are transported similarly (see **Figure 40-20**, *C*, on p. 921).

As the concentration of ions in peritubular blood increases, the blood becomes momentarily hypertonic to the tubule fluid and has a higher osmotic pressure. Through the process of osmosis, water moves rapidly from the tubule fluid into peritubular blood, thus making the two fluids isotonic. In short, transport of ions out of the proximal convoluted tubules causes osmosis of water out of the tubules as well. This is obligatory water reabsorption—obligatory because it is demanded by the principle of osmosis. Osmosis in the kidney relies on the availability and proper function of a family of water channels called *aquaporins* (see p. 101).

Proximal convoluted tubules reabsorb nutrients from the tubule fluid, notably glucose and amino acids, into peritubular blood by a special type of active transport mechanism called **sodium cotransport.**

Recall from Chapter 40 that such sodium cotransport of glucose and amino acids in the intestinal mucosa moves glucose and amino acids into the blood. In this mechanism, a carrier molecule in the cell membrane first binds to sodium and glucose (**Figure 42-21**, *B*). The carrier then passively transports both substances through the brush border of a proximal convoluted tubule cell into the cell's interior (facilitated diffusion). Sodium moves into the cell because of a concentration gradient maintained by the active transport of sodium out the other side of the cell. Glucose actually moves up its concentration gradient, but no additional energy is required because it is "riding the coattails" of sodium. Once inside the cell, the substances dissociate from the carrier molecule and diffuse to the far side of the cell. The substances move out of the epithelial cell by different mechanisms. Sodium is transported actively, and glucose is transported passively.

Normally, all the glucose that has filtered out of the glomeruli returns to the blood by this sodium cotransport mechanism. Therefore, very little glucose is lost in urine. If, however, the blood glucose level exceeds a threshold amount (usually between 130 and 300 mg/100 mL or between 7.2 and 16.7 mmol/L), not all of the glucose can be reabsorbed. The excess glucose remains in urine (**Box 42-3**). The maximum capacity for moving glucose molecules back into blood is determined by the number of cotransport carriers available. The maximum capacity for moving any substance limited by availability of carriers is called the *transport maximum (Tm* or *Tmax)* of that substance.

Urea is a nitrogen-containing waste formed as a result of protein catabolism (see Chapter 41). Actually, toxic ammonia is formed first, but much of it is quickly transformed into the less toxic urea. Urea in the tubule fluid remains in the proximal convoluted tubule as sodium, chloride, and water are reabsorbed into blood. Once these materials are gone, a tubule fluid high in urea is left. Because the urea concentration in the tubule is then greater than its concentration in peritubular blood, urea passively diffuses into the blood. About half the urea present in the tubule fluid leaves the proximal convoluted tubule this way.

Reabsorption in the proximal convoluted tubules can be summarized in the following manner:

1. Sodium is actively transported out of the tubule fluid and into blood.
2. Glucose and amino acids "hitch a ride" with sodium and passively move out of the tubule fluid by means of the sodium cotransport mechanism.
3. Chloride ions passively move into blood plasma because of an imbalance in electrical charges (positive sodium ions have already moved out, thus making the plasma positive and the tubule fluid negative).
4. Movement of sodium and chloride out of the tubule fluid into plasma creates an osmotic imbalance (the blood is hypertonic to the filtrate), so water is obliged by the principle of osmosis to passively move into blood.
5. About half the urea present in the tubule fluid passively moves out of the tubule, with half the urea thus left to move on to the loop of Henle.
6. The total content of the filtrate has been reduced greatly by the time it is ready to leave the proximal convoluted tubule. Most of the water and solutes have been recovered by the blood, and only a small volume of fluid is left to continue to the next portion of the tubule, the loop of Henle.

BOX 42-3 *health matters*
Glucose in Urine

Occasionally, the maximum cotransport capacity is greatly reduced, and glucose appears in urine *(glycosuria),* even though the blood sugar level may be normal. This condition is known as *renal diabetes* or *renal glycosuria.* It is a congenital defect.

Of course, the most common cause of glycosuria is *diabetes mellitus* (see Chapter 26). In this condition, insulin deficiency or target cell dysfunction causes glucose to accumulate in the blood, causing hyperglycaemia. The high glucose content of the filtrate formed in the renal corpuscle exceeds the maximum capacity of the cotransport mechanism. Therefore, glycosuria results. •

Quick CHECK

14. How are NaCl and water reabsorbed in the proximal convoluted tubule?
15. What is sodium cotransport?
16. What is a transport maximum?

Reabsorption in the Loop of Henle

In juxtamedullary nephrons—those low in the cortex, near the medulla—the loop of Henle and its vasa recta participate in a very unique process called a **countercurrent mechanism.** A countercurrent structure is any set of parallel passages in which the contents flow in opposite directions (**Figure 42-22**). The loop of Henle is a countercurrent structure because the contents of the ascending limb travel in a direction opposite to the flow of urine in the descending limb. The vasa recta also have a countercurrent structure because arterial blood flows down into the medulla and venous blood flows up toward the cortex. The kidney's countercurrent mechanism functions to keep the solute concentration of the medulla's IF extremely high.

Note, in the explanation that follows *osmolality* is the concentration of a solution expressed as milliosmoles of solute per kg of water (mOsm/kg H_2O). It depends on the total number of osmotically active particles per kg of water. The higher a solution's osmolality, the higher its concentration and the greater its osmotic effect.

(Compare this with *osmolarity*—the concentration of a solution expressed as the total number of solute particles per litre (mOsm/L.)

The descending limb of the loop of Henle has a much thinner wall than the thick part of the ascending limb (see **Figure 42-10**).

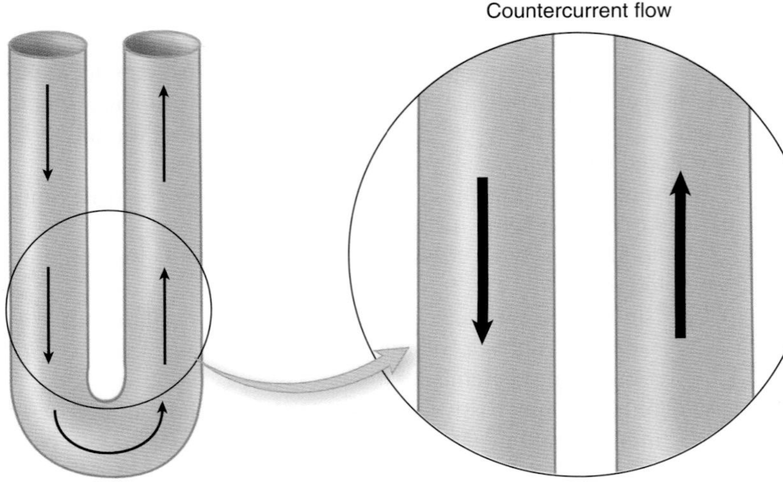

FIGURE 42-22 Concept of countercurrent flow. Countercurrent flow simply refers to flow in opposite directions, as the *inset* shows. Tubule filtrate in the loop of Henle flows in a countercurrent manner, as does blood flowing through vasa recta of the peritubular blood supply.

Even more important, the permeability and transport abilities of the two walls are very different. The thin-walled descending limb allows water and urea to pass freely into or out of the tubule, depending on their concentration gradients. The thick-walled ascending limb, however, limits the passive movement of most molecules (including water, sodium, chloride, and urea) while actively transporting selected molecules out of the tubule and into the interstitial fluid.

Given the characteristics of each limb, we can see how the system illustrated in **Figure 42-23** can develop in the loop of Henle. Look at the thick ascending limb. You will see that this limb is actively pumping sodium and chloride out of the tubule fluid and into interstitial fluid. This probably occurs by the same mechanism that operates in the proximal convoluted tubule. Normally, sodium and chloride ions simply diffuse right back into the tubule fluid to achieve equilibrium. The ascending limb prevents the diffusion of these ions, so they are "trapped" in the interstitial area. In normal circumstances, water moves from the tubule fluid to the interstitial fluid to achieve osmotic balance. However, the wall of the ascending limb is relatively impermeable to water. In short, salt ions are pumped out of the ascending limb, water is prevented from following osmotically, and thus the tubule fluid develops a low solute concentration (low osmotic pressure) and interstitial fluid develops a high solute concentration (high osmotic pressure).

The ion pumps in the ascending limb can maintain an osmotic difference of 200 mOsm/kg H_2O across the wall of the tubule. Notice in **Figure 42-23** that the movement of salt out of the tubule at any horizontal level creates a difference of 200 mOsm/kg H_2O between the tubule fluid and interstitial fluid. Because salt is continually added to the interstitial fluid, the interstitial fluid becomes very concentrated (up to 1200 mOsm/kg H_2O in our model). This high solute concentration of the interstitial fluid of the medulla is created and maintained by the constant pumping of salt by the ascending limb. For this reason, this process is often called a *countercurrent multiplier mechanism*.

You will notice that the tubule fluid in the descending limb equilibrates easily with the interstitial fluid. Because interstitial fluid has a high solute concentration (created by the ion pumps in the ascending limb), the fluid in the descending limb loses water osmotically. Thus the solute concentration of the tubule fluid becomes increasingly higher. Urea, a solute that is also highly concentrated in the renal medulla, diffuses into the tubule fluid in the descending limb—thereby increasing the solute concentration of the tubule fluid even more. However, as the fluid "rounds the bend" and begins moving into the thick portion of the ascending limb, its Na^+ and Cl^- are removed and it becomes increasingly lower in solute concentration.

When tubule fluid enters the loop of Henle, it is about 300 mOsm/kg H_2O (isotonic to most body fluids). When it leaves the loop of Henle, it is about 100 mOsm/kg H_2O (hypotonic to most body fluids). Because water is reabsorbed from the fluid in the descending limb, there is a net reduction of tubule fluid volume. And because urea entered the tubule fluid in the descending limb, there is a net increase in urea concentration in the tubule fluid.

You might think that the blood of the vasa recta (a portion of the peritubular blood supply) would remove the excess solute from

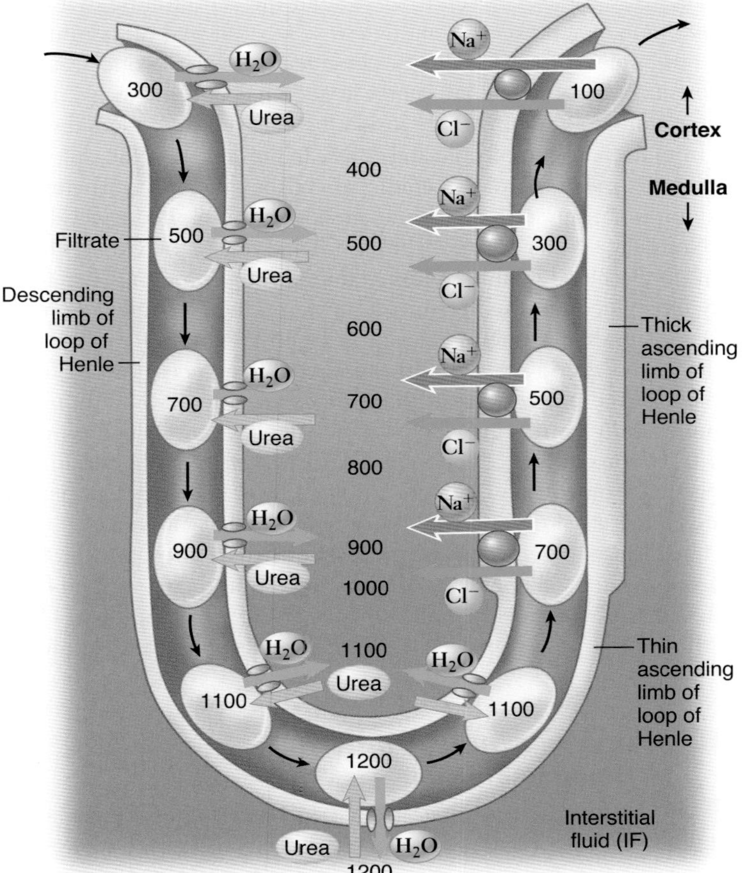

FIGURE 42-23 The countercurrent multiplier system in the Henle loop. Na^+ and Cl^- are pumped from the ascending limb and moved into interstitial fluid (IF) to maintain high osmolality there. Because the salt content of the medullary IF increases, this is called a "multiplier" mechanism. Ion pumping also lowers the tubule fluid's osmolality by 200 mOsm/kg, so fluid leaving the loop of Henle is only 100 mOsm/kg (hypotonic), as compared with 300 mOsm/kg (isotonic) when it entered the loop. Numbers in the diagram are expressed in milliosmoles per kilogram (mOsm/kg) of water.

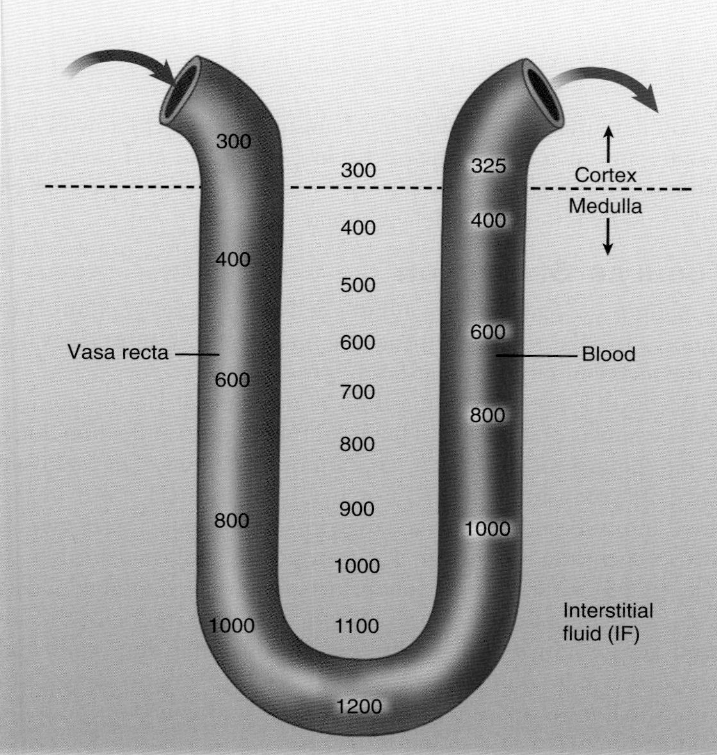

FIGURE 42-24 Countercurrent exchange mechanism in a vas rectum. Because a vas rectum forms a countercurrent loop, blood leaving the capillary bed has only a slightly higher solute content than when it entered. Thus the high osmolality of medullary tissue fluid is maintained. If peritubular blood instead travelled straight through the tissue, all excess solute in the medulla would be removed, and the osmolality of medullary interstitial fluid (IF) would be equivalent to that of the cortex. Numbers in the diagram are expressed in milliosmoles per kilogram (mOsm/kg) of water.

the medulla's interstitial fluid as it flows through the tissue. Usually it would, but the vasa recta have their own countercurrent mechanism—often called the *countercurrent exchange mechanism.* **Figure 42-24** shows how the looping of a vas rectum, down into the medulla, then back up to the cortex, prevents it from accumulating too much solute. Consider also that blood flow through a vas rectum is sluggish; it cannot remove anything very efficiently. Just enough solute is removed to prevent the medulla from crystallizing completely because of a high solute concentration. Thus the tissues of the medulla have the benefits of a blood supply without much loss of its high solute concentration.

The primary functions of the loop of Henle are summarized as follows:

- The loop of Henle reabsorbs water from the tubule fluid (and picks up urea from the interstitial fluid) in its descending limb. It reabsorbs sodium and chloride from the tubule fluid in the ascending limb.
- By reabsorbing salt from its ascending limb, it makes the tubule fluid dilute (hypotonic).
- Reabsorption of salt in the ascending limb also creates and maintains a high osmotic pressure, or high solute concentration, of the medulla's interstitial fluid.

Quick CHECK

17. What is a countercurrent mechanism?
18. How does the function of the descending limb of the loop of Henle differ from the function of the thick ascending limb?
19. What is the purpose of the countercurrent multiplier mechanism of the loop of Henle?

Reabsorption in the Distal Tubules and Collecting Ducts

The distal convoluted tubule is similar to the proximal convoluted tubule in that it also reabsorbs some sodium by active transport, but in much smaller amounts. Left to themselves, the cells that form the distal tubule's walls are relatively impermeable to water. This means that sodium can be removed, but water cannot follow osmotically, so the solute concentration of the tubule fluid continues to decrease. Recall that the tubule fluid is already hypotonic to most body fluids at this point because of the countercurrent system in the loop of Henle.

The cells that form the wall of the collecting duct also prevent water from leaving the filtrate by osmosis. Even though the collecting duct conducts the tubule fluid through the hypertonic medullary region, equilibration does not occur.

Given no other circumstances, the kidney produces and excretes only very dilute (hypotonic) urine (**Figure 42-25**). This would be

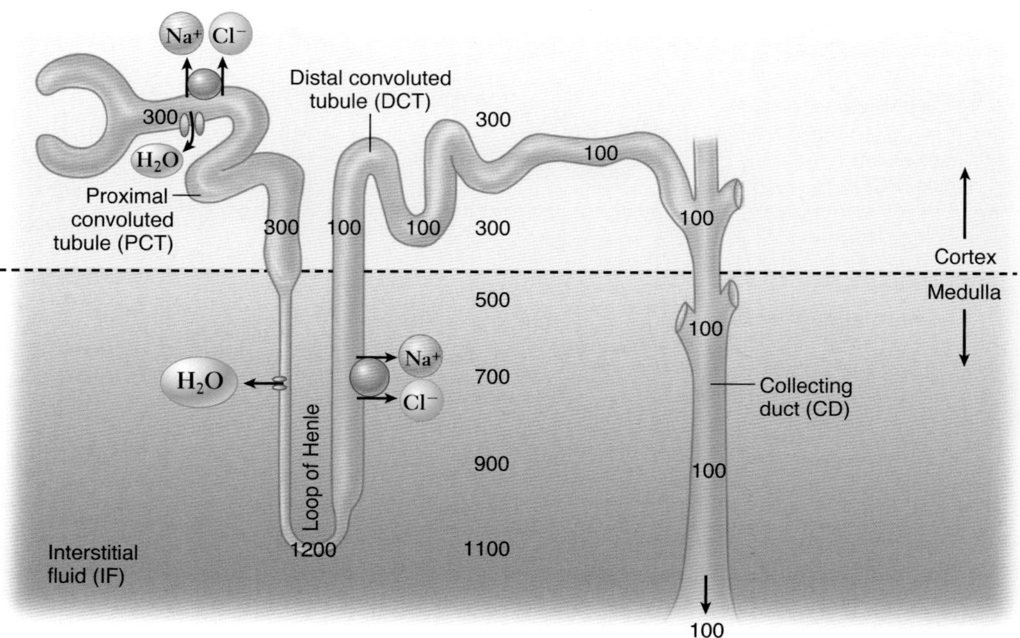

FIGURE 42-25 Production of hypotonic urine. Hypotonic urine is produced by the nephron by the mechanism shown here. The isotonic (300 mOsm/kg) tubule fluid that enters the loop of Henle becomes hypotonic (100 mOsm/kg) by the time it enters the distal convoluted tubule. The tubule fluid remains hypotonic as it is conducted out of the kidney because the walls of the distal tubule and collecting duct are impermeable to H_2O, Na^+, and Cl^-. Values are expressed in milliosmoles per kilogram (mOsm/kg) of water.

UNIT 5

catastrophic because the body would soon dehydrate. A regulatory mechanism centred outside the kidney normally prevents excessive loss of water. This mechanism, illustrated in **Figure 42-26**, involves *antidiuretic hormone (ADH)*, a hormone secreted by the neurohypophysis (posterior pituitary).

ADH targets cells of the distal tubules and collecting ducts and triggers the cells to move aquaporins to the plasma membrane. These aquaporins allow the tubule wall to become more permeable to water. Water is thereby permitted to flow osmotically out of the tubule and into the interstitial fluid, toward equilibrium. The more ADH present, the more aquaporins are available to allow more water out of the tubule, and the closer the tubule fluid's solute concentration matches that of the surrounding tissue fluid. In this way, the tubule fluid's osmotic pressure could go as high as 1200 mOsm/kg H_2O, because the medulla's interstitial fluid can be that high. The solute concentration of the urine excreted depends in large part on the amount of ADH present.

Note in **Figure 42-26** that reabsorption of urea also occurs in the collecting duct when water is reabsorbed under the influence of ADH. As water is reabsorbed from the fluid descending through the collecting duct, the urea concentration of the fluid rises. Because the urea concentration is higher inside the lower part of the collecting duct than it is in the surrounding interstitial fluid, urea diffuses out of the lower collecting duct. The addition of urea to the medullary interstitial fluid assists in maintaining a high solute concentration in the medulla. Less than half the urea that leaves the collecting duct is removed by the vasa recta. The long arrow near the bottom of **Figure 42-26** shows that much of the urea in the medullary interstitial fluid diffuses into the descending limb of the loop of Henle. Thus urea participates in a sort of countercurrent multiplier mechanism that, together with the countercurrent mechanisms of the loop of Henle and vasa recta, maintains the high osmotic pressure needed to form concentrated urine and therefore avoid dehydration.

TUBULAR SECRETION

In addition to reabsorption, tubule cells also secrete certain substances. Tubular secretion means the movement of substances out of the blood and into tubular fluid.

Recall that the descending limb of the loop of Henle removes urea by means of diffusion. The distal tubules and collecting ducts secrete potassium, hydrogen, and ammonium ions. They actively transport potassium ions (K^-) or hydrogen ions (H^+) out of the blood into tubule fluid in exchange for sodium ions (Na^+), which diffuse back into the blood (H^+ transport is discussed further in Chapter 44). Potassium secretion increases when the blood aldosterone concentration increases. *Aldosterone*, a hormone of the adrenal cortex, targets distal tubule and collecting duct cells and causes them to increase the activity of the sodium–potassium pumps that move sodium out of the tubule and potassium into the tubule. Hydrogen ion secretion increases when the blood hydrogen ion concentration increases. Ammonium ions are secreted into the tubule fluid by diffusing out of the tubule cells where they are synthesized.

Tubule cells also secrete various organic ions and compounds. Various toxins and many drugs such as penicillin (an antibiotic) and the PAH (para-aminohippurate) sometimes used in renal perfusion tests can be cleared from the blood plasma this way.

Table 42-1 summarizes the functions of the different parts of the nephron in forming urine.

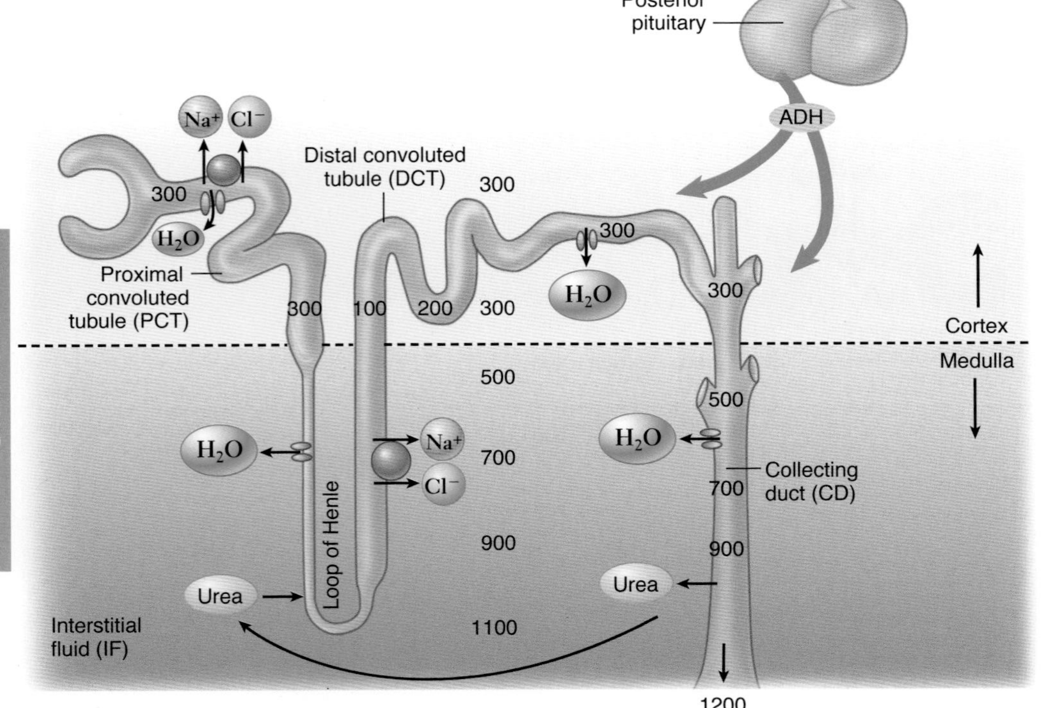

FIGURE 42-26 Production of hypertonic urine. Hypertonic urine can be formed when antidiuretic hormone (ADH) is present. ADH, a posterior pituitary hormone, increases the water permeability of the distal tubule and collecting duct. Thus hypotonic (100 mOsm/kg) tubule fluid leaving the loop of Henle can equilibrate first with the isotonic (300 mOsm/kg) interstitial fluid (IF) of the cortex, then with the increasingly hypertonic (400 to 1200 mOsm/kg) IF of the medulla. As H_2O leaves the collecting duct by osmosis, the filtrate becomes more concentrated with the solutes left behind. The concentration gradient causes urea to diffuse into the IF, where some of it is eventually picked up by tubule fluid in the descending limb of the loop of Henle *(long arrow)*. This countercurrent movement of urea helps maintain a high solute concentration in the medulla. Values are expressed in milliosmoles per kilogram (mOsm/kg) of water.

TABLE 42-1 Summary of Nephron Function

PART OF NEPHRON	FUNCTION	SUBSTANCE MOVED
Renal corpuscle	Filtration (passive)	Water Smaller solute particles (ions, glucose, etc.)
Proximal convoluted tubule (PCT)	Reabsorption (active)	Active transport: Na^+ Cotransport: glucose and amino acids
	Reabsorption (passive)	Diffusion: Cl^-, $PO_4^{\equiv}$, urea, other solutes Osmosis: water
Loop of Henle		
Descending limb (DLH) and thin ascending limb (tALH)	Reabsorption (passive)	Osmosis: water
	Secretion (passive)	Diffusion: urea
Thick ascending limb (TAL)	Reabsorption (active)	Active transport: Na^+
	Reabsorption (passive)	Diffusion: Cl^-
Distal convoluted tubule (DCT)	Reabsorption (active)	Active transport: Na^+
	Reabsorption (passive)	Diffusion: Cl^-, other anions Osmosis: water (only in the presence of ADH)
	Secretion (passive)	Diffusion: ammonia
	Secretion (active)	Active transport: K^+, H^+, some drugs
Collecting duct (CD)	Reabsorption (active)	Active transport: Na^+
	Reabsorption (passive)	Diffusion: urea Osmosis: water (only in the presence of ADH)
	Secretion (passive)	Diffusion: ammonia
	Secretion (active)	Active transport: K^+, H^+, some drugs

ADH, Antidiuretic hormone.

Regulation of Urine Volume

ADH has a central role in the regulation of urine volume. Control of the solute concentration of urine translates into control of urine volume. If no water is reabsorbed by the distal tubule and collecting ducts, urine volume is relatively high—and water loss from the body is high. As water is reabsorbed under the influence of ADH, the total volume of urine is reduced by the amount of water removed from the tubules. Thus ADH reduces water loss by the body.

Another hormone that tends to decrease urine volume—and thus conserves water—is aldosterone, a secretion of the adrenal cortex. It increases distal tubule and collecting duct absorption of sodium, which in turn causes an osmotic imbalance that drives the reabsorption of water from the tubule. Because water reabsorption in the distal tubule and collecting duct portions requires ADH, the aldosterone mechanism must work in concert with the ADH mechanism if homeostasis of the fluid content in the body is to be maintained. The cooperative roles of ADH and aldosterone in regulating urine volume—and thus regulating fluid balance in the whole body—are summarized in **Figure 42-27**.

You may recall from Chapters 26 and 30 that another hormone, specifically, **atrial natriuretic hormone (ANH),** also influences water reabsorption in the kidney. ANH is secreted by specialized muscle fibres in the atrial wall of the heart. Its name implies its function: ANH promotes natriuresis (loss of Na^+ via urine). ANH indirectly acts as an antagonist of aldosterone, by promoting the secretion of sodium into the kidney tubules rather than sodium reabsorption. Thus ANH reduces the plasma and interstitial fluid Na^+ concentration, which in turn reduces the reabsorption of water by having the effect opposite that of aldosterone. ANH also inhibits the secretion of aldosterone and opposes the aldosterone–ADH mechanism to reabsorb less water and therefore produce more urine. In short, ANH inhibits the ADH mechanism—thus inhibiting water conservation by the internal environment and increasing urine volume. Urine volume also relates to the total amount of solutes other than sodium excreted in urine. Generally, the more solutes, the more urine. Probably the best-known example of this principle occurs in untreated diabetes mellitus. The symptom that often brings a person with undiagnosed diabetes to a physician is the voiding of abnormally large amounts of urine. Excess glucose "spills over" into urine, thereby increasing the solute concentration of urine (and decreasing the solute concentration of plasma), which in turn leads to diuresis.

Urine volume is not normally altered by changes in the GFR, which remains remarkably constant in healthy individuals over extended periods. A process called *autoregulation* of glomerular filtration by **tubuloglomerular feedback** is dependent on proper functioning of the macula densa cells and the juxtaglomerular apparatus (see p. 976 and **Figure 42-12**). This regulatory mechanism helps protect the kidney from rapid systemic arterial pressure variations that would otherwise cause large GFR changes. It does so by regulating resistance in both afferent and efferent arterioles. **Figure 42-28**, *A*, summarizes the major steps of this process. As systemic blood pressure varies, chemoreceptors sensitive to the flow rate and osmolality of the filtrate can either speed up or slow down the GFR, thus allowing more or less time for chemical processing of tubular filtrate.

In addition, the feedback regulatory response also influences the renin–angiotensin mechanism and systemic blood pressure levels (see **Figure 42-27**).

The autoregulatory **myogenic mechanism** is yet another rapid and effective way to help maintain a constant GFR during systemic changes in arterial blood pressure (**Figure 42-28**, *B*). If blood pressure increases, for example, during muscular exertion, the stretched walls of the afferent arterioles automatically contract more strongly to decrease blood flow and return the GFR to resting levels. In circumstances causing a decrease in systemic blood pressure, the smooth muscle in the then relaxed walls of the afferent arterioles will cause dilation, thus increasing blood flow and the GFR to normal setpoint levels.

Urine Composition

The physical characteristics of normal urine are listed in **Table 42-2**. Notice that normal and abnormal characteristics are listed.

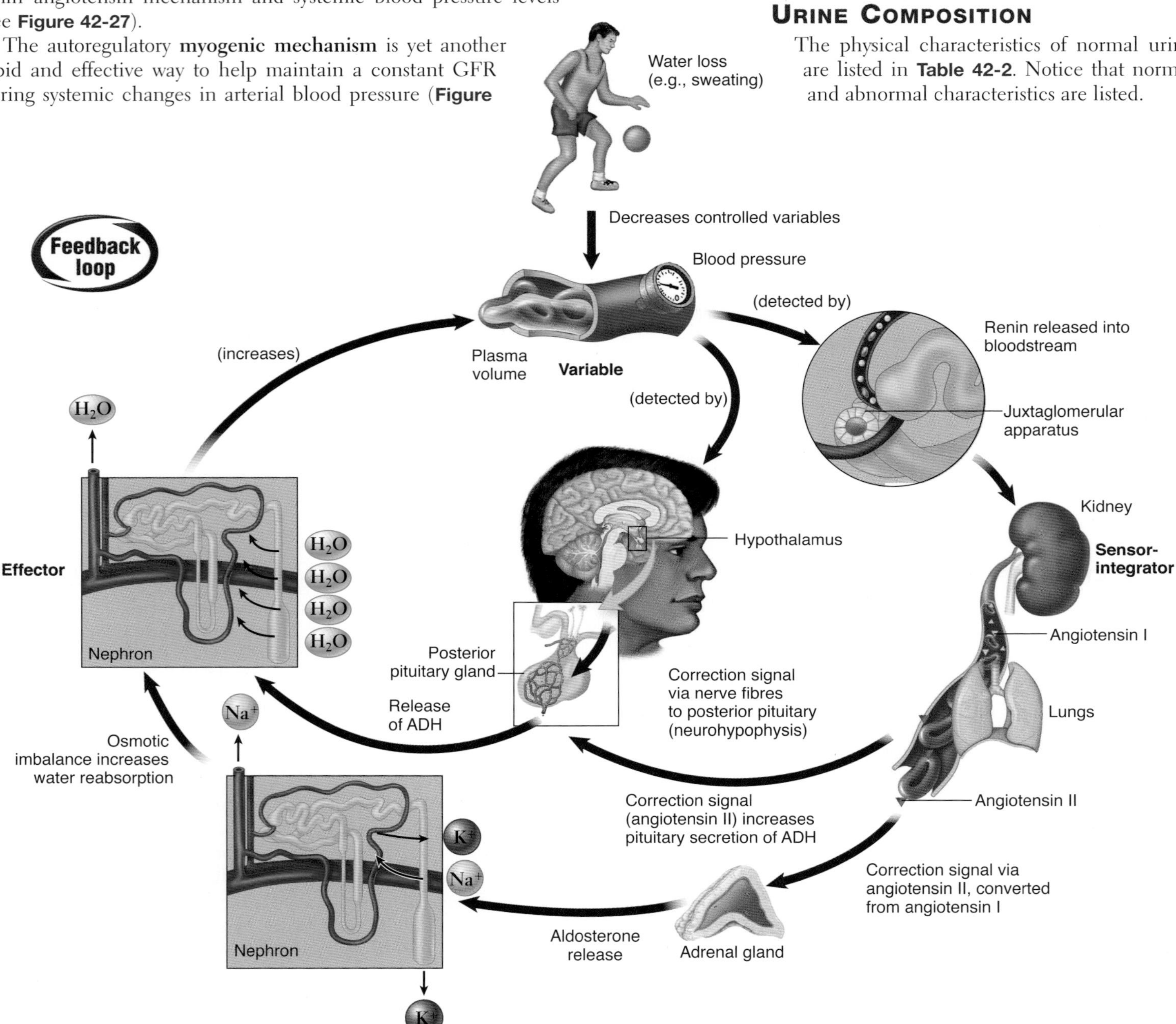

FIGURE 42-27 Cooperative roles of ADH and aldosterone in regulating urine and plasma volume. The drop in blood pressure that accompanies loss of fluid from the internal environment triggers the hypothalamus to rapidly release antidiuretic hormone (ADH) from the posterior pituitary gland. ADH increases water reabsorption by the kidney by increasing the water permeability of the distal tubules and collecting ducts. The drop in blood pressure is also detected by each nephron's juxtaglomerular apparatus, which responds by secreting renin. Recall from Chapter 26 that renin triggers the formation of angiotensin II, which stimulates the release of aldosterone from the adrenal cortex. Aldosterone then slowly boosts water reabsorption by the kidneys by increasing reabsorption of Na^+. Because angiotensin II also stimulates the secretion of ADH, it serves as an additional link between the ADH and aldosterone mechanisms.

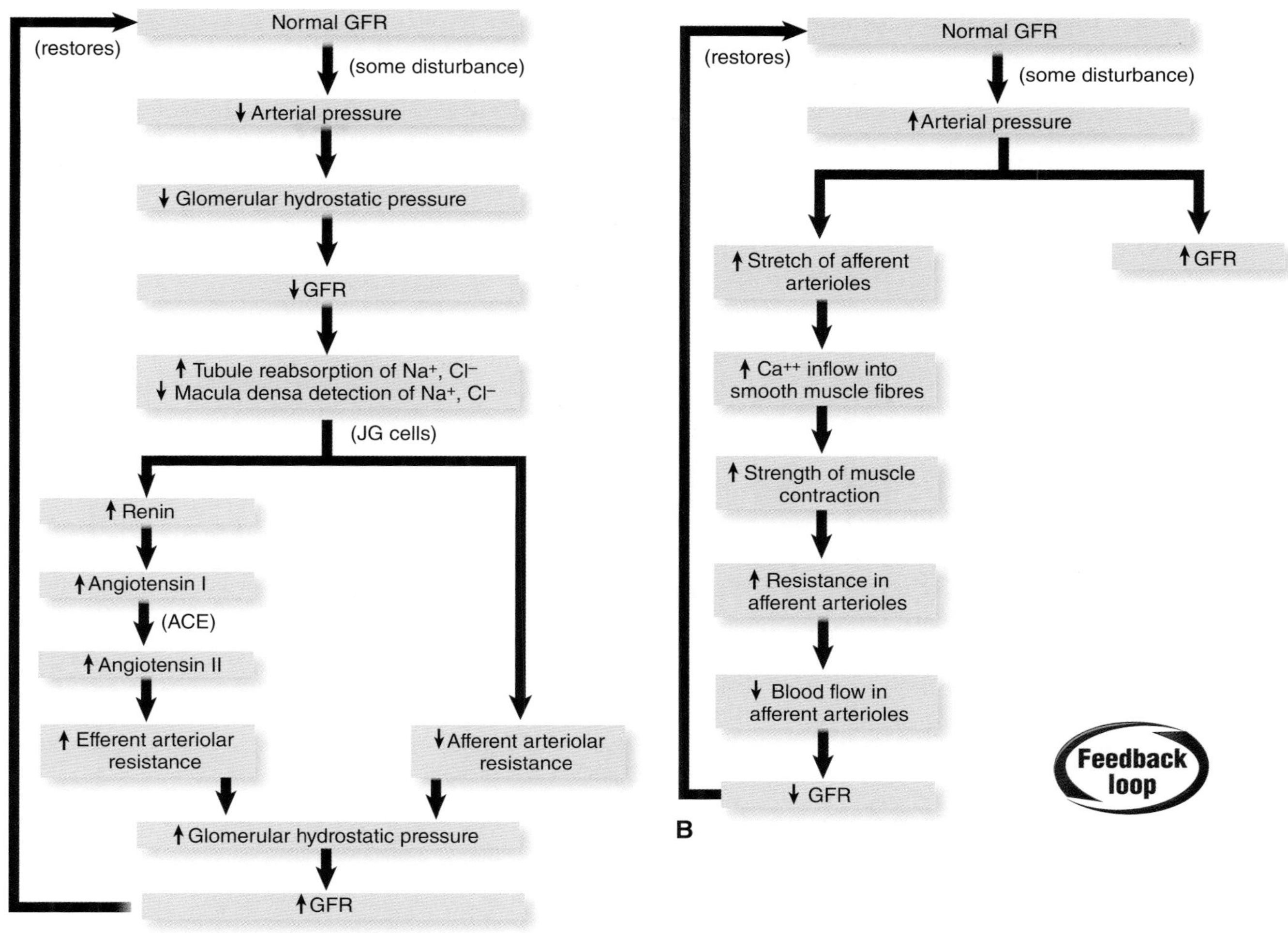

FIGURE 42-28 Autoregulation of renal blood flow and GFR. A, Tubuloglomerular feedback mechanism triggered by a disturbance that decreases renal arterial blood pressure and thus lowers glomerular filtration rate (GFR) below normal. Normal GFR is restored when juxtaglomerular (JG) cells trigger an increase of hydrostatic (blood) pressure in the glomerulus. *ACE,* Angiotensin-converting enzyme. **B,** Myogenic mechanism triggered by a disturbance that increases renal arterial blood pressure and thus increases GFR above normal. Afferent arterioles stretch and automatically contract to increase resistance and decrease blood flow, thereby reducing GFR back toward normal.

Urine is approximately 95% water, in which are dissolved several kinds of substances; the most important are discussed later in this chapter:

Nitrogenous wastes—(resulting from protein catabolism) such as urea (the most abundant solute in urine), uric acid, ammonia, and creatinine (**Box 42-4**).

Electrolytes—mainly the following ions: sodium, potassium, ammonium, chloride, bicarbonate, phosphate, and sulphate. The amounts and kinds of minerals vary with diet and other factors.

Toxins—during disease, bacterial poisons leave the body in urine. One reason for "forcing fluids" on patients suffering with infectious diseases is the need to dilute the toxins that might damage the kidney cells if eliminated in a concentrated form.

Pigments (especially *urochromes*)—yellowish bile pigments derived from products of the breakdown of old red blood cells in the liver and elsewhere. Various foods and drugs may contain, or be converted to, pigments that are cleared from plasma by the kidneys and are therefore found in the urine.

BOX 42-4 *diagnostic study*

Blood Indicators of Renal Dysfunction

Renal clearance is the volume of plasma from which a substance is removed from the blood by the kidneys per minute. Elevated urea levels in blood, as measured in a blood urea nitrogen (BUN) test, was one of the earliest clinical measurements of kidney dysfunction. Elevated BUN levels indicate failure of the kidney to clear urea and, therefore, other substances as well (see Mechanisms of Disease, p. 991, for further discussion).

Blood plasma levels of creatinine are also used to test renal function. Creatinine levels in blood seldom change significantly because they are determined by skeletal muscle mass—which seldom changes much. Therefore, an increase in the blood level of plasma creatinine is considered to be a fairly reliable indicator of depressed renal function. •

TABLE 42-2 Characteristics of Urine

	NORMAL CHARACTERISTICS	ABNORMAL CHARACTERISTICS
Colour and Clarity	Normal urine should be clear; colour varies with specific gravity Dilute urine: Transparent straw colour Concentrated urine: Deep yellow amber (Occasionally, normal urine may be cloudy because of high dietary levels of fat or phosphate)	Abnormally coloured urine may result from (1) pathologic conditions; (2) certain foods; and (3) numerous drugs: 1. Pathologic conditions (examples): Kidney cancer (haemorrhage)—red (red blood cells [RBCs]) Bile duct obstruction (gallstones)—orange/yellow (bilirubin) Pseudomonas infection—green (bacterial toxins) 2. Foods (examples): Beets—red Rhubarb—brown Carrots—dark yellow 3. Drugs (examples): Rifampicin (antimicrobial)—orange Phenytoin (anticonvulsant)—pink/red brown Triamterene (diuretic)—pale blue Cloudy urine may result from (examples): 1. Bacteria—active infection of urinary system organs 2. Blood cells RBCs—haemorrhage from kidney cancer WBCs—pus from urinary tract infection (UTI) 3. Casts—various types of tubelike clumps (blood cell, epithelial, hyaline, waxy, etc.) that form in diseased renal tubes 4. Proteinuria—(protein—usually albumin) in urine 5. Crystals—usually uric acid or phosphate/calcium oxalate in concentrated urine
Compounds	Mineral ions (for example, Na^+, Cl^-, K^+) Nitrogenous wastes: ammonia, creatinine, urea, uric acid Urine pigment: urochrome (product of bilirubin metabolism)	Ketones—generally acetone Protein—generally albumin Glucose Crystals—generally uric acid and phosphate or calcium oxalate Pigments—abnormal levels of bilirubin metabolites
Odour	Slight aromatic Some foods produce a characteristic odour (asparagus) Ammonia-like odour on standing may result from decomposition in stored urine	Strong, sweet, fruity (acetone) odour—uncontrolled diabetes mellitus Foul odour—urinary tract infections (UTIs) Musty odour—phenylketonuria Maple syrup odour—congenital defect in protein metabolism
pH	4.6–8.0 (average 6.0) Toward low normal: some foods (meat & cranberries) and drugs (chlorothiazide diuretics) Toward high normal: some foods (citrus fruits, dairy products) and drugs (bicarbonate antacids)	High in alkalosis (kidneys compensate by excreting excess base) Low in acidosis (kidneys compensate by excreting excess H^+)
Specific Gravity	Adult: 1.005–1.030 (usually, 1.010–1.025) Elderly: values decrease with age Newborn: 1.001–1.020	Above normal limits: glycosuria, proteinuria, dehydration, high solute load (may result in precipitation of solutes and kidney stone formation) Below normal limits: chronic renal diseases (inability to concentrate urine), overhydration

Hormones—high hormone levels sometimes result in significant amounts of hormone in the filtrate (and therefore in urine).

Abnormal constituents—such as blood, glucose, albumin (a plasma protein), casts (chunks of material, such as mucus, that harden inside the urinary passages and then are washed out in urine), or calculi (small stones).

CONNECT IT! 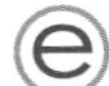

Monitoring for changes in the urine is a way to monitor overall body health. For potential signs of health dangers in urine, check out ***Toilet Signs*** online at ***Connect It!***

Quick **CHECK**

20. Does ADH promote water loss from the internal environment *or* water conservation by the internal environment?
21. How does aldosterone influence secretion in the kidney tubules?
22. How does aldosterone cause the body to conserve water?
23. What gives urine its characteristic yellowish colour?

cycle of ***life***

Urinary System The kidney plays a critical role in homeostasis by regulating the levels of many substances in blood. Primary renal functions include filtration, reabsorption, and secretion. All are interrelated by complex control systems involving central nervous system activity and hormonal secretions. More than 1 million nephron units in each kidney serve as the structural framework permitting normal function to occur.

Normally, life cycle changes in kidney structure and function occur only within rather narrow limits. Significant structural changes, such as dramatic decreases in the number of nephron units, almost always indicate serious disease or result from trauma such as crush injuries. Functionally, the kidney is able to operate normally throughout life under a wide array of conditions. If, however, the kidneys cannot cope with extreme conditions, such as water deprivation or disease, death will occur from the buildup of toxins in blood.

Initially, kidney function in a newborn is less efficient than in an older child or adult. As a result, the urine is less concentrated because the regulatory mechanisms required to retain water are not fully operative. Incontinence, or an inability to control urination, is normal in very young children. Reflex emptying occurs when the bladder fills, but normal sphincter activity keeps urine in the bladder until filling occurs. In contrast, many older adults have problems with incontinence because of loss of sphincter tone, or control.

Renal clearance is the ability of the kidneys to clear, or cleanse, the blood of a certain substance in a given unit of time, generally 1 minute. This value for certain substances tends to decrease with advanced age, thus indicating deterioration of kidney function. Changes in the porosity of the filtration membrane also occur in the elderly. Loss of functional nephron units is yet another consequence of ageing. It contributes to the gradual decline in renal function in this age group. •

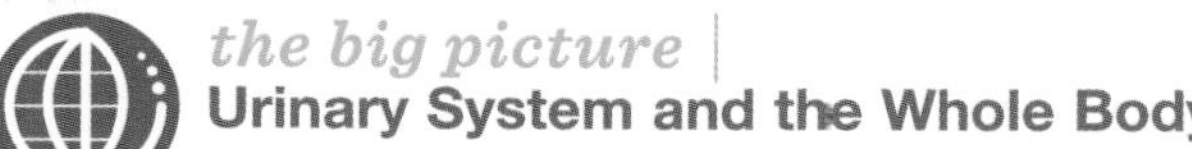

the big picture | Urinary System and the Whole Body

As our study of the urinary system has shown us, homeostasis of water and electrolytes in body fluids depends largely on proper functioning of the kidneys. Each nephron within the kidney processes blood plasma in a way that adjusts its content to maintain a dynamic constancy of the internal environment of the body. Without renal processing, blood plasma characteristics would soon move out of their setpoint range. On the other hand, without the blood pressure generated by cardiovascular mechanisms, the kidney could not filter blood plasma and therefore could not process blood plasma. Thus the urinary system and the cardiovascular system are interdependent.

Regulation of urinary function, we have seen, is often centred outside the kidney—mainly in the form of endocrine hormone action. Urinary function is also regulated to some extent by nerve reflexes. Thus both the endocrine system and the nervous system must operate properly to ensure efficient kidney function. The urinary system also interacts with many other body systems and tissues. For example, the kidneys clear the blood plasma of nitrogenous wastes and excess metabolic acids produced by the chemical activity of nearly every cell in the body. The kidneys also can clear some toxins and other compounds that enter the blood via the digestive tract, skin, or respiratory tract.

In the next chapter, we apply some of what we know about urinary function to a broader study of water and ion homeostasis within the human body's internal environment. After that, we discuss the role of the urinary system and other body systems in maintaining a relatively constant pH in the body's internal environment. •

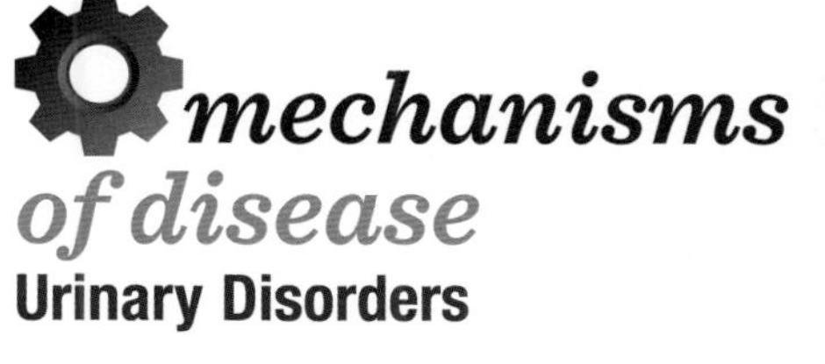

mechanisms of disease
Urinary Disorders

You may have experienced the discomfort and pain of a bladder infection or know someone who has. Bladder infection is the most common urinary disorder, but it is not usually serious if promptly treated. However, numerous renal and urinary disorders *are* very serious. Any disorder that significantly reduces the effectiveness of the kidneys is immediately life-threatening. In this section, we discuss some life-threatening kidney diseases, as well as a few of the less serious, but more common, disorders.

Renal Hypertension

Recall from Chapter 30 (p. 722) that hypertension is abnormally high blood pressure. So-called *renal hypertension* is a common type of secondary hypertension that may be caused by stenosis (narrowing) of the renal artery, often caused by the accumulation of atherosclerotic plaque. In these cases, the elevation is secondary to reduced blood flow, resulting in ischaemia of kidney tissues. When this occurs, the cells of the juxtaglomerular apparatus secrete renin, which in turn results in angiotensin production and increased blood pressure (see **Figures 30-20** and **42-27** for a review of renin–angiotensin effects). Testing of renal vein blood for increased renin levels is performed to confirm the diagnosis, and insertion of a stent into the lumen of the renal artery to increase blood flow to the kidney may be curative.

Obstructive Disorders

Obstructive urinary disorders are abnormalities that interfere with normal urine flow anywhere in the urinary tract (**Box 42-5**). The severity of obstructive disorders depends on where the interference occurs and to what degree the flow of urine is impaired. Obstruction of urine flow usually results in "backing up" of the

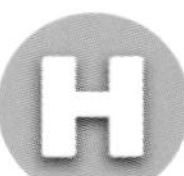

BOX 42-5 *health matters* | **Clinical Terms Associated with Urine Abnormalities**

Glycosuria or **glucosuria**—Sugar (glucose) in urine
Haematuria—Blood in urine
Pyuria—Pus in urine
Dysuria—Painful urination
Polyuria—Unusually large amounts of urine
Oliguria—Scant urine
Anuria—Absence of urine

urine, perhaps all the way to the kidney itself. When urine backs up into the kidney, causing swelling of the renal pelvis and calyces, the condition is called **hydronephrosis** (**Figure 42-29**). A few of the more important obstructive conditions are summarized here.

Renal Calculi

Renal calculi, or *kidney stones,* are crystallized mineral chunks that develop in the renal pelvis or calyces. Many calculi develop as calcium and other minerals crystallize on the renal papillae, then break off into the urine. Blood uric acid levels become elevated in those with *gout,* and deposits of uric acid in the kidneys produce uric acid stones or calculi. *Staghorn calculi* are large, branched stones that form in the pelvis and branched calyces.

If the stones are small enough, they simply pass through the ureters and urethra and are eventually voided with the urine. Larger stones may obstruct the ureters, causing intense pain called *renal colic* as rhythmic muscle contractions of the ureter attempt to dislodge it. Hydronephrosis may occur if the stone does not move from its obstructing position. In the past, only traditional surgical procedures were effective in removing relatively large stones that formed in the calyces and renal pelvis of the kidney. A technique called **lithotripsy,** which uses an ultrasound generator called a **lithotriptor,** is now used quite often to pulverize stones so that they can be flushed out of the urinary tract without surgery.

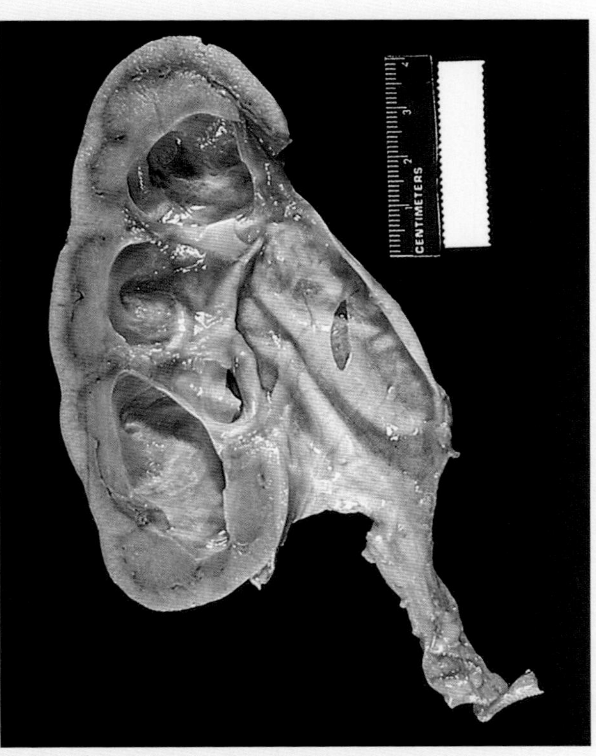

FIGURE 42-29 Hydronephrosis. Note the marked dilation of the renal pelvis and calyces caused by the blockage and "backing up" of urine.

Neurogenic and Overactive Bladder

Disruption of nervous input to the bladder results in loss of normal control of voiding. The condition is called **neurogenic bladder.** Depending on the nature and severity of the lack of nervous control, various signs and symptoms of bladder paralysis or abnormal activity result. Involuntary retention of urine, subsequent distention (bulging) of the bladder, and perhaps a burning sensation or fever with chills are common symptoms. The end result is often *urinary incontinence*—leakage of urine or some degree of involuntary urination. Serious stroke or spinal cord injury often results in a type of neurogenic bladder characterized by total loss of normal control of voiding. Called *reflex incontinence,* this is characterized by periodic but unpredictable and involuntary urination that occurs in the absence of any sensory warning or awareness.

CONNECT IT! 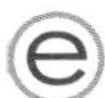

Urinary catheterization is the insertion of a flexible tube into the bladder to facilitate its emptying. To see illustrations and a brief description, check out ***Urinary Catheterization*** online at ***Connect It!***

Overactive bladder refers to the need for frequent urination because of abnormally strong or frequent micturition contractions of the bladder. If you look back to **Figure 42-9** on p. 971, you see that these contractions normally do not get strong until there is about 200 to 250 mL of urine in the bladder. With an overactive bladder, the contractions can begin to get stronger with a much lower volume of urine, which is sooner than expected. Therefore the amount voided at any one time is generally small, and feelings of extreme urgency and pain with each voiding are common. Although serious medical outcomes are rare, incontinence associated with overactive bladder is an often embarrassing and frustrating problem for those who are plagued with symptoms. In the past, treatments for this rather common problem were limited to behavioural techniques and in some cases, surgery. Now, medications are available that reduce the involuntary contractions and incontinence associated with overactive bladder. Commonly used drugs include so-called anticholinergic medications such as solifenacin and alpha-adrenergic blocker drugs that promote smooth muscle relaxation in the bladder and urethra.

Tumours and Other Obstructions

Tumours of the urinary system typically obstruct urine flow, possibly causing hydronephrosis in one or both kidneys. Most kidney tumours are malignant neoplasms called **renal cell carcinomas.** They usually occur only in one kidney. Bladder cancer occurs about as commonly as renal cancer (each accounts for about 3 in every 100 cancer cases). Renal and bladder cancer have few symptoms early in their development, other than traces of blood in the urine, or **haematuria.** As the cancer develops, pelvic pain and symptoms of urinary obstruction may occur. Insertion of a **cystoscope** through the urethra and into the bladder permits direct inspection of bladder and other lower urinary tract lesions (**Figure 42-30**). The hollow tube allows the passage of a light, a viewing lens, and various catheters and operative devices.

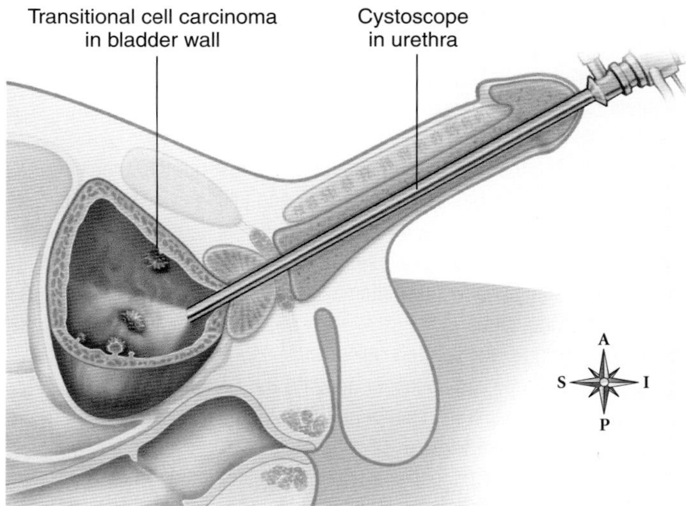

FIGURE 42-30 Cystoscopic view of bladder cancer. The cystoscope inserted through the urethra to view a male bladder.

Various other conditions can obstruct the normal flow of urine. For example, a person with a low proportion of body fat may lack the pad of fat that normally surrounds the kidneys. One or both kidneys may then drop, a condition called **renal ptosis.** In renal ptosis, the ureters that drain urine out of the kidney may kink and thus obstruct the normal flow of urine. Urinary passages may also be abnormally narrowed through scarring, inflammation, or external pressure—a condition known as a **stricture.**

Urinary Tract Infections

Most *urinary tract infections (UTIs)* are caused by bacteria, usually gram-negative types. UTIs can involve the urethra, bladder, ureter, and kidneys. Common types of urinary tract infections are summarized here.

Urethritis is an inflammation of the urethra that commonly results from bacterial infection, often *gonorrhoea.* Nongonococcal urethritis is usually caused by a *Chlamydia* infection. Males suffer from urethritis more often than females do.

Cystitis is a term that refers to any inflammation of the bladder. Cystitis commonly occurs as a result of infection but also can accompany calculi, tumours, or other conditions. Bacteria usually enter the bladder through the urethra. Cystitis occurs more commonly in women than in men because the female urethra is shorter and closer to the anus (a source of bacteria) than in males. Bladder infections are characterized by pelvic pain, an urge to urinate frequently, and haematuria. **Interstitial cystitis** is a form of bladder inflammation that occurs without evidence of bacterial infection. It is a persistent and often very painful form of cystitis that is characterized by feelings of urgency, pain on urination, and the appearance of blood in the urine. The bladder wall often shows patches of chronic mucosal ulceration. Anti-inflammatory drugs and supportive treatment of symptoms are often coupled with infusion of sterile fluid to distend the bladder and reduce feelings of urgency. Although the cause is unknown, many physicians believe an autoimmune response is involved. Interstitial cystitis is often associated with lupus erythematosus and other autoimmune disease conditions.

Nephritis is a general term referring to kidney disease, especially inflammatory conditions. **Pyelonephritis** is literally "pelvis nephritis" and refers to inflammation of the renal pelvis and connective tissues of the kidney. As with cystitis, pyelonephritis is usually caused by bacterial infection but can also result from viral infection, mycosis (fungal infection), calculi, tumours, pregnancy, and other conditions.

CONNECT IT! 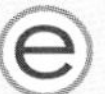

Mycotic (fungal) infections most often occur in individuals with a weakened immune system, such as the sick and elderly. To see the effects of fungal growth in the urinary tract, check out the image of an *aspergillosis* infection in ***Visualizing the Urinary Tract*** online at ***Connect It!***

Glomerular Disorders

Glomerular disorders, collectively called **glomerulonephritis,** result from damage to the glomerular capsular membrane. This damage can be caused by immune mechanisms, heredity, and other factors. Without successful treatment, glomerular disorders can progress to kidney failure.

Nephrotic syndrome is a collection of signs and symptoms that accompany various glomerular disorders. This syndrome is characterized by the following:

- Proteinuria—presence of proteins (especially *albumin*) in urine. Protein, normally absent from urine, filters through damaged glomerular capsular membranes and is not reabsorbed by the kidney tubules.
- Hypoalbuminaemia—low albumin concentration in the blood, resulting from loss of albumin from the blood through holes in the damaged glomeruli. Albumin is the most abundant plasma protein. Because it normally cannot leave the blood vessels, it usually remains as a "permanent" solute in plasma. This keeps the plasma water concentration low and thus prevents the osmosis of large amounts of water out of the blood and into tissue spaces. In hypoalbuminaemia, this function is lost and fluid leaks out of the blood vessels and into tissue spaces, thereby causing widespread oedema.
- Oedema—general tissue swelling caused by the accumulation of fluids in the tissue spaces. The oedema associated with nephrotic syndrome is caused by the loss of plasma protein (albumin), which reduces the osmotic gradient for the movement of water by osmosis from the interstitial fluid into the blood. Consequently, water accumulates in the tissue spaces.

Acute glomerulonephritis is the most common form of kidney disease. It may be caused by a delayed immune response to streptococcal infection—the same mechanism that causes valve damage in rheumatic heart disease (see Chapter 28). For this reason, it is sometimes called **postinfectious glomerulonephritis.** If antibiotic treatment is not successful, it may progress to a chronic form of glomerulonephritis.

Chronic glomerulonephritis is the general name for various noninfectious glomerular disorders that are characterized by progressive kidney damage leading to renal failure. Immune mechanisms are believed to be the major causes of chronic glomerulonephritis. One immune mechanism involves antigen–antibody complexes that form in the blood when antibodies bind with foreign antigens (or possible self-antigens). These antigen–antibody complexes lodge in the glomerular capsular membrane and trigger an inflammation response. Less commonly, the formation of antibodies that directly attack the glomerular capsular membrane causes chronic glomerulonephritis.

Kidney Failure

Kidney failure, or **renal failure,** is simply failure of the kidney to properly process blood plasma and form urine. Renal failure can be classified as acute or chronic.

Acute renal failure is an abrupt reduction in kidney function that is characterized by oliguria and a sharp rise in nitrogenous compounds in the blood. The concentration of nitrogenous wastes in blood is often assessed by the **blood urea nitrogen (BUN) test**—a high BUN result indicates failure of the kidneys to remove urea from the blood. Acute renal failure can be caused by various factors that alter blood pressure or otherwise affect glomerular filtration. For example, haemorrhage, severe burns, acute glomerulonephritis or pyelonephritis, and obstruction of the lower urinary tract may each progress to kidney failure. If the underlying cause of renal failure is attended to, recovery is usually rapid and complete.

Chronic renal failure is a slow, progressive condition resulting from the gradual loss of nephrons. There are dozens of diseases that may result in the gradual loss of nephron function, including infections, diabetes, glomerulonephritis, tumours, systemic autoimmune disorders, and obstructive disorders.

Polycystic kidney disease (PKD) is a genetic disorder in which large, fluid-filled pockets (cysts) develop in the epithelium of the kidney tubules. In this condition, *primary cilia* in the plasma membrane epithelial cells fail to do their normal job of regulating cell growth—thus allowing cells to overpopulate and obstruct the kidney tubules. The obstructions result in pockets of backed-up urine. Eventually, the kidney fails.

As kidney function is lost as a result of any of these chronic conditions, the glomerular filtration rate (GFR) decreases, causing the BUN levels to climb (**Figure 42-31**). Chronic renal failure can be described as progressing through three stages:

Stage 1. During the first stage, some nephrons are lost but the remaining healthy nephrons compensate by enlarging and taking over the function of the lost nephrons. As **Figure 42-31** shows, BUN is kept within normal limits even though up to 75% of the nephrons are lost (as indicated by a 75% drop in GFR). This stage is often asymptomatic and may last for years, depending on the underlying cause.

Stage 2. The second stage is often called *renal insufficiency.* It is during this stage that the kidney can no longer adapt to the loss of nephrons. The remaining healthy nephrons cannot handle the urea load, and BUN levels climb dramatically (see **Figure 42-31**). Because the kidney's ability to concentrate urine is impaired, polyuria and dehydration may occur.

BOX 42-6 *health matters* | Artificial Kidney

The artificial kidney is a mechanical device that uses the principle of dialysis to remove or separate waste products from the blood. In the event of kidney failure, the process called **haemodialysis** can provide a reprieve from death for the patient. During a haemodialysis treatment, a semipermeable membrane is used to separate large (nondiffusible) particles such as blood cells from small (diffusible) ones such as urea and other wastes. Part *A* of the figure shows blood from the radial artery passing through a porous (semipermeable) cellophane tube that is housed in a tanklike container. The tube is surrounded by a bath, or dialysis solution, containing varying concentrations of electrolytes and other chemicals. The pores in the membrane are small and allow only very small molecules, such as urea, to escape into the surrounding fluid. Larger molecules and blood cells cannot escape and are returned through the tube to reenter the patient via a wrist or leg vein. By constantly replacing the bath solution in the dialysis tank with freshly mixed solution, levels of waste materials can be kept at low levels. As a result, wastes such as urea in the blood rapidly pass into the surrounding wash solution. For a patient with complete kidney failure, two or three haemodialysis treatments a week are required. New dialysis methods are now being developed, and dramatic advances in treatment are expected in the next few years.

Another technique used in the treatment of renal failure is called **continuous ambulatory peritoneal dialysis (CAPD).** In this procedure, 1 to 3 litres of sterile dialysis fluid is introduced directly into the peritoneal cavity through an opening in the abdominal wall (part *B* of the figure). Peritoneal membranes in the abdominal cavity transfer waste products from blood into the dialysis fluid, which is then drained back into a plastic container after about 2 hours. This technique is less expensive than haemodialysis and does not require the use of complex equipment.

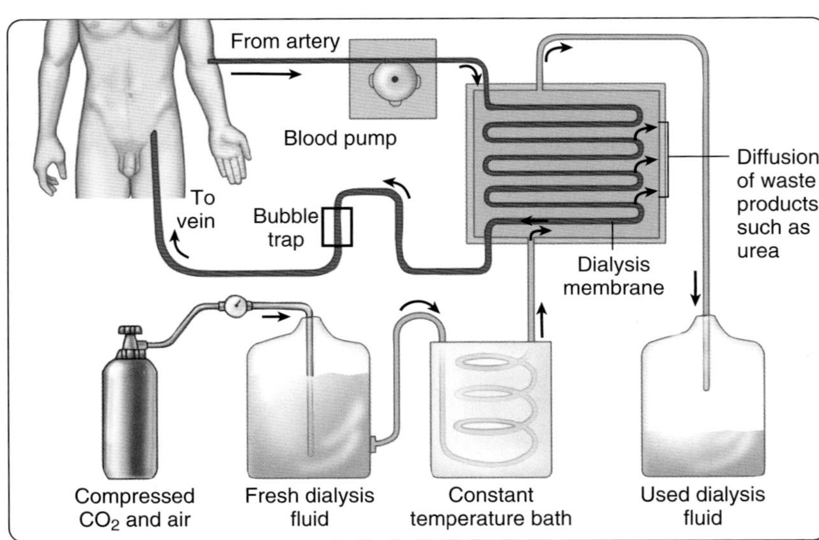

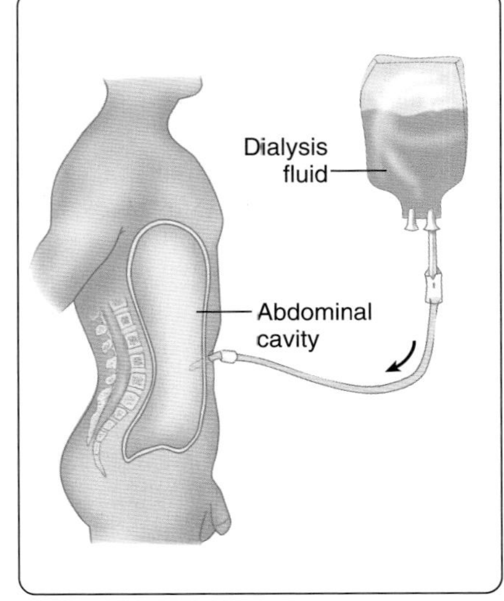

Haemodialysis.

Stage 3. The final stage of chronic renal failure is called **uraemia,** or **uraemic syndrome.** Uraemia literally means "high blood urea" and is characterized by a very high BUN value caused by loss of kidney function (see **Figure 42-31**). During this stage, a low GFR causes low urine production and oliguria. Because fluids are retained by the body rather than eliminated by the kidneys, oedema and hypertension often occur. The uraemic syndrome includes a long list of other symptoms caused directly or indirectly by the loss of kidney function. Unless an artificial kidney (**Box 42-6**) is used or a new kidney is transplanted, the progressive loss of kidney function will eventually cause death.

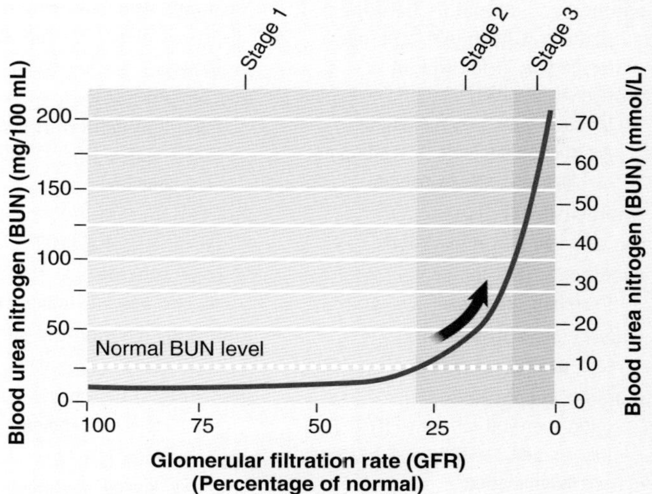

FIGURE 42-31 The three stages of chronic renal failure. Stage 1: As nephrons are lost (indicated by decreasing glomerular filtration rate [GFR]), the remaining healthy nephrons compensate—keeping blood urea nitrogen (BUN) values within the normal range. **Stage 2:** As more than 75% of kidney function is lost, BUN levels begin to climb. **Stage 3:** Uraemia (elevated BUN) results from massive loss of kidney function.

LANGUAGE OF SCIENCE *(continued from p. 966)*

juxtaglomerular cell (jux-tah-gloh-MAIR-yoo-lar)
[*juxta-* **near or adjoining,** *-glomer-* **ball,** *-ul-* **little,** *-ar* **relating to,** *cell* **storeroom**]

juxtamedullary nephron (jux-tah-MED-uh-lair-ee NEF-ron)
[*juxta-* **near or adjoining,** *-medulla-* **marrow or pith (middle),** *-ary* **relating to,** *nephro-* **kidney,** *-on* **unit**]

Loop of Henle (HEN-lee)
[*Friedrich Gustave Henle* **German anatomist**]

macula densa (MAK-yoo-lah DEN-sah)
[*macula* **spot,** *densa* **thick**] *pl.,* maculae densae

mesangial cell (mess-AN-jee-al)
[*mes-* **middle,** *-angi-* **vessel,** *-al* **relating to**]

myogenic mechanism (my-oh-JEN-ik)
[*myo-* **muscle,** *-gen-* **produce,** *-ic* **relating to**]

nephron (NEF-ron)
[*nephro-* **kidney,** *-on* **unit**]

perirenal fat capsule (pair-ee-REE-nal KAP-sul)
[*peri-* **around,** *ren-* **kidney,** *-al* **relating to,** *caps-* **box,** *-ul-* **little**]

peritubular capillary (pair-ee-TYOOB-yoo-lar KAP-ih-lair-ee)
[*peri-* **around,** *-tub-* **tube,** *-ul-* **little,** *-ar* **relating to,** *capill-* **hair,** *-ary* **relating to**]

proximal convoluted tubule (PCT) (PROK-sih-mal KON-voh-LOO-ted TYOO-byool)
[*proxima-* **near,** *-al* **relating to,** *con-* **together,** *-volut-* **roll,** *tub-* **tube,** *-ul-* **little**]

reabsorption (ree-ab-SORP-shun)
[*re-* **back again,** *-ab-* **from,** *-sorp-* **suck,** *-tion* **process**]

renal clearance (REE-nal)
[*ren-* **kidney,** *-al* **relating to**]

renal column (REE-nal)
[*ren-* **kidney,** *-al* **relating to**]

renal corpuscle (REE-nal KOR-pus-ul)
[*ren-* **kidney,** *-al* **relating to,** *corpus-* **body,** *-cle* **little**]

renal cortex (REE-nal KOR-teks)
[*ren-* **kidney,** *-al* **relating to,** *cortex* **bark**] *pl.,* cortices

renal medulla (REE-nal meh-DUL-ah)
[*ren-* **kidney,** *-al* **relating to,** *medulla* **marrow or pith (middle)**] *pl.,* medullae or medullas

renal pelvis (REE-nal PEL-vis)
[*ren-* **kidney,** *-al* **relating to,** *pelvis* **basin**]

renal pyramid (REE-nal PIR-ah-mid)
[*ren-* **kidney,** *-al* **relating to**]

renin (REE-nin)
[*ren-* **kidney,** *-in* **substance**]

sodium cotransport (SO-dee-um koh-TRANZ-port)
[*sod-* **soda,** *-ium* **chemical ending,** *co-* **with,** *-trans-* **across,** *-port* **carry**]

trigone (TRY-gohn)
[*tri-* **three,** *-gon* **corner**]

tubular reabsorption (TYOOB-yoo-lar ree-ab-SORP-shun)
[*tub-* **tube,** *-ul-* **little,** *-ar* **relating to,** *re-* **back again,** *-ab-* **from,** *-sorp-* **suck,** *-tion* **process**]

tubular secretion (TYOOB-yoo-lar seh-KREE-shun)
[*tub-* **tube,** *-ul-* **little,** *-ar* **relating to,** *secret-* **separate,** *-tion* **process**]

tubuloglomerular feedback (tyoob-yoo-loh-glow-MER-yoo-lar)
[*tub-* **tube,** *-ul-* **little,** *-glomer-* **ball,** *-ul-* **little,** *-ar* **relating to**]

ureter (YOOR-eh-ter)
[*ure-* **urine,** *-ter-* **agent or channel**]

urethra (yoo-REE-thrah)
[*ure-* **urine,** *-thr-* **agent or channel**]

urothelium (yoo-roh-THEE-lee-um)
[*uro-* **urine,** *-theli-* **nipple,** *-um* **thing**]

vasa recta (VAH-sah REK-tah)
[*vas-* **vessel,** *rect-* **straight or upright**] *sing.,* vas rectum

LANGUAGE OF MEDICINE

acute glomerulonephritis (ah-KYOOT gloh-mer-yoo-loh-neh-FRY-tis)
[*acut-* **sharp,** *glomer-* **ball,** *-ul-* **little,** *-nephr-* **kidney,** *-itis* **inflammation**]

anuria (ah-NYOO-ree-ah)
[*a-* **not,** *-ur-* **urine,** *-ia* **condition**]

blood urea nitrogen (BUN) test (yoo-REE-ah NYE-troh-jen)
[*ure-* **urine,** *nitro-* **soda,** *-gen* **produce**]

chronic glomerulonephritis (KRON-ik gloh-mer-yoo-loh-neh-FRY-tis)
[*chron-* **time,** *-ic* **relating to,** *glomer-* **ball,** *-ul-* **little,** *-nephr-* **kidney,** *-itis* **inflammation**]

chronic renal failure (KRON-ik REE-nal FAIL-yoor)
[*chron-* **time,** *-ic* **relating to,** *ren-* **kidney,** *-al* **relating to**]

UNIT 5

continuous ambulatory peritoneal dialysis (CAPD) (AM-byoo-lah-tor-ee pair-ih-toh-NEE-al dye-AL-ih-sis) [*ambulat-* **walk,** *-ory* **relating to,** *peritone-* **peritoneum,** *-al* **relating to,** *dia-* **through,** *-lysis* **loosening**]

cystitis (sis-TYE-tis) [*cyst-* **bag,** *-itis* **inflammation**]

cystoscope (SIS-toh-skohp) [*cyst-* **bag,** *-scop-* **see**]

dysuria (dis-YOO-ree-ah) [*dys-* **painful,** *-ur-* **urine,** *-ia* **condition**]

glomerulonephritis (gloh-mer-yoo-loh-neh-FRY-tis) [*glomer-* **ball,** *-ul-* **little,** *-nephr-* **kidney,** *-itis* **inflammation**]

glycosuria (glye-koh-SOO-ree-ah) [*glyco-* **sweet (glucose),** *-ur-* **urine,** *-ia* **condition**]

haematuria (hem-ah-TOO-ree-ah) [*haema-* **blood,** *-ur-* **urine,** *-ia* **condition**]

haemodialysis (hee-moh-dye-AL-ih-sis) [*haemo-* **blood,** *-dia-* **through or between,** *-lysis* **loosening**]

hydronephrosis (hye-droh-neh-FROH-sis) [*hydro-* **water,** *-nephr-* **kidney,** *-osis* **condition**]

interstitial cystitis (in-ter-STISH-al sis-TYE-tis) [*inter-* **between,** *-stit-* **stand,** *-al* **relating to,** *cyst-* **bag,** *-itis* **inflammation**]

lithotripsy (LITH-oh-trip-see) [*litho-* **stone,** *-trips-* **pound,** *-y* **action**]

lithotriptor (LITH-oh-trip-tor) [*litho-* **stone,** *-trip-* **pound,** *-or* **agent**]

nephritis (neh-FRY-tis) [*nephr-* **kidney,** *-itis* **inflammation**]

nephrotic syndrome (neh-FROT-ik SIN-drohm) [*nephr-* **kidney,** *-ic* **relating to**]

neurogenic bladder (nyoor-oh-JEN-ik BLAD-er) [*neuro-* **nerves,** *-gen-* **produce,** *-ic* **relating to**]

oliguria (ohl-ih-GOO-ree-ah) [*olig-* **few or little,** *-ur-* **urine,** *-ia* **condition**]

polyuria (pol-ee-YOO-ree-ah) [*poly-* **many,** *-ur-* **urine,** *-ia* **condition**]

postinfectious glomerulonephritis (post-in-FEK-shus gloh-mer-yoo-loh-neh-FRY-tis) [*post-* **after,** *-infec-* **stain,** *-ous* **relating to,** *glomer-* **ball,** *-ul-* **little,** *-nephr-* **kidney,** *-itis* **inflammation**]

pyelonephritis (pye-eh-loh-neh-FRY-tis) [*pyel-* **renal pelvis,** *-nephr-* **kidney,** *-itis* **inflammation**]

pyuria (pye-YOO-ree-ah) [*py-* **pus,** *-ur-* **urine,** *-ia* **condition**]

renal calculus (REE-nal KAL-kyoo-lus) [*ren-* **kidney,** *-al* **relating to,** *calculi* **little stone**] *pl.,* calculi

renal cell carcinoma (REE-nal cell kar-sih-NO-mah) [*ren-* **kidney,** *-al* **relating to,** *cell* **storeroom,** *carcino-* **cancer,** *-oma* **tumour**]

renal ptosis (REE-nal TOH-sis) [*ren-* **kidney,** *-al* **relating to,** *pto-* **fall,** *-osis* **condition**]

stricture (STRIK-chur) [*stric-* **tighten,** *-ture* **condition**]

uraemia (yoo-REE-mee-ah) [*ur-* **urine,** *-aem-* **blood,** *-ia* **condition**]

uraemic syndrome (yoo-REE-mik SIN-drohm) [*ur-* **urine,** *-aem-* **blood,** *-ic* **relating to,** *syn-* **together,** *-drome* **running or (race)course**]

urethritis (yoo-reh-THRY-tis) [*ure-* **urine,** *-thr-* **agent or channel (urethra),** *-itis* **inflammation**]

case study

William was suddenly aware of a pain in his back and groin that radiated down into his testes. The pain steadily increased and reached a maximum after about an hour, and he was sweating and nauseous. The pain then subsided slightly but continued throughout the day, so he made an urgent appointment with his GP the following morning. The GP suspected William had stones in his kidney or ureter, and a urine test showed the presence of red blood cells (haematuria) and protein.

An appointment was made for William to have an intravenous urogram (IVU). He was provided with analgesics and advised to drink 2 litres of water each day and take some bed rest until his consultation at the main hospital.

1. The GP suspects William has kidney stones. What is the most likely cause of William's pain?
   a. Kidney failure
   b. Spasm of muscles in the wall of a ureter
   c. Blockage of the urethra
   d. Irritation of the urinary bladder
2. For a kidney stone to pass naturally from the body it will have to navigate through the following structures in which order?
   a. Ureter, calyces, urethra, renal pelvis, bladder
   b. Urethra, renal pelvis, bladder, ureter, calyces
   c. Bladder, ureter, urethra, calyces, renal pelvis
   d. Calyces, renal pelvis, ureter, bladder urethra
3. The GP advised William to increase his daily intake of water to at least 2 litres. How will this affect his urinary system?
   a. His GFR will increase
   b. His volume of urine will increase
   c. He will experience temporary polyuria
   d. All of the above
4. Which of the following should not be present in a normal urine sample?
   a. Electrolytes
   b. Hormones
   c. Glucose
   d. Pigments

Hint To solve a case study, you may have to refer to the glossary or index, other chapters in this textbook, ***Connect It!,*** and other resources.

UNIT 5

CHAPTER SUMMARY

To download an MP3 version of the chapter summary for use with your mobile device, access the **Audio Chapter Summaries** *online at evolve.elsevier.com.*

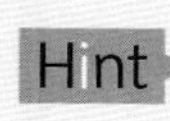

Scan this summary after reading the chapter to help you reinforce the key concepts. Later, use the summary as a quick review before your class or before a test.

Overview of the Urinary System

A. Kidneys—principal organs of the urinary system; accessory organs are the ureters, urinary bladder, and urethra (**Figure 42-1**)
B. Urinary system—regulates the content of blood plasma to maintain "dynamic constancy" or homeostasis of the internal fluid environment within normal limits

Anatomy of the Urinary System

A. Gross structure (**Figure 42-2**)
  1. Kidney
    a. Shape, size, and location
      (1) Roughly oval with a medial indentation
      (2) Approximately 11 cm by 7 cm by 3 cm
      (3) Left kidney often larger than the right; the right kidney located a little lower
      (4) Both kidneys located in a retroperitoneal position
      (5) Lie on either side of the vertebral column between T12 and L3
      (6) Superior poles of both kidneys extend above the level of the twelfth rib and the lower edge of the thoracic parietal pleura
      (7) Renal fasciae anchor the kidneys to surrounding structures
      (8) Perirenal fat capsule (renal fat pad)—heavy cushion of fat that surrounds each kidney
      (9) Hilum—concave notch on medial surface where vessels and tubes enter kidney
    b. Internal structures of the kidney
      (1) Cortex and medulla—outer and inner regions
      (2) Renal pyramids—make up much of the medullary tissue; papilla at the tip of each pyramid releases urine through multiple ducts
      (3) Renal columns—where cortical tissue dips into the medulla between the pyramids
      (4) Calyx—cuplike structure at each renal papilla that collects urine; minor calyces join to form major calyces, which in turn join together to form the renal pelvis
      (5) Renal pelvis—narrows as it exits the kidney to become the ureter; acts as a collection basin to drain urine from the kidney
    c. Blood vessels of the kidneys—kidneys are highly vascular (**Figure 42-3**)
      (1) Renal artery—large branch of the abdominal aorta; brings blood into each kidney
      (2) Interlobular arteries—between the pyramids of the medulla, the renal artery branches; interlobular arteries extend toward the cortex, arch over the bases of the pyramids, and form the arcuate arteries; from the arcuate arteries, the interlobular arteries penetrate the cortex and thus are sometimes called cortical radiate arteries
      (3) Afferent arterioles extend to the nephrons (microscopic functional units of kidney tissue)
  2. Ureter—tube running from each kidney to the urinary bladder; composed of three layers: mucous lining, muscular middle layer, and fibrous outer layer (**Figures 42-4** and **42-7**)
  3. Urinary bladder (**Figures 42-5** and **42-6**)
    a. Structure—collapsible bag located behind the pubic symphysis
      (1) Made mostly of smooth muscle tissue
      (2) Lining forms rugae
      (3) Bladder can distend considerably
    b. Functions
      (1) Reservoir for urine before it leaves the body
      (2) Aided by the urethra, it expels urine from the body
  4. Urethra
    a. Small mucous membrane–lined tube extending from the trigone to the exterior of the body
    b. In females, lies posterior to the pubic symphysis and anterior to the vagina; approximately 3 cm long (**Figure 42-8**)
    c. In males, after leaving the bladder, passes through the prostate gland where it is joined by two ejaculatory ducts; from the prostate, it extends to the base of the penis, then through the centre of the penis, and ends as the urinary meatus; approximately 20 cm long; the male urethra is part of the urinary system, as well as part of the reproductive system
  5. Mechanism for voiding bladder (urination or micturition)
    a. As bladder volume increases, micturition contractions (of detrusor muscle) increase and the internal urethral sphincter relaxes (**Figure 42-9**)
    b. External urethral sphincter muscle contracts at first, then at appropriate time relaxes to release urine
B. Microscopic structure
  1. Nephrons, the microscopic functional units, make up the bulk of the kidney; each nephron is made up of two regions (renal corpuscle and renal tubule) and connects to a shared collecting duct (**Figure 42-10**)
    a. Renal corpuscle—made up of the glomerulus tucked inside a Bowman capsule (**Figures 42-11**, **42-12**, and **42-13**); located within the cortex of the kidney
      (1) Bowman (glomerular) capsule—cup-shaped mouth of the nephron
        (a) Formed by parietal and visceral walls with a space between them
        (b) Pedicels in the visceral layer are packed closely together to form filtration slits; a slit diaphragm prevents the filtration slits from enlarging under pressure (**Figures 42-14** and **42-15**)
      (2) Glomerulus—network of fine capillaries surrounded by Bowman capsule
        (a) Fenestrations—pores in capillary walls that permit filtration

UNIT 5

(b) Mesangial cells—cells located between glomerular capillaries; various structural and functional support functions (**Figure 42-13**)
(3) Basement membrane lies between the glomerulus and Bowman capsule
(4) Glomerular capsular membrane—formed by glomerular endothelium, basement membrane, and the visceral layer of Bowman capsule; function is filtration (**Figure 42-15**)

b. Renal tubule
(1) Simple cuboidal and simple squamous epithelium
(a) Epithelial cells each possess a primary cilium
(b) Primary cilia monitor fluid chemistry and rate of flow, thus allowing regulation of tubule growth and other functions
(2) Proximal convoluted tubule (PCT)—first part of the renal tubule nearest to Bowman capsule; follows a winding, convoluted course; also known as the proximal tubule
(3) Loop of Henle (nephron loop) (**Figure 42-10**)
(a) Renal tubule segment just beyond the proximal tubule
(b) Consists of a thin descending limb, a sharp turn, and an ascending limb; ascending limb made up of thin ascending limb (tALH) followed by thick ascending limb (TAL)
(4) Distal convoluted tubule (DCT)—convoluted tubule beyond the loop of Henle; also known as the distal tubule
(a) Juxtaglomerular apparatus—located where the afferent arteriole brushes past the distal convoluted tubule
(i) Made up of macula densa (wall of distal tubule) and juxtaglomerular (JG) cells surrounding afferent arteriole
(ii) Important to maintenance of blood flow homeostasis by reflexively secreting renin when blood pressure in the afferent arteriole drops
(b) Along with other distal tubules, it joins a common collecting duct

c. Collecting duct (CD)
(1) Straight duct joined by the renal tubules of several nephrons
(2) Collecting ducts of one renal pyramid converge to form one tube that opens at a renal papilla into a minor calyx (**Figure 42-16**)

d. Blood supply of the nephron (**Figure 42-17**)
(1) Afferent arteriole enters glomerular capillary network
(2) Efferent arteriole leaves glomerulus and extends to the peritubular blood supply
(a) Vasa recta—straight arterioles that run alongside the loop of Henle
(b) Peritubular capillaries—surround renal tubule

e. Types of nephrons
(1) Juxtamedullary nephron—a nephron with a renal corpuscle near the medulla and a loop of Henle that dips far into the medulla
(2) Cortical nephron—a nephron with a loop of Henle that does not dip into the medulla but remains almost entirely within the cortex; constitutes about 85% of the total nephrons

Physiology of the Urinary System

A. Overview of kidney function
1. Chief functions of the kidney are to process blood and form urine
2. Basic functional unit of the kidney is the nephron; forms urine through three processes (**Figure 42-18**)
a. Filtration—movement of water and protein-free solutes from plasma in the glomerulus into the capsular space of Bowman capsule
b. Tubular reabsorption—movement of molecules out of the tubule and into peritubular blood
c. Tubular secretion—movement of molecules out of peritubular blood and into the tubule for excretion

B. Filtration—first step in blood processing; occurs in renal corpuscles
1. Mechanism of filtration
a. Occurs as a result of a pressure gradient (effective filtration pressure [EFP]) (**Figure 42-20**)
b. From blood in the glomerular capillaries, about 180 litres of water and solutes filter into Bowman capsules each day; takes place through the glomerular capsular membrane (**Figure 42-19**)
c. Glomerular capillary filtration occurs rapidly due to the increased number of fenestrations
2. Glomerular filtration rate (GFR)—rate of movement of fluid out of glomerulus
a. Determined mainly by glomerular hydrostatic pressure and therefore directly related to systemic blood pressure
b. Altered indirectly by changes in efficiency of cardiac contraction
c. Clinically, GFR can be estimated by renal clearance—the rate at which a substance is cleared out of blood by the kidneys

C. Reabsorption—second step in urine formation; occurs as a result of passive and active transport mechanisms from all parts of the renal tubules; major portion of reabsorption occurs in the proximal convoluted tubules (**Figure 42-19**)
1. Reabsorption in the proximal convoluted tubule—most water and solutes are recovered by the blood, leaving only a small volume of tubule fluid left to move on to the loop of Henle
a. Sodium—actively transported out of tubule fluid and into blood (**Figure 42-21**)
b. Glucose and amino acids—passively transported out of tubule fluid by sodium cotransport mechanisms; transport maximum (Tm or Tmax) is the maximum capacity of reabsorption and depends on carrier availability

c. Chloride, phosphate, and bicarbonate ions passively move into blood because of an imbalance in electrical charge
d. Water—movement of sodium and chloride into blood causes an osmotic imbalance, moving water passively into blood
e. Urea—approximately half of urea passively moves out of the tubule with the remaining urea moving on to the loop of Henle

2. Reabsorption in the loop of Henle (**Figure 42-23**)
   a. Two countercurrent mechanisms (**Figure 42-22**)
      (1) Countercurrent multiplier mechanism in loop of Henle concentrates sodium and chloride in the interstitial fluid (IF) of renal medulla (**Figure 42-23**)
      (2) Countercurrent exchange mechanism in vasa recta maintains high solute concentration in medullary IF (**Figure 42-24**)
   b. Water reabsorbed from the tubule fluid, and urea picked up from the interstitial fluid in the descending limb
   c. Sodium and chloride reabsorbed from the filtrate in the ascending limb, where the reabsorption of salt makes the tubule fluid dilute and creates and maintains a high osmotic pressure of the medulla's interstitial fluid

D. Reabsorption in the distal tubules and collecting ducts
   1. Distal convoluted tubule reabsorbs sodium by active transport but in smaller amounts than in the proximal convoluted tubule (**Figure 42-25**)
   2. ADH is secreted by the posterior pituitary and targets the cells of distal tubules and collecting ducts to make them more permeable to water (**Figure 42-26**)
   3. With reabsorption of water in the collecting duct, the urea concentration of the tubule fluid increases, which causes urea to diffuse out of the collecting duct into the medullary interstitial fluid
   4. Urea participates in a countercurrent multiplier mechanism that, along with the countercurrent mechanisms of the loop of Henle and vasa recta, maintains the high osmotic pressure needed to form concentrated urine and avoid dehydration

E. Tubular secretion
   1. Tubular secretion—the movement of substances out of the blood and into tubular fluid
   2. Descending limb of the loop of Henle secretes urea via diffusion
   3. Distal tubule and collecting ducts secrete potassium, hydrogen, and ammonium ions
   4. Aldosterone—hormone that targets the cells of the distal tubule and collecting duct cells; causes increased activity of the sodium–potassium pumps
   5. Secretion of hydrogen ions increases with increased blood hydrogen ion concentration

F. Regulation of urine volume (**Figure 42-27**)
   1. ADH influences water reabsorption; as water is reabsorbed, the total volume of urine is reduced by the amount of water removed by the tubules; ADH reduces water loss
   2. Aldosterone, secreted by the adrenal cortex, increases distal tubule absorption of sodium, thereby raising the sodium concentration of blood and thus promoting reabsorption of water
   3. Atrial natriuretic hormone (ANH), secreted by atrial muscle fibres, promotes loss of sodium via urine; opposes aldosterone, thus causing the kidneys to reabsorb less water and thereby produce more urine
   4. Tubuloglomerular feedback mechanism maintains a constant GFR by regulating resistance in afferent arterioles. Protects GFR function from rapid blood pressure variations; dependent on macula densa cells and the juxtaglomerular apparatus; may influence renin–angiotensin mechanism (**Figure 42-28**, *A*)
   5. Myogenic mechanism—rapid and effective regulation of GFR via changes in afferent arteriole smooth muscle contraction and relaxation (**Figure 42-28**, *B*)
   6. Urine volume—also related to the total amount of solutes other than sodium excreted in urine; generally, the more solutes, the more urine

G. Urine composition—approximately 95% water with several substances dissolved in it; the most important are the following:
   1. Nitrogenous wastes—result of protein metabolism; include urea, uric acid, ammonia, and creatinine
   2. Electrolytes—mainly the following ions: sodium, potassium, ammonium, chloride, bicarbonate, phosphate, and sulphate; amounts and kinds of minerals vary with diet and other factors
   3. Toxins—during disease, bacterial poisons leave the body in urine
   4. Pigments—especially urochromes
   5. Hormones—high hormone levels may spill into the filtrate
   6. Abnormal constituents—such as blood, bacteria, glucose, albumin, casts, or calculi

Cycle of Life: Urinary System

A. Life cycle changes in kidney structure and function normally occur within rather narrow limits
B. Significant structural changes almost always indicate serious disease or result from trauma
C. Kidney function in a newborn is less efficient than in an older child or adult
D. Deterioration of kidney function may occur with advanced age
   1. Renal clearance decreases
   2. Loss of functional nephron units
   3. Incontinence may occur because of a loss of sphincter tone or control

The Big Picture: Urinary System and the Whole Body

A. Homeostasis of water and electrolytes in body fluids relies on proper functioning of the kidneys; nephrons process blood to adjust its content to maintain a relatively constant internal environment
B. Urinary and cardiovascular systems are interdependent
C. Endocrine and nervous systems must operate properly to ensure efficient kidney function

REVIEW QUESTIONS

Hint

Write out the answers to these questions after reading the chapter and reviewing the Chapter Summary. Note—writing out your answers will consolidate learning and provide a valuable resource of information.

1. List the principal and accessory organs of the urinary system.
2. Name, locate, and give the main function(s) of each organ of the urinary system.
3. Identify the beginnings of the "plumbing system" of the urinary system.
4. How does the mechanism for voiding urine start?
5. The male urethra is part of two different systems. Identify them.
6. Describe the microscopic structure of the kidney.
7. Diagram the flow of blood through the kidney.
8. Define the terms *filtration, tubular reabsorption*, and *tubular secretion*.
9. How is effective filtration pressure calculated?
10. Describe the solute concentration of the interstitial fluid of the medulla.
11. What happens to sodium and chloride in the ascending limb of the loop of Henle?
12. What happens to potassium secretion when the blood aldosterone concentration increases?
13. Identify two drugs secreted by tubule cells.
14. What is the normal pH range for freshly voided urine?
15. Identify three body systems in addition to the urinary system that also excrete unneeded substances.
16. Define *retention*.
17. What is the most common cause of glycosuria?
18. What do elevated BUN levels indicate?
19. Define the term *osmolality*.

CRITICAL THINKING QUESTIONS

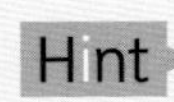

After finishing the Review Questions, write out the answers to these more in-depth questions to help you apply your new knowledge. Go back to sections of the chapter that relate to concepts that you find difficult.

1. What would result if the nerves supplying the bladder and urethra were damaged?
2. Describe the mechanism of urine formation. How is each step related to the part of the nephron that performs it?
3. If the proximal convoluted tubules were unable to transport sodium ions into blood, why would you expect to find high concentrations of both sodium and chloride ions in urine?
4. Why does ADH secretion prevent rapid dehydration of the body?
5. How is the function of ANH related to the increase in urine volume?
6. What is the relationship between age and kidney function?
7. What can you state about a person's renal clearance of creatinine if lab results show that the blood concentration of creatinine is abnormally high? What can you conclude about that person's GFR?
8. Who is most likely to experience cystitis, a man or a woman? Give reasons for your answer.
9. Predict the effects of drinking 0.5 L of water.

43 Fluid and Electrolyte Balance

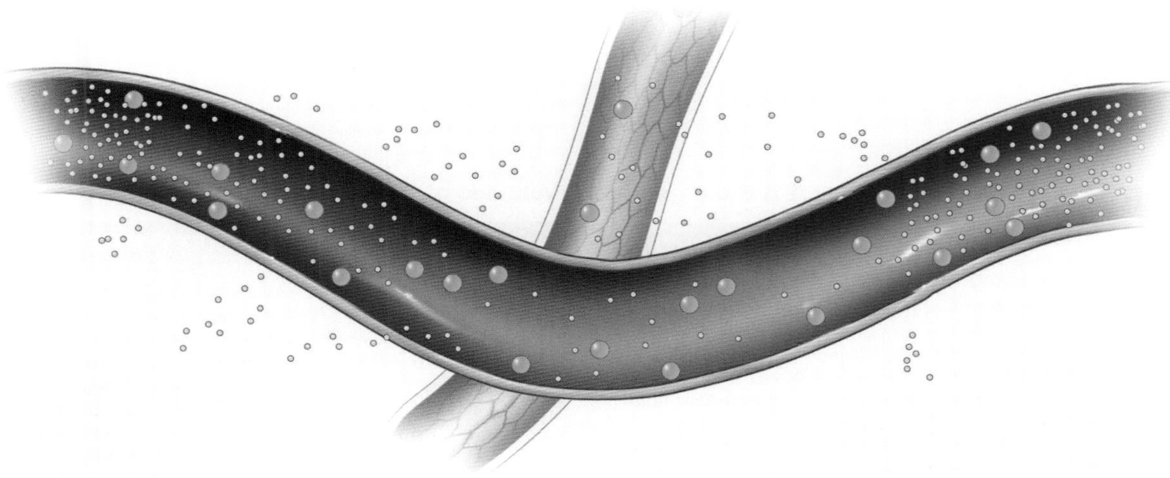

CHAPTER OUTLINE

Hint *Scan this outline before you begin to read the chapter, as a preview of how the concepts are organized.*

LANGUAGE OF SCIENCE

Hint *Use this list to aid your pronunciation of unfamiliar words.*

anion (AN-eye-on)
[*ana-* **up,** *-ion* **to go (ion)**]

blood colloid osmotic pressure (BCOP) (KOL-oyd os-MOT-ik)
[*coll-* **glue,** *-oid* **like,** *osmo-* **push,** *-ic* **relating to**]

blood hydrostatic pressure (BHP) (hye-droh-STAT-ik)
[*hydro-* **water,** *-stat-* **standing,** *-ic* **relating to**]

cation (KAT-eye-on)
[*cat-* **down,** *-ion* **to go (ion)**]

colloid osmotic pressure (KOL-oyd os-MOT-ik)
[*coll-* **glue,** *-oid* **like,** *osmo-* **push,** *-ic* **relating to**]

dehydration (dee-hye-DRAY-shun)
[*de-* **remove,** *-hydro* **water,** *-ation* **process**]

dissociate (dih-SOH-see-ayt)
[*dis-* **apart,** *-socia-* **unite,** *-ate* **action**]

electrolyte (e-LEK-troh-lyte)
[*electro-* **electricity,** *-lyt-* **loosening**]

extracellular fluid compartment (eks-trah-SELL-yoo-lar)
[*extra-* **outside,** *-cell-* **storeroom,** *-ular* **relating to**]

extracellular fluid (ECF) (eks-trah-SELL-yoo-lar)
[*extra-* **outside,** *-cell-* **storeroom,** *-ular* **relating to**]

fluid and electrolyte balance (e-LEK-troh-lyte)
[*electro-* **electricity,** *-lyt-* **loosening**]

interstitial (in-ter-STISH-al)
[*inter-* **between,** *-stit-* **stand,** *-al* **relating to**]

interstitial fluid colloid osmotic pressure (IFCOP) (in-ter-STISH-al KOL-oyd os-MAH-tik)
[*inter-* **between,** *-stit-* **stand,** *-al* **relating to,** *coll-* **glue,** *-oid* **like,** *osmo-* **push,** *-ic* **relating to**]

interstitial fluid hydrostatic pressure (IFHP) (in-ter-STISH-al hye-droh-STAT-ik)
[*inter-* **between,** *-stit-* **stand,** *-al* **relating to,** *hydro-* **water,** *-stat-* **stand,** *-ic* **relating to**]

continued on p. 1015

The phrase **fluid and electrolyte balance** implies homeostasis, or constancy, of body fluid and electrolyte levels. It means that both the amount and distribution of body fluids and electrolytes are normal and constant. For homeostasis to be maintained, body "input" of water and electrolytes must be balanced by "output". If water and electrolytes enter the body in excess of requirements, they must be selectively eliminated, and if excess losses occur, prompt replacement is critical. The volume of fluid and the electrolyte concentrations inside the cells, in the interstitial spaces, and in the blood vessels all remain relatively constant when a condition of homeostasis exists. Fluid and electrolyte imbalance, then, means that both the total volume of water and the level of electrolytes in the body or the amounts in one or more of its fluid compartments have increased or decreased beyond normal limits.

INTERRELATIONSHIP OF FLUID AND ELECTROLYTE BALANCE

Several of the basic physical properties of matter discussed in Chapter 3 help explain the mechanisms of fluid and electrolyte balance. The concept of chemical bonding is a good example. The type of chemical bonds between molecules of certain chemical compounds, such as sodium chloride (NaCl), permits breakup, or dissociation, into separate particles (Na^+ and Cl^-). Recall that such compounds are known as **electrolytes.** The dissociated particles of an electrolyte are called **ions** and carry an electrical charge. Organic substances such as glucose, however, have a type of bond that does not permit the compound to break up, or **dissociate**, in solution. Such compounds are known as **nonelectrolytes.**

Many electrolytes and their dissociated ions are of critical importance in fluid balance. Fluid balance and electrolyte balance are so interdependent that if one deviates from normal, so does the other. A discussion of one therefore necessitates a discussion of the other.

CONNECT IT! ⓔ

To ensure that we are getting sufficient input of both fluids and electrolytes into our body, we must have the ability to detect their presence in what we eat and drink. Review ***Sensing Food*** online at ***Connect It!*** to explore the mechanisms that provide such water and ion analysis.

TABLE 43-1 Volumes of Body Fluid Compartments*

BODY FLUID	INFANT	ADULT MALE	ADULT FEMALE
Extracellular fluid			
Plasma	4	4	4
Interstitial fluid	26	16	11
Intracellular fluid	45	40	35
TOTAL	75	60	50

*Percentage of body weight.

TOTAL BODY WATER

Normal values for total body water expressed as a percentage of total body weight will vary between 45% and 75%. Differences occur because of age, fat content of the body, and gender. In newborn infants, total body water represents about 75% of body weight. This percentage then decreases rapidly during the first 10 years of life. At adolescence, adult values are reached and gender differences, which account for about a 10% variation in body fluid volumes between the sexes, appear. In young, nonobese adults, males weighing 70 kg will have on average about 60% of their body weight as water (nearly 40 litres) and females about 50% (**Table 43-1**). Adipose, or fat, tissue contains the least amount of water of any tissue

TABLE 43-2 Commonly Used Abbreviations for Body Fluids and Fluid Pressures

ABBREVIATION	TERM	MEANING
BCOP	Blood colloid osmotic pressure	Force that draws water into the plasma (from the presence of colloid particles in plasma)
BHP	Blood hydrostatic pressure	Force of the blood pushing outward on blood vessel walls; blood pressure
ECF	Extracellular fluid	Any fluid outside cells, such as interstitial fluid (IF) or blood plasma
ICF	Intracellular fluid	Fluid inside the cell (cytosol)
IF	Interstitial fluid	Fluid between tissue cells
IFCOP	Interstitial fluid colloid osmotic pressure	Force that draws water out of the blood and into tissue spaces (from the presence of colloid particles in IF)
IFHP	Interstitial fluid hydrostatic pressure	Force (pressure) of the fluid between tissue cells

(including bone) in the body. Therefore, regardless of age, obese individuals, with their high body fat content, have less body water per kilogram of weight than slender people do. In aged individuals of either sex, body water content may decrease to 45% of total body weight. One reason for this is that old age is often accompanied by a decrease in muscle mass (65% water) and an increase in fat (20% water). In addition, with advancing age the kidneys are less able to produce concentrated urine, and sodium-conserving responses become less effective.

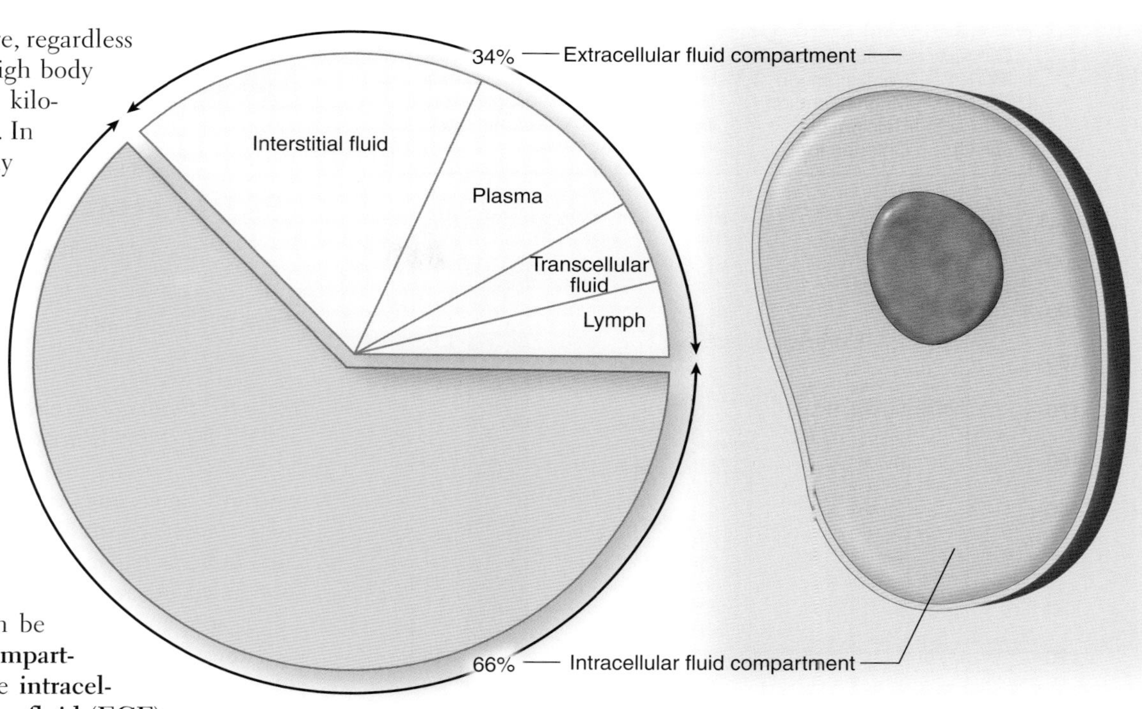

FIGURE 43-1 Distribution of total body water.

BODY FLUID COMPARTMENTS

Functionally, the total body water can be subdivided into two major **fluid compartments** called the **extracellular** and the **intracellular fluid compartments. Extracellular fluid (ECF)** consists mainly of the *plasma* found in the blood vessels and the *interstitial fluid* that surrounds the cells (**Table 43-2**). In addition, the lymph and so-called *transcellular fluid*—such as cerebrospinal fluid, joint fluids, and humours of the eye—are also considered extracellular fluid. The distribution of body water by compartment is shown in **Figure 43-1**. **Intracellular fluid (ICF)** refers to the water inside the cells.

Extracellular fluid makes up the internal environment of the body. It therefore serves the dual vital functions of providing a relatively constant environment for cells and transporting substances to and from them. Intracellular fluid, on the other hand, because it is a solvent, functions to facilitate intracellular chemical reactions that maintain life. When compared according to volume, intracellular fluid is the largest (25 L), plasma the smallest (3 L), and interstitial fluid in between (12 L). **Figure 43-2** illustrates the typical normal fluid volumes in a young adult male, and **Table 43-1** lists volumes of the body fluid compartments for both sexes as a percentage of body weight.

CHEMICAL CONTENT, DISTRIBUTION, AND MEASUREMENT OF ELECTROLYTES IN BODY FLUIDS

We have defined an electrolyte as a compound that will break up or dissociate into charged particles called *ions* when placed in solution. Sodium chloride, when dissolved in water, provides a positively charged sodium ion (Na^+) and a negatively charged chloride ion (Cl^-).

If two electrodes charged with a weak current are placed in an electrolyte solution, the ions will move, or migrate, in opposite directions according to their charge. Positive ions such as Na^+ will be attracted to the negative electrode (cathode) and are called **cations.** Negative ions such as Cl^- will migrate to the positive electrode (anode) and are called **anions.** Various anions and cations serve critical nutrient or regulatory roles in the body. Important cations include sodium (Na^+), calcium (Ca^{++}), potassium (K^+), and magnesium (Mg^{++}). Important anions include chloride (Cl^-), bicarbonate (HCO_3^-), phosphate ($HPO_4^=$), and many proteins.

The importance of electrolytes in controlling the movement of water between the body fluid compartments is discussed in this chapter. Their role in maintaining acid–base balance is examined in Chapter 44.

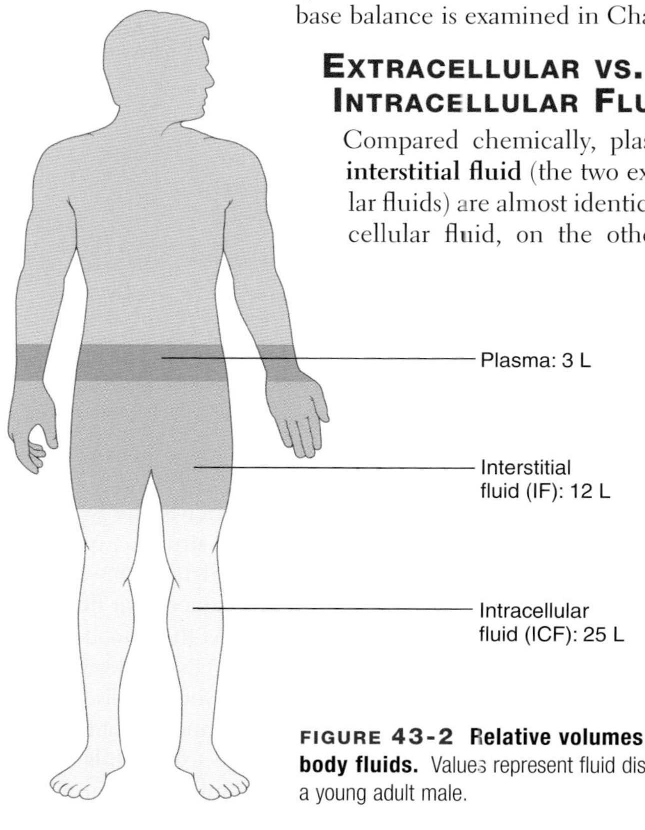

EXTRACELLULAR VS. INTRACELLULAR FLUIDS

Compared chemically, plasma and **interstitial fluid** (the two extracellular fluids) are almost identical. Intracellular fluid, on the other hand,

FIGURE 43-2 Relative volumes of three body fluids. Values represent fluid distribution in a young adult male.

UNIT 5

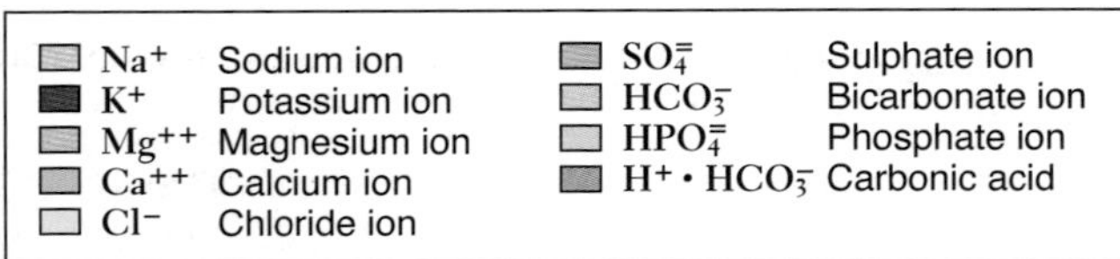

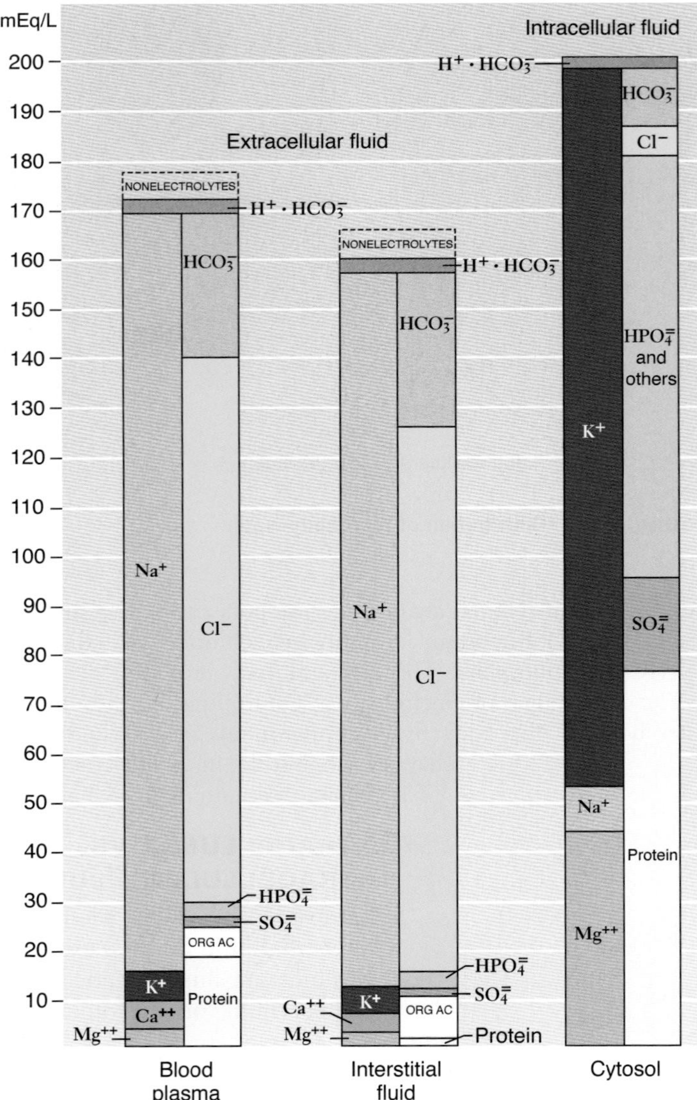

FIGURE 43-3 Chief chemical constituents of three fluid compartments. The left component of each bar in the graph shows the amounts of each *cation* (postive ion) and the right component of each bar shows the amounts of each *anion* (negative ion). *ORG AC,* Organic acid.

shows striking differences as compared with either of the two extracellular fluids. Let us examine first the chemical structure of plasma and interstitial fluid as shown in **Figure 43-3** and **Table 43-3**.

Perhaps the first difference between the two extracellular fluids that you notice (see **Figure 43-3** and **Figure 43-4**) is that blood plasma contains a slightly larger total of electrolytes (ions) than interstitial fluids do. If you compare the two fluids, ion for ion, you will discover the most important difference between blood plasma and interstitial fluid. Look at the anions (negative ions) in these two extracellular fluids. Note that blood contains an appreciable amount of protein anions.

TABLE 43-3 Electrolyte Composition of Blood Plasma

	CATIONS	ANIONS
	142 mEq Na^+	102 mEq Cl^-
	4 mEq K^+	26 HCO_3^-
	5 mEq Ca^{++}	17 protein⁻
	2 mEq Mg^{++}	6 other
		2 $HPO_4^=$
TOTAL	153 mEq/L plasma	153 mEq/L plasma

Interstitial fluid, in contrast, contains hardly any protein anions. This is the only functionally important difference between blood and interstitial fluid. It exists because the normal capillary membrane is practically impermeable to proteins. Hence, almost all protein anions remain behind in the blood instead of filtering out into the interstitial fluid. Because proteins remain in the blood, certain other differences also exist between blood and interstitial fluid—notably, blood contains more sodium ions and fewer chloride ions than interstitial fluid does.

Extracellular fluids and intracellular fluid are more unlike than alike chemically. Chemical difference predominates between the extracellular and intracellular fluids. Chemical similarity predominates between the two extracellular fluids. Study **Figures 43-3** and **43-4** and make some generalizations about the main chemical differences between the extracellular and intracellular fluids. For example: What is the most abundant cation in extracellular fluids? In intracellular fluid? What is the most abundant anion in extracellular fluids? In intracellular fluid? What about the relative concentrations of protein anions in extracellular fluids and intracellular fluid?

The reason we call attention to the chemical structure of the three body fluids is that here, as elsewhere, structure determines function. In this instance the chemical structure of the three fluids helps control water and electrolyte movement between them. Or, phrased differently, the chemical structure of body fluids, if normal, functions to maintain homeostasis of fluid distribution; if abnormal, it results in fluid imbalance. Hypervolaemia (excess blood volume) is a case in point. Oedema (discussed in detail on p. 1009), too, often stems from changes in the chemical structure of body fluids.

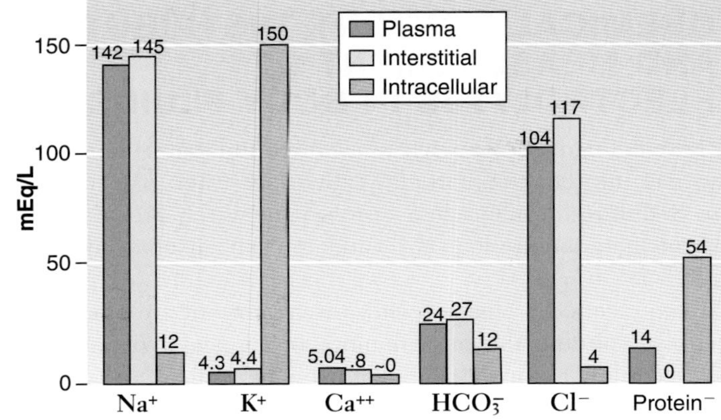

FIGURE 43-4 Electrolyte and protein concentrations in body fluid compartments. This illustration compares individual electrolyte and anionic protein concentration in the three fluid compartments.

UNIT 5

CONNECT IT! 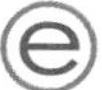

The term **parenteral therapy** is used to describe the administration by injection of special fluids that contain nutrients or electrolytes. The term implies that whatever is administered enters the body by injection and not through the alimentary canal. Examples of **parenteral** routes, including **intravenous injection** (into veins) and **subcutaneous injection** (under the skin), and how they are used to correct fluid and electrolyte imbalances are briefly outlined in ***Fluid and Electrolyte Therapy*** online at ***Connect It!***

Before discussing mechanisms that control water and electrolyte movement among blood, interstitial fluid, and intracellular fluid, it is important to understand the units used for measuring electrolytes.

MEASURING ELECTROLYTE REACTIVITY

After the important electrolytes and their constituent ions in the body fluid compartments had been established, physiologists needed to measure changes in their levels to understand the mechanisms of fluid balance. To have meaning, measurement units used to report electrolyte levels must be related to actual physiological activity.

In the past, only the weight of an electrolyte in a given amount of solution—its *concentration*—was measured. The number of milligrams per 100 mL of solution was one of the most commonly used units of measurement. However, simply reporting the concentration of an important electrolyte such as sodium or calcium in milligrams per 100 mL of blood gives no direct information about its chemical combining power or physiological activity in body fluids. The importance of valence and electrovalent or ionic bonding in chemical reactions was discussed in Chapter 3. The reactivity or combining power of an electrolyte depends not just on the number of molecular particles present but also on the total number of ionic charges (valence). Univalent ions such as sodium (Na^+) carry only a single charge, but the divalent calcium ion (Ca^{++}) carries two units of electrical charge.

The need for a unit of measurement more related to activity has resulted in increasing use of a more meaningful measurement yardstick—the **milliequivalent (mEq).** Milliequivalents measure the number of ionic charges or electrovalent bonds in a solution and therefore serve as an accurate measure of the chemical (physiological) combining power, or *reactivity*, of a particular electrolyte solution. The number of milliequivalents of an ion in a litre of solution (mEq/L) can be calculated from its weight in 100 mL by using a convenient conversion formula.

Conversion of milligrams per 100 mL to milliequivalents per litre (mEq/L):

$$\text{mEq/L} = \frac{\text{mg/100 mL} \times 10 \times \text{Valence}}{\text{Atomic weight}}$$

Example: Convert 15.6 mg/100 mL K^+ to mEq/L

$$\text{Atomic weight of } K^+ = 39$$

$$\text{Valence of } K^+ = 1$$

$$\text{mEq/L} = \frac{15.6 \times 10 \times 1}{39} = \frac{156}{39} = 4$$

Therefore, 15.6 mg/100 mL K^+ = 4 mEq/L.

***Quick* CHECK**

1. List three important cations and anions that serve critical nutrient or regulatory roles in the body.
2. Name the most abundant chemical constituent in blood plasma, interstitial fluid, and intracellular fluid.
3. Identify the units used to describe electrolyte concentration and electrolyte reactivity.

AVENUES BY WHICH WATER ENTERS AND LEAVES THE BODY

Water enters the body, as everyone knows, by way of the digestive tract—in the liquids one drinks and in the foods one eats (**Figure 43-5**). But, in addition, and less universally known, water enters the body—that is, is added to its total fluid volume—by way of its billions of cells. Each cell produces water as it catabolizes foods, and this water enters the bloodstream. Water normally leaves the body by four exits: kidneys (urine), lungs (water in expired air), skin (by diffusion and by sweat), and intestines (faeces). In accord with the cardinal principle of fluid balance, the total volume of water entering the body normally equals the total volume leaving. In short, fluid intake normally equals fluid output. **Figure 43-5** illustrates the portals of water entry and exit, and **Table 43-4** gives their normal volumes. These volumes, however, can vary considerably and still be considered normal.

***Quick* CHECK**

4. Name the type of chemical compound that breaks up, or dissociates, in solution to form ions.
5. Plasma and interstitial fluid are subdivisions of what major body fluid compartment?
6. List the volumes of body fluid compartments in a young adult female as a percentage of body weight.
7. List the major "portals" of water entry and exit from the body.

SOME GENERAL PRINCIPLES ABOUT FLUID BALANCE

The cardinal principle of fluid balance is this: fluid balance can be maintained only if intake equals output. Obviously, if more water or less leaves the body than enters it, imbalance will result. Total fluid

TABLE 43-4 Typical Normal Values (24 Hours) for Each Portal of Water Entry and Exit (with Wide Variations)

INTAKE		OUTPUT	
Water in foods	700 mL	Lungs	350 mL
Ingested liquids	1500 mL	Skin	
Water formed by catabolism	200 mL	By diffusion	350 mL
		By sweat	100 mL
		Kidneys (urine)	1400 mL
		Intestines (in faeces)	200 mL
TOTAL	2400 mL		2400 mL

UNIT 5

volume will increase or decrease but cannot remain constant under these conditions.

Mechanisms for varying output so that it equals intake are the most crucial means of maintaining fluid balance, but mechanisms for adjusting intake to output also operate. **Figure 43-6** summarizes the role of the *renin–angiotensin–aldosterone system (RAAS)* in decreasing fluid output (urine volume) to compensate for decreased intake.

Recall from Chapter 42 that cells in the outer zone of the adrenal cortex that secrete aldosterone are also influenced by *juxtaglomerular (JG) cells* in the kidney. If blood pressure decreases or if increased levels of plasma K^+ occur, additional aldosterone will be secreted. When stimulated, juxtaglomerular cells in the kidney secrete renin, which, in turn, acts on angiotensinogen in the bloodstream to form angiotensin I, which is eventually converted in lung tissue to angiotensin II (see **Figure 26-19**, p. 594). Angiotensin I and II increase aldosterone secretion and also act on the brain to stimulate the sensation of thirst. Thirst is associated with any factor that decreases the total volume of body water, such as blood loss or haemorrhage. Simple dehydration caused by sweating also results in reduced saliva secretion and thirst. Additional details of the renin–angiotensin–aldosterone system are discussed in Chapter 26. **Figure 43-7** diagrams a mechanism for adjusting intake to compensate for excess output.

Mechanisms for controlling water movement between the fluid compartments of the body are the most rapid-acting fluid balance processes. They serve first of all to maintain normal blood volume at the expense of interstitial fluid volume.

MECHANISMS THAT MAINTAIN HOMEOSTASIS OF TOTAL FLUID VOLUME

In normal conditions, homeostasis of the total volume of water in the body is maintained or restored primarily by mechanisms that adjust output (urine volume) to intake and secondarily by mechanisms that adjust fluid intake.

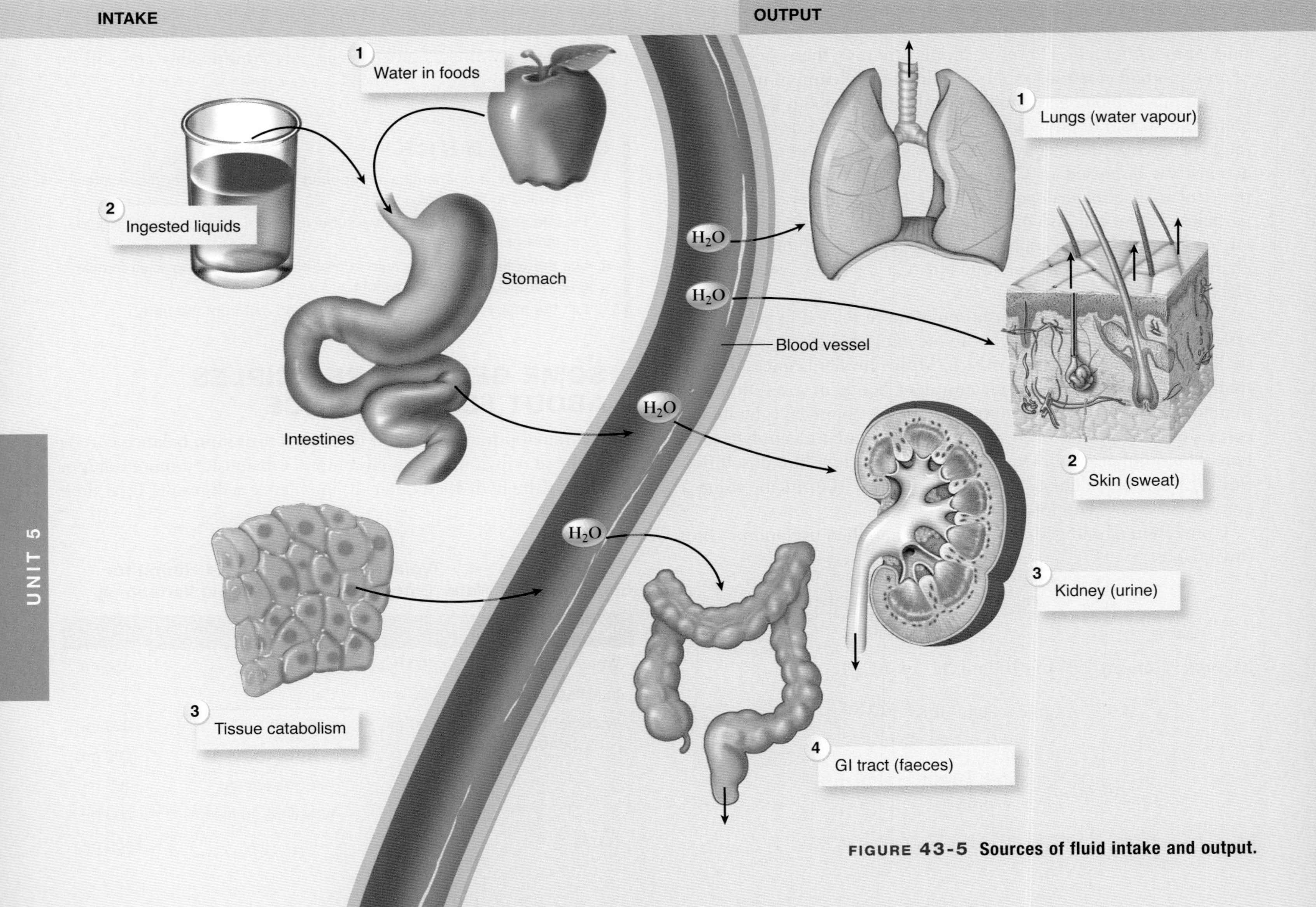

FIGURE 43-5 Sources of fluid intake and output.

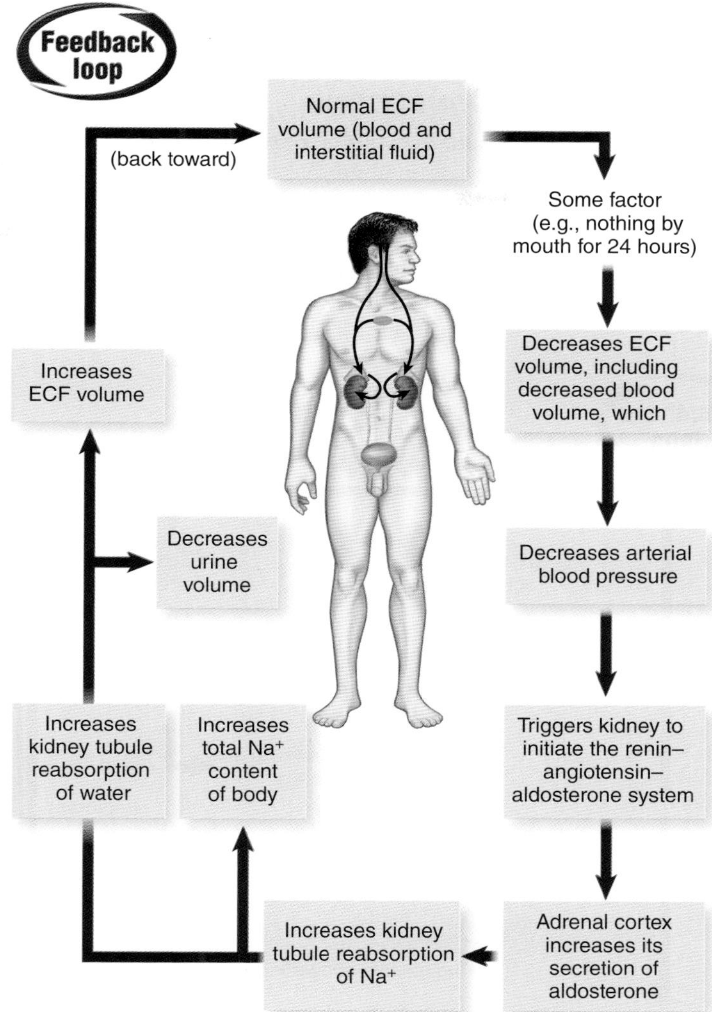

FIGURE 43-6 Role of aldosterone in ECF homeostasis. Aldosterone tends to restore normal extracellular fluid (ECF) volume when it decreases below normal. Excess aldosterone, however, leads to excess ECF volume—that is, excess blood volume (hypervolaemia) and excess interstitial fluid volume (oedema)—as well as an excess of the total Na^+ content of the body. Details of the renin–angiotensin–aldosterone system (RAAS) are shown in **Figure 26-19**.

Regulation of Fluid Intake

A detailed explanation of the mechanism for controlling fluid intake so that it increases when output increases and decreases when output decreases is not yet available. However, research has shown that nerve cells located in the roof of the third ventricle of the brain, in a structure called the **subfornical organ**, or **SFO**, act as critical regulators of fluid homeostasis. Nervous connections exist between SFO cells and other areas of the brain, including the cerebrum and the supraoptic and paraventricular nuclei of the hypothalamus. These nuclei are involved in antidiuretic hormone (ADH) production, which is important in conservation of body water when fluid intake is restricted (see Chapter 26, p. 585, and **Figure 43-16**).

Physiologists now identify both SFO and ADH-secreting cells in the hypothalamus as important **osmoreceptors**, which together make up the functional **thirst centre** of the brain. Osmoreceptors are cells able to detect an increase in solute concentration (osmolality) in extracellular fluid caused by water loss. Signals generated by osmoreceptors in the SFO and hypothalamus stimulate ADH secretion and also affect a number of other body functions, including a decrease in the secretion of saliva.

Signals from the SFO are also sent directly to the cerebrum, where they trigger a conscious sense of dry mouth and thirst and initiate complex behaviours and thought processes, which in many individuals include a perceived need to increase the consumption of water especially. Have you ever heard someone say, "Cola tastes good but nothing satisfies my thirst like a glass of water"? The end result is an overall increase in fluid intake to offset increased loss, regardless of cause, and this tends to restore fluid balance (see **Figure 43-7**). If, however, an individual takes nothing by mouth for several days, fluid balance cannot be maintained despite every effort of homeostatic mechanisms to compensate for the zero intake. Obviously, in this condition, the only way balance could be maintained would be for fluid output to also decrease to zero. But this cannot occur. Some output is obligatory. Why? Because as long as respirations continue, some water leaves the body by way of expired air. Also, as long as life continues, an irreducible minimum of water diffuses through the skin.

Regulation of Urine Volume

Two factors together determine urine volume: the glomerular filtration rate and the rate of water reabsorption by the renal tubules. The glomerular filtration rate, except under abnormal conditions, remains fairly constant—hence it does not normally cause urine volume to fluctuate. The rate of tubular reabsorption of water, on the other hand, fluctuates considerably. The rate of tubular reabsorption, therefore, rather than the glomerular filtration rate, normally adjusts urine volume to fluid intake. The amount of ADH and aldosterone secreted regulates the amount of water reabsorbed by the kidney tubules (discussed on p. 984; see also **Figure 43-6**). In other words, urine volume is regulated chiefly by hormones secreted by the posterior

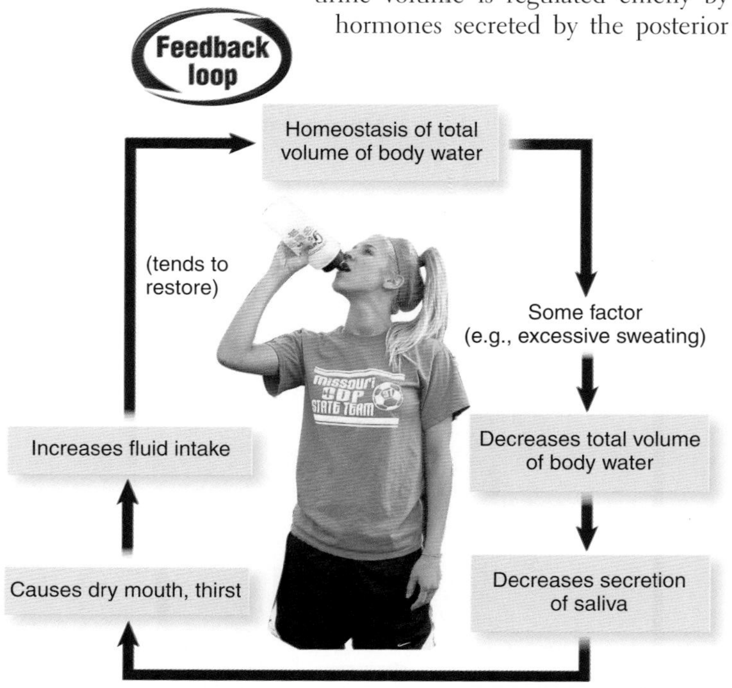

Feedback loop

Homeostasis of total volume of body water

(tends to restore)

Some factor (e.g., excessive sweating)

Decreases total volume of body water

Decreases secretion of saliva

Causes dry mouth, thirst

Increases fluid intake

FIGURE 43-7 Homeostasis of the total volume of body water. A basic mechanism for adjusting intake to compensate for excess output of body fluid is diagrammed.

pituitary (ADH) and by the adrenal cortex (aldosterone) and by atrial natriuretic hormone (ANH). Regulation of aldosterone secretion by the renin–angiotensin mechanism has also been discussed.

Although changes in the volume of fluid loss via the skin, the lungs, and the intestines also affect the fluid intake/output ratio, these volumes are not automatically adjusted to intake volume, as is the volume of urine. **Figure 43-8** summarizes the fluid and electrolyte regulation mechanisms that involve ADH, aldosterone, and ANH.

Factors That Alter Fluid Loss In Abnormal Conditions

The rate of respiration and the volume of sweat secreted may greatly alter fluid output under certain abnormal conditions. For example, a patient who hyperventilates for an extended time loses an excessive amount of water via the expired air. If, as often happens, the individual also takes in less water by mouth than normal, the fluid output then exceeds intake and a fluid imbalance develops—namely, **dehydration**

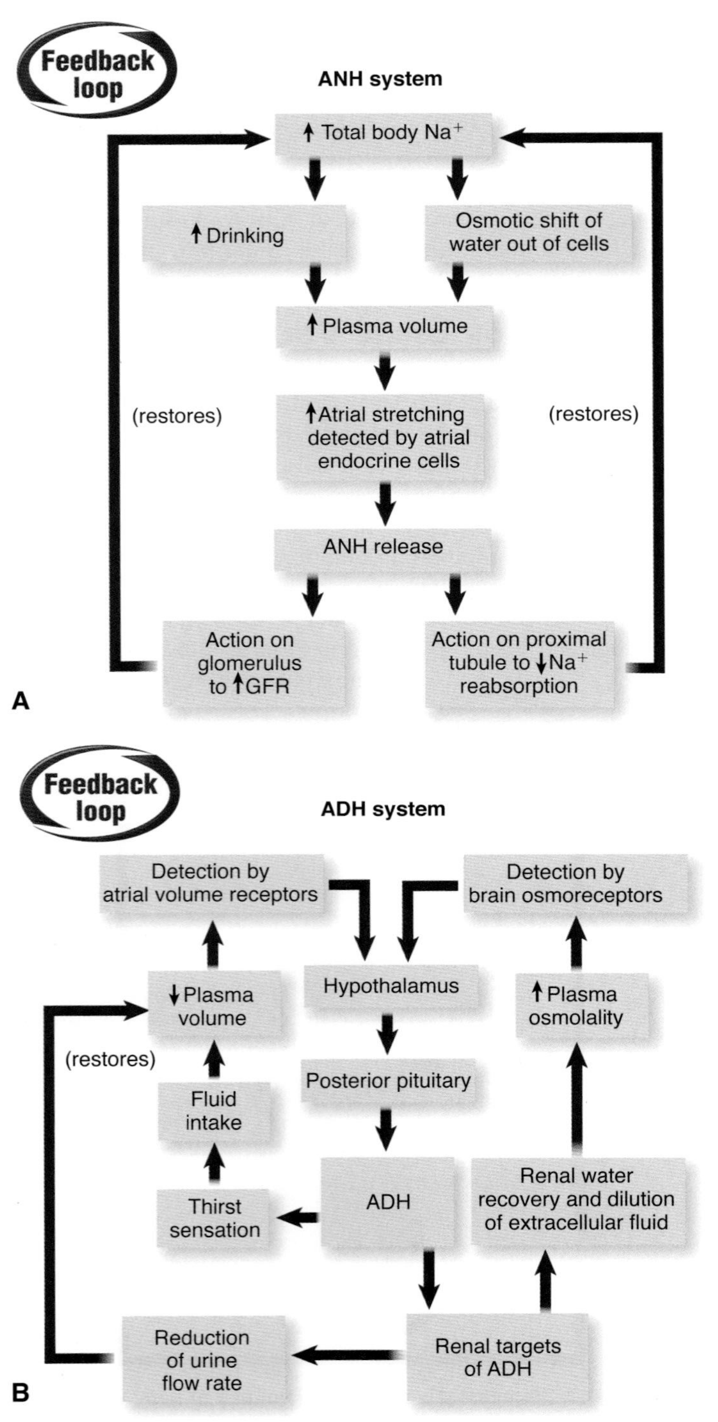

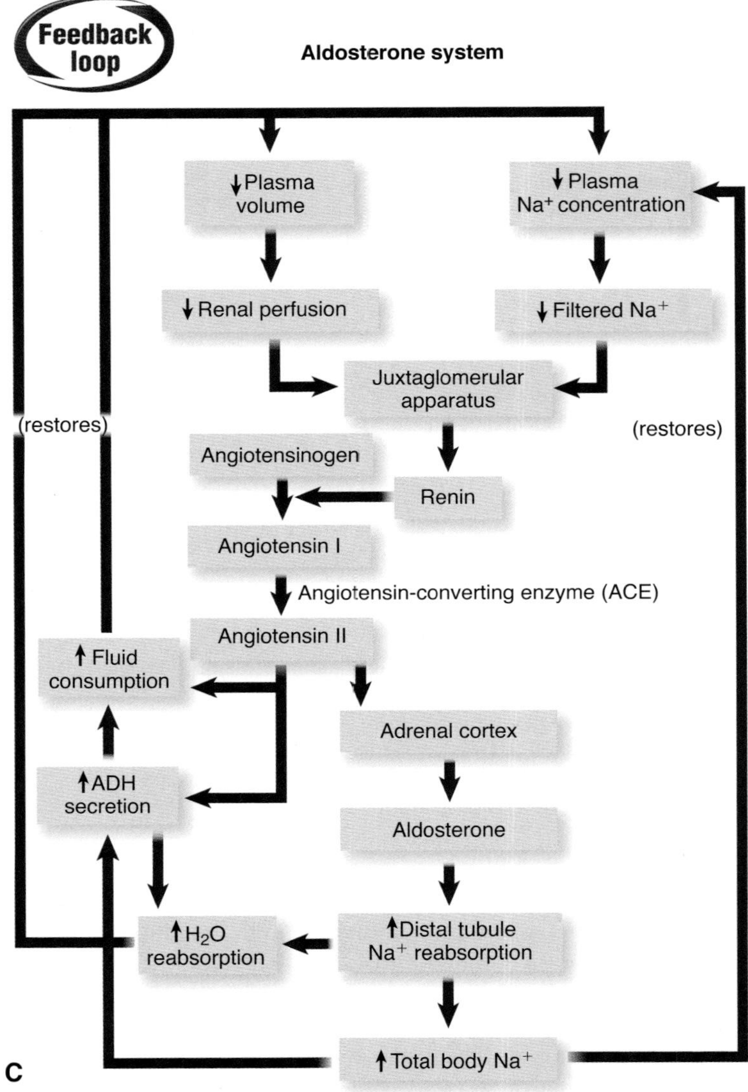

FIGURE 43-8 Mechanisms of fluid and electrolyte regulation. A, The ANH system. **B,** The ADH system. **C,** The aldosterone system. *ADH,* Antidiuretic hormone; *ANH,* atrial natriuretic hormone; *GFR,* glomerular filtration rate.

(i.e., a decrease in total body water). The severity of dehydration can be measured by weight loss as a percentage of the normal (hydrated) body weight (**Figure 43-9**). Symptoms range from simple thirst to muscle weakness and kidney failure. Clinically, dehydration is often detected by loss of skin elasticity or *turgor.* If a fold of skin, when pinched, returns to its original shape slowly—a condition called "tenting"—dehydration is suspected. Dehydration is more fully discussed in **Box 43-1**. Other abnormal conditions such as vomiting, diarrhoea, or intestinal drainage also cause fluid and electrolyte output to exceed intake and thus produce fluid and electrolyte imbalances.

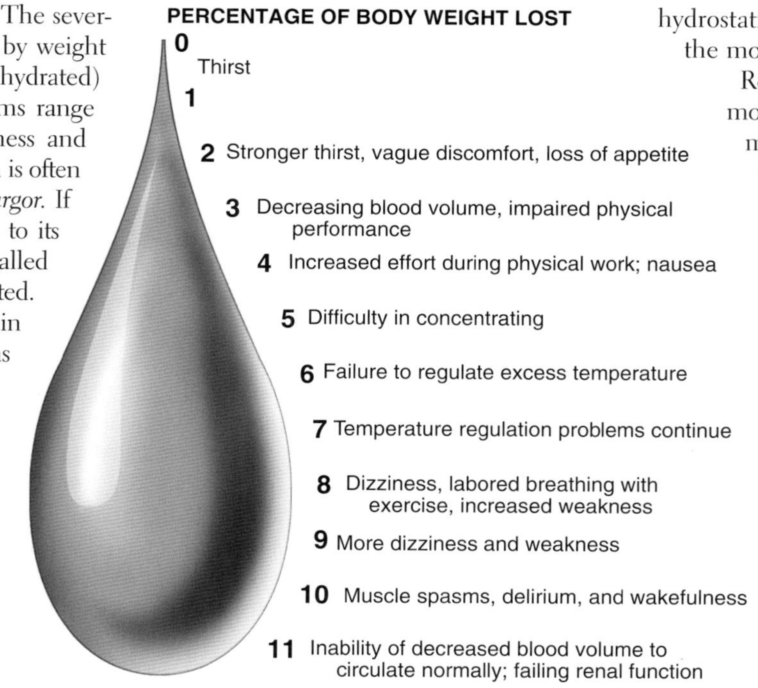

FIGURE 43-9 The effects of dehydration.

Quick CHECK

8. How does aldosterone secretion restore normal extracellular fluid (ECF) volume when it decreases below normal?
9. Identify the two substances that are most important in regulating the amount of water reabsorbed by the kidney tubules.
10. Name the two most important factors that alter fluid loss under abnormal conditions.

REGULATION OF WATER AND ELECTROLYTE LEVELS IN PLASMA AND INTERSTITIAL FLUID

More than 70 years ago, the English physiologist Ernest Starling advanced a hypothesis about the nature of the mechanisms that control water movement between plasma and interstitial fluid (extracellular fluid)—that is, across the capillary membrane. This hypothesis has since become one of the major premises of physiology and is often spoken of as *Starling's law of the capillaries,* illustrated in **Figure 30-19** on p. 713. According to this law, the control mechanism for water exchange between plasma and interstitial fluid consists of four types of pressure: *blood hydrostatic* and *colloid osmotic pressures* on one side of the capillary membrane and *interstitial fluid hydrostatic* and *colloid osmotic pressures* on the other side. Note—in the sections that follow pressures are expressed in kilopascals (kPa) and millimetres of mercury (mmHg) (1 mmHg = 0.13 kPa).

We are ready now to try to answer the following question: how does the nature of body fluids affect water movement between them, thereby influencing fluid distribution in the body?

According to this law, water exchange between plasma and interstitial fluid is determined by two opposing forces: filtration due to a hydrostatic pressure gradient, and osmosis due to osmotic pressure. The **blood hydrostatic pressure (BHP)**, which is the pressure in the capillaries, is higher than the **interstitial fluid hydrostatic pressure (IFHP)**, which is the pressure in the tissues. Fluid moves across a membrane from a higher to a lower pressure. Therefore filtration moves fluid out of the blood into the tissues, and the greater the hydrostatic pressure difference, the greater the movement of fluid.

Recall from Chapter 6 that fluid moves across a selectively permeable membrane from an area of lower osmotic pressure to an area of higher osmotic pressure. The osmotic pressure of plasma is called the **blood colloid osmotic pressure (BCOP)**, and the osmotic pressure of interstitial fluid is called the **interstitial fluid colloid osmotic pressure (IFCOP)**. Colloid osmotic pressure is due to impermeant proteins. Water moves by osmosis out of the tissues into the blood because BCOP is greater than IFCOP. The greater the osmotic pressure difference, the greater the movement of water by osmosis.

The difference between these opposing forces is the effective filtration pressure (EFP)—in other words, the net force moving fluid between the blood and interstitial fluid. In general terms, we may state Starling's law of the capillaries this way: the rate and direction of fluid exchange between capillaries and interstitial fluid are determined by the hydrostatic and colloid osmotic pressures of the two fluids. Or, we may state it more specifically as a formula:

$$\text{EFP} = \text{Filtration} - \text{Osmosis}$$
$$\text{EFP} = (\text{BHP} - \text{IFHP}) - (\text{BCOP} - \text{IFCOP})$$

To illustrate the operation of Starling's law, let us consider how it controls water exchange at the arterial ends of tissue capillaries. The lower left-hand portion of **Figure 43-10** gives normal pressures at the arterial end of capillaries. Using these figures in Starling's law of the capillaries, we get an EFP of (35 − 2) − (24 − 0) = 9 mmHg or using kilopascals (4.7 − 0.3) − (3.2 − 0) = 1.2 kPa. The movement of water into tissues due to a hydrostatic pressure difference (33 mmHg or 4.4 kPa) is greater than the movement of water out of tissues due to an osmotic pressure difference (24 mmHg or 3.2 kPa). The result is a net movement of water into tissues.

The same law operates at the venous end of capillaries (see the lower right-hand portion of **Figure 43-10**). Note that resistance to blood flow through capillaries causes BHP at the venous ends of capillaries to be lower than at the arterial ends. The movement of water changes osmotic pressure values. A gain of water by the interstitial fluid at the arterial ends of capillaries dilutes interstitial fluid concentration, lowering IFCOP to essentially zero. A loss of water from the interstitial fluid at the venous ends of capillaries increases interstitial fluid concentration and IFCOP. A loss of water from blood as it passes through the capillaries slightly increases BCOP.

Using **Figure 43-10** again, the EFP at the venous ends of capillaries is (15 − 1) − (25 − 3) = −8 mmHg or using kilopascals (2.0 − 0.1) − (3.3 − 0.4) = −1.0 kPa. The movement of water out of tissues due to an osmotic pressure difference (22 mmHg or 2.9 kPa) is greater than

BOX 43-1 *dehydration*

The term **dehydration** is used to describe the condition that results from excessive loss of body water. Loss of skin resiliency or pressure—often described as a loss of **turgor**—is a sign of dehydration (Figure *A*). Water deprivation or loss triggers a complex series of protective responses designed to maintain homeostasis of water and electrolyte levels.

Unfortunately, the term *dehydration* is incomplete. It does not, by definition, include the loss of electrolytes. To understand the control mechanisms that ensure fluid and electrolyte balance or properly interpret the clinical signs and symptoms of dehydration in disease states, it is important to realize that in any process of dehydration, water loss is always accompanied by loss of electrolytes. If water intake is reduced to the point of dehydration, a corresponding quantity of electrolytes must be removed to maintain the normal ionic content of body fluids. The same is true in the case of electrolyte loss when an accompanying loss of water must occur to maintain homeostasis of both fluid and electrolyte levels. Understanding the close interrelationships of water and electrolyte loss in dehydration provides the rationale for effective treatment. Water alone is inadequate; treatment of dehydration also requires appropriate electrolyte replacement therapy.

As discussed in Chapter 10, maintaining a constant core body temperature in a hot environment is an important function of the skin. As sweat evaporates, excess body heat can be eliminated. In hot weather or during extended periods of strenuous physical activity, the volume of water lost because of sweat production can reach 15 litres per day (Figure *B*). If water intake is inadequate, signs of dehydration will appear very rapidly. As body water levels decrease, the initial defence mechanisms are directed toward maintaining an adequate blood volume.

In addition to water, sweat contains significant quantities of sodium and chloride. However, the relative loss of water in sweat is greater than the loss of electrolytes. Therefore, as water is shifted from the interstitial fluid compartment to the plasma to compensate for fluid loss, the kidneys excrete the excess electrolytes to preserve normal ionic concentrations in the two compartments.

The chemical composition and actual volume of fluids lost from the body will also affect the type and effectiveness of defence mechanisms that occur. For example, fluids lost through vomiting or diarrhoea will have differing ratios of fluid to electrolytes than sweat has, and the actual electrolyte composition and concentration will also be different. As a result, the type of electrolyte excretion or retention by the kidneys that will be needed to maintain ionic balance in the fluid compartments will also change.

There is a lag in the volume–electrolyte adjustment mechanism triggered by dehydration. Shifts in fluid occur more quickly between compartments than does the adjustment in electrolyte levels. However, if water and electrolyte losses are limited and the interval between loss and replacement is short, the symptoms of dehydration will be mild and transitory.

In severe and prolonged water deprivation or loss, the initial shift of interstitial fluid to plasma will be followed by movement of water from the intracellular compartment as well. Over time, the extracellular and intracellular fluid losses are about equal.

Extracellular (interstitial) water is more "expendable" and quickly accessible as a fluid source to maintain blood volume in the early stages of body fluid loss. It is said to serve as the "first line of defence" against dehydration. As extracellular fluid is depleted, intracellular water must be used to prolong survival time. Ultimately, the volume of extracellular fluid can be reduced by almost 60% and intracellular fluid by 30% before death occurs. •

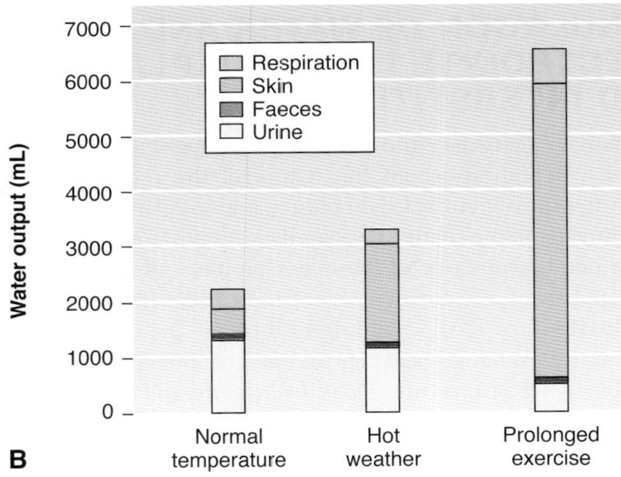

A, Testing for dehydration. Loss of skin elasticity or turgor is a sign of dehydration. Skin that does not return quickly to its normal shape after being pinched indicates interstitial water loss. **B, Water loss during varying conditions.** During hot weather or prolonged exercise, there is a dramatic increase in water output—mostly from the skin in the form of sweat. Water intake must also dramatically increase to offset the difference; otherwise, dehydration will occur.

the movement of water into tissues due to a hydrostatic pressure difference (14 mmHg or 1.9 kPa). Thus, there is net movement of water out of the tissues into the blood, which is indicated by a negative number.

Because the magnitude of the EFP moving fluid into the tissues (9 mmHg or 1.2 kPa) is greater than the EFP moving fluid out (−8 mmHg or 1.0 kPa), more fluid enters the tissues at the arterial ends of capillaries than leaves at the venous ends. Note in **Figure 43-10** that the blind-ended lymphatic capillaries in the tissue serve as a mechanism for the drainage of excess interstitial fluid. Pressure changes result in the movement of interstitial fluid and small proteins into the lymphatic system. Approximately $^{9}/_{10}$ of the fluid volume entering the tissues returns to the blood at the venous ends of capillaries. The remaining $^{1}/_{10}$ enters the lymphatic capillaries and returns to the blood.

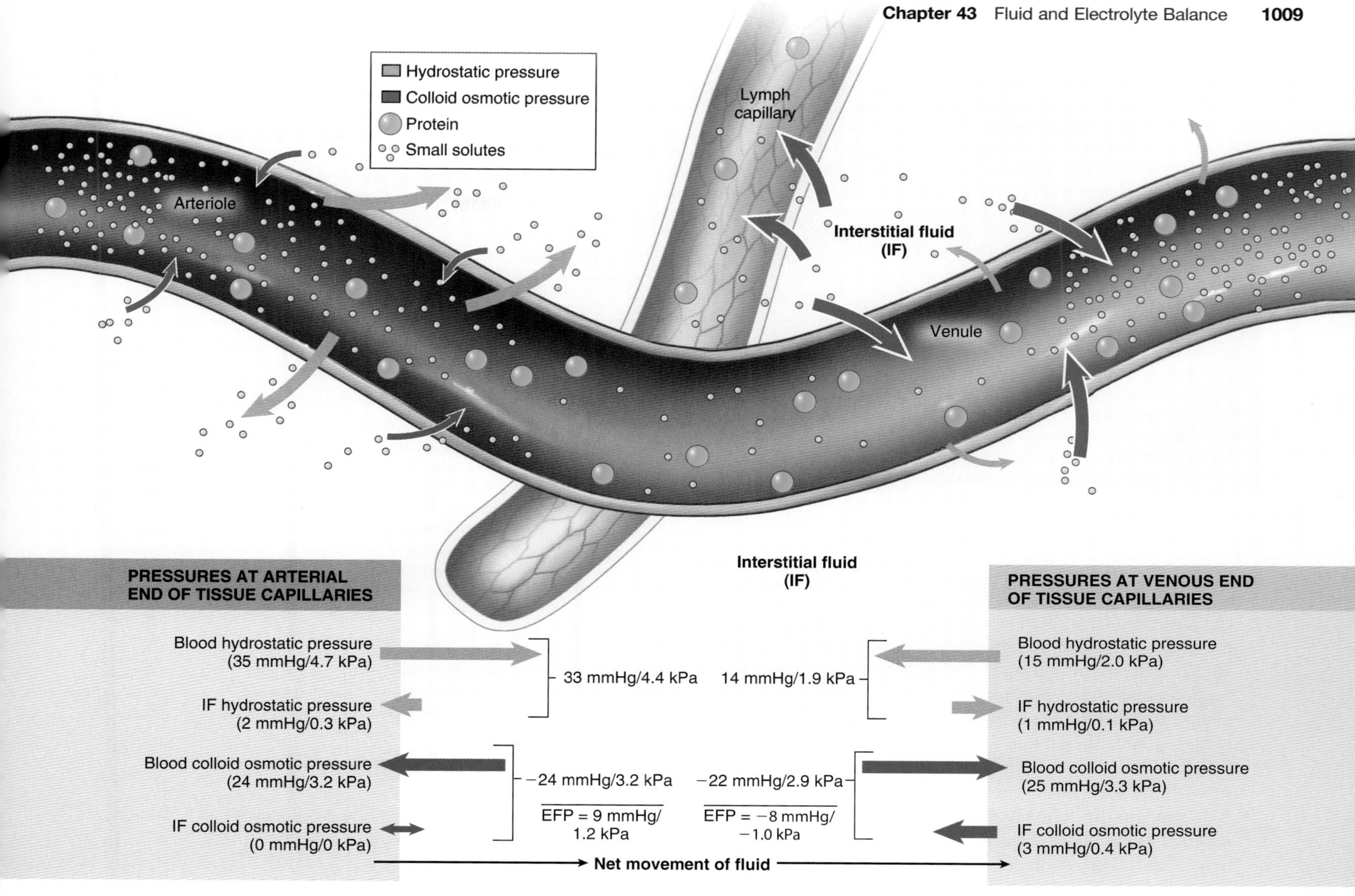

FIGURE 43-10 Movement of fluids and electrolytes between plasma and interstitial fluid caused by hydrostatic and colloid osmotic pressure. *EFP,* Effective filtration pressure. See text for discussion.

Now that you understand Starling's law of the capillaries, you will be able to understand how changes from normal hydrostatic and osmotic pressures affect the movement of water between blood and interstitial fluid. If the hydrostatic pressure difference increases above normal, or if the osmotic pressure difference decreases below normal, more fluid than normal enters the tissues at the arterial ends of capillaries and less fluid than normal leaves the tissues at the venous ends. More fluid in and less fluid out results in a "fluid shift" from the blood into the tissues. If the lymphatic system cannot remove this excess fluid, oedema results.

If the hydrostatic pressure difference decreases below normal, or the osmotic pressure difference increases above normal, less fluid than normal enters the tissues at the arterial ends of capillaries and more fluid than normal leaves the tissues at the venous ends. Less fluid in and more fluid out results in a "fluid shift" from the tissues into the blood. Note, during hypovolaemic shock from loss of blood, such a "fluid shift" can increase blood volume and help restore BP.

Oedema

Oedema is a classic example of fluid imbalance and may be defined as the presence of abnormally large amounts of fluid in the intercellular tissue spaces of the body. Oedema may occur in any organ or tissue of the body. However, the lungs, brain, and dependent body areas such as the legs and lower part of the back are affected most often. One of the most common areas for swelling to occur is in the subcutaneous tissues of the ankle and foot. The term **pitting oedema** is used to describe depressions in swollen subcutaneous tissue in this area that do not rapidly refill after an examiner has exerted finger pressure (**Figure 43-11**). The condition may be caused by disturbances in any of the factors that govern the interchange between blood plasma and the interstitial fluid compartments. Examples include the following:

- Retention of electrolytes (especially Na^+) in the extracellular fluid as a result of increased aldosterone secretion or after serious renal disease such as acute glomerulonephritis.
- An increase in capillary blood pressure. Normally, fluid is drawn from the tissue spaces into the venous end of a tissue

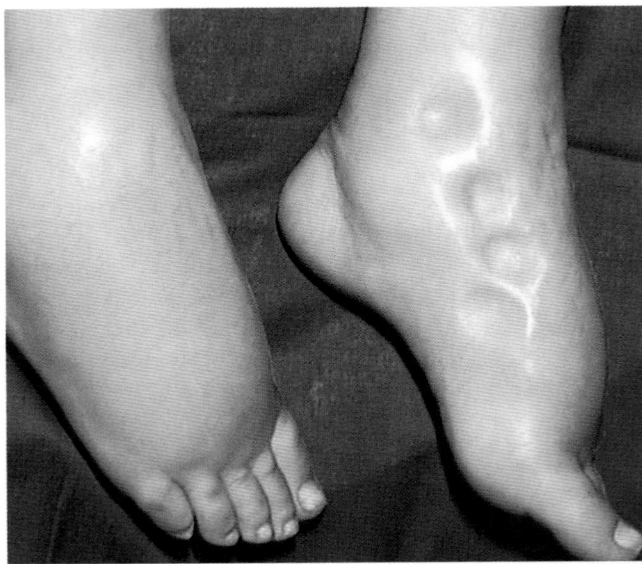

FIGURE 43-11 Pitting oedema. Note the finger-shaped depressions that do not rapidly refill after an examiner has exerted pressure.

capillary because of the low venous hydrostatic pressure and the high water-pulling force of plasma proteins (**Figure 43-12**). This balance is upset by anything that increases the capillary hydrostatic pressure. The generalized venous congestion of heart failure is the most common cause of widespread oedema. In patients with this condition, blood cannot flow freely through the capillary beds, and therefore the pressure will increase until venous return of blood improves.

- A decrease in the concentration of plasma proteins normally retained in the blood (**Figure 43-12** and **Figure 43-13**). This may occur as a result of increased capillary permeability caused by infection, burns, or shock.

FIGURE 43-12 Oedema formation. The mechanism of oedema formation can be initiated by a decrease in blood protein concentration and, therefore, a decrease in blood colloid osmotic pressure *(BCOP)*. In the diagram on the left, blood osmotic pressure has just decreased to 2.7 kPa (20 mmHg) from the normal 3.3 kPa (25 mmHg). This increases the effective filtration pressure *(EFP)* to 0.7 kPa (5 mmHg) from a normal of 0 (see Starling's formula, p. 1007). The EFP of 0.7 kPa (5 mmHg) causes fluid to shift out of blood into interstitial fluid *(IF)* until the EFP again equals 0—in this case, when the interstitial fluid volume has increased enough to raise interstitial fluid hydrostatic pressure *(HP)* to 1.2 kPa (9 mmHg), as shown in the diagram on the right. At this point a new equilibrium is established, and equal amounts of water once more are exchanged between blood and interstitial fluid. Thus the increased interstitial fluid volume—that is, the oedema—becomes stabilized.

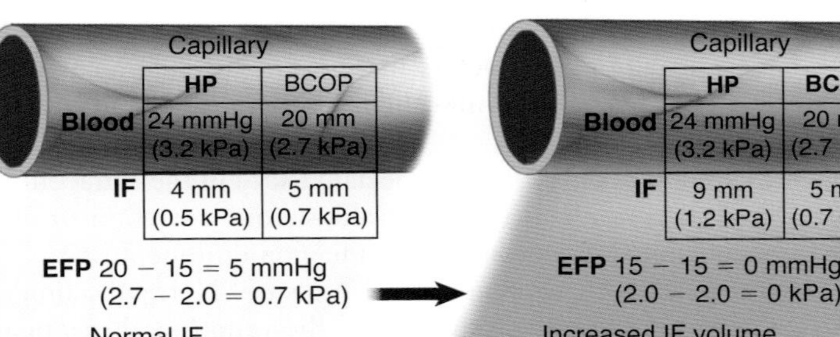

Capillary
HP
BCOP
Blood
24 mmHg (3.2 kPa)
20 mm (2.7 kPa)
IF
4 mm (0.5 kPa)
5 mm (0.7 kPa)
EFP 20 − 15 = 5 mmHg (2.7 − 2.0 = 0.7 kPa)
Normal IF fluid volume
Capillary
HP
BCOP
Blood
24 mmHg (3.2 kPa)
20 mm (2.7 kPa)
IF
9 mm (1.2 kPa)
5 mm (0.7 kPa)
EFP 15 − 15 = 0 mmHg (2.0 − 2.0 = 0 kPa)
Increased IF volume (stabilized oedema)

Quick CHECK

11. Name the four pressures that control water exchange between plasma and interstitial fluid.
12. Define the term *oedema.* How can tissue inflammation or burns cause oedema?
13. List the mechanisms that regulate movement of solutes and water between the ECF and ICF spaces.
14. Why does fluid balance depend on electrolyte balance?

REGULATION OF WATER AND ELECTROLYTE LEVELS IN ICF

It is the plasma membrane that separates the intracellular and extracellular fluid compartments. We know that a chemical difference predominates between these two fluids, and it is the plasma

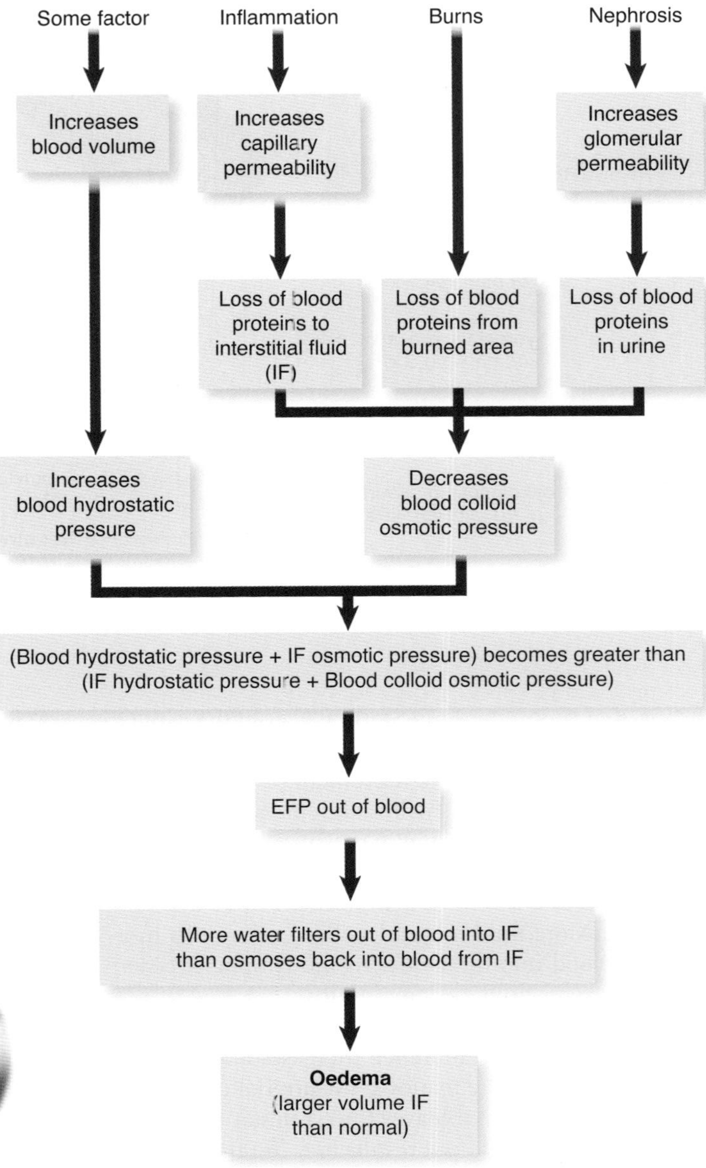

FIGURE 43-13 Mechanisms of oedema formation in some common conditions. *EFP,* Effective, or net, filtration pressure; *IF,* interstitial fluid (see also **Figure 43-6**).

membrane that plays a critical role in the regulation of intracellular fluid composition.

The mechanism that regulates water movement through cell membranes is similar to the one that regulates water movement through capillary membranes. In other words, interstitial fluid and intracellular fluid hydrostatic and colloid osmotic pressure regulate water transfer between these two fluids. But because the colloid osmotic pressure of interstitial and intracellular fluids varies more than their hydrostatic pressure, their colloid osmotic pressure serves as the chief regulator of water transfer across cell membranes. Their colloid osmotic pressure, in turn, is directly related to the electrolyte concentration gradients—notably sodium and potassium—maintained across cell membranes. As **Figures 43-3** and **43-4** show, most of the body sodium is outside the cells. A concentration of 138 to 143 mEq/L makes sodium the chief electrolyte by far in interstitial fluid. The main electrolyte of intracellular fluid is potassium. Therefore, a change in the sodium or the potassium concentration of either of these fluids causes the exchange of fluid between them to become unbalanced.

Pores in the selectively permeable cell membrane retain large molecules, such as proteins, inside the cell but permit many smaller ions such as sodium and potassium to either diffuse through or be selectively transported across the membrane. The electrical charge difference that is created by the unequal concentration of electrolytes on either side of the cell membrane also influences the composition of intracellular fluid. Mechanisms that regulate the movement of solutes and water between extracellular and intracellular fluid spaces are summarized in **Figure 43-14**.

Any change in the solute concentration of extracellular fluid will have a direct effect on water movement across the cell membrane in one direction or another. If for any reason dehydration occurs, the concentration of solutes in the extracellular fluid will increase, and osmosis will cause water to move from the intracellular space into the extracellular space (see **Box 43-1**). In severe dehydration, the increasing concentration of intracellular fluid caused by water loss to the extracellular space results in abnormal metabolism or cellular death. Increased movement of water into the cell is caused by a decreased concentration of solutes in the extracellular fluids.

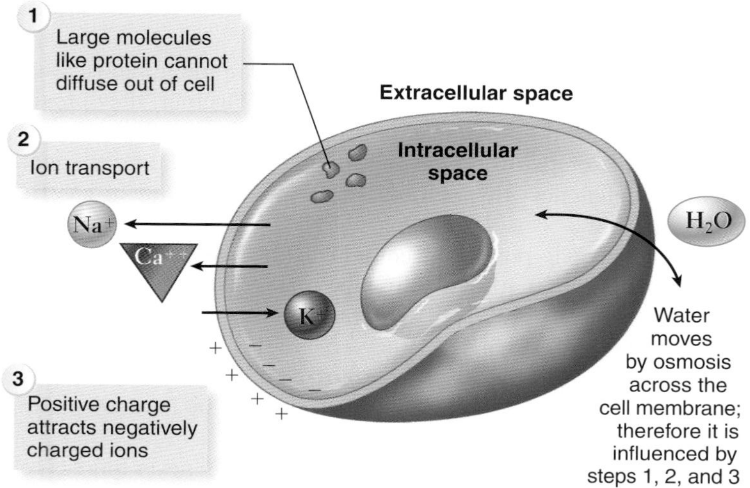

FIGURE 43-14 Mechanisms regulating movement of water and solutes between ECF and ICF spaces. *1,* Osmotic pressure is influenced by large protein molecules in the ICF, which cannot diffuse through the small pores of the cell membrane. *2,* In addition, electrolyte transport and, *3,* diffusion and the charge difference across the cell membrane also influence water movement by osmosis. *ECF,* Extracellular fluid; *ICF,* intracellular fluid.

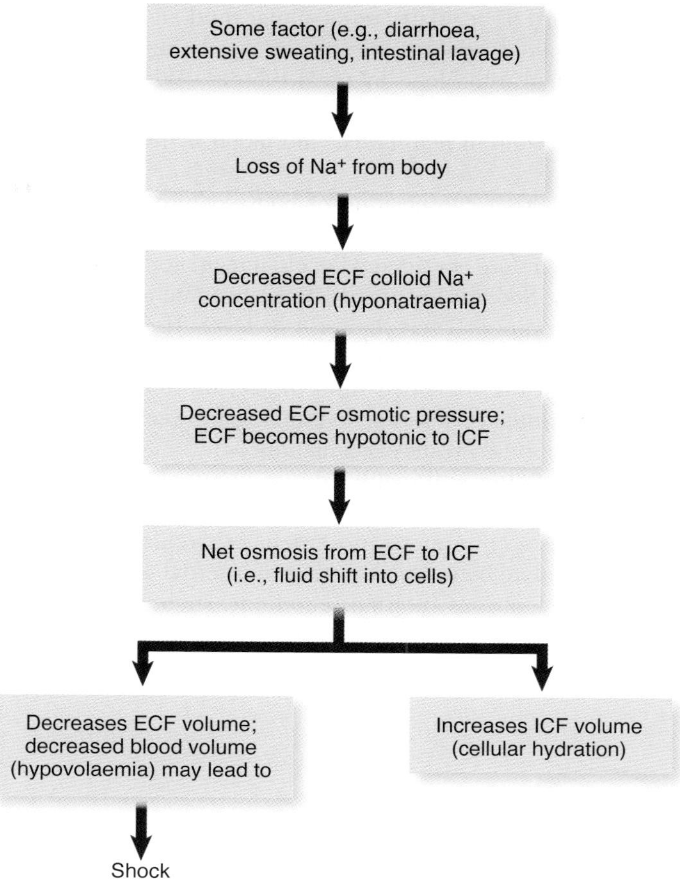

FIGURE 43-15 How electrolyte imbalance leads to fluid imbalances. The schematic uses the example of sodium deficit (hyponatraemia) and resulting hypovolaemia (cellular hydration). *ECF,* Extracellular fluid; *ICF,* intracellular fluid.

A decrease in interstitial fluid sodium concentration immediately decreases interstitial fluid colloid osmotic pressure, thus making it hypotonic to intracellular fluid colloid osmotic pressure. In other words, a decrease in interstitial fluid sodium concentration establishes a colloid osmotic pressure gradient between interstitial and intracellular fluid. This gradient causes net osmosis of fluid to occur—that is, fluid moves out of interstitial fluid into cells. In short, interstitial fluid and intracellular fluid electrolyte concentrations are the main determinants of their colloid osmotic pressure; their colloid osmotic pressure regulates the amount and direction of water transfer between the two fluids, and this regulates their volumes. Hence, fluid balance depends on electrolyte balance. Conversely, electrolyte balance depends on fluid balance. An imbalance in one produces an imbalance in the other (**Figure 43-15**).

REGULATION OF SODIUM AND POTASSIUM LEVELS IN BODY FLUIDS

A normal sodium concentration in interstitial fluid and potassium concentration in intracellular fluid depend on many factors, especially on the amount of ADH and aldosterone secreted. As shown in

Figure 43-16, ADH regulates extracellular fluid electrolyte concentration and colloid osmotic pressure by regulating the amount of water reabsorbed into blood by renal tubules. Aldosterone, on the other hand, regulates extracellular fluid volume by regulating the amount of sodium reabsorbed into blood by renal tubules (see **Figure 43-6**).

If for any reason conservation of body sodium is required, the normal kidney is capable of excreting an essentially sodium-free urine and is therefore considered the chief regulator of sodium levels in body fluids. Sodium lost in sweat can become appreciable with elevated environmental temperatures or fever. However, the thirst that results may lead to replacement of water but not the lost sodium, and because of the increased fluid intake, the remaining sodium pool may be diluted even more. Sodium loss in sweat is not therefore considered a normal means of regulation.

In addition to the well-regulated movement of sodium into and out of the body and between the three primary fluid compartments, there is a continuous movement or circulation of this important electrolyte between a number of internal secretions. More than 8 *litres* of various internal secretions, such as saliva, gastric and intestinal secretions, bile, and pancreatic fluid, are produced every day (**Figure 43-17**). The total daily secretion of sodium into these alimentary tract fluids alone will average between 1200 and 1400 mEq. A 70-kg adult has a total body sodium pool of only 2800 to 3000 mEq. Precise regulatory and conservation mechanisms for sodium are required for survival.

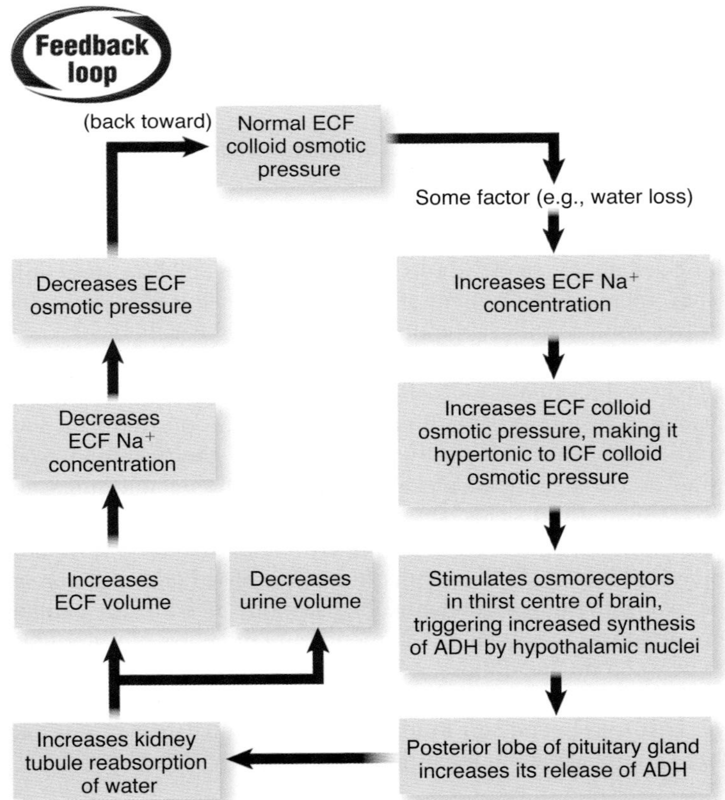

FIGURE 43-16 Antidiuretic hormone (ADH) mechanism for ECF homeostasis. The ADH mechanism helps maintain homeostasis of extracellular fluid (*ECF*) colloid osmotic pressure by regulating its volume and thereby its electrolyte concentration, that is, mainly ECF Na$^+$ concentration. *ICF,* Intracellular fluid.

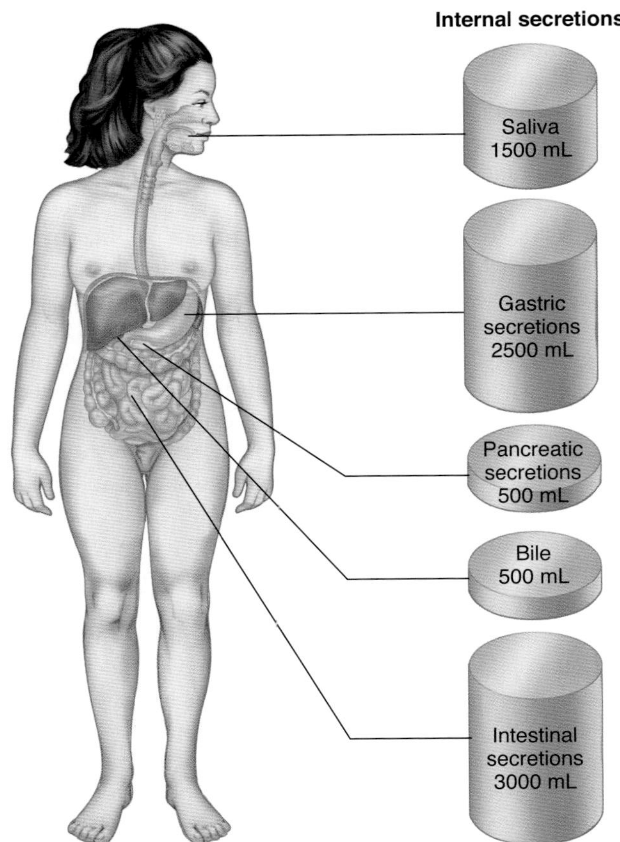

FIGURE 43-17 Sodium-containing internal secretions. Average volumes are shown. Depending on circumstances, the actual total volume of these secretions may reach 8000 mL or more in a 24-hour period.

Chloride is the most important extracellular anion and is almost always linked to sodium. Generally ingested together, they provide in large part for the isotonicity of extracellular fluid. Chloride ions are usually excreted in the urine as a potassium salt, and therefore chloride deficiency—**hypochloraemia**—is often found in cases of potassium loss.

The total body potassium content in the average-sized adult is approximately 4000 mEq. Because the majority of body potassium is intracellular, plasma (serum) determinations, which normally fall between 4.0 and 5.0 mEq/L, may not be the best index to reflect imbalances. The body may lose a third to a half of its intracellular potassium reserves before the loss is reflected in lowered plasma potassium levels.

Potassium deficit, or **hypokalaemia,** occurs whenever there is cell breakdown, as in starvation, burns, trauma, or dehydration. As individual cells disintegrate, potassium enters the extracellular fluid and is rapidly excreted because it is not reabsorbed efficiently by the kidney.

cycle of life

Fluid and Electrolyte Balance Although the amount of total water in the body does not vary much from day to day, the proportions of water to fat and dry solids in the body changes noticeably over the life span. **Figure 43-18** shows the shift in water percentages (of body mass) over the life span. As the diagram clearly shows, we start life with over two thirds of our body mass being water and progress to about half of body mass being water in adulthood. Because muscles and other metabolically active cells are high in water content, active adults have more water content than nonactive adults. Often, we become less active during late adulthood—a factor that contributes to less water in our bodies as we age. Advanced age can also bring on some of the kidney problems mentioned earlier in this chapter that can affect our ion balance as well. •

Fat and dry solids (%)
Intracellular water (%)
Extracellular water (%)

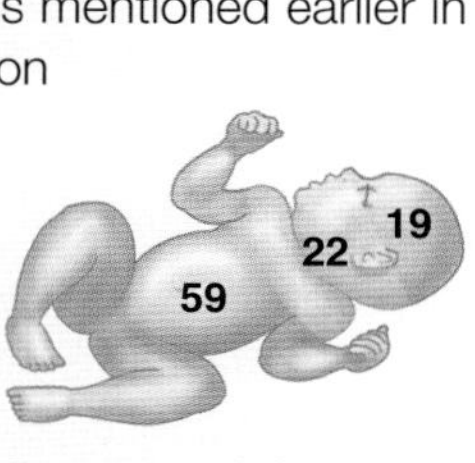

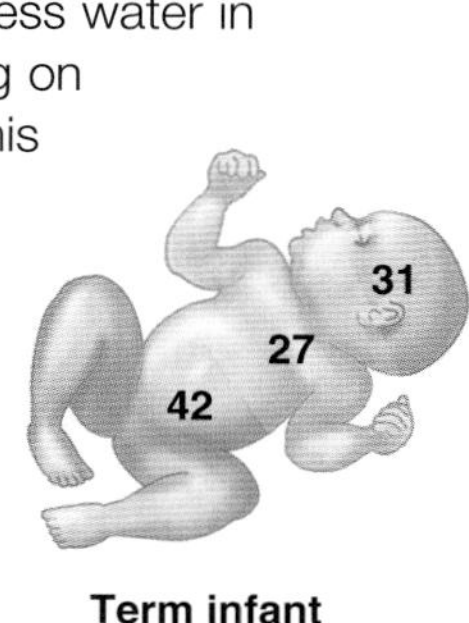

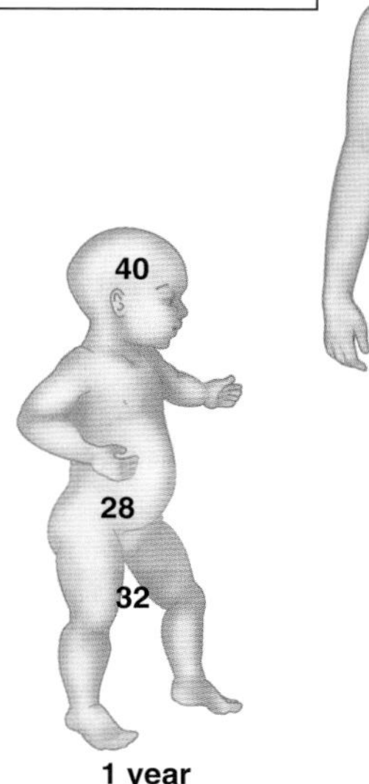

Adult female 60 kg: 51.4, 25.9, 22.7

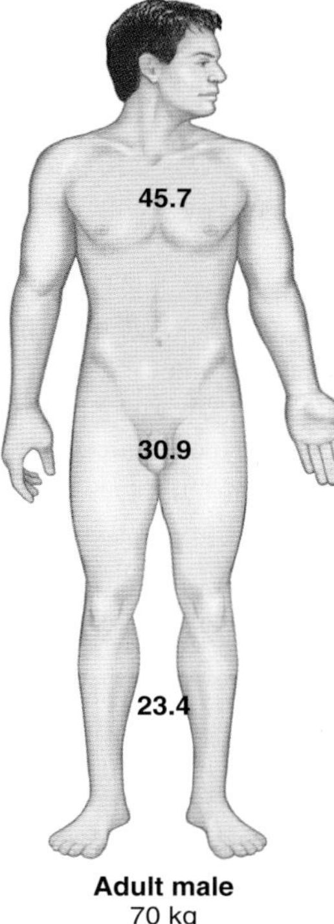

FIGURE 43-18 Body water over the life span. Fluid and nonfluid components of the body expressed as percentage of body weight.

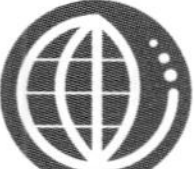

the big picture | Fluid and Electrolyte Balance

In discussing the chemical basis for life in Chapter 3, water was described as the "cradle of life". Each of the more than 37 trillion cells that make up the human body must be bathed in a precisely controlled and homeostatically regulated fluid medium. That medium, ever-changing and yet remarkably constant when a condition of homeostasis exists, fills the cells, interstitial spaces, and blood vessels of the body.

Although unique differences in many variables, such as specific fluid volumes, buffers, electrolyte levels, nutrients, circulating wastes, and protein concentrations, exist in each of the body's fluid compartments at any point in time, these changing concentrations and volumes remain within amazingly narrow ranges of their normal setpoint values in a healthy individual.

Recall from previous chapters that many ions must exist in precise balances within various fluid compartments of the body for normal operation of many vital functions. For example, proper calcium ion balance is required in bone formation or reabsorption, contraction of all three muscle types, synaptic transmission, some types of endocrine signal transduction, and other potentially vital functions. Sodium and potassium concentrations directly affect impulses in nerves and muscles. Chloride balance can affect sodium balance and thus also affect nerve and muscle function. And also recall that acids and bases are ions, and thus pH homeostasis is related to ion homeostasis.

Disease states, atypical circumstances such as fluid deprivation or specific electrolyte losses, and normal day-to-day variation in our fluid and nutrient intake, cause the body to initiate "compensatory activities" that help restore or maintain homeostasis. These activities often involve complex neuroendocrine responses that affect multiple body organ systems, including the muscular, digestive, cardiovascular, respiratory, and urinary systems. Homeostasis of fluid and electrolyte levels is one of the most crucial "big picture" requirements for the maintenance of life itself. Every cell and organ system in the body—every physiological response—depends on maintenance of homeostasis in these critical areas. •

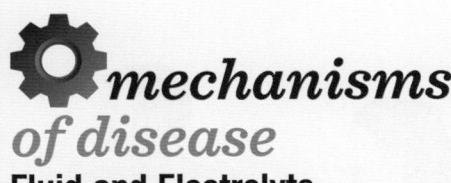

Fluid and Electrolyte Disorders

Fluid Imbalances

Fluid Volume Deficit

Total body water makes up 40% to 60% of body weight in adults and is regulated by homeostatic mechanisms of the neuroendocrine system, heart, kidneys, and blood vessels. Normal water losses, known as insensible water losses, occur through expired air from the lungs and from the skin, making up about 0.4 to 0.5 mL/hr/kg body weight. Abnormally excessive water losses produce a decline in the volume of body fluid and can lead to a state of dehydration, or **hypovolaemia,** in which there is inadequate fluid volume in the extracellular compartment (see **Box 43-1**). If left untreated, it can result in hypovolaemic shock.

Many causes of dehydration exist. The most common cause of dehydration is fluid loss from the gastrointestinal tract as a result of vomiting or diarrhoea. Dehydration also occurs when an individual fails to take in sufficient oral fluid because of depression, nausea, or oral trauma. *Diaphoresis,* or excessive perspiration, may also cause dehydration, with rapid respirations leading to water vapour losses. Any disorder of the kidneys that increases urine excretion, such as nephritis, can lead to dehydration. Fluid can also shift into a space outside the normal fluid compartments during certain disease states, including ascites, burns, pancreatitis, and traumatic injuries.

Regardless of the cause, fluid volume deficits cause low blood pressure and cardiac output, electrolyte disturbances, or acid–base abnormalities. Symptoms include dizziness, lightheadedness, weakness, poor skin turgor, and tachycardia. Restoration of the fluid losses is the main goal of therapy. If the deficit is mild, volume can be replaced orally. If the dehydration is severe, fluid volume is replaced intravenously. Examining the person's weight, skin turgor, blood pressure, and urine output will provide important data on fluid volume stability.

Fluid Volume Excess

Fluid volume excess, or **hypervolaemia,** is an expansion of fluid volume in the body. This can occur if the kidneys retain a large amount of sodium and water, as in congestive heart failure, nephrotic syndrome, renal failure, and liver failure. Manifestations include weight gain (the most consistent sign), oedema, dyspnoea, tachycardia, and pulmonary congestion. Approaches to this disorder are to treat the original pathological process (e.g., renal failure), monitor the person's weight closely, and use diuretics cautiously to remove the excess fluid (**Box 43-2**).

Water intoxication may result from rapidly drinking large volumes of water or giving hypotonic solutions to persons unable to dilute and excrete urine normally. This may occur in patients with kidney insufficiency or abnormal "thirst" mechanisms resulting from neurological disorders. Water content is elevated, and plasma sodium levels are diluted. Development of subtle mental changes such as confusion and lethargy occur. If intoxication is severe, stupor, seizures, and coma may result. Correction of the neurological impairment along with water restriction can reverse the symptoms.

Water intoxication can happen in normal individuals if water intake is rapid enough that the urinary mechanisms of water loss cannot keep up. Although this is unusual, it can happen—as witnessed by millions a few years ago when a radio station in the United States held a "water drinking race" on the air and a contestant died from the effects of severe water intoxication.

Electrolyte Imbalances

Sodium Imbalance

Disturbances in electrolytes can occur in fluid volume abnormalities and many different disease states. **Hyponatraemia** is a condition of decreased plasma sodium concentration below the normal range (less than 136 mEq/L) and is usually the result of an excess of water relative to solute. It may also result from excessive losses of sodium. Causes of hyponatraemia include skin losses via profuse perspiration, overzealous use of salt-wasting diuretics, adrenal insufficiency, renal or liver failure, low salt intake, or excessive water intake (diluting sodium content).

Signs and symptoms of hyponatraemia include muscle cramps, nausea and vomiting, postural blood pressure changes, poor skin turgor, fatigue, and difficulty breathing. Cerebral swelling can occur in severe cases, causing confusion, hemiparesis (motor weakness on one side of the body), seizures, and coma. Management includes neurological assessment and the administration of sodium orally or intravenously. Water restriction may also suffice.

Hypernatraemia is elevation of the plasma sodium concentration higher than 145 mEq/L. It is usually indicative of a body water deficit relative to sodium but can also result from grossly elevated sodium intake. Causes include lack of

---

BOX 43-2 *health matters* | **Diuretics**

The word **diuretic** is from the Greek word *diouretikos,* meaning "causing urine". By definition, a diuretic drug is a substance that promotes or stimulates the production of urine.

As a group, diuretics are among the most commonly used drugs in medicine. They are used because of their role in influencing water and electrolyte balance, especially sodium, in the body. Diuretics have their effect on tubular function in the nephron, and the differing types of diuretics are often classified according to their major site of action. Examples include (1) *proximal tubule diuretics* such as acetazolamide, (2) *Henle loop diuretics* such as bumetanide or furosemide, and (3) *distal tubule diuretics* such as chlortalidone.

Diuretics can also be classified according to the effect the drug has on the level or concentration of sodium (Na^+), chloride (Cl^-), potassium (K^+), and bicarbonate (HCO_3^-) ions in the tubular fluid.

Implications for caregivers monitoring patients receiving diuretics both in hospitals and in home health care environments include keeping a careful record of fluid intake and output and assessing the patient for signs and symptoms of electrolyte and water imbalance. For example, diuretic-induced dehydration resulting in a loss of only 6% of initial body weight will cause tingling in the extremities, stumbling gait, headache, fever, and an increase in both pulse and respiratory rates.

fluid intake, diarrhoea, diabetes insipidus, loss of water via the respiratory tract, heart disease or congestive heart failure, renal failure, or ingestion of salt in abnormal amounts.

Signs and symptoms of hypernatraemia are similar to those of dehydration and include thirst, disorientation, lethargy, and seizures. The neurological symptoms are thought to be due to cellular dehydration. Replacement with a hypotonic solution will help lower the sodium level slowly, thereby reducing the risk for cerebral oedema.

Potassium Imbalance

A common type of electrolyte imbalance is hypokalaemia, a condition in which potassium is lost from the body, resulting in a plasma potassium level below 3.5 mEq/L. Causes include potassium-wasting diuretics, increased urine output with loss of potassium, and vomiting or gastric suctioning without potassium replacement. Hypokalaemia can be life-threatening and includes manifestations of anorexia, muscle weakness, decreased reflexes, low blood pressure, and cardiac dysrhythmias. Potassium can be replaced through the diet, with potassium-rich foods, or intravenously with caution.

The opposite of hypokalaemia is **hyperkalaemia,** or a plasma potassium level above 5.5 mEq/L. This can be even more dangerous than hypokalaemia because myocardial muscle can be profoundly affected. The common cause of hyperkalaemia is kidney disease, but other factors such as vomiting, diarrhoea, potassium-conserving diuretics, extensive tissue damage as in burn or trauma patients, severe infections, and Cushing syndrome are also cited.

In hyperkalaemia, notable changes can be seen on the electrocardiogram, such as peaked T waves. Hyperkalaemia can induce ventricular dysrhythmias, thereby leading to possible cardiac arrest. Because potassium is a part of neuromuscular functions, the person may experience extremity muscle weakness or failure of the respiratory muscles. Intermittent diarrhoea, nausea, and intestinal colic are also manifested.

Dietary restriction of potassium is sufficient in mild cases, but emergency intravenous administration of calcium gluconate may be required to correct cardiac symptoms. Also, correction of the underlying condition (e.g., trauma) and dialysis to remove the excess potassium can be instituted to correct severe hyperkalaemia.

LANGUAGE OF SCIENCE *(continued from p. 999)*

intracellular fluid compartment (in-trah-SELL-yoo-lar FLOO-id) [*intra-* **occurring within,** *-cell-* **storeroom,** *-ular* **relating to**]

intracellular fluid (ICF) (in-trah-SELL-yoo-lar FLOO-id) [*intra-* **occurring within,** *-cell-* **storeroom,** *-ular* **relating to**]

ion (EYE-on) [*ion* **to go**]

milliequivalent (mEq) (mil-ee-ee-KWIV-ah-lent) [*milli-* 1/1000 **part,** *-equi-* **equal,** *-val-* **strength,** *-ent* **state**]

nonelectrolyte (non-eh-LEK-troh-lyte) [*non-* **not,** *-electro-* **electricity,** *-lyt-* **loosening**]

osmoreceptor (os-moh-ree-SEP-tor) [*osmo-* **push,** *-recept-* **receive,** *-or* **agent**]

parenteral (pah-REN-ter-al) [*par-* **beside,** *-enter-* **intestine,** *-al* **relating to**]

subfornical organ (SFO) (sub-FOR-nih-kal) [*sub-* **under,** *-fornic-* **arch,** *-al* **relating to**]

LANGUAGE OF MEDICINE

diuretic (dye-yoo-RET-ik) [*dia-* **through,** *-ure-* **urine,** *-ic* **relating to**]

hyperkalaemia (hye-per-kah-LEE-mee-ah) [*hyper-* **excessive,** *-kali-* **potassium,** *-aem-* **blood,** *-ia* **condition**]

hypernatraemia (hye-per-nah-TREE-mee-ah) [*hyper-* **excessive,** *-natri-* **sodium,** *-aem-* **blood,** *-ia* **condition**]

hypervolaemia (hye-per-voh-LEE-mee-ah) [*hyper-* **excessive,** *-vol-* **volume,** *-aem-* **blood,** *-ia* **condition**]

hypochloraemia (hye-poh-kloh-REE-mee-ah) [*hypo-* **under or below,** *-chlor-* **green (chlorine),** *-aem-* **blood,** *-ia* **condition**]

hypokalaemia (hye-poh-kah-LEE-mee-ah) [*hypo-* **under or below,** *-kal-* **potassium,** *-aem-* **blood,** *-ia* **condition**]

hyponatraemia (hye-poh-nah-TREE-mee-ah) [*hypo-* **under or below,** *-natri-* **sodium,** *-aem-* **blood,** *-ia* **condition**]

hypovolaemia (hye-poh-voh-LEE-mee-ah) [*hypo-* **under or below,** *-vol-* **volume,** *-aem-* **blood,** *-ia* **condition**]

parenteral therapy (pah-REN-ter-al) [*par-* **beside,** *-enter-* **intestine,** *-al* **relating to**]

pitting oedema (eh-DEE-mah)

subcutaneous injection (sub-kyoo-TAY-nee-us in-JEK-shun) [*sub-* **under,** *cut-* **skin,** *-aneous* **relating to,** *in-* **in,** *-ject-* **throw,** *-tion* **process**]

turgor (TUR-ger) [*turg-* **swollen,** *-or* **condition**]

case study

Chloe was enjoying her summer holiday in Crete. To make sure she could visit the whole of the archaeological site at Knossos, she stayed out in the sun at midday when the temperature peaked at 37°C. Her shirt was soaked with sweat and she had to wipe her forehead as sweat dripped into her eyes. Chloe knew she should take a break, seek shade, and have a drink, but it was her last opportunity to see everything. As she stepped off a ramp she suddenly felt faint and sat down quickly.

1. What condition was likely to have caused Chloe's faint?
   a. Hypervolaemia
   b. Ascites
   c. Hypovolaemia
   d. Hypokalaemia

A first-aider rushed over to Chloe, felt her skin and checked her pulse. He suspected Chloe was dehydrated and asked her when she had last had a drink of water.

2. What would be the most suitable fluid to give to Chloe?
   a. Distilled water
   b. Cold beer
   c. Cold soda
   d. An isotonic sports drink

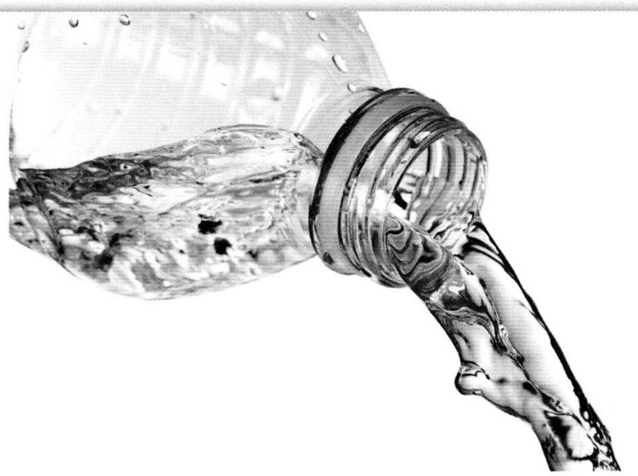

3. If Chloe's faint was due to dehydration, which hormones would be released to compensate for her lack of water?
   a. ADH and aldosterone
   b. Oestrogen and renin
   c. Aldosterone and TSH
   d. Renin and cortisol

Hint To solve a case study, you may have to refer to the glossary or index, other chapters in this textbook, ***Connect It!,*** and other resources.

CHAPTER SUMMARY

To download an MP3 version of the chapter summary for use with your mobile device, access the ***Audio Chapter Summaries*** *online at evolve.elsevier.com.*

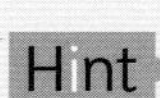

Scan this summary after reading the chapter to help you reinforce the key concepts. Later, use the summary as a quick review before your class or before a test.

Interrelationship of Fluid and Electrolyte Balance

A. Fluid and electrolyte balance—implies homeostasis
B. Electrolytes have chemical bonds that allow dissociation into ions, which carry an electrical charge; of critical importance in fluid balance
C. Fluid balance and electrolyte balance are interdependent

Total Body Water

A. Fluid content of the human body ranges from 45% to 75% of its total weight
B. Fluid content varies according to age, gender, weight, and fat content of the body

Body Fluid Compartments

A. Two major fluid compartments (**Figure 43-1**)
B. Extracellular fluid (ECF) makes up the internal environment of the body
   1. Consists mainly of plasma and interstitial fluid
   2. Lymph, cerebrospinal fluid, and joint fluids are considered extracellular
   3. ECF provides a relatively constant environment for cells and transports substances to and from the cells
C. Intracellular fluid (ICF)—water inside the cells
   1. ICF facilitates intracellular chemical reactions that maintain life
   2. By volume, ICF is the largest body fluid compartment

Chemical Content, Distribution, and Measurement of Electrolytes in Body Fluids

A. Extracellular vs. intracellular fluids
   1. Plasma and interstitial fluid (ECFs) are almost identical in chemical make-up; intracellular fluid quite different in comparison (**Figure 43-3**)
   2. Differences between extracellular fluids (blood and interstitial fluid)
      a. Blood contains a slightly larger total of ions than interstitial fluid does
      b. Functionally important difference between blood and interstitial fluid
         (1) Blood has appreciable amount of protein anions, whereas interstitial fluid has hardly any
         (2) Because the capillary membrane is practically impermeable to proteins, almost all protein anions remain in the blood
   3. Chemical structure of plasma, interstitial fluid, and intracellular fluid helps control water and electrolyte movement between them

B. Measuring electrolyte reactivity
   1. Concentration or weight of an electrolyte can be expressed as the number of milligrams per 100 mL of solution; conversion to milliequivalents per litre (mEq/L) provides information on actual physiological activity
   2. Milliequivalent—measures the number of ionic charges or electrocovalent bonds in a solution; accurately measures the physiological combining power of an electrolyte solution

Avenues by Which Water Enters and Leaves the Body

A. Water enters the body via the digestive tract; water is also added to the total fluid volume from each cell as it catabolizes food, and the resulting water enters the bloodstream (**Figure 43-5**)
B. Water leaves the body via four exits (**Figure 43-5**):
   1. As urine through the kidney
   2. As water in expired air through the lungs
   3. As sweat through the skin
   4. As faeces from the intestine

Some General Principles About Fluid Balance

A. Cardinal principle of fluid balance: fluid balance can be maintained only if intake equals output
B. Mechanisms are available to adjust output and intake to maintain fluid balance, such as the renin–angiotensin–aldosterone system (RAAS) (**Figures 43-6** and **43-8**)
C. Most rapid fluid balance mechanisms are those for controlling water movement between fluid compartments of the body; will maintain normal blood volume at the expense of interstitial fluid volume

Mechanisms That Maintain Homeostasis of Total Fluid Volume

A. Under normal conditions, homeostasis of total volume of water is maintained or restored primarily by adjusting urine volume and secondarily by fluid intake (**Figure 43-7**)
B. Regulation of fluid intake—decrease in fluid intake causes osmoreceptors in "thirst centre"—wall of third ventricle (subfornical organ) and in supraoptic and paraventricular nuclei of hypothalamus—to increase secretion of ADH (**Figure 43-16**)
C. Regulation of urine volume—determined by two factors
   1. Glomerular filtration rate, except under abnormal conditions, remains fairly constant
   2. Rate of tubular reabsorption of water fluctuates considerably; normally adjusts urine volume to fluid intake; influenced by amount of antidiuretic hormone and aldosterone
D. Factors that alter fluid loss under abnormal conditions
   1. Rate of respiration and volume of sweat secreted may alter fluid output under certain abnormal conditions
   2. Vomiting, diarrhoea, or intestinal drainage can produce fluid and electrolyte imbalances; symptoms range from simple thirst to muscle weakness and kidney failure

Regulation of Water and Electrolyte Levels in Plasma and Interstitial Fluid

A. Starling's law of the capillaries
   1. The control mechanism for water exchange between plasma and interstitial fluid consists of four types of pressure, two on one side of the capillary membrane (wall) and two on the other side
      a. Pressures on internal side of capillary membrane
         (1) Blood hydrostatic pressure (BHP)
         (2) Blood colloid osmotic pressure (BCOP)
      b. Pressures on external side of capillary membrane
         (1) Interstitial fluid hydrostatic pressure (IFHP)
         (2) Interstitial fluid colloid osmotic pressure (IFCOP)
B. The rate and direction of fluid exchange between capillaries and interstitial fluid are determined by the hydrostatic and colloid osmotic pressures of the two fluids (**Figure 43-10**)
   1. Filtration—moves water from higher hydrostatic pressure to lower hydrostatic pressure; filtration moves water out of the blood and into the IF
   2. Osmosis—moves water from lower osmotic pressure to higher osmotic pressure; osmosis moves water into the blood from the IF
   3. Effective filtration pressure (EFP)
      a. EFP is the difference between the opposing pressures of filtration and osmosis
      b. $EFP = Filtration - Osmosis = (BHP - IFHP) - (BCOP - IFCOP)$
   4. Fluid shifts may occur as a result of changes in hydrostatic or osmotic pressures
      a. Fluid shifts from blood into tissues if hydrostatic pressure difference goes up or osmotic pressure difference goes down (unless the lymphatic system cannot remove excess tissue fluid)
      b. Fluid shifts from tissues into blood if hydrostatic pressure difference goes down or osmotic pressure difference goes up
C. Oedema—classic example of fluid imbalance
   1. Defined as presence of abnormally large amounts of fluid in the intercellular tissue spaces of the body (**Figure 43-11**)
   2. Can be caused by disturbances in any factors that govern interchange between blood plasma and interstitial fluid compartments
      a. Retention of electrolytes in the extracellular fluid
      b. Increase in capillary blood pressure
      c. Decrease in the concentration of plasma proteins normally retained in the blood (**Figure 43-12**)

Regulation of Water and Electrolyte Levels in ICF

A. Plasma membrane plays critical role in regulating ICF composition
B. IF and ICF hydrostatic and colloid pressures regulate water transfer between ECF and ICF
   1. Colloid osmotic pressure is the chief regulator of water transfer across cell membranes
   2. Colloid osmotic pressure is directly related to the electrolyte concentration gradients maintained across cell membranes (**Figure 43-14**)

Regulation of Sodium and Potassium Levels in Body Fluids

A. Normal sodium concentration in IF and potassium concentration in ICF depend on various factors, especially the amount of ADH and aldosterone secreted
   1. ADH regulates ECF electrolyte concentration and colloid osmotic pressure by regulating amount of water reabsorbed into blood by renal tubules
   2. Aldosterone regulates ECF volume by regulating the amount of sodium reabsorbed into blood by renal tubules

B. Kidneys are considered the chief regulator of sodium levels; when conservation of body sodium is required, the kidneys excrete an essentially sodium-free urine

C. Chloride—most important extracellular anion and almost always linked to sodium
   1. Chloride ions generally excreted in urine in association with potassium
   2. Thus hypochloraemia is often associated with cases of potassium loss

D. Hypokalaemia (potassium deficit) occurs where there is cell breakdown
   1. Examples: starvation, burns, trauma, dehydration
   2. As cells disintegrate, potassium enters the ECF and is rapidly excreted because it is not reabsorbed efficiently by the kidney

Cycle of Life: Fluid and Electrolyte Balance

A. The total amount of water in the body does not vary much from day to day; proportions of water to fat and dry solids in the body change noticeably over the life span

B. Because muscles and other metabolically active cells are high in water content, active adults have more water content than nonactive adults

C. Advanced age may result in kidney problems that affect our ion balance

The Big Picture: Fluid and Electrolyte Balance

A. When homeostasis exists, water fills the cells, interstitial spaces, and blood vessels of the body

B. Specific fluid volumes, buffers, electrolyte levels, nutrients, circulating wastes, and protein concentrations exist in each of the body's fluid compartments

C. Ions must exist in precise balances within various fluid compartments of the body for normal operation of many vital functions
   1. Calcium ion balance is required for bone formation, muscle contraction, synaptic transmission, and some types of endocrine signal transduction
   2. Sodium and potassium concentrations directly affect impulses in nerves and muscles
   3. Chloride balance can affect sodium balance

D. Homeostasis of fluid and electrolyte levels are among the most crucial "big picture" requirements for the maintenance of life

REVIEW QUESTIONS

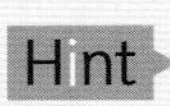

Write out the answers to these questions after reading the chapter and reviewing the Chapter Summary. Note—writing out your answers will consolidate learning and provide a valuable resource of information.

1. Discuss the changes in total body water content from infancy to adulthood. Explain the lower water content in the bodies of older adults.
2. How does total body water content differ in men and women?
3. List the compartments of extracellular fluid.
4. How does water normally leave the body?
5. What is the cardinal principle regarding fluid balance?
6. How is urine volume regulated?
7. Define the terms *cation* and *anion*.
8. Are plasma and interstitial fluid chemically similar or different? Explain.
9. Describe the electrolyte composition of blood plasma.
10. Define the term *milliequivalent*. How is it used to measure electrolyte reactivity?
11. What are the four pressures involved in Starling's law?
12. When effective filtration pressure equals 0, what is the net transfer of water between blood and interstitial fluid?
13. When does a "fluid shift" occur between blood and interstitial fluid?
14. Identify various mechanisms that may lead to oedema.
15. What role does the plasma membrane play in the regulation of intracellular fluid composition?
16. How does the antidiuretic hormone mechanism maintain homeostasis of extracellular fluid colloid osmotic pressure?
17. In your own words, define *dehydration*.
18. What role does the hypothalamus play in water regulation?

CRITICAL THINKING QUESTIONS

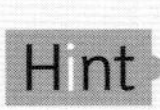

After finishing the Review Questions, write out the answers to these more in-depth questions to help you apply your new knowledge. Go back to sections of the chapter that relate to concepts that you find difficult.

1. Define *fluid and electrolyte balance*. Based on what you know, what would be the impact of glucose deficiency on the electrolyte balance of the body?
2. Summarize the role of aldosterone in thirst.
3. Are ADH and aldosterone considered antagonists or synergists in their regulation of water balance? Explain your answer.
4. Make a distinction between anions in the two extracellular fluids. What causes this difference?
5. Explain Starling's law of the capillaries.
6. How does hyponatraemia lead to fluid imbalance? Identify the possible causes.
7. Where are osmoreceptors located, and how are they related to the maintenance of fluid balance?
8. What information would you use to support the view that the homeostasis of fluid and electrolyte levels is one of the most crucial requirements for the maintenance of life itself?

44 Acid–Base Balance

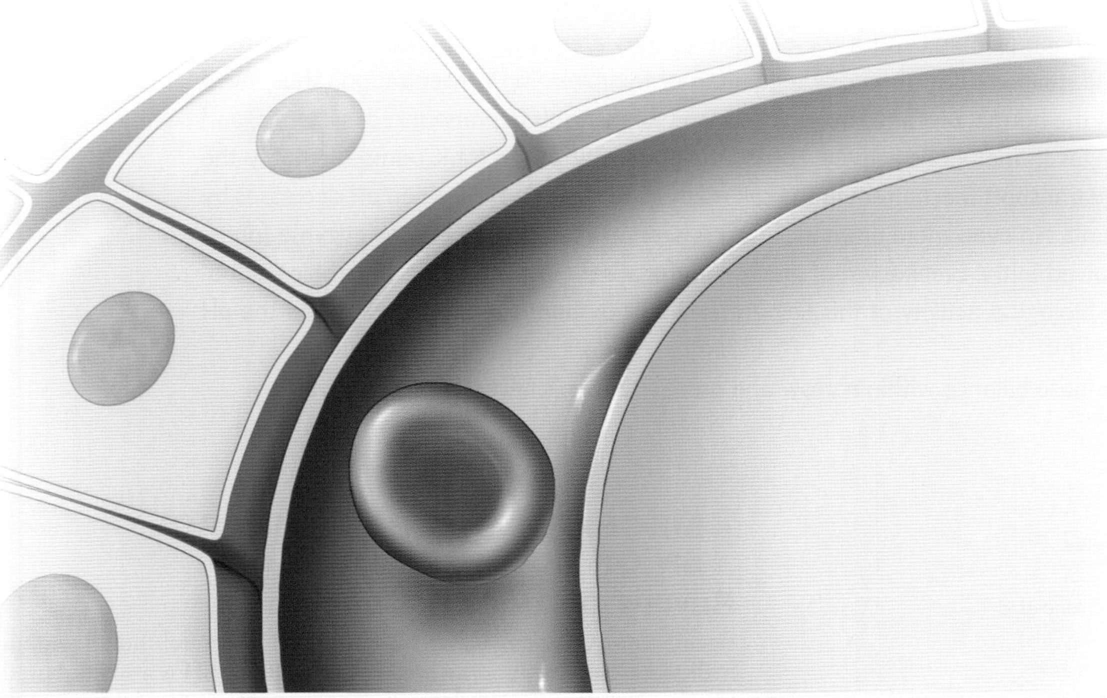

CHAPTER OUTLINE

Hint Scan this outline before you begin to read the chapter, as a preview of how the concepts are organized.

LANGUAGE OF SCIENCE

Hint Use this list to aid your pronunciation of unfamiliar words.

acid (ASS-id)
[*acid* **sour**]

acidity (ah-SID-ih-tee)
[*acid-* **sour,** *-ity* **state**]

acidosis (ass-ih-DOH-sis)
[*acid-* **sour,** *-osis* **condition**]

alkaline (AL-kah-lin)
[*alkal-* **ashes,** *-ine* **relating to**]

alkalinity (al-kah-LIN-ih-tee)
[*alkal-* **ashes,** *-in-* **relating to,** *-ity* **state**]

alkalosis (al-kah-LOH-sis)
[*alkal-* **ashes,** *-osis* **condition**]

arterial blood gas (ABG)
(ar-TEER-ee-al blud gas)
[*arteri-* **airpipe (artery),** *-al* **relating to**]

base
[*bas-* **foundation**]

buffer (BUFF-er)
[*buffe-* **cushion,** *-er* **agent**]

buffer pair (BUFF-er)
[*buffe-* **cushion,** *-er* **agent**]

carbonic anhydrase
(kar-BON-ik an-HYE-drays)
[*carbon-* **coal (carbon),** *-ic* **relating to,** *an-* **not,** *-hydr-* **water,** *-ase* **enzyme**]

chemical buffer (KEM-ih-kal BUFF-er)
[*buffe-* **cushion,** *-er* **agent**]

chloride shift (KLOR-ide shift)
[*chlor-* **green,** *-ide* **chemical**]

compensation (kom-pen-SAY-shun)

normal saline
[*sal-* **salt,** *-ine* **relating to**]

pH (pee-AYCH)
[**abbreviation for** *potenz* **power,** *hydrogen* **hydrogen**]

physiological buffer
(fiz-ee-oh-LOJ-ih-kal BUFF-er)
[*physio-* **nature (function),** *-o-* **combining form,** *-log-* **words (study of),** *-ical* **relating to,** *buffe-* **cushion,** *-er* **agent**]

ratio (RAY-shee-oh)
[*ratio* **a reckoning**]

uncompensated acidosis (un-KOM-pen-say-ted ass-ih-DOH-sis)
[*acid-* **sour,** *-osis* **condition**]

uncompensated alkalosis (un-KOM-pen-say-ted al-kah-LOH-sis)
[*alkal-* **ashes,** *-osis* **condition**]

continued on p. 1033

Acid–base balance is one of the most important of the body's homeostatic mechanisms. The term refers to regulation of hydrogen ion concentration in the body fluid. Therefore the study of acid–base physiology is, in a very real sense, the study of the hydrogen ion (H^+).

Many of the body's most biologically important molecules contain chemical groups that can either "donate" or "accept" a hydrogen ion (H^+) and thus behave as a weak acid or base. As a molecule's pH changes so does its shape and biological activity. The shape and functional ability of ion channels, membrane receptors, haemoglobin, and a variety of enzymes and other important body proteins closely depend on the maintenance of precise regulation of hydrogen ion concentration. Thus, even slight deviations from the normal pH range in body cells and fluids result in pronounced, systemic, and potentially fatal changes in metabolic activity. For example, activity of the Na-K pump, arguably the most important active transport mechanism in the cell membrane, falls by 50% when pH decreases by approximately 1 pH unit. An even more dramatic effect is seen in the activity of a key enzyme (phosphofructokinase) involved in the breakdown of glucose in the absence of O_2 during anaerobic catabolism (glycolysis). The biological activity of this key enzyme falls by approximately 90% when the pH decreases by only 0.1 unit!

Maintaining acid–base balance within narrow and precise ranges is necessary for survival.

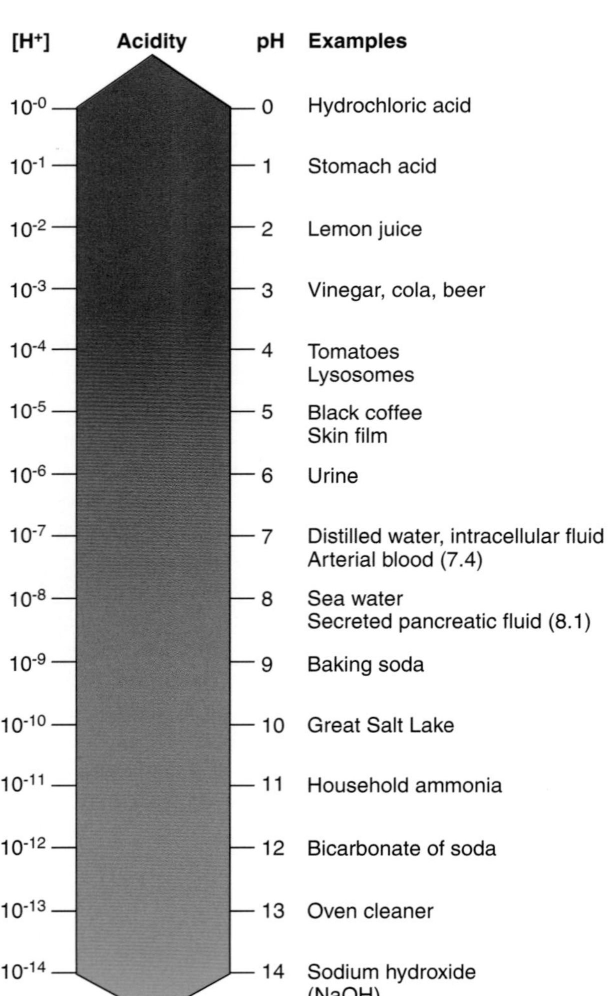

FIGURE 44-1 The pH range. Customarily acids are colour-coded red in diagrams and bases are colour-coded blue or purple, based on the *litmus test* of pH.

MECHANISMS THAT CONTROL pH OF BODY FLUIDS

REVIEW OF THE pH CONCEPT

Recall from Chapter 3 that water and all water solutions contain hydrogen ions (H^+) and hydroxide ions (OH^-). pH is a symbol used to represent the negative logarithm (exponent of 10) of the number of hydrogen ions (H^+) present in 1 litre of a solution. It is expressed as a number between 0 and 14. In **Figure 44-1** the pH value is shown on the right side of the scale and the corresponding logarithmic value is on the left.

Take a moment to review the concept of the pH unit. **pH** indicates the degree of **acidity** or **alkalinity** of a solution. As the concentration of hydrogen ions increases, the pH goes down and the solution becomes more acid; a decrease in hydrogen ion concentration makes the solution more **alkaline** and the pH goes up. A pH of 7 indicates neutrality (equal amounts of H^+ and OH^-), a pH of less than 7 indicates acidity (more H^+ than OH^-) and a pH greater than 7 indicates alkalinity (more OH^- than H^+). With a pH of about 1, gastric juice is the most acidic substance in the body.

With a pH of 7.0, intracellular fluid is essentially neutral. Arterial and venous blood are slightly alkaline because both have a pH slightly higher than 7.0. The slight increase in acidity of venous blood (pH 7.36) compared with arterial blood (pH 7.40) results primarily from carbon dioxide entering venous blood as a waste product of cellular metabolism. Although any pH value above 7.0 is considered chemically basic, in clinical medicine the term **acidosis** is used to describe an arterial blood pH of less than 7.35 and **alkalosis** is used to describe an arterial blood pH greater than 7.45.

The lungs remove the equivalent of more than 30 litres of carbonic acid each day from the venous blood by elimination of carbon dioxide, and yet 1 litre of venous blood contains only about 1/100,000,000 of a gram more hydrogen ions than does 1 litre of arterial blood. What incredible constancy! The pH homeostatic mechanism does indeed control effectively—astonishingly so.

Sources of pH-Influencing Chemicals

Acids and **bases** continually enter the blood as a result of absorbed foods and the metabolism of nutrients at the cellular level. Therefore, some kind of mechanism for neutralizing or eliminating these substances is necessary if blood pH is to remain constant.

Although both acidic and basic components are important, the homeostasis of body pH depends largely on the control of overall hydrogen ion concentration in the extracellular fluid. Hydrogen ions are continually entering the body fluids from (1) carbonic acid, (2) lactic acid, (3) sulphuric acid, (4) phosphoric acid, and (5) acidic ketone bodies.

Carbonic acid forms in the blood when cells produce waste CO_2 through catabolism of glucose. Lactic acid is produced when lactate and free H^+ ions form in the anaerobic pathway of glucose metabolism and fail to enter the aerobic pathway because of oxygen shortage. Sulphuric acid is produced when sulphur-containing amino acids are oxidized, and phosphoric acid accumulates when certain phosphoproteins and ribonucleotides are broken down for energy purposes. Acidic ketone bodies, which include *acetone*, *acetoacetic acid*, and *beta-hydroxybutyric acid*, accumulate during the incomplete breakdown of fats. Each of these acids contributes hydrogen ions in varying amounts to the extracellular fluid and influences acid–base balance. Toxic accumulation of acidic ketone bodies is a common complication of untreated diabetes mellitus.

Minerals that remain after food has been metabolized are said to be either acid-forming minerals or base-forming minerals, depending on whether they contribute to formation of an acidic or basic medium when in solution. Acid-forming elements include chlorine, sulphur, and phosphorus—all are abundant in high-protein foods such as meat, fish, poultry, and eggs. They are also present in some grains such as wheat, corn, and oats. These foods are often designated as acid-forming foods.

After metabolism is complete, most mixed diets contain a surplus of acid-forming mineral elements that must be continually buffered to maintain acid–base balance. Extremely high-protein diets that produce a predominantly *acid mineral residue* when metabolized may tax the body's ability to remain in acid–base balance if consumed over prolonged periods.

Mineral elements that are alkaline, or basic, in solution include *potassium*, *calcium*, *sodium*, and *magnesium*. All these elements are found in fruits and vegetables, which nutritionists often label as *base-forming foods*. The predominantly *basic residue* that results after metabolism of a strict vegetarian diet may also tax the ability of the body to maintain acid–base balance because of a high influx of alkaline components into the extracellular fluid.

Foods containing acids that cannot be metabolized, such as rhubarb (oxalic acid) and cranberries (benzoic acid), are said to be direct acid-forming foods, whereas antacids such as sodium bicarbonate and calcium carbonate are examples of direct base-forming substances. **Box 44-1** gives some examples of acid-forming and base-forming foods.

BOX 44-1 *fyi* | Acid-Forming and Base-Forming Potential of Foods

Examples of foods that have acid-forming characteristics include corn and corn oil, olives and olive oil, blueberries (see figure), cranberries, oats, wheat, rice, peanuts, red beans, black beans, butter, cheese, beef, fish, pork, turkey, canola oil, and sugar. On the other hand, many of the foods we eat may have base-forming characteristics, such as peppers, sea salt, tofu, almonds, mineral water, citrus fruits, grapes, blackberries, bananas, tomatoes, apples, green beans, lettuce, garlic, broccoli, carrots, and avocado. •

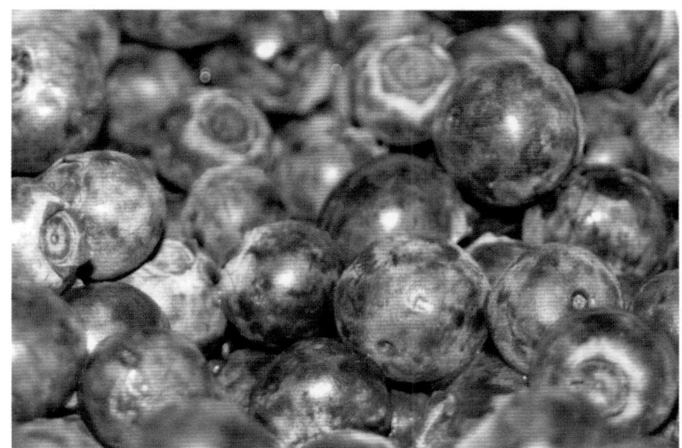

Blueberries. Blueberries have an acid-forming effect.

Quick CHECK

1. Define the term *pH.*
2. Is a solution with a pH above 7 acid or alkaline?
3. Identify three acid-forming and three base-forming elements.
4. Does CO_2 entering venous blood increase or decrease the pH level?

Types of pH Control Mechanisms

The two major types of control systems listed in **Table 44-1**—chemical and physiological—operate to maintain the constancy of body pH.

In the discussion that follows, buffer action is defined and the specific types of *chemical* and *physiological buffer systems* are discussed. The rapid-acting **chemical buffers** immediately combine with any added acid or alkali that enters the body fluids and thus prevent drastic changes in hydrogen ion concentration and pH. As explained later, all buffers act to prevent swings in pH even if

TABLE 44-1 pH Control Systems

TYPE	RESPONSE TIME	EXAMPLE
Chemical buffer systems	Immediate	Bicarbonate buffer system Phosphate buffer system Protein buffer system
Physiological buffer systems	Minutes	Respiratory response system
	Hours	Renal response system

UNIT 5

hydrogen ion concentrations change. If the immediate action of chemical buffers cannot stabilize pH, the **physiological buffers** serve as a secondary defence against harmful shifts in pH of body fluids.

pH shifts that are not halted by the immediate effects of chemical buffering cause the respiratory system to respond in 1 to 2 minutes, and changes in the rate and depth of breathing occur. For reasons explained later, such changes in carbon dioxide levels alter hydrogen ion concentration and help stabilize pH. If respiratory mechanisms are unable to stop the pH shift, a more powerful, but slower-acting, renal physiological buffer system involving the excretion of either an acid or alkaline urine will be initiated within 24 hours.

Collectively, these mechanisms—buffers, respirations, and kidney excretion of acids and bases—might be said to make up the *pH homeostatic mechanism*. One example of the relationship between these three mechanisms is shown in **Figure 44-2**. The equilibrium between hydrogen ions, carbonic acid, bicarbonate, and carbon dioxide within red blood cells illustrates the interrelated nature of the pH control mechanisms. Note that an increase in body carbon dioxide levels results in excess acid formation in red blood cells, which is counteracted by a corresponding increase in elimination of both carbon dioxide by the lungs and excess hydrogen ion in the urine.

Effectiveness of pH Control Mechanisms—Range of pH

The most convincing evidence of the effectiveness of the pH control mechanism is the extremely narrow range of blood pH—normally 7.36 to 7.41. Maintaining the body's pH within this narrow range is essential to sustain healthy life. Moving outside this pH range causes disruption of many of the body's essential chemical processes.

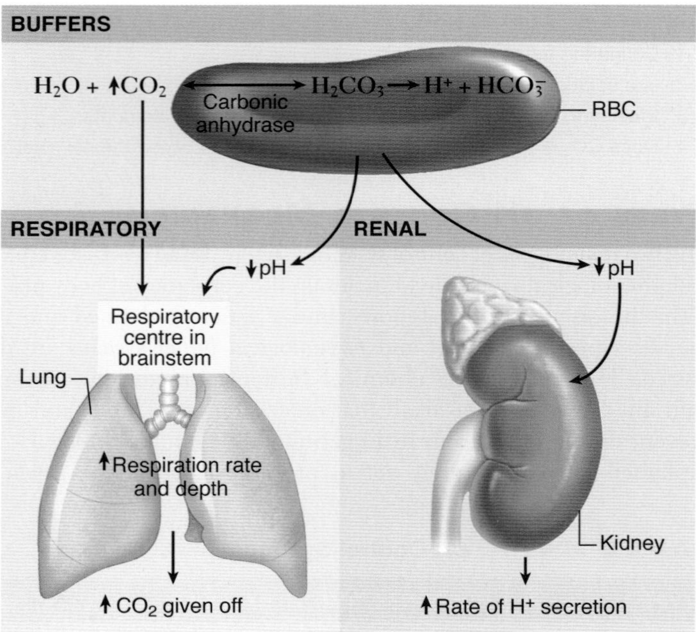

FIGURE 44-2 Integration of pH control mechanisms. Elevated carbon dioxide (CO_2) levels result in increased formation of carbonic acid in red blood cells. The resulting increase in hydrogen ions, coupled with elevated CO_2 levels, results in an increase in respiratory rate and secretion of hydrogen ions (H^+) by the kidneys, thus helping regulate the pH of body fluids.

BUFFER MECHANISMS FOR CONTROLLING pH OF BODY FLUIDS

Buffers Defined

In terms of action, a **buffer** is a substance that prevents marked changes in the pH of a solution when an acid or a base is added to it. Let us suppose that a small amount of a strong acid, hydrochloric acid, is added to a solution that contains a buffer (e.g., blood) and that its pH decreases from 7.41 to 7.27. If the same amount of hydrochloric acid were added to pure water containing no buffers, its pH would decrease much more markedly, from 7 to perhaps 3.4. In both instances, pH decreased after addition of the acid, but much less so with buffers present than without them. Stated another way, buffers do not prevent pH changes, but they do help to minimize them.

In terms of chemical composition, buffers consist of two kinds of substances and are therefore often referred to as **buffer pairs.**

Buffer Pairs Present in Body Fluids

Most of the body fluid buffer pairs consist of a weak acid and a salt of that acid. The main buffer pairs in body fluids are the following:

$$\text{Bicarbonate pairs: } \frac{NaHCO_3}{H_2CO_3}, \frac{KHCO_3}{H_2CO_3}, \text{ etc.}$$

$$\text{Plasma} \bullet \text{protein pair: } \frac{Na \bullet \text{Proteinate}}{\text{Proteins (weak acids)}}$$

$$\text{Haemoglobin pairs: } \frac{K \bullet Hb}{Hb} \text{ and } \frac{K \bullet HbHO_2}{HbO_2}$$

(Hb and HbO_2 are weak acids)

$$\text{Phosphate buffer pair: } \frac{Na_2HPO_4 \text{ (basic phosphate)}}{NaH_2PO_4 \text{ (acid phosphate)}}$$

Buffer Actions That Prevent Marked Changes in pH of Body Fluids

Buffers react with a relatively strong acid (or base) to transform it into a relatively weak acid (or base). That is, an acid that highly dissociates to yield many hydrogen ions is changed into a weaker acid that dissociates less highly to yield fewer hydrogen ions. Thus by way of the buffer reaction, instead of the strong acid remaining in the solution and contributing many hydrogen ions that would drastically lower the pH of the solution, the newly formed weaker acid takes its place, contributes fewer additional hydrogen ions to the solution, and thereby lowers its pH only slightly. Because blood contains buffer pairs, its pH fluctuates much less widely than it would without them. In other words, blood buffers act as one of the mechanisms for preventing marked changes in blood pH.

Let us consider, as a specific example of buffer action, how the sodium bicarbonate ($NaHCO_3$)–carbonic acid (H_2CO_3) system works in the presence of a strong acid or base.

The addition of a strong acid, such as hydrochloric acid (HCl), to the sodium bicarbonate–carbonic acid buffer system would initiate the reaction shown in **Figure 44-3**. Note how this reaction between HCl and the base bicarbonate ($NaHCO_3$) applies the principle of buffering. As a result of the buffering action of $NaHCO_3$, the weak acid, $H \bullet HCO_3$, replaces the very strong acid HCl, and therefore the

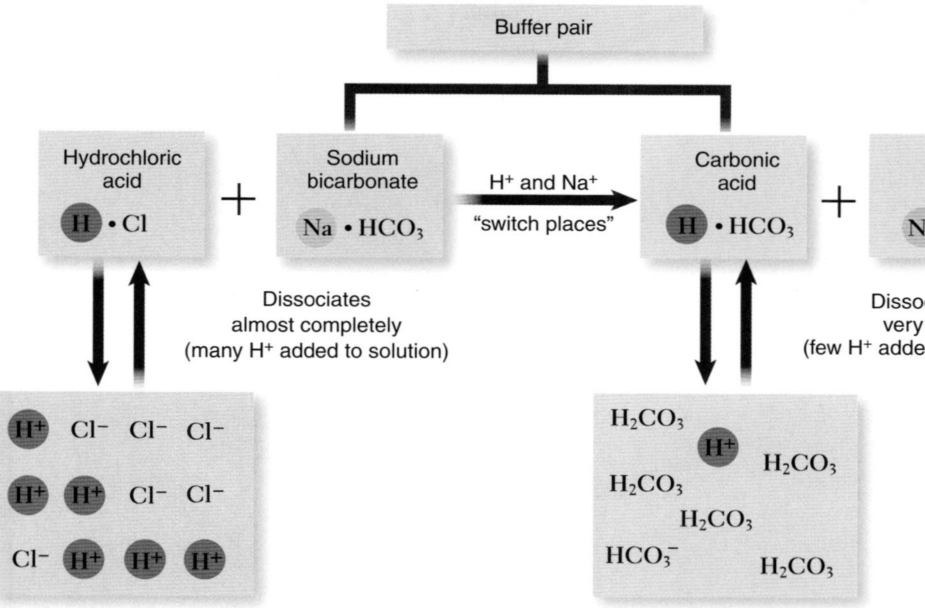

FIGURE 44-3 Buffering action of sodium bicarbonate. Buffering of acid HCl by $NaHCO_3$. As a result of the buffer action, the strong acid (HCl) is replaced by a weaker acid (H • HCO_3). Note that HCl, as a strong acid, "dissociates" almost completely and releases more H^+ than does H_2CO_3. Buffering decreases the number of H^+ in the system.

hydrogen ion concentration of the blood increases much less than it would have if HCl were not buffered.

If, on the other hand, a strong base such as sodium hydroxide (NaOH) is added to the same buffer system, the reaction shown in **Figure 44-4** would take place. The hydrogen ion of H • HCO_3, the weak acid of the buffer pair, combines with hydroxide ion (OH^-) of the strong base NaOH to form water. Note what this accomplishes. It decreases the number of hydroxide ions added to the solution, and this in turn prevents the drastic rise in pH that would occur in the absence of buffering.

Box 44-2 discusses how loss of chloride during severe vomiting could affect the balance of buffers in the body and thus increase the body's pH above normal levels.

The principles of buffer action illustrated by the reaction of HCl and NaOH with the sodium bicarbonate buffer pair can be applied equally to the plasma protein, haemoglobin, and phosphate buffer systems.

Carbon dioxide and other acid waste products are being formed continuously as a result of cellular metabolism. The formation of carbonic acid from carbon dioxide and water requires the enzyme **carbonic anhydrase** (see **Figure 44-2**), which is found in the red blood cells (RBCs). Although there are numerous types of zinc-containing carbonic anhydrases in the body, it is carbonic anhydrase 1, or CA1, that is present in the cytoplasm of erythrocytes and is primarily responsible for the formation of carbonic acid from CO_2 and water in the RBC. Carbonic acid is buffered primarily by

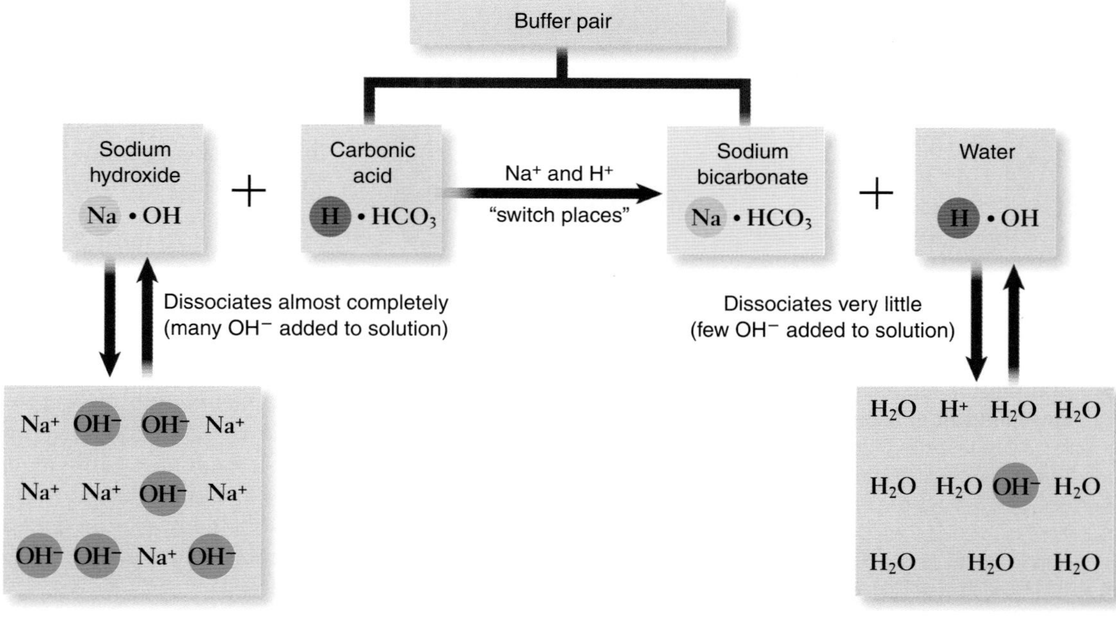

FIGURE 44-4 Buffering action of carbonic acid. Buffering of the base NaOH by H_2CO_3. As a result of buffer action, the strong base (NaOH) is replaced by $NaHCO_3$ and H_2O. As a strong base, NaOH "dissociates" almost completely and releases large quantities of OH^-. Dissociation of H_2O is minimal. Buffering decreases the number of OH^- ions in the system.

BOX 44-2 *health matters*
Metabolic Alkalosis Caused by Vomiting

Vomiting, sometimes referred to as **emesis,** is the forcible emptying or expulsion of gastric and occasionally intestinal contents through the mouth. It occurs as a result of many stimuli, including foul odours or tastes, irritation of the stomach or intestinal mucosa, and some vomitive or *emetic* drugs such as ipecac. A "vomiting centre" in the brain regulates the many coordinated (but primarily involuntary) steps involved (see **Figure 38-20**, p. 876). Severe vomiting such as the **pernicious vomiting** of pregnancy or the repeated vomiting associated with pyloric obstruction in infants can be life-threatening. One of the most common and serious complications of vomiting is metabolic alkalosis. The bicarbonate excess of metabolic alkalosis results because of the massive loss of chloride from the stomach as hydrochloric acid. It is the loss of chloride that causes a compensatory increase of bicarbonate in the extracellular fluid. The result is *metabolic alkalosis.* Therapy includes intravenous administration of chloride-containing solutions such as **normal saline** (0.9% NaCl in water). The chloride ions of the solution replace bicarbonate ions and thus help relieve the bicarbonate excess responsible for the imbalance.

Note—regular misuse of ipecac (ipecacuanha) by individuals with bulimia nervosa to induce vomiting has been linked to damage to the heart and muscles.

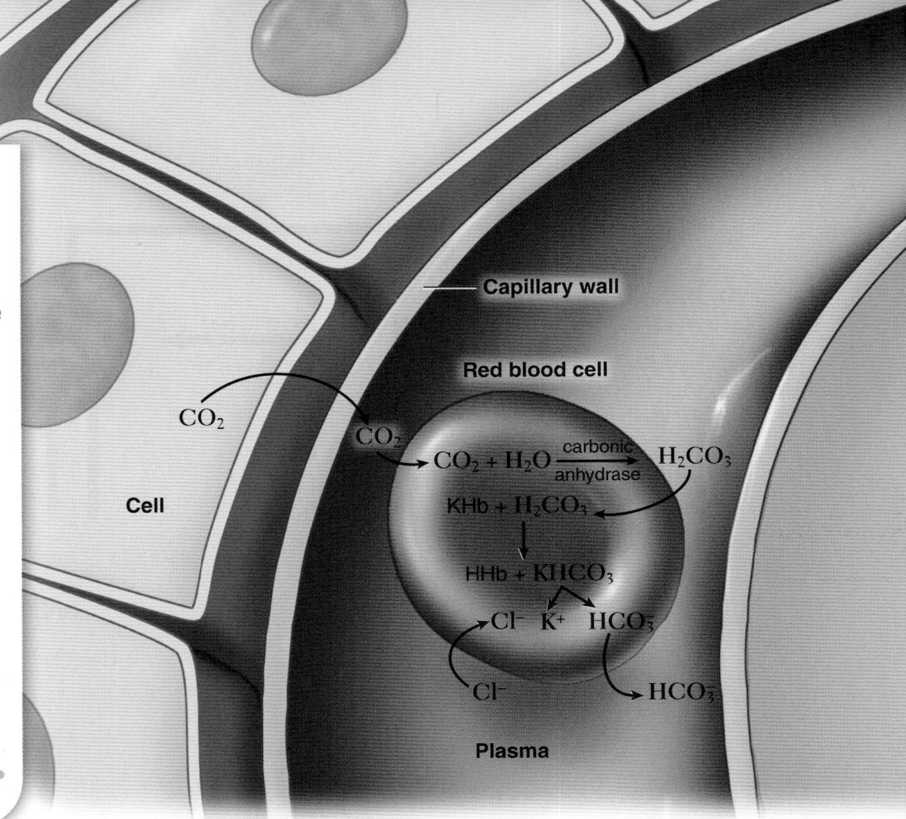

FIGURE 44-6 Chloride shift. The concentration of chloride ions (Cl^-) in red blood cells increases as bicarbonate ions (HCO_3^-) diffuse out of the cell. Bicarbonate ions form as a result of the buffering of carbonic acid by the potassium salt of haemoglobin.

the potassium salt of haemoglobin inside the RBC, as shown in **Figure 44-5**.

It is interesting to note that the $KHCO_3$ formed by the buffering of carbonic acid dissociates in the RBC, and the bicarbonate ion diffuses down its concentration gradient into the blood plasma. Because of the movement of these negatively charged ions out of the RBC, chloride ions move into the cell from the plasma to maintain the electrical balance on both sides of the RBC membrane. The process of exchanging a bicarbonate ion formed in the red blood cell with a chloride ion from the plasma is called the **chloride shift.** This process makes it possible for carbon dioxide to be buffered in the RBC and then carried as bicarbonate in the plasma. **Figure 44-6** summarizes the reactions of the chloride shift.

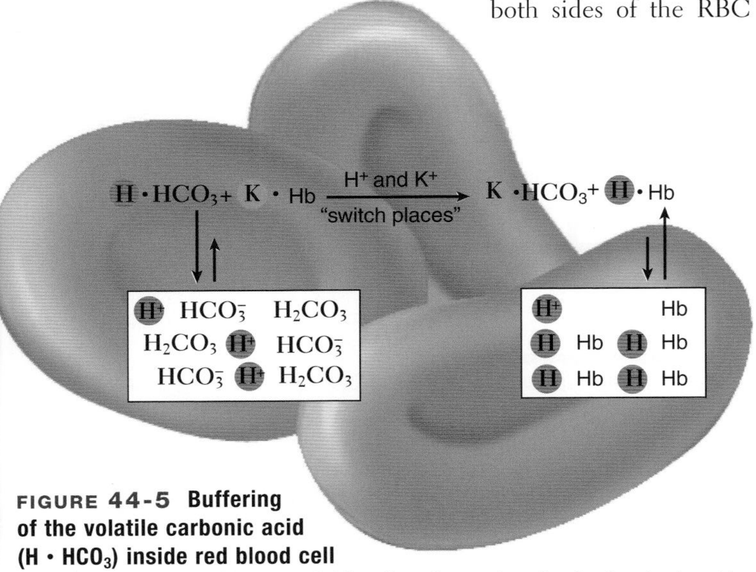

FIGURE 44-5 Buffering of the volatile carbonic acid (H • HCO_3) inside red blood cell by potassium salt of haemoglobin. Note that each molecule of carbonic acid is replaced by a molecule of acid haemoglobin. Because haemoglobin is a weaker acid than carbonic acid, fewer of these haemoglobin molecules dissociate to form hydrogen ions (H^+). Hence, fewer hydrogen ions are added to red blood cell intracellular fluid than would be added by unbuffered carbonic acid. Also, because some of the carbonic acid in the red blood cell has come from plasma, fewer hydrogen ions remain in blood than would have if there were no buffering of carbonic acid.

Nonvolatile, or fixed, acids, such as hydrochloric acid, lactic acid, and ketone bodies, are buffered mainly by sodium bicarbonate (**Figure 44-7**). **Box 44-3** discusses why some athletes consume bicarbonate to counteract the effects of lactic acid produced by exercise. **Box 44-4** discusses how lactic acidosis can result from the use of a popular diabetes drug.

Normal blood pH and acid–base balance depend on a base bicarbonate–to–carbonic acid buffer pair ratio of 20 : 1 in the extracellular fluid. Actually, in a state of acid–base balance (pH 7.4), a litre of plasma may contain 26 mEq of $NaHCO_3$ as base bicarbonate (BB)—ordinary baking soda—and 1.3 mEq of carbonic acid (CA):

$$\frac{26 \text{ mEq NaHCO}_3}{1.3 \text{ mEq H}_2\text{CO}_3} = \frac{\text{BB}}{\text{CA}} = \frac{20}{1} = \text{pH } 7.4$$

The **ratio** of base to acid is critical. If the ratio is maintained, acid–base balance (pH) remains near normal despite changes in the absolute amounts of either component of the buffer pair. This type of adjustment is called **compensation.**

For example, a BB/CA ratio of 40 : 2 or 10 : 0.5 would result in a compensated state of acid–base balance. However, an increase in the ratio causes an increase in pH (**uncompensated alkalosis**), and a decrease in the ratio causes a decrease in pH (**uncompensated acidosis**).

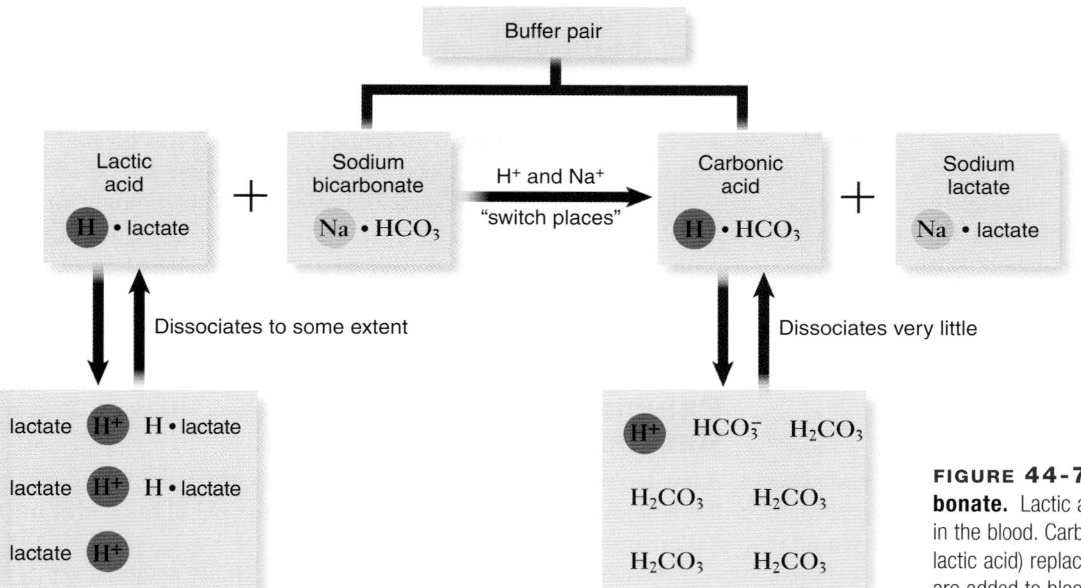

FIGURE 44-7 Lactic acid buffered by sodium bicarbonate. Lactic acid and other "fixed" acids are buffered by $NaHCO_3$ in the blood. Carbonic acid (H • HCO_3 or H_2CO_3, a weaker acid than lactic acid) replaces lactic acid. As a result, fewer hydrogen ions (H^+) are added to blood than would be if lactic acid were not buffered.

The ability of the body to regulate the amount of either component of the bicarbonate buffer pair—to maintain the correct ratio for acid–base balance—makes this system one of the most important for controlling pH of body fluids. **Correction** of acid–base balance is said to occur when components of the buffer pair return to a normal 20 : 1 ratio.

Evaluation of the Role of Buffers in pH Control

Buffering alone cannot maintain homeostasis of pH. As we have seen, hydrogen ions are added continually to capillary blood despite buffering. If even a few hydrogen ions were added every time blood circulated and no way was provided for eliminating them, blood hydrogen ion concentration would necessarily increase and thereby decrease blood pH. "Acid blood", in other words, would soon develop. Respiratory and urinary mechanisms must therefore function concurrently with buffers to remove from the blood and from the body the hydrogen ions continually being added to blood. Only then can the body maintain constancy of pH over time.

Quick CHECK

5. Define the term *buffer.*
6. Identify the two major types of buffer systems in the body. Which buffer system is the most rapid-acting?
7. Using equations, explain the buffering of HCl by sodium bicarbonate and NaOH by carbonic acid.
8. Define the term *chloride shift.*

RESPIRATORY MECHANISMS OF pH CONTROL

Explanation of Respiratory Mechanisms

Respirations play a vital role in controlling pH. With every expiration, carbon dioxide and water leave the body in the expired air. The carbon dioxide comes from the pulmonary blood and diffuses out of it as it moves through the lung capillaries. Therefore, less carbon dioxide remains in the arterial blood leaving the lung capillaries. The lower P_{CO_2} in arterial blood reduces the amount of carbonic

BOX 44-3 *sports and fitness*
Bicarbonate Loading

The buildup of lactic acid in the blood, released as excess lactate and H^+ from anaerobic catabolism in working muscles, has been blamed for the soreness and fatigue that sometimes accompany strenuous exercise. Some athletes adopt a technique called **bicarbonate loading,** in which large amounts of sodium bicarbonate ($NaHCO_3$) are ingested to counteract the effects of lactic acid buildup. Their theory is that fatigue is avoided because the $NaHCO_3$, a base, buffers the lactic acid. However, we now know that lactic acid buildup is not the primary mechanism of fatigue. Unfortunately, the excess bicarbonate intake and diarrhoea that often result can trigger fluid and electrolyte imbalances. Long-term $NaHCO_3$ abuse can lead to metabolic alkalosis and its disastrous effects. •

BOX 44-4 *lactic acidosis and metformin*

Metformin is one of the most widely used and effective of the oral antidiabetic drugs. It is used with diet and exercise to lower blood glucose levels in type 2 diabetes mellitus. A rare but very serious complication of metformin therapy is **lactic acidosis.** It is characterized by elevated blood lactate levels, electrolyte disturbances, and decreased blood pH. A maximum of 8.1 cases per 100,000 patient-years has been reported in patients taking metformin. Symptoms include a variety of gastrointestinal and respiratory complaints and feelings of weakness and muscle pain. Patients with kidney and liver disease are known to be at higher risk for lactic acidosis while taking the drug. •

acid and the number of hydrogen ions that can be formed in red blood cells by the following reactions:

$$CO_2 + H_2O \xrightarrow{\text{(carbonic anhydrase)}} H_2CO_3$$

$$H_2CO_3 \longrightarrow H^+ + HCO_3^-$$

Arterial blood leaving the pulmonary capillaries therefore has a lower hydrogen ion concentration and a higher pH than does deoxygenated blood entering the pulmonary circulation. A typical average pH for systemic venous blood is 7.36, and 7.41 is a typical average pH for systemic arterial blood.

Respiratory Adjustment to Counter pH Imbalance of Arterial Blood

For respirations to serve as a mechanism of pH control, there must be some mechanism for changing the rate or depth of respirations as needed to maintain or restore normal pH. Suppose that blood pH has decreased; that is, the hydrogen ion concentration has increased. Respirations then need to increase in rate or depth to eliminate more carbon dioxide from the body and thereby leave less carbonic acid and fewer hydrogen ions in the blood.

One mechanism for adjusting respirations to counter arterial blood carbon dioxide content or pH operates in the following way: Neurons of the respiratory centre are sensitive to changes in arterial blood carbon dioxide content and to changes in its pH. If the amount of carbon dioxide in arterial blood increases beyond a certain level, or if arterial blood pH decreases below about 7.38, the respiratory centre is stimulated and respirations accordingly increase in rate and depth. This, in turn, eliminates more carbon dioxide, reduces carbonic acid and hydrogen ions, and increases pH back toward the normal level (**Figure 44-8**).

The carotid chemoreflexes are also mechanisms by which respirations adjust to blood pH and, in turn, adjust pH.

Principles That Relate Respirations to pH Value

A few basic principles, summarized briefly here, help us understand the relationship of respiratory function to the pH of the body's internal environment.

- A decrease in blood pH below normal (acidosis) tends to stimulate increased respirations (hyperventilation), which tends to increase pH back toward normal. In other words,

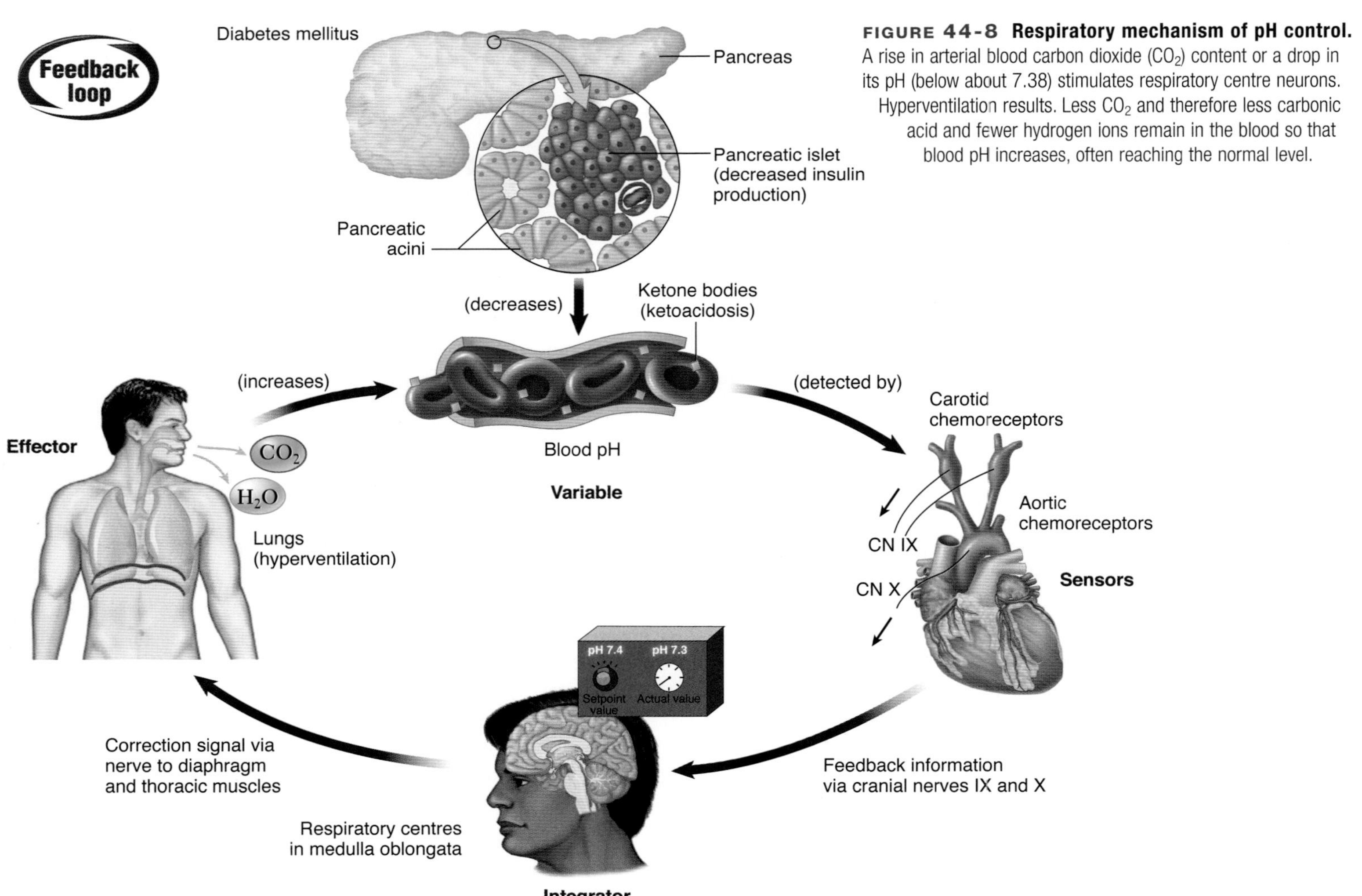

FIGURE 44-8 Respiratory mechanism of pH control. A rise in arterial blood carbon dioxide (CO_2) content or a drop in its pH (below about 7.38) stimulates respiratory centre neurons. Hyperventilation results. Less CO_2 and therefore less carbonic acid and fewer hydrogen ions remain in the blood so that blood pH increases, often reaching the normal level.

acidosis causes hyperventilation, which in turn acts as a compensating mechanism for the acidosis.

- Prolonged hyperventilation—beyond that needed to restore normal pH—may increase blood pH enough to produce alkalosis.
- An increase in blood pH above normal (or alkalosis) triggers hypoventilation, which serves as a compensating mechanism for the alkalosis by decreasing blood pH back toward normal.
- Prolonged hypoventilation—beyond that needed to restore normal pH—may decrease blood pH enough to produce acidosis.

ARTERIAL BLOOD GAS ANALYSIS

Clinically, assessment of primary acid–base imbalances often involves an analysis of the **arterial blood gases (ABGs).** This is a laboratory test of blood taken from an artery (most blood samples are taken from a vein). As the name suggests, this test shows the key characteristics of blood related to respiratory function:

1. Oxygen partial pressure or PO_2
2. Oxygen saturation of haemoglobin or $\%SO_2$
3. pH
4. Concentration of bicarbonate ions or $[HCO_3^-]$
5. Carbon dioxide partial pressure or PCO_2

Sometimes these values are listed with an "a" to emphasize that these are "arterial" values, as in P_aO_2 or P_aCO_2. Note that although not all these values are actually "gases", they are affected by blood gases. ABG test results not only reveal a patient's respiratory status, the pH, PCO_2, and $[HCO_3^-]$ components can also give key information about status of acid–base homeostasis (**Table 44-2**).

pH is the first result to look at when assessing pH status. If the result is below 7.35, there is *acidosis*, and if it's above 7.45, there is *alkalosis*.

To determine the primary status, one next looks at the PCO_2 result. If the pH is low and PCO_2 is above 6.0 kPa (45 mmHg), the primary status is *respiratory* acidosis. If pH is high and PCO_2 is below 4.7 kPa (35 mmHg), the status is *respiratory* alkalosis.

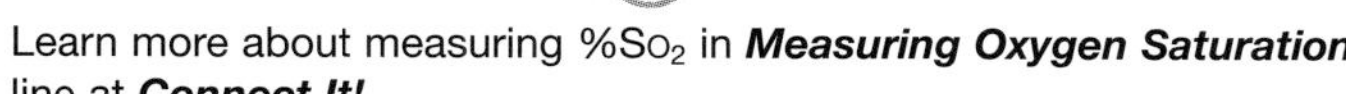

Learn more about measuring $\%SO_2$ in ***Measuring Oxygen Saturation*** online at ***Connect It!***

Next, look at the $[HCO_3^-]$ result. If pH is low and $[HCO_3^-]$ is below 22 mEq/L, the primary status is *metabolic* acidosis. If the pH is high and the $[HCO_3^-]$ is above 26 mEq/L, the primary status is *metabolic* alkalosis.

One may then try to determine whether compensation is occurring in the body. This can be done by looking at the pH-balancing mechanism *not* directly involved in determining the primary status to see if it has changed in a way that counterbalances—or *compensates* for—the primary problem. For example, if the arterial pH is low (acidotic) and the PCO_2 (acid) is high, as in respiratory acidosis, the body may compensate by increasing the $[HCO_3^-]$ (base). Likewise, if the arterial pH is low (alkalotic) and the $[HCO_3^-]$ (base) is high, as in metabolic alkalosis, the body may compensate by increasing the PCO_2 (acid).

URINARY MECHANISMS THAT CONTROL pH

GENERAL PRINCIPLES CONCERNING URINARY MECHANISMS

Because the kidneys can excrete varying amounts of acid and base, they, like the lungs, play a vital role in pH control. Kidney tubules, by excreting many or few hydrogen ions in exchange for reabsorbing many or few sodium ions, control urine pH and thereby help control blood pH.

If, for example, blood pH decreases below normal, the kidney tubules secrete more hydrogen ions from blood to urine and, in exchange for each hydrogen ion, reabsorb a sodium ion from the urine back into the blood. This, of course, decreases urine pH. But simultaneously—and of far more importance—it increases blood pH back toward normal. This urinary mechanism of pH control is a process for excreting varying amounts of hydrogen ions from the body to match the amounts entering the blood.

The urinary mechanism is a much more effective process for adjusting hydrogen output to hydrogen input than the body's only other mechanism for expelling hydrogen ions—namely, the respiratory mechanisms previously described. But abnormalities of any one of the three pH control mechanisms soon throw the body into a state of acid–base imbalance. Only when all three parts of this complex mechanism—buffering, respirations, and urine secretion—function adequately can acid–base balance be maintained.

Let us turn now to mechanisms that adjust urine pH to counteract changes in blood pH.

TABLE 44-2 Arterial Blood Gas Analysis for Acid–Base Status

ABG COMPONENT	NORMAL VALUES	ACIDOSIS		ALKALOSIS	
		Respiratory	Metabolic	Respiratory	Metabolic
pH	7.35–7.45	↓ < 7.35	↓ < 7.35	↑ > 7.45	↑ > 7.45
PCO_2	4.7–6.0 kPa	↑ > 6 kPa	Uncompensated: = 4.7–6.0 kPa Compensated: ↓ < 4.7 kPa	↓ < 4.7 kPa	↑ > 6.0 kPa
$[HCO_3^-]$	22–26 mEq/L	Uncompensated: = 22–26 Compensated: ↑ > 26	↓ < 22	Uncompensated: = 22–26 Compensated: ↓ < 22	↑ > 26

↓, Decrease; ↑, increase; *ABG*, arterial blood gas; *$[HCO_3^-]$*, bicarbonate concentration; *PCO_2*, carbon dioxide pressure.

MECHANISMS THAT CONTROL URINE pH

A decrease in blood pH accelerates the renal tubule ion exchange mechanisms that acidify urine and conserve blood's base, thereby tending to increase blood pH back to normal. Several different such mechanisms work together to remove acid from the body's internal environment.

In one urinary acidification mechanism, the distal tubules and collecting ducts secrete hydrogen ions into the urine in exchange for basic ions, which they reabsorb. Refer to **Figure 44-9** as

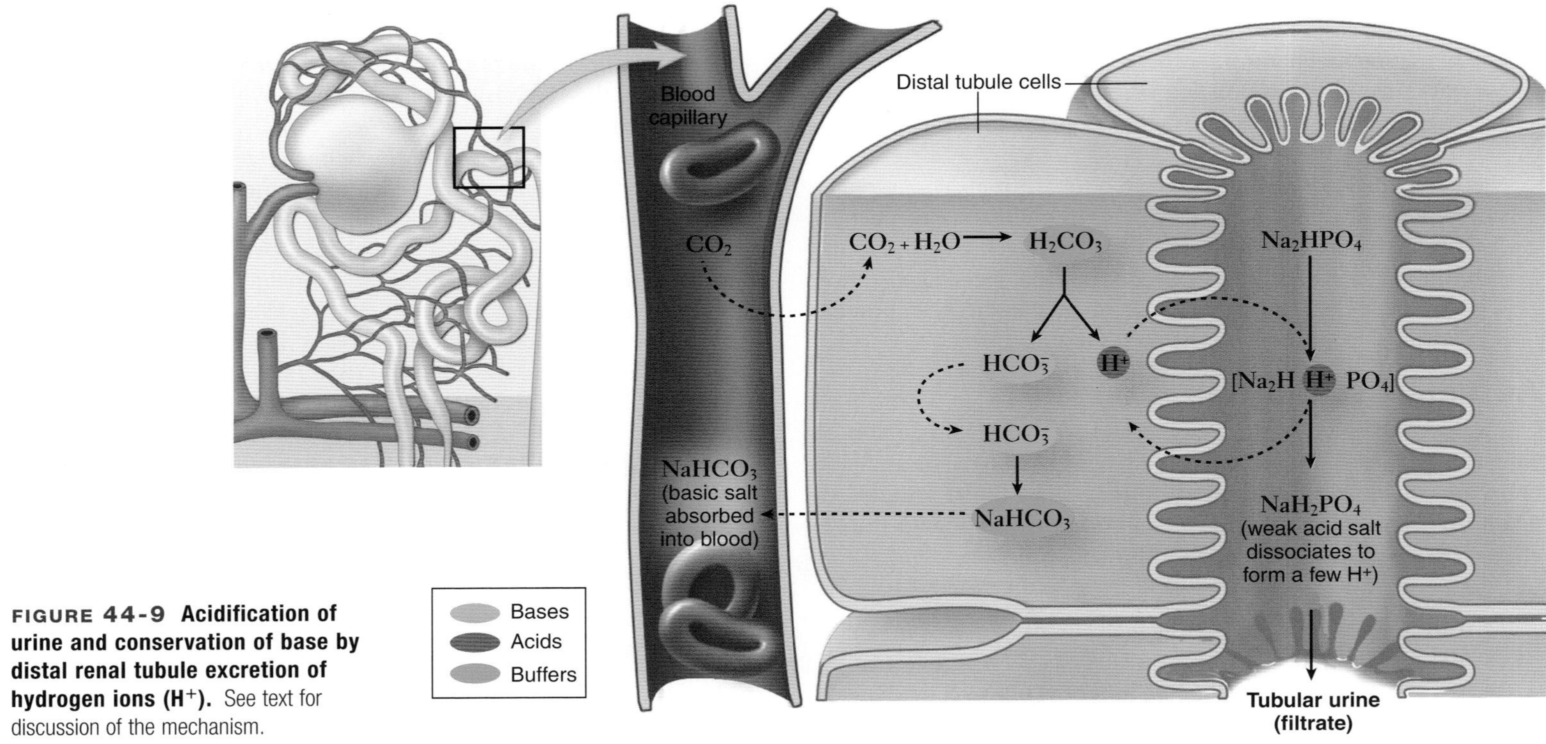

FIGURE 44-9 Acidification of urine and conservation of base by distal renal tubule excretion of hydrogen ions (H^+). See text for discussion of the mechanism.

you read the rest of this paragraph. Note that carbon dioxide diffuses from tubule capillaries into distal tubule cells, where the enzyme carbonic anhydrase accelerates the combining of carbon dioxide with water to form carbonic acid. The carbonic acid dissociates into hydrogen ions and bicarbonate ions. The hydrogen ions then move into the tubular urine, where they displace basic ions (most often sodium) from a basic salt of a weak acid and thereby change the basic salt to an acid salt or to a weak acid that is eliminated in the urine. While this is happening, the displaced sodium or other basic ion diffuses into a tubule cell. There it combines

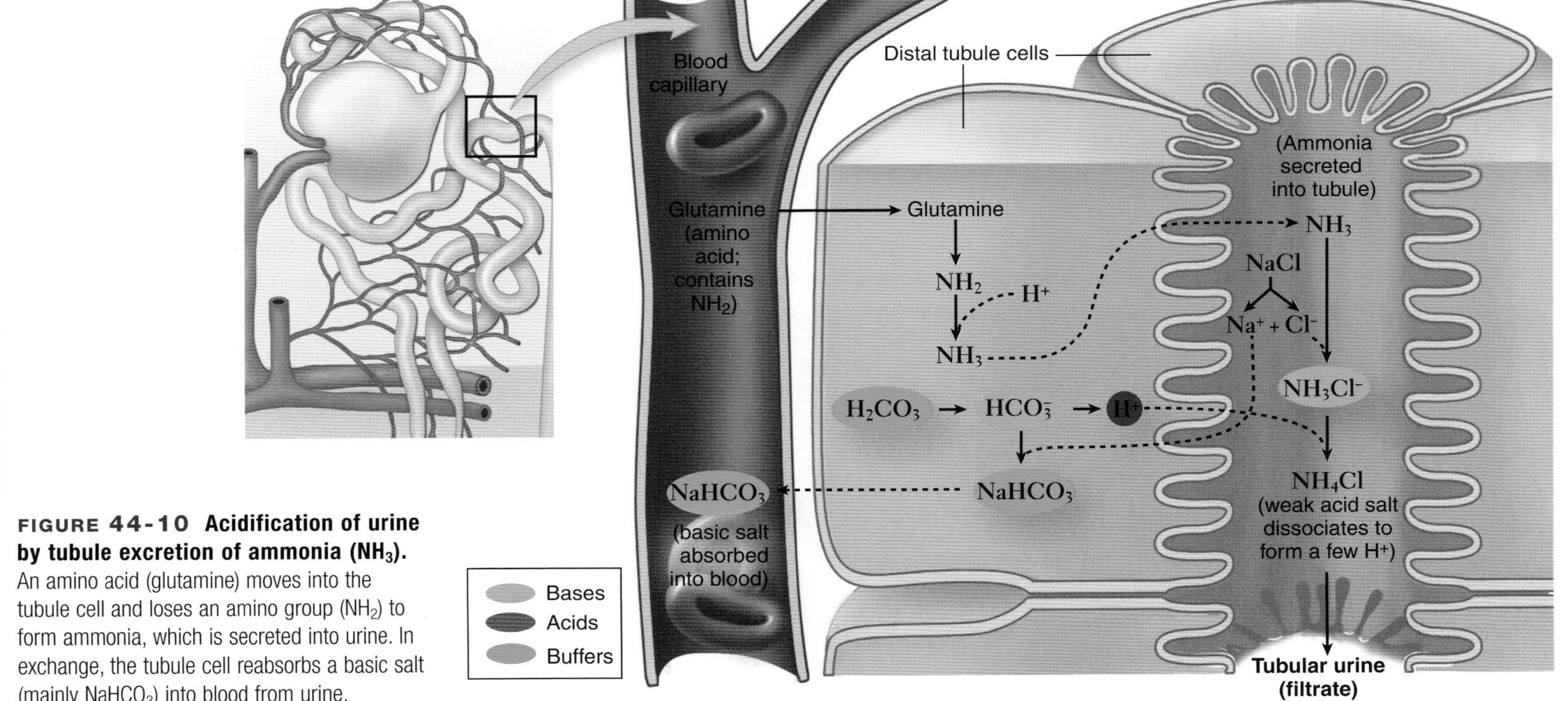

FIGURE 44-10 Acidification of urine by tubule excretion of ammonia (NH_3). An amino acid (glutamine) moves into the tubule cell and loses an amino group (NH_2) to form ammonia, which is secreted into urine. In exchange, the tubule cell reabsorbs a basic salt (mainly $NaHCO_3$) into blood from urine.

with the bicarbonate ion left over from the carbonic acid dissociation to form sodium bicarbonate. The sodium bicarbonate then diffuses—is reabsorbed—into the blood.

Consider the various results of this mechanism. Sodium bicarbonate (or other base bicarbonate) is conserved for the body. Instead of all the basic salts that filter out of glomerular blood leaving the body in the urine, considerable amounts are recovered into peritubular capillary blood. In addition, extra hydrogen ions are added to the urine and thereby eliminated from the body. Both the reabsorption of base bicarbonate into blood and the excretion of hydrogen ions into urine tend to increase the ratio of the bicarbonate buffer pair $B \bullet HCO_3/H \bullet HCO_3$ (BB/CA) present in blood. This automatically increases blood pH. In short, kidney tubule base bicarbonate reabsorption and hydrogen ion excretion both tend to alkalinize blood by acidifying urine.

In another urinary mechanism, the renal tubules can excrete hydrogen or potassium in exchange for the sodium they reabsorb. Therefore, in general, the more hydrogen ions they excrete, the fewer potassium ions they can excrete. In acidosis, tubule excretion of hydrogen ions increases markedly and potassium ion excretion decreases—an important factor because it may lead to **hyperkalaemia** (excessive blood potassium), a condition that can cause heart block and death.

In yet another urinary mechanism, the proximal tubule cells secrete ammonia into the filtrate. As **Figure 44-10** shows, in the distal tubule and collecting duct, the ammonia combines with secreted hydrogen to form an ammonium ion (NH_4). The ammonium ion displaces sodium or some other basic ion from a salt of a fixed (nonvolatile) acid to form an ammonium salt. The basic ion then diffuses back into a tubule cell and combines with a bicarbonate ion to form a basic salt, which in turn diffuses into tubular blood. Thus, like the renal tubules' excretion of hydrogen ions, their excretion of ammonia and its combining with hydrogen to form ammonium ions also tend to increase the blood bicarbonate buffer pair ratio and therefore tend to increase blood pH. Quantitatively, however, ammonium ion excretion is more important than hydrogen ion excretion.

Renal tubule excretion of hydrogen and ammonia is controlled at least in part by the blood pH level. As indicated in **Figure 44-11**, a decrease in blood pH accelerates tubule excretion of both hydrogen and ammonia. An increase in blood pH produces the opposite effects.

Quick CHECK

9. What is the function of carbonic anhydrase in buffer action?
10. How does respiratory rate affect blood pH levels?
11. Identify the test that shows the key characteristics of blood as it is related to respiratory function.
12. List two ways in which acidification of urine occurs.

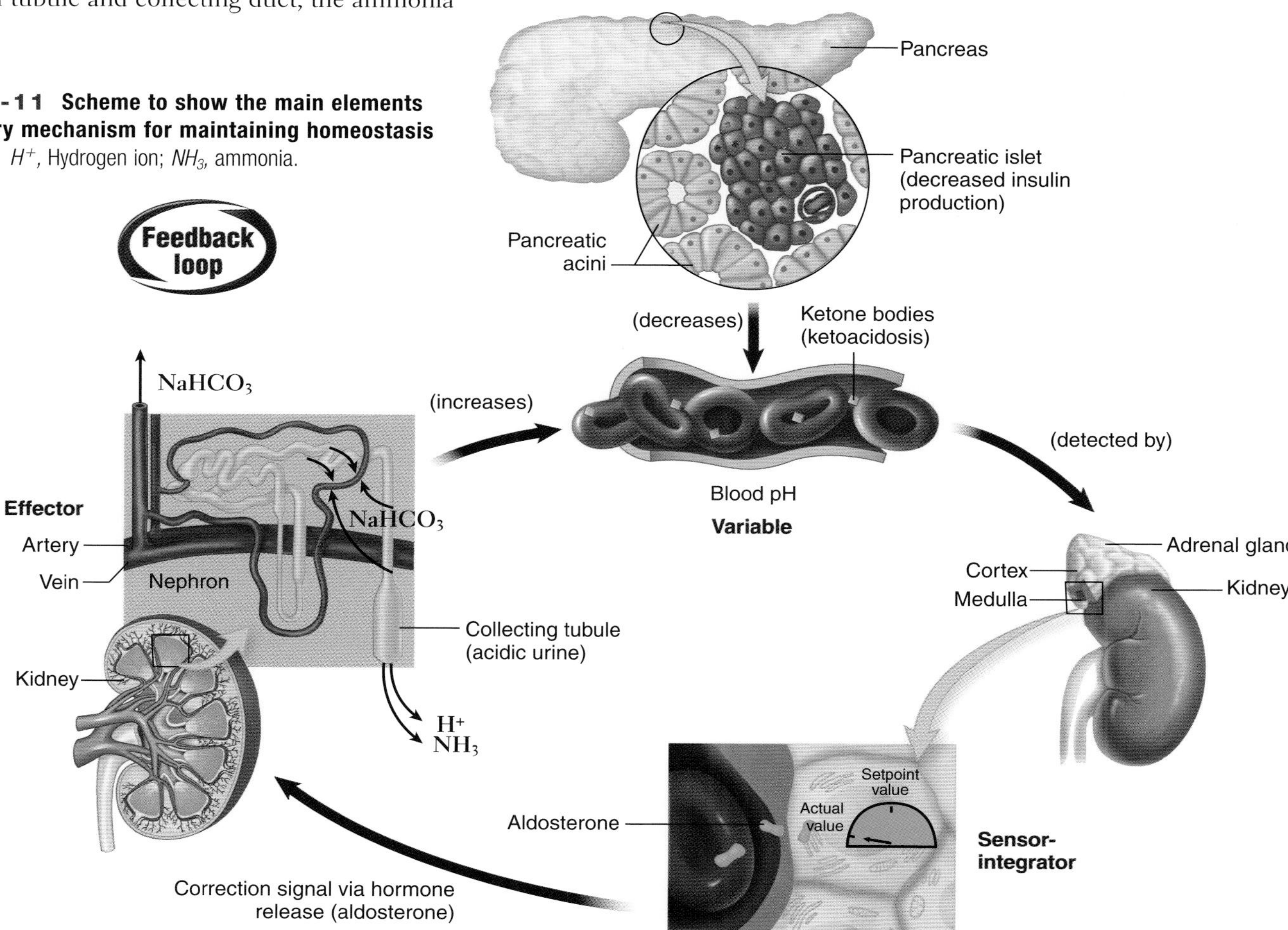

FIGURE 44-11 Scheme to show the main elements of the urinary mechanism for maintaining homeostasis of blood pH. *H^+*, Hydrogen ion; *NH_3*, ammonia.

UNIT 5

the big picture | **Acid–Base Balance**

Ultimately, all functions occur at the cellular level and, without exception, each vital physiological function depends on the maintenance of an appropriate, stable, and tightly regulated acid–base environment. Regulating chemical reactions at the cellular level permits us to control the flow of energy in the body. We need to control energy flow to accomplish cellular work and to store and transfer energy so that we can meet our immediate and long-term needs. Enzymes are the biological catalysts that permit or assist our cells in the regulation of all energy-based metabolic reactions required for the maintenance of life.

Enzymes involved in metabolic reactions have both optimal pH ranges for maximal activity and limited pH ranges in which activity is maintained. Therefore, anything that disrupts the homeostasis of acid–base balance by disrupting enzyme activity is immediately life-threatening because it affects our ability to initiate and regulate the metabolic activity required to sustain life.

The elaborate and highly sensitive pH control mechanisms intended to provide homeostasis of our acid–base environment are critical for the enzymatic action necessary for healthy metabolism and for life itself.

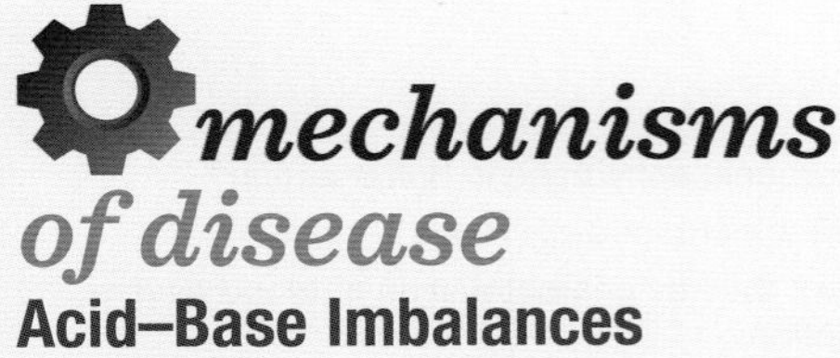

Acid–Base Imbalances

The chemistry of life can operate only within the range pH 6.8 to 8.0. The range of optimal human function is much narrower than that—pH 7.35 to 7.45. Acidosis and alkalosis are the two kinds of pH or acid–base imbalance that threaten our health and survival. All of the buffer pairs in body fluids play an important role in acid–base balance. However, only in the bicarbonate system can the body regulate quickly and precisely the levels of both chemical components in the buffer pair. Carbonic acid levels can be regulated by the respiratory system and bicarbonate ion by the kidneys. Recall that a 20 : 1 ratio of base bicarbonate to carbonic acid (BB/CA) maintains acid–base balance and normal blood pH. Therefore, from a clinical standpoint, disturbances in acid–base balance depend on the relative quantities of carbonic acid and base bicarbonate in the extracellular fluid. Two types of disturbances, metabolic and respiratory, can alter the proper ratio of these components. Metabolic disturbances affect the bicarbonate element, and respiratory disturbances affect the carbonic acid element of the buffer pair.

Metabolic acidosis and *respiratory acidosis,* for example, are separate and very different types of acid–base imbalances. Both are treated by the intravenous infusion of solutions containing **sodium lactate.** The infused lactate ions are metabolized by liver cells and converted to bicarbonate ions. This therapy helps replace the depleted bicarbonate reserves required to restore acid–base balance in metabolic acidosis. In respiratory acidosis, the additional bicarbonate ions function to offset elevated carbonic acid levels.

Metabolic Disturbances

Metabolic Acidosis (Bicarbonate Deficit)

During the course of certain diseases such as untreated diabetes mellitus or during starvation, abnormally large amounts of acids enter the blood. The ratio of BB/CA is altered as the base bicarbonate component of the buffer pair reacts with the acids. The result may be a new ratio near 10 : 1. The decreasing ratio lowers the blood pH, and the respiratory centre is stimulated (**Figure 44-12**). The resulting hyperventilation results in a "blow-off" of carbon dioxide, with a decrease in carbonic acid. This compensatory action of the respiratory system, coupled with excretion of H^+ and NH_3 in exchange for Na^+ reabsorbed by the kidneys, may be sufficient to adjust the ratio of BB/CA, and therefore blood pH, to normal. (The compensated BB/CA ratio may approach 10 : 0.5.) If, despite these compensating homeostatic processes, the ratio and pH cannot be corrected, uncompensated **metabolic acidosis** develops. Drug use (see **Box 44-4**) or metabolic conditions (such as hypoxia caused by circulatory shock) that increase lactate and protons (H^+) in the blood can also cause acidosis.

An increased blood hydrogen ion concentration—that is, decreased blood pH—as we have noted, stimulates the respiratory centre. For this reason, hyperventilation is an outstanding clinical sign of acidosis. Increases in hydrogen ion concentration above a certain level depress the central nervous system and therefore produce such symptoms as disorientation and coma. In a terminal illness, death from acidosis is likely to follow coma, whereas death from alkalosis generally follows tetany and convulsions.

Metabolic Alkalosis (Bicarbonate Excess)

Patients with chronic stomach problems such as hyperacidity sometimes ingest large quantities of alkali—often plain baking soda, or sodium bicarbonate—for extended periods. Such improper use of antacids or excessive vomiting (see **Box 44-2**) can produce **metabolic alkalosis.** Initially, the condition results in an increase in the BB/CA ratio to perhaps 40 : 1 (**Figure 44-13**). Compensatory mechanisms are aimed at increasing carbonic acid and decreasing the bicarbonate load. With breathing suppressed and the kidneys excreting bicarbonate ions, a compensated ratio of 30 : 1.25 might result. Such a ratio would restore acid–base balance and blood pH to normal. In uncompensated metabolic alkalosis, the ratio, and therefore the pH, remain increased.

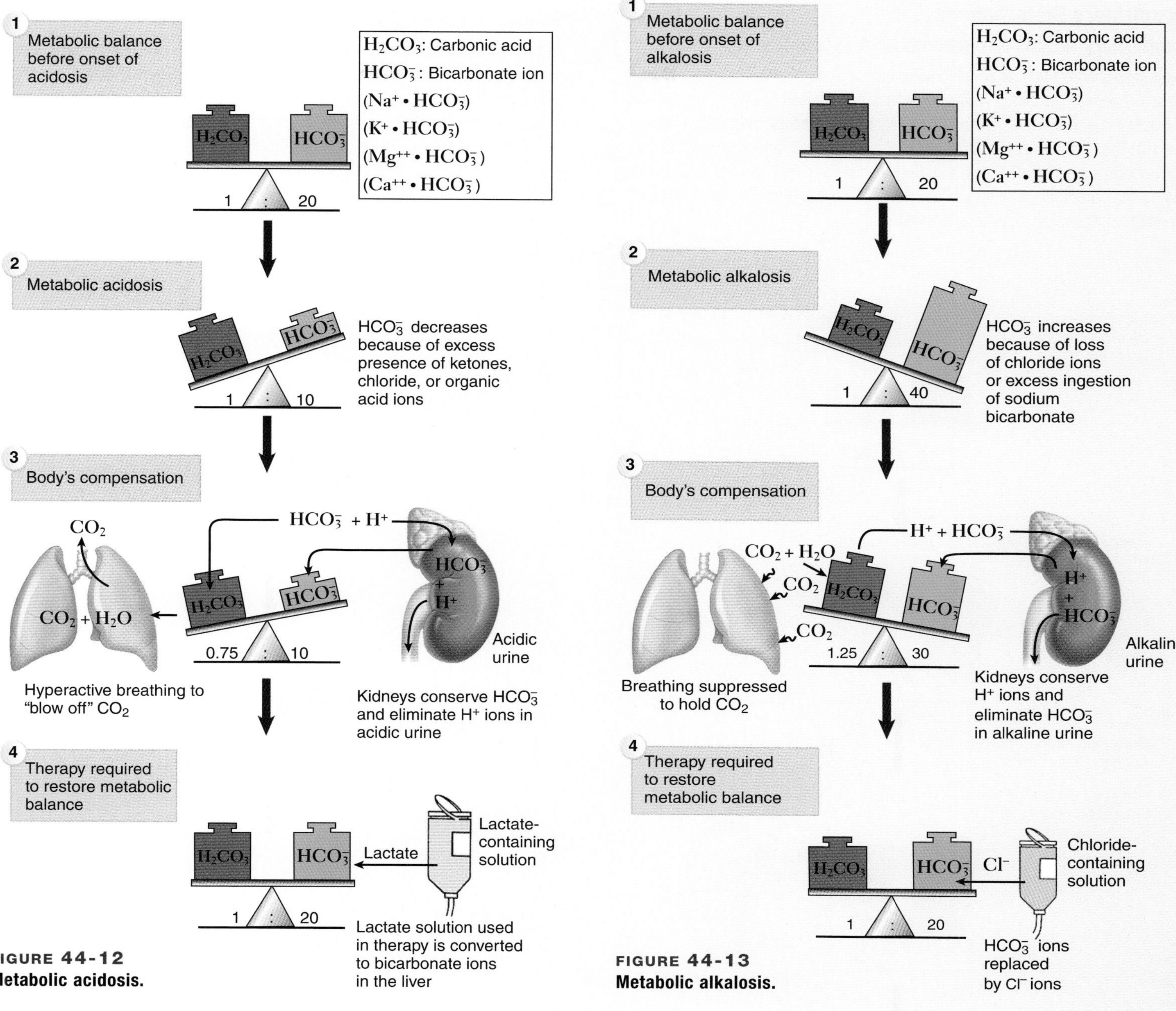

FIGURE 44-12
Metabolic acidosis.

FIGURE 44-13
Metabolic alkalosis.

Respiratory Disturbances

Respiratory Acidosis (Carbonic Acid Excess)

Clinical conditions such as pneumonia or emphysema tend to cause retention of carbon dioxide in the blood. Also, drug abuse or overdose, such as barbiturate poisoning, suppresses breathing and results in **respiratory acidosis** (**Figure 44-14**). The carbonic acid component of the bicarbonate buffer pair increases above normal in respiratory acidosis. Body compensation, if successful, increases the bicarbonate fraction so that a new BB/CA ratio (perhaps 23 : 0) will return blood pH to normal or near-normal levels.

1 Metabolic balance before onset of acidosis

H_2CO_3: Carbonic acid
HCO_3^-: Bicarbonate ion
($Na^+ \cdot HCO_3^-$)
($K^+ \cdot HCO_3^-$)
($Mg^{++} \cdot HCO_3^-$)
($Ca^{++} \cdot HCO_3^-$)

H_2CO_3 HCO_3^- 1 : 20

2 Respiratory acidosis

CO_2 CO_2 CO_2 H_2CO_3 HCO_3^- 2 : 20

Breathing is suppressed, holding CO_2 in body

3 Body's compensation

H_2CO_3 HCO_3^- ← HCO_3^- H_2CO_3 HCO_3^- + H^+ Acidic urine 2 : 30

Kidneys conserve HCO_3^- ions and eliminate H^+ ions in acidic urine

4 Therapy required to restore metabolic balance

H_2CO_3 HCO_3^- ← Lactate Lactate-containing solution 1 : 20

Lactate solution used in therapy is converted to bicarbonate ions in the liver

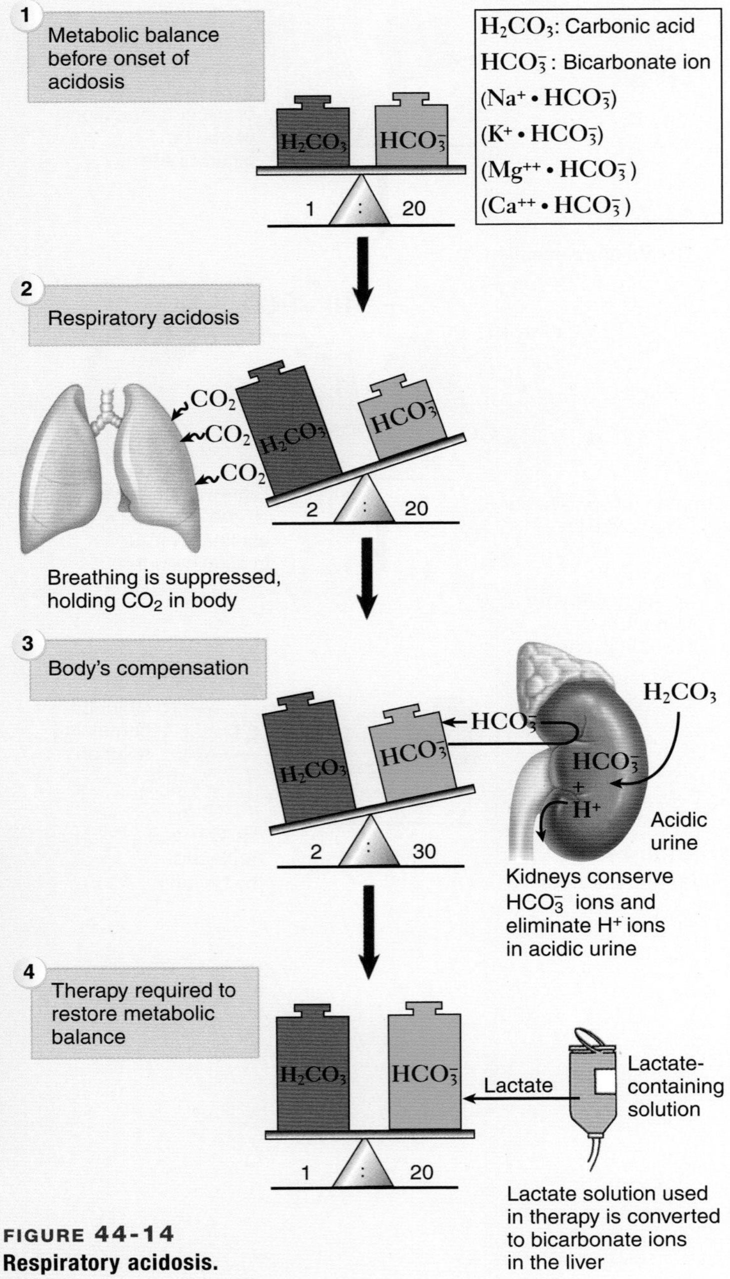

FIGURE 44-14
Respiratory acidosis.

Respiratory Alkalosis (Carbonic Acid Deficit)

Hyperventilation caused by fever or mental disease (hysteria) can result in excessive loss of carbonic acid and lead to **respiratory alkalosis** (**Figure 44-15**) with a bicarbonate buffer pair ratio of 20 : 0.5. Compensatory mechanisms may adjust the ratio to 10 : 0.5 and return blood pH to near normal.

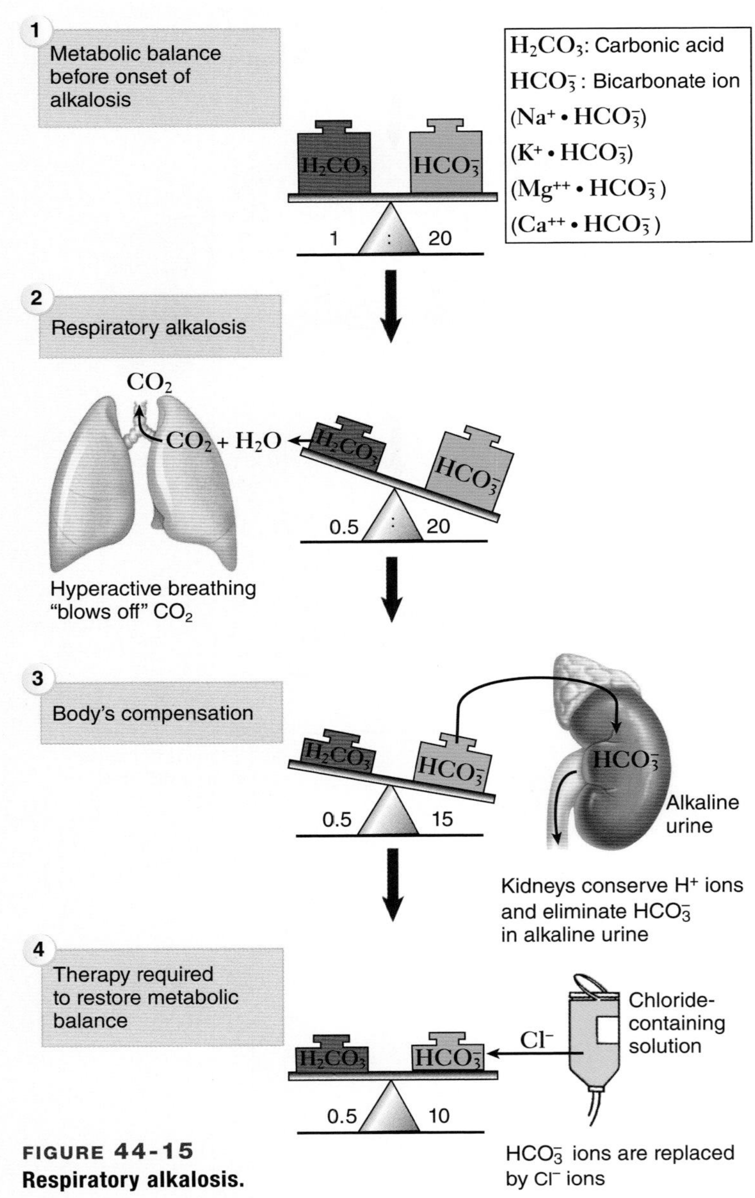

FIGURE 44-15
Respiratory alkalosis.

LANGUAGE OF MEDICINE *(continued from p. 1019)*

bicarbonate loading
(bye-KAR-boh-net)
[*bi-* **two,** *-carbon-* **coal (carbon),** *-ate* **oxygen**]

emesis (EM-eh-sis)
[*emesis* **vomiting**]

hyperkalaemia
(hye-per-kah-LEE-mee-ah)
[*hyper-* **excessive,** *-kal-* **potassium,** *-aem-* **blood,** *-ia* **condition**]

lactic acidosis
(LAK-tik ass-ih-DOH-sis)
[*lac-* **milk,** *-ic* **relating to,** *acid-* **sour,** *-osis* **condition**]

metabolic acidosis
(met-ah-BOL-ik ass-ih-DOH-sis)
[*meta-* **over,** *-bol-* **throw,** *-ic* **relating to,** *acid-* **sour,** *-osis* **condition**]

metabolic alkalosis
(met-ah-BOL-ik al-kah-LOH-sis)
[*meta-* **over,** *-bol-* **throw,** *-ic* **relating to,** *alkal-* **ashes,** *-osis* **condition**]

pernicious vomiting (per-NISH-us)
[*pernici-* **destruction,** *-ous* **relating to**]

respiratory acidosis
(RES-pih-rah-tor-ee ass-ih-DOH-sis)
[*re-* **again,** *-spir-* **breathe,** *-tory* **relating to,** *acid-* **sour,** *-osis* **condition**]

respiratory alkalosis
(RES-pih-rah-tor-ee al-kah-LOH-sis)
[*re-* **again,** *-spir-* **breathe,** *-tory* **relating to,** *alkal-* **ashes,** *-osis* **condition**]

sodium lactate (SO-dee-um LAK-tayt)
[*sod-* **soda,** *-um* **thing or substance,** *lact-* **milk,** *-ate* **chemical**]

case study

"Come on—take a deep breath for me." Coming out of anaesthesia, Jane heard the nurse talking, trying to get her to take some deep breaths. But she just couldn't. The pain was so much more than she had expected. Having had a total hip replacement (arthroplasty) in the past, Jane knew her hip would hurt after the surgery, but why did everything else ache so much? It hurt to take even a shallow breath. She continued breathing in short, shallow gasps; she was hypoventilating.

1. As Jane continued to gasp, her normal acid–base balance was disrupted by the development of which condition?
   a. Respiratory acidosis
   b. Metabolic acidosis
   c. Respiratory alkalosis
   d. Metabolic alkalosis
2. If this situation continued, which body system would make adjustments to bring her pH back toward normal?
   a. Respiratory
   b. Digestive
   c. Urinary
   d. Cardiovascular
3. Which is the most likely chemical trade-off to occur because of Jane's hypoventilation?
   a. Secretion of hydrogen ions and absorption of sodium ions
   b. Excretion of hydrogen ions and reabsorption of sodium ions
   c. Absorption of hydrogen ions and excretion of chloride ions
   d. Excretion of bicarbonate and reabsorption of hydrogen ions
4. What is the normal pH range of blood?
   a. 7.0–10.0
   b. 6.0–7.0
   c. 7.1–7.5
   d. 7.35–7.45

Hint To solve a case study, you may have to refer to the glossary or index, other chapters in this textbook, ***Connect It!,*** and other resources.

CHAPTER SUMMARY

To download an MP3 version of the chapter summary for use with your mobile device, access the ***Audio Chapter Summaries*** *online at evolve.elsevier.com.*

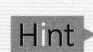

Scan this summary after reading the chapter to help you reinforce the key concepts. Later, use the summary as a quick review before your class or before a test.

Introduction

A. Acid–base balance is one of the most important of the body's homeostatic mechanisms
B. *Acid–base balance* refers to regulation of hydrogen ion concentration in body fluids
C. Precise regulation of pH at the cellular level is necessary for survival
D. Slight pH changes have dramatic effects on cellular metabolism

Mechanisms That Control pH of Body Fluids

A. Review of pH concept—negative logarithm of hydrogen ion concentration of a solution (**Figure 44-1**)
   1. pH indicates degree of acidity or alkalinity of a solution
   2. Acidosis describes arterial blood pH of less than 7.35
   3. Alkalosis describes arterial blood pH greater than 7.45
B. Sources of pH-influencing chemicals
   1. Carbonic acid—formed by CO_2 from aerobic glucose catabolism
   2. Lactic acid—thought to be formed by the lactate and excess protons (H^+) from anaerobic glucose catabolism
   3. Sulphuric acid—formed by oxidation of sulphur-containing amino acids
   4. Phosphoric acid—formed in the breakdown of phosphoproteins and ribonucleotides
   5. Acidic ketone bodies—formed in the breakdown of fats
      a. Acetone
      b. Acetoacetic acid
      c. β-hydroxybutyric acid
   6. Acid-forming potential of foods—determined by chloride, sulphur, and phosphorus content
C. Types of pH control mechanisms (**Figure 44-2**)
   1. Chemical—rapid-action buffers
      a. Bicarbonate buffer system
      b. Phosphate buffer system
      c. Protein buffer system
   2. Physiological—delayed-action buffers
      a. Respiratory response
      b. Renal response
   3. Summary of pH control mechanisms
      a. Buffers
      b. Respiration
      c. Kidney excretion of acids and bases
D. Effectiveness of pH control mechanisms—range of pH—extremely effective, normally maintain pH within a very narrow range of 7.36 to 7.40

Buffer Mechanisms for Controlling pH of Body Fluids

A. Buffers defined
   1. Substances that prevent a marked change in pH of a solution when an acid or base is added to it
   2. Consist of a weak acid (or its acid salt) and a basic salt of that acid
B. Buffer pairs present in body fluids—mainly carbonic acid, proteins, haemoglobin, acid phosphate, and sodium and potassium salts of these weak acids (**Figure 44-3** and **Figure 44-4**)
C. Buffer actions that prevent marked changes in pH of body fluids
   1. The chloride shift makes it possible for carbonic acid to be buffered in the red blood cell and then carried as bicarbonate in the plasma (**Figure 44-6**)
   2. Nonvolatile acids, such as hydrochloric acid, lactic acid, and ketone bodies, buffered mainly by sodium bicarbonate (**Figure 44-7**)
   3. Volatile acids, chiefly carbonic acid, buffered mainly by potassium salts of haemoglobin and oxyhaemoglobin (**Figure 44-5**)
   4. Bases buffered mainly by carbonic acid (when homeostasis of pH at 7.4 exists)

$$\text{Ratio } \frac{B \bullet HCO_3}{H_2CO_3} = \frac{20}{1}$$

   5. Base/acid ratio of 20:1 is critical
      a. Compensation—process of adjustment of pH balance to maintain ratio, such as 40:2 or 10:0.5
      b. Uncompensated alkalosis or acidosis—occurs when base/acid ratio is abnormal (unbalanced at a proper ratio)

   c. Correction—occurs when components of buffer pair return to normal 20:1 ratio

D. Evaluation of the role of buffers in pH control—cannot maintain normal pH without adequate functioning of the respiratory and urinary pH control mechanisms

Respiratory Mechanisms of pH Control

A. Explanation of respiratory mechanisms (**Figure 44-8**)
   1. Amount of blood carbon dioxide directly relates to the amount of carbonic acid and therefore to the concentration of H^+
   2. With increased respirations, less carbon dioxide remains in blood, hence less carbonic acid and fewer H^+ ions; with decreased respirations, more carbon dioxide remains in blood, hence more carbonic acid and more H^+ ions

B. Respiratory adjustment to counter pH imbalance of arterial blood
   1. If CO_2 in systemic arterial blood increases or decreases beyond setpoint level, respiratory centre is stimulated and respiration increases in rate and/or depth
   2. Carotid chemoreflexes also cause respiration adjustments

C. Principles that relate respirations to pH value
   1. Acidosis triggers hyperventilation, which increases rate of CO_2/H_2CO_3 loss from the body and thus reduces blood H^+ and restores homeostasis
   2. Prolonged hyperventilation, by decreasing blood H^+ excessively, may produce alkalosis
   3. Alkalosis triggers hypoventilation, which tends to correct alkalosis by increasing blood CO_2 and therefore blood H_2CO_3 and H^+
   4. Prolonged hypoventilation, by eliminating too little CO_2, causes an increase in blood H_2CO_3 and consequently in blood H^+, thereby producing acidosis

D. Arterial blood gas (ABG) analysis
   1. Laboratory test that shows the key characteristics of blood related to respiratory function
      a. Oxygen partial pressure (Po_2)
      b. Oxygen saturation of haemoglobin ($\%So_2$)
      c. pH
      d. Concentration of bicarbonate ions (HCO_3^-)
      e. Carbon dioxide partial pressure (Pco_2)
   2. Analysis of balance of ABGs can be used to assess primary acid–base imbalances (**Table 44-2**)
      a. pH < 7.35 indicates acidosis; pH > 7.45 indicates alkalosis
      b. $Pco_2 > 6.0$ kPa (45 mmHg) and low pH indicates *respiratory* acidosis; $Pco_2 < 4.7$ kPa (35 mmHg) and high pH indicates *respiratory* alkalosis
      c. [HCO_3^-] below 22 mEq/L and low pH indicates *metabolic* acidosis; [HCO_3^-] above 26 mEq/L and high pH indicates *metabolic* alkalosis

Urinary Mechanisms That Control pH

A. General principles concerning urinary mechanisms—play vital role in acid–base balance because kidneys can eliminate more H^+ from the body while reabsorbing more base when pH tends toward the acid side and eliminates fewer H^+ while reabsorbing less base when pH tends toward the alkaline side (**Figure 44-8**)

B. Mechanisms that control urine pH (**Figure 44-11**)
   1. Secretion of H^+ into urine—when blood CO_2, H_2CO_3, and H^+ increase above normal, distal tubules secrete more H^+ into urine to displace basic ion (mainly sodium) from a urine salt and then reabsorb sodium into blood in exchange for the H^+ excreted (**Figure 44-9**)
   2. Secretion of NH_3—when blood hydrogen ion concentration increases, distal tubules secrete more NH_3, which combines with the H^+ of urine to form ammonium ion (NH_4^+), which displaces a basic ion (mainly sodium) from a salt; the basic ion is then reabsorbed back into blood in exchange for the ammonium ion excreted (**Figure 44-10**)

The Big Picture: Acid–Base Balance

A. Each vital physiological function depends on the maintenance of a stable and tightly regulated acid–base environment

B. Elaborate and highly sensitive pH control mechanisms that provide homeostasis of our acid–base environment are critical for the enzymatic action necessary for a healthy metabolism and for life itself

REVIEW QUESTIONS

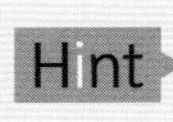

Write out the answers to these questions after reading the chapter and reviewing the Chapter Summary. Note—writing out your answers will consolidate learning and provide a valuable resource of information.

1. How are carbonic acid and lactic acid produced?
2. Are most fruits and vegetables acid-forming or base-forming foods?
3. Identify several acid-forming elements.
4. What is a physiological buffer?
5. What is the normal range of blood pH?
6. Describe the buffering action of sodium bicarbonate.
7. Identify the main buffer pairs in body fluids.
8. What key characteristics are revealed in an arterial blood gas (ABG) test?
9. How is the distal renal tubule involved in the acidification of urine and the conservation of base?
10. How can sodium lactate be useful in the treatment of both metabolic acidosis and respiratory acidosis?
11. Discuss hyperventilation in relation to the development of an acid–base imbalance.

CRITICAL THINKING QUESTIONS

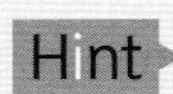

After finishing the Review Questions, write out the answers to these more in-depth questions to help you apply your new knowledge. Go back to sections of the chapter that relate to concepts that you find difficult.

1. Explain pH in terms of the ions involved. What would be the hydrogen ion concentration of a solution with a pH of 4? With a pH of 6?
2. Define and summarize the purpose of the chloride shift.
3. Predict what might happen to the pH if a drug is administered that lowers the $NaHCO_3$ concentration to 23.8 mEq but maintains the H_2CO_3 concentration at 1.3 mEq.
4. Explain the role of the respiratory system in maintaining proper blood pH.
5. A patient has ABG values of pH = 7.3, P_{CO_2} = 5.3 kPa (40 mmHg), $[HCO_3^-]$ = 20 mEq/L. What is your assessment of the patient's acid–base status?
6. How would you describe the causes and a possible treatment of the acid–base imbalance that occurs with prolonged vomiting?

UNIT 6

Reproduction and Development

The chapters of Unit 6 deal with human reproduction, growth, development, genetics, and heredity. The anatomical structures and complex control mechanisms characteristic of the male and female reproductive systems are intended to ensure survival of our genes. These systems in men and women are adapted structurally and functionally for the specific sequence of events that permit development of sperm or ova, followed by fertilization, normal development, and birth of a baby. Chapter 47 details the developmental changes that occur from fertilization to death. Chapter 48 discusses the scientific study of genetics and heredity along with medical applications.

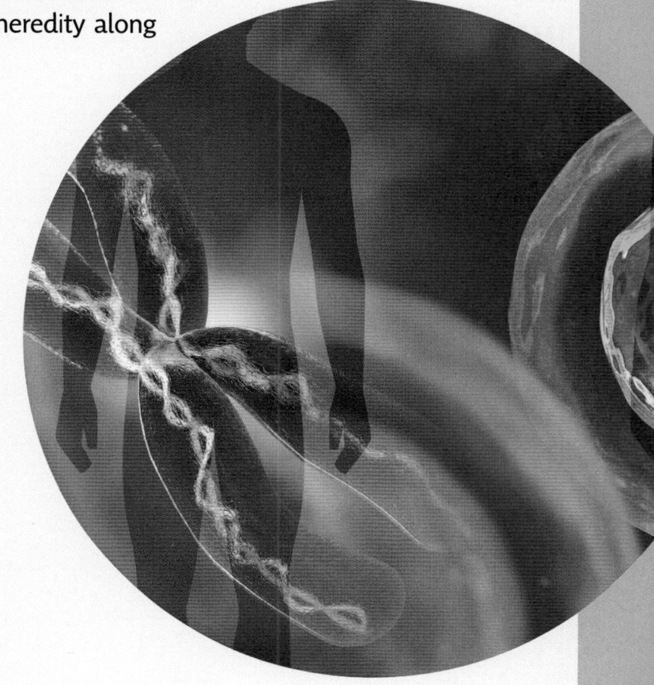

45 Male Reproductive System

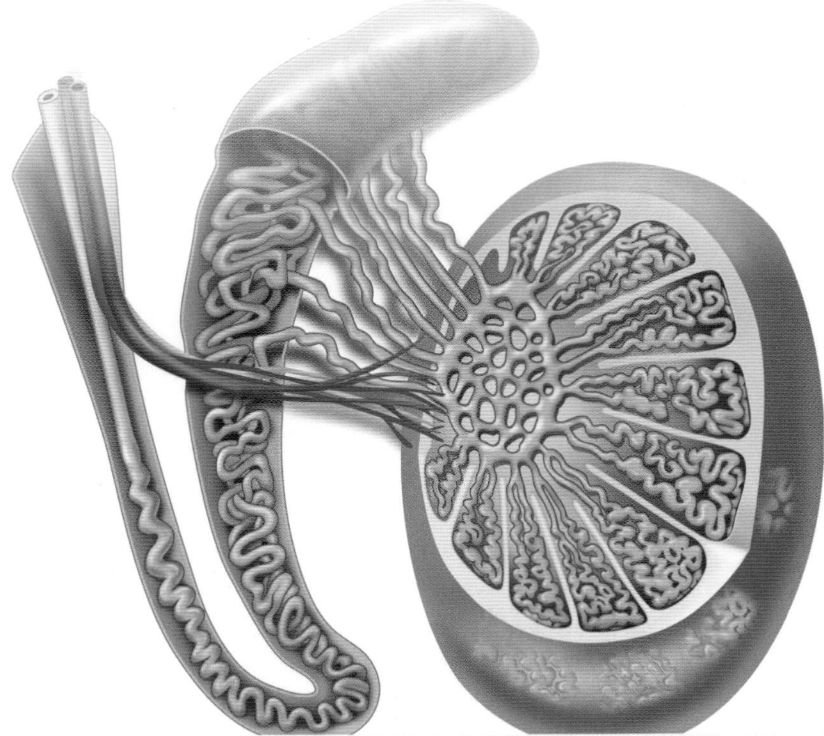

CHAPTER OUTLINE

Hint ▸ *Scan this outline before you begin to read the chapter, as a preview of how the concepts are organized.*

LANGUAGE OF SCIENCE

Hint ▸ *Use this list to aid your pronunciation of unfamiliar words.*

androgen (AN-droh-jen)
[*andro-* **male,** *-gen* **produce**]

androgen-binding protein (ABP) (AN-droh-jen-BYND-ing)
[*andro-* **male,** *-gen* **produce,** *prote-* **first rank,** *-in* **substance**]

blood–testis barrier (BTB) (blud TES-tis BAYR-ee-er)

bulbourethral gland (BUL-boh-yoo-REE-thral)
[*bulb-* **swollen root,** *-ure-* **urine,** *-thr-* **agent or channel (urethra),** *-al* **relating to**]

capacitation (kah-pas-ih-TAY-shun)

corpus cavernosum (KOHR-pus kav-er-NO-sum)
[*corpus* **body,** *cavern-* **large hollow,** *-os-* **relating to,** *-um* **thing**] *pl.,* corpora cavernosa

corpus spongiosum (KOHR-pus spun-jee-OH-sum)
[*corpus* **body,** *spong-* **sponge,** *-os-* **relating to,** *-um* **thing**] *pl.,* corpora spongiosa

ejaculation (ee-jak-yoo-LAY-shun)
[*e-* **out or away,** *-jacula-* **throw,** *-ation* **process**]

emission (ee-MISH-un)
[*e-* **out or away,** *-mis-* **send,** *-sion* **process**]

epididymis (ep-ih-DID-ih-mis)
[*epi-* **upon,** *-didymis* **pair**] *pl.,* epididymes

erection (ee-REK-shun)

gamete (GAM-eet)
[*gamete* **marriage partner**]

genital (JEN-ih-tal)
[*gen-* **produce,** *-al* **relating to**] *pl.,* genitals or genitalia

glans penis (glans PEE-nis)
[*glans* **acorn,** *penis* **male sex organ**] *pl.,* glandes penes

gonad (GO-nad)
[*gon-* **offspring,** *-ad* **relating to**]

interstitial cell (in-ter-STISH-al sell)
[*inter-* **between,** *-stit-* **stand,** *-al* **relating to,** *cell* **storeroom**]

orgasm (OR-gaz-um)
[*orgasm* **excitement**]

penis (PEE-nis)
[*penis* **male sex organ**] *pl.,* penes or penises

continued on p. 1053

The importance of reproductive system function is notably different from that of any other organ system of the body. Ordinarily, systems function to maintain the relative stability and survival of the individual organism. The reproductive system, on the other hand, ensures survival not of the individual but of the genes that characterize the human species. In both sexes, organs of the reproductive system are adapted for the specific sequence of functions that are concerned primarily with transferring genes to a new generation of offspring. A male reproductive system in one parent and a female reproductive system in another parent are needed to reproduce. This chapter begins with a brief description of the male reproductive system. Chapter 46 then follows with the story of the female reproductive system.

SEXUAL REPRODUCTION

Sexual reproduction requires two parent organisms, a male and female, each of which contributes half of the nuclear chromosomes needed to form the first cell of an offspring organism. *Asexual reproduction*, on the other hand, requires only one parent who produces an offspring genetically identical to itself. An advantage of sexual reproduction is that a new mixture of genes in each offspring increases the variety of genetic characteristics in the population. This variety of characteristics makes it more likely that in the case of infectious disease or environmental changes, such as natural disaster or shifting climatic conditions, there will be at least some individuals likely to survive and carry on the reproductive line.

Besides producing the cells needed to form the offspring, each reproductive system produces hormones that regulate development of the secondary sex characteristics that promote successful reproduction. For example, hormones create structural and behavioural differences in the sexes that permit adults to recognize and form sexual attractions with the opposite sex. Reproductive hormones and other regulatory mechanisms give us the urge to have sex, which is often reinforced with the pleasant sensations that sexual activity can produce. This sex drive is essential to success in producing offspring.

Sexual maturity and the ability to reproduce are achieved by the end of puberty. The male reproductive system consists of organs whose functions are to produce, transfer, and ultimately introduce mature sperm into the female reproductive tract, where the nuclear chromosomes from each parent can unite to form a new offspring.

MALE REPRODUCTIVE ORGANS

Organs of the reproductive system (**Figure 45-1**) make up the reproductive tract. These organs may be classified as *essential organs* for the production of **gametes** (sex cells) or as *accessory organs* that play some type of supportive role in the reproductive process.

In both sexes the essential organs of reproduction that produce the gametes, or sex cells (sperm or ova), are called **gonads.** In Chapter 47, we will explore the development of male and female reproductive organs more thoroughly. The gonads of the male are the **testes,** which produce sperm and the hormone testosterone.

The accessory organs of reproduction in the male include genital ducts, glands, and supporting structures.

Reproductive ducts convey sperm to the outside of the body. They are also called *genital ducts.* The ducts are a pair of *epididymides* (*singular*, epididymis), the paired *vasa deferentia* (*singular*, vas deferens), a pair of *ejaculatory ducts*, and the *urethra. Accessory glands* in the reproductive system produce secretions that serve to nourish, transport, and mature sperm. The glands are a pair of *seminal vesicles*, one *prostate*, and a pair of *bulbourethral glands. Supporting structures* include the *scrotum*, the *penis*, and a pair of *spermatic cords.*

Note—the term urogenital tract is sometimes used in place of reproductive tract to indicate the dual role of the urethra in males. The urethra serves as a passageway for both urine and semen to exit the body.

PERINEUM

The **perineum** in the male is an area between the thighs shaped roughly like a diamond (**Figure 45-2**). It extends from the pubic symphysis anteriorly to the coccyx posteriorly. Its most lateral boundary on either side is the ischial tuberosity. A line drawn between the two ischial tuberosities divides the area into a larger *urogenital triangle*, which contains the external genitals (penis and scrotum), and the *anal triangle*, which surrounds the anus.

Quick CHECK

1. How is the normal function of the reproductive system different from the end result of "normal function" in other organ systems?
2. Identify the essential and accessory organs of reproduction.
3. Describe the location, shape, and subdivisions of the perineum.

TESTES

STRUCTURE AND LOCATION

The testes are small, ovoid glands that are somewhat flattened from side to side, measure about 4 or 5 cm in length, and weigh 10 to 15 grams each. They are both located in a supporting sac called the *scrotum.* The left testis is generally located about 1 cm lower in the scrotal sac than the right. Both testes are suspended in the pouch by attachment to scrotal tissue and by the spermatic cords (**Figure 45-3**). Note in **Figure 45-3**, *B*, that testicular blood vessels reach the testes by passing through the spermatic cord.

A dense, white, fibrous capsule called the **tunica albuginea** encases each testis and then enters the gland, sending out partitions (septa) that radiate through its interior, dividing it into 200 or more cone-shaped *lobules.*

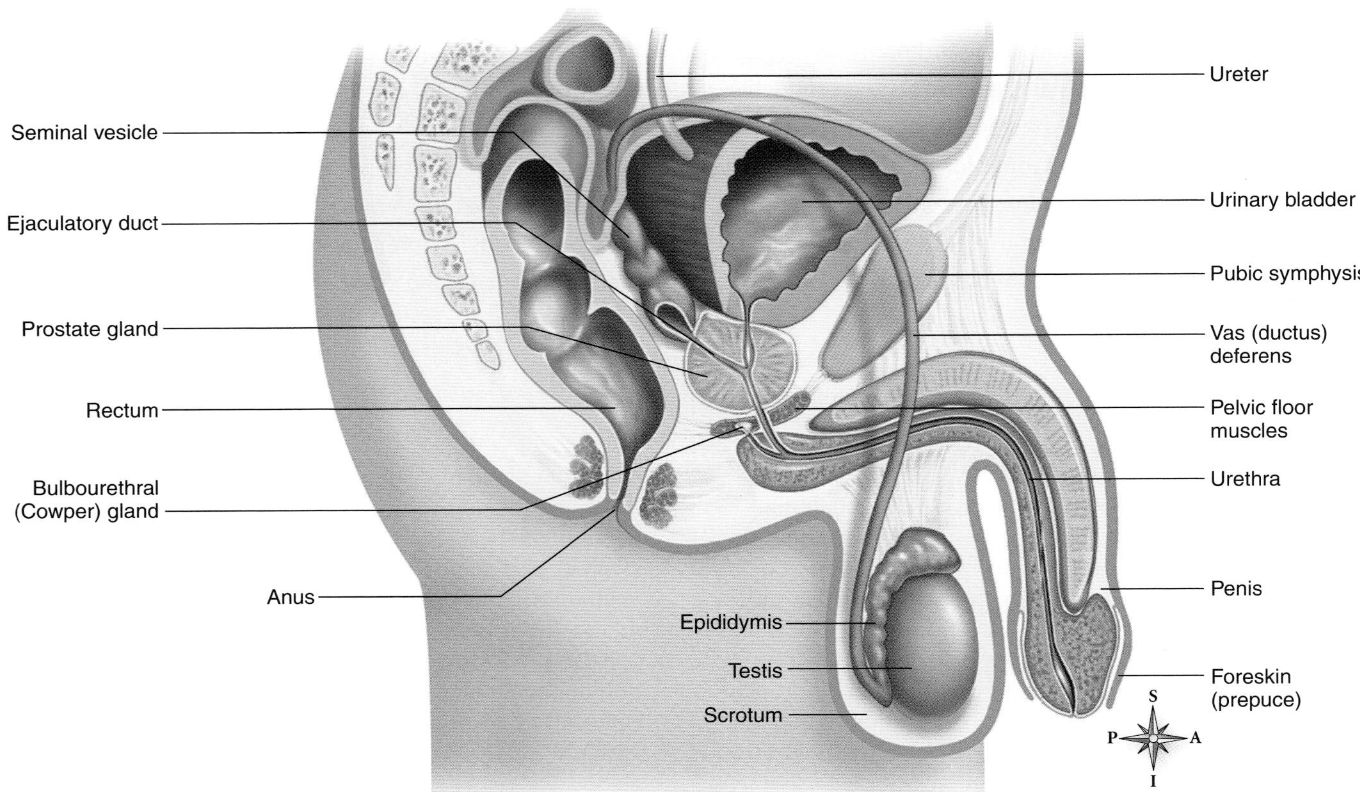

FIGURE 45-1 Male reproductive organs. Sagittal section of inferior abdominopelvic cavity showing placement of male reproductive organs.

Each lobule of the testis contains scattered *interstitial cells* and one to three tiny, coiled **seminiferous tubules,** which, if unravelled, would measure about 75 cm in length. The tubules from each lobule come together to form a plexus called the *rete testis.* A series of sperm ducts called *efferent ductules* then drain the rete testis and pierce the tunica albuginea to enter the head of the epididymis (see **Figure 45-3**).

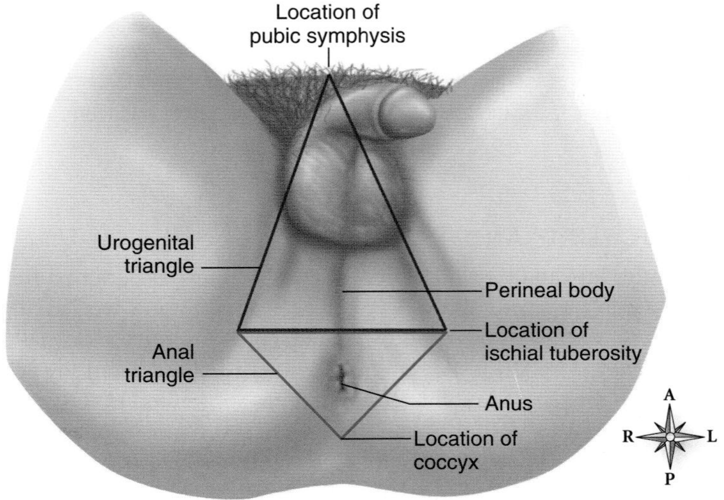

FIGURE 45-2 Male perineum. Inferior view showing an outline of the urogenital triangle *(red)* and anal triangle *(blue)*.

Microscopic Anatomy of the Testis

Figure 45-4, A is a low-power (×70) micrograph of testicular tissue showing a number of cut seminiferous tubules and numerous **interstitial cells,** or *Leydig cells,* in the surrounding connective tissue septa. In this figure, maturing sperm appear as dense nuclei with their tails projecting into the lumen of the tubule. The wall of each seminiferous tubule may contain five or more layers of cells. At puberty, when sexual maturity begins, spermatogenic cells in diverse stages of development appear, and the hormone-producing interstitial cells become more prominent in the surrounding septa. **Figure 45-4**, *B,* is a high-power micrograph showing a group of typically round interstitial cells clustered between seminiferous tubules. Also see the micrograph in Figure 5-49 in the Brief Atlas of the Human Body.

A unique cellular feature often visible in interstitial cells is an elongated rectangular-shaped mass called a *crystalloid.* Also called *Reinke crystalloids,* these masses are absent before puberty and then increase in number during the reproductive years into old age. The functional significance of these structures remains uncertain.

Irregular elongated **sustentacular cells** have a supportive and regulatory function important for the developing germ cells. Sustentacular cells of the testis are also called *nurse cells* or *Sertoli cells.*

FIGURE 45-3 Tubules of the testis and epididymis. **A,** Transilluminated photograph; the testis is the darker sphere in the centre. **B,** Illustration showing epididymis lifted free of testis. The ducts and tubules are exaggerated in size.

These cells provide mechanical support and protection for spermatids attached to their luminal surface and are visible in **Figure 45-5** within a section of seminiferous epithelium.

Sustentacular cells also secrete the hormone *inhibin,* which inhibits gonadotropin-releasing hormone (GnRH) production in the hypothalamus and follicle-stimulating hormone (FSH) production in the anterior pituitary. A drop in FSH lowers the rate of sperm production. This sets up a negative feedback mechanism in which the supportive sustentacular cells can slow down sperm production to manageable levels if needed.

At sexual maturity, sustentacular cells begin to secrete **androgen-binding protein,** or **ABP,** that binds to testosterone, a steroid lipid hormone, to make it more water-soluble. This increases the testosterone concentration within the seminiferous tubules. High

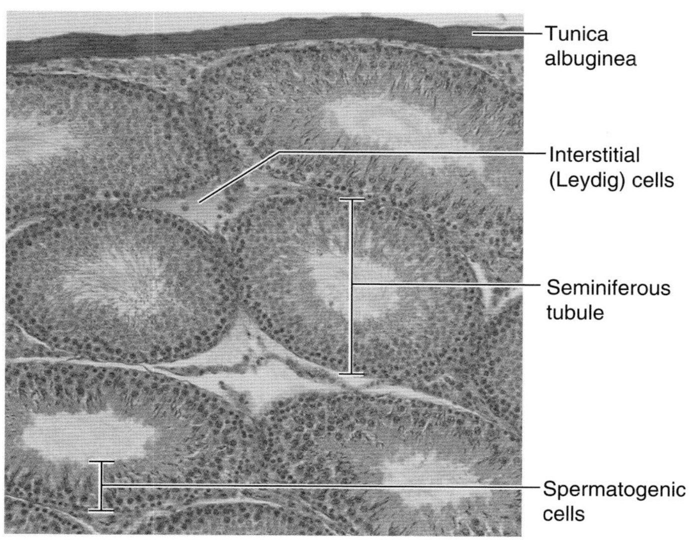

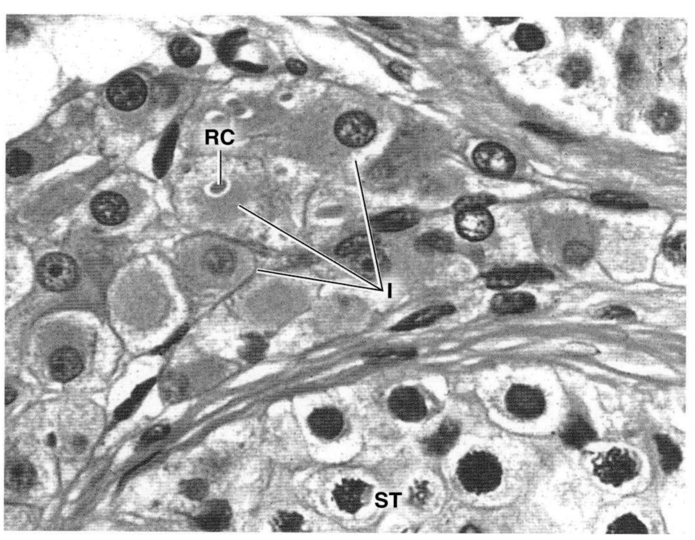

FIGURE 45-4 Testis. **A,** Low-power micrograph showing several seminiferous tubules surrounded by septa containing interstitial (Leydig) cells. **B,** High-power micrograph showing a cluster of interstitial cells *(I)* between seminiferous tubules *(ST)*. Spermatogenic cells can be identified in the wall of a seminiferous tubule. Note the presence of a Reinke crystalloid *(RC)* in an interstitial cell.

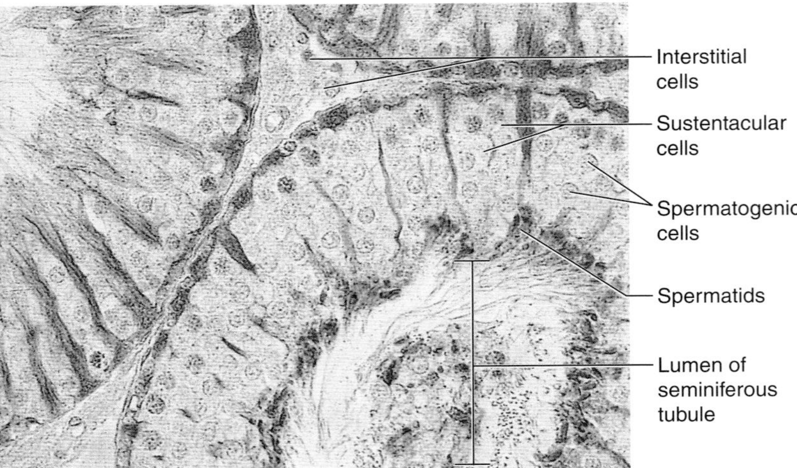

FIGURE 45-5 Sustentacular cells within seminiferous epithelium. Sustentacular cells are columnar in shape, extending from basement membrane to lumen of the tubule. Spermatids can be seen attached to the luminal surface of the sustentacular cells. Sustentacular cells are also called *nurse cells* or *Sertoli cells.*

concentrations of testosterone are required for normal germ cell maturation. Thus sustentacular cells play an important role in spermatogenesis (sperm production).

Sustentacular cells are columnar in shape and extend from the basement membrane to the luminal surface of the seminiferous tubule (**Figure 45-5** and **Figure 45-6**). *Tight junctions* exist between adjacent sustentacular cells and divide the wall of the tubule into two compartments that house either meiotically active cells near the luminal surface or spermatogonia near the basement membrane.

FIGURE 45-6 Seminiferous tubule. Wedge from a cross-section of the tubule, showing spermatogenesis and the relationship of the developing spermatozoa (sperm cells) to the sustentacular (Sertoli) cells.

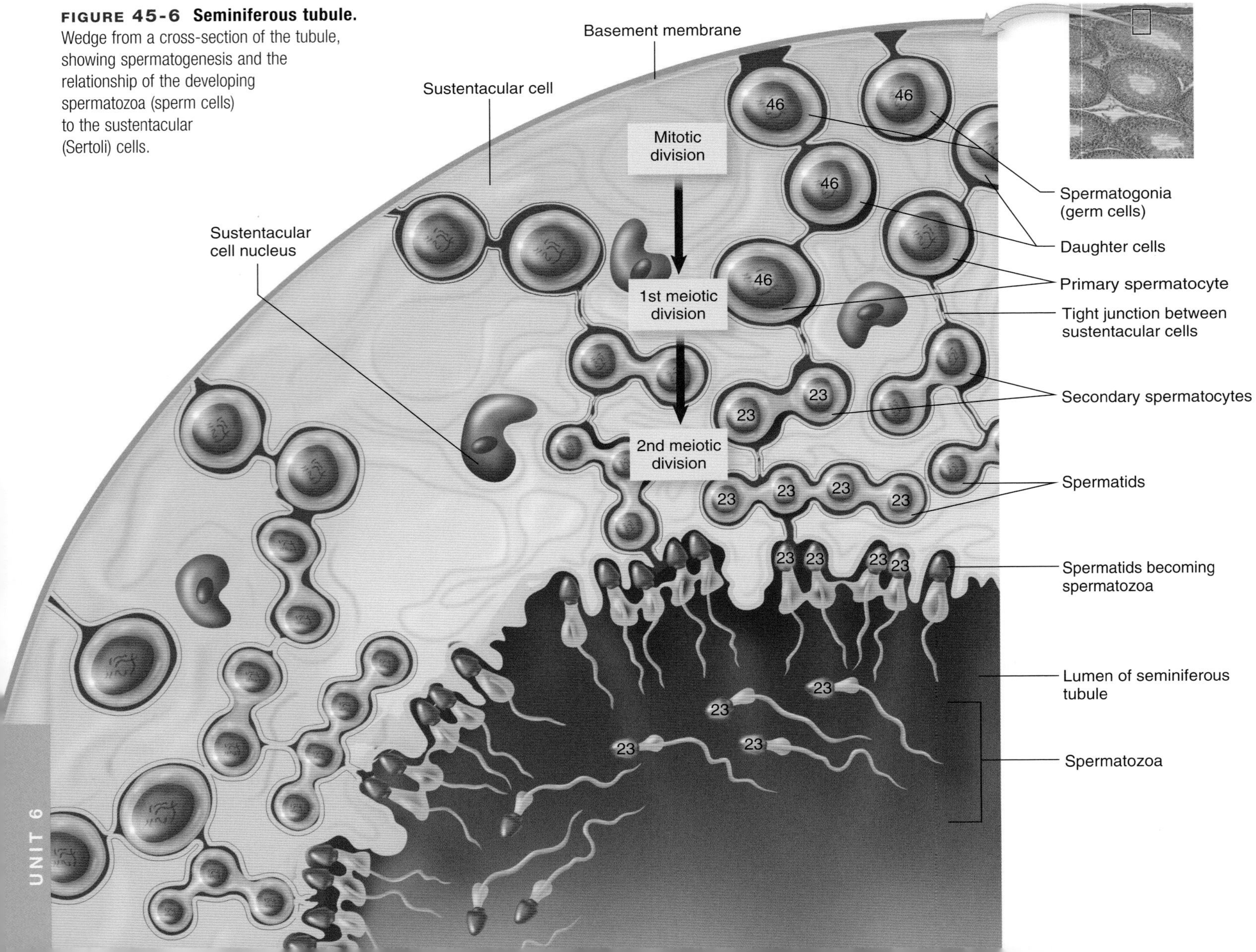

Tight junctions between sustentacular cells form the **blood–testis barrier (BTB).** This structure isolates the developing sperm cells, which have active surface antigens different from somatic body cells, from the body immune system. If these antigens were to escape from the tubule epithelium and enter the bloodstream by breaking through the basement membrane, an autoimmune reaction could occur.

Testes Functions

The testes perform two primary functions: spermatogenesis and secretion of hormones.

Spermatogenesis is the production of spermatozoa (sperm), the male gametes, or reproductive cells. The seminiferous tubules produce the sperm. **Figure 45-6** shows a cross-section of a seminiferous tubule in which two meiotic divisions result in a reduction of chromosomes from 46 in the spermatogonia to 23 in the spermatids and mature sperm. Details of spermatogenesis are discussed in Chapter 47.

Testosterone is the major **androgen** (masculinizing hormone) produced in humans. Testosterone is a steroid hormone produced by interstitial cells. Another hormone, inhibin, is produced by sustentacular cells of the testis.

Testosterone has several functions. One important group of functions is that it promotes "maleness", or development and maintenance of male secondary sex characteristics, accessory organs such as the prostate, seminal vesicles, and adult male sexual behaviour.

Testosterone also helps regulate metabolism. It is usually classified as an anabolic hormone because it stimulates the protein anabolism. By stimulating protein anabolism, testosterone promotes growth of skeletal muscles (responsible for greater male muscular development and strength). This effect has tempted some athletes to take various synthetic versions of testosterone or testosterone promoters to enhance muscular strength. Testosterone also stimulates bone growth and promotes closure of the epiphyses (see Chapter 11, p. 220). Early sexual maturation leads to early epiphyseal closure. The converse also holds true: late sexual maturation, delayed epiphyseal closure, and tallness tend to go together.

Testosterone also plays a part in fluid and electrolyte balance. Testosterone has a mild stimulating effect on kidney tubule reabsorption of sodium and water; it also promotes kidney tubule excretion of potassium.

The anterior pituitary gland controls the testes by means of its gonadotropic hormones—specifically, FSH and luteinizing hormone (LH). FSH stimulates the seminiferous tubules to produce sperm more rapidly. In the male, LH stimulates interstitial cells to increase their secretion of testosterone.

If the blood concentration of testosterone reaches a high level, it will inhibit hypothalamic secretion of gonadotropin-releasing hormone (GnRH). As a result, anterior pituitary secretion of LH will decrease and testosterone levels will return to the normal setpoint value (**Figure 45-7**). Increasing blood levels of *inhibin* will selectively decrease GnRH secretion by the hypothalamus and FSH secretion by the anterior pituitary—thus decreasing the rate of sperm

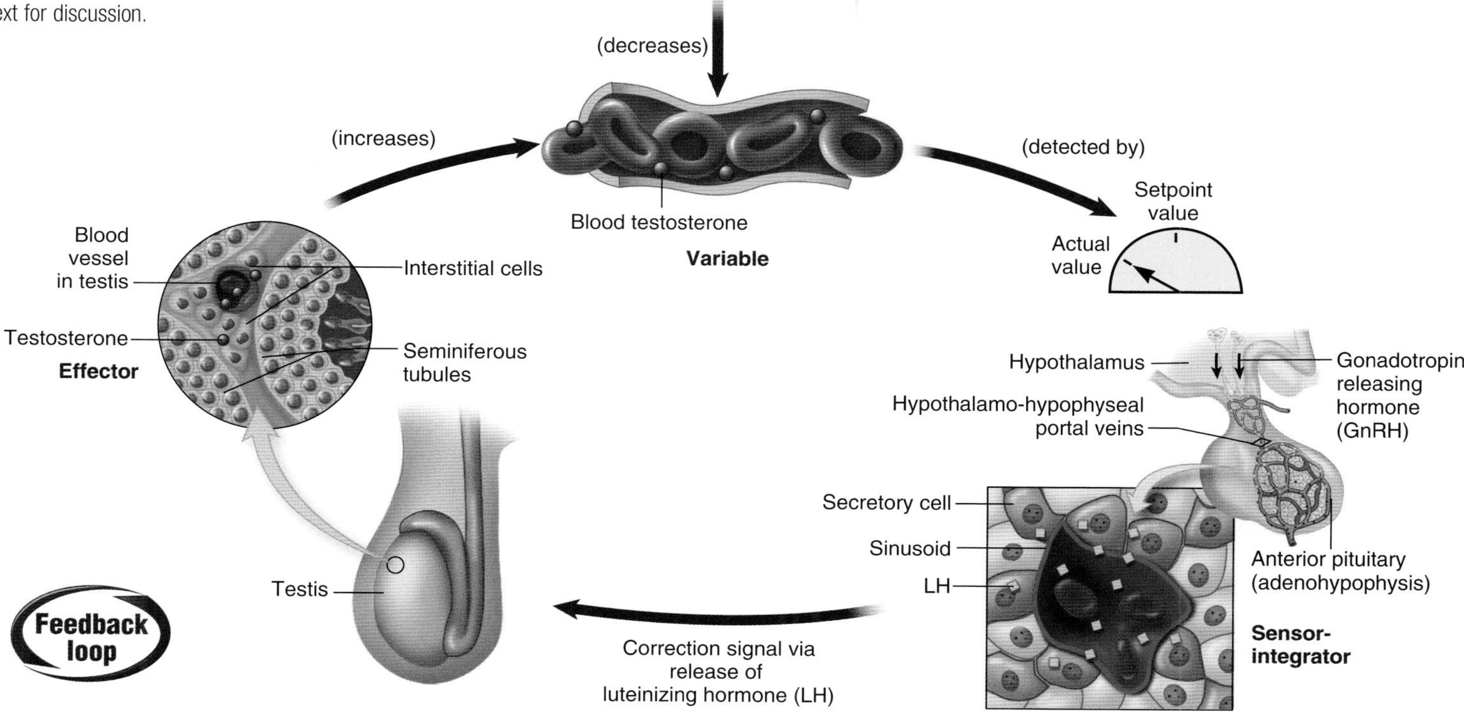

FIGURE 45-7 Negative feedback loop controlling testosterone secretion. Diagram shows the negative feedback mechanism that controls anterior pituitary gland secretion of LH and interstitial cell secretion of testosterone. A similar negative feedback loop exists between inhibin-secreting sustentacular cells in the testis and FSH-secreting cells in the anterior pituitary gland. See text for discussion.

TABLE 45-1 **Male Reproductive Hormones**

HORMONE	SOURCE	TARGET	ACTION
Dehydroepiandrosterone (DHEA)	Adrenal gland, testis, other tissues	Converted to other hormones	Eventually converted to oestrogens, testosterone, or both (see **Figure 25-5** on p. 566)
Oestrogen	Testis (interstitial cells), liver, other tissues	Testis (spermatogenic tissue), other tissues	Role of oestrogen in men is still uncertain; may play role in spermatogenesis, inhibition of gonadotropins, and male sexual behaviour
Follicle-stimulating hormone (FSH)	Anterior pituitary (gonadotroph cells)	Testis (spermatogenic tissue)	Gonadotropin; promotes development of testes and stimulates spermatogenesis
Gonadotropin-releasing hormone (GnRH)	Hypothalamus (neuroendocrine cells)	Anterior pituitary (gonadotroph cells)	Stimulates production and release of gonadotropins (FSH and LH) from anterior pituitary
Inhibin	Testis (sustentacular cells)	Hypothalamus Anterior pituitary (gonadotroph cells)	Inhibits GnRH secretion by the hypothalamus and FSH production in the anterior pituitary
Luteinizing hormone (LH)	Anterior pituitary (gonadotroph cells)	Testis (interstitial cells)	Gonadotropin; stimulates production of testosterone by interstitial cells of testis
Testosterone	Testis (interstitial cells)	Spermatogenic cells, skeletal muscle, bone, other tissues	Stimulates spermatogenesis, stimulates development of primary and secondary sexual characteristics, promotes growth of muscle and bone (anabolic effect)

production. However, if sperm counts decrease below the normal set point, inhibin secretion will drop, FSH secretion will increase, and sperm numbers will increase to normal levels. Thus a negative feedback mechanism operates between the hypothalamus, the anterior pituitary gland, and the hormone-producing cells of the testes—interstitial cells producing testosterone and sustentacular cells producing inhibin. The end result is homeostatic control of the full range of effects influenced by testosterone levels—including a direct influence on sperm numbers.

Small but measurable amounts of *oestrogen* are present in healthy adult males. More research is needed to explore its role in normal male physiology. Some of the oestrogen, a steroid hormone derived from testosterone, is made in interstitial cells (see **Figure 25-5** on p. 566). However, most of the oestrogen in males is probably made in the liver and other tissues. Possible roles for oestrogen in men include regulation of spermatogenesis, feedback inhibition of FSH and LH, and promotion of male sexual behaviour.

Table 45-1 summarizes some of the reproductive hormones in males.

Spermatozoa

The elongated tail-bearing **spermatozoa** seen in the seminiferous tubules (**Figure 45-8**, *B*) appear fully formed. We know, however, that they undergo a process of "ripening", or maturation, as they pass through the genital ducts before ejaculation. Although anatomically complete and highly motile when ejaculated, sperm must still undergo a complex process called **capacitation** before they are actually capable of fertilizing an egg cell or ovum (female gamete). Normally, capacitation occurs in sperm only after they have been introduced into the vagina of the female.

Figure 45-8, *C*, shows the characteristic parts of a spermatozoon: head, middle piece, and elongated, lashlike tail.

The head of a spermatozoon is, in essence, a highly compact package of genetic chromatin material, about 5 μm long, covered by an *acrosome* and *acrosomal (head) cap*. The acrosome contains hydrolytic (splitting) enzymes, which are released during capacitation. During the process of capacitation, the acrosomal enzymes first break down cervical mucus, allowing sperm to pass into the uterus and uterine tubes. If an ovum is present in the female reproductive tract when **semen** is introduced, continued release of acrosomal enzymes assists the sperm cells to digest and penetrate the outer covering of the egg and initiate fertilization. This is the primary reason a high sperm count is essential for male fertility. The process of fertilization is explored further in Chapter 47.

The sperm nucleus, which takes up most of the room inside the sperm head, is released into the ovum during the process of fertilization. When the genetic material of the sperm nucleus and egg nucleus unite, they form the nucleus of a new offspring cell.

The cylindrical middle piece or *midpiece* of the sperm is connected to the sperm head by a narrow *neck*. The midpiece is about 7 μm long, is characterized by a helical arrangement of mitochondria arranged end to end around a central core. It is this mitochondrial sheath that provides energy for sperm locomotion. Within the core are the ends of the microtubules that extend all the way through the sperm tail. Motor molecules within the core of the midpiece cause the microtubules to move in their typical, propellerlike fashion.

The tail is divided into a principal piece, about 40 μm long, and a short end piece, 5 to 10 μm in length. If the tail portion of a spermatozoon is cut in cross-section and viewed with an electron microscope (**Figure 45-8**, *F*), its microstructure looks like other flagella capable of motility (see Chapter 5, p. 91). Note in **Figure 45-8**, *F*, that the central portion of the sectioned sperm tail is a cylinder composed of nine double microtubules arranged around two single microtubules in the centre.

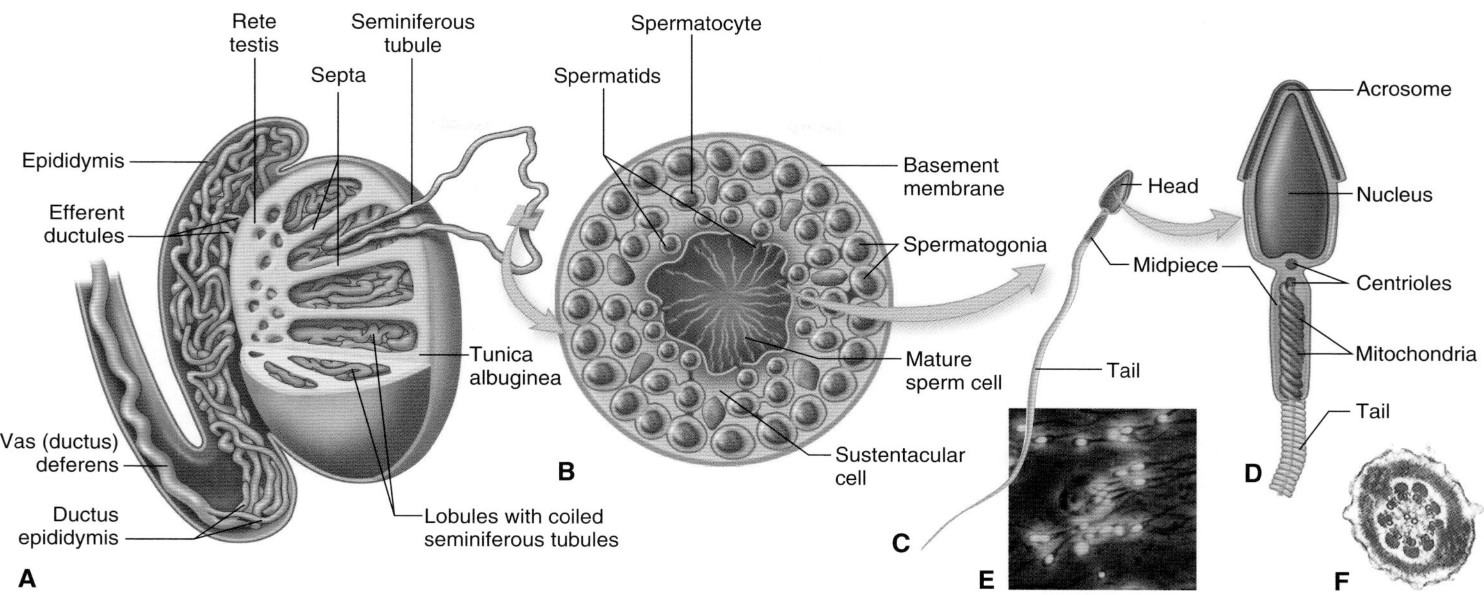

FIGURE 45-8 Development and structure of sperm. A, View of testis and seminiferous tubules. **B,** Spermatid cells in a seminiferous tubule. **C,** Mature sperm. **D,** Enlarged view of head and midpiece. **E,** Micrograph of sperm that shows taken-up nuclear material that glows with a fluorescent dye. **F,** Electron micrograph (EM) of a cross-section of sperm tail showing nine double microtubules arranged around two single central microtubules.

Progesterone and other molecules released by cells that surround the ovum trigger increased sperm motility and attract sperm toward the ovum.

Quick CHECK

4. Describe the location, the size, and the shape of the testes.
5. List the two primary functions of the testes and identify the cell type or structure involved in each function.
6. List the general functions of testosterone.
7. Identify the structural components of a spermatozoon and give the function of each.

REPRODUCTIVE DUCTS

EPIDIDYMIS

Structure and Location

Each **epididymis** consists of a single, tightly coiled tube enclosed in a fibrous casing. The tube has a very small diameter (just barely macroscopic) but measures approximately 6 metres in length. It lies along the top and behind the testis (see **Figure 45-3**). The comma-shaped epididymis is divided into a blunt superior *head* (which is connected to the testis by the efferent ductules), a central *body*, and a tapered inferior portion that is continuous with the vas deferens, called the *tail.* If the epididymis is cut or sectioned and a slide prepared as in **Figure 45-9**, the compact and highly coiled nature of the tubule is apparent.

Functions

The epididymis serves as one of the ducts through which sperm pass in their journey from the testis to the exterior. Each epididymis stores sperm, which spend from 1 to 3 weeks in this segment of the duct system. While there, the sperm continue to mature with the support of nutrients from the epididymis. Cells lining the epididymis secrete nutrients for developing sperm and remove excess testicular fluid as the developing sex cells pass through this highly coiled tube. The epididymal secretions also eventually become a small part of the seminal fluid (semen) that is eventually ejaculated with the sperm during the male sexual response. After about 3 weeks, any unused sperm in the epididymis break down and are reabsorbed by the body.

VAS DEFERENS

Structure and Location

The **vas deferens,** like the epididymis, is a tube. Also called the *ductus deferens,* the vas deferens is a duct that extends from the tail

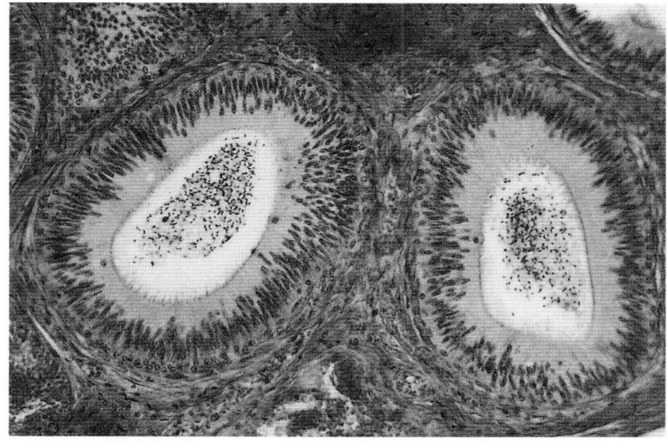

FIGURE 45-9 Epididymis section. Two cross-sections of this extensively coiled tubule are visible. Note the presence of spermatozoa within the lumina of the tubule cross-sections.

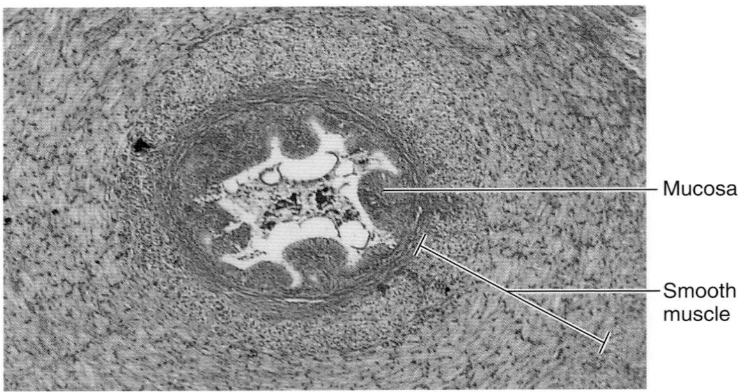

FIGURE 45-10 Transverse section of vas deferens. Mucosa protrudes into the lumen in several low folds. Note the thick muscular coat surrounding the mucosa.

of the epididymis. The vas deferens has thick, muscular walls (**Figure 45-10**) and can be palpated in the scrotal sac as a smooth, movable cord. Note in **Figure 45-10** that the muscular layer of the vas deferens has three layers: a thick intermediate circular layer of muscle fibres and inner and outer longitudinal layers. The muscular layers of the vas deferens help in propelling sperm through the duct system.

The vas deferens from each testis ascends from the scrotum and passes through the inguinal canal as part of the spermatic cord—enclosed by fibrous connective tissue with blood vessels, nerves, and lymphatics—into the abdominal cavity. Here it extends over the top and down the posterior surface of the bladder, where an enlarged and tortuous portion called the *ampulla* joins the duct from the seminal vesicle to form the ejaculatory duct (**Figures 45-1**, **45-11**, and **45-12**).

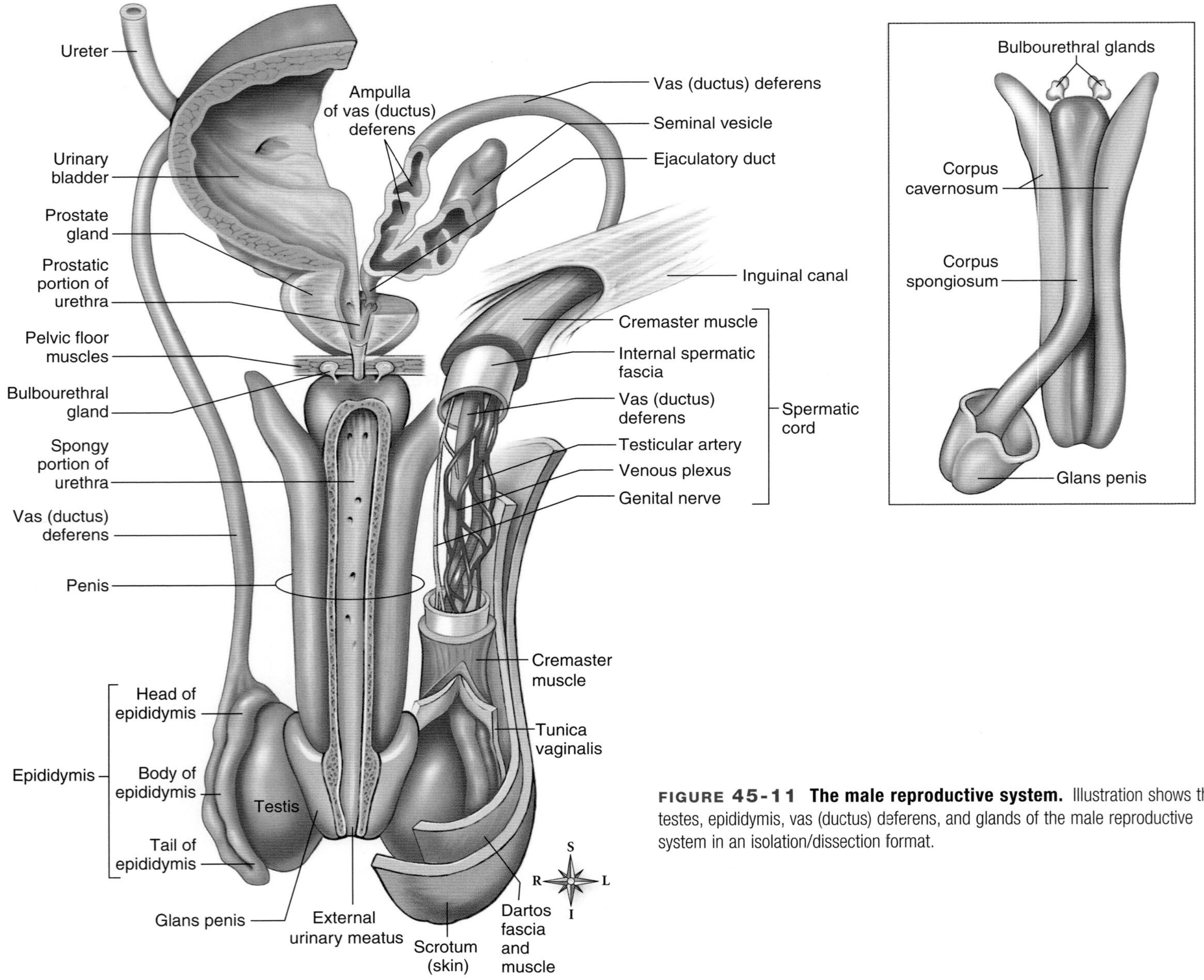

FIGURE 45-11 The male reproductive system. Illustration shows the testes, epididymis, vas (ductus) deferens, and glands of the male reproductive system in an isolation/dissection format.

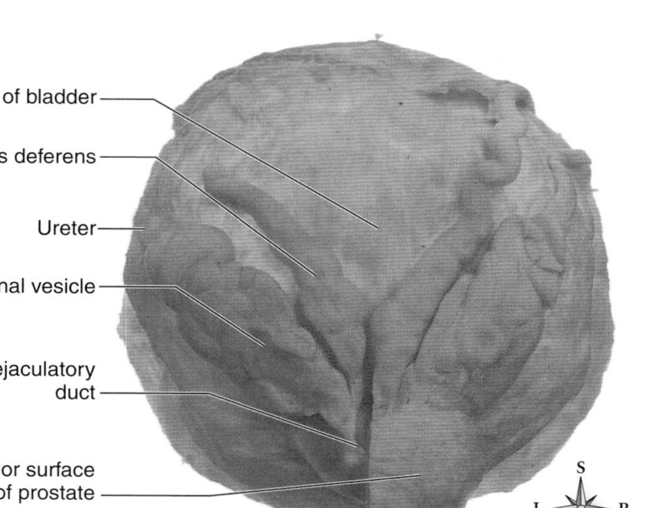

FIGURE 45-12 Prostate and related structures. Cadaver dissection showing the prostate gland and other male reproductive structures viewed from behind. The prostate has been sectioned on the left side to reveal the ejaculatory duct.

Function

The vas deferens serves as one of the male genital ducts connecting the epididymis with the ejaculatory duct. Sperm remain in the vas deferens for varying periods depending on the degree of sexual activity and frequency of ejaculation. Storage time may exceed 1 month with no loss of fertility.

Severing or clamping off the vas deferens—that is, performing a **vasectomy,** usually done through an incision in the scrotum—makes a man sterile. Why? Because it interrupts the route to the exterior from the epididymis. To leave the body, sperm must journey in succession through the epididymis, vas deferens, ejaculatory duct, and urethra.

Ejaculatory Duct

The two ejaculatory ducts are short tubes about 1 cm long that pass through the prostate gland to terminate in the urethra. As **Figures 45-11** and **45-12** show, they are formed by the union of the vas deferens distal to the ampulla with the ducts from the seminal vesicles.

Urethra

The urethra in males serves a dual function, which involves both the reproductive system and the urinary system. Refer to Chapter 42, pp. 970–971, for a discussion of this duct.

CONNECT IT! 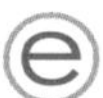

Maintaining healthy communities of microorganisms in the mucosa of the urinary and reproductive tracts helps prevent infections and other disorders. Review the human *microbiome* in ***The Human Microbiome*** at ***Connect It!***

ACCESSORY REPRODUCTIVE GLANDS

Seminal Vesicles

Structure and Location

The **seminal vesicles** are highly convoluted pouches that, when fully extended, are about 15 cm in length. Each is a tubular diverticulum of the vas deferens on one side and is coiled on itself so that it forms a body about 5 to 7 cm in length. The two vasa deferentia lie along the lower part of the posterior surface of the bladder, directly in front of the rectum (see **Figures 45-1**, **45-11**, and **45-12**). **Figure 45-12** is an isolated cadaver specimen showing the relationships of a number of the male reproductive structures, including the seminal vesicles, when viewed from behind. The highly branched and convoluted nature of the secretory epithelium filling the lumen of the seminal vesicles is apparent in **Figure 45-13**.

Function

The seminal vesicles secrete an alkaline, viscous, creamy-yellow liquid that constitutes about 60% of semen volume. The alkalinity helps neutralize the acid pH environment of the terminal urethra and in the vagina. Fructose found in this component of the semen serves as an energy source for sperm motility after ejaculation. Other components include prostaglandins, which are involved in cyclic AMP formation, and a non–blood type coagulating enzyme called *vesiculase.*

Prostate Gland

Structure and Location

The **prostate** is a compound tubuloalveolar gland that lies just below the bladder and is shaped like a doughnut. The fact that the urethra passes through the small hole in the centre of the prostate is a matter of considerable clinical significance. Most older men develop a noncancerous enlargement of this gland called **benign prostatic hypertrophy** (see p. 1052). As the prostate enlarges, it squeezes the urethra, sometimes closing it so completely that urination becomes difficult or impossible. Urinary retention results. Surgical removal of all or part of the gland (prostatectomy) is required as a cure for this condition when other less radical methods of treatment fail.

Function

The prostate secretes a watery, milky-looking, and slightly acidic fluid that constitutes about 30% of the seminal fluid volume. Citrate, found in prostatic fluid, serves as a nutrient for sperm. Other constituents include enzymes such as hyaluronidase and *prostate-specific antigen (PSA)* (**Box 45-1**). Prostatic fluid plays an important role in sperm activation, viability, and motility.

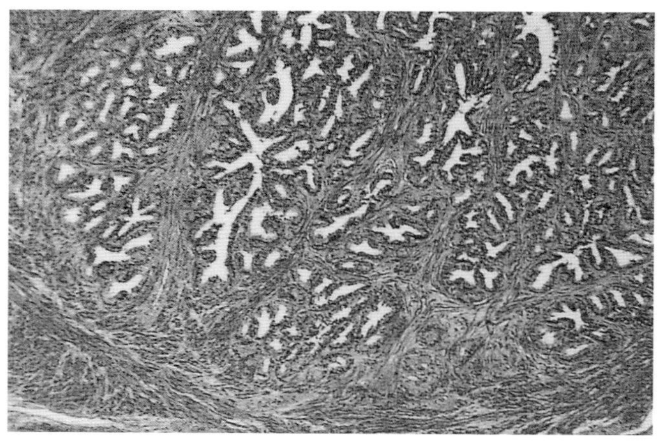

FIGURE 45-13 Seminal vesicle. Note the highly branched and convoluted nature of the secretory epithelium.

BOX 45-1 *diagnostic study* | Prostate Cancer Screening

Prostate cancer accounts for 13% of all cancer deaths in males in the UK. It is the fourth most common cause of cancer death with around 11,000 deaths reported every year. Many men could be saved if the cancer is detected early enough for effective treatment. Several screening tests are available for the detection of prostate cancer once it develops. Cancerous growths in the gland can often be palpated through the wall of the rectum (see figure).

Sometimes, rectal examinations are performed in conjunction with a screening test called the *PSA test.* This test is a type of blood analysis that screens for *prostate-specific antigen (PSA),* a substance sometimes found to be elevated in the blood of men with prostate cancer. Unfortunately, PSA levels may not be elevated with prostate cancer and may be high in some men without prostate cancer. Thus the PSA test is most useful when used with other screening methods.

A nuclear medicine *bone scan* is often used either to exclude metastatic spread of prostate cancer or to locate areas of the body where secondary prostate cancer tumours have already developed. An image of a bone scan showing the metastasis of prostate cancer can be viewed in ***Bone Scans*** online at ***Connect It!*** •

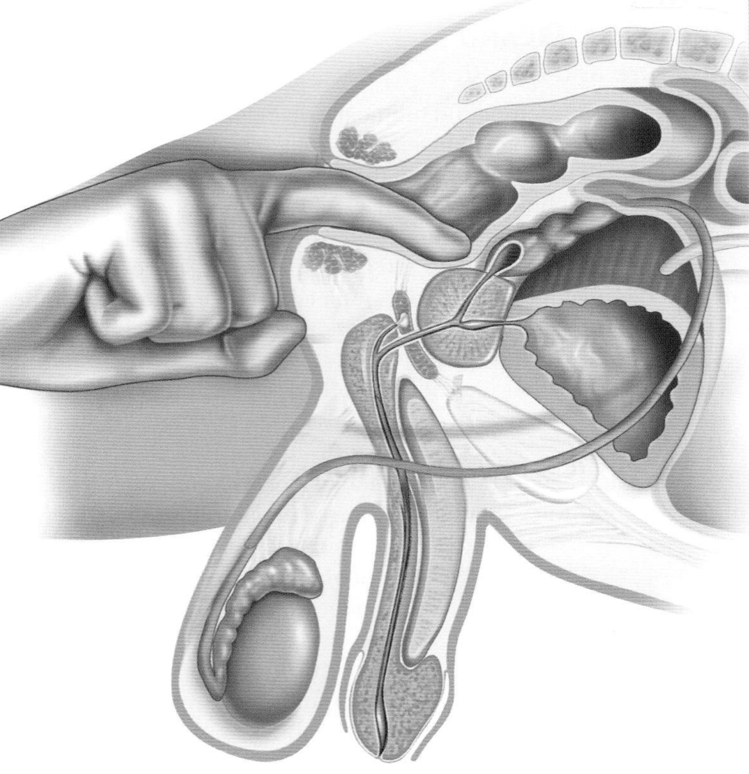

Palpation of the prostate gland. A physician inserts a lubricated, gloved finger through the anus to feel the prostate through the thin anterior wall of the rectum.

Bulbourethral Glands

Structure and Location

The two **bulbourethral glands** *(Cowper glands)* resemble peas in size and shape. You can see the location of these compound tubuloalveolar glands in **Figure 45-11**. A duct approximately 2.5 cm long connects them with the penile portion of the urethra.

Function

Like the seminal vesicles, the bulbourethral glands secrete an alkaline fluid that is important for counteracting the acid present in the male urethra and the female vagina. Mucus produced in these glands serves to lubricate the urethra and helps protect sperm from friction damage during ejaculation.

The bulbourethral glands contribute less than 5% of the seminal fluid volume ejaculated from the urethra.

Quick CHECK

8. List, in sequence, the reproductive ducts sperm pass through from formation to ejaculation.
9. What is the structural relationship between the prostate gland and the urethra?
10. Compare the volume, viscosity, pH, and composition of the secretions produced by the accessory reproductive glands.

SUPPORTING STRUCTURES

Scrotum

The **scrotum** is a skin-covered pouch suspended from the perineal region. Internally, it is divided into two sacs by a septum, each sac containing a testis, an epididymis, and the lower part of a spermatic cord.

The *dartos* fascia and muscle are located just below the skin of the scrotum (see **Figure 45-11**). Contraction of the dartos muscle fibres causes slight elevation of the testes and wrinkling of the scrotal pouch. In addition, contraction of the *cremaster muscle,* also seen in **Figure 45-11**, causes significant elevation of the testes. The cremaster muscle forms an elongated pouch for each testis within the scrotum. Each pouch containing one testis is lined with a doubled serous membrane called the *tunica vaginalis,* which permits the testis within to slide around. This testicular sliding protects against possible injury by allowing the testes to move out of harm's way when the scrotum is pressed or pinched. When the cremaster muscle contracts, the testes are pulled upward against the perineum. Sexual arousal, cold temperature, and threat of injury provide the stimulus for contraction of both the dartos and cremaster muscles.

The temperature required for optimum sperm formation is about 3°C below normal body temperature. This is the "functional" reason that justifies placement of the testes outside the body cavity where they are exposed and subject to traumatic injury. In a warm environment the scrotum becomes elongated and its skin appears loose and wrinkle-free, permitting the testes to descend away from the body. In the cold, the scrotum elevates and becomes heavily wrinkled, effectively pulling the testes upward toward the body wall. Both actions help maintain the temperature of the testes at a more constant level. Factors other than temperature, including blood flow dynamics and tissue oxygen levels, are also suggested as "reasons" for scrotal placement of the testes.

Penis

Structure

Three cylindrical masses of erectile, or cavernous, tissue, enclosed in separate fibrous coverings and held together by a covering of skin, compose the **penis** (**Figure 45-14**). The two larger and uppermost of these cylinders are named the **corpora cavernosa,** whereas the smaller, lower one, which contains the urethra, is called the **corpus spongiosum.**

The distal part of the corpus spongiosum overlaps the terminal end of the two corpora cavernosa to form a slightly bulging structure, the **glans penis,** over which the skin is folded doubly to form a more or less loose-fitting, retractable casing known as the **prepuce,** or foreskin. The opening of the urethra at the tip of the glans is called the *external urinary meatus.*

CONNECT IT!

Removal of the foreskin is called circumcision. Learn more about how and why this procedure is done in ***Male Circumcision*** online at ***Connect It!***

Functions

The penis contains the urethra, the terminal duct for both urinary and reproductive tracts. During sexual arousal, the erectile tissue of the penis fills with blood, causing the organ to become rigid and enlarge in both diameter and length. The result, called an **erection,** permits the penis to serve as a penetrating copulatory organ during sexual intercourse. The scrotum and penis constitute the external **genitals,** or *genitalia,* of the male.

Spermatic Cords

The **spermatic cords** are cylindrical casings of white, fibrous tissue located in the inguinal canals between the scrotum and the abdominal cavity. They enclose the vasa deferentia, blood vessels, lymphatics, and nerves (see **Figure 45-11**).

Composition and Course of Seminal Fluid

The following structures secrete the substances that, together, make up the *seminal fluid,* or semen:

- Testes and epididymis—secretions constitute less than 5% of the seminal fluid volume.
- Seminal vesicles—combined secretions are reported to contribute about 60% of the seminal fluid volume.
- Prostate gland—secretions constitute about 30% of the seminal fluid volume.
- Bulbourethral glands—secretions are said to constitute less than 5% of the seminal fluid volume.

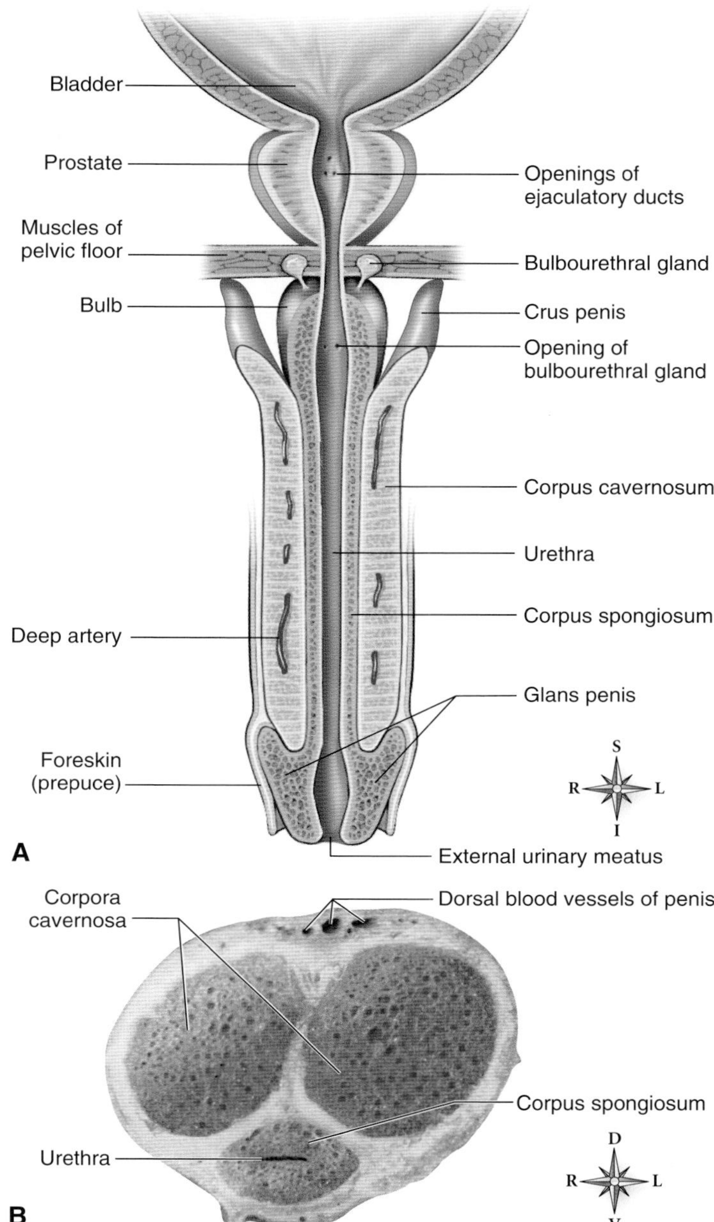

FIGURE 45-14 The penis. A, In this sagittal section of the penis viewed from above, the urethra is exposed throughout its length and can be seen exiting from the bladder and passing through the prostate gland before entering the penis to end at the external urinary meatus (urethral orifice). **B,** Photograph of a cross-section of the shaft of the penis showing the three columns of erectile, or cavernous, tissue. Note the urethra within the substance of the corpus spongiosum.

Besides contributing slightly to the seminal fluid, the testes also add hundreds of millions of sperm. In traversing the distance from their place of origin to the exterior, the sperm must pass from the testis through the epididymis, vas deferens, ejaculatory duct, and urethra. Note that sperm originate in the testes, glands located

BOX 45-2 *fyi*

Neural Control of the Male Sexual Response

Recall that all body functions but one have the ultimate goal of survival of the individual. Only the function of reproduction serves a different, a longer-range, and no doubt in nature's scheme, a more important purpose—survival of the human species. Male functions in reproduction consist of the production of male sex cells (spermatogenesis) and introduction of these cells into the female body (*coitus, copulation,* or *sexual intercourse*). For coitus to take place, erection of the penis must first occur, and for sperm to enter the female body, both the sex cells and secretions from the accessory glands must be introduced into the urethra (emission) and semen must be ejaculated from the penis.

Erection is a parasympathetic reflex initiated mainly by certain tactile, visual, and mental stimuli. It consists of dilation of the arteries and arterioles of the penis, which in turn floods and distends spaces in its erectile tissue and compresses its veins. Therefore more blood enters the penis through the dilated arteries than leaves it through the constricted veins. Hence it becomes larger and rigid, or in other words, erection occurs.

Emission is the reflex movement of sex cells, or spermatozoa, and secretions from the genital ducts and accessory glands into the prostatic urethra. Once emission has occurred, ejaculation will follow.

Ejaculation of semen is also a reflex response. It is the usual outcome of the same stimuli that initiate erection. Ejaculation and various other responses—notably accelerated heart rate, increased blood pressure, hyperventilation, dilated skin blood vessels, and intense sexual excitement—characterize the male **orgasm,** or sexual climax.

Oxytocin (OT) released by neuroendocrine tissue in the posterior pituitary during the male sexual response may enhance muscular contractions that power ejaculation and accompany orgasm. •

outside the body (i.e., not within a body cavity), travel to the inside of the body, and finally are expelled to the outside (external environment) by way of ejaculation.

Box 45-2 summarizes important elements of the male sexual response.

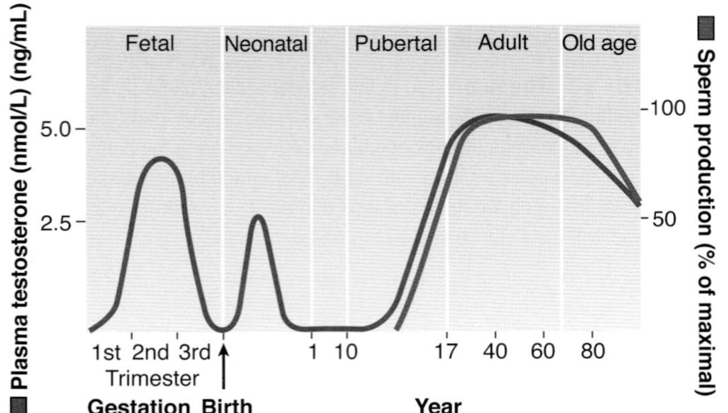

FIGURE 45-15 Testosterone levels and sperm production. Plasma testosterone levels *(red line)* rise during fetal development, when it stimulates early development of male sexual organs. Testosterone rises again briefly around the time of birth, which facilitates descent of the testes into the scrotum. At puberty testosterone rises enough to support sperm production *(blue line)*; it later tapers off in advanced old age.

MALE FERTILITY

Male fertility relates to many factors—most of all to the number of sperm ejaculated but also to their size, shape, and motility. Fertile sperm have a uniform size and shape. They are highly motile. Although only one sperm fertilizes an ovum, millions of sperm seem to be necessary for fertilization to occur. The minimum sperm concentration that is now considered within the normal range is 15 million per mL of semen. When the sperm count falls below this level, functional sterility results.

One hypothesis suggested to explain the puzzling fact that millions of sperm are necessary is as follows. Semen that contains an adequate number of sperm also contains enough hyaluronidase and other hydrolytic enzymes to liquefy the intercellular substance between the cells that encase each ovum. Without this, a single sperm cannot penetrate the layers of cells around the ovum and hence cannot fertilize it. Infertility may also be caused by production of antibodies some men make against their own sperm. This type of sperm destruction or inactivation, called *immune infertility*, is caused by an antigen–antibody reaction. A

cycle of ***life***

Male Reproductive System The reproductive system is unlike all other systems of the male body with regard to normal changes that occur throughout the life span. All other systems perform their functions from the time they develop in utero until advanced old age, when degeneration may cause loss of function and, perhaps, death. The male reproductive system, however, does not begin to perform its functions until puberty—usually during the early teenage years. Of course, the biological advantage of this "late start" is that a person does not have the biological, psychological, or social maturity to become a parent before that time.

Initial development of the male reproductive organs begins before birth, when the reproductive tract differentiates into the male form rather than the female form (see **Figures 47-17** and **47-18** on p. 1107). At about the seventh week of embryonic development, genes in the Y chromosome in males trigger the production of enough testosterone to stimulate the development of male reproductive organs. Without this early spurt of testosterone (see **Figure 45-15**), the organs would instead develop into the female form.

A couple of months before birth, the immature testes descend behind the parietal peritoneum into the scrotum (**Figure 45-16**). The testes are guided in their descent by a threadlike, fibrous gubernaculum. It is not uncommon for them to be late in completing the descent, perhaps not arriving in the scrotum until several weeks after birth. **Figure 45-15** shows a spurt in testosterone levels around the time of birth that can then stimulate descent of the testes.

The testes and other reproductive organs remain in an immature form—and thus remain incapable of providing reproductive function—until puberty, when high levels of reproductive hormones stimulate the final stages of their development (see **Figure 45-15**). From puberty until advanced old age the male reproductive system continues to operate efficiently enough to permit successful reproduction. A gradual decline in hormone production during late adulthood may decrease sexual desire and fertility to some degree, but a man may be able to father a child until the time of death. •

sperm surface protein called *fertilization antigen (FA-1)* triggers antibody production, which results in infertility.

Figure 45-15 shows that as average plasma testosterone levels increase during puberty, sperm production begins. Testosterone levels—and thus sperm production—reach a peak in early adulthood and remain high into old age. In advanced old age, testosterone production tapers off—and thus so does fertility, as seen in the dropping sperm count.

Quick CHECK

11. What two structures constitute the external genitals of the male?
12. What is the function of the dartos and cremaster muscles? How does this function influence fertility?
13. Identify by name the three cylindrical masses of erectile tissue in the penis.
14. What factors influence male fertility?

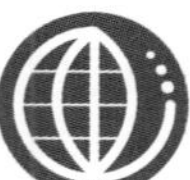

the big picture | Male Reproductive System

Propagation of the genes of a species is truly a "big picture" outcome related to functioning of the reproductive system in both sexes.

In males, the reproductive and urinary tracts are partly shared—causing some to group them together as the *genitourinary tract.* Such structural sharing also means functional sharing. For example, the urethra conducts urine during micturition but instead conducts semen during ejaculation. Changes to muscular control of the bladder, urethra, and ejaculatory duct prevent flow of urine—and backflow of semen into the bladder—during the sexual response.

Both the primary and secondary sexual functions in males depend on complex interrelationships involving nervous, endocrine, muscular, urinary, and circulatory system structures. Even the skin is a sexual organ, receiving some of the stimuli needed to produce the sexual response.

mechanisms of disease

Disorders of the Male Reproductive System

Several disorders of the male reproductive system cause **infertility**. Infertility is an abnormally low ability to reproduce. If there is a complete inability to reproduce, the condition is called **sterility.** Infertility or sterility involves an abnormally reduced capacity to deliver healthy sperm to the female reproductive tract. Reduced reproductive capacity may result from factors such as a decrease in the testes' production of sperm, structural abnormalities in the sperm, or obstruction of the reproductive ducts.

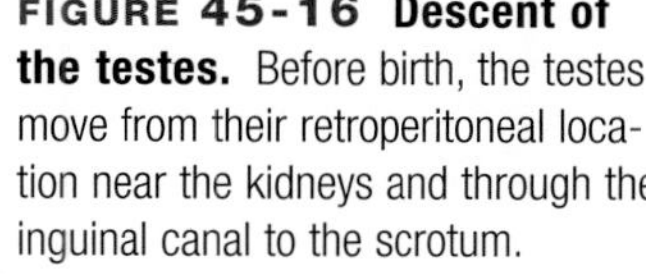

CONNECT IT!

Infections of the reproductive tract, often acquired through sexual contact with infected individuals, can progress into conditions that may cause sterility—or even death. These *sexually transmitted diseases (STDs)* are discussed in ***Sexually Transmitted Diseases*** online at **Connect It!**

Males in general do not have a well-defined andropause, or cessation of fertility in late adulthood that closely parallels the female menopause. However, sensitivity of the testis to luteinizing hormone (LH) may begin to decline after 50, causing testosterone levels to drop. Low testosterone (lowT) can cause sperm production to decline, but many men remain fertile throughout life.

Disorders of the Testes

Disruption of the sperm-producing function of the seminiferous tubules can result in decreased sperm production, a condition called **oligospermia**. If the *sperm count* is too low, infertility may result. A large number of sperm is needed to ensure that many sperm will reach the ovum and dissolve its coating—allowing a single sperm to unite with the ovum. Oligospermia can result from factors such as infection, fever, radiation, malnutrition, and high temperature in the testes. In some cases, oligospermia is temporary—as in some acute infections. Oligospermia is a leading cause of infertility. Of course, total absence of sperm production results in sterility.

Early in fetal life the testes are located in the abdominal cavity near the kidneys but normally descend into the scrotum about 2 months before birth (see **Figure 45-16**). Occasionally a baby is born with undescended testes, a condition called **cryptorchidism**, which is readily observed by palpation of the

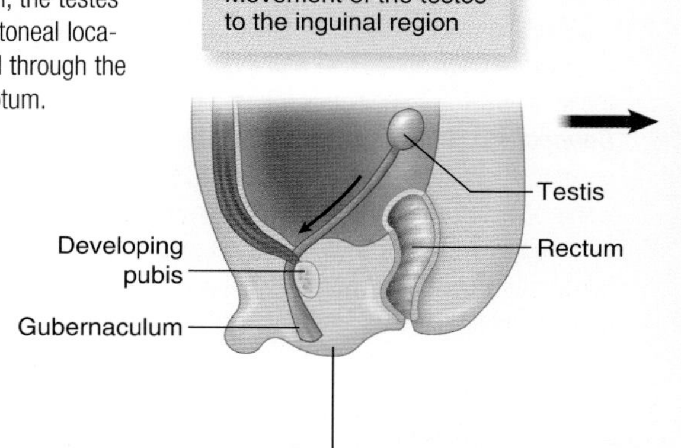

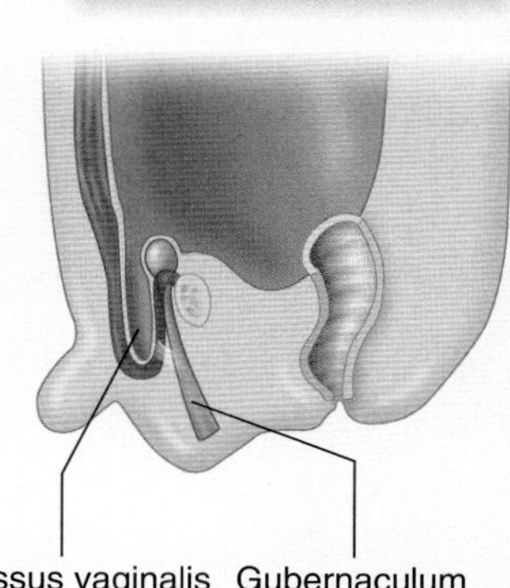

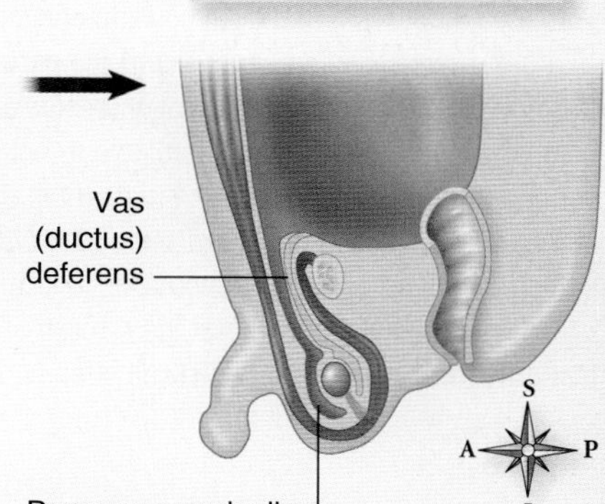

FIGURE 45-16 Descent of the testes. Before birth, the testes move from their retroperitoneal location near the kidneys and through the inguinal canal to the scrotum.

UNIT 6

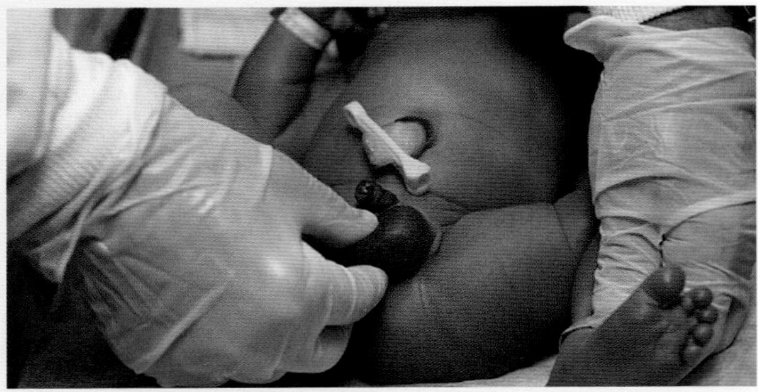

FIGURE 45-17 Screening for cryptorchidism in a newborn infant. Properly descended testes can be palpated easily in the scrotal sac at birth.

scrotum at delivery (**Figure 45-17**). The word *cryptorchidism* is from the Greek words *kryptikos* ("hidden") and *orchis* ("testis"). Failure of the testes to descend may be caused by hormonal imbalances in the developing fetus or by a physical deficiency or obstruction. Regardless of cause, in the cryptorchid infant the testes remain "hidden" in the abdominopelvic cavity. Because the higher temperature inside the body cavity inhibits spermatogenesis, measures must be taken to bring the testes down into the scrotum to prevent permanent sterility. Early treatment of this condition by surgery or by injection of testosterone, which stimulates the testes to descend (see **Figure 45-15**), may result in normal testicular and sexual development.

Most testicular cancers arise from the sperm-producing cells of the seminiferous tubules. Malignancies of the testes are most common among men 20 to 35 years old. Besides age, this type of cancer is associated with genetic predisposition, trauma or infection of the testis, and cryptorchidism. Treatment of testicular cancer is most effective when the diagnosis is made early in the development of the tumour.

CONNECT IT! ⓔ

Many physicians encourage male patients to perform regular self-examination of their testes, especially if they are in a high-risk group. Check out ***Male Genital Self-Examination*** online at ***Connect It!***

Disorders of the Prostate

A noncancerous condition called **benign prostatic hypertrophy (BPH)** occurs in 75% of men older than 50 years and in more than 90% of men older than 80 years. As the name suggests, the condition is characterized by an enlargement, or hypertrophy, of the prostate gland. As discussed earlier in the chapter, the fact that the urethra passes through the centre of the prostate after exiting from the bladder is a matter of considerable clinical significance. As the prostate enlarges, it squeezes and may distort the normal passage of the urethra, often closing it so completely that urination becomes very difficult or even impossible. Commonly the first area of the prostate to enlarge in BPH involves the so-called *periurethral glandular tissue* surrounding the urethra. Tissue near the periphery of the prostate, called *peripheral zone glandular tissue,* may remain normal even though the gland as a whole increases in size.

Surgical removal of some of the swollen tissue surrounding the urethra in a **transurethral resection (TUR)** will often be effective in reducing symptoms and improving urine flow rates. In this procedure, a tubelike instrument called a *cystoscope*—which contains operative devices, a lighting system, and viewing lenses—is inserted through the penis and into the prostatic urethra to surgically remove (resect) prostatic tissue surrounding the lumen. Alternative procedures using laser therapy, focused ultrasound, or the insertion of urethral stents may also be employed. The use of robotic devices to assist in TURs has helped improve accuracy and thus reduce surgical complications. In severe cases total removal of the gland, a procedure called **prostatectomy,** may become necessary.

Disorders of the Penis and Scrotum

The penis is subject to numerous sexually transmitted infections, as well as structural abnormalities. One such structural abnormality is **phimosis,** a condition in which the foreskin fits so tightly over the glans that it cannot retract. The usual treatment for this condition is **circumcision**—a procedure in which the foreskin is cut along the base of the glans and removed. Severe phimosis can obstruct the flow of urine, possibly causing the death of an infant born with this condition. Milder phimosis can result in accumulation of dirt and organic matter under the foreskin, possibly causing severe infections.

Failure to achieve an erection of the penis adequate enough to permit sexual intercourse is called *impotence* or **erectile dysfunction (ED).** ED affects men of all ages but is experienced most often after age 65 years. ED does not affect sperm production, but infertility often results because normal intercourse may not be possible. In the past, psychological problems such as anxiety, depression, and stress were often cited as the most important causes of impotence in sexually active men. There is no doubt that such conditions contribute to ED. However, current research suggests that purely psychological problems account for far fewer cases of impotence than previously thought. We now know that ED is often caused by medical problems related to abnormal vascular or neural control of penile blood flow. Arteriosclerosis, diabetes, alcohol abuse, numerous medications, radiation therapy, tumours, spinal cord trauma, and surgery, especially if pelvic organs such as the prostate are involved, may all cause ED.

The most common treatment option is the use of drugs that increase blood flow to the spongy cavernous tissue of the penis, causing it to stiffen and become erect. Most of the ED drugs affect the levels of nitric oxide, a local regulator and neurotransmitter that controls tension of the smooth muscles in the vessels of the penis. Other possible treatments involve vacuum pumps, internal penile supports, and other methods.

Swelling of the scrotum can be caused by various conditions. One of the most common causes of scrotal swelling is an accumulation of fluid called **hydrocele.** Hydroceles may be congenital, resulting from structural abnormalities present at birth. In adults, hydrocele often occurs when fluid produced by the serous membrane lining the scrotum is not absorbed properly. The cause of adult hydrocele is not always known, but in some cases it can be linked to trauma or infection.

Swelling of the scrotum may also occur when the intestines push through the weak area of the abdominal wall that separates the abdominopelvic cavity from the scrotum. This condition is a form of **inguinal hernia** (see ***Hernias*** online at ***Connect It!***). If the intestines protrude into the scrotum, the digestive tract may become obstructed—resulting in death. Inguinal hernia often occurs while lifting heavy objects because of the high internal pressure generated by the contraction of abdominal muscles. Inguinal hernia may also be congenital. Small inguinal hernias may be treated with external supports that prevent organs from protruding into the scrotum; more serious hernias must be repaired surgically.

LANGUAGE OF SCIENCE *(continued from p. 1038)*

perineum (pair-ih-NEE-um)
[*peri-* **around,** *-ine-* **excrete,** *-um* **thing**] *pl.,* perinea

prepuce (PREE-pus)
[*pre-* **before,** *-puc-* **penis**]

prostate (PROSS-tayt)
[*pro-* **before,** *-stat-* **set or place**]

scrotum (SKROH-tum)
[*scrotum* **bag**] *pl.,* scrota or scrotums

semen (SEE-men)
[*semen* **seed**]

seminal vesicle (SEM-ih-nal VES-ih-kul)
[*semen-* **seed,** *-al* **relating to,** *vesic-* **blister,** *-cle* **little**]

seminiferous tubule (seh-mih-NIF-er-us TYOOB-yool)
[*semin-* **seed,** *-fer-* **bear or carry,** *-ous* **relating to,** *tub-* **tube,** *-ul-* **little**]

spermatic cord (sper-MAT-ik kord)
[*sperma-* **seed,** *-ic* **relating to**]

spermatogenesis (sper-mah-toh-JEN-eh-sis)
[*sperma-* **seed,** *-gen-* **produce,** *-esis* **process**]

spermatozoon (sper-mah-tah-ZOH-on)
[*sperma-* **seed,** *-zoon* **animal**] *pl.,* spermatozoa

sustentacular cell (sus-ten-TAK-yoo-lar)
[*sustent-* **support,** *-acular* **relating to**]

testis (TES-tis)
[*testis* **witness (male gonad)**] *pl.,* testes

testosterone (tes-TOS-teh-rohn)
[*test-* **witness (testis),** *-stero-* **solid or steroid derivative,** *-one* **chemical**]

tunica albuginea (TYOO-nih-kah al-byoo-JIN-ee-ah)
[*tunica* **tunic or coat,** *albuginea* **white**] *pl.,* tunicae albuginea

vas deferens (vas DEF-er-enz)
[*vas* **duct or vessel,** *deferens* **carrying away**] *pl.,* vasa deferentia

LANGUAGE OF MEDICINE

benign prostatic hypertrophy (BPH) (be-NYNE pro-STAT-ik hye-PER-troh-fee)
[*benign* **kind,** *pro-* **before,** *-stat-* **set or place,** *-ic* **relating to,** *hyper-* **excessive or above,** *-troph-* **nourishment,** *-y* **state**]

circumcision (sir-kum-SIH-zhun)
[*circum-* **around,** *-cis-* **cut,** *-ion* **process**]

cryptorchidism (krip-TOR-kih-diz-em)
[*crypt-* **hidden,** *-orchid-* **testis,** *-ism* **condition**]

erectile dysfunction (ED) (ee-REK-tyle dis-FUNGK-shun)
[*erect* **make upright,** *-ile* **relating to,** *dys-* **bad or painful,** *-function* **performance**]

hydrocele (HYE-dro-seel)
[*hydro-* **water,** *-cele* **tumour**]

infertility (in-fer-TIL-ih-tee)
[*in-* **not,** *-fertil-* **fruitful,** *-ity* **state**]

inguinal hernia (IN-gwih-nal HER-nee-ah)
[*inguin-* **groin,** *-al* **relating to,** *hernia* **rupture**] *pl.,* herniae or hernias

oligospermia (ol-ih-goh-SPER-mee-ah)
[*oligo-* **few or little,** *-sperm-* **seed,** *-ia* **condition**]

phimosis (fih-MOH-sis)
[*phimos-* **muzzle,** *-osis* **condition**]

prostatectomy (pros-ta-TEK-toh-mee)
[*pro-* **before,** *-stat-* **set or place (prostate gland),** *-ec-* **out,** *-tom-* **cut,** *-y* **action**]

sterility (steh-RIL-ih-tee)
[*steril-* **barren,** *-ity* **state**]

transurethral resection (TUR) (tranz-yoor-REE-thral rih-SEK-shun)
[*trans-* **across or through,** *-ure-* **urine,** *-thr-* **agent or channel (urethra),** *-al* **relating to,** *re-* **again,** *-sect-* **cut,** *-tion* **process**]

vasectomy (va-SEK-toh-mee)
[*vas-* **duct or vessel (vas deferens),** *-ec-* **out,** *-tom-* **cut,** *-y* **action**]

case study

David, a professional cyclist, and his wife Karen had been trying for two years to start a family with no success. Karen's menstrual cycle was regular and seemed to be normal. They finally decided to consult their GP who referred them to an infertility specialist. At the clinic David was asked to provide a semen sample for analysis to assess the quality and quantity of his sperm (a sperm count). To David's surprise he was also asked about the amount of time he spent in his tight-fitting cycling outfit. The specialist explained that some studies have indicated that tight-fitting clothing can raise the temperature of the testes and interfere with sperm development.

1. Sperm production occurs normally at what temperature?
   a. 3°C above body temperature
   b. At body temperature
   c. 3°C below body temperature
   d. An optimal temperature that changes with the seasons
2. A low sperm count could make it difficult for Karen to conceive. What number should David's sperm count be above to be sure he is not suffering from oligospermia (condition of few sperm)?
   a. 150 million/mL
   b. 15 million/mL
   c. 1500/mL
   d. 150/mL
3. Which is the correct pathway the sperm take during ejaculation?
   a. Seminiferous tubules, rete testis, efferent ductules, epididymis, vas deferens, ejaculatory duct, urethra
   b. Rete testis, seminiferous tubules, efferent ductules, epididymis, vas deferens, urethra, ejaculatory duct
   c. Epididymis, vas deferens, seminiferous tubules, rete testis, ejaculatory duct, urethra
   d. Seminiferous tubules, rete testis, epididymis, vas deferens, efferent ductules, urethra, ejaculatory duct
4. Which hormone directly stimulates sperm production?
   a. Oestrogen
   b. Progesterone
   c. LH
   d. Testosterone

Hint To solve a case study, you may have to refer to the glossary or index, other chapters in this textbook, ***Connect It!,*** and other resources.

CHAPTER SUMMARY

To download an MP3 version of the chapter summary for use with your mobile device, access the **Audio Chapter Summaries** *online at evolve.elsevier.com.*

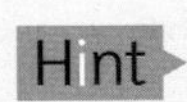

Scan this summary after reading the chapter to help you reinforce the key concepts. Later, use the summary as a quick review before your class or before a test.

Sexual Reproduction

A. Functioning of the reproductive system ensures the survival of the genetic characteristics of a species
B. Male reproductive system consists of organs whose functions are to produce, transfer, and introduce mature sperm into the female reproductive tract where fertilization can occur

Male Reproductive Organs

A. Classified as essential organs for production of gametes or accessory organs that support the reproductive process (**Figure 45-1**)
   1. Essential organs—gonads of the male; testes
   2. Accessory organs of reproduction
      a. Reproductive (genital) ducts convey sperm to outside of body; include pair of epididymides, paired vasa deferentia, pair of ejaculatory ducts, and the urethra
      b. Accessory glands produce secretions that nourish, transport, and mature sperm; include pair of seminal vesicles, the prostate, and pair of bulbourethral glands
      c. Supporting structures—scrotum, penis, and pair of spermatic cords
B. Perineum—in males, roughly diamond-shaped area between thighs
   1. Extends anteriorly from pubic symphysis to coccyx posteriorly
   2. Lateral boundary is the ischial tuberosity on either side
   3. Divided into the urogenital triangle and the anal triangle (**Figure 45-2**)

Testes

A. Structure and location
   1. Several lobules composed of seminiferous tubules and interstitial cells (Leydig cells), separated by septa, encased in fibrous capsule called the *tunica albuginea* (**Figure 45-3**)
   2. Seminiferous tubules in testis open into a plexus called *rete testis,* which is drained by a series of efferent ductules that emerge from the top of the organ and enter the head of epididymis
   3. Located in scrotum, one testis in each of two scrotal compartments
B. Microscopic anatomy (**Figures 45-4, 45-5, 45-6**)
   1. Interstitial (Leydig) cells—endocrine cells between the seminiferous tubules
   2. Seminiferous tubules
      a. Spermatogenic cells produce sperm
      b. Sustentacular cells—also called *nurse* or *Sertoli cells*
         (1) Support and regulate sperm-producing functions of the testis
         (2) Produce androgen-binding protein (ABP) that binds to testosterone to make it more soluble and thus increase its concentration, supporting sperm production
         (3) Inhibin—inhibits release of GnRH by the hypothalamus and FSH by anterior pituitary, thus allowing the testis to have some control over spermatogenesis
         (4) Tight junctions between sustentacular cells form the blood–testis barrier (BTB) that protects developing sperm from the immune system
C. Testis functions
   1. Spermatogenesis—formation of mature male gametes (spermatozoa) by seminiferous tubules; stimulated by follicle-stimulating hormone (FSH) from the anterior pituitary (and also GnRH from hypothalamus)
   2. Secretion of hormones by interstitial cells (**Figure 45-7**)
      a. Testosterone
         (1) Type of androgen—maleness hormone
         (2) Multiple functions, including promoting primary and secondary male sexual characteristics, promoting anabolism, affecting fluid and electrolyte balance
         (3) Regulated by luteinizing hormone (LH) from anterior pituitary
      b. Oestrogen—small amounts secreted by interstitial cells, liver, and other organs; role in males uncertain but may influence spermatogenesis and other functions
D. Spermatozoa (**Figure 45-8**)
   1. Structure—consist of a head (covered by acrosome), neck, midpiece, and tail; tail is divided into a principal piece and a short end piece
   2. Function—capacitation in the female tract releases acrosomal enzymes that digest barrier around ovum and promote sperm motility; sperm nucleus unites with egg nucleus to form first cell of new offspring

Reproductive Ducts

A. Epididymis
   1. Structure and location
      a. Single tightly coiled tube enclosed in fibrous casing (**Figure 45-9**)
      b. Lies along top and side of each testis
      c. Anatomical divisions include head, body, and tail
   2. Functions
      a. Duct for seminal fluid
      b. Also secretes part of seminal fluid
      c. Sperm become capable of motility while they are passing through the epididymis

B. Vas deferens (ductus deferens) (**Figures 45-10** and **45-11**)
  1. Structure and location
    a. Tube, extension of epididymis
    b. Extends through inguinal canal, into abdominal cavity, over top and down posterior surface of bladder
    c. Enlarged terminal portion called *ampulla*—joins duct of seminal vesicle
  2. Function
    a. One of excretory ducts for seminal fluid
    b. Connects epididymis with ejaculatory duct

C. Ejaculatory duct (**Figure 45-12**)
  1. Formed by union of vas deferens with duct from seminal vesicle
  2. Passes through prostate gland, terminating in urethra

D. Urethra—serves a dual function (see Chapter 42, pp. 970–971)

Accessory Reproductive Glands

A. Seminal vesicles (**Figure 45-13**)
  1. Structure and location—convoluted pouches about 5 to 7 cm long on posterior surface of bladder
  2. Function—secrete the viscous, nutrient-rich part of seminal fluid (60% of semen volume)

B. Prostate gland (**Figure 45-14**)
  1. Structure and location
    a. Doughnut shaped
    b. Encircles urethra just below bladder
  2. Function—adds slightly acidic, watery, milky-looking secretion to seminal fluid (30% of semen volume)

C. Bulbourethral glands
  1. Structure and location
    a. Small, pea-shaped structures with about 2.5-cm long ducts leading into urethra
    b. Lie below prostate gland
  2. Function—secrete alkaline fluid that is part of semen (5% of semen volume)

Supporting Structures

A. Scrotum
  1. Skin-covered pouch suspended from perineal region into which the testes descend near the time of birth (**Figure 45-11**)
  2. Divided into two compartments
  3. Contains testis, epididymis, and lower part of a spermatic cord
  4. Dartos and cremaster muscles elevate the scrotal pouch

B. Penis (**Figure 45-14**)
  1. Structure—composed of three cylindrical masses of erectile tissue, one of which contains urethra
  2. Functions—penis contains the urethra, the terminal duct for both urinary and reproductive tracts; during sexual arousal, penis becomes erect, serving as a penetrating copulatory organ during sexual intercourse

C. Spermatic cords (internal)
  1. Fibrous cylinders located in inguinal canals
  2. Enclose seminal ducts, blood vessels, lymphatics, and nerves

Composition and Course of Seminal Fluid

A. Consists of secretions from testes, epididymides, seminal vesicles, prostate, and bulbourethral glands

B. Each millilitre contains millions of sperm

C. Passes from testes through epididymis, vas deferens, ejaculatory duct, and urethra

Male Fertility

A. Relates to many factors—number of sperm; size, shape, and motility

B. Infertility may be caused by antibodies some men make against their own sperm

C. Male fertility begins at puberty and extends into old age (**Figure 45-15**)

Cycle of Life: Male Reproductive System

A. Reproductive functions begin at time of puberty

B. Development of organs begins before birth; immature testes descend into scrotum before or shortly after birth (**Figure 45-16**)

C. Puberty—high levels of hormones stimulate final stages of development

D. System operates to permit reproduction until advanced old age

E. Late adulthood—gradual decline in hormone production may decrease sexual appetite and fertility

The Big Picture: Male Reproductive System

A. Propagation of the genes of a species is related to the functioning of the reproductive system in both sexes

B. In males, the reproductive and urinary tracts are partly shared

C. Both the primary and secondary sexual functions in males depend on complex interrelationships involving nervous, endocrine, muscular, urinary, and circulatory system structures

REVIEW QUESTIONS

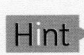

Write out the answers to these questions after reading the chapter and reviewing the Chapter Summary. Note—writing out your answers will consolidate learning and provide a valuable resource of information.

1. Name the accessory glands of the male reproductive system.
2. Name the essential organs of the male reproductive system.
3. List the supporting structures of the male reproductive system.
4. What is the tunica albuginea? How does it aid in dividing the testis into lobules?
5. Name the two primary functions of the testes.
6. What are the general functions of testosterone?
7. Discuss the structure of a mature spermatozoon.
8. What is meant by the term *capacitation?*
9. List the three functions of the epididymis.
10. List the anatomical divisions of the epididymis.
11. Discuss the formation of the ejaculatory ducts.
12. Describe the secretions typical of the prostate gland and seminal vesicles.
13. What and where are the bulbourethral glands?
14. Describe the structure, location, and function or functions of the scrotum.
15. Name the three cylindrical masses of erectile, or cavernous, tissue in the penis.
16. What and where is the glans penis? What is the role of the prepuce, or foreskin?
17. What is the spermatic cord? From what does it extend, and what does it contain?
18. Identify and define the male functions in reproduction.

CRITICAL THINKING QUESTIONS

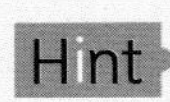

After finishing the Review Questions, write out the answers to these more in-depth questions to help you apply your new knowledge. Go back to sections of the chapter that relate to concepts that you find difficult.

1. How does the function of reproduction differ from all other body functions?
2. Identify two functions of the testes.
3. What is the relationship between the rete testis, seminiferous tubules, and efferent ductules?
4. How is the prostate gland related to the urethra? What problems can result from this relationship?
5. List the structures in the reproductive system that contribute to the formation of seminal fluid.
6. Trace the course of seminal fluid from its formation to ejaculation.
7. What is the chemical in seminal fluid that is important to fertility? What is its function?
8. How is the structure of the spermatozoon related to its function?
9. A man with a sperm count of 10,000 sperm/mL is considered to be sterile. If only one sperm is required to fertilize an egg, explain how this number signifies sterility.

46 Female Reproductive System

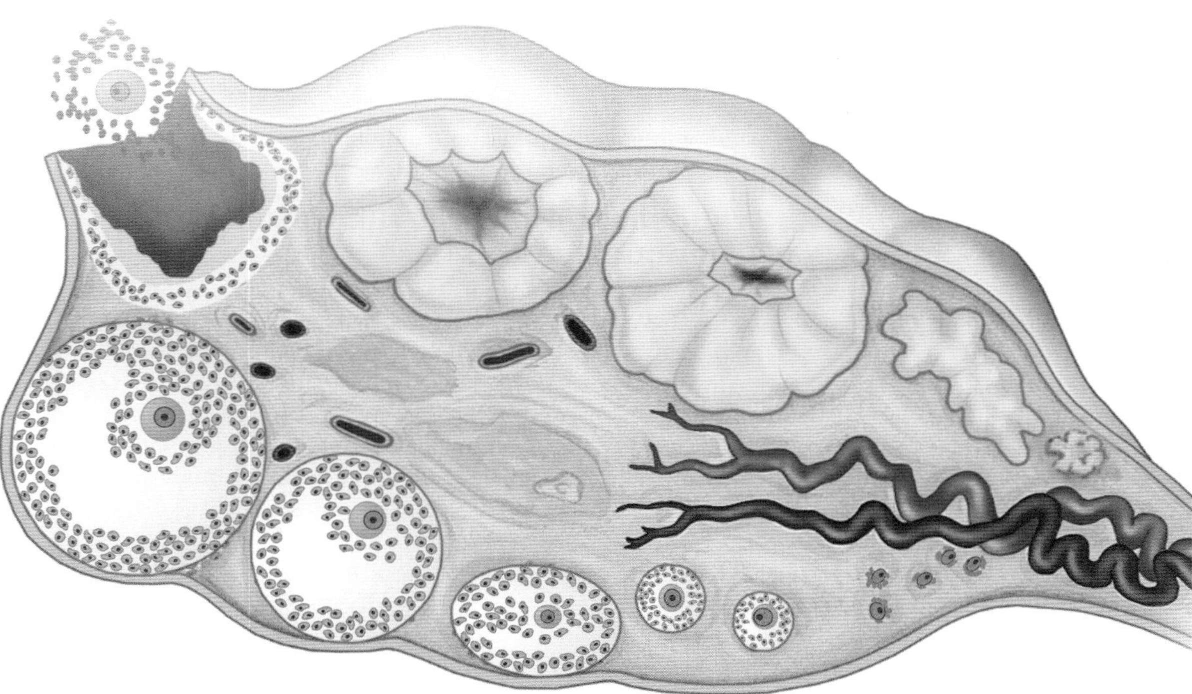

CHAPTER OUTLINE

Hint ▸ *Scan this outline before you begin to read the chapter, as a preview of how the concepts are organized.*

LANGUAGE OF SCIENCE

Hint ▸ *Use this list to aid your pronunciation of unfamiliar words.*

accessory organ (ak-SES-oh-ree OR-gan)
[*access-* **extra,** *-ory* **relating to,** *organ* **instrument**]

ampulla (am-PUL-ah)
[*ampu-* **flask,** *-ulla* **little**] *pl.,* ampullae

anal triangle
[*an-* **ring (anus),** *-al* **relating to**]

anterior fornix (an-TEER-ee-or FOR-niks)
[*ante-* **front,** *-er-* **more,** *-or* **quality,** *fornix* **arch**] *pl.,* fornices

anterior ligament (an-TEER-ee-or LIG-ah-ment)
[*ante-* **front,** *-er-* **more,** *-or* **quality,** *liga-* **bind,** *-ment* **condition**]

areola (ah-REE-oh-lah)
[*are-* **area or space,** *-ola* **little**] *pl.,* areolae, areoles, or areolas

atresia (ah-TREE-zha)
[*a-* **without,** *-tres-* **perforation,** *-ia* **process**]

body of uterus (YOO-ter-us)
[*uterus* **womb**]

broad ligament (LIG-ah-ment)
[*liga-* **bind,** *-ment* **condition**]

cervical canal (SER-vih-kal kah-NAL)
[*cervic-* **neck,** *-al* **relating to**]

cervix (SER-viks)
[*cervix* **neck**] *pl.,* cervices or cervixes

climacteric (klye-MAK-ter-ik)
[*climacter-* **critical point,** *-ic* **relating to**]

clitoris (KLIT-oh-ris)
[*clitoris* **small key or latch**] *pl.,* clitorides

corpus albicans (KOHR-pus AL-bih-kanz)
[*corpus* **body,** *albicans* **whitening**] *pl.,* corpora albicantia

corpus luteum (KOHR-pus LOO-tee-um)
[*corpus* **body,** *lute-* **yellow,** *-um* **thing**] *pl.,* corpora lutea

cortex (KOHR-teks)
[*cortex* **bark**] *pl.,* cortices

endometrium (en-doh-MEE-tree-um)
[*endo-* **within,** *-metr-* **womb,** *-um* **thing**] *pl.,* endometria

external os
[*extern-* **outside,** *-al* **relating to,** *os* **mouth or opening**] *pl.,* ora

continued on p. 1084

In the previous chapter, we discussed the structure and function of the male reproductive system. In this chapter, we discuss the structure and function of the female reproductive system. As you study this chapter, keep in mind that both systems must function properly if successful reproduction and survival of offspring are to occur. The next chapter explores the processes of development of offspring.

OVERVIEW OF THE FEMALE REPRODUCTIVE SYSTEM

FUNCTION OF THE FEMALE REPRODUCTIVE SYSTEM

The physiological importance of the female reproductive system is best understood in terms of its final outcome: production of offspring and continued existence of the genetic code. The female reproductive system produces gametes that may unite with a male gamete to form the first cell of the offspring. The function of conception emphasizes the similarity between the male and female reproductive systems. Unlike the male system, however, the female reproductive system also provides protection and nutrition to the developing offspring for up to several years after conception, as we shall see.

STRUCTURAL PLAN OF THE FEMALE REPRODUCTIVE SYSTEM

So many organs make up the female reproductive system that we need to look first at the structural plan of the system as a whole (**Figure 46-1**). As we stated in the previous chapter, reproductive organs can be classified as **essential organs** or **accessory organs,** depending on how directly they are involved in producing offspring. The essential organs of reproduction in women, the *gonads,* are the paired **ovaries.** The female gametes, or **ova,** are produced by the

FIGURE 46-1 Female reproductive organs. A, Diagram (sagittal section) of pelvis showing location of female reproductive organs. **B** (on following page), Magnetic resonance imaging (MRI) scan (sagittal view) of female pelvic viscera.

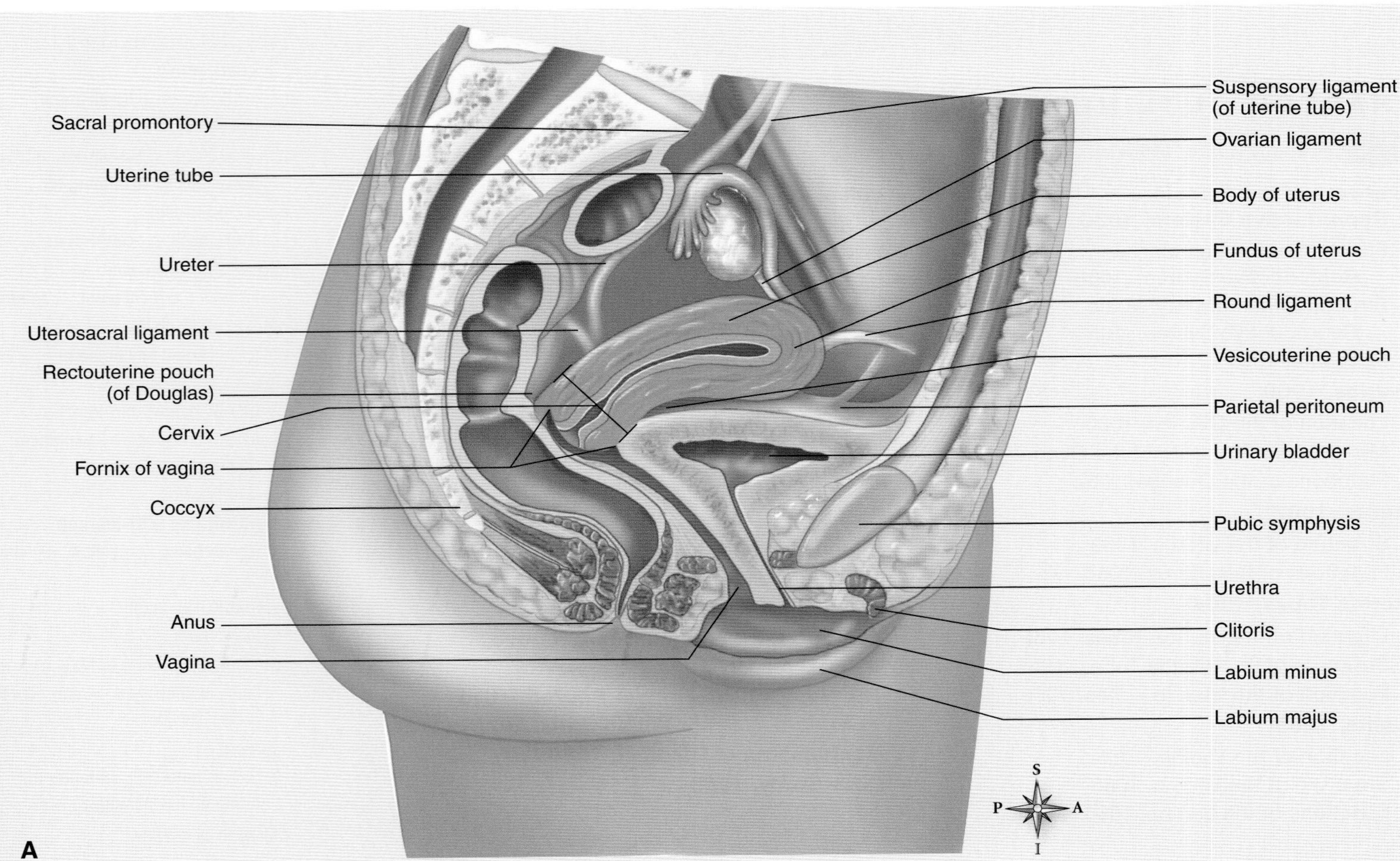

ovaries. The ovaries also produce the hormones oestrogen and progesterone. The accessory organs of reproduction in women consist of the following structures:

- A series of ducts or modified duct structures that extend from near the ovaries to the exterior. This group of organs includes the *uterine tubes*, *uterus*, and *vagina*. Along with the ovaries, these organs are sometimes collectively called the "internal genitals".
- The *vulva*, or external reproductive organs. These organs are often called the "external genitals" of the female.
- Additional glands, including the *mammary glands*, which secrete milk to provide nourishment for developing offspring.

Most of the essential and accessory organs of the female reproductive system can be seen in **Figures 46-1**, **46-2**, and **46-3**. Refer to these illustrations often as you read about each structure in the pages that follow.

PERINEUM

The perineum is the skin-covered muscular region between the vaginal orifice and the anus (see **Figure 46-2**). It is a roughly diamond-shaped area between the thighs. The perineum extends from the pubic symphysis anteriorly to the coccyx posteriorly. Its most lateral

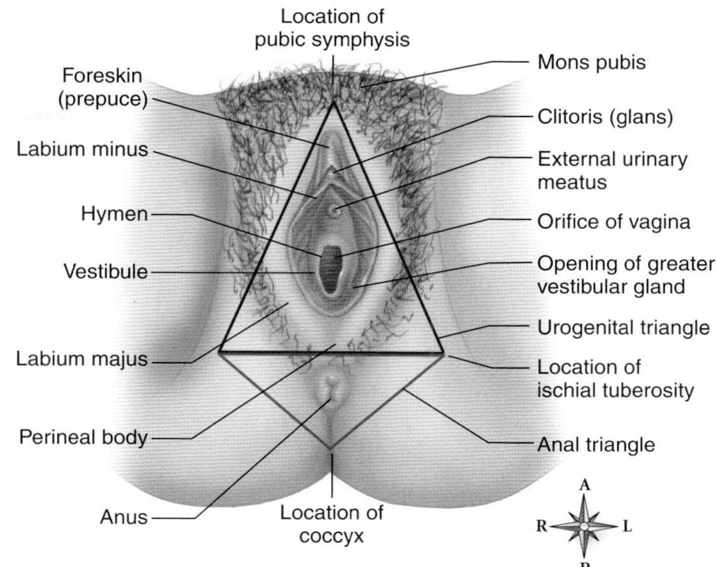

FIGURE 46-2 Female perineum. Inferior view. Sketch showing outline of the urogenital triangle *(red)* and anal triangle *(blue)*.

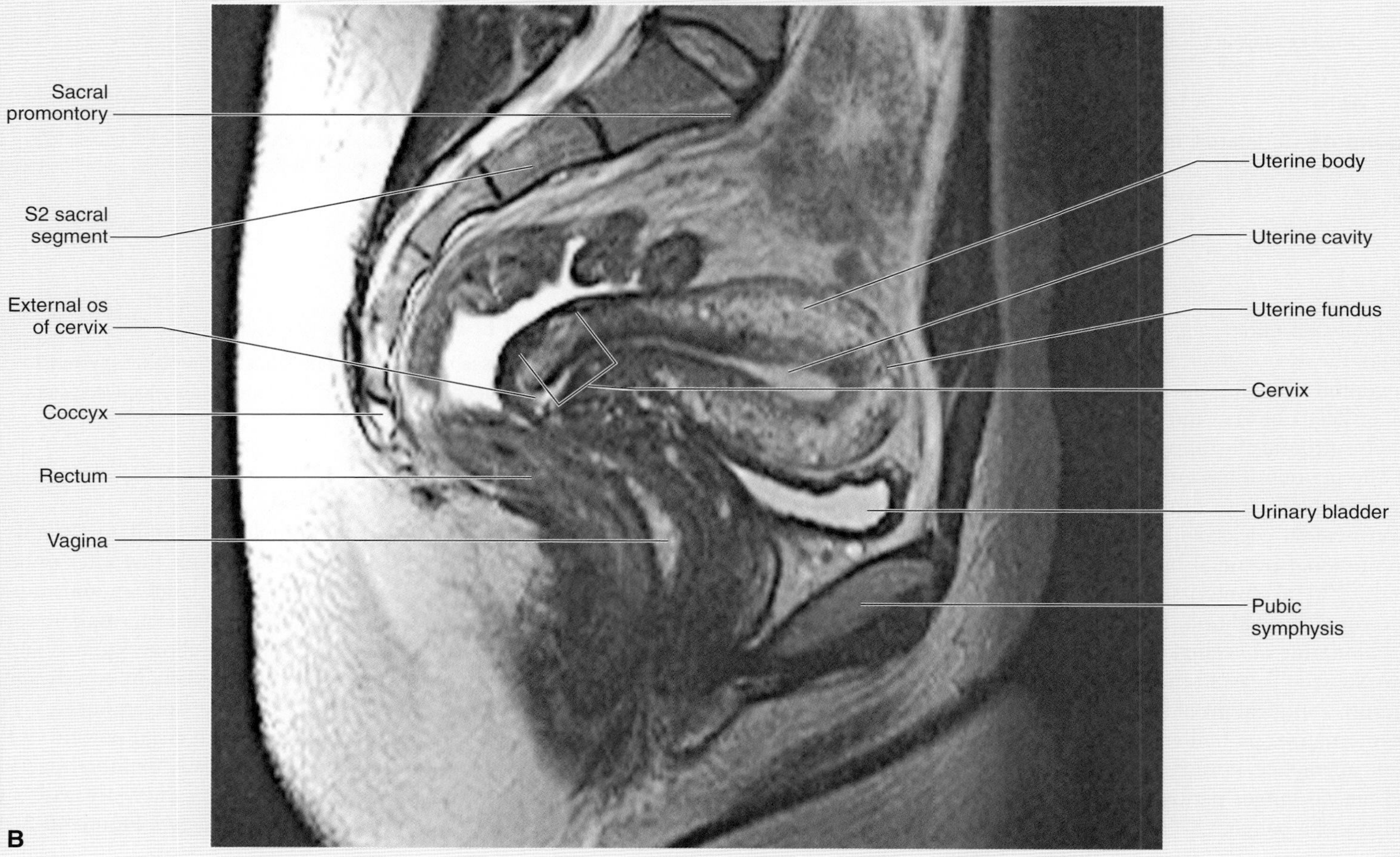

Sacral promontory
S2 sacral segment
External os of cervix
Coccyx
Rectum
Vagina
Uterine body
Uterine cavity
Uterine fundus
Cervix
Urinary bladder
Pubic symphysis
B

UNIT 6

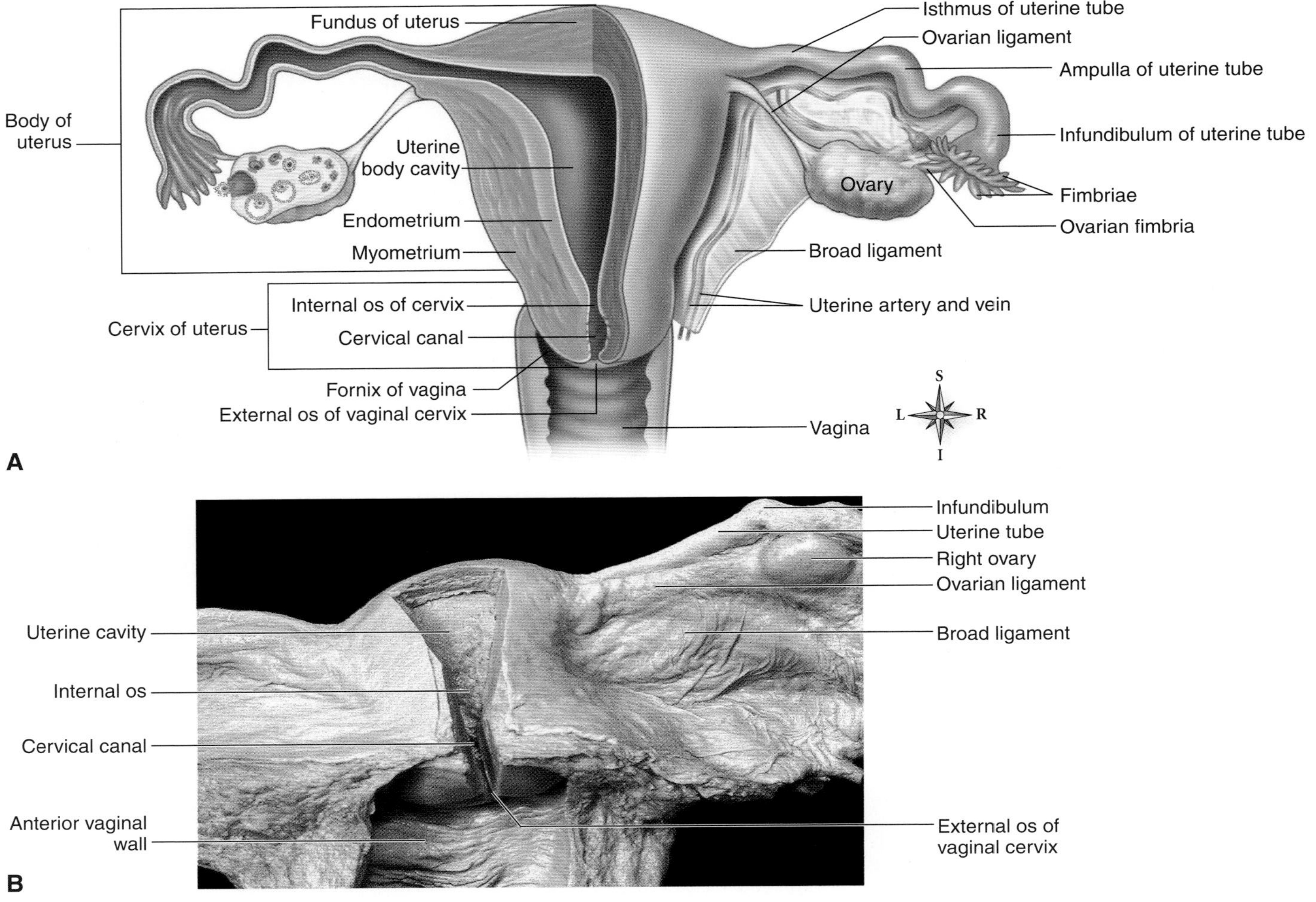

FIGURE 46-3 Internal female reproductive organs. Posterior view. **A,** Diagram shows left side of uterus and upper portion of the vagina and the left uterine tube and ovary in a coronal (frontal) section. The broad ligament has been removed from the posterior surface of the uterus and adjacent structures. **B,** Cadaver dissection showing uterine cavity and cervical canal, exposed by removal of parts of their posterior walls.

boundary on either side is the ischial tuberosity. A line drawn between the two ischial tuberosities divides the area into a larger **urogenital triangle,** which contains the external genitals (labia, vaginal orifice, clitoris) and urinary opening, and the **anal triangle,** which surrounds the anus.

The perineum has great clinical importance because of the danger of its being torn during childbirth. Such tears are often deep, have irregular edges, and extend all the way through the perineum, the muscular **perineal body,** and even through the anal sphincter, resulting in involuntary seepage from the rectum until the laceration is repaired. In addition, injuries to the perineal body can result in partial uterine or vaginal prolapse if this important support structure is weakened. To avoid these possibilities in a woman prone to such injuries, a surgical incision known as an **episiotomy** may be made in the perineum, particularly at the birth of a first baby. In current medical practice, episiotomy procedures are decreasing in frequency and are no longer performed on a routine basis preceding vaginal delivery of a baby.

Quick CHECK

1. What are the *essential organs* of the female reproductive system?
2. List the *major accessory organs* of the female reproductive system.

OVARIES

Location of the Ovaries

The female gonads, or ovaries, are homologous (similar in origin) to the testes in the male. They are nodular glands that after puberty present a puckered, uneven surface, resemble large almonds in size and shape, and are located one on each side of the uterus, below and behind the uterine tubes. Each ovary weighs about 3 grams and is attached to the posterior surface of the broad ligament by a structure called the *mesovarium,* which contains blood vessels and nerves. The *ovarian ligament* anchors it to the uterus. The distal portion of the uterine tube curves about the ovary in such a way that the fingerlike fimbriae at the end of the uterine tube cup over the ovary, with only one fimbria actually being attached to the ovary (see **Figure 46-3**, A).

This loose configuration makes it possible for a pregnancy to begin in the pelvic cavity instead of in the uterus as is normal. Development of the fetus in a location other than the uterus is referred to as an **ectopic pregnancy** (from the Greek *ektopos,* "displaced"). In the cadaver dissection specimen of the internal female reproductive organs shown in **Figure 46-3**, *B*, removal of parts of the posterior wall of the body of the uterus and cervix exposes a triangular uterine cavity communicating by way of the internal os with the cervical canal.

Microscopic Structure of the Ovaries

The ovary, like a number of other organs in the body, consists of two major layers of tissue—an outer **cortex** and inner **medulla.** Covering the outer cortex is a surface layer of slightly raised squamous-shaped epithelial cells called the *germinal epithelium.* The term *germinal* is misleading because the epithelial cells of this layer do not give rise to ova. Deep to the surface layer of epithelial cells is a tough grey-white connective tissue layer called the *tunica albuginea* that covers the **ovarian cortex.**

Scattered throughout and embedded in the connective tissue matrix of the cortex are hundreds of thousands of microscopic structures called **ovarian follicles.** Ovarian follicles contain the immature female sex cells, or *oocytes,* and their surrounding cells. After puberty, the oocytes and the specialized cells that surround them are present in varying stages of development. The **ovarian medulla** contains supportive connective tissue cells, blood vessels, nerves, and lymphatics. You may find the micrograph in Figure 5-50 of the Brief Atlas of the Human Body helpful in visualizing the basic structure of the ovary.

Refer to **Figure 46-4**, and trace the development of a female sex cell from its most primitive state through ovulation. **Figure 46-5**

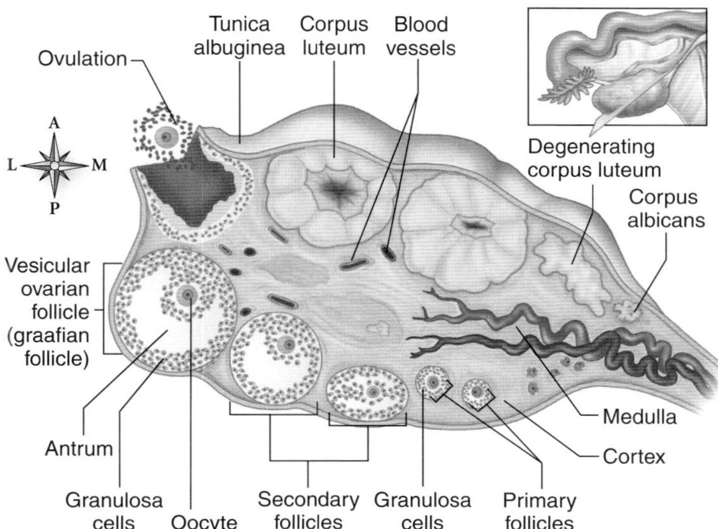

FIGURE 46-4 Stages of ovarian follicle development. Artist's rendition shows the successive stages of ovarian follicle and oocyte development. Begin with the first stage (primary follicle) and follow around clockwise to the final stage that is labelled *degenerating corpus luteum.* Remember, however, that all the stages shown occur over time to a *single* follicle, and the presence of all these stages at a single point in time is an artificial construct for learning purposes only.

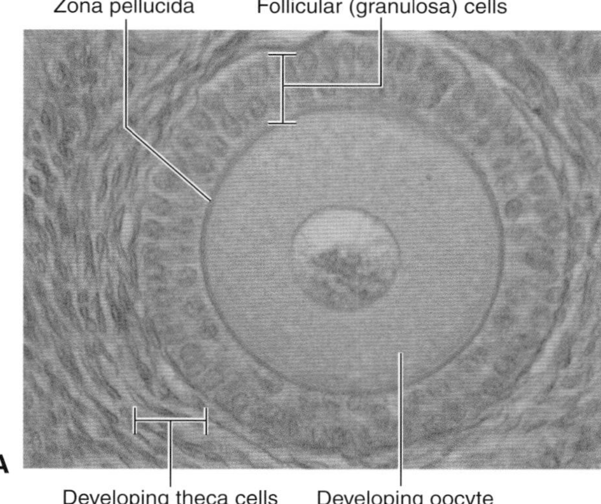

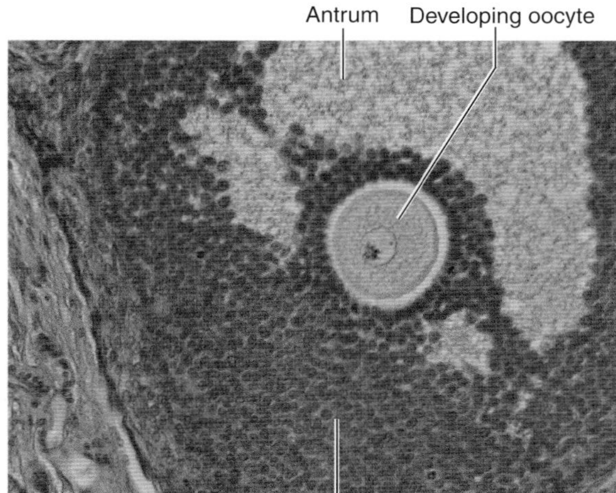

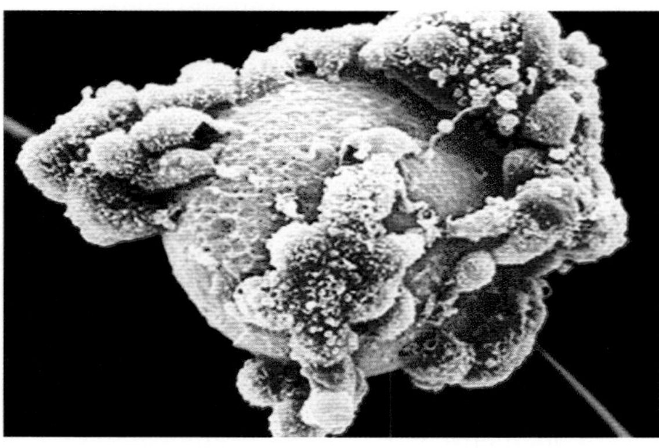

FIGURE 46-5 Developing ova. Female gametes mature within follicles in the outer region of an ovary. Follicles in early stages of development, **A,** and late stages of development, **B,** exhibit a developing oocyte (immature ovum) surrounded by hormone-secreting follicular (granulosa) cells. Notice that the more mature ovarian follicle in **B** has a fluid-filled cavity called the *antrum.* At ovulation, a mature ovum, **C,** is released. The fibres of the gel-like zona pellucida (ZP) can be seen coating the ovum, which also has many cumulus cells clinging to it. At ovulation, the ovum typically has a mass of about 20,000 cumulus cells that slowly slough away.

shows more detail of the structural differences that appear during follicle maturation. Throughout the process the oocyte grows in size. So, too, does the number of cell layers surrounding it.

Initially, the primary follicle is surrounded by a single layer of *granulosa cells*. As maturation proceeds, the number of granulosa cell layers increases and the cells begin secreting increasing amounts of an oestrogen-rich fluid that pools around the oocyte in a space called an *antrum*. The outer layer of granulosa cells in a developing follicle condenses into a layer of *theca cells* (**Figure 46-5**, A). The theca cell layer soon separates into an outer layer, or *theca externa*, which transforms into a fibrous capsule surrounding the follicle and a *theca interna* layer of cells, which secrete a precursor androgen hormone that granulosa cells ultimately convert into additional oestrogen.

As the primary follicle matures into a secondary, then eventually into a mature *vesicular ovarian follicle* or **graafian follicle,** a clump of granulosa cells called *cumulus cells* attaches the oocyte to the follicle wall where it is surrounded by fluid in the antrum. This mass of cells continues to cover the mature *ovum*, as it is called, after its release from the follicle. Cumulus cells secrete progesterone, which helps attract sperm cells toward the ovum and promotes sperm motility.

The developing oocyte also secretes the *zona pellucida (ZP)* (see **Figure 46-5**), a clear gel-like matrix that coats the ovum (underneath the cumulus cells).

The release of an ovum at the end of oogenesis is an event called **ovulation.** When ovulation occurs, blood haemorrhages from the highly vascular theca interna cell layer and fills the antrum. A small quantity of blood may also enter the peritoneal cavity and irritate its pain-sensitive surface, causing the transient lower abdominal pain many women experience at the time of ovulation (**Box 46-1**).

The blood clot filling the antrum, sometimes called the *corpus haemorrhagicum*, is soon replaced by proliferating granulosa and theca interna cells to form a yellow body called the **corpus luteum.** The corpus luteum secretes the hormones progesterone, inhibin, relaxin, and limited amounts of oestrogen. Progesterone and inhibin, a peptide hormone, suppress follicle-stimulating hormone secretion and prevent the continued development of new follicles during the functional life of the corpus luteum. The small amounts of relaxin secreted by the corpus luteum each month help "quiet" or "calm" uterine contractions, thus improving the chances for successful implantation if fertilization should occur. If pregnancy does occur, larger amounts of these hormones continue to be produced by the placenta.

Functions of the Ovaries

Recall that the ovaries are considered to be the essential organs of the female reproductive system. This means that it is the ovaries that produce female gametes, or ova. The process that culminates in the release of an ovum is called *oogenesis*, a term that literally means "egg production". As **Figure 46-4** shows, ovulation involves the rupture of an ovarian follicle and the subsequent release of fluid and an ovum. The ovum, surrounded by a coat of follicular cells, moves into the uterine tube, where it may draw a sperm cell into it and thus become the first cell of an offspring.

The ovaries are also endocrine organs, secreting the female sex hormones. **Oestrogens** (chiefly oestradiol and oestrone) and **progesterone** are secreted by cells of ovarian tissues. These hormones help regulate reproductive function in the female—making the ovaries even more essential to female reproductive function.

More details of oogenesis and fertilization are discussed in Chapter 47. Further discussion of hormonal regulation of reproductive functions, as well as associated changes within the ovaries, appears later in this chapter.

> **BOX 46-1** *fyi* | **Mittelschmerz**
>
> A few women experience pain within a few hours after ovulation. This is referred to as **mittelschmerz**—German for "middle pain" and generally occurs during days 14 to 16 in a 28-day cycle. It has been ascribed to irritation of the peritoneum by haemorrhage from the ruptured follicle. •

Quick CHECK

3. Briefly describe the location of the ovaries.
4. What are ovarian follicles?
5. List the two major functions of the ovaries.

UTERUS

Structure of the Uterus

Size and Shape of the Uterus

In a woman who has never been pregnant, the **uterus** is pear-shaped and measures approximately 7.5 cm in length, 5 cm in width at its widest part, and 3 cm in thickness. Note in **Figure 46-3** that the uterus has two main parts: a wide, upper portion, the **body**, and a lower, narrow "neck", the **cervix.** Did you notice that the body of the uterus rounds into a bulging prominence above the level at which the uterine tubes enter? This bulging upper component of the body is called the **fundus.**

Location of the Uterus

The uterus is located in the pelvic cavity between the urinary bladder in front and the rectum behind. Age, pregnancy, and distention of related pelvic viscera such as the bladder alter the position of the uterus (see **Figure 46-1**).

Between birth and puberty the uterus descends gradually from the lower abdomen into the true pelvis. At **menopause** the uterus begins a process of involution that results in a decrease in size and a position deep in the pelvis. Some variation among women in uterine placement within the pelvis is common.

Position of the Uterus

Normally the uterus is said to be *anteflexed*—or "bent forward"—between the body and cervix, with the body lying over the superior surface of the bladder, pointing forward and slightly upward (see **Figure 46-1**). The cervix points downward and backward from the point of flexion, joining the vagina at approximately a right angle (**Figure 46-6**).

Protrusion of the cervix into the lumen of the vagina creates corner spaces called the **anterior fornix** and **posterior fornix** (see **Figure 46-6**). These corners help increase the probability of reproductive success (fertilization) by retaining and pooling seminal fluid near the

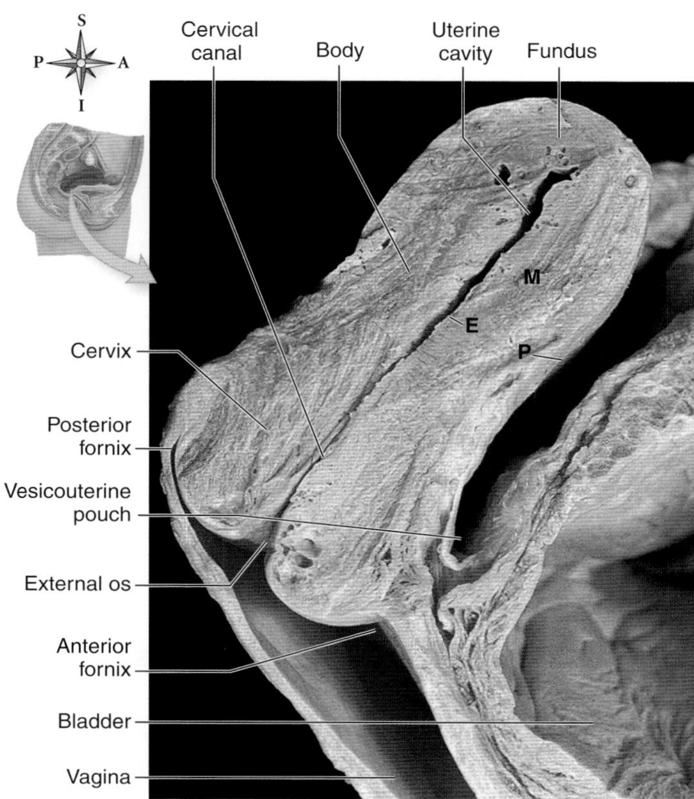

FIGURE 46-6 Uterus and vagina in sagittal section. Note that (1) the body of the uterus is "anteflexed" over the superior surface of the bladder pointing forward and slightly upward, and (2) the cervix protrudes into the vagina at approximately a right angle. *E,* Endometrium; *M,* myometrium; *P,* perimetrium.

external os for a brief period after intercourse—especially if the female remains in a supine position with knees flexed. This in turn helps increase the numbers of spermatozoa that enter the uterus and, ultimately, the uterine tubes where fertilization occurs.

Several ligaments hold the uterus in place but allow its body considerable movement, a characteristic that often leads to malpositions of the organ. Fibres from several muscles that form the pelvic floor (see **Figure 15-16**, p. 333) converge to form a node called the **perineal body** (see **Figure 46-2**), which also serves an important role in support of the uterus.

The uterus may lie in any one of several abnormal positions. A common one is *retroflexion*, or backward tilting, of the entire organ. Retroflexion may allow the uterus to prolapse, or descend, into the vaginal canal.

Eight *uterine ligaments* (three pairs, two single ones) hold the uterus in its normal position by anchoring it in the pelvic cavity. These ligaments include the broad (paired), uterosacral (paired), posterior (single), anterior (single), and round (paired) ligaments. Six of these so-called ligaments are actually extensions of the parietal peritoneum in different directions. The round ligaments are fibromuscular cords. Many of the structures listed on the next page can be identified in **Figures 46-1** and **46-3**.

- The *two* **broad ligaments** are double folds of parietal peritoneum that form a kind of partition across the pelvic cavity. The uterus is suspended between these two folds.
- The *two* **uterosacral ligaments** are foldlike extensions of the peritoneum from the posterior surface of the uterus to the sacrum, one on each side of the rectum.
- The **posterior ligament** is a fold of peritoneum extending from the posterior surface of the uterus to the rectum. This ligament forms a deep pouch posteriorly known as the **rectouterine pouch (of Douglas)**, between the uterus and rectum. Because this is the lowest point in the pelvic cavity, pus collects here when pelvic inflammations develop. To secure drainage, an incision may be made at the top of the posterior wall of the vagina. The procedure is called a *posterior colpotomy*.
- The **anterior ligament** is the fold of peritoneum formed by the extension of the peritoneum on the anterior surface of the uterus to the posterior surface of the bladder. This fold is located anteriorly and forms the **vesicouterine pouch,** which is less deep than the rectouterine pouch (see **Figures 46-1** and **46-6**).
- The *two* **round ligaments** are fibromuscular cords extending from the upper, outer angles of the uterus through the inguinal canals and terminating in the labia majora.

Wall of the Uterus

Three layers compose the walls of the uterus: the inner endometrium, a middle myometrium, and an outer incomplete layer of visceral peritoneum called the perimetrium.

Endometrium

The lining of mucous membrane, called the **endometrium,** is composed of three layers of tissues:

- *Compact layer*—a compact surface layer of partially ciliated, simple columnar epithelium
- *Spongy layer*—a spongy middle, or intermediate, layer of loose fibrous connective tissue; also called *functional layer*
- *Basal layer*—a dense inner layer that attaches the endometrium to the underlying myometrium.

During menstruation and after delivery of a baby, the compact and spongy layers slough off. The endometrium varies in thickness from 0.5 mm just after the menstrual flow to about 5 mm near the end of the endometrial cycle.

The endometrium has a rich supply of blood capillaries, as well as numerous exocrine *uterine glands* that secrete mucus and other substances onto the endometrial surface. The mucous glands in the lining of the cervix produce mucus that changes in consistency during the female reproductive cycle. Most of the time, cervical mucus acts as a barrier to sperm. Around the time of ovulation, however, cervical mucus becomes more slippery and actually facilitates the movement of sperm through the cervix and into the body of the uterus.

Myometrium

The **myometrium** is the thick, middle layer of the uterine wall. It consists of three layers of smooth muscle fibres that extend in all directions, longitudinally, transversely, and obliquely, and give the uterus great strength. The bundles of smooth muscle fibres interlace with elastic and connective tissue components and generally blend into the endometrial lining with no sharp line of demarcation between the two layers. The myometrium is thickest in the fundus and thinnest in the cervix—a good example of the principle of structural adaptation to function. To expel a fetus—that is, move it down and out of the uterus—the fundus must contract more forcibly than the lower part of the uterine wall and the cervix must be stretched or dilated.

Perimetrium

The **perimetrium** is an external layer of serous membrane that forms part of the visceral peritoneum. This serous covering of the uterus is incomplete because it covers none of the cervix and only part of the body (all except the lower one quarter of its anterior surface). The fact that the entire uterus is not covered with peritoneum has clinical significance because it makes it possible to perform operations on this organ without the same risk of infection that occurs in procedures that cut through the peritoneum.

Cavities of the Uterus

The cavities of the uterus are small because of the thickness of its walls (see **Figure 46-3**). The cavity of the body is flat and triangular. Its apex is directed downward and constitutes the **internal os,** which opens into the **cervical canal.** The cervical canal is constricted on its lower end also, forming the **external os,** which opens into the vagina. The uterine tubes open into the cavity of the uterine body at its upper, outer angles.

Blood Supply of the Uterus

The uterus receives a generous supply of blood from uterine arteries, branches of the internal iliac arteries (see **Figure 46-3**). In addition, blood from the ovarian and vaginal arteries reaches the uterus by anastomosis with the uterine vessels. Tortuous arterial vessels enter the layers of the uterine wall as arterioles and then break up into capillaries between the endometrial glands.

Uterine, ovarian, and vaginal veins return venous blood from the uterus to the internal iliac veins.

Functions of the Uterus

The uterus, or womb, has many functions important to successful reproductive function. The uterus serves as part of the female reproductive tract, permitting sperm from the male to ascend toward the uterine tubes. If fusion of gametes (*fertilization,* or *conception*) occurs, the developing offspring implants in the endometrial lining of the uterus and continues its development during the term of pregnancy *(gestation)*.

The tiny endometrial glands produce nutrient secretions—sometimes called "uterine milk"—to sustain the developing offspring until a *placenta* can be produced. The placenta is a unique organ that permits the exchange of materials between the offspring's blood and the maternal blood. The rich network of endometrial capillaries promotes efficiency of this exchange function.

Rhythmic contractions of the myometrium are inhibited during gestation but are allowed to occur as the time of delivery approaches. Myometrial contractions are the "labour contractions" that help push the offspring out of the mother's body.

If conception or the implantation of the offspring does not occur successfully, the outer layers of the endometrium are shed during *menstruation.* **Menstruation** is a regular event of the female reproductive cycle that permits the endometrium to renew itself in anticipation of conception and implantation during the next cycle. The myometrial contractions seem to aid menstruation by promoting the complete sloughing of the outer endometrial layers. Fatigue of the myometrial muscle tissues may contribute to the abdominal cramping sometimes associated with menstruation.

UTERINE TUBES

The uterine tubes are also sometimes called *fallopian tubes* (after Gabriele Fallopio, Italian anatomist b.1523), or *oviducts.*

Location of the Uterine Tubes

The uterine tubes are about 10 cm long and are attached to the uterus at its upper outer angles (see **Figures 46-1** and **46-3**). They lie in the upper free margin of the broad ligaments and extend upward and outward toward the sides of the pelvis and then curve downward and backward.

Structure of the Uterine Tubes

Wall of the Uterine Tubes

The same three layers (mucous, smooth muscle, and serous) of the uterus compose the tubes (**Figure 46-7**). The mucosal lining of the tubes, however, is directly continuous with the peritoneum lining the pelvic cavity. This has great clinical significance because the tubal mucosa is also continuous with that of the uterus and vagina and therefore often becomes infected by gonococci or other organisms introduced into the vagina.

Inflammation of the tubes **(salpingitis)** may readily spread to become inflammation of the peritoneum **(peritonitis),** a serious condition. Inflammation of the uterine tubes may also lead to scarring and partial or complete closure of the lumen, even if the original infection is cured with antibiotics (see Mechanisms of Disease, p. 1081).

In the male, there is no such direct route by which microorganisms can reach the peritoneum from the exterior.

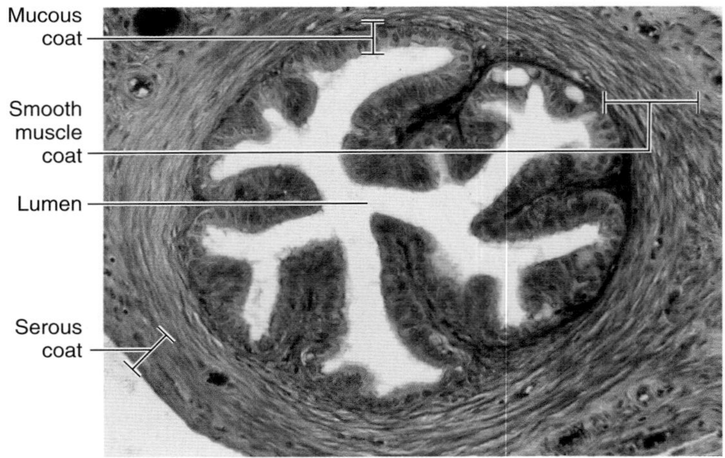

FIGURE 46-7 Transverse section of uterine tube. This micrograph shows a section of the uterine (fallopian) tube in the isthmus region. Notice the highly folded nature of the epithelial, mucous lining of the tube. The folding is even more exaggerated in the ampulla region (see **Figure 46-3** on p. 1060).

Divisions of the Uterine Tubes

Each uterine tube consists of three divisions (see **Figure 46-3**):

1. A medial third that extends from the upper outer angle of the uterus called the **isthmus.**
2. An intermediate dilated portion called the **ampulla** that follows a winding path over the ovary.
3. A funnel-shaped terminal part called the **infundibulum** that lies just above and extends laterally over the ovary and opens directly into the peritoneal cavity. The open outer margin of the infundibulum resembles a fringe in its irregular outline. The fringelike projections are known as **fimbriae** (see **Figure 46-3**). The *ovarian fimbria* is the only one of the fimbriae of each uterine tube that actually attaches directly to the ovary, helping anchor the distal end of the tube in place.

Histology of the Uterine Tubes

Figure 46-7 is a low-power micrograph that illustrates the mucosal lining of the uterine tube cut in cross section. These shapes are typical of the appearance of the mucosal lining throughout most of the duct. Note the extensive folds of mucosa that project as shelves into the lumen of the tube. An area of smooth muscle (muscularis layer) can be seen surrounding the mucosa in this section. Cilia, which are important in maintaining currents within the tube that move the ovum toward the uterus, can be seen projecting from the luminal surface in **Figure 46-8**.

Function of the Uterine Tubes

The uterine tubes are extensions of the uterus that communicate loosely with the ovaries. This arrangement allows an ovum released from the surface of the ovary to be collected by the fimbriae and swept along the uterine tube toward the body of the uterus by ciliary action.

The uterine tubes serve as more than mere transport channels, however. The uterine tube is also the site of fertilization. Sperm and ova most often meet, and fertilization occurs, in the ampulla of the uterine tube. A relatively small number of the sperm deposited in the vagina during sexual intercourse move up the uterine tube, where they meet the ovum travelling toward them. It is generally there, within the ampulla of the uterine tube, that the primary function of human sexual reproduction occurs: recombination of the genetic information from both parents in the first cell of the offspring.

Totally blocking the openings into either the distal (abdominal) or proximal (uterine) ends of both uterine tubes, for any reason, results in sterility (**Box 46-2**).

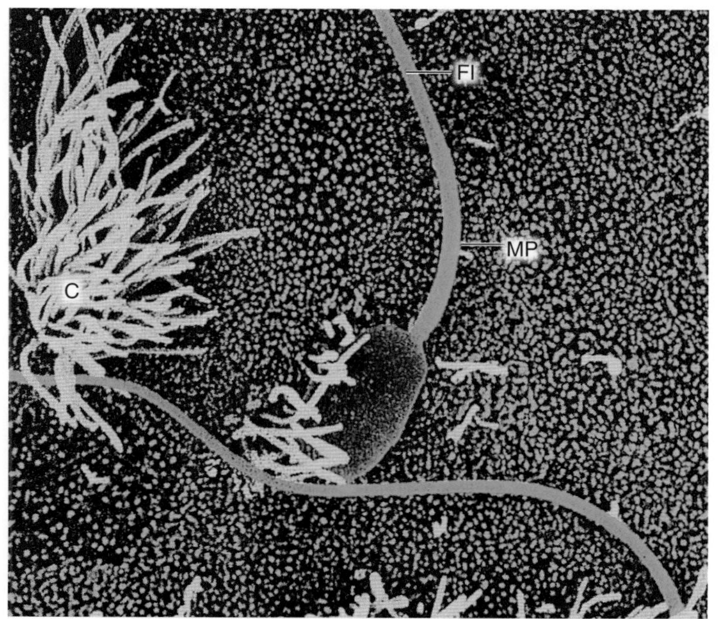

FIGURE 46-8 Luminal surface of the uterine tube. This scanning electron micrograph shows the surface of the uterine tube wall that faces the lumen, as well as some spermatozoa that are present (*Fl*, flagellum; *MP*, midpiece). The smaller, raised projections are microvilli, and the larger projections, found in clumps, are cilia *(C)*.

BOX 46-2 *fyi* | Tubal Ligation

Tubal ligation literally means "tying a tube", and thus this surgical procedure is often referred to as "having one's tubes tied". Tubal ligation involves tying a piece of suture material around each uterine tube in two places, then cutting each tube between these two points (see the figure). Other methods using clips or bands instead of cutting and tying the tubes are also used. Because sperm and eggs are thus blocked from meeting, fertilization and subsequent pregnancy are prevented. For this reason, tubal ligation is also called *surgical sterilization* and is functionally comparable to vasectomy in the male. However, vasectomy can be done under local anaesthetic in a medical office and therefore is a minor procedure when compared with tubal ligation.

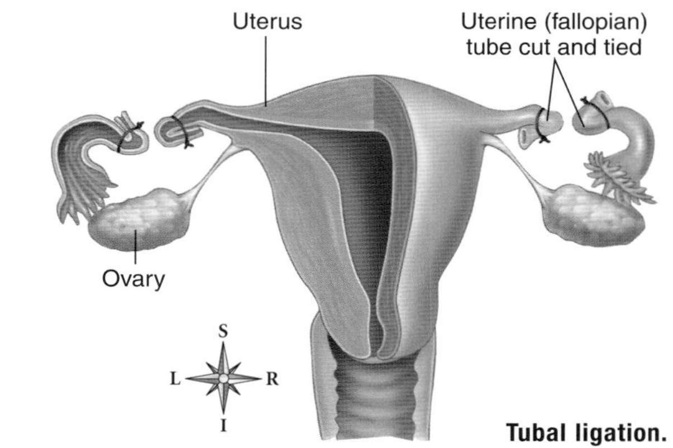

Tubal ligation.

Quick CHECK

6. Name the three principal layers of the uterine wall.
7. Describe the anatomical position of the uterus. How is it held in place?
8. List the chief functions of the uterus.
9. What are the functions of the uterine (fallopian) tubes?

Vagina

Location of the Vagina

The vagina is a tubular organ situated between the rectum, which lies posterior to it, and the urethra and bladder, which lie anterior to it (see **Figure 46-6** and **Figure 42-8** on p. 971). It extends upward and backward from its external orifice in the vestibule between the labia minora of the vulva to the cervix (see **Figures 46-1**, **46-2**, and **46-3**).

The right and left *levator ani* muscles (**Figure 15-16**, p. 333, and **Figure 42-8**, p. 971) unite at the midline to form a hammock-shaped muscular sheet often referred to as the "floor of the pelvis". In the female, the anatomical relationships between the various parts of this supportive muscular sheet and the perineal body, vagina, rectum, and urethra have clinical significance. Fibres of the levator ani insert into and become a part of all these structures.

It is not an uncommon occurrence for at least some fibres of the levator ani to become stretched or damaged in women who have experienced vaginal delivery of a full-term infant. The unfortunate result is often the appearance of a number of troublesome and often chronic symptoms. For example, damage to muscle fibres of the levator ani that constitute a part of the urethral or anal sphincters may result in urinary or faecal *incontinence*. If leakage of urine or faecal material after damage to the sphincter is associated with—or precipitated by—an increase in abdominal pressure caused by events such as coughing, laughing, or lifting weight, the condition is called *stress incontinence*.

When muscle fibres in the vagina or perineal body are significantly weakened, the vaginal walls will lose tone and the important role of the perineal body in providing support of pelvic viscera will be affected. The result may involve prolapse of the uterus into the vagina or some degree of rectal prolapse through the anus.

In severe cases of prolapse, surgery or other treatments may be required to raise or support the pelvic floor or to repair structural damage. However, in less severe cases where symptoms are limited to occasional leakage of urine, many women benefit from a noninvasive treatment option called *Kegel exercise*. Designed primarily to reduce urinary stress incontinence, Kegel exercises consist of an ongoing exercise program that involves a repetitive series of voluntary contractions of the muscles of the pelvic floor and perineum, similar to that required to stop the flow of urine when voiding. In time, the exercise program will strengthen the external urethral sphincter and improve retention of urine.

Structure of the Vagina

The vagina is a collapsible tube about 7 or 8 cm long that is capable of great distention. It is composed mainly of smooth muscle and is lined with mucous membrane arranged in rugae. The vaginal mucosa contains numerous tiny exocrine mucous glands that secrete lubricating fluid during the female sexual response. **Box 46-3** discusses the "G spot" on the anterior wall of the vagina.

Note that the anterior wall of the vagina is shorter than the posterior wall because of the way the cervix protrudes into the uppermost portion of the tube (see **Figures 46-1** and **46-6**). In some cases—especially in young girls—a fold of mucous membrane, the **hymen,** forms a border around the external opening of the vagina, partially closing the orifice. Occasionally, this structure completely covers the vaginal outlet, a condition referred to as **imperforate hymen.** Perforation must be performed at puberty before the menstrual flow can escape.

Functions of the Vagina

The **vagina** is a portion of the female reproductive tract that has several important functions. During sexual intercourse, the lining of the vagina lubricates and stimulates the glans penis, which in turn triggers the ejaculation of semen. Thus the vagina also serves as a receptacle for semen, which often pools in the anterior or posterior fornix of the vagina where it meets the cervix of the uterus (see **Figure 46-6**). Sperm within the semen may move further into the female reproductive tract by "climbing" along fibrous strands of mucus in the cervical canal.

The vagina also serves as the lower portion of the birth canal. At the time of delivery, the offspring is pushed from the body of the uterus, through the cervical canal, and finally through the vagina and out of the mother's body. The placenta, or "afterbirth", is also expelled through the vagina.

Another important function of the vagina is transport of blood and tissue shed from the lining of the uterus during menstruation.

VULVA

Structure of the Vulva

Figure 46-9, A, shows the structures that, together, constitute the female external genitals (reproductive organs). Collectively, these structures are called the **vulva** or *pudendum*. They are described in the following paragraphs.

The **mons pubis** is a skin-covered pad of fat over the pubic symphysis. Coarse pubic hairs appear on this structure at puberty and persist throughout life.

BOX 46-3 *fyi* | The "G Spot"

In 1950, Dr. Ernest Gräfenberg described what he called an "erotic zone" about 20 mm in diameter on the anterior wall of the vagina midway between the pubic symphysis and cervix (see figure). The area was later named the "Gräfenberg spot", or "G spot". In fact, this was a rediscovery of the "prostatae" in female anatomy originally described by Dutch anatomist Regnier de Graaf in 1672.

The G spot is located at the site of the spongy lesser vestibular (Skene) glands and nearby erectile tissue between the wall of the vagina and the urethra. This set of structures is now often called the *female prostate.* Not all women seem to have the same amount of glandular tissue and not all are equally sensitive in this area of the vaginal wall, so the concept of a G spot continues to be controversial among scientists. •

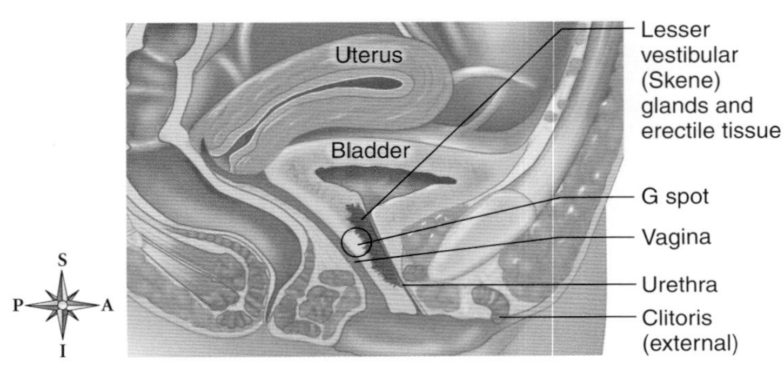

G spot (female prostate).

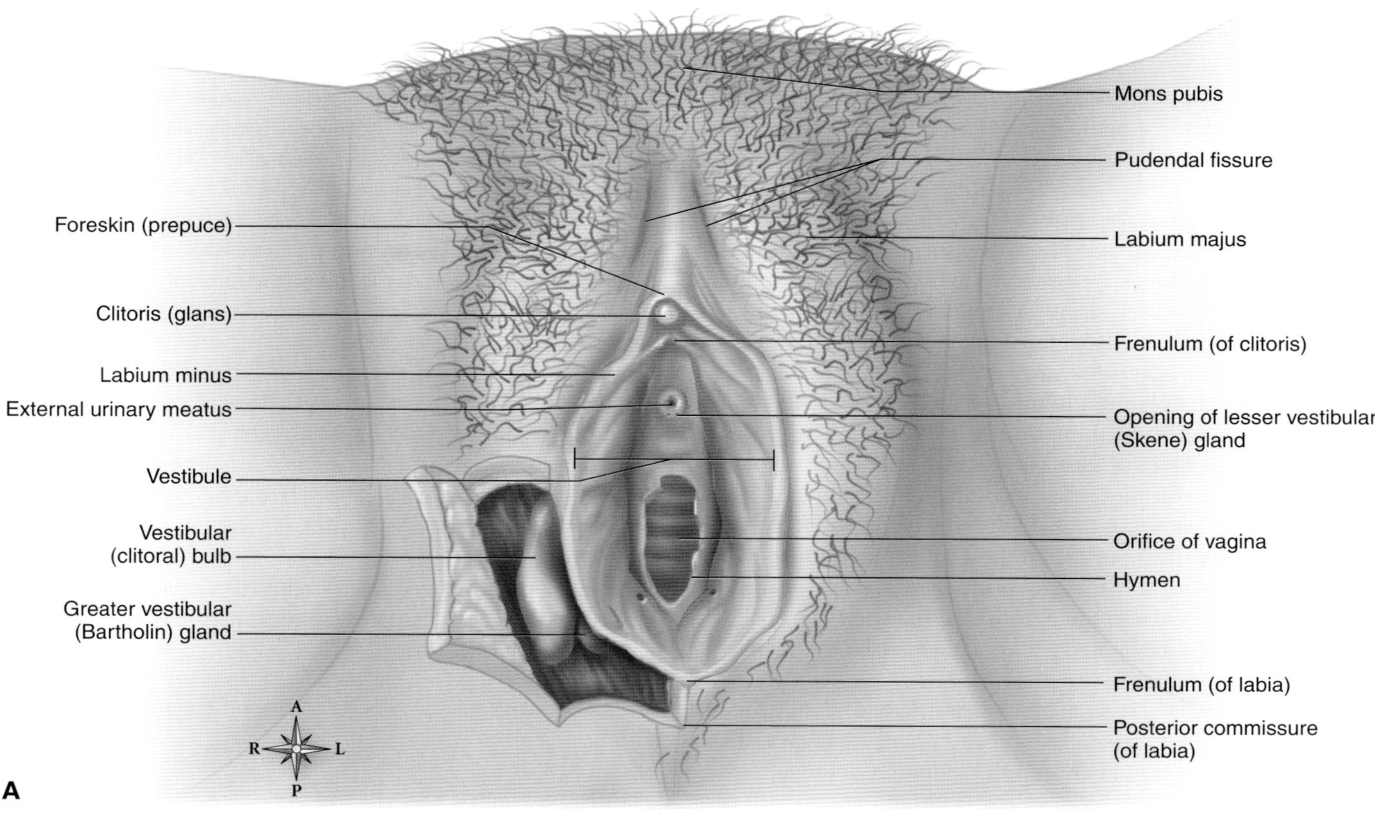

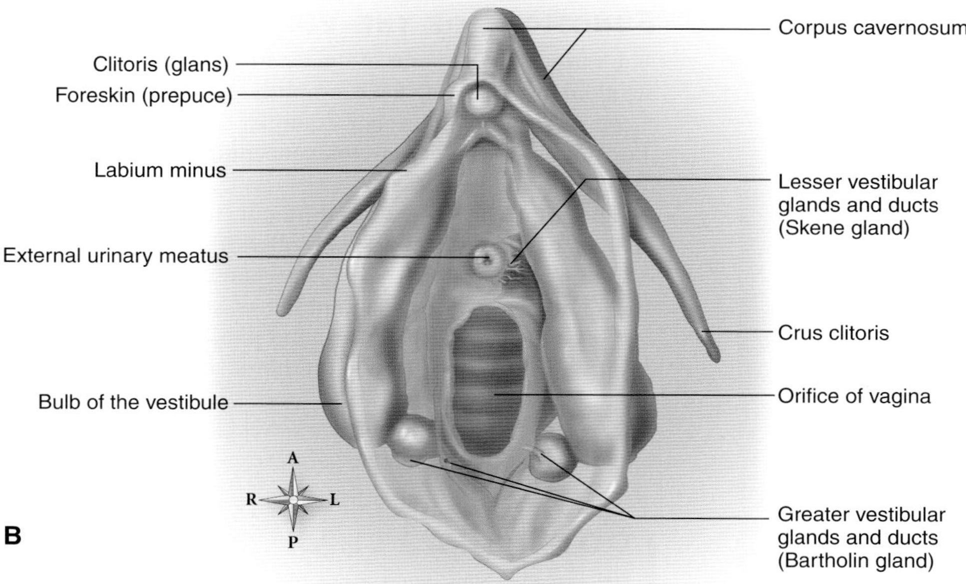

FIGURE 46-9 Vulva (pudendum). **A,** Sketch showing major features of the external female genitals (genitalia). Compare with **Figure 46-2** on p. 1059). **B,** Sketch showing the full structure of the clitoris, which in life is mostly hidden by overlying external tissue.

The **labia majora** (Latin, "large lips") are covered with pigmented skin and hair on the outer surface and are smooth and free from hair on the inner surface. Each labium majus is composed mainly of fat and connective tissue with numerous sweat and sebaceous glands on the inner surface. The labia majora are homologous to the scrotum in the male.

The **labia minora** (Latin, "small lips") are located medial to the labia majora. Each labium minus is covered with hairless skin. The two labia minora come together anteriorly in the midline. The area between the labia minora is the **vestibule.**

The **clitoris** is composed of erectile tissue, a portion of which is visible just behind the junction of the labia minora. The structure of this organ is homologous to penile structure in the male. Look again at **Figure 45-11** on p. 1046, and compare the erectile tissues of the penis in that illustration with the sketch of the clitoris shown in **Figure 46-9**, *B*. The micrograph of the clitoris in **Figure 46-10** shows a similar "spongy" structure seen in the erectile tissues of the penis. Like the erectile tissue of the male, the clitoris becomes engorged with blood during the sexual response.

The *glans clitoris* is the only visible part of the erectile structures of the clitoris. The glans clitoris is equivalent to the *glans penis* in the male. The glans clitoris is covered with highly sensitive skin involved in sexual stimulation that produces the female sexual response. In the female, the corpora cavernosa are separated into an inverted Y shape. Underneath each labium majus is a *bulb (of vestibule)* that corresponds to the male corpus spongiosum.

A clitoral *foreskin* or *prepuce* forms a hood over the superior surface of the glans clitoris. On the inferior surface of the glans clitoris there is a thin midline *frenulum* that is the female equivalent of the frenulum visible on the undersurface of the glans of the penis.

The *external urinary meatus* (urethral orifice) is the small opening of the urethra, situated between the clitoris and the vaginal orifice.

The **vaginal orifice** is an opening that is larger than the urinary meatus. It is located posterior to the meatus.

The **greater vestibular glands** are two bean-shaped glands, one on each side of the vaginal orifice. Each gland opens by means of a single, long duct into the space between the hymen and the labium minus. These glands, which are also called *Bartholin glands*, are of clinical importance because they can be infected (bartholinitis or Bartholin abscess), particularly by gonococci. They are homologous to the bulbourethral glands in the male.

Opening into the vestibule near the urinary meatus by way of two small ducts is a group of tiny mucous glands, the **lesser vestibular glands.** Also called *Skene glands*, they are of clinical interest because gonococci that lodge there are difficult to eradicate.

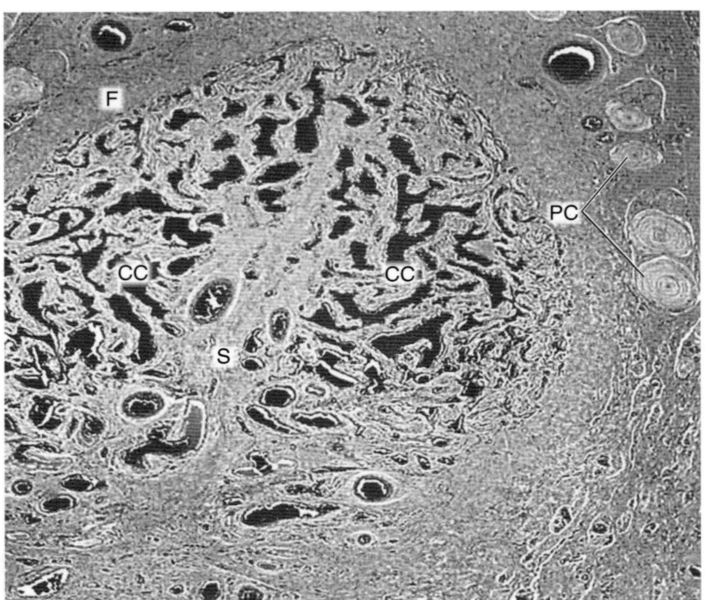

FIGURE 46-10 Micrograph of clitoris. Note the two corpora cavernosa *(CC)* separated by an incomplete central septum *(S)*. Sectioned lamellar (Pacini) corpuscles *(PC)* are visible just outside the surrounding fibrocollagenous sheath *(F)*. (Compare with **Figure 45-14**, *B*, on p. 1049.)

BOX 46-4 *fyi* | **Female Sexual Responses**

In the previous chapter, we briefly reviewed some physiological changes that occur during the male sexual response (**Box 45-2**, p. 1050). The sexual responses in females have many similarities, based on the developmental and structural similarities already mentioned. But there are many differences, as we have already discussed in the text.

For example, sexual stimuli trigger autonomic reflexes in both sexes. In males, the sexual response enables successful penetration of the female vagina during coitus and ejaculation of sperm. In females, some responses also facilitate successful penetration by producing lubricating fluids and gently squeezing the penis to maintain stimulation of both partners. The mechanisms that produce *erection* of the penis also produce engorgement of the clitoris—and in both sexes, the sensitivity of the *glans* helps sustain sexual reflex responses.

As in males, sexual climax or *orgasm* may occur that is accompanied by accelerated heart rate, increased blood pressure, hyperventilation, dilated skin vessels, and intense sexual excitement. Internally, muscular contractions that in the male ejaculate semen instead facilitate movement of sperm into and through the uterus. As in males, *oxytocin (OT)* released by neuroendocrine tissue in the posterior pituitary during the sexual response may enhance muscular contractions that accompany orgasm. •

Functions of the Vulva

The various components of the external genitals of the female operate alone or separately to accomplish several functions important to successful reproduction. For example, the protective features of the mons pubis and labia help prevent injury to the delicate tissues of the clitoris and vestibule.

The clitoris becomes erect during sexual stimulation and, like the male glans, possesses a large number of sensory receptors that feed back information to the sexual response areas of the brain (**Box 46-4**). In **Figure 46-10**, a number of sectioned lamellar (Pacini) corpuscles, encapsulated touch and pressure receptors (see Chapter 23), can be seen just outside the fibrocollagenous sheath surrounding the clitoris.

Of course, the vaginal orifice serves as the boundary between the internal and external female genitals.

CONNECT IT! 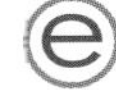

Maintaining healthy communities of microorganisms in the mucosa of the urinary and reproductive tracts helps prevent infections and other disorders. For example, even small changes in the environment of the vulva or vagina can allow for yeasts already present to bloom into an infection. Review the human microbiome in ***The Human Microbiome*** at ***Connect It!***

Quick CHECK

10. List three functions of the vagina.
11. What is another name for the external genitals of the female?
12. How are the clitoris of the female and the glans penis of the male similar in structure and function?

FEMALE REPRODUCTIVE CYCLES

RECURRING CYCLES

Many changes recur periodically in the female during the years between the onset of the menses (**menarche**) and their cessation (**menopause,** or **climacteric**). Most obvious, of course, is menstruation—the outward sign of changes in the endometrium. Most women also note periodic changes in their breasts. But these are only two of many changes that occur over and over again at fairly uniform intervals during the approximately three decades of female reproductive maturity.

First we shall describe the major cyclical changes, and then we shall discuss the mechanisms that produce them.

Ovarian Cycle

Before a female child is born, precursor cells in her ovarian tissue, called **oogonia,** begin a type of cell division characterized as *meiosis.* Meiotic cell division differs from mitotic cell division in that it reduces the number of chromosomes in the daughter cells by half (recall Chapter 7, p. 129). By the time the child is born, her ovaries contain many primary follicles, each containing an oocyte that has temporarily suspended the meiotic process before it is complete.

On a daily basis after puberty, about 20 or so oocytes within several primary follicles resume meiosis. At the same time, the follicular cells surrounding them proliferate and start to secrete oestrogens (and tiny amounts of progesterone). Over the course of almost a year, these ovarian follicles develop and mature. As development proceeds, most of the follicles undergo degeneration—or **atresia**—and disappear. Usually, only one of the developing follicles eventually matures and migrates to the surface of the ovary during any one ovarian cycle.

Just before ovulation, the meiosis within the oocyte of the mature follicle halts again. It is this cell, which has not quite completed meiosis, that is expelled from the ruptured wall of the mature follicle during ovulation. Meiosis is completed only when, and if, the head of a sperm cell is later drawn into the ovum during the process of fertilization.

When does ovulation occur? This is a question of great practical importance and one that in the past was given many answers. Today it is known that ovulation usually occurs 14 days before the next menstrual period begins. (Only in a 28-day menstrual cycle is this also 14 days after the beginning of the preceding menstrual cycle, as explained later.)

Immediately after ovulation, cells of the ruptured follicle enlarge and, because of the appearance of lipoid substances in them, become transformed into a golden-coloured body, the corpus luteum. The corpus luteum grows for 7 or 8 days. During this time, it secretes progesterone in increasing amounts. Then, provided fertilization of the ovum has not taken place, the size of the corpus luteum and the amount of its secretions gradually diminish. In time, the last components of each nonfunctional corpus luteum are reduced to a white scar called the **corpus albicans,** which moves into the central portion of the ovary and eventually disappears (see **Figure 46-4**).

Endometrial (Menstrual) Cycle

During menstruation, bits of the compact and spongy layers of the endometrium slough off, leaving denuded bleeding areas. The dark menstrual discharge generally does not clot and may vary from about 30 to 100 mL, with a majority lost during the first 3 days of the menses. As with the length of the cycle, considerable variation is considered normal.

After menstruation, the cells of these layers proliferate, causing the endometrium to reach a thickness of 2 or 3 mm by the time of ovulation. During this period, endometrial glands and arterioles grow longer and more coiled—two factors that also contribute to the thickening of the endometrium.

After ovulation, the endometrium grows still thicker, reaching a maximum of about 4 to 6 mm. Most of this increase, however, is believed to be caused by swelling produced by fluid retention rather than by further proliferation of endometrial cells. The increasingly coiled endometrial glands start to secrete their nutrient fluid during the time between ovulation and the next menses.

Then, the day before menstruation starts again, a drop in progesterone causes muscle in the walls of the tightly coiled arterioles to constrict, producing endometrial ischaemia. This leads to death of the tissue, sloughing, and once again, menstrual bleeding.

The menstrual cycle is customarily divided into phases, named for major events occurring in each: menses, postmenstrual phase, ovulation, and premenstrual phase.

Menses

The **menses,** or **menstrual period,** occurs on days 1 to 5 of a new cycle. There is some individual variation, however.

Postmenstrual Phase

The **postmenstrual phase** occurs between the end of the menses and ovulation. Therefore it is the **preovulatory phase,** as well as the postmenstrual phase. In a 28-day cycle, it usually includes cycle days 6 to 13 or 14. However, the length of this phase varies more than the others. It lasts longer in long cycles and ends sooner in short cycles.

This phase is also called the **oestrogenic phase,** or **follicular phase,** because of the high blood oestrogen level resulting from secretion by the developing follicle. Increases in oestrogen levels cause predictable changes in the appearance, amount, and consistency of cervical mucus. Collectively, these changes can be used as a fertility sign to predict ovulation (**Box 46-5**).

Increasing oestrogen levels cause cervical mucus to become elastic, a property that can be observed by placing the mucus between and then separating two glass microscope slides. The clear, watery cervical mucus found at the time of ovulation will stretch 8 cm or more before the resulting thread will break. This stretchiness is called **spinnbarkeit.**

Furthermore, if left to dry on a clean glass slide, cervical mucus produced at or near the time of ovulation will dry in a characteristic featherlike or "fern" pattern (**Figure 46-11**).

Proliferative phase is yet another name for this phase because proliferation of endometrial cells occurs at this time.

Ovulation

Ovulation, that is, rupture of the mature follicle with expulsion of its ovum into the pelvic cavity (**Figure 46-12**), occurs most often on cycle day 14 in a 28-day cycle. However, it occurs on different days in different-length cycles, depending on the length of the preovulatory phase. For example, in a 32-day cycle the preovulatory phase

BOX 46-5 *fyi* | Fertility Signs Used in Predicting the Time of Ovulation

Many rhythmic and recurring events that a woman may recognize on almost a monthly schedule during her reproductive years are called *fertility signs* and are manifestations of the body changes required for successful reproductive function. They include cyclical changes in the ovaries, in the amount and consistency of the cervical mucus produced during each cycle, in the myometrium, in the vagina, in gonadotropin secretion, in body temperature, and even in mood or "emotional tone".

Accurately predicting the time of ovulation in any given menstrual cycle by recognizing one or more of these recurring fertility signs would obviously be of help in either avoiding or achieving conception. However, knowing the length of a previous cycle or even a series of cycles cannot ensure with any degree of accuracy the time of appearance of other fertility signs in a current cycle or how many days the preovulatory phase will last in the next or some future cycle.

Simply put, prior cycle length is not an accurate fertility sign. This fact accounts for most of the unreliability of the *calendar rhythm method* of fertility planning.

Other more sophisticated *natural family planning (NFP)* methods are available that are not based on a knowledge of previous cycle lengths to predict the day of ovulation. Instead, such natural methods base their judgments about fertility at any point in a woman's cycle on other changes; for example, measurement of basal body temperature and recognition of cyclical changes in the amount and consistency of cervical mucus, both of which occur in response to changes in circulating hormones that control ovulation. Typically, use of NFP for 1 year to avoid pregnancy will result in approximately 25 of every 100 women becoming pregnant.

The time of ovulation also can be approximated by over-the-counter urine tests that detect the high levels of luteinizing hormone (LH) associated with ovulation (LH surge). •

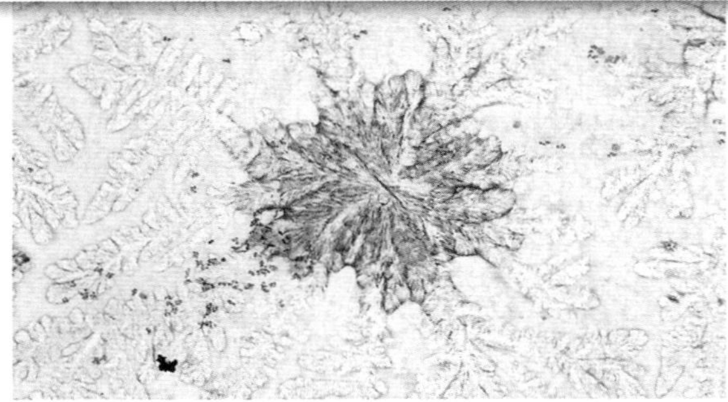

FIGURE 46-11 Ferning of cervical mucus. Stretchy cervical mucus near the time of ovulation is watery with dissolved sodium chloride that crystallizes into fernlike patterns when dried on a glass microscope slide.

probably lasts until cycle day 18, and ovulation would then occur on cycle day 19 instead of 14.

In short, because the majority of women show some month-to-month variation in the length of their cycles, the day of ovulation in a current or future cycle cannot be predicted with accuracy based on the length of previous cycles (see **Box 46-5**).

Typically, there is a decrease in basal body temperature just before ovulation and a rise in temperature at the time of ovulation. This constitutes yet another "fertility sign" (see **Figure 46-15**).

Premenstrual Phase

The **premenstrual phase,** or **postovulatory phase,** occurs between ovulation and the onset of the menses. This phase is also called the **luteal phase,** or more simply, the **secretory phase,** because the corpus luteum secretes only during this time. It is also called the **progesterone phase** because the corpus luteum secretes mainly this hormone.

The length of the premenstrual phase is fairly constant, lasting usually 14 days—or cycle days 15 to 28 in a 28-day cycle. Differences in length of the total menstrual cycle therefore exist mainly because of differences in duration of the postmenstrual rather than of the premenstrual phase.

Myometrial Cycle

The myometrium contracts mildly but with increasing frequency during the 2 weeks preceding ovulation. Contractions decrease or disappear between ovulation and the next menses, thereby lessening the probability of expulsion of a fertilized ovum that may have implanted in the endometrium.

Gonadotropic Cycle

The adenohypophysis (anterior pituitary gland) secretes two hormones called *gonadotropins* that influence female reproductive cycles. Their names are **follicle-stimulating hormone (FSH)** and **luteinizing hormone (LH).** The amount of each gonadotropin secreted varies with a rhythmic regularity that can be related, as we shall see, to the rhythmic ovarian and uterine changes just described.

Recall from Chapter 26 that pituitary secretion of gonadotropins is influenced by the pulsing release of *gonadotropin-releasing hormone (GnRH)* from the hypothalamus (see p. 584). If GnRH is

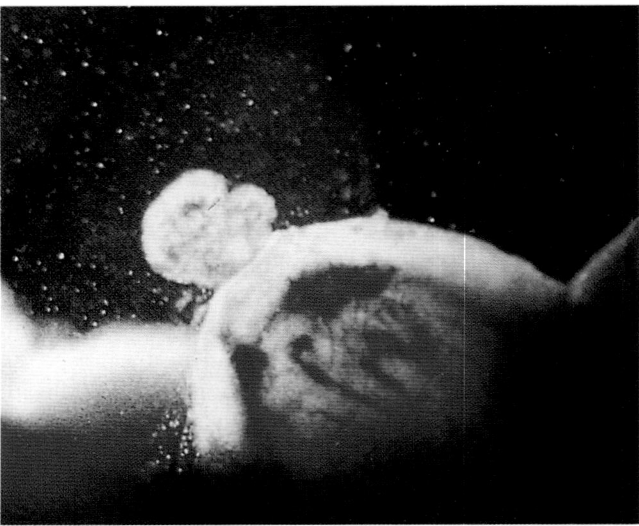

FIGURE 46-12 Ovulation. The rupture of a mature follicle on the surface of an ovary results in the release of an ovum into the pelvic cavity. This process of *ovulation* often occurs on day 14 in a 28-day menstrual cycle, but its exact timing depends on the length of the postmenstrual (preovulatory) phase. Notice in this photograph that the ovum released during ovulation is surrounded by a mass of cells.

released in pulses about once every 3 hours, FSH will be secreted. If the GnRH pulse rate increases to about once per hour, then instead LH will be secreted. In females, the pulse rate of GnRH varies throughout the reproductive cycle, thus promoting cyclic fluctuations in the release of FSH and LH.

Quick **CHECK**

13. What is the function of the corpus luteum?
14. How is the corpus luteum formed?
15. What is the difference between the ovarian cycle and the menstrual (endometrial) cycle?
16. Why is the postmenstrual phase of the menstrual cycle sometimes called the *proliferative phase?*

Control of Female Reproductive Cycles

Physiologists agree that hormones play a major role in producing the cyclical changes characteristic in women during the reproductive years. The development of a method called *radioimmunoassay* has made it possible to measure blood levels of gonadotropins. By correlating these with the monthly ovarian and uterine changes, investigators have worked out the main features of the control mechanism.

A brief description follows of the mechanisms that produce cyclical changes in the ovaries and uterus and in the amounts of gonadotropins secreted.

Control of Cyclical Changes in the Ovaries

Cyclical changes in the ovaries result from cyclical changes in the amounts of gonadotropins secreted by the anterior pituitary gland.

An increasing FSH blood level has several effects. FSH stimulates the development of primary ovarian follicles. FSH also stimulates the granulosa cells of the preovulatory follicles to begin secreting oestrogens. (Developing follicles also secrete very small amounts of progesterone.) FSH also has a permissive effect for LH, causing up-regulation of LH receptors on granulosa cells in the preovulatory follicles.

Because of the influence of FSH on follicular hormone secretion, the level of oestrogens in blood increases gradually for a few days during the postmenstrual phase. Then suddenly, on about the twelfth cycle day, it leaps upward to a maximum peak. Scarcely 12 hours after this "oestrogen surge", an "LH surge" occurs and presumably triggers ovulation a day or two later. This hormone surge is the basis of the over-the-counter "ovulation test" (see **Box 46-5**, p. 1070).

The control of cyclical ovarian changes by the gonadotropins FSH and LH is summarized in **Figure 46-13**. As **Figure 46-13** shows, LH brings about the following changes:

1. Completion of growth of preovulatory follicles and oocyte maturation. Granulosa cells in these follicles, which had begun secreting oestrogen under the influence of FSH, continue oestrogen secretion under the influence of LH (after up-regulation of LH receptors by FSH).
2. Sets in motion processes that break down connective tissue of the ovarian cortex and the wall of the follicle, rupturing the mature follicle and expelling its ovum (ovulation). Because of this function, LH is sometimes also called "the ovulating hormone".
3. Formation of a golden body, the corpus luteum, in the ruptured follicle (a process called **luteinization**). The name *luteinizing hormone* refers, obviously, to this LH function—a function to which, experiments have shown, FSH also contributes.

The corpus luteum functions as a temporary endocrine gland. It secretes only during the luteal (postovulatory, or premenstrual) phase of the menstrual cycle. Its hormones are progestins (the important one of which is progesterone) and also oestrogens.

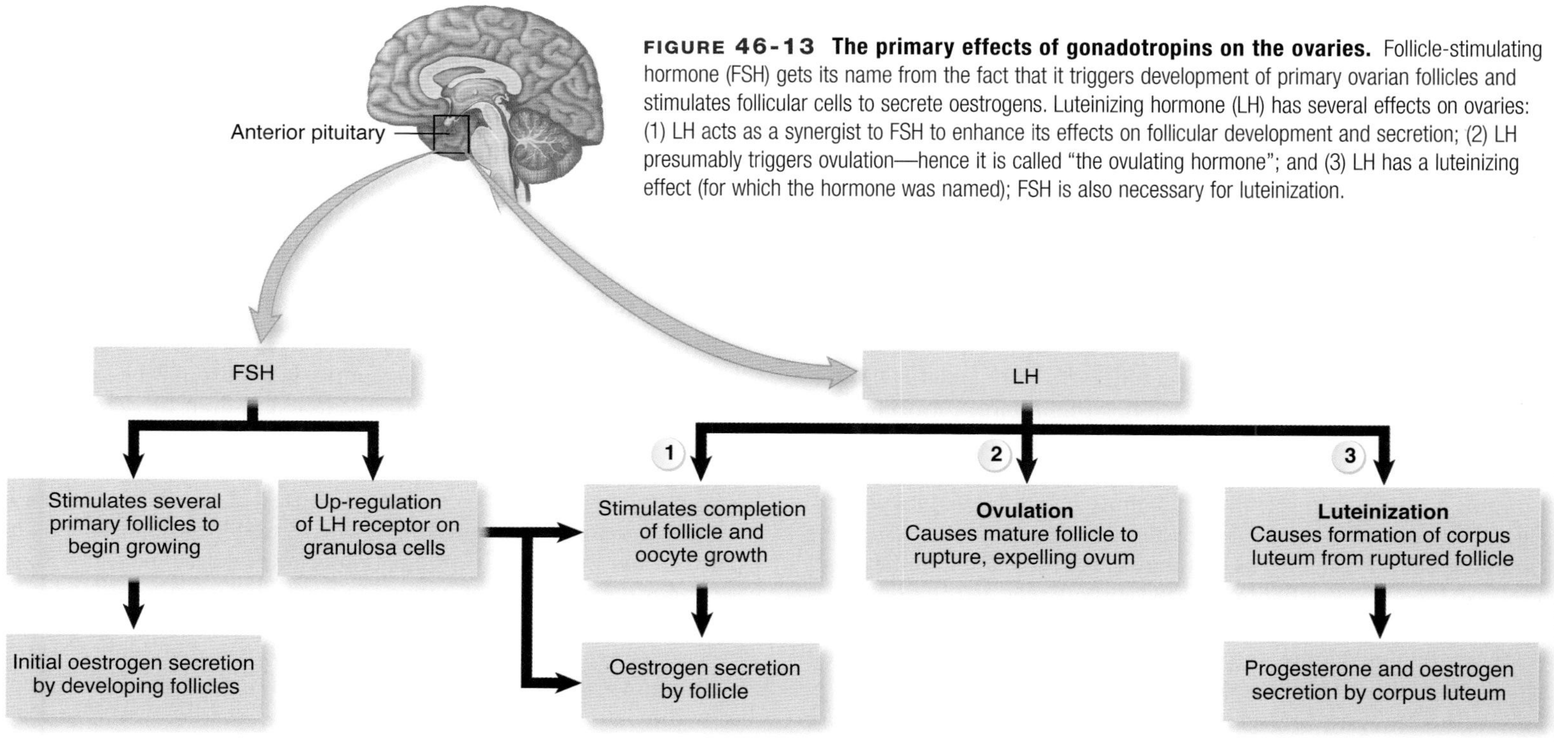

Anterior pituitary
FSH
LH
Stimulates several primary follicles to begin growing
Up-regulation of LH receptor on granulosa cells
Initial oestrogen secretion by developing follicles
1
Stimulates completion of follicle and oocyte growth
Oestrogen secretion by follicle
2
Ovulation
Causes mature follicle to rupture, expelling ovum
3
Luteinization
Causes formation of corpus luteum from ruptured follicle
Progesterone and oestrogen secretion by corpus luteum

FIGURE 46-13 The primary effects of gonadotropins on the ovaries. Follicle-stimulating hormone (FSH) gets its name from the fact that it triggers development of primary ovarian follicles and stimulates follicular cells to secrete oestrogens. Luteinizing hormone (LH) has several effects on ovaries: (1) LH acts as a synergist to FSH to enhance its effects on follicular development and secretion; (2) LH presumably triggers ovulation—hence it is called "the ovulating hormone"; and (3) LH has a luteinizing effect (for which the hormone was named); FSH is also necessary for luteinization.

UNIT 6

The blood level of progesterone rises rapidly after the "LH surge" described earlier. It remains at a high level for about a week, then decreases to a very low level approximately 3 days before menstruation begins again. This low blood level of progesterone persists during both the menstrual and the postmenstrual phases. What are its sources? Not the corpus luteum, which secretes only during the luteal phase, but the developing follicles and the adrenal cortex. The blood's oestrogen content increases during the luteal phase but to a lower level than develops before ovulation.

If pregnancy does not occur, lack of sufficient LH and FSH causes the corpus luteum to regress in about 14 days. The corpus luteum is then replaced by the corpus albicans. Review **Figure 46-4**, which shows the cyclical changes in the ovarian follicles.

Control of Cyclical Changes in the Uterus

Cyclical changes in the uterus are brought about by changing blood concentrations of oestrogens and progesterone. As blood oestrogens increase during the postmenstrual phase of the menstrual cycle, they produce the following main changes in the uterus:

- Proliferation of endometrial cells, producing a thickening of the endometrium
- Growth of endometrial glands and of the spiral arteries of the endometrium
- Increase in the water content of the endometrium
- Increased myometrial contractions

Increasing blood progesterone concentration during the premenstrual phase of the menstrual cycle produces progestational changes in the uterus—that is, changes favourable for pregnancy, specifically the following:

- Secretion by endometrial glands, thereby preparing the endometrium for implantation of a fertilized ovum
- Increase in the water content of the endometrium
- Decreased myometrial contractions

As mentioned earlier, low levels of FSH and LH cause regression of the corpus luteum if pregnancy does not occur. This in turn causes a drop in oestrogen and progesterone levels, with the result that their maintenance of a thick, vascular endometrium ceases. Thus a drop in oestrogen and progesterone levels at the end of the premenstrual phase triggers the endometrial sloughing that characterizes the menstrual phase.

Control of Cyclical Changes in Gonadotropin Secretion

Both negative and positive feedback mechanisms help control anterior pituitary secretion of the gonadotropins FSH and LH. These mechanisms involve the ovaries' secretion of inhibin, oestrogens, and progesterone and secretion of releasing hormones by the hypothalamus. **Figure 46-14** describes a negative feedback mechanism that controls gonadotropin secretion. Examine it carefully. Note particularly the effects of a sustained high blood concentration of oestrogens and progesterone on anterior pituitary gland secretion and the effect of a low blood concentration of FSH on follicular development: essentially, follicles do not mature and ovulation does not occur.

Several observations and animal experiments strongly suggest that sustained high blood levels of oestrogens, progesterone, and inhibin decrease pituitary secretion of FSH and LH. These ovarian hormones appear to inhibit certain neurons of the hypothalamus (part of the central nervous system) from secreting gonadotropin-releasing hormone (GnRH) into the hypophyseal portal vessels (see **Figure 46-14**). Without the stimulating effects of these releasing hormones, the pituitary's secretion of FSH and LH decreases.

A positive feedback mechanism has also been postulated to control LH secretion. The sudden and marked increase in blood's oestrogen content that occurs late in the follicular phase of the menstrual cycle is thought to stimulate the hypothalamus to secrete GnRH into the hypophyseal portal vessels. GnRH stimulates the release of LH by the anterior pituitary, which in turn accounts for the "LH surge" that triggers ovulation. The fact that a part of the brain—the hypothalamus—secretes gonadotropin-releasing hormones has interesting implications. This may be part of the pathway by which changes in a woman's environment or in her emotional state can alter her menstrual cycle. That this occurs is a matter of common observation. Stress, for example—such as intense fear of either becoming or not becoming pregnant—often delays menstruation.

Importance of Female Reproductive Cycles

Several important functional roles are played by the female reproductive cycles. As **Figure 46-15** shows, the changes associated with the different cycles are all closely interrelated.

The primary role of the ovarian cycle, for example, is to produce an ovum at regular enough intervals to make reproductive success likely. The ovarian cycle's secondary role is to regulate the endometrial (menstrual) cycle by means of the sex hormones oestrogen and progesterone. The role of the endometrial cycle, in turn, is to ensure that the lining of the uterus is suitable for the implantation of an embryo if fertilization of the ovum occurs. The constant renewal of the endometrium makes successful implantation more likely.

The cyclical mechanisms of female reproductive function, and the fact that an ovum must unite with a sperm during the first 24 hours or so after ovulation to reach the uterus at the proper stage of development to implant, result in the fact that a woman is fertile only a few days out of each monthly cycle. Human fertility is further limited by the fact that sperm usually cannot survive in the female reproductive tract for more than a few days. Such limited fertility increases the likelihood that conception will occur only when the woman's body is at its reproductive peak.

Box 46-6 discusses some common methods for managing fertility.

Infertility and Use of Fertility Drugs

Infertility in a couple is often defined as failure to conceive after 1 year of regular unprotected intercourse. Infertility may be caused by a wide variety of medical, environmental, and even lifestyle factors, such as smoking or alcohol abuse. Causal factors for infertility may be traced to various problems in either the male or female partner, each accounting for about 40% of cases. Of the remaining 20% of affected couples, infertility in about 10% is due to problems shared by both partners and in about 10% the reason is never determined. If testing identifies the female member of the couple as infertile, she joins a subset of about 25% of women in the overall population who will experience some period of infertility during their reproductive years.

In many cases, infertility results from a failure to ovulate—often caused by a medical condition such as *polycystic ovary syndrome* or

PCOS (see Mechanisms of Disease). Significant numbers of infertile women experiencing ovulatory dysfunction desire to become pregnant and, after a sometimes long and complex medical "workup" and selection process, become candidates to receive so-called *fertility drugs*—either alone or in combination with other assisted reproductive procedures such as artificial insemination.

An orally administered fertility drug called *clomifene* may be used to treat women who have anovulatory cycles. It is an anti-oestrogen agent that competes with oestrogen for oestrogen-receptor binding sites. By blocking oestrogen it acts as an ovulatory stimulant. How? By effectively "tricking" the pituitary gland into producing FSH and LH. The gonadotropin surge causes normal follicle growth and subsequent ovulation. Clomifene is given in daily doses of 50 or 100 mg for 5 days, generally starting on day 5 of the menstrual cycle. In a successful treatment program, ovulation most often occurs from 5 to 10 days after a course of the drug. The incidence of multiple births is about 5% to 7% (mostly twins), a percentage much lower than what is observed after direct administration (injection) of FSH and LH, where the intent is to produce multiple follicles before inducing ovulation.

Supraovulation, or simultaneous rupture of multiple mature follicles, is an infertility treatment option that may be employed if clomifene use proves ineffective or if multiple ova are deemed desirable in *assisted reproductive technologies* such as **in vitro fertilization (IVF).** It most often involves self-administered injections of either (1) drugs called **menotropins** or (2) genetically developed (recombinant) gonadotropins.

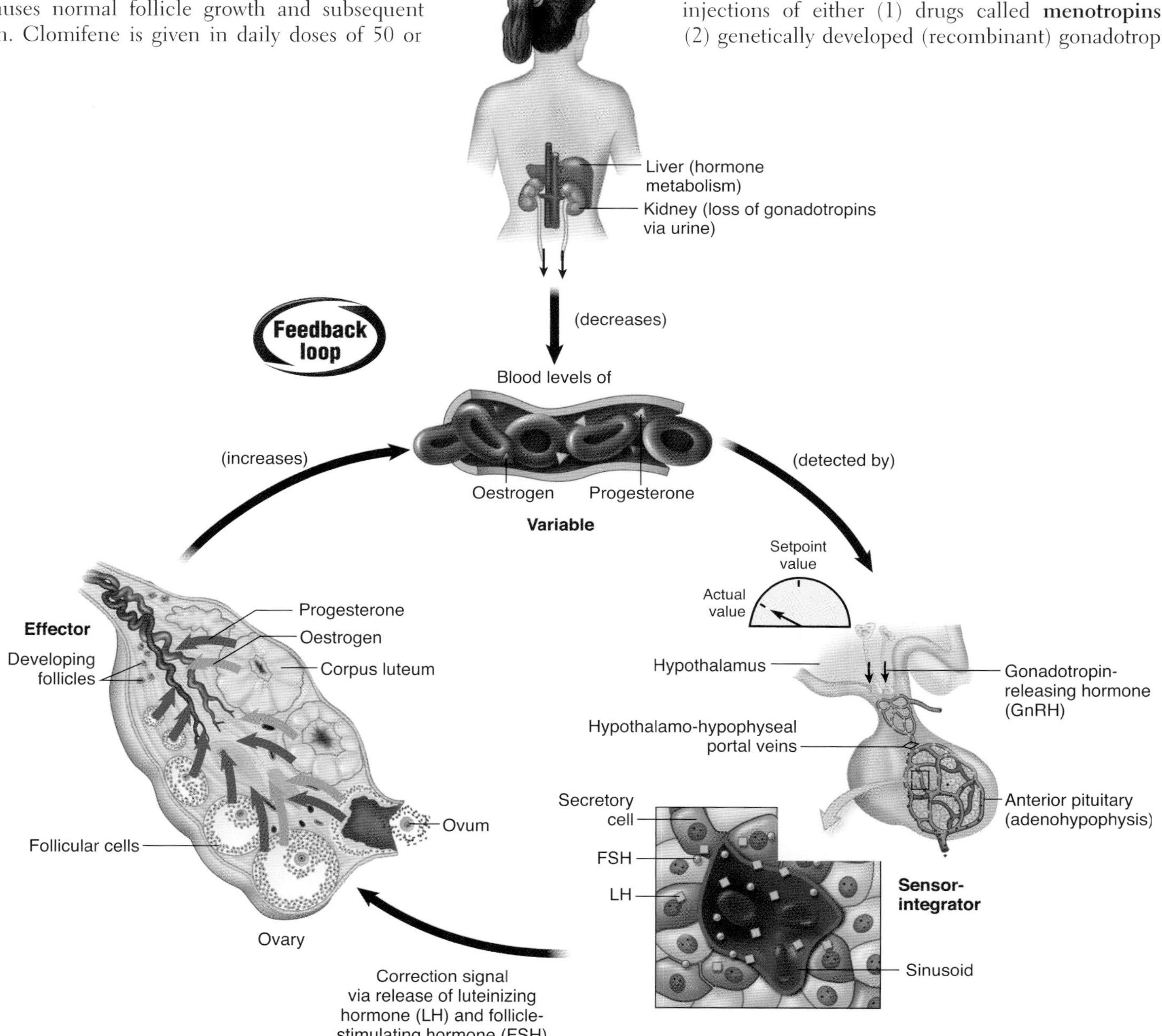

FIGURE 46-14 Control of FSH and oestrogen secretion. A negative feedback mechanism controls anterior pituitary secretion of follicle-stimulating hormone (FSH) and ovarian secretion of oestrogens. A high blood level of FSH stimulates oestrogen secretion, whereas the resulting high oestrogen level inhibits FSH secretion. How does this compare with the LH testosterone feedback mechanism in the male? (See **Figure 45-7**, p. 1043, if you want to check your answer.) According to the diagram, what effect does a high blood concentration of oestrogens have on anterior pituitary secretion of FSH? of LH?

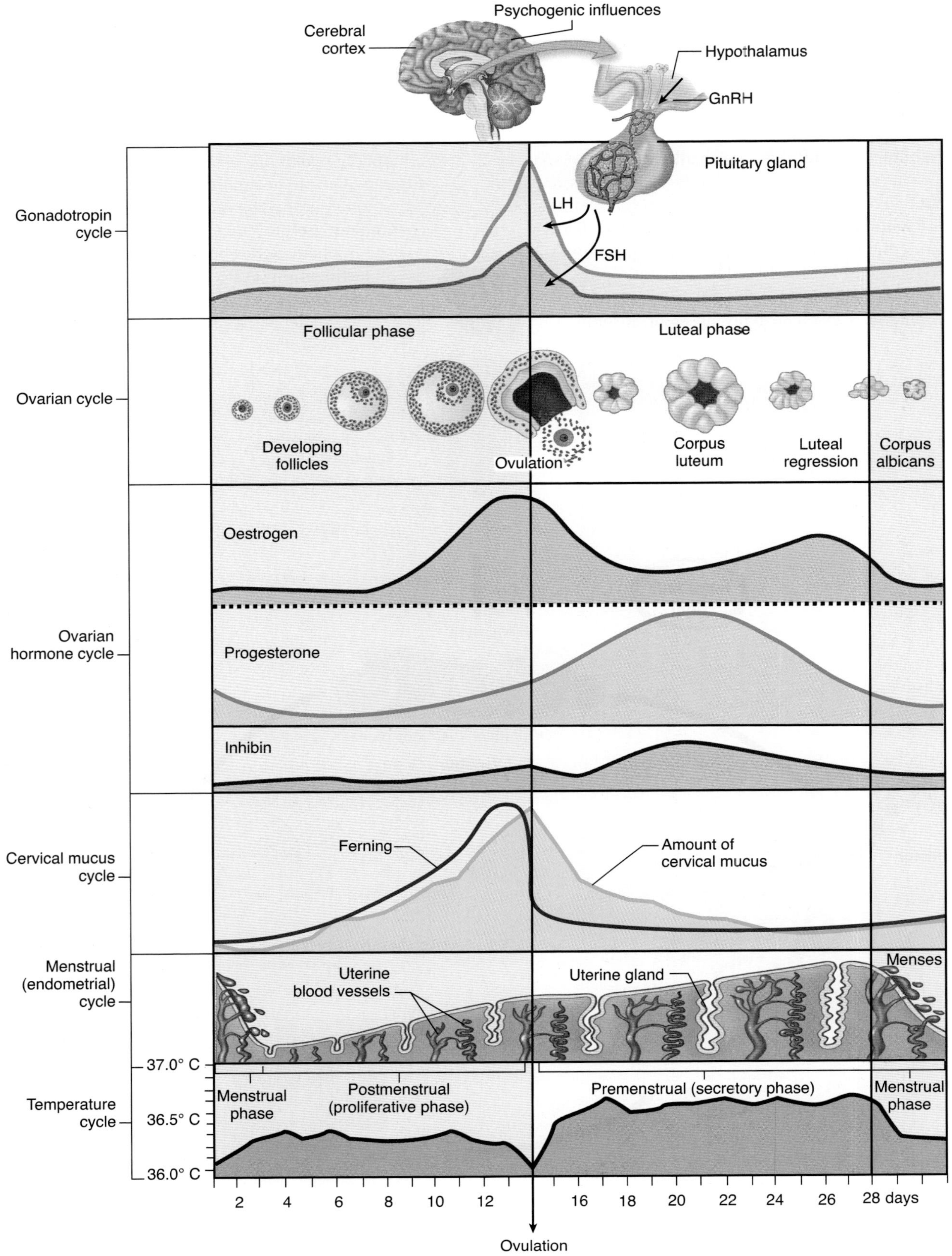

Psychogenic influences
Cerebral cortex
Hypothalamus
GnRH
Pituitary gland
LH
FSH
Gonadotropin cycle
Follicular phase
Luteal phase
Ovarian cycle
Developing follicles
Ovulation
Corpus luteum
Luteal regression
Corpus albicans
Oestrogen
Ovarian hormone cycle
Progesterone
Inhibin
Cervical mucus cycle
Ferning
Amount of cervical mucus
Menstrual (endometrial) cycle
Uterine blood vessels
Uterine gland
Menses
37.0° C
36.5° C
36.0° C
Temperature cycle
Menstrual phase
Postmenstrual (proliferative phase)
Premenstrual (secretory phase)
Menstrual phase
2 4 6 8 10 12 16 18 20 22 24 26 28 days
Ovulation

FIGURE 46-15 Female reproductive cycles. This diagram illustrates the interrelationships among the cerebral, hypothalamic, pituitary, ovarian, and uterine/cervical functions throughout a 28-day menstrual cycle. The variations in basal body temperature are also illustrated.

BOX 46-6 *health matters* | Methods of Contraception

Hormonal methods of contraception began with establishment of the relationship between sex hormone levels and ovulation. Continuing research in this area led to the development of **oral contraceptives**—often collectively called "the Pill". Numerous oral contraceptive products are now available that contain different types, combinations, and dosages of oestrogen and progesterone.

The so-called minipill contains only synthetic progesterone. Most hormonal contraceptives were developed to prevent pregnancy by initiating negative feedback inhibition of follicle-stimulating hormone (FSH) and luteinizing hormone (LH) secretion. As a result, mature follicles do not develop, and LH levels required to initiate ovulation do not occur. The next menses, however, does take place if the progesterone and oestrogen dosage is stopped in time to allow their blood levels to decrease as they normally do near the end of the cycle to bring on menstruation. For this reason, "the pill" can be used to regulate the menstrual cycle, as well as prevent pregnancy. If used correctly and consistently, "the pill" is an extremely effective contraceptive with an unintended pregnancy rate estimated at between 0.1% and 3%. The higher percentage reflects "typical" rather than "ideal" use, and underscores the impact of human error in using any form of birth control.

In addition to oral contraceptives taken in pill form, other types of hormonal birth control "delivery mechanisms" are available in some parts of the world. They include hormone-impregnated vaginal inserts, hormone injections, transcutaneous administration using skin "patches", and surgical insertion of hormone-containing implants under the skin.

The effects of hormonal contraceptives—indeed, of oestrogens and progesterone—are much more complex than our explanation here indicates. They have widespread effects on the body quite independent of their action on the reproductive and endocrine systems and are still not completely understood. Possible side effects—some extremely serious, including stroke and heart attack—may limit or prohibit use of these birth control methods by some women. Side effects of hormonal contraceptives are especially troublesome if these products are used for extended periods, by older women, by women who smoke, and in women with blood clotting problems or cardiovascular disease. On the other hand, long-term use has also been shown to have some beneficial health effects such as protection against uterine and **ovarian cancer.**

In addition to hormonal methods of contraception, many other methods, each with differing rates of effectiveness and unique advantages and disadvantages, are available. For example, *spermicidal methods* involve use of preparations (foams, jellies, and creams) that act to kill sperm, and *mechanical barrier methods* use devices such as condoms, diaphragms, and cervical caps to block sperm from entering the uterus. So-called *surgical methods* such as tubal ligation (see **Box 46-2**) and male vasectomy result in permanent sterility.

An **intrauterine device** or **IUD** is usually a small, copper-wrapped object (pictured) inserted into the lumen of the uterine body, where it remains for months or years. IUDs trigger an inflammatory response called the *foreign body reaction,* which is toxic to sperm and probably also ova. By thus inhibiting gametes, the IUD works by preventing fertilization. Some IUDs also release progesterone and thus have an action similar to other hormonal contraceptives. A common misconception not supported by research is that IUDs work by triggering abortions.

Decision making concerning the use of contraceptive methods to regulate reproductive function involves many complex interactions that are uniquely human—and very personal. The decision to use or avoid contraception—or employ any particular contraceptive method—at any point in time is often influenced by differing medical, social, cultural, ethical, and religious factors as well as by the cost, reliability, safety, or ease of use of a particular method. Informed and thoughtful decision making regarding this human behaviour is critically important. It will often be necessary for some individuals to seek out a variety of information—from different but credible and knowledgeable sources—in order to make an informed decision that is "right" for those individuals. Regardless, seeking counsel and advice from a trusted health care provider early in the process is always recommended.

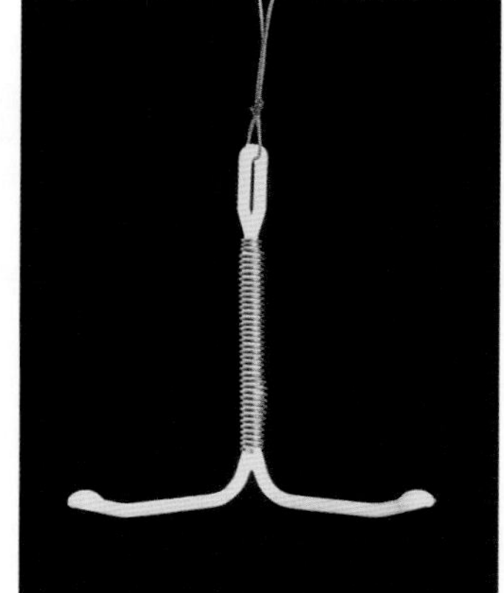

Intrauterine device (IUD).

Menotropins contain high concentrations of FSH and LH that are extracted from the urine of pregnant women or from postmenopausal women. Recombinant gonadotropins include human menopausal gonadotropins (hMGs) and FSH.

CONNECT IT! 

Artificial fertilization outside the body is sometimes used to enhance reproductive success. Read a brief description of this strategy and other *assisted reproductive technologies (ARTs)* in ***In Vitro Fertilization*** online at ***Connect It!***

Menarche and Menopause

The menstrual flow first occurs (menarche) at puberty, at about the age of 13 years, although there is individual variation according to ethnicity, nutrition, health, and heredity. Normally, it recurs about every 28 days for about 3 decades, except during pregnancy, and then ceases (menopause, or climacteric). The average age at which menstruation ceases is reported to have increased markedly—from about age 40 years a few decades ago to between ages 45 and 50 years more recently.

Recall that gonadotropins extracted from the urine of menopausal women (menotropins) are used as fertility drugs. **Figure 46-16** shows how the changes just described relate to changes in hormone levels over the life span. Relatively low concentrations of gonadotropins (FSH and LH) sustain a peak of oestrogen secretion from menarche to menopause. After menopause, oestrogen concentration decreases dramatically—which causes a negative feedback response that increases the gonadotropin levels. Because the follicular cells are no longer sensitive to gonadotropins after menopause, the increased gonadotropin level has no effect on oestrogen secretion.

Table 46-1 summarizes some of the hormones important in female reproductive function.

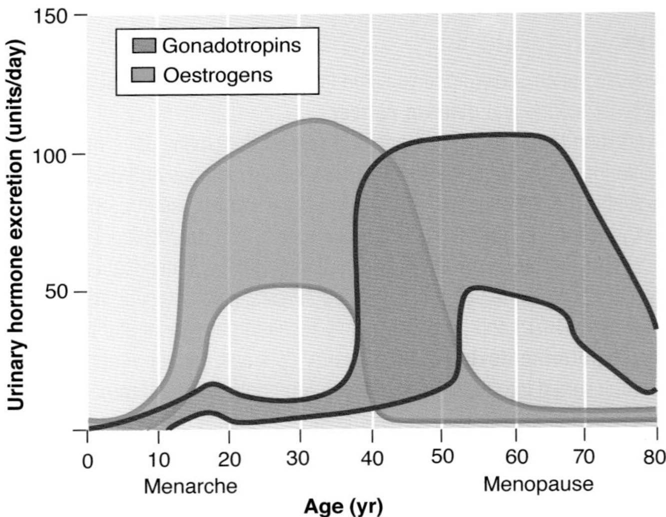

FIGURE 46-16 Gonadotropin and oestrogen levels over the life span. This graph shows changes in hormone levels as reflected in urinary excretion rates from birth to advanced old age. Note that an increase in the gonadotropin level at the time of menarche sustains a high but variable level of oestrogens until the time of menopause, when ovarian follicular cells cease to respond to gonadotropins. A negative feedback mechanism tries to increase oestrogen levels to their former high levels by increasing the gonadotropin levels—a strategy that always fails.

Quick **CHECK**

17. A surge in FSH and LH is associated with what major event of the ovarian cycle?
18. How does an increase in oestrogen level affect the uterine lining?
19. What is *menopause*? What causes menopause to occur?

BREASTS

Location and Size of the Breasts

Two breasts lie over the pectoral muscles and are attached to them by a layer of connective tissue (fascia) (**Figure 46-17**). Breasts are made up of milk-producing **mammary glands,** which are present in all mammals, along with extensive supporting tissues. Breasts are present in both males and females—but only infrequently develop or produce milk in males.

Oestrogens and progesterone, two types of ovarian hormones, control breast development during puberty. Oestrogens stimulate growth of the ducts of the mammary glands, whereas progesterone stimulates development of the actual secreting cells. Breast size is determined more by the amount of fat around the glandular tissue than by the amount of glandular tissue itself. Hence the size of the breast is not related to its ability to produce milk.

TABLE 46-1 Some Female Reproductive Hormones*

HORMONE	SOURCE	TARGET	ACTION
Dehydroepiandrosterone (DHEA)	Adrenal gland, ovary, other tissues	Converted to other hormones	Eventually converted to oestrogens, testosterone, or both (see **Figure 25-5** on p. 566)
Oestrogens (including oestradiol [E_2] and oestrone)	Ovary and placenta (small amounts in other tissues)	Uterus, breast, other tissues	Stimulates development of female sexual characteristics and breast development and promotes bone and nervous system maintenance
Follicle-stimulating hormone (FSH)	Anterior pituitary (gonadotroph cells)	Ovary	Gonadotropin; promotes development of ovarian follicle; stimulates oestrogen secretion
Gonadotropin-releasing hormone (GnRH)	Hypothalamus (neuroendocrine cells)	Anterior pituitary (gonadotroph cells)	Stimulates production and release of gonadotropins (FSH and LH) from anterior pituitary
Human chorionic gonadotropin (hCG)	Placenta	Ovary	Stimulates secretion of oestrogen and progesterone during pregnancy
Inhibin	Ovary	Hypothalamus Anterior pituitary (gonadotroph cells)	Inhibits GnRH production in the hypothalamus and FSH production in the anterior pituitary
Luteinizing hormone (LH)	Anterior pituitary (gonadotroph cells)	Ovary	Gonadotropin; triggers ovulation; promotes development of corpus luteum
Oxytocin (OT)	Posterior pituitary	Uterus and mammary glands	Stimulates uterine contractions; stimulates ejection of milk into ducts of mammary glands; involved in social bonding
Progesterone	Ovary and placenta	Uterus, mammary glands, other tissues	Helps maintain proper conditions for pregnancy
Prolactin (PRL) (lactogenic hormone)	Anterior pituitary (lactotroph cells)	Mammary glands (alveolar secretory cells)	Promotes milk secretion
Relaxin	Placenta	Uterus and joints	Inhibits uterine contractions during pregnancy and softens pelvic joints to facilitate childbirth
Testosterone	Adrenal glands, ovaries	Nervous tissue, bone tissue, other tissues	May affect mood, sex drive, learning, sleep, protein anabolism, other functions

*The role of some hormones related to pregnancy, labour, and delivery are discussed in more detail in the next chapter (Chapter 47, Growth, Development, and Ageing).

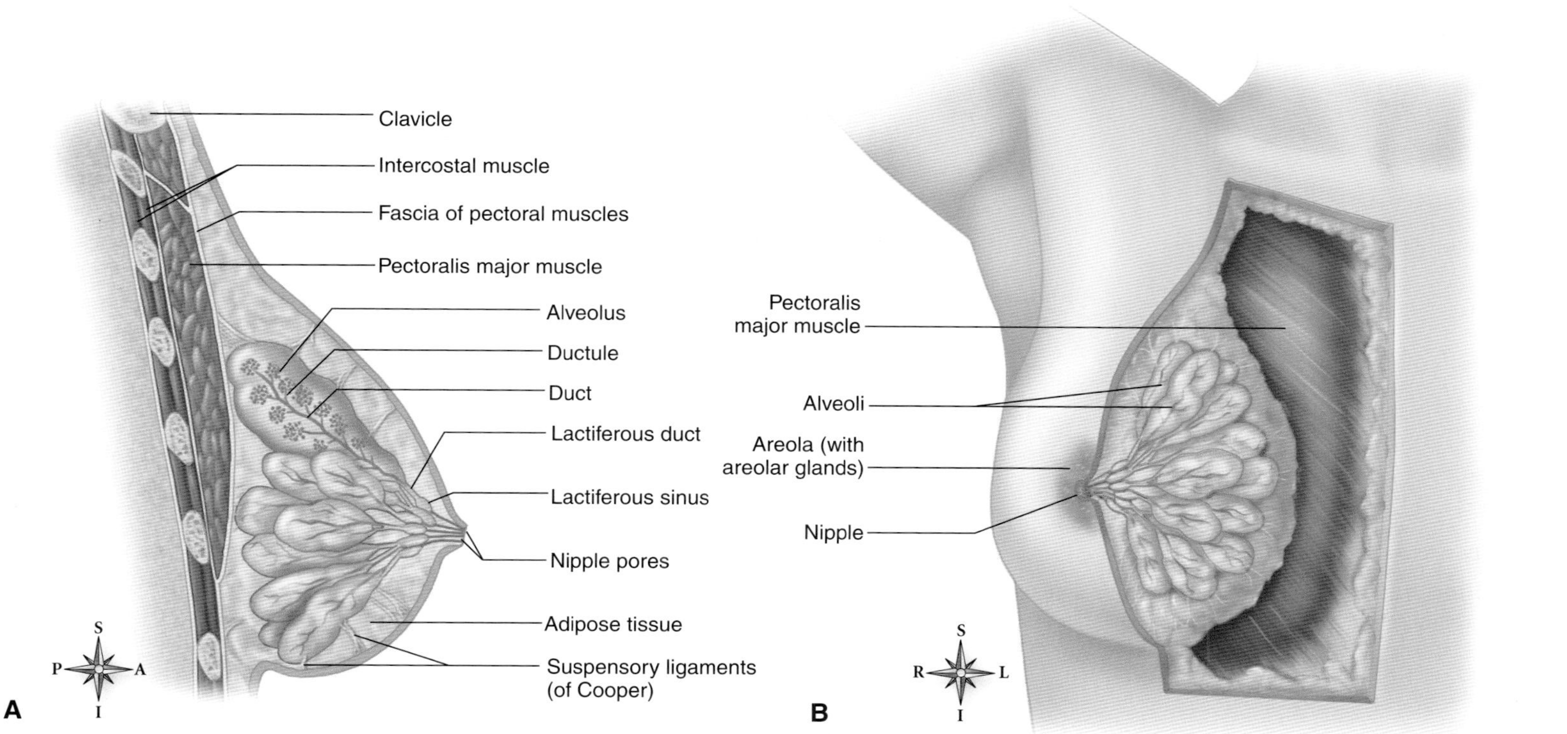

FIGURE 46-17 The female breast. A, Sagittal section of a lactating breast. Note how the glandular structures are anchored to the overlying skin and to the pectoral muscles by the suspensory ligaments of Cooper. Each lobule of glandular tissue is drained by a lactiferous duct that eventually opens through the nipple. **B,** Anterior view of a lactating breast. Overlying skin and connective tissue have been removed from the medial side to show the internal structure of the breast and underlying skeletal muscle. In nonlactating breasts, the glandular tissue is much less prominent, with adipose tissue making up most of each breast.

Structure of the Breasts

Each breast consists of several lobes separated by septa (walls) of connective tissue. Each lobe consists of several *lobules,* which, in turn, are composed of connective tissues in which are embedded the pouches of milk-secreting cells. These pouches, or *alveoli,* are arranged in grapelike clusters around the tiny ductule. **Figure 46-18** shows one of the mammary alveoli and the milk-producing cells that form its walls. Notice that a special type of epithelial cell called a *myoepithelial cell* is present around the outside of the alveolus. This type of cell contracts slightly, as if it were a muscle cell, thus squeezing milk out into the secretory duct.

The ductules from the various lobules unite, forming a single *lactiferous duct* for each lobe, or between 15 and 20 in each breast. The term *lactiferous* simply means "milk carrying". These main lactiferous ducts converge toward the nipple, like the spokes of a wheel. They enlarge slightly into small *lactiferous sinuses* before reaching the **nipple** (see **Figure 46-17**, *A*). The lactiferous sinuses are positioned to be squeezed by the suckling motion of a baby's jaws during breastfeeding—thus allowing the sinuses to act as little pumping chambers that help move milk out of the breast (**Figure 46-19**). Each of the main ducts terminates in a tiny opening on the surface of the nipple.

A comparatively large amount of adipose tissue is deposited around the surface of the gland, just under the skin, and between the lobes. *Suspensory ligaments (of Cooper)* throughout the connective tissue of the breast help support the glandular and connective tissues of the entire structure, anchoring them to the coverings of the underlying pectoral muscles.

The nipples are bordered by a circular pigmented area, the **areola** (see **Figure 46-17**, *B*). It contains numerous sebaceous glands that appear as small nodules under the skin. Sebum produced by these *areolar glands* helps reduce irritating dryness of the areolar skin associated with nursing. Areolar secretions also contain pheromones that enhance the mother–infant social bond. In some lighter-skinned women, the areola and nipple change colour from pink to brown early in pregnancy—a fact of value in diagnosing a first pregnancy. The colour decreases after lactation has ceased but never entirely returns

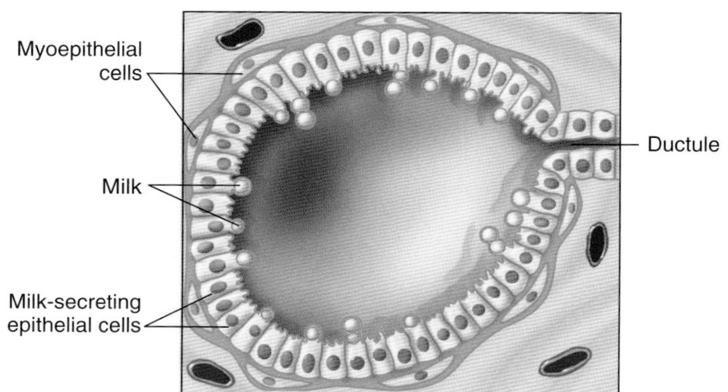

FIGURE 46-18 Alveolus of the mammary gland. Notice the contractile myoepithelial cells that surround the milk-producing cells. Milk is released by apocrine secretion, in which vesicles of fluid pinch off the cell (see **Figure 9-11** on p. 162).

FIGURE 46-19 Function of lactiferous sinuses. When an infant is properly latched on to the breast, its jaws squeeze the lactiferous sinuses rhythmically, thus pumping milk out of the breast and into the back of the infant's mouth.

to the original hue. In some darker-skinned women, no noticeable colour change in the areola or nipple heralds the first pregnancy.

Knowledge of the lymphatic drainage of the breast is important in clinical medicine because cancerous cells from malignant breast tumours often spread to other areas of the body through the lymphatics. Lymphatic drainage of the breast is presented in Chapter 31.

FUNCTION OF THE BREASTS

The function of the mammary glands is lactation—that is, the secretion of milk for the nourishment of newborn infants.

Mechanism Controlling Lactation

Very briefly, **lactation** is controlled as follows and as shown in **Figure 46-20**:

- The ovarian hormones, oestrogens and progesterone, act on the breasts to make them structurally ready to secrete milk. Oestrogens promote development of the ducts of the breasts. Progesterone acts on the oestrogen-primed breasts to promote completion of the development of the ducts and development of the alveoli, the secreting cells of the breasts. This is an example of hormonal *permissiveness;* oestrogen permits progesterone to have its full effect. A high blood concentration of oestrogens during pregnancy also inhibits anterior pituitary secretion of prolactin.
- Shedding of the placenta after delivery of the baby cuts off a major source of oestrogens. The resulting rapid drop in the blood concentration of oestrogens stimulates anterior pituitary secretion of prolactin. Also, the suckling movements of a nursing baby stimulate anterior pituitary secretion of prolactin and posterior pituitary secretion of oxytocin.
- Prolactin stimulates lactation—that is, stimulates alveoli of the mammary glands to secrete milk. Milk secretion starts about the third or fourth day after delivery of a baby, supplanting a thin, yellowish secretion called *colostrum.* With repeated stimulation by the suckling infant, plus various favourable mental and physical conditions, lactation may continue for extended periods.
- Oxytocin stimulates myoepithelial cells in the alveoli of the breasts to eject milk into the ducts, thereby making it accessible for the infant to remove by suckling.

This summary highlights only the major hormonal mechanisms that regulate lactation. **Table 46-2** shows that there are *many* hormones that support the processes needed for successful lactation and

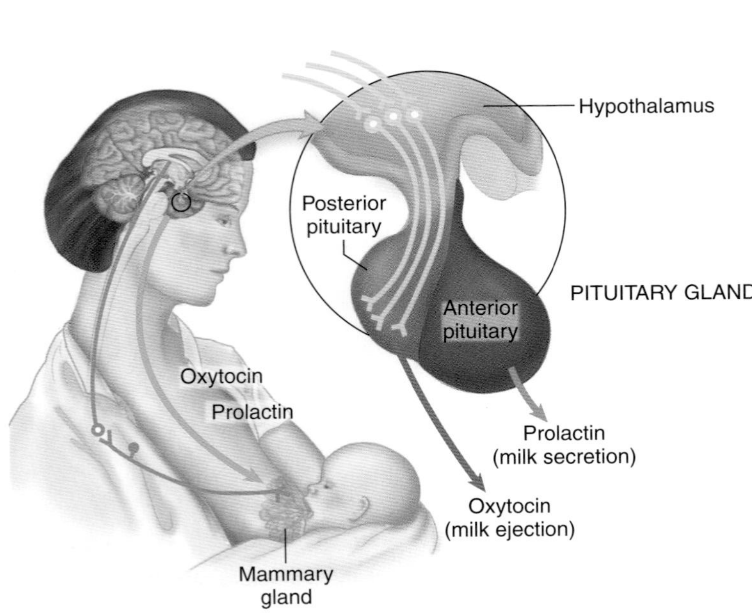

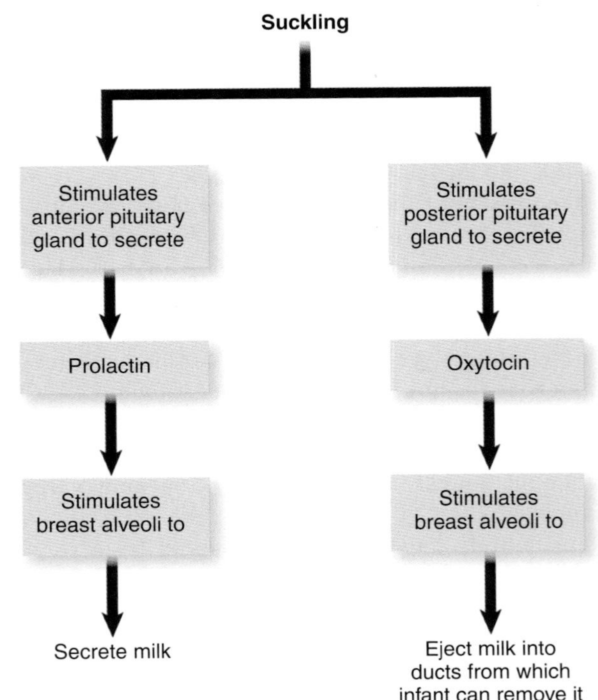

FIGURE 46-20 Lactation. The illustration and accompanying flowchart summarize the mechanisms that control the secretion and ejection of milk.

defines the major roles that these hormones play. Many of these mechanisms are adaptations of hormonal processes discussed earlier, such as insulin's ability to get glucose into cells—a function clearly needed in cells that produce sugar-rich milk.

The Importance of Lactation

The process of lactation plays an important role in the ultimate success of the reproductive system. The biological goal of human reproduction does not lie solely in delivering a healthy infant—the infant must also survive until reproductive age. If a child does not survive to reproduce, then the genetic code cannot be passed on to successive generations and the ultimate goal of reproduction has not been met. Humans and other mammals help ensure the survival of offspring for up to several years by producing nutrient-rich milk. Nursing from the mother's breast provides several advantages for human offspring, including the following:

- Milk is a rich source of proteins, fat, calcium, vitamins, and other nutrients in proportions needed by a young, developing body.
- Human milk provides passive immunity to the offspring in the form of maternal antibodies present in both colostrum and the milk.
- Nursing enhances the emotional bond between mother and child. Such bonding fosters healthy psychological development in the child and strengthens family relationships that contribute to successful human development.

Quick CHECK

20. Briefly describe the network of ducts and secreting cells that form the mammary glands.
21. List the hormones that prepare the breast structurally for lactation.
22. Which hormone causes milk to be ejected into the lactiferous ducts?

TABLE 46-2 Hormones That Support Milk Production

CATEGORY	ROLE IN LACTATION	HORMONES*
Mammogenic hormones	Promote tissue growth and development	↑ Oestrogens ↑ Growth hormone (GH) ↑ Insulin-like growth factor (IGF-1) ↑ Insulin ↑ Cortisol ↑ Prolactin (PRL) ↑ Relaxin ↑ Epidermal growth factor (EGF)
Lactogenic hormones	Initiate milk production by secretory cells of alveolus	↑ Prolactin (PRL) ↑ Placental lactogen (hPL) ↑ Cortisol ↑ Insulin ↑ Insulin-like growth factor (IGF-I) ↑ Thyroid hormones (T_3, T_4) ↑ Growth hormone (GH) ↓ Oestrogens ↓ Progesterone
Galactokinetic hormones	Promote milk ejection by stimulating myoepithelial cells surrounding alveoli	↑ Oxytocin (OT) ↑ Antidiuretic hormone (ADH) (vasopressin [AVP])
Galactopoietic hormones	Maintain milk production (after it has already started)	↑ PRL ↑ Cortisol ↑ Insulin ↑ IGF-1 ↑ (T_3, T_4)

*↑, Increased hormone produces lactation effect.
↓, Increased hormone produces lactation effect.

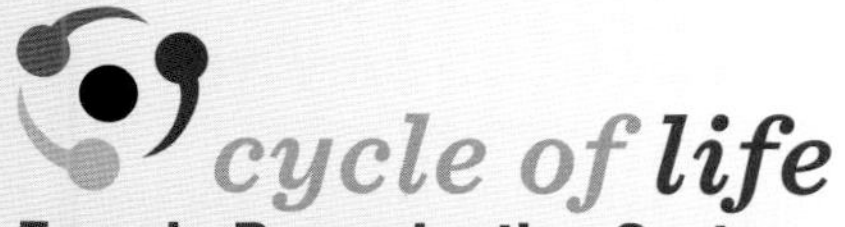

cycle of life

Female Reproductive System As mentioned in Chapter 45, the reproductive system is unlike any other body system with regard to the normal changes that occur during the life span. Unlike other systems, the female reproductive system does not begin to perform its functions until the teenage years (puberty), and unlike the male reproductive system, the female reproductive system ceases its principal functions in middle adulthood.

The female organs begin their initial stages of development in the womb. As a matter of fact, the first stage of meiotic development of all the ova that will ever be produced by a woman is completed by the time she is born. However, full development of the reproductive organs—and the gametes within the ovaries—does not resume until puberty. At puberty, reproductive hormones stimulate the organs of the reproductive tract to become functional and produce a mature ovum one at a time. Reproductive function then continues in a cyclical fashion until menopause. Menopause is an event that is usually marked by the passage of at least 1 full year without menstruation. After that time, a woman may continue to participate in normal sexual activity, but she cannot produce more offspring. •

the big picture | Female Reproductive System and the Whole Body

As stated several times in this chapter, the importance of reproductive function lies in the fact that it imparts virtual immortality to our genes. This is important not only to the survival of the human species but also to the survival of life itself. After all, life as we know it could not exist without a genetic code. The "big picture" of human reproduction requires two systems, one reproductive system in each parent. The combined roles of the male and female reproductive systems will be explored as a single topic in the early part of the next chapter.

For now, we will take a closer look at the female reproductive system and its relationships with other systems within a woman's body. As with any system, the female reproductive system cannot function without the maintenance functions of the circulatory, immune, respiratory, digestive, and urinary systems. The female reproductive system shares a special anatomical relationship with the urinary system. These two systems develop in close proximity to each other and thus share a common structure: the vulva. A special anatomical relationship with the skeletal muscular system is evident in the structure known as the *perineum*. Of course the skeletal and muscular systems both support and protect the internal organs of the female reproductive system. An even more special relationship with the integumentary system should be noted. The breasts, containing the milk-producing mammary glands, are actually modifications of the skin. Although structurally the breasts can be thought of as belonging to the integumentary system, functionally they are best considered as a part of the reproductive system. Nervous and endocrine regulation of female reproductive function has been outlined in this chapter and is explored further in the next chapter. •

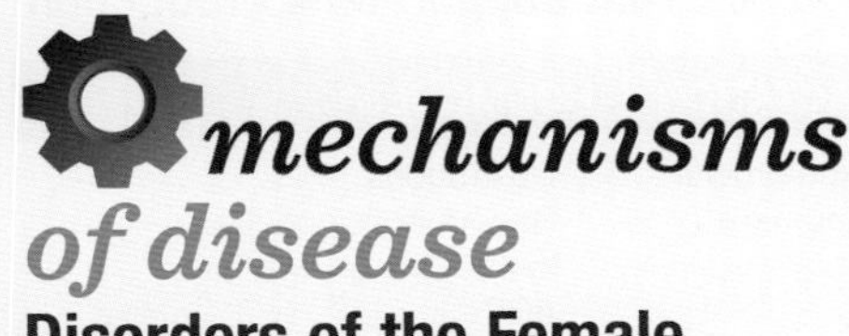

Disorders of the Female Reproductive System

Hormonal and Menstrual Disorders

Dysmenorrhoea, meaning "painful menstruation", is the term used to describe *menstrual cramps,* the painful periods that affect 75% to 80% of women at some time during their reproductive years. For significant numbers of those affected, severe lower abdominal cramping and back pain accompanied by headache, nausea, and vomiting will disrupt their school, work, athletic, or other activities. *Primary dysmenorrhoea* is the most common type, occurring primarily in adolescents and young women. Symptoms, which can last from hours to days and vary in severity from cycle to cycle, are caused by an abnormally increased concentration of certain prostaglandins produced by the uterine lining. High concentrations of prostaglandin E_2 (PGE_2) and prostaglandin F_2 (PGF_2) cause painful spasms by decreasing blood flow and oxygen delivery to uterine muscle. Fortunately, primary dysmenorrhoea is not associated with pelvic disease, such as an infection or tumour, and can generally be treated effectively with over-the-counter antiinflammatory and prostaglandin-inhibiting drugs such as ibuprofen and naproxen. In more severe cases a physician may prescribe more powerful antiinflammatory drugs or certain hormones, including oral contraceptives, to alter menstrual cycle activity or reduce the level or frequency of cyclical uterine contractions.

Secondary dysmenorrhoea refers to menstruation-related pain caused by some type of pelvic pathological condition, including inflammatory conditions and cervical stenosis. Treatment of secondary dysmenorrhoea conditions and cervical stenosis involves treating the underlying disorder.

Amenorrhoea is the absence of normal menstruation. *Primary amenorrhoea* is the failure of menstrual cycles to begin and may be caused by various factors, such as hormone imbalances, genetic disorders, brain lesions, or structural deformities of the reproductive organs. *Secondary amenorrhoea* occurs when a woman who has previously menstruated slows to three or fewer cycles per year. Secondary amenorrhoea may be a symptom of weight loss, pregnancy, lactation, menopause, or disease of the reproductive organs. Treatment of amenorrhoea involves treating the underlying disorder or condition. If amenorrhoea occurs as a component of the "sports triad" (**Box 46-7**), treatment may become part of extensive and long-term therapy needed to address a number of complex nutritional, hormonal, and self-image issues.

Dysfunctional uterine bleeding (DUB) is irregular or excessive uterine bleeding that most often results from either a structural problem or some type of hormonal imbalance that causes a disruption of blood supply rather than from an infection or other disease condition. Excessive uterine bleeding from any cause can result in life-threatening anaemia. Among UK women aged 30 to 40 years, approximately 1 in 20 presents to her GP with menorrhagia. This makes DUB one of the most often encountered gynaecological problems and is a major indication for referral to a specialist out-patient clinic. To diagnose the cause, a physician may employ ultrasound or x-ray studies, look directly inside the uterus using a scope inserted through the vagina and cervix, or examine tissue obtained by biopsy to exclude cancer.

Transabdominal pelvic ultrasound is perhaps the most widely used and useful imaging technique to look at the uterus and adjacent reproductive structures. During this procedure a transducer is placed on the lower anterior abdominal wall and high-frequency sound waves are transmitted into the pelvic viscera. The returning echoes are then viewed on a screen similar to that of a sonar receiver or "fish-finder". The resulting image, a "slice picture", may be enhanced by filling the uterus with saline solution (**Figure 46-21**). Structural problems, such as growth of a uterine malignancy or benign tumour, may cause DUB by injuring the blood vessels of the uterine wall or lining as the tissue mass grows in size and the normal contours of the organ are distorted. **Figure 46-21**, *A,* shows a normal longitudinal pelvic ultrasound image. It was taken "looking down" through the anterior abdominal wall in the mid-portion of the pelvis. Note how the bladder was used as a "window" to view the uterus and adjacent reproductive structures below. The bladder, uterus, contours of the uterine cavity, cervix, and vagina are all visible. **Figure 46-21**, *B,* shows the appearance of a similar ultrasound image in a patient suffering from DUB caused by a structural problem—abnormal muscular growths called **uterine fibroids** (discussed on pp. 1082–1083). The uterus is enlarged and pushing into the bladder, it appears "lumpy", and the cavity contours are obviously distorted. Surgical removal or treatment to shrink the fibroid growths is usually curative.

If hormonal imbalance is the cause of DUB, it is the excessive growth (hyperplasia) and breakdown of delicate endometrial tissue that results in heavy bleeding. In these cases, treatment generally begins with administration of nonsteroidal antiinflammatory drugs and hormonal manipulation using low-dose birth

BOX 46-7 *sports and fitness* | The "Sports Triad" in Elite Female Athletes

A disturbing trend among some elite female athletes involves development of a so-called triad of undesirable outcomes. In an attempt to improve performance, these athletes couple severe caloric restriction with overtraining. The result is often a flawed sense of body image that equates thinness with athletic potential. The triad involves (1) low energy availability, (2) menstrual disorders, and (3) low bone mineral density.

Low energy availability often results from disordered eating and weight loss. *Amenorrhoea* (failure to have a menstrual period) and other menstrual problems are caused by a drastic decrease in oestrogen secretion as the body attempts to conserve energy by closing down the reproductive function. It is the decrease in oestrogen levels that triggers early loss of bone density—perhaps even *osteoporosis* and permanent skeletal damage. As it progresses, the *sports triad* may also be accompanied by development of other serious and potentially fatal outcomes. •

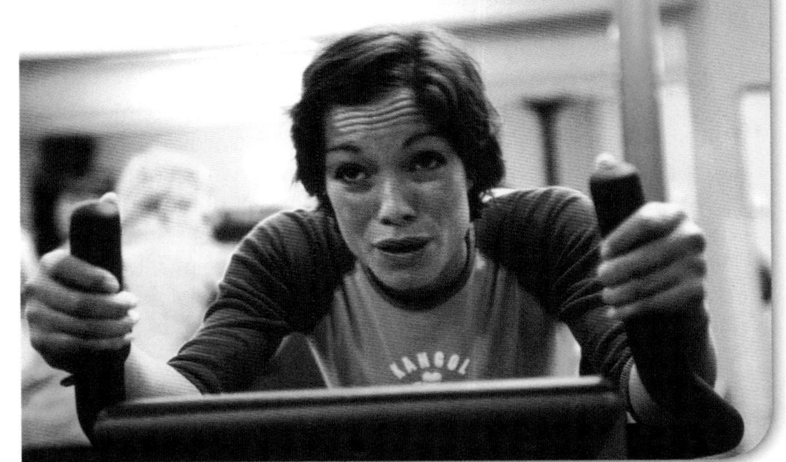

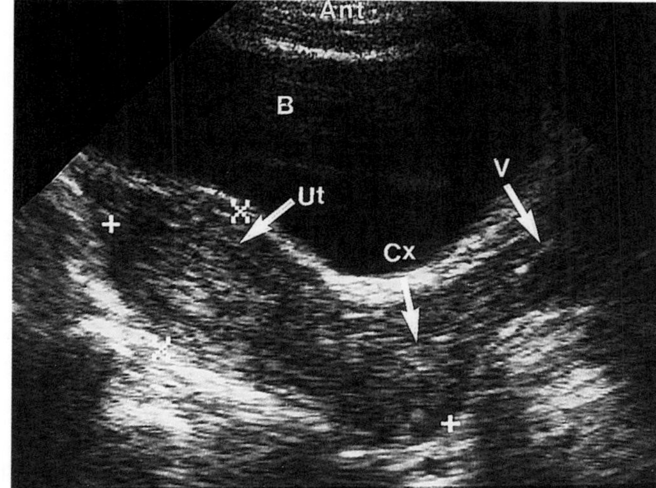

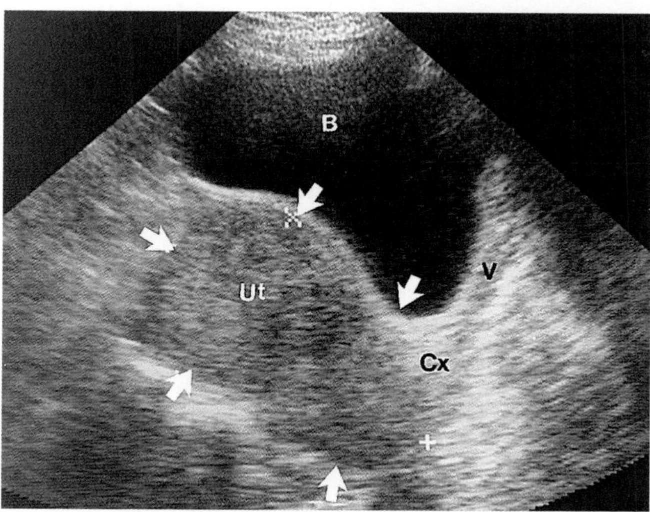

FIGURE 46-21 Female pelvic transabdominal ultrasound. A, Normal longitudinal ultrasound image. The bladder *(B)*, uterus *(Ut)*, cervix *(Cx)*, and vagina *(V)*, are visible. **B,** Longitudinal ultrasound image of uterine fibroids causing dysfunctional uterine bleeding *(DUB)*. Echo pattern shows an enlarged and "lumpy"-appearing *(arrows)* uterus *(Ut)* protruding into the bladder *(B)*. The cervix *(Cx)* and vagina *(V)* are visible.

control pills. If conservative treatment fails to stop the endometrial lining from haemorrhaging, hysterectomy remains one of the most effective curative options. However, less invasive procedures, including *endometrial ablation* techniques, are now being used more commonly to destroy the endometrial lining and halt or permanently reduce excessive menstrual blood loss in many women with DUB. In *thermal ablation,* a balloon is inserted into the uterus and filled with fluid. A heat probe is then inserted into the balloon and the fluid is heated to a temperature that will destroy the endometrium. In *radiofrequency ablation,* a gold-plated mesh fabric is used to fill the uterine cavity and is then charged with radiofrequency energy that destroys the friable and bleeding endometrial cells. Both procedures carry less risk and have shorter recovery periods than does a hysterectomy.

Premenstrual syndrome (PMS) is a condition that involves a collection of symptoms that regularly occur in many women during the premenstrual phase of their reproductive cycles. Symptoms include headache, irritability, fatigue, nervousness, weight gain, sleep changes, depression, and other problems that are often distressing enough to limit activity and affect personal relationships. Because the cause of PMS is still unclear, current treatments focus on relieving the symptoms.

Infection and Inflammation

Infections of the female reproductive tract are often classified as *exogenous* or *endogenous.* Exogenous infections result from pathogenic organisms transmitted from another person, such as *sexually transmitted diseases (STDs).* Endogenous infections result from pathogens that normally inhabit the intestines, vulva, or vagina. You may recall from Chapter 2 that many areas of the body are normally inhabited by pathogenic microorganisms but that they cause infection only when there is a change in conditions or they are moved to a new area.

CONNECT IT! ⓔ

Review examples of important STDs in ***Sexually Transmitted Diseases*** online at ***Connect It!***

Pelvic inflammatory disease (PID) occurs as either an acute or chronic inflammatory condition that can be caused by several different pathogens, which usually spread upward from the vagina. PID is a major cause of infertility and sterility in the UK and is diagnosed in approximately 1.7% of presentations to GPs by women aged 16 to 46 years. PID mainly affects sexually active women aged 15 to 24 years, but the true incidence is unknown because it can be asymptomatic or atypical, making diagnosis difficult. It is a common complication after infection by chlamydial and gonococcal STD organisms. Infection involving the uterus, uterine tubes, ovaries, and other pelvic organs often results in development of scar tissue and adhesions. Direct laparoscopic examination is often used to determine the severity of the PID infection and the reproductive organs involved (**Figure 46-22**).

PID that results in uterine tube inflammation, a condition called salpingitis, is often characterized by obstruction of the lumen and marked dilation at the end of the tube caused by accumulation of fluid that cannot escape—a condition

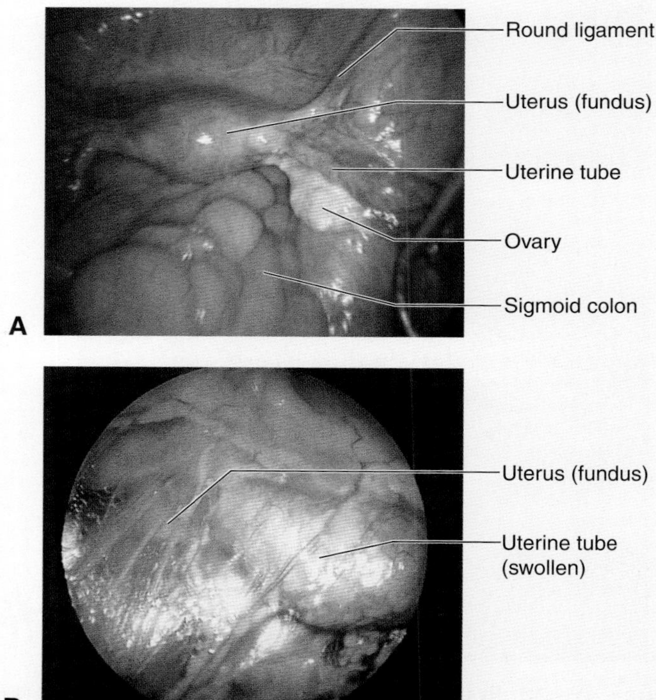

FIGURE 46-22 Laparoscopic views of the female pelvis. A, Laparoscopic image shows normal female pelvic reproductive organs. **B,** Laparoscopic view of pelvic inflammatory disease (PID). Note the clear reddish inflammatory membrane that covers and fixes the ovary, uterine tube, and uterus to the surrounding structures. The inflamed and dilated end of the fluid-filled uterine tube (hydrosalpinx) is clearly visible.

physicians refer to as **hydrosalpinx** (see **Figure 46-22**, *B*). Because ultrasound images cannot show whether the lumen of the uterine tube is open or obstructed, other imaging techniques are required to make a definitive diagnosis of infertility caused by tubal obstruction. **Figure 46-23** shows two x-ray images of the uterus and uterine tubes called **hysterosalpingograms**. In the x-ray technique used to produce these images, a cannula is inserted into the cervical canal and contrast material is injected into the uterine cavity and allowed to fill the uterine tubes. In the normal image shown in **Figure 46-23**, *A,* the contrast material has filled the uterine tubes and flowed out into the peritoneal cavity, demonstrating that the tubes are not obstructed.

Figure 46-23, *B,* is an abnormal hysterosalpingogram of a woman who was treated for salpingitis at an earlier date and later experienced infertility. Note how the contrast material fills and then collects in the dilated portion of the uterine tube (hydrosalpinx) but does not spill into the pelvis. In this case the radiograph allows the physician to make a definitive diagnosis—infertility caused by uterine tube obstruction—and treat it appropriately.

Although some chlamydial infections may not cause symptoms, most cases of PID are accompanied by fever, pelvic tenderness, and pain. Unfortunately, because of scarring and adhesions, pain may continue even after antibiotic therapy has eliminated the active infection. If left untreated, PID infections may spread to other tissues, including the blood, resulting in septic shock and death.

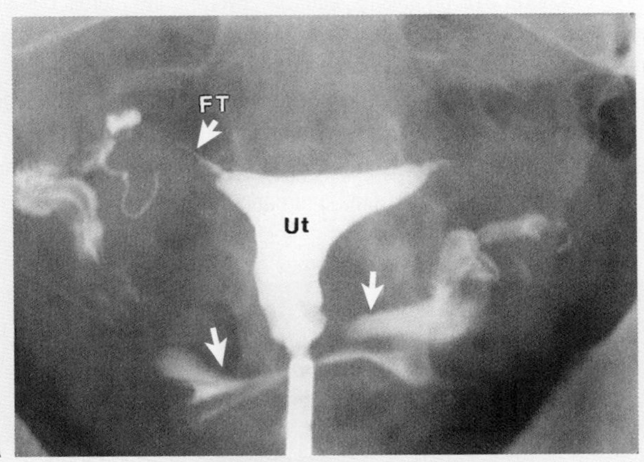

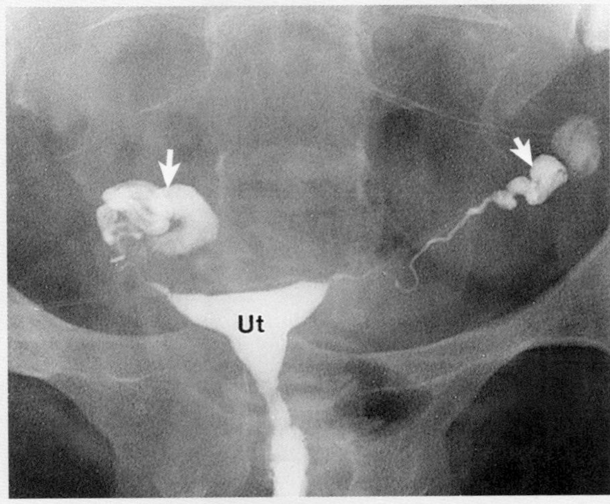

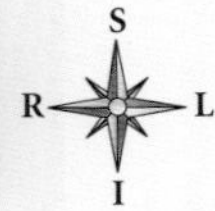

FIGURE 46-23 Hysterosalpingogram. A, Normal image. A tube is inserted in the uterine cervix, and contrast material has filled the uterus *(Ut)* and uterine (fallopian) tubes *(FT). Arrows* indicate contrast material that has flowed out into the peritoneal cavity, indicating that the tubes are not obstructed. **B,** Abnormal image. Contrast material fills the uterine cavity and tubes with no spill into the pelvis. *Arrows* point to the dilated ends of the uterine tubes (hydrosalpinx). Image confirms distal obstruction of the uterine tubes.

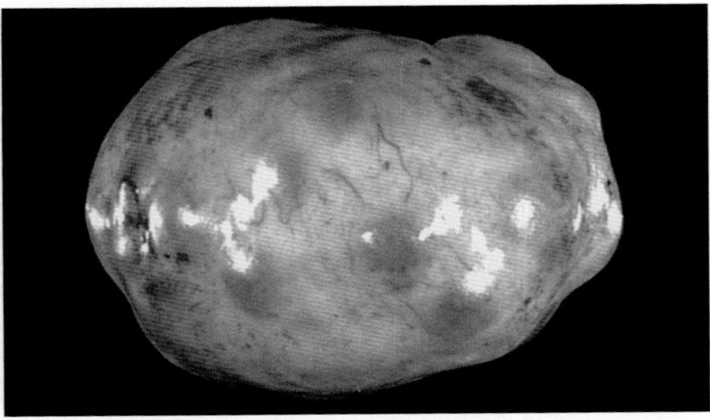

FIGURE 46-24 Polycystic ovary syndrome (PCOS). The ovary is studded with fluid-filled cysts developed from follicles that have failed to rupture.

Vaginitis is inflammation or infection of the vaginal lining. Vaginitis most often results from STDs or from a "yeast infection". So-called yeast infections are usually opportunistic infections of the fungus *Candida albicans,* producing **candidiasis**. Candidiasis infections are characterized by a whitish discharge—a symptom known as **leucorrhoea.**

Tumours and Related Conditions

Fibroid, myoma, and **fibromyoma** are all terms used to describe benign (noncancerous) tumours of uterine fibrous or smooth muscle tissue. Individual fibroids may occur, but multiple growths are not unusual. Fibroids are common in women during their reproductive years and develop most often in the myometrium of the uterine body and rarely in the cervix. The fact that they are seldom seen before puberty, increase in size during pregnancy, and tend to shrink in postmenopausal women suggests that age and oestrogen levels may play a role in their development. Fibroids range in size from small asymptomatic nodules to massive tumours that may be painful and exert pressure on other pelvic organs. Growth during pregnancy may result in placental haemorrhage or malpresentation of the fetus, complicating labour and delivery. In addition to pain, symptoms will vary depending on the size and location of the tumour. Even small tumours developing beneath the endometrium can cause severe haemorrhage (dysfunctional uterine bleeding, DUB). Tumour size, location, and severity of symptoms will determine treatment options. A technique similar to a heart catheterization, called *uterine artery embolization,* involves snaking a small catheter through an artery in the groin into the arterial vessel supplying blood to the fibroid. Tiny inert pellets are then injected into the artery, blocking the flow of blood. The procedure results in dramatic shrinkage of the treated fibroid and a reduction in symptoms, including haemorrhage. Surgical removal of individual fibroids or, in more severe cases, hysterectomy may be indicated.

Polycystic ovary syndrome (PCOS) is a condition that affects 10% of reproductive-age women but can also affect girls as young as 11 years old. It is characterized by enlarged ovaries that usually are studded with fluid-filled cysts about 0.5 to 1.5 cm in diameter (**Figure 46-24**). The cysts are found on both ovaries and develop from mature follicles that fail to rupture completely. Corpora lutea are generally absent. Women with PCOS often have numerous endocrine abnormalities, including high levels of androgens, infrequent menstrual cycles, and persistent anovulation. PCOS is the most common cause of female infertility.

Ovarian cysts are very common fluid-filled cysts that develop either from follicles that fail to rupture completely *(follicular cysts)* or from corpora lutea that fail to degenerate *(luteal cysts).* Most women develop a number of these cysts during their reproductive years and their presence does not constitute a diagnosis of polycystic ovary syndrome. Although ovarian cysts are often multiple, they rarely become dangerous. However, on occasion they may become quite large and painful, and may be diagnosed by palpation or ultrasonography. Luteal cysts are less common than follicular cysts but tend to cause more symptoms, such as pelvic pain and menstrual irregularities. Rarely, rupture of a large luteal cyst will result in internal bleeding that requires surgical intervention. The vast majority of all ovarian cysts will disappear within a few months of their appearance, most within 60 days.

Endometriosis is a benign but often painful condition that commonly affects the female reproductive tract. It is characterized by the presence of functioning endometrial tissue outside the uterus. The displaced endometrial tissue is most often found attached to an ovary or to the pelvic or abdominal organs and is occasionally found in other places throughout the body. Just how endometrial tissue spreads from the uterine cavity into the peritoneal cavity has not yet been determined. One theory suggests "retrograde menstruation" or backward movement of some endometrial tissue through the uterine tubes into the peritoneal cavity during the menstrual period. Although rare, the almost bizarre appearance of endometrial tissue in the lungs and lymph nodes has led some researchers to speculate that endometrial tissue "seeds" pass through vascular or lymphatic channels. Regardless of how the movement occurs, the development of endometriosis is a significant clinical condition that often causes infertility, dysmenorrhoea, and severe pain. Symptoms reflect the fact that displaced endometrial tissue reacts to ovarian hormones in the same way as the normal endometrium—exhibiting a cycle of growth and sloughing off. The disorder afflicts approximately 10% of women, a majority between 30 and 45 years of age.

Breast cancer, often a form of adenocarcinoma, is the most common cancer in the UK and affects approximately 55,000 women and 400 men every year. The incidence of breast cancer has risen over the past decade and is highest in people aged 85+. The incidence of this disease is projected to rise in the UK to 210 cases per 100,000 women by 2035. Fortunately, treatment of breast cancer is often successful if the cancerous tumour is detected early. Because such tumours are often painless, most physicians recommend monthly breast self-examinations and annual mammograms.

CONNECT IT!

Self-examination of breasts is a recommended routine to monitor breast health. Learn more in ***Breast Self-Examination*** online at ***Connect It!***

Treatments for breast cancer often involve surgery, chemotherapy, and radiation therapy. Surgeries can be very conservative, as with a simple lump removal or **lumpectomy.** If metastasis to surrounding tissue is suspected, a modified **radical mastectomy** may be performed. In this procedure the entire breast, with nearby lymph nodes, is removed. Just as lumpectomy results in less trauma than modified radical mastectomy, so-called *limited-field radiation* can provide effective treatment for clearly defined early-stage cancers that have not spread. It does so with shorter treatment cycles and fewer side effects than whole-breast radiation.

In the past, after women had completed their initial treatment for breast cancer they had few options available to lessen the possibility of recurrence. For a number of years the drug *tamoxifen* has been used extensively to prevent the recurrence of breast cancers fuelled by oestrogen. It does so by blocking the oestrogen receptor sites on the cancer cell membrane. Unfortunately, tamoxifen's effectiveness is limited to about 5 years. Another class of drugs called *aromatase inhibitors* (letrozole and others) are now being given to breast cancer patients to prevent recurrence of the disease. Instead of blocking oestrogen receptor sites, these drugs block oestrogen production. They may replace tamoxifen or be prescribed for use after 5 years of tamoxifen therapy. Other "rational" drugs such as trastuzumab are now being used to successfully manage recurring forms of breast cancer that in the past were very difficult to treat.

Cancer of the uterus can affect the body of the uterus or the cervix. Cancers of the uterine body most often involve the endometrium **(endometrial cancer)** and mostly affect women beyond childbearing years; a common symptom is postmenopausal uterine bleeding. Risk factors for this type of cancer include obesity, prolonged oestrogen therapy, and infertility. **Cervical cancer** occurs most often in women between the ages of 30 and 50 years. *Human papillomavirus (HPV)* infections, for which a vaccine is available, can cause cervical cancer. Cervical cancer is often diagnosed early, through screening tests such as the **Papanicolaou test (Pap smear)** (**Figure 46-25**). In this test, cells swabbed from the cervix are smeared on a glass slide, stained, and examined microscopically to determine whether any abnormalities exist. Because screening tests and other early detection methods have been so successful, the death rates for uterine cancers have dropped dramatically over the last few decades.

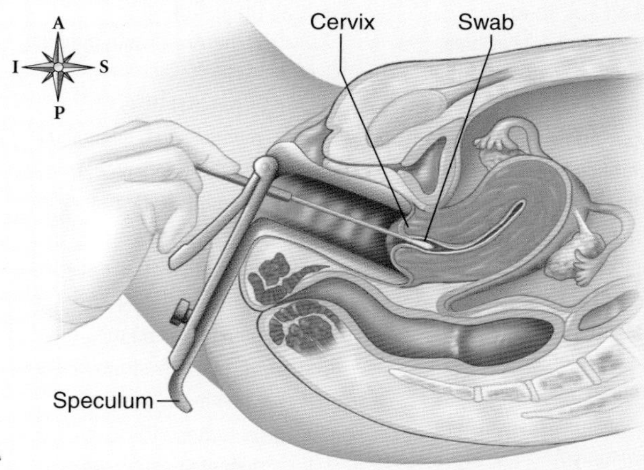

A

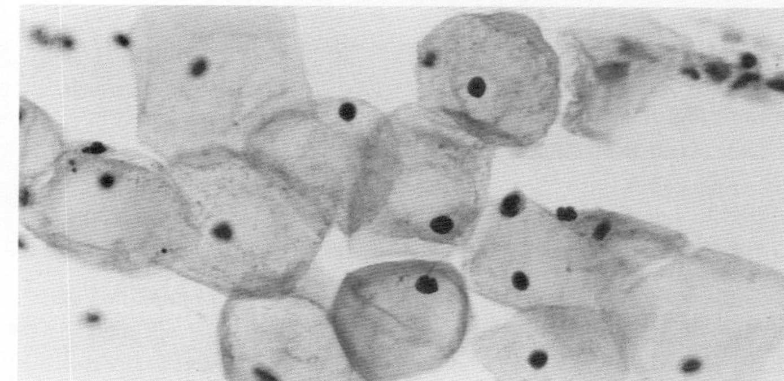

B

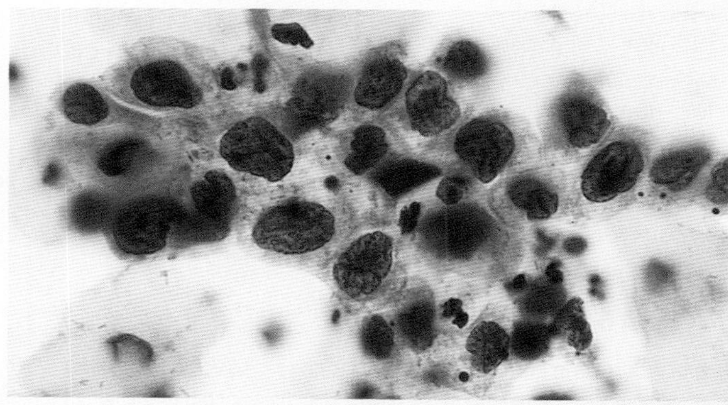

C

FIGURE 46-25 Papanicolaou (Pap) smear. A, Obtaining a Pap smear. **B,** Appearance of normal cervical epithelial cells in Pap smear. **C,** Appearance of cervical cancer cells in Pap smear. Note the reduction in cytoplasm and increased prominence of the nuclei compared with normal epithelial cells.

LANGUAGE OF SCIENCE (continued from p. 1057)

fimbria (FIM-bree-ah)
[*fimbria* **fringe**] *pl.*, fimbriae

follicle-stimulating hormone (FSH)
(FOL-ih-kul-STIM-yoo-lay-ting HOR-mohn)
[*foll-* **bag,** *-icle* **little,** *hormon-* **excite**]

follicular phase (foh-LIK-yoo-lar fayz)
[*foll-* **bag,** *-icul-* **little,** *-ar* **relating to**]

fundus (FUN-duss)
[*fundus* **bottom**] *pl.*, fundi

graafian follicle
(GRAH-fee-en FOL-ih-kul)
[*Reijnier de Graaf* **Dutch physician,** *-an* **relating to,** *foll-* **bag,** *-icle* **little**]

greater vestibular gland
(ves-TIB-yoo-lar)
[*vestibul-* **entrance hall,** *-ar* **relating to,** *gland* **acorn**]

hymen (HYE-men)
[*hymen* **membrane**]

imperforate hymen
(im-PER-fah-rayt HYE-men)
[*im-* **not,** *-perfor-* **pierce,** *-ate* **state,** *hymen* **membrane**]

infundibulum (in-fun-DIB-yoo-lum)
[*infundibulum* **funnel**]

internal os
[*intern-* **inside,** *-al* **relating to,** *os* **mouth or opening**] *pl.*, ora

isthmus (ISS-muss)
[*isthmus* **narrow connection or passage**]

labia majora
(LAY-bee-ah mah-JOH-rah)
[*labia* **lips,** *majora* **large**] *sing.*, labium majus

labia minora (LAY-bee-ah mih-NO-rah)
[*labia* **lips,** *minora* **small**] *sing.*, labium minor

lactation (lak-TAY-shun)
[*lact-* **milk,** *-ation* **process**]

lesser vestibular gland
(ves-TIB-yoo-lar)
[*vestibul-* **entrance hall,** *-ar* **relating to,** *gland* **acorn**]

luteal phase (LOO-tee-al fayz)
[*lute-* **yellow,** *-al* **relating to**]

luteinization (loo-tee-in-ih-ZAY-shun)
[*lute-* **yellow,** *-ization* **process**]

luteinizing hormone (LH)
(loo-tee-in-EYE-zing HOR-mohn)
[*lute-* **yellow,** *-izing* **process,** *hormon-* **excite**]

mammary gland (MAM-mah-ree)
[*mamma-* **breast,** *-ry* **relating to,** *gland* **acorn**]

medulla (meh-DUL-ah)
[*medulla* **marrow or pith (middle)**] *pl.*, medullae or medullas

menarche (meh-NAR-kee)
[*men-* **month,** *-arche* **beginning**]

menopause (MEN-oh-pawz)
[*meno-* **month,** *-paus-* **cease**]

menses (MEN-seez)
[*menses* **months**] *pl.*, menses

menstrual period (MEN-stroo-al)
[*mens-* **month,** *-al* **relating to**]

menstruation (men-stroo-AY-shun)
[*mens-* **month,** *-ation* **process**]

mons pubis (monz PYOO-bis)
[*mons* **mountain,** *pubis* **groin**] *pl.*, montes pubis

myometrium (my-oh-MEE-tree-um)
[*myo-* **muscle,** *-metr-* **womb,** *-um* **thing**]

nipple (NIP-el)
[*nip-* **beak,** *-le* **small**]

oestrogenic phase (es-troh-JEN-ik fayz)
[*oestro-* **frenzy,** *-gen-* **produce,** *-ic* **relating to**]

oogonium (oh-oh-GO-nee-um)
[*oo-* **egg,** *-gon-* **offspring,** *-um* **thing**] *pl.*, oogonia

ovarian cortex
(oh-VAIR-ee-an KOHR-teks)
[*ov-* **egg,** *-arian* **relating to,** *cortex* **bark**] *pl.*, cortices

ovarian follicle
(oh-VAIR-ee-an FOL-ih-kul)
[*ov-* **egg,** *-arian* **relating to,** *foll-* **bag,** *-icle* **little**]

ovarian medulla
(oh-VAIR-ee-an meh-DUL-ah)
[*ov-* **egg,** *-arian* **relating to,** *medulla* **marrow or pith (middle)**] *pl.*, medullae or medullas

ovary (OH-var-ee)
[*ov-* **egg,** *-ar-* **relating to,** *-y* **location of process**]

ovulation (ov-yoo-LAY-shun)
[*ov-* **egg,** *-ation* **process**]

ovum (OH-vum)
[*ovum* **egg**] *pl.*, ova

perimetrium (pair-ih-MEE-tree-um)
[*peri-* **around,** *-metr-* **womb,** *-um* **thing**]

perineal body (pair-ih-NEE-al)
[*peri-* **around,** *-ine-* **excrete (perineum),** *-al* **relating to**]

posterior fornix
(pohs-teer-ee-or FOR-niks)
[*poster-* **behind,** *-or* **quality,** *fornix* **arch**]

posterior ligament
(pohs-TEER-ee-or LIG-ah-ment)
[*poster-* **behind,** *-or* **quality,** *liga-* **bind,** *-ment* **condition**]

postmenstrual phase
(post-MEN-stroo-al fayz)
[*post-* **after,** *-mens-* **month,** *-al* **relating to**]

postovulatory phase
(post-ov-yoo-lah-TOR-ee fayz)
[*post-* **after,** *-ov-* **egg,** *-ory* **relating to**]

premenstrual phase
(pree-MEN-stroo-al fayz)
[*pre-* **before,** *-mens-* **month,** *-al* **relating to**]

preovulatory phase
(pree-ov-yoo-lah-TOR-ee fayz)
[*pre-* **before,** *-ov-* **egg,** *-ory* **relating to**]

progesterone (pro-JES-ter-ohn)
[*pro-* **before,** *-gester-* **bearing (pregnancy),** *-stero-* **solid or steroid derivative,** *-one* **chemical**]

progesterone phase
(proh-JES-ter-ohn fayz)
[*pro-* **before,** *-gester-* **bearing (pregnancy),** *-stero-* **solid or steroid derivative,** *-one* **chemical**]

proliferative phase
(proh-LIF-er-ah-tiv fayz)
[*proli-* **offspring,** *-fer-* **bear or carry,** *-at-* **process,** *-ive* **relating to**]

rectouterine pouch (of Douglas)
(rek-toh-YOO-ter-in)
[*recto-* **straight,** *-uter-* **womb,** *-ine* **relating to,** *James Douglas* **Scots anatomist**]

round ligament (LIG-ah-ment)
[*liga-* **bind,** *-ment* **condition**]

secretory phase
(SEEK-reh-toh-ree fayz)
[*secret-* **separate,** *-ory* **relating to**]

spinnbarkeit (SPIN-bahr-kyte)
[*spinnbarkeit* **spinnability (German)**]

urogenital triangle
(yoor-oh-GEN-ih-tal)
[*uro-* **urine,** *-gen-* **produce,** *-al* **relating to**]

uterine tube (YOO-ter-in tyoob)
[*uter-* **womb,** *-ine* **relating to**]

uterosacral ligament
(yoo-ter-oh-SAK-ral LIG-ah-ment)
[*uter-* **womb,** *sacr-* **sacred (sacrum),** *-al* **relating to,** *liga-* **bind,** *-ment* **condition**]

uterus (YOO-ter-us)
[*uterus* **womb**]

vagina (vah-JYE-nah)
[*vagina* **sheath**]

vaginal orifice (VAH-jih-nal OR-ih-fis)
[*vagina-* **sheath,** *-al* **relating to,** *ori-* **mouth,** *-fice-* **something made**]

vesicouterine pouch
(ves-ih-koh-YOO-ter-in)
[*vesic-* **blister,** *-uter-* **womb,** *-ine* **relating to**]

vestibule (VES-tih-byool)
[*vestibul-* **entrance hall**]

vulva (VUL-vah)
[*vulva* **wrapper**]

LANGUAGE OF MEDICINE

amenorrhoea (ah-men-oh-REE-ah)
[*a-* **without,** *-meno-* **month,** *-rrhoea* **flow**]

breast cancer
[*cancer* **crab or malignant tumour**]

cancer of the uterus
[*cancer* **crab or malignant tumour**]

candidiasis (kan-dih-DYE-eh-sis)
[*candid-* **white,** *-asis* **condition**]

cervical cancer (SER-vih-kal)
[*cervic-* **neck,** *-al* **relating to,** *cancer* **crab or malignant tumour**]

dysfunctional uterine bleeding (DUB)
(dis-FUNK-shun-al YOO-ter-in)
[*dys-* **difficult,** *-function-* **performance,** *-al* **relating to,** *uter-* **womb,** *-ine* **relating to**]

dysmenorrhoea (dis-men-oh-REE-ah)
[*dys-* **painful,** *-meno-* **month,** *-rrhoea* **flow**]

ectopic pregnancy (ek-TOP-ik)
[*ec-* **out of,** *-top-* **place,** *-ic* **relating to**]

endometrial cancer
(en-doh-MEE-tree-al KAN-ser)
[*endo-* **within,** *-metr-* **womb,** *-al* **relating to,** *cancer* **crab or malignant tumour**]

endometriosis
(en-doh-mee-tree-OH-sis)
[*endo-* **within,** *-metri-* **womb,** *-osis* **condition**]

episiotomy (eh-piz-ee-OT-oh-mee)
[*episio-* **vulva,** *-tom-* **cut,** *-y* **action**]

fibroid (FYE-broyd)
[*fibr-* **thread or fibre,** *-oid* **of or like**]

fibromyoma (fye-broh-my-OH-mah)
[*fibro-* **thread or fibre,** *-my-* **muscle,** *-oma* **tumour**]

hydrosalpinx (hye-droh-SAL-pinks)
[*hydro-* **water,** *-salpinx* **tube**]
pl., hydrosalpinges

hysterosalpingogram
(his-ter-oh-sal-PING-go-gram)
[*hystero-* **uterus,** *-salping-* **tube,** *-gram* **drawing**]

intrauterine device (IUD)
(in-trah-YOU-ter-in)
[*intra-* **inside or within,** *-uter-* **womb,** *-ine* **relating to**]

in vitro fertilization (IVF)
(in VEE-troh FER-tih-lih-ZAY-shun)
[*in* **within,** *vitro* **glass,** *fertil-* **fruitful,** *-iz-* **action,** *-ation* **process**]

infertility (in-fer-TIL-ih-tee)
[*in-* **not,** *-fertil-* **fruitful,** *-ity* **state**]

leucorrhoea (loo-koh-REE-ah)
[*leuco-* **white,** *-rrhoea* **flow**]

lumpectomy (lump-EK-toh-mee)
[*lump-* **mass,** *-ec-* **out,** *-tom-* **cut,** *-y* **action**]

menotropin (men-oh-TROHP-in)
[*meno-* **month,** *-trop-* **turn or change,** *-in* **substance**]

mittelschmerz (MIT-el-schmertz)
[*mittel-* **middle,** *-schmerz* **pain**]

myoma (my-OH-mah)
[*my-* **muscle,** *-oma* **tumour**]

oral contraceptive (kon-tra-SEP-tiv)
[*contra-* **against,** *-cept-* **take or receive (conception),** *-ive* **agent**]

ovarian cancer (oh-VAIR-ee-an)
[*ov-* **egg,** *-arian* **relating to,** *cancer* **crab or malignant tumour**]

ovarian cyst (oh-VAIR-ee-an SIST)
[*ov-* **egg,** *-arian* **relating to,** *cyst-* **bag**]

Papanicolaou test (Pap smear)
(pah-peh-nih-koh-LAH-oo)
[*George N. Papanicolaou* **Greek physician**]

pelvic inflammatory disease (PID)
(PEL-vik in-FLAM-ah-tor-ee)
[*pelv-* **basin,** *-ic* **relating to,** *inflam-* **set afire,** *-ory* **relating to**]

peritonitis (pair-ih-toh-NYE-tis)
[*peri-* **around,** *-ton-* **stretch (peritoneum),** *-itis* **inflammation**]

polycystic ovary syndrome (PCOS)
(pol-ee-SIS-tik OH-var-ee)
[*poly-* **many,** *-cyst-* **bag,** *-ic* **relating to,** *ov-* **egg,** *-ar-* **relating to,** *-y* **location of process**]

premenstrual syndrome (PMS)
(pree-MEN-stroo-all SIN-drohm)
[*pre-* **before,** *-mens-* **month,** *-al* **relating to,** *syn-* **together,** *-drome* **running or (race) course**]

radical mastectomy
(RAD-ih-kal mas-TEK-toh-mee)
[*radic-* **root,** *-al* **relating to,** *mast-* **breast,** *-ec-* **out,** *-tom-* **cut,** *-y* **action**]

salpingitis (sal-pin-JYE-tis)
[*salping-* **tube,** *-itis* **inflammation**]

supraovulation
(soo-prah-ov-yoo-LAY-shun)
[*supra-* **above or over,** *-ov-* **egg,** *-ation* **process**]

transabdominal pelvic ultrasound
(tranz-ab-DOM-ih-nal PEL-vik UL-trah-sound)
[*trans-* **across,** *-abdomin-* **belly,** *-al* **relating to,** *pelv-* **basin (pelvis),** *-ic* **relating to,** *ultra-* **beyond, sound**]

uterine fibroid (YOO-ter-in FYE-broyd)
[*uter-* **womb,** *-ine* **relating to,** *fibr-* **thread or fibre,** *-oid* **of or like**]

vaginitis (vaj-ih-NYE-tis)
[*vagin-* **sheath (vagina),** *-itis* **inflammation**]

case study

David, a professional cyclist, and his wife Karen had been trying for two years to start a family with no success. After a visit to an infertility specialist, they found that David had a low sperm count. However, before coming to a diagnosis, the specialist also needed to check Karen's reproductive system, and he recommended she should undergo hysterosalpingography to confirm patency of her uterine tubes.

1. Assuming no obstruction, which areas should the dye used to make the hysterosalpingogram enter?
   a. Cervix, uterus, uterine tube, ovaries
   b. Cervix, uterine tube, uterus, vulva
   c. Cervix, uterine tube, ovaries, peritoneal cavity
   d. Cervix, uterus, uterine tube, peritoneal cavity

Finding no blockage in Karen's uterine tubes, the infertility specialist recommended intrauterine insemination. To increase the chances of a sperm encountering an egg, a medication called clomifene was prescribed for Karen. Clomifene works as an anti-oestrogenic agent, causing the body to perceive low oestrogen levels; it is given on days 5 to 10 of the menstrual cycle.

2. What effect will clomifene have on FSH production?
   a. Increase in FSH production
   b. Decrease FSH production
   c. No change in FSH production
   d. A slight increase in FSH production followed by a sharp decrease

3. After ovulation, the follicular cells transform into what?
   a. Corpus lucidum
   b. Corpus luteum
   c. Corpus rubrum
   d. Corpus albicans

4. Where in the female reproductive tract does fertilization normally take place?
   a. In the cervix
   b. In the uterus
   c. In the uterine tubes
   d. In the ovaries

Hint To solve a case study, you may have to refer to the glossary or index, other chapters in this textbook, ***Connect It!,*** and other resources.

CHAPTER SUMMARY

To download an MP3 version of the chapter summary for use with your mobile device, access the ***Audio Chapter Summaries*** *online at evolve.elsevier.com.*

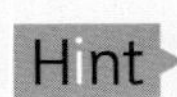

Scan this summary after reading the chapter to help you reinforce the key concepts. Later, use the summary as a quick review before your class or before a test.

Overview of the Female Reproductive System

A. Function of the female reproductive system
  1. To produce offspring and thereby ensure continuity of the genetic code
  2. To produce eggs, or female gametes, each of which has the potential to unite with a male gamete to form the first cell of an offspring
  3. To provide nutrition and protection to the offspring for up to several years after conception

B. Structural plan of the female reproductive system
  1. Reproductive organs are classified as essential or accessory (**Figure 46-1**)
     a. Essential organs—gonads are the paired ovaries; gametes are ova produced by the ovaries—the ovaries are also internal genitals
     b. Accessory organs
        (1) Internal genitals—uterine tubes, uterus, and vagina—ducts or duct structures that extend from the ovaries to the exterior
        (2) External genitals—the vulva
        (3) Additional sex glands such as the mammary glands

C. Perineum (**Figure 46-2**)
  1. Skin-covered region between the vaginal orifice and the rectum
  2. Area that may be torn during childbirth

Ovaries

A. Location of the ovaries
  1. Nodular glands located on each side of the uterus, below and behind the uterine tubes (**Figure 46-3**)
  2. Ectopic pregnancy—development of the fetus in a place other than the uterus

B. Microscopic structure of the ovaries (**Figure 46-4**)
  1. Surface of the ovaries is covered by the germinal epithelium
  2. Ovarian follicles contain the developing female sex cells
  3. Ovum—an oocyte released from the ovary

C. Functions of the ovaries
  1. Ovaries produce ova—the female gametes
  2. Oogenesis—process that results in formation of a mature egg (**Figure 46-5**)
  3. Ovaries are endocrine organs that secrete the female sex hormones (oestrogens and progesterone)

Uterus

A. Structure of the uterus (**Figure 46-3**)
  1. Size and shape of the uterus
     a. Pear-shaped structure with two main parts—the cervix and the body
     b. Bulging upper part of the body called the fundus
  2. Location of the uterus
     a. Located in the pelvic cavity between the urinary bladder and the rectum (**Figure 46-1**)
     b. Uterus position (**Figure 46-6**) is altered by age, pregnancy, and distention of related pelvic viscera
     c. Uterus descends, between birth and puberty, from the lower abdomen to the true pelvis
     d. Uterus begins to decrease in size at menopause
  3. Position of the uterus
     a. Body lies flexed over the bladder
     b. Cervix points downward and backward, joining the vagina at a right angle
     c. Several ligaments hold the uterus in place but allow some movement
  4. Wall of the uterus—composed of three layers—the inner endometrium (mucous membrane), the middle myometrium (smooth muscle), and the perimetrium (outer serous incomplete layer of visceral peritoneum)
  5. Cavities of the uterus—small because of the thickness of the uterine walls
     a. The body cavity's apex constitutes the internal os and opens into the cervical canal
     b. Cervical canal is constricted at its lower end and forms the external os that opens into the vagina
  6. Blood supply of the uterus—supplied by uterine arteries

B. Functions of the uterus
  1. Uterus is part of the reproductive tract and permits sperm to ascend toward the uterine tubes
  2. If conception occurs, an offspring develops in the uterus
     a. Embryo is supplied with nutrients by endometrial glands until the production of the placenta
     b. Placenta is an organ that permits the exchange of materials between the mother's blood and the fetal blood but keeps the two circulations separate
     c. Myometrial contractions occur during labour and help push the offspring out of the mother's body
  3. If conception does not occur, outer layers of endometrium are shed during menstruation—a cyclical event that allows the endometrium to renew itself

Uterine Tubes

A. Uterine tubes also called fallopian tubes, or oviducts

B. Location of uterine tubes
  1. Attached to the uterus at its upper outer angles
  2. Extend upward and outward toward the sides of the pelvis and then curve downward and backward

C. Structure of the uterine tubes
   1. Uterine tubes consist of mucous membrane, smooth muscle, and serous lining (**Figure 46-7**)
   2. Mucosal lining is directly continuous with the peritoneum lining the pelvic cavity
      a. Tubal mucosa is continuous with that of the vagina and uterus, which means it may become infected with organisms introduced into the vagina and thereby cause salpingitis or peritonitis
      b. Inflammation of uterine tubes may lead to scarring and partial or complete closure of the lumen
   3. Each uterine tube has three divisions: isthmus, ampulla, and infundibulum

D. Function of the uterine tubes—serve as transport channels for ova and as the site of fertilization (**Figure 46-8**)

Vagina

A. Location of the vagina—a tubular organ located between the rectum, urethra, and bladder

B. Structure of the vagina
   1. A collapsible tube capable of distention, composed of smooth muscle, and lined with mucous membrane arranged in rugae
   2. Anterior wall shorter than the posterior wall because the cervix protrudes into its uppermost portion
   3. Hymen—a mucous membrane that typically forms a border around the vagina in young premenstrual girls

C. Functions of the vagina
   1. Lining of the vagina lubricates and stimulates the penis during sexual intercourse and acts as a receptacle for semen
   2. Vagina is the lower portion of the birth canal
   3. Vagina transports tissue and blood shed during menstruation to the exterior

Vulva

A. Structure of the vulva (pudendum; the female external genitals)—mons pubis, labia majora, labia minora, clitoris, urinary meatus, vaginal orifice, and greater vestibular glands (**Figure 46-9**)

B. Functions of the vulva
   1. Mons pubis and labia protect the clitoris and vestibule
   2. Clitoris contains sensory receptors that send information to the sexual response area of the brain (**Figure 46-10**)
   3. Vaginal orifice is the boundary between the internal and external genitals

Female Reproductive Cycles

A. Female reproductive system has many cyclical, recurring changes that start with the beginning of menses
   1. Ovarian cycle
      a. Ovaries at time of birth contain oocytes in primary follicles in which the meiotic process has been suspended
      b. After puberty, about 20 or so of the oocytes resume meiosis each day; most of these will undergo atresia (degeneration) and disappear
      c. Meiosis will stop again just before an ovum (usually just one) is released during ovulation (**Figures 46-11** and **46-12**)
   2. Menstrual cycle (endometrial cycle) is divided into four phases
      a. Menses
      b. Postmenstrual phase
      c. Ovulation
      d. Premenstrual phase
   3. Myometrial cycle
   4. Gonadotropic cycle

B. Control of female reproductive cycles
   1. Hormones control cyclical changes
   2. Cyclical changes in the ovaries result from changes in the gonadotropins secreted by the pituitary gland (**Figures 46-13** and **46-14**)
   3. Cyclical changes in the uterus are caused by changes in oestrogens and progesterone (**Figure 46-15**)
   4. Low levels of FSH and LH cause regression of the corpus luteum if pregnancy does not occur; this causes a decrease in oestrogen and progesterone, which triggers endometrial sloughing of the menstrual phase
   5. Control of cyclical changes in gonadotropin secretion is caused by positive and negative feedback mechanisms and involves oestrogens, progesterone, and secretion of releasing hormones by the hypothalamus

C. Importance of the female reproductive cycles
   1. Ovarian cycle
      a. Primary function is to produce ova at regular intervals
      b. Secondary function is to regulate the endometrial cycle through oestrogen and progesterone
   2. Endometrial cycle—functions to make the uterus suitable for implantation of a new offspring
   3. Cyclical nature of the reproductive system and the fact that fertilization will occur within 24 hours after ovulation mean that a woman is fertile for only a few days of each month

D. Infertility—failure to conceive after 1 year of regular unprotected intercourse
   1. Causes are varied and can involve either or both partners
   2. Fertility drugs and other assisted reproductive procedures such as IVF (in vitro fertilization) are available

E. Menstrual flow begins at puberty, and the menstrual cycle continues for about 3 decades (**Figure 46-16**)

Breasts

A. Location and size of the breasts
   1. Breasts lie over the pectoral muscles
   2. Oestrogens and progesterone control breast development
   3. Breast size is determined by the amount of fat around glandular tissue (**Figure 46-17**)

4. Alveoli of the mammary gland produce milk (**Figure 46-18**), and a system of lactiferous ducts carries it to the nipple (**Figure 46-19**), surrounded by an areola

B. Structure of the breasts
   1. Each consists of several lobes separated by septa of connective tissue
   2. Lobes consist of several lobules, composed of connective tissue embedded with pouches of milk-secreting cells (alveoli)
   3. Lactiferous duct from each lobe converges toward nipple
   4. Suspensory ligaments help support the breast

C. Function of the breasts
   1. Function of mammary glands is lactation
   2. Mechanism controlling lactation (**Figure 46-20**)
      a. Ovarian hormones make the breasts structurally ready to produce milk
      b. Shedding of the placenta results in a decrease of oestrogens and thus stimulates prolactin
      c. Prolactin stimulates lactation
      d. Additional hormones (e.g., oxytocin) also support lactation (**Table 46-2**)
   3. Importance of lactation
      a. Can provide nutrient-rich milk to offspring for up to several years from birth
      b. Some advantages of breast milk
         (1) Nutrients
         (2) Passive immunity from antibodies present in the colostrum and milk
         (3) Emotional bonding between mother and child

Cycle of Life: Female Reproductive System

A. Unlike other systems, the female reproductive system does not begin to perform its functions until the teenage years (puberty) and ceases its principal function in middle adulthood.

B. Female organs begin their initial stages of development in the womb with the full development of the reproductive organs resuming during puberty

C. Reproductive function continues until menopause

The Big Picture: Female Reproductive System and the Whole Body

A. Reproductive system imparts immortality to genes and ensures survival of the species

B. Relationship of the female reproductive system with other body systems
   1. Close proximity to the urinary system; share a common structure: the vulva
   2. Anatomical relationship with the skeletal muscles in the perineum
   3. Breasts are actually modifications of the skin in the integumentary system

REVIEW QUESTIONS

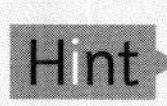

Write out the answers to these questions after reading the chapter and reviewing the Chapter Summary. Note—writing out your answers will consolidate learning and provide a valuable resource of information.

1. Create a table identifying the essential and accessory organs in the female reproductive system.
2. Describe the three layers that compose the wall of the uterus.
3. Identify the vessels that supply blood to the uterus.
4. List the eight ligaments that hold the uterus in a normal position.
5. How does the uterus serve as part of the female reproductive tract?
6. What and where are the uterine tubes? Approximately how long are they? What lines the uterine tubes? Their lining is continuous on their distal ends with what? With what on their proximal ends?
7. Trace the development of a female sex cell from its most primitive state through ovulation.
8. What hormones are secreted by the cells in ovarian tissue?
9. List all vaginal functions.
10. List all the structures that make up the female external genitals.
11. Define the term *episiotomy*.
12. Identify the advantages that nursing from the mother's breast provides offspring.
13. What method makes it possible to measure blood levels of gonadotropins?
14. Describe the hormonal changes during menopause.
15. Define the term *mittelschmerz*.

CRITICAL THINKING QUESTIONS

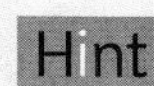

After finishing the Review Questions, write out the answers to these more in-depth questions to help you apply your new knowledge. Go back to sections of the chapter that relate to concepts that you find difficult.

1. Name and explain the function of the various hormones that regulate lactation. Where are they produced, and how would you summarize their function and their influence on lactation?
2. List the phases of the menstrual cycle. Which of these phases shows the most variance in length of time? How do the events in each phase contribute to the overall function of the reproductive system?
3. Explain the interaction of the hormones that result in ovulation. From what is the name "luteinizing" hormone derived?
4. State in your own words the control of cyclical ovarian changes brought on by FSH and LH.
5. Explain, in your own words, the control of cyclical uterine changes brought on by the ovarian hormones. The drop in the level of these hormones triggers what event?
6. Regarding hormone functions, what is the reason contraceptive pills and implants are effective in preventing pregnancy?
7. Correlate the events of the ovarian cycle with the events of the uterine cycle.
8. Female athletes may experience an undesirable condition called *amenorrhoea*. What evidence can you find to support this statement?
9. It is not uncommon for women with eating disorders, such as anorexia, to develop amenorrhoea. Explain the link between these two conditions.

47 Growth, Development, and Ageing

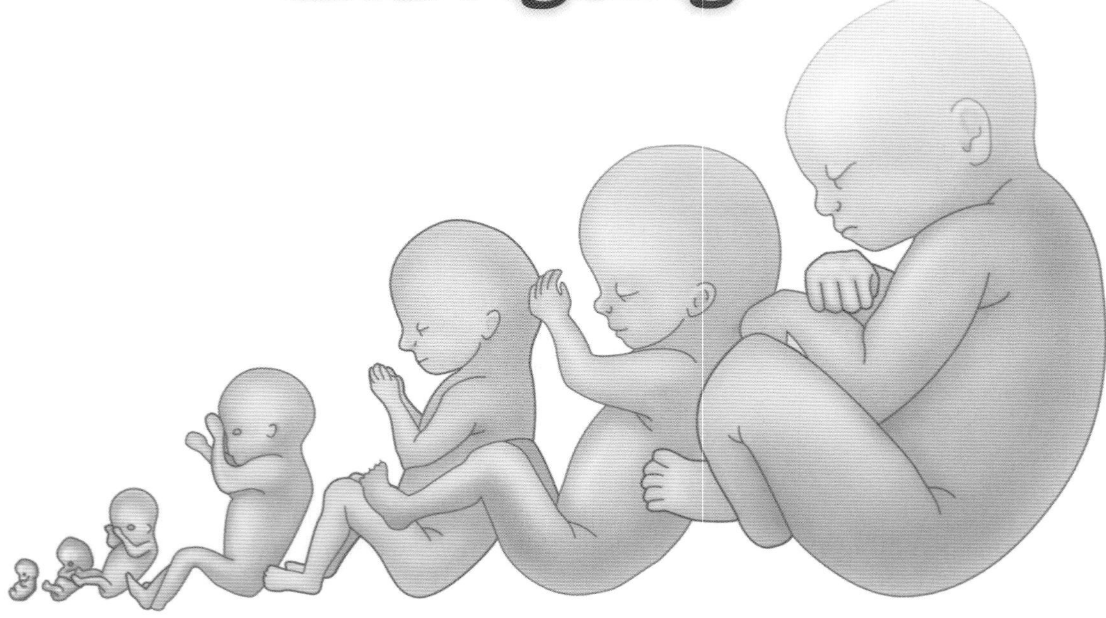

CHAPTER OUTLINE

Hint *Scan this outline before you begin to read the chapter, as a preview of how the concepts are organized.*

LANGUAGE OF SCIENCE

Hint *Use this list to aid your pronunciation of unfamiliar words.*

acrosome reaction (AK-roh-sohm)
[*acro-* **top or tip,** *-some* **body**]

adolescence (ad-oh-LESS-ens)
[*adolesc-* **grow up,** *-ence* **state**]

amniotic cavity
(am-nee-OT-ik KAV-ih-tee)
[*amnio-* **fetal membrane,** *-ic* **relating to,** *cav-* **hollow,** *-ity* **state**]

blastocyst (BLASS-toh-sist)
[*blasto-* **bud,** *-cyst* **pouch**]

chorion (KOH-ree-on)
[*chorion* **skin**]

corona radiata
(ko-ROHN-ah ray-dee-AH-tah)
[*corona* **crown,** *radiata* **radiant (with rays)**]

diploid (DIP-loyd)
[*diplo-* **twofold,** *-oid* **of or like**]

ectoderm (EK-toh-derm)
[*ecto-* **outside,** *-derm* **skin**]

endoderm (EN-doh-derm)
[*endo-* **within,** *-derm* **skin**]

fertilization (FER-tih-lih-ZAY-shun)
[*fertil-* **fruitful,** *-ation* **process**]

first polar body
[*pol-* **pole,** *-ar* **relating to**]

fraternal twin
[*frater-* **brother,** *-al* **relating to,** *twin* **twofold**]

gestation period (jes-TAY-shun)
[*gesta-* **bear,** *-tion* **process**]

granulosa cell (gran-yoo-LOH-sah)
[*gran-* **grain,** *-ul-* **little,** *-os-* **relating to,** *-a* **thing,** *cell* **storeroom**]

haploid (HAP-loyd)
[*haplo-* **single,** *-oid* **of or like**]

histogenesis (hiss-toh-JEN-eh-sis)
[*histo-* **tissue,** *-gen-* **produce,** *-esis* **process**]

human chorionic gonadotropin (hCG)
(koh-ree-ON-ik go-nah-doh-TROH-pin)
[*chorion-* **skin,** *-ic* **relating to,** *gon-* **offspring,** *-ad-* **relating to,** *-trop-* **nourishment,** *-in* **substance**]

implantation (im-plan-TAY-shun)
[*im-* **in,** *-planta-* **set or place,** *-ation* **process**]

infancy
[*infan-* **unable to speak,** *-y* **state**]

continued on p. 1120

Many of your fondest and most vivid memories are probably associated with your birthdays. The day of birth is an important milestone of life. Most people continue to remember their birthday in some special way each year; birthdays are pleasant and convenient reference points to mark periods of transition or change in our lives. The actual day of birth marks the end of one phase of development called the **prenatal period** and the beginning of a second called the **postnatal period.** The prenatal period begins at conception and ends at birth; the postnatal period begins at birth and continues until death. Although important periods in our lives such as childhood and adolescence often are remembered as a series of individual and isolated events, they are in reality part of an ongoing and continuous process. In reviewing the field of human developmental biology—study of the many changes that occur during the cycle of life from conception to death—it is often convenient to isolate certain periods such as infancy or old age for study. However, the life cycle is not a series of stop-and-start events or individual and isolated periods of time. Instead, it is a biological process that is characterized by continuous modification and change.

This chapter discusses some of the basic concepts of important events and changes that occur in the ongoing development of the individual from conception to death. Study of development during the prenatal period is followed by a review of changes occurring during infancy and adulthood, and finally, by some of the more important changes that occur in the individual organ systems of the body as a result of ageing.

HUMAN REPRODUCTION

Production of Sex Cells

Before a new human life can begin, some preliminary processes must occur. Of utmost importance is the production of mature *gametes*, or sex cells, by each parent. Spermatozoa, gametes of the male parent, are produced by a process called **spermatogenesis.** Ova, gametes of the female parent, are produced by a process called **oogenesis.**

Meiosis

Both types of gamete production require a special form of cell division characterized by **meiosis.** Recall from Chapter 7 that meiosis is the orderly arrangement and distribution of chromosomes that, unlike *mitosis*, reduces the number of chromosomes in each daughter cell to half the number present in the parent cell.

The necessity for chromosome reduction as a preliminary step to union of the sex cells is explained by the fact that the cells of each species of living organisms contain a specific number of chromosomes. Human cells, for example, contain 23 pairs, or a total of 46 chromosomes. This total of 46 chromosomes per body cell is known as the **diploid** number of chromosomes. Diploid comes from the Greek *diploos*, meaning "twofold". If the male and female cells united without first halving their respective chromosomes, the resulting cell would contain twice as many chromosomes as is normal for human beings. Mature ova and sperm therefore contain only 23 chromosomes, or half as many, as other human cells. This total of 23 chromosomes per sex cell is known as the **haploid** number of chromosomes (from the Greek *haploos*, meaning "single").

Meiotic division consists of two cell divisions that take place one after the other in succession. They are referred to as meiotic division I and meiotic division II, and in both, prophase, metaphase, anaphase, and telophase occur (**Figure 47-1**).

In the interphase that precedes prophase I (of meiotic division I) the same events occur as take place in the interphase preceding mitotic division. Specifically, each DNA molecule replicates and thereby becomes a pair of chromatids, attached to each other only at the centromere. The term *chromosome* applies to any condensed chromatin with its own centromere. For simplicity's sake, in both **Figure 47-1** and **Figure 47-2**, only 4 of the 46 chromosomes are shown. Notice that early in meiosis I, homologous pairs of chromosomes are moved together to form groupings called *tetrads*. During anaphase I the tetrads split (recall that in mitosis it is the chromosomes that split during anaphase).

In meiosis I the phenomenon of *crossing over* occurs. During crossing over a chromatid segment of each chromosome crosses over and becomes part of the adjacent chromosome in the pair (see **Figure 48-4** on p. 1131). This is a highly significant event and is discussed in some detail in the next chapter. Because each chromatid segment consists of specific genes, the crossing over of chromatids reshuffles the genes—that is, it transfers some of them from one chromosome to another. This exchange of genetic material can add almost infinite variety to the ultimate genetic makeup of an individual.

Metaphase I follows the last stage of prophase I, and as in mitosis, the chromosomes align themselves along the equator of the spindle fibres, as **Figure 47-1** shows. But in anaphase I the two chromatids that make up each chromosome do not separate from each other as they do in mitosis to form two new chromosomes out of each original one. In anaphase I, only one of each pair of chromosomes moves to each pole of the parent cell.

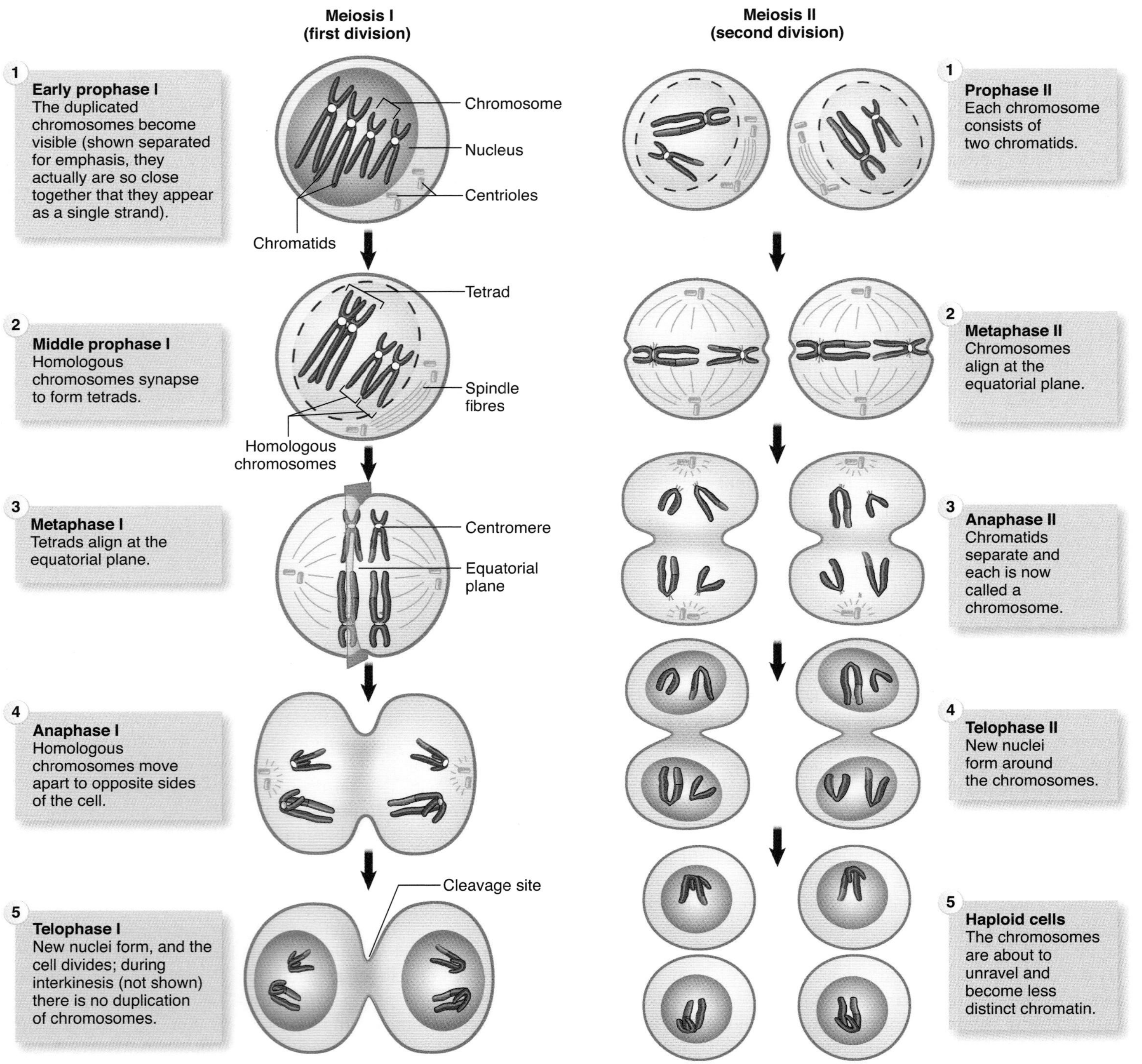

Meiosis I
(first division)
Meiosis II
(second division)
1
Early prophase I
The duplicated chromosomes become visible (shown separated for emphasis, they actually are so close together that they appear as a single strand).
Chromosome
Nucleus
Centrioles
Chromatids
1
Prophase II
Each chromosome consists of two chromatids.
2
Middle prophase I
Homologous chromosomes synapse to form tetrads.
Tetrad
Spindle fibres
Homologous chromosomes
2
Metaphase II
Chromosomes align at the equatorial plane.
3
Metaphase I
Tetrads align at the equatorial plane.
Centromere
Equatorial plane
3
Anaphase II
Chromatids separate and each is now called a chromosome.
4
Anaphase I
Homologous chromosomes move apart to opposite sides of the cell.
4
Telophase II
New nuclei form around the chromosomes.
5
Telophase I
New nuclei form, and the cell divides; during interkinesis (not shown) there is no duplication of chromosomes.
Cleavage site
5
Haploid cells
The chromosomes are about to unravel and become less distinct chromatin.

FIGURE 47-1 Meiotic cell division. Meiosis is a series of events that involves two separate division processes called *meiosis I* and *meiosis II.* Note that four daughter cells, each with the haploid number of chromosomes, are produced from each parent cell that enters meiotic cell division. For simplicity's sake, only four chromosomes are shown in the parent cell instead of the usual 46.

As you can see in **Figures 47-1** and **47-2**, when the parent cell divides to form two cells in meiotic division I, each daughter cell contains two chromosomes or half as many as the parent cell had. Remember that each chromosome still consists of two sister chromatids joined at the centromere. Thus the daughter cells formed by meiotic division I contain a haploid number of chromosomes, or half as many as the diploid number in the parent cell.

As you can see in **Figure 47-1**, meiotic division II is essentially the same as mitotic division. In both spermatogenesis and oogenesis, the second meiotic division reproduces each of the two cells formed by

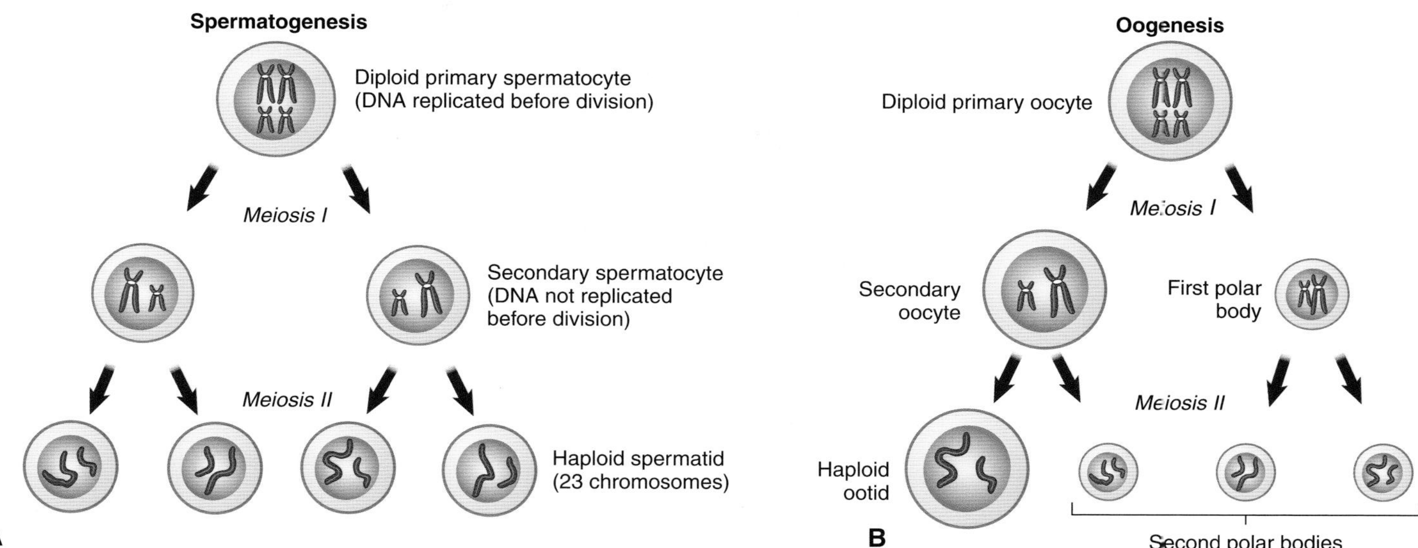

FIGURE 47-2 Overview of gamete production. A, Spermatogenesis. A primary spermatocyte (diploid) undergoes meiotic division to produce four haploid daughter spermatids. **B,** Oogenesis. A primary oocyte undergoes meiotic division to produce a single ovum and three small polar bodies.

meiotic division I and so forms four cells, each with the haploid number of chromosomes.

Spermatogenesis

Spermatogenesis is the process by which the primitive sex cells, or **spermatogonia,** already formed in the seminiferous tubules of a newborn baby boy, can later become transformed into mature sperm, or *spermatozoa*. Spermatogenesis begins at about the time of puberty and usually continues throughout a man's life. **Figure 47-3** shows some of the major steps of spermatogenesis. Trace each step in this diagram with your finger as you read the following paragraph.

Each primary spermatocyte undergoes meiotic division I to form two secondary spermatocytes, each with a haploid number of chromosomes (23). Each secondary spermatocyte undergoes meiotic division II to form a total of four spermatids. Spermatids then differentiate to form heads and tails, eventually becoming mature *spermatozoa*. Thus spermatogenesis forms four spermatozoa (singular, *spermatozoon*)—each with only 23 chromosomes—from one primary spermatocyte that had 23 pairs, or 46 total chromosomes.

Oogenesis

Oogenesis is the process by which primitive female sex cells, or **oogonia,** become mature ova. As you read through the following paragraphs, trace the steps of oogenesis in **Figure 47-4**.

During the fetal period, oogonia in the ovaries undergo mitotic division to form **primary oocytes**—about a half million of them by the time a baby girl is born. Most of the primary oocytes develop to prophase I of meiosis before birth. There they stay until puberty.

CONNECT IT! 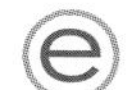

What physiological advantage is gained by postponing the completion of meiotic division as an ovum matures? The surprising answer is found in ***Arrest of Oocyte Development*** online at ***Connect It!***

During childhood, **granulosa cells** develop around each primary oocyte, forming a **primary follicle.** Although several thousand primary oocytes do not survive into puberty, by the time a girl reaches sexual maturity, about 400,000 primary oocytes remain.

Beginning at puberty, a cohort of around 20 or so primary oocytes resume meiosis each day. Their surrounding follicles begin to mature and some of the outer granulosa cells differentiate to become **theca cells.** Theca cells produce *androgen*, a steroid that is converted by granulosa cells into oestrogen. At this point, the follicles are known as **secondary follicles.**

As the secondary follicles mature, they migrate toward the surface of the ovary—sometimes in several waves during one cycle. Usually only one preovulatory follicle per cycle survives and matures enough to reach the surface of the ovary, where it can be seen as a fluid-filled bump. The fluid-filled space within each mature follicle is called the *antrum*. A mature *vesicular ovarian follicle* ready to burst open from the ovary's surface is also called a *graafian follicle*.

By that time, meiosis has resumed inside the primary oocyte within the mature follicle. Meiosis I produces a **secondary oocyte** and the **first polar body** (see **Figure 47-2**, *B*). Just before ovulation, meiosis again halts—this time at metaphase II. Under the influence of LH (luteinizing hormone), ovulation occurs. Ovulation, you may recall, is the release of an oocyte from a burst follicle.

Meiosis II in the released oocyte resumes only when, and if, the head of a sperm cell enters the secondary oocyte (ovum). If fertilization does not occur, then the ovum simply degenerates. If fertilization does occur, however, then meiotic division of the secondary oocyte produces a second polar body and a mature, fertilized ovum called the **zygote.**

Note that during oogenesis, the cytoplasm is *not* equally divided among the daughter cells. Of the four daughter cells produced, only one is large enough to survive. Thus each primary oocyte produces only one mature ovum, plus three tiny *polar bodies*. These polar bodies quickly break down and are reabsorbed into nearby cells. By

FIGURE 47-3 Spermatogenesis. First, spermatogonia in the outer rim of the seminiferous tubule produce daughter cells by mitotic division. These daughter cells, each with 46 chromosomes, become primary spermatocytes. A primary spermatocyte then undergoes meiotic division I to form two secondary spermatocytes, each with a haploid number of chromosomes (23). Each of the two secondary spermatocytes undergoes meiotic division II to form a total of four spermatids. Spermatids then differentiate to form heads and tails, eventually becoming mature spermatozoa—all with 23 chromosomes. Recall the role of the sustentacular cells (Sertoli cells), which support the developing male gametes structurally (by physically supporting them) and functionally (by releasing nutrients to them and by secretion of the hormone inhibin).

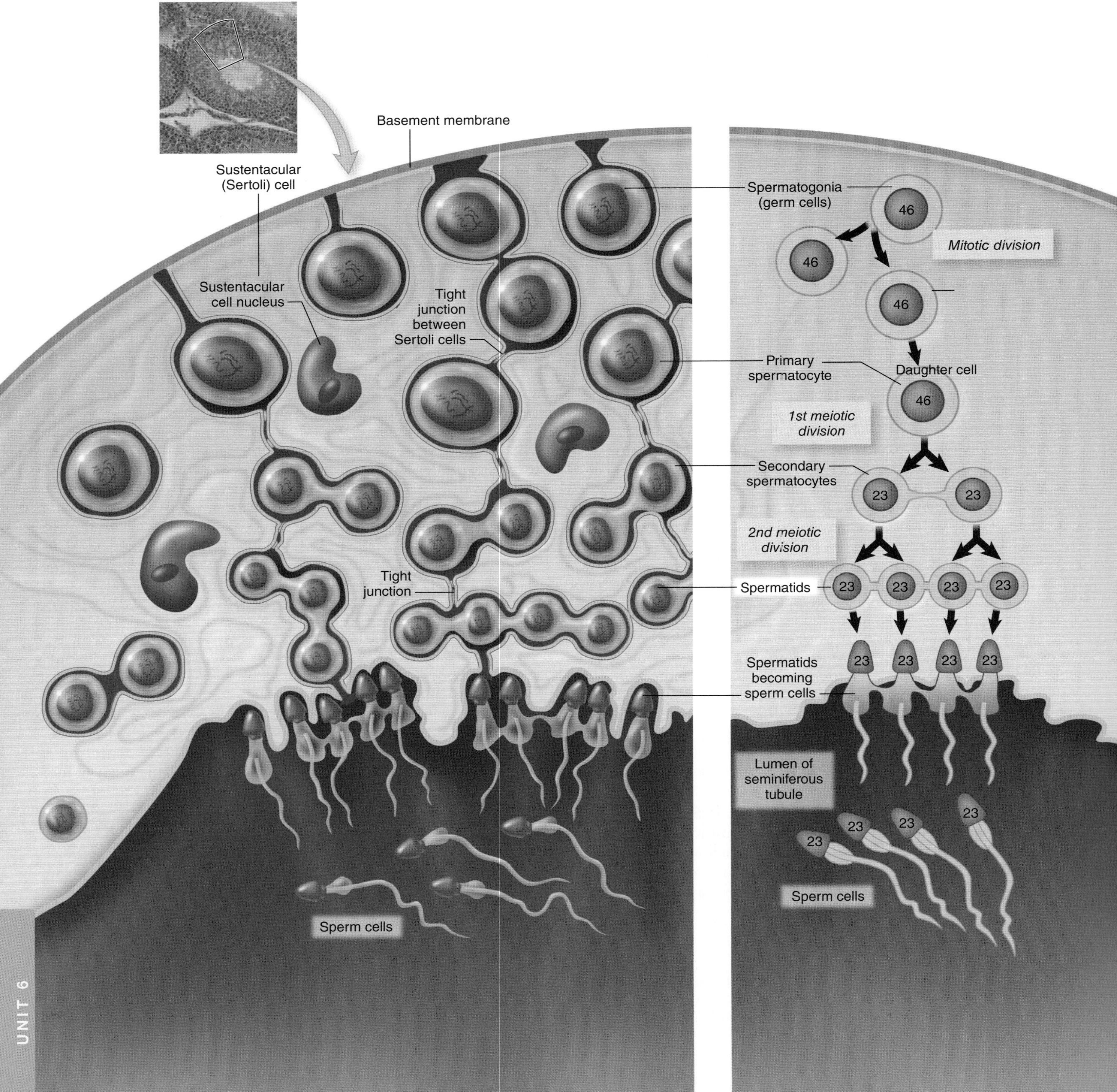

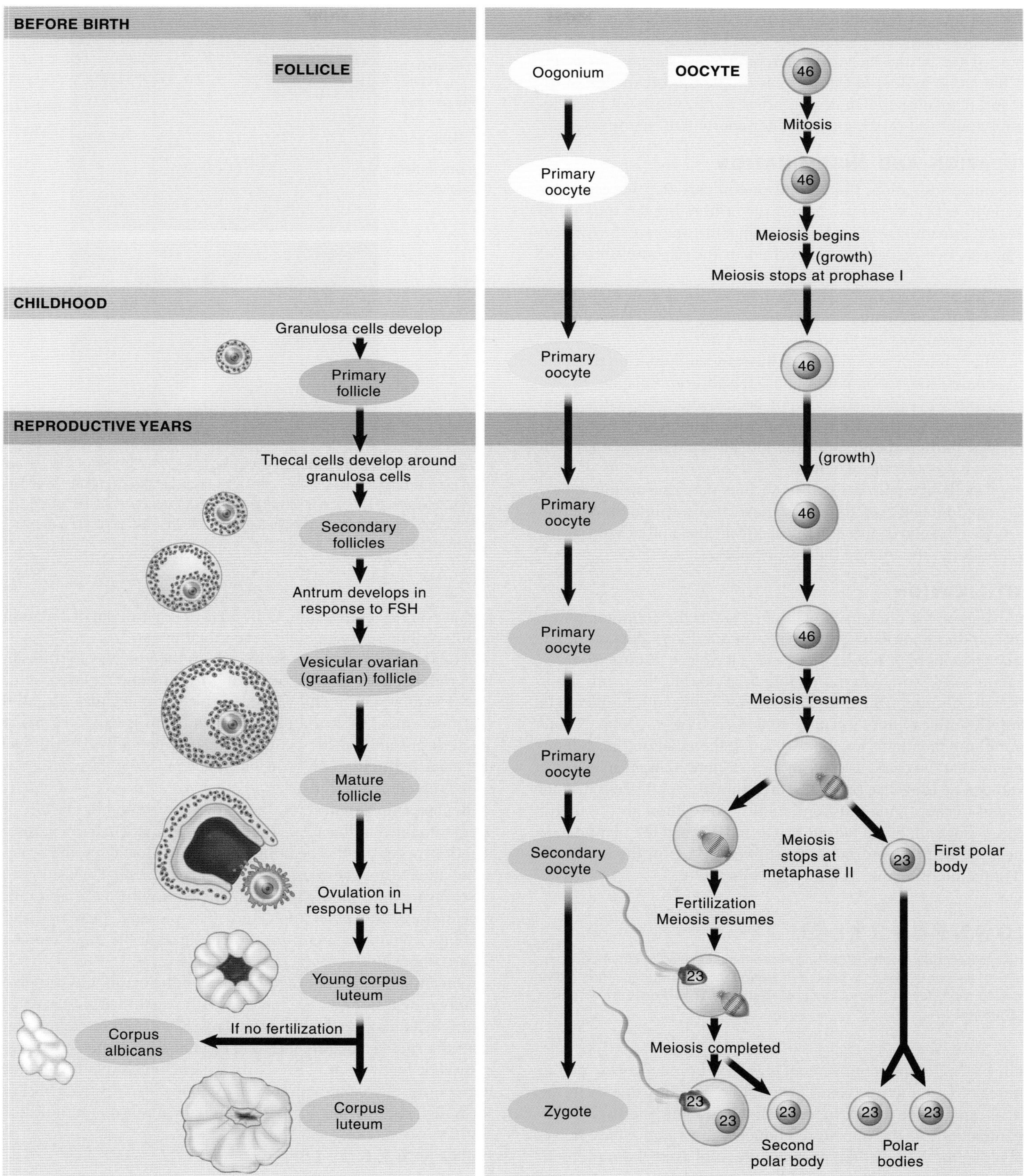

FIGURE 47-4 Oogenesis. Production of a mature ovum (oocyte) and subsequent fertilization are shown on the right as a series of cell divisions and on the left as a series of changes in the ovarian follicle. *FSH,* Follicle-stimulating hormone; *LH,* luteinizing hormone.

contrast, a total of four mature sperm cells are formed from each primary spermatocyte in spermatogenesis. This difference may be accounted for by the fact that for reproductive success, an ovum must have a huge store of cytoplasm with all of its organelles, nutrients, and regulatory molecules. In other words, nearly all the cytoplasm is conserved by the one daughter oocyte that survives.

Ovulation and Insemination

After gamete formation, the second preliminary step necessary for conception of a new individual consists of bringing the sperm and ovum into proximity with each other so that the union of the two can take place. Two processes are involved in the accomplishment of this step:

1. Ovulation or expulsion of the mature ovum from the mature ovarian follicle into the abdominopelvic cavity, from which it enters one of the uterine (fallopian) tubes.
2. Insemination or expulsion of the seminal fluid from the male urethra into the female vagina. Recall from Chapter 45 that a process called *capacitation* occurs after ejaculation, and this enables the sperm to eventually unite with an egg. Several million sperm enter the female reproductive tract with each ejaculation of semen. By lashing movements of their flagella-like tails, assisted by various processes in the female reproductive tract, the sperm make their way into the external os of the cervix, through the cervical canal and uterine cavity, and into the uterine (fallopian) tubes.

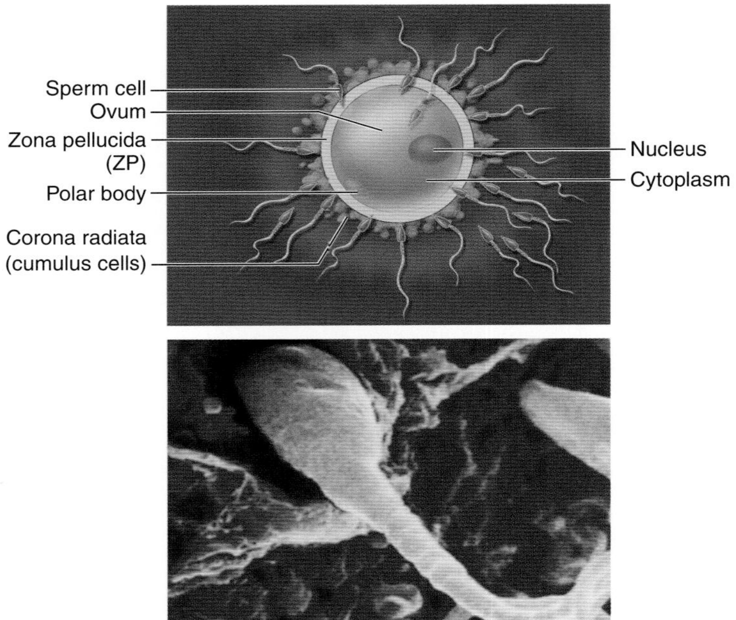

FIGURE 47-5 Fertilization. Fertilization is a specific biological event. It occurs when the male and female sex cells fuse. After union between a sperm cell and the ovum has occurred, the cycle of life begins. The scanning electron micrograph shows spermatozoa beginning to burrow into the surface of the zona pellucida *(ZP)* layer surrounding the ovum. Only one sperm may enter the ovum.

Fertilization

After ovulation the discharged ovum first enters the abdominopelvic cavity and then soon finds its way into the uterine (fallopian) tubes, where conception, or **fertilization,** may take place (**Figure 47-5**).

Sperm cells "swim" up the uterine tubes toward the ovum. Look at the relationship of the ovary, the uterine tube, and the uterus in **Figure 47-6**. Recall from Chapter 46 that each uterine tube extends outward from the uterus for about 10 cm. It then ends in the abdominal cavity near the ovary, as you can see in **Figure 47-6**, in an opening surrounded by fringelike processes, the fimbriae. Sperm cells that are deposited in the vagina must enter and "swim" through the uterus and then move out of the uterine cavity and through the uterine tube to meet the ovum. Fertilization most often occurs in the outer one third of the uterine tube, as shown in **Figure 47-6**.

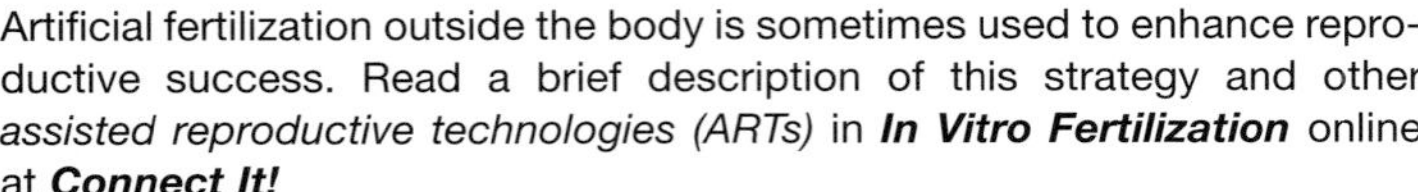

CONNECT IT!

Artificial fertilization outside the body is sometimes used to enhance reproductive success. Read a brief description of this strategy and other *assisted reproductive technologies (ARTs)* in ***In Vitro Fertilization*** online at ***Connect It!***

The process of sperm movement is assisted by mechanisms within the female reproductive tract. For example, mucous strands in the cervical canal guide the sperm on their way into the uterus. Peristaltic contractions of the female reproductive tract and ciliary movement along the lining of the uterine tubes also assist the movement of sperm. Sperm are attracted to the warmer temperatures of the uterine tubes—a process of attraction called **thermotaxis.** Despite all this, however, only a small fraction of the sperm deposited in the vagina ever reach the ovum. Only 50 to 100 sperm out of 250 million to 500 million sperm actually reach their target.

The ovum also takes an active role in the process of fertilization. Experiments show that the ovum and its surrounding layers actually attract nearby sperm with various regulatory molecules. Recall that such movement toward a chemical attractant is called *chemotaxis.* These layers around the ovum include a thick jellylike film called the **zona pellucida (ZP)** with an outer envelope of *cumulus cells* called the **corona radiata.**

Receptor molecules on these ovum-surrounding layers bind sperm attracted to the area. Once bound to a receptor, an **acrosome reaction** occurs at the head of the sperm. This acrosome reaction allows the release of enzymes from the acrosome that break down the outer layers surrounding the ovum. The cumulus cells also release progesterone and other molecules that promote increased sperm motility, which aids sperm movement through the outer layers and toward the ovum.

Once the sperm reaches the surface of the ovum, the two plasma membranes fuse and the nucleus of the sperm moves inside the ovum. In addition to the sperm nucleus, RNA and protein molecules from the sperm cell also enter the egg. The RNA molecules apparently code for proteins needed early in development—thus adding to the ovum's cellular resources. RNA molecules involved in "gene silencing" may also be released into the ovum during fertilization.

CONNECT IT!

The illustrated article ***The RNA Revolution***—available online at ***Connect It!***—details the concept of *gene silencing,* which can help regulate protein synthesis in cells.

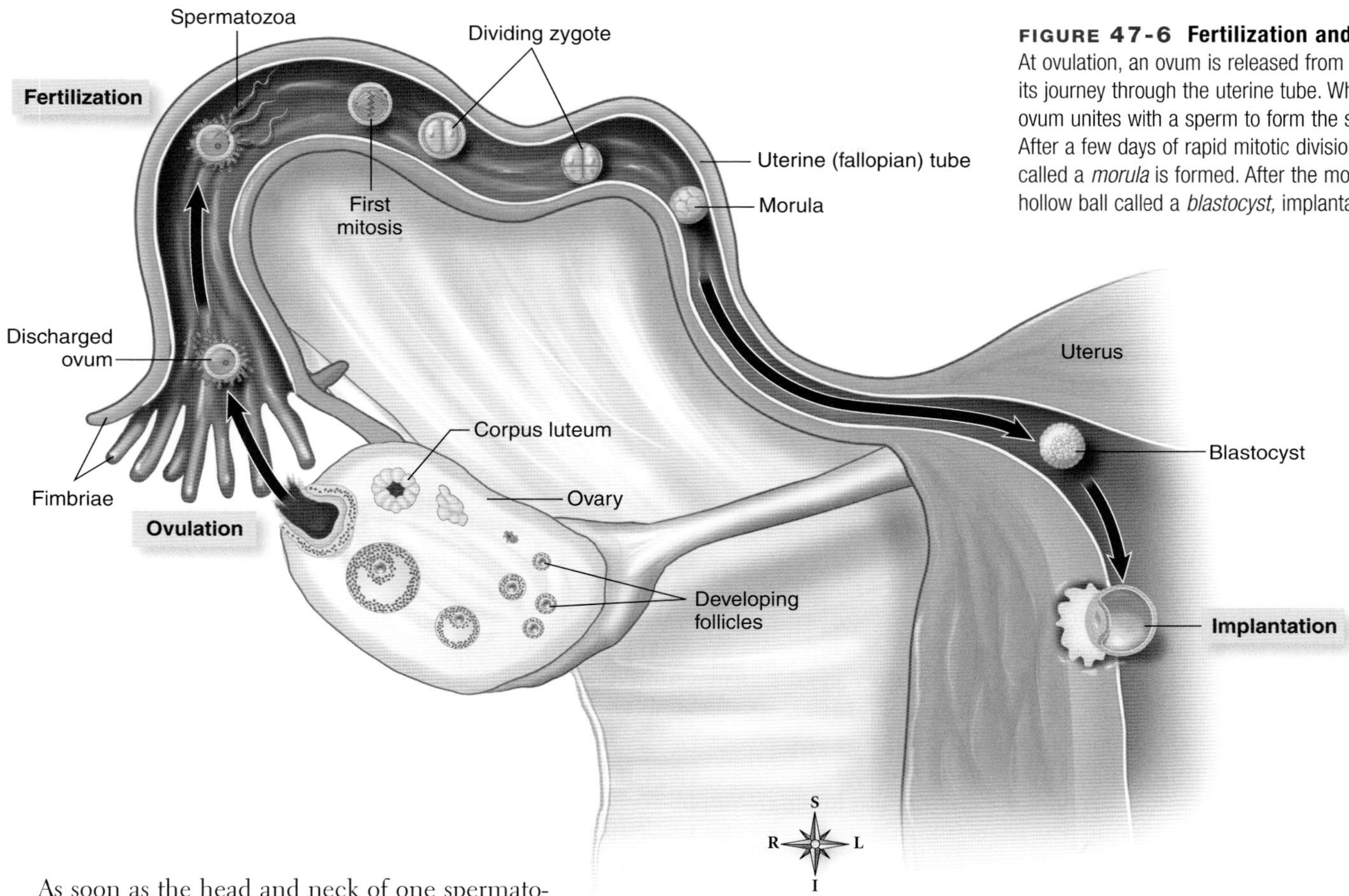

FIGURE 47-6 Fertilization and implantation. At ovulation, an ovum is released from the ovary and begins its journey through the uterine tube. While in the tube, the ovum unites with a sperm to form the single-celled zygote. After a few days of rapid mitotic division, a ball of cells called a *morula* is formed. After the morula develops into a hollow ball called a *blastocyst,* implantation occurs.

As soon as the head and neck of one spermatozoon fuse with the ovum (the tail degenerates), complex mechanisms in the egg are activated by sperm proteins to ensure that no more sperm enter. Specifically, sperm proteins trigger an increase in calcium concentration that causes vesicles just inside the ovum's plasma membrane to release enzymes that inactivate the sperm receptors on the ZP. This thick film, then, becomes an impenetrable barrier sometimes called the *fertilization membrane.* The 23 chromosomes from the sperm nucleus combine with the 23 chromosomes already in the ovum to restore the diploid number of 46 chromosomes.

In as much as the ovum lives only a short time (probably only a day or so) after leaving the ruptured follicle, the fertilization "window" occurs around the time of ovulation. Because sperm may live up to a few days after entering the female tract, sexual intercourse any time from about 3 days before ovulation to a day or so after ovulation may result in fertilization.

The fertilized ovum, or zygote, is genetically complete; it represents the first cell of a genetically new individual. Time, nourishment, and a proper prenatal environment are all that are needed for expression of characteristics such as sex, hair, and skin colour that were determined at the time of fertilization.

Quick CHECK

1. What is the function of meiotic division?
2. How does meiosis differ from mitosis?
3. Where in the female reproductive tract does fertilization usually occur?
4. What is the technical name for the fertilized ovum?

PRENATAL PERIOD

The **prenatal period** of development begins at the time of conception, or fertilization (i.e., at the moment the female ovum and the male sperm cell unite). However, a pregnancy does not begin until successful implantation in the uterus. The period of prenatal development continues until the birth of the child about 39 weeks later. The science of the development of the individual before birth is called **embryology**. It is a story of biological marvels, describing the means by which a new human life is begun and the steps by which a single microscopic cell is transformed into a complex human being.

Cleavage and Implantation

As you can see in **Figure 47-6**, once the zygote is formed, it immediately begins to cleave, or divide, and in about 3 days a solid mass of cells called a **morula** is formed. The cells of the morula begin to form an inner cavity as they continue to divide, and by the time the developing embryo reaches the uterus, it is a hollow ball of cells called a **blastocyst.** At about 1 week after fertilization, the process of **implantation** begins. In about 10 days from the time of fertilization, the blastocyst is completely implanted in the uterine lining—before nutrients from the mother are available to nourish it. Successful implantation is the start of pregnancy. Of course, problems in development or implantation may occur at any stage—resulting in loss of the offspring and termination of the developmental process.

The rapid cell division taking place up to the blastocyst stage occurs with no significant increase in total mass compared with the

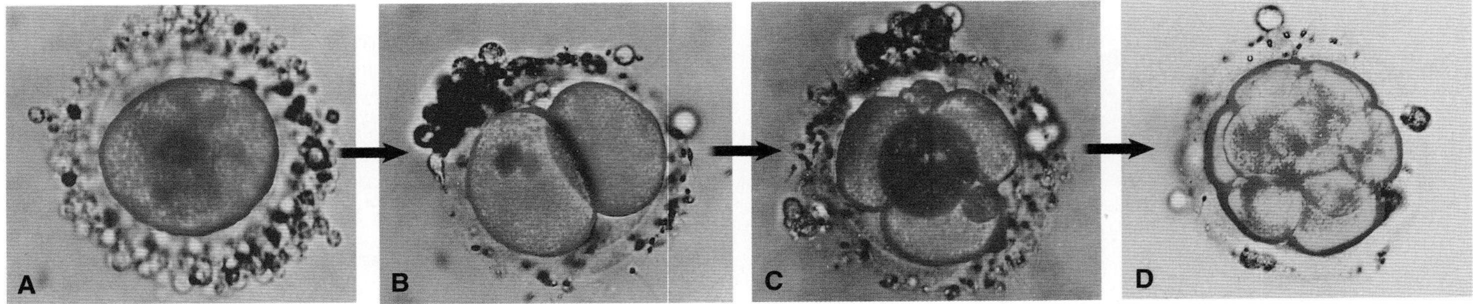

FIGURE 47-7 Initial rapid cell division in human development. A, Fertilized ovum, or zygote. **B** to **D,** Early cell divisions produce more and more cells. The solid mass of cells shown in **D** forms the morula—an early stage in embryonic development.

zygote (**Figure 47-7**). One of the specializations of the ovum (and its surrounding layers) is its incredible store of nutrients that support this embryonic development until implantation has occurred.

Note in **Figure 47-8** that the blastocyst consists of an outer layer of cells and an **inner cell mass.** The outer wall of the blastocyst is called the **trophoblast** (see **Figure 47-8**). As the blastocyst develops further, the inner cell mass forms a structure with two cavities called the **yolk sac** and **amniotic cavity** (**Figure 47-9** and **Figure 47-10**).

The yolk sac is most important in animals such as birds that depend heavily on yolk as a nutrient for the developing embryo. In these animals the yolk sac digests the yolk and provides the resulting nutrients to the embryo. Because the uterine lining provides nutrients to the developing embryo in humans, the function of the yolk sac is not a nutritive one. Instead, it has other functions. For example, it is an important site of *haematopoiesis* during embryonic development. It also produces the stem cells that migrate from the yolk sac to the two embryonic gonads that later develop into oogonia in females and spermatogonia in males.

CONNECT IT!

Review the illustration in ***Sites of Haematopoiesis*** online at ***Connect It!*** to help you visualize the important role of the yolk sac in blood cell production during early development.

It is the inner cell mass that eventually forms the tissues of the offspring's body. The trophoblast, on the other hand, forms the support structures described in the following paragraphs. (**Box 47-1** discusses the field of *developmental biology.*)

The amniotic cavity becomes a fluid-filled, shock-absorbing sac, sometimes called the "bag of waters", in which the embryo floats during development. The **chorion,** shown in **Figures 47-9** to **47-11**, develops from the trophoblast to become an important fetal membrane in the **placenta.** The *chorionic villi* shown in **Figures 47-10** and **47-11** are extensions of the blood vessels of the chorion that bring the embryonic circulation to the placenta. The placenta (see **Figure 47-11**) anchors the developing offspring to the uterus and provides a "bridge" for the exchange of nutrients and waste products between mother and baby.

PLACENTA

The placenta is a unique structure that has a temporary but very important set of functions during pregnancy. It is composed of tissues from mother and offspring and functions not only as a structural "anchor" and nutritive bridge but also as an excretory, respiratory, and endocrine organ.

Placental tissue normally separates the maternal and fetal blood supplies so that no intermixing occurs. The very thin layer of placental tissue that separates maternal and fetal blood also serves as an effective "barrier" that can protect the developing baby from many harmful substances that may enter the mother's bloodstream. Unfortunately, toxic substances such as alcohol and some infectious organisms may penetrate this protective placental barrier and possibly injure the developing fetus (see **Box 29-1** on p. 690). The virus responsible for German measles (rubella), for example, can easily pass through the placenta and cause tragic developmental defects in the fetus.

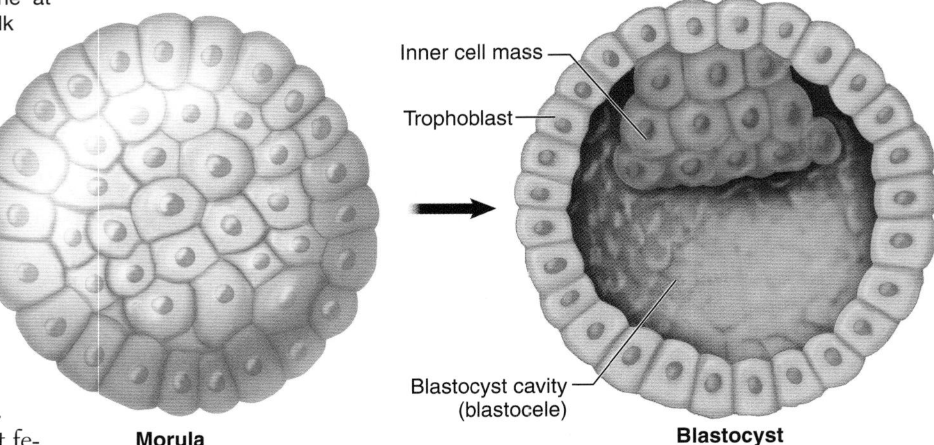

FIGURE 47-8 Early stages in the development of the human embryo. The morula consists of an almost solid spherical mass of cells. The embryo reaches this stage about 3 days after fertilization. The blastocyst (hollowing) stage develops next, before implantation in the uterine lining.

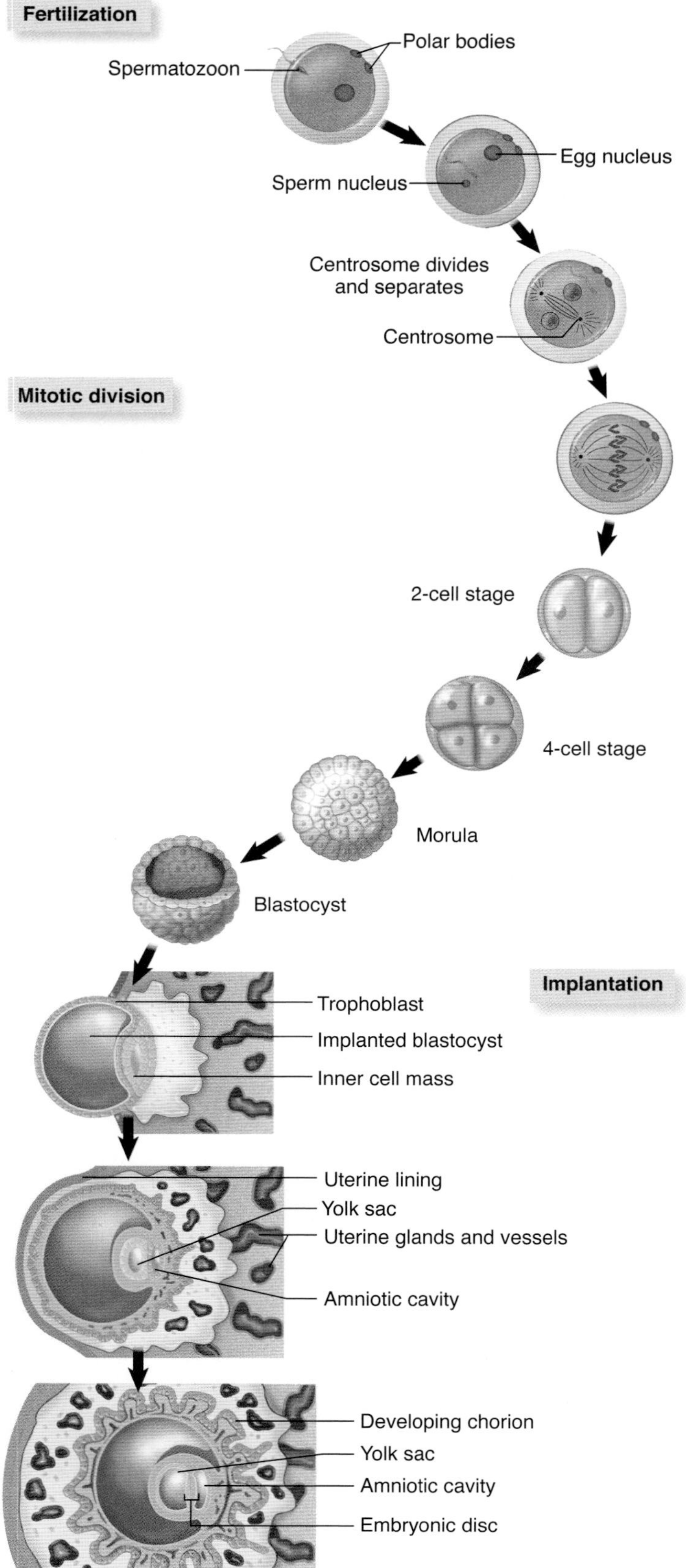

FIGURE 47-9 From fertilization to implantation and development of the yolk sac. Rapid growth of uterine glands and vessels covers the developing blastocyst at the time of implantation.

Placental tissue also has important endocrine functions. As **Figure 47-12**, A, shows, placental tissue secretes large amounts of **human chorionic gonadotropin (hCG)** early in pregnancy. hCG secretion peaks about 8 or 9 weeks after fertilization, then drops to a continuous low level by about week 16. The function of hCG, as its name implies, is to act as a gonadotropin and stimulate the corpus luteum to continue its secretion of

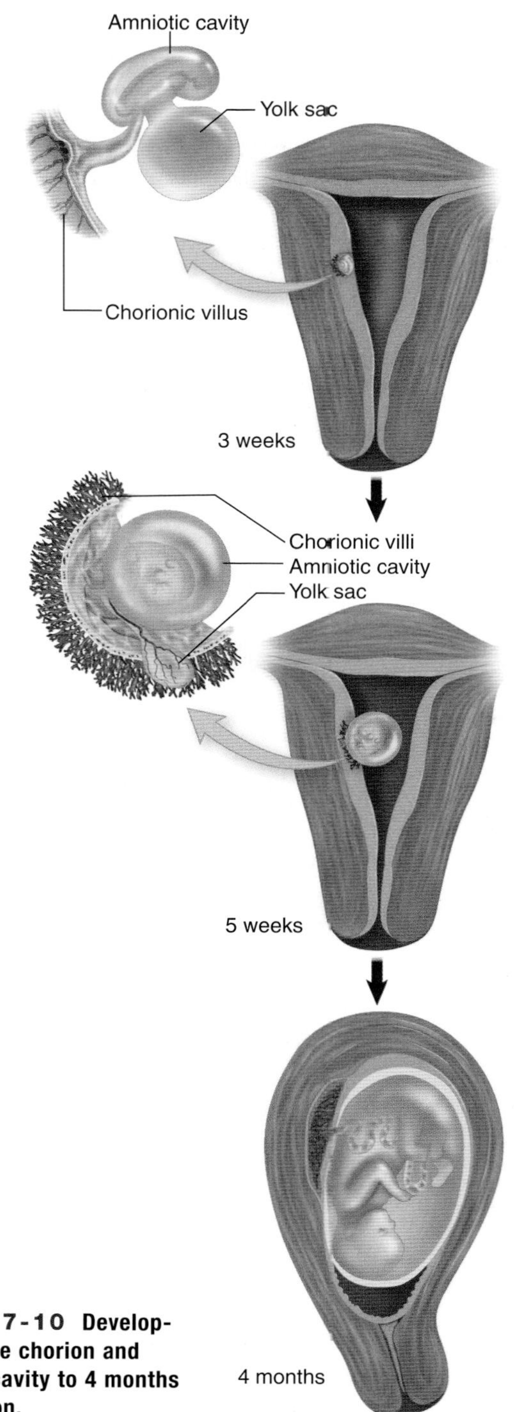

FIGURE 47-10 Development of the chorion and amniotic cavity to 4 months of gestation.

BOX 47-1 *fyi* | Developmental Biology

Developmental biology is the name given to the branch of life science that studies the process of change over the life cycle. This process of change is called *development.* It is important to realize that in developmental biology, the terms *growth* and *development* do not mean the same thing. Growth is simply an increase in body mass. Development, on the other hand, refers to the complex series of changes that occur at various times of life. Early stages of development—particularly the prenatal stages—are characterized by rapid growth, whereas later stages of development are characterized by little, if any, growth of body tissues.

In this chapter, we briefly discuss various subtopics within the field of human developmental biology. For example, prenatal development is studied by a branch of developmental biology called embryology. The biological changes observed during late adulthood are studied by a branch of developmental biology called gerontology.

Basic concepts of embryology, gerontology, and other subdisciplines of developmental biology seem to have taken on a greater practical importance during the past few decades than ever before. One reason is the explosion in knowledge of developmental processes and our ability to treat the abnormalities that we can now find. Procedures such as fetal surgery, electrocardiography, and ultrasound permit physicians to diagnose and treat the fetus much like any other patient. Ongoing discoveries about the processes of ageing—as well as the rapidly growing population of aged individuals—have spawned new methods of recognizing and treating physical and psychological problems in the elderly. Another reason developmental biology has taken on great practical importance is that it is a field that serves to unify human biology into a framework that integrates anatomy, physiology, cell biology, molecular biology, medicine, and other disciplines. Thus developmental biology gives us an excellent view of the "big picture" of the human body. •

oestrogen and progesterone. Recall from Chapter 46 (see **Figure 46-15** on p. 1074) that reduced levels of the anterior pituitary gonadotropins (FSH and LH) after ovulation normally cause a corresponding reduction in luteal secretion of the oestrogen and progesterone needed to sustain the uterine lining. The drop in oestrogen and progesterone secretion results from the fact that the FSH and LH needed to maintain the corpus luteum are now in short supply. To prevent menstruation and to allow successful implantation and development of the offspring, the cells of the trophoblast and, later, the placenta secrete enough hCG to maintain the corpus luteum and thus keep luteal oestrogen and progesterone levels high.

As the placenta develops, it begins to secrete its own oestrogen and progesterone. As **Figure 47-12**, A, shows, as more oestrogen and progesterone are secreted from the placenta, a corresponding decrease in hCG secretion produces a drop in luteal secretion of these hormones. After about 3 months, the corpus luteum has degenerated and the placenta has completely taken over the job of secreting the oestrogen and progesterone needed to sustain the pregnancy.

Over-the-counter "early pregnancy" tests detect the presence of the hCG that is excreted in the urine during the first couple of months of a pregnancy. Such tests can detect hCG in the urine as early as 1 or 2 days after implantation occurs.

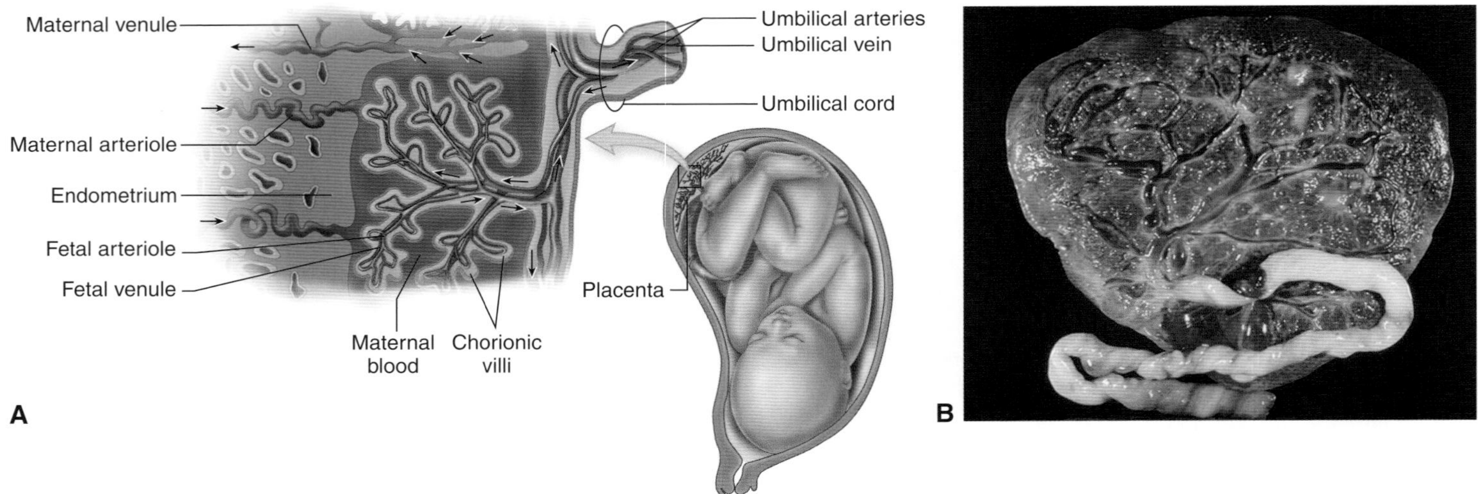

FIGURE 47-11 Structural features of the placenta. The close proximity of the fetal blood supply and the maternal blood supply permits diffusion of nutrients and other substances. The placenta also forms a thin barrier that prevents diffusion of most harmful substances. No mixing of fetal and maternal blood occurs. **A,** Diagram showing a cross-section of the placental structure. **B,** Photograph of a normal, full-term placenta (fetal side) showing the branching of the placental blood vessels and umbilical cord.

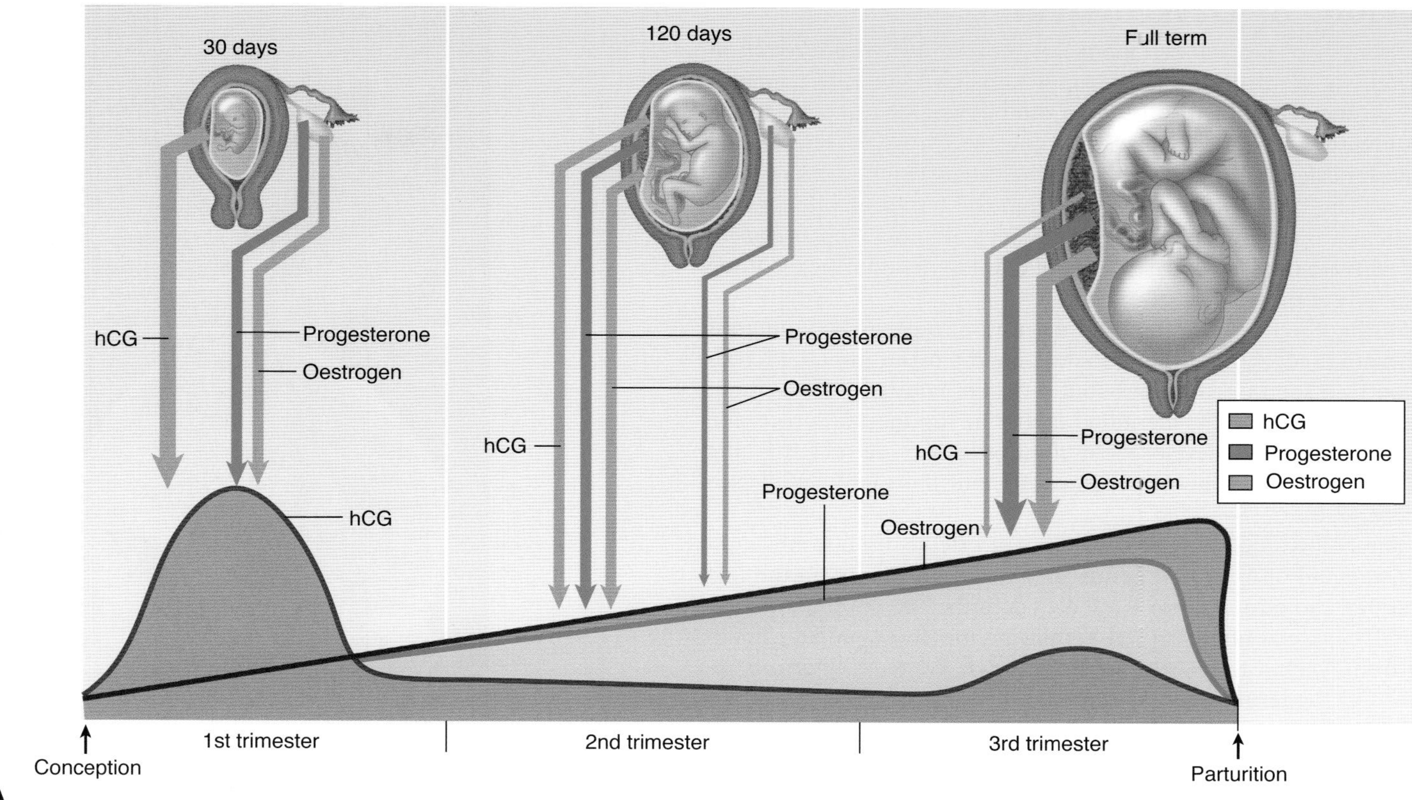

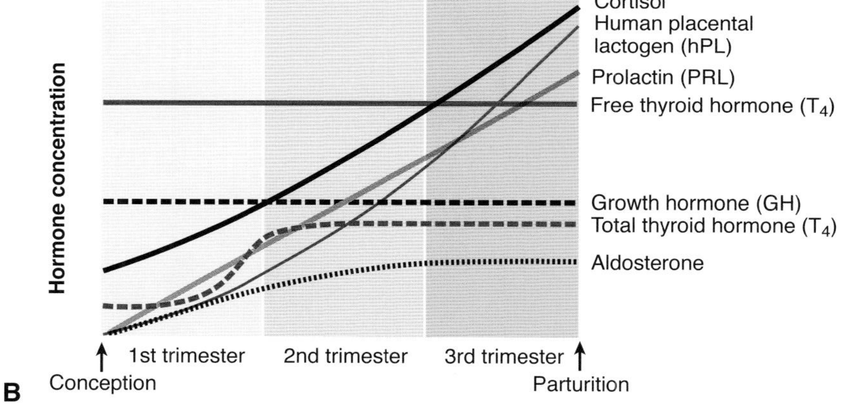

FIGURE 47-12 Hormone levels during pregnancy. **A,** Diagram showing the changes that occur in the blood concentration of human chorionic gonadotropin (hCG), oestrogen, and progesterone during gestation. Note that high hCG levels produced by placental tissue early in pregnancy maintain oestrogen and progesterone secretion by the corpus luteum. This prevents menstruation and promotes maintenance of the uterine lining. As the placenta takes over the job of secreting oestrogen and progesterone, hCG levels drop, and the corpus luteum subsequently ceases secreting these hormones. **B,** Graph showing other hormones important in supporting pregnancy and lactation. Growth hormone remains stable, as does free T_4 (although total T_4 rises).

Figure 47-12, *B*, shows some other hormones that help support pregnancy. The functions of these hormones were discussed in previous chapters. During pregnancy some hormones, such as growth hormone (GH), remain stable, but others *increase* during pregnancy. All these hormones directly or indirectly promote the physiological processes of fetal development and lactation. Cortisol, for example, also helps trigger important events during pregnancy—including the onset of labour.

Quick CHECK

5. What is a morula? What is a blastocyst?
6. What structures are derived from the trophoblast (outer wall) of the blastocyst?
7. What placental hormone maintains the corpus luteum during the early weeks of pregnancy?

Periods of Development

The length of pregnancy (about 39 weeks)—called the **gestation period**—is divided into three approximately 3-month segments called *trimesters*. The first trimester extends from the first day of the last menstrual period to the end of the twelfth week. The second trimester extends from the twelfth to the twenty-eighth week of pregnancy. The third trimester extends from the twenty-eighth week of pregnancy until the baby is delivered. Several terms such as *embryo* and *fetus* are used to describe stages of development during the three trimesters of pregnancy.

During the first trimester, or 3 months, of pregnancy, numerous terms are used. Zygote is used to describe the ovum just after fertilization by a sperm cell. After about 3 days of constant cell division, the solid mass of cells, identified earlier as the morula, enters the uterus. Continued development transforms the morula into the hollow blastocyst, which then implants into the uterine wall (see **Figure 47-9**).

The embryonic phase of development extends from fertilization until the end of week 8 of gestation. During this period in the first trimester, the term *embryo* is used to describe the developing individual. The fetal phase is used to indicate the development extending from week 8 to 39. During this period, the term *embryo* is replaced by the term *fetus*.

By day 35 of gestation (**Figure 47-13**, *A*), the heart is beating and, although the embryo is only 8 mm long, the eyes and so-called *limb buds*, which ultimately form the arms and legs, are clearly visible. **Figure 47-13**, *C*, shows the stage of development at the end of the first trimester of gestation, when the offspring becomes known as a fetus. Body size is about 7 to 8 cm long (**Figure 47-14**). The facial features of the fetus are apparent, the limbs are complete, and sex can be identified. By month 4 (**Figure 47-13**, *D*), all organ systems are formed and functioning to some extent. Growth of the embryo to 4 months is summarized in the photographs in **Figures 47-13** and **47-14**; growth to full term is summarized in the graph in **Figure 47-15**. **Box 47-2** discusses methods of diagnosis and treatment in these early developmental stages.

Stem Cells

Stem cells are unspecialized cells that reproduce to form specific lines of specialized cells. At the very beginning of the embryonic stage, all the cells are stem cells. At this stage, they have their highest "stemness" or potency—that is, they are capable of producing many different kinds of cells in the body.

Scientists call the single cell of the zygote *totipotent*, meaning "totally potent", because it is the ancestor to all the body's cell types. After the zygote cell divides, many *pluripotent* cells are formed—cells that can produce many (but not all) kinds of cells. It is these early pluripotent cells that are commonly referred to as *embryonic stem cells*. It is the embryonic stem cells that form the germ layers described in the next section.

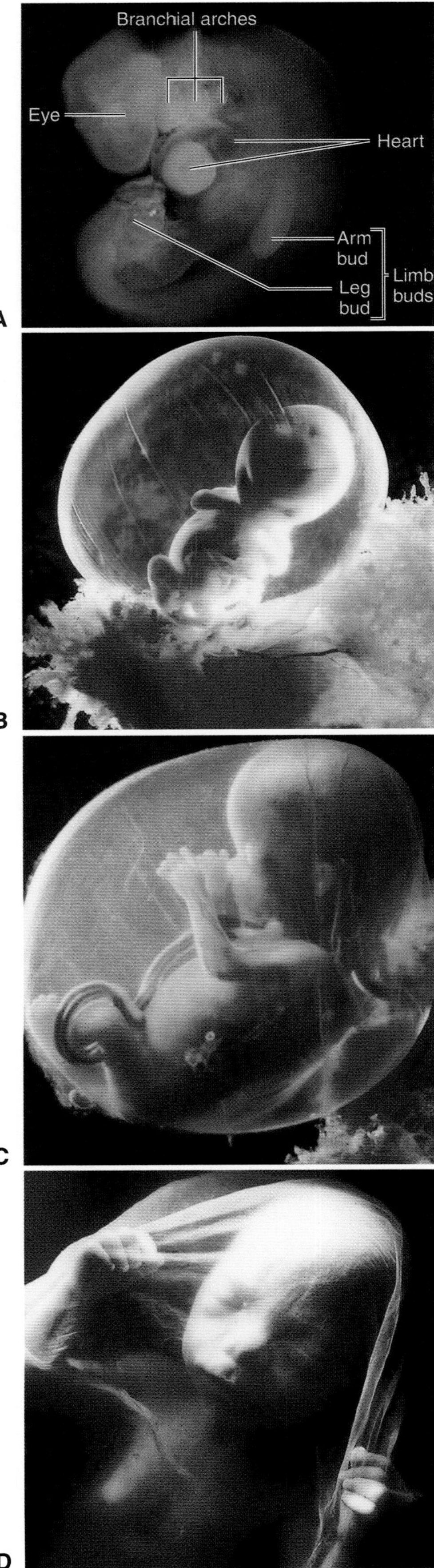

FIGURE 47-13 Human embryos and fetuses. A, At 35 days. **B,** At 49 days. **C,** At the end of the first trimester. **D,** At 4 months.

BOX 47-2 ***diagnostic study*** | **Antenatal Diagnosis and Treatment**

Advances in **antenatal medicine**—before-birth medicine—now permit extensive diagnosis and treatment of disease in the fetus much like any other patient. This new dimension in medicine began with techniques by which Rh-positive babies could be given transfusions before birth.

Current procedures using images provided by **ultrasonography** equipment (see the figure) allow physicians to prepare for and perform, before the birth of a baby, corrective surgical procedures such as bladder repair. These procedures also allow physicians to monitor the progress of other types of treatment on a developing fetus. Part A of the figure shows placement of the ultrasound transducer on the abdominal wall. The resulting image (see part B of the figure), called an *ultrasonogram,* shows a 20-week-old fetus. •

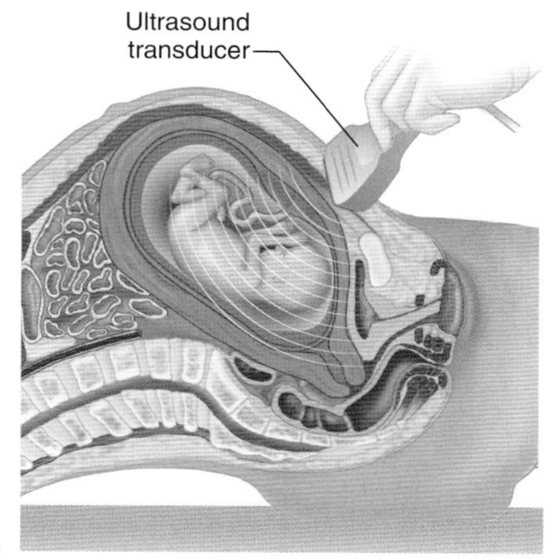

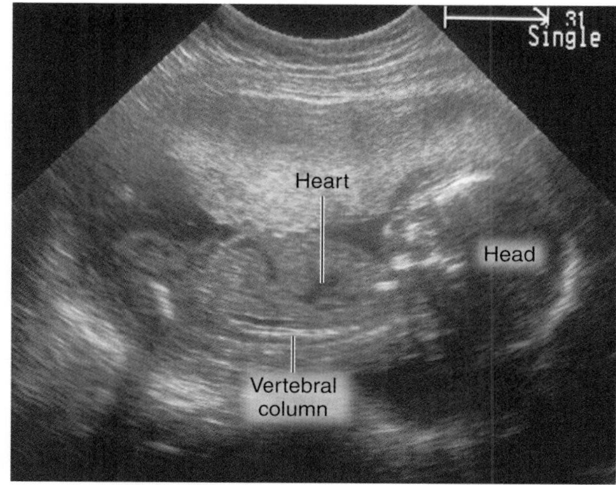

Ultrasonography. A, Placement of the ultrasound transducer on the abdominal wall. **B,** Ultrasonogram showing a midsagittal view of a 20-week-old fetus.

Some stem cells remain throughout development and maturity. These *multipotent* stem cells, such as the haematopoietic stem cells found in adult bone marrow, can only produce a few types of cells. *Adult stem cells,* as these multipotent cells are usually called, are found in many tissues of the body. For example, adult stem cells are found in the skin, fat, many glands, muscles, nerve tissue, bone, and the gastrointestinal (GI) tract. Adult stem cells replace the specialized cells in a tissue and thus ensure stable, functional populations of the cell types needed for survival.

CONNECT IT!

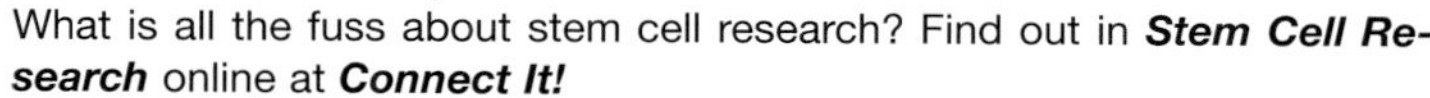

What is all the fuss about stem cell research? Find out in ***Stem Cell Research*** online at ***Connect It!***

Formation of the Primary Germ Layers

Early in the first trimester of pregnancy, three layers of unique cells develop that embryologists call the **primary germ layers.** Cells of the *embryonic disc* seen in **Figure 47-9** differentiate into distinct types that form each of these three primary germ layers. Pluripotent stem cells in each layer continue to differentiate and thus give rise to the various specific organs and systems of the body, such as the skin, nervous tissue, muscles, or digestive organs (**Figure 47-16**). As new tissues and organs develop, older cells often die through the process of apoptosis (see Chapter 7) and thus make room for newer, more specialized cells. Each primary germ layer is called, respectively, **endoderm,** or inside layer; **ectoderm,** or outside layer; and **mesoderm,** or middle layer.

Endoderm

The inner germ layer, or *endoderm,* forms the linings of various tracts, as well as several glands. For example, the lining of the respiratory tract and GI tract, including some of the accessory structures such as tonsils, is derived from the endoderm. The linings of the pancreatic ducts, hepatic ducts, and urinary tract also have an endodermal origin. The glandular epithelium of the thymus, thyroid, and parathyroid glands is also derived from the endoderm.

Ectoderm

The outer germ layer, or *ectoderm,* forms many of the structures around the periphery of the body. For example, the epidermis of the skin, enamel of the teeth, and cornea and lens of the eye are derived from the ectoderm. Besides these peripheral structures, various components of the nervous system—including the brain and the spinal cord—also have an ectodermal origin.

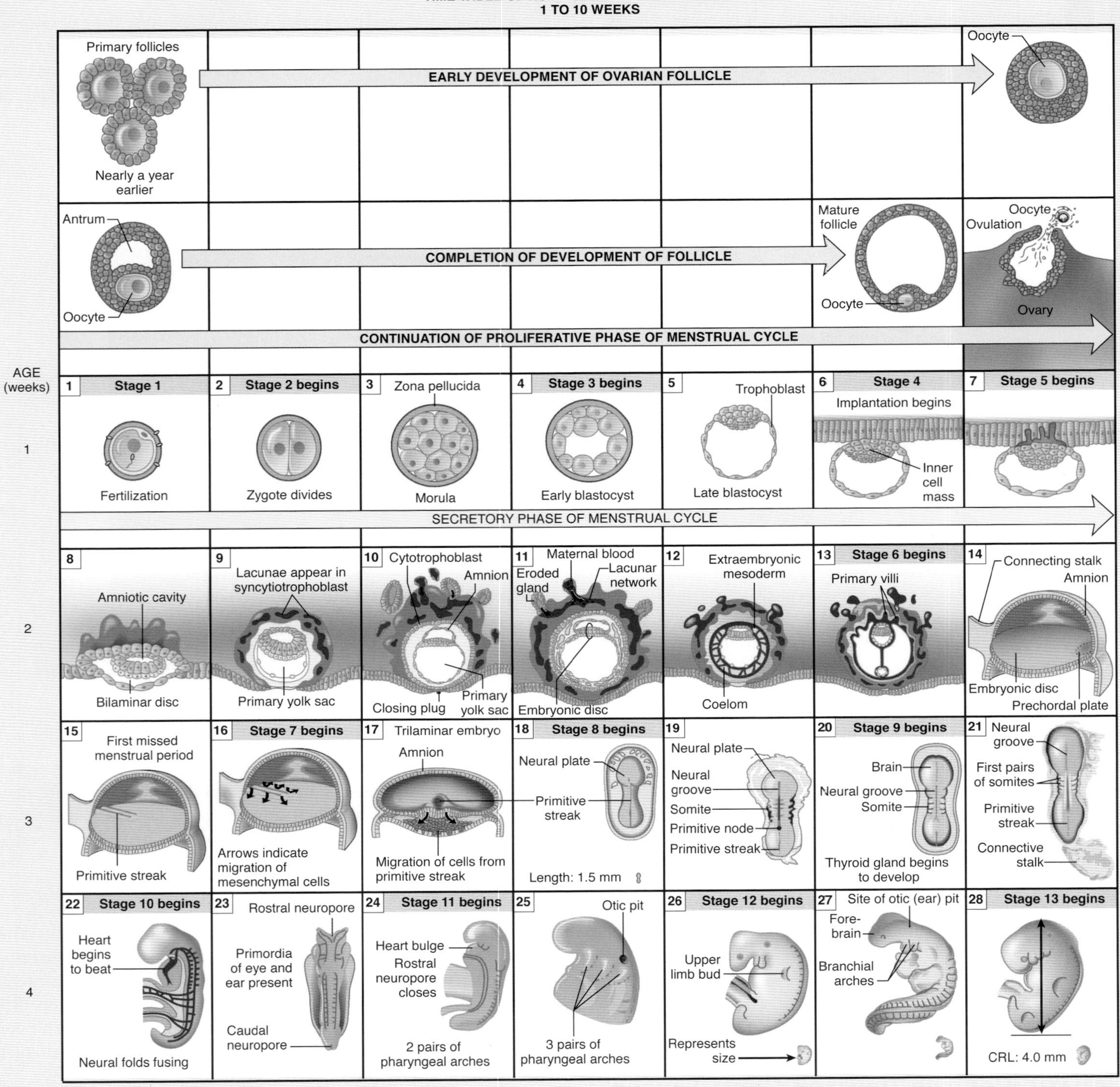

FIGURE 47-14 Developmental events during the first trimester of pregnancy. Each box represents a day, and each row represents a week. Compare this timetable with the preceding figures of this chapter. *CRL,* Crown-to-rump length.

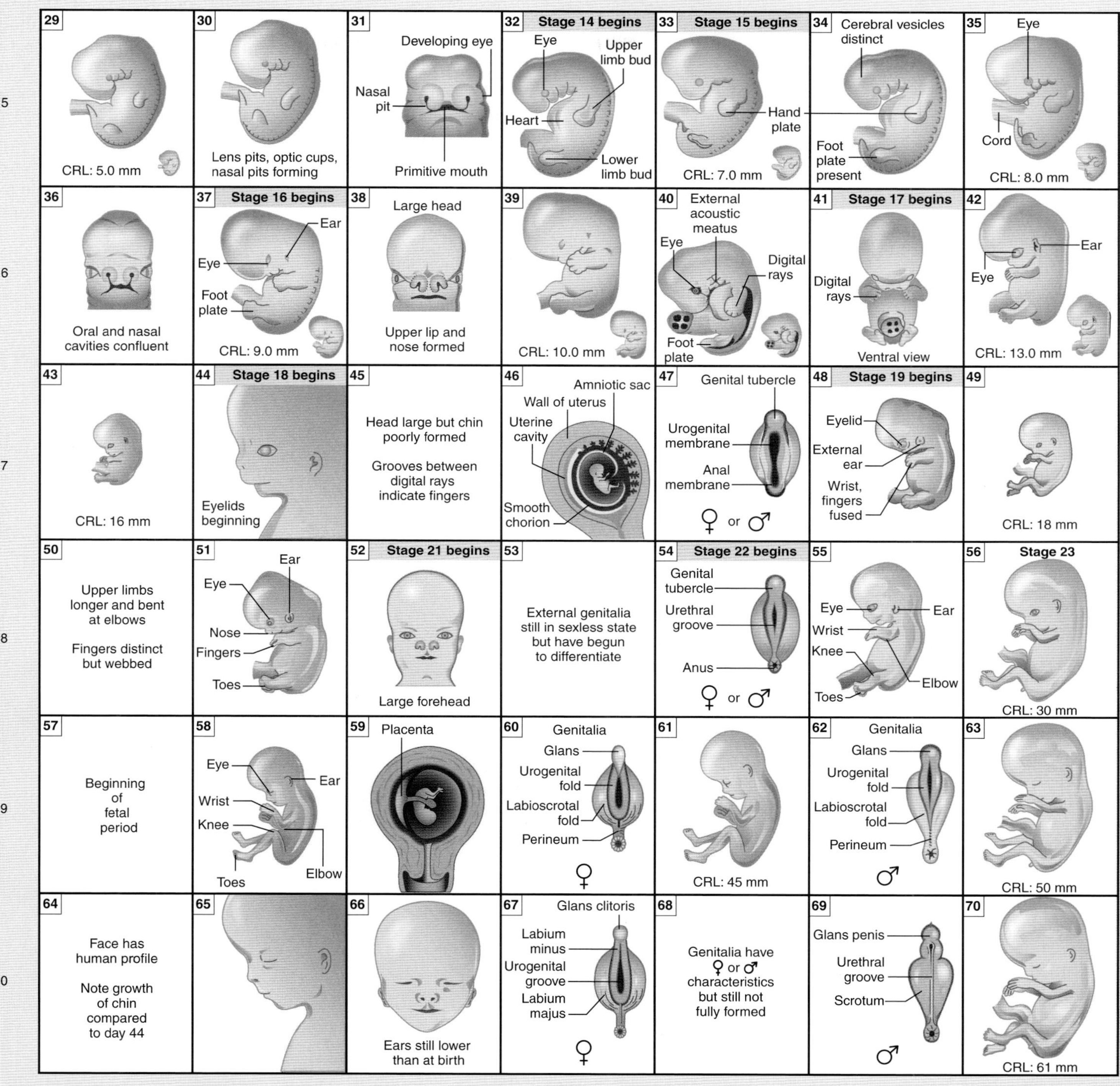
5
6
7
8
9
10
29
CRL: 5.0 mm
30
Lens pits, optic cups, nasal pits forming
31
Developing eye
Nasal pit
Primitive mouth
32 Stage 14 begins
Eye
Upper limb bud
Heart
Lower limb bud
33 Stage 15 begins
Hand plate
CRL: 7.0 mm
34 Cerebral vesicles distinct
Foot plate present
35
Eye
Cord
CRL: 8.0 mm
36
Oral and nasal cavities confluent
37 Stage 16 begins
Ear
Eye
Foot plate
CRL: 9.0 mm
38
Large head
Upper lip and nose formed
39
CRL: 10.0 mm
40
External acoustic meatus
Eye
Digital rays
Foot plate
41 Stage 17 begins
Digital rays
Ventral view
42
Ear
Eye
CRL: 13.0 mm
43
CRL: 16 mm
44 Stage 18 begins
Eyelids beginning
45
Head large but chin poorly formed
Grooves between digital rays indicate fingers
46
Amniotic sac
Wall of uterus
Uterine cavity
Smooth chorion
47
Genital tubercle
Urogenital membrane
Anal membrane
♀ or ♂
48 Stage 19 begins
Eyelid
External ear
Wrist, fingers fused
49
CRL: 18 mm
50
Upper limbs longer and bent at elbows
Fingers distinct but webbed
51
Ear
Eye
Nose
Fingers
Toes
52 Stage 21 begins
Large forehead
53
External genitalia still in sexless state but have begun to differentiate
54 Stage 22 begins
Genital tubercle
Urethral groove
Anus
♀ or ♂
55
Eye
Ear
Wrist
Knee
Elbow
Toes
56 Stage 23
CRL: 30 mm
57
Beginning of fetal period
58
Eye
Ear
Wrist
Knee
Toes
Elbow
59
Placenta
60
Genitalia
Glans
Urogenital fold
Labioscrotal fold
Perineum
♀
61
CRL: 45 mm
62
Genitalia
Glans
Urogenital fold
Labioscrotal fold
Perineum
♂
63
CRL: 50 mm
64
Face has human profile
Note growth of chin compared to day 44
65
66
Ears still lower than at birth
67
Glans clitoris
Labium minus
Urogenital groove
Labium majus
♀
68
Genitalia have ♀ or ♂ characteristics but still not fully formed
69
Glans penis
Urethral groove
Scrotum
♂
70
CRL: 61 mm

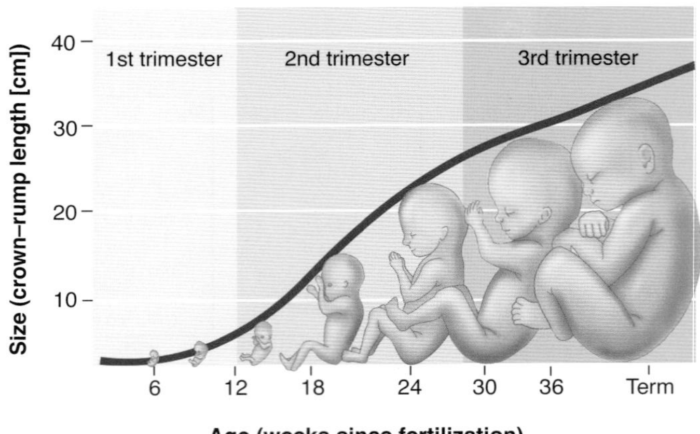

FIGURE 47-15 Increase in size during prenatal development. This graph shows the usual progression in size and body shape during the three trimesters of fetal development.

Mesoderm

The middle germ layer, or *mesoderm*, forms most of the organs and other structures between those formed by the endoderm and ectoderm. For example, the dermis of the skin, the skeletal muscles and bones, many of the glands of the body, kidneys, gonads, and components of the circulatory system are derived from the mesoderm. Look carefully at **Figure 47-16** to discern the logical pattern exhibited by germ layer development and differentiation.

HISTOGENESIS AND ORGANOGENESIS

The process by which the primary germ layers develop into many different kinds of tissues is called **histogenesis.** The way these tissues arrange themselves into organs is called **organogenesis.**

The fascinating story of histogenesis and organogenesis in human development is long and complicated; its telling belongs to the science of embryology. However, a brief example of organogenesis that is particularly useful in our current discussion of reproduction and development is the differentiation and development of the sex organs.

As **Figure 47-17** shows, the reproductive tracts of both the male and the female begin their development as sets of undifferentiated ducts and gonads. But as embryonic development continues in the male, the gonads attach to the *mesonephric (wolffian) duct*—which along with the urethra develops into the male reproductive tract (**Figure 47-17**, *B*). In the female embryo, by contrast, it is the nearby *paramesonephric (müllerian) duct* that instead develops into a female reproductive tract separate from the urinary tract (**Figure 47-17**, *C*). The female gonads (ovaries) do not attach to their ducts during development. **Figure 47-18** outlines the development of the male and female genitals. Note how they develop along slightly different paths to eventually become distinct types of structures.

A complete outline of the embryonic development of each organ and system is beyond the scope of this book. For the beginning student of anatomy and physiology, it seems sufficient to appreciate that human development begins when two sex cells unite to form a single-celled zygote and that the new offspring's body evolves by a series of processes consisting of cell differentiation, multiplication, growth, apoptosis, and rearrangement, all of which take place in a definite, orderly sequence. Development of structure and function go hand in hand, and from 4 months of gestation, when every organ system is in place and functioning to some extent, until term (about 280 days), development of the fetus is mainly a matter of growth.

Figure 47-19 shows the normal intrauterine position of a fetus just before birth in a full-term pregnancy. The large size of the pregnant uterus toward the end of pregnancy affects the normal function of the mother's body greatly. For example, you might be able to tell from **Figure 47-19** that a woman's centre of gravity is shifted forward. This can make walking and other movements of the body difficult—or even hazardous—because the sensory and motor control systems often do not compensate completely for this shift. The pregnant uterus presses on the

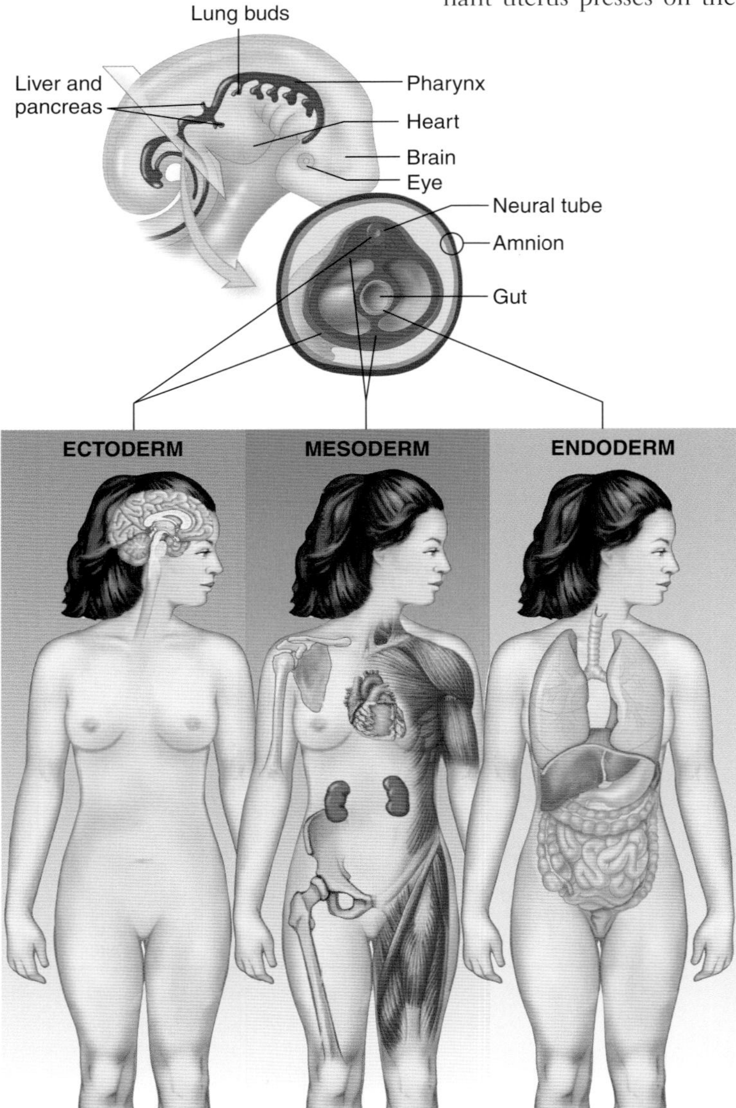

FIGURE 47-16 The primary germ layers. Illustration shows the primary germ layers and the body systems into which they develop.

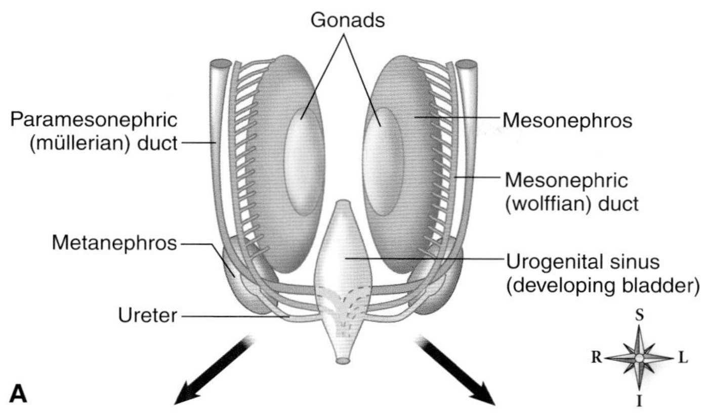

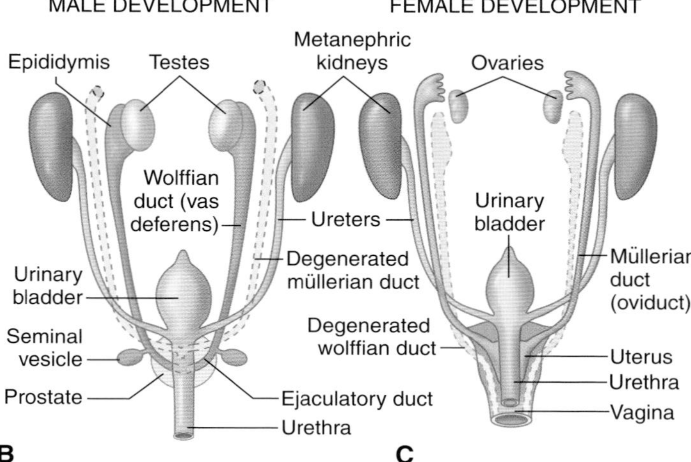

FIGURE 47-17 Development of the reproductive tracts. Both the male and female adult reproductive tracts are similar in their basic outline because they have a shared early development. **A,** Early in embryonic development, an undifferentiated set of gonads and ducts develops in both males and females. **B,** In males, the gonads (now testes) attach to the mesonephric (wolffian) ducts, which develop into the main part of the male reproductive tract. The paramesonephric ducts degenerate in males. **C,** In females, the gonads do not attach directly to a duct. It is the paramesonephric (müllerian) ducts that develop into the female reproductive tract and the mesonephric ducts that degenerate.

rectum, sometimes adversely affecting intestinal motility and thus may cause constipation and/or haemorrhoids. Pressure on the bladder reduces its urine-storing capacity, which results in frequent urination. Upward pressure pushes the abdominal organs against the diaphragm, making deep breathing difficult and sometimes causing the stomach to protrude into the thoracic cavity—a condition called *hiatal hernia*.

Quick CHECK

8. What is a *trimester*?
9. What is the difference between an *embryo* and a *fetus*?
10. Name the three primary germ layers.
11. What is histogenesis?

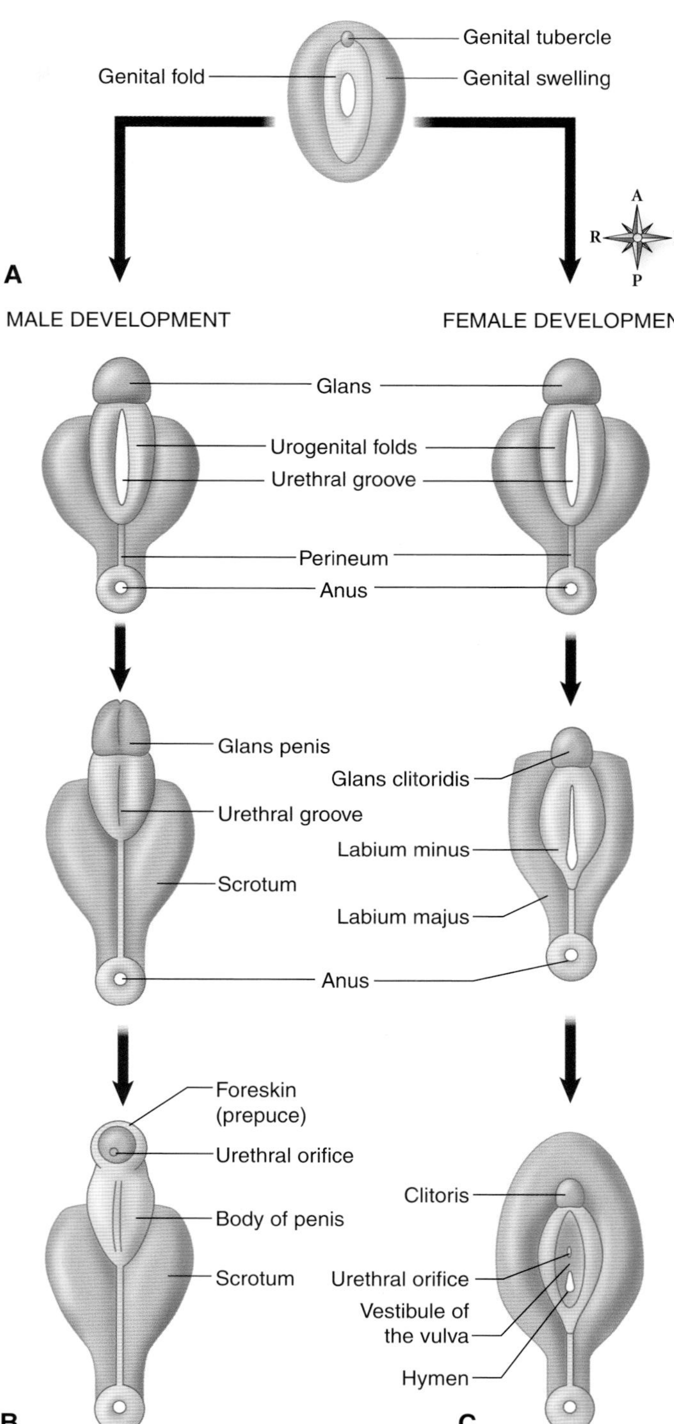

FIGURE 47-18 Development of the genitals. A, In early stages of development, the genitals are indifferent (not yet distinguishable). **B,** In the male, the genital tubercle eventually becomes the glans of the penis and the folds become the penis shaft and scrotum. **C,** In the female, the genital tubercle becomes the clitoris and the folds become the labia.

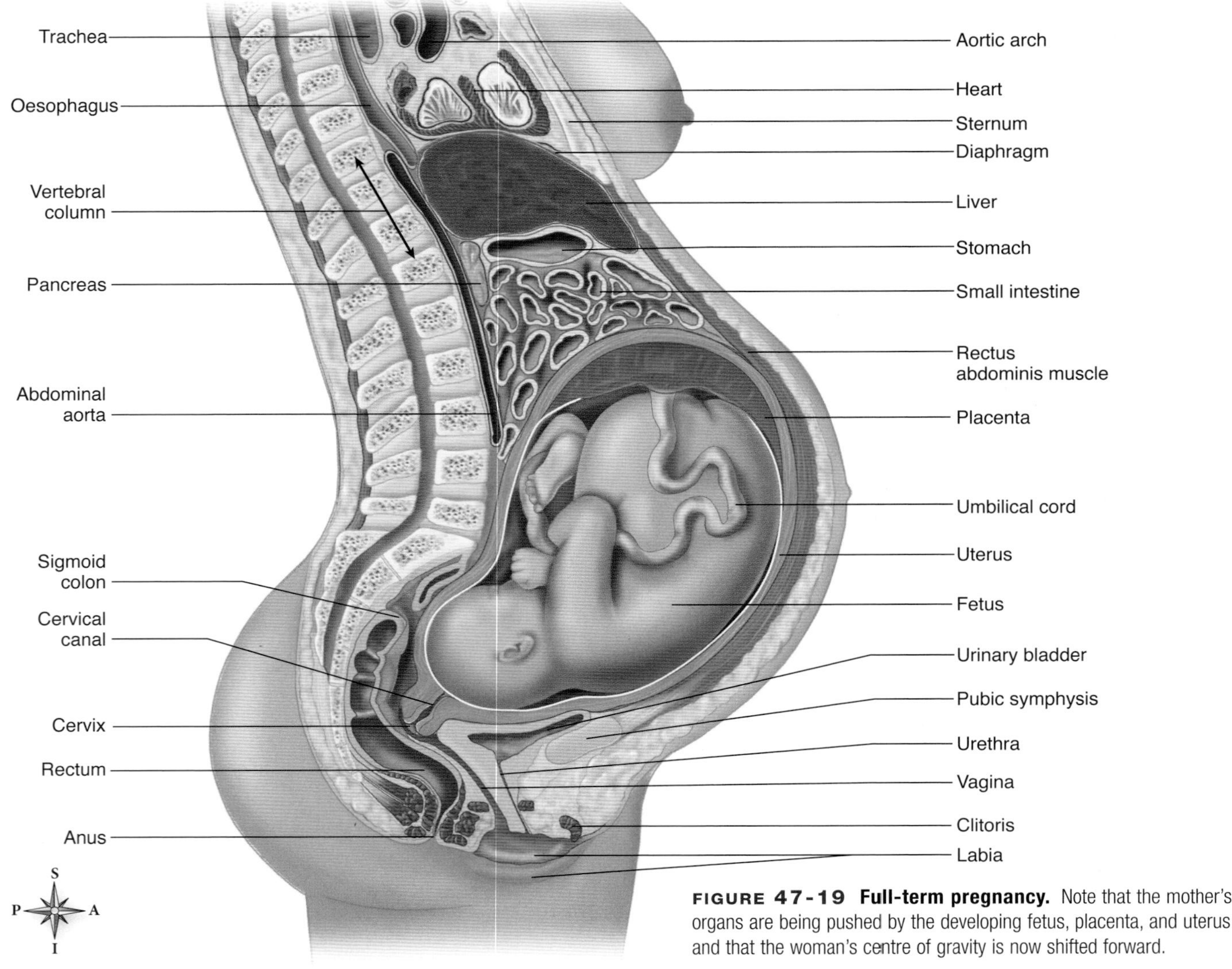

FIGURE 47-19 Full-term pregnancy. Note that the mother's organs are being pushed by the developing fetus, placenta, and uterus and that the woman's centre of gravity is now shifted forward.

BIRTH, OR PARTURITION

Birth, or **parturition**, is the point of transition between the prenatal and postnatal periods of life. As the fetus signals the end of pregnancy, the uterus becomes "irritable" and, ultimately, muscular contractions begin and cause the cervix to dilate (open), thus permitting the fetus to move from the uterus through the vagina or "birth canal" to the exterior. The process normally begins with the fetus taking a head-down position fully against the cervix (**Figure 47-20**, *1*). When contractions occur, the amniotic sac, or "bag of waters", usually ruptures, and labour begins.

Several hormones help to signal the time of labour and promote the processes needed for successful delivery. High levels of cortisol at the end of pregnancy trigger a drop in hCG, which in turn causes a drop in progesterone levels (see **Figure 47-12**). Progesterone inhibits the release of oxytocin (OT) earlier in the pregnancy—but at this point, the "brake" on the uterine muscle is released. Recall from Chapter 2 that OT is released in a positive feedback mechanism that amplifies the rate and strength of labour contractions (see **Figure 2-4** on p. 29). An injection of an OT preparation can stimulate labour contractions in a difficult or delayed delivery. Prostaglandins E_2 and F_2 (PGE_2, PGF_2) released by the placenta also play a role in the onset of labour by further sensitizing the myometrium of the uterus to OT.

STAGES OF LABOUR

Labour is the term used to describe the process that results in the birth of the baby. It is divided into three stages (see **Figure 47-20**, *2* to *5*):

1. *Stage one*—period from onset of uterine contractions until dilation of the cervix is complete
2. *Stage two*—period from the time of maximal cervical dilation until the baby exits through the vagina
3. *Stage three*—process of expulsion of the placenta through the vagina

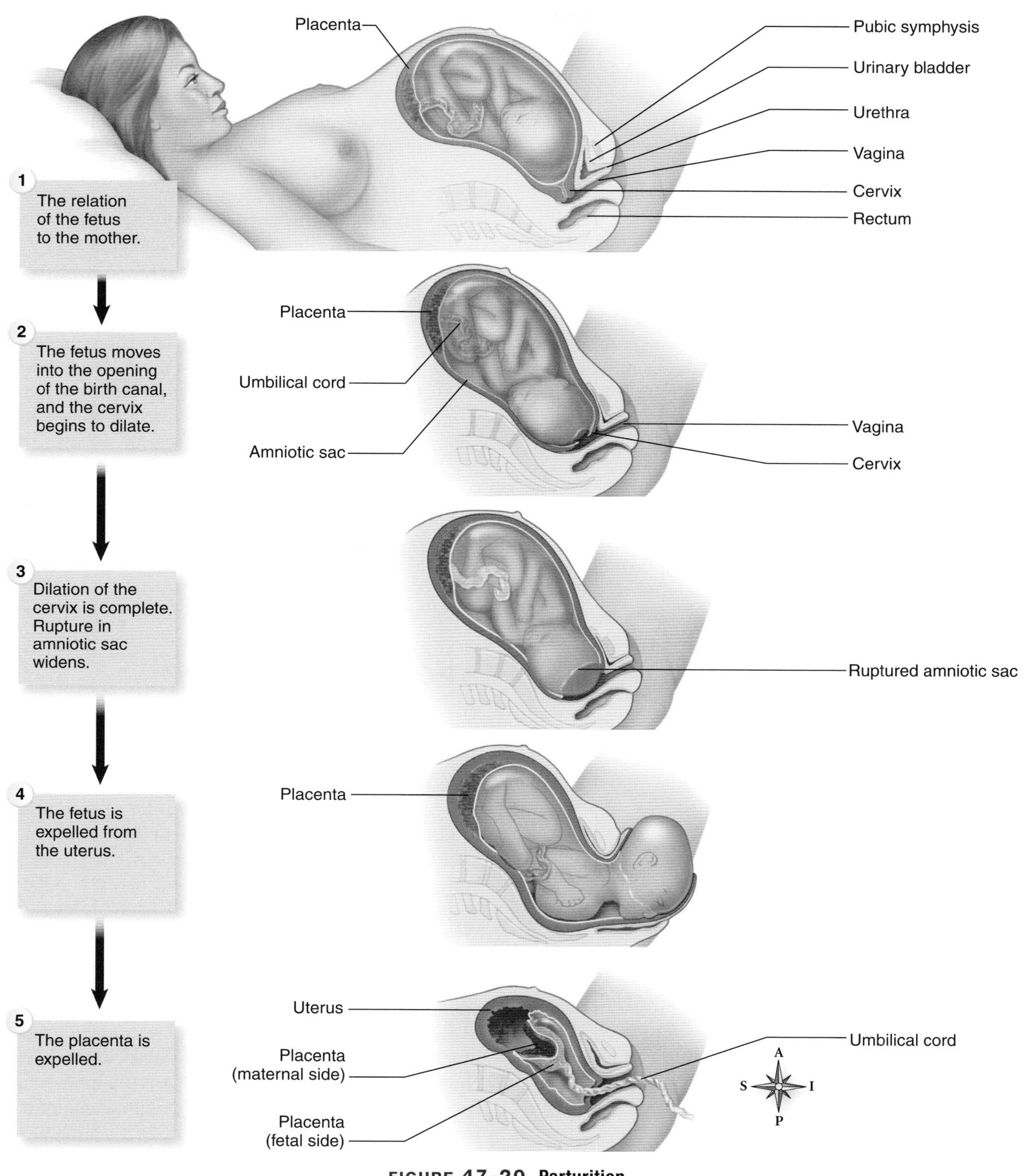
1
The relation of the fetus to the mother.
Placenta
Pubic symphysis
Urinary bladder
Urethra
Vagina
Cervix
Rectum
2
The fetus moves into the opening of the birth canal, and the cervix begins to dilate.
Placenta
Umbilical cord
Amniotic sac
Vagina
Cervix
3
Dilation of the cervix is complete. Rupture in amniotic sac widens.
Ruptured amniotic sac
4
The fetus is expelled from the uterus.
Placenta
5
The placenta is expelled.
Uterus
Placenta (maternal side)
Placenta (fetal side)
Umbilical cord
A
S
I
P

FIGURE 47-20 Parturition.

The time required for normal vaginal birth varies widely and may be influenced by many variables, including whether the woman has previously had a child. In most cases, stage one of labour lasts from 6 to 24 hours, and stage two lasts from a few minutes to an hour. Delivery of the placenta (stage three) is normally within 15 minutes after the birth of the baby. If abnormal conditions of the mother or fetus (or both) make normal vaginal delivery hazardous or impossible, physicians may suggest a **caesarean section.** Often called simply a *C-section,* it is a surgical procedure in which the newborn is delivered through an incision in the abdomen and uterine wall.

Immediately after birth, the umbilical cord is cut and clamped. Recall from Chapter 29 that at birth, the circulatory route of the infant changes as the placenta is lost and the lungs begin to function (see **Figure 29-25** on p. 691). Eventually, the remainder of the cord sloughs off—leaving the umbilicus or navel as an abdominal landmark.

CONNECT IT!

Blood from the umbilical cord is often saved for future use. Learn what it is used for in ***Freezing Umbilical Cord Blood*** online at ***Connect It!***

MULTIPLE BIRTHS

The term *multiple birth* refers to the birth of two or more infants from the same pregnancy. The birth of twins is more common than the birth of triplets, quadruplets, or quintuplets. Multiple-birth babies are often born prematurely, so they are at a greater than normal risk of complications in infancy. However, premature infants who have modern medical care available have a much lower risk of complications than those without such care.

Twinning, or double births, can result from either of two different processes:

1. **Identical twins** result from the splitting of embryonic tissue from the same zygote early in development. One way this happens is that, during the blastocyst stage of development, the inner cell mass divides into two masses. Each inner cell mass thus formed develops into a separate individual. As **Figure 47-21**, *A*, shows, identical twins usually share the same placenta but have separate umbilical cords. This is not surprising because in this type of twinning there is a single, shared trophoblast. Because they develop from the same fertilized egg, identical twins have the same genetic code. Despite this, identical twins are not absolutely identical in terms of structure and function. Different environmental factors and personal experiences lead to individuality even in genetically identical twins.
2. **Fraternal twins** result from the fertilization of two different ova by two different spermatozoa (**Figure 47-21**, *B*). Fraternal twinning requires the production of more than one mature ovum during a single menstrual cycle, a trait that is often inherited. Multiple ovulation may also occur in response to certain fertility drugs, especially the gonadotropin preparations. Fraternal twins are no more closely related genetically than any other brother–sister relationship. Because two separate fertilizations must occur, it is even possible for fraternal twins to have different biological fathers. Triplets, quadruplets, and other multiple births may be identical, fraternal, or any combination.

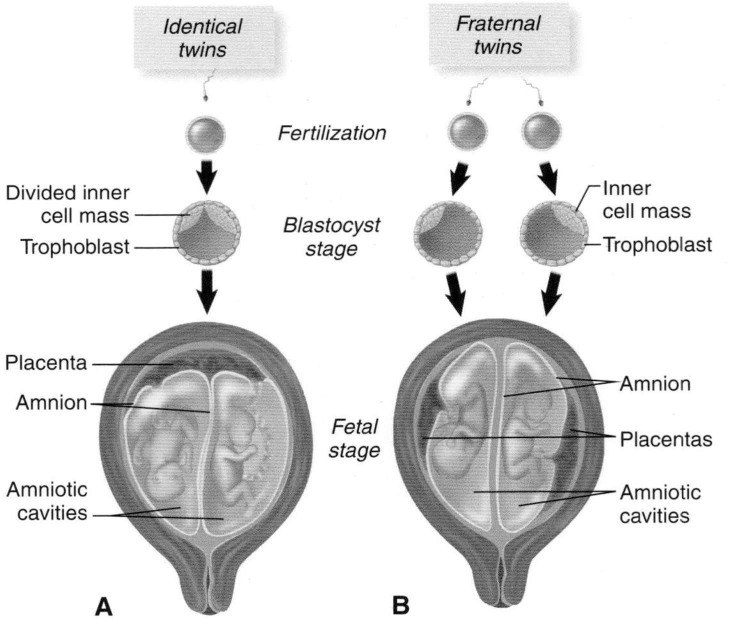

Identical twins
Fraternal twins
Fertilization
Divided inner cell mass
Trophoblast
Blastocyst stage
Inner cell mass
Trophoblast
Placenta
Amnion
Amniotic cavities
Fetal stage
Amnion
Placentas
Amniotic cavities
A
B

FIGURE 47-21 Multiple births. A, Identical twins develop when embryonic tissue from a single zygote splits to form two individuals. Note that, because the trophoblast is shared, the placenta and the part of the amnion separating the amniotic cavities are shared by the twins. **B,** Fraternal twins develop when two ova are fertilized at the same time, producing two separate zygotes. Notice that each fraternal twin has its own placenta and amnion.

Quick CHECK

12. Briefly describe the three stages of labour.
13. How does identical twinning differ from fraternal twinning?

POSTNATAL PERIOD

The **postnatal period** begins at birth and lasts until death. It is often divided into major periods for study, but we must appreciate the fact that growth and development are continuous processes that occur throughout the life cycle. Gradual changes in the physical appearance of the body as a whole and in the relative proportions of the head, trunk, and limbs are quite noticeable between birth and adolescence. Note in **Figure 47-22** the obvious changes in the size of bones and in the proportionate sizes between different bones and body areas. The head, for example, becomes proportionately smaller. Whereas the infant head is approximately one fourth the total height of the body, the adult head is only about one eighth the total height. The facial bones also show several changes between infancy and adulthood. In an infant the face is one eighth of the skull surface, but in an adult the face is half of the skull surface. Another change in proportion involves the trunk and lower extremities. The legs become proportionately longer and the trunk proportionately shorter. In addition, the thoracic and abdominal contours change from round to elliptical.

Such changes are good examples of the ever-changing and ongoing nature of growth, development, and ageing. It is unfortunate that many of the changes that occur in the later years of life do not result in an increased function. These degenerative changes are certainly important, however, and will be discussed later in this chapter (see pp. 1113–1117).

The following are the most common postnatal periods: (1) **infancy,** (2) **childhood,** (3) **adolescence** and **adulthood,** and (4) **older adulthood. Table 47-1** summarizes the projected changes in the UK population in selected age groups from 2014–2039. Note

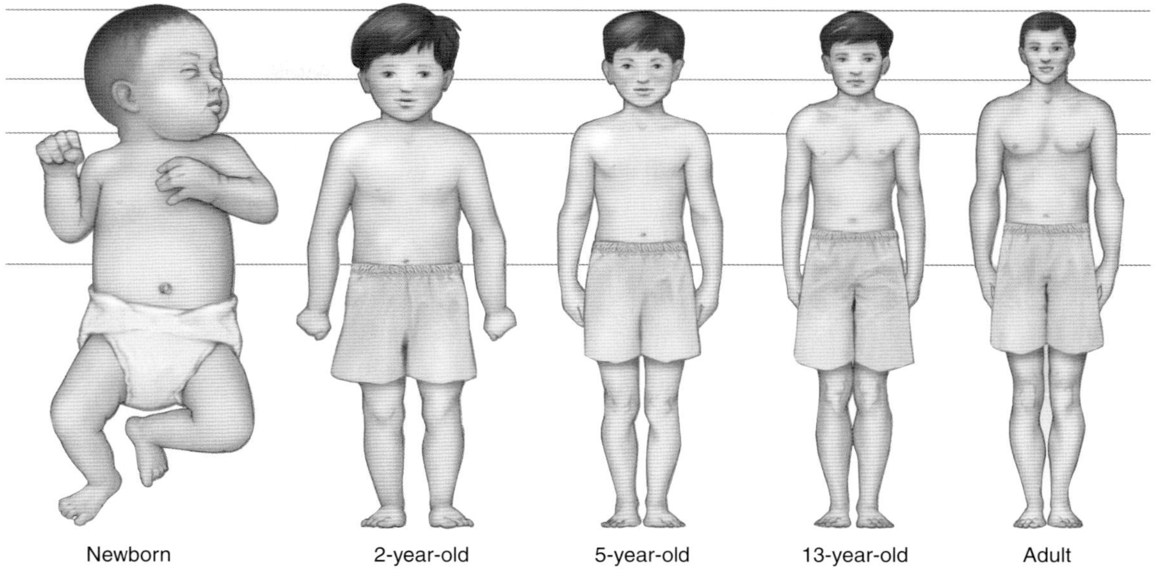

FIGURE 47-22 Changes in the proportions of body parts from birth to maturity. Note the dramatic differences in relative head size.

the proportionally higher rise in older age groups, particularly in people older than age 85 years.

INFANCY

The period of infancy begins abruptly at birth and lasts about 18 months. (Note—infancy is also regarded by some UK specialists as the first 12 months and by the World Health Organization (WHO) as the first 24 months). The first 4 weeks of infancy are often referred to as the **neonatal period.** Dramatic changes occur at a rapid rate during this short but critical period. **Neonatology** is the medical and nursing specialty concerned with the diagnosis and treatment of disorders of the newborn. Advances in this area have resulted in dramatically reduced infant mortality.

Many of the changes that occur in the cardiovascular and respiratory systems at birth are necessary for survival (see **Figures 29-24**, p. 690, and **Figure 29-25**, p. 691). Whereas the fetus totally depended on the mother for life support, the newborn infant, to survive, must become totally self-supporting in terms of blood circulation and respiration immediately after birth. A baby's first breath is deep and forceful. The stimulus to breathe results primarily from the increasing amounts of carbon dioxide (CO_2) that accumulate in the blood after the umbilical cord is cut shortly after delivery.

To assess the general condition of a newborn, a system that scores five health criteria is often used. The criteria are heart rate (HR), respiration, muscle tone, skin colour, and response to stimuli. Each aspect is scored as 0, 1, or 2—depending on the condition of the infant. The resulting total score is called the **Apgar score.** The Apgar score in a completely healthy newborn is 10.

TABLE 47-1 Projected Population by Age, United Kingdom, mid-2014 to mid 2039*

Ages	2014	2019	2024	2029	2034	2039	% CHANGE
0–14	11.4	12.0	12.3	12.3	12.3	12.4	8.8
15–29	12.6	12.4	12.3	12.6	13.2	13.5	7.1
30–44	12.7	12.9	13.6	13.7	13.3	13.2	3.9
45–59	13.0	13.4	12.9	12.6	12.7	13.4	3.1
60–74	9.7	10.4	11.1	12.0	12.4	12.0	23.7
75 & over	5.2	5.8	7.0	7.8	8.7	9.9	90.1
75–84	3.7	4.1	4.9	5.4	5.6	6.3	70.3
85 & over	1.5	1.7	2.0	2.4	3.2	3.6	140.0
All ages	64.6	66.9	69.0	71.0	72.7	74.3	15.0

*Numbers in millions.

CONNECT IT!

A fetus receives its first "doses" of the microorganisms that will form its microbiome from the mother's blood supply through the placenta. A newborn baby also receives microorganisms from the mother's birth canal during delivery, from breast milk, and contact with the skin of its parents and siblings. Review the importance of establishing these microorganisms in the human microbiome in ***The Human Microbiome*** at ***Connect It!***

Many developmental changes occur between the end of the neonatal period and 12 months of age. Birth weight generally doubles during the first 4 to 6 months and then triples by 1 year. The baby also increases in length by 50% by the twelfth month. The "baby fat" that accumulated under the skin during the first year begins to decrease, and the plump infant becomes leaner.

Early in infancy the baby has only one spinal curvature (**Figure 47-23**). The cervical curve appears as the infant begins holding up her head. The lumbar curvature appears between 12 and 18 months, as the once-helpless infant becomes a toddler who can stand (**Figure 47-24**). One of the most striking changes to occur during infancy is the rapid development of the nervous and muscular systems. This permits the infant to follow a moving object with the eyes (2 months); lift the head and raise the chest (3 months); sit when well supported (4 months); crawl (10 months); stand alone (12 months); and run, although a bit stiffly (18 months).

Childhood

Childhood extends from the end of infancy to sexual maturity, or puberty—11 to 13 years in girls and 12 to 14 years in boys. Overall, growth during early childhood continues at a rather rapid pace, but month-to-month gains become less consistent. By the age of 6 years the child appears more like a preadolescent than an infant or toddler. The child becomes less chubby, the potbelly becomes flatter, and the face loses its babyish look. The nervous and muscular systems continue to develop rapidly during the middle years of childhood; by 10 years of age the child has developed numerous motor and coordination skills.

The *deciduous teeth,* which began to appear at about 6 months of age, are lost during childhood, beginning at about 6 years of age. The *permanent teeth,* with the possible exception of the third molars (wisdom teeth), have all erupted by age 14 years.

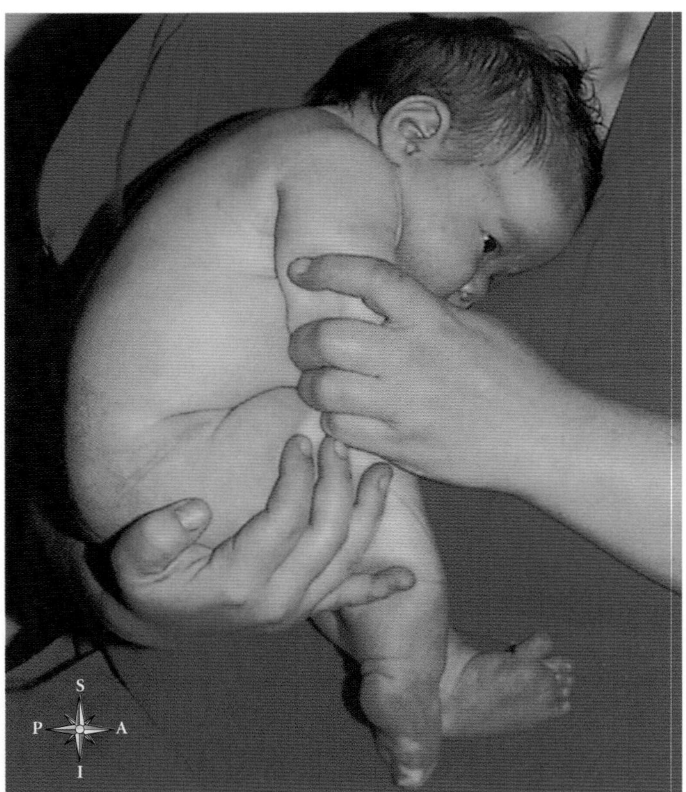

FIGURE 47-23 The infant spine. Photograph showing the normal rounded curvature of the vertebral column in an infant.

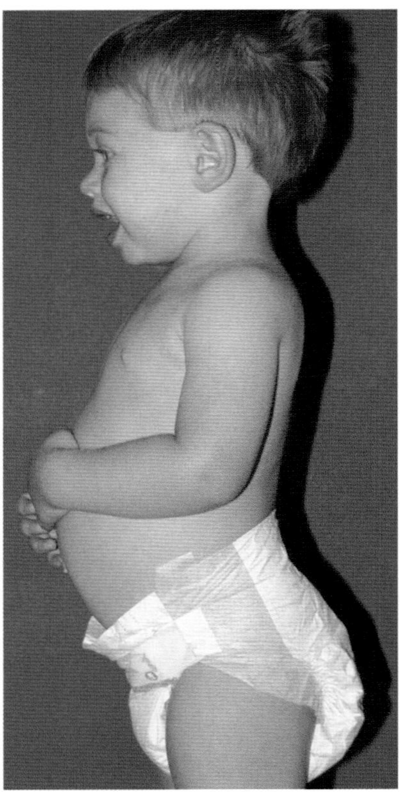

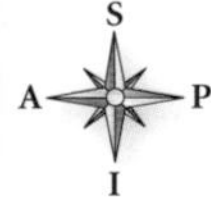

FIGURE 47-24 The toddler spine. Photograph showing the normal curvature of the vertebral column in a toddler. The dark shadow emphasizes the distinct lumbar curvature that develops with the ability to walk (compare with **Figure 47-23**).

Adolescence and Adulthood

The average age range of adolescence varies but generally the teenage years (13 to 19) are used as the standard age range. The period is marked by rapid and intense physical growth, which ultimately results in sexual maturity. Note that WHO defines an adolescent as any person between the ages of 10 and 19. Recent guidelines given to psychologists in the UK suggest it should be increased to the age of 25!

The stage of adolescence in which a person becomes sexually mature is called **puberty.** Many of the developmental changes that occur during this period are controlled by the secretion of gonadotropins (FSH and LH) and sex hormones such as testosterone and oestrogen (**Figure 47-25**). Some of these changes involve development of the gonads themselves and are called **primary sex characteristics.** However, most of the more visible changes involve development of the **secondary sex characteristics** such as skeletal changes, fat distribution patterns, growth of pubic and body hair, and growth of the larynx.

Breast development is often the first sign of approaching puberty in girls, beginning about age 9 or 10 years. Most girls begin to menstruate at 12 to 14 years of age. In boys the first sign of puberty is often enlargement of the testes, which begins between 10 and 14 years of age. Both sexes show a spurt in height during adolescence (**Figure 47-26**). In girls the spurt in height begins between the ages of 10 and 12 years and is nearly complete by 14 or 15 years. In boys the period of rapid growth begins between 12 and 13 years and is generally complete by 16 or 17 years.

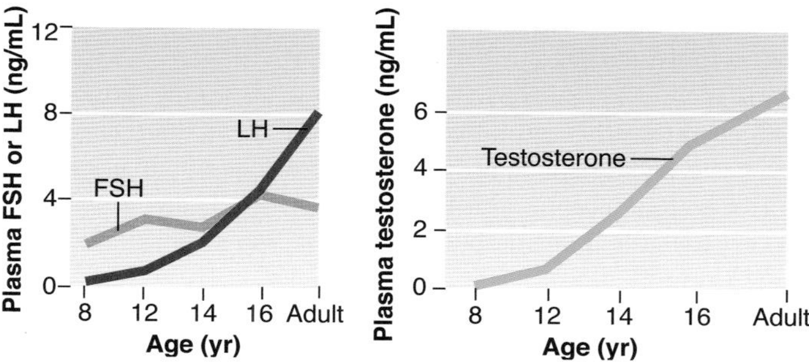

FIGURE 47-25 Hormone changes during puberty. The left graph shows the increase in gonadotropin (LH and FSH) secretion during puberty. The right graph shows changes in testosterone levels (in males) during puberty that result from increased gonadotropin levels. Female hormones show a similar change within a monthly cycle of dramatic highs and lows (see **Figures 46-14** and **46-15**). *FSH,* Follicle-stimulating hormone; *LH,* luteinizing hormone.

CONNECT IT! 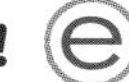

A person's body shape or *somatotype* can change during adolescence and sometimes produces anxiety because of social pressures that seem to favour certain body shapes. To learn more about this, check out ***Body Types and Disease*** at ***Connect It!***

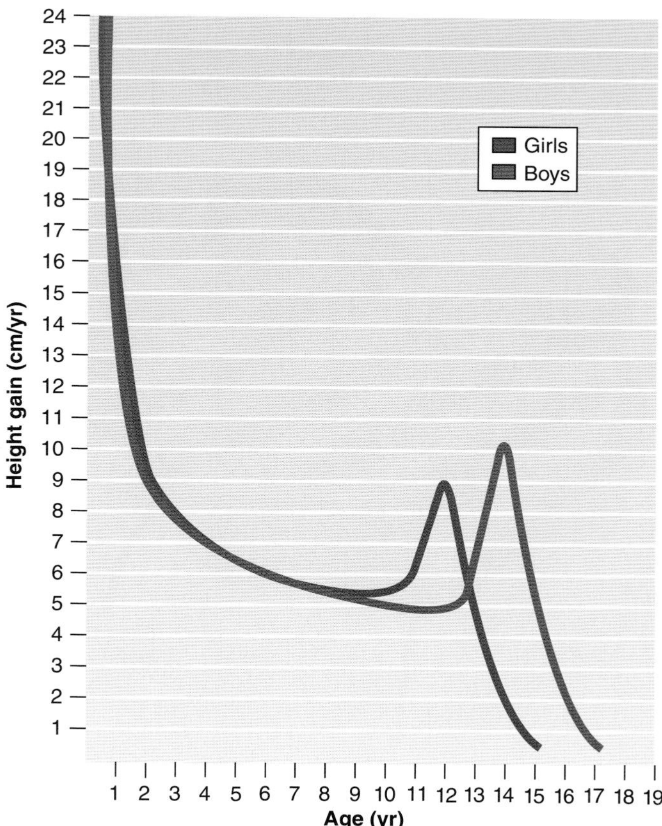

FIGURE 47-26 Growth in height. The graph shows typical patterns of gain in height from birth to adulthood for girls and boys. Note the rapid gain in height during the first few years, a period of slower growth, then another burst of growth during adolescence—finally ending at the beginning of adulthood.

Many developmental changes that begin early in childhood are not completed until the early or middle years of adulthood. Examples include the maturation of bone, resulting in the full closure of the growth plates, and changes in the size and placement of other body components such as the sinuses. Many body traits do not become apparent for years after birth. Normal balding patterns, for example, are determined at the time of fertilization by heredity but do not appear until maturity. As a rule, adulthood is characterized by the maintenance of existing body tissues. With the passage of years the ongoing effort of maintenance and repair of body tissues becomes more and more difficult. As a result, degeneration begins. This is part of the process of ageing, and it culminates in death.

Older Adulthood and Senescence

Most body systems are in peak condition and function at a high level of efficiency during early adulthood. As a person grows older, a gradual but certain decline takes place in the functioning of every major organ system in the body. The study of ageing is called **gerontology.** Older adulthood is characterized by the processes of senescence, or degenerative ageing. Unfortunately, the mechanisms and causes of ageing are not well understood.

Some gerontologists believe that an important ageing mechanism is the limit on cell reproduction. Laboratory experiments show that many types of human cells cannot reproduce more than 50 times—thus limiting the maximum life span. Cells die continually in a process called *apoptosis,* no matter what a person's age, but in older adulthood, many dead cells are not replaced—causing degeneration of tissues. Perhaps the cells are not replaced because the surrounding cells have reached their limit of reproduction. Perhaps differences in each adult's ageing process result from differences in the reproductive capacity of cells. The cellular death mechanism seems to operate in individuals with **progeria,** a rare, genetic condition in which a person appears to age rapidly (**Box 47-3**).

BOX 47-3 *diagnostic study* | Progeria

Progeria, also called *Hutchinson–Gilford progeria syndrome,* is a rare, fatal condition in which children appear to age rapidly. In progeria, the reproductive capacity of cells seems to be diminished due to a toxic protein called *progerin,* which is also found in normal cells at much lower levels and increases as we age. Thus the tissues of children with progeria fail to maintain or repair themselves normally, and many of the degenerative conditions more commonly seen in elderly individuals appear. Some of these conditions can be seen in this photograph of a boy with progeria: thin, tightened skin with stippled colouration; hair loss; loss of subcutaneous fat; and stiff, partially flexed, and swollen joints. Children with progeria die of cardiovascular disease at an average age of 14 years. •

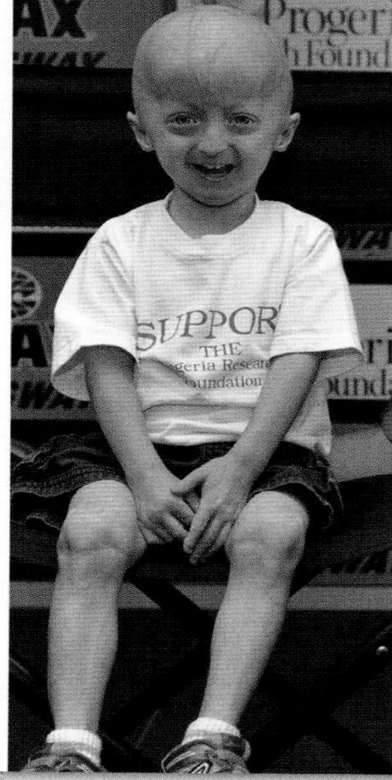

Various factors that affect the rates of cell death and cell reproduction have been cited as causes of ageing. Some gerontologists believe that nutrition, injury, disease, and other environmental factors affect the ageing process. A few have even proposed that ageing results from cellular changes caused by slow-acting "ageing" viruses found in all living cells. Other gerontologists have proposed that ageing is caused by "ageing" genes that regulate apoptosis or other cell functions—genes in which ageing is "preprogrammed".

Another proposed cause of ageing is autoimmunity. You may recall from Chapter 33 that autoimmunity occurs when the immune system attacks a person's own tissues. Yet another theory of ageing suggests that as a person ages, mitochondria become less able to shuttle adenosine triphosphate (ATP) out to the cytosol. Decreasing ATP availability renders cells less able to perform their functions and even causes them to degenerate—hallmarks of the ageing process. One popular theory of ageing states that oxygen *free radicals* play a major role in cellular ageing (see **Figure 41-23**, p. 950). Free radicals are highly reactive forms of oxygen that normally result from mitochondrial activity, but in excess may damage the cell. As a person's cells produce more and more free radicals during the later years, more damage happens to cellular structures and functions. In addition, as free-radical production increases, mitochondrial function decreases and therefore availability of ATP decreases (**Figure 47-27**).

Many different genes have been put forth as having direct or indirect effects on ageing and longevity. Most of them operate in one or more of the ageing mechanisms already discussed. It is clear that there is a genetic component to how we age and how long we live. However, the mechanisms by which these genes influence ageing still remain unclear.

Although the causes and basic mechanisms of ageing are yet to be understood, at least many of the signs of ageing are obvious. The remainder of this chapter deals with some of the more common degenerative changes that frequently characterize **senescence,** or older adulthood.

Quick CHECK

14. Name the four major phases of the postnatal period.
15. When does the *neonatal period* of human development occur?
16. What signs characterize the *adolescent period* of human development?
17. Briefly describe one of the proposed mechanisms of the ageing process.

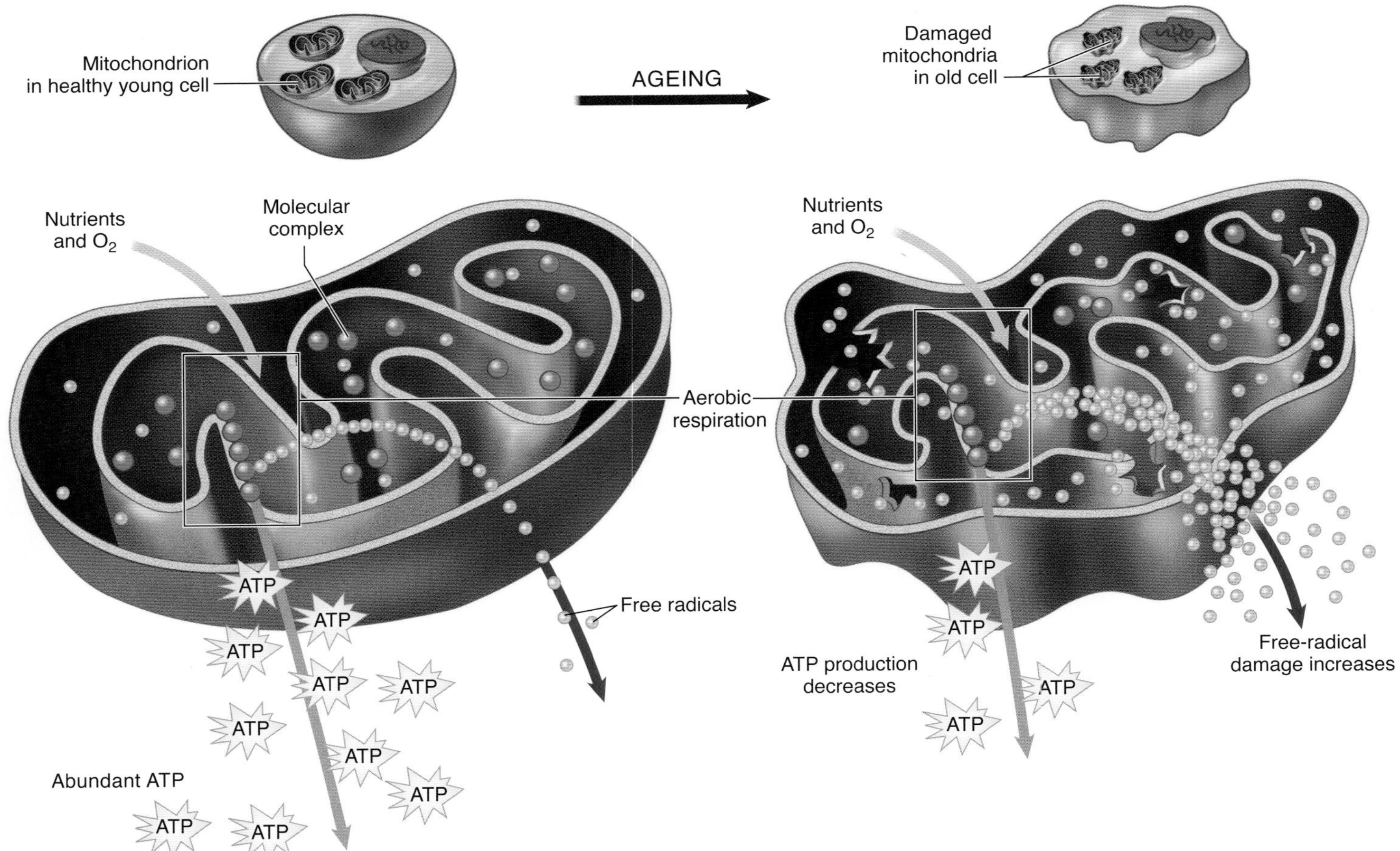

FIGURE 47-27 Free-radical theory of ageing. Being one of many possible mechanisms of the ageing processes, free-radical production by cells may increase as a person gets older, thereby increasing the amount of cellular damage. Free radicals are highly reactive forms of oxygen that are normal byproducts of cellular respiration in the mitochondria (shown) and other cell processes. As one ages, the number of free radicals increases as cellular efficiency decreases. Thus more cellular damage occurs, especially damage to cellular membranes, causing degeneration of the cell.

EFFECTS OF AGEING

Ageing affects each individual in different ways. Environment, genetics, and perhaps even attitude may affect the degree to which the structure and function of a person's body change through older adulthood. Despite advances in understanding how some of the effects of ageing can be minimized or even avoided, one cannot completely avoid the fact that body structures degenerate and functions decrease as we get older. **Figure 47-28** summarizes a few of the many biological changes that occur by the time we reach late adulthood.

SKELETAL SYSTEM

In older adulthood, bones undergo changes in texture, degree of calcification, and shape. Instead of clean-cut margins, older bones develop indistinct and shaggy-appearing margins with spurs—a process called *lipping*. This type of degenerative change restricts movement because of the piling up of bone tissue around the joints.

With advancing age, changes in calcification of bones reduce the *bone mineral density (BMD)*, as you can see in **Figure 47-29**, *A*. This may result in reduction of bone size and in bones that are porous and subject to fracture. The lower cervical and thoracic vertebrae are the site of frequent fractures. The result is curvature of the spine and the shortened stature so typical of late adulthood (**Figure 47-29**, *B*). The onset of *osteoporosis* and other types of bone loss associated with ageing may be avoided—at least to some extent—by maintaining a high BMD through exercise and sufficient calcium in the diet.

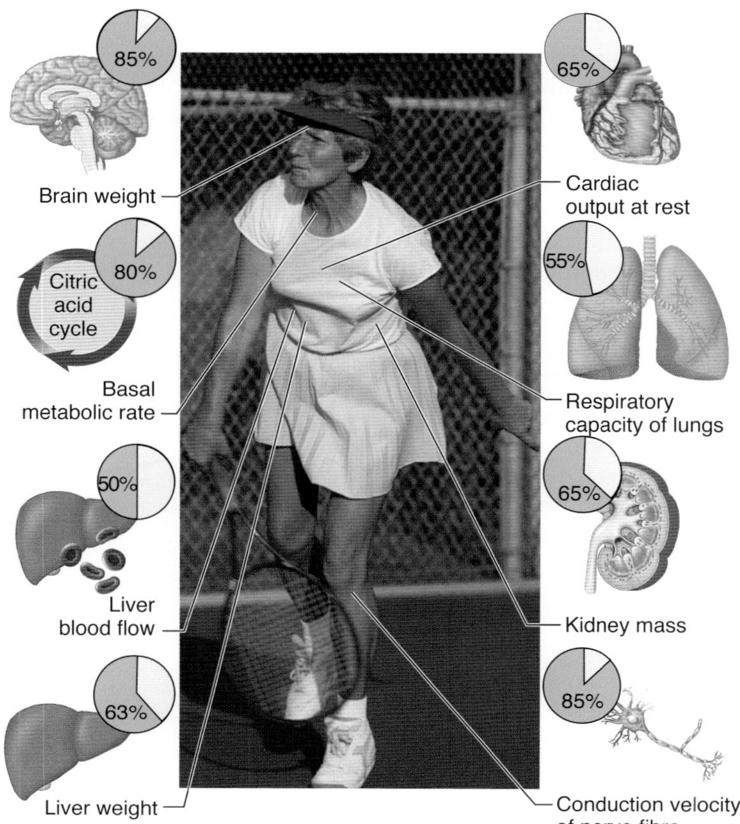

FIGURE 47-28 Some biological changes associated with maturity and ageing. Insets show proportion of remaining function in the organs of a person in late adulthood (green) compared with a 20-year-old person (yellow).

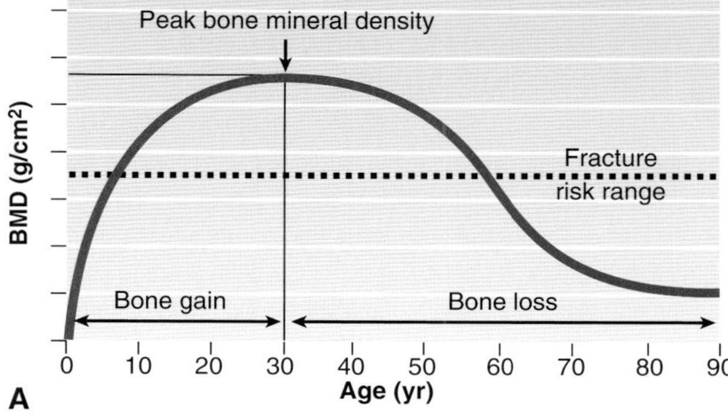

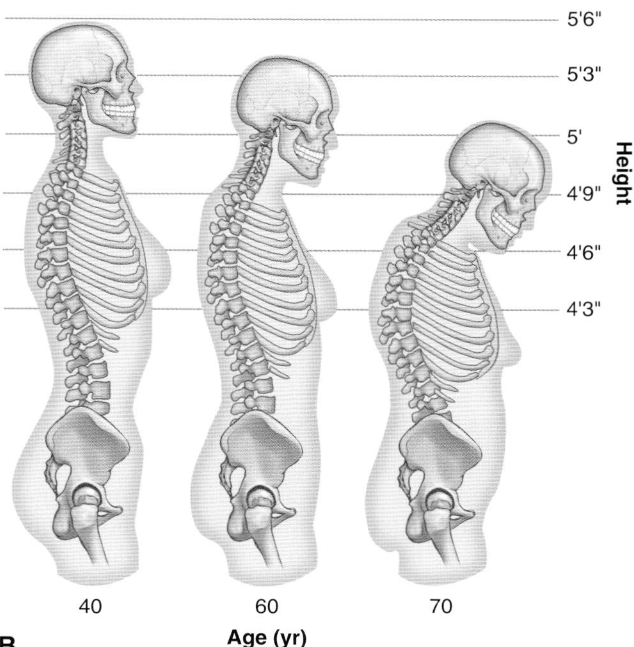

FIGURE 47-29 Loss of bone mineral density (BMD) in late adulthood. **A,** Graph showing changes in BMD over the life span in females. BMD peaks in young adulthood and decreases in late adulthood to a point at which there is an increased risk of bone fracture. Males also have a decrease in BMD beginning around age 50 years, but the decline is more gradual than in women. **B,** The normal spinal curvatures of young adulthood give way to possible changes later in life because of a decrease in BMD.

Degenerative joint diseases such as **osteoarthritis** are also common in elderly adults.

CONNECT IT!

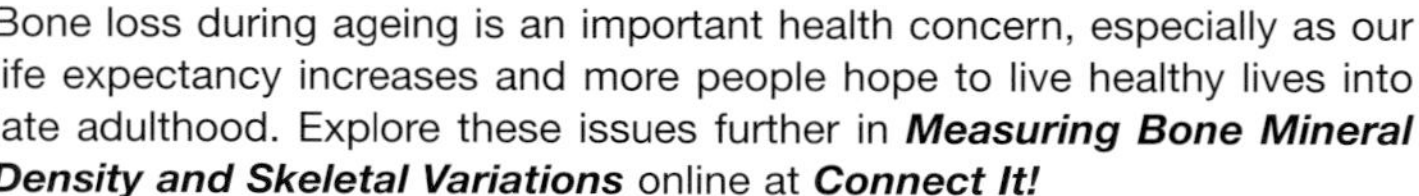
Bone loss during ageing is an important health concern, especially as our life expectancy increases and more people hope to live healthy lives into late adulthood. Explore these issues further in ***Measuring Bone Mineral Density and Skeletal Variations*** online at ***Connect It!***

MUSCULAR SYSTEM

Getting older usually involves losing muscle mass. This can begin as early as age 25 years but does not usually reach 10% loss in muscle mass until 50 years of age or so. By age 80 years, many people have lost about 50% of their skeletal muscle mass. Most of the age-related loss of muscle mass is due to a loss of muscle fibres. However, weight

BOX 47-4 *sports and fitness*

Exercise and Ageing

A sound exercise programme throughout life can reduce some of the common effects of ageing. The improved cardiovascular condition associated with aerobic training can prevent or reduce the effects of several age-related circulatory problems. The loss of bone mass that occurs in older adulthood is less troublesome if one enters this period with a higher than average bone density developed through exercising. Finally, the relatively high ratio of body fat to muscle often seen in the elderly can be reduced or avoided entirely by a lifelong fitness programme. •

training before and during one's later years can increase the mass of the remaining fibres and thus counteract at least some of the reduction in the number of muscle fibres (**Box 47-4**).

Another change in our muscles as we age is that many muscle fibres develop into slower type fibres or into an intermediate form between the "fast type" and "slow type" of muscle fibre. This usually means that the overall ratio of "fast" to "slow" function decreases—that is, our muscle function becomes relatively "slower". As **Figure 47-30** shows, the different fibre types also begin to group together in bunches and change their shape slightly. These effects seem unavoidable—even with exercise.

Integumentary System (Skin)

With advancing age the skin becomes dry, thin, and inelastic. It "sags" on the body because of increased wrinkling and skinfolds—as well as a loss of body fat under the skin. Pigmentation changes and the thinning or loss of hair are also common conditions associated with ageing.

Urinary System

The number of functioning nephron units in the kidney decreases by almost 50% between the ages of 30 and 75 years. Also, because less blood flows through the kidneys as an individual ages, there is a reduction in overall function and excretory capacity or the ability to produce urine. In the bladder, significant age-related problems often occur because of diminished muscle tone. Muscle atrophy (wasting) in the bladder wall results in decreased capacity and inability to empty, or void, completely.

Respiratory System

In older adulthood the costal cartilages that connect the ribs to the sternum become hardened or calcified. This makes it difficult for the ribcage to expand and contract as it normally does during inspiration and expiration. In time the ribs gradually become "fixed" to the sternum, and chest movements become difficult. When this occurs the ribcage remains in a more expanded position, respiratory efficiency decreases, and a condition called "barrel chest" results. With advancing years a generalized atrophy, or wasting, of muscle tissue takes place as the contractile muscle cells are replaced by connective tissue. This loss of muscle cells decreases the strength of the muscles associated with inspiration and expiration.

Although there is a moderate decline in lung function because of ageing, factors such as smoking can profoundly increase the rate and severity of the decline, as you can see in **Figure 47-31**.

Cardiovascular System

Degenerative heart and blood vessel disease is one of the most common and serious effects of ageing. Fatty deposits build up in blood vessel walls and narrow the passageway for the movement of blood, much as the buildup of scale in a water pipe decreases flow and pressure. The resulting condition, called **atherosclerosis,** often leads to eventual blockage of the coronary arteries and a "heart attack" (myocardial infarction [MI]). If fatty accumulations or other substances in blood vessels calcify, actual hardening of the arteries, or **arteriosclerosis,** occurs. Rupture of a hardened vessel in the brain (stroke) is a common cause of serious disability or death in the older adult. **Hypertension (HTN),** or high blood pressure, is also more common.

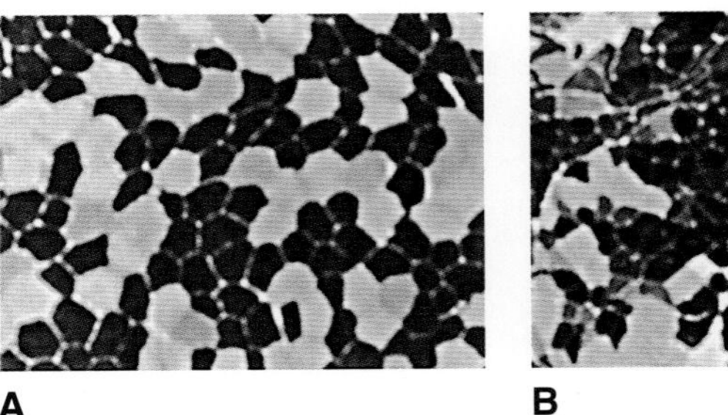

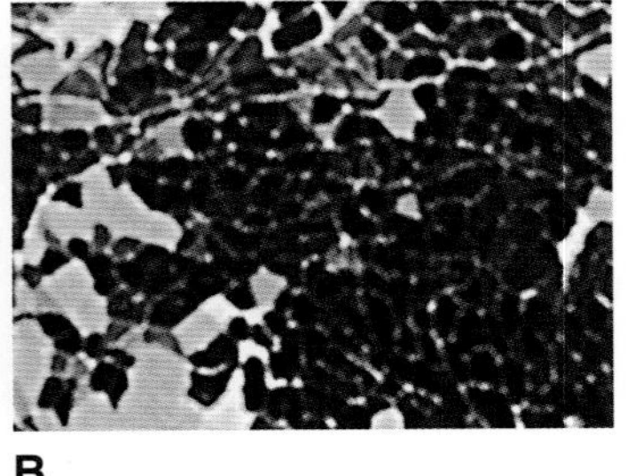

FIGURE 47-30 Muscle changes in late adulthood. Skeletal muscle tissue changes as we age. **A,** Younger muscle shows a typical "chequerboard" pattern of fast and slow fibres (distinguished by stains here). **B,** However, in the elderly the fast and slow fibres tend to group together rather than remain distributed evenly throughout the muscle organ. Note the overall increase in the slower fibres, which appear darker than the other fibres here. Also, the more angular appearance of each muscle fibre cross-section in the young changes to a more rounded cross-section in the elderly.

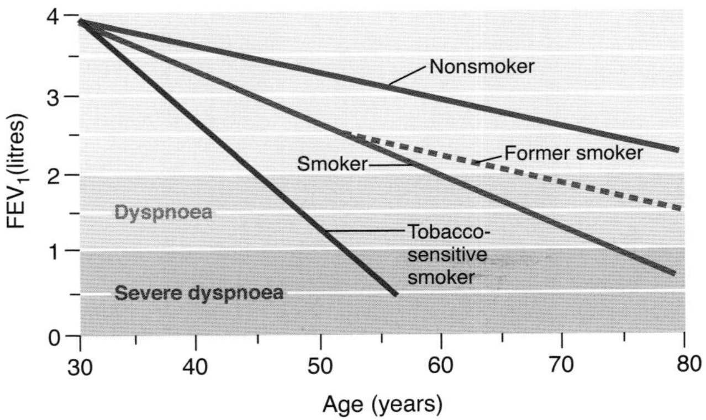

FIGURE 47-31 Lung function changes in adulthood. Graph showing changes in forced expiratory volume at one second (FEV_1), a common measure of lung function (see **Figure 36-11** on p. 837). Note that both age and exposure to cigarette smoke are factors in the decline in lung function over the life span. *Dyspnoea* is laboured or difficult breathing.

Special Senses

The sense organs, as a group, all show a gradual decline in performance and capacity as a person ages.

Most people are farsighted by age 65 years because eye lenses become hardened and lose elasticity; the lenses cannot become curved to accommodate for near vision. This hardening of the lens is called **presbyopia**, which means "old eye". Many individuals first notice the change at about 40 or 45 years of age, when it becomes difficult to do close-up work or read without holding printed material at arm's length. This explains the increased need, with advancing age, for bifocals (glasses that incorporate two lenses) to automatically accommodate for near and distant vision.

Loss of transparency of the lens or its covering capsule is another common age-related eye change. If the lens actually becomes cloudy and significantly impairs vision, it is called a **cataract** and must be removed surgically. The incidence of **glaucoma**, the most serious age-related eye disorder, increases with age. Glaucoma causes an increase in the pressure within the eyeball and, unless treated, often results in blindness.

In many elderly people a very significant loss of hair cells in the organ of Corti (spiral organ of the inner ear) causes a serious decline in the ability to hear certain frequencies. In addition, the eardrum and attached ossicles become more fixed and less able to transmit mechanical sound waves. Some degree of hearing impairment is universally present in the older adult.

The sense of taste is also decreased. Loss of appetite may be caused, at least in part, by the replacement of taste buds with connective tissue cells. Only about 40% of the taste buds present at age 30 years remain fully functional in an individual at age 75 years.

Interestingly, not everything in the sensory system diminishes with age. Evidence shows that older people are much better than younger people at spotting small movements in a visual scene. This is more a matter of interpreting sensory information in the brain than it is a matter of sensory reception. This should not be surprising, as a growing body of evidence supports our longstanding cultural notion that older adults have a sort of "wisdom" or improved thinking abilities that develop over time.

Reproductive Systems

Although most men and women remain sexually active throughout their later years, mechanisms of sexual response may change, and fertility declines. In men, erection may be more difficult to achieve and maintain. Urgency for sex may decline—perhaps from reduced blood testosterone. In women, lubrication of the vagina may decrease. Although men can continue to produce gametes as they age, women experience a cessation of reproductive cycling between the ages of 45 and 60 years called **menopause.** Menopause results from a decrease in the cyclical production of the primary sex hormones, especially oestrogen, with advancing age. The decrease in oestrogen accounts for the common symptoms of menopause: cessation of menstrual cycles, hot flashes, and thinning of the vaginal wall. The exact mechanism of hot flashes is not clearly understood, but it is related to the hormonal changes that occur during menopause. Rarely serious, hot flashes usually subside over time. Oestrogen therapy may be used to relieve menopause symptoms in some cases.

The decrease in oestrogen levels associated with menopause may also contribute to *osteoporosis*. This condition is characterized by loss of bone mass (see Chapter 11). Osteoporosis is often treated with short-term, low-dose oestrogen hormone replacement therapy (HRT) and nonhormonal bone-building drugs. Therapy to restore or maintain bone mineral density may also include high doses of vitamin D, calcium supplements, and weight-bearing exercise.

Benefits of Ageing

It is easy to see the "downside" of ageing—degradation of structures and loss of functions—but there is an "upside" to ageing. For example, studies show that as one ages, anxiety and hostility lessen, control over fear increases, and resistance to happiness decreases. And even though the image quality of vision may decrease as we age, we actually improve in our ability to interpret what we see—such as the ability to detect and track motion in our visual field.

Of course, there is the accumulation of learning over time, and problem-solving ability often improves. Historically, we have attributed wisdom mainly to our elders—a concept that has been supported by neurological research of the traits that characterize wisdom.

There may be a few social advantages to ageing if we live in a culture and a social network that values and provides for the aged.

CAUSES OF DEATH

No matter what your age, death of the individual is also part of the human life cycle. **Figure 47-32** shows the leading causes of death in England. These figures are consistent with causes of death in other economically developed countries. Note that some of these causes of death have been diminishing over the years (such as heart diseases and stroke), some have remained roughly stable (such as cancer), and some have increased (such as Alzheimer disease, Parkinson disease, and kidney disease).

CONNECT IT! ⓔ

The human life span has been increasing over time—even more so in developed areas of the world. Read about the role of genetics in this phenomenon in ***Genes and Longevity*** online at ***Connect It!***

Although heart disease, cancer, stroke, and so on are the leading killers in developed nations, it is a somewhat different story among the developing nations. In developing nations around the world, infectious diseases such as HIV/AIDS, diarrhoeal diseases, malaria, and measles are among the top killers. But even so, in developing areas heart disease and stroke are also near the very top of the list.

Quick CHECK

18. What kinds of changes occur in the skeleton as one ages?
19. List some age-related changes in the cardiovascular system.
20. How can age affect a person's vision?
21. What are some of the leading causes of death in the United Kingdom?

	Males (% of all male deaths)		Females (% of all female deaths)	
1	Heart disease	14.2%	Dementia and Alzheimer's disease	15.3%
2	Dementia and Alzheimer's disease	8.0%	Heart disease	8.8%
3	Lung cancer	6.5%	Stroke	7.5%
4	Chronic lower respiratory diseases	6.2%	Influenza and pneumonia	6.0%
5	Stroke	5.6%	Chronic lower respiratory diseases	6.0%
6	Influenza and pneumonia	5.1%	Lung cancer	5.1%
7	Prostate cancer	4.2%	Breast cancer	3.7%
8	Colorectal cancer	3.0%	Colorectal cancer	2.4%
9	Leukaemia and lymphomas	2.6%	Kidney disease and other diseases of the urinary system	1.9%
10	Cirrhosis and other liver disease	1.9%	Leukaemia and lymphomas	1.9%

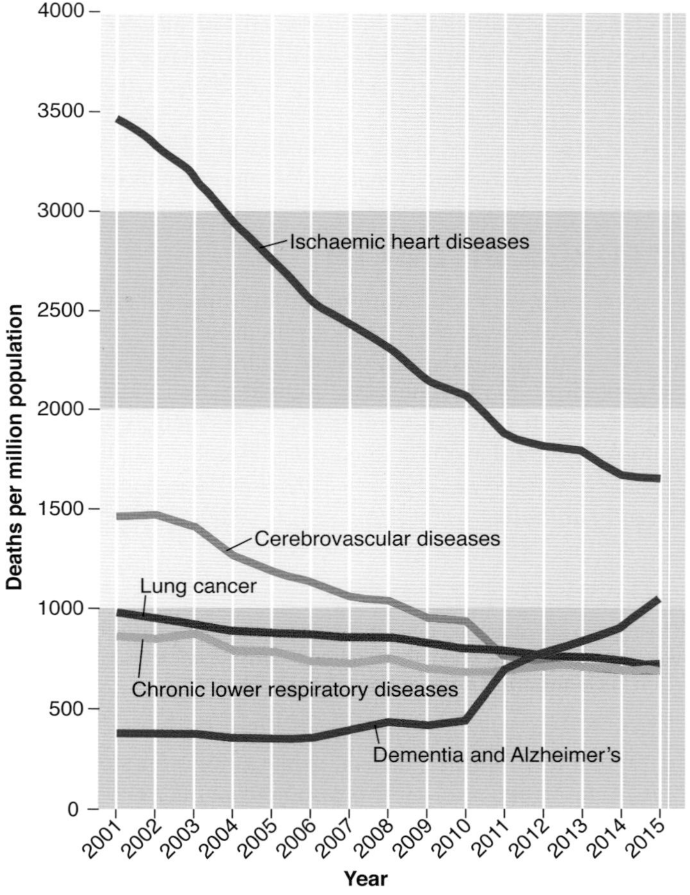

FIGURE 47-32 Leading causes of death. The 10 leading causes of death in England are listed in the inset. The trends in the main causes of death in males are shown in the graph.

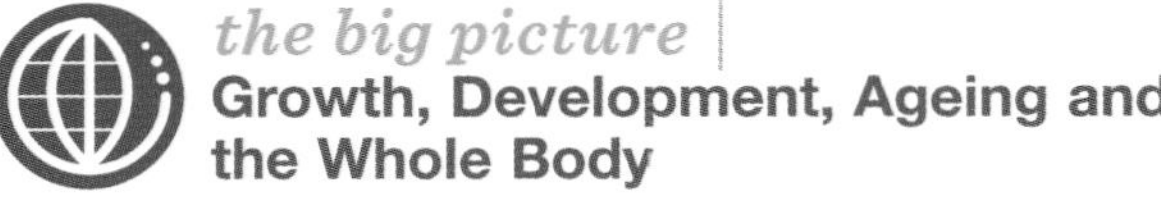

the big picture

Growth, Development, Ageing and the Whole Body

Understanding basic concepts of human growth, development, and ageing is essential for understanding the dynamic, ever-changing nature of the human body. It is important to remember that life is a biological process characterized by continuous change in the structure and function of our body.

As we discussed in this and earlier chapters, production of offspring is vital to the survival of the genetic code. Many biologists believe that this gives an important biological meaning to life in general—continued flow of genetic information from one generation to the next. Production of offspring in humans is not successful unless and until a person grows and develops for many years—more than a decade—to the point at which viable gametes can be produced. Gametogenesis, then, is the first process necessary to ready the genetic material of the parent to be passed along to the offspring.

Once gametes are available, the sexual union of a male and female may result in fusion of the gametes of the two adults to form the first cell of the offspring. Thus genetic information from two different individuals is now united in a new and unique way in the zygote.

The first cell of the offspring—the zygote—quickly divides again and again to eventually produce a mass of cells that will hopefully implant in the wall of the mother's uterus. Then a process unlike any other we have discussed takes over. The offspring and mother biologically connect to each other so that the mother's physiological mechanisms can sustain the offspring until its own systems are developed sufficiently. All the mother's systems alter their function to some degree to maintain the homeostatic balance of both the mother and the offspring.

After many weeks of growth and development—including histogenesis and organogenesis of a full complement of human structures—delivery of the offspring occurs. This event marks the beginning of a continuing series of changes: infancy, childhood, puberty, adolescence, adulthood, senescence, and death.

At some point in adolescence or adulthood many of us have the opportunity to complete the "circle of life" by passing some of the genetic code we received from our parents on to yet another human generation.

mechanisms of disease

Disorders of Pregnancy and Early Development

Implantation Disorders

A pregnancy has the best chance of a successful outcome, the birth of a healthy baby, if the blastocyst is implanted properly in the uterine wall. However, proper implantation does not always occur. Many offspring are lost before implantation occurs, often for unknown reasons. As mentioned in this chapter and the previous chapter, implantation outside the uterus results in an ectopic pregnancy. If the blastocyst implants in a region of endometriosis or normal peritoneal membrane, the pregnancy may be successful if there is room for the developing fetus to grow. Ectopic pregnancies that do succeed must be delivered by C-section rather than by normal vaginal birth. If an ectopic pregnancy occurs in a uterine tube, which cannot stretch to accommodate the developing offspring, the tube may rupture and cause life-threatening haemorrhaging. So-called **tubal pregnancies** are the most common type of ectopic pregnancy.

Occasionally, the blastocyst implants in the uterine wall near the cervix. This in itself may present no problem, but if the placenta grows too close to the cervical opening a condition called **placenta praevia** results. The normal dilation and softening of the cervix that occur in the third trimester often cause painless bleeding as the placenta near the cervix separates from the uterine wall. The massive blood loss that may result can be life-threatening for both mother and offspring (**Figure 47-33**, *A*).

Separation of the placenta from the uterine wall can occur even when implantation takes place in the upper part of the uterus. When this occurs in a pregnancy of 20 weeks or more, the condition is called **abruptio placentae.** Complete separation of the placenta causes the immediate death of the fetus. The severe haemorrhaging that often results, sometimes hidden in the uterus, may cause circulatory shock and death of the mother within minutes. A caesarean section and perhaps also a hysterectomy must be performed immediately to prevent blood loss and death (**Figure 47-33**, *B*).

Pregnancy-induced Hypertension and Preeclampsia

It is not uncommon for a woman's blood pressure to rise during pregnancy and remain elevated until the end of pregnancy—a condition often called **pregnancy-induced hypertension (PIH).** In about 6% to 8% of all pregnancies, PIH may progress to a condition called **preeclampsia.** Formerly known as *toxaemia of pregnancy,* preeclampsia is a serious disorder characterized by the onset of acute hypertension after the twenty-fourth week, accompanied by proteinuria and oedema. The causes of PIH and preeclampsia are largely unknown, but intense research efforts have led to the discovery of a gene that regulates how the kidney handles salt and that may also be involved in raising blood pressure during pregnancy. Preeclampsia can result in complications such as abruptio placentae, stroke, haemorrhage, fetal malnutrition, and low birth weight. This condition can progress to **eclampsia,** a life-threatening form of toxaemia that causes severe convulsions, coma, kidney failure, and perhaps death of the fetus and mother.

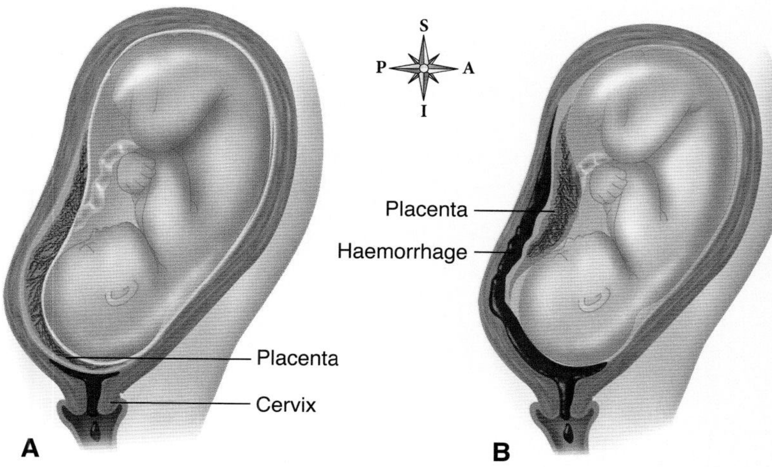

FIGURE 47-33 Implantation disorders. A, Placenta praevia. **B,** Abruptio placentae.

Gestational Diabetes

The term gestational diabetes mellitus (GDM) is applied in cases of hyperglycaemia that first occur during pregnancy.

High blood glucose in the fetus can lead to weight gain, which results in delivery of a large infant—a risk factor for complications during labour and delivery.

Fetal Death

A **miscarriage** is the loss of an embryo or fetus before the twentieth week (or a fetus weighing less than 500 grams). Technically known as a **spontaneous abortion** or *fetal demise*, the most common cause of such a loss is a structural or functional defect in the developing offspring. Abnormalities of the mother, such as hypertension, uterine abnormalities, and hormonal imbalances, can also cause spontaneous abortions. After 20 weeks, delivery of a lifeless infant is termed a **stillbirth.**

Birth Defects

Birth defects, also called **congenital abnormalities,** include any structural or functional abnormality present at birth. Congenital defects may be inherited or may be acquired during gestation or delivery. Acquired defects result from agents called **teratogens** that disrupt normal histogenesis and organogenesis. Some teratogens are chemicals such as alcohol, antibiotics, and other drugs. Microorganisms, such as those that cause rubella (a viral infection), can also cross the placental barrier and disrupt normal embryonic development. Radiation and other physical factors can also cause birth defects. Some teratogens are mutagens because they do their damage by changing the genetic code in cells of the developing embryo.

Postpartum Disorders

Puerperal fever, or *childbed fever,* is a syndrome of postpartum mothers characterized by bacterial infection that progresses to septicaemia (blood infection) and possibly death. Until the 1930s, puerperal fever was the leading cause of maternal death—claiming the lives of more than 20% of postpartum women. Modern antiseptic techniques and antibiotics now prevent most postpartum infections.

After a child is born, it needs the nourishment of milk to survive. However, several disorders of lactation (milk production) may occur to prevent a mother from nursing her infant. For example, anaemia, malnutrition, emotional stress, and structural abnormalities of the breast can all interfere with normal lactation. **Mastitis,** or breast inflammation, often caused by infection, can result in lactation problems or production of milk contaminated with pathogenic organisms. In many cultures, the availability of other nursing mothers or breast milk substitutes allows proper nourishment of the infant, even when lactation problems develop. Most breast milk substitutes are formulations of milk from another mammal such as the cow. Infants who lack the enzyme *lactase* may not be able to digest the lactose present in human or animal milk, resulting in a condition called **lactose intolerance.** Infants with lactose intolerance are sometimes given a lactose-free milk substitute made from soy or other plant products.

LANGUAGE OF SCIENCE (continued from p. 1090)

meiosis (my-OH-sis)
[*meiosis* **becoming smaller**]

mesoderm (MEZ-oh-derm)
[*meso-* **middle,** *-derm* **skin**]

morula (MOR-yoo-lah)
[*mor-* **mulberry,** *-ula* **little**] *pl.,* morulae

neonatal period (nee-oh-NAY-tal)
[*neo-* **new,** *-nat-* **birth,** *-al* **relating to**]

oogenesis (oh-oh-JEN-eh-sis)
[*oo-* **egg,** *-gen-* **produce,** *-esis* **process**]

oogonium (oh-oh-GO-nee-um)
[*oo-* **egg,** *-gonium* **offspring**] *pl.,* oogonia

organogenesis (or-gah-no-JEN-eh-sis)
[*organ-* **instrument (organ),** *-gen-* **produce,** *-esis* **process**]

parturition (pahr-tyoo-RIH-shun)
[*parturi-* **give birth,** *-tion* **process**]

placenta (plah-SEN-tah)
[*placenta* **flat cake**] *pl.,* placentae or placentas

postnatal period (POST-nay-tal)
[*post-* **after,** *-nat-* **birth,** *-al* **relating to**]

prenatal period (PREE-nay-tal)
[*pre-* **before,** *-nat-* **birth,** *-al* **relating to**]

primary follicle (FOL-ih-kul)
[*prim-* **first,** *-ary* **relating to,** *folli-* **bag,** *-cle* **small**]

primary germ layer
[*prim-* **first,** *-ary* **relating to,** *germ* **sprout**]

primary oocyte (OH-oh-syte or OH-uh-syte)
[*prim-* **first,** *-ary* **relating to,** *oo-* **egg,** *-cyte* **cell**]

primary sex characteristic
[*prim-* **first,** *-ary* **relating to,** *character-* **engraved mark**]

puberty (PYOO-ber-tee)
[*pubert-* **age of maturity,** *-y* **state**]

secondary follicle (FOL-ih-kul)
[*second-* **second,** *-ary* **relating to,** *folli-* **bag,** *-cle* **small**]

secondary oocyte
(OH-oh-site or OH-uh-syte)
[*second-* **second,** *-ary* **relating to,** *oo-* **egg,** *-cyte* **cell**]

secondary sex characteristics
[*second-* **second,** *-ary* **relating to,** *character-* **engraved mark**]

senescence (seh-NES-ens)
[*senesc-* **grow old,** *-ence* **state**]

spermatogenesis
(sper-mah-toh-JEN-eh-sis)
[*sperm-* **seed,** *-gen-* **produce,** *-esis* **process**]

spermatogonium
(sper-mah-toh-GO-nee-um)
[*sperm-* **seed,** *-gonia* **offspring**] *pl.,* spermatogonia

theca cell (THEE-kah)
[*theca* **sheath,** *cell* **storeroom**]

thermotaxis (ther-moh-TAK-sis)
[*therm-* **heat,** *-taxis* **movement or reaction**]

trophoblast (TROH-foh-blast)
[*tropho-* **nourishment,** *-blast* **sprout**]

zona pellucida (ZP)
(ZOH-nah pah-LOO-sih-dah)
[*zona* **belt or girdle,** *pellucida* **transparent**] *pl.,* zonae pellucidae

zygote (ZYE-goht)
[*zygot-* **union or yoke**]

LANGUAGE OF MEDICINE

abruptio placentae
(ab-RUP-shee-oh plah-SEN-tay)
[*ab-* **away from,** *-ruptio* **rupture,** *placentae* **of flat cake (placenta)**]

antenatal medicine (an-tee-NAY-tal)
[*ante-* **before,** *-nat-* **birth,** *-al* **relating to**]

Apgar score (AP-gar)
[*Virginia Apgar* **American physician**]

arteriosclerosis
(ar-tee-ree-oh-skleh-ROH-sis)
[*arteri-* **vessel (artery),** *-sclero-* **harden,** *-osis* **condition**]

atherosclerosis
(ath-er-oh-skleh-ROH-sis)
[*ather-* **porridge,** *-sclero-* **harden,** *-osis* **condition**]

cataract (KAT-ah-rakt)
[*cataract* **waterfall**]

caesarean section
(seh-ZAIR-ee-an SEK-shun)
[*Julius Caesar* **Roman emperor,** *-ean* **of**]

congenital abnormality
(kon-JEN-ih-tal ab-nor-MAL-ih-tee)
[*con-* **with,** *-genit-* **born,** *-al* **relating to**]

eclampsia (eh-KLAMP-see-ah)
[*ec-* **out,** *-lamp-* **shine forth,** *-sia* **condition**]

embryology (em-bree-OL-oh-gee)
[*em-* **in,** *-bryo-* **fill to bursting,** *-log-* **words (study of),** *-y* **activity**]

gerontology (jair-on-TOL-oh-jee)
[*geronto-* **old age,** *-log-* **words (study of),** *-y* **activity**]

glaucoma (glaw-KOH-mah)
[*glauco-* **grey,** *-oma* **growth**]

hypertension (HTN)
(hye-per-TEN-shun)
[*hyper-* **excessive,** *-tens-* **stretch or pull tight,** *-sion* **state**]

lactose intolerance
(LAK-tohs in-TOL-er-ans)
[*lact-* **milk,** *-ose* **carbohydrate (sugar),** *in-* **not,** *-toler-* **bear,** *-ance* **state**]

mastitis (mas-TYE-tis)
[*mast-* **breast,** *-itis* **inflammation**]

menopause (MEN-oh-pawz)
[*men-* **month,** *-pause* **cease**]

miscarriage
[*mis-* **wrongly,** *-carriage* **carry**]

neonatology (nee-oh-nay-TOL-oh-jee)
[*neo-* **new,** *-nat-* **born,** *-log-* **words (study of),** *-y* **activity**]

osteoarthritis (os-tee-oh-ar-THRY-tis)
[*osteo-* **bone,** *-arthr-* **joint,** *-itis* **inflammation**]

placenta praevia
(plah-SEN-tah PREE-vee-ah)
[*placenta* **flat cake,** *praevia* **gone before**]

preeclampsia (pree-ee-KLAMP-see-ah)
[*pre-* **before,** *-lamp-* **shine forth,** *-sia* **condition**]

pregnancy-induced hypertension (PIH) (PREG-nan-see-in-DYOOST hye-per-TEN-shun)
[*hyper-* **excessive,** *-tens-* **stretch or pull tight,** *-sion* **state**]

presbyopia (pres-bee-OH-pee-ah)
[*presby-* **ageing,** *-op-* **vision,** *-ia* **condition**]

progeria (proh-JEER-ee-ah)
[*pro-* **early,** *-ger-* **old age,** *-ia* **condition**]

puerperal fever
(pyoo-ER-per-al FEE-ver)
[*puerp-* **childbirth,** *-al* **relating to**]

spontaneous abortion
(spon-TAY-nee-us ah-BOR-shun)
[*ab-* **away from,** *-or-* **be born,** *-tion* **process**]

teratogen (TER-ah-toh-jen)
[*terato-* **monster,** *-gen* **produce**]

tubal pregnancy (TYOO-bal)
[*tub-* **tube,** *-al* **relating to**]

ultrasonography
(ul-trah-son-OG-rah-fee)
[*ultra-* **beyond,** *-sono-* **sound,** *-graph-* **draw,** *-y* **process**]

case study

David and his wife Karen had been trying for two years to start a family with no success. Following a visit to an infertility specialist, they discovered David had a low sperm count. After discussing all options, they decided to try intra-uterine insemination with David's sperm. A day or so after the procedure a sperm successfully penetrated an ovum (fertilization) in one of Karen's uterine tubes.

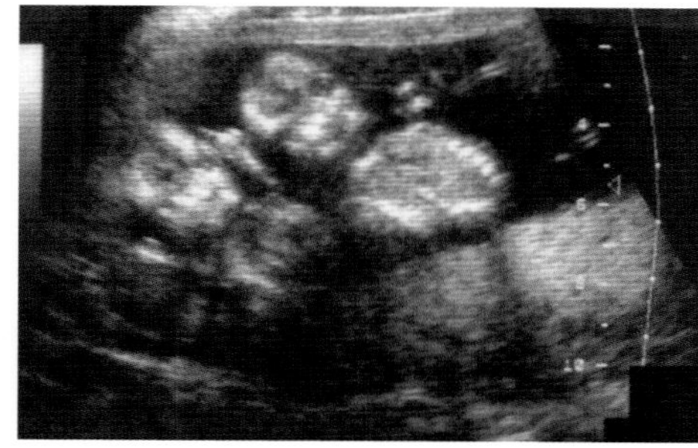

1. What is a newly fertilized ovum called?
   a. A zygote
   b. An embryo
   c. A fetus
   d. A blastocyst
2. How much time will elapse from fertilization to full implantation?
   a. 2 days
   b. 4 days
   c. 24 hours
   d. 10 days

At 13 weeks Karen had a dating ultrasound scan so her date of delivery could be estimated from the fetus measurements. The fluid at the back of the fetal head was also to be measured at the same time as part of the screening test for Down syndrome (a nuchal transparency scan). To her surprise Karen saw what appeared to be two separate images on the screen, and the sonographer confirmed she was expecting twins, one boy and one girl.

3. What type of twins was Karen expecting?
   a. Maternal
   b. Fraternal
   c. Identical
   d. Sibling

At 37 weeks Karen started feeling slight contractions, but she initially dismissed them as indigestion. Shortly afterwards she noticed a thin, watery fluid leaking from her vagina. Two hours later the contractions suddenly became stronger, so she woke her husband and they left for the maternity unit at the local hospital.

4. What was the watery fluid Karen noticed?
   a. Placental fluid
   b. Chorionic fluid
   c. Amniotic fluid
   d. Urine

Hint To solve a case study, you may have to refer to the glossary or index, other chapters in this textbook, ***Connect It!,*** and other resources.

CHAPTER SUMMARY

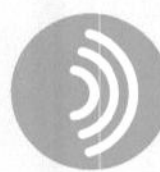

To download an MP3 version of the chapter summary for use with your mobile device, access the ***Audio Chapter Summaries*** *online at evolve.elsevier.com.*

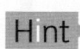

Scan this summary after reading the chapter to help you reinforce the key concepts. Later, use the summary as a quick review before your class or before a test.

Introduction

A. Prenatal period—period beginning with conception and ending at birth
B. Postnatal period—period beginning with birth and continuing until death
C. Human developmental biology—study of changes occurring during the cycles of life from conception to death

A New Human Life

A. Production of sex cells—spermatozoa are produced by spermatogenesis; ova are produced by oogenesis
   1. Meiosis (**Figures 47-1** and **47-2**)
      a. Special form of cell division that reduces the number of chromosomes in each daughter cell to one half of those in the parent cell
      b. Mature ova and sperm contain only 23 chromosomes, half as many as other human cells
      c. Meiotic division—two cell divisions that occur one after another in succession
         (1) Meiotic division I and meiotic division II
         (2) Both divisions made up of an interphase, prophase, metaphase, anaphase, and telophase
      d. During prophase I of meiosis, "crossover" occurs in which genetic material is "shuffled"

UNIT 6

e. Daughter cells formed by meiotic division I contain a haploid number of chromosomes
f. Meiotic division II—essentially the same as mitotic division; reproduces each of the two cells formed by meiotic division I and forms four cells, each with the haploid number of chromosomes
2. Spermatogenesis (**Figure 47-3**)—process by which primitive male sex cells become transformed into mature sperm; begins at approximately puberty and continues throughout a man's life
 a. Meiotic division I—one primary spermatocyte forms two secondary spermatocytes, each with 23 chromosomes
 b. Meiotic division II—each of the two secondary spermatocytes forms a total of four spermatids
3. Oogenesis (**Figure 47-4**)—process by which primitive female sex cells become transformed into mature ova
 a. Mitosis—oogonia reproduce to form primary oocytes; most primary oocytes begin meiosis and develop to prophase I before birth; there they stay until puberty
 b. Once during each menstrual cycle, a few primary oocytes resume meiosis and migrate toward the surface of the ovary; usually only one oocyte matures enough for ovulation, and meiosis again halts at metaphase II
 c. Meiosis resumes only if the head of a sperm cell enters the ovum

B. Ovulation and insemination
1. Ovulation—expulsion of the mature ovum from the mature ovarian follicle, into the abdominopelvic cavity, and then into the uterine (fallopian) tube
2. Insemination—expulsion of seminal fluid from the male into the female vagina; capacitation renders sperm able to fertilize; sperm travel through the cervix and uterus and into the uterine (fallopian) tubes

C. Fertilization—also known as *conception* (**Figure 47-5**)
1. Most often occurs in the outer one third of the uterine tube
2. Thermotaxis—sperm are attracted to warmth of uterine tubes
3. Chemotaxis—ovum attracts and "traps" sperm with special molecules
4. Acrosome reaction permits the release of enzymes that burrow through the outer layers of ovum (zona pellucida and corona radiata)
5. When one spermatozoon enters the ovum, the ovum stops collecting sperm on its surface
6. The sperm releases its nuclear chromosomes into the ovum; proteins and RNA from the sperm enter the ovum to assist with early development
7. 23 chromosomes from the sperm head and 23 chromosomes in the ovum make up a total of 46 chromosomes
8. Zygote—fertilized ovum; genetically complete

Prenatal Period

A. Begins with conception and continues until the birth of a child

B. Cleavage and implantation (**Figure 47-6**)—once zygote is formed, it immediately begins to divide
1. Morula—solid mass of cells formed from zygote; takes approximately 3 days; continues to divide (**Figure 47-7**)
2. Blastocyst—a hollow ball of cells that develops by the time the embryo reaches the uterus, where it implants into the uterine lining (**Figure 47-8**)
3. A store of nutrients in the ovum supports embryonic development until implantation has occurred (approximately 10 days from fertilization to implantation)
4. Blastocyst has an outer layer of cells and an inner cell mass
 a. Trophoblast—outer wall of the blastocyst
 b. Inner cell mass—as blastocyst develops, yolk sac and amniotic cavity are formed (**Figure 47-9**)
  (1) In humans, yolk sac's functions are largely non-nutritive (e.g., serves as a site of prenatal haematopoiesis)
  (2) Amniotic cavity becomes a fluid-filled, shock-absorbing sac (bag of waters) in which the embryo floats during development (**Figure 47-10**)
 c. Chorion develops from trophoblast to become an important fetal membrane in the placenta

C. Placenta (**Figure 47-11**)
1. Anchors fetus to the uterus and provides a "bridge" for the exchange of nutrients and waste products between mother and baby
2. Also serves as an excretory, respiratory, and endocrine organ
3. Placental tissue normally separates maternal and fetal blood supplies
4. Has important endocrine functions—secretes large amounts of hCG, which stimulate the corpus luteum to continue its secretion of oestrogen and progesterone (**Figure 47-12**)

D. Periods of development (**Figures 47-13** to **47-15**)
1. Gestation period—approximately 39 weeks; divided into three 3-month segments called trimesters
2. Embryonic phase extends from fertilization until the end of week 8 of gestation
3. Fetal phase—weeks 8 to 39

E. Stem cells
1. Stem cell—unspecialized cell that produces lines of specialized cells; has a certain level of potency (range of types it can produce)
2. Totipotent stem cell—can produce any type of cell; found in zygote
3. Pluripotent stem cell—embryonic stem cell that can produce a broad range of cell types; found in embryonic germ layers
4. Multipotent stem cell—adult stem cell found in some tissues can produce a few cell types and thus maintain functional populations of specialized cells

F. Formation of the primary germ layers
   1. Three layers of developmental cells arise early in the first trimester of pregnancy
   2. Cells of embryonic disc differentiate and form each of the three primary germ layers
   3. Each of the three primary germ layers gives rise to specific organs and systems of the body (**Figure 47-16**)
      a. Endoderm—inside layer
      b. Ectoderm—outside layer
      c. Mesoderm—middle layer

G. Histogenesis and organogenesis (**Figure 47-16**)
   1. Histogenesis—process by which primary germ layers develop into different kinds of tissues
   2. Organogenesis—how tissues arrange themselves into organs
   3. Differentiation and development of the reproductive systems are an example
      a. Reproductive tract (**Figure 47-17**)
         (1) Gonads attach to mesonephric (wolffian) ducts, which become the male reproductive tract
         (2) Gonads (unattached) and paramesonephric (müllerian) ducts develop into the female reproductive tract
      b. External genitals (**Figure 47-18**)
         (1) In the male, the genital tubercle eventually becomes the glans of the penis and the folds become the penis shaft and scrotum
         (2) In the female, the genital tubercle becomes the clitoris and the folds become the labia

Birth, or Parturition

A. Transition between prenatal and postnatal periods of life; full-term fetus is delivered as an infant (**Figure 47-19**)

B. Cortisol triggers labour by reducing hCG and thus also progesterone, removing the "brake" on oxytocin (OT), which stimulates the uterine muscles to produce labour contractions (amplified by a positive feedback effect); prostaglandins (PGs) enhance OT's effects

C. Stages of labour (**Figure 47-20**)
   1. Stage one—period from onset of uterine contractions until cervical dilation is complete
   2. Stage two—period from maximal cervical dilation until the baby exits through the vagina
   3. Stage three—process of expulsion of the placenta through the vagina

D. Multiple births—birth of two or more infants from the same pregnancy; twins are most common (**Figure 47-21**)
   1. Identical twins result from the splitting of embryonic tissue from the same zygote early in development
   2. Fraternal twins result from the fertilization of two different ova by two different spermatozoa

Postnatal Period

A. Begins at birth and continues until death; commonly divided into a number of periods (**Figure 47-22**)

B. Infancy begins at birth and lasts until approximately 18 months
   1. Neonatal period—first 4 weeks of infancy; dramatic changes occur at a rapid rate (**Figure 47-23**)
   2. Changes allow the infant to become totally self-supporting, especially the respiratory and cardiovascular systems (**Figure 47-24**)
   3. Apgar score assesses general condition of a newborn infant

C. Childhood extends from end of infancy to sexual maturity, or puberty
   1. Early childhood—growth continues at a rapid pace but month-to-month gains are less consistent
   2. By age 6 years, child looks more like a preadolescent than an infant or toddler
   3. Nervous and muscular systems develop rapidly during the middle years of childhood
   4. Deciduous teeth are lost during childhood, beginning at approximately 6 years of age
   5. Permanent teeth have erupted by age 14 years, except for the third molars (wisdom teeth)

D. Adolescence and adulthood
   1. Adolescence is considered to be the teenage years (from 13 to 19); marked by rapid and intense physical growth, resulting in sexual maturity
      a. Puberty—stage of adolescence during which a person becomes sexually mature
      b. Changes triggered by increases in reproductive hormones (**Figure 47-25**)
      c. Primary sexual characteristics—maturation of gonads and reproductive tract
      d. Secondary sexual characteristics—fat and hair distribution, skeletal changes, growth of larynx (**Figure 47-26**)
   2. Adulthood—characterized by maintenance of existing body tissues

E. Older adulthood and senescence
   1. As a person grows older, a gradual decline occurs in every major organ system in the body
   2. Gerontologists theorize a number of different ageing mechanisms, all of which may be involved in the processes of ageing
      a. Limit on cell reproduction
      b. Environmental factors
      c. Viruses
      d. Ageing genes
      e. Degeneration of mitochondria—perhaps associated with progressive damage by oxygen free radicals (**Figure 47-27**)

Effects of Ageing

A. Common degenerative changes often characterize senescence (**Figure 47-28**)

B. Skeletal system (**Figure 47-29**)
   1. Bones decrease in BMD (bone mineral density) and thus change in texture, degree of calcification, and shape

2. Lipping occurs, which can limit range of motion
3. Decreased bone size and density lead to increased risk of fracture
4. Decreased BMD can be avoided (at least partly) by exercise and adequate calcium intake

C. Muscular system (**Figure 47-30**)
1. Muscle mass decreases to about 90% by age 50 years and around 50% by age 80 years
2. The number of muscle fibres decreases as we age but can be offset by an increase in muscle fibre size through exercise
3. Ratio of "fast" to "slow" functioning in muscle fibres decreases, slowing the function of muscle organs

D. Integumentary system (skin)
1. Skin becomes dry, thin, and inelastic
2. Pigmentation changes and thinning hair are common problems associated with ageing

E. Urinary system
1. Number of nephron units in the kidney decreases by almost 50% between the ages of 30 and 75 years
2. Decreased blood flow through kidneys reduces overall function and excretory capacity
3. Diminished muscle tone in bladder results in decreased capacity and inability to empty, or void, completely

F. Respiratory system
1. Costal cartilages become calcified
2. Respiratory efficiency decreases (**Figure 47-31**)
3. Decreased strength of respiratory muscles

G. Cardiovascular system
1. Degenerative heart and blood vessel disease—one of the most common and serious effects of ageing
2. Atherosclerosis—buildup of fatty deposits on blood vessel walls narrows the passageway for blood
3. Arteriosclerosis—"hardening" of the arteries
4. Hypertension—high blood pressure

H. Special senses
1. Sense organs—gradual decline in performance and capacity with ageing
2. Presbyopia—farsightedness caused by hardening of lens
3. Cataract—cloudy lens, which impairs vision
4. Glaucoma—increased pressure within the eyeball; if left untreated, often results in blindness
5. Decreased hearing
6. Decreased taste

I. Reproductive systems
1. Mechanism of sexual response may change
2. Fertility decreases
3. In females, menopause occurs between ages 45 and 60 years

J. Benefits of ageing—mostly improved brain functions: less anxious or fearful, less resistant to happiness, better interpretation of visual information, improved problem solving and wisdom

Causes of Death

A. In developed countries such as the United Kingdom, heart disease, cancer, and stroke (cerebrovascular accident [CVA]) are among the leading causes of death (**Figure 47-32**)

B. In developing countries, heart disease and stroke are also leading causes of death, along with infectious diseases such as HIV/AIDS, diarrhoeal disorders, and malaria

The Big Picture: Growth, Development, Ageing, and the Whole Body

A. Understanding the basic concepts of human growth, development, and ageing is essential for understanding the ever-changing nature of the human body

B. Production of offspring in humans is not successful unless and until a person grows and develops for many years to the point at which viable gametes can be produced

C. At some point in adolescence or adulthood many of us have the opportunity to complete the "circle of life" by passing the genetic code we received to another human generation

REVIEW QUESTIONS

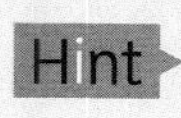

Write out the answers to these questions after reading the chapter and reviewing the Chapter Summary. Note—writing out your answers will consolidate learning and provide a valuable resource of information.

1. Define the terms *developmental biology*, *growth*, and *development*.
2. Outline the major steps in spermatogenesis. Do the same for oogenesis.
3. Identify the two processes necessary to bring the sperm and ovum into proximity with each other.
4. During fertilization, how does the ovum attract sperm?
5. At what developmental stage does implantation occur?
6. Describe the structural differences between a morula and a blastocyst.
7. Use these terms to describe the development of the placenta: blastocyst, trophoblast, chorion and chorionic villi.
8. What functions does the placenta provide?
9. Outline the hormonal levels of human chorionic gonadotropin (hCG), oestrogen, and progesterone at various stages during gestation.
10. During what period of growth is the term *embryo* replaced by the term *fetus*?
11. List the various structures derived from each of the three primary germ layers.
12. Describe the three stages of labour.
13. What is the difference between identical and fraternal twins?
14. From birth to maturity, how does the size of the head compare with the rest of the body?
15. Draw a time line showing the time spans of the following postnatal periods: infancy, childhood, adolescence.
16. During what postnatal period do the secondary sex characteristics develop? What initiates this development?
17. What structural changes may result from the changes in bone calcification because of ageing?
18. Define the terms *atherosclerosis*, *arteriosclerosis*, and *hypertension*, and describe how they can negatively impact on healthy ageing.
19. Identify and describe the most serious age-related eye disorder.
20. Discuss several benefits of ageing.

CRITICAL THINKING QUESTIONS

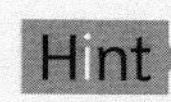

After finishing the Review Questions, write out the answers to these more in-depth questions to help you apply your new knowledge. Go back to sections of the chapter that relate to concepts that you find difficult.

1. How is the process of meiosis different from mitosis?
2. If a diploid cell rather than a haploid cell were used for human reproduction, what would the number of chromosomes per cell be after three generations?
3. How do histogenesis and organogenesis differ? Which of these occurs first in development?
4. Explain the procedure a physician might use if a normal vaginal delivery would be dangerous for the mother or baby.
5. What are the symptoms of the drop in oestrogen that occurs during menopause? To what skeletal disorder might this drop be related?
6. Explain the process of in vitro fertilization. What is the probability of the success of this procedure—that is, resulting in a full-term birth?
7. Using physiological principles, explain how a sound exercise programme can reduce some of the common effects of ageing.

48 Genetics and Heredity

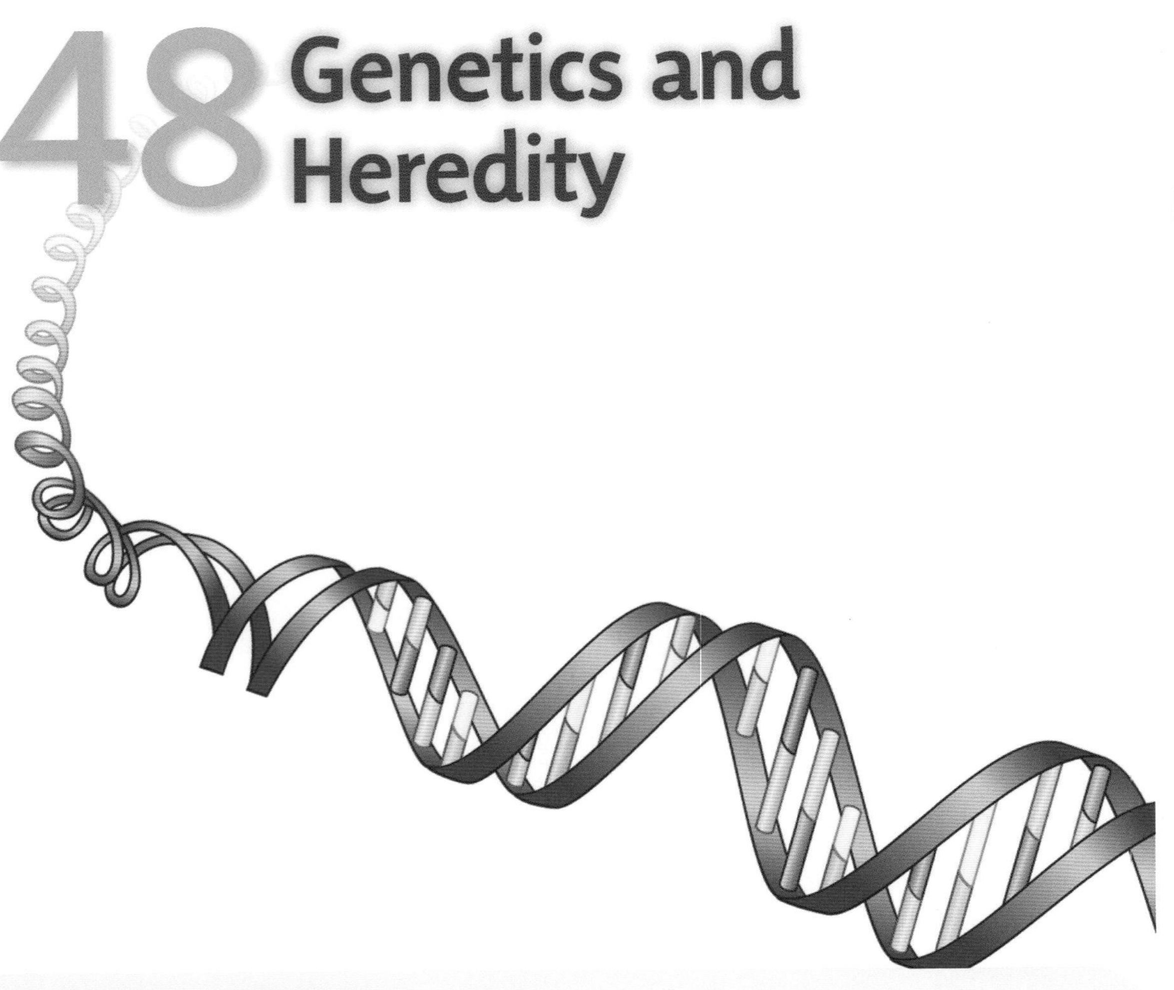

CHAPTER OUTLINE

Hint ▸ *Scan this outline before you begin to read the chapter, as a preview of how the concepts are organized.*

LANGUAGE OF SCIENCE

Hint ▸ *Use this list to aid your pronunciation of unfamiliar words.*

autosome (AW-toh-sohm)
[*auto-* **self,** *-som-* **body**]

chromatin (KROH-mah-tin)
[*chrom-* **colour,** *-in* **substance**]

chromosome (KROH-meh-sohm)
[*chrom-* **colour,** *-som-* **body**]

chromosome territory (CT)
(KROH-meh-sohm TAIR-ih-tor-ee)
[*chrom-* **colour,** *-som-* **body,** *terri-* **land,** *-ory* **place**]

codominance (koh-DOM-ih-nans)
[*co-* **together,** *-domina-* **rule,** *-ance* **state**]

diploid (DIP-loyd)
[*diplo-* **twofold,** *-oid* **form of**]

dominant gene
[*domina-* **rule,** *-ant* **characterized by,** *gen-* **produce or generate**]

epigenetics (ep-ih-jeh-NET-iks)
[*epi-* **upon,** *gen-* **produce,** *-ic* **relating to**]

gametes (GAM-eets)
[*gamete* **marriage partner**]

gene
[*gen-* **produce or generate**]

gene linkage
[*gen-* **produce or generate**]

genetic mutation
(jeh-NET-ik myoo-TAY-shun)
[*gene-* **produce,** *-ic* **relating to,** *muta* **-change,** *-ation* **process**]

genetics (jeh-NET-iks)
[*gen-* **produce,** *-ic* **relating to**]

genome (JEE-nohm)
[*gen-* **produce (gene),** *-ome* **entire collection**]

genomics (jeh-NO-miks)
[*gen-* **produce (gene),** *-om-* **entire collection,** *-ic* **relating to**]

genotype (JEN-oh-type)
[*gen-* **produce (gene),** *-type* **kind**]

haploid (HAP-loyd)
[*haplo-* **single,** *-oid* **of or like**]

heterozygous (het-er-oh-ZYE-gus)
[*hetero-* **different,** *-zygo-* **union or yoke,** *-ous* **characterized by**]

histone (HISS-tohn)
[*histo-* **tissue,** *-one* **unit**]

homozygous (hoh-moh-ZYE-gus)
[*homo-* **same,** *-zygo-* **union or yoke,** *-ous* **characterized by**]

continued on p. 1144

It seems that today we are hearing more and more about the importance of **genetics,** the scientific study of inheritance, to all fields of human biology— especially anatomy, physiology, and medicine. Popular news magazines are running story after story on the revolution in treating fatal inherited disorders by using something called gene therapy. Health and science articles in newspapers and online keep us informed of the latest discoveries of genes involved with disease, human behaviour, and even longevity. Various media keep track of the progress of the largest coordinated biological quest that anyone can remember: mapping the entire human genetic code and listing all the proteins encoded there. Even commercial ads call attention to genetic health risks. Clearly, one cannot be informed about human biology today without some knowledge of basic genetics and heredity. In this chapter, we briefly review the essential concepts of genetics and explain how heredity affects every structure and function in the body.

THE SCIENCE OF GENETICS

History shows that humans have been aware of patterns of inheritance—or *heredity*—for thousands of years, but it was not until the 1860s that the scientific study of these patterns—genetics—was born. At that time, a monk living in Brno, Moravia (now the Czech Republic) became the first to discover the basic mechanism by which traits are transmitted from parents to offspring. That man, Gregor Mendel, proved that independent units (which we now call **genes**) are responsible for the inheritance of biological traits.

The science of genetics developed from Mendel's quest to explain how normal biological characteristics are inherited. As time went by and more genetic studies were done, it became clear that certain diseases also have a genetic basis. As you may recall from Chapter 2, some diseases are inherited directly. For example, the group of blood-clotting disorders called *haemophilia* can be inherited by children from parents who have the genetic code for haemophilia. Directly inherited diseases such as haemophilia are often called "hereditary diseases". Other diseases are only partly determined by genetics—that is, they involve genetic risk factors (see Chapter 2, p. 34). For example, certain forms of skin cancer are thought to have a genetic basis. A person who inherits the genetic code associated with skin cancer will develop the disease only if the skin is also heavily exposed to the ultraviolet radiation in sunlight.

CHROMOSOMES AND GENES

Mechanism of Gene Function

Mendel proposed that the genetic code is transmitted to offspring in discrete, independent units that we now call genes. Recall from Chapters 4 and 7 that each gene is a sequence of nucleotide bases in the deoxyribonucleic acid (DNA) molecule.

Figure 48-1 shows a detailed view of human DNA. Beginning at the left of the diagram, you can see a fully condensed **chromosome** unfold toward the right, where a single double-helix strand of DNA is visible. As the genetic codes of a DNA molecule's genes are being actively transcribed in a cell's nucleus, the DNA is in the threadlike form called **chromatin.** Chromatin, as you can see in **Figure 48-1**, is actually a thread of DNA wound around little spools made of proteins called **histones.** The chromatin is thus organized into little "thread on spool" subunits called **nucleosomes.**

During cell division, each replicated strand of chromatin coils on itself to form a compact chromosome (see **Figure 48-1**). Each DNA molecule can be called either a chromatin strand or a chromosome, depending on what form it is in. Throughout this chapter we will use the term *chromosome* for DNA, regardless of its actual form, and the term *gene* for each distinct encoding segment within a DNA molecule.

CONNECT IT! ⓔ

In nondividing cells, chromosomes are found in the form of chromatin strands that occupy specific **chromosome territories (CTs)** within the nucleus. See an example of a CT map in ***Chromosome Territories*** online at ***Connect It!***

Each gene in a chromosome contains a genetic code that the cell transcribes to a ribonucleic acid (RNA) molecule. Some RNA molecules do not code for polypeptides but have a functional role—for example, ribosomal RNA (rRNA) and transfer RNA (tRNA). A transcribed messenger RNA (mRNA) molecule, however, associates with a ribosome in which the code is translated to form a specific polypeptide molecule. By way of slight differences in editing of mRNA, one mRNA may perhaps actually produce several specific polypeptides. And the polypeptides may be complete tertiary proteins by themselves—or they may combine with any of several other polypeptides to form several different specific large quaternary proteins (see **Figure 4-14** on p. 64).

CONNECT IT! ⓔ

Review the illustrated article ***The RNA Revolution***—available online at ***Connect It!***—which details the concept of *gene silencing* using *siRNA (short interfering RNA).*

Many of the protein molecules formed from the polypeptides encoded by genes are *enzymes,* functional proteins that help regulate the various metabolic pathways of the body by catalyzing specific chemical reactions. Because enzymes and other functional proteins such as haemoglobin regulate the biochemistry of the body, they regulate the entire structure and function of the body. Some proteins, such as collagen and keratin, are important structural components of the body—and thus determine important structural characteristics of various body parts.

As you can see, genes determine the structure and function of the human body by producing a set of specific structural proteins, along with many functional proteins and RNA molecules.

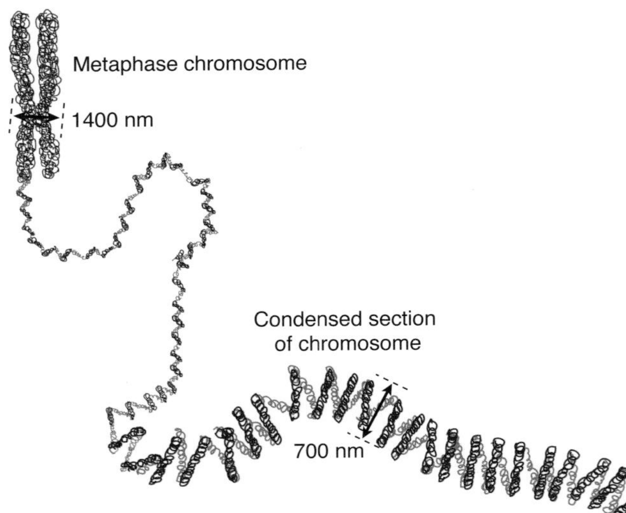

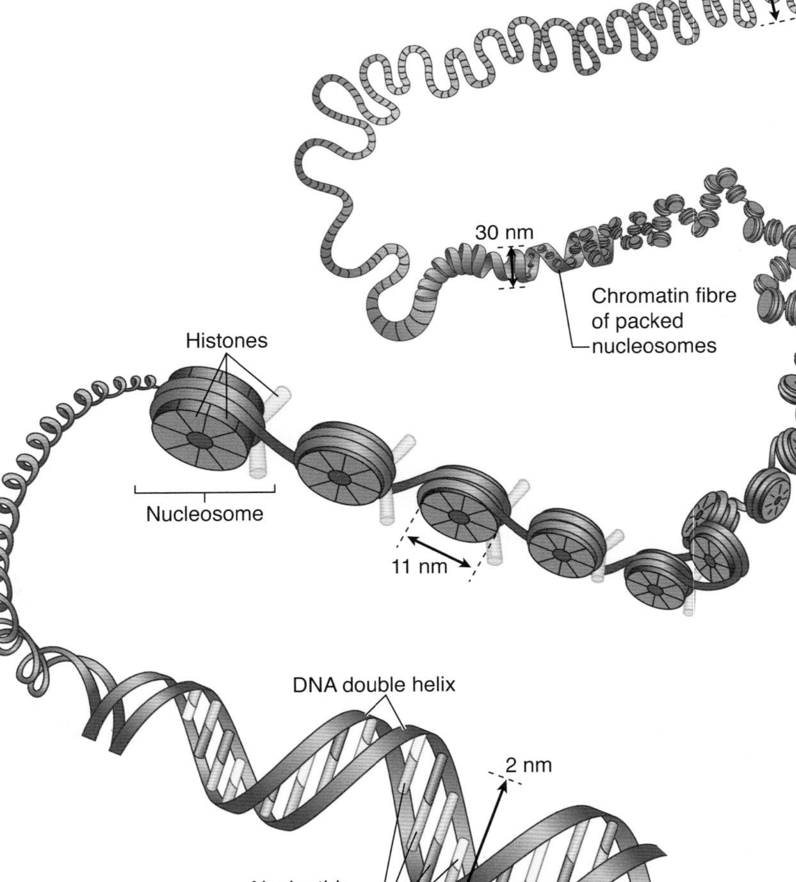

FIGURE 48-1 Human DNA. This artist's depiction of human DNA shows a fully condensed chromosome above and the unfolding of it on the right and below—unfolded to the point of a single DNA strand (double helix). Note that the scale changes dramatically as you progress from one loop of the diagram to the next.

CONNECT IT! 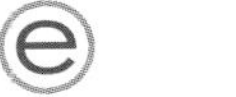

How many different kinds of amino acids are needed to form the proteins of the body? Find out in ***Amazing Amino Acids*** online at ***Connect It!***

The Human Genome

The entire collection of genetic material in each typical cell of the human body is called the **genome.** The structure of the human genome is summarized in **Figure 48-2**. The typical human genome includes 46 individual nuclear chromosomes and one mitochondrial chromosome. In 2003, the **Human Genome Project (HGP)**—a publicly funded, worldwide collaboration to map all the genes in the human genome—was completed. This landmark event coincided exactly with the fiftieth anniversary of the discovery of DNA.

We now know that the human genome contains only about 19,000 or so genes. This is about one fifth of the number originally estimated and among the smallest genomes of any animal.

We also know that less than 2% of the DNA carries protein-coding genes. A bit more of the DNA carries code for functional RNAs, such as rRNA, tRNA, and ribozymes (see **Figure 7-2** on p. 122). The rest has been called "junk DNA", or "noncoding DNA", because it is not used directly to make proteins.

A small portion of this noncoding DNA seems to be made up of broken bits of genes that are no longer functional—remnants of our evolutionary past called **pseudogenes.** According to the ongoing HGP offshoot *ENCODE (Encyclopedia of DNA Elements)*, however, about 80% of the noncoding DNA is made up of regions that regulate the timely switching of genes on and off.

The current draft of the human genome shows us that most coding genes tend to lie in clusters rich in C (cytosine) and G (guanine), separated by long stretches of noncoding DNA rich in A (adenine) and T (thymine). Chromosome 1 has the most genes, with nearly 3000 genes, and the Y chromosome has the fewest, with just over 200 genes. Hundreds of the newly discovered genes in the human genome seem to be bacterial in origin, perhaps inserted there by bacteria in our distant ancestors.

CONNECT IT! 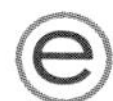

We cannot survive without the bacteria that live on and in us. Many scientists think of them as "part of" our body—at least in terms of overall function. No wonder, then, that they are busy with huge efforts at analyzing the genomes of all the bacteria that inhabit our bodies. Review the human microbiome in ***The Human Microbiome*** at ***Connect It!***

An important thing to remember about genes is that they are not each just one sequence that codes for one protein. Besides possibly coding for a nonprotein such as RNA, each gene is made up of several separated exons that join together before protein synthesis (see **Figure 7-4** on p. 123). In some cases, different combinations of some of the same exons can make up genes for different products. Recall also that some proteins are quaternary proteins made up of polypeptides that may be made from different genes. So the definition of a gene is less straightforward than it first appears!

Although we now have the essential picture of the details of the human genome, much work still lies ahead in the field of **genomics**, the analysis of the genome's code. Besides filling in the remaining details of the rough draft, we have much work to do in discovering all the possible mutations that might exist (see the discussion later in this chapter) and all the proteins encoded by the genes that make up the human genome (**Box 48-1**).

In fact, this quest has generated several other fields related to the genetic code. For example, **transcriptomics** is the analysis of all the mRNA codes actually transcribed from the human genome—the

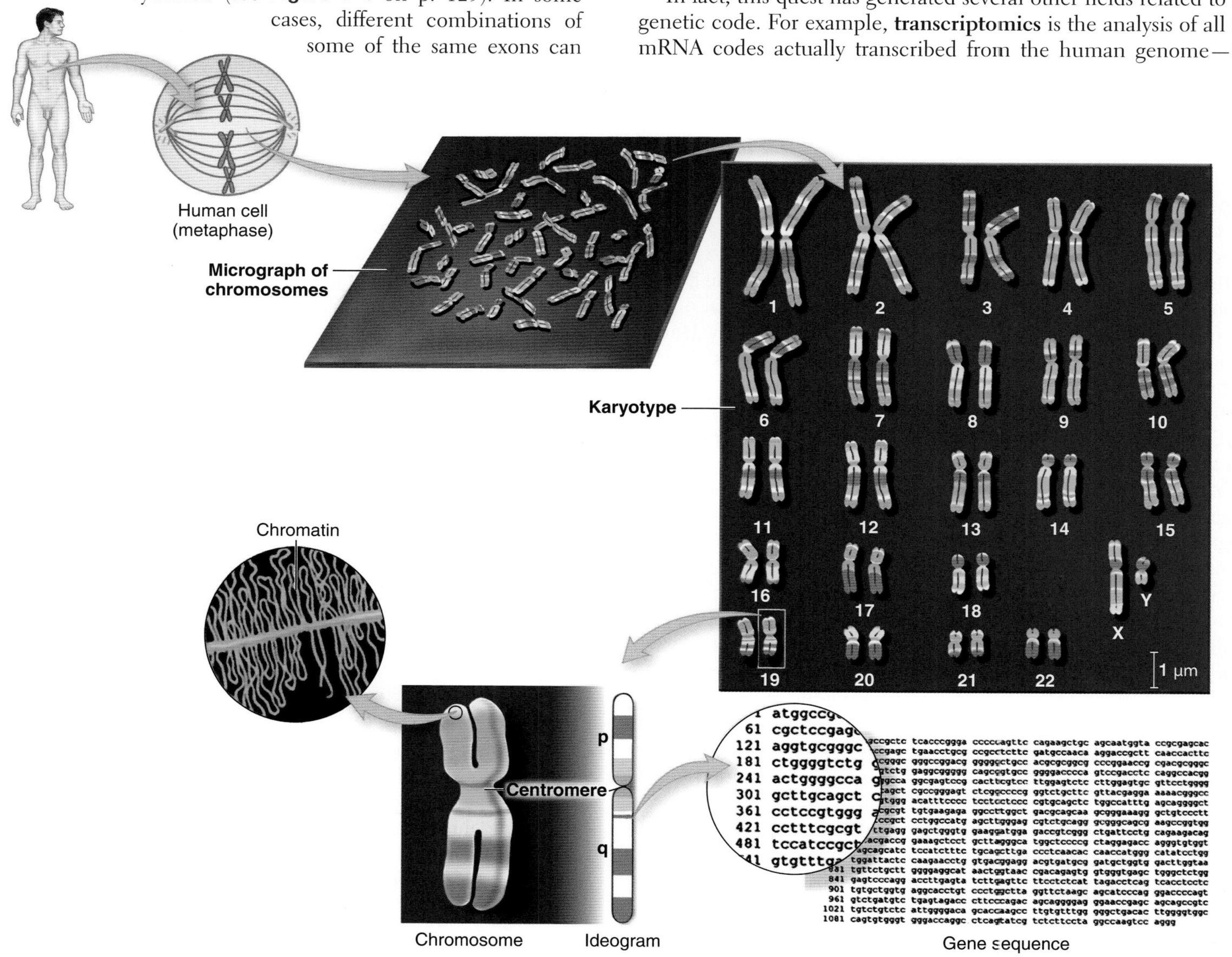

FIGURE 48-2 Human genome. A cell taken from the body is stained and photographed. A photograph of nuclear chromosomes is then cut and pasted, arranging each of the 46 chromosomes into numbered pairs of decreasing size to form a chart called the karyotype. Each chromosome is a coiled mass of chromatin (DNA). In this figure, differentially stained bands in each chromosome appear as different, bright colours. Such bands are useful as reference points when identifying the locations of specific genes within a chromosome. The staining bands are also represented on an ideogram, or simple graph, of the chromosome as reference points to locate specific genes. The genes themselves are usually represented as the actual sequence of nucleotide bases, abbreviated here as *a, c, g,* and *t.* In this figure, the sequence of one exon (segment) of a gene called *GPI* from chromosome 19 is shown. Each of the different images in this figure can be thought of as a different type of "genetic map".

UNIT 6

BOX 48-1 *fyi* | **1000 Genomes Project**

An international research partnership sponsored in part by the United States government is currently building a catalogue of at least 1000 individual human genomes. This effort, called the *1000 Genomes Project,* promises to reveal the many variant forms of genes present in the whole human genome. Although thousands of complete individual genomes have already been catalogued—most notably the genomes of gene pioneers Craig Venter and James Watson—much more information is needed. An initial phase provided about 2500 individual genomes from 26 different populations. The project catalogues the many small DNA-coding variations called *single nucleotide polymorphisms (SNPs)* as well as the larger structural variations in the human genome. Such information could lead to better understanding of the genetic basis of disease—and ultimately to effective treatments or cures. •

transcriptome. This field may eventually shed light on which genes are expressed and in what conditions.

A field called **proteomics** is the analysis of the proteins encoded by the genome. The entire group of proteins encoded by the human genome is called the human **proteome.** The ultimate goal of proteomics is to understand the role of each protein in the body. Understanding the roles of every single protein in the body will certainly go a long way toward improving our knowledge of the normal function of the body as well as mechanisms for many diseases.

The analysis of the human genome, transcriptome, and proteome has surged forward in this century with the widespread use of *RNA interference (RNAi)* techniques that silence particular genes in the laboratory setting as a means to find out what they do in the body—what proteins are transcribed from them.

Another proven technique that "knocks out" individual genes has been used for some time to demonstrate the effects of specific genes. Using embryonic stem cells from laboratory mice in which specific genes are targeted and disabled, a generation of genetically altered "knockout mice" can be produced. The mice are then studied to find out the effects of the gene(s) missing from the mouse genome.

Information obtained about the human genome can be expressed in a variety of ways. As you can see in **Figure 48-2**, an **ideogram,** or simple cartoon of a chromosome, is often used in genomics to show the overall physical structure of a chromosome. The constriction in the ideogram shows the relative position of the chromosome's centromere. The shorter segment of the chromosome is called the **p-arm** and the longer segment is called the **q-arm.**

The bands in an ideogram of a chromosome show staining landmarks and help identify the regions of the chromosome. Sometimes physical maps of genes will show exact positions of individual genes on the p-arm and q-arm of a chromosome. A more detailed representation of a gene would show the actual sequence of nucleotide bases, abbreviated here *a, c, g,* and *t* for *adenine, cytosine, guanine,* and *thymine,* as shown in **Figure 48-2**.

Distribution of Chromosomes to Offspring

Meiosis

Each cell of the human body contains 46 chromosomes. The only exceptions to this principle are the **gametes**—male *spermatozoa* and female *ova.* Recall from Chapter 47 that a special form of nuclear division called **meiosis** (see **Figure 47-1** on p. 1092) produces gametes with only 23 chromosomes—exactly one half the usual number. This number is called the **haploid** number. This process follows a basic principle of genetics first discovered by Gregor Mendel called the **principle of segregation.** This principle simply states that the two members of a pair of chromosomes separate, or *segregate,* during meiosis.

When a sperm (with its 23 chromosomes) unites with an ovum (with its 23 chromosomes) at conception, a *zygote* with 46 chromosomes is formed. Thus the zygote has the same number of chromosomes (46, the **diploid** number) as each typical body cell in the parents.

As the karyotype in **Figure 48-2** shows, the 46 human chromosomes can be arranged in 23 pairs according to size. One pair called the **sex chromosomes** may not match, but the remaining 22 pairs of **autosomes** always appear to be nearly identical to each other.

Principle of Independent Assortment

Because one half of an offspring's chromosomes are from the mother and one half are from the father, a unique blend of inherited traits is formed. According to another of Mendel's principles, each chromosome assorts itself independently during meiosis. This **principle of independent assortment** states that as sperm are formed, and chromosome pairs separate (the principle of segregation), the maternal and paternal chromosomes get mixed up and redistribute themselves independently of the other chromosome pairs (**Figure 48-3**). Thus each sperm is likely to have a *different* set of 23 chromosomes. Because the ova are formed in the same manner, each ovum is likely to be genetically different from the ovum that preceded it. Independent assortment of chromosomes ensures that each offspring from a single set of parents is very likely to be genetically unique—a phenomenon known as *genetic variation.*

According to the principle of **gene linkage,** genes on an individual chromosome tend to stay together. An important application of this principle occurs during one phase of meiosis, when pairs of matching chromosomes line up along the equator of the cell and exchange genes or groups of linked genes with one another. This process is called **crossing over** because genes from a particular location cross over to the same location on the matching chromosome (**Figure 48-4**). Crossing over introduces additional opportunities for genetic variation among the offspring of a single set of parents.

When one considers the genetic variation that is produced by independent assortment and crossing over, it is easy to understand the tremendous variation seen in the human population.

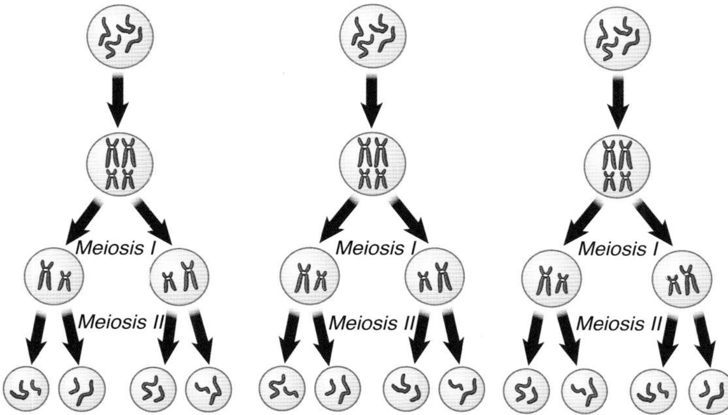

FIGURE 48-3 Meiosis and the principle of independent assortment. In meiosis, a series of two divisions results in the production of gametes with one half the number of chromosomes of the original parent cell. In both meiotic divisions shown here, the original cell has four chromosomes and the gametes each have two chromosomes. During the first division of meiosis, pairs of similar chromosomes line up along the cell's equator for even distribution to daughter cells. Because different pairs assort independently of each other, four (2^2) different alignments of chromosomes can occur. Because human cells have 23 pairs of chromosomes, more than 8 million (2^{23}) different combinations are possible.

Quick CHECK

1. How do genes produce biological traits?
2. Who might be considered the founder of the scientific study of genetics?
3. What is the difference between an autosome and a sex chromosome?
4. List some mechanisms that increase genetic variation among human offspring.

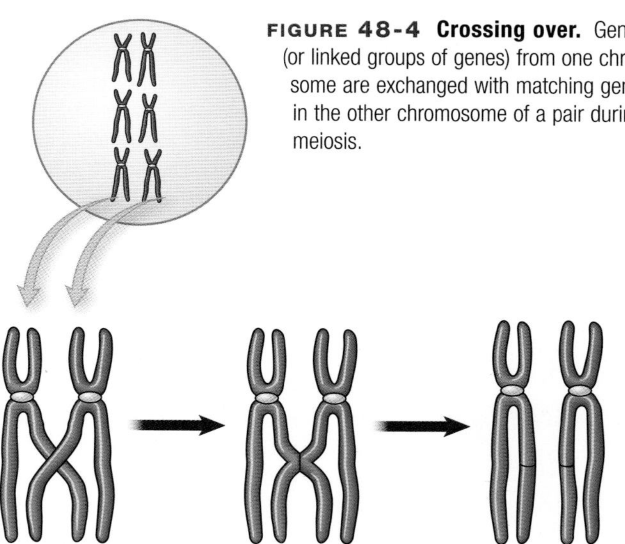

FIGURE 48-4 Crossing over. Genes (or linked groups of genes) from one chromosome are exchanged with matching genes in the other chromosome of a pair during meiosis.

GENE EXPRESSION

HEREDITARY TRAITS

Dominant and Recessive Traits

Mendel discovered that the genetic units we now call genes may be expressed differently among individual offspring. After rigorous experimentation with pea plants, he discovered that each inherited trait is controlled by two sets of similar genes, one from each parent. Each autosome in a pair matches its partner in the type of genes it contains. In other words, if one autosome has a gene for hair colour, its partner will also have a gene for hair colour—in the same location on the autosome. Although both genes specify hair colour, they may not specify the *same* hair colour. Mendel also discovered that some genes are *dominant* and some are *recessive*. A **dominant gene** is one whose effects are seen and whose effects are capable of masking the effects of a **recessive gene** for the same trait.

Consider the example of **albinism,** a total lack of melanin pigment in the skin and eyes (**Figure 48-5**). Because people with this condition lack dark pigmentation, they have difficulty seeing in bright light and must avoid direct sunlight to protect themselves from burns. The genes that cause albinism are recessive; the genes that cause normal melanin production are dominant. By convention, dominant genes are represented by uppercase letters and recessive genes by lowercase letters. One can represent the gene for albinism as *a* and one of the genes for normal skin pigmentation as *A*. An individual with the gene combination *AA* has two dominant genes—and so will exhibit a normal skin colour. The code *AA* is called a **genotype.** A person with a genotype of two identical forms of a trait is said to be **homozygous** for that trait.

The manner in which a genotype is expressed is called the **phenotype.** Thus a person who is homozygous dominant (*AA*) for skin colour will have a normal phenotype (i.e., normal skin pigmentation). Someone with the gene combination *Aa* will also have normal skin colour because the normal gene *A* is dominant over the

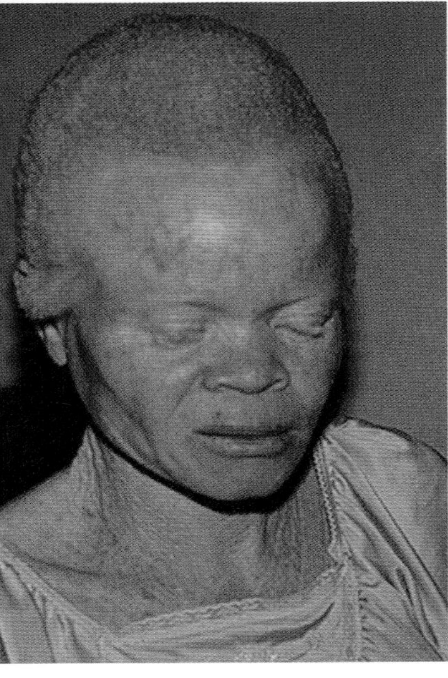

FIGURE 48-5 Albinism. There are several forms of albinism in humans. The type shown here, tyrosinase-negative oculocutaneous albinism, results from the inheritance of two abnormal genes for tyrosinase—the enzymes required to convert tyrosine to melanin pigments. Melanin is normally present in the skin as well as in the eye, where its absence produces vision problems that include sensitivity to light. This African woman would otherwise have dark skin, dark hair, and normal vision. However, as she looks away from the bright camera light as she is photographed, you can see the abnormally light hair and skin typical of this type of albinism.

recessive albinism gene *a*. A person with genotype *Aa* is said to be **heterozygous** and will express the normal phenotype. Only a person with the homozygous recessive genotype of *aa* will have the abnormal phenotype, albinism, because there is no dominant gene to mask the effects of the two recessive genes.

In the example of albinism, a person with the heterozygous genotype of *Aa* is said to be a genetic **carrier** of albinism. This means that the person can transmit the albinism gene, *a*, to offspring. Thus two normal parents, each having the heterozygous genotype *Aa*, can produce both normal children and children who have albinism (**Figure 48-6**).

Polygenic Traits

It is important to note that melanin pigmentation in human skin is actually governed by several different pairs of genes. The gene for the form of albinism discussed here, *tyrosinase-negative oculocutaneous albinism*, involves just one of the gene pairs that regulate skin colour. Inherited characteristics, such as skin colour and height, which are determined by the combined effect of many different gene pairs, are often called **polygenic** ("many genes") traits to distinguish them from **monogenic**, or single-gene, traits.

Polygenic traits are often hard to study in the phenotype because they are so variable. You can think of a polygenic trait as a "combined trait" because it results from the combined activity of several different genes. Each gene may be dominant or recessive in character. Because each gene is only one of several that govern the combined trait, however, the phenotype may be any of a large number of different variations of the trait. Using skin colour as an example, the form of albinism described earlier involves only one of several genes that govern pigmentation of the skin and eyes. But that one gene is critical; it negates the effects of all the other genes that govern skin colour. However, if the dominant form of that critical gene is in place, then it is possible for variations in any of the other genes that regulate skin colour to exert influence on skin pigmentation.

Codominant Traits

What happens if two different dominant genes occur together? Suppose there is a gene A^1 for light skin and a gene A^2 for dark skin. In a form of dominance called **codominance,** they will simply have equal effects, and a person with the heterozygous genotype A^1A^2 will exhibit a phenotype of skin colour that is something between light and dark.

Recall from ***Sickle Cell Anaemia*** online at ***Connect It!*** that the genes for sickle cell anaemia behave this way. A person with two sickle cell genes will have *sickle cell anaemia,* whereas a person with one normal gene and one sickle cell gene will have a milder form of the disease called *sickle cell trait.*

The case of sickle cell inheritance is a good example of how the mechanism of codominance works. The haemoglobin molecules within all red blood cells (RBCs) are quaternary proteins that each include four polypeptide chains—two alpha chains and two beta

FIGURE 48-6 Inheritance of albinism. Albinism is a recessive trait, producing abnormalities only in those with two recessive genes (a). Presence of the dominant gene (A) prevents albinism.

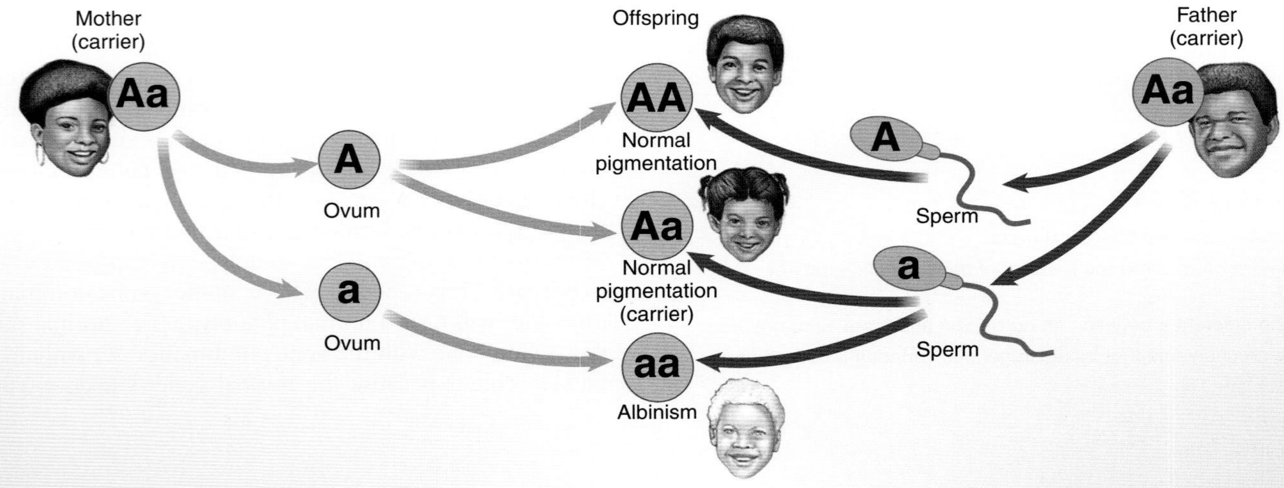

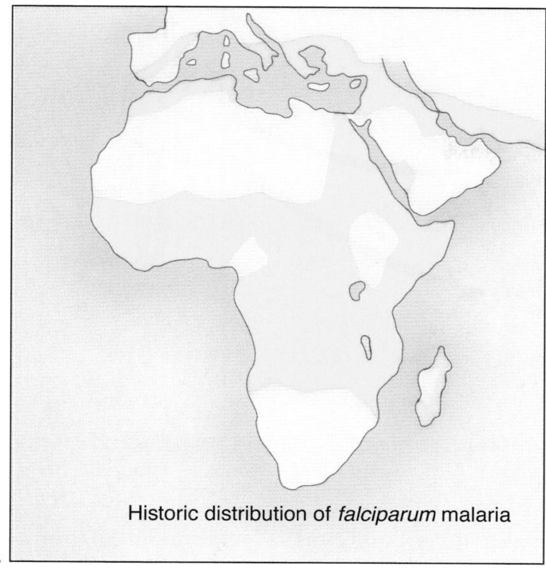

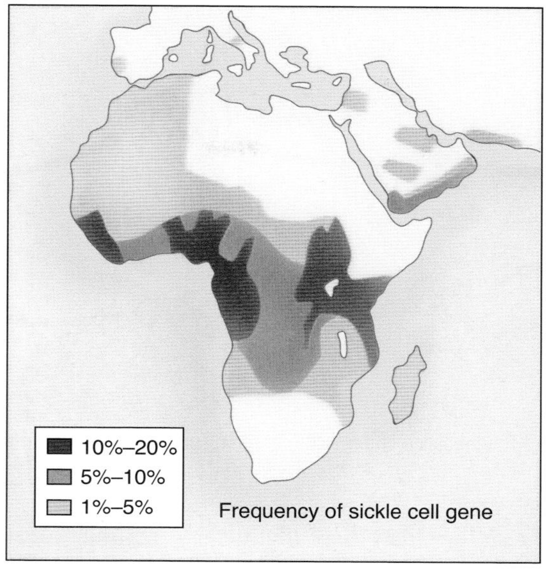

FIGURE 48-7 Relationship between the frequency of sickle cell trait and the distribution of malaria. A, The distribution of the most deadly form of malaria in Africa correlates closely with the frequency of occurrence of the sickle cell gene. **B,** The sickle cell trait provides resistance to malaria, and thus heterozygous individuals are more likely than homozygous individuals to survive and reproduce—spreading the abnormal gene further in the population.

chains (see **Figure 27-5** on p. 615). The sickle cell gene is actually an abnormal version of the gene that contains the code for the beta chains of the haemoglobin molecule. Any beta chain that is produced by this code has one (of 146) amino acid replaced by the wrong amino acid—making it different enough to drastically alter its function. The RBCs of a person with one sickle cell gene and one normal beta-chain gene contain haemoglobin in which about one half the total number of beta chains are abnormal and about one half are normal. The RBCs of a person with two sickle cell genes contain haemoglobin in which all the beta chains are abnormal. Thus in sickle cell trait only some haemoglobin molecules are defective, but in sickle cell anaemia *all* of the haemoglobin molecules are defective.

The frequency of occurrence of the abnormal sickle cell gene is an example of an interesting epidemiological phenomenon. Because sickle cell trait provides resistance to the parasite that causes the most deadly form of **malaria** (*Plasmodium falciparum* malaria), sickle cell disorders persist in areas of the world in which malaria is still prevalent (**Figure 48-7**). Malaria is a sometimes fatal condition caused by blood cell parasites (*Plasmodium* species) and is characterized by fever, **anaemia,** swollen spleen, and possible relapse months or years later. The unique distribution of *P. falciparum* malaria results from the fact that people without sickle cell trait more often die of this condition before producing offspring than those with the malaria-resistant sickle cell trait. Thus the "bad" sickle cell gene is more likely to be transmitted to the next generation than the "good" genes for normal haemoglobin.

The sickle cell/malaria relationship points to an important concept in medical genetics: "disease" genes often provide some biological advantage for a human population in certain circumstances. It is only when circumstances change that the gene is seen to do more harm than good. Genes for many other hereditary diseases (e.g., *thalassaemia* and *Tay–Sachs disease*) are now known to impart protection against pathogenic conditions in heterozygous individuals.

Sex-Linked Traits

Recall from our earlier discussion that besides the 22 pairs of autosomes, there is one pair of sex chromosomes. Note in the lower right portion of the karyotype in **Figure 48-2** that the chromosomes of this pair do not have matching structures. The larger sex chromosome is called the X *chromosome,* and the smaller one is called the Y *chromosome.* The X chromosome is sometimes called the "female chromosome" because it includes genes that determine female sexual characteristics. If a person has only X chromosomes, she is genetically a female. The Y chromosome is often called the "male chromosome" because anyone possessing a Y chromosome is genetically a male. Thus all genetically normal females have the sex chromosome combination XX, and all genetically normal males have the combination XY (**Box 48-2**). Because men produce both X-bearing and Y-bearing sperm, any two parents can produce male or female children (**Figure 48-8**).

The large X chromosome contains many genes besides those needed for female sexual traits. Genes for producing certain clotting factors, photopigments in the retina of the eye, and many other proteins are also found on the X chromosome. The tiny Y chromosome,

BOX 48-2 *fyi* | Timing and Sex Determination

Research has shown that X-bearing sperm swim more slowly than Y-bearing sperm. An interesting hypothesis stems from this fact. If insemination occurs on the day of ovulation, Y-bearing sperm, being faster than X-bearing sperm, should reach the ovum first. Therefore a Y-bearing sperm would be more apt to fertilize the ovum. And because Y-bearing sperm produce males, there should be a greater probability of having a baby boy when insemination occurs on the day of ovulation. Statistical evidence supports this view. •

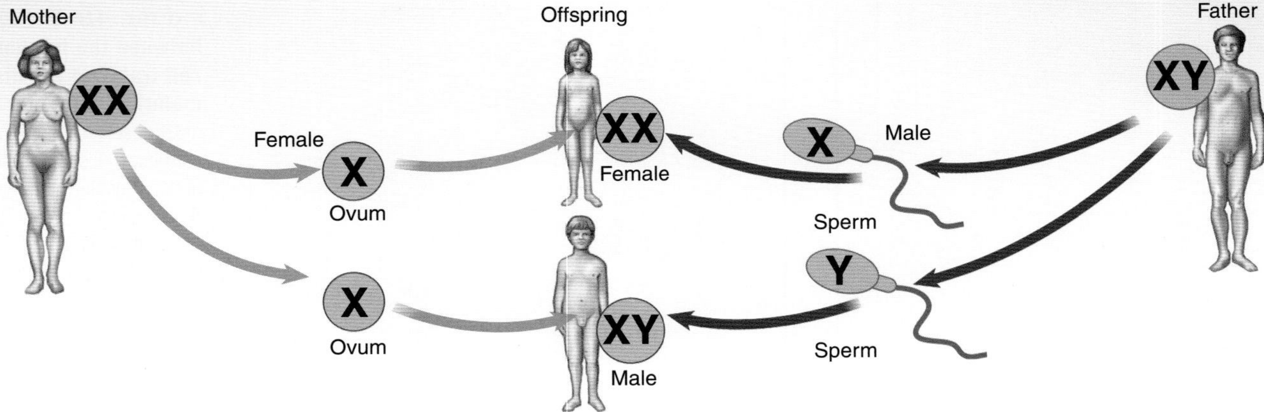

FIGURE 48-8 Sex determination. The presence of the Y chromosome specifies maleness. In the absence of a Y chromosome, an individual develops into a female.

on the other hand, contains few genes other than those that determine male sexual characteristics. Thus both males and females need at least one normal X chromosome—otherwise genes for clotting factors and other essential proteins would be missing. Traits carried on sex chromosomes are called **sex-linked traits.** Some sex-linked traits are called *X-linked traits* because they are determined by genes in the large X chromosome. Other sex-linked traits are called *Y-linked traits* because they are determined by genes in the tiny Y chromosome.

Dominant X-linked traits appear in each person, as one would expect for any dominant trait. In females, recessive X-linked genes are masked by dominant genes in the other X chromosome. Only females with two recessive X-linked genes can exhibit the recessive trait. Because males inherit only one X chromosome (from the mother), the presence of only one recessive X-linked gene is enough to produce the recessive trait. In short, in males there are no matching genes in the Y chromosome to mask recessive genes in the X chromosome. For this reason, X-linked recessive traits appear much more commonly in males than in females.

An example of a recessive X-linked condition is *red-green colour blindness*, which involves a deficiency of normal photopigments in the retina (see **Box 24-3**, p. 550). In this condition, male children of a parent who carries the recessive abnormal gene on an X chromosome may be colour blind (**Figure 48-9**). A female can inherit this form of colour blindness only if her father is colour blind *and* her mother is either colour blind (homozygous recessive) or a colour-blindness

FIGURE 48-9 Sex-linked inheritance. Some forms of colour blindness involve recessive X-linked genes. In this case, a female carrier of the abnormal gene can produce male children who are colour-blind.

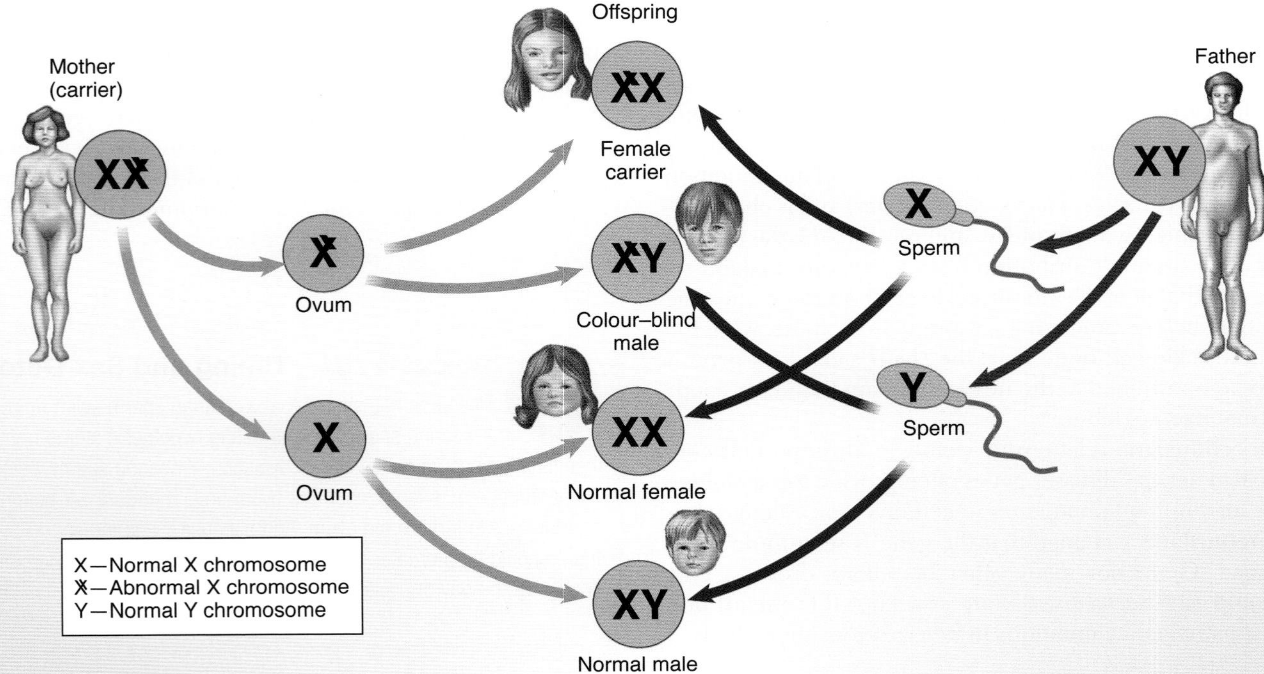

carrier (heterozygous). The X chromosome has been studied in great detail, and general locations for genes causing dozens of distinct X-linked diseases have been identified (**Figure 48-10**).

CONNECT IT!

Review the illustrated article ***Colour Blindness*** online at ***Connect It!***

Only one clinically significant Y-linked condition has been identified by geneticists. A missing part of q-arm of the Y chromosome may cause inheritable problems with spermatogenesis—and possible reduced fertility. Such a Y-linked condition may be passed from father to son.

Genetic Mutations

The term *mutation* simply means "change". A **genetic mutation** is a change in an individual's genetic code. Some mutations involve a change in the genetic code within a single gene, perhaps a slight rearrangement of the nucleotide sequence. A mutation called a **deletion** occurs when one or more nucleotide bases in a sequence are missing. An **insertion** mutation occurs when one or more nucleotides appear within the usual sequence of nucleotide bases in a gene. With either type of mutation, the cell cannot read the genetic code normally, and thus the encoded protein cannot be made in its usual form. Other mutations involve damage to a portion of a chromosome or a whole chromosome. For example, a portion of a chromosome may completely break away.

Mutations may occur spontaneously without the influence of factors outside the DNA itself. However, most genetic mutations are believed to be caused by **mutagens**—agents that cause changes in the genetic code by damaging DNA molecules. Genetic mutagens include chemicals, some forms of radiation, and even viruses.

If mutations occur in reproductive cells or their precursors, they may be inherited by offspring. Beneficial mutations allow organisms to adapt to their environments. Because such mutant genes benefit survival, they tend to spread throughout a population over the course of several generations.

Harmful mutations inhibit survival and therefore are not likely to spread widely through the population. Most harmful mutations kill the organism in which they occur or at least prevent successful reproduction—and so are never passed to offspring. Harmful mutations that are recessive, however, may persist at low frequencies in a population indefinitely because they do not cause problems for individuals who inherit just one of these genes. If a harmful dominant mutation is only mildly harmful, it may persist in a population over many generations.

Consider also the case of the mutations that cause sickle cell anaemia, thalassaemia, and Tay–Sachs disease—the heterozygous genotype produces a phenotype that resists a specific disease, and the homozygous genotype produces a phenotype characterized by emergence of a completely different disease condition.

Quick CHECK

5. What is a dominant genetic trait? A recessive trait?
6. What is codominance?
7. How can a mutant gene benefit a human population?
8. What is X-linked inheritance?

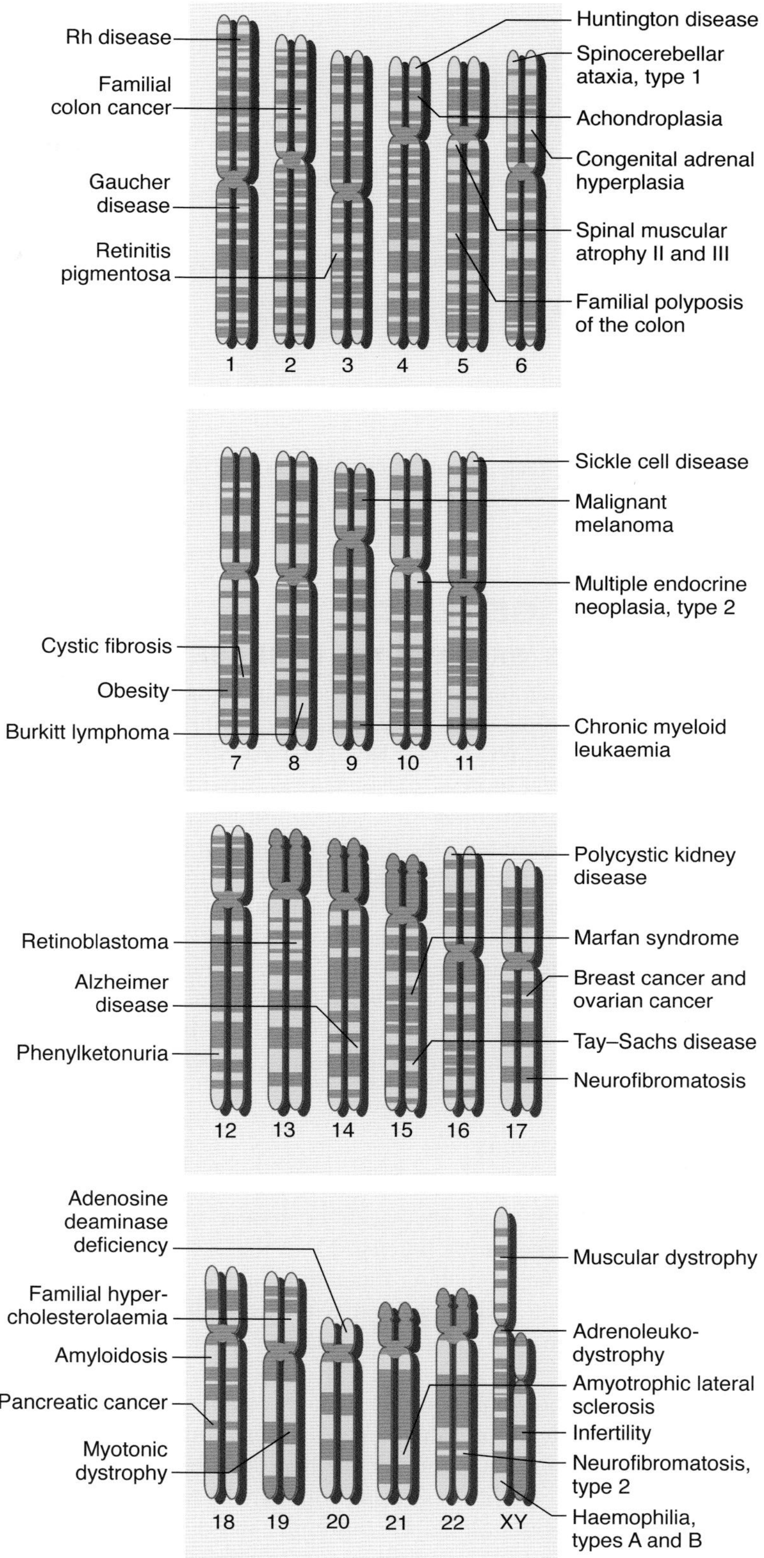

FIGURE 48-10 Disease map of chromosomes. This ideogram of each chromosome outlines just a few locations of the many genes whose mutations are responsible for genetic disorders.

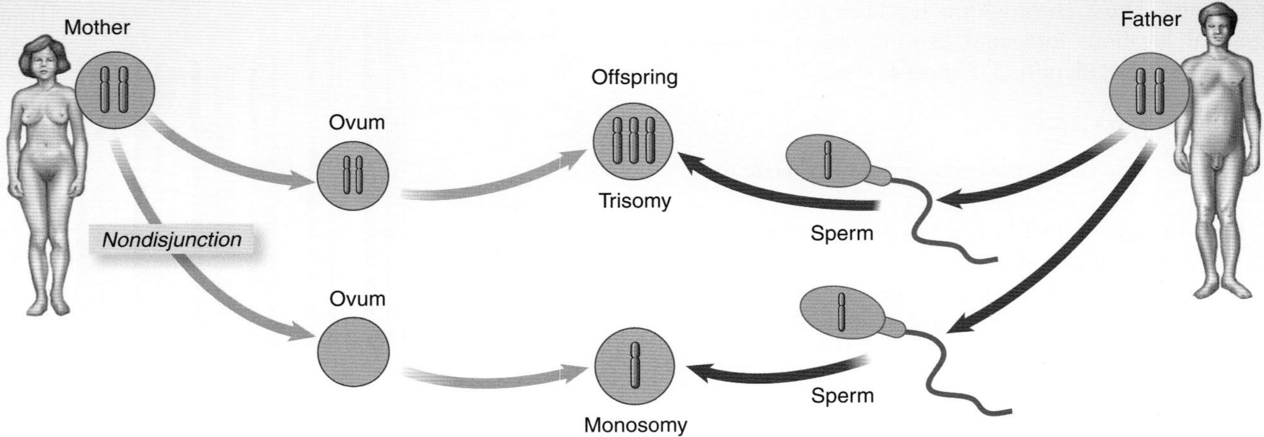

FIGURE 48-11 Effects of nondisjunction. Nondisjunction, failure of a chromosome pair to separate during gamete production, may result in trisomy or monosomy in the offspring.

MEDICAL GENETICS

Mechanisms of Genetic Diseases

As science writer Matt Ridley repeatedly and emphatically stated in his bestselling book *Genome: The Autobiography of a Species in 23 Chapters*, "GENES ARE NOT THERE TO CAUSE DISEASE." Although we often hear of new "disease genes" being discovered—and the pace is rapidly increasing—the function of these genes is not to cause disease any more than the function of an arm is to cause bone fractures. If you break an arm, a normal bone is broken and fails to serve its usual function. In genetic disorders, a normal gene or chromosome is broken (mutated) and fails to serve its usual adaptive function. Such a gene is sometimes called a "disease gene" because when it is broken, or functioning in a non-adaptive manner, it is involved in the mechanism of a particular disease. Keep this simple—but often overlooked—principle in mind as you read the following paragraphs.

Nuclear Inheritance

Single-Gene Diseases

As we just stated, genetic diseases are diseases produced by an abnormality in the genetic code. Many genetic diseases are caused by individual mutant genes in the nuclear DNA that is passed from one generation to the next—making them **single-gene diseases.** In single-gene diseases, the mutant gene may make an abnormal product that causes disease or it may fail to make a product required for normal function.

As discussed previously, some disease conditions result from the combined effects of inheritance and environmental factors. **Epigenetics** (*imprinting*) is the science that describes how environmental factors may result in offspring with genetic traits that cannot be explained by genes alone. For example, the diet of parents or grandparents may attach chemical groups to the chromosomes that may turn a certain gene either on or off. Thus the genes may be imprinted or chemically marked, and certain diseases may or may not be seen in the offspring. The effect of the environment on genes also explains why identical twins may not always share the same disease traits. Because they are not solely caused by genetic mechanisms, such conditions are not genetic diseases in the usual sense of the word; they are instead said to involve a *genetic predisposition.*

Chromosomal Genetic Diseases

Some genetic diseases do not result from an abnormality in a single gene. Instead, these diseases result from chromosome breakage or from the abnormal presence or absence of entire chromosomes. For example, a condition called **trisomy** may occur in which there is a triplet of autosomes rather than a pair. Trisomy results from a mistake in meiosis called **nondisjunction,** in which a pair of chromosomes fails to separate. This produces a gamete with two autosomes that are "stuck together" instead of the usual one. When this abnormal gamete joins with a normal gamete to form a zygote, the zygote has a triplet of autosomes (**Figure 48-11**). Trisomy of any autosome pair is usually fatal. However, if trisomy occurs in autosome pair 13, 15, 18, 21, or 22, a person may survive for a time—but with profound developmental defects. **Monosomy,** the presence of only one autosome instead of a pair, may also result from conception involving a gamete produced by nondisjunction (see **Figure 48-11**). As with trisomy, monosomy may produce life-threatening abnormalities. Because most trisomic and monosomic individuals are sterile, or do not survive long enough to reproduce, these conditions are not usually passed from generation to generation. Trisomy and monosomy are congenital conditions that are sometimes referred to as **chromosomal genetic diseases** (**Box 48-3**).

BOX 48-3 *fyi* | **Congenital Disorders**

A congenital disorder is any pathological condition present at birth. As explained in Chapter 47, congenital disorders may have a genetic cause. For example, one form of a facial deformity known as cleft palate is an X-linked inherited condition (see **Figure 48-9**). However, some congenital disorders are not inherited. For example, fetal alcohol syndrome is a group of congenital deformities that result from exposing a developing fetus to alcohol consumed by the mother (see **Box 29-1**, p. 690). Thus not all congenital disorders are inherited disorders. •

Mitochondrial Inheritance

Mitochondria are tiny, bacteria-like organelles present in every cell of the body (see **Figure 5-11** on p. 86). The major exception, of course, is the red blood cell, which does not reproduce itself. As with a bacterium, each mitochondrion has its own circular version of a DNA molecule with only 16,569 base pairs, sometimes called **mitochondrial DNA (mDNA** or **mtDNA). Figure 48-12** shows an ideogram of the structure of a mitochondrial chromosome.

Besides being a simple circle, mtDNA differs slightly from nuclear DNA in other ways. For example, there are usually 2 to 10 copies of mtDNA in each mitochondrion, unlike the single copy of each (of 46) DNA molecules in a nucleus. Each cell may have hundreds to thousands of mitochondria but generally only one nucleus. Also, a usual stop codon (UGA) instead codes for the amino acid tryptophan in mitochondria (see **Figure 7-6** on p. 125).

Each mtDNA has 37 genes, all of which are needed for the mitochondrion to function properly. Thirteen of these mitochondrial genes encode enzymes needed for *oxidative phosphorylation*—a key step in the metabolic pathway that "recharges" ATP in our cells. Two genes encode ribosomal RNA (rRNA) and 22 genes encode transfer RNA (tRNA) needed to translate the 13 protein-coding genes. All the mitochondrial proteins are translated in the cytoplasm, then imported into the mitochondria.

Inheritance of mtDNA occurs only through one's mother because the few mitochondria that a sperm may contribute to the ovum during fertilization do not survive. Because mtDNA contains the only genetic code for several important enzymes, it has the potential for carrying mutations that produce disease.

Mitochondrial inheritance is known to transmit genes for several degenerative nerve and muscle disorders. One such disease is *Leber hereditary optic neuropathy.* In this disease, young adults begin losing their eyesight as the optic nerve degenerates—resulting in total blindness by 30 years of age. Some medical researchers believe that at least some forms of several other diseases are associated with mtDNA mutations. These diseases include **Parkinson disease, Alzheimer disease (AD), diabetes mellitus (DM)** with deafness, and maternally inherited forms of deafness, myopathy, and cardiomyopathy.

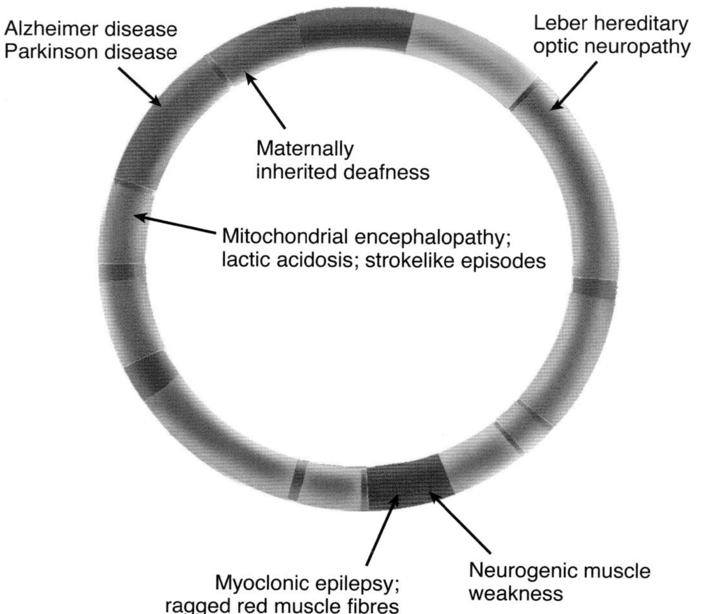

FIGURE 48-12 Map of mitochondrial DNA (mtDNA). Ideogram showing locations of some mtDNA genes associated with various diseases.

Researchers are developing experimental protocols for in vitro fertilization (IVF) in which mitochondrial inheritance of disease may be avoided by using an egg donor with normal mitochondria but using the egg nucleus from a mother with mutated mtDNA.

CONNECT IT!

Using IVF to avoid mitochondrial inheritance of disease will, in effect, produce offspring with *three* biological parents! Review this strategy in ***In Vitro Fertilization*** online at ***Connect It!***

Quick CHECK

9. How are single-gene diseases different from chromosomal conditions?
10. What is *nondisjunction?* How can it cause trisomy?
11. What is mitochondrial inheritance?

Single-Gene Diseases

There are many examples of single-gene diseases. Only a few of the many single-gene diseases are discussed here and summarized in **Table 48-1**.

Cystic fibrosis (CF), briefly mentioned in Chapter 6 (p. 116), is caused by a recessive gene in chromosome 7 that codes for *CFTR (CF transmembrane conductance regulator).* CFTR normally regulates the transfer of sodium across cell membranes and serves as a chloride channel. When this gene has a deletion of a single codon, the abnormal version of CFTR causes impairment of chloride ion transport across cell membranes. Disruption of chloride transport causes exocrine cells to secrete thick mucus and concentrated sweat. The thickened mucus is especially troublesome in the gastrointestinal (GI) and respiratory tracts, where it can cause obstruction that leads to death. This condition is often treated by the continuous use of drugs and other therapies that relieve the symptoms. CF occurs most commonly among Caucasians. The mutation that causes CF is thought to protect carriers of the gene from potentially fatal cases of diarrhoea, as in cholera and serious *Escherichia coli* infections.

Phenylketonuria (PKU) is caused by a recessive gene that fails to produce the enzyme *phenylalanine hydroxylase.* This enzyme is needed to convert the amino acid phenylalanine into another amino acid, tyrosine. Thus phenylalanine absorbed from ingested food accumulates in the body—resulting in the abnormal presence of phenylketone in the urine (hence the name phenylketonuria). A high concentration of phenylalanine in the body destroys brain tissue; babies born with this condition are at risk of progressive intellectual disability and, perhaps, death. Many PKU patients are identified at birth by state-mandated screening tests. After being identified, PKU patients are put on diets low in phenylalanine—thus avoiding a toxic accumulation of this amino acid. You may be familiar with the printed warning for people with phenylketonuria commonly seen on artificial sweetener packets that contain aspartame or other substances made from phenylalanine. The mutant PKU gene may have originated among the Celts in western

TABLE 48-1 **Examples of Genetic Conditions**

CHROMOSOME LOCATION	DISEASE	DESCRIPTION
Single-Gene Inheritance (Nuclear DNA)		
Dominant		
1p, or 3p, or 7q, or 17q	Osteogenesis imperfecta	Group of connective tissue disorders is characterized by imperfect skeletal development that produces brittle bones
17q	Neurofibromatosis	Disorder is characterized by multiple, sometimes disfiguring, benign tumours of the neuroglia that surround nerve fibres
1p, or 2p, or 19p	Hypercholesterolaemia (familial)	High blood cholesterol may lead to atherosclerosis and other cardiovascular problems
4p	Huntington disease (HD)	Degenerative brain disorder is characterized by chorea (purposeless movements) progressing to severe dementia and death generally by age 55 years
4q or 16p	Polycystic kidney disease, autosomal dominant form (ADPKD)	Polycystic kidney disease or PKD (both dominant and recessive forms) is the most common single-gene genetic disorder; clusters of fluid-filled sacs occur in kidneys and other organs, causing kidney failure, hypertension, liver problems, and heart valve problems
Codominant		
11p	Sickle cell anaemia Sickle cell trait	Blood disorder in which abnormal haemoglobin causes red blood cells (RBCs) to deform into a sickle shape; sickle cell anaemia is the severe form, and sickle cell trait the milder form
11p or 16p	Thalassaemia (a or b type)	Group of inherited haemoglobin disorders is characterized by production of hypochromic, abnormal RBCs
Recessive (Autosomal)		
7q	Cystic fibrosis (CF)	Condition is characterized by excessive secretion of thick mucus and concentrated sweat, often causing obstruction of gastrointestinal or respiratory ducts
15q	Tay–Sachs disease (TSD)	Fatal condition in which abnormal lipids accumulate in the brain and cause tissue damage leading to death by age 4 years
12q	Phenylketonuria (PKU)	Excess of phenylketones in the urine is caused by accumulation of phenylalanine in the tissues; it may cause brain injury and death if phenylalanine (amino acid) intake is not restricted
11q	Albinism (total)	Lack of the dark brown pigment *melanin* in the skin and eyes results in vision problems and susceptibility to sunburn and skin cancer
20q	Severe combined immune deficiency (SCID)	Failure of the lymphocytes to develop properly causes failure of the immune system's defence of the body; it is usually caused by adenosine deaminase (ADA) deficiency
6p	Polycystic kidney disease, autosomal recessive form (ARPKD)	Polycystic kidney disease or PKD (both dominant and recessive forms) is the most common single-gene genetic disorder; clusters of fluid-filled sacs occur in kidneys and other organs, causing kidney failure, hypertension, liver problems, and heart valve problems
Recessive (X Linked)		
23(X)q	Haemophilia	Group of blood clotting disorders is caused by failure to form clotting factor VIII, IX, or XI
23(X)p	Duchenne muscular dystrophy (DMD)	Muscle disorder is characterized by progressive atrophy of skeletal muscle without nerve involvement
23(X)q	Red-green colour blindness	Inability to distinguish red and green light results from a deficiency of photopigments in the cone cells of the retina
23(X)q	Fragile X syndrome (FSX)	Intellectual disability results from breakage of X chromosome in males
23(X)p	Ocular albinism	Form of albinism in which the pigmented layers of the eyeball lack melanin results in hypersensitivity to light and other problems
23(X)q	Androgen insensitivity	Inherited insensitivity to androgens (steroid sex hormones associated with maleness) results in reduced effects of these hormones
23(X)q	Cleft palate, X-linked form (CPX)	One form of a congenital deformity in which the skull fails to develop properly, characterized by a gap in the palate (plate separating mouth from nasal cavity)
23(X)p	Retinitis pigmentosa (RP, X-1 form)	Condition causes blindness, characterized by clumps of melanin in retina of eyes
Single-Gene Inheritance (Mitochondrial DNA [mtDNA])		
mtDNA	Leber hereditary optic neuropathy	Optic nerve degeneration in young adults results in total blindness by age 30 years
mtDNA	Parkinson disease	Nervous disorder is characterized by involuntary trembling and muscle rigidity

Europe, where it offered protection against the toxic effects of moulds growing on grains stored in cold, damp climates.

Tay–Sachs disease (TSD) is a recessive condition involving failure to make a subunit of an essential lipid-processing enzyme, hexosaminidase. Abnormal lipids accumulate in the brain tissue of Tay–Sachs patients, causing severe mental impairment and death by 4 years of age. There is currently no specific therapy for this condition.

TSD is most prevalent among certain Jewish populations. Some epidemiologists believe that this ethnic distribution is related to the hypothesis that heterozygous carriers of the Tay–Sachs gene have a higher than normal resistance to tuberculosis (TB)—a potentially fatal disease that once killed millions in the crowded Jewish ghettos of many large cities. Residents of these TB-infested areas who carried the Tay–Sachs gene apparently survived longer—and reproduced more frequently—than noncarriers.

Tay–Sachs is also found in higher than average frequencies in French Canadians in southeastern Quebec and Cajun French families in southern Louisiana—probably because of the gene's presence in several founders of these family groups, rather than natural selection by the threat of TB.

Osteogenesis imperfecta is a dominant genetic disorder of connective tissues. Its name, which means "imperfect bone formation", describes its chief characteristic. The bones of people with osteogenesis imperfecta do not have normal collagen and thus are often so brittle that the slightest trauma can result in serious fractures. There are different forms of the disease. In its most severe form, it results in fractures of the fetal skeleton in utero—often progressing to death shortly after birth. In a form seen in infancy, this disease is characterized by short, deformed limbs, a thin, enlarged skull, and easily fractured bones (**Figure 48-13**). In a less severe form, symptoms appear when a child begins to walk and become milder until after puberty—when the symptoms usually disappear.

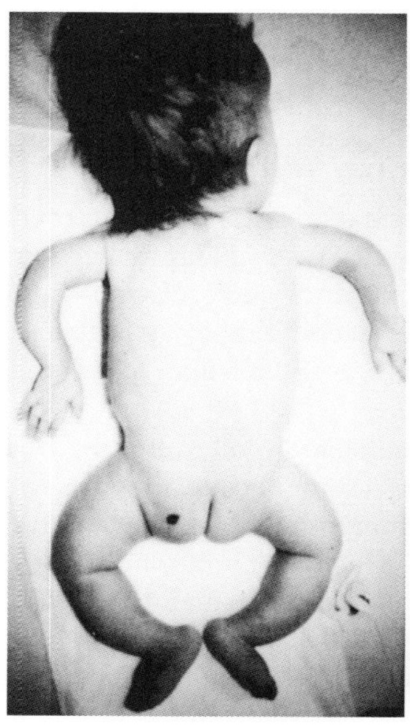

A

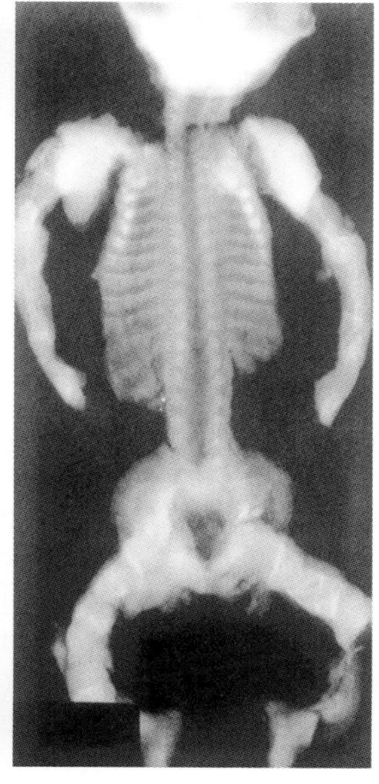

B

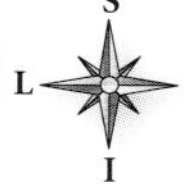

FIGURE 48-13 Osteogenesis imperfecta. A, The infantile form of this inherited disease is characterized by imperfect bone development that results in the appearance of this child: curved, brittle bones in the limbs and a thin, enlarged skull. **B,** This radiograph of a fetus with osteogenesis imperfecta shows the many bone fractures that produce an accordion-like shortening of the limbs.

Neurofibromatosis is a dominant genetic disorder discussed in Chapter 18 (p. 407). This disorder is characterized by multiple, sometimes disfiguring, skin spots and benign tumours of the glial cells that surround nerve fibres. Although usually inherited, it often arises from spontaneous mutations of DNA—which can then be inherited by offspring.

Other important inherited disorders include **Duchenne muscular dystrophy (DMD), hypercholesterolaemia, sickle cell anaemia, albinism,** certain forms of **haemophilia,** and **Huntington disease (HD).** These and other conditions are summarized in **Table 48-1**.

Multiple-Gene Diseases

It is becoming clear that most genetic disorders involve the dysfunction of more than one gene.

The omnigenic (*omni-* = "all") model of genetic disease holds that most genetic disorders involve the interaction of large numbers of genes in affected cells. The dysfunctional activity of one gene can affect the activity of many others with widespread effects.

Epigenetic Conditions

The study of how the environment may influence the genes—**epigenetics** (imprinting)—is rapidly growing. Regulation of many functions is thought to be the result of epigenetic changes that alter gene activity—sometimes producing disease. The number of epigenetic diseases may actually be huge.

Some cancers have been shown to be related to a reduction in chemical markers known as methyl groups ($—CH_3$). Other cancers are associated with too much *methylation*, which may inhibit genes that normally prevent cancer growth. Treatment of cancers with agents that either increase or decrease methylation of abnormal cells is being researched. However, not all epigenetic conditions are associated with methylation. Acetyl groups ($—COCH_3$) or ubiquitin protein also may mark the DNA, whereas other mechanisms involve the RNA molecules that regulate the production of proteins in the cell.

Fragile X syndrome (FXS) is a disease that is thought to be associated with overmethylation of a section of the DNA in the X chromosome. Methylation may occur when a string of repeating gene components, known as CGG in the normal protein gene, gets too long. The longer length of the repeating CGG nucleotides results in a greater severity of the syndrome. This area of the DNA may become overmethylated, which results in turning off the gene for a protein that normally prevents this genetic form of intellectual disability. The disorder is more common in males because they only inherit one copy of the X chromosome. Females may have a milder form because they may inherit a normal X chromosome that is able to make some of the normal protein.

CONNECT IT! 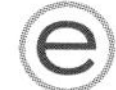

Find out more about epigenetic inheritance and Huntington disease in ***Epigenetics*** online at ***Connect It!***

Chromosomal Diseases

As described earlier, some genetic disorders are not inherited in the usual sense but result from nondisjunction during formation of the gametes. As **Figure 48-11** shows, nondisjunction results in gametes that produce either trisomy or monosomy in the cells of offspring. At least 10% of all human sperm and at least 25% of all mature oocytes have extra, missing, or broken chromosomes. Most zygotes and embryos with chromosomal abnormalities do not survive beyond a few days—and thus the mother is not even aware that conception occurred. Of the pregnancies that last long enough to become aware of, between 15% and 20% are spontaneously aborted (miscarried)—with about one half of those having chromosomal abnormalities.

A few of the major chromosomal disorders are summarized here and in **Table 48-1**.

The most well-known chromosomal disorder is *trisomy 21*, which produces a group of symptoms called **Down syndrome.** As **Figure 48-14**, A, shows, in this condition there is a triplet of chromosome 21 rather than the usual pair. In the general population, trisomy 21 occurs in only 1 of every 600 or so live births. After age 35 years, however, a mother's chances of producing a trisomic child increase dramatically—to as high as 1 in 80 births by age 40 years. One hypothesis that explains this phenomenon states that as a woman ages, her reproductive system becomes less likely to spontaneously abort abnormal blastocysts that have implanted in the endometrium. Thus nondisjunction may occur equally among young and middle-aged women, even though the number of live births may differ.

Down syndrome results from trisomy 21 and rarely from other genetic abnormalities (which can be inherited). This syndrome is characterized by intellectual disability (ranging from mild to severe) and multiple defects that include distinctive facial appearance (**Figure 48-14**, *B*), enlarged tongue, short hands and feet with stubby digits, congenital heart disease, and susceptibility to acute leukaemia. People with Down syndrome have a shorter than average life expectancy but can survive to old age.

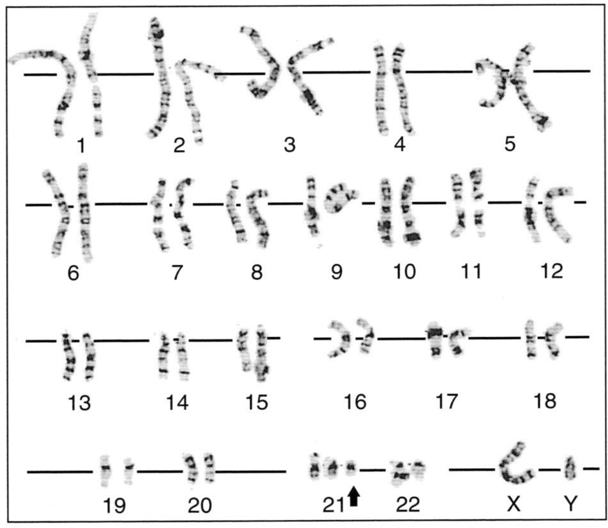

A

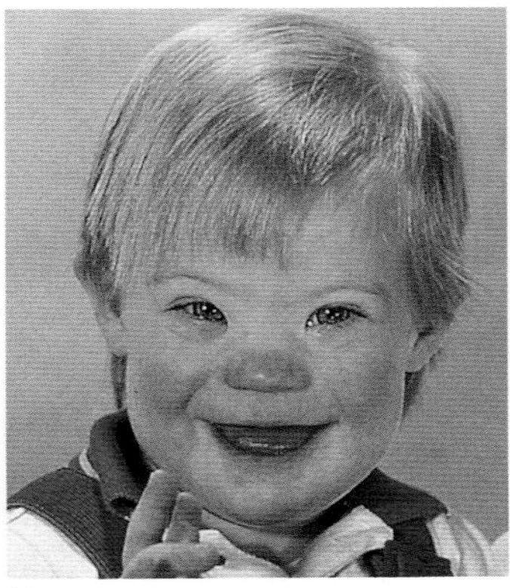

B

FIGURE 48-14 Down syndrome. **A,** Down syndrome is usually associated with trisomy of chromosome 21 (see **Figure 48-11**). **B,** A child with Down syndrome. Notice the distinctive anatomical features: exaggerated epicanthal folds around the eyes, flattened nose, round face, and short fingers.

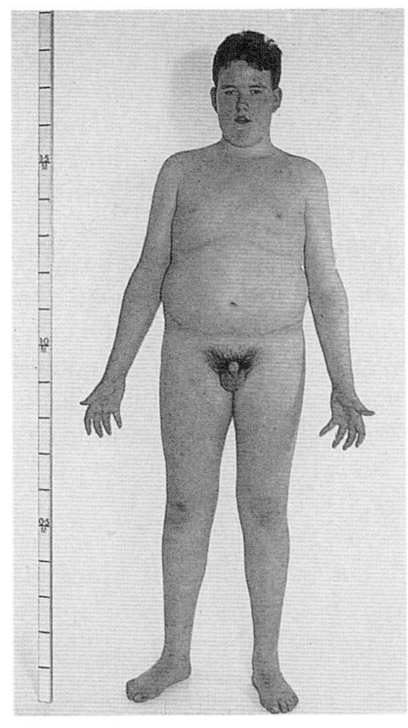

A

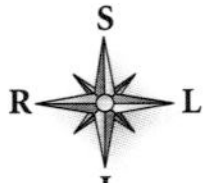

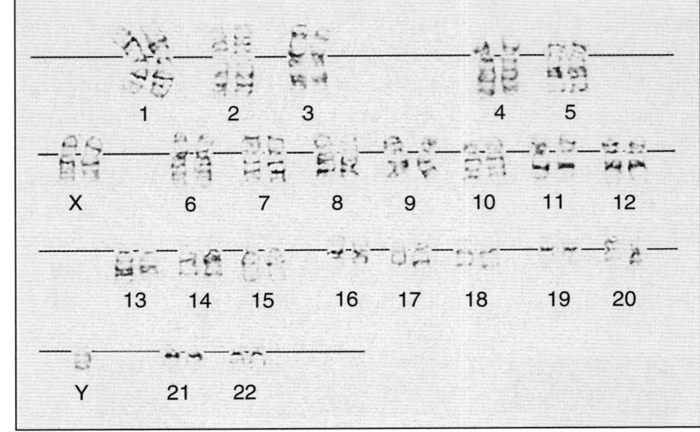

B

FIGURE 48-15 Klinefelter syndrome. **A,** This young man exhibits many of the characteristics of Klinefelter syndrome: small testes, some development of the breasts, sparse body hair, and long limbs. **B,** This syndrome results from the presence of two or more X chromosomes with a Y chromosome (genotypes XXY or XXXY, for example).

Klinefelter syndrome is another genetic disorder resulting from nondisjunction of chromosomes. This disorder occurs in males with a Y chromosome and at least two X chromosomes, typically the XXY genotype. Characteristics typical of Klinefelter syndrome include long legs, enlarged breasts, intellectual disability, small testes, sterility, and chronic pulmonary disease (**Figure 48-15**).

Turner syndrome, sometimes called *XO syndrome,* occurs in females with a single sex chromosome, X. As with the conditions described previously, the syndrome results from nondisjunction during gamete formation. Turner syndrome is characterized by failure of the ovaries and other sex organs to mature (causing sterility), cardiovascular defects, dwarfism or short stature, a webbed neck, and possible learning disorders (**Figure 48-16**). Symptoms of

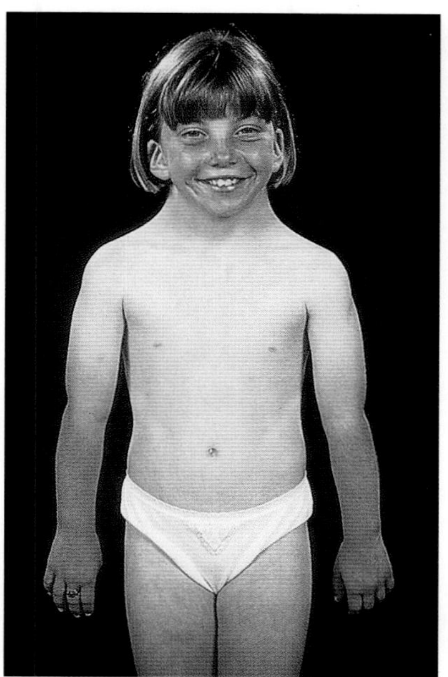

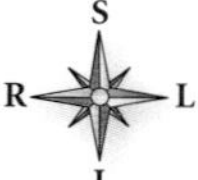

A

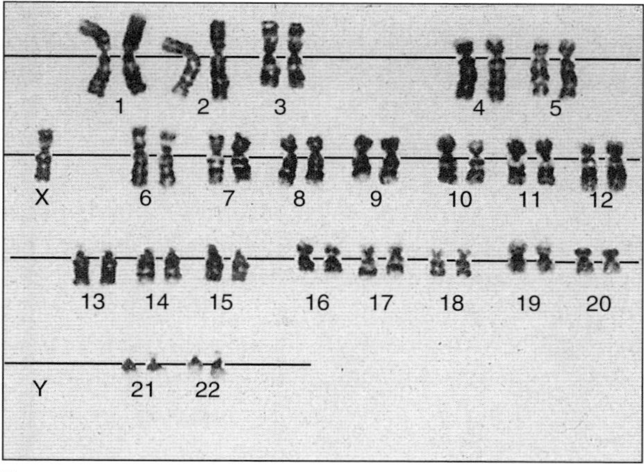

B

FIGURE 48-16 Turner syndrome. A, This young woman exhibits many of the characteristics of Turner syndrome, including short stature, webbed neck, and sexual immaturity. **B,** As this karyotype shows, Turner syndrome results from monosomy of sex chromosomes (genotype XO).

Turner syndrome can be reduced by hormone therapy using oestrogens and growth hormone. Cardiovascular defects may be repaired surgically.

Genetic Basis of Cancer

Recall from Chapter 8 that some forms of cancer are thought to be caused, at least in part, by abnormal genes called **oncogenes.** Oncogenes are altered (mutated) forms of normal genes.

One hypothesis states that most normal cells contain such cancer-causing genes. However, it is uncertain how these genes become activated and produce cancer. Perhaps oncogenes can transform a cell into a cancer cell only when certain environmental conditions occur. It has also been shown that viruses can transmit oncogenes to human cells.

Another hypothesis states that normal cells contain another class of genes, sometimes called **tumour suppressor genes.** According to this hypothesis, such genes regulate cell division so that it proceeds normally. When a tumour suppressor gene is nonfunctional because of a genetic mutation, it then allows cells to divide abnormally (or fail to die)—possibly producing cancer.

Yet another possible genetic basis for cancer relates to the genes that govern the cell's ability to repair damaged DNA. For example, a rare genetic disorder called **xeroderma pigmentosum** is characterized by the inability of skin cells to repair genetic damage caused by the ultraviolet (UV) radiation in sunlight. Individuals with this condition nearly always develop skin cancer when exposed to direct sunlight. In this condition, the genetic abnormality does not cause skin cancer directly but inhibits the cell's cancer-preventing mechanisms.

These three hypotheses regarding the genetic basis of cancer are not mutually exclusive. They are undoubtedly all important factors in the genesis of cancer. Cancer researchers are now working intensely to determine the exact role various genes play in the development of cancer. The more we understand the genetic basis of cancer, the more likely it is that we will find effective treatments—or even cures.

Quick CHECK

12. How does avoidance of phenylalanine in the diet reduce the problems associated with phenylketonuria (PKU)?
13. Briefly describe the mechanism of Tay–Sachs disease.
14. What is trisomy 21?
15. How might the genetic code be involved in the development of cancer?

PREVENTION AND TREATMENT OF GENETIC DISEASES

Genetic Counselling

The term *genetic counselling* refers to professional consultations with families regarding genetic diseases. Trained genetic counsellors may help a family determine the risk of producing children with genetic diseases.

Genetic counsellors may also help evaluate whether any offspring already have a genetic disorder and offer advice on treatment or care. A growing list of tools is available to genetic counsellors, some of which are described in the following section.

Pedigree

A **pedigree** is a chart that illustrates genetic relationships in a family over several generations (**Figure 48-17**). Using medical records and family histories, genetic counsellors assemble the chart beginning with the client and moving backward through as many generations as are known. Squares represent males; circles represent females. Fully shaded symbols represent affected individuals, and unshaded symbols represent normal individuals. Partially shaded symbols represent carriers of a recessive trait. A horizontal line between symbols designates a sexual relationship that produced offspring.

The pedigree is useful in determining the possibility of producing offspring with certain genetic disorders. It also may tell a person whether he or she might have a genetic disorder that appears late in life, such as Huntington disease. In either case, a family can prepare emotionally, financially, and medically before a crisis occurs.

Punnett Square

The **Punnett square,** named after the English geneticist Reginald Punnett, is a grid used to determine the mathematical *probability* of

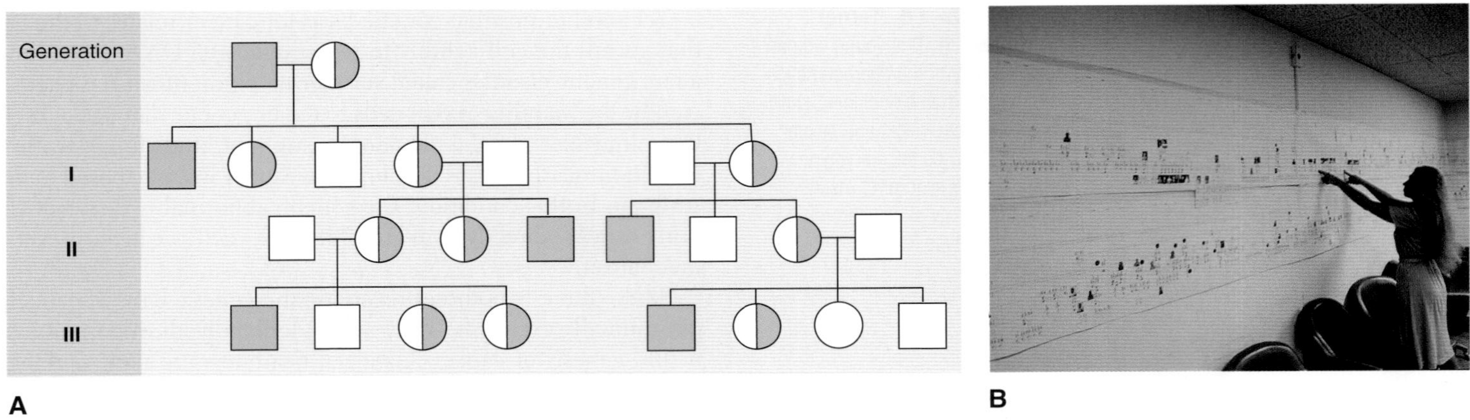

FIGURE 48-17 Pedigree. **A,** Pedigrees chart the genetic history of family lines. Squares represent males, and circles represent females. Fully shaded symbols indicate affected individuals, partly shaded symbols indicate carriers, and unshaded symbols indicate unaffected noncarriers. Roman numerals indicate the order of generations. This pedigree reveals the presence of an X-linked recessive trait. **B,** This huge pedigree compiled by Dr. Nancy Wexler of Columbia University and the Hereditary Disease Foundation traces Huntington disease (HD) over several generations of a large family in Venezuela. Dr. Wexler and other researchers collaborated in using information from this pedigree, along with techniques of molecular biology, to find the gene responsible for this disease and develop a test to detect the presence of the gene before the disease becomes apparent. Dr. Wexler became interested in this disease after her mother's death from HD.

inheriting genetic traits. As **Figure 48-18**, *A*, shows, genes in the mother's gametes are represented along the horizontal axis of the grid and genes in the father's gametes along the vertical axis. The ratio of different gene combinations in the offspring predicts their probability of occurrence in the next generation. Thus offspring produced by two carriers of PKU (a recessive disorder) have a one in four (25%) chance of inheriting this recessive condition (see **Figure 48-18**, *A*).

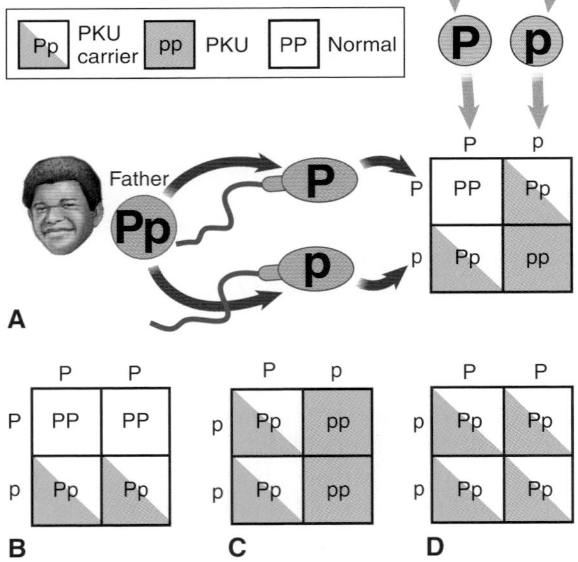

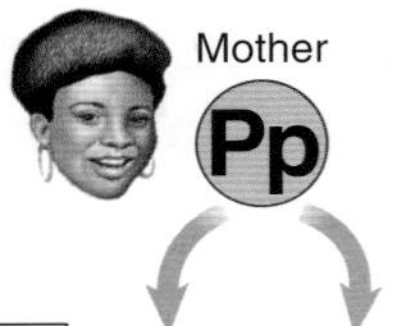

The same grid shows that there is a two in four (50%) chance that a child produced will be a PKU carrier. **Figure 48-18**, *B*, however, shows that offspring of a carrier and a noncarrier cannot inherit PKU. What is the chance of an individual offspring being a PKU carrier in this case? The grid in **Figure 48-18**, *C*, shows the probability of producing an affected offspring when a PKU patient and a PKU carrier have children. **Figure 48-18**, *D*, shows the genetic probability when a PKU patient and a noncarrier produce children.

FIGURE 48-18 Punnett square. The Punnett square is a grid used to determine relative probabilities of producing offspring with specific gene combinations. Phenylketonuria (PKU) is a recessive disorder caused by the gene *p*. *P* is the normal gene. **A,** Possible results of cross between two PKU carriers. Because one in four of the offspring represented in the grid have PKU, a genetic counsellor would predict a 25% chance that this couple will produce a PKU baby at each birth. **B,** Cross between a PKU carrier and a normal noncarrier. **C,** Cross between a PKU patient and a PKU carrier. **D,** Cross between a PKU patient and a normal noncarrier.

Karyotype

Disorders that involve trisomy (extra chromosomes), monosomy (missing chromosomes), and broken chromosomes can be detected after a **karyotype** is produced.

The first step in producing a karyotype is getting a sample of cells from the individual to be tested. This can be done by scraping cells from the lining of the cheek or from a blood sample containing white blood cells (WBCs). Fetal tissue can be collected by **amniocentesis**, a procedure in which fetal cells floating in the amniotic fluid are collected with a syringe (**Figure 48-19**). **Chorionic villus sampling (CVS)** is a newer procedure in which cells from chorionic villi that surround a young embryo (see Chapter 47, p. 1098) are collected through the opening of the cervix.

Collected cells are grown in a special culture medium and allowed to reproduce. Cells in metaphase (when the chromosomes are most distinct) are stained and photographed using a microscope. The chromosomes are cut out of the photo and pasted on a chart in pairs according to size, as in **Figures 48-2** and **48-15**, *B*. More advanced techniques use digital imaging and computers to automatically generate a karyotype.

Genetic counsellors then examine the karyotype, looking for chromosome abnormalities. What chromosome abnormality is visible in **Figure 48-15**, *B*? Is this a male or female karyotype?

FIGURE 48-19 Amniocentesis. In amniocentesis, a syringe is used to collect amniotic fluid. Ultrasound imaging is used to guide the tip of the syringe needle to prevent damage to the placenta and fetus. Fetal cells in the collected amniotic fluid can then be chemically tested or used to produce a karyotype of the developing baby.

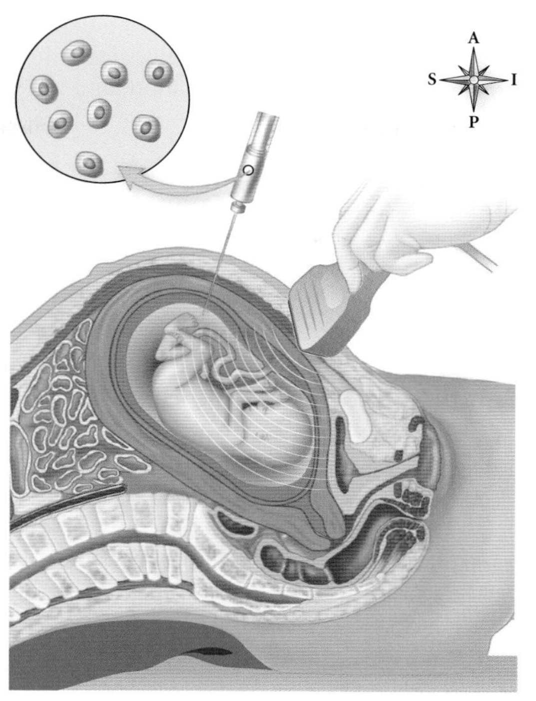

CONNECT IT! 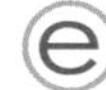

Many tools for discovering the secrets of a particular sample of DNA are available, such as **DNA fingerprinting** and **gene chips.** To see how these techniques work, check out ***DNA Analysis*** online at ***Connect It!***

***Quick* CHECK**

16. What is genetic counselling?
17. How are pedigrees used by genetic counsellors?
18. How is a Punnett square used to predict mathematical probabilities of inheriting specific genes?
19. How is a karyotype prepared? What is its purpose?

Treating Genetic Diseases

Until this century, the only hope of treating any genetic disease was to treat the symptoms. In some diseases, such as PKU, this works well. If PKU patients simply avoid large amounts of phenylalanine in their diets, especially during critical stages of development, severe complications can be avoided. In Klinefelter syndrome and Turner syndrome, hormone therapy and surgery can alleviate some symptoms. However, there are no effective treatments for a majority of genetic disorders. Fortunately, medical science now offers us some hope of treating genetic disorders through **gene therapy.**

In a therapy sometimes called **gene replacement,** genes that specify production of abnormal, disease-causing proteins are replaced by normal or "therapeutic" genes. To get the therapeutic genes to cells that need them, researchers are using genetically altered viruses as carriers. Recall that viruses are easily capable of inserting new genes into the human genome. If the therapeutic genes behave as expected, a cure may result. Thus the goal of gene replacement therapy is to genetically alter existing body cells in the hope of eliminating the cause of a genetic disease. Although called *gene replacement,* this therapy does not actually replace the defective genes—it instead inserts normal genes so that normal proteins can "replace" abnormal or missing proteins in the body's metabolic pathways.

In a therapy called **gene augmentation,** normal genes are introduced with the hope that they will augment (add to) the production of the needed protein. In one form of gene augmentation, virus-altered cells are injected into the blood or implanted under the skin of a patient to produce increased amounts of the missing protein. Some researchers have proposed grafting synthetic skin containing cells with therapeutic genes. Another approach is to use bacterial DNA rings called **plasmids** that have been altered by recombinant DNA techniques to carry the therapeutic gene or genes. Yet another approach uses the **human engineered chromosome (HEC).** In the HEC strategy, a set of therapeutic genes is incorporated into a separate strand of DNA that is inserted into a cell's nucleus, thus acting like an extra, or forty-seventh, chromosome. Gene augmentation attempts to add genetically altered cells to the body, rather than change existing body cells, as in gene replacement therapy.

CONNECT IT! 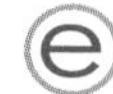

Can gene therapy be used to extend the human life span? Check out ***Genes and Longevity*** online at ***Connect It!***

There have been many disappointing results from clinical trials of cell and gene therapies. By 2016, only 8 had been approved for use in the European Union. Despite setbacks and concerns, there are currently hundreds of ongoing gene therapy trials for diverse genetic disorders, cancer, and even ageing. Thousands of laboratory experiments in anticipation of human trials are also currently under way. Hurdles that must be overcome before we will see widespread success of gene therapies include our lack of detailed knowledge regarding many of the "disease genes" and how best to effectively treat multiple-gene diseases—not to mention the high costs and risks involved with these therapies. It is too early to say for sure, but there may soon come a time when many genetic diseases are routinely treated—or even cured—with gene therapy.

CONNECT IT! 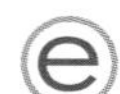

Experimentation with gene therapy in humans began as far back as 1990. Learn more about the early efforts at gene therapy in ***Using Gene Therapy and Sickle Cell Anaemia*** online at ***Connect It!***

RNA interference (RNAi) may also become a weapon against genetic disorders in an approach called **RNAi therapy.** Recall from the ***Connect It!*** article ***The RNA Revolution*** that RNAi is a method of silencing particular genes. When harnessed in the laboratory, RNAi can turn off one gene at a time—greatly increasing the chances of figuring out which protein is encoded by that gene and what the function of that protein is.

The possibilities of RNAi therapy are very exciting. Work is already under way to find an effective means of using RNAi for creating antiviral creams containing short interfering RNA (siRNA) to protect against HIV and other viruses. Some researchers are using RNAi to knock out genes that permit permanent tissue damage during heart attacks, kidney failure, and stroke. In one proposal, RNAi would be used to silence the abnormal huntingtin gene that causes Huntington disease (HD). In animal studies, RNAi successfully blocked a gene causing high blood cholesterol—without any apparent side effects. Researchers are also attempting to harness the power of RNAi to treat cancer and many types of infection. However, developing a large set of RNAi therapies may be thwarted by the possibility that they may also silence genes needed for normal function or trigger unwanted side effects in the body's immune defences.

RNA interference is also being used to develop other treatments for genetic disorders. By silencing the expression of specific genes in laboratory models (cells, tissues, animals), scientists can more precisely investigate the nature of genetic disorders and thus provide a foundation for a variety of possible therapies.

Quick CHECK

20. How are most genetic disorders treated today?
21. How does gene replacement therapy work?

the big picture | Genetics, Heredity, and the Whole Body

The study of human genetics and heredity provides an amazingly clear view of the "big picture" of the structure and function of the human body. In fact, the genetic view extends from the molecular level all the way to the context of the whole human species and beyond.

At the molecular level, the genetic perspective reveals the importance of nucleic acids—especially DNA. DNA molecules serve as tiny data storage devices that contain *all* the information needed to manufacture the molecules needed to build and maintain the human body. Each cell, tissue, organ, and system in the body is built of, and directed by, molecules that have been synthesized with recipes contained in the genes of each of our DNA molecules.

At the molecular level, we see that DNA in concert with various forms of RNA directs the synthesis of structural and functional proteins. Some of the functional proteins, in turn, trigger and direct the synthesis of all other biomolecules that form and regulate the body—lipids, carbohydrates, and so on.

This vast collection of different kinds of molecules also includes the enzymes and other molecules needed to gather and assimilate chemicals from the external environment outside the body. These external chemicals include water, oxygen, vitamins, minerals, sugars, starches, amino acids, fats, and other nutrients. Some of the molecules that ultimately owe their existence in the body to DNA also include those that help us rid the body of wastes such as urea, carbon dioxide, and bile.

If DNA directs all the chemical activity of the body, then it certainly directs cellular metabolism. And, of course, cellular metabolism is the foundation of the function of each tissue, organ, and system in the body. Our study of medical genetics has shown us that even one mistake in one codon of a gene can upset the chemistry of the body enough to shut down an entire system—and thus threaten the survival of the entire body. •

LANGUAGE OF SCIENCE *(continued from p. 1126)*

Human Genome Project (HGP)
[*gen-* **produce (gene),** *-ome* **entire collection**]

ideogram (ID-ee-oh-gram)
[*ide-* **idea,** *-gram* **drawing**]

karyotype (KAIR-ee-oh-type)
[*karyo-* **nucleus,** *-type* **kind**]

meiosis (my-OH-sis)
[*meiosis* **becoming smaller**]

mitochondrial DNA (mDNA, mtDNA) (my-toh-KON-dree-al D N A)
[*mito-* **thread,** *-chondrion-* **granule,** *-al* **relating to)**

monogenic (mon-oh-JEN-ik)
[*mono-* **single,** *-gen-* **produce (gene),** *-ic* **relating to**]

monosomy (MON-oh-so-mee)
[*mono-* **single,** *-som-* **body (chromosome),** *-y* **state**]

mutagen (MYOO-tah-jen)
[*muta-* **change,** *-gen* **produce**]

nucleosome (NYOO-klee-oh-sohm)
[*nucleo-* **kernel (nucleus),** *-som-* **body**]

p-arm
[*p* **petite (small)**]

pedigree (PED-ih-gree)
[*pied de grue* **crane's foot pattern**]

phenotype (FEE-noh-type)
[*pheno-* **appear,** *-type* **kind**]

polygenic (pol-ee-JEN-ik)
[*poly-* **many,** *-gen-* **produce,** *-ic* **relating to**]

principle of independent assortment
[*princip-* **foundation,** *in-* **not,** *-de-* **upon,** *-pend-* **hang,** *-ent* **state,** *assort-* **match into groups,** *-ment* **process**]

principle of segregation
[*princip-* **foundation,** *segrega-* **divide,** *-ation* **process**]

proteome (PRO-tee-ohm)
[*prote-* **protein,** *-ome* **entire collection**]

proteomics (proh-tee-OH-miks)
[*prote-* **first rank (protein),** *-om-* **entire collection,** *-ic* **relating to**]

pseudogene (SOOD-oh-jeen)
[*pseudo-* **false,** *-gene* **produce (gene)**]

Punnett square (PUN-it)
[*Reginald C. Punnett* **English geneticist**]

q-arm
[*q* **follows p in Roman alphabet**]

recessive gene
[*recess-* **retreat,** *-ive* **relating to,** *gene* **produce**]

sex chromosome (KROH-moh-sohm)
[*chrom-* **colour,** *-som-* **body**]

transcriptome (tran-SKRIPT-ome)
[*trans-* **across,** *-script-* **written document,** *-ome* **entire collection**]

transcriptomics (tran-skript-OHM-iks)
[*trans-* **across,** *-script-* **written document,** *-om-* **entire collection,** *-ic* **relating to**]

trisomy (TRY-soh-mee)
[*tri-* **three,** *-som-* **body (chromosome),** *-y* **state**]

LANGUAGE OF MEDICINE

albinism (AL-bih-niz-em)
[*alb-* **white,** *-in-* **characterized by,** *-ism* **state**]

Alzheimer disease (AD) (AHLZ-hye-mer)
[*Alois Alzheimer* **German neurologist**]

amniocentesis
(AM-nee-oh-sen-TEE-sis)
[*amnio-* **birth membrane,** *-centesis* **a pricking**]

anaemia (ah-NEE-mee-ah)
[*an-* **without,** *-aem-* **blood,** *-ia* **condition**]

chorionic villus sampling (CVS)
(koh-ree-ON-ik VIL-lus)
[*chorion-* **skin,** *-ic* **relating to,** *villus* **shaggy hair**]

chromosomal genetic disease
(kroh-moh-SOH-mal jeh-NET-ik)
[*chrom-* **colour,** *-soma-* **body,** *-al* **relating to,** *gen-* **produce,** *-ic* **relating to**]

cystic fibrosis (CF)
(SIS-tik fye-BROH-sis)
[*cyst-* **sac,** *-ic* **relating to,** *fibr-* **thread or fibre,** *-osis* **condition**]

diabetes mellitus (DM)
(dye-ah-BEE-teez mell-EYE-tus)
[*diabetes* **pass-through or siphon,** *mellitus* **honey-sweet**]

Down syndrome (SIN-drohm)
[*John L. Down* **English physician,** *syn-* **together,** *-drome* **running or (race) course**]

Duchenne muscular dystrophy (DMD)
(doo-SHEN MUSS-kyoo-lar DISS-troh-fee)
[*Guillaume B. A. Duchenne de Boulogne* **French neurologist,** *mus-* **mouse,** *-cul-* **little,** *-ar* **relating to,** *dys-* **bad,** *-troph-* **nourishment,** *-y* **state**]

fragile X syndrome (FXS)
(FRAJ-il eks SIN-drohm)
[*fragil-* **frail,** *X* **sex chromosome X,** *syn-* **together,** *-drome* **running or (race) course**]

gene augmentation
(jeen awg-men-TAY-shun)
[*gen-* **produce or generate**]

gene chip (jeen chip)
[*gen-* **produce or generate**]

gene replacement
[*gen-* **produce or generate**]

gene therapy (jeen THER-ah-pee)
[*gen-* **produce or generate**]

haemophilia (hee-moh-FIL-ee-ah)
[*haemo-* **blood,** *-phil-* **love,** *-ia* **condition**]

human engineered chromosome (HEC)
[*chrom-* **colour,** *-som-* **body**]

Huntington disease (HD)
(HUNT-ing-ton)
[*George S. Huntington* **American physician**]

hypercholesterolaemia
(hye-per-koh-les-ter-ohl-EE-mee-ah)
[*hyper-* **excessive,** *-chole-* **bile,** *-stero-* **solid,** *-ol-* **alcohol,** *-aem-* **blood,** *-ia* **condition**]

Klinefelter syndrome
(KLINE-fel-ter SIN-drohm)
[*Harry F. Klinefelter* **American physician,** *syn-* **together,** *-drome* **running or (race) course**]

malaria (mah-LAIR-ee-ah)
[*mal-* **bad,** *-ar-* **air,** *-ia* **condition**]

neurofibromatosis
(nyoo-roh-fye-broh-mah-TOH-sis)
[*neuro-* **nerve,** *-fibr-* **thread or fibre,** *-oma-* **tumour,** *-t-* **combining form,** *-osis* **condition**]

nondisjunction (non-dis-JUNK-shun)
[*non-* **not,** *-dis-* **split in two,** *-junction* **joint**]

oncogene (ON-koh-jeen)
[*onco-* **swelling or mass (cancer),** *-gen-* **produce or generate**]

osteogenesis imperfecta
(os-tee-oh-JEN-eh-sis im-per-FEK-tah)
[*osteo-* **bone,** *-gen-* **produce,** *-esis* **process,** *imperfecta* **not perfect**]

Parkinson disease (PARK-in-son)
[*James Parkinson* **English physician**]

phenylketonuria (PKU)
(fen-il-kee-toh-NOO-ree-ah)
[*phen-* **shining (phenol),** *-yl-* **chemical,** *-keton-* **acetone,** *-ur-* **urine,** *-ia* **condition**]

plasmid (PLAS-mid)
[*plasmid* **formed substance**]

RNAi therapy
[*RNA* **ribonucleic acid,** *i* **interference,** *therapy* **treatment**]

sickle cell anaemia
(SIK-ul sell ah-NEE-mee-ah)
[*sickle* **crescent,** *cell* **storeroom,** *an-* **without,** *-aem-* **blood,** *-ia* **condition**]

single-gene disease
[*gen-* **produce or generate**]

Tay–Sachs disease (TSD) (TAY-saks)
[*Warren Tay* **English ophthalmologist,** *Bernard Sachs* **American neurologist**]

tumour suppressor gene
[*tumour* **swelling,** *suppress-* **press down,** *-or* **agent,** *gen-* **produce or generate**]

Turner syndrome (TUR-ner SIN-drohm)
[*Harry H. Turner* **American endocrinologist,** *syn-* **together,** *-drome* **running or (race) course**]

xeroderma pigmentosum
(zeer-oh-DER-mah pig-men-TOH-sum)
[*xero-* **dry,** *-derma* **skin,** *pigment-* **paint,** *-osum* **characterized by**]

case study

David and Karen were ecstatic to have two healthy babies. Within the first hour, the babies had been cleaned and measured and their heels pricked for blood samples. These initial blood tests were to assess for PKU (phenylketonuria), thyroid hormone levels, cystic fibrosis, and several other metabolic disorders. To their surprise, their new daughter tested positive for PKU. Neither David nor Karen had PKU.

1. What is the chance their son will have PKU as well?
   a. 25%
   b. 50%
   c. 75%
   d. 0%

Thankfully, their son tested negative for PKU. When they were discussing her daughter's condition with the genetic counsellor, Karen remembered that her father had been colour-blind. Although she was not affected, Karen wondered whether her son could also be colour-blind.

2. It isn't possible to determine whether their son is colour-blind as a baby, but his chance of inheriting the condition from his grandfather can be worked out. What is the chance of David and Karen's son being colour-blind?
   a. 25%
   b. 50%
   c. 75%
   d. 0%

David and Karen were so happy with their new twins, they were thinking about trying to have more children, maybe in a few years.

3. Having had one boy and one girl, David and Karen's chance of having another boy is?
   a. Depends on the timing of the fertilization
   b. 25%
   c. 50%
   d. 75%

Hint To solve a case study, you may have to refer to the glossary or index, other chapters in this textbook, ***Connect It!,*** and other resources.

CHAPTER SUMMARY

To download an MP3 version of the chapter summary for use with your mobile device, access the ***Audio Chapter Summaries*** *online at evolve.elsevier.com.*

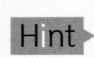

Scan this summary after reading the chapter to help you reinforce the key concepts. Later, use the summary as a quick review before your class or before a test.

The Science of Genetics

A. Genetics—scientific study of inheritance; developed to explain how normal biological characteristics are inherited
B. Directly inherited diseases are often called *hereditary diseases*

Chromosomes and Genes

A. Mechanism of gene function
   1. Genetic code transmitted by way of genes, which are segments of DNA
   2. DNA (deoxyribonucleic acid) (**Figure 48-1**)
      a. Chromosome—compact form of DNA that exists only during cell division
      b. Chromatin—strand form of DNA made up of subunits called *nucleosomes,* which are like small spools of DNA wound around proteins called *histones*
   3. Each gene is a sequence of nucleotide bases in the DNA molecule, which the cell transcribes to an RNA molecule
   4. Each mRNA molecule associates with a ribosome, which translates the code to form one or more specific polypeptide molecules
   5. Genes determine the structure and function of the human body by producing a set of specific regulatory RNA and protein molecules—along with specific structural proteins
B. The human genome (**Figure 48-2**)
   1. Genome—entire set of human chromosomes (46 in nucleus of each cell, 1 mitochondrial chromosome)
      a. Map of the entire human genome (nearly all nucleotides in sequence) was completed in 2003
      b. Contains about 19,000 or so genes and large amounts of noncoding DNA
         (1) Genes can encode proteins or other functional products such as tRNA, rRNA, ribozymes
         (2) DNA sequences called *exons* join to form a gene; the same exons may be part of different genes
         (3) Pseudogenes—bits of formerly functional genes that make up part of noncoding "junk" DNA
      c. Fewer than 2% of genome codes for proteins
         (1) Some DNA codes for regulatory RNAs
         (2) Much of the DNA ("junk DNA") includes pseudogenes that are remnants of functional genes
   2. Genomics—analysis of the sequence contained in the genome
   3. Transcriptomics—analysis of the mRNA codes actually transcribed from genes in the genome
   4. Proteomics—analysis of the entire group of proteins encoded by the genome and transcriptome, a group of proteins called the *human proteome*
   5. Genomic information can be expressed in various ways
      a. Ideogram—cartoon of a chromosome showing the centromere as a constriction and the short segment (p-arm) and long segment (q-arm)
      b. Genes are often represented as their actual sequence of nucleotide bases expressed by the letters a, c, g, and t
C. Distribution of chromosomes to offspring
   1. Meiosis (see **Figure 47-1**)
      a. Produces gametes with the haploid number of chromosomes (23)
      b. When a sperm and an ovum unite at conception, they form a zygote with 46 chromosomes
   2. Principle of independent assortment
      a. As sperm and ovum are formed during meiosis, two members of a pair of homologous chromosomes separate (the principle of segregation) and the maternal and paternal chromosomes get mixed up and redistributed independently in each gamete, with each thus having a different set of 23 chromosomes (**Figure 48-3**)
      b. Genetic variation—independent assortment of chromosomes ensures that each offspring from a single set of parents is genetically unique
      c. Applies to individual genes or groups of genes
      d. Crossing over—during one phase of meiosis, pairs of matching chromosomes line up along the equator and exchange genes with one another (**Figure 48-4**)
      e. Gene linkage—sometimes an entire group of genes stays together and crosses over as a single unit

Gene Expression

A. Hereditary traits
   1. Dominant and recessive traits
      a. Each inherited trait is controlled by two sets of similar genes, one from each parent
      b. Each autosome in a pair matches its partner in the type of gene it contains
      c. Different types of genes (**Figures 48-5** and **48-6**)
         (1) Dominant gene—effects are seen; capable of masking the effects of a recessive gene for the same trait
         (2) Recessive gene—effects are masked by the effects of a dominant gene for the same trait
      d. Genotype—combination of genes within the cells of an individual
         (1) Homozygous—genotype with two identical forms of a gene
         (2) Heterozygous—genotype with two different forms of a gene
      e. Phenotype—manner in which genotype is expressed; how an individual looks because of genotype
      f. Carrier—person who possesses the gene for a recessive trait but does not exhibit the trait
   2. Polygenic traits—when more than one gene is involved in producing a particular trait; a "combined trait" because it results from a combination of genes

3. Codominant traits—when two different dominant genes occur together, each will have an equal effect
4. Abnormal "disease" genes that persist in a population often provide some biological advantage, as in the case of the sickle gene that protects against malaria (**Figure 48-7**)

B. Sex-linked traits (**Figures 48-8** and **48-9**)
1. X chromosome—"female chromosome"; larger than Y chromosome; includes genes that determine female sexual characteristics, as well as nonsexual characteristics (**Figure 48-10**)
2. Y chromosome—"male chromosome"; smaller than X chromosome; contains few genes other than male sexual characteristics
3. Sex-linked traits—traits carried on sex chromosomes; also known as X-linked traits

C. Genetic mutations
1. Mutation—change in the genetic code
   a. Deletion—missing information in the genetic code
   b. Insertion—extra information in the genetic code
   c. Insertions and deletions result in a failure to make the usual protein encoded by a particular gene
2. Mutations can occur without outside influence
3. Mutagens—agents that cause most genetic mutations

Medical Genetics

A. Mechanisms of genetic disorders
1. Nuclear inheritance mechanisms
   a. Single-gene diseases—caused by individual mutant genes in nuclear DNA that pass from one generation to the next
   b. Genetic predisposition—disease occurring because of combined effects of inheritance and environmental factors
   c. Chromosomal genetic diseases—congenital conditions such as trisomy and monosomy that often produce life-threatening abnormalities; trisomic and monosomic individuals may die before they can reproduce (**Figure 48-11**)
   d. Epigenetic (imprinting)—how environmental factors may result in offspring with genetic traits that can't be explained by genes alone
2. Mitochondrial inheritance
   a. Mitochondrial DNA (mtDNA)—each mitochondrion has its own DNA molecule (**Figure 48-12**)
   b. Inheritance of mtDNA occurs through one's mother because sperm does not contribute mitochondria to the ovum during fertilization
   c. mtDNA contains the only genetic code for several important enzymes

B. Single-gene diseases
1. Cystic fibrosis
   a. Results because of recessive genes in chromosome pair 7
   b. Impairment of chloride ion transport across cell membranes causes exocrine cells to secrete thick mucus and concentrated sweat; thickened mucus may obstruct respiratory and gastrointestinal tracts, leading to death
   c. Treatment—use of drugs and other therapies
2. Phenylketonuria (PKU)
   a. Results from recessive genes that fail to produce phenylalanine hydroxylase
   b. Phenylalanine cannot be converted into tyrosine and thus accumulates
   c. High concentrations of phenylalanine destroy brain tissue
   d. Treatment—diets low in phenylalanine
3. Tay–Sachs disease (TSD)
   a. Recessive condition involving failure to make an essential lipid-processing enzyme; carrying one TSD gene may be protective against TB
   b. Abnormal lipids accumulate in the brain, causing severe mental impairment and death by 4 years of age
   c. No specific therapy available
4. Osteogenesis imperfecta (**Figure 48-13**)
   a. Dominant genetic disorder of connective tissues resulting in imperfect bone formation
   b. Bones do not have normal collagen and are very brittle
5. Neurofibromatosis
   a. Group of dominant genetic disorders; often inherited but can result from spontaneous mutations of DNA
   b. Characterized by multiple spots and benign tumours of glial cells that surround nerve fibres

C. Multiple-gene disorders
1. Polygenic disease
   a. Caused by more than one abnormal gene
   b. Examples include hypertension, coronary artery disease, and diabetes mellitus
2. Omnigenic model—holds that some (perhaps most) genetic conditions involve the interaction of large numbers of genes as one abnormal gene can alter the activity of many others in affected cells

D. Epigenetic conditions—alter gene activity that causes disorders
1. Fragile X syndrome—thought to be associated with overmethylation of a section of DNA in the X chromosome
2. Other diseases may include type 2 diabetes and cardiovascular disease
3. Huntington disease (HD) occurs when epigenetic changes to DNA are passed along to offspring

E. Chromosomal diseases—genetic disorders resulting from nondisjunction during formation of the gametes; produce either trisomy or monosomy
1. Trisomy 21—triplet of chromosome 21 rather than a pair; characterized by Down syndrome's intellectual disability and multiple defects (**Figure 48-14**)
2. Klinefelter syndrome—occurs in males with a Y chromosome and at least two X chromosomes; characteristics include long legs, enlarged breasts, learning difficulties, small testes, sterility, and chronic pulmonary disease (**Figure 48-15**)
3. Turner syndrome—XO syndrome; occurs in females with a single X chromosome; characterized by failure of ovaries and other organs to mature, sterility, cardiovascular defects, dwarfism, webbed neck, and learning difficulties; symptoms can be reduced by hormone therapy (**Figure 48-16**)

F. Genetic basis of cancer
   1. Oncogenes—abnormal genes thought to cause some forms of cancer
   2. Tumour suppressor genes regulate cell division so it proceeds normally; when nonfunctional because of a genetic mutation, it allows cells to divide abnormally
   3. Also, genetic abnormalities may inhibit the cell's cancer-preventing mechanisms

Prevention and Treatment of Genetic Diseases

A. Genetic counselling—professional consultations with families regarding genetic diseases
   1. Pedigree—chart that illustrates genetic relationships in a family over several generations; helpful in determining the possibility of producing offspring with certain genetic disorders (**Figure 48-17**)
   2. Punnett square—grid used to determine the mathematical probability of inheriting genetic traits (**Figure 48-18**)
   3. Karyotype—ordered arrangement of photographs of chromosomes from a single cell; used in genetic counselling to identify chromosomal disorders
B. Treating genetic diseases
   1. A few genetic conditions can be alleviated by avoiding triggers or treating symptoms
   2. Gene therapy involves changing the genetic code of cells to replace normal proteins that are absent in genetic disorders; still experimental
      a. Gene replacement—abnormal, disease-causing proteins are replaced by "therapeutic" genes; goal is to genetically alter existing body cells in the hope of eliminating the cause of a genetic disease
      b. Gene augmentation—normal genes are introduced to augment the production of the needed protein
   3. RNA interference (RNAi) therapy—disease-causing genes can be "silenced" by introducing specific short interfering RNA (siRNA) sequences into the body; still experimental

The Big Picture: Genetics, Heredity, and the Whole Body

A. The study of human genetics and heredity provides a clear view of the "big picture" of the structure and function of the human body
B. DNA in concert with RNA directs the synthesis of structural and functional proteins
   1. Some of the functional proteins direct the synthesis of biomolecules: lipids, carbohydrates, and so on
C. DNA directs cellular metabolism
   1. Cellular metabolism is the foundation of each tissue, organ, and system in the body
D. One mistake in one codon of a gene can upset the chemistry of the body and threaten the survival of the entire body

REVIEW QUESTIONS

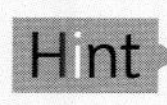

Write out the answers to these questions after reading the chapter and reviewing the Chapter Summary. Note—writing out your answers will consolidate learning and provide a valuable resource of information.

1. Who was the first person to discover the basic mechanism by which traits are transmitted from parents to offspring?
2. Describe albinism in relation to dominance, recessiveness, and genotype.
3. Explain the difference between a genotype and a phenotype.
4. Define *codominance*, and give an example of a condition that demonstrates codominance.
5. If a certain trait is identified as X-linked recessive, describe the genotype of a female expressing the given trait.
6. Identify several genetic mutagens.
7. How can mutations be beneficial to a species?
8. What role do environmental factors play in relation to certain genetic diseases?
9. Explain the "mistake" in meiosis that results in the condition called *trisomy*.
10. Describe the genetic inheritance of cystic fibrosis, phenylketonuria (PKU), and Tay–Sachs disease.
11. Identify the chromosomal disorder that involves trisomy 21.
12. Differentiate between oncogenes and tumour suppressor genes.
13. How are gene replacement and gene augmentation therapies used to treat genetic diseases?
14. Define the term *genome*.
15. When is a disorder classified as congenital?

CRITICAL THINKING QUESTIONS

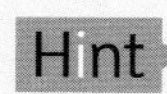

After finishing the Review Questions, write out the answers to these more in-depth questions to help you apply your new knowledge. Go back to sections of the chapter that relate to concepts that you find difficult.

1. Genes regulate protein synthesis. Why is the production of specific proteins so important to the structure and function of the body?
2. Differentiate among the text usage of chromatin, chromosomes, and genes.
3. Explain the processes that increase the variability of the genetic code in the offspring.
4. Explain why the structure of the X and Y chromosomes would predict a greater occurrence of sex-linked disorders in males.
5. Explain what is meant by a pedigree. Explain what is meant by a karyotype. Which of these would be most helpful in the diagnosis of Down syndrome? In the diagnosis of Huntington disease?

Glossary of Anatomy & Physiology

A

A band the segment of a muscle fibre's sarcomere that runs the entire length of the thick filaments; also called *anisotropic band* [A anisotropic]
abdominal (ab-DOM-ih-nal) relating to the abdomen or belly of the body [*abdomin-* belly, *-al* relating to]
abdominal aorta (ab-DOM-ih-nal ay-OR-tah) portion of the descending aorta that passes through the abdominal cavity [*abdomin-* belly, *-al* relating to, *aort-* lifted, *-a* thing] *pl.*, aortae or aortas
abdominal reflex (ab-DOM-ih-nal REE-fleks) drawing in of the abdominal wall in response to stroking the side of the abdomen [*abdomin-* belly, *-al* relating to, *re-* again, *-flex* bend]
abdominal thrusts (ab-DOM-ih-nal) lifesaving technique that can be used to open a windpipe that suddenly becomes obstructed; sometimes called *Heimlich manoeuvre* [*abdomin-* belly, *-al* relating to]
abdominopelvic cavity (ab-DOM-ih-no-PEL-vik KAV-ih-tee) term used to describe the single cavity containing the abdominal and pelvic organs [*abdomin-* belly, *-pelv-* basin, *cav-* hollow, *-ity* state]
abducens nerve (ab-DYOO-sens nerv) cranial nerve VI; motor nerve; controls movement of the eye and proprioception [*ab-* away, *-duc-* lead, *-ens* process]
abduct (ab-DUKT) to move a part away from the midline of the body; opposite motion of adduct [*ab-* away, *-duct-* lead]
abduction (ab-DUK-shun) moving away from the midline of the body; opposite motion of adduction [*ab-* away, *-duct-* lead, *-tion* process]
abnormal constituent (ab-NOR-mal kon-STICH-yoo-ent) any substance present in a body fluid that is not normally found there [*ab-* away from, *-norma* the rule]
abruptio placentae (ab-RUP-shee-oh plah-SEN-tee) separation of normally positioned placenta from the uterine wall; may result in haemorrhage and death of the fetus and/or mother [*ab-* away from, *-ruptio* rupture, *placentae* of flat cake (placenta)]
abscess (AB-ses) cavity, often pus-filled, formed by disintegration of tissues [*ab-* away, *-cess* go]
absolute refractory period (AB-so-loot ree-FRAK-toh-ree) time during which the local area of the membrane has surpassed the threshold potential and will not respond to any stimulus [*absolut-* unrestricted, *re-* back or again, *-fract-* break, *-ory* relating to, *period* circuit]
absorption (ab-SORP-shun) passage of a substance through a membrane such as skin or mucosa; often refers to passage of nutrients into blood [*ab-* from, *-sorp-* suck, *-tion* process]
accessory gland (ak-SES-oh-ree) a gland that assists organs in accomplishing their functions [*access-* extra, *-ory* relating to, *gland* acorn]
accessory hemiazygos vein (ak-SES-oh-ree hem-ee-ah-ZYE-gos vayn) connects some of the superior intercostal veins with the azygos vein [*hemi-* half, *-a-* without, *-zygo-* union or yoke, *vena* blood vessel]
accessory nerve (ak-SES-oh-ree nerv) cranial nerve XI (motor nerve) [*access-* extra, *-ory* relating to]
accessory organ (ak-SES-oh-ree) an organ that assists other organs in accomplishing their functions [*access-* extra, *-ory* relating to, *organ* instrument]
accessory spleen (ak-SES-oh-ree) a small version of the spleen commonly found in the mesentery that connects the spleen and stomach (the gastrosplenic ligament); *see* **spleen** [*access-* extra, *-ory* relating to]
accommodation (ah-kom-oh-DAY-shun) mechanism that allows the normal eye to focus on objects closer than 6 m [*accommoda-* adjust, *-ation* process]
acetoacetic acid (ass-ih-toh-ah-SEE-tik ASS-id) an acidic ketone body that accumulates during the incomplete breakdown of fats; influences acid–base balance [*acet-* vinegar, *-acid-* sour, *-ic* relating to]
acetone (ASS-ah-tohn) an acidic ketone body that accumulates during the incomplete breakdown of fats; influences acid–base balance [*acet-* vinegar, *-one* chemical]
acetylcholine (ACh) (ass-ee-til-KOH-leen) type of neurotransmitter used by motor neurons at neuromuscular junctions to stimulate muscle contraction at or in some autonomic synapses (in ganglionic synapses, at all parasympathetic effectors, and at some sympathetic effectors) [*acetyl-* vinegar, *-chole-* bile, *-ine* made of]
acetylcholinesterase (ass-ee-til-koh-lin-ES-ter-ase) enzyme that rapidly inactivates acetylcholine bound to postsynaptic receptors [*acetyl-* vinegar, *-chole-* bile, *-in-* made of, *-ester-* vinegar, *-ase* enzyme]
acid (ASS-id) substance that ionizes in water to release hydrogen ions; substance with a pH of less than 7.0 [*acid* sour]
acid-forming food (ASS-id) any food that lowers the pH after it is absorbed into the body [*acid-* sour]
acidic ketone body (ah-SID-ik KEE-tohn) contributes hydrogen ions to the extracellular fluid; influences acid–base balance [*acid-* sour, *-ic* relating to, *keto-* acetone, *-one* chemical]
acidity (ah-SID-ih-tee) the amount of acid in a solution or the state of having a low pH [*acid-* sour, *-ity* state]
acidophil (ASS-id-oh-fil) cell that stains easily with acid dyes [*acid-* sour, *-phil* love]
acidosis (ass-i-DOH-sis) condition in which there is an excessive proportion of acid in the blood and thus an abnormally low blood pH; opposite of alkalosis [*acid-* sour, *-osis* condition]
acini (ASS-i-nee) any cells of a compound gland that secretes a watery fluid; also called *acinar cells* [*acin-* grapelike] *sing.*, acinus (ASS-i-nus)
acne (AK-nee) *see* **acne vulgaris** [*acne* point]
acne vulgaris (AK-nee vul-GAR-is) inflammatory skin condition affecting sebaceous gland ducts; occurs most commonly in adolescent years; *see* **comedo** [*acne* point, *vulg-* common people, *-aris* relating to]
acoustic nerve (ah-KOOS-tik nerv) cranial nerve VIII; *see* **vestibulocochlear nerve** [*acoust-* hear, *-ic* relating to]
acoustic neuroma ah-KOOS-tik nyoo-ROH-mah) glial tumour of the Schwann cells surrounding cranial nerve VIII, causing progressive hearing loss and dizziness [*acoust-* hear, *-ic* relating to, *neuro-* nerve, *-oma* tumour]
acquired cortical colour blindness (ah-KWY-erd KOHR-tih-kahl) loss of normal colour vision caused by damage to the cortex of the cerebrum [*cortic-* cortex (bark), *-al* relating to]
acquired immunodeficiency syndrome (AIDS) (ah-KWY-erd ih-MYOON deh-FISH-en-see SIN-drohm) collection of abnormalities caused by advanced HIV infection and characterized by a depression of T-cell immunity [*-immun* free, *-de-* down, *-fic-* perform, *-ency* state, *syn-* together, *-drome* running or (race) course]
acquired immunity (ah-KWYERD im-YOO-nih-tee) immunity that is obtained after birth through exposure to a specific harmful agent; *see* **adaptive immunity** [*-immun* free, *-ity* state]
acromegaly (ak-roh-MEG-ah-lee) condition caused by hypersecretion of growth hormone after puberty, resulting in enlargement of facial features (e.g., jaw, nose), fingers, and toes [*acro-* extremities, *-mega-* great, *-aly* state]
acromial (ah-KRO-mee-al) relating to the shoulder or the acromion (process) at the high point of scapula bone [*acro-* high, *-omi-* shoulder, *-on* thing]
acrosome (AK-roh-sohm) structure on the tip of the sperm head containing enzymes that break down the covering of the ovum to facilitate conception [*acro-* top or tip, *-some* body]
acrosome reaction (AK-roh-sohm) biochemical reaction that releases digestive enzymes from the sperm head (acrosome) after it attaches to the outer layers of an ovum [*acro-* top or tip, *-some* body]
actin (AK-tin) contractile protein found in the thin myofilaments of skeletal muscle; *see* **sliding filament model** [*act-* act or do, *-in* substance]
action potential (AK-shun poh-TEN-shal) nerve impulse; membrane potential fluctuation of an actively conducting axon [*potent-* power, *-ial* relating to]
active site any location on the surface of a molecule that reacts with another molecule [*act-* move, *-ive* relating to]
active transport movement of a substance into or out of a living cell requiring the use of cellular energy [*act-* move, *-ive* relating to, *trans-* across, *-port* carry]
actual osmotic pressure (os-MOT-ik) current osmotic pressure of a solution; *see* **osmotic pressure** [*osmo-* push, *-ic* relating to]
acuity (ah-KYOO-ih-tee) sharpness of visual perception [*acu-* sharp, *-ity* state]
acute (ah-KYOOT) intense; short in duration, as in acute disease [*acut-* sharp]
acute anaemia (ah-KYOOT ah-NEE-mee-ah) condition of a precipitous drop in the red blood cell count [*acut-* sharp, *an-* without, *-(h)aem-* blood, *-ia* condition]
acute bronchitis (ah-KYOOT brong-KYE-tiss) acute form of inflammation of the bronchi of the pulmonary tract [*acut-* sharp, *bronch-* windpipe, *-itis* inflammation]
acute glomerulonephritis (ah-KYOOT gloh-mer-yoo-loh-neh-FRY-tis) most common form of kidney disease; may be caused by a delayed immune response to streptococcal infection [*acut-* sharp, *glomer-* ball, *-ul-* little, *-nephr-* kidney, *-itis* inflammation]
acute lymphocytic leukaemia (ALL) (ah-KYOOT LIM-foh-sit-ik loo-KEE-mee-ah) blood cancer that decreases the production of red blood cells, platelets, and nonmalignant lymphocyte cells [*acu-* sharp, *lymph-* water (lymphatic system), *-cyt-* cell, *-ic* relating to, *leuk-* white, *-(h)em-* blood, *-ia* condition]
acute myeloid leukaemia (AML) (ah-KYOOT MY-eh-loyd loo-KEE-mee-ah) blood cancer that is caused by pathologic transformation of myeloid stem cells [*acu-* sharp, *myel-* marrow, *-oid* like, *leuk-* white, *-(h)aem-* blood, *-ia* condition]
acute pain (ah-KYOOT) intense pain [*acut-* sharp]
adaptation (ad-ap-TAY-shun) condition of many sensory receptors in which the magnitude of a receptor potential decreases over a period of time in response to a continuous stimulus [*adapt-* fit to, *-tion* process]
adaptive immunity (ah-DAP-tiv im-YOO-nih-tee) type of immunity in which specific antigens or particles are recognized, then targeted for destruction; also called *acquired immunity* or *specific immunity* [*adapt-* fit to, *-ive* relating to, *immun-* free, *-ity* state]
Addison disease (AD-ih-son) life-threatening condition caused by the hyposecretion of adrenal cortical hormones; caused by tuberculosis, autoimmunity, or other factors [*Thomas Addison* English physician]
adduct (ad-DUKT) move a part toward the midline of the body; opposite motion of abduct [*ad-* toward, *-duct-* lead]
adduction (ad-DUK-shun) moving toward the midline of the body; opposite motion of abduction [*ad-* toward, *-duct-* lead, *-tion* process]
adenine (AD-eh-neen) one of the nitrogenous bases of the nucleotides in RNA, DNA, and related molecules [*aden-* gland]
adenocarcinoma (ad-eh-no-kar-sih-NO-mah) cancer of glandular epithelium [*adeno-* gland, *-carcin-* cancer, *-oma* tumour]
adenofibroma (ad-eh-no-fye-BROH-mah) benign neoplasm formed in epithelial and connective tissues [*adeno-* gland, *-fibra* fibre, *-oma* tumour]
adenohypophysis (ad-eh-no-hye-POF-ih-sis) anterior pituitary gland, which has the structure of an endocrine gland [*adeno-* gland, *-hypo-* under or below, *-physis* growth] *pl.*, adenohypophyses
adenoid (AD-eh-noyd) literally, glandlike; adenoids, or enlarged pharyngeal tonsils, are paired lymphoid structures in the nasopharynx [*adeno-* gland, *-oid* like]
adenoma (ad-eh-NO-mah) benign tumour of glandular epithelium [*adeno-* gland, *-oma* tumour]
adenosine deaminase deficiency (ah-DEN-oh-seen dee-AM-ih-nayse) inherited condition that produces immunodeficiency [*adenosine* blend of adenine and ribose, *de-* remove, *-amin-* ammonia, *-ase* enzyme, *-de-* down, *-fic-* perform, *-ency* state]
adenosine triphosphate (ATP) (ah-DEN-oh-seen try-FOS-fayt) chemical compound that

provides energy for use by body cells [blend of *adenine* and *ribose*, *tri-* three, *-phosph-* phosphorus, *-ate* oxygen]

adenyl cyclase (AD-eh-nil SYE-klays) enzyme that promotes ATP change into cyclic AMP [*cycl-* recurring, *-ase* enzyme]

adipocyte (AD-ih-poh-syte) fat-storing cell [*adipo-* fat, *-cyte* cell]

adipose tissue (AD-ih-pohs) fat tissue [*adipo-* fat, *-ose* full of, *tissu-* fabric]

adolescence (ad-oh-LESS-ens) period between puberty (the onset of reproductive maturity) and adulthood [*adolesc-* grow up, *-ence* state]

adrenal (ah-DREE-nal) near the kidney, as in adrenal gland [*ad-* toward, *-ren-* kidney, *-al* relating to]

adrenal cortex (ah-DREE-nal KOR-teks) outer portion of adrenal gland that secretes hormones called *corticoids* [*ad-* toward, *-ren-* kidney, *-al* relating to, *cortex* bark] *pl.*, cortices (KOR-tis-eez)

adrenal gland (ah-DREE-nal) endocrine gland that rests on the top of each kidney; made up of cortex and medulla regions [*ad-* toward, *-ren-* kidney, *-al* relating to, *gland* acorn]

adrenal medulla (ah-DREE-nal meh-DUL-ah) inner portion of adrenal gland that secretes epinephrine and norepinephrine [*ad-* toward, *-ren-* kidney, *-al* relating to, *medulla* marrow or pith (middle)] *pl.*, medullae (meh-DUL-ee) or medullas

adrenaline (ah-DREN-ah-len) *see* **epinephrine** [*ad-* to, *-ren-* kidney, *-al* relating to, *-ine* chemical]

adrenergic (ad-ren-ER-jik) describes a structure that functions with norepinephrine (NE) and epinephrine (Epi), as in a nerve fibre that releases NE or a receptor triggered by NE [*ad-* toward, *-ren-* kidney, *-erg-* work, *-ic* relating to]

adrenocorticotropic hormone (ACTH) (ah-dree-no-kor-teh-koh-TROH-pik HOR-mohn) hormone that stimulates the adrenal cortex to secrete larger amounts of hormones [*adreno-* gland, *-cortic-* cortex (bark), *-trop-* turn or change, *-ic* relating to, *hormon-* excite]

adult respiratory distress syndrome (ARDS) (RES-per-ah-tohr-ee dis-TRESS SIN-drohm) syndrome resulting from impairment or removal of surfactant in the alveoli [*re-* again, *-spir-* breathe, *-tory* relating to, *syn-* together, *-drome* running or (race) course]

adult stem cell undifferentiated cell found in adults that is capable of producing specialized daughter cells

adulthood (ah-DULT-hood) developmental period after adolescence

adventitia (ad-ven-TISH-ah) shortened form of *tunica adventitia* [*adventitia* coming from abroad]

aerobic (air-OH-bik) relating to the use of oxygen, as in aerobic respiration [*aer-* air, *-bi-* life, *-ic* relating to]

aerobic respiration (air-OH-bik res-pih-RAY-shun) catabolic process; the stage of cellular respiration requiring oxygen [*aero-* air, *-bi-* (from *-bio-*) life, *-ic* relating to, *re-* again, *-spir-* breathe, *-tion* process]

aerobic training (air-OH-bik) continuous vigorous exercise requiring the body to increase its consumption of oxygen and develop the muscles' ability to sustain activity over a long time; also known as *endurance training* [*aer-* air, *-bi-* life, *-ic* relating to]

aetiology (e-tee-OL-oh-jee) theory, or study, of the factors involved in causing a disease [*aetio-* cause, *-o-* combining form, *-log-* words (study of), *-y* activity]

afferent (AF-fer-ent) travelling, conducting, or carrying toward [*a[d]-* toward, *-fer-* carry, *-ent* relating to]

afferent (sensory) neuron (AF-fer-ent NYOO-ron) neuron that carries impulses toward the central nervous system from the periphery; sensory neuron [*a[d]-* toward, *-fer-* carry, *-ent* relating to, *neuron-* nerve]

afferent division (AF-fer-ent) sensory division (incoming pathways) of the nervous system [*a[d]-* toward, *-fer-* carry, *-ent* relating to]

afferent impulse (AF-fer-ent IM-pulse) impulse travelling toward the central nervous system [*a[d]-* toward, *-fer-* carry, *-ent* relating to]

afferent nervous system (AF-fer-ent) subdivision of the peripheral nervous system; consists of all incoming sensory nerves [*a[d]-* toward, *-fer-* carry, *-ent* relating to]

afterload (AF-ter-lohd) the pumping work of the heart to move blood against arterial pressure; the load on the heart produced by the blood after it leaves the heart; compare to **preload**

agglutinogen (ah-gloo-TIN-oh-jen) substance that stimulates agglutination (clumping), particularly of red blood cells; antigens present on red blood cell membranes [*agglutin-* glue, *-gen* produce]

aggregated lymphoid nodules (ag-rah-GAYT-ed LIM-foyd NOD-yools) isolated nodules of lymphatic tissue in the intestinal wall; also called *Peyer's patches* [*a[d]-* to, *-grega-* collect, *lymph-* water (lymphatic system), *-oid* like, *nod-* knot, *-ule* small]

agonist (AG-ah-nist) agent that works like or with (rather than against) another agent [*agon-* struggle, *-ist* agent]

agranulocyte (ah-GRAN-yoo-loh-syte) white blood cells without cytoplasmic granules [*a-* without, *-granul-* little grains or granules, *-cyte* cell]

air-contrast barium enema study (BAHR-eeum EN-e-mah) diagnostic study that outlines the bowel with barium and then adds air to enhance the presence of lesions [*bari-* heavy, *-um* substance, *enema* injection]

alarm reaction (uh-LARM ree-AK-shun) the initial response to stress [*al-* toward, *-arm* weapon, *re-* again, *-action*]

albinism (AL-bi-niz-em) recessive, inherited condition characterized by a lack of the dark brown pigment melanin in the skin, eyes, and hair, resulting in vision problems and susceptibility to sunburn and skin cancer; ocular albinism is a lack of pigment in the layers of the eyeball [*alb-* white, *-in-*characterized by, *-ism* state]

albumin (AL-byoo-min) plasma protein that aids in the regulation of the osmotic concentration of the blood [*alb-* white]

aldosterone (AL-doh-steh-rohn *or* al-DOS-tair-ohn) hormone that stimulates the kidney to retain sodium, ions, and water; only physiologically important mineralocorticoid [*aldo-* aldehyde, *-stero-* solid or steroid derivative, *-one* chemical]

aldosterone mechanism (al-DOS-ter-ohn MEK-ah-niz-em) homeostatic mechanism that restores normal extracellular fluid volume when it decreases below normal [*aldo-* aldehyde, *-stero-* solid or steroid derivative, *-one* chemical, *mechan-* machine, *-ism* state]

aldosteronism (al-doh-STAIR-on-iz-em) hypersecretion of aldosterone [*aldo-* aldehyde, *-stero-* solid or steroid derivative, *-on-* chemical, *-ism* state]

alimentary canal (al-uh-MEN-tar-ee kah-NAL) the digestive tract as a whole [*aliment-* nourishment, *-ary* relating to]

alkaline (AL-kah-lin) refers to a substance that in solution has a pH of greater than 7.0 [*alkal-* ashes, *-ine* relating to]

alkalinity (al-kah-LIN-ih-tee) state of having a high pH; amount of base or alkaline in a solution [*alkal-* ashes, *-in-* relating to, *-ity* state]

alkalosis (al-kah-LOH-sis) condition in which there is an excessive proportion of alkali (base) in the blood; opposite of acidosis [*alkal-* ashes, *-osis* condition]

allergen (AL-er-jen) any substance that produces an allergic reaction [*all-* other, *-erg-* work, *-gen* produce]

allergy (AL-er-jee) a type of hyperimmunity [*all-* other, *-erg-* work, *-y* state]

allostasis (al-lo-STAY-sis) the physiological processes used by the body to restore homeostasis during stress [*allo-* different, *-stasis* standing still]

allosteric effector (al-oh-STEER-ik ee-FEKT-or) an agent that alters the function of an enzyme by changing the shape of the enzyme's active site [*allo-* another or different, *-ster-* solid, *-ic* relating to, *effect-* accomplish, *-or* agent]

alopecia (al-o-PEE-sha) loss of hair; baldness [*alopec-* fox, *-ia* condition]

alpha (α) receptor (AL-fah ree-SEP-tor) adrenergic receptor for norepinephrine [*alpha (α)* first letter of Greek alphabet, *recept-* receive, *-or* agent]

alpha cell (AL-fah) pancreatic islet cell that secretes glucagon; also called *A cell* [*alpha (α)* first letter of Greek alphabet, *cell* storeroom]

alpha motor neuron (al-fah MOH-tor NYOO-ron) generator of efferent impulses that stimulate regular muscle fibres to contract [*alpha (α)* first letter of Greek alphabet, *mot-* move, *-or* agent, *neuron* string or nerve]

alpha particle (AL-fah PAR-tih-kul) radioactive particle consisting of two protons plus two neutrons [*alpha (α)* first letter of Greek alphabet]

alpha-fetoprotein (AFP) (AL-fah-fee-toh-PRO-teen) normal fetal protein; presence in adult suggests liver or germ cell cancer [*alpha (α)* first letter of Greek alphabet, *feto-* offspring (fetus)]

alveolar (al-VEE-oh-lar) relating to a small cavity, such as an alveolus of lung [*alveo-* hollow, *-ola-* little, *-ar* relating to]

alveolar cell (al-VEE-oh-lar) milk-producing cell that releases secretions into ducts of the breast [*alveo- hollow*, *-ola-* little, *-ar* relating to]

alveolar duct (al-VEE-oh-lar) airway that branches from the smallest bronchioles; alveolar sacs arise from alveolar ducts [*alve-* hollow, *-ol-* little, *-ar* relating to]

alveolar ventilation (al-VEE-oh-lar ven-tih-LAY-shun) volume of inspired air that actually reaches the alveoli [*alve-* hollow, *-ol-* little, *-ar* relating to, *vent-* fan or create wind, *-tion* process]

alveolus (al-VEE-oh-lus) literally, a small cavity; alveoli of lungs are microscopic saclike dilations of terminal bronchioles; gas exchange in the lungs occurs across the membranes of the alveoli [*alve-* hollow, *-olus* little] *pl.*, alveoli (al-VEE-oh-lye)

Alzheimer disease (AD) (AHLTZ-hye-mer) syndrome characterized by dementia, usually beginning in mid to late adulthood and caused by a combination of factors, including genetic and environmental [*Alois Alzheimer* German neurologist, *dis-* opposite of, *-ease* comfort]

amenorrhoea (ah-men-oh-REE-ah) absence of normal menstruation [*a-* without, *-men-* month, *-rrhoea* flow]

amine (AM-een) organic compound containing nitrogen; neurotransmitter synthesized from amino acid molecules [*amine* ammonia compound]

amino acid (ah-MEE-no ASS-id) type of chemical unit from which proteins are built; also have other functions made up of a carbon atom to which are bonded an amino group and carboxyl group [*amino* NH_2, *acid* sour]

amino acid derivative hormone (ah-MEE-no ASS-id deh-RIV-ah-tiv HOR-mohn) category of nonsteroid hormones; each hormone is derived from a single amino acid molecule [*amino* NH_2, *acid* sour, *hormon-* excite]

amniocentesis (am-nee-oh-sen-TEE-sis) procedure in which a sample of amniotic fluid is removed with a syringe for use in genetic testing, often to produce a karyotype of the fetus [*amnio-* birth membrane, *-centesis* a pricking]

amniotic cavity (am-nee-OT-ik KAV-ih-tee) cavity within the blastocyst that eventually becomes a fluid-filled sac in which the embryo will float during development [*amnio-* fetal membrane, *-ic* relating to, *cav-* hollow, *-ity* state]

amphiarthrosis (am-fee-ar-THROH-sis) slightly movable joint such as the one that connects the two pubic bones [*amphi-* both sides, *-arthr-* joint, *-osis* condition] *pl.*, amphiarthroses (am-fee-ar-THROH-seez)

ampulla (am-PUL-ah) saclike dilation of a tube or duct; found at end of each semicircular duct, contains crista ampullaris [*ampu-* flask, *-ulla* little] *pl.*, ampullae (am-PUL-ee)

amygdaloid nucleus (ah-MIG-dah-loyd NYOO-klee-us) basal nucleus (region of grey matter of the deep cerebrum) at the tip of the caudate nucleus [*amygdal-* almond, *-oid* like] *pl.*, nuclei (NYOO-klee-eye)

amylase (AM-eh-lays) enzyme that digests carbohydrates [*amyl-* starch, *-ase* enzyme]

anabolic hormone (an-ah-BOL-ik HOR-mohn) hormone that stimulates anabolism in the target organ [*anabol-* build up, *-ic* relating to, *hormon-* excite]

anabolic steroid (an-ah-BOL-ik STEHR-oyd) any steroid (lipid) hormone that promotes anabolism, such as testosterone [*anabol-* build up, *-ic* relating to, *stero-* solid, *-oid* like]

anabolism (ah-NAB-oh-liz-im) cells making complex molecules (e.g., hormones) from simpler compounds (e.g., amino acids); opposite of catabolism [*anabol-* build up, *-ism* action]

anaemia (ah-NEE-me-ah) deficient number of red blood cells, or deficient haemoglobin [*an-* without, *-(h)aem-* blood, *-ia* condition]

anaemia of chronic disease (ah-NEE-mee-ah KRON-ik) condition of abnormally low haemoglobin secondary to a long-lasting illness [*an-* without, *-(h)aem-* blood, *-ia* condition, *chron-* time, *-ic* relating to]

anaerobic (an-air-OH-bik) relating to a process that requires no oxygen [*an-* without, *-aer-* air, *-bi-* life, *-ic* relating to]

anaerobic pathway (an-air-OH-bik) catabolic process; stage of cellular respiration not requiring oxygen; although it is actually a type of fermentation, it is often called "anaerobic respiration" [*an-* without, *-aero-* air, *-bi-* (from *-bio-*) life, *-ic* relating to]

anaesthesia (an-es-THEE-zhah) state in which a person lacks the feeling of pain [*an-* absence, *-aesthesia* feeling]

anaesthetic (an-es-THET-ik) substance that reduces or eliminates the sensation of pain [*an-* absence, *-aesthesia* feeling, *-ic* relating to]

anal canal (AY-nal kah-NAL) passage from the colon to the outside of the body [*an-* ring (anus), *-al* relating to]

anal fissure (AY-nal FISH-ur) minor lacerations in the lining of the anus or anal canal [*an-* ring (anus), *-al* relating to, *fissur-* cleft]

anal fistula (AY-nal FISS-tyoo-lah) passageway that often develops between the rectal wall and skin surrounding the anus [*an-* ring (anus), *-al* relating to, *fistula* pipe] *pl.*, fistulae *or* fistulas

anal triangle (AY-nal TRY-ang-gul) area surrounding anus [*an-* ring (anus), *-al* relating to]

anaphase (AN-ah-fayz) latter stage of mitosis; duplicate chromosomes move to poles of dividing cell [*ana-* apart, *-phase* stage]

anaphylactic shock (an-ah-fih-LAK-tik) type of severe allergic reaction characterized by severe circulatory failure [*ana-* without, *-phylact-* protection, *-ic* relating to]

anaplasia (an-ah-PLAY-zee-ah) growth of abnormal (undifferentiated) cells, as in a tumour or neoplasm [*ana-* without, *-plas(m)-* substance or form, *-ia* condition]

anastomosis (ah-nas-tuh-MOH-sis) connection between vessels that allows collateral circulation [*ana-* again or anew, *-stomo-* mouth, *-osis* condition] *pl.*, anastomoses (ah-nas-toh-MOH-seez)

anatomical dead space (an-ah-TOM-ih-kal) air passageways that contain air that does not reach the alveoli [*ana-* apart, *-tom-* cut, *-ical* relating to]

anatomical position (an-ah-TOM-ih-kal po-ZISH-un) the standard reference position for the body; standing with arms hanging at sides with palms forward, gives meaning to directional terms [*ana-* apart, *-tom-* cut, *-ical-* relating to, *posit-* place, *-tion* state]

anatomy (ah-NAT-oh-mee) study of the structure of an organism and the relationships of its parts [*ana-* apart, *-tom-* cut, *-y* action]

androgen (AN-droh-jen) hormone that promotes development and maintenance of male characteristics [*andro-* male, *-gen* produce]

androgen-binding protein (ABP) (AN-droh-jen-BYND-ing PRO-teen) specialized protein that binds to testosterone and increases concentration within the seminiferous tubules [*andro-* male, *-gen* produce, *prote-* first rank, *-in* substance]

aneurysm (AN-yoo-riz-em) abnormal widening of the arterial wall; aneurysms promote formation of thrombi and also tend to burst [*aneurysm* widening]

angina pectoris (an-JYE-nah PEK-tor-iss) severe chest pain resulting when the myocardium is deprived of sufficient oxygen [*angina* strangling, *pector-* breast, *-is* relating to]

angiogenesis (an-jee-oh-JEN-eh-sis) physiological process in which new blood vessels are formed [*angi-* vessel *-gen-* produce, *-esis* process]

angiography (an-jee-OG-raf-ee) radiography in which radiopaque contrast medium is injected into a vessel to make it more visible in a medical image (angiogram); in arteries the image is called *arteriogram*; in veins, a *venogram* or *phlebogram*; in lymphatic vessels, a *lymphangiogram* [*angi-* vessel, *-graph-* draw, *-y* process]

angioplasty (AN-jee-oh-plass-tee) medical procedure in which vessels occluded by arteriosclerosis are opened (i.e., the channel for blood flow is widened) [*angio-* vessel, *-plasty* surgical repair]

angiotensin I (an-jee-oh-TEN-sin) substance formed by conversion of angiotensinogen by renin; causes vasoconstriction and an increase in blood pressure [*angio-* vessel, *-tens-* pressure or stretch, *-in* substance, *I* Roman numeral one]

angiotensin II (an-jee-oh-TEN-sin) substance formed in the lungs by enzyme conversion of angiotensin I; ultimately stimulates secretion of aldosterone; causes vasoconstriction [*angio-* vessel, *-tens-* pressure or stretch, *-in* substance, *II* Roman numeral two]

angiotensinogen (an-jee-oh-TEN-sin-oh-jen) normal constituent of blood; a precursor to angiotensin [*angio-* vessel, *-tens-* pressure or stretch, *-in-* substance, *-gen* produce]

angular movement (ANG-gyoo-lar MOOV-ment) body movement that increases or decreases the angle of a joint

anion (AN-eye-on) negatively charged molecule (negative ion) [*ana-* up, *-ion* to go (ion)]

ankle jerk reflex (ANG-kel jerk REE-fleks) extension of the foot in response to tapping of the Achilles tendon [*re-* again, *-flex* bend]

annulus fibrosis (AN-yoo-lus fye-BROH-sis) tough outer edge of intervertebral disc; surrounds nucleus pulposus [*annulus* ring, *fibrosis* fibrous]

anorexia (an-oh-REK-see-ah) loss of appetite (a symptom, rather than a distinct disorder) [*an-* without, *-orex-* appetite, *-ia* condition]

anorexia nervosa (an-oh-REK-see-ah ner-VOH-sah) behavioural eating disorder characterized by chronic refusal to eat, often related to an abnormal fear of becoming obese [*an-* without, *-orex-* appetite, *-ia* condition, *nerv-* nerve, *-os-* relating to, *-a* thing]

anorexigenic (an-oh-rek-sih-JEN-ik) relating to an agent that reduces appetite [*an-* without, *-orex-* appetite, *-gen-* produce, *-ic* relating to]

anosmia (an-OZ-mee-ah) inability to smell [*an-* without, *-osm-* smell, *-ia* condition]

antagonism (an-TAG-oh-niz-em) situation in which one agent (such as a hormone or muscle) produces the opposite effect of another agent [*ant-* against, *-agon-* struggle, *-ism* condition]

antagonist (an-TAG-oh-nist) agent that has an opposing effect or works against another agent [*ant-* against, *-agon-* struggle, *-ist* agent]

antagonist muscle (an-TAG-oh-nist) muscle that directly opposes prime movers; for example, muscles that flex the arm are antagonists to muscles that extend it [*ant-* against, *-agon-* struggle, *-ist* agent, *mus-* mouse, *-cle* small]

antebrachial (an-tee-BRAY-kee-al) relating to the forearm [*ante-* before, *-brachi-* arm, *-al* relating to]

antecubital (an-tee-KYOO-bih-tal) relating to the depressed area just in front of elbow (cubital fossa) [*ante-* before, *-cubit-* elbow, *-al* relating to]

antenatal medicine (an-tee-NAY-tal) therapy used on an embryo or fetus [*ante-* before, *-nat-* birth, *-al* relating to]

anterior (an-TEER-ee-or) front, or ventral; opposite of posterior, or dorsal [*ante-* front, *-er-* more, *-or* quality]

anterior cavity (of eye) (an-TEER-ee-or) entire space located in front of the lens of the eye; divided into anterior and posterior chambers [*ante-* front, *-er-* more, *-or* quality, *cav-* hollow, *-ity* state]

anterior corticospinal tract (an-TEER-ee-or KOR-tih-koh-spy-nal trakt) coordinates individual or small groups of muscles (hands, fingers, feet, toes) of the same side [*ante-* front, *-er-* more, *-or* quality, *cortic-* cortex (bark), *-spin-* backbone, *-al* relating to, *tract* trail]

anterior cul-de-sac (an-TEER-ee-or kul-deh-sak) space created by the protrusion of the cervix into the lumen of the vagina; formed by the anterior ligament [*ante-* front, *-er-* more, *-or* quality, *cul-de-sac* bottom of the bag] *pl.*, culs-de-sac or cul-de-sacs

anterior fornix (an-TEER-ee-or FOR-niks) space created by the protrusion of the cervix into the lumen of the vagina; increases probability of reproductive success by retaining seminal fluid [*ante-* front, *-er-* more, *-or* quality, *fornix* arch] *pl.*, fornices (FOR-nis-eez)

anterior ligament (an-TEER-ee-or LIG-ah-ment) fold of peritoneum formed by the extension of the peritoneum on the anterior surface of the uterus to the posterior surface of the bladder [*ante-* front, *-er-* more, *-or* quality, *liga-* bind, *-ment* condition]

anterior spinothalamic tract (an-TEER-ee-or SPY-no-tha-lam-ik trakt) responds to crude touch and pressure [*ante-* front, *-er-* more, *-or* quality, *spino-* backbone, *-thalam-* inner chamber, *-ic* relating to]

anterior tibial vein (an-TEER-ee-or TIB-ee-al vayn) vein along the front of the leg (shin) [*ante-* front, *-er-* more, *-or* quality, *tibia* shin bone, *-al* relating to, *vena* blood vessel]

anthrax (AN-thraks) bacterial infection caused by *Bacillus anthracis*, ordinarily affecting herbivores (sheep, cattle, goats, antelope) and often killing them; occurs rarely in humans through accidental or intentional exposure to bacterial spores through inhalation or skin contact; inhalation anthrax is life-threatening but can be treated successfully with drugs; cutaneous anthrax is less serious, characterized by a reddish-brown patch on the skin that ulcerates and then forms a dark, nearly black scab, followed by muscle pain, internal haemorrhage (bleeding), headache, fever, nausea, and vomiting [*anthrax* boil]

antianaemic principle (an-tee-ah-NEE-mik) factor that maintains a normal number of red blood cells; vitamin B_{12} [*anti-* against, *-an-* without, *-(h)aem-* blood, *-ia* condition, *-ic* relating to]

antiangiogenesis agent (AN-tee-AN-jee-oh-jen-eh-sis) class of chemotherapy drugs used in cancer treatment that inhibits development of new blood vessels in a tumour; *see* **rational drugs** [*anti-* against, *angi-* vessel, *-gen-* produce, *-esis* process]

antibody (AN-tih-bod-ee) plasma protein produced by B lymphocytes that destroys or inactivates a specific substance (antigen) that has entered the body [*anti-* against]

antibody titre (AN-tih-bod-ee TYE-ter) measurement of the amount of antibody in the plasma [*anti-* against, *titre* proportion (in a solution)]

antibody-mediated immunity (AN-tih-bod-ee-MEE-dee-ayt-ed ih-MYOO-nih-tee) immunity that is produced when antibodies render antigens unable to harm the body; also called *humoral immunity* [*anti-* against, *medi-* middle, *-ate* process, *immun-* free, *-ity* state]

anticoagulant (an-tee-koh-AG-yoo-lant) agent that opposes blood clotting [*anti-* against, *-coagul-* curdle, *-ant* agent]

anticoagulant drug treatment (an-tee-koh-AG-yoo-lant) therapy involving the use of anticlotting agents in the blood [*anti-* against, *-coagul-* curdle, *-ant* agent]

antidepressant (an-tee-deh-PRESS-ant) drug that inhibits feelings of depression or sadness [*anti-* against, *-de-* down, *-press-* press, *-ant* agent]

antidiuresis (an-tee-dye-yoo-REE-sis) opposing the production of a large urine volume [*anti-* against, *-dia-* through, *-uret-* urination, *-esis* condition]

antidiuretic hormone (ADH) (an-tee-dye-yoo-RET-ik HOR-mohn) hormone produced in the posterior pituitary gland to regulate the balance of water in the body by accelerating reabsorption of water in the kidney tubules; also called *arginine vasopressin (AVP)* [*anti-* against, *-dia-* through, *-uret-* urination, *-ic* relating to, *hormon-* excite]

antigen (AN-tih-jen) substance, usually a protein fragment, that causes an immune response [*anti-* against, *-gen* produce]

antigen–antibody complex (AN-ti-jen-AN-tih-bod-ee KOM-pleks) combination of an antigen with its complementary antibody [*anti-* against, *-gen* produce, *anti-* against, body, *com-* together, *-plex* weave or braid]

antigenic determinant (AN-tih-jen-ik deh-TUR-mih-nant) region of an antibody molecule that binds to an antigen particle [*anti-* against, *-gen* produce, *-ic* relating to, *determin-* limit, *-ant* agent of]

antigen-presenting cell (APC) (AN-tih-jen) any of a variety of immune cells that present protein fragments (antigens) on their surface and thus allow recognition and reaction by other immune system cells; include macrophages and dendritic cells (DCs) and B cells [*anti-* against, *-gen* produce, *presenting*, *cell* storeroom]

antihistamine (an-tih-HISS-tah-meen) agent that inhibits histamine, an inflammation agent [*anti-* against, *-histo-* tissue, *-amine* ammonia compound]

antioxidant (an-tee-OK-sih-dent) agent that inhibits chemical oxidation [*anti-* against, *-oxi-* sharp (oxygen), *-ant* agent]

antiplatelet drug treatment (an-tee-PLAYT-let) therapy that inhibits platelets [*anti-* against, *-plate-* flat, *-let* small]

anuria (ah-NYOO-ree-ah) lack or failure to produce urine [*a-* not, *-ur-* urine, *-ia* condition]

aorta (ay-OR-tah) largest systemic artery; extends directly from the left ventricle [*aort-* lifted, *-a* thing] *pl.*, aortae (ay-OR-tee) *or* aortas

aortic arch (ay-OR-tik) 180-degree curve of the aorta, shortly after it leaves the left ventricle [*aort-* lifted, *-ic* relating to]

aortic baroreceptor (ay-OR-tik bar-oh-ree-SEP-tor) stretch receptor located in the aorta that is sensitive to changes in blood pressure [*aort-* lifted, *-ic* relating to, *baro-* pressure, *-recept-* receive, *-or* agent]

aortic body (ay-OR-tik) small cluster of chemosensitive cells that respond to changes in blood levels of carbon dioxide and oxygen [*aort-* lifted, *-ic* relating to]

aortic reflex (ay-OR-tik REE-fleks) increase or decrease in heart rate as a result of sensory nerve fibres in the wall of aorta, responding to blood pressure [*aort-* lifted, *-ic* relating to, *re-* back or again, *-flex* bend]

aortic regurgitation (ay-OR-tik ree-gur-jih-TAY-shun) reflux of blood from the aorta to the ventricle [*aort-* lifted, *-ic* relating to, *re-* again, *-gurgit-* flow, *-ation* process]

aortic (semilunar) valve (ay-OR-tik [sem-ih-LOO-nar]) valve between the aorta and left ventricle that prevents blood from flowing back into the ventricle [*aort-* lifted, *-ic* relating to]

apatite (AP-ah-tyte) crystals of calcium and phosphate that contribute to the hardness of bone [*apat-* deceit, *-ite* mineral]

Apgar score (AP-gar) system of assessing general health of newborn infant, in which heart rate, respiration, muscle tone, skin colour and response to stimuli are scored (a perfect total score is 10) [*Virginia Apgar* American physician]

apex (AY-peks) the point or tip of a structure; *see also* **apical** [*apex* tip] *pl.*, apices

aphasia (ah-FAY-zee-ah) language deficit caused by damage in speech centres of the brain [*a-* without, *-phasia* speech]

apical (AY-pik-al) relating to the apex (tip) of an organ, cell, or other structure; in a cell, often refers to the surface facing the lumen of the organ [*apic-* tip, *-al* relating to]

aplastic anaemia (a-PLAS-tik ah-NEE-meeah) abnormally low number of red blood cells caused by destruction of bone marrow by drugs, toxic chemicals, or radiation [*a-* without, *-plast-* form, *-ic* relating to, *an-* without, *-(h)aem-* blood, *-ia* condition]

apneusis (ap-NYOO-sis) cessation of breathing in the inspiratory position [*a-* not, *-pneu-* breathe, *-sis* condition]

apneustic centre (ap-NYOO-stik) regulatory area located in the pons; stimulates the inspiratory centre to increase the length and depth of inspiration [*a-* not, *-pneus-* breathing, *-ic* relating to]

apnoea (AP-nee-ah) temporary cessation of breathing [*a-* not, *-pnoe-* breathe, *-a* condition]

apocrine gland (AP-oh-krin) gland that collects its secretions near the apex of the cell and then releases them by pinching off the distended end; for example, mammary gland [*apo-* from, *-crin-* secrete, *gland* acorn]

apocrine sweat gland (AP-oh-krin) sweat glands located in the axillae and genital regions; these glands enlarge and begin to function at puberty [*apo-* from, *-crin-* secrete, *gland* acorn]

aponeurosis (ap-oh-nyoo-ROH-sis) broad, flat sheet of connective tissue [*apo-* from, *-neur-* sinew, *-osis* condition] *pl.*, aponeuroses (ap-oh-nyoo-ROH-seez)

apoptosis (ap-o-TOH-sis *or* app-op-TOH-sis) nonpathological, programmed cell death in which specific biochemical steps within the cell lead to the fragmentation of the cell and removal of the pieces by phagocytic cells; occurs when cells are no longer needed and is the normal process by which our tissues remodel themselves [*apo-* away, *-pto-* fall, *-osis* condition or process]

appendicitis (ah-pen-dih-SYE-tis) inflammation of the vermiform appendix [*appendic-* hang upon, *-itis* inflammation]

appendicolith (ah-pen-DIK-oh-lith) hardened nodule that may form within the appendix [*appendic-* hang upon, *-lith* stone]

appendicular skeleton (ah-pen-DIK-yoo-lar SKEL-eh-ton) bones of the upper and lower extremities of the body [*append-* hang upon, *-ic-* relating to , *-ul-* little, *-ar* relating to]

appetite centre (AP-ih-tyte) cluster of neurons in the lateral hypothalamus whose impulses cause an increase in appetite [*a(d)-* toward, *-pet-* seek out, *-ite* relating to]

appositional growth (ap-oh-ZISH-un-al) process by which a flat bone or cartilage grows in size by addition of bony cartilage at its surface; also called *exogenous growth* [*ap-* toward, *-posit-* put or place, *-ion-* process, *-al* relating to]

aqueous humour (AY-kwee-us HYOO-mor) watery fluid that fills the anterior chamber of the eye, in front of the lens [*aqu-* water, *-ous* relating to]

arachnoid (ah-RAK-noyd) weblike; particularly the middle layer of the meninges [*arachn-* spider (web), *-oid* like]

arbor vitae (AR-bor VI-tay) internal white matter of the cerebellum [*arbor* tree, *vitae* of life] *pl.*, arbores vitae

areola (ah-REE-oh-lah) region of skin of the breast that surrounds the nipple [*are-* area or space, *-ola* little] *pl.*, areolae (ah-REE-oh-lee), areoles (ah-REE-oh-leez), *or* areolas

areolar tissue (ah-REE-oh-lar) a type of connective tissue consisting of fibres and a variety of cells embedded in a loose matrix of soft, sticky gel [*are-* open space, *-ola-* little, *-ar* relating to, *tissue-* fabric]

arginine vasopressin (AVP) (AHR-jih-neen vas-oh-PRES-in) see **antidiuretic hormone** [*arginine* type of amino acid, *vaso-* vessel, *-press-* pressure, *-in* substance]

arrector pili muscle (ah-REK-tor PYE-lye) smooth muscles of the skin, attached to hair follicles; when contraction occurs, the hair stands up, resulting in "goose bumps" [*arrector* raiser, *pili* of hair, *mus-* mouse, *-cle* small]

arrhythmia (ah-RITH-mee-ah) term referring to any abnormality of cardiac rhythm; also called **dysrhythmia** [*a-* without, *-rhythm-* movement in time, *-ia* condition]

arterial anastomosis (ar-TEER-ee-al ah-nas-tuh-MOH-sis) junction between two or more arteries [*arteria-* vessel, *-al* relating to, *ana-* again or anew, *-stomo-* mouth, *-osis* condition] *pl.*, anastomoses (ah-nas-toh-MOH-seez)

arterial blood Po_2 (ar-TEER-ee-al blud PEE-oh-too) partial pressure of oxygen in the blood of arteries [*arteri-* airpipe (artery), *-al* relating to, *P* pressure, O_2 oxygen]

arterial blood gas (ABG) (ar-TEER-ee-al blud gas) any of the blood characteristics related to respiratory gases normally measured in a lab analysis of arterial blood (Po_2, Pco_2, $\%SO_2$, pH, [HCO_3^-]) [*arteri-* airpipe (artery), *-al* relating to]

arterial blood pressure (ar-TEER-ee-al blud PRESH-er) hydrostatic pressure of the blood in the arteries [*arteri-* airpipe (artery), *-al* relating to]

arteriogram (ar-TEER-ee-oh-gram) *see* angiography [*arteri-* artery, *-gram* drawing]

arteriole (ar-TEER-ee-ohl) small branch of an artery [*arteri-* vessel, *-ole* little]

arteriosclerosis (ar-tee-ree-oh-skleh-ROH-sis) hardening of arteries; materials such as lipids (as in atherosclerosis) accumulate in arterial walls, often becoming hardened via calcification [*arteri-* vessel (artery), *-sclero-* harden, *-osis* condition]

arteriovenous anastomosis (ar-teer-ee-oh-VEE-nus ah-nas-teh-MOH-sis) connection between an artery and a vein [*arteri-* vessel, *-ven-* vein, *-ous* relating to, *ana-* again or anew, *-stomo-* mouth, *-osis* condition] *pl.*, anastomoses

artery (AR-ter-ee) vessel carrying blood away from the heart [*arteri-* vessel]

arthritis (ar-THRY-tis) inflammation of joint structures [*arthr-* joint, *-itis* inflammation]

arthroplasty (AR-throh-plas-tee) the total or partial replacement of a diseased joint with an artificial device (prosthesis) [*arthr-* joint, *-plasty* surgical repair]

articular cartilage (ar-TIK-yoo-lar KAR-tih-lij) layer of hyaline cartilage covering the joint surfaces of epiphyses [*artic-* joint, *-ul-* little, *-ar* relating to, *cartilag-* cartilage]

articulation (ar-tik-yoo-LAY-shun) joint [*artic-* joint, *-ul-* little, *-ation* state]

artificial immunity (ar-tih-FISH-al ih-MYOO-nih-tee) immunization; deliberate exposure to potentially harmful antigens; as opposed to natural immunity [*artific-* not natural, *-al* relating to; *immun-* free, *-ity* state of]

artificial pacemaker (ar-tih-FISH-al PAYS-may-ker) an electrical device that is implanted into the heart to treat problems with heart conduction [*artific-* not natural, *-al* relating to]

arytenoid cartilage (ah-RIT-en-oyd or ar-ih-TEE-noyd KAR-tih-lij) either of a pair of cartilages found in the supporting framework of the larynx [*aryten-* ladle, *-oid* like]

ascending aorta (ah-SEND-ing ay-OR-tah) portion of the aorta extending from the aortic valve to the aortic arch [*a[d]-* toward, *-scend-* climb, *aort-* lifted, *-a* thing] *pl.*, aortae *or* aortas

ascending colon (ah-SEND-ing KOH-lon) portion of the colon extending from the caecum to the hepatic flexure [*a[d]-* toward, *-scend-* climb, *colon* large intestine]

ascending tract (ah-SEND-ing trakt) spinal cord tract that conducts impulses up the cord to the brain [*a[d]-* toward, *-scend-* climb, *tract* trail]

ascites (ah-SYE-tees) effusion (inflow of watery fluid) in the abdominal cavity; abdominal bloating [*asc-* belly, *-ites* swelling]

aspiration biopsy cytology (ass-pih-RAY-shun BYE-op-see sye-TOL-oh-jee) procedure that draws myeloid tissue into a syringe; allows for examination of tissue to confirm or reject diagnosis [*a-* act of, *-spir-* breathe, *-ation* process, *bio-* life, *-ops-* view, *-y* act of, *cyt-* cell, *-o-* combining form, *-log-* words (study of), *-y* activity]

assimilation (ah-sim-ih-LAY-shun) the process of incorporation of a substance into the body [*assimila-* make alike, *-tion* process]

association tract (ah-so-see-AY-shun) most common cerebral tract; extends from one convolution to another in the same hemisphere [*a(d)-* to or toward, *-socia-* unite, *-ation* process, *tract* trail]

aster (AS-ter) a starlike formation of microtubules (astral fibres) radiating outward from the centrosome (containing centrioles) during cell division; astral fibres anchor the centrosome and the spindle as chromosomes are pulled apart [*aster* star]

asthma (AZ-mah) chronic obstructive pulmonary disorder characterized by recurring spasms of muscles in bronchial walls accompanied by oedema and mucus production, making breathing difficult [*asthma* panting]

astigmatism (ah-STIG-mah-tiz-em) irregular curvature of the cornea or lens that impairs formation of a well-focused image in the eye [*a-* not, *-stigma-* point, *-ism* condition]

astrocyte (ASS-troh-syte) star-shaped neuroglial cell [*astro-* star-shaped, *-cyte* cell]

astrocytoma (ass-troh-sye-TOH-mah) slow-growing neoplasm of astrocyte cells in the central nervous system [*astro-* star, *-cyt-* cell, *-oma* tumour]

atherectomy (ath-er-EK-to-mee) type of percutaneous coronary intervention (PCI) that uses a catheter to introduce lasers, drills, or spinning loops of wire to remove atherosclerotic plaque from an artery and thus clear the way for normal blood flow [*ather-* porridge or gruel, *-ec-* out, *-tom-* cut, *-y* action]

atherosclerosis (ath-er-oh-skleh-ROH-sis) type of "hardening of the arteries" in which lipids and other substances build up on the inside wall of blood vessels [*ather-* porridge or gruel, *-sclero-* harden, *-osis* condition]

atom (AT-om) smallest particle of a chemical element that retains the properties of that element; particles that combine to form molecules (chemical building blocks) [*atom* indivisible]

atomic force microscopy (AFM) (ah-TOM-ik fors my-KROS-kah-pee) form of microscopy in which an extremely fine-tipped needle drags over the surface to reveal the outer limits of the atoms and molecules that make up the surface [*atom-* indivisible, *-ic* relating to, *micro-* small, *-scop-* see, *-y* activity]

atomic mass (ah-TOM-ik) number of protons plus the number of neutrons in an atom of an element; also called *mass number* [*atom* -indivisible, *-ic* relating to]

atomic number (ah-TOM-ik) number of protons in an atom of an element [*atom-* indivisible, *-ic* relating to]

atomic weight (ah-TOM-ik) average (or range of) atomic mass of an atom of an element as it is found in nature; atomic weights are usually found in the periodic table of elements [*atom-* indivisible, *-ic* relating to]

ATP synthase (SIN-thays) enzyme that produces ATP molecules [*ATP* adenosine triphosphate, *syn-* together, *-ase* enzyme]

atresia (ah-TREE-zha) blockage of a duct or follicle; disappearance of follicle by degeneration [*a-* without, *-tres-* perforation, *-ia* process]

atrial fibrillation (A-fib or AF) (AY-tree-al fib-ril-LAY-shun) frequent, chaotic premature contractions of the atrium [*atri-* entrance courtyard, *-al* relating to, *fibr-* thread or fibre, *-illa-* little, *-ation* process]

atrial natriuretic hormone (ANH) (AY-tree-al nay-tree-yoo-RET-ik HOR-mohn) hormone produced by the atrium that promotes secretion of sodium into the urine and therefore loss of water from the body [*atria-* entrance courtyard (atrium of heart), *-al* relating to, *natri-* natrium (sodium), *-uret-* urination, *-ic* relating to, *hormon-* excite]

atrioventricular (AV) bundle (ay-tree-oh-ven-TRIK-yoo-lar BUN-del) bundle of specialized cardiac muscle fibres that extend from the AV node to the subendocardial branches (Purkinje fibres); involved in coordination of heart muscle contraction [*atrio-* entrance courtyard, *-ventr-* belly, *-icul-* little, *-ar* relating to]

atrioventricular (AV) node (ay-tree-oh-ven-TRIK-yoo-lar) a small mass of special cardiac muscle tissue; part of the conduction system of the heart [*atrio-* entrance courtyard, *-ventr-* belly, *-icul-* little, *-ar* relating to, *nod-* knot]

atrioventricular (AV) valve (ay-tree-oh-ven-TRIK-yoo-lar) either of two valves that separate the atrial chambers from the ventricles; also called *cuspid valve* [*atrio-* entrance courtyard, *-ventr-* belly, *-icul-* little, *-ar* relating to]

atrium (AY-tree-um) one of the upper chambers of the heart; receives blood from either the systemic or pulmonary circulation [*atrium* entrance courtyard] *pl.*, atria (AY-tree-ah)

atrophy (AT-ro-fee) wasting away of tissue; decrease in size of a part; sometimes referred to as *disuse atrophy* [*a-* without, *-troph-* nourishment, *-y* state]

auditory (AW-di-toh-ree) relating to hearing or the ear [*audit-* hear, *-ory* relating to]

auditory nerve (AW-di-toh-ree nerv) cranial nerve VIII; *see* **vestibulocochlear nerve** [*audit-* hear, *-ory* relating to]

auditory ossicle (AW-dih-toh-ree OS-ik-ul) any of the tiny bones in middle ear: malleus, incus, and stapes; they function to amplify sound waves passing from the eardrum to the membranes of inner ear [*audit-* hear, *-ory* relating to, *os-* bone, *-icle* little]

auditory tube (AW-dih-toh-ree tyoob) tube that connects the throat with the middle ear and equalizes pressure between the middle ear and the exterior; also known as *Eustachian tube* [*audit-* hear, *-ory* relating to]

augmented lead (AWG-men-ted) one of three electrocardiogram leads based on combinations of the standard (appendicular) cardiogram leads [*augment* increase, *lead* guide or conduct]

auricle (AW-rih-kul) part of the ear attached to the side of the head; earlike appendage of each atrium of the heart [*auri-* ear, *-icle* little]

autism spectrum disorder (ASD) (AWT-iz-em SPEK-trum dis-OR-der) group of neurological disorders characterized by various combinations and severity of difficulties in social interactions, verbal/nonverbal communication, and repetitive behaviours; also called autism [*aut-* self, *-ism* condition, *spectrum* appearance (range), *dis-* opposite of, *-order* order]

autocrine (AW-toh-krin) a type of hormone that regulates activity in the secreting cell itself [*auto-* self, *-crin* secrete]

autoimmune disease (aw-toh-ih-MYOON) disorder in which the immune system reacts against cells of one's body [*auto-* self, *-immun-* free (immunity), *dis-* opposite of, *-ease* comfort]

autoimmunity (aw-toh-ih-MYOO-nih-tee) immune system reaction against normal body structures (self-antigens) [*auto-* self, *-immun-* free, *-ity* state]

autologous transfusion (aw-TOL-eh-gus) re-infusion of blood into your own body [*auto-* self, *-log-* word or proportion, *-ous* relating to]

autonomic (visceral) reflex (aw-toh-NOM-ik [VISS-er-al] REE-fleks) feedback regulatory mechanism of the autonomic nervous system in which autonomic (visceral) sensory receptors trigger a regulatory response [*auto-* self, *-nomo-* law, *-ic* relating to, *viscer-* internal organ, *-al* relating to, *re-* again, *-flex* bend]

autonomic effector (aw-toh-NOM-ik ef-FEK-tor) tissues to which efferent (motor) autonomic neurons conduct impulses [*auto-* self, *-nomo* law, *-ic* relating to, *effect-* accomplish, *-or* agent]

autonomic nervous system (ANS) (aw-toh-NOM-ik) division of the nervous system that monitors and regulates subconscious (involuntary) functions [*auto-* self, *-nom-* rule, *-ic* relating to, *nerv-* nerve, *-ous* relating to]

autopoiesis (aw-toh-poy-EE-sis) concept of self-organization and self-maintenance as a characteristic of all living organisms [*auto-* self, *-poiesis* making]

autoregulation (aw-toh-reg-yoo-LAY-shun) *see* intrinsic control [*auto-* self, *regula-* rule, *-tion* process]

autorhythmic (aw-toh-RITH-mic) relating to the characteristic of certain cells (such as involuntary muscle fibres) to display a self-regulated repeating pattern of action, as when heart cells beat in a rhythm without external stimulation [*auto-* self, *-rhythm-* movement in time, *-ic* relating to]

autosome (AW-toh-sohm) one of the 44 (22 pairs) chromosomes in the human genome besides the two sex chromosomes; means "same body", in reference to each member of a pair of autosomes matching the other in size and other structural features [*auto-* self, *-som-* body]

avascular (ah-VAS-kyoo-lar) free of blood vessels [*a-* without, *-vas-* vessel, *-ula-* little, *-ar* relating to]

avitaminosis (ay-vye-tah-mih-NO-sis) general name for any condition resulting from a vitamin deficiency [*a-* without, *-vita-* life, *-amin-* ammonia compound, *-osis* condition]

avulsion fracture (ah-VUL-shun) type of bone fracture in which bone fragments have pulled away from the underlying bone surface or bone is torn completely from the body part [*avuls-* pull away, *-sion* process, *fracture* a breaking]

axial skeleton (AK-see-all SKEL-eh-ton) the bones of the head, neck, and torso [*axi-* axis, *-al* relating to]

axillary (AK-sil-lair-ee) relating to the armpit [*axilla-* wing, *-ary* relating to]

axillary lymph node (AK-sil-lair-ee limf nohd) lymph node in the region at or near the armpit [*axilla-* wing, *-ary* relating to, *lymph* water, *nod-* knot]

axillary tail (of Spence) (AK-sih-lar-ee tail of Spens) lateral extension of breast tissue that is in physical contact with several very large lymph nodes [*axilla-* wing, *-ary* relating to]

axillary vein (AK-sih-lair-ee vayn) vein of the armpit region [*axilla* wing, *-ary* relating to, *vena* blood vessel]

axon (AK-son) in a neuron, the single process that extends from the axon hillock and transmits impulses away from the cell body [*axon* axle]

axon collateral (AK-son koh-LAT-er-al) one or more side branches from the axon [*axon-* axle, *co-* with, together, *-later-* side, *-al* relating to]

axon hillock (AK-son HILL-ok) portion of the cell body from which the axon extends [*axon* axle, *hill-* hill, *-ock* little]

axonal transport (AK-soh-nal TRANS-port) process of transporting vesicles, small organelles, and other structures along pathways inside the axon of a neuron [*axon* axle, *-al* relating to, *trans-* across, *-port* carry]

azygos vein (AZ-ih-gohs vayn) vein in the thorax [*a-* without, *-zygo-* union or yoke, *vena* blood vessel]

B

B cell immune system cell that produces antibodies against specific antigens; same as *B lymphocyte* [*B* bursa-equivalent tissue, *cell* storeroom]

B lymphocyte (B LIM-foh-syte) immune system cell that produces antibodies against specific antigens [*B* bursa-equivalent tissue, *lympho-* lymph, *-cyte* cell]

Babinski reflex (bah-BIN-skee REE-fleks) *see* **plantar reflex** [*Joseph F. F. Babinski* French neurologist, *re-* again, *-flex* bend]

Babinski sign (bah-BIN-skee) extension of the great toe (with or without fanning of the other toes) in response to stimulation of the outer margin of the foot, instead of the usual plantar reflex in which the toes curl in flexion; normal in infants but a sign of nerve dysfunction in adults [*Joseph F. F. Babinski* French neurologist]

bacterium (bak-TEE-ree-um) primitive, single-celled organism without membranous organelles; a normal component of the human microbiome, but may be pathogenic [*bacterium* small staff] *pl.*, bacteria (bak-TEE-ree-ah)

ball-and-socket joint spheroid joint, such as shoulder or hip joint; most movable type of joint

balloon angioplasty (AN-jee-oh-plas-tee) medical procedure in which vessels occluded by arteriosclerosis are opened (i.e., the channel for blood flow is widened) by use of a balloon at the tip of a catheter (tube) inside the affected vessel; as the balloon is inflated, the blockage is pushed aside; *see* **angioplasty** [*angio-* vessel, *-plasty* surgical repair]

balloon kyphoplasty (KYE-foh-plas-tee) orthopaedic procedure used to treat vertebral compression fracture [*kypho-* hump, *-plasty* surgical repair]

Bard endoscopic suturing system (en-doh-SKOP-ic) minimally invasive procedure used for treating serious cases of GORD [*endo-* within, *-scop-* look, *-y* activity, *sutur-* seam, *system* organized whole]

baroreceptor (bar-oh-ree-SEP-tor) sensory neuron sensitive to changes in blood pressure [*baro-* pressure, *-recept-* receive, *-or* agent]

baroreflex (bar-oh-REE-fleks) feedback loop in which feedback from pressure receptors in arteries produces a regulatory effect such as a change in heart rate to restore normal blood pressure; also called *pressoreflex* [*baro-* pressure, *re-* again, *-flex* bend]

barrel (BARE-ul) cell organelle that resembles a tiny capsule and is thought to shuttle substances from place to place within a cell; also called *vault*

Barrett oesophagus (eh-SOF-ah-gus) condition related to untreated gastro-oesophageal reflux disease; may develop precancerous changes in the oesophageal lining [*Norman R. Barrett* English surgeon, *oes-* will carry, *-phag-* food (eat)] *pl.*, oesophagi (eh-SOF-ah-jye)

basal (BAY-sal) relating to the base or widest part of an organ or other structure; in a cell, pertains to the surface facing away from the lumen of an organ [*bas-* base, *-al* relating to]

basal cell (BAY-sal) cell of the base layer of a structure [*bas-* foundation, *-al* relating to, *cell* storeroom]

basal cell carcinoma (BAY-sal cell kar-si-NOH-mah) one of the most common forms of skin cancer; usually occurs on the upper face [*bas-* base, *-al* relating to, *cell* storeroom, *carcin-* cancer, *-oma* tumour]

basal ganglion (BAY-sal GANG-glee-on) any of several islands of grey matter located in the cerebrum of the brain that are responsible for repetitive movements and postures; now known more properly as *basal nucleus* [*bas-* foundation, *-al* relating to, *gangli-* knot, *-on* unit] *pl.*, ganglia

basal lamina (BAY-sal LAM-ih-nah) complex layer of protein, glycoprotein, and proteoglycan material secreted by epithelial cells that forms part of the basement membrane [*bas-* foundation, *-al* relating to, *lamina* thin plate]

basal metabolic rate (BMR) (BAY-sal met-ah-BOL-ik) number of calories of heat that must be produced per hour by catabolism to keep the body alive, awake, and comfortably warm [*bas-* basis, *-al* relating to, *meta-* over, *-bol-* throw, *-ic* relating to]

basal nucleus (BAY-sal NYOO-klee-us) any of the islands of grey matter located in the cerebrum of the brain that are responsible for repetitive movements and postures; formerly known as *basal ganglion*; also known as *cerebral nucleus* [*bas-* foundation, *-al* relating to, *nucle-* nut or kernel] *pl.*, nuclei (NYOO-klee-eye)

base substance that ionizes in water to decrease the number of hydrogen ions; also known as *alkaline* [*bas-* foundation]

base pair adenine–thymine or cytosine–guanine; occurs when complementary bases from each helical chain of DNA are held together by hydrogen bonds [*bas-* foundation]

base-forming food food that produces a rise in pH inside the body [*bas-* foundation]

basement membrane the connective tissue layer of the serous membrane that holds and supports epithelial cells [*base-* base, *-ment,* thing, *membrane* thin skin]

basic residue (BAYS-ick REHZ-ih-doo) remains or product of a chemical process that have a high pH [*bas-* foundation, *-ic* relating to, *residu-* remainder]

basilar membrane (BAYS-ih-lar) *see* **spiral membrane** [*bas-* foundation, *-ar* relating to, *membrane* thin skin]

basilic vein (bah-SIL-ik vayn) a vein of the forearm [*bas-* foundation, *-ic* relating to, *vena* blood vessel]

basophil (BAY-so-fil) white blood cell that stains readily with basic (alkaline) dyes [*bas-* foundation, *-phil* love]

basophilic erythroblast (BAY-so-fil-ik eh-RITH-roh-blast) produced during red blood cell formation; results from the mitotic division of proerythroblast [*bas-* foundation, *-phil-* love, *-ic* relating to, *erythro-* red, *-blast* bud]

belly (BELL-ee) the central portion of a organ, such as a skeletal muscle

benign (bee-NYNE) refers to a tumour, neoplasm, or other condition that does not metastasize (spread to different tissues) or otherwise cause serious harm [*benign* kind]

benign paroxysmal positional vertigo (BPPV) (be-NYNE par-ock-SIZ-mul poh-ZISH-ih-nal VER-tih-go) type of vertigo associated with inner ear problems [*benign* kind, *paroxysm-* irritation, *-al* relating to, *vertigo* turning]

benign prostatic hypertrophy (BPH) (be-NYNE pro-STAT-ik hye-PER-troh-fee) a nonmalignant enlargement of the prostate gland [*benign* kind, *pro-* before, *-stat-* set or place, *-ic* relating to, *hyper-* excessive or above, *-troph-* nourishment, *-y* state]

beta (β) blocker (BAY-tah) drug that blocks beta receptors and therefore prevents dilation of blood vessels and increased contraction of heart muscle [*beta (β)* second letter of Greek alphabet]

beta (β)-carotene (bay-tah KAR-oh-teen) precursor of vitamin A in the body; may contribute to skin colour [*beta (β)* second letter of Greek alphabet, *-carot-* carrot, *-ene* unsaturated hydrocarbon]

beta (β) cell (BAY-tah sel) pancreatic islet cell that secretes insulin; also called *B cell* [*beta (β)* second letter of Greek alphabet, *cell* storeroom]

beta (β) particle (BAY-tah PAR-tih-kul) electrons formed in a radioactive atom's nucleus by a neutron breaking down into a proton and an electron [*beta (β)* second letter of Greek alphabet]

beta (β) receptor (BAY-tah ree-SEP-tor) adrenergic receptor that, when stimulated, causes vessels to dilate and heart muscle to contract faster and stronger [*beta (β)* second letter of Greek alphabet, *recept-* receive, *-or* agent]

beta (β)-adrenergic blocker (BAY-tah-ad-ren-ER-jik) *see* **beta blocker** [*beta (β)* second letter of Greek alphabet, *ad-* toward, *-ren-* kidney, *-erg-* work, -ic relating to]

beta (β)-hydroxybutyric acid (BAY-tah-hye-DROK-see-boo-teh-rik ASS-id) acidic ketone body that accumulates during the incomplete breakdown of fats [*beta (β)* second letter of Greek alphabet, *-hydro-* hydrogen, *-oxy-* sharp (oxygen), *-butyr-* butter, *-ic* relating to, *acid-* sour]

biaxial joint (bye-AK-see-al) skeletal articulation that has two axes of movement [*bi-* two, *-axi-* axle, *-al* relating to]

bicarbonate (bye-KAR-boh-nayt) *see* **bicarbonate ion** [*bi-* two, *-carbon,* coal (carbon), *-ate* oxygen compound]

bicarbonate ion (bye-KAR-boh-nayte EYE-on) HCO_3^-; an ion that serves an important role in maintaining normal blood pH [*bi-* twice, *-carbo-* coal, *-ate* oxygen]

bicarbonate loading (bye-KAR-boh-net) practice in which a person ingests bicarbonates to counteract the buildup of acids in the body [*bi-* two, *-carbon-* coal (carbon), *-ate* oxygen]

bicuspid (bye-KUSS-pid) having two cusps [*bi-* double, *-cusp-* point, *-id* characterized by]

bilateral symmetry (bye-LAT-er-al SIM-eh-tree) concept of the right and left sides of the body being approximate mirror images of each other [*bi-* two, *-later-* side, *-al* relating to, *sym-* together, *-metr-* measure, *-ry* condition of]

bile (byle) mixture of excretions and secretions produced by the liver and released into the digestive tract; also called *gall*

bile salt (byle) a type of emulsifying agent found in bile

bilirubin (bil-ih-ROO-bin) yellowish pigment formed when the haem group is removed from the haemoglobin molecule and stripped of its iron atom; a product of the breakdown of red blood cells [*bili-* bile, *-rub-* red, *-in* substance]

binge–purge syndrome (binj-purj SIN-drohm) eating disorder in which a person overeats and then induces vomiting [*syn-* together, *-drome* running or (race) course]

biochemistry (bye-oh-KEM-is-tree) science of chemistry of living organisms [*bio-* life, *-chemeia* alchemy]

biofeedback (bye-oh-FEED-bak) method of learning to consciously control autonomic effectors by monitoring autonomic biological functions [*bio-* life]

biological clock (bye-oh-LOJ-ih-kal) internal timing mechanism that governs hunger, sleeping, reproduction, and behaviour [*bio-* life, *-log-* words (study of), *-ical* relating to]

biomolecule (bye-oh-MOL-eh-kyool) organic molecule, usually a macromolecule, often made up of smaller subunits [*bio-* life, *-molec-* mass, *-ule* small]

biopsy (BYE-op-see) procedure in which living tissue is removed from a patient for laboratory examination, as in determining the presence of cancer cells [*bio-* life, *-ops-* view, *-y* act of]

Biot's breathing (bee-OHS) breathing pattern characterized by repeated sequences of deep gasps and apnoea caused by increased intracranial pressure [*Camille Biot* French physician]

bioterrorism (bye-oh-TAIR-or-iz-em) act of using biological weapons such as disease pathogens to spread terror among civilian populations for the purpose of creating fear, panic, and general social disruption [*bio-* life, *-terror-* frighten, *-ism* action or doctrine]

bipolar neuron (bye-POH-lar NYOO-ron) neuron with only one dendrite and only one axon [*bi-* two, *-pol-* pole, *-ar* relating to, *neuron* string or nerve]

blackhead sebum that accumulates, darkens, and enlarges a duct of the sebaceous glands, as in the case of acne; also known as a *comedo*

blastocyst (BLASS-toh-sist) stage of developing embryo that implants in uterine wall; consists of hollow ball of cells plus an inner cell mass [*blasto-* bud, *-cyst* pouch]

bleaching (BLEECH-ing) process when opsin and retinal open and separate in the presence of light

blepharoplasty (blef-ar-oh-PLAS-tee) surgical procedure that corrects a drooping eyelid [*blepharo-* eyelid or eyelash, *-plasty* surgical repair]

blind spot point on retina where blood vessels and nerves exit the eyeball; "blind" portion of visual field resulting from no photoreceptors present in that portion of retina; also known as *optic disc*

blister (BLIS-ter) fluid-filled skin lesion; *see* **vesicle**

blood boosting (blud BOOST-ing) *see* **blood doping**

blood clotting (blud KLOT-ing) *see* **blood coagulation**

blood coagulation (koh-ag-yoo-LAY-shun) process by which ruptured vessels are plugged up to stop bleeding and prevent loss of precious body fluids [*coagula-* curdle, *-ation* process]

blood colloid osmotic pressure (BCOP) (blud KOL-loyd os-MOT-ik) filtration pressure that tends to draw fluid back to the capillaries [*coll-* glue, *-oid* like, *osmo-* push, *-ic* relating to]

blood doping (blud DOH-ping) practice of increasing the haematocrit by transfusing additional blood or by the use of erythropoietin to boost haematocrit

blood hydrostatic pressure (BHP) (hye-droh-STAT-ik) pressure of blood against the wall of a blood vessel [*hydro-* water, *-stat-* standing, *-ic* relating to]

blood loss anaemia (ah-NEE-mee-ah) deficiency of red blood cells and haemoglobin caused by a loss of blood from the cardiovascular system [*an-* without, *-(h)aem-* blood, *-ia* condition]

blood serum (SEER-um) in a sample of blood, the pale yellowish liquid left after a clot forms [*serum* watery fluid] *pl.*, sera (SEER-ah)

blood test clinical laboratory examination of blood components

blood type category of blood cell identified by certain antigens on the cell membrane; ABO system applies to red blood cells, but other typing systems exist

blood urea nitrogen (BUN) test (yoo-REE-ah NYE-troh-jen) clinical laboratory measurement of the amount of nitrogen in urea present in the blood and used as a measure of the efficiency of the kidney's ability to clear urea from the body [*ure-* urine, *nitro-* soda, *-gen* produce]

blood–brain barrier (BBB) (blud brayn BAYR-ee-er) structural and functional barrier formed by astrocytes and blood vessel walls in the brain; it prevents some substances from diffusing from the blood into brain tissue

blood–nerve barrier (BNB) (blud nerv BAYR-ee-er) structural and functional barrier formed by the perineurium surrounding fascicles (bundles) of nerve fibres; regulates movement of substances between the bloodstream and nerve tissue

blood–testis barrier (BTB) (blud TES-tis BAYR-ee-er) functional barrier between the testis and the rest of the body, thus protecting developing sperm from attack by the immune system

blowout fracture bone fracture of the eye orbit [*fracture* a breaking]

body the structure of the entire organism; also, the main part of an organ, cell, or other structure

body composition (com-poh-ZISH-un) percentages of the body made of lean tissue and fat tissue

body mass index (BMI) method used to assess whether a person's body weight is proportional to height

body plane imagined flat surface that cuts through the body at any of various angles; *see* **coronal plane, sagittal plane, transverse plane** [*plan-* flat surface]

Bohr effect (bor ef-FEKT) when increased P_{CO_2} decreases the affinity between haemoglobin and oxygen [*Christian Bohr* Danish physiologist, *effect* accomplishment]

boil (BOY-el) carbuncle; pus-filled lesion of the skin [*boil* bubble]

bolus (BOW-lus) a mass of substance, such as the rounded lump of food and saliva that is swallowed [*bolus* lump]

bone age method using the number of ossification centres visible on a radiograph to determine the maturation of bone

bone marking (bohn MARK-ing) specific structural feature on an individual bone

bone marrow transplant (bohn MAIR-oh TRANZ-plant) medical procedure in which bone marrow tissue from a donor is placed in a recipient in hopes that it will produce healthy blood cells [*trans-* across, *-plant* set or place]

bone matrix (bohn MAY-triks) intercellular material of the bone tissue [*matrix* womb] *pl.*, matrices (MAY-trih-seez)

bone scan (bohn skan) medical imaging technique in which the density of bone is visualized

bone tamp (bohn tamp) inflatable balloon-like device used in balloon kyphoplasty; stabilizes and seals fractures [*tamp* pack down]

bone (bohn) type of connective tissue whose matrix is hard and calcified

bone-seeking isotope (bohn SEEK-ing EYE-soh-tohp) radioactive element that will substitute for calcium in apatite crystals of bone; causes damage to red marrow and other tissues by radioactive emissions [*iso-* equal, *-tope* place]

booster shot additional vaccination that boosts the immune response against a particular antigen

Bouchard node (boo-SHAR) swelling deformity of the proximal interphalangeal joint [*Charles J. Bouchard* French physician, *nod-* knot]

bovine spongiform encephalopathy (BOH-vyne SPUNJ-ih-form en-SEF-al-OP-ath-ee) also known as *BSE* or "mad cow disease"; a degenerative disease of the central nervous system caused by prions that convert normal proteins of the nervous system into abnormal proteins, causing loss of nervous system function; the abnormal form of the protein also may be inherited; *see* **prion** [*bos-* ox, *spongi-* like a sponge, *form* specialized shape, *encephal-* brain, *-pathy* disease]

Bowman capsule (BOH-mun KAP-sul) in the kidney, the cup-shaped top of a nephron that surrounds the glomerulus; also called *glomerular capsule* [*William Bowman* English anatomist, *caps-* box, *-ul* little]

Boyle's law (boils) principle of physics that states that the pressure of a gas is proportional to its volume [*Robert Boyle* English scientist]

brachial (BRAY-kee-al) relating to the arm [*brachi-* arm, *-al* relating to]

brachial plexus (BRAY-kee-al PLEK-sus) nerve plexus located deep in the shoulder that innervates the lower part of the shoulder and the entire arm [*brachi-* arm, *-al* relating to, *plexus* braid or network] *pl.*, plexi (PLEK-sye) or plexuses (PLEK-sus-eez)

brachial vein (BRAY-kee-al vayn) vein of the arm [*brachi-* arm, *-al* relating to, *vena* blood vessel]

brachiocephalic artery (brayk-ee-oh-seh-FAL-ik AR-ter-ee) artery of the upper thorax [*brachi-* arm, *-cephal-* head, *-ic* relating to, *arteri-* vessel]

brachiocephalic vein (brayk-ee-oh-seh-FAL-ik vayn) vein of the upper thorax [*brachi-* arm, *-cephal-* head, *-ic* relating to, *vena* blood vessel]

bradycardia (bray-dee-KAR-dee-ah) slow heart rhythm (less than 50 beats/min) [*brady-* slow, *-cardi-* heart, *-ia* condition]

bradykinin (brad-ee-KYE-nin) chemical mediator released after tissue injury and cellular death [*brady-* slow or dull, *-kinin* move]

brain (brayn) part of central nervous system contained within the cranium; consists of medulla oblongata, cerebellum, and cerebrum

brain electrical activity map (BEAM) colour-coded graphic image of the brain generated on a video screen

brain waves (brayn waivz) fluctuating electrical activity occurring in the brain

brainstem (BRAYN-stem) part of brain containing the midbrain, pons, and medulla oblongata

breast cancer (brest KAN-ser) malignant neoplasm (tumour) of the breast [*cancer* crab or malignant tumour]

broad ligament (LIG-ah-ment) double fold of parietal peritoneum that forms a partition across the pelvic cavity [*liga-* bind, *-ment* condition]

bronchial tree (BRONG-kee-al) the trachea, two primary bronchi, and their many branches [*bronch-* windpipe, *-al* relating to]

bronchial vein (BRONK-kee-al vayn) vein of the pulmonary airways [*bronch-* windpipe, *-al* relating to, *vena* blood vessel]

bronchiole (BRONG-kee-ohl) small branch of a bronchus [*bronch-* windpipe, *-ol* little]

bronchitis (brong-KYE-tis) inflammation of the bronchi of the lungs, characterized by oedema and excessive mucus production that causes coughing and difficulty in breathing (especially expiration) [*bronch-* windpipe, *-itis* inflammation]

bronchogram (BRONG-koh-gram) medical image of the pulmonary airways [*bronch-* windpipe, *-gram* drawing]

bronchopulmonary segment (brong-koh-PUL-moh-nair-ee) region of the lung supplied by a tertiary bronchus [*bronch-* windpipe, *-pulmon-* lung, *-ary* relating to]

bruits (BROO-eez) blood vessel noise caused by turbulence of blood flow [*bruits* noise]

brush border lining of small intestine that resembles bristles of a brush; formed by microvilli

buccal (BUK-al) relating to the cheek; often refers specifically to the inside of the cheek [*bucca-* cheek, *-al* relating to]

buccal cavity (BUK-al KAV-ih-tee) oral cavity [*bucca-* cheek, *-al* relating to]

buccinator muscle (BUK-si-NAY-tor) muscle of the cheek [*buccinator* trumpeter, *mus-* mouse, *-cle* little]

buffer (BUFF-er) compound that combines with an acid or with a base to form a weaker acid or base, thereby lessening the change in hydrogen ion concentration that would occur without the buffer; often operates as buffer pairs [*buffe-* cushion, *-er* actor]

buffer pair (BUFF-er) a chemical system of two chemicals that together act as a buffer, minimizing changes in pH of a solution [*buffe-* cushion, *-er* agent]

buffy coat (BUFF-ee koht) found in a centrifuged sample of blood, the thin layer of leucocytes and platelets located at the interface between packed red cells and plasma [*buffe-* cushion, *-y* of or like]

bulboid corpuscle (BUL-boyd KOR-pus-ul) skin receptor that detects sensations of touch, low-frequency vibration, and texture differences; also known as *Krause end bulb* [*bulb-* swollen root, *-oid* like, *corpus-* body, *-cle* little]

bulbospongiosus muscle (bul-boh-spun-jee-OH-ses) muscle of the base of the penis [*bulbo-* swollen root (bulb), *-spongiosus* spongy, *mus-* mouse, *-cle* little]

bulbourethral gland (BUL-boh-yoo-REE-thral) either of two small glands at the base of the penis that contributes a small amount of fluid to semen; also called *Cowper gland* [*bulb-* swollen root, *-ure-* urine, *-thr-* agent or channel (urethra), *-al* relating to]

bulbous corpuscle (BUL-bus KOR-pus-ul) sensory receptor that senses deep pressure and continuous touch; located in dermis of the skin; also known as *Ruffini corpuscle* [*bulb-* swollen root, *-ous* relating to, *corpus-* body, *-cle* little]

bulimia (boo-LEE-mee-ah) eating disorder characterized by intentional purging of food by induced vomiting, laxatives, or other means [*bu-* ox, *-lim-* hunger, *-ia* condition]

bursa (BER-sah) small, cushion-like sac found between moving body parts, making movement easier [*bursa* purse] *pl.*, bursae (BER-see or BER-say)

bursitis (ber-SYE-tiss) inflammation of a bursa [*bursa-* purse, *-itis* inflammation]

bypass surgery (BYE-pass SUR-jah-ree) *see* **coronary bypass surgery** [*bi-* alongside, *sur-* hand, *-urger-* work, *-y* activity]

C

C cell type of cell of the thyroid gland that produces calcitonin [C for calcitonin, *cell* storeroom]

CA-125 tumour antigen associated with ovarian cancer [C cancer, A antigen]

cachexia (kah-KEKS-ee-ah) syndrome involving loss of weight, loss of appetite, and general weakness; usually associated with cancer [*cache-* bad, *-exia* state]

cadaver (kah-DAV-er) corpse preserved for anatomical study [*cadaver* dead body]

caesarean section (seh-SAIR-ee-an SEK-shun) surgical removal of a fetus through an incision of the skin and uterine wall; also called *C-section* [*Julius Caesar* Roman emperor, *-ean* of]

calcaneal (kal-KAH-nee-al) relating to the heel of the foot or calcaneus (heel) bone [*calcane-* heel, *-al* relating to]

calcaneal tendon (kal-KAH-nee-al TEN-den) connects gastrocnemius to calcaneus; Achilles tendon [*calcane-* heel, *-al* relating to, *tend-* pulled tight, *-on* unit]

calcitonin (CT) (kal-sih-TOH-nin) hormone secreted by the thyroid that decreases calcium levels in the blood [*calci-* lime (calcium), *-ton-* tone, *-in* substance]

calcitriol (kal-SIT-ree-ol) active form of vitamin D_3 that acts as a hormone that regulates calcium homeostasis in the body [*calci-* lime (calcium), *-tri-* three, *-ol* alcohol (after *1,25-*D_3 or *1,25-dihydroxycholecalciferol*)]

calcium (KAL-see-um) important mineral involved in bone formation, tooth formation, muscle contraction, synaptic transmission, and other vital processes of the body [*calc-* lime, *-um* thing or substance]

calcium channel blocker (KAL-see-um CHAN-al) agent that inhibits the opening of calcium channels in cell membranes [*calc-* lime, *-um* thing or substance]

calcium pump (KAL-see-um) energy-consuming structure embedded in a cell membrane that moves calcium ions through the membrane against their concentration gradient (i.e., from an area of low concentration to an area of high concentration) [*calc-* lime, *-um* thing or substance]

calendar rhythm method method of fertility management based on timing of the female reproductive cycle [*rhythm* movement in time]

callus (KAL-us) bony tissue that forms a sort of collar around the broken ends of fractured bone during the healing process; in the skin, abnormally thick stratum corneum found at points of friction [*callus* hard skin]

Calorie (C) (KAL-or-ree) heat unit; kilocalorie (kcal); the amount of heat needed to raise the temperature of 1 kilogram of water 1° C [*calor-* heat, *-ie* full of]

calorie (cal) (KAL-or-ee) heat unit; the amount of heat needed to raise the temperature of 1 gram of water 1° C [*calor-* heat, *-ie* full of]

calvarium (kal-VAIR-ee-um) name for the upper dome of the cranium of the skull [*calvarium* skull] *pl.*, calvaria or calvariums

calyx (KAY-liks) cup-shaped branch of the renal pelvis [*calyx* cuplike] *pl.*, calyces (KAY-lis-eez)

canal of Schlemm (kah-NAL of shlem) *see* **scleral venous sinus** [*canal-* channel, *Friedrich Schlemm* German anatomist]

canaliculi (kan-ah-LIK-yoo-lye) an extremely narrow tubular passage or channel in compact bone; radiates from lacunae and connects with other lacunae and the central (Haversian) canal of the osteon [*canal-* channel, *-iculi* little] *sing.*, canaliculus

canaliculus (kan-ah-LIK-yoo-lus) singular of **canaliculi** [*canal-* channel, *-uculus* little]

canalith (KAN-ah-lith) crystalline structure of the semicircular canals of the inner ear [*canal-* channel, *-lith* stone]

canalith repositioning procedure (KAN-ah-lith) procedure to restore the proper position of crystalline structures of the semicircular canals of the ear and thus eliminate balance perception problems such as vertigo [*canal-* channel, *-lith* stone]

cancellous bone (KAN-seh-lus) bone containing tiny, branchlike trabeculae; also known as *spongy bone* or *trabecular bone* [*cancel-* lattice, *-ous* characterized by]

cancellous bone tissue (KAN-seh-lus) *see* **cancellous bone** [*cancel-* lattice, *-ous* characterized by, *tissu-* fabric]
cancer malignant cellular neoplasm (tumour) that invades other cells and often metastasizes to many parts of the body [*cancer* crab or malignant tumour]
cancer of the uterus (YOO-ter-us) malignancy of uterine tissue [*cancer* crab or malignant tumour]
candidiasis (kan-dih-DYE-eh-sis) infection caused by *Candida* yeast [*candid-* white, *-asis* condition]
capacitance (kah-PASS-i-tens) the ease of stretch (distensibility) of a blood vessel wall [*capacit-* space or volume, *-ance* state]
capacitation (kah-pass-ih-TAY-shun) process occurring after ejaculation of semen and needed for a mature sperm to become capable of fertilizing an ovum [*capacit-* space or volume, *-tion* process]
capillary (KAP-ih-lair-ee) tiny vessels that connect arterioles and venules; gas exchange from blood to tissues occurs in capillaries [*capill-* hair, *-ary* relating to]
capillary exchange (KAP-ih-lair-ee) process of moving molecules into and out of the blood of a capillary [*capill-* hair, *-ary* relating to]
capitulum (kah-PITCH-uh-lum) rounded knob on the humerus bone below the lateral epicondyle [*capit-* head, *-ulum* little]
carbaminohaemoglobin (kahr-bam-ih-no-hee-moh-GLOH-bin) carbonated form of haemoglobin [*carb-* coal (carbon), *-amino-* ammonia compound (amino acid), *-haemo-* blood, *-glob-* ball, *-in* substance]
carbohydrate (kar-bo-HYE-drate) organic compounds containing carbon, hydrogen, and oxygen in certain specific proportions; for example, sugars, starches, and cellulose [*carbo-* carbon, *-hydr-* hydrogen, *-ate* oxygen]
carbon monoxide (CO) (KAR-bon mon-OKS-side) molecule made up of one carbon atom and one oxygen atom [*mono-* single, *-ox-* sharp (oxygen), *-ide* chemical]
carbon monoxide poisoning (KAR-bon mon-OK-side POY-son-ing) condition in which exposure to carbon monoxide results in the molecule tightly binding to haemoglobin and thereby preventing oxygen transport by the blood [*carbon* coal, *mono-* single, *-ox-* sharp (oxygen)]
carbonic acid (kar-BON-ik ASS-id) product of the reaction between carbon dioxide and water [*carbon-* coal (carbon), *-ic* relating to, *acid* sour]
carbonic anhydrase (CA) (kar-BON-ik an-HYE-drays) the enzyme that converts carbon dioxide into carbonic acid (and also reverses the reaction) [*carbon-* coal, *-ic* relating to, *a-* without, *-hydr-* water, *-ase* enzyme]
carbuncle (KAR-bung-kul) a mass of connected boils, pus-filled lesions associated with hair follicle infections; *see* **furuncle** [*carbun-* coal, *-cle* little]
carcinoembryonic antigen (CEA) (kar-sin-oh-em-bree-ON-ik AN-tih-jen) tumour marker found normally in the fetus and elevated colorectal and other adult cancers [*carcino-* cancer, *-em-* in, *-bryo-* fill to bursting, *-ic* relating to, *anti-* against, *-gen* produce]
carcinogen (kar-SIN-oh-jen) substance that promotes the development of cancer [*carcino-* cancer, *-gen* produce]
carcinoma (kar-sih-NO-mah) malignant tumour that arises from epithelial tissue [*carcin-* cancer, *-oma* tumour]
cardia (KAR-dee-ah) small collarlike section of the stomach near the junction with the oesophagus, so called because of its nearness to the heart; also called *cardiac part* or *cardial part* [*cardia* heart]
cardiac cycle (KAR-dee-ak SYE-kul) complete heartbeat consisting of diastole and systole of both atria and both ventricles [*cardi-* heart, *-ac* relating to, *cycl-* circle]
cardiac muscle tissue (KAR-dee-ak) muscle tissue type that makes up the heart [*cardia-* heart, *-ac* relating to, *mus-* mouse, *-cle* small, *tissu-* fabric]
cardiac nuclear scanning (KAR-dee-ak NYOO-klee-ar) medical image of the heart produced when radioactive materials flow through the coronary vessels [*cardi-* heart, *-ac* relating to, *nucle-* nut or kernel, *-ar* relating to]
cardiac output (CO) (KAR-dee-ak) volume of blood pumped by one ventricle per minute (e.g., L/min or mL/min) [*cardi-* heart, *-ac* relating to]
cardiac part (KAR-dee-ak) see **cardia** [*cardi-* heart, *-ic* relating to]
cardiac plexus (KAR-dee-ak PLEK-sus) combination of sympathetic and parasympathetic nerves that are located near the aortic arch [*cardi-* heart, *-ac* relating to, *plexus-* network]
cardiac pressoreflex (KAR-dee-ak pres-oh-REE-fleks) feedback regulatory mechanism in which pressure receptors in arteries trigger a change in heart rate to restore normal blood pressure [*cardi-* heart, *-ac* relating to, *press-* pressure, *-re-* back or again, *-flex* bend]
cardiac reserve (KAR-dee-ak ree-ZERV) amount the cardiac output can increase above resting output, usually expressed in percent above resting value [*cardi-* heart, *-ic* relating to]
cardiac sphincter (KAR-dee-ak SFINGK-ter) a ring of muscle between the stomach and oesophagus that prevents food from reentering the oesophagus when the stomach contracts [*cardi-* heart, *-ic* relating to, *sphinc-* bind tight, *-er* agent]
cardiac tamponade (KAR-dee-ak tam-puh-NOD or tam-puh-NAYD) compression of the heart caused by fluid buildup in the pericardial space, as in pericarditis or mechanical damage to the pericardium [*cardi-* heart, *-ac* relating to, *tampon-* plug, *-ade* process]
cardiogenic shock (kar-dee-oh-JEN-ik) condition characterized by low cardiac output; can result from any type of heart failure [*cardi-* heart, *-gen-* produce, *-ic* relating to]
cardiomyopathy (kar-dee-oh-my-OP-ah-thee) general term for disease of the myocardium (heart muscle) causing enlargement [*cardi-* heart, *-myo-* muscle, *-path-* disease, *-y* state]
cardiopulmonary resuscitation (CPR) (kar-dee-oh-PUL-moh-nair-ree ree-sus-ih-TAY-shun) combined external cardiac (heart) massage and artificial respiration [*cardio-* heart, *-pulmon-* lung, *-ary* relating to, *resuscita-* revive, *-ation* process]
caries (KAIR-eez) decay of teeth or of bone [*caries* decay]
carotene (KAR-oh-teen) yellowish-to-orangish pigment; precursor of vitamin A in the body (beta-carotene, especially); may contribute to skin colour [*carot-* carrot, *-ene* unsaturated hydrocarbon]
carotid sinus reflex (kah-ROT-id SYE-nus REE-fleks) homeostatic mechanism that involves baroreceptors that relay feedback information to cardiac control centre; maintains blood pressure [*caro-* heavy sleep, *-id* relating to, *sinus* hollow, *re-* back or again, *-flex* bend]
carpal (KAR-pul) relating to the wrist [*carp-* wrist, *-al* relating to]
carpal bone (KAR-pul bohn) any of the bones of the wrist [*carp-* wrist, *-al* relating to]
carpal tunnel syndrome (KAR-pul TUN-el SIN-drohm) muscle weakness, pain, and tingling in the radial side (thumb side) of the wrist, hand, and fingers, perhaps radiating to the forearm and shoulder; caused by compression of the median nerve within the carpal tunnel (a passage along the ventral concavity of the wrist) [*carp-* wrist, *-al* relating to, *syn-* together, *-drome* running or (race) course]
carpometacarpal joint (kar-po-met-ah-KAR-pal) skeletal articulation between a wrist (carpal) bone and hand (metacarpal) bone [*carpo-* wrist, *-meta-* beyond, *-carp-* wrist, *-al* relating to]
carrier (KARE-ee-er) in genetics, a person who possesses the gene for a recessive trait but who does not actually exhibit the trait; in cell biology, a protein structure in the membrane that facilitates transport of ions and other molecules
carrier-mediated passive transport (KARE-ee-er MEE-dee-ayt-ed PASS-iv TRANS-port) type of facilitated diffusion, in which solutes move down their concentration gradient through carrier mechanisms in the membrane wall [*trans-* across, *-port* carry]
cartilage (KAR-tih-lij) connective tissue type that has the consistency of a firm plastic or gristle-like gel [*cartilag-* cartilage]
cartilaginous joint (kar-tih-LAJ-in-us joynt) articulation between bones that is primarily composed of cartilage [*cartilag-* cartilage, *-in-* substance, *-ous* characterized by]
catabolism (kah-TAB-oh-liz-im) breakdown of food compounds or cytoplasmic constituents into simpler compounds; opposite of anabolism [*cata-* against, *-bol-* to throw, *-ism* condition]
catalyst (KAT-ah-list) chemical that speeds up reactions without being changed itself [*cata-* lower, *-lys-* loosen, *-(i)st* agent]
cataracts (KAT-ah-rakts) areas of opacity in the lens of the eye [*cataract* waterfall]
catecholamine (kat-eh-KOHL-ah-meen) chemical category of neurotransmitters that include norepinephrine, epinephrine, and dopamine [*catech-* melt, *-ol-* alcohol, *-amine* ammonia compound]
catheter (KATH-eh-ter) thin, flexible tube often used in medical procedures [*cathe-* send down, *-er* agent]
catheterization (kath-eh-ter-ih-ZAY-shun) passage of a flexible tube (catheter) into the body through an exterior opening (as into the bladder through the urethra for the withdrawal of urine) [*cathe-* send down, *-er* agent, *-tion* process]
cation (KAT-eye-on) positively charged particle [*cat-* down, *-ion* to go (ion)]
cauda equina (KAW-da eh-KWY-nah) lower end of spinal cord with its attached spinal nerve roots [*caud-* tail, *equina* of a horse] *pl.*, caudae equinae
caudate nucleus (KAW-dayt NYOO-klee-us) one of the basal nuclei, grey matter areas in the inner region of the cerebrum of the brain [*caud-* tail, *-ate* of or like, *nucleus* nut or kernel] *pl.*, nuclei
caveola (kav-ee-OH-la) tiny indentation of a raft in the cell's plasma membrane that traps substances and shuttles them into or through the cell [*cave-* hollow, *-ola* little] *pl.*, caveolae
CD system international system for naming surface markers on blood cells [C cluster, D differentiation]
cell (sel) basic biological and structural unit of the body consisting of a nucleus surrounded by cytoplasm and enclosed by a membrane [*cell* storeroom]
cell body (sel BOD-ee) the main part of a cell, ordinarily containing the nucleus; in the neuron, the cell body is also called the *soma* or *perikaryon* [*cell* storeroom]
cell cycle *see* **cell life cycle** [*cell* storeroom, *cycl-* circle]
cell life cycle (sel lyfe SYE-kul) the repeating process of a cell's growth and reproduction, producing successive generations of cells and proceeding through the first growth (gap) phase (G_1), DNA replication (S), second growth (gap) phase (G_2), and mitotic cell division (M); also called *cell cycle* [*cell* storeroom, *cycl-* circle]
cell theory (sel THEE-ree) concept proposed more than 100 years ago that all living organisms are made up of biological units called *cells*; *see* **cell** [*cell* storeroom, *theor-* look at, *-y* act of]
cell-mediated immunity (sell MEE-dee-ayted ih-MYOO-nih-tee) type of adaptive immunity in which T lymphocytes act directly on antigens to protect the body [*cell-* storeroom, *-medi-* middle, *-ate* process, *immun-* free, *-ity* state]
cellular immunity (SEL-yoo-lar ih-MYOO-nih-tee) see **cell-mediated immunity** [*cell* storeroom, *-ular* relating to, *immun-* free, *-ity* state]
cellular respiration (SEL-yoo-lar res-pih-RAY-shun) set of biochemical reactions of a cell that transfer energy from nutrient molecules to ATP molecules [*cell* storeroom, *-ular* relating to, *respire-* breathe, *-ation* process]
cellulose (SEL-yoo-lohs) dietary fibre; major component of most plant tissue; nondigestible by humans [*cell-* storeroom (cell), *-ul-* small, *-ose* carbohydrate]
cementum (sih-MEN-tum) hard, mineralized connective tissue similar to bone that forms a coat around the root of the tooth and helps connect the tooth to the jaw bone by serving as an anchor for periodontal ligaments [*cement-* mortar, *-um* matter]
central relating to the centre of the body, as in *central nervous system* [*centr-* centre, *-al* relating to]
central canal canal in the osteon (Haversian system) of bone that runs parallel to the long axis; contains blood vessels and nerves; also called *osteonal canal* or *Haversian canal* [*centr-* centre, *-al* relating to, *canal-* channel]
central chemoreceptor (SEN-tral kee-moh-ree-SEP-tor) sensory receptor in the brain (central nervous system) that detects changes in chemical concentrations such as oxygen, carbon dioxide, or pH [*centr-* centre, *-al* relating to, *chemo-* chemical, *-recept-* receive, *-or* agent]
central nervous system (CNS) the brain and spinal cord [*centr-* centre, *-al* relating to, *nerv-* nerves, *-ous* relating to]
central sulcus (Rolando fissure) (SUL-kus [roh-LAHN-doh FISH-ur]) groove between frontal and parietal lobes of the cerebrum [*sulcus* trench, *Luigi Rolando* Italian physician] *pl.*, sulci (SUL-kye)
centriole (SEN-tree-ohl) one of a pair of tiny cylinders in the centrosome of a cell; believed to be involved with the spindle fibres formed during mitosis [*centr-* centre, *-ole* small]
centromere (SEN-troh-meer) a beadlike structure that attaches one chromatid to another during the early stages of mitosis [*centro-* centre, *-mere* part]
centrosome (SEN-troh-sohm) area of the cytoplasm near the nucleus that coordinates the building and breaking up of microtubules in the cell [*centr-* centre, *-som-* body]
cephalic (seh-FAL-ik) relating to the head [*cephal-* head, *-ic* relating to]
cephalic phase (seh-FAL-ik fayz) stage in regulation of stomach secretion in which mental factors stimulate gastric juice secretion [*cephal-* head, *-ic* relating to]
cephalic vein (seh-FAL-ik vayn) vein of the head [*cephal-* head, *-ic* relating to, *vena* blood vessel]
cerebellum (sair-eh-BELL-um) second largest part of the human brain; plays an essential role in the production of normal movements [*cereb-* brain, *-ellum* small thing] *pl.*, cerebella or cerebellums
cerebral arterial circle (of Willis) (seh-REE-bral ar-TEER-ee-al SIR-kul [ov WILL-is]) circular network of connected arteries at the base of the brain; also called by eponym *circle of Willis* or *Willis circle* [*cerebr-* brain (cerebrum), *-al* relating to, *arteria-* vessel, *-al* relating to (*Thomas Willis* English physician)]
cerebral cortex (seh-REE-bral KOR-teks) thin layer of grey matter made up of neuron dendrites and cell bodies that compose the surface of the cerebrum [*cerebr-* brain

(cerebrum), *-al* relating to, *cortex* bark] *pl.*, cortices (KOR-tis-eez)

cerebral hemisphere (seh-REE-bral HEM-is-feer) either of the two right and left halves of the cerebrum [*cerebr-* brain, *-al* relating to, *hemi-* half, *-sphere* globe]

cerebral localization (seh-REE-bral) principle of brain function that states that specific cerebral functions are likely to be located in the cerebral cortex at specific, often predictable, locations [*cerebr-* brain, *-al* relating to, *loc-* place, *-al-* relating to, *-ization* process]

cerebral nuclei (seh-REE-bral NYOO-klee-eye) *see* **basal nuclei** [*cerebr-* brain, *-al* relating to, *nucleus-* nut or kernel]

cerebral palsy (seh-REE-bral PAWL-zee) disorder in which damage to motor control areas of the brain cause abnormally high skeletal muscle tone (and thus, mobility problems) in one or more areas of the body [*cerebr-* brain, *-al* relating to, *palsy* paralysis (*para-* beyond, *-lysis* loosening)]

cerebral peduncle (seh-REE-bral peh-DUNG-kul) white matter tracts in the brain connecting the cerebellum to the cerebrum [*cerebr-* brain, *-al* relating to, *ped- foot*, *-uncl-* little]

cerebral plasticity (seh-REE-bral plas-TIS-ih-tee) characteristic of the cerebrum that permits the relocation of functions from one area of the cerebral cortex to another area [*cerebr-* brain, *-al* relating to, *plastic-* mouldable, *-ity* state]

cerebrospinal fluid (CSF) (seh-ree-broh-SPY-nal FLOO-id) plasmalike fluid that fills the subarachnoid space in the brain and spinal cord and in the cerebral ventricles [*cerebr-* brain, *-spin-* backbone, *-al* relating to]

cerebrovascular accident (CVA) (SAIR-eh-broh-VAS-kyoo-lar) event in which haemorrhage or cessation of blood flow caused by an embolism or ruptured aneurysm in brain blood vessel results in ischaemia of brain tissue and destruction of neurons; commonly called a *stroke* [*cerebr-* brain, *-vas-* vessel, *-cul-* little, *-ar* relating to]

cerebrum (SAIR-eh-brum) largest and uppermost part of the human brain that controls consciousness, memory, sensations, emotions, and voluntary movements [*cerebrum* brain] *pl.*, cerebra (SAIR-eh-brah) or cerebrums

cerumen (seh-ROO-men) ear wax [*cer(a)-* wax, *-men* formed of]

ceruminous gland (seh-ROO-mi-nus) gland that produces a waxy substance called *cerumen* (ear wax) [*cer(a)-* wax, *-min-* formed of, *-ous* relating to, *gland* acorn]

cervical (SER-vi-kal) relating to a neck, such as the neck of the human body or the neck (or cervix) of an organ (such as the uterus) [*cervic-* neck, *-al* relating to]

cervical cancer (SER-vi-kal) malignancy of the neck (cervix) of the uterus [*cervic-* neck, *-al* relating to, *cancer* crab or malignant tumour]

cervical plexus (SER-vih-kal PLEK-sus) plexus located deep within the neck; innervates muscles and skin of the neck, upper shoulder, and part of the head [*cervic-* neck, *-al* relating to, *plexus* braid or network] *pl.*, plexi (PLEK-sye) or plexuses (PLEK-sus-eez)

cervical vertebra (SER-vi-kal VER-teh-bra) one of the seven spinal (vertebral) bones of the neck [*cervi-* neck, *-al* relating to, *vertebra* that which turns] *pl.*, vertebrae (VER-teh-bree or VER-teh-bray)

cervix (SER-viks) neck; may refer to the neck of the human body or the neck of an organ (such as the uterus) [*cervix* neck] *pl.*, cervices (SER-vis-eez) or cervixes

channel-mediated passive transport (CHAN-al MEE-dee-ayt-ed PASS-iv TRANS-port) any membrane transport mechanism in which molecules move down a concentration gradient through membrane channels

chaperonin (shap-er-OHN-in) any of a group of globular proteins that are present in every body cell and direct the intracellular steps required for other proteins to achieve the often twisted and convoluted shape required for them to function [*chaperon-* protector (escort), *-in* substance]

Charles's law (CHARLZ-ez law) gas law that states that volume is directly proportional to temperature when pressure is held constant; sometimes called *Gay-Lussac's law* (gay lus-SAKS law) after French physical scientist Joseph L. Gay-Lussac who first published it, crediting Jacques Charles with its discovery [*Jacques Alexandre César Charles* French physicist]

cheek facial prominence shaped by the underlying zygomatic bone

chemical bond energy relationship joining two or more atoms; involves sharing or exchange of electrons [*chemica-* alchemy, *-al* relating to]

chemical buffer combines with added acids or alkali in the body; changes hydrogen ion concentration and pH [*chemica-* alchemy, *-al* relating to, *buffe-* cushion, *-er* agent]

chemical digestion (dye-JES-chun) changes in chemical composition of food as it passes through the alimentary canal [*chemica-* alchemy, *-al* relating to, *digest-* break apart, *-tion* process]

chemoreceptor (kee-moh-ree-SEP-tor) receptor that responds to chemicals; responsible for taste and smell and monitoring concentration of specific chemicals in the blood [*chemo-* chemical, *-recept-* receive, *-or* agent]

chemoreceptor reflex (kee-moh-ree-SEP-tor REE-fleks) nerve reflex in which chemical changes such as a change in blood pH trigger a reflexive change in physiology, such as a change in heart rate or respiratory rate, to restore a homeostatic balance [*chemo-* chemical, *-recept-* receive, *-or* agent, *re-* back or again, *-flex* bend]

chemotactic factor (kee-moh-TAK-tik) chemical that attracts a mobile cell such as a neutrophil or macrophage to a specific location, as in an immune response [*chemo-* chemical, *-tact-* movement, *-ic* relating to]

chemotaxin (kee-moh-TAK-sin) chemotactic factor [*chemo-* chemical, *-tax-* movement or reaction, *-in* substance]

chemotaxis (kee-moh-TAK-sis) process by which a substance attracts cells or organisms into (or away from) its vicinity; for example, when inflammation mediators attract white blood cells; sometimes called *positive chemotaxis*; *see* **chemotactic factor** [*chemo-* chemical, *-taxis* movement or reaction]

chemotherapy (kee-moh-THAYR-ah-pee) technique of using chemicals to treat disease (e.g., infections, cancer) [*chemo-* chemical, *-therapy* treatment]

chest lead (leed) arrangement of ECG electrodes on the chest to test heart function; also called *precordial lead* [*chest* box, *lead* guide or conduct]

chest x-ray diagnostic procedure that examines the lungs, mediastinal contents, and bony thorax [*chest* box, *x-* unknown, *-ray* spoke or rod]

Cheyne–Stokes respiration (chain stokes respih-RAY-shun) pattern of breathing associated with critical conditions such as brain injury or drug overdose and characterized by cycles of apnoea and hyperventilation [*John Cheyne* Scots physician, *William Stokes* Irish physician, *re-* again, *-spir-* breathe, *-ation* process]

chief cell (cheef sel) cells lining the gastric glands of the stomach that secrete pepsinogen and intrinsic factor; also called *zymogenic cells* [*chief* head, *cell* storeroom]

childhood period of human development from infancy to puberty

chiropractic (kye-roh-PRAK-tik) system of therapy based on principle that alignment of the skeleton promotes healing [*chiro-* hand, *-practic* practical]

chloride channel (KLOR-ide CHAN-nul) a pore in a cell membrane that allows only chloride ions to permeate, or pass through, the membrane [*chlor-* green, *-ide* chemical]

chloride shift (KLOR-ide) diffusion of chloride ions into red blood cells as bicarbonate ions diffuse out; maintains electrical neutrality of red blood cells [*chlor-* green, *-ide* chemical]

chlorine (KLOR-een) important negative ion surrounding cells; has one unpaired electron plus three paired electrons [*chlor-* green, *-ine* chemical]

cholecystectomy (koh-leh-sis-TEK-toh-mee) surgical removal of the gallbladder [*chole-* bile, *-cyst-* bag, *-ec-* out, *-tom-* cut, *-y* action]

cholecystitis (koh-leh-sis-TYE-tis) inflammation of the gallbladder [*chole-* bile, *-cyst-* bag, *-itis* inflammation]

cholecystokinin (CCK) (koh-leh-sis-tuh-KYE-nin) hormone secreted from the intestinal mucosa of the duodenum that stimulates contraction of the gallbladder, resulting in bile flowing into the duodenum [*chole-* bile, *-cyst-* bag, *-kin-* movement, *-in* substance]

cholelithiasis (koh-leh-lih-THYE-ah-sis) gallstone formation [*chole-* bile, *-lith-* stone, *-iasis* condition]

cholera (KOL-er-ah) potentially fatal, infectious bacterial disease characterized by severe diarrhoea, vomiting, cramps, dehydration [*chole-* bile, *-a* state]

cholesterol (koh-LESS-ter-ol) steroid lipid found in many body tissues and in animal fats [*chole-* bile, *-stero-* solid, *-ol* alcohol]

cholinergic (koh-lin-ER-jik) describes a structure that functions with acetylcholine (ACh), as a nerve fibre that releases ACh or a receptor triggered by ACh [*chole-* bile, *-erg-* work, *-ic* relating to]

chondral fracture (KON-dral) fracture of an articular (cartilage) surface in a synovial joint [*condr-* cartilage, *-al* relating to, *fracture* a breaking]

chondrification centre (kon-dri-fi-KAY-shun) area of specialized mesenchymal cells; site of future cartilage formation [*chondr-* cartilage, *-fic-* make, *-ation* process]

chondrocyte (KON-droh-syte) cartilage cell [*chondro-* cartilage, *-cyte* cell]

chondroitin sulphate (kon-DROY-tin SUHL-fayt) type of proteoglycan that helps thicken and hold together the matrix of connective tissue; *see* **proteoglycan** [*chondr-* cartilage, *-oid* of or like, *-in* substance, *sulph-* sulphur, *-ate* oxygen]

chondroma (kon-DROH-mah) benign tumour of cartilage [*chondr-* cartilage, *-oma* tumour]

chondromalacia patellae (kon-droh-mah-LAY-shee-ah pah-TEL-ee) degenerative process that results in a softening of the articular surface of the patella [*chondro-* cartilage, *-malacia* softening, *pat-* dish, *-ella* small]

chordae tendineae (KOR-dee ten-DIN-ee-ee) stringlike structures that attach the AV valves to the wall of the heart [*chorda* string or cord, *tendinea* pulled tight] *sing.*, chorda tendinea

chorion (KOH-ree-on) outermost fetal membrane; contributes to tissues in the placenta [*chorion* skin]

chorionic villi (koh-ree-ON-ik VIL-eye) connection between blood vessels of the chorion and those of the placenta [*chorion-* skin, *-ic* relating to]

chorionic villus sampling (CVS) (koh-ree-ON-ik VIL-lus) procedure in which a tube is inserted through the (uterine) cervical opening and a sample of the chorionic tissue surrounding a developing embryo is removed for karyotyping [*chorion-* skin, *-ic* relating to, *villus* shaggy hair]

choroid (KOH-royd) middle layer of the eyeball; contains a dark pigment that prevents the scattering of incoming light rays [*chorio-* skin, *-oid* like]

choroid plexus (KOH-royd PLEK-sus) tuft of capillaries in ventricles of the brain that secrete cerebrospinal fluid [*chorio-* skin, *-oid* like, *plexus* braid or network] *pl.*, plexi (PLEK-sye) or plexuses (PLEK-sus-eez)

chromatid (KROH-mah-tid) either of the two DNA strands joined by a centromere existing after DNA has replicated (before cell division) but before the centromere has divided [*chrom-* colour, *-id* structure or body]

chromatin (KROH-mah-tin) threadlike form of DNA, making up the genetic material in the nucleus [*chrom-* colour, *-in* substance]

chromosomal genetic disease (kroh-moh-SOH-mal jeh-NET-ik) disease that results from chromosomal breakage or from abnormal presence or absence of entire chromosomes [*chrom-* colour, *-soma-* body, *-al* relating to, *gen-* produce, *-ic* relating to, *dis-* opposite of, *-ease* comfort]

chromosome (KROH-meh-sohm) compact, barlike bodies of chromatin (DNA) that have coiled to form a compact mass during mitosis or meiosis; each chromosome is composed of regions called *genes*, each of which transmits hereditary information [*chrom-* colour, *-som-* body]

chromosome territory (CT) (KROH-meh-sohm TAIR-ih-tor-ee) defined location within a cell's nucleus for a specific chromosome (chromatin strand) [*chrom-* colour, *-som-* body, *terri-* land, *-ory* place]

chronic (KRON-ik) long-lasting, as in "chronic disease" [*chron-* time, *-ic* relating to]

chronic glomerulonephritis (KRON-ik gloh-mer-yoo-loh-neh-FRY-tis) noninfectious glomerular disorder characterized by progressive kidney damage leading to renal failure [*chron-* time, *-ic* relating to, *glomer-* ball, *-ul-* little, *-nephr-* kidney, *-itis* inflammation]

chronic lymphocytic leukaemia (CLL) (KRON-ik LIM-foh-sit-ik loo-KEE-mee-ah) white blood cell disorder that produces large numbers of malignant precursor B lymphocytes [*chron-* time, *-ic* relating to, *lymph-* water (lymphatic system), *-cyte* cell, *leuk-* white, *-(h)aem-* blood, *-ia* condition]

chronic myeloid leukaemia (CML) (KRON-ik MY-eh-loyd loo-KEE-mee-ah) white blood cell disorder that results from cancerous transformation of granulocytic precursor cells in the bone marrow [*chronos-* time, *-ic* relating to, *myel-* bone marrow, *leuk-* white, *-(h)aem-* blood, *-ia* condition]

chronic obstructive pulmonary disease (COPD) (KRON-ik ob-STRUK-tiv PUL-moh-nair-ee) general term referring to a group of disorders characterized by progressive, irreversible obstruction of airflow in the lungs; *see* asthma, bronchitis, emphysema [*chron-* time, *-ic* relating to, *pulmon-* lung, *-ary* relating to, *dis-* opposite of, *-ease* comfort]

chronic pain (KRON-ik) pain that continues over a prolonged time [*chron-* time, *-ic* relating to]

chronic renal failure (KRON-ik REE-nal FAYL-yoor) slow, progressive condition resulting from gradual loss of nephrons [*chron-* time, *-ic* relating to, *ren-* kidney, *-al* relating to]

chronological age (kroh-noh-LODJ-ih-kul ayj) age of an individual expressed in years [*chrono-* time, *-log-* words (study of), *-ical* relating to]

chronotropic (kroh-noh-TROH-pik) refers to anything that affects the rate of myocardial contractions (heart rate) [*chron-* time, *-trop-* turn or change, *-ic* relating to]

chyle (kile) milky fluid; the fat-containing lymph in the lymphatics of the intestine [*chyl-* juice]

chylomicron (kye-loh-MY-kron) small fat droplet [*chylo-* juice (chyle), *-micro-* small, *-on* particle]

chyme (kyme) partially digested food mixture leaving the stomach [*chym-* juice]

chymotrypsin (kye-moh-TRIP-sin) pancreatic enzyme that digests proteins in the digestive tract [*chymo-* juice, *-tryps-* pound, *-in* substance]

cilia (SIL-ee-ah) hairlike projections of cells [*cili-* eyelid, *-a* things (eyelashes)] *sing.*, cilium

ciliary body (SIL-ee-air-ee) thickening of the choroid that is located between the anterior margin of the retina and the posterior margin of the iris [*cilia-* eyelashes, *-ary* relating to]

ciliary muscle (SIL-ee-air-ee) smooth muscle in the ciliary body of the eye that suspends the lens and functions in accommodation [*ciliary* eyelids or eyelashes, *mus-* mouse, *-cle* little]

cilium (SIL-ee-um) *see* **cilia** [*cili-* eyelid, *-um* thing (eyelash)] *pl.*, cilia (SIL-ee-ah)

circadian (sir-KAY-dee-en) occurring in a daily cycle [*circa-* around, *-di-* day, *-an* relating to]

circular movement (SUR-kyoo-ler MOOV-ment) arclike rotation of structure around an axis [*circul-* round, *-ar* relating to]

circular muscle (SUR-kyoo-ler MUSS-el) muscle that circles a body tube or opening; sometimes called *sphincter* [*circul-* round, *-ar* relating to, *mus-* mouse, *-cle* little]

circulatory shock (SUR-kyoo-lah-tor-ee) failure of the circulatory system to adequately deliver oxygen to the tissues [*circulat-* go around, *-ory* relating to]

circulatory system (SUR-kyoo-lah-tor-ee) system composed of the heart, blood vessels, and lymphatic vessels; permits transportation of material to and from all the cells of the body [*circulat-* go around, *-ory* relating to]

circumcision (sur-kum-SIH-zhun) surgical removal of the foreskin, or prepuce, of the penis [*circum-* around, *-cis-* cut, *-ion* process]

circumduction (sur-kum-DUK-shun) moving a part so its distal end moves in a circle [*circum-* around, *-duct-* lead, *-tion* process]

circumvallate papilla (sur-kum-VAL-ayt pah-PIL-ah) any of the huge domelike bumps with central posts on the posterior surface of the tongue mucosa that form a transverse row; each one contains thousands of taste buds [*circum-* around, *-vall-* post or stake, *-ate* relating to, *papilla* nipple] *pl.*, papillae (pah-PIL-ee)

cirrhosis (sih-ROH-sis) degeneration of liver tissue characterized by the replacement of damaged liver tissue with fibrous or fatty connective tissue [*cirrhos-* yellow-orange, *-osis* condition]

cisterna (sis-TER-na) tiny, membranous sacs, such as those that make up the Golgi apparatus [*cisterna* vessel] *pl.*, cisternae (sis-TER-nee)

cisterna chyli (sis-TER-nah KYE-lye) an enlarged pouch on the thoracic duct that serves as a storage area for lymph moving toward its point of entry into the venous system [*cisterna* vessel, *chyli* of juice]

citric acid cycle (SIT-rik ASS-id SYE-kul) second series of chemical reactions in the process of glucose metabolism in which carbon dioxide is formed and energy is released; it is an aerobic process; *see* **Krebs cycle** [*citr-* lemony, *-ic* relating to, *acid* sour, *cycl-* circle]

clavicle (KLAV-ih-kul) collar bone [*clavi-* key, *-cle* little]

cleavage line (KLEEV-ij) pattern of dense bundles of white collagenous fibres that characterize the reticular layers of dermis; also called *Langer lines* [*cleave* to split]

cleft lip (kleft) a congenital defect that affects the mouth; failure of structures in the upper lip to fuse properly during embryonic development [*cleft* split]

cleft palate (kleft PAL-ett) facial deformity that is an X-linked inherited condition; when the palatine bones fail to unite completely [*cleft* split, *palate* plate]

climacteric (klye-MAK-ter-ik) *see* **menopause** [*climacter-* critical point, *-ic* relating to]

clitoris (KLIT-oh-ris) small, erectile body located within the vestibule of the vagina; also called *glans clitoris* [*clitoris* small key or latch] *pl.*, clitorides (KLIT-oh-rid-eez)

clonal selection theory (KLOH-nal) process through which a B or T cell, once sensitized through contact with an antigen, divides rapidly to create a colony of clones that destroys the "selecting" antigen [*clon-* (plant) cutting, *-al* relating to, *theor-* look at, *-y* act of]

clone (klohn) any of a family of many identical cells descended from a single "parent" cell [*clone* a (plant) cutting]

closed fracture (klohzd FRAK-chur) *see* **simple fracture** [*fracture* a breaking]

closed reduction process by which a fracture is properly aligned without the need for surgery [*re-* again or back, *-duc-* lead, *-tion* process]

coagulation (koh-ag-yoo-LAY-shun) *see* **blood coagulation** [*coagul-* curdle, *-ation* process]

cocaine (koh-KAYN) drug that blocks the uptake of dopamine (neurotransmitter) by neurons, thus inhibiting pain signals or producing a temporary feeling of well-being [*coca-* type of shrub, *-ine* made of]

coccygeus muscle (kohk-SIJ-ee-us) one of the muscles that form the pelvic floor [*coccygeus* coccyx (cuckoo), *mus-* mouse, *-cle* little]

coccyx (KOK-sis) last bone of the vertebral column, made up of four or five vertebrae that have fused together [*coccyx* cuckoo (beak)]

cochlea (KOHK-lee-ah) snail shell–like structure in the inner ear that houses the spiral organ (organ of Corti), which is responsible for sense of hearing [*cochlea* snail shell]

cochlear duct (KOHK-lee-ar dukt) membranous tube within the bony cochlea; only part of the internal ear concerned with hearing [*cochlea-* snail shell, *-ar* relating to, *duct* path]

cochlear nerve (KOHK-lee-ar nerv) part of vestibulocochlear nerve (cranial nerve VIII); sensory nerve responsible for hearing [*cochlea-* snail shell, *-ar* relating to]

codominance (koh-DOM-ih-nance) in genetics, a form of dominance in which two dominant versions of a trait are both expressed in the same individual [*co-* together, *-domina-* rule, *-ance* state]

codon (KOH-don) in RNA, a triplet of three base pairs that codes for a particular amino acid; subunit of a protein-coding gene [*cod-* book, *-on* unit]

coeliac ganglion (SEE-lee-ak GANG-glee-on) solar plexus; collateral ganglion that lies just below the diaphragm [*cel-* belly, *-ac* relating to, *ganglion* knot]

coenzyme (koh-EN-zyme) organic, nonprotein catalyst that acts as molecule carrier [*co-* together, *-en-* in, *-zyme* ferment]

coenzyme A (CoA) (koh-EN-zyme) molecule that is converted from pyruvic acid in cell respiration; allows for the transition to the citric acid cycle from glycolysis [*co-* together, *-en-* in, *-zyme* ferment, A first letter of Roman alphabet]

cofactor (KOH-fak-ter) a nonprotein unit attached to an enzyme molecule than enables the enzyme to function properly [*co-* together, *-factor* maker]

colipase (koh-LYE-payz) coenzyme that assists the hydrolysis of lipids by the enzyme lipase [*co-* with, *lip-* fat, *-ase* enzyme]

colitis (koh-LYE-tis) any inflammatory condition of the colon and/or rectum [*col-* colon, *-itis* inflammation]

collagen (KOL-ah-jen) principal organic constituent of connective tissue [*colla-* glue, *-gen* produce]

collagenous dense fibrous tissue (kah-LAJ-eh-nus dense FYE-brus TISH-yoo) flexible but strong connective tissue; for example, tendons [*colla-* glue, *-gen* produce, *dense* thick, *fibr-* thread or fibre, *-ous* relating to, *tissu-* fabric]

collateral ganglion (koh-LAT-er-al GANG-glee-on) sympathetic, prevertebral ganglion; named for nearby blood vessels [*co-* together, *-later-* side, *-al* relating to, *gangli-* knot, *-on* unit] *pl.*, ganglia (GANG-glee-ah)

collecting duct (koh-LEK-ting) in the kidney, straight tubule joined by the distal tubules of several nephrons [*co-* together, *-lect-* gather, *duct* path]

Colles fracture (KOL-ez) fracture of the distal end of the radius [*Abraham Colles*, Irish surgeon, *fracture* a breaking]

colloid (KOL-oyd) dissolved particles that resist separation from the gas, liquid, or solid medium in which they are dissolved [*coll-* glue, *-oid* resembling]

colloid osmotic pressure (KOL-oyd os-MOT-ik) *see* **blood colloid osmotic pressure** [*coll-* glue, *-oid* like, *osmo-* push, *-ic* relating to]

colon (KOH-lon) division of the large intestine; divided into ascending, transverse, descending, and sigmoid portions [*colon* large intestine]

colonoscopy (koh-lon-OS-kah-pee) medical procedure in which the lining of the colon is checked for colorectal cancer or other abnormalities by inserting a flexible scope through the anus and into the colon [*colon* large intestine, *-scop-* see, *-y* activity]

colour Doppler mapping (DOP-ler) variation of ultrasonography that converts recorded flow frequencies into different colours; colour images are then superimposed on M-mode or two-dimensional echocardiograms [*Christian Doppler* Australian physicist/mathematician]

colorectal cancer (koh-loh-REK-tal) malignancy of the colon or rectum [*colo-* colon, *-rect-* straight or upright, *-al* relating to, *cancer* crab or malignant tumour]

columnar (koh-LUM-nar) cell classification by shape in which cells are higher than they are wide [*column-* column, *-ar* relating to]

coma (KOH-mah) altered state of consciousness from which an individual cannot be aroused [*coma* deep sleep]

combining site (kom-BYNE-ing syte) either of two small concave regions on the surface of an antibody molecule to which other molecules attach; any molecular attachment site [*com-* together, *-bine* two at a time]

comedo (KOM-ee-doh) inflamed, plugged sebaceous gland duct, common in acne conditions; *see also* **blackhead** [*comedo* glutton (applied to secretions that resemble body-devouring worms)]

comminuted fracture (kom-ih-NOO-ted) fracture that results in small, crushed bone fragments between or near the broken ends of the bone [*commin-* break into pieces, *-ute* perform action, *fracture* a breaking]

commissural tract (kom-MIS-yoo-ral) nerve tissue that connects the left and right hemispheres of the brain; *see* **corpus callosum** [*commissura-* a connection, *-al* relating to, *tract* trail]

common bile duct (KOM-on byle) duct from the liver that empties into the duodenum; made up of the merging of the hepatic duct with the cystic duct [*duct* path]

common carotid artery (kah-ROT-id AR-ter-ee) blood vessel that supplies the region of the head and neck [*caro-* heavy sleep, *-id* relating to, *arteri-* vessel]

communicable (kom-MYOO-nih-kah-bil) able to spread from one individual to another [*communic-* common, *-able* capacity for]

compact bone tissue dense bone; contains structural units called *osteons* or *Haversian systems* [*tissu-* fabric]

compensation (kom-pen-SAY-shun) physiological process in which the body's functions compensate, or counterbalance, a deviation from the normal set-point value of a characteristic of the body's internal environment—for example, pH [*compens-* balance, *-tion* process]

complement (KOM-pleh-ment) any of several proteins normally present in blood plasma that when activated kill foreign cells by puncturing them [*comple-* complete, *-ment* process]

complementary (base) pairing bonding purines and pyrimidines in DNA; adenine always binds with thymine, and cytosine always binds with guanine [*comple-* complete, *-ment-* process, *-ary* relating to]

complete blood cell count (CBC) (kom-PLEET blud sel kownt) clinical blood test that usually includes standard red blood cell, white blood cell, thrombocyte counts, the differential white blood cell count, haematocrit, and haemoglobin content [*cell* storeroom]

complete fracture (kom-PLEET FRAK-chur) fracture that totally divides a bone into separate pieces [*fracture* a breaking]

compliance (kom-PLY-ans) the ease of stretch of a material—as in lung compliance, the ease of stretch of the lung tissues [*compli-* fill up, *-ance* act of]

composite cell (KOM-pah-zit) artistic representation of a cell that includes features from many different types of cells [*cell* storeroom]

compound a chemical combination of two or more elements [*compound* put together]

compound fracture type of bone fracture in which broken bone projects through surrounding tissue and skin, thereby inviting the possibility of osteomyelitis; also called *displaced* or *open fracture* [*compound* put together, *fracture* a breaking]

computed tomography (CT) (kom-PYOO-ted toh-MOG-rah-fee) x-ray technique that produces an image representing a detailed cross-section of a body structure [*tomo-* cut, *-graph-* draw, *-y* process]

concentration gradient (kon-sen-TRAY-shun GRAY-dee-ent) measurable difference in concentration from one area to another [*con-* together, *-centr-* centre, *-ation* process, *gradi-* step, *-ent* state]

concentric contraction (kon-SEN-trik kon-TRAK-shun) contraction in which the movement results in shortening of the muscle; type of isotonic contraction or dynamic tension [*con-* together, *-centr-* centre, *-ic* relating to, *con-* together, *-tract-* drag or draw, *-tion* process]

concha (KONG-kah) scroll-shaped bone that forms a ledge projecting into the nasal cavity from its lateral wall [*concha* sea shell] *pl.*, conchae (KONG-kee or KONG-kay)

concussion (kon-KUHSH-un) damage to the brain from a blow to the head or violent shakings; sometimes called *mild traumatic brain injury (MTBI)* [*con-* with, *-cuss-* shake, *-ion* condition]

condensation (kon-den-SAY-shun) see **dehydration synthesis** [*con-* together, *-dense-* thick or crowded, *-tion* process]

conduction in human anatomy, the transfer of heat energy to the skin and then the external environment [*con-* with, *duct-* lead, *-tion* process]

conductive keratoplasty (CK) (kon-DUK-tiv ker-ah-toh-PLAS-tee) treatment for the correction of farsightedness [*con-* with, *duct-* lead, *-ive* relating to, *kera-* horn, *-plasty* surgical repair]

conductivity (kon-duk-TIV-uh-tee) ability of living cells and tissues to selectively transmit a wave of excitation from one point to another within the body [*con-* with, *duct-* lead, *-iv-* relating to, *-ity* state]

condyloid joint (KON-dih-loyd) ellipsoidal joint [*condylo-* knuckle, *-oid* resembling, *jungere-* to join]

cone receptor cell located in the retina that is stimulated by bright light

congenital abnormality (kon-JEN-ih-tal ab-nor-MAL-ih-tee) *see* **congenital disorder** [*con-* with, *-genit-* born, *-al* relating to]

congenital disorder (kon-JEN-ih-tal) refers to a condition present at birth; congenital conditions may be inherited or may be acquired in

the womb or during delivery [*con-* with, *-ge-nit-* born, -al relating to]
congestive heart failure (CHF) (kon-JES-tive) left-sided heart failure; inability of the left ventricle to pump effectively, resulting in congestion in the systemic and pulmonary circulations [*congest-* crowd together, *-ive* relating to]
conjunctiva (kon-junk-TIH-vah) mucous membrane that lines the eyelids and covers the sclera (white portion of the eye) [*con-* together, *-junct-* join, *-iv-* relating to, *-a* thing]
conjunctivitis (kon-junk-tih-VYE-tis) inflammation of the conjunctiva, usually caused by irritation, infection, or allergy [*con-* together, *-junct-* join, *-iv-* relating to, *-itis* inflammation]
connective tissue most abundant and widely distributed tissue in the body [*con-* together, *-nect-* bind, *-ive* relating to, *tissu-* fabric]
connective tissue membrane body membrane that lines movable joint cavities; for example, synovial [*con-* together, *-nect-* bind, *-ive* relating to, *tissu-* fabric, *membrane* thin skin]
connectome (kon-NEK-tohm) map of all the neural connections of the brain [*con-* together, *-nect-* bind, *-ome* complete set]
consciousness state of awareness of one's self and environment and other beings [*conscire-* to know wrong]
constipation (kon-stih-PAY-shun) condition that results when extra water is absorbed from the faecal mass, producing a hardened stool [*con-stipa-* crowd together, *-ation* process]
contact dermatitis (der-mah-TYE-tis) local skin inflammation lasting a few hours or days after being exposed to an antigen [*derma-* skin, *-itis* inflammation]
contact digestion (dye-JES-chun) when substrates bind onto enzymes located on the surface of the brush border and complete carbohydrate digestion [*digest-* break apart, *-tion* process]
continuous ambulatory peritoneal dialysis (CAPD) (AM-byoo-lah-tor-ee pair-ih-toh-NEE-al dye-AL-ih-sis) technique used in the treatment of renal failure [*ambulat-* walk, *-ory* relating to, *peritone-* peritoneum, *-al* relating to, *dia-* through, *-lysis* loosening]
continuous capillary (kah-PIL-air-ee) capillaries that have a continuous lining of endothelial cells with only small openings between them [*capill-* hair, *-ary* relating to]
continuous positive airway pressure (CPAP) special type of mechanical respirator used to treat infant respiratory distress syndrome
contractility (kon-trak-TIL-ih-tee) ability, as of muscle cell, to contract or shorten to produce movement [*con-* together, *-tract-* drag or draw, *-il-* of or like, *-ity* quality of]
contraction (kon-TRAK-shun) tension of muscle fibres produced by sliding of cytoskeletal filaments and producing either shortening of the muscle fibre, pull on a load, or both [*con-* together, *-tract-* drag or draw, *-tion* process]
contralateral (kon-trah-LAT-er-al) on the opposite side of the body [*contra-* against, *-later-* side, *-al* relating to]
contralateral reflex arc (kon-trah-LAT-er-al REE-fleks ark) reflex arc whose receptor and effectors are located on opposite sides of the body [*contra-* against, *-later-* side, *-al* relating to, *re-* again, *-flex* bend]
contusion (kon-TYOO-zhun) a bruise; an injury in which the skin or surface of an organ is not broken but underlying blood vessels rupture and leak into interstitial space [*contus-* bruise, *-sion* result]
conus medullaris (KOH-nus med-yoo-LAIR-is) tapered end of the spinal cord [*conus* cone, *medulla* marrow or pith (middle), *-ar-* relating to, *-is* thing] *pl.*, coni medullares (KOH-nye med-yoo-LAIR-eez)
convection (kon-VEK-shun) in human anatomy, transfer of heat energy to air that is flowing away from the skin [*con-* together, *-vect-* carry, *-tion* process]
convergence (kon-VER-jens) a coming together, as in movement of the two eyeballs inward so that their visual axes come together at the same point on the object viewed; also, when more than one presynaptic axon synapses with a single postsynaptic neuron [*con-* together, *-verg-* incline, *-ence* state]
convergent muscle (kon-VER-jent) muscle that radiates out from a small to a wider point of attachment; for example, pectoralis major [*con-* together, *-verg-* incline, *-ent* state, *mus-* mouse, *-cle* little]
convolution (kon-voh-LOO-shun) *see* **gyrus** [*con-* together, *-volut-* roll, *-tion* process]
convulsion (kon-VUL-shun) abnormal, uncoordinated tetanic contractions of varying groups of muscles; also called *seizure* [*con-vuls-* pull violently, *-sion* result]
cor pulmonale (kohr pul-mah-NAL-ee) failure of the right atrium and ventricle to pump blood effectively, resulting from obstruction of pulmonary blood flow [*cor* heart, *pulmon-* lung, *-ale* relating to]
Cori cycle (KOR-ee SYE-kul) circular metabolic pathway in which lactate produced by anaerobic glycolysis in skeletal muscles is carried to liver cells, where it is converted back to glucose and stored as liver glycogen or returned to the bloodstream [*Carl Ferdinand Cori and Gerty Radnitz Cori* Czech-American biochemists, *cycl-* circle]
cornea (KOR-nee-ah) transparent, anterior portion of the fibrous layer of the eye [*corn-* horn, *-a* thing]
corneal reflex (KOR-nee-al REE-fleks) blinking in response to the cornea being touched [*corn-* horn, *-al* relating to, *re-* again, *-flex* bend]
corneocyte (KOR-nee-o-site) dead, flattened keratinocyte (epidermal cell of skin) that has filled with keratin and formed a dense, waterproof epidermal layer called *stratum corneum* [*corn-* horn, *-cyte* cell]
corona radiata (ko-ROHN-ah ray-dee-AH-tah) layer surrounding ovum and its zona pellucida; made up of cumulus cells derived from the ovarian follicle [*corona* crown, *radiata* radiant (with rays)]
coronal plane (ko-RO-nal) frontal plane; divides the body into front and back portions [*corona-* crown, *-al* relating to, *plan-* flat surface]
coronary artery (KOHR-oh-nair-ee AR-ter-ee) blood vessel that provides blood to the myocardial cells [*corona-* crown, *-ary* relating to, *arteri-* vessel]
coronary artery disease (CAD) (KOHR-oh-nair-ee AR-ter-ee) condition that results from reduced blood flow to the myocardial tissue [*corona-* crown, *-ary* relating to, *arteri-* vessel, *dis-* opposite of, *-ease* comfort]
coronary bypass surgery (KOHR-oh-nair-ee) surgery to relieve severely restricted coronary blood flow; veins are taken from other parts of the body and grafted in to bypass the blockage [*corona-* crown, *-ary* relating to, *sur-* hand, *-urger-* work, *-y* activity]
coronary sinus (KOHR-oh-nair-ee SYE-nus) area that receives deoxygenated blood from the coronary veins and empties into the right atrium [*corona-* crown, *-ary* relating to, *sinus* hollow]
coronoid fossa (KOHR-uh-noyd FOSS-ah) depression at the distal end of the humerus bone, into which the coronoid process of the ulna fits (last part of the humerus-ulna articulation) [*coron-* crown, *-oid* like, *fossa* ditch] *pl.* fossae (FOSS-ee)
corpora cavernosa (KOHR-pohr-ah kav-er-NO-sah) *see* **corpus cavernosum** [*corpora-* bodies, *cavern-* hollow space]
corpora quadrigemina (KOHR-pohr-ah kwod-rih-JEM-ih-nah) midbrain landmark composed of inferior and superior colliculi [*corpora* bodies, *quadri-* fourfold, *-gemina* twin]
corpus albicans (KOHR-pus AL-bih-kans) white scar on ovary that replaces the degenerated corpus luteum [*corpus* body, *albicans* white] *pl.*, corpora albicantia (KOHR-pohr-ah al-bi-KAN-sha)
corpus callosum (KOHR-pus kah-LOH-sum) nerve tissue connecting the right and left cerebral hemispheres; also called *commissural tract* [*corpus* body, *callosum* callous or tough] *pl.*, corpora callosa (KOHR-por-ah kah-LOH-sah)
corpus cavernosum (KOHR-pus kav-er-NO-sum) either of two columns of erectile tissue in the shaft of the penis [*corpus* body, *cavern-* large hollow, *-os-* relating to, *-um* thing] *pl.*, corpora cavernosa (KOHR-por-ah kav-er-NO-sah)
corpus luteum (KOHR-pus LOO-tee-um) a hormone-secreting glandular structure formed after ovulation at the site of the ruptured follicle; it secretes chiefly progesterone with some oestrogen [*corpus* body, *lute-* yellow, *-um* thing] *pl.*, corpora lutea (KOHR-pohr-ah LOO-tee-ah)
corpus spongiosum (KOHR-pus spun-jee-OH-sum) a column of erectile tissue surrounding the urethra in the penis [*corpus* body, *spong-* sponge,*-os-* relating to, *-um* thing] *pl.*, corpora spongiosa (KOHR-pohr-ah spun-jee-OH-sah)
correction process in which a function is made to work properly, as in adjusting refraction of light in the eye to improve focusing an image on the retina
corrugator supercilii muscle (COR-uh-gaytor soo-per-SIL-ee-eye) muscle that draws the eyebrows together [*corrugator* wrinkler, *super-* above, *-cilli-* eyelash, *mus-* mouse, *-cle* little]
cortex (KOHR-teks) outer part of an internal organ; for example, the outer part of the cerebrum or the outer portion of the kidneys [*cortex* bark] *pl.*, cortices (KORT-is-eez)
cortical (KOHR-tih-kal) to the cortex, or outer area of an organ or structure [*cortic-* cortex (bark), *-al* relating to]
cortical nephron (KOHR-tih-kal NEF-rons) nephron located in the renal cortex [*cortic-* cortex (bark), *-al* relating to, *nephro-* kidney, *-on* unit]
cortical nodule (KOHR-tih-kal NOD-yool) located within sinuses along the cortex of the lymph node; packed with lymphocytes surrounding the germinal centre [*cortic-* cortex (bark), *-al* relating to, *nod-* knot, *-ule* small]
corticoid (KOHR-tih-koyd) hormone secreted by the adrenal cortex [*cortic-* cortex or bark, *-oid* like]
corticosteroid (kohr-tih-koh-STER-royd) glucocorticoid secreted by zona fasciculata of the adrenal cortex [*cortico-* cortex (bark), *-stero-* solid, *-oid* resembling]
corticotroph (kohr-tih-koh-TROHF) cell type of the adenohypophysis (anterior pituitary) that secretes ACTH (adrenocorticotropic hormone) and tiny amounts of melanocortins such as a-MSH (alpha melanocyte-stimulating hormone) [*cortic-* cortex (bark), *-troph* nourish]
cortisol (KOHR-tih-sol) glucocorticoid secreted by zona fasciculata of the adrenal cortex; also known as *hydrocortisone* [*cortis-* cortex (bark), *-ol* alcohol]
cortisone (KOHR-tih-sohn) *see* **cortisol** [*corti-* cortex (bark)]
costal cartilage (KOS-tal KAR-tih-lij) cartilage that attaches ribs two through ten to the body of the sternum [*costa-* rib, *-al* relating to, *cartilag-* cartilage]
costal surface (KOS-tal) region of the lungs that lies against the ribs; rounded to match contour of thoracic cavity [*costa-* rib, *-al* relating to]
cotransmission (koh-tranz-MISH-un) theory of efferent autonomic synaptic transmission that states that all or most postganglionic fibres release either norepinephrine or acetylcholine along with NANC (nonadrenergic-noncholinergic) transmitters or modulators and that each substance combines with post-synaptic and/or presynaptic receptors to produce regulatory effects [*co-* together, *-trans-* across, *-miss-* send, *-ion* process]
cotransport (koh-TRANZ-port) carrier that moves two or more solute types across the plasma membrane in the same direction; also called *symport* [*co-* together, *-trans-* across, *-port* carry]
cough reflex (kawf REE-fleks) epiglottis and glottis close and contract in response to foreign matter in the trachea or bronchi [*re-* back or again, *-flex* bend]
coumarin (KOO-mar-in) compound that retards blood coagulation; often given as medication to prevent heart attacks [*coumar-* tonka bean tree, *-in* substance]
countercurrent mechanism (KOWN-ter-kerrent MEK-a-niz-em) system in which renal tubule filtrate flows in opposite directions; facilitates urine concentration [*counter-* against, *-current* flow]
countertransport (KOWN-ter-tranz-port) carrier that moves two different types of molecules in opposite directions across the plasma membrane; also called *antiport* [*counter-* against, *-trans-* across, *-port* carry]
covalent bond (ko-VAYL-ent) chemical bond formed by two atoms sharing one or more pairs of electrons [*co-* with, *-valen-* power, *bond* band]
Cowper gland (KOW-per) *see* **bulbourethral gland** [*William Cowper* English anatomist]
COX inhibitor (KOKS in-HIB-it-or) drug that slows or stops the activity of the COX enzyme, which produces prostaglandins that stimulate an inflammatory response [*COX* acronym for *cycloxygenase*]
coxal (KOK-sal) relating to the hip [*coxa-* hip, *-al* relating to]
coxal bone (KOK-sal bohn) hip bone [*coxa-* hip, *-al* relating to]
CPL (C P L) a submicroscopic vesicle (bubble or membrane) within cells that acts as a "compartment for peptide loading (CPL)", in which proteins are altered in structure [shortened form of *compartment for peptide loading*]
cramp painful muscle spasm (involuntary twitch) that results from irritating stimuli, as in mild inflammation, or from ion imbalances (as in fatigue) [*cramp* bent]
cranial (KRAY-nee-al) relating to the skull [*crani-* skull, *-al* relating to]
cranial nerve (KRAY-nee-al nerv) any of twelve pairs of nerves that attach to the undersurface of the brain and conduct impulses between the brain and structures in the head, neck, and thorax [*crani-* skull, *-al* relating to]
cranial reflex (KRAY-nee-al REE-fleks) reflex response mediated within the brain [*crani-* skull, *-al* relating to, *re-* again, *-flex* bend]
craniosacral division (kray-nee-oh-SAY-kral) parasympathetic division of the autonomic nervous system [*cranio-* skull, *-sacer* sacred, *-al* relating to]
cranium (KRAY-nee-um) bony vault, made up of eight bones, that encases the brain [*cra-nium* skull]
C-reactive protein (CRP) (see re-AK-tiv PRO-teen) blood marker for inflammation; elevated levels suggest cardiac disease [C C-polysaccharide of *Pneumococcus* bacteria, *re-* again, *-act-* act, *-ive* characterized by, *prote-* first rank, *-in* substance]
creatine phosphate (CP) (KREE-ah-tin FOS-fayt) substance found in muscle cells and used for the temporary storage of chemical energy to supply ATP and ultimately for muscle contraction [*creat-* flesh, *-ine* relating to, *phosph-* phosphorus, *-ate* oxygen]
cremaster muscle (kreh-MASS-ter) muscle responsible for elevating the testes [*cremaster* hanger, *mus-* mouse, *-cle* little]
crepitus (KREP-ih-tus) sound of bone fragments rubbing together [*crepitus* crackling]

Creutzfeldt–Jakob Disease (CJD) (KROYTS-felt YAH-kobe) *see* **variant Creutzfeldt–Jakob disease (vCJD)** [*Hans* G. *Creutzfeldt* German neurologist, *Alfons* M. *Jakob* German neurologist, *dis-* opposite of, *-ease* comfort]
cribriform plate (KRIB-rih-form) perforated portion of ethmoid bone that separates the nasal and cranial cavities [*cribr-* sieve, *-form* shape]
crista (KRIS-tah) fold, for example, any of the folds of the inner membrane of a mitochondrion [*crista* crest or fold] *pl.*, cristae (KRIS-tee)
crista ampullaris (KRIS-tah am-pyoo-LAIR-iss) fold that serves as a sensory receptor organ located within the ampulla of the semicircular ducts; detects head movements [*crista* ridge, *ampu-* flask, *-ulla-* little, *-ar-* relating to, *-is* thing] *pl.*, cristae ampulares (KRIS-tee am-pyoo-LAIR-eez)
Crohn disease (krohn) type of autoimmune colitis affecting the small intestine [*Burrill B. Crohn* American physician, *dis-* opposite of, *-ease* comfort]
cross bridge junction of a thick myofilament with a thin myofilament in the myofibril of a muscle fibre, where the head of a myosin molecule in the thick filament binds to the active site of an actin molecule in the thin filament
cross-section (kraws SEK-shun) any cut made in a body part along a plane parallel to the short axis of that body part [*cross-* across, *sect-* cut, *-tion* process]
crossing over phenomenon that occurs during meiosis when pairs of homologous chromosomes synapse and exchange genes
croup (kroop) syndrome characterized by laboured inspiration and a harsh vibrating cough [*croup* croak]
crown topmost part of an organ or other structure
cruciate ligament (KRU-shee-ayt) either of two crossed ligaments inside the knee joint cavity that connect the tibia to the femur; the *anterior cruciate ligament (ACL)* and the *posterior cruciate ligament (PCL)* [*cruci-* cross, *-ate* of or like]
crural (KROO-ral) relating to the leg; sometimes instead refers to the thigh or to the thigh and leg together [*crur-* leg, *-al* relating to]
cryopreservation (krye-oh-prez-er-VAY-shun) deep freezing technique; used for reimplantation of parathyroid tissue [*cryo-* cold, *-preserv-* to keep, *-tion* process]
cryptorchidism (krip-TOR-kih-diz-em) condition resulting in undescended testes [*crypt-* hidden, *-orchid-* testis, *-ism* condition]
cubital (KYOO-bi-tal) relating to the elbow; sometimes instead refers to forearm [*cubit-* elbow, *-al* relating to]
cuboidal (KYOO-boyd-al) cell classification by shape in which cells resemble a cube [*cub-* cube, *-oid* like, *-al* relating to]
cupula (KYOO-pyoo-lah) structure found within the crista ampullaris of the semicircular duct; the gelatinous ridge in which the hair cells are embedded [*cup-* tub, *-ula* little] *pl.*, cupulae (KYOO-pyoo-lee)
Cushing syndrome (KOOSH-ing SIN-drohm) condition caused by hypersecretion of glucocorticoids from the adrenal cortex [*Harvey* W. *Cushing* American neurosurgeon, *syn-* together, *-drome* running or (race) course]
cuspid valve (KUS-pid) *see* **atrioventricular valve** [*cusp-* point, *-id* characterized by]
cutaneous (kyoo-TAYN-ee-us) relating to the skin [*cut-* skin, *-aneous* relating to]
cutaneous membrane (kyoo-TAYN-ee-us MEM-brayn) primary organ of the integumentary system; the skin [*cut-* skin, *-aneous* relating to, *membran-* thin skin]
cuticle (KYOO-tih-kul) skin fold covering the root of the nail [*cut-* skin, *-icle* little]
cyanosis (sye-ah-NO-sis) condition of blueness, particularly of the skin, resulting from inadequate oxygenation of the blood [*cyan-* blue, *-osis* condition]
cyclic AMP (SIK-lik A M P) one of several second messengers that delivers information inside the cell and thus regulates the cell's activity [*cycl-* circle, *-ic* relating to]
cyclin (SYE-klin) any of several regulatory proteins in the cell that influence the function of activating enzymes called *cyclin-dependent kinases* that drive the cell forward from phase to phase in the cell life cycle and thus regulate the cell's growth and reproduction [*cycl-* circle, *-in* substance]
cyclin-dependent kinase (CDK) (SYE-klin dee-PEND-ent KIE-nays) any of several activating enzymes that drive the cell through the various phases of its life cycle; "cyclin-dependent" refers to the CDK itself being regulated by cellular proteins called *cyclins* [*cycl-* circle, *-in* substance, *de-* from, *-pend-* hang, *-ent* relating to, *kin-* motion, *-ase* enzyme]
cystic duct (SIS-tik dukt) joins with the common hepatic duct to form the common bile duct [*cyst-* sac, *-ic* relating to, *duct* path]
cystic fibrosis (CF) (SIS-tik fye-BROH-sis) inherited disease involving abnormal chloride ion (Cl^-) transport (CFTR chloride channel); causes secretion of abnormally thick mucus and other problems [*cyst-* sac, *-ic* relating to; *fibr-* thread or fibre, *-osis* condition]
cystitis (sis-TYE-tis) inflammation of a saclike structure such as the urinary bladder [*cyst-* bag, *-itis* inflammation]
cystoscope (SIS-toh-skohp) device used to look into a bladder, such as the urinary bladder [*cyst-* bag, *-scop-* see]
cytokine (SYE-toh-kyne) chemical released from cells to trigger or regulate innate and adaptive immune responses [*cyto-* cell, *-kine* movement]
cytokinesis (sye-toh-kin-EE-sis) process by which a dividing cell splits its cytoplasm and plasma membrane into two distinct daughter cells; cytokinesis happens along with mitosis (or meiosis) during the cell division process [*cyto-* cell, *-kinesis* movement]
cytology (sye-TOL-oh-jee) study of cells [*cyto-* cell, *-log-* words (study of), *-y* activity]
cytolysis (sye-TOL-ih-sis) literally, "cell bursting"; often occurs when ions and water rush into a cell, causing it to burst [*cyto-* cell, *-lysis* loosening]
cytoplasm (SYE-toh-plaz-em) gel-like substance of a cell exclusive of the nucleus and plasma membrane; includes organelles (except nucleus) and cytosol (intracellular fluid) [*cyto-* cell, *-plasm* substance]
cytoskeleton (sye-toh-SKEL-eh-ton) cell's internal supporting, moving framework [*cyto-* cell, *-skeleton* dried body]
cytosol (SYE-toh-sawl) solution of water and other substances of a cell (outside the nucleus) in which the organelles and cellular inclusions are suspended; it is the liquid portion of the living cell substance known as *cytoplasm* [*cyto-* cell, *-sol* solution]
cytotoxic T cell (sye-toh-TOK-sik) "cell killing" T cell [*cyto-* cell, *-toxic* poison, *T* thymus gland, *cell* storeroom]

D

Dalton's law (DAL-tenz) gas law that states that the total pressure exerted by a mixture of gases is the sum of the pressure of each individual gas; also called *law of partial pressure* [*John Dalton* English chemist and physicist]
deamination (dee-am-ih-NAY-shun) removal of an amino group from an amino acid to form a molecule of ammonia and one of keto acid; occurs in the liver as first step in protein catabolism [*de-* undo, *-amin-* ammonia compound, *-ation* process]
decarboxylase (dee-kar-BOK-sih-lays) enzyme that removes carbon dioxide [*de-* undo, *-carbo* carbon, *-oxy* sour, *-ase* enzyme]
deciduous teeth (deh-SID-yoo-us) commonly referred to as "baby teeth"; 20 teeth that are shed at a certain age before development of permanent teeth [*decid-* fall off, *-ous* relating to]
decomposition reaction (dee-kom-poh-SIH-shun ree-AK-shun) chemical reaction that breaks down a substance into two or more simpler substances [*de-* opposite of, *-compo-* to assemble, *-tion* process, *re-* again, *-action* action]
decubitus ulcer (deh-KYOO-bih-tus UL-ser) area of destroyed tissue resulting from inadequate blood supply that often develops when body lies in one position for prolonged periods [*decubitus* lying-down position, *ulcer* sore]
deep further away from the body's surface, as opposed to superficial
deep vein (deep vayn) vein that is further away from the surface, as opposed to a superficial vein [*vena* blood vessel]
defaecation (def-eh-KAY-shun) expelling faeces from the digestive tract [*de-* remove, *-faeca-* waste (faeces), *-tion* process]
defibrillation (deh-fib-rih-LAY-shun) application of an electric shock to force cardiac muscle fibres to contract in unison [*de-* undo, *-fibr-* thread or fibre, *-illa-* little, *-tion* process]
deglutition (deg-loo-TISH-un) swallowing [*de-glut-* swallow, *-tion* process]
dehydration (dee-hye-DRAY-shun) an abnormal loss of fluid from the body's internal environment [*de-* remove, *-hydr-* water, *-ation* process]
dehydration synthesis (dee-hye-DRAY-shun SIN-the-sis) anabolic process by which molecules are joined to form larger molecules; often called *condensation reaction* because it joins molecules together into a denser mass [*de-* from, *-hydr-* water, *-ation* process, *synthesis* putting together]
deletion (deh-LEE-shun) genetic mutation that occurs within a DNA molecule when one or more nucleotide bases in a sequence are missing, causing a misreading of the genetic code and a failure to produce a normal protein needed for body function
delta (Δ) cell (DEL-tah) pancreatic islet cell that secretes somatostatin; also called *D cell* [*delta (Δ)* fourth letter of Greek alphabet, *cell* storeroom]
deltoid (DEL-toyd) triangular muscle that covers the shoulder joint, abducting the arm [*delta (Δ)* fourth letter of Greek alphabet, *-oid* like]
dementia (de-MEN-shah) degenerative disease that can result in destruction of neurons in the brain [*de-* off, *-ment-* mind, *-ia* condition of]
denature (de-NAYT-shur) to alter the shape of a protein by a change in pH, heat, or some other manner to change its chemical properties [*de-* remove, *-nature* nature]
dendrite (DEN-dryte) branching or treelike nerve cell process that receives input from other neurons and transmits toward the cell body (or toward the axon in a unipolar neuron) [*dendr-* tree, *-ite* part (branch) of]
dendritic cell (DC) (den-DRIH-tik) phagocytic cells in the immune system [*dendr-* tree, *-it-* part (branch) of, *-ic* relating to, *cell* storeroom]
dens (denz) upward projection from the body of the second cervical vertebra that furnishes an axis for rotating the head; also called *odontoid process* [*dens* tooth]
dense fibrous tissue (FYE-brus) tissue consisting of fibres packed densely in the matrix [*dense* thick, *fibr-* thread or fibre, *-ous* relating to, *connect-* bind, *-ive* relating to, *tissu-* fabric]
dentate fracture (DEN-tayt) type of bone fracture in which fracture components are jagged and fit together like teeth on a gear [*dent-* tooth, *-ate* of or like, *fracture* a breaking]
dentate nucleus (DEN-tayt NYOO-klee-us) either of paired cerebellar grey matter structures that are connected by tracts with the thalamus, as well as motor areas of the cerebral cortex [*dent-* tooth, *-ate* of or like, *nucleus* nut or kernel] *pl.*, nuclei (NYOO-klee-eye)
dentin (DEN-tin) hard, mineralized connective tissue similar to bone forming the body of the tooth [*dent-* tooth, *-in* substance]
deoxyribonucleic acid (DNA) (dee-OK-see-rye-boh-nyoo-KLAY-ik ASS-id) genetic material of the cell that carries the chemical "blueprint" of the body [*de-* removed, *-oxy-* oxygen, *-ribo-* ribose, *-nucle-* nucleus (kernel), *-ic* relating to, *acid* sour]
deoxyribonucleotide (dee-OK-see-rye-boh-NYOO-klee-oh-tide) type of nucleotide in DNA, consisting of the pentose sugar named *deoxyribose*, a nitrogenous base (either adenine, cytosine, guanine, or thymine), and a phosphate group [*de-* removed, *-oxy-* oxygen, *-ribo-* ribose, *-nucle-* nucleus (kernel), *nucleo-* nut or kernel, *-ide* chemical]
deoxyribose (dee-ok-see-RYE-bohs) sugar in DNA whose molecules contain only five carbons [*deoxy-* containing a decreased amount of oxygen, *-ribose* five-carbon sugar]
depolarization (dee-poh-lar-ih-ZAY-shun) electrical activity that triggers a contraction of the heart muscle [*de-* opposite, *-pol-* pole, *-ar-* relating to, *-ization* process]
depressed fracture (dee-PREST) type of bone fracture in which skull bone is partly "caved in" [*fracture* a breaking]
depression (dee-PRESH-un) movement that lowers or depresses a part, moving it in the opposite direction from elevation [*de-* down, *-press-* press, *-sion* process]
dermal papilla (DER-mal pah-PIL-ah) any of the many small bumps in the surface of the papillary layer of the dermis and which form the ridges and grooves of fingerprints [*derma-* skin, *-al* relating to, *papilla* nipple] *pl.*, papillae (pah-PIL-ee)
dermatitis (der-mah-TYE-tis) general term referring to any inflammation of the skin [*derma-* skin, *-itis* inflammation]
dermatology (der-mah-TOL-oh-jee) study of the integument and its diseases [*derma-* skin, *-to-* combining form, *-log-* words (study of), *-y* activity]
dermatome (DER-mah-tohm) skin surface areas supplied by a single spinal nerve [*derma-* skin, *-tome* cut segment or region]
dermatosis (der-mah-TOH-sis) general term meaning "skin condition" [*derma-* skin, *-osis* condition]
dermis (DER-mis) the deeper of the two major layers of the skin, composed of dense fibrous connective tissue interspersed with glands, nerve endings, and blood vessels [*dermis* skin]
dermoepidermal junction (DEJ) (DER-mo-EP-ih-der-mal JUNK-shun) thin, gluelike layer that binds the epidermis of the skin to the underlying dermis; also called *dermal-epidermal junction* [*derma-* skin, *-al* relating to, *epi-* on or upon]
descending aorta (dih-SEND-ing ay-OR-tah) conducts blood downward from the arch of the aorta to the abdominal cavity [*de-* down, *-scend-* climb, *aort-* lifted, *-a* thing] *pl.*, aortae or aortas
descending colon (dih-SEND-ing KOH-lon) portion of the colon that lies in the vertical position, on the left side of the abdomen; extends from below the stomach to the iliac crest [*de-* down, *-scend-* climb, *colon* large intestine]
descending tract (dih-SEND-ing trakt) bundle of axons in the spinal cord that conducts impulses down the cord from the brain [*de-* down, *-scend-* climb, *tract* trail]
desmosome (DES-moh-sohm) category of cell junction that holds adjacent cells together; consists of dense plate or band of connecting structures at point of adhesion [*desmo-* band, *-som-* body]
desquamation (des-kwah-MAY-shun) shedding of epithelial elements from the skin surface [*de-* to remove, *-squama-* scale, *-tion* process]

detrusor muscle (dee-TROO-sor) smooth muscle tissue making up the wall of the bladder [*detrus-* thrust, *-or* agent, *mus-* mouse, *-cle* little]
developmental anatomy *see* **developmental biology** [*ana-* not or without, *-tomy* a cut]
developmental biology branch of biology that studies the process of change over the life cycle [*bio-* life, *-log-* words (study of), *-y* activity]
deviated septum (DEE-vee-ay-ted SEP-tum) abnormal condition in which the nasal septum is far from its normal position, possibly obstructing normal nasal breathing [*devia-* turn aside, *-ate* process, *septum* partition] *pl.*, septa (SEP-tah)
diabetes insipidus (dye-ah-BEE-teez in-SIP-idus) condition resulting from hyposecretion of ADH in which large volumes of urine are formed [*diabetes* pass-through or siphon, *insipidus* without zest]
diabetes mellitus (DM) (dye-ah-BEE-teez mell-EYE-tus) condition resulting when the pancreatic islets secrete too little insulin, resulting in increased levels of blood glucose [*diabetes* pass-through or siphon, *mellitus* honey-sweet]
diabetic ketoacidosis (dye-ah-BET-ik kee-toh-ass-ih-DOH-sis) low blood pH resulting from an accumulation of ketone bodies in the blood in diabetes mellitus [*diabet-* pass-through or siphon (diabetes mellitus), *-ic* relating to, *keto-* acetone, *-acid-* sour, *-osis* condition]
diabetic neuropathy (dye-ah-BET-ik nyoo-ROP-ah-thee) nerve damage caused by diabetes mellitus [*diabet-* pass-through or siphon (diabetes mellitus), *-ic* relating to, *neuro-* nerve, *-path-* disease, *-y* state]
diabetic retinopathy (dye-ah-BET-ik ret-in-OP-ath-ee) retinal damage caused by diabetes mellitus [*diabet-* pass-through or siphon (diabetes mellitus), *-ic* relating to, *ret-* net, *-in* relating to, *-path-* disease, *-y* state]
diad (dye-AD) double structure of sarcoplasmic reticulum and T tubules in cardiac muscle fibre; also *dyad* [*diad* group of two]
dialysis (dye-AL-ih-sis) separation of smaller (diffusible) particles from larger (nondiffusible) particles through a semipermeable membrane [*dia-* apart, *-lysis* loosening]
diapedesis (dye-ah-peh-DEE-sis) passage of any formed elements within blood through the vessel wall, as in movement of white cells into an area of injury and infection [*dia-* apart or through, *-pedesis* oozing]
diaphragm (DYE-ah-fram) the flat muscular sheet that separates the thorax and abdomen; a major muscle of respiration [*dia-* across, *-phrag-* enclose, *-(u)m* thing]
diaphysis (dye-AF-ih-sis) shaft of a long bone [*dia-* through or apart, *-physis* growth] *pl.*, diaphyses (dye-AF-ih-seez)
diarrhoea (dye-ah-REE-ah) abnormally frequent defaecation of liquid or semi-liquid faeces [*dia-* through, *-rrhoea* flow]
diarthrosis (dye-ar-THROH-sis) freely movable joint [*dia-* between, *-arthr-* joint, *-osis* condition] *pl.*, diarthroses (dye-ar-THROH-seez)
diastasis (dye-ASS-tah-sis) reduced ventricular filling of the heart [*dia-* apart or through, *-stasis* standing]
diastole (dye-ASS-toh-lee) relaxation of the heart (especially the ventricles), during which it fills with blood; opposite of systole [*dia-* through, *-stol-* position]
diastolic blood pressure (dye-ah-STOL-ik blud PRESH-ur) blood pressure in arteries during diastole (relaxation) of the heart; clinically more important than systolic pressure [*dia-* apart or through, *-stol-* position, *-ic* relating to]
diencephalon (dye-en-SEF-ah-lon) "between" brain; parts of the brain between the cerebral hemispheres and the mesencephalon, or midbrain [*di-* between, *-en-* within, *-cephalon* head] *pl.*, diencephala or diencephalons
differential white blood cell count (dif-er-EN-shal) percentage enumeration of the different types of leucocytes in a stained blood smear [*different-* difference, *-al* relating to, *cell-* storeroom]
differentiate (dif-er-EN-shee-ayt) act of *differentiation*, the process of the development of diverse types of cells with specialized structures and functions [*different-* difference, *-iate* act of]
differentiation (dif-er-EN-shee-AY-shun) *see* **differentiate** [*different-* difference, *-ation* process]
diffusion (dih-FYOO-shun) spreading; natural tendency of small particles to spread out evenly within any given space; for example, scattering of dissolved particles [*diffus-* spread out, *-sion* process]
digestion (dye-JES-chun) breakdown of food materials either mechanically (through chewing) or chemically (via digestive enzymes) [*digest-* break apart, *-tion* process]
digestive system (dye-JES-tiv SIS-tem) system composed of mouth, pharynx, oesophagus, stomach, small intestine, large intestine, rectum, and anal canal [*digest-* break apart, *-ive* relating to]
digestive tract (dye-JES-tiv trakt) tube made up of the main organs of digestion, from mouth to anus [*digest-* break apart, *-ive* relating to, *tract* trail]
digital (DIJ-ih-tal) relating to a finger [*digit-* finger, *-al* relating to]
digitalis (dij-ih-TAL-is) *see* **digoxin** [*digit-* finger, *-al-* relating to, *-is* thing (from finger-shaped flowers of foxglove plant)]
digoxin (dih-JOK-sin) drug used to treat atrial fibrillation [*dig-* finger (from digitalis or foxglove), *-oxin* poison or toxin]
diploe (DIP-lo-EE) region of cancellous (spongy) bone within the wall of a flat bone of the cranium; also spelled *diploë* [*diploe* folded over (doubled)]
diploid number (DIP-loyd) normal number of chromosomes per somatic cell (46 in humans) [*diplo-* twofold, *-oid* of or like]
diplopia (dih-PLOH-pee-ah) double vision [*di-* double, *-op-* vision, *-ia* condition]
disaccharide (dye-SAK-ah-ride) double sugar, such as sucrose or lactose; made up of two monosaccharides [*di-* two, *-sacchar-* sugar, *-ide* chemical]
dislocation (dis-low-KAY-shun) condition in which the articular surfaces of bones forming a joint are no longer in proper contact [*dis-* apart, *-locat-* to place, *-tion* process]
displaced fracture (dis-PLAYSD FRAK-chur) also called *open fracture*; *see* **compound fracture** [*displace-* to remove, *fracture* a breaking]
dissection (di-SEK-shun) cutting technique used to separate body parts for study [*dissect-* to cut apart, *-tion* process]
dissociate (dih-SOH-see-ayt) when a compound breaks apart in solution forming ions that are surrounded by solvent molecules [*dis-* apart, *-socia-* unite, *-ate* action]
distal (DIS-tal) toward the end of a structure; opposite of proximal [*dist-* distance, *-al* relating to]
distal convoluted tubule (DCT) (DIS-tal KON-voh-LOO-ted TYOO-byool) in the kidney, the part of the tubule distal to the ascending limb of the Henle loop that terminates in a collecting duct; main portion of *distal tubule* [*dist-* distance, *-al* relating to, *con-* together, *-volut-* roll, *tub-* tube, *-ul-* little]
distal interphalangeal (DIP) (DIS-tal in-ter-fah-LAN-gee-al) joint between the middle and distal phalanges [*dist-* distance, *-al* relating to, *inter-* between, *-phalang-* finger bones (ref. from rows of soldiers), *-al* relating to]
distal tubule (DIS-tal TYOO-byool) *see* **distal convoluted tubule** [*dist-* distance, *-al* relating to, *tub-* tube, *-ul-* little]
disuse atrophy (DIS-yoos AT-roh-fee) loss of muscle tissue mass after a period of few or no contractions, resulting in weakness [*dis-* absence of, *a-* without, *-troph-* nourishment, *-y* state]
diuretic (dye-yoo-RET-ik) substance that promotes or stimulates the production of urine [*dia-* through, *-ure-* urine, *-ic* relating to]
divergence (dye-VER-jens) when a single presynaptic axon synapses with more than one different postsynaptic neuron [*di-* separate, *-verg-* incline, *-ence* state]
diverticulitis (dye-ver-tik-yoo-LYE-tis) inflammation of diverticula (abnormal outpouchings) of the large intestine, possibly causing constipation [*diverticul-* turn aside, *-itis* inflammation]
diverticulosis (dye-ver-tik-yoo-LOH-sis) condition resulting in the presence of abnormal saclike outpouchings of the intestinal wall [*diverticul-* turn aside, *-osis* condition]
diving reflex (DYE-ving REE-fleks) protective physiological response of the body to cold water immersion [*re-* back or again, *-flex* bend]
DNA fingerprinting technique used to analyze the genetic makeup of individuals; compares nucleotide sequences using electrophoresis
domain (doh-mayn) a specific three-dimensional region within a tertiary protein that acts as a functional unit [*doma-* house or estate]
dominant (DOM-ih-nant) in genetics, term referring to genes that have effects that appear in the offspring (dominant forms of a gene are often represented by upper case letters); *see* **recessive** [*domina-* rule, *-ant* characterized by]
dominant gene (DOM-ih-nant jeen) gene whose effects are seen; capable of masking the effects of a recessive gene for the same trait [*domina-* rule, *-ant* characterized by, *gen-* produce]
dopamine (DA) (DOH-pah-meen) chatecholamine neurotransmitter [*dopa-* contraction of dioxyphenylalanine, *-amine* ammonia compound]
dopaminergic (doh-pah-min-ER-jik) relating to a neuron that releases dopamine (neurotransmitter) or to a receptor molecule that is activated by dopamine [*dopa-* contraction of dioxyphenylalanine, *-amin-* ammonia compound, *-erg-* work, *-ic* relating to]
Doppler ultrasonography (ul-trah-son-OG-rah-fee) diagnostic study that uses sound or frequency ultrasound to record the direction of blood flow through the heart [*Christian Doppler* Austrian physicist/mathematician, *ultra-* beyond, *-sono-* sound, *-graph-* draw, *-y* process]
dorsal (DOR-sal) relating to the back; in a direction toward the back of the body; see **posterior** [*dors-* back, *-al* relating to]
dorsal (posterior) nerve root (DOR-sal) bundle of nerve fibres that carry sensory information into the spinal cord [*dors-* back, *-al* relating to]
dorsal cavities (DOR-sal KAV-ih-teez) body cavities on the dorsal side of the body, which include the cranial cavity and the spinal cavity; not a standard anatomical term, but used here to help organize the body for the beginning student [*dors-* the back, *-al* relating to, *cav-* hollow, *-ity* state]
dorsal ramus (DOR-sal RAY-mus) branch of spinal nerve that supplies somatic motor and sensory fibres to several smaller nerves [*dors-* the back, *-al* relating to, *ramus* branch] *pl.*, rami (RAY-mye)
dorsal root (DOR-sal) posterior branch of the attachment of a spinal nerve to the spinal cord [*dors-* the back, *-al* relating to]
dorsal root ganglion (DOR-sal root GANG-glee-on) small region of grey matter in dorsal nerve root made up of cell bodies of unipolar sensory neurons [*dors-* the back, *-al* relating to, *ganglion* knot]
dorsiflexion (dor-sih-FLEK-shun) ankle movement in which the top of the foot is elevated (brought toward the front of the leg) with toes pointing upward [*dorsi-* back, *-flex-* bend, *-ion* process]
double bond covalent chemical bond in which two pairs of electrons are shared
Down syndrome (SIN-drohm) group of symptoms usually caused by trisomy of chromosome 21; characterized by intellectual disability and multiple structural defects, including facial, skeletal, and cardiovascular abnormalities [*John L. Down* English physician, *syn-* together, *-drome* running or (race) course]
down-regulation (down reg-yuh-LAY-shun) process in which hormone receptors in a target cell are reduced in number by some stimulus [*regula-* rule, *-tion* process]
Duchenne muscular dystrophy (DMD) (doo-SHEN MUSS-kyoo-lar DISS-troh-fee) common form of muscular dystrophy also called *pseudohypertrophy* (meaning "false muscle growth") because the atrophy of muscle is masked by excessive replacement of muscle by fat and fibrous tissue; characterized by mild leg muscle weakness that progresses rapidly to include the shoulder muscles; caused by mutated gene for dystrophin (needed to hold muscle fibre together during contraction) on the X chromosome, thus making DMD more common in boys than girls [*Duchenne* Guillaume B.A. Duchenne de Boulogne, French neurologist, *muscul-* little mouse (muscle), *-ar* relating to, *dys-* bad, *-troph-* nourishment, *-y* state]
ductus arteriosus (DA) (DUK-tus ar-teer-ee-OH-sus) in the developing fetus, this arterial duct connects the aorta and the pulmonary artery, allowing most blood to bypass the fetus' developing lungs [*ductus* duct, *arteri-* vessel, *-osus* relating to]
ductus deferens (DUK-tus DEF-er-enz) vas deferens [*ductus* duct, *deferens* carrying away]
ductus venosus (DUK-tus veh-NO-sus) continuation of the umbilical vein that shunts blood returning from the placenta past the fetus' developing liver directly into the inferior vena cava [*ductus* duct, *ven-* vein, *-osus* relating to]
duodenum (dyoo-oh-DEE-num or dyoo-AH-de-num) first subdivision of the small intestine; where most chemical digestion occurs [*duodeni-* 12 fingers, shortened from *intestinum duodenum digitorum* intestine of 12 fingerwidths] *pl.*, duodena (dyoo-AH-de-nah) or duodenums
dura mater (DYOO-rah MAH-ter) literally "strong mother" or "tough mother"; outermost layer of the meninges [*dura* hard or tough, *mater* mother]
dural sinus (DYOO-ral SYE-nus) name for a large vein of cranial cavity [*dura-* tough, *-al* relating to, *sinus* hollow]
dwarfism (DWARF-iz-em) condition of abnormally small stature, sometimes resulting from hyposecretion of growth hormone [*dwar-* tiny, *-ism* condition]
dynamic equilibrium (dye-NAM-ik ee-kwih-LIB-ree-um) maintaining balance when the head or body is rotated or suddenly moved [*dynam-* moving force, *-ic* relating to, *equi-* equal, *-libr-* balance]
dynamic tension (dye-NAM-ik TEN-shun) another name for isotonic contraction [*dynam-* moving force, *-ic* relating to]
dysfunctional uterine bleeding (DUB) (dis-FUNK-shun-al YOO-ter-in) irregular or excessive uterine bleeding; results from structural problem or hormonal imbalance [*dys-* difficult, *-function-* performance, *-al* relating to, *uter-* womb, *-ine* relating to]
dysmenorrhoea (dis-men-oh-REE-ah) menstrual cramps [*dys-* painful, *-men-* month, *-rhoea* flow]

dysplasia (diss-PLAY-zha) abnormal changes in size, shape, and organization of cells in a tissue associated with neoplasms (tumours) [*dys-* disordered, *-plas(m)-* substance or form, *-ia* condition]
dyspnoea (DISP-nee-ah) difficult or laboured breathing [*dys-* painful, *-pnoe-* breathe, *-a* condition]
dysrhythmia (dis-RITH-mee-ah) abnormal heart rhythm; also called **arrhythmia** [*dys-* disordered, *-rhythm-* movement in time, *-ia* condition]
dystrophin (DIS-trof-in) protein molecule that forms strands in each skeletal muscle fibre and helps to hold the cytoskeleton to the sarcolemma to keep the muscle fibre from breaking during contractions; normal dystrophin is missing in Duchenne muscular dystrophy (DMD) and related conditions and thus cells break apart more easily, causing the symptoms of DMD [*dys-* bad, *-troph-* nourishment, *-in* substance]
dysuria (dis-YOO-ree-ah) painful urination

E

eardrum *see* **tympanic membrane** [*eare-* ear]
eccentric contraction (ek-SENT-rik kon-TRAK-shun) type of isotonic muscle contraction in which muscle lengthens while it is contracting [*ec-* out of, *-centr-* centre, *-ic* relating to, *con-* together, *-tract-* drag or draw, *-tion* process]
eccrine sweat gland (EK-rin) water-producing exocrine sweat glands widely dispersed throughout the skin [*ec-* out, *-crin-* secrete, *gland* acorn]
echocardiography (ek-oh-kar-dee-OG-rah-fee) diagnostic technique that uses ultrasound waves that reflect off the heart to produce images of heart function [*echo-* reflect sound, *-cardi-* heart, *-graph-* draw, *-y* activity]
eclampsia (eh-KLAMP-see-ah) potentially fatal condition associated with toxaemia of pregnancy; characterized by convulsions and coma [*ec-* out, *-lamp-* shine forth, *-sia* condition]
ectoderm (EK-toh-derm) outermost of the primary germ layers that develops early in the first trimester of pregnancy; gives rise to the skin and the nervous system [*ecto-* outside, *-derm* skin]
ectomorph (EK-toh-morf) thin, lean body type [*ecto-* outside, *-morph* form]
ectopic pacemaker (ek-TOP-ik PAYS-may-ker) pacemaker other than the SA node [*ec-* out of, *-top-* place, *-ic* relating to]
ectopic pregnancy (ek-TOP-ik) pregnancy in which the fertilized ovum develops in some place other than in the uterus [*ec-* out of, *-top-* place, *-ic* relating to]
eczema (EK-zeh-mah) inflammatory skin condition associated with various diseases and characterized by erythema, papules, vesicles, and crusts [*ec-* out, *-zema* boiling]
Edmonton protocol (ED-mon-ton PRO-toh-kol) islet cell transplant technique used in the treatment of type 1 diabetes [*Edmonton* city in Canada]
effector (ef-FEK-tor) organ, gland, or muscle that responds to a regulatory control signal, such as a nerve stimulus or hormone [*effect-* accomplish, *-or* agent]
effector B cell (ef-FEK-tor bee sel) cell that differentiates from a B cell; synthesizes and secretes huge amounts of antibodies [*effect-* accomplish, *-or* agent, *B* bursa-equivalent tissue, *cell* storeroom]
effector cell (ef-FEK-tor sel) type of lymphocyte that attacks antigens [*effect-* accomplish, *-or* agent, *cell* storeroom]
effector T cell (ef-FEK-tor tee sel) cell that differentiates from a T cell; causes contact killing of a target cell [*effect-* accomplish, *-or* agent, *T* thymus gland, *cell* storeroom]
efferent (EF-fer-ent) transporting, conducting, or carrying away from [*e-* away, *-fer-* carry, *-ent* relating to]
efferent division (EF-fer-ent di-VI-shun) the motor division (outgoing pathways) of the nervous system [*e-* away, *-fer-* carry, *-ent* relating to]
efferent ductule (EF-fer-ent DUKT-yool) series of sperm ducts that drain the rete testis and pierce the tunica albuginea [*e-* away, *-fer* carry, *duct-* path, *-ule* small one]
efferent (motor) neuron (EF-fer-ent NYOO-ron) nerve cell that transmits impulses away from the central nervous system to or toward muscles or glands [*e-* away, *-fer-* carry, *-ent* relating to]
efferent nervous system (EF-fer-ent) subdivision of the peripheral nervous system (PNS) that consists of all outgoing motor nerves [*e-* away, *-fer-* carry, *-ent* relating to, *nerv-* nerve, *-ous* relating to]
eicosanoid (eye-KOH-sah-noyd) family of compounds derived from 20-carbon fatty acid molecules that serve as chemical signals in the body; examples include prostaglandins, thromboxane, leukotrienes; also called *icosanoid* [*eicosa-* twenty, *-an(e)-* chemical, *-oid* of or like]
Einthoven's triangle (EYN-to-venz) three-angle view of the heart's electrical activity [*Willem Einthoven* Dutch physiologist]
ejaculation (ee-jak-yoo-LAY-shun) sudden discharging of semen from the body [*e-* out or away, *-jacula-* throw, *-ation* process]
ejaculatory duct (ee-JAK-yoo-lah-toh-ree) duct formed by the joining of the ductus deferens and the duct from the seminal vesicle that allows sperm to enter the urethra [*e-* out or away, *-jacula-* throw, *-ory* relating to, *duct* path]
ejection fraction (EF) (ee-JEK-shun) ratio of stroke volume (SV) of the heart to the end-diastolic volume (EDV); expressed as a percentage: EF = (SV/EDV) × 100; the EF refers to the ejection fraction of the left ventricle, unless specified otherwise, and decreases below 55% as the myocardium fails to contract normally—thus making EF an indicator of heart failure [*eject-* to cast out, *-tion* process, *fract-* a breaking, *-tion* process]
elastic artery (eh-LAS-tik AR-ter-ee) largest artery; includes aorta and some of its branches [*elast-* to drive or propel, *-ic* relating to, *arteri-* vessel]
elastic cartilage (eh-LAS-tik KAR-ti-lij) cartilage with elastic, as well as collagenous, fibres; provides elasticity and firmness, as in, for example, the cartilage of the external ear [*elast-* drive or propel, *-ic* relating to, *cartilag-* cartilage]
elastic dense fibrous tissue form of dense (regular) fibrous tissue that contains mostly elastic fibres [*elast-* drive or propel, *-ic* relating to, *dense* thick, *fibr-* fibre, *tissu-* fabric]
elastic filament in muscle fibres, microscopic protein filaments composed of *titin (connectin)* that anchor the ends of the thick filaments to the Z disc and give myofibrils their characteristic elasticity [*elas-* drive or propel, *-ic* relating to, *fila-* thread, *-ment* thing]
elastic recoil (e-LAS-tik REE-koyl) tendency of the thorax and lungs to return to their preinspiration volume [*elast-* drive or propel, *-ic* relating to]
elastin (e-LAS-tin) stretchy protein found in elastic fibre [*elast-* to drive or propel, *-in* substance]
electrocardiogram (ECG [written] or EKG [spoken]) (eh-lek-troh-KAR-dee-oh-gram) graphic record of the heart's action potentials [*electro-* electricity, *-cardio-* heart, *-gram* drawing]
electrocardiograph (eh-lek-troh-KAR-dee-oh-graf) machine that produces electrocardiograms [*electro-* electricity, *-cardio-* heart, *-graph* draw]
electrocardiography (eh-lek-troh-kar-dee-OG-rah-fee) process or technology that produces electrocardiograms [*electro-* electricity, *-cardio-* heart, *-graph-* draw, *-y* process]
electroencephalogram (EEG) (eh-lek-troh-en-SEF-ah-loh-gram) graphic representation of voltage changes in brain tissue used to evaluate nerve tissue function [*electro-* electricity, *-en-* within, *-cephal-* head, *-gram* drawing]
electroencephalography (eh-lek-troh-en-SEF-ah-lo-grah-fee) diagnostic study that measures electrical activity produced by the brain [*electro-* electricity, *-en-* inside, *-cephal-* head, *-graph-* draw, *-y* activity]
electrolyte (e-LEK-troh-lyte) substance that dissociates into ions in solution, rendering the solution capable of conducting an electric current [*electro-* electricity, *-lyt-* loosening]
electromyography (eh-lek-troh-my-OG-rah-fee) process or technology that records electrical impulses from muscles as they contract [*electro-* electricity, *-myo-* muscle, *-graph* draw, *-y* activity]
electron (eh-LEK-tron) small, negatively charged subatomic particle [*electr-* electric, *-on* unit]
electron microscopy (EM) (eh-LEK-tron my-KROS-kah-pee) technique of observing small structures by either passing a beam of electrons through a specimen (transmission electron microscopy, TEM) or reflecting a beam of electrons off a specimen (scanning electron microscopy, SEM) and focusing the resulting electron beam(s) to form a magnified image of the specimen [*electr-* electric, *-on* unit, *micro-* small, *-scop-* see, *-y* activity]
electron transport system (ETS) (eh-LEK-tron) carrier molecules embedded in the inner membrane of the mitochondria that take high-energy electrons from the citric acid cycle and form water and energy for oxidative phosphorylation; also called *electron transport chain (ETC)* [*electro-* electricity, *-on* subatomic particle, *trans-* across, *-port* carry]
electrophoresis (eh-lek-troh-foh-REE-sis) laboratory procedure in which different types of charged molecules are separated according to molecular weight using a weak electric current [*electro-* electricity, *-phoresis* a carrying]
eleidin (eh-LEE-din or eh-LEE-ih-din) substance found in the dying cells of the stratum lucidum; transforms to keratin [*elei-* olive tree, *-in* substance]
element (EL-eh-ment) substance composed of only one type of atom that cannot be broken into simpler constituents by chemical means [*element* first principle]
elephantiasis (el-eh-fan-TYE-ah-sis) extreme lymphoedema (swelling resulting from lymphatic blockage) in the limbs caused by a parasitic worm infestation; so called because the limbs swell to "elephantine proportions" [*elephant-* elephant, *-iasis* condition]
elevation (el-eh-VAY-shun) action that moves a part up [*e(x)-* up, *-lev-* raise, *-at-* perform, *-tion* process]
elimination defaecation [*e-* out, *-limen-* threshold, *-ation* process]
embolism (EM-boh-liz-em) condition that results from a moving blood clot circulating in the bloodstream [*embol-* plug, *-ism* condition]
embolus (EM-boh-lus) a moving blood clot circulating in the bloodstream [*embolus* plug]
embryo (EM-bree-oh) animal in early stages of intrauterine development; in humans, the embryonic stage is the first 8 weeks after conception [*em-* in, *-bryo* fill to bursting]
embryology (em-bree-OL-oh-gee) study of the development of an individual from conception to birth [*em-* in, *-bryo-* fill to bursting, *-log-* words (study of), *-y* activity]
embryonic disc (em-bree-ON-ik) cells of the early embryo that differentiate into the three primary germ layers [*em-* in, *-bryo-* fill to bursting, *-ic* relating to]
embryonic stem cell (em-bree-ON-ik) nondifferentiated cells found in the embryo [*em-* in, *-bryo-* fill to bursting, *-ic* relating to]
emesis (EM-eh-sis) vomiting [*emesis* vomiting]
emission (ee-MISH-un) reflex movement of spermatozoa and secretions from genital ducts and accessory glands into prostatic urethra; precedes ejaculation [*e-* out or away, *-mis-* send, *-sion* process]
emmetropic (em-eh-TROHP-ik) relating to the relaxed, normal eye [*emmetr-* correct measure, *-op-* eye, *-ic* relating to]
emphysema (em-fih-SEE-mah) abnormal condition characterized by trapping of air in alveoli of the lung that causes them to rupture and fuse to other alveoli; see also **chronic obstructive pulmonary disease** [*em-* in, *-physema* blowing or puffing up]
emulsified (ee-MULL-seh-fyde) dispersed fat molecules formed into tiny droplets before they can be digested [*e-* out, *-muls-* milk, *-i-* combining form, *-fy* process]
enamel (ih-NA-mel) hard, mineralized connective tissue, harder than bone, forms hard covering of exposed tooth surfaces; hardest substance in body [*en-* in, *-amel* melt]
end artery (end AR-ter-ee) artery that diverges into a capillary [end *-arteri-* vessel]
end-diastolic volume (EDV) (end-dye-ah-STOL-lik) the amount of blood in the heart at the end of diastole [*dia-* through, *-stol-* position, *-ic* relating to]
endemic (en-DEM-ik) refers to a disease native to a local region of the world [*en-* in, *-dem-* people, *-ic* relating to]
endocardium (en-doh-KAR-dee-um) thin layer of very smooth tissue lining each chamber of the heart [*endo-* within, *-cardi-* heart, *-um* thing]
endochondral ossification (en-doh-KON-dral os-ih-fih-KAY-shun) process by which bones are formed by replacement of cartilage models [*endo-* inward or within, *-chondr-* cartilage, *-al* relating to, *oss-* bone, *-fic-* make, *-ation* process]
endocrine (EN-doh-krin) secreting into blood or tissue fluid rather than into a duct; opposite of exocrine [*endo-* within, *-crin-* secrete]
endocrine cell (EN-doh-krin) glandular secretory cells located in the pancreas; found in pancreatic islets [*endo-* within, *-crin-* secrete, *cell* storeroom]
endocrine gland (EN-doh-krin) secretory structure that discharges hormones directly into the blood [*endo-* inward or within, *-crin-* secrete, *gland* acorn]
endocrine hormone (EN-doh-krin HOR-mohn) substance secreted by an endocrine gland into the bloodstream that acts on a specific target tissue to produce a given response [*endo-* inward or within, *-crin-* secrete, *hormon-* excite]
endocrine reflex (EN-doh-krin REE-fleks) response that results from feedback loops within the endocrine system [*endo-* within, *-crin-* secrete, *re-* again, *-flex* bend]
endocrine system (EN-doh-krin) system composed of glands that secrete chemicals known as *hormones* directly into the blood [*endo-* inward or within, *-crin-* secrete]
endocrinology (en-doh-krin-OL-oh-jee) study of the endocrine glands and their hormones [*endo-* within, *-crin-* secrete, *-log-* words (study of), *-y* activity]
endocytosis (en-doh-sye-TOH-sis) process that allows extracellular material to enter the cell without actually passing through the plasma membrane [*endo-* inward or within, *-cyto-* cell, *-osis* condition]
endoderm (EN-doh-derm) innermost layer of the primary germ layers that develops early in the first trimester of pregnancy; gives rise to digestive and urinary structures, as well as many other glands and organ parts [*endo-* within, *-derm* skin]

endogenous growth (en-DOJ-en-us) *see* **interstitial growth** [*endo-* within, *-gen-* produce, *-ous* relating to]
endolymph (EN-doh-limf) clear potassium-rich fluid that fills the membranous labyrinth of the inner ear [*endo-* within, *-lymph* water]
endometrial ablation (en-doh-MEE-tree-al ab-LAY-shun) minimally invasive technique used to destroy the endometrial lining and reduce excessive blood loss among women suffering from dysfunctional uterine bleeding [*endo-* within, *-metr-* womb, *-al* relating to, *ab-* away from, *-lat-* carry, *-tion* process]
endometrial cancer (en-doh-MEE-tree-al) cancer of the endometrium [*endo-* within, *-metr-* womb, *-al* relating to, *cancer* crab or malignant tumour]
endometriosis (en-doh-mee-tree-OH-sis) benign condition that affects the female reproductive tract; characterized by functioning endometrial tissue outside the uterus [*endo-* within, *-metr-* womb, *-osis* condition]
endometrium (en-doh-MEE-tree-um) mucous membrane lining the uterus [*endo-* within, *-metr-* womb, *-um* thing] *pl.*, endometria (en-doh-MEE-tree-ah)
endomorph (EN-doh-morf) body type characterized by excessive fat [*endo-* within, *-morph* shape]
endomysium (en-doh-MEE-see-um) delicate connective tissue membrane covering the skeletal muscle fibres in a skeletal muscle organ [*endo-* within, *-mys-* muscle, *-um* thing]
endoneurium (en-doh-NYOO-ree-um) thin wrapping of fibrous connective tissue that surrounds each axon in a nerve [*endo-* inward, *-neuri-* nerve, *-um* thing] *pl.*, endoneuria
endoplasm (en-doh-PLAZ-im) material within a cell [*endo-* within, *-plasm* cell or tissue substance]
endoplasmic reticulum (ER) (en-doh-PLAZ-mik reh-TIK-yoo-lum) network of tubules and vesicles in cytoplasm that contributes to cellular protein manufacture (via attached ribosomes) and distribution [*endo-* inward or within, *-plasm-* substance, *-ic* relating to, *ret-* net, *-ic-* relating to, *-ul-* little, *-um* thing] *pl.*, endoplasmic reticula (reh-TIK-yoo-lah)
endorphin (en-DOR-fin) chemical in central nervous system that influences pain perception; a natural painkiller [*endo-* within, *-(m) orph- Morpheus* (Roman god of dreams), *–in* substance]
endoscopic cholangiography (en-doh-SKOP-ik koh-lan-jee-OG-rah-fee) procedure that uses x-rays to visualize the gallbladder and ducts that carry bile [*endo-* within, *-scop-* see, *chol-* bile, *angi-* vessel, *-graph-* draw, *-y* process]
endosteum (en-DOS-tee-um) fibrous membrane that lines the medullary cavity of long bones [*end-* within, *-osteum* bone]
endothelium (en-doh-THEE-lee-um) squamous epithelial cells that line the inner surface of the entire circulatory system and the vessels of the lymphatic system [*endo-* within, *-theli-* nipple, *-um* thing]
endotracheal intubation (en-doh-TRAY-kee-al in-tyoo-BAY-shun) placing a tube in the trachea to ensure an open airway [*endo-* within, *-trache-* rough duct, *-al* relating to, *in-* within, *-tub-* tube, *-ation* process]
end-product inhibition (end-PROD-ukt inhib-ISH-un) process in a biochemical pathway in which the chemical product at the end of the pathway (the end product) becomes an allosteric effector, inhibiting the function of one or more enzymes in the pathway and thus inhibiting further production of the end product [end, *-pro-* forward, *-duct* bring, *inhib-* restrain, *-tion* process]
endurance training continuous vigorous exercise requiring the body to increase its consumption of oxygen and develop the muscles' ability to sustain activity over a prolonged period
energy level limited region surrounding the nucleus of an atom at a certain distance containing electrons; also called a *shell* [*en-* within, *-erg-* work, *-y* state]
enkephalin (en-KEF-ah-lin) peptide chemical in the central nervous system that acts as a natural painkiller [*en-* within, *-kephal-* head, *-in* substance]
enteric nervous system (ENS) (en-TER-ik) complex arrangement of neurons that are interconnected with the central nervous system and with various divisions of the autonomic nervous system; for example, gastrointestinal muscles and mucous membranes [*enter-* intestine, *-ic* relating to]
enterocyte (EN-ter-oh-syte) absorptive epithelial cell within the mucosa lining the small intestine [*entero-* intestine, *-cyte* cell]
enteroendocrine cell (EN-ter-oh-EN-doh-krin cell) endocrine cell of the intestinal mucosa [*entero-* intestine, *-endo-* within, *-crin* secrete, *cell* storeroom]
enterogastric reflex (en-ter-oh-GAS-trik REE-fleks) nervous reflex causing inhibition of gastric peristalsis in response to the presence of acid and distention of duodenal mucosa; also may inhibit gastric secretion [*entero-* intestine, *-gastr-* stomach, *-ic* relating to, *re-* back or again, *-flex* bend]
enterogastrone (en-ter-oh-GAS-trown) hormone involved with decreasing gastric peristalsis [*entero-* intestine, *-gastr-* stomach, *-one* hormone]
enterokinase (en-ter-oh-KYE-nays) enzyme that activates trypsin in the intestinal lumen [*entero-* intestine, *-kin-* movement, *-ase* enzyme]
enzyme (EN-zyme) biochemical catalyst that allows chemical reactions to take place; functional proteins that regulate various metabolic pathways of the body [*en-* in, *-zyme* ferment]
eosinophil (ee-oh-SIN-oh-fil) white blood cell, readily stained by eosin (a reddish acid dye) that attacks large parasites and produces some allergic responses [*eosin-* reddish colour, *-phil* love]
ependymal cell (eh-PEN-dih-mal) cells that line the ventricles of the brain and the central canal of the spinal cord [*ep-* over, *-en-* on, *-dyma-* put, *-al* relating to, *cell* storeroom]
ependymoma (eh-pen-dih-MOH-mah) tumour of glial cells called *ependyma* that line fluid spaces of the central nervous system [*ep-* over, *-en-* on, *-dyma-* put, *-oma* tumour]
epicardium (ep-ih-KAR-dee-um) inner layer of the pericardium that covers the surface of the heart; it is also called the *visceral pericardium* [*epi-* on or upon, *-cardi-* heart, *-um* thing]
epidemic (ep-ih-DEM-ik) refers to a disease that occurs in many individuals at the same time [*epi-* upon, *-dem-* people, *-ic* relating to]
epidemiology (EP-ih-dee-mee-OL-oh-jee) study of the occurrence, distribution, and transmission of diseases in human populations [*epi-* upon, *-dem-* people, *-o-* combining form, *-log-* words (study of), *-y* activity]
epidermis (ep-ih-DER-mis) outermost layer of the skin; sometimes called the "false" skin [*epi-* on or upon, *-dermis* skin]
epididymis (ep-ih-DID-ih-miss) one of a pair of tightly coiled male reproductive tubes that carry sperm to the vas deferens [*epi-* upon, *-didymis* pair] *pl.*, epididymes (ep-ih-DID-ih-meez)
epidural space (ep-ih-DYOO-ral) in the brain, the space above the dura mater [*epi-* upon, *-dura-* hard, *-al* relating to]
epigenetics (ep-ih-jeh-NET-iks) any process of inheritance other than direct DNA inheritance, sometimes by adding a methyl group (or other chemical) to DNA, as in maternal/paternal imprinting of genes [*epi-* upon, *gen-* produce, *-ic* relating to]
epiglottis (ep-ih-GLOT-iss) lidlike cartilage overhanging the entrance to the larynx [*epi-* upon, *-glottis* mouth of windpipe] *pl.*, epiglottides (ep-ih-GLOT-id-eez) or epiglottises
epiglottitis (EPP-ih-glaw-TYE-tiss) form of laryngeal oedema [*epi-* upon, *-glotti-* mouth of windpipe (glottis), *-itis* inflammation]
epilepsy (EP-ih-lep-see) chronic seizure disorder [*epi-* upon, *-lep(t)-* seize, *-sy* state or condition]
epimysium (ep-ih-MIS-ee-um) coarse sheet of connective tissue that covers a muscle as a whole [*epi-* upon, *-mys-* muscle, *-um* thing]
epinephrine (epi) (ep-ih-NEF-rin) adrenaline; neurotransmitter related to norepinephrine; neurohormone secreted by the adrenal medulla [*epi-* upon, *-nephr-* kidney, *-ine* substance]
epineurium (ep-ih-NYOO-ree-um) fibrous coat surrounding a bundle of nerve fibres (tough fibrous sheath that covers the whole nerve) [*epi-* upon, *-neuri-* nerve, *-um* thing] *pl.*, epineuria
epiphyseal fracture (ep-ih-FEEZ-ee-al) when the epiphyseal plate is separated from the epiphysis or diaphysis; this type of fracture can disrupt normal growth of the bone [*epi-* on, *-phys-* growth, *-al* relating to, *fracture* a breaking]
epiphyseal plate (ep-ih-FEEZ-ee-al) cartilage plate that is between the epiphysis and the diaphysis and allows growth to occur; sometimes referred to as a *growth plate* [*epi-* on, *-phys-* growth, *-al* relating to]
epiphysis (eh-PIF-ih-sis) end of a long bone; also, the pineal body of the brain [*epi-* on, *-physis* growth] *pl.*, epiphyses (eh-PIF-ih-seez)
epiploic appendage (eh-pih-PLOH-ik ah-FEN-daj) fatty extension of the periteum on the outer surface of the colon [*epiplo-* omentum, *-ic* relating to, *append-* hang upon, *-age* thing]
episiotomy (eh-piz-ee-OT-oh-mee) surgical procedure used during birth to prevent a laceration of the mother's perineum or the vagina [*episi-* vulva, *-tom-* cut, *-y* action]
epispadias (ep-ih-SPAY-dee-us) congenital defect that involves the opening of the urethral meatus on the dorsal surface of the glans or penile shaft [*epi-* on or above, *-spad-* rip or split]
epistaxis (ep-ih-STAK-sis) clinical term referring to a bloody nose [*epi-* upon, *-staxis* drip]
epithalamus (ep-ih-THAL-ah-mus) small nuclei located outside the thalamus and hypothalamus; considered to be one of the structures of the diencephalon [*epi-* upon, *-thalamus* inner chamber] *pl.*, epithalami (ep-ih-THAL-ah-mye)
epithelial membrane (ep-ih-THEE-lee-al) membrane composed of epithelial tissue with an underlying layer of connective tissue [*epi-* on or upon, *-theli-* nipple, *-al* relating to, *membrane* thin skin]
epithelial support cell (ep-ih-THEE-lee-al) one of the types of cells that makes up the olfactory epithelium [*epi-* upon, *-theli-* nipple, *-al* relating to]
epithelial tissue (ep-ih-THEE-lee-al) tissue type that covers the body and its parts; lines various parts of the body; forms continuous sheets that contain no blood vessels; classified according to shape and arrangement [*epi-* on or upon, *-theli-* nipple, *-al* relating to, *tissu-* fabric]
epithelium (ep-ih-THEE-lee-um) epithelial tissue [*epi-* on or upon, *-theli-* nipple, *-um* thing] *pl.*, epithelia (ep-ih-THEE-lee-ah)
epitope (EP-ih-tohp) specific portion of an antigen that elicits an immune response [*epi-* on or upon, *-tope* place]
eponym (EP-o-nim) scientific term based on a person's name, such as *islets of Langerhans* (equivalent to *pancreatic islets*); eponyms are avoided in modern usage [*epo-* above, *-nym* name]
epsilon (ϵ) cell (EP-sih-lon) type of endocrine cell found in the pancreatic islet and which secretes the hormone ghrelin [*epsilon (ϵ)* fifth letter of Greek alphabet, *cell* storeroom]
equatorial plate (eh-kwah-TOH-ree-al) plane at the "equator" or middle of a cell during metaphase where the chromosomes align [*equat-* make even, *-or-* agent, *-al* relating to]
equilibration (eh-kwih-lih-BRAY-shun) process of achieving equilibrium, a balance between opposing elements [*equilibr-* equal, *-ation* process]
equilibrium (e-kwih-LIB-ree-um) a balance between opposing elements [*equi-* equal, *-libr-* balance] *pl.*, equilibria [*equilibr-* equal, *-um* state]
erectile dysfunction (ED) (eh-REK-tyle) failure to achieve an erection of the penis adequate enough to permit sexual intercourse [*erect-* upright, *-ile* relating to, *dys-* bad or painful, *-func-* perform, *-tion* process]
erection (eh-REK-shun) condition of erectile tissue when filled with blood; often refers to enlargement of the penis during sexual arousal [*erect-* upright, *-tion* process]
erector spinae muscle (eh-REK-tor SPYNE-ee) muscle group in the back consisting of a number of long, thin muscles that travel all the way down the back; the muscles extend (straighten or pull back) the vertebral column and rotate and flex the back laterally [*erector* that which makes rigid or upright, *spinae* of the spine, *mus-* mouse, *-cle* little]
erosive oesophagitis (eh-ROH-siv eh-SOF-ah-jye-tis) narrowing or chronic inflammation of the oesophagus [*oes-* will carry, *-phag-* food (eat), *-itis* inflammation]
erythema (er-ih-THEE-mah) reddening of the skin [*erythem-* become red, *-a* condition]
erythroblastosis fetalis (eh-rith-roh-blas-TOH-sis feh-TAL-is) condition of a fetus or infant caused by the mother's Rh antibodies reacting with the baby's Rh-positive red blood cells, characterized by massive agglutination of the blood and resulting in life-threatening circulatory problems for the infant [*erythro-* red, *-blast-* bud, *-osis* condition, *fet-* offspring, *-al* relating to, *-is* thing]
erythrocyte (eh-RITH-roh-syte) red blood cell [*erythro-* red, *-cyte* cell]
erythrocyte sedimentation rate (ESR) (eh-RITH-roh-syte sed-ih-men-TAY-shun) the rate at which formed elements settle in a tube in 1 hour [*erythro-* red, *-cyte* cell]
erythropoiesis (eh-rith-roh-poy-EE-sis) process of red blood cell formation [*erythro-* red, *-poiesis* making]
erythropoietin (eh-RITH-roh-POY-eh-tin) glycoprotein secreted to increase red blood cell production in response to oxygen deficiency [*erythro-* red, *-poiet-* make, *-in* substance]
essential fatty acid unsaturated fatty acid that must be provided by the diet; serves as a source within the body for prostaglandin synthesis [*acid* sour]
essential hypertension (hye-per-TEN-shun) high blood pressure condition with no identifiable pathological mechanism or reason [*hyper-* excessive, *-tens-* stretch or pull tight, *-sion* state]
essential organ primary organ; organ needed for the essential functions of a system [*organ* instrument]
essential reproductive organ reproductive organ that must be present for reproduction to occur; the gonads [*re-* again, *-pro-* forward, *-duct-* bring or carry, *-ive* relating to, *organ* instrument]
ethmoid (ETH-moyd) irregular cranial bone that lies anterior to the sphenoid and posterior to the nasal bones [*ethmo-* sieve, *-oid* like]
eumelanin (yoo-MEL-ah-nin) type of melanin pigment that is dark brown in colour [*eu-* true, *-melan-* black, *-in* substance]
eupnoea (YOOP-nee-ah) normal respiration [*eu-* easily, *-pnoe-* breathe, *-a* condition]
eustachian tube (yoo-STAY-shun) auditory tube [*Bartolomeo Eustachio* Italian anatomist, *-an* relating to]

evaporation (ee-vap-oh-RAY-shun) in anatomy and physiology, heat lost from the body by vaporization of liquid (sweat) from the skin [*e-* out from, *-vapour* steam, *-ation* process]
eversion (ee-VER-shun) movement that turns a body part (such as the foot) outward [*e(x)-* outward, *-ver-* turn, *-sion* process]
evert (ee-VERT) to turn outward [*e(x)-* outward, *-vert* turn]
evoked potential (EP) measurement of the electrical activity of the brain; information can be analyzed by a computer and generated on a video screen (brain electrical activity map) [*potent-* power, *-ial* relating to]
excess postexercise oxygen consumption (EPOC) *see* **oxygen debt**
exchange reaction chemical reaction that breaks down a compound and then synthesizes a new compound by switching portions of the molecules; for example, AB + CD → AD + BC [*ex-* from, *-change* to change, *re-* again, *-action* action]
excitability (ek-syte-eh-BIL-ih-tee) ability of a muscle to be stimulated; also known as *irritability* [*excit-* arouse, *-abil-* capable, *-ity* state]
excitation (ek-sye-TAY-shun) electrical fluctuation (increase in voltage) occurring when a neuron or muscle fibre is stimulated and additional Na^+ channels open [*excit-* arouse, *-ation* process]
excitatory neurotransmitter (ek-SYE-tah-toh-ree nyoo-roh-TRANZ-mit-er) neurotransmitter that causes excitation (and thus depolarization) of the postsynaptic neuron [*excita-* arouse, *-ory* relating to, *neuro-* nerves, *-trans- across*, *-mitt-* send, *-er* agent]
excitatory postsynaptic potential (EPSP) (ek-SYE-tah-toh-ree post-sih-NAP-tik poh-TEN-shal) temporary depolarization of postsynaptic membrane following stimulation [*excita-* arouse, *-ory* relating to, *post-* after, *-syn-* together, *-apt-* join, *-ic* relating to, *potent-* power, *-ial* relating to]
excitotoxin (ek-SYE-toh-TAWK-sin) glutamate or other substance that has an excessive stimulatory effect on neurons or other cells, thus causing damage or cell death [*excit-* arouse, *-tox-* poison, *-in* substance]
excretion (eks-KREE-shun) removal of waste products produced during body functions; occurs by defaecation, urination, and respiration and through the skin [*excret-* separate, *-tion* process]
exocrine (EKS-oh-krin) secreting into a duct, as in glands that secrete their products via ducts onto a surface or into a cavity; opposite of endocrine [*exo-* outside or outward, *-crin-* secrete]
exocrine gland (EK-soh-krin) secretory structure that discharges products into ducts [*exo-* outside or outward, *-crin-* secrete, *gland* acorn]
exocytosis (eks-oh-sye-TOH-sis) process that allows large molecules to leave the cell without actually passing through the plasma membrane [*exo-* outside or outward, *-cyto* cell, *-osis* condition]
exogenous growth (eks-OJ-eh-nus) *see* **appositional growth** [*exo-* outside or outward, *-gen-* produce, *-ous* relating to]
exosome (EKS-oh-sohm) vesicle outside a cell produced by exocytosis [*exo-* outside or outward, *-some* body]
experiment test (or series of tests) of a proposed scientific idea or hypothesis; a controlled experiment is one that accounts for, and eliminates, effects of influences other than those being tested [*exo-* outside, *-gen* produce, *-ous* relating to]
exon (EKS-on) segment of a gene in DNA that is used directly for protein synthesis; in the mRNA transcript of a gene, the intervening intron (noncoding) segments are removed and the remaining exon (coding) segments are spliced together to form the final, edited version of the mRNA transcript; *see* **ribonucleic acid (RNA), transcription** [*exo-* outside, *-on* unit]
exophthalmos (ek-soff-THAL-mus) protrusion of the eyeballs resulting, in part, from oedema of tissue at the back of the eye socket [*ex-* outside, *-oph-* eye, *-thalm-* inner chamber, *-ic* relating to]
expiration (eks-pih-RAY-shun) exhaling [*ex-* out, *-pir-* breathe, *-tion* process]
expiratory centre (eks-PYE-rah-tor-ee) one of the two most important respiratory control centres, located in the medulla [*ex-* out of, *-[s]pir-* breathe, *-tory* relating to]
expiratory muscles (eks-PYE-rah-tor-ee) muscles that allow more forceful expiration to increase the rate and depth of ventilation; internal intercostals and abdominal muscles [*ex-* out of, *-[s]pir-* breathe, *-tory* relating to, *musc-* mouse, *-cle* little]
expiratory reserve volume (ERV) (eks-PYE-rah-tor-ee) amount of air that can be forcibly exhaled after expiring the tidal volume (TV) [*ex-* out of, *-[s]pir-* breathe, *-tory* relating to]
extensibility (ek-STEN-sih-BIL-ih-tee) ability of a muscle to extend or stretch and return to resting length [*ex- outward*, *-tens-* stretch, *-abil-* capable, *-ity* state]
extend (ek-STEND) stretch or unbend, as when increasing the angle between two bones at a joint; as opposed to flex [*ex-* outward, *-tens-* stretch]
extension (ek-STEN-shun) increasing the angle between two bones at a joint; as opposed to flexion [*ex-* outward, *-tens-* stretch, *-sion* process]
extensor digitorum longus muscle (ek-STEN-ser dij-ih-TOH-rum) dorsal flexor muscle on the anterior surface of the foot [*extensor* stretcher, *digit* of the finger or toe, *-orum* relating to *longus* long, *mus-* mouse, *-cle* little]
external anal sphincter muscle (AY-nal SFINGK-ter) circular muscle located around the anus [*extern-* outside, *-al* relating to, *an-* ring (anus), *-al* relating to, *sphinc-* bind tight, *-er* agent, *mus-* mouse, *-cle* little]
external acoustic meatus (ak-OOS-tik mee-AY-tus) ear canal; a curved tube (approximately 2.5 cm) extending from the auricle into the temporal bone, ending at the tympanic membrane [*extern-* outside, *acust-* hearing, *-ic* relating to, *meatus* channel or passage] *pl.*, meatus or meatuses
external ear outer part of the ear: auricle and external auditory canal [*extern-* outside, *-al* relating to]
external genital (JEN-ih-tal) any of the reproductive organs (usually the external organs); penis, scrotum, and related structures in males; vagina, vulva, and related structures in females [*extern-* outside, *-al* relating to, *genit-* birth or reproduction, *-al* relating to]
external iliac vein (IL-ee-ak vayn) vein of the lower extremity [*extern-* outside, *-al* relating to, *ilium* flank, *vena* blood vessel]
external intercostal muscle (in-ter-KOS-tal) muscle of the thorax; elevates the ribs [*extern-* outside, *-al* relating to, *inter-* between, *-costa-* rib, *-al* relating to, *mus-* mouse, *-cle* little]
external jugular vein (JUG-yoo-lar vayn) vein of the neck [*extern-* outside, *-al* relating to, *jugul-* neck, *-ar* relating to, *vena* blood vessel]
external oblique muscle (o-BLEEK) muscle of the abdominal wall [*extern-* outside, *-al* relating to, *obliq-* slanted, *mus-* mouse, *-cle* little]
external os constricted end of the uterus [*extern-* outside, *-al* relating to, *os* mouth or opening] *pl.*, ora
external table outer wall of a flat bone of the cranium, made of compact bone; compare to **internal table** [*extern-* outside, *-al* relating to]
exteroceptor (eks-ter-oh-SEP-tor) somatic sense receptor located on the body surface [*exter-* outside, *-cept-* receive, *-or* agent]
extracellular (eks-trah-SELL-yoo-lar) space outside the cell [*extra-* outside, *-cell-* storeroom, *-ular* relating to]
extracellular fluid (ECF) (eks-trah-SELL-yoo-lar) liquid found outside of cells, located in two compartments: between cells (interstitial fluid) and in blood (plasma); lymph, cerebrospinal fluid, and joint fluids are also *extracellular fluids* [*extra-* outside, *-cell-* storeroom, *-ular* relating to]
extracellular matrix (ECM) (eks-trah-SEL-yoo-lar MAY-triks) material between cells in a tissue, made up of water and a variety of proteins and other molecules [*extra-* beyond, *-cell-* storeroom, *-ular* relating to, *matrix* womb] *pl.*, matrices (MAY-tris-eez)
extraperitoneal (eks-trah-pair-ih-toh-NEE-al) relating to the space outside the parietal peritoneum [*extra-* outside, *peri-* around, *-tone-* stretched, *-al* relating to]
extrapyramidal tract (eks-trah-pih-RAH-mih-dal trakt) motor tract from the brain to the spinal cord anterior horn motor neurons, except for the corticospinal tract [*extra-* outside, *-pyramid-* pyramid, *-al* relating to, *tract* trail]
extrinsic clotting pathway (eks-TRIN-sik) clotting mechanism that involves chemicals released from damaged tissue outside of the blood [*extr-* outside, *-sic* beside]
extrinsic control (eks-TRIN-sik) style of physiological regulation in which the control centre (regulatory centre) is outside, or extrinsic to, the tissue being regulated; for example, the brain's control of a leg muscle or the pituitary gland's regulation of the thyroid gland [*extr-* outside or beyond, *-sic* beside]
extrinsic eye muscle (eks-TRIN-sik) voluntary muscle that attaches the eyeball to the socket and produces movement of the eyeball [*extr-* outside, *-sic* beside, *mus-* mouse, *-cle* small]
extrinsic factor (eks-TRIN-sik) substance secreted in the stomach that allows vitamin B_{12} to be absorbed by the body [*extr-* outside, *-sic* beside]
extrinsic foot muscle (eks-TRIN-sik) leg muscle responsible for movement of the ankle and foot [*extr-* outside, *-sic* beside, *mus-* mouse, *-cle* little]
extrinsic muscle (eks-TRIN-sik) muscle originating from outside of the part of the skeleton moved [*extr-* outside, *-sic* beside, *mus-* mouse, *-cle* little]

F

face front of the head
facet (fah-SET or FASS-et) flat, rounded face on a bone projection (as in vertebrae) [*fac-* appearance (face), *-et* small]
facial (FAY-shal) relating to the face [*faci-* face, *-al* relating to]
facial nerve (FAY-shal nerv) cranial nerve VII, mixed nerve [*faci-* face, *-al* relating to]
facilitated diffusion (fah-SIL-ih-tay-ted dih-FYOO-zhun) special type of diffusion; when movement of a molecule is made more efficient by action of carrier or channel mechanisms in the plasma membrane [*facili-* easy, *-ate* act of, *diffuse-* spread out, *-sion* process]
faecal transplant (FEE-kal TRANZ-plant) medical prodedure in which bacteria from faeces of a healthy donor are transplanted to the colon of a recipient suffering from a severe intestinal disorder to restore a healthy balance to the recipient's gut microbiome [*faec(es)-* waste, *-al* relating to, *trans-* across, *-plant* set or place]
faeces (FEE-seez) waste material discharged from the intestines [*faeces* waste]
fallen arches (flatfoot) (FALL-en ARCH-ez [FLAT-foot]) condition in which the tendons and ligaments of the foot weaken, allowing the normally curved arch to flatten out
fallopian tube (fal-LOH-pee-an) uterine tube; either of a pair of tubes that conduct the ovum from the ovary to the uterus [*Gabriello Fallopio*]
false pelvis (PEL-vis) structure above the pelvic inlet [*pelvis* basin] *pl.*, pelves (PEL-veez) or pelvises (PEL-vis-ez)
false vocal fold upper pair of folds of mucous membrane in the larynx; also called *vestibular fold* [*voca-* voice, *-al* relating to]
falx cerebelli (falks ser-eh-BEL-lee) small fold in the dura mater in the posterior cranial fossa, between the cerebellum and cerebrum [*falx* sickle, *cerebelli* of the cerebellum (small brain)] *pl.*, falces cerebelli (FAL-seez)
falx cerebri (falks SER-eh-bree) fold in the dura mater that separates the two cerebral hemispheres [*falx* sickle, *cerebri* of the cerebrum] *pl.*, falces cerebri (FAL-seez)
farsightedness *see* **hyperopia**
fascicle (FAS-ih-kul) small bundle or cluster, as in groups of skeletal muscle fibres bound together by perimysium or groups of nerve fibres held together by perineurium [*fasci-* band or bundle, *-cle* small]
fascia (FASH-ee-ah) general name for the fibrous connective tissue masses located throughout the body [*fascia* band or bundle]
fasciculus cuneatus (fah-SIK-yoo-lus KYOO-nee-ay-tus) wedgelike bundle of spinal cord sensory tracts; carries information regarding discrimination touch and conscious sensation of body position and movement [*fasci-* bundles, *-iculus* little, *cuneatus* wedgelike] *pl.*, fasciculi
fasciculus gracilis (fah-SIK-yoo-lus GRAH-sil-iss) thin bundle of spinal cord sensory tracts that carry information for detecting touch and conscious sensation of position and movement of the body [*fasci-* bundles, *-iculus* little, *gracilis* thin]
fast (A) pain fibre type of nerve fibre that carries pain impulses that result in sharp pain; associated with superficial injury or trauma [*fast* quickly, swiftly, *poena-* punishment, *fibr-* thread or fibre]
fast fibre *see* **fast muscle fibre** [*fibr-* thread or fibre]
fast muscle fibre white muscle fibre; primarily relies on anaerobic processes to produce ATP; responds quickly [*mus-* mouse, *-cle* little, *fibr-* thread or fibre]
fatty acid (FAT-tee ASS-id) product of fat digestion; building block of fat molecules [*fat-* fat, *-ty* state, *acid* sour]
fauces (FAW-seez) opening from the mouth into the oropharynx [from *faux* throat]
febrile (FEB-ril) referring to fever [*febri-* fever, *-ile* characterized by]
feedback control loop highly complex and integrated communication control network, classified as negative or positive; negative feedback loops are the most important and numerous homeostatic control mechanisms
feed-forward (feed-FOR-ward) concept that information may flow ahead to another process to trigger a change in anticipation of an event that will follow
femoral (FEM-or-al) relating to the thigh [*femor-* thigh, *-al* relating to]
femoral hernia (FEM-or-al HER-nee-ah) rupture of the lower abdominal wall at the femoral ring [*femor-* femur, *-al* relating to, *hernia* rupture] *pl.*, herniae or hernias (HER-nee-ee)
femoral vein (FEM-or-al vayn) vein of the thigh [*femor-* thigh, *-al* relating to, *vena* blood vessel]
femur (FEE-mur) thigh bone [*femur* thigh]
fenestrated capillary (fen-es-TRAY-tid KAP-ih-lair-ee) type of capillary that has intercellular clefts between the lining of endothelial cells and small holes through the plasma membrane [*fenestra-* window, *-ate* characterized by, *capill-* hair, *-ary* relating to]
fenestration (fen-es-TRAY-shun) perforation in the endothelium of a capillary, as in the glomerulus [*fenestra-* window, *-ation* process]
fertility drug (fer-TIL-ih-tee) drug taken to correct ovulatory dysfunction [*fertil-* fruitful, *-ity* state]
fertility sign (fer-TIL-ih-tee) structural or functional change in the body used to predict ovulation [*fertil-* fruitful, *-ity* state]

fertilization (FER-tih-lih-ZAY-shun) union of an ovum and a sperm; conception [*fertil-* fruitful, *-ation* process]

fetal alcohol syndrome (FAS) (FEE-tal AL-koh-hol SIN-drohm) a condition that may cause congenital abnormalities in a baby; it results from a woman consuming alcohol during pregnancy [*fet-* offspring, *-al* relating to, *syn-* together, *-drome* running or (race) course]

fetal haemoglobin (FEE-tal hee-moh-GLOH-bin) oxygen-binding protein present in the fetus that is made up of two alpha chains and two gamma chains [*fet-* offspring, *-al* relating to, *haemo-* blood, *-glob-* ball, *-in* substance]

fetal programming (FEE-tal) process that refers to the relationship between events occurring during the course of fetal development and the appearance of specific anatomical, physiological, or disease states that develop later in life [*fet-* offspring, *-al* relating to]

fetus (FEE-tus) unborn young, especially in the later stages; in human beings, the fetal stage is from the third month of the intrauterine period until birth [*fetus* fruitful]

fever unusually high body temperature

fibre (FYE-ber) threadlike structure, as in a muscle fibre (a threadlike cell) or a collagen fibre (a threadlike protein strand) [*fibr-* thread or fibre]

fibrillation (fih-brih-LAY-shun) condition in which individual muscle fibres, or small groups of fibres, contract asynchronously (out of time) with other muscle fibres in an organ (especially the heart), producing no effective movement [*fibr-* thread or fibre, *-illa-* small, *-ation* process]

fibrin (FYE-brin) insoluble protein in clotted blood [*fibr-* thread or fibre, *-in* substance]

fibrinogen (fye-BRIN-oh-jen) soluble blood protein that is converted to insoluble fibrin during clotting [*fibr-* thread or fibre, *-gen* produce]

fibrinolysis (fye-brin-OL-ih-sis) physiological mechanism that dissolves clots [*fibr-* thread or fibre, *-lysis* loosening]

fibroblast (FYE-broh-blast) connective tissue cell that synthesizes interstitial fibres and gels [*fibr-* thread or fibre, *-blast* bud]

fibrocartilage (fye-broh-KAR-tih-lij) cartilage with the greatest number of collagenous fibres; strongest and most durable type of cartilage [*fibr-* thread or fibre, *-cartilag-* cartilage]

fibroid (FYE-broyd) *see* **fibromyoma** [*fibr-* thread or fibre, *-oid* of or like]

fibromyalgia (FM) (fye-broh-my-AL-jah) syndrome of chronic, widespread musculoskeletal pain accompanied by distress and other symptoms; resulting primarily from overamplification of pain in the central nervous system [*fibr-* thread or fibre, *-my-* muscle, *-algia* pain]

fibromyoma (fye-broh-my-OH-mah) benign tumour of uterine fibrous or smooth muscle tissue [*fibr-* thread or fibre, *-my-* muscle, *-oma* tumour]

fibromyositis (fye-broh-my-oh-SYE-tis) tendon inflammation with myositis (muscle inflammation), as in a charley horse [*fibr-* thread or fibre, *-myos-* muscle, *-itis* inflammation]

fibrosarcoma (fye-broh-sar-KOH-mah) cancer of fibrous connective tissue [*fibr-* thread or fibre, *-sarco-* flesh, *-oma* tumour]

fibrous connective tissue (FYE-brus) strong, nonstretchable, white collagen fibres that make up tendons [*fibr-* thread or fibre, *-ous* relating to, *connect-* bind, *-ive* relating to, *tissu-* fabric]

fibrous joint (FYE-brus joynt) connection between bones made primarily by bands of fibrous connective tissue [*fibr-* thread or fibre, *-ous* relating to]

fibrous pericardium (FYE-brus pair-ih-KAR-dee-um) tough, loose-fitting, and inelastic sac around the heart [*fibr-* thread or fibre, *-ous* relating to, *peri-* around, *-cardi-* heart, *-um* thing]

fibula (FIB-yoo-lah) leg bone; lateral to tibia [*fibula* clasp] *pl.*, fibulae or fibulas (FIB-yoo-lee)

fibular (peroneal) vein (FIB-yoo-lar [per-oh-NEE-al] vayn) vein of the leg [*fibula-* clasp (fibula), *-ar* relating to, *perone-* brooch, *-al* relating to, *vena* blood vessel]

fibularis tertius muscle (fib-yoo-LAR-is TER-shee-us) leg muscle that flexes and everts the foot; also **peroneous tertius** [*fibula-* clasp (fibula), *-ar-* relating to, *-is* thing, *tertius* third, *mus-* mouse, *-cle* little]

Fick's law (fiks law) a set of principles that together describe diffusion and factors that affect diffusion; also called *Fick's law of diffusion* [*Adolph Eugen Fick* German physiologist]

fight-or-flight reaction (fyte or flyte ree-AK-shun) changes produced by increased sympathetic impulses allowing the body to deal with any type of stress [*re-* again, *-action* action]

filaria (fih-LAR-ee-ah) taxonomic group of organisms that includes parasitic worms [*fila-* thread, *-ar-* like, *-ia* things] *pl.*, filariae (fih-LAR-ee-ee)

filiform papilla (FIL-ih-form pah-PIL-ah) bumps of the tongue mucosa with tiny, threadlike projections; these papillae are scattered among the fungiform papillae; they do not contain taste buds but allow us to experience food texture and "feel" [*fili-* thread, *-form* shape, *papilla* nipple] *pl.*, papillae (pah-PIL-ee)

filtrate (FIL-trayt) substance remaining in a liquid after it has passed through a filter [*filtr-* strain, *-ate* result]

filtration (fil-TRAY-shun) movement of water and solutes through a membrane because of a higher hydrostatic pressure on one side [*filtr-* strain, *-ation* process]

filum terminale (FYE-lum ter-mih-NAL-ee) slender filament formed by the pia mater that blends with the dura mater and then the periosteum of the coccyx [*filum* thread, *termin-* boundary, *-al* relating to] *pl.*, fila terminales (FYE-lah ter-mih-NAL-eez)

fimbria (FIM-bree-ah) fringe of tiny fingerlike projections around the opening of each fallopian (uterine) tube; the projections help move an ovum into the fallopian tube [*fimbria* fringe] *pl.*, fimbriae (FIM-bree-ee)

first polar body small, nonfunctional cell produced during meiotic divisions in the formation of the female gamete [*pol-* pole, *-ar* relating to]

fissure (FISH-ur) groove [*fissure* cleft]

fixator muscle (fik-SAY-tor) muscle that functions as a joint stabilizer [*fixator* fastener, *mus-* mouse, *-cle* little]

fixed-membrane-receptor model *see* **second-messenger model** [*figere-* to fasten, *membran-* thin skin, *recept-* receive, *-or* agent]

flaccid muscle (FLAK-sid) muscle with less tone than normal [*flac-* flabby, *-id* structure or body, *mus-* mouse, *-cle* little]

flagellum (flah-JEL-um) single projection extending from the cell surface similar to a cilium; only example in human is the "tail" of the male sperm [*flagellum* whip] *pl.*, flagella

flat bone broad and thin bone with a flattened and often curved surface

flavin adenine dinucleotide (FAD) (FLAY-vin AD-en-een dye-NYOO-klee-oh-tyde) molecule that serves as an electron carrier in the electron transport system [*flav-* yellow, *-in* substance, *aden-* gland, *-ine* chemical, *di-* two, *nucleo-* kernel (nucleus), *-t-* combining form, *-ide* chemical]

flex (FLEKS) to bend a part, as in decreasing the angle between two bones at the joint; opposite of extend [*flex* bend]

flexion (FLEK-shun) act of bending; decreasing the angle between two bones at the joint; opposite of extension [*flex-* bend, *-ion* process]

flexure (FLEK-shur) a bending; as in any of the bends that occur in the colon [*flex-* bend, *-ure* result of action]

flow–volume loop a type of spirogram (breathing graph) that shows the flow rate (L/min) of breathing along one axis and volume of breathing (L) along the other axis, thus forming a loop or circle with each respiratory cycle

fluid and electrolyte balance (eh-LEK-troh-lyte) constancy of body fluid and electrolyte levels [*electro-* electricity, *-lyt-* loosening]

fluid balance homeostasis of fluids; the volumes of interstitial fluid, intracellular fluid, and plasma and total volume of water remain relatively constant

fluid compartment area in the body where fluid is located; interstitial fluid, plasma, and intracellular fluid compartments are the major fluid compartments of the body

fluid mosaic model (moh-ZAY-ik) theory of plasma membrane composition in which molecules of the membrane are bound tightly enough to form a continuous layer but loosely enough so molecules can slip past one another

fluorescence microscopy (FM) (flor-ESS-ens my-KROS-kah-pee) type of light microscopy that uses a certain wavelength of light (such as UV) to trigger special fluorescent stains in a microscopic specimen to glow brightly [*fluor-* fluorite (fluorescent mineral), *-escence* state, *micro-* small, *-scop-* see, *-y* activity]

folate deficiency anaemia (FOH-layt deh-FISH-en-see ah-NEE-mee-ah) condition in which there is a decrease in the red blood cell count resulting from a vitamin deficiency [*fol-* leaf, *-ate* relating to, *-de-* down, *-fic-* perform, *-ency* state, *an-* without, *-(h)aem-* blood, *-ia* condition]

folia (FOH-lee-ah) thin, delicate gyri (raised ridges) of the surface of the cerebellum [*folia* leaves] *sing.*, folium

foliate papilla (FOL-ee-ayt pah-PIL-ah) red, leaflike ridges of mucosa on the lateral edges of the posterior tongue surface; each contains about a hundred or so taste buds [*foli-* leaf, *-ate* relating to, *papilla* nipple] *pl.*, papillae

follicle (FOL-lih-kul) general name for a pocket or bubble structure; for example, ovarian structure consisting of oocyte surrounded by numerous supporting cells (follicle cells); also, pocketlike structures from which a hair grows; also, a small hollow sphere with a wall of glandular epithelium, found in thyroid tissue [*foll-* bag, *-icle* little]

follicle-stimulating hormone (FSH) (FOL-lih-kul-STIM-yoo-lay-ting HOR-mohn) hormone present in males and females; in males, FSH stimulates the production of sperm; in females, FSH stimulates the ovarian follicles to mature and follicle cells to secrete oestrogen [*foll-* bag, *-icle* little, *hormon-* excite]

follicular cell (foh-LIK-yoo-lar) cell that produces thyroid colloid [*foll-* bag, *-icul-* small, *-ar* relating to, *cell* storeroom]

follicular phase (foh-LIK-yoo-lar) postmenstrual phase of the female reproductive cycle; also called *preovulatory* or *estrogenic phase* [*foll-* bag, *-icul-* little, *-ar* relating to]

fontanelle (FON-tah-nel) "soft spot" where ossification in the cranium is incomplete at birth [*fontam-* fountain, *-el* little]

foot distal extremity of the leg specially adapted to supporting weight

foramen (foh-RAY-men) hole or opening, as in a bone (for blood vessels and nerves) [*foramen* opening] *pl.*, foramina (foh-RAM-in-ah) or foramens (foh-RAY-menz)

foramen ovale (foh-RAY-men oh-VAL-ee) in the developing fetus, opening that shunts blood from the right atrium directly into the left atrium, allowing most blood to bypass the baby's developing lungs [*foramen* opening, *ovale* egg shaped] *pl.*, foramina ovales (foh-RAM-in-ah oh-VAL-eez)

forced expiratory volume (FEV) (eks-PYE-rah-tor-ee) maximum volume (mL or L) of air that can be breathed out; also called *forced vital capacity (FVC)* [*ex-* out of, *-[s] pir-* breathe, *-tory* relating to]

formed element (formd EL-eh-ment) any of the cells of the blood tissue: red blood cells, white blood cells, and platelets in blood [*element* first principle]

fornix (FOR-niks) corner of the vagina where it meets the cervix of the uterus [*fornix* arch]

fossa (FOSS-ah) slight depression, as in a bone [*fossa* ditch] *pl.*, fossae (FOSS-ee)

fovea centralis (FOH-vee-ah sen-TRAL-is) small depression in the macula lutea where cones are most densely packed; vision is sharpest where light rays focus on the fovea [*fovea* pit, *centralis* centre] *pl.*, foveae centrales (FOH-vee-ee sen-TRAL-eez)

fractal geometry (FRAK-tal jee-OM-eh-tree) study of surfaces with a seemingly infinite area, such as the lining of the small intestine [*fract-* a breaking, *-al* relating to, *geo-* earth or land, *-metr-* measure, *-y* activity]

fundoplication (fun-doh-plih-KAY-shun) surgical procedure performed to strengthen the lower oesophageal sphincter [*fund-* bottom, *-plica-* fold, *-tion* state]

fragile X syndrome (FXS) (FRAJ-il eks SIN-drohm) condition in which intellectual disability results from breakage of X chromosome in males [*fragil-* frail; X sex chromosome X; *syn-* together, *-drome* running or (race) course]

fraternal twin (frah-TERN-al) offspring that results from the fertilization of two different ova by two different spermatozoa [*frater-* brother, *-al* relating to, *twin* twofold]

free fatty acid (FFA) fatty acid combined with albumin to be transported by the blood to other cells [*acid* sour]

free nerve ending any of the sensory receptors in the skin that respond to pain

free radical (RAD-ih-kal) the temporarily uncombined and highly reactive form of any radical (functional group of atoms); compare to **radical** [*radic-* root, *-al* relating to]

friction ridge raised underlying dermal papillae; form fingerprints [*fric-* rub, *-tion* process]

frontal relating to the forehead [*front-* forehead, *-al* relating to]

frontal bone forehead bone [*front-* forehead, *-al* relating to]

frontal plane lengthwise plane running from side to side, dividing the body into anterior and posterior portions [*front-* forehead, *-al* relating to, *plan-* flat surface]

frostbite local damage to tissues caused by extremely low temperature

full-thickness burn a burn involving the entire thickness of the skin and possibly subcutaneous tissue skin is severely damaged and nerve endings are destroyed [*thick-* not thin, *-ness* state of]

functional group (FUNK-shun-al groop) small cluster of atoms in an organic molecule that gives the molecule particular functional characteristics such as certain chemical binding properties; also called *radical* and thus often represented generically by the letter R [*function-* perform, *-al* relating to]

functional MRI (fMRI) (FUNK-shun-al M R I) procedure that detects which areas of the brain are most active by measuring oxygen consumption by neurons [*function-* perform, *-al* relating to, *MRI* magnetic resonance imaging]

functional protein (FUNK-shun-al PRO-teen) category of proteins that affect the functional operations of a cell; contrast to **structural protein** [*function-* perform, *-al* relating to, *prote-* primary, *-in* substance]

functional residual capacity (FRC) (FUNK-shun-al reh-ZID-yoo-al kah-PAS-ih-tee) amount of air left in the lungs at the end of a normal expiration [*function-* perform, *-al*, *residu-* left over, *-al* relating to, *capac-* hold, *-ity* state]

fundus (FUN-duss) base of an organ, often opposite a major opening; the fundus of the stomach is the outpouching next to the oesophageal opening and opposite the pyloric opening at the apex of the stomach; the fundus of the uterus is the portion between the uterine tube openings and opposite the cervix at the apex of the uterus [*fundus* bottom] *pl.*, fundi (FUN-dye)

fungiform papilla (FUN-jih-form pah-PIL-ah) large, mushroom-shaped bumps of the tongue mucosa found in the anterior two thirds of the tongue surface; each one contains one or a few taste buds [*fungi-* mushroom, *-form* shape, *papilla* nipple] *pl.*, papillae (pah-PIL-ee)

fungus (FUNG-us) organism similar to plants but lacking chlorophyll and capable of producing mycotic (fungal) infections [*fungus* mushroom] *pl.*, fungi (FUNJ-eye)

funiculus (fuh-NIK-yoo-lus) large bundle of nerve fibres divided into smaller bundles called *spinal tracts* [*funi-* rope, *-icul-* little] *pl.*, funiculi (fuh-NIK-yoo-lye)

furuncle (FUR-un-kul) boil; pus-filled cavity formed by some hair follicle infections; see also **carbuncle** [*furuncle-* little thief]

fusiform muscle (FYOO-sih-form) muscle that has fascicles close to parallel in the centre of the muscle but converge to a tendon at one or both ends [*fusi-* spindle, *-form* shape, *mus-* mouse, *-cle* little]

G

G protein protein in the plasma membrane of a target cell (such as a postsynaptic cell) involved in signal transduction of a message from outside the cell [G for guanine-nucleotide binding, *prote-* first rank, *-in* substance]

G protein–coupled receptor (GPCR) (jee-PROH-teen–kup-eld ree-SEP-ter) receptor mechanism embedded in plasma membranes of cells that receives chemical messengers (such as neurotransmitters and nonsteroid hormones) and initiates signal transduction to the cell by way of a G protein, which triggers the resulting changes in the cell [G for guanine-nucleotide binding, *-prote-* first rank, *-in* substance, *recept-* receive, *-or* agent]

G_0 phase step of the cell life cycle in which a newly formed daughter cell grows in size and then maintains itself for some time, but fails to proceed onward to prepare for later reproduction (cell division); G_0 phase follows the M phase (mitotic division) and represents the cell "opting out" of further reproduction; *see* **cell life cycle** [G- growth or gap, *phase* appearance]

G_1 phase step of the cell life cycle in which a newly formed daughter cell grows in size, in anticipation of later reproduction (cell division); G_1 phase follows the M phase (mitotic division) and precedes the S phase (DNA replication); *see* **cell life cycle** [G- growth or gap, *phase* appearance]

G_2 phase step of the cell life cycle in which a cell grows in size after having replicated its DNA and prepares for mitotic reproduction (cell division); G_2 phase follows the S phase (DNA replication) and precedes the M phase (mitotic division); *see* **cell life cycle** [G- growth or gap, *phase* appearance]

galactokinetic hormone (gal-ak-toh-kih-NET-ik HOR-mohn) any hormone that promotes milk ejection into ducts of the breast by stimulating myoepithelial cells surrounding alveoli [*galact-* milk, *-kinesis* motion, *-ic* relating to, *hormon-* excite]

galactopoietic hormone (gal-ak-toh-poy-ET-ik HOR-mohn) any hormone that maintains milk production in the breast (after it has already started) [*galact-* milk, *-poiet-* make, *-ic* relating to, *hormon-* excite]

gamete (GAM-eet) sex cells; spermatozoa and ova [*gamet-* sexual union or marriage partner]

gamma (γ) motor neuron (GAM-mah MOH-tor NYOO-ron) stimulate contraction of the striated ends of the muscle spindle fibre (intrafusal fibre) [*gamma (γ)* third letter of Greek alphabet, *mot-* move, *-or* agent, *neuron* string or nerve]

gamma (γ) ray (GAM-mah) electromagnetic radiation; more penetrating than alpha and beta particles [*gamma (γ)* third letter of Greek alphabet]

ganglion (GANG-lee-on) in peripheral nerves, a region of grey matter made up of unmyelinated fibres [*gangli-* knot, *-on* unit] *pl.*, ganglia (GANG-lee-ah)

ganglion neuron (GANG-glee-ON) sensory neurons in the retina of the eye that collect information from rods and cones and also act as photoreceptors themselves [*gangli-* knot, *-on* unit, *neuron* string or nerve]

gangrene (GANG-green) tissue death (necrosis) that involves decay of tissue [*gangren-* gnawing sore]

gap junction (gap JUNK-shun) cell connection formed when membrane channels of adjacent plasma membranes adhere to each other [*junction* to join]

gastric inhibitory peptide (GIP) (GAS-trik in-HIB-ih-tor-ee PEP-tyde) hormone produced by the intestinal mucosa that inhibits gastric secretion and motility; because it also enhances pancreatic insulin secretion in the presence of high plasma glucose, it has been more recently called *glucose-dependent insulinotropic polypeptide (GIP)* [*gastr-* stomach, *-ic* relating to, *inhibit-* restrain, *-ory* relating to, *pept-* digest, *-ide* chemical]

gastric juice (GAS-trik) stomach secretion containing acid and enzymes; aids in the digestion of food [*gastr-* stomach, *-ic* relating to]

gastric phase (GAS-trik) during this phase the stomach releases gastrin, which accelerates secretion of gastric juice [*gastr-* stomach, *-ic* relating to]

gastrin (GAS-trin) gastrointestinal (GI) hormone that plays an important regulatory role in the digestive process by stimulating gastric secretion [*gastr-* stomach, *-in* substance]

gastrocnemius muscle (GAS-trok-NEE-mee-us) calf muscle [*gastro-* belly, *-cnemius* leg, *mus-* mouse, *-cle* little]

gastroenteritis (gas-troh-en-ter-EYE-tis) inflammation of the stomach and intestines [*gastr-* stomach, *-enter-* intestine, *-itis* inflammation]

gastroenterology (gas-troh-en-ter-OL-oh-jee) study of the stomach and intestines and their diseases [*gastr-* stomach, *-entero-* intestine, *-o-* combining form, *-log-* words (study of), *-y* activity]

gastrointestinal (GI) tract (gas-troh-in-TES-tih-nul trakt) alimentary canal; tube formed by the major organs of digestion [*gastr-* stomach, *-intestin-* intestine, *-al* relating to, *tract* trail]

gastro-oesophageal reflux disease (GORD) (gas-troh-eh-sof-eh-JEE-all REE-fluks) condition that results when stomach acid enters into the oesophagus [*gastro-* stomach, *-oes-* will carry, *-phag-* food (eat), *-al* relating to, *re-* again or back, *-flux* flow, *dis-* opposite of, *-ease* comfort]

gastrulation (gas-troo-LAY-shun) process by which blastocyst cells move and then differentiate into the three primary germ layers [*gastr-* belly, *-ula-* little, *-tion* process]

gated channel channel in the plasma membrane that can be opened and closed to alter membrane permeability

gene one of many segments of a chromosome (DNA molecule); each gene contains the genetic code for synthesizing a protein molecule such as an enzyme or hormone or to make a functional RNA molecule such as tRNA or rRNA [*gen-* produce or generate]

gene augmentation (awg-men-TAY-shun) therapeutic technique that introduces genes with the hope that they will add to the production of a needed protein [*gen-* produce or generate]

gene chip DNA analysis technique [*gen-* produce or generate]

gene linkage when a whole group of genes stay together during the crossing-over process [*gen-* produce or generate]

gene replacement therapeutic technique that replaces genes that specify production of abnormal proteins with normal genes [*gen-* produce or generate]

gene therapy manipulation of genes to cure genetic problems; most forms of gene therapy have not yet proven to be effective in humans [*gen-* produce or generate]

general adaptation syndrome (GAS) (JEN-er-al ad-ap-TAY-shun SIN-drohm) group of changes that make the presence of stress in the body known [*adapt-* fit to, *-ation* process, *syn-* together, *-drome* running or (race) course]

general sense organ structure that consists of microscopic receptors widely distributed throughout the body [*organ* instrument]

genetic counselling (jeh-NET-ik) professional consultations with families regarding genetic diseases [*gene-* produce, *-ic* relating to, *council-* plan]

genetic factor (jeh-NET-ik) inherited trait [*gene-* produce, *-ic* relating to]

genetic mutation (jeh-NET-ik myoo-TAY-shun) change in the genetic material within a genome; may occur spontaneously or as a result of mutagens [*gene-* produce, *-ic* relating to, *muta-* change, *-ation* process]

genetic predisposition (jeh-NET-ik pree-dispoh-ZIH-shun) likelihood because of inherited genes of developing a condition even though the condition itself may not be solely caused by genetic mechanisms [*gene-* produce, *-ic* relating to, *pre-* before, *dispos-* put in order, *-tion* process]

genetics (jeh-NET-iks) scientific study of heredity and the genetic code [*gene-* produce, *-ic* relating to]

geniculate body (jeh-NIK-yoo-layt BOD-ee) either of two groups of cerebral nuclei comprising the thalamus; located in posterior region of each lateral mass; play role in processing auditory and visual input [*gen-* knee or knot, *-icul-* small, *-ate* of or like]

genital (JEN-ih-tal) reproductive organ [*gen-* produce, *-al* relating to] *pl.*, genitals or genitalia

genital duct (JEN-ih-tal) conveys sperm to the outside of the body; also called *reproductive duct* [*gen-* produce, *-al* relating to]

genitalia (jen-ih-TAIL-yah) reproductive organs (*see* **genital**) [*gen-* produce, *-al-* relating to, *-ia* things]

genome (JEE-nohm) entire set of chromosomes in a cell; the *human genome* refers to the entire set of human chromosomes [*gen-* produce (gene), *-ome* entire collection]

genomics (jeh-NO-miks) field of endeavour involving the analysis of the genetic code contained in the human or another species' genome [*gen-* produce (gene), *-om-* entire collection, *-ic* relating to]

genotype (JEN-oh-type) alleles present at one or more specific loci on a chromosome of a given individual; *see* **phenotype** [*gen-* produce (gene), *-type* kind]

germinal epithelium (JER-mih-nal ep-ih-THEE-lee-um) small epithelial cells that are on the surface of the ovaries [*germ* sprout, *-al* relating to, *epi-* on or upon, *-theli-* nipple, *-al* relating to]

germinal matrix (JER-mih-nal MAY-triks) cap-shaped cluster of cells at the bottom of a hair follicle [*germ* sprout, *-al* relating to, *matrix* womb] *pl.*, matrices (MAY-tris-eez)

gerontology (jair-on-TOL-oh-jee) study of the ageing process [*geronto-* old age, *-log-* words (study of), *-y* activity]

gestation period (jes-TAY-shun) length of pregnancy, approximately 9 months in humans [*gesta-* bear, *-tion* process]

ghrelin (GHRL) (GRAY-lin) hormone secreted by epithelial cells lining the stomach; ghrelin boosts appetite, slows metabolism, and reduces fat burning; may be involved in the development of obesity [*ghrel-* grow (also acronym for growth-hormone-releasing peptide), *-in* substance]

gigantism (jye-GAN-tiz-em) condition produced by hypersecretion of growth hormone during the early years of life; results in a child who grows to gigantic size [*gigant-* great, *-ism* condition]

gingiva (JIN-jih-vah) mucous membrane that surrounds the teeth; also known as *gums* [*gingiv-* gum] *pl.*, gingivae (JIN-jih-vee)

gingivitis (jin-ji-VYE-tis) inflammation of the gum (gingiva), often as a result of poor oral hygiene [*gingiv-* gum, *-itis* inflammation]

gland secreting structure [*gland* acorn]

glandular (GLAN-dyoo-lar) resembling a gland [*gland-* acorn (gland), *-ula-* little, *-ar* relating to]

glans penis (glans PEE-nis) slightly bulging structure formed by the distal end of the corpus spongiosum; head of the penis; covered by the foreskin in uncircumcised males [*glans* acorn, *penis* male sex organ] *pl.*, glandes penes (GLAN-deez PEE-neez)

glans clitoris (glans KLIT-oh-ris) *see* **clitoris** [*glans* acorn, *clitoris* small key or latch]

glaucoma (glaw-KOH-mah) disorder characterized by elevated pressure in the eye; can lead to permanent blindness [*glauco-* grey or silver, *-oma* tumour (growth)]

glia (GLEE-ah) nonexcitable supporting cells of nervous tissue; formerly called *neuroglia* [*glia* glue] *sing.*, glial cell

gliding joint (GLYDE-ing joynt) type of synovial joint that allow multiaxial gliding movement between flat planes of bone

gliding movement (GLYDE-ing MOOV-ment) movement that results when the articular surface of one bone moves over the articular surface of another without any angular or circular movement

glioblastoma multiforme (glye-oh-blas-TOH-ma mul-tih-FOR-mee) malignant tumour of astrocyte cells of the brain [*glia-* glue, *-blasto-* bud, *-oma* tumour, *multi-* many, *-form-* shape]

glioma (glee-OH-mah) any tumour of neuroglia (glial) cells in nerve tissue [*glio-* neuroglia, *-oma* tumour]

globin (GLOH-bin) chain of four proteins; binds to a red pigment (haem) to form haemoglobin [*glob-* ball, *-in* substance]

glomerular capsular membrane (gloh-MER-yoo-lar KAP-syoo-lahr) membrane made up of glomerular endothelium, basement membrane, and visceral layer of the Bowman capsule; function is filtration [*glomer-* ball, *-ul-* little, *-ar* relating to, *caps-* box, *-ula-* little, *-ar* relating to, *membran-* thin skin]

glomerular filtration rate (GFR) (gloh-MER-yoo-lar fil-TRAY-shun) the rate of movement of fluid out of the glomerulus and into the capsular space [*glomer-* ball, *-ul-* little, *-ar* relating to, *filtr-* strain, *-ation* process]

glomerulonephritis (gloh-mer-yoo-loh-neh-FRY-tis) inflammatory disease of the glomerular-capsular membranes of the kidney [*glomer-* ball, *-ul-* little, *-nephr-* kidney, *-itis* inflammation]

glomerulus (gloh-MAIR-yoo-lus) compact cluster, particularly when referring to the tuft of capillaries forming part of the nephron [*glomer-* ball, *-ulus* little] *pl.*, glomeruli

glossopharyngeal nerve (glos-oh-fah-RIN-jee-al) cranial nerve IX; mixed nerve [*glosso-* tongue, *-pharyng-* throat, *-al* relating to]

glottis (GLOT-iss) composed of the true vocal cords and the space between them [*glottis* mouth of windpipe] *pl.*, glottides (GLOT-id-eez) or glottises

glucagon (GLOO-kah-gon) hormone secreted by alpha cells of the pancreatic islets; increases activity of phosphorylase [*gluca-* sweet (glucose), *-agon* lead or bring]
glucocorticoid (GC) (gloo-koh-KOR-tih-koyd) hormone that influences food metabolism; secreted by the adrenal cortex [*gluco-* sweet (glucose), *-cortic* cortex (bark), *-oid* like]
gluconeogenesis (gloo-koh-nee-oh-JEN-eh-sis) formulation of glucose or glycogen from protein or fat compounds [*gluco-* sweet (glucose), *-neo-* new, *-gen-* produce, *-esis* process]
glucosamine (gloo-KOHS-ah-meen) component of some proteoglycans that thicken and hold together connective tissues such as cartilage [*gluco-* sweetness or glucose, *-amine* ammonia compound]
glucose (GLOO-kohs) monosaccharide, or simple sugar; principal blood sugar used by cells [*gluco-* sweet, *-ose* carbohydrate (sugar)]
glucose-dependent insulinotropic polypeptide (GIP) (GLOO-kohs dih-PEN-dent insuh-LIN-oh-troph-ik poh-lee-PEP-tyde) *see* **gastric inhibitory peptide** [*gluco-* sweet, *-ose* carbohydrate (sugar), *depend-* to hang upon, *insula-* island, *-troph* nourishment, *-ic* relating to]
glucose phosphorylation (GLOO-kohs fos-for-ih-LAY-shun) process of converting glucose to glucose-6-phosphate; prepares glucose for further metabolic reactions [*gluco-* sweet, *-ose* carbohydrate (sugar), *phos-* light, *-phor-* carry, *-yl-* chemical, *-ation* process]
glutamate (GLOO-tah-mayt) glutamic acid; amino acid that when acting as a neurotransmitter is believed to be responsible for up to 75% of the excitatory signals in the brain [*glut-* glue, *-am-* ammonia compound, *-ate* salt of acid]
gluteal (GLOO-tee-al) relating to the buttock [*glut-* buttock, *-al* relating to, *mus-* mouse, *-cle* little]
gluteal muscle (GLOO-tee-al) buttock muscle; moves the thigh [*glut-* buttocks, *-al* relating to, *mus-* mouse, *-cle* little]
glycerol (GLIS-er-ol) sugar alcohol subunit of some lipid molecules; product of fat digestion [*glyce-* sweet, *-ol* alcohol]
glycine (GLYE-seen) amino acid; most widely distributed inhibitory neurotransmitter in the spinal cord [*gly-* sweet, *-amine* ammonia]
glycogen (GLYE-koh-jen) polysaccharide (complex carbohydrate); main carbohydrate stored in animal cells [*glyco-* sweet, *-gen* produce]
glycogenesis (glye-koh-JEN-eh-sis) anabolic pathway of glycogen formation; formation of glycogen from glucose or from other monosaccharides, fructose, or galactose [*glyco-* sweet, *-gen-* produce, *-esis* process]
glycogenolysis (glye-koh-jeh-NOL-ih-sis) hydrolysis of glycogen to glucose-6-phosphate or to glucose [*glyco-* sweet (glucose), *-gen-* produce, *-o-* combining form, *-lysis* loosening]
glycolipid (glye-koh-LIP-id) lipid molecule with attached carbohydrate group [*glyco-* sweet (glucose), *-lipid* fat]
glycolysis (glye-KOHL-ih-sis) first series of chemical reactions in carbohydrate catabolism; changes glucose to pyruvic acid in a series of anaerobic reactions [*glyco-* sweet (glucose), *-o-* combining form, *-lysis* loosening]
glycophospholipid (glye-koh-fos-foh-LIP-id) molecule that is part sugar and part phospholipid; formed in epidermal cells of the skin to produce a waterproof barrier [*glyco-* sweet (glucose), *phos-* light, *-pho-* bear, *-lipid* fat]
glycoprotein (glye-koh-PROH-teen) substance made of molecules that are a combined form of carbohydrate and protein [*glyco-* sweet (glucose), *-prote-* first rank, *-in* substance, *hormon-* excite]
glycoprotein hormone (glye-koh-PRO-teen HOR-mohn) hormone made of molecules that are a combined form of carbohydrate and protein [*glyco-* sweet (glucose), *-prote-* first rank, *-in* substance, *hormon-* excite]
glycosuria (glye-koh-SOO-ree-ah) glucose in urine; a sign of diabetes mellitus [*glyco-* sweet (glucose), *-ur-* urine, *-ia* condition]
goblet cell (GOB-let sel) epithelial cell that produces and secretes large amounts of mucus [*gobl-* bowl, *-et* small, *cell* storeroom]
Golgi apparatus (GOL-jee ap-ah-RA-tus) organelle consisting of small sacs stacked on one another near the nucleus that makes carbohydrate compounds, combines them with protein molecules, and packages the product for distribution from the cell [*Camillo Golgi* Italian histologist]
Golgi tendon organ (GOL-jee TEN-don OR-gan) sensory organ imbedded in muscle tendons made up of sensory neurons (Golgi tendon receptors) that are encapsulated with collagen bundles; also called *tendon organ* [*Camillo Golgi* Italian histologist, *tend-* pulled tight, *-on* unit]
Golgi tendon receptor (GOL-jee TEN-don ree-SEP-tor) sensory stretch receptor neuron (part of the Golgi tendon organ) that is responsible for proprioception (muscle tension); stimulated by excessive muscle contraction; also called *tendon receptor* [*Camillo Golgi* Italian histologist, *tend-* pulled tight, *-on* unit, *recept-* receive, *-or* agent]
Golgi tendon reflex (GOL-jee TEN-den REE-fleks) spinal nerve reflex that protects muscles from tearing internally or pulling away from their tendinous points of attachment to bone because of excessive contractile force by relaxing a muscle when its tension becomes too great; also called *tendon reflex* [*Camillo Golgi* Italian histologist, *tend-* pulled tight, *-on* unit, *re-* back or again, *-flex* bend]
gomphosis (gom-FOH-sis) fibrous joint where a process is inserted into a socket; for example, the joint between the tooth and mandible [*gomphos-* bolt, *-osis* condition] *pl.*, gomphoses (gom-FOH-seez)
gonad (GO-nad) sex gland in which reproductive cells are formed; ovary in women, testis in men [*gon-* offspring, *-ad* relating to]
gonadotroph (go-NAD-oh-trohf) cell type of the adenohypophysis (anterior pituitary) that secretes the gonadotropins luteinizing hormone (LH) and follicle-stimulating hormone (FSH) [*gon-* offspring, *-ad-* relating to, *-troph* nourish]
gonadotropin (go-nah-doh-TROH-pin) any of the hormones (FSH and LSH) produced by the anterior pituitary or embryonic tissue (hCG) that stimulate growth and maintenance of the testes or ovaries [*gon-* offspring, *-ad-* relating to, *-trop-* turn or change, *-in* substance]
goniometer (gon-ee-OM-eh-ter) instrument used to measure range of motion (ROM) angles of a joint [*gonio-* angle, *-meter* measure]
gout (gowt) condition characterized by excessive levels of uric acid in the blood that are deposited in the joints [*gout* drop]
gouty arthritis (gow-TEE ar-THRY-tis) metabolic disorder in which excess blood levels of uric acid are deposited within the synovial fluid of joints and other tissues [*gout-* drop, *-y* of or like, *arthr-* joint, *-itis* inflammation]
graafian follicle (GRAH-fee-en FOL-lih-kul) a secondary follicle; consists of a mature ovum surrounded by granulosa cells at boundary of fluid-filled antrum [*Reijnier de Graaf* Dutch physician, *-an* relating to, *foll-* bag, *-icle* little]
graded potential local potentials that vary according to strength of stimulus and distance of membrane from source [*grad-* step, *potent-* power, *-ial* relating to]
graded strength principle skeletal muscles contract with varying degrees of strength at different times
gradient (GRAY-dee-ent) measurable difference between two points of a given variable such as molecular concentration, pressure, or electrical charge [*grad-* step, *-ent* state]
graft-versus-host rejection (graft VUR-suhz host reh-JEK-shun) rejection of grafted tissue that occurs when donated tissue attacks the recipient's human leucocyte antigens [*graft-* stylus, *-versus-* turned toward or against, *-host* guest, *re-* again, *-ject-* throw, *ion* process]
granulation tissue (gran-yool-AY-shun TISH-yoo) fibrous connective tissue with a rich blood supply and high number of immune cells that forms in a wound as a blood clot dissolves; it is a normal tissue present during the healing process [*gran-* grain, *-ul-* little, *-ation* process, *tissue* fabric]
granule cell (GRAN-yool) inhibits action potentials in the olfactory bulb [*gran-* grain, *-ule* little, *cell* storeroom]
granulocyte (GRAN-yoo-loh-syte) leucocyte with granules in cytoplasm [*gran-* grain, *-ul-* little, *-cyte* cell]
granulosa cell (gran-yoo-LOH-sah) develops around each primary oocyte forming a primary follicle [*gran-* grain, *-ul-* little, *-os-* relating to, *-a* thing, *cell* storeroom]
Graves disease (grayvz) inherited, possibly autoimmune endocrine disorder characterized by hyperthyroidism accompanied by exophthalmos (protruding eyes) [*Robert J. Graves* Irish physician, *dis-* opposite of, *-ease* comfort]
great saphenous vein (grayt sah-FEE-nus vayn) vein of the lower extremity; drains much of the superficial leg and foot [*saphen-* manifest, *-ous* relating to, *vena* blood vessel]
greater omentum (oh-MEN-tum) pouchlike extension of the visceral peritoneum extending from greater curvature of the stomach to the transverse colon; often called "the lace apron" [*omentum* fatty covering of intestines] *pl.*, omenta (oh-MEN-tah)
greater vestibular gland (ves-TIB-yoo-lar) either of the glands on each side of the vaginal orifice that secrete a lubricating fluid; also called *Bartholin glands* [*vestibul-* entrance hall, *-ar* relating to, *gland* acorn]
greenstick fracture (GREEN-stik FRAK-chur) type of incomplete bone fracture in which bone is bent but broken only on one side (common in children) [*fracture* a breaking]
grey column (gray KOL-um) any one of the three longitudinal areas (anterior, lateral, posterior) of the spinal cord that contain grey matter
grey commissure (gray KOHM-is-shoor) middle band of grey matter that joins the left and right columns [*commiss-* join, *-ur-* result of process]
grey fibre (gray FYE-ber) unmyelinated nerve fibre; component of grey matter [*fibre* thread]
grey matter (gray MAT-ter) type of nerve tissue characterized by a relative lack of myelin; often includes many neuron cell bodies and synapses that process information; contrast with *white matter* [*materia-* something from which something is made]
grey ramus (gray RAY-muss) short branch by which some postganglionic axons return to a spinal nerve [*ramus* branch]
gross anatomy the study of the larger structures of an organism, such as organs and systems, that are large enough to be seen without magnification; also called *macroscopic anatomy*; compare to **microscopic anatomy** [*gross* large, *ana-* apart, *-tom-* cut, *-y* action]
ground substance organic matrix of bone and cartilage
growth hormone (GH) (HOR-mohn) hormone secreted by the anterior pituitary gland that controls the rate of skeletal and visceral growth [*hormon-* excite]
growth normal increase in size or number of cells
gustatory (GUS-tah-tor-ee) refers to taste [*gusta-* taste, *-ory* relating to]
gustatory cell (GUS-tah-tor-ee) chemoreceptors in tongue that sense taste [*gusta-* taste, *-ory* relating to, *cell* storeroom]
gustatory hair (GUS-tah-tor-ee) cilia-like structure projecting from gustatory cells and into taste pores [*gusta-* taste, *-ory* relating to]
Guthrie test (GUH-three) blood test to detect phenylketonuria (PKU) [*Robert Guthrie* American microbiologist]
gynaecology (gye-neh-KOL-oh-jee) study of the female reproductive system [*gynaeco-* woman or female gender, *-logy* study of]
gyrus (JYE-rus) convoluted ridge, usually refers to rounded elevations of the brain surface; also called *convolution* [*gyrus* circle]

H

haematocrit (Hct) (hee-MAT-oh-krit) volume percent of blood cells in whole blood; packed cell volume [*haemato-* blood, *-crit* separate]
haematopoiesis (hee-mah-toh-poy-EE-sis) process of blood cell formation [*haemo-* blood, *-poiesis* making]
haematopoietic stem cell (hee-mah-toh-poy-ET-ik) nucleated cell in the red bone marrow that develops into a red blood cell [*haem-* blood, *-poiesis* making, *stem-* tree or trunk, *cell* storeroom]
haematopoietic tissue (hee-mah-toh-poy-ET-ik) connective tissue type that is responsible for formation of blood cells and lymphatic system cells; in red bone marrow, spleen, tonsils, and lymph nodes [*haem-* blood, *-poie-* to make, *-ic* relating to, *tissu-* fabric]
haematuria (hem-ah-TOO-ree-ah) blood in the urine [*haema-* blood, *-ur-* urine, *-ia* condition]
haem (heem) iron-containing chemical group found in haemoglobin; temporarily binds to oxygen [*haem-* blood]
haem group (heem) *see* **haeme** [*haem-* blood]
haemocytoblast (hee-moh-SYE-toh-blast) bone marrow stem cell from which all formed elements of blood arise [*haemo-* blood, *-cyto* cell, *-blast* embryonic state of development]
haemodialysis (hee-moh-dye-AL-ih-sis) therapy involving separation of smaller (diffusible) particles from larger (nondiffusible) particles in blood through a semipermeable membrane, usually employed when a patient's kidneys fail to remove these particles from the blood [*haemo-* blood, *-dia-* through or between, *-lysis* loosening]
haemodynamics (hee-moh-dye-NAM-iks) study of the mechanisms that influence dynamic circulation of blood [*haemo-* blood, *-dynam-* moving force, *-ic* relating to]
haemoglobin (hee-moh-GLOH-bin) iron-containing protein in red blood cells responsible for their oxygen-carrying capacity [*haemo-*blood, *-glob-* ball, *-in* substance]
haemolytic anaemia (hee-moh-LIT-ik ah-NEE-mee-ah) inherited blood disorder that is characterized by abnormal types of haemoglobin [*haemo-* blood, *-lyt-* loosen, *-ic* relating to, *an-* without, *-(h)aem-* blood, *-ia* condition]
haemophilia (hee-moh-FIL-ee-ah) X-linked inherited disorder that decreases the production of one or more plasma proteins responsible for blood clotting [*haemo-* blood, *-phil-* love, *-ia* condition]
haemorrhoid (HEM-uh-royd) varicose vein in the rectum; also called *piles* [*haemo-* blood, *-rrh-* flow, *-oid* of or like]
haemostasis (hee-moh-STAY-sis) stoppage of blood flow [*haemo-* blood, *-stasis* standing]
H band in a muscle fibre's sarcomere, refers to the middle region of the thick filaments where they do not overlap the thin filaments [*H heller* bright]
hair cell mechanoreceptor cells with sensory cilia or "hairs" in the ear that are responsible for balance and hearing [*cell* storeroom]
hair follicle (FOHL-ih-kul) small blind-end tube extending from the dermis through the epidermis that contains the hair root and where hair growth occurs; sebaceous and

apocrine skin glands have ducts leading into the follicle [*foll-* bag, *-icle* little]

hair papilla (pah-PIL-ah) small, cap-shaped cluster of cells located at the base of the follicle where hair growth begins [*papilla* nipple] *pl.*, papillae (pah-PIL-ee)

hairline fracture type of bone fracture common in the skull—fracture components are small and aligned; if the fracture is pushed downward, called a *depressed fracture* [*fracture* a breaking]

Haldane effect (HAWL-dayn ef-FEKT) phenomenon that refers to the increased CO_2 loading caused by a decrease in Po_2 [*John Scott Haldane* Scots physiologist, *effect* accomplishment]

hallux (HAL-luks) great toe [*hallux* great toe] *pl.*, halluces (HAL-lus-eez)

hangman's fracture bone fracture of the posterior elements in the upper cervical spine, especially the axis [*fracture* a breaking]

haploid (number) (HAP-loyd) halved number of chromosomes in gametes resulting from meiosis; in humans, 23 chromosomes per sex cell [*haplo-* single, *-oid* of or like]

hard palate (PAL-et) portions of four bones (two maxillae and two palatines) that make up the roof of the mouth [*palat-* palate (roof of the mouth)]

haustra (HAW-strah) pouchlike segments of the colon formed by dense rings of circular muscle in the colon wall [*haustr-* scoop of a waterwheel] *sing.*, haustrum (HAW-strum)

Haversian canal (hah-VER-shun) *see* **central canal** (of bone) [*Clopton Havers*, English physician]

Haversian system (hah-VER-shun) *see* **osteon** [*Clopton Havers*, English physician]

heart organ of circulatory system that pumps the blood; composed of cardiac muscle tissue

heart block blockage of impulse conduction from atria to ventricles so that the heart beats at a slower rate than normal

heart failure inability of the heart to pump returned blood sufficiently

heart murmur abnormal heart sound that may indicate valvular insufficiency or stenosing of the valve [*murmur* mutter]

heat exhaustion condition caused by fluid loss resulting from activity of thermoregulatory mechanisms in a warm external environment

heat stroke life-threatening condition characterized by high body temperature; failure of thermoregulatory mechanisms to maintain homeostasis in a very warm external environment

Heberden node (HEB-er-den) swelling deformity of the distal interphalangeal joints [*William Heberden* English physician, *nod-* knot]

Heimlich manoeuvre (HYME-lik mah-NOO-ver) see **abdominal thrusts** [*Henry J. Heimlich* American physician]

helper T cell (T_H cell) immune system cells that help B cells differentiate into antibody-secreting plasma cells; also help coordinate cellular immunity through direct contact with other immune cells [helper, *T* thymus gland, *cell* storeroom]

hemiazygos vein (hem-ee-AZ-ih-gohs vayn) vein of the thorax [*hemi-* half, *-a-* without, *-zygo-*union or yoke, *vena* blood vessel]

hemiplegia (hem-ee-PLEE-jee-ah) condition that refers to paralysis of one whole side of the body [*hemi-* half, *-pleg-* stricken, *-ia* condition]

hemisphere (HEM-iss-feer) one half of a generally spherical structure, as in the left and right hemispheres of the cerebellum or cerebrum [*hemi-* half, *-sphere* globe]

hemisphericity (HEM-ih-sfeer-is-ih-tee) different specialization of function in each hemisphere of an organ, as in the cerebral hemispheres [*hemi-* half, *-spher-* globe, *-ic-* relating to, *-ity* state]

Henry's law gas law that describes how the pressure of a gas relates to the concentration of that gas in a liquid solution [*William Henry* English chemist]

heparin (HEP-ah-rin) substance obtained from the liver; inhibits blood clotting [*hepar-* liver, *-in* substance]

hepatic (heh-PAT-ik) relating to the liver [*hepat-* liver, *-ic* relating to]

hepatic duct (heh-PAT-ik) one of two ducts that drains bile out of the liver [*hepa-* liver, *-ic* relating to, *duct* path]

hepatic lobule (heh-PAT-ik LOB-yool) anatomical units of the liver [*hepa-* liver, *-ic* relating to, *lob-* pod, *-ule* small]

hepatic portal circulation (heh-PAT-ik POR-tal) the route of blood flow through the liver [*hepa-* liver, *-ic* relating to, *port-* doorway, *-al* relating to, *circulat-* go around, *-tion* process]

hepatitis (hep-ah-TYE-tis) inflammation of the liver; may be caused by toxins, viruses (e.g., hepatitis A, hepatitis B), bacteria, or parasites [*hepat-* liver, *-itis* inflammation]

hepatocyte (heh-PAT-oh-syte) relating to the liver [*hepat-* liver, *-cyte* cell]

heredity (heh-RED-ih-tee) transmission of characteristics from parents to offspring [*heredity-* inheritance]

Hering–Breuer reflex (HER-ing BROO-er REE-fleks) stretch reflex to control respirations—especially rate and rhythmicity [*Heinrich E. Hering* German physiologist, *Joseph Breuer* Australian physician, *re-* back or again, *-flex* bend]

herniated disc (HER-nee-ayt-ed) condition of the vertebral disc when the annulus fibrosis becomes disrupted, allowing the nucleus pulposus to protrude [*hernia-* rupture, *-ate* act of]

herpes zoster (HER-peez ZOS-ter) "shingles", viral infection that affects the skin of a single dermatome [*herpe* creep, *zoster* girdle]

heterozygous (het-er-oh-ZYE-gus) genotype with two different forms of a trait [*hetero-* different, *-zygo-* union or yoke, *-ous* characterized by]

hexose (HEK-sohs) monosaccharide molecule with six carbons [*hex-* six, *-ose* sugar]

hiatal hernia (hye-AY-tal HER-nee-ah) condition in which a portion of the stomach is pushed through the hiatus (opening) of the diaphragm, often weakening or expanding the cardiac sphincter at the inferior end of the oesophagus [*hiat-* gap, *-al* relating to, *hernia* rupture] *pl.*, herniae (HER-nee-ee) or hernias

hiccup (HIK-up) involuntary spasmodic contraction of the diaphragm [*hiccup* imitation of sound made when hiccupping]

high-density lipoprotein (lip-oh-PROH-teen) a blood lipid fraction (plasma protein) composed of cholesterol, about 50% protein, and triglycerides; often called "good cholesterol" because it carries cholesterol out of the blood to the liver for elimination [*dense-* thick, *-ity* state, *lipo-* fat, *-protein* first rank]

high-energy bond chemical bond that requires an input of energy to form and when broken can result in the transfer of useful energy to cellular processes, as in ATP [*en-* in, *-erg* work, *-y* state, *bond* band]

hilum (HYE-lum) slit on medial surface of each lung where primary bronchi and pulmonary vessels enter; slit on medial surface of each kidney where blood vessels and other structures enter the kidney [*hilum* least bit] *pl.*, hila

hinge joint (hinj joynt) type of diarthrotic synovial joint that allows movement around a single axis in the manner of a hinge

histamine (HIS-tah-meen) inflammatory chemical [*hist-* tissue, *-amine* ammonia compound]

histogenesis (hiss-toh-JEN-eh-sis) formation of tissues from primary germ layers of embryo [*histo-* tissue, *-gen-* produce, *-esis* process]

histology (his-TOL-oh-jee) branch of microscopic anatomy that studies tissues; biology of tissues [*histo-* tissue, *-o-* combining form, *-log-* words (study of), *-y* activity]

histone (HISS-tohn) protein that organizes chromatin into nucleosomes [*histo-* tissue, *-one* unit]

histophysiology (his-toh-fiz-ee-OL-oh-jee) study of microscopic anatomy of cells and tissues and how structural information correlates with function [*histo-* tissue, *-o-* combining form, *-physio-* nature (function), *-o-* combining form, *-log-* words (study of), *-y* activity]

H-K pump ion pump in the gastric parietal cells [*H* hydrogen, *K* potassium]

Hodgkin disease (HOJ-kin) type of lymphoma (malignant lymph tumour) characterized by painless swelling of lymph nodes in the neck, progressing to other regions [*Thomas Hodgkin* English physician, *dis-* opposite of, *-ease* comfort]

Hodgkin lymphoma (HOJ-kin lim-FOH-mah) *see* **Hodgkin disease** [*Thomas Hodgkin* English physician, *lymph-* water (lymphatic system), *-oma* tumour]

holocrine gland (HOH-loh-krin) gland that collects secretory product inside its cells, which then rupture completely to release it; for example, sebaceous glands of the skin [*holo-* whole, *-crine* to secrete]

homeostasis (ho-me-oh-STAY-sis) relative constancy of the normal body's internal (fluid) environment [*homeo-* same or equal, *-stasis* standing still]

homeostatic control mechanisms (hoh-mee-oh-STAH-tik) devices for maintaining or restoring homeostasis [*homeo-* same or equal, *-stat-* stand, *-ic* relating to]

homologous transfusion (ho-MOL-oh-gus) blood transfused into the body of another individual [*homo-* same, *-log-* word or proportion, *-ous* relating to]

homozygous (hoh-moh-ZYE-gus) genotype with two identical forms of a trait [*homo-* same, *-zygo-* union or yoke, *-ous* characterized by]

horizontal fissure (hor-ih-ZON-tal FISH-ur) separates the superior lobe of the right lung from the middle lobe [*fissur-* cleft]

horizontal plane (hor-ih-ZON-tal) transverse plane; divides the body into superior and inferior portions [*plan-* flat surface]

hormone (HOR-mohn) substance secreted by an endocrine gland into the bloodstream that acts on a specific target tissue to produce a given response [*hormon-* excite]

hormone-receptor complex (HOR-mohn ree-SEP-tor) when a steroid hormone combines to a receptor site in the target cell and then moves into the nucleus of the target cell [*hormon-* excite, *recept-* receive, *-or* agent, *com-* together, *-plex* weave or braid]

host-versus-graft rejection (host VUR-suhz graft reh-JEK-shun) rejection of grafted tissue that occurs when the recipient's immune system recognizes foreign human leucocyte antigens and attacks them, destroying the donated tissue [*host-* guest, *-versus-* turned toward or against, *-graft* stylus, *re-* again, *-ject-* to throw, *-tion* process]

human chorionic gonadotropin (HCG or hCG) (koh-ree-ON-ik go-nah-doh-TROH-pin) hormone secreted early in pregnancy by the placenta that serves to maintain the uterine lining [*human-* of or belonging to a man, *chorion-* skin, *-ic* relating to, *gon-* offspring, *-ad-* relating to, *-trop-* nourish, *-in* substance]

human engineered chromosome (HEC) (KROH-meh-sohm) gene augmentation procedure that inserts therapeutic genes into a separate strand of DNA that is inserted into nucleus of cell [*chrom-* colour, *-som-* body]

Human Genome Project (HGP) (JEE-nome) a worldwide collaborative effort of scientists and others to map out the entire human genome and study the biological, medical, and ethical aspects of their discoveries; the HGP is largely funded by U.S. government sources such as the DOE (Department of Energy) and the NIH (National Institutes of Health); a currently active HGP offshoot is *ENCODE (The Encyclopedia of DNA Elements)*; *see* **genome, genomics** (*gen-* to produce, *-om(e)-* whole collection, *-ic* relating to]

human immunodeficiency virus (HIV) (ih-myoo-noh-deh-FISH-en-see) a retrovirus that contains RNA that produces its own DNA inside infected cells; results in acquired immunodeficiency syndrome (AIDS) [*immuno-* free (immunity), *-de-* down, *-fic-* perform, *-ency* state, *virus* poison]

human leucocyte antigen (HLA) (LOO-koh-syte AN-tih-jen) protein involved in transplant rejection [*leuco-* white, *-cyte* cell, *anti-* against, *-gen* produce]

human placental lactogen (hPL) (plah-SEN-tal LAK-toh-jen) hormone released by the placenta; promotes development of mammary glands during pregnancy and regulates energy balance in fetus [*placenta-* flat cake, *-al* relating to, *lacto-* milk, *-gen* produce]

humerus (HYOO-mer-us) arm bone [*humerus* arm] *pl.*, humeri

humoral immunity (HYOO-mor-al ih-MYOO-nih-tee) antibody-mediated immunity occurring within blood plasma and other body fluids [*humor-* liquid, *-al* relating to, *immun-* free, *-ity* state]

huntingtin (HUN-ting-tin) a protein normally present in all cells; an abnormal version of huntingtin is produced in people with Huntington disease (HD), clinging to molecules too tightly in the brain and thus preventing normal function [*George S. Huntington* American physician]

Huntington disease (HD) (HUN-ting-ton) an inherited disease characterized by chorea (involuntary, purposeless movements) that progresses to severe dementia and death; *see* **huntingtin** [*George S. Huntington* American physician, *dis-* opposite of, *-ease* comfort]

hyaline cartilage (HYE-ah-lin KAR-tih-lij) most common type of cartilage; appears gelatinous and glossy [*hyal-* glass, *-ine* of or like, *cartilag-* cartilage]

hyaline membrane disease (HMD) (HYE-ah-lin) condition that results from a deficiency of surfactant in premature infants [*hyal-* glass, *-ine* of or like, *membrane-* thin skin, *dis-* opposite of, *-ease* comfort]

hyaluronic acid (hye-al-yoo-RON-ik ASS-id) type of proteoglycan that helps thicken and hold together the matrix of connective tissue; *see* **proteoglycan** [*hyal-* glass, *-uron-* urine, *-ic* relating to, *acid* sour]

hybridoma (hye-brid-OH-mah) hybrid cell formed by fusion of cancerous cell with a lymphocyte to mass-produce a specific antibody (monoclonal antibodies) [*hybrid-* mixed offspring, *-oma* tumour]

hydrase (HYE-drays) enzyme that adds water to a molecule without splitting it [*hydr-* water, *-ase* enzyme]

hydrocele (HYE-dro-seel) accumulation of fluid that causes scrotal swelling [*hydro-* water, *-cele* tumour]

hydrocephalus (hye-droh-SEF-ah-lus) condition that results from an accumulation of cerebrospinal fluid in the subarachnoid space around the brain [*hydro-* water, *-cephalus* head]

hydrocortisone (hye-droh-KOHR-tih-zohn) hormone secreted by the adrenal cortex; cortisol; compound [*hydro-* water, *-cortisone* cortex of adrenal gland]

hydrogen bond (HYE-droh-jen) weak chemical bond that occurs between the partial positive charge on a hydrogen atom covalently bound to a nitrogen or oxygen atom and the partial negative charge of another polar molecule [*hydro-* water, *-gen* produce]

hydrogen ion (HYE-droh-jen EYE-on) a proton or a hydrogen atom without its electron; occurs in water and water solutions; produces an acidic solution; has a positive charge (H^+) [*hydro-* water, *-gen* produce, *ion* to go]

hydrolase (HYE-droh-lays) hydrolyzing enzyme [*hydro-* water, *-ase* enzyme]

hydrolysis (hye-DROHL-ih-sis) chemical process in which a compound is split by addition of H and OH^- portions of a water molecule [*hydro-* water, *-lysis* loosening]

hydronephrosis (hye-droh-neh-FROH-sis) condition resulting when urine backs up into the kidney, causing a swelling of the renal pelvis and calyces [*hydro-* water, *-nephr-* kidney, *-osis* condition]

hydrophilic (hye-dro-FIL-ik) describes a particle or substance that is attracted to water [*hydro-* water, *-phil-* love, *-ic* relating to]

hydrophobic (hye-droh-FOH-bik) describes a particle or substance that is not attracted to (or is repelled by) water [*hydro-* water, *-phob-* fear, *-ic* relating to]

hydrosalpinx (hye-droh-SAL-pinks) condition that results from obstruction of the uterine tube and marked dilation at the end of the tube caused by accumulation of fluid that cannot escape [*hydro-* water, *-salpinx* tube] *pl.*, hydrosalpinges (hye-droh-SAL-pin-jeez)

hydrostatic pressure (hye-droh-STAT-ik) force of a fluid pushing against some surface [*hydro-* water, *-stat-* stand, -ic relating to]

hydrostatic pressure gradient (hye-droh-STAT-ik PRESH-ur GRAY-dee-ent) situation in which a difference in pressure is caused by the force of a fluid as it moves from one point to another [*hydro-* water, *-stat-* stand, -ic relating to, *grad-* step, *-ent* state]

hymen (HYE-men) Greek for "membrane"; mucous membrane that may partially or entirely occlude the vaginal outlet [*hymen* membrane]

hyoid bone (HYE-oyd bohn) U-shaped bone of the neck between the mandible and the larynx [*hy-* Greek letter upsilon (Υ or υ), *-oid* like]

hypercapnia (hye-per-KAP-nee-ah) excessive carbon dioxide in the blood [*hyper-* above, *-capn-* vapour (CO_2), *-ia* condition]

hypercholesterolaemia (hye-per-koh-les-ter-ohl-EE-mee-ah) elevated blood concentration of cholesterol [*hyper-* excessive, *-chole-* bile, *-stero-* solid, *-ol-* alcohol, *-(h)aem-* blood, *-ia* condition]

hyperchromic (hye-per-KROH-mik) abnormally high haemoglobin content in a red blood cell, producing a more saturated red colouration [*hyper-* excessive, *-chrom-* colour, *-ic* relating to]

hyperextension (hye-per-ek-STEN-shun) stretching an extended part beyond its anatomical position; may clinically refer to abnormal extension beyond normal range of motion [*hyper-* excessive, *-ex-* out, *-ten-* stretch, *-sion* process]

hyperglycaemia (hye-per-glye-SEE-mee-ah) higher than normal blood glucose concentration [*hyper-* excessive, *-glyc-* sweet (glucose), *-(h)aem-* blood, *-ia* condition]

hyperkalaemia (hye-per-kah-LEE-mee-ah) excessive potassium in the blood [*hyper* excessive, *-kal-* potassium, *-(h)aem-* blood, *-ia* condition]

hyperkeratosis (hye-per-ker-ah-TOH-sis) thickening of the horny layer of the skin [*hyper* excessive, *-kera-* horn, *-osis* condition]

hyperlipidaemia (hye-per-lip-id-EE-mee-ah) elevated blood concentration of lipids (e.g., cholesterol, triglycerides) [*hyper-* excessive, *-lipi-* fat, *-id-* form, *-(h)aem-* blood, *-ia* condition]

hypernatraemia (hye-per-nah-TREE-mee-ah) excessive sodium in the blood [*hyper-* excessive, *-natri-* sodium, *-(h)aem-* blood, *-ia* condition]

hyperopia (hye-per-OH-pee-ah) refractive disorder of the eye caused by a shorter-than-normal eyeball; results in ability to see objects at a distance better than objects nearer; also called *farsightedness* [*hyper-* excessive or above, *-op-* vision, *-ia* condition]

hyperpituitarism (hye-per-pih-TYOO-ih-tar-iz-em) disorder that results from benign tumours in the pituitary gland [*hyper-* excessive, *-pituitar-* phlegm (pituitary gland), *-ism* condition]

hyperplasia (hye-per-PLAY-zee-ah) growth of an abnormally large number of cells at a local site, as in a neoplasm or tumour [*hyper-* excessive, *-plas(m)-* substance or form, *-ia* condition]

hyperpnoea (hye-PERP-nee-ah) abnormal increase in respiratory rate and depth [*hyper-* excessive, *-pnoe-* breathe, *-a* condition]

hyperpolarization (hye-per-pol-lar-ih-ZAY-shun) increase in electrical charges separated by the cell membrane; causes change further below 0 mV [*hyper-* excessive, *-pol-* pole, *-ar-* relating to, *-ization* process]

hypersecretion (hye-per-seh-KREE-shun) too much secretion of a substance [*hyper-* excessive, *-secret-* separate, *-tion* process]

hypersensitivity (hye-per-sen-sih-TIV-ih-tee) type of inappropriate or excessive response of the immune system [*hyper-* excessive, *-sensitiv-* able to feel, *-ity* state]

hypertension (HTN) (hye-per-TEN-shun) abnormally high blood pressure [*hyper-* excessive, *-tens-* stretch or pull tight, *-sion* state]

hyperthyroidism (hye-per-THYE-royd-iz-em) hypersecretion of thyroid hormone [*hyper-* excessive, *-thyr-* shield (thyroid gland), *-oid* like, *-ism* condition]

hypertonic (hye-per-TON-ik) adjective used to describe a solution that has a higher potential osmotic pressure than a solution to which it is being compared; a hypertonic solution tends to have high osmolality and thus tends to gain water (by way of osmosis) from the solution to which it is compared; solution containing a higher level of salt (NaCl) than is found in a living red blood cell (more than 0.9% NaCl); causes cells to shrink [*hyper-* excessive, *-ton-* tension, *-ic* relating to]

hypertriglyceridaemia (hye-per-try-gliss-er-ih-DEE-mee-ah) elevated blood concentration of triglycerides [*hyper-* excessive, *-tri-* three, *-glycer-* sweet (glycerine), *-id-* chemical, *-(h)aem-* blood, *-ia* condition]

hypertrophic cardiomyopathy (hye-PER-troh-fik kar-dee-oh-my-OP-ah-thee) genetic condition that causes an abnormal enlargement of the heart [*hyper-* excessive, *-troph-* nourishment, *-ic* relating to, *cardi-* heart, *-myo-* muscle, *-path-* disease, *-y* state]

hypertrophy (hye-PER-tro-fee) increased size of an organ or part caused by an increase in the size of its cells [*hyper-* excessive, *-troph-* nourishment, *-y* state]

hyperventilation (hye-per-ven-tih-LAY-shun) very rapid, deep respirations [*hyper-* excessive, *-vent-* fan or create wind, *-tion* process]

hypervitaminosis (hye-per-vye-tah-mih-NO-sis) general name for any condition resulting from an abnormally high intake of vitamins [*hyper-* excessive, *-vita-* life, *-amin-* ammonia compound, *-osis* condition]

hypervolaemia (hye-per-voh-LEE-mee-ah) abnormally increased blood volume [*hyper-* excessive, *-vol-* volume, *-(h)aem-* blood, *-ia* condition]

hypoallergenic (hye-poh-al-er-JEN-ik) refers to having a lower potential for producing allergic reactions [*hypo-* under or below, *-aller-* other, *-gen-* produce, *-ic* relating to]

hypocalcaemia (hye-poh-kal-SEE-mee-ah) abnormally low calcium levels in the blood [*hypo-* under or below, *-calc-* lime (calcium), *-(h)aem-* blood, *-ia* condition]

hypochloraemia (hye-poh-kloh-REE-mee-ah) abnormally low levels of chloride in the blood associated with potassium loss [*hypo-* under or below, *-chlor-* green (chlorine), *-(h)aem-* blood, *-ia* condition]

hypochromic (hye-poh-KROH-mik) abnormally low haemoglobin content in a red blood cell, producing a less saturated red colouration [*hyper-* under or below, *-chrom-* colour, *-ic* relating to]

hypodermis (hye-poh-DER-mis) loose layer fascia under the skin, rich in fat and areolar tissue located beneath the dermis; also called *subcutaneous layer* or *superficial fascia* [*hypo-* under or below, *-dermis* skin]

hypoglossal (hye-poh-GLOS-al) under the tongue [*hypo-* under or below, *-gloss-* tongue, *-al* relating to]

hypoglossal nerve (hye-poh-GLOS-al nerv) cranial nerve XII; motor nerve; responsible for tongue movement [*hypo-* under or below, *-gloss-* tongue, *-al* relating to]

hypoglycaemia (hye-poh-gly-SEE-mee-ah) lower than normal blood glucose concentration [*hypo-* under or below, *-glyc-* sweet (glucose), *-(h)aem-* blood, *-ia* condition]

hypokalaemia (hye-poh-kah-LEE-mee-ah) abnormally low serum potassium level [*hypo-* under or below, *-kal-* potassium, *-(h)aem-* blood, *-ia* condition]

hyponatraemia (hye-poh-nah-TREE-mee-ah) abnormally low sodium levels in the blood [*hypo-* under or below, *-natri-* sodium, *-(h)aem-* blood, *-ia* condition]

hypophyseal portal system (hye-poh-FIZ-ee-al POR-tal) complex of small blood vessels through which releasing hormones travel from the hypothalamus to the pituitary [*hypo-* under or below, *-physis-* growth, *-al* relating to, *portal* doorway]

hypophysectomy (hye-pof-ih-SEK-toh-mee) surgical removal of the pituitary gland [*hypo-* under or below, *-phys-* growth, *-ec-* out, *-tom-* cut, *-y* action]

hypophysis (hye-POF-ih-sis) pituitary gland; also called *hypophysis cerebri* [*hypo-* under or below, *-physis-* growth]

hypopotassaemia (hye-poh-poh-tah-SEE-mee-ah) potassium deficit [*hypo-* under or below, *-potass* potassium, *-(h)aem-* blood, *-ia* condition]

hyposecretion (hye-poh-seh-KREE-shun) too little secretion of a substance [*hypo-* under or below, *-secret-* separate, *-tion* process]

hypospadias (hye-poh-SPAY-dee-us) congenital condition that is characterized by the opening of the urethral meatus on the underside or ventral surface of the glans or penile shaft [*hypo-* under or below, *-spad-* rip or split, *-ias* condition]

hypothalamic–pituitary–adrenal axis (HPA axis) (hye-poh-THAL-ah-mik pih-TYOO-ih-tair-ee ah-DREE-nal AK-sis) process that activates a stress mechanism that stimulates the sympathetic nervous system and pituitary gland [*hypo-* under or below, *-thalam-* inner chamber, *-ic* relating to, *pituit-* phlegm, *-ary* relating to, *ad-* toward, *-ren-* kidney, *-al* relating to, *- axis* axle]

hypothalamus (hye-poh-THAL-ah-muss) important autonomic and neuroendocrine control centre located inferior to the thalamus in the brain [*hypo-* under or below, *-thalamus* inner chamber] *pl.*, hypothalami

hypothermia (hye-poh-THER-mee-ah) failure of thermoregulatory mechanisms to maintain homeostasis in a very cold external environment; results in abnormally—sometimes life-threatening—low body temperature [*hypo-* under or below, *-therm-* heat, *-ia* abnormal condition]

hypothesis (hye-POTH-eh-sis) idea or scientific concept, usually based on previous ideas or observations, that is proposed as a possible explanation of nature or a natural process; hypotheses undergo intense testing before being accepted widely in the scientific community; *see also* **law, science, theory** [*hypo-* under or below, *-thesis* placing or proposition] *pl.*, hypotheses (hye-POTH-eh-seez)

hypotonic (hye-poh-TON-ik) adjective used to describe a solution that has a lower potential osmotic pressure than a solution to which it is being compared; a hypotonic solution tends to have low osmolality and thus tends to lose water (by way of osmosis) to the solution to which it is compared [*hypo-* under or below, *-ton-* tension, *-ic* relating to]

hypoventilation (hye-poh-ven-tih-LAY-shun) slow and shallow respirations [*hypo-* under or below, *-vent-* fan or create wind, *-tion* process]

hypovolaemia (hye-poh-voh-LEE-mee-ah) inadequate fluid volume in the extracellular compartment; dehydration [*hypo-* under or below, *-vol-* volume, *-(h)aem-* blood, *-ia* condition]

hypovolaemic shock (hye-poh-voh-LEE-mik) condition when dehydration results in multiple organ failure [*hypo-* under or below, *-vol-* whirl, *-aemi(a)-* blood condition, *-ic* relating to]

hypoxia (hye-POK-see-ah) deficiency of oxygen in the blood [*hypo-* under or below, *-ox-* oxygen, *-ia* condition]

hysterosalpingogram (his-ter-oh-sal-PING-go-gram) x-ray technique used to produce images of the uterus and uterine tube [*hyster-* uterus, *-salping-* tube, *-gram* drawing]

I

I band the segment of a muscle fibre's sarcomere that includes the Z disc (Z line) and the ends of the thin filaments where they do not overlap the thick filaments; also called *isotropic band* [*I* isotropic]

ideal gas gas whose molecules are so far apart that the molecules rarely collide with one another

identical twin one of two siblings born as a result of the splitting of embryonic tissue from the same zygote early in development

ideogram (ID-ee-oh-gram) a graphic representation of any idea; in genomics, a simple cartoon of a chromosome often used to show the overall physical structure of a chromosome; *see also* **chromosome, genomics** [*ide-* idea, *-gram* drawing]

idiopathic (id-ee-oh-PATH-ik) refers to a disease of undetermined cause [*idio-* peculiar, *-path-* disease, *-ic* relating to]

ileum (IL-ee-um) distal portion of the small intestine [*ileum* groin or flank] *pl.*, ilea

iliac lymph node (ILL-ee-ak limf nohd) pelvic and groin lymph node [*ilia-* loin or gut (ileum), *-ac* relating to, *lymph* water, *nod-* knot]

ilium (IL-ee-um) largest and uppermost coxal bone (fuses with other coxal bones by adulthood) [*ilium* flank] *pl.*, ilia (IL-ee-ah)

immune deficiency (im-YOON deh-FISH-en-see) failure of immune system mechanisms to defend against pathogens; also called *immunodeficiency* [*immun* free (immunity), *de-* down, *-fic-* perform, *-ency* state]

immune system (im-YOON) body's defence system against disease [*immun-* free (immunity)]

immunization (im-yoo-nih-ZAY-shun) deliberate artificial exposure to disease for the purpose of producing acquired immunity [*immun-* free (immunity), *-tion* process]

immunocompetence (ih-myoo-noh-KOM-peh-tens) ability of our adaptive mechanisms (antibodies and/or T cells) to activate an effective response to an antigen; also called *immunologic competence* or *immune competence* [*immuno-* free (immunity), *-competence* capability]

immunoglobulin (Ig) (ih-myoo-noh-GLOB-yoo-lin) antibody [*immuno-* free (immunity), *-glob-* ball, *-ul-* small, *-in* substance]

immunological synapse (IS) (ih-myoo-no-LOJ-ih-kal SIN-aps) temporary junction between an immune cell and another cell, such as another immune cell or a target cell to be destroyed; compare to **synapse** [*immuno-* free (immunity), *-log-* words (study of), *-ical* relating to, *syn-* together, *-aps-* join]

immunology (im-yoo-NOL-oh-jee) study of immune system functions and mechanisms [*immuno-* free (immunity), *-logy* study of]

immunosuppressive drugs (ih-myoo-no-soo-PRES-iv) drugs that suppress the immune system's ability to attack the foreign antigens in the donated tissue [*immuno-* free (immunity), *-suppress-* press down, *-ive* relating to]

immunotherapy (im-yoo-no-THAYR-ah-pee) therapeutic technique that bolsters a person's immune system in an attempt to control a disease [*immuno-* free, *-therapy* treatment]

impacted fracture (im-PAK-ted FRAK-chur) type of bone fracture in which one end of the fracture is driven into the diaphysis of the other fragment [*im-* into, *-pact-* push, *fracture* a breaking]

imperforate hymen (im-PER-fah-rayt HYE-men) condition in which the hymen completely covers the vaginal outlet [*im-* not, *-perfor-* pierce, *-ate* state, *hymen* membrane]

impermeable (im-PERM-ee-ah-bul) adjective used to describe a membrane that does not allow substances to pass through (permeate) it [*im-* not, *-per-* through, *-mea(t)-* pass, *-able* capable of]

impermeant (im-PERM-ee-ent) adjective used to describe a substance that is not able to pass through (permeate) a membrane [*im-* not, *-per-* through, *-mea(t)-* pass, *-ant* characterized by]

impetigo (im-peh-TYE-go) highly contagious bacterial skin infection that occurs most often in children [*impetigo* an attack]

implantation (im-plan-TAY-shun) process in which developing offspring tissue connects to the uterine wall of the mother [*im-* in, *-planta-* set or place, *-ation* process]

impotence (IM-poh-tense) *see* **erectile dysfunction (ED)** [*im-* not, *-poten-* power, *-ence* state]

impulse (IM-puls) an electrical signal; *see* **action potential** [*impuls-* drive or push]

in vitro fertilization (IVF) (in VEE-troh FER-tih-lih-ZAY-shun) artificial union of sperm and egg "in glass" in a laboratory dish [*in* in, *vitro* glass, *fertil-* fruitful, *-ation* process]

inborn errors of metabolism (IN-born AIR-ors meh-TAB-oh-liz-em) group of genetic conditions involving a deficiency or absence of a particular enzyme [*meta-* over, *-bol-* throw, *-ism* action]

inborn immunity (IN-born im-YOO-nih-tee) inherited immunity to disease [*in-* within, *-born* brought forth, *immuno-* free (immunity)]

inclusion an unidentified particle within a cell or other structure [*in-* within, *-clus-* shut, *-ion* process]

incomplete fracture (in-kom-PLEET FRAK-chur) type of bone fracture in which some fracture components are still partially joined [*fracture* a breaking]

incomplete tetanus (in-kom-PLEET TET-ah-nus) tetanus with very short periods of relaxation occurring between peaks of muscle tension [*tetanus* tension]

incontinence (in-KON-tih-nens) involuntary voiding of urine [*in-* not, *-contin-* contain, *-ence* state]

incretin (in-KREE-tin) any GI hormone that triggers the release of insulin from the pancreatic islets; examples, glucagon-like peptide 1 (GLP-1) and gastric inhibitory peptide [glucose-dependent insulinotropic peptide] (GIP) [*in-* in, *-cret-* secrete, *-in* substance]

incubation (in-kyoo-BAY-shun) early, latent stage of an infection, during which an infection has begun but signs or symptoms have not yet developed in the host [*in-* in or on, *-cubat-* lie, *-tion* process]

indirect calorimetry (kal-oh-RIM-eh-tree) method used to determine body mass index (BMR) [*in-* not, direct, *calor-* heat, *-metr-* measuring, *-y* process]

infancy period of human development from birth to about 18 months of age [*infan-* unable to speak, *-y* state]

infant respiratory distress syndrome (IRDS) (RES-per-ah-toh-ree dis-TRESS SIN-drohm) leading cause of death in premature babies, caused by a lack of surfactant in the alveolar air sacs, inferior lower portion; opposite of superior [*infan-* unable to speak, *re-* again, *-spir-* breathe, *-tory* relating to, *syn-* together, *-drome* course]

infectious mononucleosis (in-FEK-shuss mon-oh-nyoo-klee-OH-sis) a viral (noncancerous) white blood cell (WBC) disorder common in young adults; characterized by leucocytosis of atypical lymphocytes and severe fatigue [*in-fect-* stain, *-ous* relating to, *mono-* single, *-nucle-* nut, *-osis* condition]

inferior; opposite of superior [*infer-* lower, *-or* quality]

inferior cerebellar peduncle (SAIR-eh-bell-ar peh-DUNG-kul) tract that enters the cerebellum from the medulla and cord [*infer-* lower, *-or* quality, *cerebell-* cerebellum (small brain), *-ar* relating to, *ped-* foot, *-uncl-* little]

inferior colliculi (koh-LIK-yoo-lee) form the posterior, upper part of the midbrain [*infer-* lower, *-or* quality, *colli-* hill, *-iculus* small] *sing.*, colliculus (koh-LIK-yoo-lus)

inferior nasal concha (KONG-kah) *see* **concha** [*infer-* lower, *-or* quality, *nas-* nose, *-al* relating to, *concha* sea shell] *pl.*, conchae (KONG-kee or KONG-kay)

inferior vena cava (VEE-nah KAY-vah) vein of the thorax; drains blood from the lower trunk and extremity [*infer-* lower, *-or* quality, *vena* vein, *cava* hollow] *pl.*, venae cavae (VEE-nee KAY-vee)

infertility (in-fer-TIL-ih-tee) failure to conceive after 1 year of regular unprotected intercourse [*in-* not, *-fertil-* fruitful, *-ity* state]

inflammation (in-flah-MAY-shun) group of responses to a tissue irritant marked by signs of redness, heat, swelling, and pain [*inflam-* set afire, *-tion* process]

inflammatory exudate (in-FLAM-ah-toh-ree EK-soo-dayt) substance that accumulates in the interstitial spaces as a result of increased permeability of blood vessels, increased blood flow, and migration and accumulation of white blood cells [*inflam-* set afire, *-ory* relating to, *exud-* sweat out, *-ate* thing]

inflammatory joint disease (in-FLAM-ah-toh-ree) joint condition that involves inflammation of the synovial fluid [*inflam-* set afire, *-ory* relating to, *dis-* opposite of, *-ease* comfort]

inflammatory response (in-FLAM-ah-toh-ree) specific process involving tissues and blood vessels in response to injury [*inflam-* set afire, *-ory* relating to]

infraspinatus muscle (IN-frah-spy-nah-tus) one of the four rotator cuff muscles around the shoulder joint [*infra-* below, *-spina-* spine, *mus-* mouse, *-cle* little]

infundibulum (in-fun-DIB-yoo-lum) stalk that connects the pituitary gland to the hypothalamus [*infundibulum* funnel] *pl.*, infundibula (in-fun-DIB-yoo-lah)

ingestion (in-JES-chun) taking in of complex foods, usually by mouth [*in-* within, *-gest-* carry, *-tion* process]

inguinal (ING-gwih-nal) relating to the groin [*inguin-* groin, *-al* relating to]

inguinal hernia (ING-gwih-nal HER-nee-ah) rupture of the lower abdominal wall at the inguinal canal [*inguin-* groin, *-al* relating to, *hernia* rupture] *pl.*, herniae (HER-nee-ee) or hernias

inguinal lymph node (ING-gwih-nal limf nohd) pelvic and groin lymph node [*inguin-* groin, *-al* relating to, *lymph* water, *-atic* relating to, *nod-* knot]

inherited immunity (in-HAIR-ih-ted ih-MYOO-nih-tee) inborn immunity; occurs when immune mechanisms are put in place by genetic mechanisms during the early stages of human development [*in-* within, *-herit* to make an heir, *immun-* free (immunity)]

inhibin (in-HIB-in) glycoprotein hormone produced by the ovary to regulate FSH secretion by the anterior pituitary (adenohypophysis) [*inhib-* inhibit, *-in* substance]

inhibitory (in-HIB-ih-tor-ee) something that slows or stops a process [*inhib-* to restrain, *-ory* relating to]

inhibitory neurotransmitter (in-HIB-ih-tor-ee nyoo-roh-TRANZ-mit-er) neurotransmitter that causes hyperpolarization of the postsynaptic membrane, thereby decreasing chances of impulse propagation [*inhib-* restrain, *-ory* relating to, *neuro-* nerve, *-trans-* across, *-mitt-* send, *-er* agent]

inhibitory postsynaptic potential (IPSP) (in-HIB-ih-tor-ee post-sih-NAP-tik poh-TEN-shal) temporary hyperpolarization that makes the inside of the membrane even more negative than at the resting potential [*inhib-* restrain, *-ory* relating to, *post-* after, *-syn-* together, *-apt-* join, *-ic* relating to, *potent-* power, *-ial* relating to]

innate immunity (IN-ayt im-YOO-nih-tee) type of immunity that exists prior to exposure to a specific antigen and that can recognize and destroy a variety of harmful agents or conditions; also called *nonspecific immunity* [*innat-* inborn, *immun-* free, *-ity* state]

inner cell mass layer of cells in the blastocyst [*cell* storeroom]

inner ear region of the ear consisting of a bony labyrinth and a membranous labyrinth; also called *labyrinth*

inorganic compounds (in-or-GAN-ik) chemical constituents that do not contain both carbon and hydrogen; for example, water, carbon dioxide, and oxygen [*in-* not, *-organic* natural, *compound-* to assemble]

inotropic (ee-noh-TROH-pik) refers to anything that affects the strength of myocardial contractions [*in-* sinew, *-trop-* turn or change, *-ic* relating to]

insertion (muscle insertion) attachment of a muscle to the bone that it moves when contraction occurs (as distinguished from its origin); (insertion mutation) a type of genetic mutation that occurs when one or more nucleotide bases appear within the usual sequence of nucleotide bases in a gene; in insertion mutations, the cell cannot read the genetic code normally and thus the encoded protein cannot be made in its usual form; *see* **deletion** [*in-* in, *-ser-* join, *-tion* process]

inspiration (in-spih-RAY-shun) process of bringing air into the lungs [*in-* in, *-spir-*breathe, *-ation* process]

inspiratory capacity (IC) (in-SPY-rah-tor-ee kah-PASS-ih-tee) maximum amount of air an individual can inspire after a normal expiration [*in-* in, *-spir-* breathe, *-tory* relating to, *capac-* hold, *-ity* state]

inspiratory centre (in-SPY-rah-tor-ee) one of the two most important control centres located in the medulla; the other is the expiratory centre [*in-* in, *-spir-* breathe, *-tory* relating to]

inspiratory muscle (in-SPY-rah-tor-ee MUSS-el) any of the muscles that expand the thorax to enable movement of air into lungs (inspiration); for example, diaphragm, external intercostals [*in-* in, *-spir-* breathe, *-tory* relating to, *mus-* mouse, *-cle* little]

inspiratory reserve volume (IRV) (in-SPY-rah-tor-ee) amount of air that can be forcibly inspired over and above a normal inspiration [*in-* in, *-spir-* breathe, *-tory* relating to]

insula (IN-soo-lah) lobe of the cerebral cortex; lies hidden from view in the lateral fissure [*insula* island] *pl.*, insulae

insulin (IN-suh-lin) hormone secreted by beta cells of the pancreatic islets that increases the uptake of glucose and amino acids by most body cells [*insul-* island, *-in* substance]

integral membrane protein (IMP) (IN-teh-grel MEM-brayn PROH-teen) any of the numerous kinds of proteins embedded within cellular membranes [*integr-* whole, *-al* relating to, *membran-* thin skin, *prote-* primary, *-in* substance]

integrator (IN-teh-gray-ter) an integration centre or control centre that receives sensed information and compares that to stored or set-point information, possibly sending a response to an effector that will act to change the value of the sensed information [*integr-* whole, *-at(e)-* process, *-or* agent]

integrin (in-TEG-rin) type of protein that acts as a connector to bind structural proteins in a way that connects a cell's cytoskeleton to surrounding structures such as other cells [*integr-* whole, *-in* substance]

integument (in-TEG-yoo-ment) skin; the body's largest organ [*in-* on, *-teg-* cover, *-ment* result of action]

integumentary system (in-teg-yoo-MEN-taree) skin and its related structures [*in-* on, *-teg-* cover, *-ment* result of action, *-ary* relating to]

interatrial bundle (in-ter-AT-tree-al) conducting fibres that facilitate rapid conduction to the left atrium [*inter-* between, *-atri-* entrance courtyard, *-al* relating to]

intercalated disc (in-TER-kah-lay-ted) any of the disclike connections between ends of adjacent cardiac muscle fibres characterized by gap junctions and often appearing as tiny, darkly stained lines in micrographs [*intercalate-* to insert]

intercarpal joint (in-ter-KAR-pal) articulation between the eight carpal bones [*inter-* between, *-carp-* wrist, *-al* relating to]

interferon (IFN) (in-ter-FEER-on) small protein produced by the immune system that inhibits virus multiplication [*inter-* between, *-fer-* strike, *-on* substance]

interleukin (IL) (in-ter-LOO-kin) any of a class of about a dozen cytokines, regulatory chemicals secreted by leucocytes and other cells, that are involved in regulating a wide variety of immune functions in different cell types; each interleukin is named by the IL acronym with its number, such as IL-1, IL-2, and so on [*inter-* between, *-leuko-* white (blood cell), *-in* substance]

intermediate fibre (in-ter-MEE-dee-it) muscle fibre exhibiting characteristics between fast and slow fibres [*inter-* between, *-medi-* middle, *-ate* of or like]

intermediate filament (in-ter-MEE-dee-it FIL-ah-ment) twisted strands of protein, slightly larger than microfilaments that make up part of the cell's internal skeleton (the cytoskeleton) [*inter-* between, *-mediate* to divide, *fila-* threadlike, *-ment* process]

intermittent claudication (in-ter-MIT-tent klaw-dih-KAY-shun) condition that causes cramplike pain in the calves after walking and is caused by intermittent arterial occlusion by platelet plugs [*inter-* between, *-mitt-* send, *-ent* state, *claudica-* limping, *-ation* process]

internal capsule (in-TERN-al KAP-sul) large mass of white matter associated with the basal nuclei [*intern-* inside, *-al* relating to, *caps-* box, *-ul-* little]

internal environment (in-TERN-al en-VI-ron-ment) the conditions inside the body, particularly the fluids that surround the cells of the body, which are distinct from conditions in the external environment [*intern-* inside, *-al* relating to, *environ-* surround, *-ment* condition]

internal intercostal muscle (in-TERN-al in-ter-KOS-tal) muscle attached to ribs; contraction depresses ribs [*intern-* inside, *-al* relating to, *inter-* between, *-costal-* rib, *-al* relating to, *mus-* mouse, *-cle* little]
internal jugular vein (in-TERN-al en-VI-ron-ment) JUG-yoo-lar vayn) deep vein of the neck [*intern-* inside, *-al* relating to, *jugul-* neck, *-ar* relating to, *vena* blood vessel]
internal oblique muscle (in-TERN-al oh-BLEEK) abdominal muscle [*intern-* inside, *-al* relating to, *obliq-* slanted, *mus-* mouse, *-cle* little]
internal os (in-TERN-al os) cavity of the uterus that opens into the cervical canal [*intern-* inside, *-al* relating to, *os* mouth or opening] *pl.*, ora
internal table (in-TERN-al TAY-bel) inner wall of a flat bone of the cranium, made of compact bone; compare to **external table** [*intern-* inside, *-al* relating to]
interneuron (in-ter-NYOO-ron) in a three-neuron reflex arc, nerve cell that conducts impulses from a sensory neuron to a motor neuron [*inter-* between, *-neuron* string or nerve]
internodal bundle (in-ter-NOH-dal) conducting fibres that allow for complete contraction of both atrial chambers before the impulse reaches the ventricles [*inter-* between, *-nod-* knot, *-al* relating to]
interoceptor (in-ter-oh-SEP-tor) *see* **visceroceptor** [*inter-* inward, *-cept-* receive, *-or* agent]
interosseous muscles (in-ter-OSS-ee-us MUSS-elz) muscles of the hand found between the metacarpal bones; the dorsal interossei abduct the fingers and the palmar interossei adduct the fingers [*inter-* between, *-os-* bone, *-ous* relating to, *mus-* mouse, *-cle* little]
interphalangeal joint (in-ter-fah-LAN-jee-al) articulation that exists between the heads of the phalanges and the bases of the more distal phalanges [*inter-* between, *-phalang-* finger bones (ref. from rows of soldiers), *-al* relating to]
interphase (IN-ter-fayz) mitotic phase immediately before visible condensation of the chromosomes during which the DNA of each chromosome replicates itself [*inter-* between, *-phase* stage]
interspinales group (in-ter-spy-NAH-leez) group of back muscles that connect one vertebra to the next—also helping to extend the back and neck or flex them to the side [*inter-* between, *-spina-* spine, *-al* relating to]
interstitial (in-ter-STISH-al) in an in-between location, as between tissue cells [*inter-* between, *-stit-* stand, *-al* relating to]
interstitial cell (in-ter-STISH-al) any of the small cells in the testes found between seminiferous tubules and that secrete the male sex hormone, testosterone; also called *Leydig cell* [*inter-* between, *-stit-* stand, *-al* relating to, *cell* storeroom]
interstitial cystitis (in-ter-STISH-al sis-TYE-tis) form of bladder inflammation that occurs without evidence of bacterial infection [*inter-* between, *-stit-* stand, *-al* relating to, *cyst-* bag, *-itis* inflammation]
interstitial fluid (IF) (in-ter-STISH-al) fluid located in microscopic spaces between cells [*inter-* between, *-stit-* stand, *-al* relating to]
interstitial fluid colloid osmotic pressure (IFCOP) (in-ter-STISH-al KOL-oyd os-MAH-tik) one of four types of pressure that serve as a control mechanism for water exchange between plasma and interstitial fluid; draws fluid back out of the capillaries [*inter-* between, *-stit-* stand, *-al* relating to, *coll-* glue, *-oid* like, *osmo-* push, *-ic* relating to]
interstitial fluid hydrostatic pressure (IFHP) (in-ter-STISH-al hye-droh-STAT-ik) one of four types of pressure that serves as a control mechanism for water exchange between plasma and interstitial fluid; tends to force fluid out of the interstitial fluid into the capillaries [*inter-* between, *-stit-* stand, *-al* relating to, *hydro-* water, *-stat-* stand, -ic relating to]
interstitial growth (in-ter-STISH-al) cartilage growth following mitosis and secretion of matrix by chondrocytes; interstitial growth of epiphyseal plate results in growth in length of long bones; also called *endogenous growth* [*inter-* between, *-stit-* stand, *-al* relating to]
intestinal crypt (of Lieberkühn) (in-TES-tih-nal kript [LEE-ber-kyoon]) deep pit in the intestinal mucosa between adjacent villi serving as a source of new mucosal cells, mucus, and other secretions; also called *Lieberkühn crypt* or *intestinal gland* [*intestin-* intestine, *-al* relating to, *crypt* hidden cave (*Johannes Lieberkühn* German anatomist)]
intestinal flora (in-TES-tih-nal FLOR-ah) community of various bacterial populations that normally inhabit the colon [*intestin-* intestine, *-al* relating to, *flora-* flowers]
intestinal juice (in-TES-tih-nal) refers to the sum total of intestinal secretions [*intestin-* intestine, *-al* relating to]
intestinal phase (in-TES-tih-nal) stage of gastric secretion triggered when material leaves the stomach and enters the small intestine [*intestin-* intestine, *-al* relating to, *phase* appearance]
intestine (in-TES-tin) part of the digestive tract into which food passes after it leaves the stomach; separated into two segments, the small and the large intestine [*intestin-* intestine]
intracellular (in-trah-SELL-yoo-lar) relating to the interior of the cell [*intra-* occurring within, *-cell-* storeroom, *-ular* relating to]
intracellular control (in-tra-SELL-yoo-lar) level of homeostatic control of body processes that occurs within cells, as in genetic regulation or enzymatic regulation of the cell [*intra-* inside or within, *-cell* storeroom]
intracellular fluid (ICF) (in-trah-SELL-yoo-lar) fluid located within cells [*intra-* occurring within, *-cell-* storeroom, *-ular* relating to]
intracellular fluid (ICF) compartment (in-trah-SELL-yoo-lar) largest fluid compartment [*intra-* occurring within, *-cell-* storeroom, *-ular* relating to, *com-* together, *-partiri* to share]
intramembranous ossification (in-trah-MEM-brah-nus os-ih-fih-KAY-shun) process by which most flat bones are formed within connective tissue membranes [*intra-* within, *-membran-* thin skin, *-ous* characterized by, *os-* bone, *-fic-* make, *-ation* process]
intramural plexus (in-trah-MYOO-ral PLEK-sus) complex arrangement of neurons in the gastrointestinal tract [*intra-* within, *-mura-*wall, *-al* relating to, *plexus* braid or network] *pl.*, plexi (PLEK-sye) or plexuses (PLEK-sus-eez)
intramuscular injection (in-trah-MUSS-kyoo-lar in-JEK-shun) administration of medication into the muscle [*intra-* within, *mus-* mouse, *-cle* little, *-ar* relating to, *in-* in, *-ject-* throw, *-tion* process]
intraocular pressure (in-trah-OK-yoo-lar PRESH-ur) fluid pressure within the eyeball [*intra-* within, *-ocul-* eye, *-ar* relating to]
intraperitoneal (in-trah pair-ih-toh-NEE-al) relating to the space within the visceral peritoneum [*intra-* within, *peri-* around, *-tone-* stretched, *-al* relating to]
intratracheal injection (in-trah-TRAY-kee-al in-JEK-shun) administration of surfactant through a tube directly into the airways [*intra-* within, *-trache-* rough duct, *-al* relating to, *in-* in, *-ject-* throw, *-tion* process]
intrauterine device (IUD) (in-trah-YOO-ter-in) contraceptive device that works by inducing an immune response toxic to gametes; some IUDs also release progesterone and thus have an action similar to other hormonal contraceptives [*intra-* inside or within, *-uter-* womb, *-ine* relating to]
intravenous injection (in-trah-VEE-nus in-JEK-shun) administration of medication into veins [*intra-* within, *-ven-* vein, *-ous* relating to, *in-* in, *-ject* throw, *-tion* process]
intrinsic clotting pathway (in-TRIN-sik) series of reactions that begin with factors normally present in the blood [*intr-* within, *-sic* beside]
intrinsic control (in-TRIN-sik) level of homeostatic control of body processes that occurs within a particular tissue or organ, as when local regulators such as prostaglandins regulate local physiology; may be called *local control* or *autoregulation* [*intr-* inside or within, *-insic* beside]
intrinsic eye muscle (in-TRIN-sik) involuntary muscle located within the eye; responsible for size of the iris and shape of the lens [*intr-* within, *-sic* beside, *mus-* mouse, *-cle* small]
intrinsic factor (in-TRIN-sik) binds to molecules of B_{12}, protecting them from the acids and enzymes of the stomach; secreted by parietal cells [*intr-* inside or within, *-insic* beside]
intrinsic foot muscle (in-TRIN-sik) muscle located within the foot [*intrins-* inward, *-ic* relating to, *mus-* mouse, *-cle* little]
intrinsic muscle (in-TRIN-sik) muscle that is actually within the part moved [*instrins-* inward, *-ic* relating to, *mus-* mouse, *-cle* little]
intrinsic rhythm (in-TRIN-sik RITH-em) phenomenon of specialized cells in the sinoatrial (SA) node that produce regular impulses without stimulation from the brain or spinal cord [*instrins-* inward, *-ic* relating to, *rhythm-* measure flow or movement]
intron (IN-tron) segment of a gene in a DNA molecule that is not used to code for a protein; introns are removed from mRNA transcripts of the gene and the remaining exons are spliced together to form the final, edited version of the mRNA transcript; *see also* **exon, RNA** [*intra-* within, *-on* unit]
inversion (in-VER-shun) movement that turns the sole of the foot inward, toward the median [*in-* inward, *-ver-* turn, *-sion* process]
invert (in-VERT) to move a part inward [*in-* inward, *-vert* turn]
involuntary muscle (in-VOL-un-tair-ee) smooth muscle not under conscious control; found in organs such as the stomach, small intestine, and ureters [*in-* not, *volunt-* will, *mus-* mouse, *-cle* little]
involution (in-voh-LOO-shun) return of an organ to its normal size after enlargement; also after retrograde or degenerative change [*in-* in, *-volu-* roll, *-tion* state]
ion (EYE-on) electrically charged atom or group of atoms [*ion* to go]
ion channel (EYE-on) transport proteins in the plasma membrane that move sodium or potassium ions [*ion* to go, *channel* water pipe]
ionic bond (eye-ON-ik) electrocovalent bond; bond formed by transferring of electrons from one atom to another [*ion* to go, *bond* band]
ionizing radiation (EYE-on-eyz-ing) form of radioactivity, or radiation energy, resulting from alpha or beta particles or gamma rays emitted from radioactive atoms scoring direct hits on other atoms and thus ionizing the atoms by knocking electrons out of their outer energy levels; the effect of ionization may injure, kill, or change living cells; *see also* **radiation, radiation sickness** [*ion-* to go, *-ize* make, *radiat-* emit rays, *-tion* process]
ionotropic receptor (eye-on-eh-TROH-pik ree-SEP-tor) membrane receptor that includes a ion channel that opens or closes in response to stimulation (binding) of the receptor site [*ion-* to go (ion), *-trop-* turn or change, *-ic* relating to, *recept-* receive, *-or* agent]
ipsilateral (ip-sih-LAT-er-al) on the same side [*ipsi-* same, *-later* side, *-al* relating to]
ipsilateral reflex arc (ip-sih-LAT-er-al REE-fleks ark) reflex arc whose receptors and effectors are located on the same side of the body [*ipsi-* same, *-later* side, *-al* relating to, *re-* again, *-flex* bend, *arc-* bow]
iris (EYE-ris) coloured portion of the eye [*iris* rainbow]
irisin (EYE-ris-in) hormone produced by skeletal muscle tissue during exercise that triggers white fat to convert to brown fat; classified as a *myokine* (signal molecule from muscle) [*iris-* Greek messenger goddess, *-in* substance]
iron deficiency anaemia (deh-FISH-en-see ah-NEE-mee-ah) condition in which there are inadequate levels of iron in the diet causing less haemoglobin to be produced [*iron* strong metal, *de-* down, *-fic-* perform, *-ency* state, *an-* without, *-(h)aem-* blood, *-ia* condition]
irregular bone bone that has no particular size or shape [*ir-* not, *-regula-* rule, -ar relating to]
irritability ability of a muscle to be stimulated; *see* **excitability** [*irrita-* tease, *-ble* capable, *-ity* state]
irritable bowel syndrome (SIN-drohm) common chronic noninflammatory condition that is often caused by stress; characterized by diarrhoea or constipation with or without pain [*irrita-* tease, *-ble* capable, *bowel* sausage, *syn-* together, *-drome* running or (race) course]
ischaemia (is-KEE-mee-ah) decreased blood supply to a tissue resulting in impairment of cell function [*ische-* hold back, *-(h)aem-* blood, *-ia* condition]
ischaemic (is-KEE-mik) relating to ischaemia [*ischaem-* hold back, *-ic* relating to]
ischiocavernosus muscle (iss-kee-oh-KAV-er-no-sus) muscle of the pelvic floor; forms the urogenital triangle [*ischio-* hip joint, *-cavern-* hollow space, *-osus* relating to, *mus-* mouse, *-cle* little]
ischium (IS-kee-um) lowermost coxal bone (fuses with other coxal bones by adulthood) [*ischium* hip joint] *pl.*, ischia (IS-kee-ah)
islets of Langerhans (EYE-lets of LAHNG-er-hahnz) pancreatic islets [*isl-* island, *-et* little, *Paul Langerhans* German pathologist]
isoimmunity (eye-soh-ih-MYOO-nih-tee) normal but undesirable reaction of the immune system to antigens from a different individual of the same species [*iso-* equal, *-immun-* free, *-ity* state]
isometric contraction (eye-soh-MET-rik kon-TRAK-shun) type of muscle contraction in which muscle does not alter the distance between two bones; *see* **isotonic contraction**
isotonic (eye-soh-TON-ik) two fluids that have the same potential osmotic pressure [*iso-* equal, *-ton-* tension, *-ic* relating to]
isotonic contraction (eye-soh-TON-ik kon-TRAK-shun) type of muscle contraction in which the muscle sustains the same tension or pressure and a change in the distance between two bones occurs [*iso-* equal, *ton-* stretch or tension, *-ic* relating to, *con-* together, *-tract-* drag or draw, *-tion* process]
isotope (EYE-so-tohp) atoms with the same atomic number but different atomic masses [*iso-* equal, *-tope* place]
isthmus (ISS-muss) constriction between two larger parts of an organ; for example, isthmus of thyroid [*isthmus* narrow connection or passage]

J

jaundice (JAWN-dis) abnormal yellowing of skin, mucous membranes, and whites of eyes [*jaun-* yellow, *-ice* state]
jejunum (jeh-JOO-num) middle third of the small intestine [*jejun-* empty, *-um* thing]
joint capsule (joynt KAP-sool) sleevelike extension of the periosteum of each of the bones at an articulation [*joint* a joining, *caps-* box, *-ule* little]
joint cavity (joynt KAV-i-tee) small space between articulating surfaces of the two bones of the joint [*joint* a joining, *cav-* hollow, *-ity* state]

joint (joynt) junction between two or more bones; articulation [*joint* a joining]

joule (J or j) (jool) unit of measuring energy; *see* calorie [*James Prescott Joule* English physicist]

juvenile rheumatoid arthritis (JRA) (JOO-veh-nye-el ROO-mah-toyd ar-THRY-tis) systemic autoimmune disease that results in severe deterioration and deformity of joints [*juven-* youth, *-ile* of or like, *rheuma-* flow, *-oid* like, *arthr-* joint, *-itis* inflammation]

juxtaglomerular apparatus (juks-tah-gloh-MER-yoo-lar app-ah-RAT-us) in the nephron, the complex of cells from the distal tubule and the afferent arteriole, which helps regulate blood pressure by secreting renin in response to blood pressure changes in the kidney; located near the glomerulus; also called *juxtaglomular complex* [*juxta-* near or adjoining, *-glomer-* ball, *-ul-* little, *-ar* relating to]

juxtaglomerular (JG) cell (jux-tah-gloh-MER-yoo-lar) cell of the juxtaglomerular apparatus [*juxta-* near or adjoining, *-glomer-* ball, *-ul-* little, *-ar* relating to, *cell* storeroom]

juxtamedullary nephron (jux-tah-MED-uh-lair-ee NEF-ron) region of the nephron that lies near the junction of the cortical and medullary layers of the kidney [*juxta-* near or adjoining, *-medulla-* marrow or pith (middle), *-ary* relating to, *nephro-* kidney, *-on* unit]

K

Kaposi sarcoma (KS) (KAH-poh-see sar-KOH-mah) rare malignant neoplasm of the skin that often spreads to lymph nodes and internal organs; Kaposi sarcoma is often found in people with AIDS [*Moritz K. Kaposi* Hungarian dermatologist, *sarco-* flesh, *-oma* tumour]

karyotype (KAIR-ee-oh-type) ordered arrangement of photographs of chromosomes from a single cell used in genetic counselling to identify chromosomal disorders such as trisomy or monosomy [*karyo-* nucleus, *-type* kind]

Kegel exercise (KEE-gel) noninvasive treatment used to reduce urinary stress incontinence [*Arnold Kegel* American gynaecologist]

keloid (KEE-loyd) unusually thick fibrous scar on the skin [*kel-* claw, *-oid* like]

keratin (KER-ah-tin) tough, fibrous protein substance in hair, nails, outer skin cells, and horny tissues [*kera-* horn, *-in* substance]

keratinization (ker-ah-tin-ih-ZAY-shun) process by which cells of the stratum corneum become fitted with keratin and move to the surface [*kera-* horn, *-in-* substance, *-iz-* to cause, *-ation* process]

keratinocyte (keh-RAT-ih-no-syte) epidermal cell responsible for synthesizing keratin [*kera-* horn, *-in-* substance, *-cyte* cell]

keratohyalin (ker-ah-toh-HYE-ah-lin) staining granules located within the stratum lucidum; required for surface keratin formation [*kera-* horn, *-hyal-* glass, *-in* substance]

ketogenesis (kee-toh-JEN-eh-sis) process that produces ketone bodies [*keto-* acetone, *-gen-* produce, *-esis* process]

ketone body (KEE-tohn) acid produced during fat catabolism [*keto-* acetone, *-one* chemical]

ketosis (kee-TOH-sis) large amount of ketone bodies present in the blood of a person with uncontrolled diabetes mellitus [*keto-* acetone, *-osis* condition]

kidney (KID-nee) one of the two organs that cleanses the blood of waste products continually produced by metabolism; the kidneys produce urine

killer T cell cytotoxic T lymphocyte [killer, *T* thymus, *cell* storeroom]

kilocalorie (Kcal) (KIL-oh-kal-oh-ree) 1000 calories; *see* Calorie [*kilo-* one thousand, *-calor* heat]

kinaesthesia (kin-es-THEE-zee-ah) "muscle sense"; that is, sense of position and movement of body parts [*kin-* movement, *aesthesia* feeling]

kinase (KYE-nayz) substance that converts proenzymes to active enzymes [*kin-* motion, *-ase* enzyme]

kinesiopathology (kih-nee-see-oh-PA-thol-oh-jee) existence of or study of any abnormality of motion of the musculoskeletal system of the body [*kinesio-* movement, *-path-* disease, *-o-* combining form, *-log-* words (study of), *-y* activity]

kinin (KYE-nin) chemical compound that is released from injured tissues; results in vasodilation and increases the permeability of blood vessels [*kin-* move, *-in* substance]

Klinefelter syndrome (KLINE-fel-ter SIN-drohm) genetic disorder caused by the presence of two or more X chromosomes in a male (typically trisomy XXY); characterized by long legs, enlarged breasts, low intelligence, small testes, sterility, and chronic pulmonary disease [*Harry F. Klinefelter* American physician, *syn-* together, *-drome* running or (race) course]

knee jerk reflex (nee jerk REE-fleks) extension of the leg in response to tapping of the patellar tendon; also called *patellar reflex* [*re-* again, *-flex* bend]

Korotkoff sound (kor-ROT-koff) sound of blood turbulence heard when measuring arterial blood pressure with a sphygmomanometer [*Nicolai Korotkoff* Russian physician]

Krause end bulb (krows end bulb) *see* bulboid corpuscle [*Wilhelm J. F. Krause* German anatomist]

Krebs cycle (krebz SYE-kul) also called *tricarboxylic acid (TCA) cycle*; *see* citric acid cycle [*Sir Hans Adolf Krebs* British biochemist, *cycl-* circle]

Kupffer cell (KOOP-fer sel) eponym for the *stellate macrophage* found in spaces between liver cells [*Karl W. von Kupffer* German surgeon, *cell* storeroom]

kwashiorkor (kwah-shee-OR-kor) nutritional disorder that results from a protein deficiency in the presence of sufficient calories [*kwashiorkor* one who is displaced (from the breast)]

kyphosis (kye-FOH-sis) abnormally exaggerated thoracic curvature of the vertebral column [*kypho-* hump, *-osis* condition]

L

labia majora (LAY-bee-ah mah-JOH-rah) large lateral folds of the vulva [*labia* lips, *majora* large] *sing.*, labium majus (LAY-bee-um MAY-jus)

labia minora (LAY-bee-ah mih-NO-rah) small medial folds of the vulva [*labia* lips, *minora* small] *sing.*, labium minor (LAY-bee-um MYE-nor)

labour process of expulsion of the fetus and the placenta; childbirth

labyrinth (LAB-ih-rinth) bony cavities and membranes of the inner ear [*labyrinth* maze]

lacrimal apparatus (LAK-rih-mal app-ah-RAT-us) in the eye, the tear (lacrimal) gland plus associated ducts that form tears [*lacrima-* tear, *-al* relating to, *apparatus* equipment]

lacrimal bone (LAK-rih-mal bohn) facial bone that joins the maxilla, frontal bone, and ethmoid bone [*lacrima-* tear, *-al* relating to]

lactase (LAK-tayse) enzyme needed to digest lactose [*lact-* milk, *-ase* enzyme]

lactation (lak-TAY-shun) milk production [*lact-* milk, *-ation* process]

lacteal (LAK-tee-al) lymphatic vessel located in each villus of the intestine; serves to absorb fat materials from chyme passing through the small intestine [*lact-* milk, *-al* relating to]

lactic acid (LAK-tik ASS-id) product of anaerobic energy metabolism that accumulates in muscle tissue during exercise and causes a burning sensation [*lac-* milk, *-ic* relating to, *acid* sour]

lactic acidosis (LAK-tik ass-ih-DOH-sis) condition characterized by elevated blood lactate levels, electrolyte imbalances, and decreased blood pH [*lac-* milk, *-ic* relating to, *acid-* sour, *-osis* condition]

lactogenic hormone (lak-toh-JEN-ik HOR-mohn) any hormone that initiates milk production by secretory cells of breast alveoli [*lact-* milk, *-gen-* produce, *-ic* relating to, *hormon-* excite]

lactose intolerance (LAK-tohs in-TOL-er-ans) condition in which one lacks the enzyme lactase, resulting in an inability to digest lactose (a disaccharide in milk and dairy products) [*lact-* milk, *-ose* carbohydrate (sugar), *in-* not, *-toler-* bear, *-ance* state]

lactotroph (lak-toh-TROHF) cell type of the adenohypophysis (anterior pituitary) that secretes prolactin [*lacto-* milk, *-troph* nourish]

lacuna (lah-KOO-nah) space or cavity; for example, lacunae in bone contain bone cells [*lacuna* pit] *pl.*, lacunae (lah-KOO-nee)

lamella (lah-MEL-ah) thin layer, as of bone [*lam-* plate, *-ella* little] *pl.*, lamellae (lah-MEL-ee)

lamellar corpuscle (lah-MEL-ar KOR-pus-ul) sensory receptor with a layered encapsulation found deep in the dermis that detects pressure on the skin surface; also known as *Pacini corpuscle* [*lam-* plate, *-ella-* little, *-ar* relating to, *corpus-* body, *-cle* little]

lamina propria (LAM-in-ah PROH-pree-ah) fibrous connective tissue underlying the epithelium in mucous membranes (*lamina* thin plate, *propria* proper]

laminar flow (LAM-ih-nar) the manner in which blood flows through a smooth vessel [*lamina-* plate, *-ar* relating to]

Langer lines (LANG-er) pattern of dense bundles of white collagenous fibres that characterize the reticular layers of dermis; also called *cleavage lines* [*Karl Langer* Austrian anatomist]

Langerhans cell (LAHNG-er-hahnz) epidermal dendritic cell; cell that plays a role in immunology of the skin and thus serves as defence mechanism for the body [*Paul Langerhans* German pathologist, *cell* storeroom]

lanugo (lah-NOO-go) extremely fine and soft hair coat on developing fetus [*lanugo* down]

laparoscope (LAP-ah-roh-skope) fibre-optic viewing instrument [*laparo-* abdomen, *-scop-* see]

Laplace, law of (lah-PLAHS) *see* **Young-Laplace law** [*Pierre S. de Laplace* French physicist]

laryngitis (lar-in-JYE-tis) inflammation of the mucous tissues of the larynx (voice box) [*laryng-* voice box (larynx), *-itis* inflammation]

laryngopharynx (lah-ring-go-FAIR-inks) lowest part of the pharynx [*laryng-* voice box (larynx), *-pharynx* throat] *pl.*, laryngopharynges (lah-ring-go-FAIR-in-jeez) or laryngopharynxes

larynx (LAIR-inks) voice box located just below the pharynx; the largest piece of cartilage making up the larynx is the thyroid cartilage, commonly known as the *Adam's apple* [*larynx* voice box] *pl.*, larynges (LAIR-in-jeez) or larynxes

laser therapy (LAY-zer) procedure that uses an intense beam of light to destroy a tumour [*laser* shortened "light amplification by stimulated emission of radiation"]

laser-assisted *in situ* keratomileusis (LASIK) (LAY-zer ah-SIS-ted in-SIT-yoo kair-at-oh-mill-YOO-sis) refractive eye surgery to correct myopia [*laser* shortened "light amplification by stimulated emission of radiation", *in* in, *situ* place, *kera-* horn, *-mileusis* carving]

latent period (LAY-tent) period between time a muscle fibre is stimulated and when it contracts; precedes the contraction phase [*latent* hidden]

lateral (LAT-er-al) of or toward the side; opposite of medial [*later-* side, *-al* relating to]

lateral corticospinal tract (LAT-er-al kohr-tih-koh-SPY-nal trakt) spinal motor tract that controls the contraction of individual or small group of muscles, particularly those moving hands, fingers, feet, and toes on opposite side of the body [*later-* side, *-al* relating to, *cortico-* cortex (bark), *-spin-* backbone, *-al* relating to, *tract* trail]

lateral fissure (Sylvius fissure) (LAT-er-al FISH-ur [SIL-vee-us FISH-ur]) deep groove between the temporal lobe below and the frontal and parietal lobes of the brain [*later-* side, *-al* relating to, *Franciscus Sylvius* German medical professor]

lateral lobe (LAT-er-al) one of two large lobes of the thyroid gland [*later-* side, *-al* relating to]

lateral longitudinal arch (LAT-er-al lon-jih-TYOO-dih-nal) supportive arch of the foot; shaped by the calcaneus, cuboid tarsals, and the fourth and fifth metacarpals [*later-* side, *-al* relating to, *longitud-* length, *-al* relating to]

lateral spinothalamic tract (LAT-er-al spy-no-tha-LAM-ik trakt) sensory tract that integrates crude touch, pain, and temperature [*later-* side, *-al* relating to, *spino-* backbone, *-thalam-* inner chamber, *-ic* relating to, *tract* trail]

law scientific idea or explanation that is viewed with a very high degree of confidence or certainty after rigorous testing and observation; compare to **hypothesis** and **theory**

law of partial pressures *see* Dalton's law [*pars-* parts, *-al* relating to]

lecithin (LES-ih-thin) substance in bile that emulsifies dietary oils and fats in the lumen of the small intestine [*lecith-* yolk, *-in* substance]

Le Fort fracture (leh-FOHR) bone fracture of the face and/or base of the skull (also called *Guérin fracture*) [*Rene Le Fort* French surgeon, *Alphonse F.M. Guérin*, French surgeon, *fracture* a breaking]

legionnaires' disease (LEE-jen-airs) form of bacterial pneumonia caused by infection with the *Legionella pneumophila* organism [originally named for American Legion, at whose convention location the first outbreak was noted]

length–tension relationship maximum strength that a muscle can develop bears a direct relationship to the initial length of its fibres

lens refracting mechanism of the eye that is located directly behind the pupil [*lens* lentil]

lentiform nucleus (LEN-tih-form NYOO-klee-us) mass of grey matter in the interior of each cerebral hemisphere; consists of the putamen and the pallidum [*lent-* lentil (lens), *-form* shape, *nucleus* nut or kernel] *pl.*, nuclei (NYOO-klee-eye)

leptin (LEP-tin) a protein hormone produced by fat-storing cells in adipose tissue that plays a role in inhibiting food intake by regulating the satiety centre in the hypothalamus; leptin also plays a role in reducing fat storage in nonadipose cells in the liver and skeletal muscles; because of its role in fat storage, it may play a role in future treatments for diabetes, obesity, and other conditions related to fat metabolism; *see* **satiety centre**; leptin also helps regulate some immune and neuroendocrine functions and plays a role in development [*lept-* thin, *-in* substance]

lesser omentum (oh-MEN-tum) extension of the peritoneum that is attached from the liver to the lesser curvature of the stomach and the first part of the duodenum [*omentum* fatty covering of intestines]

lesser vestibular gland (ves-TIB-yoo-lar) tiny mucous gland located near the female's urinary meatus by way of two small ducts; also called *Skene glands* [*vestibul-* entrance hall, *-ar* relating to, *gland* acorn]

leucocyte (LOO-koh-syte) white blood cell [*leuco-* white, *-cyte* cell]

leucocytosis (loo-koh-sye-TOH-sis) abnormally high white blood cell numbers in the blood [*leuco-* white, *-cyt-* cell, *-osis* condition]

leucocytosis-promoting (LP) factor (look-oh-sye-TOH-sis) substance released by injured tissue; stimulates the release of white cells from storage areas and increases the number of circulating white blood cells [*leuco-* white, *-cyto-* cell, *-osis* condition]

leucopenia (loo-koh-PEE-nee-ah) abnormally low white blood cell numbers in the blood [*leuco-* white, *-penia* lack]

leucoplakia (loo-koh-PLAY-kee-ah) precancerous change in the mucous membrane characterized by thickened, white, and slightly raised patches of tissue [*leuco-* white, *-plak-* flat area, *-ia* condition]

leucopoiesis (loo-koh-poy-EE-sis) process of producing new white blood cells (leucocytes) [*leuco-* white, *-poiesis* making]

leucoreduction (loo-koh-ree-DUK-shun) filtering process that removes leucocytes from blood [*leuco-* white, *-re-* back, *-duc-* lead, *-tion* process]

leucorrhoea (loo-koh-REE-ah) whitish vaginal discharge [*leuco-* white, *-rrhoea* flow]

leukaemia (loo-KEE-mee-ah) blood cancer; affects white blood cells [*leuk-* white, *-(h)aem-* blood, *-ia* condition]

leukotriene (loo-koh-TRY-een) cytokine compound that functions as an inflammation mediator [*leuko-* white, *-tri-* three, *-ene* chemical]

levator ani muscle (leh-VAY-tor AY-nye) muscle of the pelvic floor [*levator* lifter, *ani* of the anus, *mus-* mouse, *-cle* little]

levator scapulae (leh-VAY-tor SCAP-yoo-lee) shoulder girdle muscle that elevates the scapula [*levator* lifter, *scapulae* of the shoulder blade]

lever (LEEV-er) any rigid bar free to turn about a fixed point [*lev-* lift, *-er* agent]

lever system (LEEV-er) simple mechanical device that makes the work of moving a weight or other load easier [*lev-* lift, *-er* agent]

levodopa (L-dopa) (LEEV-oh-doh-pah) a molecule derived from tyrosine in neurons that is used to produce the neurotransmitter dopamine [*levo-* left (form of molecule), *-dopa* acronym denoting 3,4- *d*ihydroxy *p*henyl*a*lanine]

Leydig cell (LYE-dig) *see* interstitial cell [*Franz von Leydig* German anatomist, *cell* storeroom]

ligament (LIG-ah-ment) band of white fibrous tissue connecting bones to other bones [*liga-* bind, *-ment* result of action]

light micrograph (LM) (MYK-roh-graf) photographic image of a microscopic structure using a light microscope [*micro-* small, *-graph* drawing]

light microscope (LM) (MYK-roh-skope) magnifying device made of glass lenses that uses light transmitted through or reflected from a specimen [*micro-* small, *-scop-* see]

limb lead (lim leed) electrode placed on limbs during electrocardiography

limbic system (LIM-bik) parts of the brain involved in emotions and sense of smell; play key role in coupling sensory inputs to short- and long-term memory; consist of the hippocampus, the hypothalamus, and several other structures [*limb-* edge, *-ic* relating to]

limited-field radiation treatment procedure for early-stage cancers that have not spread [*radiat-* emit rays, *-tion* process]

linea alba (LIN-ee-ah AL-bah) tough band of connective tissue that covers the rectus abdominis muscle [*linea* line, *alba* white]

linear fracture (LIN-ee-ar) type of bone fracture in which fracture line is parallel to the bone's long axis [*linea-* line, *-ar* relating to, *fracture* a breaking]

lingual tonsil (LING-gwal TON-sil) tonsil located at the base of the tongue [*lingua-* tongue, *-al* relating to, *tons-* goitre, *-il* little]

lip region that lines the mouth and continues into the oral cavity [*lip-* edge]

lipase (LYE-payz) fat-digesting enzyme [*lip-* fat, *-ase* enzyme]

lipid (LIP-id) class of organic compounds that includes fats, oils, and related substances [*lip-* fat, *-id* form]

lipogenesis (lip-oh-JEN-eh-sis) formation of body fat from food sources [*lipo-* fat, *-gen-* produce, *-esis* process]

lipokine (LIP-oh-kyne) lipid hormone molecule released by adipose tissue to regulate metabolism in other tissues; primary example is **lipokine palmiteolate** [*lipo-* fat, *-kine* motion]

lipoma (lih-POH-mah) benign tumour of adipose (fat) tissue [*lip-* fat, *-oma* tumour]

lipoprotein (lip-oh-PROH-teen) substance that is part lipid and part protein; produced mainly in the liver [*lipo-* fat, *prote-* primary, *-in* substance]

lithotripsy (LITH-oh-trip-see) technique that pulverizes kidney stones [*litho-* stone, *-trips-* pound, *-y* action]

lithotriptor (LITH-oh-trip-tor) ultrasound generator used in lithotripsy; also spelled "lithotripter" [*litho-* stone, *-trip-* pound, *-or* agent]

litmus (LIT-mus) pigment used to test for acidity and alkalinity [*litmus-* coloured herb]

lobar (LOH-bar) referring to a lobe [*lob-* lobe, *-ar* relating to]

lobectomy (loh-BEK-toh-mee) surgical removal of a single lobe of an organ, as in the removal of one lobe of a lung [*lob-* lobe, *-ec-tomy* surgical removal]

local potential (poh-TEN-shal) slight shift from resting membrane potential in a specific region of the plasma membrane [*potent-* power, *-ial* relating to]

lock-and-key model description of how a specific enzyme will fit into only a specific substrate, like a key fits into a lock [*lock-* fastening, *model-* mode]

long bone bone that is characterized by its extended longitudinal axis and unique articular ends

longissimus capitis muscle (lon-JIS-ih-mus KAP-ih-tis) muscle of the head [*longissimus* longest or very long, *capit-* head, *-is* thing, *mus-* mouse, *-cle* little]

longitudinal arch (lon-jih-TYOO-dih-nal) two arches, the medial and lateral, that extend lengthwise in the foot [*longitud-* length, *-al* relating to]

longitudinal fissure (lon-jih-TYOO-dih-nal FISH-ur) deepest groove in the cerebrum; divides the cerebrum into two hemispheres [*longitud-* length, *-al* relating to]

longitudinal section (lon-jih-TYOO-dih-nal SEK-shun) any cut made in a body part along a plane parallel to the long axis of the body part [*longitud-* length, *-al* relating to, *sect-* cut, *-tion* process]

Loop of Henle (HEN-lee) extension of the proximal tubule of the nephron; also called *loop of Henle, Henle loop* or *nephron loop* [*Friedrich Gustave Henle* German anatomist]

loose fibrous connective tissue *see* **areolar tissue** [*loose-* free, *con-* together, *-nect-* bind, *-ive* relating to, *fibr-* thread or fibre, *-ous,* characterized by, *tissu-* fabric]

lordosis (lor-DOH-sis) abnormally exaggerated lumbar curvature of the vertebral column [*lordos-* bent backward, *-osis* condition]

low-density lipoprotein (lip-oh-PROH-teen) a blood lipid fraction (plasma protein) composed of relatively more cholesterol and triglycerides than protein; often called "bad cholesterol" because high levels contribute to atherosclerotic plaque formation and arterial wall damage [*lipo-* fat, *-protein* first rank]

lower oesophageal sphincter (LES) (eh-SOF-eh-JEE-ul SFINGK-ter) muscle located at the junction between the terminal portion of the oesophagus and the stomach; also called *cardiac sphincter* [*oes-* will carry, *-phag-* food (eat), *-al* relating to, *sphinc-* bind tight, *-er* agent]

lower respiratory tract (RES-pih-rah-tor-ee) region of the respiratory tract that consists of the trachea, all segments of the bronchial tree, and the lungs [*re-* again, *-spir-* breathe, *-tory* relating to, *tract* trail]

lumbar (LUM-bar) relating to the loin or lower part of back (between ribs and pelvis) [*lumb-* loin, *-ar* relating to]

lumbar plexus (LUM-bar PLEK-sus) spinal nerve plexus located in the low back [*lumb-* loin, *-ar* relating to, *plexus* braid or network] *pl.*, plexi (PLEK-sye) or plexuses (PLEK-sus-eez)

lumbar puncture (LUM-bar) clinical procedure in which some cerebrospinal fluid is withdrawn from the subarachnoid space in the lumbar region of the spinal cord for analysis [*lumb-* loin, *-ar* relating to]

lumbar vertebra (LUM-bar VER-teh-bra) lower five bones of the vertebral column; support the small of the back [*lumb-* loin, *-ar* relating to, *vertebra* that which turns] *pl.*, vertebrae

lumbrical muscle (LUM-brih-kal) intrinsic muscle of the foot [*lumbric-* worm, *-al* relating to, *mus-* mouse, *-cle* little]

lumen (LOO-men) the hollow area of a hollow organ such as the stomach, blood vessel, or urinary bladder; *see also* **luminal** [*lumen* light] *pl.*, lumina

luminal (LOO-min-al) relating to the hollow part, or lumen, of a hollow organ such as the urinary bladder or small intestine; *see also* **lumen** [*lumin-* light, *-al* relating to]

lumpectomy (lump-EK-toh-mee) surgical removal of a tumour from breast tissue [*lump-* mass, *-ec-* out, *-tom-* cut, *-y* action]

lung cancer malignancy of pulmonary tissue [*cancer* crab or malignant tumour]

lunula (LOO-nyoo-lah) crescent-shaped white area under the proximal nail bed [*luna-* moon, *-ula* small]

luteal phase (LOO-tee-al) phase of the menstrual cycle that occurs between ovulation and the onset of menses; also called *premenstrual phase, postovulatory phase,* or *secretory phase* [*lute-* yellow, *-al* relating to]

luteinization (loo-tee-in-ih-ZAY-shun) formation of a golden body (corpus luteum) in the ruptured follicle [*lute-* yellow, *-ization* process]

luteinizing hormone (LH) (loo-tee-in-EYE-zing HOR-mohn) in females, acts in conjunction with follicle-stimulating hormone (FSH) to stimulate follicle and ovum maturation, release of oestrogen, and ovulation; known as the *ovulating hormone*; in males, causes testes to develop and secrete testosterone [*lute-* yellow, *-izing* process, *hormon-* excite]

lymph (limf) watery fluid drained from the tissue spaces that returns excess fluid and protein molecules to the blood via the lymphatic vessels [*lymph* water]

lymph node (limf nohd) small structure that performs biological filtration of lymph on its way to the circulatory system [*lymph* water, *nod-* knot]

lymphangiography (lim-fan-jee-OG-rah-fee) method using x-rays and radiopaque material to examine lymphatic vessels [*lymph-* water, *-angi-* vessel, *-graph-* draw, *-y* process]

lymphangitis (lim-fan-JYE-tis) inflammation of lymph vessels, usually caused by infection, characterized by fine red streaks extending from the site of infection; may progress to septicaemia (blood infection) [*lymph-* water, *-angi-* vessel, *-itis* inflammation]

lymphatic capillary (lim-FAT-ik KAP-ILL-air-ee) microscopic blind-ended vessels that transport lymph [*lymph-* water, *-atic* relating to, *capill-* hair, *-ary* relating to]

lymphatic vessel (lim-FAT-ik) any vessel of a system of blind-ended vessels that collect lymph and deliver it to the circulatory system via the thoracic duct and the right lymphatic duct [*lymph-* water, *-atic* relating to]

lymphocyte (LIM-foh-syte) one type of white blood cell; *see* **B lymphocyte, T lymphocyte** [*lymph-* water (lymphatic system), *-cyte* cell]

lymphoedema (lim-fah-DEE-mah) swelling caused by lymphatic vessel blockage [*lymph-* water, *-oedema* swelling]

lymphokine (LIM-foh-kyne) chemical compounds released by antigen-bound sensitized T cells [*lymph-* water (lymphatic system), *-kine* motion]

lymphoid neoplasm (LIM-foyd NEE-oh-plazem) *see* **lymphoma** [*lymph-* water (lymphatic system), *-oid* like, *neo-* new, *-plasm* substance]

lymphoid tissue (LIM-foyd) type of reticular tissue that contains lymphocytes and other specialized cells [*lymph-* water (lymphatic system), *-oid* like, *tissu* fabric]

lymphokinesis (lim-foh-kih-NEE-sis) flow of lymph [*lymph-* water, *-kinesis* activation]

lymphoma (lim-FOH-mah) cancer of lymphatic tissue [*lymph-* water (lymphatic system), *-oma* tumour]

lymphotoxin (lim-foh-TOK-sin) powerful poison that quickly kills any cells it attacks [*lympho-* water (lymphocyte), *-tox-* poison, *-in* substance]

lysosome (LYE-so-sohm) membranous organelle containing various enzymes that can dissolve most cellular compounds; called *digestive bags* or *suicide bags of cell* [*lyso-* loosen, *-som-* body]

M

M line region of the sarcomere where myosin filaments are held together and stabilized by protein molecules [*M mittel* middle]

M phase step of the cell life cycle in which a cell divides through the process of mitosis (mitotic cell division); M phase follows the G_2 phase (second growth phase) and occurs along with cytokinesis (splitting of the cell's cytoplasm into two daughter cells); *see* **cell life cycle** [*phase* appearance]

macromineral (mak-roh-MIN-er-al) dietary mineral needed in large daily quantities of at least 100 mg per day (e.g., calcium, phosphorus) [*macro-* large, *-miner-* mine, *-al* relating to]

macromolecule (mak-roh-MOL-eh-kyool) large, complex chemical made of combinations of molecules [*macro-* large, *-molec-* mass, *-ule* small]

macronutrient (MAK-roh-NYOO-tree-ent) nutrient needed in large amounts; carbohydrates, fats, and proteins [*macro-* large, *-nutri-* nourish, *-ent* agent]

macrophage (MAK-roh-fayj) phagocytic cell in the immune system [*macro-* large, *-phag-* eat]

macula (MAK-yoo-lah) strip of sensory epithelium in the utricle and saccule; provides information related to head position or acceleration [*macula* spot] *pl.*, maculae (MAK-yoo-lee) or maculas

macula densa (MAK-yoo-lah DEN-sah) distal tubule cells in the juxtaglomerular apparatus that are dense and tightly packed [*macula* spot, *densa* thick] *pl.*, maculae densae (MAK-yoo-lee DEN-see)

macula lutea (MAK-yoo-lah LOO-tee-ah) yellowish area near centre of the retina where cones are densely distributed; also called simply "macula" [*macula* spot, *lutea* yellow] *pl.*, maculae luteae (MAK-yoo-lee LOO-tee-ee)

magnesium (mag-NEE-see-um) element that is a component of many energy-transferring enzymes [*magne-* lodestone, *-um* thing or substance]

magnetic resonance imaging (MRI) (mag-NET-ik REZ-ah-nens IM-ah-jing) scanning technique that uses a magnetic field to induce tissues to emit radio waves that can be used by computer to construct a sectional view of a patient's body [*magnet-* lodestone, *-ic* relating to, *re-* again, *-sona-* sound, *-ance* state]

magnetoencephalography (MEG) (mag-NET-oh-en-sef-eh-LOG-reh-fee) method of measuring brain activity using a sensitivity machine called a *biomagnetometer*; detects very small magnetic fields generated by neural activity [*magneto-* lodestone, *-en-* within, *-cephalo-* head, *-graph-* draw, *-y* activity]

major histocompatibility complex (MHC) (MAY-jer HIST-oh-kom-PAT-ih-bil-it-ee KOM-pleks) set of genes in chromosome 6 that all code for antigen-presenting proteins and other immune system proteins; proteins produced by MHC genes in class I and class II also are called *human leucocyte antigens (HLAs)*; MHC proteins present different protein fragments (peptides) at the surface of the cell for possible recognition as either self or nonself antigens by immune system cells [*histo-* tissue, *-compatibil-* agreeable, *-ity* state, *com-* together, *-plex* weave or braid]

malabsorption syndrome (mal-ab-SORP-shun SIN-drohm) refers to a group of symptoms resulting from the failure of the small intestine to absorb nutrients properly [*mal-* bad, *-ab-* from, *-sorp-* suck, *-tion* process, *syn-* together, *-drome* running or (race) course]

malaria (mah-LAIR-ee-ah) sometimes fatal condition caused by blood parasites [*mal-* bad, *-ar-* air, *-ia* condition]

male pattern baldness common type of baldness that results when the gene for baldness is present and testosterone is present

malignant (mah-LIG-nant) refers to a tumour or neoplasm that is capable of metastasizing, or spreading, to new tissues; cancer [*malign-* bad, *-ant* state]

malignant hyperthermia (MH) (mah-LIG-nant hye-per-THERM-ee-ah) inherited condition characterized by abnormally increased body temperature and muscle rigidity when exposed to certain anaesthetics or muscle relaxants [*malign-* bad, *-ant* state, *hyper-* excessive, *-therm-* heat, *-ia* abnormal condition]

malignant melanoma (mah-LIG-nant mel-ah-NO-mah) most deadly type of skin cancer [*malign-* bad, *-ant* state, *melan-* black, *-oma* tumour]

malignant tumour (mah-LIG-nant TYOO-mer) cancer that is not encapsulated and tends to spread to other regions of the body [*malign* bad, *-ant* state, *tumour* swelling]

malocclusion (mal-oh-CLEW-zhun) condition that occurs when missing teeth create wide spaces in the dentition, when teeth overlap, or when one or more teeth prevents correct alignment [*mal-* bad, *-occlu-* close up, *-sion* state]

maltase (MAL-tays) enzyme that catalyzes the final steps of carbohydrate digestion [*malt-* grain, *-ase* enzyme]

mammary (MAM-mah-ree) relating to the breast [*mamma-* breast, *-ry* relating to]

mammary gland (MAM-mah-ree) milk-producing glands of the breasts; classified as external accessory sex organs in females (they are present but usually nonfunctional in males) [*mamma-* breast, *-ry* relating to, *gland* acorn]

mammogenic hormone (mam-moh-JEN-ik HOR-mohn) any hormone that promotes breast tissue growth and development [*mammo-* breast, *-gen-* produce, *-ic* relating to, *hormon-* excite]

mammography (mam-OG-rah-fee) x-ray photography of the breast [*mammo-* breast, *-graphy* kind of printing or recording]

mandible (MAN-di-bal) jaw bone; largest and strongest bone of the face [*mandi-* chew, *-ible* capable]

mandibular nerve (man-DIB-yoo-lar) part of the trigeminal nerve [*mandibl-* jaw, *-ar* relating to]

manual (MAN-yoo-al) relating to the hand [*manu-* hand, *-al* relating to]

marasmus (mah-RAZ-mus) form of protein-calorie malnutrition; results from an overall lack of calories and protein [*marasmus* a wasting]

marrow cavity (MAIR-oh KAV-ih-tee) *see* medullary cavity [*marrow* pith (middle), *cav-* hollow, *-ity* state]

mass number see **atomic mass**

masseter (mah-SEE-ter) facial muscle responsible for chewing [*masseter* chewer]

mast cell immune system cell to which antibodies become attached in early stages of inflammation [*mast* fattening, *cell* storeroom]

mastectomy (mas-TEK-toh-mee) surgical removal of the breast [*mast-* breast, *-ectomy* surgical removal]

mastication (mass-tih-KAY-shun) chewing [*mastica-* chew, *-ation* process]

mastitis (mass-TYE-tis) breast inflammation [*mast-* breast, *-itis* inflammation]

mastoidectomy (mass-toyd-EK-toh-mee) inflammation of the air spaces within the mastoid portion of the temporal bone [*mast-* breast, *-oid-* like, *-ec-* out, *-tom-* cut, *-y* action]

mastoiditis (mas-toyd-EYE-tis) inflammation of the air cells within the mastoid portion of the temporal bone; usually caused by infection [*mast-* breast, *-oid-* like, *-itis* inflammation]

matrix (MAY-triks) extracellular substance of a tissue; for example, the matrix of bone is calcified, whereas that of blood is liquid; *see also* **extracellular matrix** (ECM) [*matrix* womb] *pl.*, matrices

matter anything that has mass and occupies space [*matter-* something from which something is made]

maxilla (mak-SIH-lah) upper jaw bone [*maxilla* upper jaw] *pl.*, maxillae (mak-SIH-lee)

maxillary nerve (MAK-sih-lair-ee) branch of the trigeminal nerve [*maxilla-* upper jaw, *-ary* relating to]

maximum oxygen consumption ($Vo_{2\ max}$) the maximum amount of oxygen that a person can take up by the lungs, transport to the tissues, and use to do work in cells of the body [*maximum* greatest, *oxy-* sharp, *-gen* produce, *con-* with or in, *-sum-* take, *-tion* process]

McBurney point (mak-BUR-nee) a point on the abdominal wall midway between the right anterior superior iliac spine and the umbilicus; site of pain in acute appendicitis [*Charles McBurney* American surgeon]

mean arterial pressure (MAP) (meen ar-TEER-ee-al PRESH-er) average blood pressure in the arteries used to determine perfusion pressure to the organs [*mean* average, *arteri-* vessel, *-al* relating to]

meatus (mee-AYT-us) any tubelike passageway or opening [*meatus* channel or passage] *pl.*, meatus or meatuses

mechanical digestion process through which food is broken into smaller portions through chewing and movements of the alimentary canal; enables enzymes to act on a larger surface area to accomplish chemical digestion [*digest-* break apart, *-tion* process]

mechanoreceptor (mek-an-oh-ree-SEP-tor) receptors that respond to physical movement in the environment, such as sound waves; for example, equilibrium and balance sensors in the ears [*mechano-* machine (mechanical), *-cept-* receive, *-or* agent]

medial (MEE-dee-al) of or toward the middle; opposite of lateral [*media-* middle, *-al* relating to]

medial lemniscal system (MEE-dee-al lem-NIS-kal) posterior white columns of the spinal cord plus the medial lemniscus; functions in touch sensations and conscious proprioception [*media-* middle, *-al* relating to, *lemnis-* fillet, *cal-* relating to, *system* arrangement]

medial longitudinal arch (MEE-dee-al lon-jih-TYOO-dih-nal) inner lengthwise (antero-posterior) support structure of the foot [*medial* middle, *-al* relating to, *longitudo-* length, *-al* relating to]

median (MEE-dee-an) relating to the medial (middle) aspect of the body or a body structure; midline of the body or a body structure [*medi-* middle, *-an* relating to]

median cubital vein (MEE-dee-an KYOO-bih-tal vayn) forearm vein [*medi-* middle, *-an* relating to, *cubit-* elbow, *-al* relating to, *vena* blood vessel]

mediastinum (MEE-dee-as-TYE-num) a portion of the thorax cavity in the middle of the thorax [*mediastin-* midway, *-um* thing]

medical imaging techniques that visualize tissues for medical study [*medic-* heal, *-al* relating to]

medulla (meh-DUL-ah) Latin for "marrow"; the inner portion of an organ in contrast to the outer portion, or cortex [*medulla* marrow or pith (middle)] *pl.*, medullae or medullas

medulla oblongata (meh-DUL-ah ob-long-GAH-tah) lowest part of the brainstem; an enlarged extension of the spinal cord; the vital centres are located within this area [*medulla* marrow or pith (middle), *oblongata* oblong] *pl.*, medullae oblongatae (meh-DUL-ee ob-long-GAH-tee)

medullary (meh-DUL-ar-ee) relating to the middle or centre of an organ or structure [*medulla-* marrow or pith (middle), *-ary* relating to]

medullary cavity (meh-DUL-ar-ee) hollow area inside the diaphysis of the bone that contains yellow marrow [*medulla-* marrow or pith (middle), *-ary* relating to, *cav-* hollow, *-ity* state]

medullary ischaemic reflex (meh-DUL-ar-ee is-KEE-mik REE-fleks) mechanism that exerts powerful control of blood vessels during emergency situations when blood flow to the brain drops below normal [*medulla-* middle, *-ary* relating to, *ischaem-* hold back, *-ic* relating to, *re-* back or again, *-flex* bend]

medullary rhythmicity area (meh-DUL-ar-ee rith-MIH-sih-tee) area in the brainstem that generates the basic rhythm of the respiratory cycle of inspiration and expiration [*medulla-* marrow or pith (middle), *-ary* relating to, *rhythm-* movement in time, *-ic* relating to, *-ity* condition]

megakaryocyte (meg-ah-KAIR-ee-oh-syte) large cell in the spleen that contributes to formation of platelets [*mega-* huge, *-karyo* nut, *-cyte* cell]

meiosis (my-OH-sis) nuclear division in which the number of chromosomes is reduced to half their original number through separation of homologous pairs; produces gametes [*meiosis* becoming smaller]

Meissner corpuscle (MYZ-ner KOR-pus-ul) *see* **tactile corpuscle** [*George Meissner* German physiologist]

melacine (MEL-ah-seen) vaccine made from melanoma cancer cells; used for prevention of recurrence of malignant melanoma following initial treatment and as a less toxic alternative to chemotherapy for treatment of advanced melanoma [*mela-* black, *-cine* from vaccine]

melanin (MEL-ah-nin) brown pigment primarily in skin and hair [*melan-* black, *-in* substance]

melanocyte (MEL-ah-noh-syte) cell type in the stratum basale of the skin that produces melanin pigment granules, releasing them to other nearby skin cells [*melan-* black, *-cyte* cell]

melanocyte-stimulating hormone (MSH) (MEL-ah-noh-syte-STIM-yoo-lay-ting HOR-mohn) hormone secreted by the pituitary that increases production of melanin, leading to darker skin colour [*melan-* black, *-cyte* cell, *hormon-* excite]

melanoma (mel-ah-NO-mah) cancer of pigmented epithelial cells [*melan-* black, *-oma* tumour]

melanosome (MEL-ah-no-sohm) pigment granule released by melanocytes [*melan-* black, *-som-* body]

melatonin (mel-ah-TOH-nin) important hormone produced by the pineal gland; it is believed to regulate onset of puberty and the menstrual cycle; also referred to as the *third eye* because it responds to levels of light and is thought to be involved with the body's internal clock [*mela-* black, *-ton-* tone, *-in* substance]

membrane thin, sheetlike structure [*membran-* thin skin]

membrane attack complex (MAC) (MEM-brayn at-TAK KOM-pleks) molecules formed by the complement cascade; leads to cell lysis [*membran-* thin skin, *com-* together, *-plex* weave or braid]

membrane bone bone formed within membranous tissues, such as the flat bones of the skull, instead of indirectly through endochondral ossification [*membran-* thin skin]

membrane channel pores within the cell membrane through which specific ions or other small, water-soluble molecules can pass [*membran-* thin skin, *channel* water pipe]

membrane potential difference in electrical charge between inside and outside of the plasma membrane [*membran-* thin skin, *potent-* power, *-ial* relating to]

membranous (MEM-brah-nus) resembling a membrane [*membran-* thin skin, *-ous* characterized by]

membranous organelle (MEM-brah-nus or-gah-NELL) cell organ that is defined or bordered by a membrane [*membran-* thin skin, *-ous* characterized by, *organ-* instrument, *-elle* small]

memory B cell (MEM-oh-ree bee sel) B cell that has been activated but is not an effector cell producing an active response [memory, *B* bursa-equivalent tissue, *cell* storeroom]

memory cell (MEM-oh-ree sel) cell that remains in reserve in the lymph nodes until their ability to secrete antibodies is needed [*cell* storeroom]

memory T cell (MEM-oh-ree tee sel) T cell that has been activated but is not an effector cell producing an active response [memory, *T* thymus gland, *cell* storeroom]

menarche (meh-NAR-kee) first menses occurring at the onset of puberty [*men-* month, *-arche* beginning]

Ménière disease (men-ee-AIR) chronic inner ear disease of unknown cause [*Prosper Ménière* French physician, *dis-* opposite of, *-ease* comfort]

meninges (meh-NIN-jeez) fluid-containing membranes surrounding the brain and spinal cord [*meninx* membrane] *sing.*, meninx (meh-NINKS)

meningitis (men-in-JYE-tis) inflammation of the meninges caused by various factors, including bacterial infection, mycosis, viral infection, and tumours [*mening-* membrane, *-itis* inflammation]

meniscus (meh-NIS-kus) articular cartilage disc [*meniscus* crescent] *pl.*, menisci (meh-NIS-keye or meh-NIS-kye)

menopause (MEN-oh-pawz) termination of menstrual cycles; also called *climacteric* [*men-* month, *-paus-* cease]

menotropin (men-oh-TROHP-in) drug used as an infertility treatment [*men-* month, *-trop-* nourish, *-in* substance]

menses (MEN-seez) periodic shedding of endometrial lining in uterus; occurs in cycles of about 28 days [*menses* months] *pl.*, menses (MEN-ses)

menstrual cycle (MEN-stroo-al SYE-kul) series of changes that regularly occurs in sexually mature, nonpregnant women that results in shedding of the uterine lining approximately once a month [*mens-* month, *-al* relating to, *cycl-* circle]

menstrual period (MEN-stroo-al) *see* **menses** [*mens-* month, *-al* relating to]

menstruation (men-stroo-AY-shun) menses; regular event of the female reproductive cycle that allows the endometrium to renew itself [*mens-* month, *-ation* process]

mental (MEN-tal) relating to the chin [*ment-* chin, *-al* relating to]

Merkel cell (MER-kuhl) *see* **tactile epithelial cell** [*Friedrich Sigmund Merkel* German anatomist]

merocrine gland (MER-oh-krin) gland that discharges secretions directly through the cell or plasma membrane [*mero-* part, *-crine* to separate]

mesangial cell (mess-AN-jee-al) irregular cell that functions as a support and phagocytic cell; unique to renal corpuscles [*mes-* middle, *-angi-* vessel, *-al* relating to, *cell-* storeroom]

mesencephalon (mez-en-SEF-ah-lon) primary or secondary vesicle of the neural tube during embryonic development that eventually becomes the midbrain; often used as a synonym for *midbrain* [*mes-* middle, *-en-* within, *-cephalon* head]

mesentery (MEZ-en-tair-ee) large double fold of peritoneal tissue that anchors the loops of the digestive tract to the posterior wall of the abdominal cavity [*mes-* middle, *-enter-* intestine, *-y* location]

mesoderm (MEZ-oh-derm) middle layer of the primary germ layers; gives rise to such structures as muscle, bones, and blood vessels [*meso-* middle, *-derm* skin]

mesomorph (MEZ-oh-morf) body type characterized by a muscular build [*meso-* middle, *-morph* form]

mesothelium (mez-oh-THEE-lee-um) epithelial lining of the pleura, pericardium, and peritoneum [*meso-* middle or median, *-theli-* nipple, *-um* thing] *pl.*, mesothelia

messenger RNA (mRNA) duplicate copy of a gene sequence on the DNA that passes from the nucleus to the cytoplasm; used by ribosomes to create specific proteins [*RNA*-ribonucleic acid]

metabolic acidosis (met-ah-BOL-ik ass-ih-DOH-sis) disturbance affecting the bicarbonate element of the bicarbonate-carbonic acid buffer pair in the blood; bicarbonate deficit [*meta-* over, *-bol-* throw, *-ic* relating to, *acid-* sour, *-osis* condition]

metabolic alkalosis (met-ah-BOL-ik al-kah-LOH-sis) disturbance affecting the bicarbonate element of the bicarbonate-carbonic acid buffer pair in the blood; bicarbonate excess [*meta-* over, *-bol-* throw, *-ic* relating to, *alkal-* ashes, *-osis* condition]

metabolic pathway (met-ah-BOL-ik) sequence of chemical reactions [*meta-* over, *-bol-* throw, *-ic* relating to]

metabolic rate (met-ah-BOL-ik) amount of energy released by catabolism in the body over a given period [*meta-* over, *-bol-* throw, *-ic* relating to]

metabolic syndrome (met-ah-BOL-ik SIN-drohm) collection of risk factors that together increase the risk of coronary heart disease, stroke, and type 2 diabetes mellitus (e.g., central obesity, insulin resistance, high blood lipids, hypertension) [*meta-* over, *-bol-* throw, *-ic* relating to, *syn-* together, *-drome* running or (race) course]

metabolism (meh-TAB-oh-liz-im) complex, intertwining set of chemical processes by which life is made possible for a living organism; *see* **anabolism, catabolism** [*meta-* over, *-bol-* throw, *-ism* action]

metabotropic receptor (meh-TAB-eh-TROH-pik ree-SEP-tor) a G protein–coupled receptor (GPCR) that triggers cell metabolic pathways when stimulated, rather than directly opening a membrane channel [*meta-* over, *-bo-* throw, *-trop-* turn or change, *-ic* relating to, *recept-* receive, *-or* agent]

metacarpal bone (met-ah-KAR-pal) bone of the hand [*meta-* beyond,*-carp-* wrist, *-al* relating to]

metacarpophalangeal joint (met-ah-KAR-poh-fah-LAN-jee-al) type of joint with the rounded heads of the metacarpals and the concave bases of the proximal phalanges articulating with each other [*meta-* beyond, *-carpo-* wrist, *-phalang-* finger bones (ref. from rows of soldiers), *-al* relating to]

metaphase (MET-ah-fayz) second stage of mitosis, during which the nuclear membrane and nucleolus disappear and the chromosomes align on the equatorial plane [*meta-* change or middle, *-phase* stage]

metaphysis (meh-TAF-ih-sis) in a long bone, the region between the epiphyses and diaphysis (in a mature bone) or the epiphyseal plate region (in a growing bone) [*meta-* middle, *-physis* growth]

metarteriole (met-ar-TEER-ee-ohl) short connecting blood vessel that connects a true arteriole with the proximal end of dozens of capillaries [*meta-* middle, *arteri-* vessel, *-ole* little]

metastasis (meh-TAS-tah-sis) process characteristic of cancer by which malignant tumour cells separate from a primary tumour and then migrate to a new tissue to initiate a secondary tumour [*meta-* change, *-stasis* standing]

metastasize (meh-TAS-tah-size) undergo metastasis; see **metastasis** [*meta-* change, *-stas-* standing, *-ize* make]

metencephalon (met-en-SEF-ah-lon) secondary vesicle of the neural tube during embryonic development that forms from the hindbrain (rhombencephalon) and eventually becomes the pons and cerebellum [*met-* behind or middle, *-en-* within, *-cephalon* head]

micelle (my-SELL) droplet of lipid surrounded by bile salts, which makes the lipid temporarily water-soluble [*mic-* grain, *-elle* small]

microarray (my-kroh-ar-RAY) DNA biotechnology technique that uses a tiny silicon plate with a grid made up of tiny wells [*micro-* small, *-array* arrangement in rows]

microbe (MY-krohb) general name for any microscopic organism (bacteria, fungi, etc.) in nature [*micro-* small, *-b(io)-* life]

microbiome (my-kroh-BYE-ohm) all the interacting ecosystems of microbes (bacteria, fungi, etc.) that live on or in the human body; also called the *human microbiome* or *human microbial system* [*micro-* small, *-bio-* life, *-ome* entire collection]

microcephaly (my-kroh-SEF-ah-lee) congenital abnormality in which an infant is born with an abnormally small head [*micro-* small, *-ceph-* head, *-aly* relating to]

microcirculation (my-kroh-sir-kyoo-LAY-shun) flow of blood through the capillary bed [*micro-* small, *circulat-* go around, *-tion* process]

microfilament (my-kroh-FIL-ah-ment) smallest cell fibres; "cellular muscles" [*micro* small, *-fila-* threadlike, *-ment* thing]

microglia (my-KROG-lee-ah) type of small neuroglial cell of nerve tissue that serves an immune system function by becoming an active phagocyte when stimulated [*micro-* small, *-glia* glue] *sing.*, microglial cell (my-kroh-GLEE-al sel)

microkeratome (my-kroh-KAR-ah-tohm) surgical device used in automated lamellar keratoplasty (ALK) [*micro-* small, *-kera-* horn, *-tom-* cut]

micromineral (my-kroh-MIN-er-al) dietary mineral needed in small daily quantities of less than 15 mg per day [*micro-* small, *-miner-* mine, *-al* relating to]

micronutrient (MY-kroh-NYOO-tree-ent) nutrient needed by the body in very small quantity [*micro-* small, *nutri-* nourish, *-ent* agent]

microscopic anatomy (my-kroh-SKOP-ik ah-NAT-oh-mee) the study of the smaller structures of an organism, such as cells and tissues, that are small enough to require significant magnification; compare to **gross anatomy** [*micro-* small, *-scop-* see, *-ic* relating to, *ana-* apart, *-tom-* cut, *-y* action]

microscopy (my-KROS-kah-pee) any of several techniques used to visualize structures too small to be seen by the unaided human eye [*micro-* small, *-scop-* see, *-y* activity]

microtubule (my-kroh-TYOOB-yool) thick cell fibre (compared to microfilament); hollow tube responsible for movement of substances within the cell or movement of the cell itself [*micro-* small, *-tubule* little tube]

microvillus (my-kroh-VIL-us) brushlike border made up of epithelial cells on each villus in the small intestine; increases the surface area for absorption of nutrients [*micro-* small, *-villi* shaggy hairs] *pl.*, microvilli (my-kroh-VIL-eye or my-kroh-VIL-ee)

micturition (mik-too-RISH-un) urination, voiding [*mictur-* urinate, *-tion* process]

midbrain (MID-brayn) region of the brainstem between the pons and the diencephalon [*mid-* middle]

middle cerebellar peduncle (SAIR-eh-bell-ar peh-DUNG-kul) tracts that enter the cerebellum from the pons [*cerebell-* cerebellum (small brain), -ar relating to, *ped-* foot, *-uncl-* little]

middle ear tiny and very thin epithelium-lined cavity in the temporal bone that houses the ossicles; in the middle ear, sound waves are amplified

midsagittal plane (mid-SAJ-ih-tal) cut, or plane, that divides the body or any of its parts into two equal (mirror-image) halves [*mid-* middle, *-sagitta-* arrow, *-al* relating to, *plan-* flat surface]

migrating motor complex (MMC) (my-GRAYT-ing MOH-ter KOM-pleks) wave of rhythmic contractions of the smooth muscle in the gastrointestinal tract during the fasting state [*migra-* wander, *-at-* process, *motor* move, *com-* together, *-plex* weave or braid]

milliequivalent (mil-ih-ee-KWIV-ah-lent) number of ionic charges or electrocovalent bonds in a solution; abbreviated mEq [*milli-* 1/1000 part, *-equi-* equal, *-val-* strength, *-ent* state]

Milwaukee brace (mil-WAWK-ee) supportive brace used to correct scoliosis [*Milwaukee* after the city in Wisconsin, U.S.A.]

mineralocorticoid (MC) (MIN-er-al-oh-KOR-tih-koyd) hormone that influences mineral salt metabolism; secreted by adrenal cortex; aldosterone is the chief mineralocorticoid [*miner-* mine, *-al* relating to, *-cortic* cortex (bark), *-oid* like]

mineral inorganic element or salts occurring naturally in the earth, many of which are vital to proper functioning of the body and must be obtained in the diet [*miner-* mine, *-al* relating to]

minute volume (MI-nit VOL-yoom) volume of blood circulating through the body per minute

mirror neuron (MEER-or NYOO-ron) type of nerve cell in the cerebral cortex of the brain that is stimulated both when a person performs an action or when *another* person performs an action, thus enabling the brain to "mirror" the activity of another person's brain; may be partly responsible for the ability to imitate actions of others and to empathize with the feelings of others [*mirror-* to look at, *neuron-* nerve]

miscarriage (mis-KARE-ij) loss of an embryo or fetus before the twentieth week of pregnancy; after 20 weeks, the event is termed a *stillbirth* [*mis-* wrongly, *-carriage* carry]

mitochondrial DNA (mDNA, mtDNA) (my-toh-KON-dree-al D N A) DNA specifically in the mitochondrion that has the only genetic code for several important enzymes [*mito-* thread, *-chondrion-* granule, *-al* relating to]

mitochondrion (my-toh-KON-dree-on) organelle in which ATP generation occurs; often termed "powerhouse of cell" [*mito-* thread, *-chondrion* granule] *pl.*, mitochondria (my-toh-KON-dree-ah)

mitosis (my-TOH-sis) complex process in which a cell's DNA is replicated and divided equally between two daughter cells [*mitos-* thread, *-osis* condition]

mitral valve (MY-tral) located between the left atrium and ventricle, this valve prevents backflow of blood into the left atrium; named for its resemblance to a bishop's hat (miter); also known as the *bicuspid valve* [*mitr-* bishop's hat, *-al* relating to]

mitral valve prolapse (MVP) (MY-tral valv PROH-laps) condition in which the bicuspid (mitral) valve extends into the left atrium, causing incompetence (leaking) of the valve [*mitr-* bishop's hat, *-al* relating to, *pro-* forward, *-laps-* fall]

mittelschmerz (MIT-el-schmertz) abdominal discomfort experienced by many women at the time of ovulation [*mittel-* middle, *-schmerz* pain]

mixed cranial nerve (KRAY-nee-al) bundle of axons that contain both sensory and motor neurons [*crani-* skull, *-al* relating to]

mixed nerve (mikst nerv) nerve with axons of both sensory and motor neurons

M-mode echocardiogram (ek-oh-KAR-dee-oh-gram) method of echocardiography that shows motion of the heart walls and valves over time as a transducer is held in a stable position [*M-* motion, *-mode* manner, *echo-* reflected sound, *-cardio-* heart, *-gram* drawing]

mobile-receptor model theory that a hormone enters a target cell where it binds to a free (nonstationary) receptor, thereby activating a gene and thus the beginning of mRNA transcription [*recept-* receive, *-or* agent]

modiolus (moh-DI-oh-lus) cone-shaped core of bone around which the tube of the cochlea is wound [*modiolus* hub]

molar (MOHL-ar) a tricuspid tooth, which is a relatively flat-topped tooth near the posterior of the jaw [*mola-* millstone, *-ar* relating to]

mole (mohl) standard unit of measuring amount of a substance; one mole of a substance is made up of 6.02×10^{23} particles of that substance; moles per litre as a concentration of a solute in a solvent is expressed as "molar concentration" or M [*mole* mass]

molecular genetics (moh-LEK-yoo-lar jeh-NET-iks) branch of genetics that studies DNA and RNA and the mechanisms by which they store and transmit hereditary information [*mole-* mass, *-cul-* small, *-ar* relating to]

molecular motor (mo-LEK-yoo-lar) small structures in the cell made up of one or two molecules and that act as mechanisms of movement [*mole-* mass, *-cul-* small, *-ar* relating to, *mot-* move, *-or* agent]

molecule (MOL-eh-kyool) formed when two or more atoms join [*mole-* mass, *-cul-* small]

monoamine (mon-oh-ah-MEEN) category of small neurotransmitter molecule derived from a single amino acid [*mono-* single, *-amine* ammonia compound (amino acid)]

monoamine oxidase (MAO) (mon-oh-ah-MEEN OK-sih-dase) enzyme located in synaptic knobs of postganglionic neurons; responsible for breaking down neurotransmitters [*mono-* single, *-amine* ammonia compound (amino acid), *oxi-* oxygen, *-ase* enzyme]

monoamine oxidase inhibitor (MAOI) (mon-oh-ah-MEEN OK-sih-dase in-HIB-ih-tor) class of antidepressant drugs that block the action of monoamine oxidase, the enzyme that inactivates dopamine and serotonin [*mono-* single, *-amine* ammonia compound (amino acid), *oxid-* oxygen compound, *-ase* enzyme, *inhibit-* prevent, *-or* agent]

monoclonal (mon-oh-KLONE-al) genetically identical; member of the same family or clone of cells [*mono-* single, *-clon-* (plant) cutting, *-al* relating to]

monoclonal antibody (MAb) (mon-oh-KLONE-al AN-tih-bod-ee) specific antibody produced from a population of identical cells; *see* **hybridoma** [*mono-* single, *-clon-* plant cutting, *-al* relating to, *anti-* against]

monocyte (MON-oh-syte) large white blood cell; an agranular leucocyte [*mono-* single, *-cyte* cell]

monogenic (mon-oh-JEN-ik) single-gene [*mono-* single, *-gen-* produce (gene), *-ic* relating to]
monosaccharide (mon-oh-SAK-ah-ride) simple sugar, such as glucose or fructose; building block of carbohydrates [*mono-* one, *-sacchar-* sugar, *-ide* chemical]
monosomy (MON-oh-so-mee) abnormal genetic condition in which cells have only one chromosome instead of a pair; usually caused by nondisjunction (failure of chromosome pairs to separate) during gamete production [*mono-* single, *-som-* body (chromosome), *-y* state]
monounsaturated fatty acid (mon-oh-un-SACH-ur-ayt-ed FAT-tee ASS-id) hydrocarbon chain (fatty acid) in which all but one available bonds are filled (saturated) with hydrogen [*mono-* single, *-un-* not, *-saturat-* fill, *acid* sour]
mons pubis (monz PYOO-bis) skin-covered pad of fat over the pubic symphysis in the female [*mons* mountain, *pubis* groin] *pl.*, montes pubis (MON-teez PYOO-beez)
morula (MOR-yoo-lah) solid mass of cells formed by the divisions of a fertilized egg [*mor-* mulberry, *-ula* little] *pl.*, morulae
motif (moh-TEEF) specific pattern of structure within the secondary structure of a protein, such as a particular set of helices and/or folds, that imparts certain structural or functional characteristics in each protein where it appears; also called *supersecondary structure* [*motif* theme]
motilin (moh-TIL-in) hormone released from the endocrine cells in the duodenum; triggers the migrating motor complex [*mot-* move, *-il-* relating to, *-in* substance]
motility (moh-TIL-ih-tee) ability to move spontaneously [*mot-* move, *-il-* relating to, *-ity* state]
motor cranial nerve (MOH-tor KRAY-nee-al nerv) nerve that consists mainly of motor neurons [*mot-* move, *-or* agent, *crani-* skull, *-al* relating to]
motor endplate (MOH-ter END-playt) point at which motor neurons connect to the sarcolemma to form the neuromuscular junction [*mot-* move, *-or* agent]
motor nerve (MOH-ter nerv) nerve containing motor neurons that transmits nerve impulses from the brain and spinal cord to muscles and glandular epithelial tissues [*mot-* move, *-or* agent]
motor neuron (MOH-ter NYOO-ron) nerve cell that transmits nerve impulses from the brain and spinal cord to muscles and glandular epithelial tissues [*mot-* move, *-or* agent, *neuron* string or nerve]
motor program (MOH-ter PROH-gram) set of coordinated commands that control the programmed muscle activity mediated by extrapyramidal pathways [*mot-* move, *-or* agent]
motor unit (MOH-ter YOO-nit) functional unit composed of a single motor neuron with the muscle cells it innervates [*mot-* move, *-or* agent]
mouth oral cavity
mucosa (myoo-KOH-sah) innermost layer of the gastrointestinal wall [*muc-* slime, *-os-* relating to, *-a* thing] *pl.*, mucosae (myoo-KOH-see)
mucosal immune system (myoo-KOH-sal im-YOON) immune system in the mucous membranes, protecting the external boundaries of the body [*muc-* slime, *-osal* relating to, *immun-* free]
mucosal-associated lymphoid tissue (MALT) (myoo-KOH-sal-ah-soh-she-AYT-ed LIM-foyd) location of the immune cells that make up the mucosal immune system [*muc-* slime, *-osal* relating to, *associa-* unite, *-ate* process, *lymph-* water (lymphatic system), *-oid* like, *tissue* fabric]
mucous membrane (MYOO-kus) epithelial membrane that lines body surfaces opening directly to the exterior and secretes mucus [*muc-* slime, *-ous* characterized by, *membran-* thin skin]
mucus (MYOO-kus) thick, slippery material secreted by mucous membranes that keeps the membrane moist and protected [*mucus* slime]
multiaxial joint (mul-tee-AK-see-al) joint that permits movement around three or more axes and in three or more planes [*multi-* many, *-axon* axle]
multicellular gland (mul-tih-SELL-yoo-lar) cluster or group of glandular epithelial cells [*multi-* many, *-cell-* storeroom, *-ular* relating to, *gland* acorn]
multifides group (mul-TIF-ih-deez) group of back muscles that each connect one vertebra to the next, also helping to extend the back and neck or flex them to the side [*multi-* many, *-fides* split (into pieces)]
multiple myeloma (my-eh-LOH-mah) cancer of antibody-secreting B lymphocytes [*myel-* marrow, *-oma* tumour]
multiple sclerosis (MS) (skleh-ROH-sis) most common primary disease of the central nervous system, MS leads to demyelination of nerves, which commonly causes problems with vision, muscle control, and incontinence [*multi-* many, *-pl-* fold, *sclera-* hard, *-osis* condition]
multiple wave summation (sum-MAY-shun) condition in which a series of stimuli come in rapid enough succession that the muscle is not able to relax completely, and sustained or more forceful contraction results [*multi-* many, *-pl-* fold, *wave*, *summa-* total, *-tion* process]
multipolar neuron (NYOO-ron) neuron with only one axon but several dendrites [*multi-* many, *-pol-* pole, *-ar* relating to, *neuron* string or nerve]
multiunit smooth muscle type of smooth muscle tissue composed of many independent single-fibre units that does not usually generate its own impulse but rather responds only to nervous input and is often found in bundles [*multi-* many, *mus-* mouse, *-cle* little]
mumps acute viral disease characterized by swelling of the parotid salivary glands [*mumps* grimace]
muscarinic (M) receptor (mus-kah-RIN-ik ree-SEP-tor) type of cholinergic receptor responding to muscarine, as well as acetylcholine [*musca-* fly, *-in-* substance, *-ic* relating to (after the toxic mushroom *A. muscaria*), *recept-* receive, *-or* agent]
muscle fatigue state of exhaustion produced by strenuous muscular activity [*mus-* mouse, *-cle* little, *fatig-* tire]
muscle spindle stretch receptor in muscle cells involved in maintaining muscle tone [*mus-* mouse, *-cle* small]
muscle strain muscle injury resulting from overexertion or trauma and involving overstretching or tearing of muscle fibres [*mus-* mouse, *-cle* small]
muscle tissue tissue type that produces movement [*mus-* mouse, *-cle* small, *tissu-* fabric]
muscle tone tonic contraction; characteristic of muscle of a normal individual who is awake [*mus-* mouse, *-cle* little, *ton-* stretch or tension]
muscular artery (MUSS-kyoo-lar AR-ter-ee) carries blood farther away from the heart to specific organs and areas of the body; also called *distributing artery* [*mus-* mouse, *-cul-* little, *-ar* relating to, *arteri-* vessel]
muscular dystrophy (MUSS-kyoo-lar DISS-troh-fee) group of genetic diseases characterized by atrophy of skeletal muscle tissue [*mus-* mouse, *-cul-* little, *-ar* relating to, *dys-* bad, *-troph-* nourishment, *-y* state]
muscular system (MUSS-kyoo-lar SIS-tem) the muscles of the body [*mus-* mouse, *-cul-* little, *-ar* relating to]
muscularis (mus-kyoo-LAIR-is) two layers of muscle surrounding the digestive tube that produce wavelike, rhythmic contractions, called *peristalsis*, that move food material along the digestive tract [*mus-* mouse, *-cul-* little, *-ar-* relating to, *-is* thing] *pl.*, musculares (mus-kyoo-LAIR-eez)
mutagen (MYOO-tah-jen) agent capable of causing mutation (alteration) of DNA [*muta-* change, *-gen* produce]
mutation (myoo-TAY-shun) change in genetic material within a cell [*mutat-* change, *-tion* state]
myalgia (my-AL-jee-ah) muscle pain [*my-* muscle, *-algia* pain]
myasthenia gravis (my-es-THEE-nee-ah GRAH-vis) chronic autoimmune disease characterized by muscle weakness, especially in the face and throat, caused by immune attacks at the neuromuscular junction [*my-* muscle, *-asthenia* weakness, *gravis* severe]
myelencephalon (my-el-en-SEF-ah-lon) secondary vesicle of the neural tube during embryonic development formed from the hindbrain (rhombencephalon) and that eventually becomes the medulla oblongata [*myel-* marrow, *-en-* within, *-cephalon* head]
myelin (MY-eh-lin) lipoprotein substance in the myelin sheath around many nerve fibres that contributes to high-speed conductivity of impulses [*myel-* marrow, *-in* substance]
myelin disorder (MY-eh-lin) any of several disorders characterized by loss or improper development of the myelin sheath that surrounds many axons of the nervous system [*myel-* marrow, *-in* substance]
myelin sheath (MY-eh-lin sheeth) whitish, fatty sheath surrounding nerve fibres; substance produced by Schwann cells [*myel-* marrow, *-in* substance]
myelin sheath gap (MY-eh-lin sheeth) *see* **node of Ranvier** [*myel-* marrow, *-in* substance]
myelinated fibre (MY-eh-li-nay-ted) axon surrounded by a sheath of myelin formed by Schwann cells (PNS) or oligodendrocytes (CNS) [*myel-* marrow, *-in-* substance, *-ate* act of]
myeloid neoplasm (MY-eh-loyd NEE-oh-plazem) blood-related cancer [*myel-* marrow, *-oid* like, *neo-* new, *-plasm* substance]
myeloid tissue (MY-eh-loyd) red bone marrow; type of soft, diffuse connective tissue; the site of haematopoiesis [*myel-* marrow, *-oid* of or like, *tissu-* fabric]
myocardial infarction (MI) (my-oh-KAR-dee-al in-FARK-shun) death of cardiac muscle cells resulting from inadequate blood supply, as in coronary thrombosis; also called "heart attack" [*myo-* muscle, *-cardi-* heart, *-al* relating to, *in-* in, *-farc-* stuff or block, *-tion* process]
myocardium (my-oh-KAR-dee-um) muscle of the heart [*myo-* muscle, *-cardi-* heart, *-um* thing] *pl.*, myocardia (my-oh-KAR-dee-ah)
myofascial meridian (my-oh-FAY-shul mer-ID-ee-an) line or chain of force or tension in the body formed by the continuous structures of a group of skeletal muscles and connective tissue (fascia) that are structurally and functionally linked [*myo-* muscle, *-fasci-* bundle, *-al* relating to, *meridi-* midday, *-an* relating to]
myofibril (my-oh-FYE-bril) very fine longitudinal fibres found in skeletal muscle cells; composed of thick and thin filaments [*myo-* muscle, *-fibr-* thread or fibre, *-il* little]
myofilament (my-oh-FIL-ah-ment) ultramicroscopic, threadlike structures found in myofibrils; composed of myosin (thick) and actin (thin) [*myo-* muscle, *-fila-* thread, *-ment* thing]
myogenic mechanism (my-oh-JEN-ik) smooth muscle autoregulatory mechanism that helps to maintain glomerular filtration rate [*myo-* muscle, *-gen-* produce, *-ic* relating to]
myoglobin (my-oh-GLO-bin) large protein molecule in the sarcoplasm of muscle cells that attracts oxygen and holds it temporarily [*myo-* muscle, *-glob-* ball, *-in* substance]
myography (my-OG-rah-fee) procedure in which the contraction of an isolated muscle is recorded [*myo-* muscle, *-graphy* process of recording]
myoma (my-OH-mah) benign tumour of the uterine fibrous or smooth muscle tissue [*my-* muscle, *-oma* tumour]
myometrium (my-oh-MEE-tree-um) middle muscle layer in the uterus [*myo-* muscle, *-metr-* womb, *-um* thing]
myopathology (my-oh-path-OL-oh-jee) existence of or study of any abnormality of muscle tissue or muscle function [*myo-* muscle, *-path-* disease, *-o-* combining form, *-log-* words (study of), *-y* activity]
myopathy (my-OP-ah-thee) general term referring to any muscle disease [*myo-* muscle, *-path-* disease, *-y* state]
myopia (my-OH-pee-ah) refractive disorder of the eye caused by an elongated eyeball; nearsightedness [*myops-* nearsighted, *-op-* vision, *-ia* condition]
myosin (MY-oh-sin) contractile protein found in the thick filaments of skeletal muscle myofilaments [*myos-* muscle, *-in* substance]
myositis (my-oh-SYE-tis) inflammation of muscle tissue [*myos-* muscle, *-itis* inflammation]
myotome (MY-oh-tohm) skeletal muscle or group of muscles that receives motor axons from a given spinal nerve [*myo-* muscle, *-tome* cut segment or region]
myxoedema (mik-seh-DEE-mah) firm swelling (oedema) of the skin caused by deficiency of thyroid hormone in adults [*myx-* mucus, *-oedema* swelling]

N

naevus (NEE-vus) small, pigmented benign tumour of the skin; a mole [*naevus-* birthmark]
nail bed layer of epithelium under the nail
nail body visible part of the nail
nail multilayered, protective structure composed of epithelial cells containing hard keratin; located at the distal ends of fingers and toes
nail root part of the nail hidden by the cuticle
naïve (nye-EEV) refers to a B or T cell that is inactive [*naïve* natural]
naïve B cell (nye-EEV) *see* naïve [*naïve* natural, *B* bursa-equivalent tissue, *cell* storeroom]
nanobody (NAN-oh-bod-ee) antibody fragment [*nano-* small, body]
nasal (NAY-zal) relating to the nose [*nas-* nose, *-al* relating to]
nasal bone (NAY-zal bohn) bone that gives shape to the nose; forms upper bridge of the nose [*nas-* nose, *-al* relating to]
nasal mucosa (NAY-zal myoo-KOH-sah) mucous membrane in the nose that air passes over [*nas-* nose, *-al* relating to, *muc-* slime, *-os-* relating to, *-a* thing] *pl.*, mucosae (myoo-KOH-see)
nasolacrimal duct (nay-zoh-LAK-rih-mal) tube that extends from lacrimal sac into the inferior meatus of the nose [*naso-* nose, *-lacrim* tear, *-al* relating to, *duct* path]
nasopharynx (nay-zoh-FAIR-inks) uppermost portion of the tube just behind the nasal cavities [*naso-* nose, *-pharynx* throat] *pl.*, nasopharynges (nay-zoh-FAIR-in-jeez) or nasopharynxes
native state the final, folded and functional shape of a complete protein molecule [*native-* produced by birth]
natural family planning method of predicting the time of ovulation based on the woman's cyclical changes
natural immunity (im-YOO-nih-tee) acquired immunity resulting from exposure to disease-causing agents in the course of daily living [*immun-* free, *-ity* state]

natural killer cell (NK cell) (NACH-er-ul KIL-er sel) type of lymphocyte that kills many types of tumour cells [*cell* storeroom]
nausea (NAW-zee-ah) unpleasant sensation of the gastrointestinal tract that commonly precedes the urge to vomit; upset stomach [*nausea* seasickness]
navel (NAY-vel) relating to the umbilicus, the round depression near the centre of the abdomen through which the umbilical vessels once entered the abdominopelvic cavity; the umbilicus itself [*nave-* wheel hub or umbilicus, *-(a)l* relating to]
near reflex (neer REE-fleks) constriction of the pupil for near vision [*re-* again, *-flex* bend]
necrosis (neh-KROH-sis) death of cells in a tissue, often resulting from ischaemia (reduced blood flow) [*necr-* death, *-osis* condition]
negative feedback (NEG-ah-tiv FEED-bak) feedback control system in which the level of a variable is changed in the direction opposite to that of the initial stimulus [*negat-* deny, *-ive* relating to]
negative nitrogen balance (NEG-ah-tiv NYE-troh-jen) condition in which the amount of nitrogen in the urine exceeds the amount of nitrogen in the protein food ingested [*negat-* deny, *-ive* relating to, *nitro-* soda, *-gen* produce]
neonatal period (nee-oh-NAY-tal) period of development immediately after birth [*neo-* new, *-nat-* birth, *-al* relating to]
neonatology (nee-oh-nay-TOL-oh-jee) diagnosis and treatment of disorders of the newborn [*neo-* new, *-nat-* born, *-log-* words (study of), *-y* activity]
neoplasm (NEE-oh-plaz-em) tumour or abnormal growth; may be benign or malignant [*neo-* new, *-plasm* substance or tissue]
nephritis (neh-FRY-tis) inflammatory kidney disease [*nephr-* kidney, *-itis* inflammation]
nephron (NEF-ron) anatomical and functional unit of the kidney, consisting of the renal corpuscle and the renal tubule [*nephro-* kidney, *-on* unit]
nephrotic syndrome (neh-FROT-ik SIN-drohm) collection of signs and symptoms that accompany various glomerular disorders [*nephr-* kidney, *-ic* relating to, *syn-* together, *-drome* running or (race) course]
nerve bundle of nerve fibres, plus surrounding connective tissue, located outside the brain or spinal cord
nerve fibre axon of neuron in the nervous system
nerve impulse self-propagating wave of electrical depolarization that carries information along nerves; also called *action potential* [*impuls-* drive or push]
nerve zero very thin nerve near each olfactory nerve; *see* **terminal nerve**
nervous system brain, spinal cord, and nerves [*nerv-* nerve, *-ous* relating to]
nervous tissue tissue type consisting of neurons and glia that provides rapid communication and control of body function [*nerv-* nerve, *-ous* relating to, *tissu-* fabric]
neural network (NYOOR-al) a network of interconnected neurons in nervous tissue, forming a web of pathways to process information [*neur-* nerve, *-al* relating to]
neural tube (NYOOR-al tyoob) invagination of the embryonic ectoderm layer that forms a fluid-filled canal that eventually becomes a series of vesicles in the embryo, then develops further into the brain and spinal cord [*neur-* nerve, *-al* relating to]
neuralgia (nyoo-RAL-jee-ah) general term referring to nerve pain [*neur-* nerve, *-algia* pain]
neurilemma (nyoo-rih-LEM-mah) sheath of Schwann; formed by the nonmyelinated outer layer of the Schwann cell (neurilemmocyte) around the axon of a neuron; also *neurolemma* [*neuri-* neuron, *-lemma* sheath] *pl.*, neurilemmae (noo-rih-LEM-mee)
neurilemmocyte (nyoo-rih-LEM-moh-syte) another name for the Schwann cell; also spelled *neurolemmocyte* [*neuro-* neuron, *-lemmo* sheath, *-cyte* cell]
neurobiology (nyoo-roh-bye-OL-oh-jee) branch of biology that studies the basic science of the nervous system; compare to **neurology** [*neuro-* nerve, *-bio-* life, *-log-* words (study of), *-y* activity]
neuroblastoma (nyoo-roh-blas-TOH-mah) malignant tumour of sympathetic nervous tissue, found mainly in young children [*neuro-* nerve, *-blast* germ, *-oma* tumour]
neuroendocrine system (nyoo-roh-EN-doh-krin) endocrine and nervous systems working in concert to perform communication, integration, and control within the body [*neuro-* nerve, *-endo-* within, *-crin-* secrete]
neurofibril (nyoo-roh-FYE-bril) fine strands extending through the cytoplasm of each neuron; formed by cell's cytoskeleton [*neuro-* nerve, *-fibr-* thread or fibre, *-il* small]
neurofibromatosis (nyoo-roh-fye-broh-mah-TOH-sis) group of genetic disorders characterized by multiple, sometimes disfiguring, benign tumours of the glia that surround nerve fibres [*neuro-* nerve, *-fibr-* thread or fibre, *-oma-* tumour, *-osis* condition]
neurogenic bladder (nyoor-oh-JEN-ik) disorder of the bladder that results in loss of control of normal voiding; due to disruption of nervous input to the bladder [*neuro-* nerve, *-gen-* produce, *-ic* relating to]
neurogenic shock (nyoo-roh-JEN-ik) condition that results from widespread dilation of blood vessels caused by an imbalance in autonomic stimulation of smooth muscle in vessel walls [*neuro-* nerve, *-gen-* produce, *-ic* relating to]
neuroglia (nyoo-ROG-lee-ah) nonexcitable supporting cells of nervous tissue; more properly called *glia* [*neuro-* nerve, *-glia* glue] *sing.*, neuroglial cell
neuroglobin (Ngb) (NYOO-roh-gloh-bin) protein in neurons similar to haemoglobin used to temporarily store a "back up" supply of oxygen [neuro- nerve, *-glob-* ball, *-in* substance]
neurohypophysis (nyoo-roh-hye-POF-ih-sis) posterior pituitary gland [*neuro-* nerve, *-hypo-* under or below, *-physis* growth] *pl.*, neurohypophyses (noo-roh-hye-POF-ih-seez)
neurology (nyoo-ROL-oh-jee) branch of medical science that deals with the nervous system, especially its disorders and their treatments; compare to **neurobiology** [*neur-* nerve, *-log-* words (study of), *-y* activity]
neuroma (nyoo-ROH-mah) any tumour arising from nervous tissue [*neur-* nerve, *-oma* tumour]
neuromodulator (nyoo-roh-MOD-yoo-lay-tor) "cotransmitter" that regulates the effects of neurotransmitter(s) released along with it [*neuro-* nerve, *-modul-* regulate, *at(e)-* act of, *-or* agent]
neuromuscular junction (NMJ) (nyoo-roh-MUSS-kyoo-lar JUNK-shun) point of contact between nerve endings and muscle fibres; *see* **motor endplate** [*neuro-* nerve, *-mus-* mouse, *-cul-* little, *-ar* relating to]
neuron (NYOO-ron) nerve cell, including its processes (axons and dendrites) [*neuron* string or nerve]
neuron doctrine (NYOO-ron DOK-trin) theory stating that the neuron is the basic structural and functional unit of the nervous system and that neurons are independent units connected by chemical synapses; now includes concepts of a larger neural network [*neuron* string or nerve]
neuropeptide (nyoo-roh-PEP-tyde) neurotransmitter with short strands of polypeptides [*neuro-* nerve, *-pept-* digest, *-ide* chemical]
neuropeptide Y (NPY) (nyoor-oh-PEP-tyde) type of neurotransmitter; enhances blood vessel constriction, regulates energy balance, and learning and memory [*neuro-* nerve, *-pept-* digest, *-ide* chemical, Y 25th letter of the Roman alphabet]
neurosecretory tissue (nyoo-roh-SEK-reh-toree) modified neurons that secrete chemical messengers that diffuse into the bloodstream rather than across a synapse; for example, in the hypothalamus [*neuro-* nerve, *-secret-* separate, *-ory* relating to, *tissu-* fabric]
neurotransmitter (nyoo-roh-tranz-MIT-ter) chemicals by which neurons communicate; the substance is released by a neuron, diffuses across the synapse, and binds to the postsynaptic neuron [*neuro-* nerve, *-trans-* across, *-mitt-* send, *-er* agent]
neurotrophin (nyoo-roh-TROF-in) nerve growth factor [*neuro-* nerve, *-troph-* nutrition, *-in* substance]
neutron (NYOO-tron) neutral subatomic particle located in the nucleus of an atom [*neutr-* neither]
neutrophil (NYOO-troh-fil) white blood cell that stains readily with neutral dyes [*neutr-* neither, *-phil* love]
nicotinamide adenine dinucleotide (NAD) (nik-oh-TIN-ah-myde AD-eh-neen dye-NYOO-klee-oh-tyde) molecule that serves as an electron carrier in the electron transport system [*Jean Nicot de Villemain* French diplomat (brought tobacco to France), *-in-* substance (after plant genus *Nicotiana*), *-am-* ammonia, *-ide* chemical, *aden-* gland, *-ine* derived substance, *di-* two, *nucleo-* kernel (nucleus), *-t-* combining form, *-ide* chemical]
nicotinic (N) receptor (NIK-oh-tin-ik) type of cholinergic receptor [*Jean Nicot de Villemain* French diplomat (brought tobacco to France), *-in-* substance, *-ic* relating to (after plant genus *Nicotiana*), *recept-* receive, *-or* agent]
nipple small projection at the centre of the areola on the anterior surface of the breast where the lactiferous ducts release milk [*nip-* beak, *-le* small]
Nissl substance (NISS-ul SUB-stans) granular bodies in neurons made of rough endoplasmic reticulum along with free polyribosomes, provide protein molecules needed for transmission of nerve impulses from one neuron to another; also called *Nissl bodies, chromatophilic substance,* or *tigroid substance* [*Franz Nissl* German neurologist]
nitric oxide (NO) (NYE-trik AWK-side) small gas molecule used as a neurotransmitter that *diffuses backward* from a postsynaptic cell toward the presynaptic neuron, where it has its biochemical effects and gives the opportunity for feedback [*nitr-* nitrogen, *-ic* relating to, *ox-* oxygen, *-ide* chemical]
nitrogen balance (NYE-troh-jen) state in which the amount of nitrogen taken into the body equals the amount of nitrogen excreted [*nitro-* soda, *-gen* produce]
nitrogenous waste (nye-TROJ-ih–nes) waste from protein catabolism; for example, urea, uric acid, ammonia, and creatinine [*nitro-* soda, *-gen- produce, -ous* relating to]
nitroglycerin (nye-troh-GLIS-eh-rin) heart medication that dilates coronary blood vessels thus improving supply of oxygen to myocardium [*nitro-* nitrogen, *-glyc-* sweet (sugar), *-in* substance]
nociceptor (noh-see-SEP-tor) receptor activated by intense stimuli of any type that results in tissue damage; pain receptor [*noci-* harm, *-cept-* receive, *-or* agent]
node of Ranvier (node of rahn-vee-AY) short space in the myelin sheath between adjacent Schwann cells; also called *myelin sheath gap* [*nod-* knot, *Louis A. Ranvier* French pathologist]
nonadrenergic-noncholinergic (NANC) transmission (non-AD-ren-er-jik non-KOHL-in-er-jik tranz-MISH-un) neural synaptic transmission in the efferent autonomic pathways that involves transmitters other than the classical autonomic neurotransmitters norepinephrine and acetylcholine; NANC transmitters include GABA, ATP, NPY, and others [*non-* not, *-ad-* toward, *-ren-* kidney, *-erg-* work, *-ic* relating to, *-non-* not, *-chole-* bile, *-erg-* work, *-ic* relating to]
nondisjunction (non-dis-JUNK-shun) occurs during meiosis when a pair of chromosomes fails to separate [*non-* not, *-dis-* split in two, *-junction* joint]
nondisplaced fracture (non-dis-PLAYSD FRAK-chur) *see* **simple fracture** [*non-* not, *-displace* remove, *fracture* a breaking]
nonelectrolyte (non-ee-LEK-troh-lyte) compound that does not dissociate in solution; for example, glucose [*non-* not, *-electro-* electricity, *-lyt-* loosening]
noninflammatory joint disease (non-in-FLAM-ah-toh-ree joynt DIS-eez) joint disorder that does not involve inflammation of the synovial membrane [*non-* not, *-inflam-* set afire, *-ory* relating to, *joint* a joining, *dis-* opposite of, *-ease* comfort]
nonmembranous organelle (NON-mem-bra-nus or-gah-NELL) cell organ that is not defined or bordered by a membrane [*non-* without, *membran-* thin skin, *organ-* instrument, *-elle* small]
nonpolar describes a covalent chemical bond (or covalently bonded molecule) in which there is equal sharing of electrons and therefore no distinct areas of electrical charge [*non-* not, *-pol-* pole, *-ar* relating to]
nonself (NON-self) concept in immunology that the immune system agents can recognize certain cell-surface molecules or other molecules as not belonging to that individual and thus being a potential target for destruction or damage by the immune system [*non-* not, *-self* one's own person]
nonself antigens (NON-self AN-tih-jens) foreign and tumour cell markers that a body's immune cells can recognize as being different from the self; also called *nonself markers* [*non-* not, *-self* one's own person, *anti-* against, *-gen* produce]
nonspecific immunity (non-speh-SIF-ik im-YOO-nih-tee) mechanisms that resist various threatening agents or conditions, not just certain specific agents; *see* **innate immunity** [*non-* not, *-spec-* form or kind, *-ific* relating to, *immun-* free, *-ity* state]
nonsteroid (non-STAYR-oyd) hormone synthesized primarily from amino acids rather than from cholesterol [*non-* not, *-stero-* solid, *-oid* like]
nonsteroidal antiinflammatory drug (NSAID) (non-steh-ROID-al an-tee-in-FLAM-ah-tor-ee drug [EN-SAYD or EN-SED]) pain medication; for example, aspirin and ibuprofen [*non-* not, *-stero-* solid, *-oid-* like, *-al* relating to, *anti-* against, *-inflamm-* set afire, *-ory* relating to]
norepinephrine (NE, NR) (nor-ep-ih-NEF-rin) hormone secreted by adrenal medulla that increases cardiac output; neurotransmitter released by sympathetic postganglionic neurons of the ANS; also called *noradrenaline* [*nor-* chemical prefix (unbranched C chain), *-epi-* upon, *-nephr-* kidney, *-ine* substance]
norepinephrine reuptake inhibitor (NRI) (nor-ep-ih-NEF-rin ree-UP-tayk in-HIB-it-or) type of drug that stops the return of norepinephrine (neurotransmitter) to the presynaptic neuron, thus increasing the baseline amount of norepinephrine in the synapse and restoring the baseline to a normal neurotransmitter level [*nor-* chemical prefix (unbranched C chain), *-epi-* upon, *-nephr-* kidney, *-ine* substance, *re-* again, *inhib-* restrain, *-or* agent]
normal saline (SAY-leen) chloride-containing solution [*norm-* rule, *-al* relating to, *sal-* salt, *-ine* relating to]
nuclear envelope (NYOO-klee-ar) the boundary of a cell's nucleus, made up of a double layer of cellular membrane [*nucle-* nucleus, *-ar* relating to]

nuclear magnetic resonance (NMR) (NYOO-klee-ar mag-NET-ik REH-son-ans) *see* **magnetic resonance imaging** [*nucle-* nucleus, *-ar* relating to, *magnet-* lodestone, *-ic* relating to, *re-* again, *-sona-* sound, *-ance* state]

nuclear pore complex (NPC) (NYOO-klee-ar poor KOM-plex) complicated, channel-like structure in the nuclear envelope; the nuclear pore (as it is sometimes called) selectively transports molecules into or out of the nucleus [*nucle-* nucleus, *-ar* relating to, *pore* passage, *com-* together, *-plex* weave or braid]

nuclease (NYOO-klee-ayz) RNA and DNA digesting enzyme [*nucle-* nut or kernel (nucleic acid),*-ase* enzyme]

nucleic acid (nyoo-KLAY-ik ASS-id) any of the high-molecular-weight organic compounds composed of nucleotides, a ribose or deoxyribose sugar, and a phosphate group. See as examples deoxyribonucleic acid (DNA) and ribonucleic acid (RNA) [*nucle-* nut kernel, *-ic* relating to, *acid* sour]

nucleic acid test (NAT) (nyoo-KLAY-ik ASS-id) blood-safety screening procedure that detects minute particles of genetic material found in infectious agents [*nucle-* nut or kernel, *-ic* relating to, *acid* sour]

nucleolus (nyoo-KLEE-oh-lus) dense, well-defined but membraneless body within the nucleus; critical to protein formation because it "programs" the formation of ribosomes in the nucleus [*nucleo-* nucleus (kernel), *-olus* little] *pl.*, nucleoli (nyoo-KLEE-oh-lye)

nucleoplasm (NYOO-klee-oh-plaz-im) substance inside a cell's nucleus [*nucleo-* kernel (nucleus), *-plasm* substance]

nucleosome (NYOO-klee-oh-sohm) tightly wound subunit of chromatin and proteins (histones) [*nucleo-* kernel (nucleus), *-som-* body]

nucleotide (NYOO-klee-oh-tide) monomer made up of three types of chemical groups (sugar, phosphate, nitrogen base) that can act alone or to make up a polymer (nucleic acid) [*nucleo-* nut or kernel, *-ide* chemical]

nucleus (NYOO-klee-us) membranous organelle that contains most of the genetic material of the cell; also, group of neuron cell bodies in the brain or spinal cord [*nucleus* kernel] *pl.*, nuclei (NYOO-klee-eye)

nucleus pulposus (NYOO-klee-us pul-POH-sus) gel-like centre of the intervertebral disc; surrounded by annulus fibrosis [*nucleus* kernel, *pulposus* fleshy or pulpy]

nurse cell *see* **Sertoli cell** [*nurse-* that suckles, nourishes, *cell* storeroom]

nutrition foods we eat and the nutrients they contain [*nutri-* nourish, *-tion* process]

nyctalopia (nik-tah-LOH-pee-ah) disorder of the retina that causes difficulty seeing at night or in dim light; also called *night blindness* [*nyct-* night, *-op-* vision, *-ia* condition]

O

obesity (oh-BEES-ih-tee) abnormal increase in the proportion of fat in the body [*obes-* fatness, *-ity* state]

obligatory base pairing (oh-BLIG-ah-tor-ee) same nitrogen bases in the DNA structure pairing off with each other; adenine to thymine and cytosine to guanine [*oblig-* bind, *-tory* relating to]

oblique fissure (oh-BLEEK FISH-ur) fissure in the lungs that separates the inferior and medial lobes [*obliqu-* slanted, *fissur-* cleft]

oblique fracture (oh-BLEEK FRAK-sher) type of bone fracture in which fracture line is slanted or diagonal to the longitudinal axis [*obliq-* slanted, *fracture* a breaking]

oblique section (oh-BLEEK SEK-shun) cut in the body or a body part that follows a diagonal plane; a diagonal or slanted cut [*obliq-* slanted, *sect-* cut, *-tion* process]

occipital (ok-SIP-it-al) relating to the back, lower part of skull or head [*occipit-* back of head, *-al* relating to]

occipital bone (ok-SIP-it-al bohn) posterior and inferior bone of the skull [*occipit-* back of head, *-al* relating to]

occipital lobe (ok-SIP-it-al) posterior and inferior lobe of the cerebrum [*occipit-* back of head, *-al* relating to]

occipitofrontalis (ok-sip-ih-toh-fron-TAL-is) muscle that covers the frontal bone and occipital bone [*occipit-* back of head, *front-* forehead, *-al* relating to, *-is* thing]

octet rule (ok-TET) general principle in chemistry whereby atoms usually form bonds in ways that will provide each atom with an outer shell of eight electrons [*octet* group of eight]

oculomotor nerve (ok-yoo-loh-MOH-tor nerv) cranial nerve III; motor nerve; controls eye movements [*oculo-* eye, *-mot-* move, *-or* agent]

oedema (eh-DEE-mah) accumulation of fluid in a tissue, as in inflammation; swelling [*edema* a swelling]

oesophageal endoscope (eh-sof-ah-JEE-ul EN-doh-skohp) flexible tube used to insert and then remove the necessary electrode or suturing device required for treatment of gastro-oesophageal reflux disease [*oes-* will carry, *-phag-* food (eat), *-al* relating to, *endo-* within, *-scop-* see]

oesophageal vein (eh-sof-ah-JEE-al vayn) small vein that returns blood from thoracic organs to the superior vena cava or azgos vein [*oes-* will carry, *-phag-* food (eat), *-al* relating to, *vena* blood vessel]

oesophagus (eh-SOF-ah-gus) muscular, mucus-lined tube that connects the pharynx with the stomach; also known as the *food pipe* [*oes-* will carry, *-phagus* food] *pl.*, oesophagi (eh-SOF-ah-jye)

oestrogen (ES-troh-jen) sex hormone secreted by the ovary that causes development and maintenance of female secondary sex characteristics and stimulates growth of the epithelial cells lining the uterus [*oestro-* frenzy, *-gen* produce]

oestrogenic phase (es-troh-JEN-ik) menstrual cycle phase that occurs between the end of menses and ovulation; also called *postmenstrual, preovulatory phase,* or *follicular phase* [*oestr-* frenzy, *-gen-* produce, *-ic* relating to]

older adulthood postnatal period after adulthood

olecranal (oh-LEK-rahn-al) relating to the back of the elbow at the olecranon (distal end of ulna) [*olecran-* elbow, *-al* relating to]

olecranon (oh-LEK-rah-non) scoop-shaped process at distal end of ulna that articulates with the humerus at the elbow joint [*olecranon* elbow]

olecranon bursa (oh-LEK-rah-non BER-sah) cushion-like sac located just under the skin overlying the olecranon of the ulna [*olecranon* elbow, *bursa* purse] *pl.*, bursae

olecranon bursitis (oh-LEK-rah-non ber-SYE-tis) inflammation of the olecranon bursa [*olecranon* elbow, *burs-* purse, *-itis* inflammation]

olecranon fossa (oh-LEK-rah-non FOSS-ah) depression in the posterior surface of the humerus bone to allow room for the olecranon of the ulna when the elbow joint extends [*olecranon* elbow, *fossa* ditch] *pl.*, fossae (FOSS-ee)

olfactory (ohl-FAK-tor-ee) relating to the sense of smell [*olfact-* smell, *-ory* relating to]

olfactory epithelium (ohl-FAK-tor-ee ep-ih-THEE-lee-um) lining of the upper surface of the nasal cavity [*olfact-* smell, *-ory* relating to, *epi-* upon, *theli-* nipple, *-um* thing] *pl.*, epithelia (ep-ih-THEE-lee-ah)

olfactory nerve (ol-FAK-tor-ee nerv) cranial nerve I; sensory nerve; responsible for the sense of smell [*olfact-* smell, *-ory* relating to]

olfactory receptor neuron (ol-FAK-tor-ee ree-SEP-tor NYOO-ron) *see* **olfactory sensory neuron** [*olfact-* smell, *-ory* relating to, *recept-* receive, *-or* agent, *neuron* string or nerve]

olfactory sensory neuron (ol-FAK-tor-ee SEN-so-ree NYOO-ron) afferent neuron in the roof of the nose mucosa that is adapted to detect odours [*olfact-* smell, *-ory* relating to, *neuron* string or nerve]

oligodendrocyte (oh-lih-go-DEN-droh-syte) small astrocyte with few cell processes; helps to form myelin sheaths around axons within the central nervous system [*oligo-* few, *-dendr-* part (branch) of, *-cyte* cell]

oligodendroglioma (oh-lih-go-DEN-droh-glee-OH-mah) tumour arising from oligodendrocytes (neuroglia of central nervous tracts) [*oligo-* few, *-dendro-* part (branch) of, *-glio-* glue, *-oma* tumour]

oligospermia (oh-lih-goh-SPER-mee-ah) disruption of the sperm-producing function of the seminiferous tubules [*oligo-* few or little, *-sperm-* seed, *-ia* condition]

oliguria (oh-lih-GOO-ree-ah) condition of reduced urine production [*olig-* few or little, *-ur-* urine, *-ia* condition]

olive (OL-iv) oval projection located lateral to the pyramids

oncogene (ON-koh-jeen) gene (DNA segment) thought to be responsible for the development of a cancer [*onco-* swelling or mass (cancer), *-gen-* produce or generate]

oncologist (ong-KOL-oh-jist) cancer specialist [*onco-* swelling or mass (cancer), *-log-* words (study of), *-ist* agent]

onycholysis (on-ik-oh-LYE-sis) separation of the nail from the nail bed [*onycho-* nail, *-lysis* loosen]

oocyte (O-o-syte or o-uh-syte) developing female sex cell contained within ovarian follicles [*oo-* egg, *-cyte* cell]

oogenesis (o-o-JEN-eh-sis or o-uh-JEN-eh-sis) production of female gametes [*oo-* egg, *-gen-* produce, *-esis* process]

oogonium (oh-oh-GO-nee-um or o-uh-GO-nee-um) primitive cell from which oocytes derive meiosis [*oo-* egg, *-gon-* offspring, *-um* thing] *pl.*, oogonia (o-o-GO-nee-ah or o-uh-GO-nee-ah)

open fracture *see* **compound fracture** [*open* uncovered, *fracture* a breaking]

open reduction surgical procedure that aligns the broken ends of the bone [*open* uncovered, *re-* again or back, *-duc-* lead, *-tion* process]

ophthalmic (opff-THAL-mik or off-THAL-mik) relating to the eye or visual function of the eye [*oph-* eye or vision, *-thalm-* inner chamber, *-ic* relating to]

ophthalmic nerve (opff-THAL-mik or off-THAL-mik nerv) part of the trigeminal nerve [*oph-* eye or vision, *-thalm-* inner chamber, *-ic* relating to]

ophthalmology (op-thal-MOL-eh-jee or off-thal-MOL-eh-jee) medical practice specialty concerned with pathological conditions of the eye and the diagnosis and treatment of eye disorders [*oph-* eye or vision, *-thalm-* inner chamber, *-o-* combining form, *-log-* words (study of), *-y* activity]

ophthalmoscope (op-THAL-mah-skohp or off-THAL-mah-skohp) instrument used to examine the retinal surface and internal eye structures [*oph-* eye or vision, *-thalmo-* inner chamber, *-scop-* see]

opponens pollicis muscle (oh-POH-nenz POL-ih-sis) thumb muscle [*opponens* opposing, *pollicis* pole, *mus-* mouse, *-cle* little]

opsin (OP-sin) protein produced by the breakdown of rhodopsin in rods and cones of the retina; involved in a chemical reaction that initiates an impulse that results in interpretation of light energy as vision [*ops-* vision, *-in* substance]

opsonin (OP-so-nin) any agent that marks a pathogen for destruction by the immune system, a process called opsinization [*opsoni-* supply food, *-in* substance]

opsonization (OP-so-nih-ZAY-shen) process that marks a pathogen for destruction by the immune system [*opsoni-* supply food, *-ation process*]

optic chiasma (OP-tik kye-AS-mah) region where right and left optic nerves enter the brain and cross each other, exchanging fibres; also called *optic chiasm* [*opti-* vision, *-ic* relating to, *chiasma* crossed lines (from Greek letter chi [X])] *pl.*, chiasmata (kye-as-MAH-tah), chiasms, or chiasmas

optic disc (OP-tik disc) area in the retina where the optic nerve fibres exit the eye and where therefore no rods or cones are present; also known as a *blind spot* [*opti-* vision, *-ic* relating to]

optic nerve (OP-tik nerv) cranial nerve II; sensory nerve; nerves that conduct visual information to the brain [*opt-* vision, *-ic* relating to]

optic tract (OP-tik trakt) bundles of fibres formed after the optic nerves pass through the optic chiasma [*opt-* vision, *-ic* relating to, *tract* trail]

oral (OR-al) related to the mouth [*or-* mouth, *-al* relating to]

oral contraceptive (OR-al kon-tra-SEP-tiv) medication that controls sex hormone levels and ovulation [*or-* mouth, *-al* relating to, *contra-* against, *-cept-* take or receive (conception), *-ive* agent]

oral hypoglycaemic agent (OR-al hye-poh-glye-SEE-mik) treatment for type 2 diabetes that stimulates beta cells to increase insulin supplies [*or-* mouth, *-al* relating to, *hypo-* under or below, *-glyc-* sweet, *-(h)aem-* blood, *-ia* condition]

oral rehydration therapy (ORT) treatment of infant diarrhoea by the administration of a liberal dose of sugar and salt solution [*or-* mouth, *-alis* relating to, *re-* back again, *-hydra-* water, *-ation* process]

orbicularis oculi muscle (or-bik-yoo-LAR-is OK-yoo-lye) muscle that encircles each eye and allows it to close [*orbi-* circle, *-cul-* little, *-ar* relating to, *ocul-* eye, *mus-* mouse, *-cle* little]

orbicularis oris muscle (or-bik-yoo-LAIR-is OR-iss) muscle that encircles and closes the eye [*orbi-* circle, *-cul-* little, *-ar* relating to, *oris* mouth, *mus-* mouse, *-cle* little]

orbital (OR-bih-tal) relating to the eye region or orbit (socket) of the eye [*orbit-* circle, *-al* relating to]

orchitis (or-KYE-tis) testicular inflammation [*orchi-* testis, *-itis* inflammation]

orexigenic (oh-rek-sih-JEN-ik) appetite producing [*orex-* appetite, *-gen-* produce, *-ic* relating to]

orexin (oh-REK-sin) factor that stimulates appetite [*orex-* appetite, *-in* substance]

organ group of several tissue types that together perform a special function [*organ* tool or instrument]

organ of Corti (KOR-tee) *see* **spiral organ;** also *Corti organ* [*organ* tool or instrument, *Alfonso Corti* Italian anatomist]

organelle (or-gah-NELL) any of many cell "organs" or organized structures; for example, a ribosome or mitochondrion [*organ-* tool or instrument, *-elle* small]

organic (or-GAN-ik) referring to chemicals that contain covalently bound carbon and hydrogen atoms and are involved in metabolic reactions [*organ-* tool or instrument, *-ic* relating to]

organism (OR-gah-niz-im) any living entity considered as a whole; may be unicellular (one-celled) or composed of many different cells and body systems working together to maintain life [*organ-* instrument, *-ism* condition]

organogenesis (or-gah-no-JEN-eh-sis) formation of organs from the primary germ layers of the embryo [*organ-* instrument (organ), *-gen-* produce, *-esis* process]

orgasm (OR-gaz-um) sexual climax [*orgasm* excitement]

origin attachment of a muscle to the bone, which does not move when contraction occurs; compare to **insertion** [*origin* source]

oropharynx (or-oh-FAIR-inks) portion of the pharynx that is located behind the mouth [*oro-* mouth, *-pharynx* throat] *pl.*, oropharynges (or-oh-FAIR-in-jeez) or oropharynxes

orthodontics (or-thoh-DON-tiks) branch of dentistry that deals with the prevention and correction of positioning irregularities of the teeth and malocclusion [*ortho-* straight or upright, *-odont-* tooth, *-ic* relating to]

orthopaedics (or-thoh-PEE-diks) medical specialty dealing with skeletal injury and disease [*ortho-* straight or normal, *-paed-* feet, *-ic* relating to]

orthopnoea (or-THOP-nee-ah) dyspnoea (difficulty in breathing) that is relieved after moving into an upright or sitting position [*ortho-* straight or upright, *-pnoe-* breathe, *-a* condition]

orthostatic effect (or-thoh-STAT-ik) shift of the blood reservoir to the veins in the legs when standing [*ortho-* upright, *-stat-* standing, *-ic* relating to, *effect* accomplishment]

Osgood–Schlatter disease (OZ-good SCHLAYT-er) avulsion fracture of bone fragments from the surface of the tibial tuberosity [*Robert B. Osgood* American surgeon, *Carl Schlatter* Swiss surgeon]

osmolality (os-moh-LAL-ih-tee) osmotic concentration of a solution; the number of moles of a substance per kilogram times the number of particles into which the solute dissociates [*osmo-* push (osmosis), *-al* relating to, *-ity* state]

osmoreceptor (os-moh-ree-SEP-tor) special receptors near the supraoptic nucleus that detect decreased osmotic pressure of blood when the body dehydrates [*osmo-* push (osmosis), *-cept-* receive, *-or* agent]

osmosis (os-MO-sis) passive movement of water through a semipermeable membrane from an area of lesser solute concentration to an area of greater concentration due to an imbalance of impermeant solutes across the membrane [*osmos-* push, *-osis* condition]

osmotic pressure (os-MOT-ik) water pressure that develops in a solution across a semipermeable membrane as a result of osmosis [*osmo-* push, *-ic* relating to]

osseous tissue (OS-ee-us) bone tissue [*os-* bone, *-ous* relating to]

ossification (os-ih-fih-KAY-shun) bone formation [*os-* bone, *-fic-* make, *-ation* process]

osteitis fibrosa cystica (os-tee-EYE-tis fye-BROH-sah SIS-tih-kah) bone disease caused by hypercalcaemia [*oste-* bone, *-itis* inflammation, *fibr-* thread or fibre, *cyst-* cyst, *-ica* relating to]

osteoarthritis (os-tee-oh-ar-THRY-tis) degenerative joint disease; a noninflammatory disorder of a joint characterized by degeneration of articular cartilage [*osteo-* bone, *-arthr-* joint, *-itis* inflammation]

osteoblast (OS-tee-oh-blast) bone-forming cell [*osteo-* bone, *-blast* bud]

osteoclast (OS-tee-oh-klast) bone-absorbing cell [*osteo-* bone, *-clast* break]

osteocyte (OS-tee-oh-syte) bone cell [*osteo*-bone, *-cyte* cell]

osteogenic stem cell (os-tee-oh-JEN-ik stem sel) cell that differentiates to produce different types of bone cells; *see also* **stem cell** [*osteo-* bone, *-gen-* produce, *-ic* relating to]

osteogenesis (os-tee-oh-JEN-eh-sis) combined action of osteoblasts and osteoclasts to mould bones into adult shape [*osteo-* bone, *-gen-* produce, *-esis* process]

osteogenesis imperfecta (os-tee-oh-JEN-eh-sis im-per-FEK-tah) dominant, inherited disorder of connective tissue characterized by imperfect skeletal development, resulting in brittle bones [*osteo-* bone, *-gen-* produce, *-esis* process, *imperfecta* not perfect]

osteoid (OS-tee-oid) organic matrix of bone [*oste-* bone, *-oid* like]

osteoma (os-tee-OH-mah) benign bone tumour [*oste-* bone, *-oma* tumour]

osteomalacia (os-tee-oh-mah-LAY-shah) metabolic skeletal disease [*osteo-* bone, *-malacia* softening]

osteomyelitis (os-tee-oh-my-eh-LYE-tis) bacterial (usually staphylococcal) infection of bone tissue [*osteo-* bone, *myel-* marrow, *-itis* inflammation]

osteon (OS-tee-on) unit of compact bone tissue made up of a tapered cylinder with layered, concentric arrangements of calcified matrix and cells around a central canal for nerves and blood vessels; also called *Haversian system* [*osteo-* bone, *-on* unit]

osteonal canal (OS-tee-on) *see* **central canal (of bone)** [*osteo-* bone, *-on-* unit, *-al* relating to]

osteoporosis (os-tee-oh-poh-ROH-sis) bone disorder characterized by loss of minerals and collagen from bone matrix, reducing the volume and strength of skeletal bone [*osteo-* bone, *-poro-* pore, *-osis* condition]

osteosarcoma (os-tee-oh-sar-KOH-mah) bone cancer [*osteo-* bone, *-sarc* flesh, *-oma* tumour]

otic (O-tik) relating to the ear [*ot-* ear, *-ic* relating to]

otitis (o-TYE-tis) general term referring to inflammation or infection of the ear [*ot-* ear, *-itis* inflammation]

otitis media (oh-TYE-tis MEE-dee-ah) middle ear infection [*ot-* ear, *-itis* inflammation, *medi-* middle, *-al* relating to]

otolith (O-toh-lith) tiny "ear stones" composed of protein and calcium carbonate in the maculae of the ear, which, by responding to gravity and changes in body position, trigger hair cells that initiate impulses resulting in sense of balance [*oto-* ear, *-lith* stone]

otosclerosis (o-toh-skleh-ROH-sis) inherited bone disorder; impairs sound conduction by causing structural irregularities in the stapes; *see also* **tinnitus** [*oto-* ear, *-sclero-* hard, *-sis* condition]

otoscope (O-toh-skohp) lighted instrument used to examine the external ear canal and outer surface of the tympanic membrane [*oto-* ear, *-scop-* see]

oval window small, membrane-covered opening that separates the middle and inner ear [*oval-* egg-shaped]

ovarian cancer (oh-VAIR-ee-an) cancer of the ovary [*ovum* egg, *cancer* crab or malignant tumour]

ovarian cortex (oh-VAIR-ee-an KOHR-teks) outer region of the ovary [*ov-* egg, *-arian* relating to, *cortex* bark] *pl.*, cortices (KOHR-tis-eez)

ovarian cyst (oh-VAIR-ee-an SIST) fluid-filled cyst on the ovary that develops from follicles that fail to rupture completely or from corpora lutea that fail to degenerate [*ov-* egg, *-arian* relating to, *cyst-* bag]

ovarian follicle (oh-VAIR-ee-an FOL-ih-kul) spherical configuration of cells in the ovary that contains a single oocyte [*ov-* egg, *-arian* relating to, *foll-* bag, *-icle* little]

ovarian medulla (oh-VAIR-ee-an meh-DUL-ah) inner region of the ovary; contains supportive connective tissue cells, blood vessels, nerves, and lymphatics [*ov-* egg, *-arian* relating to, *medulla* marrow or pith (middle)] *pl.*, medullae (meh-DUL-ee) or medullas

ovary (OH-var-ee) female gonad that produces ova (sex cells) [*ov-* egg, *-ar-* relating to, *-y* location of process]

overactive bladder refers to frequent urination characterized by urgency

oviduct (OH-vih-dukt) *see* **fallopian tube, uterine tube** [*ovi-* egg, *-duct* path]

ovulation (ov-yoo-LAY-shun) release of an ovum from the ovary at the end of oogenesis [*ov-* egg, *-ation* process]

ovum (OH-vum) female sex cell (gamete) [*ovum* egg] *pl.*, ova

oxidative phosphorylation (ok-sih-DAY-tiv fos-for-ih-LAY-shun) reaction that joins a phosphate group to ADP to form ATP [*oxi-* sharp (oxygen), *-id-* chemical (*-ide*), *-at-* action of (*-ate*), *-ive* relating to, *phos-* light, *-phor-* carry, *-yl-* chemical, *-ation* process]

oxygen debt (OK-sih-jen) additional oxygen required for ATP synthesis to remove excess lactic acid following anaerobic exercise; also called *excess postexercise oxygen consumption (EPOC)* [*oxy-* sharp, *-gen* produce, *debt* something owed]

oxygen–haemoglobin dissociation curve (AHK-sih-jen hee-moh-GLOH-bin dih-soh-see-AY-shun) graph representing the relationship between Po_2 and O_2 saturation of haemoglobin [*oxy-* sharp, *-gen* produce, *haemo-* blood, *-glob-* ball, *-in* substance, *dis-* reverse, *-socia-* unite, *-ation* process]

oxyhaemoglobin (ok-see-hee-moh-GLOH-bin) haemoglobin combined with oxygen [*oxy-* sharp (oxygen), *-haemo-* blood, *-glob-* ball, *-in* substance]

oxytocin (OT) (ok-see-TOH-sin) hormone secreted by the posterior pituitary gland before and after delivering a baby; thought to initiate and maintain labour, as well as cause the release of breast milk into ducts of the mammary glands [*-oxy-* sharp (oxygen), *-toc-* birth, *-in* substance]

P

P wave electrocardiogram deflection that represents depolarization of the atria [named for 16th letter of Roman alphabet]

p53 gene (pee fif-tee-three jeen) type of "tumour suppressor" gene that codes for proteins that act to slow or stop the progress of the cell cycle, thus limiting tissue growth; is abnormal in some cancers, allowing formation of a tumour [*p-* p-arm of chrosome, -53 position on chromosome]

pacemaker (PAYS-may-ker) *see* **sinoatrial node**

Pacini corpuscle (pah-SIN-ee KOHR-pus-ul) *see* **lamellar corpuscle** [*Filippo Pacini* Italian anatomist, *corpus-* body, *-cle* little]

packed cell volume (PCV) *see* **haematocrit** [*pack-* bundle, *cell* storeroom]

pain control area place in the pain conduction pathway where impulses from pain receptors can be inhibited [*pain-* punishment, *control-* regulate, *area-* open space]

palatine bone (PAL-ah-tyne) bone that forms the posterior part of the hard palate and the lateral wall of the posterior part of each nasal cavity [*palat-* palate (roof of mouth), *-ine* relating to]

palatine tonsil (PAL-ah-tyne TON-sil) either of a pair of tonsils located behind and below the pillars of the fauces [*palat-* palate (roof of mouth), *-ine* relating to, *tons-* goitre, *-il* little]

palmar (PAHL-mar) relating to the palm (anterior surface) of the hand [*palm-* palm of hand, *-ar* relating to]

palmar venous arch (PAHL-mar VEE-nus) superficial vein of the hand [*palm-* palm of hand, *-ar* relating to, *ven-* vein, *-ous* relating to]

palmiteolate (pal-mih-TOH-lee-ayt) type of lipokine secreted by adipose tissue that regulates metabolism in other tissues; also called C16:1n7-palmitoleate [*palmit-* palm oil, *-ole-* oil, *-ate* chemical]

palpable (PAL-pah-bul) can be identified by touch, such as bony landmarks located beneath the skin [*palp-* touch gently, *-able* capable]

palpebrae (PAL-peh-bree) eyelids [*palpebra* eyelid] *sing.*, palpebra

palpebral fissure (PAL-peh-bral FISH-ur) opening between the two eyelids [*palpebra-* eyelid, *-al* relating to, *fissure* cleft]

pancreas (PAN-kree-ass) endocrine gland located in the abdominal cavity; contains pancreatic islets that secrete glucagon and insulin [*pan-* all, *-creas* flesh]

pancreatic cancer (pan-kree-AT-ik) cancer of the pancreas; usually a form of adenocarcinoma [*pan-* all, *-creat-* flesh, *-ic* relating to, *cancer* crab or malignant tumour]

pancreatic islet (pan-kree-AT-ik eye-let) endocrine portion of the pancreas; made up of alpha and beta cells, among others; source of insulin and glucagon; *also called* islets of Langerhans [*pan-* all, *-creat-* flesh, *-ic* relating to, *isl-* island, *-et* little]

pancreatic juice (pan-kree-AT-ik) digestive secretion; secreted by the exocrine acinar cells of the pancreas [*pan-* all, *-creat-* flesh, *-ic* relating to]

pancreatic polypeptide (pan-kree-AT-ik pol-ee-PEP-tyde) hormone produced in the periphery of the pancreatic islets; influences digestion and distribution of food molecules [*pan-* all, *-creat-* flesh, *-ic* relating to, *poly-* many, *-pept-* to digest, *-ide* chemical, *cell* storeroom]

pancreatitis (pan-kree-ah-TYE-tiss) inflammation of the pancreas [*pan-* all, *-creat*-flesh, *-itis* inflammation]

panda eyes (pan-dah eyes) condition that may occur as a result of the fracture of the fragile bones of the eye orbit

pandemic (pan-DEM-ik) refers to a disease that affects many people worldwide [*pan-* all, *-dem-* people, *-ic* relating to]

Paneth cell (PAH-net sel) cell located deep within intestinal crypt that produces antimicrobial enzymes [*Josef Paneth* Austrian physiologist]

pannus (PAN-us) aggregation of inflammatory cells, granulation tissue, and fibroblasts that adheres to the articular cartilage; destroys articular cartilage and bridges the opposing bones [*pannus* tattered cloth]

Papanicolaou test (Pap smear) (pah-peh-NIK-oh-lah-oo) cancer-screening test in which cells swabbed from the uterine cervix are smeared on a glass slide and examined for abnormalities; also called *Pap smear* or *Pap test* [*George N. Papanicolaou* Greek physician]

papilla (pah-PIL-ah) small, nipple-shaped elevation [*papilla* nipple] *pl.*, papillae (pah-PIL-ee)

papillary (PAP-ih-lair-ee) relating to papillae, as in the papillary layer of the dermis located at the dermal papillae [*papilla-* nipple, *-ary* relating to]

papilloma (pap-ih-LOH-mah) benign skin tumour characterized by fingerlike projections (e.g., a wart) [*papilla-* nipple, *-oma* tumour]

paracrine [agent or hormone] (PAIR-ah-krin) hormone that regulates activity in nearby cells within the same tissue as their source [*para-* beside, *-crin-* secrete]

parallel muscle long straplike muscles with parallel fascicles [*para-* beside, *-llel* one another, *mus-* mouse, *-cle* little]

paralysis (pah-RAL-ih-sis) loss of power of motion, especially voluntary motion [*para-* beside, *-lysis* loosening]

paramyxovirus (pair-ah-MIK-soh-VYE-rus) virus responsible for mumps [*para-* beside, *-myx-* mucus, *-virus* poison]

paranasal sinus (pair-ah-NAY-zal SYE-nus) air-containing spaces that are connected by channels to the nasal cavity [*para-* beside, *-nas-* nose, *-al* relating to, *sinus* hollow]

paraplegia (pair-ah-PLEE-jee-ah) spastic paralysis that affects both legs [*para-* beside, *-pleg-* stricken, *-ia* condition]

parasympathetic division (pair-ah-sim-pah-THET-ik) part of the autonomic nervous system; ganglia are connected to the brainstem and the sacral segments of the spinal cord; controls many autonomic effectors under normal ("rest and repair") conditions [*para-* beside, *-sym- together*, *-pathe-* feel, *-ic* relating to]

parathyroid gland (pair-ah-THYE-royd) endocrine gland located in the neck on the posterior aspect of the thyroid gland; secretes parathyroid hormone [*para-* beside, *-thyr-* shield, *-oid* like, *gland* acorn]

parathyroid hormone (PTH) (pair-ah-THYE-royd HOR-mohn) hormone released by the parathyroid gland that increases concentration of calcium in the blood [*para-* besides, *-thyr-* shield, *-oid* like, *hormon-* excite]

parenteral (therapy) (pah-REN-ter-al) administration of nutrients, special fluids, and/or electrolytes by injection [*par-* beside, *-enter-* intestine, *-al* relating to]

parietal (pah-RYE-ih-tal) refers to the walls of an organ or cavity [*parie-* wall, *-al* relating to]

parietal bone (pah-RYE-ih-tal) cranial bone [*parie-* wall, *-al* relating to]

parietal cell (pah-RYE-ih-tal) cell located on the basement membrane of gastric glands of the stomach that secretes hydrochloric acid [*parie-* wall, *-al* relating to, *cell* storeroom]

parietal lobe (pah-RYE-ih-tal) lobe that occupies the lateral and medial surface of the cerebrum [*parie-* wall, *-al* relating to]

parietal membrane (pah-RYE-ih-tal) portion of the serous membrane that lines the wall of a body cavity [*parie-* wall, *-al* relating to, *membran-* thin skin]

parietal peritoneum (pah-RYE-ih-tal pair-ih-TOH-nee-um) serous membrane that covers organs of the abdomen, pelvis, and thorax [*parie-* wall, *-al* relating to, *peri-* around, *-tone-* stretched, *-um* thing]

parietal pleura (pah-RYE-ih-tal PLOO-rah) serous membrane that lines the entire thoracic cavity [*parie-* wall, *-al* relating to, *pleura* side of body] *pl.*, pleurae (PLOO-ree)

parietooccipital sulcus (pah-RYE-eh-toh-ok-SIP-ih-tal SUL-kus) groove in the cerebrum that separates the occipital lobe from the parietal lobe; also *parietooccipital fissure* [*parieto-* wall, *-occipit-* back of head, *-al* relating to, *sulcus* trench] *pl.*, sulci (SUL-kye)

Parkinson disease (PD) (PARK-in-son) nervous disorder characterized by abnormally low levels of the neurotransmitter dopamine in parts of the brain that control voluntary movement—patients usually exhibit involuntary trembling and muscle rigidity [*James Parkinson* English physician]

p-arm the shorter segment of the chromosome, which is divided into two "arms" by the centromere (the longer segment is called the *q-arm*) [*p* petite (small), arm]

parotid (gland) (peh-ROT-id) largest of the paired salivary glands [*par-* beside, *-ot-* ear, *-id* relating to]

parotitis (pair-oh-TYE-tis) *see* **mumps** [*par-* beside, *-ot-* ear (parotid salivary gland), *-itis* inflammation]

pars anterior (parz an-TEER-ee-or) major part of the anterior pituitary gland [*pars* part, *ante-* front, *-er-* more, *-or* quality]

pars intermedia (PARS in-ter-MEE-dee-ah) forms a small part of the anterior pituitary gland [*pars* part, *inter-* between, *-media* to divide]

partial pressure (PAR-shal) pressure exerted by any one gas in a mixture of gases or in a liquid

partial thickness, deep dermal burn a burn involving the epidermis, papillary and reticular layers of the dermis

partial-thickness, superficial dermal burn (PAR-shal) a burn involving the epidermis and papillary layer of the demis

parturition (pahr-too-RIH-shun) act of giving birth [*parturi-* give birth, *-tion* process]

passive transport cellular process in which substances move through a cellular membrane with the energy supplied directly by the cell or its membrane [*trans-* across, *-port* carry]

patella (pah-TEL-ah) knee cap [*pat-* dish, *-ella* small] *pl.*, patellae (pah-TEL-ee)

patellar (pah-TEL-ar) relating to the knee cap [*pat-* dish, *-ella-* small, *-ar* relating to]

pathogen (PATH-oh-jen) microorganism that causes disease [*patho-* disease, *-gen* produce]

pathogenesis (path-oh-JEN-eh-sis) pattern of a disease's development [*patho-* disease, *-gen-* produce, *-esis* process]

pathogenic animal (path-oh-JEN-ik) animal, such as an insect, that causes disease in humans; *see also* **vector** [*patho-* disease, *-gen-* produce, *-ic* condition of]

pathological fracture (path-o-LOJ-ik-al) bone fracture caused by weakening of the bone by a disease, thus making normal movements too stressful for the bone to bear; also called *spontaneous fracture* [*patho-* disease, *-log-* words (study of), *-ical* relating to, *fracture* a breaking]

pathology (path-OL-o-jee) study of diseased body structures [*patho-* disease, *-o-* combining form, *-log-* words (study of), *-y* activity]

pathophysiology (path-oh-fiz-ee-OL-oh-jee) study of the underlying physiological aspects of disease [*patho-* disease, *-physio-* nature (function), *-o-* combining form, *-log-* words (study of), *-y* activity]

pattern-recognition receptor (PRR) (PAT-urn rek-ug-NISH-un ree-SEP-tor) receptor on human cells that can recognize patterns of molecules that exist on microbes, thus acting as a nonspecific screening mechanism in immunity

pavementing (PAYV-ment-ing) adherence of neutrophils and other phagocytes to a vessel's endothelial lining [*pave-* cover with stones, *-ment-* process]

pectoral girdle (PEK-toh-ral GIRD-el) incomplete ring of bones formed by the scapulae and clavicles and providing structural support for the upper limbs; the shoulder girdle [*pector-* breast, *-al* relating to, *girdle* belt]

pectoralis minor (pek-toh-RAL-is) muscle that pulls the shoulder down and forward [*pector-* breast, *-al* relating to, *-is* thing, *minor* lesser]

pedal (PEED-al) relating to the foot (*ped-* foot, *-al* relating to]

pedicel (PED-ih-cel) branches of the podocytes of the Bowman capsule, packed tightly together with only filtration slits between them [*pedic-* feet, *-el* small]

pedigree (PED-ih-gree) chart used in genetic counselling to illustrate genetic relationships over several generations [*pied de grue* crane's foot pattern]

pelvic (PEL-vik) relating to the hip (pelvic) bones or lower portion of the abdominopelvic cavity (pelvis) [*pelvi-* basin, *-ic* relating to]

pelvic girdle (PEL-vik GER-dul) bony structure formed by the coxal bones; supports the trunk and attaches the lower extremities to it [*pelvi-* basin, *-ic* relating to, *girdle* belt]

pelvic inflammatory disease (PID) (PEL-vik in-FLAM-ah-tor-ee) inflammatory condition caused by several pathogens that spreads upward from the vagina [*pelv-* basin, *-ic* relating to, *inflam-* set afire, *-ory* relating to]

pelvis (PEL-vis) relating to the hip (pelvic) region or the basinlike lower portion of the abdominopelvic cavity [*pelvis* basin]

penis (PEE-nis) mass of erectile tissue; forms part of the male genitalia; when sexually aroused, becomes stiff to enable it to enter and deposit sperm in the vagina [*penis* male sex organ] *pl.*, penes (PEE-neez) or penises (PEE-nis-ez)

pennate muscle (PEN-ayt) muscle with fascicle attachments that appear "featherlike" [*penn-* feather, *-ate* of or like, *mus-* mouse, *-cle* little]

pentose (PEN-tohs) five-carbon sugar such as ribose or deoxyribose [*pent-* five, *-ose* sugar]

pepsin (PEP-sin) protein-digesting enzyme of the stomach [*peps-* digestion, *-in* substance]

pepsinogen (pep-SIN-oh-jen) proenzyme that is converted to pepsin by hydrochloric acid [*peps-* digestion, *-in* substance, *-o-* combining form, *-gen* produce]

peptidase (PEP-tyd-ayz) protease found in the intestinal brush border; hydrolyzes peptides to amino acids [*pept-* digestion, *-ide* chemical, *-ase* enzyme]

peptide (PEP-tyde) compound made of two or more amino acids connected by peptide bonds (compare to **polypeptide**)

peptide bond (PEP-tyde) bond that forms between the amino group of one amino acid and the carboxyl group of another [*pept-* digest, *-ide* chemical]

peptide hormone (PEP-tyde HOR-mohn) major category of nonsteroid hormones; smaller than protein hormones; made up of a short chain of amino acids; for example, antidiuretic hormone (ADH) [*pept-* to digest, *-ide* chemical, *hormon-* excite]

perception (per-SEP-shun) interpreting a sensation [*per-* through, *-cept-* receive, *-ion* process]

percutaneous coronary intervention (PCI) (per-kyoo-TAYN-ee-us KOR-oh-nair-ee inter-VEN-shun) a group of procedures in which a catheter is inserted through the skin and along an artery to an atherosclerotic plaque and instruments are then passed along the catheter to push away or remove the plaque; examples include angioplasty and atherectomy [*per-* through, *cut-* skin, *-aneous* relating to, *corona-* crown, *-ary* relating to, *inter-* between, *-ven-* go, *-tion* process]

perfusion pressure (per-FYOO-shun) local pressure gradient needed to maintain blood flow in a tissue [*per-* through, *-fus-* pour, *-sion* process]

pericardial effusion (pair-ih-KAR-dee-all ef-FYOO-shen) accumulation of pericardial fluid, pus, or blood in the space between the two pericardial layers [*peri-* around, *-cardi-* heart, *-al* relating to, *e(x)-* outside, *-fus-* pour, *-sion* process]

pericardial fluid (pair-ih-KAR-dee-al) lubricating fluid secreted by the serous membrane; in pericardial space [*peri-* around, *-cardi-* heart, *-al* relating to]

pericardial space (pair-ih-KAR-dee-al) space between the visceral layer and the parietal layer surrounding the heart, filled with pericardial fluid [*peri-* around, *-cardi-* heart, *-al* relating to]

pericardial vein (pair-ih-KAR-dee-al vayn) vein of the thorax [*peri-* around, *-cardi-* heart, *-al* relating to, *vena* blood vessel]

pericardiocentesis (pair-ee-KAR-dee-oh-sen-TEE-sis) pericardial drainage [*peri-* around, *-cardi-* heart, *-centesis* pricking]

pericarditis (pair-ih-kar-DYE-tis) inflammation of the pericardium [*peri-* around, *-cardi-* heart, *-itis* inflammation]

pericardium (pair-ih-KAR-dee-um) membrane that surrounds the heart [*peri-* around, *-cardi-* heart, *-um* thing] *pl.*, pericardia (pair-ih-KAR-dee-ah)

perichondrium (pair-ih-KON-dree-um) fibrous covering of cartilage structures [*peri-* around, *-chondr-* cartilage, *-um* thing] *pl.*, perichondria (pair-ih-KON-dree-ah)

perikaryon (pair-ih-KAR-ee-on) *see* **cell body** [*peri-* around, *-karyon* nut or kernel]

perilymph (PAIR-ih-limf) watery fluid that fills the bony labyrinth of the ear [*peri-* around, *-lymph* water]

perimetrium (pair-ih-MEE-tree-um) serous covering that partly covers the uterus; a portion of the parietal peritoneum [*peri-* around, *-metr-* womb, *-um* thing]

perimysium (pair-ih-MEE-see-um) tough, connective tissue surrounding fascicles [*peri-* around, *-mys-* muscle, *-um* thing]

perineal (pair-ih-NEE-al) relating to the perineum (the area between the anus and genitals) [*peri-* around, *-ine-* excrete (perineum), *-al* relating to]

perineal body (pair-ih-NEE-al) node formed by fibres from several muscles that form the pelvic floor [*peri-* around, *-ine-* excrete (perineum), *-al* relating to]

perineum (pair-ih-NEE-um) area between anus and genitals [*peri-* around, *-ine-* excrete, *-um* thing] *pl.*, perinea (pair-IH-nee-ah)

perineurium (pair-ih-NYOO-ree-um) connective tissue that encircles a bundle of nerve fibres within a nerve [*peri-* around, *-neuri-* nerve, *-um* thing] *pl.*, perineuria (pair-ih-NYOO-ree-ah)

periodontitis (pair-ee-oh-don-TYE-tis) inflammation of the periodontal membrane that anchors teeth to jaw bone; common cause of tooth loss among adults [*peri-* around, *-odont-* tooth, *-itis* inflammation]

periosteum (pair-ee-OS-tee-um) tough, connective tissue covering the bone [*peri-* around, *-osteum* bone] *pl.*, periostea (pair-ee-OS-tee-ah)

peripheral (pe-RIF-er-al) relating to the periphery, or outer boundaries of the body, as in peripheral nervous system [*peri-* around, *-phera-* boundary, *-al* relating to]

peripheral chemoreceptor (pe-RIF-er-al kee-moh-ree-SEP-tor) sensory receptor in a peripheral nerve that detects changes in chemical concentrations such as oxygen, carbon dioxide, or pH [*centr-* centre, *-al* relating to, *chemo-* chemical, *-recept-* receive, *-or* agent]

peripheral nervous system (PNS) (peh-RIF-er-al) nerves connecting brain and spinal cord to other parts of the body [*peri-* around, *-phera-* boundary, *-al* relating to, *nerv-* nerves, *-ous* relating to]

peripheral neuropathy (peh-RIF-er-al nyoo-ROP-ah-thee) general term for any disease or disorder that involves damage to peripheral nerves; also called *peripheral neuritis*, or if many nerves are involved, *polyneuropathy* or *polyneuritis* [*peri-* around, *-phera-* boundary, *-al* relating to, *neuro-* nerves, *-path-* disease, *-y* state]

peripheral resistance (peh-RIF-er-al ree-ZIS-tens) resistance to blood flow caused by friction of blood passing through blood vessels [*peri-* around, *-phera-* boundary, *-al* relating to, *resist-* withstand, *-ance* act of]

peripheral vascular disease (PVD) (peh-RIF-er-al VAS-kyoo-lar) decrease in blood flow in the hands, legs, or feet [*peri-* around, *-pher-* boundary, *-al* relating to, *-vas-* vessel, *-ular* relating to, *dis-* opposite of, *-ease* comfort]

perirenal fat capsule (pair-ee-REE-nal KAP-sul) pad of fat that surrounds each kidney and holds it in position; also called *renal fat pad* [*peri-* around, *ren-* kidney, *-al* relating to, *caps-* box, *-ul-* little]

peristalsis (pair-ih-STAL-sis) wavelike, rhythmic contractions of the stomach and intestines that move food material along the digestive tract [*peri-* around, *-stalsis* contraction]

peritoneum (pair-ih-toh-NEE-um) large, moist, slippery sheet of serous membrane that lines the abdominopelvic cavity (parietal layer) and its organs (visceral layer) [*peri-* around, *-tone-* stretched, *-um* thing] *pl.*, peritonea (pair-ih-toh-NEE-ah)

peritonitis (pair-ih-toh-NYE-tis) inflammation of the serous membranes in the abdominopelvic cavity; sometimes a serious complication of an infected appendix [*peri-* around, *-ton-* stretch (peritoneum), *-itis* inflammation]

peritubular capillary (pair-ee-TYOOB-yoo-lar cap-IL-ar-ee) capillaries around the tubules in the kidney [*peri-* around, *-tub-* tube, *-ul-* little, *-ar* relating to, *capill-* hair, *-ary* relating to]

permanent teeth set of 32 teeth that replaces deciduous teeth

permeable (PERM-ee-ah-bil) adjective used to describe a membrane that allows substances to move through (permeate) it [*per-* through, *-mea(t)-* pass, *-able* capable of]

permeant (PERM-ee-ent) adjective used to describe a substance that is able to move through (permeate) a membrane [*per-* through, *-mea(t)-* pass, *-ant* characterized by]

permeate (PERM-ee-ayt) to move through or soak through, as water moving through the pores of a fabric or molecules diffusing through the pores of a cellular membrane [*per-* through, *-meat-* pass]

permissiveness (per-MISS-iv-ness) hormone action that occurs when a small amount of one hormone allows a second hormone to have its full effect on a target cell

pernicious anaemia (per-NISH-us ah-NEE-mee-ah) blood disorder characterized by a low number of red blood cells as a result of a dietary deficiency of vitamin B_{12} [*pernici-* destruction, *-ous* relating to, *an-* without, *-(h)aem-* blood, *-ia* condition]

pernicious vomiting (per-NISH-us) severe vomiting [*pernici-* destruction, *-ous* relating to]

peroneus tertius muscle (per-oh-NEE-us TER-shee-us) leg muscle that flexes and everts the foot; also *fibularis tertius* [*peroneus* pin (of brooch or buckle), *tertius* third, *mus-* mouse, *-cle* little]

peroxisome (pe-ROKS-ih-sohm) organelles that detoxify harmful substances that have entered cells [*peroxi-* hydrogen peroxide, *-soma* body]

perspiration transparent, watery liquid released by glands in the skin that eliminates ammonia and uric acid and helps maintain body temperature; also known as *sweating* [*per-* through, *-spir-* breathe, *-ation* process]

pH units by which acid and base concentrations (relative H ion concentrations) are measured; scale ranges from 0 (extremely acidic; high H concentration) to 14 (extremely basic, or alkaline; low H concentration) [abbreviation for *potenz* power, *hydrogen* hydrogen]

phalanx (FAH-lanks) any of the bones of the fingers or toes [*phalanx* formation of soldiers in rows] *pl.*, phalanges (fah-LAN-jeez)

phagocyte (FAG-oh-syte) type of cell, especially a white blood cell, that engulfs microorganisms and digests them [*phago-* eat, *-cyte* cell]

phagocytosis (fag-oh-sye-TOH-sis) ingestion and digestion of particles by a cell [*phago-* eat, *-cyte-* cell, *-osis* condition]

pharmacology (far-mah-KOL-oh-jee) study of drug actions [*pharmaco-* drug, *-log-* words (study of), *-y* activity]

pharyngeal tonsil (fah-RIN-jee-al TON-sil) tonsil located in the nasopharynx on its posterior wall; when enlarged, referred to as *adenoids* [*pharyng-* throat, *-al* relating to, *tons-* goitre, *-il* little]

pharyngitis (fair-in-JYE-tis) sore throat; inflammation or infection of the pharynx [*pharyng-* throat (pharynx), *-itis* inflammation]

pharynx (FAIR-inks) tubelike structure that extends from the base of the skull to the oesophagus; also called *throat* [*pharynx* throat] *pl.*, pharynges (fair-IN-jeez) or pharynxes

phenotype (FEE-no-type) overt, observable expression of a genotype [*pheno-* appear, *-type* kind]

phenylalanine hydroxylase (fen-il-AL-ah-neen hye-DROK-seh-lays) enzyme needed to convert phenylalanine into tyrosine; its absence causes phenylketonuria [*phen-* shining (phenol), *-yl-* chemical, *-alanine* amino acid, *hydro-* water, *-oxy-* oxygen, *-ase* enzyme]

phenylketonuria (PKU) (fen-il-kee-toh-NYOO-ree-ah) recessive, inherited condition characterized by excess of phenylketone in the urine, caused by accumulation of phenylalanine (an amino acid) in the tissues; may cause brain injury and death if phenylalanine intake is not managed properly [*phen-* shining (phenol), *-yl-* chemical, *-keton-* acetone, *-ur-* urine, *-ia* condition]

pheomelanin (fee-oh-MEL-ah-nin) type of melanin pigment that is reddish in colour [*pheo-* dusky, *-melan-* black, *-in* substance]

pheromone (FAIR-o-mohn) class of organic molecules found in apocrine sweat (possibly in urine and other excretions) and which acts as sexual (or other) signals to other individuals [*pher-* carry, *-mone* hormone (excite)]

phimosis (fi-MOH-sis) condition in which the foreskin of the penis fits so tightly over the glans that it cannot be retracted [*phimos-* muzzle, *-osis* condition]

phlebitis (fleh-BYE-tis) inflammation of a vein [*phleb-* vein, *-itis* inflammation]

phosphatase (FOS-fah-tayse) enzyme that removes phosphate groups [*phospho-* phosphorus, *-ase* enzyme]

phosphoinositide (PI) (fos-foh-in-OH-sih-tide) any of a small subgroup of phospholipid molecules in a cell acting as regulators of a variety of cell functions [*phospho-* phosphorus, *-ino-* muscle, *-os(e)-* sugar, *-ide* chemical]

phospholipid (fos-fo-LIP-id) phosphate-containing fat molecule; an important constituent of cell membranes [*phospho-* phosphorus, *-lip-* fat, *-id* form]

phosphoric acid (foss-FOR-ik ASS-id) contributes hydrogen ions to the extracellular fluid; influences acid–base balance [*phos-* light, *-phor-* bear (phosphorus), *-ic* relating to, *acid* sour]

phosphorus (FOS-for-us) element that is the principal component in the backbone of nucleic acids; important in energy transfer [*phos-* light, *-phorus* bearer]

phosphorylase (fos-FOR-ih-layse) enzyme that adds phosphate groups [*phos-* light, *-phor-* carry, *-yl-* chemical, *-ase* enzyme]

phosphorylation (fos-for-ih-LAY-shun) process of adding a phosphate group to a molecule [*phos-* light, *-phor-* carry, *-yl-* chemical, *-ation* process]

photodynamic therapy (PDT) (foh-toh-dye-NAM-ik) less invasive treatment of certain types of lung cancer [*photo-* light, *-dynam-* moving force, *-ic* relating to]

photopigment (foh-toh-PIG-ment) chemicals in retinal cells that are sensitive to light [*photo-* light, *-pigment* paint]

photopupil reflex (foh-toh-PYOO-pul REE-fleks) constriction of the pupil in bright light to protect the retina from too intense or too sudden stimulation; also known as *pupillary light reflex* [*photo-* light, *-pupil* centre of eye, *re-* again, *-flex* to bend]

photoreceptor (foh-toh-ree-SEP-tor) receptor only in the eye; responds to light stimuli if the intensity is great enough to generate a receptor potential [*photo-* light, *-cept-* receive, *-or* agent]

photorefractive keratectomy (foh-toh-ree-FRAK-tiv kair-ah-TEK-toh-mee) laser surgery that uses a "cool" excimer laser beam to vaporize corneal tissue [*photo-* light, *re-* back or again, *-fract-* break, *-ive* relating to, *kera-* hard, *-ec-* out, *-tom-* cut, *-y* action]

phrenic nerve (FREN-ik nerv) nerve that stimulates the diaphragm to contract [*phren-* mind, *-ic* relating to]

physiological buffer (fiz-ee-oh-LOJ-ih-kal BUFF-er) secondary defence against harmful shifts in pH of body fluids; comes into play after the chemical buffer system [*physio-* nature (function), *-o-* combining form, *-log-* words (study of), *-ical* relating to, *buffe-* cushion, *-er* agent]

physiological dead space (fiz-ee-oh-LOJ-ih-kal) the anatomical dead space (pulmonary airway volume outside the alveoli) plus any alveolar dead space (i.e., obstructed or diseased alveoli); *see* **anatomical dead space** [*physio-* nature, *-log-* words (study of), *-ical* relating to]

physiological fatigue (fiz-ee-oh-LOJ-ih-kal fah-TEEG) fatigue caused by a relative lack of ATP, rendering the myosin cross bridges incapable of producing the force required for further muscle contractions [*physio-* nature, *-log-* words (study of), *-ical* relating to, *fatigue-* to tire]

physiological polycythaemia (fiz-ee-oh-LOJ-ih-kal pol-ee-sye-THEE-mee-ah) elevated red blood cell numbers and haematocrit values in healthy individuals who live and work in high altitudes [*physi-* nature, *-o-* combining form, *-log-* words (study of), *-y* activity, *poly-* many, *-cyt-* cell, *-(h)aem-* blood, *-ia* condition]

physiology (fiz-ee-OL-oh-jee) scientific study of an organism's body function [*physio-* nature (function), *-o-* combining form, *-log-* words (study of), *-y* activity]

physique (fi-ZEEK) body build [*physique-* natural, physics]

pia mater (PEE-ah MAH-ter) vascular innermost covering (meninx) of the brain and spinal cord [*pia-* tender, *mater* mother]

pigment colouring material produced in the body; for example, melanin [*pigment* paint]

pimple (PIM-pul) pustule on the skin, usually associated with acne

pineal body (PIN-ee-al) endocrine gland located in the diencephalon and thought to be involved with regulating the body's biological clock; produces melatonin; also called *pineal gland* [*pine-* pine, *-al* relating to, *gland* acorn]

pineal gland (PIN-ee-al) *see* **pineal body** [*pine-* pine, *-al* relating to, *gland* acorn]

pinna (PIN-nah) flap of the external ear [*pinna* wing or fin]

pinocytosis (pin-oh-sye-TOE-sis) active transport mechanism used to transfer fluids or dissolved substances into cells [*pino-* drink, *-cyto-* cell, *-osis* condition]

pitch number of sound waves that occur during a specific time unit (frequency)

pitting oedema (PIT-ing eh-DEE-mah) depressions in swollen subcutaneous tissue [*oedema* swelling]

pituitary dwarfism (pih-TYOO-ih-tair-ee DWARF-iz-em) condition resulting from hyposecretion of growth hormone during the growth years [*pituit-* phlegm, *-ary* relating to, *dwar-* tiny, *-ism* condition]

pituitary gland (pih-TYOO-ih-tair-ee) neuroendocrine gland located near base of the brain that has numerous and important regulatory functions; also called the *hypophysis* [*pituit-* phlegm, *-ary* relating to, *gland* acorn]

pivot joint (PIV-it joynt) type of diarthrotic synovial joint in which a projection from one bone articulates with a ring or notch in another bone, allowing rotational movement

placenta (plah-SEN-tah) structure that anchors the developing fetus to the uterus and provides a "bridge" for the exchange of nutrients and waste products between the mother and developing baby [*placenta* flat cake] *pl.*, placentae (plah-SEN-tee) or placentas

placenta previa (plah-SEN-tah PREE-vee-ah) abnormal condition in which a blastocyst implants in the lower uterus, developing a placenta that approaches or covers the cervical opening; placenta previa involves risk of placental separation and haemorrhage [*placenta* flat cake, *previa* gone before]

plantar (PLAN-tar) relating to the bottom (sole) of the foot [*planta-* sole, *-ar* relating to]

plantar flexion (PLAN-tar FLEK-shun) the bottom of the foot is directed downward; this motion allows a person to stand on tiptoe [*planta-* sole, *-ar* relating to, *flex-* bend, *-ion* process]

plantar reflex (PLAN-tar REE-fleks) reflex in which the toes curl in flexion in response to stimulation of the outer margin of the foot; the Babinski sign is extension of the great toe (with or without fanning of the other toes) instead (normal in infants) [*planta-* sole, *-ar* relating to, *re-* again, *-flex* bend]

plaque (plak) raised skin lesion greater than 1 cm in diameter [*plaque* patch]

plasma (PLAZ-mah) liquid part of the blood [*plasma* substance]

plasma cell (PLAZ-mah) *see* **B lymphocyte** [*plasma* substance (blood plasma), *cell* storeroom]

plasma membrane (PLAZ-mah) membrane that separates the contents of a cell from the tissue fluid, encloses the cytoplasm, and forms the outer boundary of the cell [*plasma* substance, *membrane* thin skin]

plasmid (PLAS-mid) small circular ring of bacterial DNA [*plasmid* formed substance]

platelet (PLAYT-let) flattened cell fragment found in the blood that functions in haemostasis; thrombocyte [*plate-* flat, *-let* small]

platelet plug (PLAYT-let) results when platelets undergo a change caused by an encounter with a damaged capillary wall, or with underlying connective tissue fibres; helps to stop the flow of blood into the tissues [*plate-* flat, *-let* small]

pleura (PLOO-rah) serous membrane in the thoracic cavity [*pleura* side of body] *pl.*, pleurae

pleurisy (PLOOR-ih-see) inflammation of the pleura [*pleur-* side of body, *-isy* condition]

plexus (PLEK-sus) complex network formed by converging and diverging nerves, blood vessels, or lymphatics [*plexus* braid or network] *pl.*, plexi (PLEK-sye) or plexuses (PLEK-sus-eez)

plica (PLYE-ka) fold or ridge of tissue [*plica* fold] *pl.*, plicae (PLYE-kee) or plicas

pneumonectomy (nyoo-moh-NEK-toh-mee) surgical procedure in which an entire lung is removed [*pneumon-* lung, *-ec-* out, *-tom-* cut, *-y* action]

pneumonia (nyoo-MOH-nee-ah) abnormal condition characterized by acute inflammation of the lungs in which alveoli and bronchial passages become plugged with thick fluid (exudate) [*pneumon-* lung, *-ia* condition]

pneumotaxic centre (nyoo-moh-TAK-sik) group of cells in the pons of the brain that affects the rate of respiration by inhibiting the inspiration centre [*pneumo-* wind (breath), *-taxi-* movement or reaction, *-ic* relating to]

pneumothorax (nyoo-moh-THOH-raks) abnormal condition in which air is present in the pleural space surrounding the lung, possibly causing collapse of the lung [*pneumo-* air or wind, *-thorax* chest]

podocyte (POD-oh-syte) special epithelial cells making up the visceral layer of the Bowman capsule [*pod-* foot, *-cyte* cell]

Poiseuille's law (pwah-ZWEE-ez) volume of blood circulated per minute is directly related to mean arterial pressure minus central venous pressure and inversely related to resistance [*Jean L.M. Poiseuille* French physiologist]

polar molecule (POH-lar MOL-eh-kyool) molecule in which the electrical charge is not evenly distributed, causing one side of the molecule to be more positive or negative than the other [*pol-* pole, *-ar* relating to]

polarity (poh-LAIR-ih-tee) condition of having two opposite faces or ends; e.g., molecules and membranes can exhibit polar faces with different charges and epithelial cells have basal and apical poles [*pol-* pole, *-ar-* relating to, *-ity* state]

poliomyelitis (pol-ee-oh-my-eh-LYE-tis) viral disease that damages motor nerves, often progressing to paralysis of skeletal muscles [*polio-* grey, *-mye-* marrow, *-itis* inflammation]

pollex (POL-lex) thumb [*pollex* thumb] *pl.*, pollices (POL-lis-eez)

polychromatic erythroblast (pol-ee-kroh-MAT-ik ee-RITH-roh-blast) produced during red blood cell formation; produces haemoglobin [*poly-* many, *-chrom-* colour, *-ic* relating to, *erythro-* red, *-blast* bud]

polycystic ovary disease (PCOD) (pol-ee-SIS-tik OH-var-ee) condition that is characterized by ovaries usually twice the normal size and that are studded with fluid-filled cysts [*poly-* many, *-cyst-* bag, *-ic* relating to, *ov-* egg, *-ar-* relating to, *-y* location of process]

polycythaemia (pol-ee-sye-THEE-mee-ah) excess of red blood cells [*poly-* many, *-cyt-* cell, *-(h)aem-* blood, *-ia* condition]

polydipsia (pol-ee-DIP-see-ah) excessive and ongoing thirst [*poly-* many. *-dipsa-* thirst, *-ia* condition]

polygenic (pol-ee-JEN-ik) refers to traits that are determined by the combined effect of many different pairs of genes [*poly-* many, *-gen-* produce, *-ic* relating to]

polymer (POL-ih-mer) large molecule made up of many identical smaller molecules joined together in sequence [*poly-* many, *-mer* parts]

polymorphonuclear leucocyte (pol-ee-mohr-foh-NYOO-klee-er LOO-koh-syte) another name for neutrophil, describing the two, three, or more lobes of their nuclei [*poly-* many, *-morph-* form , *-nucle-* nut or kernel, *-ar* relating to, *leuco-* white, *-cyte* cell]

polynucleotide (pol-ee-NYOOK-lee-oh-tyde) strand of nucleotides bound to each other by chemical bonds, as in the polynucleotide strand that makes up an mRNA molecule [*poly-* many, *nucleo-* nut or kernel, *-ide* chemical]

polypeptide (pol-ee-PEP-tyde) compound made of many amino acids connected by peptide bonds [*poly-* many, *pept-* digest, *-ide* chemical]

polyphagia (pol-ee-FAY-jee-ah) intense and continuous hunger [*poly-* many, *-phag-* eat, *-ia* condition]

polyribosome (POL-ee-RYE-bo-sohm) temporary structure formed within a cell by many ribosomes following one another along a strand of mRNA during the process of translation [*poly-* many, *-som-* body]

polysaccharide (pol-ee-SAK-ah-ride) complex sugar or starch, such as glycogen and plant starches; made up of many monosaccharides [*poly-* many, *-sacchar-* sugar, *-ide* chemical]

polyunsaturated fatty acid (pol-ee-un-SACH-ur-ayt-ed FAT-tee ASS-id) hydrocarbon chain (fatty acid) in which several available bonds are not filled (saturated) with hydrogen [*poly-* many, *-un-* not, *-saturat-* fill, *acid* sour]

polyuria (pol-ee-YOO-ree-ah) frequent urination [*poly-* many, *-ur-* urine, *-ia* condition]

pons (ponz) part of the brainstem between the medulla oblongata and the midbrain [*pons* bridge] *pl.*, pontes (PON-tees)

popliteal (pop-LIT-ee-al) relating to the area behind the knee joint [*poplit-* back of knee, *-al* relating to]

popliteal vein (pop-LIT-ee-al vayn) vein that runs behind the knee joint [*poplit-* back of knee, *-al* relating to, *vena* blood vessel]

portal system (PORT-al SIS-tem) arrangement of blood vessels in which blood exiting one tissue is immediately carried to a second tissue before being returned to the heart and lungs for oxygenation and redistribution [*port-* doorway, *-al* relating to]

portal triad (PORT-al TRY-ad) arrangement of three primary ducts (interlobular artery, interlobular portal vein, interlobular bile duct) plus a lymphatic vessel and vagus nerve branch at each corner of every hepatic lobule of the liver [*port-* doorway, *-al* relating to, *triad* group of three]

positive feedback (POZ-ih-tiv FEED-bak) feedback control system that is stimulatory; tends to amplify or reinforce a change in the internal environment [*posit-* put or place, *-ive* relating to]

positive nitrogen balance (POZ-ih-tiv NYE-troh-jen) nitrogen intake in foods is greater than nitrogen output in urine [*posit-* put or place, *-ive* relating to, *nitro-* soda, *-gen* produce]

positron-emission tomography (PET) (POZ-ih-tron eh-MISH-un toh-MOG-rah-fee) variation of computed tomography scanning; radioactive substance is introduced into the blood supply of the brain, projecting a bright spot on the image [*positron* positive electron, *e-* out, *-mission* send, *tomo-* cut, *-graph-* draw, *-y* activity]

posterior (pohs-TEER-ee-or) located behind; opposite of anterior [*poster-* behind, *-or* quality]

posterior cavity (of eye) (pohs-TEER-ee-or KAV-ih-tee) all the space posterior to the lens of the eye; contains vitreous body [*poster-* behind, *-or* quality, *cav-* hollow, *-ity* state]

posterior chamber (of eye) (pohs-TEER-ee-or CHAIM-ber) subdivision of the anterior cavity of the eye; small space behind the iris and anterior to the lens [*poster-* behind, *-or* quality, *chamber* vaulted enclosure]

posterior cul-de-sac (of Douglas) (pohs-TEER-ee-or kul-deh-sak) a deep pouch between the uterus and the anus; formed by the posterior ligament [*poster-* behind, *-or* quality, *cul-de-sac* end of the pouch, *James Douglas* Scots anatomist] *pl.*, culs-de-sac or cul-de-sacs

posterior fornix (pohs-teer-ee-or FOR-niks) space created by the protrusion of the cervix into the lumen of the vagina; increases probability of reproductive success by retaining seminal fluid [*poster-* behind, *-or* quality, *fornix* arch]

posterior ligament (pohs-TEER-ee-or LIG-ah-ment) fold of peritoneum extending from the posterior surface of the uterus to the rectum [*poster-* behind, *-or* quality, *liga-* bind, *-ment* condition]

posterior tibial vein (pohs-TEER-ee-or TIB-ee-al vayn) deep vein of the leg [*poster-* behind, *-or* quality, *tibia-* shin bone, *-al* relating to, *vena* blood vessel]

postganglionic neuron (post-gang-glee-ON-ik NYOO-ron) efferent autonomic neuron that conducts nerve impulses from a ganglion to effectors such as cardiac or smooth muscle or glandular epithelial tissue [*post-* after, *-ganglion-* knot, *-ic* relating to, *neuron* string or nerve]

postinfectious glomerulonephritis (post-in-FEK-shus gloh-mer-yoo-loh-neh-FRY-tis) *see* **acute glomerulonephritis** [*post-* after, *-infec-* stain, *-ous* relating to, *glomer-* ball, *-ul-* little, *-nephr-* kidney, *-itis* inflammation]

postmenstrual phase (post-MEN-stroo-al) phase in the menstrual cycle that occurs between the end of menses and ovulation; also called *preovulatory phase* and *proliferative phase* [*post-* after, *-mens-* month, *-al* relating to]

postnatal period (POST-nay-tal) period after birth, ending at death [*post-* after, *-nat-* birth, *-al* relating to]

postovulatory phase (post-ov-yoo-lah-TOR-ee) *see* **premenstrual phase** [*post-* after, *-ov-* egg, *-ory* relating to]

postsynaptic (post-sih-NAP-tik) adjective describing any structure after a synapse (junction) of one neuron to another or any function that occurs after synaptic transmission [*post-* after, *-syn-* together, *-apt-* join, *-ic* relating to]

postsynaptic neuron (post-sih-NAP-tik NYOO-ron) in neuron-to-neuron communication, the neuron that receives a stimulus via an adjacent neuron's transmission of neurotransmitters across the synapse [*post-* after, *-syn-* together, *-apt-* join, *-ic* relating to]

postsynaptic potential (post-sih-NAP-tik poh-TEN-shal) local potential produced by opening of ion channels in the postsynaptic membrane [*post-* after, *-syn-* together, *-apt-* join, *-ic* relating to, *potent-* power, *-ial* relating to]

posture (POS-chur) position of the body; often refers to the erect position of the body maintained unconsciously [*pos(i)t-* position, *-ure* state]

potassium (poh-TASS-ee-um) mineral element that forms the ion K [*potass-* potash, *-um* thing or substance]

potassium channel (poh-TASS-ee-um CHAN-el) a pore in a cell membrane that allows only potassium ions to permeate, or pass through, the membrane [*potass-* potash, *-um* thing or substance, *channel-* groove]

potential osmotic pressure (po-TEN-shal os-MOT-ik) maximum osmotic pressure that could develop in a solution when it is separated from pure water by a selectively permeable membrane [*potent-* power, *-ial* relating to, *osmo-* push, *-ic* relating to]

Pott fracture fracture of the lower part of the tibia [*Percival Pott*, English physician, *fracture* a breaking]

preauricular lymph node (pree-ah-RIK-yoo-lar limf nohd) lymphatic tissue located just in front of the ear [*pre-* before, *-auri-* ear, *-cula-* little, *-ar* relating to, *lymph* water, *nod-* knot]

prebiotic (pree-bye-OT-ik) substance or preparation that does not contain microorganisms but affects the growth and activity of normal microorganisms of the body and used to prevent or correct unhealthy disruptions to the human microbiome; compare to **probiotic** [*pre-* before, *-bio-* life, *-ic* relating to]

precapillary sphincter (pree-cap-IL-ar-ee SFINGK-ter) smooth muscle cells that regulate the entrance to the capillary; probably exist as a discrete structure only in capillaries of the mesenteries [*pre-* before, *-capill-* hair, *-ary* relating to, *sphinc-* bind tight, *-er* agent]

precapillary tone (pree-cap-IL-ar-ee tohn) smooth muscle tension around the arterioles, which can be altered to regulate local blood flow in capillary beds [*pre-* before, *-capill-* hair, *-ary* relating to, *tone* tension]

precordial lead (pree-KOR-dee-al) *see* **chest lead** [*pre-* before, *-cordi-* heart, *-al* relating to, *lead* guide or conduct]

preeclampsia (pree-ee-KLAMP-see-ah) syndrome of abnormal conditions of uncertain cause in pregnancy; symptoms include hypertension, proteinuria, and oedema; also called *toxaemia of pregnancy*, it may progress to eclampsia—severe toxaemia that may cause death [*pre-* before, *-lamp-* shine forth, *-sia* condition]

preganglionic neuron (pree-gang-glee-ON-ik NYOO-ron) efferent autonomic neuron that conducts nerve impulses between the spinal cord and a ganglion [*pre-* before, *-ganglion-* knot, *-ic* relating to, *neuron* string or nerve]

pregnancy-induced hypertension (PIH) (PREG-nan-see-in-DYOOST hye-per-TEN-shun) a condition in which a woman's blood pressure rises after the twentieth week of pregnancy and remains elevated until the end of pregnancy; PIH may have a genetic component and may progress to *preeclampsia* [*hyper-* excessive, *-tens-* stretch or pull tight, *-sion* state]

preload (PREE-lohd) the pumping work of the heart to move blood received from venous return; the load on the heart produced by the blood before it leaves the heart; compare to **afterload**

premature contraction (pree-muh-CHOOR kon-TRAK-shun) contraction that occurs before the next expected contraction in a series of cardiac cycles; also called *extrasystole* [*pre-* before, *-mature* to ripen, *con-* together, *-tract* to draw, *-tion* process]

premenstrual phase (pree-MEN-stroo-al) phase of the menstrual cycle that occurs between ovulation and the onset of the menses; also called *postovulatory phase*, *progesterone phase*, *luteal phase*, or *secretory phase* [*pre-* before, *-mens-* month, *-al* relating to]

premenstrual syndrome (PMS) (pree-MEN-stroo-all SIN-drohm) condition that involves a collection of symptoms that regularly occur in many women during the premenstrual phase [*pre-* before, *-mens-* month, *-al* relating to, *syn-* together, *-drome* running or (race) course]

prenatal period (PREE-nay-tal) developmental period after conception until birth [*pre-* before, *-nat-* birth, *-al* relating to]

preovulatory phase (pree-ov-yoo-lah-TOR-ee) *see* **postmenstrual phase** [*pre-* before, *-ov-* egg, *-ory* relating to]

prepatellar bursitis (pree-pah-TEL-er ber-SYE-tis) inflammation of the prepatellar bursa; also called "housemaid's knee" [*pre-* in front of, *-pat-* dish, *-ella* small, *-ar* relating to, *bursa-* purse, *-itis* inflammation]

prepuce (PREE-pus) foreskin, especially covering fold of skin over the glans penis [*pre-* before, *-puc-* penis]

presbycusis (pres-bih-KYOO-sis) progressive hearing loss as a result of nerve impairment; common among elderly [*presby-* elderly, *-cusis* hearing]

presbyopia (pres-bee-OH-pee-ah) farsightedness of old age [*presby-* ageing, *-op-* vision, *-ia* condition]

pressoreflex (pres-oh-REE-fleks) *see* **baroreflex pressure**

pressure gradient (PRESH-ur GRAY-dee-ent) any measurable difference in pressure between two points [*grad-* step, *-ent* state]

presynaptic (pree-sih-NAP-tik) adjective describing any structure before a synapse (junction) of one neuron to another or any function that occurs before synaptic transmission [*press-* pressure, *-re-* back or again, *-flex* bend]

presynaptic neuron (pree-sih-NAP-tik NYOO-ron) in neuron-to-neuron communication, the neuron that transmits a signal to an adjacent neuron via release of neurotransmitters that cross the synapse and bind to the postsynaptic neuron [*pre-* before, *-syn-* together, *-apt-* join, *-ic* relating to]

prevertebral ganglion (pree-VER-teb-ral GANG-glee-on) collateral ganglion; pairs of sympathetic ganglia located a short distance from the spinal cord [*pre-* before, *-vertebra-* that which turns, *-al* relating to, *ganglion* knot]

primary bronchus (PRY-mair-ee BRONG-kus) either of the two branches of the trachea that enter the lungs [*prim-* first, *-ary* relating to, *bronchus* windpipe] *pl.*, bronchi (BRONG-kye)

primary follicle (PRY-mair-ee FOL-ih-kul) follicles present at puberty; formed from granulosa cell [*prim-* first, *-ary* relating to, *folli-* *bag*, *-cle* small]

primary germ layer (PRY-mair-ee jerm LAY-er) any of the three layers of developmental cells that give rise to definite structures as the embryo develops; *see also* **ectoderm, endoderm, mesoderm** [*prim-* first, *-ary* relating to, *germ* sprout]

primary hyperparathyroidism (PRY-mair-ee hye-per-pair-ah-THY-royd-iz-em) condition that results when parathyroid gland fails to adjust its hormone output to compensate for changes in blood calcium levels [*prim-* first, *-ary* relating to, *hyper-* excessive, *-para-* beside, *-thyr-* shield (thyroid), *-oid* like, *-ism* condition]

primary oocyte (PRY-mair-ee OH-oh-syte or OH-ah-syte) developmental stage of the ova; formed from oogonia during the fetal period [*prim-* first, *-ary* relating to, *oo-* egg, *-cyte* cell]

primary ossification centre (PRY-mair-ee osi-fih-KAY-shun) where a blood vessel enters the cartilage of a developing bone at the midpoint of the diaphysis to initiate bone formation [*prim-* first, *-ary* relating to, *os-* bone, *-fic-* make, *-ation* process]

primary principle of ventilation (PRY-mair-ee) movement of air in the pulmonary airways from the area where the pressure is higher to the area where the pressure is lower [*prim-* first, *-ary* relating to, *princip-* foundation, *vent-* fan or create wind, *-tion* process]

primary protein structure (PRY-mair-ee PRO-teen STRUK-cher) simplest level of protein structure, it is the sequence of amino acids that will eventually curl into a more complex structure [*prim-* first, *-ary* relating to, *prote-* primary, *-in* substance, *structur-* arrangement]

primary sex characteristics (PRY-mair-ee) changes that involve the development of the gonads [*prim-* first, *-ary* relating to, *character-* engraved mark, *-istic* relating to]

prime mover main muscle responsible for producing a particular movement [*prime* first order]

principle of independent assortment genetic principle that states as chromosome pairs separate, the maternal and paternal chromosomes redistribute themselves independently of the other chromosome pairs [*princip-* foundation, *in-* not, *-de-* upon, *-pend-* hang, *-ent* state, *assort-* match into groups, *-ment* process]

principle of segregation genetic principle that states that the two members of a pair of chromosomes separate during meiosis [*princip-* foundation, *segrega-* divide, *-ation* process]

prion (PREE-on) a term that is short for "proteinaceous infectious particles", which are proteins that convert proteins of the cell into different proteins and the altered form of the protein may then be inherited; may act as a pathogen, forming abnormal protein tangles in brain cells; *see also* **bovine spongiform encephalopathy, variant Creutzfeldt–Jakob Disease (vCJD)** [condensed from proteinaceous infectious particle]

probiotic (proh-bye-OT-ik) preparation of specific bacteria used to prevent or treat imbalances in the human microbiome or confer other health benefits; compare to **prebiotic** [*pro-* favoring, *-bio-* life, *-ic* relating to]

process (PRO-sess) 1. A series of actions having a result 2. A projection from a structure such as a bone [*process* advance or project (from)]

product molecules or atoms that result from a chemical reaction [*produc-* bring forth]

proctitis (prok-TYE-tis) inflammation of the rectal mucosa [*proct-* anus, *-itis* inflammation]

proencephalon (pro-en-SEF-ah-lon) primary vesicle of the neural tube during embryonic development that eventually becomes the cerebrum (telencephalon) and diencephalon; also called *forebrain*; often used as a synonym for the most superior part of the brain [*pro-* first, *-en-* within, *-cephalon* head]

proenzyme (pro-EN-zime) inactive form in which many enzymes are synthesized [*pro-* first, *-en-* in, *-zyme* ferment]

proerythroblast (proh-eh-RITH-roh-blast) maturation stage of the red blood cell; appearance of this cell begins differentiation in red blood cells [*pro-* first, *-erythro-* red, *-blast* bud]

progeria (proh-JEER-ee-ah) rare, inherited condition in which a young child appears to age rapidly, also called *Hutchinson–Gilford disease* [*pro-* early, *-ger-* old age, *-ia* condition]

progesterone (proh-JES-ter-ohn) steroid hormone produced by the ovaries (particularly the corpus luteum) that helps prepare the uterus for implantation; along with oestrogen, helps maintain normal uterine and mammary gland function [*pro-* before, *-gester-* bearing (pregnancy), *-stero-* solid or steroid derivative, *-one* chemical]

progesterone phase (proh-JES-ter-ohn) *see* **premenstrual phase** [*pro-* before, *-gester-* bearing (pregnancy), *-stero-* solid or steroid derivative, *-one* chemical]

prohormone (proh-HOR-mohn) hormone precursor [*pro-* first, *hormon-* excite]

projection tract extension of the sensory spinothalamic tracts and descending corticospinal tracts in the brain [*project-* thrown forward, *-ion* process, *tract* trail]

prolactin (PRL) (proh-LAK-tin) hormone secreted by the anterior pituitary gland during pregnancy to stimulate the breast development needed for lactation [*pro-* before, *-lact-* milk, *-in* substance]

proliferative phase (PROH-lif-er-eh-tiv) *see* **postmenstrual phase** [*proli-* offspring, *-fer-* bear or carry, *-at-* process, *-ive* relating to]

pronation (proh-NAY-shun) movement that turns the palm of the hand down [*pronat-* bend forward, *-tion* process]

prophase (PRO-fayz) first stage of mitosis during which chromosomes become visible [*pro-* first, *-phase* stage]

proprioception (proh-pree-oh-SEP-shun) perception of movement and position of the body [*propri-* one's own, *-cept-* receive, *-tion* process]

proprioceptor (proh-pree-oh-SEP-tor) receptor located in the muscles, tendons, and joints; allows the body to perceive its position relative to surroundings [*propri-* one's own, *-cept-* receive, *-or* agent]

propulsion (proh-PUL-shun) continual pushing of chyme in the stomach toward the pyloric sphincter by peristaltic contractions [*pro-* in front, *-pul-* drive, *-sion* process]

prostaglandin (PG) (pross-tah-GLAN-din) any of a group of naturally occurring lipid-based substances that act in a hormone-like way to affect many body functions, including vasodilation, uterine smooth muscle contraction, and the inflammatory response [*pro-* before, *-stat-* set or place (prostate), *-gland-* acorn (gland), *-in* substance]

prostate (PROSS-tayt) exocrine gland that lies just below the bladder in the male; secretes a fluid that constitutes about 30% of the seminal fluid volume; helps activate sperm and helps them maintain motility [*pro-* before, *-stat-* set or place]

prostatectomy (pros-tah-TEK-toh-mee) surgical removal all or part of the prostate [*pro-* before, *-stat-* set or place (prostate gland), *-ec-* out, *-tom-* cut, *-y* action]

prostate-specific antigen (PSA) (PROSS-tayt speh-SIF-ik AN-tih-jen) blood protein sometimes associated with prostate cancer [*pro-* before, *-stat-* set or place (prostate gland), *specif-* form, *-ic* relating to, *anti-* against, *-gen* produce]

prosthesis (pros-THEE-sis) artificial device that is used in the partial or total replacement of a diseased joint [*prosthesis* addition] *pl.*, prostheses (pros-THEE-seez)

protease (PRO-tee-ayz) enzyme that catalyzes the hydrolysis of proteins into intermediate compounds (proteoses and peptides) [*prote-* protein, *-ase* enzyme]

proteasome (PRO-tee-ah-sohm) cell structure that breaks down individual proteins [*protea-* protein, *-som-* body]

protein (PRO-teen) large molecules formed by linkage of amino acids by peptide bonds; one of the basic building blocks of the body [*prote-* primary, *-in* substance]

protein balance (PRO-teen) rate of protein anabolism equals or balances the rate of protein catabolism [*prote-* primary, *-in* substance]

protein hormone (PRO-teen HOR-mohn) long, folded chain of amino acids; for example, insulin and parathyroid hormone [*prote-* first rank, *-in* substance, *hormon-* excite]

protein–calorie malnutrition (PCM) (PRO-teen KAHL-ah-ree mal-nyoo-TRISH-un) abnormal condition resulting from a deficiency of calories in general and protein in particular [*mal-* poor, *-nutri-* nourish, *-tion* process]

proteoglycan (PRO-tee-oh-GLYE-kan) large molecule made up of a protein strand that forms a backbone to which are attached many carbohydrate molecules [*proteo-* protein, *-glycan* polysaccharide (from *-glyc-* sweet)]

proteome (PRO-tee-ohm) the entire group of proteins produced by a cell or by the entire body [*prote-* protein, *-ome* entire collection]

proteomics (proh-tee-OH-miks) the endeavour that involves the analysis of the proteins encoded by the genome, with the ultimate goal of understanding the role of each protein in the body [*prote-* first rank (protein), *-om-* entire collection, *-ic* relating to]

proton (PROH-ton) positively charged subatomic particle [*protos-* first, *-on* elementary atomic particle]

protozoan (pro-toe-ZO-an) single-celled organism with a nucleus and other membranous organelles that can infect humans [*proto-* first, *-zoan* animal] *pl.*, protozoa (pro-toe-ZO-ah)

protraction (proh-TRAK-shun) movement that moves a part forward [*pro-* forward, *-tract-* drag, *-tion* process]

proximal (PROK-sih-mal) next or nearest; located nearest the centre of the body or the point of attachment of a structure; opposite of distal [*proxima-* near, *-al* relating to]

proximal convoluted tubule (PROK-sih-mal KON-voh-LOO-ted TYOO-byool) second part of the nephron and the first segment of a renal tubule; major portion of the *proximal tubule* [*proxima-* near, *-al* relating to, *con-* together, *-volut-* roll, *tub-* tube, *-ul-* little]

proximal interphalangeal (PIP) joint (PROK-sih-mal in-ter-fah-LAN-gee-al) joint between the proximal and middle phalanges [*proxima-* near, *-al* relating to, *inter-* between, *-phalang-* finger bones (ref. from rows of soldiers), *-al* relating to]

proximal tubule (PROK-sih-mal TYOO-byool) *see* **proximal convoluted tubule** [*proxima-* near, *-al* relating to, *tub-* tube, *-ul-* little]

pseudogene (SOOD-oh-jeen) nonfunctional "broken" genetic code found in "junk DNA" located between the functioning, coding genes of a DNA molecule; pseudo genes are thought to be genetic "fossils" remaining from our evolutionary past [*pseudo-* false, *-gene* produce (gene)]

pseudostratified columnar epithelium (SOOD-oh-STRAT-ih-fyed KOL-um-nar ep-ih-THEE-lee-um) type of tissue similar to simple columnar epithelium; forms a membrane made up of single layer of cells that are tall and narrow but have been squeezed together in a way that pushes the nuclei into two layers and thus gives the appearance that it is stratified [*pseudo-* false, *-strati-* layer, *-fied* made, *column-* column, *-ar* characterized by] *pl.*, epithelia (ep-ih-THEE-lee-ah)

psoriasis (so-RYE-ah-sis) chronic, inflammatory skin disorder characterized by cutaneous inflammation and scaly plaques [*psor-* itching, *-iasis* condition]

psychological stressor (sye-koh-LOJ-ih-kal STRESS-or) anything an individual perceives as a threat [*psycho-* the mind, *-log-* words (study of), *-al* relating to, *stress-* tighten, *-or* agent]

psychophysiology (sye-koh-fiz-ee-OL-oh-jee) scientific discipline that studies physiological responses of individuals being subjected to psychological stressors [*psycho-* the mind, *-physio* nature (function), *-o-* combining form, *-log-* words (study of), *-y* activity]

psychosomatic (sye-koh-soh-MAT-ik) mind influencing the body [*psycho-* the mind, *-soma* body, *-ic* relating to]

ptosis (TOH-sis) downward displacement of an organ; for example the lowered kidneys of very thin individuals [*pto-* fall, *-osis* condition]

pterygoid muscle (TER-ih-goid) muscle of mastication; opens and protrudes the mandible while causing sideways movement [*ptery-* wing, *-oid* like, *mus-* mouse, *-cle* little]

puberty (PYOO-ber-tee) stage of adolescence in which a person becomes sexually mature [*pubert-* age of maturity, *-y* state]

pubic (PYOO-bik) relating to the groin area or (more specifically) to the most anterior coxal bone (pubis, which fuses with other coxal bones by adulthood) [*pubis* groin]

pubis (PYOO-biss) most anterior coxal bone (fuses with other coxal bones by adulthood) [*pubis* groin] *pl.*, pubes (PYOO-beez)

puerperal fever (pyoo-ER-per-al) condition caused by bacterial infection in a woman after delivery of an infant, possibly progressing to septicaemia and death; also called "childbed fever" [*puerp-* childbirth, *-al* relating to]

pulmonary artery (PUL-moh-nair-ee AR-ter-ee) artery that carries deoxygenated blood from the right ventricle of the heart to the lungs; exiting the heart is the trunk of the pulmonary artery (pulmonary trunk), which branches into a left and right pulmonary artery [*pulmon-* lung, *-ary* relating to, *arteri-* vessel]

pulmonary circulation (PUL-moh-nair-ee) blood flow from the right ventricle to the lung and returning to the left atrium [*pulmon-* lung, *-ary* relating to, *circulat-* go around, *-tion* process]

pulmonary oedema (PUL-moh-nair-ee eh-DEE-mah) congestion of blood in the pulmonary circulation [*pulmon-* lung, *-ary* relating to, *oedema* swelling]

pulmonary embolism (PUL-moh-nair-ee EM-boh-liz-em) blockage of the pulmonary circulation by a thrombus or other matter; may lead to death if blockage of pulmonary blood flow is significant [*pulmon-* lung, *-ary* relating to, *embol-* plug, *-ism* condition]

pulmonary radiology (PUL-moh-nair-ee ray-dee-OHL-oh-gee) chest x-ray examination [*pulmon-* lung, *-ary* relating to, *radi-* ray or radiation, *-o-* combining form, *-log-* words (study of), *-y* activity]

pulmonary trunk (PUL-moh-nair-ee trunk) initial segment of the pulmonary artery, before it splits into left and right branches [*pulmon-* lung, *-ary* relating to]

pulmonary (semilunar) valve (PUL-moh-nair-ee [semi-LOO-nar]) valve located at the beginning of the pulmonary artery [*pulmon-* lung, *-ary* relating to, *semi-* half, *-luna* moon, *-ar* relating to

pulmonary vein (PUL-moh-nair-ee vayn) any vein that carries oxygenated blood from the lungs to the left atrium [*pulmon-* lung, *-ary* relating to, *vena* blood vessel]

pulmonary ventilation (PUL-moh-nair-ee ven-tih-LAY-shun) breathing; process that moves air in and out of the lungs [*pulmon-* lung, *-ary* relating to, *vent-* fan or create wind, *-tion* process]

pulp dental tissue that is a subtype of loose, fibrous connective tissue with blood and lymphatic vessels and sensory nerves within the interior pulp cavity of a tooth [*pulp* flesh]

pulp cavity cavity in the dentin of a tooth that contains connective tissue, blood and lymphatic vessels, and sensory nerves [*pulp* flesh, *cav-* hollow, *-ity* condition]

pulse point point where the pulse can be palpated; that is, wherever an artery lies near the surface and over a bone or other firm background; for example, radial artery [*pulse* beat]

pulse pressure (PP) difference between systolic and diastolic blood pressure [*pulse* beat]

puncta (PUNK-ta) *see* **punctum**

punctum (PUNK-tum) opening into the lacrimal canals located at the inner canthus of the eye [*punctum* small point] *pl.*, puncta (PUNK-tah)

Punnett square (PUN-it) grid used in genetic counselling to determine the probability of inheriting genetic traits [*Reginald C. Punnett* English geneticist]

pupil opening in the centre of the iris that regulates the amount of light entering the eye [*pup-* doll, *-il* little]

pupillary light reflex (PYOO-pih-lair-ee lyte REE-fleks) photopupil reflex [*pup-* doll, *-il* little, *-ary* relating to, *re-* again, *-flex* bend]

purine base (PYOO-reen) one of two types of nitrogenous bases that are vital components of DNA derived from purine; adenine and guanine [*pur-* pure, *-ine* chemical]

purine neurotransmitter (PYOO-reen nyoo-roh-tranz-MIT-ter) a small-molecule neurotransmitter that contains the purine group adenine; for example ATP and adenosine [*pur-* pure, *-ine* chemical]

purinergic (pyoo-rin-ER-jik) describes a structure that functions with purine molecules (such as ATP or adenosine) as in a receptor that is triggered by a purine [*chole-* bile, *-erg* to work, *-ic* relating to]

Purkinje fibres (pur-KIN-jee) *see* **subendocardial branches** [*Johannes E. Purkinje* Czech physiologist]

pus (puhs) accumulation of white blood cells, dead bacterial cells, and damaged tissue cells at site of an infection [*pus* corrupt matter]

pustule (PUS-tyool) small, raised skin lesion filled with pus [*pustul-* blister or pimple]

pyelonephritis (pye-eh-loh-neh-FRY-tis) inflammation of the renal pelvis and connective tissues of the kidney [*pyel-* renal pelvis, *-nephr-* kidney, *-itis* inflammation]

pyloric sphincter (pye-LOR-ik SFINGK-ter) sphincter (muscular valve) that prevents food from leaving the stomach and entering the duodenum [*pyl-* gate, *-or-* to guard, *-ic* relating to, *sphinc-* bind tight, *-er* agent]

pyloric stenosis (pye-LOR-ik steh-NO-sis) obstructive narrowing of the pylorus [*pyl-* gate, *-or-* guard, *-ic* relating to, *stenos-* narrow, *-osis* condition] *pl.*, stenoses (steh-NO-seez)

pylorospasm (pye-LOHR-oh-spaz-um) condition occurring in infants when the pyloric fibres do not relax normally to allow food to leave the stomach, and the infant vomits food instead of digesting and absorbing it [*pyl-* gate, *-or-* guard, *-spasm* twitch or involuntary contraction]

pylorus (pye-LOR-us) lower part of the stomach [*pyl-* gate, *-orus* guard]

pyramid (PEER-ah-mid) one of two bulges of white matter located on the ventral surface of the medulla [*pyramis-* pyramid]

pyramidal tract (pih-RAM-ih-dal trakt) fibres that come together in the medulla to form the pyramids; also called *corticospinal tract* [*pyrami-* pyramid, *-al* relating to, *tract* trail]

pyramids (PEER-ah-mids) triangular-shaped divisions of the medulla of the kidney [*pyramis-* pyramid]

pyrimidine base (pih-RIM-ih-deen) one of two types of nitrogenous bases that are vital components of DNA derived from pyrimidine; cytosine and thymine [*pyrimid-* nitrogen compound, *-ine* chemical]

pyrogen (PYE-roh-jen) systemic inflammatory response chemical that causes the thermostatic control centres of the hypothalamus to produce a fever [*pyro-* heat, *-gen* produce]

pyuria (pye-YOO-ree-ah) pus in urine [*py-* pus, *-ur-* urine, *-ia* condition]

Q

q-arm the longer segment of the chromosome, which is divided into two "arms" by the centromere (the shorter segment is called the p-arm) [*q* follows *p* in Roman alphabet]

QRS complex electrocardiogram deflection that represents depolarization of the ventricles [named for 17th-19th letters of Roman alphabet]

quadriplegia (kwod-rih-PLEE-jee-ah) paralysis that affects all four extremities [*quadri-* fourfold, *-pleg-* stricken, *-ia* condition]

quaternary protein structure (KWAH-ter-nair-ee PRO-teen STRUK-cher) fourth level of complexity in the structure of a protein molecule, made up of several tertiary protein structures in combination; a *quaternary protein* is a protein possessing a fourth level of complexity in its molecular structure [*quatern-* fourth, *-ary* relating to, *prote-* primary, *-in* substance, *structur-* arrangement]

R

radial keratotomy (RAY-dee-al kar-ah-TOT-oh-mee) surgical placement of six or more radial slits in a spoke-like pattern around the cornea; flattens cornea and improves focus [*radi-* ray, *-al* relating to, *kera-* horn, *-tom-* cut, *-y* action]

radiation (ray-dee-AY-shun) electromagnetic energy, including light, x-rays, heat; in physiology, often refers to flow of excess heat energy away from the body via the blood [*radiat-* send out rays, *-ion* process]

radiation sickness (ray-dee-AY-shun) a condition caused by ionizing radiation that can be mild to severe, or even fatal, depending on the level of radiation exposure and the length of time exposed; exposure at lower doses of radiation can result in headache, nausea and vomiting, appetite loss, and diarrhoea; exposure to low doses for a longer period of time or a single high-level exposure may cause sterility, damage to fetal development, cancer (including leukaemia), cataracts, hair loss (alopecia), and skin damage (radiation dermatitis); *see* **ionizing radiation** [*radiat-* send out rays, *-ion* process]

radiation therapy (ray-dee-AY-shun) treatment often used to combat cancer; high-intensity (x-ray or gamma) radiation is used to destroy cancer cells; also called *radiotherapy* [*radiat-* emit rays, *-tion* process, *therapy* treatment]

radical (RAD-ih-kal) group of atoms that stays together and combines and uncombines with other molecules; often designated with the symbol R; also called *functional group*; compare to **free radical** [*radic-* root, -al relating to]

radical mastectomy (RAD-ih-kal mas-TEK-toh-mee) procedure that removes the entire breast, nearby muscles and lymph nodes [*radic-* root, -al relating to, *mast-* breast, *-ec-* out, *-tom-* cut, *-y* action]

radioactive isotope (ray-dee-oh-AK-tiv EYE-so-tohp) unstable isotope that spontaneously emits subatomic particles and electromagnetic radiation [*radi(at)-* emit rays, *-act-* to do, drive, *-iv-* state, *iso-* equal, *-tope* place]

radioactivity (ray-dee-oh-ak-TIV-it-ee) the ongoing process of emitting subatomic particles and electromagnetic radiation [*radi(at)-* emit rays, *act-* to do, drive, *-ivity* state]

radiocarpal joint (RAY-dee-oh-KAR-pal) the point of articulation where the radius distally articulates directly with the carpal bones [*radi-* ray, *-carp-* wrist, *-al* relating to]

radiofrequency ablation (RAY-dee-oh-FREE-kwen-see ab-LAY-shun) procedure that uses a gold-plated mesh fabric to fill the uterine cavity, which is then charged with radiofrequency energy to destroy bleeding endometrial cells [*radi-* ray, frequency, *ab-* away from, *-lat-* carry, *-tion* process]

radiography (ray-dee-OG-rah-fee) imaging technique using x-rays that pass through certain tissues more easily than others, allowing an image of tissues to form on a photographic plate [*radi-* ray, frequency, *-graphy* drawing]

radioisotope (ray-dee-oh-EYE-so-tohp) an isotope that is unstable and undergoes nuclear breakdown [*radi-* ray, *-iso-* equal, *-tope* place]

radiotherapy (ray-dee-oh-THER-ah-pee) radiation therapy [*radi-* ray, *-therapy* treatment]

radioulnar joint (RAY-dee-oh-UL-nur) articulation of the head of the radius and the radial notch of the ulna [*radi-* ray, *-ulna-* elbow or arm, *-ar* relating to]

radius (RAY-dee-us) forearm bone; located on thumb side [*radius* ray] *pl.*, radii (RAY-dee-eye)

raft a structure made up of groupings of molecules (cholesterol, certain phospholipids, proteins) within a cell membrane that travel together on the surface of the cell, something like a log raft on a lake; also called *lipid raft*

ramus (RAY-mus) large branch of a spinal nerve as it emerges from the spinal cavity [*ramus* branch] *pl.*, rami (RAY-mye)

range of motion (ROM) (raynj ov MOH-shun) extent of movement of a joint [*range-* placed in a row, *mot-* to move, *-ion* process]

rapid eye movement (REM) sleep stage of sleep characterized by rapid movements of the eye; associated with vivid dreaming

rate law law of mass action

ratio (RAY-shee-oh) the relationship of one quantity to one or more other quantities expressed as a proportion of one to the others

rational drugs chemotherapy drugs that target only those specific molecules, enzymes, or receptors unique to cancer cells or tumour growth, thereby affecting only the cancer and sparing normal cells, increasing efficiency and reducing side effects [*ration-* reason, *-al* relating to]

reabsorption (ree-ab-SORP-shun) movement of substances back into the bloodstream, as when bone calcium is dissolved by osteoclasts and diffuses into the bloodstream, or when solutes in renal filtrate (in the nephron) move back into the bloodstream [*re-* back again, *-ab-* from, *-sorp-* suck, *-tion* process]

reactant (ree-AK-tant) participant in a chemical reaction that is changed by the reaction [*re-* again, *-act-* act, *-ant* agent]

receptor portion of a sensory neuron that responds to an external stimulus; also, any molecule on the surface of a cell that binds specifically to other molecules (such as cell markers, hormones, neurotransmitters) [*re-cept-* receive, *-or* agent]

receptor potential potential that develops in the receptor's membrane when an adequate stimulus has been received [*recept-* receive, *-or* agent, *potent-* power, *-ial* relating to]

recessive (ree-SES-iv) in genetics, refers to genes that have effects that do not appear in the offspring when they are masked by a dominant gene (recessive forms of a gene are represented by lowercase letters); *see* **dominant** [*recess-* retreat, *-ive* relating to]

recombinant DNA (ree-KOM-bih-nant D N A) joining together of hereditary material into new, biologically functional combinations [*re-* again, *-comb* together, *-bini* two by two]

recessive gene (ree-SES-iv jeen) gene that has effects that do not appear in the offspring when they are masked by the dominant gene [*recess-* retreat, *-ive* relating to, *gene* produce]

recruit (ree-KROOT) to supply with new members, as in stimulating additional muscle fibres to contract simultaneously in a muscle in order to strengthen the contraction force [*re-* again, *-cruit* grow]

rectouterine pouch (rek-toh-YOO-ter-in) *see* **posterior cul-de-sac (of Douglas)** [*recto-* straight, *-uter-* womb, *-ine* relating to]

rectum (REK-tum) distal region of the intestinal tube [*rect-* straight or upright, *-um* thing]

rectus abdominis muscle (REK-tus ab-DOM-ih-nus) muscle that runs down the middle of the abdomen; compresses abdomen [*rectus* straight or upright, *abdominis* abdomen, *mus-* mouse, *-cle* little]

rectus sheath (REK-tus sheeth) layer of aponeuroses that cover the rectus abdominis muscle [*rectus* straight or upright]

red fibre muscle fibres that contain large amounts of myoglobin and have a deep red appearance [*fibr-* thread or fibre]

red marrow (MAIR-oh) bone marrow found in the ends of long bones and in flat bones; so named because of its function in the production of red blood cells [*marrow* pith (middle)]

reduction division meiosis when the diploid chromosome number (46) is reduced to the haploid number (23) [*re-* again or back, *-duc-* lead, *-tion* process, *divis-* divide, *-ion* process, *meiosis* becoming smaller]

reduction proper alignment of a fractured bone; in chemistry, the gain of one or more electrons by a molecule (as in oxidation-reduction reactions) [*re-* again or back, *-duc-* lead, *-tion* process]

referred pain pain felt on or near the surface of the body that results from stimulation of nociceptors in deep structures; for example, experiencing pain in the left arm when heart muscle receptors signal pain, as during a heart attack [*referre-* to bring back, *poena-* punishment]

reflex (REE-fleks) automatic involuntary reaction to a stimulus resulting from a nerve impulse passing over a reflex arc [*re-* again, *-flex* bend]

reflex arc (REE-fleks ark) impulse conduction route to and from the central nervous system; smallest portion of nervous system that can receive a stimulus and generate a response [*re-* back or again, *-flex* bend, *arc* curve]

refraction (ree-FRAK-shun) bending of a ray of light as it passes from a medium of one density to one of a different density; occurs as light rays pass through the eye [*re-* back or again, *-fract-* break, *-tion* process]

regeneration (ree-jen-er-AY-shun) process of replacing missing tissue with new tissue by means of cell division [*re-* again, *generat-* produce, *-tion* process]

regulator T cell (T-reg) *see* **suppressor T cell** [*regula-* rule, *T* thymus gland, *cell* storeroom]

Reissner membrane (RYZ-ner) *see* **vestibular membrane** [*Ernst Reissner* German anatomist, *membran-* thin skin]

rejection syndrome (reh-JEK-shun SIN-drohm) reaction of immune system against foreign antigens in grafted tissue [*re-* again, *-ject* to throw, *-tion* process, *syn-* together, *-drome* running or (race) course]

relative refractory period (ree-FRAK-tor-ee) in muscle cell contraction, the few milliseconds after the absolute refractory period; time during which the membrane is repolarizing and restoring the resting membrane potential [*re-* back or again, *-fract-* break, *-ory* relating to, *period* circuit]

relaxation state of lessened tension [*relax-* loosen or soften, *-ation* process]

relaxin (reh-LAK-sin) hormone that inhibits contractions during pregnancy and softens pelvic joints to facilitate childbirth [*relax-* loosen or soften, *-in* substance]

releasing hormone (HOR-mohn) hormone produced by the hypothalamus that causes the pituitary gland to release its hormones [*hormon-* excite]

remission (ree-MISH-un) stage of a disease during which a temporary recovery from symptoms occurs [*re-* back or again, *-miss-* to send, *-sion* condition of]

renal artery (REE-nal AR-ter-ee) large branch of the abdominal aorta that brings blood into each kidney [*ren-* kidney, *-al* relating to, *arteri-* vessel]

renal calculus (REE-nal KAL-kyoo-lus) crystallized mineral chunks that develop in the renal pelvis or calyces; also called *kidney stones* [*ren-* kidney, *-al* relating to, *calculi* little stone] *pl.*, calculi

renal cell carcinoma (REE-nal sel kar-si-NO-mah) malignant neoplasm of the kidney [*ren-* kidney, *-al* relating to, *cell* storeroom, *carcino-* cancer, *-oma* tumour]

renal clearance (REE-nal KLEER-ents) amount of blood plasma cleared of a particular substance by the kidneys per minute [*ren-* kidney, *-al* relating to]

renal columns (REE-nal) within the kidneys, the cortical tissue in the medulla between the pyramids [*ren-* kidney, *-al* relating to]

renal corpuscle (REE-nal KOR-pus-ul) within the nephron, the glomerulus plus the Bowman capsule surrounding it [*ren-* kidney, *-al* relating to, *corpus-* body, *-cle* little]

renal cortex (REE-nal KOR-teks) outer portion of the kidney [*ren-* kidney, *-al* relating to, *cortex* bark] *pl.*, cortices (KOR-tis-eez)

renal diabetes (REE-nal dye-ah-BEE-teez) when the maximum cotransport capacity of the kidney is greatly reduced and glucose appears in the urine even though the blood sugar level may be normal; also called *renal glycosuria* [*ren-* kidney, *-al* relating to, *diabetes* pass-through or siphon]

renal failure (REE-nal) failure of the kidney to properly process blood plasma and form urine [*ren-* kidney, *-al* relating to]

renal medulla (REE-nal meh-DUL-ah) inner portion of the kidney [*ren-* kidney, *-al* relating to, *medulla* marrow or pith (middle)] *pl.*, medullae (meh-DUL-ee) or medullas

renal pelvis (REE-nal PEL-vis) basinlike upper end of the ureter that is located inside the kidney into which the calyces drain [*ren-* kidney, *-al* relating to, *pelvis* basin] *pl.*, pelves (PEL-veez) or pelvises (PEL-vis-eez)

renal ptosis (REE-nal TOH-sis) condition in which one or both kidneys drop from their normal position [*ren-* kidney, *-al* relating to, *pto-* fall, *-osis* condition]

renal pyramid (REE-nal PIR-ah-mid) any of the distinct triangular wedges that make up most of the medullary tissue in the kidney [*ren-* kidney, *-al* relating to]

renal tubule (REE-nal TYOOB-yool) a principal part of the nephron; consists of the proximal convoluted tubule, the Henle loop, and the distal tubule; receives filtrate from Bowman capsule and transports it to collecting ducts while filtrate is reabsorbed and additional substances are secreted into it in the process of urine formation [*ren-* kidney, *-al* relating to, *tube-* pipe, *-ule* small]

renal vein (REE-nal vayn) kidney vein [*ren-* kidney, *-al* relating to, *vena* blood vessel]

renature (ree-NAYT-shur) to reverse the alteration (denaturation) of a protein and thus restore its normal shape and chemical properties [*re-* again, *-nature* born]

renin (REE-nin) enzyme produced by the juxtaglomerular apparatus of the kidney nephrons that catalyzes the formation of angiotensin, a substance that increases blood pressure; *see* **renin–angiotensin–aldosterone system (RAAS)** [*ren-* kidney, *-in* substance]

renin–angiotensin mechanism (REE-nin an-jee-oh-TEN-sin) *see* **renin–angiotensin–aldosterone system (RAAS)** [*ren-* kidney, *-in-* substance, *-angio-* vessel, *-tens-* pressure or stretch, *-in* substance, *mechan-* machine, *-ism* state]

renin–angiotensin–aldosterone system (RAAS) (REE-nin–an-jee-oh-TEN-sin–al-DOS-tair-ohn) causes changes in blood plasma volume mainly by controlling aldosterone secretion [*ren-* kidney, *-in* substance, *angio-* vessel, *-tens-* pressure or stretch, *-in* substance, *aldo-* aldehyde, *-stero-* solid or steroid derivative, *-one* chemical]

repolarization (ree-poh-lah-rih-ZAY-shun) phase of the action potential in which the membrane potential changes from its maximum degree of depolarization toward the resting state potential [*re-* back or again, *-pol-* pole, *-ar-* relating to, *-ization* process]

reproduction formation of a new individual; formation of new cells in the body to permit growth [*re-* again, *-produc-* bring forth, *-tion* process]

reproductive system system in both sexes that is composed of the gonads, genital ducts, accessory glands, and genitals [*re-* again, *-produc-* bring forth, *-tive* relating to]

residual volume (ree-ZID-yoo-al) amount of air that remains in the lungs after the most forceful expiration [*residu-* remainder, *-al* relating to]

resistin (reh-SIS-tin) hormone that reduces sensitivity to insulin and thus raises blood glucose levels [*resist-* withstand, *-in* substance]

respiration (res-pi-RAY-shun) processes that result in the absorption, transport, and utilization or exchange of respiratory gases between an organism and its environment [*re-* again, *-spir-* breathe, *-ation* process]

respiratory acidosis (RES-pih-rah-tor-ee ass-ih-DOH-sis) retention of carbon dioxide in the blood [*re-* again, *-spir-* breathe, *-tory* relating to, *acid-* sour, *-osis* condition]

respiratory alkalosis (RES-pih-rah-tor-ee al-kah-LOH-sis) excessive loss of carbonic acid from the blood [*re-* again, *-spir-* breathe, *-tory* relating to, *alkal-* ashes; *-osis* condition]

respiratory arrest (RES-pih-rah-tor-ee ah-REST) cessation of breathing without resumption [*re-* again, *-spir-* breathe, *-tory* relating to]

respiratory centre (RES-pih-rah-tor-ee) control centre located in the medulla and pons that stimulates muscles of respiration [*re-* again, *-spir-* breathe, *-tory* relating to]

respiratory cycle (RES-pih-rah-tor-ee SYE-kul) the alternating pattern of inspiration and expiration (inhalation/exhalation) of breathing [*re-* again, *-spir-* breathe, *-tory* relating to, *cycle-* circle]

respiratory distress syndrome (RDS) (RES-pih-rah-tor-ee di-STRESS SIN-drohm) difficulty in breathing caused by absence or failure of the surfactant in fluid lining the alveoli of the lung; IRDS is infant respiratory distress syndrome; ARDS is adult respiratory distress syndrome [*re-* again, *-spir-* breathe, *-tory* relating to, *syn-* together, *-drome* running or (race) course]

respiratory membrane (RES-pih-rah-tor-ee) single layer of cells that makes up the wall of the alveoli [*re-* again, *-spir-* breathe, *-tory* relating to, *membran-* thin skin]

respiratory mucosa (RES-pih-rah-tor-ee myoo-KOH-sah) mucus-covered membrane that lines tubes of the respiratory tree [*re-* again, *-spir-* breathe, *-tory* relating to, *muc-* slime, *-os-* characterized by, *-a* thing] *pl.*, mucosae (myoo-KOH-see)

respiratory physiology (RES-pih-rah-tor-ee fiz-ee-OL-oh-jee) study of the function of the respiratory system [*re-* again, *-spir-* breathe, *-tory* relating to, *physio-* nature, *-log-* words (study), *-y* process]

respiratory portion (of nasal passage) (RES-pih-rah-tor-ee) area within the nasal passage that extends from the inferior meatus to the small funnel-shaped orifices of the *posterior nares* [*re-* again, *-spir-* breathe, *-tory* relating to]

respiratory system (RES-pih-rah-tor-ee) system composed of the nose, pharynx, larynx, trachea, bronchi, and lungs [*re-* again, *-spir-* breathe, *-tory* relating to]

respiratory tract (RES-pih-rah-tor-ee trakt) organs of the respiratory system, divided into lower and upper respiratory tracts [*re-* again, *-spir-* breathe, *-tory* relating to, *tract* trail]

response (ree-SPONS) reaction to a stimulus [*respons-* reply]

responsiveness (ree-SPON-siv-ness) characteristic of life that permits an organism to sense, monitor, and react to changes in its external environment [*respons-* reply, *-ive-* relating to, *-ness* state or condition]

resting membrane potential (RMP) membrane potential maintained by a nonconducting neuron's plasma membrane; approximately 70 mV [*membran-* thin skin, *potent-* power, *-ial* relating to]

retention (ree-TEN-shun) inability to void urine even though the bladder contains an excessive amount of urine [*reten-* hold, *-ion* process]

reticular (reh-TIK-yoo-lar) resembling a netlike pattern [*ret-* net, *-icul-* little, *-ar* relating to]

reticular activating system (RAS) (reh-TIK-yoo-lar) complex processing system in the neural network (reticular formation) in the brain responsible for maintaining consciousness [*ret-* net, *-ic-* relating to, *-ul-* little, *-ar* characterized by]

reticular formation (reh-TIK-yoo-lar) neural network located in the brainstem where it is involved in arousal (reticular activating system) [*ret-* net, *-ic-* relating to, *-ul-* little, *-ar* characterized by]

reticular theory (reh-TIK-yoo-lar) concept that the nervous system is best understood as a large integrated network—one endless piece [*ret-* net, *-ic-* relating to, *-ul-* little, *-ar* characterized by, *theor-* look at, *-y* act of]

reticular tissue (reh-TIK-yoo-lar) meshwork of netlike tissue that forms the framework of the spleen, lymph nodes, and bone marrow [*ret-* net, *-ic-* relating to, *-ul-* little, *-ar* characterized by, *tissu-* fabric]

reticulin (reh-TIK-yoo-lin) type of collagen found in reticular fibres; also called *collagen III* [*ret-* net, *-ic-* relating to, *-ul-* little, *-in* substance]

reticulocyte (reh-TIK-yoo-loh-syte) immature red blood cells [*ret-* net, *-ic-* relating to, *-ul-* little, *-cyte* cell]

reticulocyte count (reh-TIK-yoo-loh-syte) medical procedure used to determine the rate of erythropoiesis cells [*ret-* net, *-ic-* relating to, *-ul-* little, *-cyte* cell]

reticulospinal tract (reh-TIK-yoo-loh-SPY-nal trakt) spinal cord motor tract that helps maintain posture during skeletal muscle movement [*ret-* net, *-ic-* relating to, *-ul-* little, *-spin-* backbone, *-al* relating to, *tract* trail]

reticulum (reh-TIK-yoo-lum) intricate network of fibres [*ret-* net, *-ic-* relating to, *-ul-* little, *-um* thing]

retina (RET-ih-nah) innermost layer of the eyeball; contains rods and cones and continues posteriorly with the optic nerve [*ret-* net, *-in-* relating to, *-a* thing]

retinal (RET-ih-nal) light-absorbing portion of all photopigments [*ret-* net, *-in-* relating to, *-al* relating to]

retinal detachment (RET-ih-nal) condition that occurs when part of the retina falls away from the tissue supporting it [*ret-* net, *-in-* relating to, *-al* relating to]

retraction (re-TRAK-shun) movement that moves a part back [*re-* back, *-tract-* drag, *-tion* process]

retrograde pyelogram (RET-roh-grayd PYE-eh-loh-gram) an x-ray image produced as a result of contrast material injected through a catheter [*retro-* backward, *-grad-* step, *pyelo-* renal pelvis, *-gram* drawing]

retrograde signalling (RET-roh-grayd SIG-nah-ling) type of synaptic transmission in which chemical signals are sent from the postsynaptic neuron back to the presynaptic neuron, usually to facilitate or inhibit further presynaptic signals [*retro-* backward, *-grad-* step, *sign-* mark, *-al* relating to]

retroperitoneal (reh-troh-pair-ih-toh-NEE-al) relating to the area outside of and posterior to the parietal peritoneum [*retro-* backward, *peri-* around, *-tone-* stretched, *-al* relating to]

retropulsion (ret-roh-PUL-shun) process of chyme being forced to move backward behind a closed pyloric sphincter [*retro-* backward, *-pul-* drive, *-sion* process]

reversible reaction (ree-VER-sih-bul ree-AK-shun) when the products of a chemical reaction change back to the original reactants; generally, an equilibrium of products and reactants exists [*re-* again, *-vers-* turn, *-ible* capable, *re-* again, *-action* action]

Rh factor (R h FAK-tor) antigen present on the red blood cells of Rh^+ individuals; so named because it was first studied in the rhesus monkey [*Rh* for *rhesus monkey]*

rheumatic fever (roo-MAT-ik) delayed inflammatory response to streptococcal infection that, if not properly treated, may allow the cardiac valves to become inflamed [*rheuma-* flow, *-ic* relating to]

rheumatic heart disease (roo-MAT-ik) cardiac damage (especially to the endocardium, including the valves) resulting from a delayed inflammatory response to streptococcal infection; *see* **rheumatic fever** [*rheuma-* flow, *-ic* relating to, *dis-* opposite of, *-ease* comfort]

rheumatoid arthritis (RA) (ROO-mah-toyd ar-THRY-tis) form of systemic autoimmune disease that involves chronic inflammation of many different tissues and organs of the body [*rheuma-* flow, *-oid* like, *arthr-* joint, *-itis* inflammation]

rhinitis (rye-NYE-tis) inflammation of the nasal mucosa often caused by nasal infections [*rhin-* nose, *-itis* inflammation]

rhodopsin (roh-DOP-sin) photopigment in rods [*rhodo-* red, *-ops-* vision, *-in* substance]

rhombencephalon (rom-ben-SEF-ah-lon) primary vesicle of the neural tube during embryonic development that eventually becomes the pons, medulla, and cerebellum; also called the *hindbrain* [*rhombo-* flatfish or equilateral parallelogram (rhombus), *-en-* within, *-cephalon* head]

rhomboid major/minor muscle (ROM-boyd) upper limb muscle that adducts and elevates the scapula [*rhombo-* flatfish or equilateral parallelogram (rhombus), *-oid* like, *major* greater, *minor* lesser, *-oid* like, *mus-* mouse, *-cle* little]

ribonucleic acid (RNA) (rye-boh-nyoo-KLAY-ik ASS-id) nucleic acid found in both nucleus and cytoplasm of cells; involved in transmission of genetic information from nucleus to cytoplasm and in cytoplasmic assembly of proteins [*ribo-* ribose (sugar), *nucle-* nucleus, *-ic* relating to, *acid-* sour]

ribonucleotide (rye-boh-NYOO-klee-oh-tide) type of nucleotide in RNA, consisting of the pentose sugar named *ribose*, a nitrogenous base (either adenine, cytosine, guanine, or uracil), and a phosphate group [*ribo-* ribose, *-nucle-* nucleus (kernel), *nucleo-* nut or kernel, *-ide* chemical]

ribose (RYE-bohse) five-carbon sugar; the sugar in RNA [*rib-* rearranged from gum arabic, *-ose* sugar]

ribosome (RYE-boh-sohm) organelle in the cytoplasm of cells that synthesizes proteins; sometimes called "protein factory" [*ribo-* ribose or RNA, *-som-* body]

ribozyme (RYE-boh-zyme) form of RNA (ribonucleic acid) that acts like an enzyme to promote or regulate chemical reactions in the cell [*ribo-* ribose or RNA, *-zyme* enzyme]

rickets (RIK-ets) condition primarily seen in infants and children caused by vitamin D deficiency; disease results in soft, pliable bones and skeletal deformities caused by abnormal calcium metabolism [unknown origin]

right lobe the right portion of an organ, such as the liver [*lob-* pod or hull, husk]

right lymphatic duct (lim-FAT-ik) main lymphatic duct that drains lymph ino the right subclavian vein [*lymph-* water, *-atic* relating to, *duct* path]

righting reflexes (RYTE-ing REE-fleks-ez) muscular responses that restore the body and its parts to their normal position when they have been displaced [*re-* again, *-flex* to bend]

rigor mortis (RIG-or MOR-tis) literally "stiffness of death"; the permanent contraction of muscle tissue after death caused by the depletion of ATP during the actin-myosin reaction, preventing myosin from releasing actin to allow relaxation of the muscle [*rigor* stiffness, *mortis* of death]

RNA *see* **ribonucleic acid** [*RNA-* ribonucleic acid]

RNA interference (RNAi) (RNA in-ter-FEER-enz) a regulatory process of the cell in which a small molecule of dsRNA (double-stranded RNA) called *siRNA* (small interfering RNA) joins with a RISC (RNA-induced silencing complex) protein structure to break down a specific mRNA (messenger RNA) transcript and thus effectively silence the gene encoded by the mRNA; RNAi is a natural regulatory process thought to be involved with regulating gene expression, as in inhibiting viral infections, but is also used as a research technique to study the human genome [*RNA* ribonucleic acid]

RNAi therapy any medical procedure in which RNAi techniques are used to silence (disable) the effects of a disease-causing gene; *see also* **RNA interference** [*RNA-* ribonucleic acid, *-i* interference, *therapy* treatment]

rod photoreceptor cell responsible for night vision [*rod* pole]

root blunt tip of the tongue; portion of the tooth that fits into the socket of the alveolar process of either the upper or lower jaw [*root* underground part of plant]

rotate (roh-TAYT) move in a circle around a central point [*rot-* turn, *-ate* process]

rotation joint movement around a longitudinal axis; for example, shaking your head "no" [*rot-* turn, *-ation* process]

rotator cuff (ROH-tay-tor) musculotendinous cuff resulting from fusion of the tendons of the supraspinatus, infraspinatus, teres minor, and subscapularis (SITS muscles); adds to the stability of the glenohumeral (shoulder) joint [*rot-* turn, *-ator* agent, *mus-* mouse, *-cle* little]

rotator cuff muscle (roh-TAY-tor) a muscle of the rotator cuff group [*rot-* turn, *-ator* agent, *mus-* mouse, *-cle* little]

round ligament (LIG-ah-ment) fibromuscular cord that extends from the upper, outer angles of the uterus through the inguinal canals and terminating in the labia majora [*liga-* bind, *-ment* condition]

round window opening into inner ear; covered by a membrane

rubrospinal tract (roo-broh-SPY-nal trakt) spinal cord nerves that transmit impulses that coordinate body movements and maintain posture [*rubro-* red, *-spin-* backbone, *-al* relating to, *tract* trail]

Ruffini corpuscle (roo-FEE-nee KOR-pus-ul) *see* **bulbous corpuscle** [*Angelo Ruffini* Italian anatomist, *corpus-* body, *-cle* little]

rule of nines frequently used method to estimate extent of a burn injury in an adult; the body is divided into areas that are multiples and fractions of 9%

S

S phase step of the cell life cycle in which a growing cell synthesizes a second copy of its nuclear DNA molecules, a process also called *DNA replication*, in anticipation of later reproduction (cell division); S phase follows the G_1 phase (first growth phase) and precedes the G_2 phase (second growth phase); *see* **cell life cycle** [*S* synthesis, *phase* appearance]

saccule (SAK-yool) part of the membranous labyrinth in the inner ear; contains sensory structure called a *macula*, which functions in sensation of static equilibrium [*sac-* bag, *-ule* small]

sacral plexus (SAY-kral PLEK-sus) plexus formed by fibres from the fourth and fifth lumbar nerves and the first four sacral nerves [*sacr-* sacred, *-al* relating to (sacrum), *plexus* braid or network] *pl.*, plexi (PLEK-sye) or plexuses (PLEK-sus-ez)

sacrum (SAY-krum) bone of the lower vertebral column between the last lumbar vertebra and the coccyx, formed by the fusion of five sacral vertebrae [*sacr-* sacred, *-um* thing]

sagittal plane (SAJ-ih-tal) longitudinal plane that divides the body or a part into left and right sides [*sagitta-* arrow, *-al* relating to, *plan-* flat surface]

saliva (sah-LYE-vah) secretion of the salivary glands that is made up of water, mucus, amylase, sodium bicarbonate, and lipase [*saliva* spittle]

salpingitis (sal-pin-JYE-tis) inflammation of the uterine tubes [*salping-* tube, *-itis* inflammation]

saltatory conduction (SAL-tah-tor-ee) process in which a nerve impulse travels along a myelinated fibre by jumping from one node of Ranvier to the next [*salta-* leap, *-ory* relating to]

sarcolemma (sar-koh-LEM-ah) plasma membrane of a striated muscle fibre [*sarco-* flesh, *-lemma* sheath] *pl.*, sarcolemmae (sar-koh-LEM-ee)

sarcoma (sar-KOH-mah) tumour of muscle tissue [*sarco-* flesh, *-oma* tumour]

sarcomere (SAR-koh-meer) contractile unit of muscle cells; length of a myofibril between two Z discs [*sarco-* flesh, *-mere* part]

sarcoplasm (SAR-koh-plaz-em) cytoplasm of muscle fibres [*sarco-* flesh, *-plasm* substance]

sarcoplasmic reticulum (SR) (sar-koh-PLAZ-mik reh-TIK-yoo-lum) network of tubules and sacs in muscle cells; similar to endoplasmic reticulum of other cells [*sarco-* flesh, *-plasm-* substance, *-ic* relating to, *ret-* net, *-ic-* relating to, *-ul-* little, *-um* thing] *pl.*, reticula

satellite cell a type of Schwann cell (neuroglial cell) that surrounds the cell bodies of neurons of the peripheral nervous system [*satell-* attendant, *-ite* relating to, *cell* storeroom]

satiety centre (sah-TYE-eh-tee) cells in the hypothalamus that send impulses to decrease appetite so that an individual feels satisfied; *see also* **leptin** [*sati-* enough or full, *-ety* state]

saturated condition when all available bonds of a hydrocarbon chain are filled with hydrogen atoms [*saturat-* fill]

saturated fat fats containing triglycerides in which fatty acid chains contain no double bonds (because they are "saturated" with hydrogen atoms) [*saturat-* fill]

scala tympani (SKAH-lah TIM-pah-nee) lower portion of the cochlear duct lying below the basilar membrane [*scala-* to climb, *tympani-* drum]

scala vestibuli (SKAH-lah ves-TIB-yoo-lye) upper portion of the cochlear duct scar-thickened mass of tissue, usually fibrous connective tissue, that remains after a damaged tissue has been repaired [*scala-* to climb, *vestibuli-* courtyard]

scanning electron microscopy (SEM) (eh-LEK-tron my-KROS-kah-pee) procedure that uses a beam of electrons to scan the surface of a specimen; the electrons reflected from, or knocked off, the surface are detected by a special sensor producing an image of the specimen's surface on a video monitor [*electro-* electric, *-on* subatomic particle, *micro-* small, *-scop-* see, *-y* activity]

scapula (SKAP-yoo-lah) upper extremity bone; shoulder blade [*scapula* shoulder blade] *pl.*, scapulae (SKAP-yoo-lee)

scar dense fibrous mass of tissue that remains after a damaged tissue has been repaired

Scheuermann disease (SHOY-er-man) abnormal skeletal condition developing in puberty that is characterized by increased roundness in the thoracic curvature (kyphosis) [*Holger W. Scheuermann*, Danish surgeon]

Schwann cell (shwon *or* shvon) any of the large nucleated cells that form myelin around the axons of neurons; also called *neurilemmocyte* [*Theodor Schwann* German anatomist]

sciatic nerve (sye-AT-ik nerv) largest nerve in the body [*(i)sci-* hip joint, *-atic* relating to]

sciatica (sye-AT-ih-kah) neuralgia of the sciatic nerve [*sciatica* hip pain]

science field of inquiry that uses rational or logical methods to determine the nature of the universe; biology is the branch of science that specifically studies the living organisms of the universe [*scienc-* knowledge]

sclera (SKLEH-rah) dense white lateral and posterior portion of the outer fibrous layer of the eyeball [*scler-* hard, *-a* thing or substance]

scleral venous sinus (SKLEH-ral VEE-nus SYE-nus) a ring-shaped venous sinus located deep within the anterior portion of the sclera; also called *canal of Schlemm* [*scler-* hard, *-al* relating to, *ven-* vein, *-ous* of or like, *sinus* hollow]

scleroderma (skleer-oh-DER-mah) rare disorder affecting vessels and connective tissue of skin and other tissues, characterized by tissue hardening [*sclero-* hard, *-derma* skin]

scoliosis (skoh-lee-OH-sis) abnormal lateral (side-to-side) curvature of the vertebral column [*scolio-* twisted or crooked, *-osis* condition]

scotoma (skoh-TOH-mah) form of neuritis (nerve inflammation), often associated with multiple sclerosis; can cause loss of only the centre of the visual field [*scoto-* darkness, *-oma* tumour]

scrotum (SKROH-tum) pouchlike sac that contains the testes [*scrotum* bag] *pl.*, scrota or scrotums

seasonal affective disorder (SAD) mental disorder in which a patient suffers severe depression only in winter; linked to the pineal gland [*season-* period of year, *-al* relating to, *affect-* act on, *-ive* relating to, *dis-* without, *-order* arrangement]

sebaceous gland (seh-BAY-shus) any of the oil-producing glands in the skin [*seb-* tallow (hard animal fat), *-ous* relating to, *gland* acorn]

sebum (SEE-bum) secretion of sebaceous glands [*sebum* tallow (hard animal fat)]

second messenger model theory of signal transduction (of hormones or neurotransmitters) in which the signal molecule binds to receptors of the target cell, which then triggers a second molecule within the cell (such as cyclic AMP) to accomplish its function; also called *fixed-membrane receptor model*

secondary bronchi (SEK-on-dair-ee BRONG-kye) *see* **secondary bronchus** [*second-* second, *-ary* relating to, *bronch-* windpipe]

secondary bronchus (SEK-on-dair-ee BRONG-kus) branch of the pulmonary airway formed when the primary bronchus enters the lung on its respective side and immediately splits into smaller bronchioles [*second-* second, *-ary* relating to, *bronchus* windpipe] *pl.*, bronchi (BRONG-kye)

secondary follicle (SEK-on-dair-ee FOL-ih-kul) *see* **graafian follicle** [*second-* second, *-ary* relating to, *folli-* bag, *-cle* small]

secondary hypertension (SEK-on-dair-ee hye-per-TEN-shun) high blood pressure resulting from a specific condition [*second-* second, *-ary* relating to, *hyper-* excessive, *-tens-* stretch or pull tight, *-sion* state]

secondary oocyte (SEK-on-dair-ee OH-oh-site or OH-uh-syte) oocyte that arises from a primary oocyte after it completes meiosis I [*second-* second, *-ary* relating to, *oo-* egg, *-cyte* cell]

secondary ossification centre (SEK-on-dair-ee os-ih-fih-KAY-shun) growth centre located in the epiphyses of long bones; *see* **primary ossification centre** [*second-* second, *-ary* relating to, *os-* bone, *-fic-* make, *-ation* process]

secondary protein structure (SEK-on-dair-ee PRO-teen STRUK-cher) second level of protein structure, formed after the primary structure (a strand of amino acids) curls and folds into a more complex structure; commonly occurring patterns of twists or folds with a specifc function are called *motifs* [*second-* second, *-ary* relating to, *prote-* primary, *-in* substance, *structur-* arrangement]

secondary sexual characteristics external physical characteristics of sexual maturity resulting from action of sex hormones; include male and female patterns of body hair and fat distribution, as well as development of external genitals [*secondary-* second, *-ary* relating to, *sexual-* relating to sex, *character-* engraved mark, *-istic* relating to]

second-messenger model (SEK-und MESS-en-jer MOD-el) model that explains nonsteroid hormone mechanism of action; nonsteroid hormone is "first messenger" acting on cell membrane; intracellular "second messenger"—often cyclic AMP—triggers specific cellular action; also called *fixed-membrane-receptor model*

secretin (seh-KREE-tin) gastrointestinal hormone; first hormone discovered [*secret-* separate, *-in* substance]

secretion process by which a substance is released outside the cell [*secret-* separate, *-tion* process]

secretory phase (SEEK-reh-toh-ree) *see* **premenstrual phase** [*secret-* separate, *-ory* relating to, *phase-* appearance]

section (SEK-shun) any cut made in the body or any of its parts; some sections are identified by the anatomical plane along which the cut was made (e.g., sagittal, coronal, transverse) [*sect-* cut, *-tion* process]

secretory vesicle (SEEK-reh-toh-ree VES-ih-kil) bubble made of cellular membrane; contains products of cell metabolism that move from inside the cell to the plasma membrane, where it breaks open and secretes the products outside of the cell [*secret-* separate, *-ory* relating to, *vesi-* bladder or blister, *-cle* small]

segmental reflex (seg-MEN-tal REE-fleks) reflex whose mediating reflexes enter and leave the same segment of the spinal cord [*segment-* cut section, *-al* relating to, *re-* again, *-flex* bend]

segmentation (seg-men-TAY-shun) occurs when digestive reflexes cause a forward-and-backward movement within a single region of the GI tract [*segment-* cut section, *-ation* process]

seizure (SEE-zhur) *see* **convulsion** [*seiz-* grasp suddenly, *-ure* result of action]

selectively permeable (sel-EK-tiv-lee PERM-ee-ah-bil) adjective used to describe a living membrane that allows only certain substances to move through (permeate) it and only at certain times [*select-* to choose, *-ive* relating to, *per-* through, *-mea(t)-* pass, *-able* capable of]

self concept in immunology that proposes the immune system agents can recognize certain cell surface molecules as belonging to that individual, which thus makes them "safe" from destruction or damage from the immune system [*self* one's own person]

self-antigen (AN-tih-jen) molecule located on the plasma membrane of all body cells that identifies all normal cells of the body for the immune system; also called *self-marker* [*self-* one's own person, *anti-* against, *-gen* produce]

self-examination process of looking at one's own body to screen for health abnormalities, as in breast self-examination or testicular self-examination [*self-* one's own person, *exam-* test or try, *-ation* process]

self-tolerance (self-TOL-er-unts) ability of our immune system to attack abnormal or foreign cells but spare our own normal cells [*self-* one's own person, *tolerare-* to endure]

semen (SEE-men) ejaculate from the penis that contains spermatozoa plus fluids from the testes, seminal vesicles, bulbourethral glands, and prostate [*semen* seed]

semicircular canal (sem-ih-SIR-kyoo-lar) three bony, tubelike structures located in the temporal bone, making up part of the inner ear; each structure contains a membranous semicircular duct that functions in the sense of equilibrium [*semi-* half, *-circul-* round, *-ar* relating to, *canal* channel]

semilunar (SL) valve (sem-ih-LOO-nar) valve located between each ventricle and the large artery that carries blood away from it; valves in the veins are sometimes referred to as *semilunar valves* [*semi-* half, *-luna* moon]

seminal vesicle (SEM-ih-nal VES-ih-kul) highly convoluted pouch that secretes an alkaline, viscous, creamy-yellow liquid that constitutes about 60% of semen volume [*semen-* seed, *-al* relating to, *vesic-* blister, *-cle* little]

seminiferous tubule (seh-mih-NIF-er-us TYOOB-yool) long, coiled structure that forms the bulk of the testicular mass and in which spermatozoa develop [*semin-* seed,

-fer- bear or carry, *-ous* relating to, *tub-* tube, *-ul-* little]

semipermeable (sem-ee-PERM-ee-ah-bil) adjective used to describe a membrane that allows only certain substances to move through (permeate) it; compare to **selectively permeable** [*semi-* half, *-per-* through, *-mea(t)-* pass, *-able* capable of]

semispinalis capitis muscle (sem-ee-spih-NAL-is KAP-ih-tis MUSS-el) broad muscle that extends the head at the neck and bends it laterally (adducts) [*semi-* half, *-spin-* thorn (spine), *-al-* relating to, *-is* thing, *capit-* head, *-is* thing, *mus-* mouse, *-cle* little]

senescence (seh-NES-enz) older adulthood; ageing [*senesc-* grow old, *-ence* state]

sensation interpretation of sensory nerve impulses by the brain as an awareness of an internal or external event; for example, feeling pain [*sens-* feel, *-ation* process]

sensor (SEN-ser) any agent or mechanism that detects a change in conditions (or stimulus) inside or outside the body, such as a sensory receptor [*sens-* feel, *-ory* relating to, *crani-* skull, *-al* relating to]

sensory cranial nerve (SEN-soh-ree KRAY-nee-al nerv) cranial nerve that consists of only sensory axons [*sens-* feel, *-ory* relating to, *crani-* skull, *-al* relating to]

sensory nerve (SEN-soh-ree nerv) nerve that contains primarily sensory neurons [*sens-* feel, *-ory* relating to]

sensory neuron (SEN-soh-ree NYOO-ron) neuron that transmits impulses to the spinal cord and brain from any part of the body [*sens-* feel, *-ory* relating to, *neuron* string or nerve]

sensory projection (SEN-soh-ree proh-JEK-shen) brain function that pinpoints the area of the body from which a receptor potential was initiated [*sens-* feel, *-ory* relating to, *project-* thrown forward, *-ion* process]

sensory receptor (SEN-soh-ree ree-SEP-ter) sense organs in the peripheral nervous system that enable the body to respond to stimuli caused by changes in its internal or external environment [*sens-* feel, *-ory* relating to, *recept-* receive, *-or* agent]

sentinel lymph node (SLN) (SEN-tin-el limf nohd) lymph node that is the first to receive a metastasized cancer cell from a nearby tumour [*sentinel* lookout, *lymph* water, *nod-* knot]

septic shock (SEP-tik) condition that results from complications of septicaemia [*septi-* putrid, *-ic* relating to]

septicaemia (sep-tih-SEE-mee-ah) blood poisoning [*septic-* putrid, *-(h)aem-* blood, *-ia* condition]

septum (SEP-tum) a wall that divides two areas; for example, nasal septum [*septum* wall] *pl.*, septa

serosa (see-ROH-sah) outermost covering of the digestive tract; composed of the parietal pleura in the abdominal cavity [*ser-* watery fluid, *-os-* relating to, *-a* thing] *pl.*, serosae (see-ROH-see)

serotonin (5-HT) (sair-oh-TOH-nin) neurotransmitter that belongs to a group of compounds called *monoamines*; also known as 5-hydroxytryptamine [*sero-* watery body fluid, *-ton-* tension, *-in* substance]

serotonin and norepinephrine reuptake inhibitor (SNRI) (sair-oh-TOH-nin and norep-ih-NEF-rin ree-UP-tayk in-HIB-it-or) type of drug that stops the return of serotonin and norepinephrine (neurotransmitters) to the presynaptic neuron, thus increasing the baseline amount of serotonin and/or norepinephrine in the synapse and restoring the baseline to a normal neurotransmitter level [*sero-* serum (watery fluid), *-ton-* tension, *-in* substance, *nor-* chemical prefix (unbranched C chain), *-epi-* upon, *-nephr-* kidney, *-ine* substance, *re-* again, *inhib-* restrain, *-or* agent]

serotonin-specific reuptake inhibitor (SSRI) (sair-oh-TOH-nin speh-SIF-ik ree-UP-tayk in-HIB-it-or) type of drug that stops the return of serotonin (neurotransmitter) to the presynaptic neuron, thus increasing the baseline amount of serotonin in the synapse and restoring the baseline to a normal serotonin level [*sero-* serum (watery fluid), *-ton-* tension, *-in-* substance, *-specif-* kind, *-ic* relating to, *re-* again, *inhib-* restrain, *-or* agent]

serous membrane (SEE-rus) two-layer epithelial membrane that lines body cavities and covers surfaces of organs [*sero-* watery body fluid, *-ous* characterized by, *membran-* thin skin]

serous pericardium (SEER-us pair-ih-KAR-dee-um) part of pericardial coverings of the heart; made up of a parietal layer and a visceral layer [*sero-* watery fluid, *-ous* relating to, *peri-* around, *-cardi-* heart, *-um* thing] *pl.*, pericardia

serratus anterior muscle (ser-RAY-tus) anterior chest wall muscle [*serra-* saw teeth, *ante-* front, *-er-* more, *-or* quality, *mus-* mouse, *-cle* little, *-us* thing]

Sertoli cell (ser-TOH-lee) testis cell found within walls of the seminiferous tubules; provides mechanical support and protection for the developing sperm; also called *sustentacular cell* or *nurse cell* [*Enrico Sertoli* Italian histologist, *cell* storeroom]

sesamoid bone (SES-ah-moyd) small seed-shaped bones imbedded in tendons; the patella is the largest and most consistently found in the human skeleton [*sesam-* sesame seed, *-oid* like]

set point normal reading or range of normal; also called *setpoint range* [*point-* distinguishing feature]

severe combined immunodeficiency (SCID) (ih-MYOON deh-FISH-en-see) condition in which stem cells are missing or are unable to grow properly; humoral immunity and cell-mediated immunity are defective [*immun-* free, *-de-* down, *-fic-* perform, *-ency* state]

sex chromosome (KROH-moh-sohm) pair of chromosomes in the human genome that determine gender; normal males have one X chromosome and one Y chromosome (XY); normal females have two X chromosomes (XX) [*chrom-* colour, *-som-* body]

sex hormone (seks HOR-mohn) hormone that targets reproductive tissue; examples include oestrogen, progesterone, and testosterone [*hormon-* excite]

sex-linked trait nonsexual, inherited trait governed by genes located in a sex chromosome (X or Y); most known sex-linked traits are X-linked [*link-* joint, *trait-* feature]

sexually transmitted diseases (STDs) any communicable disease that is commonly transmitted through sexual contact [*sexual-* relating to sex, *transmit-* transfer, *dis-* opposite of, *ease*]

shaft *see* **diaphysis** [*shaft* slender rod]

shingles (SHING-guls) *see* **herpes zoster** [from *cingulum* girdle (inflammation often extends around the middle of the body, like a girdle]

short bone cube- or box-shaped bone that is about as broad as it is long; for example, carpals and tarsals [*short* stunted]

shoulder girdle clavicle and scapula, which form the only bony attachment of the upper extremity to the trunk [*girdle* belt or sash]

shunt tube used to drain the flow of a body fluid from one cavity or vessel to another [*shunt* to shun]

sickle cell anaemia (SIK-ul sell ah-NEE-mee-ah) severe, possibly fatal, hereditary disease in which red blood cells become sickle-shaped because of presence of an abnormal type of haemoglobin [*sickle* crescent, *cell* storeroom, *an-* without, *-(h)aem-* blood, *-ia* condition]

sickle cell trait (SIK-ul sell trayt) condition that occurs when only one gene for sickle cell is inherited and only a small amount of abnormal haemoglobin is produced [*sickle* crescent, *cell* storeroom, *trait-* feature]

sigmoid colon (SIG-moyd) portion of the large intestine that courses downward below the iliac crest [*sigm-* sigma (Σ or σ) 18th letter of Greek alphabet (Roman S), *-oid* like, *colon* colon]

sign objective deviation from normal that marks the presence of a disease [*sign* mark]

signal transduction (tranz-DUK-shun) process of changing a signal such as a hormone or neurotransmitter into another form such as enzymatic reaction within the cell receiving the signal (thus the extracellular hormone signal is transduced, or changed, to an intracellular enzymatic signal) [*trans-* across, *-duc-* transfer, *-tion* process]

signal transduction inhibitor (tranz-DUK-shun in-HIB-ih-tor) any agent that blocks normal processing (transduction) of physiological signalling at a membrane receptor [*trans-* across, *-duc-* transfer, *-tion* process, *inhibit-* prevent, *-or* agent]

silent gallstone gallstone that does not cause a problem [*gall* bile]

simple diffusion movement of molecules through a membrane by means of the natural tendency of the molecules to spread and the ability of the spreading molecules to move through, or permeate [*simple* not mixed, *diffus-* spread out, *-sion* process]

simple epithelium (ep-ih-THEE-lee-um) arrangement of epithelial cells in a single layer [*simple* not mixed, *epi-* on, *-theli-* nipple, *-um* thing] *pl.*, epithelia (ep-ih-THEE-lee-ah)

simple fracture type of bone fracture in which broken bone does not project through surrounding tissue and skin; also called *nondisplaced* or *closed fracture* [*simple* not mixed, *fracture* a breaking]

simple goitre (GOY-ter) condition in which the thyroid enlarges because iodine is lacking in the diet [*simple* not mixed, from *gutter* throat]

single unit smooth muscle most common type of smooth muscle tissue; smooth muscle tissue in which gap junctions join individual smooth muscle fibres into large, continuous sheets that contract together in an autorhythmic fashion; also called *visceral muscle* [*mus-* mouse, *-cle* little]

single-gene disease disease caused by individual mutant genes in nuclear DNA that pass from one generation to the next [*gen-* produce or generate, *dis-* opposite of, *-ease* comfort]

single-photon emission computed tomography (SPECT) (toh-MOG-rah-fee) method of scanning that is used to visualize blood flow patterns in the brain [*photo-* light, *e-* out, *-mission* send, *tomo-* cut, *-graph-* draw, *-y* activity]

sinoatrial (SA) node (sye-no-AY-tree-al) the heart's pacemaker; where the impulse conduction of the heart normally starts; located in the wall of the right atrium near the opening of the superior vena cava [*sin-* hollow (sinus), *atri-* entrance courtyard, *-al* relating to, *nod-* knot]

sinus (SYE-nus) space or cavity [*sinus* hollow]

sinus dysrhythmia (SYE-nus dis-RITH-mee-ah) variation in rhythm of heart rate during the breathing cycle (inspiration and expiration) [*sinus* hollow, *dys-* disordered, *-rhythm-* movement in time, *-ia* condition]

sinusitis (sye-nus-SYE-tis) sinus inflammation [*sinus-* hollow, *-itis* inflammation]

sinusoid (SYE-nuh-soyd) capillary that has a much larger lumen and more winding or tortuous course than other capillary vessels [*sinus-* hollow, *-oid* like]

Sjögren syndrome (SHOW-grin SIN-drohm) autoimmune disease in which the body's immune system targets salivary and tear glands for destruction [*Henrik S. C. Sjögren* Swedish ophthalmologist, *syn-* together, *-drome* running or (race) course]

skeletal muscle (SKEL-et-al or skeh-LEET-al) muscle organ or muscle tissue under willed or voluntary control; *see* **skeletal muscle tissue** [*skeleto-* dried body, *-al* relating to, *mus-* mouse, *-cle* small]

skeletal muscle tissue (SKEL-et-al or skeh-LEET-al) also known as *voluntary* or *striated voluntary muscle*; includes muscle fibres under willed or voluntary control [*skeleto-* dried body, *-al* relating to, *mus-* mouse, *-cle* small, *tissu-* fabric]

skeletal system (SKEL-et-al) interconnected system of bones, cartilage, and ligaments that provide the body with a rigid framework for support and protection [*skeleto-* dried body, *-al* relating to]

skin *see* **cutaneous membrane**

sleep apnoea (APP-nee-ah) transitional period of sleep characterized by loud snoring to variable periods of complete cessation of breathing [*a-* not, *-pnoea* breathe]

sliding filament model theory of muscle contraction in which sliding of thin filaments toward the centre of each sarcomere quickly shortens the muscle fibre and thereby the entire muscle

slow (B) pain fibre type of nerve fibre that carries impulses that result in dull, aching pain; originates in deep body structures [*slow-* inactive, sluggish, *poena-* punishment]

slow muscle fibre red muscle fibre; also called *slow-twitch muscle fibre* [*mus-* mouse, *-cle* small, *fibre-* thread]

slow-wave sleep (SWS) stage of sleep that is characterized by slow-frequency, high-voltage delta rays seen in the EEG during deep sleep

small saphenous vein (sah-FEE-nus vayn) superficial vein of the lower extremity [*saphen-* manifest, *-ous* relating to, *vena* blood vessel]

smooth muscle muscle fibres that are not under conscious control; also known as *involuntary* or *visceral muscle*; forms the walls of blood vessels and hollow organs [*mus-* mouse, *-cle* small]

smooth muscle tissue *see* **smooth muscle** [*mus-* mouse, *-cle* small, *tissu-* fabric]

sneeze reflex (sneez REE-fleks) a burst of air directed through the nose and mouth; stimulated by contaminants in the nasal cavity [*re-* back or again, *-flex* bend]

sodium (SO-dee-um) important positive ion surrounding cells [*sod-* soda, *-um* thing or substance]

sodium channel (SO-dee-um CHAN-el) pore in a cell membrane that allows only sodium ions to permeate, or pass through, the membrane [*sod-* soda, *-um* thing or substance, *channel-* water pipe]

sodium cotransport (SO-dee-um koh-TRANS-port) complex transport process in which carriers that bind both sodium ions and glucose molecules passively transport the molecules together out of the GI lumen [*sod-* soda, *-ium* chemical ending, *co-* with, *-trans-* across, *-port* carry]

sodium lactate (SO-dee-um LAK-tayt) compound used to treat metabolic and respiratory acidosis [*sod-* soda, -um thing or substance, *lact-* milk, *-ate* chemical]

sodium–potassium pump (SO-dee-um poh-TAS-ee-um pump) active transport pump that operates in the plasma membrane of all human cells; transports both sodium ions and potassium ions but in opposite directions and in a 3:2 ratio, thereby maintaining a gradient across the plasma membrane [*sod-* soda, *-um* thing or substance, *potass-* potash, *-um* thing or substance]

soft palate (soft PAL-et) partition between the mouth and nasopharynx [*palate-* roof of mouth]

soleus muscle (SOH-lee-us MUSS-el) leg muscle that extends the foot [*soleus* sole of foot, *mus-* mouse, *-cle* little]

solubility (sol-yoo-BIL-ih-tee) relative ability to dissolve [*solu-* dissolve, *-bil-* capable, *-ity* state]

solute (SOL-yoot) dissolved particles in solution [*solut-* dissolved]

solution liquid made up of a mixture of molecule types, usually made of solutes (solids) scattered in a solvent (liquid), such as salt in water [*solut-* dissolved, *-ion* process]

solvent (SOL-vent) liquid portion of a solution in which a solute is dissolved [*solv-* dissolve, *-ent* agent]

soma (SO-mah) body; for example, the body of a neuron; also called *perikaryon* [*soma* body]

somatic (so-MAH-tik) referring to the body [*soma-* body, *-ic* relating to]

somatic motor neuron (so-MAH-tik MOH-tor NYOO-ron) motor neuron that stimulates a muscle fibre [*soma-* body, *-ic* relating to, *mot-* move, *-or* agent, *neuron-* nerve]

somatic nervous system (SNS) (so-MAH-tik) motor neurons that control voluntary actions of skeletal muscles [*soma-* body, *-ic* relating to, *nerv-* nerves, *-ous* relating to]

somatic pain (so-MAH-tik) sharp "take your breath away" type of pain associated with superficial injury or trauma; also called *fast pain* [*soma-* body, *-ic* relating to]

somatic reflex (so-MAH-tik REE-fleks) reflexive contraction of skeletal muscles [*soma-* body, *-ic* relating to, *re-* again, *-flex* bend]

somatic sense (so-MAH-tik) sense that enables an individual to detect sensations such as pain, temperature, and proprioception [*soma-* body, *-ic* relating to, *sens-* feel]

somatic sensory division (so-MAH-tik) division of the nervous system made up of afferent (incoming) pathways from somatic sensory receptors (receptors involved in conscious perception) [*soma-* body, *-ic* relating to, *sens-* feel, *-ory* relating to]

somatopsychic (so-mah-toh-SYE-kik) refers to the body affecting the mind; physical disorder that produces mental symptoms; *see* **psychosomatic** [*soma-* body, *-psychic* relation between mind and body]

somatostatin (soh-mah-toh-STAT-in) hormone produced by delta cells of the pancreas that inhibits secretion of glucagon, insulin, and pancreatic polypeptide [*soma-* body, *-stat-* stand, *-in* substance]

somatotroph (soh-mah-toh-TROHF) cell type of the adenohypophysis (anterior pituitary) that secretes growth hormone (somatotropin) [*soma-* body, *-troph* nourish]

somatotropin (STH) (soh-mah-toh-TROH-pin) growth hormone [*soma-* body, *-trop-* nourish, *-in* substance]

somatotype (so-MAT-oh-type) classification of body type determined on the basis of certain physical characteristics; *see also* **ectomorph, endomorph, mesomorph** [*soma-* body, *-type* kind]

snRNP (snurp) small nuclear ribonucleoprotein particle; it forms subunits of the spliceosome used in editing mRNA in a cell's nucleus [acronym for small nuclear ribonucleoprotein particle]

spastic paralysis (SPAS-tik pah-RAL-ih-sis) type of paralysis characterized by involuntary contractions of affected muscles [*spast-* pull, *-ic* relating to, *para-* beyond, *-lysis* loosening]

spatial summation (SPAY-shal sum-MAY-shun) ability of the postsynaptic neuron to add together the inhibitory and stimulatory input received from numerous different presynaptic neurons and produce an action potential based on that collation of information [*spati-* space, *-al* relating to, *summa-* total, *-tion* process]

special movement (SPESH-ul MOOV-ment) unique or unusual movement that occurs only in a very limited number of joints [*spec-* form or kind, *-al* relating to]

special sense characterized by receptors grouped closely together or grouped in a complex sensory organ; for example, sense of smell, taste, hearing, equilibrium, or vision [*spec-* form or kind, *-al* relating to]

species resistance (SPEE-sheez ree-ZIS-tens) genetic characteristics common to all organisms of a particular species that provide natural inborn immunity to a certain disease [*species* form or kind, *resist-* withstand, *-ance* act of]

specific heat the ratio of the heat capacity of a substance to the heat capacity of water, equivalent to the amount of heat required to raise 1 gram of substance 1 degree centigrade [*spec-* form or kind, *-ific* relating to]

specific immunity (im-YOO-nih-tee) protective mechanisms by which the immune system is able to recognize, remember, and destroy specific types of bacteria or toxins; *see* **adaptive immunity** [*spec-* form or kind, *-ific* relating to, *immun-* free, *-ity* state]

spectrin (SPEK-trin) unique protein on red blood cells that makes it possible for them to be flexible enough to pass through small blood capillaries [*spect-* look, *-in* substance]

sperm mature male gamete; sperm cell or spermatozoon [*sperm* seed] *pl.*, sperms or sperm

spermatic cord (sper-MAT-ik) cylindrical casings of white fibrous tissue formed by the ductus deferens and located in the inguinal canal between the scrotum and the abdominal cavity [*sperma-* seed, *-ic* relating to]

spermatogenesis (sper-mah-toh-JEN-eh-sis) production of sperm cells [*sperm-* seed, *-gen-* produce, *-esis* process]

spermatogonium (sper-mah-toh-GO-nee-um) stem cell of a population that gives rise to sperm cells [*sperm-* seed, *-gonia* offspring] *pl.*, spermatogonia (sper-mah-toh-GO-nee-ah)

spermatozoon (sper-mah-tah-ZOH-on) mature male gamete; sperm cell [*sperma-* seed, *-zoon* animal] *pl.*, spermatozoa (sper-mah-tah-ZOH-ah)

sphenoid bone (SFEE-noyd) keystone bone of the cranium; resembles a bat [*spheno-* wedge, *-oid* like]

sphincter urethrae muscle (SFINGK-ter yoo-REE-three) *see* **urethral sphincter** [*sphinc-* bind tight, *-er* agent, *ure-* urine, *-thr-* agent or channel (urethra), *mus-* mouse, *-cle* little]

sphygmomanometer (sfig-moh-mah-NOM-eh-ter) device for measuring blood pressure in the arteries of a limb [*sphygmo-* pulse, *-mano-* thin, *-meter* measure]

spinal cord (SPY-nul kord) portion of central nervous system that provides two-way conduction from the brain; major reflex centre [*spin-* backbone, *-al* relating to]

spinal ganglion (SPY-nul GANG-glee-on) enlarged portion of the dorsal root of the spinal cord, where afferent nerve fibres from sensory receptors synapse with associated sensory neurons on their way to the brain or lower reflex centres [*spin-* backbone, *-al* relating to, *ganglion* knot]

spinal meningitis (SPY-nul men-in-JYE-tis) inflammation of the spinal meninges [*spin-* backbone, *-al* relating to, *meninx-* membrane, *-itis* inflammation]

spinal nerve (SPY-nul nerv) nerve that connects the spinal cord to peripheral structures such as the skin and skeletal muscles [*spin-* backbone, *-al* relating to]

spinal reflex (SPY-nul REE-fleks) reflex arc whose centre is located in the spinal cord [*spine-* backbone, *-al* relating to, *re-* again, *-flex* bend]

spinal tract (SPY-nul trakt) white columns of the spinal cord that provide conduction paths to and from the brain; ascending tracts carry information to the brain, whereas descending tracts conduct impulses from the brain [*spin-* backbone, *-al* relating to, *tract* trail]

spindle fibre (SPIN-dul FYE-ber) network of tubules formed in the cytoplasm between the centrioles as they are moving away from each other during mitosis [*spind-* spin, *-le* agent, *fibre* thread]

spinnbarkeit (SPIN-bahr-kyte) characteristic of fluids that allow them to be stretched into a fibre; fibrosity; observed cervical mucus around the time of ovulation [*spinnbarkeit* spinnability (German)]

spinocerebellar tract (SPY-no-sair-eh-BELL-ar trakt) sensory tract that conveys information about subconscious kinaesthesia [*spino-* backbone, *-cerebell-* cerebellum (small brain), *-ar* relating to, *tract* trail]

spinotectal tract (SPY-no-TEK-tal trakt) sensory tract that conveys information about touch that triggers visual reflexes [*spino-* backbone, *-tect-* roof, *-al* relating to, *tract* trail]

spinothalamic pathway (spy-no-thah-LAM-ik) pathway that conducts impulses that produce sensations of crude touch and pressure [*spino-* backbone, *-thalam-* inner chamber, *-ic* relating to]

spinothalamic tract (spy-no-thah-LAM-ik trakt) ascending tracts of the spinal cord that convey information about pain, temperature, deep pressure, and coarse touch; these tracts cross over in the spinal cord [*spino-* backbone, *-thalam-* inner chamber, *-ic* relating to, *tract* trail]

spinous process (SPY-nus PRO-ses) sharp projection from the laminae of vertebral bones, pointing posteriorly and inferiorly [*spino-* thorn or backbone, *-ous* relating to, *process* project (from)] *pl.*, processes (PRO-ses-eez)

spiral fracture type of bone fracture in which fracture line spirals around the long axis [*spir-* coiled, *-al* relating to, *fracture* a breaking]

spiral membrane floor of the cochlear duct; this structure's vibrating response to sound frequencies leads to the transduction of sound waves into nerve impulses; also called *basilar membrane* [*spir-* coiled, *-al* relating to, *membran-* thin skin]

spiral muscle muscle that has fibres twisted between their points of attachment; for example, latissimus dorsi [*spir-* coiled, *-al* relating to, *mus-* mouse, *-cle* little]

spiral organ organ of hearing located in the cochlea; consists of membranes and embedded hair cells capable of converting mechanical motion of sound waves into neural impulses; also called *organ of Corti* [*spir-* coiled, *-al* relating to, *organ* tool or instrument]

spirogram (SPY-roh-gram) graphic recording of the changing pulmonary volumes observed during breathing [*spir-* breathe, *-gram* drawing]

spirometer (spih-ROM-eh-ter) instrument used to measure the amount of air exchanged in breathing [*spir-* breathe, *-meter* measure]

splanchnic nerve (SPLANK-nik nerv) nerve that innervates the viscera [*splanchn-* internal organ, *-ic* relating to]

spleen largest lymphoid organ; filters blood, destroys worn out red blood cells, salvages iron from haemoglobin, and serves as a blood reservoir

splenectomy (spleh-NEK-toh-mee) surgical removal of the spleen [*splen-* spleen, *-ec-* out, *-tom-* cut, *-y* action]

splenius capitis (SPLEH-nee-us KAP-ih-tis) deep muscle of the neck; extends the head [*splen-* patch, *capit-* head, *-is* thing]

splenomegaly (spleh-no-MEG-ah-lee) condition of enlargement of the spleen [*splen-* spleen, *-mega* large, *-ly* relating to]

spliceosome (SPLISE-oh-sohm) small structure within the nucleus, about the size of a ribosome and made up of snRNPs (small nuclear ribonucleotides) along with polypeptides; removes introns from mRNA transcript and splices remaining exons into final version of mRNA [*splice-* cut rope and join remaining ends, *-som-* body]

spongy bone net-like arrangement of bone tissue found inside bones and which is often filled with red marrow; also called *cancellous bone* or *trabecular bone*

spontaneous abortion (spon-TAY-nee-us ah-BOR-shun) *see* **miscarriage** [*ab-* away from, *-or-* be born, *-tion* process]

spontaneous fracture (spon-TAY-nee-us FRAK-chur) *see* **pathological fracture** [*fracture* a breaking]

spore form assumed by a bacterium that is resistant to heat, drying, and chemicals but can later become active to cause infection [*spore* seed]

sprain injury to ligamentous joint structures often caused by twisting or wrenching movements [unknown origin]

squamous (SKWAY-muss) scalelike [*squam-* scale, *-ous* characterized by]

squamous cell carcinoma (SKWAY-muss sell kar-sih-NO-mah) slow-growing skin cancer that arises in the epidermis [*squam-* scale, *-ous* characterized by, *cell* storeroom, *carcin-* cancer, *-oma* tumour]

stage of exhaustion (stayj ov eg-ZAWS-chun) third stage of the general adaptation syndrome; when the body can no longer cope or adapt to stressors [*exhaust-* drain away, *-ion* process]

stage of resistance (stayj ov ree-ZIS-tens) second stage of the general adaptation syndrome [*resist-* withstand, *-ance* state]

staircase phenomenon (feh-NOM-eh-non) *see* **treppe** [*stair-* single step, *-case* box, *phenomenon-* that which appears or is seen]

standard lead one of three electrodes (lead *I*, lead *II*, or lead *III*) used in electrocardiography

Starling's law of the capillaries (STAR-lingz cap-IL-air-eez) principle that states that a balance between inwardly directed forces and outwardly directed forces will determine whether fluids will move into or out of the plasma in the capillaries at any particular point [*Ernest H. Starling* English physiologist, *capill-* hair, *-ary* relating to]

Starling's law of the heart (STAR-lingz) principle stating that as myocardial fibres are stretched, the force of contraction is increased [*Ernest H. Starling* English physiologist]

static equilibrium (STAT-ik ee-kwih-LIB-ree-um) sensing the position of the head relative to gravity; compare with **dynamic equilibrium** [*stat-* stand, *-ic* relating to, *equi-* equal, *-libr-* balance]

static tension another name for isometric (muscle) contraction [*stat-* stand, *-ic* relating to, *tendere-* to stretch]

steatorrhoea (stee-ah-toh-REE-ah) foul-smelling stool as a result of impaired fat absorption [*steat-* fat, *-o-* combining form, *-rrhoea* flow]

stellate macrophage (of the liver) (STEL-ayt MAK-roh-fayj) macrophage found in spaces between liver cells; a type of dendritic cell (DC) of innate immunity; commonly known as *Kupffer cell* [*stell-* star, *-ate* of or like, *macro-* large, *-phag-* eat]

stem cell cells that have the ability to maintain a constant population of newly differentiating cells [*stem* tree trunk, *cell* storeroom]

stenosed valve (steh-NOSD) valve that is narrower than normal, slowing blood flow from a heart chamber [*stenos-* narrow, *-osis* condition]

stent (stent) metal spring or mesh tube inserted into an affected artery to keep it open [*Charles Stent* English dentist]

stereognosis (steh-ree-og-NO-sis) awareness of an object's size, shape, and texture [*steros-* solid, *-gnosis* knowledge]

sterility (steh-RIL-ih-tee) loss of reproductive function [*steril-* barren, *-ity* state]

sternocleidomastoid muscle (STERN-oh-KLYE-doh-MAS-toyd) muscle that flexes the head; "prayer" muscle [*sterno-* breast-bone (sternum), *-cleid-* key (clavicle), *-masto-* breast (mastoid process), *-oid* like, *mus-* mouse, *-cle* little]

sternum (STER-num) breastbone [*sternum* breastbone] *pl.*, sterna (STER-nah) or sternums

steroid (STAYR-oid) any of a class of lipids related to sterols and forming numerous reproductive and adrenal hormones [*ster-* sterol, *-oid* like]

steroid hormone (STAYR-oyd HOR-mohn) lipid-soluble hormone that passes intact through the cell membrane of the target cell and influences cell activity by acting on specific genes [*ster-* sterol, *-oid* like, *hormon-* excite]

stillbirth delivery of a dead fetus after the twentieth week of gestation; before 20 weeks it is termed a *spontaneous abortion*

stimulus (STIM-yoo-lus) any change, often an excitant or irritating agent, that induces a response [*stimulus* incitement]

stimulus-gated channel type of cell-membrane channel for the transport of molecules that is controlled by a gate that responds to a stimulus such as a sensory stimulus or chemical (neurotransmitter) stimulus [*stimulus* incitement, *channel* water pipe]

stomach organ of the digestive system; an expansion of the digestive tract between the oesophagus and small intestine, where some protein digestion begins and where food is churned and mixed with gastric juices before entering the small intestine [*stomach* opening]

stomach cancer gastric carcinoma [*stomach* opening, *cancer* crab or malignant tumour]

strabismus (strah-BIS-mus) abnormal condition in which lack of coordination of, or weakness in, the muscles that control the eye causes improper focusing of images on the retina, making depth perception difficult [*strab-* squinting, *-ismus* condition]

strain overexertion or trauma-type injury resulting in tearing of skeletal muscle fibres [*strain* stretch]

stratified epithelium (STRAT-ih-fyde ep-ih-THEE-lee-um) epithelial cells layered one on another [*strati-* layer, *-fied* made, *epi-* on, *-theli-* nipple, *-um* thing] *pl.*, epithelia (ep-ih-THEE-lee-ah)

stratum (STRAH-tum) layer [*stratum* layer] *pl.*, strata (STRAH-tah)

stratum basale (STRAH-tum bay-SAH-lee) "base layer"; deepest layer of the epidermis; cells in this layer are able to reproduce themselves [*stratum* layer, *bas-* base, *-ale* relating to] *pl.*, strata basales (STRAH-tah bay-SAH-leez)

stratum compactum (STRAH-tum kom-PAKT-um) surface layer of the endometrium in the uterus [*stratum* layer, *compact-* concentrated, *-um* thing] *pl.*, strata compacta (STRAH-tah kom-PAKT-ah)

stratum corneum (STRAH-tum KOR-nee-um) tough outer layer of the epidermis; cells are filled with keratin [*stratum* layer, *corneum* horn] *pl.*, strata (STRAH-tah KOR-nee-ah)

stratum germinativum (STRAH-tum jer-min-ah-TIV-um) synonym for stratum basale of the skin epidermis; sometimes used to denote stratum basale and stratum spinosum together [*stratum* layer, *germinativum* something that sprouts] *pl.*, strata germinativa (STRAH-tah jer-min-ah-TIV-ah)

stratum granulosum (STRAH-tum gran-yoo-LOH-sum) "granular layer"; layer in which the process of keratinization begins [*stratum* layer, *gran-* grain, *-ul-* little, *-osum* thing] *pl.*, strata granulosa (STRAH-tah gran-yoo-LOH-sah)

stratum lucidum (STRAH-tum LOO-see-dum) "clear" layer of the epidermis, in thick skin between the stratum granulosum and the stratum corneum [*stratum* layer, *lucid-* clear, *-um* thing] *pl.*, strata lucida (STRAH-tah LOO-see-dah)

stratum spinosum (STRAH-tum spih-NO-sum) "spiny layer"; layer of epidermis that is rich in RNA to aid in protein synthesis required for keratin production [*stratum* layer, *spino-* spine, *-um* thing] *pl.*, strata spinosa (STRAH-tah spih-NO-sah)

stratum spongiosum (STRA-tum spon-gee-OH-sum) middle layer of the endometrium (of uterus), composed of loose fibrous connective tissue [*stratum* layer, *spongia-* sponge, *-um* thing] *pl.*, strata spongiosa (STRAH-tah spon-gee-OH-sah)

strength training contracting muscles against resistance to enhance muscle hypertrophy; *see also* **aerobic training, endurance training** [*strength-* power, *train-* instruct]

stress (stres) any stimulus that directly or indirectly stimulates neurons of the hypothalamus to release corticotropin-releasing hormone [*stress* tighten]

stress fracture (stres FRAK-chur) bone fracture caused by mechanical stress (pressure) [*stress* tighten, *fracture* a breaking]

stress response (stres ree-SPONS) *see* **stress syndrome** [*stress* tighten, *response* reply]

stress syndrome (stres SIN-drohm) signs and symptoms associated with the body's frequently maladaptive response to stressors; diverse changes initiated by a threat [*stress* tighten, *syn-* together, *-drome* running or (race) course]

stress triad (stres TRYE-ad) three changes (hypertrophied adrenals, atrophied lymphatic organs, and bleeding gastrointestinal ulcers) as described by Selye that occur together characterize not any one particular kind of injury but all kinds of harmful stimuli [*stress* tighten, *triad* group of three]

stress–age syndrome (stres-AYJ SIN-drohm) refers to a group of anatomical, neurohormonal, and immune system changes related to ageing that influence both physiological and psychological stress responses [*stress-* tighten, *syn-* together, *-drome* running or (race) course]

stressor (STRES-er) any agent or stimulus that produces stress [*stress-* tighten, *-or* agent]

stress–relaxation effect (stres-ree-laks-AY-shun ef-FEKT) effect that occurs when overall blood pressure rises and the elastic nature of blood vessels allows them to expand and adapt to the higher pressure to maintain normal blood flow [*stress-* tighten, *relax-* loosen, *-ation* process, *effect* accomplishment]

stretch marks tiny silver-white scars resulting when elastic fibres in the dermis are stretched too much; also called *striae* [*stretch-* pull tight, *mark-* appearance]

stretch reflex (stretch REE-fleks) automatic response in which the muscle reacts and tries to maintain a constancy of muscle length when a load is applied [*re-* again, *-flex* bend]

Stretta procedure (STRETT-ah) procedure for treating serious cases of GORD; uses radiofrequency energy emitted by a special electrode to produce small burns that tighten the muscular wall of the lower oesophageal sphincter and reduce acid reflux from the stomach; *Stretta* is a brand name [*stretta* tight]

striated involuntary muscle (STRYE-ay-ted) cardiac muscle [*stri-* stripe, *-ate-* characterized by, *mus-* mouse, *-cle* little]

striated muscle (STRYE-ay-ted) *see* **skeletal muscle** [*stri-* stripe, *-ate-* characterized by, *mus-* mouse, *-cle* little]

stricture (STRIK-chur) abnormally narrowed passage [*stric-* tighten, *-ture* condition]

stroke event in which haemorrhage or cessation of blood flow caused by an embolism or ruptured aneurysm in brain blood vessel results in ischaemia of brain tissue and destruction of neurons; *see* **cerebrovascular accident (CVA)** [*stroke* a strike]

stroke volume (SV) amount of blood that is ejected from the ventricles of the heart with each beat [*stroke* a strike]

structural protein any of a category of proteins with the primary function of forming structures of the cell or tissue; contrast with *functional protein* [*structura-* arrangement, *-al* relating to, *prote-* primary, *-in* substance]

subarachnoid space (sub-ah-RAK-noyd) within the meninges, space under the arachnoid and outside the pia mater [*sub-* beneath, *-arachn-* spider, *-oid* like]

subareolar plexus (sub-ah-REE-oh-lar PLEKS-us) where the cutaneous plexus and large lymphatics that drain the secretory tissue and ducts of the breast come together [*sub-* beneath, *areola-* little space, *-ar* relating to, *plexus* braid or network]

subatomic particle (sub-ah-TOM-ik PART-ih-kul) any of the particles that make up atoms; for example, neutrons, protons, and electrons [*sub-* beneath, *-atom* indivisible, *-ic* relating to, *part-* bit, *-icle* little]

subclavian artery (sub-KLAY-vee-an AR-ter-ee) artery of the upper extremity [*sub-* below, *-clavi-* key, *-ula* little, *arteri-* vessel]

subclavian vein (sub-KLAY-vee-an vayn) deep vein of the upper extremity [*sub-* below, *-clavi-* key (clavicle bone), *-an* relating to, *vena* blood vessel]

subcutaneous injection (sub-kyoo-TAY-nee-us in-JEK-shun) administration of nutrients, special fluids, and/or electrolytes into the spongy and porous subcutaneous layer beneath the skin [*sub-* under, *cut-* skin, *-aneous* relating to, *in-* in, *-ject-* throw, *-tion* process]

subcutaneous layer (sub-kyoo-TAY-nee-us) *see* **hypodermis** [*sub-* beneath, *-cut-* skin, *-ous* relating to]

subdural space (sub-DYOO-ral) within the meninges; the space between the dura mater and the arachnoid membrane [*sub-* beneath, *-dura-* hard or tough, *-al* relating to]

subendocardial branches (sub-en-doh-KAR-dee-al) conductive cardiac muscle fibres located in the walls of the ventricles; relay impulses from the AV node to the ventricles, causing them to contract; also called *Purkinje fibres* [*sub-* under, *-endo-* within, *-cardi-* heart, *-al* relating to]

subfornical organ (SFO) (sub-FOR-nih-kal) highly specialized nerve cells located in the roof of the third ventricle in the brain; critical regulator of fluid homeostasis [*sub-* under, *-fornic-* arch, *-al* relating to]

sublingual gland (sub-LING-gwall) smallest of the three major salivary glands; produces a mucous type of saliva [*sub-* under, *-lingua-* tongue, *-al* relating to, *gland* acorn]

submandibular gland (sub-man-DIB-yoo-lar) salivary gland located just below the mandibular angle; contains enzyme and mucus-producing elements [*sub-* under, *-mandibul-* chew (mandible or jawbone), *-ar* relating to, *gland* acorn]

submandibular group (sub-man-DIB-yoo-lar) group of lymph nodes under the mandible [*sub-* beneath, *-mandibul-* chew (mandible or jawbone), *-ar* relating to]

submaxillary group (sub-MAK-sih-lair-ee) alternate name for *submandibular group* [*sub-* beneath, *-maxilla-* upper jaw, *-ary* relating to]

submental group (sub-MEN-tal) group of lymph nodes located in the floor of the mouth; lymph from the nose, lips, and teeth drains through these nodes [*sub-* beneath, *-ment-* chin, *-al* relating to]

submucosa (sub-myoo-KOH-sah) connective tissue layer containing blood vessels and nerves in the wall of the digestive tract [*sub-* under, *-muc-* slime, *-os-* relating to, *-a* thing] *pl.*, submucosae (sub-myoo-KOH-see)

subscapularis muscle (sub-skap-yoo-LAR-is) one of a group of muscles (rotator cuff) that serve as both a structural and functional cuff around the shoulder joint [*sub-* beneath, *-scapula-* shoulder blades, *-ar* relating to, *mus-* mouse, *-cle* little]

substantia nigra (sub-STAN-shee-ah NYE-grah) midbrain structure that consists of clusters of cell bodies of neurons involved in muscular control [*substantia* substance, *nigra* black]

substrate (SUB-strayt) substance on which an enzyme acts [*sub-* below, *-strat-* layer]

subtalar joint (sub-TAY-ler joynt) diarthrotic synovial joint formed by the talus bone of the ankle overlying the calcaneus bone; permits side-to-side motion of the foot [*sub-* below, *-tal-* ankle (talus), *-ar* relating to]

sucrase (soo-krays) enzyme that catalyzes the hydrolysis of sucrose and maltose [*sucr-* sugar, *-ase* enzyme]

sudoriferous gland (soo-doh-RIF-er-us) epidermal sweat glands [*sudo-* sweat, *-fer-* bear or carry, *-ous* relating to, *gland* acorn]

sulcus (SUL-kus) furrow, or groove, often associated with the cerebral cortex [*sulcus* furrow]

sulphur (SUL-fur) component of many energy-transferring enzymes [*sulphur* brimstone]

sulphuric acid (sul-FYOOR-ik ASS-id) contributes hydrogen ions to the extracellular fluid; influences acid-base balance [*sulphur-* brimstone (sulphur), *-ic* relating to]

superficial (soo-per-FISH-al) relating to (toward) the body surface; opposite of deep [*super-* over or above, *-fici-* face, *-al* relating to]

superficial cervical lymph node (soo-per-FISH-al SER-vih-kal limf nohd) lymph node that drains lymph from the head and neck; located in the neck along the sternocleidomastoid muscle [*super-* over or above, *-fici-* face, *-al* relating to, *cervic-* neck, *-al* relating to, *lymph* water, *nod-* knot]

superficial cubital lymph node (soo-per-FISH-al KYOO-bih-tal limf nohd) lymph node located just above the bend of the elbow; lymph from the forearm passes through this node [*super-* over or above, *-fici-* face, *-al* relating to, *cubit-* elbow, *-al* relating to, *lymph* water, *nod-* knot]

superficial fascia (soo-per-FISH-al FAH-shah) hypodermis; subcutaneous layer beneath the dermis [*super-* over or above, *-fici-* face, *-al* relating to, *fascia* band]

superficial reflex (soo-per-FISH-al REE-fleks) reflexes elicited by stimulation of receptors located in the skin or mucosa [*super-* over or above, *-fici-* face, *-al* relating to, *re-* again, *-flex* bend]

superficial vein (soo-per-FISH-al vayn) vein that lies near the surface [*super-* over or above, *-fici-* face, *-al* relating to, *vena* blood vessel]

superior (soo-PEER-ee-or) higher; opposite of inferior [*super-* over or above, *-or* quality]

superior cerebellar peduncle (soo-PEER-ee-or SAIR-eh-bell-ar peh-DUNG-kul) internal white matter of the cerebellum composed principally of tracts from dentate nuclei in the cerebellum through the red nucleus of the midbrain to the thalamus [*super-* over or above, *-or* quality, *cerebell-* cerebellum (small brain), *-ar* relating to, *ped-* foot, *-uncl-* little]

superior colliculi (soo-PEER-ee-or koh-LIK-yoo-lee) superior region of the corpora quadrigemina [*super-* over or above, *-or* quality, *colli-* hill, *-iculus* small] *sing.*, colliculus

superior intercostal vein (soo-PEER-ee-or in-ter-KOS-tal vayn) vein of the thorax [*super-* over or above, *-or* quality, *inter-* between, *-costa-* rib, *-al* relating to, *vena* blood vessel]

superior vena cava (soo-PEER-ee-or VEE-nah KAY-vah) large vein of the upper extremity; drains blood into the right atrium of the heart [*super-* over or above, *-or* quality, *vena* vein, *cava* hollow] *pl.*, venae cavae

supination (soo-pih-NAY-shun) movement that turns the hand palm side up [*supin-* lying on the back, *-ation* process]

suppressor T cell (suh-PRESS-er tee sel) T lymphocyte of the immune system that suppresses B-cell differentiation into plasma cells, allowing fine-tuning of antibody-mediated immune responses; often called *regulator T cell (T-reg)* [*suppress-* press down, *-or* agent, *T* thymus gland, *cell* storeroom]

supraclavicular (soo-pra-cla-VIK-yoo-lar) relating to the area above the clavicle (collarbone)

[*supra-* above or over, *-clavi-* key, *-ula-* little, *-ar* relating to]

supraovulation (soo-prah-oh-vyoo-LAY-shun) simultaneous rupture of multiple mature follicles [*supra-* above or over, *-ov-* egg, *-ation* process]

suprarenal (soo-prah-REE-nal) situated above a kidney [*supra-* above or over, *ren-* kidney, *-al* relating to]

suprarenal vein (soo-prah-REE-nal vayn) abdominal vein; drains blood into the adrenal gland [*supra-* above or over, *-ren-* kidney, *-al* relating to, *vena* blood vessel]

supraspinatus muscle (SOO-prah-spy-nah-tus) one of a group of muscles (rotator cuff) that serve as both a structural and functional cuff around the shoulder joint [*supra-* above, *-spina-* spine, *mus-* mouse, *-cle* little]

supratrochlear lymph node (soo-prah-TROHK-lee-ar limf) *see* **superficial cubital lymph node** [*supra-* above, *-trochlea-* pulley, *-ar* relating to, *lymph* water, *nod-* knot]

sural (SUR-al) relating to the calf of the leg [*sura-* calf of leg, *-al* relating to]

surface film layer on the outer surface of skin made up of a mixture of secretions from sweat and sebaceous glands along with epithelial cells being shed from the epidermis; works as a protective barrier [*sur-* above, *-face* form]

surface tension the force of attraction between water molecules [*sur-* above, *-face* form, *tendere-* to stretch]

surfactant (sur-FAK-tant) substance covering the surface of the respiratory membrane inside the alveolus; it reduces surface tension and prevents the alveoli from collapsing [combination of *surf(ace) act(ive) a(ge)nt*]

surgical neck (SER-jik-el nek) region of the humerus bone of the arm just below the tubercles, so named because of its liability to fracture (*surg-* handwork, *-ical* relating to)

suspensory ligament (sus-PEN-so-ree LIG-ah-ment) fibres attached to the capsule of the lens that help hold it in place [*suspendere-* to hang, *-ory* relating to, *ligare-* to bind]

sustentacular cell (sus-ten-TAK-yoo-lar) *see* **Sertoli cell** [*sustent-* support, *-acular* relating to]

suture (SOO-chur) immovable joint, such as those between the bones of the skull [*sutur-* seam]

sweat gland gland in the skin that produces a transparent, watery liquid that eliminates ammonia and uric acid and helps maintain body temperature [*gland* acorn]

sympathetic division (sim-pah-THET-ik) part of the autonomic nervous system; ganglia are connected to the thoracic and lumbar regions of the spinal cord; functions in "fight or flight" response [*sym- together, -pathe-* feel, *-ic* relating to]

sympathetic trunk (sim-pah-THET-ik) arrangement of sympathetic axon collaterals that bridge the gap between adjacent ganglia that lie on the same side of the vertebral column [*sym-* together, *-pathe-* feel, *-ic* relating to]

symphysis (SIM-fih-sis) joint characterized by the presence of a pad or disc of fibrocartilage connecting the two bones [*sym-* together, *-physis* growth] *pl.*, symphyses (SIM-fi-seez)

symptom subjective deviation from normal that marks the presence of a disease; sometimes used synonymously with *sign* [*sym-* together, *-tom* fall]

symptomatic gallstone (simp-toh-MAT-ik) gallstone that produces painful symptoms or other medical complications [*sym-* together, *-tom* fall, *-ic* relating to, *gall* bile]

synapse (SIN-aps) membrane-to-membrane junction between a neuron and another neuron, effector cell, or sensory cell; functions to propagate nerve impulses (via neurotransmitters); two types: electrical and chemical; compare to **immunological synapse** [*syn-* together, *-aps-* join]

synaptic cleft (sih-NAP-tik kleft) space between a synaptic knob and the plasma membrane of a postsynaptic neuron [*syn-* together, *-apt-*join, *-ic* relating to]

synaptic knob (sih-NAP-tik nob) tiny bulge at the end of a terminal branch of a presynaptic neuron's axon that contains vesicles with neurotransmitters [*syn-* together, *-apt-* join, *-ic* relating to]

synarthrosis (sin-ar-THROH-sis) joint in which fibrous connective tissue joins bones and holds them together tightly; commonly called *sutures* [*syn-* together, *-arthr-* joint, *-osis* condition] *pl.*, synarthroses (sin-ar-THROH-seez)

synchondrosis (SIN-kon-DROH-sis) joint characterized by the presence of hyaline cartilage between articulating bones [*syn-* together, *-chondr-* cartilage, *-osis* condition] *pl.*, synchondroses

syncytium (sin-SISH-ee-em) continuous, electrically coupled mass of cardiac fibres; allows an efficient, coordinated pumping action [*syn-* together, *-cyt-* cell, *-um* a thing] *pl.*, syncytia (sin-SISH-ah)

syndesmosis (SIN-dez-MO-sis) fibrous joint [*syn-* together, *-desmo-* bond, *-osis* condition] *pl.*, syndesmoses (SIN-dez-MO-seez)

syndrome (SIN-drome) collection of signs or symptoms, usually with a common cause, that defines or gives a clear picture of a pathological condition [*syn-* together, *-drome* running or (race) course]

synergism (SIN-er-jiz-em) with hormones, a combination of hormones has a greater effect on a target than the sum of effects that each would have if acting alone [*syn-* together, *-erg-* work, *-ism* condition]

synergist (SIN-er-jist) muscle that assists a prime mover [*syn-* together, *-erg-* to work, *-ist* agent]

synovial fluid (sih-NO-vee-all) thick, colourless lubricating fluid secreted by the synovial membrane in synovial joints [*syn-* together, *-ovi-* egg (white),*-al* relating to, *fluid* flow]

synovial membrane (sih-NO-vee-all) connective tissue membrane lining spaces between bones and joints that secretes synovial fluid [*syn-* together, *-ovi-* egg (white), *-al* relating to, *membran-* thin skin]

synthesis (SIN-the-sis) combination, as in the combination of molecules to form a larger molecule [*synthes-* put together, *-is* process]

synthesis reaction (SIN-the-sis ree-AK-shun) chemical reaction that combines two or more reactants to form a more complex structure [*synthes-* put together, *-is* process, *re-* again, *-action* action]

system a group of organs that functions as a coordinated team; also called a *body system* [*system* organized whole]

systemic anatomy (sis-TEM-ik ah-NAT-oh-mee) study of anatomy that focuses on learning about body systems [*system* organized whole, *-ic* relating to, *ana-* apart, *-tom-* cut, *-y* action]

systemic circulation (sis-TEM-ik sur-kyoo-LAY-shun) blood flow from the left ventricle to all parts of the body and back to the right atrium [*system-* organized whole, *-ic* relating to, *circulat-* go around, *-tion* process]

systemic lupus erythematosus (SLE) (sis-TEM-ik LOO-pus er-ih-them-ah-TOH-sus) autoimmune disease that affects many tissues in the body; red rash often develops on the faces of those afflicted with SLE [*system-* organized whole, *-ic* relating to, *lupus* wolf, *erythema-* redness, *-osus* condition]

systole (SIS-toh-lee) contraction of heart muscle [*sy(n)-* together, *-stol-* position]

systolic blood pressure (sis-TOL-ik blud PRESH-ur) force with which blood pushes against artery walls when ventricles contract [*sy(n)-* together, *-stol-* position, *-ic* relating to]

systolic discharge (sis-TOL-ik) volume of blood pumped by one contraction [*sy(n)-* together, *-stol-* position, *-ic* relating to]

T

T cell *see* **T lymphocyte** [*T* thymus gland, *cell* storeroom]

T lymphocyte (LIM-foh-syte) cells of the immune system that have undergone maturation in the thymus; produce cell-mediated immunity [*T* thymus gland, *lymph-* water (lymphatic system), *-cyte* cell]

T tubule (TYOOB-yool) transverse tubules unique to muscle cells; formed by inward extensions of the sarcolemma that allow electrical impulses to move deeper into the cell [*T* transverse, *tub-* tube, *-ul-* little]

T wave electrocardiogram deflection that reflects the repolarization of the ventricles [named for 20th letter of Roman alphabet]

tachycardia (tak-ih-KAR-dee-ah) rapid heart rhythm (more than 100 beats/min) [*tachy-* rapid, *-cardi-* heart, *-ia* condition]

tactile corpuscle (TAK-tyle KOR-pus-ul) large, encapsulated sensory neuron of the skin for light or discriminative touch; also known as *Meissner corpuscle* [*tact-* touch, *-ile* relating to, *corpus-* body, *-cle* little]

tactile disc (TAK-tyle) flat-ended, unencapsulated sensory neuron of the skin for light or discriminative touch; also known as *Merkel disc* or *tactile meniscus* [*tact-* touch, *-ile* relating to]

tactile epithelial cell (TAK-tyle ep-ih-THEE-lee-al) stiff epithelial cell of the epidermis of the skin that passes compression of the skin on to the sensory tactile disc neuron; also known as *Merkel cell* [*tact-* touch, *-ile* relating to, *cell* storeroom]

taeniae coli (TEE-nee-ee KOH-lye) flat bands of dense longitudinal muscle fibres in the wall of the colon; [*taenia* ribbon or tape, *coli* relating to the large intestine] *sing.*, taenia coli (TEE-nee-ah KOH-lye)

talus (TAY-lus) bone overlying the calcaneus bone and articulating with the tibia and fibula of the leg to form the ankle joint [*talus* ankle] *pl.*, tali (TAY-lye)

tamoxifen (teh-MOK-seh-fin) drug used extensively to prevent the recurrence of breast cancers fueled by oestrogen. [*t-* trans (across), *-am-* amino (ammonia compound), *-oxi-* oxygen, *-fen* phenol (shining)]

target destination of a physiological agent such as a hormone or neurotransmitter [*targuete-* small shield]

target cell cell that, when acted on by a particular hormone, responds because it has receptors to which the hormone can bind [*targuete-* small shield, *cell* storeroom]

target organ organ that is acted on and responds to a particular hormone [*targuete-* small shield, *organ* instrument]

tarsal (TAR-sal) relating to the ankle (posterior) portion of the foot [*tars-* ankle, *-al* relating to]

tarsal bone (TAR-sal bohn) any of the bones of the posterior region of the foot [*tars-* ankle, *-al* relating to]

tarsal plate (TAR-sal) border of thick connective tissue at the free edge of each eyelid [*tarsos-* flat surface, *plate-* flat, or broad]

taste bud chemical receptors in the tongue that generate nerve impulses, resulting in the sense of taste

Tay–Sachs disease (TSD) (TAY-saks) recessive, inherited condition in which abnormal lipids accumulate in the brain and cause tissue damage that leads to death by age 4 years [*Warren Tay* English ophthalmologist, *Bernard Sachs* American neurologist]

tectorial membrane (tek-TOH-ree-al) gelatinous membrane of inner ear that tops hair cells in the spiral organ (organ of Corti) [*tect-* roof, *-or-* quality, *-al* relating to, *membran-* thin skin]

tectospinal tract (tek-toh-SPY-nal trakt) motor tract that conveys messages for head and neck movement related to visual reflexes [*tecto-* roof, *-spin-* backbone, *-al* relating to, *tract* trail]

telencephalon (tel-en-SEF-ah-lon) secondary vesicle of the neural tube during embryonic development formed from the proencephalon and that eventually becomes the cerebrum; sometimes used as a synonym for *cerebrum* [*tele-* end, *-en-* within, *-cephalon* head]

telodendrion (tel-oh-DEN-dree-on or tee-loh-DEN-dree-on) any of the distal tips of axons that form branches; each branch terminates in a synaptic knob [*telo-* end, *-dendr-* part (branch) of] *pl.*, telodendria (tel-oh-DEN-dree-ah)

telomere (TEL-oh-meer or TEE-loh-meer) a strand of additional noncoding nucleotides that can be lost during normal DNA replication without affecting the coding part of the chromosome [*telo-* end, *-mer-* root]

telophase (TEL-oh-fayz or TEE-loh-fayz) last stage of mitosis [*telo-* end, *-phase* stage]

temporal (TEM-poh-ral) relating to the side (temple) of the head or skull [*tempora-* temple (of head), *-al* relating to]

temporal bone (TEM-poh-ral bohn) cranial bone located on lower side of cranium and part of its floor [*tempora-* temple (of head), *-al* relating to]

temporal summation (TEM-poh-ral sum-MAY-shun) when synaptic knobs stimulate a postsynaptic neuron in rapid succession and the effects add up over time to produce an action potential (also spatial summation) [*tempor-* time, *-al* relating to]

temporalis muscle (tem-poh-RAL-is) muscle of mastication; elevates and retracts the mandible [*tempo-* temple of head, *-al* relating to, *-is* thing, *mus-* mouse, *-cle* little]

tendon (TEN-den) bands or cords of fibrous connective tissue that attach a muscle to a bone or other structure [*tend-* pulled tight, *-on* unit]

tendon organ (TEN-den OR-gun) *see* **Golgi tendon organ** [*tend-* pulled tight, *-on* unit]

tendon receptor (TEN-den ree-SEP-tor) *see* **Golgi tendon receptor** [*tend-* pulled tight, *-on* unit, *recept-* receive, *-or* agent]

tendon reflex (TEN-den REE-fleks) reflex stimulated by tapping on a tendon; *see also* **Golgi tendon reflex** [*tend-* pulled tight, *-on* unit, *re-* again, *-flex* bend]

tendon sheath (sheeth) tube-shaped structure lined with synovial membrane that encloses certain tendons [*tend-* pulled tight, *-on* unit]

tenosynovitis (ten-oh-sin-oh-VYE-tis) inflammation of a tendon sheath [*teno-* pulled tight (tendon), *-syn-* together, *-ovi-* egg white (joint fluid), *-itis* inflammation]

tension (TEN-shun) pressure or force, as in muscle contraction force or osmotic force [*tens-* stretch, *-ion* state]

tensor fasciae latae muscle (TEN-sor FASH-ee LAT-tee) muscle that moves the thigh and leg [*tensor* stretcher, *fascia* band or bundle, *lat-* side, *mus-* mouse, *-cle* little]

tentorium cerebelli (ten-TOR-ee-um sair-eh-BEL-lee) inward extension of the dura mater that separates the cerebellum from the cerebrum [*tentorium* tent, *cerebelli* of the cerebellum (small brain)] *pl.*, tentoria cerebelli (ten-TOR-ee-ah sair-eh-BEL-lee)

teratogen (TER-ah-toh-jen) physical or chemical agent that disrupts normal embryonic development and thus causes congenital defects [*terato-* monster, *-gen* produce]

teres minor (TER-eez) one of four rotator cuff muscles; forms a structural and functional cuff around the shoulder joint [*teres* rounded, *minor* lesser]

terminal ganglion (GANG-glee-on) ganglia that consists of parasympathetic fibres near or in the effectors in the chest and abdomen [*termin-* boundary, *-al* relating to, *gangli-* knot, *-on* unit] *pl.*, ganglia

terminal hair coarse pubic and axillary hair that develops at puberty [*termin-* boundary, *-al* relating to]

terminal nerve (TER-mih-nal nerv) pair of cranial nerves alongside the olfactory nerves, thought to be involved in sensing pheromones (sex signals); often called *nerve zero*, not usually found in the classic list of 12 cranial nerves [*termin-* boundary, *-al* relating to]

Terminologia anatomica (Ta or TA) (ter-mih-noh-LOJ-ee-ah an-ah-TOM-ik-ah) literally "Terminology of Anatomy"; the official list of anatomical terms related to gross anatomy sponsored by the International Federation of Associations of Anatomists; lists all terms by number and name (in both Latin and English) as well as general principles of usage

Terminologia histologica (Th or TH) (termih-noh-LOJ-ee-ah his-to-LO-jik-ah) literally "Terminology of Histology"; the official list of anatomical terms related to microscopic anatomy sponsored by the International Federation of Associations of Anatomists; lists all terms by number and name (in both Latin and English) as well as general principles of usage

tertiary protein structure (TER-shee-air-ee PRO-teen STRUK-cher) third level of protein structure, formed after the secondary structure (a curled, folded strand of amino acids) folds into an even more complex three-dimensional structure; may include several complicated "knots" called *domains*; a *tertiary protein* is a complete protein possessing the third (but not fourth) level of complexity in its molecular structure [*tert-* third, *-ary* relating to, *prote-* primary, *-in* substance, *structur-* arrangement]

testicle (TES-tik-ul) informal synonym of *testis*; male gonad [*testi-* witness (male gonad), *-cle* little]

testicular self-examination (tes-TIK-yoo-lar) recommended procedure that involves palpating each testis, preferably after a warm shower or bath when the scrotum is relaxed and the testes are descended and accessible [*testi-* witness (testis), *-cul-* small, *-ar* relating to]

testis (TES-tis) male gonad [*testis* witness (male gonad)] *pl.*, testes (TES-teez)

testosterone (tes-TOS-teh-rohn) male sex hormone produced by interstitial cells in the testes; the "masculinizing hormone" [*testo-* witness (testis), *-stero-* solid or steroid derivative, *-one* chemical]

tetanus (TET-ah-nus) smooth, sustained muscular contraction caused by high-frequency stimulation [*tetanus* tension]

tetraiodothyronine (T_4) (tet-rah-eye-oh-doh-THY-roh-neen) one of two hormones that compose the thyroid hormone; also called *thyroxine* [*tetra-* four, *-iodo-* violet (iodine), *-thyro-* shield (thyroid gland), *-ine* chemical]

thalamus (THAL-ah-muss) mass of grey matter located in diencephalon just above the hypothalamus; helps produce sensations, associates sensations with emotions, and plays a part in the arousal mechanism [*thalamus* inner chamber] *pl.*, thalami (THAL-ah-mye)

thalassaemia (thal-ah-SEE-mee-ah) group of inherited haemoglobin disorders characterized by production of abnormal red blood cells [*thalass-* sea, *-(h)aem-* blood, *-ia* condition]

theca cell (THEE-kah) specialized cell formed from the outer layer of granulosa cells; transforms into a fibrous capsule that secretes a hormone that ultimately converts into additional oestrogen [*theca* sheath, *cell* storeroom]

theory a scientific idea or explanation that has a reasonably high degree of confidence after rigorous testing or observation; compare to **hypothesis** and **law** [*theor-* look at, *-y* act of]

thermal ablation (THUR-mal ab-LAY-shun) procedure that is used to treat women who suffer from dysfunctional uterine bleeding (DUB) [*therm-* heat, *-al* relating to, *ab-* away from, *-lat-* carry, *-tion* process]

thermogenesis (ther-moh-JEN-eh-sis) process of generating heat, as in *shivering* thermogenesis muscles or *nonshivering* thermogenesis in active brown adipose tissue [*thermo-* heat, *-gen-* produce, *-esis* process]

thermoreceptor (ther-moh-ree-SEP-tor) sensory receptor activated by heat or cold [*thermo-* heat, *-cept-* receive, *-or* agent]

thermotaxis (ther-moh-TAK-sis) process in which a cell, such as a sperm cell, is attracted to heat and moves toward the source of heat [*therm-* heat, *-taxis* movement or reaction]

thick ascending limb (TAL) (thik ah-SEND-ing lim) thick-walled region of the limbs of the hairpin nephron loop (loop of Henle) that conducts filtrate toward the distal tubule [*ascend-* climb, *Friedrich Gustave Henle* German anatomist]

thin ascending limb of Henle (tALH) (thin ah-SEND-ing lim ov HEN-lee) thin-walled region of the limbs of the hairpin nephron loop (loop of Henle) that conducts filtrate toward the distal tubule [*ascend-* climb, *Friedrich Gustave Henle* German anatomist]

thirst centre region of the hypothalamus containing osmoreceptors that can detect an increase in solute concentration in extracellular fluid caused by water loss

thoracic (thoh-RASS-ik) related to the thorax [*thorac-* chest, *-ic* relating to]

thoracic aorta (thoh-RASS-ik ay-OR-tah) downward arch of the aorta through the thorax and ending at the diaphragm [*thorac-*chest, *-ic* relating to, *aort-* lifted, *-a* thing] *pl.*, aortae (ay-OR-tee) or aortas

thoracic cavity (thoh-RASS-ik KAV-ih-tee) hollow space within the larger ventral body cavity that contains the lungs (in pleural cavities) and heart (in the mediastinum) [*thorac-* chest (thorax), *-ic* relating to, *cav-* hollow, *-ity* state]

thoracic duct (thoh-RASS-ik) largest lymphatic vessel in the body [*thorac-* chest (thorax), *-ic* relating to, *duct* path]

thoracic vertebra (thoh-RASS-ik VER-te-bra) vertebral bone located in the posterior part of the chest [*thorac-* chest, *-ic* relating to, *vertebra* that which turns] *pl.*, vertebrae (VER-te-bree)

thoracolumbar division (thoh-rah-koh-LUM-bar) sympathetic division of the autonomic nervous system [*thoraco-* chest, *lumb-* loin, *-ar* relating to]

thorax (THOH-raks) chest [*thorax* chest] *pl.*, thoraces (THOH-rah-seez)

thoroughfare channel (THUR-oh-fair CHAN-el) the distal end of a metarteriole that is devoid of precapillary sphincters, allowing blood to bypass a capillary bed

threshold potential (THRESH-hold poh-TEN-shal) magnitude of voltage across a membrane at which an action potential, or nerve impulse, is produced [*potent-* power, *-ial* relating to]

threshold stimulus (THRESH-hold STIM-yoo-lus) minimal level of stimulation required to cause a muscle fibre to contract [*stimul-* excite, *-us* thing] *pl.*, stimuli (STIM-yoo-lye)

thrombocyte (THROM-boh-syte) cell fragments that play a role in blood clotting; also called *platelets* [*thrombo-* clot, *-cyte* cell]

thrombocytopenia (throm-boh-sye-toh-PEE-nee-ah) condition resulting from a decreased platelet count [*thrombo-* clot, *-cyto-* cell, *-penia* lack]

thrombophlebitis (throm-boh-fleh-BYE-tis) vein inflammation (phlebitis) accompanied by clot formation [*thrombo-* clot, *-phleb-* vein, *-itis* inflammation]

thrombopoiesis (throm-boh-poy-EE-sis) formation of platelets [*thromb-* clot, *-poiesis* making]

thrombosis (throm-BOH-sis) condition resulting from a clot (thrombus) that stays in one place [*thrombo-* clot, *-osis* condition]

thromboxane (throm-BOKS-ayne) prostaglandin-like substance in platelets that plays a role in haemostasis and blood clotting [*thrombo-* clot, *-oxa-* oxygen, *-ane* chemical]

thrombus (THROM-bus) a nonmoving or fixed blood clot attached to the lining of a vein or artery [*thrombus* clot] *pl.*, thrombi (THROM-bye)

thymic corpuscle (THYE-mik KOR-pus-ul) any of the laminated spherical structures found in the thymus; composed of concentric layers of keratinized epithelial cells; also called *Hassall corpuscle* [*thym-* thyme flower (thymus gland), *-ic* relating to, *corpus-* body, *-cle* little]

thymocyte (THY-moh-syte) cell in the thymus that develops into T lymphocytes [*thymo-* thyme flower (thymus gland), *-cyte* cell]

thymopoietin (thy-moh-POY-eh-tin) peptide that has a critical role in the development of the immune system; thought to stimulate the production of specialized lymphocytes involved in the immune response called *T cells* [*thymo-* thymus gland, *-poiet-* make, *-in* substance]

thymosin (THY-moh-sin) hormone produced by the thymus that is vital to the development and functioning of the body's immune system [*thymos-* thyme flower (thymus gland), *-in* substance]

thymus (THY-muss) endocrine gland located in the mediastinum; vital part of the body's immune system [*thymus* thyme flower] *pl.*, thymuses

thyroglobulin (thy-roh-GLOB-yoo-lin) protein-iodine complex that is a precursor of thyroid hormones [*thyro-* shield (thyroid gland), *-glob-* ball, *-ul-* small, *-in* substance]

thyroid cartilage (THY-royd KAR-tih-lij) largest cartilage of the larynx; Adam's apple [*thyr-* shield, *-oid* like]

thyroid colloid (THY-royd KOL-oyd) thick fluid that fills the interior of thyroid follicles [*thyro-* shield (thyroid gland), *-oid* like, *coll-* glue, *-oid* like]

thyroid gland (THY-royd) endocrine gland located in the neck that stores its hormones until needed; thyroid hormones regulate cellular metabolism [*thyro-* shield, *-oid* like, *gland* acorn]

thyroid hormone (THY-royd HOR-mohn) hormone that accelerates catabolism of glucose [*thyro-* shield, *-oid* like, *hormon-* excite]

thyroid-stimulating hormone (TSH) (THY-royd STIM-yoo-lay-ting HOR-mohn) a tropic hormone secreted by the anterior pituitary gland that stimulates the thyroid gland to increase its secretion of thyroid hormone [*thyro-* shield, *-oid* like, *hormon-* excite]

thyrotroph (thy-roh-TROHF) cell type of the adenohypophysis (anterior pituitary) that secretes thyroid-stimulating hormone (TSH) [*thyro-* shield (thyroid gland), *-troph* nourish]

thyroxine (thy-ROK-sin) thyroid hormone that stimulates cellular metabolism [*thyro-* shield (thyroid gland), *-ox-* oxygen, *-ine* chemical]

tibia (TIB-ee-ah) larger, stronger and more medially and superficially located of the two leg bones [*tibia* shin bone] *pl.*, tibiae (TIB-ee-ee) or tibias (TIB-ee-ahz)

tibialis anterior muscle (tib-ee-AL-is) dorsal flexor muscle of the foot; located on the anterior surface of the leg [*tibia* shinbone, *-al* relating to, *-is* thing, *ante-* front, *-er-* more, *-or* quality, *mus-* mouse, *-cle* little]

tic douloureux (tik doo-loo-ROO) *see* **trigeminal neuralgia** [*tic* spasm, *douloureux* painful (French)]

tidal volume (TV) (TYE-dal) amount of air breathed in and out with each breath [*tid-* time, *-al* relating to]

tight junction (tyte JUNK-shun) connection between cells in which they are joined by "collars" of tightly fused membrane [*tight-* strong, *junct-* to join, *-ion* process]

tinea (TIN-ee-ah) fungal infection of the skin [*tinea* worm]

tinnitus (tih-NYE-tus or TIN-nit-us) "ringing in the ear"; *see* **otosclerosis** [*tinnitis* a ringing or tinkling]

tissue group of similar cells that performs a common function [*tissu-* fabric]

tissue plasminogen activator (t-PA) (plaz-MIN-oh-jen AK-tih-vay-tor) clot-dissolving substance [*tissue-* fabric, *plasm-* substance (plasma), *-in-* substance, *-gen* produce]

TMR *see* **transmyocardial laser revascularization** [abbreviation *of* transmyocardial laser revascularization]

TNF blocker (TEE-EN-EF [TYOO-mer ne-KRO-sis FAK-tor] BLOK-er) drug used in the treatment of rheumatoid arthritis [*TNF* tumour necrosis factor]

Toll-like receptor (TLR) family of membrane receptors that act as pattern-recognition receptors in immunity to identify any of a large, nonspecific group of microbial antigen molecules and then trigger an innate immune response [*toll-* weird or amazing, *-like*, *recept-* receive, *-or* agent]

tongue solid mass of skeletal muscle components covered by a mucous membrane; manipulates food in the mouth and contains taste buds

tonic contraction (TON-ik kon-TRAK-shun) type of skeletal muscle contraction used to maintain posture [*ton-* to stretch, *-ic* relating to, *con-* together, *-tract-* drag or draw, *-tion* process]

tonicity (toh-NIS-ih-tee) potential osmotic pressure [*ton-* stretch or tension, *-ic* relating to, *-ty* state]

tonsil (TON-sil) masses of lymphoid tissue; protect against bacteria; three types: palatine tonsils, located on each side of the throat; pharyngeal tonsils (adenoids), near the posterior opening of the nasal cavity; and lingual tonsils, near the base of the tongue [*tons-* goitre, *-il* little]

tonsillectomy (ton-sih-LEK-toh-mee) surgical removal of the tonsils [*tons-* goitre, *-il-* little, *-ec-* out, *-tom-* cut, *-y* action]

tonsillitis (ton-sih-LYE-tis) inflammation of the tonsils, usually because of infection [*tons-* goitre, *-il* little, *-itis* inflammation]

tophus (TOH-fus) sodium urate crystal deposited within the synovial fluid of joints and in other tissues [*tophus* porous rock] *pl.*, tophi (TOH-fye)

total lung capacity (TLC) (TOHT-il lung kah-PASS-ih-tee) total volume of air a lung can hold [*capac-* hold, *-ity* state]

total metabolic rate (TMR) (TOHT-il met-ah-BOL-ik) total amount of energy used by the body per day [*meta-* over, *-bol-* throw, *-ic* relating to]

total minute volume (TOHT-il MIN-it VOL-yoom) rate of pulmonary ventilation per minute [*minute-* sixtieth part of an hour]

total peripheral resistance (TPR) (TOHT-il peh-RIF-er-al ree-ZIS-tens) cumulative arterial resistance to blood flow [*peri-* around, *-phera-* boundary, *-al* relating to, *resist-* withstand, *-ance* act of]

toxin (TOK-sin) poison; chemical that can cause sickness or damage in the body [*toxin* poison]

toxoid (TOK-soyd) form of bacterial toxin that stimulates production of antibodies [*tox-* poison, *-oid* like]

trabecula (trah-BEK-yoo-la) tiny branchlike threads in a tissue, such as the beams of spongy (cancellous) bone, that surround a network of spaces [*trab-* beam, *-ula* little] *pl.*, trabeculae (trah-BEK-yoo-lee)

trabecula carnea (trah-BEK-yoo-la KAR-nee-ah) any of the branched columns of muscle visible in the lining of the ventricles of the heart [*trab-* beam, *-ula* little, *carne-* flesh (muscle)] *pl.*, trabeculae carneae (trah-BEK-yoo-lee KAR-nee-ee)

trabecular bone (trah-BEK-yoo-lar) *see* **spongy bone, cancellous bone** [*trab-* beam, *-ula-* little, *-ar* relating to]

trace element elements found in small amounts in the body [*element* first principle]

trachea (TRAY-kee-ah) windpipe; the tube extending from the larynx to the bronchi [*trachea* rough duct] *pl.*, tracheae (TRAY-kee-ee) or tracheas

tracheostomy (tray-kee-OS-toh-mee) surgical procedure in which an opening is cut into the trachea [*trache-* rough duct, *-os-* mouth or opening, *-tom-* cut, *-y* action]

trachoma (trah-KOH-mah) chronic infection of the conjunctiva and cornea [*trach-* rough, *-oma* tumour]

tract (trakt) bundle of nerve fibres within the central nervous system; unlike a nerve, a tract does not have connective tissue coverings [*trac-* course]

transabdominal pelvic ultrasound (tranz-ab-DOM-ih-nal PEL-vik UL-trah-sound) imaging technique used to look at the uterus and adjacent reproductive structures [*trans-* across, *-abdomin-* belly, *-al* relating to, *pelv-* basin (pelvis), *-ic* relating to, *ultra-* beyond, sound]

transcription (tran-SKRIP-shun) process in which DNA molecule is used as template to form mRNA, thus making a temporary "working copy" of the gene [*trans-* across, *-script-* write, *-tion* process]

transcriptome (tran-SKRIPT-ome) mRNA codes transcribed from the human genome [*trans-* across, *-script-* written document, *-ome* entire collection]

transcriptomics (tran-skript-OHM-iks) analysis of all the mRNA codes actually transcribed from the human genome (transcriptome) [*trans-* across, *-script-* written document, *-om-* entire collection, *-ic* relating to]

transcutaneous electrical nerve stimulation (TENS) unit (tranz-kyoo-TAY-nee-us) device used to stimulate skin touch receptors in a painful area; results in closure of the spinal cord pain gate and relief of pain [*trans-* across, *-cutan-* skin, *-ous* relating to]

transduction (tranz-DUK-shun) process of changing one form of energy or other physical event to another form, as when sound energy is changed to electrical energy in a microphone [*trans-*through, *-duct-* path, *-ion* process]

transfer RNA (tRNA) RNA involved with protein synthesis; tRNA molecules carry amino acids to the ribosome for placement in the sequence prescribed by mRNA [*trans-* across, *-fer* carry, *RNA* ribonucleic acid]

transfusion reaction (tranz-FYOO-zhun ree-AK-shun) fatal event resulting from a mixture of agglutinogens (antigens) and agglutinins (antibodies) resulting in the agglutination of the donor and recipient blood [*trans-* across, *-fus-* pour, *-sion* process, *re-* again, *-action* action]

transient ischaemic attack (TIA) (is-KEE-mik) brief (transient) episode of brain dysfunction caused by interruption of blood flow (ischaemia) to the affected area; often referred to as a mini-stroke [*trans-* across, *-ent* state, *ischaem-* hold back, *-ic* relating to]

transitional epithelium (tran-ZISH-en-al epi-THEE-lee-um) stratified tissue typically found in body areas that are subjected to stress and tension changes, such as the urinary tract, where it is called *urothelium* [*trans-* across, *-tion* process, *-al* relating to, *epi-* on, *-theli-* nipple, *-um* thing] *pl.*, epithelia (epi-THEE-lee-ah)

translation (trans-LAY-shun) process in which mRNA is used by ribosomes in the synthesis of a protein [*translat-* a bringing over, *-tion* process]

transmission electron micrograph (TEM) (MY-kroh-graf) photograph of an image produced by a transmission electron microscope [*trans-* across, *-miss-* send, *-ion* process, *electro-* electric, *-on* subatomic particle, *micro-* small, *-graph* drawing]

transmyocardial laser revascularization (TMR) (tranz-my-oh-KARD-ee-al LAY-zer ree-VAS-kyoo-lar-i-zay-shun) heart surgery used with patients suffering from severe angina (chest/heart pain) in which a laser beam makes toothpick-sized holes in the myocardium, which stimulates the growth of new blood vessels (angiogenesis) that relieves the angina [*trans-* across, *-myo* muscle, *-cardi* heart, *-al* relating to, *laser* abbreviation for light amplification by stimulated emission of radiation, re-again, *-vasculum* little vessel, *-ar* relating to, *-ation* process]

transplant tranz-PLANT [verb] or TRANZ-plant [noun] v. medical procedure in which tissue from a donor is surgically grafted into the body of another; *n.* the grafted tissue [*trans-* across, *-plant* set or place]

transportation process of carrying essential materials within the body [*trans-* across, *-port-* carry, *-tion* process]

transpulmonary pressure (tranz-PUHL-moh-nair-ee) the pressure difference between the alveolar air pressure in the lungs and the fluid pressure in the intrapleural space, that is, the pressure difference across the wall of the lung [*trans-* across, *-pulmon-* lung, *-ary* relating to]

transurethral resection (TUR) (tranz-yoor-REE-thral rih-SEK-shun) surgical removal of swollen tissue surrounding the urethra [*trans-* across or through, *-ure-* urine, *-thr-* agent or channel (urethra), *-al* relating to, *re-* again, *-sect-* cut, *-tion* process]

transvenous approach (tranz-VEE-nus) method of inserting a permanent pacemaker [*trans-* across, *-ven-* vein, *-ous* relating to]

transverse arch (tranz-VERS arch) curve of the foot from medial to lateral that helps stabilize the foot's support of the body's weight [*trans-* across, *-vers-* turn]

transverse canal (tranz-VERS kah-NAL) communicating canal between central (Haversian) canals that contains vessels to carry blood to the osteons; also carries nerves and lymphatic vessels; also called *Volkmann canal* [*trans-* across, *-vers-* turn]

transverse colon (tranz-VERS KOH-lon) division of the colon that passes horizontally across the abdomen [*trans-* across, *-vers-* turn, *colon* large intestine]

transverse fracture (tranz-VERS FRAK-sher) type of bone fracture in which fracture line is at a right angle to the long axis of the bone [*trans-* across, *-verse* turn, *fracture* a breaking]

transverse mesocolon (tranz-VERS MEZ-oh-koh-lon) fold of peritoneum that attaches the transverse colon to the posterior abdominal wall [*trans-* across, *-vers-* turn, *meso-* middle, *-colon* large intestine]

transverse plane (tranz-VERS) horizontal plane that divides the body or any of its parts into upper and lower parts [*trans-* across or through, *-vers* turn, *plan-* flat surface]

transverse process (tranz-VERS PRO-ses) any of the lateral projections of a vertebral bone [*trans-* across or through, *-vers* turn, *process* project (from)] *pl.*, processes (PRO-ses-eez)

transversus abdominis muscle (tranz-VERS-us ab-DOM-in-us) innermost muscle of the anterolateral wall of the abdomen [*trans-* across, *-vers-* turn, *abdomin-* belly]

trapezius muscle (trah-PEE-zee-us) upper limb muscle that raises or lowers the shoulders and shrugs them [*trapezi-* small table, *mus-* mouse, *-cle* little]

traumatic brain injury (TBI) (truh-MAT-ik brayn IN-jur-ee) damage to the brain caused by an external force; also see **concussion** [*trauma-* wound, *-atic* relating to]

treppe (TREP-ee) gradual increase in the extent of muscular contraction following rapidly repeated stimulation; also called *staircase phenomenon* [*treppe* staircase]

triad (TRY-ad) triplet of tubules; allows an electrical impulse travelling along a T tubule to stimulate the membranes of adjacent sacs of the sarcoplasmic reticulum [*triad* group of three]

tricarboxylic acid (TCA) cycle (try-kar-bok-SIL-ik ASS-id SYE-kul) aerobic metabolic pathway in which acetyl CoA (from other metabolic pathways) is converted into CO_2 and H_2O with the formation of ATP; also known as *citric acid cycle*, or *Krebs cycle* [*tri-* three, *-carbo-* carbon, *-oxy-* sharp (oxygen), *-yl-* chemical, *-ic* relating to, *acid* sour, *cyclo-* circle]

tricuspid valve (try-KUS-pid valv) heart valve located between right atrium and ventricle [*tri-* three, *-cusp-* point, *-id* characterized by]

trigeminal nerve (try-JEM-ih-nal nerv) cranial nerve V; responsible for chewing movements and sensations of the head and face [*tri-* three, *-gemina-* twin or pair, *-al* relating to]

trigeminal neuralgia (try-JEM-ih-nal nyoo-RAL-jee-ah) pain in one or more (of three) branches of the fifth cranial nerve (trigeminal nerve) that runs along the face; also called *tic douloureux* [*tri-* three, *-gemina-* twins or pair, *-al* relating to, *neur-* nerves, *-algia* pain]

triglyceride (try-GLIH-ser-ide) lipid that is synthesized from fatty acids and glycerol or from excess glucose or amino acids; stored mainly in adipose tissue cells [*tri-* three, *-glycer-* sweet, *-ide* chemical]

trigone (TRY-gohn) triangular structure, as in the three-cornered floor of the urinary bladder [*tri-* three, *-gon* corner]

triiodothyronine (T_3) (try-eye-oh-doh-THY-roh-neen) thyroid hormone that stimulates cellular metabolism [*tri-* three, *-iodo-* violet (iodine), *-thyro-* shield (thyroid gland), *-nine* chemical]

trimester three-month segments of the gestation period [*tri-* three, *-me(n)s-* month, *-ster* thing]

triplegia (try-PLEE-jee-ah) paralysis that affects both legs and one arm [*tri-* three, *-pleg-* stricken, *-ia* condition]

trisomy (TRY-so-mee) abnormal genetic condition in which cells have three chromosomes (a triplet) where there should be a pair; usually caused by nondisjunction (failure of chromosome pairs to separate) during gamete production [*tri-* three, *-som-* body (chromosome), *-y* state]

trochlea (TROK-lee-ah) spool-shaped projection on the distal end of the humerus bone of the arm that articulates with the olecranon of the ulna [*trochlea* pulley] *pl.*, trochleae (TROK-lee-ee)

trochlear nerve (TROK-lee-ar nerv) cranial nerve IV; motor nerve; responsible for eye movements [*trochlea-* pulley, *-ar* relating to]

trophoblast (TROH-foh-blast) outer wall of the blastocyst; contributes in formation of the placenta [*tropho-* nourishment, *-blast* sprout]

tropic hormone (TROH-pik HOR-mohn) hormone that stimulates another endocrine gland to secrete its hormones [*trop-* turn or change, *-ic* relating to, *hormon-* excite]

tropomyosin (troh-poh-MY-oh-sin) in sliding-filament theory of muscle cell contraction, the long protein molecule that covers the active sites of myosin; myofilament [*tropo-* to turn, *-myo-* muscle, *-in* substance]

troponin (troh-POH-nin) the protein molecule in the thin filament of a muscle fibre spaced at intervals along tropomyosin strands that blocks actin's active sites when the myofilament is at rest [*tropo-* turn, *-in* substance]

troponins test (TROH-poh-nins) diagnostic aid used to identify a specific biochemical marker present in cardiac disease [*tropo-* turn, *-in* substance]

true ankle joint (tru ANG-kel joynt) diarthrotic synovial joint formed at the distal ends of the medial malleolus of the tibia and the lateral malleolus of the fibula embracing the underlying talus, allowing up-and-down movement of the foot

true capillary (tru cap-IL-air-ee) blood vessel that receives blood flowing out of metarterioles or other small arterioles [*capill-* hair, *-ary* relating to]

true pelvis (tru PEL-vis) structure forming a bony ring between the pelvic inlet and the pelvic outlet of the skeleton [pelvic basin] *pl.*, pelves (PEL-veez) or pelvises (PEL-vis-ez)

true vocal cord *see* **vocal fold** [*voca-* voice, *-al* relating to]

trypsin (TRIP-sin) protein-digesting enzyme (protease) [*tryps-* pound, *-in* substance]

trypsinogen (trip-SIN-oh-gen) inactive proenzyme that is subsequently converted to active trypsin by enterokinase in the intestinal lumen [*tryps-* pound, *-in* substance, *-o-* combining form, *-gen* produce]

tubal pregnancy (TYOO-bal PREG-nen-see) ectopic pregnancy that occurs in a uterine tube [*tub-* tube, *-al* relating to, *pre-* before, *-g-* related to, *-na(t)-* birth, *-ancy* state]

tuberculosis (TB) (too-ber-kyoo-LOH-sis) chronic bacterial (bacillus) infection of the lungs or other tissues caused by *Mycobacterium tuberculosis* organisms [*tuber-* swelling, *-cul-* little, *-osis* condition]

tubular (TYOOB-yoo-lar) relating to a tube or resembling a tube [*tub-* tube, *-ul-* little, *-ar* relating to]

tubular reabsorption (TYOOB-yoo-lar ree-ab-SORP-shun) movement of molecules out of the various segments of the renal tubule and into the peritubular blood [*tub-* tube, *-ul-* little, *-ar* relating to, *re-* back again, *-ab-* from, *-sorp-* suck, *-tion* process]

tubular secretion (TYOOB-yoo-lar seh-KREE-shun) movement of molecules out of the peritubular blood and into the renal tubule for excretion [*tub-* tube, *-ul-* little, *-ar* relating to, *secret-* separate, *-tion* process]

tubuloglomerular feedback (tyoob-yoo-loh-glow-MER-yoo-lar) regulatory mechanism that helps protect the kidney from rapid systemic arterial pressure variations [*tub-* tube, *-ul-* little, *-glomer-*ball, *-ul-* little, *-ar* relating to]

tuft cell cell of the intestinal mucosa with an apical tuft or cluster of microvilli that secretes prostaglandins and opioids (endorphins); also called *brush cell*

tumour growth of tissues in which cell proliferation is uncontrolled and progressive [*tumour* swelling]

tumour marker abnormal antigen on cancer cells; also called *tumour-specific antigen* [*tumour* swelling]

tumour suppressor gene gene that works against the development of cancerous cells [*tumour* swelling, *suppress-* press down, *-or* agent, *gen-* produce or generate]

tumour-specific antigen (TYOO-mer-speh-SIF-ik AN-tih-jen) *see* **tumour marker** [*tumour* swelling, *specif-* form, *-ic* relating to, *anti-* against, *-gen* produce]

tunica adventitia (TYOO-nih-kah ad-ven-TISH-ah) outermost layer of arteries, veins, lymphatic vessels, and other organs; made of strong, flexible fibrous connective tissue; usually called *tunica externa* or simply *adventitia* [*tunica* tunic or coat, *adventitia* coming from abroad] *pl.*, tunicae adventitiae (TYOO-nih-kee ad-ven-TISH-ahe)

tunica albuginea (TYOO-nih-kah al-byoo-JIN-ee-ah) tough, whitish membrane that surrounds each testis and enters the gland to divide it into lobules [*tunica* tunic or coat, *albuginea* white] *pl.*, tunicae albuginea (TYOO-nih-kee al-byoo-JIN-ee-ah)

tunica externa (TYOO-nih-kah ex-TER-nah) outermost layer of arteries, veins, lymphatic vessels, and other organs; made of strong, flexible fibrous connective tissue; sometimes called *tunica adventitia* [*tunica* tunic or coat, *extern-* outside] *pl.*, tunicae externae (TYOO-nih-kee ex-TER-nee)

tunica interna (TYOO-nih-kah in-TER-nah) *see* **tunica intima** [*tunica* tunic or coat, *intern-* inside] *pl.*, tunicae internae (TYOO-nih-kee in-TER-nee)

tunica intima (TYOO-nih-kah IN-tih-mah) layer made up of endothelium that lines blood vessels; also called *tunica interna* [*tunica* tunic or coat, *intima* innermost] *pl.*, tunicae intimae (TYOO-nih-kee IN-tih-mee)

tunica media (TYOO-nih-kah MEE-dee-ah) muscular middle layer in blood vessels; the tunica media of arteries is more muscular than that of veins [*tunica* tunic or coat, *media* middle] *pl.*, tunicae mediae (TYOO-nih-kee MEE-dee-ee)

turbinate (TUR-bih-nayt) *see* **concha** [*turbin-* top (spinning toy), *-ate* of or like]

turbulent flow (TUR-byoo-lent flo) flow of blood that occurs normally at heart valves; contributes to the first and second heart sounds [*turb-* turmoil, *-ulent* characterized by]

turgor (TUR-ger) resiliency or fluid pressure in the cells of the skin, often lost during dehydration [*turg-* swollen, *-or* condition]

Turner syndrome (TUR-ner SIN-drohm) genetic disorder caused by monosomy of the X chromosome (XO) in females; characterized by immaturity of sex organs (causing sterility), webbed neck, cardiovascular defects, and learning disorders [*Harry H. Turner* American endocrinologist, *syn-* together, *-drome* running or (race) course]

twitch contraction (twich kon-TRAK-shun) quick jerk of a muscle produced by a single, brief threshold stimulus [*con-* together, *-tract-* drag or draw, *-tion* process]

two-point discrimination test procedure that tests the distribution of touch receptors in the skin [*discrimina-* separate, *-ation* process]

tympanic membrane (tim-PAN-ik) eardrum [*tympan-* drum, *-ic* relating to, *membran-* thin skin]

tympanotomy tube (tim-pah-NOT-eh-mee) surgical tool used to relieve pressure and permit drainage of the ear [*tympan-* drum, *-tom-* cut, *-y* action]

type 1 diabetes mellitus (dye-ah-BEE-teez mell-EYE-tus) condition resulting when the pancreatic islets secrete too little insulin, resulting in increased blood glucose [*diabetes* pass-through or siphon, *mellitus* honey sweet]

type 2 diabetes mellitus (dye-ah-BEE-teez mell-EYE-tus) condition resulting when cells of the body become less sensitive to the hormone insulin and perhaps the pancreatic islets secrete too little insulin, resulting in increased levels of blood glucose [*diabetes* pass-through or siphon, *mellitus* honey sweet]

Type A blood type that has antigen A on red blood cells

Type AB blood type that has both antigen A and antigen B on red blood cells

Type B blood type that has antigen B on red blood cells

type II cell produces surfactant in the alveoli [*II* Roman numeral two, *cell* storeroom]

Type O blood type that has neither antigen A nor antigen B on red blood cells

tyrosine kinase inhibitor (TYE-roh-seen KIN-ayz in-HIB-it-er) class of chemotherapy drugs that inhibit tyrosine-activating enzymes in cancer cells [*tyro-* cheese, *-sine* chemical, *kinesis-* motion, *-ase* enzyme, *inhibit-* restrain, *-or* agent]

U

U wave electrocardiogram deflection that results from late repolarization of Purkinje fibres in the papillary muscle of the ventricular myocardium, or possibly from different durations of action potential in the ventricular myocardium producing a two-part T wave [named for 21st letter of Roman alphabet]

ubiquitin (yoo-BIK-wit-in) a class of numerous, very small proteins used by the cell to tag proteins for destruction by the proteasome [*ubiqui-* everywhere, *-in* substance]

ulcer (UL-ser) necrotic open sore or lesion [*ulc-* sore]

ulna (UL-nah) forearm bone [*ulna* elbow] *pl.*, ulnae (UL-nee) or ulnas (UL-nahz)

ulnar deviation (UL-nur dee-vee-AY-shun) deformity of the hands as a result of rheumatoid arthritis [*ulna-* elbow, *-ar* relating to, *de-* out of, *-via-* road or path, *-ation* process]

ultrasonography (ul-trah-son-OG-rah-fee) imaging technique in which high-frequency sound waves are reflected off tissue to form an image [*ultra-* beyond, *-sono-* sound, *-graph-* draw, *-y* process]

ultrasound lithotripsy (UL-trah-sound LITH-oh-trip-see) procedure that uses an ultrasound generator to pulverize stones so that they can be flushed out of the urinary tract without surgery [*ultra-* beyond, sound, *litho-* stone, *-trips-* pound, *-y* action]

umbilical artery (um-BIL-ih-kul AR-ter-ee) two small arteries that carry oxygen-poor blood from the developing fetus to the placenta [*umbilic-* navel, *-al* relating to, *arteri-* vessel]

umbilical cord (um-BIL-ih-kul) flexible structure connecting the fetus with the placenta; contains umbilical arteries and vein [*umbilic-* navel, *-al* relating to]

umbilical hernia (um-BIL-ih-kul HER-nee-ah) rupture of the anterior abdominal wall at the navel [*umbilic-* navel, *-al* relating to, *hernia* rupture] *pl.*, herniae (HER-nee-ee) or hernias

umbilical vein (um-BIL-ih-kul vayn) large vein carrying oxygen-rich blood from the placenta to the developing fetus [*umbilic-* navel, *-al* relating to, *vena* blood vessel]

umbilicus (um-BIL-ih-kus) navel [*umbilic-* navel, *-us* thing]

uncompensated acidosis (un-KOM-pen-say-ted ass-ih-DOH-sis) decrease in the ratio of base to acid; causes a decrease in pH [*acid-* sour, *-osis* condition]

uncompensated alkalosis (un-KOM-pen-say-ted al-kah-LOH-sis) increase in the ratio of base to acid; causes an increase in pH [*alkal-* ashes, *-osis* condition]

uniaxial joint (yoo-nee-AK-see-al) synovial joint that permits movement around only one axis and in only one plane [*uni-* one, *-axi-* axle, *-al* relating to]

unicellular gland (yoo-nee-SEL-yoo-lar) single glandular epithelial cell [*uni-* one, *-cell-* storeroom, *-ular* relating to, *gland* acorn]

unipolar (pseudounipolar) **neuron** (yoo-nee-POH-lar [SOO-doh-yoo-nee-POH-lar] NYOO-ron) structural category of neurons made up of cells that appear to have only one extension from the cell body [*uni-* single, *-pol-* pole, *-ar* relating to, *pseudo-* false, *neuron* string or nerve]

unmyelinated fibre (un-MY-eh-lin-ay-ted) nerve fibre that does not have a myelin sheath; also referred to as *grey fibre* [*un-* not, *-myel-* marrow, *-in-* substance, *-ate* act of, *fibre-* thread]

unsaturated fat (un-SATCH-yoo-ray-ted) fat-containing fatty acid chains in which there are some double bonds, not all sites for hydrogen are filled; usually liquid at room temperature [*un-* not, *-saturat-* fill, *-ate* act of]

upper oesophageal sphincter (UES) (eh-SOF-ah-JEE-ul SFINGK-ter) ring of muscular tissue at proximal end of oesophagus; helps prevent air from entering the oesophagus during respiration [*oes-* will carry, *-phag-* food (eat), *-al* relating to, *sphinc-* bind tight, *-er* agent]

upper respiratory infection (RES-pih-rah-to-ree) infection localized in the muscosa of the upper respiratory tract [*re-* again, *-spir-* breathe, *-tory* relating to, *infec-* stain, *-tion* process]

upper respiratory tract (RES-pih-rah-tor-ee trakt) respiratory organs that are not contained within the thorax; includes nasal cavity, pharynx, and associated structures [*re-* again, *-spir-* breathe, *-tory* relating to, *tract* trail]

up-regulation (uhp reg-yuh-LAY-shun) phenomenon that occurs when a target cell has more receptors and thus can be more sensitive to a hormone [*up-* increase, *-regula-* rule, *-tion* process]

urea (yoo-REE-ah) nitrogen-containing waste product [*urea-* urine]

uraemia (yoo-REE-mee-ah) condition in which blood urea concentration is abnormally elevated, expressed as a high blood urea nitrogen (BUN) value; uraemia is often caused by renal failure; also called *uraemic syndrome* [*ur-* urine, *-(h)aem-* blood, *-ia* condition]

uraemic syndrome (yoo-REE-mik SIN-drohm) *see* **uraemia** [*ur-* urine, *-(h)aem-* blood, *-ic* relating to, *syn-* together, *-drome* running or (race) course]

ureter (YOOR-eh-ter) long tube that carries urine from kidney to bladder [*ure-* urine, *-ter* agent or channel]

urethra (yoo-REE-thrah) passageway from bladder to exterior; functions in elimination of urine; in males, also acts as a genital duct that carries sperm to the exterior [*ure-* urine, *-thr-* agent or channel]

urethral sphincter (yoo-REE-thral SFINGK-ter) circular muscle of the pelvic floor that constricts around the urethra, thus regulating urine flow from the bladder and out of the body [*ure-* urine, *-thr-* agent or channel (urethra), *-al* relating to, *sphinc-* bind tight, *-er* agent]

urethral stricture (yoo-REE-thral STRIK-chur) narrowing or blockage of the urethra [*ure-* urine, *-thr-* agent or channel (urethra), *-al* relating to, *stric-* tighten, *-ture* condition]

urethritis (yoo-reh-THRY-tis) inflammation or infection of the urethra [*ure-* urine, *-thr-* agent or channel (urethra), *-itis* inflammation]

urinary bladder (YOOR-ih-nair-ee) collapsible saclike organ that collects urine from the kidneys and stores it before elimination [*urin-* urine, *-ary* relating to]

urinary meatus (YOOR-ih-nair-ee mee-AY-tus) external opening of the urethra [*urin-* urine, *-ary* relating to, *meatus* channel or passage] *pl.*, meatus or meatuses

urinary system (YOOR-ih-nair-ee) system responsible for excreting most liquid wastes from the body [*urin-* urine, *-ary* relating to]

urination (yoor-ih-NAY-shun) passage of urine from the body; emptying of the bladder; also called *micturition* [*urin-* urine, *-ation* process]

urine (YOOR-in) fluid waste excreted by kidneys [*ur-* urine, *-ine* chemical]

urochrome (YOOR-oh-krohm) pigments from the breakdown of old red blood cells in the liver and elsewhere that are found in the urine [*uro-* urine, *-chroma* colour]

urodynamics (yoo-roh-dye-NAM-iks) force of urine flow in the urinary tract [*uro-* urine, *dynam-* moving force, *-ic* relating to]

urogenital triangle (YOO-roh-JEN-ih-tal) region of the perineum that contains the external genitals (labia, vaginal orifice, clitoris) and urinary opening, and the anal triangle, which surrounds the anus [*uro-* urine, *-genit-* reproduction, *-al* relating to, *tri-* three, *-angle* corner]

urothelium (yoo-roh-THEE-lee-um) another name for transitional epithelium, the stretchable stratified epithelium that lines the urinary tract [*uro-* urine, *-theli-* nipple, *-um* thing]

urticaria (er-tih-KAIR-ee-ah) hives; allergic or hypersensitive response characterized by raised red lesions [*urtica-* nettle, *-ia* abnormal condition]

uterine artery embolization (YOO-ter-in AR-ter-ee em-boh-lih-ZAY-shun) technique that involves snaking a small catheter through an artery in the groin into the arterial vessel supplying blood to a fibroid; procedure results in dramatic shrinkage of the treated fibroid and a reduction in symptoms, including haemorrhage [*uter-* womb, *-ine* relating to, *arteri-* vessel, *embol-* plug, *-ation* process]

uterine fibroid (YOO-ter-in FYE-broyd) abnormal muscular growth in the uterus that may result in dysfunctional uterine bleeding [*uter-* womb, *-ine* relating to, *fibr-* thread or fibre, *-oid* of or like]

uterine tube (YOO-ter-in) fallopian tube [*uter-* womb, *-ine* relating to]

uterosacral ligament (yoo-ter-oh-SAK-ral LIG-ah-ment) foldlike extension of the peritoneum from the posterior surface of the uterus to the sacrum [*uter-* womb, *sacr-* sacred (sacrum), *-al* relating to (sacrum), *liga-* bind, *-ment* condition]

uterus (YOO-ter-us) hollow, muscular organ that holds and sustains developing offspring until birth [*uterus* womb]

utricle (YOO-tri-kul) part of membranous labyrinth of inner ear; involved with sensation of static equilibrium [*uter-* bag, *-cle* little]

uvula (YOO-vyoo-lah) cone-shaped process hanging from the soft palate that helps prevent food and liquid from entering the nasal cavities [*uva-* grape, *-ul-* little, *-a* thing]

V

vaccination (vak-sih-NAY-shun) method used to achieve active immunity by triggering the body to form antibodies against specific pathogens [*vaccin-* cow (cowpox), *-ation* process]

vaccine (VAK-seen) application of killed or attenuated (weakened) pathogens (or portions of pathogens) to a patient to stimulate immunity against that pathogen [*vaccin-* cow (cowpox)]

vagina (vah-JYE-nah) internal tube from uterus to vulva [*vagina* sheath]

vaginal orifice (VAj-ih-nal OR-ih-fis) opening of the vagina to the outside of the body [*vagina-* sheath, *-al* relating to, *ori-* mouth, *-fice-* something made]

vaginitis (vaj-ih-NYE-tis) inflammation of the vagina [*vagin-* sheath (vagina), *-itis* inflammation]

vagus nerve (VAY-gus nerv) cranial nerve X; mixed nerve; sensations and movements of organs [*vagus* wanderer]

Valsalva manoeuvre (VAL-sahl-vah mah-NOO-ver) procedure in which one closes the mouth, pinches the nose shut, and exhales moderately to push air into the auditory tube if needed to equalize pressure on the tympanic membrane; straining during defaecation is a modification of the Valsalva manoeuvre [*Antonio Maria Valsalva* Italian anatomist]

valvuloplasty (VAL-vyoo-loh-plas-tee) procedure that replaces damaged or defective cardiac valves [*valv-* valve, *-plasty* surgical repair]

variable (VAIR-ee-ah-bil) anything that varies or changes; a physiological variable is any condition or state inside the body that can change and is controlled or kept relatively constant by homeostatic mechanisms [*vari-* change, *-able* capable]

variant Creutzfeldt–Jakob Disease (vCJ) (VAIR-ee-ant KROYTS-felt YAH-kobe) degenerative disease of the central nervous system caused by prions (*pro*teinaceous *in*fectious particles) that convert normal proteins of the nervous system into abnormal proteins, causing loss of function; *see* **prion** [*Hans G.*

Creutzfeldt German neurologist, *Alfons M. Jakob* German neurologist]

varicose vein (VAIR-ih-kohse vayn) enlarged vein in which blood pools; also called *varix* [*varic-* swollen vein, *-ose* characterized by, *vena* blood vessel] *pl.*, varices

varix (VAIR-ix) varicose vein [*varix* swollen vein] *pl.*, varices

vas deferens (vas DEF-er-enz) reproductive duct that extends from the epididymis to the ejaculatory duct; also called *ductus deferens* [*vas* duct or vessel, *deferens* carrying away] *pl.*, vasa deferentia

vasa recta (VAH-sah REK-tah) the long, hairpin-shaped arterioles of the kidney leading from the efferent arteriole and following the nephron loop; also called *straight arterioles (of kidney)* [*vas-* vessel, *rect-* straight or upright] *sing.*, vas rectum

vasa vasorum (VAS-ah vah-SOR-um) tiny blood vessels that supply the smooth muscles that surround the walls of larger blood vessels [*vasa* vessel, *vaso-* vessel or duct, *-um* small one]

vascular anastomosis (VAS-kyoo-lar ah-nas-toh-MOH-sis) condition when blood moves from veins to other veins or arteries to other arteries without passing through an intervening capillary network [*vas-* vessel, *-ular* relating to, *ana-* again or anew, *-stomo-* mouth, *-osis* condition] *pl.*, anatomoses

vasectomy (va-SEK-toh-mee) surgical severing of the vas deferens to render a male sterile [*vaso-* vessel (vas deferens), *-ec-* out, *-tom-* cut, *-y* action]

vasoactive intestinal peptide (VIP) (vay-so-AK-tiv in-TES-tih-nal PEP-tyde) hormone involved with controlling intestinal secretion [*vas-* vessel, *-act* to do, drive, *-tive* state, *intestin-* intestine, *-al* relating to, *pept-* digest, *-ide* chemical]

vasoconstriction (vay-soh-kon-STRIK-shun) reduction in vessel diameter caused by increased contraction of the muscular coat [*vaso-* vessel, *-constrict-* draw tight, *-tion* state]

vasodilation (vay-soh-dye-LAY-shun) increase in vessel diameter caused by relaxation of vascular muscles [*vaso-* vessel, *-dilat-* widen, *-tion* state]

vasodilator (vay-so-DYE-lay-tor) class of drugs that trigger the smooth muscles of arterial walls to relax, causing the arteries to dilate [*vaso-* vessel or duct, *-dilat-* widen, *-or* agent]

vasodilatory shock (vay-soh-DYE-lah-tor-ee) *see* **neurogenic shock** [*vaso-* vessel, *-dilat-* widen, *-ory* relating to]

vasomotor chemoreflex (vay-so-MOH-tor kee-moh-REE-fleks) chemoreceptors located in the aortic and carotid bodies are sensitive to hypercapnia, hypoxia, and decreased arterial blood pH [*vaso-* vessel, *-motor* move, *chemo-* chemical, *-re-* back or again, *-flex* bend]

vasomotor mechanism (vay-so-MOH-tor) feedback regulation of the diameter of arterioles [*vaso-* vessel, *-motor* move, *mechan-* machine, *-ism* state]

vasomotor pressoreflex (vay-so-MOH-tor press-oh-REE-fleks) reflex that occurs in response to a change in arterial blood pressure [*vaso-* vessel, *-motor* move, *press-* pressure, *-re-* back or again, *-flex* bend]

vault *see* **barrel**

vector (VEK-tor) arthropod that carries an infectious pathogen from one organism to another [*vect-* carry, *-or* agent]

vein (vayn) vessel carrying blood from capillaries toward the heart [*vena* blood vessel]

vellus (VEL-us) strong, fine, and less pigmented hair found in skin before puberty [*vellus* wool]

venoconstriction (vee-noh-kon-STRIK-shun) type of vasoconstriction (vessel wall constriction by smooth muscles) in veins [*ven-* vein, *-constrict-* draw tight, *-tion* state]

venous pump (VEE-nus) blood-pumping action of respirations and skeletal muscle contractions facilitate venous return by increasing pressure gradient between peripheral veins and venae cavae [*ven-* vein, *-ous* relating to]

venous return (VEE-nus) amount of blood returned to the heart by the veins [*ven-* vein, *-ous* relating to]

venous sinus (VEE-nus SYE-nus) large specialized venous structures that have very thin endothelial walls [*ven-* vein, *-ous* relating to, *sinus* hollow]

ventilation (ven-tih-LAY-shun) rate and depth of breathing [*vent-* fan or create wind, *-tion* process]

ventral (anterior) nerve root (VEN-tral) bundle of nerve fibres that carry motor information out of the spinal cord [*ventr-* belly, *-al* relating to]

ventral (VEN-tral) of or near the belly; in humans, front or anterior; opposite of dorsal or posterior [*ventr-* belly, *-al* relating to]

ventral cavities (VEN-tral KAV-ih-teez) body cavities on the ventral side of the body, which include the thoracic cavity and abdominopelvic cavity; not a standard anatomical term, but used here to help organize the body for the beginning student [*ventr-* belly, *-al* relating to, *cav-* hollow, *-ity* state]

ventral ramus (VEN-tral RAY-mus) large, complex branch of each spinal nerve [*ventr-* belly, *-al* relating to *ramus* branch] *pl.*, rami

ventral root (VEN-tral) motor branch of a spinal nerve, by which it is attached to the spinal cord [*ventr-* belly, *-al* relating to]

ventricle (VEN-trih-kul) a cavity, such as the large, fluid-filled spaces within the brain or the chambers of the heart [*ventr-* belly, *-icle* little]

ventricular fibrillation (ven-TRIK-yoo-lar fib-ril-LAY-shun) an immediately life-threatening condition caused by the lack of ventricular pumping suddenly stopping flow of blood to vital organs [*ventr-* belly, *-icul-* little, *-ar* relating to, *fibr-* thread or fibre, *-illa-* little, *-ation* process]

venule (VEN-yool) small blood vessels that collect blood from capillaries and join to form veins [*ven-* vein, *-ule* little]

vermiform appendix (VERM-ih-form ah-PEN-diks) hollow, tubular structure attached to the caecum (of the colon) and thought to be a breeding ground for beneficial intestinal bacteria [*vermi-* worm, *-form* shape, *append-* hang upon, *-ix* thing] *pl.*, appendices (ah-PEN-dis-eez)

vermis (VER-mis) central section of the cerebellum [*vermis* worm] *pl.*, vermes (VER-meez)

vertebra (VER-teh-bra) any of the bones that make up the spinal column [*vertebra* that which turns] *pl.*, vertebrae (VER-teh-bray or VER-teh-bree)

vertebral column (ver-TEE-bral) the spinal column, made up of a series of separate vertebrae that form a flexible, curved rod; made up of the cervical, thoracic, lumbar, sacral, and coccygeal segments [*vertebra-* that which turns, *-al* relating to, *column* pillar]

vertebral foramen (ver-TEE-bral for-AY-men) the central opening in the vertebral column that contains the spinal cord [*vertebra* that which turns, *-al* relating to, *foramen* hole]

vertebroplasty (ver-tee-broh-PLAS-tee) orthopaedic procedure used to treat the vertebral compression fractures that occur in osteoporosis; involves injecting bone cement, but without using a balloon [*vertebr-* that which turns, *-plasty* surgical repair]

vertigo (VER-tih-go) abnormal sensation of spinning; dizziness [*vertigo* turning]

vesicle (VES-ih-kul) any tiny membranous bubble within a cell; clinical term referring to blisters, fluid-filled skin lesions; *see also* **blister** [*vesic-* blister, *-cle* little]

vesicouterine pouch (ves-ih-koh-YOO-ter-in) *see* **anterior cul-de-sac** [*vesic-* blister, *-uter-* womb, *-ine* relating to]

vestibular fold (ves-TIB-yoo-lar) either of the lower of two pairs of lateral folds of the mucosa in the larynx, just above the vocal folds; also called *false vocal fold* or *false vocal cord*; compare to **vocal fold** [*vestibul-* entrance hall, *-ar* relating to]

vestibular membrane (ves-TIB-yoo-lar) roof of the cochlear duct; also called *Reissner's membrane* [*vestibul-* entrance hall, *-ar* relating to, *membran-* thin skin]

vestibular nerve (ves-TIB-yoo-lar nerv) division of the vestibulocochlear nerve (eighth cranial nerve)

vestibule (VES-tih-byool) located in the bony labyrinth of the inner ear; portion adjacent to the oval window between the semicircular canals and the cochlea [*vestibul-* entrance hall]

vestibulocochlear nerve (ves-TIB-yoo-loh-kok-lee-ar nerv) cranial nerve VIII; sensory nerve; responsible for hearing and equilibrium [*vestibulo-* entrance hall, *-cochle-* snail shell, *-ar* relating to]

vestibulospinal tract (ves-TIB-yoo-loh-SPY-nal) descending, or motor, tract that conveys neural messages that coordinate posture and balance [*vestibul-* entrance hall, *-spino-* backbone, *-al* relating to, *tract* trail]

vibrissa (vye-BRISS-ah) coarse hair found in the skin of the vestibule of the nose [*vibrissa* nostril hair] *pl.*, vibrissae (vye-BRISS-ee)

villus (VIL-us) any of the fingerlike folds covering the plicae of the small intestines [*villus* shaggy hair], *pl.*, villi (VIL-eye or VIL-ee)

Vincent infection (VIN-sent) bacterial (spirochete) infection of the gum, producing gingivitis; also called *Vincent angina* and *trench mouth* [*Henri Vincent* French physician]

virion (VYE-ree-on) a complete viral particle (genetic material and protein capsule) [*vir-* poison, *-on* unit]

virus (VYE-rus) microscopic, intracellular parasitic entity consisting of a nucleic acid bound by a protein coat and sometimes a lipoprotein envelope [*virus* poison]

viscera (VISS-er-ah) internal organs [*visc-* internal organ] *sing.*, viscus (VISS-kus)

visceral (VISS-er-al) relating to the viscera (internal organs); toward or on the internal organs (opposite of parietal) [*viscer-* internal organ, *-al* relating to]

visceral membrane (VISS-er-al) serous membrane that covers the surface of the viscera [*viscer-* internal organ, *-al* relating to, *membran-* thin skin]

visceral pericardium (VISS-er-al pair-ih-KAR-dee-um) the serous membrane that adheres to and covers the heart; also called the *epicardium* [*viscer-* internal organ, *-al* relating to, *peri-* around, *-cardi-* heart, *-um* thing]

visceral pleura (VISS-er-al PLOO-rah) the serous membrane that adheres to and covers the lung [*viscer-* internal organ, *-al* relating to, *pleura* side of body] *pl.*, pleurae (PLOO-ree)

visceral portion (VISS-er-al) serous membrane that covers the surfaces of organs in the body cavity [*viscer-* internal organ, *-al* relating to]

visceral reflex (VISS-er-al REE-fleks) autonomic reflex; contractions of smooth or cardiac muscles or secretion by glands [*viscer-* internal organ, *-al* relating to, *re-* again, *-flex* bend]

visceral sensory division (VISS-er-al) division of the nervous system made up of afferent (incoming) pathways from autonomic sensory receptors (receptors involved in subconscious perception) of the internal organs (viscera) [*viscer-* internal organs, *-al* relating to, *sens-* feel, *-ory* relating to]

visceroceptor (viss-er-oh-SEP-tor) somatic sense receptor located in the internal visceral organs; also called *interoceptor* [*viscero-* internal organs, *-cept-* receive, *-or* agent]

viscosity (vis-KOS-ih-tee) thickness of a fluid [*viscos-* sticky, *-ity* state]

vital capacity (VC) (largest amount of air that can be moved in and out of the lungs in one inspiration and expiration [*vita-* life, *-al* relating to. *capac-* hold, *-ity* state]

vitamin organic molecules needed in small quantities to help enzymes operate effectively [*vita-* life, *-amin(e)* ammonia compound]

vitamin D compound that influences several important chemical reactions in the body; for example, formation of bones and teeth [*vit-* life, *-amin(e)* ammonia compound]

vitiligo (vit-ih-LYE-go) acquired condition that results in loss of pigment in certain areas of the skin [*vitiligo* blemish]

vitreous body (VIT-ree-us) sac filled with jelly-like fluid in the eye, posterior to the lens [*vitre-* glassy, *-ous* of or like]

vocal cord *see* **vocal fold** [*voca-* voice, *-al* relating to]

vocal fold lower pair of lateral folds of mucosa in the larynx, responsible for vocalization; also called *true vocal fold* or *true vocal cord* or *vocal cord*; compare to **false vocal fold** [*voca-* voice *-al* relating to]

voiding (VOYD-ing) emptying the bladder [*void-* empty]

volar (VOH-lar) palm of the hand or sole of the foot [*vola-* palm, sole, *-ar* relating to]

Volkmann canal (VOLK-man) *see* **transverse canal (of bone)** [*Richard von Volkmann*, German surgeon]

voltage-gated channel type of cell-membrane channel for the transport of molecules that is controlled by a gate that responds to a change in voltage (difference in charge across the cell membrane) [*volt-* unit of electrical force (after *Alessandro Volta* Italian physicist), *-age* amount]

volume measurement of the amount of space taken up by a substance

voluntary muscle *see* **skeletal muscle** [*mus-* mouse, *-cle* little]

vomer bone (VOH-mer) bone that forms the lower and posterior part of the nasal septum [*vomer* plowshare]

vomeronasal organ (VNO) (voh-mer-oh-NAY-sal) sensory organ for detecting pheromones (sex signal molecules) located in the muscosa of the nasal septum [*vomer-* plowshare (vomer bone), *nas-* nose, *-al* relating to, *organ* instrument]

vulva (VUL-vah) external genitals of the female [*vulva* wrapper]

vulvitis (vul-VYE-tis) inflammation of the vulva (external female genitals) [*vulv-* wrapper (vulva), *-itis* inflammation]

W

wart nipplelike neoplasm of the skin; caused by papilloma virus [*wart* swelling]

white fibres muscle fibres containing little myoglobin; also called *fast fibres*; nerve fibres with a thick myelin sheath [*fibre* thread]

white matter (wyte MAT-ter) nerves covered with white myelin sheath

white ramus (wyte RAY-mus) small branch of myelinated sympathetic preganglionic fibres [*ramus* branch]

windpipe informal synonym for *trachea*

withdrawal reflex (with-DRAW-ul REE-fleks) reflex that moves a body part away from an irritating stimulus [*with-* away, *-draw-* draw, *-al* relating to, *re-* again, *-flex* bend]

X

X chromosome (KROH-moh-sohm) sex chromosome, which, in females, is paired with another X chromosome; as opposed to being paired to a Y chromosome as in males [*chromo-* colour, *-some* body]

xeroderma pigmentosum (zeer-oh-DER-mah pig-men-TOH-sum) rare genetic disorder characterized by the inability of skin cells to repair genetic damage caused by the ultraviolet (UV) radiation in sunlight [*xero-* dry, *-derma* skin, *pigment-* paint, *-osum* characterized by]

xerostomia (zee-roh-STOH-mee-ah) condition that results from a dramatic reduction of production of saliva and tears; dry mouth [*xero-* dryness, *-stom-* mouth, *-ia* condition]

X-linked trait genetic trait associated with the female (X) chromosome

x-ray photography method of noninvasive imaging of internal body structures; uses energy in the x band of the radiation spectrum beamed through the body to photographic film; also called *radiography* [*x-* unknown, *-ray* spoke or rod, *photo-* light, *-graph-* draw, *-y* activity]

Y

Y chromosome (KROH-moh-sohm) sex chromosome that contains genes that determine maleness [*chromo-* colour, *-some* body]

yawn slow, deep inspiration through an unusually widened mouth

yeast (yeest) single-celled fungus; may be a normal or pathogenic component of the human microbiome (compared to mould, which is a multicellular fungus) [*yeast* foam or froth]

yellow marrow (MAIR-oh) connective tissue rich in fat that is found in the medullary cavity of the long bones of an adult; inactive in red cell production [*marrow* pith (middle)]

Y-linked trait genetic trait associated with the male (Y) chromosome

yolk sac in humans, involved with production of blood cells in the developing embryo [*yoke* joining]

Young–Laplace law (law of Laplace) (yung lah-PLAHS) principle that states that air pressure (P) in a bubble is inversely proportional to the radius (r) and directly proportional to the surface tension (T) summarized by the equation $P = 2T/r$ [*Thomas Young* English physician, *Pierre Simon de Laplace* French physicist]

Z

Z disc also called Z *line*; microscopic structure within the myofibril of a muscle fibre where the thin filaments unite with each other and form a netlike disc; serves as boundary of sarcomere unit [Z *zwischen* between]

zona fasciculata (ZOH-nah fas-sic-yoo-LAY-tah) middle zone of the adrenal cortex that secretes glucocorticoids [*zona* belt, *fasci-* bundle, *-cul-* little, *-ata* characterized by] *pl.*, zonae fasciculatae (ZOH-nee fas-sic-yoo-LAY-tee)

zona glomerulosa (ZOH-nah gloh-mair-yoo-LOH-sah) outer zone of the adrenal cortex that secretes mineralocorticoids [*zona* belt, *glomerulosa* having small balls] *pl.*, zonae glomerulosae (ZOH-nee gloh-mair-yoo-LOH-see)

zona pellucida (ZP) (ZOH-nah pah-LOO-sih-dah) thick, clear jelly-like film surrounding the ovum, beneath the cumulus cells of the corona radiata [*zona* belt or girdle, *pellucida* transparent] *pl.*, zonae pellucidae (ZOH-nee pah-LOO-sih-dee)

zona reticularis (ZOH-nah reh-tik-yoo-LAIR-is) inner zone of the adrenal cortex that secretes small amounts of sex hormones [*zona* belt, *reticularis* having little nets] *pl.*, zonae reticulares (ZOH-nee reh-tik-yoo-LAIR-eez)

zone of calcification (kal-sih-fih-KAY-shun) deepest layer of the epiphyseal plate; composed of cartilage undergoing rapid calcification [*calc-* lime, *-fica-* make, *-tion* process]

zone of hypertrophy (hye-PER-troh-fee) third layer of the epiphyseal plate; composed of older, enlarged cartilage cells that are undergoing degenerative changes associated with calcium deposition [*hyper-* excessive, *-troph-* nourishment, *-y* state]

zone of proliferation (proh-LIF-er-ay-shun) second layer of the epiphyseal plate; composed of cartilage cells undergoing active mitosis [*prol-* offspring, *-fer-* carry, *-ation* process]

zygomatic (zye-goh-MAT-ik) relating to the cheek bone or outside of cheek [*zygo-* union or yoke, *-ic* relating to]

zygomatic bone (zye-goh-MAT-ik bohn) cheek bone; also called *malar bone* [*zygo-* union or yoke, *-ic* relating to]

zygomaticus major muscle (zye-goh-MAT-ih-kus) muscle that elevates corners of the mouth and lips; also known as the "smiling muscle" [*zygo-* union or yoke, *-ic* relating to, *major* greater, *mus-* mouse, *-cle* little]

zygote (ZYE-goht) original cell of an offspring, formed by the union of an ovum and sperm [*zygot-* union or yoke]

zymogenic cell (zye-moh-JEN-ik) *see* **chief cell** [*zym-* ferment (enzyme), *-o-* combining form, *-gen-* produce, *-ic* relating to, *cell* storeroom]

Index

Page numbers followed by *b*, *t*, and *f* indicate boxes, tables, and figures, respectively.

H

CONNECT IT!

***Connecting anatomy and physiology topics with current research and bonus material in the field! Visit the Evolve website for the full articles:* evolve.elsevier.com/Patton/AP/**

Abdominal Thrusts: Outlines the steps of the Heimlich Manoeuvre, also called abdominal thrusts, for situations when the patient is standing, laying on the ground, or an infant.

Amazing Amino Acids: Summarizes the importance of amino acids in the body by highlighting some of the uses made of them in the body. Clarifies which amino acids are used for protein synthesis.

Arrest of Oocyte Development: Explains the advantage of arresting the development of the oocyte during meiosis and how meiosis resumes.

Artificial Cardiac Pacemakers: Discusses the artificial pacemaker, a device implanted into patients whose own natural pacemakers fail to maintain healthy heart rhythms.

Barium Enema Study: Explains how the commonly performed "lower GI series" is done, including illustrations of radiographic positioning and example medical images.

Biomimicry: Describes the research being done in mimicking cell functions in order to efficiently manufacture synthetic versions of natural substances, drugs, and other complex molecules.

Blood Doping: Explains how blood transfusions, hormones, or drugs can boost red blood cell counts and thus boost athletic endurance, but at great medical risk.

Blood Transfusions: Discusses the concepts behind blood transfusions, artificial blood, and converting one type of blood to another.

Bone Fractures: Describes the many types of bone fractures, how they occur, and how they are treated.

Bone Scans: Explains how radioactive compounds can be used in imaging of the bones.

Brain Studies: Discusses medical imaging techniques that can identify brain disorders and can further studies of the science of the brain.

Brain Wrinkles: Shows how the wrinkles on the brain's surface actually increase the amount of work the brain can do. Also includes a numbered map of Brodmann areas, which are commonly used to pinpoint functional areas on the brain's wrinkled surface.

Breast Self-Examination: Illustrates the process of breast self-examination, something both men and women should perform regularly to detect changes that might indicate mastitis or breast cancer.

Broken Heart: Discusses "broken heart syndrome", also called stress cardiomyopathy, a condition induced by intense physical or emotional stress.

Cardiac Marker Studies: Explains how substances released when heart muscle is damaged or inflamed can be detected in common medical blood tests to assess heart disease and heart attacks.

Cardiac Nuclear Scanning: Explains the method of evaluating the heart by injecting the patient with a radioactive substance and using a gamma-ray detector to create an image.

Chromosome Territories: Illustrates and summarizes the concept of localization of chromosomes within a cell's nucleus.

Clinical and Laboratory Values: Lists data on substances in the body that are commonly measured and how to convert some of these values into the International System (SI) of units.

Cochlear Implants: Describes a type of medical device commonly implanted to alleviate certain types of deafness. Illustrates how these devices work.

Colour Blindness: Text and images illustrating how colours are actually seen by colour blind individuals. Also included are samples of images used to screen for this condition.

Corneal Transplants: Describes how corneas are transplanted to restore clear vision to many patients. Photographs illustrate a recently transplanted cornea and a case of transplant rejection.

Deep Breathing after Exercise: Discusses the factors that trigger rapid, deep breathing following strenuous exercise.

Detailed Map of the Nephron: Expands on the simplified scheme of microscopic renal anatomy that is presented in the book by providing a detailed illustration of the nephron.

Diabetes Mellitus: Describes one of the most common endocrine disorders, how it affects a person's health, and how to treat it.

Disease as a Weapon: Describes how the intentional transmission of disease, such as anthrax, can be used as a weapon of terror.

DNA Analysis: Outlines some of the methods available for analyzing the genetic makeup of individuals, including electrophoresis, DNA fingerprinting, and the gene chip.

Echocardiography: Explains how ultrasound beams directed into the patient's chest can be used to evaluate the internal structures and motions of the heart and great vessels.

Electrocardiography: Describes electrocardiography and how different placements of electrodes, or leads, can show electrical activity of the heart from different angles.

Embryonic Development of Tissues: Illustrates the concept of the primary germ layers and what body structures these layers eventually give rise to.

Epigenetics: Explains epigenetics, the inheritance of traits by means other than a DNA sequence, and how it leads to different methods of disease transmission.

Erythrocyte Sedimentation Rate: Discusses the frequently performed diagnostic blood test that can reveal inflammatory conditions in the body, illustrating how the test is performed.

Faecal Fat Test: Explains how a stool sample can be analyzed to determine if dietary fats are being absorbed properly.

Fluid and Electrolyte Therapy: Discusses parenteral therapy—a strategy to bypass the digestive tract by injecting fluids, electrolytes, and nutrients directly into the bloodstream by intravenous or subcutaneous injection.

Freezing Umbilical Cord Blood: Discusses how freezing umbilical cord blood can have clinical significance because stem cells from this blood can be used in place of bone marrow transplants.

Functional Foods: Explains one of the hottest fields in nutrition, functional foods, which are foods thought to prevent disease.

Gallstones and Weight Loss: Discusses gallstones, how they are formed and treated, and their association with weight loss and dieting.

Genes and Longevity: Discusses the possibility of using the genetic discovery of "longevity genes" to lengthen the lives of people using gene therapy.

Heart Attack: Illustrates the steps of a heart attack, or myocardial infarction, a common cause of death in middle to late adulthood.

Heart Sounds: Explains more about heart sounds and what they sound like.

Hernias: Describes the common types of hernias, protrusions of organs through body cavity walls.

How to Trace the Flow of Blood: Outlines how to trace blood flow through the body and provides a diagram for a visual reference.

Hydrocephalus: Describes hydrocephalus, a condition in which the cerebrospinal fluid produces abnormal fluid pressure in the brain, and how it can be treated.

The Human Microbiome: Explains the various important roles played by microorganisms in and on our body, showing locations and types of microbial communities of the human body.

Immunotherapy: Reviews treatments that can be used to bolster the body's immune defences, and explains how antibodies can be introduced into the body to target tumour cells.

In Vitro Fertilization: Describes some of the many assistive reproductive techniques, including in vitro fertilization, that are available to promote reproductive success.

Infant Diarrhoea: Discusses the global impact of rotavirus infections and the role of vaccines and oral rehydration therapy in alleviating this disease.

Inflammation: Outlines the events of the inflammatory response and its effects on the tissues of the body.

Interferon Therapy: Describes the therapeutic use of one of the body's own immunity proteins.

Kidney Biopsy: Illustrates how tissue is removed from a possibly diseased kidney for clinical laboratory examination.

Learning Cranial Nerves: Focuses on methods of learning the names of the cranial nerves and their functions.

Leverage: Explains the mechanical advantage gained in a lever system, and how muscles, joints, and bones form lever systems in the body.

Lung Volume Reduction Surgery: Dramatic photos of a lung with emphysema punctuate this discussion of surgical procedures used to remove diseased portions of a lung in emphysema patients.

Male Circumcision: Discusses male circumcision, including why it is done, how it is performed, and the controversy that surrounds it.

Male Genital Self-Examination: Explains male genital self-examination, which should be done regularly to look for lumps, changes in size, changes in texture of a testis, and surface abnormalities.

Measuring Bone Mineral Density: Describes osteoporosis, a disease characterized by increased bone porosity and reduced mineral density and mass, and explains how to measure bone mineral density.

Measuring Energy: Explains the units of measuring energy, the joule or calorie depending on where you are, and the energy values of selected nutrients and activities.

Measuring Oxygen Saturation: Learn about the pulse oximeter, a medical device that measures the oxygen saturation of the blood (%SO2) passing through a fingertip, and what it tells you about a patient's blood.

Medical Imaging of the Body: Describes medical imaging techniques that allow physicians to visualize internal structures of the body without risking the trauma or other complications associated with extensive surgery.

Meningitis: Discusses types of conditions that involve inflammation of the brain's coverings, which can range from mild to life-threatening. Illustrated with photographs.

Meth Mouth: Summarizes the disorder caused by methamphetamine abuse.

Metric Measurements and Their Equivalents: Provides tables showing metric units of measurement, the prefixes used with metric units, and some common conversion factors that can be used in anatomy and physiology studies.

Monoclonal Antibodies and Nanobodies: Describes how scientists are able to produce large quantities of pure antibodies, monoclonal antibodies, and tiny antibody fragments called nanobodies that can be used to treat disease.

Nerve Zero: Discusses the very thin nerve discovered after the classic list of twelve, the terminal nerve, or nerve zero.

New Model of ANS Pathway: Addresses recent proposals that the sacral efferent pathways are sympathetic not parasympathetic as the classic model holds.

The Nobel Legacy: Lists the major physiology and medicine breakthroughs of the past century that have earned Nobel Prizes.

Osmotic Pressure of a Solution: Provides explanations, equations, and examples for calculating the osmotic pressure of a solution.

The Oxygen Debt: Outlines the factors that produce the oxygen debt, the excess oxygen needed after anaerobic exercise.

Oxygen Supplements: Explains how oxygen therapy can be used to treat disease and improve athletic performance and even used recreationally at "oxygen bars".

Oxygen-Binding Proteins: Explains the oxygen-binding proteins other than haemoglobin that are important to human physiology.

Pain Control Areas: Discusses pain control areas, areas where pain signals heading toward the conscious brain can be inhibited, and how they have led to pain-reducing therapies.

Phenylketonuria (PKU): Illustrates the concept of genetic disorders called "inborn errors of metabolism" by discussing what happens when a single enzyme is not present in the body, how this is detected in newborns, and how it can be treated.

Pheromones and the Vomeronasal Organ: Describes pheromones, signalling molecules that other individuals detect, and the vomeronasal organ, which is thought to detect them.

Photodynamic Therapy: Outlines this treatment of certain lung cancers, in which photosensitizing drugs are injected into the patient and a laser causes a chemical reaction with the drugs that destroys cancerous cells.

CONNECT IT!—continued from previous page

Protective Strategies of the Respiratory Tract: Provides a table summarizing the important protective mechanisms that operate in each segment of the respiratory airways.

Prothrombin Time: Explains the common laboratory test used to assess the body's ability to form blood clots

Pulmonary Radiology: Explains the types of x-ray studies that can be done to detect bronchial and lung disorders, including standard x-rays, bronchiograms, and arteriograms.

Radioactivity: Describes how radioactivity works and what effects it can have on the human body.

Refractive Eye Surgery: Discusses the common refractive eye surgeries and how they are performed.

The RNA Revolution: Discusses scientific advances in understanding the many roles of RNA in human health and disease, including illustrations of RNA interference or "gene silencing".

Retrograde Signalling: Explains the process of retrograde signalling, or signals being sent backward at a synapse.

Rhabdomyolysis: Describes the effects of crushing injuries to skeletal muscle that can release massive amounts of intracellular substances into the bloodstream with life-threatening consequences.

Sensing Food: Besides our various senses of taste, we also use smell, temperature, touch, and even pain sensations to construct a complete sensory experience of food.

Sexually Transmitted Diseases: Illustrates and describes some of the sexually transmitted diseases that occur in both males and females.

Sickle Cell Anaemia: Illustrated discussion of genetic disorders of red blood cells that affect both the structure and function of the blood.

Sites of Haematopoiesis: Heavily illustrated summary of where in the body blood cells are formed, including changes over the life span.

Skeletal Radiography: Illustrates skeletal radiography, or x-ray photography, with a description and radiographs of several parts of the body.

Skeletal Variations: Describes the natural variations in the human skeleton, including male and female variations and age-related variations.

Skin Cancer: Explains and illustrates the different types of skin cancer and how they are treated.

Sleep: Outlines the stages of the sleep cycle, including what happens to the body during each of the stages.

Specialization of Cerebral Hemispheres: Explains the specialization of the two hemispheres of the brain, and illustrates some of the suggested "special talents" attributed to each side of the brain.

Stem Cell Research: Discusses a controversial topic of scientific research, including the different types of stem cells and how stem cell research could help in cell therapy, the use of special cells to treat disease.

Summary of Gas Exchange: Summarizes some of the essential concepts of gas exchange with a description and a simplified illustration.

Swollen Larynx: Describes and illustrates syndromes that involve a swollen larynx, a potentially lethal condition.

Sympathetic Stimulation of Skeletal Muscle: The sympathetic nervous system is often thought to regulate only smooth or cardiac muscle tissues, but during a stress response, sympathetic stimulation of skeletal muscle can reduce muscle fatigue as a threat is avoided or resisted.

Synaesthesia: Learn about this sensory phenomenon where the experience of one sense stimulates a second sensory pathway, for example, the association of sounds or numbers with visual perception of colours.

The Timekeeping Hormone: Illustrates how melatonin plays a role in keeping our internal clocks synchronized.

Toilet Signs: A summary of how changes in our urine and faeces, including changes in elimination patterns, can reveal important information about our health.

Tools of Microscopic Anatomy: Explains and gives examples of the most common tools in microscopic anatomy: light microscopy, scanning and transmission electron microscopy, and atomic force microscopy.

Tracing Blood Flow in the Kidney: Summarizes the flow of blood in the kidney by providing a simplified flow chart and comparing it to the flow of the blood through the body.

Types of Leukaemia: Describes and illustrates several major varieties of cancers that affect human white blood cells.

Urinary Catheterization: Illustrates a commonly performed procedure in which a tube inserted into the bladder allows urine to escape.

Using Gene Therapy: Summarizes the origins and early history of using gene therapy to treat genetic disorders.

Vaults: Shows the structure of a tiny cell organelle that may hold the key to mysteries of how molecules are shuttled around the cell in an organized way.

Vertigo and Ear Rocks: Describes the sensation of vertigo, how "ear rocks" can cause this, and how to treat the problem.

Visualizing the Urinary Tract: Explains two methods of medical imaging used to examine the urinary tract: retrograde pyelogram and intravenous pyelogram.

Whole-Body Muscle Mechanics: Discusses how muscles are made up of muscle fibres and many layers of connective tissues, all working together to provide movement and maintain posture.